NURSING CARE OF INFANTS AND CHILDREN

LUCILLE F. WHALEY, R.N., M.S.

Associate Professor of Nursing,
San Jose State University,
San Jose, California

DONNA L. WONG, R.N., M.N., P.N.P.

Nurse Counselor in Private Practice,
Totowa, New Jersey;
formerly Assistant Professor of Nursing,
Seton Hall University,
School of Nursing,
South Orange, New Jersey

With 746 illustrations

The C. V. Mosby Company

ST. LOUIS • TORONTO • LONDON 1979

Printed in the United States of America

The C. V. Mosby Company
11830 Westline Industrial Drive, St. Louis, Missouri 63141

Library of Congress Cataloging in Publication Data

Whaley, Lucille F 1923-
Nursing care of infants and children.

Bibliography: p.
Includes index.
1. Pediatric nursing. I. Wong, Donna Lee, 1948- joint author. II. Title. [DNLM: 1. Pediatric nursing. WY159 W552n]
RJ245.W47 610.73′62 78-31225
ISBN 0-8016-5417-3

GW/VH/VH 9 8 7 6 5 4 3 02/D/215

CONTRIBUTORS

MARCENE L. ERICKSON, R.N., M.N.
Associate Professor,
University of Washington School of Nursing,
University of Washington,
Seattle, Washington

DIANA W. GUTHRIE, R.N., M.S.P.H., F.A.A.N.
Department of Nursing,
Wichita State University,
University of Kansas School of Medicine,
Wichita Branch, Wichita, Kansas

RICHARD A. GUTHRIE, M.D., F.A.A.P.
University of Kansas School of Medicine,
Wichita Branch, Wichita, Kansas

DOROTHY SMILEY SIEGELE, R.N., M.S.N.
Associate Professor,
Department of Nursing,
San Jose State University,
San Jose, California

Lt. FREDA WARREN, R.N., M.S., M.A.
Maternal-Child Clinical Coordinator,
Balboa Naval Hospital,
San Diego, California

To

Bert

devoted husband and father

To

Kathy and Reen

everything a parent could wish for

L. F. W.

To my husband

Ting Kin Wong

to whom there are no words to express my deepest love and appreciation

D. L. W.

PREFACE

Several dilemmas are immediately encountered when one contemplates writing a pediatric nursing textbook, such as the amount of content to include, the content to exclude, the depth to which the content should be covered, and the organization of that content. In attempting to solve these dilemmas, we have chosen to include content that will enable the nurse to provide care for both well and ill children. In order to plan, implement, and evaluate comprehensive and individualized nursing care, this care must be based on a firm understanding of facts and principles derived from biologic, physical, and behavioral sciences. Incorporating these concepts into a single volume has necessitated a lengthy book.

The topics chosen for discussion are those that we believe are relevant, common, or complex and in which nursing care plays a prominent role. Although some rare health problems or disorders have been deleted in light of book size, the principles and concepts of nursing practice have been elaborated on to allow both beginning students and practitioners of nursing an opportunity to expand and refine their nursing care. Summaries, using a conceptual approach to nursing care, are found throughout the text and are related to the more significant and multifaceted problems requiring nursing intervention. They are designed to serve as a concise guide to the most relevant goals for nursing care with the associated nursing responsibilities. It is hoped that the summaries will help the nurse appreciate the medical and psychologic needs of the child and family and the immediate as well as long-range goals necessary to restore and promote health.

There are two general approaches to the material presented. In Units one to nine the health problems of infancy and childhood are considered in a developmental framework, stressing the importance of the nurse's role in health promotion and maintenance. Unit one provides a longitudinal view of the child as an individual on a continuum of developmental changes from birth through adolescence and as a member of a family unit maturing within a culture and a community. Unit two is concerned with the principles and skills of nursing assessment, including interviewing, observation, physical and behavioral assessment, and health guidance. An in-depth discussion of health assessment is included in this unit to enable the nurse to use assessment skills to promote wellness and prevent illness in the child and family. History taking and physical examination are presented in detail to allow students, graduate nurses, and educators the opportunity to refine their knowledge in this expanded area of nursing practice.

Unit three is concerned with preconceptual and prenatal influences on child health and well-being; Unit four stresses the importance of the neonatal period, a time of greatest risk to survival. Units five to eight present the major developmental stages outlined in Unit one, which are expanded to provide the reader with a broader concept of these stages and the health problems most often associated with them. Special emphasis is placed on the preventive aspects of care. Unit nine deals with children who have the same developmental needs as growing children but who, because of congenital or early-acquired physical or mental impairment, require alternative interventions to facilitate development.

The second part of the book, consisting of Units ten to sixteen, is concerned with the more serious health problems of infants and children that frequently necessitate hospitalization. It follows a biologic systems orientation, which has the practical organizational value of permitting health problems and nursing considerations to relate to specific pathophysiologic disturbances. It also is a convenient method of presenting those health deviations that are not peculiar to one particular age-group. It is expected that the reader will incorporate into the discussions of various medical conditions the principles of growth and development from the earlier chapters to formulate a care plan that is individualized to the needs of each child.

Regardless of the way in which a book is organized, a certain amount of repetition of content is inevitable, but we have attempted to minimize this through the use of a conceptual approach to common problems whenever possible and through cross-references. We recognize that many of the clinical conditions selected represent more than one problem. Therefore, we have placed them according to the major problem or where they serve to illustrate a problem. For example, although diarrhea is a gastrointestinal disorder, the fluid and electrolyte disturbance is the primary threat to the child's well-being. Likewise, the pulmonary implications of cystic fibrosis of the pancreas are more life-threatening than the problem of maldigestion. References and an extensive bibliography follow each chapter to supplement the text and to serve as a guide and stimulus for further investigation.

Just as children and their families bring with them a vast and unique background that affects their role within the health care system, so it is that each nurse brings to each child and family an individual set of characteristics and values that will affect their relationship. Although we have attempted to present a total picture of the child in each age-group in wellness and in illness, no one child, family, or nurse will be found in this book. We hope that each page, chapter, and unit builds a foundation on which the nurse can begin to construct the ideal of comprehensive individualized nursing care for children.

The successful completion of a project such as this is never solely the effort of its authors. This book represents the contributions of numerous friends, colleagues, and family members. Many of its refinements are the result of suggestions from anonymous reviewers and colleagues who have graciously contributed their expertise. This book also reflects the education and inspiration we received as students, practitioners, and teachers of nursing. It has been enriched by many children, their families, and our students, from whom we have learned much. To all who have shared in this project we wish to convey our thanks and our gratitude.

We are especially grateful to each of our friends and colleagues who somehow found time to examine portions of the manuscript and offer constructive suggestions and encouragement: Margaret Jensen, Martha Thompson, Marsha Heims, and Sharon Raj, San Jose State University; Marie Jenkins, Pam Edwards, Sharon Bornstein (who also contributed original photographs), and Lois Dawson, Santa Clara Valley Medical Center, San Jose; Constance Petrucelli, Sr. Ellen Farrell, and the pediatric nursing staff of St. Joseph's Medical Center, Paterson, New Jersey, for their assistance in securing many of the photographs; Jean Barres Rollin, Rose Kayden, and Michael A. Baker, for his assistance regarding pharmacologic agents. We wish to express special appreciation to Joan Ballard and Robyn Nayyar for their collaboration in compiling the original outline and to Kathleen Whaley, Paula Thommen, Bob McGee, and Jack Tandy for their patience and cooperation in putting our ideas regarding illustrations into reality. Thanks to Barbara Wilson, Eldora Pollax, and Caroline Plank, librarians at Santa Clara Valley Medical Center, for their assistance and forbearance. A very warm and special thanks is extended to the nursing staff and administration of the pediatric and neonatal units at Santa Clara Valley Medical Center for their cooperation in this project and their friendship through the years.

This book truly embodies the concept of "family-centered" care. It represents the support, sacrifice, and productive efforts of both our families. Madeline Mitchko and Maureen Whaley (who also served as photographer) cheerfully typed and retyped thousands of manuscript pages. They also contributed valuable criticism and advice regarding editing of first and second drafts. Without their tireless, consistent efforts, this book could not have been completed. The original photography has been primarily the efforts of Kathleen and Bert Whaley and Ting Kin Wong who spent many long hours on their days off in unfamiliar surroundings to capture the expressions and effects we wished to illustrate. For Ting and Kathy it also represents hours in their respective darkrooms. A special word of gratitude is due Fran Potwora, who has become Nina Lee Wong's "surrogate mother" while her real mother spent most of her time in the "library, writing a book." We wish to thank all of them for their love and encouragement, and, last of all, we wish to thank each other for a pleasant working relationship and the beginning of a lifelong friendship.

Lucille F. Whaley

Donna L. Wong

CONTENTS

APPENDIXES

UNIT ONE
Children, their families, and the nurse

The ultimate goal of infant and child care is the promotion of optimum health and development for children at any stage of health or illness. To accomplish this purpose, nurses need an understanding of children and the way in which they grow and relate with significant persons in their environment, as well as an awareness of the multiple factors that contribute to the uniqueness of each child. To assess and evaluate the health and development of children, it is essential to be aware that the child is in the process of becoming.

Chapter 1, *Perspectives of Pediatric Nursing,* directs the focus for the remainder of the book, which emphasizes a child-centered rather than a disease-centered approach to nursing of infants and children. It presents the child as a unique individual on a life-long developmental continuum, whose needs are the same as, yet different from, those of all other children. Nursing is viewed as a process and the nurse as a person who can work effectively with infants and children and a person who can help create the kind of conditions in which others, particularly the parents, can function more effectively in child care.

Chapter 2, *The Interpersonal Environment of the Child,* is concerned with children in their family setting. It includes cultural, psychologic, and sociologic forces in the family situation that determine, to some extent, the way the family influences development. It examines various aspects of the family and the child's place within it with emphasis on the role of parents in shaping the child's attitudes and behavior.

Chapter 3, *The Child: the Wonder of Unfolding,* is a vertical or longitudinal view of the alterations that take place during growth and development and serves as a preface to the horizontal view of the various age-related units that follow. It is important to recognize that at each stage children differ physiologically, morphologically, and emotionally from adults, from other children, and from the children they were or will be. This chapter includes general body changes, specific organ and system alterations, and a brief overview of the major theories of development.

1

Perspectives of pediatric nursing

Throughout the ages the care of children has been influenced by their importance to society. In primitive times children were valued not for themselves but for their potential productivity both as children and as adults. Sickly or malformed infants and children were destroyed because the price of their survival would tax the resources of the total community. Although ancient civilizations gradually began to regard children as an asset, societies such as the Spartan Greeks would tolerate only healthy well-built children, leaving weak or deformed infants to die on the hillside. Even in modern times, history records a period of gross injustice and neglect for the welfare of children. During the Industrial Revolution of the nineteenth century child labor was quite common because it was cheap, plentiful, and efficient. The living conditions of the family unit also changed during this period from farm life to crowded city slums rife with unsanitary food supplies and overcrowded quarters. Children then became a burden rather than an asset. In the wake of worsening conditions, humanitarian and economic concerns called for a better quality of life for children. This attitude, as well as our fascination with the spontaneity and vigor of youth, has continued to grow so much that the twentieth century may well be called the "era of youth."

Today in most cultures children are more highly valued and coveted for themselves than in previous generations. What we now take for granted as the life-style of children was once a luxury. For example, the manufacture of toys is a multimillion-dollar industry. The variety of games, toys, dolls, and crafts seems limitless, in contrast to earlier times when play articles were made by the family or invented through the child's infinite imagination. In the past, groups such as the Puritans denied their children any opportunity for recreation because they believed that work was an essential requisite for holiness. Now play is recognized as children's natural medium of expression about themselves and their world and is frequently the only window into a child's thoughts, fantasies, and fears.

Paralleling society's changing view of children as valuable assets in the present as well as their potential for the future has been a changing focus in health care. Through increased strides in the physical and social sciences and with recent advances in the widespread use of immunizations and antibiotics, health care for children has shifted from the treatment of disease to the prevention of illness. The nurse is no longer merely involved in the episodic care of children but is obligated to provide comprehensive care that attends to the needs of children and their families. This necessitates that today's pediatric nurse be a student of developmental psychology and family dynamics as well as a specialist in the medical and surgical problems encountered in a group of patients whose physical and emotional responses are remarkably variable. Although total patient care is the goal of health care, it remains only an ideal because of the multitude of influences affecting a child that no one nurse can understand and assimilate. Yet the very fact that prevents the full realization of this design for total care also mandates the interdependent function of health professionals for the provision of improved and refined health care.

ROLE OF THE PEDIATRIC NURSE

Nursing of infants and children is based on the premise that its purpose is to promote the highest possible state of health in each child. It consists of preventing disease or injury; assisting children, including those with a permanent handicap or health problem, to achieve and maintain an optimum level of health and development; and treating or rehabilitating children who have health deviations. Health has been defined by the World Health Organization as "a state of complete physical, mental, and social well-being and not merely the absence of disease." This implies that nursing is involved in every aspect of a child's growth and development. Nursing functions vary according to regional job structures, individual education and experience, and personal expectations of their profession. Just as clients (children and their families) present a vast and unique background, so it is that each nurse will bring to the clients an individual set of variables that will affect their relationship. No matter where pediatric nurses practice, their primary concern is the welfare of the child and his family.

Family advocacy

Although the nurse is responsible to self, the profession, and the institution of employment, primary responsibility is to the recipient of nursing services, the child and family. The nurse must work with members of the family, identifying their goals and needs, and plan interventions that best meet the defined problems. As a consumer advocate the goal of the nurse is to ensure that families are aware of all available health services, informed adequately of treatments and procedures, involved in the child's care when possible, and encouraged to change or support existing health-care practices. The pediatric nurse is aware of the United Nations Declaration of the Rights of the Child (see Appendix H) and practices within these guidelines to ensure that every child receives optimal care.

Of special significance is the nurse's role as child advocate. The following Pediatric Bill of Rights, composed by a 10-year-old child, clearly states the child's views regarding true "rights."

1. Any person regardless of age has the right to refuse pedeatric care.
2. Any person regardless of age has the right to pick there own pedeatrision, if there a girl they can pick a girl, if there a boy they can pick a boy.
3. Any person regardless of age has the right to not take there medicen if they dont want to.
4. Any person regardless of age has the right not to wear those paperthings at the doctors office.
5. Any person regardless of age has the right not to get weighed at the doctors office.*

Unfortunately, most of these "rights" are not in the child's best interest when health care is needed. However, they emphasize the need for nurses to consider the child's feelings and to individualize care to allow for personal preferences, fears, dislikes, and so on. Throughout this text there are innumerable examples relating to special needs of children in various age-groups. As child advocate the nurse utilizes this knowledge to adapt care for the child's optimum physical and emotional well-being. Examples of this may be fostering the parent-child relationship during hospitalization, preparing the child prior to *any* unfamiliar treatment or procedure, allowing the child privacy, providing play activities for expression of fear, aggression, or loss of control, and respecting cultural differences relating to feeding or child-rearing practices.

The nurse is aware of the needs of children and works with all care givers to ensure that these fundamental requirements are met. This often necessitates that the nurse expand the boundaries of practice to less traditional settings. As a child advocate the nurse may be involved in education, political/legislative change, rehabilitation, screening, administration, and even engineering and architecture. Regardless of how removed from direct patient care individual nurses become, they continue to foster health-care practices that promote the optimum well-being of children by incorporating knowledge of child growth and development into particular roles of practice. For example, as educator the nurse has the primary responsibility of helping others learn about and care for children. The audience for this information may be other nurses, parents, schoolteachers, other members of the health team, or the general public. In some states nurses are involved in mass media programs for immunization of all children.

Not infrequently, the role of family advocate conflicts with other roles of the nurse, such as those imposed by the institution. Inflexible rules, regulations designed for purposes of administration rather than optimal child welfare,

*Andreasen, S.: Pediatrics **55**(3):370, March 1975. Copyright American Academy of Pediatrics 1975.

Code for nurses*

1. The nurse provides services with respect for human dignity and the uniqueness of the client unrestricted by considerations of social or economic status, personal attributes, or the nature of health problems.
2. The nurse safeguards the client's right to privacy by judiciously protecting information of a confidential nature.
3. The nurse acts to safeguard the client and the public when health care and safety are affected by the incompetent, unethical, or illegal practice of any person.
4. The nurse assumes responsibility and accountability for individual nursing judgments and actions.
5. The nurse maintains competence in nursing.
6. The nurse exercises informed judgment and uses individual competence and qualifications as criteria in seeking consultation, accepting responsibilities, and delegating nursing activities to others.
7. The nurse participates in activities that contribute to the ongoing development of the profession's body of knowledge.
8. The nurse participates in the profession's efforts to implement and improve standards of nursing.
9. The nurse participates in the profession's efforts to establish and maintain conditions of employment conducive to high quality nursing care.
10. The nurse participates in the profession's effort to protect the public from misinformation and misrepresentation and to maintain the integrity of nursing.
11. The nurse collaborates with members of the health professions and other citizens in promoting community and national efforts to meet the health needs of the public.

*American Nurses' Association, 1976. Reproduced with permission of the American Nurses' Association.

and relationships with other professionals who are not knowledgeable of children's needs can create tremendous conflicts and challenges for the nurse who is dedicated to caring for the family in light of individual needs. Although there are rarely easy solutions to such dilemmas, the nurse can turn to the professional Code of Ethics for guidance (see boxed material). A code of ethics provides one means for professional self-regulation. In the past the Code for Nurses, adopted by the American Nurses' Association in 1950, was more prescriptive, identifying codes of both personal and professional behavior, describing appropriate relationships with physicians and other health team members, and identifying certain responsibilities of the nurse as a citizen and employee. The present code focuses on the nurse's accountability and responsibility to the client and emphasizes the nursing role as an independent professional role that upholds its own legal liability.

Prevention

The emerging trend toward health care has been prevention of illness and maintenance of health, rather than treatment of disease or disability. Nursing has kept pace with this change, especially in the area of child care. In 1965 specialized programs for pediatric nurse associates/practitioners began to develop that have led to several specialized ambulatory or primary care roles for nurses. The thrust of these programs has been to educate nurses beyond the basic preparational stage in areas of child health maintenance in order for all children to receive high-quality care. An outgrowth of the practitioner programs has been expanded programs for school nurses. Although the curriculum design varies from program to program, the course content generally includes history taking, physical diagnosis, growth and development, health education, counseling, common childhood problems, and planning care for individuals and groups.

Obviously, the thrust of these nurse practitioner programs is prevention. However, it is not limited to them. Every nurse involved with child care must practice within the overall dimension of preventive health. Regardless of the identified problem, the role of the nurse is to plan care that fosters every aspect of growth and development. Based on a thorough assessment process, problems related to nutrition, immunizations, safety, dental care, development, socialization, discipline, or schooling frequently become obvious. Once the problem is identified, the nurse acts to intervene directly or to refer the family to other health persons or agencies.

The best approach to prevention is education and anticipatory guidance. Each chapter on growth and development includes sections on anticipatory guidance. With an appreciation of the hazards or conflicts of each developmental period, the nurse is able to guide parents regarding child-rearing practices aimed at preventing potential problems. One of the most significant examples is safety. Since each age-group is at risk for special types of accidents, with preventive teaching, most accidents can be prevented, thus significantly lowering the permanent disability and mortality from accidental injuries in children.

Prevention involves less obvious aspects of child care. Besides preventing physical disease or injury, the nurse's role is also to promote mental health. For example, it is not sufficient to administer immunizations without regard for the psychologic trauma associated with the procedure. Optimum health involves the practice of good medicine with a humane approach to health care; the nurse is often the one professional capable of ensuring "humanity." Because of current educational emphasis on the total person, the extended and less formal interaction with the family, and the nursing role within the health team, the nurse's role is often one of *facilitator* of care rather than direct intervenor.

Health teaching

Health teaching is inseparable from family advocacy and prevention. Health teaching may be a direct goal of the nurse, such as during parenting classes, or may be indirect, such as informing parents and children of a diagnosis or medical treatment, encouraging children to ask questions about their bodies, referring families to health-related professional or lay groups, and supplying patients with appropriate literature.

Health teaching is often one area in which nurses feel competent because it involves translating information rather than receiving messages, translating them, and planning intervention. In other words, it is a concrete, structured type of communication as opposed to other emotionally laden, nondirected types of interaction. However, the nurse focuses on giving appropriate health teaching with generous feedback and evaluation to promote learning.

Support/counseling

Attention to emotional needs necessitates support and sometimes counseling. Frequently, the role of child advocate or health teacher is supportive by the very nature of the individualized approach. Support can be offered in many ways, the most common of which include listening, touching, and physical presence. The last two are most helpful with children because they facilitate nonverbal communication.

Counseling involves a mutual exchange of ideas and opinions that provides the basis for mutual problem solving. It usually culminates in giving advice based on the content of the discussion. Although it is similar to health teaching, its focus is broader and more intense because it frequently implies some crisis or upsetting event that needs intervention. It involves support as well as teaching, techniques to foster expression of feelings or thoughts, and approaches to help the family cope with stress. Although counseling is often the role of more specialized nurses, counseling techniques are discussed in various sections of the text to help students and nurses cope with immediate crises about them and refer families for additional professional assistance.

Restoration

The most basic of all nurses' roles is the restoration of health through care-giving activities. Nurses are intimately involved with meeting the physical and emotional needs of children, including feeding, bathing, toileting, dressing, security, and socialization. They are primarily responsible for instituting physician's prescriptions; they are also held singularly accountable for their own actions and judgments regardless of written orders.

A significant aspect of restoration of health is continual assessment and evaluation of physical status. Indeed, the concentrated focus throughout the text on physical assessment, pathophysiology, and scientific rationale for therapy is to assist the nurse in decision making regarding health status. Only when aware of normal findings can the nurse intelligently identify and document deviations. In addition the pediatric nurse never loses sight of the emotional and developmental needs of the individual child, which can significantly influence the course of the disease process.

Restoration frequently implies habilitation and rehabilitation. Through expanding roles nurses are increasingly responsible for health care of handicapped children. For example, school nurses or pediatric nurse practitioners are involved in programs for severely developmentally disabled children in order to facilitate their attendance in regular classes.

Coordination/collaboration

The nurse as a member of the health team collaborates and coordinates nurses' services with other professionals' activities. Working in isolation does not serve the child's best interest. First, the concept of "total care" can only be realized through a unified interdisciplinary approach. Second, aware of individual contributions and limitations to the child's care, the nurse must collaborate with other specialists to provide for high-quality health services. Failure to recognize limitations can be nontherapeutic at best and destructive at worst. For example, the nurse who feels competent in counseling when really inadequate in this area may not only prevent the child from dealing with a crisis but may also retard his future success with a qualified professional.

Even nurses who practice in isolated geographic areas widely separated from other health professionals cannot be considered independent. Every nurse works interdependently with the child and family, collaborating on needs and interventions so that the final care plan is one that truly meets the child's needs. Unfortunately, this is one aspect of collaboration and coordination that is lacking in health care planning. Often numerous disciplines work together to formulate a comprehensive approach without consulting with clients regarding their ideas or preferences. The nurse is in a vital position to include consumers in their care, either directly or indirectly, by communicating their thoughts to the group.

Health care planning

So far, the nurse's role has been viewed through the nucleus of a family. However, the nursing role is far more extensive and includes the community or society as a whole. Traditionally nurses have been involved in public health care, either on a distributive or episodic basis. Rarely, however, have nurses been involved in health care planning, especially on a political or legislative level. Their role must also involve the decision-making body of government. Nursing, as the largest health profession, needs to have a voice, especially as family/consumer advocate. This does not mean that the nurse must hold public office. Rather it refers to knowledge and awareness of community needs, interest in government formulation of bills and support of politicians to assure passage (or rejection) of significant legislation, and active involvement in groups dedicated to the welfare of children, such as professional nursing societies, Parent-Teacher Organizations, parent support groups, religious affiliations, and voluntary organizations.

Health care planning involves not only providing new services but also promoting the highest quality of existing ones. Nursing needs to ensure the excellence of its own profession through each individual member, who practices according to the Code of Ethics and Standards of Practice. Pediatric nurses are obligated to follow the Standards of Maternal and Child Health Nursing. They should also be involved in assuring that their colleagues implement the standards, through education, role modeling, and/or supervision.

Throughout the text the standards of nursing practice are continually reflected in the emphasis on thorough assessment, focus on scientific rationale as the basis for care, summary of nursing care goals and responsibilities, and comprehensive discussion of growth and development. Family-centered principles are continually evident in the consideration of dynamics affecting the child, parents, siblings, and extended members. The nurse is viewed as a vital component of the health care delivery system. Although nursing functions are clearly outlined, nursing responsibilities must be equally emphasized. It is hoped that the roles briefly described here will be studied, practiced, and implemented to the ultimate benefit of all children.

BEHAVIORS OF THE PEDIATRIC NURSE

Nursing behaviors can be categorized into three major types—protective, nurturing, and generative behaviors—that are operative at any stage of health or illness.

Protective behaviors encompass all those activities and interactions that are directed toward shielding an infant or child from injury or harm. These are the behaviors that anticipate problems. They are preventive or precautionary measures that are designed and carried out to ward off undesired consequences, to hinder the progress of deleterious forces, or to promote and maintain health.

Nurturing behaviors are those that promote, support, and comfort. These are the expression of the curative or therapeutic aspect of the nursing process. To nurture means to care for, to nourish (in the broad sense as well as the narrow), and to promote growth through all those ministering activities that meet the ever-changing and ongoing processes of life.

Generative behaviors are those that bring into being or cause to be produced activities or attitudes conducive to health. This is sometimes seen as the rehabilitative component of nursing. For example, motivating and assisting a family to carry out a therapeutic regimen is a generative nursing behavior.

These behaviors of nursing are neither mutually inclusive nor exclusive. Many behaviors that prevent problems can also be therapeutic and/or rehabilitative, such as range of motion exercises, administration of oxygen, or therapeutic communication. In addition to upholding the goals to which these behaviors aim, the nurse also focuses these behaviors on individuals or groups of individuals—the child, the child and the primary care giver, or the child and his family.

Focus of nursing behaviors

Nursing activities that promote health in an individual child are directed to the individual life processes: the process of growth and development, cognitive development, personality formation and expression, and the evolution of a self-concept. Since the child's stage of development has a significant effect on the health hazards to which he is vulnerable, the nurse must be able to discern the inner and outer forces that influence his overall development.

Nursing activities are also directed toward promoting optimum functioning of two or more persons, usually a family. They are concerned with the individuality of family members, the family situation, and the goals and resources of the family complex. Particularly significant for nursing is the relationship between the child and the care giver, usually the mother. So intimate and dependent is this relationship that, although separate entities, the child cannot be considered apart from the mother. Nursing of the family involves assessment of the way in which the child functions within the family and the way in which others affect the development and welfare of the child. Relationships within the family may include child-parent, child-nurse, child-parent-nurse, child-child, and the total family complex. Often the family complex includes small subgroups (extended family, religious groups, day-care center) or the relationship of the family and child with other professionals (physicians, teachers, social workers).

A community is a group of persons who participate in a common organization for mutual interests and goals. To promote child health within the community, nurses may become involved with many groups that contribute knowledge and services for the attainment of child and community health. This involvement may be limited to local groups or may extend to international organizations or agencies. Protective, nurturing, and generative nursing activities within a community are directed toward reducing threats to the health of an entire community, promoting optimal community health, and supporting the coping skills of a community.

PROCESS OF NURSING CHILDREN

Planning and implementing nursing care to meet the needs of infants and children requires a systematic approach to decision making. The problem-solving process consists of five operational phases: assessment, problem identification, plan formulation, implementation, and evaluation. It involves both cognitive and operational skills. How successfully the process is carried out depends on such factors as the nurse's level of competence, the formation of the nurse-child-family relationship, and the goals and capabilities of the family members.

Summary of decision-making process

Assessment is a continuous process that is operative at all phases of problem solving. Derived through multiple nursing skills, it consists of the purposeful collection, classification, and analysis of data from a variety of sources. Assessment is the foundation for decision making. It is from the interrelatedness of the pertinent data that the nurse is able to arrive at an interpretation for problem identification.

Reflection on the assessment should result in *problem identification*. In order to solve a problem it is essential to acknowledge that it exists and describe its nature. The problem may involve an unmet need, an unrealized expectation, an interrupted process, or a community crisis. The nursing problem arises from the child's problem, and the statement of the nursing problem defines the nursing goal.

Plan formulation is the decision-making phase of the process. Armed with a specific problem statement, the nurse is able to design a plan of action. A design for action involves the selection of a plan that is based on scientific principles derived from a variety of disciplines. The nurse chooses an alternative for intervention that is most likely to achieve the desired consequence with a minimum of risk to the persons involved.

The phase of *implementation* begins when the nurse puts the selected intervention into action and accumulates feedback regarding its effects. The feedback returns in the form of observation and communication and provides a data base on which to evaluate the outcome of the nursing intervention.

To complete the decision-making process, the nurse gathers, sorts, and analyzes data to determine if (1) the goal has been met, (2) the plan requires modification, or (3) another alternative should be considered. This *evaluation* either completes the nursing process or serves as the basis for selection of other alternatives for intervention in solving the specific problem.

Adaptability

The process of nursing children and the attendant behaviors that nurses exhibit describe the structure and function by which optimal health care occurs. Permeating the process of nursing is the ever-present element of *change*. Science and technology are creating rapid changes that extend to all aspects of daily life. New knowledge is acquired at a phenomenal rate. To keep pace with these advances in knowledge and in answer to the increased demand for health services from a better informed and influential consumer, nurses are encouraged to continue and refine their education, heighten their level of practice, and be attentive to the interrelatedness of the knowledge flow between the various disciplines.

In addition to the increased information available to the nurse are the changes that occur within the profession itself. An ever-maturing sense of professionalism and an open attitude toward the goals and practices of nursing have led to expanded roles for the pediatric nurse. Whereas pediatric nurses once functioned only in hospitals or physician's offices, they now assume major roles in well-child clinics, special education facilities, and independent practice.

Finally, the nurse who cares for children not only utilizes innovations from society and the profession itself but perfects an individual mode for change in terms of flexibility and creativity. The needs of children often demand creative responses, so that this too becomes a personal responsibility of the pediatric nurse.

THE CHILD

All children are basically alike. They follow the same pattern of development and maturation, whereas, at the same time, their hereditary, cultural, and experiential backgrounds make each a distinct and unique individual. They differ in their rate of growth, their ultimate size and capabilities, and the way in which they respond to their environment. However, regardless of their stage of development, their state of health, or the situation in which they are encountered, *the child is first of all a child.*

Children are born with certain traits, the core of their uniqueness, that are continually influenced and modified by family, cultural, and subcultural factors. The type of family in which they are reared, their racial or ethnic background, religion, social status, the type of food they eat, patterns of living, and their attitudes toward and relationships with others are just a few of these influences. Initially society does not act directly on its infant and child members, but it profoundly influences the direction and course of their development through the process of cultural learning that is mediated primarily through the family. It is the parents or other care givers who supply the value system first, most intimately, and during the child's most formative years.

In most instances parents assume the responsibility of child rearing with the intent to produce a well-adjusted member of society. Most succeed. The exceptional failures are usually attributed to faulty parenting in which the level of maturity, cultural background, and the quality of the parents' own upbringing influence their ability to provide for the care and nurture of their children. Parents and child can seldom be separated one from the other in child care. Anything that affects the parents will also affect the child. It is not uncommon for a child to develop physical symptoms as a response to intrafamily stress or disharmony. Nurses who assist parents to a successful relationship with their children will assure a healthier environment for the children.

Needs of infants and children

Every society and every generation has regulated child-care practices and used children for its own purposes. Child rearing has been based on traditional beliefs and practices and dictated by cultural and religious values, political and economic requirements, and a variety of ideas and purposes that were often remote from the children themselves. Today the trend in the care and nurture of children is based on their developmental needs. Children need plenty of physical room in which to grow as well as support from the adults in their environment. Because they do not have the resources for coping with the world, children need to be surrounded by friendly people who are willing to share their pleasures and help them through troubling times.

Although the emphasis and classification may vary according to the interpreter, the essential needs of children during all stages of development are physical, biologic, and emotional needs, including love, emotional security, discipline, independence, and self-esteem.

Physical and biologic needs. First of all, children's basic physical and biologic needs for food, water, air, warmth, elimination, and shelter must be met. Infants, except for limited reflex responses, are totally dependent on adults for satisfaction of even the most basic needs. As development proceeds, children begin to communicate their needs, through both verbal and nonverbal means, then gradually to assume increasing responsibility for their own basic need gratification.

Those who care for children come to understand the physical changes that take place during the process of development and the special needs generated by these changes, for example, the nature and quantity of the food intake, the method and frequency of feeding, and the amount of sleep and activity that change during childhood. Health and safety hazards associated with every phase of development require implementation of measures to provide for the child's physical safety, including prevention of accidents and disease and education of children, families, and communities regarding these potential threats to health and well-being.

Love and affection. The single most important emotional need of children is to be loved and to feel secure in that love. Children strive above all else to gain the love and acceptance of those who are significant in their lives. When they feel secure in this love they are able to withstand the normal crises associated with growing up and those unexpected crises (illness, loss, and so on) that are superimposed on the anticipated course of development.

Children cannot receive too much love. However, this love must be communicated to them through words and actions that tell them that they are loved, not for their actions or achievement, but for what they are or simply *because they are*. Although love is closely associated with discipline, independence, and other factors that influence the child's self-concept, it is an undemanding, accepting love that is indispensible to the development of a healthy personality. Unconditional love, freely bestowed, helps establish a sense of security and a positive sense of self within children that will persist throughout their lifetime. It is important that children know they are loved and that whatever happens they can depend on this love. Without the security of such a loving relationship, children may become tense, insecure, and develop undesirable behavior patterns as they attempt to obtain that love or try to compensate for its loss.

The primary source of love, particularly during infancy, is the mother or mothering person. The importance of establishing this early love attachment (or bonding) profoundly influences subsequent interpersonal relationships. With ever-widening relationships, children need the love and acceptance of others. They need to feel they are wanted, accepted, and belong in whatever relationships are important to them at each stage of development.

Parents, with few exceptions, want to be "good" parents and ordinarily do not need to be told to love their children. In all likelihood they *will* love them; however, the quality and extent of the manifestations of their love depend on the love that they, the parents, received in their own childhood. Parents may truly love their children but be unable to communicate this love to them. Parents who are insecure of their parenting skills frequently seek advice and reassurance from health professionals. Nurses who are aware of indications of parental insecurity will be able to provide assistance and reassurance that can preserve and enhance the parent-child relationship and build a sense of confidence in the parent.

Security. Closely allied to the need for love is the need for a sense of security. As they grow and develop in a complex world, children encounter many threats to their sense of security. Indeed, most behavior problems of childhood are associated with an element of insecurity. Every change in themselves or their environment creates a feeling of uncertainty. Faced with a jumble of confusing, conflicting adjustments, young children need the security provided by relatively stable situations and dependable human relationships. The degree to which they can cope with these stresses depends on the patience and support they receive from those most closely involved in their care.

There are a multitude of factors that generate a feeling of insecurity in children. Ordinarily the parents, who are sources of comfort, guidance, and encouragement, provide a measure of security in an insecure world. To achieve this security children need the warm acceptance of loving parents, a stable family unit, and judicious handling of stress-provoking situations such as sibling rivalry, relocation to a new neighborhood, and illness in themselves or other members of the family. A disturbed home environment caused by such factors as marital discord, illness of a parent or family member, or death of a family member can shatter their equilibrium.

Infants are disturbed by physical threats, such as hunger, cold, or discomfort; small children are physiologically disturbed by emotions such as anger, fear, and grief, which they can release only in overt behavior. A measure of relief from these feelings can be obtained by the reassurance that their physical needs will be met, restraints will be placed on their behavior, and expectations that keep pace with their inner controls will be held. Rejection by significant persons, social ineptitude, and physical handicaps often produce insecurity in a child. The number and variety of factors originating within or outside the child are often difficult to determine; therefore those responsible for the child's care must be alert for cues that reveal threats to this sense of security.

Discipline and authority. Because children live in an organized society, they must be prepared to accept restrictions on their behavior. Discipline is not punishment. Rather, it is the teaching of desirable behavior. Children need to learn the rules governing behavior in the home, the neighborhood, the school, and the community at large. To learn acceptable behavior that permits them to live enjoyably with themselves and others, children need the steady, firm guidance of loving parents and others in authority roles. Good discipline provides children with protection from dangers (from within and without) and relieves them of the burden of decisions that they are not prepared to make, yet allows them to develop independence of thought and action within a secure framework.

Children who learn to live within reasonable rules are happier and more secure children. Without the stabilizing influence of controls, children feel uncertain and insecure. Too often, inexperienced and insecure parents fear the loss of a child's love, suffer feelings of guilt over disciplinary action, or may even relinguish their authority to the child. To discipline is to teach reality. Sensible, mature parents establish fair rules and regulations in the home and then see that they are carried out. Parents should never exploit children's love for them as a means to control their children. Children's anxiety lest they lose that love is already great. Discipline based on love of the child and carried out with conviction, confidence, and consistency will produce a self-reliant, bouyant, and self-controlled child.

Dependence and independence. As children grow and mature, they are increasingly able to direct their own activities and to make more and more independent decisions. However, there are great fluctuations in their ability to function independently. Even with a compelling inner drive to master and achieve, they are not always able to cope with difficult and frustrating problems or conflicts. All children feel the urge to grow up and move forward toward maturity, but they have at their disposal only those energies that are not being used to maintain their mastery over old conflicts. Independence should be permitted to grow at its own rate.

Periods of regression and dependence are not only normal but are often necessary and helpful. If children feel sufficiently comfortable and content in a situation or relationship and reasonably certain that they can return to this safety and security, they will venture into the untried and untested on their own. If they feel doubtful concerning their abilities to cope, regression to a more comfortable level of competence allows them to replenish their inner resources and prepare to move ahead once again. Independence grows out of dependence; one cannot be considered as distinct from the other.

Children will learn independence of thought and decision making provided the opportunity is not withheld from them. If they are pushed into acting independently before they feel themselves ready, they may withdraw from independence. When they choose not to relinquish the joys of independence and autonomy or move ahead to new worlds of independence, they will dawdle. Parents, teachers, nurses, and others responsible for child care must be able to adjust their expectations and support to meet the child's needs of the moment. It is important to recognize when to help and when not to help children to experiment with their immature and imperfect self-control, when to make demands that require children's utmost ability, and when to allow them to function temporarily on a more immature level. They need these freedoms and controls in the process of becoming mature, self-reliant adults.

Self-esteem. Self-esteem is children's personal, subjective judgment of their worthiness. It is the result of self-evaluation, principally in the areas of competence and social acceptance.

The content of self-esteem changes with children's development. Highly egocentric toddlers are unaware of any difference between competence and social approval. They are the center of their world and, to them, all positive experiences are evidence of their importance and value. Preschool and early school-age children, on the other hand, are increasingly aware of the discrepancy between their competencies and the abilities of more advanced children. They are expected to evaluate a situation and anticipate the consequences of their behavior before they act. The acceptance of adults and peers outside the family group become more important to them. Since these valued persons may not be as proud of their achievements or as understanding of their limitations as their families are, their recently acquired capacity for guilt may lead to anxiety over failure, and they will be more vulnerable to feelings of worthlessness and depression. As their competencies increase and they develop meaningful relationships, their self-esteem rises. Their self-esteem is again at risk during early adolescence when they are defining an identity and sense of self in the context of their peer group.

Unless children are continually made to feel incompetent and of little worth, a decrease in self-esteem during vulnerable periods is only temporary. It can be expected that there will be transitory periods of lowered self-esteem at the stages of development when they must set new goals or where there are very obvious discrepancies in competence. A constant source of anxiety arises from the endless number of separations that occur in the process of acquiring autonomy, independence, and individuality. As an expression of their own urgencies, parents often set overambitious goals for their children and expect them to perform beyond the limits of their capacity. Also, children's attempts at autonomy and achievement are often thwarted by parental overprotection, either because the parents fear that they will be hurt or because it is more convenient for the parents to do things for them.

In order to develop and preserve self-esteem, children need to feel that they are worthwhile individuals who are in *some* way different from, superior to, and more lovable than, any other individual in the world. They need recognition for their achievements and the approval of parents and peers. Parents and other authority figures can foster a positive self-concept by providing appropriate encouragement and recognition for achievement and by discouraging inappropriate behaviors. However, when disapproval is being expressed, it is imperative to convey to a child that it is the *behavior* that is unacceptable, not the child.

Children who experience warm, affectionate relationships with parents, who are accepted by their parents, and who are aware of their parents' positive attitudes toward them are more accepting of themselves. Children who have a strong sense of their own worth are confident, able to initiate activities, explore their environment, and take risks in their behavior when confronted with new or novel situations. They approach tasks and relationships with the expectation that they will be well received and successful.

COMMUNICATION

Essential to the nursing of children is communication. It is the most important skill used in assessment of children and their families and the most important feature in forming trusting relationships with them. Communication consists of all those behaviors by which one person, consciously or unconsciously, affects another. One cannot *not* communicate. All behavior transmits a message: even the attempt not to communicate creates a particular impression. Inherent in communication are the power of observation, the use of all the senses, and the intangible reaction of intuition.

The forms of communication may be verbal, nonverbal, or abstract. Verbal communication may involve language and its expression, vocalizations in the forms of laughs, moans, squalls, and so on, or the implications of what is *not* said in light of what has been said. Nonverbal communication is often called body language and includes gestures, movements, facial expressions, postures, and reactions. Communication that is abstract takes the form of play, artistic expression, symbols, photographs, choice of clothing, and so on. Because it is possible to exert greater conscious control over verbal communication, it becomes the least reliable indicator of true feelings and is particularly irrelevant in relationships with children. It is through the process of observation that one actively, consciously, and deliberately perceives messages communicated through nonverbal behavior.

Communication is a circular interdependent pattern of action-reaction and validation. It consists of three essential operations: perception, evaluation, and transmission. Perception is the reception of expressive action; evaluation is the analysis or interpretation of the information provided that leads to prediction and decision making; and transmission is the expressive action by gesture, speech, or movement. Feedback is provided when the expressed action of a sender is perceived by another who reacts to the message and then, in some manner, relays back to the sender that the message was received. Feedback serves to verify that the expressed action was indeed perceived as well as to clarify, extend, or alter the sender's original idea[1] (Fig. 1-1).

There are many factors that influence the communication system. To be successful (gratifying), communication must be appropriate to the situation, properly timed, and clearly delivered. This implies that nurses understand and use techniques of effective communication, including listening. Verbal and nonverbal messages must be congruent, that is, two or more messages sent via different levels must not be contradictory. Those elements that create disturbed communication, such as overloading the system with input that is too intense or underloading it with nonresponsive or malfunctioning communication apparatus (deafness, blindness, mental retardation), faulty or erroneous perception or interpretation of messages, or misuse of communication through poor timing, inappropriateness, or double messages, must be altered or avoided.

Nurses need to recognize their own feelings and attempt

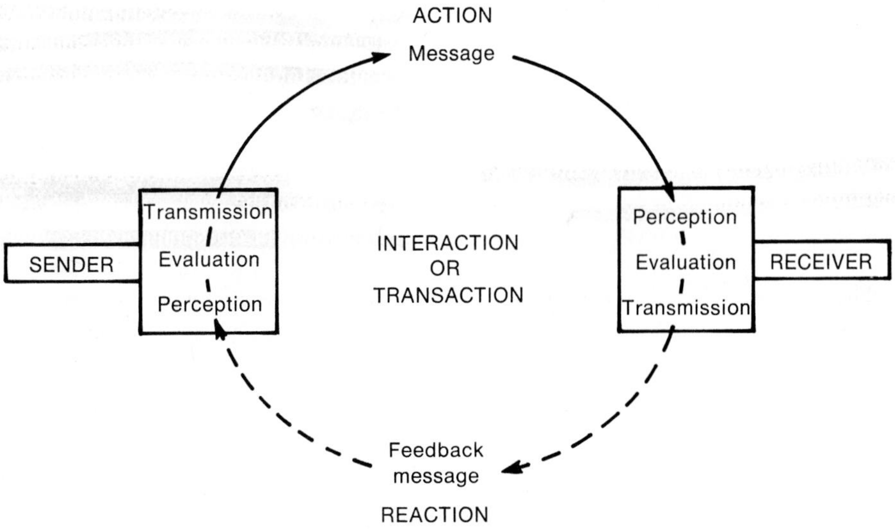

Fig. 1-1. Interdependent pattern of communication.

to recognize those of the persons with whom the communicative interchange takes place. Biases and judgments interfere with all aspects of the process. The tendency to approve or disapprove of another's statements inhibits positive reactions. In addition, the transmission and reception of messages may be altered by influences of intimacy or distance, dependence and independence, trust and mistrust, security and insecurity, or caring and not caring on the part of the participants. The value of effective communication is increased understanding between the nurse, the child, and the family. Since nursing of infants and children always involves the inclusion of a care giver, nurses must be able to communicate not only with children of all ages but with the adults in their lives as well.

Communicating with parents

Although the parent and child are separate and distinct entities, relationships with the child are frequently mediated via the parent—particularly in the case of younger children. For the most part, information about the child is acquired by direct observation or is communicated to the nurse by the parents. Usually it can be assumed that because of the close contact with the child, the information imparted by the parent is reliable. To make an assessment of the child requires input from the child (verbal and nonverbal), information from the parent, and the nurse's own observations, including assessment of the child and interpretation of the relationship between the child and the parent. Counseling and guidance must be directed to the care giver of infants and small children; when children are old enough to be active participants in their own health maintenance, the parent becomes a collaborator in health care. Usually mothers' communication concerning children will be used throughout most of this discussion. However, the communication might involve both parents, the father, or other care givers.

Interviewing. Since nurses' effectiveness in practice depends to a large extent on their ability to relate to others, they use the communication process to help children and their parents make use of the nurse's professional knowledge and skill. The most widely used method of communicating with parents on a professional basis is the interview process. Interviewing, unlike much social conversation, is a specific form of goal-directed communication. As nurses converse with parents, they endeavor to focus on the parents to determine the kind of persons they are, their usual mode of handling problems, if help is needed, and the way in which they react to counseling. It requires time and patience to develop interviewing skills, but there are some guiding principles and some pitfalls to be avoided that facilitate this process.

The attitude and approach of the interviewer set the tone and pace of the interaction. A warm, accepting environment is conducive to the reduction of anxiety and the expression of feelings. Parents assume that the nurse is a competent professional, and, therefore, they expect to receive accurate information. Parents often respond to personal qualities such as friendliness, interest, and the desire to understand to a greater degree than to information provided by the nurse. All too often troubled mothers will turn to the most sympathetic listener rather than to the person who has the most information.

The attitudes and feelings of the nurse are easily injected into an interview. It is important that nurses understand and recognize their own reactions in order to minimize their potential impact on a parent. It is not uncommon for nurses (and parents) to react to emotions related to past experiences instead of the circumstances of the present situation and then convey a false impression to the other person. Often nurses' perception of a parent's behavior is influenced by their own perceptions, prejudices, and assumptions, which may include racial, religious, and cultural stereotypes. What may be interpreted as passive hostility or disinterest in a parent may, in fact, be shyness or an expression of anxiety. Although it is necessary for nurses to make some preliminary judgments, they must attempt to "hear" the parent with as much objectivity as possible by clarifying meanings and attempting to see the situation from the parent's point of view. Effective interviewers use conscious control over their reactions, responses, and the techniques they employ.

When nurses attempt to elicit information, it is tempting to use direct and pointed questioning in order to cover all areas in the interview, particularly when there are a specified number of items that must be covered. Nurses have a tendency to rush the interview along for fear that the information may be incomplete. Most nurses are more comfortable with structured and pointed interviews. They feel the need to categorize the information and follow a set pattern. An unstructured interview is uncomfortable, and it takes time and effort to develop a more leisurely approach. The most successful interviews are, indeed, not unstructured, but the questions and direction are such that they allow for maximum parent participation without loss of the focus. The interviewer picks up and follows cues and signals that permit exploration while maintaining the overall focus. It is best to avoid phrasing a question in such a way that it can be answered with "yes" or "no," because this tends to cut off spontaneous conversation.

Encourage the parent to talk. Interviewing parents offers the nurse the opportunity to determine not only the health and developmental status of the child but also offers cues and guides to all those factors that influence the child's life. The mother is usually the most influential factor in the child's growth and adjustment; therefore, anything that affects her will necessarily affect the child. Whatever the mother sees as a problem should be a concern of the nurse. These problems are not always easy to identify. Nurses will need to be alert for clues and signals by which a mother communicates worries and anxieties. Careful phrasing of inquiries is rewarded with the specific information needed and the feelings and attitudes of the parent. For example, one broad open-ended question such as "What is Jimmy eating now?" will provide more information than several single-answer questions such as "Is Jimmy eating what the rest of the family eats?" that can be answered with "yes" or "no."

Allow the mother to take the initiative and provide the direction, then assist her to move ahead. An initial question such as "How are things with Julie today?" or "How are things today?" allows the mother to take the lead and may provide clues to a problem area and the present status of the parent-child relationship. This approach may be more uncomfortable for the novice interviewer and may create a feeling of loss of control, but use of carefully structured, leading questions allows the interviewer to maintain command and, at the same time, direct the course of the interview.

Sometimes the mother will take the lead without stimulation. Other times it may be necessary for the nurse to direct another question based on an observation such as "Connie seems unhappy today," or "Does it bother you when David cries?" If the mother appears to be tired or distraught, the nurse might ask, "What do you do to relax?" or "Do you get any help with the children?" A comment such as "You handle the baby very well. Have you had a lot of experience with babies?" to a new mother who appears comfortable with her first child gives her positive reinforcement and provides an opening for any questions she might have regarding the care of her infant. Mothers who are relaxed and spontaneous are more likely to bring out useful information than are tense, defensive parents. Often all that is required to keep the mother talking is a nod, saying "yes," "uh-huh," and so on, to let the mother know the nurse is listening and interested.

Use of open-ended, leading questions encourages spontaneous expression of feelings and concerns. It is more comfortable to use a questionnaire-type technique in which the nurse asks a series of questions that elicit simple, direct answers. Uncomfortable interviewers will ask practical questions as a defense against expression of feelings. It is easier for nurses to respond to a mother's overt questions about diet, physical health, and so on, than it is to deal with her feelings. A question that requires a simple, direct answer provides little information, tends to sound final, and closes off communication, whereas the open-ended technique tends to focus on the mother and her more immediate needs and concerns, for example, "Do you get any help in the care of the children?" "How do you manage?" "How bad is it?" "How do you feel about it?" or "Why does that trouble you?"

When attempting to elicit feelings and covert problem areas, it is best to avoid beginning a question with "Does . . .," "Did . . .," or "Its . . .," which usually require only a single response. Instead, it is helpful to use "What . . .," "How . . .," "Tell me about . . .," and encourage elaboration with "You were saying . . .," "You say that . . .," or reflecting back a key word. Open-ended questions are nonthreatening and encourage description.

When nurses do not speak the language of the family, the communication process is severely hampered. If the parents understand some words it is doubly important that nurses listen carefully and speak clearly, slowly, and with a vocabulary that is simple to understand. This is true even when using an interpreter. Cultural differences in meanings of words can easily create misunderstanding in either direction of communication. A nod to indicate understanding is insufficient evidence of comprehension. If nurses repeat their perception of what was said directly or through the interpreter and have the parent do the same, the interpretation of the message is more apt to be accurate. It is not uncommon for an interpreter to be embarrassed or otherwise hesitant to ask a parent questions that they feel may be embarrassing to the parent or an invasion of privacy. Sometimes they reword the questions or answers to convey a distorted meaning.

Another hazard related to communication with persons from another culture is in regard to verbal style or words that have different meanings. A word in one culture may have an entirely different meaning in another. A word or phrase spoken figuratively might be interpreted literally by an unknowing parent.

Use of minimal verbal activity with active listening facilitates parent involvement. Nurses are prone to become quite verbal when health education and advice are indicated. It is tempting to spend time explaining, describing, and interpreting health information when the opportunity presents itself. However, it is possible to provide effective health education by properly timing the information and presenting only as much as is necessary at the moment.

Allow time for the mother to respond. Rapid-fire questioning is apt to lead to inhibition or withdrawal on her part. This sometimes happens when nurses are unable to relax, are uncomfortable with silence or long pauses, or are fearful that they may not acquire or provide the information needed to accomplish a given purpose. A high rate of questioning decreases the level of interaction.

Listening is an active process that requires concentration and attention to all aspects of conversation. Too often listeners attend to only that which they *wish* to hear and in so doing fail to grasp all the meanings conveyed by the informant. This limits the communication process and inhibits identification of parental concerns.

Other forms of verbal activity that tend to cut off communication include socializing, giving unrestricted advice, premature or inappropriate reassurance, overready encouragement, jumping to conclusions, changing the subject to a less significant aspect of conversation, or asking a specific, structured, practical question.

Use of clues, verbal leads, or signals from the mother helps to move the interview along. Previous comments or behaviors serve as guides to questions or comments, whereas irrelevant questions tend to confine or sidetrack the person being interviewed. Frequent references to an area, repetition of certain key words, or a special emphasis on something or someone serve as cues to the interviewer for the direction of inquiry. Concerns and anxieties are usually mentioned in a casual, offhand manner. Even though they are casual, they are of importance to the mother and deserve more careful scrutiny. This serves to identify problem areas and helps nurses to pursue the investigation and solution of a problem with systematic questioning. For example, a mother who is concerned about a child's habit of bed-wetting may casually mention that his bed was "wet this morning."

Listening also provides a means to assess the education and intellectual level of the mother. Taking time to provide a mother with information she already has and how to handle a situation that she can manage very well is a waste of time that can be spent on problems she *does* have.

Concerns of parents. Most parents want to be "good" parents and have at least some anxiety about their ability to function in this role. Questionable behavior on the part of children tends to cast doubt on their success as parents. A mother's worries revolve around herself and her adequacy as a mother, as well as concern over the health and development of her children. When her feelings of maternal adequacy are threatened, her anxiety rises. She wants and needs reassurance that she is handling the task of parenthood, thus it is important that nurses do not communicate to the mother in a manner that is threatening to her self-esteem. For example, the statement, "Johnny is sleeping in his own room, of course," injects the interviewer's values into the situation. The mother is most likely to respond affirmatively because she feels that the nurse wants to hear this or else that she is not behaving correctly as a mother.

The mother needs to have the nurse show an interest in her as an individual as well as in her children. Questions such as "How do you manage?" "How bad is it?" or "What do you do when things get difficult?" provide an opportunity for her to express those things that concern her but that are not directly related to the children. Being able to vent feelings to an accepting and impartial listener assists the mother to recoup her resources for problem solving and coping.

The expectations of the mother are significant factors in determining the progress and outcome of an interview. She expects to receive guidance regarding health matters but is usually not prepared for the nurse's concern for her emotional problems. Even though she is aware of her needs, a mother does not believe that she ought to "take up time" with what she considers to be nonhealth-related concerns. One objective of nursing is to help mothers to be better mothers. In the process of assessing the mother's capabilities and needs, nurses can provide the mother with reassurance that she is doing well when this is appropriate. A mother may not have a specific problem but may need only to be reassured that everything is alright—that her child is well and that her performance is appropriate.

It is comforting to concerned mothers to know that they have feelings and problems that are shared by other mothers. All want to be assured that their children are developing normally, and most have some problems or concerns about feeding, sleep, behavior, and discipline. Occasionally women do have negative feelings toward their children and need to know that such ambivalence is normal. If the nurse has determined that there is no pathology or emotional problem underlying the reaction, parents can gain a measure of reassurance in knowing that this is a common feeling. The mother and nurse can work together to find possible avenues for coping with these feelings.

Problem solving. In order to arrive at a solution to a problem, the nurse and the parent must agree that a problem exists. If neither believes that there is a problem, there is certainly no need to create one. Sometimes the parent may believe that there is a problem that the nurse is unable to see. For example, a mother was overly concerned about every small sniffle, sneeze, or cough in her infant who had been carefully examined and found to be healthy with no evidence of a respiratory problem. On careful questioning, the nurse discovered that a previous child had died of pneumonia in infancy. Consequently the nurse was able to better understand the mother's concern. Once the nurse acknowledges the mother's fear, he or she can help the mother deal with her special anxieties about her infant and teach her how to recognize when there is need for concern.

Occasionally the nurse identifies a problem that the parent denies exists. In this case the nurse should pursue the situation and either find a way to deal with the situation or enlist the aid of other health team members. For example, the parents of a child with Down's syndrome may refuse to believe that their child is different from any other child of the same age. They may say, "He is just a little slow" and "All the child needs to do is to try harder." A child with an obvious behavior problem may be described by the parents as "just stubborn" or "just behaving that way to spite us." Such statements may be clues to disturbed relationships in the family.

Once the problem is identified and agreed upon by parent and nurse, they can begin to arrive at a solution. A parent who is included in the problem-solving process is more apt to follow through with a course of action. Such questions as "What have you tried so far?" or "What have you thought about doing?" provide leads for exploration and give the parents the feeling that their ideas and solutions are worthwhile. These can be followed by "What prevents you from trying that?" "That sounds like a good plan," and "You seem to be stumped. Have you considered trying this?" Such approaches reinforce rather than belittle parents' efforts to solve their problems and encourage active participation.

Sometimes a parent arrives at a solution that the nurse does not consider to be the best alternative. If it can be ascertained that it will do no harm and the parents are convinced of its merits, it is usually best to allow them to continue with the plan. A course of action is much more likely to be carried out when parents can reach their own conclusions. Parents believe, and rightly so, that they know what is best for their children. Decisions should be theirs with the nurse serving as a facilitator in problem solving.

Anticipatory guidance. The ideal way to handle a problem is to prevent it—to deal with it *before* it becomes a problem. The best preventive measure is anticipatory guidance. Parents who know what to expect will be prepared for a behavior when it appears. For example, a fussy, irritable infant will not worry parents who have been advised that the infant is at an age when he will normally cut a first tooth. Parents of a toddler will be prepared for his behavior when he is confronted with a new brother or sister. Some developmental changes that may disturb unprepared parents are beginning locomotion, diminished appetite, altered sleeping patterns, and anxiety toward strangers.

Communicating with children

Although the greatest amount of verbal communication is usually carried out with the parent, the child should not be excluded during the interview. Periodic attention to infants and younger children through play or by occasionally directing questions or remarks to them make children participants in the interview. Older children can be actively included as informants.

When relating with children of all ages it is the nonverbal components of the communication process that convey the most significant messages to children. It is difficult to disguise feelings, attitudes, and anxiety when relating to children. They are very alert to surroundings and attach meaning to every gesture and move the nurse makes. This is particularly true with very young children. It is best to avoid rushing in on a child—with gestures or with words. Allow the child time to make the first move when possible. Sudden or rapid movements are frightening to a child. So are threatening gestures such as facial contortions, including very broad smiles. Although these are usually intended as friendly gestures, they frequently have the opposite effect.

Children are uncomfortable or even frightened when they are stared at. It is best to refrain from extended eye contact with a child. Active attempts to make friends with children before they have had an opportunity to evaluate an unfamiliar person tend to increase their anxiety. It is best to wait for the child to make the first move, if possible. A helpful tactic is to continue to talk to the child but go about activities that do not involve him directly, thus allowing him to carry out his observations from a safe position. Sometimes nurses feel uncomfortable under this silent, intense scrutiny of a small child.

Children should be met on their own eye level since communicating down to children emphasizes their smallness. Adults in strange places may assume overwhelming proportions to children who believe themselves to be in helpless positions. Sitting on a low chair, kneeling, squatting, or even sitting on the floor, if appropriate, places the nurse in a more favorable and less threatening position when relating to small children.

At any age children respond best to a quiet, unhurried, and confident voice. Children attend to softly spoken words; they tend to withdraw when a voice is raised. Even a crying, distressed child will be more apt to "hear" a voice that speaks quietly than one that is attempting to compete with the child's own volume. This is the most successful approach to calming even an uncooperative child.

When giving directions to or seeking cooperation from a child, the nurse should speak clearly, be specific, and use as few words as possible. Simple language is more easily understood. Also, children's language comprehension precedes their use of words. Although they may not yet talk, it does not mean that they do not understand. The same concept applies when nurses and parents discuss children in their presence. It is more effective to use a positive approach in relating with children. Directions and suggestions are best stated in a positive way. An easy way to do this is to avoid using the word "don't." There is more likelihood that a child's cooperation will be gained by saying "The crayon is for writing" instead of "Don't eat the crayon."

The nurse should be honest with children and make no promises that are impossible to carry out. To assure them that a procedure, such as an injection, will not hurt is no measure of comfort to children who have either experienced the discomfort previously or who discover that indeed it *does* hurt. Any trust that has been built between the child and the nurse will be damaged by the deception, and the child will be justifiably angry.

Children should be told in advance what is going to happen to them. They are fearful of the unknown, and their active imaginations can fantasize images out of proportion to the actual event. The explanation or warning should immediately precede the action. Once the child has been told what to expect, follow through without delay. Too much advance warning will be either nullified by intervening activities or will allow time for anxiety about the anticipated event to mount. When fearful procedures are being carried out, the child should be approached with confidence and the procedure executed swiftly and immediately following a brief warning. The child should be comforted with physical contact after a painful or stressful event. The mother, who has always been the source of comfort to the child, is an ideal person to provide consolation for her infant or child.

It is confusing to children when they are offered a choice when there actually is none. Again, a positive approach is most successful. For example, when clothes must be removed for an examination, "Would you like to take off your dress?" offers the child an alternative she in fact does not have. "We need the dress off so that I can listen to your chest. Shall I help you take it off?" gives the child an explanation, a choice, and some measure of control in the situation.

Communication related to development of thought processes. The normal development of language and thought offers a frame of reference for nurses in knowing how to communicate with children. Thought processes progress from concrete to functional and finally to abstract, formal operations.

Because they are unable to use words, infants primarily use and understand nonverbal communication. Infants communicate their needs and feelings through nonverbal behaviors and vocalizations that can be interpreted by someone who is around them for a sufficient amount of time. Infants smile and coo when content and cry when distressed. Crying is provoked by unpleasant stimuli from inside or outside, such as hunger, pain, body restraint, or loneliness. Adults interpret this to mean that an infant needs something and consequently try to alleviate the discomfort and reduce tension. Crying (or the desire to cry) persists as a part of everyone's communication repertory.

Infants respond to adults' nonverbal behaviors. They become quiet when they are cuddled, patted, or receive other forms of gentle, physical contact. They derive comfort from the sound of a voice even though they do not understand the words that are spoken. Until infants reach the age where they experience stranger anxiety, they readily respond to any firm, gentle handling and quiet, calm speech. Loud, harsh sounds and sudden movements are frightening.

Older infants' attentions are centered on themselves and their mothers; therefore, any stranger is a potential threat until proved otherwise. Holding out the hands and asking the infant to "come" is seldom successful, especially if the infant is with the mother. If infants must be handled, the best approach is simply to pick them up firmly without gestures. It is helpful to observe the position in which the mother holds her infant. Most infants have learned to prefer a particular position and manner of handling. In general, infants are more at ease in an upright position than in a horizontal one. Also it is best to hold infants in such a way that they can keep their mothers in view. Until they have developed the understanding that an object (in this case the mother) removed from sight can still be present, they have no way of knowing that the object is still there.

Children less than 5 years of age are almost completely egocentric. They see things only in relation to themselves and from their point of view. Therefore, any communication to them should be focused on *them*. They need to be told what they can do or how they will feel. Experiences of others are of no interest to them. It is futile to use another child's experience as an attempt to gain the cooperation of very small children. They should be allowed to touch, examine, and familiarize themselves with articles that will come in contact with them. A stethoscope bell will feel cold; palpating a neck might tickle. Although they have not yet acquired sufficient language skills to express their feelings and wants, toddlers are able to communicate effectively with their hands to transmit ideas without words. They push an unwanted object away, pull another person to show them something, point, and cover the mouth that is saying something they do not wish to hear.

Everything to small children is direct and concrete. They are unable to work with abstractions and base all deductions on literal formulations. Analogies escape them because they are unable to separate fact from fantasy. For example, they attach literal meaning to such common phrases as "two-faced," "sticky fingers," or "coughing your head off." Children who are told they will get "a little stick in the arm" may not be able to envision an injection. These literal interpretations are an appealing part of this phase of development, but nurses must beware of inadvertently using a phrase that might be misinterpreted by a small child.

Children in this age category assign human attributes to inanimate objects. They endow mechanical devices and instruments with living characteristics. Consequently, they fear that these objects may jump, bite, cut, or pinch all by themselves. Children do not know that these devices are unable to perform without human direction. Unfamiliar devices need to be simply explained without building the child's fantasies. Understanding comes slowly and is not usually achieved with one explanation, so the nurse should be prepared to explain and describe things over and over again. If the child does understand, he may be seeking affirmation.

Children ages 5 to 8 years rely less on what they see and more on what they know when faced with new problems. They want explanations and reasons for everything but require no verification beyond that. They are interested in the functional aspect of all procedures, objects, and activities. They want to know why an object exists, why it is used, how it works, and the intent and purpose of its instigator. They need to know what is going to take place and why it is being done to *them* specifically. Again they need to know what is going to be done and why it is being done to *them* specifically. For example, to explain a procedure such as taking a blood pressure, the nurse might show the child how squeezing the bulb pushes air into the cuff and makes the "silver" in the tube go up. Permit the child to operate the bulb. An explanation for the reason might be as simple as "I want to see how far the silver goes up when the cuff squeezes your arm." Consequently the child becomes an enthusiastic participant. Allowing children to ask questions about what is happening to them and maintaining a permissive climate is conducive to questioning.

Children at this age have a heightened concern about body integrity. Because of the special importance and value they place on their body, they are overly sensitive to anything that constitutes a threat or suggestion of injury to it. This concern extends to their possessions also, so that they may appear to overreact to loss or threatened loss of those objects that they treasure. Helping children to voice their concerns enables the nurse to provide reassurance and to implement activities that reduce their anxiety. For example, if a reticent child fears being the single object of probing inquiry, the nurse can ignore that particular child by talking and relating to other children in the family or group. When the child no longer feels like a single target, he will usually interject his ideas, feelings, and interpretations of events.

Older children have an adequate and satisfactory use of language. They still require relatively simple explanations, but their ability to think abstractly can facilitate communication and explanation. Commonly, they have sufficient experience with health and health workers to understand what is transpiring and, generally, what is expected of them. They also need to know what is expected of them and to be told in advance what to anticipate.

As children move into adolescence they fluctuate between child and adult thinking and behavior. They are riding a current that is rapidly driving them toward a maturity that may be beyond their ability to cope. Therefore, when tensions rise, they may seek the security of the more familiar and comfortable expectations of childhood. Anticipating these shifts in identity focus allows the nurse to adjust the course of interaction to meet the needs of the moment. No single approach can be relied on consistently, and one can expect to encounter hostility, anger, bravado, and a variety of other behaviors and attitudes. It is as much a mistake to regard the adolescent as an adult with an adult's wisdom and control as it is to confine him to the concerns and expectations of a child.

Frequently adolescents are more willing to discuss their concerns with an adult outside the family and welcome the opportunity to interact with a nurse. They are more verbal than children and are extremely susceptible to the advances of anyone who displays a genuine interest in them. However, adolescents are quick to reject persons who attempt to impose their values on them, whose interest is feigned, or who appear to have little respect for who they are and what they think or say.

As with all children, adolescents need to express their feelings, so they should be allowed to talk. Generally they will talk quite freely when given an opportunity. Remember that what adolescents say cannot always be taken at face value. When emotional factors are involved, the feelings that are injected into words are as significant as the words that are used. The best way to give support is to be attentive, try not to interrupt, and avoid comments or expressions that convey disapproval or surprise. Prying and asking embarrassing questions should be avoided, and any impulse to give advice should be resisted. Frequently adolescents will reveal their feelings or a source of concern or will ask a question when they are involved in routine matters such as a physical assessment.

Teenagers characteristically have a language and culture all their own that further sets them apart from others. Since it is usually futile to attempt to keep abreast of the current vocabulary, frequent clarification of terms is advisable. Occasionally adolescents will be reticent and answer only in monosyllables. Usually this happens when they are opposed to the contact with the nurse or do not yet feel safe enough to reveal themselves. In this instance the best approach is to confine discussions to irrelevant topics to reduce the element of threat until such time as they feel more secure. Be alert for signals that indicate they are ready to talk. The major sources of concern for adolescents are attitudes and feelings toward sex, relationships with parents, peer group acceptance, and developing a sense of identity.

Play as a medium of communication. Play is a universal language of children. It is one of the most important forms of communication and can be an effective technique in relating with them. Clues about physical, intellectual, and social developmental progress can often be gleaned from the form and complexity of a child's play behaviors. This requires a minimum of equipment or none at all. Therapeutic play is often used to reduce the trauma of illness and hospitalization as is discussed in Chapter 26.

Because their ability to perceive precedes their ability to transmit, small infants respond to activities that register on their senses. Patting, stroking, and other skin play convey messages. Repetitive actions such as stretching an infant's arms out to the side while he is lying on his back and then folding them across his chest or raising and revolving his legs in a bicycling motion will elicit pleasurable sounds. Colorful items to catch the eye or interesting sounds such as a ticking clock, chimes, bells, or singing can be used to attract the child's attention.

Older infants respond to simple games. The old game of peekaboo is an excellent means of initiating communication with infants while maintaining a "safe" nonthreatening distance. After this intermittent eye-to-eye contact, the nurse is no longer viewed as a stranger but as someone who is no longer threatening. This can be followed by touch games. Clapping an infant's hands together for pat-a-cake or wiggling his toes for "this little piggy" delights an infant or small child. Much of the nursing assessment can be carried out with the use of games and simple play equipment while the infant remains in the safety of the mother's arms or lap. Talking to a foot or other part of the child's body is an effective tactic.

The nurse can capitalize on the natural curiosity of small children by playing games such as "Which hand do you take?" and "Guess what I have in my hand" or by manipulating items such as a flashlight or stethoscope. Finger games are very useful. More elaborate materials, such as puppets and replicas of familiar or unfamiliar items, serve as excellent means to communicate with small children. The variety and extent are limited only by the nurse's imagination.

Communication with the health team

Since much of infant and child care involves other members of the health team, communicating nursing action is a crucial and intrinsic part of the nursing process. Relating nursing care involves all the elements and modalities of communication (records, referrals, letters, conferences, reports, conversation) as well as an understanding of appropriate channels for communication. The success or failure of health care may depend on the effectiveness of this interchange. The type of communication is less important than that the data acquired regarding the child are communicated to other members of the team. In this way the health team can provide comprehensive care without duplication of effort or omission of essential services.

REFERENCE

1. Reusch, J.: Communication and human relations: an interdisciplinary approach. In Griffin, K., and Patton, B. R., editors: Basic readings in interpersonal communication, New York, 1971, Harper & Row, Publishers.

BIBLIOGRAPHY

Bird, B.: Talking with patients, ed. 2, Philadelphia, 1974, J. B. Lippincott Co.

Bower, F. L.: The process of planning nursing care: a model for practice, ed. 2, St. Louis, 1977, The C. V. Mosby Co.

Brammer, L. M.: The helping relationship, Englewood Cliffs, N.J., 1973, Prentice-Hall, Inc.

Byrne, M. L., and Thompson, L. F.: Key concepts for the study and practice of nursing, ed. 2, St. Louis, 1978, The C. V. Mosby Co.

Campbell, J. H., and Helper, H. W., editors: Dimensions in communications: readings, ed. 2, Belmont, Calif., 1970, Wadsworth Publishing Co., Inc.

Cantril, H.: Perception and interpersonal relations. In Griffin, K., and Patton, B. R., editors: Basic readings in interpersonal communication, New York, 1971, Harper & Row, Publishers.

Carrieri, V. K., and Sitzman, J.: Components of the nursing process, Nurs. Clin. North Am. **6:**115-124, March 1971.

Chinn, P. L., and Leitch, C. J.: Child health maintenance: a guide to clinical assessment, ed. 2, St. Louis, 1979, The C. V. Mosby Co.

Daubenmire, M. J., and King, I. M.: Nursing process models: a systems approach, Nurs. Outlook **21:**512-517, August 1973.

Davis, A. J.: The skills of communication, Am. J. Nurs. **63:**66-71, January 1963.

Department of Health, Education and Welfare: Secretary's Committee to Study Extended Roles for Nurses: extending the scope of nursing practice, Nurs. Outlook **20:**46-52, January 1972.

Douglass, L. M., and Bevis, E. O.: Nursing leadership in action, ed. 3, St. Louis, 1979, The C. V. Mosby Co.

Fast, J.: Body language, New York, 1970, J. B. Lippincott Co.

Fleming, A. W.: Our children—without them there is no future! Clin. Pediatr. **14:**92-95, January 1975.

Gallagher, J. R.: The care of adolescents. In Gallagher, J. R., Heald, F. P., and Garell, D. C.: Medical care of the adolescent, ed. 3, New York, 1975, Appleton-Century-Crofts.

Gebbie, K., and Lavin, M. A.: Classifying nursing diagnoses, Am. J. Nurs. **74:**250-253, 1974.

Gero, S. V., and Haffke, E. D.: A new formula for solving nursing problems, Nurs. '73 **3**(3):32-35, 1973.

Grant, W. W.: The child plus the parent equal one patient: an important lesson, Clin. Pediatr. **11:**433, August 1972.

Griffin, K., and Patton, B. R.: Basic readings in interpersonal communication, New York, 1971, Harper & Row, Publishers.

Haney, W. V.: Perception and communication. In Griffin, K., and Patton, B. R., editors: Basic readings in interpersonal communication, New York, 1971, Harper & Row, Publishers.

Hardiman, M. A.: Interviewing or social chit-chat, Am. J. Nurs. **71:**1379-1381, July 1971.

Hazzard, M. E.: An overview of systems theory, Nurs. Clin. North Am. **6:**385-393, September 1971.

Hughes, J. C.: Synopsis of pediatrics, ed. 4, St. Louis, 1975, The C. V. Mosby Co.

Interaction Associates: Strategy notebook, San Francisco, 1971, Interaction Associates, Inc.

Jakobson, R.: Verbal communication, Sci. Am. **227:**73-80, March 1972.

Johnson, R. C., and Medinnus, G. R.: Child psychology, ed. 3, New York, 1974, John Wiley & Sons, Inc.

King, I. M.: Toward a theory for nursing, New York, 1972, John Wiley & Sons, Inc.

Kramer, M.: The consumer's influence on health care, Nurs. Outlook **20:**574-578, September 1972.

Lewis, G. K.: Nurse-patient communication, ed. 2, Dubuque, Iowa, 1973, William C. Brown Co., Publishers.

Little, D., and Carnevalli, D.: The nursing care planning system, Nurs. Outlook **19:**164-167, 1971.

Marram, G. D.: The group approach in nursing practice, ed. 2, St. Louis, 1978, The C. V. Mosby Co.

Muencke, M.: Overcoming the language barrier, Nurs. Outlook **18:**53-54, April 1970.

Murphy, J. F.: Role expansion or role extension: some conceptual differences, Nurs. Forum **9**(4):380-390, 1970.

Murray, R., and Zentner, J.: Nursing concepts for health promotion, Englewood Cliffs, N.J., 1975, Prentice-Hall, Inc.

Pardee, G., and associates: Patient care evaluation is every nurse's job, Am. J. Nurs. **71:**1958-1960, 1971.

Purtilo, R.: The allied health professional and the patient: techniques of effective interaction, Philadelphia, 1973, W. B. Saunders Co.

Reusch, J.: Communication and human relations: an interdisciplinary approach. In Griffin, K., and Patton, B. R., editors: Basic readings in interpersonal communication, New York, 1971, Harper & Row, Publishers.

Rogers, M.: An introduction to the theoretical basis of nursing, Philadelphia, 1970, F. A. Davis Co.

Satir, V.: Communication: a process of making requests of the receiver. In Griffin, K., and Patton, B. R., editors: Basic readings in interpersonal communication, New York, 1971, Harper & Row, Publishers.

Satir, V.: Peoplemaking, Palo Alto, Calif., 1972, Science and Behavior Books, Inc.

Saunders, L.: Permanence and change. In Lewis, E. P.: Changing patterns of nursing practice, New York, 1971, The American Journal of Nursing Co.

Schumaker, C. J.: Change in health sponsorship. II. Cohesiveness, compactness and family constellation of medical care patterns, Am. J. Public Health **62:**931, July 1972.

Standeven, M.: The relevant "who" of problem solving, Nurs. Forum **10**(2):166-175, 1971.

Stoeffler, V. R., Meyer, R., and Smith, S. C.: Lessons to be learned from new child health programs: where do we go from here? Am. J. Public Health **62:**1444, November 1972.

Thoma, D., and Pittman, K.: Evaluation of problem-oriented nursing notes, Nurs. Admin. **2:**50, May-June 1972.

Travelbee, J.: Interpersonal aspects of nursing, ed. 2, Philadelphia, 1971, F. A. Davis Co.

Underwood, P.: Communication through role playing, Am. J. Nurs. **71:**1184-1186, June 1971.

Wilson, L. M.: Listening. In Carlson, C. E., editor: Behavioral concepts and nursing intervention, Philadelphia, 1970, J. B. Lippincott Co.

2

The interpersonal environment of the child

The future of any society depends on its children. If it is to survive, the society must make provision for their care and nurture. Cultural survival depends on whether the customs and values of the culture are transmitted from one generation to the next. To fulfill this critical need, societies have established institutions designed for the express purpose of rearing and educating their children. The primary institution that accepts this responsibility is the family, and, as the basic interpersonal group, it is a universal characteristic of all human societies. Although the structure and subordinate goals of the family vary among and within cultures and change at different times and in different places, the overall purpose of the family is to provide for the future of the society and the stability of the culture.

The culture into which children are born outlines the roles of their parents, structures their relationships with other people, and determines much of the behavior they acquire. A holistic view of any child requires that nurses develop some understanding of the ways that culture contributes to the development of social and emotional relationships and influences child-rearing practices and attitudes toward health. This includes an awareness of the nurse's own cultural frame of reference and a concerted effort to recognize and appreciate the views and beliefs of the health care recipients.

THE CHILD, THE CULTURE, AND CONFORMITY

A culture is composed of individuals who share a set of values, beliefs, practices, and information. It is, essentially, the way of life of a group of people that incorporates experiences of the past, influences thought and action in the present, and transmits these traditions to future group members. Culture is not a surface veneer that covers a basic outlook shared by all human beings, but an ingrained orientation to life that serves as a frame of reference for individual perception and judgment. People from one culture differ from those in other cultures in the ways they think, solve problems, perceive, and structure the world. The culture in which children are reared determines the type of food they will eat, the language they will speak, the ideals of behavior, and the way in which social roles should be conducted. To be acceptable members of the culture, children must learn how the culture expects them to behave toward others in the group. In turn, they learn how they can expect others to behave toward them. Cultures and subcultures contribute to the uniqueness of the child members in such a subtle way and at such an early age that the child grows up to feel that his beliefs, attitudes, values, and practices are the "correct" or "normal" ones; those of others may be viewed as "deviant" or "wrong." A set of values learned in childhood is apt to characterize children's attitudes and behavior for life—to guide their long-range strivings and monitor their short-range, impulse-driven inclinations.

The manner and sequence of the growth and development phenomenon are universal and fundamental features of all children; however, the variations in behavioral responses that children display to similar events are believed to be determined by cultures. Inborn temperament and modes of behavior that prompt children to behave in their own preferred and highly individual manner may be in harmony or in conflict with the culture. Such forces as heredity and maturation impose limits on the influence that parents and other social groups may bring to bear. The culture fosters and reinforces those behaviors deemed desirable and appropriate; it attempts to depress or extinguish those that are at conflict with cultural norms. Some cultures encourage aggressive behaviors in their children, others favor amiability and compliance; some foster individual resourcefulness and competition; others emphasize cooperation and submission to group interest. Since standards and norms vary from location to location, a practice that is accepted in one area may meet with disapproval or create tension in another. The extent to which cultures tolerate divergence from the established norm varies among cultures and subcultural groups. Although conformity provides a degree of security, it is a decided deterrent to change.

Background for the family: primary- and secondary-group influences[11]

Much of children's self-concept is derived from their ideas about their social roles. Because the culture delineates and clarifies roles, it is a significant influence on the development of children's self-concept, that is, the attitudes and beliefs they have about themselves. A concept of social role also depends a great deal on whether a child is reared in a primary- or secondary-group community. Children are subjected to perceptively different forms of parental training in these two types of environments. A *primary group* is characterized by intimate, continued, face-to-face contact and mutual support of the members and the ability to order or constrain a considerable proportion of the individual members' behavior. Two such groups are the family and the peer group, both of whom exert a great deal of influence on the American child. *Secondary groups* are groups that involve limited, intermittent contact and in which there is generally little concern for the members' behavior. These groups offer little in terms of support or pressure toward conformity except in rigidly limited areas. Examples of secondary groups are professional associations, church organizations, and so on.

In a primary-group community (for example, some contemporary rural, religious, or ethnic communities), all members are known to each other, most belong to the same subgroups, and all are concerned about each member's behavior. There is a high degree of material and psychologic support among the community members, and, since there is one traditional set of values that the entire group agrees on and supports, there is little conflict of values. In a stable community where the members remain within comparatively defined limits and relatives are likely to live close together, there is ample opportunity for young members to observe and absorb the practices and customs of the culture. Any member of the community feels justified in evaluating and censuring the conduct of another member. Children reared in a primary-group community learn that there is only one acceptable way to respond to any given situation. The entire group agrees, and any tendency to deviate is met with collective disapproval. It is the duty of the parents to see that the children learn and adhere to social roles and modes of behavior defined and strengthened by the views of the community.

The child-rearing orientation in a secondary-group environment, such as urban communities, differs considerably from that of a primary-group community. An urban community is dynamic and rapidly changing. Many of the traditional behaviors and values do not meet the needs of a changing society. Consequently parents are often uncertain what to teach their children. They may wish to rear their children with values consistent with their own, but the differences in experience between the generations are too great. As a result, they often grant their children autonomy in some areas of decision making early in the developmental process, and the other groups assume a greater influence. The children are exposed to an assortment of social groups with diverse sets of values and expectations. None of the groups is highly dominant in its influence; therefore, the children are exposed to an eclectic set of values, some in agreement and some at conflict with the others. From these they must ultimately select those that they determine to be best for them and adopt them to form a consistent set of roles and behaviors to be incorporated into the self-concept.

Guilt and shame. Conditioning the children to feel either guilt or shame for misdeeds is used by a culture to control social behavior. Some cultural groups value a well-developed conscience (superego) and condition their children to feel guilt following wrongdoing. Since guilt is based within the individual, successful conditioning produces self-regulated persons who punish themselves without their being caught in the act of wrongdoing. In many cultural groups guilt is lacking and social controls are based on the use of shame. Children in these groups learn that anything is acceptable as long as one is not caught; the shame results when the forbidden act is found out by others. Although both techniques are used by members of both primary- and secondary-group communities, shame is apt to be more successful in a primary-group community since most behaviors are quite public. In secondary-group communities it is less effective; persons are not as apt to be caught and, if caught, can join a group that is unaware of the misdeed. Guilt probably has a greater influence on behavior in urban communities and, although it is characteristic of most American cultures, many authorities believe that the trend in urban America is shifting away from a guilt orientation. Rapid changes in the American culture leave parents unsure of their own values; therefore, much of their function is abandoned to the school and peers. Peers are notorious for the use of shame as a disciplinary technique.

Background for the family: subcultural influence

Except in rare situations, children grow in a blend of cultures and subcultures, those smaller groups within a culture that possess many characteristics of the larger culture while contributing their own particular values. In a large, complex society such as America, there are different groups that have their own set of standards, values, and expectations within the collective ways of the large culture. Most were formed when groups of people clustered together by preference, by external pressures from the majority culture, or by geographic isolation. Although many cultural differences are related to geographic boundaries, subcultures are not always restricted by location. There are even subcultures related to the age stages of development that have traditions, games, loyalties, and rules. This is easily identified in the behavior of school-age children and adolescents. The culture is handed down by word of mouth from one "generation" to the next with its rituals and behavior standards that are highly resistant to outside influence.

Children's membership in a cultural subgroup is, for the most part, involuntary. They are born into a family with a specific ethnic or racial heritage, socioeconomic level, and religious beliefs. Although in the complex American society there are countless subcultures and considerable variation in the way of life between regions, ethnic groups, and social classes, those that seem to exert the greatest influence on child rearing are ethnicity, social class, and occupational role.

Ethnicity. Ethnic differences extend to many areas that include such manifestations as family structure, language, food preferences, moral codes, and expression of emotion. Some standards of behavior result from the cultural heritage of the specific ethnic group as, for example, the traditional role of the father. Others reflect the interaction between subcultures, most notably between members of the majority culture and a minority subculture. To establish their place in the group, children learn how to adhere to a mode of behavior that is in accordance with standards distinctive to the group and how they can expect others to behave toward them. They take their cues from observing and imitating those to whom they are exposed. For example, children of a racial minority form a perception of their role as a group member by observing the manner in which role models within the subgroup respond to treatment by people outside the subgroup. When they see group members display an attitude of inferiority, they assume this to be the appropriate behavior. These perceptions are then incorporated into their own self-concept.

In America the cross-cultural lines are becoming blurred as subcultures are being assimilated and blended into the large culture. Although ethnic differences in child rearing are probably diminishing, they remain important. It is particularly difficult for persons to attempt to maintain an identity with a subculture while living and conforming to the requirements of the larger culture. Universal customs and language of the dominant culture used in commercial and educational systems are different from those of the minority culture. Often the values are in conflict. Consequently children reared in this environment are confused about roles and values, and they usually adopt those of the more influential or higher-status culture.

The religious orientation of the family dictates a code of morality and a meaning for life's mysteries as well as behavior standards. The religious affiliation influences the family's attitudes toward education, male and female role identity, and attitudes regarding their ultimate destiny. It may determine the school that the children attend, the companions with whom they associate, and often their mate selection. In many cultures the religious beliefs are such an integral part of the culture that it is difficult to distinguish one from the other. In a few instances religion is the basis of a common way of life that determines where the children are reared and a totally individualistic life-style.

Social class. Those who have made extensive studies conclude that probably the greatest influence on child-rearing practices and its results is the social class of the family into which a child is born. Differences in child-rearing goals and practices as well as attitudes toward health have been found to be greater between social classes than between races or ethnic groups. In America social class and socioeconomic level are essentially synonymous, inasmuch as the factors by which a social class is defined are education, occupation, area of residence, and family income. Since children are reared differently by parents who vary in respect to these factors, social class can be expected to produce substantial variation in their upbringing.

Upper and middle class children live in an enriched environment that provides material comforts and broader opportunities. The parents are usually educated, and other authority figures such as teachers with whom the children are routinely in contact are usually from a middle class background and have activities and expectations for the children that are similar to those of the parents. Parents have occupations that require judgment, creativity, and resourcefulness, and these attributes are fostered in their children.

Members of the upper classes do not participate in studies; therefore, information on child-rearing practices in these groups is limited. Attitudes toward children appear to be generally permissive; however, much of the actual child care is delegated to surrogates, such as housekeepers, governesses, or private schools. The mother serves as an arbitrator between the children and the servants.

Although differences in parental behavior in different social classes are less marked than they have been in the past, one of the distinctions that is observed in middle classes but not in lower classes is the willingness to delay gratification. The uncertainty of their life leads members of the lower classes to take advantage of gratifications when they are available. This characteristic has caused lower classes to be labeled as present oriented, whereas middle classes seem to be future oriented. With better job security through unionization, unemployment compensation, and other welfare features, some segments of the lower classes are finding life more predictable. They are less apt to seize gratifications lest the opportunity vanish and are beginning to develop long-range goals, including an increased interest in education for their children. Middle class parents have higher educational and occupational aspirations for their children and use long-range planning to meet these goals.

There appear to be differences in intellectual skills and scholastic achievement between children in the upper and middle classes and those in the lower classes. The more apparent differences lie in the areas of abstract thinking and manipulation. Although the relative merits of testing techniques and standards are a matter of question, it is known that there is a higher incidence of academic failure in children from the lower class with its attendant dropout rate. It has been found that lower class parents value the concrete and tangible rather than the abstract and are, therefore, less inclined to encourage these qualities in their children. Their own educational level discourages these parents from reading to their children and providing other means for learning in the home. There are no role models in the family to support the value of education, and numerous provisions for intellectual growth are restricted by cost. To compound this, lower class neighborhoods have the poorest schools, and the children are often hampered in their learning by poor health and inadequate nutrition.[20]

Middle class parents are positively oriented toward change, whereas working class parents remain tradition oriented. Consequently the working class emphasizes conformity to parental values and external regulations, whereas middle class parents are more concerned with producing self-directed children. This may reflect the occupation orientation of the different classes. Middle class occupations tend to involve more self-direction and getting ahead; lower class occupations tend to be standardized with direct supervision. Middle class parents encourage their children in activities that foster achievement and that they believe will make them well-rounded adults. They involve their children in dancing lessons, athletic activities such as Little League, and scouting. Working class parents are more concerned that their children grow up to be moral, upright, and religious. Lower class parents are less interested in the direction of the children's activities than with their conduct. They are more concerned that the children stay out of trouble.[18,20]

With few exceptions, parents in all classes love their children and, in a broad sense, have similar goals regarding child rearing. Differences lie in the parental behavior toward the children in attempting to help them to reach these goals. Lower class parents are more restrictive and rely on coercive techniques in child training. They stress obedience and conformity, and the most frequently used form of discipline for undesirable behavior is physical punishment. Middle class parents are more apt to make use of manipulative techniques such as reasoning and drawing on the child's sense of guilt. They tend to scold and use isolation rather than physical punishment. There is more concern regarding the *intent* of the act than the *consequence* of the act. It is believed that upper class parents are more permissive and foster desirable behavior through positive reinforcement. Overall these differences tend to be small, and the general trend is in the direction of less coerciveness at all levels.

The very poor in the society who consistently exist on or below the poverty level live in a perpetual state of despair. Their limited skills give them no bargaining power in the job market, and the education needed to improve their status is beyond them. The poor desire better things for their children but are trapped in a circular pattern that perpetuates their life condition. Their powerlessness to control their fate or condition is a source of fatalism and resignation that is characteristic of the group in general. Optimism, when it is manifest, is more likely to be expressed in terms of luck or chance. This fatalistic attitude is a significant impediment to occupational and educational aspirations and to seeking health care.

One of the most disadvantaged groups are the children of migrant farm workers. Their family's low position on the economic scale and their rootless, mobile existence are especially deleterious to the children. Because both parents work in the fields, children receive little adult supervision; therefore, accident rates are high and meals are erratic. Schooling and health care are inadequate. Children are apt to live in a number of localities and attend a variety of schools in the course of a year with no continuity in either education or health care. Except where it is prohibited by law, the children are even recruited to work in the fields along with the adults.[11]

Occupational role. Some authorities believe that the occupational environment of the family head correlates more closely than does social class with the direction of child rearing and the values parents attempt to convey to their children. There appear to be differences in the way of life between "entrepreneurial" and "bureaucratic" parents. Entrepreneurial occupations include the smaller and more traditional enterprises, such as small businessmen, salesmen, physicians, and so on, that require self-reliance and independence. Income depends on hard work, individual initiative, and risk taking. The term "bureaucrat" is applied to the "organization man" with a position in a large organizational structure where job security is high and risk taking is minimal; where there is more adjustment to and dependence on others.

Entrepreneurs believe the world to be harsher than do bureaucrats and rear their children in a more authoritarian manner. They emphasize self-control, self-denial, and responsible independence with a vigorous and control-oriented approach to life. They lean toward more rigid delineation of sex roles and a more traditional orientation to family life. Bureaucratic parents tend to foster passivity, dependency, and some degree of impulse expression. A concern for group approval (outer-directedness) takes precedence over development of the individual (inner-directedness). They are more socially minded and usually allow their children more freedom. The general trend toward passivity and outer-directedness among young Americans may be rooted in this philosophy.

Cultural influence on health and health services

To begin to understand and to deal with families in a multicultural community, it is most important that nurses be aware of their own attitudes and values regarding a way of life, including health practices. Nurses, too, are a product of their own cultural background and education. Those who are aware of their own culturally founded behavior are more sensitive to cultural behavior in others. To recognize that a behavior may be characteristic of a culture rather than an "abnormal" behavior places nurses at an advantage in their relationships with families. When nurses respect cultural differences of a family, they are able to postpone judgment until it is determined whether the behavior is distinctive to the individual or a characteristic of the culture. What appears to be puzzling behavior may, in fact, be the customary response in the culture (for example, expression of emotion). It is all too easy to label another person according to one's own value system. Cultural standards and values, the family structure and function, and past experiences with health care influence parents' feelings and attitudes toward health, their children, and health-care delivery systems. It is often difficult for nurses to be nonjudgmental and objective in working with families whose behaviors and attitudes differ from or conflict with their own. To be aware of one's own feelings and attitudes as well as to respect those of the parents are essential to a helping relationship and achievement of nursing goals. To rely on one's own values and experiences for guidance can result only in frustration and disappointment. It is one thing to know what is needed to deal with a health problem; it is often quite another to implement a fruitful course of action.

Cultural beliefs and practices are an important part of data gathering in the nursing assessment. Nurses continually encounter beliefs and practices that may facilitate or impede nursing interventions, including attitudes toward family planning, food habits, and folkways that are firmly entrenched in the culture. The language of the client may be different from that of the larger culture, or there may be regional or ethnic peculiarities in the use of the basic English. Subcultural influences, such as some religious beliefs and practices, may be in conflict with standard health practices and therapeutic interventions.

The most overwhelming adverse influence on health is socioeconomic status. A higher percentage of individuals are suffering from some health problem at any one time in lower classes than in any other group. The sum of all aspects of their situation contributes to and compounds health problems, such as crowded living conditions and poor sanitation, which facilitate transfer of disease. In the lower classes, children are less likely to be immunized against preventable diseases than they are in the upper and middle classes. Lack of funds or inaccessibility to health services inhibits treatment for any but severe illness or accident. Sometimes health care is inadequate because of ignorance. In some areas a disorder is so commonplace that it is looked upon as unavoidable and is not recognized as something out of the ordinary that requires (or is amenable to) treatment. The parents may not have information regarding causes, treatment, outcome of the illness, or preventive measures. Upper and middle class parents are more apt to seek treatment for many more types of symptoms than are lower class parents, and they are more concerned with detecting and preventing illness in their children. The disinclination to utilize preventive health services is probably another symptom of the fatalistic approach to problems and a time orientation that is concentrated on the present rather than the future. Preventive dental care, immunization, and prenatal care are examples of such health services. The incidence of prematurity is highest in the lower classes. Significantly, lower class parents have a low rate of participation in community health programs and are more likely to practice home treatment.[11,18]

Nurses should make themselves aware of any specific attitudes regarding the manner of approach to a child in a given culture. Navajo Indians do not like a stranger near their infants. It is feared that the stranger may "witch" the child and produce harmful effects on his life. On the other hand, if a stranger, particularly a woman, lavishes attention on a Mexican-American infant but fails to touch him, he will develop symptoms of the "evil-eye," or *mal ojo,* that include restlessness, crying, diarrhea, vomiting, and fever. The concept of the "evil-eye" is common to many cultures throughout the world and serves to explain inexplicable onset of illness, particularly in infants and small children.[1,4]

Nurses who are members of a majority culture may encounter tension and distrust in a child from a minority culture as a result of the child's prior learned conception or relationships with other persons in the majority group. Based on these perceptions, minority children often suspect that nurses may have hostile feelings toward them and fear ill treatment. When such children are hospitalized, this feeling compounds their feelings of loneliness, helplessness, and retribution that accompany fearful happenings and separation from families. The reverse situation may be encountered by a nurse from a minority culture attempting to meet the needs of a child who has been conditioned to view the nurse's cultural or ethnic group as inferior.

To aid their efforts to understand and respect the cultural beliefs of families, it is helpful for nurses to have an available resource file containing pertinent information about the cultural and subcultural characteristics of the community in which they practice. To bridge cultural gaps in delivery of health care to children requires the establishment of a close relationship with the influential persons in the community, such as the local health healer. In this way good health practice can be presented and carried out within the framework of the culture.

THE FAMILY: THE FOLD FOR NURTURE

The family provides each newborn member of a society with legitimacy, that is, a family connection (usually symbolized by a family name), and an ascribed position in the societal strata. To maintain the viability of the family, each culture has devised standards of behavior (for example, parental role models and marriage rituals), systems that reward those who support or conform to these standards (for example, legal and moral sanctions of marriage, "Mother's Day," and other recognition that gives the participants fulfillment), and systems that punish those who do not conform to the established standards (for example, the legal and moral ostracism of homosexuals and the banishment of unwed mothers). Family is traditionally conceptualized as a group, and the belief has been held that both the mother and the father are needed to rear a child. A great deal of emotion has been generated about some of the newer concepts of family.

By and large, families fall into the following two major categories:

1. The basic reproductive unit composed of a man and a woman with a fertile sexual relationship, and their offspring
2. The family of procreation—the family that an individual helps to form, usually by marriage, and in which he or she may become a parent

Family has many meanings and has provided a fertile field for study by both sociologists and anthropologists. The family has been defined in a number of ways and for a number of purposes according to the individual's own frame of reference or in terms of what a family ought to be. During the long period of time required for human infants to reach a level of independence, families assume the responsibility for their rearing, although they differ considerably in form, complexity, and goals for socialization.

Functions of the family[11]

Authorities agree that the basic function of the family is to replace dying members of the society. To maintain its continuity, the knowledge, customs, values, and beliefs of the society must be transmitted to the young. Where children are not an economic necessity, their primary function is to receive and to give love. They are not only loved more, but they are loved as children for a longer period of time. Children bring very little predetermined behavior into the world with them; therefore, they depend on their parents to meet the primary requirements for growth and development and to establish for them an atmosphere of security. Although goals for socialization and child-rearing practices differ from one culture to another, in most societies the family appears to serve three principal functions in relation to children: (1) to provide physical care for children; (2) to educate and train children for adjustment to the culture; and (3) to accept responsibility for children's psychologic and emotional welfare.

Physical care. Human infants are totally helpless and require a long period of time to reach a level of independence, which makes them dependent on adults for their survival. The family takes responsibility for providing the child's basic needs for food, clothing, shelter, protection from harm, and health care.

Education and training. One of the major functions of the family is to socialize children. It is through the family that infants receive their contact with culture directly. They learn the language, appropriate role behavior, and the value system and ethical standards of the culture. Later, school, peers, and others will exert influence, but the family remains the primary socializing influence during childhood.

Training consists of teaching children acceptable methods of gratifying physical needs such as feeding, elimination, and self-help skills, such as dressing, tidiness, and so on. *Education* is directed toward indoctrination into their position within the family and the society. They learn the standards of responsibility to individuals. Relationships begin with siblings and adults in the family, then with peers and other authority figures, and finally with social institutions, such as school and law-enforcement agencies. Children are taught cultural sanctions and prohibitions that range from disapproval of biting another person to more rigid taboos such as incest.

Psychologic and emotional welfare. Only recently has this been stressed as a major family function. Relatively recent studies have emphasized the importance of the early psychologic relationship between parents and child to later emotional adjustment of the child. It has been shown that children are most susceptible to psychologic influences in their environment during early childhood, although the extent to which these early influences exert long-range effects is still somewhat controversial.

It is within the family setting that children test their emotions and responses to others. Through relationships with family members they learn patterns of behavior that are extended to other persons and other situations. It is these interactions with others that contribute most to formation of the self-concept, social competence, and the ability to form warm relationships later. The foundation of a health personality is laid within the family unit.

Family structure

A structure is a manner of organization or the arrangement of a number of parts that are interrelated in specified, recurring ways. The family structure consists of individuals with socially recognized statuses and positions who interact with one another on a regular, recurring basis in socially sanctioned ways. When members are gained or lost through marriage, divorce, birth, death, and so on, positions are lost or added. The family structure is altered, and roles must be redefined or redistributed.

Traditionally the family structure is referred to as either *nuclear* or *extended,* and the predominant pattern in any society depends to a large extent on the mobility of the families as they pursue economic goals. In general, extended families are associated with agricultural societies, whereas small conjugal units are characteristic of the more advanced, industrialized societies.

Nuclear family. The nuclear or conjugal family structure consists of a man, his wife, and their children (natural or adopted) who live in a common household. This is the reproductive unit in which the marital tie (legally or otherwise sanctioned) is the chief binding force. In some instances one or more additional persons (such as a relative, friend, foster child, or others) may reside in the same household. Also some authorities classify childless couples as a nuclear family because it is a conjugal alliance with the theoretical potential for reproduction. The strongly functional nuclear family is the prototype of human relationships and the basic unit from which more complex familial forms are composed.

The nuclear family, the predominant structure in America, is more characteristic of an urban mobile society. It is highly adaptable with the ability to adjust and reshape its structure when needed. It is free to move where there is opportunity for higher incomes with concomitant improvement in other areas such as social class and prestige. It is not economically bound to a geographic area nor dependent on the cooperative efforts of other members. The family members are employed on an individual basis, and economic resources are in the form of money. The present-day family must purchase the services of specialized individuals and groups, whereas previously these needs and services were met on a cooperative basis by the extended family members. With no relatives readily available for advice and assistance with child care, parents turn to the "experts" for child-rearing guidance. Although extended families residing in the same household are rapidly disappearing in American society, the isolated nuclear family without relatives within easy visiting distance is rare. This is most often seen where there has been extreme mobility of separate generations, such as wide geographic separations or marriages into different social strata, religions, or roles. Most consanguineous family members maintain contact through visits, telephone calls, letters, and gift exchanges.

The majority of nuclear families in America are associated with an extended kinship network of nuclear families living in separate households but in close geographic proximity. This concept, sometimes referred to as a modified extended family, is a meaningful aspect of daily existence as reflected in frequent visiting and the exchange of services and financial aid. This family association meets the psychologic needs to a greater extent than do experts, friends, or organizations. It is not uncommon for families to reject opportunity for social or economic advancement rather than leave the kinship associations.

Extended family. The extended, or consanguineous, family consists of the nuclear family plus lineal or collateral kinsmen. More often it is composed of two or more nuclear families affiliated through extension of the parent-child relationship, that is, grandparents, parents, and grandchildren. Broader views recognize the affiliation of collateral kinsmen as an extended family—not necessarily organized into nuclear families.

Extended family structure is more functional in areas where land is the basis of wealth and sustenance. Today the best examples of extended family units can be found in groups of individuals with great wealth, successful farmers, American Indians, and certain recent immigrants. Here the family serves as the basic social, educational, and productive unit providing services and sharing resources. Extended families direct cooperative efforts for the common goals; the needs of the individual are sublimated for the welfare of the family enterprise and survival. Children are an asset and are essential to the goals, survival, and continuation of the family. In contrast to the isolated nuclear family, the extended family is adult oriented rather than child oriented. The children learn early in life to respect their elders, and this value is reinforced through observation of their parents' behavior toward the older family members. Because of the prolonged close association, parents' responsibility for the children continues in some form throughout the children's lifetime.

In the extended family, child rearing is often a shared responsibility. Relatives are always present and available to help young mothers with household chores and child-care activities. Authority in the nuclear unit is vested in the father, and sex roles are clearly delineated. Daily lives of the children are organized around the needs and requirements of the family with assigned tasks and obligations. Family ties between the nuclear unit and the main extended family are strong, although there is a high degree of competition between individual nuclear units for acquisition of power and resources. Children also become skillful at maneuvering the favor of certain elder members of the larger unit.

Structure and social class.[20] In family structure, as with other aspects of child rearing, there are greater differences related to social class than any other variable. In the upper-upper class, or the old aristocracy, the nuclear family is firmly imbedded in an extended kinship structure. It is primarily patrifocal in that the older husband and father is the unilateral authority. The family's source of wealth is supervised by male family members, controlled by the eldest, and handed down from one generation to the next. In the lower-upper and upper-middle classes the family ties are most loosely attached. This is the most highly mobile element of the population both socially, economically, and geographically, all of which encourage the separation of extended family relationships.

The tendency in the lower-lower class is toward matrifocal family units. Since the family unit is often torn apart by continual economic stress, the mother-child relationship is the strongest and most intimate tie. There is a higher rate of divorce, illegitimacy, and desertion in this segment of society. Husband and wife are often emotionally separated by unfulfilled expectations. The father, who has few personal or economic assets (and who is more often an economic burden), has difficulty establishing a dominant role in the family. In this class the mother is often more easily employed than the father, and she is eligible for welfare benefits when there are minor dependent children; therefore, the mother-child dyad is predominant. Frequently there are three generations—grandmother, mother, and children—living in an extended structure to share the economic burden and child care.

Variant structures. Present-day America is undergoing rapid changes in relation to family form. Variations on the traditional nuclear family have come about as a result of some recent social phenomena. For example, the *single-parent family* is now recognized as a family and has emerged partially as a consequence of women's rights movements wherein more women have established separate households as a result of divorce, death, desertion, or illegitimacy. Also the more liberal attitude of the courts has made it possible for single persons to adopt children, whereas, previously, rigid prerequisites specified that both a father and a mother must be present in the home.

Predominantly female-headed, the incidence of the single-parent family occurs more often in the lower classes, particularly in the lower-lower class in which absence of a father in the home is more frequent. Unmarried mothers, choosing to keep and raise their children rather than place them for adoption or marry, are absorbed into the extended family. In the lower-lower class of the United States where the incidence of illegitimacy is highest, the maternal grandmother is usually available to care for the children. Although illegitimacy is more accepted now than previously, the general social response is disapproval at all levels, including the poor, and the unwed mother experiences lowered self-esteem. However, with the increased psychologic independence of women as a whole and as illegitimacy becomes increasingly acceptable to society, more unmarried women are deliberately choosing mother-child families.

An alternative life-style, the *communal family,* has seemed to emerge, as have all previous experimental communities, from a disenchantment with most contemporary life choices. Although they may have divergent beliefs, practices, and organization, the basic impetus has been dissatisfaction with social systems and life goals of the larger communities and with the nuclear family structure as it exists—either from an ideologic or a practical perspective.[12]

The increase in the formation of communal groups and collectives is one representation of the counterculture in America and a reversion to the values provided by the cooperative efforts of an extended family group. In communes there is common ownership of property and goods; in cooperatives there is private ownership of property, but certain goods and services are shared and exchanged cooperatively without monetary consideration. They are located in urban, suburban, and rural settings. Members of some recreate a primitive, self-reliant life-style; others prefer a modernistic approach. Members of both types seem to be committed to experimentation with the definition of the family unit with various forms of child rearing and education and sharing of endeavors that allow individual members greater opportunities for leisure time. There is strong reliance on group members and material interdependence. Both provide collective security for nonproductive members, share homemaking and child-rearing functions, and help overcome the problem of interpersonal isolation or loneliness. Although communes and cooperatives are proposed as a "new" family form, they are actually a form of the traditional extended family and may be meeting a need for close family ties.[11,15]

Most communes in America, characterized by lack of planning or planners, seem to have originated spontaneously. Consequently, they more nearly resemble way stations for "searching, alienated youth." Unlike the traditional extended family, nuclear units in a commune may come and go at will. There is no consanguineous tie between the units. The mother-child tie is strong during infancy and early childhood, but many parents are happy to relinquish the older child to the care of others. Although the parents maintain primary responsibility for the health and well-being of the children, the children are free to form close relationships with a number of adults in the commune and are encouraged to do so. As opposed to the traditional family systems where the total responsibility for child rearing is left to the parents and the school, in the commune the parental role is deemphasized and all children are the collective responsibility of the adult members. This is one of the major attractions of communal living—it frees the parent from total responsibility for the child. Children are not viewed as an extension of or a reflection on the parents and their abilities—another attractive aspect of communal child rearing. Children are provided freedom to be themselves and are viewed as a product of their own natural growth and inclinations.

There are other family forms that are relatively rare. Although it is not legally sanctioned, sometimes the conjugal unit can be extended by the addition of spouses in polygamous matings. Most often mothers and their children share a husband and father, usually with each mother and her children maintaining a separate household. Another form that has yet to be evaluated is the homosexual family in which there is a marital or common-law tie between two persons of the same sex who have adopted children or in which one or both partners have natural children from a prior heterosexual mating.

Familial factors affecting children

Numerous familial factors can alter the childhood environment. No two children grow in exactly the same environment, although identical twins more nearly approximate this. For example, in a nuclear family with two children—even of the same sex—one will live in a family with an older sibling whereas the other will be reared in a family with a younger sibling. Or in a family where there is a 10-year age span in the children, one may be born to a 20-year-old mother, the other to a 30-year-old mother. For the child in each situation the environment is different.

Family size. The size of the family of orientation has a decided impact on the child. In the small family more emphasis is placed on the individual development of the children. Parenting is intensive rather than extensive, and there is constant pressure to measure up to family expectations. Children's development and achievement are measured against that of other children in the neighborhood and social class. In small families there is more democratic participation by the children than in larger families. Adolescents in small families identify more strongly with their parents and rely more on parents for advice. They have well-developed, autonomous inner controls as contrasted with adolescents from larger families who rely more on adult authority. In small families there is more opportunity for democratic participation by all the children.

Children in a large family are able to adjust to a variety of changes and crises. There is more emphasis on the group and less on the individual. Cooperation is essential, often because of economic necessity. The large number of persons sharing a limited amount of space requires a greater degree of organization, administration, and authoritarian control. The control is wielded by a dominant family member—a parent or an older child. The number of children reduces the intimate, one-to-one contact between the parent and any individual child. Consequently, children turn to each other for what they cannot get from their parents. The reduced parent-child contact encourages individual children to adopt specialized roles in an attempt at recognition in the family.

Discipline is often administered by older siblings in large families. Siblings are usually better attuned to what constitutes misbehavior, and sibling disapproval or ostracism is frequently a more meaningful disciplinary measure than parental spankings. In situations such as death or illness of a parent, an older sibling assumes responsibility for the family at considerable personal sacrifice. Large families seem to generate a sense of security in the children fostered by sibling support and cooperation. However, adolescents from a large family are more peer oriented than family oriented.

A greater amount of contact and interaction with parents is enjoyed by only children. With adults as speech models, they are consistently advanced in language development, and the close contact with interested adults motivates them to higher intellectual achievement. The relative isolation from other children encourages a rich fantasy life, independence, and originality. There is no evidence to indicate that there are significant differences in adjustment and personality based on the fact that they have no siblings.

Sibling position and sex. Relationships between siblings in the family group duplicate, to some extent, many of the social interaction experiences of later years. Through relationships with siblings, children learn patterns of loyalty, competition, dominance, and so on. Such factors as whether a child is the firstborn, a middle child, or the youngest child or whether there is 1 or 6 years separating him from his sibling affect his view of the world and his relationship with others inside and outside the family. None of these characteristics are absolute, nor do they apply to all children and all parents. The potential effects depend on all intrafamilial factors such as parenting practices, the number of children in a family, the age differences between siblings, and the sex and birth order of older and younger siblings.

Firstborn children are more achievement oriented than children born later and exhibit strong drive and ambition. They usually receive more physical punishment than younger children and are allowed to show more aggression toward their younger siblings. They have stronger consciences and are usually more self-disciplined, inner-directed, and prone to feelings of guilt, which may account for a higher intellectual achievement. Firstborn children are better represented in college populations than are younger siblings. Although they are more likely to have tasks imposed on them, the oldest child seems to experience fewer frustrations in the family setting than does a younger sibling. They are better planners and tend to identify with parents and to measure themselves by adult standards.

Younger children reflect the decrease in the amount of parental attention and anxieties. On the whole, mothers are warmer toward the youngest child than the oldest and middle child, and the youngest child receives little physical punishment. The youngest child is less dependent than a firstborn and more apt to be left to manage things for himself. Younger children are usually more backward than the firstborn in language development and articulation. They appear to be less tense, more affectionate, and more good-natured than the firstborn, and they tend to identify more with the peer group than with parents. Second-born children seem to have more numerous interests. The older and middle children are usually assigned more tasks in the family than are younger ones, and the middle children more so than the older ones. The middle children appear to occupy the most difficult position. There are more demands on them for help with household tasks, they are praised less often for good behavior, and they receive less of the mother's time for pleasurable activities.[17]

One of the reasons for these differences is that the first child is most likely to be the most wanted child. The first-born child, born to relatively inexperienced parents, is the recipient of all the parental uncertainties, unskilled experimentation, and a great deal of adult attention and pressure. Parents expect more from him than from later children, tend to be more tense, and worry more about him. Parents, having had the experience of one child, are more relaxed when the second arrives, and they tend to be less strict and less preoccupied with the parental role. The close, intense attention that the eldest receives contributes to his adult orientation.

The age difference between siblings affects the childhood environment but to a lesser extent than does the sex of the siblings. The arrival of a sibling has the greatest impact on the older child, and a 2- to 4-year difference in age appears to be most threatening. When the older child is very young, his self-image is too immature to be threatened. At an older age he is better able to understand the situation and, therefore, less likely to see the newcomer as a threat, although he does feel the loss of his only-child status.

In general the narrower the spacing between siblings the more the children influence one another, especially in emotional characteristics; the wider the spacing, the greater the influence of the parents. Also, younger children tend to identify with older siblings. Consequently they assume some of the personality characteristics of the older child. Girls with brothers have more masculine characteristics than girls raised with sisters. They are, on the whole, more aggressive, ambitious, and perform better on tests of intellectual ability, probably related to the more stimulating environment created by competitive, aggressive boys. Boys with older sisters, especially if the age difference is slight, are generally less aggressive and daring than boys raised with older boys, probably a reflection of the identification process and the more power exerted by the older sibling.

Working mothers. A great deal has been written and a variety of conclusions arrived at regarding the effects of mothers working outside the home. The number of women in the labor force has increased steadily during the past 2 decades and shows every indication of continuing. Mothers work for several reasons. Most work for purely economic reasons, either because they are the sole support of the family, to supplement a husband's inadequate income, or to provide the family with a higher standard of living. Others work as a response to the boredom of housework or simply to meet their own ego needs. No matter what the mother's motivation, the consensus is that deleterious effects on the children are related to the *quality* of the mother-child interaction rather than the *quantity* of time spent with the children.[19]

The mother's relationship to the rest of the family depends to a large extent on her own feelings and reactions to working and to her job. Although most mothers feel some guilt about leaving their children in the care of others, those who feel secure and happy in their work usually reflect this attitude in the home and in relationships with other members of the family. Sometimes, however, the mother feels guilty about leaving the children so that she can pursue a career or a job, particularly if she enjoys the outside activity. If she compensates for guilt feelings with overindulgence toward the children, they may feel more insecure and take advantage of her vulnerability with demanding behavior. On the whole, children of working mothers are self-reliant, do better in school, and show relatively few ill effects of the separation.

Many factors are related to the effect that a mother's absence has on the children: the age of the child (very young children feel the impact of the mother's absence more than older children), the attitude of the father toward the wife's employment, and the regularity with which she is away from the family. Delinquency rates appear to be highest in families where the mother works sporadically. However, these are predominantly children from the lower classes where other factors are also in operation. The mother's emotional stability is a more important factor in these situations.

Absent father. Fathers have been referred to as "absentee fathers" because they are away from the home for the greater part of the day. Even though the trend is toward equilateral responsibility for home and family, chances are that when he is at home he is fatigued and only too glad to abdicate all responsibility for the children to the mother (unless she, too, is working outside the home). Our concern here, however, is with the family without a father because of death, divorce, desertion, illegitimacy, or involuntary separation such as military service, job demands, jail, and so on.[9]

The most serious consequences of parent absence are related to separation of the child from the mother (see p. 881) in infancy and early childhood. However, there are some effects on child development when a parent (usually the father) is absent during childhood. The primary effect of absence of either parent from the home is in the difficulty in adjustment and development of a sexual identity. This is more marked when the parental absence occurs early in the child's life and when it is the same sex parent. Girls from homes where fathers are absent are more dependent on their mothers and show some anxiety about relationships with males during adolescence. Boys from homes without fathers tend to be less aggressive, are more apt to have emotional and social problems, and demonstrate cognitive patterning more similar to that of girls. Overprotectiveness, extreme indulgence, and often prolonged physical contact with the mother over a period of years may contribute to serious sex identity problems in male children.[10]

Children from homes in which one or both parents are frequently absent are highly susceptible to peer group influence; this appears to be related to lack of attention and concern at home rather than to a positive attraction of the peer group. Also, the peer group serves a role identification function for young males from homes where the father is absent or ineffectual.

Divorce. Authorities agree that marital factors within the home contribute to children's development. Children from a happy, relaxed atmosphere in the home are less likely to have a negative outlook than are those from stressed homes. The causes of marital strife are varied, but the effect of the parents' inability to adapt influence the adjustment and personality growth of young children. It is difficult to determine to what extent the child's maladjustment is related to the family atmosphere leading to a divorce or to the divorce itself.

It is known that divorce is not good for children; however, children who are under the continual stress of intact but unhappy homes feel more secure and happy after the marital relationship is dissolved. Children who felt that their homes were happy before the divorce have a more difficult adjustment. Factors present in the divorce situation itself exert harmful influences on children's psychologic adjustment. The child who becomes involved in divorce has feelings of terror and abandonment. As the parents become involved with their own feelings and concerns, they are less available and have less to give the children. The children see themselves apart from the family, feel alone and isolated, and long for consistency and order in their lives.

Since a function of parenthood is to provide for the emotional welfare of the child, disruption of the family structure often engenders strong feelings of guilt in the parents. Some may feel resentment toward the child who makes the situation more difficult, and they may attempt to compensate in overprotective behavior and excessive concern for the child's welfare. The child, also, has guilt feelings as though he has failed or is being punished for past misbehavior. The interpersonal tension created by parental insecurity and anxiety is communicated to the child who does not have the ego resources to cope with these feelings of tension and the vague threat of a change in his world. Although there are counseling services available to parents, very little such help is available for children. Children need to be taught that relationships change and how to deal with the new form that the relationship takes.

During a divorce the parental capacity is diminished. The parents are much too preoccupied with their own needs and life changes to be supportive to their children. Moreover, they need to know what to do, and there are no acceptable models on which they can rely. Many parents do not tell their children about the divorce either because they do not know what to tell the children or because they believe that the children will not understand.

The impact of divorce on children depends on the age of the child and the quality of parental care during the years following the divorce. Although a child at any age is profoundly affected by divorce, the greatest amount of stress is suffered by preschool children; adolescents and school-age children are better able to cope with the separation. Egocentric preschoolers, who see and understand things only in relation to themselves, assume themselves to be the cause of parental distress and interpret the separation as punishment. They feel a sadness and a strong feeling of responsibility for the loss of the absent parent. Moreover, they consciously fear that they may be abandoned by the remaining parent. Consequently it is essential to establish some kind of stability for these children; otherwise they will convert their energies to restabilization rather than to growth and development. They need frequent, repeated, and concrete explanations of what is going to happen to them, how they will be cared for, and assurance that something new will take the place of the old and that they will not be deserted. In order that they will not imagine things, explanations, such as where they will live, who will prepare their meals when the parent is at work, and when they will see the absent parent again, should be specific. They need a focus on reality.

School-age children and adolescents are able to deal with parental separation better than younger children. They feel intense pain and loneliness; their ability to learn is affected since they are unable to focus on learning; and somatic complaints, especially in school-age children, and emotional disturbances in adolescents are observed. Often they must move to an unfamiliar environment and a new neighborhood and form new relationships in addition to coping with the alteration in their family structure. They almost invariably wish for the parents to reunite.

To predict the impact of divorce on any specific child it is important to anticipate how much love and understanding will continue after the parent separation and how much genuine concern and affection exist for the child. Other complications include efforts on the part of one parent to subvert the child's loyalties to the other, abandonment to other care givers, and adjustment to a stepparent. In 90% of divorce cases the mother receives custody of the child; this has an effect on the male child's identification with a father figure in addition to all the other ramifications of the family without a father and the single-parent family. Many divorced mothers with small children move in with parents, other relatives, or friends in some kind of dependent or sharing arrangement. In general, better educated parents and those in the upper strata of society are less apt to divorce, separate, or desert each other; the incidence is highest in the lower social classes.

There are numerous other factors that significantly influence the childhood environment such as a handicapped or chronically ill child in the family (see Chapter 22), death of a sibling or parent (see Chapter 27), the advent of a stepparent and sometimes stepsiblings, and the experience of a foster child, who often must adjust to several families.

Family roles and relationships[14]

The way in which persons are located in the family system constitutes the family structure. Each individual has a position, or status, in this structure, and each occupant of a position plays culturally and socially defined roles in interactions within the group. Cultural norms specify the rights and obligations of the individual who occupies a particular position. Within prescribed guidelines for behavior set by the culture, subcultures (including the family group) establish variations in role definition and may specify different requirements for playing the same role. Each family has its own traditions and values, and each sets its own standards for interaction within and outside the family group. Each determines the experiences the children should have, those they are to be shielded from, and how each of these experiences meets the needs of family members.

Roles are mutually interactive, that is, each role is enacted in relation to persons occupying other positions in the family. The behaviors of others within the group provide cues by which one determines his position and role within the group. For example, the behaviors that are expected of someone in the role of mother are enacted in relation to the complementary behaviors of an infant or child; the cues that are provided by her infant guide the mother in appropriate behaviors toward that child. Once the person locates the position of others in the structure and attributes role expectations to them and their position, he is able to determine the reciprocal position and can enact a corresponding role.

Family roles are continually changing, emerging, being modified, and terminating. The infant has only one role, that of child. Each successive developmental stage requires the individual to assume a variety of roles within the family and to participate in roles and relationships within the context of other social groups. A situation or event that requires a person to alter a role and act accordingly is interpreted as a crisis. For example, a new child in the family expands the role of son or daughter to that of an older sibling; a child on the first day of school assumes the role of student.

Although individuals bring their own temperaments, abilities, philosophies, and value orientations to the enactment of the roles they play, most roles exist independently of the persons who play them. Everyone has expectations about the role of nurse that guide their evaluation of each nurse whom they meet. These same expectations influence the way the person who performs the role of nurse behaves in the role. Role performance is influenced by the knowledge of role behaviors associated with the role and responses of all those who interact with the performer. Individuals are strongly disposed to perform roles assigned to them—even when the role may be damaging to self-esteem.

Roles are learned through the socialization process. During all stages of development children are learning and practicing, through interaction with others and in their play, a set of social roles and something of the characteristics of other roles. They will behave in patterned and more or less predictable ways because they learn roles that define mutual expectations in typical and recurring social relationships. Role conceptions are transmitted by socializing agents (parents, peers, authority figures) who use positive and negative sanctions to ensure conformity to their norms. Role behaviors positively reinforced by rewards such as love, affection, friendship, and honors are strengthened. Negative reinforcement takes the form of ridicule, withdrawal of love, expressions of disapproval, or banishment. Conformity to group norms is directly related to the strength and nature of group ties. Where family ties are strong, social control is highly effective, and most members play their roles willingly and with commitment.

Children are influenced in many other ways. For example, individuals may look outside the family environment and pattern behavior after role models of a position or status they hope to achieve. A person in a lower class may adopt behaviors of middle class persons, using persons outside his group or persons in the mass media as role models.

Parental roles. In all family groups the socially recognized statuses of father and mother exist with socially sanctioned roles that prescribe appropriate sexual behavior and child-rearing responsibilities. The guides for behavior in these roles serve to control sexual conflict in society and provide for prolonged care of children. The degree to which parents are committed to and the way they play their respective roles are influenced by a number of variables. Each individual is affected by his own unique socialization experience. In addition the rate of social change that is accompanied by alterations, modifications, and contradictions in role definitions continually exerts an influence on role expectations and performance. Because of the biologic attachment, the woman has assumed the role of nurturer and sustainer. Consequently the traditional role concept of the married woman and mother in the Western culture has been to remain in the home to bear and raise children, perform household chores, and accept the authority of the husband. For this she received the love and gratitude of her husband and children and the approval of society. Female characteristics in America and elsewhere tend toward the passive and nurturing, with less independence and achievement orientation than is seen in males. Males are expected to be aggressive, self-reliant, and high achievers.

Role definitions are changing as a result of the changing economy and the women's liberation movement. Women are achieving equality with men in education, more of them are entering the labor force, and the number of women who choose to have fewer children or none at all is increasing. During childhood, particularly in the upper and middle classes, the trend is toward deemphasizing the basic male-female characteristics of aggression, dependence, and achievement. As the role of the woman changes there must be, necessarily, a change in the complementary role of the male. Fathers are taking a more active role in the child-rearing and household activities. This is most evident in middle class families. Marital roles are most segregated in the lower classes. Redefinition of sex roles in the American family is taking place, but there is still a cultural lag of the persisting traditional role definitions that create role conflict in many of these families.

Role structure. In every family there is a pattern for assigning power and responsibility. Although it can be distributed in many different ways, the family member who controls the resources is usually (but not always) perceived as having the most power. The way this power is allocated has implications for the psychologic development of family members, especially the children.

The first pattern is one in which the power is invested in one person—either the father or the mother. This comes about because one adult either controls family resources, one parent perceives himself or herself as superior, one adult is absent, or one parent abdicates decision making to the other and is willing to accept the decisions of the other. The pattern of authority can be either patricentric, in which the father has greatest power (a common pattern in traditional and old-world families) or matricentric, where the mother exercises greatest control (frequently seen in lower class black families). In either situation the demands on the authority figure are heavy and constant and the success of relationships rests on whether or not other family members accept this authority as legitimate. A single authority produces maximum efficiency in decision making and provides the person in power with a personal sense of competence, but others may resent this power and then this person becomes an easy target for blame. This adult is most likely to be the primary source of rewards and punishment in the family and, consequently, a strong identification model for the children.

A second pattern of authority allocation is one in which the adults in the family jointly assume the decision making and assignment of tasks. More often this is a husband-wife executive dyad, although it may include other adults who live in the household, such as a grandparent. There is more diversity of ideas and opinions in this pattern, and decisions are less apt to be impulsive than those resulting from a single-executive power. In this pattern children are subordinate to the adults and are viewed as incapable of making decisions; this is sometimes a cause for rebellious action on the part of the children. The adults make joint decisions and, therefore, share responsibility for misjudgments and incorrect decisions. This is probably characteristic of most families in America.

In the third pattern the family as a whole shares the responsibility of decision making. Problems are brought to the entire family, including children, and each member is given the opportunity to offer opinions, suggestions, or solutions. Although slower and more cumbersome, this process provides a diversity of ideas and opinions, results in a learning experience for the children in problem solving, and assures that the needs of all members, if not met, are at least considered. This model probably has shortcomings in terms of efficiency, but it also has long-term gains in group cooperation, mutual satisfaction, and the preparation of the children for decision making in adulthood.

One can readily envision the role relationships of parents who have been reared where the role expectations and role structure in their respective families may be either in agreement or in conflict. For instance, a husband who is accustomed to a subordinate role in relationships with persons in his family (an authoritarian mother or older sisters) will expect similar behavior in his wife. If his wife has a similar background there should be no role conflict—she will in all likelihood assume the leadership role. If, on the other hand, the wife expects her husband to be authoritarian or to share in decision making, one or both of them will need to redefine and adjust role expectations in order to avoid conflict.

Role learning in children

One responsibility of the family is to develop in the children culturally appropriate role behavior. Very early, children learn to perform in expected ways consistent with their position in the family and the culture. The observed behavior of each child is a single manifestation—a combination of social influences and individual psychologic processes. Thus the uniting of the child's intrapersonal system (the self) with the interpersonal system (the family) is comprehended simultaneously as the conduct of the child.

Children respond to life situations according to behaviors learned in reciprocal transactions with others. Initially this takes place within the family unit where the children perform a set of roles and respond to the complementary roles of their parents and other family members. The roles of the children are shaped primarily by the parents who may or may not be aware of their influence.

Types of roles.[14] The types of roles that are learned can be broadly classified as ascribed, achieved, adopted, and assumed roles.

An *ascribed role* is one that is strictly defined by the culture and very little deviation is allowed to modify it. Ascribed roles apply to general traits such as sex, age, kinship, social class, and ethnic origin. There are culturally determined behaviors that must be adhered to in respect to these roles, and they are expected to be learned in the home. For example, a child who attempts to change an ascribed role (such as sex) will be confronted with serious problems.

An *achieved role* is acquired through effort, and the child must do something to attain it. Achieved roles include educational, occupational, religious, and recreational roles.

These are based on performance and are acquired through satisfaction of specified requirements. The direction of these role achievements is strongly influenced by values conveyed to the children by the parents. For example, some parents believe that a college education is essential; others encourage children to seek occupational gratification. Achievement of athletic prowess is highly valued by some parents; musical accomplishment is esteemed by others.

Adopted roles are sometimes transient in nature, such as the role of patient or traveler. More often, adopted behavior patterns become more fixed into what are known as character roles and apply to the unique behaviors that the child displays in a given situation. Such roles as the leader, the follower, the prankster, the deceiver, the show-off, or the honest one are examples of adopted roles. They are often adopted when playing the role meets a need or is the response to a complementary role in another.

Assumed roles are related to fantasy and are especially important in childhood. This is one of the dominant means for children's adjustment and socialization. Children continually assume roles of persons they observe in their environment. The environment is a primary resource for learning the conduct that befits their position or status. Assumed roles only become a problem if they persist into the world of reality. For example, a child who persistently plays an infantile role is severely hampered in relationships with peers; a girl who consistently fantasizes that she is a boy may be unable to achieve motherliness at the appropriate time.

In order to structure desired role responses in children, parents and others use various techniques. Parents may apply direct or indirect pressures in an attempt to induce or force children into the desired patterns of behavior, or they may direct their efforts toward modification of the role responses of the child on a mutually acceptable basis. Each set of parents has their own techniques, and each will determine the course that the process of socialization is to follow.

Induction techniques. When parents force the child into submission to their wishes, they use induction techniques. The most common of these, *coercion,* represents a hostile, aggressive threat of punishment (physical or verbal) if the child does not acquiesce to the parents' demands. A child responds to this type of technique either with defiance or with submission as an expression of futility. With *coaxing,* parents attempt to elicit desired behavior by enticing the child with the promise of rewards in exchange for compliance. This may tend to create a false sense of power in the child, he may respond with defiance, or he may comply in order to receive the gratification. By *postponing,* parents attempt to delay dealing with the conflict in hopes that it will resolve without further action. It may provide time to further assess the situation, but intervening factors may reduce or intensify the difficulty. Parents use *evaluation* when they express approval, disapproval, praise, or blame; compare; or otherwise place a value judgment on the child's behavior. The child is uncomfortable because if he is "good" he will be expected to remain good; if he is "bad" he will be expected to change. Parents may attempt to manipulate a situation by *masking,* that is, withholding information or substituting incorrect information to resolve a conflict. This technique tends to create an atmosphere of distrust and insecurity in the relationship. Parents sometimes try *role reversal* as an attempt to control the child's behavior. The parent may say, "I think I see what you mean, but. . ."

Role modification. Role-modification procedures help to achieve a measure of understanding between family members and, unlike induction techniques, are based on a reciprocal role relationship. *Humor* enables one to appreciate and adapt to the other's point of view with a minimum of discomfort. When the parent can expose the inconsistencies in a situation or appeal to the child's sense of the absurd, this is usually effective in relieving tension. Sometimes it becomes necessary to enlist the aid of a third party to explore the problem with them. *Arbitration* or mediation is best performed by a person who has skills not available to the parent or child but who has information regarding the dynamics of the situation. *Exploration* of the various aspects of the problem provides both parent and child with the opportunity to look at alternatives and to propose and reject possible solutions in their attempt to arrive at an agreement. Use of this technique demonstrates a respect for the wishes and goals of the other and a willingness to search for a mutually satisfactory solution to the problem. *Compromise* usually follows arbitration or exploration and refers to a problem solution that involves concessions on the part of both parties but to the detriment of neither. It requires the appraisal of each person's position and goals and the ability to reach a reasonable agreement without submission by one in order to "keep the peace." *Role clarification* is probably the most successful approach to establish complementary role relationships in the family. In situations requiring role adjustment or modification, parents are the persons who determine appropriate role responses in relation to cultural and family expectations. If they can appropriately evaluate the child's role position and their reciprocal role responses, they can assist the child to manage the specific role situation with a minimum of disequilibrium.

Consolidation is the integrated effect of redistribution of goals and rewards as a consequence of the various role-modification techniques. Successful consolidation as a result of learning to work through and synthesize new roles brings a closer unity and a higher level of complementariness to the relationships of family members.

Continuity and discontinuity.[11] Anthropologists who make a study of societies throughout the world have determined that there are decided differences from culture to culture in the continuity with which young children are prepared for adult roles. In some cultures the children begin to learn adult roles and behaviors at a very early age and continue to do so throughout childhood. In others, children are taught roles and behaviors that are in direct opposition to those they are expected to assume as adults. For example, cultures that value courage and aggressiveness continuously encourage these behaviors in their children. In others, including America, children are expected to be submissive in childhood but dominant as adults. The continuity in the rearing of females in the Western cultures has been more continuous in terms of role identification than is generally experienced by males. With expanding female roles, this continuity is becoming less apparent. Another example is in regard to attitudes toward sexuality. Many cultures are highly restrictive regarding sexual activity throughout childhood but become permissive or even demanding in adulthood; others are thoroughly permissive at all ages.

Sex role identification. From the moment of birth a child is treated differently by the parents based on the biologic sex of the infant. Almost immediately the infant is placed in a male or female category with a given name that clearly indicates a sex, dressed in pink if a girl or blue if a boy, and referred to as either "he" or "she." Thus information regarding a sexual identity is conveyed to the child and to the world, and along with these overt messages a set of sex-related attitudes toward the child emerges.

Parents recognize the importance of sex differences and, even in infancy, treat boys differently from girls. Parental attitudes and expectations regarding sex-appropriate behaviors, acquired from their own upbringing, influence the manner in which they react to the infant. These attitudes and expectations are transmitted to the infant first in subtle, then in more obvious, ways. Parents handle little girls more tenderly than they do little boys, who are stimulated with boisterous activity and vigorous motor play. They provide sex-appropriate toys and encourage play consistent with the sex-role expectations of the child.[13]

Four dimensions appear to be involved in the development of sex-role identification. Children (1) learn to apply appropriate gender label to themselves, (2) acquire sex-appropriate standards of behavior, (3) develop a preference for being the sex that they are, and (4) identify with their parent of the same sex.

The *gender label* is achieved early and subtly through imitation of the parents' expressions as they refer to the child's gender, for example, "That's a good girl" or "That's a good boy." Since it is such an important and basic component of the child's total identity, it is vital that the appropriate gender be assigned as soon as possible in rare cases where the sex of the infant is in doubt (p. 417). The gender orientation has more effect on development than does chromosomal determination of sex.[13]

Beginning when a child is a toddler, *sex-role standards* are differentiated and continuously developed throughout childhood. By the time children are 3 years old, they know whether they are boys or girls and have acquired considerable knowledge of and a preference for sex-appropriate behaviors. They can differentiate one sex from the other even before they learn anatomic differences; a 2-year-old child can identify others as girls or boys based on external appearances. Toddlers are given sex-appropriate toys and objects and are encouraged in activities that are appropriate to their sex.

Preschool children have definite impressions of masculinity and femininity, which are reflected in overt play. Most children in this age-group engage in stereotyped sex-appropriate play activities. Little girls play at housekeeping, taking care of dolls, dressing up, and cooking; boys choose trucks, blocks, and more physically active play. Boys are generally more aggressive in their play and, in disagreements with peers, they are more apt to react with shouting or fighting. Girls tend to be more dependent and introverted in their play. With the strong women's movement, more liberal views regarding sex role typing, and the unisex trend in all areas of interaction, these sex-associated characteristics are less apparent than they have been in the past. However, this country, as in most cultures, still remains heavily masculine oriented with males accorded more privileges than females.

Parents expect children to learn appropriate sex-role behavior early and to deviate little from it. From parents, teachers, and peers, children acquire information about how they are expected to behave in relation to their sex. Each set of parents has their own concept of what constitutes male or female attributes and the types of sex-linked behavior they wish to cultivate in their children. These are conveyed to the children by a variety of means, and parents exert special efforts to gain compliance with their expectations. Experiences the children are exposed to, toys that are selected for them, and activities in which they are encouraged to participate all reflect some aspect of the parents' sex-role conformity to standards of achievement, competition, self-assertiveness, and independence with control of feelings and repression of emotions. With little girls, more emphasis is placed on passive activities and development of interpersonal sensitivity, docility, interrelatedness with others, and nurturance.

In the case of little boys, the prohibition against effeminate behavior is very strong. Boys are rewarded less often for displaying behavior considered appropriate for their sex, but they are discouraged from exhibiting undesirable behavior by negative reinforcement. Parents emphasize the things that boys should *not* do or be, that is, those things that might label them as "sissies." Avoidance of the opposite sex-role behavior is a major means of sex-role learning in the American culture, especially for boys. This emphasis seems to be stronger in lower class families, where sex roles are more clearly defined and segregated. In middle class homes sex-role differentiation is less clear-cut. Mothers often work outside the home and male role models are more apt to help with behaviors that have been traditionally assigned to the female, such as housework and baby-sitting. The family situation may be more influential for sex-role development of girls than of boys since a boy is more apt to learn much of his masculine behaviors from role models outside the home. For example, in lower class black families in which the father is frequently absent, a male child often associates with gangs to learn a masculine role, whereas a Mexican-American youth who has a male model in the home may join such gangs to escape the paternal dominance in order to be free to express his masculine role.

Girls, on the other hand, are dealt with more leniently in America. Their role is less rigidly defined than that of boys. They are permitted to engage in masculine games and activities, to wear pants, and to be a tomboy without strong cultural disapproval. This greater variance may create some confusion in establishing a sex-role identity. A girl's acceptance of a parental role model depends a great deal on whether the role model of the mother is congruent with the girl's concept of a sex role.

A *gender preference* for the sex into which the child is born is acquired over a long period of time and depends on several things. Children will prefer to be a member of their own sex when their own behaviors and competence closely approximate the sex-role standards, when they like their parent of the same sex, and when they believe that their sex is valued. The sexes are not always valued equally in all cultures nor in all families. In cultures where males are more highly valued and are given higher status, boys are likely to develop a firm preference for their sex. However, girls in these cultures may be less certain regarding their gender assignment, even to the point of rejecting their sex group. A deterrent to sex-role preference by the child can exist in a family where the parents, at a specific birth, had hoped strongly for a child of the opposite sex. The environmental cues within the family will convey to this child that the opposite sex is a preferred one.

The process by which children come to style themselves after the parent of the same sex and to internalize their values and outlook is *identification*. Most children wish to be like their parent of the same sex, and, although the motivation for identification is still unsettled, children are more willing to share these parental attributes when they are able to see a degree of similarity between themselves and their parents. Children become aware of the similarity when they perceive actual physical and psychologic similarities, adopt parental behaviors, and are told of similarities by others. Once this identification is formed, it can be strengthened by the continued positive conception of the role model or weakened if the child does not perceive the model as desirable. Identification is not a total, all-or-nothing happening. To some extent children identify with both parents, and, as their sphere of social contacts widens, they identify with peers and other adults outside the family.

The formation of a sexual identity and role is influenced by a number of factors and is an enduring part of the personality that affects behavior, attitudes, and relationships in many aspects of daily life. The outcome of the identification process depends on the characteristics of the parents and other role models, the innate capacities and preferences of the child, and the value (cultural and familial) placed on his or her particular sex.

PARENTHOOD

The biologic route to parenthood is the same regardless of cultural background, age, or the motivation of the couple. Although the impulse for sexual union is spontaneous and not seasonally limited, the union for purposes of procreation can be timed according to needs and desires of the family and based on rational attachment to and the care and welfare of another individual, a great deal of which involves total dependency. It is a developmental stage in the life cycle, the end of which may be viewed by the parents as an endurance contest, a dismal failure, or the most rewarding and pleasurable experience of their lives.

Motivation

It is a characteristic in all societies that the adults are expected to become parents and to be gratified by the experience. Pressures of tradition, sentiment regarding the state of motherhood, and religious exhortations to fulfill divine commands of fertility profoundly influence decision making, because conformity to social-role expectations is a strong influence in family planning.

Conscious and unconscious motivation may enter into the decision to initiate a pregnancy. For a number of parents the motivation is based on the simple assumption that all normal people get married and have children. For many it provides proof of their biologic adequacy or demonstrates their adulthood. Some may wish to fulfill a parent's wish for grandchildren or to perpetuate the family name and fortune. To have a child in an attempt to cement a tenuous marriage is a hazardous motive. A corollary to this is the woman who desires a child to compensate for the lack of a meaningful relationship with her husband and to combat a feeling of inner loneliness and boredom. A child may be the only means for some persons to fulfill the urge to create something of value. Some persons have children in order to experience the full potential of their sexuality. In a few societies childless persons are not considered to have reached full maturity until they have children. Other motivating factors are to seek stimulation and novelty, to have power, to influence life, or to compete with others. However, in most instances the couple sincerely wishes to become parents.

The decisions for second and subsequent children may be as varied as the initial motivation for parenthood. Parents may reason that a single child will benefit from interaction with a sibling to provide companionship, sharing, and experience with conflict in human relationships. Occasionally disappointment with a first child may prompt parents to try again in the hope for a more gratifying experience. Many find parenthood a satisfying experience and enjoy the presence of children. In other families, the advent of a child is an unplanned event that is met with mixed emotions or, in many lower class families, with a passive fatalism.

The number of children that a couple chooses to have is an individual matter. Whether this choice is fulfilled may depend on how effectively the couple practices contraception as well as on their changing values and attitudes toward more or fewer children. Family size preferences do not remain the same throughout the marriage. Factors that are more likely to influence family size are social class, religion, race, type of conjugal role relationships, and the social-psychologic aspects of sexual relations. If a time comes when all parenthood becomes a matter of choice without religious, societal, or family pressures, it might be interesting to speculate on what types of people will choose to become parents.

Preparation for parenthood

There is little evidence to support the existence of a "parental instinct" or a "maternal instinct." There appear to be no internal mechanisms to guide parental behavior; therefore, parental behaviors must be learned. Adults in America as a whole are ill-prepared for the monumental task of parenthood. Education in American schools is notably deficient in courses that are relevant to most aspects of family life, such as sex, child care, home management, and interpersonal relationships. There are programs designed for preparation for childbirth during pregnancy, but few that prepare young adults for this life process. There are some courses that help prepare young people to be husbands and wives, but not to be parents. A few new parents have had limited experience caring for younger siblings or for siblings' children, and the experience of others has been confined to occasional baby-sitting for neighbors during adolescence. New parents approach parenthood with meager experience and scant knowledge, although no other task can compare, in the overall consequences, with that of rearing a human being. Parents learn by trial and error, committing the same mistakes that have been committed by countless other parents, but they somehow manage to accomplish the task, while becoming more skilled with each additional child. Tradition rather than rational planning furnishes the chief norms for child rearing.

The empirical preparation for parenthood is begun in the parent's own childhood. It has been established that the amount and quality of mothering that individuals have experienced in their own childhood significantly influence their later relationships with others and their ability to assume the role of parents in adulthood. By observation and imitation of their own parents and other role models, such as acquaintances, married siblings, and persons in the mass media, individuals learn culturally defined, sex-appropriate roles. Their own parents are probably the only persons that parents observe intimately in the parental role; this results in a *generational continuity*—parents rear their own children in very much the same way as they themselves were reared—which is evident in the way that individuals fulfill their parental role.

Parenthood as a developmental process[2]

The transition to parenthood is abrupt. Although a couple has anticipated the child's arrival, the fact of the birth means the sudden imposition of totally dependent care 24 hours a day for the new member of the family. Some have described the birth of an infant as a crisis. If the event is perceived as disturbing old habits and relationships and eliciting new responses, then childbirth might be termed a crisis. It requires role changes, destroys former relationships, and means adjusting to role realignments. Whereas previously the roles of a couple were husband and wife, they now become, in addition, father and mother. It is difficult to adjust to being parents, but it is a normal human experience and a tool for personal growth.

Erikson,[5] in describing the process of developing a healthy personality, places the period encompassing parenthood as one of the eight stages of man (see p. 69). Following the development of a sense of intimacy with another, an individual moves toward a sense of generativity; for most persons this means establishing and guiding the next generation. It is a time of production and creativity indicated best by (but not limited to) interest in producing and caring for children. Individuals who have successfully mastered the preceding stages of development will move into and through the stage of generativity with confidence. Failure to develop this vital component is one factor in disturbed family relationships that have a significant impact on the children's physical and emotional growth and well-being.

The ways in which the child and the parents influence one another are discussed at greater length in relation to each major stage of child development in subsequent chapters. Briefly, development of a parental sense can be divided into four phases[6]:

1. *Anticipation*. Looking forward to parenthood, a young couple thinks about and discusses becoming parents and the way in which they will rear their children. They wonder what changes will develop in their relationship and what kind of parents they will be.
2. *Honeymoon*. This is the early interpersonal adjustment to the infant in which an attachment is formed between the parents and the child and new role learning takes place.

The transition in self-image from a nonparent to a parent is made.

3. *Plateau.* The long middle period of parental development parallels child development:

The child is an infant—parents learn to interpret his needs.
The child is a toddler—parents learn to accept growth and development.
The child is a preschooler—parents and child learn to separate.
The child goes to school—parents learn to accept rejection and still be supportive.
The child is a teenager—parents begin to rebuild their lives.

4. *Disengagement.* This phase ends the active parental role, usually at the time of the child's marriage.

Parenthood never truly ends until the death of the parent. There are ties that bind the parents to their children throughout a lifetime. Parenthood, like all stages of development, is influenced by past experiences, and current events affect the future of the parents. Many events and feelings regarding the past are brought out as parents care for their own children. In addition, the child is a reflection of the parent. If parents like what they see in the child, their own self-esteem is increased. A successful relationship with a child builds the parents' self-image and contributes to a better acceptance of themselves.

Special parenting situations

The complexities of parenthood and the long-term effects on children are numerous and varied. Many will be considered elsewhere, for example, the problems related to the birth and care of a handicapped or chronically ill child (Chapter 22) or dying child (Chapter 27). Also there are relatively commonplace situations that may alter relationships between parent and child, such as families with a single parent or a stepparent or the family with an adopted child.

The single parent.[7] The problem of the single parent is closely related to the problems of the child with a single parent. The acquisition of single-parent status is accompanied by an altered self-image as well as by the need for another realignment of role. The physical separation is not accompanied by psychologic separation. There are many unresolved feelings associated with the separation. Feelings of anger, remorse, guilt, retaliation, mixed feelings of hatred and love, and sorrow for oneself can maintain an emotional relationship for some time following the physical separation. For each parent this separation is accompanied by mourning and resolving and facing true feelings about oneself. It takes time but can be facilitated by working through these feelings with understanding friends, relatives, or professionals, such as psychologists, social workers, or nurse practitioners.

Being the sole provider in all areas of child care places a stress on the parent both economically and emotionally. In the process of resolution, the single parent must cope with loneliness and fewer family interactions. The feeling of being isolated from all but the children may create parent-child relationships in which the parent and child are either overly attached to each other or in constant conflict. The reaction of the parent is to devote extra attention to the child because of feelings of guilt, lowered self-esteem, and as a protection against intimacy with other adults. Children feel that the burden of the parent's happiness or unhappiness is on their shoulders. There is a need on the part of the parent for social contacts and a life separate from the children for the emotional growth of both parent and child.

The stepparent. The role of stepparent is unclear and often confusing. The stepparent is in the awkward position of having to share a role with the parent who is missing from the original family in such functions as financial support, education, and coordinating visits when the parent is living and in carrying out moral, religious, and other responsibilities if the parent is dead. The reality of the natural parent's presence, be he or she dead or alive, is important to the stepchildren's development of their own identity, but this complicates the role of stepparent.

A stepparent plays three roles, and it is difficult to determine which role to assume in the process of rearing a stepchild. One is the role of *parent* in matters of discipline, planning family experiences, and setting limits on behavior; another is *stepparent* when plans and activities must be shared with the absent natural parent; and a third is that of a *nonparent* when the stepparent steps aside to allow the spouse to manage those things of which the stepparent is not or does not wish to be a part.

The stereotype of wicked stepmother and cruel stepfather has done little to foster healthy relationships with stepchildren, and stepparents usually go to great lengths in an attempt to avoid this image. They studiously avoid taking positions with stepchildren or minimize involvement with them as much as possible. Sometimes the natural parent at home feels guilty about separating the children from their other parent and restrains the stepparent from an authority position, thus rendering the stepparent powerless in a parental role. Sometimes the parent may wish that the stepparent would totally assume the parental role. Many factors that affect child rearing can interfere with the relationship between parent and stepparent. The child may serve to constantly remind the parent of the previous relationship; an unresolved relationship between the natural parents may interfere with full development of the new relationship; and feelings and attitudes of the stepchild toward the stepparent may inhibit relationships. A stepchild may feel guilty about liking a stepparent better than the absent parent, especially when the outside parent "uses" the child as a go-between in an attempt to destroy the new family relationship. In this situation the best approach is to tell the child that the natural parent failed as a marriage partner, not as a parent, although children eventually realize this.

The stepparent who has replaced a dead parent is in a more difficult position. In this situation, guilt and idealization, part of the normal grief process, may become intensified in the children. Overidealization and an attempt to hold onto the dead parent cause some children to make unfair and discriminating comparisons. Probably the best approach on the part of the stepparent is to be frank about the good points of the deceased parent but not to agree with the comparison and to avoid defensiveness.

In many situations the relationship produces satisfaction for both the children and the stepparent. The children have warm feelings toward the stepparent and gain understanding and maturity that they would not have achieved without a stepparent.

Adoptive parents. "Adoption is the method provided by law to establish the legal relationship of parent and child between persons who are not so related by birth, with the same rights and obligations that exist between children and their natural parents."[3] Adoptive parents are those who, by whatever motivation, assume the sociologic and ethical responsibility of biologic parents, and these ties of affection are just as strong as biologic ties.[16]

Persons are motivated to adopt a child for different reasons. Most instances involve an adopting couple who find it impossible to have children of their own, and agencies in the past regarded this as the major criterion for placement of adoptable children. However, today many people consider adoption for other reasons. There are some who feel a responsibility to provide a home for a child who needs one; others who are able to have more children of their own but are seriously concerned about overpopulation elect to increase their family through adoption; many with families are finding room for "one more" with whom to share their love. In addition, single, divorced, and widowed persons who believe that they have love and security to offer a child are seeking to adopt. Unfortunately for persons wishing to adopt a child, the demand for white infants with no physical or mental problems far exceeds the supply of these children. However, there has been an increase in the number of children, formerly considered to be unadoptable, who are finding homes through the adoptive process. These include physically handicapped children, older children, and children who are of a minority or mixed racial ancestry.

The major source of infants for adoption has been socially unsanctioned pregnancies, primarily unwed mothers. Society grants a very high rating to the married status. Although adoption as a means of creating a family is openly acceptable, having children outside the marriage state is generally met with societal disapproval. Consequently, unwed mothers have been the primary source of adoptable infants. With the widespread use of contraception, more liberalized abortion laws, and more liberal attitudes toward out-of-wedlock parents, the number of these children available for adoption has significantly decreased.

Almost half the adoptable children in the United States are adopted by relatives. Nonrelative adoptions are primarily arranged through licensed social agencies. A small proportion are arranged independently by individuals such

Table 2-1. Advantages and disadvantages of agency and independent adoptions

Definition	Advantages	Disadvantages
Agency adoption—placement by a certified or authorized public agency	Legal safeguards for both relinquishing and adoptive parents Natural parents and adoptive parents are unknown to each other Relinquishing parent receives counseling services Careful social study of adoptive family Agency services to adoptive parents extend through the adjustment period Agency, which maintains custody of medical and other information, remains an available resource to parents and medical personnel Cost minimal	Delay in placement Placement policies of individual agencies may limit opportunities for placement of some children Not available in all areas Legal and health services vary in quality from place to place and depend on availability of legal and medical staff supervision
Independent adoption—placement by persons other than an authorized agency, such as physicians, lawyers, nurses, clergymen	Faster than agency adoptions No investigation of adopting family An alternative when unable to secure agency adoption	No guarantee of child's anonymity Limited number or lack of safeguards (legal, medical, social) Limited opportunity for selective placement Cost may be high; this may even be a profit-making venture of the intermediaries Frequently the child is not legally free for adoption at the time of placement

as physicians, nurses, clergymen, and lawyers. It is well-recognized that the safest and most satisfactory adoptions are those conducted through a licensed social agency, either public or voluntary. Some of the advantages and disadvantages of independent and agency adoptions are summarized in Table 2-1.

Risks related to adoption are usually less than those encountered in family life. Careful screening of infants can detect all but the more obscure defects, and subsequent development of defects or illnesses is no less predictable than in natural families. However, inherent emotional difficulties may be intensified in the case of adoption.

The decision to adopt should be mutual, and various attitudes and feelings must be examined before the couple can assume the responsibility for an adopted child. Most adults assume that they will be able to have children of their own. To discover that they are unable to do so is often accompanied by feelings of inferiority, doubts about masculinity or femininity, and feelings of guilt or blame in relation to the spouse. These feelings and frustrations superimposed on the anxious waiting for pregnancies, feelings of loss, and the endless medical procedures to establish infertility, provide an adoptive couple with their own unique preparation for parenthood.

Most problems faced by adoptive parents are no different from those encountered by natural parents. All parents want to be good parents, but this desire is often intensified in adoptive parents. The mother, in particular, believes that she must be a better parent than the biologic mother would have been and, if she harbors any feelings about unmarried parents who relinquish children, this may affect her feelings toward the child.

One of the major tasks in rearing adopted children is helping them to deal with the fact that they have had another set of parents. If the children are adopted after the age of 2 years, they maintain an image of the previous parenting persons that may cause the adopting parents some insecurity. The parents may not feel as close to these children as they would to those who are adopted in infancy. It is necessary that the children maintain the image of the natural parents. As they grow, the children are able to clearly distinguish between the parents who loved and cared for them and those who were merely responsible for their birth. Some of the early difficulties of adaptation are related to the change in surroundings, a change that is difficult for all children.

The task of telling children that they are adopted is a cause of deep concern and anxiety. Unfortunately there are no clear-cut guidelines for parents to follow in determining precisely when and at what age children are ready for the information, and parents are naturally reluctant to present the children with such unsettling news. However, it is an important aspect of their parental responsibilities, and, although they may be tempted to withhold the fact from a child, it is an essential component of the child's identity.

The timing seems to arise naturally as parents become aware of the child's readiness. Some authorities believe that the best time is between ages 7 and 10 years; others recommend an earlier age.[8] The time must be right for both the parents and the child and is highly individual. One such time is when children ask where babies come from. At the same time children can be told the facts of their adoption. If they are told in such a way as to convey the idea that they were active participants in the selection process, they will be less apt to feel that they were abandoned victims in a helpless situation. For example, the parents can tell a child that his behavior when they were looking for a child led them to believe that he wanted to go with them. Complete honesty between parents and child usually strengthens the relationship, and children should be encouraged to ask questions.

The time of adolescence may be an especially trying time for parents of adopted children. The normal confrontations of adolescents and parents may assume more painful aspects in adoptive families. Adolescents may use the fact of their adoption as a tool in defying parental authority or as a justification of aberrant behavior. As they attempt to master the task of identity formation, the feeling of abandonment by their natural parents may come to awareness or may be intensified. The children fantasize about their parents, and they may feel the need to discover the identity of their natural parents. In some states birth certificates are made legally available to adopted children when they become of age. In such situations it is important for parents to be honest with questioning adolescents and to tell them of this possibility (the parents themselves are unable to provide this for them; it is the children's responsibility if they wish).

Whatever motivates a couple to seek adoption as an alternative means to acquire a family, the decision should be based on emotionally healthy needs. The welfare of the child should be the primary consideration in placement, and such motives as the need to strengthen an unstable marriage, to treat emotional problems (including grief over death of a child), or to treat psychogenic sterility should be carefully explored. When the adoption satisfies the needs of only one of the two parents, the outcome is questionable.

Parent behavior

It is impossible to discuss parent personalities and all the parental attitudes and behaviors that influence the personality development of their children; volumes have been written of the significance of interactions between parents and their children. The parents' overall acceptance of a child and their disciplinary orientation have a profound impact on the way in which children view themselves and relate with others. Adults' attitudes as parents are influenced by their conception of their roles in relation to the children.

Child rearing may be viewed as restricting and controlling child behavior, as taming the child's innate rebellious and uncivilized nature, or as guidance, providing a suitable role model for the child to emulate. Much depends on the parents' own background, their mental health, their attitudes toward child rearing in general, and their attitudes toward any individual child. A parent sees each child differently, and feedback provided by certain types of children may inadvertently create undesired attitudes in a parent.

Acceptance vs rejection.[11] A warm relationship between parent and child creates the healthiest environment for the child. Children who come from homes in which they are loved and accepted display socially acceptable behavior and are generally good natured, cheerful, friendly, cooperative, and emotionally stable. Because they are loved and accepted themselves, they are able to form satisfactory relationships with others.

Parents' rejection of their children appears in a number of forms and for a number of reasons. Rejection may be subtle or blatant; manifestations may be extensive, from neglect and belittling to physical abuse. Children who are rejected develop feelings of insecurity and inferiority; they believe that if they are unworthy of parental love, they must be of no value. Consequently they attempt to win parental affection through attention-getting behaviors that frequently serve only to compound the rejective behavior of the parents. When these tactics fail, the child may become either hostile and aggressive or withdrawn and submissive. Sometimes rejected children find social acceptance and adjustment with identification with peers, but more often they develop feelings of isolation, inadequacy, and generally lowered self-esteem. A persistent pattern of rejection can have pervasive and long-range effects on a child's personality. The problems of disturbed parent-child relationships that are severely damaging to children are discussed in relation to failure-to-thrive syndrome (p. 494), the abused child (p. 594), and some of the emotional problems of childhood (p. 649).

Control vs autonomy. The extent to which parents restrict children's behavior or allow them autonomy and freedom significantly affects the psychologic atmosphere in the home.

Dominant, authoritarian parents demand absolute obedience and submission. Power is expressed openly, and the children are not allowed to express aggression within the family. Their activities are closely supervised, and criticism and overconcern are expressed over trifles. Careful training often results in rigidly conforming behavior in the children, who tend to be sensitive, shy, self-conscious, retiring, and submissive. They are more apt to be courteous, loyal, honest, and dependable but docile.

Submissive or overly permissive parents allow the children to have their own way; well-meaning parents sometimes confuse permissiveness with license. They employ lax, inconsistent discipline, do not set sensible limits, and do not prevent the children from upsetting the home routine. In effect the children control the parents. Children of submissive parents are often disobedient, disrespectful, irresponsible, aggressive, and generally defiant of authority.

These are extremes on the dominance-submission scale. The personality characteristics of both the children and the parents influence the degree to which these approaches produce an effect on personality development. Also, differences between the behaviors of the two parents are important factors. For instance, restrictiveness combined with hostility may produce passivity and dependence, whereas restrictiveness and warm involvement may prove to be beneficial. Rebelliousness in children is linked with highly authoritarian control. Sometimes children who feel hostility but are unable to express it at home may transfer these feelings to those in subordinate positions, strangers, and members of minority groups. Bullies and sadists are frequently the products of authoritarian upbringing.

The current philosophy of child rearing favors a rational, issue-oriented approach to directing the child's activities and behaviors. Parents should not set rigid, arbitrary limits but should maintain firm control, particularly in areas of parent-child disagreement. Permissiveness, necessary for children to develop their full potential, is tempered with reasonable and consistent setting of limits. There is more flexibility in decisions and demands on the children, and discipline is more apt to be based on reasoning with encouragement of verbal give-and-take. This approach to child rearing is more likely to facilitate the development of competence in children that will be displayed by independent and responsible behavior on the part of the children.

THE CHILD IN AMERICA

America is an aggregate of numerous old- and new-world cultures that are blended with the unique heritage of pioneering frontiersmen. Models of child rearing appear to reflect the history of the country. The early philosophic standards of the Protestant ethic, which resulted in that pleasureless, hard-driven, independent individual represented to some extent by the entrepreneurial philosophy discussed earlier, is gradually being replaced in contemporary American society by the social ethic, which emphasizes a group-oriented and other-directed philosophy.

The frontier background of the American culture has also contributed to the overall orientation to life and child rearing. There has always been a basic optimistic view of the world and a belief that things can be better and that the children can and will be better off than the parents. This hopeful outlook and a general future orientation together with the possibility of upward social mobility has created a pervasive overall attitude of optimism. Increasing development of self-confidence and autonomy in children is fostered and encouraged. Children are, in general, permitted a greater degree of freedom than in more tradition-oriented cultures where a child who is born in one social class will remain in that class for a lifetime.

Family life in America is characterized by increasing geographic and economic mobility. Here there is less reliance on tradition, families are fragmented, and there is limited opportunity to transmit and acquire the traditional and accepted customs of a culture. Consequently young adults rely to a greater extent on the professed experts, peers, and the mass media for acquisition of acceptable patterns of behavior, including child-rearing practices. Each generation, as it adapts to the new, discards the inadequacies of previous generations. This often constitutes a source of confusion and frustration as parents attempt to adjust to rapid changes; tradition and precedent no longer meet needs and challenges of rapid change that require new approaches and innovation for problem solving. Competent parents attempt to determine the comparatively stable, essential components of the culture and transmit these to their children. Awareness of an attention to changing cultural norms during child rearing helps the parent to adapt to the new demands of the culture that are different from those they learned as children.

Children in America grow up with a number of adults who differ from one another but who all provide input to them as role models, teachers, and standards for behavior. Most of the children live in nuclear families located in sharply differentiated neighborhoods determined by income and ethnic status within a highly technical, largely urban society. Class differences in child rearing still persist, but they are becoming less divergent as a result of the increased homogeneity of the culture. Working classes still tend to be more tradition oriented, whereas the middle classes are more positively oriented toward social change. There are still differences in time orientation and attitudes toward education and in maternal behavior, but the differences are changing perceptively.

Influence of "experts"

Evidence indicates that there have been decided shifts in the overall philosophy of child rearing during the twentieth century. Directions on child rearing, with parental roles and practices defined by the experts, have been transmitted as advice to parents through a steady flow of pamphlets, books, and articles. The influences have reflected the ideals of the culture and have differed among social classes at various times. The impact has begun with the upper and middle classes and has gradually filtered down to parents in the lower classes. The changes in the opinions of these experts are the result of alterations in the concept of child development and behavior and of research into the effects of parent-child interaction.

The early view of child care advocated rigid scheduling, early weaning and toilet training, and prohibition of devices that provided the child with passive pleasures, such as pacifiers. Cautions were issued regarding behaviors that might "spoil the child," such as fondling, cuddling, and other forms of bodily contact between parent and child. This approach was stressful to parents and, fortunately, most were unable to adhere to these rigid, impersonal guidelines.

These severe techniques were replaced by an easier, warmer, and more relaxed approach toward coping with child behavior that emphasized "tender loving care" as the basis for satisfactory physical and emotional well-being. It has been argued by some that this method generated too much permissiveness, which may have had some long-range adverse effects.

Now there are indications that the trend is again reversing toward a more firm, though less rigid, approach. No doubt the opinions of experts will continue to influence adult relationships with children, although members of a better-informed and wary generation are less likely to be totally accepting of any formula. Nurses can help parents choose the practices and approaches to child rearing that best meet their needs based on the personalities of the persons involved and the needs and goals of the family, thereby helping them function effectively in the day-to-day care of their children.

Influence of schools

When children enter school their radius of relationships extends to include a wider variety of peers and a new focus of authority. Although parents continue to exert the major influence on the children, in the school environment teachers have the most significant psychologic impact on their development. The function of teachers is primarily limited to teaching, but, like parents, they are concerned about the emotional welfare of the children. Both parents and teachers must constrain behavior, and both are in a position to enforce standards of conduct.

Teachers stimulate and guide the intellectual development of children, but equally important is their influence on personality development. The differential systems of reward and punishment administered by teachers affect the emotional adjustment and the self-concept of children as well as the way in which they respond to school in general. The interaction between the teacher and any given child also affects the child's acceptance by peers. Praise by a teacher stimulates positive reactions toward the child by the other children. In this way teachers are able to influence values and attitudes of children in a variety of areas, such as attitudes toward minority group, handicapped, or less favorably endowed, children.

Influence of mass media of communication

There is no doubt that the communications media provide children with a means for extending their knowledge about the world in which they live and have contributed to narrowing the differences between classes.

Reading material. The oldest of the mass media—books, newspapers, and magazines—contribute to a child's competence in almost every direction, as well as provide enjoyment. Recognition of the impact that reading matter in the schools has on the value system and socialization processes has prompted reevaluation of the content of textbooks, for example, the biased presentation of male and female role models, the unrealistic, sugar-coated view of life situations, and an unrealistic, biased history of minority groups.

Fairy tales, for generations the mainstay of young children's literature, have suffered condemnation as sexist, overly violent in content, and riddled with unfavorable stereotypes, such as the wicked stepmother, dwarfs, and physical unattractiveness associated with evil. Recently this attitude is being questioned, however.

Comic books and other "trash" reading material have been popular in every generation, usually at the expense of literature provided by schools, libraries, and parents. Many children have nothing else to read. The easy reading, quick action, and adventure in brief episodes seem to fulfill a need for children who are striving to understand both aggression in others and their own impulses. Reading ability, intelligence, and school adjustment seem to have no relationship with the number and type of comic books read. The vocabulary level of comic books is relatively high. Most comic books appear to be relatively harmless to the majority of children and in some ways even beneficial. Comic books seem to have only a minor influence on acquisition of beliefs, values, and behaviors.

Movies. Movies not closely bound to reality and often portraying an assortment of socially approved behaviors perhaps make a contribution to children's value systems, but they also provide opportunities for desirable social learning. On the other hand, children, especially adolescents, flock to the "macho" movies and those whose heroes resort to violent resolution of problems, such as the use of karate techniques and wild automobile chases. The carryover of these influences into daily life and relationships may account, in part, for the increase in violent behavior of young persons.

Television. The medium that has the most impact on children in America today is television, which has become one of the most significant socializing agents in the life of young children. The content of programs and commercials provides multiple sources for acquiring information, modeling behaviors, and observing value orientations. Besides producing a leveling effect on class differences in general information and vocabulary, television exposes children to a wider variety of topics and events than they encounter in day-to-day life. Television always has time to talk to children and is a form of access to the adult world.

Television is a solitary activity and, as such, increases passivity and decreases physical activity and peer group interaction. Controversy continues regarding the favorable vs deleterious effects of television viewing. There is ample documentation to implicate television as a source for learning antisocial, aggressive behavior, but there is also evidence to indicate that television is a positive reinforcement for prosocial behavior. Most programming stresses the triumph of good over evil, but with an unrealistically rapid resolution of problems, including moral dilemmas, often accompanied by pain or violence.

Much of the adverse influence of the communications media (in any form) depends on the susceptibility of the individual child. Many experts believe that adequately designed studies show no appreciable overall effect of the mass media on most children but that insecure children with strong feelings of rejection may become addicted to the media in order to meet a need that they are unable to satisfy in other ways. It encourages low energy and apathy and contributes to development of obesity in susceptible children.

Influence of minority group membership

In addition to the problems and risks encountered by all children in the course of development, there are a small percentage of children who are particularly vulnerable to hostility, derogation, and discrimination from children and adults of the majority group. America abounds with racial, ethnic, and religious minority groups. Although the effects of a minority status can apply to any of them, the one on whom the impact is greatest is the black minority. This group is the largest minority and is one whose members are distinguished by the color of their skin, which renders them readily identifiable.

Studies in the past indicate that early in life children become aware of their racial or ethnic status and of the discriminatory attitudes of the majority culture toward their group. Reflecting these attitudes, minority group children react by viewing their own group as undesirable and by adopting the majority judgments about the group. The direct effects of discrimination are anger and low self-esteem, which become manifest in a variety of behaviors. Inner conflicts and suppressed hostility that focus children's attention inward may be a factor in the failure of many children to achieve in other areas.

Because of many factors, for most blacks membership in the black minority also implies membership in the lower levels of the social structure. This lower class, lower-caste status is characterized by broken homes, dominance of maternal authority, impoverished and deteriorating neighborhoods, environmental encouragement of delinquency, and, frequently, parent-child friction and antagonism.

Evidence indicates that changes in attitudes are slowly taking place in some groups and in some places. With growing awareness, interest, and understanding by increasing numbers of the majority group, which has accompanied the recent emergence of racial and ethnic pride, minority-group children are becoming more secure and confident in their racial or ethnic identity. Individuals vary in their reactions to membership in a minority group, and much of this variation can be attributed to familial factors. As with all children, the most important influences on development of a positive self-image are warm, understanding parents who take an active interest in fostering their children's growth. Parents who accept their children and react positively and constructively rather than in a negative and self-defeating manner will help their children develop feelings of self-worth, self-esteem, and self-acceptance. The more adequate that children feel, the more positive will be their attitudes toward both majority and minority children, the greater will be their ability to withstand prejudice and intolerance, and the less will be their need for counteraggressive behavior.

REFERENCES

1. Abril, I. F.: Mexican-American folk beliefs: how they affect health care, Am. J. Maternal Child Nurs. **2**(3):168-173, 1977.
2. Anthony, E. J., and Benedik, T., editors: Parenthood, its psychology and psychopathology, Boston, 1970, Little, Brown and Co.
3. Child Welfare League of America: Standard for adoption services, New York, 1968, Child Welfare League of America.
4. Clark, M.: Health in the Mexican-American culture, a community study, ed. 2, Berkeley, 1970, University of California Press.
5. Erikson, E.: Childhood and society, New York, 1963, W. W. Norton & Co., Inc.
6. Friedman, D.: Parent development, Calif. Med. **86**:25-28, January 1957.
7. Group for the Advancement of Psychiatry: The joys and sorrows of parenthood, New York, 1973, Charles Scribner's Sons.
8. Hammons, C.: The adoptive family, Am. J. Nurs. **76**:251-260, 1976.
9. Hetherington, E. M.: Effects of father absence on personality development in adolescent daughters, Dev. Psychol. **7**:327-336, 1972.
10. Hetherington, E. M., and Deur, J.: The effects of father absence on child development, Young Child. **26**:233-248, 1971.
11. Johnson, R. C., and Medinnus, G. R.: Child psychology: behavior and development, ed. 3, New York, 1974, John Wiley & Sons, Inc., Chapter 7.
12. Johnston, C. M., and Deisher, R. W.: Contemporary communal child rearing, Pediatrics **52**:319-326, 1973.
13. Newman, B. M., and Newman, P. R.: Development through life: a psychosocial approach, Homewood, Ill., 1975, Dorsey Press.
14. Robischon, P., and Scott, D.: Role theory and its application to nursing, Nurs. Outlook **17**:52-57, 1969.
15. Sands, R. M.: Toward communal child rearing, Social Work **18**:54-59, 1973.
16. Schechter, M. D.: About adoptive parents. In Anthony, E. J., and Benedik, T., editors: Parenthood, its psychology and psychopathology, Boston, 1970, Little, Brown and Co.
17. Schooler, C.: Birth order effects: not here, not now! Psychol. Bull. **78**:161-175, 1972.
18. Schulz, D.: The changing family: its function and future, Englewood Cliffs, N.J., 1972, Prentice-Hall, Inc.
19. Wallston, B.: The effects of maternal employment on children, J. Child Psychol. Psychiatry **14**:81-95, 1973.
20. Yorburg, B.: The changing family, New York, 1973, Columbia University Press.

BIBLIOGRAPHY

Adams, B.: The American family: a sociological interpretation, Chicago, 1973, Markham/Rand McNally & Co.

Aichlmayr, R.: Cultural understanding: a key to acceptance, Nurs. Outlook **17**:20-23, July 1969.

Anderson, R. E., and Carter, I. E.: Human behavior in the social environment: a social systems approach, Chicago, 1974, Aldine Publishing Co.

Anthony, E. J., and Doupernik, C., editors: The child in his family, New York, 1970, Wiley-Interscience.

Arasteh, J.: Parenthood: some antecedents and consequences: a preliminary survey of the mental health literature, J. Genet. Psychol. **118**:179-202, 1971.

Bandura, A., and Wittenberg, C.: The impact of visual media on personality. In Segal, J., editor: The mental health of the child, Washington, D.C., 1971, U.S. Government Printing Office, P.H. pamphlet no. 2168.

Barnard, M. U.: Supportive care for the adoptive family, Iss. Compr. Pediatr. Nurs. **2**(3):22-29, 1977.

Baumrind, D.: Current patterns of parental authority, Dev. Psychol. Monograph, vol. 4, no. 1, part 2, 1971.

Bell, R. R.: Studies in marriage and the family, ed. 2, New York, 1973, Thomas Y. Crowell Co., Inc.

Bennett, M. B., Hackett, B. M., and Millar, R. M.: Child rearing in communes. In Howe, L. K., editor: The future of the family, New York, 1972, Simon & Schuster, Inc.

Bettelheim, B.: The children of the dream: communal child-rearing and American education, New York, 1970, Avon Books.

Bierman, S.: The role of children in the family. In Liebman, S., editor: Emotional forces in the family, Philadelphia, 1959, J. B. Lippincott Co.

Biller, H. B.: Father absence and the personality development of the male child, Dev. Psychol. **2**:181-201, 1970.

Biller, H. B., and Davids, A.: Parent-child relations, personality development and psychopathology. In Davids, A., editor: Abnormal child psychology, Belmont, Calif., 1973, Brooks/Cole Publishing Co.

Block, J.: Conceptions of sex role: some cross-cultural and longitudinal perspectives, Am. Psychol. **28**:512-526, 1973.

Boukling, E.: The family as an agent of social change, Futurist **6**:186-191, October 1972.

Braff, A. M.: Telling children about their adoption: new alternatives for parents, Am. J. Maternal Child Nurs. **2**:254-259, 1977.

Branch, M. F., and Paxton, P. P.: Providing safe nursing care for ethnic people of color, New York, 1976, Appleton-Century-Crofts.

Branham, E.: One parent adoptions, Children **17:**103-107, May/June 1970.

Brink, P. J.: Transcultural nursing: a book of readings, Englewood Cliffs, N.J., 1976, Prentice-Hall, Inc.

Brinton, D.: Health center milieu: interaction of nurses and low income families, Nurs. Res. **21:**46-52, 1972.

Brinton, D.: Value differences between nurses and low-income families, Nurs. Res. **21:**46-52, 1972.

Brody, G. F.: Socioeconomic differences in stated child-rearing practices and in observed maternal behavior, J. Marriage Fam. **30:**656-660, 1968.

Brown, J. B.: Infant temperament: a clue to childbearing for parents and nurses, Am. J. Maternal Child Nurs. **2:**228-232, 1977.

Bullough, B., and Bullough, V. L.: Poverty, ethnic identity, and health care, New York, 1972, Appleton-Century-Crofts.

Cantoni, L.: The family: a conceptual framework, Child Fam. **9:**73, 1970.

Child Welfare League of America: CWLA standards for adoption services, New York, 1968, Child Welfare League of America.

Clemmens, R. L., and Denny, T. J.: Prevention of emotional problems in childhood: a philosophy for child rearing (commentary), Clin. Pediatr. **16:**122-123, 1977.

Cole, M., and Bruner, J. S.: Cultural differences and inferences about psychological processes, Am. Psychol. **26:**867-876, 1971.

Cole, M. and associates: The cultural context of learning and thinking, New York, 1971, Basic Books, Inc., Publishers.

Cominos, H.: Teaching infant care to adopting parents, Nurs. Outlook **19:**421, June 1971.

Committee on Adoption and Dependent Care: Adoption of children, ed. 3, Evanston, Ill., 1973, American Academy of Pediatrics.

Committee on Adoptions: Identity development in adopted children, Pediatrics **47:**948-949, 1971.

Cronenwett, L. R.: Transition to parenthood. In McNall, L. K., and Galeener, J. T.: Current practice in obstetric and gynecologic nursing, St. Louis, 1976, The C. V. Mosby Co.

Derdeyn, A. P.: Children in divorce: intervention in the phase of separation, Pediatrics **60:**20-27, 1977.

Dombaugh, M. M.: A personal experience in single-parent adoption. In McNall, L. K., and Galeener, J. T.: Current practice in obstetric and gynecologic nursing, St. Louis, 1976, The C. V. Mosby Co.

Dresden, S.: The young adult: adjusting to single parenting, Am. J. Nurs. **76:**1286-1289, 1976.

Dudding, G. S.: Counseling children through their parents' divorce, Iss. Compr. Pediatr. Nurs. **2**(3):40-51, 1977.

Eiduson, B. T.: Looking at children in emergent family styles, Child. Today **3:**2-6, 1974.

Feldman, S. D., and Thielbar, G. W., editors: Life styles: diversity in American society, Boston, 1972, Little, Brown and Co.

Fleming, A. W.: Our children—without them there is no future, Clin. Pediatr. **14:**92-95, January 1975.

Ford, F. R., and Herrick, J.: Family roles: family life styles, Am. J. Orthopsychiatry **94:**61-69, January 1974.

Fuentes, J. A.: The need for effective and comprehensive planning for migrant workers, Am. J. Public Health **64:**2-10, 1974.

Fulcomer, D. M.: The nuclear family. In Clausen, J. P., and associates: Maternity nursing today, New York, 1973, McGraw-Hill Book Co.

Gallagher, U. M.: Adoption in a changing society, Child. Today **1:**2-6, September/October 1972.

Gustin, K.: The adopting family. In Hymovich, D. P., and Barnard, M. U., editors: Family health care, New York, 1973, McGraw-Hill Book Co.

Hall, J. E., and Weaver, B. R., editors: Nursing of families in crisis, Philadelphia, 1974, J. B. Lippincott Co.

Handel, G.: Sociological aspects of parenthood. In Anthony, E. J., and Benedik, T., editors: Parenthood, its psychology and psychopathology, Boston, 1970, Little, Brown and Co.

Herrera, T., and Wagner, N. N.: Behavioral approaches to delivering health services in a Chicano community. In Reinhardt, A. M., and Quinn, M. D., editors: Current practice in family-centered community nursing, St. Louis, 1977, The C. V. Mosby Co.

Herzog, E., and Sudea, C.: Boys in fatherless families, Washington, D.C., 1971, U.S. Department of Health, Education and Welfare.

Hochbaum, G. M.: Social influences on health behavior, Belmont, Calif., 1970, Wadsworth Publishing Co., Inc.

Horowitz, J. A., and Perdue, B. J.: Single-parent families, Nurs. Clin. North Am. **12:**503-511, 1977.

Howe, L. K.: The future of the family, New York, 1972, Simon & Schuster, Inc.

Howell, M. C.: Employed mothers and their families, Pediatrics **52:**252 and 327, 1973.

Hrobsky, D. M.: Transition to parenthood: a balancing of needs, Nurs. Clin. North Am. **12:**457-468, 1977.

Hurley, J., and Hohn, R.: Shifts in child-rearing attitudes linked with parenthood and occupation, Dev. Psychol. **4:**324-328, 1971.

Hymovich, D., and Barnard, M. U.: Family health care, New York, 1973, McGraw-Hill Book Co.

Irelan, L. M., editor: Low-income life styles, Washington, D.C., 1967, U.S. Department of Health, Education and Welfare.

Irvine, J.: On not being upper class, N. Engl. J. Med. **282:**453, February 19, 1970.

Jack, M. S.: The single-parent family: an issue in nursing, Iss. Compr. Pediatr. Nurs. **2**(3):30-39, 1977.

Jackson, D.: The study of the family. In Ackerman, N.: Family process, New York, 1970, Basic Books, Inc., Publishers.

Jessner, J., Weigert, E., and Foy, J. L.: The development of parental attitudes during pregnancy. In Anthony, E. J., and Benedik, T., editors: Parenthood, its psychology and psychopathology, Boston, 1970, Little, Brown and Co.

Johnston, M.: Folk beliefs and ethnocultural behavior in pediatrics, medicine or magic, Nurs. Clin. North Am. **12:**77-84, 1977.

Johnston, M., Dayne, M., and Mittleider, K.: Putting more PEP in parenting, Am. J. Nurs. **77:**994-995, 1977.

Kantor, R. M.: Communes, Psychol. Today **4:**53-57, February 1970.

Kelly, J., and Wallerstein, J.: The effects of parental divorce: experiences of the child in early latency, Am. J. Orthopsychiatry **46:**20-32, 1976.

Kelly, J., and Wallerstein, J.: Brief interventions with children in divorcing families, Am. J. Orthopsychiatry **47:**23-39, 1977.

Kessler, S.: The American way of divorce, Chicago, 1975, Nelson-Hall Co.

Kiernan, B., and Scoloveno, M. A.: Fathering, Nurs. Clin. North Am. **12:**481-490, 1977.

Klein, C.: The single family experience, New York, 1973, Avon Books.

Kruger, W. S.: Education for parenthood and the schools, Child. Today **2:**4-7, January 1973.

Latham, H. C., and associates: Pediatric nursing, ed. 3, St. Louis, 1977, The C. V. Mosby Co., Chapter 1.

Leininger, M.: Transcultural nursing: concepts, theories, and practices, New York, 1978, John Wiley & Sons, Inc.

Leininger, M.: Cultural diversities of health and nursing care, Nurs. Clin. North Am. **12:**5-18, 1977.

Leininger, M. M.: Nursing and anthropology, New York, 1970, John Wiley & Sons, Inc.

LeMasters, E. E.: Parents in modern America: a sociological analysis, Homewood, Ill., 1970, Dorsey Press.

McBride, A. B.: Can family life survive? Am. J. Nurs. **75:**1648-1653, October 1975.

McKeighen, R. J.: Basic counseling for children, Iss. Compr. Pediatr. Nurs., November/December 1976.

McRae, M.: An approach to the single parent dilemma, Am. J. Maternal Child Nurs. **2**(3):164-167, 1977.

Messer, A.: The individual in his family: an adaptational study, Springfield, Ill., 1970, Charles C Thomas, Publisher.

Mevis, E. J.: The extended family. In Clausen, J. P., and associates: Maternity nursing today, New York, 1973, McGraw-Hill Book Co.

Mock, R., and Tuddenham, R.: Race and conformity among children, Dev. Psychol. **4:**349-365, 1971.

Murray, R., and Zentner, J.: Nursing concepts for health promotion, Englewood Cliffs, N.J., 1975, Prentice-Hall, Inc., Chapters 10, 12, and 13.

Mussen, P. H., Conger, J., and Kagen, J.: Child development and personality, New York, 1974, Harper & Row, Publishers.

Nadelman, L.: Sex identity in American children: memory, knowledge and preference tests, Dev. Psychol. **10:**413-417, 1974.

Palceszny, M.: Sexual identity and role in children, Clin. Pediatr. **13:**154-158, February 1974.

Parsons, T.: Definitions of health and illness in the light of American values and social structure. In Jaco, E. G.: Patients, physicians, and illness, ed. 2, New York, 1972, The Free Press.

Patterson, J.: If you're a woman and head a family, J. Home Economics **65:**20-22, 1973.

Perdue, B. J., Horowitz, J. A., and Herz, F.: Mothering, Nurs. Clin. North Am. **12:**491-502, 1977.

Perkins, M. R.: Does availability of health services ensure their use? Nurs. Outlook **22:**496-498, 1974.

Pratt, L.: Relationship of socioeconomic status to health, Am. J. Public Health **61:**281-291, February 1971.

Pratt, L.: Family structure and effective health behavior, Boston, 1976, Houghton Mifflin Co.

Primeaux, M. H.: American Indian health care practices: a cross-cultural perspective, Nurs. Clin. North Am. **12:**55-65, 1977.

Rodgers, J. A.: Struggling out of the feminine pluperfect, Am. J. Nurs. **75:**1655-1659, October 1975.

Rohr, F.: How parents tell their children they are adopted, Child Welfare **50:**298-300, 1971.

Russell, B., and Lofstrom, L.: Health clinic for the alienated, Am. J. Nurs. **71:**80-83, January 1971.

Russell, C. S.: Transitions to parenthood: problems and gratifications, J. Marriage Fam. **36:**294-301, 1974.

Santrock, J. W.: Paternal absence, sex typing, and identification, Dev. Psychol. **2:**264-272, 1970.

Sayre, J. W., and Sayre, R. F.: American children and the "children of nature," Am. J. Dis. Child. **130:**716-723, 1976.

Scherz, F. H.: Maturational crisis and parent-child relationships, Social casework **52:**362-369, June 1971.

Schulz, D. A., and Wilson, R. A.: Readings on the changing family, Englewood Cliffs, N.J., 1973, Prentice-Hall, Inc.

Scott, R. B., and Winston, M. R.: The health and welfare of the black family in the United States, Am. J. Dis. Child. **130:**704-708, 1976.

Smoyak, S. A.: Introduction: symposium on parenting, Nurs. Clin. North Am. **12:**447-445, 1977.

Sobol, E. G., and Robischon, P.: Family nursing, ed. 2, St. Louis, 1975, The C. V. Mosby Co.

Starr, B. D., and Goldstein, H. S.: Human development and behavior: psychology in nursing, New York, 1975, Springer Publishing Co., Inc., Chapter 13.

Steinbroner, M.: The commune. In Calusen, J. P., and associates: Maternity nursing today, New York, 1973, McGraw-Hill Book Co.

Stokes, L. G.: Delivering health services in a black community. In Reinhardt, A. M., and Quinn, M. D., editors: Current practice in family-centered community nursing, St. Louis, 1977, The C. V. Mosby Co.

Stone, L. J., and Church, J.: Childhood and adolescence: a psychology of the growing person, ed. 3, New York, 1973, Random House, Inc., Chapter 3 and 8.

Suchman, E.: Social patterns of illness and medical care. In Jaco, E. G.: Patients, physicians, and illness, ed. 2, New York, 1972, The Free Press.

Sugar, M.: Children of divorce. Pediatrics **46:**588-595, 1970.

Tapia, J. A.: The nursing process in family health, Nurs. Outlook **20:**267-270, April 1972.

Taylor, C.: The nurse and cultural barriers. In Hymovich, D. P., and Barnard, M. U.: Family health care, New York, 1973, McGraw-Hill Book Co.

Tizard, J.: Early malnutrition, growth and mental development in man, Br. Med. Bull. **30:**169-174, 1974.

Toffler, A.: Future shock, New York, 1970, Random House, Inc.

Torbett, D. S.: The single-parent family. In Clausen, J. P. and associates: Maternity nursing today, New York, 1973, McGraw-Hill Book Co.

Veevers, J. E.: The social meanings of parenthood, Psychiatry **36:**291-310, 1973.

Vogel, S. and associates: Maternal employment and perception of sex roles among college students, Dev. Psychol. **3:**384-391, 1970.

Vroegh, K.: The relationship of birth order and sex of siblings to gender role identity, Dev. Psychol. **4:**407-411, 1971.

Wallerstein, J., and Keeley, J.: Divorce counseling: a community service for families in the midst of divorce, Am. J. Orthopsychiatry **47:**4-22, 1977.

Weiss, M. O.: Cultural shock, Nurs. Outlook **19:**40-43, January 1971.

Westman, J.: Effects of divorce on a child's personality development, Med. Aspects Hum. Sexuality **6:**38-55, 1972.

Willerman, L., Broman, S. H., and Fielder, M. F.: Infant development, preschool IQ and social class, Child Dev. **41:**69-77, 1970.

Williams, S. R.: Nutrition and diet therapy, ed. 3, St. Louis, 1977, The C. V. Mosby Co., Chapter 13.

Williams, T. M.: Childrearing practices of young mothers, Am. J. Orthopsychiatry **44:**70-75, 1974.

Winch, R. F.: Permanence and change in the history of the American family and some speculations as to its future. J. Marriage Fam. **1:**8-16, January 1970.

Winch, R. G.: The modern family, ed. 3, New York, 1971, Holt, Rinehart and Winston, Inc.

Women workers today, Nurs. Outlook **22:**191, 1974.

Woods, M.: The unsupervised child of the working mother, Dev. Psychol. **6:**14-25, 1972.

Wuerger, M.: The young adult—stepping into parenthood, Am. J. Nurs. **76:**1283-1289, 1976.

Zicklin, G.: Communal child-rearing: a report on three cases. In Dreitzel, H. P., editor: Childhood and socialization, New York, 1973, Macmillan, Inc.

Zimmerman, B. M.: The exceptional stresses of adoptive parenthood, Am. J. Maternal Child Nurs. **2**(3):191-197, 1977.

3

The child: the wonder of unfolding

Every child grows and develops in response to a predetermined plan. Established at the time of his conception, this plan governs the physical and, to some extent, behavioral changes that continually take place within his body and mind. At any point in time on a lifelong continuum the child is the product of past events and relationships, whereas all present events and relationships will affect his future development and well-being. Nursing care of infants and children requires an awareness of the forces within the child that push him onward and the forces in the environment that aid or impede that progress.

Growth and development are complex processes involving numerous components that are subject to a wide variety of influences. All facets of the child's body, mind, and personality develop simultaneously, with varying rates and sequences, but not independently. Development of one part may be controlled or influenced by the activity of another part. Physical growth begins at the time of conception; behavior and personality do not develop until after birth, and they mature as the child is increasingly able to control his physical structure. Each aspect of development, such as the organ systems and personality components, has a timetable for growth, maturation, or elaboration. Because of the dynamic, ever-changing nature of the developmental process, a condition or behavior that is normal at one age is considered to be abnormal if it persists into subsequent stages of development.

HEREDITY AND ENVIRONMENT

Human beings begin their existence with a physical, biochemical, and mental potential that is determined by the genes they receive from each of their parents. The blueprint contained within these genes establishes the plan that determines their ultimate developmental capacity; however, the genes are unable to work independently. There is no assurance that this plan will be fulfilled, because equally influential in shaping the individual throughout a lifetime is the environment, which is neither constant nor dependable. This includes the intracellular and intercellular environments within the organism, the intrauterine environment before birth, and the extrauterine environment from birth until death. Heredity and environment are so interrelated that they become inseparable. A given hereditary trait will present varying manifestations under different environmental conditions. Similarly the relative contribution of the environment will differ under different hereditary conditions. At the present time hereditary factors cannot be altered, but the environment is subject to varying degrees of manipulation.

For decades the relative importance of heredity and environment in molding development has been deliberated by scientists, educators, and health professionals. It is now commonly accepted that the end product is not a result of the *action* of one or the other of these processes but the *interaction* of one with the other. For example, children who receive genes for above-average height can only achieve full potential with an optimum environment including good diet, love, and freedom from disease. On the other hand, children who inherit genes for less than average height will never attain greater than their programmed stature even in a superior environment. Children with limited intellectual capability can never excel in a field that requires highly intellectual skills, no matter to what extent they are pushed. But children with superior mentality will be wasted without an environment that stimulates and encourages their innate capacity. It can be said that heredity determines the limits to which children *can* achieve; the environment determines the extent to which they actually *do* achieve.

The areas that have stimulated the greatest controversy are in regard to the contribution of each (heredity and environment) to behavior characteristics and intelligence. Intellectual diversity of individuals is undisputed, but the extent to which large human groups differ in intelligence on a genetic basis is continually challenged. There is a significant relationship between the intelligence of genetically similar persons (even those reared in dissimilar environments) and certain aspects of intellectual functioning (for example, verbal, spatial, and number abilities, clerical speed and accuracy, reasoning, and memory). There is evidence that hereditary influence on intellectual functioning is most marked in girls, whereas environment has a greater impact on boys.[17] Infant and early childhood stimulation programs and innovative techniques in education at all levels of intellectual endowment have substantiated the positive influence of environmental stimulation on achievement. On the other hand, early childhood deprivation and the alarming effects of inadequate nutrition during critical periods of development are areas of concern to health professionals.

The influences on behavior traits are more difficult to assess. The culture dictates that some hereditary characteristics (for example, sex) imply conformity to specific behavioral expectations. Many dimensions of personality that appear to be hereditary (such as the degree of responsiveness or unresponsiveness, activity level, extroversion-introversion, and the degree to which an individual plans ahead or reacts impulsively) and various constitutional traits (such as beauty, ugliness, physical deformity, sensory handicaps, or learning impairment) affect the way in which others react to children and the interpersonal behavior children display in response. When a child displays undesirable behavior, careful evaluation is required to determine the degree to which the behavior can be attributed to his interpersonal environment or to hereditary influences. It becomes a significant factor in assessing whether or not he would profit from therapy or if he should be removed from that environment. Children will react in different ways according to the composition of their environment and the innate resources with which they confront that environment.

GROWTH AND DEVELOPMENT OF THE CHILD

Growth and development, usually referred to as a unit, express the sum of the numerous changes that take place during the lifetime of an individual. The entire course is a dynamic process that encompasses several interrelated dimensions.

Growth implies a change in quantity and results when cells divide and synthesize new proteins. This increase in number and size of cells is reflected in increased size and weight of the whole or any of its parts.

Maturation, which literally means to ripen, is described as aging or as an increase in competence and adaptability. It is usually used to describe a qualitative change, that is, a change in the complexity of a structure that makes it possible for that structure to begin functioning or to function at a higher level. Sometimes maturation designates the unfolding of traits inherent in the organism.

Differentiation is primarily a biologic description of the processes by which early cells and structures are systematically modified and altered to achieve specific and characteristic physical and chemical properties (see p. 211), although it is sometimes a term used to describe one of the trends in development, that is, mass to specific.

Development is a gradual growth and expansion. It, too, involves a change, in this case from a lower to a more advanced stage of complexity. Development is the emerging and expanding of capacities of the individual to provide progressively greater facility in functioning and is achieved through growth, maturation, and learning.

All of these processes are interrelated. Although they are simultaneous, ongoing processes, none occurs apart from the others. The child's body becomes larger and more complex; the personality simultaneously expands in scope and complexity. Very simply, growth can be viewed as a *quantitative* change, development as a *qualitative* change. Children "grow" by maintaining a positive balance of increase over loss in size; they "grow up" by maturing in structure and function.

Stages of development

Most authorities in the field of child development conveniently categorize child growth and behavior into approximate age stages or in terms that describe the features of an age-group. The age ranges of these stages are admittedly arbitrary and, since they do not take into account individual differences, cannot be applied to all children with any degree of precision. However, this categorization affords a convenient means to describe the characteristics associated with the majority of children at periods when distinctive developmental changes appear and specific developmental tasks* must be accomplished. It is also significant for nurses to know that there are characteristic health problems peculiar to each major phase of development. The sequence of descriptive age periods and subperiods that are used here and elaborated in subsequent chapters include:

Prenatal period: conception to birth
- EMBRYONIC: conception to 8 weeks
- FETAL: 8 to 40 weeks (birth)

A rapid growth rate and total dependency makes this one of the most crucial periods in the developmental process. The relationship between maternal health and certain manifestations in the newborn emphasizes the importance of adequate prenatal care to the health and well-being of the infant.

Infancy period: birth to 12 or 18 months
- NEONATAL: birth to 28 days
- INFANCY: 2 to approximately 12 months

The infancy period is one of rapid motor, cognitive, and social development. Through mutuality with the care giver (mother), the infant establishes a basic trust in the world and the foundation for future interpersonal relationships. The critical first month of life, although part of the infancy period, is often differentiated from the remainder because of the major physical adjustments to extrauterine existence and the psychologic adjustment of the mother.

Early childhood: 1 to 6 years
- TODDLER: 1 to 3 years
- PRESCHOOL: 3 to 6 years

*A developmental task is a set of skills and competencies peculiar to each developmental stage that children must accomplish or master in order to deal effectively with their environment.[8]

This period, which extends from the time children attain upright locomotion until they enter school, is characterized by intense activity and discovery. It is a time of marked physical and personality development. Motor development advances steadily. Children at this age acquire language and wider social relationships, learn role standards, gain self-control and mastery, develop increasing awareness of dependence and independence, and begin to develop a self-concept.

Middle childhood: 6 to 11 or 12 years

Frequently referred to as the "school age," this period of development is one in which the child is directed away from the family group and is centered around the wider world of peer relationships. There is steady advancement in physical, mental, and social development with emphasis on developing skill competencies. Social cooperation and early moral development take on more importance with relevance for later life stages. This is a critical period in the development of a self-concept.

Later childhood: 11 to 18 years

PREPUBERTAL: 10 to 13 years

ADOLESCENCE: 13 to approximately 18 years

The tumultuous period of rapid maturation and change known as adolescence has been described in various ways. It is considered to be a transitional period that begins at the onset of puberty and extends to the point of entry into the adult world—usually high school graduation. Biologic and personality maturation are accompanied by physical and emotional turmoil, and there is redefining of the self-concept. In the late adolescent period the child begins to internalize all the previously learned values and to focus on an individual, rather than a group, identity.

Methods of studying growth and development

The early growth period in the human being extends over a longer period of time than that of any other mammalian species. The long period of childhood allows for more elaborate brain development, body growth, and the development of those characteristics of personality that distinguish man from lower animals. During these early years children prepare for adulthood in several dimensions—they increase in size and acquire increasingly intricate motor capacities, their personality emerges, and they assimilate their culture.

To determine whether or not growth and development have taken place, the child can be compared to a representative group of children at the same point in time (cross-sectional method), or the same child can be measured and compared at different points in time (longitudinal method). Standards or norms for the study of developmental progress have been established by these two contrasting methods.

The *cross-sectional* method, which tests or measures the characteristics of a number of children representing the various ages or stages of development, is the more common. The observations are made of children at the same point in time. For example, a group of school children, ages 6 to 12 years, are measured for specific characteristics such as height, weight, mental ability, motor ability, or vocabulary. The data that are collected and averaged on a group of 6-year-old children, 7-year-old children, and so on provide information on the expected achievement of a child in that age-group. If large groups are used, the results are expressed as averages, but the meaning of these results is directly related to the similarities within the groups, such as race, sex, socioeconomic level, and so on. Most norms or averages are determined in this way and are useful in comparing groups. For instance, the average height of 8-year-old children in Chicago can be compared with the average height of 8-year-old Mexican children. This method is especially useful to establish norms for a given age-group with or without other factors.

The *longitudinal* method is often used to determine growth trends and rates. Each child in a group of children is observed and measured periodically over a number of years and through successive stages of growth and development. This approach is also useful in assessing the long-term or delayed effects of an early experience, such as a prolonged illness, malnutrition, or maternal rejection. Although the longitudinal method is more difficult to carry out, the growth and development of a child can be compared at any moment with a representative group of children and can be followed through successive stages to determine the speed and direction of that child's distinctive growth.

Patterns of development

There are definite and predictable patterns in growth and development that are continuous, orderly, and progressive. These patterns, sometimes referred to as trends or principles, are universal and basic to all human beings. Although they are more apparent with respect to physical growth, most of these patterns apply to psychologic and social growth as well. Growth and development follow predetermined trends in direction, sequence, and pace, but each human being accomplishes these in a manner and time unique to that individual.

Directional trends. Growth and development proceed in regular, related directions or gradients and reflect the physical development and maturation of neuromuscular functions (Fig. 3-1). The first pattern is the *cephalocaudal,* or head-to-tail, direction. That is, the head end of the organism develops first and is very large and complex, whereas the lower end is small and simple and takes shape at a later period. The physical evidence of this trend is most apparent during the period before birth, but it also applies to postnatal behavior development. Infants achieve structural control of the head before the trunk and extremities, hold their back erect before they stand, use their eyes before their hands, and gain control of their hands before they have control of their feet.

Second, the *proximodistal,* or near-to-far, trend applies

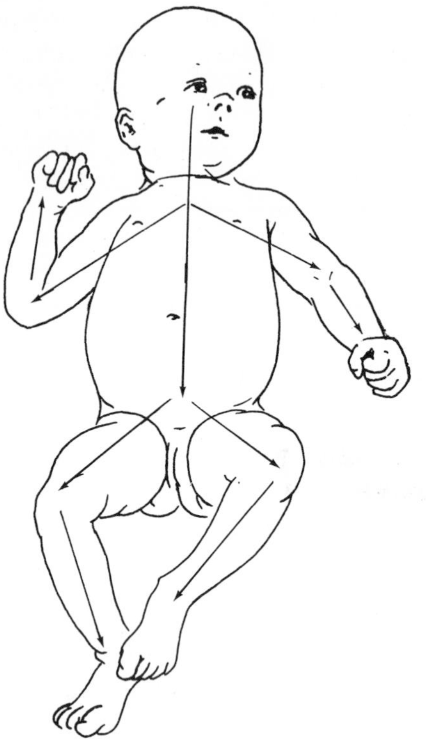

Fig. 3-1. Directional trends in growth.

to the midline-to-peripheral concept. A conspicuous illustration is the early embryonic development of limb buds, which is followed by rudimentary fingers and toes. In the infant, shoulder control precedes mastery of hands, the whole hand is used as a unit before the fingers can be manipulated, and the central nervous system develops more rapidly than the peripheral nervous system.

These trends or patterns are bilateral and appear to be symmetric—each side develops in the same direction and at the same rate as the other. For some of the neurologic functions, this symmetry is only external because of unilateral differentiation of function at an early stage of postnatal development. For example, by the age of approximately 5 years the child has demonstrated a decided preference for the use of one hand over the other, although previously he has used either one.

The third trend in the direction growth, *mass to specific* (sometimes referred to as differentiation), describes development from simple operations to more complex activities and functions. From very broad, global patterns of behavior, more specific, refined patterns emerge. All areas of development (physical, mental, social, and emotional) proceed in this direction. Through the processes of development and differentiation, early embryonal cells with vague, undifferentiated functions progress to an immensely complex organism composed of highly specialized and diversified cells, tissues, and organs. Generalized development will precede specific or specialized development. Physically there are gross, random muscle movements before fine muscle control takes place. The child will at first run and jump for the sake of motion, but eventually these activities take the more complex form of a race or hopscotch. Infants will respond to people in general before they recognize and prefer their mothers.

Sequential trends. In all dimensions of growth and development there is a definite, predictable sequence. It is orderly and continuous, with each child normally passing through every stage. Children crawl before they creep, creep before they stand, and stand before they walk. Each stage is affected by those preceding it and affects those that follow. For example, children must stand on their feet before they can move them in locomotion. Sequential patterns have been described for motor skills such as locomotion and use of hands, language, social, and other types of behavior. A child first plays alone, then with others in increasing numbers and increasingly complex activities.

New parts or behaviors arise out of and build on those already established. This continuity with the past that serves as a foundation for the future is *epigenesis,* and it requires interaction with a suitable environment at the proper time. In very early physical development, fingers arise from webbed appendages on limb buds, the nervous system develops from a neural tube derived from a primitive streak in the embryo, and sexual organs differentiate from a morphologically neutral primitive gonad. Later facets of the personality are built on the early foundation of trust. The child babbles, then forms words and, finally, sentences; writing emerges from scribbling.

Critical periods. There are limited times during the process of growth when the organism will interact with a particular environment in a specific manner. The quality of interactions during these critical periods determines whether the effects on the organism will be beneficial or harmful. The character and extent of the consequences of the interaction depend on the nature of the environmental influences and the stage of development. For example, physiologic maturation of the central nervous system is influenced by adequacy and timing of contributions from the environment, such as stimulation and nutrition. The first 3 months of prenatal life are critical periods for physical growth. It is during this period of accelerated growth and differentiation that specific organs and systems are most vulnerable to environmental influences, and the earlier the impact, the more far-reaching are its effects.

Psychologic development also appears to have critical periods when an environmental event has maximal influence on the developing personality. Observers have identified periods in development when behavior patterns are most readily acquired. For example, primary socialization occurs during the first year when the infant makes the initial social attachments and establishes a basic trust in the world.

It is at this time that a warm relationship with a mother figure is fundamental to a healthy personality. The same concept might be applied to readiness for learning skills such as toilet training or reading. In these instances there appears to be a sensitive period in development, that is, an opportune time when the skill is best learned. However, if the skill is not learned at this time, acquisition at a later time is still possible.

Developmental pace. Although there is a fixed, precise order to development, it does not progress at the same rate or pace. There are periods of accelerated growth and periods of decelerated growth. This includes both total body growth and growth of subsystems. The very rapid growth rate before and after birth gradually levels off through early childhood. The rate is relatively slow during middle childhood, but there is a marked increase at the beginning of adolescence followed by a leveling off in early adulthood. Also, the focus of development and growth shifts at successive stages in development. The growth of various organs and subsystems develops at different times. That is, the head grows most rapidly before birth, whereas other body parts grow more slowly; after birth the other structures grow faster than the head. This accounts for the shifts in body proportion, facial characteristics, voice, and so forth. Similarly, one type of development seems to take precedence over another. At times of rapid physical growth, other development may reach a pleateau. For example, when the child begins to walk, the thrills of upright locomotion take precedence over other activity such as speech, and he may not learn any new words for 3 to 4 months. Schoolwork may suffer during the early adolescent growth spurt.

Cycles of behavior.[10] Observation of child behavior over the course of development indicates that behavioral trends follow a more or less regular cyclic pattern of equilibrium and disequilibrium; this sequence of behavior appears to occur repeatedly as children mature. Periods in which children appear to be relatively tranquil and untroubled are followed by periods of disequilibrium (Table 3-1). At about ages 2, 5, and 10 years they have little difficulty within themselves or with the world around them.

Each of these relatively smooth stages are followed at 2½, 5½ to 6, and 11 years of age by a brief period of disturbed, troubled, and generally "broken-up" behavior in which children are at odds with the environment and with themselves. These stages are followed again by periods of relative calm at 3, 6½, and 12 years of age when the children seem to be in good balance and happy with themselves and their environment.

The next phase, in which there is a very pronounced focus of the child's attention inward, children become introspective and thoughtful. They incorporate outer impressions and experiences to mull over, think about, and digest. At these ages, about 3½, 7, and 13 years, the inner process may be expressed differently at the various age stages. Children 3½ years old may exhibit general emotional instability, such as a variety of fears, hand tremor, stumbling, poor spatial orientation, whining, and a high, tremulous voice. Older children, better able to withstand the stresses of this inwardizing, are more apt to express this stage in marked sensitivity and touchiness, excessive withdrawal and moroseness, and a pessimistic attitude toward life in general.

Extreme expansiveness is characteristic of the ages 4, 8, and 14 years. Children at these ages are markedly outgoing so much so that they may be in danger of expanding too much. For example, the 4-year-old child may wander from home, the 8-year-old child may attempt hazardous activities (such as bicycle riding in the street) and get hurt, and the 14-year-old adolescent may become tangled in multiple and conflicting social plans. Less is known about ages 4½, 9, and 15 years, although each is characterized by behavior that is less outgoing than in the previous stage. During these periods children are less well balanced and have been frequently described as "neurotic." Following this again come ages of relative stability and equilibrium at 5, 10, and 16 years of age.

Table 3-1. Summary of behavior cycles[10]

Ages (years)	Behaviors
2, 5, 10	Smooth, consolidated
2½, 5½-6, 11	Breaking up
3, 6½, 12	Rounded, balanced
3½, 7, 13	Inwardized
4, 8, 14	Vigorous, expansive
4½, 9, 15	Inwardized-outwardized, troubled, "neurotic"
5, 10, 16	Smooth, consolidated

Individual differences

Each child grows in his or her own unique and personal way. There is great individual variation in the age at which developmental milestones are reached. The sequence is predictable; the exact timing is not. Rates of growth vary from one individual to another, and measurements are defined in terms of ranges to allow for individual differences between children. There are some children who are fast growers, others are moderate, and some are slower to reach maturity. Periods of fast growth, such as the pubescent growth spurt, may begin earlier or later in some children than in others. The child may grow fast or slow during the spurt and may finish sooner or later than other children. The sex of the child is an influential factor because girls seem to be more advanced in physiologic growth at all ages.

Optimal tendency and terminal points. The terminal points in growth vary immensely from one child to another. For example, one individual will grow until he reaches a height of over 6 feet, another will cease growing at 5 feet, while the majority will achieve varying points between the two. The average female will reach both height and weight terminals before the average male, with the average terminal height in males exceeding that for females.

There appears to be a tendency for the organism to strive for optimum developmental potential in both structure and function. When environmental factors interfere with normal development for a time (for example, during periods of inadequate food supply or illness), children will usually make up for the interrupted period and return to their characteristic pattern of growth. However, if the deprivation is severe or occurs throughout a critical period, development may be permanently impaired. Children born prematurely will demonstrate retarded development during the early months but will usually "catch up" to others of the same age by the time they enter school.

Interrelatedness. Children develop as whole beings, not in pieces and parts. They are a product of the past environment in which they have grown and the current stresses and satisfactions. Factors that affect one part will influence the others. For example, a child deprived of love and affection will be delayed in physical and mental development. Although there are exceptions, a child who deviates from the average with respect to one aspect of growth will probably deviate in others.

Secular trend in growth

From measurements and observations recorded over the past century, there appears to be a significant world-wide trend in the rate and age of maturation. Children from widely different populations are maturing earlier and becoming larger at each age. There appears to be a slight but not so marked increase in average adult height, because although children are growing faster they also stop growing sooner. The average young man reaches his full height at approximately age 20 years, whereas in 1900 he did not reach his final height until about 25 years of age. The average size increase since 1900 is near 1 cm (0.4 inch) per decade in height and 1 kg (2.2 pounds) in weight in preschool children and 2.5 cm (1 inch) and 2.5 kg (5.5 pounds) per decade during puberty. In girls the age of menarche has advanced progressively. The trend appears to reach a plateau in populations with optimum environments, which suggests that there is a maximum end point. Many theories have been advanced to explain this phenomenon. Improved environmental factors, such as nutrition and socioeconomic conditions, are important factors as well as the sharp decrease in infant mortality during this century. Since body size is an inherited trait, the tendency toward the selection of mates from wider geographic areas is an important factor.

PHYSICAL DEVELOPMENT

As children grow, their external dimensions change. These changes are accompanied by corresponding alterations in structure and function of internal organs and tissues that reflect the gradual acquisition of physiologic competence. These alterations, although progressive and interdependent, are not a uniform process, but are characterized by cycles of accelerated and slow development that vary from organ to organ and system to system within the organism. Each part has its own rate of growth, and many are directly related to alterations in the size of the child (for example, heart rate). Skeletal muscle growth approximates whole body growth; brain, lymphoid, adrenal, and reproductive tissues follow distinct and individual patterns (Fig. 3-2).

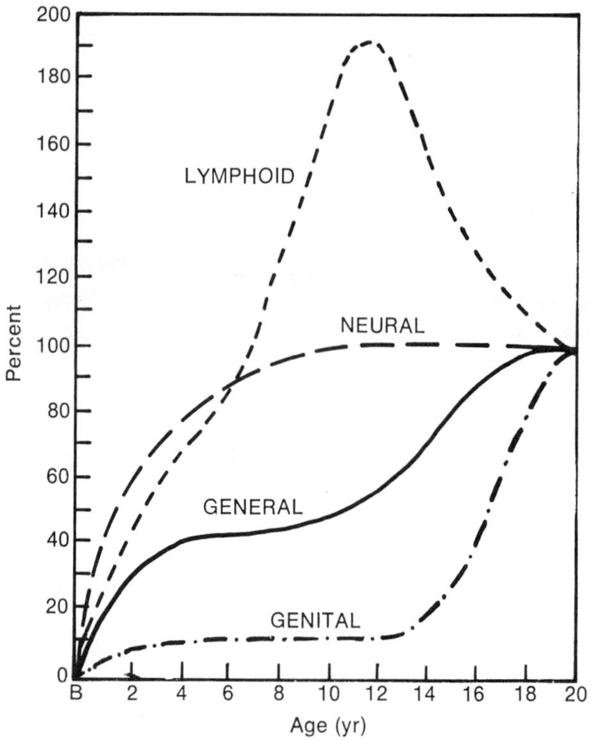

Fig. 3-2. Growth rates for the body as a whole and three types of tissues. *Lymphoid type,* thymus, lymph nodes, and intestinal lymph masses; *neural type,* brain, dura, spinal cord, optic apparatus, and head dimensions; *general type,* body as a whole, external dimensions, and respiratory, digestive, renal, circulatory, and musculoskeletal systems. (Adapted from Harris, J. A., and associates: The measurement of man, Minneapolis, 1930, University of Minnesota Press.)

External proportions

The changes in external dimensions as a child matures that are so clear in the present day were not always so obvious. Early paintings and replicas of children depict them as miniature adults. They appeared with the typical chubby outlines of small children but with adult proportions. Variations in the growth rate of different tissues and organ sys-

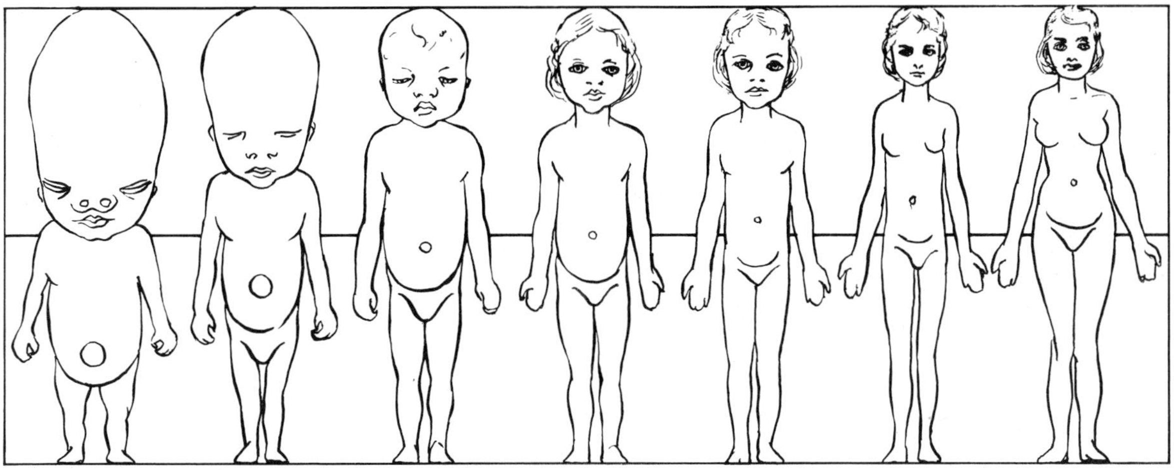

Fig. 3-3. Changes in relative proportions of head, trunk, and extremities from the second fetal month to maturity.

tems produce significant changes in body proportions during childhood. The cephalocaudal trend of development is most evident in total body growth as indicated by these changes (Fig. 3-3). During fetal development the head is the fastest growing part, and at 2 months of gestation the head comprises 50% of total body length. During infancy growth of the trunk predominates; the legs are the most rapidly growing part during childhood; then, in adolescence, the trunk once again elongates. In the newborn infant the lower limbs are one third the total body length but only 15% of the total body weight; in the adult the lower limbs comprise one half the total body height and 30% of total body weight. As growth proceeds, the midpoint in head-to-toe measurements gradually descends from a level even with the umbilicus at birth to the level of the symphysis pubis at maturity.[15]

The first year is a period of rapid growth dominated by lengthening of the trunk and the accumulation of subcutaneous fat. The legs are bowed. When infants begin to walk, their large head, heavy trunk, and protruberant addomen atop short legs force them to walk with a wide stance, outward rotation of the hips, and everted feet. The high center of gravity created by this disproportionate bulk causes them to walk unsteadily and contributes to frequent falls.

After the first year and extending to puberty, the legs grow more rapidly than any other part. The bowlegged appearance disappears with locomotion, the abdomen is held in, and the body becomes slender and elongated. Until puberty this slender, long-legged build is characteristic of both sexes. In fact, in similar clothes and hairstyle the two sexes are indistinguishable. With the onset of puberty there is a marked alteration in body proportion when all structures show the effects of the pubertal "growth spurt." The feet and hands are first to increase in rate of growth; therefore, during this transient period they appear large and ungainly in relation to the rest of the body, often creating a source of embarrassment to the adolescent. The trunk again grows faster than the legs so that a large portion of the increase in height at adolescence is a result of trunk growth.

Since the legs continue to grow until puberty, early-maturing children have shorter than average legs, and the legs of later-maturing children are longer. Inasmuch as the onset of puberty is approximately 2½ years earlier in girls, for awhile girls are larger than boys and girls' legs are shorter than boys'. Following rapid linear growth there is a laterality of growth—both boys and girls proceed to "fill out" during the later stages of adolescent growth.

One of the more outstanding features of changing body proportion is related to shoulder and hip breadth as a result of hormone secretion from the maturing gonads. Shoulder and hip growth increases in both sexes, but the shoulder width in boys is considerably greater than it is in girls. The anterior-posterior hip diameter increases in girls and the female pelvis becomes wider, shallower, and roomier than the male pelvis. The differences in deposition of fat produce the distinctive feminine contours in girls, whereas boys lose subcutaneous fat.

Facial proportion. Facial proportions show characteristic changes during childhood. In infancy and early childhood the face is small in relation to the skull (Fig. 3-4). The size of the cranial vault reflects the advanced development of the brain. The brain has achieved 25% of its adult size at birth and 66% at the end of 1 year. Over 90% of the growth of the brain cavity has been achieved by the end of the fifth year, and 98% has been achieved at age 15 years.

After the first year of life the facial skeleton grows more rapidly than the brain case. The principle growth is in the jaws as they enlarge to accommodate the teeth and in development of the muscles of mastication. The face grows first in width and then in length so that the child's face ap-

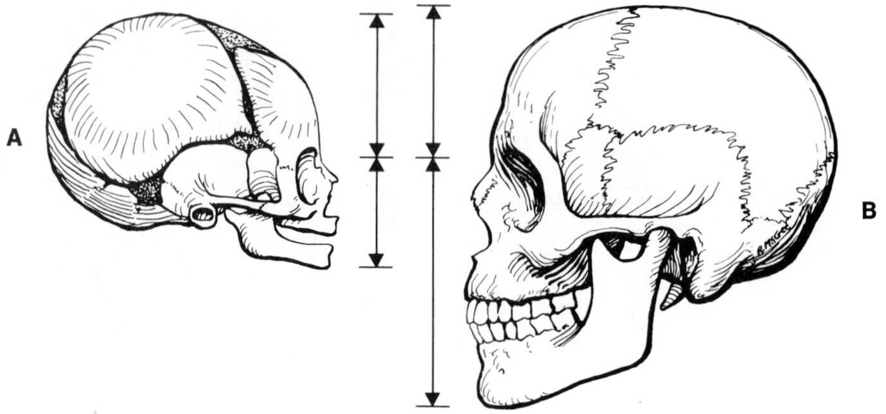

Fig. 3-4. Comparison of face and cranial proportions in infant and adult skull. **A,** Infant; **B,** adult. Note differences in relative size of face and angle of mandible, absence of mastoid sinus in infant, and absence of fontanels in adult.

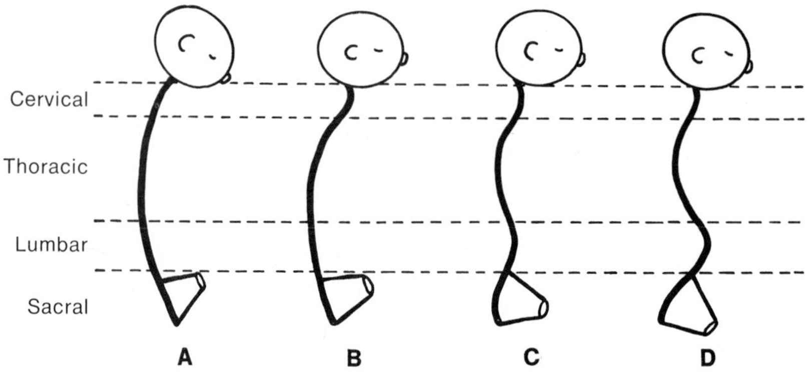

Fig. 3-5. Development of spinal curvatures. **A,** Newborn infant; **B,** cervical secondary curvature; **C,** lumbar secondary curvature; **D,** lordosis.

pears to emerge from underneath his skull, particularly during adolescence.[15]

The size of the face relative to the skull has implications for child health in the infant and young child. The large, heavy cranium is the primary site of injury in falls. The changing dimensions of the face alter the diameter and angle of ear structures, particularly the external auditory meatus and the eustachian tube. The latter contributes significantly to the incidence of middle ear infection (see p. 575).

Posture. Posture is also altered by concomitant growth and maturation of various structures. Within the narrow confines of the uterus the prenatal posture is one of total flexion. The spine is curved with the head and extremities bent upon the child. The bones in the vertebral column of the newborn infant form two primary curvatures, one in the thoracic region and one in the sacral region (Fig. 3-5, *A*). Both are forward, concave curvatures that rely largely on the shape of their component bones. The thoracic curve is relatively stable, and movement is limited in scope and amount by thin intervertebral discs and oblique spinous processes. The sacral curve eventually becomes fused and permanently fixed.

As the infant gains control of his head, at approximately 3 months of age, a secondary curvature appears in the cervical region (Fig. 3-5, *B*). This curve, unlike the primary curvatures, is convex forward, and its mobility is maintained by thick intervertebral discs and tension of muscles stretched across its convexity.

To maintain a sitting posture another secondary curvature is created in the lumbar region (Fig. 3-5, *C*). Like the cervical curve the lumbar curve is convex, mobile, depends largely on intervertebral discs, and is controlled by the large postural muscles of the spine. When children first assume an upright posture in their initial efforts to walk, they compensate for a high center of gravity and the weight of a large liver by an exaggerated lumbar curvature or *lordosis* (Fig. 3-5, *D*). With advancing skill in locomotion

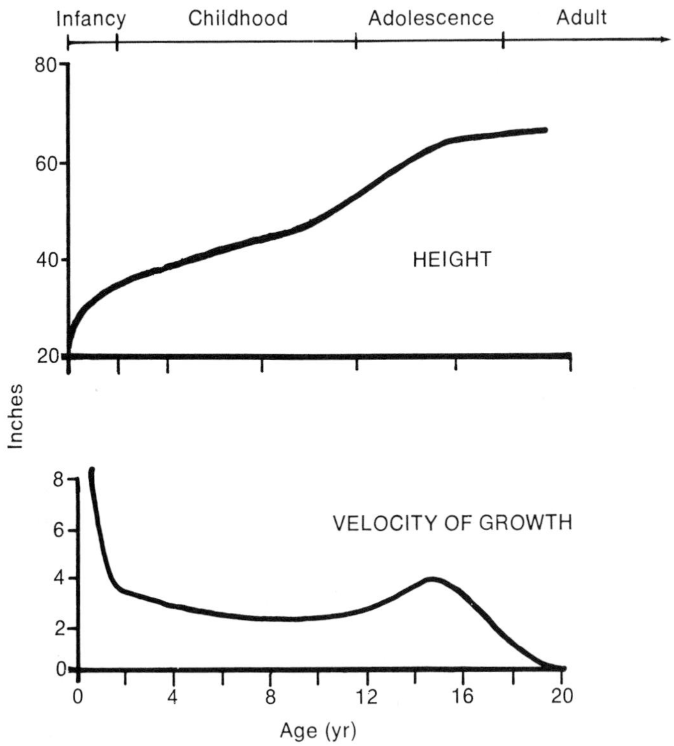

Fig. 3-6. Linear growth of one boy, expressed as increments per year. (Adapted from Falkner, F.: The physical development of children, Pediatrics **29:**448, 1962.)

there is a gradual progression toward normal upright posture. When situations cause a delay in holding up the head or sitting, the secondary curvatures may fail to develop at the expected time.

Growth in height and weight

Linear growth occurs almost entirely as a result of skeletal growth and is considered to be a stable measure of general growth. Growth in height is not uniform throughout life, but when maturation of the skeleton is complete, linear growth ceases. The maximum growth in length occurs before birth, but the newborn continues to grow at a rapid, though slower, rate. As the months pass, the growth rate rapidly decelerates (Fig. 3-6). By 2 years of age the child normally has achieved 50% of his adult height. By age 4 years birth length has usually doubled.

At approximately 3 years of age the child begins a relatively stable and steady growth rate of 5 to 6 cm (2 to 2.5 inches) per year that continues for the next 9 years. (Occasionally a child will exhibit a transitory midgrowth height increase at the age of 6 or 7 years.) This long midgrowth period is ended by a sudden and marked acceleration—the adolescent growth spurt. Although there is wide variation, this increase, which begins about ages 10½ to 11 years in girls and 12½ to 13 years in boys, lasts approximately 2 to 2½ years. During this time a boy may add 20 cm (8 inches) to his height and a girl 16 cm (6.5 inches). Usually, 98% of the terminal height is reached by age 16½ years in girls but not until 17¾ years in boys.

Serial measurements of growth are plotted periodically on standard growth charts to determine the pattern of growth and to compare the individual child with the norm for that particular age-group (see Appendix E). As a whole, children usually can be categorized into one of the following six groups according to their pattern of maturation:

1. Average children—closely approximate the mean for height and weight at all ages
2. Early-maturing children—tall in childhood but not unusually tall adults
3. Early-maturing children who are also genetically tall—above the mean at all ages
4. Late-maturing children—shorter than average in childhood but not necessarily short adults
5. Late-maturing children who are also genetically short—below the mean at all ages
6. Children who deviate significantly from the normal growth curve—very rapid- and early-maturing children; much later- and slower-maturing children

Deviations from the normal pattern of linear growth may indicate a health problem, especially in relation to hormonal imbalances. However, most children who represent points at the upper or lower percentiles merely reflect hereditary factors. When assessing children in the extremes of height ranges, it is important to compare their height with the height of their parents and siblings.

From analysis of data derived from longitudinal studies, it is possible to state the percentage of terminal height that has been achieved at any given age and to predict the future height of an individual from measurements taken in childhood (Table 3-2). Birth length is influenced considerably by the prenatal environment and gestational age; therefore, prediction of height is of little worth until the second year of life. By this time the child has usually compensated for prenatally influenced deviations. Variability in the onset of puberty may also alter the predictive value in this age-group. Such predictions are valuable as a tool to help parents and their slow-maturing children accept the child's unique pattern of growth and to help these puzzled children to understand why they are different from their taller age-mates. These predictions are sometimes useful in order to avoid possible disappointment in the preparation for occupations or careers that have height restrictions and require early beginning preparation (for example, ballet dancing). More important, if parents are satisfied that a child's apparently small size merely reflects the normal expectations based on their own adult size, they will be less likely to force feed the child, which can result in obesity or food refusal and poor appetite. For the young girl whose predicted adult height is excessively tall, this early indication provides time to initiate therapy, if advisable, and to help the

Table 3-2. Percentage of mature height attained at different ages

Chronologic age (years)	Percentage of eventual height	
	Boys	Girls
1	42.2	44.7
2	49.5	52.8
3	53.8	57.0
4	58.0	61.8
5	61.8	66.2
6	65.2	70.3
7	69.0	74.0
8	72.0	77.5
9	75.0	80.7
10	78.0	84.4
11	81.1	88.4
12	84.2	92.9
13	87.3	96.5
14	91.5	98.3
15	96.1	99.1
16	98.3	99.6
17	99.3	100.0
18	99.8	100.0

From Bayley, N.: Growth curves of height and weight for boys and girls, scaled according to physical maturity, J. Pediatr. **48:**187-194, 1956.

child develop the capacity to deal with the potential problems associated with this trait.

Weight at birth is more variable than height at birth and is, to a greater extent, a reflection of the intrauterine environment. The average newborn weighs 3175 to 3400 g (7 to 7.5 pounds), which is an increase of approximately 3 billion times the weight of the fertilized ovum. The rate of weight gain increases rapidly for a short time after birth but soon decreases markedly. By the time the individual reaches maturity the birth weight has only increased about twenty times (to 68 kg or 150 pounds). In general, the birth weight doubles by 5 to 6 months of age and triples by the end of the first year. By the end of the second year it usually quadruples. After this point the "normal" rate of weight gain, just as the growth in height, assumes a steady annual increase of approximately 2 to 2.75 kg (4.4 to 6 pounds) per year until the adolescent growth spurt. Although the weight gain usually lags behind the gain in height by about 3 months, boys may add 20 kg (44 pounds) and girls 15 kg (33 pounds) during the growth spurt.

The factors that influence body weight are so numerous and varied that they cannot be adequately dealt with in this overview. For example, birth weight alone is influenced by such factors as heredity, length of gestation, and other variables related to the maternal state (see p. 322). Lifetime postnatal weight gain is subject to equally numerous intrinsic and extrinsic factors that will be discussed as they apply to specific situations or conditions. Growth responses become apparent by changes in weight before they appear in other aspects of growth. Weight gain is usually considered to be an indication of satisfactory growth progress in a child and is probably the best index of nutrition and growth. However, it may be difficult to determine if this increase in weight is caused by healthy tissue development or by an unhealthy deposition of fat or accumulation of fluid.

Tissue composition and development

Throughout the developmental process various tissues in the body undergo changes in composition and structure. In some tissues the changes are continuous; in others significant alterations occur only at specific times. For example, the changes in bone growth and dentition are continuous and are useful in the assessment of growth and maturation of the child. An overview of these changes will be presented as part of the overview of growth and development. The relationship of surface area to body mass is of primary importance during very early development (see p. 257). Similarly the physical characteristics related to hormonal changes are most significant during the adolescent period and will be discussed as they apply to problems associated with this phase of development.

Water content

The embryo is composed primarily of water with little tissue substance. As the organism grows and develops, there is a progressive decrease in total body water with the fastest rate of decline during fetal life. The changes in water content and distribution that occur with age reflect the changes that take place in the relative amounts of bone, muscle, and fat of which the body is composed. The percentage of total body water falls from 90% in the 1-month-old embryo to 75% or 80% of total body weight at birth. At 3 years of age body water comprises 63% of body weight and decreases slowly until age 12 years, when it reaches approximately 58%. At maturity the percentage of total body water is somewhat higher in the male than in the female and is probably a result of the differences in body composition, particularly fat and muscle content.

Another important aspect of growth changes in water distribution is related to the intracellular and extracellular fluid compartments. In the fetus and prematurely born infant, the largest proportion of body water is contained in the extracellular compartment. As growth and development proceed, the proportion within this fluid compartment decreases as the intracellular fluid and cell solids increase. The extracellular fluid decreases from approximately 40% of body weight at birth to 25% at 2 years of age and 20% at maturity. The significance of these fluid compartments and their regulation will be discussed with problems of fluid and electrolyte balance in Chapter 29.

Growth of cartilage and bone

Growth of the skeleton follows a genetically programmed developmental plan that furnishes not only the best indicator of general growth progress, but also provides the best estimate of biologic age. Some degree of assessment can be achieved by observation of facial bone development (that is, nasal bridge height, prominence of malar eminences, and mandibular size), but the most accurate measure of general development is the determination of osseous maturation by roentgenography. Skeletal age appears to correlate more closely with other measures of physiologic maturity (such as onset of menarche) than with chronologic age or height. This ''bone age'' is determined by comparing the mineralization of ossification centers and advancing bony form to age-related standards. Skeletal maturation begins with the appearance of centers of ossification in the embryo and ends when the last epiphysis is firmly fused to the shaft of its bone.

In the healthy child skeletal growth and development consist of two concurrent processes: (1) the creation of new cells and tissues (growth), and (2) the consolidation of these tissues into a permanent form (maturation). Early in fetal life embryonic connective tissues begin to differentiate and become more closely packed to form cartilage. This cartilage enlarges by cell division and expansion within the forming structures and by the laying down of successive layers on the surface of the mass. During the second month of fetal life, bone formation begins when calcium salts are deposited in the intercellular substance (matrix) to form calcified cartilage first and then true bone. There are some differences in this bone formation. In small bones, the bone continues to form in the center and cartilage continues to be laid down on the surfaces. Bones of the face and cranium are laid out in a tough membrane and directly ossified into bone during fetal life.

In long bones the ossification takes place in two centers. It begins in the *diaphysis* (the long central portion of the bone) from a ''primary'' center and continues in the epiphysis (the end portions of the bone) at ''secondary'' centers of ossification. Situated between the diaphysis and the epiphysis is an epiphyseal cartilage plate that is united to the diaphysis by columns of spongy tissue, the metaphysis (Fig. 3-7). It is at this site that active growth in length takes place, and interference with this growth site by trauma or infection can result in deformity (p. 1559). Under the influence of hormones, primarily pituitary growth hormone and thyroid hormone, bones increase in circumference by the formation of new bone tissue beneath the membrane that surrounds the bone (periosteum) and in length by proliferation of cartilage.

Over the growth period of approximately 19 to 20 years, this development can be divided into three distinct but overlapping phases: (1) ossification of the diaphysis, (2) ossification of the epiphysis, and (3) invasion and subsequent replacement of growth cartilage plates with bony fusion of epiphysis and diaphysis. These changes do not take place in all bones simultaneously but appear in a specific order and at a specific time. Although the speed of bone growth and amount of maturity at specific ages vary from one child to another, the order of ossification is constant. The first centers of ossification appear in the 2-month-old embryo, and at birth the number is approximately 400, about half the number at maturity. New centers appear at regular intervals during the growth period and provide the basis for assessment of ''bone age.'' Postnatally, the earliest centers to appear (at 5 to 6 months of age) are those of the capitate and hamate bones in the wrist. Therefore, x-rays of the hand and wrist provide the most useful areas for screening to determine skeletal age, especially before age 6 years. A common rule of thumb is: *age in years + 1 = number of ossification centers in the wrist.*[9] These centers appear earlier in girls than in boys.

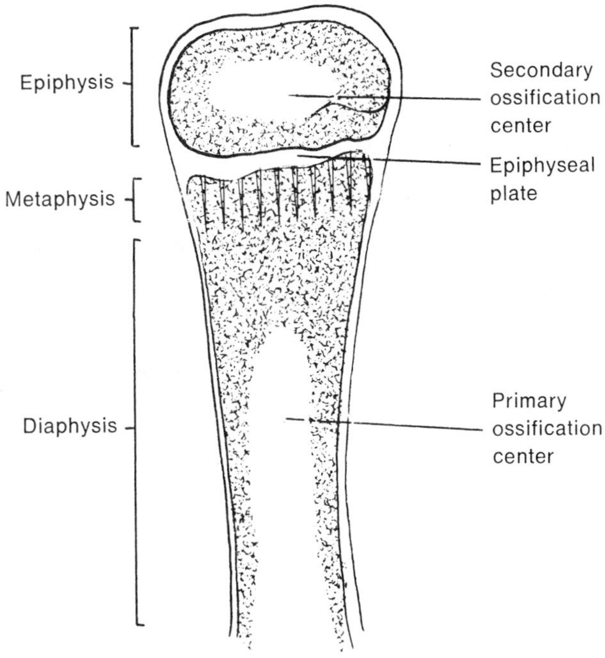

Fig. 3-7. Model of a long bone.

Skeletal development advances until maturity through growth of ossification centers and lengthening of long bones at the metaphysis and cartilage plates. Linear growth can continue as long as the epiphysis is separated from the diaphysis by the cartilage plate; when the cartilage disappears, the epiphysis unites with the diaphysis and growth ceases. Epiphyseal fusion also follows an orderly sequence, thus the timing of epiphyseal closure furnishes another medium for measuring skeletal age.

Investigation and assessment based on bone growth furnish a reliable index of growth rate in the individual child. In addition to the assessment of general developmental and nutritional status of the child, the findings are of value in the diagnosis of many metabolic and endocrine disturbances affecting growth as well as some congenital conditions.

Growth of muscle

As skeletal development is responsible for linear growth, muscle growth accounts for a significant portion of the increase in body weight. The number of muscle fibers is established by the fourth or fifth month of fetal life and remains constant throughout life. Differences in muscle size between individuals and differences in one person at various times during a lifetime are a result of the ability of the separate muscle fibers to increase in size. The increase in muscle fiber length that accompanies growth is also associated with an increase in the number of nuclei in the fibers. This increase is most apparent during the adolescent growth spurt. At this time the increase in secretion of growth hormone and adrenal androgens stimulates the growth of muscle fibers in both sexes, but the growth in boys is further stimulated by the secretion of testosterone. At about 6 months of prenatal life, muscle mass constitutes approximately one sixth of the body weight; at birth, about one fourth, and, at adolescence, one third. The variability in size and strength of muscle is influenced by genetic constitution, nutrition, and exercise. At all ages muscles increase in size with use and shrink when inactive. Consequently, maintaining muscle tone to minimize the amount of atrophy in skeletal muscle through active or passive range of motion exercises is an important protective nursing function.

Lymphoid tissues

Lymphoid tissues contained in the lymph nodes, thymus, spleen, tonsils, adenoids, and blood lymphocytes follow a distinctive growth pattern unlike that of other body tissues. These tissues are small in relation to total body size, but they are well developed at birth. They increase rapidly to reach adult dimensions by 6 years of age and continue to grow. About age 10 to 12 years they reach a maximum development that is approximately twice their adult size. This is followed by a rapid decline to stable adult dimensions by the end of adolescence.

Lymph nodes are large, and the superficially located nodes are often palpable. The tonsils, massive during early childhood, become inconspicuous in the adult. The thymus gland beneath the sternum, a prominent feature in infancy, may be impossible to detect in an adult. The growth pattern of lymphatic tissues parallels the development of immunity and probably reflects the repeated exposure to new infectious agents.

Adipose tissue

There is wide variation in the degree of fatness or thinness between individuals at all ages because of a multitude of factors. Fat is contained in connective tissue cells that are usually referred to as adipose tissue, which has a distinct lifetime pattern of development and distribution. Fat is characteristicically found in subcutaneous tissues (except those of the eyelids, external ear, nose, scrotum, and backs of hands and feet, which contain very little), the omentum, and in close relation to some viscera, such as the heart and kidneys. Although it contributes substantially to the body weight, whether fat "grows" like other tissues is uncertain. The deposits of fat throughout the body function primarily as a means for storing energy. Therefore, it is a labile tissue markedly affected by the nutrition of the individual (see p. 754).

Normal fat distribution during childhood follows a definite pattern. Fat first appears in the subcutaneous tissues of the fetus at approximately the sixth month of prenatal life. There is a rapid accumulation from the seventh month through the first six postnatal months, and the amount of subcutaneous fat present in the newborn correlates with the weight of the infant. However, at the end of the first year the infant who was lean at birth has approximately the same length and muscle mass as infants who were fatter initially. The significance of subcutaneous fat related to both the specialized "brown fat" and gestational age is discussed in relation to problems of prematurity (p. 336) and temperature regulation in the newborn (pp. 252 and 257).

After 6 months of age the rate of fat accumulation declines rapidly and then decreases steadily in both sexes until 6 to 8 years of age. All children begin to slim down soon after the first birthday, but the decrease is somewhat less in girls than in boys; thus at any age girls are slightly fatter than boys. From the ages of 6 to 8 years, fat again begins to accumulate slowly. It is during this period that obesity may begin to appear in some children. Many children also put on excess fat just prior to the adolescent growth spurt. Up to the time of the onset of puberty there is very little difference in fat accumulation and distribution in boys and girls. During the adolescent growth spurt the amount of fat in boys decreases sharply (especially in the limbs) and is not regained until early adulthood. Their increase in body weight and mass is primarily the result of accelerated bone and muscle growth. In many boys a preadolescent period of fat growth, often a source of social concern to both the child and his parents, precedes the general changes of adolescence. In girls the fat accumulation continues but assumes a typical distribution pattern that produces the feminine curves of the mature female.

The amount and distribution of fat is also correlated with genetically controlled body build that appears to be unrelated to caloric intake. In addition culturally determined diets, amount of exercise, emotions, and numerous other factors that influence caloric consumption are reflected in increased fat deposits. It is now believed that the number of fat cells is established at an early age and that overfeeding

A

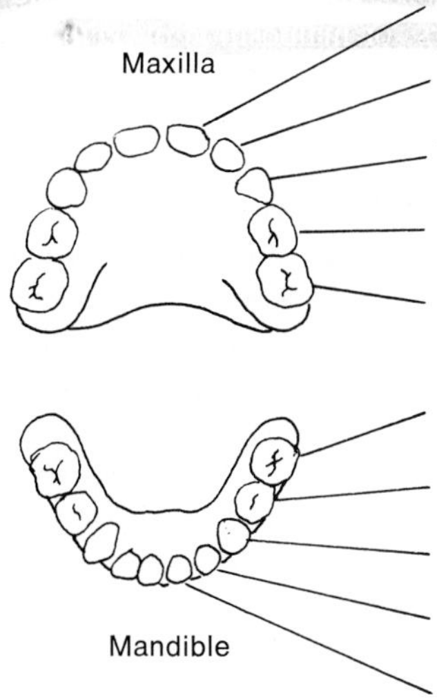

	Age of eruption (mo) Early	Average	Late	Average age of shedding (yr)
Maxilla	6	9.6	12	7.5
	7	12.4	18	8
	11	18.3	24	11.5
	10	15.7	20	10.5
	13	26.2	31	10.5
Mandible	13	26.0	31	11
	10	15.1	30	10
	11	18.2	24	9.5
	7	11.5	15	7
	5	7.8	11	6

B

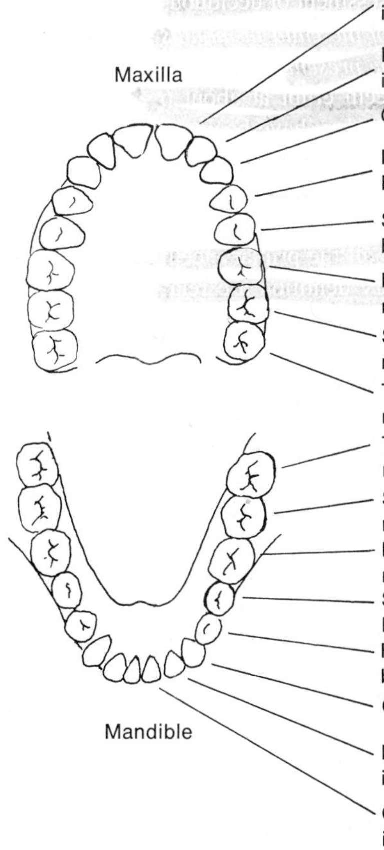

		Average age of eruption (yr) Boys	Girls
Maxilla	Central incisor	7.5	7.2
	Lateral incisor	8.7	8.2
	Cuspid	11.7	11.0
	First bicuspid	10.4	10.0
	Second bicuspid	11.2	10.9
	First molar	6.4	6.2
	Second molar	12.7	12.2
	Third molar	Variable 17-21	
Mandible	Third molar	Variable 17-21	
	Second molar	12.1	11.7
	First molar	6.2	5.9
	Second bicuspid	11.5	10.9
	First bicuspid	10.8	10.2
	Cuspid	10.8	9.9
	Lateral incisor	7.7	7.3
	Central incisor	6.5	6.3

Fig. 3-8. Sequence of eruption and shedding of **A,** primary, and **B,** secondary, teeth.

during this time may have a significant influence on obesity at a later age (p. 754). It has been shown that obese adolescents were significantly heavier than average at 1 year of age and that a large number of obese adults were also obese in childhood. These problems will be discussed as they apply to specific aspects of health promotion.

Dentition

The course of dentition is sometimes divided into four major stages: (1) growth, (2) calcification, (3) eruption, and (4) attrition. The primary teeth begin to form about the sixth week of gestation and begin to calcify during the fourth to sixth months. About the middle of the first year the primary (deciduous) teeth begin to erupt, although calcification is not completed until sometime during the third year. The age of tooth eruption shows considerable variation among all children, but the order of their appearance is fairly regular and predictable (Fig. 3-8, *A* and *B*). The first primary teeth to erupt are the lower central incisors, which appear at approximately 6 to 8 months of age. This may vary from 4 months to 1 year in normal children, and infants may even be born with teeth. The total of twenty primary teeth are acquired in characteristic sequence by 30 months of age. Calcification of the primary teeth is complete at this time. A quick guide to assessment of deciduous teeth during the first 2 years is: *age of the child in months − 6 = number of teeth that should be present*.[9]

The first permanent (secondary) teeth erupt at about 6 years of age. Prior to their appearance they have been developing in the jaw beneath the deciduous (primary) teeth. Meanwhile, the roots of the latter are gradually being absorbed so that at the time a deciduous tooth is shed, only the crown remains. At 6 years of age all the primary teeth are present and those of the secondary dentition are relatively well formed. At this time, eruption of the permanent teeth begins, usually starting with the 6-year molar, which erupts posterior to the deciduous molars. The others appear in approximately the same order as eruption of the primary teeth and follow shedding of the deciduous teeth. The pattern of shedding primary teeth and the eruption of secondary teeth are subject to wide variation among children. To allow the larger permanent teeth to occupy the limited space left by shed primary teeth, a series of complicated changes must take place in the jaws. It is at this time that many of the difficulties created by crowding of teeth become apparent. With the appearance of the second permanent (12-year) molar, most of the permanent teeth are present. The third permanent molars, or wisdom teeth, may erupt from 18 to 25 years of age or later. Permanent dentition, as in other aspects of development, is somewhat more advanced in girls than it is in boys. The eruption of teeth is sometimes used as a criterion for developmental assessment, especially the 6-year molar, which seems to be the most universally consistent in timing. However, dental maturation does not correlate well with bone age and is less reliable as an index of biologic age. Retarded eruption is more frequent than accelerated eruption and may be caused by heredity or may indicate health problems, such as endocrine disturbance, nutritional factors, or malposition of teeth.

Catch-up growth

When there is a secondary cause of growth deficiency, such as severe illness or acute malnutrition, the establishment of an adequate diet or recovery from the illness will result in a dramatic acceleration of the growth rate that usually continues until the child's individual growth pattern is resumed. Although the phenomenon has not been satisfactorily explained, apparently during this period the biologic timing mechanism is unaffected. When the problem is corrected the child will tend to catch up to the developmental stage at which he would normally be. For example, the newborn exhibits a transitory weight loss during the neonatal period, which is rapidly regained. Also, during the early months of life the developmental achievements of the prematurely born infant will lag behind those of full-term infants of the same chronologic age. The deficit in the attainment of developmental landmarks closely corresponds to the degree of prematurity; however, the differences become less conspicuous as the infant matures. The child will usually catch up to age-mates during the preschool years.

Catch-up growth involves growth in both length and weight, but the extent of inadequacy will depend on the timing, severity, duration, and character of the source of the secondary deficiency. In general any *serious* interruption in progress will have an impact, although small, on the ultimate size of the individual. Growth retardation that is prolonged or that occurs during a critical period may not be compensated. Catch-up growth applies to those tissues that can increase in size and to those that still retain the capacity to increase cell numbers. Growth deficiency in tissues such as the brain will result in a permanent deficit when the problem occurs during a critical period in its development.

GROWTH AND DEVELOPMENT OF MAJOR BODY SYSTEMS

The physiologic competence of the major organ systems also develops at varying rates and stages. All major systems are established early in fetal life and achieve varying degrees of refinement during the remainder of the prenatal period. At birth they are prepared to meet the requirements of a relatively independent existence, that is, they can function independently of the maternal system.

Temperature and metabolism

Metabolism. Metabolism—all chemical and energy transformations in the body—is affected by an assortment of intrinsic and extrinsic factors (for example, body size, age, sex, emotions, exercise, climate, hormones, environmental temperature). Therefore, metabolic needs vary among individuals and within each individual. The rate of metabolism when the body is at rest (basal metabolic rate [BMR]) demonstrates a distinctive change throughout childhood. It is highest in the newborn infant and is closely related to the proportion of surface area to body mass, which changes as the body increases in size. Most authorities consider surface area to be the best estimate of the amount of functioning protoplasm present in the organism (see p. 932 for computation of surface area). In both sexes the proportion decreases progressively to maturity. The basal metabolic rate is slightly higher in boys at all ages and further increases over that of girls during pubescence.

Table 3-3. Average daily requirements of children for calories, water, and protein

Age (years)	Energy (kcal/kg)	Water (ml/kg)	Protein (g/kg)
Infant	110-120	150	3.5-2.0
1 to 3	100	125	2.5-2.0
4 to 6	90	100	3.0
7 to 9	80	75	2.8
10 to 12	70	75	2.0
13 to 15	60	50	1.7
16 to 19	50	50	1.5
Adult	40	50	1.0

The rate of metabolism determines the caloric requirements of the child. The basal requirement of infants is about 110 to 120 kcal/kg (50 to 55 kcal/pound) of body weight and decreases to 40 to 50 kcal/kg (18 to 25 kcal/pound) at maturity (Table 3-3). Children's energy needs vary considerably at different ages and with changing circumstances. The greatest proportion of calories in infancy is utilized for basal metabolic needs and growth. The energy requirement to build tissue steadily decreases with age, following the general growth curve; however, exercise needs vary with the individual child and may be considerably more. The change in distribution of calorie expenditure during childhood is shown in Fig. 3-9. For short periods of time (such as during strenuous exercise) and more prolonged periods of time (such as illness), the needs can be very high. For example, each degree of fever increases the basal metabolism 10% with a corresponding fluid requirement. The term specific dynamic action (SDA) refers to the energy required to ingest and assimilate food. A very small portion of ingested calories is lost in stools during normal metabolism, but much more may be lost in this way in conditions that impair digestion or absorption.

Temperature. Body temperature, reflecting metabolism, displays the same decrement from infancy to maturity (Table 3-4). Following the unstable regulatory ability in the neonatal periods, heat production (as reflected in body temperature) steadily declines as the infant grows into childhood. Individual differences of ½° to 1° are normal, and occasionally a child will normally display an unusually high or low temperature. Beginning at approximately 12 years

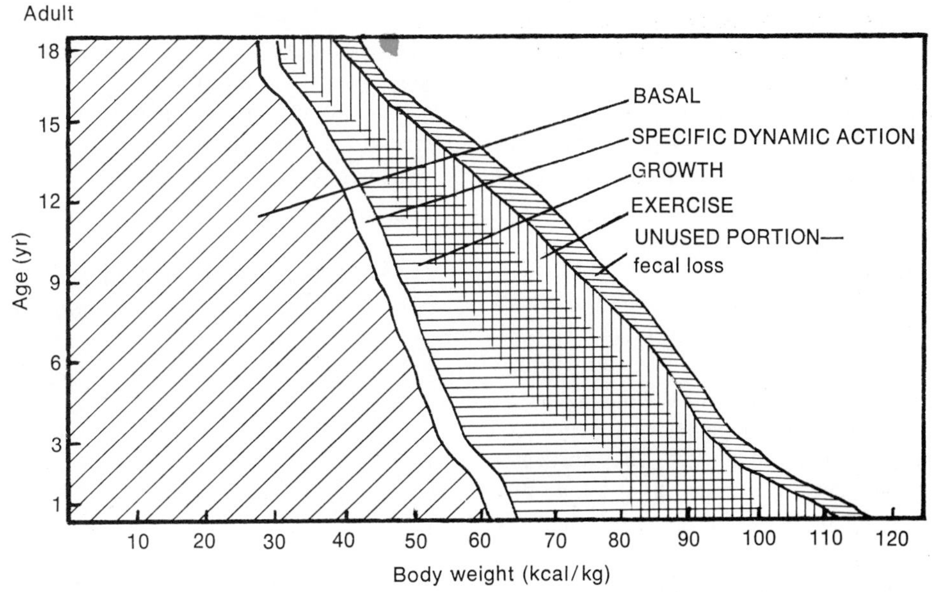

Fig. 3-9. Total daily expenditure of calories among individual factors in relation to age. (From Vaughn, V. C., and McKay, R. J.: Textbook of pediatrics, ed. 10, Philadelphia, 1975, W. B. Saunders Co.)

Table 3-4. Average body temperatures in well children under basal conditions

Age	Temperature	
	F	C
3 months	99.4	37.5
6 months	99.5	37.5
1 year	99.7	37.7
3 years	99.0	37.2
5 years	98.6	37.0
7 years	98.3	36.8
9 years	98.1	36.7
11 years	98.0	36.7
13 years	97.8	36.6

Modified from Lowrey, G. H.: Growth and development of children, ed. 6, Chicago, 1973, Year Book Medical Publishers, Inc.

of age the temperature in girls remains relatively stable, whereas in boys it continues to fall for a few years longer. Females maintain a temperature slightly above that of males throughout life.

Even with improved temperature regulation, infants and young children are highly susceptible to temperature fluctuations. Body temperature responds to changes in environmental temperature and is increased with active exercise, crying, and emotional upset. Infections can cause a higher and more rapid temperature increase in infants and young children than in older children. In relation to body weight, an infant produces more heat per unit than children near maturity. Consequently, during active play or when heavily clothed, an infant or small child is likely to become overheated.

Gastrointestinal system

The gastrointestinal (GI) system serves to process and absorb nutrients necessary to maintain metabolic processes and to support growth and development. It also performs an excretory function for both digestive residue and other waste products that pour into the intestine from the blood or are excreted in the bile. The role of the gastrointestinal tract is important for detoxification while other routes of elimination (kidneys, liver, skin) are still immature. It also participates in maintaining fluid and electrolyte balance in infancy. All actions of the gastrointestinal tract are subject to a variety of outside influences at all ages. They are sensitive to tensions and anxieties, and many diseases and disorders are reflected in altered gastrointestinal function.

The primitive digestive system forms during the fourth week of gestation, but the most rapid and extensive development occurs just before birth. As a result, most biochemical and physiologic functions are established at the time of birth. Prior to this time the exchange of nutrients and waste is assumed by the placenta; therefore, the demands on the alimentary tract are minimal. However, the presence in the intestine of a thick, sticky, greenish-black material (meconium) composed of cast-off epithelial cells, digestive tract secretions (such as mucus and bile), and residue from swallowed amniotic fluid attests to prenatal activity. The passage of this meconium after birth provides evidence of the patency of the tract.

The mechanical functions of digestion are relatively immature at birth. Sucking and swallowing are established prenatally but do not become fully developed until after birth. Swallowing is an automatic reflex action for the first 3 months, and the infant has no voluntary control of swallowing until the striated muscles in the throat establish their cerebral connections. This begins at approximately 6 weeks of age. By 6 months the infant is capable of swallowing, holding food in the mouth, or spitting it out at will. The mechanism of sucking is also a reflexive activity in the newborn, and the muscular action of the tongue has a typical forward thrust. With neural and muscular development, the infant gradually acquires the ability to perform the coordinated muscular action typical of the adult type of swallowing (see p. 451). The chewing function is facilitated by eruption of the primary teeth. The timing of dietary changes closely parallels these progressive capabilities. First to develop are those that require merely swallowing, then those that need no mastication, and, finally, those that require biting and chewing.

The stomach, lying horizontally, is round until approximately 2 years of age. It then gradually elongates until it assumes the shape and anatomic position of the adult at about 7 years of age. This anatomic placement of the stomach in infancy influences positioning practices during and after feeding (p. 287). At birth, capacity of the stomach is only about 10 to 20 ml, but, a distensible organ, the stomach rapidly expands to triple its capacity in 3 weeks and to reach five to ten times its original birth capacity at the age of 1 month (see box below).

Stomach capacity (approximate) at various stages of development

Age	*Capacity (ml)*
Newborn	10-20
1 week	30-90
2-3 weeks	75-100
1 month	90-150
3 months	150-200
1 year	210-360
2 years	500
10 years	750-900
16 years	1500
Adult	2000-3000

The immaturity of the digestive system in the infant is demonstrated by the rapidity with which swallowed food is propelled through the entire tract. The frequency and character of stools is affected by the rate of peristalsis and the nature of ingested food. For example, the frequent, yellow stools of the neonate gradually assume a more adult regularity and character in the infant. The emptying time of the stomach increases from 2½ to 3 hours in the newborn to 3 to 6 hours in older infants and children. The small stomach capacity with a rapid transit time has implications for determining the amount and frequency of feedings during this period of growth. In addition, peristalsis is more rapid in infancy than at other periods of life, and it is not uncommon for peristaltic waves to reverse and cause spitting up or, if vigorous, vomiting of stomach contents. An immature, relaxed cardiac sphincter in infancy and early childhood contributes to this ease of regurgitation.

During the prenatal period the large intestine grows more rapidly than the small intestine, but after birth this rate is reversed. The length of the intestine in infants is six times the body length and is proportionately greater than that of the full-grown individual, which is four to five times the body length. There are two periods of accelerated growth of the intestine that correlate with nutritional and physiologic changes that are taking place—the first, between 1 and 3 years of age, during a period of diet transition, and the second, between 10 and 15 years of age, which coincides with the adolescent growth spurt.

The secretory cells of the gastrointestinal tract are believed to be functional at birth. However, since most of the digestive enzymes depend on a specific pH relationship that is gradually acquired with age, their efficiency may be impaired. The newborn produces only small amounts of saliva, which contains some of the starch-splitting enzyme ptyalin; therefore, its primary purpose at this time is to moisten the mouth and throat. It has little time to act on starches in the rapidly swallowed food. By the end of the second year the salivary glands have increased in size about five times to reach their full size and function.

Gastric acidity varies during childhood. The acidity of gastric juice is low during infancy and rises during childhood to level off at approximately 10 years of age. At the time of the adolescent growth spurt there is an increase in free hydrochloric acid. It is particularly marked in males, which probably contributes to the simultaneous increase in consumption of food. Most of the chemical activity is functional within these limitations and to the extent that it is dependent on the development of hormonal and neurologic maturation.

The significant aspects of gastrointestinal function as related to the physiology and nutritional needs of the newborn, premature infant, and full-term infant as well as problems related to gastrointestinal function will be discussed as they apply to these situations.

Respiratory system

The respiratory tract consists of a complex of structures that function under neural and hormonal control. At birth the respiratory system is relatively small, but after the first breath the lungs grow rapidly. Changes take place in the air passages that increase respiratory surface area. For example, during the first year the alveoli in the terminal units rapidly increase in number. In addition, the early globular alveoli develop septa that cause them to become more lobular, thus enlarging the area available for gas exchange. They continue to increase steadily until, at age 12 years, there are approximately nine times as many as were present at birth. In later stages of growth the structures lengthen and enlarge.

After the early weeks of life the respiratory tract follows the general growth curve. However, the respiratory apparatus grows faster than the vertebral column, resulting in alterations in the relationships between these structures. The bifurcation of the trachea lies opposite the third thoracic vertebra in the infant and gradually descends to a position opposite the fourth vertebra in the adult; the cricoid cartilage descends from the level of the fourth cervical vertebra in the infant to that of the sixth in the adult. These anatomic changes produce differences in the angle of access to the trachea at various ages and must be considered when the infant or child is to be positioned for purposes of resuscitation and airway clearance (see Chapter 32). The larynx grows slowly until puberty, when its accelerated growth produces changes in the voice that are particularly marked in boys.

Respiratory movements are first evident at approximately 20 weeks gestation, and throughout fetal life there is an exchange of amniotic fluid in the alveoli. In the neonate the respiratory rate is rapid to meet the needs of a high metabolism. During growth, the rate steadily decreases in both boys and girls until it levels off at maturity (see Appendix E). The volume of air inhaled increases with the growth of the lungs and is closely related to body size. In addition, there is a qualitative difference in expired air at different ages. The amount of oxygen in the expired air gradually decreases and the amount of carbon dioxide increases during growth. Other important aspects of respiratory function are discussed as they relate to prenatal life and perinatal adjustments, the newborn infant, and acute and chronic respiratory problems of infants and children.

Cardiovascular system

The fetal heart begins to beat at approximately 4 weeks gestation. During prenatal life it distributes oxygen and nutrients, supplied via the placenta, to the developing fetus through an efficient system of shunts that partially bypass the nonfunctioning lungs. With the initiation of independent respiration at the time of birth, the altered pressures within the vascular system functionally close the shunts and postnatal circulation is established (p. 222).

In infancy the size of the heart in relation to total body size is larger, and it occupies a larger space within the lung enclosure. It lies at a transverse angle, but with growth and the enlarging lungs it comes to lie lower and more obliquely at maturity. The ventricle walls are more or less equal in thickness (some believe that the right ventricle may be somewhat larger) at birth. With the increased demand of the postnatal peripheral circulation, the left side becomes thicker than the right. An increase in heart size accompanies the adolescent growth spurt with a resulting increase in blood pressure and decrease in heart rate.

Heart rate. Heart action is controlled by the autonomic nervous system, but the rate is influenced by the needs of other organs and tissues and emotional states. The heart rate at any age shows an inverse relationship to body size. In the neonate the rate is rapid, and it decreases steadily throughout life (see Appendix A, Table A-1).

The arteries and veins elongate to keep pace with expanding body dimensions, and the vessel walls thicken to cope with the increased pressure. The systolic blood pressure after birth is low (40 mm Hg), reflecting the weaker left ventricle of the neonate. With the developing strength and power of the left side of the heart, the systolic pressure rises to 70 mm Hg at 2 weeks of age and to 80 mm at 1 month. It continues to rise, although at a slower pace, until it reaches approximately 100 mm Hg just prior to puberty. At puberty the blood pressure rises rapidly to adult levels (see Appendix A, Table A-3).

Problems of cardiac malfunction and changes in blood composition are discussed in Unit 14.

Renal system

Development of the kidney begins within the first weeks of embryonic life but is not completed until about the end of the first year after birth. The functional units of the kidney—the nephrons—increase in number throughout gestation and reach their full complement by birth. However, they are immature. Many of the tubular sections are not fully formed, and the glomeruli enlarge considerably after birth. The epithelial cells of both tubules are cubical in the newborn, whereas they are flat and thin in the mature nephrons. As a result, filtration and absorption are relatively poor during the first year. All parts of the nephron increase in size and complexity with growth. Lengthening of the loop of Henle, the site of the urine-concentrating mechanism, produces a gradual increase in the ability to concentrate urine, which is very dilute in the newborn.

Because of the small, conical pelvis, the urinary bladder is an abdominal organ in infancy, but, as the pelvis expands with growth, the bladder settles into it to become a pelvic organ. The kidney functions during fetal life and produces urine that contributes to the amniotic fluid volume. The 24-hour urine volume is low at birth, rapidly increases in the neonatal period, and steadily increases with normal growth (see Appendix B). Problems related to renal structure and function are discussed in Chapter 31 and with the specific age-groups in which they are most prevalent.

Neurologic system

In contrast to other body tissues, which grow rapidly after birth, the nervous system grows proportionately more rapidly before birth. Two periods of rapid brain cell growth occur during fetal life. There is a dramatic increase in the number of neurons between 15 and 20 weeks gestation, and another increase in rate begins at 30 weeks gestation and extends to 1 year of age. At birth the brain has achieved about two thirds of its mature size; 82% of the adult size has been attained by 1 year of age. Brain volume is readily reflected in head circumference, which increases six times as much during the first year as it does in the second year of life (see Appendix E). It is believed that no new nerve cells appear after the sixth month of fetal life. Postnatal growth consists of increasing the amount of cytoplasm around the nuclei of existing cells, increasing the number and intricacy of communications with other cells, and advancing their peripheral axons to keep pace with expanding body dimensions.

The brain comprises 12% of the body weight at birth. It doubles this weight in the first year, and by the age of 5 or 6 years its weight at birth has tripled. Thereafter, growth slows until in adulthood the brain is only about 2% of the total body weight. The surface configuration also changes with development. The early embryonic brain surface is smooth, but with advancing development the sulci deepen. This process continues throughout childhood. At birth the cortex is only about one half its adult thickness, although all the major surface features are present. There is very little cortical control over body movements at birth, with the movements guided principally by primitive reflexes (see p. 273). With advancing development and maturation, the brain, through association pathways, exercises increasing control over much of the reflex activity. This allows the growing child to perform progressively complex tasks requiring coordinated movements. Persistence of primitive reflexes may suggest defective cortical development.

Cortical control is closely associated with the acquisition of a myelin coating on the nerves. Although nerve fibers are able to conduct impulses without this myelin sheath, the impulses travel at a slower rate and with more likelihood of diffusion. Myelinization of the various nerve tracts in the central nervous system, which allows progressive neuromotor function, follows the cephalocaudal and proximodistal sequence. It appears first with the fibers of the spinal cord and cranial nerves, then in the brain stem and corticospinal tracts. The rate of myelogenesis accelerates rapidly after birth. In general, the pathways concerned with sensation are myelinated early, before the motor pathways. The acquisition of motor skills depends on the maturation and myelination of the nervous system, and no amount of special training or practice will hasten the process. Most of the advancing performance in an infant is a direct result of brain development and only indirectly dependent on environmental stimuli.

Neurophysiologic changes also provide the foundation for language, learning, and behavior development. Neurologic and electroencephalographic development are sometimes used as indicators of maturational age in the early weeks of life.

Development of vision

All the special senses are present at birth, although discrimination is probably lacking until neural pathways are myelinated and the vast elaboration of dendrite processes is accomplished. However, the visual mechanism is relatively immature and physiologic changes in the eye alter the visual acuity during childhood. The eye of the infant is small and hyperopic, that is, the short diameter of the eye causes an image to focus behind the retina. However, since the lens is soft and pliable, the infant is able to accommodate easily. In fact, most small children are able to see an object clearly at very close range. The visual function becomes increasingly organized with growth. Binocular vision is established by 4 months of age and mature function of the eye muscles is attained by 1 year of age. The hyperopia of infancy is gradually replaced by emmetropia (normal accommodation and refraction) at about age 6 years. The development of central visual acuity is outlined in Table 3-5.

Integumentary system

The skin with its component structures (nails, hair, sebaceous glands, eccrine and apocrine sweat glands) and associated structures (nervous and vascular networks, muscles, and connective and adipose tissues) constitute the integumentary system. The largest organ in the body, the skin, is a thin structure only about 1 mm thick at birth that increases to approximately twice that thickness at maturity. It consists of three layers: (1) an outer layer, the epidermis, composed of epithelial cells that provide a relatively impenetrable barrier to the loss of body contents and the entrance of environmental hazards; (2) a middle layer, the corium or dermis, that constitutes the bulk of the organ and contains the masses of glands, hair follicles, blood vessels, nerves, and muscles; and, (3) an inner layer composed of fatty tissue of varying thickness that separates the skin from the subcutaneous tissues. The activity of the skin is controlled by the autonomic nervous system and the endocrine glands.

The major skin layers arise from different embryologic origins. Early in the embryonic period, a single layer of epithelium forms from the ectoderm, while, simultaneously, the corium develops from the mesenchyme. In the infant and small child the epidermis is still loosely bound to the corium. Consequently the layers may easily separate during an inflammatory process to form blisters or during careless handling (such as removal of adhesive tape).

The efficiency with which the skin layers prevent evaporative loss of water (independent of sweat) increases with development. A transitional zone between the epidermal layers allows more of the larger fluid content (70%) of the lower layers to enter the outer, drier layers (15% water), where it is lost in greater or lesser amounts depending on environmental temperature and humidity. In the young child the transitional zone is less effective than in an older child or adult. Consequently the small child's skin chaps more easily. The fluid loss is most marked in the prematurely born infant.

Hair. The various skin appendages develop at different times and at different rates. An extensive growth of fine body hair, lanugo, begins to appear at the end of the second intrauterine month, reaches its maximum development between the seventh and eight months of fetal life, and begins to decrease before birth. It continues to regress steadily during early infancy and is replaced by a less extensive distribution of hair. The amount and texture of scalp hair vary between individual infants at birth and the scalp hair is lost during the first few months after birth. It is slowly replaced by permanent hair, which gradually thickens and often darkens as the child grows. At puberty the secretion of androgenic hormones stimulates an increase in the thickening and darkening of scalp hair, the growth of hair in the axilla and pubic regions of both sexes, and the growth of facial hair in boys. Late in the adolescent period some boys acquire additional amounts and distribution of body hair such as hair on the chest.

Sebaceous glands. The sebaceous glands form in connection with hair follicles. Their function is to produce a fatty secretion called sebum that helps keep the skin supple by decreasing water loss. The sebaceous activity is maintained at a relatively constant rate by the secretion of androgens; an increase in androgens causes an increase in sebum production. Sebaceous glands have a regional distribution and are most abundant on the scalp, the face, and the genitals; are less numerous on the trunk; are sparce on the extremities; and do not appear on the palms and soles.

Table 3-5. Visual acuity at various ages

Age	Vision
16 weeks	20/200
36 weeks	20/200+
1 year	20/100
2 years	20/40
3 years	20/30
4 years	Nearly 20/20

Sebaceous glands begin to form during the fifth month of fetal life and are very active during the month prior to birth, when they produce the protective *vernix caseosa*. The sebaceous activity slowly subsides after birth and continues to decrease throughout infancy. In the newborn period and early infancy, sebaceous secretion may cause minor problems such as "cradle cap" in some infants (see p. 492). The secretion gradually rises in childhood to increase markedly at puberty where it remains constant and contributes greatly to the disturbing skin problems of adolescence (see p. 720).

Sweat glands. The sweat glands, both eccrine and apocrine, are present at birth. They appear between the fifth and seventh months of fetal life, but their activity is scant. The eccrine sweat glands function primarily as a part of the body heat–regulating mechanism of the body and to some extent in maintaining electrolyte balance. At birth the eccrine glands function poorly but produce more sweat as childhood advances to reach full potential at puberty. There are individual differences in the amount of sweat produced, and there are no sex differences until after puberty, when males sweat more than females. Numerous factors influence the amount and chemical content of the sweat, for example, emotions and some disease states such as congestive heart failure in infancy and cystic fibrosis.

The apocrine sweat glands are located primarily in the axilla and the genital and anal areas. They are inactive throughout infancy and childhood and mature during puberty.

Sleep and rest

Sleep, a protective function in all organisms, allows for repair and recovery of tissues following activity. As in most aspects of development, there is wide variation between individual children and ages of children in the amount and distribution of sleep during childhood. As the child matures, not only is there a change in the quantity of time the child spends in sleep but there is also a change in the quality of that sleep. The length of time spent in sleep decreases throughout childhood. Newborn infants sleep nearly all the time that is not occupied with feeding and other aspects of their care. Larger newborn infants sleep for longer periods of time than smaller infants because of their larger stomach capacity. Gradually, the total time spent in sleep decreases, infants remain awake for longer periods of time, and they sleep longer at night. During the second year most children sleep through the night and take one or two naps during the day. By the time they are 3 years old, most children have eliminated the second nap; this pattern continues

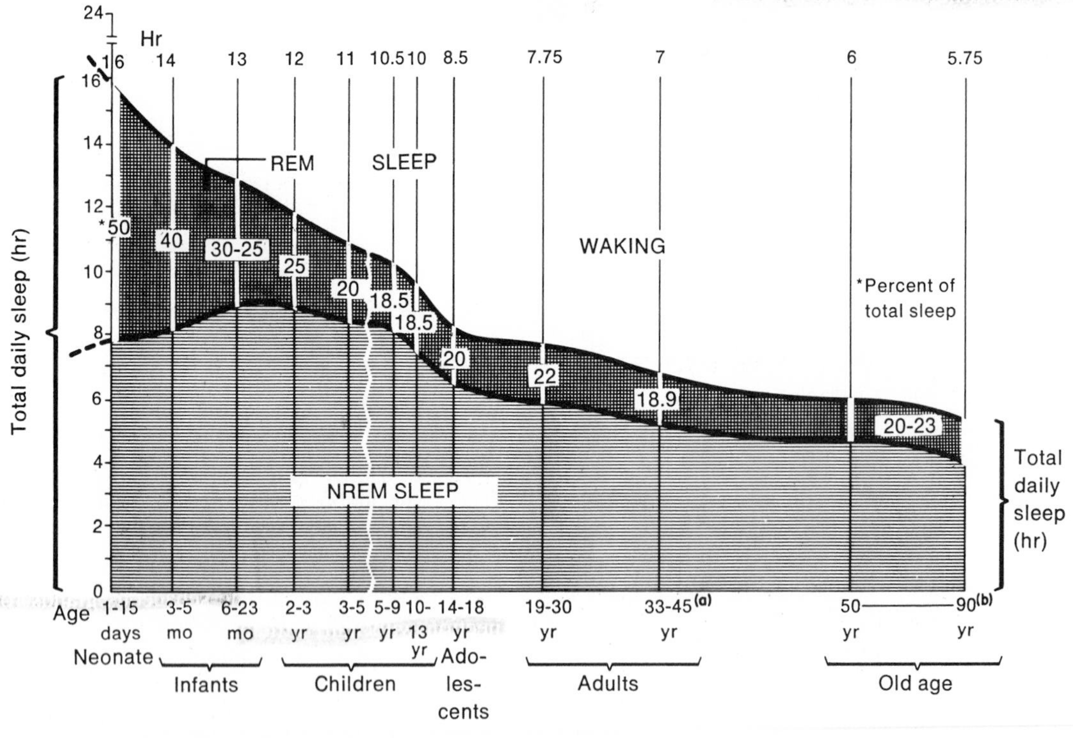

Fig. 3-10. Age changes in total amounts of daily sleep, daily REM sleep, and percentage of REM sleep. (From Roffwarg, H. P., Muzio, J. N., and Dement, W. C.: Ontogenetic development of the human sleep-dream cycle. Revised by the authors since publication in Science **152:**604-619, April 1966. Copyright 1966 by the American Association for the Advancement of Science.)

until 4 or 5 years of age. After 5 years of age the child has usually given up daytime naps except in those cultures in which an afternoon nap or siesta is customary. During ages 5 to 10 years, sleep time remains relatively constant, then declines sharply during adolescence.

Development takes place in the percentage of sleep time spent in each of the two different identified sleep cycles: (1) active sleep characterized by irregular pulse and respirations, many body movements, and short, rapid eye movements (paradoxic or REM sleep); and (2) quiet sleep in which breathing and heart beat are regular and body and eye movements are absent (slow-wave or non-REM sleep). The sleep of the newborn infant consists of approximately 50% REM sleep in contrast to approximately 20% in the older child. The changes in total sleep and proportion of REM to non-REM sleep are illustrated in Fig. 3-10. The large amount of active, REM sleep in early infancy is believed to serve as an endogenous source of stimulation to the higher brain centers and is important for normal development at a time when exogenous sources are minimal because of the short periods of arousal. The decrease in REM sleep as development progresses may indicate that, with longer periods of wakefulness, the more mature brain has less need for this endogenous stimulation. The deep, restful non-REM sleep increases proportionately with age, and the fact that children who have recently given up napping take a longer time to get into REM sleep during the initial sleep cycle than do either older or younger children suggests that they are more fatigued. Spontaneous awakening during sleep is relatively infrequent in childhood and adolescence.

DEVELOPMENT OF MENTAL FUNCTION

Personality and cognitive skills develop in the same manner as biologic growth, and many aspects depend on physical growth and maturation of their accomplishment. This is not a comprehensive account of the multiple facets of personality and behavior development. Many aspects will be integrated with the child's emotional and social development in later discussions of the various age-groups.

Learning

Learning occurs when behavior changes as a result of experience, and learning theories attempt to explain the ways in which controlled changes in the environment produce predictable changes in behavior. Basically, the mechanisms by which children acquire new behaviors and produce alterations in existing behaviors are: (1) forming associations through conditioning and (2) observation of models.

Conditioning. Conditioning is learning by association, that is, establishing a connection between a stimulus and a response. In *classical* conditioning, two events that occur simultaneously or close together in time come to have similar meanings to the child and thus evoke the same response. For example, infants learn very early to associate the sight of the mother's face and the sound of her voice with feeding or other pleasant sensations. Consequently, the infant will cease crying or otherwise indicate pleasure when she speaks or enters the infant's visual field. This type of learning appears to be the predominant form that takes place during infancy, particularly in the first 6 months, before the development of motor control.

Operant or *instrumental* conditioning involves the use of rewards or reinforcements to encourage the performance of specific behaviors. Reinforcing desired responses whenever they happen to occur increases the likelihood that they will be repeated. These reinforcements can be inner satisfactions or externally applied reward systems. Behavior that is not in some way reinforced or rewarded will be extinguished. The principles of instrumental conditioning are especially applicable to learning that takes place naturally in toddlers and preschool children. They can appreciate the significance of rewards and punishments even though they may not be able to conceptualize the context or framework in which they are operating. A substantial proportion of early childhood learning, such as acquisition of motor skills, consists of simple operant conditioning.

Avoidance conditioning discourages undesired behaviors through the use of punishment and fear of punishment. The effectiveness of rewards and punishments depends on the child's subjective assessment of the reward or punishment. Some rewards are not reinforcing, and punishments do not generate fear if they are inappropriate to the developmental level, emotional state, or value system of the individual child. Punishment is effective in controlling behavior, but it must be correctly timed, brief, appropriate to the child and the undesired behavior, and tempered with love.

Operant conditioning is the basis of behavior-modification procedures that have achieved varying degrees of success in speech therapy and in modifying behavior in overly aggressive children and mentally retarded children. Behavior is shaped by reinforcing closer and closer approximations of the behavior being taught.

Observation. Much of childhood learning takes place because of the innate tendency to observe and imitate the behavior of others, sometimes called social learning. Children imitate the behavior of those who are significant in their lives (such as parents, siblings, peers, teachers, and so on), and they are more apt to imitate those whom they believe to be prestigious and those whom they see being rewarded for their behavior. Imitative behavior requires no external reinforcement. Apparently, modeling is its own reward.

As children gain more complex cognitive skills and the use of language, learning assumes broader dimensions involving creativity, problem solving, and abstract conceptualization.

Cognitive development

The term cognition refers to the process by which the developing individual becomes acquainted with the world and the objects it contains. Children are born with inherited potentialities for intellectual growth, but they must develop into that potential through interaction with the environment. By assimilating information through the senses, processing it, and acting on it, they come to understand relationships between objects and between themselves and their world. With cognitive development, individuals acquire the ability to reason abstractly, to think in a logical manner, and to organize intellectual functions or performances into higher-order structures. The best known and more comprehensive theory regarding children's thinking has been developed by the Swiss psychologist Jean Piaget.[14] He believes that intelligence enables individuals to make adaptations to the environment that increase the probability of survival and that through their behavior they establish and maintain an equilibrium with that environment.

According to Piaget, children progress through a series of stages of mental activity in an orderly and sequential manner. The mechanisms that enable them to adapt to new situations and to move from one stage to the next are assimilation and accommodation. By *assimilation* the child incorporates new knowledges, skills, ideas, and insights into a cognitive scheme (Piaget uses the term "schema"*) that the child already has and can deal with. To new situations that do not fit into an established schema the child *accommodates*. He changes and organizes an existing schema to solve a more difficult task and form a new schema. The child's understanding of a new experience is based on all relevant previous experiences. The child achieves equilibrium over and over again by applying schemas already available to him (Fig. 3-11). Thus the child achieves an accurate understanding of reality and comes to deal with increasingly complex problems in an increasingly effective manner.

*A schema is a pattern of action and/or thought.

Piaget believes that there are four major stages in the development of logical thinking. Each is derived from and builds on the accomplishments of the previous stage in a continuous, orderly process. The course of intellectual development is both maturational and invariant and is divided into periods, subperiods, and stages (ages are approximate):

Sensorimotor (0 to 2 years). The sensorimotor stage of intellectual development consists of six substages (see p. 441) that are governed by sensations in which simple learning takes place. Children progress from reflex activity through simple repetitive behaviors to imitative behavior. They develop a sense of "cause-and-effect" as they direct behavior toward objects, and problem solving is primarily trial and error. They display a high level of curiosity, experimentation, and enjoyment of novelty. As a result of interactions with their environment, children begin to develop a sense of self as they are able to differentiate themselves from their environment. They become aware that

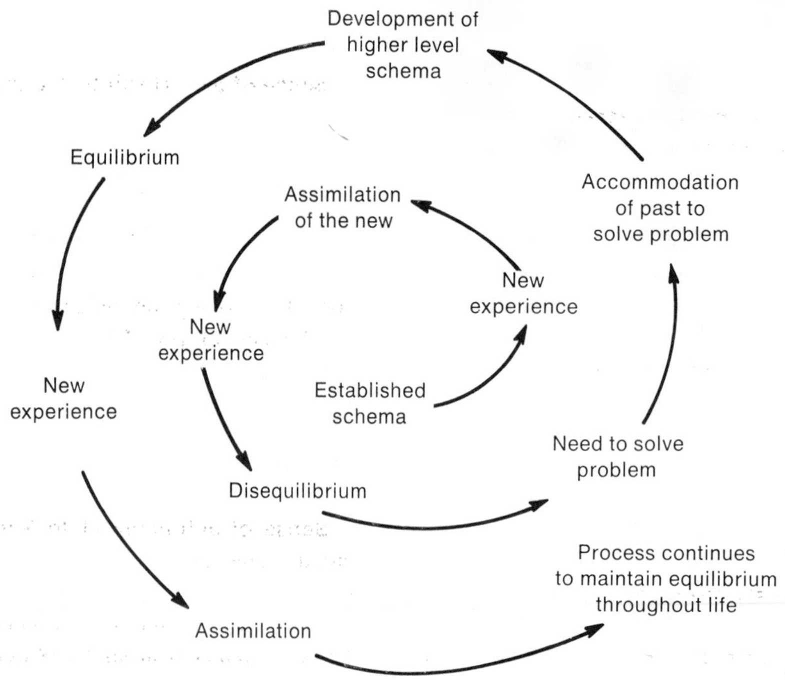

Fig. 3-11. Mechanisms for adaptation to new situations: assimilation and accommodation.

objects have permanence—that an object exists even though it is no longer visible. Toward the end of the sensorimotor period children begin to use language and representational thought appears as they imitate the behavior of others—even in the absence of these other persons.

Preoperational (2 to 7 years). The predominant characteristic of this period of intellectual development is *egocentricity*. Egocentricity in this sense does not mean selfishness or self-centeredness, but, rather, the inability to put oneself in the place of another. Children interpret objects and events, not in terms of general properties, but in terms of the relationships or use to them. They are unable to see things from any perspective other than their own; they cannot see another's point of view, nor can they see any reason to do so.

Preoperational thinking is concrete and tangible. Children cannot reason beyond the observable, and they lack the ability to make deductions or generalizations. Thought is dominated by what they see, hear, or otherwise experience. However, they are increasingly able to use language and symbols to represent objects in their environment. Through imaginative play, questioning, and otherwise interacting, they begin to elaborate concepts more and to make simple associations between ideas. One of the most salient features of preoperational thought is lack of conservation or reversibility. That is, for every action or operation there is an action or operation that cancels it. For example, children in this age-group are unable to grasp the idea that a ball of clay can be changed and brought back to the original shape. In the latter stage of this period their reasoning is *intuitive* (for example, the stars have to go to bed just as they do) and they are only beginning to deal with problems of weight, length, size, and time.

Concrete operations (7 to 11 years). At this age, thought becomes increasingly logical and coherent. Children are able to classify, sort, order, and otherwise organize facts about the world to use in problem solving. They develop a new concept of permanence—conservation. That is, they realize that volume, weight, number, etc. remain the same even though outward appearances are changed. They are able to deal with a number of different aspects of a situation simultaneously. They do not have the capacity to deal in abstraction; they solve problems in a concrete, systematic fashion based on that which they can perceive. Reasoning is inductive. Through progressive changes in thought processes and relationships with others, thought becomes decentered. They can consider points of view other than their own. Thinking has become socialized.

Formal operations (12 to 15 years). Formal operational thought is characterized by adaptability and flexibility. Adolescents can think in abstract terms, use abstract symbols, and draw logical conclusions from a set of observations. They can make hypotheses and test them; they consider abstract, theoretic, and philosophic matters. Although they may confuse the ideal with the practical, most contradictions in the world can be dealt with and resolved.

Personality development

The personality evolves as children react to their changing bodies and to the environment. Personality development can be described by predictable age-related stages during which specific changes are assumed to take place. The most widely accepted and used is Erik Erikson's theory of personality development. Built on Freudian theory, it emphasizes a healthy personality as opposed to a pathologic approach. In his theory, Erikson also utilizes the biologic concepts of critical periods and epigenesis. Erikson describes key conflicts or core problems that the individual strives to master during critical periods in personality development. Successful completion or mastery of each of these core conflicts is built on the satisfactory completion or mastery of the previous core.

Each stage has two components, the favorable and unfavorable aspects of the core conflict, and progress to the next stage is dependent on resolution of this conflict. No core problem is ever solved in its entirety; each new situation will present this conflict in a new form. For example, when children who have satisfactorily achieved a sense of trust and other tasks require hospitalization, they must, again, develop a sense of trust in those responsible for their care in order to master the situation.

Erikson's description of the core conflicts in the eight stages of personality development, which coincides with Freud's psychosexual stages, contains distinctive goals with lasting outcomes of their successful attainment (all ages are approximate). (See Table 3-6.)

Sense of trust (birth to 1 year). The first and most important attribute of a healthy personality to develop is a basic trust. Establishment of basic trust dominates the first year of life and describes all the child's satisfying experiences at this age. Corresponding to Freud's oral stage, it is a time of "getting" and "taking in" through all the senses. It exists only in relation to something or someone; therefore, consistent, loving care by a mothering person is essential to development of trust. *Mistrust* develops when trust-promoting experiences are deficient or lacking or when basic needs are inconsistently or inadequately met. Although shreds of mistrust are sprinkled throughout the personality, from a basic trust in parents stems a basic trust in the world, other people, and oneself. The result is faith and optimism.

Sense of autonomy (1 to 3 years). Corresponding to Freud's anal stage, the problem of autonomy can be symbolized by the holding on and letting go of the sphincter muscles. The development of autonomy during the toddler period is centered around children's increasing ability to control their bodies, themselves, and their environment. They want to use their powers to do for themselves—these newly acquired motor skills of walking, climbing, and

Table 3-6. Summary of cognitive and personality development

	Stage	Age (years)	Radius of significant relationships	Psychosexual stages	Cognitive sphere
I	Infancy	Birth to 1	Maternal person (unipolar-bipolar)	Oral sensory	Sensorimotor (birth to 18 years)
II	Toddlerhood	1-3	Parental persons (tripolar)	Anal-urethral	Preoperational thought, preconceptual phase (transductive reasoning, for example, specific to specific) (2-4 years)
III	Early childhood	3-6	Basic family	Phallic-locomotion	Preoperational thought, intuitive phase (transductive reasoning) (4-7 years)
IV	Middle childhood	6-12	Neighborhood, school	Latency	Concrete operations (inductive reasoning and beginning logic)
V	Adolescence	13-18	Peer groups and outgroups Models of leadership	Puberty	Formal operations (deductive and abstract reasoning)
VI	Early adulthood		Partners in friendship, sex, competition, cooperation	Genitality	
VII	Young and middle adulthood		Divided labor and shared household		
VIII	Later adulthood		Mankind "My kind"		

Data from Erikson, E. H.: Childhood and society, ed. 2, New York, 1963, W. W. Norton & Co.; Newman, B. M., and Newman, P. R.: Development through

manipulating and mental powers of selection and decision making. Negative feelings of *doubt* and *shame* arise when children are made to feel small and self-conscious, when their choices are disastrous, when others shame them, or when they are forced to be dependent in areas in which they are capable of assuming control. The favorable outcome of this stage is self-control and willpower.

Sense of initiative (3 to 6 years). This stage is characterized by vigorous, intrusive behavior, enterprise, and a strong imagination. Children explore the physical world with all their senses and powers. They develop a conscience. No longer guided only by outsiders, there is an inner voice that warns and threatens. Being made to feel that their activities or imaginings are bad produces a sense of *guilt*. This stage corresponds to Freud's infantile genital or phallic stage, and an outstanding feature of this stage is the Oedipal phase when the child forms an attachment to the parent of the opposite sex. The outcome is direction and purpose.

Sense of industry (6 to 12 years). Having achieved the more crucial stages in personality development, children are now ready to be workers and producers. They want to engage in tasks and activities that they can carry through to completion. They need and want real achievement. They learn to compete with others and to cooperate, and they learn the rules. It is a decisive period in their social relationships with others. Feelings of inadequacy and *inferiority* may develop if too much is expected of them or they believe that they cannot measure up to the standards set for them by others. This is the latency period of Freud. The favorable outcome of a sense of industry is method and competence.

Sense of identity (12 to 18 years). Corresponding to Freud's puberty, this period is characterized by rapid and marked physical changes. Previous trust in their bodies is shaken, and children become overly preoccupied with the way they appear in the eyes of others as compared with their own self-concept. Adolescents struggle to fit the roles they have played and those they hope to play with the current style, to integrate their concepts and values with those of society, and to come to a decision regarding an occupation. Inability to solve the core conflict results in *role diffusion*. The outcome of successful mastery is devotion and fidelity.

Sense of intimacy (early adulthood). A sense of intimacy is established on a sense of identity. It is the capacity to develop an intimate love relationship with another and intimate interpersonal relationships with friends, partners, and so on. This is Freud's stage of genitality. Without intimacy, the individual feels *isolated* and alone. The favorable outcome is affiliation and love.

Sense of generativity (young and middle adulthood). Central to this stage of development is the creation and care of the next generation. The essential element is to nourish

Psychosocial stages	Central process	Social modalities	Lasting outcomes	Related elements of social order
Trust vs mistrust	Mutuality with care giver	To get To give in return	Drive and hope	Faith Cosmic order
Autonomy vs shame and doubt	Imitation	To hold (on) To let (go)	Self-control and willpower	Law and order
Initiative vs guilt	Identification	To make (going after) To "make like" (playing)	Direction and purpose	Ideal prototype
Industry vs inferiority	Education	To make things (completing) To make things (together)	Method and competence	Technical fundamentals
Identity and repudiation vs identity confusion	Peer pressure Role experimentation	To be oneself (or not to be) To share being oneself	Devotion and fidelity	Ideologic perspectives
Intimacy and solidarity vs isolation	Mutuality among peers	To lose and find oneself in another	Affiliation and love	Patterns of cooperation and competition
Generativity vs self-absorption	Creativity	To make being To take care	Production and care	Currents of education and tradition
Ego integrity vs despair	Introspection	To be by having been To face not being	Renunciation and wisdom	Wisdom and philosophy

life, Homewood, Ill., 1975, Dorsey Press; Smart, M. S., and Smart, R. C.: Children: development and relationships, ed. 3, New York, 1977, Macmillan, Inc.

and nurture that which has been produced. It may be directed toward one's own children, children of others, or products of creativity of other sorts. The individual who fails in this component of personality development becomes *self-absorbed* and stagnant. The favorable outcome is production and care.

Sense of ego integrity (old age). A sense of integrity results from satisfaction with life and acceptance of what has been; despair arises from remorse for that which might have been. The favorable outcome is renunciation and wisdom.

Language development

Children are born with the mechanism and capacity to develop speech and language skills. However, they will not speak spontaneously. The environment must provide a means for them to acquire these skills. Speech requires intact physiologic function of (1) the respiratory system, (2) speech control centers in the cerebral cortex, and (3) articulation and resonance structures of the mouth and nasal cavities. In addition acquisition of language requires (1) an intact and discriminating auditory apparatus, (2) intelligence, (3) a need to communicate, and (4) stimulation.

The rate of speech development varies from child to child and is directly related to neurologic competence and intellectual development. All children go through the same sequence of stages in prelingual speech. These stages are summarized in Table 3-7. Gesture precedes speech, and in this way a small child communicates satisfactorily. As speech develops, gesture recedes but never disappears entirely. Evidence has shown that early speech stimulation is important to the development of normal speech; therefore, those responsible for the child's care should provide auditory stimulation and verbal feedback. Continual relationships with others enhance the desire to acquire greater vocabulary and communication skills.

At all stages of language development, children's understanding vocabulary is greater than their expressed vocabulary. The acquisition of vocabulary and language keeps pace with cognitive advancement, and children begin to use words as substitutes for action. The growth of children's vocabulary reflects a continuing process of modification that involves both the acquisition of new words and the expanding and refining of word meanings previously learned. By the time they begin to walk, children are able to attach a name to objects and persons. The first parts of speech used are nouns, sometimes verbs (for example, go), and combination words (such as bye-bye). Following the use of the first meaningful words, children begin to relate words to one another to form simple and then more complex sentences. Responses are usually structurally incomplete during the preschool period, although the meaning is clear. Next they begin to use adjectives and adverbs to qualify nouns, followed by adverbs to qualify nouns and

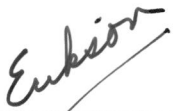

Table 3-7. Stages of prelingual speech development

Stage	Approximate age (months)	Characteristics	Significant aspects
1. Reflex vocalization	0-1	Isolated sound Undifferentiated cry with total body response	Colic cry and cerebral cry are higher pitched Used to express needs
	1-4	Differentiated cry Still total body response Nature of cry varies with the need	Used to express needs
2. Babbling	3½-6	Primarily vocal play Variety of random sounds	Persists in congenitally deaf child
3. Lallation (imperfect imitation)	6-9	Awareness and repetition Repetition and self-produced sounds	
4. Echolalia (correct imitation)	9-10	Imitation of sounds made by others Emotional elements of communication are interjected	Believed to be an important period of speech development
5. Verbal utterance	10-18	First words at this time Association of words with objects Jargon (language of his own)	Beginning of true language

Table 3-8. Language development

Age (years)	Vocabulary	Characteristics	Significant aspects
1-2	One to three words at age 1 year to 200 to 300 words at age 2 years	Names of familiar objects and persons Relating of symbol and object meanings, but usually as by-products of action Nouns, some verbs, and "pivot words," such as "more" and "off"	Following of initiating commands Reflection of egocentricity
2-3	300 to 500 words	Complete, simple sentences of two to three words	Response to both initiating and inhibiting commands May be frustrated because speech is inadequate for communication needs Objects acquire stability and permanence by being named
3-4	600 to 1000 words	Use of adjectives, adverbs, and prepositions Complete sentences of at least four words Use of pronouns and gender words	Use of speech to stop and start own actions Culturally related grammar and structure can be erroneously viewed as language deficits Normal stumbling and hesitant speech may become a fixed pattern of stuttering if others force him or otherwise generate self-consciousness about speech
4-5	1100 to 1600 words	Increased use of adjectives, adverbs, prepositions, and conjunctions Beginning of use of articles Use of plural forms	Many questions Name calling and some profanities
5-6	1500 to 2500 words	Use of five- to six-word sentences Use of complex sentences Syntax near normal	Fewer questions Production of 88% of all sounds correctly

verbs. Later, pronouns and gender words are added (such as he and she). By the time children enter school they are able to use simple structurally complete sentences that average five to seven words (Table 3-8).

A common rule of thumb that is helpful in evaluation of early speech acquisition is: *the number of words in an average response should correspond to the chronologic age of the child.*[5] For example, a 2-year-old child might say, "Me do"; a 3-year-old might add a word, "Me do it"; and a 4-year-old child might say, "Let me do it."

Girls are more advanced in language development than are boys; this is probably related to the slower neurophysiologic maturation of boys. Firstborn children develop language earlier than do later-born children, and children of multiple births (twins, triplets) develop language later than children of single births. Delayed, lack of, or impaired speech can result from a variety of sources, including congenital structural defects of the mouth and nasopharynx, a hearing deficit, neurologic dysfunction (including mental retardation), maternal deprivation, and emotional factors. Some of these will be discussed in relation to health problems in which impaired speech is a symptom or a consequence. It is also important to note that some of the organ systems on which speech depends, such as the respiratory system for gas exchange and the tongue for eating, are responsible for higher priority functions that take precedence over the lesser important function of communication. During illness or trauma, children may direct their limited energy to the more vital functions of these systems, that is, breathing and eating.

FACTORS THAT INFLUENCE DEVELOPMENT

Children are engaged in a continuous, dynamic, and reciprocal relationship with their environment in order to achieve and maintain an equilibrium. This equilibrium, or balance, is continually upset and regained through numerous and varied complex interactions. It is impossible to include a discussion of all the complex and interrelated factors that influence the development of children as unique individuals. Children are affected by physical factors such as the climate in which they live, physiologic influences such as their innate characteristics and susceptibilities, the value system of their families and culture, and psychologic influences such as the quality of parenting and the number, sex, and personalities of the significant persons in their lives. Some factors that may be facilitated, modified, or otherwise influenced by nursing interventions will be mentioned, although specific activities and elaboration will be discussed elsewhere as appropriate.

Heredity

Inherited characteristics have a profound influence on development. The sex of the child, determined by random selection at the time of conception, directs both his pattern of growth and the behavior of others toward him. In all cultures, attitudes and expectations are different with respect to the sex of the child. Sex plus other hereditary determinants strongly affect the end result of growth and the rate of progress toward it. There is a high correlation between parent and child with regard to traits such as height, weight, and rate of growth. Most physical characteristics, including shape and form of features, body build, and physical peculiarities, are inherited and can influence the way in which children grow and interact with their environment. The child's heritage may cause a deviation from established physical standards for growth and development. For example, Japanese children are smaller than average at all ages. Black children, although they are on the average smaller at birth, are somewhat taller and heavier than white children during the school-age and pubescent periods (ages approximately 5 to 14 years).

Differences in health and vigor of children may be attributed to hereditary traits. An inherited physical or mental defect or disorder will alter or modify a child's physical and/or emotional growth and interactions. The extent to which handicapping conditions interfere with the child's growth and well-being will be considered in relation to numerous disabilities throughout the remainder of the book.

Neuroendocrine

It has been suggested that there may be a growth center in the region of the hypothalamus that is responsible for maintaining developing individuals on their genetically determined growth patterns. It is believed that there is probably some functional relationship between the hypothalamus and the endocrine system that influences growth. There is also evidence, based on observations of denervated skeletal muscles, that the peripheral nervous system may influence growth, because muscles deprived of nerve supply degenerate. Many of these effects are not sufficiently explained by disuse or diminished blood supply. For example, nail growth on an extremity with a severed nerve will lag behind the nail growth on the corresponding extremity, but the growth returns to normal with regeneration of the nerve. There is no satisfactory explanation for this; but the process may involve a chemical substance secreted by nerve cells that modifies the growth and repair processes.

Hormones. Probably all hormones affect growth in some fashion. Three hormones—somatotrophic hormone, thyroid hormone, and androgens—when given to persons in whom these hormones are deficient, stimulate protein anabolism and thereby produce retention of elements essential for building protoplasm and bony tissue. It appears that each of the hormones that has significant influence on growth manifests its major effect at a different period of growth (Table 3-9).

Table 3-9. Effect of hormones on growth and development

Hormone	Source	Age of maximum effect	Effect	Deficiency	Excess
Somatotrophic hormone (STH) or growth hormone (GH)	Adenohypophysis	Childhood	Main effect is on linear growth Maintains a normal rate of protein synthesis Inhibits fat and oxidation of carbohydrates Essential for proliferation of cartilage cells at epiphyseal plate Ineffective after epiphyseal closure	Epiphyseal fusion with cessation of growth Dwarfism	Giantism
Thyrotropic hormone (TH)	Adenohypophysis	Major effect in early childhood	Stimulates thyroid hormone secretion	Hypothyroidism	Hyperthyroidism
Thyroxine (T_4) and triiodothyronine (T_3)	Thyroid	Continuous	Essential to normal postnatal growth and development Stimulates general metabolism Especially important for growth of bones, teeth, and brain	Cretinism Stunted growth Mental retardation	Accelerated linear growth Advanced skeletal maturation
Adrenocorticotrophic hormone (ACTH)	Adenohypophysis	Adolescence	Stimulates adrenal cortex to secrete androgens Stimulates hypothalamus, which causes adenohypophysis to secrete gonadotropic hormones	Delayed maturation	Precocious puberty
Gonadotropic hormones	Adenohypophysis	Adolescence	Stimulates interstitial cells of gonads—testes and ovaries	Delayed sexual development	Precocious puberty
Testosterone	Testes	Adolescence	Stimulates testes to produce spermatozoa Stimulates development of secondary sex characteristics	Delayed sexual development	Precocious puberty Accelerated skeletal maturation
Estrogen	Ovaries	Adolescence	Stimulates ripening of ova Stimulates development of secondary sex characteristics	Delayed sexual development	Precocious puberty Premature epiphyseal closure
Insulin	Islands of Langerhans of pancreas	Continuous	Essential for carbohydrate, fat, and protein metabolism Decreases gluconeogenesis Increases glycolysis Facilitates protein synthesis from amino acids	Stunted growth	
Parathormone	Parathyroids	Continuous	Influences ossification and development of bone	Uncertain	Bone demineralization
Calcitonin	Thyroid	Continuous	Influences ossification and development of bone	Uncertain	Uncertain
Cortisol	Adrenal cortex	Continuous	Stimulates gluconeogenesis Decreases protein synthesis Increases catabolism of cellular protein	Impaired growth and sexual function	Severe impairment of growth with slowing of skeletal maturation Excess fat deposition

Nutrition

Probably the single most important influence on growth is nutrition. Dietary factors regulate growth at *all* stages of development, and their effects are exerted in numerous and complex ways. Adequate nutrition provides the essential nutrients in the amount and balance necessary to sustain physiologic needs. These needs vary widely according to age, level of activity, and environmental conditions. Inadequacies in any or all of these essential nutrients will be reflected in altered growth.

The nutritional requirements of childhood are directly related to the rate and direction of growth. During the rapid prenatal growth period, faulty nutrition may influence development from the time of implantation of the ovum until birth. The nutritional needs are met entirely through the maternal system; as a result, maternal deficiencies or abnormalities in the supplementary intrauterine structures will be manifest in fetal development (see Chapter 7).

During infancy and childhood, the demand for calories is relatively great, as evidenced by the rapid increase in both height and weight. At this time, protein and caloric requirements are higher than at almost any period of postnatal development. As the growth rate slows with its concomitant decrease in metabolism, there is a corresponding reduction in caloric and protein requirement (see Table 3-3). Growth is uneven during the periods of childhood between infancy and adolescence, when there are plateaus and small growth spurts. The child's appetite will fluctuate in response to these variations until the turbulent growth spurt of adolescence, when adequate nutrition is extremely important but may be subject to numerous emotional influences. The child's caloric intake must equal his energy output plus that needed for growth. It is estimated that the average child (for example, the 6- to 10-year-old child) will expend 55% of his energy for metabolic maintenance, 25% for physical activity, 8% in fecal loss, and 12% for growth (see Fig. 3-9).

The most predominant feature of childhood and adolescence is physical growth; satisfactory growth achievement is most frequently judged in terms of increase in body weight, height, and skeletal growth. Adequate nutrition is closely related to good health throughout life, and an overall improvement in nourishment is evidenced by the gradual increase in size and early maturation of children in this century. In the growing child, inadequate nutrition is dangerous, particularly during those periods identified as critical for growth (see pp. 50 and 233). Inadequate nutrition has the greatest impact during the critical periods of rapid cell division. For example, normal development of the central nervous system depends on adequate nutrition during fetal life and throughout the first 2 years of postnatal life.

Malnutrition. The term malnutrition in its strictest sense is usually used to describe undernutrition, primarily that resulting from insufficient caloric intake. However, malnutrition may result from the following: (1) a dietary intake that is quantitatively or qualitatively inadequate, or both, including overnutrition; (2) disease that interferes with appetite, digestion, or absorption while increasing nutritional requirements; (3) excessive physical activity or inadequate rest; or (4) disturbed interpersonal relationships and other environmental or psychologic factors. Severe malnutrition during the critical periods of development, particularly the first 6 months of life, are positively correlated with diminished height, weight, and intelligence scores. The importance of nutrition as a vital aspect of health promotion during all phases of the illness-wellness continuum is included as it relates to developmental phases and to specific health problems.

Season, climate, and oxygen concentration

There is some evidence that season and climate may have an influence on growth. Growth in height appears to be faster in the spring and summer months, whereas growth in weight proceeds more rapidly during the autumn and winter. These observations have not been satisfactorily explained. This phenomenon may have a hormonal basis, or it may be related to seasonal differences in activity levels.

Formerly, it was believed that individuals living in a warm climate were smaller than those from a cold climate. However, it is much too difficult to separate the effects of climate from other factors such as race, nutrition, or disease. There does seem to be more evidence regarding the effects of hypoxia on growth. Children with disorders that produce a chronic hypoxia are characteristically small when compared with children of the same chronologic age. Also, children native to high altitudes are smaller than those living at sea level. These observations have been supported by animal studies, although there are no substantiating studies with human subjects.

Disease

Altered growth and development is one of the clinical manifestations in a number of hereditary disorders. Growth impairment is particularly marked in skeletal disorders, such as the various forms of dwarfism and at least one of the chromosomal anomalies (Turner's syndrome). Many of the disorders of metabolism, such as vitamin D–resistant rickets, mucopolysaccharidoses, and the numerous endocrine disorders, interfere with the normal growth pattern. In other disorders the tendency is toward the upper percentile of height, for example, Klinefelter's syndrome and Marfan's syndrome.

Many chronic illnesses that are associated with varying degrees of growth failure are congenital cardiac anomalies and respiratory disorders such as cystic fibrosis. Any disorder characterized by the inability to digest and absorb body nutrients will have an adverse effect on growth and development. These include the malabsorption syndromes and defects in digestive enzyme systems. Almost any disorder or disease state that persists over an extended period, particularly during a critical period of development, may have a permanent effect on growth.

Children who are in a prolonged state of disequilibrium caused by illness, such as chronic infections, are under a constant inner stress that inhibits their response to adult demands and contributes to their difficulty in managing stimulating environmental experiences. Behaviors that these children display as they cope with outside stimuli as well as inner irritations can be misinterpreted as distractibility and lack of persistence toward a goal. A prolonged illness that occurs in the second year during the phase of rapid acquisition of motor control and autonomy may cause a child to lose the natural impetus peculiar to this stage of development. Such a child may remain passive and require special stimulation to develop the independence, which, under normal circumstances, would have developed spontaneously.

Interpersonal relationships

It is well established that relationships with significant others play an important role in development, particularly in emotional, intellectual, and personality development. Not only do the quality and quantity of contacts with other persons exert an influence on the growing child, but the widening range of contacts is essential to learning and the development of a healthy personality. During the formative years, culturally determined, age-appropriate behaviors are reinforced and, consequently, repeated. Thus patterns of reward and punishment, modeling, etc. continually modify the child's individuality of character and temperament. The child behaves in a manner that elicits rewards from the person most significant in his life at a given point in time.

Significant others. The mother or mothering person is unquestionably the single most influential person during early infancy. She is the one who meets the infant's basic needs of food, warmth, comfort, and love. She provides stimulation for his senses and facilitates his expanding capacities. Through her, the child learns to trust the world and feel secure to venture in increasingly wider relationships. The child learns, through her constant reinforcement, the behaviors that bring satisfaction to the mother and incorporates them. Eventually, these behaviors become self-motivating. For example, children learn that evacuating the bowel in a proper receptacle produces a positive response from the mother that results in a lifetime behavioral pattern.

The sphere of persons from whom children seek approval widens to include other members of their family, their peers, and, to a lesser extent, other authority figures (for example, teachers). The increasing importance of the peer group in determining the behavior of school-age children and adolescents is well documented. However, it is the quality of the parent-child relationship that determines, to a large extent, the impact of peer influence on a child.

It is generally the parents who are most influential in assisting the child to assume sex-role identification. Parents define and reinforce acceptable sex-role behavior and provide sex-appropriate role models for the child. In the absence of a sex-role model in the family setting, the child may adopt some characteristics of the opposite sex parent or sibling. Frequently, the child identifies with a teacher or other significant person of the same sex.

Siblings are the child's first peers, and the way in which he learns to relate to them affects later interactions with peers outside the family group. For example, a firstborn child who is accustomed to a position of leadership with siblings will tend to assume the same position with peers; younger children are more often followers. Ease in relationships with peers of the same or opposite sex is frequently associated with similar associations in the home.

Emotional deprivation. The most prominent feature of emotional deprivation, particularly during the first year, is developmental retardation. Much of the information regarding the adverse effects of interpersonal influences on development has been acquired through retrospective studies of gross deprivation and trauma. The most notable instances involved homeless infants who were placed in institutions for care. These infants, who did not receive consistent mothering care, failed to gain weight even with an adequate diet; were pale, listless, and immobile; and were unresponsive to stimuli that usually elicits a response in the normal infant, such as a smile, cooing, and so on. It has been found that if the emotional deprivation continues for a sufficient length of time, the child does not survive infancy.

Dr. Harlow's[7] classic experiments with infant monkeys illustrate the far-reaching effects of emotional and social deprivation in infancy. In these experiments the monkeys were raised by substitute, inanimate "mothers" made of cloth-covered wire from whom they derived nourishment and a measure of comfort but no mothering. These monkeys developed abnormal play and sex behavior. The few who bore offspring were unable to "mother" them. However, those who were allowed peer associations developed normal play and social-sex behavior. By correlating these findings with retrospective studies of human infants in comparable age-groups, attempts are made to explain some of the behaviors observed in these children in later interpersonal relationships. Although the most remarkable examples of emotional deprivation were first recognized among infants in institutions, the term "masked deprivation" has been used to describe children who are reared in homes where there is a distorted mother-child relationship or otherwise disordered home environment. Infants do not thrive if the mothering person is hostile, fearful of handling them, or indifferent to them and their needs. Such children exhibit poor growth even though apparently free of physical disease. Children past the age of infancy who evidence physical underdevelopment are also retarded in "bone age." Growth retardation in these children is believed to be caused by a psychologically induced endocrine imbalance that interferes with growth. These same infants and children display "catch-up" growth in a changed environment.

ROLE OF PLAY IN DEVELOPMENT

It is through the universal medium of play that children learn what no one can teach them. They learn about their world and how to deal with this environment of objects, time, space, structure, and people. They learn about themselves operating within that environment—what they can do, how to relate to things and situations, and how to adapt themselves to the demands society makes on them. It has been said that play is the *work* of the child. In play, children continually practice the complicated, stressful processes of living, communicating, and achieving satisfactory relationships with other people. In addition, while promoting and advancing development and relationships, play is its own reward.

Classification of play

From a developmental point of view, patterns of children's play can be categorized according to *content* and the *social character* of play. In both there is an additive effect. Each builds on past accomplishments, and some element of each is maintained throughout life. At each stage in development the new predominates.

Content of play. Play begins with *social-affective* play, wherein the infant takes pleasure in relationships with people. As adults talk, fondle, nuzzle, and in various ways elicit a response from the infant, he soon learns to provoke parental emotions and responses with such behaviors as smiling, cooing, or initiating games and activities. The type and intensity of the adult behavior with children vary among cultures.

Sense-pleasure play is a nonsocial stimulating experience that originates from without. Objects in the environment—light and color, tastes and odors, textures and consistencies—attract a child's attention, stimulate his senses, and give pleasure. Pleasurable experiences are derived from handling raw materials (water, sand, food), from body motion (swinging, bouncing, rocking), and from other uses of senses and abilities, such as smelling, humming, and so on.

Once infants have developed the ability to grasp and manipulate, they persistently demonstrate and exercise their newly acquired abilities through *skill play,* repeating an action over and over again. The element of sense-pleasure play is often evident in the practicing of a new ability, but all too frequently the determination to conquer the elusive skill produces pain and frustration (for example, learning to ride a bicycle).

One of the vital elements in the child's process of identification is *dramatic* play. It begins in toddlerhood and is the predominant form of play in the preschool child. Once children begin to invest situations and people with meanings and to attribute affective significance to the world, they can pretend and fantasize almost anything. By acting out events of daily life, children learn and practice the roles and identities modeled by the members of their family and society. Their small toys, replicas of the tools of the society in which they live, provide a medium for learning about these adult roles and activities that may be both puzzling and frustrating to them. Interacting with the world is one of the ways in which children get to know it. The simple, imitative, dramatic play of the toddler, such as using the telephone, driving a car, or rocking a doll, evolves into more complex, sustained dramas of the preschooler that extend beyond common domestic matters to the wider aspects of the world and the society, such as playing policeman, storekeeper, teacher, nurse, and so on. Older children work out elaborate themes, act out stories, and compose plays.

Very young children participate in simple, *imitative games* such as pat-a-cake and peekaboo. Preschool children learn and enjoy *formal games* that begin with ritualistic, self-sustaining games, such as ring-around-a-rosy and London Bridge, then progress to *competitive games,* such as cards, Parcheesi, or baseball.

Social character of play. The play interactions of infancy are between the child and an adult. Children continue to enjoy the company of an adult but are increasingly able to play alone. As age advances, interaction with agemates increases in importance and becomes an essential part of the socialization process. Through it, the highly egocentric infant, unable to tolerate delay or interference, ultimately acquires concern for others and the ability to delay gratification or even to reject gratification at the expense of another. A pair of toddlers will engage in a good deal of combat since their personal needs cannot stand delay or compromise. By the time they reach age 5 or 6 years, children are able to arrive at a compromise or make use of arbitration—usually after each child has attempted but failed to gain his own way. Through continued interaction with peers and the growth of conceptual abilities and social skills, children are able to increase participation with others.

Social involvement during play can be categorized by the following:

Solitary play
Children play alone and independently with toys different from those used by other children within the same area. They enjoy the presence of other children but make no effort to get close to or speak to them. Their interest is centered on their own activity, which they pursue with no reference to the activities of the others.

Parallel play
Children play independently but among other children. They play with toys that are like those that the children around

them are using, but as each sees fit, neither influencing nor being influenced by the other children. Each plays beside, but not with, other children. Parallel play is the characteristic play of the toddler.

Associative play

Children play together and are engaged in a similar or even identical activity, but there is no organization, division of labor, or interchange. There is borrowing and lending of play materials, following one another with wagons and tricycles, and sometimes attempts to control who may or may not play in the group. Each child acts according to his own wishes; there is no group goal. There is a great deal of behavioral contagion—when one child initiates an activity, the entire group follows the example.

Cooperative play

Play is organized. The children discuss and plan activities for the purposes of accomplishing an end—to make something, to attain a competitive goal, to dramatize situations of adult or group life, or to play formal games. There is a marked sense of belonging or not belonging to the group. The goal and its attainment require organization of activities, division of labor, and playing roles. One or two members of the group usually control the group situations, assign roles, and direct the activity of the others.

Functions of play

The specific values of play or the functions that it serves throughout childhood include sensorimotor development, intellectual development, socialization, creativity, self-awareness, and therapeutic and moral value.

Sensorimotor development. Sensorimotor activity is a major component of play at all ages and is the predominant form in infancy. Active play is essential for muscle development and serves a useful purpose as a release for surplus energy. Through sensorimotor play children explore the nature of the physical world. Infants gain impressions of themselves and their world through tactile, auditory, visual, and kinesthetic stimulation. Toddlers and preschoolers revel in body movement and exploration of things in space. Children continue to engage in sensorimotor play, although with increasing maturity the play becomes more differentiated and involved. While very young children run for the sheer joy of body movement, older children incorporate or modify the motions into increasingly complex and coordinated activities such as races, games, roller skating, and bicycle riding.

Intellectual development. Through exploration and manipulation, children learn colors, shapes, sizes, textures, and the significance of objects. They learn the significance of numbers and how to use them, they learn to associate words with objects, and they develop an understanding of abstract concepts and spatial relationships, such as up, down, under, over, and so on. Activities such as puzzles and games help them develop problem-solving skills. Books, stories, films, and collections expand knowledge and provide enjoyment as well. Play provides a means to practice and expand language skills. Through play, children continually rehearse past experiences to assimilate them into new perceptions and relationships. Play helps children to comprehend the world in which they live and to distinguish between fantasy and reality.

Socialization. From very early infancy, children show interest and pleasure in the company of others. Their initial social contact is with the mothering person, but through play with other children they learn to establish social relationships and solve the problems associated with these relationships. They learn to give and take, which is more readily learned from critical peers than from the more tolerant adults. They learn the sex role that society expects them to fulfill as well as approved patterns of behavior and deportment. Closely associated with socialization is development of moral values and ethics. Children learn right from wrong, the standards of the society, and to assume responsibility for their actions.

Creativity. In no other situation is there more opportunity to be creative than in play. Children can experiment and try out their ideas in play through every medium at their disposal, including raw materials, fantasy, and exploration. Creativity is stifled by pressure toward conformity; therefore, striving for peer approval may inhibit creative endeavors in the school-age or adolescent child. Creativity is primarily a product of solitary, as opposed to group, activity. Once children feel the satisfaction of creating something new and different, they transfer this creative interest to situations outside the world of play.

Self-awareness. Beginning with active explorations of their bodies and awareness of themselves as separate from the mother, the process of self-identity is facilitated through play activities. Children learn who they are and what their place is in the world. They become increasingly able to regulate their own behavior, to learn what their abilities are, and to compare their abilities with those of others. Through play, children are able to test their abilities, assume and try out various roles, and learn the effect that their behavior has on others.

Therapeutic value. There is no doubt that play is therapeutic at any age. It provides a means for release from the tension and stress encountered through the environment. In play, children can express emotions and release unacceptable impulses in a socially acceptable fashion. Children are able to experiment and test fearful situations and can assume and vicariously master the roles and positions that they are unable to perform in the world of reality. Children reveal much about themselves in play. Through play, children are able to communicate to the alert observer the needs, fears, and desires that they are unable to express with their limited language skills. Throughout their play, children need the acceptance of adults and their presence to help them control aggression and to channel their destructive tendencies.

Moral value. Although children learn at home and at school those behaviors that are considered right and wrong in the culture, the interaction with peers during play contributes significantly to their moral training. Nowhere is the enforcement of moral standards so rigid as in the play situation. If they are to be acceptable members of the group, children must adhere to the accepted codes of behavior of the culture—fairness, honesty, self-control, consideration for others, and so on. Children soon learn that their peers are less tolerant of violations than are adults and that to maintain a place in the play group they must conform to the standards of the group.

Characteristics of play

There are several aspects of play that display developmental changes and that differentiate children's play from adult play.

Tradition. In general, the play of small children varies little from generation to generation within a culture. Each generation of children imitates the play of the preceding generation, in this way the more satisfying forms of play are perpetuated. Many types of play are characteristic of all cultures, for example, playing with balls, some form of doll, or some form of walking toy to help a child just beginning to walk to maintain balance.

Seasonal changes are accompanied by traditional forms of toys and play activities. Sledding and ice skating are popular in winter; jump rope, marbles, and jacks are played in spring and summer.

Time and age. The amount of time that children spend in play decreases with age. Older children have less time available for play because of an increase in schoolwork and other responsibilities for which they are accountable. With advancing age and development, the number and variety of play activities diminish and become less physically active, but the time spent in specific activities increases as interests narrow and the attention span lengthens. The number of playmates decreases with age as children progress from play with anyone available to play with a few selected and special age-mates.

Children's play can be divided into the following four categories: (1) imitative, (2) exploratory, (3) testing, and (4) model building. At all ages each of these types is evident in children's play, but one type will predominate over the others at specific ages. For example, imitative play can be seen in the infant who mimics the actions of another (pat-a-cake), but it reaches its peak in the dramatic play of preschoolers who play "house," "astronaut," "cowboy," or "school." It can also be observed in circular group singing and rhythmic games such as ring-around-a-rosy.

As children grow older, play activities become less spontaneous, more formal and structured, and increasingly sex appropriate. Whereas infants and small children of both sexes play in much the same way, by the time they enter school, children engage in activities deemed appropriate for their sex. Little boys, in particular, are clearly aware that they do not play with certain toys, and they avoid their girl playmates.

Patterns of development. Throughout childhood certain play activities are popular at one age and not at another. These activities are so consistent and predictable that childhood is sometimes divided into age stages according to the types of play characteristic of each particular phase of development.

Exploratory stage
: This stage lasts from approximately 3 months of age to near the end of the first year. It consists mostly of grasping, holding, and examining articles, and exploration via creeping or crawling.

Toy stage
: The toy stage begins in the first year and reaches a maximum at 7 to 8 years of age.

Play stage
: During this stage school-age children's play repertory increases. Interest in toys diminishes, whereas interest in games, sports, and hobbies increases.

Daydreaming stage
: This stage is characteristic of older children and pubescents who play the martyr who is misunderstood and mistreated by everyone or the hero or beauty who is admired by everyone.

As they grow older, children also use materials in more meaningful ways. For example, an infant or small child first uses a block as something to handle or throw, then as something to represent another object, such as an airplane or car. To older children a block is a building material with which they can construct increasingly complex structures. They require replicas of cars and airplanes. Eventually these materials are discarded altogether.

Accidents

Accidents are the leading cause of death in children at all ages, and the type of injury and the circumstances surrounding the accident are closely related to normal growth and development behavior. As the child develops, his innate curiosity impels him to investigate activities and to mimic the behavior of others. This is essential in order to acquire competency as an adult, but "curiosity and mimicry precede their skill in dealing with the new and their cognition of dangers in acting according to what they see."[11] The developmental stage of the child partially determines the types of accidents that are most likely to occur at a specific age and thus helps provide clues to preventive measures that might be implemented. For example, small infants are helpless in any environment, and when they begin to roll over or otherwise propel themselves, they can fall from unprotected surfaces. The creeping infant with a natural tendency to place objects in the mouth is at risk of aspiration or poisoning. The mobile toddler with the instinct to explore and investigate and the ability to run and climb is subject to a variety of accidents, including falls, burns, and collision with objects. As children grow older their absorption with play often makes them oblivious to environmental hazards such as street traffic or water, and the need to conform and gain acceptance compels older children and adolescents to accept challenges and dares. At all ages children are continually in contact with toys, tools, and an infinite variety of mechanical devices that are easily accessible and that they may explore without proper guidance or supervision. Although the highest incidence of accidental injury is in children less than 9 years of age (especially ages 2 and 3 years, with ages 5 and 6 years next), most fatal injuries occur in later childhood and adolescence. Older children have more accidents outside the home; younger children are more often injured in or around the home.

The personality of a child can be a factor in his susceptibility to accidents. The bright, alert, and adventuresome child is apt to have more accidents than the dull, passive, or less curious child. Boys, at all ages, have more accidents than girls, and this tendency increases as the child gets older. Because they are usually more closely supervised and have been taught to be more cautious, firstborn and only children seem to have fewer accidents than younger siblings.

A number of unrelated and seemingly ordinary things appear to contribute to accidents. Very often an accident occurs when there is a minor family illness and especially when the mother is ill, pregnant, or just about to begin a menstrual period. Accidents frequently occur when the mother is rushed, tells the child, "Don't do that!" but is too busy to see that the direction is carried out. An overly tired parent has difficulty setting limits on behavior. A higher incidence of accidents takes place from Thursday through Saturday. On Saturday when both parents are

Table 3-10. Typical accidents related to developmental level

Behavioral characteristics	Type of accident	Preventive measures
Infant		
Increasing acquisition of mobility such as ability to squirm, roll over, creep, crawl, and pull self erect	Falls	Do not leave infant alone on tables, etc., from which the infant can fall Keep crib sides raised Keep stairs fenced
Exploration of environment with touch, movement (locomotion), taste Oral stage of development; placing anything and everything in mouth	Aspiration or ingestion of foreign objects Poisoning	Do not give small items to infant Check items carefully for removable parts Do not feed small solid items, such as peanuts, whole-kernel corn, etc. Keep harmful substances out of reach
Reaching for items such as an appliance cord, table cover Placing objects into openings	Burns	Keep hot items out of reach Keep handles of pans on stove out of reach Cover electrical outlets
Helpless in water	Drowning	Do not leave alone in tub or water or near a pool, lake, or stream when able to crawl or creep
Toddler		
Increased mobility with upright posture Unaware of danger Climbing with ease Navigation of stairways Curious Imitative Placing almost anything in mouth Almost helpless in water Investigation of drawers and cupboards	Falls Burns Drowning Motor vehicle accidents Pedestrian Passenger Ingestion and/or aspiration of harmful substances or items Suffocation	Provide adequate supervision Place gate at head of stairs Place screens on windows Keep in enclosed space when outdoors and/or not in company of adult Place handles of pots and pans on stove out of reach and containers of hot foods away from table Keep harmful substances (medicines, cleaners) and items (scissors) out of reach Avoid demonstrating unsafe behaviors Cover unused electrical outlets; keep cords out of reach Use safety belt or selected infant car seats Examine toys for presence of safety Protect from water in tub, pool, or other area Purchase fire-retardant clothing Make certain any enclosed container large enough to hold child has airway or is unable to be tightly closed (for example, discarded refrigerator)

usually at home, the routine is disrupted and each parent thinks the other is watching the child. Accidents are lowest on Sunday when adults have more leisure time and are able to supervise children more carefully. Accidents are more apt to occur when the child is in the care of an unfamiliar person or a sibling who is too young for such responsibility, when the child changes surroundings, or when he is on a trip. With increased stress on the part of either the child or the person taking care of him, there is more risk of an accident.

Accidents are also more apt to occur when the child is hungry. The majority of accidents take place about an hour before a meal when the mother is busy and cannot supervise the child carefully. The child is hypoglycemic, tired, fretful, and quarrelsome. It is often better to give the child a snack than to make him wait until the meal is ready. The highest concentration of accidents takes place during the hours between 3 and 6 PM.

Development and accidents. Accidents are amenable to control, and the preventive aspects of child care should be an ongoing part of health promotion throughout childhood. This necessitates protection, education, and legislation. To protect the child from accidental injury, persons who are responsible for children need to be aware of the normal behavior characteristics that render them vulnerable to accidents and to be alert to factors in the environment that create a hazard to their safety. Parents and others are often surprisingly out of tune with their child's developmental progress and seem unaware of their capabilities. Anticipatory guidance regarding developmental expectations serves to alert the parents to the type of accidents that are most likely to occur at any given age and to environmental circumstances that might precipitate an accident. For example, infants must not be left where they can fall or roll over and toddlers must not be given objects or toys with small removable parts or sharp edges nor given unsupervised access

Table 3-10. Typical accidents related to developmental level—cont'd

Behavioral characteristics	Type of accident	Preventive measures
Preschooler		
Ability to open doors Running and climbing with ease Investigation of drawers, cupboards, closets Riding tricycle Playing with mechanical gadgets Ability to throw	Falls Drowning Ingestion or aspiration of harmful substances or items Burns Motor vehicle accidents Pedestrian Passenger	Keep doors locked if danger of falls Place screen guards on windows Teach safety: watch out for automobiles in driveways and streets, play in approved areas Keep harmful items (knifes, medicines, electrical equipment) out of reach Teach swimming and water safety Examine toys for safety Keep firearms locked up Provide safe play equipment for use Caution against talking to strangers Teach safety with matches, lighters, etc.
School-age child		
Daring and adventurous Increased motor skills Playing in hazardous places Need for strenuous physical activity Need for peer approval Attempting hazardous feats Accompanying peers to hazardous facilities	Falls Sports injuries Drowning Burns Motor vehicle accidents Pedestrian Passenger Bicycle	Teach safety rules for pedestrians, bicycles, skateboarding, and sports activities Encourage playing in safe places Teach swimming and water safety Keep firearms safely locked up except during adult supervision Teach safety with fires, matches, lighters, barbecues, bonfires Provide safe sports and other equipment and teach their proper use Provide facilities for supervised recreation
Adolescent		
Strong need for peer approval may lead to attempting hazardous feats Increased strength and agility Age permitted to drive automobile	Motor vehicle accidents Pedestrian Passenger Driver Drowning Suicide Poisoning (drug abuse)	Teach motor vehicle safety; provide supervised instruction Provide safe recreational facilities Teach safe use of sports equipment Instruct in safe use of firearms Recognize signs of depression Educate regarding hazards of drug abuse

to places where they can fall, drown, or get burned. Of course, much depends on the characteristics of the individual children and their families.

Toys. Selection of toys and play equipment is a joint effort between parents and children, but evaluation of their safety is the responsibility of the adult. Government agencies do not inspect and police all toys on the market. Therefore, adults who purchase, supervise purchases, or allow the child to use play equipment need to evaluate such equipment for its safety. This often includes toys that are gifts or those that are purchased by the children themselves. Children need toys and activities that increase their sense of competence but that do not create a threat to their health and safety.

Accident prevention

Theoretically, all accidents are preventable, and one of the chief nursing responsibilities is to anticipate and recognize where safety measures are applicable. Safety should be an intrinsic element of nursing practice. Nurses who themselves practice safety, who are alert to safety needs in the environment, and who recognize the need for safety education contribute to accident reduction. Three major areas of focus for accident prevention in children are:

1. Improving the quality of child care
2. Instructing those concerned about measures to safeguard the environment so that *exogenous* factors are removed, such as attractive hazards
3. Being attentive and alert to the *endogenous* factors that are intrinsic in the behavioral characteristics of the developing child

Very early in the parent-child relationship, the parents need to learn how to provide a safe environment for their child, what kinds of behaviors they can expect of the child at various stages in their development, and their responsibility for the safety of their children. Adult negligence contributes in some way to most accidental injuries sustained by children during infancy and early childhood. Parents need to be attuned to the changing capabilities of their children and alert to the new hazards that are inherent in normal development. This is particularly important for first-time parents. Safety responsibility in such areas as purchase of the infant layette and nursery furniture, including infant seat and car seat, should begin before the child is born.

It cannot be assumed that parents of one or more children are familiar with all areas of child safety. Often, no one has discussed with them the problems of safety. Moreover, the addition of a new child brings up the issue of sibling rivalry and the unwelcome but realistic possibility that the new child may be at risk from a jealous older sibling. For example, the parents should be cautioned against leaving the infant alone with the older child who feels threatened by the newcomer. It is not uncommon for a jealous child to inflict injury on a younger sibling.

To provide a safe environment for the child involves the combined efforts of family, nurses, and community. At each age level there are environmental attractions that are hazardous to the safety of the child. The specific hazards vary according to season (drowning, accidents related to winter heating devices), geographic area (water accidents in areas with swimming pools, rivers, lakes, etc.; heater burns in cold climates), and socioeconomic level (lead poisoning and street injuries in slum areas, bicycle accidents in middle class areas). The special problems and preventive measures are discussed as appropriate throughout the book and are related to the various age levels and conditions that predispose to specific hazards. Major developmental characteristics, hazards that are related to these developmental characteristics, and preventive measures to implement are listed in Table 3-10.

In addition to risks related to the normal growth and development process, individual differences in children influence the extent to which they are prone to accidental injury. Some children are more curious, adventuresome, and hostile, whereas others tend to be more passive and amenable to discipline. Children from more closely knit families have fewer accidents than those from families where there is discord. The behavioral characteristics associated with accidents in childhood are listed below (see boxed material).

Checklist of behavioral characteristics related to accident liability*

Characteristics that increase exposure to hazards
- Higher levels of general activity
- Daring
- Excessive curiosity
- Mimicry of older persons' behaviors
- Gregariousness
- Happy-go-lucky personality
- Inability to delay gratification
- Exaggerated oral tendencies, including pica
- Easily overstimulated

Characteristics that reduce ability to cope with hazards
- High-strung or "hot-headed"
- Stubborn or "hard-headed"
- Easily irritated or frustrated
- Poor concentration or attention
- Heedless or careless in play
- Lack of self-control
- Aggressive

*From Matheny, A. P., Brown, A. M., and Wilson, R. S.: Assessment of children's behavioral characteristics: a tool in accident prevention, Clin. Pediatr. **11**:437-439, 1972.

REFERENCES

1. Conway, B. L.: Pediatric neurologic nursing, St. Louis, 1977, The C. V. Mosby Co.
2. Erikson, E. H.: Childhood and society, ed. 2, New York, 1963, W. W. Norton & Co., Inc.
3. Falkner, R., editor: Human development, Philadelphia, 1966, W. B. Saunders Co.
4. Gardner, L. I.: Deprivation dwarfism, Sci. Am. **229:**76-82, July 1972.
5. Goda, S.: Speech development in children, Am. J. Nurs. **70:**276-278, February 1970.
6. Guyton, A.: Textbook of medical physiology, ed. 5, Philadelphia, 1976, W. B. Saunders Co.
7. Harlow, H. F., and Harlow, M. K.: Social deprivation in monkeys, Sci. Am. **203:**136-146, November 1962.
8. Havighurst, R. J.: Developmental tasks and education, ed. 3, New York, 1972, David McKay Co., Inc.
9. Hughes, J. G.: Synopsis of pediatrics, ed. 4, St. Louis, 1975, The C. V. Mosby Co.
10. Ilg, F. L., and Ames, L. B.: Child behavior. New York, 1955, Harper & Brothers.
11. Matheney, A P., Brown, A. M., and Wilson, R. S.: Assessment of children's behavior characteristics—a tool in prevention. Clin. Pediatr. **11:**437-439, 1972.
12. Mussen, P. H., Conger, J. J., and Kagan, J.: Child development and personality, ed. 4, New York, 1974, Harper & Row, Publishers.
13. Newman, B. M., and Newman, P. R.: Development through life, Homewood, Ill., 1975, Dorsey Press.
14. Phillips, J. L.: The origins of intellect: Piaget's theory, San Francisco, 1969, W. H. Freeman and Co. Publishers.
15. Sinclair, D.: Human growth after birth, New York, 1969, Oxford University Press, Inc.
16. Smart, M. S., and Smart, R. C.: Children: development and relationships, ed. 3, New York, 1977, Macmillan, Inc.
17. Stone, L. J., and Church, J.: Childhood and adolescence, ed. 3, New York, 1973, Random House, Inc.

BIBLIOGRAPHY

Ames, L. B.: Child care and development, Philadelphia, 1970, J. B. Lippincott Co.

Bakwin, H., and Bakwin, R. M.: Behavior disorders in children, ed. 4, Philadelphia, 1972, W. B. Saunders Co.

Bandura, A., editor: Psychological modeling, Chicago, 1971, Aldine Publishing Co.

Bird, B.: Talking with patients, ed. 2, Philadelphia, 1973, J. B. Lippincott Co.

Bolles, R. C.: Reinforcement, expectancy, and learning, Psychol. Rev. **79:**294-309, 1972.

Brown, V.: Providing a safe environment for children, Am. J. Maternal Child Nurs. **3**(1):53-55, 1978.

Chase, H. P., and Martin, H. P.: Undernutrition and child development, N. Engl. J. Med. **282:**933, 1970.

Children are different, Columbus, Ohio, 1970, Ross Laboratories.

Chinn, P. L.: Child health maintenance, ed. 2, St. Louis, 1979, The C. V. Mosby Co.

Coplan, F., and Coplan, T.: The power of play, New York, 1973, Anchor Press.

Cullinan, T. R.: Children at risk of accident, Community Health **2:**175-178, 1971.

Ellison, C. W., and Firestone, I. J.: Development of international trust as a function of self-esteem, target status and target style, J. Pers. Soc. Psychol. **29:**655-663, 1975.

Erikson, E. H.: Childhood and society, ed. 2, New York, 1963, W. W. Norton & Co., Inc.

Erikson, E. H.: Identity, youth and crisis, New York, 1968, W. W. Norton & Co., Inc.

Falkner, R., editor: Human development, Philadelphia, 1966, W. B. Saunders Co.

Frank, D. J., and Drobish, N. L.: Toy safety in hospitals—or beware of parents bearing gifts, Clin. Pediatr. **14:**400-442, 1975.

Gardner, L. I.: Deprivation dwarfism, Sci. Am. **229:**76-82, July 1972.

Goda, S.: Speech development in children, Am. J. Nurs. **70:**276-278, February 1970.

Guyton, A.: Textbook of medical physiology, ed. 5, Philadelphia, 1976, W. B. Saunders Co.

Hall, C. S., and Lindzey, G.: Theories of personality, ed. 2, New York, 1970, John Wiley & Sons, Inc.

Harlow, H. F., and Harlow, M. K.: Learning to love, Am. Sci. **54:**244-272, 1966.

Havighurst, R. J.: Developmental tasks and education, ed. 3, New York, 1972, David McKay Co., Inc.

de Hirsch, K.: A review of early language development, Dev. Med. Child Neurol. **12:**87-97, February 1970.

Hughes, J. G.: Synopsis of pediatrics, ed. 4, St. Louis, 1975, The C. V. Mosby Co.

Hurlock, E. B.: Child development, New York, 1972, McGraw-Hill Book Co.

Illingworth, R. S.: The development of the infant and young child, ed. 5, Edinburgh, 1972, Churchill Livingstone.

Johnson, R. C., and Medinnus, G. R.: Child psychology, ed. 3, New York, 1974, John Wiley & Sons, Inc.

Kagan, J.: Understanding children: behavior, motives and thought, New York, 1971, Harcourt Brace Jovanovich, Inc.

Kaluger, G., and Kaluger, M. F.: Human development: the span of life, ed. 2, St. Louis, 1979, The C. V. Mosby Co.

Kosslyn, S. M., Pick, H. L., and Fariello, G. R.: Cognitive maps in children and men, Child Dev. **45:**707-716, 1974.

Lash, J., and Whittaker, J. R.: Concepts of development, Stamford, Conn., 1974, Sinauer Associates, Inc.

Lowrey, G. H.: Growth and development of children, ed. 6, Chicago, 1973, Year Book Medical Publishers, Inc.

Lewis, M.: Clinical aspects of child development, Philadelphia, 1971, Lea & Febiger.

McNeill, D.: The development of language. In Mussen, P., editor: Carmichael's manual of child psychology, New York, 1970, John Wiley & Sons, Inc.

Maslow, A. H.: Toward a psychology of being, ed. 2, New York, 1968, Van Nostrand Reinhold Co.

Mussen, P. H., Conger, J. J., and Kagan, J.: Child development and personality, ed. 4, New York, 1974, Harper & Row, Publishers.

Newman, B. M., and Newman, P. R.: Development through life, Homewood, Ill., 1975, Dorsey Press.

Paluszny, M.: Sexual identity and role in children, Clin. Pediatr. **13:**154-158, February 1974.
Petrillo, M., and Sangay, S.: Emotional care of the hospitalized child, Philadelphia, 1972, J. B. Lippincott Co.
Phillips, J. L.: The origins of intellect: Piaget's theory, San Francisco, 1969, W. H. Freeman and Co. Publishers.
Piaget, J.: The theory of stages in cognitive development, New York, 1969, McGraw-Hill Book Co.
Piaget, J., and Inhelder, B.: The psychology of the child, New York, 1969, Basic Books, Inc., Publishers.
Piers, M. W.: Play and development, New York, 1972, W. W. Norton & Co., Inc.
Reed, C. E., editor: The learning of language, New York, 1971, Appleton-Century-Crofts.
Slobin, D. I.: They learn the same way all around the world, Psychol. Today **6:**71-82, 1972.
Smart, M. S., and Smart, R. C.: Children: development and relationships, ed. 3, New York, 1977, Macmillan, Inc.
Smith, D. W., and Bierman, E. L.: The biologic ages of man, Philadelphia, 1973, W. B. Saunders Co.
Smith, D. W., and Marshall, R. E., editors: Introduction to clinical pediatrics, Philadelphia, 1972, W. B. Saunders Co.
Smolensky, J.: A guide to child growth and development, Dubuque, Iowa, 1973, Kendall/Hunt Publishing Co.
Stevenson, H. W.: Learning and reinforcement effects. In Spencer, T. D., and Kass, N., editors: Perspectives in child psychology, New York, 1970, McGraw-Hill Book Co.
Stone, L. J., and Church, J.: Childhood and adolescence, ed. 3, New York, 1973, Random House, Inc.
Sutterly, D. C., and Donnelly, G. G.: Perspectives in human development, Philadelphia, 1973, J. B. Lippincott Co.
Thomson, A. M.: The evaluation of human growth patterns, Am. J. Dis. Child. **120:**398-403, November 1970.
Timiras, P. S.: Developmental physiology and aging, New York, 1972, Macmillan, Inc.
Toman, W.: Family constellation, ed. 2, New York, 1969, Springer Publishing Co., Inc.
Whitten, C. F.: T.L.C. and the hungry child, Nutr. Today **7:**10-14, January/December 1972.
Williams, S. R.: Nutrition and diet therapy, ed. 3, St. Louis, 1977, The C. V. Mosby Co.
Wipple, D. V.: Dynamics of development: euthenic pediatrics, New York, 1966, McGraw-Hill Book Co.
Wu, R.: Child development: a basis for nursing care. In Bergersen, B., and associates, editors: Current concepts in clinical nursing, vol. 2, St. Louis, 1969, The C. V. Mosby Co.

UNIT TWO

Assessment of child and family

Fundamental to the nursing process is assessment. Establishing a data base on which to formulate a nursing diagnosis, base plans of intervention, and evaluate outcomes of care is essential whether the nurse is involved with a well or an ill child. Assessment facilitates identification of present problems and prevention of future ones. Although the assessment process primarily focuses on the child, it permits an exploration into the family dynamics and often is the first clue to cultural, environmental, socioeconomic, or religious traditions that influence the child's total well-being.

Traditionally the skills of history taking and physical examination have been sharply defined between the medical and nursing professions. With the trend toward expanded roles in nursing, these activities are gradually being assumed by an increasing number of nurses. Chapter 4, *History Taking of the Child and Family,* is concerned primarily with history taking of the child and family. Chapter 5, *Physical Assessment of the Child,* deals with the procedures and skills required to perform a complete pediatric physical assessment, including sensory and developmental testing. Findings primarily related to normal structure and function are emphasized, with notation of those deviations that require further evaluation.

4

History taking of the child and family

This chapter is mainly concerned with assessment through history taking. Each section of the history is discussed in considerable detail to allow the reader an opportunity to learn what constitutes a thorough assessment. The precise depth and extent of a nursing history vary with its intended purpose. In primary health care, all areas need to be complete. During the hospital admission interview, personal/social and past history are of primary importance. For nurses involved in genetic counseling, a review of systems and the family history take precedence. The nurse uses judgment in deciding what data are necessary and relevant for the identification of problems.

The format used resembles a medical history, but the objective of each assessment area is the identification of nursing diagnoses or patient problems. The value in following the well-established medical approach is that it is systematic and familiar in sequence and intent to members of the health team. Although different titles can be used for organization of the data, the following categories encompass the person's current and past health status and information about his or her psychosocial environment[5]:

1. Chief complaint (CC): to establish the major *specific* reason for the individual's seeking professional health attention
2. Present illness (PI): to obtain *all* details related to the chief complaint
3. Past history (PH): to elicit a profile of the individual's previous illnesses, injuries, or operations
4. Review of systems (ROS): to elicit information concerning any potential health problem
5. Family history (FH): to identify the presence of genetic traits or diseases that have familial tendencies, to assess exposure to a communicable disease in a family member, and potentially to assess the individual's reactions to disease or death in the family
6. Personal/social history (P/SH): to develop an understanding of the person as an individual and as a member of a family and a community
7. Patient profile (P/P): to summarize the interviewer's overall impression of the individual's physical, psychologic, and socioeconomic background

The major subdivisions included in each of the categories in a pediatric health history are listed in the boxed ma-

Outline of a pediatric health history

Identifying information
1. Name
2. Address
3. Telephone
4. Age and birthdate
5. Race
6. Sex
7. Religion
8. Nationality
9. Date of interview
10. Informant

Chief complaint

Present illness

Past history
1. Birth history
2. Feeding history
3. Previous illnesses, injuries, or operations
4. Allergies
5. Current medications
6. Immunizations
7. Growth and development
8. Habits

Review of systems
1. General
2. Integument
3. Head
4. Eyes
5. Ears
6. Nose
7. Mouth, teeth, tongue, and gums
8. Throat and neck
9. Chest
10. Respiratory
11. Cardiovascular
12. Gastrointestinal
13. Genitourinary
14. Gynecologic (obstetric)
15. Musculoskeletal
16. Neuropsychiatric
17. Lymphatic and hematologic
18. Endocrine

Family history
1. Family pedigree
2. Familial diseases and congenital anomalies

Personal/social history
1. Home and community environment
2. Occupation and education of family members
3. Cultural and religious traditions
4. Marital and sexual history

Patient profile (summary)
1. Health status
2. Psychologic status
3. Socioeconomic status

terial. This format is a general plan for organization of data. Areas such as "habits" can also be placed under personal/social history, especially if inquiry into habits may be more anxiety provoking, such as questions about drug abuse or alcoholism. Depending on the age of the child, some categories will assume more or less importance, such as birth history, feeding schedule, immunization, growth and development, and sexual history.

APPROACHES TO TAKING A HEALTH HISTORY

Establishing the setting

Part of the success in taking a complete and detailed health history depends on the type of physical and psychologic setting that the interviewer constructs. Appropriate introduction, role clarification, explanation of the reason for the history, preliminary acquaintance with the family, and assurance of privacy and confidentiality are prerequisites for establishing a setting conducive to communication.

Appropriate introduction. Nurses introduce themselves to, and ask the name of, each family member who is present. During the history and physical examination, each person is addressed by name. In this way the nurse immediately conveys respect for each person and communicates a personal interest in him.

During the introduction the nurse attempts to identify the most reliable informant. If one parent accompanies the child, there is no choice of informant, unless the child is old enough to answer for himself. However, if more than one adult is present, which one is the primary care giver is determined. This is particularly important if the mother and grandmother accompany the child. Often, in young single-parent families, the maternal grandmother assumes some or all of the child-care responsibilities. The nurse can indirectly assess this information during the preliminary acquaintance by asking who is home with the child during the day, who lives with the child, if the mother works or goes to school, or who spends the most time with the child. It is especially important to ask such questions in a nonjudgmental, casual manner, because many parents may feel insecure of their part-time or shared parenting responsibilities.

At the very beginning of the visit, the nurse includes the child in the interaction by asking him his name, age, and other information. Often, nurses direct all questions to the adult, even when the child is old enough to speak for himself. This serves to terminate one extremely valuable source of information, the patient himself. When including the child, the general rules for communicating with children are followed (see p. 11).

Role clarification and explanation of the history. During the introduction it is also necessary to clarify the nurse's particular role in the health setting. Nurses performing histories may be pediatric nurse practitioners, inpatient staff nurses, clinic staff nurses, office nurses, visiting nurses, or school nurses. Since the format resembles a medical history, the nurse needs to clarify the reason for eliciting this information. A nurse is much more likely to induce a parent to reveal personal information about the child and family if the relevance and importance of a history are stressed. If this is not done, parents may refuse to elaborate on certain areas because they feel it has no bearing on the "problem." Also, since more than one member of the health team may take a history during the course of a hospital admission, it is important to clarify the reason for each history. For example, the staff nurse who performs an admission history needs to explain why similar questions such as feeding, elimination, etc. are repeated. The redundancy of several histories during a clinic or hospital visit also supports the need for collaboration among health personnel.

Another reason for role clarification is education of the health consumer. With expanded roles in nursing, it is not unusual for families to think that the examiner is a physician, not a nurse. Role clarification is especially important because some parents may feel deceived if they later are made aware of the nurse's identity. Since the general consumer acceptance of pediatric nurse practitioners has been very favorable, it is also important to acknowledge the expertise of the nurse by emphasizing the nurses' role.

Preliminary acquaintance. When one contemplates the personal and private nature of a complex, detailed health history, one also wonders at the human trust the person being interviewed needs to have for the interviewer in order to reveal such extensive information. Therefore, it is best to commence the history with some general conversation. This should not be lengthy because a health history demands considerable time. However, the opening statements can be general, but still informative. Comments such as, "How have things been since your last visit?" "Tell me about Johnny," or (to the child) "What do you think is going to happen today?" allow the parent or child to express his main concern in a casual, relaxed atmosphere.

The preliminary acquaintance conversation also reveals how responsive the informant may be to questions. For example, using open-ended statements, such as, "Tell me about the baby," may lead the parent into a lengthy detailed discussion. In this case the nurse may find it more beneficial to direct questions toward specific answers in order to avoid tangential remarks. At other times a parent may respond to open-ended questions with only minimal information, in which case the continued use of open-ended questions probably reveals more data than "yes" or "no" type questions.

Assurance of privacy and confidentiality. The place where the interview is conducted is almost as important as the interview itself. The physical environment should allow for at least sound privacy during the history and visual privacy during the examination. There should be minimal distractions during the interview, such as interruptions, ambient noise, or other visible activity. The environment should also have some play provision for young children to keep them occupied during the parent-nurse interview. Parents who are constantly interrupted by their children are unable to concentrate fully on the questions asked of them. As a result, they tend to give short, brief answers to terminate the visit as quickly as possible.

Confidentiality is also an essential component of the initial phase of the interview. Since the history is usually shared with others, such as other members of the nursing staff, the physician, or the teacher (as in the case of students), it is the interviewer's responsibility and obligation to establish the confidential limits of the history. The way in which the nurse establishes the setting for the interview communicates to families how confidential and respected their history will be. Assuring privacy, communicating concern, and temporarily terminating questioning if interrupted bespeak confidentiality and, therefore, trust in the relationship.

Communicating effectively

No history can be reliable unless communication is effective. Although it is not the intent of this discussion to elaborate on effective communication, several points are particularly important for history taking. (1) Avoid judgment; use the person's words (in quotes whenever possible) or statements of fact, rather than interpretation. (2) Clarify words or questions; do not assume that the person knows what is asked. For example, when asking about "immunizations," substitute the phrase "baby shots" if the parent does not give specific answers. (3) Observe the person's emotional state. Anxiety can markedly reduce the reliability of information. (4) Be aware of personal attitudes or anxieties. Questioning parents about their marital status may arouse personal feelings in the nurse if the nurse is having difficulty in private life in this area. (5) Avoid premature offers of advice. Doing so may immediately terminate parents' willingness to reveal information if they feel judged or criticized.

Listening. Listening is the most important ingredient for effective communication. Because the interview is almost always triangular—nurse, child, and parent—the parent may wish to convey information in such a way as to prevent the child from hearing it. The following example illustrates this point:

During a routine health visit, the nurse performed a complete history and physical examination on a 4-year-old girl. The child was accompanied by her mother, who appeared to be a reliable, well-informed, and talkative informant. During the child's birth history, the mother gave all the information asked. However, during the family history, the mother stated to the nurse, "I had a hysterectomy 6 years ago." Because the nurse gave no indication of acknowledging the significance of this statement, the mother repeated it, only this time she stressed the "6 years." The nurse, who had not been listening as attentively as she should have, realized that the mother was telling her something very important. The mother raised her eyebrows and gently shook her head "no," warning the nurse not to explore this area too openly. The nurse correctly read the cues and stated, "Let's return to your health history later."

At the completion of the physical examination, the nurse brought the child to the Health Center's playroom and took the opportunity to investigate this contradictory information of a "4-year-old child born to a woman with a hysterectomy 6 years ago." The mother revealed that this child was adopted. The mother was greatly concerned about the fact that the child was unaware of this and requested the nurse's advice.

Fortunately, the nurse had "listened" carefully enough to realize the significance of this woman's concern and allowed her the opportunity to discuss it in private.

Listening is also helpful in assessing reliability. For example, the answers elicited at the beginning of the history may differ from those at the end of the interview, when the parent feels more confident in revealing problems. It is important to identify any discrepancies and reintroduce those topics for further investigation.

Directing the focus. One of the hazards in listening is that the parent will talk at great length about a subject that has little relevance to the history. Ability to direct the focus of the interview, while allowing for maximum freedom of expression, is one of the most difficult goals in effective communication. One approach toward directing the focus or avoiding tangential statements is using fact-finding questions, such as, "Do you have other children?" Although this type of question certainly has its function, the answer may be very limiting and usually requires additional questions to elicit sufficient data. Using open-ended statements, such as, "Tell me about your other children," often allows for more than the desired information but provides the parent the opportunity to voice concerns that otherwise may not have been revealed.

One approach that directs the focus but allows an opportunity for expanded discussion is the use of open-ended or broad questions, followed with guiding statements. For example, if the parent proceeds to list the other children by name, the nurse can also say, "Tell me their ages, too." If the parent continues on this theme by describing each child in depth, which is not the purpose of the interview, the nurse can redirect the focus by stating, "Let's talk about the other children later. You were beginning to tell me about Paul's activities at school." This approach conveys interest in the other children but focuses the data collection on the identified patient.

In the event that the parent has suggested that a problem exists with one of the other children, the nurse should reintroduce this subject at the end of the interview to assess the need for further family follow-up. Saying to the parent, "Before, you were mentioning that your older son is having trouble in school. Tell me what you see as the problem,'' reintroduces this subject but only in terms of the possible problem. If the nurse fails to focus on one aspect, it is likely that another lengthy complete history could be initiated, which may not be appropriate for the present interview.

Assessing reliability. Once the informant has been identified, the nurse must make some judgment regarding the individual's reliability, or accuracy of the revealed data in terms of repeatability. A totally reliable informant will always give the same answers to questions. Because it has been shown that the reliability of maternal recall is often deficient,[2] it is important for nurses to compare the data from a verbal history with another source of recorded information to ensure some degree of accuracy. For example, recall data concerning immunizations should be checked against actual vaccination records. The mother's description of previous developmental milestones should be compared to objective findings from a current developmental screening test. The exact nature of previous illnesses and treatments should be evaluated against recorded hospital charts.

Several generalizations are also worthy in considering the parent's reliability.[2] (1) Concrete facts, such as birth weight, length, and date are recalled most accurately. (2) Minor illnesses are forgotten more easily than major ones. The high level of anxiety associated with a stressful event facilitates accurate recall. (3) Mothers, particularly those of firstborns, tend to exaggerate the child's achievement of developmental skills. (4) Mothers of several children tend to be less accurate in their recall of most items than mothers of single children. (5) The mother's educational level is directly related to the accuracy of recall for some items, such as immunizations. (6) More specific and detailed questioning considerably increases the accuracy of recall.

The last generalization is particularly significant to the discussion of effective communication. Nurses who utilize the suggestions for approaches to history taking are more likely to positively influence reliable parent recall than are those who fail to consider such factors.

Using an interpreter. Sometimes effective communication is blocked because two people speak different languages. In this case, it is necessary to obtain information through a third party, the interpreter. Because this is not an infrequent situation, it is important to discuss effective ways of communicating via interpreters.[3]

Role clarification and explanation of the interview. The nurse introduces herself to the interpreter and explains the reason for the interview and the type of questions she will ask. An interpreter should know whether a detailed or brief answer is required and whether the translated response can be general or literal.

Introduction and preliminary acquaintance. The nurse introduces the interpreter to each family member. Ideally, the interpreter and parent are allowed some time together before the actual interview so that they can become acquainted.

Communicate directly with the parent. When asking questions, the nurse addresses the parent directly in order to reinforce interest in the parent. The nurse observes carefully for nonverbal expressions and mentally notes to ask the interpreter about these later. It is important to refrain from interrupting the parent and interpreter while they are conversing. If the parent answers statements with lengthy discussions, it may be necessary to use more direct questions, rather than open-ended ones. If the translation is shorter than the actual answer, do not assume that the interpreter is withholding information. He or she may have had difficulty in understanding the explanation and needed time for clarification.

Avoid commenting to the interpreter about the patient. It is best to presume that the parent understands some English.

Respect cultural differences. It is often necessary to pose questions about sex, marriage, or pregnancy indirectly. For example, it is best to ask about the child's ''father'' rather than the mother's ''husband.'' Be aware of difficulty on the part of the interpreter in asking such questions.

Communicate directly with the interpreter. Following the interview, allow time to share information with the interpreter in private. This is the time to ask about nonverbal clues to communication, to ask for personal interpretations of the parent's reliability, ease in revealing information, and so on, and to allow the interpreter an opportunity to share something that he or she felt could not be said earlier.

Continuity. Whenever possible, arrange for the parent to speak with the same interpreter on subsequent visits. This helps all three parties feel more comfortable and facilitates effective translation of both words and feelings.

These guidelines apply primarily to the use of an adult interpreter. Often, no one other than an older child is available to help translate. In this situation it is important to stress *literal* translation of parent responses. To maximize correct translations, it may be necessary to interrupt the parent and ask the child to translate every few sentences. When children are used as interpreters, the nurse needs to ask questions directed at specific answers and must assess the interpreted translation in terms of nonverbal expressions of communication.

Using a systematic approach

A systematic approach to data collection has several important functions: (1) it assures consistency and completeness, (2) it allows for individualized nursing care based on a large number of variables, (3) it maximizes the amount and quality of data collection within a short period of time, (4) it provides baseline data for future evaluation of health status and efficacy of care, and (5) it provides an immediate basis for decisions making regarding the planning of nursing care.[4]

Using the direct or indirect approach. The format used for history taking may be (1) direct—the nurse asks the information via direct interview with the informant, or (2) indirect—the informant supplies the information by completing some type of questionnaire. The direct method is superior to the indirect approach or a combination of both. However, in view of time constraints, the nurse may find that the direct approach is not always practical. If so, it is important to review informants' written responses and question parents regarding any unusual answers.

The direct method can lose its value if the nurse asks questions directly from a form. In essence, the parent is completing the form by listening to it, rather than reading it. Using a systematic approach does not imply rote memory of a specific outline. Rather, it denotes the use of categories to define what areas of information are required. If nurses use as a model the seven basic categories outlined on p. 87 and understand the objective of each, they can then obtain the required information as it arises during the course of the conversation. However, the nurse should record the history using the specified format.

PERFORMING A HEALTH HISTORY

The following discussion focuses primarily on the types of information that should be elicited under each major category. The general outline of a pediatric health history (boxed material on p. 87) is used as one example of a systematic approach.

Identifying information

Much of the identifying information may already be available to the nurse from other recorded sources. However, if the parent seems anxious, the nurse may well use this opportunity to ask about such information to help the parent feel more comfortable.

Informant. Although most of the required information is self-explanatory, the nurse should record certain data under informant, such as the identified person, the subjective impression of reliability, his or her willingness to communicate, his or her general state or attitude, and any special circumstances, such as the use of an interpreter. An example of a statement for informant is: "Mother, reliability questionable, answers items with hesitation, speaks primarily Spanish, interpreter (Mrs. ______) present for history."

Chief complaint

The chief complaint represents the specific reason for the child's visit to the clinic, office, or hospital. The chief complaint may be viewed as the theme with the present illness as the description of the problem. Six guidelines determine appropriate recording of the chief complaint: (1) it is limited to a brief statement, (2) it is restricted to one or two symptoms, (3) it refers to a concrete complaint, (4) it is recorded in the child's or parent's own words, (5) it avoids the use of diagnostic terms or translations, and (6) it states the duration of the symptoms.

The nurse elicits the chief complaint by asking open-ended neutral questions, such as, "Tell me what seems to be the matter," "How may I help you?" or "What brings you here?" Labeling-type questions, such as, "How are you sick?" should be avoided, since it is possible that the reason for the visit is not because of illness. For example, the visit may be for a routine health assessment, or the chief complaint may be of a nonphysical nature. Examples of properly recorded chief complaints for a variety of situations may be: (1) ambulatory clinic—"My child has had a runny nose and sore throat for 4 days, but today it is worse," (2) hospital admission—"I need to have my tonsils fixed," sore throat and repeated earaches for 5 years, and (3) health center—"We are here for a routine checkup," last visit 1 year ago.

Occasionally it is difficult to isolate one symptom or problem as the chief complaint because the parent may identify many. In this situation it is important to be as specific as possible when asking questions. For example, asking informants to state which *one* problem or symptom caused them to seek help now may help them focus on the most immediate concern.

Present illness

The history of the present illness* is a narrative of the chief complaint from its earliest onset through its progression to the present. Its four major components are: (1) details of onset, (2) complete *interval* history, (3) *present* status, and (4) reason for seeking help *now*.[5] The focus of the present illness is on all those factors that are relevant to the main problem, even if they have disappeared or changed during the onset, interval, and present.

Analyzing a symptom. Since pain is often the most characteristic symptom denoting onset of a physical problem, the nurse should assess pain for (1) type, (2) location, (3) severity, (4) duration, and (5) influencing factors.[5] The *type* or character of pain should be as specific as possible. However, with young children, it is almost always impossible for them to describe the pain. Asking the parents how they know the child is in pain may help describe its type, location, and severity. For example, a mother stated, "My child must have a severe earache because she pulls at her ears, rolls her head on the floor, and screams. Nothing seems to help."

The nurse can help older children describe the pain by asking them if it is sharp, throbbing, dull, aching, stabbing, and so on. Whatever words they use should be recorded in quotes.

---

*NOTE: The term "illness" is used in its broadest sense to denote any problem of a physical, emotional, or psychosocial nature. It is actually a history of the chief complaint.

The location of the pain also must be specific. "Stomach pains" is too general a description. Children can better localize the pain if the nurse asks them to "point with one finger to where it hurts." The nurse can also determine if the pain radiates by asking, "Does the pain stay there or move? Show me where it goes with your finger."

The *severity* of pain is best determined by finding out how it affects the child's usual behavior. Pain that prevents a child from playing, interacting with others, sleeping, and eating is most often severe. It is preferable to record pain in terms of interference with activity, rather than to quote the parent's or child's adjectives.

Duration of pain should include the duration, onset, and frequency of attacks. It may be necessary to describe this in terms of activity and behavior, such as "pain lasted all night because child refused to sleep and cried intermittently."

Influencing factors are anything that causes a change in the type, location, severity, or duration of the pain. These include (1) precipitating events (those that cause or increase the pain), (2) relieving events (those that lessen the pain, such as medications), (3) temporal events (times when the pain is relieved or increased), (4) positional events (standing, sitting, lying down, and so on), and (5) associated events (meals, stress, coughing, and so on).

A standard method of analyzing a symptom is listed below. These three categories—onset, characteristics, and course since onset—comprise the essential data for the present illness. Although the analysis of a symptom has concentrated on discussion of physical complaints, the same process of description and investigation can be used for emotional or psychosocial problems.

*Analysis of a symptom**

1. Onset
- **a.** Date of onset
- **b.** Manner of onset (gradual or sudden)
- **c.** Precipitating and predisposing factors related to onset (emotional disturbance, physical exertion, fatigue, bodily function, pregnancy, environment, injury, infection, toxins and allergens, therapeutic agents, and so on)

2. Characteristics
- **a.** Character (quality, quantity, consistency, or other)
- **b.** Location and radiation (of pain)
- **c.** Intensity or severity
- **d.** Timing (continuous or intermittent, duration of each, temporal relationship to other events)
- **e.** Aggravating and relieving factors
- **f.** Associated symptoms

3. Course since onset
- **a.** Incidence
  - **1.** Single acute attack
  - **2.** Recurrent acute attacks
  - **3.** Daily occurrences
  - **4.** Periodic occurrences
  - **5.** Continuous chronic episode
- **b.** Progress (better, worse, unchanged)
- **c.** Effect of therapy

*From Hochstein, E., and Rubin, A.: Physical diagnosis: a textbook and workbook in methods of clinical examination, New York. Copyright 1964, McGraw-Hill Book Co. Used with permission of McGraw-Hill Book Co.

Determining the reason for seeking help. The preceding discussion deals primarily with the description of the problem. However, from the fact that most chief complaints have a "duration," it follows that something significant must have occurred to motivate the person to seek help at this time. Such factors may be a change in physical status, a change in behavioral reaction, or a result of social pressure. Eliciting such information may alter the possible nursing diagnoses and plan of care. The following example illustrates the potential significance of determining why a person seeks help at a particular time:

Chief complaint: "I can't control my son. It's been a problem, but for the past year and a half it has become worse."

Present history: Child has had temper tantrums since infancy. He "throws things, hits and kicks people, yells and screams." It occurs whenever he "doesn't get his way." They usually last "a minute or two" and occur at least weekly. Mother has responded to them in a variety of ways: hits him, ignores him, takes a special object or privilege away, insults him. Nothing seems to work. Mother admits that ignoring the behavior is the most difficult approach, and she rarely can do so without eventually hitting or scolding him.

Mother is not able to identify why she sought help now.

Further physical history revealed nothing unusual. Family history disclosed several significant facts, especially that (1) the father had died 2 months earlier, and (2) he had been ill for 1½ years prior to his death. The nurse focused the history on events that had occurred since the beginning of the father's illness, which coincided with the son's increased behavior problems. The mother revealed that during her husband's illness she had had too little time to concern herself with her son's behavior, other than realizing that it was a problem. However, after his death, she could no longer ignore its severity or disruptive effect on the family. As she verbalized these thoughts, she began to identify the specific reason for seeking help now. She stated, "I used to wait for my husband to come home to take the children off my hands. When he was sick, I was too busy worrying about him. But now I am home all alone. When dinnertime comes, there is no one to relieve me."

Although the interventions included several approaches to managing the problem, one of them focused on providing the mother with some freedom from the responsibility of total parenting. Had the nurse not concentrated on uncovering the mother's reason for seeking help at this particular time, a very important clue in planning care might have been missed.

Past history

The past history contains information relating to all previous aspects of the child's health status and concentrates on several areas that are ordinarily deleted in the history of an adult, such as birth history, detailed feeding history, immunizations, and growth and development. Since a great deal of data is included in this section, it is more efficient for nurses to use a combination of open-ended and fact-finding questions. For example, the nurse may begin interviewing for each section with an open-ended statement, such as "Tell me about your child's birth," in order to provide the informant with the opportunity to relate what he or she thinks is most important. Fact-finding questions related to specific details are asked whenever necessary to focus the interview on certain topics.

Open-ended questions also allow the informant an opportunity for control in the disclosure of personal information. For example, in the beginning of the interview, the parent may reveal purely factual data about the birth history. However, as the interview continues, the parent may be willing to disclose other significant data, such as the presence or absence of the child's father during and after delivery. The voluntary willingness to reveal such information is generally an indication of the increasing trust and developing rapport between the nurse and parent. It may also be a signal that the parent feels confident enough to discuss other aspects of his or her personal life. The nurse may at this point focus on the social history, particularly as it relates to the present topic. At no time should the nurse insinuate or directly admonish the parent for not disclosing certain information earlier in the history. It is important to remember that although the history is written according to a specific format, the order of questioning may vary considerably.

Birth history. Birth history includes all data concerning (1) the mother's health during pregnancy, (2) the labor and delivery, and (3) the infant's condition immediately after birth. Since prenatal influences have significant effects on a child's physical and emotional development, a thorough investigation of birth history is essential. Since parents may question what relevance pregnancy and birth have on the child's present condition, particularly if the child is past infancy, it is best to explain why such questions are included. The nurse may state to the parents: "I will be asking you some questions about your pregnancy and ________'s (refer to child by name) birth. Your answers will give me a more complete picture of his overall health."

Pregnancy and labor and delivery. Pregnancy history should begin with an overview of the pregnancy, preferably by an open-ended question, such as, "How was your pregnancy?" This allows the mother to state what she thought was most significant. Most importantly, the nurse should ask about the use of medications or other remedies that the mother used to relieve the physical symptoms. For example, one mother, whose 3-year-old child had obviously discolored teeth, revealed that she had taken tetracycline during her pregnancy. She was unaware of the drug's effect on the formation of tooth enamel and thought that the child's brown teeth were the result of inadequate oral hygiene. For specific guidelines determining the pregnancy and labor and delivery history, refer to p. 235.

Because emotional factors also affect the outcome of pregnancy and the subsequent parent-child relationship, it is important for the nurse to investigate (1) concurrent crises during pregnancy and (2) prenatal attitudes toward the fetus. One way of assessing the former is to inquire about the mother's activities during pregnancy. For example, one mother stated, "I worked all during my pregnancy. I had to work. I have two other children to support. It was a constant worry to me." The nurse was able to use this information to ask about the mother's feelings concerning another child by stating in a questioning tone, "Working was a constant worry during your last pregnancy?" The mother replied, "Yes. In fact, I thought of having an abortion because this child was a mistake." The nurse then asked, "How do you feel now?" The mother answered, "As soon as I felt him move inside me, I knew I could never give him up. Now, of course, I love him. But after that pregnancy I had my tubes tied." Had the mother not disclosed the particular type of birth control she was using, the nurse could have focused on the subject of contraception. Although the history is primarily about the child, for effective, comprehensive care planning, it must focus on the child as a member of the family.

It is best to approach the topic of parental acceptance of pregnancy through indirect questioning. Asking parents if the pregnancy was planned is a leading statement because they may respond affirmatively for fear of criticism if the pregnancy was unexpected. The nurse can encourage parents to disclose their true reactions by referring to specific facts relating to the pregnancy, such as the spacing between offspring, an extended or short interval between marriage and conception, or the concurrent experience of pregnancy and adolescence. The parent can choose to explore such statements with further explanations or, for the moment, may not be able to reveal such feelings. Silence should alert the nurse to the importance of refocusing on this topic later in the interview.

Perinatal history. The perinatal period refers to the first 28 days of extrauterine life, but the primary focus is on the immediate period after birth and during hospitalization. Specific data include: weight and length at birth, loss of weight following delivery, time of regaining birth weight, and condition of health immediately after birth, such as quality of cry, level of activity (feeble or vigorous), Apgar score (some mothers may be aware of this), color of skin, and possible problems, such as fever, convulsions, hemorrhage, snuffles, skin eruptions, desquamation, paralysis, birth injuries, deformities, or congenital anomalies. If any birth problems are reported, medical treatment or correction and the parents' emotional response to the event should be inquired about.

Feeding history. The exact question the nurse asks to elicit a feeding history depends on the child's age. In general, the younger the child, the more specific and detailed the feeding history should be. In regard to infant feeding, the following information is important: type of feeding (breast, commercial preparation, home preparation, special formulas), time and reason for changing feeding habits (breast to bottle, bottle to cup, one type of formula to another, formula to regular milk, introduction of solid foods), interval of feedings, time required for one feeding, apparent appetite, quantity consumed, addition of vitamins, weight change, any problems associated with feeding (vomiting, diarrhea, colic, "spitting up," rumination, refusal to eat), and remedies used for each problem.

For older children it is best to use a "diet diary" approach for eliciting a feeding history by asking the parent to list "what the child ate yesterday" and ascertaining if that menu was typical of most days. The nurse should ask specific questions about snacks between meals, special likes and dislikes, changes in the appetite, and eating habits, such as time at the table. The nurse should then analyze the daily food diary by comparing it to the four basic food groups. For example, if the list includes no vegetables, the nurse should ask the reason for this, rather than assume that the child dislikes vegetables, because it may be that the mother failed to serve any on that day. Based on the specific details of the nutrition history, the nurse would then plan appropriate counseling following completion of the assessment.

Because cultural practices are very prevalent in food preparation, it is important to consider carefully the kind of questions that the nurse asks and the judgment made in regard to counseling. For example, some cultures, such as Puerto Rican, Mexican, black, and American Indian, include many vegetables, legumes, and starches in their diet that together provide sufficient amounts of essential amino acids, even though the actual amount of meat or dairy protein may be low.

Also, many cultures believe in feeding the infant formula, cow's milk, or human milk for extended periods of time. Since iron-deficiency anemia is the most prevalent nutritional problem in the United States, it is essential that the nurse assess the total number of ounces of milk consumed by the child. However, the way in which one gathers this information may influence the reliability of the data. For example, many parents are aware of the fact that "doctors say babies shouldn't drink too much milk." Therefore, if the nurse asks, "How much milk does your child drink?" the parent may know the correct "medical" answer. If the nurse suspects a greater quantity than what the parent states, the next question can be, "Are you sure he drinks enough milk?" This gives parents the opportunity to change their answer, because the nurse has altered the perceived "expected" response. The nurse should accept all subsequent information neutrally and, throughout the history, refrain from initiating counseling until the assessment is completed. Otherwise, the informant's willingness to disclose other data may be prematurely terminated.

Previous illnesses, injuries, and operations. When inquiring about past medical illnesses, the nurse can begin with a general statement, such as, "What other illnesses has your child had?" Since parents are most likely to recall serious health problems, it is important to specifically ask about colds, earaches, and common childhood diseases, such as measles, rubella (German measles), chickenpox, mumps, pertussis (whooping cough), diphtheria, scarlet fever, strep throat, tonsillitis, or allergic manifestations. It is best not to accept simple statements from the parents regarding the nature of the disease. Rather, encourage them to give onset, symptoms, course, and termination. For example, it is not uncommon for parents to confuse measles with rubella or strep throat with tonsillitis. Other important information concerning previous illnesses includes occurrence of similar symptoms in other children at the same time, course of convalescence with or without complications or sequelae, and geographic incidence of the disease.

In addition to illnesses, the nurse also questions the parent about injuries that required medical intervention, operations, and any other reason for hospitalization, including dates of each incident. It is important to focus on injuries such as accidental falls, poisonings, choking, or burns, since this may be a potential area for parental guidance. While obtaining a history of the injury, what happened prior to the accident (who was the child with, where were the parents, had this ever happened before) should be ascertained as well as what immediate action the parent took. For example, if the child ingested a foreign substance, specific questions should be asked about how the parents identified the incident, how they reacted to it, where they called for help, and what emergency measures they instituted.

The nurse also inquires about the child's emotional reactions to each experience, since this may have significant relevance. For example, one mother stated that her 4-year-old daughter had recently been admitted to the hospital for respiratory distress. She added that the child reacted poorly to the experience and that since then she had been very afraid of all medical personnel, procedures, and equipment. The nurse realized from this information that the child needed special preparation for the physical examination.

Allergies. The nurse asks about commonly known allergic disorders, such as hay fever and asthma, as well as unusual reactions to food, drugs, or contact agents, such as poisonous plants, animals, household products, or fabrics. It is especially important to have the parent describe the allergic reactions to drugs, since a known side effect can be confused with an allergic reaction. If the child has a known allergy to eggs, it is important to inquire about reactions to specific immunizations, such as measles or rubella.

Current medications. In addition to any allergies to drugs, the nurse asks about current drug regimens, including vitamins, aspirin, antibiotics, antihistamines, decongestants, or antitussives. All medications should be listed, including name, dose, schedule, duration, and reason for administration. Not infrequently, parents are unaware of the actual name of the drug. Whenever possible, it is advisable to ask parents to bring the containers to the hospital during the next visit. It is also possible to ask them for the name of the pharmacy and to call directly for a list of all the child's recent prescription medications. However, this approach does not uncover over-the-counter medications.

Immunizations. A record of all immunizations or "baby shots" is essential. Since many parents are unaware of the exact name and date of each immunization, the most reliable source of information is a hospital, clinic, or private physician's record. All immunizations and "boosters" should be listed, stating name of the specific disease, number of injections, dosage (sometimes lesser amounts are given if a reaction is anticipated), ages when administered, and the occurrence of any reaction following the immunization. The nurse should also inquire about the previous administration of any horse or other foreign serum, recent administration of gamma globulin or blood transfusion, or sensitivity to egg albumin.

Since tuberculin testing is commonly performed in conjunction with certain immunizations, the nurse should also inquire about this. If parents are not sure if testing was done, the nurse should explain the usual procedure to increase their recall of the event. If testing was done, the nurse also records the child's positive or negative intradermal reaction.

Growth and development. The reliability of parents' recall of physical growth and developmental milestones is frequently questionable. Whenever possible, the responses should be compared to existing health records or to current evaluation of actual growth (height, weight, and dentition) and developmental performance (screening tests such as Denver Developmental Screening Test, grade in school, scholastic achievement, play activities, and social relationships).

The most important previous growth patterns to record are: (1) approximate weight at 6 months, 1 year, 2 years, and 5 years of age, (2) approximate length at ages 1 and 4 years, and (3) dentition, including age of onset, number of teeth, and symptoms during teething. Developmental milestones include: (1) age of holding up head steadily, (2) age of sitting alone without support, (3) age of walking without assistance, (4) age of saying first words with meaning, (5) present grade in school, (6) scholastic grades, and (7) interaction with other children, peers, and adults.

The nurse should use specific and detailed questions when inquiring about each developmental milestone. For example, "sitting up" can mean many different activities, such as sitting propped up, sitting in one's lap, sitting with support, sitting up alone but in a hyperflexed position for assisted balance, or sitting up unsupported with the back slightly rounded. The clue to misunderstanding of the requested activity is an unusually early age of achievement. For instance, one mother claimed that her daughter could sit up at 2 months of age. When the nurse asked her to describe what the child did, the mother explained that the infant "sat up" in a high chair, in a person's lap, or in the stroller. When the nurse inquired if the infant could sit without help, the mother quickly replied, "The baby would fall over unless we padded her in or supported her in our arms; she couldn't sit alone until 8 months!" Had the nurse clarified exactly which activity was asked for, the mother would have responded correctly.

Occasionally, probing the area of developmental or intellectual performance is a delicate one for parents, especially if there is a question concerning the child's progress. Therefore, it is best to approach such questioning with broad questions, such as, "How is Jimmy doing in school?" rather than with qualifying statements, such as, "Does Jimmy do well in school?" If the parents' response is vague and general, it is advisable to follow with questions such as, "How does he do in spelling, reading, or math?" Since these questions are appropriate for older children, the nurse addresses them directly to the child, as well as to the parent, for comparison of responses and increased reliability.

Habits. Habits include (1) behavior patterns, such as nail biting, thumb-sucking, pica, rituals ("security" blanket or toy), and unusual movements (head banging, rocking, overt masturbation, walking on toes, and so on); (2) activities of daily living, such as hour of sleep and arising, duration of nighttime sleep and naps, type and duration of exercise, regularity of stools and urination, age of toilet training, and occurrences of daytime or nighttime bedwetting; (3) usual disposition as well as response to frustration; and (4) use or abuse of alcohol, drugs, coffee, and cigarettes.

The latter category is primarily applicable to adolescents, although nurses must be aware of the increasingly juvenile experimentation and use of potentially harmful substances. If a youngster admits to smoking, drinking, or drug use, the nurse records a specific average amount, such as one cigarette a week or two cans of beer on weekends. A statement such as "I pop pills once in awhile" has tremendously wide variations in meaning. Following this response with, "How many pills and when is once in a while?" yields a measurable intake of drugs. If older children deny use of such substances, it is advisable to inquire about past experimentation. Asking, "You mean you never tried to smoke or drink?'' implies that the nurse expects some such activity and consequently is likely to be nonjudgmental of an affirmative answer. She should also be aware of the confidential nature of such questioning and the adverse effect that the parents' presence may have on the adolescent's willingness to answer.

Review of systems

Review of systems is exactly what the title implies—a specific review of each body system, similar to the order of the physical examination. Often the history of the present illness provides a complete review of the system involved in the chief complaint. Since asking questions about other body systems may appear unrelated and irrelevant to the parents or child, it is important to precede the questioning with an explanation of why the nurse needs these data (similar to the explanation concerning relevance of birth history) and reassurance that the child's main problem has not been forgotten.

Although the items listed in each system review mainly physical deviations from health, their investigation is warranted even if the chief complaint is not directly related to illness. For example, one family who brought their 5-year-old child to the health center stated the main concern as ''inattentiveness, disinterest, and sullenness since toddlerhood.'' A review of systems revealed several episodes of earaches and sore throats and some delayed milestones in speech. Further auditory testing confirmed the diagnosis of partial hearing loss, which was the basis of the child's behavior problems.

The inclusion of data in review of systems is somewhat arbitrary. Some of the information recorded under ''Habits'' could also be included under the appropriate system, such as bowel and bladder habits under genitourinary system. The specific questions asked also vary according to the child's age. The gynecologic and/or obstetric review will necessarily be more detailed for the adolescent and young adult than for the child.

Interviewing is most efficient if a combination of open-ended and fact-finding questions are used. For example, it is beneficial to begin reviewing a specific system with a broad statement, such as, ''How has your child's general health been?'' or ''Has your child had any problems with his eyes?'' If the parent states that there have been past problems with some body function, the nurse should pursue this with an encouraging statement, such as, ''Tell me more about that.'' If the parent denies any problems, it is best to query for specific symptoms, such as, ''No headaches, bumping into objects, or squinting?'' If the parent reconfirms the absence of such symptoms, the nurse should make positive statements to this effect in the history, such as, ''Mother denies headaches, bumping into objects, or squinting.'' In this way, anyone who reviews the health history is aware of exactly what symptoms were investigated.

The following is an outline of suggested areas for review of each body system. Although medical terminology may be used to record a symptom during the interview, the nurse should use terms that are clearly understood by the parent or child.

general overall state of health, fatigue, recent and/or unexplained weight gain or loss, period of time for either, contributing factors (change of diet, illness, altered appetite), exercise tolerance, fevers (time of day), chills, night sweats (unrelated to climatic conditions), frequent infections, general ability to carry out activities of daily living

integument pruritus, pigment or other color changes, acne, eruptions, rashes (location), tendency to bruising, petechiae, excessive dryness, general texture, disorders or deformities of nails, hair growth or loss, hair color change (for adolescent, use of hair dyes or other potentially toxic substances, such as hair straighteners)

head headaches, dizziness, injury (specific details)

eyes visual problems (ask about behaviors indicative of blurred vision, such as bumping into objects, clumsiness, sitting very close to television, holding a book close to the face, writing with head near desk, squinting, rubbing the eyes, bending the head in an awkward position), ''cross-eye'' (strabismus), eye infections, edema of lids, excessive tearing, use of glasses or contact lenses, date of last optic examination

nose nosebleeds (epistaxis), constant or frequent running or stuffy nose, nasal obstruction (difficulty in breathing), sense of smell

ears earaches, discharge, evidence of hearing loss (ask about behaviors, such as need to repeat requests, loud speech, inattentive behavior), results of any previous auditory testing

mouth mouth breathing, gum bleeding, toothaches, problems with toothbrushing, difficulty with teething (symptoms), last visit to dentist (especially if temporary dentition is complete)

throat sore throats, difficulty in swallowing, choking (especially when chewing food—may be from poor chewing habits), hoarseness or other voice irregularities

neck pain, limitation of movement, stiffness, difficulty in holding head straight (torticollis), thyroid enlargement, enlarged nodes or other masses

chest breast enlargement, discharge, masses, enlarged axillary nodes (for adolescent female, ask about self-breast examination)

respiratory chronic cough, frequent colds (number per year), wheezing, shortness of breath at rest or on exertion, difficulty in breathing, sputum production, infections (pneumonia, tuberculosis), date of last chest x-ray examination

cardiovascular cyanosis or fatigue on exertion, history of heart murmur or rheumatic fever, anemia, date of last blood count, blood type, recent transfusion

gastrointestinal (much of this in regard to appetite, food tolerance, and elimination habits has been asked elsewhere), concentrate on nausea, vomiting (not associated with eating may be indicative of brain tumor or increased intracranial pressure), jaundice or yellowing skin or sclera, belching, flatulence, recent change in bowel habits (blood in stools, change of color, diarrhea, or constipation)

genitourinary pain on urination, frequency, hesitancy, urgency, hematuria, nocturia, polyuria, unpleasant odor to urine, force of stream, discharge, change in size of scrotum, (for adolescent, venereal disease, type of treatment), date of last urinalysis

gynecologic menarche, date of last menstrual period, regularity or problems with menstruation, vaginal discharge, pruritus, date and result of last Pap smear (include obstetric history as discussed under birth history when applicable), if sexually active, type of contraception

musculoskeletal weakness, clumsiness, lack of coordination, unusual movements, back or joint stiffness, muscle pains or cramps, abnormal gait, deformity, fractures, serious sprains, activity level

neurologic seizures, tremors, dizziness, loss of memory, general affect, fears, nightmares, speech problems, any unusual habits

endocrine intolerance to weather changes, excessive thirst, excessive sweating, salty taste to skin, signs of early puberty

Family history

The medical family history is primarily for the purpose of discovering the potential existence of hereditary or familial diseases in the parents and child. However, it affords much more information for nursing consideration in terms of status of the marital relationship, availability of support systems in extended relatives, and age relationships among siblings.

In general, the family tree or pedigree chart is confined to first-degree relatives. In the case of children, this includes the maternal and paternal parents, siblings, and offspring. Information for each includes age, state of health if living, cause of death if deceased, and any evidence of the following conditions: heart disease, hypertension, cancer, diabetes mellitus, obesity, congenital anomalies, allergy, asthma, tuberculosis, sickle cell disease, mental retardation, convulsions, insanity or other emotional problems, syphilis, or rheumatic fever. The nurse confirms accuracy of the reported incidence by inquiring as to the symptoms, course, treatment, and sequelae of each diagnosis.

Construction of a pedigree chart (see p. 202) requires accurate information from both the child's mother and father. Sometimes this is not possible because of the absence of one parent. It is important when asking about family members that the nurse choose terms wisely. For example, every child has a father, but not every mother has a husband. Therefore, it is best to inquire about the paternal history by referring to "the child's father." Since the pedigree includes the outcome of all the mother's pregnancies (viable births, stillborns, or miscarriages), it is not unlikely for more than one father to be listed. Nurses must be careful of their reaction to the mother's reporting of different sexual partners. It may be difficult for the mother to reveal illegitimacy if she fears reproach or criticism.

Personal/social history

This section of the history includes all the personal, social, and economic factors that influence the child's and family's overall psychobiologic health. It focuses on (1) home and community environment, (2) occupation and education of family members, (3) cultural and religious traditions, (4) geographic location, and (5) marital and sexual history of the parents and child. Since the information elicited in this part of the history is often the most personal and confidential, it is left to the end of the interview, when the nurse-parent-child rapport should be well established.

Home and community environment. Information about the home environment includes type of dwelling (private home, apartment, multiple dwelling, and so on), number of rooms, number of occupants, sleeping arrangements, number of floors and accessibility of stairs or elevators, ventilation, exposure to sunlight, type of heating and other utilities, safety features (fire escape, windows with bars, fire alarms, and so on), and housing problems (insects, poor sanitation, flaking paint, and so on).

Information regarding the community environment may vary according to geographic location, such as an urban or rural setting. It is the nurse's responsibility to have at least a general knowledge of the locality in order to focus questions on specific areas of significance. However, some general topics for investigation include type of neighborhood (residential or industrial, relative age of neighboring families, willingness of neighbors to help one another, interracial or ethnic problems), availability of age-mates for the child, location and distance of school, usual transportation to school, and available play areas. It is also important to focus on potential dangers in the community environment, such as proximity to industrial centers (for example, an asbestos or chemical factory), incidence of crime, and potential accident sources such as a swimming pool or other adjacent body of water, steep hill or cliff, or heavy street traffic.

Occupation and education of family members. The occupational history of the parents is more than a listing of their career and place of employment. It should focus on type of activity (manual or sedentary, individual-paced or highly pressured), number of hours away from the home, exposure to environmental hazards (chemicals, coal, radiation, lead, carbon monoxide, fire, etc.), and satisfaction associated with the employment.

The occupational history should also lead into a discussion of the family's financial status. Since some parents may resist disclosing their yearly income, the nurse can assess the adequacy of financial resources by inquiring about source of income when unemployed, usual housing expenses, and expenditures for food, shelter, clothing, and recreation. The nurse can also make a general statement, such as, "The cost of living is certainly high today. How do you make ends meet?" to encourage parents to discuss any financial hardships without fear of criticism or debasement. The nurse also investigates the type of medical coverage or insurance the family has.

Ascertaining the parents' educational preparation usually follows a discussion of occupation. By the end of the interview the nurse has probably made some personal judgment regarding the parent's level of formal and informal education. However, since many people feel embarrassed to admit failure to complete the usual academic learning, it is best to approach the area of years in school indirectly whenever possible. For example, the nurse can ask about the type of training, education, or acquisition of special skills that may be required for the parents' vocation. This information is highly valuable in planning implementation of care, such as counseling, guidance, or teaching, and is another reason why the nurse should refrain from actual intervention until the history (and physical examination whenever warranted) is completed.

Cultural and religious traditions. Although the nurse usually asks about nationality and religious affiliation at the beginning of the interview as part of the identifying information, specific cultural traditions and religious practices should again be referred to in the social/personal history. Generally by the end of the interview the nurse has formed some assumptions about the influence of culture and religion on the family, such as specific nutritional practices, child-rearing beliefs, attitudes toward health care, or personal faith in God. If the nurse fails to consider the tremendous impact such traditions play in a family's life-style, nursing care will probably also end in failure.

The nurse can encourage parents to verbalize about their heritage by posing questions such as, "How do your beliefs regarding ______ differ from those of your parents?" "How is your religion a part of your life?" "What special ______ (name of culture of nationality) traditions do you practice in your home?" "What language do you use in the home?" "How does American school education differ from what you teach your children?" or "Do you think American children act differently from children in your country?"

Geographic location. Geographic location, including birthplace and travel to different areas in or outside of the country, is important for identification of possible exposure to indigenous diseases. Although the primary interest concerns the child's temporary residence in various localities, the nurse also inquires about close family members' travel, especially during tours of military service or business trips. Children are especially susceptible to parasitic infestation in areas of poor sanitary conditions and to vector-borne diseases, such as those from mosquitoes or ticks, in warm and humid or heavily wooded regions.

Marital and sexual history. This last area requires the most interviewing skill from the nurse and the greatest trust and confidence from the informant (parent or child). One way of approaching the topic of marital relationships is to ascertain the identity of household members. If the parent fails to mention the other parent, the nurse can then ask, "Where is the child's father (or mother)?" It is best to avoid the term husband or wife because that precludes the existence of nonmarital relationships. If the parent states that the child's father (or mother) is not part of the family constellation, the nurse can explore this by inquiring about his or her continued relationship with the child and the presence of any other significant male (or female) within the household. The nurse should also inquire about previous marriages, separations, death of spouses, or divorces. It is important to also ask about the child's reaction to any of these events, which usually have a tremendous effect on his general physical and emotional health status.

If some type of consenting adult relationship exists, the nurse also attempts to assess its stability, strength, and support for each parent and the children. One way of evaluating this is to ask, "Who do you talk to when you have something on your mind?" The answer opens doors to further exploration of the type of communication, understanding, mutuality, and respect between the partners.

The degree of inquiry into the parents' sexual activity is dependent on many factors. For example, it may be limited to a brief discussion of their plans regarding future children and the methods used to ensure their wishes, such as type of contraception. In instances where overt adult sexual activity may be having an adverse effect on the children, a more detailed exploration of this area is warranted. The nurse must make this decision based on facts learned during the interview, because this line of questioning should never be wanton prying. If parents ask the relevance of revealing such matters, the nurse must be prepared to offer a sound and logical explanation. It is every person's right to refuse to disclose personal information, especially if he or she is not informed of its significance or value.

A sexual history is an essential component of all adolescents' health assessments. It is warranted regardless of their degree of sexual activity, since concerns about sexual matters may bear heavily on older children's physical and psychologic well-being.

One way of initiating a conversation about sexual concerns is asking adolescents to describe their sex education and attitudes[1] toward such areas as premarital sex, masturbation, "going steady," and so on. It is best to begin interviewing for a sexual history with open-ended, expansive statements, such as, "Tell me about your social life" or "Who are your closest friends?" and gradually narrow the focus of the discussion to relationships with the opposite sex. Since homosexual experimentation is not infrequent during adolescence, this is also a recommended area for investigation. Because homosexual experimentation can cause much concern and anxiety among older children, it is preferable to probe into this area late in the interview.

The nurse must be aware of the language each participant

uses in either eliciting or conveying sexual information. For example, when the nurse directly asks if the adolescent is "sexually active" or "having sex," what either phrase means should be clarified. To some, it may signify foreplay, self-stimulation, erotic visual stimulation, or intercourse. Adolescents' fantasies and strong sexual desires are alone sufficient to cause them concern. Therefore, the nurse not only wants to know the incidence of intimate sexual contacts but also looks for areas of sexual concern for the adolescent.

The following example illustrates the importance of the latter area:

Mary, 14 years old, had come to the health center for a "physical checkup, with chief complaint of 'cramping' for 1 week." A complete history and physical examination revealed normal findings. When the nurse attempted to elicit a sexual history, Mary became physically anxious (wringing her hands, biting her lip, sitting more rigidly), but denied any sexual activity. Noting this behavior, the nurse stated: "Sometimes being a teenager is difficult, because you have things on your mind that you feel nobody will understand, yet at the same time you feel you must talk about. Has that ever happened to you?" Mary shook her head in affirmation, but offered no further explanation.

At the end of the visit, the nurse discussed with Mary the results of the physical examination, stating to her that if the cramps returned, she should revisit the health center. She also stressed that anytime Mary wanted to talk, she should come in to see the nurse. As Mary reached the door, she suddenly blurted out, "Would you do a VD test?" The nurse responded, "If you wish. Why don't you come back and tell me about it?" Mary proceeded to explain that she had been dating a boy for a few months. They had never "gone all the way" but had engaged in "kissing and touching everywhere." A week ago she had learned from a friend that this boy had VD. Mary was positive she had it also.

Although genital and/or oral genital transmission had not occurred, the nurse agreed to perform the VDRL test as objective evidence of lack of disease. She also discussed with Mary the type of sexual contact necessary for transmission of venereal disease, and Mary's present attitude toward her boyfriend. When she returned to the center the following week, Mary stated that her cramps were gone, she had talked to the boyfriend about her knowledge of his having venereal disease, which he confirmed, and had decided not to see him anymore. As she stated to the nurse, "I really think I only went out with him because all my friends were dating. But I was always afraid of going too far. I am so glad I talked to you about the VD. I think I would have gone crazy from worry if I didn't. I think I'm too young to date right now."

Patient profile

The patient profile is a summary of the nurse's impression of the child's health status and the psychologic-socioeconomic variables that influence his total well-being. It is sometimes written after completion of the physical examination and includes pertinent physical findings regarding the child's present state of health.

A well-written patient profile is actually the beginning of a problem list or nursing diagnoses of both objective findings and subjective impressions. Frequently, physical findings during the examination yield supportive data of initial concerns identified during the history. Some of the more common health problems discovered during the interview include visual disturbances, delayed speech development, need for dental hygiene, nutritional inadequacy, the impact of family problems such as divorce or separation on the child, and discipline or behavioral concerns.[6]

The following is an example of a patient profile for the adolescent described in the preceding section: "A 14-year-old white female, dressed neatly, apparent physical hygiene, lives with parents and two younger brothers in private home; attends junior high school; initially shy, alert, responsive to direct questions, obviously anxious regarding sexual activity; at end of interview, voluntarily voiced main concern regarding contact with VD victim."

REFERENCES

1. Adams, G.: The sexual history as an integral part of the patient history, Am. J. Maternal Child Nurs. **1**(3):170-175, May/June 1976.
2. Hoekelman, R. A., Kelly, J., and Zimmer, A. W.: The reliability of maternal recall, Clin. Pediatr. **15**(3):261-265, March 1976.
3. Kohut, S. A.: Guidelines for using interpreters, Hosp. Prog. **56**(4):39-40, April 1975.
4. Sana, J. M., and Judge, R. D.: Physical appraisal methods in nursing practice, Boston, 1975, Little, Brown and Co.
5. Sherman, J. L., and Fields, S. K.: Guide to patient evaluation, New York, 1976, Medical Examination Publishing Co., Inc.
6. Wong, D.: Providing experience in physical assessment for students in basic programs, Am. J. Nurs. **75**(6):974-975, June 1975.

BIBLIOGRAPHY

Alexander, M. M., and Brown, M. S.: Physical examination. Part I. The why and the how of the examination, Nursing '73 **3**(7):25-28, July 1973.

Alexander, M. M., and Brown, M. S.: Physical examination. Part II. History taking, Nursing '73 **3**(8):35-39, August 1973.

Baer, E. D., McGowan, M. N., and McGivern, D. O.: Taking a health history, Am. J. Nurs. **7**(77):1190-1193, July 1977.

Bates, B., and Lynaugh, J. E.: Laying the foundation for medical nursing practice, Am. J. Nurs. **73**(8):1375-1379, August 1973.

Berni, R., and Readey, H.: Problem-oriented medical record implementation: allied health review, ed. 2, St. Louis, 1978, The C. V. Mosby Co.

Bouchier, I. A., and Morris, J. S.: Clinical skills: a system of clinical examination, Philadelphia, 1976, W. B. Saunders Co.

Brown, M. S., and Murphy, M. A.: Ambulatory pediatrics for nurses, New York, 1975, McGraw-Hill Book Co.

DeAngelis, C.: Basic pediatrics for the primary health care provider, Boston, 1975, Little, Brown and Co.

Faigel, H. C.: Getting patients to follow advice: the art of communication, Clin. Pediatr. **11**(12):666-667, December 1972.

Fox, D. J.: Fundamentals of research in nursing, New York, 1970, Meredith Corp.

Froelich, R. E., and Bishop, F. M.: Clinical interviewing skills: a programmed manual for data gathering, evaluation, and patient management, ed. 3, St. Louis, 1977, The C. V. Mosby Co.

Gozzi, E.: We plan ahead what to ask, Nurs. Outlook **13**(6):30-33, June 1965.

Gulbrandsen, M. W.: Guide to health assessment, Am. J. Nurs. **76**(8):1276-1277, August 1976.

Hochstein, E., and Rubin, A.: Physical diagnosis: a textbook and workbook in methods of clinical examination, New York, 1964, McGraw-Hill Book Co.

Hofman, A. D.: Identifying and counseling the sexually active adolescent is every physician's responsibility, Clin. Pediatr. **11**(11):625-629, November 1972.

Manthey, M.: A guide for interviewing, Am. J. Nurs. **67**(10): 2088-2090, October 1967.

McBride, M. M.: Can you tell me where it hurts? Pediatr. Nurs. **3**(4):7-8, July/August 1977.

McCain, F.: Nursing by assessment—not intuition, Am. J. Nurs. **65**(4):82-84, April 1965.

McPhetridge, L. M.: Nursing history: one means to personalized care, Am. J. Nurs. **68**(1):68-75, January 1968.

Prior, J. A., and Silberstein, J. S.: Physical diagnosis: the history and examination of the patient, St. Louis, 1977, The C. V. Mosby Co.

Programmed instruction: patient assessment: taking a patient's history, Am. J. Nurs. **74**(2):293-324, February 1974.

Roznoy, M. S.: How to take a sexual history, Am. J. Nurs. **76**(8): 1279-1282, August 1976.

Smith, D. M.: A clinical nursing tool, Am. J. Nurs. **68**(11):2384-2388, November 1968.

Stillman, P. L., Sabers, D. L., and Redfield, D. L.: The use of paraprofessionals to teach interviewing skills, Pediatrics **57** (5):749-774, May 1976.

Snyder, J. C., and Wilson, M. F.: Elements of a psychological assessment, Am. J. Nurs. **77**(2):235-239, February 1977.

Whaley, L. F.: Understanding inherited disorders, St. Louis, 1974, The C. V. Mosby Co.

5

Physical assessment of the child

Physical assessment is a continuous process that begins during the interview, primarily by use of the tool of inspection or observation, and continues to some degree throughout the professional relationship. Although the format for organization of a systematic approach resembles that of a medical physical examination, the objective of each assessment area is to formulate nursing diagnoses and evaluate the effectiveness of interventions. Although the nurse may diagnose or assist in the establishment of a medical diagnosis, this is secondary to the primary goal of identifying nursing problems.

This chapter discusses the influence of age in the preparation of children for physical examination, the tools used for assessment of health status, and the performance of the examination.

The "systems" approach with children

The systematic approach for organization of physical assessment affords the same general advantages as for the history in terms of data collection (p. 90). However, its main function is to serve as a general guideline for completeness and consistency in performing and recording physical findings. Few errors in physical diagnosis occur as a result of ignorance. Most are caused primarily by careless omission of simple procedures.[4]

For adults the physical examination proceeds in a head-to-toe direction and from general inspection to detailed investigation. The typical body-systems approach followed during physical assessment of adults is listed below.

General outline for nursing assessment

- **A.** General
  - **1.** Measurements
    - **a.** Height
    - **b.** Weight
    - **c.** Head circumference
    - **d.** Vital signs
    - **e.** Blood pressure
  - **2.** General appearance
  - **3.** Skin
  - **4.** Lymph glands
- **B.** Head
- **C.** Neck
- **D.** Eyes
- **E.** Ears
- **F.** Mouth and throat
- **G.** Chest
- **H.** Lungs
- **I.** Heart
- **J.** Abdomen
- **K.** Genitalia
- **L.** Back and extremities
- **M.** Neurologic
  - **1.** Behavior
  - **2.** Cognitive-perceptual development
  - **3.** Motor functioning
  - **4.** Sensory functioning
    - **a.** Hearing
    - **b.** Vision
  - **5.** Cerebellar functioning
  - **6.** Reflexes
  - **7.** Cranial nerves
  - **8.** "Soft" signs
- **N.** Developmental screening

In pediatrics the age of the child frequently alters this sequence of performance, although written recording follows the traditional model. Using developmental and chronologic age as the main criteria for assessing each body system accomplishes several goals: (1) minimization of stress and anxiety associated with assessment of various body parts, (2) fostering of a trusting nurse-child-parent relationship, (3) allowance for maximum preparation of the child, (4) preservation of the essential security of the parent-child relationship, especially with young children, and (5) maximization of the accuracy and reliability of assessment findings.

Most of the suggestions for performing a physical assessment according to different ages are based on logic and developmental principles. Since no child fits precisely into one age category, the guidelines for positioning, sequence, and preparation as shown in Table 5-1 must be based on the

Table 5-1. General approaches to physical examination during childhood

Age	Position	Sequence of examination	Preparation
Infants	Before child sits alone unsupported, examination can be done while infant is supine or prone, but preferably in parent's lap After child sits by himself, examination is best accomplished in this position, whenever possible, and preferably in parent's lap	If infant is quiet, auscultate heart, lungs, and abdomen first and record pulse and respirations. Palpate and percuss these areas if infant remains quiet and relaxed. Proceed with examination in usual head-to-toe direction, using inspection as main tool. Terminate examination with most traumatic procedures, such as examination of eyes, ears and mouth. Although rectal or axillary temperature and blood pressure monitoring may not disturb a young infant, these procedures usually distress the older infant. If vital signs are taken while child is crying, record the behavior with the measurement. Most primitive reflexes can be elicited when specific body part is examined (such as grasp reflex with upper extremities), but general reflexes such as Moro reflex should be done at end of examination.	Completely undress infant if room temperature permits, leaving diaper in place, especially in males, to eliminate accidents during urination Gain infant's cooperation by (a) distracting him with brightly colored toys, talking to him, or encouraging parent to play with him, or (b) giving the infant sugar water or his regular bottle feeding. Gain parent's cooperation to assist as much as possible during examination, especially with necessary immobilization of the head for otoscopic, optic, and oral examination. If this is not possible, use a mummy restraint (p. 000).
Toddlers	Prefer sitting or standing position, preferably very close to parent Generally resist lying down position under all circumstances Any position of restraint or immobility, even in parent's arms, causes great distress	Similar to infant in that *all* traumatic procedures are left to end of examination. Inspect body areas as much as possibly by playing with child, initially using little touch, and gradually proceeding toward trunk and head for percussion and palpation. Toward end of examination, perform auscultation, which requires little ambient noise, record pulse and respiration, then proceed with blood pressure and examination of eyes, ears, and mouth. Rectal temperature, if not part of routine initial screening with height and weight, is usually done at end of examination. Record activity with vital signs if child is crying.	Since removing clothing may be very upsetting to toddler, have parent remove articles of clothing as each body part is examined. Ideally, parent can begin removing heavy outerclothing during the interview, leaving diaper, undershirt, and socks on. In this way, undressing is not associated with the physical examination. Make as much of the examination natural and spontaneous as possible, for example, instead of asking child to walk, observe this activity as it occurs. Allow child to see, feel, and play with stethoscope, blood pressure machine, and otoscope. It may be best to just present these objects for child's inspection rather than demonstrate their use. For example, toddlers usually do not like having the stethoscope in their ears, but they enjoy putting it around their neck and playing with it (see Fig. 5-1). Watching the nurse look in parent's ear or take parent's blood pressure presents a nonthreatening model of the activity. If this approach increases anxiety, perform each procedure quickly, using whatever restraint necessary—prolonging the inevitable increases resistance and anxiety. Although verbal skills may still be poorly developed, comprehension is quite

Table 5-1. General approaches to physical examination during childhood—cont'd

Age	Position	Sequence of examination	Preparation
Toddlers—cont'd			extensive. Briefly explain to toddlers what you will be doing, for example, tell them that you will be feeling their tummy, looking in their ear, or listening to their "heart make noise." Although it may not decrease their anxiety during this visit, it helps prepare them for future visits.
Preschoolers	Ideally position of their choice, although, in general, sitting or standing is preferable Usually like to be on a table or "stage," although some still prefer parent's lap and most desire parent's presence	Usually preschoolers are cooperative and responsive to preparation, allowing examination to proceed in usual head-to-toe sequence. It may still be preferable to use all instruments at end of examination after children have had ample opportunity to play with them.	Preschoolers usually do not mind undressing but prefer to leave their underpants on. Eliciting their cooperation by letting them undress themselves is preferable to doing it for them and offers the opportunity to assess self-help skills. Before beginning examination, briefly explain what you will be doing, for example, saying to them, "I want to see how everything is working. I am going to look, feel, and listen, like this (place hand on abdomen). These things will help me hear and see better." Show the equipment to them, ask them what they think it is for, and then demonstrate appropriate use, such as putting the stethoscope in their ears and listening to the heart. Capitalize on their egocentrism and magical thicking. For example, mirrors not only distract them, thereby lessening any fear, but usually increase their willingness to cooperate and perform. Making a story out of inspecting the ears, such as, looking for "elephants," usually entices their imagination enough to make them want you to look again. Similarly, present the blood pressure machine in terms of watching the "silver line climb up the pole" or "seeing how strong their muscles are when pumping the bulb." When actually performing procedures such as otoscopy, *tell* child what to do, rather *asking* him to do something.
School-age children	Although they generally prefer sitting up, they are usually cooperative in any position Older children, such as preadolescents, may prefer the privacy of having parents wait outside the room; younger school-age children may still prefer their parents' presence, but enjoy being the center of attention, with directions and questions directed toward them	Usually examination can proceed in head-to-toe direction, although examination of genitalia for older child may be done last.	School-age children usually do not mind undressing if they are given some type of covering, such as a loose gown or sheet. When these are not available, their underclothes should be removed as necessary. Although privacy may not be an overtly expressed concern, respect for it usually increases their cooperativeness. If as preschoolers they were appropriately prepared for a physical examination, school-age children are familiar with the equipment and prefer to learn about its technical use, rather than just playing with it. Older children may be more concerned with the findings and significance of normalcy than with the instruments' mechanical functioning.

Continued.

Table 5-1. General approaches to physical examination during childhood—cont'd

Age	Position	Sequence of examination	Preparation
School-age children —cont'd			If older children demonstrate minimal or incorrect knowledge concerning the instruments, it is best to do some preliminary preparation similar to that done for preschoolers. The explanation focuses on actual significance of procedure, such as otoscopic examination for inspection of the eardrum, which is necessary for hearing. Throughout examination, nurse should use the opportunity to teach older children about their bodies.
Adolescents	Same as for school-age children, although most adolescents prefer the privacy of having parents wait outside the room until examination is completed (this may include history, as well)	Proceed same as in adult, although examination of genitalia is usually done last.	Adolescents' chief concern with body image is reflected in their needs for preparation. Although they do not mind undressing, they prefer to do so in private, to wear a gown, and to have only one body area exposed at a time. Concerns for privacy are usually paramount during this period. Although they are cooperative for any assessment procedures, their concerns focus primarily on the results. It is helpful for the nurse to report evidence of normal findings as she examines each area. For example, she may state while palpating the abdomen, "Everything is soft, of good size, and your muscles are well developed." Since concerns for sexual maturity are of prime importance but may not be voiced, the nurse casually and matter-of-factly comments about development of secondary sex characteristics, such as, "Your breasts are developing just as they should be for your age." She follows such statements with inquiries into the adolescent's feelings about sexual body development. Since even the most superficial examination of male genitalia may cause an involuntary erection and be a source of tremendous embarrassment for the boy, the nurse should proceed quickly and matter-of-factly with examination and call as little attention as possible to the occurrence.

preliminary assessment made by the nurse during the interview of the child's developmental achievements and needs. For example, even when the best approach is used, many toddlers seem to be uncooperative and unable to be consoled for almost all of the physical examination. However, some seem intrigued by the new surroundings and unusual equipment and respond more like preschoolers than like toddlers. Likewise, some early preschoolers may require more of the "security measures" employed with younger children, such as continued mother-child contact, and less of the preparatory measures used with preschoolers, such as playing with the equipment before and during the actual examination (see Fig. 5-1).

Although the variations in the general approaches are numerous, some of them are elaborated here because they are not infrequent. For example, the suggested sequence may change considerably when the child is in pain or when obvious physical defects are present. In either situation it is

A 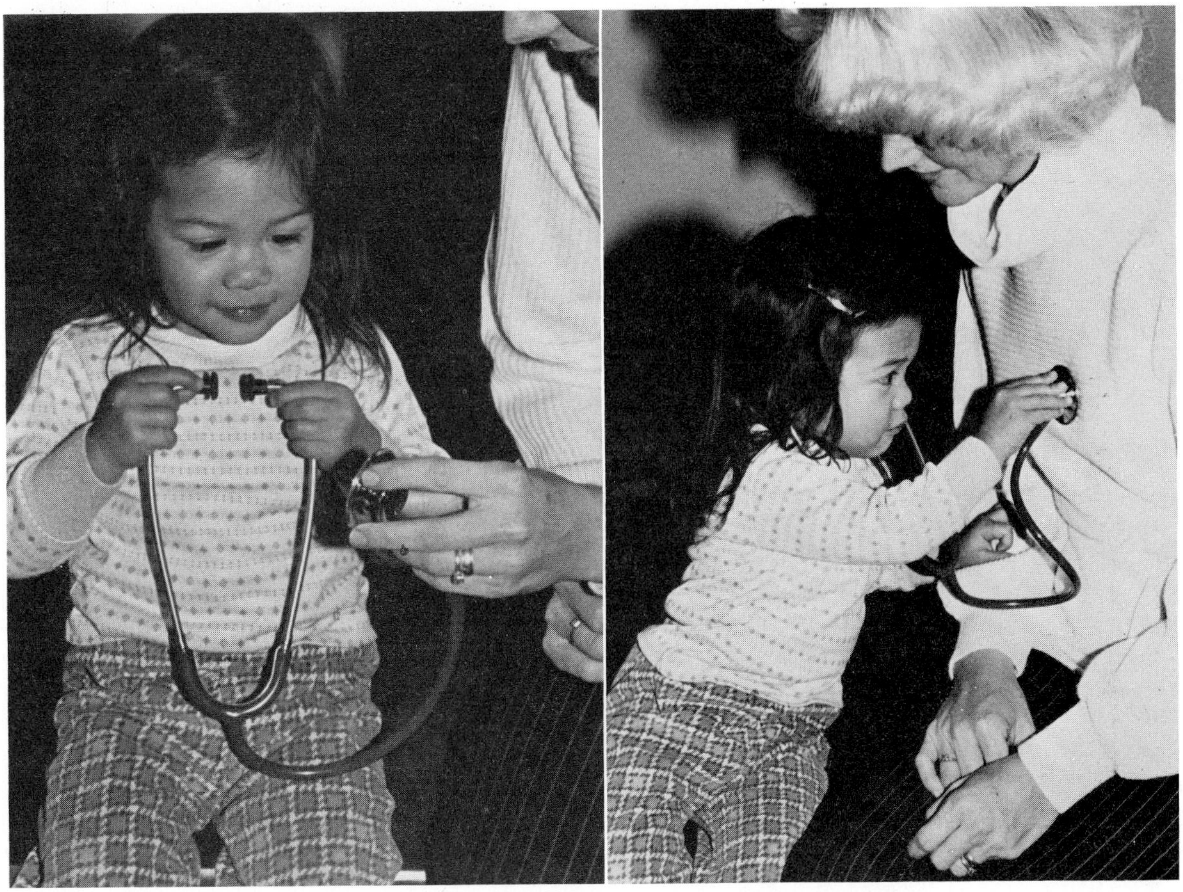 B

Fig. 5-1. A and **B,** Preparing a child for physical examination.

preferable to examine the affected area last, in order to minimize distress early in the examination and to focus on normal, healthy, or functioning body parts, rather than defective ones. Positioning may also be altered because of physical distress. For example, the child who is having difficulty in breathing may not be able to lie down, necessitating that as much of the physical examination as possible be performed in a sitting or slightly reclining position or that the examination be completed at another time.

Although parental presence is almost always conducive to a child's cooperation and sense of security, there are occasions when parents' anxiety increases the child's emotional distress. In those rare instances when it is preferable for parents to leave the room, it is best to request this before the examination begins. When the nurse and child are alone, the nurse should begin establishing rapport on a one-to-one basis by talking to or playing with the child and using appropriate preparatory measures, rather than immediately initiating the examination. If the nurse judges that assistance will be needed during some of the procedures, another person's help should be enlisted, rather than trying to succeed alone, probably at the expense of safety and prolonged trauma to the child.

With skill and the child's cooperation, the physical examination should be completed rapidly. The time consideration is important because an adequate initial interview may require as much as an hour, and a developmental screening test, about 10 to 20 minutes. When combined with an unnecessarily prolonged physical assessment, the child and parent can become exhausted and less cooperative. Establishing one's own systematic sequence of performance for each age-group will greatly enhance one's ability to skillfully and thoroughly execute a complete physical appraisal.

ASSESSMENT SKILLS

The traditional four categories of assessment skills include inspection, palpation, percussion, and auscultation. Each of these involves a set of tools to facilitate its performance, usefulness, and accuracy. Although the trend has been to incorporate more specialized and technical equipment into nursing assessment, the nurse is equipped with all of the tools necessary for a fairly comprehensive and detailed physical examination. The use of the senses of sight, smell, hearing, and sometimes taste are necessary for inspection. The hands and fingers are the main tools of palpation and percussion, and the ear is an excellent instrument for auscultation. Although several specific instruments refine the examination, it is important to remember that few of them can replace the human tools of skill, knowledge, and interpretation.

Besides these four traditional categories of skills, measurements are an essential component of every physical assessment and include such areas as height, weight (length), head circumference, vital signs, and blood pressure. Although such clinical measurements are routine simple procedures that may be performed by other paraprofessionals, it is the nurse's responsibility to check their accuracy and compare the findings against other physical parameters.

Inspection

Inspection is the most valuable, least mechanical, and most difficult skill to learn. It involves the use of the senses, primarily vision, to make judgments, comparisons, and decisions. Because inspection is a highly subjective process, it requires skill, repetition, and practice to establish reliable findings for distinguishing among ranges of normal, borderline, and abnormal.

Methods of inspection. One of the keys to competent inspection is the conscious, systematic, and active use of one's senses. As the nurse examines each body part, the visible areas are deliberately inspected for color, texture, firmness, hygiene, masses, hair distribution, tone, movement, behavior, tension, flaccidity, symmetry, location, position, temperature, and so on. As each of these is observed, it is compared to what constitutes normal anatomy and physiology. Although it is not the nurse's objective to "diagnose" an abnormality by labeling it as a specific disorder, defect, or disease, it is the nurse's responsibility to recognize and record its presence.

Inspection may be combined with specific instruments for better visualization, such as the otoscope for the ear (p. 133), and with measurements to validate subjective impressions. For example, the nurse may observe that the child appears thin for his age; this impression is substantiated by recording height and weight on a growth chart, comparing the values, and judging those measurements in terms of genetic background, previous growth trends, physical status, and nutritional intake. After establishing a thorough data base, the nurse then proceeds to draw conclusions and formulate nursing diagnoses.

Frequently, competent inspection involves intangible skills for which no yardstick exists. The most common example relates to measuring emotional state or behavior. An experienced nurse may look at a child and know that he is ill without any further assessment. Often, however, the nurse is unable to specifically state what behaviors have led to that conclusion. One way of developing skill is to consciously analyze behaviors, such as appearance, movement, relationships, activity, verbal interaction, mood, and orientation, and to record what is observed, not what is interpreted.[6] For example, observation or inspection is a factual statement, such as, "An 11-year-old Oriental male, color is pale, moves slowly, holds right lower quadrant of abdomen, occasional facial grimaces, answers questions slowly and briefly." An interpretative statement is, "An 11-year-old Oriental male in distress, pain in lower right abdomen, and refuses to talk." The later statement is much more liable to erroneous or altered interpretations by others than the former statement, which is a list of what is seen.

Palpation

Palpation is primarily the use of touch or the tactile sense to detect both superficial and deeper characteristics of the body. It is combined with inspection, because in many instances it validates a visual impression, such as texture of the skin. Palpation uses touch to assess temperature, position, form, size, consistency, moisture, and movement, such as vibration or pulsation. It is used to examine all accessible parts of the body, such as organs, glands, blood vessels, bones, muscles, hair, skin, and mucosa. A thorough knowledge of anatomy is essential in differentiating palpation of normal body structures from abnormal ones, such as masses.

Methods of palpation. Palpation involves the use of the fingers and hands for superficial and deep examination of body parts. When small areas are palpated, such as the neck for lymph glands or the infant's skull for fontanels, or when fine tactile discriminations are made, such as texture of the skin, the fingertips are most useful and precise. For evaluating temperature, the tips of the fingers and dorsa (back) of the hands are most accurate because the skin is thin and sensitive to temperature differences. For detecting vibration, such as heart thrills or the point of maximum impulse of the heart on the chest wall, the palmar surfaces of the fingers and hand are most sensitive. To evaluate consistency, position, and size, the grasping action of the fingers is best. When palpating deeper organs, particularly those in the abdomen, a bimanual maneuver may be used. One hand is placed on the abdomen, and the other hand applies pressure to the first hand. Palpation is done with the cushions and palmar surfaces of the contact hand, not with the fingernails. In small children the distal palmar surfaces of the fingers are directly applied to the skin, and the other hand may or may not be used to apply pressure to the contact hand. Frequently the nonpalpating hand is placed against the child's back directly underneath the area to be palpated. In this way the organ is "caught" or felt between both hands (Fig. 5-2).

For any type of palpation to be effective, but especially for deep palpation of internal organs, the child must be relaxed, otherwise the tense muscles act like a wall between the hand and the organ. Helping the child relax includes positioning him comfortably, for example, in a semireclining position in a parent's lap, warming the hands before

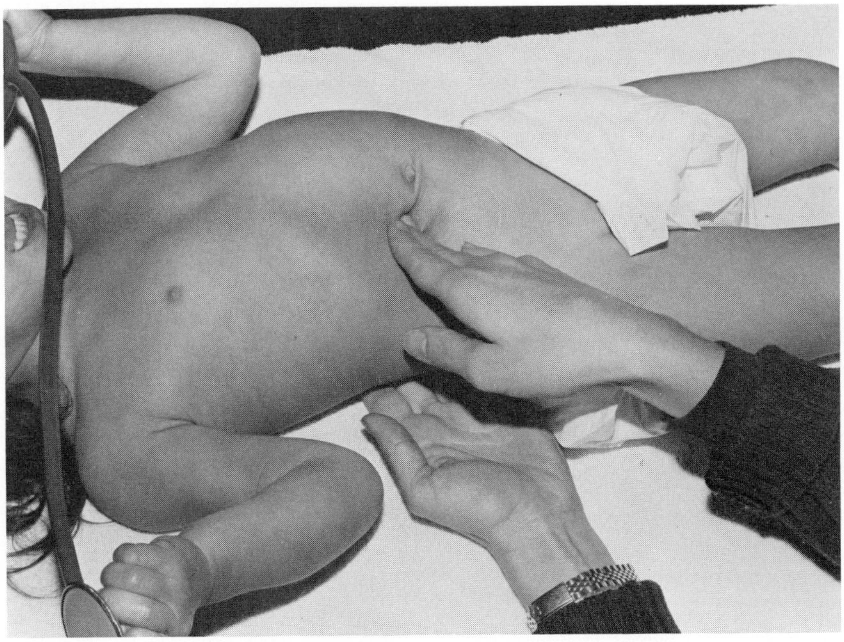

Fig. 5-2. Palpation.

touching him, using distraction, beginning with light superficial palpation and gradually progressing to deeper palpation, giving the infant a bottle or pacifier, and palpating any tender or painful areas last. Deep breathing and concentrating on a fixed object may help older children relax. Although the sequence generally follows suggestions in Table 5-1, the nurse should use a bilateral and symmetric approach in order to compare the findings on one side of the body with those on the other side.

Percussion

Percussion is the striking or tapping of the body surface to produce sounds that correlate with the type of underlying tissue density. The principles of percussion are the same as those used to produce sounds in a musical instrument, such as the drum. For example, hollow, air-filled spaces, such as the lungs, create a low-pitched, well-sustained note called *resonance*. Dense, solid objects, such as organs or masses, create a high-pitched, short, thudding sound called *dullness*. Percussion sounds are described in terms of *tones* and *notes* (Table 5-2). Because sounds are difficult to describe in words, practice in percussing different areas of the body and comparing the emitted sounds is fundamental to developing skill and competence.

Methods of percussion. Techniques for percussion may be direct or indirect. *Direct* percussion is striking or tapping the body surface directly with the finger (Fig. 5-3, *A*). It is useful for percussing well-defined areas, such as a bone or the borders of an organ. It is also advantageous for greater accuracy when examining infants or small children, where body organs are in close proximity.

In the *indirect* method, the tapping is done by striking a stationary finger positioned on the body. Some practitioners prefer this method because there is less perception by the patient of being hit or struck than in the direct approach. The nurse performs this technique by (1) placing the index or middle finger against the body area to be percussed and (2) using the tip of the middle finger of the other hand to strike the base of the distal phalanx of the nonpercussing finger (Fig. 5-3, *B*). No other fingers of the nonpercussing hand should touch the chest wall. In order for the sound produced to be clear and not damped or muffled, quick, firm, sharp taps are necessary, similar to playing staccato notes on the piano. The nurse holds the forearm stationary and delivers the blows by using a loose hinge-joint action of the wrist. An excellent way of practicing correct percussion is by striking keys on a piano. If the blow is not sharp with a quick rebound of the finger, the note will be of a distinctly different sound than one that is staccato-like.

Auscultation

Auscultation is similar to percussion in that it involves evaluation of body sounds. It differs in that the nurse listens for those sounds produced by the body, such as sounds arising from the heart, lungs, and abdomen, not for those that are exogenously produced. The characteristics of auscultatory sounds are the same as those used to describe percussion tones, that is, intensity, pitch, duration, and quality (see Table 5-2).

Methods of auscultation and types of stethoscopes. As with percussion, the nurse can use the direct or indirect method of listening for sounds. In the *direct* meth-

Table 5-2. Definition of percussion sounds

Percussion sounds	Examples
Tones*	
Intensity—amplitude or loudness of tone	Loud tones—produced by more hollow, air-filled spaces, such as the lungs Soft tones—produced by more dense or solid masses, such as the heart
Pitch—frequency or number of vibrations per second; the greater the number of vibrations, the higher the pitch; the fewer the number, the lower the pitch	Low-pitched—air-filled lungs High-pitched—consolidated lung
Duration—time period of vibrations and length of time the sound lasts	Long duration—normal lungs Short duration—high-density organ, such as the heart
Quality or timbre—subjective evaluation that depends on the source of the sound	The same musical note from two different instruments produces a different quality or timbre of sound, for example, sounds of equal loudness and pitch from different organs, such as the lungs and heart, produce sounds of varying quality
Notes	
Resonance—clear hollow note, low pitch, long duration, relatively loud (heard with ease)	Normal lungs
Tympany—clear hollow note, higher pitched than resonance, musical with rich overtones (quality), long duration	Tympanic sound can be produced by lightly tapping an air-filled cheek with the finger; similar sound when percussing an air-filled stomach
Hyperresonance—cross between resonance and tympany; lower pitch than normal resonance, high intensity, and long duration	Usually indicates less density, such as increased amount of of air or decreased amount of tissue; usually pathologic, such as pneumothorax or asthma
Dullness—high-pitched, short duration, soft (low intensity), and thudding	Related to increased density and solidarity, such as the heart
Flatness—absolute dullness, high-pitched, very short, non-musical in quality	Solid tissue, such as the thigh

Adapted from Sana, J. M., and Judge, R. D.: Physical appraisal methods in nursing practice, Boston, 1975, Little, Brown and Co.
*These same terms are used to describe any sound and are used in physical assessment to record auscultatory sounds.

A

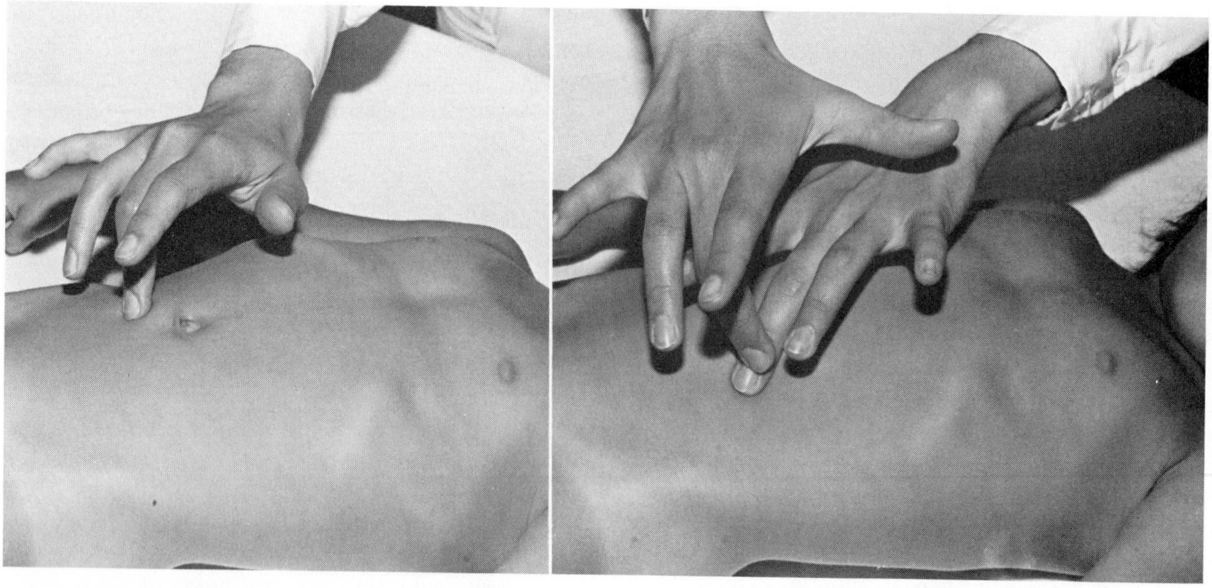

B

Fig. 5-3. Two examples of percussion. **A,** Direct percussion; **B,** indirect percussion.

od the nurse applies the ear directly to the body surface. In some instances loud sounds, such as grade VI murmurs or expiratory wheezes, can be heard by placing the ear in close proximity to the child, but not directly against the skin. The direct approach has disadvantages in terms of patient modesty, aversion to skin-to-skin contact, or possible infection to the examiner from skin lesions.

Indirect auscultation involves the use of a stethoscope to transmit internal body sounds to the nurse's ear. There are two main types of stethoscopes: the open bell and the closed diaphragm.[17] The *open-bell* or Ford chestpiece consists of a short cone or funnel-shaped horn joined to a binaural headset and eartips with flexible tubing. The open-bell chestpiece has the advantage of conducting sounds with virtually no distortion of pitch or timbre and is better for the perception of certain low-pitched sounds, such as diastolic murmurs. However, it must be placed firmly against the body surface for an airtight seal. Normally the diameter of the bell does not exceed 1 inch. A larger width bell would not permit a tight seal on bony or small surfaces, resulting in admittance of ambient sounds. This restriction in size limits the volume of sound it can accumulate.

The *closed-diaphragm* or Bowles chestpiece is larger but flatter and not as bulky as the open-bell chestpiece; it is sealed by its own diaphragm. These features afford it several advantages. Its larger diaphragm admits a greater quantity of sound and is more sensitive to high-pitched sounds. The diaphragm filters out and suppresses low-frequency vibrations, so that sounds appear to be of higher pitch than when heard through the bell. The self-sealing diaphragm obviates the need for an airtight skin seal, so that a larger diaphragm is still accurate when placed on a bony or small chest. However, a close-fitting seal is still recommended in order to decrease the admittance of environmental sounds. In infants and small children, especially premature infants, the use of a specially sized pediatric diaphragm is recommended both to achieve sufficient skin contact and to localize sounds in segmented areas of the chest. For example, an adult-size diaphragm almost completely covers the landmarks used to localize heart sounds, whereas a smaller-size diaphragm permits placement of the stethoscope over appropriate thoracic sites, facilitating differentiation of heart sounds (Fig. 5-4).

Although the length of the flexible tubing may vary considerably without significantly affecting the transmission of sound, it should not be unnecessarily long or impractically short. A sufficient length is about 50 cm (20 inches).[17] The binaural headset should be light, flexible, and comfortable, and the earpieces should fit snugly to occlude the ear canals and prevent intrusion of extraneous noise. The ear tubes are inclined anteriorly in order to conform to the natural direction of the auditory canals. If they are positioned incorrectly, they are usually uncomfortable and decrease the perception of transmitted body sounds. The importance of comfortable, close-fitting earpieces cannot be overemphasized.

Use of the stethoscope. Using the stethoscope properly involves knowledge of how it works and factors that interfere with its performance. As with percussion, skill requires considerable practice, particularly in listening to normal body sounds. Although descriptions of auscultatory sounds are discussed in examination of the specific body system, the nurse should employ several practical measures when using a stethoscope. For example,

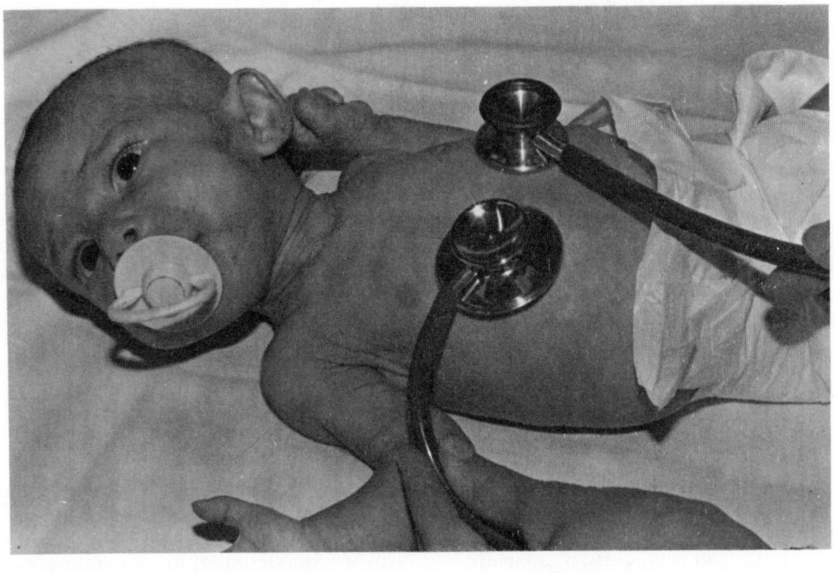

Fig. 5-4. Comparison of pediatric- and adult-size stethoscope on infant's chest.

the child should be relaxed and not crying, talking, or laughing. The room should be of a comfortable temperature and as quiet as possible. The nurse should warm the stethoscope before placing it against the skin. Although applying firm pressure on the chestpiece may improve auscultation, too much pressure forces the chamber of the chestpiece against the diaphragm, preventing vibrations and transmission of sound. Placing the stethoscope over hair or clothing, moving it against the skin, breathing on the tubing, or sliding one's fingers over the chestpiece may cause sounds that falsely resemble pathologic findings. The nurse should practice deliberately producing these sounds in order to differentiate them from actual auscultatory sounds during an examination.

Auscultation, like inspection, requires the mental discipline of concentrating on one aspect of many simultaneous stimuli. The nurse must consciously listen for one sound, such as breathing, while deliberately disregarding other presenting sounds, such as the heartbeat or environmental noises. This is particularly important in children, whose thin chest wall effectively transmits sounds throughout the thoracic cavity. The nurse must also establish a systematic, symmetric approach to auscultation that proceeds from one area of the body to another. Because accurate auscultation requires additional time for the beginning practitioner, it is always thoughtful to explain to parents or older children why one is listening for so long, in order to allay their fears that some abnormality is suspected.

PHYSICAL EXAMINATION

Although the approach to and sequence of the physical examination differ according to the child's age, the following discussion outlines the traditional model for physical assessment. It emphasizes normal findings, variations from the norm that may cause parents or children concern but that require little or no intervention, and abnormalities that necessitate appropriate referral. Although the focus includes all age-groups, the reader is referred to Chapter 8 for a detailed discussion of a newborn assessment, because procedures or findings peculiar to the neonate are not included here.

Growth measurements

Measurement of physical growth in children is a key element in evaluation of the health status of children. Physical growth parameters include weight, height (length), and head circumference. Although not a usual part of the physical examination, assessment of bone growth and dentition may be used to further evaluate body growth.

Values for weight, length, and head circumference are plotted on growth charts, and the child's measurements in percentiles are compared to those of the general population. Studies show that differences in height and weight among well-nourished children of different ethnic backgrounds are relatively small (3% for height and about 6% for weight), but the differences between these children and those of poorer socioeconomic standards of living, regardless of ethnic background, are high (about 12% for height and 30% for weight).[10] Such findings dictate that the present growth charts can be used for all racial or ethnic groups with similar socioeconomic level but that differing environmental factors significantly affect the reliability of standard growth percentiles. The growth charts listed in Appendix E, Fig. E-5, use the fifth and ninety-fifth percentiles as criteria for determining which children fall outside the normal limits for growth. In general those whose height or weight fall below the fifth percentile are considered underweight or small in stature; those above the ninety-fifth percentile are considered overweight or large in stature. Other growth charts, such as those by Stuart and associates from The Children's Hospital Medical Center, Boston, Massachusetts (Appendix E, Figs. E-1 to E-4), use the third and ninety-seventh percentiles as lower and upper limits of normal.

Overall evaluation of growth requires judgment in interpretation of growth percentiles. Children who fall above or below the standard deviation in both height and weight may not be abnormal but may reflect a genetically small or large frame. Comparing their growth trends with those of their parents and siblings is essential in evaluating adequate growth. Children whose growth may be questionable include (1) children whose height and weight percentiles are widely disparate, for example, height in the tenth percentile and weight in the ninetieth percentile is most likely indicative of overweight, (2) children who fail to show the expected gain in height and weight, especially during the rapid growth periods of infancy and adolescence, and (3) children who show a sudden increase or decrease in a previously steady growth pattern. Since growth is a continuous but uneven process, the most reliable evaluation lies in comparison of growth measurements over a prolonged period of time.

Tables for standard height and weight are listed in Appendix E. Table 5-3 summarizes the usual expected growth trends in height and weight during childhood and serves as a reference guide for quickly estimating expected growth.

Techniques for measuring growth

Length. Until children are 24 months old, recumbent height or length is measured in the supine position. Because of their normally flexed position during infancy, measuring length requires full extension of the legs. Although several methods can be used for measuring the fully extended length, the nurse must position the infant correctly by (1) holding the head in midline, (2) grasp-

Table 5-3. General trends in physical growth during childhood

Age	Weight*	Height*
Infants		
Birth-6 months	Weekly gain: 140-200 g (5-7 ounces) Birth weight doubles by end of first 6 months†	Monthly gain: 2.5 cm (1 inch)
6-12 months	Weekly gain: 85-140 g (3-5 ounces) Birth weight triples by end of first year	Monthly gain: 1.25 cm (0.5 inch) Birth length increases by approximately 50% by end of first year
Toddlers	Birth weight quadruples by age 2½ years Yearly gain: 2-3 kg (4.4-6.6 pounds)	Height at 2 years is approximately 50% of eventual adult height Gain during second year: about 12 cm (4.8 inches) Gain during third year: about 6-8 cm (2.4-3.2 inches)
Preschoolers	Yearly gain: 2-3 kg (4.4-6.6 pounds)	Birth length doubles by 4 years of age Yearly gain: 6-8 cm (2.4-3.2 inches)
School-age children	Yearly gain: 2-3 kg (4.4-6.6 pounds)	Yearly gain after age 7 years: 5.0 cm (2 inches) Birth length triples by about 13 years of age
Pubertal growth spurt		
Females—between 10 and 14 years	Weight gain: 7-25 kg (15-55 pounds) Mean: 17.5 kg (38.1 pounds)	Height gain: 5-25 cm (2-10 inches); approximately 95% of mature height achieved by onset of menarche or skeletal age of 13 years Mean: 20.5 cm (8.2 inches)
Males—between 11 and 16 years	Weight gain: 7-30 kg (15-65 pounds) Mean: 23.7 kg (52.1 pounds)	Height gain: 10-30 cm (4-12 inches); approximately 95% of mature height achieved by skeletal age of 15 years Mean: 27.5 cm (11 inches)

*Yearly height and weight gains for each age-group represent averaged estimates from a variety of sources.
†A recent study has shown the mean time for doubling of birth weight to be 3.8 months.[19]

ing the knees together gently, and (3) pushing down on them until the legs are fully extended and flat against the table. If a measuring board is used (Fig. 5-5), the head is placed firmly at the top of the board and the heels of the feet are placed firmly against the footboard.

If such a measuring device is not available, the nurse measures the child's length by placing him on a paper-covered surface and marking the end points of the vertex of the head and heel of the feet. The nurse then removes the child and measures between these two points. Accurate measurement necessitates that the writing utensil be held at a right angle to the table when the cephalic point is marked and that the feet be positioned with the toes pointing directly to the ceiling when the heel point is marked. Regardless of the method used, the parent's assistance in holding the child's head in midline should be enlisted while the nurse extends the legs and takes the measurements.

Height. Recumbent or standing height may be taken in children who are over 24 months of age, although the latter is the usual procedure for those 3 years of age or older. The nurse measures standing height by having the child remove his shoes and socks and stand as tall and straight as possible, with the head in midline and the line of vision parallel to the ceiling or floor. The child's back should be to the wall or other vertical flat surface, with the heels, buttocks, and back of the shoulders touching the wall. The nurse checks for any flexion of the knees, slumping of the shoulders, or raising of the heels of the feet. Height is measured by placing a firm, flat surface against the vertex or crown of the head. The movable measuring rod of platform scales is inaccurate if it does not maintain a parallel position to the floor or rest securely on the topmost part of the crown (Fig. 5-6, *A*). One way of improvising a flat surface for measuring length is to attach a paper or metal tape or yardstick to the wall, position the child adjacent to the tape, and place a thick book on his head, making sure that the end of the book rests firmly against the wall to form a right angle. The nurse marks the point of juncture of the underside of the book and the tape or yardstick (Fig. 5-6, *B*). Length or stature should be measured to the nearest ⅛ inch or 1 mm.[20]

Occasionally special length measurements are taken, such as the *crown-to-rump length* or *sitting height* (see p. 264 for the newborn). In older infants and children, length is most easily determined by having the child sit against the wall and measuring between the vertex of the

A

B

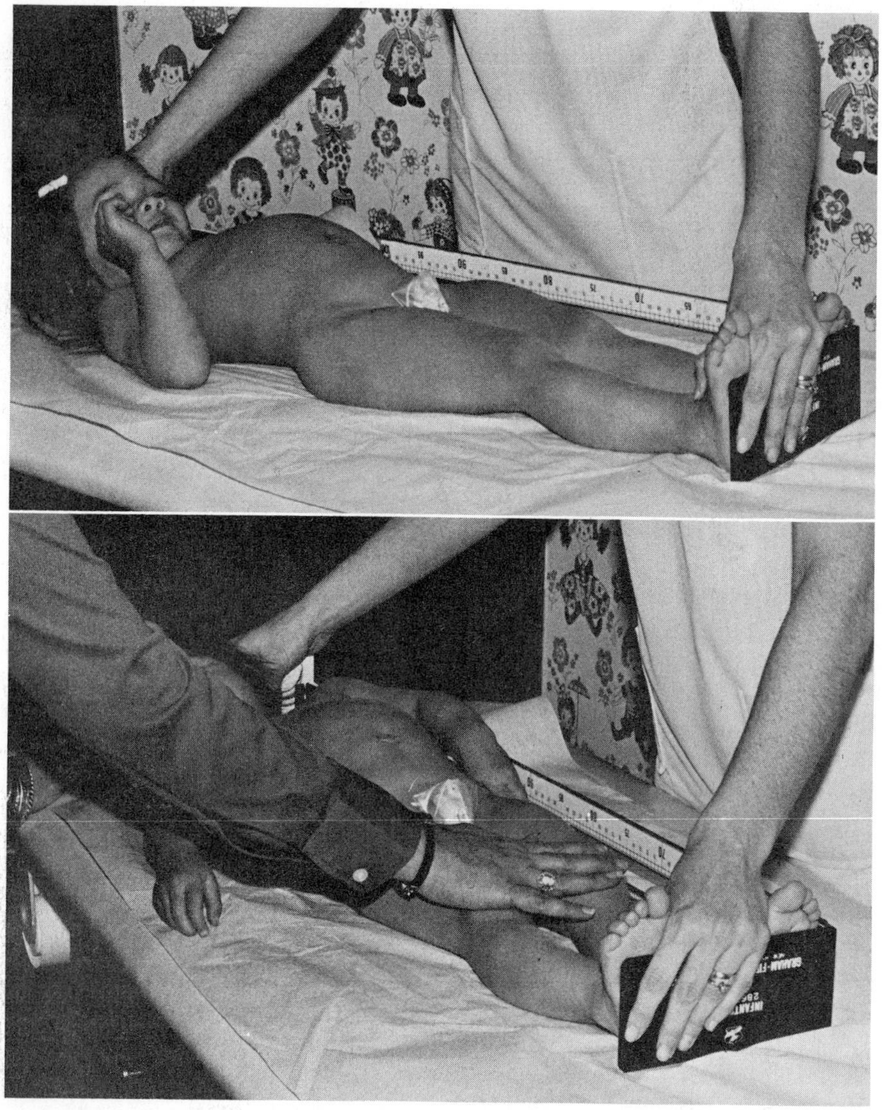

Fig. 5-5. Measurement of child's length. **A,** Incorrect procedure because knees are not firmly pressed for full extension of legs. **B,** Correct procedure of firmly pressing down the knees resulted in ½ inch addition in length.

head and the sitting surface. Although not a usual measurement, this is used in children suspected of being dwarfs. It can help distinguish true dwarfism from small stature. Normally, sitting height accounts for 70% of total body length at birth, 60% at 2 years of age, and about 52% at age 10 years.[4]

Weight. Weight is measured using an appropriate-sized beam balance scale, which measures weights to the nearest 10 g or ½ ounce for infants and 100 g or ¼ pound for children.[20] Before weighing children, the nurse checks to see that the scale is balanced by setting it at zero and noting if the balance registers exactly in the middle of the mark. If the end of the balance beam rises to the top or bottom of the mark, more or less weight, respectively, must be added. Some scales are designed to allow for self-correction, while others need to be recalibrated by the manufacturer.

Measurements should be made in a comfortably warm room. Infants are weighed nude; older children are usually weighed while wearing their underpants or a light gown. It is essential to always respect their need for privacy. If the child must be weighed wearing some article of clothing or some type of special device, such as a prosthesis, this should be noted when the weight is recorded. Children who are measured for recumbent height are usually weighed on a large platform-type infant scale and

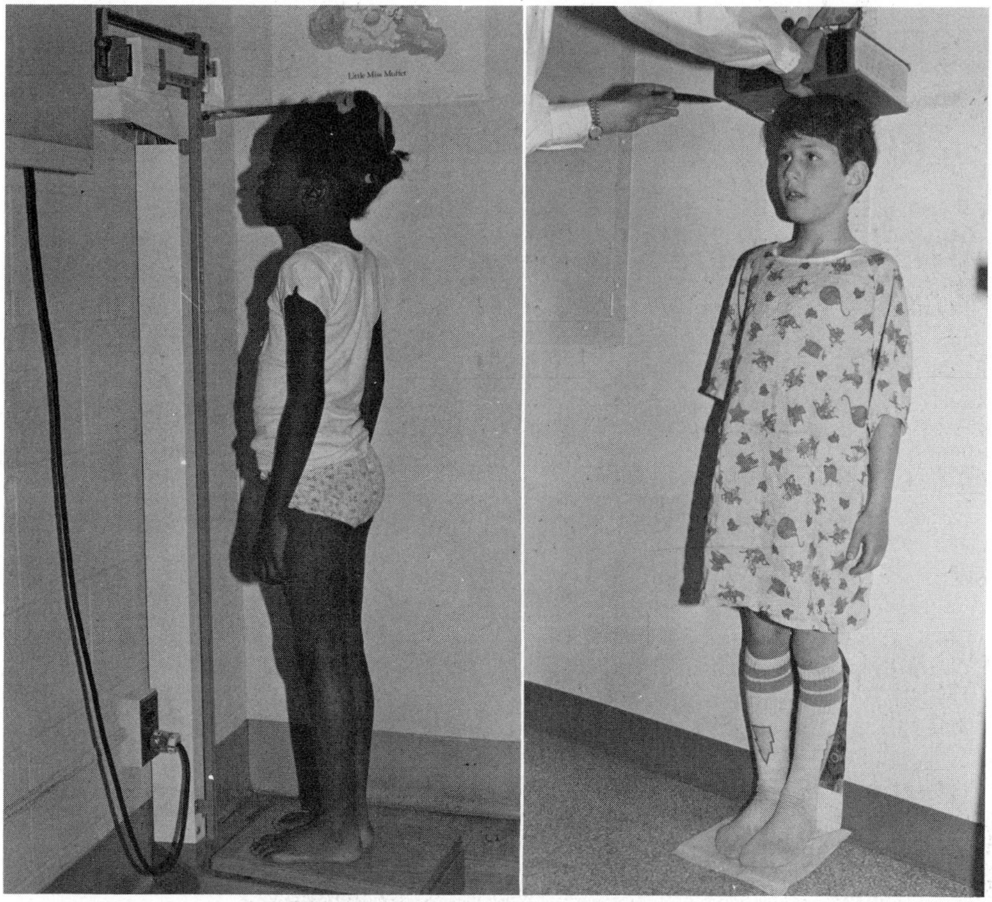

Fig. 5-6. A, Measuring height on a stand-up scale. **B,** Improvising for accurate measurement of height.

placed in a lying-down or sitting position. When weighing infants, the nurse places the hand lightly above the infant to prevent him from accidentally falling off the scale. Once standing height is taken, weight can also be done on a standing-type upright platform scale. For maximum asepsis, either scale is usually covered with a clean sheet of paper that is changed between each child's measurement. (See Figs. 5-6 and 5-7.)

Head circumference. Head circumference is usually taken in all children up to 36 months of age and in any child whose head size is questionable, such as a child with hydrocephalus. The nurse measures the head at its greatest circumference, that is, slightly above the eyebrows and pinna of the ears and around the occipital prominence at the back of the skull (Fig. 5-8). A paper or metal tape is used, not a cloth tape, which can stretch, giving a falsely small measurement. The head size is plotted on the growth chart under head circumference (see Appendix E, Fig. E-12). Generally (1) head circumference in newborns is between 33 and 35.5 cm (13 to 14 inches), (2) at birth head circumference exceeds chest circumference by about 2 to 3 cm or 1 inch, (3) head and chest circumference are equal at about 1 to 2 years of age, and (4) during childhood chest circumference exceeds head size by about 5 to 7 cm (2 to 3 inches).

Physiologic measurements

Physiologic measurements, key elements in evaluating physical status of vital functions, include temperature, pulse, respiration, and blood pressure. Although not usually recorded on a graph similar to growth charts for determination of percentiles, the nurse should compare each physiologic recording with normal values for that age-group (see Appendix A). In addition, the nurse compares the values taken on preceding health visits with present recordings. For example, a spuriously elevated blood pressure reading may not indicate hypertension if previous recent readings have been within normal limits. The isolated recording may be indicative of some other physiologic or psychologic event in the child's life at the time of the present visit.

A

B

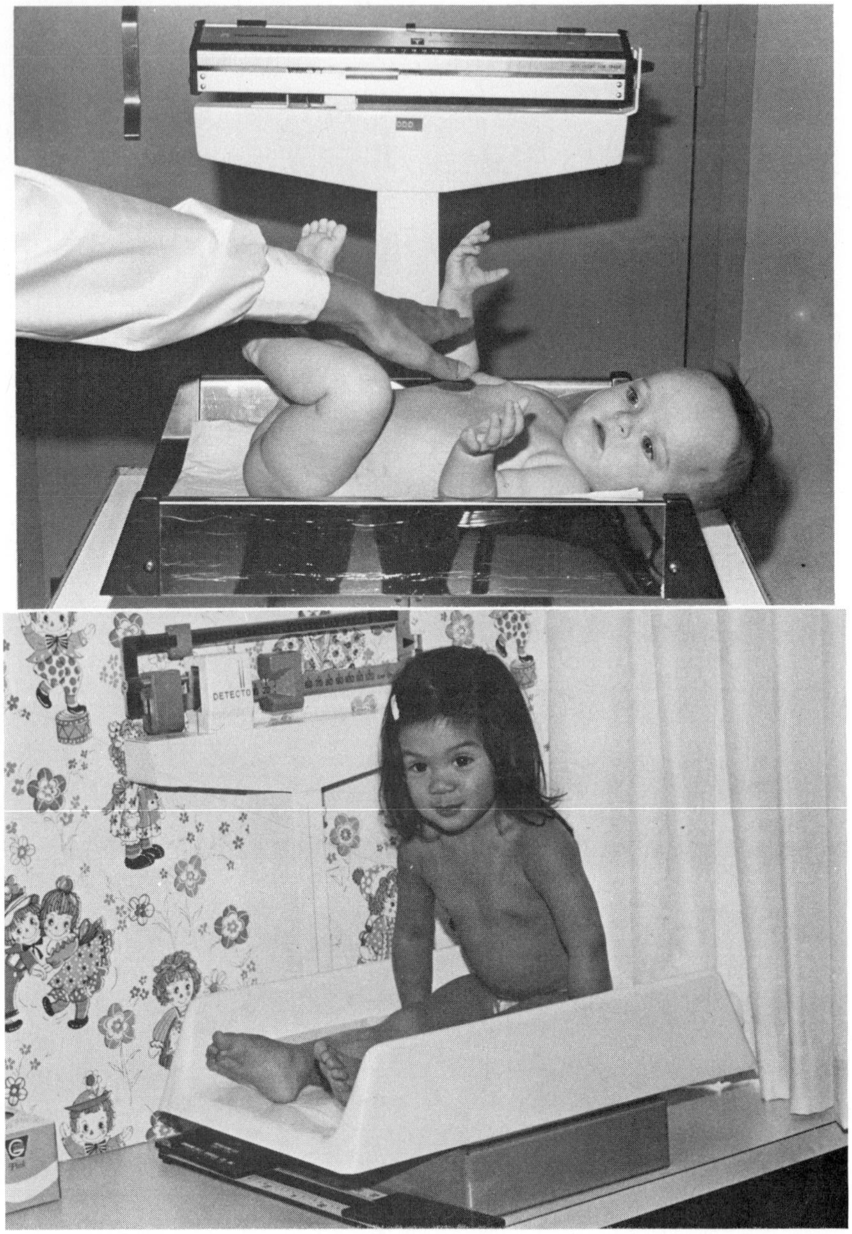

Fig. 5-7. A, Infant on scale. **B,** Weighing a toddler on infant platform scale.

Techniques for measuring vital signs

As in most procedures carried out with children, older children and adolescents in particular are treated much the same as are adult patients. School-age children cooperate better when they understand what is being done, what they will experience personally, and if they are allowed to manipulate the equipment when feasible. For example, they can be allowed to operate a blood pressure apparatus and to watch the mercury (or needle) move as they pump the cuff, listen to their own or another's heartbeat with a stethoscope, and hold the watch while a pulse is being counted.

Special consideration must be given to preschool children, whose fear of body mutilation is intensified with any intrusive procedure (p. 886). Rectal temperatures are particularly threatening. For best results in taking vital signs on infants, the usual order of approach is reversed. That is, respirations are counted first, before the infant is disturbed, the pulse rate next, and the rectal or axillary temperature last. The temperature, if taken first, is likely to precipitate crying and an abnormally high reading of respiratory rate and pulse. If the vital signs cannot be taken without disturbing the child, the child's behavior (for example, cry-

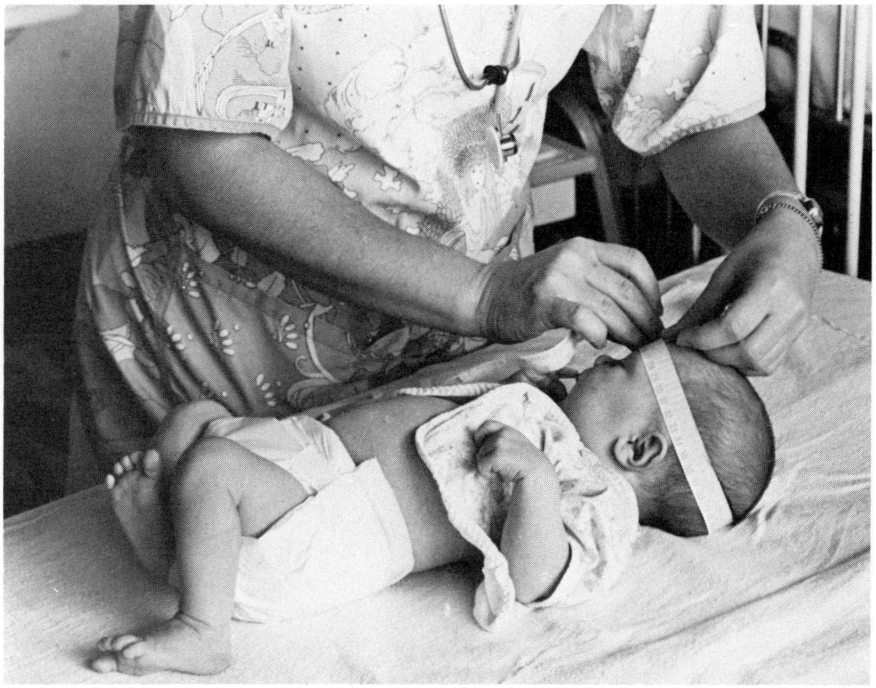

Fig. 5-8. Measuring head circumference.

ing) at the time should be recorded with the vital signs.

Temperature. Temperatures are taken by the oral route on children who can be trusted to maintain the thermometer in position and not bite down on it. Some hospitals and clinics have set a specific age limit (usually 5 or 6 years) at which oral temperatures are permitted. In many instances this may be as young as 4 years of age if the child is alert, not seriously ill, or if there are no other contraindications. The newer electronic temperature-measuring equipment is ideally suited to pediatric use because the plastic sheath is unbreakable, the child's mouth can remain open, and the temperature registers almost immediately.

Axillary temperatures are often recommended for children who object strongly to a rectal temperature but on whom an oral temperature is not feasible. Temperatures on newborn and premature infants are taken by the axillary route (p. 265).

On children less than 5 or 6 years old, rectal temperatures are taken unless contraindicated. Children are positioned in the side-lying or prone position for insertion, and infants are positioned either prone or supine. In the supine position with knees flexed, the nurse holds the infant's feet in one hand and inserts the thermometer with the other. The lightly lubricated or moistened thermometer is inserted only the length of the bulb and left in place for at least 1 full minute. It is advisable to cover the penis of little boys because this procedure often stimulates them to urinate. Rectal temperatures are indicated in children with oral injuries or surgery, children whose mental age contraindicates use of an oral thermometer, unconscious or agitated children, and those who are so seriously ill that it is difficult for them to hold a thermometer in their mouth.

A characteristic of some small children is the tendency toward a rapid temperature elevation with the associated risk of precipitating seizures. Whenever a child feels extra warm to the touch, his temperature should be taken, even if it was found to be normal or of little concern only a short time before. Children under 3 years of age are especially vulnerable to febrile seizures.

Pulse. A satisfactory pulse can be taken radially in children over 2 years of age. However, in infants and young children the apical pulse (heard through a stethoscope held to the chest at the level of the apex of the heart) is more reliable. In infants the point of maximum intensity is located just lateral to the nipple at the third or fourth interspace. With growth, this point gradually assumes a lower, more medial position to reach the fourth or fifth interspace at the midclavicular line. (See Appendix A, Table A-1 for normal rates for pediatric age-groups.) Because infants are disturbed by these common procedures and may become restless or cry and as a result the pulse rate may be elevated, the activity of the child should be recorded with the findings.

Respiration. The respiratory rate is counted in the same manner as it is in the adult patient except that, in infants, the movements are primarily diaphragmatic and, therefore, observed by abdominal movement. Since they are irregular, they should be counted for 1 full minute for accuracy. (See Appendix A, Table A-2 for normal respiratory rates in children.)

Blood pressure. Blood pressure measurements should be considered part of a routine vital sign determination. They can be obtained by several techniques: palpation, auscultation, flush method, Doppler instrument, or an electronic monitoring device. The child should be quiet and relaxed during the procedure; therefore, the blood pressure should be measured before any anxiety-producing procedures are performed or injections given, and techniques for putting the child at ease must be employed. Infants and small children may be more quiet if the reading is taken while they are sitting in the mother's lap. There are no definite data to indicate that one position, sitting or supine, is superior to the other. Children's cooperation can be enlisted if the equipment and each step of the procedure are explained and if they are told how it will feel to them.

Selection of cuff. Accurate measurement requires the use of an appropriately size cuff. The width of the cuff should cover approximately two thirds of the upper arm (or thigh) or be 20% greater than the diameter of the extremity without causing pressure in the axilla or impinging on the anticubital fossa. Ill-fitting cuffs are the most frequent cause of false blood pressure readings: a cuff too narrow will cause a falsely elevated reading; a cuff too wide will result in a lower reading. Compression of the brachial artery in the axilla by clothing pushed up the arm will also produce a false low reading. The length of the bladder of the cuff should be long enough to sufficiently encircle the extremity. A cuff too short to adequately compress the tissues overlying the brachial artery will significantly alter the measurement. This may be a problem in the very obese child. Sometimes an adult thigh cuff may be needed for the severely obese adolescent. Approximate guidelines for selection of cuff sizes are listed below, although the selection of a cuff must be individualized for each child.

Measurement. The technique of blood pressure measurement in children is generally the same as that used for adults. Systolic pressure is the point at which the sound is first apparent, and diastolic pressure is the point at which the sound becomes muffled, not the point at which it disappears. In children less than 1 year of age the thigh pressure is equal to the arm blood pressure, but in children over age 1 year the thigh pressure normally averages 20 mm Hg higher than the arm pressure. A lower pressure in the lower extremities may indicate some interference with circulation such as coarctation of the aorta. Appendix A, Table A-3 gives the average blood pressure readings at various ages throughout childhood.

The blood pressure can be taken by the conventional *auscultation* method by listening for the sound at the brachial artery in the anticubital fossa. A systolic reading can be obtained by *palpation* and is measured as the point at which the pulse at the radial, or other distal, artery reappears as the cuff is deflated. A pediatric stethoscope with a small-diameter diaphragm and amplification is helpful for hearing blood pressure sounds in small children and infants. In some cases the *Doppler* instrument is used. This apparatus translates changes in ultrasound frequency caused by blood movement within the artery to audible sound by means of a transducer in the cuff.

In newborns (including the premature infants) or in small infants whose pressure is difficult or impossible to obtain by other techniques, the *flush* method is employed. Although the flush blood pressure reflects the *mean* blood pressure, it has been found to correlate well with the mean aortic pressure in comparison tests. Current standards for flush blood pressure readings have not been established for infants at all weights. A range of 30 to 60 mm Hg is considered normal for infants over 2500 g (5.5 pounds). The pressure of most larger infants is outlined in Appendix A, Table A-4. A flush blood pressure determination is performed as follows:

1. Apply blood pressure cuff (usually 5 cm) to extremity.
2. Wrap portion of extremity distal to cuff snuggly with elastic bandage. Wrap from fingers or toes toward cuff for complete capillary emptying.
3. Inflate cuff to 120 to 140 mm Hg.
4. Remove elastic bandage.
5. Gradually deflate cuff at the rate of approximately 5 mm/second.

The point at which the earliest discernible flush is observed in the blanched extremity is considered to be the flush end point (Fig. 5-9). Although many nurses can blanch the extremity satisfactorily by applying compression with one hand while inflating the cuff with the other, greatest accuracy is achieved with the use of an elastic bandage.

Guidelines for selection of standard blood pressure cuffs

Age	*Size (cm)*
Newborn (premature or full-term)	2.5-3
Infants (less than 1 year)	4-5
Children	
Less than 4 years	6-7
5 to 10 years	8-10
10 years and older	10-12

General appearance

The general appearance of the child is a cumulative, subjective impression of the child's physical appearance, state of nutrition, behavior, personality, interactions with parents and nurse (also siblings if present), posture, development, and speech. Although general appearance is recorded in the beginning of the physical examination, it encompasses all

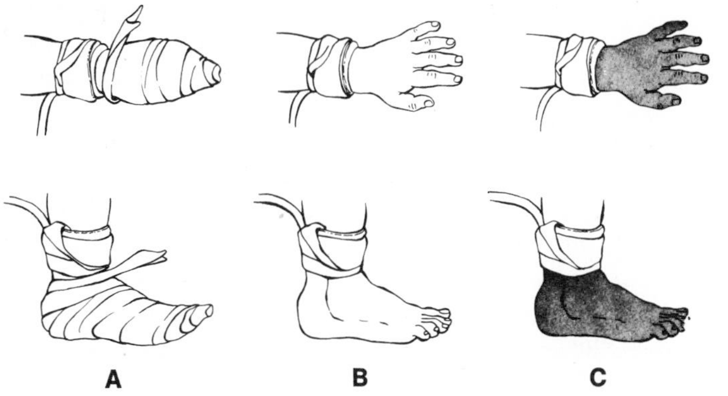

Fig. 5-9. Indirect method to determine blood pressure measurement. **A,** Extremity wrapped with elastic bandage. **B,** Cuff inflated. **C,** Flush indicates return of circulation to extremity. (From Moss, A. J., and Adams, F. H.: Problems of blood pressure in childhood, 1962. Courtesy of Charles C Thomas, Publisher, Springfield, Ill.)

the nurse's observations of the child during the interview and physical assessment. It is similar to the "patient profile" discussed on p. 99 but focuses more on physical characteristics of appearance.

Physical appearance. The description of physical appearance should make special note of *facies,* the facial expression and appearance of the child. For example, the facies may give clues to children who are in pain, have difficulty in breathing, feel frightened, discontent, or happy, are mentally deficient, or are acutely ill.

Posture, position, and types of body movement also are important in the overall assessment of physical appearance. The child with hearing or vision loss may characteristically tilt his head in an awkward position to facilitate perception of sound or sight. The child in pain may favor a body part. The child with low self-esteem or a feeling of rejection may assume a slumped, careless, and apathetic type pose or posture. Likewise, a child with confidence, a feeling of self-worth, and a sense of security usually demonstrates a tall, straight, well-balanced posture. Although the nurse observes such "body language," it must not be interpreted too freely but rather recorded objectively.

The nurse also takes note of the child's state of cleanliness or *hygiene,* the appropriateness of dress for climatic conditions, unusual odor, the condition of the hair, neck, nails, teeth, and feet, and the condition of the clothing. Such observations give excellent clues to possible instances of neglect, inadequate financial resources, housing difficulties such as no running water, or lack of knowledge of children's needs.

Nutrition. General appearance includes an overall impression of the child's state of nutrition. This impression is more than a statement describing body weight or stature, such as "slender and tall." It is an estimation of the quality, as well as quantity, of nutritional intake. For example, two children can be of the same height and weight, yet one can appear overweight because of flabby, loose skin, while the other child appears strong, robust, and well built because of firm, well-defined musculature. Likewise, a small, slender child may be well-nourished, with no signs of chronic undernutrition, such as bony prominences, protuberant abdomen, flat buttocks, gaunt facies, and poor muscle tone with evidence of wasting.

The nurse's impression of nutritional state should be compared with the parents' history of feeding practices. Discrepancies between the two "impressions" may be a valuable area for nutritional counseling. For example, parents who believe that their child is too thin and eats too little, despite evidence of adequate growth and physical signs of proper nutrition, may find it helpful to keep a daily diary in order to calculate the child's cumulative food intake. When this is done, many parents are surprised at the quantity of food ingested, even though the amounts at each meal or snack are small.

Behavior. Behavior is so encompassing that it is difficult to discuss adequately. It includes the child's personality, level of activity, reaction to stress, requests, or frustration, interactions with others, primarily the parent and nurse, degree of alertness, and response to stimuli. It is one of the most important observations that the nurse makes during a child's health assessment.

Some mental questions that serve as reminders for observing behavior include: what is the child's overall personality—calm, anxious, tense, content, outgoing, shy, talkative, aggressive, introverted, stable, or moody; is he active, sedentary, fidgety, or restless; does he have a long attention span or is he easily distracted; does he sit quietly on the examining table or his mother's lap or does he climb, run, open doors, and explore everything; how does he react to commands—with fear or willingness to obey; how advanced is his ability to follow requests, can he follow two or three commands in succession without the need for repetition, is he attentive to requests or must they be repeated several times; is he cooperative, belligerent, or argumentive; what is his response to delayed gratification or frustration, is he able to withstand momentary discomfort and wait for his requests to be met; in what tone of voice does he make requests or talk to his parents; does he seek their approval and gain satisfaction from it; does he use eye-to-eye contact during conversation; how willingly does he answer questions; does he agree with his parents' answers or find reasons to disagree, interrupt, or argue; what is his reaction to the nurse—respectful, friendly, reserved, apprehensive, or uninterested; is he interested in his surroundings, does he look around the room, ask questions about unfamiliar objects, seem to enjoy exploring them, or attempt to break or destroy them; can he follow directions for using the instruments or imitate their use, is he quick or slow to grasp explanations?

Development. Although the nurse can usually assess gross developmental achievement from careful and detailed observation of the child, the impressions should be documented with screening tests, such as the Denver Developmental Screening Test. Various tests for assessing development, speech, vision, and hearing are discussed later in this chapter and in Chapter 24.

The nurse should record under general appearance an overall estimate of the child's speech development, motor skills, degree of coordination, and recent area of achievement. For example, the nurse may make the following statement about an 18-month-old child: "Motor development advanced for age, climbs, runs, jumps (most recent motor skill), manipulates small objects with ease, excellent coordination and balance, beginning to name many objects, uses two-word phrases, and enjoys 'talking' to self and others."

Skin

Skin is assessed for color, texture, temperature, moisture, and turgor. Hair is also inspected for color, texture, quality, distribution, and elasticity. Examination of the skin and its accessory organs primarily involves inspection and palpation.

Physical factors influencing assessment. The nurse examines the child in a well-illuminated room, with non-glare lighting. Ideally, the room should be neutral in color. Colors such as pink, blue, yellow, or orange cast deceiving glows on the skin. The room should also be comfortably warm, since air-conditioning can cause a cold-induced cyanosis and excessive heat can produce flushing. Poor hygiene and artificial paint on nails or lips also mask true determination of color. Sometimes it is necessary to clean the skin with soap and water and to remove cosmetics before beginning inspection. Although not a frequent situation in pediatrics, the nurse should remember that such factors can hide signs of ecchymoses, petechiae, pallor, or cyanosis.

Texture, temperature, moisture, and turgor can be subjectively inspected, but palpation must be done for greater accuracy. Clothing always interferes with palpation, thereby necessitating that the nurse examine each area of the body nude either as part of the general overall examination or combined with assessment of each body system. Since texture is affected by climatic exposure, such as cold, sun, wind, and so on, the nurse should compare the texture of areas of the body that are usually clothed to those that are generally exposed.

Genetic factors influencing assessment of color. The normal color in light-skinned children varies from a milky-white and rosy color to a more deep-hued pink color. In general, bluish discolorations or cyanosis are not normal, except in the newborn (see p. 266). Dark-skinned children, such as those from American Indian, Mexican, black, Latin, Mediterranean, or Oriental descent, have inherited various brown, red, yellow, olive-green, and bluish tones in their skin, which can falsely alter one's assessment. For example, some children of Mediterranean origin normally have bluish-tinged lips, suggestive of cyanosis. Oriental persons, whose skin is normally of a yellow tone, may appear to be jaundiced. Full-blooded black individuals often have normal bluish pigmentation of the gums, buccal cavity, borders of the tongue, and nail beds. The visible portion of their sclera may contain speckled deposits of brown melanin that resemble petechiae.[23]

Physiologic factors influencing assessment of color. Edema of the skin affects color in all individuals because it increases the amount of interstitial fluid, thereby increasing the distance between the outermost layers of the epidermis and the pigmented and vascular layers. Edema decreases the intensity of skin color, sometimes producing a false pallor.

Exposure to sunlight, on the other hand, stimulates the melanocytes to produce more melanin, thereby increasing the color of the skin. Individuals who are deeply suntanned require as careful observation as those who are genetically dark skinned.

In general the amount of adipose tissue does not markedly affect skin color because deposition of fat cells is below the pigmented layers of the skin. However, the nurse should be aware that overnutrition may not mean adequate nutrition, and observation of pallor that may be indicative of nutritional-iron deficiency should be carefully done.

Reliable areas for assessment of color. Color changes are most reliably assessed in those areas of the body where melanin production is least: sclera, conjunctiva, nail beds, lips, tongue, buccal mucosa, palms, and soles. In children the latter sites are usually more reliable than in adults, because the formation of calluses can give the tissue an orange or yellow hue.[23] These areas are rarely affected by edema or amount of adipose tissue but are sensitive to changes from physical factors, such as use of cosmetics or ingestion of colored food substances.

Variations in skin color. Many of the specific color changes peculiar to the newborn are described on p. 266. In general, color changes of significance include pallor, cyanosis, erythema, ecchymosis, petechiae, and jaundice.

Pallor and cyanosis. The skin receives its pigmented color of yellow, brown, and black from melanin and its shades of red or blue from the color of hemoglobin. Oxygenated hemoglobin in the superficial capillaries of the dermis gives skin a rosy, pink glow. Reduced (deoxygenated) hemoglobin reflects a bluish tone through the skin, called cyanosis, which is evident when reduced hemoglobin levels reach 5 mg/100 ml of blood or more, regardless of the total hemoglobin.[4] In general, the darker the skin pigmentation, the greater the amount of deoxygenated hemoglobin must be for cyanosis to be evident. Pallor, or paleness, is evident as a loss of the rosy glow in light-skinned individuals, an ashen-gray appearance in black-skinned children, and a more yellowish-brown color in brown-skinned people. It may be a sign of anemia, chronic disease, edema, or shock. However, it may be a normal complexion characteristic or an indication of indoor living.

Pallor or cyanosis is most evident in the palpebral conjunctiva (lower eyelid), nail beds, earlobes (mainly for light-skinned children), lips, oral membranes, soles, and palms. Pallor or cyanosis can be compared to the color change normally produced by blanching. For example, in nonpigmented nails, the nurse presses down on the free edge of the child's index or middle finger. Exerting pressure on the nail of a person with good skin color will produce marked blanching or whitening as compared to the return blood flow. In a child with pallor, the difference in color change will be slight. The blanching color change can be observed in dark-skinned individuals by gently applying pressure to their lips or gums.

Erythema. Erythema, or redness of the skin, may be the result of increased temperature from climatic conditions, local inflammation, or infection. It may also appear as a sign of skin irritation, allergy, or other dermatoses. The degree of redness reflects the amount of increased blood flow to the area. The nurse notes any reddening and describes its location, size, presence of warmth, itching, type of distribution (diffuse, clearly circumscribed, parallel to a vein, and so on), and the presence of characteristic lesions, such as macules, papules, or vesicles (see Chapter 18 for a description of skin lesions). Because erythema is much more difficult to assess in darkly pigmented individuals, the nurse must rely heavily on carefully palpating the area for evidence of associated signs, such as warmth or skin lesions.

Ecchymosis and petechiae. Ecchymosis and petechiae are caused by extravasation or hemorrhage of blood into the skin; the only difference between the two is in size. Ecchymoses are large, diffuse areas, usually black and blue in color, and are usually the result of accidental injuries in healthy, active children. Since ecchymotic areas can be indicative of systemic disorders or of child maltreatment, the nurse should always investigate the reported cause of the bruises, especially when they are located in suspicious areas, such as the back or buttocks, rather than on the knees, shins, elbows, or forearms.

Petechiae are small, distinct pinpoint hemorrhages 2 mm or less in size, which usually denote some type of blood disorder, such as decreased platelets in leukemia. Because of their size, ecchymoses are more readily observed than are petechiae, which may only be visible in areas of very light-colored skin, such as the buttocks, abdomen, and inner surfaces of the arms or legs. They are usually invisible in heavily pigmented skin, except in the oral mucosa, the palpebral conjunctiva of the eyelids, and the bulbar conjunctiva covering the eyeball.

The nurse can distinguish areas of erythema from ecchymosis or petechiae by blanching the skin. Since erythema is a result of increased blood flow *to* the area, exerting pressure will momentarily empty the engorged vessels and produce blanching. Since the other discolorations are produced by blood leaking *into* tissue spaces, blanching will not occur.

Jaundice. Jaundice, a yellow staining of the skin usually caused by bile pigments, is always a significant finding. It is most reliably observed in the sclera of the eyes in both dark- and light-skinned children, but it may also be evident in the skin, fingernails, soles, palms, and oral mucosa membranes of the latter group. If a yellow-orange cast is noted in an otherwise healthy child, the nurse should inquire about the quantity of ingested yellow vegetables, such as carrots, which in excess produce a yellow-orange color from deposits of carotene in the skin, called carotenemia.

Texture. The nurse palpates the skin for texture, noting moisture and temperature. Any marks or scars that are suggestive of healed injuries are noted, and inquiries are made about their origin. Normally the skin of young children is smooth, slightly dry to the touch, not oily or clammy, and of even exterior temperature. Any variations from these findings are noted, because they may indicate common problems of childhood such as cradle cap (scaliness on the scalp), eczema (scaliness and desquamation on the scalp, cheeks, knees, and elbows), diaper rash (redness and dryness in the genital area), or excesssive dryness all over the body from too frequent bathing, exposure to the weather, or vitamin-A deficiency. Excessively moist, clammy skin may indicate serious health problems, particularly heart disease.

Temperature. The nurse evaluates skin temperature by symmetrically feeling each part of the body and comparing upper areas with lower ones. Any distinct difference in temperature is noted. Although not a common anomaly, one of the key signs for coarctation of the aorta is warm upper extremities and cool lower ones. The nurse also observes the skin temperature of the dressed child. Young children produce heat rapidly, and they quickly become overheated if dressed too warmly. Many parents do not realize this and fail to change the amount of clothing to accomodate climactic variations.

Turgor. Tissue turgor refers to the amount of elasticity in the skin. It is best determined by grasping the skin on the abdomen between the thumb and index finger, pulling it taut, and quickly releasing it. Elastic tissue immediately assumes its normal position without residual marks or creases. In children with poor skin turgor the skin remains suspended or tented for a few seconds before slowly falling back on the abdomen. Skin turgor is one of the best estimates of adequate hydration and nutrition.

While evaluating turgor, the nurse also inspects for signs of *edema,* normally evident as swelling or puffiness. Periorbital edema is a sign of several systemic disorders, such as kidney diseases, but may normally be seen in children who have been crying, sleeping, or who have allergies. Edema should be evaluated for change according to position, its specific location, and response to pressure. For example, in pitting edema, pressing a finger into the edematous area will cause a temporary indentation.

Accessory organs. Inspection of the accessory organs of the skin, namely the hair, nails, and dermatoglyphics formed by the sweat glands of the fingers and hands, may be performed while the skin is being examined or when the scalp and extremities are being assessed.

Hair. The hair is inspected for color, texture, quality, distribution, and elasticity. Children's scalp hair is usually lustrous, silky, strong, and elastic. Genetic factors affect the appearance of hair. For example, the hair of black children is usually curlier and coarser than that of white children. Hair that is stringy, dull, brittle, dry, friable, and depigmented may suggest poor nutrition. Any bald or thinning spots are recorded. Although alopecia can be a sign of various skin disorders, such as tinea capitis, loss of hair in infants may be indicative of lying in the same position and may be a clue for counseling parents concerning the child's stimulation needs.

The nurse also inspects the hair and scalp for general cleanliness. Various ethnic groups condition their hair with oils or lubricants, which, if not thoroughly washed from the scalp, clog the sebaceous glands, causing scalp infections. The nurse also inspect hair shafts for lice, whose ova appear as grayish translucent flakes. The nurse can distinguish the ova or nits from dandruff because the eggs adhere to the hair. If pediculosis capitis is suspected, the nurse should be careful to guard against self-infestation of the lice by wearing gloves, washing the hands after the examination, and standing away from the child when looking through the hair.

The nurse also inspects the scalp for ticks, which appear as grayish or brown oval bodies. Although they can be found anywhere on the body, the most common sites are exposed parts, such as the head. They fasten themselves to the host with their teeth, embedding their head in the skin. They transmit a number of infectious diseases, such as Rocky Mountain spotted fever, through their bite, crushed tissues, feces, or blood. Nurses who suspect a tick should remove it with its body intact and be careful not to touch it with bare hands. Applying the hot tip of a match or cigarette to the tick's body may cause it to detach from the skin. If it must be manually removed, the entire body is pryed out with a needle, and the puncture site is disinfected. Although not all dog or wood ticks transmit serious disease, a notation is made on the child's chart of its removal in case symptoms appear.

Unusual hairiness anywhere on the body, such as arms, legs, trunk, or face is noted. Tufts of hair anywhere along the spine, especially over the sacrum, are significant because they can mark the site of spina bifida occulta.

In older children who are approaching puberty, the nurse observes for growth of secondary hair as signs of normally progressing pubertal changes. Pubic hair begins to appear in girls between 11 and 14 years of age, followed by axillary hair about 6 months later. Pubic and axillary hair follow the same sequence in boys but begin to appear between 12 and 16 years of age, followed by facial hair 6 months after the appearance of axillary hair. Appearance of hair in these areas indicates normal adrenal and testicular function. Precocious or delayed appearance of hair growth is noted because, although not always suggestive of hormonal dysfunction, it may be of great concern to the early- or late-maturing adolescent.

Nails. The nails are inspected for color, shape, texture, and quality. Normally the nails are pink, convex in shape, smooth, and hard but flexible, not brittle. The edges, which are usually white, should extend over the fingers. Dark-skinned individuals may have more deeply pigmented nail beds. Variation in color, such as blueness, is suggestive of cyanosis, and a yellow tint may indicate jaundice. Bluish-black discoloration usually indicates hemorrhage under the nail from trauma. Fungal infections cause the entire nail to become whitish in color, with a pitting surface. Short ragged nails are typical of habitual biting. Uncut nails with dirt accumulated under the edge are sometimes an indication of children with poor hygiene.

Changes in the shape of nails are also significant. For example, concave curves or "spoon nails," called koilonychia, are sometimes seen in iron-deficiency anemia, a frequent nutritional problem of children. Clubbing of the nails is always a significant finding and usually is associated with chronic cyanosis. In clubbing, the base of the nail becomes visibly swollen and feels springy or floating when palpated, rather than firm as in the normal nail.

Dermatoglyphics. Each individual has a distinct set of handprints and footprints created by epidermal ridges and creases formed in the third month of prenatal life and cracks that develop subsequently throughout a lifetime. The patterns, or *dermatoglyphics,* are unique to the individual and vary a great deal in detail and complexity of patterns. For example, fingerprint patterns consist of loops, swirls, and arches in highly individualized types and combinations (Fig. 5-10). Flexion creases also appear on the palm of the hand and the sole of the foot. The palm normally shows three flexion creases (Fig. 5-11, *A*). In some situations the two distal horizontal creases are fused to form a single horizontal crease called a *single palmar crease,* or *simian crease* (Fig. 5-11, *B*), which is noted in almost all conditions that are caused by chromosomal abnormalities. Another variation noted by some investigators is the *Sydney line* (Fig. 5-11, *C*), in which the transverse palmar crease extends to the ulnar margin of the palm. This is seen in a large percentage of children with rubella syndrome. If grossly abnormal lines or folds are observed, the nurse should sketch a picture to describe them and refer the finding to a specialist for further investigation.

Lymph nodes

Lymph nodes are usually assessed when the part of the body in which they are located is examined. Although the body's lymphatic drainage system is extensive, the usual sites for palpating accessible lymph nodes are shown in Fig. 5-12. Since the major function of lymph nodes is to collect and filter the lymph of bacteria and other foreign matter as it returns to the circulatory system, the nurse must have knowledge of the lymph's directional flow. Tender, enlarged warm lymph nodes are generally indicative of infection or inflammation proximal to their location. For example, occipital or postauricular adenopathy is often seen in local scalp infection, such as pediculosis, tick bite, or external otitis. Cervical adenopathy usually accompanies acute infections in or around the mouth or throat. In children, however, small, nontender, movable nodes are usually normal.

The nurse palpates for nodes by using the distal portion of the fingers, gently but firmly pressing in a circular motion

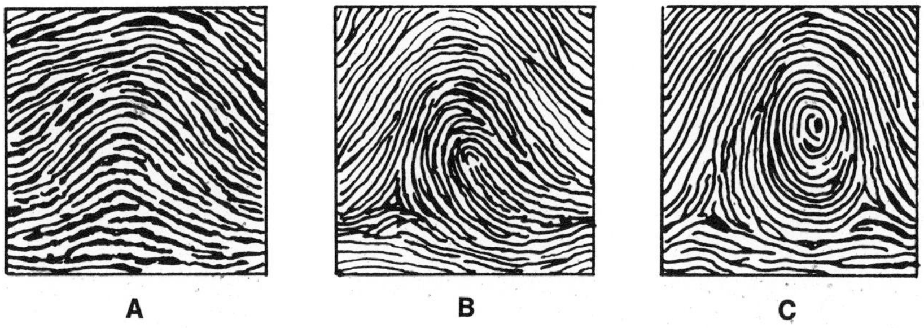

Fig. 5-10. Examples of the three basic fingerprint types. **A,** Arch; **B,** loop; and **C,** whorl. (From Whaley, L. F.: Understanding inherited disorders, St. Louis, 1974, The C. V. Mosby Co., p. 210.)

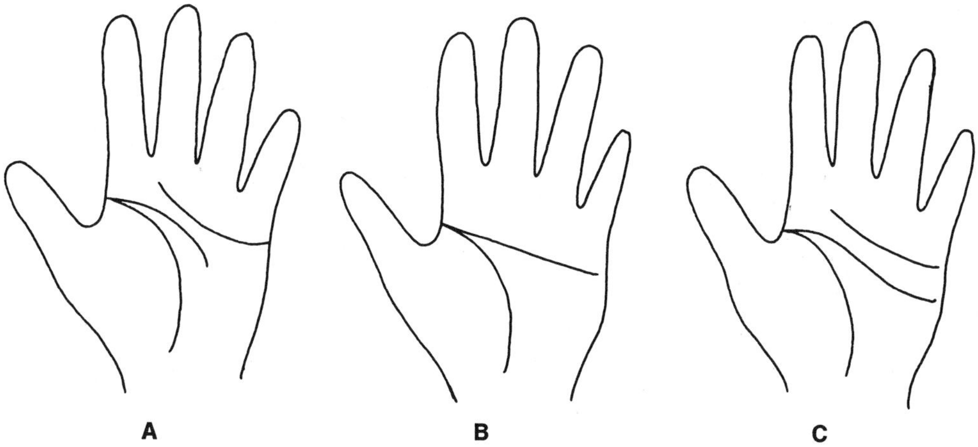

Fig. 5-11. Examples of flexion creases on the palm. **A,** Normal; **B,** simian line; **C,** Sydney line. (From Whaley, L. F.: Understanding inherited disorders, St. Louis, 1974, The C. V. Mosby Co., p. 211.)

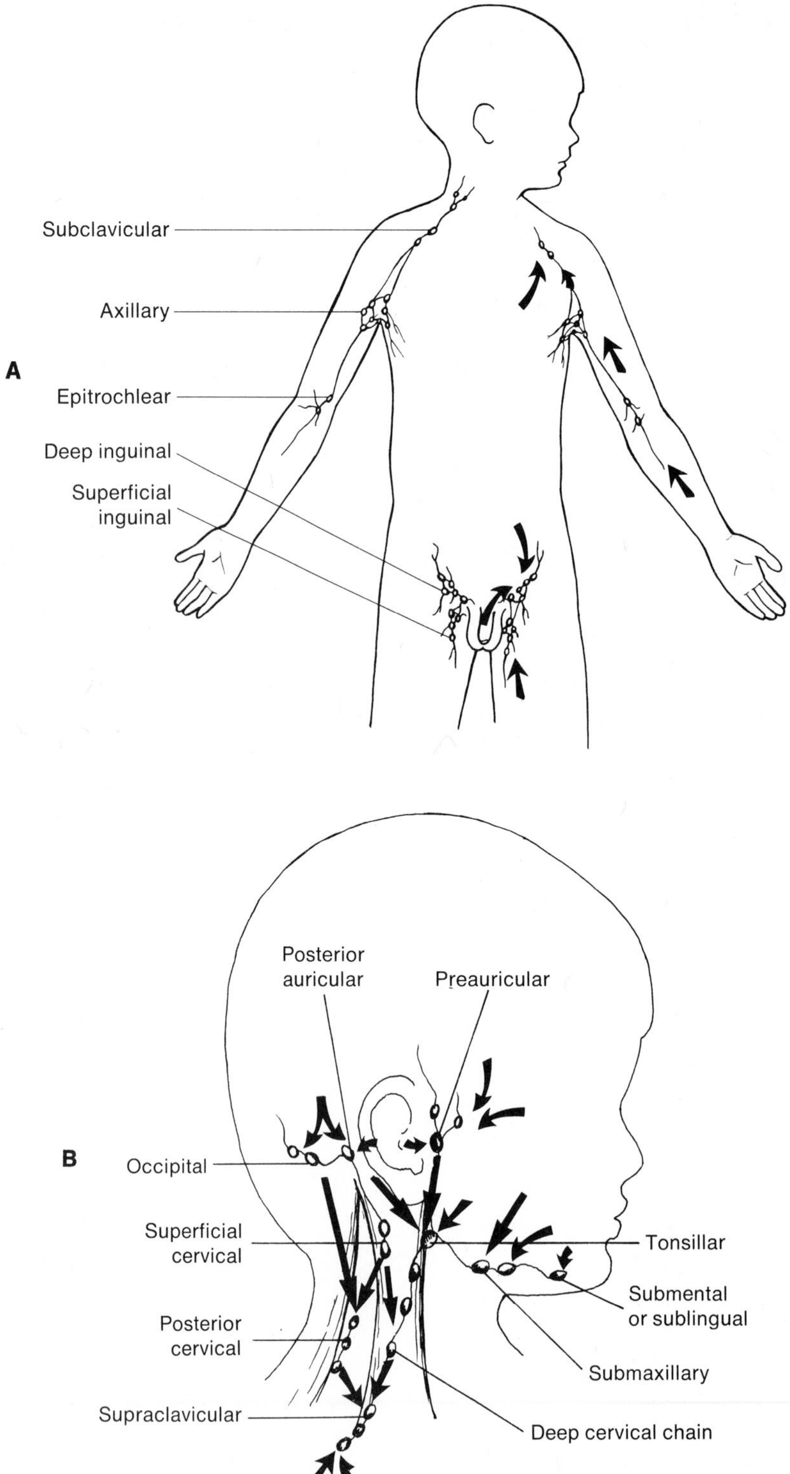

Fig. 5-12. A and **B,** Location of superficial lymph nodes. *Arrows* indicate directional flow of lymph.

along the regions where nodes are normally present. When assessing the nodes in the head and neck, the child's head is tilted upward slightly but without tensing the sternocleidomastoid or trapezius muscles. This position facilitates palpation of all surface nodes in this region. Flexing the head on the chest, which often happens when children resist this procedure, makes palpation of the submental, submaxillary, tonsillar, and cervical nodes very difficult. The axillary nodes are palpated with the arms relaxed at the side but slightly abducted. The inguinal nodes are best assessed with the child in the supine position. Size, mobility, temperature, and tenderness are noted, as well as reports by the parents regarding any visible change of enlarged nodes.

Head

The head is inspected for general *shape* and *symmetry*. A flattening of one part of the head, such as the occiput, may indicate that the child continually lies in this position. Marked asymmetry is usually abnormal and may indicate premature closure of the sutures (craniosynostosis).

The nurse also notes *head control* in infants and head posture in older children. Most infants by 4 months of age should be able to hold the head erect and in midline when in a vertical position. Significant head lag after 6 months of age is strongly indicative of cerebral injury.

The *scalp* is examined for cleanliness, lesions, scaliness, evidence of infestation, such as lice or ticks, and signs of trauma, such as ecchymosis, masses, or scars.

The *skull* is palpated for patent sutures, fontanels, fractures, and swellings. Normally the posterior fontanel closes by the second month of life and the anterior fontanel closes between 12 and 18 months of age. Early or late closure is noted, since either may be a sign of pathology. For a more detailed discussion of the cranial bones, see p. 267 under assessment of the neonate.

While the head is being examined, the nurse also inspects the face for symmetry, movement, and general appearance. Asking the child to "make a face" helps the nurse assess symmetric movement and discover any degree of paralysis. Any unusual facial proportion should be noted, such as unusually high or low forehead, wide or close-set eyes, or small, receding chin.

The nurse also notes any unusual swellings or sites of edema that may be associated with specific disorders, such as nephrosis, Cushing's syndrome, or steroid therapy. Visible and palpable swelling anterior to the earlobe and above the angle of the jaw is characteristic of parotid gland enlargement in mumps. It gives the child a characteristic "chipmunk" appearance.

The nurse also evaluates range of motion by asking the older child to look in each direction (to either side, up, and down) or manually puts the younger child through each position. Limited range of motion may indicate wry-neck or *torticollis,* a result of injury to the sternocleidomastoid muscle, in which the child usually holds his head to one side with the chin pointing toward the opposite side. Hyperextension of the head (opisthotonos) with pain on flexion is a serious indication of meningeal irritation.

Generally the head and face are not auscultated or percussed, with the exception of the sinuses. The *sinuses* are air cavities within certain bones adjacent to the nasal cavity (Fig. 5-13). The sinuses develop as the skull bones enlarge throughout childhood and adolescence. The maxillary sinus is usually present at birth but does not enlarge very much until after the teeth erupt. The frontal sinus begins to develop in early infancy, and the ethmoid and sphenoid sinuses develop later in childhood. The frontal and maxillary sinuses may be directly percussed in children over 2 years of age. Tenderness or pain usually indicates sinusitis.

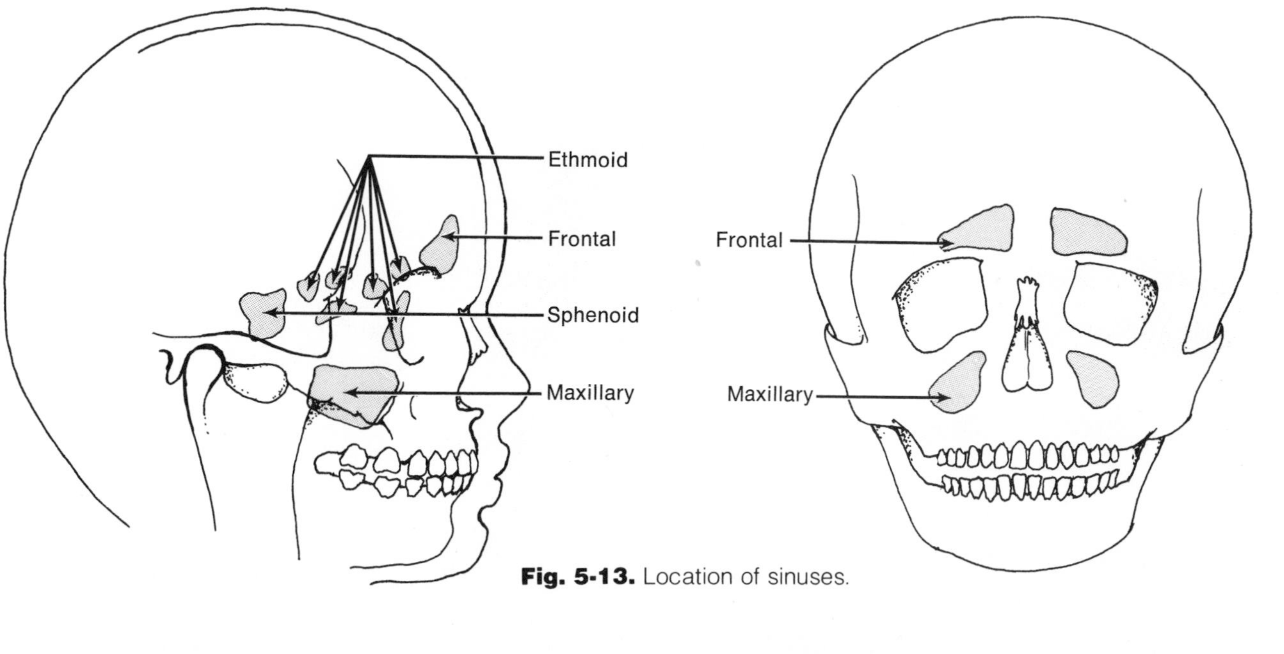

Fig. 5-13. Location of sinuses.

Neck

Besides assessing motility of the head and neck, the nurse also inspects its size and palpates it for associated structures. The neck normally is short with skin folds between the head and shoulders during infancy; however, it lengthens during the next 3 to 4 years. A short and/or webbed neck is associated with various anomalies, such as Turner's syndrome. Marked edema of the neck may indicate mumps, local throat or mouth infections, or diphtheria. Distended neck veins often indicate difficulty with breathing on expiration, such as in asthma or cystic fibrosis.

The nurse palpates the *trachea* by placing the thumb and index finger on each side and sliding them back and forth to note any masses. Normally the trachea is slightly to the right of the midline. Any shift is noted since it can signify serious lung problems, such as a tumor or foreign body in the lung. The nurse also palpates for the *thyroid gland,* which is located at the base of the neck. This butterfly-shaped gland straddles the trachea and has two large lateral lobes connected by an isthmus or band of glandular tissue. The isthmus is the only portion of the thyroid that is usually palpable, because the lobes that curve posteriorly around the trachea are partially covered by the sternocleidomastoid muscle (Fig. 5-14). Normally the thyroid rises as the child swallows. However, palpating the thyroid takes considerable practice and is especially difficult in an infant, whose neck is short and thick. If the nurse detects any masses in the neck, they are recorded and reported for further investigation.

Children who have received external irradiation to the

Fig. 5-14. Two views of thyroid gland. **A,** Front view; **B,** side view.

A

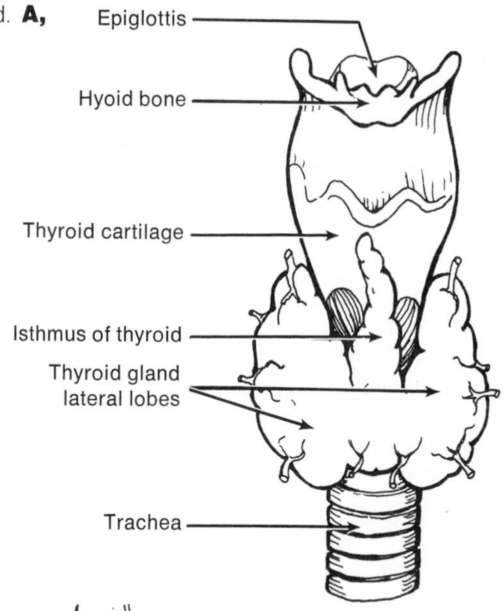

B

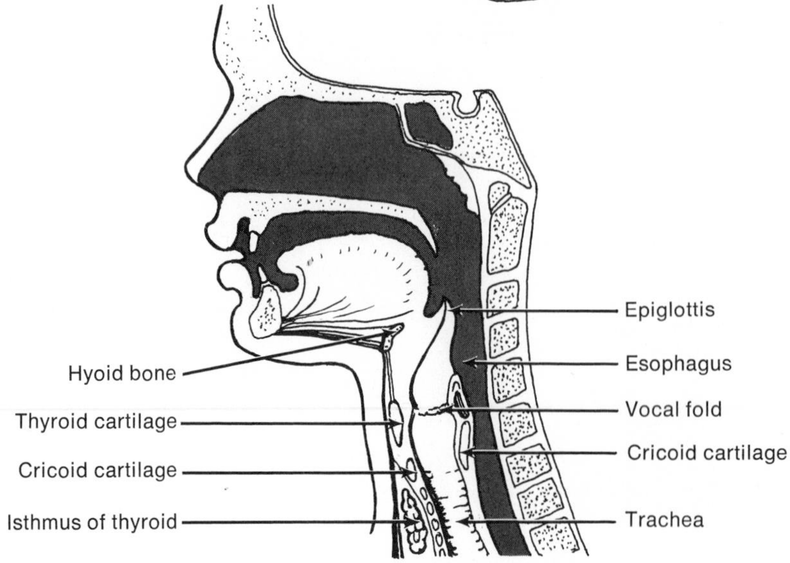

cervical or upper thoracic region in infancy or early childhood are at high risk for developing carcinoma of the thyroid.[21] Although the rate of thyroid cancer has declined since the dangers of routine radiation therapy have been discovered, the nurse should carefully question parents of those children born before 1960 for exposure to such treatment, especially for benign disorders such as enlarged thymus or tonsils, and refer these children to a physician for further evaluation of the thyroid gland.[25]

Eyes

Examination of the eyes involves inspection of all exterior structures for size, symmetry, color, and motility, and inspection of the interior surfaces for examination of retinal structures. The latter requires the use of an ophthalmoscope and is a highly skilled procedure. Discussion of the funduscopic examination includes the basic normal findings that the nurse should be able to discern with some practice in using the ophthalmoscope. The third part of the examination, testing of visual acuity, is discussed on p. 168.

General inspection. The nurse inspects the placement and alignment of the eyes on the face and observes each external structure of the eye for color, size, shape, movement, and symmetry. In order to correctly describe each structure and to measure symmetry and location, the nurse must have an understanding of the usual landmarks and visible portions of the eyeball (Fig. 5-15).

Placement and alignment. The eyes are judged for their relative placement on the face, their symmetry of location, and the general slant of the palpebral fissures or lids. (Fig. 5-16). If the nurse observes any possible abnormality of placement, these findings can be substantiated by measuring the interpupillary distance, which is approximately 3.5 to 5.5 cm (1.4 to 2.2 inches) or the inner canthal dis-

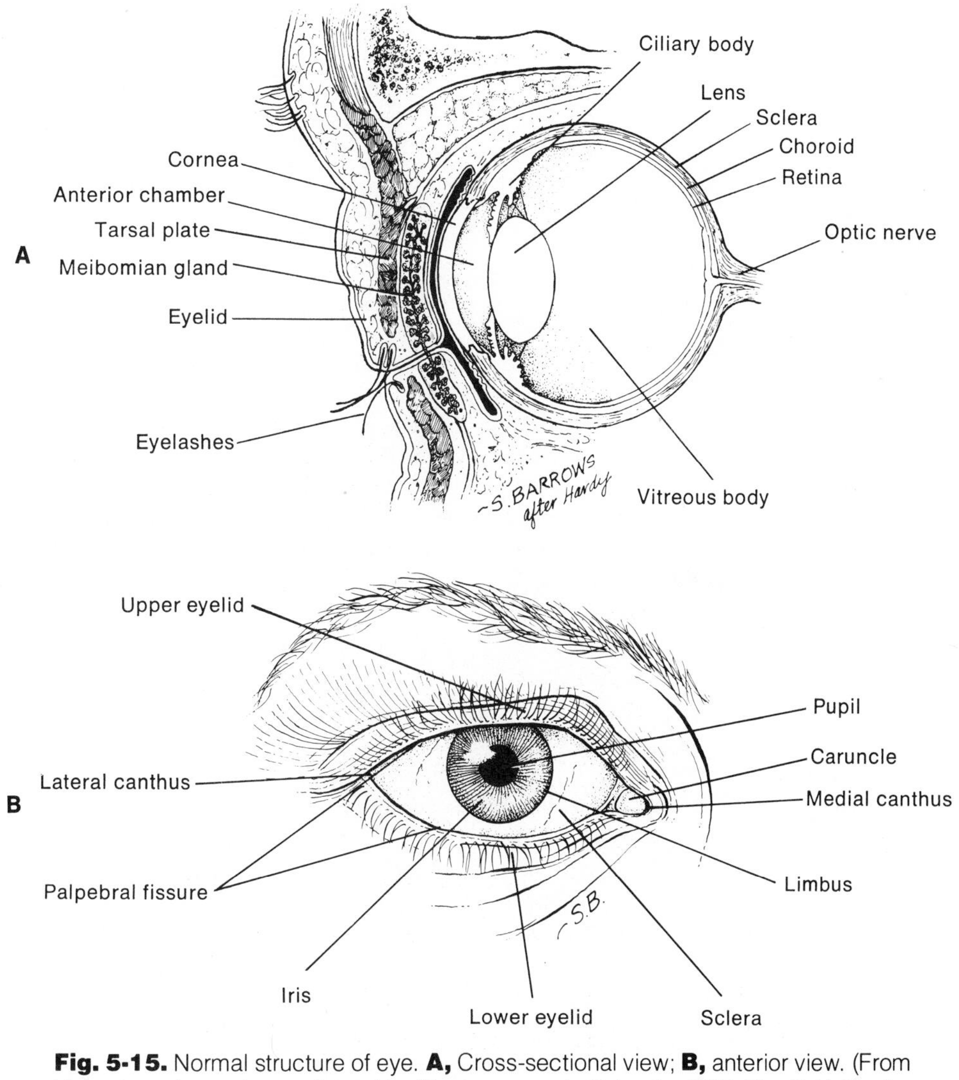

Fig. 5-15. Normal structure of eye. **A,** Cross-sectional view; **B,** anterior view. (From Malasanos, L., and associates: Health assessment, St. Louis, 1977, The C. V. Mosby Co., pp. 143-144.)

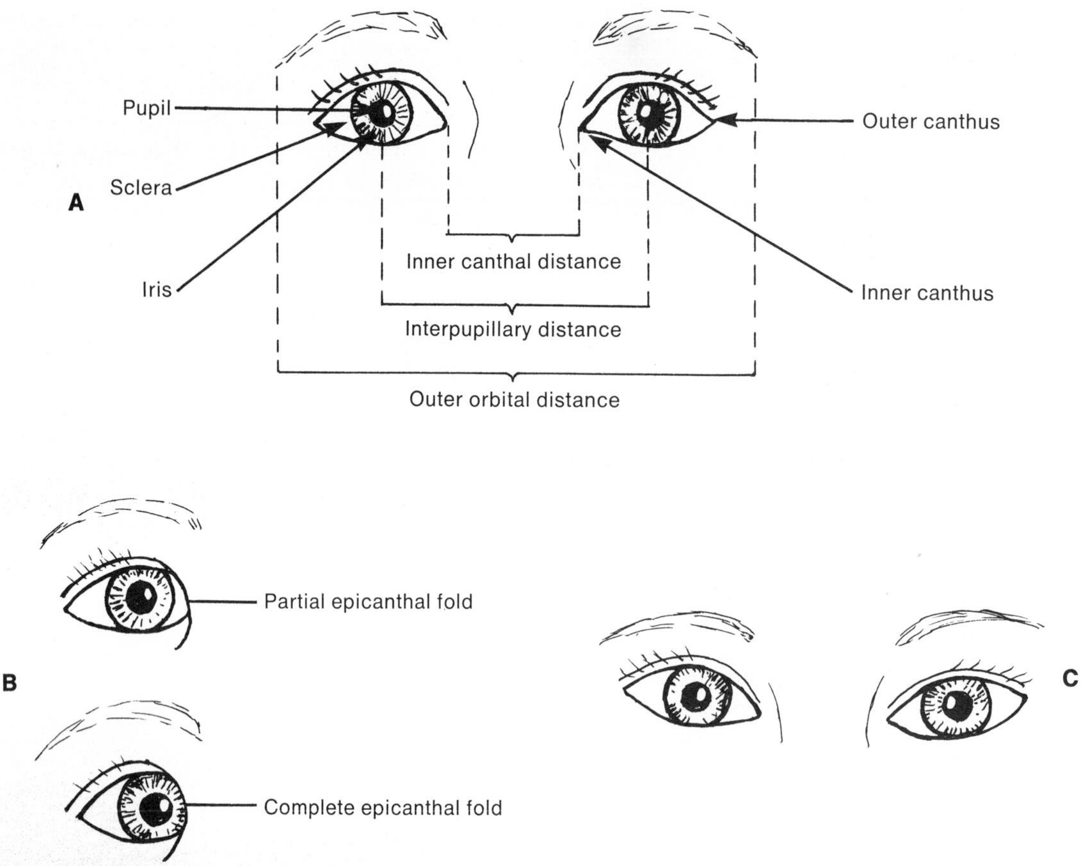

Fig. 5-16. A, Anatomic landmarks of eye. **B,** Epicanthal folds. **C,** Upward palpebral slant.

tance, which averages about 3.0 cm (1.2 inches).[14] Large spacing between the eyes is called *hypertelorism*. Although a normal variant in some children, hypertelorism with other midfacial anomalies may suggest mental retardation. Epicanthal folds, an excess fold of skin extending from the roof of the nose to the inner termination of the eyebrow and partially or completely overlapping the inner canthus of the eye, may give a false impression of hypertelorism and/or malalignment of the eyes (strabismus). Epicanthal folds are frequently found in children of Asiatic descent. They may be normally present in non-Oriental infants, but they usually disappear as the child grows older.

The *palpebral slant* is also inspected. The degree of slant is judged by drawing an imaginary line through the two points of the medial canthus and across the outer orbit of the eyes and aligning each eye on the line. Usually the palpebral fissures lie horizontally. However, in Oriental persons the slant is normally upward. Since eye abnormalities are common in many chromosomal disorders, the nurse must be careful to observe and record any deviations from the expected. For example, children with Down's syndrome characteristically demonstrate hypertelorism, epicanthal folds, and upward palpebral slant.

The nurse inspects the *lids* for proper placement on the eye. When the eye is open, the upper lid should fall somewhere between the upper iris and the pupil. If the lid covers part of the pupil or the lower part of the iris, this is called *ptosis*. If the lid falls above the iris, allowing any part of the sclera or "white-of-the-eye" to show, this is called *"sunset eyes"* or the *"setting-sun" sign*. Although either can be a normal variant of lid placement, it can also be a sign of several disorders.

When the eyes are closed, the lids should completely cover the cornea and sclera. Failure to do so can result in chronic eye irritation and infection. When the lids are opened or closed, no palpebral conjunctiva should be visible. Malposition of the eyelids includes *ectropion,* a rolling out of the lids with exposed conjunctiva, and *entropion,* a turning in of the lid. The latter is normally found in some Oriental children. The nurse should check to see if the inturned lid causes irritation of the cornea.

One of the most important tests is alignment of the eyes to detect nonbinocular vision or *strabismus*. Normally, by the age of 3 to 4 months, children achieve the ability to fixate on one visual field with both eyes simultaneously (binocularity). In some children, however, one eye deviates

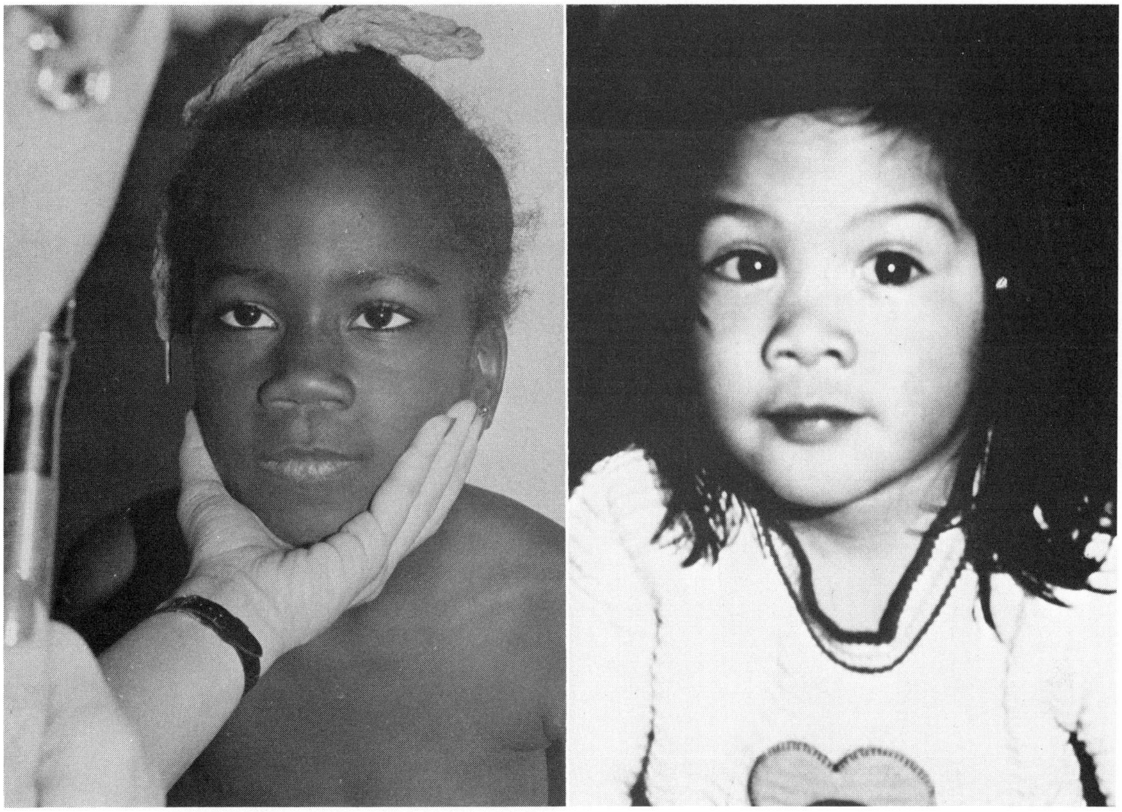

A B

Fig. 5-17. A, Corneal light reflex test demonstrating orthophoric eyes. **B,** Pseudostrabismus. The inner epicanthal folds cause the eyes to appear malaligned; however, the corneal light reflexes fall perfectly symmetric.

from the point of fixation, resulting in strabismus or "cross-eye." If the malalignment is constant, the weak eye becomes "lazy" and eventually the brain suppresses the image produced by that eye (suppression scotoma). If strabismus is not detected and corrected by age 4 to 6 years, blindness, called ambylopia, may result.

Two tests commonly used to detect malalignment are the corneal light reflex and cover test. In the *corneal light reflex test,* the nurse shines a flashlight or the light of the ophthalmoscope directly into the eyes from a distance of about 40.5 cm (16 inches). If the eyes are *orthophoric* or normal, the light falls perfectly symmetrically within each pupil (Fig. 5-17). If the light falls off center in one eye, the eyes are malaligned. Inward deviation of the eye is called *esotropia* or *esophoria*. Outward deviation of the eye is called *exotropia* or *exophoria*. A *tropia* is a constant or intermittent alignment of the eyes. A *phoria* is a malalignment that is not obvious until fusion is disrupted. A tropia is more severe and, therefore, more likely to result in amblyopia.

In the *cover test* one eye is covered and the movement of the *uncovered* eye is observed while the child fixes his gaze on a near (33 cm or 13 inches) or distant (50 cm or 20 inches) object. If the uncovered eye does not move, it is aligned. If the uncovered eye moves, a malalignment is present because when the stronger eye is temporarily covered, the weaker eye attempts to fixate on the object.

In the *alternate cover test* the nurse shifts occlusion back and forth from one eye to the other eye and observes movement of the *covered* eye while the child is fixating at a point in front of him. If normal alignment is present, shifting the cover from one eye to the other eye will not cause movement of the covered eye. If malalignment is present, the covered eye will move from its position when covered to a straight position when uncovered. This test takes more practice than the other cover test because the nurse must move the occluder back and forth quickly and accurately in order to see the eye move. Usually it is easier to perform this test by using one's hand rather than a card or other object as the occluder (Fig. 5-18, *A* to *C*). Since deviations can occur at different ranges, particularly in the case of phorias, it is important to perform the cover tests at both close and far distances.

Inspection of external structures. The nurse observes the *lids* for color (any sign of hemorrhage), size (any evidence of edema), and mobility. Normally the lids contain

A

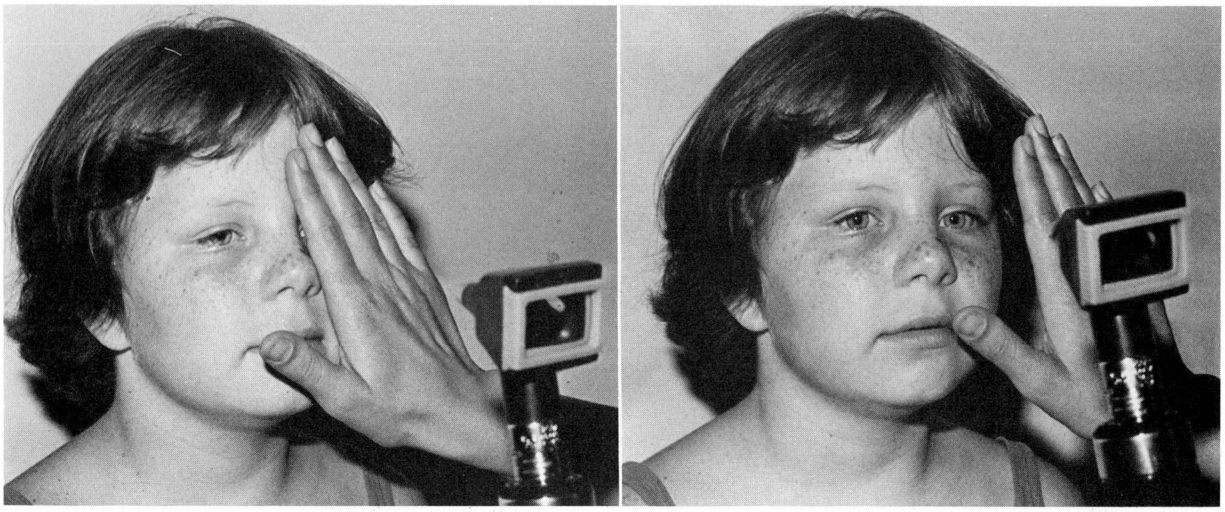

B

C

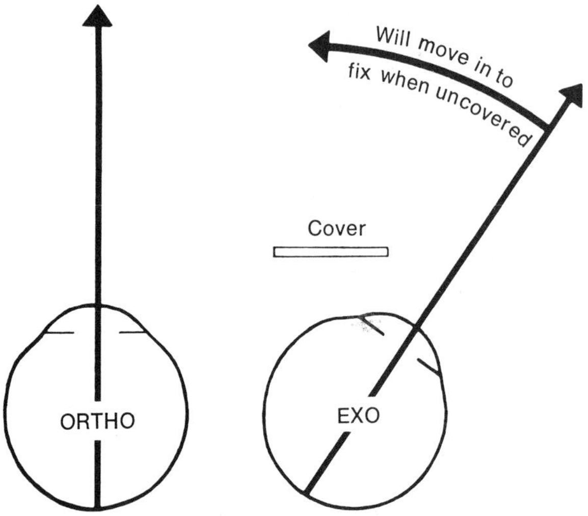

Fig. 5-18. Alternate cover test for strabismus. **A,** Eye is occluded, child is fixating on a light source. **B,** If when uncovered eye does not move, eyes are aligned. **C,** Exophoria—as eye is uncovered it shifts to fixate on an object. (**C** From Prior, J. A., and Silberstein, J. S.: Physical diagnosis: the history and examination of the patient, ed. 5, St. Louis, 1977, The C. V. Mosby Co., p. 111.)

the same amount of pigmentation as does the rest of the skin. Inflammation or erythema along the lid should be noted. Some of the more common lid disorders are listed in the boxed material.

The nurse also inspects the lining of the lids, the *palpebral conjunctiva*. Inspecting the lower conjunctival sac is easily accomplished by pulling the lid down while the patient looks up. To evert the upper lid, the child looks down while the nurse holds the upper lashes and gently pulls *down* and *forward*. If this is not successful, the nurse can place a tongue blade or stem of a cotton-tipped applicator 1 cm above the edge of the lid margin. With this in place, the nurse gently pushes down on the lid with the stick and rolls the lid upward. As soon as the lid is everted, the fingers holding the lashes are used to keep the lid everted. Normally the conjunctiva appears pink and glossy. Vertical yellow striations along the edge are the meibomian or sebaceous glands near the hair follicle. Located in the

Inflammations of the eyelid

Hordeolum or stye	Inflammation of sebaceous glands near lashes, usually on lower lid; painful, red, swollen areas
Internal stye	Acute inflammation of meibomian glands of upper lid; if upper lid is everted, stye appears as a yellow line across the tarsus (edge of eyelid)
Chalazion	Granulomas or cysts of internal sebaceous glands (meibomian glands); localized, nontender, firm, discrete swellings covered with freely movable skin
Marginal blepharitis	Inflammation of edge of lid; red, scaly, crusted lid edges, may include pustules around base of lashes and pus from meibomian glands
Dacryocystitis	Inflammation and blockage of lacrimal sac or duct; swelling, redness, and pain, below and to nasal side of inner canthus, with purulent discharge

inner or medial canthus and situated on the inner edge of the upper and lower lids is a tiny opening, called the lacrimal punctum. The nurse should note any excessive tearing or inflammation of the lacrimal apparatus.

The nurse also observes the lids for blinking movement. Excessive blinking can indicate eyestrain or a nervous habit. Asymmetric or infrequent blinking can be a sign of paralysis or muscle weakness. The nurse tests for the blink reflex by making a quick movement toward the eye.

The nurse inspects the *eyelashes* for distribution, direction of growth, and pigmentation. Normally the upper lashes curl upward and the lower lashes curve downward. Lashes that turn inward toward the eyeball can cause conjunctival irritation.

The *bulbar conjunctiva,* which covers the eye up to the limbus or junction of the cornea and sclera, is inspected next. It should be transparent and the white color of the underlying sclera. Dilation of the blood vessels in the conjunctiva makes it appear red. Although this redness is characteristic of many disorders, it can also indicate eyestrain, irritation, or fatigue.

The *sclera* or white covering of the eyeball should be clear. Any yellow staining is noted, since this is often indicative of jaundice. Tiny black marks in the sclera of heavily pigmented individuals is normal and does not indicate petechiae or the presence of a foreign body. A bluish tone may indicate disorders such as osteogenesis imperfecta or glaucoma.

The *cornea,* or covering of the iris and pupil, should be clear and transparent. Any opacities are recorded since they can be signs of scarring or ulceration, which can interfere with vision. The best way to test for opacities is to illuminate the eyeball by shining a light at an angle (obliquely) toward the cornea.

The *pupils* are compared for size, shape, and movement. They should be round, clear, and equal. The nurse tests their *reaction to light* by quickly shining a source of light toward the eye and removing it. As the light approaches, the pupils should constrict; as the light fades, the pupils should dilate. *Accommodation,* or the focusing ability of the eyes to produce clear vision at different distances, is tested by having the child look at a bright, shiny object at a distance and quickly moving the object toward his face. The pupils should constrict as the object is brought near the eye. The normal findings when examining the pupil may be recorded as PERRLA, which means "pupil equal, round, react to light and accommodation."

The *iris* is inspected for color, size, and clarity. Permanent eye color is usually established by 6 to 12 months of age. Lack of usual eye color and a pink glow to the iris is indicative of albinism. The pink color is a reflection of the red reflex of the retina. Black and white speckling of the iris, known as Brushfield's spots, is seen in Down's syndrome.

As the nurse inspects the iris and pupil, the *lens* is also examined. Normally the nurse should not see the lens while looking into the pupil. White or gray spots usually indicate opacities or cataracts in the lens. Complete opacities prevent funduscopic examination of internal retinal structures.

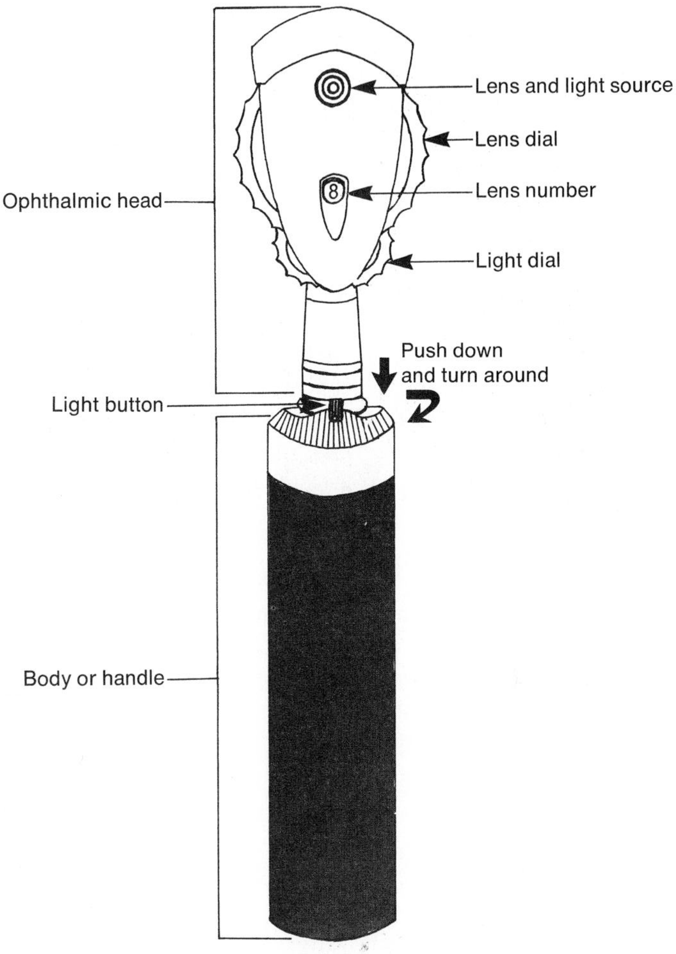

Fig. 5-19. Ophthalmoscope.

Inspection of internal structures

Use of ophthalmoscope. The ophthalmoscope permits visualization of the interior of the eyeball with a system of lenses and a high-intensity light. Fig. 5-19 illustrates the various parts of the instrument. The "ophthalmic head" contains plus lenses (magnifiers), which are usually indicated by black numbers and minus lenses (minifiers), which are indicated by red numbers. The lenses are changed by rotating a disc on the outside of the head. These lenses permit clear visualization of eye structures at different distances from the nurse's eye and correct visual acuity differences in the examiner and child.

If the nurse wears corrective lenses or glasses, they should be worn when the ophthalmoscope is being used. If the child wears glasses, these should be removed unless they are worn to correct severe astigmation, which can cause distortion of the images. The lens of the ophthalmoscope can grossly detect visual acuity problems in the child if the nurse who has 20/20 vision is forced to use plus or minus lenses to see the red reflex or retinal structures clearly. With hyperopia, or farsightedness, the nurse would use higher plus or convex lenses; with myopia, or nearsightedness, more minus or concave lenses would be used.[24] Use of the ophthalmoscope requires practice to know which lens setting produces the clearest image.

The interior of the eye is illuminated by a light source within the ophthalmic head, which shines through the lens from a small window. The light is switched on and off by pressing a button at the neck of the head downward and clockwise. There is also a light dial that changes the type of light emitted through the window. For general purposes the small white circular light is used for the undilated pupil and the larger white circular light is used for the dilated pupil. Other light settings are the white vertical slit, grid, and green filter.

The ophthalmic and otic head are usually interchangeable on one "body" or handle, which encloses the power source, which is either disposable or rechargeable batteries. The nurse should practice changing the heads, which snap on and are secured with a quarter turn, and replacing the batteries and light bulbs.

Manipulating the instrument. The nurse uses the ophthalmoscope by placing the hand around its body and resting the instrument against the nose and cheek so that the lens remains directly in front of the eye and the light shines toward the child's eye. With the instrument in position the nurse moves toward the child, approaching from the side at a 15-degree angle, not directly toward the eye. When examining the left eye, the nurse uses the left eye, and vice versa. This is to prevent eyestrain and to approach the child in the best juxtaposition. The nurse's free hand may be used to attract the child's attention away from the instrument's light source and toward a point directly in front of him or to help in guidance while moving as close as possible to the child. The examination should be done in a dimly-lit, but not necessarily dark, room.

As the nurse approaches the child from a distance of about 1 foot, the examination of the cornea, iris, and lens is begun with a lens setting of +8 to +2. As the nurse nears the child's face, the lens is changed to 0 or minus 2. At this point the nurse should see a red reflex and then details of the posterior wall of the eye or fundus. Since the light source falls on only part of the retina at a time, the nurse systematically moves the ophthalmoscope up and down and from size to side to visualize each structure within the fundus (Fig. 5-20).

Preparing the child. The nurse prepares the child for the

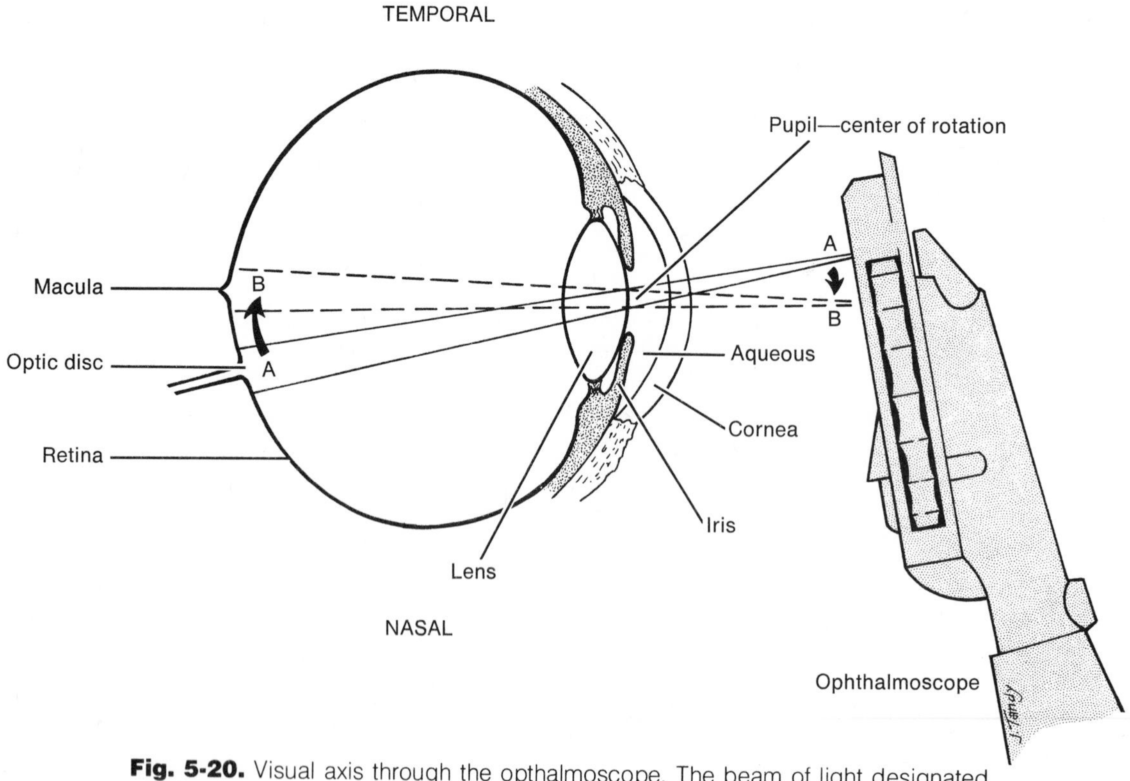

Fig. 5-20. Visual axis through the opthalmoscope. The beam of light designated *A* and its corresponding visual field is the usual view when approaching the child from the side at a 15-degree angle. View *B* represents a direct visualization with the child staring at the light.

ophthalmic examination by showing him the instrument, demonstrating the light source and how it shines in the eye, explaining the reason for darkening the room, and stressing that the procedure is not painful. For infants and young children who do not respond to such explanations, it is best to try and use distraction to encourage them to keep their eyes open. Forcibly parting the lids results in an uncooperative, watery-eyed child and a frustrated nurse. Usually, with some practice, the nurse can elicit a red reflex almost instantly while approaching the child and may also gain a momentary inspection of the blood vessels, macula, or optic disc.

The funduscopic examination. Fig. 5-21 illustrates the structures of the back of the eyeball or the fundus. In examining the interior of the eye, the nurse inspects the red reflex, the optic disc, the macula, and the blood vessels. It is important to remember that the ophthalmoscope permits only a small area of visualization. In order to perform a funduscopic examination, the nurse must move the ophthalmoscope systematically around the fundus to locate each structure.

The fundus derives its orange-red color from the inner two layers of the eye, the choroid and the retina, which is immediately apparent as the *red reflex*. The intensity of the orange-red color normally increases in darkly pigmented individuals. A brilliant, uniform red reflex is an important sign, because it virtually rules out almost all serious defects of the cornea, aqueous chamber, lens, and vitreous chamber.[11] Any dark shadows or opacities are recorded because they usually indicate some abnormality in any of these structures.

As the nurse approaches closer to the child with the ophthalmoscope, the most conspicuous feature of the fundus is the *optic disc,* the area where the blood vessels and optic nerve fibers enter and exit from the eye. The color of the disc is creamy pink, but lighter than the surrounding fundus. It derives its color from the rich capillary network. It is normally round or vertically oval. Its size is important because other structures of the fundus are measured in relationship to the disc's diameter (DD). Most discs have a small, pale depression in their center, called the *physiologic cup or depression,* which represents the blind spot of the retina. It is not always visible but, when large enough to be seen, should not extend to the disc margin. Blurring of the disc margins, loss of the depression, and a bulging disc are important signs of papilledema or swelling of the optic nerve, which is clinically indicative of increased intracranial pressure.

As the nurse locates the optic disc, the area is inspected for *blood vessels*. The central retinal artery and vein appear in the depths of the disc and emanate outward with visible branching. The *veins* are darker in color and about one fourth larger in size than the *arteries*. A narrow band of light, the *arteriolar light reflex,* is reflected from the center of an artery but does not appear in veins. Normally the branches of the arteries and veins cross each other. It is important to observe the pattern of branching for abnormalities such as notching or indenting at the crossings, tortuosity or dilatation of the vessels, or small hemorrhages (dark areas) along the branches. Any of these findings are reported for further investigation.

About 2 DD temporal to the disc is the *macula,* the area

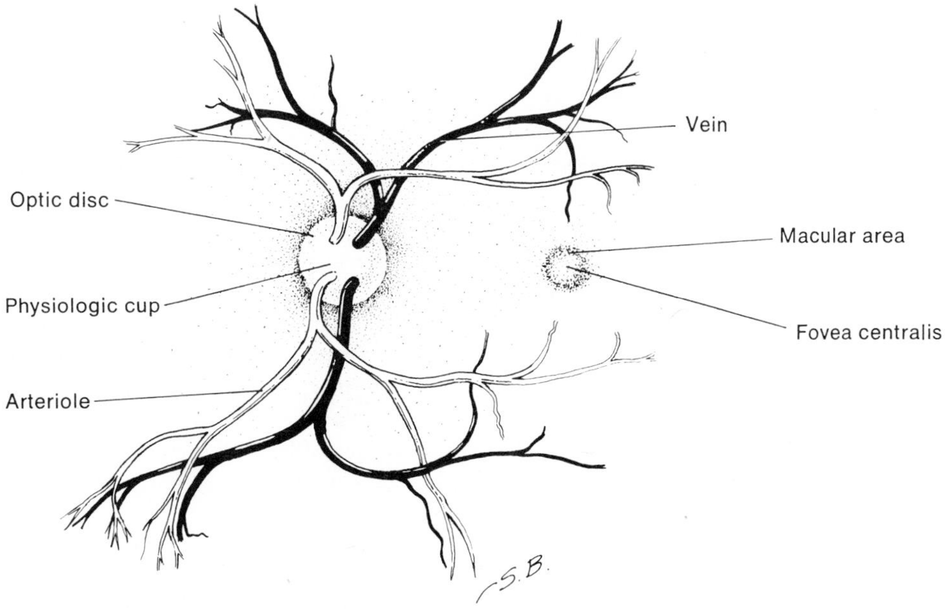

Fig. 5-21. Structures of fundus. (From Malasanos, L., and associates: Health assessment, St. Louis, 1977, The C. V. Mosby Co., p. 146.)

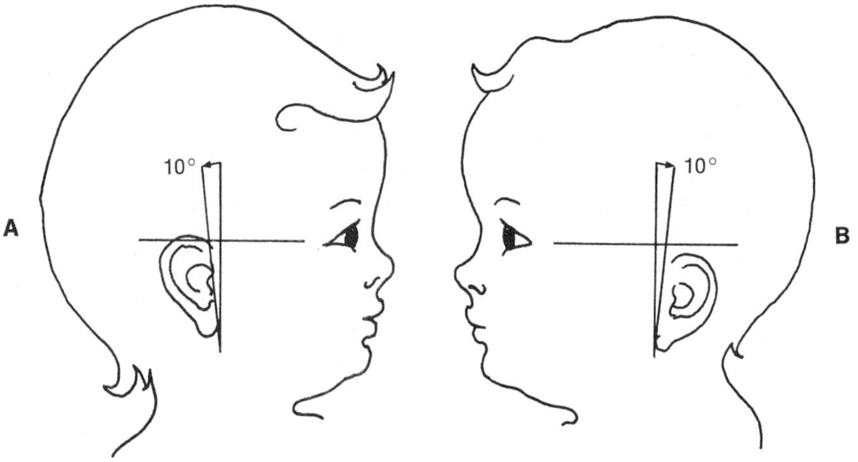

Fig. 5-22. Ear alignment. **A,** Normal; **B,** abnormal.

of the fundus with the greatest concentration of visual receptors. It is about 1 DD in size and darker in color than the fundus (red reflex) or optic disc. The intensity of the color directly correlates with the individual's skin pigmentation, that is, the darker the skin, the darker the color of the macula. In the center of the macula is a minute glistening spot of reflected light called the *fovea centralis*. It is the area of most perfect vision.

Although abnormalities of the macula are usually not apparent unless the eye is dilated and more detailed inspection is performed, the nurse should at least note its presence. If locating the macula is difficult, the child should be asked to look directly at the light. As Fig. 5-20 shows, a light shone directly into the eye falls on the fovea. However, since this is the most light/sensitive area of the retina, the nurse must be careful to focus on the macula only momentarily. If direct visualization does *not* cause the light to fall on the center of the fovea the nurse must consider the possibility of strabismus because fixation is occurring at a point adjacent to the center of the macula. Recognition of this deviation is of great importance in determining the type of treatment for strabismus, because in this situation the usual regimen of occlusive therapy (covering the stronger eye to force the weaker or deviating eye to focus) will not benefit the child.[11]

Ears

Like the eyes, examination of the ears involves inspection of the external auditory structures and visualization of the internal landmarks using a special instrument called the otoscope. Screening for hearing ability is discussed later in this chapter under neurologic assessment.

General inspection

Placement and alignment. The entire external earlobe is called the pinna or auricle and is located on each side of the head. The height alignment of the pinna is measured by drawing an imaginary line from the outer orbit of the eye to the occiput or most prominent protuberance of the skull. The top of the pinna should meet or cross this line. Low-set ears are commonly associated with renal anomalies or mental retardation. The angle of the pinna is measured by drawing a perpendicular line from the imaginary horizontal line and aligning the pinna next to this mark. Normally the pinna lies within a 10-degree angle of the vertical line (Fig. 5-22). If it falls outside this area, the nurse records the deviation and looks closely for other anomalies.

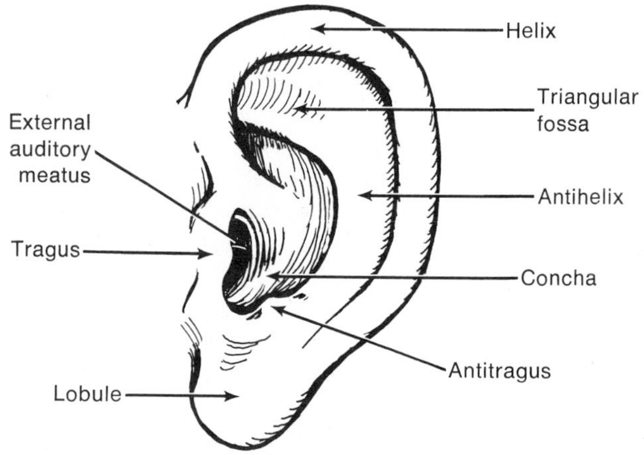

Fig. 5-23. Usual landmarks of pinna.

Normally the pinna extends slightly outward from the skull. Except in newborn infants, ears that are flat against the head or protruding away from the scalp may indicate problems. For example, masses or swelling make the pinna stand forward and may be indicative of mastoiditis, mumps, or postauricular abscesses. Flattened ears in infants may

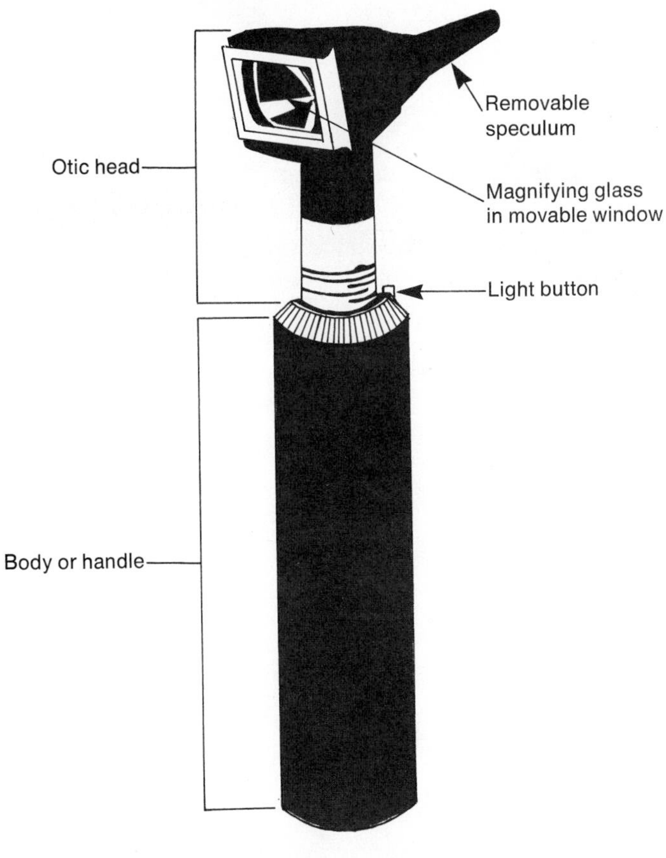

Fig. 5-24. Otoscope.

suggest a frequent side-lying position and, just as with isolated areas of hair loss, may be a clue to investigating parents' understanding of the child's stimulation needs.

Inspection of external structures. The pinna or auricle can be considered an ''oracle'' because deviations in structure can be a portentous sign of possible middle ear anomalies and resultant congenital conductive hearing loss.[12] Fig. 5-23 illustrates the usual landmarks of the pinna. The *helix* is the prominent outer rim of the pinna. The *antihelix* is a second curved rim that is adjacent and almost parallel to the helix. The *concha* is a deep cavity, within and partly surrounded by the antihelix, that leads into the external auditory canal. Lying anterior to the concha is a prominent protuberance called the *tragus,* and opposite to this is the *antitragus,* below which is the *lobule*. In some children the lobule is adherent with the helix in an upward and backward slant. An adherent lobule is considered a normal variation. Each of the major projections of the pinna form corresponding depressions. There is remarkable similarity among external pinnas, and the nurse should be familiar with the eminences and depressions in order to note deviations.

The skin surface around the ear is inspected for small openings, extra tags of skin, or sinuses. If a sinus is found, the nurse makes a special notation of this, since it may represent a fistula that drains into some area of the neck or ear. Cutaneous tags represent no pathologic process but may cause parents concern in terms of the child's appearance.

The ear is also inspected for general hygiene. An otoscope is not necessary for the nurse to look into the external canal to note the presence of cerumen, a waxy substance produced by the ceruminous glands in the outer portion of the canal. If the ear canal appears totally free of cerumen, the nurse should inquire concerning how the ears are cleaned. Occasionally parents insert cotton-tipped swabs or thin objects, such as bobby pins, into the canal to remove wax. Deep insertion of such objects can damage the drum or walls of the canal, as well as push the wax against the tympanic membrane to form a plug. It is best to question parents about ear cleaning by remarking about how clean the canals are and casually asking how they remove the wax. This approach is more likely to yield an honest answer than is direct questioning about the use of specific instruments. In general it is best to advise parents or children to clean the ears with a washcloth and, if they use a swab, to gently wipe the outermost portion of the canal. They should always avoid using any sharp, hard object in the ear. If the cerumen is hard and dry (appears dark and crusted, rather than yellow-brown and soft), it can be softened and removed by instilling a couple of drops of mineral oil into the ear for a few days and then rinsing the canal with an ear syringe. Commercial products are also available without prescription to aid in removing desiccated cerumen.

The nurse also observes the presence of any discharge from the aural canal, noting its color and odor. Bloody discharge may be the result of irritation from a foreign body within the ear. If discharge is noted in one canal, the nurse is careful not to transmit potentially infectious material to the other ear or to another child. Handwashing and changing otic speculums are essential preventive measures. Disposable speculums are also available.

Inspection of internal structures

Use of otoscope. The otic head permits visualization of the tympanic membrane by use of a bright light, a magnifying glass, and a speculum (Fig. 5-24). Some otoscopes have an attachment for a pneumonic device to insert air into the canal. The speculum, which is inserted into the external canal, comes in a variety of sizes (2, 3, 4, and 5 mm) to accommodate different canal widths. The nurse uses the largest speculum that fits comfortably into the ear in order to achieve the greatest area of visualization. The lens or magnifying glass is movable, allowing the examiner to insert an object, such as a curette, into the ear canal through the speculum while still viewing the structures through the lens. The handle is the same as for the ophthalmic head and operates similarly. The nurse should become familiar with the instrument and practice attaching the speculum securely to the head.

Positioning the child. Before beginning the otoscopic

A

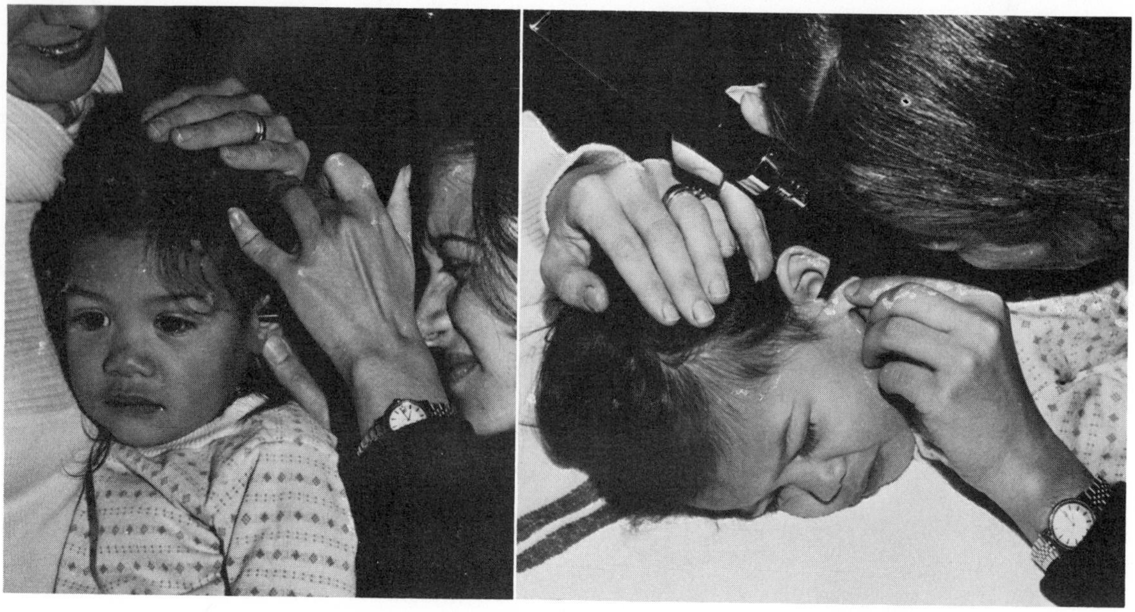

B

Fig. 5-25. A and **B,** Positions for otoscopic examination.

A

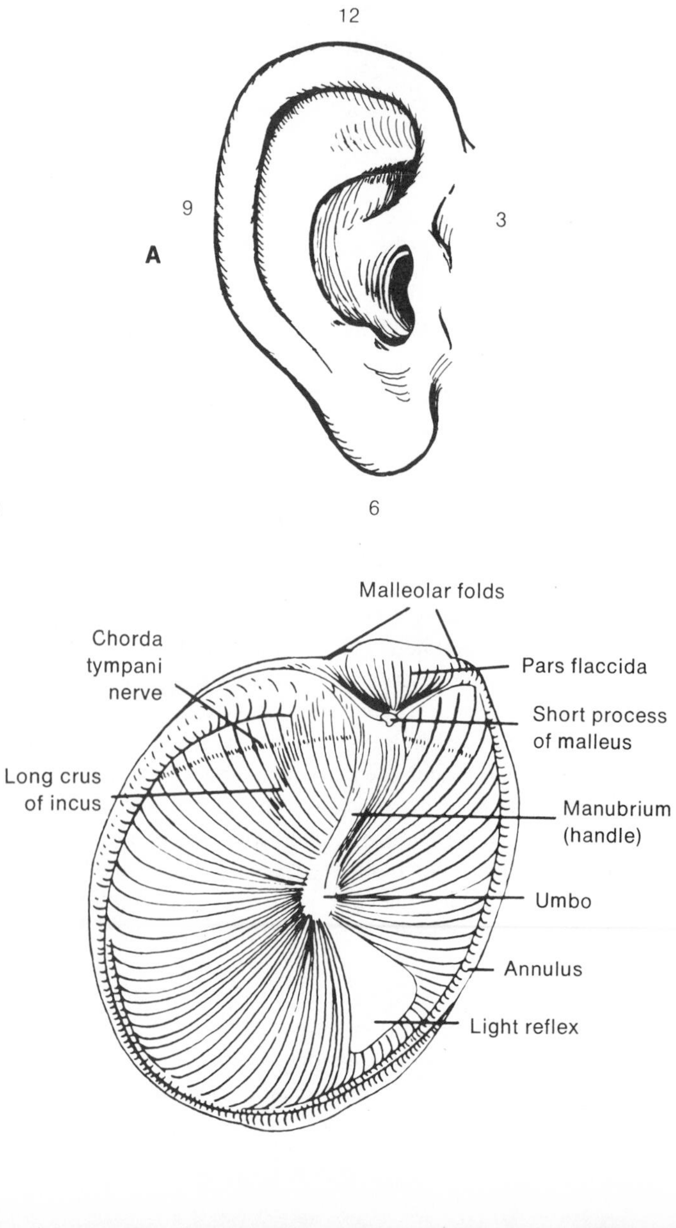

Fig. 5-26. Right tympanic membrane. **A,** Usual landmarks of pinna. **B,** Right tympanic membrane. (**B** From Prior, J. A., and Silberstein, J. S.: Physical diagnosis: the history and examination of the patient, ed. 5, St. Louis, 1977, The C. V. Mosby Co., p. 156.)

examination, the nurse positions the child. Older children usually are cooperative and need no type of restraint. They should, however, be prepared for the procedure by allowing them to play with the instrument, demonstrating how it works, and assuring them that it is not painful if they remain still. A helpful suggestion is letting them observe the nurse examining the parent's ear. The nurse can let older children view the inside of the ear. With younger children the nurse can explain that he or she is looking for a "big elephant" in the ear. This kind of "fairy tale" is an absorbing distraction and usually elicits much cooperation. As the nurse inserts the speculum into the meatus, it should be moved around the outer rim to accustom the child to the feel of something entering the ear.

For their protection and safety, infants and toddlers cannot be trusted to remain still, regardless of their former degree of cooperation. There are two general positions of restraint. In one the child is seated sideways in the parent's lap with one arm "hugging" the parents and the other arm at his side. The ear to be examined is toward the nurse. With one arm the parent holds the child's head firmly against his or her chest, and with the other arm "hugs" the child, thereby securing the child's free arm. The nurse then examines the ear using the same procedure in holding the otoscope as described below (Fig. 5-25, *A*).

The other position involves placing the child on his abdomen with his arms at his side and his head turned so that the ear to be examined points toward the ceiling. The nurse leans over the child and uses the upper part of the body to restrain his arms and upper trunk movements and the examining hand to stabilize his head. This position is practical for young infants or for older children who need minimal restraining, but it may not be feasible for other children who protest vigorously. For safety, the nurse should enlist the parent's help in immobilizing the head by firmly placing one hand above the ear (Fig. 5-25, *B*).

Manipulating the instrument. With the thumb and forefinger of the free hand, the nurse grasps the auricle and places the other three free fingers on the child's head to detect and resist sudden head movements. For either of the two positions of restraint, the nurse holds the otoscope upside down at the junction of its head and handle with the thumb and index finger. The other fingers are placed against the skull to allow the otoscope to move with the child in case he moves suddenly. In examining a cooperative child, the nurse holds the handle between the thumb and index finger with the otic head upright. The other three fingers are still placed against the child's head to detect unexpected movement.

Entering the canal. Before entering the canal, the nurse should imagine that the external ear and the tympanic membrane are superimposed on a clock (Fig. 5-26). The numbers become important geographic landmarks. The nurse introduces the speculum into the meatus between the 3 and 9 o'clock positions in a downward and forward position. Because the canal is curved, the speculum does not permit a panoramic view of the tympanic membrane unless the canal is straightened. In infants the canal curves upward and the tympanic membrane lies almost horizontally along the upper wall of the canal. The pinna must be pulled *downward* and *backward* to the 6 to 9 o'clock range, which retracts the canal and the drum downward (Fig. 5-27, *A*). With older children, usually those over 3 years of age, the canal curves downward and forward, and the drum, although more vertical, slopes inward and forward to form a 55-degree angle with the floor of the canal. Therefore, the pinna is pulled upward and back toward a 10 o'clock position, and the head is tilted slightly away from the nurse or toward the child's opposite shoulder to bring the drum into a 90-degree angle (Fig. 5-27, *B*). Proper positioning of the head is essential in achieving a full view of the membrane (Fig. 5-27, *C* and *D*).

In neonates and young infants, the walls of the canals are pliable and floppy because of the underdeveloped cartilaginous and bony structures. Therefore, the very small 2-mm speculum usually needs to be inserted deeper into the canal than in older children. Great care must be exercised not to damage the walls or drum. Because the small opening of the speculum permits a limited view, the nurse must systematically inspect each quadrant of the membrane. In older children the speculum need not be inserted past the membranous portion of the canal, usually a distance of 0.60 to 1.25 cm (0.25 to 0.50 inch). The entire length of the canal is approximately 2.5 cm (1 inch). Insertion of the speculum into the posterior or bony portion of the canal causes pain (Fig. 5-28).

Ostoscopic examination. As the nurse introduces the speculum into the external canal, the walls of the canal, the color of the tympanic membrane, the light reflex, and the usual landmarks of the bony prominences of the middle ear are inspected. Fig. 5-26, *B* illustrates the usual view of the tympanic membrane.

The *walls* of the external auditory canal are usually pink in color, although they are normally more pigmented in dark-skinned children. Minute hairs are evident in the outermost portion, where cerumen is produced. The nurse should note signs of irritation, foreign bodies, or evidence of infection.

The *color* of the *tympanic membrane* is normally a translucent light pearly pink or gray color. The nurse should note marked erythema, which may indicate suppurative otitis media, a dull nontransparent grayish color, sometimes suggestive of serous otitis media, or ashen gray areas, signs of scarring from a previous perforation. A black area usually suggests a perforation of the membrane that has not healed. Slight redness is normal in the newborn because of increased vascularity and is often seen in older infants and young children as a result of crying.

The characteristic tenseness and slope of the tympanic membrane causes the light of the otoscope to reflect at about

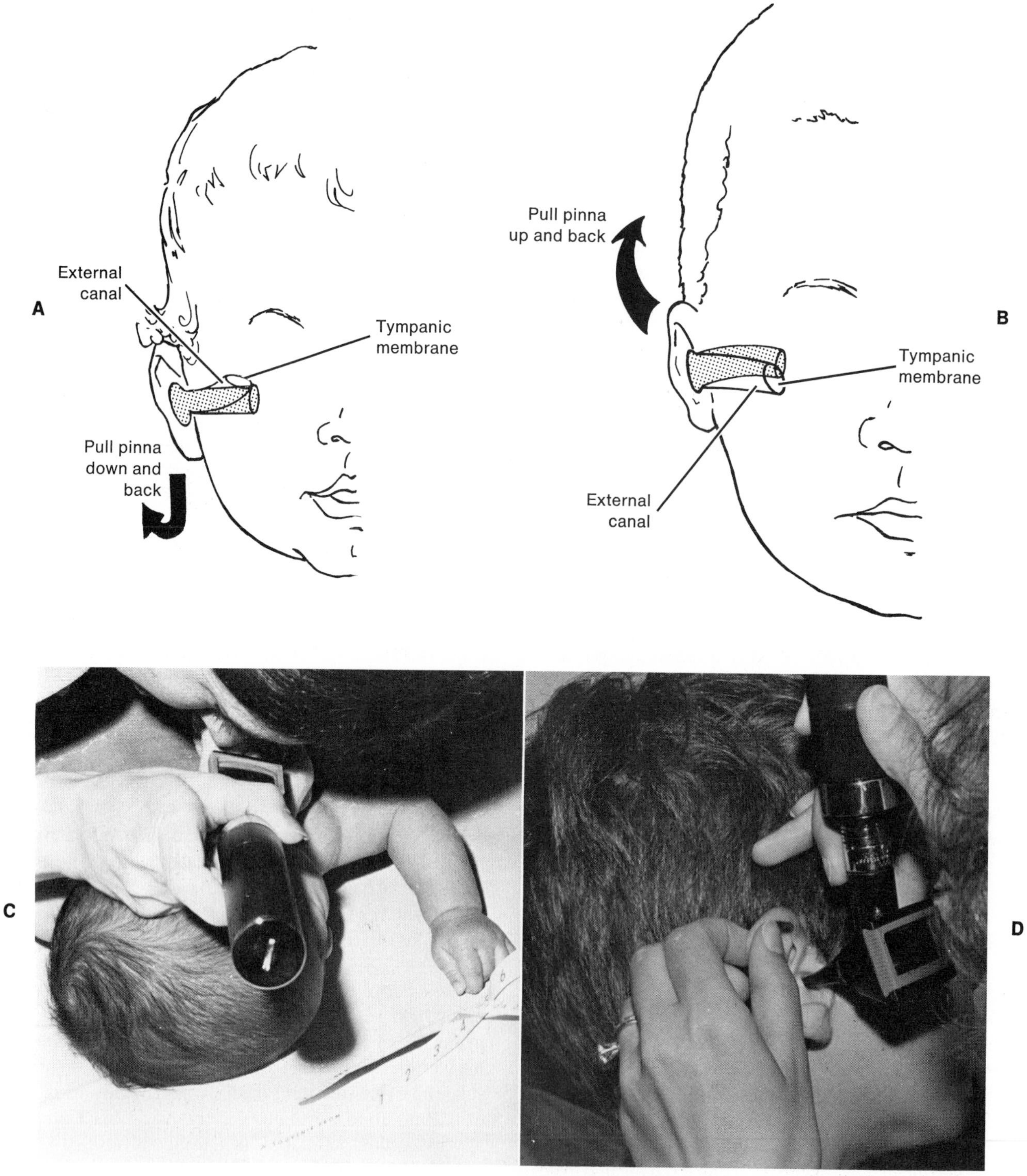

Fig. 5-27. Techniques for examining child's ear. **A,** Infant; **B,** older child. **C** and **D,** Proper positioning of the head is essential in achieving a full view of the membrane. **D,** Note that the child's head is tilted slightly away from the nurse.

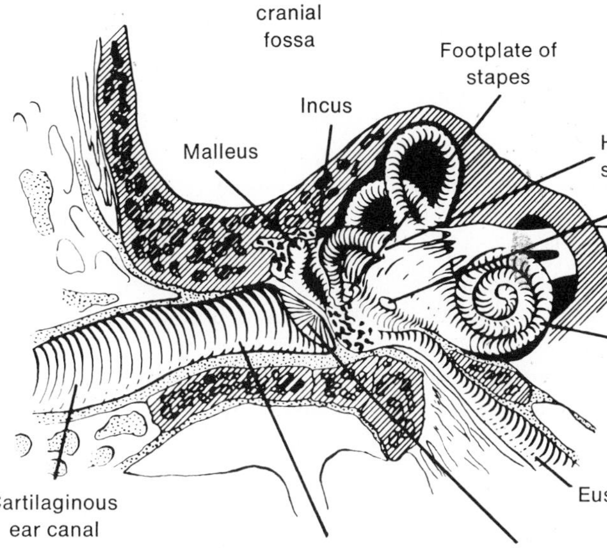

Fig. 5-28. External auditory canal and middle and inner ear. (From Prior, J. A., and Silberstein, J. S.: Physical diagnosis: the history and examination of the patient, ed. 5, St. Louis, 1977, The C. V. Mosby Co., p. 155.)

the 5 or 7 o'clock position. The *light reflex* is a fairly well-defined cone-shaped reflection, which normally points away from the face. Absence of the light reflex is always recorded, because it usually signifies bulging of the membrane and loss of its usual contours.

The *bony landmarks* of the drum are formed by the *umbo,* or long arm of the malleus bone, which appears as a small, round, opaque concave spot near the center of the drum. The *manubrium* (long process or handle) of the malleus appears as a whitish line extending from the umbo upward to the margin of the membrane. At the upper end of the long process near the 1 o'clock position is a sharp knob-like protuberance, representing the *short process* of the malleus. The *annulus* is the fibrous ring surrounding the periphery of the membrane, except for an area at the anterior and posterior *malleolar folds*. The annulus should be carefully inspected because it is a frequent location of perforations. Above the malleolar folds, the membrane is thin and slack and is called the *pars flaccida*. The remainder of the membrane, such as the area of the light reflex, is taut and is called the *pars tensa*. Loss of any of these landmarks is noted, because it is probably a result of bulging of the membrane as a result of fluid accumulation in the middle ear. Retraction of the drum with abnormal prominence of the bony landmarks is suggestive of serous otitis media.

Although not always a routine assessment procedure, the membrane is sometimes tested for mobility or compliance. A normal drum covering only air in the middle ear moves easily when negative or positive pressure is applied. Measurements of compliance can be done objectively with a device called the *tympanometer* or subjectively by blowing air gently in the ear with a pneumonic device attached to the otoscope. Decreased or low compliance usually indicates middle ear effusion. This is an important test for confirming the diagnosis of serous otitis media, a potential cause of conductive hearing loss.

Nose

The nose marks the beginning of the passageway through the respiratory tract. It is an important organ for filtration, temperature control, and humidification of inspired air, as well as a sensory organ for olfaction (smell). Each of these functions is dependent on the patency of the passageways and the mucosal lining of the nasal cavity. The nurse uses primarily inspection for assessing the external and internal structures.

Inspection of external structures. The nose is located in the middle of the face just below the eyes and above the lips. Its placement and alignment can be compared by drawing an imaginary vertical line from the center point between the eyes down to the notch of the upper lip. The nose should lie exactly vertical to this line, with each side exactly symmetric. The nurse notes its location, any deviation to one side, and asymmetry in overall size and in diameter of the nares (nostrils). The bridge of the nose is sometimes flat in black children or children of Asiatic descent. The alae nasi are noted for any sign of flaring, which is usually indicative of respiratory difficulty. Fig. 5-29 illustrates the usual landmarks used in describing the external structures of the nose.

Inspection of internal structures. The nurse can inspect the anterior vestibule of the nose by pushing the tip upward, tilting the head backward, and illuminating the cavity with a flashlight or otoscope without the attached ear speculum. For a deeper view of the inferior and middle turbinates and the middle meatus, the nurse uses a nasal speculum, such as a 9 mm speculum with a very short barrel that attaches to the otoscope head. Forceps speculums are not routinely used in children. The short, wide speculum is inserted into the nares, slightly away from the septum, and the otoscope is tilted upward to straighten the passageway toward the posterior wall of the cavity. Pushing against the septum causes pain. Generally inspection is adequate without the speculum, unless the nurse decides that a closer examination of the nasal membranes is warranted. If the nurse uses the nose speculum, the process should be explained to the child, similar to the type of preparation for using the otoscope.

The nurse notes the *color* of the *mucosal lining,* which is normally redder than the oral membranes, as well as any swelling, discharge, dryness, or bleeding. Nasal membranes that are abnormally pale, grayish-pink, and swollen may indicate nasal allergies. Red, swollen membranes are usually characteristic of the common cold. These differences in appearance are important diagnostic clues to differentiating between allergy and cold symptoms.

Normally, there should be no *discharge* from the nose. However, if the child has been crying, a watery discharge is normal. At other times a thin, clear exudate may indicate allergies, chronic rhinitis, or sinusitis. Purulent discharge is caused by infection and can indicate upper respiratory tract infections resulting from a viral or bacterial agent.

As the nurse looks deeper into the nose, the *turbinates* or *concha,* plates of bone enveloped by mucous membrane that jut into the nasal cavity, are inspected. The turbinates greatly increase the surface area of the nasal cavity as air is inhaled. The spaces or channels between the turbinates are called *meatus* and correspond to each of the three turbinates. Normally the nurse may be able to see the front end of the inferior and middle turbinate and the middle meatus. They should be the same color as the lining of the vestibule. Enlarged, boggy, pale, grayish mucosa should be noted. Swollen turbinates greatly occlude the passageways for entry of air.

As the nurse looks inside the nose, the *septum,* which should equally divide the vestibules, is also inspected. Any deviation is noted, especially if it causes an occlusion of one side of the nose. A perforation may be evident within the septum. If this is suspected, the nurse can shine the light of the otoscope into one nare and look for admittance of light through the perforation to the other nostril.

Since olfaction is an important function of the nose, the nurse asks older children about their *sense of smell.* Testing for smell is part of the assessment of the cranial nerves (see p. 172).

Mouth and throat

The mouth is the beginning of the passageway to the digestive tract, but it also functions in the entry or exit of air. The major structure of the exterior of the mouth is the *lips.* Inspection of the lips for color has been discussed in the section on skin (p. 118). The nurse should note the presence of painful, inflamed, and dried cracks or fissures of the lips, called cheilitis. These may be caused by exposure to harsh climatic conditions, habitual licking or biting of the lips,

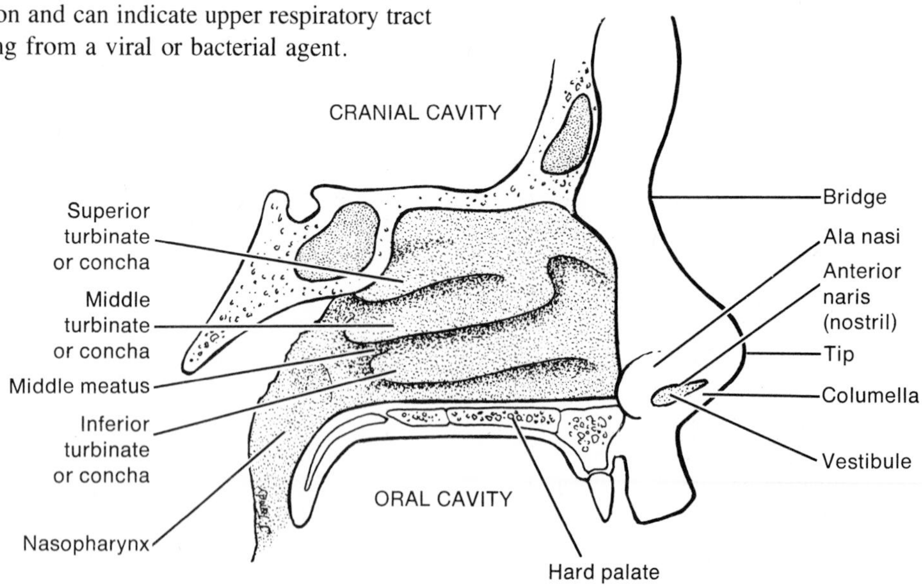

Fig. 5-29. External landmarks and internal structures of nose.

mouth breathing from respiratory distress, or dehydration, particularly with fever in systemic disease. Cheilosis, or angular stomatitis, is fissuring at the angles or corners of the lips and may indicate vitamin deficiencies of riboflavin or niacin.

The nurse also notes any lesions on the lips. The herpes simplex virus produces singular or clusters of vesicular eruptions on the lip, which are often called "cold sores." The lip may also be the site of a primary syphilitic chancre, which appears as a firm nodule that ulcerates and crusts. If the nurse suspects a chancre, it should be examined with a gloved hand for the nurse's protection.

Inspection of internal structures. The mouth and throat are divided into three areas: (1) the oral cavity, which extends from the lips to the palatopharyngeal arches, (2) the oropharynx, which extends from the epiglottis to the lower edge of the adenoids, and (3) the nasopharynx, which extends from above the lower edge of the adenoids to the nasal cavity. The major structures that are visible on examination within the oral cavity and oropharynx are the mucosal lining of the lips and cheeks, gums or gingiva, teeth, tongue, palate, uvula, tonsils, and posterior oropharynx (Fig. 5-30). Other pharyngeal structures that are not visible on examination are the epiglottis, lingual tonsils, and pharyngeal tonsils or adenoids.

With a cooperative child, almost the entire examination can be done without the use of a tongue blade. The nurse asks the child to open his mouth wide, requests that he move his tongue in different directions for full visualization, and has him say "Ahh" in order to depress the tongue for full view of the back of the mouth (tonsils, uvula, and oropharynx). For a closer look at the buccal mucosa or lining of the cheeks, the nurse can ask the child to use his fingers to move the outer lip and cheek to one side. Performing the examination in front of a mirror is a great aid in enlisting children's cooperation.

Infants and toddlers, however, usually resist attempts to keep the mouth open. Because it is an upsetting part of the examination, the nurse should reserve it until last (with examination of the ears) or take any opportunity during episodes of crying to view the oral cavity. However, the use of a tongue blade to depress the tongue is necessary. Depressing the tongue at the center back area elicits the gag reflex, which should be avoided, but depressing it toward the side does not. Fig. 5-31 illustrates proper positioning of the child for oral examination. If the child resists in opening his mouth, pinching the nostrils closed forces the child to breathe by mouth and, therefore, open the mouth.

The nurse inspects all areas lined with *mucous membranes* (inside the lips and cheeks, gingiva, underside of tongue, palate, and back of pharynx), noting its color, any areas of white patches or ulceration, bleeding, sensitivity, and moisture. The membranes should be bright pink, smooth, glistening, uniform, and moist. Any deviations are noted. For example, reddened areas with white ulcerated centers may be canker sores (aphthae), which may be caused by trauma to the gums during toothbrushing or chewing. Koplik's spots, indicative of measles during the prodromal stage, appear as grayish areas surrounded with a red, irregular areola. They first appear on the buccal mucosa opposite the lower molars. White curdy plaques or patches anywhere on the oral mucosa, but particularly on the surface of the tongue and hard palate, that bleed when scraped are signs of moniliasis or thrush.

As the nurse observes the lining of the mouth, any odor (halitosis) is noted. Mouth odors are characteristic of a num-

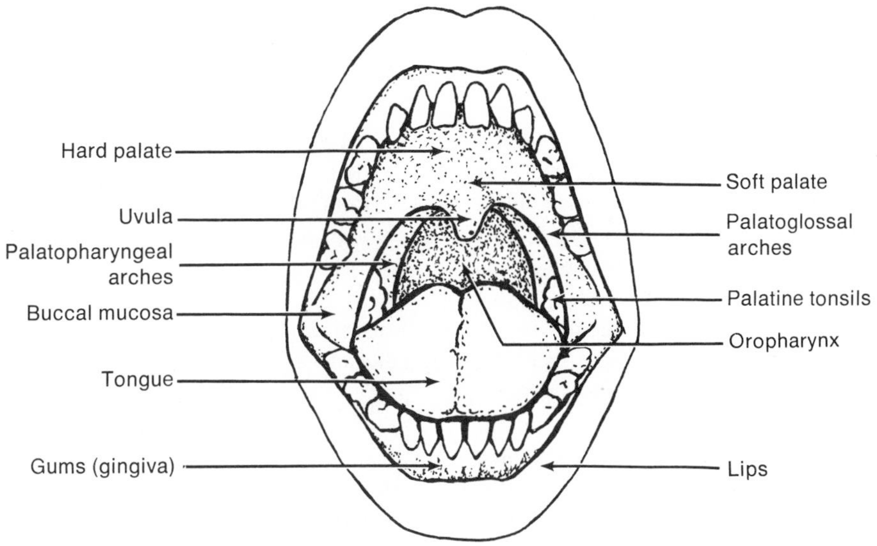

Fig. 5-30. Interior structure of mouth.

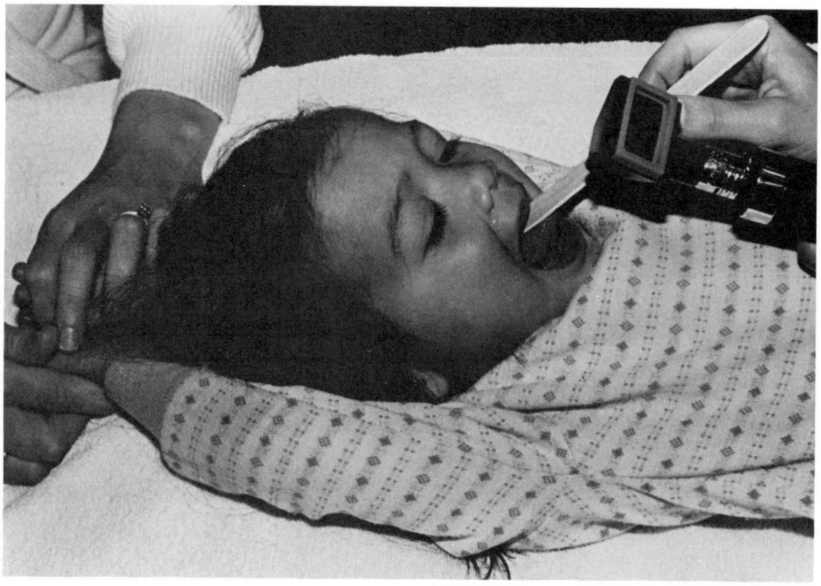

Fig. 5-31. Positioning child for examination of mouth.

ber of important health problems, such as poor dental hygiene, gingival disease, chronic constipation, dehydration, malnutrition, or systemic illness. A sudden, foul odor in the mouth may indicate a foreign body in the nose, particularly a bean or pea. The nurse should inspect the nose carefully and, if possible, remove the object with tweezers. If it is deep in the cavity, the child should be referred to a physician.

The *teeth* are inspected for number in each dental arch, hygiene, and occlusion or bite. The general rule for estimating the number of temporary teeth in children who are 2 years of age or younger consists of: *the child's age in months minus 6 months equals the number of teeth.* Discoloration of tooth enamel with obvious plaque (whitish coating on the surface of the teeth) is a sign of poor dental hygiene. Brown spots in the crevices of the crown of the tooth or between the teeth may be caries. Teeth that appear greenish-black may be stained from oral ingestion of supplemental iron. Although unsightly, this disappears after the iron is no longer given. Malocclusion or poor biting relationship of the teeth is evaluated in terms of (1) how the jaws relate to each other in vertical, transverse, and anterior-posterior directions, for example, the "buck-toothed" appearance that results when the maxilla is forward in relation to the mandible, (2) how the teeth are aligned, and (3) how the teeth interdigitate when in occlusion. Although parents frequently express concern regarding thumb-sucking and the development of orthodontic problems, thumb-sucking that ceases before the age of 6 years probably does little harm.[29]

The *gums* surrounding the teeth are examined. The color is normally a pale red with stippled appearance. In dark-skinned children a brownish melanin pigmentation is often observed along the gum line.

The *tongue* is inspected for the presence of papillae, small projections that contain several taste buds each and give the tongue its characteristic rough appearance. The nurse should note any changes in the surface texture, such as (1) "geographic tongue," unusual patterns of papillae formation and denuded areas, (2) coated tongue, such as in thrush, or (3) an exceptionally beefy red and swollen tongue, which is a sign of various systemic diseases.

The nurse also notes the size and mobility of the tongue, especially protrusion, which is frequently seen in children with mental retardation. Normally the tip of the tongue should extend to the lips. If the child is unable to move the tongue forward to this point, the frenulum, or central band of mucous membrane, which attaches the tongue to the floor of the mouth, may be too short. "Tongue-tie" can result in speech problems.

The roof of the mouth consists of the *hard palate,* near the front of the cavity, and the *soft palate,* toward the back of the pharynx, which has a small midline protrusion called the *uvula.* The nurse should carefully inspect them to be sure that both palates are intact. Sometimes there is a pin-point cleft in the soft palate, which may go undetected unless carefully inspected. Such a cleft is especially important if the uvula is bifid or separated into two appendages. A submucosal cleft may result in speech problems later on, since air cannot be effectively trapped for vocalization. The arch of the palate should be dome shaped. A narrow-flat roof or high-arched palate affects the placement of the tongue and can cause feeding and speech problems. Movement of the uvula should be tested by eliciting a gag reflex.

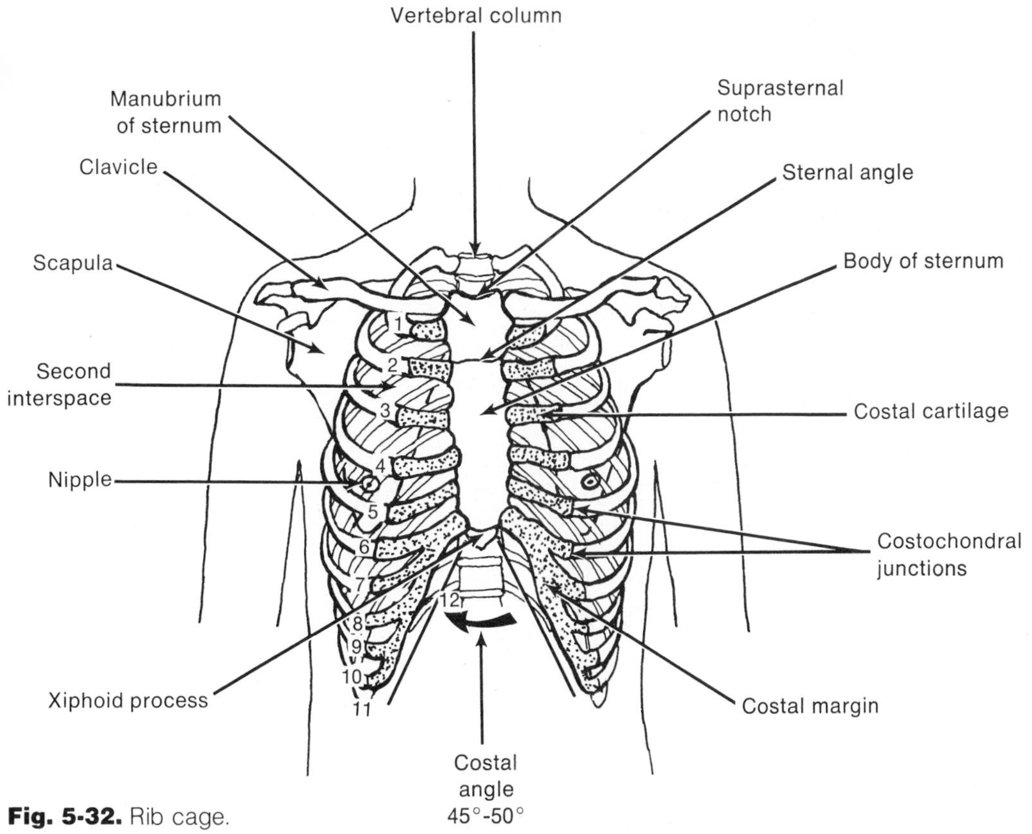

Fig. 5-32. Rib cage.

It should move upward to close off the nasopharynx from the oropharynx.

As the nurse inspects the recesses of the oropharynx, the size and color of the *palatine tonsils* are also noted. They are normally the same color as the surrounding mucosa, glandular, rather than smooth in appearance, and barely visible over the edge of the palatoglossal arches. Enlargement, redness, and white patches on the tonsils and surrounding area are recorded. Such signs are indicative of suppurative tonsillitis or pharyngitis.

Chest

Although the thoracic cavity houses two vital organs, the heart and lungs, the anatomic structures of the chest wall are important sources of information concerning cardiac and pulmonary function, skeletal formation, and secondary sexual development. The nurse inspects the chest for size, shape, symmetry, movement, breast development, and the presence of the bony landmarks formed by the ribs and sternum.

The *rib cage* consists of twelve ribs and the sternum, or breast bone, located in the midline of the trunk (Fig. 5-32). The first seven ribs, often called "true ribs," attach directly to the costal cartilages of the sternum at the costochondral junction. The next five ribs are called "false ribs" because they do not attach directly to the costal cartilages of the sternum. The eighth, ninth, and tenth ribs attach to the costal cartilages below the seventh rib, and the last two ribs, often called "floaters," have no direct attachment to the sternum or anterior ribs, other than their posterior attachment to the vertebral column.

The *sternum* is composed of three main parts. The *manubrium,* the uppermost portion, can be felt at the base of the neck at the *suprasternal notch.* The largest segment of the sternum is the *body,* which forms the *sternal angle* as it articulates with the manubrium. At the end of the body is a small, movable process called the *xiphoid.* The angle of the costal margin as it attaches to the sternum is called the *costal angle* and is normally about 45 to 50 degrees. These bony structures are important landmarks in the location of ribs and intercostal spaces. The first rib attaches directly to the manubrium. The second rib attaches directly to the body of the sternum below the sternal angle. The sternal angle is felt as a ridge a few centimeters below the suprasternal notch. The space immediately below the second rib is the second interspace.

The nurse must become familiar with locating and properly numbering each rib, because they are geographic landmarks for palpating, percussing, and auscultating underlying organs. Normally all the ribs can be counted by palpating inferiorily from the second rib. The tip of the eleventh rib can be felt laterally, and the tip of the twelfth rib can be felt posteriorily. Other helpful landmarks include the nipples, which are usually located between the fourth and fifth ribs or at the fourth interspace and, posteriorly, the tip of the scapula, which is located at the level of the eighth rib or interspace. In children with thin chest walls, correctly locating the ribs presents little difficulty.

The *thoracic cavity* is also divided into segments by drawing imaginary lines on the chest and back. Fig. 5-33 illustrates the anterior, lateral, and posterior divisions. The nurse should become familiar with each imaginary landmark, as well as with the rib number and corresponding interspace.

The *size* of the chest is measured by placing the tape around the rib cage at the nipple line (Fig. 5-34). For greatest accuracy at least two measurements should be taken, one during inspiration and the other during expiration, and the average recorded. Chest size is important mainly in comparison to its relationship with head circumference, which

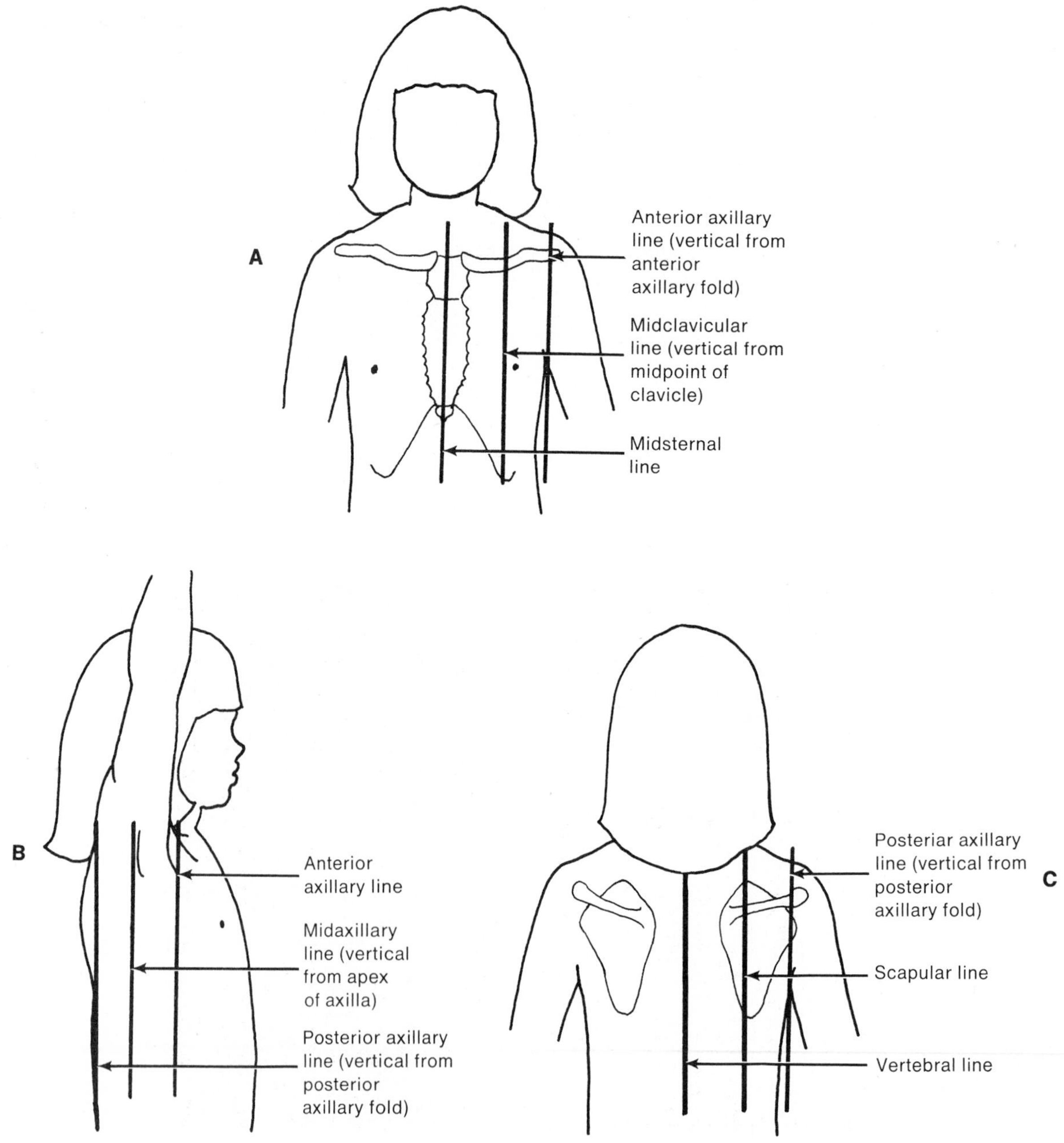

Fig. 5-33. Imaginary landmarks of chest. **A,** Anterior; **B,** right lateral; **C,** posterior.

has been discussed on p. 113. Marked disproportions are always recorded, because most are caused by abnormal head growth, although some may be the result of altered chest shape, such as barrel chest or pigeon chest.

During infancy the *shape* of the chest is almost circular, with the anteroposterior diameter equaling the transverse or lateral diameter. As the child grows the chest normally increases in the transverse direction, causing the anteroposterior diameter to be less than the lateral diameter. In an older child the characteristic barrel shape of an infant's chest is a significant sign of chronic obstructive lung disease, such as asthma or cystic fibrosis. Other variations in shape that are usually variants of the normal configuration are *pigeon breast,* or *pectus carinatum,* in which the sternum protrudes outward, increasing the anteroposterior diameter, and *funnel chest,* or *pectus excavatum,* in which the lower portion of the sternum is depressed. A severe depression may impair cardiac function, but in general neither condition causes pathologic dysfunction. However, these conditions often cause parents and children concern regarding acceptable physical appearance.

The nurse also notes the *angle* made by the lower costal margin and the sternum, which ordinarily is about 45 degrees. A larger angle is characteristic of lung diseases that also cause a barrel shape of the chest. A smaller angle may be a sign of malnutrition. As the nurse inspects the rib cage, the junction of the ribs to the costal cartilage (costochondral junction) and sternum is noted. Normally the points of attachment are fairly smooth. Swellings or blunt knobs along either side of the sternum are known as the *rachitic rosary* and may indicate vitamin D deficiency. Another variation in shape that may either be normal or may suggest rickets (vitamin D deficiency) is *Harrison's groove,* which appears as a depression or horizontal groove where the diaphragm leaves the chest wall. Usually marked flaring of the rib cage below the groove is significant of an abnormal finding.

Body *symmetry* is always an important notation during inspection. Asymmetry in the chest may indicate serious underlying problems, such as cardiac enlargement (bulging on the left side of rib cage) or pulmonary dysfunction. However, asymmetry is most often a sign of scoliosis, lateral curvature of the spine (p. 1528). Asymmetry always warrants further medical investigation.

All of the preceding characteristics of the chest are affected by *movement.* With normal inspiration the chest expands, the sternal angle increases, and the diaphragm descends. With normal expiration the reverse occurs, that is, the chest decreases in size, the sternal angle decreases, and the diaphragm rises.

Paradoxical respirations occur when the diaphragm rises on inspiration and descends on expiration. These respirations are indicative of several disease states and always warrant further investigation. In children under 6 or 7 years of age, respiratory movements are mainly abdominal because of the more horizontal positioning of the ribs (see p. 256). In older children thoracic movements are mainly responsible for the exchange of air. Marked *retraction* of muscles either between the ribs (intercostal), above the sternum (suprasternal), or above the clavicles (supraclavicular) is always noted and reported, because it is a sign of respiratory difficulty. Any asymmetry of movement is also an important pathologic sign. Decreased movement on

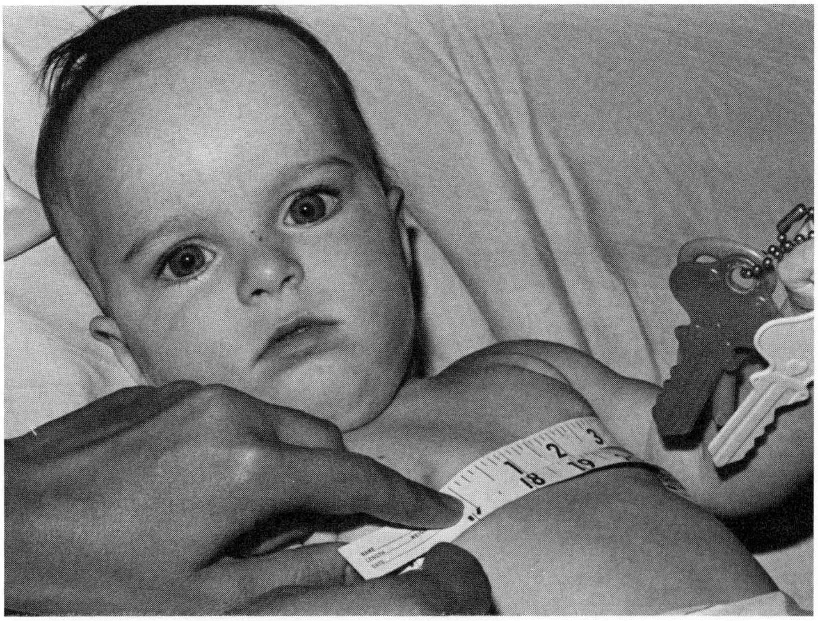

Fig. 5-34. Measuring chest circumference.

one side of the chest may indicate pneumonia, pneumothorax, atelectasis, or an obstructive foreign body.

As the nurse inspects the skin surface of the chest, the position of the *nipples* is observed as well as any evidence of *breast* development (Fig. 5-35). Normally the nipples are located slightly lateral to the midclavicular line between the fourth and fifth ribs. The nurse notes symmetry of nipple placement and the normal configuration of a darker pigmented areola surrounding a flat nipple in the prepubertal child.

Pubertal breast development usually begins in girls between 10 and 14 years of age. The nurse should note evidence of breast enlargement, which is discussed in Chapter 19. Precocious or delayed breast development is recorded, as well as evidence of any other secondary sexual characteristics. In males gynecomastia may be caused by hormonal or systemic disorders, but more commonly it is the result of adipose tissue from obesity or a transitory body change during early puberty. In either case the nurse should investigate the child's feelings regarding breast enlargement.

In adolescent females who have achieved sexual maturity, the nurse should palpate the breasts for evidence of any masses or hard nodules. This opportunity should also be taken to discuss the importance of routine self-breast examination. Although carcinoma of the breast is rare in women under 20 years of age, it is advisable to stress the value of routine self-breast examination so that it becomes a practiced habit during later years. If a mass is palpable, the vast majority are benign fibroadenomas.[30] The nurse should emphasize this fact in order to decrease any fear or concern that results when a mass is felt.

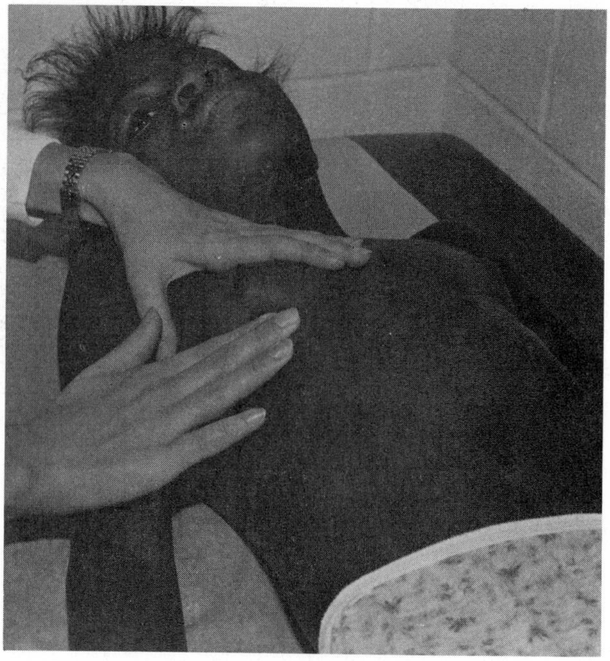

Fig. 5-35. Palpating the breast.

Lungs

The lungs are situated inside the thoracic cavity, with one lung on each side of the sternum. Each lung is divided into an *apex,* which is slightly pointed and rises above the first rib, a *base,* which is wide and concave and rides on the dome-shaped diaphragm, and a body, which is divided into *lobes*. The right lung has three lobes: the upper, middle, and lower. The left lobe has only two lobes, the upper and lower, because of the space occupied by the heart. The two surfaces of the lung are the *costal surface,* which faces the chest wall and backs up to the vertebral column, and the *mediastinal surface,* which faces the space lying between the lungs, the mediastinum. The center of the mediastinal surface is called the *hilus,* where the bronchus and blood vessels enter the lung (Fig. 5-36, *A*).

Examination of the lungs requires knowledge of their location and their relationship to the rib cage. The trachea bifurcates slightly below the level of the sternal angle. The apex of each lung rises about 2 to 4 cm above the inner third of the clavicles. The lower costal margin crosses the sixth rib at the midclavicular line and the eighth rib at the midaxillary line. The posterior base of the lungs crosses the eleventh rib at the vertebral line. The upper border of the right middle lobe parallels the inferior surface of the fourth rib. Fig. 5-36 illustrates the position of the lobes within the thoracic cavity during relaxation. Respiration will cause characteristic displacement of the lobes upward (expiration) or downward (inspiration).

Inspection. Inspection of the lungs involves primarily observation of respiratory movements, which have been discussed on p. 143. Respirations are evaluated for rate (number per minute), rhythm (regular, irregular, or periodic), depth (deep or shallow), and quality (effortless, automatic, difficult, or labored). The nurse also notes the character of breath sounds based on inspection without the aid of auscultation, such as noisy, grunting, snoring, or heavy. Usual terms for describing various patterns of respiration are listed in Table 5-4.

Respiratory rate is always evaluated in relation to general physical status. For example, tachypnea is expected with fever, because for every degree Fahrenheit elevation in temperature, the respiratory rate increases 4 breaths/minute. The usual ratio of breaths to heartbeats is 1:4 (see Appendix A for normal respiratory rates at various ages).

Palpation. Respiratory movements are felt by placing each hand flat against the back or chest with the thumbs in midline along the lower costal margin of the lungs. The child should be sitting during this procedure and, if cooperative, should take several deep breaths. During respiration the nurse's hands will move with the chest wall. The nurse evaluates the amount and speed of respiratory excursion,

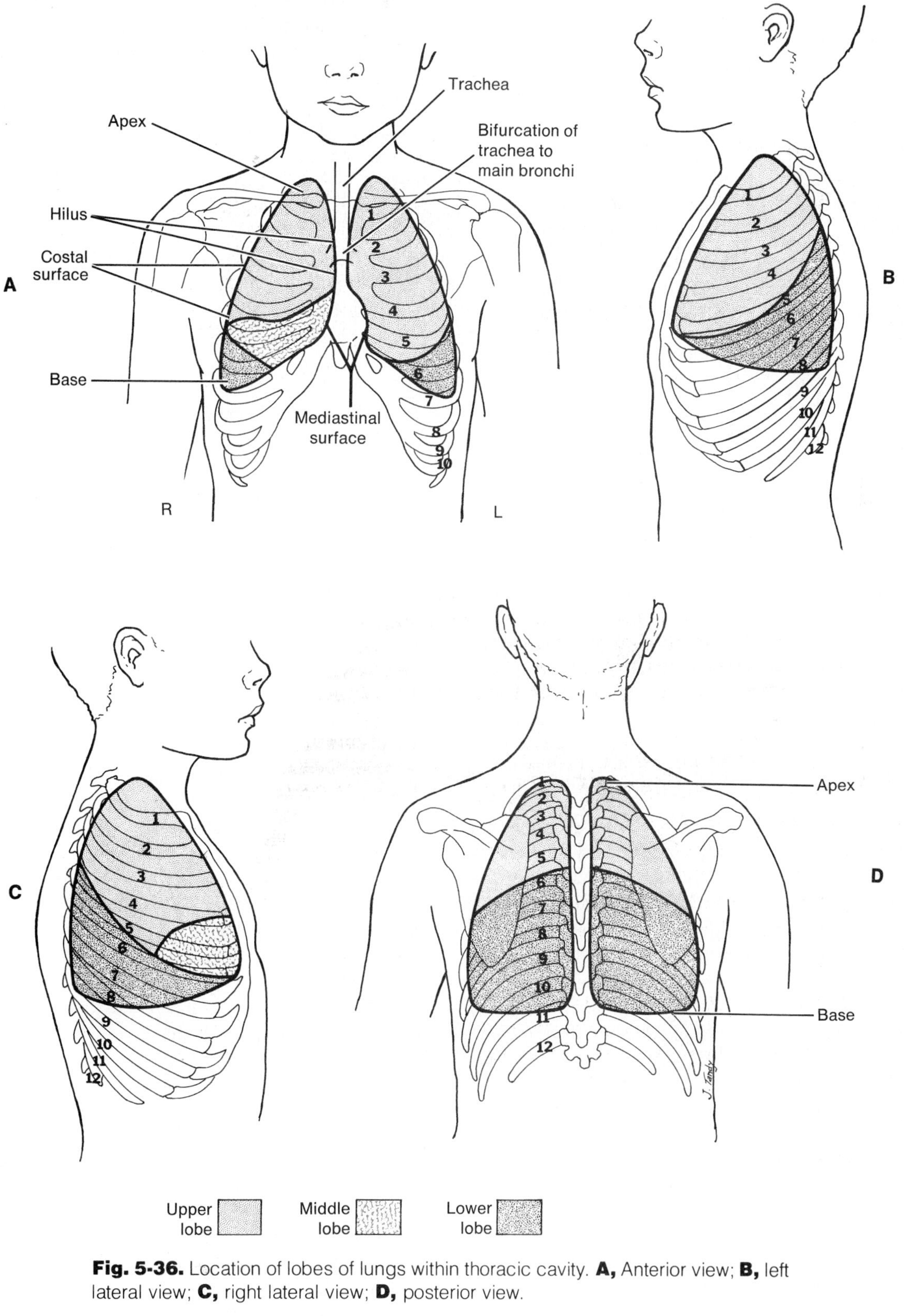

Fig. 5-36. Location of lobes of lungs within thoracic cavity. **A,** Anterior view; **B,** left lateral view; **C,** right lateral view; **D,** posterior view.

Table 5-4. Various patterns of respiration

Term	Description
Tachypnea	Increased rate
Bradypnea	Decreased rate
Dyspnea	Distress during breathing
Apnea	Cessation of breathing
Hyperpnea	Increased depth
Hypoventilation	Decreased depth (shallow) and irregular rhythm
Hyperventilation	Increased rate and depth
Kussmaul breathing	Hyperventilation, gasping and labored respiration, usually seen in diabetic coma or other states of respiratory acidosis
Cheyne-Stokes respirations	Gradually increasing rate and depth with periods of apnea
Biot's breathing	Periods of hyperpnea alternating with apnea (similar to Cheyne-Stokes except that the depth remains constant)
Seesaw (paradoxical) respirations	Chest rises while the abdomen falls

noting any asymmetry of movement. Normally the posterior base of the lungs descends 5 to 6 cm (2 to 2.3 inches) during a deep inspiration.

The nurse also palpates for *vocal fremitus,* the conduction of voice sounds through the respiratory tract. With the palmar surfaces of each hand on the chest, the nurse asks the child to repeat words, such as "ninety-nine," "one, two, three," or "eee-eee." The child should speak the words with a voice of uniform intensity. The nurse feels the vibrations as the hands are moved symmetrically on either side of the sternum and vertebral column. In general, vocal fremitus is most intense in the regions of the thorax where the trachea and bronchi are closest to the surface, particularly along the sternum between the first and second ribs and posteriorly between the scapula. Progressing downward, the sound decreases and is least prominent at the base of the lungs. Decreased vocal fremitus in the upper airway may indicate several gross pulmonary changes. Absence of fremitus usually indicates obstruction of a major bronchus, which may occur as a result of aspiration of a foreign body. Decreased or absent fremitus is always recorded and reported for further investigation.

During palpation the nurse notes other vibrations that indicate pathology. One is a *pleural friction rub,* which feels like a grating sensation. It is usually synchronous with respiratory movements and is the result of opposing surfaces of the inflamed pleural lining rubbing against one another.

Crepitation is felt as a coarse, cracking sensation as the nurse presses the hand over the affected area. It is the result of the escape of air from the lungs into the subcutaneous tissues as a result of injury of surgical intervention. Both pleural friction rubs and crepitation can usually be heard as well as felt.

Percussion. The lungs are percussed in order to evaluate the densities of the underlying organs. Fig. 5-37 illustrates the usual percussion sounds within the thorax. Resonance is usually heard over all the lobes of the lungs that are not adjacent to other organs. Dullness is usually heard beginning at the fifth interspace in the right midclavicular line. Percussing downward to the end of the liver, the sound becomes flat, because the liver no longer overlies the air-filled lung. Cardiac dullness is normally felt over the left sternal border from the second to the fifth interspace medially to the midclavicular line. Below the fifth interspace on the left side, tympany results from the air-filled stomach. Deviations from these expected sounds are always recorded and reported.

In percussing the chest, the anterior lung is percussed from apex to base, usually with the child in the supine or sitting position. The nurse percusses each side of the chest in sequence in order to compare the sounds, such as the dullness of the liver on the right side with the tympany of the stomach on the left side. When percussing the posterior lung, the procedure and sequence are the same, although the child should be sitting. Normally, only resonance is heard when percussing the posterior thorax from the shoulder to the eighth or tenth rib. At the base of the lungs dullness is heard as the diaphragm is percussed. Normally the diaphragm should descend about 5 to 6 cm (2 to 2.3 inches) during inspiration.

Auscultation. Auscultation involves using the stethoscope to evaluate breath and voice sounds. In the normal lungs breath sounds are classified as vesicular or bronchovesicular. *Vesicular breath sounds* are normally heard over the entire surface of the lungs with the exception of the upper intrascapular area and the area beneath the manubrium. Inspiration is louder, longer, and higher-pitched than expiration. Sometimes the expiratory phase seems nearly absent in comparison to the long inspiratory phase. The sound is usually a soft swishing noise.

Bronchovesicular breath sounds are normally heard over the manubrium and in the upper intrascapular regions where there are bifurcations of large airways, such as the trachea and bronchi. Inspiration and expiration are of almost equal duration, quality, pitch, and intensity. Inspiration is normally louder and higher in pitch than that heard in vesicular breathing.

Another type of breathing that is normal only over the trachea near the suprasternal notch is *bronchial breath sounds.* They are almost the reverse of vesicular sounds; the inspiratory phase is short and the expiratory phase is longer, louder, and of higher pitch. They are usually louder than any of the normal breath sounds and have a hollow, blowing character. Bronchial breathing anywhere in the lung except

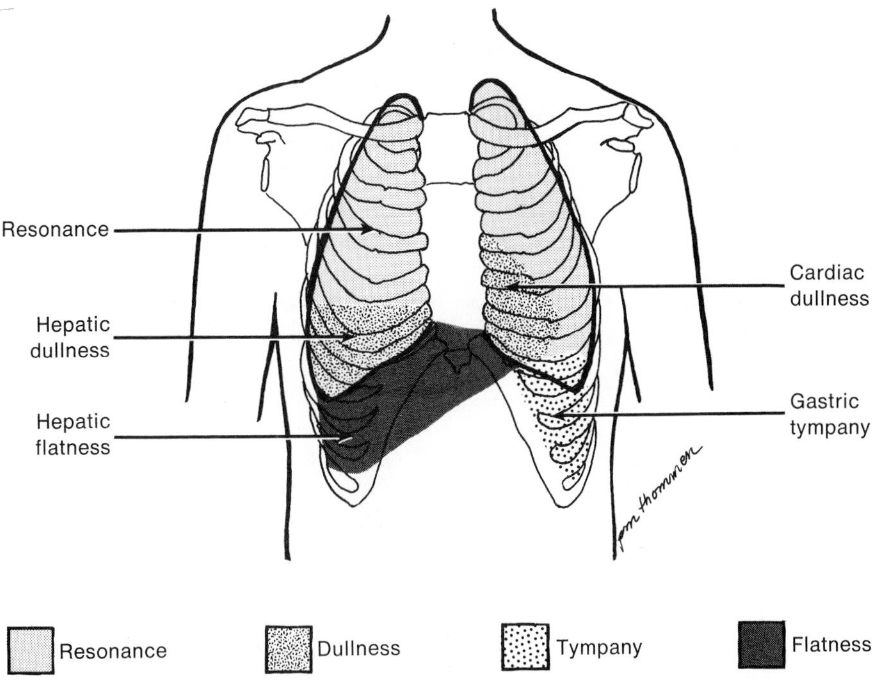

Fig. 5-37. Percussion sounds found in normal thorax.

over the trachea denotes some abnormality, such as consolidation or compression of lung tissue.

Absent or diminished breath sounds are always an abnormal finding warranting investigation. Fluid, air, or solid masses in the pleural space all interfere with the conduction of breath sounds. Diminished breath sounds in certain segments of the lung can alert the nurse to pulmonary areas that may benefit from postural drainage and percussion. Increased breath sounds following pulmonary therapy indicate improved passage of air through the respiratory tract.

Voice sounds are also part of the normal auscultation of the lungs. Normally voice sounds or vocal resonance are heard, but the syllables are indistinct. They are elicited in the same manner as vocal fremitus, except that the nurse listens with the stethoscope. Consolidation of lung tissue produces three types of abnormal voice sounds: (1) *whispered pectoriloquy,* in which the child whispers words and the nurse hears the syllables, (2) *bronchophony,* in which the child speaks words that are not distinguishable but the vocal resonance is increased in intensity and clarity, and (3) *egophony,* in which the child says the letter "ee," which is heard as the nasal sound "ay" through the stethoscope. Decreased or absent vocal resonance is caused by the same conditions that affect vocal fremitus.

Various pulmonary abnormalities produce *adventitious sounds* that are not normally heard over the chest. They are not alterations of normal breath sounds but rather sounds that occur in addition to normal or abnormal breath sounds. They are classified into two main groups: rales (from the French word meaning "rattle") and rhonchi. Considerable practice with an experienced tutor is necessary to differentiate the various types of rales and rhonchi. Often it is best to describe the type of sound heard in the lungs rather than to try and label it correctly.

Rales result from the passage of air through fluid or moisture. The type of rales is determined by the size of the passageway and the type of exudate the air passes through. Rales are similar to the sound of the "fizz" from a recently opened carbonated drink, such as a bottle of soda. They are roughly divided into three categories: fine, medium, and coarse.

Fine rales (sometimes called crepitant rales) can be simulated by rubbing a few strands of hair between the thumb and index finger close to the ear or by slowly separating the thumb and index finger after they have been moistened with saliva. The result is a series of fine crackling sounds. Fine rales are most prominent at the end of inspiration and are not cleared by coughing. They occur in the smallest passageways, the alveoli and bronchioles.

Medium rales are not as delicate as fine rales and can be simulated by listening to the "fizz" of carbonated drinks or by rolling a dry cigar between the fingers. They are prominent earlier during inspiration and occur in the larger passages of the bronchioles and small bronchi.

Coarse rales are relatively loud, coarse, bubbling, gurgling sounds that occur in the large airways of the trachea, bronchi, and smaller bronchi. Often they clear partially during coughing.

Rhonchi are sounds produced as air passes through narrowed passageways, regardless of the cause, such as exudate, inflammation, spasm, or tumor. Rhonchi are more continuous sounds than rales and, although often more prominent during expirations, are usually present during both phases of respiration. Rhonchi are classified according to pitch as sibilant or sonorous.

Sibilant rhonchi are high-pitched, musical, wheezing, or squeaking in character. The wheezing quality is often more pronounced on forced expiration. Sibilant rhonchi are produced in the smaller bronchi and bronchioles.

Sonorous rhonchi are low-pitched and often snoring or moaning in character. They are produced in the large passages of the trachea and bronchi. Like coarse rales, they can be partly cleared by coughing. Some clinicians classify sonorous rhonchi as coarse rales, or vice versa.

The other adventitious sound of importance is the *pleural friction rub,* discussed on p. 146. Its sound can be simulated by cupping one hand to the ear and rubbing a finger of the other hand across the cupped hand. The most common site for a friction rub to be heard is the lower anterolateral chest wall (between the midaxillary and midclavicular lines), the area of greatest thoracic mobility.

Heart

Examination of the heart involves the skills of inspection, palpation, percussion, and auscultation, although the latter is the most significant. Overall assessment of cardiac function involves a comprehensive evaluation of pulse, blood pressure, respiratory function, and general physical growth and development. The nurse must be familiar with the anatomy and physiology of the normal heart in order to properly evaluate the findings. Chapter 35 discusses the normal circulation of the blood through the heart chambers, major blood vessesl, and valves.

The heart is situated in the thoracic cavity between the lungs in the mediastinum and above the diaphragm. About two thirds of the heart lies within the left side of the rib cage, with the other third on the right side as it crosses the sternum. Knowledge of the location of the heart in relation to the rib cage is essential for evaluating and describing findings. Fig. 5-38 illustrates the usual position of the heart in the thorax.

The heart is situated almost like a triangle. One side extends vertically along the right sternal border (RSB) from the second to the fifth rib, one side extends from the lower right sternum horizontally to the fifth rib at the left midclavicular line (LMCL), and the longest side extends diagonally from the right sternal border at the second rib to the left midclavicular line at the fifth rib. The *base* of the heart, which is actually the top of the triangle, is located at the right and left sternal borders and second intercostal space (ICS) or pulmonic and aortic areas. The *apex* is located at the left midclavicular line and fifth intercostal space or mitral area. The heart of the infant is normally more horizontally positioned; therefore, the apex is usually higher

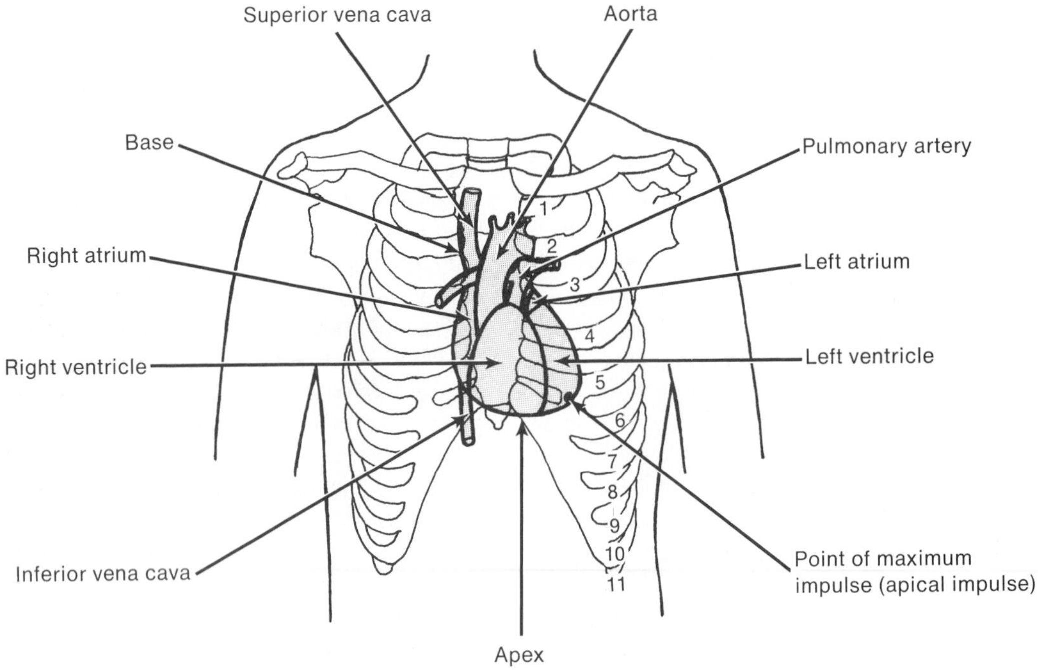

Fig. 5-38. Position of heart within thorax.

(third to fourth intercostal space) and to the left of the midclavicular line. The apical impulse or *point of maximum impulse* (PMI) (area where the heartbeat is loudest) is usually located at the apex. Most of the anterior cardiac surface is occupied by the right ventricle. Part of the right atrium and left ventricle also face anteriorly, whereas the left atrium lies primarily in a posterior position.

Inspection. As the nurse is examining the chest, any obvious bulging is noted, especially on the left side, which may indicate cardiac enlargement. This is best done by observing the child sitting in a semi-Fowler's position and looking at the anterior chest wall from an angle, comparing both sides of the rib cage to each other. Normally they should be symmetric. In children with thin chest walls, the point of maximum impulse or apical pulse is sometimes apparent as a pulsation. Noting the location of the impulse may give some indication of the size and positioning of the heart, especially if it deviates from the expected apical site.

Since comprehensive evaluation of cardiac function is not limited to the heart, the nurse also considers other findings, such as presence of all pulses (especially the femoral pulses), distended neck veins, clubbing of the fingers, peripheral cyanosis, edema, blood pressure, and respiratory status.

Palpation. Palpation is useful in determing the size of the heart by feeling for the point of maximum impulse, which ordinarily corresponds to the apex. The apex is usually at a lower interspace and more lateral in a child with cardiac enlargement. The apex is felt by placing the fingertips or the palmar aspect of the fingers and hand at the fifth intercostal space and left midclavicular line.

As the nurse feels for the point of maximum impulse, the presence of vibratory thrills and pericardial friction rubs is noted. *Thrills* are palpable vibrations most commonly produced by the flow of blood from one chamber of the heart to another through a narrowed or abnormal opening, such as a stenotic valve or a septal defect. Thrills feel similar to the placing of one's hand on a purring cat.

Pericardial friction rubs are scratchy, high-pitched grating sounds, similar to pleural friction rubs, except that they are not affected by changes in respiration. This is a useful clue in differentiating the two rubs, because the pleural rub will cease if the child holds his breath, but the pericardial rub will not. Both thrills and rubs are abnormal and must be reported for further evaluation.

Percussion. Percussion is used mainly to determine the size of the heart by outlining its borders. Dullness is normally heard over the left area of the heart and partially over the right, although dullness on the right side descends past the border of the heart to the nearby liver (Fig. 5-37). The most important area of percussion is dullness along the lower sternal border to the left midclavicular line. This finding is often referred to as *left border of cardiac dullness* (LBCD). Deviation from the expected finding may indicate cardiac enlargement or displacement and warrants further study.

Auscultation. Auscultation involves listening for heart sounds with the stethoscope, similar to the procedure used in assessing breath sounds.

Origin of heart sounds. The heart sounds are produced by the opening and closing of the valves and the vibration of blood against the walls of the heart and vessels. Normally two sounds—S_1 and S_2—are heard, which correspond respectively to the familiar "lub dub" often used to describe the sounds. S_1 is caused by the closure of the *tricuspid* and *mitral valves* (sometimes called the atrioventricular valves). Right ventricular contraction follows tricuspid valve closure, and left ventricular contraction follows mitral valve closure. The contractions (systole) occur almost simultaneously, although the mitral valve (left side) closes slightly before the tricuspid valve (right side). Normally this split of the sounds is so close that it is not audible, except occasionally at the apex of the heart.

S_2 is the result of the closure of the *pulmonic* and *aortic* valves (sometimes called semilunar valves). Aortic valve closing (left side) occurs slightly before pulmonic valve closing (right side). The flow of blood into the aorta and pulmonary artery occurs following closure of their respective valves. The interval between S_2 and S_1 is diastole or relaxation of the heart. Normally the split of the two sounds in S_2 is distinguishable and widens during inspiration, because inspiration prolongs right ventricular filling and delays pulmonary valve closure. "Physiologic splitting" is a significant normal finding that should be elicited. "Fixed splitting," in which the split in S_2 does not change during inspiration, is an important diagnostic sign of atrial septal defect (see p. 1316).

Fig. 5-39 illustrates the approximate anatomic position of the valves within the heart chambers. It is important to note that the anatomic location of valves does not correspond to the area where the sounds are heard best. The auscultatory sites are located in the direction of the blood flow through the valves.

Two other heart sounds—S_3 and S_4—may be produced. S_3 is the result of vibrations produced during ventricular filling. It is normally heard only in some children and young adults, but it is considered abnormal in older individuals. S_4 is caused by the recoil of vibrations between the atria and ventricles following atrial contraction at the end of diastole. It is rarely heard as a normal heart sound; usually it is considered indicative of further cardiac evaluation.

Another important category of heart sounds is *murmurs*, which are produced by vibrations within the heart chambers or in the major arteries from the back and forth flow of blood (see Chapter 35 for a more detailed discussion). Murmurs are classified as (1) innocent or functional (no organic cause) and (2) organic (a result of some cardiac defect). The description and classification of murmurs are skills that re-

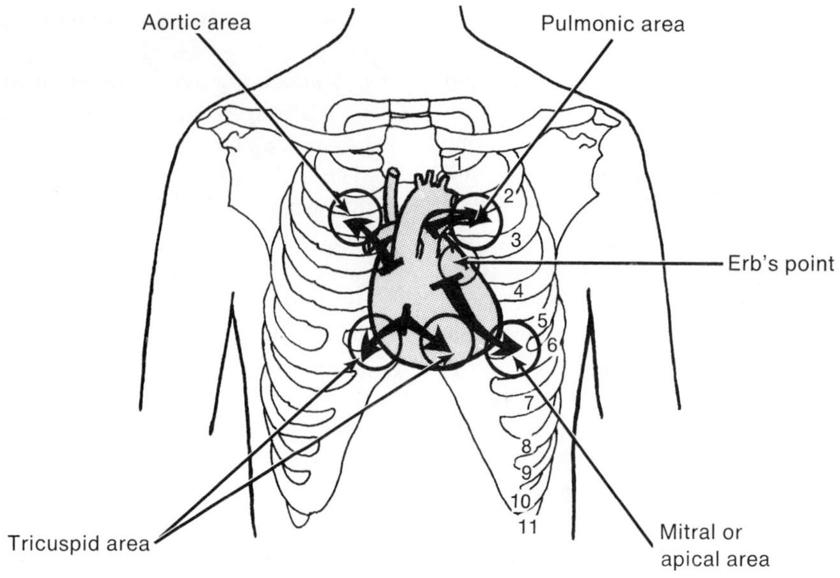

Fig. 5-39. Direction of heart sounds from anatomic valve sites.

Table 5-5. Grading of the intensity of heart murmurs

Grade	Description
I	Very faint, frequently not heard if child sits up or after he exercises
II	Usually readily heard, slightly louder than grade I, audible in all positions and after exercise
III	Loud, but not accompanied by a thrill
IV	Loud, accompanied by a thrill
V	Loud enough to be heard with the stethoscope barely on the chest, accompanied by a thrill
VI	Loud enough to be heard with the stethoscope not touching the chest; often heard with the human ear close to the chest, accompanied by a thrill

quire considerable practice and training. In general the nurse should be able to recognize murmurs as distinct swishing sounds that occur in addition to the normal heart sounds. The following information should be found: (1) location of the area of the heart where the murmur is heard best, (2) time of the occurrence of the murmur within the S_1S_2 cycle, (3) evaluation of its intensity in relationship to the child's position, and (4) estimation of its loudness. The usual subjective method of grading the loudness or intensity of a murmur is listed in Table 5-5.

Although the nurse should consult with a physician whenever a murmur is identified, the following guidelines can be used in distinguishing between innocent and organic murmurs. Innocent murmurs generally are (1) systolic, that is, they occur with or after S_1, (2) of short duration and have no transmission to other areas of the heart, (3) grade III or less in intensity and do not increase over time, (4) usually loudest in the pulmonic area (second or third intercostal space along the left sternal border), (5) variable in relationship to position, respiration, and activity (for example, audible in the supine position but absent in the sitting position), (6) not associated with any physical signs of cardiac disease, and (7) usually of a low-pitched, musical, or groaning quality.

There are a number of other abnormal sounds, such as ejection clicks, snaps, gallops, hums, and so on. It is beyond the scope of this discussion to elaborate on the gamut of adventitious heart sounds. The best approach is for the nurse to become familiar with normal heart sounds and to refer any questionable heart sound to a physician for further medical evaluation.

Differentiating normal heart sounds. In referring to Figure 5-39, it is apparent that normally S_1 is louder at the apex of the heart in the mitral and tricuspid area and that S_2 is louder near the base of the heart in the pulmonic and aortic area. The nurse listens to each sound by inching down the chest in the sequence outlined in Table 5-6. If the nurse has difficulty in deciding which sound is S_1 or S_2, especially when the rate is rapid, the carotid pulse should be simultaneously palpated with the index and middle finger and the heart sounds should be listened to. S_1 is synchronous with the carotid pulse. In addition to the areas listed in Table 5-6, the nurse should also listen in the sternoclavicular area above the clavicles and manubrium, along the sternal border, along the left midaxillary line, and below the scapulae

Table 5-6. Sequence of auscultating heart sounds*

Auscultatory site	Chest location	Characteristics of heart sounds
Aortic area	Second right intercostal space close to sternum	S_2 heard louder than S_1; Aortic closure heard loudest
Pulmonic area	Second left intercostal space close to sternum	Splitting of S_2 heard best, normally widens on inspiration; pulmonic closure heard best
Erb's point	Second and third left intercostal space close to sternum	Frequent site of innocent murmurs and those of aortic or pulmonic origin
Tricuspid area	Fifth right and left intercostal space close to sternum	S_1 heard as louder sound preceding S_2 (S_1 synchronous with carotid pulse)
Mitral or apical area	Fifth intercostal space, left midclavicular line (third to fourth intercostal space and lateral to left midclavicular line in infants)	S_1 heard loudest; splitting of S_1 may be audible because mitral closure is louder than tricuspid closure S_3 heard best at beginning of expiration with child in recumbent or left side-lying position, occurs immediately after S_2, sounds like word "Ken-tuc-ky" S_1 S_2 S_3 S_4 heard best during expiration with child in recumbent position (left side-lying position decreases sound), occurs immediately before S_1, sounds like word "Ten-nes-see" S_4 S_1 S_2

*Use both diaphragm and bell chestpieces when auscultating heart sounds. Bell chestpiece is necessary for low-pitched sounds of murmurs, S_3, and S_4.

for sounds, such as murmurs, which may radiate to these areas.

The nurse listens to the heart with the child in at least two positions, sitting and reclining (Fig. 5-40). If adventitious sounds are detected, the nurse should further evaluate them with the child standing, sitting and leaning forward, and lying on his left side. For example, atrial sounds such as S_4 are heard best with the person in a recumbent position and usually fade if the person sits or stands. The nurse also uses both the diaphragm and bell chestpieces when listening to each auscultatory area. The diaphragm chestpiece is better for the detection of high-pitched sounds, such as S_1 and S_2. The bell chestpiece is used for low-pitched sounds, such as S_3, S_4, or murmurs. If the nurse fails to listen to each normal heart sound with both chestpieces, it is not unlikely for a grade I murmur to be missed.

Heart sounds are evaluated for (1) *quality,* which should be clear and distinct, not muffled, diffuse, or distant, (2) *intensity,* especially in relation to location or auscultatory site, (3) *rate,* which should be the same as the radial pulse, and (4) *rhythm,* which should be regular and even. A particular arrhythmia that occurs normally in many children is *sinus arrhythmia,* in which the heart rate increases with inspiration and decreases with expiration. This can be differentiated from a truly abnormal arrhythmia by having the child hold his breath. In sinus arrhythmia cessation of breathing causes the heart rate to remain steady. Table 5-7 lists variations in patterns of heart rate or pulse. Like respiratory rate, heart rate is always evaluated in relation to the child's general physical status. For example, the pulse rate is usually increased by 8 to 10 beats/minute for each degree Fahrenheit elevation in temperature. Athletic children occasionally have lowered heart rates that may even reach rates suggestive of bradycardia (below 60 beats/minute) but that represent a highly developed and efficient heart muscle (see Appendix A, Table A-1 for normal heart rates at various ages).

Abdomen

Examination of the abdomen involves the usual four skills, except that the order is significantly changed. Inspection is followed by auscultation, percussion, and then palpation, which may distort the normal abdominal sounds. The nurse must have knowledge of the anatomic placement of the abdominal organs in order to differentiate normal, expected findings from abnormal ones (Fig. 5-41).

The sequence of examining the abdomen changes according to the age and cooperativeness of the child. Frequently all four types of assessment are performed at different times. For example, the nurse may auscultate for bowel sounds following evaluation of heart and lung sounds at the

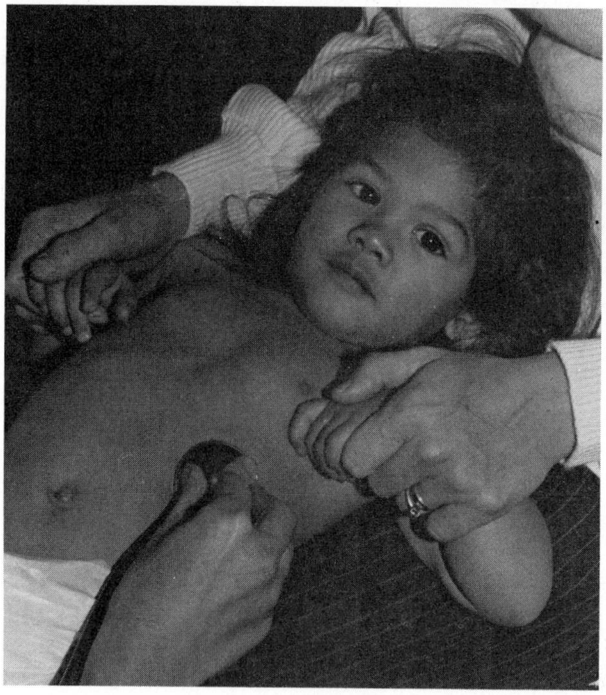

Fig. 5-40. Reclining position in parent's lap for auscultation of heart.

Table 5-7. Various patterns of heart rate or pulse

Term	Description
Tachycardia	Increased rate
Bradycardia	Decreased rate
Pulsus alternans	Strong beat followed by weak beat
Pulsus bigeminus	Coupled rhythm in which beat is felt in pairs because of premature beat
Pulsus paradoxus	Intensity or force of pulse decreases with inspiration
Sinus arrhythmia	Rate increases with inspiration, decreases with expiration
Water-hammer or Corrigan's pulse	Especially forceful beat caused by a very wide pulse pressure (systolic blood pressure minus diastolic blood pressure)
Dicrotic pulse	Double radial pulse for every apical beat
Thready pulse	Rapid, weak pulse that seems to appear and disappear

beginning of the examination when the child is quiet. Inspection may occur at any time during the examination. Percussion usually follows lung percussion, and palpation may be done toward the end of the examination when the child is relaxed and more trusting of the nurse. Although examination of the anal area is included in discussion of the abdomen, this part of the assessment may be done when the back and spine are inspected or when a rectal temperature is taken.

The *abdominal cavity* is the portion of the trunk from directly beneath the diaphragm and thoracic cavity to the region of the pelvic cavity (Fig. 5-42). No definitive structures separate the abdominal from the pelvic cavity, although the demarcation is formed by the junction of the pelvic bones anteriorly and the sacrum posteriorly. The abdominal cavity contains the major organs of digestion, and the pelvic cavity houses the internal reproductive organs, the urinary bladder, and the lower parts of the digestive tract. The abdominal cavity is divided into four quadrants for descriptive purposes by drawing a vertical line midway from the sternum to the pubic symphysis and a horizontal line across the abdomen through the umbilicus. This method of division actually includes the pelvic cavity. The major structures located in each of the four quadrants are listed in the boxed material on p. 154.

Inspection. The nurse inspects the *contour* of the abdomen both while the child is erect and supine. Normally the abdomen of infants and young children is quite cylindric and, in the erect position, fairly prominent because of the physiologic lordosis of the spine. In the supine position the abdomen appears flat. During adolescence the usual male and female contours of the pelvic cavity change the shape of the abdomen to form characteristic adult curves, especially in the female.

The *size* and *tone* of the abdomen also give some indication of general nutritional status and muscular development. A large, prominent, flabby abdomen is often seen in obese children, whereas a concave abdomen is frequently sugges-

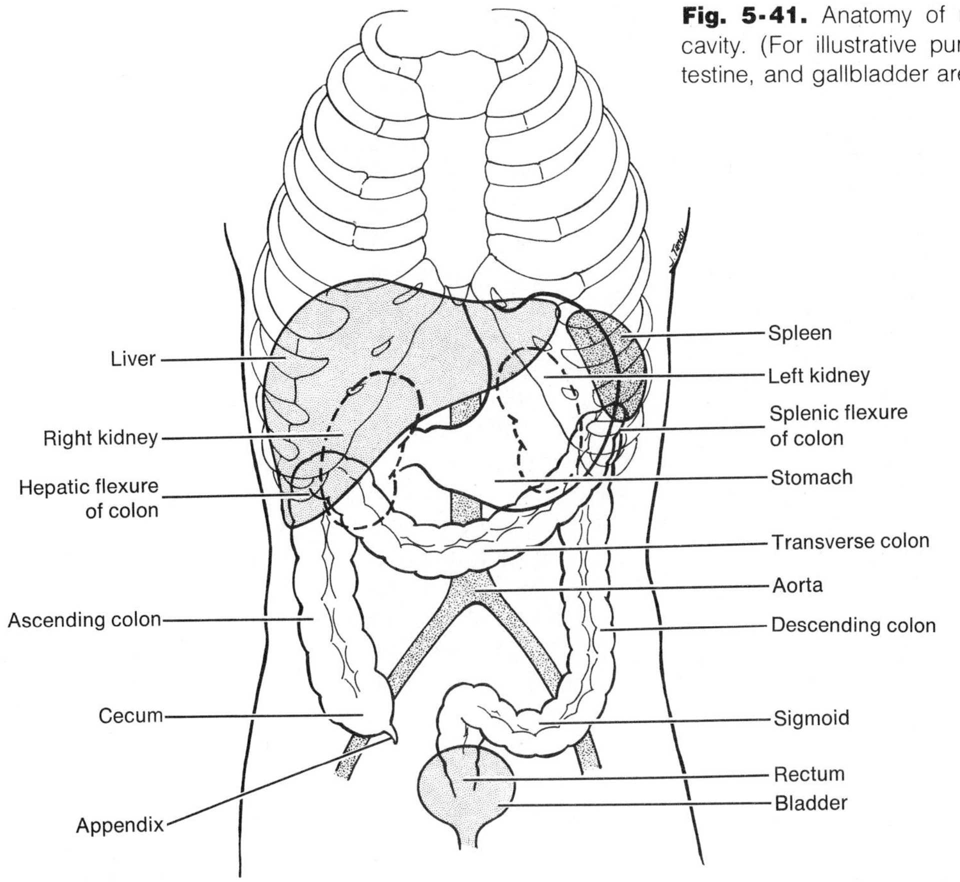

Fig. 5-41. Anatomy of major organs within abdominal cavity. (For illustrative purposes, the pancreas, small intestine, and gallbladder are not shown.)

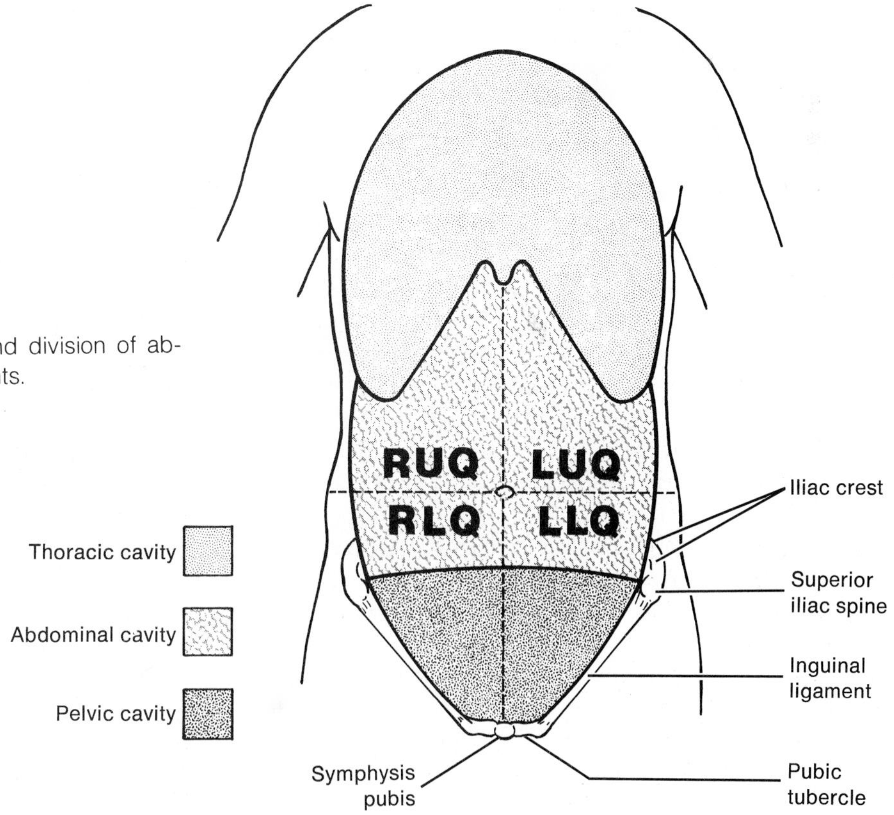

Fig. 5-42. Major cavities of trunk and division of abdominal cavity into respective quadrants.

Location of major structures in each abdominal quadrant

Right upper quadrant (RUQ)
- Liver*
- Duodenum
- Pylorus
- Pancreas
- Gallbladder
- Hepatic flexure of colon
- Part of transverse and ascending colon

Left upper quadrant (LUQ)
- Stomach
- Spleen*
- Pancreas
- Left kidney
- Splenic flexure of colon
- Part of transverse and descending colon

Right lower quadrant (RLQ)
- Cecum
- Appendix
- Part of ascending colon
- Right overy and fallopian tube
- Right femoral pulse*

Left lower quadrant (LLQ)
- Sigmoid colon
- Part of descending colon
- Left ovary and fallopian tubes
- Left femoral pulse*

Midline
- Umbilicus*
- Aorta*
- Bladder
- Rectum
- Uterus

*Organs that are usually palpable.

tive of undernutrition. However, the nurse should make careful note of a protruding abdomen, which may indicate pathologic states such as abdominal distention, ascites, tumors, or organomegaly. A protuberant abdomen with spindly extremities and flat wasted buttocks suggests severe malnutrition that may occur from inadequate nutritional intake such as kwashiorkor or from diseases such as cystic fibrosis. Likewise, a scaphoid abdomen may indicate dehydration or diaphragmatic hernia, in which the abdominal organs rise into the thoracic cavity, or a "scaphoid-like" abdomen that only appears sunken in relationship to pneumothorax or high intestinal obstruction. A midline protrusion from the xiphoid to the umbilicus or pubic symphysis is usually *diastasis recti,* or failure of the rectus abdominis muscles to join in utero. In a healthy child a midline protrusion is usually a variation of normal muscular development. A tense, boardlike abdomen is a serious sign of paralytic ileus and intestinal obstruction.

The nurse also notes the condition of the *skin* covering the abdomen. It should be uniformily taut, without wrinkles or creases. Sometimes silvery, whitish striae are seen, especially if the skin has been stretched as in obesity or with distention resulting from ascites. The nurse should note and record any scars, ecchymotic areas, excessive hair distribution, or distended veins.

The nurse also notes *movement* of the abdomen. In infants and thin children, *peristaltic waves* may be visible through the abdominal wall, although they always warrant careful evaluation. They are best observed by standing at eye level to and across from the abdomen. Visible peristaltic waves most often indicate pathologic states, particularly intestinal obstruction such as pyloric stenosis.

The nurse may observe *pulsation* of the descending *aorta* in the epigastric region (midline and below the xiphoid). Although visible pulsations are normally seen, especially in thin children, the nurse should auscultate and palpate the aorta for any evidence of an aneurysm, a sac-like enlargement of the vessel.

In children under 7 or 8 years of age, breathing is primarily abdominal. If the abdomen fails to move with respiration, even in older children, this may indicate serious abdominal problems. Conversely if the thoracic muscles fail to move, so that breathing is confined to abdominal movement, pulmonary problems may be at fault. Normally chest and abdominal movements are synchronous. In *seesaw or paradoxical respiration,* the abdomen falls as the chest rises during inspiration and the reverse movements occur during expiration. This is seen in children with neuromuscular diseases and some pulmonary disorders, such as pneumothorax.

The nurse also inspects the *umbilicus* for any herniation, fistulas, such as a patent urachus (an abnormal connection between the umbilicus and bladder), discharge, and hygiene. If a herniation is present the nurse also palpates the sac for abdominal contents and estimates the approximate size of the opening. Umbilical hernias are common in infants, especially in black children. Since "home remedies" for treatment such as taping coins over the umbilicus or using "belly binders" may be harmful to the skin and actually delay natural closure, the nurse should ask parents whether such procedures have been used. Umbilical hernias normally protrude and expand when the child coughs, cries, or strains.

The nurse observes for *hernias* elsewhere on the abdominal wall, such as in the inguinal or femoral region. An *inguinal hernia* is a protrusion of peritoneum through the abdominal wall in the inguinal canal. It most often occurs in males, is frequently bilateral, and may be visible as a mass in the scrotum. It is palpated for by sliding the little finger into the external inguinal ring at the base of the scrotum. The nurse asks the child to cough, and if a hernia is present it will hit the tip of the finger. A *femoral hernia,* which occurs more frequently in girls, is felt or seen as a small mass on the anterior surface of the thigh just below the inguinal ligament. Its location can be estimated by placing the index finger of the right hand on the child's right femoral pulse (left hand for left pulse) and the middle ring finger flat against the skin toward the midline. The ring finger lies over the femoral canal, where the herniation occurs. Palpation of hernias in the pelvic region, particularly inguinal ones, is often part of the examination of genitalia.

The nurse also inspects the *anal* region. Normally a rectal examination by finger palpation is not routinely done in children. The anal area is inspected for general firmness of the buttocks and sphincter tone. The *anal reflex* is elicited by stimulating the perianal area, either by scratching or pricking it gently. The normal response is an obvious quick contraction of the external anal sphincter. The nurse inspects the sphincter area for *fissures,* small cuts or tears in the mucosa that are painful and often lead to constipation as the child refrains from defecating; *prolapse* of the rectum, which is evident as a tube-like protrusion that can be retracted manually; *polyps,* cherry-red protrusions that often cause bleeding; and *hemorrhoids,* dark protrusions of blood vessels. Each of these, although not common, is reported for further medical investigation. Benign protrusions are small *mucosal tabs* of skin attached to the anal sphincter.

The nurse inspects the skin around the anal area for lesions, the most common of which are caused by diaper rash. If this is a finding, the nurse discusses with the parent general toileting hygiene. If the child complains of perianal itching, the nurse should look for pinworms, although these may not be evident after passage of the first daily stool (see p. 654).

Auscultation. The most important sound to listen for is *peristalsis* or *bowel sounds,* which sound like short metallic clicks and gurgles. Loud grumbling noises, known as borborygmi, are the familiar "stomach growls" usually denoting hunger. A sound may be heard every 10 to 30 seconds and its frequency per minute should be recorded (for example, 5 bowel sounds/minute). The normal rate has been estimated to be 15 to 34 sounds/minute. However, frequently the nurse must listen for several minutes before audible peristalsis can be heard. Each of the four quadrants should be auscultated using the diaphragm and bell chestpieces. Unlike listening to the heart or lungs, in which the stethoscope rests gently on the skin, to hear bowel sounds the stethoscope must be pressed firmly against the abdominal surface. With the diaphragm chestpiece this usually presents no difficulty, but with the bell chestpiece, especially one with a short cone, the skin may occlude the opening and prevent transmission of sound. Bowel sounds may be stimulated by stroking the abdominal surface with a fingernail. Absent bowel sounds or hyperperistalsis is recorded and reported, since either usually denotes abdominal pathology.

Various other sounds may be heard in the abdominal cavity. Normally the pulsation of the aorta is heard in the epigastrium. Sounds that resemble murmurs (called bruits), hums, or rubs are always referred for further evaluation. Bruits along the descending aorta may indicate an aneurysm.

Percussion. Percussion of the abdomen is performed in the same manner as percussion of the lungs and heart (see Fig. 5-37). Normally dullness or flatness is heard on the right side at the lower costal margin because of the location of the liver. Tympany is typically heard over the stomach on the left side and usually in the rest of the abdomen. An unusually tympanitic sound, like the beating of a tight drum, usually denotes air in the stomach, a common cause of which is mouth breathing. However, it can also denote pathology such as low intestinal obstruction or paralytic ileus. Lack of tympany may occur normally when the stomach is full after a meal, but in other situations it may denote the presence of fluid or solid masses. Normally the area of hepatic dullness varies only slightly if the child's position changes from supine to side lying. Marked *shifting dullness* usually indicates free abdominal fluid, or ascites. Variation in percussion tones not explained by normal physiologic processes warrants referral for further investigation.

Palpation. Two types of palpation are performed, superficial and deep. In *superficial palpation* the nurse lightly places the hand against the skin and feels each quadrant, noting any areas of tenderness, muscle tone, and superficial lesions, such as cysts. Skin turgor, discussed on p. 120, is also tested.

Superficial palpation is often perceived as "tickling" by the child, which can interfere with its effectiveness. The nurse can avoid this problem in the older child by using the distraction of telling stories or by having him "help" with the palpation by placing his hand over the nurse's palpating hand. Admonishing the child to stop laughing only draws attention to the sensation and decreases cooperation. In a younger child, using the parent's lap as the examining surface, distracting him with toys or mobiles, or giving him a bottle or pacifier often increases relaxation and cooperation.

Tenderness anywhere in the abdomen during superficial palpation is always noted. There are two types of abdominal pain: (1) *visceral,* which arises from the viscera or internal organs such as the intestines, and (2) *somatic,* which arises from the walls or linings of the abdominal cavity such as the peritoneum. Visceral pain is usually dull, poorly localized, and difficult for the patient to describe. Somatic pain is generally sharp, well localized, and more easily described. A special phenomenon called *rebound tenderness* or Blumberg's sign is performed if the child complains of abdominal pain. It is produced by pressing firmly over part of the abdomen distal to the area of tenderness. When the pressure is suddenly released, the child feels pain in the original area of tenderness. This response is only found when the peritoneum overlying a diseased viscus or organ is inflamed, such as in appendicitis.

Deep palpation is used for palpating organs and large blood vessels, and for detecting masses and tenderness that were not discovered during superficial palpation. If the child complains of abdominal pain, that area of the abdomen is palpated last. Normally palpation of the midepigastrium causes pain as pressure is exerted over the aorta, but this should not be confused with visceral or somatic tenderness.

The nurse palpates the abdominal organs by pressing them against the free hand, which is placed on the child's back (see Fig. 5-2). Palpation usually begins in the lower quadrants and proceeds upward. In this way the edge of an enlarged liver or spleen is not missed. Except for palpating the liver, successful identification of other organs, such as the spleen, kidney, and part of the colon, requires considerable practice with tutored supervision.

The lower edge of the *liver* is sometimes palpable in infants and young children as a superficial mass 1 to 2 cm (0.4 to 0.8 inch) below the right costal margin (the distance is sometimes measured in fingerbreadths). If the liver is palpable 3 cm (1.2 inches) or 2 fingerbreadths below the costal margin, it is considered enlarged and this finding must be referred to a physician. Normally the liver descends during inspiration as the diaphragm moves downward. The nurse should not mistake this downward displacement as a sign of hepatomegaly. In older children the liver frequently is not palpable, although its lower edge can be estimated by percussing dullness at the costal margin.

The nurse palpates the *spleen* by feeling it between the hand placed against the back and the one palpating the left upper quadrant. The spleen is much smaller than the liver and positioned behind the fundus of the stomach. The tip of the spleen is normally felt during inspiration as it descends within the abdominal cavity. It is sometimes palpable 1 to 2 cm below the left costal margin in infants and young children. A spleen that is readily palpated more than 2 cm below the right costal margin is enlarged and is always reported for further medical investigation.

Other anatomic structures that are sometimes palpable in children include the kidney, bladder, cecum, and sigmoid colon. Palpation of the *kidney,* which is discussed under assessment of the neonate (p. 272), is quite difficult because of its deep position within the abdominal cavity. Normally only the tip of the right kidney is palpable due to its lower placement within the cavity. It is best felt during inspiration. The nurse should attempt to palpate the kidneys because failure to do so rules out such problems as hydronephrosis or Wilms' tumor. The *bladder* may be palpated slightly above the pubic symphysis in infants and young children. It descends deeper into the pelvic cavity during adolescence, when it is not palpable except if distended. Occasionally parts of the colon are palpable. The *cecum* is a soft, gas-filled mass in the right lower quadrant. The *sigmoid colon* is felt as a sausage-shaped mass that is freely movable over the pelvic brim in the left lower quadrant and is normally tender.

Although most of these structures are not routinely felt, the nurse should be aware of their relative location and characteristics in order not to mistake them for abnormal masses. The most common palpable mass in children is feces. However, any questionable mass must be referred to a physician before it can be ruled out as benign. In sexually active pubescent females, a palpable mass in the lower abdomen may be an enlarged uterus caused by pregnancy.

During palpation of the abdomen the nurse also checks for the aortic and femoral pulses. The transmitted pulsation of the *aorta* may be normally felt in the epigastrium and/or umbilical area. In thin children the descending aorta may be palpable. The nurse should gently palpate along the aorta for any evidence of an outpocketing of its thin wall. If the nurse has any questions concerning the existence of an abnormality, the findings are referred to a physician.

The *femoral pulses* are best felt by placing the tips of two or three fingers (index, middle, and/or ring) along the inguinal ligament about midway between the iliac crest and pubic symphysis. The nurse should feel both pulses simultaneously to make certain that they are equal and strong (Fig. 5-43). Absence of femoral pulses is a significant sign of coarctation of the aorta.

While examining the abdomen, the nurse may decide to test for *abdominal reflexes,* which are obtained by scratching the skin in four directions as shown in Fig. 5-44. The normal response is for the umbilicus to move toward the stimulus or quadrant that was stroked. Normally the response may be absent in children under 1 year of age. Asymmetry or absence of response is noted and reported, although there is great variability in correctly eliciting a response.

Genitalia

Examination of genitalia conveniently follows assessment of the abdomen while the child is still supine. In adolescents inspection of the genitalia may be left to the end of the examination. This part of the physical appraisal is usually uneventful for infants or toddlers but begins to be anxiety-producing for some preschoolers and most older children and adolescents, mainly because of their concern for modesty and privacy. The best approach is to examine the genitals quickly, placing no more emphasis on this part of the assessment than on any other segment. It helps to relieve children's and parents' anxiety by telling them the results of the findings as the nurse proceeds, for example, by stating, "Everything looks fine here." If the nurse finds it necessary to ask questions, such as about discharge, difficulty in urinating, and so on, consideration should be shown at all times and the child's privacy should be observed by covering the lower abdomen with the gown or underpants.

In examining the genitalia of adolescents it is sometimes advisable to wear gloves to guard against contamination from venereal disease. It might be helpful for the adolescent to know that this also prevents skin-to-skin contact.[7] The nurse explains each step of the examination before performing it, such as checking the scrotum for an inguinal hernia

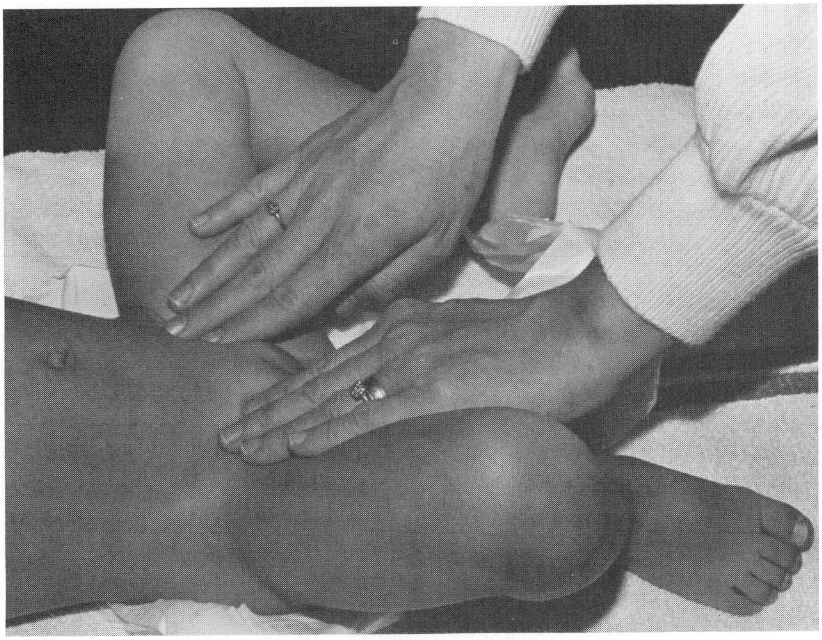

Fig. 5-43. Palpating for femoral pulses.

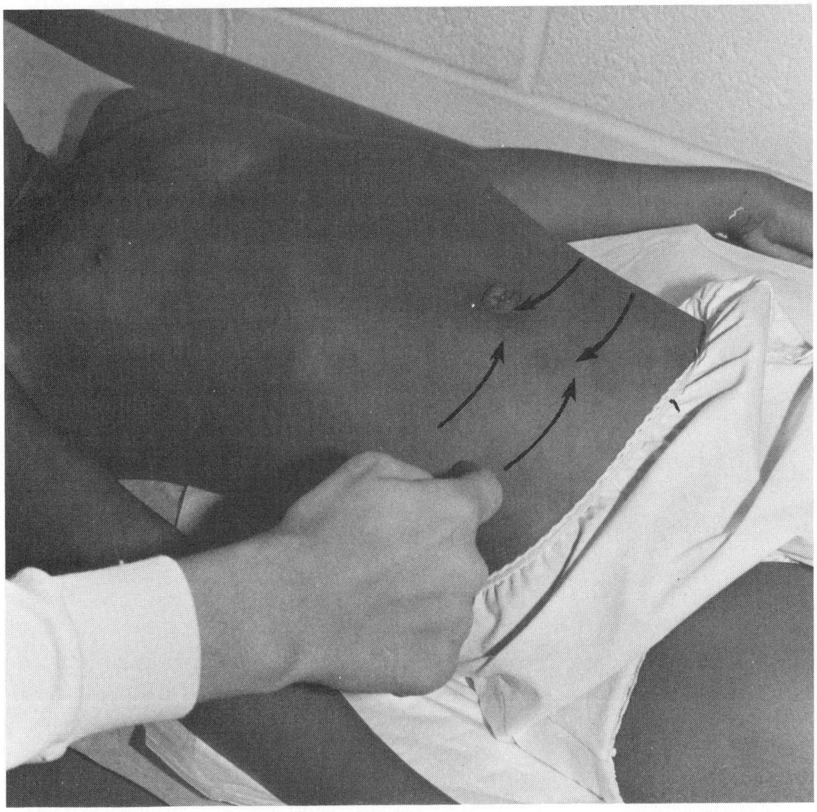

Fig. 5-44. Eliciting abdominal reflex.

(discussed on p. 154) and the reason for asking the boy to cough. If the male adolescent does have an erection during the examination, the nurse assures him that this is a normal involuntary physiologic response to touch. However, the nurse should focus on the erection only momentarily while proceeding with the remainder of the examination.

In the female, examination of the genitalia is only external. Need for a gynecologic examination is referred or performed if the nurse has the required training. The adolescent female has the same needs for preparation, reassurance, and privacy as the male. For both sexes this part of the examination is an excellent time for eliciting questions of concern about body functioning or sexual activity. The nurse can also use this opportunity to increase or reinforce the child's knowledge of reproductive anatomy by naming each body part and explaining its function. For example, many females are unaware of the existence of two openings within the vulva. They assume that the passage of urine occurs from the vagina.

One of the most important factors in successfully performing the examination is that the nurse recognize any personal fears or anxieties and deal with them. Transfer of anxiety, especially in the beginning practitioner, can be the greatest deterrent to preparing the older child in order to lessen his or her fear.

Male genitalia—inspection. The nurse notes the external appearance of the glans and shaft of the penis, the prepuce, the urethral meatus, and the scrotum (Fig. 5-45). The nurse notes the general *size* of the *penis*. A very small penis may actually be an enlarged clitoris in a genetically female child. In an obese child the penis often looks abnormally small because of the folds of skin partially covering it at the base. An enlarged penis in a young child may denote precocious puberty. The nurse should be familiar with normal pubertal growth of the external male genitalia in order to compare the findings with the expected sequence of maturation (see p. 691).

The nurse examines the *glans* (head of the penis) and *shaft* (portion between the perineum and prepuce) for signs of swelling, skin lesions, inflammation, or other irregulari-

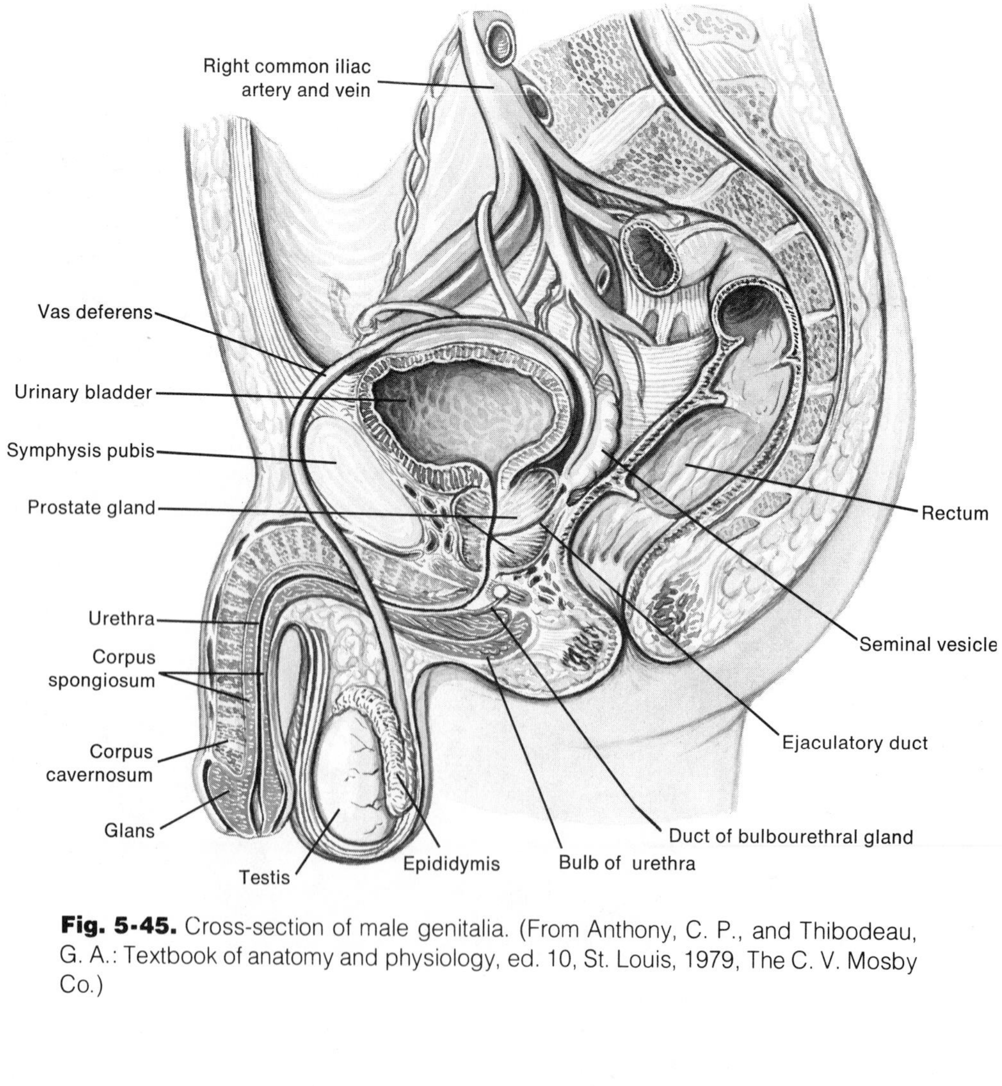

Fig. 5-45. Cross-section of male genitalia. (From Anthony, C. P., and Thibodeau, G. A.: Textbook of anatomy and physiology, ed. 10, St. Louis, 1979, The C. V. Mosby Co.)

ties. Any of these signs may denote underlying urinary or reproductive disorders. A *syphilitic chancre* appears as an oval or round, dark red, painless erosion or ulcer with an indurated base. Caution should be exercised in examining such lesions if the nurse is not wearing gloves. Warts on the penis, perineum, or anal area, called *condyloma acuminata,* are usually benign growths, although they can be caused by the irritating discharges of venereal disease.

If the child is uncircumsized, the nurse inspects the *prepuce* or foreskin covering the glans or head of the penis. In infants the prepuce is normally tight for the first 2 to 3 months of life and probably should not be retracted for examination, since accidental tearing of the thin membrane may cause scarring and adhesion formation later on.[1] In older infants and children the foreskin should be gently retracted for examination of the glans and the meatus. A tight foreskin that cannot be retracted is called *phimosis*.

The *urethral meatus* is carefully inspected for location and evidence of discharge. Normally it is centered at the tip of the shaft. If it opens on the ventral or underneath side of the glans or shaft, it is called *hypospadias*. An opening on the dorsal or top part of the penis is termed *epispadias*. If the urethral meatus opens into the perineum at the junction of the scrotum, the nurse carefully inspects for signs suggestive of ambiguous genitalia (Table 5-8). If feasible, the nurse notes the strength and direction of the urinary stream during micturition.

The nurse notes the *size* of the *scrotum,* which should hang freely from the perineum behind the penis. In infants the scrota appear large in relation to the rest of the genitalia. Normally one scrotum hangs lower than the other. The nurse notes scrota that are small, close to the perineum, or with evidence of any midline separation, which could be enlarged labia. An abnormally large scrotal sac may indicate an inguinal hernia, a hydrocele, or inflammation of the internal reproductive structures, particularly the epididymis.

The nurse also inspects the *skin* of the *scrotum,* which is usually loose and highly rugated (wrinkled). Well-formed rugae usually mean that the testes have descended at some time, even when they are not palpable.[1] During early adolescence the skin normally becomes redder and coarser. In dark-skinned children the scrota are usually more deeply pigmented. A smooth, shiny surface with pigmentation that varies markedly from the surrounding skin should be reported.

Hair distribution is also noted. Normally before puberty no pubic hair is present. Soft downy hair at the base of the penis is an early sign of pubertal maturation. In older adolescents the nurse notes the typical male pattern of hair distribution, which is usually triangular as it extends from the base of the penis along the midline to the umbilicus.

Palpation. Palpation of the scrotum includes identification of the testes, epididymis, spermatic cords, and, if present, inguinal hernias. The two testes are felt as small ovoid bodies, about 1.5 to 2 cm (0.6 to 0.8 inch) long—one in each scrotal sac. They do not enlarge until puberty, when they approximately double in size. Normally the testes descend during the last trimester of uterine development, usually by the eighth month of gestation. Therefore, undescended testes (cryptorchidism) is a common finding in premature infants.

Palpating for the presence of the testes requires an under-

Table 5-8. Findings suggestive of ambiguous genitalia

Sex	Normal finding	Variation suggestive of possible ambiguous genitalia
Male	Penile shaft protrudes from perineum and hangs freely	Small penis (less than 2-3 cm [0.8-1.2 inches] in newborn) may be enlarged clitoris
	Urethral meatus centered at tip of glans penis	Urethral meatus anywhere along dorsal or ventral surface of penis, but especially on perineum
	Two scrotal sacs hang freely, covered with loose, wrinkled skin	Small scrotum with smoother, tighter skin with any degree of separation in midline may be enlarged labia
	Palpable testes in each scrotum	Absent testes may be undescended, but if combined with small scrotum, may be further evidence of enlarged labia
Female	Small clitoris at anterior end of labia	Enlarged clitoris that protrudes from labia may be small penis
	Urethral meatus located between clitoris and vagina	Urethral meatus located in clitoris may suggest small penis
	Labia minora prominent in newborn but atrophy and almost absent in prepubertal female; completely separated from clitoris to posterior vault of vagina; on palpation, no masses in labia	Prominent labia, partially or completely fused with palpable masses on each side, may be small scrotum with testes

standing of the normal anatomy and physiology of the coverings of the testes and scrotal sac. The scrotum and testes are surrounded by fascia called the cremaster muscle, which attaches to a point in the abdomen and extends downward along the inner surface of the thigh. The muscle or *cremasteric reflex* is stimulated by cold, touch, emotional excitement, or exercise. It causes the skin of the scrotum to shrink and pulls the testes higher into the pelvic cavity. Therefore, the nurse must be careful not to elicit this reflex.

Several measures are useful in preventing the cremasteric reflex during palpation of the scrotum. First the hands should be warm, not cold. Second, if old enough, the child should be examined while sitting in a tailor or ''Indian'' position, which stretches the muscle, preventing its contraction. Third the normal pathway of ascent of the testes can be blocked by placing the thumb and index finger over the upper part of the scrotal sac along the inguinal canal (Fig. 5-46). The site is the same as that described for locating the internal inguinal ring when palpating for hernias. The nurse should also place the index and middle finger in a scissor fashion to separate the right and left scrotum if there is any question concerning the existence of two testes. If after each of these precautions the testes have not been palpated, the nurse feels along the inguinal canal and perineum to locate masses that may be incompletely descended testes. True undescended testes are reported and referred, although they may descend at any time during childhood and, therefore, are checked at each visit.

The *epididymis* is palpated as a vertical ridge of soft nodular tissue behind the testes. The *spermatic cord* consists of the blood vessels, nerves, lymphatic glands, and the ductus deferens of the testes. It should be traced from its origin in the testes up into the pelvic cavity. Any masses, swelling, or tenderness is noted and reported.

Female genitalia—inspection and palpation. A convenient position for examination of the genitalia involves placing the young child in a semireclining position on the parent's lap with the feet supported on the nurse's knees as the nurse sits facing the child. The child's attention is diverted from the examination by instructing her to try to keep the soles of her feet in apposition.[22] The nurse grasps the labia majora between the thumb and index finger and retracts them outward in order to expose the labia minora, urethral meatus, and vaginal orifice.

The nurse inspects the female genitalia for size and location of the structures of the *vulva* or *pudendum* (Fig. 5-47). The *mons pubis* is a pad of adipose tissue over the symphysis pubis. At puberty the mons is covered with hair, which extends along the labia. The usual pattern of female *hair distribution* is an inverted triangle. Any extension of hair along the linea alba to the umbilicus is noted. The appearance of soft downy hair along the labia majora is an early sign of sexual maturation.

The *clitoris* is an erectile organ located at the anterior end of the labia minora. It is covered by a small flap of skin, the prepuce. The nurse should note its *size,* because, although variable, a large protruding clitoris may represent an underdeveloped phallus.

The *labia majora* are two thick folds of skin running posteriorly from the mons to the posterior commissure of the vagina. Internal to the labia majora are two folds of skin called the *labia minora*. Although the labia minora are usually prominent in the newborn, they gradually atrophy,

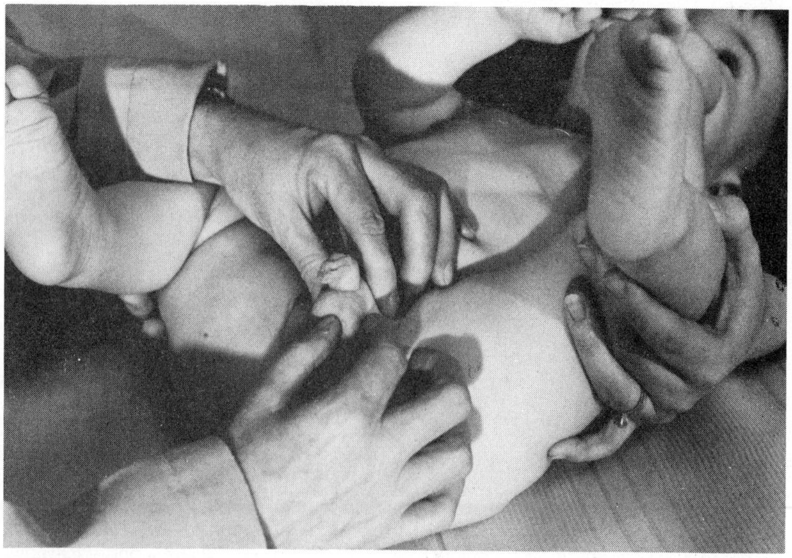

Fig. 5-46. Palpation of scrotum to determine if testes are descended. (From Malasanos, L., and associates: Health assessment, St. Louis, 1977, The C. V. Mosby Co., p. 432.)

A

B

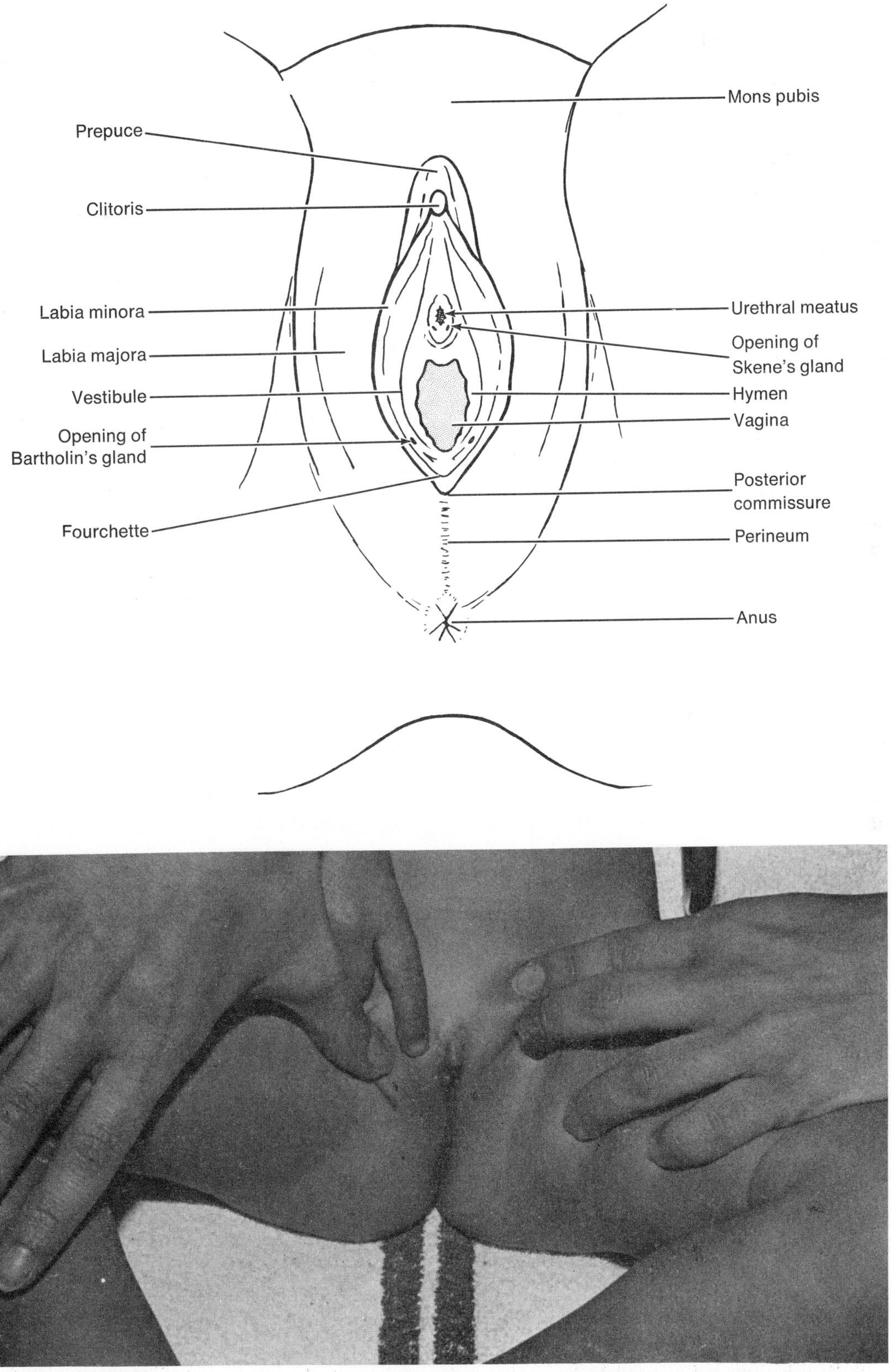

Fig. 5-47. A, Anatomy of external female genitalia, or vulva. **B,** Positioning the child for examination.

which makes them almost invisible until their enlargement during puberty.

The nurse inspects the inner surface of the labia, which should be pink and moist. Any skin lesions such as chancres or warts (condyloma acuminatum) are noted. Any lesion suggestive of chancres, such as sores, blisters, or pimples, is investigated as a possible sign of acquired syphilis. The nurse notes the size of the labia and any evidence of fusion, which may suggest male scrota. Normally no masses are palpable within the labia. However, in genitalia of an ambiguous nature, palpable masses may represent descended testes.

The urethral meatus and vaginal orifice are located in the space between the labia, the *vestibule*. The *urethral meatus* is located posterior to the clitoris and is surrounded by Skene's glands and ducts. Although not a prominent structure, the meatus can be more readily identified by wiping downward along the vestibule toward the perineum. It will appear as a small V-shaped slit. The nurse notes its location, especially if it opens from the clitoris or inside the vagina. The glands, which are common sites of cysts and venereal lesions, are gently palpated.

The *vaginal orifice* is located posterior to the urethral meatus. Its appearance is variable depending on individual anatomy and sexual activity. Ordinarily examination of the vagina is limited to inspection. However, in the presence of other signs suggestive of ambiguous genitalia, the nurse may decide to refer or perform a manual examination to determine if a vaginal vault exists.

In virgins a thin crescent-shaped or circular membrane, called the *hymen,* may cover part of the vaginal opening. At times it completely occludes the orifice. After rupture, small rounded pieces of tissue called caruncles remain. Although an imperforate hymen denotes lack of penile intercourse, a perforate one does not necessarily indicate such activity. However, the information can be very useful as is demonstrated in the following example:

A 14-year-old girl accompanied by her mother visited the clinic with chief complaint of nausea, stomach pains, and fatigue for the past 6 weeks. During the history she denied any sexual activity. She stated that she had missed her menstrual periods lately but that this was normal for her. On physical examination a mass was palpated in the suprapubic area. Examination of the genitalia revealed a perforated hymen.

At the end of the visit, the nurse requested to talk with the adolescent alone. The mother agreed to wait outside. The nurse began a casual conversation about the girl's friends, social life, activities, and so on. The girl talked freely but never mentioned any boyfriends. The nurse directly posed the question about a special boyfriend, but again the child denied any such relationship. Finally the nurse asked, "Has anything happened lately between you and a boy who is not your boyfriend?" The girl hesitantly said "No," but the nurse, sensing the change of tone, prodded further, stating, "Are you sure?" The child began to fidget and tears came into her eyes. The nurse gently moved closer to her and said, "Tell me about it." The girl revealed that about 3 months earlier an older boy from school had attacked her. He had forced intercourse on her, but she was so ashamed that she had told no one.

The nurse talked with her for some time about the findings from the examination and the possibility of her being pregnant. She also discussed the alternative choices concerning continuing or terminating the pregnancy and the importance of telling her parents. She continually emphasized that the feelings of shame and guilt were normal but that in no way was the girl responsible. At the end of the visit, the child agreed to tell her mother with the nurse's help. The mother reacted with support, concern, and empathy for her child. They discussed the feasibility of an abortion, and, following a positive pregnancy test, the adolescent's pregnancy was terminated.

Surrounding the vaginal opening are *Bartholin's glands,* which secrete a clear, mucoid fluid into the vagina for lubrication during intercourse. The nurse palpates the ducts for cysts. The discharge from the vagina is also noted, which is usually clear or whitish. Variations in the appearance, such as white and cheesy or yellow-greenish, and odor may indicate infection. Sudden, foul-smelling, and profuse discharge may suggest a foreign body inside the vaginal vault. The presence of feces or urine from the vagina usually suggests a fistula from the rectum or urethra. The nurse notes any swelling, inflammation, or prolapsed area around the vagina. Any such findings are referred for further gynecologic evaluation.

Back and extremities

Spine. Following examination of the abdomen and genitalia, the nurse may have the child lie prone in order to inspect the spine and back, although they are observed in the sitting and standing position as well. The nurse notes the general *curvature* of the spine. Normally the back of a newborn is rounded or C-shaped from the thoracic and pelvic curves. The development of the cervical and lumbar curves approximates development of various motor skills, such as cervical curvature with head control, and gives the older child the typical double-S curve (see Fig. 3-5).

Marked curvatures in posture are noted. *Lordosis,* exaggerated curvature of the lumbar vertebrae, is normal during early childhood but decreases with age. Marked lordosis may be a sign of rickets or muscular weakness. *Kyphosis,* exaggerated curvature of the thoracic vertebrae, causes a hunchback appearance. It can be the result of poor posture or various disease states. *Scoliosis,* lateral curvature of the spine, is an important childhood problem, especially in females. Although scoliosis may be palpated as one feels along the spine and notes a sideways displacement, more objective tests include: (1) having the child stand erect, clothed only in underpants (and bra if older girl) and observing from behind the child and noting asymmetry of the shoulders and hips, and (2) having the child bend forward so that the back is parallel to the floor and observing from the side and noting asymmetry or prominence of the rib cage. A slight limp, a crooked hemline, or complaints of a sore back are other signs and symptoms of scoliosis.

The nurse inspects the *back,* especially along the spine, for any tufts of hair, dimples, or discoloration. A small dimple usually with a tuft of hair called a *pilonidal cyst* may indicate an underlying spina bifida occulta. The nurse palpates the spine to identify each spiny process of the vertebrae or lack of them. Any masses, which may be meningoceles, evidence of tenderness, and swelling are noted. *Mobility* of the vertebral column is easily assessed in most children because of their propensity for constant motion during the examination. However, the nurse can specifically test for mobility by asking the child to sit up from a prone position or to do a modified sit-up exercise. Maintaining a rigid straightness when performing these maneuvers is considered abnormal and may indicate central nervous system infection or irritation. However, some individuals who are unable to relax, despite normal skeletal function, may also retain a rigid posture.

Movement of the cervical spine is an important diagnostic sign for neurologic problems, such as meningitis. Normally movement of the head in all directions is effortless. Hyperextension of the neck and spine, called *opisthotonos,* which is accompanied by pain if the nurse attempts to flex the head, is always referred for immediate medical evaluation.

Extremities. The nurse inspects each extremity for symmetry of length and size; any deviation is referred for orthopedic evaluation. The fingers and toes are counted to be certain of the normal number. This is so often taken for granted that an extra digit (polydactyly) or fusion of digits (syndactyly) may go unnoticed. The fingers and toes are also inspected for any evidence of clubbing, cyanosis, disorders of the nails (including habitual nail biting), and general hygiene. These have been discussed in more detail under assessment of the skin.

The arms and legs are inspected for *temperature, color, tenderness,* and *masses*. Temperature in each extremity should be equal, although the feet may normally be colder than the hands because they loose heat almost twice as fast as the hands.[8] Coolness denotes decreased blood circulation, such as from occlusion of a blood vessel, whereas heat denotes increased blood flow, such as an infection or inflammation. Enlargement of bone, such as from swelling, with redness, heat, and tenderness needs further evaluation. It may signify trauma, infection, or an underlying disease process, such as sickle cell anemia. Since accidental fractures are common in children, the nurse should be familiar with assessing orthopedic injuries. The five main criteria are pain, pulse, paresthesia (abnormal sensation, such as numbness), pallor, and paralysis.[32] Palpation over a possible fractured bone may elicit crepitation, a grating sound produced by movement of the broken ends of the bone. A solid mass palpable along a bone with or without pain may be a tumor. Although not all masses are malignant, they must be evaluated further by a medical specialist.

The *shape* of bones is assessed. Several different variations of bone shape may be observed in children. "Bowleg" or *genu varum* is lateral bowing of the tibia. It is clinically present when the child stands with the medial malleoli (rounded prominence on either side of the ankle) in apposition and the space between the knees is greater than 1 inch (Fig. 5-48). Toddlers are usually bowlegged after beginning to walk until all their lower back and leg muscles are well developed. Persistence of genu varum may indicate rickets from a weakening of the bone.

Knock knee or *genu valgum* appears as the opposite of bowleg, in that the knees are close together but the feet are spread apart. It is determined clinically by using the same method as for genu varum but by measuring the distance between the malleoli, which normally should be less than 1 inch (Fig. 5-49). Knock knee is normally present in children from about 2 to 3½ years of age. Persistence of this leg posture can be a result of several disorders including rickets.

Tibial torsion is abnormal rotation or bowing of the tibia. The nurse tests for tibial torsion by laying the child on his back with his hips and knees flexed and his foot flat on the examining surface. An imaginary line drawn from the tibial tuberosity to the middle of the malleoli should parallel a straight tibial shaft (Fig. 5-50). If a bowing is present it will be evident as a nonparallel curved line to the imaginary line. This test is independent of associated foot anomalies. The nurse can also screen for this abnormality by placing the infant supine with the legs in a relaxed extended position or

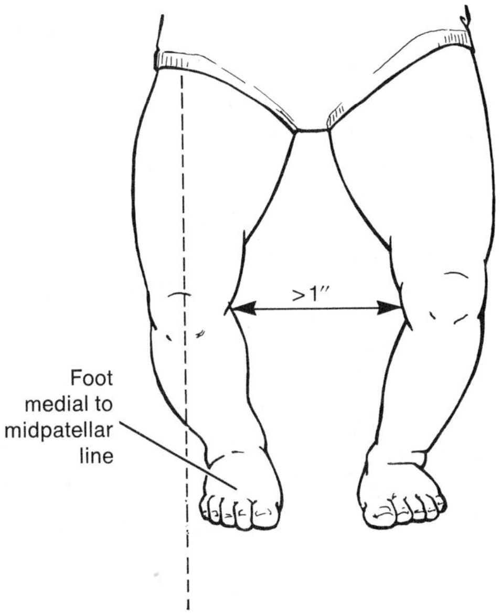

Fig. 5-48. Bowleg.

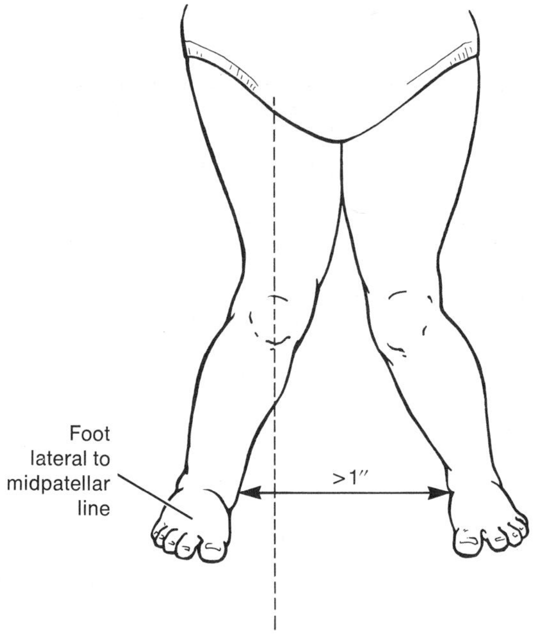

Fig. 5-49. Knock knee.

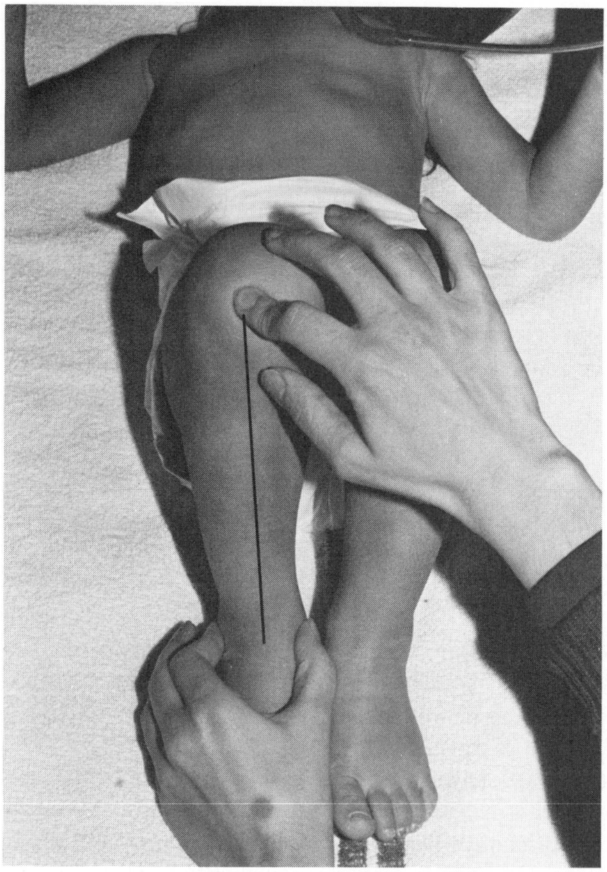

Fig. 5-50. Testing for tibial torsion.

by having an older child stand naturally with both feet together. A straight line is drawn from the anterior superior iliac spine (felt externally as the "point" of the hip) through the center of the patella (knee cap). Normally this imaginary line intersects the second toe provided the foot is in normal alignment. If it intersects the fourth or fifth toe or bypasses the lateral aspect of the foot, the child is referred for orthopedic evaluation.

The nurse next inspects the *feet.* Infants' and toddlers' feet appear flat because the foot is normally wide and the arch is covered by a fat pad. Development of the arch occurs naturally from the action of walking. Normally at birth the feet are held in a valgus (outward) or varus (inward) position. To determine if a foot deformity at birth is the result of intrauterine position or development, the nurse scratches the outer, then inner, side of the sole. If the foot position is self-correctable, it will assume a right angle to the leg. As the child begins to walk, the feet should point straight ahead. Variations in foot positions are listed in Table 5-9.

The nurse also elicits the *plantar reflex* by exerting firm but gentle pressure with the tip of the thumb against the lateral sole of the foot from the heel upward to the little toe and then across to the big toe. The normal response in children who are walking is flexion of the toes. *Babinski's sign,* dorsiflexion of the big toe and fanning of the other toes, is normal during infancy but abnormal after about 1 year of age or when locomotion begins. A positive Babinski's sign after age 1 year is an indication of spinal cord lesions and requires further neurologic evaluation.

Inspection of the lower extremities also involves observing the child's *gait.* Normally toddlers have a "toddling" or broad-based gait, which facilitates walking by lowering the center of gravity. As the child reaches preschool age, the legs are brought closer together. By school age the walking posture is much more graceful and balanced. Deviations from normal gait are recorded and reported.

The most common gait problem in young children is pigeon toe or toeing in, which may be the result of (1) metatarsus varus, (2) internal tibial torsion, or (3) anteversion (forward turning) of the neck of the femur.[16] Other gait abnormalities include (1) persistence of a broad-based gait, which may indicate problems with balancing in the cerebellum, (2) scissor gait (a characteristic sign of spastic-type cerebral palsy), in which the legs are stiff and cross over as the child tries to walk, and (3) waddling gait, which may be noted in children with a dislocated hip.

The nurse should also investigate the type of shoes the child is wearing. Shoes that are too small or too large can simulate gait or foot abnormalities. Selection of shoes for young children is discussed in Chapter 14.

Joints. The joints are evaluated for *range of motion.* Normally this requires no specific testing if the nurse has

Table 5-9. Assessment of foot and ankle deformities

Deformity	Anatomic variation
Talipes* valgus	Eversion (turning outward) of the foot so that only the inner side of the foot rests on the ground
Talipes varus	Inversion (turning inward) of the foot so that only the outer sole of the foot rests on the ground
Talipes equinus	Extension or plantar flexion of the foot so that only the ball and toes rest on the ground, commonly combined with talipes varus (most common of the clubfoot deformities)
Talipes calcaneous	Dorsal flexion of the foot so that only the heel rests on the ground
Metatarsus varus (also called metatarsus adductus, toeing in, or pigeon toe)	Inversion of the forefoot while the heel remains straight
Metatarsus valgus (also called toeing out or duck walk)	Eversion of the forefoot while the heel remains straight
Pes* valgus	Eversion of the entire foot but the sole rests on the ground
Pes varus	Inversion of the entire foot but the sole rests on the ground

*Talipes refers to ankle (talus) and foot (pes) deformity and commonly refers to "clubfoot." Pes refers only to foot deformity.

been observant of the child's movements during the examination. However, the hips should be routinely investigated in infants for congenital dislocation. Signs of congenital hip dislocation are discussed on p. 387. Any evidence of joint immobility or hyperflexibility is reported.

The joints are routinely palpated for *heat, tenderness,* and *swelling*. These signs, as well as redness over the joint, may indicate infection or any of the collagen diseases. The nurse refers such findings to a physician for further investigation.

Muscles. Much of the examination of the spine, extremities, and joints indicates mucular development. The nurse specifically notes development, tone, and strength. *Development* is observed as one looks at the shape and contour of the body both in a relaxed and tensed state. If the nurse notes asymmetry of development, the circumference of the muscle mass is measured with a tape measure and compared to the measurement of the contralateral muscle. Marked disparity between the two sizes is reported.

Development is closely associated with *tone* or the balance between muscle mass and nervous stimulation. Tone is estimated by grasping the muscle and feeling its firmness when it is relaxed and contracted. A common site for testing tone is the biceps muscle of the arm. Children usually willingly "make a muscle" by clenching their fist. The nurse tests symmetry of tone in each extremity and over the abdomen. Disuse of a muscle results in *atrophy* or decreased muscle mass. Overdevelopment of a muscle from continuous use is termed *hypertrophy*. Any evidence of atrophy, spasticity, flaccidity, or rigidity is reported.

The nurse estimates *strength* by having the child use an extremity to push or pull against resistance. For example, arm strength can be tested by having the child hold his arms outstretched in front of him. He is asked to raise his arms while the nurse applies downward pressure. Hand strength can be tested by using a "handshake" and finger strength by squeezing one or two fingers of the nurse's hand. Leg strength can be tested by having the child sit on a table or chair with the legs dangling. The nurse holds the lower leg and while applying resistance asks the child to raise his legs. The nurse estimates symmetry of strength in each extremity, hands, and fingers. Evidence of paresis or weakness is reported.

Neurologic assessment

The assessment of the nervous system is the broadest and most diverse, since every function of man, both physical and emotional, is controlled by neurologic impulses. This discussion will focus primarily on a general appraisal of behavior, cognitive-perceptual development, sensory and cerebellar functioning, deep tendon reflexes, the cranial nerves, and "soft" signs.

Assessment of neurologic function requires the use of a few additional tools. A reflex hammer, which has a small rounded rubber head, is used to test deep tendon reflexes. A pin and cotton are useful when testing sensory function. For the assessment of the cranial nerves, some flavors to taste and some odors to smell are necessary, although nothing elaborate is required (see Table 5-12). Vision and hearing testing requires the use of a flashlight (otic head without the speculum is acceptable), tuning fork, and visual acuity charts. Motor development is best evaluated with screening tests, such as the Denver Developmental Screening Test (DDST). However, simple toys such as small wooden blocks, paper and pencil, and a ball are sufficient.

Behavior. There is no special testing for behavior. Rather, it is an overall impression of the child's personality, affect, level of activity, social interaction, and attention span.

Assessing behavior has been discussed previously on p. 117. The nurse should inquire about home, school, and social behavior to identify possible problem areas that necessitate further psychologic study.

State of consciousness is a specific area for behavior under neurologic assessment. Hyperirritability, hyporeactivity, lethargy, delirium, stupor, or coma requires immediate referral. Level of consciousness can be evaluated by observing the child's response to commands, calling his name, or detecting his response to a pinprick or other painful stimuli. Lack of response indicates decreasing consciousness and increasing stupor. The nurse should always question parents' perceptions of change in behavior, which usually precedes an altered level of consciousness.

Cognitive-perceptual development. Cognitive and perceptual development is best assessed using a formal screening test such as the DDST. Adaptive and speech-comprehension development are significant indicators of intellectual functioning. If the nurse suspects intellectual or perceptual impairment or is aware of learning difficulties in school, the child should be referred to an appropriate developmental study team for further evaluation. "Soft" signs that should alert the nurse to minimal or borderline brain dysfunction are discussed at the conclusion of assessment of the neurologic system (p. 170).

Motor functioning. Motor ability primarily involves assessment of voluntary muscle contraction and acquisition of age-specific developmental milestones for gross and fine motor skills (see DDST, p. 173). The nurse evaluates *muscle development* by assessing development (size), tone, strength, and any abnormal involuntary movements, such as those listed in Table 5-10. Other signs of possible neurologic damage include hyperflexibility, rapid blinking, head nodding, the constant holding of both hands over the mouth, or a markedly asymmetric or flaccid posture in an infant.

One of the most important milestones in motor development is head control. Since development proceeds in the cephalocaudal direction, head lag suggests early brain damage. Head control is usually acquired by 4 months of age, although even the newborn demonstrates head control. For example, when held prone, the neonate is able to hold the head in a straight line with the back, and, when pulled to a sitting position, the infant attempts to flex the head and momentarily holds it erect. Inability to hold the head erect and in midline while sitting or standing past 6 months of age always requires immediate investigation.

The nurse notes fine motor skills, such as voluntary grasp, pincer control, and so on (see DDST, Appendix F). *Handedness* should also be observed. Infants and toddlers may show preference for one hand, but they usually do not display marked preference until the preschool years. Sole use of one hand may indicate paresis on the opposite side. Failure to demonstrate handedness by a school-age child suggests failure of the brain to develop dominance and is a frequent finding in children with minimal brain damage.

Sensory functioning. Sensory functioning is mainly assessed in terms of the sensory cranial nerves, in particular, vision and hearing and peripheral sensation. *Tactile sensory intactness* can be tested by touching the skin lightly with a pin and having the child point to the stimulated area while keeping his eyes closed. With older children the nurse can assess *sensory discrimation* by (1) touching the skin with a pin or piece of cotton and asking the child to describe the different sensations, (2) placing a cold or warm object on the skin (the rubber and metal heads of the reflex hammer work well) and having the child differentiate between them, and (3) touching different parts of the body simultaneously and seeing if the child can localize both points. In each of these tests the child's eyes are kept closed. Because these tests are similar to playing a game, the nurse may perform the temperature or two-point discrimination (not using a pin) tests at the beginning of the examination in order to decrease the child's anxiety and foster his trust. Decreased sensation or hyperesthesia (excessive sensation) are abnormal and must be referred for further neurologic evaluation.

Hearing tests. Several types of hearing tests are available. Some of them, such as audiometric testing, use specialized equipment that measures the degree of hearing loss. Others, such as tests for the startle reflex in neonates, are rough estimations of perception of sound. The nurse com-

Table 5-10. Description of abnormal involuntary muscular movements

Term	Description
Ataxia	Gross incoordination, which may worsen with the eyes closed
Spasm	Unusual tenseness of the muscle mass
Spasticity	Prolonged and steady contraction of a muscle characterized by clonus (alternating relaxation and contraction of the muscle) and exaggerated reflexes
Rigidity	Inability to flex a joint
Tremors	Constant small movements
Twitching	Spasmodic movements of short duration
Choreiform movements	Quick, jerky, grossly incoordinated, irregular movements that may disappear on relaxation
Athetosis	Slow, writhing, wormlike, constant, grossly incoordinated movements that increase on voluntary activity and decrease on relaxation
Dystonia	Slow twisting movements of limbs or trunk
Associated movements	Voluntary movement of one muscle accompanied by involuntary movement of another muscle
Mirroring movements	Same as associated movements except with symmetric muscle groups

bines questions from the history of review of systems concerning the ear and hearing, observations and parental statements regarding the child's behavior, and the results of screening tests to evaluate auditory function. Any child who is suspected of a hearing loss either because of (1) a high-risk birth history, (2) past medical history of recurrent otitis media, (3) delayed speech, or (4) behavior problems is referred for specialized testing. Types of hearing loss, causes, clinical manifestations, and appropriate treatment are discussed in Chapter 24.

TYPES OF HEARING TESTS. In *audiometry* an electrical instrument called an audiometer measures the threshold of hearing for pure-tone frequencies and loudness. The pure-tone audiogram provides valuable information regarding the severity of the hearing loss, the sound cycles involved, and the possible location of the defect. However, it requires specialized training of personnel, expensive equipment, and cooperation from the child in terms of confirming the perception of sound. The latter makes it especially nonapplicable to infants, toddlers, or mentally retarded children. In addition it does not show how the individual child interprets what he does hear. For example, some children with poor auditory discrimination and gross speech defects demonstrate normal audiograms, whereas other children with audiogram results that show pure-tone loss function as normally as hearing individuals.[26] Therefore, the use of a clinical speech test, such as the five-toy test, which is readily given by a nurse with minimal equipment, is advantageous.

Another specialized test that does not directly measure perception of sound but rather the status of the middle ear in terms of the conduction of sound is *acoustic impedance* measurements or *tympanometry*. This technique measures tympanic membrane compliance (or mobility) and estimates middle ear air pressure. It is suitable for infants, young children, and those who are difficult to test by other methods because little cooperation is necessary and the procedure is not painful. Like audiometry, this technique requires special equipment, although minimal training is necessary for the procedure. However, although this test detects middle ear disease and abnormalities, it does not indicate the degree of hearing loss or the interpretation of sound. Tests that are more applicable for routine screening, can be easily administered by the nurse, and indicate the perception and interpretation of sound are the following clinical hearing tests.

In newborns, hearing is best determined by eliciting the *startle reflex* (p. 275). Nurses also observe other neonatal responses to loud noises, such as facial grimaces, blinking, gross motor movements, quieting if crying or crying if quiet, opening the eyes, or ceasing sucking activity. An objective sign may be a change in heart or respiratory rate because of a loud noise, usually a quickening of the rate. Absence of such alerting behaviors suggests a hearing loss.

During infancy the nurse can test hearing by making a noise and noting the child's specific reaction to *localization of sound*. The nurse stands about 18 inches away from the child, to the side, and out of his peripheral field of vision. With the room silent and the child sitting contentedly in his parent's lap, distracted by a toy or other object, the nurse makes a voice sound, such as PS or PHTH, which is high-pitched, or OO, which is low-pitched, rings a bell or a rattle, or rustles tissue paper. The child's response in terms of localizing the sound is compared to the expected age response (see box, p. 432). This test is usually inadequate for toddlers and preschoolers because of less cooperation and the learned response to willingly inhibit sounds.

A test that can be used with young children consists of the child's identifying a series of familiar toys. For example, for children between 18 and 23 months of age, a *five-toy test* is used. A cup, ball, car, doll, and brick are placed in front of the child. The nurse sits or stands 2 to 3 feet in front of the child, shows him each toy, and has him repeat the word. The nurse then gives directions, such as "Give me the cup," and waits for the child to respond. If the child does this correctly, the nurse gives the directions from a distance of 6 feet, and then 10 feet. The same procedure is used for 2-year-old children with six toys and for 3- to 4-year-old children with seven toys. With these children, their correct duplication of sound (or articulation) is also assessed. With children 5 to 7 years of age, a picture vocabulary test is used that primarily assesses speech, since replication of speech sounds is a direct consequence of hearing.[26]

Two tests are also used to distinguish between air and bone conduction, the Rinne test and Weber's test. In air conduction, sound is transmitted to the brain through the external, middle, and inner ear structures. In bone conduction, the sound bypasses these structures and is transmitted to the brain through the mastoid bone to the inner ear structures and auditory nerve. Normally air conduction is considerably better than bone conduction.

In the *Rinne test* the stem of the tuning fork is placed against the mastoid bone until the sound ceases to be audible. It is then moved so that the prongs are held near, but not touching, the auditory meatus. The child should again hear the sound. If sound is not again audible, then some abnormality is interfering with the conduction of air through the external and middle ear chambers. This test requires the cooperation and ability of the child to signal when the sound is no longer audible and when it is again heard. It is not useful for most children before preschool age.

In *Weber's test* the stem of the tuning fork is held in the midline of the head. The child should hear the sound equally in both ears. With air conductive loss he will hear the sound better in the *affected* ear. This test is frequently not suitable for young children because of their difficulty in discriminating between "better, more, or less." Any child who is suspected of a hearing loss because of poor performance using any of these tests is referred for special audiometric testing.

Vestibular testing for inner ear function concerning equilibrium is tested in infants by holding them at a 30-degree angle and rotating them in a complete circle in each direction. The normal response is nystagmus (movement of the eyes) in the direction of the rotation while being swung and in the opposite direction when the movement stops. This same procedure can be done by using a swivel chair for older children or by having them pivot quickly to one side, then the other.

Vision testing. Vision testing mainly involves assessing light perception and screening for visual acuity. In newborns vision is tested mainly by checking for *light perception* by shining a light into the eyes and noting responses such as blinking, following the light to midline, increased alertness, or refusal to open the eyes after exposure to the light. Vision can also be tested in an alert newborn by rotating a striped drum in front of his face and noting nystagmus, which indicates that vision is present. Signs that should alert the nurse to visual loss include fixed pupils, marked strabismus, constant nystagmus, "setting-sun" sign, and slow lateral movements. Unfortunately it is very difficult to test each eye separately, but the nurse should be aware that such signs in one eye could indicate unilateral blindness.

Visual acuity refers to the ability to see near and far objects clearly. The most common and accurate test for measuring acuity is the *Snellen alphabet chart* (see Appendix F). It consists of nine lines of letters in decreasing size. Each line is given a value, for example, line 8 is "20." The person to be tested stands 20 feet from the chart and reads each line. If he can read line 8, he has 20/20 vision, the accepted standard for normal acuity. If the person can only read line 2, he has 20/100 vision. That means that what he is able to see at a distance of 20 feet, the person with 20/20 or normal eyesight can see at 100 feet. This test is suitable for most children above the third grade, who are familiar with reading the alphabet.

Another version of the Snellen chart is the *Snellen E Chart,* which uses the capital letter E pointing in four different directions. The child "reads" the chart by showing the direction of the letter E or the "legs of the table" either by pointing with his hand or by verbally identifying the direction, such as "toward ceiling, floor, window, or wall." Preschoolers may have difficulty with this test because of confusion in identifying the direction rather than inability to see clearly. This can be corrected by giving them a large duplicate letter E and having them turn it to match the letter on the chart. The Snellen E chart is available for home vision screening from the National Society for the Prevention of Blindness, Inc.,* which recommends its use for children between preschool age and 6 years of age.

Criteria for referring children when using the Snellen charts are:

Preschoolers[3]

1. Three-year-old children who have 20/50 vision or less
2. Four- to 5-year-old children who have 20/40 vision or less
3. Children with any one-line difference between the two eyes
4. Children with strabismus

School-age children[18]

1. Children in kindergarten through third grade who have 20/40 vision or less
2. Fourth-grade children and above who have 20/30 vision or less
3. Children in all grades with a one-line difference between the two eyes

It is recommended that any child who meets these criteria be rescreened once before a referral is made.[3]

Another test that is suitable for children age 2½ years and older is the *Denver Eye Screening Test* (DEST) (see Appendix F). It tests for visual acuity in children 3 years or older by using a single card for the letter E (20/30), but from a distance of 15 feet, rather than 20 feet. The large E (20/100) is used primarily for explanation and demonstration of the procedure to the child. The small E (20/30) is used for testing. Failure to correctly identify the direction of the small E over three trials is considered abnormal. As with every other vision screening test, each eye is tested separately.

For children from 2½ to 2¹¹⁄₁₂ years of age or those who are untestable with the DEST letter E test, picture cards (or Allen cards) are used. Although the DEST is recommended for children beginning at age 30 months, the Allen cards can be used reliably with cooperative children from the age of 24 months. The pictures (a tree, birthday cake, horse and rider, telephone, car, house, and teddy bear) are shown to the child at close range to make certain that he can readily identify them, and then are shown at a distance of 15 feet. If the child cannot correctly name three of the seven cards in three to five trials, his performance is considered abnormal.

The DEST also screens children from 6 to 30 months of age who may be at risk for visual problems by testing for (1) fixation (ability to follow a moving light source or spinning toy), (2) squinting (observation of the child's eyes or report by parent), and (3) strabismus (report by parent and performance on cover and pupillary light reflex tests). Abnormal is failure to fixate, presence of a squint, and/or failing two of the three procedures for strabismus.

Another test that is available for screening vision in children 2 years of age and older is the *STYCAR* (screening tests young children and retardates).[27] It uses the letters H, L, C, T, O, X, A, V, and U, which are readily recognized by young children because they follow the usual progression of drawing, that is, at age 2 years the child copies a vertical line; at age 2½ years, a horizontal line; at age 3 years, a cir-

*National Society for the Prevention of Blindness, Inc., 79 Madison Avenue, New York, N.Y. 10016.

cle; at age 4 years, a cross; at age 5 years, a square; and at age 5½ years, a triangle. The younger the age-group, the fewer letters used for testing. Young or retarded children who do not know the names of the letters are given cards to match with the letter they see.

In a child who is old enough to cooperate, the nurse estimates *peripheral vision,* or the *visual field* of each eye, as the person looks straight ahead. The nurse performs this test by having the child fixate on a specific point directly in front of him as an object, such as her finger or a pencil, is moved from beyond the field of vision into the range of peripheral vision. The nurse checks each eye separately and for each quadrant of vision. As soon as the child sees the object, he tells the nurse to stop moving the object. The nurse estimates the angle from the anteroposterior axis of the eye (straight line of vision) to the peripheral axis (point at which the object is first seen). Normally the child sees about 50 degrees upward, 70 degrees downward, 60 degrees nasalward, and 90 degrees temporally. Limitations in peripheral vision may be indicative of blindness from damage to structures within the eye or to any of the visual pathways.

Another important test is for *color vision.* It is estimated that from 6% to 8% of white males (1 in seventeen to 1 in thirteen) and about half that percentage of black males have inherited the X-linked disorder known as *color blindness.*[31] Although the severity of impaired perception of color varies considerably, the two common types are the red:blue-green type (also called *protan*) and the green:purple type (also called *deutan*). The child who tests as a strong protan confuses browns, red, and black. A strong deutan shows confusion with greens, browns, purples, and grays. Some of the difficulties encountered by these individuals in everyday life may be inability to distinguish amber or red traffic lights, failure to see a red brake light on the rear of a car, difficulty in distinguishing green traffic lights from certain types of incandescent street lamps, and a poor sense of color coordination of clothing. For school-age children the greatest difficulty lies in performance of academic skills that use color as a visual aid. Adolescents who are color blind are ineligible for certain vocational opportunities, such as electrical fields, which use color coding of wires, and for several types of military service. Obviously testing of all children to diagnose those who are affected by this disorder is of major significance.

The tests available for color vision include *Ishihara's* test and the *Hardy-Rand-Rittler* (HRR) test. Each consists of a series of cards (pseudoisochromatic) on which is printed a colored field composed of spots of a certain "confusion" color. Against the field is a letter or figure similarly printed in dots but of a color likely to be confused by the color-blind person with the field color. As a result the figure or letter is invisible to an affected individual but is clearly seen by a normal person. By using Ishihara's test, which is designed for people who cannot read, reliable testing can be done on children as young as 4 years of age.[31] Nurses administering the test must be familiar with the testing materials and should be able to inform the parents of the disorder's effects on practical areas of living, its genetic transmission, and its irreversibility.

Cerebellar functioning. The cerebellum mainly controls balance and coordination. Much of the assessment of cerebellar functioning is included in observing the child's posture, body movements, gait, and development of fine and gross motor skills. Tests such as balancing on one foot and heel-to-toe walk on the DDST assess balance. Coordination is tested by asking the child to reach for a toy, button his clothes, tie his shoes, or draw a straight line on a piece of paper, provided he is old enough to be expected to do each of these activities.

Several tests for cerebellar function that can be performed as games include: (1) *finger-to-nose test:* with the arm extended, ask the child to touch his nose with the index finger both with his eyes opened and then closed, (2) *heel-to-shin test:* with the child standing, have him run the heel of one foot down the shin or anterior aspect of the tibia of the other leg, both with his eyes opened and then closed, and (3) *Romberg test:* with the eyes closed, have the child stand with his heels together; falling or leaning to one side is abnormal and is called Romberg's sign.

School-age children should be able to perform these tests, although preschoolers normally can only bring the finger within 2 to 3 inches of their nose. Difficulty in performing these exercises indicates poor sense of position (especially with the eyes closed) and incoordination (especially with the eyes opened). Coordination can also be tested by any sequence of rapid successive movements, such as quickly touching each finger with the thumb of the same hand. Cerebellar testing is particularly significant in children with symptoms suggestive of hyperactivity or learning difficulty.

Reflexes. Testing reflexes is an important part of the neurologic examination. Persistence of primitive reflexes, loss of reflexes, or hyperactivity of deep tendon reflexes is usually the result of a cerebral insult. This discussion is primarily concerned with reflexes found in children past infancy. The primitive reflexes of the newborn are discussed in Chapter 8 under physical assessment of the neonate.

In eliciting reflexes it is important for the nurse to have some understanding of their basic physiology. A *reflex* is an involuntary response to a stimulus. However, three characteristics are important: (1) the individual is aware of the movement, (2) he may be able to inhibit it, such as by tensing the muscle, but (3) when the activity occurs, it does so without the person's conscious assistance.[15] Although reflexes are under the control of higher brain centers, they may continue to function even though the influence of the brain has been lost. This commonly occurs in spinal cord injury, when the child is unable to walk but still demonstrates the patellar reflex.

Table 5-11. Assessment of deep tendon reflexes

Reflex	Testing procedure	Normal response
Arm		
Biceps	Hold the child's arm by placing the partially flexed elbow in your hand with the thumb over the antecubital space. Strike your thumbnail with the hammer (Fig. 5-51, *A*).	Partial flexion of forearm
Triceps	Abduct the arm, supporting the upper part with your hand and letting the forearm hang freely. Strike the triceps tendon above the elbow. Alternate procedure: If the child is supine, rest his arms over his chest and strike the triceps tendon (Fig. 5-51, *B*).	Partial extension of forearm
Leg		
Patellar or quadriceps (knee jerk)	Sit the child on the edge of the examining table or on his parent's lap with the lower legs flexed at the knee and dangling freely. Tap the patellar tendon just below the knee cap (Fig. 5-51, *C*).	Partial extension of lower leg
Achilles	Use the same position as for the knee jerk. Support the foot lightly in your hand, and strike the Achilles tendon with the hammer (Fig. 5-51, *D*).	Plantar flexion of foot (foot pointing downward)

Several *superficial reflexes* are present, such as the abdominal, cremasteric, anal, and plantar. These have already been discussed throughout the chapter. *Deep tendon reflexes* are stretch reflexes of a muscle. The most common reflex in this category is the *knee jerk* or *patellar reflex* (sometimes called quadriceps reflex) (Table 5-11). The nurse can elicit reflexes by using the rubber head of the reflex hammer, flat of the finger, or side of the hand. If the child is easily frightened by equipment, it is best to use one's hand or finger. Although a simple procedure to perform, the child may inhibit the reflex by unconsciously tensing the leg. The nurse should try to distract younger children with toys or by talking to them. Older children can concentrate on the exercise of grasping their two hands in front of them and trying to pull them apart (Fig. 5-51, *C*). This diverts their attention away from what the nurse is doing and causes involuntary relaxation of the leg muscles. Other reflexes that may be elicited are listed in Table 5-11. Any diminished or hyperreflexic response is reported for further testing.

Several other reflexes are normally present or absent but are not elicited unless specific indications exist. For example, in the presence of symptoms suggestive of meningeal irritation, the nurse can attempt to elicit Kernig's or Brudzinski's sign. The former involves having the child lie supine and extending the leg with the hip flexed. Inability to extend the leg or pain on extension is abnormal and is called *Kernig's sign*. The second test is obtained by flexing the head while the child is supine. Normally this should not cause pain or associated movements. *Brudzinski's sign* is positive when the knees and hips flex involuntarily.

Cranial nerves. The twelve cranial nerves arise directly from the brain and supply the structures of the head and neck. Parts of the tenth nerve, the vagus, branch off to supply structures of the trunk. Assessment of the cranial nerves is an important area of neurologic assessment (Table 5-12). With older children most of the tests can be made into games and, because no traumatic equipment is used, may encourage trust and security at the beginning of the examination. However, if the nurse is familiar with the functions of each nerve, much of the testing can be included when each "system" is examined, such as tongue movement and strength, gag reflex, swallowing, and position of the uvula during examination of the mouth. Regardless of the system the nurse uses, the nurse must be consistent in assessing each cranial nerve function.

"Soft" signs. One of the difficulties in assessment of the nervous system is the clear-cut differentiation between normal and abnormal findings (sometimes referred to as "hard" signs). There is a gray area called "soft" signs. It is defined as "a finding that is normal in a young child but that in the normal course of maturation should go away . . . it represents a developmental delay or lag in the differentiation of a sensory or motor system."[13] Soft signs represent the persistence of a more primitive form of behavior or response and a failure to perform the age-specific activity. Although the list of soft signs is long and the controversy concerning their significance far from resolved, the nurse should be familiar with some of the more classical signs, which are listed in the boxed material on p. 173.

In evaluating the comprehensive data from the child's history and physical, the nurse must appreciate that no one sign is diagnostic of neurologic dysfunction. Rather, neurologic dysfunction is a composite profile of several such signs that collectively place the child at high risk or interfere with his performance or behavior at home, at school, or with peers that supports the need for further neuropsychologic evaluation.

A B C D

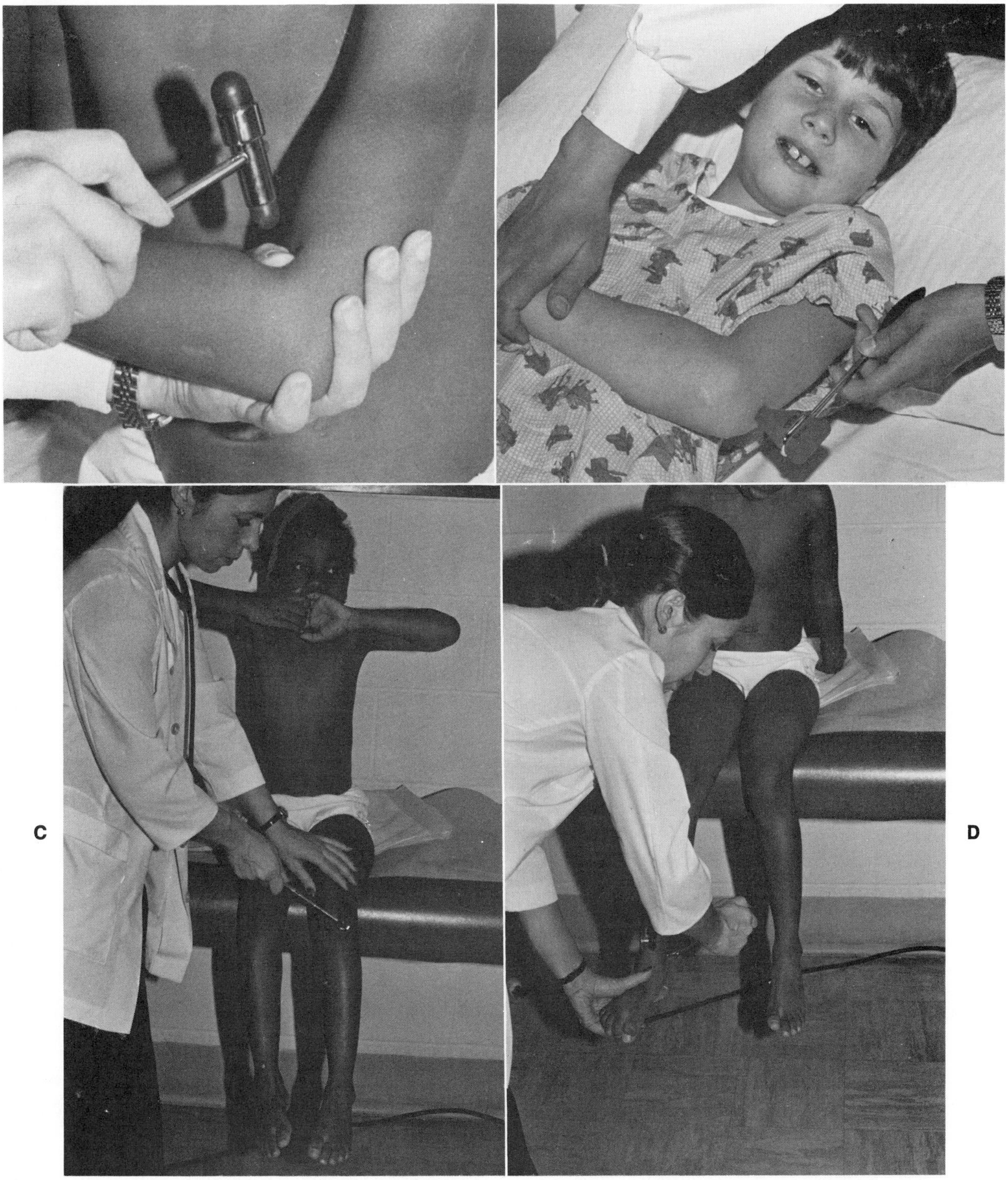

Fig. 5-51. A, Testing for biceps reflex; **B,** testing for triceps reflex; **C,** testing for knee jerk reflex, utilizing distraction; **D,** testing for Achilles tendon reflex.

Table 5-12. Assessment of cranial nerves

Nerve	Distribution	Test
I—Olfactory (S)*	Olfactory mucosa of nasal cavity	With his eyes closed, have child identify odors such as coffee, alcohol from a swab, or other smells. Test each nostril separately.
II—Optic (S)	Rods and cones of retina, optic nerve	Check for perception of light, visual acuity, peripheral vision, color vision, and normal optic disc.
III—Oculomotor (M)*	Muscles of eye	Have child follow an object such as a light or bright toy in all directions using only his eyes, not head movement.
IV—Trochlear (M)	Superior oblique muscle of eye	Have child look downward.
V—Trigeminal (M, S)	Muscles of mastication, skin of face, and two thirds of anterior scalp	Have child bite down hard and open his jaw; test symmetry and strength. With his eyes closed, see if child can detect light touch in the mandibular and maxillary regions. Test corneal and blink reflex by touching cornea lightly (approach child from the side so that he does not blink before cornea is touched).
VI—Abducens (M)	Lateral rectus muscle of eye	Have child look toward each side.
VII—Facial (M, S)	Nasal cavity and lacrimal gland, sublingual and submandibular salivary glands, muscles for facial expression, and anterior two thirds of tongue (taste)	Have child smile, make a funny face, or show his teeth to see symmetry of expression. Have child identify a sweet, sour, or bitter solution. Place each taste on anterior section and sides of protruding tongue; if child retracts tongue, solution will dissolve toward posterior part of tongue.
VIII—Auditory, acoustic, or vestibulocochlear (S)	Internal ear	Test hearing; note any loss of equilibrium or presence of vertigo.
IX—Glossopharyngeal (M, S)	Pharynx, tongue, and posterior one third of tongue for taste	Stimulate the posterior pharynx with a tongue blade; the child should gag. Test sense of taste on posterior segment of tongue.
X—Vagus (M, S)	Muscles of larynx, pharynx, some organs of gastrointestinal system, sensory fibers of root of tongue, heart, lung, and some organs of gastrointestinal system	Note hoarseness of the voice, gag reflex, and ability to swallow. Check that uvula is in midline; when stimulated with a tongue blade, should deviate upward and to the stimulated side.
XI—Accessory (M)	Sternocleidomastoid and trapezius muscles of shoulder	Have child shrug his shoulders while applying mild pressure. With the hands placed on his shoulders, have child turn his head against opposing pressure on either side. Note symmetry and strength.
XII—Hypoglossal (M)	Muscles of tongue	Have child move tongue in all directions. Have him protrude the tongue as far as possible; note any midline deviation. Test strength by placing tongue blade on one side of tongue and having child move it away.

*S—sensory; M—motor

Neurologic "soft" signs

Short attention span
Unusual body movements, such as mirroring
Poor coordination and sense of position
Excessive, sustained, and purposeless movement (hyperactivity)
Hypoactivity
Impulsiveness
Labile emotions
Distractibility
No established handedness
Language and articulation problems
Perceptual deficits (space, form, movement, and time)
Problems with learning, especially reading, writing, and arithmetic

DEVELOPMENTAL SCREENING

One of the most essential components of a complete health appraisal is assessment of developmental functioning. There are two main categories of developmental testing: (1) *screening procedures,* which are designed to identify quickly and reliably those children whose developmental level is below normal for their age and who, therefore, require further investigation, and to provide a means of recording objective measurements of present developmental functioning for failure reference, and (2) *diagnostic procedures,* namely, psychometric tests, which are designed to establish more accurately the nature, extent, and severity of the developmental disability. In this discussion the nurse's role is viewed primarily in terms of screening.

Denver Developmental Screening Test

One of the most widely used screening tests for assessing a young child's development is the *Denver Developmental Screening Test (DDST)* (see Appendix F). It is composed of four major categories: personal-social, fine motor–adaptive, language, and gross motor and is applicable for children from birth through 6 years of age. The age divisions are monthly until age 24 months and then every 6 months until 6 years of age. Allowances are made for infants who were born prematurely by subtracting the number of weeks missed gestation from their present age and testing them at the adjusted age. For example, a 9-month-old infant who was born 4 weeks prior to the expected date of confinement is tested at an 8-month level.

The DDST has been subjected to several reliability and validity tests and has been found to yield normal, questionable, and abnormal results that correlate with psychometric tests, such as the Cattell Infant Intelligence Scale and the Revised Bayley Infant Scale. Studies have also shown a predictive correlation between results of the DDST and the later development of school problems. Results showed that children with questionable scores, as well as those with abnormal scores, are at risk for developing school problems despite adequate intelligence.[5] Such findings are extremely relevant to nurses who are in an optimum position to identify high-risk children and refer them for further testing. One weakness of the DDST is its limitations in terms of predictive validity with minority ethnic groups.

The DDST is designed for administration by both professionals and paraprofessionals. The DDST is accompanied by a detailed instruction manual as well as by self-instructional units.* The kits for testing include a red wool "ball," raisins, a small clear bottle with a ⅝-inch opening, a rattle with a narrow handle, eight 1-inch square blocks in red, blue, yellow, and green colors, a small ball, a tennis ball, and a pencil. The child is tested for each item that the age line intersects, although he is not expected to pass every item.

Each item is designated by a bar that represents the ages at which 25%, 50%, 70%, and 90% of the tested population could perform the particular item. Scoring is based on the number of *delays,* which are defined as "failure to perform an item which is passed by 90% of the children who are of the same age or any item which falls completely to the *left* of the age line." *Abnormal* is determined by (1) two or more sectors with two or more delays, or (2) one sector with two or more delays plus one or more sectors with one delay and, in that same sector, no passes through the age line. *Questionable* is determined by (1) one sector with two or more delays, or (2) one or more sectors with one delay and, in that same sector, no passes through the age line. If the child refuses to cooperate with testing so that a large number of items would be scored as failures, the child is evaluated as *untestable* and, if possible, retested at a future date. *Normal* is determined by any score that does not meet these three other criteria.

Although it is not the purpose of this discussion to detail the instruction manual, there are some points concerning preparation, administration, and interpretation of the test that necessitate emphasis. Before beginning the test, both the child and parent need an explanation of the DDST. For parents this means clarifying that the DDST is *not* an intelligence test but a method of helping the nurse observe what the child can do at this age. It is best to deemphasize the word "test" while emphasizing that the child is *not* expected to perform each item on the sheet. In scoring the DDST, usually a "P" is used to denote passing, an "F" for failing, an "N. O." if the child has had no opportunity to perform the item, such as pedaling a tricycle, and an "R" for refusing to do the item. Sometimes parents become anxious when they see the nurse marking "F's" on the

*The DDST and instruction manual are available from Mead Johnson Laboratories, Evansville, Indiana 47721.

sheet. In this case the nurse should repeat that an "F" does not denote failure, because the child may not be expected to perform the item, or should use a different symbol to further allay the parent's anxiety. If a different symbol is used, the nurse must remember to note this on the sheet, so that another examiner will be able to reliably interpret the results.

The parent is told before the testing begins that the nurse will explain the results of the child's performance after all the items have been concluded. In this way the parent is aware that the results are for the child's benefit and are not to be used elsewhere. It is the nurse's responsibility to properly inform parents of any testing or screening procedure prior to its administration so that they are fully aware of its purpose and intent.

The nurse prepares toddlers and preschoolers for the test by presenting it as a game. Frequently the DDST is an excellent way to begin a health appraisal because it is nonthreatening, requires no painful or unfamiliar procedures, and capitalizes on the child's natural activity of play. Since many children are easily distracted, it is best to perform the test quickly and to present only one toy from the kit at a time. After that toy's purpose is concluded, such as building a tower of blocks or identifying its color, the toy is replaced in the bag and another one is brought out for testing purposes. Other temporary factors that may interfere with the child's performance include fatigue, illness, fear, hospitalization, separation from the parent, or general unwillingness to perform activities asked of the child. In addition, undiagnosed mental retardation, hearing loss, vision loss, neurologic impairment, or a familial pattern of slow development greatly influences the child's performance.

Following completion of the DDST, the nurse asks the parent if the child's performance was typical of his behavior at other times. If the parent replies affirmatively and the child's cooperation was satisfactory, the nurse explains the results, emphasizing all successful items first, then those items failed but which the child was not expected to pass, and, last, those items that were delays.

In explaining a normal score the nurse should focus on how well the child performed and should reinforce the parents' efforts in satisfactorily stimulating their child. Although the nurse does not wish to encourage parents to teach their child skills in order to pass the test, the DDST can be used to guide parents toward those activities that are appropriate, although not necessarily expected, for the child's age. For example, although not all 3-year-old children can button their clothes or dress with supervision, the nurse can inquire if the parent has presented such opportunities to the child. If the parent has not, the nurse can state that this is an activity that some 3-year-old children can perform, especially if encouraged and helped to do so.

In explaining delays the nurse carefully notes the parent's response, especially casual acceptance, such as, "He'll catch up." Since all children with questionable or abnormal results should be rescreened before referral for diagnostic testing, the nurse can defer some of the parents' more serious questions, such as, "Does this mean my child is retarded?" until the next screening session. The nurse must be aware of personal anxieties during these situations and refrain from giving glib reassurances, such as, "I'm sure he will do better the next time." Rather, parents' questions should be answered honestly yet with appropriate flexibility and concern by stating, "I need to observe your child again before I can give you any answers or even make assumptions concerning his developmental progress. I will retest him next week, and then possibly, I will know more. What are your thoughts about how he performed the items on the DDST?"

If the parents reply that the child's performance was not typical of his usual behavior, it is best for the nurse to defer any scoring or discussion of the test results with the parents, especially if the refusals, when marked as failures, yield a questionable or abnormal rating. In this case the nurse reschedules the DDST for a time when the child is more likely to cooperate.

Several other screening tests are available. For example, a prescreening questionnaire, the *Denver Prescreening Developmental Questionnaire* (PDQ), is designed to identify those children who require a more thorough screening with the DDST.[9] It has the advantages of being very easy and rapid to administer (it takes parents about 5 minutes to answer the questions), and it does not require the presence or cooperation of the child. Another screening test that is designed for children from birth through 12 years of age is the *Developmental Profile,* which includes the following five scales: physical age, self-help, social age, academic age, and communication age.[2] Like the Denver Prescreening Developmental Questionnaire, it relies largely on verbal responses from the child's parent, teacher, or other well-acquainted individual.

Another test that can be used to assess intellectual development is the *Goodenough Draw-A-Man Test.* The child is given a pencil with an eraser and paper and simply asked to "draw a man or a person." No further directions are supplied regarding the drawing, other than he should draw the best picture of a person that he can. He should be left alone and given as much time as needed to finish the picture.

The scoring is determined by giving 1 point for each item included in the drawing (see boxed material). Each point is equal to 3 months. The number of points are converted to months and/or years and added to the base age of 3 years. The final score in months/years is approximately equal to the child's mental age. The child's intelligence quotient (IQ) can be found by the ratio of mental age to chronologic age multiplied by 100. For example, if a 5-year-old child scores 12 points on the test, he has a mental age of 6 years (3 years + [12 × 3 months] = 6 years) and an IQ of 120 $\left(\frac{6\text{ years}}{5\text{ years}} \times 100 = 120\right)$.

Method of scoring Goodenough draw-a-man test*

1. Head present
2. Legs present
3. Arms present
4. Trunk present
5. Trunk longer than broad
6. Shoulder indicated
7. Both arms and legs attached to trunk
8. Legs and arms attached to trunk at proper level
9. Neck present
10. Outline of neck continuous with that of head or trunk or both
11. Eyes present
12. Nose present
13. Mouth present
14. Both nose and mouth in two dimensions; two lips shown
15. Nostrils indicated
16. Hair shown
17. Hair on more than circumference of head, nontransparent, better than scribble
18. Clothing present
19. Two articles of clothing, nontransparent
20. Entire clothing with sleeves and trousers shown, nontransparent
21. Four or more articles of clothing definitely indicated
22. Costume complete without incongruities
23. Fingers shown
24. Correct number of fingers
25. Fingers in two dimensions, length greater than breadth, angle subtended not greater than 180°
26. Opposition of thumbs shown
27. Hands shown distinct from fingers and arms
28. Arm joints shown (elbow or shoulder or both)
29. Head in proportion
30. Arms in proportion
31. Legs in proportion
32. Feet in proportion
33. Arms and legs in two dimensions
34. Heel shown
35. Lines somewhat controlled
36. Lines well controlled
37. Head outline well controlled
38. Trunk outline well controlled
39. Outline of arms and legs well controlled
40. Outline of features well controlled
41. Ears present
42. Ears present in correct position
43. Eyebrows or lashes present
44. Pupil shown
45. Proportion of eyes correct
46. Glance directed to front in profile drawing
47. Both chin and forehead shown
48. Projection of shin shown
49. Profile with not more than one error
50. Correct profile

*In each item listed above, give the child 1 point. The number of points multiplied by 3 months plus 3 years equals the mental age.

Although reports concerning the reliability of the Goodenough test vary, it is a valuable procedure for assessing intellectual development in children 3 to 10 years of age, particularly in screening for children with low scores who may require further measurement of mental functioning.

Although screening tests are an effective method of applying the knowledge of children's expected rate of development to a large segment of the population, they are only as successful as the individuals' expertise in administering them. Since many of the screening tests are devised to be used by paraprofessionals, there are inherent risks in screening if such individuals are not properly trained or supervised. For example, false-positives can label the child as developmentally delayed and cause problems that otherwise might not have existed.[28] It is nurses' responsibility to ensure that screening tests are properly administered and the results correctly interpreted. The complexity of mental and physical health can never be measured by any one index. Evaluation of the child's total well-being is the result of evaluating data from a comprehensive history, physical examination, and developmental screening.

REFERENCES

1. Alexander, M. M., and Brown, M. S.: Physical examination. Part 14. Male genitalia, Nursing '76 **6**(2):39-43, February 1976.
2. Alpern, G. D., and Boll, T. J.: Developmental profile, Aspen, Colo., 1972, Psychological Development Publications.
3. American Academy of Pediatrics, Committee on Children with Handicaps: Vision screening of preschool children, Pediatrics **50**(6):966-967, December 1972.
4. Barness, L. A.: Manual of pediatric physical diagnosis, Chicago, 1972, Year Book Medical Publishers, Inc.
5. Camp, B. W., and associates: Preschool developmental testing in prediction of school problems, Clin. Pediatr. **16**(3): 257-263, March 1977.
6. Carbonara, N. T.: Techniques for observing normal child behavior, Pittsburgh, 1961, University of Pittsburgh Press.
7. Chard, M.: An approach to examining the adolescent male, Am. J. Maternal Child Nurs. **1**(1):41-43, January/February 1976.
8. Fowler, M. D.: Behold the great right toe, Am. J. Nurs. **74**(10):1817-1819, October 1974.
9. Frankenburg, W. K., and associates: The Denver Prescreening Developmental Questionnaire (PDQ), Pediatrics **57**(5): 744-753, May 1976.
10. Habicht, J. P., and associates: Height and weight standards for preschool children: how relevant are ethnic differences in growth potential? Lancet **1**(7858):611-614, April 6, 1974.
11. Havener, W. H.: Synopsis of ophthalmology, ed. 5, St. Louis, 1979, The C. V. Mosby Co.
12. Jaffe, B. F.: Pinna anomalies associated with congenital conductive hearing loss, Pediatrics **57**(3):332-341, March 1976.
13. Kinsbourne, M.: School problems, Pediatrics **52**(5):697-710, November 1973.
14. Laestadius, N., Aase, J., and Smith, D.: Normal inner can-

thal and outer orbital dimensions, J. Pediatr. **74**(3):465-468, March 1969.

15. Langley, L. L., Telford, I. R., and Christensen, J. B.: Dynamic anatomy and physiology, New York, 1974, McGraw-Hill Book Co.
16. Larson, C. B., and Gould, M.: Orthopaedic nursing, ed. 9, St. Louis, 1978, The C. V. Mosby Co.
17. Littman, D.: Stethoscopes and auscultation, Am. J. Nurs. **72**(7):1238-1241, July 1972.
18. National Association for the Prevention of Blindness, Inc.: Vision screening of children, New York, 1971, The Association.
19. Neumann, C. G., and Alpaugh, M.: Birth-weight doubling time: a fresh look, Pediatrics **57**(4):469-473, April 1976.
20. Owens, G. J.: The assessment and recording of measurements of growth of children: report of a small conference, Pediatrics **51**(3):461-465, March 1973.
21. Pilch, B. Z., and associates: Thyroid cancer after radioactive iodine diagnostic procedures in childhood, Pediatrics **51**(5): 898-902, May 1973.
22. Redman, J. F., and Bissada, N. K.: How to make a good examination of the genitalia in young girls, Clin. Pediatr. **15**(10):907-908, October 1976.
23. Roach, L. B.: Color changes in dark skin, Nursing '77 **7**(1): 48-51, January 1977.
24. Sana, J. M., and Judge, R. D.: Physical appraisal methods in nursing practice, Boston, 1975, Little, Brown and Co.
25. Scott, M. D., and Crawford, J. D.: Solitary thyroid nodules: is the incidence of thyroid carcinoma declining? Pediatrics **58**(4):521-525, October 1976.
26. Sheridan, M. D.: Simple clinical hearing tests for very young or mentally retarded children, Br. Med. J. **2**:999-1004, October 25, 1958.
27. Sheridan, M. D., and Gardiner, P. A.: Sheridan-Gardiner test for visual acuity, Br. Med. J. **2**:108-109, April 11, 1970.
28. Solnit, A. J.: The risks of screening, Pediatrics **57**(5):646-647, May 1976.
29. Starnbach, H. K., and Gellin, M. E.: What should the physician know about orthodontics? Clin. Pediatr. **16**(6):552-555, June 1977.
30. Sutow, W. W., Vietti, T. J., and Fernbach, D. J.: Clinical pediatric oncology, ed. 2, St. Louis, 1977, The C. V. Mosby Co.
31. Thuline, H. C.: Color blindness in children: the importance and feasibility of early recognition, Clin. Pediatr. **11**(5):295-299, May 1972.
32. Webb, K. J.: Early assessment of orthopedic injuries, Am. J. Nurs. **74**(6):1048-1052, June 1974.

BIBLIOGRAPHY

Adler, J.: Patient assessment: abnormalities of the heartbeat, Am. J. Nurs. **77**(4):647-673, April 1977.

Alexander, M., and Brown, M. S.: Physical examination. Part 12. Examining the chest and lungs, Nursing '75 **5**(1):44-48, January 1975.

Alexander, M. M. and Brown, M. S.: Physical examination. Part 13. Examining the abdomen, Nursing '76 **6**(1):65-70, January 1976.

Alexander, M. M., and Brown, M. S.: Physical examination. Part 16. The musculoskeletal system, Nursing '76 **6**(4):51-56, April 1976.

Alexander, M. M., and Brown, M. S.: Physical examination. Part 17. Performing the neurological examination, Nursing '76 **6**(6):38-43, June 1976.

Alexander, M. M., and Brown, M. S.: Physical examination. Part 18. Neurological examination, Nursing '76 **6**(7):50-55, July 1976.

Brown, M. S.: Vision tests for preschoolers, Nursing '75 **5**(5):72-74, May 1975.

Brown, M. S., and Alexander, M. M.: Physical examination. Part 15. Female genitalia, Nursing '76 **6**(3):39-41, March 1976.

Brown, M. S., and Murphy, M. A.: Ambulatory pediatrics for nurses, New York, 1975, McGraw-Hill Book Co.

De Angelis, C.: Basic pediatrics for the primary health care provider, Boston, 1975, Little, Brown and Co.

deCastro, F. J., Rolfe, U., and Drew, J.: The pediatric nurse practitioner, ed. 2, St. Louis, 1976, The C. V. Mosby Co.

Delaney, M. T.: Examining the chest. Part II. The heart, Nursing '75 **5**(9):41-44, September 1975.

Delaney, M. T.: Examining the chest. Part I. The lungs, Nursing '75 **5**(8):12-14, August 1975.

Dessertine, P. S.: Those neglected heart sounds, Pediatr. Nurs. **3**(1):18-20, January/February 1977.

Downs, M. P., and Silver, N. K.: The "A.B.C.D." to H.E.A.R.: early identification in nursery, office, and clinic of the infant who is deaf, Clin. Pediatr. **11**(10):563-565, October 1972.

Eavey, R., and associates: How to examine the ear of the neonate, Clin. Pediatr. **15**(4):338-341, April 1976.

Ehrlich, M. A., and Tait, C. A.: The application of acoustic impedance measurements to pediatric clinical practice, Pediatrics **55**(5):666, May 1975.

Erickson, M. L.: Assessment and management of developmental changes in children, St. Louis, 1976, The C. V. Mosby Co.

Eviatar, L., and Eviatar, A.: Vertigo in children: differential diagnosis and treatment, Pediatrics **59**(6):833-838, June 1977.

Fowkes, W. C., and Hunn, V. K.: Clinical assessment for the nurse practitioner, St. Louis, 1973, The C. V. Mosby Co.

Frankenburg, W. K., and Dodds, J.: The Denver Developmental Screening Test, J. Pediatr. **71**(2):181-191, August 1967.

Frankenburg, W. K., and associates: The reliability and stability of the Denver Developmental Screening Test, Child Dev. **42:**1315, 1971.

Frankenburg, W. K., and associates: The revised Denver Developmental Screening Test: its accuracy as a screening instrument, J. Pediatr. **76**(6):988-995, December 1971.

Frankenburg, W. K., and associates: Validity of the Denver Developmental Screening Test, Child Dev. **42:**475, 1971.

Goodenough, F. L.: Measurement of intelligence by drawings, New York, 1926, World Book Co.

Hiles, D.: Strabismus, Am. J. Nurs. **74**(6):1082-1089, June 1974.

Hill, S.: The child with ambiguous genitalia, Am. J. Nurs. **77**(5): 810-814, May 1977.

Hovenden, H. G.: Rocky Mountain spotted fever, Am. J. Nurs. **76**(3):419-421, March 1976.

Illingworth, R. S.: The development of the infant and young child, Edinburgh, 1975, Churchill Livingstone.

Ireton, H., and Thwing, E.: Appraising the development of a

preschool child by means of a standardized report prepared by the mother: the Minnesota Child Development Inventory, Clin. Pediatr. **15**(10):875-882, October 1976.

Jarvis, C. M.: Vital signs: how to take them accurately . . . and understand them fully, Nursing '76 **6**(4):31-37, April 1976.

Kerr, G. R.: Physical growth during childhood, Drug Therapy **35:**49, October 1976.

Larsen, G.: Removing cerumen with a Water Pik, Am. J. Nurs. **76**(2):264-265, February 1976.

Lehman, J.: Auscultation of heart sounds, Am. J. Nurs. **72**(7): 1242-1246, July 1972.

Lynaugh, J. E., and Bates, B.: Physical diagnosis: a skill for all nurses? Am. J. Nurs. **74**(1):58-59, January 1974.

Mechner, F.: Patient assessment: examination of the eye. Part I, Am. J. Nurs. **74**(11):1-24, November 1974.

Mechner, F.: Patient assessment: examination of the eye. Part II, Am. J. Nurs. **75**(1):1-24, January 1975.

Mechner, F.: Patient assessment: examination of the ear, Am. J. Nurs. **75**(3):1-24, March 1975.

Mechner, F.: Patient assessment: examination of the head and neck, Am. J. Nurs. **75**(5):1-24, May 1975.

Mechner, F.: Patient assessment: neurological examination. Part III, Am. J. Nurs. **76**(4):608-633, April 1976.

Mechner, F.: Patient assessment: examination of the chest and lungs, Am. J. Nurs. **76**(9):1453-1475, September 1976.

Mechner, F.: Patient assessment: examination of the heart and great vessels. Part I, Am. J. Nurs. **76**(11):1807-1830, November 1976.

Mechner, F.: Patient assessment: auscultation of the heart. Part II, Am. J. Nurs. **77**(2):275-298, February 1977.

Metz, J. R., and associates: A pediatric screening examination for psychosocial problems, Pediatrics **58**(4):595-606, October 1976.

Paradise, J. L., Smith, C. G., and Bluestone, C. D.: Tympanometric detection of middle ear effusion in infants and young children, Pediatrics **58**(2):198-210, August 1976.

Park, M. K., Kawabori, I., and Guntheroth, W. G.: Need for an improved standard for blood pressure cuff size, Clin. Pediatr. **15**(9):784-787, September 1976.

Patel, R., and Groff, D. B.: Condyloma acuminata in childhood, Pediatrics **50**(1):153-154, July 1972.

Preventable Diseases and Nutrition Activity, Bureau of Smallpox Eradication, Center for Disease Control and the Maternal and Child Health Program, Bureau of Community Health Service, Health Service Administration, Public Health Service, Department of Health, Education, and Welfare: Evaluation of body size and physical growth of children, Washington, D.C., 1976, U.S. Government Printing Office.

Prior, J. A., and Silberstein, J. S.: Physical diagnosis: the history and examination of the patient, ed. 5, St. Louis, 1977, The C. V. Mosby Co.

Pryor, H. B., and Thelander, H. E.: Growth comparisons of urban and rural children in southern Mexico with randomly selected California children, Clin. Pediatr. **11**(7):411-416, July 1972.

Rajkumar, S. U., and associates: Popsicle panniculitis of the cheeks, Clin. Pediatr. **15**(7):619-621, July 1976.

Rice, A.: Common skin infections in school children, Am. J. Nurs. **73**(11):1905-1909, November 1973.

Romano, P., and Von Noorden, G. K.: Limitations of cover test in detecting strabismus, Am. J. Ophthalmol. **72**(1):10-12, July 1971.

Sells, C. J., and May, E. A.: Scoliosis screening, Am. J. Nurs. **74**(1):60-62, January 1974.

Sheridan, M. D.: Vision screening of very young or handicapped children, Br. Med. J. **2:**453-456, August 6, 1960.

Sherman, J. L., and Fields, S. K.: Guide to patient evaluation, New York, 1976, Medical Examination Publishing Co., Inc.

Sibinga, M. S., and Carey, W. B.: Dealing with unnecessary medical trauma to children, Pediatrics **57**(5):800-803, May 1976.

Stright, P. A., and Soukup, M.: How to hear it right: evaluating and choosing a stethoscope, Am. J. Nurs. **77**(9):1477, September 1977.

Swigarth, E., and Stool, S. E.: Hearing sensitivity and physical characteristics of the eardrum observed during otoscopic examination, Clin. Pediatr. **16**(6):556-560, June 1977.

Thorp, R. J.: The use of the pediatric nurse practitioner in comprehensive health care, Pediatr. Nurs. **1**(3):33-35, May/June 1975.

Traver, G. A.: Assessment of thorax and lungs, Am. J. Nurs. **73**(3):466-471, March 1973.

Wirtschafter, J. D., and Strapp, I. P.: Strabismus cover test demonstrator, Am. J. Ophthalmol. **71**(3):760-764, March 1971.

UNIT THREE
The unborn child

The period from conception to birth is the most mysterious and least known phase of the life cycle. It is the period when the fewest outside demands are placed on the organism, but, at the same time, it is fraught with dangers that may have lifelong consequences. Recognition of the tremendous importance of this period of rapid growth and change has focused interest on fetal development, the relationship between prenatal events and infant health, and the factors that influence the well-being of the individual during this and subsequent stages of life.

Chapter 6, *Hereditary Influences,* is concerned with genetic factors that affect the growth and health of children and with the nurse's role in counseling parents of children with defects of hereditary origin. Chapter 7, *Fetal Development and Prenatal Influences,* focuses on the child before birth, the way in which development progresses, maternal factors that may affect the outcome of the pregnancy, and the nurse's role in promoting fetal health. A knowledge of the prenatal stages of development aids understanding of the normal relationships of body structures and the way in which maldevelopment produces the congenital defects often encountered in pediatric nursing practice.

6

Hereditary influences

Child development consists of both genetic components and environmental factors that interact to produce the physical, biochemical, and mental characteristics of the child. These include not only those traits that create the individuality of each child, but also those characteristics that produce unpleasant symptoms or undesirable physical abnormalities that are interpreted as disease. Numerous defects and diseases are seen more frequently in the population and show an increased incidence in some families or under certain environmental conditions. Parents and health workers alike are concerned with the probability that a specific disease or disorder will recur in a family in which the condition has been known to occur. In order to be better able to counsel families and to anticipate probable problems, the nurse needs a fundamental understanding of the principles of heredity and the importance of heredity as an etiologic factor in diseases and disorders of childhood.

HEREDITY IN HEALTH PROBLEMS

There is probably a genetic component in all disease processes. In some disorders the genetic defect is known; in others the precise nature of the genetic component is more obscure. In some the disorder is apparent at birth; in others the manifestations do not appear for weeks, months, or years. All disease processes seem to fall on a continuous spectrum (Fig. 6-1). On one end are those diseases and disorders that are determined by the genetic constitution of the individual. Examples in this category are phenylketonuria, hemophilia, muscular dystrophy, sickle cell anemia, and Down's syndrome. Some diseases, although genetically determined, are not on the extreme end of the spectrum because the disease does not become clinically apparent until environmental factors precipitate the onset of symptoms. For instance, an infant with phenylketonuria, a disorder caused by lack of an enzyme essential for the metabolism of the protein phenylalanine, does not display any symptoms until a sufficient amount of milk containing the protein is ingested.

On the opposite end of the spectrum are the diseases primarily resulting from environmental factors. These include most infectious diseases and trauma. Development of the disease depends on environmental contact with the etiologic agent, but there is strong evidence to indicate a decided genetic element in the susceptibility to most diseases (for example, tuberculosis, poliomyelitis, and measles in some populations).

Between these two extremes fall the bulk of common diseases and disorders that have varying degrees of genetic influence. This category contains most of the birth defects, the allergic disorders, many neurologic defects, and some metabolic diseases, the most notable of which is diabetes mellitus. All in all, heredity influences those disorders that are primarily of environmental origin; environment influences disorders primarily of hereditary origin.

To facilitate a discussion of the genetic influence on the health of children, it will be necessary to clarify some of the terms used to describe hereditary conditions.

congenital the condition is present at birth. The disorder may be brought about by genetic causes, nongenetic causes, or a combination of these.

genetic the disorder is caused by a single deleterious gene or by a deviation in chromosomal number or structure. A genetic disorder may or may not be apparent at birth.

inherited (heritable, hereditary) synonymous with genetic, although in the past was often used to describe a disorder that had appeared in parent and offspring over several generations.

familial a disorder that "runs in families" or is present in more members of a family than would be expected by chance.

In most instances only unusual diseases can be attributed precisely to a genetic etiology and display a clear-cut inheritance pattern. Individually they are rare; collectively they constitute a sizable portion of the health problems of children. In the more common diseases and disorders the genetic component varies from disease to disease, and, although there is an increased incidence in families, no clear-cut mode of inheritance can be identified.

Genetic diseases can usually be classified into one of the

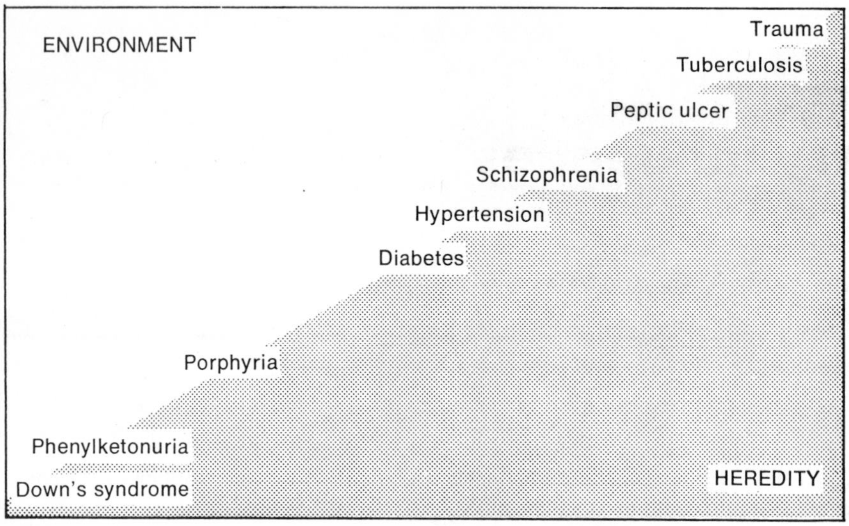

Fig. 6-1. Spectrum of diseases, indicating the relative importance of genetic and environmental factors. (From Whaley, L. F.: Understanding inherited disorders, St. Louis, 1974, The C. V. Mosby Co., p. 137.)

following three broad categories according to the hereditary factors that produce the observed effect:

1. Chromosomal aberrations in which there is addition, loss, or structural alteration of a chromosome, for example, Down's syndrome (p. 812), Klinefelter's syndrome (p. 714) and, Turner's syndrome (p. 713)
2. Disorders that are caused by mutation of a gene or genes and that are distributed in families according to the basic mendelian inheritance patterns, for example, cystic fibrosis (p. 1252), hemophilia (p. 1390), muscular dystrophy (p. 1522), and phenylketonuria (p. 316)
3. The common diseases and disorders that are multifactorial, that is, resulting from a complex interaction of both genetic and environmental factors, for example, diabetes mellitus (p. 1478) and congenital defects (Chapter 11)

In order to counsel effectively families in which there is a serious condition known to be hereditary, the nurse needs a basic understanding of the mechanisms of heredity and the manner in which a deviation from normal produces an adverse effect in the child.

Biologic basis of heredity

The physical and chemical individuality of an organism is determined by finite segments of deoxyribonucleic acid (DNA). The unique structure of DNA provides the means by which the genetic material is maintained and transferred through countless generations and by which the synthesis of appropriate proteins from amino acids is directed within the cells. In every cell there are thousands of these DNA units, called *genes,* each of which controls or regulates a specific cellular function. The term used to describe the gene constitution of the individual is the *genotype*. The appearance or observable characteristics of the person that result from the interaction of the environment on the genotype are termed the *phenotype*. Factors that alter the genotype will produce an effect on the phenotype even though the relationship between the two seems remote.

All somatic (body) cells contain two sets of genes, one set derived from each parent during the process of reproduction. Genes are arranged in linear order along highly organized structures within the cell nucleus—the *chromosomes*. Each gene has a definite position, or locus, on a specific chromosome and may take one of several different forms. These different forms, which produce varying effects, are termed *alleles;* for example, there are a number of alleles that produce eye color. When corresponding genes at a locus produce the same effect they are said to be *homozygous*. If the genes of a pair produce different effects, they are said to be *heterozygous*.

In man the entire complement of genes is contained in forty-six, or twenty-three pairs of, chromosomes—twenty-two pairs of *autosomes* and one pair of *sex chromosomes*. The autosomes are alike in both male and female; the sex chromosomes are alike in the female (XX) but are morphologically different in the male (XY). To appreciate the way in which chromosomes behave in relation to transmission of hereditary disorders, it will be helpful to review the basic elements of cell division.

Cell division. During the stage between the phases of active cell division, chromosomes in the cell nucleus appear as vague, dark-staining, amorphous granules. When the cell begins to divide, the chromosomes condense and shorten until they assume a definite configuration. They are most easily visualized under the microscope when the chromosomes are partially divided, that is, two duplicated longitudinal halves *(chromatids)* united at a constricted area (the

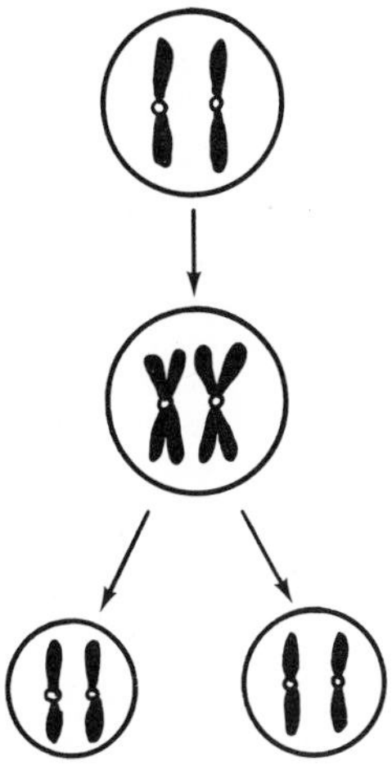

Fig. 6-2. Mitosis in a somatic cell.

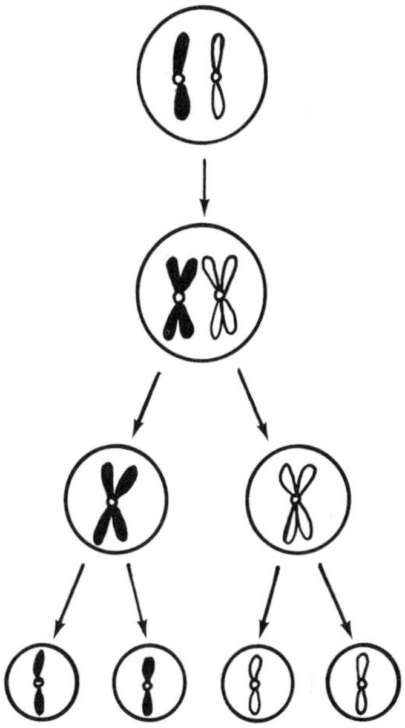

Fig. 6-3. Meiosis in a germ cell.

centromere). It is the location of this centromere that gives the chromosome its characteristic appearance—a centrally located centromere produces an X appearance; a terminal location results in a wishbone or Y shape. Complete division of the chromosome occurs when the chromatids separate longitudinally at the centromere.

Somatic cells divide via *mitosis,* an *equational division* in which cell components, particularly the genetic material, are distributed in equal amounts to two daughter cells so that each possesses the same kind and number of chromosomes found in the mother cell (Fig. 6-2).

Mitosis, a most satisfactory method for duplicating and replacing somatic cells, is totally unsatisfactory for duplication of reproductive cells, the ova and sperm. By a related process, *meiosis* or *reduction division,* the total chromosomal number in both male and female germ cells is reduced by half so that when the resulting gametes are united at fertilization the original number is restored. Meiotic division consists of two successive divisions during which an original cell with forty-six paired chromosomes becomes four cells, each with twenty-three unpaired chromosomes. The process of meiosis differs from mitosis primarily in the first division. At this time, instead of the longitudinal splitting of each chromosome, the chromosomal pairs separate intact and one member of each pair goes to each of the two newly formed cells. At a second division the twenty-three chromosomes split and distribute equally to the daughter cells (Fig. 6-3). The characteristic segregation of chromosomes during meiotic division is the basis of the statistically predictable mendelian ratios that constitute the basic principles of inheritance.

In order to observe and analyze chromosomes, somatic cells (usually leukocytes obtained from peripheral blood) are stimulated to divide. At the optimum time the cells are prepared, stained, and photographed by a camera attached to a high-powered microscope. After the photograph is enlarged, the individual chromosomes are cut out and arranged according to a standard classification system. The paired chromosomes are positioned in order of decreasing length, assigned a number, and separated into seven major groups (designated A through G) composed of morphologically similar pairs. Most individual chromosomes cannot be identified with certainty but can be readily assigned to a group. The sex chromosomes, still designated X and Y, are either individually placed with the group they resemble or paired to form a separate group. This systematic arrangement of chromosomes is termed a *karyotype* (Fig. 6-4). A chromosomal analysis is carried out to confirm or refute the probable diagnosis of a chromosomal abnormality, to identify a suspected carrier of chromosomal abnormality, or when the sex of an infant is in doubt.

DISORDERS CAUSED BY CHROMOSOMAL ABERRATIONS

An aberration is defined as a deviation from that which is normal or typical. Aberrations of chromosomes are deviations in either structure or number, and the consequences in either situation can be readily observed in the affected individual. Since the development of improved techniques for the study of chromosomes, a number of physical disabilities have been directly associated with chromosomal defects. Although the types of chromosomal disorders are not as varied as those caused by a single mutant gene, the incidence for many of the specific abnormalities is significantly higher than any of the single-gene disorders.

The complex nature of cell division makes it highly susceptible to mechanical error, particularly during the critical

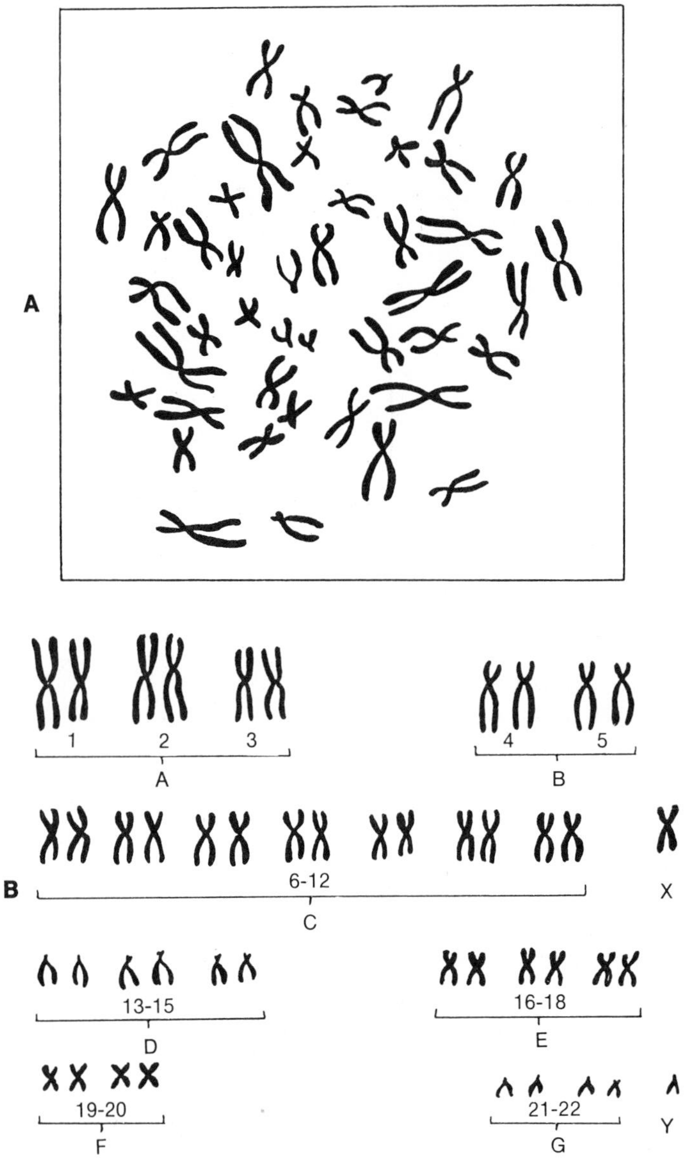

Fig. 6-4. A metaphase spread of male chromosomes. **A,** Example of a photomicrograph. **B,** Chromosomes arranged in a karyotype. (From Whaley, L. F.: Understanding inherited disorders, St. Louis, 1974, The C. V. Mosby Co., p. 9.)

processes of gamete formation and in the early divisions of the zygote following fertilization. The majority of abnormalities accounted for in the literature are related to variations in chromosomal number; however, there is evidence that, with technical advances, the structural abnormalities may assume greater significance in human disease.

A structural aberration involves loss, addition, rearrangement, or exchange of some of the genes of a chromosome. If there is sufficient remaining genetic material to render the organism viable, there can be an endless variety of clinical manifestations.

Deviations in chromosomal number involve the gain or loss of a chromosome and are designated with the suffix *-somy*. A cell that contains one less than the total number of chromosomes is called a *monosomy* because of the loss of one member of a chromosome pair; a cell that contains one more than the total number of chromosomes resulting from the addition of an extra member to a normal pair is called a *trisomy*. A number of deviations occur in man that are compatible with life, especially those involving the sex chromosomes, but the more serious outcomes are related to abnormalities of the autosomes. Trisomies are the chromosomal aberrations encountered most frequently by health workers; it is of interest that the viable trisomies seem to involve only

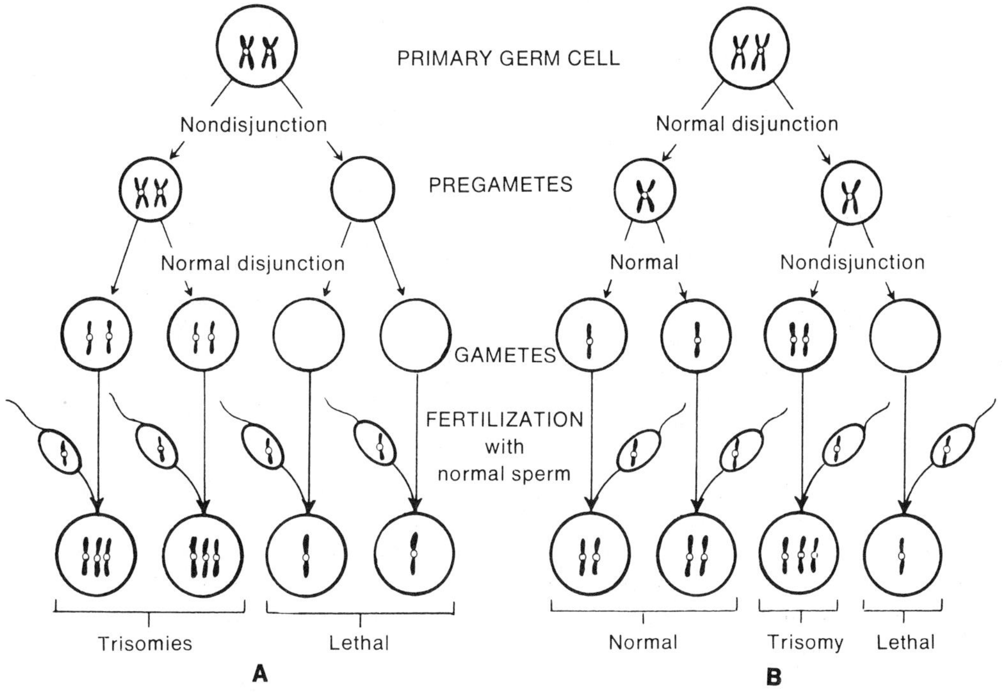

Fig. 6-5. Mechanisms of maldistribution of chromosomes during meiosis in the ovum and fertilization with normal sperm. **A,** During first meiotic division; **B,** during second meiotic division. (From Whaley, L. F.: Understanding inherited disorders, St. Louis, 1974, The C. V. Mosby Co., p. 77.)

the small chromosomes. There has been no reported trisomy for any of the large chromosomes, nor has there been a reported instance of an individual with monosomy of an autosome.

The clinical consequences that attend variations in the chromosomal complement frequently consist of discrete, identifiable syndromes, particularly in regard to the trisomies, for example, trisomy 21 (Down's syndrome), monosomy of the X chromosome (Turner's syndrome), and XXY trisomy (Klinefelter's syndrome). The chromosomal structural anomalies form a more diverse group of reported physical deviations with few recognized syndromes. A large number probably are unrecognized, especially if the variation involves only small segments of a chromosome. Some of the chromosomal disorders, such as Down's syndrome, can be identified on the basis of the physical characteristics; others require chromosomal analysis to establish a chromosomal abnormality as a causative factor. Many of these unidentified cases have been massed together and labeled with the dubious title "funny-looking kid."

Maldistribution of chromosomes

Nondisjunction. The mechanism that is considered to be responsible for maldistribution of chromosomes in the majority of cases is nondisjunction during meiosis. *Disjunction* refers to the separation and migration of chromosomes during cell division; failure of this process is termed *nondisjunction*. The consequence of this prolonged attachment of chromatids during division is an unequal distribution of chromosomes between the two daughter cells. Nondisjunction can take place during ova formation or sperm formation (rare) and can involve autosomes or sex chromosomes. The ratio of trisomic gametes that are produced depends on whether nondisjunction occurs during the first or second meiotic division. The types of germ cells (gametes) that can be formed and the results when they unite with normal gametes are illustrated in Fig. 6-5.

It is believed that nondisjunction occurs primarily, if not exclusively, during germ cell formation in the mother. This hypothesis is based on the observation that the incidence of trisomic births strongly corresponds with increasing maternal age, irregardless of the number of pregnancies, but shows no correlation with the age of the father. There is no positive explanation for these observations. However, unlike the male, who produces fresh sperm continuously throughout his lifetime, the female is born with her total supply of primitive ova that remain in a partial state of meiotic division until, beginning at puberty and extending throughout her reproductive life, once a month a cell is stimulated to complete the process. Consequently these cells are vulnerable to a variety of exogenous influences as well as to the normal effects of the aging process.

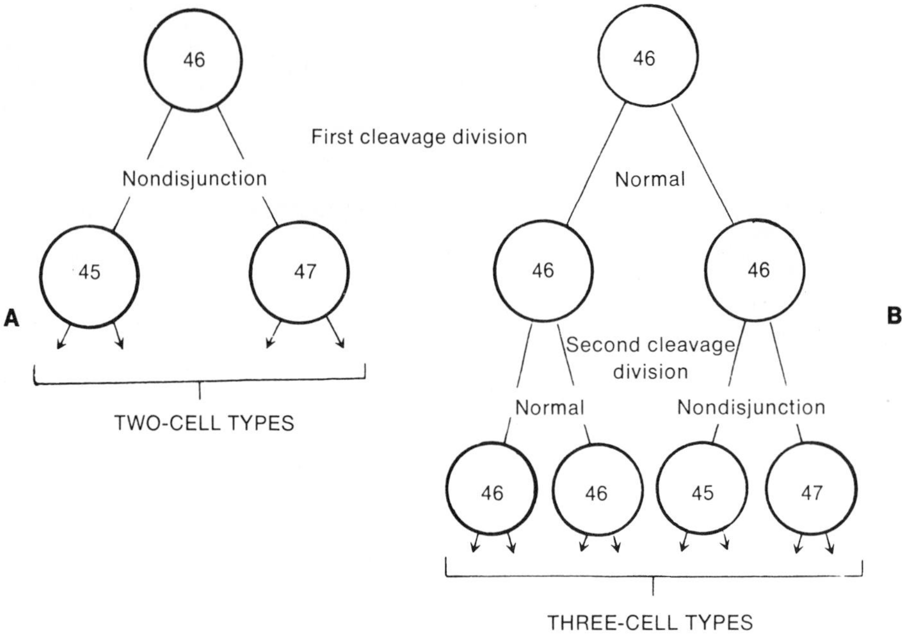

Fig. 6-6. Nondisjunction in early mitotic division of the zygote, which produces a mosaic genotype. **A,** Disjunction at first mitotic division; **B,** disjunction during second mitotic division. (From Whaley, L. F.: Understanding inherited disorders, St. Louis, 1974, The C. V. Mosby Co., p. 78.)

Nondisjunction that occurs during early cell division following fertilization will result in an individual with mixed cell lines. The types of cells and their ratio depend on whether nondisjunction occurs at the first or later divisions. Nondisjunction during the first division produces two cell types: half will contain forty-five chromosomes and half will contain forty-seven chromosomes (Fig. 6-6, *A*). Disjunction that occurs in one of the two normal cells during the second division will produce cells with both normal and abnormal chromosomal constitutions (Fig. 6-6, *B*). An individual whose cells display mixed chromosomal counts is called a *mosaic*. Since monosomic cells are nonviable (with the exception of the X monosomy, which is discussed later), most mosaics have an intermixture of normal and trisomic cells. The extent of clinical manifestations is determined by the type of tissues that contain cells with abnormal chromosomal numbers and may vary from near normal to a fully manifested syndrome.

Translocation. Translocation is a defect in chromosomal structure that occurs when one chromosome becomes attached to another to create one large chromosome. The translocations encountered most frequently are those between wishbone-shaped chromosomes, the best known being the fusion of a group D and a group G chromosome or two group G chromosomes. Because the cells of a person with a translocated chromosome have the normal amount of genetic material, there are no physical abnormalities associated with its possession even though the total chromosomal count is only forty-five. The attached chromosomes give the appearance of one large chromosome and, since they behave as a single chromosome during cell division, can be transmitted from parent to offspring. During the first meiotic division of gamete formation, there may be a balanced or an unbalanced distribution of genetic material. Fig. 6-7 shows the possible distribution of genetic material during germ cell formation and the results when these various cells combine with gametes of normal chromosomal constitution. Persons who are clinically affected because of a translocation have an extra chromosome, although their chromosomal count is forty-six.

There appears to be no correlation between parental age and a translocated chromosome. Parents of a child affected as a result of a translocated chromosome are generally in the younger age-group and have a history of spontaneous abortion of previous pregnancies or a family history of abortions. Often one parent is found to be a carrier with normal characteristics and a chromosomal complement of forty-five chromosomes. In a situation where a parent has a translocation involving a group D or G chromosome, the chances for an affected offspring are estimated to be in the order of one in five when the mother is a carrier and less than one in twenty when the father carries the translocation. An uncommon translocation occurs when the two members of chromosome 21 are fused together in a somatically normal individual. Such a person can produce nothing but affected offspring because the gametes that are formed will contain

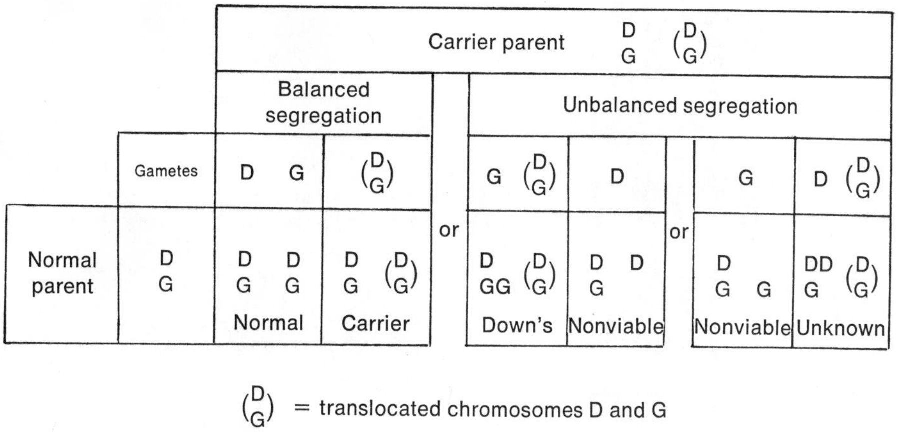

Fig. 6-7. Possible offspring from mating of a somatically normal carrier of a D/G translocation with a genetically and somatically normal individual.

only the translocated chromosome 21 or no chromosome 21 and, thus, will be nonviable.

Chromosomal nomenclature. To clarify and standardize the designating and reporting of chromosomal abnormalities, a standard nomenclature has been developed that identifies individual chromosomal complements according to chromosomal number, sex, and the addition or deletion of the specific chromosome, or part of a chromosome, involved. For example, the complement is recorded as 46,XY or 46,XX for a normal male and female, respectively. A numeric aberration such as a male with an extra group G chromosome is described as 47,XY,G+. The precise chromosome is indicated by number when it can be identified, for example, 47,XY,21+. Structural alterations are designated by the use of several lowercase symbols. The short arm of a chromosome is designated p, the long arm q, and a translocation by the letter t. A translocation between a group D and a group G chromosome would be indicated as 45,XX,D−,G−,t(DqGq)+, which signifies that there are a total of forty-five chromosomes, XX sex chromosomes, and a missing chromosome from both groups D and G, with their long arms uniting to form a D/G chromosome.

Autosomal aberrations

Both numeric and structural abnormalities of autosomes account for a variety of disorders of infancy and childhood. A few are associated with a group of characteristics that clearly indicate the precise chromosomal anomaly. The first disorder in which an associated chromosomal abnormality was demonstrated is Down's syndrome.

Heredity of Down's syndrome. Variously known as trisomy 21 syndrome, trisomy G, "mongolism," and Down's syndrome, this disorder is one of the more common of the trisomies and is a consequence of an extra group G chromosome (Fig. 6-8). The incidence is approximately one in 500 live births. Of this number approximately 95% can be attributed to nondisjunction, usually meiotic nondisjunction in the maternal gamete. A small percentage are mosaics caused by nondisjunction during mitosis following fertilization. The relationship between Down's syndrome and advancing maternal age has been well demonstrated: the frequency in mothers below 35 years of age is approximately one in 1000 to 2000 births; at the age of 35 years the incidence increases to one in 300; and from the age of 40 years the incidence rises sharply to become one in thirty to fifty women over age 45 years.

A small percentage (5%) of cases are caused by translocation in which chromosome 21 becomes attached to another chromosome, usually a group D or another group G chromosome. In this situation maternal age is no factor.

The mechanism by which the syndrome occurs has little effect on the characteristics displayed by the affected child and the management of the disorder. However, it is significant for purposes of genetic counseling. Whereas nondisjunction is usually a sporadic event with evidence of a maternal age effect, a translocation is more often hereditary. It is important to rule out the possibility of a carrier, especially in young parents.

Since the duplicated chromosome 21 is an autosome, it occurs with equal frequency in both boys and girls. Most individuals with Down's syndrome are sterile; however, there are recorded cases in which a female with the disorder passed her extra chromosome to her child, who was similarly affected. In this instance there is, theoretically, a 50% risk of an affected offspring with each pregnancy. In actuality the risk is significantly less since trisomic embryos appear to have decreased viability and are often aborted early in pregnancy.

Recognizing autosomal anomalies. The known viable trisomies (21, 18, and 13) are easily identified, and the diagnosis can nearly always be made early on physical characteristics alone—usually in the delivery room or newborn

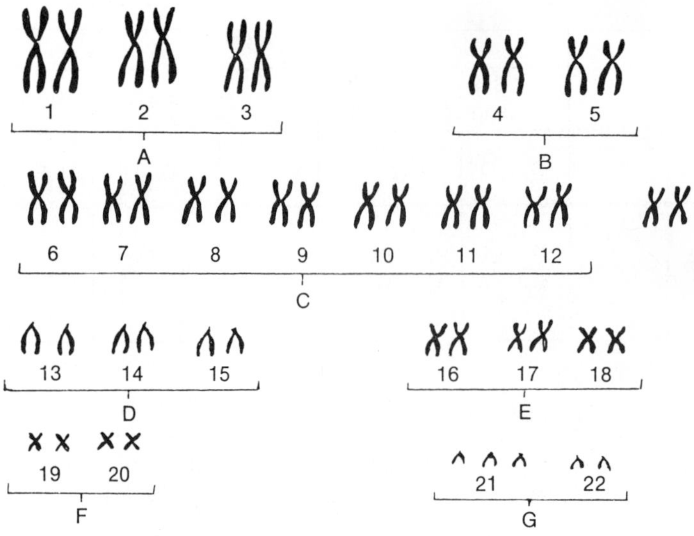

Fig. 6-8. Model of a female karyotype with trisomy of the 21 (G) chromosome group (47,XX,21+). (From Whaley, L. F.: Understanding inherited disorders, St. Louis, 1974, The C. V. Mosby Co., p. 81.)

Table 6-1. Common autosomal aberrations

Syndrome	Chromosomal abnormality and nomenclature	Average Incidence	Major clinical manifestations
Cri du chat	Deletion of short arm of a B (No. 5) chromosome—46,XY,5p−		Distinctive weak, high-pitched mewlike cry resembling the cry of a cat; small head; hypertelorism; failure to thrive; severe mental retardation—profound with age
Trisomy 13 (Patau's)	Trisomy of a group D (No. 13) chromosome—47,XY,13+	1/15,000	Multiple anomalies, including cleft lip and palate (frequently bilateral); ear malformations; microphthalmia; polydactyly; eye defects; mental retardation; early death
Trisomy 18 (Edwards')	Trisomy of a group E (No. 18) chromosome—47,XY,18+	1/5000	Deformed and low-set ears; micrognathia; rocker-bottom feet; overlapping (index over third) fingers; prominent occiput; hypertelorism; failure to thrive and early death; mental retardation
Trisomy 21 (Down's)	Trisomy of a group G (No. 21) chromosome—47,XY,21+ (trisomy); 46XY,D−,G−,(DqGq)+ (translocation); 46,XY/47,XY,21+ (mosaic)	1/500	Brachycephaly with flat occiput; inner epicanthal folds; small ears, nose, and mouth with protruding tongue; muscular hypotonia; broad, short hands with stubby fingers and transverse palmar crease; broad, stubby feet with wide space between big and second toes; mental retardation; variable life expectancy

nursery. The characteristics of the more common autosomal abnormalities are summarized in Table 6-1. The manifestations and related nursing care of children with Down's syndrome are discussed in relation to the major clinical manifestation, mental retardation (p. 812).

Often nurses in the newborn nursery see an infant who has a facial appearance that sets him apart from other infants. The infant may have no obvious congenital malformations, but on closer inspection he may evidence other variations, the sum of which disclose the specific features of known syndromes. These peculiar features or malformations are frequently the result of chromosomal abnormalities and give these infants the "funny looking" aspect that first attracts the observer's attention.

It need not be appearance only that indicates more careful scrutiny of such infants. They may exhibit strange behavior, such as an unusual cry, poor feeding behavior, or abnormal reflex responses. Strange behavior or appearance has been shown to be clinically significant in the diagnosis of infants with most of the identified chromosomal abnormalities but is also useful in recognizing many syndromes associated with other disorders with a genetic basis. As a rule,

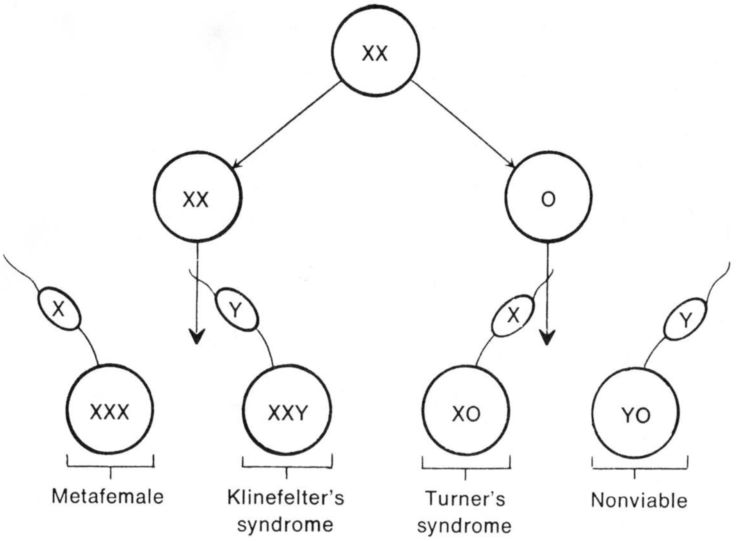

Fig. 6-9. Nondisjunction of X chromosomes in the ovum fertilized by normal sperm to produce the more common sex chromosomal aberrations. (From Whaley, L. F.: Understanding inherited disorders, St. Louis, 1974, The C. V. Mosby Co., p. 86.)

deletion syndromes are less constant in their clinical picture than are trisomies.

Abnormalities of sex chromosomes

Compared with most hereditary disorders, sex chromosomal aberrations are encountered with relatively high frequency. The possible mechanisms by which they may occur are those previously described, that is, prefertilization nondisjunction during one of the meiotic divisions of gametogenesis in either parent or in the early postfertilization divisions of the zygote. Most are a result of an increase in sex chromosomal number as a result of nondisjunction during meiosis. Fig. 6-9 illustrates the manner by which disjunction produces the more common sex chromosomal defects—Klinefelter's and Turner's syndromes. An increase in the number of sex chromosomes does not produce the profound effects that are associated with the autosomal trisomies, although some degree of mental deficiency accompanies a large percentage of them.

This reduced disability in children with multiple sex chromosomes when compared to the severe effects in children with additional autosomes is attributed to an unusual characteristic of sex chromosomes—*X inactivation*. In all body cells only one X chromosome is biologically active; the other (or others) is in some way "switched off" or *inactivated* during the very early divisions of the zygote and remains so throughout life. This inactivated chromosome can be easily observed through a microscope as a condensed dark-staining mass lying on the periphery of the cell nucleus—the *sex chromatin* or *Barr body*. It is established that the maximum number of chromatin bodies is one less than the total number of X chromosomes in that cell nucleus (Fig. 6-10); therefore, female somatic cells are normally chromatin-positive (containing one active and one inactive X chromosome), and male cells are chromatin-negative (containing only one X chromosome). Visible in 20% to 50% of cells, the sex chromatin test provides a convenient means to determine the presence or absence of inactivated X chromosomes in somatic cells. Cells scraped from the buccal mucosa are usually used for this test, which is often performed when a sex chromosomal abnormality is suspected in an infant. Sex chromatin can also be detected in polymorphonuclear leukocytes where it appears as a drumstick-like mass attached to one of the nuclear lobes of the cell.

A number of sex chromosomal abnormalities have been described, and some are listed in Table 6-2. The more common of these, Klinefelter's and Turner's syndromes, will be discussed further in relation to developmental problems of later childhood (pp. 713 and 714). Some general characteristics of sex chromosomal abnormalities are:

1. There is a direct relationship between the male or female phenotype and the presence or absence of a Y chromosome. It appears that the Y chromosome is essential for development of male characteristics.
2. The severity of defects is not related to the number of extra X chromosomes, except for mental retardation, which increases proportionately with each X chromosome.
3. The presence of more than one Y chromosome appears to have variable but as yet not well-defined effects on the phenotype.

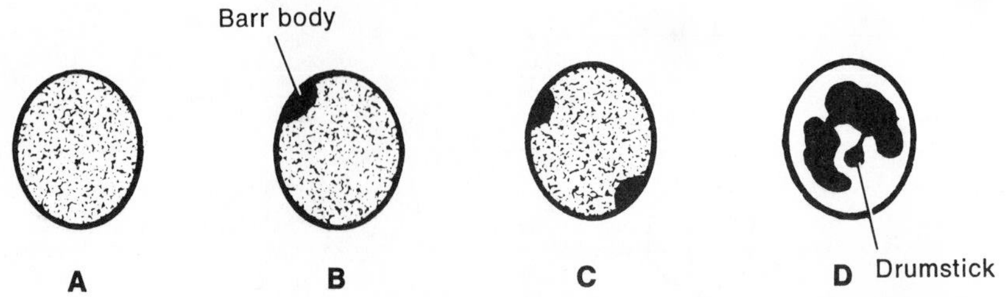

Fig. 6-10. Sex chromatin, or Barr body. **A,** No sex chromatin is found in normal male somatic cells. **B,** One Barr body is normal in female somatic cells. **C,** Two Barr bodies are found in cells with three X chromosomes (XXX or XXXY). **D,** The drumstick is found in many polymorphonuclear leukocytes of the normal female. (From Whaley, L. F.: Understanding inherited disorders, St. Louis, 1974, The C. V. Mosby Co., p. 85.)

Table 6-2. Common sex chromosomal abnormalities

Syndrome	Chromosomal nomenclature	Phenotype	X chromosome	Y chromosome	Clinical manifestations
Turner's	45,X	Female	0	0	Short stature; webbed neck; low posterior hair-line; shield-shaped chest with widely spaced nipples; sterile
Triple X or superfemale	47,XXX (can also be 48,XXXX or 49,XXXXX)	Female	+1 or more	0	Normal female characteristics; usually mentally retarded; mental deficiency in others; fertile
XYY male	47,XYY (can also be 48,XYYY or mosaic)	Male	0	+ 1 per Y	Usually normal sex development; tendency to be tall with long head; poor coordination; may demonstrate aberrant behavior
Klinefelter's	47,XXY (48,XXYY, 48,XXXY, 49,XXXXY, etc. mosaics)	Male	+ 1 or more (1 per X)	+ 1 per Y	Tall with long legs; hypogenitalism; sterile; male secondary sex characteristics may be deficient; may demonstrate aberrant behavior

DISORDERS CAUSED BY A SINGLE MUTANT GENE

Disorders for which a simple, definite inheritance pattern can be identified are rare individually, but collectively they constitute a sizable portion of health problems seen in infants and children. They can involve any system in the body. They can be of such minor importance that they have little effect on the child or so severe as to cause serious disability or be incompatible with life.

The fundamental principles of mendelian genetics, which describe the activity of genes during gamete formation and fertilization, form the basis for understanding these inherited disorders. The statistically predictable results of combinations and recombinations of genes and their distribution in families can be summarized by the following:

principles of dominance not all genes that determine a given trait operate with equal vigor. When two genes at a given locus produce a different effect (for example, the gene for eye color) they may compete for expression in the individual. As a result, one may mask or conceal the effect of the other. The characteristic that is manifest in the individual (and the gene that produces the effect) is referred to as *dominant;* that which is hidden and not manifest is *recessive*.

principle of segregation the paired chromosomes, bearing genes derived from each parent, are separated when gametes are formed during meiosis. Each gene segregates in pure form, and chance alone determines which gene (paternally derived or maternally derived) will travel to which gamete.

principle of independent assortment the members of one pair of genes are distributed in the gametes in random fashion independent of other pairs.

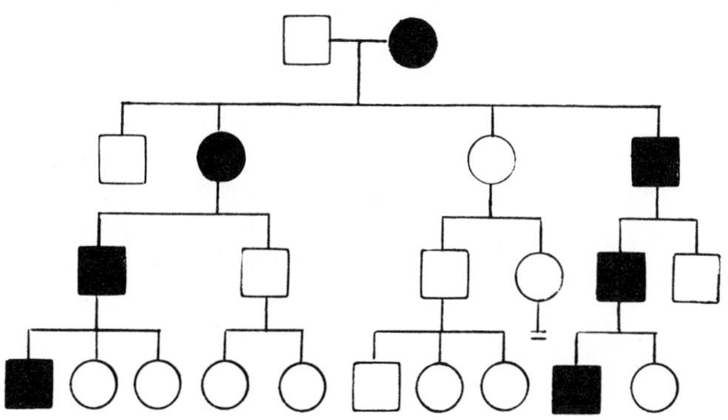

A

		Affected parent	
	Gametes	A	a
Normal parent	a	A a Affected	a a Normal
	a	A a Affected	a a Normal

B

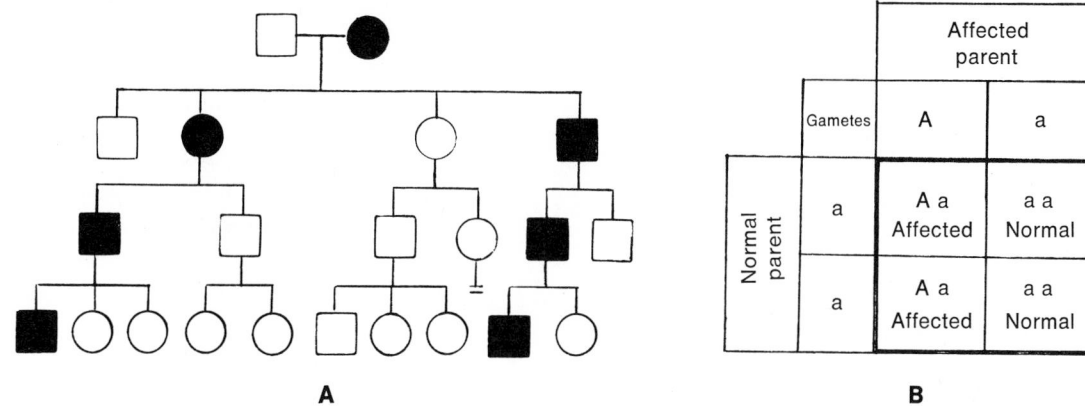

Fig. 6-11. Autosomal-dominant inheritance pattern occurring in four generations. **A,** Pedigree. **B,** Possible offspring of mating between normal parent and one with autosomal-dominant trait.

Mutation. A mutation is a change in genetic material. It can be either spontaneous or induced, and, although a rare occurrence, the genetic material becomes altered or rearranged in such a way that it no longer serves its original function. Genes are usually stable units, but when a gene changes the mutant gene is equally stable and is transmitted to future generations.

Autosomal inheritance patterns

Conditions that can be directly attributed to a single gene are distributed in families in characteristic patterns according to the basic principles just described. Genes are either dominant or recessive in their effect, and most disorders caused by a single gene can be recognized readily by the simple mendelian family patterns that they display.

Some generalizations can be made regarding diseases and malformations caused by a single gene on either the autosomes or sex chromosomes. Disorders resulting from structural defects seem to be primarily the result of dominant genes; most metabolic defects appear to be caused by recessive genes. Dominant traits are seen more frequently and are usually less severe than are recessive traits. This is probably because of the "double-dose" effect. Whereas recessive traits are only manifest when both genes are present, a dominant disorder usually involves a single gene from a heterozygous parent. The presence of a normal gene appears to overcome the effect of a recessive gene and to reduce the severity of a dominant gene.

The major inheritance patterns are described with stylized models indicating the mendelian ratios that can be predicted in each type. Since there are forty-four autosomes and only two sex chromosomes, the majority of hereditary disorders are a result of defective genes on an autosome.

Autosomal-dominant inheritance. Characteristics of a condition caused by a dominant gene on an autosome include the following (Fig. 6-11)[4]:

1. Males and females are affected with equal frequency.
2. Affected individuals will have an affected parent (unless the condition is caused by a fresh mutation).
3. Half the children of a heterozygous affected parent will be affected.
4. Normal children of affected parents will have normal children.
5. Traits can be traced vertically through previous generations—a positive family history.

Usually the first case in a family appears suddenly as the result of a fresh mutation and, depending on the degree of disability the condition imposes on the individual, will either die out or continue to be passed on through several generations. Examples of an autosomal-dominant disorder include achondroplasia, osteogenesis imperfecta, polydactyly, and Marfan's syndrome.

Autosomal-recessive inheritance. Characteristics of a condition caused by a recessive gene on an autosome include the following (Fig. 6-12)[4]:

1. Males and females are affected with equal frequency.
2. Affected individuals will have unaffected parents who are heterozygous for the trait.
3. One fourth of the children of two unaffected heterozygous parents will be affected.
4. Two affected parents will have affected children exclusively.
5. Affected individuals married to unaffected individuals will have normal children, all of whom will be carriers.
6. There is usually no evidence of the trait in antecedent generations—a negative family history.

Children who display an autosomal-recessive disorder will always be homozygous for that trait. The heterozygous person, with only one gene for a rare recessive disorder, remains undetected in the population. It is estimated that each person carries from three to eight genes for such a severe genetic disease. However, the probability of mating

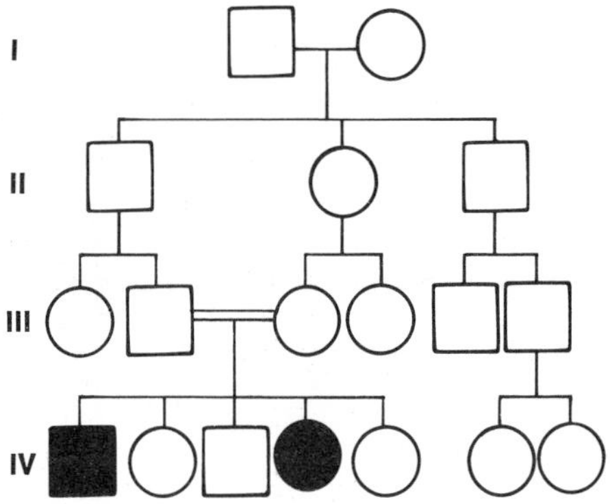

A

		Heterozygous parent A/a	
	Gametes	A	a
Heterozygous parent A/a	A	AA Normal	Aa Carrier
	a	Aa Carrier	aa Affected

B

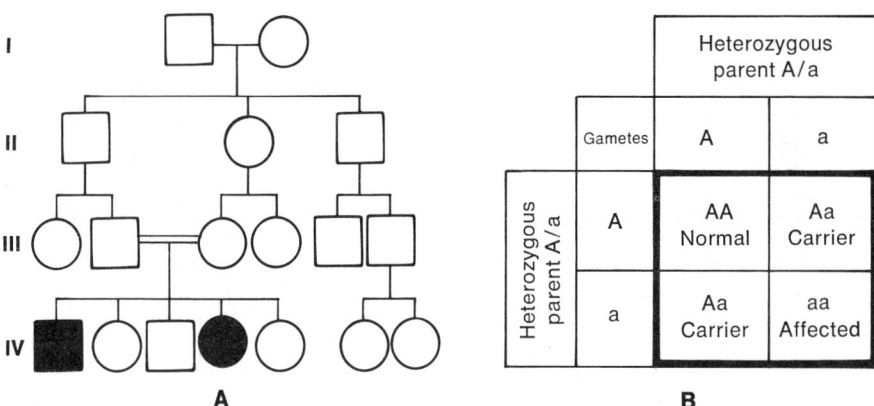

Fig. 6-12. Autosomal-recessive inheritance pattern. **A,** Pedigree. **B,** Possible offspring of mating between two parents with a recessive gene on an autosome.

between two persons who carry the same gene is highly unlikely. If they are blood relatives, the likelihood is increased. Examples of an autosomal-recessive disorder include cystic fibrosis, phenylketonuria, and galactosemia.

Codominance. In codominance both allelic genes of a pair are expressed equally; neither is recessive to the other. This is characteristic of the major blood groups, such as the ABO blood groups in which both the A and the B antigens are dominant. The O trait, without antigens, behaves as a recessive gene. This is clearly illustrated by the person who has type AB blood. The *A* or *B* phenotype can be homozygous *(AA; BB)* or heterozygous *(AO; BO)*. The individual with type O blood is always homozygous *(OO)*.

X-linked inheritance patterns

Genes on the X chromosome differ from those on the Y chromosome; therefore, the transmission of traits caused by these genes will vary according to the sex of the individual who carries the gene. The two X chromosomes in the female are alike in gene constitution with two genes for each trait. Genes in the X chromosome have no counterpart on the Y chromosome; therefore, a characteristic determined by a gene on the X chromosome is *always* expressed in the male. One of the most significant aspects of X-linked inheritance is the absence of father-to-son transmission. Although it is essential for development of the male phenotype, the Y chromosome carries no known medically significant characteristics.

X-linked dominant inheritance. Characteristics of a condition caused by a dominant gene on an X chromosome include the following (Figs. 6-13 and 6-14)[4]:

1. Affected individuals will have an affected parent.
2. All the daughters but none of the sons of an affected male will be affected.
3. Half the sons and half the daughters of an affected female will be affected.

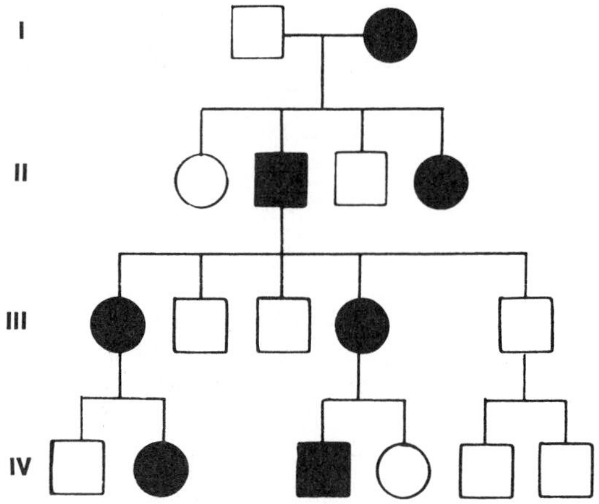

Fig. 6-13. X-linked–dominant inheritance pattern. (From Whaley, L. F.: Understanding inherited disorders, St. Louis, 1974, The C. V. Mosby Co., p. 40.)

4. Normal children of an affected parent will have normal offspring.
5. The inheritance pattern shows a positive family history.

Superficially this pattern resembles an autosomal-dominant inheritance pattern. An example of an X-linked dominant disorder is hypophosphatemic vitamin D—resistant rickets.

X-linked recessive inheritance. Characteristics of a disorder caused by a recessive gene on the X chromosome include the following (Figs. 6-15 and 6-16)[4]:

1. Affected individuals are principally males.
2. Affected individuals will have unaffected parents (except in the rare possibility that the father is affected and the mother is a carrier).
3. Half of the female siblings of an affected male will be carriers of the trait.

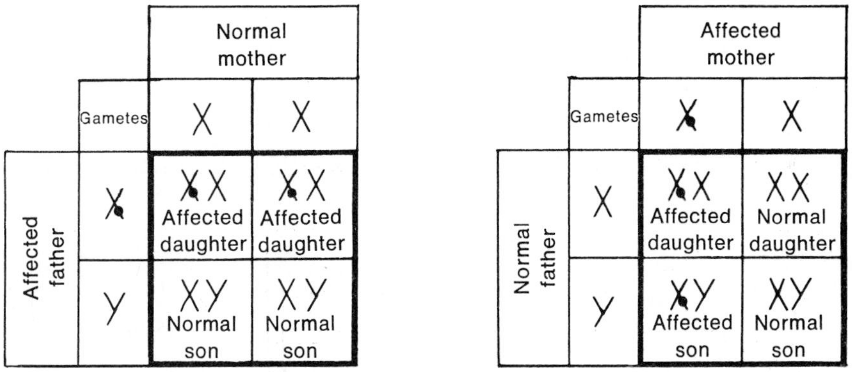

Fig. 6-14. Punnett square illustrating the sex differences in offspring ratios in X-linked–dominant inheritance. • = Dominant allele on X chromosome. (From Whaley, L. F.: Understanding inherited disorders, St. Louis, 1974, The C. V. Mosby Co., p. 40.)

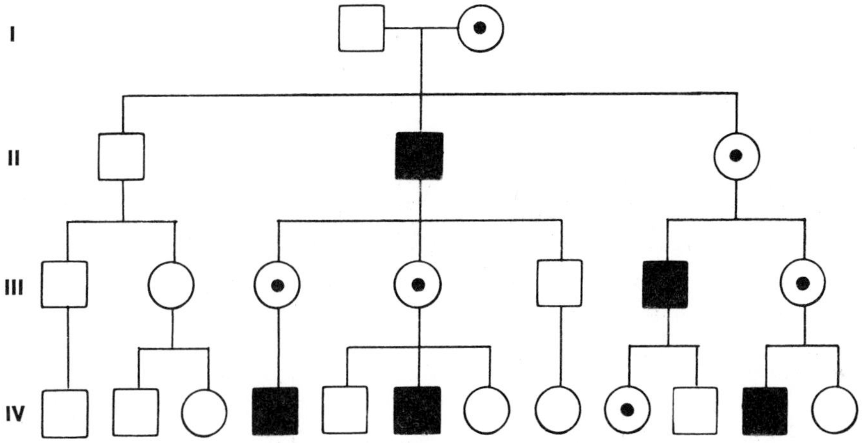

Fig. 6-15. X-linked–recessive inheritance pattern. (From Whaley, L. F.: Understanding inherited disorders, St. Louis, 1974, The C. V. Mosby Co., p. 41.)

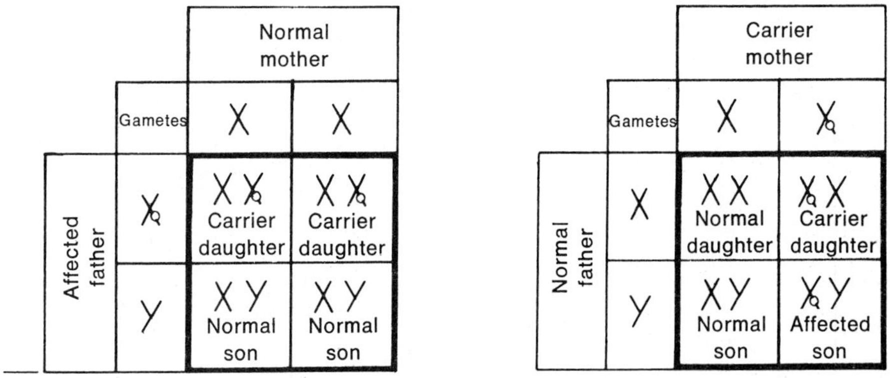

Fig. 6-16. Punnett square illustrating the sex differences in offspring ratios in X-linked–recessive inheritance. ◦ = Recessive allele on X chromosome. (From Whaley, L. F.: Understanding inherited disorders, St. Louis, 1974, The C. V. Mosby Co., p. 41.)

4. Unaffected male siblings of an affected male cannot transmit the disorder.
5. Sons of an affected male are unaffected.
6. Daughters of an affected male are carriers.
7. The unaffected male children of a carrier female do not transmit the disorder.

The abnormal gene behaves as any recessive gene, that is, its effect will be hidden by a normal dominant gene. Examples of an X-linked recessive disorder include hemophilia (p. 1390) and Duchenne type muscular dystrophy (p. 1522).

Variations of inheritance patterns

There are a number of variables, such as penetrance, expressivity, and pleiotropy, that may modify the basic inheritance patterns. The degree to which a gene exerts its effect or the differences in effects that a given gene may produce sometimes appears to contradict the established concepts of inheritance.

penetrance the regularity with which an inherited trait is manifest in the person who carries the gene. When a gene produces its effect on the phenotype each time it is present in the genotype, it is said to be *fully penetrant* or to exhibit *complete penetrance*. For example, achondroplasia (a form of dwarfism) is always evident whenever the gene is present. If a trait is not recognized in a person who carries the gene for it, it is said to be *nonpenetrant* in that individual. This accounts for what appears to be skipped generations. For instance, retinoblastoma, a tumor of the retina, is 90% penetrant because 10% of the children who carry the gene do not develop the tumor.

expressivity the degree of severity of, or the variability in, the manifestations seen in persons of a particular genotype. For instance, polydactyly can be expressed as any number of extra digits, or the extra digits may be fingers in one generation and toes in another. The severity of a disorder may be so mild as to be almost undetected or so severe that the affected individual is totally incapacitated.

pleiotropy the multiple, different, and seemingly unrelated effects associated with a particular disorder; the varied clinical features that constitute a syndrome. For example, Marfan's syndrome, a disorder of the elastic fibers of connective tissue, may be manifest in an individual by any or all of the symptoms associated with it—aortic aneurysm, dislocation of the optic lens, or any of a number of skeletal deformities.

Inborn errors of metabolism

End products of gene action are proteins—either structural cell components or enzymes. Genes are potentially mutable units; therefore, a change in a gene will disturb the synthesis of the specific protein for which it is responsible. This results in the formation of a different protein (or no protein at all), which alters the process or processes that depend on it. When the protein is absent or deficient the normal process is impaired, resulting in phenotypic effects of greater or lesser consequence to the individual. The defects in cellular enzyme formation are known as *inborn errors of metabolism,* and most are characterized by abnormal protein, carbohydrate, or fat metabolism.

All biochemical processes are under genetic control, and each consists of a complex sequence of reactions. Fig. 6-17, *A,* schematically represents a portion of a normal metabolic pathway. A substrate (the substance on which an enzyme acts) is converted to a product through the action of a specific enzyme. A metabolic pathway consists of many such reactions, or steps, each depending on the previous reaction and each catalyzed by a specific enzyme. Fig. 6-17, *B,* illustrates how a change in a gene that interferes with the synthesis of an essential enzyme interrupts this process. A block in the normal pathway can produce an accu-

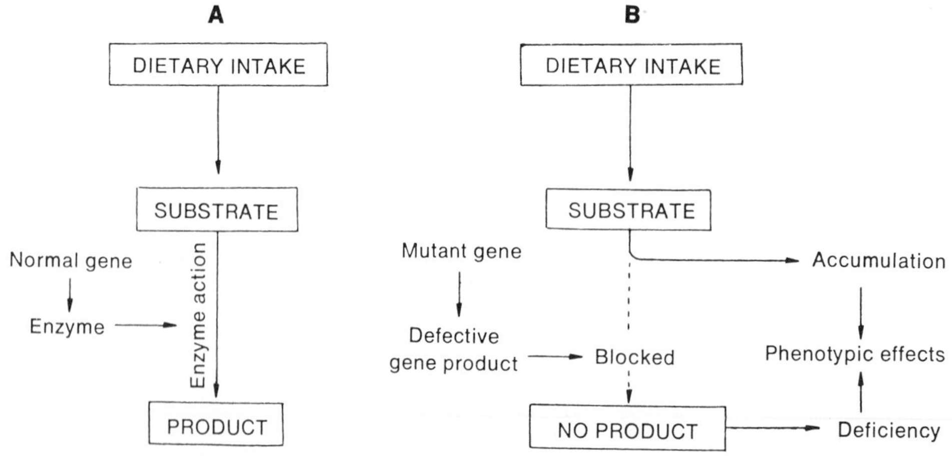

Fig. 6-17. Metabolic pathway. **A,** Normal metabolic pathway. **B,** Effect of defective gene action. (From Whaley, L. F.: Understanding inherited disorders, St. Louis, 1974, The C. V. Mosby Co., p. 48.)

mulation of the products preceding the block, such as galactose in galactosemia or phenylalanine in phenylketonuria, or might create a deficiency in the product, such as melanin in albinism or thyroxine in familial cretinism. Sometimes alternate pathways are used and there is an increase in the products of these processes, such as the production of phenylketones in phenylketonuria. These effects of defective gene action are observable in the individual as diseases.

Varying degrees of success have been achieved by attempts to alter or modify the adverse effects resulting from defects in metabolism. In some diseases the deficient product is supplied, such as thyroid extract in cretinism. Limiting the intake of a substance that the body is unable to metabolize properly decreases the accumulation of its toxic metabolites, such as phenylalanine restriction in phenylketonuria and elimination of milk sugar in galactosemia.

There are many inherited disorders caused by an inborn error of metabolism that involves either the buildup or breakdown of metabolic processes (Table 6-3). They are

Table 6-3. Partial list of single-gene disorders

Diseases	Inheritance	Basic defect	Manifestations	Therapy
Achondroplasia	Autosomal dominant	Defect in ossification at epiphyseal plate (growth portion of bones)	Very short limbs; large head; lordosis	None
Adrenogenital syndrome	Autosomal recessive	21-Hydroxylase deficiency; failure of hydrocortisone synthesis in adrenal cortex	Virilization	Hydrocortisone
Albinism	Autosomal recessive	Deficiency of tyrosinase; failure to convert tyrosine to dopa and, hence, lack of melanin synthesis	Lack of pigment in skin, hair, and eyes; eye defects	None; avoid exposure to sunlight; ophthalmologic care
Arachnodactyly (Marfan's syndrome)	Autosomal dominant	Defect in elastic fibers of connective tissues	Tall, thin individuals with long tapering fingers; poorly developed musculature; associated defects include aortic aneurysm, dislocation of optic lens, winged scapula	Surgical correction of deformities
Crigler-Najjar syndrome	Autosomal recessive	Glucuronyl transferase deficiency; inability to convert indirect bilirubin to direct bilirubin	Jaundice; spasticity; opisthotonus; early death	None
Cystic fibrosis	Autosomal recessive	Unknown; defect in mucous-secreting glands; sweat glands secrete abnormal amounts of sodium chloride	Meconium ileus in newborn; celiac syndrome; pulmonary disease; failure to thrive	Inhalation therapy; antibiotics; pancreatic enzymes
Cystinosis (Fanconi's syndrome)	Autosomal recessive	Renal transport mechanism	Skeletal abnormalities; cystine crystals in tissues; chronic acidosis; polyuria; photophobia; early death	Vitamin D; supplementary actinium and phosphorus; penicillamine (?)
Familial cretinism	Autosomal recessive	Deficiency of iodotyrosine deiodinase	Lethargy; stunted growth; mental retardation	Early administration of thyroid hormone
Galactosemia	Autosomal recessive	Deficiency of galactose-1-phosphate uridyl transferase; inability to convert galactose to glucose	Failure to thrive; mental and motor retardation; cataracts; jaundice; hepatomegaly; cirrhosis of the liver	Eliminate galactose from diet

Continued.

Table 6-3. Partial list of single-gene disorders—cont'd

Diseases	Inheritance	Basic defect	Manifestations	Therapy
Glucose-6-phosphate dehydrogenase deficiency (G-6-PD deficiency)	X-linked recessive	Deficiency of glucose-6-phosphate dehydrogenase	Asymptomatic under normal circumstances; certain drugs (primaquine, acetanilid, sulfanilamide, and naphthalene) as well as ingestion of fava beans produce hemolytic anemia and jaundice	Avoid agents that precipitate clinical symptoms
Hemophilia A	X-linked recessive	Deficiency of blood factor VIII prevents coagulation of blood	Uncontrollable bleeding after trauma, may be spontaneous; hematomas in any tissue; bleeding in joints, especially elbow, knee, and ankle, eventually causing stiffness and deformity	Blood transfusion; prophylactic administration of cryoprecipitates, lyophilized concentrates; plasma (fresh); prevention of trauma
Hemophilia B	X-linked recessive	Deficiency of blood factor IX prevents coagulation of blood	Same but less severe than hemophilia A	Plasma (fresh); lyophilized concentrates
Hunter's syndrome	X-linked recessive	Defect in metabolism of mucopolysaccharides	Gargoyle features; dwarfism; less severe than Hurler's syndrome; progressive mental deterioration	None
Hurler's syndrome	Autosomal recessive	Defect in metabolism of mucopolysaccharides	Gargoyle features; dwarfism; clouding of cornea; more severe than Hunter's syndrome; mental retardation; early death	None
Hypophosphatasia	Autosomal recessive	Deficiency of alkaline phosphatase	Skeletal abnormalities	None
Maple syrup urine disease	Autosomal recessive	Defective metabolism of branched chain amino acids	Onset in early infancy; neurologic disorders; odor of urine similar to that of maple syrup	Diet low in branched chain amino acids
McArdle syndrome	Autosomal recessive	Deficiency of muscle phosphorylase	Muscle weakness	Glucagon injections
Muscular dystrophy	Autosomal dominant; autosomal recessive; X-linked recessive	Unknown; appears to be caused by metabolic disturbance unrelated to nervous system	Progressive weakness and wasting of skeletal muscles, with increasing disability and deformity; most severe form, X-linked Duchenne type, is fatal in second or early third decade	Symptomatic; prevention of deformities
Nephrogenic diabetes insipidus	Autosomal dominant (?); X-linked recessive (?)	Failure of renal tubules to respond to antidiuretic hormone	Polyuria with low specific gravity; polydypsia	Prevent dehydration; thiazide diuretics
Niemann-Pick disease	Autosomal recessive	Disturbed lipid metabolism that leads to excessive sphingomyelin in reticuloendothelial cells in central nervous system	Progressive neurologic deterioration; blindness; hepatomegaly; death in early childhood	None

Table 6-3. Partial list of single-gene disorders—cont'd

Diseases	Inheritance	Basic defect	Manifestations	Therapy
Retinoblastoma	Autosomal dominant	Malignant tumor of retina	Onset before age 2 years; cat's eye reflex; strabismus; red, painful eye, often with glaucoma; blindness	Radiation therapy; enucleation
Sickle cell anemia	Autosomal recessive	Abnormal hemoglobin structure (Hb S instead of Hb A); deoxygenation produces changes in red blood cell shape that cause these cells to obstruct blood flow in small vessels; destruction of sickled cells	Presence of characteristic sickle-shaped red blood cells; chronic hemolytic anemia; episodes of pain from tissue ischemia caused by occulsion of small blood vessels; symptoms directly related to tissues and organs involved	No definitive treatment; palliative therapy during acute attacks
Tay-Sachs disease (amaurotic familial idiocy)	Autosomal recessive	Deficiency of hexosaminidase; defect in synthesis of gangliosides	Predominantly in Ashkenazi Jews; progressive neurologic deterioration; blindness—cherry-red spot in macula; early death	None
Thalassemias	Autosomal recessive	Impaired protein synthesis of hemoglobin that results in shortened red blood cell survival time	Severe, fatal anemia in major forms; most do not survive childhood	Palliative; blood transfusion and sometimes splenectomy
Tyrosinosis	Autosomal recessive	Deficiency of *p*-hydroxyphenylpyruvic acid oxidase	Hepatosplenomegaly	None
Vitamin D (hypophosphatemic)–resistant rickets	X-linked dominant	Defect in phosphate reabsorption in renal tubules	Rachitic symptoms; retarded linear growth	Calciferol; administration of phosphorus; megadoses of vitamin D, with care to avoid toxic effects
von Gierke's disease	Autosomal recessive (?)	Deficiency of glucose-6-phosphatase; inability to reconvert glycogen to glucose	Hepatomegaly; vomiting; hypoglycemia; convulsions; coma; usually early death	High-protein diet; no definitive therapy
Werdnig-Hoffmann disease	Autosomal recessive	Unknown; atrophy of anterior horn cells in spinal cord and motor nuclei in brain stem	Onset before age 2 years and usually apparent at birth; "floppy" infant; lies in frog position; fatal in childhood—the earlier the onset, the earlier death	Symptomatic
Wilson's disease	Autosomal recessive	Deficiency of plasma protein ceruloplasmin; disturbed copper metabolism	Progressive lenticular degeneration with neurologic deterioration; cirrhosis of liver; renal calculi	Administration of copper chelating agent penicillamine

rare diseases, and the mode of inheritance is almost always autosomal recessive. This is best understood by considering the double-dose effect as it relates to the concept that one gene is responsible for one enzyme. If a specific gene controls the formation of an essential enzyme and each individual has two such genes (the normal homozygote), then the enzyme is produced in normal amounts. The heterozygote, who has one gene with a normal effect, is still able to produce the enzyme in sufficient amounts to carry out the metabolic function under normal circumstances. Therefore, the heterozygote does not exhibit symptoms of the disorder, whereas the abnormal homozygote, who inherits a defective gene from both parents, has no functioning enzyme and is, thus, clinically affected. Some of the more significant inborn errors of metabolism and related nursing responsibilities are discussed in greater detail in other chapters.

DISORDERS CAUSED BY GENETIC AND ENVIRONMENTAL FACTORS

There are a number of diseases and defects that are frequently encountered in the population and that show an increased incidence in some families. Although this incidence is higher than would be expected by chance, no specific mode of inheritance can be identified. In some, environmental factors appear to play an important role. These are the conditions classified as *multifactorial*—disorders in which a genetic susceptibility combined with the appropriate environmental agents interact to produce a disease state. With multifactorial traits there is no clear-cut affected-unaffected classification. Rather, there is a *continuous variation* in the effects with a few persons at one end, a few at the other, and the majority of persons graded between the two extremes. Most differences between normal human beings are a result of continuous variation.

A term used in relation to, and sometimes interchangeably with, multifactorial is *polygenic* (literally meaning many genes), which is usually used to describe the genetic component of multifactorial inheritance. Polygenes are those genes that do not produce a large effect but are a number of minor genes at different positions on the chromosomes whose combined effects produce a given characteristic, each making a small contribution to the total effect. The effects of each gene are small and additive so that the trait produced is the result of the activity of many genes in the right combination.

When the laws of inheritance are applied to polygenic characteristics, it is expected that relatives will have more genes in common. Therefore, there is an increased likelihood that these genes will be expressed more often when united with a similar combination of genes. If the gene(s) is very common, relatives will receive it from different sources; if the gene is a rare one, they will seldom inherit it. Table 6-4 shows the proportion of genes that relatives have in common. The more distant the relationship, the fewer the shared genes. A very simple rule can be applied: *for each step further away in relationship the number of genes in common is reduced by one half;* that is, parent and child have half their genes in common, child and grandparent have one fourth their genes in common, etc. In families where there is an increased incidence of a disorder, the frequency in first-degree relatives may be three to fifteen times the incidence in the population as a whole. More than one affected family member indicates a greater number of polygenes in common (Table 6-5). However, socioeconomic differences or seasonal distribution might suggest environmental influences.

Table 6-4. Proportion of genes in common in various relationships

Relationship	Proportion of genes in common
First-degree relatives	
Parent, child, sibling	1/2
Second-degree relatives	
Grandparent, grandchild, uncle, aunt, nephew, niece, half-sibling	1/4
Third-degree relatives	
First cousins	1/8
Second cousins	1/32

Table 6-5. Inherited component in some common conditions

Condition	Incidence		Concordance in twins	
	General population	First-degree relatives (%)	Monozygotic (%)	Dizygotic (%)
Cleft lip and palate	1/625	5	18	2
Clubfoot	1/1000	2.5	35	3
Congenital dislocated hip	1/500	5	40	3
Congenital heart disease	1/500	3.7	25	5
Juvenile diabetes mellitus	1/500	6.7	49	1
Pyloric stenosis	3/1000	6.7	30-50	4.5
Schizophrenia	1/100	10	40-60	10-14

Traits that best illustrate a multifactorial cause are stature, intelligence, and skin color. Although a trait such as height is primarily attributed to the action of polygenes, environmental factors such as poor nutrition, assortative mating (for example, tall persons tend to marry each other), or a chronic disease may distort the picture.

The appearance of clinical manifestations of multifactorial traits requires a strong genetic predisposition that places susceptible individuals at a point of risk where environmental influences determine whether (and in some cases to what extent) they will be affected. Diseases or disorders that fall into this category are diabetes mellitus, schizophrenia, and psoriasis. The more common congenital defects, for example, cleft lip and palate, congenital dislocated hip, pyloric stenosis, and so on, appear to be consistent with polygenic inheritance.

The study of twins is a method that has been proved of value in providing information about the roles of heredity and environment in the development of specific traits. Since monozygotic (identical) twins have the same genotype, a disease or trait appearing with higher frequency in them than in dizygotic (fraternal) twins suggests a genetic etiology. Since both types normally grow up under the same or similar conditions, any differences that appear in dizgotic but not in monozygotic pairs can be attributed to differences in genotypes. Differences that appear in both monozygotic and dizygotic twins must be the result of environmental influences, although these are usually difficult to determine. If both members of a pair of twins display the trait under observation, they are said to be *concordant* for that trait; if only one of a pair of twins displays the trait, the twins are said to be *discordant* for that trait.

Congenital malformations

Congenital malformations, or birth defects, constitute a large heterogeneous group of defects and disorders that are so variable in type and causation that there is no satisfactory method for classifying them. A few are clearly caused by a single gene; others are associated with chromosomal abnormalities. There are some congenital malformations that are produced by known intrauterine environmental factors. However, many of the more common and severe malformations (for example, central nervous system malformations, cataracts, and congenital heart disease) fit in no clearly defined category. There is a high correlation between the incidence of congenital malformations and the infant who is small for gestational age. The more severe the growth retardation, the more likely the chance for malformation.

Because of the steady decline in infant mortality from other causes, congenital malformations, although not increasing in incidence, are responsible for an ever-increasing proportion of all deaths in infancy. They also constitute an increasing proportion of infants requiring intensive newborn care. Since many malformations are not readily recognized in the neonatal period or until the infants are in severe distress, early and careful observation and assessment are assuming increasing importance in neonatal nursing care.

Nongenetic factors can produce a congenital malformation that imitates, or is indistinguishable from, one genetically determined. Such a condition is termed a *phenocopy*. For example, deafness, cretinism, and cataracts can all be caused by mutant genes, but they may also be caused by exogenous agents. Deafness can be a result of a number of different agents, rubella virus can cause congenital cataracts, and lack of iodine in a child can produce cretinism. Assigning a cause of mental retardation presents a particularly difficult problem. Mental retardation is a manifestation of a variety of syndromes, both single-gene and chromosomal, and numerous environmental agents are known to be damaging to brain tissue, for example, lack of oxygen as a result of anesthesia or drugs during labor and delivery. For this reason it is extremely important that such exogenous factors be ruled out before any given congenital defect is labeled hereditary.

DETECTION OF GENETIC DISEASE

Tests to detect the presence of a defective gene are rapidly assuming greater importance in management of genetic disorders as more defects are identified and techniques are developed for easy application. A number of screening programs to identify persons who possess defective genes are now carried out for a variety of specific diseases. It is probable that, with improved technology, mass screening for numerous defects may eventually be a routine procedure. However, to be truly effective, screening programs must be accompanied by education and counseling.

Genetic screening[2]

Genetic screening is screening of a population of persons for those who possess a specific genotype. There are several purposes for this screening: (1) to detect the presence of disease, incipient or overt, (2) to provide reproductive information, and (3) to gain information concerning the incidence of a disorder in the population.

Screening for disease. The rationale for screening for disease in the general population or for specific diseases in persons at risk is to discover those persons who: (1) have the disease, either manifest or incipient; or (2) may, in time or under special circumstances, develop the disease. The purpose of this knowledge is to anticipate serious consequences and provide the individual with treatment and management that will prevent, reverse, or diminish the adverse effects of the disorder. An example is the generalized, systematic screening of all newborn infants for phenylketonuria (PKU), a disorder in which the child is unable to properly metabolize the amino acid phenylalanine. This disease eventually leads to mental retardation in perhaps 95% of affected children (see p. 316). Screening techniques are available for an increasing number of disorders and are carried out on infants suspected of having a disease such as cystic fibrosis (p. 1252), Duchenne type muscular dystrophy (p. 1522), or the diseases known collectively as inborn errors of metabolism. Another example of such screening is prenatal diagnosis by amniocentesis. Although it carries a certain amount of risk, this technique has been employed to detect affected fetuses for a variety of inborn errors of metabolism, chromosomal abnormalities, some central nervous system abnormalities, and sex of infant in sex-related disorders.

Screening for reproductive information. From a reproductive viewpoint, screening can discover healthy persons in the population who carry genes that, when they mate with an individual who carries a similar gene, have a high risk of producing an affected offspring. These individuals are thus provided with the knowledge they need for use in decisions about family planning. Carriers of a number of diseases can be detected by laboratory tests, but because of their rarity, mass screening is unfeasible except in persons known to be at risk, for example, close relatives of persons affected with an inborn error of metabolism or certain ethnic populations known to have a high incidence of a specific disease such as sickle cell anemia in blacks and Tay-Sachs disease in Ashkenazic Jews. This reproductive screening has been extended to include testing of the unborn child by amniocentesis to detect the presence of genetic disease in persons at risk.

Screening for epidemiologic information. Public health officials may use screening as a method of monitoring the incidence of diseases or malformations in a population in order to detect environmental or other causes that might be a cause of significant influence in the incidence of the disorder. For example, the observation that the incidence of a syndrome was significantly increased in a population 8 to 10 months after a German measles epidemic led to the discovery that this disease has a significant damaging impact on the unborn child during the first trimester of pregnancy.

Significance of screening. Mass screening programs have not been enthusiastically endorsed and carried out by all members of the health professions nor wholeheartedly accepted by the public. However, with the success of several well-organized and/or legislated programs and their significance in the prevention of disease or of the damaging effects of disease, an increasing number of programs are gaining acceptance and support. Much depends on education of both health professionals and the public regarding these programs.

GENETIC COUNSELING

In recent years the significance of heredity as an etiologic agent in disease and disability has assumed a more prominent place in the nursing of infants and children. Medical science has made rapid advances in the control of infectious diseases and nutritional disorders that formerly accounted for the major share of deaths in infancy. At the same time, contributions from the fields of biochemistry and cytology have established a genetic basis for an increasing number of diseases and disorders. Consequently nurses encounter a relative increase in the proportion of conditions in which genetic factors are prominent. In addition an increasingly well-informed public, assuming more responsibility for the quality of future populations, is creating a justified demand for accurate information regarding risks to present and future generations. The actual number of persons who need advice is relatively small when compared with those who have many other health problems, but their need is great. When expert counseling is not accessible, these persons may become victims of well-meaning but uninformed quasi-professionals or misguided relatives and acquaintances.

It is estimated that only a small proportion of persons who need counseling are seen by professional counselors. Many families who might benefit from counseling do not recognize the need, or this special need is not apparent to those who supervise their care. Unfortunately families who need counseling are rarely referred to counselors unless they themselves request the service. Nurses in the field of infant and child care continually encounter genetic diseases and families in which there is a risk that a disorder may be transmitted to an offspring. It is a responsibility of nurses to be alert to situations in which persons could benefit from genetic counseling, to become familiar with facilities in their areas where genetic counseling is available, and to learn the basic principles of heredity. In this way they will be able to direct individuals and families to take advantage of needed services and to be active participants in the counseling process.

A comprehensive definition of genetic counseling prepared by a group of eminent medical geneticists states that "genetic counseling is a communication process which deals with the human problems associated with the occurrence, or risk of occurrence, of a genetic disorder in a family. This process involves an attempt by one or more appropriately trained persons to help the individual or family:

1. Comprehend the medical facts, including the diagnosis, the probable course of the disorder, and the available management;
2. Appreciate the way heredity contributes to the disorder, and the risk of recurrence in specified relatives;
3. Understand the options for dealing with the risk of recurrence;
4. Choose the course of action which seems appropriate to them in view of their risk and their family goals and act in accordance with that decision; and
5. Make the best possible adjustment to the disorder in an affected family member and/or to the risk of recurrence of that disorder."[3]

Clients

The clients, or persons who seek advice, may or may not be affected themselves but may request genetic counseling about the heritability of a trait that may be deleterious, beneficial, or merely troublesome. Clients may be a young couple contemplating marriage or childbearing who are concerned about a disorder in one of their families, no matter how remote the relationship. They may seek advice because they are related. A couple who are both members of a population at risk for certain diseases may wish to determine whether they carry the harmful gene (for example, blacks and sickle cell anemia, Ashkenazic Jews and Tay-Sachs disease, or Italians and thalassemia). A couple planning adoption may seek counseling regarding a prospective child. More often persons who inquire about the possibility of recurrence of a disease or disorder are parents of a child with a specific disease or defect that significantly impairs fitness who are concerned that they might produce another similarly affected child. This advice may be sought before the couple initiate another pregnancy, after the mother is already pregnant, or after the birth of another child. There may be concern regarding the risk to unaffected siblings of the affected child or to the affected child's future children.

Some families may need counseling in regard to the advisability of sterilization, artificial insemination, prenatal diagnosis, or termination of a pregnancy. Infertility or recurrent abortion in a family may indicate a need for counseling. Occasionally a counselor becomes involved in cases of disputed paternity, rape, and incestuous matings. Delayed or abnormal sexual development may be a reason to seek genetic advice.

Objectives of genetic counseling

Carter[1] has outlined three objectives of genetic counseling: (1) to advise parents and answer questions regarding the risks of recurrence when a member of the family has a disorder that might be genetically determined; (2) to alert the medical profession to the possibility that a particular child may be born with a genetic abnormality; and (3) to prevent an increase in the number of children with a serious handicap and ultimately to reduce the proportion of these children who are born.

Advising parents. More than ever before, parents plan and feel responsible for their children. Concerned persons are entitled to accurate information regarding risks and to have this information presented to them in language that they can understand and in the proper perspective. That is, they need to know the risk in *their particular situation* and how it relates to the random risk for *any* prospective parents. It has been found that when parents understand the risks involved they normally make sensible decisions regarding family planning.

Special risk situations. When health personnel are alerted to the possibility of an inherited disease in a family, this knowledge facilitates the early detection and subsequent treatment of the disease. This is increasingly important as more treatments are becoming available for genetically determined disease and is especially true in situations where treatment is effective only when initiated early. History of a condition in an older sibling, such as phenylketonuria, galactosemia, and so on, provides a clue for specific and thorough testing for the condition in a newborn. In this way early therapy can be initiated when indicated, thus minimizing or eliminating the disease or defect.

Reducing numbers of affected children. Since it is now possible to detect the carrier state in an increasing variety of single-gene defects, this aspect of genetic counseling is assuming greater importance and offers hope in preventing disabling disease. Persons with a family history of one of these hereditary disorders, or those in an ethnic group at risk for a particular disease, are able to ascertain before initiating a pregnancy whether they are carriers of the gene for a severe defect. In these instances the genetic counselor is able to advise the couple on the risks related to any pregnancy, in regard to that specific defect, with a high degree of accuracy. New techniques for prenatal diagnosis of chromosomal aberrations and an increasing number of metabolic defects have created a means for detecting the presence of an abnormal fetus early in pregnancy, thus providing a couple with the prospect of a defective child with option to terminate the pregnancy.

Information essential for genetic counseling

Unlike a medical prognosis that predicts the outcome of a disease, a genetic prognosis directly involves other persons: the affected child, other family members, relatives, and future offspring. Effective genetic counseling requires a thorough evaluation of each situation. Information from which the counselor derives risks of recurrence is acquired from several sources, such as accurate diagnosis, family history, and knowledge of genetics.

Accurate diagnosis. The first and most important component in the counseling process is an accurate diagnosis. The disease may be diagnosed by the attending physician who refers the family for counseling, or the physician may call on the services of a counseling unit for a definitive diagnosis by special biochemical or cytogenetic tests, particularly in cases of very rare and unusual syndromes. There are about 2000 known inherited disorders, many of which have similar clinical manifestations but totally different modes of inheritance. For example, symptoms in the early stages of severe X-linked muscular dystrophy appear much like those of the more mild autosomal-recessive and autosomal-dominant varieties, autosomal-recessive neurogenic muscular atrophies, and nongenetic poliomyelitis. The significance of the risks related to each type of disorder is readily apparent. It is especially difficult to assign an etiology to deafness and mental retardation.

Family history. A careful, detailed family history is necessary to the counseling process. Not only does it provide a picture of the *proband* (the affected person or *index case*) in relation to other family members, but it may also serve to identify other persons who are similarly affected. Analyzing the pattern of affected members of the family may assist in confirming a tentative diagnosis or in determining the level of risk in multifactorial inheritance.

The person taking a family history must allow a liberal amount of time. When possible, it is best to include both parents in the interview in order to elicit information about relatives on both sides of the family. Medical records, birth and death records, family bibles, and photograph albums are helpful resources, and persons being interviewed should be instructed to bring such items if they are available. It may be necessary to consult other members of the family. The amount of education and the level of understanding vary widely among informants and influence the reliability of the information. There may be reticence on the part of informants, particularly if they view the disorder as something to be ashamed of or in some way threatening. Sometimes true relationships may be concealed, such as illegitimacy.

The family history is recorded in the form of a pedigree chart, or family tree, using standard symbols to indicate persons, relationships, and significant details related to them (Fig. 6-18). It is important to include information about births—live births, stillbirths, and abortions; marriages—consanguineous, multiple, unwed matings, and other complex relationships; and health of family members, including any diseases or disorders, death, and causes of death. Sometimes the place of birth and ethnic background are significant. For example, the incidence of Tay-Sachs disease is higher in Ashkenazic Jews from eastern Europe than in Jews from other geographic origins. Also, when a pedigree chart is being evaluated, the fact that a sister died in infancy as a "blue baby" might be genetically significant, whereas a healthy sibling who drowned at age 1 year would not. Information concerning first-degree relatives is most important, and information on these should be complete.

Construction of a pedigree chart begins with the affected child (proband), who is designated with an arrow, and the outcome of *all* the mother's pregnancies (Fig. 6-19, *A*). Significant information about a pregnancy should be noted, such as bleeding, anemia, x-ray, or infectious diseases. Marriages are represented by a bar with males usually indicated on the left. Siblings, including stillbirths and abortions, are designated by arabic numerals in order of birth. Generations are represented by roman numerals, the earliest at the top. Next the medical history of the maternal relatives is explored beginning with the mother's

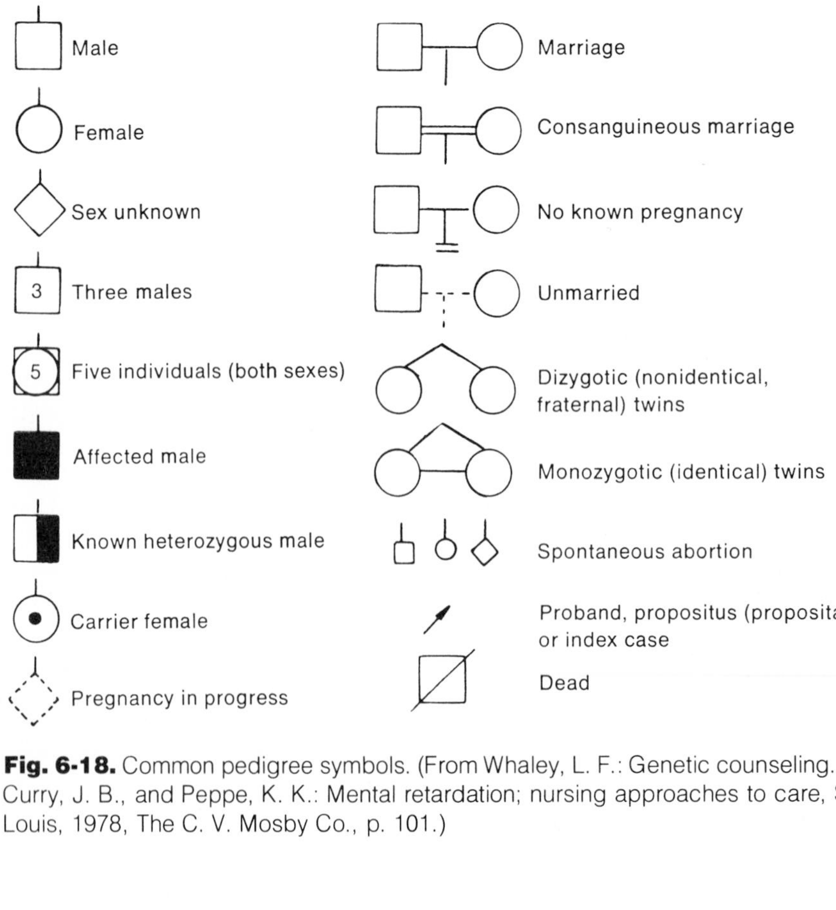

Fig. 6-18. Common pedigree symbols. (From Whaley, L. F.: Genetic counseling. In Curry, J. B., and Peppe, K. K.: Mental retardation; nursing approaches to care, St. Louis, 1978, The C. V. Mosby Co., p. 101.)

siblings and the outcome of her mother's pregnancies (Fig. 6-19, *B*). Details concerning the general health or death of maternal grandparents, nieces, nephews, uncles, aunts, and first cousins are included in a family history if the mother has information about them. Information about relatives on the father's side is gathered in the same manner (Fig. 6-19, *C*). It is important at this point to determine whether the couple might be related in any way.

When a family history is completed, the pedigree chart will reflect either a *positive family history,* in which other relatives are affected with same disorder, or a *negative family history,* in which the proband is an isolated case.

Knowledge of genetics. In order to counsel families regarding their particular problem, a counselor must have a thorough understanding of genetic principles, a knowledge of the risks related to multifactorial inheritance, and up-to-date information on genetic diseases.

Estimation of risks

The mode of inheritance determines the degree of risk in the major categories of genetic disorders. In general, the more definite and clear-cut the genetics, the greater the risks; as the causative factors become more obscure, the outlook is more hopeful. Broadly the risks can be categorized as (1) random risk, (2) high risk of one in ten or greater, and (3) moderate risk of less than one in ten and usually less than one in twenty.

Random-risk situations. The random risk for any pregnancy is considered to be in the order of one in thirty. Conditions that are caused by environmental agents and, there-

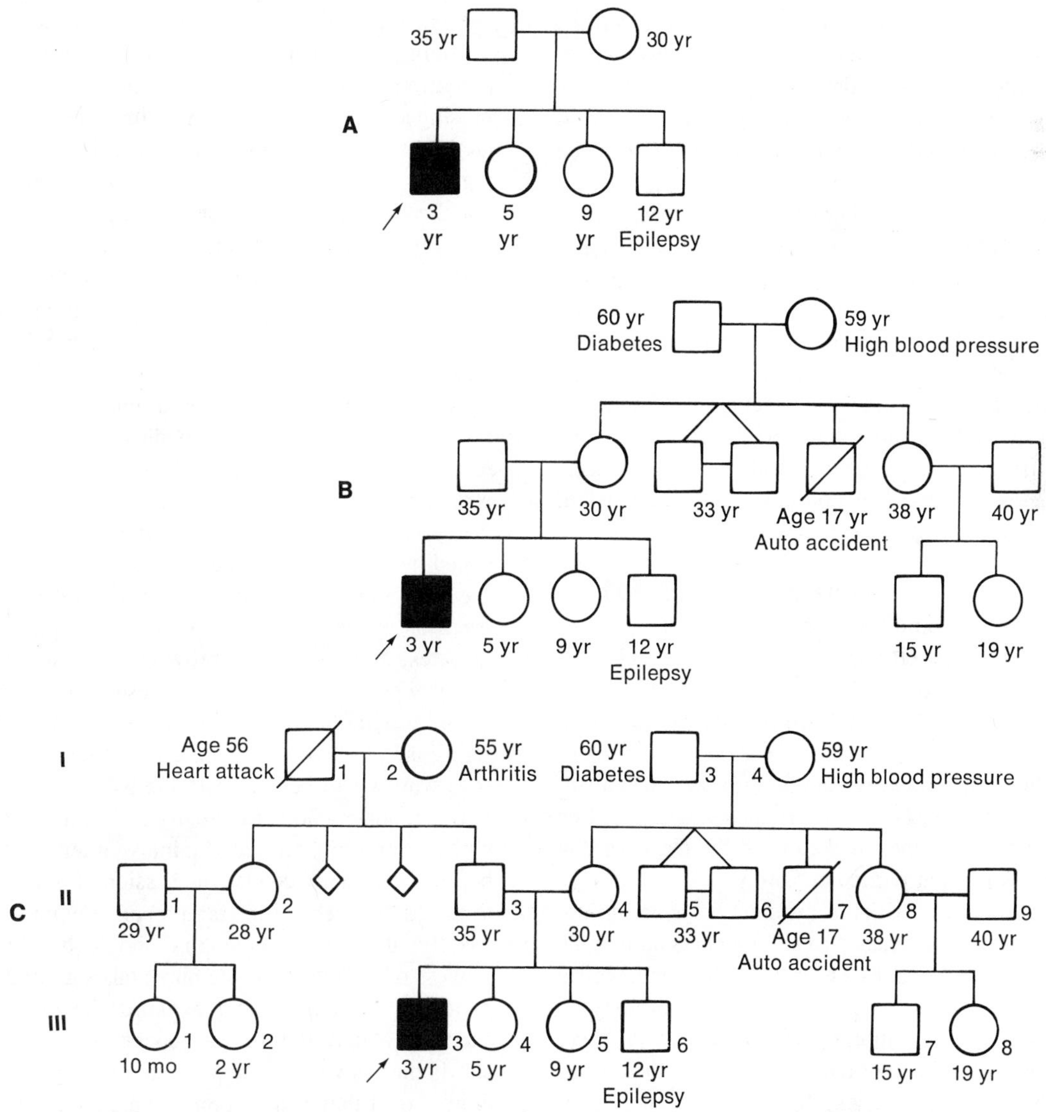

Fig. 6-19. Construction of a pedigree. **A,** Proband, siblings, and parents; **B,** maternal relatives; **C,** paternal relatives added.

fore, are not likely to recur in another pregnancy are regarded as random risks. A subsequent pregnancy would carry no more risk of the same defect than for any person in the general population. Examples of random-risk situations include conditions resulting from maternal infection (rubella, toxoplasmosis), maternal ingestion of drugs (thalidomide), a disorder due to a fresh mutation, and most chromosomal abnormalities.

High-risk situations. When the condition is caused by a factor that segregates during cell division (genes and chromosomes), the probability of an affected offspring can be predicted with a high degree of accuracy. Examples of high-risk situations include all disorders caused by a single mutant gene and Down's syndrome when caused by a translocation.

Moderate-risk situations. The largest group of conditions are considered to be moderate risks. These include the multifactorial disorders that appear to "run in families" and are greater than the risks for the population as a whole. Risk recurrence in these disorders is *empiric*. That is, it is not based on genetic theory, but on prior experience and observation of the disorder in other families that have been recorded in the literature. To arrive at an empiric risk estimate, the counselor applies a knowledge of the frequencies that have been observed in other families with a similar condition to the incidence of the disorder in the family under consideration. When more than one member of a family is affected, the risks of recurrence are substantially increased, especially if these persons are near relatives. Examples of moderate-risk situations include common disorders, such as cleft lip and palate, pyloric stenosis, spina bifida, and congenital heart defects, and common diseases, such as diabetes mellitus, schizophrenia, and hypertension.

Interpretation of risks

When explaining risk estimates, the counselor does not attempt to make recommendations or decisions for the counsultants. The counselor provides appropriate and accurate information about the nature of the disorder, the extent of the risk involved, the probable consequences, and alternative solutions but leaves the final decision to the persons concerned. In some instances genetic information will increase the family's distress; in others their anxiety will be reduced, depending on their makeup and the meaning that the disorder has for that particular family.

It is helpful to explain risks in different ways and to use examples from games of chance to aid in understanding the meaning of probabilities. Most persons do not have an adequate knowledge of genetics and human biology to fully comprehend these complex concepts. However, there are few people who have not had experience with flipping coins, baseball pools, lotteries, horse racing, and other games based on probabilities. Flipping coins can be used effectively to illustrate the probabilities in single-gene disorders, and weather reports and horse racing are well-known examples of empiric-risk estimates.

It is important to impress on the family that *each pregnancy is an independent event*. It is not uncommon for parents who are told that a recessive disorder carries a one in four risk of recurrence to feel secure with one affected child. They incorrectly reason that since they already have one affected child the next three will be unaffected. "Chance has no memory"; the risk is one in four for each and every pregnancy.

Nurse and genetic counseling

Nurses skilled in counseling techniques are in a unique position to help meet the counseling needs of families in which there is a genetic disease or disorder. Public health nurses work with a family in a close, sustained relationship and earn the family's confidence and trust; genetics nurse specialists, with advanced preparation in genetic theory, are assuming a prominent position on counseling teams; and practitioners in the specialty areas of maternity and pediatric nursing are constantly involved with genetic defects. Nurses are frequently the persons who recognize clues that indicate a genetic-related problem, who assist the family in obtaining the needed services for diagnosis and treatment, and who provide follow-up care.

Counseling services. The most efficient counseling service consists of a group of specialists that may include physicians, geneticists, psychologists, biochemists, cytologists, nurses, social workers, and other auxiliary personnel. The services are most often under the leadership of a medical physician trained in medical genetics, who assumes responsibility for the medical aspects of the group. The counseling service may serve only as a referral group, or it may conduct a regular clinic service. Most often it is associated with a large medical center. There are numerous specialty clinics that deal with specific genetic disorders (such as cystic fibrosis, muscular dystrophy, hemophilia, diabetes, and so on) and provide their own genetic counseling services. Unfortunately these units are concentrated in and around large metropolitan areas. As a result, counseling is not always accessible to the large number of persons who would benefit from the service.

It is a nurse who is frequently the family's initial contact with a counseling service. An intake interview is conducted before the primary counseling session or diagnostic workup to assess the needs of the family and attempt to reduce their anxiety; therefore, ample time should be allotted. In the process of the interview the nurse takes a family history for pertinent information and explains the clinic procedures carefully. Many families are concerned about such things as whether they will be required to undress, if blood is to be drawn, or if they can accompany the child during the visit. Families who have a relaxed and nonstressful initial discussion are able to gain more from a counseling session.

Follow-up care. The success of counseling is measured by the way in which the family utilizes the information presented to them. Maintaining contact with the family or referral to an agency that can provide a sustained relationship, usually the public health agency in their locality, is one of the most important aspects of the counseling process. Some families do not choose to have follow-up visits, but in most instances these visits make the family feel that they have not been abandoned and facilitate the process of adjustment to the problem.

Follow-up visits to the counseling service or in the home provide the family with the opportunity to ask questions that they did not ask on previous visits. Often the family has not really "heard" the information presented to them or have misinterpreted what they have heard so that it may be necessary to repeat and reinforce counseling. In some disorders a diagnosis of one family member places relatives at risk and is an indication for further screening. In a disorder such as phenylketonuria that requires conscientious diet management, it is important to make certain that the family understands and follows the advice. Children born subsequently must be carefully observed for early detection of symptoms.

Nurses should be prepared to help families arrive at tentative decisions regarding the future, including family planning, education or institutionalization of a handicapped child, plans for adoption, and many other problems related to their specific problems. Location of agencies and clinics specializing in the specific disorder that can provide services (such as equipment, medication, and rehabilitation), educational programs, and parent groups are all part of the nurses' resources.

Psychologic aspects of genetic disease[4]

It requires time and understanding to deal with the emotional tension and anxiety generated in families who are faced with the prospect of a genetic disorder. Knowledge of and the ability to deal with the range of psychologic responses and all their ramifications (such as the grief reaction, guilt, anger, and coping mechanisms) are essential components of the nursing role in genetic counseling. Many of these factors determine the degree to which a counselor's message is understood and influence the family's attitudes and the use they make of counseling information. Awareness and understanding of these feelings make the difference between a genetic informant and a genetic counselor.

Timing of the counseling requires careful evaluation. Some families may not be ready to listen immediately after a diagnosis is made; many do not listen effectively the first time information is presented to them. There may be numerous blocks to getting information across to families. Often they are so angry or frightened that they do not hear what is being said to them; they may feel guilty, embarrassed, or somehow inferior or inadequate. It is sometimes necessary to wait a week or more to allow the family sufficient time to absorb the initial impact of the situation before they are ready to assimilate any new information.

It is important early in counseling to get a clear understanding of the family's initial concerns, their state of knowledge about the disease, and their attitudes and beliefs concerning the condition and to determine the kind and amount of information they need or want. Some are not sure they should be at a counseling service. Whether the persons needing help are parents who have given birth to an affected child, relatives of an affected individual, or persons who have been identified as carriers of a deleterious gene, their feelings, attitudes, and fears must be dealt with.

Guilt and self-blame are very natural and universal reactions. Nurses must deal with parents' feelings of guilt about carrying "bad genes" or having "made my child sick." Often the counseling person is in a position to absolve the parents of guilt by explaining the random nature of segregation during both gamete formation and fertilization. Sometimes there is comfort in knowing that everyone carries defective genes and that it is mere chance that a particular couple happens to carry the same abnormal gene. Reactions may be different in situations where one member can pinpoint the "blame" (dominant or X-linked disorders), whereas there is some measure of reassurance in recessive disorders for the couple to know that it is not just one of them who carries the defective gene. Anxieties generated by old wives' tales, superstitions, and misconceptions can be dispelled.

It is important to stress the fact that there is nothing shameful about an inherited or congenital defect and to emphasize any appropriate remedy. Families have a tendency to be more ashamed of a hereditary disorder than of one caused by self-indulgence, such as obesity or alcoholism. The threat of a hereditary "taint" often creates intrafamily strife, hostility, and marital disharmony, sometimes to the point of family disintegration. Relatives frequently cease reproduction after the diagnosis of a hereditary defect, or the decision to marry may be deferred on the basis of a disorder, even a remote one, in a partner's family. While people may understand the situation on an intellectual level, this will not help them on an emotional level. A large and vital part of the nurse's role in genetic counseling is that of sympathetic and supportive listener.

Burden of genetic defect. The way in which members of a family respond to the probability of a genetic disorder will depend a great deal on the nature of the condition and the burden, actual or perceived, that it may place on them. A burden is considered to be the total amount of distress created by the birth of an affected child—the anticipated burden as well as the threat of disability. Various factors that are associated with disorders produce a burden in different ways to determine the total impact on a family. These include severity, chronicity, age of onset, mortality, morbidity, presence or absence of chronic pain, mental retardation, and cosmetic disfiguration.

Persons respond differently to probabilities. A risk that is reassuring to one may be threatening or intolerable to another. On the other hand, two individuals will respond differently to a hazard that both perceive as threatening. Some parents will choose to have children even in the face of high risk, while others believe that even a moderate risk is too much to take. Some may risk a child with a disorder that produces a minor defect or even one that causes early death but elect not to risk having a child with a life-long disability. The longer the duration of the disability, the greater the financial and emotional burden.

In some disorders, such as Down's syndrome, the burden of the disease rests primarily on the family rather than on the affected child. In diseases with severe crippling effects, such as muscular dystrophy, the impact of the disease affects both the child and the family.

All of these matters confront a family when they must make a decision about whether to risk a pregnancy that might result in a defective child, and nurses should be prepared to explore these probabilities with them. Parents who elect to have children in spite of a fairly high risk of recurrence can be helped by education. By learning about the disorder, they will be alert to signs of the disease so that early treatment can be initiated to minimize the ill effects of the disorder.

Barriers to effective counseling. Obstacles to the use of genetic counseling involve the attitudes of both the family and the counselor. Frequent obstacles to an objective use of information are religious attitudes toward conception and opposition to sterilization and to abortion in situations where there is a high risk of recurrence or where prenatal diagnosis has indicated a defective fetus. Many persons fatalistically accept "the will of God." Another obstacle is the rights of the individual—the right of the fetus to come to full term and the right of parents to conceive. A person with a high risk of producing a disabling condition in an offspring may believe that he is entitled to the same rights as anyone else, including the right of procreation.

Differences in the ability to comprehend what is said probably interfere most with effective use of counseling information. Clients vary in experiences, education, and intellectual level, and, even with careful explanation, many are still unable to understand the basic fundamentals of inheritance. They may be able to repeat information but fail to grasp its significance.

Sometimes nurses themselves create barriers with their own biases. There are some diseases that have a special impact on individual nurses, and in such cases it is difficult to be nonjudgmental. Families may become defensive if they believe that the nurse is bringing undo pressure to bear on their decision. Others may pressure the nurse to make the decision for them. "What would you do if you were in this situation?" is a common question. There are instances where some nurses (intentionally or unintentionally) do influence families. In genetic counseling the families should be given all the facts and possible consequences and then assisted in their problem solving, but the decision concerning a course of action should be left to them.

GENETICS AND SOCIETY

There is no doubt that genetic diseases constitute a significant portion of the world health deficit, and the advantages to improvement of the human race are seldom questioned. The controversy exists between those who advocate improvement in the species by selective breeding and those who recommend providing a better environment. Improvement of the race through altering the genetic make-up of the individual is termed *eugenics;* improvement of the human race by modifying the environment is called *euthenics*.

Eugenics

Eugenics is essentially planned breeding designed to alter future generations. Such practice has been successfully used for many years by animal and plant breeders in developing superior food products. For many persons any discussion of controlling heredity creates visions of Hitler's interpretation and misuse of directed evolution, for some racial groups it is a code word for genocide, and religious groups protest that it is tampering with God's creation. Eugenics can be further segregated into *positive eugenics* and *negative eugenics*.

Positive eugenics. Positive eugenics is the attempt to encourage reproduction among those individuals who are considered to possess superior or beneficial characteristics. Suggested means for accomplishing this purpose include selected mating of individuals with what are considered to be superior traits. Other methods are the establishment of sperm banks with sperm from a small, selected number of donors to be frozen and used to impregnate a large number of suitable women and the production, asexually, of replicas of desirable persons by cloning (replacing the cell nucleus of a fertilized ovum with the nucleus of a cell from the desired individual; asexual reproduction). Some of the qualifications considered superior might be physical characteristics, socially desirable behavior, and superior intellect, as well as absence of genetically determined defects or disease.

Negative eugenics. Negative eugenics is the discouragement or prohibition of reproduction among individuals who are considered to be physically or mentally handicapped. Voluntary or legal prohibition of reproduction by persons with these characteristics might be accomplished with marriage laws, sterilization, and abortion. The arguments for and against the relative merits and objections of eugenics will continue for years to come. The multiple problems inherent in either positive or negative eugenics are readily apparent.

Euthenics

An opposite point of view is taken by those who support euthenics, which advocates the modification of the environment to allow the genetically abnormal individual to live a relatively normal life. Examples of euthenic measures are prescription glasses for nearsighted persons and special schools for the deaf. Medical treatments such as special diets for children with inborn errors of metabolism, hormone replacement such as insulin for diabetic persons and thyroid for persons with cretinism, and special orthopedic appliances and prosthetic devices can be considered environmental manipulation. Providing better nutrition and home environment for children during the growing stages and educational and social stimulation are prime examples of euthenics.

REFERENCES

1. Carter, C. D.: Genetic counseling, Med. Clin. North Am. **53:** 991-999, 1969.
2. Childs, B.: Genetic screening. In Roman, H. L., Campbell, A., and Sandler, L. M., editors: Annual review of genetics, Palo Alto, Calif., 1975, Annual Reviews, Inc.
3. Fraser, F. C.: Genetic counseling, Am. J. Hum. Genet. **26:** 636-659, 1974.
4. Whaley, L. F.: Understanding inherited disorders, St. Louis, 1974, The C. V. Mosby Co.

BIBLIOGRAPHY

Bergsma, D., and Niel, J. V., editors: Contemporary genetic counseling, Birth Defects: Original Article Series, vol. IX, No. 4, 1973, The National Foundation.

Bogdanovic, S.: Prenatal detection of Down's syndrome, J. Obstet. Gynecol. Neonatal Nurs. **4**(6):35-38, 1975.

Callahan, D.: Ethics, law and genetic counseling, Science **176:** 197-200, 1972.

Childs, B.: Genetic screening. In Roman, H. L., Campbell, A., and Sandler, L. M., editors: Annual review of genetics, Palo Alto, Calif., 1975, Annual Reviews, Inc.

Clow, C. L., and associates: On the application of knowledge to the patient with genetic disease, Prog. Med. Genet. **9:**159-214, 1973.

Cowell, H. R.: Genetic aspects of orthopedic diseases, Am. J. Nurs. **70:**763, April 1970.

Ferguson-Smith, M. A.: Chromosome abnormalities. II. Sex chromosome defects. In McKusick, V. A., and Claiborn, R., editors: Medical genetics, New York, 1973, H. P. Publishing Co., Inc.

Hecht, F., and Everett, W. L.: Genetic diagnosis in the newborn, Pediatr. Clin. North Am. **17:**1039-1053, November 1970.

Hilton, B., and associates, editors: Ethical issues in human genetics, New Yrok, 1973, Plenum Press.

Hirschhorn, K.: Chromosome abnormalities. I. Autosomal defects. In McKusick, V. A., and Claiborne, R., editors: Medical genetics, New York, 1973, H. P. Publishing Co., Inc.

Infant screening for inborn errors of metabolism, Nutr. Today **9:** 105-113, November/December 1974.

Jackson, L. G.: Heterozygote detection for autosomal recessive genetic diseases, Clin. Pediatr. **13:**307-309, 1974.

Justice, P., and Smith, G. F.: Phenylketonuria, Am. J. Nurs. **75:** 1303-1305, August 1975.

Kelley, V. C., editor: Metabolic, endocrine and genetic disorders of children, vol. II, New York, 1974, Harper & Row, Publishers.

Leonard, D. O., Chase, G. A., and Childs, B.: Genetic counseling: a consumer's view, N. Engl. J. Med. **287:**433, 1972.

Levine, L.: Biology of the gene, ed. 2, St. Louis, 1973, The C. V. Mosby Co.

McKusick, V. A.: Human genetics, ed. 3, Englewood Cliffs, N.J., 1969, Prentice-Hall, Inc.

McKusick, V. A.: Genetics and disease. In Wintrobe, M. M., and associates, editors: Harrison's principles of internal medicine, ed. 6, New York, 1970, McGraw-Hill Book Co.

Neu, R. L., and Lytt, I. G.: Clinical aspects of abnormalities of the X and Y chromosomes, Clin. Obstet. Gynecol. **15:**141, 1972.

Nitowsky, H. M., and Legum, C. P.: Genetic counseling: general principles and clinical applications, Adv. Pediatr. **18:**13, 1971.

Paris Conference (1971): Standardization in human cytogenetics, Birth Defects: Original Article Series, vol. VIII, No. 7, 1972, The National Foundation.

Pearn, J. H.: Patients' subjective interpretation of risks offered in genetic counseling, J. Med. Genet. **10:**129-134, 1973.

Riccardi, V. M.: Health care and disease prevention through genetic counseling: a regional approach, Am. J. Public Health **66:** 268-272, 1976.

Roberts, J. A. F.: An introduction to medical genetics, ed. 5, London, 1970, Oxford University Press.

Sahin, S. T.: The multifaceted role of the nurse as genetic counselor, Am. J. Maternal Child Nurs. **1**(4):211-216, 1976.

Scott, C. I., and Thomas, G. H.: Genetic disorders associated with mental retardation, Pediatr. Clin. North Am. **20:**121, February 1973.

Scriver, C. R.: Inborn errors of metabolism: a new frontier of nutrition, Nutr. Today **9:**4-15, September/October 1974.

Shapiro, L. R.: The cytogenetics laboratory in pediatrics, Pediatr. Clin. North Am. **18:**209, February 1971.

Stanbury, J. B., Wyngaarden, J. B., and Fredrickson, D. S., editors: The metabolic basis of inherited disease, ed. 3., New York, 1972, McGraw-Hill Book Co.

Stern, C.: Principles of human genetics, ed. 3, San Francisco, 1972, W. H. Freeman and Co., Publishers.

Stewart, J. M.: Genetic counseling. In Clausen, J. P., and associates, editors: Maternity nursing today, New York, 1973, McGraw-Hill Book Co.

Sultz, H. A., Schlesinger, E. R., and Feldman, J.: An epidemiologic justification for genetic counseling in family planning, Am. J. Public Health **62:**1489-1492, November 1972.

Thompson, J. S., and Thompson, M. W.: Genetics in medicine, ed. 2, Philadelphia, 1973, W. B. Saunders Co.

Valentine, G. H.: The reproductive counseling process, Clin. Pediatr. **16:**233-238, 1977.

Whaley, L. F.: Understanding inherited disorders, St. Louis, 1974, The C. V. Mosby Co.

Whaley, L. F.: Genetic counseling in maternity nursing. In McNall, L. K., and Galeener, J. T., editors: Current practice in

obstetric and gynecologic nursing, vol. I., St. Louis, 1976, The C. V. Mosby Co.
Whaley, L. F.: Genetic counseling. In Curry, J. B., and Peppe, K. K., editors: Mental retardation: nursing approaches to care, St. Louis, 1978, The C. V. Mosby Co.
Wilson, M. G.: Genetic counseling, Curr. Probl. Pediatr. **5**(7):1-51, 1975.
Wolf, L.: The nurse's role in genetic counseling. In Hymovich, D. P., and Barnard, M. U., editors: Family health care, New York, 1973, McGraw-Hill Book Co.

7

Fetal development and prenatal influences

Regulation of life before birth is directed by the action of many genetic mechanisms controlled by a strict chronology. No less significant are the influences of environment, particularly during the time of critical differentiation. A knowledge, even rudimentary, of the sequence and organ relationships of early development helps nurses to appreciate the significance of disturbances during this crucial time that produce consequences in the form of congenital malformations—the source of major pediatric nursing problems. This chapter is concerned with some of the genetic factors that play a role in growth and development and some of the environmental influences that can alter the normal course of events.

A NEW LIFE

The formation of a new individual, although commonplace, is one of the most dramatic events known to man. For every human being, life begins at the time of conception when the female germ cell, with its genetic material handed down through countless generations, unites with a similar complement from the mature male germ cell to form a single, life-giving cell. From this single cell will evolve millions of cells with the diversity to carry on an enormous variety of essential functions.

Gametogenesis

Germ-cell formation (gametogenesis) takes place in the male and female gonads and consists of three major phases:

1. A period of proliferation in which primordial cells (the oogonia and spermatogonia) divide repeatedly by the process of mitosis
2. A period of growth marked by enlargement of the primitive cells into primary germ cells (oocytes and spermatocytes)
3. A period of maturation that includes the fundamental nuclear changes of the two meiotic divisions

The primordial cells are formed in embryonic life, and, although the overall process is similar in both the male and the female, there are significant differences in the timing of the divisions and in the number, size, and extranuclear composition of the mature gametes. Also, the mature male cells pass through an additional stage in their conversion to motile spermatozoa (Fig. 7-1).

Oogenesis. The process by which a mature ovum is formed begins during intrauterine life when the primordial cells, or *oogonia,* proliferate within the germinal epithelium of the ovarian cortex. At the time of birth most of the oogonia have enlarged and developed into *primary oocytes,* each surrounded by a layer of epithelial cells that together form the *primordial* (or *primary*) *follicle*. These oocytes (numbering approximately 500,000) have begun the first meiotic division. Primary oocytes remain suspended at the first meiotic division until the time of sexual maturity, when each month one or two are stimulated to complete the division simultaneously with maturation of the follicle. They then become *secondary oocytes*.

The cell division in ova is distinctive. In both meiotic divisions the nuclei of the cells divide evenly, but there is uneven distribution of the cytoplasm. The first meiotic division, which occurs about the time the ovum is released from the ovary, produces a large *secondary oocyte* that contains the bulk of the cellular contents and a small, nonfunctional cell, the *first polar body*. The second meiotic division begins at ovulation but remains suspended at the first prophase until triggered to complete the process by the entry of the sperm at fertilization. This second division produces the large *ovum* and a small *second polar body*. Polar bodies are incapable of supporting reproduction and soon disintegrate (Fig. 7-1, *B*).

Spermatogenesis. Unlike oogenesis, spermatogenesis, the formation of spermatozoa, is a continuous process that begins about the time of puberty and continues until senescence. Primitive germ cells (the *spermatogonia*), situated adjacent to the basement membrane of the seminiferous tubules, proliferate and mature into *primary spermatocytes*. These divide to form *secondary spermatocytes* and then *spermatids* that undergo gradual differentiation into active, motile sperm cells, or *spermatozoa* (Fig. 7-1, *A*). The length of time required to convert the primitive germ cells to the mature sperm is approximately 2 months.

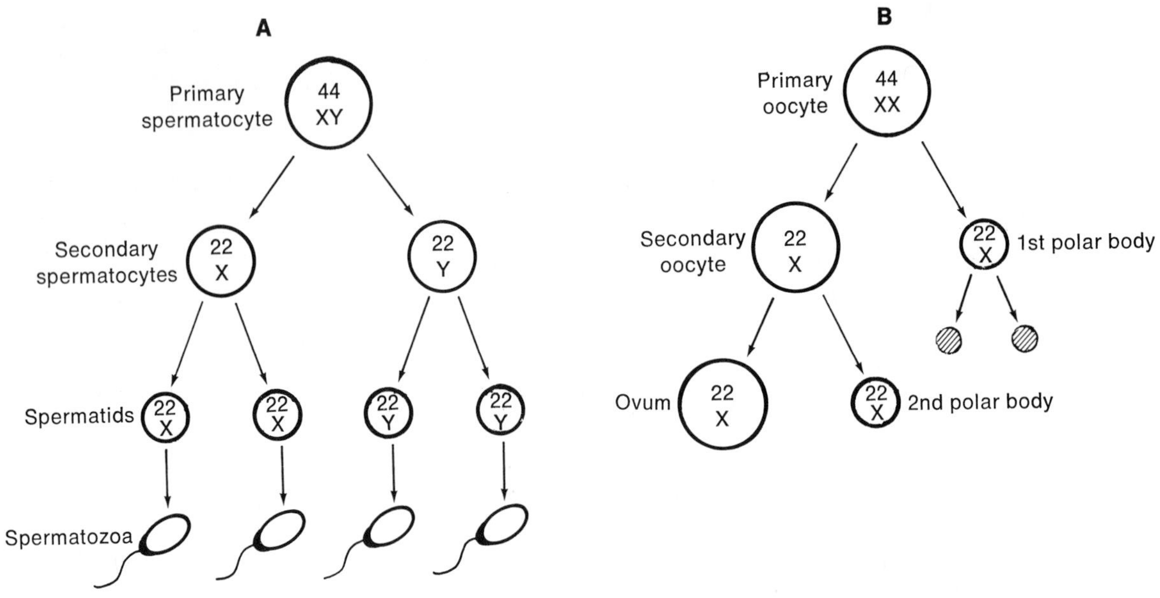

Fig. 7-1. Gametogenesis in male and female germ cells. **A,** Spermatogenesis results in four gametes (spermatozoa). **B,** Oogenesis results in only one gamete (ovum).

Fertilization

Fertilization is believed to take place in the outer third of the oviduct, or fallopian tube, within 24 hours after ovulation. From the millions of sperm deposited at the cervical opening at the time of sexual union, only one will overcome the multiple barriers to penetrate and fertilize the waiting ovum. With the entrance of the sperm through its cell wall, the ovum completes the final meiotic division and the nucleus of the sperm cell unites with the nucleus of the ovum. As a result: (1) the full chromosomal number (forty-six) is restored, (2) the sex of the future individual is determined, and (3) a series of mitotic divisions is initiated. The cell is now known as a *zygote,* literally meaning yoked together.

Length of gestation

The average length of time required to complete the transformation from single cell to newborn infant is based on (1) the menstrual age, calculated from the beginning of the mother's last menstrual period—10 lunar months, 40 weeks, or 280 days or (2) the fertilization age estimated from the average time of ovulation, presumed to be 2 weeks prior to the onset of menstruation—9 months, 38 weeks, or 266 days. Since the precise date of fertilization is seldom known with certainty and ovulation dates are variable, an estimated date of birth is always presumptive. The actual duration of gestation also varies from person to person and with different pregnancies of the same woman.

Stages of prenatal development

It has been customary to divide intrauterine life into phases, according to (1) the course of pregnancy (gestation), and (2) certain characteristics of fetal development.

Trimesters of pregnancy. From the maternal standpoint the 9-month gestation period is divided into *trimesters,* each 3 calendar months in length. The first trimester encompasses the rapid changes that take place within the developing embryo and the initial maternal emotional responses and physical adjustments to the parasitic organism. The second trimester is a relatively tranquil period of continued growth and expansion for the unborn child and one of psychologic adjustment for the mother-to-be. The third trimester is concerned with preparation for birth and a symbiotic relationship between mother and infant—for the unborn child, preparing for physiologic independence, and, for the mother, preparing to meet the needs of a new and helpless human being.

Stages of development. The *conceptus* is a general term that is frequently used to describe the fertilized ovum at all stages from implantation to birth.

The stages in the development of the unborn child are related to its biologic status. The first 10 days to 2 weeks after fertilization, or until it is well implanted in the uterine wall, the growing organism is known as a fertilized ovum or *zygote.* From the second through the eighth weeks it is an *embryo.* This period is characterized by rapid growth, differentiation of major organ primorida, and development of the main features of external form. The remainder of intrauterine life, after the organism has acquired a recognizable human form, it is termed a *fetus.* The period of the fetus is characterized by growth, further differentiation of structural detail, and development of differentiated function.

PRENATAL DEVELOPMENT

When they begin their existence, human beings bear no resemblance to the complex organisms into which they will develop. In fact, during the very early stages, they are indistinguishable from any other animal species. The early zygote contains no structures that remotely correspond to any of the organs and tissues that go to make up the fully developed individual. Development from zygote to fully formed infant consists of two distinct but interrelated processes: growth and differentiation. *Growth* results when cells divide and synthesize new proteins and is reflected in increased size and weight. *Differentiation* is the process by which these early cells are systematically modified and specialized to form all the tissues that are necessary to assure an organized, coordinated individual.

Embryogenesis

Soon after the stimulation of fertilization the zygote begins to divide with orderly precision (Fig. 7-2). It first divides by *cleavage* into two smaller, identical cells called *blastomeres*. As division continues it produces progressively smaller blastomeres that maintain the same cellular composition with each successive division until the organism consists of a cluster of cells, the *morula*. At this stage the cells are simple structures and fairly uniform in size, shape, and physiologic capabilities. If the cells are separated during these very early divisions (for example, the two-cell or the four-cell stage), each will develop into a complete embryo to form identical twins (see p. 224).

As division continues, the cells become unequal in both size and configuration. Fluid accumulates between the cells, converting the morula into a *blastocyst* consisting of a fluid-filled ball of thinned-out cells, the *trophoblast,* and a cluster of centrally located cells known as the *inner cell mass* that protrudes into the cavity. From two *formative layers* within the inner cell mass the embryo proper will develop, whereas the cells surrounding the cavity produce the extraembryonic structures.

The trophoblastic cells release enzymes that digest a small cavity in the lining of the uterus, and fingerlike projections (villi) burrow into the endometrium to attach the blastocyst to the uterine wall and seal it from the uterine cavity. This attachment, or *implantation,* occurs about the ninth day postfertilization and marks the beginning of the period of the embryo. The conceptus grows rapidly as the highly invasive trophoblastic cells tap the maternal blood supply. By the fourth month erosion of the maternal tissues has ceased and elaboration of the villous structures at the point of attachment forms the *placenta,* the essential organ for physiologic exchange between the maternal and fetal systems. The unattached trophoblastic cells become compressed and degenerate to produce a smooth lining membrane, the *chorion*. From embryonic cells another membrane, the *amnion,* containing the amniotic fluid, forms within the chorion to surround and envelope the developing embryo. The embryo, floating in its protective amniotic fluid and attached by a connecting stalk, is encased in two membrane layers.

At the same time, within the inner cell mass the cells of the early embryo rapidly differentiate into three distinct systems and organs. These three primary germ layers (the *ectoderm,* the *entoderm,* and the *mesoderm*) and the tissues to which they give origin are listed in Table 7-1. With the differentiation of these three germ layers the human embryo begins to initiate body building, and by the end of the eighth week the embryo begins to look quite human.

Fetal growth

Growth of the conceptus is accomplished by two mechanisms: (1) *hyperplasia,* an increase in cell numbers, and (2) *hypertrophy,* an increase in cell size. Hyperplasia is the predominant form of growth during the embryonic period, and, although the rate decreases during the later stages of gestation, cell division continues into the postnatal period. Hypertrophy is increasingly prominent during the later periods of growth.

There is a growth pattern that is typical for each organ and tissue, but all organs progress from a stage characterized by increase in cell number to one of growth by increase in cell size. If there is interference with the growth pattern of an organ, the overall result is a reduction in the size and weight of that organ. However, the consequences of the inhibiting factor depend on whether the insult is inflicted during a period of hyperplasia or a period of hypertrophy. Interruption of growth during cell enlargement is usually only temporary and can be overcome with proper intervention. Interference with growth during a period of cell proliferation is likely to cause irreversible growth retardation of that organ with permanent deficit in overall cell numbers.

The overall prenatal growth pattern shows that the most rapid gain in length precedes the gain in weight. The most rapid linear growth takes place during midfetal life; the most rapid gain in weight occurs in late fetal life (Fig. 7-3).

Differentiation[24,35]

All somatic cells have the same gene complement as the zygote from which they have descended, yet each cell differs measurably in form and function from the zygote and other types of body cells. The chromosomal material remains equally distributed throughout all cells; however, as cell division proceeds, the early cells gradually deviate and assort into a variety of very different cell types (for example, muscle, nerve, bone, and gland cells). Whereas early embryonal cells are vague in function, with random form and structure, later embryonal cells are less flexible in function, are diverse in size and structure, and gradually demonstrate a rigid lack of adaptability. Specialized tissues form, from which develop the organs and organ systems.

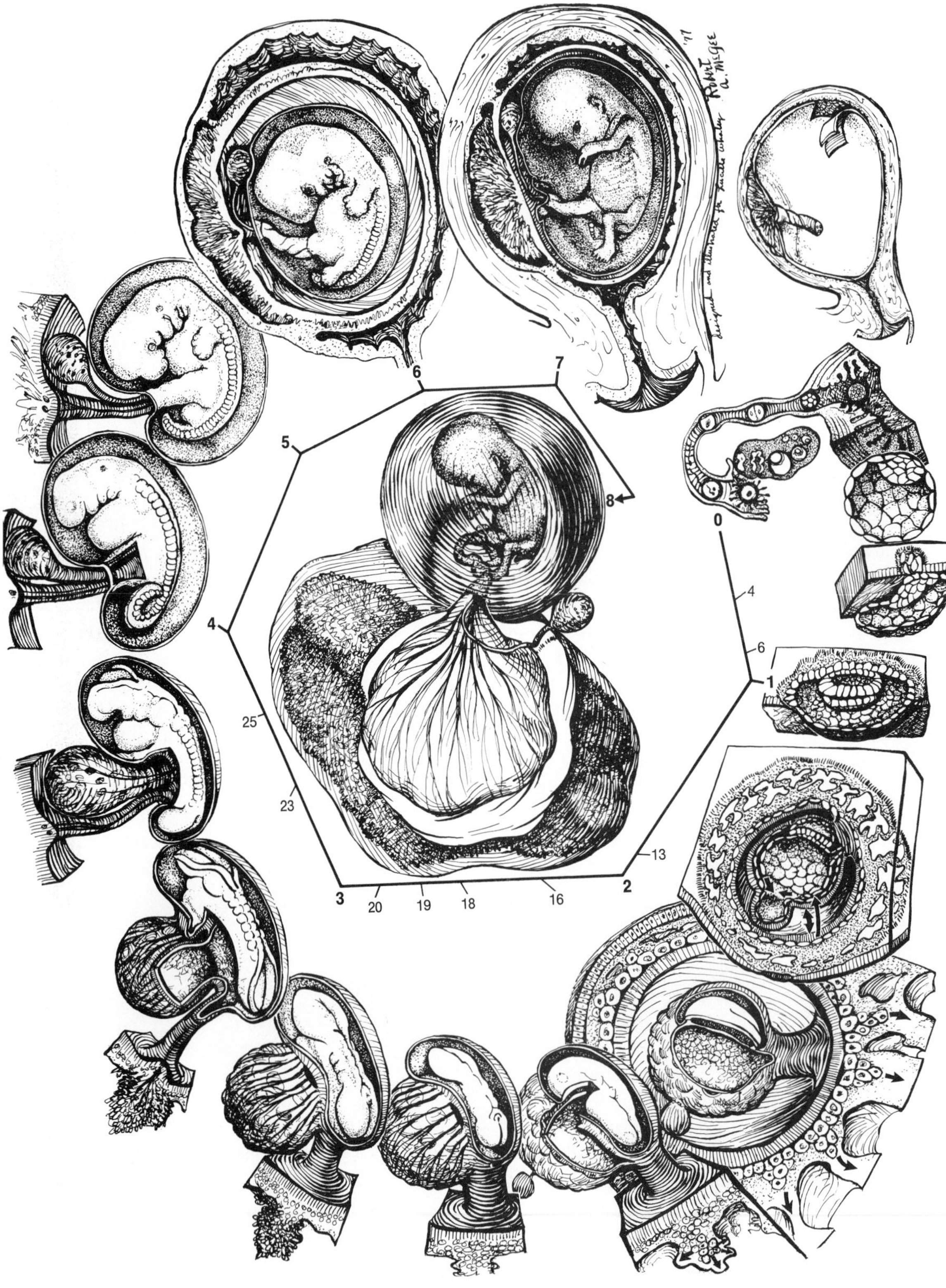

Fig. 7-2. Fertilization, implantation, and embryonic development. Large numbers indicate weeks; small numbers represent days.

Table 7-1. Organs and tissues arising from the three primary germ layers

Ectoderm	Entoderm	Mesoderm
Epidermis and its appendages, including lining cells of skin glands, hair, and nails Nervous system Pituitary gland Neuroepithelium of the sense organs Chromaffin organs, including adrenal medulla Optic lens; epithelium of the cornea, conjunctiva, and lacrimal glands; and muscles of the iris Epithelium of nasopharynx and mouth Salivary glands Tooth enamel Lining of the lower part of the anal canal	Epithelial lining of the alimentary canal (except those portions arising from the ectoderm) Lining cells of the glands that open into the alimentary canal, including the liver and pancreas (but excluding the salivary glands) Epithelial lining of the auditory canal and the tympanic membrane Epithelium of the thyroid, parathyroid, and thymus glands Epithelial lining of the larynx, trachea, and air passages, including the alveoli and air sacs Epithelium of most of the urinary bladder, urethra, and prostate	Connective and sclerous tissues Teeth (except the enamel) Body musculature—both smooth and striated (except muscles of the iris) Blood and vascular systems—blood and lymphatic vessels Urogenital system (except those portions arising from the entoderm) Adrenal cortex Mesothelial linings of pericardial, pleural, and peritoneal cavities

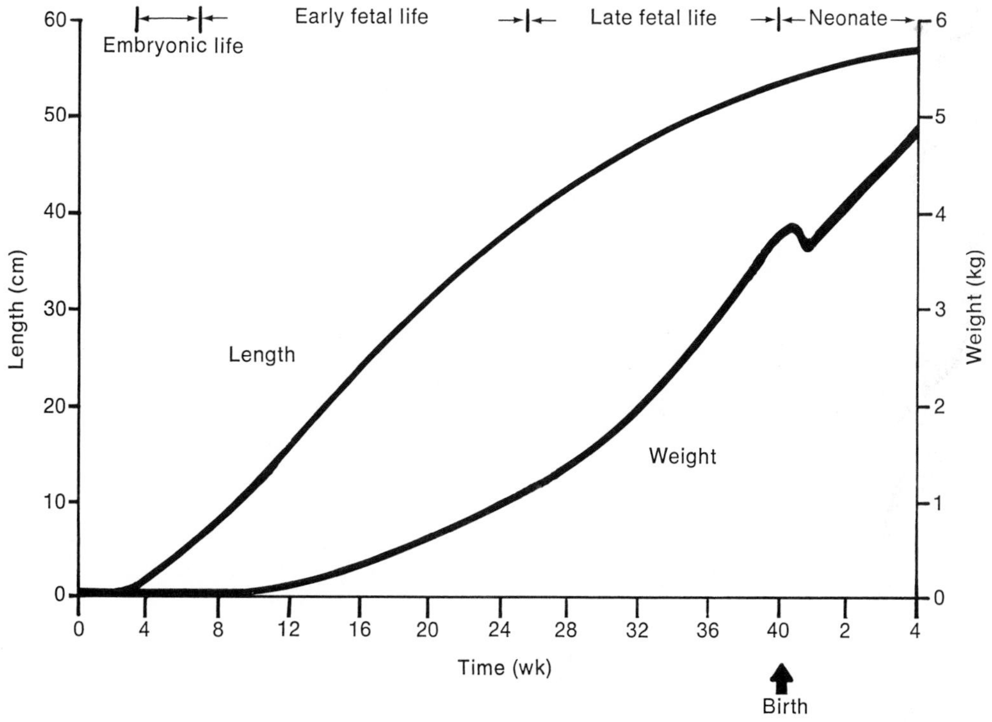

Fig. 7-3. Prenatal growth rate. (From Sinclair, D.: Human growth after birth, New York, London, 1969, Oxford University Press.)

Differentiation is the process by which cells acquire specific and characteristic properties and is accomplished by various mechanisms—controlled mitotic division, shifts in intracellular activity, tissue movement (migration), increase in size, increase in number, controlled cellular death, aggregation of like cells, and inductive interaction between different tissues—in a specified, sequential order. Each step in the differentiation process depends on successful completion of a previous step. Anything, such as a mutant gene or environmental agent, that interferes with one of these steps will cause an arrest in the development of that particular tissue or organ. Divergence from the normal course of development will result in maldevelopment of a part or, if it occurs at an early age, a sequence of distortions causing more severe or multiple malformations.

Organogenesis

The first 8 to 12 weeks of fetal life are particularly critical to the survival of the organism. During this time of extremely rapid development and change, the beginnings of all major organ systems are formed and the embryo begins to acquire the specific functions needed to integrate these organs and organ systems into an organized, coordinated whole. This is also the period during which the organism is most vulnerable to environmental hazards.

One-month-old embryo. A summary of the main features of the 4-week-old embryo serves to illustrate the extent to which early development takes place. Initially the embryo appears almost straight, but the more rapid growth and differentiation of the dorsal structures in contrast to the slower developing ventral surface produce the characteristic C-shaped curve and flexion of the embryo. The large, ventrally-flexed head and rudimentary tail exaggerate the curvature. Somites, pairs of cuboidal surface elevations that give rise to the axial skeleton and muscle, appear along the dorsal aspect, limb buds and sense organs form on the lateral surfaces, and brachial arches that eventually form the jaws are visible on the underside of the head.

Table 7-2. Milestones in human development before birth

4 weeks	8 weeks	12 weeks	16 weeks
External appearance			
Body flexed, C-shaped Arm and leg buds present Head at right angles to body	Body fairly well formed Nose flat, eyes far apart Digits well formed Head elevating Tail almost disappeared Eyes, ears, nose, and mouth recognizable	Nails appearing Resembles a human Head erect but disproportionately large Skin pink, delicate	Head still dominant Face looks human Eye, ear, and nose approach typical appearance on gross examination Arm-leg ratio proportionate Scalp hair appears Motor activity present
Crown-to-rump measurement (cm)			
0.4-0.5	2.5-3	6-8	11.5-13.5
Approximate weight (g)			
0.4	2	19	100
Musculoskeletal system			
All somites present	First indication of ossification—occiput, mandible, and humerus Fetus capable of some movement, definitive muscles of trunk, limbs, and head well represented	Some bones well outlined; ossification spreading Upper cervical to lower sacral arches and bodies ossify Smooth muscle layers indicated in hollow viscera	Most bones distinctly indicated throughout body Joint cavities appear Muscular movements can be detected
Circulatory system			
Heart develops; double chambers visible; begins to beat Aortic arches and major veins completed	Main blood vessels assume final plan Enucleated red cells predominate in blood	Blood forming in marrow	Heart muscle well developed Blood formation active in spleen

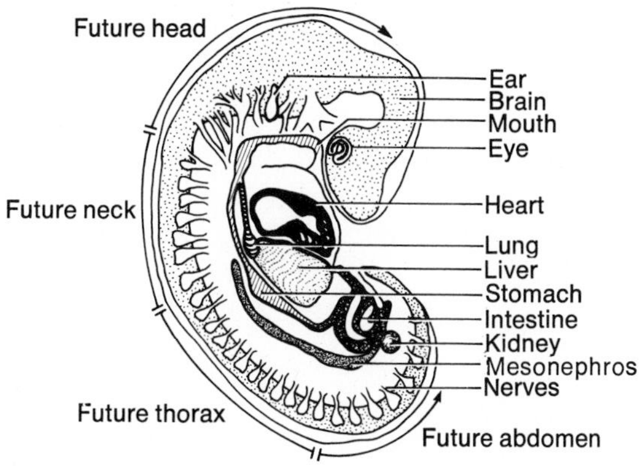

Fig. 7-4. One-month-old embryo.

20 weeks	24 weeks	28 weeks	32 weeks	36 weeks	40 weeks
Vernix caseosa appears Lanugo hair appears Legs lengthen considerably Sebaceous glands appear	Body lean but fairly well proportioned Skin red and wrinkled Vernix caseosa present Sweat glands forming	Lean body, less wrinkled and red Nails appear	Subcutaneous fat beginning to collect More rounded appearance Skin pink and smooth Has assumed delivery position	Skin pink, body rounded General lanugo disappearing Body usually plump	Skin smooth and pink; copious vernex caseosa Moderate to profuse hair Lanugo on shoulders and upper body only Nasal and alar cartilage apparent
16-18.5	23	27	31	35	40
300	600	1100	1800-2100	2200-2900	3200+
Sternum ossifies Fetal movements strong enough for mother to feel		Astragalus ossifies	Middle fourth phalanges ossify Permanent teeth primordia indicated	Distal femoral ossification centers present	
	Blood formation increases in bone marrow and decreases in liver				

Continued.

Table 7-2. Milestones in human development before birth—cont'd

4 weeks	8 weeks	12 weeks	16 weeks
Gastrointestinal system			
Stomach at midline and fusiform Conspicuous liver Esophagus short Intestine a short tube	Intestinal villi developing Small intestines coil within umbilical cord Palatal folds present Liver very large	Bile secreted Palatal fusion complete Intestines have withdrawn from cord and assume characteristic positions	Meconium in bowel Some enzyme secretion Anus open
Respiratory system			
Primary lung buds appear	Pleural and pericardial cavities forming Branching bronchioles Nostrils closed by epithelial plugs	Lungs acquire definite shape Vocal cords appear	Elastic fibers appear in lungs Terminal and respiratory bronchioles appear
Renal system			
Rudimentary ureteric buds appear	Earliest secretory tubules differentiating Bladder-urethra separates from rectum	Kidney able to secrete urine Bladder expands as a sac	Kidney in position Attains typical shape and plan
Nervous system			
Well-marked midbrain flexure No hindbrain or cervical flexures Neural groove closed	Cerebral cortex begins to acquire typical cells Differentiation of cerebral cortex, meninges, ventricular foramina, cerebrospinal fluid circulation Spinal cord extends entire length of spine	Brain structural configuration roughly complete Cord shows cervical and lumbar enlargements Fourth ventricle foramina developed	Cerebral lobes delineated Cerebellum assumes some prominence
Sense organs			
Eye and ear appearing as optic vessel and otocyst	Primordial choroid plexuses develop Ventricles large relative to cortex Development progressing Eyes converging rapidly Internal ear developing	Earliest taste buds indicated Characteristic organization of eye attained	General sense organs differentiated
Genital system			
Genital ridge appears (fifth week)	Testes and ovaries distinguishable External genitalia sexless but begin to differentiate	Sex recognizable Internal and external sex organs specific	Testes in position for descent into scrotum Vagina open

Internally the heart becomes conspicuous as a ventral bulge, and a functional circulation begins as a system of blood vessels is established. The gut elongates into a blind pouch, a prominent liver is recognizable, and a rudimentary lung and kidney begin to form. By the end of the fourth week the major body organs have begun to take shape (Fig. 7-4). Major differentiation of organs continues until the end of the eighth week; thereafter, the principal changes are growth and elaboration of organs and systems.

An overview of the major changes in development of various organs and systems is outlined in Table 7-2. Although growth and development are proportionately greater in the early weeks, the rate is somewhat uneven and variable.

FETAL NUTRITION AND RESPIRATION

In anticipation of fertilization, the maternal genital tract has made its monthly preparations to receive the new organism. Through the action of ovarian hormones, the endometrium has become thick and succulent with a rich blood supply and glands secreting nutritive substances to sustain the conceptus during the early weeks of gestation. Nutritional requirements of the organism during early cleavage divisions, although slight, are provided in part by sub-

20 weeks	24 weeks	28 weeks	32 weeks	36 weeks	40 weeks
Enamel and dentine depositing Ascending colon recognizable					
Nostrils reopen	Alveolar ducts and sacs present Primitive respiratory-like movements begin Lecithin begins to appear in amniotic fluid	Surfactant forming on alveolar surfaces	Lecithin/sphingomyelin ratio = 1.2:1	Lecithin/sphingomyelin ratio 2:1 or greater	Pulmonary branching only two thirds complete
				Formation of new nephrons ceases	
Brain grossly formed Cord myelination begins Spinal cord *ends* at level of *S1*	Cerebral cortex layered typically Neuronal proliferation in cerebral cortex ends	Appearance of cerebral fissures; convolutions rapidly appearing		End of spinal cord at level of L3	Myelination of brain begins
Nose and ear ossify		Eyelids reopen Retinal layers completed; light receptive Pupils capable of reacting to light	Sense of taste present Aware of sounds outside mother's body		
	Testes at inguinal ring in descent to scrotum		Testes descending to scrotum		Testes in scrotum Labia majora well developed

stances within the ovum but chiefly via osmosis from tubal and uterine secretions.

With implantation of the blastocyst, nutritive substances are taken up by the trophoblast and transmitted to the conceptus by direct osmosis. As the trophoblast grows, its villous projections penetrate and destroy the superficial layers of endometrium to tap the rich glycogen stores and the increasingly permeable endometrial blood vessels. The villi continue to branch and invade the endometrium until erosion of maternal vessels produces pools of blood that coalesce to form intervillous spaces. About the third week rudimentary blood vessels appear in the embryo and the cells of the trophoblast differentiate for more specialized function. By the end of the fourth month erosion of maternal tissues ceases, and the vascular pattern in the villous structure allows the direct transmission of nutritive materials through the placental filter from the maternal to the fetal system.

Placenta

Throughout prenatal life the primary source of fetal nourishment is the placenta, the large discoid organ that develops from the trophoblast and is expelled at the time of birth. The placenta serves several functions: respiration, nutrition, excretion, and protection for the fetus; however, in order to understand some of the placental functions it is helpful to describe the nature of placental structure.

Placental structure. When the trophoblast ceases invasion of the endometrium, tree-like branching blood vessels of the villi form fifteen to thirty irregular globular areas called *cotyledons* separated from each other by wedge-shaped areas from the maternal portion. Each of these richly vascularized fetal villi are surrounded by blood-filled sinuses, the intervillous spaces, fed by spiral uterine arteries. The endometrium to which the fetal structures are anchored has been transformed into loose, porous tissues at the point of placental attachment termed the *decidua basalis;* the remainder is the *decidua parietalis*. This spongy stratum of the decidua is the site of placental separation following birth, after which ruptured vessels are mechanically closed by firm uterine contractions. Fig. 7-5 illustrates the final placental structure with its fetal and maternal relationships.

Amniotic fluid. Securely linked to the placenta by the umbilical cord, the embryo (and, later, the fetus) floats freely in the amniotic fluid within the amniotic cavity. The source of this substance is probably a product of the amniotic membrane, but as pregnancy progresses the fetus is capable of modifying its volume and composition by swallowing and urinating increasingly larger amounts. Both the volume and composition of the fluid vary during the course of gestation. The volume increases rapidly during the early weeks to reach a maximum average of 1000 ml at term. The normal regulation of the fluid volume can be altered by conditions that interfere with either the absorptive activity of the gastrointestinal tract or excretion by the fetal urinary tract. An excess of fluid *(polyhydramnios)* may occur in malformations of the central nervous system in which fetal swallowing is impaired, such as anencephaly, or in malformations where the fluid is unable to pass to the intestine for absorption, such as esophageal or duodenal atresia. In fetal conditions in which little or no urine is excreted, such as renal agenesis or atresia of the urethra, the volume of amniotic fluid may be greatly diminished *(oligohydramnios)*.

The amniotic fluid serves several important functions. This buoyant medium allows the fetus to move about freely, thus facilitating musculoskeletal development. It aids in maintaining a relatively stable body temperature and provides a cushion against possible injury by equalizing pressures, thus distributing the impact of externally inflicted trauma. The fluid aids symmetric growth and development of the fetus and prevents the amnion from adhering to the organism to form adhesions. In addition, analysis of amniotic fluid contents provides a means to assess an increasing number of conditions that threaten the welfare of fetus and newborn. At the time of birth its hydrostatic action may provide a wedge to help dilate the cervix during labor.

Placental circulation. The most important feature of the

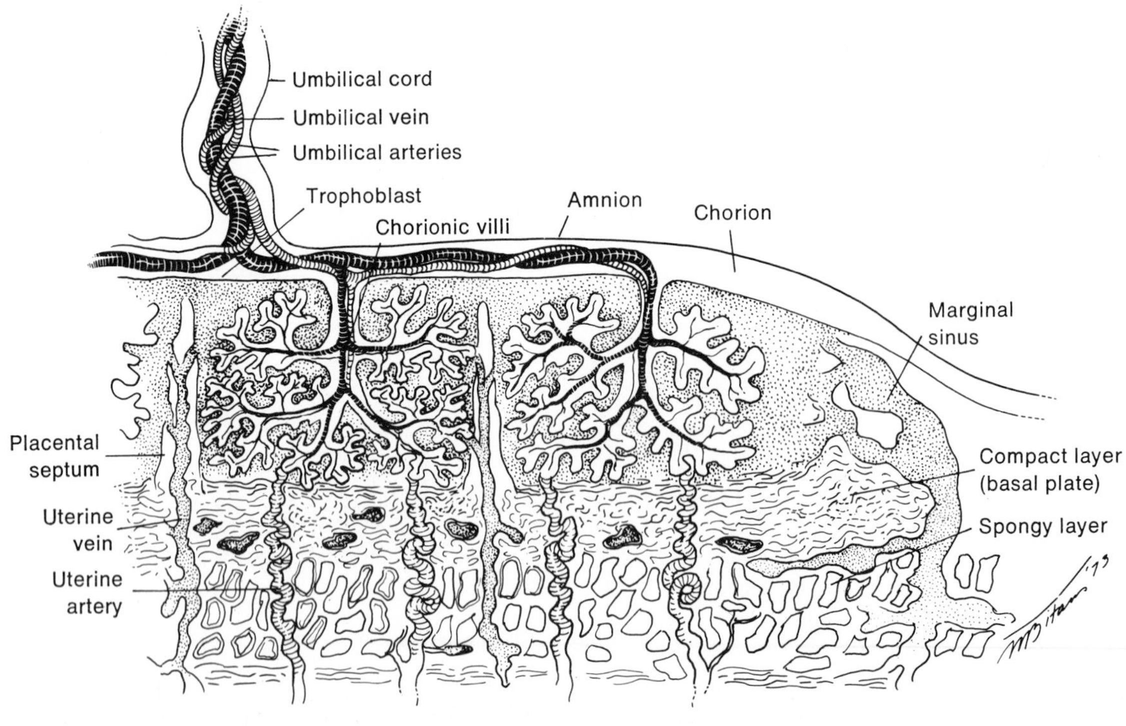

Fig. 7-5. Structure of the mature placenta. (From Chinn, P. L.: Child health maintenance: concepts in family centered care, ed. 2, St. Louis, 1979, The C. V. Mosby Co.)

placenta is the arrangement of the maternal and fetal circulatory systems and the manner of their relationship with one another. The two bloodstreams, moving in opposite directions, are separated by three layers of fetal cells that constitute the placental membrane. Sometimes called the placental barrier, it does not uniformly behave as a physical barrier, because it is across this placental membrane that the selective interchange of materials between the fetal and maternal bloodstreams takes place.

Blood from the maternal system empties into the intervillous space propelled in jet-like streams by the maternal blood pressure. This pressure directs the blood toward the chorionic plate, and from there it flows laterally. The closeness of the villi slows the flow of blood so that it seeps slowly through the peripheral portion of the cotyledon where it comes into direct contact with the villous surfaces to allow for exchange of materials. The blood then returns to the maternal surface of the placenta where it enters randomly distributed maternal veins. The arteries enter the intervillous spaces at a perpendicular angle, whereas most of the veins drain from a horizontal plane. This arrangement has the effect of closing off the *veins* during a uterine contraction and thereby prevents the squeezing out of essential maternal blood.

Deoxygenated blood from the fetal circulation enters the placenta via two umbilical arteries encased in a protective jelly within the umbilical cord—the structure that has developed from the body stalk and is normally inserted in the center of the placenta. From the umbilical arteries the blood is dispersed through the arterial-capillary-venous network within the chorionic villi. Here it comes into close proximity to the maternal blood in the intervillous space where the carbon dioxide and waste materials are exchanged for oxygen and nutrients. The oxygenated fetal blood then flows into veins that converge to form the large umbilical vein, which returns to the fetus through the umbilical cord (see Fig. 7-5). During the later weeks of gestation approximately 750 ml of blood flows through the placenta each minute.

Placental function. The placenta carries out several essential activities directed toward maintaining pregnancy and promoting normal fetal development. First it synthesizes steroid hormones (estrogen and progesterone) and protein hormones (the gonadotropins and thyrotropin) that help maintain the conceptus within the uterus and prepare auxiliary structures for birth and lactation.

One of the most important functions of the placenta is the selective transport of a variety of materials to and from the fetal and maternal blood. This transfer of substances across the placental membrane is accomplished by mechanisms similar to cellular exchanges elsewhere in the body, such as diffusion and active transport. Most substances with a small molecular weight readily cross the placental membrane by simple diffusion. The smaller the molecule, the more rapid its rate of transfer. The rates and direction of transfer are influenced by chemical forces and the degree of the membrane's permeability. During fetal life the placental membrane becomes progressively thinner and more permeable to a variety of substances, although shortly before birth the permeability may decrease somewhat because of degeneration of the aging placenta. Water crosses the membrane more rapidly than any other substance, even against a hydrostatic gradient, but the mechanism is not altogether clear.

Gases. Gases, principally oxygen and carbon dioxide, readily diffuse across the placental membrane. The direction in which gases move is determined by the differences in the partial pressures of gases (Po_2 and Pco_2) that exist between the maternal and fetal blood. Since gases diffuse in response to pressure gradients from a higher pressure to a lower one, the higher concentration of dissolved oxygen in the maternal blood of the intervillous spaces passes through the membrane to the fetal blood, and the highly soluble carbon dioxide, formed in fetal tissues, diffuses readily to the maternal system for excretion. The placental membrane seems to offer less resistance to the movement of carbon dioxide than it does to oxygen. Maintenance of these pressure gradients depends on normal gas levels in the mother and sufficient blood flow in both the maternal and fetal systems. Environmental influences that reduce the oxygen levels in the maternal blood or impair maternal circulation may pose a serious threat to the fetus. Some of these include cardiac or pulmonary disorders, convulsive episodes, and shock. Gases such as carbon monoxide and anesthetic agents also pass through the membrane by diffusion but do so at varying rates.

Nutrients. Metabolic substances for fetal nutrition cross the placental membrane in much the same manner as oxygen. Although diffusion is an important method of placental transfer, the chorionic villi exhibit a great deal of selectivity in transfer to maintain different concentrations of a variety of substances in the two systems. Facilitated diffusion, active transport, and pinocytosis are all mechanisms whereby substances are transferred across the membrane in significant quantities.

Glucose is quickly transferred and, since it is being rapidly metabolized by the fetus, its level in the fetal blood is 20% to 30% lower than in the maternal blood. Amino acids, free fatty acids, and electrolytes (such as calcium, phosphorus, sodium, and chlorides) are also transferred. As the substances are used by the fetus, their concentrations in the fetal blood decrease, which produces increased concentration gradients and causes increased movement through the membrane. Water-soluble vitamins cross the membrane more quickly than fat-soluble vitamins, and iron is actively transported from the maternal to the fetal blood.

Antibodies. Noncellular elements of the immunologic process are able to cross the placental membrane, and some passive immunity is conferred on the fetus by transplacental transfer of maternal antibodies, particularly immunoglobulin G (IgG). In this way the newborn acquires a short-term immunity to such diseases as diphtheria, smallpox, and measles.

Occasionally, and particularly during the later stages of gestation, ''breaks'' may occur in the membrane that allow fetal blood cells to pass into the maternal system. If the mother's antigens are incompatible with those of the fetus, the mother's immunologic defense mechanisms react by forming antibodies against these foreign proteins. These maternal antibodies are then able to cross to the fetal blood and attack the fetal red blood cells to produce hemolytic disease (see p. 295).

Waste materials. In addition to carbon dioxide, the placenta serves to transfer metabolic wastes, such as urea, uric acid, and creatinine, to be excreted with the mother's excretory products.

Other substances. Most drugs taken by the mother cross the placenta freely, and infectious agents, particularly viruses, may pass through the placental membrane and produce fetal infection. Some of these factors are known to cause deleterious effects on the developing organism depending on the stage of development. These and other influential factors are discussed on p. 228. Although large protein hormones such as ACTH and TSH do not cross the placental membrane, others, such as the steroids and insulin, are able to transverse the membrane freely. The extent to which these external agents affect the well-being of the organism depends on its vulnerability at the time the injurious agent comes in contact with it.

Fetal adaptive mechanisms

The fetus *in utero* has been described as living in a state of chronic hypoxia not unlike existence in the low-oxygen atmosphere at very high altitudes. Therefore, its survival under these conditions requires that its metabolic and circulatory systems have the capacity to adapt to hypoxemia without disturbing normal growth and development. Fetal mechanisms that contribute to this adaptation are the peculiar characteristics of the fetal blood and the distinctive features of fetal circulation.

Some of the characteristics of the fetal blood include the following[5,26,36]:

1. A cardiac output that is much higher when compared to that of the adult at rest (an average of 200 ml/kg/minute in the fetus and approximately 60 ml/kg/minute in the adult)
2. A hemoglobin that consists of primarily *fetal hemoglobin* (HgF), which is normally synthesized only during fetal life; fetal hemoglobin has the unique capacity to achieve a high saturation of oxygen at a lower oxygen pressure (Po_2); fetal hemoglobin has been demonstrated to carry 20% to 30% more oxygen than does the maternal hemoglobin
3. A high hemoglobin concentration (approximately 18 g/100 ml—about 50% greater than that of the mother) that increases the amount of oxygen that is carried by the fetal red blood cells
4. A higher erythrocyte count (about 5.5 million/ml)

Even though the mixture of maternal arterial and venous blood in the intervillous spaces has a decreased oxygen saturation and Po_2, the high oxygen affinity of fetal hemoglobin together with an increase in red cell volume provides the fetus with a perfectly adequate supply of oxygen under normal circumstances. In addition the fetus probably has an increased capacity to shift to anaerobic metabolism in conditions of hypoxemia.

Fetal circulation. The normal growth and development of the fetus relies on an active, independent metabolism, but it also requires an efficient circulation. During fetal life the lungs are essentially nonfunctional and the liver only partially functional; therefore, less blood is needed in these organs than is required after birth. The fetal brain requires the highest oxygen concentration, and the heart must pump a large amount of blood through the placenta. The characteristics of fetal circulation assure that the most vital organs and tissues receive the maximum concentration of vital materials for growth.

Blood carrying oxygen and nutritive materials from the placenta enters the fetal system through the umbilicus via the large umbilical vein (Fig. 7-6). The blood then travels upward to the underside of the liver where it separates—part of the blood enters the portal and hepatic circulation of the liver and the remainder travels directly to the inferior vena cava by way of the *ductus venosus*. Because of the higher pressure of blood entering the right atrium from the inferior vena cava, it is directed posteriorly in a straight pathway across the right atrium and through the *foramen ovale* to the left atrium. In this way the better-oxygenated blood enters the left atrium and ventricle to be pumped through the aorta to the head and upper extremities. Blood from the head and upper extremities entering the right atrium from the superior vena cava is directed downward through the tricuspid valve into the right ventricle. From here it is pumped through the pulmonary artery where the major portion is shunted to the descending aorta via the *ductus arteriosus*. Only a small amount flows to and from the nonfunctioning fetal lungs. Blood is returned to the placenta from the descending aorta through the two umbilical arteries.

Before birth the high pulmonary vascular resistance created by the collapsed fetal lung causes greater pressures in the right side of the heart and the pulmonary arteries. At the same time the free-flowing placental circulation and the ductus arteriosus produce a low vascular resistance in the remainder of the fetal vascular system. With the clamping of the umbilical cord and the expansion of the lungs at birth, the hemodynamics of the fetal vascular system undergo pronounced and abrupt changes. These changes are the direct result of cessation of the placental blood flow and the beginning of lung respiration. The primary and secondary changes that occur at birth are outlined in Table 7-3 and illustrated in Fig. 7-7.[7]

ABNORMAL DEVELOPMENT

The development of an organism, especially during embryogenesis, is an intricate process. Growth and development of all parts must be properly integrated to ensure a coordinated whole. The rate must be such that one part is ready when needed by another part; otherwise, either part may cease to grow or may deviate from its normal path. For example, during early development the optic lens is formed from overlying tissues only after an inductive trigger is released by the optic vessel. Some malformations result when a state, present in one phase of development as a normal condition, persists into another phase as abnormal. For example, a cleft lip is normal in a young embryo and a patent ductus arteriosus is essential during fetal life. Any agent that interferes with these complex processes will produce a defect in development ranging in severity from complete degeneration to a local anomaly.

Severe injury to the fetus at any time during prenatal development is capable of producing death or a defect that is incompatible with postnatal survival. It is estimated that 25% of all fertilized ova either fail during implantation or during early developmental processes because of some defect in the conceptus. Although the first trimester is the time of highest fetal loss, no period of pregnancy is free of detrimental forces that are hazardous to the fetus. By the time of birth almost 30% of pregnancies have ended in abortion or stillbirth; an additional 1% will succumb secondary to premature birth.

Table 7-3. Cardiovascular changes at birth

Prenatal status	Postnatal status	Associated factors
Primary changes		
Pulmonary circulation—high pulmonary vascular resistance; increased pressure in right ventricle and pulmonary arteries	Low pulmonary vascular resistance; decreased pressures in right atrium, ventricle, and pulmonary arteries	Expansion of the collapsed fetal lung
Systemic circulation—low pressures in left atrium, ventricle, and aorta	High systemic vascular resistance; increased pressure in left atrium, ventricle, and aorta	Loss of placental blood flow
Secondary changes		
Umbilical arteries—patent; carry blood from placenta to ductus venosus and liver	Functionally closed at birth; obliteration by fibrous proliferation may take 2 to 3 months; distal portions become the *lateral vesicoumbilical* ligaments; proximal portions remain open as *superior vesical arteries*	Closure precedes that of umbilical vein; probably accomplished by smooth muscle contraction in response to thermal and mechanical stimuli and alteration in oxygen tension; mechanically severed with cord at birth
Umbilical vein—patent; carries blood from placenta to ductus venosus and liver	Closed; after obliteration, it becomes *ligamentum teres hepatis*	Closure shortly after umbilical arteries; hence blood from placenta may enter neonate for short period after birth; mechanically severed with cord at birth
Ductus venosus—patent; connects umbilical vein to inferior vena cava	Closed; after obliteration, it becomes *ligamentum venosus*	Loss of blood flow from umbilical vein
Ductus arteriosus—patent; shunts blood from pulmonary artery to descending aorta	Functional closure almost immediately after birth; anatomic obliteration of the lumen by fibrous proliferation requires 1 to 3 months; becomes the *ligamentum arteriosum*	High systemic resistance increases the aortic pressure; low pulmonary resistance reduces pulmonary arterial pressure Increased oxygen content of the blood in ductus arteriosus creates vasospasm of its muscular wall
Foramen ovale—forms a valve opening that allows blood to flow from the right to the left atrium	Functionally closes at birth; constant apposition gradually leads to fusion and permanent closure within a few months or years in the majority of persons	Increased pressures in the left atrium together with decreased pressure in the right atrium cause closure of the valve over the foramen

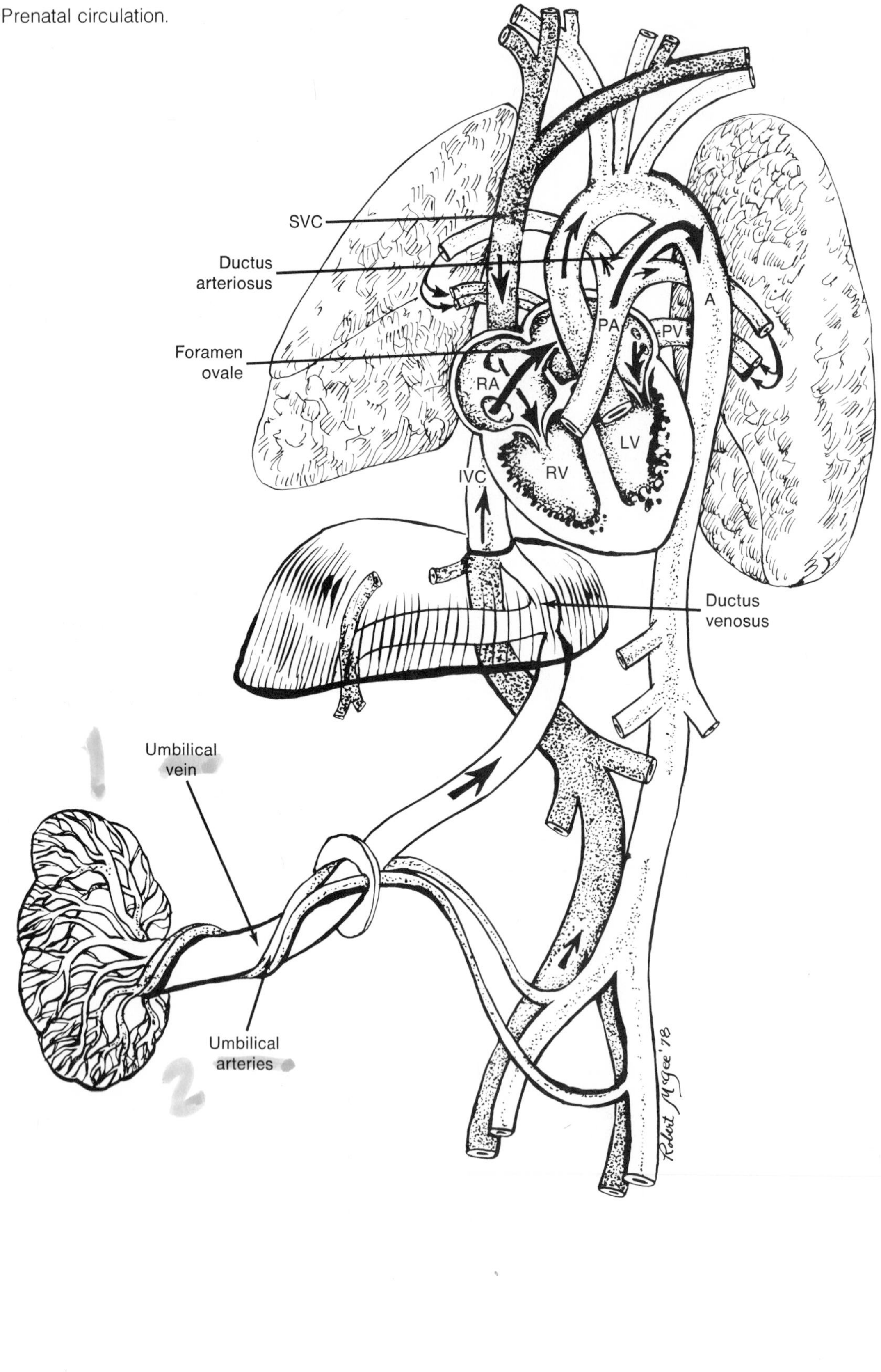

Fig. 7-6. Prenatal circulation.

Fig. 7-7. Postnatal circulation.

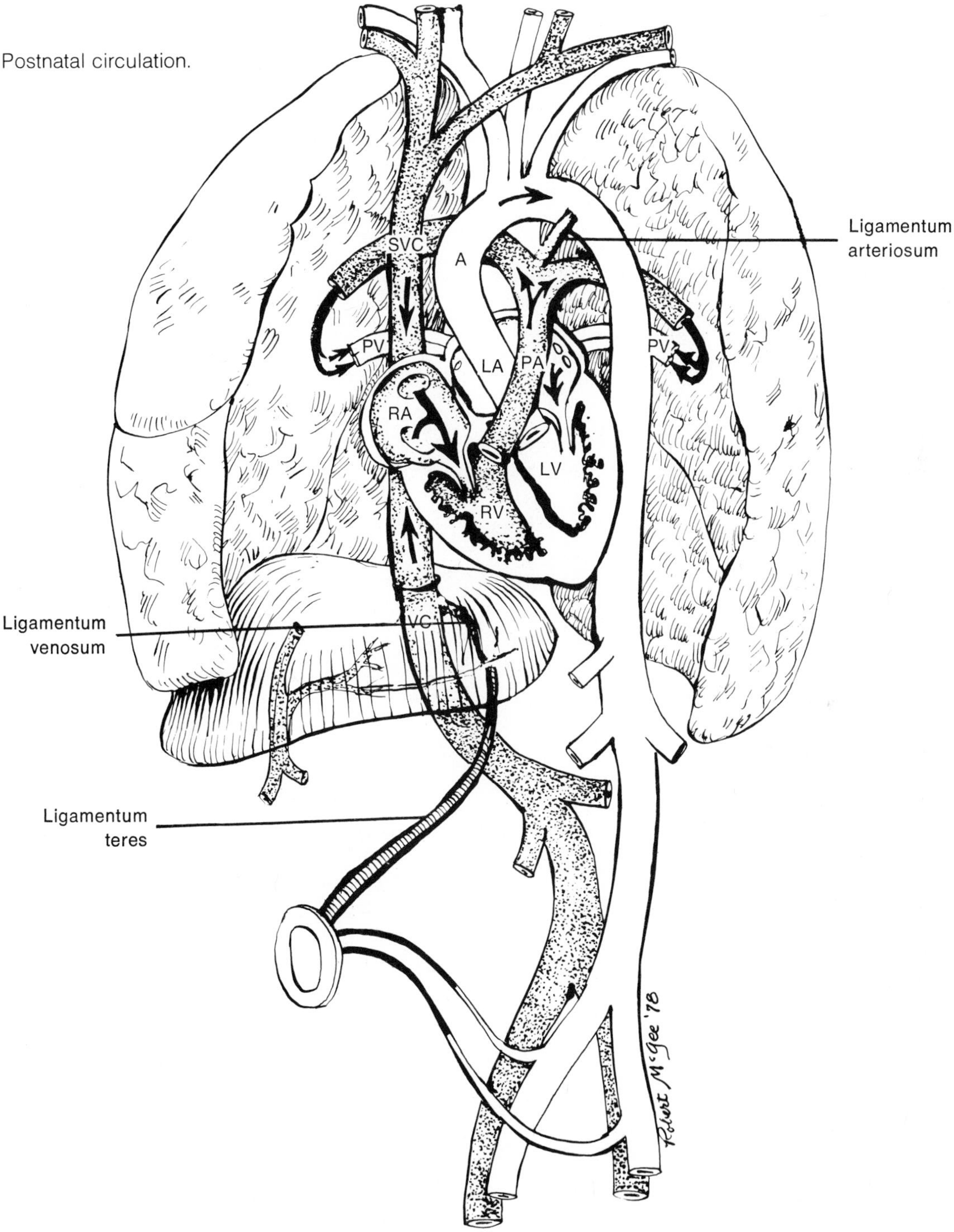

Congenital malformations

Congenital malformations, or birth defects, are defined as structural defects present at birth. The incidence is estimated to be about six in every 1000 births, but the methods of interpretation and reporting are subject to the criteria of the individual investigator or recorder. Malformations can arise at any stage of development and present wide variability in the determining factors as well as in the type, extent, and frequency of defects. Many, such as cleft lip, deformed limbs, or myelomeningocele, are readily apparent in the newborn infant; others, such as congenital heart disease or absent kidney, may not become evident until days, weeks, or even years after birth. Some defects are of such minor significance that they have little or no effect on survival or the quality of life; others are so severe as to be incompatible with life or are a serious threat to survival. There is also a high correlation between the incidence of congenital malformations and the infant who is small for gestational age. The more severe the growth retardation, the more likely the chance for malformation.

There appears to be a relationship between the incidence of one congenital anomaly and the presence of additional anomalies in an affected child. For example, there is a striking association between malformed ears and kidney abnormalities that reflects a common developmental stage. Observation of one anomaly alerts the examiner to the possibility of defective development in another tissue or organ. The knowledge of the stage of development for a variety of organs and systems and comparison of the developmental stage at which the observed anomaly occurred provide clues for closer scrutiny of other organs or anomalies that reflect the same stage of development.

Classification. Congenital malformations can be broadly classified according to their probable etiology:

1. Malformations determined by a single mutant gene on either an autosome or a sex chromosome, for example, polydactyly, deafness, and dwarfism
2. Defects caused by chromosomal aberrations, such as Down's syndrome and other autosomal trisomies
3. Defects resulting from intrauterine environmental factors, for example, heart or eye defects as a result of maternal rubella, absence of a limb from maternal ingestion of the drug thalidomide, and limb deformities caused by intrauterine positional pressures
4. Defects attributed to a complex interaction between genetic and environmental factors, for example, common malformations such as congenital dislocated hip, myelomeningocele, cleft lip and/or palate, and pyloric stenosis

Although birth injuries are a separate classification, they are often considered in conjunction with congenital malformations. They are not defects in development but are caused by mechanical or anoxic trauma during the birth process. Birth injuries include fractures, cerebral palsy, and hemorrhage.

Congenital anomalies are more often conveniently classified according to the organ system that is affected, for example, developmental defects of the nervous system and congenital heart defects. A more descriptive categorization of anomalies denotes the ways in which defective development occurs:

developmental failure tissue or organ primordia fail to appear or do not develop to a significant degree *(agenesis)*. Examples of developmental failure include absence of a limb or part of a limb, absence of an organ, or absence of skin pigment (albinism).

developmental arrest developmental progress falls short of normal completion, for instance, cleft palate, spina bifida, umbilical hernia, and most congenital heart defects. This includes conditions in which normal growth ceases, such as some types of dwarfism and infantile genitalia.

developmental excess this may involve excessive growth of a part or in general (gigantism). It may result in an increase in numbers, such as extra digits, or the process of development may exceed that which is normal, such as excessive growth of hair, a thick epidermis, or hypertrophy of the pyloric sphincter.

fusion organs that are usually separated are pushed so close together during normal migration that they fuse into one large organ, such as a horseshoe kidney, or close prematurely, such as the skull bones in craniostenosis.

splitting occasionally primordial structures are split to create partial or complete duplication of the part, for example, a double ureter or an abnormal cleft as in a lobster-claw hand.

failure to subdivide common primitive fields are retained, for example polycystic kidneys, syndactyly, or truncus arteriosus.

failure to atrophy temporary structures that normally disappear remain, such as the anal membrane of an imperforate anus.

failure to consolidate lobed or accessory organs frequently result when the mass fails to consolidate in such organs as the spleen, pancreas, or adrenal glands.

incorrect migration the normal shift in location fails in whole or in part, such as undescended testicles (cryptorchidism), or exceeds normal migration, such as ovaries in external genitalia.

misplacement organs are situated in unexpected locations, such as dextrocardia, palatine teeth, or transposed viscera.

atypical differentiation the course of development and the resulting physical manifestations are unlike those seen in the normal fetus and newborn. Examples include congenital tumors, osteogenesis imperfecta, and Down's syndrome.

atavism possession of a trait characteristic of remote rather than immediate ancestors; a reversion. An example is an elevator muscle of the clavicle that is seen in climbing primates.

Twins[4,8]

A deviation in early development that occurs with relative frequency is twinning. It is well known that twins are of two distinct types: *identical* or *monozygotic* (MZ) and *fraternal* or *dizygotic* (DZ). These two types are separate and apparently unrelated phenomena. Dizygotic twins are derived from the fertilization of two ova that are released nearly simultaneously from the ovary. They may be of like sex or opposite sexes, and they differ both physically and in genetic constitution. They are merely siblings who happen to be born at the same time. Monozygotic twins are the result of one fertilized ovum that becomes separated at a very early stage of development, with each part developing into a complete individual. Monozygotic twins are always alike in both gene complement and physical characteristics, including sex. The term identical, used to describe monozygotic twins, is not entirely accurate, because no two individuals are ever exactly alike in every detail.

The frequency of twin births varies according to ethnic origin, maternal age, and heredity, and these differences are related almost exclusively to the incidence of dizygotic twins. Monozygotic twins occur with relatively uniform frequency in all populations (approximately one in 200 to 285 births) and appear to be random events. Dizygotic twinning, on the other hand, shows variable frequency among racial populations, the highest being in the black races and the lowest in the Mongoloid races, with the white races being somewhere intermediate. In the United States the overall twinning rate is approximately one in 80 pregnancies and consists of one third monozygotic and two thirds dizygotic twins.

Dizygotic twinning becomes increasingly common with advancing maternal age, rising to a maximum between the ages of 35 and 39 years and then decreasing rapidly. Maternal age has little if any effect on the monozygotic twinning rate. Monozygotic twinning is unaffected by heredity, but dizygous twins show a marked familial tendency. The tendency toward dizygous twinning is a hereditary trait expressed only in the females. There is an increase in twins among relatives of mothers of twins (for example, female siblings and offspring of dizygotic twins) but not among relatives of the fathers (for example, brothers of dizygotic twins and offspring of a dizygotic twin). Fathers do, however, appear to transmit the disposition toward double ovulation to their daughters.

Determination of zygosity. It is important to distinguish between monozygotic and dizygotic twins for two reasons. First monozygotic twin studies serve as a useful tool in the scientific study of the influence of heredity and environment in developmental phenomena and disease processes. Second since there is an ever-increasing need for transplant donors and since truly successful organ or tissue transplantation is possible only between genetically identical individuals, identification of monozygotic twins is a very practical consideration. The earlier this distinction is made, the more useful the information will be. Methods used to determine zygosity are examination of fetal membranes or comparison and contrasting of physical similarities and differences between members of a pair of twins. It can be established that a pair of twins is not monozygotic, but not with absolute certainty.

Twins of different sexes or with obvious differences in physical characteristics such as hair or eye color or ear shape are dizygotic. Monozygotic twins are always of like sex. Blood group comparisons are the most reliable physical means to distinguish types of twins. Monozygotic twins always possess identical blood groups; dizygotic twins may be alike or may differ in any or all blood group systems. If a single difference is found, it can be concluded that the pair is dizygotic.

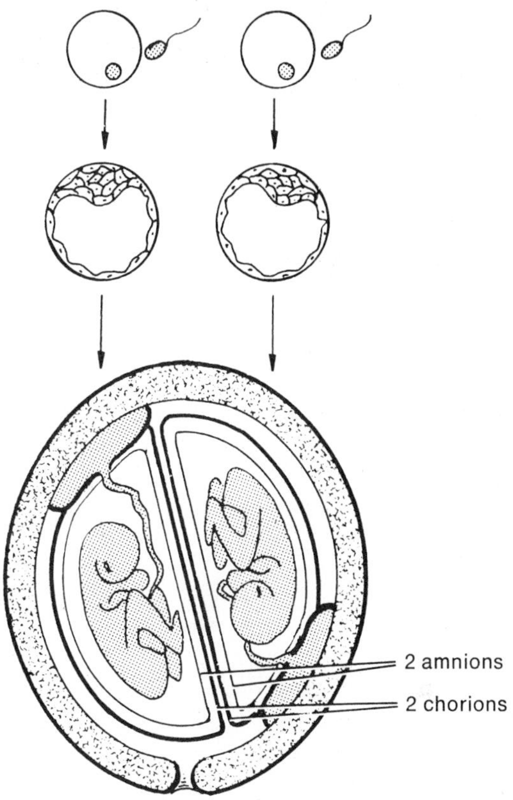

Fig. 7-8. Formation of dizygotic twins. There is fertilization of the two ova, two implantations, two placentas, two chorions, and two amnions. (From Whaley, L.: Understanding inherited disorders, St. Louis, 1974, The C. V. Mosby Co., p. 100.)

Examination of fetal membranes provides an early means of differentiating between monozygotic and dizygotic twins of like sex. Dizygotic twins have two separate and distinct placentas and membranes, both amnion and chorion (Fig. 7-8). In some instances, if the implantations are close together on the uterine wall, the placentas may grow together, giving the impression of one placenta.

Monozygotic twins may have single or separate placentas and membranes, depending on the time during early development when division has taken place. If, during the blastomere stage, the cells do not separate and two inner cell masses form, the two embryos will develop within a single chorion but with individual amnions. Rarely the embryos will develop within a single amnion. If the blastomeres

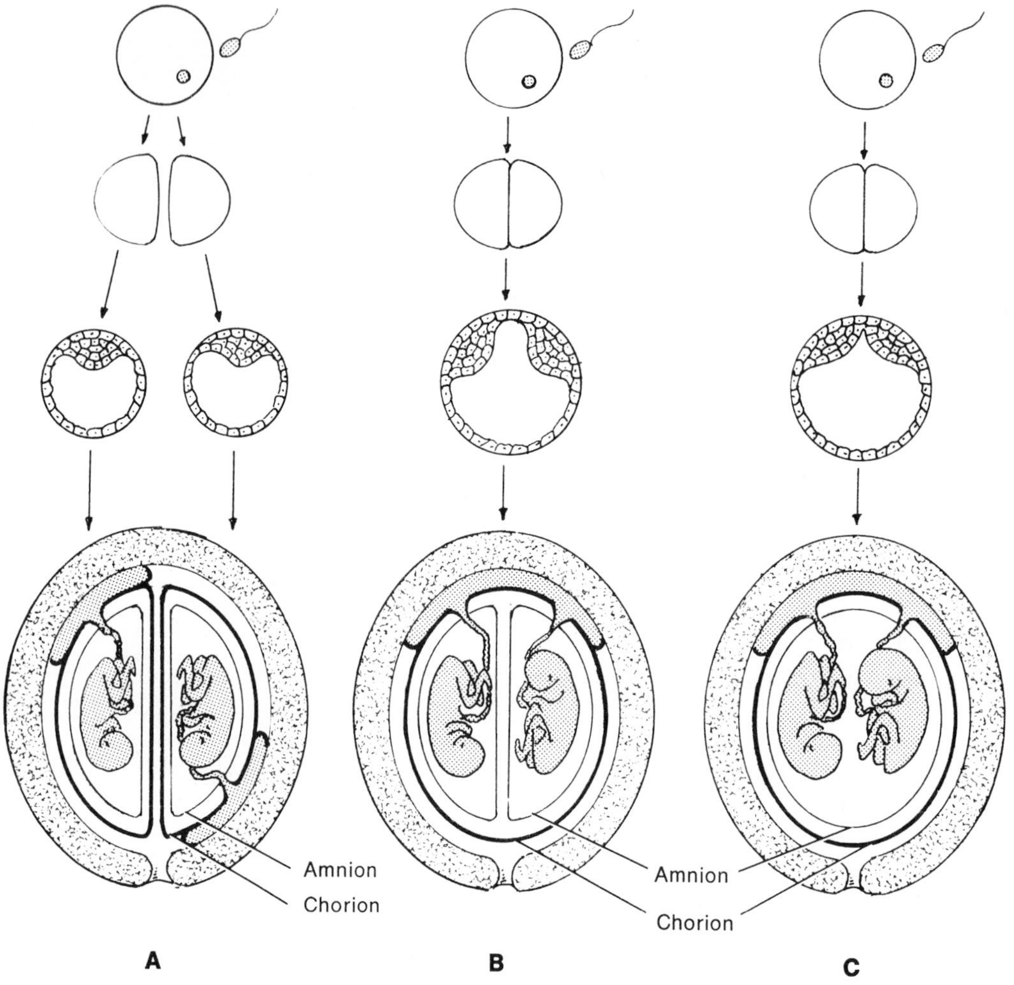

Fig. 7-9. Formation of monozygotic twins. **A,** One fertilization, blastomeres separate, resulting in two implantations, two placentas, and two sets of membranes. **B,** One blastomere with two inner cell masses, one fused placenta, one chorion, separate amnions. **C,** Later separation of inner cell masses, with fused placenta and single amnion and chorion. (From Whaley, L.: Understanding inherited disorders, St. Louis, 1974, The C. V. Mosby Co., p. 102.)

separate, the two zygotes formed from this separation will implant separately and form their own amnion and chorion in much the same manner as dizygotic twins (Fig. 7-9). When division is late and incomplete, the result is conjoined, or "Siamese," twins. Twins that are enclosed in a single chorion (monochorionic) can be regarded as monozygotic twins; however, in other cases distinction is not certain since both types of twins can have two amnions, chorions, and placentas or a single placenta.

ENVIRONMENTAL INFLUENCES ON DEVELOPMENT AND DIFFERENTIATION

During intrauterine life the developing organism is protected to a great extent by the environment provided by the mother; however, this protection is not complete. Numerous internal and external factors can produce injury to the embryo especially during periods of rapid growth or differentiation. The impact of these factors depends on the nature of the environmental change and the developmental stage of the embryo at the time of exposure.

Critical periods in prenatal development

Every organ, system, and body part goes through a period in which it experiences the most rapid cell division and differentiation. During this time of accelerated growth and differentiation, the organism displays a marked susceptibility to injurious influences. These specific stages of crucial developmental advancement are termed *critical peri-*

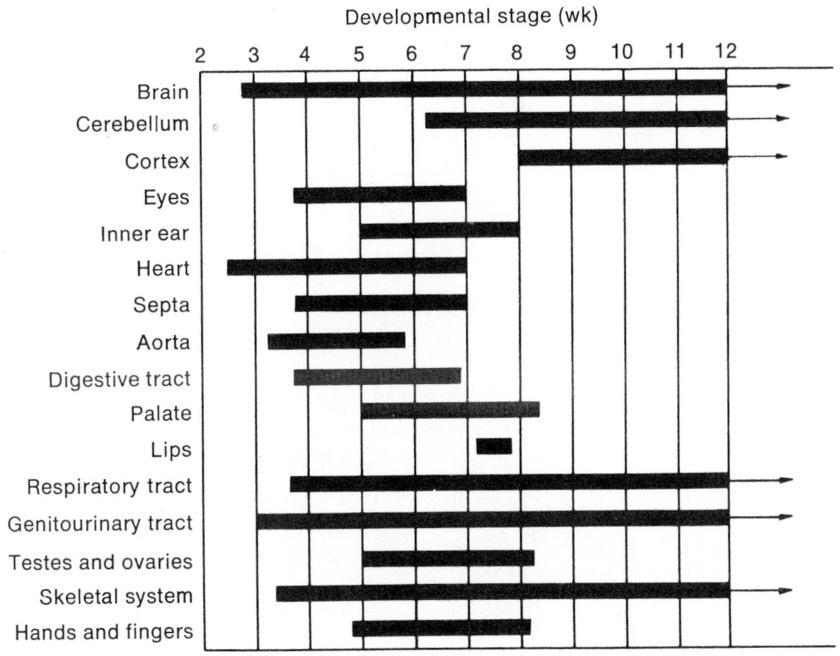

Fig. 7-10. Approximate periods of critical differentiation for some specific organs. (From Whaley, L.: Understanding inherited disorders, St. Louis, 1974, The C. V. Mosby Co., p. 109.)

ods, and the major impact of environmental factors always coincides with these periods.

Although critical periods in prenatal development are predominant during the early stages of development, the critical periods for all organs or parts do not occur simultaneously. A part that is susceptible to adverse influences at one particular time may be resistant to the same influence at other periods of development. At the same time, the impact on another part may be highly sensitive at the moment. Influences that alter or halt development at a critical period can be highly effective in producing disturbed development. Susceptibility to environmental influences decreases as organ formation advances. The younger the organism and the fewer the number of cells, the greater the extent of involvement proportionately when any cell or group of cells is injured.

Teratogenesis

The term teratogenesis (*terato,* monster; *genesis,* production) is a term that refers to the origin or method by which prenatal growth processes are disturbed to produce a physical defect, and the agents capable of producing such an adverse effect are called *teratogens*. Teratogens may act directly on the embryo or indirectly by their effect on accessory structures (for example, the placenta) or the maternal system. Since teratogens must affect a specific process in the developing organism, the *time of application* will determine the type and extent of the damage.[6]

Periods of vulnerability. During the preimplantation period, the embryo is generally considered to be relatively resistant to environmental influences. The impact at this phase either damages all or a majority of the dividing cells with subsequent abortion, or it will damage only a few. Since these are undifferentiated cells, the regulative capacities of the very early conceptus will compensate for the loss with no apparent abnormalities.

During the period of intensive differentiation most teratogenic agents are highly effective and may produce a variety of malformations. The type of malformation that is produced depends on which organ is most susceptible at the time of application. Fig. 7-10 indicates the approximate times of critical differentiation for some of the major organs and systems.

In the later periods of development, characterized by growth and elaboration of organs, the susceptibility to teratogenic influences decreases rapidly. The primary effects during this time are growth retardation, minor physical abnormalities, and physiologic or functional disturbances. In recent years the study of defective development (teratology) has been broadened to include any birth defect—morphologic, biochemical, or behavioral—induced at any stage of gestation that is detected at birth or later in life.

Principles of teratology. As a result of data gathered from retrospective studies and animal experiments, a few basic principles have emerged that present some insight into the probability of children being affected by some specific teratogens.

1. The susceptibility of the organism to teratogenic factors is determined by the stage of development.
2. The effect of a teratogen depends on the genetic predisposition. There are indications that a teratogenic agent accentuates the incidence of those defects that occur sporadically, implying underlying genetic instabilities.
3. A single teratogen may produce a variety of anomalies. For example, it has been established that rubella infection of the mother can produce a variety of defects, including cataracts, deafness, heart anomalies, and mental retardation.
4. A variety of teratogenic agents may produce similar anomalies; for example, viruses, chemicals, and radiation can all produce a mental deficit.
5. Teratogenic anomalies may be indistinguishable from hereditary malformations (phenocopies), for example, inherited deafness and deafness caused by maternal rubella.
6. Many teratogenic agents have little or no adverse effect on the maternal system and may even be beneficial to the mother. A dramatic illustration is the well-publicized defects produced in the 1960s by the drug thalidomide. This effective hypnotic drug, nontoxic to the mother, is severely teratogenic to the fetus.

Environmental factors

Before birth the maternal host determines the well-being of the fetus by the manner in which she protects, favors, or deprives it. An unfavorable maternally imposed environment may produce effects on the fetus that are of a transient nature with few, if any, deleterious consequences or serious enough to cause long-range health problems in the infant or child.

Maternal age. There appears to be a relationship between the age of the mother at the time of birth and the outcome of pregnancy. Overall, mothers less than 20 years of age encounter difficulties with greater frequency than do older mothers. Excessive weight gain, toxemia of pregnancy, and prolonged labor are experienced more frequently by women in this group. Infants born to very young mothers are more apt to fall into the low-birth weight category with an attendant increased risk of neonatal morbidity and mortality associated with these infants in general. There is not complete agreement regarding an increased incidence of malformations in infants of mothers less than 20 years of age.

Mothers who become pregnant in the later period of their biologic reproductive years (over age 35) seem to be less able to physically withstand the rigors of pregnancy and childbearing. There is an increase in maternal disease, such as hypertensive disease and toxemia, in addition to other complications, such as malposition of the fetus, uterine inertia, and pelvic disproportion. A higher incidence of spontaneous abortion has been documented in this age-group, and the number of infants with chromosomal abnormalities, primarily Down's syndrome, increases markedly in women over age 35 years. A number of fetal malformations have been reported with greater frequency in older mothers, although implication of the age factor is largely speculative. Some of these malformations include abnormalities of the central nervous system, musculoskeletal disorders, gastrointestinal anomalies, and cardiovascular defects.

Chemicals.[15, 18, 24, 40] As previously stated, the relationship of the fetal and maternal circulations allows for the interchange of chemical substances across the placental membrane. During gestation, deficiencies in the fetal metabolism (such as hypothyroidism) are usually compensated by the maternal system to afford some measure of protection to the fetus. However, the limited metabolic capabilities of the fetal liver and its immature enzyme and transport systems render the unborn child ill equipped for maintaining homeostasis when chemical disturbances are imposed by the mother. This includes both substances produced by the mother in response to a disease state (such as diabetes) and exogenous substances ingested or inhaled by the mother. The intensity and duration of drug action are affected by the age of the conceptus and the state of its ability to absorb, distribute, detoxify, and excrete the substance. The substance is likely to cause failure of a series of interrelated and interdependent functions of the fetal system rather than a single mechanism.

The thalidomide tragedy of the 1960s accelerated the interest in drugs and other environmental factors as a cause of congenital malformations. Many drugs have been suspected of having teratogenic properties and some have been definitely implicated; however, none has created the impact of thalidomide. During the few short years that it was available, it is estimated that 4000 to 5000 children were affected in Germany alone (the country in which it was most widely used). Although an efficient sleep-producing drug in the mother, it produced severe malformations in the fetus. Most cases involved malformations of the upper extremities (phocomelia or amelia), but all extremities were affected, as well as some facial defects, heart malformations, and visceral abnormalities. When the drug was taken during the sensitive period, between the thirty-fourth and fiftieth days of gestation, the incidence of malformation reached 100% even with small doses. The drug was removed from the market as soon as the relationship between administration of the drug and defects in the infants was recognized.

It has been estimated that women take an average of four or five drugs—either prescription or over-the-counter preparations—during their pregnancy. Also, hormones have been implicated in animal teratogenesis and in some disorders found in the newborn infant. Because they are frequently administered as drugs, these substances are often classified as such. Hormones originate and circulate normally in all individuals; an exogenous source simply increases the amount already present in the body. The physiologically active and chemical substances known to produce adverse effects on the fetus, neonate, or child and their physical consequences are listed in Table 7-4. The extent to which chemical agents affect the unborn child depends on the interplay of the factors mentioned previously—the nature of the agent and its accessibility to the fetus, the time of its applications, the level and duration of the dosage, and the genetic makeup of the fetus.[15,39]

Infectious factors. The range of pathology produced by infectious agents is large, and the difference between the maternal and fetal effects of any one agent is also great. Severe maternal infections, especially during early gestation, can result in fetal loss or malformations caused by the debilitating effect on the health of the mother that may interfere with her ability to maintain the pregnancy, the infectious agent crossing the placental membrane to affect fetal

Table 7-4. Effects of chemical agents on the fetus or newborn*

Chemical agent	Effect on fetus or newborn	Comments
Analgesics		
Salicylates (large amounts)	Neonatal bleeding; coagulation defects	Most vulnerable near term
Anticoagulants		
Warfarin (Coumadin, dicumarol)	Fetal death; hemorrhage; high perinatal mortality	Vulnerable throughout gestation; conclusive evidence
Anticonvulsives		
Trimethadione	Abortion; malformations; mental retardation	Conclusive evidence
Antihypertensives		
Reserpine	Drowsiness; nasal congestion in neonate; hypothermia; hypertonia	Transient
Thiazides	Neonatal thrombocytopenia	Conclusive evidence
Antimicrobials		
Chloramphenicol	"Gray syndrome," death	Vulnerable near term; fairly well documented
Nitrofurantoin	Hemolysis	Vulnerable near term; fairly well documented
Sulfonamides	Hyperbilirubinemia; kernicterus	Vulnerable near term; fairly well documented
Streptomycin	Eighth cranial nerve damage (hearing loss); skeletal anomalies	Vulnerable near term; fairly well documented
Tetracyclines	Inhibition of bone growth	Suggestive evidence only
	Teeth discoloration	Vulnerable second and third trimesters; conclusive evidence
Antineoplastic agents		
Aminopterin	Abortion; skeletal defects; central nervous system anomalies; cleft palate	Conclusive evidence
Chlorambucil	Renal agenesis	Suggestive evidence
Cyclophosphamide	Multiple malformations	Suggestive evidence
Methotrexate	Multiple malformations, especially skeletal	Vulnerable first trimester
Antithyroid drugs		
Iodides, propylthiouracil, methimazole	Goiter; hypothyroidism; mental retardation	Vulnerable fourteenth week on; conclusive evidence
Endocrine hormones		
Insulin shock	Death	Conclusive evidence
Adrenocorticoids	Cleft palate; adrenocortical failure in newborn	Suggestive evidence
Sex hormones—androgens, estrogens (oral), progestins	Masculinization of female fetus; labial fusion (early in pregnancy); clitoral enlargement (later in pregnancy)	Conclusive evidence of masculinization; suggestive evidence of labial fusion and clitoral enlargement

*Data from references 15, 24, 35, and 40.

Continued.

Table 7-4. Effects of chemical agents on the fetus or newborn—cont'd

Chemical agent	Effect on fetus or newborn	Comments
Endocrine hormones—cont'd		
Diethylstilbestrol	Vaginal adenocarcinoma in adolescence and young adulthood	Conclusive evidence
	Masculinization of female fetus	Suggestive evidence
Narcotics		
Heroin- or morphine-addicted mother	Generally impaired neonatal adjustment; withdrawal symptoms; convulsions; death	Vulnerable near term; fairly well documented
Sedatives		
Alcohol (heavy consumption during pregnancy)	Growth deficiency; fetal alcohol syndrome—flat facial profile, short eye slits, smaller brain; may be associated limb and cardiovascular defects	Suggestive evidence
Barbiturates	Nonattentiveness; may be accompanied by permanent neurologic sequelae	In excessive amounts, conclusive evidence
Thalidomide	Phocomelia; amelia	Known teratogen
Vitamins		
Vitamin K	Hyperbilirubinemia in newborn; hemolysis	In excessive amounts, conclusive evidence
Vitamin D	Excessive blood calcium; mental retardation	In excessive amounts, conclusive evidence
Other		
Lysergic acid diethylamide (LSD)	Convulsions, stunted growth, skeletal defects; chromosomal damage	Inconclusive evidence
Nicotine (smoking)	Low birth weight infants; prematurity	Conclusive evidence
Oral hypoglycemic agents—sulfonylurea derivatives	Congenital malformations	Questionable evidence

development directly, or ascending inflammation crossing the fetal membranes by way of the cervix. If the conceptus is affected, the consequences may be abortion, stillbirth, premature birth, congenital anomalies, growth retardation, or disease observable after birth. Most often maternal infection goes unrecognized, and frequently the fetus will also suffer few, if any effects of the infection. However, the ability of the fetus to handle organisms is limited. The fetal immunologic system is inadequate, and the fetus is unable to prevent the dissemination of organisms to the various tissues. For example, the fetal blood-brain barrier offers little resistance to infectious agents.

Because they are the smallest of the infectious organisms and cross the placenta more easily, viruses are important in the etiology of congenital defects.[20] However, a great deal depends on the prevalence of these agents in the population. Some, such as respiratory and gastrointestinal viruses, tend to be present in almost all communities; others, such as smallpox and poliomyelitis, have been significantly reduced in most areas of the world. Data have implicated a number of viruses in health problems of infants. The most notable of these is rubella or German measles, a mild disease in adults but one that has been definitely shown to produce a high percentage of congenital malformation in the fetus when the mother is infected during the first 10 weeks of pregnancy. This important discovery was made in the early 1940s when it was found that the increased incidence of some congenital malformations correlated with an epidemic of German measles at about the time the mothers of these infants were in their third month of pregnancy. More frequent anomalies associated with rubella are congenital cataracts, deafness, mental retardation, and congenital heart disease.[20] The incidence of fetal malformation is 10% to 15% if the infection is come into contact with during the first month, 14% to 24% in the second month, and 6% to 17% in the third month of gestation. After this time fetal abnormalities are uncommon. The chance of spontaneous abortion during the first trimester is 10% to 15%.[1] Some of the infectious agents that have been implicated in fetal malformations or disease are listed in Table 7-5.

Table 7-5. Effects of maternal infections on the mother, fetus, or newborn*

Infection	Effects on mother	Effects on fetus or newborn	Preventive measures
Coxsackie virus infection	Mild infection—influenza-like enteric or respiratory illness	Meningoencephalitis in neonate Myocarditis—congenital heart disease Digestive and urinary tract abnormalities	Avoid contact
Cytomegalic inclusion disease (CID) cytomegalovirus ("salivary gland virus")	Asymptomatic Mononucleosis-type illness 50% of mothers susceptible	Increased incidence of low birth weight and prematurity Massive hepatosplenomegaly; jaundice Central nervous system involvement—microcephaly, lethargy, seizures, severe mental and motor retardation High mortality rate in severely affected infants Infants may acquire the virus through the birth canal during birth	None
Hepatitis type A and B	Disease manifestations—jaundice, fever, malaise, nausea and vomiting, pruritus, upper right quadrant pain	Abortion Low birth weight Neonatal hepatitis	Pregnant women should avoid caring for infected infants and handling blood products
Herpes simplex virus hominis (HVH) (usually type II)	Herpetic vulvovaginitis	Fetal infection variable—subclinical to generalized viremia with multiple organ involvement and death Mild disease—recovery; severe disease—death	Cesarean section delivery where maternal genital lesions are present (prior to rupture of maternal membranes)
Influenza	Maternal disease variable	Increased incidence of abortion Increased incidence of prematurity Occasional association with central nervous system malformations, especially myelomeningocele and anencephaly	Avoid contact with affected persons Active immunization by attenuated vaccine contraindicated during pregnancy
Mumps	Maternal infection variable	Increased incidence of abortion, prematurity, and stillbirth Endocardial fibroelastosis	Hyperimmune convalescent serum prophylaxis to susceptible women (increased risk of serum hepatitis, however)
Poliomyelitis	Variable from mild symptoms to paralytic poliomyelitis Pregnant women more susceptible	Abortion Fetal or neonatal death Growth retardation	Virtually eliminated by widespread childhood immunization programs Salk vaccine safe during pregnancy Sabin live virus vaccine contraindicated during pregnancy
Rubella	Maternal infection usually mild	Abortion Congenital malformations of the heart, eye, and ear Mental retardation Low birth weight	Pregnant women should avoid contact with infected persons Immunizations or purposeful exposure of nonpregnant susceptible women Therapeutic termination of pregnancy when the mother becomes infected during the first trimester

*Data from references, 2, 9, 32, and 35.

Continued.

Table 7-5. Effects of maternal infections on the mother, fetus, or newborn—cont'd

Infection	Effects on mother	Effects on fetus or newborn	Preventive measures
Rubella—cont'd			Mandatory contraception for 2 months following immunization of sexually active women
Rubeola	Maternal disease	Increased incidence of abortion Low birth weight Maternal rubeola at any time during gestation is responsible for increased perinatal mortality Rarely, fetal malformations Majority of infants normal	Vaccination of all nonimmune women prior to but not during pregnancy
Syphilis	Maternal disease	Major cause of midtrimester abortion, fetal death in utero, or prematurity Early congenital syphilis—septicemia, skin lesions, anemia, jaundice, periostitis Late congenital syphilis	Prenatal serologic test early in pregnancy Antibiotic therapy for mothers with positive serologic findings
Toxoplasmosis	Signs of active disease practically never found in pregnant women	High incidence of abortion Intrauterine growth retardation Early manifestations—hepatosplenomegaly, jaundice, chorioretinitis, microphthalmia, convulsions Later manifestations—hydrocephalus or microcephaly, mental retardation High mortality rate	Prevention of maternal disease Encysted organisms found in some meats—especially pork and lamb—therefore thorough cooking is advised
Varicella	Maternal disease during early weeks	Skin lesions, brain damage (usually not recognized until well after birth)	Avoid contact No immunization available

Radiation. Ionizing radiation has been shown to be both mutagenic (capable of producing mutations) and teratogenic in man. Pelvic irradiation of pregnant women—from natural background radiation that is present everywhere in varying degrees, from occupational exposure, and from diagnostic or therapeutic procedures—is believed to be hazardous to the embryo, although the extent of teratogenicity and the exact dosage required to induce somatic change are still under consideration. Most of the teratogenic effects of radiation have been determined by studies carried out on children who were exposed in utero to the atomic bombs in Hiroshima and Nagasaki and by animal studies. Radiation may damage the conceptus at any time during its prenatal existence, and it is known that rapidly dividing and differentiating cells, such as those of the embryo, have increased radiosensitivity. As with other teratogens, the type of effect produced is closely correlated with the stage of development at which the radiation exposure occurs. During the preimplantation period, when there is rapid division but little differentiation, irradiation produces a high incidence of embryonic death; however, surviving embryos appear to be normal. Radiation during the period of major organogenesis, which begins shortly after implantation, can cause a whole spectrum of malformations depending on the stage of development at which the radiation is applied. Most of these malformed embryos survive and may exhibit abnormalities of the brain (especially microcephaly), eyes (microphthalmia), or skeleton.[34]

After the major organ systems have been formed, irradiation can still cause injury to the conceptus. The malformations are less severe than those brought about during the earlier periods, and the doses required to produce them are usually higher. The cells of the nervous system seem to be most sensitive at this time. Defects are primarily related to specific neural structures within the system, for example, the cerebellum and retina rather than the brain or the system as a whole. No amount of radiation can be considered absolutely safe; therefore, it is recommended that exposure to diagnostic or therapeutic radiation be carried out on women in the childbearing years only during the first half of their menstrual cycle before fertilization and implantation are likely to have occurred. Also, the harmful effects of maternal radioactive iodine (RAI) therapy on the fetal thyroid has led to the conclusion that pregnancies that occur during RAI therapy should be terminated.

Mechanical factors. The intrauterine environment minimizes the possibility of trauma to the fetus; however, during the later months of gestation the fetus may be subjected to a variety of positional abnormalities. As pregnancy advances, maintaining an attitude of complete flexion in the cramped quarters of the uterus predisposes the fetus to a number of deformities, for example, metatarsus varus, torticollis, and dislocation of the hip. Often the increased pressure from crowding is a factor as evidenced by the higher incidence of physical deformities encountered in twins (particularly monozygotic twins) than in single births. However, the incidence is not significant enough to cause undo anxiety in the mother expecting the birth of twins.

Sometimes defects occur as the result of amniotic bands or adhesions between the amnion and the fetus, such as the constriction of fetal limbs by bands of amniotic tissue that inhibit the growth of distal segments. Decrease in the production of amniotic fluid may create deformities of varying degrees as a result of the restriction of intrauterine space, for example, malformations of the jaw and ribs, asymmetry of the head, and compression marks on the body.

Although the fetus is well protected from physical trauma, severe violence inflicted to the abdomen of a pregnant woman may precipitate a spontaneous abortion, premature delivery, or traumatic injury to the unborn child with subsequent birth of a handicapped child. Deliberate violence toward a pregnant woman may constitute a form of prenatal child abuse.[37]

High-risk infant

There are a number of fetal and maternal situations in addition to those just outlined that place newborn infants at risk, that is, that threaten their extrauterine existence and place them in need of special care. Infants at risk and the special care they require are discussed in Chapter 10; specific developmental defects are considered in Chapter 11 and throughout the book as applicable.

Nutritional factors. The human conceptus has no store of nutrients to sustain vital functions during the prenatal period; therefore, it must rely on the mother as its single source of nutrition. The nutritional requirements for building fetal cells and for their functional maintenance include the calories and the properties of all the essential food substances—carbohydrates, proteins, and fats, including necessary vitamins, minerals, and water. In addition continued growth and development of the fetus depends on a number of related variables, acting alone or in combination, that influence fetal access to the nutrients. These include reduction of maternal intake of one or more nutrients that results in a decreased concentration of these substances in placental arterial blood; decreased uterine blood flow; diminished umbilical blood flow; overutilization of nutrients by the placenta; decreased efficiency of transport mechanisms for various nutrients across the placental membrane; multiple pregnancy that produces an increase in the total "litter" weight; and ureteroplacental insufficiency, that is, a decreased surface area for the exchange of nutrients.

Other factors related to the maternal system that may alter the availability of nutrients to the fetus are the general nutritional state and special needs or requirements of the mother. The chronically malnourished mother has few nutritional reserves available for fetal use, and the accumulated effects of lifetime nutritional deficiency may produce physiologic and anatomic structural defects that impair the mother's ability to support pregnancy and contribute to difficulties during labor. The teenage mother who has special nutritional requirements for meeting her own growth needs may compete with the fetus for available nutrients. Diet fads, such as the Zen macrobiotic diet and some of the new vegetarian diets, seriously compromise the health of both the mother and the fetus.

As a general rule, heavier women produce heavier infants and underweight women have lighter infants. Low birth weight infants are more common in poorly nourished mothers, but the varying degrees of malnutrition are so closely linked with socioeconomic status, subcultural diet practices, and general health that it is often difficult to determine precisely which factor is responsible for detrimental effects on the fetus. Maternal overnutrition and certain disease states (such as diabetes or maternal phenylketonuria) are also detrimental to the fetus. Although the ideal or average maternal weight gain has not been established, it appears that the greater the maternal weight gain during pregnancy (except for the obese mother), the higher the infant birth weight and the fewer the postnatal problems.[29]

During the early weeks of pregnancy, the nutritional demands of the conceptus are less and smaller amounts of essential nutrients are required to support development. As gestation advances and the fetal mass increases, the nutritional demands become progressively greater. In recent years a great deal of attention has been centered on inadequate maternal nutrition and its long-term effects on organ growth and maturation. Current information indicates that the restriction of calorie and protein during prenatal development profoundly affects the size, viability, postnatal growth, and behavior of children. The timing and duration of nutritional deprivation appears to be crucial. Of greatest concern are the consequences of dietary restriction at the time the brain is undergoing the most rapid growth and development. Insufficient nutrients to the fetus during the time of rapid brain cell division results in permanent deficiency in brain cell numbers. It appears that the critical period for increasing cell numbers in the brain takes place during the prenatal period and the first few months of life, with the greatest growth and development taking place during the third trimester of pregnancy. Although the most conclusive data have been derived from animal studies, it appears that inadequate protein-calorie intake results in reduced activity of important brain enzymes and perhaps decreased dendrite branching and synapse formation; insufficient maternal intake of essential fatty acids inhibits formation of the protective myelin sheath. The long-term consequences of nutritional deficiency may be manifest as cognitive, behavioral, and language retardation. There is a highly complicated relationship between maternal intake, postnatal environmental conditions, and the intellectual functions of offspring that is worthy of further exploration.[11,14,25,39]

Maternal health. Since the physiologic well-being of the fetus depends on the maternal environment in which it grows, any disorder that affects the maternal system will have some effect on the fetal system. Many of the specific disorders and related problems are discussed in Chapter 10 and elsewhere in the text and are, therefore, mentioned only briefly here.

Other factors capable of adversely affecting the fetus include:

1. Physical factors such as high altitude and smoking
2. Maternal disease such as toxemia of pregnancy, metabolic disorders such as diabetes and thyroid disease, and vascular diseases such as heart disease, lupus erythematosus, hypertension, and the hemoglobinopathies
3. Isoimmunization from maternal-fetal blood incompatibility
4. Prenatal diagnostic and therapeutic procedures

Folklore and maternal influences. Since ancient times the striking appearance of abnormal human development has been of concern to man as evidenced by descriptions in primitive drawings and on clay tablets and has served as the origin of numerous legendary and mythologic creatures. Consequently man has surrounded the processes of pregnancy and birth with strongly held beliefs and superstitions that involve taboos and prescriptions for behavior directed toward assuring the well-being of the unborn child. Even in the face of scientific advances, these superstitions and folkways have survived for generations and may still persist in various forms as part of a cultural heritage. The degree to which these beliefs are expressed depends on the strength of the cultural influence, the attitudes of the individual families, and the confidence and credibility engendered by the health care providers.

One of the most universal explanations of defective development has been maternal impressions. It has been a widespread belief that the appearance of the unborn child will be improved if the pregnant woman looks at beautiful people or things. The same concept in reverse has been used to explain birth defects. For example, if a pregnant woman was frightened by a rabbit, it was believed that her child would be born with a harelip, a microcephalic infant was attributed to the mother's seeing a monkey during pregnancy, and the mother's viewing a person with missing limbs would cause the unborn child to be similary affected. Activities such as a mother reaching her arms above her head, walking in circles, or tying knots were believed to cause the umbilical cord to be knotted or twisted around the neck of the fetus. Even the shape of birthmarks and other skin defects is sometimes believed to reflect maternal impressions. For example, eating strawberries by the mother is associated with nevi. Articles of apparel or adornment, food cravings, emotions such as fright and anger, undesirable thoughts, and the time and manner of announcing the pregnancy are all believed to influence the well-being of the unborn child.[3]

Expectant mothers who are able to rationalize the illogical nature of the beliefs will, through a normal fear of having an abnormal infant, conform to the superstitions. In most instances these customs are relatively harmless and are not in conflict with sound health practices. However, there are situations when conformity to cultural or subcultural beliefs may compromise the health and well-being of either mother or fetus, for example, the practice of eating clay. Understanding and judicious management on the part of nurses and other health care workers are required to explore with the mother all the ramifications of the practice without creating undo stress and guilt in the mother.

Not all of these beliefs are unfounded. There is evidence that maternal emotions may indeed affect the fetus. Prolonged stimulation of the autonomic nervous system caused by extreme stress or long-term anxiety produces physiologic changes in the maternal system such as increased heart rate, vasoconstriction, decreased gastric motility, and so on. In addition to the indirect effect produced by constriction of uterine blood flow, the stress hormones cross the placental membrane to affect the fetus directly. Assisting the expectant mother to deal with her stresses or securing counseling services for her is part of the nursing considerations.

PRENATAL CARE OF MOTHER AND FETUS

The importance of early and adequate prenatal care for the expectant mother cannot be overemphasized. Ideally preparation for childbirth begins in the mother's own childhood with a healthy physical environment and warm, affectionate parent-child relationships. It is well known that chronic exposure to substandard living conditions, poor nutrition, and inadequate health supervision are interrelated circumstances that contribute to fetal and infant morbidity and mortality, the most widely used indicator of the status of maternal and infant health care.

Nurses have always been important providers of health services to mothers and children. Now, with their expanding role as independent nurse practitioners, nurses' opportunities and responsibilities for maternal and infant health are assuming even broader dimensions. Careful assessment and monitoring of maternal health, anticipation of possible problems, and appropriate intervention will increase the likelihood of a successful outcome of pregnancy for both mother and infant.

Summary of initial maternal assessment

The general and specific aspects of health supervision during the prenatal period are well discussed in obstetric nursing textbooks, and the student is directed to these resources for comprehensive coverage of prenatal care. The major areas of concern are outlined here with particular emphasis on those that most directly affect the outcome of pregnancy for the fetus.

Maternal history

- Family history (including father's family)
  - Family constellation: number of siblings
  - Health history of family: genetic defects or diseases, multiple births, health of family members, deaths, including stillbirths, and abortions
- Maternal health history
  - Age
  - Past health: injuries and operations; serious illnesses; diseases, especially mental illness, convulsions, diabetes, and hypertension; drug sensitivities; transfusions; and extensive x-ray treatment
  - Immunizations
  - Chronic health problems: heart disease, diabetes, asthma and hypothyroidism
  - Coincidental medical disorders: phlebitis and urinary tract infections
  - Habits: smoking
  - Drug consumption, effects, and intoxicants
  - Exercise: type and amount
  - Menstrual history: time of menarche; interval and duration; amount of flow, any discomfort
- Social history
  - Marital status
  - Ethnic and geographic origin
  - Religion
  - Employment: type and amount of work
- Obstetric history
  - Number of pregnancies (gravida)
    - Dates of deliveries
  - Outcome of pregnancies (parity)
    - Full-term infants
    - Stillbirths and/or abortions: length of gestation at time of delivery
    - Premature births: length of gestation at time of delivery
  - Labor (each child)
    - Length in hours
    - Type: spontaneous, induced
  - Delivery (each child)
    - Method: natural, forceps, breech, cesarean section, spontaneous, anesthetic
    - Perineum: episiotomy, laceration, healing
    - Place of delivery: hospital, home, in transit
  - Complications
    - Pregnancy: toxemia, diseases, vascular problems, weight gain
    - Labor and delivery: hemorrhage, placental accidents, infection
    - Puerperium: hemorrhage, infection
  - Condition of each infant
    - At birth
    - Present health
- Present pregnancy
  - Date and character of last menstrual period
  - Symptoms associated with pregnancy: nausea and/or vomiting, constipation, quickening (if applicable)
  - Other symptoms: abdominal pain, bleeding, ankle swelling, headaches, varicosities, pruritus, leukorrhea, and so on
  - Contact with teratogens: infections, drug, x-ray exposure
  - Assessment of psychologic resources for coping with pregnancy

Health assessment

- General physical examination
  - Weight and height
  - Vital signs: pulse and blood pressure
  - Assessment of body systems
- Nutritional assessment[4]: factors that, if present, necessitate more intensive assessment
  - Poverty: poor nutrition is chronically associated with economic disadvantage
  - Adolescence: pregnancy superimposed on special metabolic needs of this age-group
  - Underweight: prepregnancy state may be inadequate
  - Grand multiparity: a particular risk when interval between pregnancies is short, for example, less than 1 year, or even 2 years
  - Anemia or obesity: may indicate poor diet habits
  - Unusual nutritional patterns: at special risk are food faddists, constant dieters, and pica practicers
  - Chronic systemic illness: associated with poor nutritional intake or utilization, for example, chronic infections, diabetes, alcoholism, malabsorption syndromes, drug abuse, severe emotional problems
  - Poor reproductive history: previous low birth weight or premature infants
- Pelvic examination
  - Palpation and auscultation of uterus
  - Measurement of bony pelvis
  - Visualization of cervix, vagina, and vulva
- Laboratory tests
  - Blood: hematocrit, hemoglobin, type (ABO and Rh), serology
  - Urine: protein, glucose, microscopic
  - Papanicolaou's smear from cervix
  - Unusual discharge: culture or smear

Ongoing assessment of mother and fetus

Maternal and fetal health are monitored at regular intervals during pregnancy. Those systems and areas that are most closely associated with the reproductive processes are given careful assessment, and sources of potential problems are anticipated and explored.

Summary of periodic maternal assessment

- Routine maternal assessment
  - Weight gain

Table 7-6. Fetal assessment techniques

Measurement	Description	Significance
Routine fetal assessment techniques		
Palpation of fundus	Measurement in centimeters from top of pubic bone to top of fundus divided by 4 gives age of fetus in months	Estimation of fetal growth
Measurement of fundus height		Less than expected may indicate failure to thrive or fetal anomaly such as anencephaly Greater than expected may indicate miscalculated due date, multiple pregnancy, polyhydramnios, or oversized fetus
Palpation of fetal outline	Major fetal parts (head and back) can be detected by gentle bimanual palpation of fundus—Leopold's maneuvers	Determine fetal position, for example, vertex (head) at pelvic outlet, head in fundus, and breech at outlet; anticipate difficult labor and delivery in positions such as breech or shoulder presentations
Detection of fetal movements	Fetal movement can be felt	Mother can usually detect fetal movement (quickening) at about 12-13 weeks Cessation of fetal kicking indicates fetal distress
Auscultation of fundus		
Detection of fetal movements	Auscultation of abdomen with stethoscope or fetoscope	Confirmation of maternal observations
Detection of fetal heart sounds	Auscultation of abdomen with stethoscope or Doppler-type sensory apparatus	Rate, rhythm, and quality of heart sounds provide clues to fetal well-being Can be heard with fetoscope at 16-20 weeks; with ultrasonic Doppler apparatus at 11-12 weeks
Special extrauterine techniques		
X-ray film of maternal abdomen	Anteroposterior and lateral views of abdomen	Not usually performed until term Confirms suspected multiple pregnancy Establishes fetal position May establish intrauterine fetal death—exaggerated fetal spinal curve and overriding skull bones Assesses fetal maturity by identifying ossification centers and presence of distal femoral and proximal tibial epiphyses
	Injection of radiopaque dye into amniotic fluid	Establishes patency of gastrointestinal tract when radiopaque substance is seen in fetal intestinal tract
	Intravenous injection of isotopes	Placental localization
	X-ray pelvimetry	Demonstrates adequacy of maternal pelvis in relation to size of the fetus
Maternal metabolites	Urinary excretion of estriol (estrogen) Serum estriol levels Urinary excretion of pregnanediol (progesterone)	Decreased levels are associated with a variety of fetal problems—intrauterine growth retardation, congenital anomalies, impending fetal death Decreased urinary estriol and pregnanediol levels may indicate placental insufficiency
	Serum diamine oxidase (DAO) levels	Decreased DAO levels are related to increased fetal mortality
Ultrasonography (sonar)	Intermittent high-frequency sound waves are directed toward uterus in a scanning manner; echos that bounce back from intrauterine structures are projected on a screen and recorded by timed polarizing photography	Provides accurate measurement of the fetus and placenta; determines fetal size, position, and configuration as well as location and size of placenta Safe and reliable method for placental localization and biparietal diameter of fetal skull Detection of some fetal abnormalities
Electrocardiography (external)	Application of electrocardiograph leads to maternal abdomen	Fetal electrocardiogram can be recorded from eleventh week; interference from maternal heartbeat and other muscular activity, especially during early weeks of gestation

Table 7-6. Fetal assessment techniques—cont'd

Measurement	Description	Significance
Special extrauterine techniques—cont'd		
Fetal stress testing		All methods use controlled asphyxial stress to evoke a characteristic heart rate response in the fetus with compromised placental function
Exercise stress test	Submits mother to a given amount of exercise to transiently reduce uterine blood flow by diverting blood flow to exercising skeletal muscle	
Hypoxic stress test	Mother breathes air with 25% to 50% reduction in oxygen	Determines the functional margin of reserve of the fetus by duplicating the stresses of labor Used primarily in high-risk pregnancies
Contraction stress test or oxytocin challenge test	Baseline recording of fetal heart rate and uterine activity is obtained with monitoring equipment; mother is given a controlled amount of intravenous oxytocin until three firm contractions are produced in less than 10 minutes	Fetal response is recorded and evaluated
Special intrauterine techniques		
Amniotic fluid examination	Amniocentesis—transabdominal aspiration of amniotic fluid (5 to 10 ml) from the pregnant uterus; fluid is centrifuged to separate cellular components from fluid	Can be obtained as early as the twelfth week; early amniocentesis is usually performed during the fourteenth to sixteenth weeks if therapeutic abortion is a possibility; for anticipation of postnatal problems, procedure is performed later in pregnancy
Fluid color		Yellowish color may reflect red blood cell breakdown from blood incompatibility Greenish color may suggest meconium staining
Supernatant fluid (noncellular portion)	Antibody determination	During third trimester
	Bilirubin breakdown products	Detection of presence and severity of Rh isoimmunization
	Viral and bacterial studies	Determine evidence of intrauterine infection
	Biochemical studies	Third trimester
	Creatinine level	Determines fetal age
	Lecithin-sphingomyelin ratio	Determines maturation of pulmonary surfactant system, basis for prediction of respiratory distress syndrome
	Alpha fetoprotein level	Associated with certain central nervous system abnormalities, for example, spina bifida
Cellular components (desquamated fetal cells)	Direct examination	
	Sex chromatin	Sex determination (not reliable)
	Biochemical and enzyme studies	Of limited value at present
	Cultivated fetal cells	
	Cytology	Sex determination—significant in X-linked genetic disorders, for example, hemophilia, Duchenne type muscular dystrophy Diagnosis of chromosomal aberrations, for example, Down's syndrome
	Biochemical and enzyme studies	Detection of an increasing number of genetic metabolic diseases, for example, Tay-Sachs disease, the mucopolysaccharidoses, and galactosemia
Fetoscopy	Direct visualization of fetus; fetoscope is introduced into uterine cavity through abdominal wall or cervical os	Detection of physical abnormalities Risk of infection, abortion, or premature labor with this procedure
Electrocardiography (internal)	Scalp electrodes attached to monitor fetal heart	Detection of abnormalities Detection of fetal distress
Fetal blood sampling	Blood samples taken from presenting part	Assessment of acid-base status Detection of anemia

Blood pressure measurement
Urine examination: glucose, acetone, and protein
Periodic blood analysis of hemoglobin and hematocrit (if indicated)
Monitoring of special situations
Excessive weight gain, edema
Concomitant disorders
Complications, such as rising blood titers (Rh antibodies)
Exploration of unusual symptoms or signs
Assessment of maternal psychologic resources
Past history of mental health
Response to present pregnancy
Family interpersonal relationships

Special prenatal assessment techniques

Routine assessment and monitoring procedures are usually sufficient to determine satisfactory developmental progress, and any deviations from normal alert the examiner to possible threats to fetal or maternal health. In addition to these observations there are a number of more sophisticated techniques that serve to assess fetal status more accurately.[1,17]

The nurse's role in relation to fetal testing primarily consists of education, observation, and support. The expectant parents, particularly the mother, who is directly involved, need to know what the procedure is, why it is being done, and what effect it will have on both the mother and the unborn child. The mother wants to know what she can expect to experience physically and the limitations that may be imposed on her during and after the procedure. The strange and unfamiliar machinery and diagnostic apparatus are often frightening, and there is the ever-present apprehension regarding needles and other intrusive instruments. Many women have an aversion to exposing their bodies; therefore, careful draping and efforts to minimize the length of time of needed exposure are important nursing considerations. Supportive attendance during procedures is a nursing responsibility that serves to reduce anxiety in the mother and helps secure her cooperation.

INTRAPARTAL CARE

Birth, the process by which the fetus is expelled from the mother's body, is a dramatic event that marks the beginning of a new period in the life span of each individual. At this moment the infant must be prepared to make an adjustment to a completely new manner of living in a strange and unfamiliar environment. The transition from intrauterine to extrauterine existence is accompanied by rapid physiologic changes and multiple adaptations that are essential for independent survival. It is the responsibility of the health team to provide for optimum progression through the birth process and to facilitate the transition to extrauterine life.[32]

Factors that influence neonatal adjustments

Factors that determine the degree to which the newborn adjusts to the extrauterine environment are numerous and varied. Many remain unknown, but most can be grouped into three large categories:[27] *First* are those that determine the innate constitutional structure and function of the neonate. These factors include hereditary characteristics and all those environmental factors that influence development from the time of conception. Congenital diseases and malformations caused by both hereditary and environmental factors have been discussed previously, and the specific problems related to many of these will be discussed in Chapters 10 and 11 and elsewhere throughout the book as appropriate.

The *second* category involves the state of maturity of the neonate. Although infants are able to survive before the optimum level of maturity has been reached, there is a point at which extrauterine existence is impossible even with excellent, intensive prenatal, intrapartal, and postnatal care. Statistics of postnatal survival rates provide positive evidence that the shorter the gestational age and the lower the birth weight, the higher the rate of morbidity and mortality. Except in special circumstances (such as some maternal diseases and placental accidents), the longer the fetus remains in the protection of the uterine environment, the better the adjustment to independent survival.

The *third* category consists of all those factors that produce pathologic conditions in an otherwise normal, full-term infant who has optimal genetic endowment and prenatal development. These pathologic conditions may be directly related to the birth process or may be postnatal hazards to the newborn. Among the conditions resulting from the birth process are those that are the result of direct trauma (such as fractures, soft tissue trauma, peripheral nerve damage, or intracranial injury) and those produced by anoxia from a variety of causes including placental accidents and the use of analgesic, anesthetic, and sedative drugs. Postnatal hazards such as infections, pathologic variations of normal physiologic processes (for example, hemorrhage from decrease in coagulation factors after birth), or feeding disturbances also interfere with neonatal well-being.

Effects of labor and delivery on the fetus

During the process of parturition the defenseless fetus is submitted to relentless pressure exerted by the contracting uterus against resistant maternal structures and compressed through a constricted, tortuous, but expansible, passageway. During the gestation period the mother and fetus are equipped to cope with the rigors of the birth process and the adjustment of extrauterine existence. For example, the presenting part, the portion of the fetal anatomy that leads the way through the birth canal, is usually and ideally the head. The pliable construction of this largest and least compressible part of the fetal anatomy facilitates the difficult passage, and membranous seams that unite the bones of the skull allow for molding and overlapping to accommodate the head to the changing contours of the maternal pelvic structures.

Also, the fetus, accustomed to decreased oxygen levels, is able to withstand the short periods of diminished circulatory exchange produced by the contracting uterine muscles.

At the time of delivery, when the infant is thrust from the security of a soft, dark, and warmly moist, though constricted, atmosphere into a strange, new environment, he is bombarded by a variety of foreign sensations: cold air, bright lights, loud noises, numerous textures and pressures against his skin, and unrestricted movement. Some maternity personnel have attempted in various ways to minimize the birth trauma and to facilitate initial psychologic attachment of mother and infant (see Chapter 8). Recently an attempt has been made by some to alter the delivery environment to more nearly approximate some of the intrauterine conditions, thereby providing a more gradual transition to the outside world. In a warm, darkened, quiet room the infant is delivered and immediately placed on the mother's bared abdomen where she gently strokes his skin for direct physical contact. Then, after the cord has been clamped and cut, the infant is immersed in a basin of warm water. Those who advocate this method believe that the infant, subjected to less trauma at birth, will be a more relaxed and less anxious individual.[22]

Assessment of fetal status. The most reliable indicator of fetal well-being during labor is the fetal heartbeat. Traditionally, active fetal heart monitoring by stethoscope has been, and still is, the most widely used method of assessment. Since fetal distress occurs in approximately 10% of normal labors, this important nursing function is carried out frequently (at least every 15 to 30 minutes) during the course of labor. Unfortunately, without continuous monitoring, clues to fetal distress are sometimes missed or only gross changes are detected.[10,16,30,31]

Newer methods that are designed to assess fetal heart sounds are gradually replacing this auscultatory method. Electronic devices, either external or internal, are providing continuous fetal heart rate (FHR) monitoring during labor and are particularly desirable in high-risk pregnancies. *External monitoring* is accomplished by taping a small sensoring device to the mother's abdomen that converts fetal heart sounds into audible beeps and translates them into electronic impulses on graph paper for a permanent record.

Internal monitoring is the most reliable and precise technique available for immediate detection of changes in fetal status. The fetal heart rate is monitored by an electrode attached to the fetal scalp and connected to a monitor, where it is amplified and permanently recorded on a graph. Simultaneous uterine contractions are monitored by way of a saline-filled catheter inserted vaginally into the uterine cavity (Fig. 7-11). This catheter, connected to a pressure recorder, provides a continuous record of the frequency, intensity, and duration of each contraction. In this way a correlation can be made between the fetal heart rate and the uterine contraction.[30,31]

The value of such monitoring systems depends on the ability of the nurse to understand and interpret the significance of the findings. The normal range for the fetal heart rate is considered to be between 120 and 160 beats/minute. During the process of labor the magnitude of the stress created by the uterine contractions and the ability of the fetus

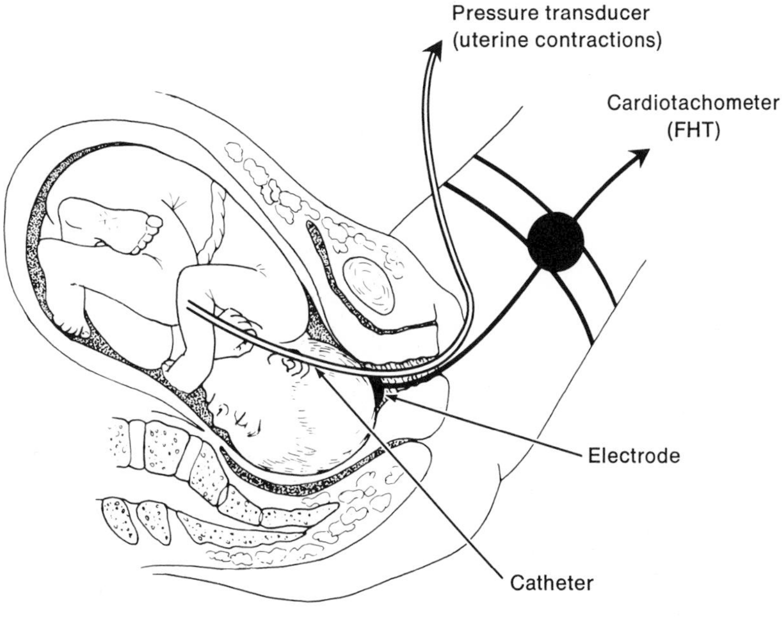

Fig. 7-11. Internal invasive fetal monitoring (membranes ruptured and cervix dilated). (From Jensen, M. D., Benson, R. C., and Bobak, I. M.: Maternity care: the nurse and the family, St. Louis, 1977, The C. V. Mosby Co., p. 302.)

to accommodate to the stress are reflected in the fetal heart rate pattern. Patterns that appear during contractions have a different significance than those that appear in the interval between contractions. Studies indicate that a drop in fetal heart rate that occurs *simultaneously* with uterine contraction and returns to the original baseline rate merely reflects the vagal response to intracranial pressure and is not unusual or indicative of distress. However, a decrease in fetal heart rate *after* the peak of the uterine contraction may be cause for concern. Also, deviations from the baseline fetal heart rate, either faster or slower, between contractions alert the observer to impending fetal distress. Fluctuations in fetal heart rate of 10 to 20 beats/minute are considered normal, but fluctuations greater than this (even if within the normal range) are considered abnormal. A baseline fetal heart rate that drops progressively after each contraction is cause for concern. Fig. 7-12 illustrates three fetal heart rate patterns and their probable causes.[21,25,31]

Fetal heart monitoring provides early warning of impending fetal compromise, thus allowing time for therapeutic intervention. Conditions that can be detected by fetal monitoring techniques in order of increasing morbidity are[10,13,16]:

1. Fetal head compression
2. Umbilical cord compression
3. Fetal intoxication by maternal drugs
4. Umbilical cord entanglement
5. Uteroplacental insufficiency

Fetal blood sampling is sometimes employed when the fetal heart rate pattern is questionable. Monitoring blood pH and blood gases from small samples of blood taken from the fetal scalp exposed by the dilating cervix provide clues to the extent of fetal anoxia.[27,35]

Other methods are continually being tested and applied in order to determine the state of the unborn child. However, during labor there is no device that can take the place of competent, conscientious nursing observations. In addition to the multiple tasks associated with the comfort and support of the laboring mother, the nurse is responsible for the continuous observation of the unborn child—monitoring contractions and fetal heart sounds and being alert for signs that indicate jeopardy to fetal well-being. For example, an elevated temperature in the mother will also affect the fetus and may indicate intrauterine infection; passage of meconium-stained amniotic fluid (unless the fetus is in breech presentation) or sudden, violent movements of the fetus may warn of fetal distress; and vaginal bleeding (other than the blood-tinged mucus that accompanies normal labor) is a threat to both mother and fetus.

Factors that influence outcome of labor. Although the full-term fetus is well prepared for the arduous process of birth, there are factors that may interfere with the normal adjustments and compromise fetal or neonatal well-being. Situations that *decrease the blood supply* to the fetus are hazards that require immediate intervention. These include:

Placental accidents
- Placenta previa—the placenta implants completely or partially over the uterine os
- Abruptio placentae—the placenta separates prematurely, before the cervix is dilated enough to permit delivery

Umbilical cord accidents
- Prolapsed cord—a loop of the umbilical cord slips down in front of the presenting part where it is compressed against the pelvic brim
- Compressed cord—the umbilical cord is compressed between fetal parts or between the fetus and the uterine wall; it may also be wound around the neck, an extremity, etc.

Hypotensive states in the mother
- Large vessel compression—weight of heavy uterus against large vessels when mother lies in supine position
- Regional anesthesia—local vasodilatation causes pooling of maternal blood in lower extremities

Any factor that *reduces the oxygen supply* to either the mother or the fetus directly will seriously compromise the intrauterine occupant. The factors mentioned above, by virtue of the diminished blood supply, also reduce the oxygen available to the fetus. Other situations that may interfere with fetal oxygen are:

Maternal medications[12]
- Analgesics such as meperedine hydrochloride or morphine sulfate readily cross the placental membrane and cause various levels of neonatal respiratory depression
- Barbiturates such as pentobarbital or secobarbital readily cross the placental membrane and may cause neonatal depression[18]

Anesthesia
- Local or regional anesthesia—usually no effect unless inadvertently injected into the fetus
- General anesthesia—degree of fetal anoxia depends on depth and amount of anesthesia and length of time administered

Other perinatal factors that can interfere with fetal or neonatal well-being include those that produce *ineffectual and prolonged labor,* such as uterine inertia and tone, rigid soft tissues, malpresentation of the fetus (shoulder, face, brow), breech presentation, and excessive fetal size; *toxemia of pregnancy;* or a *rapid and precipitous delivery.*

In situations where termination of the pregnancy enhances the likelihood of fetal (and maternal) survival, operative intervention is indicated. Facilitating normal delivery by forceps or vacuum extraction shortens the second stage of labor, and in situations that render vaginal delivery hazardous or impossible, delivery by hysterotomy (cesarean section) is the intervention of choice.

Summary of nursing role in fetal assessment during labor

Observation of uterine contractions
- Timing (by the clock)
  - Duration of contraction from the time it begins to tense until it has relaxed

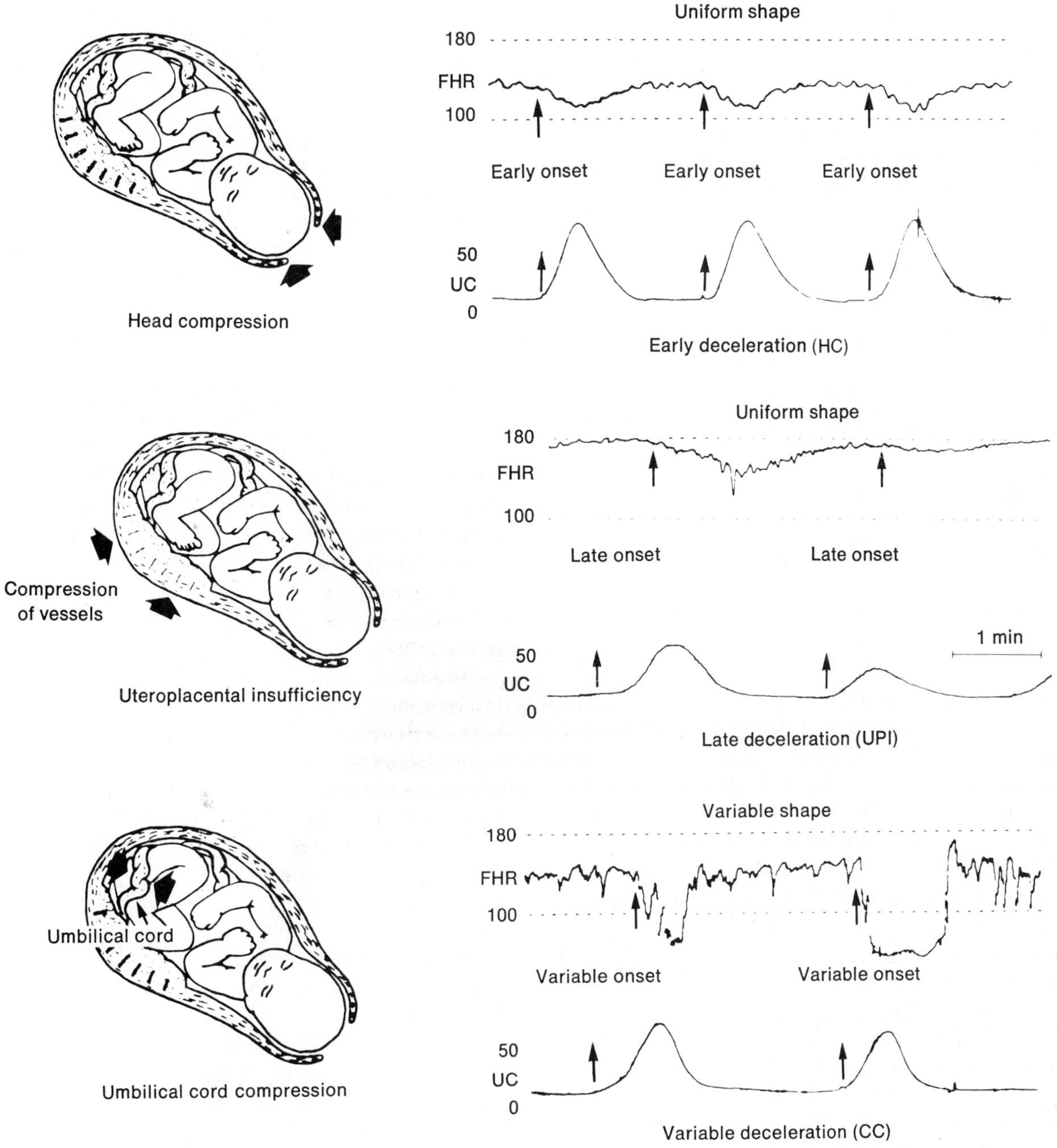

Fig. 7-12. The three major patterns of decelerated fetal heart rates. Note the relationship of onset and end of bradycardia to increased intrauterine pressures (contractions). *FHR,* Fetal heart rate; *UC,* uterine contraction; *HC,* head compression; *UPI,* uteroplacental insufficiency; *CC,* cord compression. (From Hon, E. H.: An introduction to fetal heart rate monitoring, Los Angeles, 1973, University of Southern California Press.)

Frequency of contractions timed from the beginning of one until the beginning of the next
Intensity
Mild contraction: uterus contracts but feels only mildly tense
Moderate contraction: uterus feels firm
Strong contraction: uterus feels very hard; cannot be indented with fingertips
Report contractions with duration longer than 90 seconds
Monitor fetal heart sounds
Monitor every 15 to 30 minutes during first stage of labor
Rate: bradycardia (less than 120 beats/minute); tachycardia (greater than 160 beats/minute); any deviations in baseline fetal heart rate
Rhythm: report any variations
Quality: report any changes
Check immediately following rupture of membranes
Check after every contraction during second stage of labor
Observe for untoward signs and symptoms
Vaginal bleeding
Bleeding without discomfort may warn of placenta previa
Bleeding associated with prolonged, painful, and board-like uterine contraction may indicate abruptio placentae
Ineffectual labor: continued labor with no progress
Altered vital signs
Preparation for receiving infant
Have warming and resuscitating equipment ready and in working order

REFERENCES

1. Aladjem, S.: The fetus as a patient: diagnostic and therapeutic approaches. In Aladjem, S., and Brown, A. K., editors: Clinical perinatology, St. Louis, 1974, The C. V. Mosby Co.
2. Alford, C. A., Stagno, S., and Reynolds, D. W.: Congenitally acquired toxoplasmosis: pertinent clinical, laboratory and therapeutic considerations, Bull. N.Y. Acad. Med. **50:**160, 1974.
3. Bagnall, D.: Obstetric rituals and taboos, Nurs. Times **70:** 1130-1133, 1972.
4. Benirschke, K.: Origin and clinical significance of twinning, Clin. Obstet. Gynocol. **15:**220, 1972.
5. Bertles, J. F.: The occurrence and significance of fetal hemoglobins. In Gordon, A. S., editor: Regulation of hematopoiesis, New York, 1970, Appleton-Century-Crofts.
6. Bloom, A. D.: Induced chromosomal aberrations—biological and clinical significance, J. Pediatr. **81:**1-8, July 1972.
7. Brady, J. P.: Homeostatic adjustment of the fetus and neonate. In Aladjem, S., and Brown, A. K. editors: Clinical perinatology, St. Louis, 1974, The C. V. Mosby Co.
8. Bulmer, M. G.: The biology of twinning in man, Oxford, 1970, Clarendon Press.
9. Caldwell, J. G.: Congenital syphilis: a nonvenereal disease, Am. J. Nurs. **71:**1768-1772, September 1971.
10. Chan, W. H., Paul, R. H., and Toews, J.: Intrapartum fetal monitoring: maternal and fetal morbidity and perinatal mortality, Obstet. Gynecol. **41:**7-13, 1973.
11. Cheek, D. B., Graystone, J. E., and Read, M. S.: Cellular growth, nutrition and development, Pediatrics **45:**315-334, 1970.
12. Cohen, S. N., and Olson, W. A.: Drugs that depress the newborn infant, Pediatr. Clin. North Am. **17:**835-850, November, 1970.
13. Copher, D. E.: Evaluating fetal well-being under clinical conditions by continuous electronic monitoring. Part I. Fetal monitoring—the state of the art. In Measuring for medicine and the life sciences, vol. 5, pp. 1-5, Hewlett-Packard Co.
14. Coursin, D. B.: Maternal nutrition and the offspring's development, Nutr. Today **8:**12-18, March-April 1973.
15. Eriksson, M., Catz, C. S., and Yaffe, S. J.: Drugs and pregnancy, Clin. Obstet. Gynecol. **16:**198, 1973.
16. Freeman, R. K.: Intrapartum fetal evaluation, Clin. Obstet. Gynecol **17:**83-94, September 1974.
17. Gauthier, C., Jr., Desjardins, P., and McLean, F.: Fetal maturity: amniotic fluid analysis correlated with neonatal assessment, Am. J. Obstet. Gynecol. **112:**344-350, 1972.
18. Ginsburg, J.: Placental drug transfer, Annu. Rev. Pharmacol. Toxicol. **11:**400, 1971.
19. Gumpel, S. M., Hayes, K., and Dudgeon, J. A.: Congenital perceptive deafness: role of intrauterine rubella, Br. Med. J. **2:**300, 1971.
20. Hardy, J. B.: Fetal consequences of maternal viral infections in pregnancy, Arch. Otolaryngol. **98:**218, 1973.
21. Hobel, C. J.: Intrapartum clinical assessment of fetal distress, Am. J. Obstet. Gynecol. **110:**336, 1971.
22. LeBoyer, F.: Childbirth without violence. New York, 1974, Alfred A. Knopf, Inc.
23. Markert, C. L., and Ursprung, H.: Developmental genetics, Englewood Cliffs, N.J., 1971, Prentice-Hall, Inc.
24. Marx, J. L.: Drugs during pregnancy: do they affect the unborn child? Science **180:**174-175, 1973.
25. Naeye, R. L., and associates: Effects of maternal nutrition on the human fetus, Pediatrics **52:**494, October 1973.
26. Oski, F. A.: The unique fetal red cell and its function, Pediatrics **51:**494, 1973.
27. Parmlee, A. H.: Management of the newborn, Chicago, 1961, Year Book Medical Publishers, Inc., pp. 45-50.
28. Paul, R. H., and associates: Clinical fetal monitoring: effects on perinatal outcome, Am. J. Obstet. Gynecol. **118:**529, 1974.
29. Pitkin, R. M., and associates: Maternal nutrition, Obstet. Gynecol. **40:**773, 1972.
30. Quilligan, E. J., and Paul, R. H.: Fetal monitoring: is it worth it? Obstet. Gynecol **45:**96, 1975.
31. Russin, A. W., O'Cureck, J. E., and Roux, J. F.: Electronic monitoring of the fetus, Am. J. Nurs. **74:**1294-1299, July 1974.
32. Sasmor, J. L., Castor, C. R., and Hassid, P.: The childbirth team during labor, Am. J. Nurs. **73:**444, March 1973.
33. Shafer, N.: Toxoplasmosis, N.Y. State J. Med. **75:**1049-1060, June 1975.
34. Sternberg, J.: Radiation and pregnancy, Can. Med. Assoc. J. **109:**51-57, 1973.
35. Stevenson, R. E.: The fetus and newly born infant: influences of the prenatal environment, ed. 2, St. Louis, 1977, The C. V. Mosby Co.
36. Timiras, P. S.: Developmental physiology and aging, New York, 1972, Macmillan Publishing Co., Inc.

37. Van Stolk, M.: Beaten women, battered children, Child. Today **5:**8-12, March/April 1976.
38. Weller, T. H.: The cytomegaloviruses: ubiquitous agents with protean clinical manifestations, N. Engl. J. Med. **285:**203, 267, 1971.
39. Winik, M., Brasel, J., and Velasco, E. G.: Effects of prenatal nutrition upon pregnancy risk, Clin. Obstet. Gynecol. **16:**184, 1973.
40. Yaffe, S. J., and Catz, C. S.: Drugs and the intrauterine patient. In Aladjem, S., editor: Risks in the practice of modern obstetrics, ed. 2, St. Louis, 1975, The C. V. Mosby Co.

BIBLIOGRAPHY

Aladjem, S.: Risks of antepartum diagnostic and therapeutic approaches. In Aladjem, S., editor: Risks in the practice of modern obstetrics, ed. 2, St. Louis, 1975, The C. V. Mosby Co.

Aladjem, S., and Brown, A. K., editors: Clinical perinatology, St. Louis, 1974, The C. V. Mosby Co.

Alderman, M. M.: Managing the high-risk pregnancy, Patient Care **7:**96, March 15, 1973.

Alford, C. A., Stagno, S., and Reynolds, D. W.: Perinatal infections caused by viruses, toxoplasma, and treponema pallidum. In Aladjem, S., and Brown, A. K., editors: Clinical perinatology, St. Louis, 1974, The C. V. Mosby Co.

Allen, H. H., and associates: Infants undergoing antenatal genetic diagnosis: a preliminary report, Am. J. Obstet. Gynecol. **118:** 310, 1974.

Amiel-Tison, C. I.: Neurologic disorders in neonates associated with abnormalities of pregnancy and birth, Curr. Probl. Pediatr. **3:**3-37, 1973.

Assali, N. S., Brinkman, C. R., III, and Nuwayhid, B.: Uteroplacental circulation and respiratory gas exchange. In Gluck, L., editor: Modern perinatal medicine, Chicago, 1974, Year Book Medical Publishers, Inc.

Aubrey, R. H., Roberts, A., and Cuenca, V. G.: The assessment of maternal nutrition, Clin. Perinatol. **2:**207-219, September 1975.

Babson, S. G., and Lubchenco, L. O.: Growth measurements. Section I. Fetal growth. In Frankenburg, W. F., and Camp, B. W.: Pediatric screening tests, Springfield, Ill., 1975, Charles C Thomas, Publisher.

Babson, S. G., and associates: Management of high-risk pregnancy and intensive care of the neonate, ed. 3, St. Louis, 1975, The C. V. Mosby Co.

Bancroft, A. V.: Pregnancy and the counterculture, Nurs. Clin. North Am. **8:**67-76, 1973.

Barden, T. P.: Fetal distress: find it earlier, Consultant, pp. 29-31, December 1973.

Beck, F., Moffatt, D. B., and Lloyd, J. B.: Human embryology and genetics, Oxford, 1973, Blackwell Scientific Publications, Ltd.

Beer, S.: What?! No meat?! Pediatr. Nurs. **3**(3):16-19, May/June, 1977.

Benirschke, K.: Syphilis—the placenta and the fetus, Am. J. Dis. Child **128:**142-143, 1974.

Bentrem, G. C., Perkins, P., and Waxman, B.: Newer methods of evaluating fetal maturity, Am. J. Obstet. Gynecol. **106:**917-919, 1970.

Bergner, L., and Susser, M. W.: Low birth weight and prenatal nutrition: an interpretative review, Pediatrics **46:**946, 1970.

Bibbo, M., and associates: Follow-up study of male and female offspring of DES-exposed mothers, Obstet. Gynecol. **49:**1-8, 1977.

Biggs, J. S. G.: Progress in fetal assessment, Obstet. Gynecol. **45:** 227, 1975.

Bogdanovic, S.: Prenatal detection of Down's syndrome, J. Obstet. Gynecol. Neonatal Nurs. **4:**35-38, November/December 1975.

Broome, D. L., and associates: Needle puncture of the fetus during amniocentesis, Lancet **2:**604, 1975.

Brown, G. C.: Maternal virus infection and congenital anomalies: a prospective study, Arch. Environ. Health **21:**362, 1970.

Burton, B. K., and associates: Present status of intrauterine diagnosis of genetic defects, Am. J. Obstet. Gynecol. **113:**718-746, 1974.

Butler, N. R., Goldstein, H., and Ross, E. M.: Cigarette smoking in pregnancy: its influence on birth weight and perinatal mortality, Br. Med. J. **2:**127, 1972.

Campbell, S.: The antenatal detection of fetal abnormality by ultrasonic diagnosis. In Motulsky, A. G., and associates: Birth defects: proceedings of the fourth international congress, New York, 1974, American Elsevier Publishing Co., Inc.

Campbell, S.: Fetal growth, Clin. Obstet. Gynecol. **1:**41, 1974.

Carrington, E. R.: Relationship of stilbestrol exposure in utero to vaginal lesions in adolescence, Pediatrics **85:**295-296, 1974.

Chagnon, L. J., and Heldonbrand, C. L.: Nurses undertake direct and indirect fetal monitoring at a community hospital, J. Obstet. Gynecol. Nurs. **3:**41, 1974.

Chapple, C. C.: Developmental defects: some thoughts on their causes. Birth Defects **8**(6): September 1972.

Clements, J. A., and associates: Assessment of the risk of respiratory distress syndrome by a rapid test for surfactant in amniotic fluid, N. Engl. J. Med. **286:**1077, 1972.

Crowley, L.: An introduction to clinical embryology, Chicago, 1974, Year Book Medical Publishers, Inc.

Dahn, L. S., and James, L. S.: Newborn temperature and calculated heat loss in the delivery room, Pediatrics **49:**504, 1972.

Dodson, W. E.: Neonatal drug intoxication: local anesthetics, Pediatr. Clin. North Am. **23:**399-411, 1976.

Doran, T. A., and associates: The antenatal diagnosis of genetic disease, Am. J. Obstet. Gynecol. **118:**314, 1974.

Douglas, C. P.: Perinatal implications of maternal disorders. In Aladjem, S., and Brown, A. K., editors: Clinical perinatology, St. Louis, 1974, The C. V. Mosby Co.

Dwyer, J. M.: Human reproduction. The female system and the neonate, Philadelphia, 1976, F. A. Davis Co.

Dwyer, J. T.: Family nutrition and the health care team, Issues Comprehensive Pediatr. Nurs. **1**(5):1-21, April 1977.

Edwards, R. G.: Advances in reproductive biology on human congenital defects. In Motulsky, A. G., and associates: Birth defects: proceedings of the fourth international conference, New York, 1974, American Elsevier Publishing Co., Inc.

Emery, A. E. H., editor: Antenatal diagnosis of genetic disease, Baltimore, 1973, The Williams & Wilkins Co.

Ferrier, P. E., Nicod, I., and Ferrier, S.: Fetal alcohol syndrome, Lancet **2:**1496, 1973.

Fleshman, R. P.: Eating rituals and realities, Nurs. Clin. North Am. **8:**91-106, 1973.

Florman, A. L., and associates: Intrauterine infection with herpes simplex virus: resultant congenital malformations, J.A.M.A. **225:**129, 1973.

Forbes, G. B.: Nutrition and growth, J. Pediatr. **91:**40-43, 1977.

Forfar, J. O., and Nelson, M. M.: Epidemiology of drugs taken by pregnant women. Part 2. Drugs that may affect the fetus adversely, Clin. Pharmacol. Ther. **14:**632-642, 1973.

Fredrich, J., Alberman, E. D., and Goldstein, H.: Possible teratogenic effect of cigarette smoking, Nature **231:**529, 1971.

Freeman, R. K.: The use of the oxytocin challenge test for antepartum clinical evaluation of uteroplacental respiratory function, Am. J. Obstet. Gynecol. **121**(4):481-489, February 1975.

Friedmann, T.: Prenatal diagnosis of genetic disease, Sci. Am. **225:**34-42, 1971.

Galloway, K. G.: Placental evaluation studies: the procedures, their purposes, and the nursing care involved, Am. J. Maternal Child Nurs. **1:**300-306, 1976.

Gluck, L., and Kulovich, M. V.: Lecithin/sphingomyelin ratios in amniotic fluid in normal and abnormal pregnancy, Am. J. Obstet. Gynecol. **115:**539-546, 1973.

Gluck, L., and associates: Diagnosis of the respiratory distress syndrome by amniocentesis, Am. J. Obstet. Gynecol. **109:**440-445, 1971.

Harris, J. M., III, and Pashayan, H. J.: Teratogenesis, Orthop. Clin. North Am. **7:**281-290, 1976.

Holey, E. S.: Promoting adequate weight gain in pregnant women, Am. J. Maternal Child Nurs. **2:**86-89, March/April 1977.

Hsu, L. Y., and associates: Results and pitfalls in prenatal cytogenetic diagnosis, J. Med. Genet. **10:**112-119, 1973.

Jackson, R. L.: Long-term consequences of suboptimal nutritional practices in early life, Pediatr. Clin. North Am. **24:**63-70, 1977.

Jensen, M., Benson, R. C., and Bobak, I. M.: Maternity care: the nurse and the family, St. Louis, 1977, The C. V. Mosby Co.

Johnson, P. V.: Nutrition and neural development, Food Nutr. News **45:**639-646, 1973.

Jones, K. L., and associates: Pattern of malformation in offspring of chronic alcoholic mothers, Lancet **1:**1267-1271, June 9, 1973.

Jones, M. B.: Antepartum assessment in high-risk pregnancy, J. Obstet. Gynecol. Nurs. **4**(6):23-27, 1975.

Kan, Y. W., and associates: Fetal blood-sampling in utero, Lancet **1:**79, 1974.

Kelly, J. V.: Diagnostic techniques in prepartal fetal evaluation, Clin. Obstet. Gynecol. **17:**53-82, September 1974.

Kibrick, S., and Loria, R. M.: Rubell and cytomegalovirus: current concepts of congenital and acquired infection, Pediatr. Clin. North Am. **21:**513, 1974.

Langhorne, F.: The fetal monitor: a friend or foe? Am. J. Maternal Child Nurs. **1:**313, 1976.

Langman, J.: Medical embryology. Human development—normal and abnormal, ed. 3., Baltimore, 1975, The Williams & Wilkins Co.

Lasater, C.: Electronic monitoring of mother and fetus, Am. J. Nurs. **72:**728-730, April 1972.

Leck, J., and Steward, J. K.: Incidence of neoplasms in children born after influenza epidemics, Br. Med. J. **4:**631, 1972.

Lemons, J. A., and Jaffe, R. B.: Amniotic fluid lecithin/sphingomyelin ratio in the diagnosis of hyaline membrane disease, Am. J. Obstet. Gynecol. **115:**233-237, 1973.

Lewkonia, J. K., and Jackson, A. A.: Infantile herpes zoster after intrauterine exposure to varicella, Br. Med. J. **3:**149, 1973.

Liley, A. W.: Rh hemolytic disease: can it be eradicated or are we in a war we cannot win? Mod. Med., pp. 33-48, February 1, 1977.

Lowe, C. R.: Congenital malformations and the problem of their control, Br. Med. J. **3:**515, 1972.

Luke, B.: Guide to better evaluation of antepartum nutrition, J. Obstet. Gynecol. Nurs. **5**(4):37-43, 1976.

Luke, B.: Maternal alcoholism and fetal alcohol syndrome, Am. J. Nurs. **77:**1924-1926, 1977.

Mack, H., editor: Prenatal life, Detroit, 1970, Wayne State University Press.

Macri, J. N., and associates: Antenatal diagnosis of neural-tube defects using cerebrospinal-fluid proteins, Lancet **1:**15, 1974.

Mann, L. I., Carmichael, A., and Duchin, S.: The effect of head compression on FHR, brain metabolism and function, Obstet. Gynecol. **39:**721-726, 1972.

Mann, L. I., and associates: The effect of metabolic acidosis on fetal brain function and metabolism, Am. J. Obstet. Gynecol. **111:**353-359, 1971.

Maternal nutrition and the course of pregnancy, Washington, D.C., 1970, National Academy of Sciences.

Milunsky, A.: The prenatal diagnosis of hereditary disorders, Springfield, Ill., 1973, Charles C Thomas, Publisher.

Milunsky, A., and associates: Prenatal genetic diagnosis, N. Engl. J. Med. **283:**1370-1381 (Part I), 1441-1447 (Part II), 1498-1504 (Part III), 1970.

Mocasary, P., and associates: Relationship between fetal intracranial pressure and fetal heart rate during labor, Am. J. Obstet. Gynecol. **106:**407-411, 1970.

Moore, K. L.: The developing human: clinically oriented embryology, Philadelphia, 1973, W. B. Saunders Co.

Motulsky, A. G., Fraser, G. R., and Felsenstein, J.: Public health and long-term genetic implications of intrauterine diagnosis and selective abortion, Birth Defects **7:**22-32, 1971.

Nadler, H. L.: Prenatal diagnosis of inborn defects: a status report, Hosp. Pract. **10:**41-51, June 1975.

Nahmias, A. J., Alford, C. A., and Korones, S. B.: Infection of the newborn with herpesvirus hominis, Adv. Pediatr. **17:**185, 1970.

Nahmias, A. J., and associates: Perinatal risk associated with maternal genital herpes simplex virus infection, Am. J. Obstet. Gynecol. **110:**825, 1971.

Neeson, J. D.: Herpesvirus genitalis: a nursing perspective, Nurs. Clin. North Am. **10:**598-607, 1975.

Nitowsky, H. M.: Prenatal diagnosis of genetic abnormality, Am. J. Nurs. **71:**1551-1556, August 1971.

Nora, J. J., and Nora, A. H.: Birth defects and oral contraceptives, Lancet **1:**941-942, 1973.

O'Gureck, J. E., Roux, J. F., and Neuman, M. R.: Neonatal depression and fetal heart rate patterns during labor, Obstet. Gynecol. **40:**347-355, 1972.

O'Gureck, J. E., Roux, J. F., and Neuman, M. R.: A practical classification of fetal heart patterns, Obstet. Gynecol. **40:**356-361, 1972.

Palmer, R. H., and associates: Congenital malformations in offspring of a chronic alcoholic mother, Pediatrics **53:**490-494, 1974.

Palmisano, P. A., and Polhill, R. B.: Fetal pharmacology, Pediatr. Clin. North Am. **19:**3, 1972.

Persaud, T. V. N., and Moore, K. L.: Causes and prenatal diagnosis of congenital abnormalities, J. Obstet. Gynecol. Neonatal Nurs. **3:**50-55, July/August 1974.

Phillips, C. R.: The essence of birth without violence, Am. J. Maternal Child Nurs. **1**(3)162-163, 1976.

Pierog, S. H., and Ferrara, A.: Medical care of the sick newborn, ed. 2, St. Louis, 1976, The C. V. Mosby Co.

Potter, E. L., and Craig, J. M.: Pathology of the fetus and the infant, ed. 3, Chicago, 1975, Year Book Medical Publishers, Inc.

Queenan, J. T., and Gadow, E. L.: Amniography for detection of congenital malformations, Obstet. Gynecol. **35:**648, 1970.

Ray, H., and associates: Clinical experience with the oxytocin challenge test, Am. J. Obstet. Gynecol. **114:**1, 1972.

Reed, B., Sutorius, J., and Coen, R.: Management of the infant during delivery, and in the immediate neonatal period, Nurs. Clin. North Am. **6:**3, March 1971.

Reeder, F.: Fact or fantasy? Maternal and infant nutrition affect brain development and intellectual performance. In Brandt, P. A., Chinn, P. L., and Smith, M. E.: Current practice in pediatric nursing, vol. 1, St. Louis, 1976, The C. V. Mosby Co.

Renwick, J. H.: Analysis of cause—long cut to prevention? Nature **246:**114, 1973.

Rice, G. T.: Recognition and treatment of intrapartal fetal distress, J. Obstet. Gynecol. Neonatal Nurs. **1:**15-22, July/August 1972.

Robinson, A.: Intrauterine diagnosis and ultrasounds, Lancet **2:** 1504, 1973.

Robinson, A., and associates: Intrauterine diagnosis: potential complications, Am. J. Obstet. Gynecol. **116:**937, 1973.

Robson, J. R. K.: Food fadism, Pediatr. Clin. North Am. **24:**189-201, 1977.

Rodman, M. J.: The pregnant patient: treating her without harming the baby, RN, pp. 61-75, February 1975.

Roux, J. F.: Monitoring of labor in high-risk centers. In Aladjem, S., and Brown, A. K., editors: Clinical perinatology, St. Louis, 1974, The C. V. Mosby Co.

Roux, J. F., and Nakamura, J.: Determination of fetal maturation by amniocentesis. In Aladjem, S., and Brown, A. K., editors: Clinical perinatology, St. Louis, 1974, The C. V. Mosby Co.

Saxon, S. A., and associates: Intellectual defects in children born with subclinical congenital toxoplasmosis: a preliminary report, J. Pediatr. **82:**792, 1973.

Schifrin, B. S., and associates: Contraction stress test for antepartum fetal evaluation, Obstet. Gynecol. **45:**433, 1975.

Scrimgeour, J. B.: Amniocentesis: technique and complications. In Emery, A. E. H., editor: Antenatal diagnosis of genetic disease, Baltimore, 1973, The Williams & Wilkins Co.

Senior, B., and Chernoff, H. L.: Iodide goiter in the newborn, Pediatrics **47:**510, 1971.

Shank, R. E.: A chink in our armor, Nutr. Today **5:**2-11, Summer 1970.

Spellacy, W. N.: Management of the high-risk pregnancy, Baltimore, 1976, University Park Press.

Stenchever, M. A., Kunysz, T. J., and Allen, M. A.: Chromosome breakage in users of marihuana, Am. J. Obstet. Gynecol. **118:**106, 1974.

Stiehm, E. R.: Fetal defense mechanisms, Am. J. Dis. Child. **129:** 438, 1975.

Stocker, J., and associates: Ultrasonic cephalometry, Obstet. Gynecol. **45:**275, 1975.

Stratford, B. F.: Abnormalities of early human development, Am. J. Obstet. Gynecol. **107:**1223, 1970.

Sureau, C.: The stress of labor. In Aladjem, S., and Brown, A. K., editors: Clinical perinatology, St. Louis, 1974, The C. V. Mosby Co.

Timiras, P. S.: Development physiology and aging, New York, 1972, Macmillan Publishing Co., Inc.

Tuchmann-Duplessis, H., David, G., and Haegel, P.: Illustrated human embryology. Vol. I. Embryogenesis. Vol. II. Organogenesis. Vol. III. Nervous system and endocrine glands, New York, 1972, Springer-Verlag New York, Inc.

Valenti, C.: Endoamnioscopy and fetal biopsy: a new technique, Am. J. Obstet. Gynecol. **114:**561, 1972.

Valenti, C.: Perinatal genetic studies and counseling. In Aladjem, S., and Brown, A. K., editors: Clinical perinatology, St. Louis, 1974, The C. V. Mosby Co.

Waisman, H. A., and Kerr, G. R.: Fetal growth and development, New York, 1970, McGraw-Hill Book Co.

Walker, D., Grimwade, J., and Wood, C.: Intrauterine noise: a component of the fetal environment, Am. J. Obstet. Gynecol. **109:**91-95, 1971.

Waranky, J.: Congenital malformations, Chicago, 1971, Year Book Medical Publishers, Inc.

Wilson, J. G.: Environment and birth defects, New York, 1973, Academic Press, Inc.

Wilson, J. G.: Present status of drugs as teratogens in man, Teratology **7:**7, February 1973.

Winick, M.: Fetal nutrition and growth processes, Hosp. Pract. **34:**33, May 1970.

Winick, M., and Coombs, J.: Nutrition, environment and behavioral development, Annu. Rev. Med. **23:**149, 1972.

Zelson, C.: Infant of the addicted mother, N. Engl. J. Med. **288:** 1393-1395, 1973.

Ziring, P. R.: Current status of the rubella problem, Cardiovasc. Nurs. **6:**47-50, July/August 1970.

UNIT FOUR
The neonate

Probably no event is more dramatic or miraculous than the birth of a child. It is the culmination of a 9-month gestation period during which the fetus prepares for extrauterine existence and the parents prepare for the addition of a totally dependent member to their lives. At the time of delivery, profound physiologic and psychologic reactions occur to initiate the child and parents' preparation for this experience.

In most instances the birth and perinatal period are uneventful and the infant returns home with his parents to begin developing as a vital, healthy, and loved child. Chapter 8, *The Normal Neonate,* is concerned with the infant's normal adjustment to extrauterine life, his physiologic status at birth, and the nursing knowledge required to care for the infant at and immediately following delivery, to perform a neonatal assessment, and to promote the infant-parent attachment. Chapter 9, *Health Problems of the Neonate,* deals with problems related to physical status, environmental agents, birth injury, or metabolic errors that may occur in normal newborns at or during the perinatal period. The emphasis is on the nurse's recognition, prevention, and intervention of each of these problems.

Unfortunately, not all neonates are born fully matured or perfectly developed. Chapter 10, *The High-Risk Neonate,* focuses on identification and assessment of high-risk neonates, problems common to them because of their high-risk status, physiologic conditions requiring medical and nursing intervention, and supportive care of the child and family throughout this ordeal. Chapter 11, *Conditions Caused by Defects in Physical Development,* discusses the more common malformations requiring immediate, temporary, or permanent intervention. Emphasis is on recognition of the abnormality, prevention of complications before and after correction, and emotional support of the parents who are grieving over the birth of a defective child.

8

The normal neonate

Parturition is an intense and exhausting physiologic and emotional experience for the mother and newborn. Even when this process progresses normally, the neonate is required to withstand extreme changes as he leaves a thermoconstant, aquatic, completely life-sustaining environment and enters a variable pressurized atmosphere that demands profound physiologic alteration for survival. The neonatal or perinatal period, the interval from viability until 28 days after birth, presents the greatest risk to the newborn. In fact, in the United States two thirds of all deaths that occur during the first year of life happen during these 4 weeks.

The nurse's role is one of supporting the mother and infant through the birth process, preventing physiologic complications in the neonate's adjustment to extrauterine life, and promoting the attachment process between child and parents. Expert technologic and psychologic nursing care during the immediate postpartum period lays a strong foundation for healthy parent-child development.

ADJUSTMENT TO EXTRAUTERINE LIFE

Factors affecting adjustment

The most profound physiologic change required of the neonate is transition from fetal or placental circulation to independent respiration. The loss of the placental connection means the loss of complete metabolic support, the most important and essential function being the supply of oxygen and the removal of carbon dioxide. The normal stresses of labor and delivery produce alterations of placental gas exchange patterns, acid-base balance in the blood, and cardiovascular activity in the fetus. Any factors that interfere with this normal transition or that increase fetal asphyxia (a condition of hypoxemia, hypercapnia, and acidosis) will affect the fetus's adjustment to extrauterine life.

Decreased maternal blood flow to the chorionic villi of the placenta results from a number of conditions, including (1) prolonged uterine contractions from dystocia or uterine tetany, (2) inferior vena caval or aortic compression by the uterus, (3) premature separation of the placenta (abruptio placentae), (4) abnormal implantation of the placenta in the lower uterine segment (placenta previa), (5) cord compression or prolapse before or during delivery, and (6) maternal hemorrhage. Decreased oxygenation and altered maternal acid-base balance may be caused by drugs or anesthesia, excessive muscular activity and dehydration, especially during prolonged and diffuse labor, and excessive hyperventilation during labor. Since hydrogen ions are readily exchanged across the placenta, maternal acidosis is readily reflected in the fetus.

A host of other maternal and fetal conditions also predisposes the infant to a high-risk status. Maternal factors include diabetes mellitus, which causes fetal hypoglycemia, age below 18 or above 35 years, malnutrition, chronic alcoholism, cephalopelvic disproportion, and a history of miscarriages, premature deliveries, and congenital anomalies in previous offspring. Obstetric problems such as malpresentation increase the risk of fetal trauma, prematurity, and asphyxia. In addition, fetal conditions such as prematurity, postmaturity, inappropriate weight for gestational age, and presence of congenital anomalies decrease the neonate's ability to adjust to extrauterine life. (For a more detailed discussion of maternal and fetal high-risk factors, see Chapters 7 and 10.)

Immediate adjustments

The neonate's adjustment to extrauterine life is a complex physiologic process. The first 24 hours are the most critical, since during this time respiratory distress and circulatory failure can occur rapidly and with little warning. There is a higher incidence of death during these initial 24 hours than during the entire succeeding perinatal period.

#1

Initiation of respiration. The most critical and immediate physiologic change required of the neonate is the onset of breathing. The stimuli that help initiate the first respiratory movements are primarily chemical and thermal. Following a normal delivery from a mother who has not been depressed by analgesics and anesthetics, the newborn begins to breathe after the head and chest are delivered. Often the first cry is heard before the entire body is beyond the perineum. The promptness of this transition is initiated by sudden exposure to stimuli in the exterior environment.

Sudden chilling of the infant probably excites peripheral sensory impulses in the skin, which are transmitted to the respiratory center. Undoubtedly the rapid decrease of temperature from 37°C (98.6°F) in the uterus to an ambient temperature of 21° to 23°C (70° to 75°F) in the delivery room is a powerful stimulus.

Chemical factors also trigger the respiratory center. The asphyxiant changes in the blood of low oxygen tension, high carbon dioxide tension, and low pH excite the medulla either directly or through the chemoreceptors in the carotid artery or aorta. The significance of tactile stimulation in initiating respiration is questionable. Although slapping the infant's heel or buttock usually does no harm, it is a waste of precious time in the event of respiratory difficulty. Inverting the infant and slapping the heel should be avoided in the presence of suspected cerebral trauma because dural tears and subdural hemorrhage may result.

Initial entry of air into the lungs is opposed by the surface tension of the viscid fluid that fills the alveoli. Because respiratory movements occurred before birth, fluid filled the lungs, which were largely nonfunctional since exchange of oxygen and carbon dioxide occurred through the process of diffusion via placental circulation. In order for respiration to occur, this surface tension must be opposed by a negative pressure greater than 25 mm Hg to open the alveoli for the first time. The first lusty cry of the newborn exerts a negative pressure of up to 50 mm Hg. Once the alveoli are opened, further respiration of less force maintains alveolar stability.

Another significant factor in expansion of the alveoli is the presence of surfactant, a lipoprotein film produced by the alveolar epithelium that coats the alveolar surface. Surfactant acts very much like a detergent as it decreases the surface tension of the fluids that line the alveoli and respiratory passages. Because the surface tension effect of surfactant is inversely proportional to the size of the alveoli, the effect of surfactant is several times greater when the alveoli become smaller in size during expiration. This is very fortunate since alveolar expansion is maintained at the end of expiration so that subsequent respirations can occur with relative ease. In hyaline membrane disease or respiratory distress syndrome, there is a deficiency of surfactant in the immature lung. The infant with this syndrome usually breathes satisfactorily immediately after birth but, because of deficient surfactant to maintain alveolar stability and functional residual capacity (the amount of air remaining in the lung at the end of normal expiration), develops severe respiratory distress during the ensuing few hours (usually by 6 to 8 hours after birth) or days (usually by 2 to 3 days).

Another favorable factor affecting the entry of air is the viscosity of the fluid in the respiratory tract. This fluid tends to be fairly rapidly absorbed into the alveolar capillaries and lymphatic vessels because of its lesser viscosity and lower protein content than amniotic fluid. In addition the mechanism of vaginal vertex delivery exerts a thoracic squeeze on the infant that results in the passage of as much as 20 ml of fluid through the neonate's mouth as he exits through the birth canal.

Circulatory changes. Equally as important as the initiation of respiration are the immediate circulatory changes that allow blood to flow through the lungs. Subsequent circulatory changes of a more gradual onset allow more blood to pass through the liver as well. In order to understand the circulatory changes that occur at birth, it is necessary to review fetal circulation, with emphasis on the special anatomic structures that close after birth.

The fetal heart pumps large quantities of blood through the placenta, largely bypassing the lungs and liver. As illustrated in Fig. 7-6, oxygenated blood leaves the placenta through the umbilical vein and mainly bypasses the liver through the *ductus venosus*. Most of the blood entering the right atrium from the inferior vena cava flows directly into the left atrium through the *foramen ovale*. The blood then enters the left ventricle and flows through the ascending aorta to supply the head and forelimbs.

Deoxygenated blood from the superior vena cava enters the right atrium and passes through the tricuspid valve into the right ventricle and then into the pulmonary artery. Most of the blood in the pulmonary artery bypasses the lungs and flows through the *ductus arteriosus* into the descending aorta where it mixes with some oxygenated blood from the left ventricle. Part of it supplies the abdominal viscera and lower limbs, but the majority of the blood flows through the two umbilical arteries back to the placenta for reoxygenation. During fetal life only 12% of the blood flows through the lungs.

The changes in pressure in the lungs and heart chambers during the first seconds of life cause these fetal anatomic structures, which shunted fetal blood directly to the left side of the heart and past the lungs, to close. With the first breath, almost 100% of the blood passes through the lungs. Blood returning from the pulmonary veins increases the pressure in the left atrium, resulting in functional closure of the foramen ovale. Placental transfer of blood to the infant approximately doubles the systemic vascular resistance at birth and causes increased pressures in the aorta, left atrium, and left ventricle.

Pulmonary vascular resistance is lowered as a result of lung expansion. During fetal life the blood vessels were compressed because of the small lung volume. Also, the hypoxia and hypercapnia of the fetal lungs caused vasoconstriction of the blood vessels, greatly increasing resistance to blood flow. However, with aeration of the lungs, which eliminates the hypoxia and hypercapnia, there is vasodilation. This lowered pulmonary resistance, which allows almost nine times the amount of blood to flow through the lungs, causes decreased pressure in the pulmonary artery. The decreased pulmonary arterial pressure and increased aortic pressure cause blood flow backward through the ductus arteriosus or from the aorta to the pulmonary artery. This reverse shunting of blood also increases the volume of blood flow to the lungs. Within 3 to 4 days after birth, the muscular wall of the ductus arteriosus gradually constricts to prevent all blood flow across these vessels. Sometime during the second month of life, the ductus becomes anatomically occluded by fibrotic tissue.

The cause of the functional or anatomic closure is unknown but may be a result of increased oxygenation through the ductus arteriosus, since the degree of contraction of the ductus arteriosus is directly proportional to the percentage of oxygen saturation. Because of the gradual anatomic closure of these shunts, functional murmurs are sometimes heard in newborns.

During the first few days of life the closure of the foramen ovale is reversible. In conditions such as crying that result in increased pressure in the vena cava and right atrium, there is a shunting of unoxygenated blood from the right side of the heart to the left side. This shunting of blood causes transient periods of cyanosis in the newborn.

Initial assessment: Apgar scoring

During the first seconds of the newborn's life, complex extensive physiologic changes are occurring. It is imperative that the nurse make astute observations during this time. One of the methods used to assess the newborn's immediate adjustment to extrauterine life is the Apgar scoring system, developed by Dr. Virginia Apgar in 1952. The score is based on observation of heart rate, respiratory effort, muscle tone, reflex irritability, and color (Table 8-1). Each item is given a score of 0, 1, or 2. Evaluations of all five categories are made at 1 and 5 minutes after birth and may be repeated until the infant's condition stabilizes. Total scores of 0 to 3 represent severe distress, scores of 4 to 6 signify moderate difficulty, and scores of 7 to 10 indicate absence of difficulty in adjusting to life. Studies have shown that a 5-minute score of 0 to 1 correlates with a 50% neonatal mortality rate. In terms of morbidity, children with Apgar scores of 0 to 3 exhibit three times as many neurologic abnormalities at 1 year of age as do children with a 5-minute score of 7 or better.

The *heart rate* is the most evaluative of the five items. A heart rate below 100 beats/minute is indicative of severe asphyxia and usually means that some form of resuscitation is necessary. Tachycardia, or heart rate above 160 beats/minute, indicates moderate, but recent, asphyxia and may be a poor prognostic sign. For accuracy, the heart rate should be counted for at least 30 seconds and correlated with the infant's activity. Detection of the apical pulse should be done with a stethoscope, although palpation of the umbilical cord at its junction with the abdomen is also reliable, and visible pulsations of the cord may also be counted.

Respiratory effort is evaluated as an index of adequate ventilation. If the respirations are slow, shallow, irregular, or gasping, they are indicative of respiratory distress.

Muscle tone refers to the degree of flexion and resistance offered by the infant when the nurse attempts to extend his extremities. The normal infant's position is one of flexion—the extremities are flexed and close to the body, and the fist is tightly clenched. Any attempt to alter this flexed position is generally met with resistance. At the other extreme, an asphyxiated infant is limp and offers no resistance to a change in position.

Reflex irritability is judged by the infant's response to passing a catheter through the nose after suctioning. The usual response from a healthy newborn is a loud, angry cry. A moderately depressed infant will demonstrate his annoyance by a facial grimace, but a severely depressed neonate will have no behavioral response. Reflex irritability can also be evaluated by slapping the sole of the foot with the palm of the hand. Flicking the sole of the foot with the finger or slapping the buttocks should be avoided when attempting to elicit a response.

Color is indicative of peripheral tissue oxygenation. Few newborns are completely pink at 1 minute after birth. Most infants continue to have some blueness of the extremities, whereas the rest of the body is pink. Pallor and cyanosis all over the body are indicative of a severely asphyxiated neonate. In evaluating color of nonwhite newborns, it is important to inspect the color of the mucous membranes of mouth and conjunctiva as well as the color of the lips, palms of the hands, and soles of the feet.

Table 8-1. Infant evaluation at birth—Apgar scoring system

	0	1	2
Heart rate	Absent	Slow (below 100 beats/minute)	Over 100 beats/minute
Respiratory effort	Absent	Slow or irregular	Good crying
Muscle tone	Limp	Some flexion of extremities	Active motion
Response to catheter in nostril (tested after oropharynx is clear)	No response	Grimace	Cough or sneeze
Color	Blue or pale	Body pink, extremities blue	Completely pink

Immediate care of the newborn

Maintenance of a patent airway. In addition to the respiratory and circulatory changes taking place during adjustment to extrauterine existence, several anatomic features of the neonate enhance the danger of airway obstruction. The infant is an obligatory nose breather, and the nasal passages, which are narrow, are easily occluded. The tongue is large, whereas the trachea and glottis are small. The ciliated columnar epithelium of the respiratory tract is especially susceptible to edema. In addition mucus is produced in excessive amounts during the first reactive phase (initial 10 to 30 minutes after delivery) and the second reactive phase (2 to 4 hours later).

The oropharynx and nostrils are suctioned with a bulb syringe as soon as the head is delivered. To avoid aspiration of amniotic fluid or mucus, the pharynx is cleared first, then the nasal passages. The bulb is compressed before insertion to prevent forcing secretions into the bronchi. A mucus trap can also be used. The nurse places one end of the tubing in the infant's mouth and the other end in her mouth. Air is then withdrawn through the tubing, creating suction at the other end. The mucus is trapped in the container in the middle of the tubing. The De Lee mucous trap is also an easy and efficient method of collecting an uncontaminated specimen (see Fig. 26-15, p. 931).

If more forceful removal of secretions is required, mechanical suction is used. The use of the proper size catheter and correct suctioning technique is essential in order to prevent mucosal damage and edema. Gentle suctioning is necessary to prevent reflex bradycardia, laryngospasm, and cardiac arrhythmias from vagal stimulation. Suctioning should be done for approximately 10 seconds to prevent depletion of the infant's oxygen supply.

After the infant is completely born, suctioning is performed with the child in a position that facilitates drainage of secretions, such as lying on the side or abdomen, with the head slightly lower than the chest. Gentle patting over the lung provides a form of percussion with the postural drainage. Milking the trachea is of questionable value since manipulation may cause injury to the cartilaginous rings of the trachea. In some delivery rooms the stomach is routinely lavaged to remove amniotic fluid that may cause abdominal distention, which may interfere with the establishment of respiration.

Thermoregulation and maintenance of stable body heat. At birth a major cause of heat loss is through evaporation from amniotic fluid that bathes the infant's skin. Rapid drying of the skin with a warmed towel as well as placement of the infant in a warmed environment are mandatory. Another major cause of heat loss is through radiation, or loss of heat to cooler *solid* objects in the environment that are not in direct contact with the infant. Loss of heat through radiation increases as these solid objects become colder and closer to the infant. The temperature of ambient or surrounding air in the Isolette or incubator essentially has no effect on loss of heat through radiation. This is a critical point to remember when attempting to maintain a constant temperature for the infant because even though the temperature of the ambient air is optimal, the infant can be hypothermic.

An example of radiant heat loss is the placement of the incubator in close proximity to a cold window or air conditioning unit. The cold from either source will cool the walls of the incubator and, subsequently, the body of the neonate. In order to compensate for this radiant heat loss, the infant will have to produce increased heat through accelerated metabolism. Since the amount of radiant heat loss varies inversely with the distance from cooler solid objects, the infant should be examined as far away as possible from the delivery room walls, preferably in the center of the room close to the mother.

Heat loss immediately after birth can also occur through conduction and convection. Conduction involves loss of heat from the body because of direct contact of skin with a cooler solid object. This can be minimized by placing the infant on a padded, covered surface and by providing insulation through clothes and blankets rather than by placing the infant directly on a hard table. Placing the newborn very close to his mother, such as in her arms or on her abdomen, is physically beneficial in terms of conserving heat as well as fostering maternal attachment.

Convection is similar to conduction, except that heat loss is aided by surrounding air currents. The rate of heat loss depends on ambient temperature and the velocity of airflow. For example, placing the infant in the direct flow of air from a fan or air conditioner vent will cause rapid heat loss through convection. Transporting the neonate in a crib with solid sides reduces airflow around the infant (Table 8-2).

Protection from infection and injury. Proper handwashing technique of all delivery room personnel is essential to prevent cross-contamination. The nurse washes the hands prior to and after handling the infant. In some institutions sterile gloves are worn, although hand washing is practiced outside the delivery room.

Prophylactic eye treatment against *Neisseria gonorrhoeae,* which can cause blindness in infants born of mothers with gonorrhea, is done by instilling one to two drops of 1% silver nitrate solution into each eye. Rinsing each eye with sterile normal saline is not recommended because it decreases the drug's effectiveness. Proper instillation of silver nitrate is essential because improper technique can cause a transient severe chemical conjunctivitis. Eye drops should always be placed on the conjunctival sac, never directly on the cornea, and should be allowed to flow from the inner to the outer aspect of the eye (Fig. 8-1). Other local antibiotic preparations such as penicillin or tetracycline can also be used for prophylaxis of gonorrheal ophthalmia neonatorum. Although these preparations may produce less irritation of

Table 8-2. Nursing care based on neonate's thermoregulation needs

Principle cause of heat loss	Preventive nursing action
Evaporation	Dry the skin and hair rapidly with a warmed towel after delivery. Postpone bath for first 4 to 6 hours until temperature stabilizes.
Conduction	Wrap infant snugly in a warmed blanket. Place infant in a preheated environment. (Ideally, place newborn next to mother after delivery.) Place infant on a padded, covered surface. Warm all objects used to examine or cover infant, for example, place them under radiant warmer. Uncover only one area of body for examination or procedures.
Radiation	Place newborn under a radiant heater. Keep newborn away from delivery or nursery room outside walls and windows. Monitor skin temperature and relate it to ambient air temperature; decreased skin temperature may indicate radiant heat loss.
Convection	Keep infant away from drafts, air conditioning vents, or fans. Place infant in a recessed cubicle with walls high enough to shield him from cross ventilation.

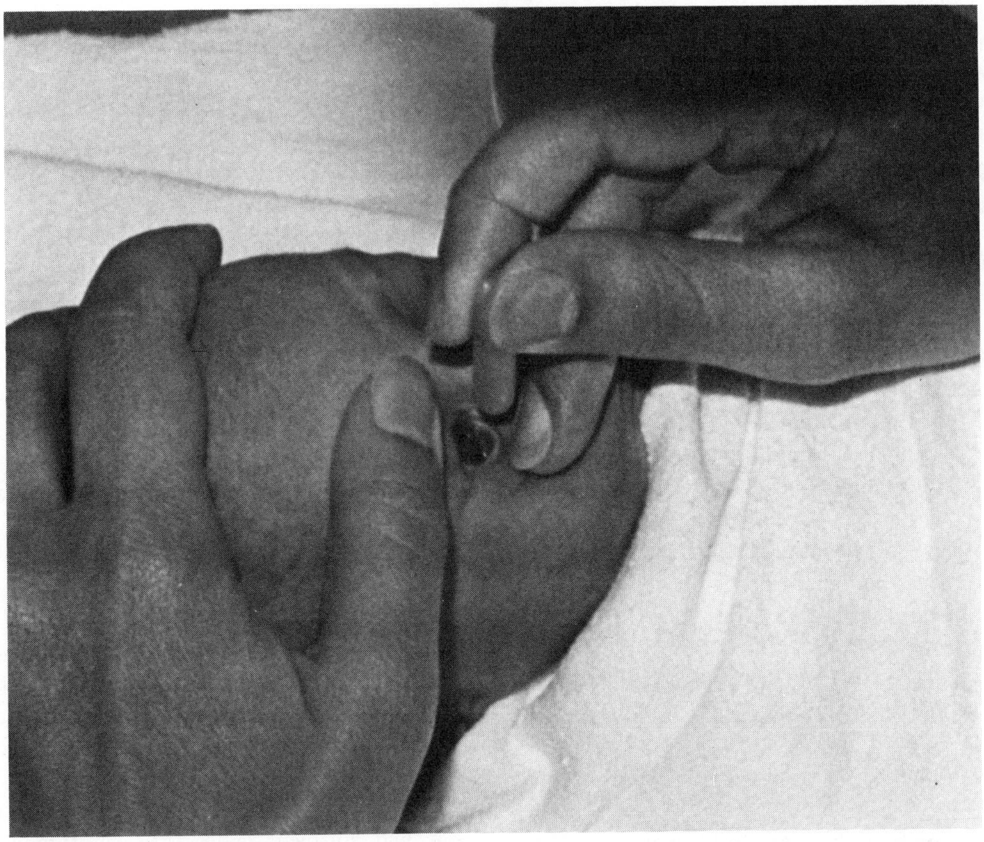

Fig. 8-1. Procedure for instilling eye drops in the neonate.

the eye, silver nitrate continues to be the drug of choice. It is very important for nurses to explain the reason for the instillation of these drops, because the resultant conjunctivitis can be upsetting for new parents.

Traditionally antimicrobial preparations have been instilled in the newborn's eyes only minutes after birth. Although the medical reason for use of such prophylactic drugs is justified, it is possible that the timing of their administration should be questioned. Studies on maternal attachment emphasize that in the first hour of life a newborn has a greater ability to focus on coordinated movement than at any other time during the next several days. This initial hour is very important in the development of maternal-infant bonding, one component of which is the establishment of eye-to-eye contact. Based on these findings, it is recommended that the routine administration of silver nitrate or antibiotics be postponed until after the parents and child have established such visual contact and bonding has begun.[11]

Another important initial observation concerns the appearance of the umbilical cord. The cord is usually clamped about 30 seconds after delivery, although much controversy surrounds this issue because of its effect on blood volume via placental transfusion. The nurse should carefully inspect the cut surface to determine the presence of two arteries, which look like two papular structures, and one vein, which has a larger lumen than the arteries and a thinner vessel wall. Absence of an artery is frequently associated with congenital anomalies, particularly of the genitourinary system. The basic principle for cord care is prevention of infection and trauma. The cord must be kept clean and dry until separation and complete healing take place, usually in about 12 to 15 days.

Shortly after birth, vitamin K is administered intramuscularly to the newborn. Vitamin K is normally synthesized by the normal intestinal flora, but, since the infant's intestine is sterile at birth, the supply of vitamin K is inadequate for at least the first 3 to 4 days. The major function of vitamin K is to catalyze the synthesis of prothrombin in the liver. A deficiency of this vitamin inhibits blood clotting and coagulation. It is important that the vastus lateralis muscle be used as the injection site because of the absence of other well-developed muscle masses (see p. 938).

Observation. The nurse notes and records the exact time of birth, which is when the infant is completely delivered from the birth canal. Besides the observations detailed in the Apgar scoring system (p. 251), the nurse notes the condition of the skin, the quality of the infant's cry, and the presence of congenital anomalies or evidence of birth trauma. The infant is weighed and his length is measured. Before the infant is removed from the delivery room, he is tagged with special identification bracelets, which are usually placed on his wrist and ankle. Some hospitals also have policies regarding handprinting and footprinting for identification purposes.

The nurse records the time of first voiding and passage of meconium. Normally full-term neonates void within the first 24 hours and pass their first stool within 36 hours. Delayed micturition is often the first clue to urinary tract pathology, whereas failure to pass meconium is a clue to alimentary obstruction.

FIRST 24 HOURS

An understanding of the complex physiologic changes that occur in both mother and infant at birth, combined with an appreciation of maternal-infant attachment, can justifiably support the idea that birth is a miracle. Without such an understanding and appreciation, those present at the time of birth cannot maintain, prevent, or anticipate those phenomena considered normal or abnormal. In fact unless nurses know what behaviors are characteristic of newborns, they will not be able to identify and hopefully prevent deviations from the normal.

Periods of reactivity

The newborn exhibits behavioral and physiologic characteristics that can at first appear to be signs of stress. However, during the initial 24 hours, changes in heart rate, respiration, motor activity, color, mucous production, and bowel activity occur in an orderly, predictable sequence, which is normal and indicative of lack of stress. Distressed infants will also progress through these stages but at a slower rate.

For the first 6 to 8 hours after birth, the newborn is in the *first period of reactivity* (Fig. 8-2). During the first 30 minutes the infant is very alert, cries vigorously, may suck his fist greedily, and appears very interested in his environment. At this time his eyes are usually open, suggesting that this is an excellent opportunity for mother, father, and child to see each other. Because he has a vigorous suck, this is also an opportune time to begin breast-feeding, because he will usually latch on quickly, satisfying both mother and infant. This is particularly important for nurses to remember, because it is not unlikely that after this initially highly active state the infant may be quite sleepy and uninterested in sucking. Physiologically the respiratory rate during this period may be as high as 82 breaths/minute, rales may be heard, heart rate may reach 180 beats/minute, bowel sounds are active, mucous secretions are increased, and temperature may decrease.

When one considers this normal behavior in a newborn, who has just passed through hours of "labor," and the mother's revitalized energy after her exhausting physiologic efforts in preparation for birth, one cannot help but wonder if nature has arranged this immediate time for introduction of mother and child. Ideally the nurse and others who participate in the birth experience should respect this critical time and enhance, rather than interfere with, the initial bonding of parents and child. In fact studies have shown that the type of maternal behavior displayed toward the in-

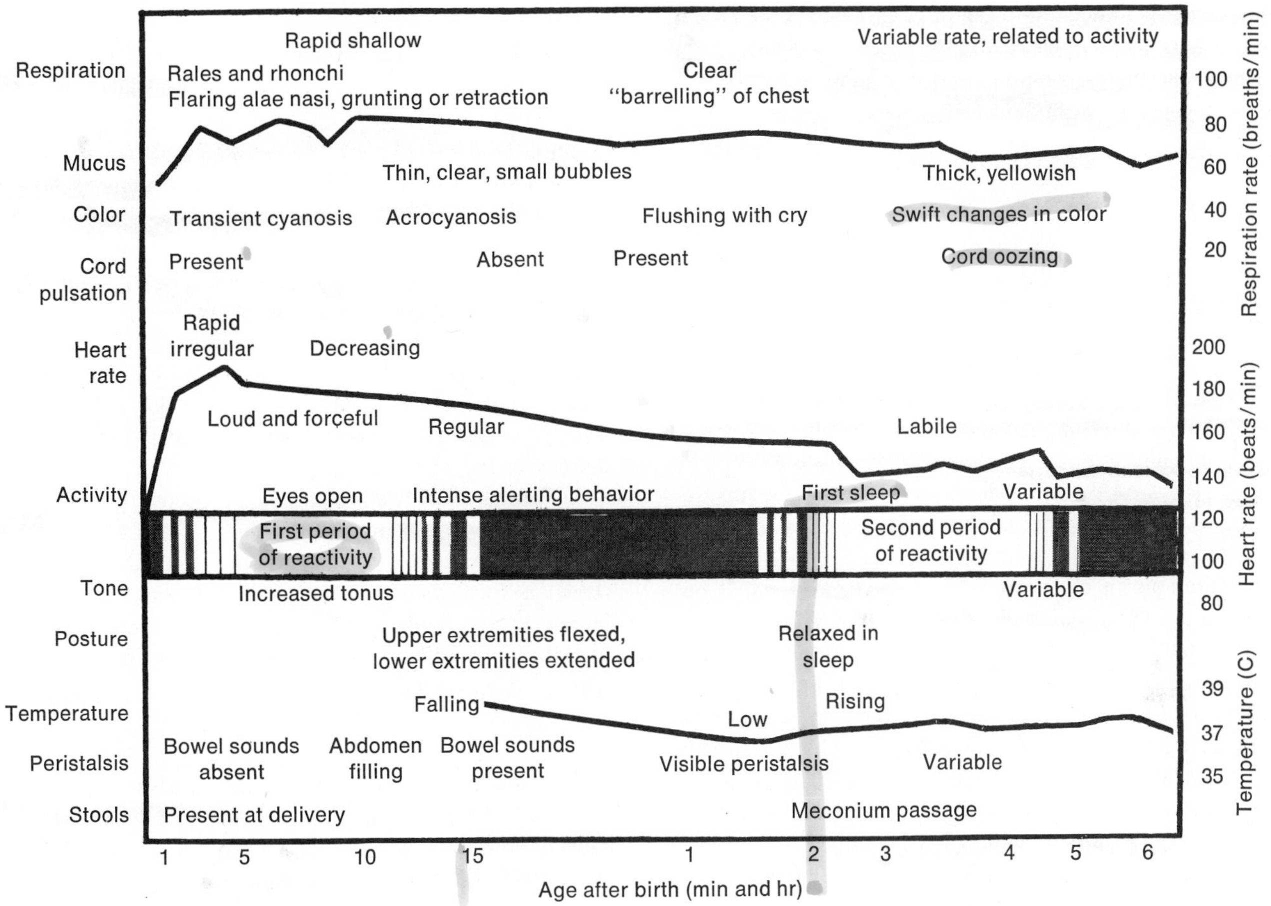

Fig. 8-2. Periods of reactivity. (From Arnold, H. W., and associates: Transition to extrauterine life. Copyright October 1965, the American Journal of Nursing Co. Reproduced with permission from the American Journal of Nursing, vol. 65, no. 10.)

fant is influenced by an extended period of initial contact with the newborn. Researchers have demonstrated that a total of 16 extra contact hours with their infant (1 hour after delivery and 5 hours each afternoon) influenced mothers to be more reluctant to leave their infant with someone else, to show greater soothing behavior and fondling, and to engage in significantly more eye-to-eye contact. These results were reaffirmed in a 1-year follow-up study.[11]

After this initial stage of alertness and activity, the infant's responsiveness diminishes. Heart and respiratory rates decrease, temperature continues to fall, mucous production decreases, and urine or stool is usually not passed. The infant is in a state of sleep and relative calm. Any attempt to stimulate him usually elicits a minimal response. This second stage of the first reactive period generally lasts 2 to 4 hours. Because of the continued decrease in body temperature, it is best to avoid undressing or bathing the infant during this time.

The *second period of reactivity* begins when the infant awakes from this deep sleep. The infant is again alert and responsive, heart and respiratory rates increase, the gag reflex is active, gastric and respiratory secretions are increased, and passage of meconium frequently occurs. This second period of reactivity lasts about 2 to 5 hours and provides another excellent opportunity for child and parents to interact. This period is usually over when the amount of respiratory mucus has decreased. Following this stage is a period of stabilization of physiologic systems and a vacillating pattern of sleep and activity.

After a discussion of the seemingly erratic patterns of behavior in the newborn, it is apparent that, in order to identify abnormalities or signs of distress in the respiratory, cardiovascular, or neurologic system, the nurse must thoroughly understand normal characteristics. Observation, not machines, is the nurse's greatest tool for assessment, and the nursing goal is anticipation and prevention of neonatal stress. The timing of nursing care is based on observation of the neonate's physiologic status. For example, the infant should be dried immediately after delivery to minimize heat loss from evaporation, the initial bath should be postponed until after body temperature has stabilized, eye drops should be instilled after parents and child have established visual contact, and breast-feeding or bottle-feeding should be initiated during one of the two periods of reactivity.

PHYSIOLOGIC STATUS OF NEWBORN

Several of the major life-dependent physiologic changes in the neonate have been discussed. Since many systems at the time of birth are still immature, each should be observed closely for possible malfunction and abnormality.

Respiratory system

The normal respirations of the newborn are usually irregular and abdominal, and the rate is generally between 30 and 50 breaths/minute. Short periods of apnea are usually considered normal. After the initial forceful breaths required to initiate respiration, subsequent breaths should be easy and fairly regular in rhythm.

Respirations in the newborn are chiefly abdominal because of the horizontal position of the ribs. The ribs of an adult articulate with the vertebrae and sternum from a downward and lateral angle. Contraction of the intercostal muscles raises the ribs to a horizontal position, causing the chest cavity to enlarge. In the infant the ribs are already horizontal and, if raised further, decrease the diameter of the chest (Fig. 8-3). Therefore, the infant relies almost entirely on diaphragmatic-abdominal breathing. During inspiration the diaphragm is forced downward, increasing the available space for lung expansion.

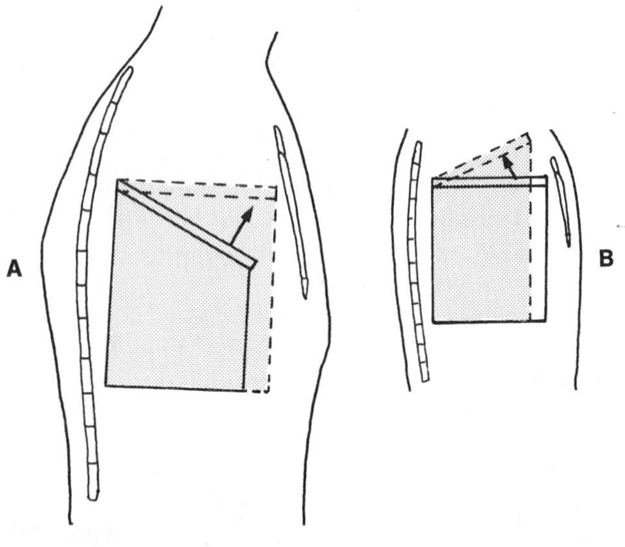

Fig. 8-3. Mechanisms of respiratory excursion. **A,** Downward and lateral position of the rib in the adult and expansion of lung capacity on thoracic inspiration. **B,** More horizontal position of the rib in infant and decreased expansion of lung capacity on thoracic inspiration.

Circulatory system

Apical rate changes in the initial newborn period. The fetal heart rate is generally considered normal at 120 to 160 beats/minute, although it changes with the stages of labor. At birth the heart rate may reach 180 beats/minute, which is typical of the first period of reactivity. During stage II of the first reactive period, the rate may fall to 100 beats/minute, then gradually rise to 120 beats/minute during the next 2 to 10 hours. Generally, by the second day, the infant's heart rate is between 90 and 160 beats/minute, depending on activity such as sleeping or crying. Auscultation will frequently reveal a soft systolic murmur caused by the functional incomplete anatomic closure of the fetal shunts. These functional or innocent murmurs usually disappear by the end of the first month.

The size of the heart is larger and occupies more space within the pleural cavity in the infant. Because of its more horizontal position, the apex or point of maximum impulse (PMI) is located at the third to fourth intercostal space, lateral to the midclavicular line. With increased chest growth, it gradually moves downward to the fifth intercostal space, midclavicular line.

Hemopoietic system

The blood volume of the neonate depends on the amount of placental transfer of blood. The blood volume of the fetus at term is about 90 ml/kg. Immediately after birth the total blood volume averages 300 ml, but, depending on how long the infant is attached to the placenta and if the cord is stripped, an additional 75 ml can be added to the blood volume. Blood flow through the umbilical arteries stops approximately 45 seconds after birth, whereas the umbilical vein remains patent longer. Gravity significantly influences the placental transfer of blood. Elevation of the infant above the mother's abdomen will decrease the blood volume from the placenta. Usually the newborn is placed below the level of the placenta and the cord is clamped approximately 30 seconds after delivery. It is important that the delivery nurse take special note of this time interval between birth and cord clamping, since blood volume affects hematocrit values, initial blood pressure, and respiratory status. Late clamping results in hypervolemia, which tends to cause an increase in the hematocrit and blood pressure and contributes to respiratory distress by causing mild pulmonary edema.

The average red blood cell (RBC) count of the newborn is 5 million/mm^3, depending on the amount of placental transfer of blood. In utero the increased number of red blood cells assures adequate oxygenation to the fetus. However, after birth few new red blood cells are produced, presumably because of the absence of the hypoxic stimulus on the hemopoietic system during neonatal life. Therefore, for about the next 8 to 10 weeks, the average red blood cell count falls to about 3 to 4 million/mm^3, resulting in a "physiologic anemia." By 2 to 3 months of age, the red blood cell count will be at a normal level of about 4 million/mm^3. There is a parallel fall in hemoglobin and hematocrit values as well, with the minimum level usually reached by age 3 months in the full-term infant. The average hemoglobin value at birth is 16 to 18 g/100 ml of blood, the average hematocrit value is between 45 and 50 ml/100 ml, and the white blood cell count averages 20,000/mm^3. However, it has been demonstrated that normal blood valves vary greatly in the newborn. (See Appendix B, Table B-4.)

Bilirubin formed in the fetus can cross the placenta and be excreted through the maternal liver. However, at birth the level of bilirubin from the breakdown of red blood cells rises because the neonate's immature liver is incapable of conjugating significant quantities of bilirubin with glucuronic acid for excretion into the bile. Consequently the plasma levels of bilirubin rise from a normal value of less than 1 mg/100 ml to an average of 5 mg/100 ml of blood during the second to fourth days of life. This normal elevation of serum bilirubin is referred to as neonatal or physiologic jaundice (see p. 294).

Fluid and electrolyte balance

Changes occur in the total body water volume, extracellular fluid volume, and intracellular fluid volume during the transition from fetal to postnatal life. The early fetus is composed almost entirely of water and at term is 73% fluid, as compared to 58% in the adult. There is also a shift in the ratio of extracellular to intracellular fluids. There is a higher level of extracellular fluid than intracellular fluid in the fetus, but this changes progressively throughout life probably because of the growth of cells at the expense of extracellular fluid. The infant has a proportionately higher ratio of extracellular fluid than the adult and consequently has a higher level of total body sodium and chloride and a lower level of potassium, magnesium, and phosphate (see Chapter 29).

A very important aspect of fluid balance in the neonate is its relationship to other systems. Besides the fact that the rate of fluid exchange is seven times greater in the infant than in the adult, the infant's rate of metabolism is twice as great in relation to body weight. As a result, twice as much acid is formed, leading to more rapid development of acidosis. In addition the immature kidneys cannot sufficiently concentrate urine to conserve body water. As a result of these three factors the infant is more prone to problems of dehydration, acidosis, and potentially overhydration.

Thermoregulation

The neonate's body temperature regulatory mechanisms are affected by several important factors. At birth the newborn's capacity for heat production is adequate but is dependent on increased metabolic activity. The normal metabolic rate per unit weight of the newborn is about twice that of the adult, but the neonate's surface area per unit weight is about three times larger than that of the adult. Therefore, the metabolic rate per unit area is less for the infant than for the adult. The crucial issue in the thermoregulation of the neonate is, therefore, to minimize the difference between heat generation and heat loss. The infant's proportionately larger surface area (15% of the adult's) in relation to body weight (5% of the adult's) provides more exposure to the environment and greater heat loss per unit of body weight. However, conservation of heat is aided by the newborn's usual position of flexion, which decreases the surface area exposed to the environment.

Another anatomic factor that retards the conservation of body heat is the newborn's thin layer of subcutaneous fat. Since core body temperature is approximately 1° higher than surface body temperature, this temperature gradient will cause a heat transfer from higher to lower temperature. A thicker layer of subcutaneous fat would increase the resistance for heat transfer, since the rate of heat transfer is equal to the temperature difference divided by the resistance.

The major sources of body heat in the newborn probably are the heart, liver, and brain. However, there is an additional source unique to the neonate. Brown fat, which owes its name to its larger content of mitochondrial cytochromes, has a greater capacity for heat production through intensified metabolic activity than does ordinary adipose tissue. Heat generated in the brown fat is distributed to other parts of the body by the blood, which is warmed as it flows through the layers of this tissue. Superficial deposits of brown fat are located between the scapula, around the neck, and behind the sternum. Deeper layers surround the kidneys and adrenals. The location of the brown fat may explain why the nape of the neck frequently feels warmer than the rest of the infant's body. It is important to remember that, regardless of the source of heat, its production is through increased metabolic activity, which will affect calorie requirements and oxygen consumption.

Gastrointestinal system

The ability of the newborn to digest, absorb, and metabolize foodstuff is adequate. The stomach has a capacity of about 90 ml, which gradually increases to about 150 ml by 1 month of age and to 360 ml by age 12 months. The emptying time is short, about 2½ to 3 hours, and peristalsis is rapid. These two factors increase transit time for food to pass through the stomach and colon. During the early weeks of life the newborn may have a bowel movement after each feeding. Also, the infant requires frequent small feedings because of limited stomach capacity.

The infant's intestine is longer in relation to body size than in the adult. Therefore, there are a larger number of secretory glands and a larger surface area for absorption as compared to the adult's intestine. Reverse peristalsis is not infrequent, and, when combined with an immature relaxed cardiac sphincter, regurgitation is a common occurrence. Some salivary glands are functioning, but the majority do not begin to secrete saliva until about age 2 to 3 months, when drooling is frequent.

Enzymes are adequate to handle the proteins and simple carbohydrates (monosaccharides and disaccharides), but deficient production of pancreatic amylase impairs utilization of complex carbohydrates (polysaccharides). Deficiency of pancreatic lipase limits the absorption of fats, especially with ingestion of foods with a high saturated fatty acid content, such as cow's milk.

The liver is the most immature of the gastrointestinal organs. It poorly conjugates bilirubin (p. 293) with glucuronic acid. It is deficient in forming plasma proteins, resulting in a decreased plasma protein concentration. This hypoproteinemia may contribute to the edema usually seen in the neonate. The liver is also deficient in its function of gluconeogenesis. As a result the blood glucose level of the unfed newborn falls to about 30 to 40 mg/100 ml. Until feeding occurs, the infant must depend on stored fat as the source of energy. However, the brain is one organ that is dependent on carbohydrate as its source of energy. Because of this, early initiation of breast- or bottle-feeding is advisable. The liver is also deficient in its formation of prothrombin and factor VII, which are needed for blood coagulation.

Renal system

All structural components are present in the renal system, but there is a functional deficiency in the kidney's ability to concentrate urine and to cope with conditions of fluid and electrolyte stress, such as dehydration or a concentrated solute load. The functional development of the nephrons is not complete until approximately 1 month of age. The tubules—in specific, the loop of Henle—are short and narrow and do not reach mature proportions until about 5 months of age. The small size of this structure affects the concentrating ability of the kidney. In addition the posterior lobe of the pituitary gland produces limited quantities of antidiuretic hormone (ADH) or vasopressin, which normally inhibits diuresis. Both of these factors render the young infant highly susceptible to dehydration. Another anatomic change occurs in the epithelium of the glomeruli and tubules. During infancy the columnar cells of the epithelium are tall and narrow; later they become flattened to form a more efficient filtering system.

The newborn is able to concentrate urine to only one and one-half the osmolality of plasma, as compared with three to four times that in the adult. Total volume per 24 hours is about 200 to 300 ml by the end of the first week, which is about seven times the rate in relation to body weight when compared to the adult. However, the bladder involuntarily empties when stretched by a volume of 15 ml, resulting in as many as twenty voidings per day. The first voiding usually occurs within 24 hours and should be noted and recorded. The neonate's urine generally is colorless and odorless and has a specific gravity of about 1.008. Limited glomerular filtration allows albumin and urates, a salt of uric acid, to be present in the urine. Poor phosphate clearance causes excessive urates to precipitate as uric acid infarcts, which can occlude the renal tubules. Urates will cause the urine to leave a brick red stain on the diaper, which may be mistaken for blood. When urates are present, fluids should be increased to prevent the formation of infarcts.

Integumentary system

At birth all the structures within the skin are present, but many of the functions of the integument are immature. The two layers of the skin, the epidermis and dermis, are loosely bound to each other and are very thin (p. 65). Slight friction across the epidermis causes separation of these layers and blister formation. During later life these layers are more tightly bound and, consequently, are more resistant to external irritation. Also, the transitional zone between the cornified and living layers of the epidermis is less effective in preventing fluid from reaching the skin surface. As fluid escapes, it is lost through evaporation, another factor that predisposes the infant to dehydration. The sebaceous glands are very active late in fetal life and in early infancy. They are most densely located on the scalp, face, and genitalia. Plugging of the glands on the face causes milia at birth, which usually resolve by age 4 to 6 weeks. Production of sebum on the scalp frequently causes cradle cap, particularly if the hair is infrequently shampooed (see p. 492). During later infancy and childhood these glands are relatively inactive, until the onset of puberty. The eccrine glands, which produce sweat in response to heat or emotional stimuli, are nonfunctional at birth but become active during the next few days, beginning with sweating on the face, then palms. However, their ability to produce sweat remains minimal until puberty, a factor that helps conserve fluid loss via evaporation.

The protective function of the skin against bacteria is fairly efficient during infancy. Because of the relative dryness of the skin from minimal sweat and sebum, bacterial growth is inhibited, except in areas such as the genitalia, where moisture from urine and feces favors growth of bacteria and fungus.

Musculoskeletal system

At birth the skeletal system contains larger amounts of cartilage than ossified bone, although the process of ossification is fairly rapid during the first year. The nose, for example, is predominantly cartilage at birth and is frequently flattened by the force of delivery. The six skull bones are relatively soft and not yet joined. Separating these bones are bands of connective tissue called sutures. Broader palpable areas at the junction of sutures are called fontanels. The sinuses are also incompletely formed in the newborn. The ethmoidal and maxillary sinuses are present as small holes, and the sphenoidal sinuses are pinpoint indentations. The frontal sinuses and the mastoid process are not present until 7 or 8 years of age.

Unlike the skeletal system, the muscular system is almost completely formed at birth. Growth in the size of muscular tissue is caused by hyperplasia, rather than hypertrophy, of cells. As the muscle increases in size, the degree of strength also increases. The progressive strength allows the infant to assume various postural adjustments during infancy, such as rolling over, sitting, crawling, and walking. The integration of the musculoskeletal and neurologic systems must also be present for adequate function to develop.

Defenses against infection

The infant is born with several defenses against infection. The first line of defense is the skin, which protects the body from invading organisms. The second line of defense is the reticuloendothelial system, which produces several types of cells capable of attacking a pathogen. The process of phagocytosis is mature at birth. The neutrophils and monocytes are phagocytes, which enables them to engulf, ingest, and destroy foreign agents. Eosinophils also probably have a phagocytic property, because in the presence of foreign protein they increase in number. The lymphocytes are capable of being converted to other cell types, such as monocytes and antibodies. Although the phagocytic properties of the blood are present in the infant, the inflammatory response of the tissues to localize an infection is immature. The exact reason for this is unknown.

The third line of defense is the formation of specific antibodies to an antigen. This process requires exposure to various foreign agents for antibody production to occur. The infant is generally not capable of producing his own gamma globulins until the beginning of the second month of life but has received considerable passive immunity from the maternal circulation. He is protected against most major childhood diseases, including diphtheria, measles, and smallpox, for approximately 6 months, provided the mother has developed antibodies to these illnesses. Immunity against pertussis is normally insufficient, necessitating that the newborn be artificially immunized against this disease before 6 months of age (see immunization schedule, p. 457). In addition breast-fed infants may derive additional immunity to such diseases as polio, mumps, influenza, and chickenpox through IgA in the early breast secretion colostrum.

Endocrine system

Ordinarily the endocrine system of the newborn is adequately developed, but its functions are immature under certain conditions. One of the most common occurrences is the effect of maternal sex hormones on the infant's breast, which may be engorged and secrete milk during the first few days of life. Female newborns may have pseudomenstruation and genital hypertrophy from the sudden drop in the level of progesterone and estrogen. An infant of a diabetic mother may have hypertrophy and hyperfunction of the islets of Langerhans. As a consequence the hyperinsulinism will produce hypoglycemia shortly after birth. (See p. 435 for development of the endocrine system during the first year.)

Neurologic system

At birth the nervous system is incompletely integrated but well enough developed to sustain extrauterine life. Most neurologic functions are primitive reflexes. The autonomic nervous system is crucial during transition because it stimulates initial respirations, helps maintain acid-base balance, and partially regulates temperature control. All cranial nerves are present and myelinated except for the optic and olfactory nerves. At birth the brain is 25% of its eventual mature size and comprises about 12% of total body weight as compared to 2.5% in the adult (Table 8-3).

Myelination of the nervous system follows the cephalocaudal-proximodistal laws of development and is closely related to observed mastery of fine and gross motor skills. Myelin is necessary for rapid and efficient transmission of nerve impulses along the neural pathway. The tracts that develop myelin earliest are the sensory, cerebellar, and extrapyramidal. This accounts for the acute senses of taste, smell, and hearing in the newborn. The cerebellum acts to coordinate gross voluntary movement and assists in maintaining equilibrium. The extrapyramidal tract also is involved in postural adjustment and gross motor movement, which is mostly reflexive. It coordinates the reciprocal flexion and extension of muscle groups to maintain smooth, coordinated movement. At birth most of the neurologic functions are primitive reflexes (Table 8-6).

Sensory functions

Vision. At birth the eye is structurally incomplete. The fovea centralis is not yet completely differentiated from the

Table 8-3. Comparison of brain growth to body growth*

Age	Brain (%)†	Height (%)	Weight (%)
Birth	25	29	5
6 months	50	38	10
1 year	66	43	15
2½ years	75	53	20
6 years	90	70	30

*As compared with average growth of a male adult.

†Data from Dobbing, J., and Sands, J.: Arch. Dis. Child. **48:**757-767, 1973.

macula. Complete differentiation generally occurs at about 4 months of age, when visual acuity is 20/200. The ciliary muscles are also immature, limiting the ability of the eyes to accommodate and fixate on an object. However, the pupils react to light, the blink reflex is responsive to a minimal stimulus, and the corneal reflex is activated by a light touch. The newborn has the ability to momentarily fixate on a bright or moving object that is within 8 inches and is in the midline of the visual field. In fact the infant's ability to fixate on coordinated movement is greater during the first hour of life than during the succeeding several days. Tear glands usually do not begin to function until the infant is 2 to 4 weeks of age. Permanent eye color may be determined at age 3 months, but pigmentation of the iris is not complete until the end of the first year. The color of most light-skinned newborns' eyes is slate gray or dark blue; dark-skinned neonates usually have brown eye color.

Hearing. Once the amniotic fluid has drained from the ears, the infant probably has auditory acuity similar to that of an adult. The neonate is able to detect a loud sound of about 90 decibels and reacts with a startle reflex. The newborn's response to sounds of low frequency vs those of high frequency differs; the former, such as the sound of a heartbeat, metronome, or lullaby, tends to decrease an infant's motor activity and crying, whereas the latter seems to elicit an alerting reaction. There also seems to be an early sensitivity to the sound of human voices, though not specifically speech sounds. As early as age 2 weeks the infant may stop crying to listen to the sound of a voice.

At birth all the structural components of the ear are fully mature. However, the cortical activity associated with hearing or with any other sense is still incomplete, because of the immature myelination of the various neural pathways beyond the midbrain. This lack of cortical integration is responsible for the infant's generalized response to sound.

Smell. Limited research has been done on the newborn's ability to smell. However, it is known that newborns will react to strong odors such as alcohol or vinegar by turning their heads away. Recent studies have demonstrated that breast-fed infants seem able to smell breast milk and will cry for their mothers when the breasts are engorged and leaking.

Taste. The newborn has the ability to distinguish between tastes. Various types of solutions elicit differing gustofacial reflexes. A tasteless solution elicits no facial expression, a sweet solution elicits an eager suck and a look of satisfaction, a sour solution causes the usual puckering of the lips, and a bitter liquid produces an angry, upset expression. During early childhood the taste buds are distributed mostly on the tip of the tongue.

Touch. At birth the infant is able to perceive tactile sensation in any part of the body, although the face, especially the mouth, hands, and soles of the feet, seems to be most sensitive. There is increasing documentation that touch and motion are essential to normal growth and development. Gentle patting of the back or rubbing of the abdomen usually elicits a calming response from the infant. However, painful stimuli, such as a pinprick, will elicit an angry, upsetting response.

ASSESSMENT OF THE NEONATE

Physical assessment

An important aspect of the care of the newborn is a thorough, detailed physical examination that identifies normal characteristics and existing abnormalities and establishes a baseline for future physiologic changes. The physical assessment of the neonate should be one of the nurse's priorities in the plan of care. As with any physical examination, the four arts of observation, percussion, palpation, and auscultation are utilized. These have been discussed in considerable detail in Chapter 5. This discussion focuses on the newborn assessment with emphasis on normal findings, variations from the norm that require little or no therapy, and specific potential danger signs that should alert the nurse to more careful observation of the infant. Table 8-4 summarizes physical assessment of the neonate.

Examination of the newborn generally presents few problems in terms of gaining his acceptance or cooperation. However, a few comments may prove helpful. In general it is best to proceed in an orderly head-to-toe progression. Since exposing an infant to the air when undressing him usually elicits crying, it is best to listen to the heart, lungs, and abdomen first. It is also helpful to take head, chest, and length measurements at the same time in order to record them accurately and to mentally make a note of their relationship to each other. Weight should be taken with the infant fully undressed. If clothing is not removed, the scale should be prebalanced to adjust for the excess weight by weighing similar articles of clothing first. If the newborn is irritable and crying during the examination, allowing him to suck on a nipple or on one's gloved finger usually pacifies him sufficiently to complete palpation and auscultation satisfactorily. Whether or not all these suggestions are followed is less important than establishing a routine that minimizes delay, haphazard organization, and omission of details.

General measurements

There are several important measurements of the newborn that have significance when compared to each other as well as when recorded over time on a graph. For the full-term infant, average *head circumference* is between 33 and 35.5 cm (13 to 14 inches). It is not unusual for head circumference to be somewhat less immediately after birth because of the molding process that occurs during a normal vaginal delivery. Usually by the second or third day the normal size and contour of the skull have replaced the molded one.

Table 8-4. Physical assessment of the neonate

Area	Usual findings	Common variations/ minor abnormalities	Potential signs of distress/ major abnormalities
General measurements	Head circumference 33-35.5 cm (13-14 inches) Chest circumference 30.5-33 cm (12-13 inches) Head circumference should be about 2-3 cm (1 inch) larger than chest circumference Crown-to-rump length 31-35 cm (12.5-14 inches) Crown-to-rump length approximately equal to head circumference Head-to-heel length 48-53 cm (19-21 inches) Birth weight 2700-4000 g (6-9 pounds)	Molding after birth may decrease head circumference Head and chest circumferences may be equal for first 1-2 days after birth	Head circumference smaller than chest circumference Head circumference more than 4 cm (1.5-2 inches) larger than chest circumference Birth weight less than 2500 g (5.5 pounds)
General appearance	Posture—flexion of head and extremities, which rest on chest and abdomen	Frank breech—extended legs, abducted and fully rotated thighs, flattened head, extended neck	Limp posture, extension of extremities
Skin	At birth, bright red, puffy, smooth Second to third day, pink, flaky, dry Vernix caseosa Lanugo Edema around eyes, face, legs, dorsa of hands, feet, and scrotum or labia	Neonatal jaundice after first 24 hours Harlequin color change Acrocyanosis Mongolian spots Ecchymoses or petechiae caused by birth trauma Milia neonatorum Sudamina Telangiectatic nevi Cutis marmorata Subcutaneous fat necrosis Erythema toxicum	Progressive jaundice, especially in first 24 hours Cracked or peeling skin Generalized cyanosis Pallor Grayness Hemorrhage, ecchymoses, or petechiae that persist Sclerema
Head	Anterior fontanel—diamond-shaped 2.5-4.0 cm (1-1.75 inches) Posterior fontanel—triangular-shaped, 0.5-1 cm (0.2-0.4 inch) Fontanels should be flat, soft, and firm	Molding following vaginal delivery Third sagittal (parietal) fontanel Bulging fontanel because of crying or coughing Craniotabes Caput succedaneum Cephalhematoma	Fused sutures Bulging or depressed fontanels Widened sutures and fontanels
Eyes	Lids usually edematous Eyes usually closed Color—slate gray, dark blue, brown Absence of tears Presence of red reflex Corneal reflex in response to touch Pupillary reflex in response to light Blink reflex in response to light or touch Rudimentary fixation on objects and ability to follow to midline	Chemical conjunctivitis Subconjunctival hemorrhages Retinal hemorrhages Searching nystagmus or strabismus Hypertelorism (3 cm or greater)	Pink color of iris Purulent discharge Mongoloid slant Congenital cataracts Constricted or dilated fixed pupil Absence of red reflex Absence of pupillary or corneal reflex Inability to follow object or bright light to midline

Continued.

Table 8-4. Physical assessment of the neonate—cont'd

Area	Usual findings	Common variations/ minor abnormalities	Potential signs of distress/ major abnormalities
Ears	Position—top of pinna on horizontal line with outer canthus of eye Startle reflex elicited by a loud, sudden noise Pinna flexible, cartilage present	Inability to visualize tympanic membrane because of filled aural canals Pinna flat against head	Low placement of ears Absence of startle reflex in response to loud noise
Nose	Nasal patency Nasal discharge—thin white mucus Sneezing	Flattened and bruised	Nonpatent canals Thick, bloody nasal discharge Flaring of nares (alae nasi)
Mouth and throat	Intact, high-arched palate Uvula in midline Frenulum of tongue Frenum of upper lip Sucking reflex Rooting reflex Gag reflex Extrusion reflex Absent or minimal salivation	Precocious teeth Inclusion cysts Epstein's pearls White patches (thrush)	Cleft lip Cleft palate Large, protruding tongue or posterior displacement of tongue Profuse salivation or drooling Inability to pass nasogastric tube
Neck	Short, thick, usually surrounded by skin folds Tonic neck reflex Neck-righting reflex Otolith-righting reflex	Torticollis Branchial cleft cysts	Excessive skin folds Resistance to flexion Absence of tonic neck, neck-righting, or otolith-righting reflex
Chest	Anteroposterior and lateral diameters equal Slight sternal retractions evident during inspiration Xiphoid process evident Breast enlargement	Funnel chest (pectus excavatum) Pigeon chest (pectus carinatum) Supernumerary nipples Secretion of milky substance from breasts	Depressed sternum Marked retractions of chin, chest, and intercostal spaces during respiration Asymmetric chest expansion or overexpansion Redness and firmness around nipples
Lungs	Rate—30-60 breaths/minute Respirations chiefly abdominal Cough reflex absent at birth, present by 1-2 days Bilateral bronchial breath sounds	Rate and depth of respirations may be irregular, momentary apneic spells Rales shortly after birth	Apnea Dyspnea Tachypnea—rate above 60 breaths/minute Persistent irregular breathing Periodic breathing with repeated apneic spells Grunting respirations Deep sighing respirations Seesaw respirations Persistent fine rales Rhonchi Diminished breath sounds Peristaltic sounds on one side, with diminished breath sounds on same side
Heart	Rate—120-140 beats/minute and regular Apex—third to fourth intercostal space, lateral to midclavicular line S_2 slightly sharper and higher in pitch than S_1	Murmurs Sinus arrhythmia	Dextrocardia Displacement of apex Cardiomegaly Abdominal shunts

Table 8-4. Physical assessment of the neonate—cont'd

Area	Usual findings	Common variations/ minor abnormalities	Potential signs of distress/ major abnormalities
Abdomen	Cylindric in shape Liver—palpable 2-3 cm below right costal margin Spleen—tip palpable at end of first week of age Kidneys—palpable 1-2 cm above umbilicus Equal bilateral femoral pulses	Visible peristalsis and veins in thin infants Umbilical hernia Diastasis recti	Abdominal distention Localized bulging Distended veins Absent bowel sounds Enlarged liver and spleen Ascites Visible peristaltic waves Scaphoid or concave abdomen Palpable bladder distention following scanty voiding Absent femoral pulses
Female genitalia	Labia and clitoris usually edematous Labia minora larger than labia majora Urethral meatus behind clitoris Hymenal tag Vernix caseosa between labia	Blood-tinged discharge (pseudomenstruation)	Enlarged clitoris with urethral meatus at tip Fused labia Absence of vaginal opening Fecal discharge from vaginal opening
Male genitalia	Urethral opening at tip of glans penis Testes palpable in each scrotum Scrotum usually large, edematous, and pendulous; usually deeply pigmented in dark-skinned ethnic groups Smegma	Urethral opening covered by prepuce Inability to retract foreskin Epithelial pearls Erection or priapism Testes palpable in inguinal canal Scrotum small Hydrocele Inguinal hernia	Hypospadias Epispadias Testes not palpable in scrotum or inguinal canal
Back and rectum	Spine intact, no openings, masses, or prominent curves Trunk incurvation reflex Patent anal opening	Pilonidal cyst or sinus Anal fissures	Spina bifida Imperforate anus
Extremities	10 fingers and toes Full range of motion Negative scarf sign—elbow does not reach midline Nail beds pink, with transient cyanosis immediately after birth Creases on anterior two thirds of sole Sole usually flat Symmetry of extremities Equal muscle tone bilaterally, especially resistance to opposing flexion	Partial syndactyly between second and third toes Clinodactyly of second toe with overlapping into third toe Wide gap between hallux and second toe Deep crease on plantar surface of foot between first and second toes Asymmetric length of toes Dorsiflexion and shortness of hallux	Polydactyly Syndactyly Hyperflexibility of joints Persistent cyanosis of nail beds Yellowing of nail beds Sole covered with creases Fractures Dislocated hip Limitation in hip abduction Unequal gluteal or leg folds Unequal leg length (Allis' sign) Audible click on abduction (Ortolani's sign) Asymmetry of extremities Unequal muscle tone or range of motion
Neuromuscular system	Extremities usually maintain some degree of flexion Extension of an extremity followed by previous position of flexion Head lag while sitting, but momentary ability to hold head erect Able to turn head from side to side when prone Able to hold head in horizontal line with back when held prone	Quivering or momentary tremors	Limp extremities Straightening of extremities Paralysis Hypotonia Tremors, twitches, and myoclonic jerks Marked head lag

Chest circumference is generally 30.5 to 33 cm (12 to 13 inches). The usual relationship between head and chest circumference is a difference of about 2 to 3 cm, or 1 inch. Because of the molding of the head during delivery, initially these measurements may appear equal. However, if the head is significantly smaller than the chest, microcephaly or premature closure of the sutures (craniostenosis) should be suspected. If the head is more than 4 cm larger than the chest and this relationship remains constant or increases over several days, then hydrocephalus must be considered. Other causes of increased head circumference are caput succedaneum, cephalhematoma, and subdural hematoma. Prematurity and malnutrition will cause the head measurement to be significantly larger than the chest circumference, but this is because of decreased chest size, not increased head circumference.[6]

Head circumference may also be compared with *crown-to-rump* length, or sitting height (Fig. 8-4). Crown-to-rump measurements are usually 31 to 35 cm (12.5 to 14 inches) and are approximately equal to head circumference. The relationship of the head and crown-to-rump measurements is probably more reliable than that of the head and chest.

Head-to-heel length is also measured in the newborn. Because of the usual flexed position of the infant, it is important to extend the leg completely when measuring total body length. The average length of the newborn is 48 to 53 cm (19 to 21 inches). *Body weight* should be taken in the delivery room, because weight loss will occur fairly rapidly after birth. Normally the neonate loses about 10% of the birth weight by 3 to 4 days of age because of loss of excessive extracellular fluid, meconium, and limited food intake. The birth weight is usually regained by the tenth day of life. Most newborns weigh 2700 to 4000 g (6 to 9 pounds), the average weight being about 3400 g (7.5 pounds). Newborns who weigh below 2500 g (5.5 pounds) are usually classified as low birth weight infants. Accurate birth weights and lengths are important because they provide a baseline for assessment of future growth.

Another category of measurements is vital signs. Axillary temperatures should be taken because insertion of a thermometer into the rectum can cause perforation of the mucosa. However, taking a rectal temperature provides an opportunity to determine patency of the anus. Core body temperature varies according to the periods of reactivity but is usually 35.5° to 37.5°C (96° to 99.5°F). Skin temperature is slightly lower than core body temperature.

Pulse and *respirations* also vary according to the periods of reactivity and to the infant's behaviors but are usually in the range of 120 to 140 beats/minute and 40 to 60 breaths/minute, respectively. Both should be counted for a full 60 seconds to detect irregularities in rate or rhythm. Heart rate should be taken apically with a stethoscope (see the boxed material on the opposite page).

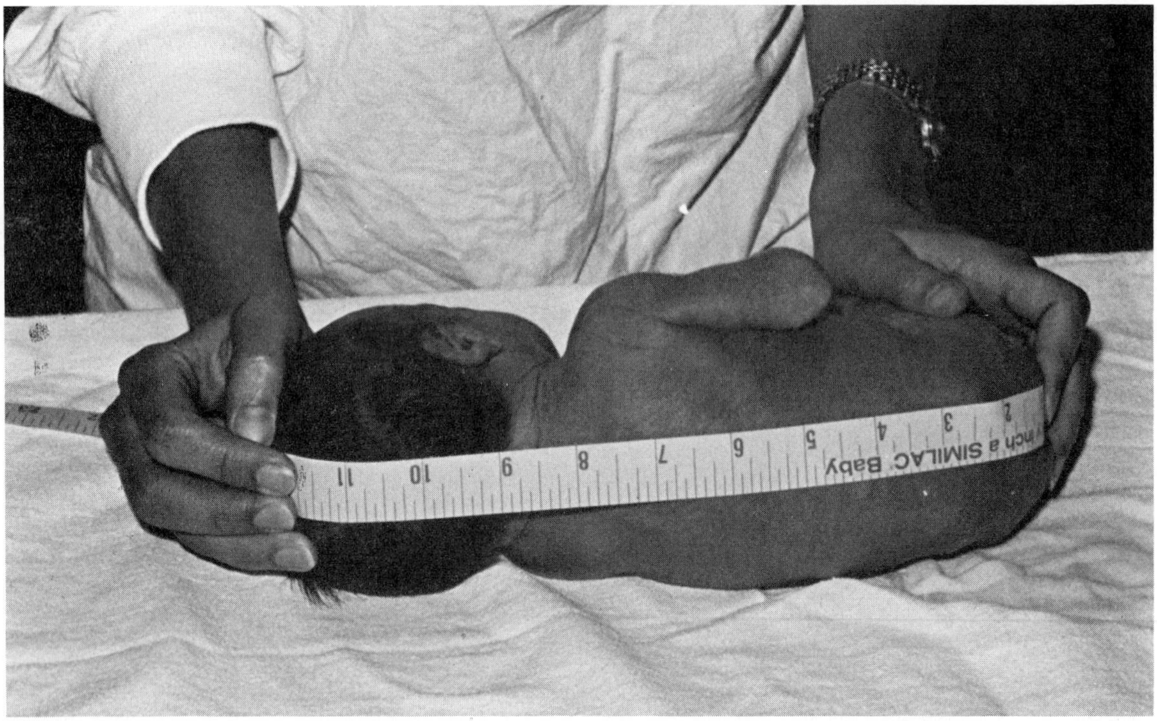

Fig. 8-4. Measurement of crown-to-rump length in appraisal of newborn.

Vital signs in the newborn

Temperature	*Nursing considerations*
Axillary—36.5° to 37°C (97.7° to 98°F) Rectal—35.5° to 37.5°C (96° to 99.5°F)	1. Axillary temperature is preferable and should be taken for at least 3 minutes. Rectal temperatures may cause perforation of the intestine. 2. Difference between axillary and rectal temperature should be slight. A higher rectal temperature may indicate a febrile state. A lower axillary reading may indicate heat loss to the ambient air. 3. Incubator temperature should be measured and compared to rectal and axillary readings. Cooler ambient air will decrease skin temperature and increase metabolic activity. 4. Crying may increase rectal temperature from 0.11° to 1.0°C (0.2° to 1.8°F), but temperature will usually return to the precrying measurement in 1 to 2½ minutes after cessation of crying.
Heart rate	
Apical—120 to 140 beats/minute	1. Heart rate should be taken apically with the use of a proper size stethoscope. 2. Heart rate should be counted for a full 60 seconds in order to detect irregularities in rate or rhythm. Tapping the finger while counting will help in establishing a rhythm and rate. 3. Heart rate should be recorded in terms of infant's activity. Crying will usually increase pulse rate. A deep sleep may decrease the rate to below 100 beats/minute. 4. Bradycardia is usually indicated by a rate below 120 beats/minute; tachycardia is usually indicated by a rate higher than 160 to 170 beats/minute.
Respirations	
Rate—40 to 60 breaths/minute	1. Respiratory rate should be counted for a full 60 seconds in order to determine irregularity in rate and occurrence of apneic spells. 2. Respirations may be observed by watching rise and fall of the abdomen or may be auscultated with a stethoscope. 3. The rise and fall of the chest and abdomen, which should be synchronous, should be observed. Seesaw movements, retractions, and asymmetric chest expansion should be carefully noted. 4. Respiratory rate should be recorded in terms of infant's activity, for example, crying will increase respiratory rate. 5. Tachypnea is usually indicated by respiratory rate above 60 breaths/minute.
Blood pressure	
At birth Systolic pressure—60 to 80 mm/Hg Diastolic pressure—40 to 50 mm/Hg By tenth day Systolic pressure—95 to 100 mm/Hg Diastolic pressure—slight rise	1. Width of blood pressure cuff affects readings. A cuff of 2.5 cm (1 inch) in width is used with palpation of the radial pulse. 2. The flush method for determination of blood pressure may be used, but for accurate readings the infant must be quiet (see p. 116 for description of this technique). 3. Fluctuations in blood pressure occur with changes in activity, such as crying or sleeping.

General appearance

Posture. Before each body system is assessed, it is important to describe the general posture, color, and behavior of the newborn. In the full-term neonate the *posture* is one of flexion, a result of in utero position (Fig. 8-5). The infant born in a vertex position keeps the head flexed, with the chin resting on the upper chest. The arms are flexed at the elbows, and they rest, folded, on the chest. The hands are held in a clenched or fisted position. The legs are flexed at the knees, and the hips are flexed in such a position that the thighs rest on the abdomen. The feet are dorsiflexed and positioned on the anterior aspect of the legs. The vertebral column is also flexed. It is important that any deviation from this very characteristic fetal position be recognized. For example, infants of preterm birth as well as hypoxic infants do not assume a posture of total flexion, but rather one of limp extension. Nonvertex presentations also result in variations in posture. In breech presentations the posture will depend on the presenting part, for example, a frank breech presentation results in extended legs, abducted and fully rotated thighs, a flattened head on top, and a neck that appears elongated.

Color. Although color is described more specifically when examining the skin, general observations are made about the color of the skin in relation to activity, position, and temperature changes. In general the infant becomes redder when crying and may demonstrate transient periods of cyanosis. Decreased temperature will increase the degree of cyanosis because of vasoconstriction. *Harlequin color change,* a benign transient blush on the dependent half of the body when the infant lies on his side, is characteristic between 48 and 96 hours after birth.

Behavior. The infant's *behavior* is carefully noted, especially the degree of alertness, drowsiness, and irritability, which are common signs of neurologic problems. Some questions that the nurse may mentally ask when assessing behavior include: is the infant awakened easily by a loud noise; is he comforted by rocking, sucking, or cuddling; do there seem to be periods of deep and light sleep; when he is awake, does he seem satisfied after a feeding; what stimili elicit responses from him; and, when he is disturbed, how much does he protest?

Skin. The skin of the newborn is usually smooth and puffy, especially about the eyes, the legs, the dorsal aspect of the hands and the feet, and the scrotum or labia.

The color depends on racial and familial background. The white infant is usually pink to red; the black newborn may appear a pinkish brown. Infants of Oriental descent may resemble a shade of tea rose; those of Latin descent may have an olive tint or a slight yellow cast to the skin. By the second or third day the skin turns to its more natural tone and is more dry and flaky.

At birth the skin is covered with a grayish-white, cheese-like substance called *vernix caseosa*. If it is not removed during the bath, it will dry and disappear by about 24 to 48 hours. It is thought to have an insulating effect against heat loss. A fine, downy hair called *lanugo* is present on the skin, especially on the forehead, cheeks, shoulders, and back. *Milia,* distended sebaceous glands, appear as tiny white papules on the cheeks, chin, and nose. They usually disappear spontaneously in a few weeks. *Sudamina* are distended sweat glands that cause minute vesicles on the skin surface, especially on the face.

Several color changes may be noted on the skin. *Jaundice,* a yellow staining of the integument resulting from excess bilirubin in the blood, is sometimes evident in newborns by the second or third day of life and usually disappears by the fifth to seventh day. Jaundice during the first 24 hours usually indicates a pathophysiologic state and requires immediate attention (p. 295). The yellow color of the skin may be more closely assessed by applying pressure to the skin with two fingers, which will cause blanching of the normally red skin and reveal an underlying yellow stain.

Acrocyanosis, or peripheral cyanosis of the hands and

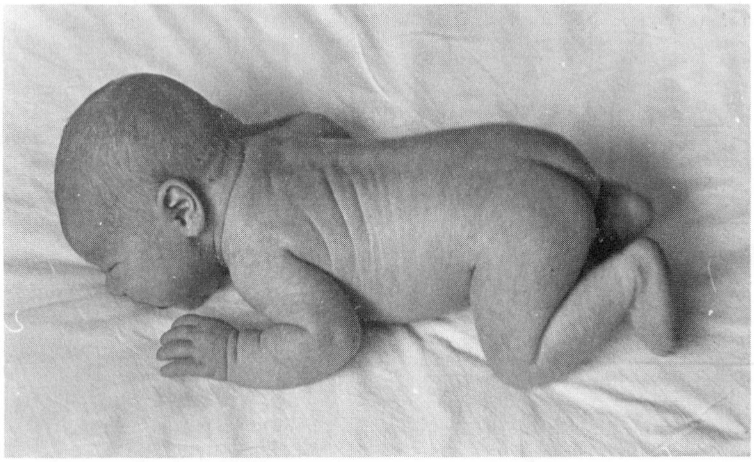

Fig. 8-5. Flexed position of neonate.

feet, is a normal condition, probably caused by venous stasis rather than by hypoxia. Localized cyanosis will also appear over presenting or dependent parts of the body, particularly when the infant is lying in unusual positions, such as when an arm is extending over the mattress. *Harlequin color change* is an unusual color discrepancy between the two longitudinal halves of the body, extending from the forehead to the pubic symphysis. When the infant lies on his side for several minutes, the dependent half of the body becomes pink and the upper half becomes pale. When the infant is placed on the opposite side, the color change reverses. This peculiar phenomenon has no known physiologic explanation and does not occur when the infant is prone or supine.

Mongolian spots are irregular areas of deep blue pigmentation in the deeper layer of the skin, usually distributed over the sacral and gluteal regions. They are very common in black infants and may be seen in newborns of Asian, Latin, or southern European descent. These harmless discolorations may begin to fade after several weeks and usually disappear by 4 years of age. *Telangiectatic nevi,* or stork bites, are flat, deep pink localized areas of capillary dilatation that are almost universal in newborns. They are most evident on the back of the neck, lower occiput, upper eyelids, upper lip, and bridge of the nose. Blanching the skin will cause them to momentarily fade. They permanently disappear by about 2 years of age but may reappear during episodes of crying.

Cutis marmorata, or transient mottling, is a purple, reticulated pattern seen on the skin when the infant is exposed to a cool environment. It disappears when the infant is covered with adequate clothing or placed in a warm atmosphere. *Pallor* in a newborn should always be noted since it is usually a sign of circulatory failure, anoxia, edema, or shock. It may also be caused by a severe neonatal anemia.

Birth trauma may result in changes on the skin. *Ecchymoses* appear as bruises anywhere on the body and may be the result of a forceps delivery or of brisk manipulation of the infant during and after birth. *Petechiae* are pinpoint hemorrhagic areas that may have been a result of increased vascular pressure that ruptured capillaries during delivery. They are particularly noted on the upper trunk and face. Ecchymoses and petechiae may also be signs of serious infection or a bleeding disorder, such as thrombocytopenia. Normally petechiae from trauma will disappear in 24 to 48 hours after delivery, and no new lesions will appear.

Hemorrhagic areas can be distinguished from rashes or skin discolorations by blanching the skin with two fingers or with a glass slide pressed against the skin. Petechiae and ecchymoses do not disappear because the extravasated blood is fixed in the tissue. Erythema from local vascular engorgement will fade because pressure causes blood to be emptied from the engorged vessels.

Subcutaneous fat necrosis is indicated by clearly outlined, firm masses of varying size that are located in the subcutaneous tissue and are fixed to overlying skin but are movable over the underlying tissue. They may appear reddish purple in color and are a result of manipulation during delivery, such as application of forceps. These lesions most often occur on the face and usually resolve in a few days.

Erythema toxicum is a pink papular rash with vesicles frequently superimposed. Since the vesicles often appear purulent, this condition is often confused with a staphylococcal infection. The rash most frequently covers the thorax, back, diaper area, and abdomen. It usually appears by 24 to 48 hours and disappears spontaneously after several days. *Sclerema* is a generalized hardening of the skin and subcutaneous tissue, probably resulting from severe cold stress. Therefore, it is most often seen in severely ill newborns.

Head. General observation of the contour of the head is important since molding occurs in almost all vaginal deliveries. In a vertex delivery the head will usually be flattened at the forehead, with the apex rising and forming a point at the end of the parietal bones and the posterior skull or occiput dropping abruptly. The usual more oval contour of the head is apparent by 1 to 2 days after birth. The change in shape occurs because the bones of the cranium are not fused, allowing for overlapping of the edges of these bones to accommodate to the size of the birth canal during delivery.

Six bones—the frontal, occipital, two parietals, and two temporals—comprise the cranium. Between the junction of these bones are bands of connective tissue called *sutures.* At the junction of the sutures are wider spaces of unossified membranous tissue called *fontanels.* The two most prominent fontanels in infants are the *anterior fontanel,* formed by the junction of the sagittal, coronal, and frontal sutures, and the *posterior fontanel,* formed by the junction of the sagittal and lambdoid sutures. One can easily remember the location of the sutures because the coronal suture "crowns" the head and the sagittal suture "separates" the head. Two other fontanels—the *sphenoidal* and *mastoid* fontanels—are normally present but are not usually palpable (Fig. 8-6). An additional fontanel located between the anterior and posterior fontanels along the sagittal suture is found in some normal neonates but is also found in some infants with Down's syndrome. The presence of this sagittal or parietal fontanel is always recorded.

The nurse palpates the skull for all patent sutures and fontanels, noting size, shape, molding, or abnormal closure. The sutures are felt as cracks between the skull bones, and the fontanels are felt as wider "soft spots" at the junction of the sutures. These are palpated by using the tip of the index finger and running it along the ends of the bones (Fig. 8-7).

The anterior fontanel is diamond-shaped, measuring 2.5 cm (1 inch) along the coronal suture and 4.0 to 5.0 cm (about 2 inches) along the sagittal suture. The nurse easily

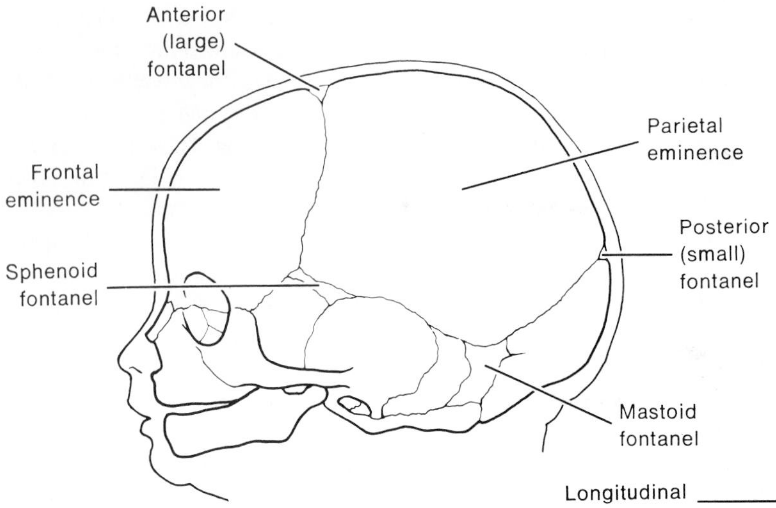

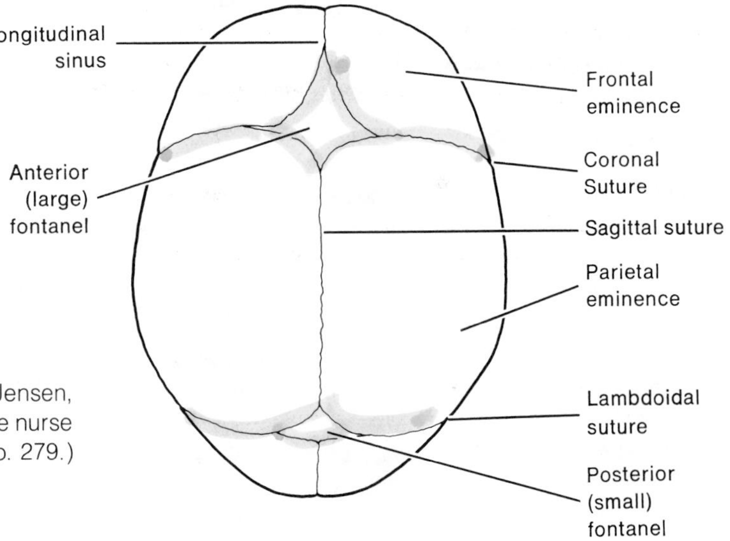

Fig. 8-6. Location of sutures and fontanels. (From Jensen, M.D., Benson, R. C., and Bobak, I. M.: Maternity care: the nurse and the family, St. Louis, 1977, The C. V. Mosby Co., p. 279.)

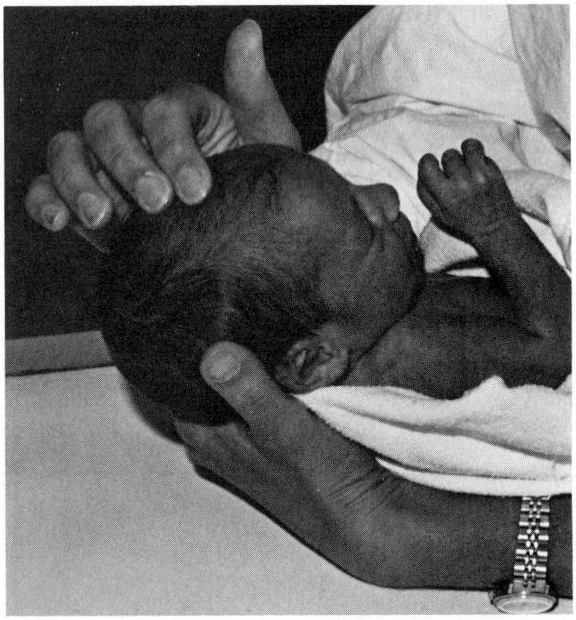

Fig. 8-7. Palpating for fontanels.

locates the posterior fontanel by following the sagittal suture toward the occiput. The posterior fontanel is triangular-shaped, usually measuring between 0.5 and 1 cm (less than 0.5 inch) at its widest part. The fontanels should feel flat, firm, and well-demarcated against the bony edges of the skull. Frequently pulsations are visible at the anterior fontanel. Coughing, crying, or lying down may temporarily cause the fontanels to bulge and become more taut. However, a widened, tense, bulging fontanel is a sign of increased intracranial pressure. A markedly sunken, depressed fontanel is an indication of dehydration. Such findings should always be recorded and reported to the physician.

The nurse also palpates the skull for any unusual masses or prominences, particularly those resulting from birth trauma, such as caput succedaneum or cephalhematoma. *Caput succedaneum* is an edematous swelling of the scalp caused by prolonged pressure of the occiput against the cervix during labor. It is usually a soft, poorly outlined mass that easily indents with pressure and is not fluctuant. It is usually present at or shortly after birth. *Cephalhematoma* is an edematous mass of the skull resulting from the extravasation of blood between the periosteum and underlying bone. It is usually soft and fluctuant and clearly outlines the side of the bone margin. It is usually not visible until 1 or 2 days after birth. It is most frequently located over the parietal bones, but it does not cross the suture line. It may take several weeks or months for the cephalhematoma to completely recede, whereas the caput succedaneum usually disappears in a few days.

Because of the pliability of the skull, exerting pressure at the margin of the parietal and occipital bones along the lambdoid suture may produce a snapping sensation similar to the identation of a Ping-Pong ball. This phenomenon is known as *physiologic craniotabes* and, although usually a normal finding, can be indicative of hydrocephalus or syphilis.

Eyes. Usually the newborn will keep his eyes tightly closed. It is best to begin the examination of the eyes by observing the lids for edema, which is normally present for the first 2 days after delivery. A mongoloid slant, the lateral upward slope of the eyes with an inner epicanthal fold, may be indicative of Down's syndrome. The eyes should be observed for symmetry and for hypertelorism. The mean distance between the inner canthi is 2 cm; 3 cm or more is considered ocular hypertelorism.[12,13] Tears usually do not appear until the first or second month of life. *Purulent* discharge from the eyes shortly after birth may signify *ophthalmia neonatorum* caused by gonorrhea. *Chemical irritation* or *conjunctivitis* may appear within 1 hour after instillation of silver nitrate. The nurse carefully notes and records any discharge.

In order to visualize the surface structures of the eye, the nurse holds the infant supine and gently lowers the head. The eyes will usually open, similar to the mechanism of dolls' eyes. The sclera should be examined for *subconjunctival hemorrhages,* which usually result from impairment of venous return and rupture of capillaries in the sclera, because of pressure on the fetal head during delivery. They are of no pathologic significance, even when the entire sclera is ecchymotic. The most common location of subconjunctival hemorrhages is the limbus of the iris. *Retinal hemorrhages* may also occur because of pressure on the fetal head during delivery. They are usually flame-shaped, irregular, or round and are generally of no significance, unless they are extensive, which may be indicative of subdural hematoma or brain trauma.

The cornea is examined for the presence of any opacities or haziness. The *corneal reflex* is normally present at birth but is generally not elicited, unless brain or eye damage is suspected. The pupil will usually respond to light by constricting. Absence of the *pupillary reflex,* particularly by 3 weeks of age, suggests blindness. A fixed, dilated, or constricted pupil may indicate anoxia or brain damage.

A searching *nystagmus* or *strabismus* is common after birth. Persistence of this type of ocular movement may, however, suggest blindness. Intermittent strabismus is common in infants until about 4 to 6 months of age. The color of the iris is noted. Most light-skinned newborns have slate gray or dark blue eyes, whereas dark-skinned infants have brown eyes. Absence of color is characteristic of albinism.

Although it is quite difficult to perform a funduscopic examination of the retina, a red reflex should be elicited. Absence of the red reflex may indicate the presence of retinal hemorrhages or *congenital cataracts*.

Ears. The ears are examined for position, structure, and auditory function. The top of the pinna of the ear should lie in a horizontal plane to the outer canthus of the eye. *Low-set ears* are often associated with mental retardation or renal anomalies. The *canals* are usually filled with vernix caseosa and amniotic fluid, making visualization of the drum difficult. Usually the drums can be examined by a few days after birth. It is best not to attempt to remove the debris unless deafness is indicated. *Auditory ability* can be assessed by making a sharp, loud noise close to the infant's head. Normally the infant will respond with a *startle reflex* or twitching of the eyelids. Absence of any behavioral response to a sudden noise may indicate congenital deafness or blocked auditory canals.

Nose. The nose is usually flattened after birth, and bruises are not uncommon. Patency of the nasal canals can be assessed by holding the hand over the infant's mouth and one canal and noting the passage of air through the unobstructed opening. If nasal patency is questionable, a soft rubber catheter may be used, as during suctioning. Congenital anomalies such as choanal atresia, deviated septum, or encephalocele may block a canal.

Thin white mucus is very common in the newborn, but a

thick bloody nasal discharge without sneezing may suggest the snuffles of congenital syphilis. *Sneezing* is very common in the newborn. *Flaring of the nares* is always noted because it is a serious sign of air hunger from respiratory distress.

Mouth and throat. The nurse inspects the mouth to identify existing structures and, in particular, to note the presence of congenital anomalies such as cleft palate. Cleft lip is readily identified as soon as the infant is born, but cleft palate must be carefully assessed because it may involve the soft and/or hard palate or only the uvula.

The palate is normally high-arched and somewhat narrow. Rarely *teeth* may be present. *Inclusion* or *retention cysts*—gray, round lesions on the gum margins—may appear to be teeth but usually disappear in a few weeks. Flat white spots that do not rub off usually indicate *Monilia* or thrush, which was contracted from the infected vaginal canal during delivery. *Epstein's pearls* are small, white, epithelial cysts along both sides of the midline of the hard palate. They are insignificant, should not be confused with thrush, and disappear in several weeks.

The tongue is attached to the lingual surface by the *frenulum*. The frenulum is a sharp, thin ridge of tissue that arises from the base of the tongue in the midline and attaches to the lingual surface in the midline. When the frenulum is attached close to the tip of the tongue, protusion of the tongue is somewhat limited but rarely interferes with sucking, feeding, or speech. A large, protruding tongue may suggest Down's syndrome.

The *frenum* of the upper lip is a band of thick, pink tissue that lies under the inner surface of the upper lip and extends to the maxillary alveolar ridge. It usually disappears as the maxilla grows. It is particularly evident when the infant yawns or smiles.

The *sucking reflex* should be elicited by placing a nipple or tongue blade in the infant's mouth. The *rooting reflex* is obtained by stroking the cheek and noting the infant's response of turning toward the stimulated side and sucking. Although the *gag reflex* is not elicited, it may be seen during pharyngeal suctioning or during passage of a nasogastric catheter. Usually saliva is scant until the second or third month of life. Profuse salivation may indicate tracheoesophageal fistula, cystic fibrosis, or tracheal aspiration or irritation.

It is difficult to examine the back of the throat. If the nurse attempts to depress the tongue, the infant will object with strong reflex protrusion of the tongue. Therefore, it is best to visualize the *uvula* while the infant is crying and the chin is depressed. However, the uvula may be retracted upward and backward during crying. Tonsillar tissue is generally not seen in the newborn.

Neck. The newborn's neck is usually covered with folds of tissue. Adequate assessment of the neck requires allowing the head to fall gently backward in hyperextension while the back is supported in a slightly raised position. The nurse observes for range of motion, shape, and any abnormal masses.

A fractured clavicle may be evident as a mass in the neck. Crepitation may be heard over the fractured bone if the area is palpated. A mass in the lower part of the sternocleidomastoid muscle with limitation of neck movement may be *torticollis*. Small cystic masses in the upper part of the muscle may be *brachial cleft cysts*. Excessive skin folds may be indicative of gonadal dysgenesis or other chromosomal aberrations, such as Turner's syndrome.

Range of motion of the neck is important in eliciting certain reflexes. When the infant is supine, the *tonic neck reflex* should be evident. As the head is turned to one side, the arm and leg will extend on the side to which the head is turned, and the opposite arm and leg will flex. The infant's posture will resemble a fencing position (Fig. 8-8). Absence of this reflex may indicate central nervous system damage.

The *neck-righting reflex* is elicited by turning the infant's head to one side. When the infant is supine, the trunk should turn to the same side as the head. Similarly if the

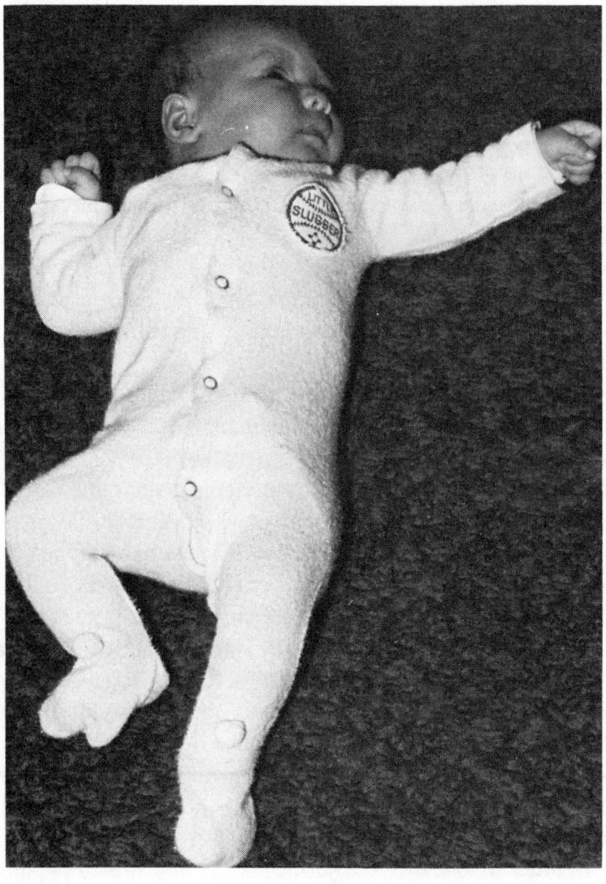

Fig. 8-8. Tonic neck reflex.

body of an erect infant is tilted, the head should return to the upright position, demonstrating the *otolith-righting reflex*.

Chest. The newborn's chest is almost circular because the *anteroposterior* and *lateral diameters* are equal. The ribs are very flexible, and slight intercostal retractions are normally seen on inspiration. Marked retractions suggest upper airway obstruction, such as laryngeal stenosis, and warrant immediate medical attention. The *xiphoid process* is commonly visible as a small protrusion at the end of the sternum. The *sternum* is generally raised and slightly curved. Forward projection of the chest may be *pigeon chest* or *pectus carinatum*. Depression of the chest may indicate an anatomic defect called *funnel chest* or *pectus excavatum*. However, it may also suggest severe problems such as respiratory distress syndrome and atelectasis. *Asymmetry* of the chest wall may indicate several pathologic conditions, such as diaphragmatic hernia, pneumothorax, pulmonary agenesis, or pneumonia. All such deviations are recorded and reported to the physician for further evaluation.

Breast enlargement appears in many newborns of either sex by the second or third day and is caused by maternal hormones. Occasionally a milky substance sometimes called "witches' milk" is secreted by the infant's breasts by the end of the first week. Redness and firmness around the nipples, although uncommon, may be signs of mastitis. *Supernumerary nipples* without glandular tissue are sometimes present and are frequently located inferior and slightly medial to the normal nipple.

Lungs. Respirations in the newborn are chiefly abdominal. Decreased abdominal respiration is frequently associated with abdominal distention. Thoracic breathing usually decreases the expansion of the chest cavity because of the horizontal position of the ribs. Intrathoracic disease may be indicated if signs such as unequal movements of the chest wall, deep retraction of the sternum, flaring nares, generalized cyanosis, or rapid, gasping, or grunting respirations are present.

The average respiratory rate varies widely, from 30 to 60 breaths/minute. In the normal infant, respirations may be irregular in depth and rate, with occasional momentary apneic spells. Irregular respirations with repeated *apneic spells* often indicate a depressed central nervous system. A *respiratory grunt* is an important sign of respiratory difficulty. It is a compensatory mechanism by which the infant attempts to retain air in the lungs to increase arterial oxygen levels. An *expiratory grunt* is an audible sign during expiration. Air hunger is usually indicated by flaring of the nares during inspirations.

It is important that the nurse learn to carefully assess the respiratory status of the newborn through observation, since auscultation is difficult because of the small size of the chest and the effective transmission of cardiac and bowel sounds to all parts of the pleural cavity. Auscultation should reveal bronchial breath sounds bilaterally, especially in the midaxillary line. *Rales* soon after birth may indicate areas of atelectasis, which represent the normal transition of the lungs to extrauterine life. However, continuous fine rales heard best at the end of a deep inspiration may indicate hyaline membrane disease, pneumonia, or pulmonary edema. *Rhonchi* are more frequently caused by fluid in the larger bronchi and are especially important in determining if aspiration of feeding or oral secretions has occurred. Peristaltic sounds may be heard in the pleural area because of the normal transmission of sounds from the abdomen. However, the presence of such sounds may indicate diaphragmatic hernia, particularly if breath sounds are absent in the same area.

Heart. Heart rate should always be auscultated and may range from 100 to 180 beats/minute shortly after birth and, when the infant has stabilized, from 120 to 140 beats/minute. The size and location of the heart should be located. The *apex* of the heart is usually palpated or auscultated at the third or fourth intercostal space, lateral to the midclavicular line, because of its more horizontal position in the newborn. Displacement of the apex is noted because it may indicate conditions such as diaphragmatic hernia or pneumothorax. If the heart is located on the right side of the body, a condition known as *dextrocardia* may exist. This should be particularly noted since the abdominal organs may also be reversed, which may or may not be associated with functional circulatory abnormalities.

Auscultation of the specific components of the heart sounds is difficult because of the rapid rate and effective transmission of respiratory sounds. However, the *first* and *second sounds* should be clear and well defined; the second sound is somewhat higher in pitch and sharper than the first. Murmurs are very frequently heard in the newborn, especially over the base of the heart or at the left sternal border in the third or fourth interspace. Ordinarily they are not associated with specific cardiac defects, since they more frequently represent the incomplete anatomic closure of fetal shunts. However, they are always recorded and reported.

Abdomen. The normal contour of the abdomen is cylindric and usually prominent with visible veins. A *distended abdomen* is characterized by a taut skin through which engorged blood vessels are easily seen. Distention should always be carefully noted and measured at the level of the umbilicus in order to obtain objective baseline data.

Bowel sounds are usually heard a few hours after birth. Absence of peristaltic sounds plus a tender distended abdomen suggest the serious condition of peritonitis. Usually, visible peristaltic waves are observable in thin newborns, but they should not be seen in well-nourished infants. Such a finding may indicate intestinal obstruction.

Localized bulging in the flank area suggests enlarged kidneys, possibly hydronephrosis. A *scaphoid* or *concave abdomen* may be noted in infants who have diaphragmatic hernia or intestinal atresia. Failure of the rectus muscles to join during uterine development results in *diastasis recti.* This is most evident when the infant cries or strains, which causes part of the abdominal organs to be pushed through the opening.

Congenital absence of the abdominal musculature, sometimes called "prune-belly syndrome," is a serious anomaly. It is usually readily identified by the characteristic appearance of the skin, which is loose and wrinkled. Also, the medial aspect of the abdomen is normally sunken, whereas the intestines, which are covered by a thin layer of subcutaneous tissue, bulge pendulously from the flanks.

The *umbilical cord* should always be carefully inspected for any signs of infection, such as purulent drainage or foul odor. At birth the cord should appear bluish white and moist. After clamping it begins to dry and appears a dull, yellowish brown. It progressively shrivels in size and turns greenish black. An *umbilical hernia* is a skin-covered protrusion at the umbilicus that is frequently found in black children.

Palpation is done after inspection of the abdomen. The *liver* is usually palpable 2 to 3 cm (about 1 inch) below the right costal margin. The tip of the *spleen* can sometimes be felt in the newborn and is usually palpable by 1 week of age. Both *kidneys* should be palpated, especially soon after delivery, when the intestines are still not filled with air. The lower half of the right kidney and the tip of the left kidney are usually felt 1 to 2 cm above the umbilicus. However, the abdomen must be relaxed for the palpation to be effective. Supporting the infant in a semi-Fowler's position with one hand and palpating the abdomen with the other hand usually causes the abdominal muscles to relax. Flexing the infant's knees toward the abdomen while the infant is supine will also increase relaxation. Often, it is necessary to use both hands to locate the kidneys. As one hand palpates the abdominal area, the other hand provides countertraction by pushing upward from the posterior flank area. The kidney is felt as an oval structure between the fingers of each hand.

The suprapubic area should also be palpated and percussed for evidence of a *distended bladder.* The neonate should void during the first 24 hours after birth. A distended bladder following a scanty voiding may indicate a urethral obstruction.

During examination of the lower abdomen, it is particularly important to palpate for *femoral pulses.* They should be strong and equal bilaterally. Absence of the femoral pulses may be a key indicator of coarctation of the aorta, a congenital heart defect.

Female genitalia. Normally the *labia minora* and *clitoris* are edematous, especially following a breech delivery. However, the labia and clitoris must be carefully inspected to identify any evidence of ambiguous genitalia. For example, a partially fused labia may suggest the presence of scrotum and should be carefully palpated to identify the existence of testes. Normally in a female the *urethral opening* should be located behind the clitoris. Any deviation from this may suggest that the clitoris may mistakenly be identified as a small penis, which can occur in conditions such as adrenal hyperplasia.

A *hymenal tag* is usually visible from the posterior opening of the vagina. It is comprised of tissue from the hymen and the labia minora. It usually disappears in several weeks. Generally the vaginal vault is not inspected. However, absence of the hymenal tag may indicate vaginal agenesis, and in this case further examination would be warranted.

Vaginal discharge may be noted during the first week of life. This *pseudomenstruation* is a manifestation of the abrupt decrease of maternal hormones and usually disappears by 2 to 4 weeks. *Fecal discharge* from the vaginal opening indicates a rectovaginal fistula and is always reported. Vernix caseosa may be present in large amounts between the labia.

Male genitalia. The penis should be inspected for the location of the *urethral opening,* which normally is located at the tip. However, the opening may be totally covered by the *prepuce,* or foreskin, which covers the glans penis. A tight prepuce is a very common finding in the newborn and usually does not indicate phimosis. It should not be forcefully retracted, except to locate the urinary opening. *Smegma,* a white cheesy substance, is commonly found around the glans penis, under the foreskin. If the urethral meatus originates anywhere along the ventral side of the penis, *hypospadias* exists. If the reverse occurs, that is, the opening is on the dorsal surface of the penis, then *epispadias* exists. *Erection* or *priapism* is not uncommon in the newborn. Small, white, firm lesions called *epithelial pearls* may be seen at the tip of the prepuce.

The *scrotum* may be large, edematous, and pendulous in the full-term neonate, especially in the infant born in breech position. It is usually deeply pigmented in dark-skinned races. A noncommunicating *hydrocele* frequently occurs unilaterally and disappears within a few months. The *testes* should always be palpated for in the scrotum. In small newborns, particularly premature infants, the testes may be palpable within the inguinal canal. Absence of the testes may also be a sign of ambiguous genitalia, especially in addition to presence of a small scrotum and penis. *Inguinal hernia* may or may not be manifested immediately after birth. Identification of a hernia is facilitated by examination when the infant is crying.

Back and rectum. With the infant prone, the *spine* should be inspected for any abnormal openings or masses. A large, protruding sac anywhere along the spine, but most commonly in the sacral area, indicates some type of *spina bifida.* A small sinus, which may or may not be communicating with the spine, is a *pilonidal sinus.* It is frequently covered with a tuft of hair. Although it may have no pathologic significance, it may indicate the existence of spina bifida occluta or be a portal of entry into the spinal column.

The shape of the spine, which should be gently rounded, with none of the characteristic S-shaped curves seen later in life, is noted. Stroking the back along one side of the vertebral column will cause the infant to move the hips toward the stimulated side (trunk incurvation reflex).

Passage of meconium during the first 24 to 48 hours of life indicates *anal patency*. If an imperforate anus is suspected, a rectal thermometer or a rubber catheter should be inserted into the anal opening. If a thermometer is used, care must be exercised in order to avoid mucosal perforation. With the infant still prone, the buttocks should gently be separated to inspect the anal area for presence of *fissures*, small cracks in the mucosa. Anal fissures are a frequent cause of constipation because the infant refuses to strain during defecation in order to avoid pain. Asymmetry of the mucosal folds around the sphincter is also suggestive of fissures.

Extremities. The extremities should be examined for symmetry, range of motion, and signs of malformation or trauma. The fingers and toes are counted, and supernumerary digits *(polydactyly)* or fusion of digits *(syndactyly)* is noted. A partial syndactyly between the second and third toes is a common variation seen in otherwise normal infants.

Range of motion of the extremities should be observed throughout the entire examination. *Hyperflexibility* of joints is characteristic of Down's syndrome. Eliciting the *scarf sign* may be helpful in identifying abnormal flexion of joints. With the infant supine, the nurse crosses the infant's hand and arm over the chest toward the opposite shoulder. In a full-term newborn the elbow should not be able to reach the midline. If the elbow reaches the midline, hyperflexibility is present. This maneuver is also helpful in establishing gestational age, since premature infants also demonstrate hyperflexible joints (p. 327).

The fingernails should also be examined. The *nail beds* should be pink, although slight blueness is evident in acrocyanosis. Persistent cyanosis of the nail beds indicates anoxia or vasoconstriction. Yellowing of the nail beds may indicate intrauterine distress, postmaturity, or hemolytic disease. Short or absent nails are seen in premature infants, whereas long nails, extending over the ends of the fingers, are characteristic of postmature newborns.

The *palms* of the hands should have the usual creases (Fig. 5-12). A transverse palmar crease, called a *simian crease,* may suggest Down's syndrome. The full-term newborn usually has creases on the anterior two thirds of the *sole* of the foot. In postmature infants the sole is covered with deep creases, and in premature infants the creases are absent. The soles of the feet are normally flat; arches develop later in life.

The nurse inspects the extremities for evidence of fractures from birth trauma. The clavicle, humerus, and femur are most frequently involved. Limitation of movement, visible deformity, asymmetry of reflexes, and malposition of the site are signs suggestive of a fracture.

The *hips* are rotated to identify a congenital dislocation. With the infant supine, the legs should be flexed at the hips and knees and abducted to almost 175 degrees. Limitation in abduction is indicative of dislocation. Other signs of this condition are unequal gluteal or leg folds, an audible click during abduction *(Ortolani's sign),* and unequal leg length *(Allis's sign)*. Shortening of the affected leg occurs as the femur rides upward above the acetabulum. It is particularly evident when the length of each leg is compared at the knees. To demonstrate this, the nurse positions the infant supine, flexes the hips and knees, and places the feet flat on the table. When the height of each knee is compared, the knee on the affected side is higher than the knee on the unaffected side (see Fig. 11-9).

Symmetry should be noted when the infant moves, particularly when a Moro reflex is elicited. Asymmetry may suggest a fracture, paralysis, or spinal cord injury or anomaly. *Muscle tone* should also be assessed. By attempting to extend a flexed extremity, the nurse determines if tone is equal bilaterally.

Neurologic assessment

A critical part of the physical assessment of the newborn is a complete neurologic examination. Observations of the infant's posture, muscle tone, and movement are one aspect of this examination; demonstration of several important reflexes is left to the end of the examination because eliciting some reflexes may disturb the infant and interfere with auscultation or palpation of other parts of the body.

As has been noted several times, *muscle tone* is extremely important. Besides the usual fetal position, the infant will normally maintain some degree of flexion of the extremities. Extension of any extremity is usually met with resistance, and, when released, the extremity will return to its previous flexed position. *Hypotonia* suggests some degree of hypoxia. Asymmetric muscle tone may indicate a degree of paralysis from brain damage. Failure to move the lower limbs suggests a spinal cord lesion or injury. *Tremors, twitches,* and *myoclonic jerks* characterize neonatal seizures or may be indicative of neonatal narcotic withdrawal syndrome. Quivering or momentary tremors are usually normal.

Assessing the degree of *head control* in the neonate is a valuable indicator of neurologic status. Although *head lag* is normal in the newborn, the degree of the ability to control the head in certain positions should be recognized. If the supine infant is pulled from the arms into a semi-Fowler's position, marked head lag and hyperextension are noted (Fig. 8-9, *A*). However, as one continues to bring the infant forward into a sitting position, the infant will attempt to

A

B

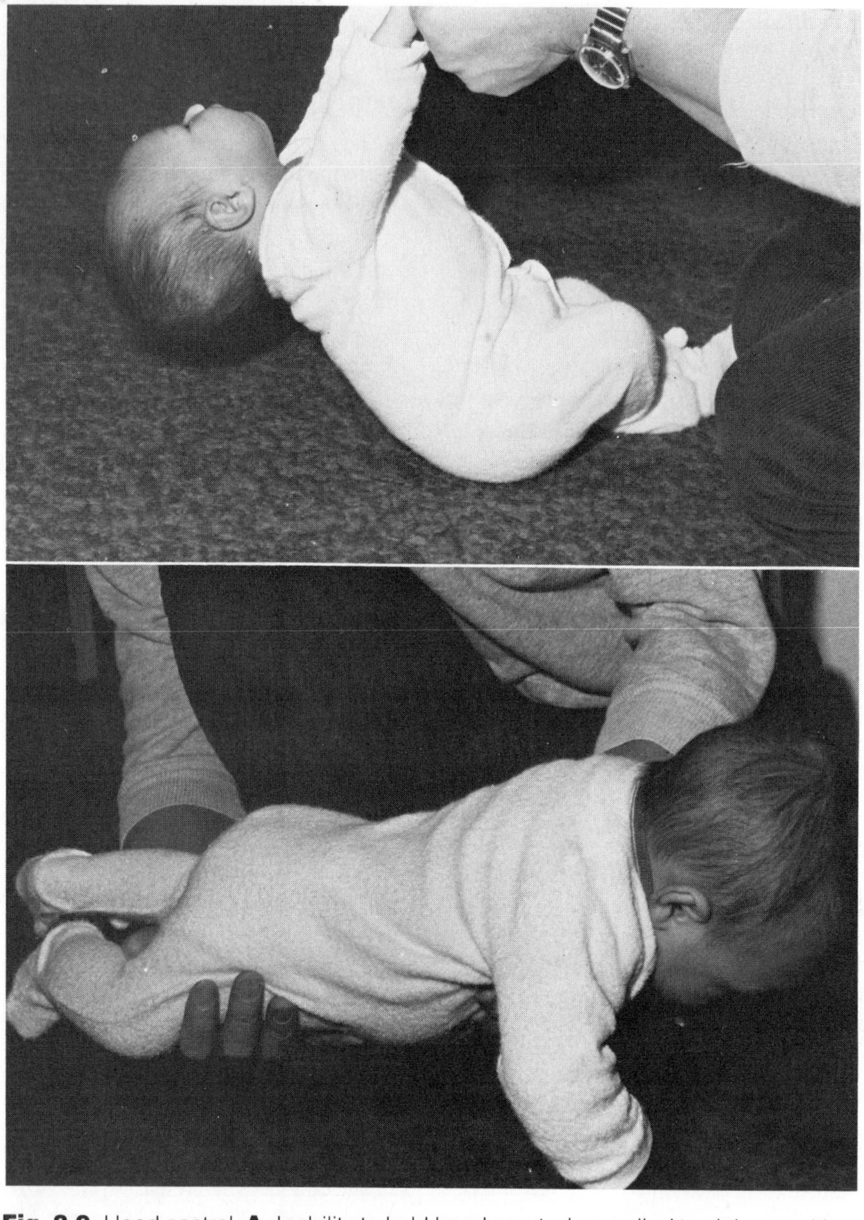

Fig. 8-9. Head control. **A,** Inability to hold head erect when pulled to sitting position. **B,** Ability to hold head erect when placed in ventral suspension.

control the head in an upright position. As the head falls forward onto the chest, many infants will attempt to right it into the erect position. Also, if the infant is held in ventral suspension, that is, held prone above and parallel to the examining surface, the infant will hold his head in a straight line with the spinal column (Fig. 8-9, *B*). When lying on the abdomen, the newborn has the ability to lift the head slightly, turning it from side to side. Marked head lag is seen in Down's syndrome, hypoxic infants, and newborns with brain damage.

Several reflexes, such as the sucking, gag, rooting, corneal, and pupillary reflexes, are usually observed during some other part of the physical examination (see Table 8-5 and Chapter 5). Several positional reflexes, such as the tonic neck and Moro reflexes, are also commonly seen. The *Moro reflex*, which is demonstrable in all normal neonates, results in valuable information regarding decreased muscle tone, bone fractures, and nerve damage. The Moro reflex should be elicited by holding the infant above the examining table in a supine position with one hand beneath the sacrum and the other supporting the upper back and head. The infant's head is then suddenly allowed to fall about 30 degrees. The normal response is extension and abduction of the extremities, wrists, and fingers, followed by an immediate flexion of the extremities on the body (Fig. 8-10). A loud, angry cry usually accompanies the infant's somatic

Table 8-5. Assessment of reflexes in the normal neonate

Reflexes	Expected behavioral responses	Deviation
Localized		
Eyes		
Blinking or corneal reflex	Infant will blink at sudden appearance of a bright light or at approach of an object toward the cornea; should persist throughout life	Absent or asymmetric blink suggests damage to cranial nerves III, IV, and V
Pupillary	Pupil constricts when a bright light shines toward it; should persist throughout life	Unequal constriction Fixed dilated pupil
Doll's eye	As the head is moved slowly to the right or left, eyes normally do not move; should disappear as fixation develops	Asymmetric in abducens paralysis
Nose		
Sneeze	Spontaneous response of nasal passages to irritation or obstruction; should persist throughout life	Absent or continuous sneezing
Mouth and throat		
Sucking	Infant should begin strong sucking movements of circumoral area in response to stimulation; should persist throughout infancy, even without stimulation, such as during sleep	Weak or absent suck
Gag	Stimulation of posterior pharynx by food, suction, or passage of a tube should cause infant to gag; should persist throughout life	Absence of gag suggests damage to glossopharyngeal nerve
Rooting	Touching or stroking the cheek along the side of the mouth will cause infant to turn the head toward that side and begin to suck; should disappear at about age 3-4 months, but may persist for up to 12 months	Absence, especially when infant is not satiated
Extrusion	When tongue is touched or depressed, infant responds by forcing it outward; should disappear by age 4 months	Constant protrusion of tongue may suggest Down's syndrome
Yawn	Spontaneous response to decreased oxygen by increasing amount of inspired air; should persist throughout life	Absence
Cough	Irritation of mucous membranes of larynx or tracheobronchial tree causes coughing; should persist throughout life; usually present after first day of birth	Absence
Extremities		
Grasp	Touching palms of hands or soles of feet near base of digits causes flexion of hands and toes (Fig. 8-11); palmar grasp should lessen after age 3 months, to be replaced by voluntary movement; plantar grasp lessens by 8 months of age	Asymmetric flexion may indicate paralysis
Babinski's	Stroking outer sole of foot upward from heel and across ball of foot causes toes to hyperextend and hallux to dorsiflex; should disappear after age 1 year	Persistence indicates a pyramidal tract lesion
Mass		
Moro	Sudden jarring or change in equilibrium causes sudden extension and abduction of extremities and fanning of fingers, with index finger and thumb forming a "C" shape, followed by flexion and adduction of extremities; legs may weakly flex; infant may cry (Fig. 8-10); should disappear after age 3-4 months, usually strongest during first 2 months	Persistence of Moro reflex past age 6 months may indicate brain damage Asymmetric Moro reflex may suggest injury to brachial plexus, clavicle, or humerus
Startle	A sudden loud noise causes abduction of the arms with flexion of the elbows; the hands remain clenched; should disappear by age 4 months	Absence indicates hearing loss
Perez	While infant is prone on a firm surface, thumb is pressed along spine from sacrum to neck; infant will respond by crying, flexing the extremities, and elevating the pelvis and head; lordosis of the spine, as well as defecation and urination, may occur; should disappear by age 4-6 months	Significance is similar to that of Moro reflex

Continued.

Table 8-5. Assessment of reflexes in the normal neonate—cont'd

Reflexes	Expected behavioral responses	Deviation
Mass—cont'd		
Asymmetric tonic neck	When infant's head is quickly turned to one side, arm and leg will extend on that side, and opposite arm and leg will flex (Fig. 8-8); should disappear by age 3-4 months, to be replaced by symmetric positioning of both sides of body	Absence or persistence may indicate central nervous system damage
Neck-righting	While infant is supine, head is turned to one side; shoulder and trunk will turn toward that side, followed by pelvis; disappears at age 10 months	Absence; significance is similar to that of asymmetric tonic neck reflex
Otolith-righting	When body of an erect infant is tilted, head is returned to upright, erect position	Absence; significance is similar to that of asymmetric tonic neck reflex
Trunk incurvation (Galant) reflex	Stroking infant's back alongside spine will cause hips to move toward stimulated side; should disappear by age 4 weeks	Absence may indicate spinal cord lesion
Dance or step	If infant is held so that sole of foot touches a hard surface, there will be a reciprocal flexion and extension of the leg, simulating walking (Fig. 8-12); should disappear after age 3-4 weeks, to be replaced by deliberate movement	Asymmetry of stepping
Crawling	When infant is placed on abdomen, he will make crawling movements with the arms and legs; should disappear at about age 6 weeks	Asymmetry of movement

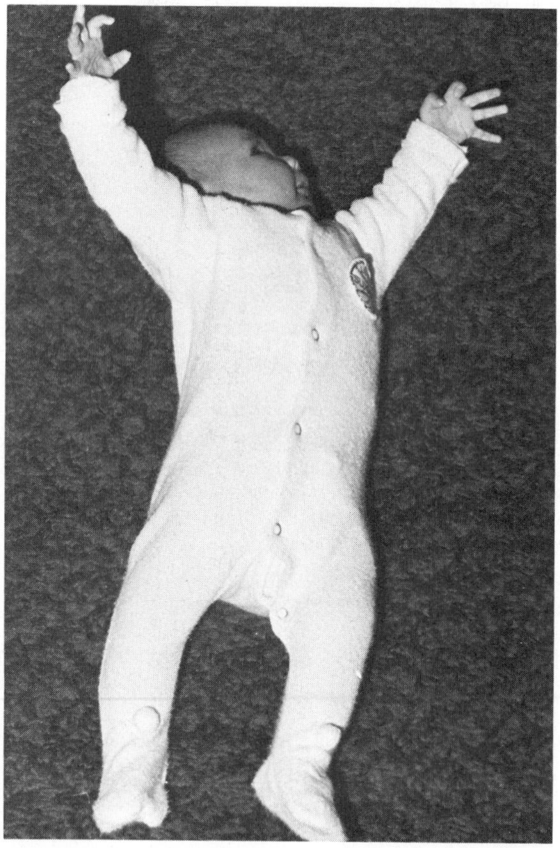

Fig. 8-10. Eliciting Moro reflex. Note the abduction of the arms, the C shape formed by the fingers, and the extension of the legs.

response. (For a more complete description of neonatal reflexes, see Table 8-5.)

Behavioral assessment

Only about a decade ago, newborns were described as primitive beings who reacted to the environment through reflexes and had little ability to influence the environment around them. Now studies are increasingly demonstrating newborns' ability to react to various stimuli willfully and to greatly affect how others relate to them. At one time parents were given standard guidelines of what to expect from their infant in regard to feeding, sleep, and wakeful activity. Now it is no longer valid to anticipate that each infant's routine will be similar, any more than it is valid to say that each adult's daily habits are alike.

Patterns of sleep and activity. Newborns begin life with a systematic schedule of sleep and activity that is initially evident during the periods of reactivity. For the first hour after birth the newborn is intensely alert, the eyes are wide open, and sucking behavior is vigorous. The infant then becomes quiet and relatively unresponsive to either internal or external stimuli. He relaxes and falls asleep for a period of a few minutes to 2 to 4 hours. On awakening, the infant may

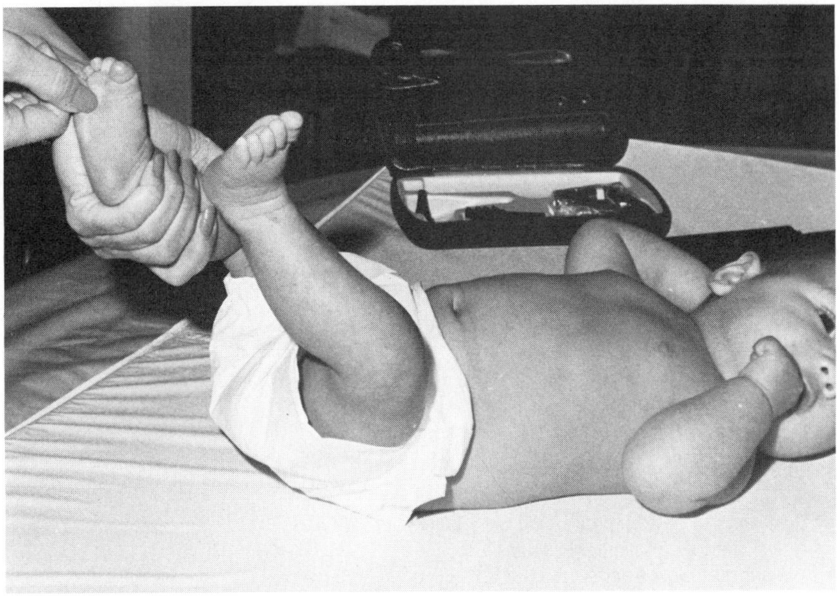

Fig. 8-11. Grasp reflex.

be hyperresponsive to stimuli. This begins the second period of reactivity, which may last from 2 to 5 hours. When the second period of reactivity is over, the infant's vital signs and patterns of sleep and activity stabilize. It is not unusual for the infant to sleep almost constantly for the next 2 to 3 days in order to recover from the exhausting birth process.

Five distinct states comprise the infant's sleep. During *regular sleep* the infant's eyes are closed, breathing is regular, and movement is absent, except for sudden generalized startles. Strong external or internal stimulation is absent or minimal, and mild stimuli, such as usual household noise, will not arouse the infant. During *irregular sleep* the eyes are still closed, but the breathing is irregular. Although the body is still quiet, the muscles twitch occasionally. The external stimuli that were subliminal during regular sleep now cause the infant to smile, cry out, or groan.

The third state of sleep is *drowsiness,* which occurs before or after regular and irregular sleep. The eyes may be open, breathing is irregular, and the body is actively moving. The infant is sensitive to such external stimuli as footsteps, voices, or the appearance of the mother. The occurrence of spontaneous discharges such as reflex smiles or startles, sucking movement, or erections are frequent. This period is followed by *alert inactivity,* provided that the infant's needs such as feeding and diapering have been satisfied. The infant will respond to environmental stimuli by moving the head, limbs, and trunk and by staring at close-

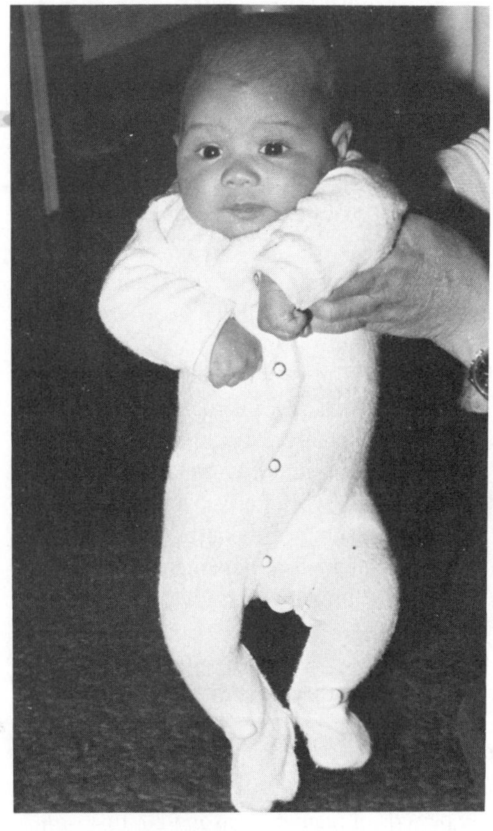

Fig. 8-12. Dance reflex.

Table 8-6. States of sleep

State	Behavior	Duration	Implications for parenting
Regular sleep	Closed eyes Regular breathing No movement except for sudden bodily jerks	4-5 hours/day, 10-20 minutes/sleep cycle	External stimuli will not arouse infant. Usual house noises should continue. If a sudden loud noise awakens infant and he cries, leave him alone; he will usually fall back to sleep.
Irregular sleep	Closed eyes Irregular breathing Slight muscular twitching of body	12-15 hours/day, 20-45 minutes/sleep cycle	External stimuli that did not arouse infant during regular sleep may minimally arouse him now. Periodic groaning or crying is usual and should not be interpreted as an indication of pain or discomfort.
Drowsiness	Eyes may be open Irregular breathing Active body movement	Variable	Most stimuli will arouse infant. He should be picked up during this time rather than left in the crib.
Alert inactivity	Responds to environment by active body movement and staring at close-range objects	2-3 hours/day	Infant's needs such as hunger must be satisfied. He should be placed in that part of home where activity is continuous. He should not be left in crib or playpen with no stimuli close by. Objects should be within 7-8 inches of viewing. Constant stimulation will initiate and prolong this state.
Waking activity and crying	May begin with whimpering and slight body movement Progresses to strong, angry crying and uncoordinated thrashing of extremities	1-4 hours/day	Behavior provoked by intense internal or external stimuli; such stimuli must be removed for termination of this state. Stimuli that were effective during alert inactivity are usually ineffective. Rocking and swaddling may decrease crying.

range objects, such as a swaying mobile or a smiling face. An interesting, stimulating environment can initiate or maintain a quiet, alert state.

The state that usually is most identifiable to parents is *waking activity and crying*. Intense internal stimuli, such as hunger, pain, or cold, or intense external stimuli, such as removing the bottle while the infant is sucking or restraining the infant's extremities, will elicit such responses as a strong, angry cry and thrashing of the arms and legs in an uncoordinated manner. Attempts at quieting the infant may be ineffective unless the primary causative stimuli is removed.

The cycle of these sleep states is highly variable and is based on the number of hours an infant sleeps per day, which may range anywhere from 16 to 22 hours. Generally about 75% of the infant's sleep is in the irregular state. Sleep cycles range from 45 minutes to 2 hours, divided into 10- to 20-minute periods of regular sleep and 20- to 45-minute periods of irregular sleep (Table 8-6). These sleep cycles also roughly correlate with periods of REM and non-REM sleep (See Chapter 3, p. 66).

States of sleep and periods of activity are highly influenced by environmental stimuli. It is especially important for parents to understand these states and the methods effective in altering them. Feeding will usually terminate the state of crying when hunger is the cause. However, an awake infant will exhibit more motor activity before feeding than after. Swaddling or wrapping an infant snugly in a blanket usually promotes sleep as well as maintains body temperature. Much study has recently focused on rocking the infant to reduce crying and induce quiet alertness or sleep. Some particularly interesting research findings regarding rocking include: rocking with the infant held in a vertical position is more effective than in a horizontal direction,[16] and higher amplitudes and higher frequencies of rocking are more effective than are lower ones.[17]

Cry. The newborn should begin extrauterine life with a strong, lusty cry. Variations in this initial cry can indicate abnormalities. A weak, groaning cry or grunt during expiration usually indicates severe respiratory disturbances. Absent, weak, or constant crying suggests brain damage. A high-pitched, shrill cry may be a sign of increased intracranial pressure. One study of supposedly normal newborns in the nursery found a basic difference in the patterns of pitch in the infant's cry. With the use of special equipment to analyze sound waves, it was possible to differentiate the normal infant from the probably abnormal infant.[15]

The sounds produced by crying can be classified into two groups, those of discomfort and comfort. Discomfort sounds consist initially of gasps and cries in which the consonant "H" is clearly distinguishable. Later the sounds of "W" and "L" are added. The almost universal "MAMA" sound is usually associated with much discomfort and is readily recognized by mothers.

The duration of crying is as highly variable in each infant as is the duration of sleep patterns. Some newborns may cry as little as 5 minutes or as much as 2 hours or more per day. Crying may continue to increase for the first several weeks of life but usually decreases at about 8 weeks when the infant is making other vocalizations, such as cooing.

Individual differences and parenting. Nurses must appreciate the individuality and uniqueness of each infant. According to the infant's temperament, he will change and shape his environment, which will undoubtedly influence his future development. Obviously an infant who sleeps 20 hours/day will be exposed to much fewer stimuli than the infant who sleeps 16 hours/day. In turn, each infant will likely effect a different response from his parents. The infant who is quiet, undemanding, and passive may receive much less attention than the infant who is responsive, alert, and active. Such behavioral characteristics have implications for parenting, because forming a relationship is based on responding to reciprocal clues from each individual. The infant who responds to cuddling, smiling, and cooing invokes an attentive, pleasurable response from the parent, which will reinforce such behavior. An infant who stiffens when held, looks away when someone approaches too closely, or cries after feedings typically invokes feelings of rejection, dissatisfaction, and insecurity in the parent. This may very well be where child abuse or the maternal deprivation syndrome has its roots.

Nurses can intervene and positively influence the attachment of parent and child. The first step is recognizing individual differences and explaining to parents that such characteristics are normal. For example, most people believe that infants sleep throughout the day, except for a half-hour feeding. For some newborns this may be true, but for many it is not. Understanding that the infant's wakefulness is part of his body rhythm and not a reflection of inadequate mothering can be crucial in promoting healthy parent-child relationships. Another aspect of helping parents concerns supplying guidelines on how to enhance the infant's development during awake periods. Placing the child in a crib to stare at the same mobile every day is not particularly exciting, but carrying him into each room as one does daily chores can be fascinating. A few simple suggestions can make life very stimulating for the infant and much more pleasurable and gratifying for the parents (see the boxed material above).

How to make the infant's world more exciting

- Objects should be placed about 8 inches away from infant.
- Infant prefers animated objects to inanimate objects.
- Infant enjoys novelty, quickly tires of seeing same objects—mobile should be changed frequently.
- Infant prefers to look at colors rather than black or white, likes patterns over straight lines and circles over squares.
- Contrasting lights are especially interesting.
- But most of all, nothing is as fascinating as the human face and voice!

One method of systematically assessing the infant's behavior is the use of the Neonatal Behavior Assessment Scale.[4] The scale is designed to assess the infant's alertness, motor maturity, irritability or consolability, and interaction with others. Besides its use as an initial and ongoing tool to assess neurologic and behavioral responses, it can be used as a predictor of initial parent-child relationships, as a guide for parents to help them focus on their infant's individuality and to develop a deeper attachment to their child, and as a preventive instrument that identifies the care giver as one who may benefit from a role model.

NURSING CARE OF THE NEONATE

Objectives of nursing care

The main nursing goal for newborns is the *promotion and maintenance of homeostasis or body equilibrium*. Objectives of care for the newborn include: (1) establishment and maintenance of a patent airway, (2) maintenance of a stable body temperature, (3) protection from infection and injury, (4) provision of adequate nutrition, and (5) promotion of infant-parent attachment (see the boxed material on pp. 280-282). Nursing care of the neonate can be divided into three periods: immediate care in the delivery room, care during the transition period, and care in the nursery until discharge. Nursing priorities in the delivery room have been discussed on p. 252.

Vital signs. Following the transition period there is a stabilization of *vital signs*. A minimal schedule for monitoring vital signs in normal neonates is every 15 minutes for at least 1 hour, every 2 hours for the next 8 hours, every 4 hours until 24 hours of age, and then twice a day until discharge. However, any change in the infant, such as in color,

Summary of nursing care of the neonate

Goals	Responsibilities
Establish and maintain patent airway	**Immediate and transitional care** Suction naso-oropharynx Lavage stomach of amniotic fluid (not routinely done in all hospitals) Position infant on side or abdomen with head slightly lower than chest (about 15 degrees) to facilitate drainage of secretions Perform as few procedures as possible on infant during first hour and have oxygen ready for use if respiratory distress should develop Take vital signs every 15 minutes until stable, and more frequently if necessary **Care in nursery** Position infant on right side or abdomen after feeding to prevent aspiration Keep diapers, clothing, and blankets loose enough to allow maximum lung expansion Clean nares of any crusted secretions during bath or when necessary
Maintain stable body temperature	**Immediate and transitional care** Dry skin rapidly with a warmed towel Wrap infant in a warm blanket immediately and place on covered surface Place infant in a warm, draft-free area that is far from sources of radiant heat loss Postpone bath for first 4 to 6 hours Monitor axillary temperature every 15 minutes until stable Be aware of signs of hypothermia or hyperthermia Postpone circumcision until after postnatal recovery period Perform procedures such as footprinting and identification with the smallest amount of body surface possible exposed **Care in nursery** Take temperature on arrival at nursery and, if stable, every 2 to 4 hours Maintain room temperature between 24.0° and 25.5°C (75° to 78°F) and humidity about 40% to 50% Dress infant in a shirt and diaper and swaddle him in a blanket Prevent chilling during daily bath If there is any question regarding stabilization of body temperature, postpone bath Keep head covered if heat loss is a problem
Protect infant from infection and trauma	**Immediate and transitional care** Use sterile gloves when handling newborn immediately after birth; afterward, employ hand washing before and after caring for each infant Instill prophylactic eye medication into conjunctival sac of each eye from inner canthus outward; do not irrigate eyes with sterile saline Ideally, perform eye care after initial meeting of infant and parents, usually about 1 hour after birth Administer vitamin K intramuscularly, using vastus lateralis muscle as site of injection Inspect cut surface of umbilical cord for presence of two arteries and one vein

Summary of nursing care of the neonate—cont'd

Goals	Responsibilities
Protect infant from infection and trauma—cont'd	**Care in nursery** Check eyes daily for any discharge; explain to parents the reason for chemical conjunctivitis Ideally, involve mother and father in bathing of infant; use plain warm water for daily bath except for the genital and rectal area, where mild soap can be used Clean vulva in posterior direction to prevent fecal contamination of vagina or urethra; stress this to parents Repeat cleansing of labia to remove the large amount of vernix caseosa While cleansing the penis, do not retract the foreskin but gently move it back to wipe away the smegma Maintain asepsis during circumcision If the infant has been circumsized, cover the area with a petrolatum jelly gauze for the first 24 hours, then remove the dressing Keep umbilical stump clean and dry; place diapers below umbilical stump
Protect infant from injury	**Immediate, transitional, and nursery care** Place identification bracelet on infant immediately after birth; check often to assure correct infant identity Never leave infant unsupervised on a raised surface without sides; newborns have been known to roll over, and the crawling reflex propels them short distances Always close diaper pins and place them away from infant's body Keep pointed or sharp objects out of infant's reach; grasp reflex can inadvertently be stimulated as hand approaches such an object and can cause damage to skin or, most importantly, to eyes
Provide adequate nutrition	**Immediate and transitional care** During first hour after delivery, put the infant to breast when possible Postpone bottle-feeding of 5% glucose water until sucking and swallowing are well coordinated, usually after the second period of reactivity; do not offer water or supplementary feedings to breast-feeding infants, since this may satiate their hunger and interfere with lactation and breast-feeding **Care in nursery** Bring breast-fed infants to their mothers on demand during day and night (stomach emptying time is about 2 to 3 hours, which does not coincide with the usual hospital feeding schedules of every 4 hours) Offer bottle-fed infants 2 to 3 ounces of formula after they have retained their glucose feeding Support and assist breast-feeding mothers during initial feedings; encourage the father to remain with the mother to help her and the infant with positioning, relaxation, and reinforcement Encourage the father to participate in bottle-feeding Place infant on the right side after feeding to prevent regurgitation Observe stool pattern
Promote infant-parent attachment	**Immediate and transitional care** As soon after delivery as possible, the parents should see and hold their infant; the newborn should be placed close to the face of the parent so that visual contact can be established

Continued.

Summary of nursing care of the neonate—cont'd

Goals	Responsibilities
Promote infant-parent attachment—cont'd	**Immediate and transitional care—cont'd** Identify for the parents specific behaviors manifested by the infant, for example, alertness, ability to see, vigorous suck, rooting behavior, and attention to the human voice **Care in nursery or mother's room** Discuss with parents their expectations of fantasy child vs real child Encourage parents to "talk-out" their labor and delivery experience; identify any events that signify loss of control to either parent, especially the mother Identify the behavioral steps in the attachment process and evaluate those aspects that could be considered positive and those that may represent inadequate or delayed parenting Observe attention–non attention cycles and assess the relating of reciprocal cues between infant and parent; assist parents in recognizing each cycle and in understanding its significance Assess variables affecting the development of attachment through observation of infant and parent and interviewing of each parent or other significant care giver

muscle tone, or behavior, necessitates more frequent monitoring of vital signs.

Axillary temperatures are preferable to rectal ones. However, if an infant is in any type of warmer or servocontrolled device, a skin sensor may be taped to the abdomen for constant temperature monitoring. The sensor must be firmly attached to the skin surface so that ambient air temperature is not measured. The sensor and tape are not allowed to get wet, which may occur during bathing or diapering, because the evaporative loss will be measured as heat loss from the infant. If the infant is positioned on the abdomen, the sensor must be retaped to the back to prevent spuriously high readings from being recorded. If a high erroneous temperature occurs the heater will automatically shut off, even though the infant may still need an increased environmental temperature. As with the use of *any* machine, nurses should rely on their own observation and periodic recording of measurements to prevent misuse of electronic devices. A motto to follow—the machine is guilty until proved innocent!

Respirations and heart rate are routinely taken with temperature. Generally blood pressure is not automatically recorded, but it should be taken at least once during the hospital stay. With increasing concern about hypertension in children and adolescents, this initial blood pressure may be a potential indicator of individuals at risk. (For a review of vital signs and nursing considerations, see the boxed material on p. 265.)

Bathing. Bathing should be done in the nursery after the vital signs have stabilized. There is no need to immediately wash a newborn, except to remove the blood from the face and head. In fact the vernix caseosa probably has bacteriostatic and insulating properties, which make leaving it on the skin advantageous. Plain warm water should be used for the bath. Oils should not be used since they clog pores and provide a medium for bacterial growth. Lotion can be used to cleanse or massage the skin to provide pleasurable tactile stimulation. This is particularly effective for a sick newborn, who is often denied the warmth and comfort of close human contact.

Cleansing proceeds in the cephalocaudal direction. The eyes are carefully wiped from the inner to the outer aspect of the lid. Plain water is used, and the cloth is turned so that a clean part touches the skin with each stroke. The face is cleansed next. The nares are carefully inspected for any crusted secretions. The scalp is usually wiped, although it is sometimes necessary to shampoo the hair. Shampooing is best accomplished by positioning the infant's head over a small basin, lathering the scalp with a mild soap, and rinsing by pouring water from a small vessel over the head into the basin. The rest of the body should be covered during this procedure. The nurse dries the head quickly in order to prevent evaporative heat loss.

The ears are cleaned with the twisted end of a washcloth or very carefully with a cotton-tipped swab. The swab is not inserted into the canal but is gently rotated around the pinna and immediate site of entry into the external canal.

The rest of the body is washed in a similar manner. Although the infant's skin requires little rubbing for adequate cleansing, certain areas such as the folds of the neck, the axillae, and creases at joints need special attention. The area around the neck is especially prone to a rash from regurgitation of feeding and should be thoroughly washed and dried.

The genitalia of both sexes require careful cleansing. In the female the labia are separated to remove the vernix caseosa, which is usually thick and adherent to the skin. Use of oil may help soften the vernix caseosa, but all the oil must be removed afterward. The nurse removes some of the vernix caseosa at each diaper change, rather than at one time, in order to avoid irritation. In some instances it is helpful to sit the infant in a few inches of warm water and let the vernix caseosa soak off. However, when the sitz bath is given, care must be taken to keep the umbilical area dry and to prevent chilling. Cleansing of the vulva is always done in a front-to-back direction. The bath is a perfect opportunity to stress this part of hygiene to the mother, both for the infant's and her protection against urinary tract infection.

Cleansing the male genitalia involves washing the penis and scrotum. Sometimes a white, cheesy secretion called smegma needs to be removed by gently pulling back on the foreskin and wiping around the glans. The foreskin is never forcibly retracted. When pulled back slightly, it is quickly returned to its original position. Because the prepuce is normally tight in newborns, leaving it in a retracted position will constrict the blood vessels supplying the glans penis, causing edema. If the infant is not to be circumsized, the nurse explains to the parents how to cleanse under and around the foreskin.

The buttocks and anal area are thoroughly cleansed of any fecal material. Mild soap, oil, or lotion can be used. As with the rest of the body, the area is dried to prevent a warm, moist environment that fosters growth of bacteria. Diaper dermatitis results from inadequate cleansing. Urine or feces on the skin causes excoriation and, if allowed to remain on the skin, may cause denudement and secondary bacterial infection. Exposing the buttocks or groin to the air and applying heat from a lamp is the best treatment for diaper rash. Plastic pants or the plastic lining of disposable diapers promotes diaper rash by increasing warmth and preventing air circulation. Infants who are sensitive to disposable diapers are usually able to wear them comfortably if the plastic backing is removed. Sensitivity to disposable diapers is distinguishable from diaper rash because the former characteristically follows the outline of the irritant, whereas diaper rash is confined to the genital-anal area. Diapers should fit snugly around the thighs and abdomen to prevent urine from leaking. They should be fastened with the back of the diaper overlapping the front so that flexion of the legs is not inhibited. In males cloth diapers should be folded with extra thickness in the front to provide greater absorbency. In females the placement of the extra fold depends on whether the infant is prone or supine.

The nurse should discuss the choice of cloth or disposable diapers with parents because of the economic difference between each. Using disposable diapers exclusively is the most expensive method, costing from three to four times more than cloth diapers laundered at home. Diaper service costs approximately two to two and a half times as much as the self-laundry method.[8] Over a 1- to 2-year period, the cost or savings can be considerable, particularly if more than one child is wearing diapers.

Daily observations. The bath time can be an opportunity for the nurse to accomplish much more than general hygiene. It is an excellent time for observations of the infant's behavior, such as irritability, state of arousal, alertness, and muscular activity.

In hospitals where there is rooming-in of infant and mother, the bath time provides an opportunity for the nurse to involve the parents in the care of their child and to learn about his individual characteristics. Parents should be encouraged to examine every finger and toe of their infant. Frequently normal variations such as Epstein's pearls, mongolian spots, or stork bites cause parents much worry because they are unaware of the insignificance of such findings. Minor birth injuries, particularly caput succedaneum, cephalhematoma, or conjunctival or retinal hemorrhage, may appear as major defects to them. Explaining how these occurred and when they will disappear reassures parents of their infant's normalcy. Where rooming-in is not allowed the nurse should initiate conversation about the infant when he is brought to the mother for feeding. The nurse will not only allay the parents' fears by talking to and showing them their infant but will also demonstrate interest and concern for them and thereby establish a relationship that will foster their acceptance of and attachment to their child.

During bath time the nurse also notes bodily functions such as voiding and defection. Voiding should occur during the first 24 hours, and the urine is usually odorless and colorless.[5] An infant may void fifteen to twenty times a day. Passage of meconium should occur within the first 36 hours.[5]

Progressive changes in the stooling pattern are indicative of a properly functioning gastrointestinal tract. The infant's first stool is *meconium,* which is usually sticky and greenish black in color. It is composed of intrauterine debris, such as bile pigments, epithelial cells, fatty acids, mucus, blood, and amniotic fluid. With the ingestion of formula or breast milk, the color, consistency, and frequency of the stools change.

Usually by the third day after the initiation of feedings,

transitional stools appear. They are greenish brown to yellowish brown in color, less sticky than meconium, and may contain some milk curds. By the fourth day a typical milk stool is passed. In breast-fed infants the stools are yellow to golden in color and pasty in consistency. They have a peculiar odor, similar to sour milk. In infants being fed cow's milk formula, the stools are pale yellow to light brown, are firmer in consistency, and have a more offensive odor. Breast-fed infants usually have more stools than do bottle-fed infants. The stool pattern can vary widely; six stools a day may be normal for one infant, whereas a stool every other day may be normal for a different infant.

Stools are observed carefully, and any deviation from the pattern is noted. A green, watery stool may indicate an intestinal infection. A white, colorless stool probably suggests some type of liver obstruction, since lack of color indicates that the bile pigments have not entered the colon.

Care of the umbilicus and circumcision. The umbilical cord is clamped and cut after delivery. The stump deteriorates through the process of dry gangrene and usually falls off in 7 to 10 days. The umbilical stump is an excellent medium for bacterial growth. Therefore, it should be kept clean and dry by exposing it to the air as much as possible and avoiding irritation against clothing. After the stump has fallen off, the cord base takes a few more weeks to heal completely. Cleansing the area with mild soap and water during the daily bath and drying it thoroughly keeps the cord free from infection.

The nurse instructs the parents regarding proper umbilical care. Any signs of infection, such as the presence of a malodorous, purulent discharge, should be reported to the physician. A constant, clear discharge from the umbilicus needs to be investigated, since it may signify a patent urachus, the fetal structure that connects the bladder to the umbilicus.

Circumcision is the surgical removal of the foreskin on the glans penis. In the Jewish culture circumcision is performed during a highly significant ceremony called a brit, which takes place on the eighth day of life. A rabbi skilled in the procedure usually performs the circumcision. However, in most instances it is routinely done in the hospital. Those who favor circumcision believe that it improves hygiene, decreases the chance of infection, and reduces the risk of cancer of the penis in men and the possibility of uterine cancer in mates of circumcized males. Opponents of circumcision refute these findings, stating that optimal hygiene prevents complications such as phimosis, removal of the foreskin lessens sexual stimulation, and the procedure presents an unnecessary risk to newborns.

Circumcision is usually performed in the nursery sometime after birth. It should not be performed immediately after delivery because of the neonate's unstabilized physiologic status and increased susceptibility to stress. Preoperative nursing care includes obtaining a signed informed consent from the parents, adequately restraining the infant, cleaning the penis with soap and water, and draping the infant with sterile towels to keep him warm and provide an aseptic field (Fig. 8-13). Even though no anesthesia is given, the infant is allowed nothing by mouth prior to the procedure to prevent aspiration of vomitus. All the equipment used for the procedure, such as gloves, instruments, alcohol wipes, dressings, and draping towels, must be sterile.

The procedure involves freeing the foreskin from the

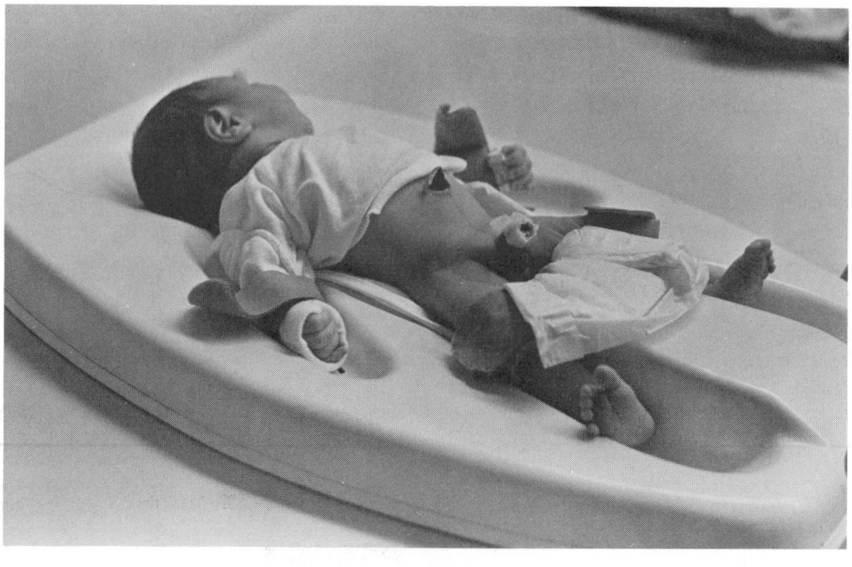

Fig. 8-13. Proper positioning of infant in Circumstraint.

glans penis by using a scalpel, a Yellen or Gomco clamp, or a Hollister plastibell. The clamp crushes the nerve endings and blood vessels, promoting hemostasis. After the procedure a petrolatum gauze dressing is applied, which is usually removed in 24 hours. However, if the dressing becomes dry, it is moistened with hydrogen peroxide before being removed. As soon as the procedure is completed, the nurse releases the infant from the restraints and comforts him. Since parents are often concerned about the infant's well-being during this time, the nurse reassures them that the infant is recovering uneventfully. As soon as the infant is calmed and stabilized, he can be brought to the parents.

No special care following circumcision is required other than ordinary cleansing and observation for bleeding when the diaper is changed. Since the area is tender, the diaper is applied loosely to prevent friction against the penis. Normally on the second day a yellowish-white exudate forms as part of the granulating process. This is not a sign of infection and should not be forcibly removed. As healing progresses, the exudate disappears.

Infant nutrition. Heredity determines the ultimate growth that a person can achieve, but nutrition influences the attainment of that growth. Much research has focused on malnutrition during fetal life and early infancy. Reduced brain size and reduction in the number of brain cells have been demonstrated in malnourished rats. Whether or not this also occurs in the human fetus is uncertain, because the human brain is the most protected organ in any survival-threatening condition. There can be no doubt, however, that optimal nutrition during fetal life and infancy should be the goal for every child.

Selection of a feeding method. During pregnancy parents ask themselves the question, "How will we feed the infant?" In general there are three acceptable choices: human milk, modified cow's milk, or commercially prepared cow's milk formula. Which is best? Human milk and modified cow's milk differ significantly in nutritional content (Table 8-7).

Protein is essential for growth. Human milk contains 1.1 g/100 ml protein; cow's milk yields 3.5 g/100 ml. When the growth of the infant is compared to the growth of a calf, it is apparent that cow's milk contains three times the amount of protein because calves grow three times as fast as human infants. Also, the type of protein differs. Human milk contains more lactalbumin, which is a more complete protein than casein because it contains a higher percentage of amino acids. The higher percentage of casein in cow's milk results in formation of large, hard curds. Human milk is more easily digested because of the presence of soft, flocculent curds. Therefore, stomach emptying time is more rapid with human milk, necessitating more frequent feedings.

Human milk also contains a higher amount of cystine, an amino acid that may be essential during the first few weeks of life, because the enzyme cystathionase, which converts methionine to cystine, is very low in newborns.

Although the amount of fat in both types of milk is similar, the type of fat differs. Human milk contains more monounsaturated fatty acids, mainly oleic acid, whereas cow's milk has more polysaturated fatty acids. Besides the fact that the unsaturated fatty acids in human milk enhance absorption of fat and calcium in the infant, human milk may also be important for decreasing the incidence of atherosclerosis in adulthood.

Cow's milk and human milk both provide 20 kcal/ounce, but human milk contains a higher amount of lactose, a disaccharide that is converted into the monosaccharides glucose and galactose. Galactose is essential for the formation of galactolipids, which is necessary for the growth of the central nervous system.

Certain minerals are important for optimal growth. Calcium and phosphorus are essential, but the proportion or ratio of these two minerals is more important than the absolute amount. In human milk there is a higher ratio of calcium to phosphorus. In cow's milk this is reversed; therefore, the infant receives a high phosphorus load. The infant is unable to eliminate this excess phosphorus because of "physiologic hypoparathyroidism." Parathyroid hormone is necessary for the excretion of phosphorus. However, as phosphorus increases in the blood, calcium is eliminated, resulting in low serum calcium or tetany.

Iron is available in insufficient quantities in both human and cow's milk. However, the full-term neonate is born with an iron reserve that should last for 5 to 6 months. Since iron deficiency in the United States is common, it is important that the infant's diet be reevaluated periodically. Iron has been added to many commercially prepared milk formulas. The Committee on Nutrition of the American Acad-

Table 8-7. Comparison of human and modified cow's milk

Substance	Protein (g/100 ml)	Lactalbumin (%)	Casein (%)	Cystine (mg/100 ml)	Fat (%)	Lactose (g/100 ml)	Calcium (%)	Phosphorus (%)
Human milk	1.1	60	40	24	3.5—4; higher percentage of unsaturated fats (oleic acid)	7	0.034-0.045	0.015-0.04
Whole cow's milk	3.5	18	82	13	3.5-5; higher percentage of saturated fats (butterfat)	4.5	0.222-0.179	0.09-0.196

emy of Pediatrics recommends the addition of 1 mg/kg/day of iron to the infant's diet.

Breast-feeding. Breast milk is certainly the most perfect form of nutrition for the infant. However, whether or not this method is chosen is based on many variables, especially when one considers that 75% to 80% of all infants in the United States are bottle fed. Rather than presenting an argument for or against breast-feeding, it is probably wiser to consider its advantages and disadvantages, because mothers will most likely make their decision based on one or more of them. Probably the most outstanding benefit of breast-feeding besides the quality of the milk is the close maternal-child relationship. The infant is nestled very close to the mother's skin, can hear the rhythm of her heartbeat, feel the warmth of her body, and sense a peaceful security. The mother has a very close feeling of union with her child and feels a sense of accomplishment and satisfaction as the infant draws milk from her. Some mothers also experience a type of sensation similar to sexual excitement.

Breast-feeding is the most economical form of feeding, although it is not ''free'' milk because the lactating mother must have a high-protein, high-calorie diet. Breast milk is always available, ready to serve at room temperature, and free of contamination. In addition there is no need to sterilize bottles. There is also less chance of overfeeding and consequent obesity because the infant nurses until satisfied. Bottle-fed infants are usually encouraged to finish all their formula. Studies show that bottle-fed infants gain weight faster than do breast-fed infants.[8]

Breast-feeding offers some important physiologic advantages. Breast milk contains antibodies against such diseases as chickenpox, mumps, measles, and polio. The incidence of respiratory infections in breast-fed infants is lower during the second 6 months of life. Colostrum and breast milk have a laxative effect; as a result, constipation is rare. Feeding difficulties such as colic, spitting up, and allergic reactions are much less common. There is a lower incidence of breast cancer in mothers who breast-feed their infants.

There are very few contraindications to breast-feeding. Any serious, debilitating illness in the mother, such as severe heart disease or advanced cancer, or infections, such as active tuberculosis, will prevent the mother from breast-feeding. Mastitis is usually not a reason to stop breast-feeding, unless the discomfort is too great. In the infant lactase deficiency, the enzyme necessary to metabolize lactose, will necessitate that a lactose-free formula, such as Isomil, Neo Mull Soy, Meat Base Formula (MBF), or Prosobee, be substituted for human or cow's milk.

Breast milk may also produce hyperbilirubinemia (jaundice) in the newborn during the second week of life, because it contains a substance (a form of pregnanediol) that inhibits the activity of glucuronyl transferase, which is necessary for conjugation of bilirubin. However, this is a temporary condition and ordinarily does not necessitate interruption of breast-feeding.

Probably the greatest disadvantage of breast-feeding to most mothers is the inconvenience of having to be home more often. Many women resume their careers shortly after their pregnancy and prefer to use bottle-feeding. However, it is usually well to emphasize to new mothers that breast milk can be manually expressed for certain feedings and that formula can be substituted for one or two feedings during the mother's absence.

It is important to remember that successful breast-feeding is probably more dependent on the mother's desire to breast-feed than on any other factor. Contrary to popular belief, breast-feeding is not instinctive. Mothers need support, encouragement, and assistance during their postpartum hospital stay to enhance their opportunities for success and satisfaction. Research increasingly supports the idea that early breast-feeding, especially during the first hour of life, increases the chances of success and mutual infant-mother satisfaction.[10]

Bottle-feeding. Bottle-feeding is the most common method of feeding used in the United States. With commercial formulas that closely approximate human milk and greatly improved conditions of sanitation, this is a perfectly acceptable method of feeding. Nurses should not assume that new mothers automatically know how to bottle-feed their infant. These mothers also need support and assistance in meeting their infant's needs. Providing the infant with nutrition is only part of feeding. Holding the infant close to the body and rocking or cuddling him help to assure the emotional component of feeding. There are a few important aspects of bottle-feeding that should be emphasized. The feeding should not be hurried. Even though the infant may suck vigorously for the first 5 minutes and seem to be satisfied, he should be allowed to continue sucking. Infants need at least 2 hours of sucking a day. If there are six feedings per day, then about 20 minutes of sucking should be allowed at each feeding for oral gratification.

Propping the bottle should be discouraged. First of all, propping denies the infant the important component of close human contact. Feeding should be associated with socialization. Also, sucking on the bottle in a dark room is associated with separation of the mother. Because infants do not have the motor control to voluntarily push the bottle away when finished, they may aspirate formula while sleeping. These infants also tend to contract more middle ear infections, since, as the infant lies flat and sucks, milk that has pooled in the pharynx is a suitable medium for bacterial growth. Bacteria then enter the eustachian tube, which leads to the middle ear, causing acute otitis media.

After feedings the infant is positioned on his right side to permit the feeding to flow toward the lower end of the stomach and to allow any swallowed air to rise above the fluid and through the esophagus (Fig. 8-14). This prevents regurgitation and distention. To maintain the side-lying position, a pillow can be propped behind the infant's back.

Five fairly distinct behavioral stages occur during suc-

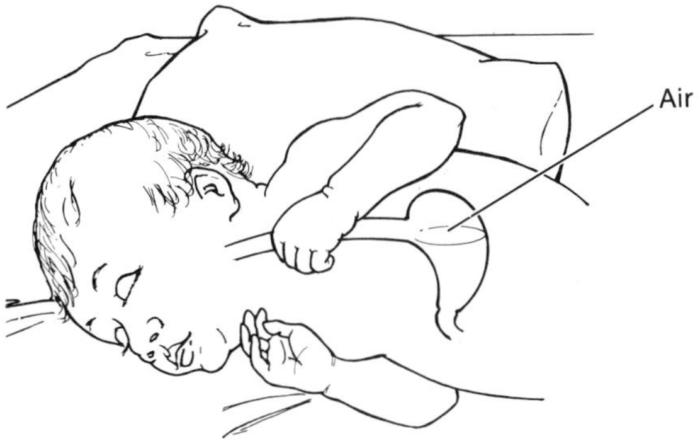

Fig. 8-14. Right side-lying position after feeding.

cessful feeding.[14] Recognizing these steps can assist nurses in identifying potential feeding problems caused by improper feeding techniques. *Prefeeding* behavior, such as crying or fussing, demonstrates the infant's level of arousal and degree of hunger. *Approach behavior* is indicated by sucking movements, the rooting reflex, or, later in infancy, recognition of the bottle. *Attachment behavior* includes those activities that occur from the time the infant receives the nipple until he latches on and sucks. Attachment behavior is sometimes more pronounced during initial attempts at breast-feeding than bottle-feeding. *Consummatory behavior* consists of coordinated sucking and swallowing. Persistent gagging might indicate unsuccessful consummatory behavior. *Satiety behavior* is observed when the infant lets the mother know that he is satisfied. The most common expression of satiation is falling asleep.

Preparation of formula. The analysis of human and cow's milk shows that whole cow's milk is unsuitable for infant nutrition. It would have to be diluted to meet the protein requirement, but, when diluted, it does not meet the caloric requirement. Therefore, evaporated whole milk is usually modified to meet the necessary nutritional demands. Evaporated milk has many advantages over whole milk. It is readily available in cans, needs no refrigeration if unopened, provides a softer, more digestible curd, and contains more lactalbumin and a higher calcium:phosphorus ratio. Evaporated milk must not be confused with condensed milk, which is a form of evaporated milk with 45% more sugar added. Because of its high carbohydrate concentration and disproportionately low fat and protein content, condensed milk should not be used for infant feeding. Likewise, skim milk should not be used because it is deficient in caloric concentration, significantly increases the renal solute load and water demands, and deprives the body of essential fatty acids.

Modification of evaporated milk is determined by daily caloric requirements, which are 110 kcal/kg (50 kcal/pound) in the full-term neonate. Undiluted evaporated milk contains about 44 kcal/ounce. Adding 15½ ounces of sterile water to the 13-ounce can will result in a solution containing 20 kcal/ounce (65 kcal/100 ml). However, sugar or Karo syrup is added to prevent constipation. Because this alters the final carbohydrate content and, therefore, the final number of calories, the following formula is used:

$$\text{13 ounces evaporated milk} + \text{17 ounces water} + \text{1 to 2 tbsp sugar} = \text{20 kcal/ounce}$$

To calculate the number of ounces of formula needed by the infant per day, the following formula should be used:

$$\frac{\text{Weight (kg)} \times \text{110 kcal/kg}}{\text{20 kcal/ounce}} = \text{total no. ounces/day}$$

Fluid requirements must also be calculated to ensure adequate tissue hydration. The newborn requires about 150 ml/kg (70 ml/pound) of fluid per day. To calculate the daily fluid requirement, the following formula should be used:

$$\text{Weight (kg)} \times \text{150 ml} = \text{total no. ml/day}$$

To convert the number of milliliters into ounces, divide by 30 (30 ml = 1 ounce). For example, a 3-kg infant will require 16.5 ounces of formula $\left(\frac{\text{3 kg} \times \text{110 kcal}}{\text{20 kcal}} = \text{16.5 ounces}\right)$ and 15 ounces of fluid (3 kg × 150 ml = $\frac{\text{450 ml}}{\text{30 ml}}$ = 15 ounces). In other words, the 16.5 ounces of formula will meet the caloric requirement and will supply 1.5 ounces of extra fluid.

Commercially prepared formulas (Similac, Enfamil, SMA) are milk-based formulas that have been modified to closely resemble human milk. Although they are not an exact substitute, they do provide an optimal source of nutrition. The formulas are available in three preparations: (1) a ready-to-use form in cans or bottles, (2) a concentrated liquid form, which must be diluted with an equal amount of water, and (3) a powdered form, which must be prepared according to the manufacturer's directions. One consideration in the use of commercially prepared formulas is their cost. In general any of these preparations costs about twice as much as does evaporated milk. It is wise to advise parents to do comparison shopping. For example, the concentrated liquid often costs less per ounce than does the powdered form, which requires more steps on the part of the parents in its preparation.

The two most common ways of preparing formula are the terminal heat method and the aseptic method. In the terminal heat method all the utensils and formula are sterilized together. In the aseptic method the equipment is sterilized separately, after which the sterilized formula is poured into the bottles. (See boxed material on p. 288 for explanation.) Because of improved sanitary conditions, it is not essential to do either of the above. Some physicians now recommend that the bottles and other equipment be washed well and that tap water and evaporated milk or formula be poured directly into the bottles.

Feeding schedules. Ideally feeding schedules should be determined by the infant's hunger. Since sleeping patterns

Methods of preparing formula

Terminal heating method

1. Wash all bottles, nipples, caps, and utensils used for preparing the formula (the dishwasher is excellent for this)
2. Measure the exact amount of water and sugar, then add to the evaporated milk or whole milk; if commercial formulas are being used, follow label directions
3. Pour formula into clean nursing bottles; attach nipples and cap loosely to allow steam to escape
4. Place bottles on rack in sterilizer or deep kettle, which contains 2 to 3 inches of water; cover utensil with a tight-fitting lid
5. After the water has begun to boil, boil gently for 25 minutes, then let bottles cool; if lid vibrates, do not remove
6. Remove bottles, tighten caps, and refrigerate

Aseptic method

1. Wash all equipment as noted above
2. Boil bottles, nipples, caps, and utensils (including measuring cup) needed for preparing formula for 5 minutes
3. Boil water for formula for 5 minutes; allow a few extra ounces for evaporation
4. Remeasure water and add exact amounts of other ingredients; mix in utensil used to boil water
5. Pour into sterilized bottles; put on nipples and caps, being careful not to touch inner surface or tip of nipples; refrigerate until ready to use

vary from one child to another, it is not illogical to assume that feeding schedules also differ. Feeding the infant when he signals his readiness is called *feeding on demand*. More frequently, parents *schedule feedings* to meet their life-style. Most hospitals routinely feed infants every 4 hours. Although this is usually satisfactory for bottle-fed infants, it usually hinders the breast-feeding process. Breast-fed infants tend to be hungry every 2 to 3 hours, and, since lactation is dependent on breast stimulation, these infants should be on demand feedings. Also, if the infant is offered supplemental feedings in the nursery, the likelihood is that he will not suck vigorously when he is brought to the mother. Lactation is also dependent on the breast being emptied at each feeding. If milk is allowed to accumulate in the ducts, causing breast engorgement, ischemia results, suppressing the activity of the acini or milk-secreting cells. Consequently milk production will be reduced.

Usually by 3 weeks of age lactation is well-established and a feeding schedule has been formed. Bottle-fed infants usually retain about 2 to 3 ounces of formula at each feeding and are fed about six times a day. Larger infants are able to retain increased amounts because of greater stomach capacity; as a result they generally will sleep through the night sooner than will smaller infants or breast-fed infants.

PROMOTING FAMILY RELATIONSHIPS

The process of parenting is based on a mutual relationship between parent and infant. Much of past research on parent-child attachment has focused on the development of "mothering" or maternal attachment to the infant. Recently attention has focused on the infant's role in this process. As one learns of the complexity of the neonate and of his potential for influencing and shaping his environment, particularly his interaction with significant others, one cannot help but realize that promoting positive parent-child relationships necessitates an understanding of factors involved in identifying behavioral steps in attachment, variables that enhance or hinder this process, and methods of teaching parents ways to develop a stronger relationship with their child, especially by recognizing potential problems.

Infant behavior and parental attachment

The infant's behavior influences and ultimately shapes the interaction between him and his parents. As has been discussed previously in this chapter, a docile, passive infant will probably receive less attention and stimulation than will an alert, active infant. The Neonatal Behavioral Assessment Scale can be utilized to assess the degree of the infant's activity. Studies have demonstrated that by showing parents the unique characteristics of their infant, there develops a more positive attitude toward the infant, less infant feeding and sleeping problems, and a consequently higher level of activity and alertness in the infant. In a 1-year follow-up study the infants in the experimental group, who received the Brazelton assessment, scored 10 to 20 points higher on the Bayley Mental and Motor Scores.[1]

Maternal attachment. Many variables affect the attachment process. Part of promoting the attachment is an understanding of some of these factors. During pregnancy, and in many cases even before conception occurs, parents develop an image of the "ideal or fantasy infant." The unborn child has an imagined appearance, pattern of behavior, expected accomplishments, and predetermined effect on the life-style of the parents. At birth the fantasy infant becomes the real infant. How closely the dream child resembles the real child will influence the acceptance process. If the parents expected an alert, active infant who sleeps little and enjoys human contact and the real infant fulfills these expectations, the attachment process will be facilitated. If parents imagine that the newborn will sleep most of the time, will need little attention except feeding and diapering, and will not disturb their life-style significantly, the birth of a very active infant may cause considerable conflicts in the emotional bonding. Assessing such expectations during pregnancy and at the time of the infant's birth will allow nurses to identify discrepancies in the parents' view of the fantasy vs real child syndrome.

The labor process also significantly affects the immediate attachment of mothers to their newborn child. In general the mother's perception of maintaining control during the labor and birth process enhances the initial attachment, which, ideally, should take place during the first hour of life. A feeling of loss of control because of factors such as a long, difficult labor, excessive medication and sedation, or unwanted medical intervention, will hinder the initial bonding process. Encouraging mothers to talk about their feelings of loss of control, particularly about the specific event that they perceive caused the lack of self-control, allows them to dissipate the emotional energy invested in these feelings. It is not until such emotional tensions and anxieties are released that parents can attend to the emotional component of the attachment process.

Mothers demonstrate a predictable and orderly pattern of behavior during the development of the attachment process. Researchers have found that when mothers were presented with their nude infants, they began examining the infant with their fingertips, concentrating on touching the extremities. In about 4 to 8 minutes they proceeded to massage and encompass the trunk with their entire hands.[11] They also found that the *en face* position, a position in which the mother's and the infant's eyes meet in visual contact in the same vertical plane, was significant in the formation of affectional ties. Observing such behavioral characteristics can assist nurses in identifying potential signs of inadequate or delayed mothering. For example, the mother who consistently feeds her infant while holding him at a distance from her body, who supports him with fingertips rather than encompassing him in her arm, and who looks away from the infant most of the time is exhibiting behavior that needs to be assessed more carefully.

Five steps occur in positive mother-infant reciprocity.[3] The first step is *initiation,* in which interaction between infant and parent begins. Next is *orientation,* which establishes the partners' expectation of each other during the interaction. Following orientation is *acceleration* of the attention cycle to a peak of excitement. The infant reaches out and coos, both arms jerk forward, the head moves backward, the eyes dilate, and the face brightens. After a short time, *deceleration* of the excitement and *turning away* occur, in which the infant shifts his eyes away from his mother's and grasps his shirt. During this cycle of nonattention, repeated verbal or visual attempts to reinitiate his attention will be ineffective. This deceleration and turning away probably prevent the infant from being overwhelmed by excessive stimuli. In a good interaction, both partners will have synchronized their attention-nonattention cycles. Parents or other care givers who do not allow the infant to turn away and who continually attempt to maintain visual contact will encourage the infant to turn off his attention cycles and prolong the nonattention phase.

Although this description of reciprocal interacting behavior is usually observable in the infant by 2 to 3 weeks of age, nurses can use this information to teach parents how to interact with their infant. Recognizing the attention cycle vs the nonattention cycle and understanding that the latter is not a rejection of the parent is one aspect in helping parents develop competence in parenting.

Paternal engrossment. Fathers also show specific behaviors during the attachment process, or what has been termed "engrossment," forming a sense of absorption, preoccupation, and interest in the infant.[7] The major characteristics of engrossment include (1) visual awareness of the newborn, especially focusing on the beauty of the child, (2) tactile awareness, often expressed in a desire to hold the infant, (3) awareness of distinct characteristics with emphasis on those features of the infant that resemble the father, (4) perception of the infant as perfect, (5) development of a strong feeling of attraction to the child that leads to intense focusing of attention on him, (6) experiencing a feeling of extreme elation, and (7) feeling a sense of deep self-esteem and satisfaction. These responses are greatest during the early contacts with the infant and are intensified by the neonate's normal reflex activity, especially the grasp reflex and visual alertness.

The development of engrossment has significant implications for nurses. Initially it is imperative that nurses recognize the importance of early father-infant contact in releasing these behaviors. Fathers need to be encouraged to express their positive feelings, especially if such emotions are contrary to the cultural belief that fathers should remain stoic. If this is not clarified, fathers may feel confused and attempt to suppress the natural sensations of absorption, preoccupation, and interest in order to conform with societal expectations.

Mothers also need to be aware of the responses of the father toward the newborn, especially since one of the consequences of paternal preoccupation with the infant is less overt attention toward the mother. If both parents are able to share their feelings, each can appreciate the process of attachment toward their child and will avoid the unfortunate conflict of being insensitive and unaware of the other's needs. In addition a father who is encouraged to form a relationship with his newborn is also less likely to feel excluded and abandoned once the family returns home and the mother directs her attention toward caring for the infant.

Ideally the process of engrossment should be discussed with parents prior to the delivery, such as in prenatal classes, to reinforce the father's awareness of his natural feelings toward the expected child. Focusing on the future experience of seeing, touching, and holding one's newborn may also help expectant fathers become more comfortable in accepting their paternal feelings toward the unborn child. This in turn can assist them in being more supportive toward their wives, especially as the labor and delivery event draws near.

At the infant's birth the nurse can play a vital role in assisting the father in release or expression of engrossment by assessing the neonate in front of the couple, pointing out normal characteristics, especially the grasp reflex, encouraging identification through consistent referral to the child by using his name, encouraging the father to cuddle, hold, talk to, and/or feed the infant, and demonstrating whenever necessary the soothing powers of caressing, stroking, and rocking the child. The nurse observes for the same indication of affectional ties from the father as were discussed for the mother, such as visual contact in the *en face* position and embracing the infant close to the body. When present, such behaviors are reinforced. If such responses are not obvious, the nurse needs to assess the father's feelings regarding this birth, cultural beliefs that may prevent his emotional expression, and other factors in order to help him facilitate a positive attachment during this critical period.

Assessment of attachment behavior

Unlike physical assessment of the neonate, which has concrete guidelines to follow, assessment of parent-child attachment requires much more skill in terms of observation and interviewing. The assessment process is even more challenging when one considers that postpartum hospital recovery is shorter and shorter. However, rooming-in of mother and infant and liberal visiting privileges for father, siblings, and grandparents facilitate recognition of behaviors that demonstrate positive or negative development of attachment.

What should the nurse observe when with the parents and the infant? Probably the most important activities to observe include feeding, bathing, and comforting. For example, when the infant is brought to the mother, does she reach out for him, call him by name, or involve the father in the greeting process? Do the parents speak about the child in terms of identification—who does he look like; what appears special about him over the other infants; how "smart" do they think he is? When the mother or father is holding the infant, what kind of body contact is there—do they feel at ease in changing the infant's position; are fingertips or whole hands used; are there parts of the body they avoid touching or parts of the body they investigate and scrutinize? When the infant is awake, what kinds of stimulation do the parents provide—do they talk to the infant, to each other, or to no one; how do they look at the infant—direct visual contact, avoidance of eye contact, or looking at other people or objects?

Talking to the parents uncovers many variables that will affect the development of attachment and parenting. What expectations do they have for this child? In other words how similar are their predictions of the fantasy child and their realizations about the real child? They should be encouraged to talk about their relationship with their parents. Mothering and fathering of one's child are probably more dependent on the type of parenting that parents received as a child than on any other variable. Is this a planned birth, how do they see the addition of a dependent family member affecting their life-style, and what arrangements have they made in terms of such changes in life-style? What "support system" or significant others are available for assistance? What are their views regarding child rearing?

Although the area of child rearing is very broad, narrowing the discussion to focus on the parents' ideas about "spoiling" the child is important. Many parents believe that they will "spoil" the infant if they promptly respond to his gestures, such as crying or fussing. Bell and Ainsworth's research suggests that the opposite is true. To ignore the infant's crying and to delay responding to his needs reinforces crying and fussing, whereas responding quickly to the child's wants helps him learn to develop more noncrying methods of seeking attention, such as bubbling or vocalizing.[2]

Although the attachment process has been discussed almost exclusively in terms of the parents and infant, it is essential that nurses be aware of other family members, such as siblings and members of the extended family, who need preparation for the acceptance of this new child. Professional support should be continued from the hospital to the home through community services, such as visiting nurse agencies. Ideally the concept of family-centered care will be practiced when the family receives consistent comprehensive care from the same health team members, beginning with preventive prenatal care and continuing through infant health maintenance.

REFERENCES

1. Barnard, K.: The acquaintance process. In Klaus, M., and associates, editors: Maternal attachment and mothering disorders, New Brunswick, N.J., 1974, Johnson & Johnson, Baby Products Co.
2. Bell, S., and Ainsworth, M.: Infant crying and maternal responsiveness, Child Dev. **43:**1171-1190, December 1972.
3. Brazelton, T.: Mother-infant reciprocity. In Klaus, M., and associates, editors: Maternal attachment and mothering disorders, New Brunswick, N.J., 1974, Johnson & Johnson, Baby Products Co.
4. Brazelton, T.: Neonatal Behavioral Assessment Scale, Clin. Dev. Med. **50:** 1974.
5. Clark, D. A.: Times of first void and first stool in 500 newborns, Pediatrics **60**(4):457-459, October 1977.
6. German, L. D., Mason, P. A., and Rosman, N. P.: Reliability of head circumference measurement in the newborn, Clin. Pediatr. **15:**891-893, 1976.
7. Greenberg, M., and Morris, N.: Engrossment: the newborn's impact upon the father, Am. J. Orthopsychiatry **44**(4):520-531, July 1974.
8. Infant nutrition: feeding the infant . . . building the man, New York, 1972, Medcom, Inc.
9. Johnson, E. S.: Diapers: cloth or disposable? Nurs. Digest **4**(2):4, March/April 1976.
10. Johnson, N.: Breast-feeding at one hour of age, A. M. J. Maternal Child Nurs. **1**(1):12-16, January/February 1976.

11. Klaus, M., and associates: Maternal attachment—importance of the first postpartum days, N. Engl. J. Med. **286:**460, 1972.
12. Laestadius, N., Aase, J., and Smith, D.: Normal inner costal and outer orbital dimensions, J. Pediatr. **74:**465-468, 1969.
13. Marden, P. M., Smith, D. W., and McDonald, M. J.: Congenital anomalies in the newborn infant, including minor variations, J. Pediatr. **64**(3):357-371, March 1964.
14. O'Grady, R.: Feeding behavior in infants, Am. J. Nurs. **71**(4):736-739, April 1971.
15. Ostwald, P., and Paltemen, P.: The cry of the human infant, Sci. Am. **230**(3):84-90, March 1974.
16. Pedersen, D. R., and associates: Relative soothing effects of vertical and horizontal rocking, Paper presented at the biennial meetings of the Society for Research in Child Development, Santa Monica, Calif., March 1969.
17. Pedersen, D. R., and Ter Vrugt, D.: The influence of amplitude and frequency of vestibular stimulation on the activity of two-month-old infants, Child Dev. **44:**122-128, March 1973.

BIBLIOGRAPHY

Abramson, H., editor: Resuscitation of the newborn infant: and related emergency procedures in the perinatal center special care nursery, ed. 3, St. Louis, 1973, The C. V. Mosby Co.

Aladjem, S., editor: Risks in the practice of modern obstetrics, ed. 2, St. Louis, 1975, The C. V. Mosby Co.

Alexander, M., and Brown, M.: Pediatric physical diagnosis for nurses, New York, 1974, McGraw-Hill Book Co.

Andrews, B., and associates: When the baby is full-term and fine, Patient Care, pp. 59-89, February 1, 1975.

Apgar, V.: The newborn (Apgar) scoring system, Pediatr. Clin. North Am. **13:**645, 1966.

Apgar, V., and associates: Evaluation of the newborn infant, second report, J.A.M.A. **168:**1985, December 13, 1958.

Arms, S.: Immaculate deception, San Francisco, 1975, San Francisco Book Co., Inc./Houghton Mifflin Books.

Arnold, H. W., and associates: The newborn: transition to extrauterine life, Am. J. Nurs. **65:**77, 1965.

Babson, S. G., and associates: Management of high-risk pregnancy and intensive care of the neonate, ed. 3, St. Louis, 1975, The C. V. Mosby Co.

Barness, L.: Manual of pediatric physical diagnosis, ed. 4, Chicago, 1972, Year Book Medical Publishers, Inc.

Bennett, S.: Infant caretaker interactions, J. Child Psychiatry **10:** 321-335, 1971.

Bergersen, B. S., and Goth, A.: Pharmacology in nursing, ed. 13, St. Louis, 1976, The C. V. Mosby Co.

Binzley, V. A.: State: an overloaded factor in newborn nursing, Am. J. Nurs. **77**(1):102-103, January 1977.

Bishop, B.: A guide to assessing parenting capabilities, Am. J. Nurs. **76**(11):1784-1787, November 1976.

Botwin, E.: Should children be screened for hypertension?, Am. J. Maternal Child Nurs. **1**(3):152-158, May/June 1976.

Brown, M., and Murphy, M.: A child grows, Pediatr. Nurs. **1:**9, January/February 1975.

Brown, M., and Murphy, M.: A child grows. Part 4. The child's perceptual and linguistic development, Pediatr. Nurs. **1**(4):9-15, July/August 1975.

Brown, M., and Murphy, M.: Ambulatory pediatrics for nurses, New York, 1975, McGraw-Hill Book Co.

Cahill, B.: The neonatal nurse specialist—new techniques for the asymptomatic newborn, J. Obstet. Gynecol. Neonatal Nurs. **3**(1):34-38, January/February 1974.

Callon, H.: Nursing responsibility in maintaining the body heat of the newborn infant. In Neonatal thermoregulation, module 1, New York, 1976, The National Foundation—March of Dimes.

Chinn, P. L.: Child health maintenance: concepts in family centered care, ed. 2, St. Louis, 1979, The C. V. Mosby Co.

Chinn, P. L., and Leitch, C.: Child health maintenance: a guide to clinical assessment, ed. 2, St. Louis, 1979, The C. V. Mosby Co.

Clark, A., and Affonso, D.: Childbearing: a nursing perspective, Philadelphia, 1976, F. A. Davis Co.

Clark, A., and Affonso, D.: Infant behavior and maternal attachment: two sides of the coin, Am. J. Maternal Child Nurs. **1**(2):94-99, March/April 1976.

Clark, L.: Introducing mother and baby, Am. J. Nurs. **74**(8):1483-1484, August 1974.

DeAngelis, C.: Basic pediatrics for the primary health care provider, Boston, 1975, Little, Brown and Co.

Desmond, M., and associates: The clinical behavior of the newly born. Part 2. The term baby, J. Pediatr. **62:**307-325, 1963.

Desmond, M., and associates: The transitional care nursery, Pediatr. Clin. North Am. **13:**656, 1966.

Devney, A., and Kingsbury, B.: Hypothermia: on fact and fantasy, Am. J. Nurs. **72:**1424, August 1972.

Dickason, E., and Schult, M., editors: Maternal and infant care, New York, 1975, McGraw-Hill Book Co.

Essoka, G., and associates: Pediatric Nursing Continuing Education Review, Flushing, N.Y., 1975, Medical Examination Publishing Co., Inc.

Evans, H., and Glass, L.: Perinatal medicine, New York, 1976, Harper & Row, Publishers.

Farhi, A., and associates: Pediatric skin care, Pediatr. Nurs. **2**(2): 18-19, March/April 1976.

Farrar, C.: A data collection procedure to assess behavioral individuality in the neonate, J. Obstet. Gynecol. Neonatal Nurs. **3**(3):15-20, May/June 1974.

Filhart, R.: Bathing the ICN baby, Pediatr. Nurs. **1**(4):17-19, July/August 1975.

Goerzen, J. L., and Chinn, P. L.: Review of maternal and child nursing, St. Louis, 1975, The C. V. Mosby Co.

Graven, S.: Temperature control in newborn babies. In Neonatal thermoregulation, module 1, New York, 1976, The National Foundation—March of Dimes.

Guyton, A. C.: Textbook of medical physiology, ed. 5, Philadelphia, 1976, W. B. Saunders Co.

Harbin, R.: Is there a place for a rocking chair in your newborn nursery? Pediatr. Nurs. **1**(4):16, July/August 1975.

Hughes, J. G.: Synopsis of pediatrics, ed. 4, St. Louis, 1975, The C. V. Mosby Co.

Illingworth, R. S.: Development of the infant and young child, Baltimore, 1963, The Williams & Wilkins Co.

Iorio, J.: Childbirth: family centered nursing, ed. 3, St. Louis, 1975, The C. V. Mosby Co.

Johnson, S., and Grubbs, J.: The premature infant's reflex behavior: effect on the maternal-child relationship, J. Obstet. Gynecol. Neonatal Nurs. **4**(3):15-21, May/June 1975.

Klaus, M., Leger, T., and Trause, M., editors: Maternal attachment and mothering disorders, New Brunswick, N.J., 1974, Johnson & Johnson, Baby Products Co.

Klaus, M., and associates: Human maternal behavior at the first contact with her young, Pediatrics **46**(2):187-192, August 1970.

Knoblich, H., and Pasamanick, B., editors: Gesell and Amatruda's developmental diagnosis, New York, 1974, Harper & Row, Publishers.

Korner, A., and Thoman, E.: Visual alertness in neonates as evoked by maternal care, J. Exp. Child Psychol. **10:**67-78, 1970.

Korones, S. B.: High risk newborn infants: the basis for intensive nursing care, St. Louis, 1976, The C. V. Mosby Co.

Lake, A.: New babies are smarter than you think, Woman's Day, pp. 9-22, June 1976.

Lutz, L., and Perlstein, P.: Temperature control in newborn babies, Nurs. Clin. North Am. **6**(1):15-23, March 1971.

McAdams, W. H.: Heat transmission, ed. 3, New York, 1954, McGraw-Hill Book Co.

McKilligan, H.: The first day of life, New York, 1970, Springer Publishing Co., Inc.

Money, J.: Sex errors of the body, Baltimore, 1968, The Johns Hopkins University Press.

Murdaugh, A., and Miller, L.: Helping the breast-feeding mother, Am. J. Nurs. **72**(8):1420-1423, August 1972.

Murphy, M.: The crying infant, Pediatr. Nurs. **1:**15-17, January/February 1975.

Nelson, W. E., Vaughan, V. C., and McKay, R. J.: Textbook of pediatrics, ed. 10, Philadelphia, 1975, W. B. Saunders Co.

Papalia, D., and Olds, S.: A child's world, infancy through adolescence, New York, 1975, McGraw-Hill Book Co.

Phillips, C.: Neonatal heat loss in heated cribs vs. mother's arms, J. Obstet. Gynecol. Neonatal Nurs. **3**(6):11-15, November 1, 1974.

Reed, B., and associates: Management of the infant during labor, delivery, and in the immediate neonatal period, Nurs. Clin. North Am. **6**(1):3-14, March 1971.

Roberts, J.: Suctioning the newborn, Am. J. Nurs. **73:**63, January 1973.

Rudolph, A. M., editor: Pediatrics, ed. 16, New York, 1977, Appleton-Century-Crofts.

Scanlon, J. W.: How is the baby: the Apgar score revisited, Clin. Pediatr. **12:**61, February 1973.

Scipien, G., and associates: Comprehensive pediatric nursing, New York, 1975, McGraw-Hill Book Co.

Silverman, W., and Parke, P.: Keep him warm, Am. J. Nurs. **65**(10):81-84, October 1965.

Sinclair, D.: Human growth after birth, New York, 1969, Oxford University Press, Inc.

Smith, N., editor: Nathan Smith on developmental nutrition: the challenge of obesity, No. 1, Columbus, Ohio, 1972, Ross Laboratories.

Standards and recommendations for hospital care of newborn infants, Chicago, 1971, The American Academy of Pediatrics.

Standley, K., and associates: Local regional anesthesia during childbirth: effect on newborn behaviors, Science **186:**634-635, November 15, 1974.

Tulkin, S., and Kagan, J.: Mother-child interaction in the first year of life, Child Dev. **43:**31-41, 1972.

Weiner, I., and Elkind, D.: Child development: a core approach, New York, 1972, John Wiley & Sons, Inc.

Williams, S. R.: Nutrition and diet therapy, ed. 3, St. Louis, 1977, The C. V. Mosby Co.

Wolman, I. J., editor: Common causes of abnormal coloration of infant skin, Clin. Pediatr. **11:**16B-C, November 1972.

The womanly art of breast feeding, Chicago, 1963, LaLeche League International.

9

Health problems of the neonate

The newborn's immature physiologic systems impose threats to his survival. Some of the conditions that result from this immaturity require no intervention other than careful assessment and continued observation to distinguish them from potential pathologic situations. Others require immediate identification and intervention to prevent future problems. The nurse's ability to recognize such conditions and institute appropriate care significantly affects the neonate's immediate survival and later development.

PROBLEMS RELATED TO PHYSICAL STATUS

Hyperbilirubinemia

Hyperbilirubinemia refers to increased bilirubin levels in the blood. Bilirubin is one of the breakdown products of hemoglobin from hemolyzed or dissolved red blood cells. As the cells reach the end of viability, they become too fragile to exist in the circulatory system, their cell membranes rupture, and the released hemoglobin is phagocytized by the reticuloendothelial cells, primarily in the liver and spleen. The hemoglobin is then split into heme and globin.

The exact pathway by which the heme complex is converted to bilirubin is not fully known. It is thought to be dependent on an enzyme, heme oxygenase, in the reticuloendothelial cells, which transforms the heme molecule after loss of iron and globin to biliverdin. Biliverdin, a water-soluble green pigment, is rapidly reduced by the enzyme biliverdin reductase to form bilirubin.

The unconjugated bilirubin, which is relatively insoluble in body fluids, is released by the reticuloendothelial cells and is rapidly bound to albumin. In the liver the bilirubin is detached from the plasma protein and in the presence of the enzyme *glucuronyl transferase* is conjugated with glucuronic acid to produce a highly soluble form, bilirubin glucuronide, which is then excreted into the bile. The bile enters the intestine where the action of the bacterial flora reduces the conjugated bilirubin to urobilinogen and stercobilin, the pigment that gives stool its characteristic color. Most of the reduced bilirubin is excreted through the feces and a small amount is eliminated as urobilinogen in the urine (Fig. 9-1).

Hyperbilirubinemia in the newborn most often results from physiologic immaturity of hepatic functions or increased erythrocyte destruction, particularly from blood group incompatibility. The main pathophysiologic damage from hyperbilirubinemia is encephalopathy or kernicterus.

Kernicterus. Kernicterus results from the deposition of unconjugated bilirubin in brain cells. The exact mechanisms responsible for brain damage are unknown. It is postulated that unconjugated bilirubin, which is lipid soluble, passes into the cell membrane of neurons and its various structures, blocking critical steps in the metabolism or transport of energy. The pathogenesis seems to be almost identical with that seen in hypoxia.[2]

There is a direct relationship between the total serum bilirubin concentration and the risk of kernicterus. In general a serum bilirubin level of 20 mg/100 ml in a full-term infant is considered the maximal level prior to the development of brain damage. However, several factors affect this relationship. Normally only minute amounts of unconjugated bilirubin that is not bound to serum albumin enter the brain. Bound unconjugated bilirubin is unable to cross the protective blood-brain barrier. However, as conditions occur that lower the binding capacity of plasma, more free unconjugated bilirubin is available for cerebral entry. Factors that enhance the development of kernicterus include metabolic acidosis, lowered albumin levels, free fatty acids, and drugs such as salicylates or sulfonamides that compete for attachment to the plasma protein. In addition any condition that increases the metabolic demands for oxygen or glucose, such as fetal distress or hypothermia, also increases the risk of brain damage despite lowered serum levels of bilirubin.

The signs of kernicterus are those of central nervous system depression or excitation. Generally the clinical symptoms appear during the first week of life. Signs of severe depression include lethargy, diminished deep tendon reflexes, absent Moro reflex, hypotonia, and absent sucking reflex. Neurologic excitation is evidenced by tremors, twitching, convulsions, opisthotonos, and high-pitched cry. The mortality rate approaches 50% during the first month. Those

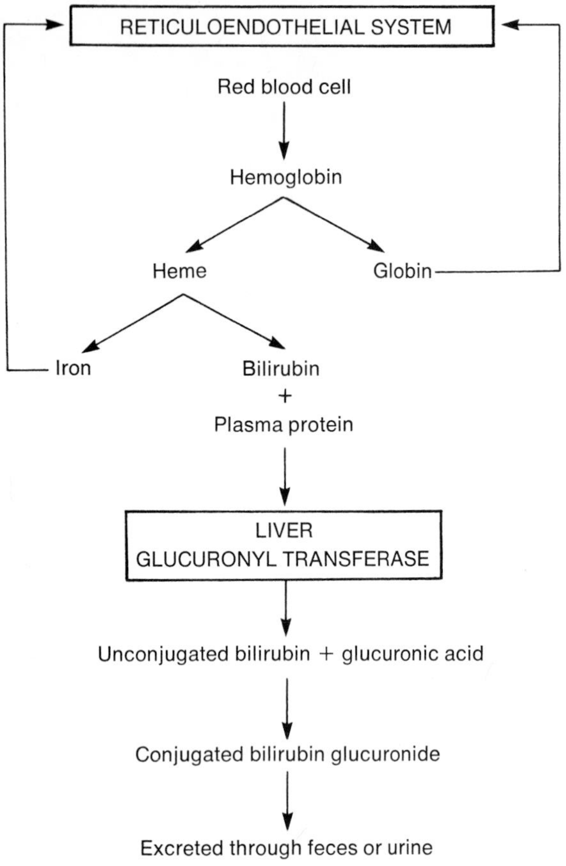

Fig. 9-1. Formation and excretion of bilirubin.

who survive may initially appear well but may eventually show evidence of neurologic damage such as mental retardation, minimal brain dysfunction, delayed motor development or abnormal motor movement, especially ataxia, or athetosis, behavior disorders, perceptual problems, or sensorineural hearing loss.[5]

Medical management. The aim of therapy for hyperbilirubinemia is prevention of kernicterus. The main forms of treatment involve phototherapy, exchange transfusion, and pharmacologic management.

Phototherapy. Phototherapy involves the use of intense fluorescent light on the infant's exposed skin. Light in the blue range decomposes bilirubin by the process of photooxidation. Although the value of phototherapy in effectively reducing or preventing rising bilirubin levels is well documented, its long-term effects are not. At the present time the recommended use of phototherapy is (1) to prevent hyperbilirubinemia in premature newborn infants in the absence of disease, when bilirubin levels reach 10 mg/100 ml and (2) to treat already established hyperbilirubinemia after determining its cause in premature and low birth weight neonates, along with other modalities of treatment, such as exchange transfusion.[1] Specific precautions during phototherapy are discussed under nursing considerations of the neonate with hemolytic disease on p. 300.

Exchange transfusion. Exchange transfusion is the standard mode of therapy for treatment of hyperbilirubinemia caused by increased erythrocyte destruction in blood group incompatibility. It is discussed in greater detail under hemolytic disease of the newborn on p. 298.

Pharmacologic management. Pharmacologic treatment of hyperbilirubinemia has focused mainly on the use of barbiturates, such as phenobarbital, which stimulates protein synthesis (increasing available albumin for binding with unconjugated bilirubin) and promotes hepatic glucuronyl transferase synthesis (increasing conjugation of bilirubin and hepatic clearance of the pigment in bile). The most effective results are observed when the drug is given to the mother 1 to 2 weeks prior to delivery. Much controversy exists regarding barbiturate therapy because of its known side effects, namely, excessive sedation, potential addiction, and other potent metabolic effects in addition to those of bilirubin metabolism.[2]

Physiologic jaundice

Physiologic jaundice is a result of the immaturity of hepatic functions in the newborn combined with an increased bilirubin load from increased hemolysis of red blood cells. Although almost all newborns experience elevated bilirubin levels (above the normal value of 0.2 to 1.4 mg/100 ml), only about half demonstrate observable signs of *jaundice,* yellow staining of the body tissues, especially subcutaneous tissue, from the accumulation of the lipid-soluble pigment unconjugated bilirubin. In the newborn, bilirubin levels must exceed 5 mg/100 ml before jaundice or icterus is reflected in the sclera, nails, or skin. This is in contrast to older children and adults who become jaundiced when bilirubin levels exceed 2 mg/100 ml.[2]

Mechanisms involved in physiologic jaundice. The normal newborn produces an average of twice as much bilirubin as does an adult, because of higher concentrations of circulating erythrocytes (especially from stripping of cord blood at delivery) and a shorter life span of red blood cells (only 60 to 80 days in contrast to 120 days in the older child and adult). In addition the liver's ability to conjugate bilirubin is impaired because of a deficiency of the enzyme glucuronyl transferase.

Other factors are also partially responsible for the elevated bilirubin levels. Newborns have a lower plasma-binding capacity for bilirubin because of reduced albumin concentrations as compared to those of older children. The profound changes in hepatic circulation may represent a major hemodynamic shock, resulting in impaired liver function. At birth closure of the ductus venosus deprives the liver of the richly oxygenated blood supplied by the umbilical vein and makes it dependent on the poorly oxygenated portal venous blood. Marked improvement in bilirubin excretion by the fourth day may represent hepatic adjustment to extrauterine circulatory changes.[9]

Another cause of increased bilirubin load on the liver cell is the reabsorption of unconjugated bilirubin from the intestine. Normally conjugated bilirubin is reduced to urobilin by the intestinal flora and excreted in feces. However, the newborn's bowel is sterile, which prevents the conversion and excretion of bilirubin via this route. Consequently some unconjugated bilirubin is reabsorbed by the intestine and circulated back to the liver. The beneficial effect of lowering bilirubin levels by introducing early feedings may be related to this mechanism because feeding stimulates peristalsis and produces more rapid passage of meconium, thus diminishing the amount of reabsorption of unconjugated bilirubin, and introduces bacteria to aid in reduction of bilirubin to urobilinogen.[9]

Clinical manifestations. In full-term infants jaundice first appears after 24 hours. Bilirubin levels peak by the second to third day (mean bilirubin level, 6 mg/100 ml), rapidly decline by the fifth day, and slowly reach normal levels by the tenth day. In premature infants jaundice is initially evident by 48 hours. Bilirubin levels reach peak concentrations (10 to 12 mg/100 ml) by the fifth day and gradually return to normal by the end of the first month. Except for the icteric appearance, these infants are well.

The severity of physiologic jaundice differs markedly among different races. Infants of Oriental descent, including the American Indian, have mean bilirubin levels almost twice those seen in whites or blacks. In addition peoples from certain geographic areas, particularly areas around Greece, demonstrate an increased incidence of hyperbilirubinemia in newborns. The exact reasons for these differences are unclear but may include environmental factors, such as maternal ingestion of certain ethnic foods or a genetic predisposition for decelerated hepatic maturation.[2]

Medical management. The approaches toward treating physiologic jaundice vary. Some institutions favor the use of phototherapy for all jaundiced infants (serum bilirubin levels of 5 mg/100 ml or more). However, such therapy does not follow recommended criteria for phototherapy. The suggested protocol involves carefully monitoring serum bilirubin levels, investigating possible pathologic causes for hyperbilirubinemia in which serum bilirubin levels exceed 5 mg/100 ml during the first 24 hours, and identifying high-risk infants who may develop kernicterus with bilirubin levels near 15 mg/100 ml, such as premature neonates experiencing hypoxia and acidosis.

Initiation of feedings during the first 6 to 12 hours has also been advocated as a preventive measure. The type of feeding does not seem to influence bilirubin levels. The atypical response of some infants to develop unconjugated hyperbilirubinemia after breast-feeding does not affect physiologic jaundice. This acquired syndrome occurs during the second week of life. It results from a substance in breast milk that inhibits the hepatic enzyme glucuronyl transferase. Provided the infant is well, gains weight, and maintains bilirubin levels under 20 mg/100 ml, breast-feeding is not interrupted, since the jaundice will resolve spontaneously.

Nursing considerations. The primary nursing consideration is recognition of jaundice and differentiation of the physiologic type from pathologic causes. Part of the routine physical assessment includes observing for evidence of jaundice at regular intervals. Jaundice is most reliably assessed by observing the color of the sclera, nails, and skin, including palms, soles, and mucous membranes. Applying direct pressure to the skin, especially over bony prominences such as the tip of the nose or the sternum, causes blanching and allows the yellow stain to be more pronounced. For dark-skinned infants, the color of the sclera, conjunctiva, and oral mucosa is the most reliable indicator. The nurse observes the infant in natural daylight for a true assessment of color. Any neonate who becomes icteric during the first 24 hours of life and has rapidly rising bilirubin levels is referred to the physician for immediate evaluation.

For infants requiring phototherapy, nurses institute the same precautions both for the neonate and themselves as discussed under hemolytic disease. They institute breast- or formula-feeding as soon as possible after delivery. The significance of this type of jaundice is discussed with the parents, and they are assured of its benign nature. Since jaundice may still be evident the day of discharge, the nurse emphasizes that the yellow discoloration of the skin will completely disappear. It is also advisable to mention to breast-feeding mothers that the infant may remain jaundiced longer than bottle-fed infants but that feeding need not be interrupted, unless the jaundice persists beyond a week, in which case the physician should be notified.

Hemolytic disease of the newborn (erythroblastosis fetalis)

Hyperbilirubinemia occurs when large numbers of erythrocytes are hemolyzed, releasing excess quantities of unconjugated bilirubin. One of the major causes of increased erythrocyte destruction is isoimmunization, primarily Rh or ABO incompatibility. At one time Rh incompatibility was a leading cause of kernicterus and a significant cause of neonatal death. With the administration of Rh_0 immune globulin (RhoGAM)* to all unsensitized Rh-negative mothers after delivery or abortion of an Rh-positive infant or fetus, the incidence of this disease has been greatly reduced. Most cases of isoimmunization are now a result of ABO incompatibility, which is generally mild.

*Orthodiagnostics, Raritan, N.J.

Rh incompatibility

The Rh blood group, so named because of the experiments done in the rhesus monkey, consists of several antigens contained in or on the outer membrane of the erythrocyte. (An antigen is a substance capable of producing an immune response if recognized by the body as a foreign substance.) The Rh system consists of no less than eight gene complexes, some of which are designated C, D, E, c, d, e. The D antigen is the strongest and most common Rh antigen and is implicated in Rh incompatibility. The D and d alleles can genetically produce three genotypes—DD, Dd, and dd. The DD and Dd genotypes are Rh positive, which means that they contain D antigens; the dd genotype is Rh negative and, therefore, contains no antigen. In the white race 85% of the population are Rh positive and 15% are Rh negative. Only 5% to 7% of blacks and less than 1% of American Indians or persons of the Mongoloid race are Rh negative.

Incompatibility results when the fetus' blood group is Rh positive and the mother's is Rh negative. Such a situation can arise from mating of a homozygous Rh-positive male (DD) and an Rh-negative female (dd) in which case all the offspring will be heterozygous Rh positive (Dd). If the male is heterozygous Rh positive (Dd), half of the offspring will be heterozygous Rh positive (Dd) and the other half will be Rh negative (dd). Obviously if the male is Rh negative (dd), all the offspring will inherit the Rh-negative genes (dd) and no incompatibility will exist between fetus and mother.

Pathophysiology. In the presence of incompatibility, fetal red blood cells cross the placenta to the Rh-negative mother. Since her red blood cells lack the antigens present on the fetal erythrocytes, maternal antibodies are produced that destroy the fetal blood cells. If these antibodies are passed back through the placenta into the fetal circulation, hemolysis of fetal erythrocytes occurs.

Ordinarily this process of isoimmunization does not affect the fetus during the first pregnancy because the initial sensitization to D antigens does not occur prior to the onset of labor. However, as larger amounts of fetal blood are transferred to the maternal circulation during placental separation, maternal antibody production is stimulated. Therefore, during a second pregnancy, maternal antibodies to the fetus' Rh-positive blood are present and, as they enter the circulation, cause destruction of fetal erythrocytes (Fig. 9-2). Since the disease begins in utero, the fetus attempts to compensate for the progressive hemolysis by accelerating the rate of erythropoiesis. As a result immature red blood cells (erythroblasts) appear in the fetal circulation, hence the term "erythroblastosis fetalis."

There is a wide variability in the development of maternal sensitization to Rh-positive antigens. Sensitization may occur during the first pregnancy if the woman had previously received an Rh-positive blood transfusion. No sensitization may occur in situations where a strong placental barrier prevents transfer of fetal blood into the maternal circulation. In about 10% to 15% of sensitized mothers, there is no hemolytic reaction in the newborn.

Clinical manifestations. The clinical manifestations of Rh incompatibility result from the hemolysis of large numbers of erythrocytes (anemia) and the liver's inability to conjugate and excrete the excess bilirubin levels (hyper-

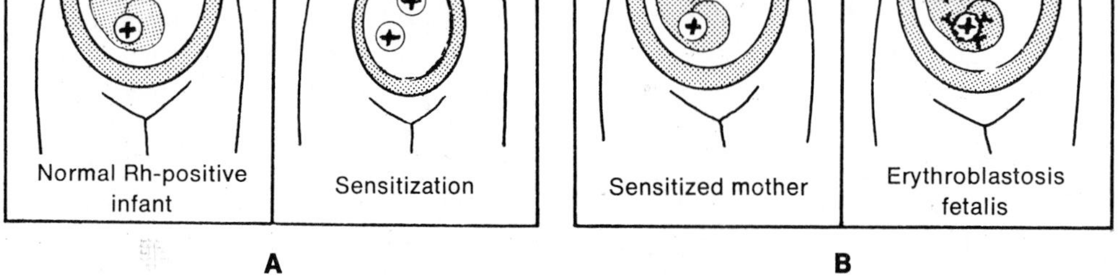

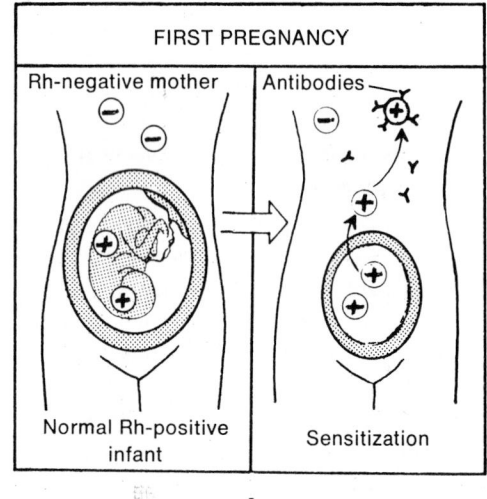

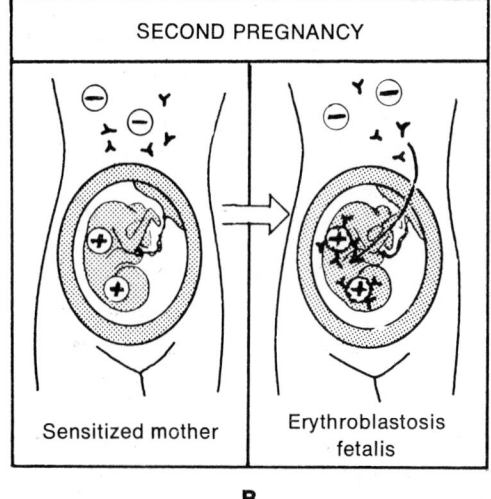

Fig. 9-2. Development of maternal sensitization to Rh antigens. **A,** Fetal Rh-positive erythrocytes enter the maternal system. Maternal anti-Rh antibodies are formed. **B,** Anti-Rh antibodies cross placental barrier and attack fetal erythrocytes. (From Whaley, L. F.: Understanding inherited disorders, St. Louis, 1974, The C. V. Mosby Co., p. 123.)

bilirubinemia, jaundice, and potentially kernicterus). The first visible indication of the severity of the disease may be the color of the amniotic fluid when the membranes break. Straw-colored fluid is associated with absent or mild fetal disease, deep yellow fluid is associated with severe disease, and green or brown-tinted fluid often signals a stillborn fetus (hydrops fetalis).[8]

Most erythroblastotic newborns are not icteric at birth because some of the unconjugated bilirubin has been transferred across the placenta to the maternal circulation. However, shortly after birth, jaundice (icterus neonatorum) is evident and unconjugated bilirubin levels rise rapidly. Hepatosplenomegaly may be evident because of the increased activity of these organs to compensate for the hemolysis by excessive production of erythroblasts. If the fetus is severely affected, signs of anemia—notably, marked pallor—are seen in the newborn. Since the hemolytic process continues after delivery, the anemia progressively worsens and represents additional hazards to the neonate because of the blood's decreased oxygen-carrying capacity and decreased blood volume, which predisposes to cardiac failure and shock.

The severest form of erythroblastosis fetalis results in *hydrops fetalis*. The progressive hemolysis causes fetal hypoxia, cardiac failure, generalized edema (anasarca), and effusions of the pericardial, pleural, and peritoneal spaces. The fetus may be delivered stillborn or in severe respiratory stress. Even with immediate exchange transfusions, few hydropic infants survive.

Diagnostic evaluation. Diagnosis of the disease before delivery is confirmed through amniocentesis and analysis of bilirubin levels in amniotic fluid. Increasing bilirubin levels indicate progressive fetal hemolysis and may indicate the need for an intrauterine transfusion or immediate termination of the pregnancy.

Erythroblastosis fetalis can also be assessed by evaluating rising anti-D antibody titers in the maternal circulation (indirect Coombs' test). The disease can be confirmed postnatally by detecting antibodies attached to the circulating erythrocytes of affected infants (direct Coombs' test).

Prevention. RhoGAM prevents the development of maternal sensitization to the Rh factor. When RhoGAM is given to unsensitized mothers within 48 hours after delivery or abortion, injected anti-D antibodies destroy the fetal erythrocytes passing into the maternal circulation before they are able to exert their immunogenic effect. To be effective, RhoGAM must be administered following the first delivery and repeated after subsequent ones. It is not effective against existing Rh-positive antibodies in the maternal circulation.

ABO incompatibility

Hemolytic disease can also occur when the major blood group antigens of the fetus are different from those of the mother. The major blood groups are A, B, AB, and O. The incidence of these blood groups varies according to race and geographic location. In the North American white population, 46% of the population have O blood group, 42% have A blood group, 9% have B blood group, and 3% have AB blood group. Persons with A blood group have antigen A on their red blood cells and anti-B antibodies in their serum; B blood group persons have antigen B on their red blood cells and anti-A antibodies in their serum. Individuals with AB blood group have both A and B antigens and no antibodies; they are referred to as universal recipients since they have no antibodies to attack antigens. Individuals with O blood group have no A or B antigens but possess both anti-A and anti-B antibodies. These persons are sometimes called universal donors because of the absence of antigens. Since the genes for type O are recessive to those for types A and B, an individual with A blood group can be genetically AA or AO (Table 9-1).

The presence or absence of antibodies and antigens determines whether agglutination will occur. Antibodies in the serum of one group (except AB blood group, which contains no antibodies) will produce an agglutination or clumping reaction when mixed with antigens of a different blood group. For example, if an individual with A blood group receives type-B blood, the donor's antibodies (anti-A) will be diluted in the recipient's circulation and cause little harm. However, the naturally occurring anti-B antibodies in the recipient's blood will cause agglutination of the donor's red blood cells. The agglutinated donor cells become trapped in the recipient's peripheral blood vessels. The cells then hemolyze, releasing large amounts of bilirubin into the circulation. Clinical manifestations of trans-

Table 9-1. ABO relationships of antigens/antibodies and donor-recipient compatibility

Blood group (phenotype	Genotype	Antigen	Antibody	Compatibility	
				As donor to type	As recipient from type
A	AA,AO	A	B	AB,A	O,A
B	BB,BO	B	A	AB,B	O,B
AB	AB	A and B	None	AB	O,A,B,AB
O	OO	None	A and B	AB,A,B,O	O

fusion reaction represent the pathophysiology of blocked blood vessels or released toxins into the vascular system. Renal shutdown is the most significant response and can cause death from kidney failure.

The most common blood group incompatibility in the neonate is between a mother with O blood group and infant with A or B blood group. (Other possible ABO incompatibilities are listed in Table 9-2). The naturally occurring anti-A or anti-B antibodies already present in the maternal circulation cross the placenta and attack the fetal red blood cells, causing hemolysis. Usually, however, the hemolytic reaction is less severe than in Rh incompatibility. Clinical manifestations are similar, such as jaundice during the initial 24 hours and enlarged liver and spleen, but severe anemia is rare. Laboratory evaluation and treatment of ABO reactions are also similar to that for Rh incompatibility. One fact that should be kept in mind is that since the anti-A or anti-B antibodies are naturally present in the serum, the number of pregnancies is insignificant in the development of ABO incompatibility.

Medical management. The aim of treatment in any blood group incompatibility is to reverse the hemolytic process. Exchange transfusion, in which the infant's blood is removed in small amounts (usually 10 to 20 ml at a time) and replaced with compatible blood (such as Rh-negative blood) is the treatment of choice. Exchange transfusion removes the sensitized erythrocytes, lowers the serum bilirubin to prevent kernicterus, corrects the anemia, and prevents cardiac failure. Indications for exchange transfusion include a positive direct Coombs' test, hemoglobin concentration of cord blood below 12 g/100 ml, and a bilirubin level of 20 mg/100 ml in the full-term infant or 15 mg/100 ml in the premature infant. An infant born with hydrops fetalis or signs of cardiac failure is an immediate candidate for exchange transfusion.

In exchange transfusion, fresh whole blood is used. It is typed and cross-matched to the mother's serum. The amount of donor blood used is usually double the blood volume of the infant, which is about 85 mg/kg, but no more than 500 ml is used. The two-volume exchange transfusion will replace approximately 85% of the neonate's blood, eliminating the bilirubin in the plasma but eliminating less effectively the bilirubin in the tissues. As a rule, serum bilirubin is about 50% lower than its preexchange level but may rise because of the migration of stored pigment in the tissues to the vascular system. Although the hemolytic process may have been reversed by the initial transfusion, the danger of kernicterus may still be present, necessitating repeated exchange transfusions.

An exchange transfusion is a sterile surgical procedure. The umbilicus is cut and a catheter is inserted into the umbilical vein and threaded into the inferior vena cava. Depending on the infant's weight, 5 to 20 ml of blood is withdrawn within 15 to 20 seconds, and the same volume of donor blood is infused over 60 to 90 seconds. If the blood has been citrated (the addition of acid citrate dextrose [ACD] to prevent coagulation), calcium gluconate may be given after infusion of each 100 ml of donor's blood. Calcium gluconate prevents hypocalcemia, which may result when the serum calcium binds with the acid citrate dextrose, making the calcium nonionizable.

Phototherapy may be used in conjunction with exchange transfusion but is not recommended for treatment of Rh incompatibility because the rate of hemolysis usually exceeds the rate of bilirubin diminution caused by photo-oxidation.[8] If used immediately following the initial exchange transfusion, phototherapy increases the rate of bilirubin removal from the tissues and may avert the need for repeated transfusions. It is indicated in ABO incompatibility when serum bilirubin levels are above 10 mg/100 ml but are below levels indicative of exchange transfusion and when anemia is absent or mild.

Nursing considerations. The initial objective is similar to that discussed under physiologic jaundice, namely early identification of jaundice and rising bilirubin levels in order to diagnose pathologic causes for the condition. Much of the nursing care of the severely jaundiced neonate is related to the treatments used to lower the bilirubin levels and reverse the hemolytic process. In instances in which blood incompatibility is suspected, the nurse keeps the cord moist with a sterile saline-soaked dressing to preserve the umbilical veins for exchange transfusion.

Exchange transfusions. Besides assisting the physician during the initial stages of the procedure, the nurse keeps accurate records of blood volumes exchanged, including amount of blood withdrawn and infused, time of each procedure, and cumulative record of the total volume exchanged. Vital signs that are monitored electronically are evaluated frequently and correlated with removal and infusion of blood. If signs of restlessness or cardiac arrhythmias occur, rate of infusion is slowed. Throughout the procedure the nurse attends to the infant's thermoregulation needs. He should be kept under a radiant warmer, and blankets should be available if he suddenly becomes chilled. Hypothermia (cold stress) increases oxygen and glucose consumption, causing metabolic acidosis. Not only do these consequences hinder the infant's overall physical ability to withstand the long procedure, but they also inhibit the binding capacity of albumin and bilirubin and the hepatic enzymatic reactions, thus increasing the risk of kernicterus. Conversely hyperthermia damages the donor

Table 9-2. Potential maternal-fetal ABO incompatibilities

Maternal blood group	Fetal blood group
O	A or B
B	A or AB
A	B or AB

erythrocytes, elevating the free potassium content and predisposing the infant to cardiac arrest.

Throughout the procedure the nurse observes for signs of exchange transfusion reactions and institutes appropriate interventions (Table 9-3). In addition all the principles of intravenous therapy are observed, namely, maintenance of a sterile, closed system to prevent air emboli and infection. After the procedure is completed, the nurse inspects the umbilical site for evidence of bleeding. Usually the catheter remains in place for use during repeated exchanges. A sterile dressing is applied and checked periodically for evidence of bleeding or infection.

Table 9-3. Possible complications of exchange transfusion

Reaction	Cause	Nursing intervention
Heart failure	Hypervolemia from too rapid infusion of blood or excessive replacement	Infuse blood slowly Keep accurate records of blood withdrawn and replaced Monitor vital signs
Cardiac arrest	Hyperkalemia (from hemolysis of old red blood cells)	Use only fresh blood whenever possible Keep blood refrigerated until ready to use Do not force blood through catheter (causes lysis of red blood cells)
Cardiac arrhythmias	Forceful injection of infused blood causes myocardial irritation	Reduce rate of infusion
Bradycardia	Too rapid infusion of calcium gluconate causes acute hypercalcemia Hypocalcemia may occur when citrated blood is given but calcium is not replaced	Infuse calcium gluconate slowly, observe for slowing of the heart rate following the procedure Observe for signs of tetany and cardiac arrhythmias; notify physician
Acidemia	Results when fresh blood is not used because donor red blood cells continue anaerobic glycolysis, resulting in production of acid metabolites	Check pH of blood before administration (should be corrected to pH of 7.1) Observe for signs of metabolic acidosis: deep rapid breathing, decreased consciousness, acid urine
Intestinal perforation (peritonitis)	Results from ischemia of the bowel, especially when catheter is threaded into portal vein; withdrawal of blood disrupts vascular pressure in the intestine, thereby decreasing blood flow and causing ischemia, necrosis, and potentially perforation	Observe for signs of perforation and peritonitis: bloody stools, bile-stained vomitus, abdominal distention, respiratory distress, hypotension, pallor, cyanosis Report signs immediately to physician (condition diagnosed by x-ray examination and corrected surgically)
Thrombocytopenia, hemorrhage	Use of overheparinized blood Use of citrated blood without calcium replacement	Observe for bleeding at catheter site Observe for evidence of petechiae (need to inspect skin carefully to note petechiae in presence of jaundice)
Hemolytic reaction	Use of mismatched donor blood	Check donor's blood type and group against infant's blood with physician prior to administration (see also Table 36-2, p. 1387)
Air emboli	Air may enter catheter when tubing is first inserted or if blood is allowed to completely infuse before turning stopcock to "off" position or to alternate saline infusion	Fill catheter with sterile normal saline solution prior to insertion Switch stopcock to alternate position before blood is completely infused Maintain closed system
Hypothermia	Infusion of cold blood	Allow blood to warm to at least room temperature before beginning infusion Run tubing from blood container through warm water bath to infant Keep infant under radiant warmer during procedure Have warmed blankets available in case of chilling
Hypoglycemia	Occurs in erythoblastosis fetalis independent of exchange transfusion Aggravated by fasting state maintained in infant prior to (3-4 hours) and during procedure	Maintain regular intravenous infusions of 5% dextrose Check blood for glucose (Dextrostix) hourly after procedure for at least 2-4 hours

Phototherapy. Several precautions are instituted to protect the nurse and infant during phototherapy. The infant's eyes are shielded by an opaque mask to prevent exposure to the light. The nurse ensures that the infant's eyelids are closed prior to applying the mask, since the corneas may become excoriated if they come in contact with the dressing. On each shift the eyes are checked for evidence of discharge, excessive pressure on the lids, or corneal irritation. If the shield allows light to enter, the area of jaundice around the eyes will be disappearing; this alerts the nurse to the need for better eye protection. The eye shield should also be properly sized and correctly positioned to prevent any occlusion of the nares.

The infant is placed nude under the fluorescent light since phototherapy must come in contact with the skin surfaces to be effective. The infant is turned frequently to expose all areas to the light. Areas that are protected from the light retain their jaundiced appearance. When the infant is placed in a supine or side-lying position, the testes are covered with a diaper (a string-type disposable face mask makes a suitable string bikini) to prevent these organs from possible damage. In some institutions a stockinette is used to cover the infant's head, although this is controversial.

Frequently the phototherapy unit is combined with a radiant heat warmer or servocontrolled incubator to provide an optimally regulated thermal environment. The thermistor should be attached to the infant in such a way that it is not exposed to direct radiation. This requires changing the sensor from the abdomen to the back according to the infant's position. Vital signs are taken at least every 4 hours to ensure that the infant's body temperature is normothermic. Sometimes it is necessary to regulate the temperature in the Isolette to maintain proper body heat.

Infants who are in an open crib should have a protective Plexiglas shield between them and the fluorescent lights to minimize the amount of undesirable ultraviolet light reaching their skin and to protect them from accidental bulb breakage. Their temperature must be closely monitored to prevent hyperthermia and, less often, hypothermia.

Phototherapy should not interfere with parental visiting. The parents should be encouraged to hold and feed their infant, during which time the lights are turned off and the infant's eye shields are removed. The nurse notes the times that phototherapy is started and stopped, including intervals when no light was applied, and also charts (1) the proper shielding of the eyes and testes, (2) the type of fluorescent lamp (by manufacturer), (3) the number of lamps, (4) the distance between surface of lamps and infant, and (5) the use of phototherapy in combination with an Isolette or open bassinet. A record should also be kept of the total hours used since bulb replacement.[1]

At the present time the long-term risks from phototherapy are not known. However, minor side effects do occur and should be observed for and recorded. These include loose greenish stools, hyperthermia, increased metabolic rate, increased evaporative loss of water, and priapism. The nurse observes for dehydration and drying of the skin, which can lead to excoriation and breakdown. These infants require up to 25% additional fluid volume to compensate for insensible and intestinal fluid loss.[2]

Another reaction to phototherapy is the "bronze-baby syndrome," in which the serum, urine, and skin become blackish brown in color several hours after the infant is placed under the light. The cause for this response is not known, although it almost always occurs in infants who have elevated conjugated hyperbilirubinemia. It is postulated that it may represent a benign cosmetic response, a sign of hepatocellular disease, an inborn error of metabolism, or an unusual toxicity to phototherapy.[2]

The effects of phototherapy on personnel working directly with the infant are also unknown. However, safety measures for nurses include wearing dark glasses to protect their eyes and a cap or bandana over their hair to prevent scorching of hair strands from contact with the bulbs (Fig. 9-3). Some facial tanning may also occur from continuous exposure to the light.

The effectiveness of phototherapy is determined by a decrease in bilirubin levels, usually a fall of 3 to 4 mg/100 ml after 8 to 12 hours of therapy. One must be careful to assess the infant's total physical status because the suppression of jaundice may mask signs of sepsis, hemolytic disease, or hepatitis. Although the bilirubin levels may be controlled in mild erythroblastosis fetalis, the hemolysis may continue, causing severe anemia.

Frequently in cases of blood group incompatibility, the parents are aware of the potential danger to their child, especially in cases of Rh incompatibility in which the initial birth was not treated with RhoGAM. Parents need constant reassurance concerning their infant's progress. All the procedures should be explained to them so that they are aware of the benefits and risks. For example, they need to be reassured that the naked infant who is under the bilirubin light is warm and comfortable. Parents may be concerned about the blindfolds since "blindness" is a frightening experience. However, the neonate is used to darkness after the uterine existence and benefits a great deal from auditory and tactile stimulation. Parents frequently feel guilty because they think they have caused the blood incompatibility. Parents should never be made to feel responsible or negligent. They should be encouraged to verbalize and express their thoughts. Actions they did to prevent any problems, such as frequent antepartum examinations and blood tests, should be supported and praised.

Unless kernicterus develops, most infants recover satisfactorily following hemolytic disease. They can usually be fed by the parents' method of choice, including breast-feeding. If several exchange transfusions were performed, oral supplemental ferrous sulfate therapy may be begun at 2 to 3

A

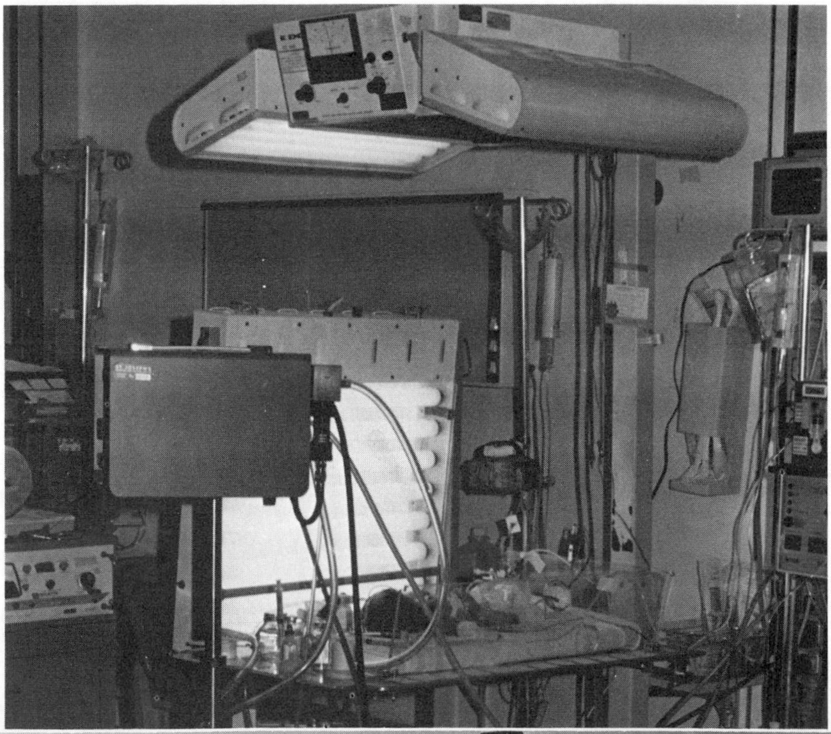

B

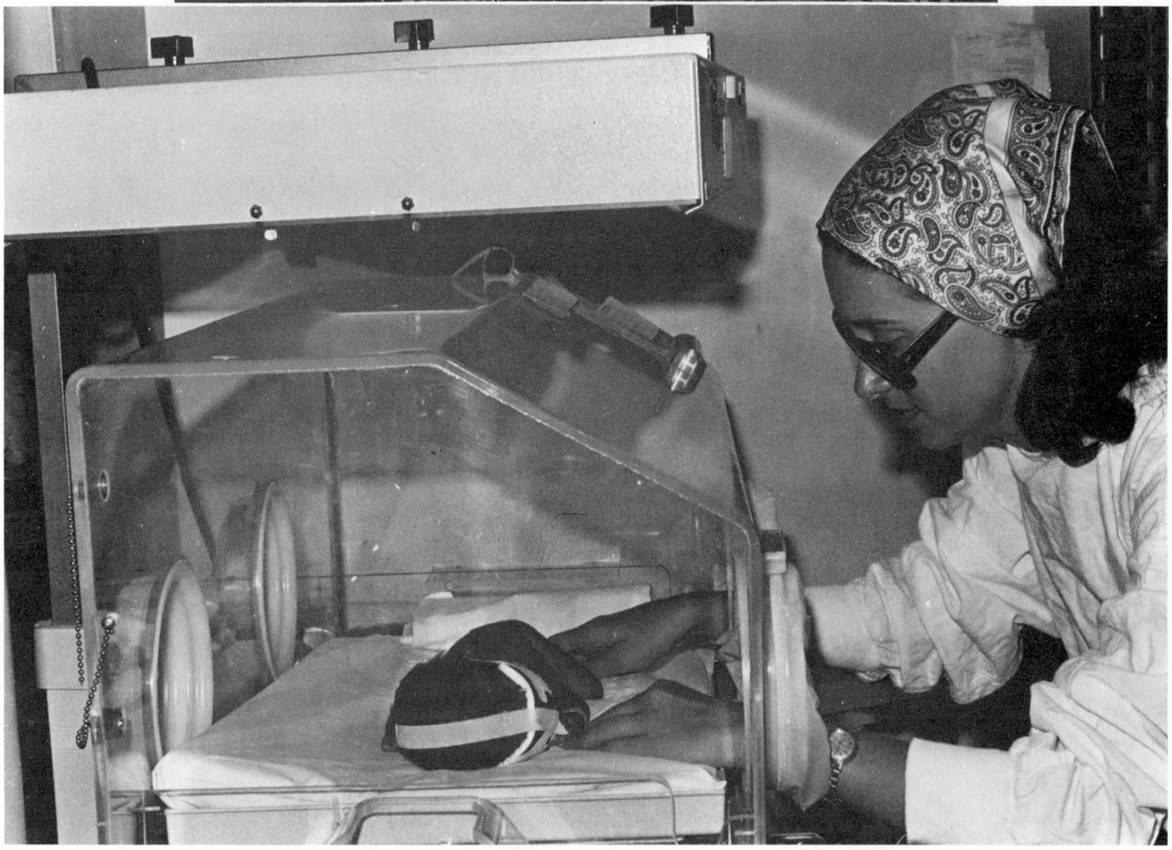

Fig. 9-3. A, Phototherapy unit combined with radiant heat warmer. Note the lateral position of the bilirubin lights to increase the intensity of phototherapy. **B,** The nurse is wearing protective dark glasses and a hair covering while caring for an infant who is under the phototherapy lights.

Summary of nursing care of the neonate with hyperbilirubinemia

Goals	Responsibilities
Prevent neonatal jaundice	Introduce feedings early
Prevent blood incompatibility	Encourage pregnant women to seek early antepartal care Determine blood group and Rh type Carefully follow all Rh-negative pregnant women with possibility of Rh-positive fetus for rising bilirubin levels (amniocentesis, indirect Coombs' test) Administer RhoGAM to Rh-negative women at delivery or time of abortion
Identify infants at risk for hyperbilirubinemia and kernicterus	Observe color of amniotic fluid at time of rupture of membranes Observe for evidence of jaundice, anemia, and central nervous system irritability Refer infant with signs of jaundice and rising bilirubin levels during first 24 hours to physician Be aware of conditions (acidosis, hypoxia, hypothermia, and so on) that increase the risk of kernicterus at lower bilirubin levels
Assist in medical therapies Phototherapy	Shield infant's eyes; check that lids are closed prior to applying shield; check eyes each shift for drainage or irritation Place infant nude under light but cover testes when positioned supine Change position frequently Monitor body temperature; check axial or rectal temperature with reading on servocontrolled unit Ensure that protective Plexiglas shield separates infant from lights Chart duration of therapy, type of lights, distance of lights to infant, use of open or closed bassinet, and shielding of infant's eyes and testes
Exchange transfusions	Give infant nothing by mouth prior to procedure (usually for 3 to 4 hours) Check donor blood with physician for correct blood group and Rh type Assist physician during procedure; ensure asepsis Keep accurate records of amounts of blood infused and withdrawn Monitor vital signs, especially following infusion of calcium gluconate Maintain optimal body temperature of infant during procedure (blankets, radiant warmer) Observe for signs of exchange transfusion reactions (Table 9-3) Have resuscitative equipment (supplemental oxygen, airway, AMBU bag, endotracheal tube, and laryngoscope) at bedside Apply sterile dressing to catheter site
Observe for complications Kernicterus	Observe for signs of central nervous system depression (lethargy, diminished or absent reflexes, hypotonia, poor sucking reflex) or excitation (irritability, tremors, convulsions, high-pitched cry, opisthotonos)
Phototherapy	Observe for hyperthermia, signs of dehydration, loose stools, priapism, and "bronze-baby" syndrome
Exchange transfusions	Check umbilical site for bleeding or infection Monitor vital signs following transfusion Observe for signs of kernicterus
Practice personal safeguards during phototherapy	Wear sunglasses when caring for infant during exposure to lights Wear hat or bandana to protect hair from scorching

Summary of nursing care of the neonate with hyperbilirubinemia—cont'd

Goals	Responsibilities
Provide emotional support to parents	Explain reason for jaundice Discontinue phototherapy during parental visiting; remove infant's eye shields
Neonatal jaundice	Emphasize benign nature of condition Assure parents that skin will regain normal pigmentation Advise breast-feeding mothers of possibility of prolonged jaundice
Blood incompatibility	Explain therapies to parents Reassure parents during various procedures Allow parents to express any feelings regarding their "causing" the blood incompatibility Reinforce parents' previous attempts to provide optimal care for their infant, such as frequent antepartal checkups
Plan for follow-up, especially if bilirubin levels approached 20 mg/100 ml in full-term neonate	Encourage parents to report the perinatal history during subsequent infant assessments, especially when the child is seen by unfamiliar health personnel Plan for early developmental and hearing assessment Check blood during first 2 months for evidence of anemia and need for supplemental iron

months of age for about 2 months. The infant should be observed frequently during the first few months for any sign of anemia. If kernicterus has occurred, the infant should be periodically assessed for sensorineural hearing loss, cerebral damage, or developmental lag. Nurses in ambulatory settings should be aware of the need for early auditory, neurologic, and developmental testing of these infants during their well-child care. (See boxed material for summary of nursing care of the neonate with hyperbilirubinemia.)

PROBLEMS RELATED TO ENVIRONMENTAL AGENTS

Hypocalcemia and neonatal tetany

Etiology. Several factors affect the development of low serum calcium in the neonate. Probably the most significant factor in neonatal hypocalcemia is decreased activity of the parathyroid gland, which normally controls the excretion of phosphorus and calcium. In the newborn the feedback system of the parathyroid gland is suppressed because of increased levels of parathyroid hormone (parathormone) from maternal sources. Difficulty usually arises when large amounts of phosphorus are ingested. However, the actual amount of phosphorus is less important than the calcium-phosphorus ratio. In cow's milk formula, such as evaporated milk, the higher phosphate load occurs because of the lower calcium:phosphorus ratio (1.35:1) as compared to human milk (2.25:1).[4] (Commercially prepared formulas have adjusted calcium:phosphorus ratios, which approximate human milk.) As phosphate levels increase, calcium is excreted because of the decreased parathyroid hormone and immature functioning of the renal tubules for phosphorus clearance. Normally parathyroid hormone would cause increased excretion of phosphate through the kidneys and increased reabsorption of calcium from the renal tubules.

Several factors increase the risk of hypocalcemia and tetany. Exchange transfusions cause hypocalcemia because of the addition of the anticoagulant citrate, which combines with the serum calcium so that the calcium becomes nonionizable. Without the presence of ionizable calcium, the coagulation process cannot occur. During exchange transfusions, 10% calcium gluconate is administered in order to replace this loss and prevent hypocalcemia. Stress, such as perinatal asphyxia, results in lowered serum calcium levels because of increased corticosteroid and thyrocalcitonin secretion, which has the opposite effect on calcium as parathyroid hormone. Treatment of acidosis with bicarbonate also decreases the ionized portion of serum calcium. Hypocalcemia occurs frequently in infants born of diabetic mothers. Prematurity is another common cause of decreased serum calcium. When hypocalcemia occurs during the first 24 to 48 hours of life, clinical signs are usually not characteristic of tetany but include such manifestations as edema, apnea, intermittent cyanosis, vomiting, and abdominal distention. It is often very difficult to recognize that such symptoms are indicative of hypocalcemia, since other pathophysiologic changes frequently occur in these infants as well.

Clinical manifestations. Classical neonatal tetany usually appears after cow's milk feedings between the fifth and tenth days of life. Symptoms represent increased nervous system excitability because a decreased extracellular fluid concentration of calcium increases neuronal membrane permeability. Clinical manifestations include twitching, tremors, exaggerated Moro response, restlessness, high-pitched cry, and focal or generalized convulsions. The symptoms, especially convulsions, may be more pronounced when the infant is handled, such as during feedings. In older children laryngospasm and carpopedal spasms (muscle spasms of the hands and feet) are common. However, such signs are rare in newborns.

Eliciting *Trousseau's sign* by occluding blood flow to the wrist for 3 minutes may be helpful in identifying latent tetany. A positive Trousseau's sign is indicated by palmar flexion. *Chvostek's sign* may not be helpful because it is usually positive in the neonate. It is demonstrated by the nurse tapping sharply over the facial nerve below the temple and anterior to the ear; the sign is positive when twitching of the mouth, nose, and eye occurs.

Diagnostic evaluation. Diagnosis should be confirmed with serum electrolyte determinations. Serum calcium values are usually 8 to 10 mg/100 ml (4 to 5 mEq/liter). Hypocalcemia in the full-term neonate is indicated at levels below 7 mg/100 ml (3.5 mEq/liter). About 30% of preterm newborns weighing less than 2000 g (4 pounds, 6.5 ounces) have serum calcium levels under 7 mg/100 ml during the first 2 days of life. In neonatal tetany there will be a corresponding hyperphosphatemia of above 8 mg/100 ml. Normal values range from 4.0 to 6.5 mg/100 ml, although up to 8 mg/100 ml is considered normal in the newborn.

Medical management. Treatment of neonatal tetany involves intravenous administration of 10% calcium gluconate, which must be administered slowly, usually over a period of 5 minutes, to prevent nausea, vomiting, bradycardia, and circulatory collapse. If the heart rate falls below 100 beats/minute, the injection should be immediately discontinued. It is advisable to monitor the heart rate electronically. After the normal rate has resumed for at least 30 minutes, the drug can be reinitiated. Care must be taken to ascertain that the needle is positioned within the vein because extravasation into surrounding tissue causes local calcification and sloughing. Intramuscular administration of calcium gluconate is contraindicated because it precipitates in the tissue, causing necrosis.

As soon as feasible, oral doses of calcium are given with formula feedings. Calcium gluconate, chloride, or lactate may be given. Calcium chloride is the most effective preparation, but it causes gastric irritation and vomiting. It should be given in concentrations of less than 2% in the formula and discontinued after 2 days, to be replaced by another calcium salt.

Nursing considerations. Ideally neonatal tetany can be prevented by counseling postpartal women about the advantages of breast-feeding or using commercially prepared formulas. Unfortunately the expense of the latter method may prevent families in lower socioeconomic levels from using them.

Since neonatal tetany typically occurs during the fifth to tenth days of life, it is rarely seen in the nursery. Nurses working in emergency rooms, ambulatory clinics, or physician's offices are more likely to see infants with symptoms of this disorder. A careful history regarding feeding practices is important in distinguishing neonatal hypocalcemia from other conditions that have similar symptoms, such as hypoglycemia or sepsis.

After the diagnosis of neonatal tetany is made, the child is hospitalized for calcium replacement therapy. Since intravenous calcium gluconate can cause tissue necrosis and scar formation, it is recommended that the scalp veins be avoided. The nurse should be familiar with the causes of necrosis, mainly, prolonged use of the same needle site, excessive movement of the needle in the vein, which allows slight leakage during infusion, and sudden extravasation of fluid into the tissues during removal of the needle. To prevent necrosis the infusion site should be changed frequently (ideally every 12 hours).[10] The nurse ensures that the needle is firmly secured by tape to the skin and during removal applies gentle pressure at the puncture site for at least 1 minute.

The nurse also observes for signs of acute hypercalcemia (nausea, vomiting, and bradycardia). If such symptoms occur the injection or infusion is discontinued and the physician is notified.

Since convulsions are common, the nurse institutes seizure precautions. Minor stimuli, such as picking the infant up for a feeding or a sudden jarring of the crib, can provoke tremors or seizures. During the acute phase the environment is manipulated to allow for maximal rest and minimal activity around the infant.

If the infant is discharged on formula feedings supplemented with calcium salts, the nurse teaches the parents the correct procedure for diluting the mineral in the formula. The possibility of changing to commercial formulas can also be discussed with the parents, although this is not essential. Since oral calcium may result in more frequent bowel movements, the parents are made aware of this fact to prevent their associating this change with diarrhea or another gastrointestinal disorder.

Once the diagnosis is made, the nurse reassures the parents that the condition is a result of nutritional imbalance of the formula. Since the restlessness, irritability, and convulsive activity of the infant are usually of much concern to the parents, the nurse supports them during the hospitalization and emphasizes that the condition will subside rapidly with no consequent ill effects. Since handling the infant stimulates neurologic excitement, the nurse discusses with the parents the necessity of not disturbing the infant. As soon as calcium levels rise, the nurse encourages the parents to hold and feed the infant in order to reestablish or promote parent-child attachment.

Neonatal hypoglycemia

The fetus receives glucose supplies from the maternal blood through the process of facilitated diffusion. During the last trimester of pregnancy, glycogen, the stored form of glucose, is deposited in the liver, heart, and skeletal muscle. At birth hepatic glycogen stores are twice the adult concentration, cardiac glycogen stores are ten times those found in the adult, and skeletal muscle glycogen stores are about four times the adult concentration.

At birth the infant must rely on the glycogen stores and exogenous sources of glucose. Any condition that decreased the glycogen stores in utero, such as malnutrition or preterm birth, will compromise the infant's ability to withstand extrauterine stress. The normal physiologic exertion of respiration, thermoregulation, and muscular activity rapidly depletes the glycogen stores in the normal full-term neonate. In fact approximately 90% of liver glycogen is utilized for these activities by the third hour after birth. Any abnormal physical exertion such as respiratory distress, asphyxia, or hypothermia will profoundly deplete the infant's reserve for energy expenditure. Fetal glycogen stores may also be depleted during a prolonged labor and/or difficult delivery, especially if the mother did not receive supplemental glucose.

In addition the liver's ability for gluconeogenesis is decreased. As the blood sugar level falls, the liver is unable to convert amino acids into glucose. As a result fat is used as the principal source of energy. In the preterm neonate, whose subcutaneous fat stores are deficient, the body is quickly deprived of this substrate for energy. The full-term infant usually has adequate sources of energy for the first 2 to 3 days of life.

Etiology. There are several main causes of hypoglycemia in the neonate. The first is a decreased amount of glycogen stores because of intrauterine malnutrition. Infants who are likely to be affected by this deficiency are premature, postmature, or small-for-gestational-age (SGA) infants, the smaller of a pair of twins, and infants born of toxemic mothers. Small-for-gestational-age infants also suffer from hypoglycemia because of increased numbers of cells per unit weight. The brain, which is an active consumer of glucose for energy, is relatively normal in size, whereas other organs, such as the liver, are proportionately smaller in size. For example, in the full-term infant the brain weighs three times as much as the liver, but in the premature infant the brain is five to seven times heavier than the liver.

Another cause of hypoglycemia is increased utilization of blood glucose, which occurs when the infant is subjected to physiologic stresses such as hypothermia, respiratory distress syndrome, cerebral trauma, or fetal asphyxia. Hypoglycemia may also be induced iatrogenically, such as during exchange transfusions, when the infant is deprived of oral feedings. Physiologic mechanisms that occur in diseases such as erythroblastosis fetalis and maternal diabetes mellitus also cause hypoglycemia. The latter will be discussed in detail in Chapter 10. Metabolic disorders such as glycogen storage disease and galactosemia also induce low blood glucose.

Clinical manifestations. The symptoms attributable to hypoglycemia are usually vague and are very similar to other conditions such as hypocalcemia, septicemia, central nervous system disorders, or cardiorespiratory problems. Because the brain is dependent on glucose for energy, cerebral signs such as jitteriness, tremors, twitches, weak or high-pitched cry, lethargy, limpness, apathy, convulsions, and coma are common. Other clinical manifestations include cyanosis, apnea, rapid and irregular respirations, sweating, eye rolling, and refusal to feed. Symptoms usually appear between 24 and 72 hours of age. Severely distressed infants may demonstrate signs of hypoglycemia within 6 hours after birth. Frequently the symptoms are transient but recurrent.

Diagnostic evaluation. Diagnosis must be confirmed by direct analysis of blood glucose concentration. Two specimens of blood should be analyzed because of the many factors that can affect correct readings. Proper handling of the specimen is essential because storage at room temperature increases glycolysis; glucose concentration decreases approximately 15 to 18 mg/100 ml/hour. Accurate readings can be facilitated by storing the blood sample in ice or removing the red blood cells by centrifugation.

Blood sugar level may also be determined with a Dextrostix test. A drop of blood from the heel placed on a special Dextrostix paper causes the paper to change color, indicating glucose concentration. Although a simple procedure, it is a very sensitive test and must be done correctly to avoid false readings. For example, the blood must remain on the dipstick for exactly 1 minute and then be compared to the color chart. Inaccurate timing will produce varying stages of the reaction. Color changes that indicate a blood glucose level of less than 45 mg/100 ml should be confirmed by a laboratory analysis of whole blood. Since hypoglycemia is a potential hazard in premature neonates, routine Dextrostix determinations should be done at least twice during the first 24 hours of life and usually more frequently for the next 2 to 3 days.

Blood glucose concentrations may range from 30 to 125 mg/100 ml in the full-term neonate and from 20 to 100 mg/100 ml in the premature infant. Hypoglycemia is generally indicated by:

1. Levels below 30 mg/100 ml in full-term infants during the first 72 hours of life

2. Levels below 40 mg/100 ml in full-term infants after the first 3 days of life
3. Levels below 20 mg/100 ml in premature neonates.[4]

Hyperglycemia is suggested at levels above 125 mg/100 ml in the full-term neonate.

Medical management. Prevention of hypoglycemia involves initiation of early feeding in newborns. Breast-fed infants should be put to breast as soon as possible after delivery. Colostrum, the precursor of breast milk, contains greater quantities of protein, minerals, and vitamin A and lesser quantities of lactose and fat than does later breast milk and provides adequate nutrition for the infant. Bottle-fed infants should be offered 5% to 10% glucose and sterile water as early as 2 hours after birth, especially if hypoglycemia is suspected, such as in premature infants. Before offering glucose or formula feedings, the nurse should begin with plain sterile water to ascertain patency of the esophagus in order to prevent aspiration of a hypertonic solution.

In cases of more severe hypoglycemia, parenteral infusion of glucose is indicated. Exact therapy for glucose administration varies but usually initially includes a dose of 2 to 4 ml/kg of body weight of a 10% to 25% dextrose solution. This is followed by a continuous 10% to 15% glucose solution at a rate that supplies 65 to 75 ml/kg of body weight per 24 hours. In situations where this therapy does not stabilize blood glucose concentration, steroids, which stimulate gluconeogenesis in the liver, may be given.

Nursing considerations. Much of the nursing responsibility of the hypoglycemic infant involves identification of the problem through careful observation of physical status. Another area of concern is to decrease those environmental factors that predispose to the development of decreased blood glucose, such as cold stress and respiratory difficulty. Proper feeding technique of the breast-fed or bottle-fed infant promotes adequate ingestion of nutrients, particularly carbohydrates.

Preventing, anticipating, and recognizing potential dangers of concentrated dextrose infusion is also a major nursing objective. Too rapid infusion of the hypertonic solution can cause circulatory overload, hyperglycemia, and intracellular dehydration. Maintaining the ordered flow rate decreases such hazards. If the intravenous transfusion has been temporarily discontinued, the nurse should not try to "catch up" or make up for the lost fluid during the interruption.

The infusion should be administered through a large vein to increase hemodilution of the concentrated solution and to prevent irritation of the vessel walls. Extravasation of the fluid into the surrounding area can cause sloughing of the tissues. Termination of the glucose solution must be gradual in order to prevent hypoglycemia caused by hyperinsulinism.

Hypoglycemia is frequently a symptom of some other underlying pathophysiologic process. Parents are usually very concerned over their infant's progress, particularly since these infants do not feed well or behave responsively. Nurses need to be aware of parents' thoughts, should allow ventilation and expression of feelings, and must keep parents aware of the infant's progress. Since neonatal hypoglycemia usually occurs fairly soon after delivery, the mother may find it difficult to visit the nursery and appreciates others keeping her informed of the infant's condition. In hospitals where there are separate nursing staffs for each area of obstetrics, communication is frequently a problem and may result in avoidance of the parents by the postpartum staff and resultant anger and frustration on the part of the parents. Realizing that such a vicious cycle can occur is part of the implementation of the solution to the problem.

Sepsis

Sepsis or septicemia refers to a generalized bacterial infection in the bloodstream. Neonates are susceptible to infection because they have diminished nonspecific (inflammatory) and specific (humoral) immunity, namely impaired phagocytosis, delayed chemotactic response, minimal or absent IgA and IgM, and decreased complement levels (see also p. 342). Because of the poor response to pathogenic agents, there is usually no local inflammatory reaction at the portal of entry to signal an infection and the resulting symptoms tend to be vague and nonspecific. Consequently diagnosis and treatment may be delayed.

The frequency of infection is almost twice as great in male infants as in females and carries a higher mortality rate for the former sex as well. Other factors increasing the risk of infection are prematurity (see p. 342) and bottle-feeding, which can introduce pathogens from environmental contamination. Breast-feeding has a protective benefit against infection. Colostrum contains agglutinins that are effective against gram-negative bacteria. Human milk contains large quantities of iron-binding protein that exert a bacteriostatic effect on *Escherichia coli*. Human milk also contains macrophages and lymphocytes that promote a local inflammatory reaction.[2]

Before the use of antibiotics, mortality rates approached 90% from sepsis. With the use of antibiotics, mortality rates have decreased considerably and are presently in the range of 13% to 45%, depending on the infecting organism. However, the incidence of septicemia has not diminished. Nursery epidemics are not infrequent, and the high-risk infant is more than four times in danger of developing septicemia than is the normal neonate.

Source of infection. Several modes of transmission contribute to the potential occurrence of septicemia. In utero the fetus may contract an organism from amnionitis, infection of the amniotic fluid. The fetus may aspirate the infected fluid, resulting in congenital pneumonia and sepsis. Prolonged rupture of the membranes always presents a risk of this type from maternal-fetal transfer of pathogenic organisms. In utero transplantal transfer of organisms can occur, such as *Treponema pallidum* (syphilis), which crosses the placenta during the latter half of pregnancy.

During birth, infection can occur as the infant descends through the birth canal. The most common infecting organism is *E. coli,* which may be present in the vagina from fecal contamination. *E. coli* accounts for about two thirds of all cases of sepsis caused by gram-negative organisms. Proper hygiene of the perineum is one method of preventing this mode of transmission. Other pathogens that are harbored in the vagina and that may infect the infant include gonococcus, *Candida albicans,* herpes simplex virus (type II), *Listeria,* and β-hemolytic streptococcus.

The infant is at risk for self-infection because of the proximity of the umbilical wound to the perineum. Bacterial invasion can also occur through sites other than the umbilical stump, such as the skin, mucous membranes of the eye, nose, pharynx, and ear, and internal systems such as respiratory, nervous, urinary, and gastrointestinal.

Another major mode of bacterial transmission is through the environment. Bacteria that are frequently called "water bugs" because they are able to grow in water and cause disease in infants are found in water supplies, humidifying apparatus, sink drains, suction machines, and most respiratory equipment. Infants who require medical intervention such as ventilating assistance or emergency cardiorespiratory measures are particularly susceptible to this type of infection. It is these same newborns, who are usually born premature or at risk, who are least capable of resisting such bacterial invasion. Frequently these organisms are transmitted by the personnel from person to person or object to person by poor hand washing and inadequate housecleaning.

Clinical manifestations. One of the major difficulties in the management of sepsis is the vagueness of the presenting symptoms. Frequently the only complaint concerning the infant's progress is "failure to do well," "not looking right," or nonspecific respiratory distress. Rarely is there any indication of a local inflammatory response, which would suggest the portal of entry into the bloodstream. The presence of some bacteria will be indicated by a specific characteristic, for example, *Pseudomonas,* which produces necrotic purplish skin lesions, or group B β-hemolytic streptococci, which usually result in severe respiratory distress and periods of apnea.

All bodily systems tend to show some indication of sepsis (see also p. 343). Respiratory distress is usually noticed by periods of apnea, irregular, grunting respirations, and retractions. Gastric distress is evidenced by signs such as vomiting, which may be bile stained, diarrhea, abdominal distention and absent stools from paralytic ileus, and poor sucking and feeding. Skin manifestations may include cyanosis, pallor, mottling, or signs of jaundice, as well as the lesions associated with specific organisms. Signs of central nervous system involvement are similar to those seen in hypocalcemia or hypoglycemia, notably irritability, apathy, tremors, convulsions, and coma. Since meningitis is a frequent sequelae of sepsis, signs of increased intracranial pressure may also be evident. Fever, which is usually characteristic of any infection, is frequently absent in neonatal sepsis. Body temperature is commonly normal or suboptimal.

Diagnostic evaluation. Isolation of the specific organism is always attempted through repeated blood cultures and analysis of potential primary sources of infection, such as the umbilicus, naso-oral-pharyngeal cavity, ear canals, skin lesions, cerebrospinal fluid, stool, and urine. Direct (conjugated) hyperbilirubinemia is frequently seen in infants with sepsis, particularly of gram-negative origin. Blood studies may show signs of anemia, leukocytosis, or leukopenia. Leukopenia is usually an ominous sign because it is frequently associated with high mortality.

Medical management. Often diagnosis of sepsis is based on suspicion of its existence, and antibiotic therapy is begun before laboratory results are available for confirmation and identification of the exact organism. Penicillin preparations such as ampicillin combined with an antibiotic such as kanamycin (Kantrex) provide a broad-spectrum antibiotic therapy that is effective against approximately 90% of all potential organisms. In cases where gram-negative bacteria, such as *Pseudomonas aeruginosa,* are resistant to these drugs, gentamicin is usually given. Drug therapy is usually continued for a minimum of 10 days and is most often administered via intravenous infusion.

Supportive therapy usually involves administration of oxygen if respiratory distress or cyanosis is evident, adequate hydration with intravenous fluid and electrolytes, and isolation of the infant in an Isolette or incubator.

Nursing considerations. Nursing care of the infant with sepsis is similar to the care of infants with hypoglycemia or hypocalcemia. Recognition of the existing problem is of paramount importance; it is usually the nurse who frequently observes and assesses the infant who identifies that "something is wrong" with the child. Awareness of the potential modes of transmission also allows the nurse to identify those infants more at risk for developing sepsis. Ideally nursery nurses should have the authority to make decisions regarding the transfer of these infants to neonatal intensive care units.

Much of the care of the infant involves the medical treatment of illness. Knowledge of the side effects of the specific antibiotic and proper regulation and administration of the drug via intravenous soluset is mandatory (Table 9-4). The nurse calculates the infusion to allow for the drug to be administered in the proper amount of time, including in the calculation the 10 ml of fluid that occupies the tubing (if extension tubing is added, the fluid occupying that space must

Table 9-4. Drugs commonly used in the treatment of sepsis

Antibiotic	Dose	Route of administration	Nursing considerations
Penicillin G	30,000 U/kg/12 hours	IM, IV	Side effects of penicillin preparation are usually mild—urticaria, skin rash, and pruritus; gastrointestinal disturbances such as nausea, vomiting, or diarrhea can occur with oral preparations; anaphylaxis and central nervous system toxicity (convulsions) are more serious potential complications
Semisynthetic penicillin			Semisynthetic preparations are more stable in gastric acid, have increased penicillinase resistance, and have extended bacterial spectrum
Ampicillin (Omnipen, Polycillin, Penbritin)	50-100 mg/kg/12 hours	IM, IV, PO	Must be used within 1 hour after the powder is reconstituted; volume and rate of infusion must be adjusted before drug loses its stability
Methicillin (Staphcillin)	50-80 mg/kg/8 hours	IM, IV	Solutions are stable for 24 hours at room temperature, 4 days at refrigeration
Nafcillin (Unipen)	40-60 mg/kg/8 hours	IM, IV, PO	After reconstitution, keep under refrigeration and use within 48 hours
Oxacillin (Prostaphlin, Resistopen)	40-60 mg/kg/8 hours	IM, IV, PO	In newborns and infants, transient renal impairment may occur (hematuria, albuminuria, and azotemia)
Kanamycin (Kantrex)	7.5 mg/kg/12 hours	IM, IV	Renal and auditory toxicity is a potential complication; urinary signs of renal irritation include casts, white or red blood cells, and albumin in the urine; adequate hydration reverses and prevents these complications; irritation and pain at side of injection is common; opened vials should be used within 48 hours
Gentamicin (Garamycin)	2.5-3.5 mg/kg/12 hours	IM, IV	Renal and auditory (vestibular and cochlear) toxicity is a potential complication; ototoxicity is a greater danger when combined with renal impairment Intravenous infusion should be administered over a period of 1 hour
Neomycin	2.5 mg/kg/6 hours	PO	Renal and auditory nerve damage can occur; should not be given in combination with other ototoxic drugs; acute systemic toxicity is manifested by a curare-like muscular paralysis and respiratory arrest; emergency treatment is with intravenous calcium gluconate
Polymyxin	2 mg/1 kg/12 hours 6 ml/kg/6 hours 1 mg/kg/24 hours	IM, IV PO Intrathecal	Nephrotoxicity may occur, characterized by albuminuria, cellular casts, and azotemia; neurotoxicity is evidenced by irritability, weakness, drowsiness, ataxia, numbness of the extremities, and transient blurring of vision; symptoms usually disappear within 24 to 48 hours after discontinuing therapy; pain and irritation at the site of injection is common; procaine with intrathecal preparation Intravenous administration should be over a period of 60-90 minutes

also be considered). For example, if ampicillin is added to 10 ml of solution and the pediatric Soluset is regulated at 10 drops/minute, by the end of 1 hour the 10 ml in the tubing and none of the antibiotic will have infused into the infant. The 10 ml of the medication will remain in the tubing. To ensure that the antibiotic is infused within the 1-hour limit, the microdropper must be set at 20 drops/minute.

As a general rule, all antibiotics administered via Soluset should infuse within 1 hour and only one antibiotic should be administered at a time. If the intravenous solution contains other medications such as electrolytes or vitamins, antibiotics are not added to this preparation because the other drugs may inactivate the antibiotic. In this situation another bottle of intravenous solution is hung and attached via a stopcock to the main infusion line. This "piggyback" setup allows antibiotics to be infused without mixing with the other solution.

Prolonged antibiotic therapy predisposes the infant to growth of resistant organisms and infection with fungal or mycotic agents, such as *Candida albicans*. The nurse observes for evidence of such infections.

Part of the total care of the infant with sepsis is to decrease any additional physiologic or environmental stress. This includes providing an optimal thermoregulated environment and anticipating potential problems such as dehydration or anoxia. Isolation of the infant prevents spread of infection to other newborns, but, in order to be effective, isolation must be carried out by all care givers. Proper hand washing, use of disposable equipment (such as linens, catheters, feeding utensils, and intravenous equipment), disposing of excretions (such as vomitus and stool), and adequate housekeeping of the environment and equipment are essential. Since nurses are the most consistent care givers involved with the sick infant, it is usually their responsibility to oversee that all aspects of isolation are maintained.

Another aspect of caring for the infant with sepsis involves observation for signs of meningitis, a frequent sequelae of septicemia. The most common indication of meningitis is a full or bulging anterior fontanel; opisthotonos is rare. Usually the infectious agent is the same for both conditions; however, antibiotic therapy chosen for treatment of sepsis may not diffuse into spinal fluid, necessitating intrathecal administration of such drugs as polymyxin.

Other complications of sepsis include pyarthrosis, which may affect any joint, but most commonly localizes in the hip. Local inflammation of the involved area is again uncommon, so that identification is difficult. Limited movement of the affected joint may be one of the few indications of infection. A severe complication of sepsis is shock, caused by the release of toxins within the bloodstream. Signs of shock are often difficult to distinguish from those of sepsis, such as rapid, irregular respirations and pulse. However, blood pressure usually falls in shock, and therefore this measurement should be a part of the infant's routine vital signs. The nurse needs to be especially aware of the importance of blood pressure, since this is one measurement that is frequently neglected in the assessment of children.

The newborn with sepsis is usually quite ill, and, as with children with hypocalcemia or hypoglycemia, parents are very concerned about recovery. Prognosis is variable, but with immediate antibiotic therapy, mortality is quite low. (See boxed material for summary of nursing care for these infants.) Mental retardation can occur with late diagnosis of meningitis. Unlike hypocalcemia and hypoglycemia, which respond rapidly to treatment, infants with sepsis require a longer hospitalization. In any situation where there is separation of the infant and parents, the parents should be encouraged to stay as much as possible with their child and should be included in care-giving activities. In this way the nurse fosters parent-child attachment, which otherwise may be affected by the separation of prolonged hospitalization.

Skin manifestations

Thrush. Thrush or moniliasis is caused by the yeast *Candida albicans*. In the presence of a vaginal monilial infection, the infant may contract the disease during descent through the birth canal. Any susceptible area of the body is at risk, most notably the mucous membranes of the oral cavity. Besides infection from the birth canal, *Candida* may also be transmitted by poor hand-washing technique and by contaminated bottles and nipples. Infants with anomalies such as cleft lip or palate are also at risk for developing persistent thrush. Infection with *Candida albicans* frequently follows prolonged antibiotic therapy and is common in children with immunologic deficiencies. Newborns of diabetic mothers are particularly vulnerable because the high-glucose content of maternal urine provides an excellent medium for growth of yeast.

Clinical manifestations. Thrush is characterized by white patches on the tongue, palate, and inner aspects of the cheeks. The patches are caused by spores that lodge between the epithelial cells, separating the layers. Later the disease spreads on the surface of the mucous membranes. It can be distinguished from coagulated milk because attempts to scrape it away will be unsuccessful, usually resulting in bleeding of the area. The infant may refuse to suck because of pain in the mouth, but this is infrequent.

Neonatal thrush is usually self-limiting but should always be treated with good hygiene, application of a fungicide, and identification of the source to prevent reinfection. Spontaneous cure may take as long as 2 months, during which time lesions may spread to the larynx, trachea, bronchi, and lungs and along the gastrointestinal tract.

Nursing considerations. Treatment of thrush involves application of nystatin (Mycostatin), 100,000 units/ml over the surfaces of the oral cavity four times a day or every 6 hours. It should be applied after feedings, and the excess should be swallowed to treat any lesions along the gastrointestinal tract. Absorption of nystatin is negligible. Continuation of therapy should be continued for about a week, even if lesions have disappeared within a few days. The suspension is stable for only 1 week.

Another treatment of the lesions is application of 1% gentian violet directly to the lesions three times a day. The infant should not swallow any excess because irritation of the trachea, larynx, or esophagus may result. After application of the solution to the patches, the infant should be placed prone to allow secretions to drool out of the mouth. One must be careful with this preparation because it stains clothing, skin, and other objects a violet color.

Other measures in controlling thrush include rinsing the mouth with plain water after each feeding for oral cleansing, boiling nipples and bottles for at least 20 minutes after thorough washing (spores are heat resistant), and treating the source. Application of 3% hydrogen peroxide three times a day may also be effective, since this chemical may

Summary of nursing care of the infant with hypocalcemia, hypoglycemia, or sepsis

Goals	Responsibilities
Recognize early signs of pathophysiologic state	Assess each system for signs and symptoms suggestive of each condition; correlate findings with general impression of progress of infant (feeding, weight gain, response to stimuli, and sleeping patterns)
Prevent or decrease potential side effects of medical intervention	
Hypocalcemia	Administer calcium gluconate slowly; if heart rate falls below 100 beats/minute, stop infusion Prevent extravasation of calcium gluconate into tissues: Avoid scalp vein Ensure placement of needle before administering drug Tape needle securely at site of insertion Apply pressure to puncture site after removal of needle Counsel mother regarding infant feeding (breast-feeding or appropriate formulas)
Hypoglycemia	Begin oral feeding as soon as possible after birth Administer glucose infusion carefully; avoid overloading the system by speeding up intravenous administration Observe for signs of hyperglycemia (acidosis) and possible need for insulin Decrease intravenous administration of glucose slowly to avoid hypoglycemia from physiologic hyperinsulinemia
Sepsis	Observe for side effects of antibiotics (Table 9-4) Regulate infusion carefully to allow for antibiotic to be administered within 1 hour Use "piggyback" setup if main intravenous solution has added drugs
Monitor environment to decrease factors that will complicate recovery from each condition	Maintain thermoregulation, hydration, and oxygenation of infant Monitor vital signs and correlate with infant's progress
Hypocalcemia	Reduce environmental stimuli Organize care to ensure minimal handling of infant Discuss with parents reasons for minimal holding Institute seizure precautions
Sepsis	Institute appropriate isolation techniques
Observe for complications of disease	
Hypocalcemia	Observe for tetany and convulsions
Hypoglycemia	Check heel blood with Dextrostix Check urine for glycosuria
Sepsis	Observe for signs of meningitis, especially bulging anterior fontanel Observe for pyarthrosis, usually evidenced by limited movement of affected joint Observe for signs of shock, especially fall in blood pressure
Provide emotional support for parents	Allow parents the opportunity to express their feelings Keep parents informed of infant's progress Encourage frequent visiting and participation in care to foster parent-child attachment

be a fungicide and provides good débridement of the membranes. Mechanically removing the patches should be avoided because additional contamination may occur.

Impetigo. Impetigo is an infectious skin condition caused by various strains of group A β-hemolytic streptococci or coagulase-positive *Staphylococcus aureus*. It is characterized by vesicular lesions that vary in size from a few millimeters to several centimeters. The blebs usually occur in the axilla, in the groin, on the undersurface of the neck, and on the face. Once the vesicles rupture, reinfection occurs on other parts of the body, contributing to the contagious nature of this disease. Yellow crusts form over the lesions, which are surrounded by erythema. These lesions are usually pruritic and, if scratched, increase the chance of further infection. Impetigo is frequently associated with conditions of suboptimal hygiene.

Nursing considerations. Treatment of impetigo involves administration of systemic and local antibiotics. Isolation of the infant and initiation of meticulous hand-washing techniques is essential since this disease is highly contagious. Wound and skin precautions are usually the isolation technique of choice. The infant may be separated in a private room. Gowns are worn when the nurse is caring for the infant. Gloves are worn when direct contact is made with the infected lesion. Masks are not necessary. Articles that have been in contact with the infant must be discarded separately.

The infant's arms may need to be restrained with elbow restraints or by pulling the undershirt sleeves over the hands and securing the openings with tape. If restraints of any kind are used, the nurse must allow the infant freedom of movement at supervised times. Even though the infant is isolated, he should be held during feeding and rocked and cuddled as much as possible. Prompt treatment of a streptococcus infection is particularly important in older children or adults because rheumatic fever and pyelonephritis are potential sequelae.

Erythema toxicum. Erythema toxicum, also known as flea bite dermatitis or newborn rash, is a benign self-limiting condition that most frequently appears after the first 24 hours. The lesions, which contain a white papule or vesicle within the lesion's center, appear as a blotchy macular erythema. The rash is transient and is more obvious during crying spells. The sites most commonly involved are the face, proximal extremities, trunk, and buttocks. The rash is probably a result of environmental irritants. Although no treatment is necessary, parents are usually concerned about the rash and need to be reassured of its benign and transient nature.

BIRTH INJURIES

The forces of labor and delivery may result in trauma to the infant during the birth process, many of which are minor and spontaneously resolve in a few days. Others, although minor, require some degree of intervention. Still others can be very serious, even fatal. Part of the nurse's responsibility is identification of such injuries so that appropriate intervention can be initiated as soon as possible. Parents' concern may be greater than the degree of injury warrants because of their lack of knowledge. For example, visual trauma such as caput succedaneum or cephalhematoma, which may appear grotesque, are in fact benign. Nurses must be aware of parents' thoughts and clarify misconceptions. Parents need adequate explanations of birth injuries to alleviate fears and anxiety.

Many of the minor birth injuries, such as cephalhematoma and caput succedaneum (p. 269), have been discussed under physical assessment of the neonate. The following discussion is concerned with more serious injuries that require medical and/or nursing intervention. Birth trauma according to the type of body structure involved is listed below. (See the boxed material.)

Facial paralysis

Pressure on the facial nerve during delivery caused by compression in the birth canal or forceps intervention may result in injury to cranial nerve VII at a point posterior to the lower end of the pinna. Clinical manifestations are primarily loss of movement on the affected side, such as inability to completely close the eye, drooping of the corner of the mouth, and absence of wrinkling of the forehead

Classification of neonatal birth injury

- Muscles and peripheral nerves
  - Facial paralysis
  - Brachial palsy (Erb-Duchenne paralysis, Klumpke's palsy)
  - Phrenic nerve palsy (diaphragmatic paralysis)
- Bones
  - Skull molding
  - Skull fracture (depressed or linear)
  - Fractures of clavicle, humerus, or femur
- Soft tissue
  - Caput succedaneum
  - Cephalhematoma
  - Subcutaneous fat necrosis (pressure necrosis)
  - Subconjunctival (scleral) hemorrhage
  - Retinal hemorrhage
  - Cyanosis and edema of buttocks and extremities
  - Ecchymoses and petechiae of skin
  - Hemorrhage into abdominal organs
- Nervous system
  - Intracranial hemorrhage
  - Subdural hematoma
  - Spinal cord injury

(Fig. 9-4). The paralysis is most noticeable when the infant cries. No medical intervention is necessary; the paralysis usually disappears spontaneously in a few days, but may take as long as several months.

Nursing considerations. Nursing care involves aiding the infant in sucking because part of the mouth cannot close tightly around the nipple. Using a soft rubber nipple with a large hole is often helpful. Sometimes the infant needs to be gavage fed to prevent aspiration. Breast-feeding is not contraindicated, but the mother will need additional assistance in helping the infant to latch on and compress the areolar area.

The eye on the affected side must be protected from injury to the cornea if the lid does not close completely. Artificial tears may need to be instilled daily to prevent drying of the conjunctiva, sclera, and cornea. The nurse teaches this procedure to the parents prior to the infant's discharge from the nursery (see p. 252).

Brachial palsy

Plexus injury results from certain forces that change the normal position and relationship of the arm, shoulder, and neck. Nerves arising from the brachial plexus supply all the muscles and skin of the upper extremity as well as the muscles on the back and chest that move the extremity. Damage to the upper plexus is called *Erb's palsy* (Erb-Duchenne paralysis) and is usually a result of stretching or pulling the shoulder away from the head, which can occur during vertex or breech deliveries. Lower plexus palsy or *Klumpke's palsy* is less common and results from severely stretching the upper extremity while the trunk is relatively immobile. Temporary paralysis results from compression caused by the hemorrhage and edema of soft tissue injury. If the nerve roots have been avulsed or torn from the spinal cord, permanent damage can result.

Clinical manifestations. Clinical manifestations of Erb's palsy are related to the paralysis of the affected extremity and muscles. The normal flexed position of the arm at the elbow is absent. The arm hangs limp alongside the body and is internally rotated, and the wrist is pronated (Fig. 9-5). The grasp reflex is present, but the deep tendon (biceps) reflex is lost. When eliciting a Moro reflex, the affected extremity will respond with decreased range of motion and flexion.

In lower plexus palsy, which is less frequent but more severe, the muscles of the hand, lower arm, and wrist are involved. The deep tendon reflex is intact, but the grasp is absent (Fig. 9-6). Sensory changes, cyanosis, and edema may be present. If the first thoracic root is involved, cervical sympathetic damage (Horner's syndrome—ptosis, miosis, and enophthalmos) may result. A fractured clavicle or phrenic nerve palsy may also be associated with either type of paralysis.

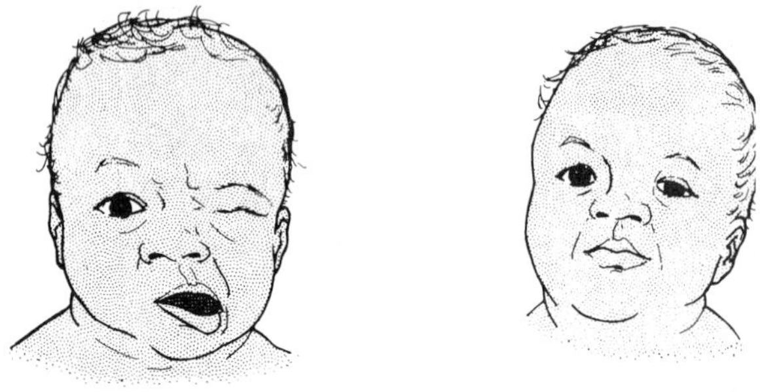

A B

Fig. 9-4. A, Paralysis of right side of face 15 minutes after forceps delivery. Absence of movement on affected side is especially noticeable when the infant cries. **B,** Same infant 24 hours later. Recovery was complete in another 24 hours. (From Jensen, M. D., Benson, R. C., and Bobak, I. M.: Maternity care: the nurse and the family, St. Louis, 1977, The C. V. Mosby Co., p. 520.)

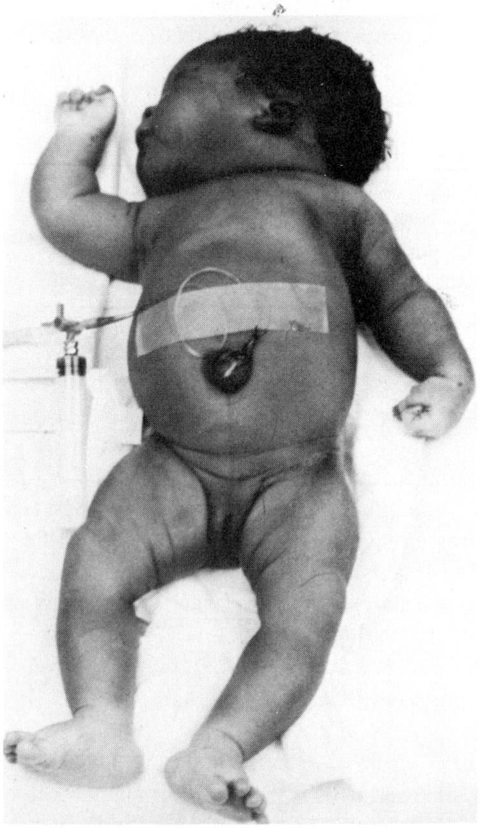

Fig. 9-5. Brachial plexus (Erb's) palsy, left-sided. Note the extended internally rotated arm and pronated wrist on the affected side. (From Korones, S. B.: High risk newborn infants: the basis for intensive nursing care, ed. 2, St. Louis, 1976, The C. V. Mosby Co., p. 48.)

Nursing considerations. Treatment of the affected arm is aimed at preventing contractures of the paralyzed muscles and maintaining correct placement of the humeral head within the glenoid fossa of the scapula. The arm is positioned in an abducted, externally rotated position to relieve pressure on the stretched nerves. Sometimes a cast or splint is applied to maintain this position. If a cast is used, the mother must be shown how to check for adequate circulation in the hands and fingers. Normal growth of the infant can quickly cause the cast to become tight, occluding blood vessels and causing pressure areas. Frequently the desired position is maintained by pinning the shirt sleeve to the mattress. A towel or diaper can be securely wrapped around the arm like a sling and attached to the mattress (Fig. 9-7).

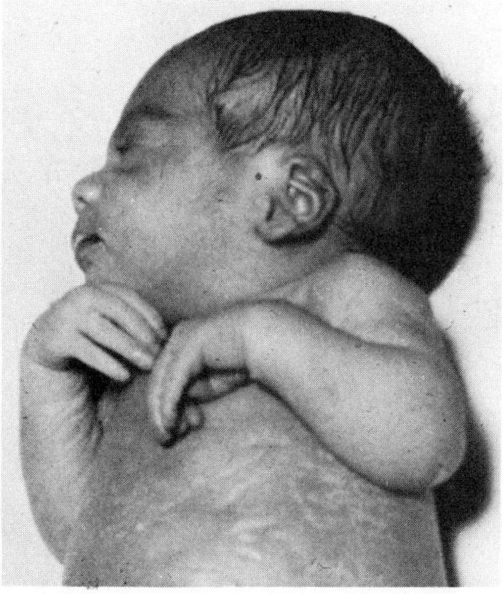

Fig. 9-6. Bilateral brachial plexus (Klumpke's) palsy. Note the wristdrop and lack of grasp reflex. (From Korones, S. B.: High risk newborn infants: the basis for intensive nursing care, ed. 2, St. Louis, 1976, The C. V. Mosby Co., p. 50.)

The arm should also be put through complete passive range of motion exercises daily to maintain muscle tone and function. When dressing the infant, the nurse should always give special preference to the affected arm. Undressing should begin with the unaffected arm and redressing should begin with the affected arm to prevent unnecessary manipulation and stress on the paralyzed muscles. Complete recovery from stretched nerves usually takes about 3 months. Avulsion of the nerves may result in permanent damage requiring surgical and orthopedic intervention. In either case the nurse must prepare the parents for discharge and should refer the family to a public health agency for follow-up care at home.

Phrenic nerve palsy

Injury to the phrenic nerve is almost always associated with brachial palsy and is a result of similar forces during delivery. The phrenic nerve is part of the cervical plexus, originates from the spinal cord, and is the only nerve that innervates the diaphragm. Therefore, respiratory distress is

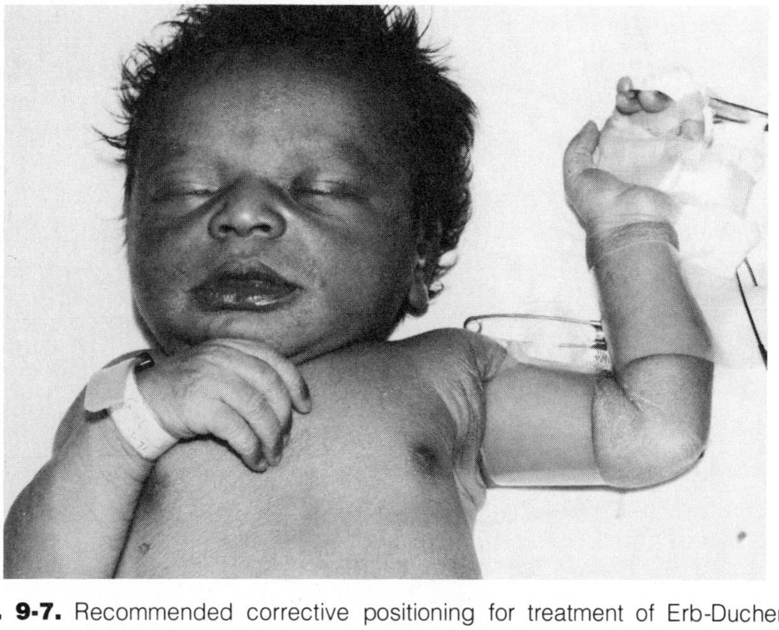

Fig. 9-7. Recommended corrective positioning for treatment of Erb-Duchenne paralysis. Note abduction and external rotation at shoulder, flexion at elbow, supination of forearm, and slight dorsiflexion at wrist. (From Behrman, R. E., editor: Neonatology: diseases of the fetus and infant, St. Louis, 1973, The C. V. Mosby Co.)

the most common and important sign of injury. Since injury to this nerve is usually unilateral, the lung on the affected side does not expand, resulting in pneumonia. Nursing care of the infant with this condition is similar to that of any neonate who is suffering from respiratory difficulty (see Chapter 10).

Fractures

Fracture of the clavicle or collar bone is the most frequent birth injury. It is associated with difficult vertex or breech birth and delivery of infants of above average weight. The fracture may be detected during delivery by an audible click or snap. It may be diagnosed during observation of the infant because spontaneous movement of the affected part is diminished and painful. The Moro reflex is asymmetric, and edema and ecchymosis may be seen at the site of injury.

Not infrequently the fracture is undiagnosed at birth and the mother discovers a hard mass along the clavicle several weeks later, which represents a callus formation. Similarly fractures of long bones, such as the femur or humerus, are undetected because the epiphysis is mostly cartilage, which is usually not dense enough to show clearly on an x-ray film.

Nursing considerations. Frequently no intervention may be prescribed other than proper body alignment, careful dressing and undressing of the infant, and handling and carrying that support the affected bone. For example, when picking up the infant who has a fractured clavicle, it is important to do so by supporting the upper and lower back rather than by pulling the infant up from under the arms. Occasionally the arm on the side of the fractured clavicle may be fixed on the body by pinning the sleeve to the shirt for immobilization and relief of pain. The parents should be involved in caring for the infant during hospitalization as part of discharge planning for care at home.

Intracranial hemorrhage

One of the severest birth injuries is hemorrhage into the cranial vault. Accumulation of blood occupies the spaces between the dura and arachnoid linings (subdural space), between the arachnoid and pia (subarachnoid space), or between the ventricles.

Etiology. Intracranial hemorrhage may be caused by hypoxia or trauma. Hemorrhage from hypoxia, which damages cerebral vessels, mostly involves the ventricular and subarachnoid spaces and is frequently not associated with trauma in premature infants. Hemorrhage from trauma most frequently involves the subdural space (subdural hematoma) and is the result of excessive pressure or force during the birth process. Precipitate delivery (less than 3 hours) results

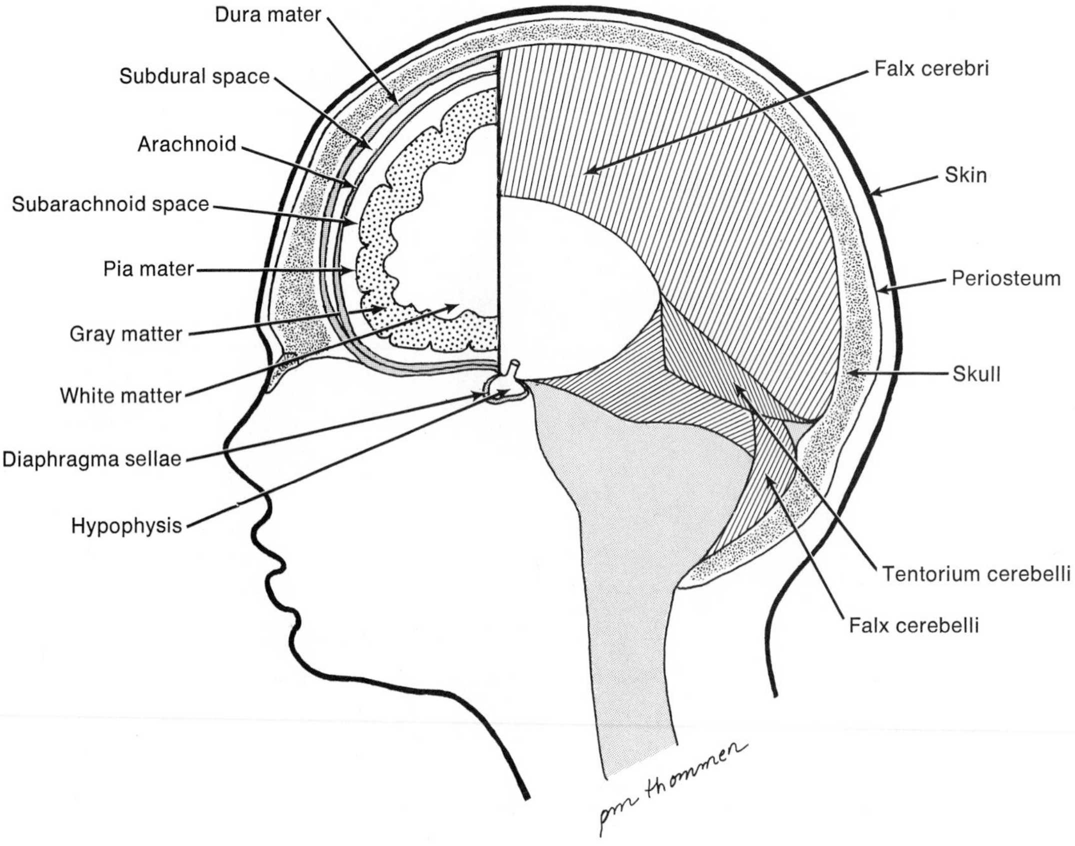

Fig. 9-8. Possible anatomic sites of intracranial hemorrhage.

in rapid changes within the fetal circulatory system, causing rupture of blood vessels. Prolonged or difficult labor causes sustained and extreme pressures against the cranium, resulting in stretching and tearing of large vessels, such as the emissary or sinus veins in the dural membrane (subdural hematoma). This most commonly occurs in the *tentorium cerebelli,* which separates the cerebral hemispheres from the cerebellum, or the *falx cerebri,* which longitudinally separates the cerebral hemispheres (Fig. 9-8).

Other causes of intracranial hemorrhage are cephalopelvic disproportion, breech presentation, high forceps deliveries, and infants with large heads (hydrocephalus). Prematurity predisposes toward hemorrhage because of fragile vessel walls and greater incidence of coagulation defects.

Pathophysiology. Pathology results as blood accumulates between the subdural spaces, exerting pressure against the brain, which decreases circulation to brain cells. About 80% of subdural hematomas are bilateral. The most severe complication is pressure against the respiratory center, causing respiratory distress. This is most likely when collection of blood is rapid, not allowing for the sutures in the skull to expand. Mental retardation is an important future complication and should be suspected in every infant who has survived this birth injury.

Clinical manifestations. Signs of intracranial hemorrhage are the result of increased intracranial pressure. Onset of the symptoms can vary from a few hours to a few days. High shrill cry, a staring expression, poor sucking reflex and feeding, irritability, and lethargy characterize the infant's behavior. Signs of respiratory distress include cyanosis, apneic spells, and irregular breathing pattern. Hypotonia, spasticity, seizures, and coma may occur. Physical assessment reveals bulging, widened fontanels and sutures. Projectile vomiting not necessarily associated with feeding indicates increasing cerebral irritation.

Medical management. The aim of intervention is to relieve the intracranial pressure. If the collection of blood is at the area of the falx cerebri, a subdural tap can be done through the anterior fontanel or coronal suture to remove the accumulated fluid. The collection of blood in the tentorium cerebelli is usually inaccessible to aspiration by this procedure. Surgical intervention may be indicated in such situations.

When bleeding into the subarachnoid space has occurred, the cerebrospinal fluid will be bloody, and pressure can be relieved by aspirating fluid during a lumbar puncture. Prognosis is variable depending on the severity of the hemorrhage, location within the brain, and success of treatment.

Nursing considerations. Besides observing for signs of this injury, especially in infants of traumatic deliveries, the nurse must be aware of the potential graveness of the outcome and appraise parents of the infant's progress. Unlike visible birth trauma such as caput succedaneum or cephalhematoma, intracranial hemorrhage is not a readily apparent injury, and parents need much explanation regarding its seriousness. Frequently one or the other of these scalp injuries is present with intracranial hematoma. The nurse must be able to recognize each and explain the various meanings to the parents. For example, cephalhematoma is first noticed a day or two following delivery but has no significance in terms of the progress of intracranial or subdural hematoma (Table 9-5 and Fig. 9-9).

Since many tests are usually done, such as blood studies for signs of anemia and rising bilirubin levels from hemorrhage and subdural and spinal taps, the nurse must be aware of the infant's need for oxygen, nutrition, and optimal warmth. The infant is usually positioned in a slight reverse Trendelenburg's position to decrease intracranial pressure and facilitate lung expansion. Since sucking is usually affected, the infant may be fed by gavage or temporarily

Table 9-5. Comparison of cephalic injuries caused by birth trauma

Injury	Time of onset	Pathology	Clinical manifestations
Caput succedaneum	Within 24 hours after birth	Edema of soft scalp tissue	Outline is ill defined; mass is soft but not fluctuant, pressure causes pitting of edema
Cephalhematoma	After initial 24 to 48 hours after birth	Hematoma between periosteum and skull bone	Outline is well defined against edge of bone margin; mass is soft and fluctuant
Subdural hematoma	Variable—from a few hours to a few days after birth	Hematoma in space between dura and arachnoid linings of the brain (tentorium cerebelli, falx cerebri, or falx cerebelli)	No mass is visible; signs are those of Increased intracranial pressure: bulging and widened fontanels and sutures, high-pitched cry, vomiting, poor sucking reflex, irritability, lethargy, weak Moro reflex, flaccidity followed by spasticity, seizures, and coma Respiratory distress: cyanosis, apnea, and irregular respirations Progressive signs of hemorrhage and shock: pale, cold, clammy skin, weak pulse, and signs of jaundice and anemia

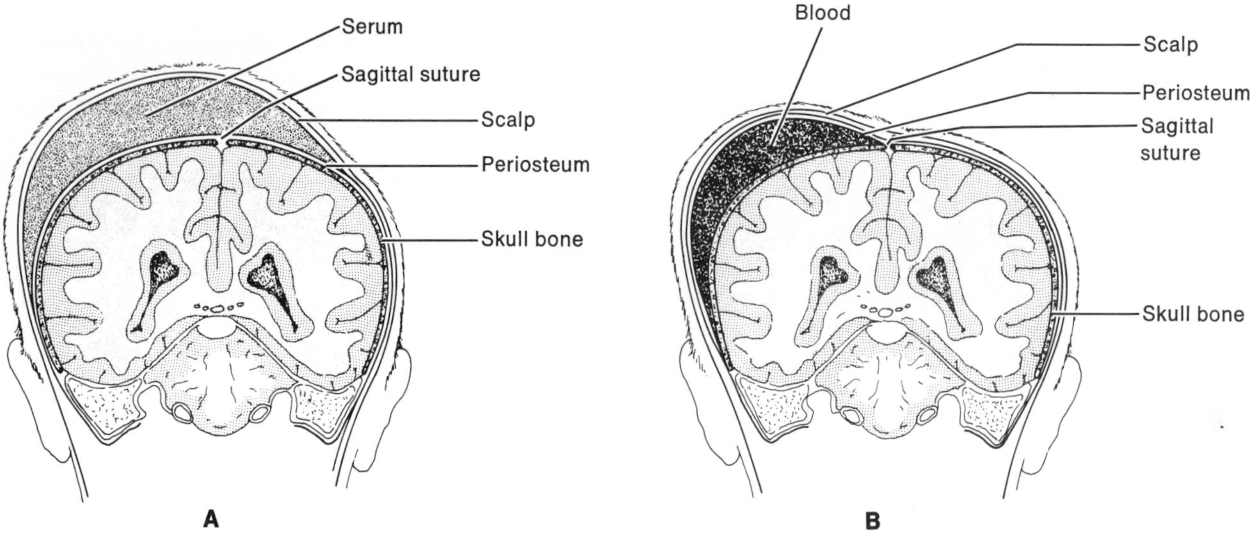

Fig. 9-9. Difference between *caput succedaneum,* **A,** and cephalhematoma, **B.** See Table 9-5 for a further comparison of these injuries. (From Jensen, M. D., Benson, R. C., and Bobak, I. M.: Maternity care: the nurse and the family, St. Louis, 1977, The C. V. Mosby Co.)

maintained by intravenous fluid and electrolytes. Fluid intake is carefully calculated and monitored to prevent hypervolemia, which increases intracranial pressure.

INBORN ERRORS OF METABOLISM

Phenylketonuria (PKU)

Phenylketonuria is an inherited genetic defect that results in the body's inability to metabolize the essential amino acid phenylalanine. It is not a common inborn error of metabolism, affecting one in every 10,000 to 20,000 live births, but it accounts for about 1% of institutionalized mentally defective individuals. It primarily affects whites, with the incidence being highest in those people living in the United States or Northern Europe. It is very rare in the African, Jewish, or Japanese population.

The disease is inherited as an autosomal-recessive trait. Based on the incidence of phenylketonuria, theoretically one person in 50 to 100 is a carrier. If two carriers mate, there is a 25% chance of having a child with the disease. With better diagnosis and treatment of individuals with phenylketonuria the chances of a person marrying an unaffected partner is greatly increased. In this case all the children will be carriers. If an affected person marries a carrier, half of the offspring will be affected and the other half will be carriers.

Pathophysiology and clinical manifestations. The hepatic enzyme phenylalanine hydroxylase, which normally controls the conversion of phenylalanine to tyrosine, is absent, resulting in the accumulation of phenylalanine in the bloodstream and urinary excretion of its abnormal metabolites, the phenyl acids (Fig. 9-10). One of these phenyl ketones, phenylpyruvic acid, which gives urine the characteristic musty odor associated with this disease, is responsible for the term phenylketonuria. In the presence of ferric chloride, phenylpyruvic acid turns urine green. The presence of the musty odor and the chemical reaction with ferric chloride led Dr. Asbjorn Fölling, a Norwegian biochemist and physician, to the discovery of this disorder.

Other metabolites that are probably formed in the liver by alternate pathways include phenylacetic acid, which also has a characteristic musty or horsey odor. It is present in the perspiration and urine of affected individuals. Phenyllactic acid, orthohydroxyphenylacetic acid, and phenylacetylglutamine are also greatly increased in the urine, blood, sweat, cerebrospinal fluid, and tissues. Accumulation of phenylalanine and its derivatives apparently prevents normal development of the brain and central nervous system. The abnormalities that result include defective myelinization, cystic degeneration of the gray and white matter, and disturbances in cortical lamination. Mental retardation occurs before the metabolites are detected in the urine and will progress if ingested phenylalanine levels are not lowered.

Besides the accumulating phenylalanine, there is also an absence of the amino acid tyrosine, which is needed for the formation of the pigment melanin and the hormones epinephrine and thyroxin. Decreased melanin production results in similar phenotypes of most phenylketonuric children. Typically they have blonde hair, blue eyes, and fair skin, which is particularly susceptible to eczema and other dermatologic problems. Other clinical manifestations of

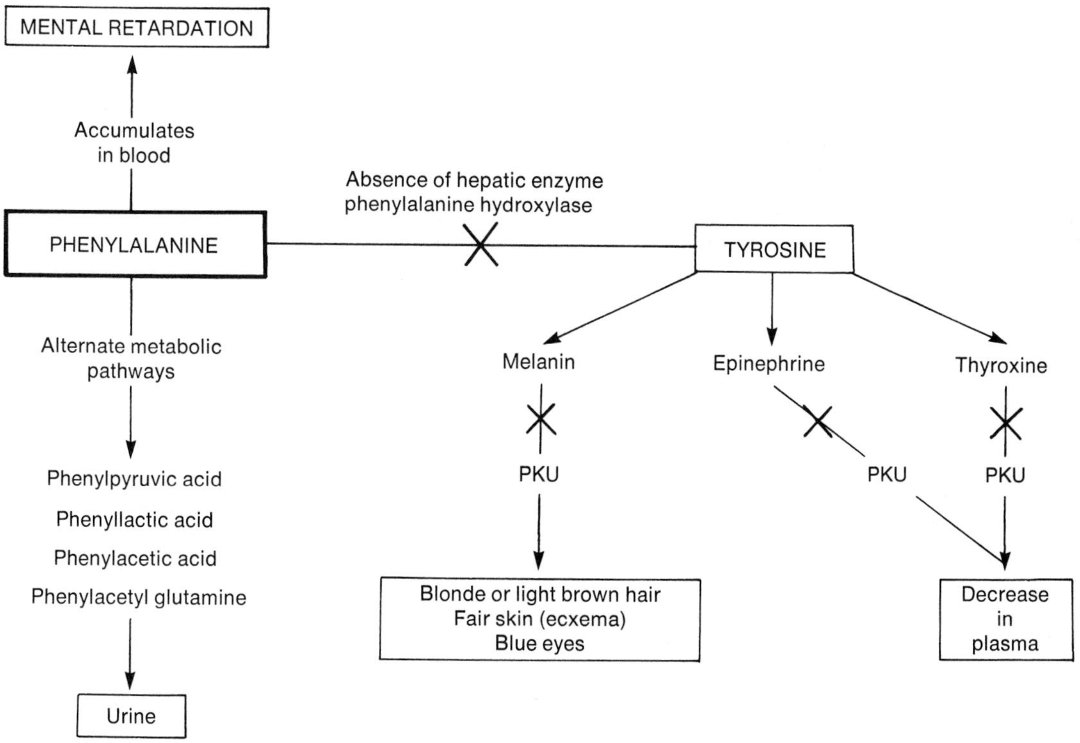

Fig. 9-10. Metabolic error and clinical effects in phenylketonuria.

phenylketonuria include failure to thrive, frequent vomiting, irritability, hyperactivity, and unpredictable, erratic behavior. Bizarre or schizoid-like behavior patterns are common, such as fright reactions, screaming episodes, disorientation, failure to respond to strong stimuli, and catatonic-like positions. Many of the severaly retarded children have convulsions, and about 80% of untreated persons with phenylketonuria demonstrate abnormal electroencephalographs, regardless of overt seizures.

Diagnostic evaluation. The objective in diagnosing or treating the disorder is to prevent mental retardation. All the tests for phenylketonuria are based on detecting increasing phenylalanine levels in the blood or alternate metabolites in the urine (Table 9-6). The most reliable test for screening newborns for phenylketonuria is the Guthrie blood test. If properly done, it will detect serum phenylalanine levels above 4 mg/100 ml. The Guthrie test is a bacterial inhibition procedure. *Bacillus subtilis,* which is present in the culture media, is dependent on a sufficient amount of phenylalanine to grow. If a drop of blood that contains abnormal quantities of phenylalanine is placed on the culture media and the bacteria grow, phenylketonuria is suspected. Since this test provides a qualitative analysis, serum phenylalanine and tyrosine levels should be taken.

Two important drawbacks exist when using this test. For this test to be effective, the newborn must have ingested a high phenylalanine substance (cow's milk or human milk) for a full 4 days for the serum phenylalanine levels to reach 4 mg/100 ml (normal value, below 2 mg/100 ml). Testing the infant before this time, delayed feeding, or vomiting can yield false-negative results. Since infants with phenylketonuria tend to vomit and refuse to eat more frequently than do normal infants, this is an important point to remember. Retesting should be done within a month or less, particularly of infants who are siblings of phenylketonuric children. False-positive results can occur if liver disease, galactosemia, or prematurity exist.

Several tests exist for detecting phenylpyruvic acid in urine. All of them utilize the reagent ferric chloride, which turns green when in contact with phenylpyruvic acid. The Phenixtix test* employs a dipstick that has a ferric salt impregnated in the filter paper. When it is dipped in urine or pressed against a wet diaper, the dipstick will turn green if abnormal phenylalanine levels are present. Fading of the color occurs within 1 minute. For reliable results, fresh urine and new filter paper must be used. False-positive results can occur if large amounts of ketones are present (diabetic acidosis). Aspirin and other salicylate-containing compounds will turn the paper a nonfading bluish purple.

The main problem in all the urine tests for phenylketo-

*Ames Company, Elkhart, Ind.

Table 9-6. Diagnostic tests for phenylketonuria

Test	Method	Use
Urine tests		
Diaper test	10% ferric chloride dropped on freshly wet diaper; green spot is positive, indicates probable PKU	Cheap; useful in screening large groups of infants but not of value until infant is at least 6 weeks of age
Phenistix test*	Prepared test stick pressed against wet diaper or dipped in urine; green color reaction indicates probable PKU	Simple; more accurate than diaper test; useful in screening large groups of infants but not of value until after infant is 6 weeks of age
Dinitrophenyl-hydrazine (DNPH) test†	0.5 to 1 ml of urine placed in test tube, and equal amount of DNPH solution added; immediate pale yellow-orange color reaction is negative; gradual change to opaque bright yellow is positive and indicates probable PKU	Cheap, accurate, but more complicated than diaper test or Phenistix; most useful in clinical setting to confirm these tests
Blood serum phenylalanine tests		
Guthrie inhibition assay method‡	Drops of blood placed on filter paper; laboratory uses a bacterial growth inhibition test; level above 8 mg phenylalanine/100 ml blood diagnostic of PKU	Effective in newborn period; used also to monitor PKU diet; blood easily obtained by heel or finger puncture; inexpensive; used for wide-scale screening
LaDu-Michael method§	5 ml of blood, serum separated and tested for phenylalanine; level above 8 mg/100 ml blood indicates PKU; in PKU patients, level above 8 to 12 mg phenylalanine/100 ml blood indicates loss of dietary control	Useful diagnostic tool and to monitor PKU diet; requires blood drawn from patient, and laboratory method is difficult (test not available in many laboratories)
McCaman and Robins fluorometric method‖	5 ml of blood, serum separated and tested for phenylalanine; level above 8 mg indicates PKU or loss of dietary control	Diagnostic and diet monitoring tool; laboratory procedure simpler than LaDu-Michael method; test not available in many laboratories

From Williams, S. R.: Nutrition and diet therapy, ed. 3, St. Louis, 1977, The C. V. Mosby Co., p. 441.
*Manufactured by Ames Company, Elkhart, Ind.
†Centerwall, W., and Centerwall, S.: Phenylketonuria, U.S. Children's Bureau, Pub. No. 338, Washington, D.C., 1961, U.S. Government Printing Office.
‡Guthrie, R.: Blood screening for phenylketonuria, J.A.M.A. **178:**863, 1961.
§LaDu, B., and Michael, P.: An enzymatic spectrophotometric method for the determination of phenylalanine in blood, J. Lab. Clin. Med. **55:**491, 1960.
‖McCaman, M., and Robins, E.: Fluorometric method for the determination of phenylalanine in the serum, J. Lab. Clin. Med. **59:**885, 1962.

nuria is that the serum phenylalanine level must exceed 10 to 15 mg/100 ml for phenylpyruvic acid to be present in urine. Such high levels usually do not occur until the affected infant is 10 to 14 days old. By this time, brain damage may have occurred. Therefore, urine testing is not a reliable method of screening in the neonate. At the present time the Guthrie blood test is mandatory for all newborns in most states.

Medical management. Treatment of phenylketonuria is dietary. Since the genetic enzyme is intracellular, systemic administration of phenylalanine hydroxylase is of no value. Phenylalanine cannot be eliminated because it is an essential amino acid, necessary for tissue growth. Therefore, dietary management must meet two criteria:

1. It must meet the child's nutritional need for optimum growth
2. It must maintain phenylalanine levels within a safe range

The diet is calculated to allow 20 to 30 mg/kg/day of phenylalanine, which should maintain blood levels between 3 and 7 mg/100 ml. Significant brain damage usually occurs when levels are above 10 to 15 mg/100 ml. At levels less than 2 mg/100 ml the body begins to catabolize its protein stores, resulting in growth retardation.

Since all natural food proteins contain about 5% phenylalanine, a specially prepared milk substitute called Lofenalac* is usually given to the infant. Lofenalac is made from specially treated enzymic casein hydrolysate, which provides 0.4% phenylalanine (28.5 mg/8 ounces). It also contains minerals and vitamins to provide a balanced nutritional formula. Since tyrosine is deficient because of the block in the metabolic conversion of phenylalanine, this amino acid, as well as several others, is supplied to the infant. When Lofenalac is mixed with the proper amount of water

*Mead Johnson & Co., Evansville, Ind.

(one measure of powder to 2 ounces of water), it supplies 20 kcal/ounce. It is usually well accepted by infants, although older children may not find it palatable.

The optimum time for beginning a low-phenylalanine diet is still uncertain, but since phenylalanine levels rise to dangerous levels (10 to 15 mg/100 ml) by 2 weeks of age, it is logical that early initiation is essential. One study demonstrated that infants who were treated within 3 weeks of birth had normal IQs. Those treated within 3 to 6 weeks had slightly lower IQs. Children who were treated at 8 months or later did not differ in IQ from children with phenylketonuria who had never been treated.[7] Other reports indicate that even when treatment begins early and is vigorously monitored, minimal intellectual impairment results.[3] It is not yet known how long the diet therapy must be continued. At present most authorities suggest continuing the diet until the child is 6 to 8 years old, when at least 90% of brain growth has occurred.[6]

If dietary management is begun after brain damage has occurred, it will not reverse the process but will limit its progress. Restricting phenylalanine in older children with phenylketonuria has proved to be of some benefit in improving behavior, motor ability, and decreasing exacerbations of eczema.

Nursing considerations. As with the birth of any child with a defect, parents of children with phenylketonuria first grieve the loss of a perfect son or daughter. However, these parents have the extra burden of knowing that they are carriers of the defect and must make serious decisions regarding future children (see Chapters 6 and 10).

Although the treatment for phenylketonuria may sound simple, the task of maintaining such a strict dietary regime is very demanding. Foods with low phenylalanine levels, such as vegetables, fruits, juices, and some cereals, breads, and starches, must be measured in order to provide the prescribed amount of phenylalanine. Most high-protein foods, such as meat or dairy products, are either eliminated or restricted to small amounts. Unfortunately Lofenalac is quite expensive, adding financial burdens. However, it is essential that it be used in place of milk products. Milk can be used in the event that Lofenalac is not available, but this must be a temporary exception.

During infancy Lofenalac is used as a formula and presents few problems. Solid foods, such as cereal, fruits, and vegetables, should be introduced as usual to the infant. As the child gets older, more difficulties can arise. Decreased appetite and refusal to eat may decrease consumption of the calculated phenylalanine requirement. The child's increasing independence may inhibit absolute control of what he eats. Either factor can result in decreased or increased phenylalanine levels. During the school years peer pressure becomes a major force in deterring the child from drinking Lofenalac or abstaining from high-protein foods, such as milk shakes or ice cream. Still further, illness or growth spurts will increase the body's need for this essential amino acid.

To evaluate the effectiveness of dietary treatment, frequent monitoring of urinary phenylpyruvic levels is necessary. Phenylalanine deficiency is associated with acidosis, hypoglycemia, extensive skin rash, anemia, and fulminating infection. Suboptimal phenylalanine levels will cause retarded growth in height and weight. A careful record should be kept of these two determinants of growth, in addition to frequent urine and blood assays of phenylalanine.

With improved dietary control of phenylketonuria, neonatal retardation can be prevented. However, the increased life span of individuals with phenylketonuria presents additional concerns. High phenylalanine blood levels in mothers with phenylketonuria seem to affect the normal embryologic development of the fetus, leading to congenital malformation, microcephaly, and/or mental retardation in the infant. For this reason the low-phenylalanine diet should be resumed during pregnancy. Since long-term results of dietary management are as yet unavailable, it is likely to assume that genetic counseling will be particularly important for families who have children with this disorder. For nursing care of the child with eczema, a frequent complication of phenylketonuria, see p. 489.

Galactosemia

Galactosemia is an inborn error of carbohydrate metabolism in which the hepatic enzyme galactose-I-phosphate uridyl transferase (UDP—galactose transferase) is absent. The enzyme is one of three needed for the conversion of galactose to glucose (Fig. 9-11). As galactose accumulates in the blood, several organs are affected. Hepatic dysfunction leads to cirrhosis, resulting in jaundice in the infant by the second week of life. The spleen subsequently becomes enlarged as a result of portal hypertension. Cataracts are usually recognizable by 1 or 2 months of age; cerebral damage is evident soon afterward, evidenced by the symptoms of lethargy and hypotonia. Infants with this disorder appear normal at birth but within a few days after ingesting milk, which has a high lactose content, begin to vomit and lose weight. Drowsiness, nausea, and diarrhea also occur, and death during the first month of life is not infrequent in untreated galactosemic infants.

Galactosemia is inherited as an autosomal-recessive trait, following the laws of mendelian inheritance, as explained in the discussion of phenylketonuria (p. 316). It is rare, however, affecting one in 25,000 to 35,000 live births. Diagnosis is made on the basis of galactosuria, increased levels of galactose in the blood, or decreased levels of galactose-I-phosphate uridyl transferase activity in erthrocytes (normal range, 2.5 to 9 units of enzyme per gram of hemoglobin). Cord blood can be analyzed at birth to establish a diagnosis in suspected infants. Carriers can also be identified by the latter test, because heterozygote individuals will have sig-

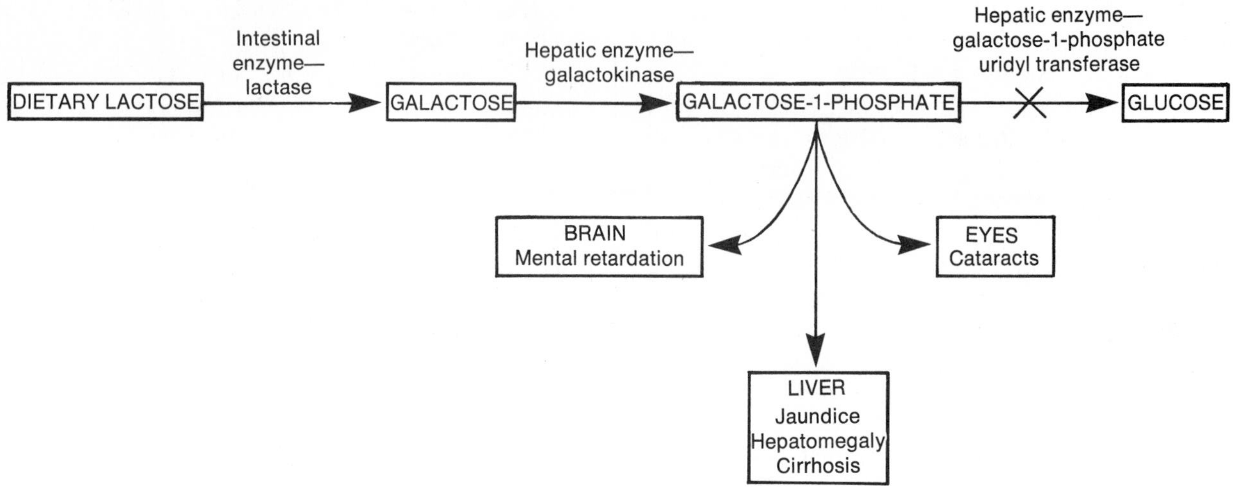

Fig. 9-11. Metabolic error and clinical effects in galactosemia. (Adapted from Williams, S. R.: Nutrition and diet therapy, ed. 3, St. Louis, 1977, The C. V. Mosby Co.)

nificantly lower levels of the enzyme. Although asymptomatic, such individuals have been noted to spontaneously dislike galactose-containing food and, therefore. limit ingestion of such substances.

Treatment of galactosemia is dietary and consists of eliminating all milk and galactose-containing foods. This involves reading food labels very carefully for the addition of any form of dairy product such as cream, yogurt, cheese, or butter. During infancy, soybean-based formulas are used. Many drugs, such as penicillin, contain lactose as fillers and must also be avoided.

Nursing considerations are similar to those for phenylketonuria.

REFERENCES

1. Behrman, R. E., chairman: Preliminary report of the committee on phototherapy in the newborn infant, J. Pediatr. **84**(1): 135-147, January 1974.
2. Behrman, R. E., editor: Neonatal-perinatal medicine: diseases of the fetus and infant, ed. 2, St. Louis, 1977, The C. V. Mosby Co.
3. Dobson, J. C., and associates: Intellectual performance of 36 phenylketonuria patients and their unaffected siblings, Pediatrics **58**(1):53-58, July 1976.
4. Hughes, J. G.: Synopsis of pediatrics, ed. 4, St. Louis, 1975, The C. V. Mosby Co.
5. Hyman, C. B., and associates: CNS abnormalities after neonatal hemolytic disease or hyperbilirubinemia, Am. J. Dis. Child. **117**:395-405, April 1969.
6. Johnson, C. F.: What is the best age to discontinue the low phenylalanine diet in phenylketonuria? Clin. Pediatr. **11**(3): 148-156, March 1972.
7. Kang, E., and associates: Results of treatment and termination of diet in phenylketonuria, Pediatrics **46**(6):881-890, June 1970.
8. Korones, S. B.: High risk newborn infants, ed. 2, St. Louis, 1976, The C. V. Mosby Co.
9. Maisels, M. J.: Bilirubin: on understanding and influencing its metabolism in the newborn infant, Pediatr. Clin. North Am. **19**(2):447-501, May 1972.
10. Weiss, Y., Ackerman, C., and Shmilovitz, L.: Localized necrosis of scalp in neonates due to calcium gluconate infusions: a cautionary note, Pediatrics **56**(6):1084-1086, December 1975.

BIBLIOGRAPHY

Abramson, H., editor: Resuscitation of the newborn infant: and related emergency procedures in the perinatal center special care nursery, ed. 3, St. Louis, 1973, The C. V. Mosby Co.

Aladjem, S., editor: Risks in the practice of modern obstetrics, St. Louis, 1975, The C. V. Mosby Co.

Babson, S. G., and associates: Management of high-risk pregnancy and intensive care of the neonate, ed. 3, St. Louis, 1975, The C. V. Mosby Co.

Bergersen, B. S., and Goth, A.: Pharmacology in nursing, ed. 13, St. Louis, 1976, The C. V. Mosby Co.

Jensen, M., Benson, R. C., and Bobak, I. M.: Maternity care: the nurse and the family, St. Louis, 1977, The C. V. Mosby Co.

Kissane, J. M.: Pathology of infancy and childhood, ed. 2, St. Louis, 1975, The C. V. Mosby Co.

Nelson, W. E., Vaughan, V. C., and McKay, R. J.: Textbook of pediatrics, Philadelphia, 1975, W. B. Saunders Co.

Rudolph, A. M., editor: Pediatrics, New York, 1977, Appleton-Century-Crofts.

Shirkey, H. C., editor: Pediatric therapy, ed. 5, St. Louis, 1975, The C. V. Mosby Co.

Smith, C. H.: Blood diseases of infancy and childhood, ed. 3, St. Louis, 1972, The C. V. Mosby Co.

Problems related to physical status

Behrman, R. E., and Fisher, D. E.: Phenobarbital for neonatal jaundice, J. Pediatr. **76:**945, 1970.

Crichton, J., and associates: Long term effects of neonatal jaundice on brain function in children of low birth weight, Pediatrics **49**(5):656-668, June 1972.

Food and Drug Administration, Department of Health, Education, and Welfare: Comment: hazard of ultraviolet radiation from fluorescent lamps to infant during phototherapy, J. Pediatr. **84:** 145, 1974.

Kopelman, A. E., Brown, R. S., and Odell, G. B.: The "bronze" baby syndrome: a complication of phototherapy, J. Pediatr. **81:** 466, 1972.

Lucey, J. F.: Comment: another view of phototherapy, J. Pediatr. **84:**145, 1974.

Page, I. H., Gartner, L. M., and Arias, I. M.: Formation, transport, metabolism and excretion of bilirubin, N. Engl. J. Med. **280:**1339, 1969.

Papageorgiades, G.: Transplacental passage of fetal red cells into the maternal circulation, Clin. Pediatr. **15**(1):42-43, January 1976.

Poland, R. I., and Odell, G. B.: Physiologic jaundice: the enterohepatic circulation of bilirubin, N. Engl. J. Med. **284:**1, 1971.

Sharma, R. K., and associates: A complication of photogherapy in the newborn: the bronze baby, Clin. Pediatr. **12:**231-233, April 1973.

Shennan, A. T.: The effect of phototherapy on the hyperbilirubinemia of rhesus incompatibility, Pediatrics **54:**417, 1974.

Whaley, L.: Understanding inherited disorders, St. Louis, 1974, The C. V. Mosby Co.

Williams, S. R.: Phototherapy in hyperbilirubinemia, Am. J. Nurs. **71**(7):1397-1399, July 1971.

Woody, N. C., and Brodkey, M. J.: Tanning from phototherapy for neonatal jaundice, J. Pediatr. **82:**1042, 1973.

Yoder, B.: Patching babies' eyes for phototherapy, Am. J. Nurs. **75**(2):266, February 1975.

Problems related to environmental agents

American Academy of Pediatrics, Committee on Fetus and Newborn: Statement: skin care of newborns, Pediatrics **54:**682, 1974.

Beard, A. G., and associates: Neonatal hypoglycemia: a discussion, J. Pediatr. **79:**314, 1971.

Chantler, C., Baum, J. D., and Norman, D. A.: Dextrostix in the diagnosis of neonatal hypoglycemia, Lancet **2:**1395, 1967.

Davies, P.: Bacterial infection in the fetus and newborn, Arch. Dis. Child. **46**(245):1, 20, January 1971.

Garner, J., and Kaiser, A.: How often is isolation needed? Am. J. Nurs. **72**(4):733, 737, April 1972.

Gehibach, S. H., and associates: Recurrence of skin disease in a nursery: ineffectuality of hexachlorophene bathing, Pediatrics **55:**422, 1975.

Gotoff, S. P.: Neonatal immunity, J. Pediatr. **85:**149, 1974.

Gotoff, S. P., and Behrman, R. E.: Neonatal septicemia, J. Pediatr. **76:**142, 1970.

Hodgman, J., and associates: Neonatal dermatology, Pediatr. Clin. North Am. **13**(3):713, 756, March 1971.

Krugman, S., Ward, R., and Katz, S. L.: Infectious diseases of children, ed. 6, St. Louis, 1977, The C. V. Mosby Co.

Lee, F. A., and Gwinn, J. L.: Roentgen patterns of extravasation of calcium gluconate in the tissues of the neonate, J. Pediatr. **86:**598, 1975.

McCracken, G. H., Jr.: Group B streptococci: the new challenge in neonatal infections, J. Pediatr. **82:**703, 1973.

McCracken, G. H., Jr., and Eichenwald, H. F.: Antimicrobial therapy: therapeutic recommendations and a review of newer drugs. I. Therapy of infectious conditions, J. Pediatr. **85:**297, 1974.

McCracken, G. H., Jr., and Eichenwald, H. F.: Antimicrobial therapy: therapeutic recommendations and a review of the newer drugs. II. The clinical pharmacology of the newer antimicrobial agents, J. Pediatr. **85:**451, 1974.

Miller, D. R., and associates: Fatal disseminated herpes simplex virus infection and hemorrhage in the neonate: coagulation studies in a case and a review, J. Pediatr. **76:**409, 1970.

Overbach, A. M., Daniel, S. J., and Cassady, G.: The value of umbilical cord histology in the management of potential perinatal infection, J. Pediatr. **76:**22, 1970.

Peter, G., Lloyd-Still, J. D., and Lovejoy, F. H., Jr.: Local infection and bacteremia from scalp vein needles and polyethylene catheters in children, J. Pediatr. **80:**78, 1972.

Rosen, F. S.: Immunity in the fetus and newborn. In Gluck, L., editor: Modern perinatal medicine, Chicago, 1974, Year Book Medical Publishers, Inc.

Tripp, A.: Hyper and hypocalcemia, Am. J. Nurs. **76**(7):1142, 1145, July 1976.

Tsang, R. C., and associates: Neonatal hypocalcemia in infants with birth asphyxia, J. Pediatr. **84:**428, 1974.

Birth injuries

Rosman, P.: Increased intracranial pressure in childhood, Pediatr. Clin. North Am. **21**(2):483-499, February 1974.

Zelson, C., Lee, S. J., and Pearl, M.: The incidence of skull fractures underlying cephalohematomas in newborn infants, J. Pediatr. **85:**371, 1974.

Inborn errors of metabolism

Dodge, P. R., Prensky, A. L., and Feigin, R. D.: Nutrition and the developing nervous system, St. Louis, 1975, The C. V. Mosby Co.

Justice, P., and Smith, G.: Phenylketonuria, Am. J. Nurs. **75**(8): 1303-1305, August 1975.

Phenylketonuria, Indiana, 1973, Mead Johnson & Co.

Rothman, K. J., and Pueschel, S. N.: Birthweight of children with phenylketonuria, Pediatrics **58**(6):842, 844, December 1976.

Schild, S.: Parents of children with phenylketonuria, Children **11**(3):92-96, May/June 1964.

Williams, S. R.: Nutrition and diet therapy, ed. 3, St. Louis, 1977, The C. V. Mosby Co.

Yu, J., and associates: False negative screening tests in phenylketonuria, Arch. Dis. Chil. **46**(1):124-125, January 1971.

10

The high-risk neonate

The high-risk neonate can be defined as the newborn, regardless of gestational age or birth weight, who has a greater than average chance of morbidity or mortality because of conditions or circumstances that are superimposed on the normal course of events associated with birth and the adjustment to extrauterine existence. This includes the periods in human growth and development from the time of viability until 28 days following birth and involves threats to life and health that occur during the prenatal, perinatal, and postnatal periods.

IDENTIFICATION OF HIGH-RISK NEONATES

When problems are anticipated, preparations can be made for intensive care during the periods of greatest threat and, through this care, the incidence of fetal and neonatal mortality can be significantly reduced. Nurses in a variety of settings play an important role in detection and intervention where high-risk factors are most likely to occur. This care begins in the preconceptual period when parents at risk for problems associated with procreation (usually genetic defects) are provided with information they need to make a judicious decision regarding childbearing. In the prenatal period the single most important aspect in anticipating or averting problems is early and consistent prenatal care. Nurses in the community are in a position to find the family in need and to arrange for ongoing prenatal observation. During labor and delivery the obstetric nurse who is alert to the signs of fetal distress and maternal conditions that contribute to neonatal morbidity can avert numerous problems related to the intrapartal period. Assessment and prompt intervention in life-threatening emergencies often make the difference between a favorable outcome and a lifetime of disability. The nurse in the newborn nursery is familiar with the characteristics of the neonate and recognizes the significance of benign and serious deviations from expected observations.

It is estimated that 5% of newborn infants will require care in special, intensive care nurseries and that only about half of the infants with potentially serious problems are identified at birth. Therefore, the nurse is in the crucial position to identify those subtle signs that indicate impending difficulties—color changes, lethargy, poor feeding, altered vital signs, and other unusual behavior. When the need for specialized care can be anticipated and planned for, the probability of successful outcome is increased.

Anticipation of problems

Many of the factors that influence the outcome of these vulnerable periods occur simultaneously and in combination. For example, infants born prematurely often suffer from perinatal anoxia, have cerebral hemorrhage during delivery, have associated congenital anomalies, and/or develop hyaline membrane disease. The list of factors associated with increased risk in the neonatal period continues to grow as applied research in the fields of perinatology and neonatology adds new data. The major situations that contribute to perinatal morbidity and mortality in infancy and, possibly, the future physical and intellectual quality of the child or that warn of impending difficulties include the following[3,21,22]:

Preconceptual

Hereditary diseases or abnormalities—inborn errors of metabolism, anomalies of heart and central nervous system, sickle cell anemia, and so on

Socioeconomic factors—poor nutrition and general health of mother; frequently teenage pregnancy

High altitude—associated with low birth weight infants

Parental age

- Maternal—over 35 or under 16 years of age
- Paternal—over 40 years of age

Maternal size—less than 5 feet; prepregnant weight less than 20% over or under standards for height and weight

Grand multiparity—more than five, especially when the mother is over 35 years of age

History of obstetric complications—prolonged period of infertility, spontaneous abortion, placental accidents, previous larger-than-average or small-for-date infants, toxemia, isoimmunization, multiple pregnancies, previous birth of abnormal infant

Uterine abnormality—tumors (fibroid, myoma), developmental anomalies (uterus bicornis), incompetent cervix

Prenatal

Maternal disease—toxemia, hypertension, malignancy, heart disease, hemoglobinopathy, renal diseases, endocrine (thyroid, diabetes)
Maternal infection—bacterial, viral, spirochetal, protozoal
Maternal disorders associated with pregnancy—toxemia, placental abnormalities, hyperemesis gravidarum
Socioeconomic problems—malnutrition, long-delayed or lack of prenatal care
Maternal addiction—narcotics, barbiturates, amphetamines, hallucinogenics
Maternal medication (see Table 7-4)
Gases—maternal smoking, anesthesia
Multiple pregnancy—smaller size and premature delivery
Isoimmunization—Rh or ABO blood incompatibility
Uterine accidents—abruptio placentae, placenta previa, ruptured uterus, trauma
Fetal size—larger or smaller than expected for age; over or under normal gestational age (premature, postmature); cephalopelvic disproportion
Polyhydramnios or oligohydramnios—often associated with fetal anomalies
Diagnostic procedures—x-ray films or treatment, amniocentesis
Surgical procedures—incidental operation during course of pregnancy

Natal (intrapartum)

Fever—may indicate maternal infection
Premature labor—preterm infant is at greater risk
Premature rupture of fetal membranes—associated with intrauterine infection and prolapse of umbilical cord
Fetal distress—tachycardia (fetal heart rate above 180 beats/minute), bradycardia (fetal heart rate below 120 beats/minute), irregular heart rate, meconium-stained amniotic fluid (in vertex presentation), abnormal deceleration curve (monitored), scalp vein pH 7.2 or less
Abnormalities of fetal position—transverse, breech, unengaged presenting part
Cesarean section—associated with higher neonatal morbidity; often performed because of adverse prenatal or natal conditions
Abnormal labor and/or delivery—precipitous, prolonged, breech, assisted (forceps), other complications
Uterine accidents—rupture, abruptio placentae
Cord accidents—knots, tight nuchal cord, prolapse
Maternal analgesia or anesthesia—may cause depression in fetus and newborn

Postnatal (immediate)

Single umbilical artery—often associated with fetal anomalies
Low Apgar score—especially 5-minute one
Abnormal placenta—massive infarction, evidence of separation, amnionitis
Prematurity—newborn less able to withstand rigors of birth and transition
Multiple birth—newborn usually small and immature at birth
Disproportion between weight or length and gestational age—may indicate intrauterine growth retardation, intrauterine malnutrition, concomitant disorders (for example, infant of diabetic mother)
Depression—may indicate central nervous system damage, hypoxia, maternal oversedation
Birth trauma—head injury, fractures, and so on
Presence of congenital anomalies—cleft palate, imperforate anus, choanal atresia, omphalocele, diaphragmatic hernia, tracheoesophageal fistula, cardiovascular defect
Severe blood loss, sepsis, meconium aspiration—adversely influence adjustment

Postnatal (warning signs)

Abnormal respiration—may indicate congenital anomalies, lung syndromes, acidosis, and so on
Apneic episodes—may be caused by central nervous system disturbance, immaturity of regulatory mechanisms, congestion, obstruction, drugs, cardiac anomalies, hypoglycemia, hypocalcemia, and so on
Tremor and/or seizures—may indicate hypoglycemia, hypocalcemia, narcotic addiction, central nervous system hemorrhage or infection, postasphyxia, or depression
Limpness and/or lethargy—may be the result of central nervous system damage, hypoxia, Down's syndrome, cretinism
Vomiting or difficulty in swallowing—central nervous system damage, immature reflexes, congenital defects
Abdominal distention—may indicate congenital anomalies
Failure to void or pass meconium in first 24 hours—associated with congenital anomalies
Pallor—may indicate anemia, hemorrhage, or cold stress
Jaundice—especially serious when appears in first 24 hours
Petechiae—a sign of thrombocytopenia
Thermal instability—central nervous system damage, immaturity, environmental factors
Failure to regain birth weight by 10 days of age, congenital anomalies, metabolic disorders, central nervous system damage, sepsis, feeding difficulties
Cyanosis—respiratory or cardiac disorders, apnea

Although not considered as high-risk situations in the usual sense, difficulties in the ability of the mother to properly care for the child or disturbances in the mother-child relationship can have serious consequences—both immediate and long term—for the infant. These difficulties may be caused by neurologic, malignant, rheumatic, or other disorders that impair the mother's ability to physically care for her infant and by psychologic illness that interferes with her ability to provide proper care for the child. These situations will not be discussed in depth here; however, nurses must be alert to indications of these special problems that profoundly influence the well-being of the infant and thus place the infant at risk.

Classification of high-risk infants

High-risk infants are most often classified according to size, gestational age, and the predominant pathophysiologic problems. The more common problems related to physiologic status are closely associated with the state of maturity of the infant and usually involve chemical disturbances (hypoglycemia, hypocalcemia) and/or consequences of immature functioning organs and systems (hyperbilirubinemia, respiratory distress, hypothermia). Since high-risk factors are common to several specialty areas, particularly obstetrics, pediatrics, and neonatology, specific terminology is needed to describe the developmental status of the newborn. Formerly, weight at birth was considered to reflect a reasonably accurate estimation of gestational age. That is, if an infant's birth weight exceeded 2500 g (5.5 pounds) he was considered mature. However, accumulated data have shown that intrauterine growth rates are not the same for all infants and that other factors (for example, heredity, placental insufficiency, and maternal disease) influence intrauterine growth and birth weight of the infant. The outgrowth of these data has been a more definitive and meaningful classification system that encompases size, gestational age, and fetal outcome. It has also been determined that the lowest perinatal mortality is found in the full-term infant who weighs between 3500 and 4000 g (approximately 7.75 to 8.8 pounds).

Classification according to size

Low birth weight (LBW) infant—an infant whose birth weight is less than 2500 g without regard to gestational age

Appropriate-for-gestational-age (AGA) infant—an infant whose intrauterine growth was normal at the moment of birth

Small-for-date (SFD) or small-for-gestational-age (SGA) infant—an infant whose rate of intrauterine growth was slowed and who was delivered at or later than term; these infants are usually 2 standard deviations below the mean for infants of appropriate weight at birth and their birth weight falls below the tenth percentile on intrauterine growth curves

Intrauterine growth retardation (IUGR)—found in infants whose intrauterine growth is retarded (sometimes used as more descriptive of small-for-gestational-age infant)

Large-for-gestational-age (LGA) infant—an infant whose birth weight falls above the ninetieth percentile on intrauterine growth curves

Classification according to gestational age

Premature (preterm) infant—an infant born before completion of the thirty-seventh week of gestation, regardless of birth weight

Term infant—an infant born between the beginning of the thirty-eighth week and the completion of the forty-second week of gestation regardless of birth weight

Postmature (postterm) infant—an infant born after completion of the forty-second week of gestational age, regardless of birth weight

Classification according to mortality

Fetal death—death of the fetus after 20 weeks of gestation and before delivery regardless of gestational age and with absence of any signs of life following birth

Neonatal death—death that occurs in the first 28 days of life; early neonatal or postnatal deaths occur in the first week of life

Perinatal mortality—describes the total number of fetal and early neonatal deaths per 1000 total births

Many problems can be anticipated prior to delivery. Prenatal testing and labor monitoring, discussed in Chapter 7, have reduced the incidence of perinatal mortality, and specialized care of the distressed newborn is increasing the survival rate of these infants. If the infant is likely to require special therapy at or soon after birth, plans should be made for delivery to take place at or near a hospital that has the facilities to provide such care. In this way there is no delay in initiating needed care and some of the hazards associated with transporting the sick newborn are averted.

INTENSIVE CARE FACILITIES

Awareness of the unique characteristics of perinatal disorders has generated the provision of special care units in major medical facilities. Rapid advances in the understanding of the pathophysiology of the neonate and the increased capacity to apply this knowledge have emphasized the need for appropriate settings in which to care for the seriously ill infant. Much of the impetus for the special care units arose in response to the emergence of neonatology and perinatology as separate disciplines of medicine and nursing as well as to advancements in electronics and biochemistry. New methods for monitoring cardiorespiratory function, microtechniques for biochemical determination from minute quantities of blood, and new methods for assisted ventilation and conservation of body heat have made it possible to effectively manage the newborn infant with serious illness.[22]

Intensive care of the ill and immature newborn requires specialized knowledge and skill in a number of areas of expertise. Much of the equipment long used in care of the critically ill adult is unsuited to the singular needs of the very small infant; therefore, commonplace apparatus must be modified to meet these needs. Examples of modifications include respirators that deliver small volumes of oxygen in the proper concentration and pressure, infusion pumps that can be regulated accurately in very small amounts, and a means to provide a constant source of warmth while, at the same time, allowing maximum access to the infant. Most important of all, intensive care has created a need for highly skilled personnel specially trained in the art of neonatal intensive care.

Special care units are designed to meet a wide range of special needs ranging from the observation of apparently well infants who have been determined to be "at risk" of serious illness to the intensive treatment of acutely ill infants whose survival is in doubt. This requires that the unit arrange for graduated care for the infant population. That is, there should be adequate facilities and skilled personnel to provide one-to-one nursing care to each seriously ill infant and a means for graduation to one-to-four or one-to-five nursing care in a "convalescent" area where the infants require less intensive care until they are ready to leave the unit.

Nurses in the neonatal intensive care unit (NICU) are highly trained in the management of a variety of sophisticated mechanical devices and educated in the art of recognizing subtle changes in the infant's behavior, interpreting observations of others, and timing interventions appropriately. Proficiency is developed through daily observation and practice under the guidance of a skilled practitioner; in-service education is one of the prime objectives in the ongoing management of a successful neonatal intensive care unit. The teaching activities of nurses in the neonatal intensive care unit are extended to include not only new nurses but also residents, interns, and parents.[16]

Transporting high-risk neonates

It is not economically feasible for every institution to have a functioning neonatal intensive care facility; therefore, most such services are organized on a regional basis. Special equipment, skilled personnel, and ancillary services are concentrated in a centralized institution that serves the needs of a number of hospitals within a given geographic area. When the infant at risk is identified or anticipated, arrangements are made for care in the intensive care facility. There is no question that the uterus is the ideal transport unit for the infant with anticipated difficulties; therefore, whenever possible the mother is delivered where special care is available. However, many infants develop difficulties after a seemingly normal pregnancy and uncomplicated labor. For these infants a coordinated system is needed to transport them to the centralized facility.

Communication is the key to success of a transport system. The neonatologist in the intensive care facility controls and directs the operation, which must be available on a 24-hour basis. The transfer is initiated by the referring physician, who communicates the problem to the neonatologist. The neonatologist, in turn, notifies the transport team and alerts the intensive care unit of the nature of the problem so that preparations can be made to receive the infant. The transport unit is dispatched to the referring institution. The infant is transported in a specially designed incubator unit, containing a complete life-support system, that can be carried by ambulance, van, or helicopter (Fig. 10-1). The team also takes along a monitor and an assortment of emergency equipment.

The transport team may consist of one or more of the highly trained persons from the neonatal intensive care unit—a neonatologist (or a Fellow in Neonatology), intern or resident, and one or more nurses. When complex problems are anticipated the neonatologist or Fellow accompanies the infant; in relatively uncomplicated cases a nurse may go alone. The person assigned to accompany the infant has to be constantly alert to every change in the infant's condition and able to intervene appropriately. The neonate who must be moved from one place to another within the hospital (to surgery, from delivery room to nursery) is transported in an incubator or radiant warmer accompanied by necessary personnel and equipment.

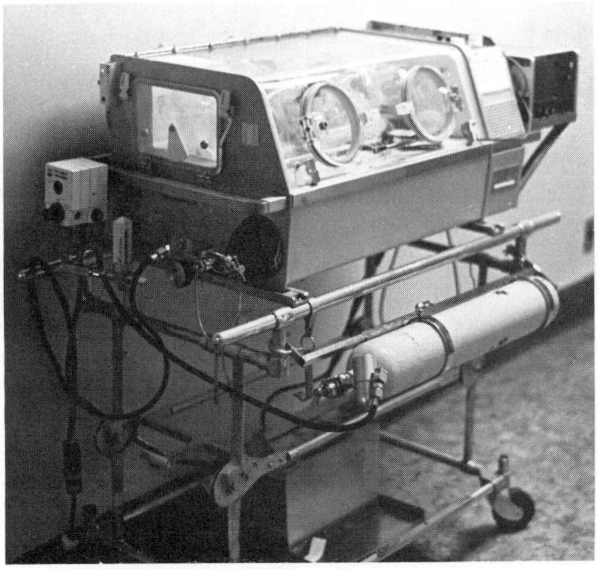

Fig. 10-1. Self-sustained infant transport unit.

Nurses in neonatal intensive care unit

Nurses in a neonatal intensive care unit are vital to the successful operation of the unit and the ultimate outcome of infant therapy. Neonatal intensive care nursing is a highly specialized area of knowledge and practice that requires lengthy supervised experience to reach a level of competence that permits independent functioning. Neonatal intensive care nursing involves an understanding of neonatal physiology and characteristics, a knowledge of the function and management of a number of mechanical devices and apparatus, the ability to recognize very subtle deviations from the expected, and the ability to implement a judicious course of action.

Baptism. The precarious nature of many high-risk infants makes death a very real and ever-present danger. Since most Christian parents wish to have their child baptized if death is anticipated or a decided possibility, this becomes a nursing responsibility. Whenever possible it is most desirable that a representative of the parent's faith that is, a Roman Catholic priest or a Protestant minister, perform such a ritual. When death is imminent a nurse or a physician can perform the baptism by simply pouring water on the infant's forehead (a medicine dropper is a convenient means) while repeating the words, "I baptize you in the name of the Father and of the Son and of the Holy Spirit."

This includes a birth of any gestational age, particularly when the parents are of the Roman Catholic faith. When the faith of the parent is uncertain, a conditional baptism can be carried out by saying, "If you are capable of receiving baptism, I baptize you in the name of the Father and of the Son and of the Holy Spirit." The fact of the baptism is recorded in the infant's chart and a notice placed on the crib or Isolette. Parents are informed at the first opportunity.

ASSESSMENT OF HIGH-RISK NEONATES

At birth the newborn is given a cursory assessment to determine any apparent problems and those that demand immediate attention. This examination is primarily concerned with evaluation of cardiopulmonary and neurologic function. The assessment includes the assignment of an Apgar score (see p. 251) and evaluation for pallor, cyanosis, prematurity, any obvious congenital anomalies, or evidence of neonatal disease. If the infant displays any need for intensive care, he is taken immediately to the neonatal intensive care nursery for initiation of therapy and more extensive assessment.

Assessment of gestational age

The weight of the infant at birth, which can be easily and reliably determined, correlates with the incidence of perinatal morbidity and mortality. Since many infants who weigh less than 2500 g are not premature by gestational age, there is often confusion between the preterm and the small-for-gestational-age infants; fetal growth, gestational age, and fetal maturity are closely related but are not synonymous. Maturity implies functional capacity—the degree to which the neonate's organ systems are able to adapt to the requirements of extrauterine life. Therefore, gestational age is more closely related to fetal maturity than is birth weight. Some infants' heredity influences their size at birth. Oriental and black infants tend to be smaller than white newborns. Small parents have smaller infants and vice versa; therefore, it is important to note the size of other family members as part of the assessment process.

Weight related to gestational age. The infant's birth weight is plotted on a standardized graph that identifies normal weights for gestational age. The graph indicates the expected weight vertically and the gestational age (derived

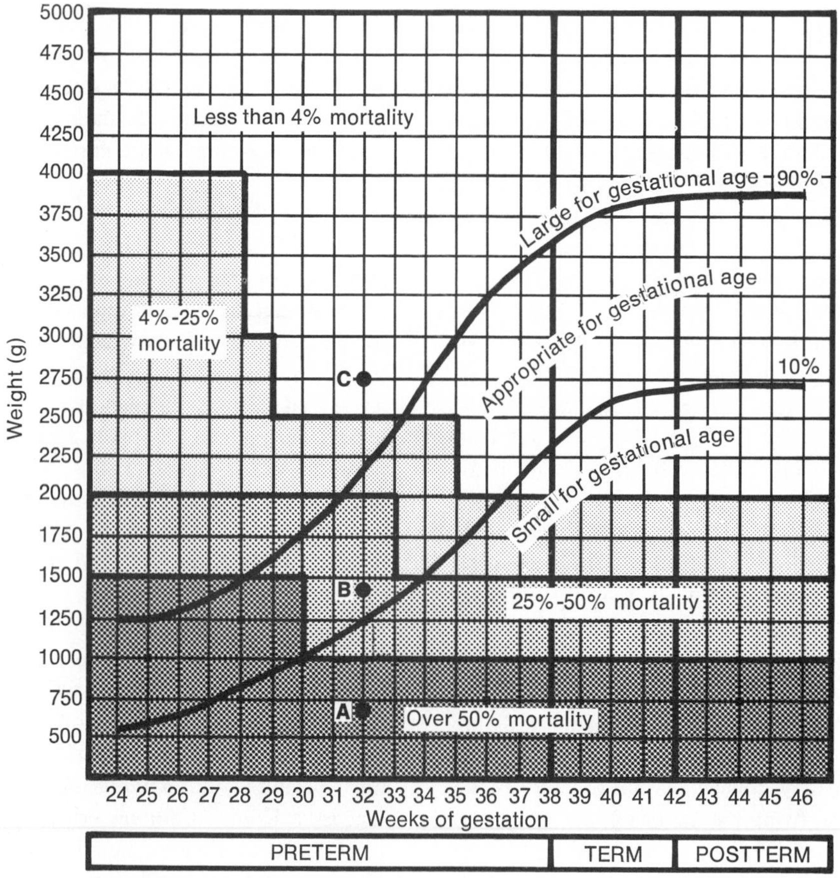

Fig. 10-2. Intrauterine growth status for gestational ages and according to appropriateness of growth. (Adapted from Battaglia, F. C., and Lubchenco, L. O.: J. Pediatrics **71:**59, 1967.)

from the date of the mother's last menstrual period) horizontally (Fig. 10-2). The infant whose weight is appropriate for gestational age can be presumed to have grown at a normal rate regardless of the time of birth—preterm, term, or postterm. The infant who is large for gestational age (above the ninetieth percentile) can be presumed to have grown at an accelerated rate during fetal life; the small-for-gestational-age infant (below the tenth percentile) can be assumed to have grown at a retarded rate during intrauterine life. Fig. 10-3 illustrates the disparity between the birth weights of three preterm infants of the same gestational age. The infant's weight at birth is not necessarily a good indicator of the state of maturity, however. Classification of infants at birth by both weight and gestational age provides a more satisfactory method for predicting mortality risks and providing guidelines for management of the high-risk neonate.

The preterm infant has a number of characteristics that are distinctive at various stages of development. Identification of these characteristics provides valuable clues to the gestational age and, hence, to the physiologic capabilities of infants. The general outward physical appearance changes as the fetus progresses to maturity. Characteristics of skin, general attitude when supine, appearance of hair, and subcutaneous fat provide cues to the newborn's physical development. Observation of spontaneous, active movements and response to stimulation and passive movement contribute to the assessment of neurologic status. The appraisal is made as soon as possible after admission to the nursery since much of the observation and management of the infant depends on this information.

The physical neurologic features of the newborn at various stages of development are assessed based on the outline in Fig. 10-4. The infant is observed first lying quietly in the supine position. The observer notes the attitude in which the child lies, including flexion, extension, and rotation of arms and legs. Muscle tone is assessed by simple testing of recoil. To facilitate the use of the assessment chart, the following tests and observations are further described:

resting posture with the infant lying in a supine position, the degree of extension and flexion of arms and legs, knees and elbows, and adduction and abduction of hips are evaluated.

recoil the arm or leg is fully flexed for 5 seconds, then extended by traction on foot or hand and the maximum response is noted. Full flexion is a maximum response. A brisk return to full extension is characteristic of a full-term infant; the preterm infant displays sluggish return, only random movements, or no movement at all.

heel-to-ear maneuver the infant's foot is drawn as near to the head as possible without the use of force. The degree of extension and the distance between the foot and the head are noted.

scarf sign the examiner attempts to place the infant's hand as far posteriorly around the neck as possible in the direction of the opposite shoulder.

square window the examiner flexes the forearm with enough pressure applied to get as full a flexion as possible to measure the angle between the hypothenar eminence and the ventral aspect of the forearm.

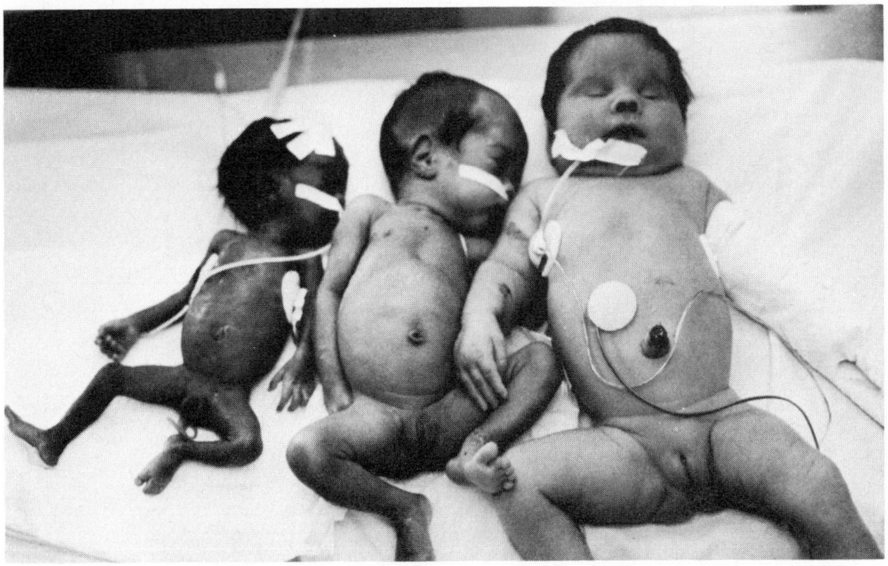

Fig. 10-3. Three babies, same gestational age, weight 600, 1400, and 2750 g, respectively, from left to right. They are plotted on Fig. 10-2 at points A, B, and C. (From Korones, S. B.: High-risk newborn infants: the basis for intensive nursing care, ed. 2, St. Louis, 1976, The C. V. Mosby Co., p. 77.)

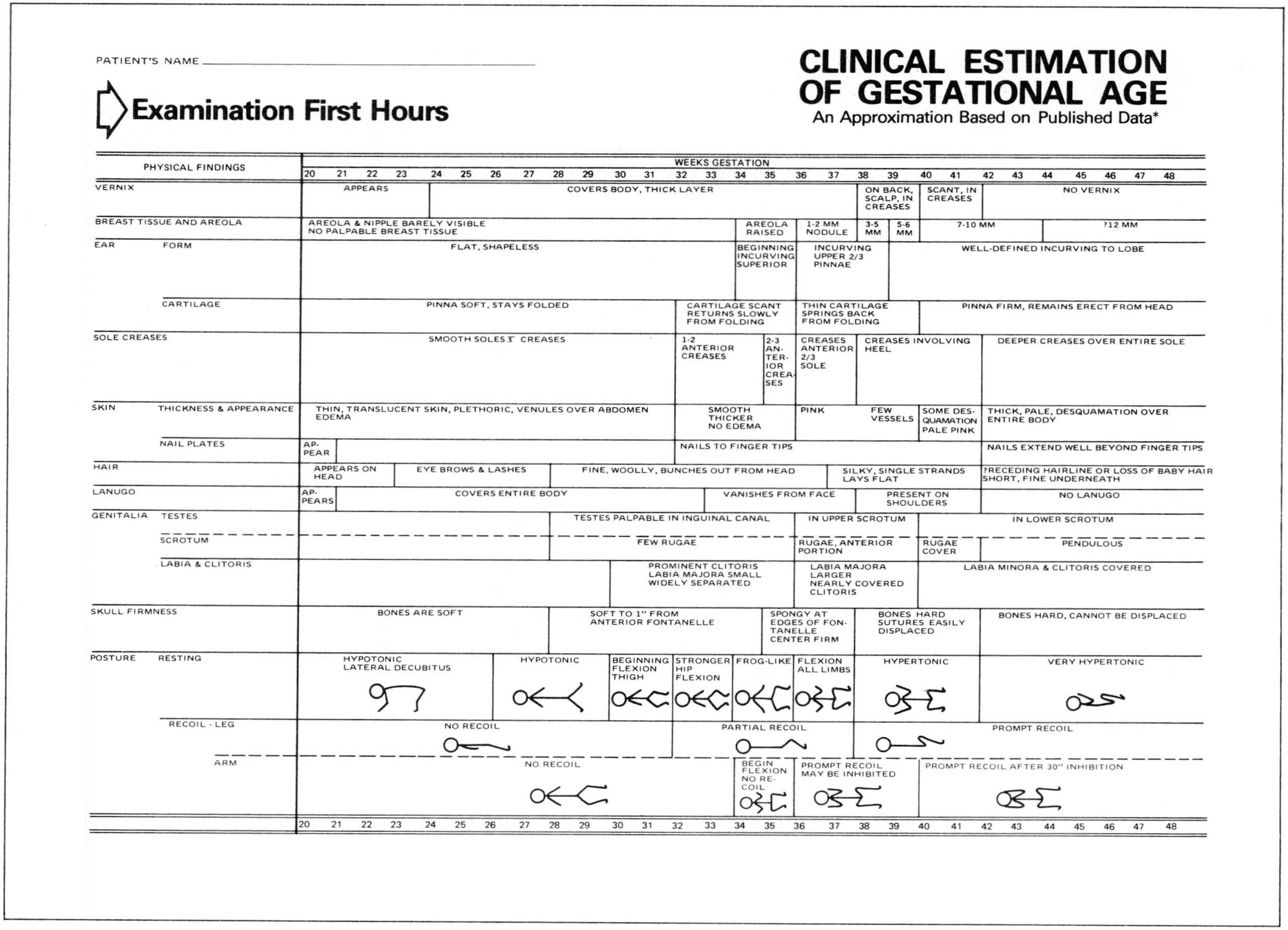
PATIENT'S NAME
Examination First Hours
CLINICAL ESTIMATION OF GESTATIONAL AGE
An Approximation Based on Published Data*
PHYSICAL FINDINGS
WEEKS GESTATION
20 21 22 23 24 25 26 27 28 29 30 31 32 33 34 35 36 37 38 39 40 41 42 43 44 45 46 47 48
VERNIX
APPEARS
COVERS BODY, THICK LAYER
ON BACK, SCALP, IN CREASES
SCANT, IN CREASES
NO VERNIX
BREAST TISSUE AND AREOLA
AREOLA & NIPPLE BARELY VISIBLE NO PALPABLE BREAST TISSUE
AREOLA RAISED
1-2 MM NODULE
3-5 MM
5-6 MM
7-10 MM
?12 MM
EAR
FORM
FLAT, SHAPELESS
BEGINNING INCURVING SUPERIOR
INCURVING UPPER 2/3 PINNAE
WELL-DEFINED INCURVING TO LOBE
CARTILAGE
PINNA SOFT, STAYS FOLDED
CARTILAGE SCANT RETURNS SLOWLY FROM FOLDING
THIN CARTILAGE SPRINGS BACK FROM FOLDING
PINNA FIRM, REMAINS ERECT FROM HEAD
SOLE CREASES
SMOOTH SOLES ∓ CREASES
1-2 ANTERIOR CREASES
2-3 ANTERIOR CREASES
CREASES ANTERIOR 2/3 SOLE
CREASES INVOLVING HEEL
DEEPER CREASES OVER ENTIRE SOLE
SKIN
THICKNESS & APPEARANCE
THIN, TRANSLUCENT SKIN, PLETHORIC, VENULES OVER ABDOMEN EDEMA
SMOOTH THICKER NO EDEMA
PINK
FEW VESSELS
SOME DESQUAMATION PALE PINK
THICK, PALE, DESQUAMATION OVER ENTIRE BODY
NAIL PLATES
APPEAR
NAILS TO FINGER TIPS
NAILS EXTEND WELL BEYOND FINGER TIPS
HAIR
APPEARS ON HEAD
EYE BROWS & LASHES
FINE, WOOLLY, BUNCHES OUT FROM HEAD
SILKY, SINGLE STRANDS LAYS FLAT
?RECEDING HAIRLINE OR LOSS OF BABY HAIR SHORT, FINE UNDERNEATH
LANUGO
APPEARS
COVERS ENTIRE BODY
VANISHES FROM FACE
PRESENT ON SHOULDERS
NO LANUGO
GENITALIA
TESTES
TESTES PALPABLE IN INGUINAL CANAL
IN UPPER SCROTUM
IN LOWER SCROTUM
SCROTUM
FEW RUGAE
RUGAE, ANTERIOR PORTION
RUGAE COVER
PENDULOUS
LABIA & CLITORIS
PROMINENT CLITORIS LABIA MAJORA SMALL WIDELY SEPARATED
LABIA MAJORA LARGER NEARLY COVERED CLITORIS
LABIA MINORA & CLITORIS COVERED
SKULL FIRMNESS
BONES ARE SOFT
SOFT TO 1" FROM ANTERIOR FONTANELLE
SPONGY AT EDGES OF FONTANELLE CENTER FIRM
BONES HARD SUTURES EASILY DISPLACED
BONES HARD, CANNOT BE DISPLACED
POSTURE
RESTING
HYPOTONIC LATERAL DECUBITUS
HYPOTONIC
BEGINNING FLEXION THIGH
STRONGER HIP FLEXION
FROG-LIKE
FLEXION ALL LIMBS
HYPERTONIC
VERY HYPERTONIC
RECOIL - LEG
NO RECOIL
PARTIAL RECOIL
PROMPT RECOIL
ARM
NO RECOIL
BEGIN FLEXION NO RECOIL
PROMPT RECOIL MAY BE INHIBITED
PROMPT RECOIL AFTER 30" INHIBITION

Fig. 10-4. Clinical estimation of gestational age. (From Kempe, C. H., Silver, H. K., and O'Brien, D., editors: Current pediatric diagnosis and treatment, ed. 5, Los Altos, Calif., 1978, Lange Medical Publications.) (See also Fig. 10-6.)

Confirmatory Neurologic Examination to be Done After 24 Hours

MeadJohnson LABORATORIES

	Physical findings	Weeks gestation (20–48)					
TONE	HEEL TO EAR	NO RESISTANCE	SOME RESISTANCE	IMPOSSIBLE			
	SCARF SIGN	NO RESISTANCE	ELBOW PASSES MIDLINE	ELBOW AT MIDLINE	ELBOW DOES NOT REACH MIDLINE		
	NECK FLEXORS (HEAD LAG)	ABSENT	HEAD IN PLANE OF BODY	HOLDS HEAD			
	NECK EXTENSORS	HEAD BEGINS TO RIGHT ITSELF FROM FLEXED POSITION	GOOD RIGHTING CANNOT HOLD IT	HOLDS HEAD FEW SECONDS	KEEPS HEAD IN LINE c̄ TRUNK > 40"	TURNS HEAD FROM SIDE TO SIDE	
	BODY EXTENSORS	STRAIGHT-ENING OF LEGS	STRAIGHT-ENING OF TRUNK	STRAIGHTENING OF HEAD & TRUNK TOGETHER			
	VERTICAL POSITIONS	WHEN HELD UNDER ARMS, BODY SLIPS THROUGH HANDS	ARMS HOLD BABY LEGS EXTENDED	LEGS FLEXED GOOD SUPPORT c̄ ARMS			
	HORIZONTAL POSITIONS	HYPOTONIC ARMS & LEGS STRAIGHT	ARMS AND LEGS FLEXED	HEAD & BACK EVEN FLEXED EXTREMITIES	HEAD ABOVE BACK		
FLEXION ANGLES	POPLITEAL	NO RESISTANCE	150°	110°	100°	90°	80°
	ANKLE	45°	20°	0	A PRE-TERM WHO HAS REACHED 40 WEEKS STILL HAS A 40° ANGLE		
	WRIST (SQUARE WINDOW)	90°	60°	45°	30°	0	
REFLEXES	SUCKING	WEAK NOT SYNCHRONIZED c̄ SWALLOWING	STRONGER SYNCHRO-NIZED	PERFECT	PERFECT HAND TO MOUTH	PERFECT	
	ROOTING	LONG LATENCY PERIOD SLOW, IMPERFECT	HAND TO MOUTH	BRISK, COMPLETE, DURABLE	COMPLETE		
	GRASP	FINGER GRASP IS GOOD STRENGTH IS POOR	STRONGER	CAN LIFT BABY OFF BED INVOLVES ARMS	HANDS OPEN		
	MORO	BARELY APPARENT	WEAK NOT ELICITED EVERY TIME	STRONGER	COMPLETE c̄ ARM EXTENSION OPEN FINGERS, CRY	ARM ADDUCTION ADDED	?BEGINS TO LOSE MORO
	CROSSED EXTENSION	FLEXION & EXTENSION IN A RANDOM, PURPOSELESS PATTERN	EXTENSION BUT NO ADDUCTION	STILL INCOMPLETE	EXTENSION ADDUCTION FANNING OF TOES	COMPLETE	
	AUTOMATIC WALK	MINIMAL	BEGINS TIPTOEING GOOD SUPPORT ON SOLE	FAST TIPTOEING	HEEL-TOE PROGRESSION WHOLE SOLE OF FOOT	A PRE-TERM WHO HAS REACHED 40 WEEKS WALKS ON TOES	?BEGINS TO LOSE AUTO-MATIC WALK
	PUPILLARY REFLEX	ABSENT	APPEARS	PRESENT			
	GLABELLAR TAP	ABSENT	APPEARS	PRESENT			
	TONIC NECK REFLEX	ABSENT	APPEARS	PRESENT			
	NECK-RIGHTING	ABSENT	APPEARS	PRESENT AFTER 37 WEEKS			

*Brazie, J.V., and Lubchenco, L.O.: The Estimation of Gestational Age Chart, in Kempe, Silver and O'Brien: Current Pediatric Diagnosis and Treatment, ed. 3, Los Altos, California, Lange Medical Publications, 1974, chapter 3.

Lit. 181, 12/74

Fig. 10-4, cont'd. For legend see opposite page.

popliteal angle with the thigh in knee-chest position, the leg is extended by gentle pressure to measure the popliteal angle.
head lag the position of the head in relation to the trunk is observed as the child is slowly pulled toward the sitting position.
ventral suspension the degree of extension of the back and the amount of flexion of arms and legs are observed when the infant is suspended prone on the examiner's hand.

The sum of observations provides the examiner with a guide for management of the infant and special problems that might be anticipated in nursing care.

Nursing observations

Many of the components of nursing observation related to care of the neonate that apply to nursing of the high-risk newborn are discussed in Chapters 8 and 9. Others will be considered throughout the remainder of this chapter and summarized in relation to specific patient problems. Detailed, ongoing records of all activities and observations are an important function of nurses in the intensive care setting. Knowledge and operation of complex pieces of equipment and mechanical devices are inherent in the care of the ill neonate. However, sophisticated monitoring and life-support systems cannot replace the vigilance and constant scrutiny of the infants by experienced personnel. Subtle changes that are not apparent on the mechanical devices can be detected by alert nurses, for example, changes in color and regurgitated formula, which will not register on a monitor until aspiration produces an apneic spell. Some of the crucial factors in observation of ill newborns cannot be detected by monitors. These are[22]:

Acceptance of feedings
Course of weight gain
Early detection of regurgitation
Abdominal distention
Frequency and character of stools
Changes in behavior (lethargy, seizure activity, hyperactivity)
Changes in color (jaundice, pallor, cyanosis)
Skin lesions
Deviations from prescribed volumes of intravenous infusions
Edema
Respiratory distress (tachypnea, retractions, flaring nares, grunting)
Quality of breath sounds
Character and location of heart sounds

Monitoring physiologic data. Most neonates under intensive observation are placed in a controlled thermal environment and monitored for heart rate, respiratory activity, and temperature. Routine monitoring of heart rate consists of a pulse rate indicator that signals each ventricular contraction by an audible beep and flashing light. The indicator is integrated with an alarm system so that a pulse rate above or below predetermined limits triggers the alarm. When the heart rate falls below or rises above the preset rate, both audio and visual alarms alert the nurse. The limits set for cardiac monitors are determined by the condition of the individual infant and the philosophy of the special care unit but are usually below 80 beats/minute and above 160 beats/minute. Each alarm requires the nurse to observe, assess the situation, and made a decision regarding the infant's status. Factors other than altered infant condition may trigger the alarm, for example, poor contact between the infant and the electrodes, loose connections, poor placement, or other interferences such as inadequate grounding, soiled electrodes, or movement. Proper placement and maintenance of electrodes and their connections are nursing responsibilities. Electrodes are either attached topically to the outer aspect of the chest wall, one on each side, by special electrode paste or jelly and adhesive discs or by needle electrodes inserted intradermally and anchored with hypoallergenic tape.

Respiratory activity is also monitored since the heart rate does not always drop with apnea, although bradycardia frequently follows an apneic spell. Apnea monitors consist of either an air-filled mattress that is sensitive to movement of air coincidental with respirations or of an impedance monitor that measures the electrical resistance across the chest as it changes with respiration. The alarm works in the same manner as the cardiac monitor. The monitor is usually set at a 10- to 15-second delay for apnea. This involves electrode placement as in cardiac monitoring, and the two are often combined in the same monitoring equipment (Fig. 10-5).

The placement of electrodes is a continual nursing problem because of lack of flat areas and limited space for alternating sites, the size of the electrodes, and irritation from the paste and/or tape. Electrodes for monitors can often be applied to the upper arms to provide relief for chest areas. It is important to follow the manufacturer's directions for care and handling of electrodes.

Blood pressure is monitored routinely in the sick neonate either by internal or external means. Direct recording with arterial catheters if often employed but carries the risks inherent in any procedure in which a needle or other implement is introduced into a blood vessel. The transcutaneous Doppler apparatus is a simple, effective means for detecting weak impulses, but it is expensive. In cases in which these methods are not available or desirable, the flush blood pressure method provides a reliable systolic reading that is readily adaptable to a variety of situations. The technique is easily learned and the equipment is inexpensive (see p. 116 for description of the technique). Flush blood pressure is adversely affected by some conditions that compromise the circulation in the extremities, such as anemia (which causes an unrecognizable end point), marked edema, and cold.

In the neonatal intensive care unit frequent laboratory examinations are an integral part of the ongoing assess-

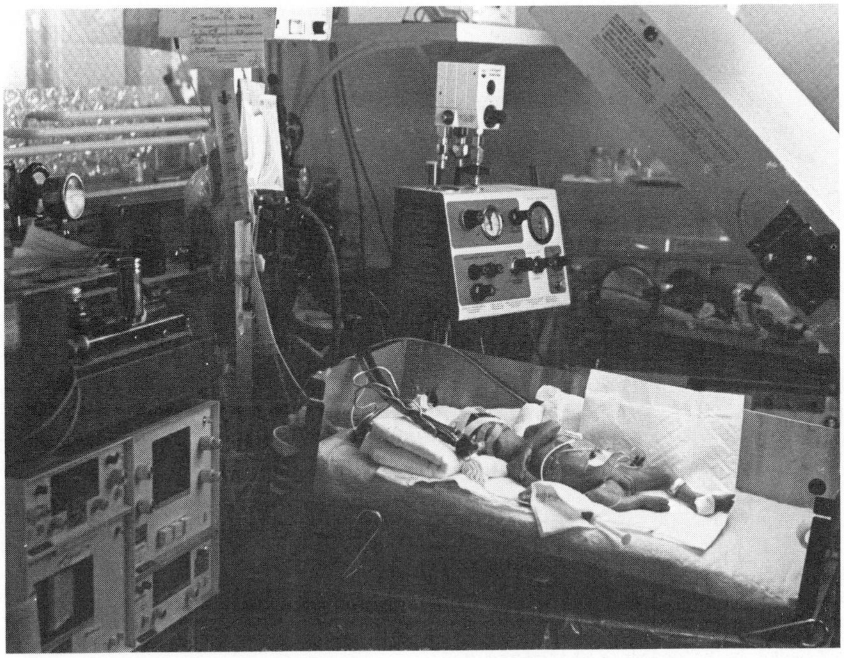

Fig. 10-5. Infant attached to cardiac and apnea monitors and receiving an intravenous infusion and assisted ventilation.

ment of infants' progress. An accurate intake and output record is kept on all infants. An accurate output can be obtained by collection of urine in a plastic urine collection bag (see p. 929) or by weighing the diapers. Weighing the diapers is the most simple and least traumatic means of measuring urine output. The preweighed wet diaper is weighed on a gram scale and the gram weight of the urine is converted directly to milliliters, for example, 25 g = 25 ml. Plastic collecting devices can be used when it is necessary to collect urine for laboratory examination. Specific gravity is measured periodically on voided urine to help assess the adequacy of hydration. Since the volume normally voided is insufficient to float the standard urometer, a refractometer requiring only a single drop of urine is standard equipment in the neonatal intensive care unit. A drop of urine is easily aspirated from the wet diaper with a syringe.

Blood examinations are a necessary part of the ongoing assessment and monitoring of the sick neonates' progress. The tests performed most often are blood glucose, bilirubin, calcium, hematocrit, and blood gases. Samples may be obtained either by blood taken from the heel, venipuncture, or an indwelling catheter in an umbilical vein. The indwelling catheter is usually connected to a heparin lock system in order to prevent clotting of blood in the needle. When the specimen is being collected, it is important to relate the type of test to the treatment the infant is receiving. For example, when an infant is receiving an intravenous infusion of glucose solution, collecting a sample of blood from the heel would provide a more accurate picture of the blood glucose level than would a sample from the intravenous catheter, and phototherapy must be discontinued while a sample is drawn for a bilirubin level or the light will alter the bilirubin in the sample. Capillary samples are usually collected from the heel after the foot has been warmed to approximately 45.5°C (110°F), which takes 5 to 10 minutes. Wrapping the foot in a warm washcloth is a simple means to create adequate vasodilatation. When numerous samples must be drawn, it is important to keep a record of the amount of blood removed since a tiny infant's blood supply can be seriously depleted over a period of time.

Systematic assessment of the infant. Nurses are usually responsible for the same infant each day, which allows for more accurate determination of day-to-day progress. During the course of daily care the nurse makes frequent systematic assessments of physical status since vital signs of small infants change several times in the period of a very few hours. It has been said that the newborn undergoes as many changes in 4 to 6 hours as an adult does in 24 hours.

In the course of an assessment the nurse ascertains whether the life-support apparatus is functioning properly—that the respiratory equipment is at the correct pressure and/or volume setting and no leaks are apparent, that the monitors are set at the desired limits and tracings are within normal limits, and that the infusion pump is delivering the correct volume and type of fluid. The assessment of the infant should proceed in a systematic manner. Each nurse develops an approach that is comfortable for him or her and follows the same pattern routinely. An observational assessment is usually performed hourly, or more frequently on very ill infants, and a synopsis is included in the charting. However, any assessment procedures that require that the infant be disturbed should be timed to allow for sufficient rest between assessments.

Respiratory assessment

Description of shape of chest—barrel, concave, and so on
Description of use of accessory muscles—nasal flaring or substernal, intercostal, or subclavicular retractions
Determination of respiratory rate and regularity
Description of breath sounds—rales, rhonchi, wheezing, grunts, areas of absence of sound
Determination of whether suctioning is needed

Cardiovascular assessment

Determination of heart rate and rhythm
Description of heart sounds, including any suspected murmurs
Determination of the point of maximum intensity (PMI), the point where the heart beat sounds loudest (a change in the point of maximum intensity may indicate a mediastinal shift)
Description of infant's color (may be of cardiac, respiratory, or hematopoietic origin)—cyanosis, pallor, plethora, jaundice
Determination of blood pressure (indicate extremity used)
Description of peripheral pulses
Determination of central venous pressure (if central venous pressure line is part of infant's apparatus)

Neurologic-musculoskeletal assessment

Description of infant's movements—random, purposeful, jittery, twitching, spontaneous, elicited
Description of infant's position or attitude
Description of reflexes observed

Temperature

Determination of axillary temperature
Determination of relationship to environmental temperature

Gastrointestinal assessment

Determination of presence of any indication of abdominal distention—increase in circumference, shiny skin
Determination of any signs of regurgitation, especially following feeding; character and amount of residual
Description of amount, color, consistency, and odor of any emesis
Description of amount, color, and consistency of stools; occult blood should be checked for if indicated by physician's order or appearance of stool
Description of bowel sounds; presence or abscence

Renal assessment

Description of amount (as determined by weight), color, and specific gravity (to determine adequacy of hydration) of urine

Skin assessment

Description of any discoloration, reddened area, or signs of irritation, especially where monitoring equipment, infusions, or other apparatus comes in contact with skin
Determination of texture and turgor of skin—dry, smooth, flaky, peeling, and so on
Description of any rash or skin lesion
Determination of whether intravenous infusion catheter or needle is in place and observation for signs of infiltration

The infant's position is changed every 1 to 2 hours, and any significant reaction to the changing or to a specific position is noted. To conserve the infant's energy, the position changing and periodic treatments should be timed to coincide with an assessment.

Safety measures. The life-saving attributes of the neonatal intensive care facility do not obviate the need for ongoing measures to avoid the imposition of additional hazards on the infant who is already at risk. Protection from infection is an integral part of all newborn care. Preterm and sick neonates are particularly susceptible; therefore, care must be exercised to avoid their contact with contaminants. Thorough, meticulous hand washing is the foundation of a preventive program and includes all persons who come in contact with the infants and/or the equipment. Special clothing (scrub outfits, uniforms, and cover gowns), furnished and laundered by the institution, is worn by everyone entering the unit. All linen and equipment used in the care of the infants are either sterile or scrupulously clean, and personnel with infectious disorders are either barred from the unit until they can no longer transmit the disease to the infants and other personnel or wear suitable shields, such as masks or gloves, to reduce the likelihood of contamination. Most of the infants are effectively isolated from airborne infective agents in the protective environment of the Isolette. However, the Isolette must be cleaned regularly as part of the infection control measures.

Administration of therapeutic agents, such as drugs, ointments, intravenous infusions, and oxygen, require judicious handling and meticulous attention to details. The computation, preparation, and administration of drugs in minute amounts often requires collaboration between nurses to reduce the chance of error. In addition the immaturity of the infant's detoxification mechanisms and inability to demonstrate symptoms of toxicity (for example, signs of auditory nerve involvement from ototoxic drugs such as kanamycin) complicate drug therapy and require that nurses be particularly alert for signs of adverse reaction. (See section on administration of medications in Chapter 26.)

A constant problem in the care of the sick neonate is related to parenteral therapy. The very small, fragile blood vessels (unless an umbilical vessel is used) are subject to rupture and subsequent infiltration. The situation is compounded by the consistent use of pump-type infusion apparatus necessary in order to deliver infusions in minute, regulated quantities. Consequently nurses are constantly on the alert for signs of infiltration, which is very difficult to ascertain, especially in the preterm infant. When the intravenous infusion is inserted into a hand vein, it is often easier to check for infiltration on the palmar surface since the back of the hand is usually obliterated by tape used to secure the needle in place. To check for scalp vein infiltration it is helpful to look in areas where fluid might pool, such as around the ears. It is important to be alert for signs of infiltration, since many infusions contain drugs that can cause severe tissue damage, and for signs of overhydration (see section on intravenous administration on p. 1084).

When adhesive tape is removed from the very small and immature infant it is unsafe to use scissors because it is easy to snip off tiny extremities or nick loosely attached skin. Adhesive tape is best removed by carefully lifting the tape while applying pressure on the skin directly beneath the tape. Rapid removal is contraindicated since the delicate skin is readily separated from understructures and can be easily pulled away with the tape. Paper or hypoallergenic tape is the only kind that should be used on infants.

The proliferation of equipment technology over the past few years has increased the dangers associated with its use, especially performance malfunction and electrical hazards. Malfunction includes such things as inaccurate monitor function, erratic delivery rates in infusion devices, and low or high suction in pumps. Electrical hazards are related to defective equipment, wiring, grounding, or improper use of equipment. One of the most effective means for assuring the safety of infant and staff is the nurse's knowledge, alertness, and common sense regarding the function of equipment. It is important to check equipment for all correct component parts, to report equipment that is not performing according to specifications, and to obey the basic rules of electrical safety—handle equipment with care, be alert to signs of trouble, and follow electrical safety guidelines.

PREMATURE INFANTS

Since the majority of infants who are admitted to intensive care facilities are born prior to the estimated date of delivery, the major discussion of problems related to the high-risk neonate will be directed toward this group. The incidence of neonatal complications, for example, hyaline membrane disease, is highest in the preterm infant, and often other high-risk factors, for example, severe congenital malformations, are found in association with prematurity. Prematurity is generally accepted as the single largest factor contributing to infant mortality.

Etiology and characteristics

Most of the factors concerning high-risk neonates listed on pp. 222 to 224 are related to the incidence of prematurity; however, the actual cause of prematurity is not known in most instances. The incidence of prematurity is lowest in the middle to high socioeconomic classes, in which pregnant women are generally in good health, are well-nourished, and receive prompt and comprehensive prenatal care; the incidence is highest in the low socioeconomic class, in which a combination of deleterious circumstances is present. Other factors such as multiple pregnancies, toxemia, and placental accidents that interrupt the normal course of gestation prior to completion of fetal development are responsible for a large number of premature births.

The outlook for a premature infant is largely, but not entirely, related to the state of physiologic and anatomic immaturity of the various organs and systems at the time of birth. The infant at term has advanced to a state of maturity sufficient to allow a successful transition to the extrauterine environment. The infant born prematurely must make the same adjustments but with functional immaturity proportional to the stage of development that has been reached at the time of birth. The degree to which the infant is prepared for extrauterine life can be predicted to some extent by weight and estimated gestational age. The landmarks of prenatal development in Table 7-2 provide some concept of the status of the systems at various stages of development that must cope with the functional changes that occur with birth. The infant with a birth weight of less than 400 g never develops effective respirations and dies shortly after birth. Infants who weigh 400 to 1000 g at birth have a very poor prognosis, but, with meticulous care and good fortune, about 10% survive. Most of the infants with a birth weight of 1000 to 1500 g have reached a stage of pulmonary maturity in which 40% to 50% can survive with intensive care, and 75% to 85% of infants weighing 1500 to 2000 g at birth are expected to survive. The physical characteristics of the infant of 2000- to 2500-g birth weight, whose survival rate is 90% to 95%, differ very little from those of the full-term infant.

Characteristics. On inspection the premature infant is very small and appears scrawny because of lack of or minimal subcutaneous fat deposits, with a proportionately large head in relation to the body, which reflects the cephalocaudal direction of growth. Of all the body measurements, the head is reduced least, and sucking pads in the cheeks are strikingly prominent. The skin is bright pink, smooth, and shiny (may be edematous) with small blood vessels clearly visible underneath the thin, transparent epidermis. The fine lanugo hair is abundant over the body but is sparse, fine, and fuzzy on the head. The ear cartilage is soft and pliable, and the soles and palms have minimal creases, resulting in a smooth appearance. The bones of the skull and the ribs feel soft, and the prominent eyes are closed. Male infants have few scrotal rugae, and the testes are undescended; labia and clitoris are prominent in the female. (See Fig. 10-6 for a comparison of the features of the normal and premature infant.)

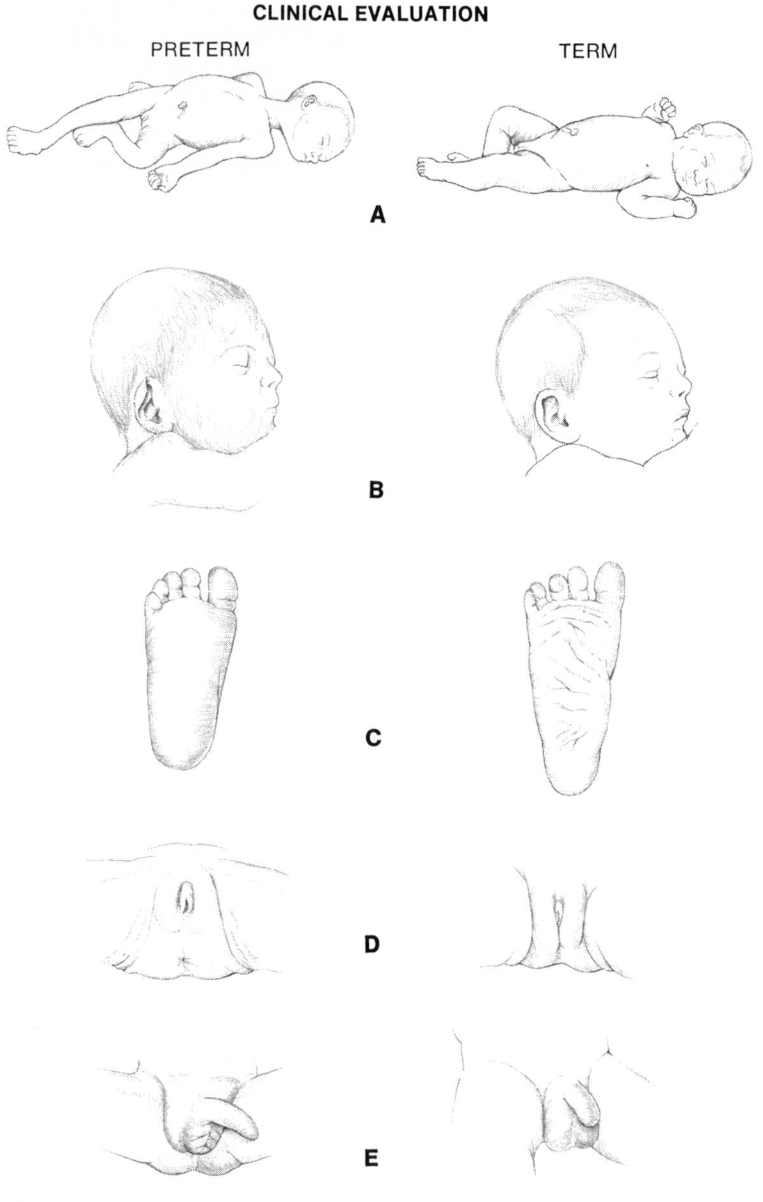

Fig. 10-6. Estimation of gestational age; some clinical and neurologic examinations. *Clinical evaluation.* **A,** The preterm infant lies in a "relaxed attitude," limbs more extended; his body size is small, and his head may appear somewhat larger in proportion to the body size. The term infant has more subcutaneous fat tissue and rests in a more flexed attitude. **B,** The preterm infant's ear cartilages are poorly developed, and the ear may fold easily; the hair is fine and feathery, and lanugo may cover the back and face. The mature infant's ear cartilages are well formed, and the hair is more likely to form firm separate strands. **C,** The sole of the foot of the preterm infant appears more turgid and may have only fine wrinkles. The mature infant's sole (foot) is well and deeply creased. **D,** The preterm female infant's clitoris is prominent, and labia majora are poorly developed and gaping. The mature female infant's labia majora are fully developed, and the clitoris is not as prominent. **E,** The preterm male infant's scrotum is undeveloped and not pendulous, minimal rugae are present, and the testes may be in the inguinal canals or in the abdominal cavity. The term male infant's scrotum is well developed, pendulous, and rugated, and the testes are well down in the scrotal sac.

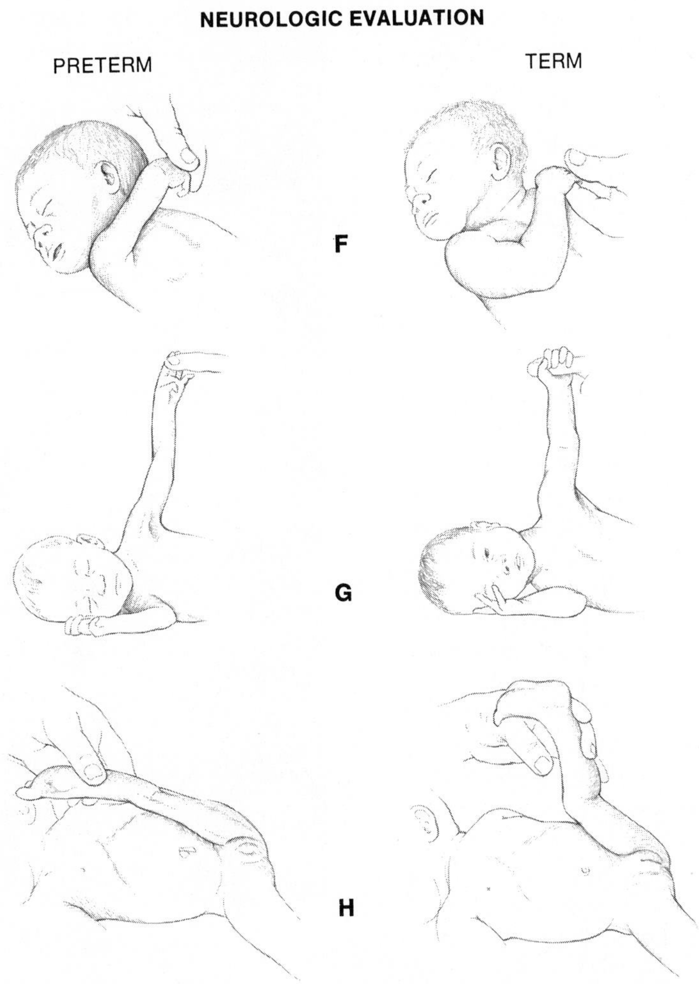

Fig. 10-6, cont'd. *Neurologic evaluation.* **F,** *Scarf sign*—The preterm infant's elbow may be easily brought across the chest with little or no resistance. The mature infant's elbow may be brought to the midline of the chest, resisting attempts to bring the elbow past the midline. **G,** *Grasp reflex*—The preterm infant's grasp is weak; the term infant's grasp is strong, allowing the infant to be lifted up from the mattress. **H,** *Heel-to-ear maneuver*—The preterm infant's heel is easily brought to the ear, meeting with no resistance. This maneuver is not possible in the term infant, since there is considerable resistance at the knee. (From Pierog, S. H., and Ferrara, A.: Medical care of the sick newborn, ed. 2, St. Louis, 1976, The C. V. Mosby Co., pp. 80-81.)

In contrast to the full-term infant's overall attitude of flexion and continuous activity, the premature infant is inactive and torpid. The extremities maintain an attitude of extension and remain in any position in which they are placed. Reflex activity is only partially developed—sucking is absent, weak, or ineffectual; swallowing, gag, and cough reflexes are weak; and other neurologic signs are absent or diminished. Physiologically immature, the preterm infant is unable to maintain body temperature, has limited ability to excrete solutes in the urine, and has an increased susceptibility to infection. A pliable thorax along with immature lung tissue and regulatory center lead to periodic breathing, hypoventilation, and frequent periods of apnea.

COMMON PROBLEMS OF PRETERM INFANTS

As a consequence of anatomic, physiologic, and biochemical inadequacies, the premature infant is prone to a variety of problems that must be anticipated and managed in the neonatal period. The naked infant is placed in a controlled microenvironment in an Isolette or incubator. A Plexiglas top affords a clear view of the infant from all aspects. There is easy access through portholes that minimize temperature and oxygen loss and a large door that provides a more extensive approach (Fig. 10-7). Maximum accessibility is provided by an open unit with an overhead radiant warming system. These units are employed for distressed infants who require extensive mechanical instrumentation, such as a ventilator, monitors, and intravenous infusions, and frequent manipulation, such as vital signs, suctioning, and chest percussion (Fig. 10-8).

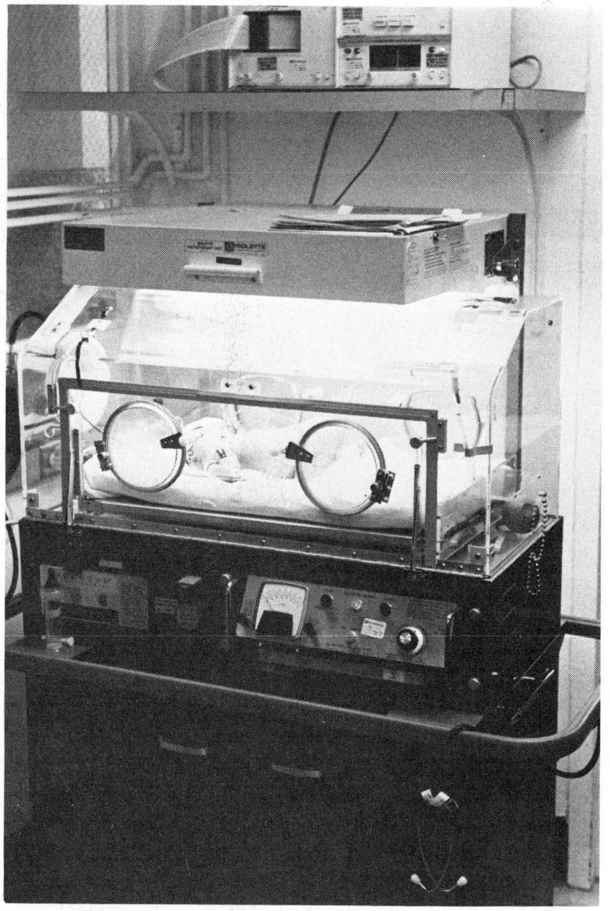

Fig. 10-7. Infant in Isolette.

Thermoregulation

After the establishment of respiration, the most crucial need of the premature is application of external warmth. Prevention of heat loss in the distressed infant is absolutely essential for survival, and maintaining a neutral thermal environment is a challenging aspect of neonatal intensive nursing care. The immature neonate has all the problems related to heat production that are faced by the full-term infant (see p. 257). However, premature infants are placed at further disadvantage by a number of additional problems. They have an even smaller muscle mass for producing heat, lack insulating subcutaneous fat, and have poor reflex control of skin capillaries. Heat production is a complicated process that involves the cardiovascular, neurologic, and metabolic systems. The immature neonate, unable to increase activity and lacking a shivering response, produces heat primarily through increased metabolic processes. Some heat continues to be generated by liver, heart, brain, and skeletal muscles, but the major source of increased production of heat during cold stress is *nonshivering thermogenesis*. Norepinephrine, secreted by the sympathetic nerve endings in response to chilling, stimulates fat metabolism in the richly vascularized brown adipose tissue to produce internal heat, which is then conducted through the blood to surface tissues. Significantly an increase in metabolism requires an increase in oxygen consumption.[21,22]

The consequences of cold stress that produce additional hazards to the neonate are hypoxia, metabolic acidosis, and hypoglycemia. Increased metabolism in response to chilling creates a compensatory increase in oxygen and calorie consumption. If available oxygen is not increased to accommodate this need, arterial oxygen tension is decreased. This is further complicated by a smaller lung volume in relation to metabolic rate that creates diminished oxygen in the blood. There is a small advantage gained by the persistence of fetal hemoglobin (HgF), with its increased capacity to carry oxygen, which allows the infant to exist for longer periods of time in conditions of lowered oxygen tension. It also appears that norepinephrine, released in response to cold stress, causes a pulmonary vasoconstriction that further reduces the effectiveness of pulmonary ventilation. This decrease in oxygen diminishes the supply available for glycose metabolism. As a result, glucose is broken down by an alternate, hypoxic pathway (anaerobic glycolysis) that generates increased lactic acid formation. This, together with acid end products of brown fat metabolism, contributes to the acidotic state. Anaerobic metabolism dissipates glycogen at a markedly increased rate over aerobic metabolism, thus precipitating hypoglycemia. This is especially marked where glycogen stores are diminished at birth and where there is inadequate caloric intake after birth.

Nursing considerations. To delay or prevent the effects of cold stress, newborns at risk are placed in a heated environment immediately following birth where they remain until they are able to maintain thermal stability (the capacity to balance heat production and conservation and heat dissipation). Since overheating produces an increase in oxygen and calorie consumption, the infant is also jeopardized in a hyperthermic environment. A *neutral thermal environment* is one that permits the infant to maintain a normal core temperature with minimal oxygen consumption and calorie expenditure. The very small infant, especially one with a meager subcutaneous fat layer, can control body heat loss or gain only within a very limited range of environmental temperature. It has been found that oxygen consumption is minimal when the ambient air temperature is 1.5°C warmer than the abdominal skin temperature. Consumption of oxy-

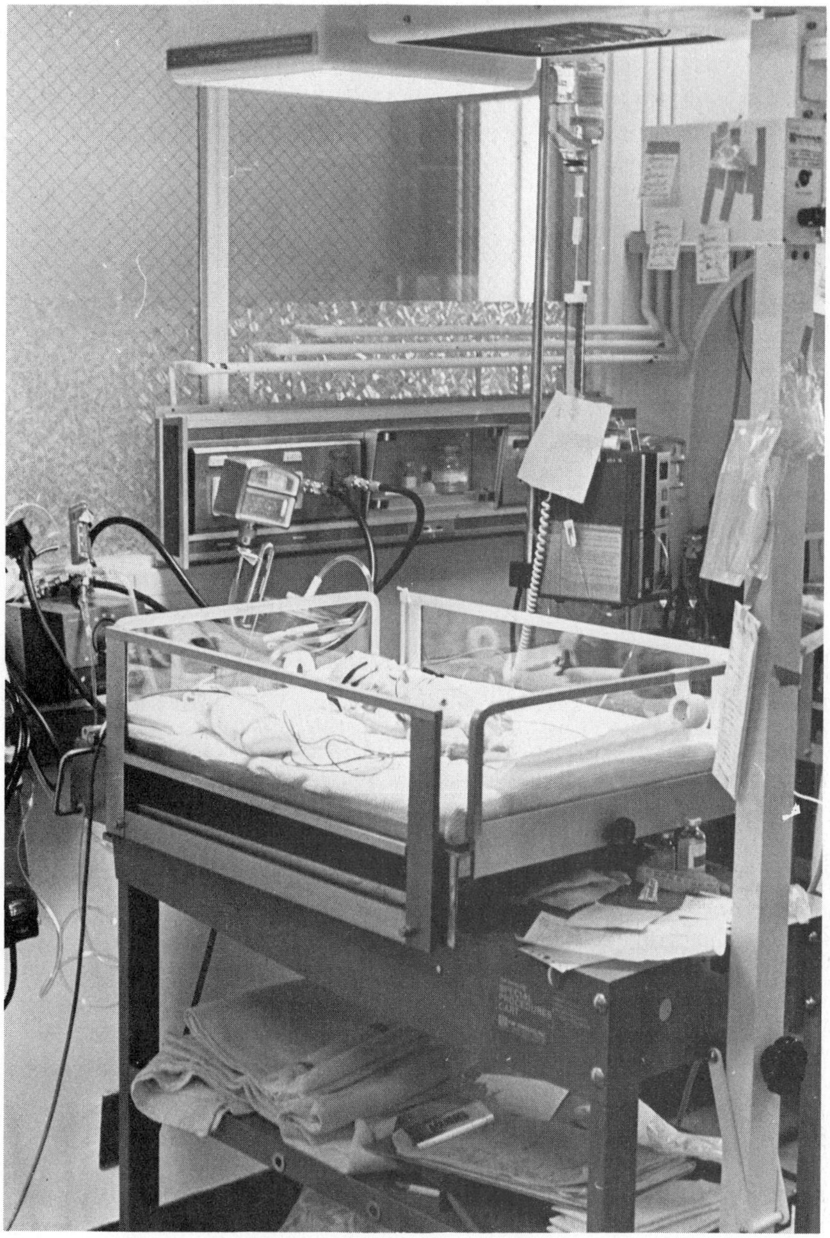

Fig. 10-8. Infant under overhead warming unit.

gen is minimal at an abdominal skin temperature of 36.5°C (97.7°F). When abdominal skin temperature increases to 37.2°C (98.9°F), the consumption of oxygen increases 6%; when skin temperature decreases to 35.9°C (96.6°F), the oxygen consumption increases by 10%. The range of abdominal temperature resulting in a neutral thermal environment is from 36.1° to 36.8°C (97° to 98.2°F).

The three methods for maintaining a neutral thermal environment are by the use of a radiant warming panel, an Isolette or incubator, and an open bassinet with cotton blankets. The dressed infant under blankets can maintain a temperature within a wider range of environmental temperatures; however, the close observations required by high-risk infants are best accomplished if the infants remain unclothed. When the infant is removed from the warm environment of the Isolette for feeding or cuddling, he is clothed and wrapped warmly in blankets. To prevent undue heat loss from the head, a small stocking cap can be fashioned from stockinette for the infant to wear outside the enclosed crib or Isolette (Fig. 10-9). The most effective means for maintaining the desired range of temperature in the naked infant is by way of a manually adjusted or automatically

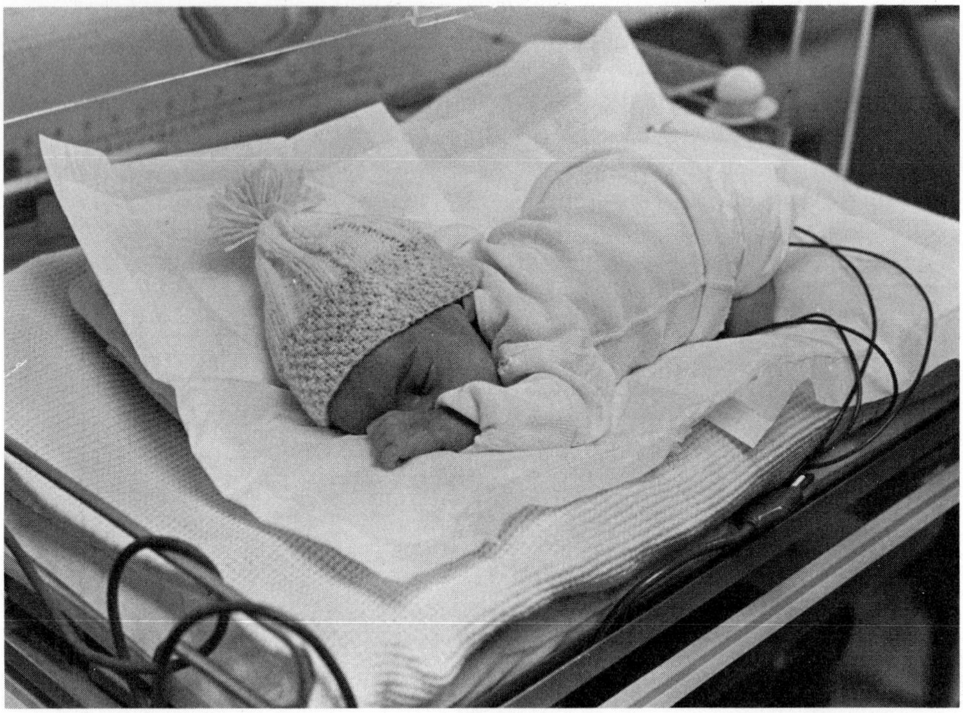

Fig. 10-9. Infant wearing cap knit for him by his mother. A satisfactory substitute can be fashioned from a piece of stockinette.

controlled (servocontrolled) heat panel or incubator. The latter mechanism, when set at the upper and lower limits of the desired circulating air temperature range, adjusts automatically in response to signals from a thermal sensor attached to the abdominal skin. If the infant's temperature drops, the warming device is triggered to increase heat output.

There are always disadvantages inherent in any mechanical device; therefore, an important part of nursing assessment is to compare the infant's temperature with the temperature in the Isolette. For example, if the infant's temperature is increased in response to sepsis or intracranial hemorrhage, the servocontrolled mechanism would respond by decreasing the ambient air temperature. Therefore, a critical observation could be easily overlooked. A heat-sensing probe attached to the abdomen registers a false high temperature when the infant is in the prone position. Either the probe should be moved to the flank area of the back when the infant is placed in the prone position or the infant should remain on the back or side or in a partial side-lying position. Body temperature regulation can also be influenced by thermal sensors located in the trigeminal area of the face and on the forehead. When the infant's face is exposed to a cool environmental temperature, even though the body is adequately warmed, these temperature-stimulation zones respond as though the infant is cold stressed. For this reason oxygen or any source of air such as an oxygen mask or tube should not blow directly on the infant's face. Oxygen concentrated around the head, such as that supplied to a hood, must be warmed.[33]

The axillary temperature provides the best indication of the infant's temperature. Rectal temperature, in addition to the possibility of injury and vagal stimulation, is misleading since it registers core temperature. Heat production is activated by a lowered skin temperature; therefore, core temperature drops only after body heat cannot be maintained by increased metabolic activity.

The physical factors that affect temperature regulation operate to influence temperature regulation in Isolettes and radiant heat units. Loss of heat by convection is a constant problem in the open units, and the skin probe should be covered with a small foam or felt disc to avoid the effect of radiant heat acting directly on the sensor itself.[22] Otherwise the heated sensor discontinues the heat source, whereas the infant remains cold. Radiant heat loss is one of the greatest threats to temperature regulation in the Isolette since the temperature of circulating air within has no influence on heat loss to cooler surfaces without, such as windows, walls, or a lower nursery temperature.

A high-humidity atmosphere contributes to body temperature maintenance by reducing evaporative heat loss. Humidity is provided in incubators by air circulating over a heated water reservoir, which has the additional advantage of decreasing heat loss by convection as the air flows over the infant. Since stagnant, warm water provides an excellent breeding medium for microorganisms, the reservoir is emptied every 8 to 24 hours and replaced with fresh distilled water containing a disinfectant (usually silver nitrate). The recommended humidity is 50% to 65%; higher humidity is recommended if the infant weighs less than 1500 g. Because of the ever-present danger of infection, most nurseries no longer use water in Isolettes. Humidity is provided from an external source such as humidified oxygen in air.

Other methods have been employed by nurses to create a neutral thermal environment when more sophisticated methods are unavailable. These include plastic or rubber gloves filled with warm water, K-pads, and goose-necked lamps; however, extreme care must be exercised when using these methods to avoid burning the infant's fragile skin. Lining the inside of the Isolette with aluminum foil may help prevent heat loss caused by radiation, and a plastic bubble wrap, similar to that used as a packing material, is sometimes used as a blanket to help preserve heat and prevent fluid loss, especially for infants under the radiant warmer.

Apnea

Apnea is a common phenomenon in the preterm infant. Approximately one third of infants less than 32 weeks of gestation and almost all apparently healthy infants less than 30 weeks of gestation have apneic spells. Characteristically, premature infants are periodic breathers, that is, they have periods of rapid respiration separated by periods of very slow breathing and, often, short periods during which there are no visible or audible respirations. Apnea is primarily an extension of this periodic breathing and can be defined as a lapse of spontaneous breathing for 20 or more seconds followed by bradycardia and color change. Apnea probably reflects the immature and poorly refined neurologic and chemical respiratory control mechanisms. These infants are not as responsive to oxygen and carbon dioxide, and their neurons have fewer dendritic associations than the more mature infant. Also, apnea is characteristically observed during periods of rapid eye movement in sleep. As the gestational age increases there is a decrease in the incidence of periodic breathing. There is usually no apnea beyond about 11 days of age, although this may vary considerably with the infant's gestational age. It has been found that oral administration of theophylline is often effective in reducing the frequency of primary apnea-bradycardia spells in newborn infants. Theophylline appears to act centrally by increasing the infant's sensitivity to carbon dioxide. The neonate who receives the drug must be closely observed for tachycardia; a rate greater than 180 to 190 beats/minute indicates a need to reduce the dosage.[38]

A number of factors appear to promote the incidence of apnea in the preterm neonate. Apnea can be anticipated in the infant with any of the following circumstances; conversely one of these disorders may be suspected in the infant with persistent apneic spells. Although apnea is an expected event in preterm neonates, its observation is cause to screen for possible causes. These conditions are:

- Airway congestion, obstruction with mucus, or poor position
- Anemia
- Dehydration
- Cooling
- Overheating
- Hypercapnia
- Hypocapnia
- Hypoglycemia
- Hypocalcemia
- Sepsis, meningitis
- Seizures
- Increased vagal tone (frequently observed in infants with very full stomachs after eating)
- Prolonged periodic breathing
- Central nervous system depression from pharmacologic agents
- Intracranial hemorrhage
- Heart failure
- Depression following maternal obstetric sedation
- Respiratory-distressed infants who are tiring

Nursing considerations

Management of periodic apnea consists of monitoring respiration and/or heart rate routinely in all small preterm infants and prevention of conditions that might precipitate it. Since tactile stimulation decreases the incidence of neonatal apnea, many advocate routine cutaneous stimulation for 5 out of every 15 minutes to prevent apneic episodes. A small shoulder roll to produce slight neck extension when the infant is in the supine position minimizes airway obstruction. Mechanical apnea monitors provide a means to alert the staff to cessation of respiration according to a preset delay time, usually 10 to 15 seconds. Effective monitoring devices do not obviate the need for alert nursing observation. Any mechanical device is subject to malfunction. When the alarm sounds, the infant is first assessed for color and for presence of respiration. If the infant displays the usual color and respirations, the nurse investigates possible causes of a false alarm, such as faulty lead placement, detached or disconnected leads, improper alarm setting, or mechanical failure. If the infant is found to be apneic, the following emergency measures are initiated:

1. Give light, tactile stimulus to the skin over the face, chest, and groin; raise and lower the shoulder roll to elicit the Moro response. Stimulation will stop most apneic spells if it is begun early.
2. Suction nose and nasopharynx; empty the stomach if full.
3. If breathing does not begin, raise the chin and *gently* apply sufficient pressure with mash and AMBU bag to lift the rib cage.
4. If bradycardia persists, the infant will require assisted (mechanical) ventilation.

After breathing is restored the infant is assessed for possible precipitating factors, such as temperature, humidity, distention (if not observed earlier), and ambient oxygen content of Isolette. Persistent and repeated periods of apnea are treated by mechanical ventilation with the respirator set at low pressure and rate.

Feeding and nutrition

There are difficulties associated with meeting the nutritional needs of the premature infant. The various mechanisms for ingestion and digestion of foods are not fully developed, and the younger the infant, the greater the problem. The infant's need for rapid growth and daily maintenance must be met in the presence of several anatomic and physiologic handicaps. Although sucking and swallowing are established before birth, coordination of these mechanisms does not occur until approximately 32 to 34 weeks of gestation and they are not fully developed until after birth. Consequently the preterm infant is highly prone to aspiration with its attendant dangers. These reflexes may also become easily exhausted. As with most full-term infants, the premature infant has poor muscle tone in the area of the inferior esophageal (cardiac) sphincter. This causes milk in the stomach to be easily regurgitated into the esophagus, where it can interfere with diaphragmatic movement. As a consequence the infant breathes more rapidly, there may be vagal stimulation, and, again, there is the ever-present danger of aspiration. The stomach itself has very limited capacity in the preterm infant and is easily overdistended to further compromise respiration (Table 10-1).

Physiologically the preterm infant has approximately the same digestive powers as does the full-term infant, except for fat absorption. Carbohydrates are handled well, but there is no doubt that saturated fats are handled less well by preterm infants. To meet the caloric requirements for growth and maintenance, the infant will need approximately 110 to 140 kcal and 120 to 150 ml/kg/day of water by 1 week of age. Daily nutritional requirements for low birth weight infants (after the first week) are listed below.

Calories	110 to 140 kcal/kg/day
Water	120 to 150 ml/kg/day
Protein	3 to 4 g/kg/day
Fat	5 to 7 g/kg/day
Carbohydrates	10 to 15 g/kg-day
Electrolytes, Minerals, Vitamins	Individualized according to condition, laboratory values, and gestational age

The caloric requirements are regulated by the increased metabolic rate, more rapid growth rate, and increased surface area of the infant but are somewhat counterbalanced by the decreased muscular activity. Since most of the nutritional stores are laid down in the final months of gestation, the preterm infant is hampered by low stores of calcium, iron, phosphorus, proteins, and vitamins A and C.

The nutritional needs vary with the size, age, and condition of the infant; therefore, the amount, interval, and method of feeding is individualized for each child. A vigorous infant can be fed with a soft nipple with little difficulty, whereas a weaker infant will require an alternate method. It is important not to tire the infant nor overtax his capacity to retain the feedings. For example, an infant with a stomach capacity of 5 ml is unable to take enough formula to meet even the minimal daily requirements. When the infant is unable to tolerate bottle feedings, intermittent feedings by gavage are instituted until he gains enough strength and coordination to handle the nipple. Breast-feeding is almost universally impossible for the small preterm infant. However, breast milk obtained from the infant's mother or a milk bank is highly desirable and frequently used. Very small or ill infants are fed by the parenteral route until their condition is stabilized and their neurologic and physical state permits oral feedings. Often oral feedings are supplemented by parenteral infusions to assure an adequate intake of carbohydrate and water. Although the timing of the first feeding has been a matter of controversy, most authorities now believe that early feeding, usually within 3 to 6 hours, reduces the incidence of complicating factors, such as hypoglycemia, dehydration, and the degree of hyperbilirubinemia. The regimen on which most stable premature infants seem to thrive is[5]:

1 ml distilled water via nasogastric tube within 3 to 6 hours after birth
2 to 4 ml of 5% glucose in water every 3 hours for 1 day
Human milk or simulated human milk formula containing 65 kcal/100 ml (20 kcal/ounce) beginning the second day; this low-sodium formula should consist of 1.7% protein, 7% lactose, and 3.5% fat, half of which is polyunsaturated fat
Vitamin supplements are added on the fifth day

Table 10-1. Average physiologic capacity of the stomach in the first days of life

Day of life	Stomach capacity (ml/kg birth weight)
1	2
2	4
3	10
4	16
5	19
6	19
7	21
8	23
9	25
10	27

From Silverman, W. A.: Dunham's premature infants, ed. 3, New York, 1961, Harper & Row, Publishers, p. 157.

Nursing considerations. The initial feeding is not attempted until the infant has adapted to extrauterine existence as evidenced by temperature neutrality, normal breathing, and good color, tone, and cry. Sterile water is offered for the initial trial feeding, the same as for any newborn infant. It causes no pulmonary reaction if aspirated as has been found with both milk and glucose water. The amount to be fed, again, is determined according to the size of the infant. Subsequent feedings are largely regulated by the infant's tolerance (Fig. 10-10). The complications of aspiration make it important that he is not overfed. If the infant takes very little and appears to be tired, the feeding may have to be repeated in a short while and then at more frequent intervals. A 3-hour interval is usually tolerated by most infants, but smaller infants may need to be fed every 2 hours before progressing to larger, less frequent feedings. The preterm infant is often a slow feeder and requires periods of rest and frequent bubbling. To determine how well the infant tolerates the feedings, the stomach contents are aspirated prior to each feeding and the residual fluid is recorded and replaced as part of the feeding. For example, if the feeding is 10 ml and 1 ml is aspirated, the 1 ml is returned to the stomach and the infant is given 9 ml of formula. A consistent residual in excess of 2 to 3 ml after a 3-hour interval may be an indication to reduce the amount for one or two feedings, or, if persistent, this should be called to the attention of the physician.

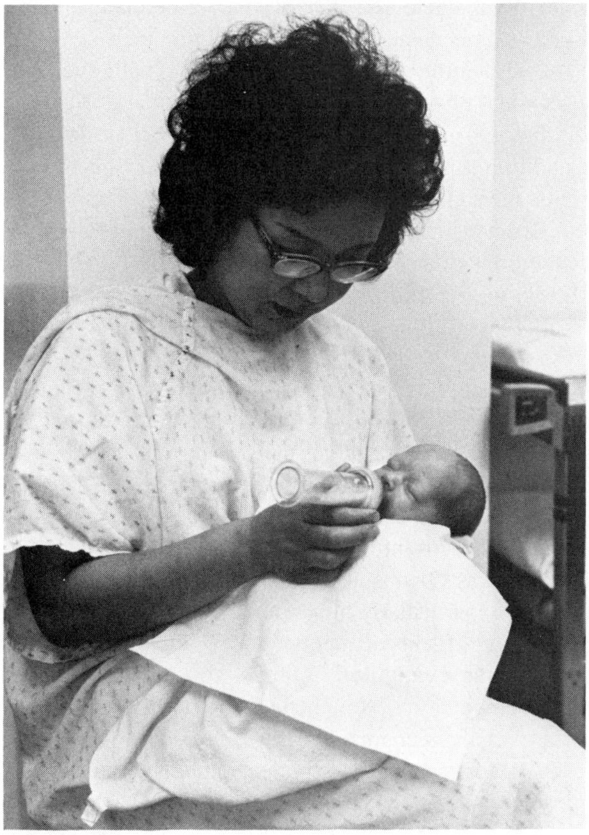

Fig. 10-10. Position for nipple-feeding the premature infant.

The amount of the initial feedings is determined largely by the infant's weight and is gradually and cautiously increased by increments of 1 to 2 ml per feeding each day until a satisfactory caloric intake is assured. The rate of increase that is well tolerated varies from one infant to another, and the decision to increase feedings is often a nursing responsibility. Sometimes supplementary calories are needed in the form of dietary additives, such as Lipomul-Oral,* which provides vegetable fat and carbohydrate, and MCT oil,† which provides fat in the form of medium-chain triglycerides.

Gavage feeding. Intermittent gavage feeding is one of the safest means for meeting the nutritional requirements of the infant who is less than 32 weeks of gestation or weighs less than 1650 g. These infants are usually too weak to suck effectively and are unable to coordinate swallowing. In larger infants who become excessively tired, are listless, or become cyanotic, gavage feeding is used as an energy-conserving technique. A 15-inch size 5 or 8 French polyethylene feeding tube is used to instill the formula, and the usual methods for determining correct placement are employed (see p. 943 for technique). Although the more relaxed cardiac sphincter makes passage of the tube easier, there may be changes in heart rate and blood pressure in response to vagal stimulation. The procedure is best accomplished with the infant in a prone or a right side-lying position with the head slightly elevated. It is preferable to insert the tube through the mouth rather than the nares. Nose insertion obstructs obligatory nose breathing and may irritate the delicate, nasal mucosa. Passage through the mouth also provides an opportunity to observe the sucking response. The formula is allowed to flow by gravity, and the length of time should approximate the time required for a nipple feeding. This procedure is not used as a timesaving method for the nurse.[36] The tube is rarely left in place between feedings because of complications such as obstructed nares, mucous plugs, purulent rhinitis, epistaxis, and possible stomach perforation that are sometimes seen with an indwelling catheter. This method is reserved for infants who cannot tolerate the intubation process.[8]

The intermittent method of gavage feeding stimulates the infant to begin making attempts at sucking and swallowing. The nurse needs to observe the premature infant closely for behaviors that indicate readiness to handle bottle feedings. These include (1) a strong, vigorous suck, (2) coordination of sucking and swallowing, (3) sucking in response to the gavage tube or other objects placed near the mouth, and (4) wakefulness before and sleeping after feedings. When these

*The Upjohn Co., Kalamazoo, Mich.

†Mead Johnson & Co., Evansville, Ind.

behaviors are noted the infant can be challenged with nipple feedings introduced slowly. It is often helpful to allow infants to suck on a pacifier during gavage feedings to assess their sucking ability and so that they associate the sucking with the feeling of food in the stomach. Bottle-feedings are continued if the infant is able to tolerate the feeding and takes the required amount. When the infant requires more than 30 minutes to complete a feeding, the next one should be given by gavage. Poor sucking in an infant who has been feeding well may indicate serious illness and should be reported to the physician.

Hydration. It is not uncommon for the preterm infant to receive supplemental parenteral fluids to supply additional calories, electrolytes, or water. The sites most frequently used in the neonate are peripheral veins on the hand or foot, scalp veins, antecubital veins, and the umbilical vessels. If these sites are exhausted by long-term therapy, a venous cutdown (usually inserted in the saphenous vein) may be employed. Adequate hydration is particularly important in the premature infant whose extracellular water content is higher than that of a full-term infant (70% in full-term infants and up to 90% in preterm infants), and the capacity for osmotic diuresis is limited in the premature infant's immature kidneys.[29] Nephrogenesis is still developing at a rapid rate during the later weeks of gestation, and early birth implies less than a full complement of functioning nephrons. As a result the preterm infant is highly vulnerable to water depletion, especially where there are increased losses through the gastrointestinal tract, lungs, and skin. There is a great deal of heat and moisture lost in rapid breathing, and the infant under a radiant warmer or phototherapy lights must be closely watched for signs of dehydration.

SERIOUS PROBLEMS OF PRETERM INFANTS

Preterm infants are prone to the same hazards as are full-term infants. In addition the immaturity of the various systems and protective mechanisms renders them even more vulnerable to a variety of life-threatening conditions. They are more easily susceptible to biochemical alterations such as hyperbilirubinemia, hypoglycemia, and electrolyte imbalances. The preterm infant has a higher extracellular water content that renders him more vulnerable to fluid and electrolyte derangements, and his small total blood volume is easily depleted by repeated withdrawals. The premature infant will exchange fully half his extracellular fluid volume every 24 hours as compared with one seventh in the adult (see p. 1062 for fluid volume comparison). In addition premature infants are prone to develop disorders, such as sepsis, respiratory distress syndrome, and necrotizing enterocolitis, more readily than are full-term infants.

Ongoing nursing assessment of the infant's physical status is essential to the early diagnosis and treatment of pathologic conditions (see p. 331 for systematic assessment guide). Frequent auscultations and scrupulous observations of external signs and behaviors provide clues to the physical state. Since the signs of illness in the preterm infant are ambiguous and vague, they will not be repeated again nor will the nursing care in relation to specific disorders except as it differs from the nursing care of the high-risk infant in general. However, careful attention to signs of impending problems facilitates the implementation of prophylactic or therapeutic regimens.

Sepsis

The premature withdrawal of the placental barrier leaves the infant vulnerable to most common viral, bacterial, fungal, and parasitic infections. Normally, immune substances, primarily immunoglobulin G (IgG), are acquired from the maternal system and stored in fetal tissues during the final weeks of gestation to provide the newborn with passive immunity to a variety of infectious agents. Early birth interrupts this transplacental transmission, thus the preterm infant has a low amount of circulating IgG with the concentration directly related to the length of gestation. Immunoglobulin A (IgA), which plays a role in defense against viral infections, and immunoglobulin M (IgM), with properties that are most efficient in dealing with gram-negative organisms, are not transferred to the fetus, leaving the infant highly vulnerable to invasion by these organisms.

The infant's defense mechanism is further hampered by a reduced number and inefficient functioning of circulating leukocytes. Furthermore, these leukocytes, with diminished motility and phagocytic capacity, are unable to concentrate their limited numbers selectively at the site of infection. In addition a hypofunctioning adrenal gland contributes only a meager antiinflammatory response. Consequently these deficiencies permit rapid invasion, spread, and multiplication of organisms.

Etiology. Sepsis in the neonatal period can be acquired prenatally or during labor from infected amniotic fluid, across the placenta from the maternal bloodstream, or by direct contact with maternal tissues during passage through the birth canal. Postnatal infection is acquired by cross-contamination from other infants, personnel, or objects in the environment, primarily life-saving apparatus such as mechanical ventilators and indwelling venous and arterial catheters used for infusions, blood sampling, and monitoring vital signs. Neonatal sepsis is most common in the infant at risk, particularly the preterm infant and the one born following a difficult or traumatic labor and delivery.

Diagnostic evaluation. A few neonatal infections (for example, pyoderma, conjunctivitis, omphalitis, and mastitis) are easily recognized. However, systemic infections are characterized by very subtle, vague, nonspecific, and almost imperceptible physical signs. Often there is little correlation between the manifestations and the etiologic agent or system involved. For example, (1) convulsions may not represent central nervous system infection and (2) fever, a universal feature of infection in the older child, may be absent in the neonate. It is usually the nurses' observation of subtle changes in the infant's appearance and behavior that leads to the detection of infection. The nonspecific early signs are changes in color, tone, activity, and feeding with poor temperature control, unabsorbed formula with abdominal distention, jaundice, lethargy, and apnea. Significantly, similar signs may be manifestations of a number of clinical conditions unrelated to sepsis, such as hypoglycemia, hypocalcemia, heroin withdrawal, or central nervous system pathology. Clinical signs that may indicate possible neonatal sepsis are listed in the boxed material below. Because sepsis is so easily confused with other neonatal disorders, the definitive diagnosis is established by laboratory and x-ray examination.

Medical management. Early recognition and diagnosis with institution of vigorous therapeutic measures are essential in order to increase the chance for survival and reduce the likelihood of permanent neurologic damage. Treatment consists of aggressive administration of antibiotics and supportive therapy, such as oxygen as indicated, careful regulation of fluids and electrolytes, and temporary discontinuation of oral feedings. Blood transfusions may be needed to correct anemia and/or shock, and electronic monitoring of vital signs and regulation of the thermal environment are mandatory (see also p. 336).

Manifestations observed in neonatal sepsis

- General signs
  - Infant generally "not doing well"
  - Poor temperature control—hyperthermia, hypothermia
- Circulatory system
  - Pallor, cyanosis, or mottling
  - Cold, clammy skin
  - Hypotension
  - Edema
  - Abnormal heartbeat—arrhythmia, tachycardia
- Respiratory system
  - Irregular respirations, apnea, or tachypnea
  - Cyanosis
  - Grunting
  - Dyspnea
  - Retractions
- Central nervous system
  - Diminished activity—lethargy, hyporeflexia, coma
  - Increased activity—irritability, tremors, seizures
  - Full fontanel
  - Increased or decreased tone
  - Abnormal eye movements
- Gastrointestinal system
  - Poor feeding
  - Vomiting
  - Diarrhea or decreased stool
  - Abdominal distention
  - Hepatomegaly
- Hematopoietic system
  - Jaundice
  - Pallor
  - Purpura, petechiae, ecchymosis
  - Splenomegaly
  - Bleeding

Respiratory distress syndrome

Respiratory distress is common to several neonatal disorders, for example, hypovolemia, hypoglycemia, congenital heart disease, and cerebral hemorrhage. However, the terms respiratory distress syndrome (RDS), idiopathic respiratory distress syndrome (IRDS), and hyaline membrane disease (HMD) are most often applied to the severe lung disorder that is not only responsible for more deaths in the pediatric age-group than any other disease but also carries the highest risk in terms of long-term neurologic complications. It is seen almost exclusively in the preterm infant, the infant of the diabetic mother, and the infant born by cesarean section. Significantly in both the latter conditions the incidence of prematurity is very high. The disorder is rare in the infant of the narcotic-addicted mother or the infant who has been subjected to intrauterine stress (for example toxemia or hypertension).[9]

Etiology and pathophysiology. The preterm infant is born before the lungs are fully prepared to serve as efficient organs for gas exchange. This appears to be a critical factor in the development of respiratory distress syndrome. Although the precise cause is still undetermined, several features in the development of the disorder are established and there are a number of interdependent relationships that complicate the situation.

Prior to birth there is evidence of respiratory activity. The lungs make feeble respiratory movements, and fluid is excreted through the alveoli during fetal life. Since the final infolding of the alveolar septa, which increases the surface area of the lungs, takes place during the last trimester of pregnancy, the premature infant is born with numerous underdeveloped and many uninflatable alveoli. There is limited pulmonary blood flow resulting from the collapsed state of the fetal lung and from poor vascular development in general and an immature capillary network in particular. Because of the increased pulmonary vascular resistance, the major portion of fetal blood is shunted from the lungs by way of the ductus arteriosus and foramen ovale (see p. 220).

At the time of birth the infant must initiate breathing and then keep the previously fluid-filled lungs inflated with air. At the same time the pulmonary capillary blood flow must be increased approximately tenfold to provide for adequate lung perfusion and to alter the intracardiac pressure that closes the fetal cardiac structures. Most full-term infants successfully accomplish these adjustments; the preterm infant with respiratory distress is unable to do so. Although a number of factors are involved, most authorities believe that the central factor responsible for this adaptation is normal development of the surfactant system. Surfactant is a surface-active phospholipid secreted by the alveolar epithelium. Acting much like a detergent, this substance reduces surface tension of fluids that line the alveoli and respiratory passages, resulting in uniform expansion and maintenance of lung expansion at low intra-alveolar pressure. Immature development of these functions produces consequences that seriously compromise respiratory efficiency. Deficient surfactant production causes unequal inflation of alveoli on inspiration and collapse of alveoli on end expiration. Without surfactant the infant is unable to keep the lungs inflated and, therefore, exerts a great deal of effort to reexpand the alveoli with each breath. It has been estimated that each breath requires as much negative pressure (60 to 75 cm water) as the initial lung expansion at birth. As a result the infant uses more oxygen to expend this energy than he takes in, which rapidly leads to exhaustion. With increasing exhaustion the number of alveoli he is able to open decreases. This inability to maintain lung expansion produces widespread atelectasis.

In the absence of alveolar stability (normal functional residual capacity) and with progressive atelectasis, the pulmonary vascular resistance is increased, whereas with normal lung expansion it would be decreased. Consequently there is hypoperfusion to the lung tissue with a decrease in effective pulmonary blood flow. The increase in pulmonary vascular resistance causes partial reversion to the fetal circulation with a right-to-left shunting of blood through the persisting fetal communications—the ductus arteriosus and foramen ovale. Inadequate pulmonary perfusion and ventilation produce hypoxemia and hypercapnia. Pulmonary arterioles, with their thick muscular layer, are markedly reactive to diminished oxygen concentration. Thus a decrease in oxygen tension causes vasospasm in the pulmonary arterioles that is further enhanced by a decrease in blood pH. This vasoconstriction contributes to a marked increase in pulmonary vascular resistance. In normal ventilation with increased oxygen concentration, the ductus arteriosus constricts and the pulmonary vessels dilate to decrease pulmonary vascular resistance (Fig. 10-11).

To compound this situation, prolonged hypoxemia activates the anaerobic glycolysis that produces increased amounts of lactic acid. Increase in lactic acid causes a metabolic acidosis; inability of the atelectatic lungs to blow off excess carbon dioxide produces a respiratory acidosis. Lowered pH causes further vasoconstriction. With deficient pulmonary circulation and alveolar perfusion, the blood oxygen concentration continues to fall, the pH falls, and materials needed for surfactant production are not circulated to the alveoli.

Deficiencies in other systems contribute to respiratory distress. For example, a high threshold of the respiratory center to afferent stimuli and weak gag and cough reflexes reflect the immaturity of the nervous system. Also the persistence of fetal hemoglobin, so beneficial in prenatal existence, may place the infant at a disadvantage in respiratory distress. Although the binding power of fetal hemoglobin for oxygen is much greater than in adult hemoglobin, this increased affinity also causes less oxygen to be released to the tissues at normal oxygen tension. In the newborn the arterial oxygen concentration must fall to a lower level for bound oxygen to be released from fetal hemoglobin.

The hyaline membrane, pathognomonic of the disorder,

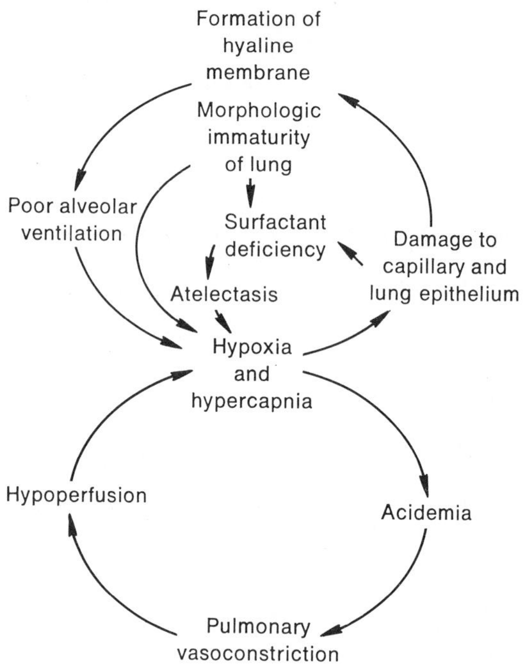

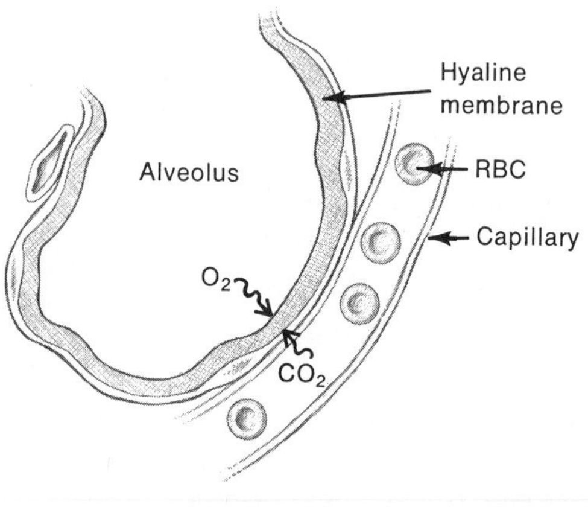

Fig. 10-11. Interdependent relationship of factors involved in the pathology of respiratory distress syndrome (hyaline membrane disease). (From Pierog, S. H., and Ferrara, A.: Medical care of the sick newborn, ed. 2, St. Louis, 1976, The C. V. Mosby Co., p. 144.)

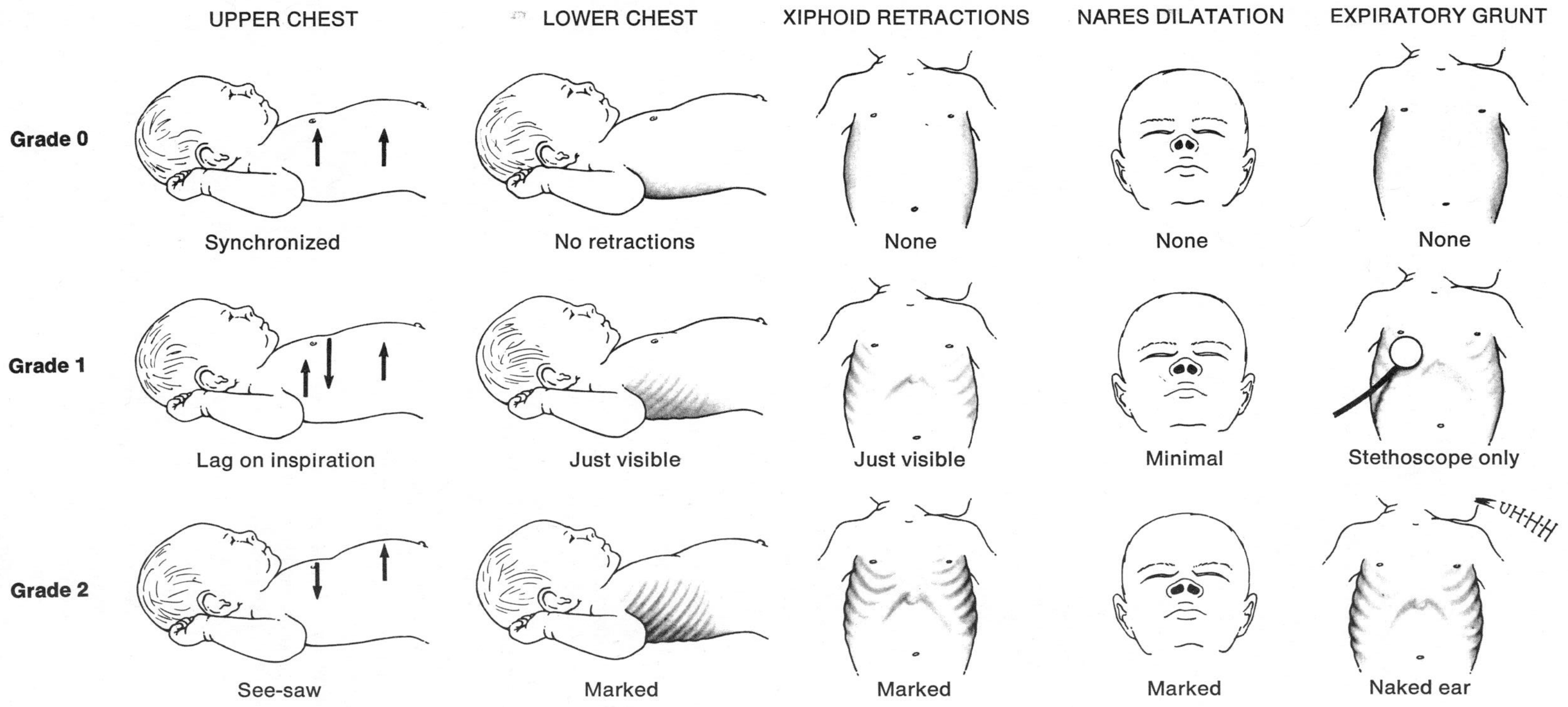

Fig. 10-12. Criteria for evaluating respiratory distress. (From Silverman, W. A., and Anderson, D. H.: Pediatrics **17:**1, 1956. Copyright American Academy of Pediatrics, 1956.)

is formed as hypoxemia and the increased pulmonary vascular pressure cause transudation of fluid into the alveoli. Necrotic cells from damaged alveoli plus the fibrin in the transudate form a membranous layer that lines the alveoli to inhibit gas exchange. Presence of the membrane contributes to respiratory difficulties by markedly diminishing lung distensibility, or compliance—the elastic quality of lung tissue that permits expansion in response to a given amount of applied pressure during inspiration. Affected lungs are stiffer and require far more pressure than do normal lungs to achieve an equal amount of expansion. The major factors that produce respiratory distress in the immature infant can be summarized[10]:

Cause	*Effect*
Increased surface tension of alveoli (surfactant deficiency)	Alveolar collapse; atelectasis Increased work of breathing Hypoxemia and hypercapnia with respiratory acidosis
Impaired gas exchange	
Increased pulmonary vascular resistance	Hypoperfusion of pulmonary circulation
Hypoperfusion (with hypoxemia)	Tissue hypoxia and metabolic acidosis
Increased transudation of fluid into lung	Hyaline membrane formation Impaired gas exchange

Clinical manifestations. The infant with respiratory distress syndrome can develop respiratory insufficiency either acutely or over a period of hours. Usually the observable signs produced by the pulmonary changes begin to appear in an infant who apparently achieves normal breathing and color soon after birth. In 30 minutes to 2 hours, breathing gradually becomes more difficult and the infant displays substernal retractions. Retractions are a prominent feature of pulmonary difficulties in preterm infants because of a compliant chest wall. Weak chest wall muscles and the highly cartilaginous nature of the rib structure produce an abnormally elastic rib cage. Thus much negative pressure is wasted as the infant attempts to develop higher intrathoracic pressure changes. During this early period the infant's color remains satisfactory and auscultation reveals good air entry.

Within a few hours, respiratory distress becomes more obvious. The respiratory rate increases (to 80 to 120 breaths/minute), and breathing becomes more labored. It is significant to note that an infant will increase the *rate* of respiration rather than the *depth* of respiration when in distress. Substernal retractions become more pronounced as the diaphragm works hard in an attempt to fill collapsed air sacs. Fine inspiratory rales can be heard over both lungs, and there is an audible expiratory grunt. This grunt, a useful mechanism observed in the earlier stages of respiratory distress syndrome, serves to increase expiratory end pressure in the lungs, thus maintaining alveolar expansion and allowing gas exchange for an additional brief period. Flaring of the external nares is also a sign that accompanies tachypnea, grunting, and retractions in respiratory distress. Cyanosis appears but can usually be abolished by a 40% to 50% ambient oxygen concentration.

At this point the respiratory distress may gradually decrease over a period of 12 to 24 hours with eventual recovery, or it may increase in severity. In this case cyanosis becomes more marked despite increases in ambient oxygen concentration. Often there is pallor caused by peripheral vasoconstriction, but it is frequently masked by the cyanosis. The infant becomes flaccid, inert, and unresponsive and begins to display frequent apneic episodes. Auscultation of the chest reveals diminished breath sounds. Now the chances of recovery without assisted ventilation are very small. Severe hyaline membrane disease is often associated with a shocklike state as manifest by diminished cardiac inflow and low arterial blood pressure. The affected lungs produce a typical ground-glass appearance on x-ray examination because of the small generalized, closely spaced densities that represent atelectatic areas.

Infants with respiratory distress syndrome who survive the first 96 hours have a reasonable chance of recovery.[10] Nursing care and assessment are crucial to the infant's survival. Nursing considerations include those outlined for all high-risk infants with special responsibilities as described in the following discussions.

Principles of medical management. The treatment of respiratory distress syndrome is largely supportive and includes all the general measures required of any premature infant. At the same time, measures are instituted to correct imbalances and irregularities. General supportive measures include minimal handling, maintaining a neutral thermal environment, and providing adequate caloric intake and hydration. Oral feedings are contraindicated in any situation that creates a marked increase in respiratory rate because of the greater hazards of aspiration. Nutrition is provided by gavage and/or parenteral feedings.

The specific supportive measures that are most crucial to a favorable outcome are (1) correction of acidosis by intravenous administration of sodium bicarbonate or tromethamine (THAM) to dilate pulmonary vessels and reduce the constriction response, (2) maintenance of a neutral temperature environment to conserve utilization of oxygen, and (3) provision of additional fractional inspired oxygen (FiO_2) content by increasing ambient oxygen concentration or by assisted ventilation. The goals of oxygen therapy are provision of adequate oxygen to the tissues, prevention of lactic acid accumulation resulting from hypoxia, and, at the same time, avoidance of toxic effects of oxygen, that is, retrolental fibroplasia and pulmonary oxygen toxicity.[1]

Oxygen therapy. Numerous methods have been devised to improve oxygenation (Table 10-2). All require that the gas be warmed and humidified before entering the respiratory tract. The most widely used method is assisted ventilation where continuous positive pressure of 3 to 10 cm

Table 10-2. Common methods for assisted and controlled ventilation in respiratory distress syndrome

Method	Description	How provided
Continuous positive airway pressure (CPAP) or continuous positive pressure breathing (CPPB)	Provides constant distending pressure to airway in spontaneously breathing infant	Mask Head box or hood Nasal prongs Endotracheal tube
Continuous negative pressure (CNP)	Exerts sustained negative pressure to thorax that prevents its collapse at end expiration in spontaneously breathing infant	Specially designed devices that envelope the chest or entire body Used in conjunction with oxygen source—usually a hood
Positive end-expiratory pressure (PEEP)	Provides increased end-expiratory transpulmonary pressure that prevents alveolar collapse during controlled ventilation	Endotracheal intubation
Continuous positive pressure ventilation (CPPV)	Maintains continuous positive pressure to airways in the infant attached to ventilator	Endotracheal intubation and either volume- or pressure-controlled ventilators

water is supplied, against which the infant must breath. This method is known as continuous positive airway pressure (CPAP) or continuous positive pressure breathing (CPPB), which takes advantage of the infant's spontaneous respiration. The objective of continuous positive airway pressure is to apply just enough pressure to open and keep open most of the alveoli and yet avoid overdistending the already expanded alveoli. If oxygen saturation (Po_2) of the blood cannot be maintained at a satisfactory level and the carbon dioxide level (Pco_2) rises, the infant will require controlled ventilation, usually positive end-expiratory pressure (PEEP).

Nursing considerations in oxygen therapy. A respiratory therapist, an important member of the neonatal intensive care team, is responsible for regulation and maintenance of respiratory equipment. However, it is a nursing responsibility to understand the function of the apparatus and to recognize when it is not functioning correctly according to the physician's specifications. The most essential nursing function is to observe and assess the infant's response to therapy. Since oxygen concentration and continuous positive airway pressure are prescribed according to the infant's color and blood gas measurements and since the infant's status can change rapidly, frequent monitoring and close observation are mandatory. Changes in oxygen concentration are based on these observations. The amount of oxygen administered, expressed as the fraction of inspired air (Fi_{O_2}), is determined on an individual basis according to arterial oxygen concentration (preferred) or capillary blood samples. Arterial samples (Pa_{O_2}) are drawn from an umbilical artery catheter or from radial, pedal, or temporal arteries by needle puncture. For capillary samples, blood is most often collected from the heel. These nursing activities are frequently carried out at least every 4 hours on sick infants and as often as every 15 minutes on acutely ill infants.

The infant receiving assisted or controlled ventilation is subject to problems associated with the therapy. Thick, tenacious mucus frequently forms in the respiratory tract and interferes with gas flow and predisposes to obstruction of the passages, including the endotracheal tube. Routine suctioning may be required every 2 hours or as needed based on assessment. Care must be exercised since the procedure may cause bronchospasm or vagal nerve stimulation that can produce bradycardia. When the nasopharyngeal passages, trachea, or endotracheal tube is being suctioned, the catheter should be inserted gently but quickly, then intermittent suction applied as the catheter is withdrawn. It is imperative that the time the airway is obstructed by the catheter is limited to no more than 5 to 10 seconds. Also, continuous suction removes air from the lungs along with the mucus. One fourth to ½ ml of sterile normal saline instilled in the endotracheal tube prior to insertion of the suction catheter aids in loosening mucus and removing secretions.

Removal of secretions can be further facilitated by application of percussion and vibration to the thoracic wall. The technique and positioning for postural drainage, percussion, and vibration are outlined in Chapter 32. The principles are the same, but the cupped hand is much too large to be used on the very small infant. An effective means to provide percussion is by the use of small plastic cups with padded rims or a small face mask with the airway opening occluded (Fig. 10-13). Vibration is even more difficult to accomplish on the infant whose respiratory rate is 60 to 80 breaths/minute. Some units have found a helpful aid in the electric toothbrush with foam padding placed over the handle. When applied to the chest, this provides effective vibrations. Percussion and vibration are performed every 2 hours, with rotation of segments of the lungs that are percussed. The preterm infant is usually unable to tolerate a full regimen each time. The length of time allotted to any given segment is also subject to the infant's tolerance and the degree of lobar involvement, which is best determined by radiologic evaluation.

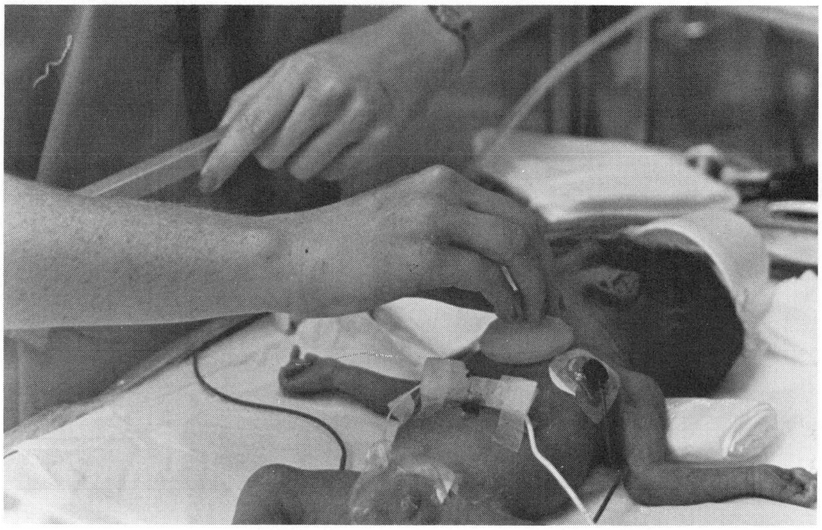

Fig. 10-13. Use of face mask for percussion of infant.

Inspection of the skin is part of routine infant assessment. Position changes and use of water pillows or fleece are helpful in guarding against skin breakdown. The most advantageous positions of the infant for facilitating an open airway are on the side with the head supported in alignment by a small folded blanket or towel or on the back with a small shoulder roll to keep the neck slightly extended. With the head in the "sniffing" position, the trachea is opened at its maximum; hyperextension reduces the tracheal diameter in the neonate.

Mouth care is especially important when the infant is receiving nothing by mouth, and the problem is often aggravated by the drying effect of oxygen therapy. Drying and cracking can be prevented by good oral hygiene using saline or glycerin swabs. Irritation to the nares or mouth that occurs from appliances used to administer oxygen may be reduced by the use of antibiotic ointment.

Complications of oxygen therapy in the preterm infant. Oxygen therapy, although lifesaving, is not without its hazards. Positive pressure introduced by mechanical apparatus has created an increase in the incidence of ruptured alveoli and subsequent *pneumothorax*. This complication can be suspected on the basis of absent or diminished breath sounds and a shift in location of maximum intensity of heart sounds; its presence is confirmed by x-ray examination. Treatment consists of monitoring and observation for increased respiratory distress, either aspiration of the accumulated air or insertion of the catheter into the pleural space and use of water-seal drainage (see p. 1336).

RETROLENTAL FIBROPLASIA (RLF). Retrolental fibroplasia is a disease of the eyes related to hypoxemia. It occurs almost exclusively in premature infants, and the incidence correlates with the degree of maturity—the shorter the gestational age, the greater the likelihood of its development. Vasoconstriction as a result of very high concentrations of oxygen in retinal capillaries causes a wild overgrowth of these developing blood vessels; veins become numerous and dilate. First the aqueous, followed by the vitreous, humor becomes turbid as new vessels proliferate toward the lens. The retina becomes edematous, and hemorrhages separate the retina from its attachment. Advanced scarring occurs from the retina to the lens, destroying the normal architecture of the eye. This extensive retinal detachment and scarring result in irreversible blindness. Unfortunately there is no documented safety level of Po_2 concentration or length of application. The best prophylaxis at present is to reduce the oxygen concentration to the minimum in terms of both amount and length of time required to relieve hypoxia. Therefore, careful monitoring of the infant and the arterial oxygen tension is essential.

BRONCHOPULMONARY DYSPLASIA (BPD). Bronchopulmonary dysplasia, also known as *chronic* or *respirator lung disease,* is a pathologic process that may develop in the lungs of infants with hyaline membrane disease who have required high concentrations of oxygen and assisted ventilation. The condition is characterized by epithelial damage with thickening and fibrotic proliferation of the alveolar walls and squamous metaplasia of the bronchiolar epithelium. Areas of atelectasis and cystlike foci of hyperaeration are visible on radiographs between 10 and 20 days of life and persist for weeks.[22,29]

The etiology of bronchopulmonary dysplasia is unknown. However, its development appears to be related to several factors: the alveolar damage caused by hyaline membrane disease, exposure to high oxygen concentrations, use of positive pressure ventilation (CPAP or PEEP), endotracheal intubation, and the prolonged use of these therapies. Bronchopulmonary dysplasia is seldom observed in infants being administered negative-pressure ventilation without endotracheal intubation. In addition the ciliary activity is paralyzed by high oxygen concentrations that interfere with the ability to clear the lung of mucus, thus aggravating airway obstruction and atelectasis.[32] The true incidence of the disorder in survivors of hyaline membrane disease is unknown. To date there is no evidence to indicate a relationship between the incidence of bronchopulmonary dysplasia and the increased survival of infants with severe hyaline membrane disease. The marked similarity between bronchopulmonary dysplasia and the *Wilson-Mikity syndrome* of alveolar thickening and cystlike patterns of hyperventilation seen in some premature infants has led some investigators to theorize that the two entities may be part of a continuous spectrum of the same lung disorder.

There is no specific treatment for bronchopulmonary dysplasia aside from oxygen therapy and other supportive measures. Most infants recover by 6 months to 1 year of age, usually with normal pulmonary function, although some appear to have minimal obstructive and restrictive pulmonary deficiency that limits the child's tolerance to exercise.

Prevention of respiratory distress syndrome. Since idiopathic respiratory distress syndrome appears to be a maturational disorder primarily related to the production of pulmonary surfactant, one approach to prevention is through stimulation of surfactant production. Limited experiments with administration of corticosteroids to mothers from 24 hours to 7 days prior to delivery has demonstrated a significant reduction in the incidence of hyaline membrane disease in their infants when compared with controls. More conclusive evidence on a broader scale will be needed before this will be accepted as common practice. There have been no beneficial effects in prevention of hyaline membrane disease by administration of corticosteroids to infants after birth.[25]

The most successful approach to prevention of hyaline membrane disease is prevention of premature delivery, especially in elective early delivery and cesarean section. Improved methods for assessing the maturity of the fetal lung by amniocentesis, although not a routine procedure, allow a reasonable prediction of adequate surfactant formation. About the time that the fetus has developed sufficient surface-active material to maintain alveolar stability, the amount of the principal constituent of surfactant (lecithin) rises markedly in relation to another phospholipid (sphingomyelin) in the amniotic fluid. Measuring the lecithin/sphingomyelin (L/S) ratio provides a basis for assessment of lung maturity. Another indication of pulmonary maturity and the presence of surfactant is the shake or "bubble" test in which stable foam or bubbles form when amniotic fluid is shaken in the presence of ethanol. These tests are used to determine whether the fetus of a high-risk pregnancy is likely to develop hyaline membrane disease. Since estimation of a date of delivery can be miscalculated by as much as a month, these tests are particularly valuable when scheduling elective cesarean section.

Necrotizing enterocolitis (NEC)

This serious condition in a premature infant may go undetected for some time because of the ambiguity of symptoms in the preterm infant and preoccupation with other life-threatening problems by members of the staff. The precise cause of the disorder is still speculative, although it appears to occur in infants whose gastrointestinal tract has suffered a vascular compromise somehow related to an episode of hypoxia or sepsis or after an exchange transfusion. There is evidence to indicate that this enteric vascular ischemia is a consequence of an earlier oxygen depletion in brain and heart that had triggered the "diving reflex." To meet the oxygen needs of these vital organs, blood is shunted away from organs better able to withstand prolonged anoxia, such as the intestines. As a result of this circulatory shunting, there is convulsive vasoconstriction of the mesenteric vessels with severe reduction of blood supply to the intestines. The damage to mucosal cells lining the bowel wall is great—diminished blood supply to these cells causes their death in large numbers, they stop secreting protective, lubricating mucus, and the thin unprotected bowel wall is attacked by proteolytic enzymes. Thus the bowel wall continues to swell and break down. Gas-forming bacteria invade the damaged areas to produce pneumatosis intestinales (presence of air in the submucosal or subserosal surfaces of the colon), a consistent and diagnostic finding.[30]

The nonspecific clinical signs of necrotizing enterocolitis include lethargy, vomiting, distended (often shiny) abdomen, blood in the stools or gastric contents, and absence of bowel sounds (ileus). A consistent relationship has been observed between the development of necrotizing enterocolitis and enteric feeding of hypertonic formula. Apparently there is a synergistic effect produced by the enteric mucosal ischemia and the hypertonic formula.[17,31] Significantly animal experiments indicate there may be an element in breast milk that protects the mucous membranes from excessive damage, although its nature and mechanism are unclear. Necrotizing enterocolitis was absent in breast-fed animals.[4]

Treatment of necrotizing enterocolitis consists of discontinuation of all oral feedings, institution of abdominal decompression via nasogastric suction, and administration of systemic antibiotics. If there is progressive deterioration under medical management or evidence of perforation, surgical resection and anastomosis are carried out. Extensive involvement may necessitate establishment of an ileostomy or colostomy.

Infants with heart disease

Congenital heart disease (CHD) is an important cause of neonatal disease and is the most common cause of death, other than problems related to prematurity, in the newborn infant. Because of its seriousness and relative frequency, congenital heart disease is discussed in Chapter 35 and, therefore, will not merit extensive discussion at this time. However, many cardiac problems constitute a high-risk situation, and early recognition and treatment of severe defects have a profound influence on survival.

The signs of heart disease may mimic signs of other neonatal problems, but the cardinal signs of severe congenital heart disease are *cyanosis* and *congestive heart failure*. Central cyanosis, involving the mucous membranes, lips and tongue, and conjunctiva, and cyanosis that persists beyond 3 hours of life in the absence of obvious causes (such as respiratory distress syndrome, tracheoesophageal fistula, diaphragmatic hernia, and so on) is highly suspicious of congenital heart disease. It is often difficult to differentiate between cyanosis from pulmonary or cardiac causes. When administered 100% oxygen, infants with cyanosis of cardiac origin will show lower arterial oxygen tension and saturation than will those with a pulmonary disorder.

Congestive heart failure is defined as a state in which the heart is unable to maintain adequate circulation to meet the needs of the body despite satisfactory venous filling pressure. The primary manifestations are tachycardia, tachypnea, and dyspnea. The respiratory rate is over 60 breaths/minute and is frequently as high as 100 to 120 breaths/minute with associated pulmonary manifestations such as flaring of the nares, subcostal retractions, and wheezing. Other signs may include poor peripheral pulses, pallor, and shock. There may or may not be significant murmurs, but hepatomegaly and venous congestion are frequently present and cardiomegaly is almost always evident on x-ray examination. Other common manifestations are poor feeding, vomiting, and cough.[28]

A number of cardiac anomalies are associated with recognizable syndromes (for example, chromosomal abnormalities), and there is a high incidence of a patent ductus arteriosus in preterm infants. Some cardiac defects associated with severe cyanosis require prompt evaluation by both invasive and noninvasive techniques to determine the type of defect so that therapy can be instigated immediately. The most classic example is transposition of the great vessels in which the pulmonary artery arises from the left ventricle and the aorta from the right. The condition is incompatible with life unless an abnormal communication is already present or is created between the two circulations by septostomy.[19]

In addition to the routine measures used in management of high-risk infants, medical care of infants with congenital heart disease consists of:

1. Digitalis to improve the strength of cardiac muscle contraction and thus cardiac output
2. Diuretic administration to reduce pulmonary congestion and, if present, peripheral edema
3. Low-salt, or moderately low-sodium, formula to reduce fluid retention; this is often given via gavage to conserve energy or to prevent aspiration in dyspneic infants
4. Oxygen administration to improve arterial oxygen concentration
5. Positioning, usually at a 20- to 30-degree tilt and sometimes a knee-chest position, to decrease the workload of the heart

See Chapter 35 for nursing care of the infant with a cardiac defect.

Associated neonatal problems of premature infants

The preterm infant is more vulnerable to disorders associated with the immature state that often complicate the neonatal adjustments or create long-term neurologic problems. The premature infant is subject to all the problems to which the full-term infant is susceptible, such as hyperbilirubinemia, hypoglycemia, and hypocalcemia, which have been discussed in relation to complications in the neonate. Premature infants are particularly vulnerable, and a number of problems are seen with greater frequency in the preterm infant, for example, hyperbilirubinemia is seen in the majority of these neonates.

Intracranial hemorrhage. Intracranial hemorrhage is a common complication of premature birth as a result of either trauma or hypoxia. Fragility and increased permeability of capillaries and prolonged prothrombin time predispose the premature infant to trauma when delicate structures are subjected to the forces of labor. Traumatic bleeding occurs into the subdural space (subdural hematoma) or into the brain substance. Subdural hematomas, life-threatening collections of blood in the subdural space, are most often produced by stretching and tearing of the large veins in the tentorium cerebelli, the dural membrane that separates the cerebrum from the cerebellum. These are especially serious because of the inaccessibility of the hematoma to aspiration by subdural tap. Less frequently, hemorrhage occurs when veins in the subdural space over the surface of the brain are torn. Intracranial hemorrhage is frequently associated with skull compression during abrupt, precipitous delivery. Hemorrhage from repeated hypoxic spells is not associated with trauma and occurs into the ventricles and subarachnoid space. Consumption of clotting factors during periventricular hemorrhage may contribute to further bleeding and ventricular hemorrhage. Increase in intracranial hemorrhage is manifest by tense, bulging anterior fontanel, separated sutures, and neurologic signs such as twitching, stupor, and convulsions.

Anemia. Preterm infants tend to develop anemia that is more severe and appears earlier than in more mature infants. It may be the result of hemorrhage during the course of labor and delivery (into brain, liver, spleen, or kidneys), blood disorders (hemolytic disease, thrombocytopenia), or conditions that produce swelling or distention of abdominal organs. Physiologic characteristics of prematurity tend to contribute to development of anemia, that is, a drop in production of fetal hemoglobin and shortened survival time of the red blood cells. This lag in hematopoiesis while growth continues results in physiologic anemia.

Disseminated intravascular coagulation (DIC). Consumption of clotting factors and thrombocytes during the course of a variety of conditions produces this relatively common disorder, also known as *consumption coagulopathy*. It does not occur as a primary disorder but is a secondary process that complicates many other disease states. Disseminated intravascular coagulation is characterized by inappropriate systemic activation and acceleration of the normal hemostatic mechanism as a result of disturbance of the equilibrium between microclot formation and destruction in the vascular system. The abnormal coagulation can be stimulated by disorders such as sepsis, shock, anoxia, respiratory distress syndrome, cyanotic heart disease, and severe antigen-antibody reactions. Introduction of the stimulus causes local and widespread fibrin deposition in the vessels, consumption of plasma proteins, aggregation and destruction of platelets, and eventual activation of the fibrinolytic system (see normal clotting mechanism, p. 1391). Without sufficient clotting factors, the infant is vulnerable to uncontrollable hemorrhage into vital organs. Disseminated intravascular coagulation is suspected when there is an increased tendency to bleed, as from venipuncture or blood taken from the heel, and bleeding from umbilicus, trachea, or gastrointestinal tract. Treatment is directed toward correcting the precipitating disorder and administration of heparin or transfusion with fresh whole plasma to halt the consumption of clotting factors and platelets.

OTHER HIGH-RISK CONDITIONS IN NEONATES

Various congenital malformations are associated with increased risk in the newborn period and may or may not be related to prematurity. Most are discussed in Chapter 11 and throughout the book as appropriate. There are several disorders that are related to maternal complications and to complications associated with other disease states that need some elaboration.

Infants of diabetic mothers

Prior to the introduction of insulin therapy, few diabetic women were able to conceive, and, for those who did, the mortality rate for both mother and infant was extremely high. As a result of effective control of diabetes, the risk to the mother is essentially unaltered by the pregnant state; however, the risk to the infant is considerable. With expert care the mortality rate for these infants is reported between 15% and 25%; where special care is not available the infant death rate may be as high as 50%. As the incidence of the disorder rises in the population as a whole, increasing numbers of these infants are admitted to intensive care nurseries.

The severity of the maternal disease affects infant and fetal survival, and there is a relationship between length of gestation and neonatal mortality. There is a higher incidence of stillborn infants in the more severe, insulin-dependent diabetic women, and their live-born infants appear to be more at risk than those of mothers with less severe diabetic involvement. Severity of maternal diabetes is classified according to the duration of the disease prior to pregnancy, the age of onset, and the extent of vascular complications. The least severe and most common group are those asymptomatic cases classified as *gestational diabetes* and *prediabetes*. Women with prediabetes are those with no clinical or chemical signs but who have a positive family history and previously have had large infants. Gestational or stress diabetes consists of an abnormal glucose tolerance test during pregnancy (or other stress situations) that returns to normal in the absence of stress. The least favorable outcome is in mothers with early-onset diabetes (onset before age 10 years) who have had the disease for 20 years or more at the time of pregnancy. The outlook is especially discouraging when vascular and renal disease complicate the clinical picture. Toxemia of pregnancy is more likely to accompany vascular disease and creates an additional risk.

It has been found that the gestational age most favorable to survival of infants of diabetic mothers is between 36 and 37 weeks. Delivery at an earlier age is associated with increased neonatal mortality, but the incidence of stillborn infants is higher in later deliveries, probably caused by failing placental competence. It is unclear whether the placenta is inadequate to meet the nurturing needs of the over-sized infant or whether vascular changes contribute to placental dysfunction. The favored approach is to induce labor or to deliver the infant by cesarean section at approximately 37 weeks; however, estimation of the gestational age is always subject to error. Monitoring the maternal uterine estriol level during the last trimester provides some indication of developing placental insufficiency. A steady decline in estriol level is an indication for termination of the pregnancy.

All infants of diabetic mothers have a characteristic appearance. They are oversized for their gestational age, very plump and full-faced, liberally coated with vernix caseosa, and plethoric. The placenta and umbilical cord, too, are larger than average. "During their first 24 or more extrauterine hours they lie on their backs, bloated and flushed, their legs flexed and abducted, their lightly closed hands on each side of their head, the abdomen prominent and their respiration sighing. They convey a distinct impression of having had such a surfeit of both food and fluid pressed upon them by an insistent hostess that they desire only peace so that they may recover from their excesses."[11]

Removal from a hostile intrauterine environment minimizes but does not eliminate the perinatal hazards to the infant. A number of conditions are associated with infants of diabetic mothers. There is an increase in congenital anomalies in this group as well as a high susceptibility to hypoglycemia, hypocalcemia, hyperbilirubinemia, and hyaline membrane disease. No satisfactory explanation has been accepted for all the abnormalities in these infants, although complications may be related to the prematurity factor in a number of cases (for example, hyaline membrane disease). Although they are large, these infants are often prematurely born in an elective early delivery or because of other reasons. Their appearance has been described as looking at a premature infant through a magnifying glass.

Hypoglycemia, defined as a blood sugar level below 30 mg/100 ml for the normal newborn and below 20 mg/100 ml for the premature infant, appears within a short period after birth and is associated with increased insulin activity in the blood. It has been demonstrated that infants of diabetic mothers have hypertrophy and hyperplasia of the pancreatic islet cells and that they are actually in a state of hyperinsulinism. It is generally agreed that during fetal life high maternal blood sugar levels provide a continual stimulus to the fetal islet cells for insulin production. This sustained state of hyperglycemia promotes fetal insulin secretion that ultimately leads to excessive growth and deposition of fat that probably accounts for the infants who are large for gestational age. When the glucose supply is removed abruptly at the time of birth, the continued production of insulin soon depletes the blood of circulating glucose, creating a state of hypoglycemia within 2 to 4 hours, especially in infants of mothers with overt diabetes. Precipitous drops in blood glucose levels can cause serious neurologic abnormality or death.

As mentioned previously, the signs of hypoglycemia that is, lethargy, episodes of apnea, cyanosis, twitching, seizures, or simply "not doing well," are very nonspecific and similar to manifestations of other disorders. However, hypoglycemia may be asymptomatic, and, since glucose is the primary source of energy for the brain, if left untreated it can cause rapid, irreversible central nervous system damage. The most effective management appears to be careful observation of all infants of diabetic mothers in the special care nursery with early feeding of 5% to 10% glucose followed by formula, if tolerated. Critically ill infants require intravenous infusions. Approximately half of these infants get along very well and adjust without complications. However, since the hypertrophied pancreas is so sensitive to blood glucose concentrations, the administration of glucose may trigger massive insulin release with a rebound hypoglycemia. Therefore, frequent blood glucose levels are needed for the first 2 days of life to assess the degree of hypoglycemia present at any given time. Blood taken from the heel tested with Dextrostix is a simple and effective screening test with confirmation by laboratory examinations several times a day. A rapid rise in blood sugar can be obtained by administration of glucagon to mobilize liver glycogen (see p. 1478), but this may also produce a rebound hypoglycemia. A more effective treatment has been intramuscular administration of epinephrine 1:10,000, which inhibits insulin release while stimulating the release of glucose from glycogen stores in liver and muscles and the release of fatty acids for glucose production.[18]

Postmaturity

Infants born of a gestation that extends beyond 42 weeks as calculated from the mother's last menstrual period are considered to be postmature or postterm, regardless of birth weight. This comprises approximately 12% of all births. The cause of delayed birth is unknown. Some infants are appropriate for gestational age, but many show the characteristics of progressive placental dysfunction. The appropriate-for-gestational-age infants are indistinguishable in appearance form term infants. Others, most often called postmature infants—display the characteristics of infants who are 1 to 3 weeks of age, such as absence of lanugo, little if any vernix caseosa, abundant scalp hair, long fingernails, and whiter skin than term newborns. Frequently the skin is cracked, parchment-like, and desquamating. A common finding in postmature infants is a wasted physical appearance that reflects intrauterine impoverishment. There is a depletion of subcutaneous fat that gives them a thin, long appearance. The little vernix caseosa that remains in skin folds is usually stained deep yellow or green.

There is a significant increase in fetal and neonatal mortality in postterm infants compared to those born at term. They are especially prone to intrauterine hypoxia associated with the decreasing efficiency of the placenta. The greatest risk occurs during the stresses of labor and delivery, particularly in infants of primigravidas (women delivering their first child). Cesarean section or induction of labor is usually recommended when the infant is significantly overdue.

Narcotic-addicted infants

Narcotics, which have a low molecular weight, readily cross the placental membrane and enter the fetal system. When the mother is a habitual user of narcotics, in particular heroin or methadone, the unborn child also becomes passively addicted to the drug, which places such infants at risk during the early neonatal period. Most passively addicted infants of drug-dependent mothers appear normal at birth but begin to exhibit signs of drug withdrawal within 12 to 24 hours if the mother has been taking heroin alone. If she has been taking methadone the signs appear somewhat later, anywhere from 1 or 2 days to a week or more after birth. The manifestations become most pronounced between 48 and 72 hours of age and may last anywhere from 6 days to 8 weeks, depending on the severity of the withdrawal.[12]

The clinical manifestations of withdrawal in the neonate, which are predominantly those of autonomic nervous system hyperirritability, may persist for 3 or 4 months. The most common acute signs are tremors, restlessness, hyperactive reflexes, increased muscle tone, sneezing, tachypnea, and a high-pitched, shrill cry. Although these infants suck avidly on fists and display an exaggerated rooting reflex, they are poor feeders with uncoordinated and ineffectual sucking and swallowing reflexes. Regurgitation and vomiting after feedings are common, and diarrhea is a later manifestation. An unusual observation in a large percentage of these infants is generalized sweating, the incidence of which is double that in normal newborns who display sweating. It is significant to note that, although passively addicted infants have some tachypnea, cyanosis, and/or apnea, they rarely develop respiratory distress syndrome. Apparently the heroin or related factors in the intrauterine environment cause accelerated lung maturation in these infants even in the face of a high incidence of prematurity.

Not all infants of heroin-addicted mothers will show signs of withdrawal. Because of irregular and varying degrees of drug use, quality of drug, and mixed drug usage by the mother, some infants display mild or variable mani-

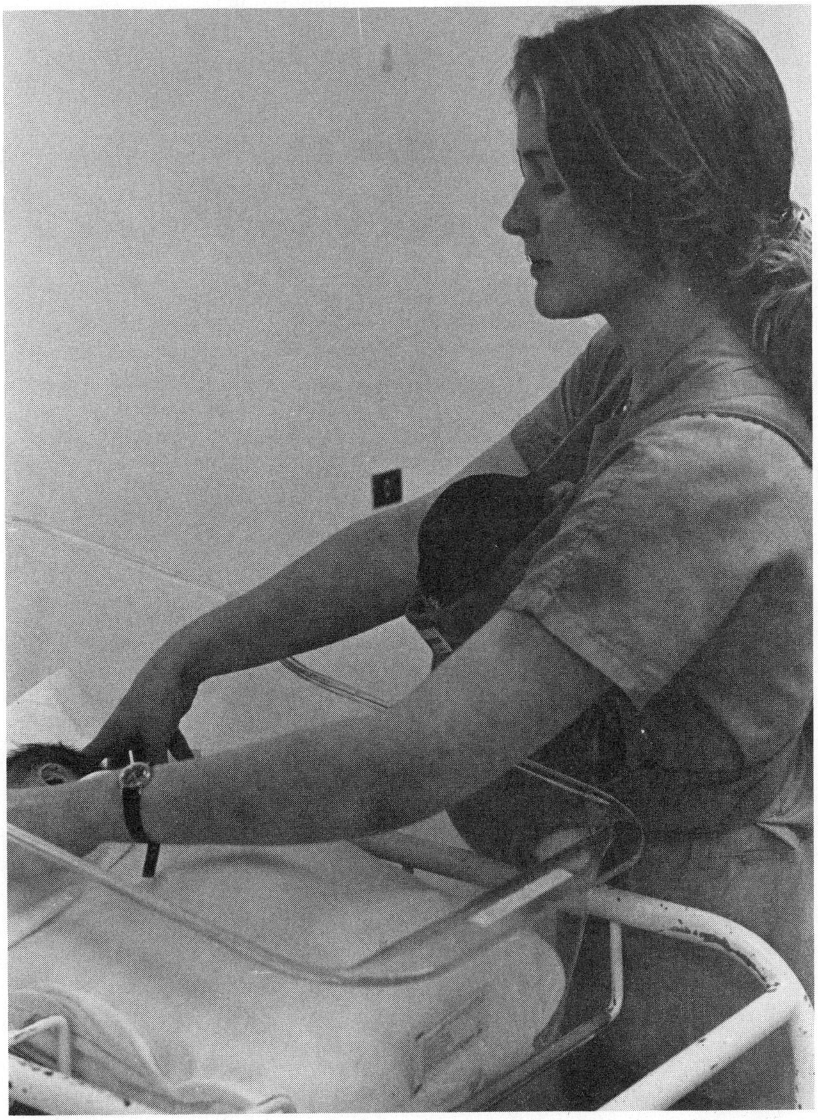

Fig. 10-14. The nurse carries the narcotic-addicted newborn to help reduce agitation associated with withdrawal symptoms.

festations. Most manifestations are the vague nonspecific signs characteristic of all infants in general; therefore, it is important to differentiate between drug withdrawal and other disorders before specific therapy is instituted. Often other states, for example, hypocalcemia, hypoglycemia, or sepsis, coexist with the drug withdrawal. Also, it is not uncommon for the mother to be taking other drugs in addition to narcotics, for example, barbiturates, amphetamines, or hallucinogens. The treatment of the infant consists of intramuscular administration of chlorpromazine or phenobarbital in four divided doses over 2 to 4 days and then orally in decreasing doses for an additional 7 to 10 days. If there are gastrointestinal symptoms such as diarrhea, paregoric may be the drug of choice.

Irritable and hyperactive infants have been found to respond to comforting, movement, and close contact. Consequently some nurseries have adopted the use of infant carriers to provide this need (Fig. 10-14).

A valuable aid to anticipating problems in the newborn is recognizing drug addiction in the mother. Unless the mother is enrolled in a methadone rehabilitation program, she seldom risks calling attention to her habit by seeking prenatal care. Consequently the infant and mother are exposed to the additional hazards of obstetric and medical complications. In addition the nature of heroin addiction predisposes the user to disorders such as infection, hepatitis, and foreign body reaction as well as the hazards of inadequate nutrition and premature birth. Methadone treatment does not prevent withdrawal reaction in the neonate, but the clinical course may be modified. Also, the intensive psychologic support of the mother is a factor in treatment and the reduction of perinatal mortality. Experience has indicated that the mother is usually anxious, depressed, lacks confidence, and has difficulty with interpersonal relationships. She has a psychologic need for the pregnancy and the infant.

There are many problems in relation to the disposition of the infant of the drug-dependent mother. Those who advocate separation of mother and child argue that the mother is not capable of assuming the responsibility for the infant's care, that child care is frustrating to her, and that her existence is too disorganized and chaotic. Others encourage the maternal-infant bond and recommend a protected environment such as a therapeutic community, a halfway house, or continuous, ongoing supportive services in the home after discharge. Each situation requires careful evaluation and the cooperative efforts of a variety of health professionals, whether the choice is foster home placement or supportive follow-up care of the mother who keeps her infant.

SUPPORTIVE CARE OF INFANT AND FAMILY

Professional health workers are often so absorbed in the life-saving physical aspects of care that the emotional needs of infants and their families are all too frequently ignored. The significance of the early mother-child interaction and infant stimulation have been documented by reliable research, and nurses, aware of these infant and family needs, must incorporate activities that facilitate their development into the nursing care plan.

Developmental correlates

Some physiologic systems in the preterm infant mature earlier than they would if the infant had remained within the uterus, for example, the function of some enzyme and immunologic systems and organs, such as kidney and gastrointestinal efficiency; others slow down, such as growth in height and weight; still others keep pace with the development of those of their counterparts still in utero, for example, reflex behaviors.[3]

Longitudinal studies of infants born prematurely indicate that there are differences in many aspects of development that may be a consequence of the immaturity at birth and related perinatal problems. It has been found that growth is generally retarded in all aspects. These children remain in the lower percentile range for height and weight, although they follow the same general growth pattern as infants born at term. There is a rapid increase in growth during the first 6 months, and growth remains somewhat accelerated until the normal growth curve is reached by age 2 to 3 years.[13]

Neurologic impairment and serious sequelae appear to correlate with the size and gestational age of the infant at birth and with the degree of intensive care instituted. The greater the degree of immaturity, the greater the degree of handicap. Small-for-gestational-age infants appear to be less at a disadvantage than appropriate-for-gestational-age infants born early, although both are at a greater disadvantage than are normal infants.[26,27] For example, in pairs of monzygotic twins where one has suffered severe intrauterine growth retardation, the smaller twin continues to be inferior to the normal sibling in both physical and intellectual development.[2] There is an increase in the incidence of neurologic sequelae in preterm infants, such as cerebral palsy and the entity termed minimal brain dysfunction (see p. 640), and intellectual functioning is affected, especially in male infants.[14] The highest incidence of neurologic handicap is found in infants who are born before 38 weeks of gestation but who weigh more than 2500 g. All infants at risk seem to benefit from special care, since undesirable sequelae appear to be decreased in infants who receive intensive medical and nursing care as opposed to those who receive routine care.[27]

Infant stimulation

Recently attention has been focused on the effects of early stimulation, or its lack, on both normal and preterm infants. Findings indicate that infants are able to respond to a greater variety of stimuli than has been previously thought. Nurses who are aware of this need incorporate a stimulation program into the nursing care plan. Tactile, visual, and auditory stimuli are provided whenever possible. Touching is a vital part of any infant stimulation program. As soon as the infant's condition will allow, rocking in a specially designed sling inside the Isolette has been used in some areas to provide kinesthetic stimulation. Holding the infant in a rocking chair is a pleasant means for meeting this need in the infant who can tolerate room atmosphere.

Visual stimulation can be provided by hanging mobiles and placing colorful toys in the infant's line of vision. Nurses and others who care for the child should hold him in such a way that he can see the care giver's face at close range and should attempt to get him to follow their head movements with his eyes. Talking to the infant is one of the best means for providing simultaneous auditory stimulation, and many parents bring small music boxes or similar audio toys to place in the infant's crib or Isolette.[7]

The effects of the intensive care environment on subsequent development has yet to be evaluated. Twenty-four–hour surveillance of sick infants implies maximum visibility. However, many units have instigated a program to help establish a night-day sleep pattern by either darkening the room, if the infant's condition allows, or by placing eye patches over the infant's eyes at night. It has been found that the sound levels are significantly higher in the neonatal intensive care unit than in the regular nursery, but the long-term effects are not known. Evaluation is complicated by unknown factors such as the immaturity of hearing mechanisms at birth and possible effects of ototoxic drugs frequently used in medical management of the high-risk neonate.[35]

Parental involvement

The birth of a premature infant is usually an unexpected and stressful event for which the family is emotionally unprepared. To compound the situation the precarious nature of the infant's condition engenders an atmosphere of apprehension and uncertainty. The frightening array of equipment and activity is stressful to parents, and they need reassurance that the infant is receiving proper care. Once they understand that the infant needs this intensive care, they are content to be kept informed of his condition. It is not necessary to share too much information with the parents, such as very technical information that does not contribute to their understanding. Considering the parents' fears, the nurse can be truthful without being unduly candid regarding the more negative aspects of the child's condition. Most infants survive despite early, worrisome problems.

Because of his insecure status, the infant is separated from the mother immediately and surrounded by a complex and impenetrable barrier of glass windows, mechanical equipment, and special care givers. There is increasing evidence to indicate that the emotional separation that accompanies the physical separation of mother and infant intereferes with the normal maternal-infant attachment process (see p. 288). Maternal attachment is a cumulative process that begins before conception, is strengthened by significant events during pregnancy, and matures through maternal-infant contact during the neonatal period. When the infant is sick, the necessary physical separation appears to be accompanied by an emotional estrangement on the part of the mother that may seriously damage her capacity for mothering the infant. This detachment is further hampered by the tenuous nature of the infant's condition. When the infant's survival is in doubt, the mother may be reluctant to establish a relationship with him. She prepares herself for the death of her infant while continuing to hope for his recovery. This anticipatory grief (see p. 976) and hesitancy to embark on a relationship is evidenced by behaviors such as delay in giving the infant a name, reluctance in visiting the nursery or, when she does visit, focusing on equipment and treatments rather than on the infant, and hesitancy to touch or handle the infant when she is provided the opportunity.

Facilitating maternal-infant relationships. The newer concept in the comprehensive management of the high-risk newborn is to encourage parental involvement rather than to isolate them from the infant and his care. This is particularly important in relation to the mother, and, to reduce the effects of physical separation, the mother is united with her newborn at the earliest opportunity. Preparing the parents to see their infant for the first time is a nursing responsibility. Prior to the first visit the parents should be prepared for the infant's appearance, the equipment that is attached to him, and some indication of the general atmosphere of the unit. At the bedside the nurse explains the function of each piece of equipment and the role it plays in facilitating recovery. Where possible, some items related to therapy can be removed, for example, phototherapy can be temporarily discontinued and eye patches removed to permit eye-to-eye contact.

Parents will usually appreciate the support of a nurse during the initial visit with the infant, but they should be left alone with the infant for a short while. It is important during the early visits to emphasize positive aspects of the infant's behavior to help the parents focus on the infant as an individual rather than on the equipment that surrounds him. For example, the nurse may describe the infant's spontaneous behaviors during care, such as grasp, swallowing, and movement, or make comments about the infant's biologic functions. Most institutions allow parents to visit their infants as often as they wish and encourage them to do so. Mothers vary greatly in the degree to which they are able to interact with their infants. Some may wish

Summary of nursing care of the preterm or other high-risk infant

Goals	Responsibilities
Determine physiologic status	Weigh and measure infant Assess gestational age based on external characteristics and neurologic signs
Ascertain infant's status	Carry out routine systematic assessment Weigh daily
Prevent infection	Carry out meticulous hand washing before handling infant Ensure that all equipment in contact with infant is scrupulously clean or sterile Prevent personnel with infections from coming into direct contact with infant Administer prophylactic antibiotics as ordered
Conserve energy	Maintain neutral thermal environment Concentrate activities to allow for longer periods of rest Administer gavage feeding when infant tires easily Ensure minimal handling of infant
Support respiratory efforts	Position for optimum air exchange (shoulder roll when on back or abdomen; head supported when on side) Observe for deviations from desired functioning; recognize signs of distress Suction as necessary to remove accumulated mucus from nasopharynx, trachea, and (where necessary) endotracheal tube Carry out percussion, vibration, and postural drainage to loosen secretions in respiratory tree Maintain ambient oxygen at level to assure satisfactory skin color with minimal respiratory effort and energy expenditure Prevent aspiration Carry out regimen prescribed for supplemental oxygen therapy (maintain ambient oxygen concentration at minimal FiO_2 level to maintain good color and energy expenditure) Observe for signs of respiratory distress—nasal flaring, retractions, tachypnea Understand functioning of respiratory support apparatus Assisted ventilation apparatus Controlled ventilation apparatus Insufflation bags with masks and/or endotracheal adaptor Oxygen hoods Humidifier warmers Correct application and management of monitoring equipment
Provide neutral thermal environment	Place infant in humidified Isolette, radiant warmer, or warmly clothed in open crib Monitor temperature hourly in unstable infants (take axillary temperature; check function of servocontrolled mechanism when used) Check temperature of infant in relation to temperature of heating unit Avoid situations that might predispose to chilling, such as exposure to cool air
Provide nutrition and hydration	Bottle-feed infant if strong sucking and swallowing reflexes are present Gavage feed if infant tires easily or has weak sucking, gag, or swallowing reflexes Measure specific gravity several times daily to help assess adequacy of hydration Maintain parenteral fluid or hyperalimentation therapy as ordered
Provide sensory stimulation	Tactile Caress, fondle, and otherwise provide skin contact; hold and cuddle infant if condition permits

Summary of nursing care of the preterm or other high-risk infant—cont'd

Goals	Responsibilities
Provide sensory stimulation—cont'd	Auditory Talk to infant during care Encourage parents and others to talk to infant Allow parents to provide musical toys Visual Place colorful mobiles and toys within visual field Hold face within 9 to 12 inches of infant's face and stimulate to follow head movements
Monitor physiologic data	Take vital signs as ordered (axillary temperature, apical pulse) Understand proper function and use of monitoring equipment and maintain at desired settings Apnea monitor Heart rate monitor, including oscilloscope and electrocardiograph printout units Temperature monitor, usually with skin probe Oxygen analyzers Collect specimens Blood for glucose, bilirubin, electrolytes, and pH determinations Blood for hemoglobin, hematocrit, microscopic examination, and culture Urine for laboratory examination
Assist in specific therapies	Phototherapy—(ensure correct application and protection of eyes from light) Administer medications as ordered Antibiotics prophylactically or therapeutically Vitamin K to prevent hemorrhage Sedatives, etc., for withdrawal symptoms, seizures, irritability Electrolyte replacement Alkali therapy in acidosis Other therapeutic measures as indicated
Encourage positive relationship with parents	Keep parents informed of infant's progress Answer questions; allow expression of concern regarding care and prognosis Encourage mother and father to visit and/or call unit Emphasize positive aspects of infant status Be honest but not overly candid or overly optimistic
Facilitate maternal-infant attachment process	Initiate mother's visit as soon as possible Encourage mothers to Visit infant frequently Touch, fondle, and caress infant Become actively involved in infant's care Bring clothing to dress up infant as soon as condition permits Reinforce mother's endeavors Be alert to signs of tension in mother Allow mother to spend time alone with infant Help mother interpret infant responses; comment regarding any positive infant response Help mother by demonstrating techniques and offer support
Prepare for infant discharge	Assess readiness of parents (especially mother) to care for infant Teach necessary techniques and observations Arrange for public health referral if indicated Reinforce follow-up care Refer to appropriate agencies or services for needed assistance

to touch or hold their infant during the first visit, whereas others may not feel comfortable enough even to enter the nursery. These reactions depend on a variety of prenatal and postnatal factors, such as the parity of the mother and her preparation before birth, the size, condition, and physical appearance of the infant, and the type of treatment he is receiving. The mother's inability to focus on the infant is a clue for the nurse to focus on the mother and allow her to express her feelings of guilt, doubt, and ambivalence. Nurses can help mothers deal with these distressing feelings and recognize that they are normal responses shared by other mothers. It is important to point out and reinforce the positive aspects of the mother's behavior and interactions with the child.[37]

Most mothers feel very "shaky" and insecure about initiating interaction with the infant. Nurses can sense the mother's level of readiness and offer encouragement in these initial efforts. Mothers of premature infants follow the same acquaintance process as do mothers of normal infants. They may quickly proceed through the process or may require several days or even weeks to complete the process. The mother begins by touching the infant's extremities with her fingertips and poking him tenderly, then proceeds to caresses and fondling. The mother needs to be prepared for the infant's exaggerated and generalized startle response to a touch so that she will not interpret this as a negative reaction to her overtures.[20] Eventually she begins to endow him with an identity—a part of the family. When he no longer resembles a "chicken" or other nonhuman counterpart and begins to take on aspects of family members, such as father's chin or sister's nose, nurses can facilitate this incorporation.[37] Parents are encouraged to bring in clothes and toys for the infant, and the nurse helps the mother set goals both for herself and the infant. Feeding schedules are discussed and the mother is encouraged to visit at times when she can become involved in the infant's care.

Throughout the maternal-infant acquaintance process, the nurse listens carefully to what the mother says in order to assess her concerns and her progress toward incorporating the infant into her life. The manner in which the mother refers to the infant and the questions she asks reveal her worries and feelings and can serve as valuable clues to future relationships with the infant. The alert nurse is attuned to these subtle indications of the mother's needs that provide guidelines for nursing intervention. Often all that the mother needs is reassurance that the behavior about which she is concerned is a normal reaction and that it will disappear as the infant matures (for example, the exaggerated Moro reflex or inability to coordinate swallowing) or that she will have the support of the nurse during care-giving activities. Knowing that members of the staff are available for telephone or personal contact when she takes the infant home provides a measure of security to an insecure mother. Above all, encouragement and reinforcement for the mother during her care-giving activities and interactions with the infant promote a healthy mother-child relationship. (See the boxed material on pp. 356-357.) Fathers, too, need support in forming a relationship with the infant. Nursing care is directed primarily toward facilitating the engrossment process (p. 289).

REFERENCES

1. Affonso, D., and Harris, T.: Continuous positive airway pressure, Am. J. Nurs. **76:**570-575, 1976.
2. Babson, S. G., and Phillips, D. S.: Growth and development of twins dissimilar in size at birth, N. Engl. J. Med. **289:**937-940, 1973.
3. Babson, S. G., and associates: Management of high-risk pregnancy and intensive care of the neonate, ed. 3, St. Louis, 1975, The C. V. Mosby Co.
4. Barlow, B., and associates: An experimental study of acute neonatal enterocolitis, J. Pediatr. Surg. **9:**587-595, 1974.
5. Barness, L. A.: Feeding the premature infant. In Wyeth Laboratories: Infant nutrition, Philadelphia, 1973, Medcom, Inc.
6. Bauer, C. H.: The low birth weight baby—special emphasis on the respiratory distress syndrome (RDS) of the newborn and early discharge, Pediatr. Ann., pp. 21-29, November 1972.
7. Brown, J., and Hepler, R.: Stimulation—a corollary to physical care, Am. J. Nurs. **76:**578-581, 1976.
8. Chinn, P. L.: Infant gavage feeding, Am. J. Nurs. **71:**1964-1967, 1971.
9. Dahms, B. B., Krauss, A. N., and Auld, P. A. M.: Pulmonary function in dysmature infants, J. Pediatr. **84:**434-437, 1974.
10. Driscoll, J. M., and Mellins, R. B.: Idiopathic respiratory distress syndrome of infancy, Respir. Care **19:**298, 1974.
11. Farquhar, J. W.: The child of the diabetic woman, Arch. Dis. Child. **34:**76, 1959.
12. Finnegan, L. P., and MacNew, B. A.: Care of the addicted infant, Am. J. Nurs. **74:**685-693, 1974.
13. Fitzhardinge, P. M.: Early growth and development in low-birth weight infants following treatment in an intensive care nursery, Pediatrics **56:**162, 1975.
14. Fitzhardinge, P. M., and Steven, E. M.: The small-for-date infant. I. Later growth patterns, Pediatrics **49:**671, 1972.
15. Fitzhardinge, P. M., and Steven, E. M.: The small-for-date infant. II. Neurological and intellectual sequelae, Pediatrics **50:**50, 1972.
16. Fogerty, S.: The nurse and the high-risk infant, Nurs. Clin. North Am. **8:**533-548, 1973.
17. Franz, I. D., III, and associates: Necrotizing enterocolitis, J. Pediatr. **86:**259-263, 1975.
18. Guthrie, D. W., and Guthrie, R. A.: The infant of the diabetic mother, Am. J. Nurs. **74:**2008-2009, 1974.
19. Gutrecht, N. M. V., and Khoury, G.: Cardiopulmonary emergencies in the newborn: diagnosis and management, Heart Lung **2:**878-883, 1973.
20. Johnson, S. H., and Grubbs, J. P.: The premature infant's reflex behaviors: effects on the maternal-child relationships, J. Obstet. Gynecol. Neonatal Nurs. **4:**15-21, May/June 1975.

21. Klaus, M. H., and Fanaroff, A. A.: Care of the high-risk neonate, Philadelphia, 1973, W. B. Saunders Co.

22. Korones, S. B.: High risk newborn infants: the basis for intensive nursing care, ed. 2, St. Louis, 1976, The C. V. Mosby Co.

23. Lancaster, J.: Impact of intensive care on the maternal-infant relationship. In Korones, S. B.: High risk newborn infants: the basis for intensive nursing care, ed. 2, St. Louis, 1976, The C. V. Mosby Co.

24. Lees, M. H.: Heart failure in the newborn infant, J. Pediatr. **75:**139-152, 1969.

25. Liggins, G. C., and Howe, R. N.: A controlled trial of antepartum glucocorticoid treatment for prevention of the respiratory distress syndrome in premature infants, Pediatrics **50:** 515, 1972.

26. Lubchenco, L. O., Delivoria-Papadopoulos, M., and Searls, D.: Long-term follow-up studies of prematurely born infants. II. Influence of birth weight and gestational age on sequelae, J. Pediatr. **80:**509, 1972.

27. Lubchenco, L. O., and associates: Newborn intensive care and long-term prognosis, Dev. Med. Child Neurol. **16:**421, 1974.

28. Nadas, A. S., Flyer, D. C., and Castaneda, A. R.: The critically ill infant with congenital heart disease, Mod. Concepts Cardiovasc. Dis. **42**(11):53-58, 1973.

29. Pierog, S. H., and Ferrara, A.: Medical care of the sick newborn, ed. 2, St. Louis, 1976, The C. V. Mosby Co.

30. Reid, D. W., and Shannon, M. P.: Necrotizing enterocolitis—a medical approach to treatment, Can. Med. Assoc. J. **108:**573-576, 1973.

31. Roback, S. A., and associates: Necrotizing enterocolitis, Arch. Surg. **109:**314-319, 1974.

32. Segal, S.: Oxygen: too much, too little, Nurs. Clin. North Am. **6:**39-53, 1971.

33. Stern, L.: The use and misuse of oxygen in the newborn infant, Pediatr. Clin. North Am. **20:**447-464, 1973.

34. Trought, E. A.: Equipment hazards, Am. J. Nurs. **73:**858-860, 1973.

35. Vidyasagar, D., Joseph, M. E., and Hamilton, L. R.: Letter to the editor: noise levels in the neonatal intensive care unit, J. Pediatr. **88:**115, 1976.

36. Warren, F. M.: Autotutorial unit on infant gavage feeding. master's thesis, Department of Nursing, San Jose State University, January 1974.

37. Warrick, L. H.: Family-centered care in the premature nursery, Am. J. Nurs. **71:**2134-2138, 1971.

38. Zenk, K. E.: Pediatric pharmacology, Crit. Care Update, pp. 5-17, August 1976.

BIBLIOGRAPHY

Alderman, M. M.: Identifying the high risk pregnancy in time, Patient Care **6:**18-50, September 30, 1972.

Alderman, M. M.: Priority care of the newborn, Patient Care **8**(13):73-152, July 4, 1974.

American Academy of Pediatrics, Committee on Fetus and Newborn: Hospital care of newborn infants, Evanston, Ind., 1971, The Academy.

Behrman, R. E., editor: Neonatal-perinatal medicine: diseases of the fetus and infant, ed. 2, St. Louis, 1977, The C. V. Mosby Co.

Black, M.: Assessment of weight and gestational age, Nurs. Clin. North Am. **13:**13-22, 1978.

Boros, S. J., and Reynolds, J. W.: Prolonged apnea of prematurity, Clin. Pediatr. **15**(2):123-134, 1976.

Brazelton, T. B.: Assessment of the infant at risk, Clin. Obstet. Gynecol. **16:**361-363, 1973.

Bresadola, C.: One infant/one nurse/one objective: quality care, Am. J. Maternal Child Nurs. **2:**287-290, 1977.

Campbell, S.: Fetal growth, Clin. Obstet. Gynecol. **1:**41, 1974.

Clatworthy, H. W., and Grosfeld, J. L.: Danger signals in the newborn, Hosp. Med. **9:**60-64, 1974.

DeMarco, J. P., and Reed, R.: Care of the high-risk infant in the intensive care unit, Nurs. Clin. North Am. **5:**375-386, 1970.

Dreszer, M.: Fluid and electrolyte requirements in the newborn infant, Pediatr. Clin. North Am. **24:**537-546, 1977.

Drillien, C. M.: The small-for-date infant, Etiology and prognosis, Pediatr. Clin. North Am. **17:**9-24, 1970.

Dubowitz, L. M. S., and associates: Clinical assessment of gestational age in the newborn infant, J. Pediatr. **77:**1-10, 1970.

DuBrow, I. W., Chen, J. W., and Wong, P. W.: Bradycardia preceding apneic attacks in low-birthweight infants, Clin. Pediatr. **15**(5):119-122, 1976.

Dweck, H. S., and associates: Early development of the tiny premature infant, Am. J. Dis. Child. **126:**28, 1973.

Edwards, N. K., and Edwards, D. S.: Are babies dying of electrocution? Nurs. Clin. North Am. **6:**81-92, 1971.

Fanaroff, A. A. and associates: Insensible water loss in low birth weight infants, Pediatrics **50:**236, 1972.

Fox, H. A.: Newborn special care—the high risk baby, Pediatr. Ann. **1:**55-59, October 1972.

Francis-Williams, J., and Davis, P. A.: Very low birth weight and later intelligence, Dev. Med. Child Nuerol. **16:**709, 1974.

Galloway, K.: Early detection of congenital anomalies, J. Obstet. Gynecol. Neonatal Nurs. **2:**37-38, 1973.

Gladder, B. E., and Buchanan, G. R.: The bleeding neonate, Pediatrics **58:**548-555, 1976.

Gluck, L.: The diagnosis of fetal maturity. In Gluck, L., editor: Modern perinatal medicine, Chicago, 1974, Year Book Medical Publishers, Inc.

Gluck, L., editor: Modern perinatal medicine, Chicago, 1974, Year Book Medical Publishers, Inc.

Green, H. L.: Hazards of electronic equipment in critical care areas: a research approach, Cardiovasc. Nurs. **9:**7-12, 1973.

Grosfeld, J. L.: The youngest surgical patient, Emergency Med. **6:**93-115, 1974.

Guy, M.: Neonatal transport, Nurs. Clin. North Am. **13:**3-12, 1978.

Guyton, A. C.: Textbook of medical physiology, ed. 5, Philadelphia, 1976, W. B. Saunders Co.

Hackel, A.: A medical transport system for the neonate, Anesthesiology **43:**258-267, 1975.

Harding, H. G.: The metabolism of brown and white adipose tissue in fetus and newborn, Clin. Obstet. Gynecol. **14:**685-709, 1971.

Heim, T.: Thermogenesis in the newborn infant, Clin. Obstet. Gynecol. **14:**790-820, 1971.

Jensen, M., Benson, R. C., and Bobak, I. M.: Maternity care:

the nurse and the family, St. Louis, 1977, The C. V. Mosby Co.

Kagan, B. M., and associates: Body composition of premature infants: relation to nutrition, Am. J. Clin. Nutr. **25**:1153, 1972.

Kress, L. M.: Transporting the sick neonate, Issues Comprehensive Pediatr. Nurs. **2**(1):8-19, 1977.

Lewis, C.: Nursing care of the neonate requiring surgery for congenital defects, Nurs. Clin. North Am. **5**:387-397, 1970.

Lubchenco, L. O.: The high risk infant, Philadelphia, 1976, W. B. Saunders Co.

Lubchenco, L. O., Searls, D. T., and Brazie, J. V.: Neonatal mortality rate: relationship to birth weight and gestational age, J. Pediatr. **81**:814, 1974.

Lutz, L., and Perlstein, P. H.: Temperature control in newborn babies, Nurs. Clin. North Am. **6**:15-23, 1971.

Marks, F. H.: Infant incubators, Nursing '72 **2**:26, November 1972.

McLean, F. H.: Significance of birthweight for gestational age in identifying infants at risk, J. Obstet. Gynecol. Neonatal Nurs. **3**:19-24, November/December 1974.

Miller, M. E.: Host defenses in the human neonate, Pediatr. Clin. North Am. **24**:413-423, 1977.

Myers, M. S.: Mature or immature? Assessment of gestational age, RN **38**:22-25, January 1975.

Mylrea, K. C., and O'Neal, L. B.: Electricity and electrical safety in the hospital, Nursing '76 **6**(1):52-59, 1976.

Parmlee, A. H., and Schulte, F. J.: Developmental testing of preterm and small-for-date infants, Pediatrics **45**:21, 1970.

Pascoe, D. J., and Grossman, M. G., editors: Pediatric emergencies, Philadelphia, 1973, J. B. Lippincott Co.

Pinneo, R.: Cardiac monitoring, Nurs. Clin. North Am. **7**:457-468, 1972.

Regionalization of perinatal care. Sixty-sixth Ross Conference on Pediatric Research, Columbus, Ohio, 1974, Ross Laboratories.

Roberts, F. B.: Perinatal nursing, New York, 1977, McGraw-Hill Book Co.

Roy, R. N., and Sinclair, J. C.: Hydration of the low birth-weight infant, Clin. Perinatol. **2**:393-417, Sepbember 1975.

Schaffer, A. J., and Avery, M. E.: Diseases of the newborn, ed. 4, Philadelphia, 1976, W. B. Saunders Co.

Schulkind, M. L., and associates: Neonatal health insurance, Clin. Pediatr. **13**:209-210, March 1974.

Shannon, D. C., and associates: Prevention of apnea and bradycardia in low birth weight infants, Pediatrics **55**:589, 1975.

Silverman, W. A.: Intensive care of the low birth weight and other at-risk infants, Clin. Obstet. Gynecol. **13**:87, 1970.

Silverman, W. A.: Diagnosis and treatment; use and misuse of temperature and humidity in care of the newborn infant, Pediatrics **33**:276, 1974.

Sinclair, J. C., and associates: Supportive management of the sick neonate, Pediatr. Clin. North Am. **17**:863, 1970.

Stewart, A. L., and Reynolds, E. O. R.: Improved prognosis for infants of very low birth weight, Pediatrics **54**:724, 1974.

Stewart, S.: The risk of handicap due to birth defect in infants of very low birth weight, Dev. Med. Child Neurol **14**:585, 1972.

St. Petery, J. R.: The high-risk infant and family. In Scipien, G. M., and associates: Comprehensive pediatric nursing, New York, 1975, McGraw-Hill Book Co.

Terris, M., and Glasser, M.: A life table analysis of the relation of prenatal care to prematurity, Am. J. Public Health **64**:869-875, 1974.

VanLeeuwen, G.: The nurse in prevention and intervention in the neonatal period, Nurs. Clin. North Am. **3**:509, 531, 1973.

Virnig, N. L., and Reynolds, J. W.: Reliability of flush blood pressure measurements in the sick newborn infant, J. Pediatr. **84**:594-598, 1974.

Waechter, E. H., Blake, F. G., and Lipp, J. P.: Nursing care of children, Philadelphia, 1976, J. B. Lippincott Co.

Warren, F. M.: Blood pressure readings; getting them quickly on an infant, Nursing '75 **5**:13, April 1975.

Yashiro, K., and associates: Preliminary studies on the thermal environment of low-birth-weight infants, J. Pediatr. **82**:991, 1973.

Zamansky, H., and Strobel, K.: Care of the critically ill newborn, Am. J. Nurs. **76**:566-569, 1976.

Intensive care facilities

Callon, H. F.: Regionalizing perinatal care in Wisconsin, Nurs. Clin. North Am. **10**:263-274, 1975.

Cunningham, M. D., and Smith, F. R.: Stabilization and transport of severely ill infants, Pediatr. Clin. North Am. **20**:359, 1973.

Duff, R., and Campbell, A.: Moral and ethical dilemmas in the special care nursery, N. Engl. J. Med. **289**:108, 1973.

Luchner, K. R.: Stress in neonatal intensive care units, Issues Comprehensive Pediatr. Nurs. **2**(1):20-35, 1977.

Meyer, H. B. P., and associates: Statewide reduction of neonatal mortality through effective regionalization of newborn intensive care, Pediatr. Res. **7**:404, 1973.

Segal, S., and Girie, G.: Equipment and personnel for neonatal special care, Pediatr. Clin. North Am. **17**:793, 1970.

Swyer, P. R.: The regional organization of special care for the neonate, Pediatr. Clin. North Am. **17**:761, 1970.

Tabor, M.: Intensive care for the newborn—everywhere, Nursing '73 **3**:33-34, 1973.

Feeding and nutrition

Altman, R. P., and Randolph, J. G.: Application and hazards of total parenteral nutrition in infants, Ann. Surg. **174**:85, 1971.

American Academy of Pediatrics: Human milk in premature infant feeding: summary of a workshop, Pediatrics **57**:741-743, 1976.

Babson, S.: Feeding the low birth weight infant, J. Pediatr. **79**: 694, 1971.

Barnes, L., and Pitkin, R. M., editors: Symposium on nutrition, Clin. Perinatol. **2**(2), 1975.

Barness, L. A.: Nutrition for the low birth weight infant, Clin. Perinatol. **2**:345-352, September 1975.

Cheek, J. A., and Staub, G. F.: Nasojejunal alimentation for premature and full-term newborn infants, J. Pediatr. **82**:955, 1973.

Choi, M. W.: Breast milk for infants who can't breast-feed, Am. J. Nurs. **78**:852-855, 1978.

Conway, A., and Williams, T.: Parenteral alimentation, Am. J. Nurs. **76**:574-577, 1976.

Dudrick, S. J., and associates: Long-term parenteral nutrition: its current status, Hosp. Pract. **10**:49, May 1975.

Fomon, S.: Infant nutrition, ed. 2, Philadelphia, 1974, W. B. Saunders Co.

Gabler, M., and Oh, W.: Nomogram for calculating caloric intake, Am. J. Nurs. **70:**816-817, 1970.
Goldman, A. S., and Smith, C. W.: Host resistance factors in human milk, J. Pediatr. **82:**1082, 1973.
Heins, W.: Feeding the premature infant, Am. J. Dis. Child. **131:** 468-469, 1977.
Heird, W. C.: Feeding the premature infant, Am. J. Dis. Child. **131:**468-469, 1977.
Heird, W. C., and Anderson, T. L.: Nutritional requirements and methods of feeding low birth weight infants, Curr. Probl. Pediatr. **7**(8):1-40, June 1977.
Heird, W. C., and Driscoll, J. M., Jr.: Newer methods for feeding low birth weight infants, Clin. Perinatol. **2:**309-325, September 1975.
Heird, W. C., and Winters, R. W.: Total parenteral nutrition, J. Pediatr. **86:**2, 1975.
Peden, V. H., and Karpel, J. T.: Total parenteral nutrition in premature infants, J. Pediatr. **81:**137, 1972.
Rothfeder, B., and Tiedeman, M.: Feeding the low-birth-weight neonate, Nursing '77 **7**(10):58-59, 1977.
Shaw, J. C. L.: Parenteral nutrition in the management of sick low birth weight infants, Pediatr. Clin. North Am. **20:**333, 1973.
Sinclair, J. C., and associates: Supportive management of the sick neonate: parenteral calories, water, and electrolytes, Pediatr. Clin. North Am. **17:**863, 1970.
Valman, H. B., Heath, C. D., and Brown, R. J. K.: Continuous intragastric milk feeds in infants of low birth weight, Br. Med. J. **2:**547, 1972.

Serious problems of preterm infants

Auld, P.: Resuscitation of the newborn infant, Am. J. Nurs. **74:** 68-70, 1974.
Comstock, G. W., and associates: Low birth weight and neonatal mortality rate related to maternal smoking and socioeconomic status, Am. J. Obstet. Gynecol. **11:**53, 1971.
DeLeon, A. S., Elliott, J. H., and Jones, D. B.: The resurgence of retrolental fibroplasia, Pediatr. Clin. North Am. **17:**309, 1970.
Elian, M.: Herpes simples encephalitis. Prognosis and long-term follow-up, Arch. Neurol. **32:**39-43, January 1975.
Freeman, J. M.: Neonatal seizures—diagnosis and management, J. Pediatr. **77:**701-708, 1970.
Gill, F. M., and Schwartz, E.: Anemia in early infancy, Pediatr. Clin. North Am. **19:**841-853, 1972.
Gotoff, S., and Behrman, R.: Neonatal septicemia, J. Pediatr. **76:**142, 1970.
Green, H. G.: Infants of alcoholic mothers, Am. J. Obstet. Gynecol. **113:**713-716, 1974.
Hecht, F., and Lovrien, E. W.: Genetic diagnosis in the newborn, Pediatr. Clin. North Am. **17:**1039-1053, 1970.
Jones, K. L., and associates: Recognition of the fetal alcohol syndrome in early infancy, Lancet **2:**1269, 1973.
McCracken, G. H.: Managing neonatal infections, Hosp. Pract., **10:**49-57, February 1976.
McCracken, G. H., Jr.: Pharmacological basis for antimicrobial therapy in newborn infants, Am. J. Dis. Child. **128:**407-419, 1974.
Miner, H.: Problems and prognosis for the small-for-gestational-age and the premature infant, Am. J. Maternal Child Nurs. **3:** 221-226, 1978.
Morrow, G., III.: Nutritional management of infants with inborn metabolic errors, Clin. Perinatol. **2:**361-372, September 1975.
Nahmias, A. J.: The TORCH complex, Hosp. Pract. **9:**65-72, May 1974.
Tokuhata, G. K.: Hospital related characteristics associated with perinatal mortality, Am. J. Public Health **63:**227-236, 1973.
Volpe, J. J.: Perinatal hypoxic-ischemic brain injury, Pediatr. Clin. North Am. **23:**383-397, 1976.
Wilson, H. D., and Eichenwald, H. F.: Sepsis neonatorum, Pediatr. Clin. North Am. **21:**571-582, 1974.
Windle, W. F.: Cerebral hemorrhage in relation to birth asphyxia, Science **167:**1000, 1970.

Respiratory distress syndrome

Ashbaugh, D. G., and Petty, T. L.: Positive end-expiratory pressure: physiology, indications, and contraindications, J. Thorac. Cardiovasc. Surg. **65:**165-170, 1973.
Avery, M. E.: What is new in our understanding of perinatal pulmonary problems? Pediatr. Res. **7:**842, 1973.
Avery, M. E., and Fletcher, B. D.: The lung and its disorders in the newborn infant, Philadelphia, 1974, W. B. Saunders Co.
Brumley, G. W.: The critically ill child; the respiratory distress syndrome of the newborn, Pediatrics **47:**758, 1971.
Clements, J. A. and associates: Assessment of the risk of the respiratory distress syndrome by a rapid test for surfactant in amniotic fluid, N. Engl. J. Med. **286:**1077, 1972.
Daily, W. J. R., and Cave-Smith, P.: Mechanical ventilation of the newborn infant. Parts I and II, Curr. Probl. Pediatr. **1**(8 and 9): entire issue, 1971.
Davis, L. A.: Neonatal respiratory emergencies, Nurs. Clin. North Am. **8:**441-446, 1973.
Doran, T. A., and associates: Amniotic fluid tests for fetal maturity, Am. J. Obstet. Gynecol. **119:**829-837, 1974.
Driscoll, J. M., Jr.: Perinatal approach to the infant with RDS, Pediatr. Ann., pp. 53-64, November 1972.
Dunn, D., and Lewis, A. T.: Some important aspects of neonatal nursing related to pulmonary disease and family involvement, Pediatr. Clin. North Am. **20:**481-497, 1973.
Ennis, S., and Harris, T. R.: Positioning infants with hyaline membrane disease, Am. J. Nurs. **78:**398-401, 1978.
Fowler, M. D.: Idiopathic respiratory distress syndrome of the newborn. In McNall, L. K., and Galeener, J. T., editors: Current practice in obstetric and gynecologic nursing, vol. 1, St. Louis, 1976, The C. V. Mosby Co.
Freeman, R. K.: The use of the oxytocin challenge test for antepartum clinical evaluation of uteroplacental respiratory function, Am. J. Obstet. Gynecol. **121:**481, 1975.
Garvey, J.: Infant respiratory distress syndrome, Am. J. Nurs. **75:**614, 1975.
Gluck, L.: Surfactant: 1972, Pediatr. Clin. North Am. **19:**325-331, 1972.
Gould, J. B., and associates: The sleep state characteristics of apnea during infancy, Pediatrics **59:**182-194, 1977.
Gregory, G. A.: Respiratory care of newborn infants, Pediatr. Clin. North Am. **19:**311-324, 1972.
Gregory, G. A., and associates: Treatment of the idiopathic respi-

ratory distress syndrome with continuous positive airway pressure, N. Engl. J. Med. **284:**1333, 1971.

Hall, R. T., and Rhodes, P. R.: Pneumothorax and pneumo-mediastinum in infants with idiopathic respiratory distress syndrome receiving continuous positive airway pressure, Pediatrics **55:**493, 1975.

Johnson, J. D., and associates: Prognosis of children surviving with the aid of mechanical ventilation in the neonatal period, Pediatr. Res. **6:**404, 1972.

Kattwinkel, J.: Neonatal apnea: pathogenesis and therapy, J. Pediatr. **90:**242-247, 1977.

Kattwinkel, J., and associates: Apnea of prematurity; comparative therapeutic effects of cutaneous stimulation and nasal continuous positive airway pressure, J. Pediatr. **86:**588-592, 1975.

Krauss, A. N., Klain, D. B., and Auld, P. A. M.: Chronic pulmonary insufficiency of prematurity, Pediatrics **55:**55, 1975.

Kumpe, M., and Kleinman, L.: Care of the infant with respiratory distress syndrome, Nurs. Clin. North Am. **6:**25, 1971.

Larroche, J.: Lung pathology in infants with RDS, Pediatr. Ann. **1:**31-44, November 1972.

Liggins, G. C., and Howie, R. N.: A controlled trial of antepartum glucocorticoid treatment on prevention of the respiratory distress syndrome in premature infants, Pediatrics **50:**515, 1972.

Naeye, R. L.: Respiratory distress syndrome. In Villee, C. A., Villee, C. B., and Zuckerman, J., editors: Respiratory distress syndrome, New York, 1973, Academic Press, Inc.

Nalepka, C. D.: The oxygen hood for newborns in respiratory distress, Am. J. Nurs. **75:**2185-2187, 1975.

Nett, L., and Petty, T. I.: Oxygen toxicity, Am. J. Nurs. **73:**1556-1558, 1973.

Philip, A. G. S.: Oxygen plus pressure plus time: the etiology of bronchopulmonary dysplasia, Pediatrics **55:**44, 1975.

Reynolds, E. O. R., and Taghizadeh, A.: Improved prognosis of infants mechanically ventilated for hyaline membrane disease, Arch. Dis. Child. **49:**505, 1974.

Roberts, J. E.: Suctioning the newborn, Am. J. Nurs. **73:**63-65, 1973.

Sham, B., and Messerly, A. M.: Apnea in the premature infant, Nurs. Clin. North Am. **13:**29-38, 1978.

Stern, L.: Therapy of the respiratory distress syndrome, Pediatr. Clin. North Am. **19:**221, 1972.

Stern, L.: The use and misuse of oxygen in the newborn infant, Pediatr. Clin. North Am. **20:**447, 1973.

Tinker, J. H., and Wehner, R.: The nurse and the ventilator, Am. J. Nurs. **74:**1276-1278, 1974.

Truog, W. E., Prueitt, J. L., and Woodrum, D. E.: Unchanged incidence of bronchopulmonary dysplasia in survivors of hyaline membrane disease, J. Pediatr. **92:**261-264, 1978.

Necrotizing enterocolitis

Barlow, B., and associates: An experimental study of acute neonatal enterocolitis—the importance of breast milk, J. Pediatr. Surg. **9:**587-595, 1974.

Bliss, V. J.: Nursing care for infants with neonatal necrotizing enterocolitis, Am. J. Maternal Child Nurs. **1:**37-40, 1976.

Book, L. S., and associates: Necrotizing enterocolitis in low-birth-weight infants fed an elemental formula, J. Pediatr. **87:**602, 1975.

Flores, R. N.: Necrotizing enterocolitis, Nurs. Clin. North Am. **13:**39-46, 1978.

Holt, S. A., and Friedland, G. W.: Neonatal necrotizing enterocolitis, West. J. Med. **120:**110, 1974.

Hopkins, G. B., and associates: Necrotizing enterocolitis in premature infants, Am. J. Dis. Child. **120:**229, 1970.

Polin, R. A., and associates: Necrotizing enterocolitis in term infants, J. Pediatr. **89:**460-462, 1976.

Torma, M. J., and associates: Necrotizing enterocolitis in infants, Am. J. Surg. **126:**758-761, 1973.

Infants of diabetic mothers

Cranley, M. S., and Frazier, S. A.: Preventive intensive care of the diabetic mother and her fetus, Nurs. Clin. North Am. **8:**489-500, 1973.

Dunn, P.: The infant of the diabetic mother, Issues Comprehensive Pediatr. Nurs. **2**(1):36-48, 1977.

Haworth, J. C., Dilling, L. A., and Vidyasagar, D.: Hypoglycemia in infants of diabetic mothers; effect of epinephrine therapy, J. Pediatr. **82:**94, 1974.

Horger, E. O., III., Miller, G., III., and Conner, E. D.: Relation of large birthweight to maternal diabetes mellitus, Obstet. Gynecol. **45:**150, 1975.

Jasper, M. L.: Pregnancy complicated by diabetes—a case study, Am. J. Maternal Child Nurs. **1:**307-312, 1976.

Kinch, E. A.: Management of the diabetic pregnancy, J. Reprod. Med. **7:**40, 1971.

King, K. C., and associates: Infants of diabetic mothers, Pediatrics **45:**889, 1970.

Krouskop, R. W., Brown, E. G., and Sweet, A. Y.: The relationship of feeding to necrotizing enterocolitis, Pediatr. Res. **8:**383, 1974.

Obenshain, S. S., and associates: Human fetal insulin response to sustained maternal hyperglycemia, N. Engl. J. Med. **283:**566, 1970.

Pildes, R. S.: Infants of diabetic mothers, N. Engl. J. Med. **289:**902-904, 1973.

Priestly, B. L.: Neurological assessment of infants with diabetic mothers in the first week of life, Pediatrics **50:**578, 1972.

Roberts, M. F., and associates: Maternal diabetes and the respiratory distress syndrome, N. Engl. J. Med. **294:**357, 1976.

White, M., and Keenan, W.: Recognition and management of hypoglycemia in the newborn infant, Nurs. Clin. North Am. **6:**67, 1971.

Infants with heart disease

Clarkson, P. M., and Orgill, A. A.: Continuous murmurs in infants of low birth weight, J. Pediatr. **84:**208-211, 1974.

Friedberg, D. Z., and Caldart, L.: A center for pediatric cardiovascular patients, Am. J. Nurs. **75:**1480-1482, 1975.

Gillon, J. E.: Behavior of newborns with cardiac distress, Am. J. Nurs. **73:**254-257, 1973.

Kitterman, J. A., and associates: Patent ductus arteriosus in premature infants, N. Engl. J. Med. **287:**473, 1972.

Meyer, R. A., and Lindower, B.: Management of the symptomatic neonate with congenital heart disease, Heart Lung **3:**392-395, 1974.

Neal, W. A., and associates: Patent ductus arteriosus complicating RDS in preterm infants, J. Pediatr. **86:**127-131, 1975.

Posey, R. A.: Creative nursing care of babies with heart disease, Nursing '74 **4**(10):40-45, October 1974.

Robert, M. F., and associates: Maternal diabetes and the respiratory distress syndrome, N. Engl. J. Med. **294:**357, 1976.

Striker, T. W., and Schreiber, M. J.: Respiratory problems associated with congenital heart disease, Heart Lung **3:**401-406, 1974.

Thibeault, D. W., and associates: Patent ductus arteriosus complicating RDS in preterm infants, J. Pediatr. **86:**120-126, 1975.

Narcotic-addicted infants

Blinick, G., and associates: Methadone maintenance, pregnancy and progeny, J.A.M.A. **225:**477-479, 1973.

Carroll, M. H.: Preventing newborn deaths from drug withdrawal, RN **34:**34, 1971.

Eriksson, M., Catz, C. S., and Yaffe, S. J.: Drugs and pregnancy, Clin. Obstet. Gynecol. **16:**198, 1973.

Glass, L., and associates: Effect of heroin withdrawal on respiratory rate and acid-base status in the newborn, N. Engl. J. Med. **286:**746, 1972.

Kandall, S. R., and Gartner, L. M.: Late presentation of drug with drawal symptoms in newborns, Am. J. Dis. Child. **127:**58-61, 1974.

Lipsitz, P. J.: A proposed narcotic withdrawal score for use with newborn infants. A pragmatic evaluation of its efficacy, Clin. Pediatr. **14:**592, 1975.

Naeye, R. L., and associates: Fetal complications of maternal heroin addiction, J. Pediatr. **83:**1055-1061, 1973.

Rothstein, P., and Gould, J.: Born with a habit: infants to drug addicted mothers, Pediatrics **51:**5, 1972.

Stone, M. L., and associates: Narcotic addiction in pregnancy, Am. J. Obstet. Gynecol. **109:**716, 1971.

Zaslow, S. S.: Nursing care of the addicted newborn, RN **37:**50-51, May 1974.

Zelson, C.: Current concepts. Infants of the addicted mother, N. Engl. J. Med. **228:**1393, 1974.

Zelson, C., Rubio, E., and Wasserman, E.: Neonatal narcotic addiction: 10 year observation, Pediatrics **48:**178, 1971.

Parental involvement

Aab, C. A.: Assessment of maternal behavior during early mother-infant interaction. In Brandt, P. A., Chinn, P. L., and Smith, M. L., editors: Current practice in pediatric nursing, vol. 1, St. Louis, 1976, The C. V. Mosby Co.

Barnard, M. U.: Supportive nursing care for the mother and newborn who are separated from each other, Am. J. Maternal Child Nurs. **1**(2):107-110, March/April 1976.

Burnett, C., and associates: Neonatal separation: the maternal side of interactional deprivation, Pediatrics **45:**197, 1970.

Christensen, A. Z.: Coping with the crisis of a premature brith—one couple's story, Am. J. Maternal Child Nurs. **2**(1):33-37, January/February 1977.

Clark, A. L., and Affonso, D. D.: Infant behavior and maternal attachment: two sides to the coin, Am. J. Maternal Child Nurs. **1**(2):94-99, March/April 1976.

Dubois, D. R.: Indications of an unhealthy relationship between parents and premature infant, J. Obstet. Gynecol. Neonatal Nurs. **4:**21, 1975.

Eager, M.: Long-distance nurturing of the family bond, Am. J. Maternal Child Nurs. **2:**293-294, 1977.

Eckes, S.: The significance of increased early contact between mother and newborn infant, J. Obstet. Gynecol. Neonatal Nurs. **3:**42-44, July/August 1974.

Erdman, D.: Parent-to-parent support: the best for those with sick newborns, Am. J. Maternal Child Nurs. **2:**291-292, 1977.

Fanaroff, A. A., Kennell, J. H., and Klaus, M.: Follow-up of low birth weight infants: the predictive value of maternal visiting patterns, Pediatrics **49:**287, 1972.

Harper, R. G., and associates: Observation on unrestricted parental contact with infants in the neonatal intensive care unit, J. Pediatr. **89:**441-445, 1976.

Kennedy, J. C.: The high-risk maternal-infant acquaintance process, Nurs. Clin. North Am. **8:**549, 1973.

Klaus, M. H., and Kennell, J. H.: Mothers separated from their newborn infants, Pediatr. Clin. North Am. **17:**1015, 1970.

Klaus, M. H., and associates: Human maternal behavior at the first contact with her young, Pediatrics **46:**187, 1970.

Klaus, M. H., and associates: Maternal attachment: importance of the first postpartum days, N. Engl. J. Med. **286:**460, 1972.

Leifer, A. D., and associates: Effects of mother-infant separation on maternal attachment behavior, Child. Dev. **43:**1203, 1972.

Miller, C.: Working with parents of high-risk infants, Am. J. Nurs. **78:**1228-1230, 1978.

Scarr-Salapatick, S., and Williams, M.: The effects of early stimulation on low birth weight infants, Child. Deve. **44:**94-101, 1973.

Seashore, M. J., and associates: The effects of denial of early mother-infant interaction on maternal self-confidence, J. Pers. Soc. Psychol. **26:**369-378, 1973.

Tempesta, L. D.: The importance of touch in the care of newborns, J. Obstet. Gynecol. Neonatal Nurs. **1:**27-28, September/October 1972.

Follow-up

Abbey, B. L., and associates: Nursing responsibility in referring the convalescent newborn, Am. J. Maternal Child Nurs. **2:** 295-297, 1977.

Beargie, R. A., James, V. L., and Greene, J. W.: Growth and development of small-for-dates newborns, Pediatr. Clin. North Am. **17:**159, 1970.

Cassady, G.: Impact of neonatal intensive care on quality of life. In Aladjem, S., and Brown, A. K., editors: Clinical perinatology, St. Louis, 1974, The C. V. Mosby Co.

Dweck, H. S., and associates: Developmental sequelae in infants having suffered severe perinatal asphyxia, Am. J. Obstet. Gynecol. **229:**811-828, 1974.

Eaves, L. C., and associates: Developmental and psycological test scores in children of low birth weight, Pediatrics **45:**9, 1970.

Grassy, R. G., Jr., and associates: The growth and development of low birth weight infants receiving intensive neonatal care, Clin. Pediatr. **15**(6):549-553, 1976.

Hardy, J. B.: Birth weight and subsequent physical and intellectual development, N. Engl. J. Med. **289:**973-974, 1973.

Harrod, J. R., and associates: Long-term follow-up of severe respiratory distress syndrome treated with IPPB, J. Pediatr. **84:** 277-286, 1974.

Johnson, L. H., and associates: Survivors of respiratory distress syndrome (RDS)—a 4 year follow-up, Pediatr. Res. **6:**411, 1972.

Komich, M. P., and associates: The sequential development of infants of low birthweight, Am. J. Occup. Ther. **27:**396-402, 1973.

Outerbridge, E. W., and Stern, L.: Developmental follow-up of artificially-ventilated infants with neonatal respiratory failure, Pediatr. Res. **6:**412, 1972.

Schlesinger, E. R.: Neonatal intensive care: planning for services and outcomes following care, J. Pediatr. **82:**916, 1973.

Sherman, N.: High-risk newborns: continuity of care between hospitals and communities, Fam. Comm. Health **1:**47-59, 1978.

Stahlman, M., and associates: A six-year follow-up of clinical hyaline membrane disease, Pediatr. Clin. North Am. **20:**433, 1973.

Stewart, A. L., and Reynolds, E. O.: Improved prognosis for infants of very low birth weight, Pediatrics **54:**724, 1974.

11

Conditions caused by defects in physical development

Congenital malformations constitute a large percentage of the health problems of infants and children, and, although many severe disorders of childhood can either be prevented or effectively treated, very little progress has been achieved in prevention of congenital defects. Anyone who works in a children's unit of a hospital cannot help but be impressed by the number of children who are there because of a congenital defect. It is calculated that approximately one third of hospitalized children suffer from a congenital defect or its sequelae. Not all congenital defects are considered to be malformations, for example, inborn errors of metabolism and mental retardation. However, this chapter is primarily concerned with structural defects, most of which are apparent at birth.

BIRTH OF A DEFECTIVE CHILD

The parents are the most significant influences in the life of the child, and the initial maternal-infant attachment is the relationship on which future interactions are based. The birth of any child is considered by some to constitute a crisis situation, but when the newborn suffers from a physical or mental defect the parents' need for understanding and supportive care from health professionals is magnified. The manner in which nurses and other health personnel work with the parents immediately after the birth profoundly influences the situation for all persons concerned.

Parental responses

Preparation for childbirth involves fantasies and images of the expected infant. Normally every mother wishes for a perfect child, but, at the same time, she fears that the infant will be abnormal. This fear is often expressed by the expectant mother when she states that her concern is not whether the child is to be a girl or a boy, just that it is healthy. One of the first things the mother wishes confirmed at the time of birth is, "Is my baby all right?" In most instances there is some discrepancy between the mother's idealized child and the infant she delivers, for example, the birth of a boy when she has hoped for a girl. Resolution of this discrepancy is a developmental task of motherhood and is essential to the establishment of a healthy mother-child relationship. If this discrepancy is too great, as with the birth of an infant with a gross defect or where the wishes of the mother are unrealistic, the resulting emotional stress may be overwhelming, and the more severe the defect, the greater the impact of the experience.

The birth of a defective child abruptly ends the psychologic attachment the mother has formed for the child she has idealized during pregnancy. She must now deal with loss of this wished-for, healthy child. Her fears have been realized, and she is faced with meeting the demands of the defective child for care and affection. The need for the mother to grieve for the loss of the expected child while adapting to the care of the handicapped child places overwhelming demands on her at a time when her own psychologic and physiologic resources have been depleted by the birth experience.[18]

The grief reaction experienced by mothers at the birth of a defective child is the same as the response that follows the loss of any valued or significant object (see section on grief process, p. 970). The mothers experience shock, frustration, and anger at what has happened to them, and they ask themselves, "Why? Why me?" Parents may feel shame and embarrassment, often with feelings of personal failure and guilt. Frequently the mother believes that she might have caused harm to the child, and she may associate the condition with wrongdoing or evil thoughts, especially if the pregnancy was unwanted initially.[21]

To deal with stress and anxiety, parents use defense mechanisms that have provided protection in their past. A very common response is *denial,* which may be short-lived or may last for many months. They do not appear to "hear" what is told to them about their child, and they behave as though nothing is wrong with the child. Denial during the shock phase of the grief process can serve as a constructive means for parents to deal with the sudden and profound impact of the initial stress until they are better able to cope with the situation.[12]

When parents are unable to face the reality of the infant's condition, they *withdraw* from the situation either physically or emotionally. They frequently become incapacitated and unable to function in their usual manner. They avoid interpersonal contacts. Unable to face relatives and friends for fear of the reactions they may encounter, parents choose the protection of isolation. They feel as though they are alone in a world all their own. Avoidance behaviors on the part of others, including health workers, contribute to this withdrawal and compound the feelings of loneliness that are so common in parents of a defective infant.

Parents often extend this avoidance behavior to include the infant. They seem to be unable to face the infant and do not visit the child in the nursery or the pediatric unit. Sometimes it takes time for the parents to master their own feelings before they are able to deal constructively with the situation. A more subtle form of isolation is seen in parents who are very objective in their behavior toward the infant and his defect. They are intellectually concerned with their infant's medical care but display no emotional involvement. Their attention is focused on the abnormality, not on the infant.

Parental reactions depend to a large extent on the type and severity of the defect. A gross, visible anomaly, especially one involving the face, elicits a more intense emotional response than one that is less apparent, such as a heart defect. The extent of the impairment cannot be used as a criterion to determine the degree of parental depressive reactions.[9] Also, because of their limited contact with congenital defects, parents' perception of the situation may be distorted, and much depends on previous feelings they may have experienced with a similar abnormality. Therefore, their reactions may seem out of proportion to the actual extent and severity of the impairment as viewed by health professionals.[21]

Nursing considerations

The attitudes and behaviors of nurses and other health personnel at the birth of a defective child significantly influence the effect that the situation has on the parents. During this time parents are particularly sensitive and responsive to the behaviors of those with whom they are in contact. Therefore, the reactions of the health professionals toward the infant and the parents provide cues to the parents that can affect their feelings toward the infant and themselves.

Initial contact. The first indication that all is not well occurs at the time of delivery. The atmosphere of happy anticipation suddenly changes to one laden with anxiety. Even when the mother is unable to see the infant, she senses with terrifying awareness the heightened and prolonged tension in the room, which conveys to her that something is seriously wrong. Personnel, unprepared for this disturbing experience, find it difficult to cope with their own feelings and react with feelings of frustration and resentment toward a situation that they are powerless to change. As a result they may forget about or retreat from the parents, who, at this moment, are suffering the most.

Most physicians believe that it is their responsibility to inform the parents of a congenital anomaly. At the time of delivery, unless a pediatrician is in attendance, there is a delay while the physician is involved with the mother's care. During this period the mother, unable to see her child and feeling the tense atmosphere, will believe either that the child is normal but that others do not share her enthusiasm or that the child is so terrible that the professional people in the room are unable to talk about it. A nurse, the person who is most likely to be free to support the mother and who is familiar with most common congenital anomalies, can make truthful statements about the defect.

The manner in which nurses present the infant to the parents may well set the tone for the early parent-child relationship. It is probably best to explain briefly to them in simple language what the defect is and something concerning the prognosis before the infant is shown to them, when they are more apt to "hear" what is said. Parents attach a great deal of meaning to the behavior of others during this critical period and will watch the facial expressions of others closely for signs of revulsion or rejection. Presenting the infant as something precious, although incomplete, and emphasizing the well-formed aspects of the infant's body provide some reassurance to parents in this crisis period. It is important to allow time and opportunity for the parents to express their initial response to the situation. They need to be encouraged to ask questions and to receive honest, straightforward answers without undo optimism or pessimism.

Supportive care. Nurses who understand the grief response will be prepared to support the parents through this necessary process. This is particularly important with the birth of a defective child because the parents cannot begin to invest any feeling for the child until they are able to talk about and work through their feelings of disappointment, resentment, guilt, and helplessness. Parents need to talk, and the supportive nurse is one who creates and maintains an atmosphere that encourages expression of feelings. Open expression is difficult for many people, and the parent(s) may hesitate to display intense feelings. Containing those feelings utilizes a great deal of energy that would be better used a little later on to develop a relationship with the infant. Nurses, therefore, need to listen closely for cues that indicate areas of discomfort or readiness to talk. They can initiate a discussion about matters that were of concern to others in a similar situation and help the parents to know that their feelings are natural. Parents need to be allowed silence and solitude if this is their wish. Most of all, nurses need to promote communication within the family and help strengthen family interpersonal relationships. Family disintegration is a sequel that is all too common to the birth of a defective child.

Mothers are very uneasy about handling their infant and will require support and encouragement in their mothering tasks. A longer period of dependency is needed by these mothers to regroup their resources for coping. Although the mother should not feel forced to care for the infant until she is ready for the responsibility, she can be given opportunities to assume care of the infant as soon as possible to help her deal with the reality of the infant's condition. Mothers' responses are highly individual and must be evaluated on this premise. However, all mothers need sympathetic, patient, and understanding help to gain feelings of adequacy in the care of their children and facilitate development of a positive relationship with the infant later on. Nurses must be prepared to accept any or all of the parental reactions and defenses—anger, hostility, rejection, dependency—without anger and without withdrawing from the situation. If nurses make themselves available to the parents for support, they can often find nonthreatening ways of help, comfort, and support.

Supplying information. Parents need to have accurate, up-to-date information given to them early and in language they can understand. Since they do not hear all that is said the first time it is told to them, they want careful explanations about the child's defect, the treatments outlined, and what will be expected of them. Parents often misinterpret information and, therefore, require repeated explanations. Often the nurse's responsibility is to explain, interpret, and clarify information that has been given by the physician and to answer questions. Following basic concepts of interviewing, the nurse determines what the parents know and proceeds from that point. One cannot assume that the parents' failure to ask questions means they understand. Most parents have little or no knowledge of basic anatomy or physiology; therefore, pictures and other visual aids can be used effectively to explain both normal and deviant structures.

Teaching the parents to provide the special care that is frequently required for an infant with a developmental defect is an important nursing responsibility. Special feeding, holding, and positioning techniques need to be explained and demonstrated. Anticipatory guidance regarding problems that are peculiar to each abnormality reduce apprehension and stimulate the parents to institute preventive measures and to make alert observations.

Referral to agencies and organizations that offer services for the specific defect can provide parents with help to deal with ongoing problems and to plan for those they will encounter in raising a child with a defect, including financial burdens. Public health agencies, social services, mental health clinics, and parent groups all have unique and specialized services that are designed to help support the family and aid parents in their problem solving.

Summary

Parents are the persons who exert the greatest influence on the growth and development of the defective child, and the initial relationship with the child significantly affects the subsequent course of interaction. They must be allowed ample time to grieve for the loss of the expected child before they are able to form an emotional attachment to the child they have. However, as long as the defective child remains a living reminder of their loss, parents may never be able to totally resolve their grief. It is a nursing responsibility to help parents with their grief work and to facilitate the formation of a satisfactory adjustment to the child with a defect. They need help to see their infant as a *person,* support in coping with their situation, and guidance in physical care of the child.

Malformations of the central nervous system

Defects of the central nervous system are usually the result of embryologic developmental failures. Some can be attributed to prenatal insults (caused by factors such as maternal infections or radiation), anoxia, or genetic factors; others may be a result of postnatal infections; however, in most cases the etiology is obscure. The defects that will be discussed are (1) cranial deformities caused by failure of cranial sutures to remain open during the period of brain growth, (2) defects of neural tube closure, and (3) those characterized by an increase of free fluid in the cranial cavity, such as hydrocephalus.

CRANIAL DEFORMITIES

Various types of cranial deformities are encountered in early infancy. These include the enlarged head with frontal protrusion or bossing characteristic of hydrocephalus, the parietal bossing that is seen in chronic subdural hematoma, the small head, and a variety of skull deformities (Fig. 11-1). Some occur during prenatal development; in others, head circumference is usually within normal limits at birth and the defective development becomes apparent with advancing age.

In the normal newborn the cranial sutures are separated by membranous seams several millimeters wide. For the first few hours to 1 to 2 days after birth, the cranial bones may override one another and are highly mobile in relationship to one another. This mobility allows the cranial bones to mold and slide over one another, adjusting the circumference of the head to accommodate to the changing shape and character of the birth canal. The principal sutures in the infant's skull are the sagittal, coronal, and lambdoid sutures, and the major soft areas at the juncture of these sutures are the anterior and posterior fontanels. Following birth, growth occurs in a direction perpendicular to the line of the suture and normal closure occurs in a regular and predictable order. Although there are wide variations in the age at which closure takes place in individual children, normally all sutures and fontanels should be ossified by the following ages:

3 months—posterior fontanel closed
6 months—fibrous union of suture lines and interlocking of serrated edges
20 months—anterior fontanel closed

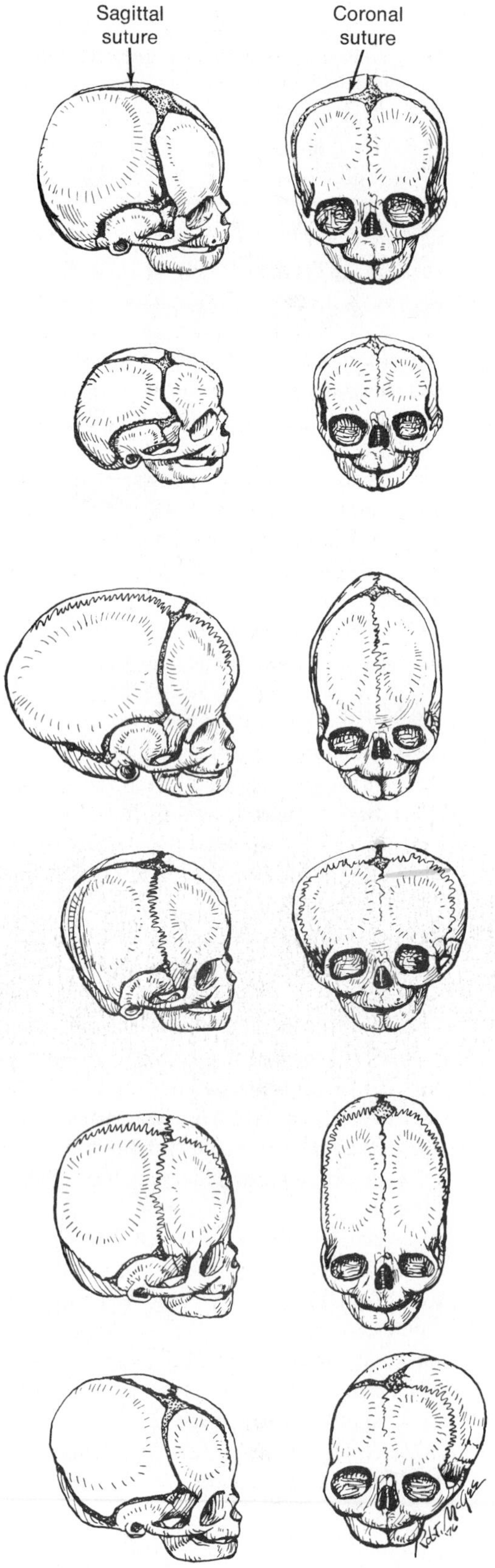
Sagittal suture
Coronal suture
NORMAL SKULL: bones separated by membranous seams until sutures gradually close
MICROCEPHALY AND CRANIOSTENOSIS: microcephaly is head circumference more than 2 standard deviations below the mean for age, sex, race, and gestation and reflects a small brain; craniosynostosis is premature closure of sutures
SCAPHROCEPHALY OR DOLICHOCEPHALY: premature closure of sagittal suture resulting in restricted lateral growth
BRACHYCEPHALY: premature closure of coronal suture resulting in excessive lateral growth
OXYCEPHALY OR ACROCEPHALY: premature closure of all coronal and sagittal sutures resulting in accelerated upward growth and small head circumference
PLAGIOCEPHALY: unilateral premature closure of coronal suture resulting in asymmetric growth

Fig. 11-1. Craniostenosis. Abnormal head configuration resulting from premature closing of cranial sutures.

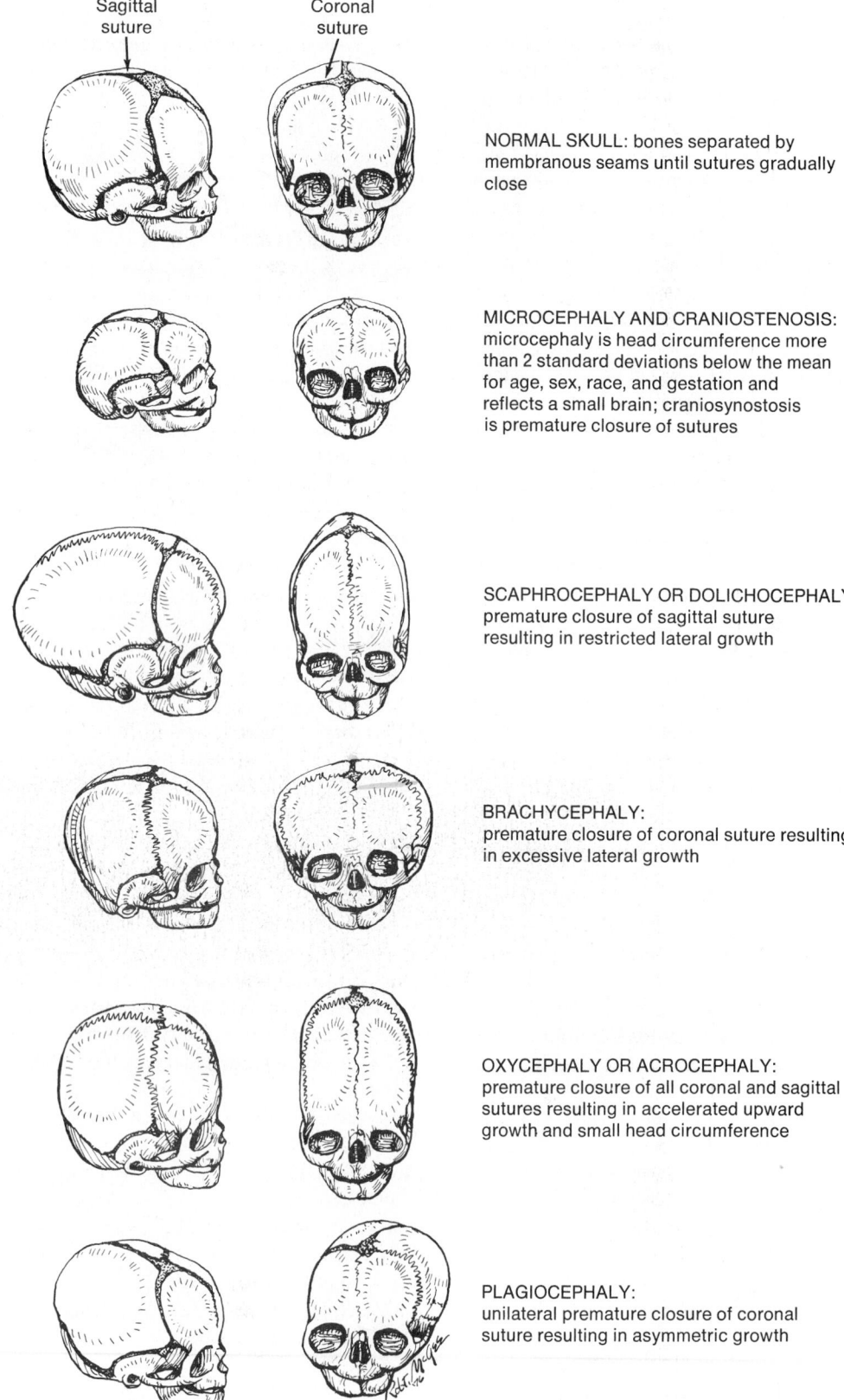

12 years—sutures unable to be separated by increased intracranial pressure

Solid union of all sutures is not completed until very late childhood.

Closure of a suture before the expected time inhibits growth of the skull *perpendicular* to the line of fusion. Since normal increase in brain volume requires expansion, the skull is forced to grow in a direction *parallel* to the fused suture. This alteration in the growth pattern of the skull always produces a distortion of the head shape when the underlying brain growth is normal. The small head with closed and normal shape is the result of deficient brain growth; the suture closure is secondary to this brain growth failure. Failure of brain growth is not secondary to suture closure.

Microcephaly

Primary microcephaly reflects a small brain and may be caused by an autosomal-recessive disorder, a chromosomal abnormality, or the result of application of a toxic stimulus during the period of induction and major cell migration in prenatal development (see Chapter 7). These stimuli may be irradiation (especially between 4 and 20 weeks of gestation), maternal infection (notably toxoplasmosis, rubella, or cytomegalovirus), or chemical agents. *Secondary microcephaly* can result from a variety of insults that occur during the third trimester of pregnancy, the perinatal period, or early infancy. Infection, trauma, metabolic disorders, and anoxia are all capable of causing decreased brain growth and early closure of cranial sutures.

In both types the neurologic manifestations range from decerebration, complete unresponsiveness, and/or autistic behavior to mild motor impairment, educable mental retardation, and/or mild hyperkinesis. There appears to be a decided relationship between microcephaly and mental retardation of varying degrees. There is no treatment. Nursing care is directed toward helping parents adjust to rearing a brain-damaged child (see Chapter 23).

Craniostenosis (craniosynostosis)

Premature closure of the sutures of the skull produces deformities of the head, frequently with damage to the brain and eyes. In contrast to microcephaly, suture closure is the primary defect and is not the result of impaired brain growth. Consequently brain growth continues and the clinical picture depends on which sutures close, the duration of the closure process, and the success or failure of the other sutures to compensate by expansion. Usually the skull growth is inhibited in a direction at right angles to the closed sutures (see Fig. 11-1). The most common form is premature closure of the sagittal suture with consequent elongation of the skull in the anterioposterior direction. (A similar head shape is seen as a result of postnatal position maintenance in some premature infants.)

Treatment, if any, involves surgical excision of long bars of bone along or parallel to the fused suture and placement of a polyethylene- or silicone-coated film over the bony margins to delay closure. Surgery is performed for cosmetic reasons or, when multiple sutures are fused, to relieve cerebral pressure symptoms and complications.

DEFECTS OF NEURAL TUBE CLOSURE

Abnormalities along the neural axis constitute a significant portion of congenital malformations. The defects may extend the entire length of the neural tube or may be restricted to a small area only. The amount of deformity and disability depends on the degree of neural involvement. *Myelodysplasia* is an all-inclusive term that refers to defective development of any part of the spinal cord, but it is usually used to describe abnormalities without gross superficial defects, especially those of the lower segment. The more severe defects are *rachischisis,* a fissure in the spinal column that leaves the meninges and spinal cord exposed, and *anencephaly,* absence of the brain with only an exposed vascular mass and no bony covering. The majority of neural tube malformations consist of defects in closure of the vertebral column with varying degrees of tissue protrusion through the bony cleft called *spinal dysrhaphia* or *spina bifida.* If the anomaly is not visible externally it is termed *spina bifida occulta;* if there is an external saccular protrusion the defect is termed *spina bifida cystica* and is further classified according to the extent of neural involvement (Fig. 11-2). A herniation of brain and meninges through a defect in the skull producing a saclike structure is termed *encephalocele.*

Etiology and pathophysiology

Malformations that are derived from the embryonic neural tube, primarily anencephaly and spina bifida, constitute the largest group of congenital anomalies that is consistent with multifactorial inheritance. Two of the defects, anencephaly and spina bifida, occur in association with one another more often than would be expected by chance, suggesting a common origin. The central nervous system defects may alternate in siblings, which also tends to bear out the theory of a common origin. In a family who has had a child with either anencephaly or spina bifida, the possibility of having a subsequent child with either anomaly is higher than in the general population (p. 198). There is some speculation regarding a viral cause of spina bifida since there appears to be an increased incidence of the defect in the early winter months. Radiation and other environmental influences have also been implicated, based on animal experiments.

Pathophysiology. The pathophysiology of spina bifida is best understood when related to the normal formative stages of the nervous system. At approximately 20 days of gestation a decided depression, the neural groove, appears

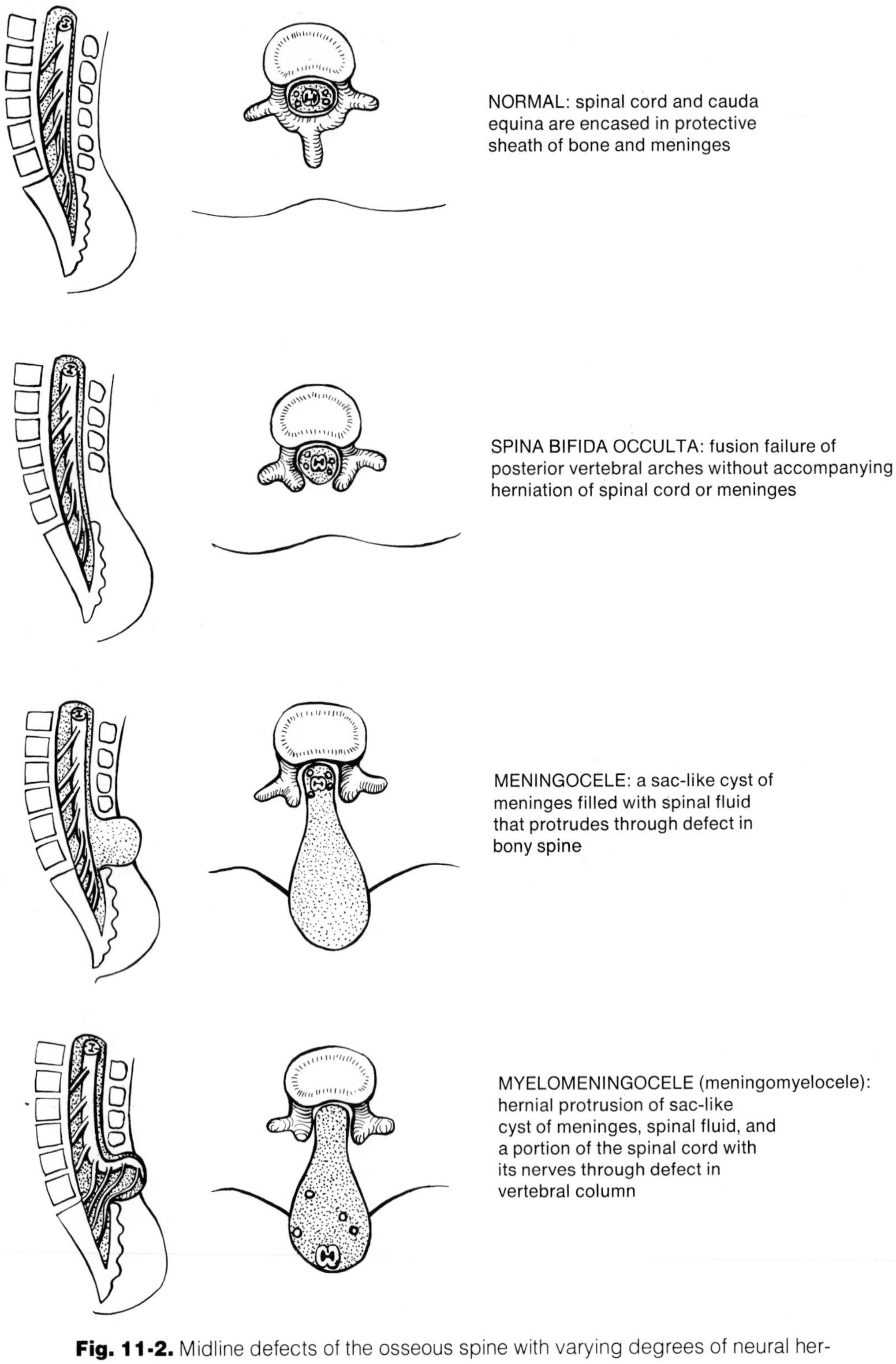
NORMAL: spinal cord and cauda equina are encased in protective sheath of bone and meninges
SPINA BIFIDA OCCULTA: fusion failure of posterior vertebral arches without accompanying herniation of spinal cord or meninges
MENINGOCELE: a sac-like cyst of meninges filled with spinal fluid that protrudes through defect in bony spine
MYELOMENINGOCELE (meningomyelocele): hernial protrusion of sac-like cyst of meninges, spinal fluid, and a portion of the spinal cord with its nerves through defect in vertebral column

Fig. 11-2. Midline defects of the osseous spine with varying degrees of neural herniations.

in the dorsal ectoderm of the embryo. During the fourth week of gestation the groove deepens rapidly and its elevated margins develop laterally and then fuse dorsally to form the neural tube. Neural tube formation begins in the cervical region near the center of the embryo and advances in both directions—caudally and cephalically—until by the end of the fourth week of gestation the ends of the neural tube, the anterior and posterior neuropores, are closed. The primary defect in neural tube malformations is believed by most authorities to be a failure of neural tube closure. However, there is evidence to indicate that the defects are a result of splitting of the already closed neural tube as a result of an abnormal increase in cerebrospinal fluid pressure during the first trimester.[11]

Prenatal detection. It is possible to determine the presence of some major open neural tube defects prenatally. Ultrasonic scanning of the uterus and elevated concentrations of alpha-fetoprotein (AFP), a fetal-specific alpha-1 globulin, in amniotic fluid can indicate the presence of anencephaly or myelomeningocele. The optimal time for these diagnostic tests to be carried out is between the fourteenth and sixteenth weeks of gestation before alpha-fetoprotein concentrations normally diminish and in sufficient time to permit a therapeutic abortion. It is recommended that such diagnostic procedures be considered for all mothers at risk.[16]

Diagnostic evaluation

Spina bifida cystica. The cystic defect affects 0.2 to 4.2 in every 1000 live births, is readily apparent, and is usually detected at birth. Most commonly it appears as a sac-like structure that may be located at any point along the spinal column. Usually the sac is encased in a fine membrane that is prone to tears through which cerebrospinal fluid leaks. In other instances the sac may be covered by dura, meninges, or skin, in which instances there is rapid and spontaneous epithelialization. If the mass can be transilluminated (that is, becomes translucent when a light is held behind it), the defect is probably a meningocele. In these cases there is rarely disturbed neurologic function even though the nerve roots are somewhat displaced. If the mass does not transilluminate it is more likely a myelomeningocele as are 75% of defects, about one in every 800 births.[19] The degree of neurologic dysfunction is directly related to the anatomic level of the defect and, thus, the nerves involved.

Since it is the last segment of the neural tube to close, the largest number of myelomeningoceles are found in the lumbar or lumbosacral area (Fig. 11-3). When the defect is located below the second lumbar vertebra, the nerves of the cauda equina are involved, giving rise to symptoms such as flaccid, areflexic partial paralysis of the lower extremities and varying degrees of sensory deficit. Sensory disturbances usually parallel motor dysfunction. The upper level of sensory and motor impairment can be determined by observation of the infant's response to a pinprick over the legs and trunk. The infant will respond to the sensory stimulus with limb movement, arousal, and crying. When withdrawal activity is employed to determine the lowest level of spinal cord function, the response to pinprick should begin above the lesion.[19] It is important to observe the infant's behavior in conjunction with the stimulus since limb movements can be induced in response to spinal cord reflex activity that has no connection with the higher centers. Defective nerve supply to the bladder affects both sphincter and detrusor tone to produce overflow incontinence with constant dribbling of urine. Often there is poor anal sphincter tone and poor anal skin reflex, which result in lack of bowel control and, sometimes, rectal prolapse. If the defect is located below the third sacral vertebra, there is no motor impairment but there may be saddle anesthesia with bladder and anal sphincter paralysis.

Sometimes the denervation to the muscles of the lower extremities will produce in utero joint deformities, primarily flexion or extension contractures, talipes valgus or varus contractures, kyphosis, lumbosacral scoliosis, and hip dislocations. The extent and severity of these associated deformities again depends on the degree of nerve involvement. Most flexion deformities result from the pull of stronger, fully innervated muscles acting without the counterpull of their nonfunctioning, paralyzed antagonists.

The anomaly most frequently associated with myelomeningocele is hydrocephalus, which complicates approximately 90% of lumbosacral myelomeningoceles. This is usually some form of the defect involving the brain stem and cerebellum known as the *Arnold-Chiari malformation* (p. 380). In most cases hydrocephalus is apparent at birth; in other children it appears shortly thereafter as evidenced by increasing occipitofrontal circumference measurements.

Spina bifida occulta. Noncystic spina bifida is failure of the spinous processes to join posteriorly in the lumbosacral area (L5 and S1). Routine x-ray examinations indicate that the disorder is quite common, but it may not be apparent unless there are associated cutaneous manifestations or neuromuscular disturbances. The incidence is estimated to occur in up to 25% of younger children in whom there is eventual fusion of the vertebral arches and in approximately 5% of all individuals. Superficial indications include a skin depression or dimple (which may also mark the outlet of a dermal sinus tract that extends to the subarachnoid space), port-wine angiomatous nevi, dark tufts of hair, or soft, subcutaneous lipomas. These signs may be absent, appear singly, or be present in combination. Neuromuscular disturbances usually consist of progressive disturbance of gait with foot weakness and/or bowel and bladder sphincter disturbances caused by abnormal adhesion of the spinal cord to the area of the malformation, resulting in traction on the spinal cord and cauda equina with growth. See

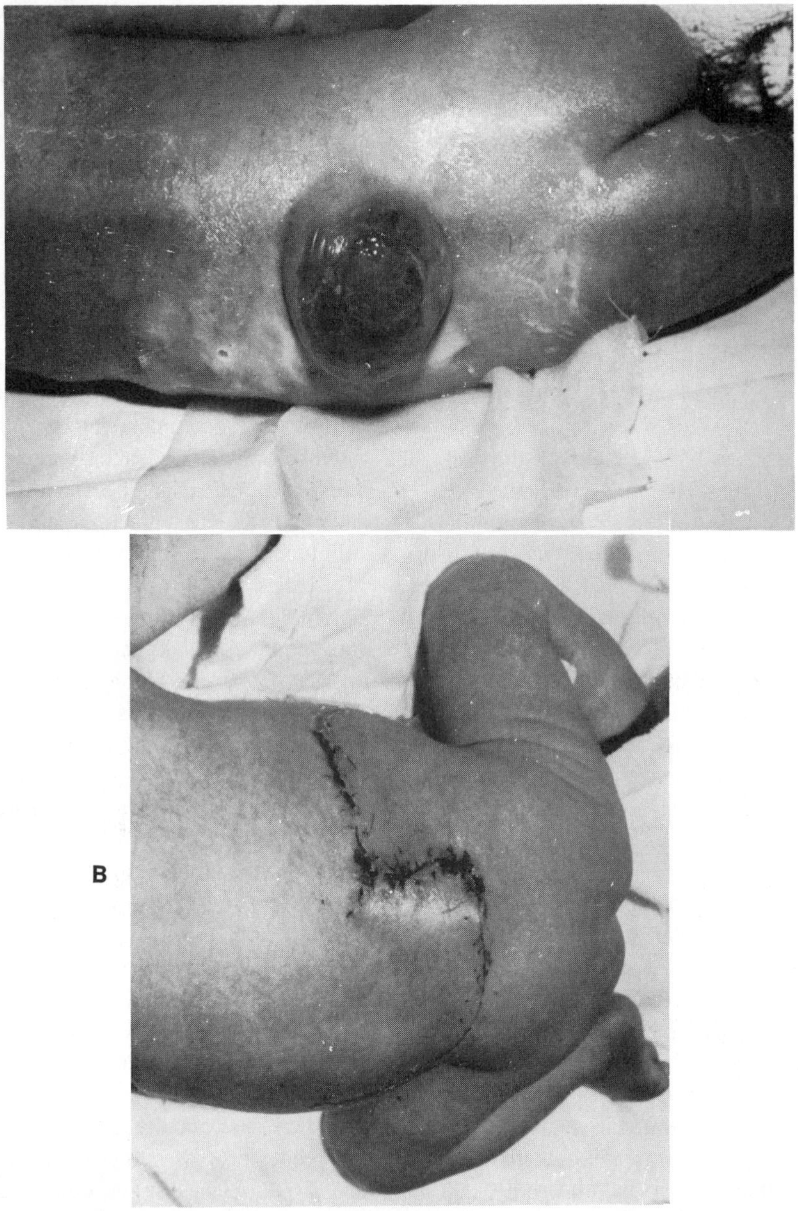

A

B

Fig. 11-3. A, Myelomeningocele before surgery. (An antibacterial dressing was used.) **B,** Repair of the same patient. (Courtesy M. C. Gleason, M. D., San Diego, Calif. From Ingalls, A. J., and Salerno, M. C.: Maternal and child health nursing, ed. 3, St. Louis, 1975, The C. V. Mosby Co., p. 236.)

Fig. 40-22 for areas innervated by specific spinal nerves.

Other diagnostic procedures. Supplementary diagnostic measures include plain x-ray films to disclose the precise bony defect in symptomatic lesions and to establish the diagnosis in the suspected, nonsymptomatic occult variety. Occasionally spinal tomograms and myelography are employed to differentiate between spina bifida occulta and other spinal pathology. Skull films and air encephalography help establish the presence or absence of hydrocephalus in spina bifida cystica.

Laboratory examinations are used primarily to determine causative organisms in the major complications of spina bifida—meningitis and urinary tract infections. Children with urinary tract incontinence require urine analysis, culture, blood urea nitrogen (BUN) evaluation, and creatinine clearance evaluation.

Medical management

Care and management of the child who has spina bifida with myelomeningocele require a multidisciplinary approach involving the specialties of neurology, neurosurgery, pediatrics, urology, orthopedics, and rehabilitation and physical therapy, as well as intensive nursing care in a variety of specialty areas. The collaborative efforts of these specialists are directed toward the five major problems associated with this serious defect—myelomeningocele, hydrocephalus, urinary tract paralysis, locomotion, and rehabilitation and education of both child and family. (See Chapter 40.)

Surgical treatment. Initial care involves prevention of infection, neurologic assessment, including observation for associated anomalies, and dealing with the impact of the anomaly on the parents. Although meningoceles are repaired early, especially if there is danger of rupture of the sac, the philosophy regarding skin closure of myelomeningoceles varies radically among authorities. At the present time, however, most authorities believe that early closure, within the first 24 to 48 hours, offers the most favorable outcome, especially in regard to morbidity and mortality from serious infection. Proponents of early closure argue that early closure, preferably in the first 12 to 18 hours, not only prevents local infection and trauma to the exposed tissues but also avoids stretching of other nerve roots that may occur as the meningeal sac expands during the first 24 hours after birth, thus preventing further motor impairment. There are those who recommend that surgical repair is best delayed for further assessment of neurologic function, intellectual potential, and extent of complications. They believe that, in addition to increased ability of the infant to tolerate the surgical procedure, delay allows for better epithelialization of the sac (thus reducing the risk of infection) and permits easier mobilization of skin for closure. Delay is also believed to be beneficial by some because early closure contributes to the development of hydrocephalus by reducing the absorptive surface provided by the meningocele. Others believe that the hydrocephalus is preexistent and unrelated to the time of closure. The preferred method of surgical repair of the lesion employs skin grafts or Z closure without disturbing the neural elements or removal of any portion of the sac (see Fig. 11-3, *B*). Wide excision of the large membranous covering may damage functioning neural tissue. Where the skin over the defect is intact, as often occurs with meningocele, surgical intervention may be performed for cosmetic reasons.

Recently some experimentation has been carried out using small, individual oxygen chambers that fit over the lesion. There is evidence to indicate that this relatively simple procedure hastens healing and prevents spread of infection in infants already infected or in those who are otherwise unable to undergo immediate surgery.

Associated problems are assessed and managed by appropriate surgical and supportive measures. Shunt procedures provide relief from imminent or progressive hydrocephalus. Often, in instances where a shunt procedure is performed before closure of the spinal defect, relief of the hydrocephalus also produces a collapse of the myelomeningocele with subsequent epithelialization of the sac. Meningitis, urinary tract infection, and pneumonia are treated with vigorous antibiotic therapy and supportive measures.

Orthopedic considerations. According to most orthopedists, musculoskeletal problems that will affect later locomotion should be evaluated early, and treatment, where indicated, should be instituted without delay. In collaboration with appropriate members of the team, the infant is evaluated in regard to the true level of neurologic functioning and corrective measures are carried out in coordination with the activities of the neurosurgeon. Casting, bracing, traction, and surgical techniques for correction of hip, knee, and foot deformities are employed when they may aid later ambulation. The minimal degree of future handicap can usually be ascertained although the maximum degree of disability is impossible to predict.[10] Corrective procedures, when indicated, are best initiated at an early age in order that the infant will not lag significantly behind age-mates in developmental progress. Where there is little hope for lower extremity functioning, surgery is seldom recommended.

Management of excretory function. Myelomeningocele is one of the most frequent causes of neurogenic bladder dysfunction in childhood. The prognosis for children who survive the early hazards of meningitis and hydrocephalus ultimately depends on the severity of their renal disease. Not only does renal failure pose a threat to life, but the lack of bladder control is important to the development of self-image and the social acceptability of the child. Ongoing assessment and monitoring of urologic status is a lifelong problem in management of the myelodysplastic child with or without surgical repair of the spinal defect. Since the majority of these children suffer from incontinence and are subject to recurrent or persistent pyuria, prevention and treatment of renal complications are a constant goal. Treatment of renal disorders includes (1) lifetime administration of urinary tract antiseptic drugs, (2) reduction of urinary stasis with suprapubic manual expression of urine (Credé maneuver), and (3) a system for bladder drainage, such as an indwelling catheter or collecting device, to reduce vesicoureteral reflux and hydronephrosis. Drugs such as bethanechol (Urecholine), propantheline (Pro-Banthine), phenoxybenzamine (Dibenzyline), and ephedrine prove useful in some cases, and in many areas the surgically implanted artificial urinary sphincter and bladder pacemaker are being used with increasing frequency.[14] In cases of intractable severe hydronephrosis or incontinence, urinary diversion such as a ureteroileostomy, ureterostomy, or cystostomy may be necessary.

Fecal incontinence can usually be controlled with diet modification and bowel training. Colostomy may prove more convenient for social reasons in children who are otherwise able to function.

Outcome. The early prognosis for the child with myelomeningocele depends on the neurologic deficit present at birth, including motor ability and bladder innervation and the presence of associated cerebral anomalies. Early surgical repair of the spinal defect, antibiotic therapy to reduce the incidence of total meningitis and ventriculitis, and correction of hydrocephalus have significantly increased the survival rate. Untreated, 45% of affected children die by 3 months of age and 84% to 90% do not survive past the second year of life. A large percentage of children (30% to 50%) are left with total flaccid paralysis and incontinence, and the remainder have significant motor disability. Approximately 50% are mentally retarded.[2] Improved surgical techniques do not alter the major physical disability and deformity, retardation, and chronic urinary tract and pulmonary infections that alter the quality of life for these children. Superimposed on these physical problems are the effect that the disorder has on family life and finances, on school and hospital services, and so on. There are those who question whether operative procedures should be considered for children with overwhelming neurologic deficit or whether the disorder should be allowed to assume its natural course. Such controversies present serious ethical problems.

Death during early months is caused by central nervous system infection or hydrocephalus. Mortality in later childhood is the result of urinary tract infection with sepsis and renal failure, complications of shunt therapy for hydrocephalus, or pulmonary disease resulting from progressive kyphoscoliosis.

Nursing considerations

Care of the infant and child with defective development of the spinal cord requires both immediate and long-term nursing and medical supervision. At the time of delivery an examination is performed to assess the intactness of the membranous cyst, and every effort is made to prevent trauma to this protective covering. It is inspected for possible spinal fluid leaks through tears in the membrane, and a moist saline dressing is applied. In the newborn period nursing responsibilities are directed toward preventing infection of and trauma to the fragile cyst, observation for complications, and providing support for and education of parents. Long-term management is directed toward preventing complications and improving the quality of life for the child and family.

Care of myelomeningocele sac. The infant is usually placed in an Isolette or warmer so that his temperature can be maintained without clothing or covers that might irritate the delicate lesion. When an overhead warmer is used, the dressings over the defect require more frequent moistening because of the dehydrating effect of the dry heat.

Prior to surgical closure the myelomeningocele is prevented from drying by the application of a sterile, moist gauze dressing over the defect. The moistening solution is usually sterile normal saline, although soaks with antibacterial solutions such as silver nitrate or bacitracin are also advocated. Soaks are changed frequently (every 2 to 4 hours), and the sac is closely inspected for leaks, abrasions, irritation, or any signs of infection. Any opening in the sac greatly increases the risk of infection to the central nervous system. The area must be carefully cleansed with hydrogen peroxide solution if it becomes soiled or contaminated. If surgical closure is to be delayed, measures are directed toward facilitating the drying and epithelialization of the sac. In this instance the sac is usually left exposed to the air or covered with a dry gauze or nonadherent dressing.

Special measures to toughen the skin or membrane such as application of benzoin tincture may be indicated, but care must be taken to prevent a dressing from adhering to and damaging the sac. Prolonged use of ointments or moist dressings is usually contraindicated in order to avoid maceration and breakdown of the tissues. A large doughnut-shaped piece of foam rubber or other spongy material can be fashioned to provide a protective shield for the sac. The edges should be left sufficiently wide to allow for adequate anchoring with strips of bandage or paper tape. A sterile drape or gauze cover can form a roof over the opening but should not come in contact with the sac. When surgery is delayed or the defect unrepaired, a ''bubble'' individually molded from lightweight orthopedic splinting material can be prepared and secured around the abdomen, shoulders, and chest with adjustable bands.[13]

Positioning. One of the most difficult, important, and challenging aspects in the early care of the infant with myelomeningocele is positioning. Prior to surgery the infant is kept in the prone position to minimize tension on the sac and the risk of trauma. The prone position also allows for optimal positioning of legs, especially in cases of associated hip dysplasia. Ideally the infant is placed in a low Trendelenburg's position to reduce spinal fluid pressure in the defect with the hips only slightly flexed to reduce tension on the defect. The legs are maintained in abduction with a pad between the knees to counteract hip subluxation, and a small roll is placed under the ankles to maintain a neutral foot position. Sometimes, however, positioning with the head of the bed elevated is desirable and preferred by the neurosurgeon, especially after closure of the defect and where there is increased intracranial pressure from impending hydrocephalus. A variety of aids, including diaper rolls, pads, small sandbags, or specially designed frames and appliances, can be used to maintain the desired position.

The prone position affects other aspects of the infant's care. For example, in this position the infant is more difficult to keep clean, pressure areas are a constant threat, and feeding becomes a problem. The infant's head is turned to one side and tilted upward for bottle-feeding. Until the child is able to lift the head and shoulders from the bed, solid foods are best mixed with formula and fed through a nipple with an enlarged hole. Fortunately most defects are repaired early and the infant can be held for feeding as soon as the surgical site is sufficiently healed to permit handling.

The prone position is maintained after operative closure, although many neurosurgeons allow a side-lying or partial side-lying position unless it aggravates a coexisting hip dysplasia or permits undesirable hip flexion. This offers an opportunity for position changes, which reduces the risk of pressure sores and facilitates feeding. If permitted by the physician, the infant can be held upright against the body as one would normally do with care to avoid pressure on the operative site.

General care. Diapering the infant is contraindicated until the defect has been repaired and healing is well advanced or epithelialization has taken place. The padding beneath the diaper area is changed as needed to keep the skin dry and free of irritation. When urinary retention is present, gentle pressure applied to the suprapubic area will facilitate emptying of the bladder which is still an abdominal organ in early infancy.

Since the bowel sphincter is frequently affected, there is continual passage of stool, often misinterpreted as diarrhea, which is a constant irritant to the skin and a source of infection to the spinal lesion. This provides another rationale for closure before the infant's first feeding while the meconium is still free of organisms.

Areas of sensory and motor impairment are subject to skin breakdown and, therefore, require meticulous care. Placing the infant on a soft foam or fleece pad reduces pressure on the knees and ankles. Periodic cleansing with application of lotion and gentle massage aid circulation. Changing linen is best accomplished by two persons—one changes the linen while the other holds the infant, assuring that the spine is maintained in good alignment without tension in the area of the defect.

Gentle range of motion exercises are sometimes carried out to prevent contractures plus stretching of contractures when indicated. However, these exercises may be restricted to the foot, ankle, and knee joint. Where the hip joints are unstable, stretching against tight hip flexors or adductor muscles, which act much like bowstrings, may aggravate a tendency toward subluxation. In addition the bones of these infants tend to be fragile and subject to fractures.

Since infants with myelomeningocele are unable to be held in the arms and cuddled for some time as unaffected infants are, their need for tactile stimulation is met by fondling, stroking, and other comfort measures. Bright mobiles or other objects can be placed within the infant's view, and other stimulating activities usually provided for infants are appropriate. All infants respond to pleasant sounds.

Observation. The nurse is in a position to aid the physician in determining the extent of neuromuscular involvement. Movement of the extremities or skin response, especially an anal reflex, that might provide additional cues to the degree of motor or sensory status is noted. The head circumference is measured daily (see p. 113), and the fontanels are examined for signs of tension or bulging. The nurse is also alert to early signs of infection, such as elevated temperature (axillary), irritability, lethargy, and nuchal rigidity, and to signs of increased intracranial pressure.

Parent education and long-term supervision. As soon as the parents are emotionally able to cope with the infant's condition, they should become actively involved in his care. They need to learn how to continue at home the care that has been initiated in the hospital—positioning, feeding, the importance of skin care, manual expression of urine, and range-of-motion exercises when appropriate. In cases in which the defect has not been repaired, they are taught to care for the lesion and to observe for signs of complications.

As the child grows and develops it is important that the parents encourage and stimulate the infant to accomplish developmental tasks of his age level within the limits imposed by his disabilities. Upper limb movement can be stimulated early by placing the infant on the floor in a prone position with toys in front of him. Activities that encourage body consciousness, such as rolling over and pulling to a sitting position, should be encouraged at the appropriate times. Creeping and crawling, even in a limited way, help the child to explore his environment. The parents may need help to modify appliances and activities normally expected of a growing child. For example, the paraplegic infant should be encouraged to use arms and shoulders as much as possible. When sitting in an infant seat, stroller, high chair, or feeding table, the infant's hips can be supported, and he should have a footrest and wear hard-soled shoes to maintain the feet in correct alignment and to protect the insensitive feet from trauma. A standing table is helpful for a variety of activities, and it is best for the child to begin supported weight bearing and standing as close as possible to the time expected for normal children.

The long-range planning with and support of parents and child begins in the hospital and extends throughout childhood and even beyond. Long-term care of these children is of uncertain length. Nurses assume an important role as a central member of the health team. As a coordinator the nurse reviews information with the family, takes responsibility for family teaching, and acts as liaison between inpatient and outpatient services. The child will need numerous hospitalizations over the years, and each one will be a source of stress to which the younger child is especially vulnerable.

Habilitation involves not only solving problems of self help and locomotion but also the most distressing problem of incontinence, which threatens the child's social acceptability. Assistance with placement in schools designed to accommodate the deficiencies and special needs of handicapped children helps provide a better initial adjustment to

Summary of nursing care related to management of the infant with myelomeningocele

Goals	Responsibilities
Prevent local infection	Cleanse myelomeningocele carefully with sterile saline or hydrogen peroxide solution as ordered Inspect myelomeningocele for any changes in appearance, for example, abrasions, tears, signs of infection Apply sterile dressings (moisten with sterile solution as ordered [saline, silver nitrate, antibiotic]) Report any change in appearance Position infant to prevent contamination from urine and stool Administer antibiotics as ordered Administer similar care of operative site postoperatively
Prevent local trauma	Handle infant carefully Place infant in prone position or side-lying position, if permitted Apply protective devices Modify routine nursing activities, for example, feeding, making bed, comforting activities
Prevent complications	Observe for signs of hydrocephalus: Measure head circumference daily Check fontanels for tenseness or bulging Note irritability, lethargy, difficulty in feeding, high-pitched cry Observe for signs of meningeal irritation and inflammation, for example, fever, nuchal rigidity, irritability (take vital signs every 2 to 4 hours as ordered)
Prevent urinary tract infection	Avoid contamination with stool Empty bladder periodically (apply gentle, downward pressure to bladder [Credé])
Prevent skin breakdown	Change position frequently Place soft foam or fleece pad under infant Rub skin with lotion periodically to stimulate circulation Maintain meticulous skin cleanliness Apply protective lotion to areas where excoriation is most likely—anal and perineal areas, knees, elbows, ankles, chin, and so on
Prevent or minimize hip and lower extremity deformity	Carry out passive range-of-motion exercises Carry out muscle stretching when indicated Carry out exercises with care to avoid fracturing fragile bones Maintain hips in slight to moderate abduction to prevent dislocation
Maintain hydration and electrolyte balance	Measure intake and output Administer fluids as ordered Observe for signs of dehydration

broader social experiences. It would be difficult to enumerate all that the condition entails in terms of suffering, frustration, family stress, and economic burden. The multiple aspects in care of the child with a handicapping condition are discussed in Chapter 22 and need not be elaborated here nor will the complex problems associated with partial or complete lower extremity paralysis, which are discussed in Chapter 40. These include bowel and bladder control, orthopedic appliances, and the observation and management of complications, especially urinary tract infections and pressure necrosis. (For a summary of nursing care related to management of the infant with myelomeningocele, see the boxed material above.)

HYDROCEPHALUS

Hydrocephalus is a pathologic entity characterized by an excessive accumulation of cerebrospinal fluid (CSF), usually under increased pressure, as a consequence of obstructed

Summary of nursing care related to management of the infant with myelomeningocele—cont'd

Goals	Responsibilities
Maintain warmth	Place infant in Isolette or overhead warmer
Provide nutrition	Provide diet for age Devise feeding techniques to assure adequate intake
Provide tender, loving care	Fondle and caress Speak to child Encourage parents to visit and fondle infant Use an *en face* position as often as possible
Deal with parental anxiety about recurrence in future children	Refer parents to genetic counseling service
Prepare parents for discharge of child	Assess ability of parents to care for infant Teach parents essential aspects of infant's physical care Allow ample time for preparation Encourage questions and expression of feelings Allow for supervised practice in care Refer for evaluation of foster-care placement when parents are unable or unwilling to care for child
Give anticipatory guidance	Give anticipatory guidance regarding development expectations Teach parents to observe for signs of complications Signs of infection Signs of possible shunt failure (when shunt procedure has been performed for hydrocephalus)
Facilitate developmental progress	Help parents plan activities appropriate to developmental level Assist with nursery school and educational placement
Support parents	Provide or arrange for ongoing contact with family Refer to parent groups
Coordinate services	Plan for home visits where needed Maintain contact with family Make appointments for follow-up care Make referrals to special agencies as needed Act as liaison between inpatient and outpatient services

drainage that produces passive dilatation of the ventricles. The variations in manifestations depend primarily on the site of obstruction and the age at which obstruction develops.

Etiology and pathophysiology

In order to improve the condition, an understanding of the dynamics of cerebrospinal fluid and the relationship between the various structures that make up the ventricular and subarachnoid spaces is necessary (Fig. 11-4). The primary site of cerebrospinal fluid formation is believed to be the choroid plexi of the ventricles. It flows from the lateral ventricles through the *foramen of Monro* to the third ventricle, where it combines with fluid secreted by the third ventricle. From there it flows through the *aqueduct of Sylvius* into the fourth ventricle where more fluid is formed; it then leaves the fourth ventricle by way of the lateral *foramen of Luschka* and the midline *foramen of Magendie* into the *cis-*

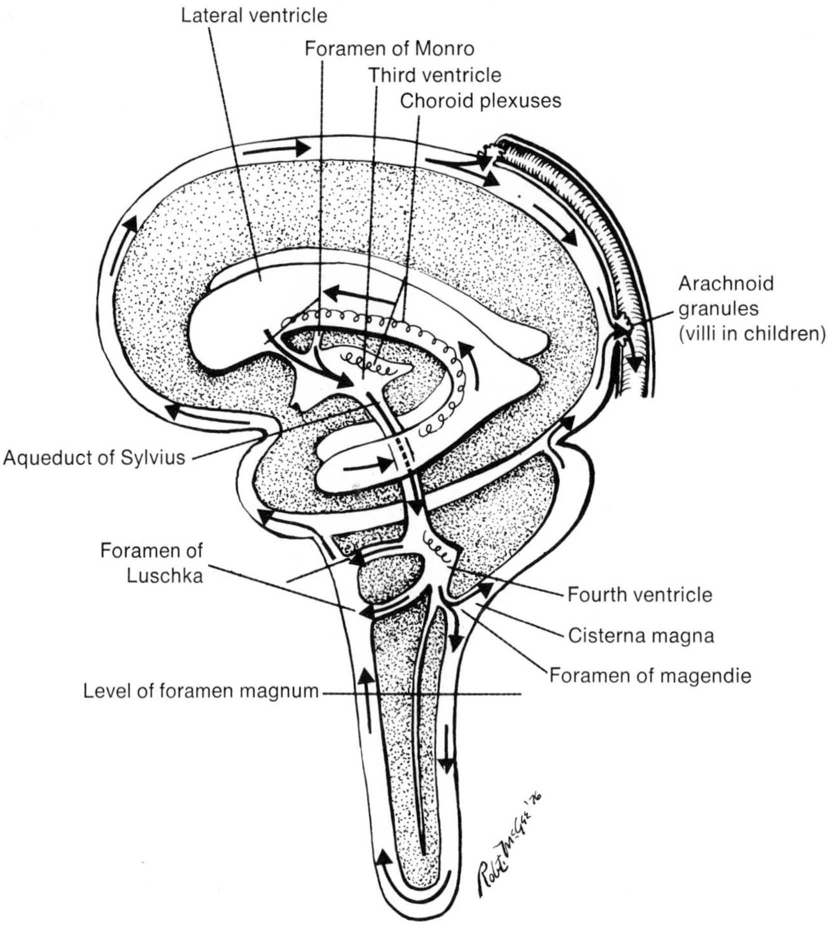

Fig. 11-4. Cerebrospinal fluid circulation.

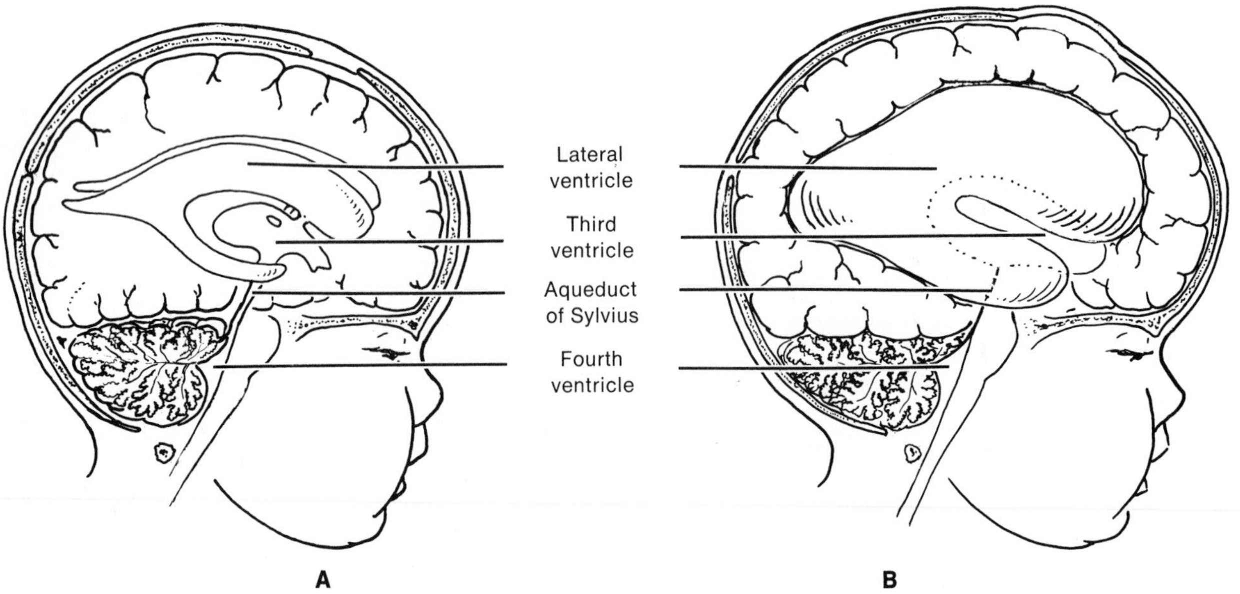

Fig. 11-5. Hydrocephalus: a block in the flow of cerebrospinal fluid. **A,** Patent cerebrospinal fluid circulation. **B,** Enlarged lateral and third ventricles caused by obstruction of circulation—stenosis of the aqueduct of Sylvius.

terna magna. From there it flows to the cerebral and cerebellar subarachnoid spaces, although the precise mechanism of its absorption is not entirely clear. There is evidence to indicate that a large portion is absorbed through the arachnoid villi, but the sinuses, veins, brain substance, and dura also participate in absorption. Hydrocephalus is almost always a result of interference with the circulation or absorption of cerebrospinal fluid.

A block in the cerebrospinal fluid pathway from the foramen of Monro to the arachnoid villi of the subarachnoid space will cause an increased amount of cerebrospinal fluid under increased pressure. Consequently the ventricles become dilated and the brain substance is compressed against the surrounding rigid bony cranium. When this occurs prior to fusion of the cranial sutures, it produces enlargement of the skull as well as dilatation of the ventricles.

Pathophysiology. The causes of hydrocephalus can be classified into three general categories:

1. Excess secretion: caused by a choroid plexus papilloma, a tumor composed of a large aggregate of choroidal fronds structurally similar to the choroid plexus that produces large quantities of cerebrospinal fluid.
2. Noncommunicating (intraventricular): The circulation of cerebrospinal fluid is blocked somewhere within the ventricular system, preventing its flow to the subarachnoid spaces. This is sometimes referred to as obstructive hydrocephalus or by the older term "internal hydrocephalus" (Fig. 11-5).
3. Communicating (extraventricular): No interference to the flow of cerebrospinal fluid within the ventricular system. Fluid pathways are open so that fluid moves freely into the spinal subarachnoid space but is not absorbed from the cerebral subarachnoid space.

Most cases of noncommunicating hydrocephalus are a result of developmental malformations and, although the defect usually becomes apparent in early infancy, it may become evident at any time from the prenatal period to late childhood or early adulthood. Other causes include neoplasms, infections, and trauma. An obstruction to the normal flow can occur at any point in the cerebrospinal fluid pathway to produce increased pressure and dilatation of the pathways proximal to the site of obstruction. Table 11-1 describes the most frequent sites of obstruction and the consequences.

During infancy hydrocephalus is usually a major developmental defect. For example, Arnold-Chiari malformations, aqueduct stenosis, and aqueduct gliosis account for most cases of hydrocephalus from birth to 2 years of age. Hydrocephalus is so often associated with myelomeningocele that all such infants should be observed for its development. In the remainder of cases there is a history of intrauterine infection, perinatal hemorrhage (anoxic or traumatic), and neonatal meningoencephalitis (bacterial or viral). In older children hydrocephalus is most often the result of space-occupying lesions, preexisting developmental defects (aqueduct stenosis, Arnold-Chiari malformations), intracranial infections, or hemorrhage.

Diagnostic evaluation

The two factors that influence the clinical picture in hydrocephalus are the time of onset and preexisting structural lesions. In infancy prior to closure of the cranial sutures, head enlargement is the predominant sign of hydrocephalus, whereas in older infants and children the lesions responsible for hydrocephalus produce other neurologic signs through pressure on adjacent structures before causing cerebrospinal fluid obstruction.

In infants the head grows at an abnormal rate, although the first signs may be bulging fontanels without head enlargement (Fig. 11-6). With the increase in intracranial volume the bones of the skull become thin and the sutures become palpably separated to produce the "cracked-pot" sound (Macewen's sign) on percussion of the skull. The anterior fontanel is tense, often bulging, and nonpulsatile. Scalp veins are dilated and markedly so when the infant cries. There may be frontal enlargement or "bossing" with depressed eyes and a "setting-sun" sign in which the sclera are visible above the iris because of pressure on a thinned orbital roof or the third ventricle on the tectum of mesencephalon. Typical behaviors include irritability, opisthotonos (often extreme), and lower extremity spasticity. Early infantile nonreflex acts may persist, and normally expected responses fail to appear, indicating failure in the development of normal cortical inhibition.

If hydrocephalus is allowed to progress, development of lower brain stem functions is disrupted as manifested by difficulty in sucking and feeding and a shrill, brief, and high-pitched cry. Eventually the skull becomes enormous and the cortex is destroyed. If the hydrocephalus is rapidly progressive, the infant may display emesis, somnolence, seizures, and cardiopulmonary embarrassment. Severely affected infants usually do not survive the neonatal period.

The signs and symptoms in early to late childhood are caused by increased intracranial pressure, and specific manifestations are related to the focal lesion. Most commonly resulting from posterior fossa neoplasms and aqueduct stenosis, the clinical manifestations are primarily those associated with space-occupying lesions, that is, headache on awakening with improvement following emesis or upright posture, papilledema, strabismus, and extrapyramidal tract signs such as ataxia (see p. 1024). In one of the congenital defects with later onset, the Dandy-Walker syndrome, characteristic manifestations are bulging occiput, nystagmus, ataxia, and cranial nerve deficits.

Diagnostic studies. In infancy the diagnosis of hydrocephalus is based on head circumference that crosses one or more grid lines on the measurement chart within a period of 2 to 4 weeks and on associated neurologic signs that are present and progressive. However, other diagnostic studies are needed to localize the site of cerebrospinal fluid obstruction. Routine daily head circumference measurements are carried out in infants with myelomeningocele and intracranial infections. In evaluation of a premature infant, spe-

Table 11-1. Sites of obstruction in hydrocephalus

Site of obstruction	Type	Etiology	Comment
Noncommunicating hydrocephalus			
Aqueduct of Sylvius	Stenosis or atresia	Congenital	Insidious onset of symptoms from birth to adulthood
		X-linked recessive inheritance in a small number	
	Gliosis	Postinflammatory, usually secondary to a perinatal infection or hemorrhage	
		Prenatal maternal infection	Toxoplasmosis
	Obstructive	Tumors of the third ventricle or midbrain	Aqueduct stenosis accounts for 20% of hydrocephalus
		Ependymitis from maternal toxoplasmosis	
		Congenital aneurysm of the vein of Galen	
Fourth ventricle and foramen magnum	Obstruction of foramen magnum	Chiari malformations	Fourth ventricle obstruction accounts for 50% of all hydrocephalus in children, with 40% resulting from Chiari defects
		Type I	A neural tube defect with herniation of the lower brain stem and cerebellum through the foramen magnum; may be asymptomatic in childhood
		Type II (Arnold-Chiari malformation)	Same as for Type I but more severe, with greater downward displacement and fixed attachment of spinal cord at site of myelomeningocele
	Absence or occlusion of the outlets of the fourth ventricle	Congenital (Dandy-Walker syndrome)	Obstruction of foramina of Luschka and Magendie, causing cystic enlargement of the ventricle
		Tumors of the posterior fossa	Medulloblastoma, for example
		Less often, subdural hematoma, bacterial or granulomatous meningitis	Space-occupying lesions cause pressure on surrounding tissues, obstructing cerebrospinal fluid flow
Communicating hydrocephalus			
Arachnoid villi and cisterna magna	Obstruction by thick arachnoid membrane or meninges	Subarachnoid hemorrhage	Secondary to hypoxia in premature infants Trauma in full-term infants
		Meningitis	Bacterial or granulomatous In acute phase, by clumping of purulent fluid in drainage channels In chronic phase, by organization of blood and exudate that results in fibrosis of the subarachnoid spaces
		Prenatal maternal infections	Toxoplasmosis, cytomegalic inclusion disease (CID), mumps
		Meningeal malignancy	Caused by leukemia or lymphoma
		Arachnoid cyst	Located in basal cystern or (uncommon) over cerebral cortex
		Tuberculosis, fungal or parasitic infection	More common in children age 2 to 10 years

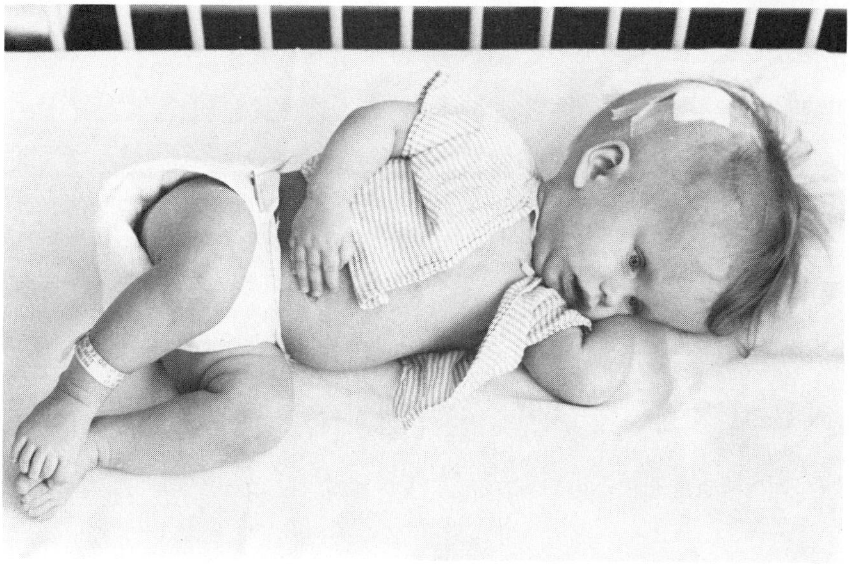

Fig. 11-6. Child with enlarged head caused by hydrocephalus.

cially adapted head circumference charts are consulted to distinguish abnormal head growth from rapid head growth that takes place normally.

Problems in differential diagnosis are related to the child whose head circumference is greater than the ninety-seventh percentile but whose head growth parallels the normal growth curve. In these children air encephalography is contraindicated as an early diagnostic tool since partially or completely arrested hydrocephalus may be reactivated by these procedures. The diagnostic tool of choice is computerized axial tomography. The child is sedated prior to the test since he must remain absolutely still for an accurate picture. Diagnostic evaluation of children who have symptoms of hydrocephalus after infancy is similar to that employed in those with suspected intracranial tumor. The most frequently employed diagnostic, laboratory, and x-ray examinations are outlined in Table 11-2.

Medical management

The treatment of hydrocephalus is almost exclusively surgical. Medical therapy directed toward reduction of the production of cerebrospinal fluid has proved to be ineffective in all but a few selected cases that involve overproduction. In these instances acetazolamide (Diamox) has been only modestly successful in reestablishing equilibrium between cerebrospinal fluid production and absorption.

Surgical treatment. Improved techniques have established surgical treatment as the therapy of choice in almost all cases of hydrocephalus. The general principles underlying surgical intervention are[10]:

1. Correction of cerebrospinal fluid obstruction—direct removal of the obstruction, for example, resection of neoplasm, cyst, or hematoma
2. Reduction of cerebrospinal fluid production—endoscopic choroid plexus extirpation (plexectomy or electric coagulation) or third or fourth ventriculostomy
3. Ventricular bypass into a normal intracranial channel, for example, shunting of cerebrospinal fluid from the lateral ventricle to the cisterna magna (Torkildsen procedure) in noncommunicating hydrocephalus
4. Ventricular bypass into an extracranial compartment, for example, ventriculoatrial or ventriculoperitoneal shunts in either noncommunicating or communicating hydrocephalus

Generally the ventricular bypass procedure is used in older children with noncommunicating hydrocephalus caused by aqueduct stenosis or posterior fossa masses (for example, medulloblastoma). Technical difficulties preclude its use in infants since these spaces are poorly developed in the infant. At present the most widely used procedure and the treatment of choice for communicating hydrocephalus and infantile noncommunicating hydrocephalus is drainage of the fluid from a lateral ventricle into an extracranial compartment (the most common being the right atrium and peritoneum) by way of an artificial passage, or shunt (Fig. 11-7, *A* and *B*). Shunts from the lateral ventricle are accomplished with plastic tubing and one-way valves. Slit one-way valves are designed to open at a predetermined intraventricular pressure and close when the pressure falls below that level. Thus back flow of blood or other secretions is prevented. Two types of valves are most widely used at present. The Holter valve consists of two fish-mouth stainless steel check valves connected by a short length of silicone tubing. The Pudenz-Heyer-Schulte valve is a plastic bubble pump with the distal end connected to a slit valve. When the latter is used it can be "pumped" for patency and to clear partial obstructions. In both mechanisms the initial success rate is

Table 11-2. Diagnostic tests used in hydrocephalus

Test	Description	Comments
Transillumination	Flashlight with a rubber adapter is held snugly against the infant's head in a totally darkened room	Normally in a full-term infant, a halo of light extends 1 to 2 cm from rim of light source; varying degrees of localized glowing may be seen in abnormal fluid accumulation in various areas of the head
Cerebrospinal fluid examination	Ventricular or spinal tap (dangers attending the spinal puncture should be weighed against value of information gained)	Elevated cerebrospinal fluid protein level in choroid plexus papilloma and occasionally after central nervous system infection or hemorrhage Decreased cerebrospinal fluid glucose level in postinfectious hydrocephalus or meningeal invasion of tumor Increased 5-dehydroxyindoleacetic acid in obstructive hydrocephalus Tumor cells may appear in cerebrospinal fluid
Radiography	Anteroposterior and lateral skull films	Indicates thinning of bones with separation of sutures and widening of fontanels; disproportionately large cranium
Computerized axial tomography	Pinpoint x-ray beam is directed on a horizontal or vertical plane to provide a series of longitudinal "cuts" that are fed into the computer, assembled in an image displayed on a videoscreen, and transferred to a permanent record	Visualizes horizontal or vertical cross section of brain at any axis, which distinguishes the density of various brain tissues
Air encephalography	X-ray visualization of ventricular system and subarachnoid spaces after injection of air or oxygen into the cerebrospinal fluid pathways	Defines site of obstruction; sufficient air is introduced to visualize entire cerebrospinal fluid space May cause exacerbation of hydrocephalus
Pneumoencephalography	Air or oxygen is injected into the lumbar subarachnoid space	Used only where intracranial pressure is normal or only slightly elevated; preferred procedure for older children
Ventriculography	Air or oxygen is injected into the lateral ventricle through the anterior fontanel in infants and through a burr hole in older children	Preferred study in young infant and in presence of significantly increased intracranial pressure Should include radiographs taken with child's head in an inverted position to visualize aqueduct, fourth ventricle, and cisterna magna
Dye	Contrast medium is introduced into the lateral ventricles via ventricular puncture	Dye appears in spinal fluid in 2 to 12 minutes in communicating hydrocephalus
Brain scan	Isotope scan for gamma emission follows injection of radioiodinated human serum albumin into the lumbar or cisternal subarachnoid space	Visualizes cerebrospinal fluid pathways In normal children or noncommunicating hydrocephalus there is no retrograde filling of the ventricles
Arteriography	Visualization of cerebral blood vessels by percutaneous injection of radiopaque dyes into the carotid arteries (or by reflux from cannulization of brachial or femoral arteries)	Tumors are localized by distortion of normal vascular pattern Requires general anesthesia
Echoencephalography	Reflection of ultrasound from reflecting surfaces	May show ventricular dilatation Detects major shifts of midline structures

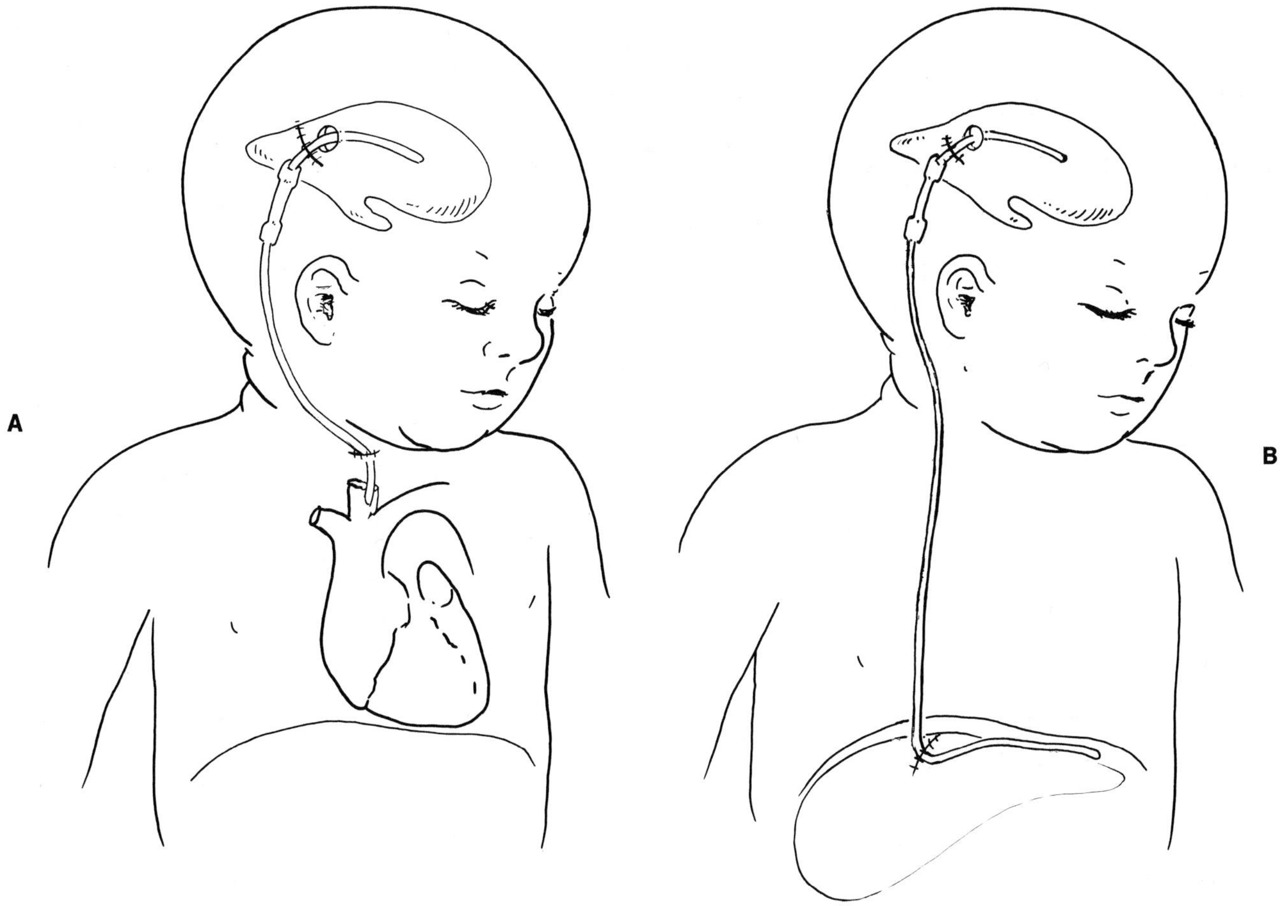

Fig. 11-7. A, Ventriculoarterial shunt; **B,** ventriculoperitoneal shunt.

relatively high; however, they are associated with complications that interfere with continued shunt function or that threaten the life of the child. All are subject to mechanical difficulties, such as kinking, plugging, or separation of the tubing, and to bacterial infection, the most common serious complication. In case of infection, massive doses of antibiotics are administered by the intravenous route or directly into the ventricles. A persistent infection necessitates removal of the shunt until the infection is controlled. Table 11-3 outlines the shunt procedures employed to reduce increased intracranial pressure.

Prognosis. Untreated, hydrocephalus has a 50% to 60% mortality rate to the disorder or intercurrent illnesses. Of the survivors, very few (less than 10%) are intellectually normal and a large majority have major physical and/or disabling neurologic handicaps such as ataxia, spastic diplegia, poor fine motor coordination, and perceptual deficits. Spontaneous arrest occurs occasionally in approximately 40% of these with near-normal intelligence.

The prognosis of children with treated hydrocephalus depends largely on the cause of the condition. Malignant tumors have a high mortality rate regardless of other complicating factors.

Surgically treated hydrocephalus with continued neurosurgical and medical management has a survival rate of about 80% with the highest incidence of mortality occurring within the first year of treatment. Of the surviving children approximately one third are both intellectually and neurologically normal and one half have neurologic disabilities. Hydrocephalus complicating a myelomeningocele carries an even less favorable prognosis. In some children irreversible damage may have been produced by the hydrocephalus or from the original infection; in addition there are sometimes coincidental cerebral defects. Generally noninfective hydrocephalus appears to carry the best prognosis.

Nursing considerations

Preoperatively the infant with diagnosed or suspected hydrocephalus is observed carefully for signs of increasing intracranial pressure. In infants the head is measured daily at the point of largest measurement—the occipitofrontal circumference (OFC). Ideally the measurement should be

Table 11-3. Extracranial shunt procedures

Cerebrospinal fluid reservoir	Extracranial compartment	Comments	Complications
Lateral ventricle	Right atrium via internal jugular vein	Most widely used shunt Requires repeated revision with growth	Endocardial contusions and clotting, resulting in bacterial endocarditis, bacteremia, and ventriculitis Shunt infection more common
Lateral ventricle	Peritoneum	Requires revision with growth May or may not use one-way valve	Less serious complications but higher incidence of obstruction than ventriculoatrial shunt
Lateral ventricle or lumbar subarachnoid space	Ureter and drained into urinary bladder	Requires nephrectomy Cerebrospinal fluid not reabsorbed into the body Seldom-used procedures—used only in older children and when other shunts fail	Loss of electrolytes to cause hyponatremic-hypochloremic dehydration
Lateral ventricle	Pleural cavity	May require revision with age	May develop serious hydrothorax, requiring thoracentesis or removal of shunt
Lumbar subarachnoid space	Peritoneum or pleural cavity	Can be used only with communicating hydrocephalus	
Lateral ventricle	Mastoid cells to drain via eustachian tube into posterior pharynx	Seldom used	High risk of infection and meningitis

taken by the same person to reduce the likelihood of wide discrepancies. Fontanels and suture lines are gently palpated for size, signs of bulging, tenseness, and separation. However, an infant with normal intracranial pressure will display bulging under certain circumstances such as straining or crying; therefore, such accompanying behavior should be noted. Irritability, lethargy, or seizure activity as well as altered vital signs and feeding behavior may indicate advancing pathology.

General nursing care of the infant with hydrocephalus may present special problems. Maintaining adequate nutrition often requires flexible feeding schedules to accommodate diagnostic procedures since feeding before or after handling can precipitate an episode of vomiting. Small feedings at more frequent intervals are frequently better tolerated than are larger ones spaced farther apart. These infants are often difficult to feed and require extra time and innovation. Care must be exercised to see that the large head is well supported when the infant is fed or moved to prevent extra strain on the infant's neck, and measures must be taken to prevent development of pressure areas. As the hydrocephaly progresses, untreated children become increasingly helpless and prone to the multiple problems of immobility, for example, pressure sores, contracture deformities, and so on. Not infrequently infants with irreversible brain damage or with severe developmental defects such as hydranencephaly, in which both cerebral hemispheres fail to develop and are replaced with a membranous sac filled with cerebrospinal fluid, are placed in long-term institutions specially designed for care of these infants.

In addition to measuring head circumference and observation of neurologic signs, the nurse is responsible for preparation of the child for diagnostic tests and assisting the physician with procedures such as a ventricular tap, which is often performed to relieve excessive pressure during the preoperative period, and cerebrospinal fluid examination.

Postoperative care. In addition to routine postoperative care and observation, the infant or child is positioned on the unoperated side to prevent pressure on the shunt valve with care to avoid pressure areas and is kept flat to help avert complications resulting from too rapid reduction of intracranial fluid. When the ventricular size is reduced too rapidly, the cerebral cortex may pull away from the dura and tear the small interlacing veins, producing a subdural hematoma. This is not a problem in children with elective shunt revision since their intraventricular size and pressure have been normal.[1] Sedation is avoided since the level of consciousness is an important observation.

Observation for signs of increased intracranial pressure, which indicate obstruction of the shunt, is continued. Sometimes the valve can be pumped several times to relieve the pressure and the procedure is repeated routinely a pre-

Summary of nursing care of the child with hydrocephalus

Goals	Responsibilities
Assess hydrocephalus	Assist with diagnostic evaluation Measure head circumference daily Observe for signs of increased intracranial pressure Prepare for procedures Assist with diagnostic procedures when appropriate, for example, ventricular tap, transillumination
Prevent pressure sore on head	Administer skin care and general hygiene measures Change position every 2 hours
Prevent postoperative complications	Position flat to prevent subdural hematoma Turn every 2 hours to prevent hypostatic pneumonia Position on unoperated side Observe for signs of infection or increased intracranial pressure Maintain care of and observe shunt and operative sites Observe and evaluate state of consciousness
Maintain nutrition and hydration	Institute flexible feeding schedule Give small, frequent feedings
Administer comfort measures	Administer general hygiene Provide tactile stimulation Encourage parental involvement in care
Reduce parental anxiety	Support parents Explain procedures and medical plan Answer questions Give anticipatory guidance
Guide posthospital care	Refer to appropriate agencies (public health, crippled children's services, social service) If parents are unable or unwilling to care for child, arrange placement in long-term care facility or refer to social service for foster home care

scribed number of times every hour or two as ordered. If these measures are unsuccessful, the shunt may require replacement.

Since infection is the greatest hazard of the postoperative period, nurses are continually on the alert for the usual manifestations of cerebrospinal fluid infection, which may include elevated vital signs, poor feeding, vomiting, decreased responsiveness, and seizure activity. There may be signs of local inflammation at the operative sites and along the shunt tract. Antibiotics are administered by the intravenous route as ordered, and the nurse may also need to assist the physician with intraventricular instillation.

Parental support. Helping parents cope with the hydrocephalic child or the child with a functioning shunt is an important nursing responsibility. Specific needs and concerns of parents during periods of hospitalization are related to the reason for the child's hospitalization (that is, shunt revision, infection, diagnosis) and the diagnostic and/or surgical procedures to which the child must be submitted. Often parents have very little understanding of anatomy; therefore, they need further exploration and reinforcement of information that was given to them by the physician and neurosurgeon as well as information about what they can expect. They are especially frightened of any procedure that involves the brain, and the fear of retardation or brain damage is very real and pervasive. Nurses can do much to allay their anxiety with explanations of the rationale underlying the various nursing and medical activities such as positioning or testing and by simply being available and willing to listen to their concerns.

To prepare for the child's discharge and home care, the parents are instructed how to recognize signs that indicate shunt malfunction or infection and how to pump the shunt, if necessary. Active children may have accidents, such as a fall, that can damage the shunt, and the tubing may pull out of the distal insertion site or become disconnected during normal growth. Anticipatory guidance will prepare parents for such eventualities and help them to avoid being overprotective of the child. There need be few restrictions placed on the child's activities (mainly contact sports), and he should be encouraged to live as would any child of the same age and abilities. Parents need support and encouragement in coping with the child and problems he may encounter in relationships with peers and others. Reactions of other children when the child has a noticeably enlarged head or requires shaving at the times of revision are stress situations for both child and parents (see Chapter 22 for problems and coping of the handicapped child). (For a summary of nursing care of the child with hydrocephalus, see the boxed material on p. 385.)

Skeletal defects

The types and variations of deformity in developmental skeletal defects are numerous and display an equally diverse spectrum of physical disability. Some skeletal deformities constitute one or more of the manifestations associated with a syndrome, for example, the short extremities of the various forms of dwarfism, the long, thin extremities and sternal deformities of arachnodactyly (Marfan's syndrome), and somatic defects in chromosomal aberrations. Many are isolated defects with hereditary (clawhand, polydactyly), environmental (thalidomide phocomelia or amelia), or multifactorial (congenital hip dysplasia) etiology. This discussion is limited to those defects in development that are most common, amenable to therapy, and involve nurses to a considerable extent. Less common defects are listed in Table 11-4.

CONGENITAL HIP DYSPLASIA

The broad term "congenital hip dysplasia" is applied to malformations of the hip with various degrees of deformity that are present at birth. Three degrees of congenital dysplasia can be identified (Fig. 11-8):

acetabular dysplasia (or preluxation) the mildest form in which there is neither subluxation nor dislocation. The dysplasia reflects an apparent delay in acetabular development evidenced by osseous hypoplasia of the acetabular roof that is oblique and shallow although the cartilaginous roof is comparatively intact. The femoral head remains in the acetabulum.

subluxation accounts for the largest percentage of congenital hip dysplasias. Subluxation implies incomplete dislocation or dislocatable hip and is sometimes regarded as an intermediate stage in the development from primary dysplasia to complete dislocation. The femoral head remains in contact with the acetabulum, but a stretched capsule and ligamentum teres cause the head of the femur to be partially displaced. Pressure on the cartilaginous roof inhibits ossification and produces a flattening of the socket.

dislocation the femoral head loses contact with the acetabulum and is displaced posteriorly and superiorly over the fibrocartilaginous rim. The ligamentum teres is elongated and taut.

Etiology and pathophysiology

The cause of hip dysplasia, one of the most common congenital defects, is unknown. The incidence is about one in 500 to 1000 births, and it occurs more frequently in females than in males (7:1). The disorder occurs twenty-five to thirty times more often in first-degree relatives than in the general population, and the concordance in monozygotic twins is 40% but only 3% in dizygotic twins, which suggests that genetic factors play a role in the etiology. One fourth of cases involve both hips, and when only one hip is involved the left hip is affected three times more often than the right. Congenital hip dysplasia is frequently associated with other conditions, such as spina bifida.

There appear to be intrauterine, racial, and cultural factors associated with congenital hip disorders. The disorder is virtually unknown in the Far East and relatively common among Navajo Indians and Canadian Eskimos. There appears to be a striking relationship between the development of dislocation and methods of handling infants. Among the cultures with the highest incidence of dislocation, newly born infants are tightly wrapped in blankets or other swaddling material or are strapped to cradle boards. In cultures where mothers traditionally carry infants on their backs or hips in the widely abducted straddle position, the incidence is lowest.

Prenatal factors that are considered to influence development of hip abnormalities are maternal hormone secretion and mechanical factors of intrauterine posture. Toward the end of pregnancy there is increased maternal pelvic laxity mediated by maternal hormone secretion (principally estrogen). All joints have been noted to be more lax in the newborn period, and the increased incidence of hip dislocation in females may be explained by their greater reactivity to the maternal hormones. Also a reliable association exists between a higher incidence of congenital hip deformities and breech presentations and cesarean section (often necessitated by abnormal intrauterine position). The position of the legs in frank breech position, that is, with the hips acutely flexed and knees extended, is an important factor in the etiology of hip dislocation. The excess of firstborn

Table 11-4. Congenital defects involving the skeleton

Disorder	Description	Therapy
Achondroplasia	Inherited (autosomal dominant) Defect in ossification at the epiphyseal plate, resulting in very short limbs, large head, and lordosis	None
Osteogenesis imperfecta	Inherited (autosomal dominant, autosomal recessive) Characterized by brittle, fragile, and easily fractured bones Intrauterine fractures may produce congenital deformities	Reduction of fractures Careful handling of extremities
Pes planus (flatfoot)	Normal finding in infancy May be result of muscular weakness in older child	Rarely indicated Wedge on inner side of heel and sole for persistent or severe cases
Metatarsus varus	Often confused with talipes varus	Passive exercises carried out by care giver Corrective shoes If persistent, may require casting
Supernumerary digits (polydactyly)	Excessive number of fingers, toes, or both; usually inherited (autosomal dominant)	No treatment, or amputation of extra digits to improve function or for cosmetic reasons
Genu varum (bowleg)	May be congenital, result of rickets, or caused by osteochondrosis of proximal tibial epiphysis	Corrective splinting Osteotomy in severe or neglected cases
Genu recurvatum (back knee)	Congenital, result of prenatal developmental defect or abnormal intrauterine position Developmental, result of postnatal trauma or infection	Repeated corrective casting Corrective shoes Exercises
Klippel-Feil syndrome	Absence of one or more cervical vertebrae and two or more fused together Neck short and limited in motion Sometimes kyphosis and scoliosis	Rarely indicated Scapula brought down and fixed if marked deformity or loss of function Bracing of spinal deformities
Arachnodactyly (Marfan's syndrome)	Inherited (autosomal dominant) Abnormal length of fingers, toes, and extremities; hypermobility of joints; defects of spine and chest (pigeon breast); other associated abnormalities	Supportive measures
Congenital spine deformities	Kyphosis, scoliosis, lordosis, or a combination of these	Prevention of progression of defect with growth Casting and/or bracing Operative stabilization of affected vertebra
Arthrogryposis multiplex congenita	Incomplete fibrous ankylosis of many or all joints (except spine and jaw) associated with hypoplasia of attached muscles Contracture deformities—some extension, others flexion	Bracing, splinting, corrective surgery, and rehabilitation efforts

children may be related to this factor since the breech position in first deliveries is nearly always a frank breech.

Diagnostic evaluation

The diagnosis of congenital hip dysplasia should be made in the newborn period if possible since treatment initiated before 2 months of age achieves the highest rate of success. In the newborn period dysplasia usually appears as hip joint laxity rather than as outright dislocation. Subluxation and the tendency to dislocate can be demonstrated by Ortolani's manipulation or Barlow's modification of the maneuver. With the infant in the supine position and the legs facing the examiner, the hips are flexed to a right angle and the knees are flexed. The examiner places the middle finger of each hand over the greater trochanter and the thumbs on the inner side of the thigh at a point opposite the lesser trochanter. The knees are carried to midabduction and each hip joint in turn is submitted first to forward pressure exerted behind the trochanter and second to backward pressure exerted from the thumbs in front as the opposite joint is held steady. If the femoral head can be felt to slip forward into the acetabulum on pressure from behind, it

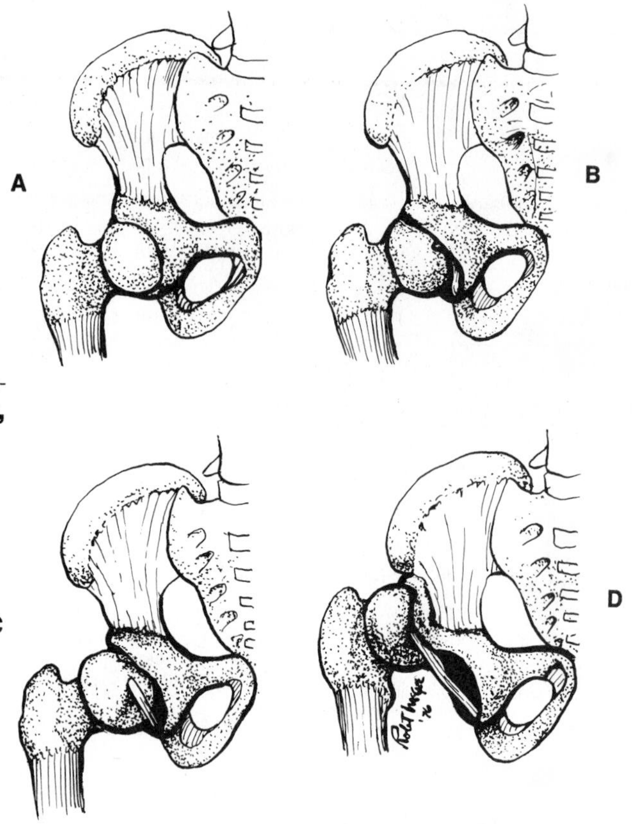

Fig. 11-8. Configuration and relationship of structure in congenital hip deformities. **A,** Normal; **B,** dysplasia; **C,** subluxation; **D,** dislocation.

has been dislocated (Ortolani's sign). If, on pressure from the front, the femoral head is felt to slip out over the posterior lip of the acetabulum and immediately slips back in place when pressure is released, the hip is said to be dislocatable or "unstable" (Barlow's modification). Sometimes an audible click can be heard on exit or entry of the femur out of or into the acetabulum.

The infant with hip dislocation manifests other physical signs such as restricted abduction of the affected hip, shortening of the limb on the affected side (Allis's sign), asymmetric thigh and gluteal folds, and broadening of the perineum (in bilateral dislocation) (Fig. 11-9). Sometimes weight bearing will precipitate a transition from subluxation to dislocation in unrecognized cases. Often the disorder is not apparent at birth.

In the older infant and child the affected leg will be shorter than the other with telescoping or piston mobility, that is, the head of the femur can be felt to move up and down in the buttock when the extended thigh is pushed first toward the child's head and then pulled distally. Instability of the hip on weight bearing delays walking and produces a characteristic limp. When the child stands first on one foot and then on the other (holding onto a chair, rail, or someone's hands) bearing weight on the affected hip, the pelvis tilts downward on the normal side instead of upward as it would with normal stability (Trendelenburg's sign). In both unilateral and bilateral dislocations the greater trochanter is prominent and appears above a line from the anterior superior iliac spine to the tuberosity of the ischium. The child with bilateral dislocations has marked lordosis and a peculiar waddling gait.

In older infants and children x-ray examination is useful in confirming the diagnosis. An upward slope in the roof of the acetabulum (the acetabular angle) greater than 40 degrees with upward and outward displacement of the femoral head is a frequent finding in older children. Radiographic examination in early infancy is not reliable. The bones are largely cartilaginous and difficult to visualize.

Medical management

Treatment is begun as soon as the condition is recognized since early intervention is more favorable to the restoration of normal bony architecture and function. The longer treatment is delayed, the more severe the deformity, the more difficult the treatment, and the less favorable the prognosis. The treatment varies with the age of the child and the extent of the dysplasia.

Infancy. In the child less than 1 year of age a dislocated hip securely held in full abduction is usually sufficient to produce a stable joint. In many instances where the defect

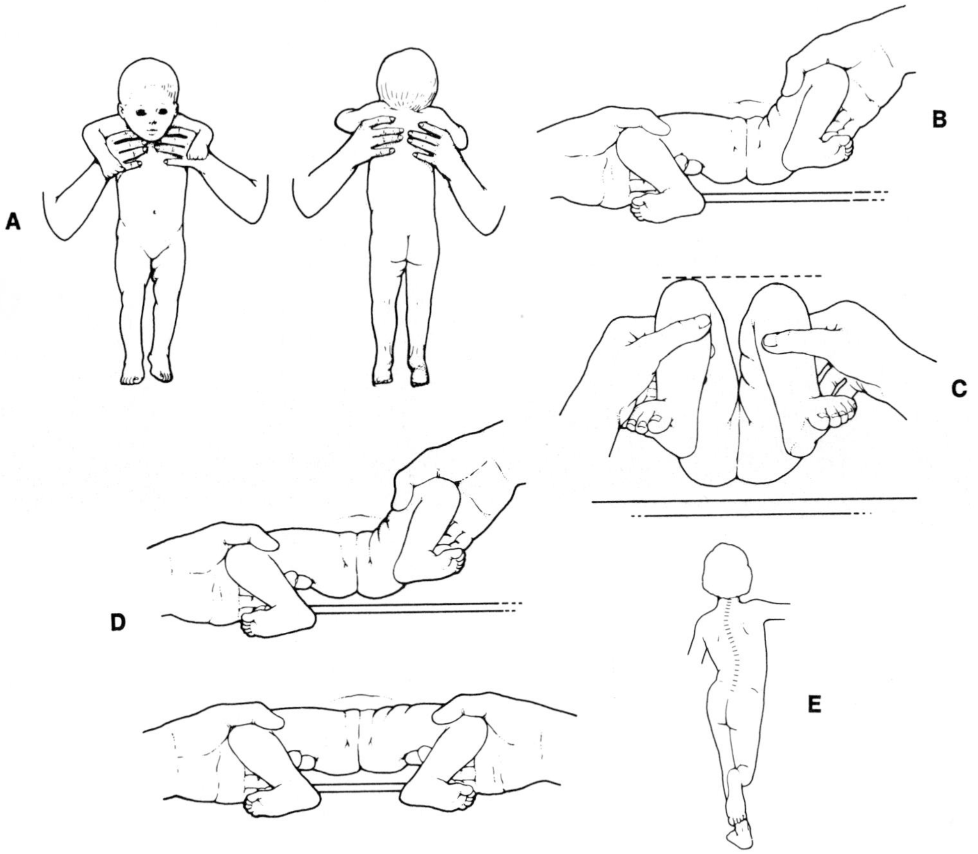

Fig. 11-9. Signs of congenital dislocation of the hip. **A,** Asymmetry of gluteal and thigh folds. **B,** Limited hip abduction, as seen in flexion. **C,** Apparent shortening of the femur, as indicated by the level of the knees in flexion. **D,** Ortolani click if infant is under 4 weeks of age. **E,** Positive Trendelenburg sign or gait if child is weight bearing. (From Hilt, N. E., and Schmitt, E. W., Jr.: Pediatric orthopedic nursing, St. Louis, 1975, The C. V. Mosby Co., p. 31.)

is recognized within the first week of life, simple abduction by way of double diapering is sufficient to create secure positioning that will produce a stable joint and prevent dislocation. For infants beyond the neonatal period an abduction device, which may be constructed from plastic, metal, leather, or a soft pillow (Frejka pillow splint), is worn that can be removed for bathing (Fig. 11-10). When adduction contracture is present, the hips are slowly and gently stretched to full abduction, after which wide abduction is maintained until stability is attained. This is accomplished by devices that can be adjusted as the amount of abduction is gradually increased. The device is worn anywhere from days (in the newborn) to several weeks.

When there is difficulty in maintaining stable reduction, a plaster hip spica cast is applied and changed periodically to accommodate the child's growth. After 3 to 6 months, sufficient stability is acquired to allow transfer to a removable protective abduction brace. The duration of treatment depends on development of the acetabulum but is usually accomplished within the first year.

Toddler. In this age-group the dislocation is not recognized until the child begins to walk, when attendant shortening of the limb and contractures of hip adductor and flexor muscles becomes apparent. Gradual reduction by traction is followed by plaster cast immobilization, which is maintained until x-ray examination confirms a stable joint. Often soft tissue may obstruct and complicate reduction and subsequent joint development. In this case open reduction is performed to remove the obstruction with postoperative spica cast immobilization and, after 4 to 6 months, replacement with an abduction splint.

Older child. Correction of the hip deformity in the older child is inherently more difficult than in the preceding age-groups since secondary adaptive changes complicate the condition. Operative reduction, which may involve preoperative traction, tenotomy of contracted muscles, and

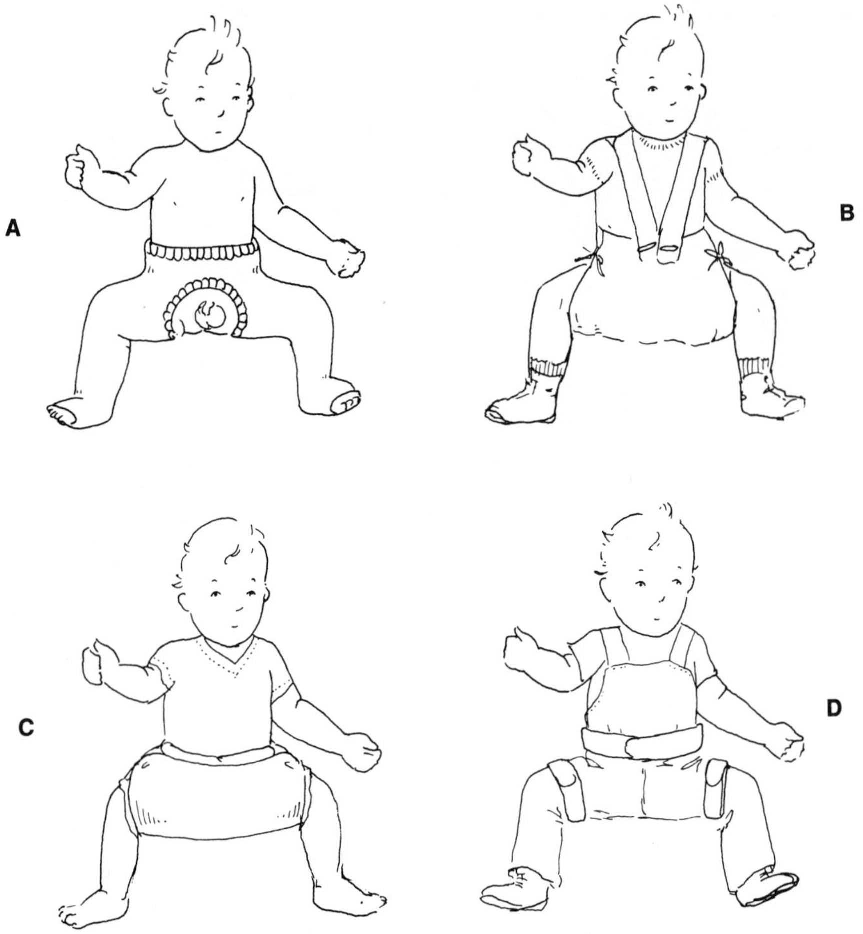

Fig. 11-10. Various devices used to reduce congenitally dislocated hip. **A,** Cast; **B,** Frejka pillow splint; **C,** abduction splint; **D,** brace.

any one of several innominate osteotomy procedures designed to construct an acetabular roof, is usually required. After cast removal and before weight bearing is permitted, range-of-motion exercises help restore movement. Next, rehabilitative measures are instituted. Successful reduction and reconstruction become increasingly difficult after the age of 4 years and are usually impossible or inadvisable over 6 years of age because of severe shortening and contracture of muscles and deformity of the femoral and acetabular structures.

Nursing considerations

Nurses are in a unique position to detect congenital dislocation of the hip in the newborn. During the infant assessment process (p. 260) and routine nurturing activities the hips and extremities are inspected for any deviations from the normal. Usually only nurses specially trained in the technique are permitted to perform Barlow's maneuver, but any nurse can be alert to other signs such as leg shortening, gluteal folds, and limited abduction. Diapering, for example, provides an excellent opportunity to observe for limited movement and a wide perineum. These observations are reported to the attending physician, and the ambulatory child who displays a limp or an unusual gait should be referred for evaluation. This may indicate an orthopedic or neurologic problem.

Care of the child in a reduction device. The major nursing problems in the care of an infant or child in a cast or other device are related to maintenance of the device and adapting nurturing activities to meet the needs of the infant or child. Generally treatment and follow-up care of these children are carried out in a clinic, physician's office, or outpatient unit. However, hospitalization may be necessary for cast application or brace fitting but seldom exceeds 24 to 48 hours. Longer hospitalization is required for open reduction procedures or if the child is hospitalized for a concurrent illness.

The simplest devices to care for are multiple diapers

Summary of nursing care of the child with congenital dislocation of the hip (CDH)

Goals	Responsibilities
Recognize congenital dislocation of the hip	Inspect and assess infant Repeat hip inspection at every postnatal well-baby check for undetected or overlooked signs
Maintain corrective positioning of hip	Apply reduction device correctly Maintain care of reduction device Assist with application of cast
Prevent complications	Observe for tightness of cast or apparatus, which indicates need for change or adjustment Check for evidence of impaired circulation Check for skin irritation and carry out appropriate skin care
Maintain care of corrective device	Maintain care of cast to prevent soiling or damage Administer correct care of braces or splints Position with suitable arrangement of pillows
Maintain nutrition	Feed in upright position whenever possible (appetite is seldom affected by the disorder or treatment) Avoid soiling cast or appliance with food Allow self-help as child is able
Provide comfort	Encourage parents to fondle and hold infant or child Maintain accustomed routine at home and, when possible, if hospitalized
Facilitate developmental progress	Provide appropriate stimulation and activities for stage of development
Provide ongoing and follow-up care	Refer to public health agency and crippled children's services Teach parents care of cast or appliance Help devise modifications for routine activities

and the Frejka pillow splint. With diapers, two or more are applied in the routine manner and maintained in position to achieve the desired abduction. They should fit snugly but not tightly. The pillow splint, a firm, rectangular pillow held in place by a romper-like outer garment, must be removed and reapplied with each diaper change. Although plastic pants worn over the diaper reduces the chance of soiling, it is necessary to have a second cover for the pillow to permit removal for laundering. These devices allow for easy handling of the infant and usually produce less apprehension in the mother.

Casts and braces offer more challenging nursing problems since they cannot be removed for routine care, although sometimes the physician allows a brace to be removed for bathing. Care of an infant or small child with a cast requires nursing innovation to reduce irritation and to maintain cleanliness of both the child and the cast, particularly in the diaper area. Cast care and observation are covered in Chapter 40 and, therefore, will not be elaborated here. However, inasmuch as congenital dislocated hip (CDH) is almost the exclusive reason for application of casts in early infancy, some of the problems specific to that age-group will be mentioned.

Parents are taught the proper care of the cast (or brace) and are helped to devise means for maintaining cleanliness. Plastic film or other waterproof material is applied around the edges of the cast in the peritoneal area to protect the cast from becoming wet and soiled. This material is removed, washed, dried, and replaced at least once a day. The skin must be kept clean and dry around and under the cast and checked frequently for evidence or irritation or pressure. Foam rubber can be used to provide extra protection if needed. Since older infants and small children may stuff bits of food, small toys, or other items under the cast, parents should be alerted to this possibility and suitable preventive measures should be instigated.

Feeding the infant in a hip spica cast or brace offers problems of positioning. Very young infants can be fed in the supine position with head elevated, and, with the infant's hips and legs supported on a pillow at her side, the mother can cuddle the infant in her arms during feeding. A somewhat similar position can be used for breast-feeding, that is, with the infant supported on pillows or held in a "football" hold facing the mother and with the legs behind her. An alternate position is to hold the infant upright on the mother's lap. When the infant is able to sit up, he can be fed in a feeding table or a modified high chair. The parents may be able to fashion a tilt board with a padded seat or an adjustable chair.

It is important for nurses, parents, and other care givers to understand that these children need to be involved in all the activities of any child in the same age-group. Confinement in a cast should not exclude children from family (or unit) activities. They can be held astride a lap for comfort and transported to areas of activity, for example. The child may be allowed to walk in the cast. (For a summary of nursing care of the child with congenital dislocation of the hip, see the boxed material on p. 391.)

CONGENITAL CLUBFOOT

Clubfoot is a general term used to describe a common deformity in which the foot is twisted out of shape or position. Any foot deformity involving the ankle is called *talipes,* derived from *talus,* meaning ankle, and *pes,* meaning foot. Deformities of foot and ankle are conveniently described according to the position of the ankle and foot. The more common positions involve the variations: *talipes varus,* an inversion or a bending inward; *talipes valgus,* an eversion or bending outward; *talipes equinus,* plantar flexion in which the toes are lower than the heel; and *talipes calcaneus,* or dorsiflexion, in which the toes are higher than the heel. Most clubfeet are a combination of these positions, and the most frequently occurring type of clubfoot (approximately 95%) is the composite deformity *talipes equinovarus,* in which the foot is pointed downward and inward in varying degrees of severity (Fig. 11-11). Unilateral clubfoot is somewhat more common than bilateral clubfoot and may occur as an isolated defect or in association with other disorders or syndromes such as chromosomal aberrations, arthrogryposis (a generalized immobility of the joints), cerebral palsy, or spina bifida.

Etiology and pathophysiology

The frequency of clubfoot in the general population is one in every 700 to 1000 live births, with boys affected twice as often as girls. There is a 35% concordance in monozygotic twins as opposed to a 3% concordance in dizygotic twins, which indicates a hereditary component.

The precise cause is unknown. There are those who attribute the defect to abnormal positioning and restricted movement in utero, although the evidence is not conclusive. Others implicate arrested or anomalous embryonic development since the foot normally goes through a flexion and eversion during early development and gradually assumes a normal attitude by the seventh month. Arrested development during this early stage tends to result in a rigid deformity, whereas mechanical pressures from intrauterine position are more likely to be operating in the more flexible deformities. Embryologists are divided in acceptance of the embryonic arrest theory.

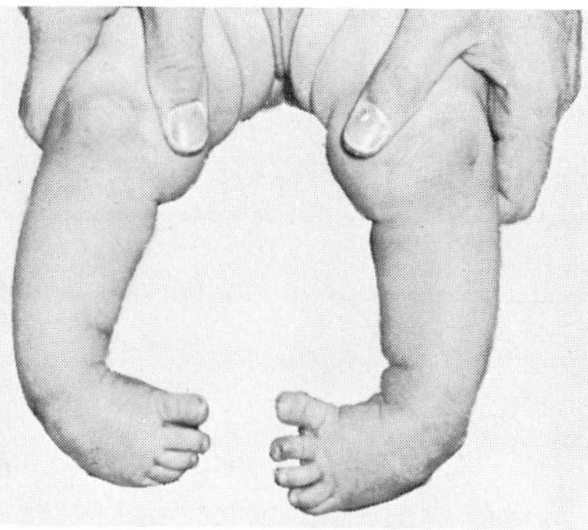

Fig. 11-11. Bilateral congenital talipes equinovarus (congenital clubfoot) in 2-month-old infant. (From Brashear, H. R., Jr., and Raney, R. B.: Shands' handbook of orthopaedic surgery, ed. 9, St. Louis, 1978, The C. V. Mosby Co., p. 33.)

Diagnostic evaluation

The deformity is readily apparent and easily detected at birth. However, it must be differentiated from some positional deformities that can be passively corrected or overcorrected. The true clubfoot is fixed. Paralytic changes in the lower extremity of children with neuromuscular involvement often produce equinovarus deformity.

Medical management

Treatment, which is begun as soon as the deformity is recognized, involves three stages: first, correction of the deformity; second, maintenance of the correction until normal muscle balance is regained; and third, follow-up observation to avert possible recurrence of the deformity. Some feet respond to treatment readily, some respond only to prolonged, vigorous, and sustained efforts, and the improvement in others remains disappointing even with maximal effort on the part of all concerned.

Correction of talipes equinovarus is most reliably accomplished by the application of a series of casts begun immediately or shortly after birth and continued until marked overcorrection is reached (Fig. 11-12). Successive casts allow for gradual stretching of tight structures on the medial side and gradual contraction of lax structures on the lateral side of the foot. The adduction deformity is corrected first, the inversion deformity next, and the plantar flexion deformity last. Weekly manipulations and cast

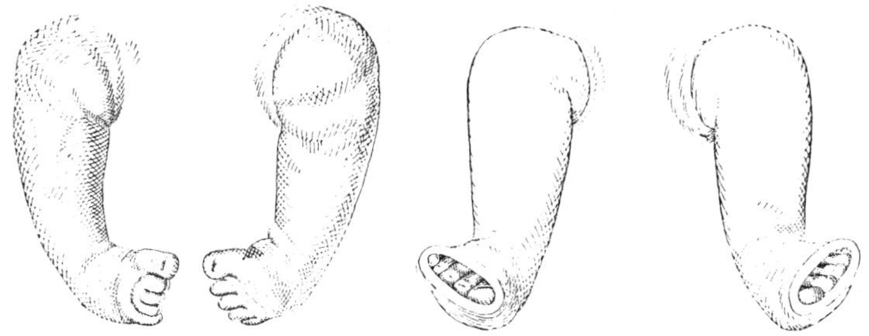

Fig. 11-12. Feet casted for correction of bilateral congenital talipes equinovarus. **A,** Before correction. **B,** Undergoing correction in plaster casts. (From Brashear, H. R., Jr., and Raney, R. B.: Shands' handbook of orthopaedic surgery, ed. 9, St. Louis, 1978, The C. V. Mosby Co., p. 34.)

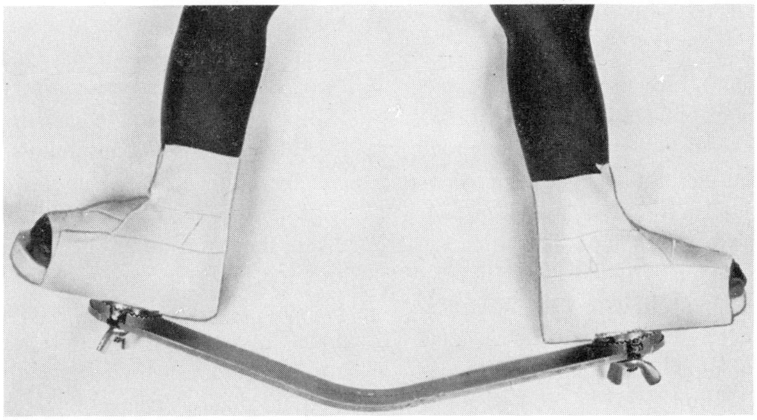

Fig. 11-13. Denis Browne splint for correction of clubfoot. Felt-padded plates are strapped to feet in corrected position with adhesive tape. Control of rotation, eversion, and dorsiflexion is adjustable. (From Brashear, H. R., Jr., and Raney, R. B.: Shands' handbook of orthopaedic surgery, ed. 9, St. Louis, 1978, The C. V. Mosby Co., p. 35.)

changes are needed in the beginning to accommodate the rapid growth of early infancy.

Some physicians favor the use of gentle but firm manipulations for 1 or 2 weeks prior to applying a cast to a newborn to take advantage of the pliability of the infant's foot at this early age. Much of the correction can be obtained during this period, but the success of treatment is based on its early initiation and consistent application. Manipulations are carried out on a regular basis (at least five to six times per day) by the nursery staff and the mother according to detailed instruction.[22]

An alternative method is use of the Denis Browne splint, a device that consists of two padded metal plates to which the infant's feet are securely fastened with adhesive tape and connected to a metal crossbar. Another device uses shoes affixed to the metal crossbar. The foot plates are adjusted to achieve the desired positioning. This device makes use of the infant's natural kicking movements to accelerate the correction process (Fig. 11-13).

Maintaining the correction is accomplished by use of special clubfoot shoes designed to maintain the correction (Fig. 11-14). The lateral side of the shoe is raised to maintain correction of the varus deformity and the front portion of the shoe turns outward to maintain forefoot abduction. Sometimes corrective shoes or splints are worn at night, and walking is encouraged to help strengthen the muscles. It is important for the feet to be observed throughout childhood since there is frequently a tendency for recurrence, which demands prompt attention.

Surgical intervention is sometimes required for children

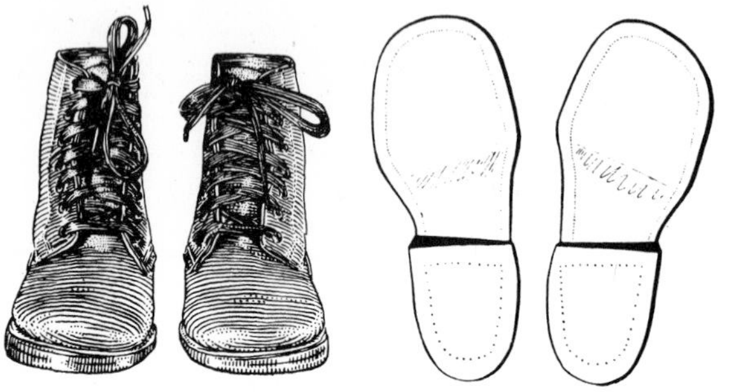

Fig. 11-14. Clubfoot shoes. The lateral side of the soles and heels is raised to maintain correction of varus deformity, and the front half of the shoes is turned out to maintain correction of forefoot adduction. (From Brashear, H. R., Jr., and Raney, R. B.: Shands' handbook of orthopaedic surgery, ed. 9, St. Louis, 1978, The C. V. Mosby Co., p. 36.)

with recurrent deformity or in cases that are resistant to more conservative measures. Surgery may be performed to correct bony deformity, to release tight ligaments, or to lengthen or transplant tendons. Again the extremity (or extremities) are casted until the desired result is achieved.

Nursing considerations

Nursing care of the child with nonsurgical correction of clubfoot is the same as it is for any child who has limited mobility and whose limbs are confined with casts or braces (pp. 1564 and 1549). The child will spend a considerable time in a corrective device; therefore, nursing care plans include both long-term and short-term goals. Conscientious observation of skin and circulation is particularly important in young infants because of their normally rapid growth rate. Since treatment and follow-up care are carried out in the orthopedist's office, clinic, or outpatient department, parent education and support are important aspects in nursing care of these children. Parents need to understand the overall treatment program, the importance of regular cast changes, and the role they play in the long-term effectiveness of the therapy. Reinforcing and clarifying the orthopedist's explanations and instructions, teaching parents about care of a cast or appliance, including vigilant observation for potential problems, and encouraging them to facilitate normal development within the limitations imposed by the deformity or therapy are all part of nursing responsibilities.

SKELETAL LIMB DEFICIENCY

Congenital limb deficiencies, or reduction malformations, are manifest by a variety of degree of loss of functional capacity. They are characterized by underdevelopment of skeletal elements of the extremities. The range of malformation can extend from minor defects of the digits to serious abnormalities such as *amelia,* absence of an entire extremity, or *meromelia,* partial absence of an extremity including *phocomelia* (seal limbs) an intercalary deficiency of long bones with relatively good development of hands and feet attached at or near the shoulder or the hips.

In rare instances prenatal destruction of limbs has been reported, but most reduction deformities are primary defects of development (agenesis, aplasia). Therefore, congenital amputations, in the literal sense, are not amputations since nonexistent limbs cannot be amputated.

Etiology and pathophysiology

Limb deficiencies can be attributed to both heredity and environment. The upper limb appears first as a limb bud in the fourth week of gestation, and its entire skeleton can be recognized in its early stages by the fifth week of gestation. During the sixth week of gestation cartilage forms the structural model of the bones and ossification from humerus to phalanges begins between the sixth and seventh weeks of gestation. The development of the upper limbs precedes that of the lower limbs slightly, and the cartilaginous structure appears in a proximodistal sequence. By 8 weeks of gestation the digits are well formed and their number determined; by 12 weeks of gestation primary centers of ossification can be detected in nearly all bones of the extremities.

Malformations can originate at any stage of limb development. Formation of limbs may be suppressed at the time of limb bud formation, or there may be interference in later stages of differentiation and growth. Heredity appears to play a prominent role, and prenatal environmental insults have been implicated in a number of cases. The well-publicized thalidomide tragedy is a dramatic illustration of the effects of environmental interference with limb development. Children damaged by maternal ingestion of the drug displayed a variety of serious limb anomalies that demonstrated a clear relationship between the time of exposure and the presence and type of limb deformity.

Medical management

It is generally agreed that children with congenital limb deficiencies should be fitted with prosthetic devices whenever possible and that such a functional replacement should be applied at the earliest possible stage of development in an attempt to match the motor readiness of the infant. This favors natural progression of prosthetic use. For example, an infant with an upper extremity deficiency is fitted with a simple passive device, such as a mitten prosthesis, between 3 and 6 months of age when limb exploration is active, sitting is beginning with the extremities needed for support, and bilateral hand activities are to be encouraged. Lower limb prostheses are applied when the infant is ready to pull himself to a standing position. In preparation for prosthetic devices, surgical modification is often necessary to assure the most favorable use of the device since severe deformity can interfere with its effective use. Phocomelic digits are preserved for controlling switches of externally powered appliances in upper extremities. Digits (in both upper and lower extremities) provide the child with surfaces for tactile exploration and stimulation. Prostheses are replaced to accommodate growth and increasing capabilities of the child.[7]

Prosthetic application training and habilitation involve a team of health professionals including the parents, who must encourage the child in making age-commensurate adjustments to the environment. Although these children need assistance, excessive overprotection may produce overdependency with later maladjustment to school and other situations.[22]

Cleft lip and/or palate

Clefts of the lip and palate are facial malformations that are common to all human populations and constitute a severe handicap to the affected individual. The defects are classified into two major groups. The first includes those clefts that involve the lip and anterior maxilla regardless of whether the defect involves the remaining portions of the hard and soft palate (sometimes called harelip). The second group consists of those clefts that involve only the hard and soft palate. Although there are differences in the severity and extent of deformities within each category, the terms and their abbreviations associated with these groups are:

CL clefts that involve the lip.
CLP clefts that involve the lip and palate.
CL(P) clefts that involve the lip with or without cleft palate.
CP clefts that involve the hard and soft palate only.
CL/P all types of clefts that involve the lip and/or palate.

The term ''complete cleft'' indicates the maximum degree of clefting.

Etiology and pathophysiology

Many factors appear to be involved in the etiology of clefts of the lip and/or palate, and evidence indicates that cleft lip with or without cleft palate is developmentally and genetically different from cleft palate. Defective development of the embryonic *primary* palate may result in clefts of the lip and anterior maxilla; clefts of the hard and soft palate are caused by defective development of the embryonic *secondary* palate and often appear in persons with cleft lip. There are no less than fifty recognized syndromes that include cleft lip and/or palate as a feature: some are caused by mutant genes, others result from chromosomal abnormalities, and teratogens have been implicated in a very small number. The great majority of cases appear to be consistent with the concept of multifactoral inheritance as evidenced by an increased incidence in relatives and a higher concordance in monozygotic than in dizygotic twins. However, there is apparently no relationship between the incidence of cleft lip with or without cleft palate and the incidence of cleft palate among relatives, that is, relatives of persons with cleft palate have an increased incidence of cleft palate but not cleft lip with or without cleft palate and vice versa.

The incidence of cleft lip and/or cleft palate shows a wide variation in races: it occurs in about one in 1000 live births in whites, twice that in Japan, and less than half as many in American blacks. The incidence of cleft palate is about one is 2500. There is less racial difference in cleft palate. Affected males outnumber females with cleft lip with or without cleft palate, particularly in the more severe defects (that is, greater for cleft lip), with or without cleft palate than isolated cleft lips, but cleft palate occurs more often in females. Cleft lip and palate is the most common of the facial malformations (50%), whereas cleft lip and cleft palate each account for half that number (25%).[5]

Pathophysiology. Development of the primary and secondary palates takes place at different times and involves different developmental processes. Cleft lip with or without cleft palate results from failure of the maxillary processes to fuse with the nasal elevations on the frontal prominence, which normally occurs during the sixth week of gestation (Fig. 11-15, *A*). Merging of the upper lip at the midline is completed between the seventh and eighth weeks of gestation. There is evidence that in some cases separation may be the result of rupture subsequent to fusion, however.

Fusion of the secondary palate (hard and soft palate) takes place later in development, between the seventh and twelfth weeks of gestation (Fig. 11-15, *B* to *D*). At the time the primary palate is completed, the two lateral palatine processes are situated in a vertical position at the side of the tongue. In the process of migrating to a horizontal position they are, for a short time, separated by the tongue. With development of the neck and jaws, the tongue moves downward, allowing the palatine processes to fuse with each other and with the primary palate to form the roof of the mouth. If there is delay in this movement or if the tongue fails to descend soon enough, the remainder of development proceeds and the palate never fuses.

Diagnostic evaluation

The cleft that involves the lip with or without cleft palate is readily apparent at birth and is one of the defects that elicits the most severe emotional reactions in parents. Incomplete fusion of the primary palate produces a variation in the degree of malformation (Fig. 11-16). Clefts of the lip may be unilateral or bilateral and may range from a notch

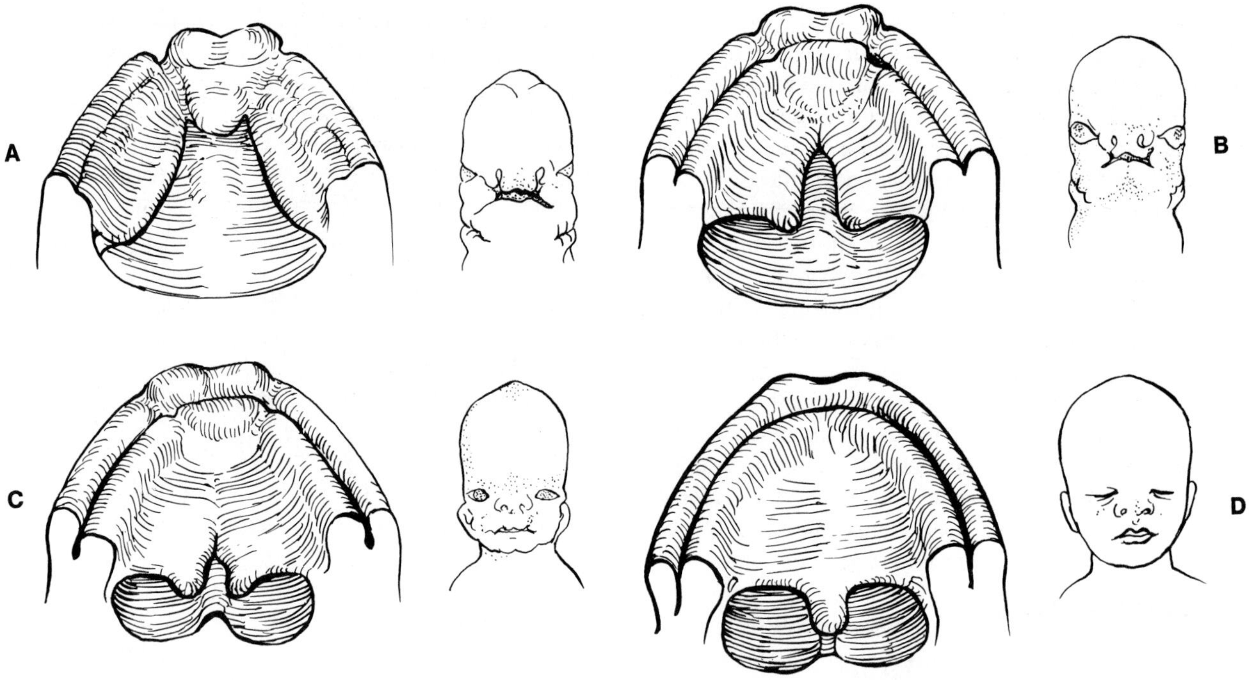

Fig. 11-15. Stages in palatine development.

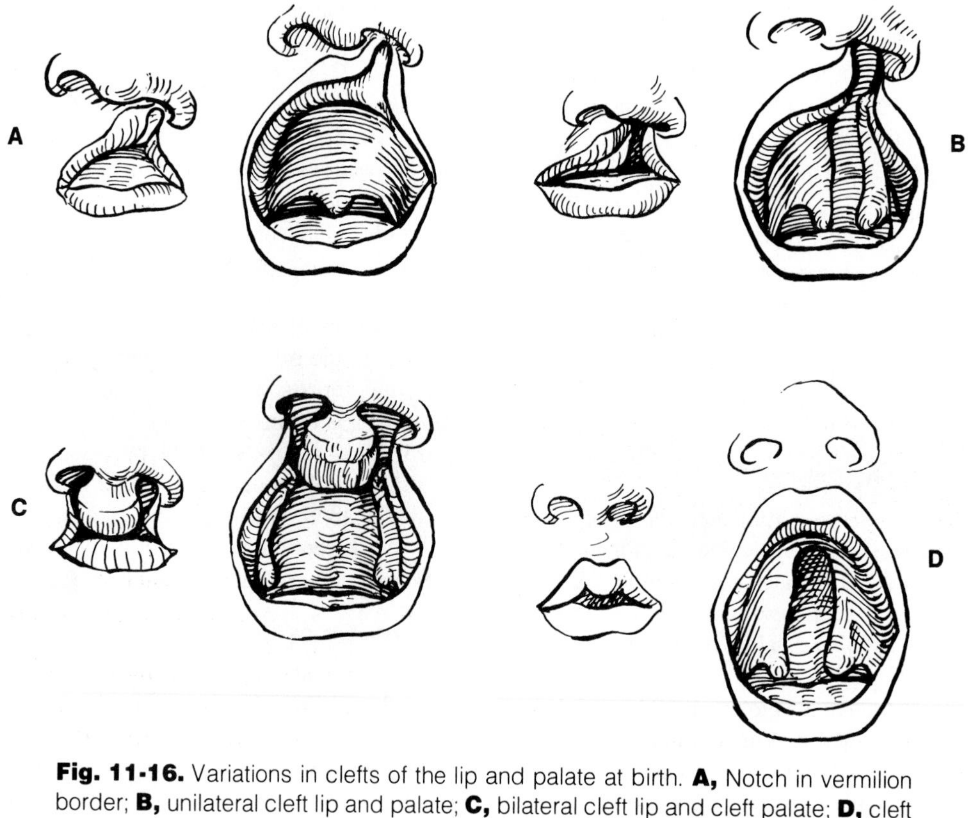

Fig. 11-16. Variations in clefts of the lip and palate at birth. **A,** Notch in vermilion border; **B,** unilateral cleft lip and palate; **C,** bilateral cleft lip and cleft palate; **D,** cleft palate.

in the vermilion border of the lip to complete separation extending to the floor of the nose. Where the cleft is unilateral, about two thirds is on the left side, and an associated cleft palate is found more often with bilateral than with unilateral cleft lip. Varying degrees of nasal distortion usually accompany cleft lip with or without cleft palate, and the defect frequently involves supernumerary, deformed, or absent teeth.

Clefts of the palate may occur as an isolated defect or in association with cleft lip. Less obvious than cleft lip, the defect may not be detected without a thorough assessment of the mouth. The deformity can be identified by placing the examiner's fingers directly on the palate. Without a proper evaluation, the defect may not be detected until the infant has difficulty with initial feedings. As with cleft lip, the degree of deformity varies and may involve only the uvula or may extend through both the soft and hard palates to the incisive foramen. The isolated cleft palate occurs in the midline, but, when associated with cleft lip, it may involve the midline of the soft palate and extend into the hard palate on the side of the lip cleft or on both sides in bilateral clefts. Clefts of the hard palate form a continuous opening between the mouth and the nasal cavity. This creates special feeding problems. The infant is unable to develop suction because of the defect and has difficulty in swallowing. The open pathway must be closed in order to provide sufficient pressure for the swallowing sequence.

Medical management

Treatment of the child with cleft lip and palate involves the cooperative efforts of a number of specialists—pediatrician, nurses, plastic surgeon, orthodontist, prosthodentist, otolaryngologist, speech therapist, and, sometimes, a psychiatrist. Treatment continues over a long period of time, but even after completion of a program of health care the child will probably retain defects of speech, facial appearance, or other problems related to the cleft. Medical management is directed toward closure of the cleft(s), prevention of complications, habilitation, and facilitation of normal growth and development of the child.

Surgical correction. Closure of the lip defect precedes that of the palate, although the optimal times for surgery are still being debated. Those who favor immediate repair of the lip argue that it makes the infant more acceptable to the parents before discharge from the hospital, thereby improving establishment of satisfactory parent-child relationships. Others prefer to wait until the infant shows a steady weight gain and a hemoglobin level of at least 10 g/100 ml, usually at 6 to 12 weeks of age. They believe that the delay helps the infant better withstand the surgery, offers time to detect any associated serious anomalies unrecognized at birth, and reduces parental disappointment with surgical repair. That is, parents ordinarily adjust to the defect during this time and more fully appreciate the cosmetic effects of the surgical correction. Technical repair of the cleft lip and/or palate can be done quite successfully at any age.

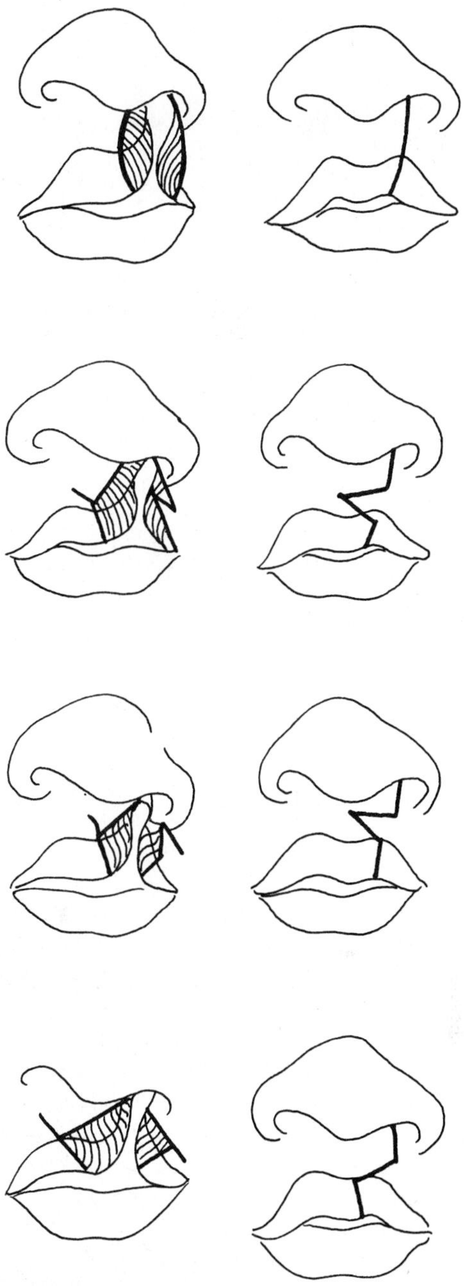

Fig. 11-17. Basic cleft lip operations indicating line of incision and approximation of suture lines.

The method most commonly used in repair of the lip cleft involves one of several staggered or Z-shaped suture lines to minimize notching of the lip from retraction of scar tissue (Fig. 11-17). Immediately after surgery the suture line is protected from tension by a thin, arched metal device (the Logan bow) (Fig. 11-18) taped to the cheeks or a butterfly-type adhesive restraint, and the arms are restrained at the el-

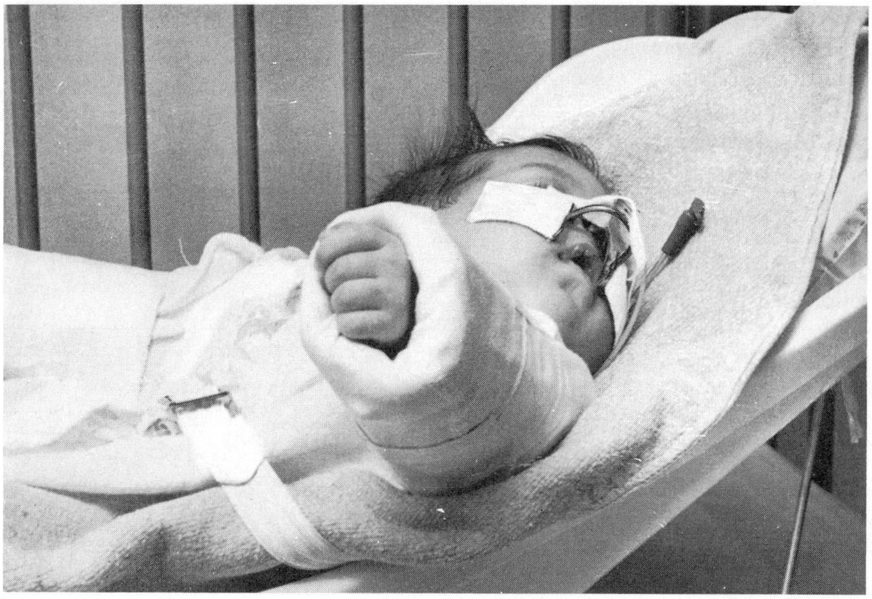

Fig. 11-18. Infant with Logan bow in place to prevent tension on suture line and elbow restraints. (Courtesy Children's Health Center, San Diego, Calif. From Ingalls, A. J., and Salerno, M. C.: Maternal and child health nursing, ed. 3, St. Louis, 1975, The C. V. Mosby Co., p. 240.)

bows to prevent the infant from rubbing the incision with his hands. Improved surgical techniques have minimized deformity related to scar retraction, but good cosmetic results are difficult to obtain in defects that are more severe initially. In the absence of infection or trauma, healing takes place with little scar formation; however, in some instances the results are less than satisfactory from the parents' (and, later, the child's) viewpoint. Characteristics of the older child are residual nasal deformity, mildly protruding lower lip, and a somewhat flattened lower third of the upper lip usually with an abnormally shaped red lip margin. Not infrequently revisions may be required at a later age.

Cleft palate repair is generally postponed until later in order to take advantage of palatal changes that take place with normal growth, sometime between the ages of 6 months and 5 years. Most surgeons prefer to close the cleft between 1 and 2 years of age, before the child develops faulty speech habits. If surgery is delayed beyond 3 years of age a special denture plate helps occlude the cleft to assist in development of normal speech patterns.

Long-term problems. The team concept in the delivery of health care is exemplified in the habilitation of the child with cleft lip and/or palate. Treatment of individual patients is integrated by a group of specialists who meet periodically to examine the child and consult with each other and with the parents. The majority of children with cleft lip and/or cleft palate have some degree of speech impairment, even with good anatomic closure, that requires speech therapy. The physical problems are the result of inefficient functioning of the muscles of the soft palate and nasopharynx, improper tooth alignment, and varying degrees of hearing loss. Improper drainage of the middle ear, as the result of inefficient function of the eustachian tube, contributes to recurrent otitis media with scarring of the tympanic membrane, which leads to hearing impairment in a large proportion of children with palatal clefts. The problem may be easily overlooked in the infant and young child, thereby contributing to permanent impairment. Upper respiratory infections require immediate and meticulous attention, and polyethylene drainage tubes are inserted to facilitate drainage in chronic serous otitis media (see p. 375). Extensive orthodontics and prosthodontics are needed to correct problems of malposition of teeth and maxillary arches. In addition a significant number of these children have an inadequate nasal airway that forces them to breathe through their mouths, which also contributes to oral deformity.

Some of the more difficult long-term problems are related to social adjustment of the child. The better the physical habilitation, the better the chance for emotional and social adjustment, although the presence of the defect and the degree of residual disability are not directly related to a satisfactory adjustment. Physical defects are always a threat to the self-image, and abnormal speech quality is an impediment to social expression.

Nursing considerations

The immediate nursing problems in the care of an infant with cleft lip and palate deformities are related to feeding the infant and dealing with the severe parental reaction to the defect. Facial deformities are particularly disturbing to parents. A cleft lip is the most disfiguring of the visible defects and one that generates strong negative responses in both nurses and parents. It is especially important for nurses to emphasize the positive aspects of the infant's physical appearance and optimism regarding surgical correction. The manner of the nurse in handling the infant should convey to the parents that the infant is indeed a precious, although incomplete, human being.

Unless there are associated, complicating anomalies, nursing care of these children offers no significant differences from that of any newborn except in modification of feeding techniques.

Feeding. Feeding the infant offers a special challenge to nurses. Clefts of lip or palate reduce the infant's ability to suck, which interferes with compression of the areola and usually renders breast-feeding impossible and makes bottle-feeding difficult. Liquid taken into the mouth has a tendency to escape via the cleft through the nose. Feeding is usually best accomplished with the infant's head in an upright position, either held in the nurse's hand or cradled in the arm. Normal nipples are unsuitable for these infants, who are unable to generate the suction required; therefore, special nipples or other feeding devices are needed. A variety of special "cleft palate" nipples have been devised and used with some success. However, large, soft nipples with large holes, Nursettes, or the long, soft lamb's nipples appear to offer the best means for nipple feeding. These also have the advantage of helping to meet the infant's sucking needs and, when placed in the normal sucking position (not through the cleft), encourage use of the sucking muscles. Muscle development is especially important for development of speech later on. Gentle, steady pressure on the base of the bottle reduces the chance of choking or coughing, and the person feeding should resist the temptation to remove the nipple frequently because of the noise the infant makes or for fear that he will choke.[17] Since these infants have a tendency to swallow excessive amounts of air, they require frequently bubbling.

When the infant has trouble with nipple feeding, either a rubber-tipped medicine dropper, Asepto syringe, or "breck feeder" often provides an efficient, safe feeding device. The rubber extension should be sufficiently long to extend well back into the mouth to reduce the likelihood of regurgitation through the nose. The formula is deposited on the back of the tongue and the flow controlled by bulb compression that is adjusted to the infant's capacity to handle it.

With some infants, spoon feeding works best. The mother should begin to feed the infant as soon as possible, preferably after the initial nursery feeding. In this way she is able to help determine the method best suited to her and the infant and to become adept in the technique before they are discharged from the hospital.

Preoperative care. In preparation for surgical repair, the mother is frequently instructed to accustom the infant to some of the needs of the early postoperative period, particularly if surgery is delayed several months. Since it is mandatory for the infant to be positioned on the back postoperatively, it is helpful to train him to lie in this position a great deal of the time to reduce the irritability and resistance associated with any change in routine. It is also helpful to place the infant or child in arm restraints periodically prior to admission and, after admission, to feed him with a rubber-tipped Asepto syringe or other device in the manner to be used postoperatively. No special formula is required, and the infant is usually allowed to eat up to about 6 hours preoperatively. Preoperative preparation, including medication, is determined by the surgeon and anesthesiologist.

Postoperative care. The major efforts in the postoperative period are directed toward protecting the operative site. Before the infant leaves the operating room the metal appliance is securely taped to the cheeks to relax the operative site and prevent tension on the suture line caused by crying or other facial movement. Arm restraints (see p. 922) are needed to prevent the infant from rubbing or otherwise disturbing the suture line and are ready at the bedside for immediate application on his arrival at the unit. It is advisable to pin the cuff of the restraints to the infant's clothing or bed to prevent rubbing the face with the upper arms. The older infant who is able to roll over will require a jacket restraint in addition to restricting arm movement to prevent his rolling on the abdomen and rubbing his face on the sheet. It is important to remove the restraints periodically to exercise the arms, to provide relief from restrictions, and to observe the skin for signs of irritation. It is advisable to release the restraints one at a time, especially in a very vigorous, active infant. Removing restraints also offers an opportunity for cuddling and body contact. Sitting him in an infant seat provides a change of position and a different perspective of the environment. Sedation is sometimes needed for a very restless, anxious infant.

Feeding is essentially the same as previous to surgery. It is safe to offer clear liquids when the infant has fully recovered from the anesthesia, and formula feeding is usually resumed when tolerated. Asepto-syringe feeding is preferred in most cases. Care should be taken to slip the rubber tip in from the side of the mouth to avoid the operative area and to prevent the infant from sucking on the tubing. This method is continued until the lip is well healed, after which bottle-feeding can be resumed if this has been the infant's mode of feeding. The mouth should be rinsed with water before and after each feeding. The suture site is carefully cleansed of formula or serosanguineous drainage as needed with a gauze- or cotton-tipped swab dipped in saline or hydrogen peroxide. Meticulous care of the suture line is a nursing responsibility since inflammation or sloughing will

Summary of postoperative hospital nursing care of the child with cleft lip and/or palate

Goals	Responsibilities
Prevent trauma to suture line	Do not allow to suck Position on back or side (on abdomen for cleft palate) Maintain lip protective device Use nontraumatic feeding techniques Restrain arms to prevent access to operative site Use jacket restraints on older infant
Prevent tissue infection and breakdown	Cleanse suture line gently after feeding and as necessary in manner ordered by surgeon Keep suture line dry
Facilitate breathing	Position to allow for mucus drainage (partial side-lying position)
Provide adequate nutritional intake	Administer diet appropriate for age Modify feeding techniques to adjust to defect Feed in sitting position Use special appliances Encourage frequent bubbling
Provide comfort measures	Remove restraints periodically Provide cuddling and tactile stimulation Involve parents in infant's care
Facilitate parents' acceptance of infant	Allow expression of feelings Convey attitude of acceptance of infant and parents Indicate by conduct that child is a valuable human being
Educate parents	Involve parents in determining best feeding methods Teach feeding and suctioning techniques Teach cleansing and restraining procedures especially when infant will be discharged before suture removal
Meet parents' concerns about recurrence in future children	Refer to genetic counseling services
Provide for continued support	Refer to public health agency for continuity of care Refer to social service Refer to crippled children's services for financial assistance Refer to local cleft palate parent group

interfere with optimum healing and the ultimate cosmetic effect of the surgical repair.

Gentle aspiration of mouth and nasopharynx secretions may be necessary to prevent aspiration and respiratory complications. A side-lying or partial side-lying position is helpful for the infant in the immediate postoperative period and for one who has difficulty in handling secretions. As with any infant, the child with cleft palate repair is placed on the right side after feedings to reduce the chance of aspirating regurgitated formula.

The child with a cleft palate repair is allowed to lie on the abdomen, especially immediately postoperatively. The nurse avoids the use of suction or other objects in the mouth, such as a tongue depressor when the suture lines are being checked or straws when the child is given liquids. Moreover, spoons should not be allowed in the mouth. The child with a cleft palate repair may be fed with a wide-bowl spoon (such as a soup spoon) that cannot enter the mouth.

Sometimes the child will have difficulty in breathing following surgery—especially the child with cleft palate repair who must alter an established pattern of breathing and adjust to breathing through the nose. This is frustrating but seldom requires more than positioning and support. Sometimes the infant or child is placed in a mist tent for a short period after surgery.

For a summary of postoperative hospital nursing care of the child with cleft lip and/or cleft palate, see the boxed material on the opposite page.

Gastrointestinal tract atresias

Atresia is absence or closure of a normal body orifice. Closure at any point along the length of the gastrointestinal tract creates an obstruction to the normal progress of nutrients and secretions through the gastrointestinal passages. The most common are atresias of the esophagus, intestine, and anus, all of which require surgical intervention. The diagnosis and management of intestinal atresia are similar to that of intestinal obstruction from other factors and will be outlined but not elaborated in this discussion (see Chapter 34). Intestinal obstruction in the neonatal period may be caused by:

atresia complete obstruction because of developmental arrest during the second and third months of fetal life. The duodenum and lower ileum are the most common sites.

stenosis partial closure of the gut. Pyloric stenosis is discussed on p. 1108.

annular pancreas the head of the pancreas surrounds and constricts the second segment of duodenum.

malrotation of the colon the colon fails to rotate during the tenth week of fetal life. Before this time the cecum is situated in the lower left quadrant, then normally rotates ventrally in a counterclockwise direction to the right upper quadrant, and finally moves to the lower right quadrant. At the same time the mesentery of the ascending colon becomes fixed posteriorly and laterally to the parietal peritoneum. In malrotation the cecum remains in the upper right quadrant and the posterior fixation of the mesentery is inadequate and allows twisting of the small intestine, or *volvulus,* to create an obstruction. Obstruction can also be caused by *peritoneal bands* or *folds* that cross the duodenum as they attach the abnormally placed cecum to the right peritoneum. Thus the duodenum is partially obstructed by the external pressure of the bands.

meconium ileus the intestine becomes obstructed by thick, inspissated, impacted meconium—the earliest manifestation of cystic fibrosis (p. 1252).

congenital megacolon (Hirschsprung's disease) absence or deficiency of innervation to the musculature of the rectum and distal colon. This produces a functional obstruction caused by propulsive peristalsis (p. 1273).

ESOPHAGEAL ATRESIA WITH TRACHEOESOPHAGEAL FISTULA

Congenital atresia of the esophagus and tracheoesophageal (T-E) fistula are rare malformations that represent a failure of the esophagus to develop as a continuous passage. These defects may occur as separate entities or in combination (Fig. 11-19) and, without early diagnosis and treatment, are rapidly fatal.

Etiology and pathophysiology

The incidence of esophageal atresia and tracheoesophageal fistula is not known. Various authorities have estimated the incidence to be from one in 800 to one in 5000 live births. There appear to be no sex differences, but the birth weight of most affected infants is significantly lower than average and there is an unusually high percentage of prematurity. A history of maternal hydramnios is common, and approximately half the infants with esophageal defects have associated anomalies, especially congenital heart disease, anorectal malformations, and genitourinary anomalies. There is little evidence to implicate heredity as a factor.

Pathophysiology. The esophagus develops from the first segment of the embryonic gut. During the fourth and fifth weeks of gestation, this foregut normally lengthens and separates longitudinally and each longitudinal portion fuses to form two parallel channels that are joined only at the larynx. Anomalies involving the trachea and esophagus are caused by defective separation, incomplete fusion of the tracheal folds following this separation, or altered cellular growth during the process. The esophagus may consist merely of two blind pouches, one at the pharyngeal end and one at the gastric end. More often one portion ends in a blind pouch and the other is connected to the trachea by way of a fistula.

The most commonly encountered form of esophageal atresia and tracheoesophageal fistula (80% to 95% of cases) is one in which the proximal esophageal segment terminates in a blind pouch and the distal segment is connected to the trachea or primary bronchus by a short fistula at or near the bifurcation (Fig. 11-19, *C*). The second most common variety (5% to 8%) consists of a blind pouch at each end, widely separated and with no communication to the trachea (Fig. 11-19, *A*). Less frequently an otherwise normal trachea and esophagus are connected by a common fistula (Fig. 11-19, *E*). Extremely rare anomalies involve a fistula from the trachea to the upper esophageal segment (Fig. 11-19, *B*). or to both the upper and lower segments (Fig. 11-19, *D*).

Diagnostic evaluation

The presence of esophageal atresia is suspected in an infant with excessive salivation and in a newborn with drooling that is frequently accompanied by choking, coughing, and sneezing. If fed, the infant swallows normally but suddenly coughs and struggles and the fluid returns through the nose and mouth. He becomes cyanotic and may stop breathing as the overflow of fluid from the blind pouch is aspirated into the trachea or bronchus. The cyanosis is the result of laryngospasm, the protective mechanism that operates to prevent aspiration into the trachea.

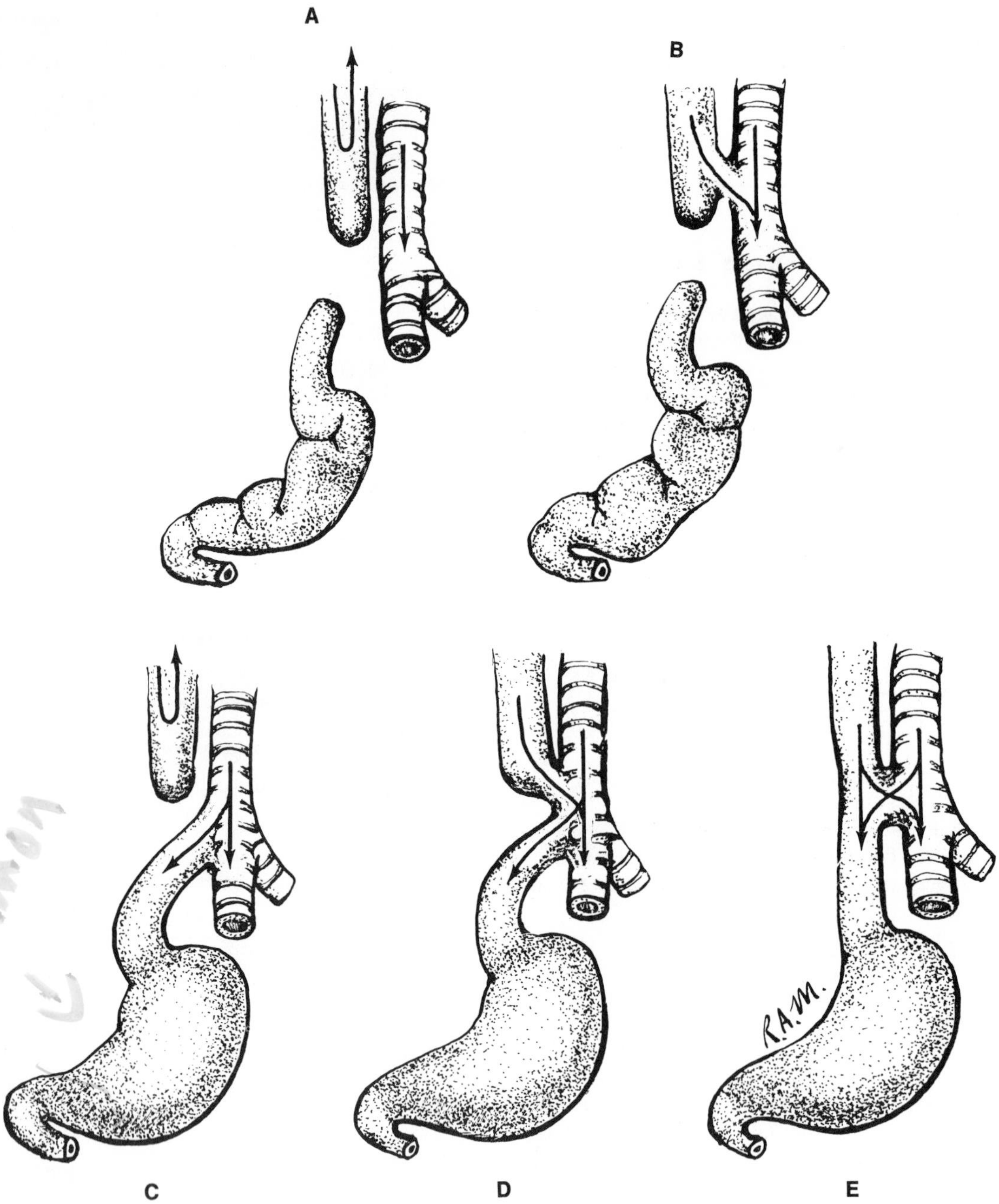

Fig. 11-19. The five most common types of esophageal atresia and tracheoesophageal fistula.

In the infant with type C malformation, the stomach becomes distended with air and thoracic and abdominal compression (especially during crying) cause the gastric contents to be regurgitated through the fistula into the trachea, producing a chemical pneumonitis. When the upper segment of the esophagus opens directly into the trachea (types B and D), the infant is in danger of drowning immediately from any swallowed material. Cyanosis or choking during feeding may be the only symptom of type E fistula.

To rule out esophageal atresia a catheter is gently passed into the esophagus. It will meet with resistance if the lumen is blocked but will pass unobstructed if the lumen is patent. A moderately stiff catheter is used to avoid coiling in the esophageal pouch. Aspiration of stomach contents or auscultation over the stomach as air is introduced through the catheter confirms a patent esophagus. Gastric lavage immediately after delivery, although not a universal practice, offers earlier diagnosis of esophageal fistula as well as reducing gastric distension to assist respiration.

The exact type of anomaly is determined by x-ray studies. Radiopaque fluid carefully instilled in the esophagus under fluoroscopy will readily establish the diagnosis. Sometimes fistulas are not patent, which makes their presence more difficult to diagnose.

Medical management

The treatment of esophageal atresia and tracheoesophageal fistula includes prevention of pneumonia and surgical repair of the anomaly. Since type C anomaly is the most common, the discussion will be directed primarily toward it.

When a tracheoesophageal fistula is suspected, the infant is immediately deprived of oral intake, started on intravenous fluids, and placed in the most advantageous position to decrease the likelihood of aspiration. Accumulated secretions are suctioned frequently from the mouth and pharynx. A catheter is placed into the upper esophageal pouch and the infant's head is kept in an upright position, so that fluid collected in the pouch is easily removed. A gastrostomy is usually performed to decompress the stomach and prevent further aspiration of gastric contents by way of the fistula. Since aspiration pneumonia is almost inevitable and appears early, broad-spectrum antibiotic therapy is instituted.

Surgical correction. Most malformations can be corrected surgically in one operation or staged with two or more procedures. The success depends to a great extent on early diagnosis before complicating factors (pneumonia, dehydration, and inanition) have progressed to an irreversible stage as well as on skilled nursing care and the technical skill and judgment of the surgeon. With measures instituted to prevent aspiration pneumonia and to assure adequate hydration and nutrition, surgery can be postponed to allow for more effective treatment of pneumonia so that the infant can better withstand the complex surgery. The delay also offers an opportunity for further evaluation and assessment for any concomitant anomalies.

The surgery consists of a thoracotomy with division and ligation of the tracheoesophageal fistula and an end-to-end anastomosis of the esophagus. For infants who are premature, have multiple anomalies, or are in very poor condition, a staged operation is preferred that involves palliative measures including gastrostomy, ligation of the tracheoesophageal fistula, and provision of constant drainage of the esophageal pouch.

There are rare instances in which a primary anastomosis cannot be accomplished because of insufficient length of the two segments of esophagus. In these cases the defect must be bridged with a segment of intestine. This esophageal replacement is usually deferred until the child is 18 to 24 months old. In the meantime the fistula is closed and the child fed directly by gastrostomy, whereas the upper esophageal segment is drained by means of a cervical esophagostomy. When the time is right for esophageal replacement, a segment of either the right or the transverse colon is dissected and transplanted, along with its undisturbed blood and nerve supply, through a surgical opening in the diaphragm and ligated to the esophageal pouches maintaining the proximodistal orientation. At this time the gastrostomy and esophagostomy are closed.

In all surgical procedures involving the esophagus there may be problems with stricture caused by scar tissue contraction that require evaluation by barium x-ray studies, esophagoscopy, and mechanical dilatation. Many surgeons routinely perform dilatation at regularly scheduled intervals for some time after surgery. The procedure may need to be repeated several times during growth. Strictures that do not respond to dilatation require surgical intervention.

Nursing considerations

Nursing responsibility for detection of this serious malformation begins *immediately* after birth. Nurses should suspect any infant who has an excessive amount of mucus or difficulty with secretions and unexplained episodes of cyanosis. Ideally the condition is diagnosed before the initial feeding, but often it is not. For this reason it is customary for the nurse to give the infant the first feeding in order to observe his reactions. Poor handling of mucus is characteristic of other problems, for example, the infant with central nervous system damage and the preterm infant with weak or absent cough and swallowing reflexes. This is often a cause of confusion, especially with the premature infant who may also have a tracheoesophageal fistula.

Cyanosis is usually the result of laryngospasm caused by overflow of saliva into the larynx from the proximal esophageal pouch, and it normally clears after removal of the secretions from the oropharynx by suctioning. These two signs, excessive mucus and unexplained episodes of cyanosis, should alert nursery nurses to the possibility of a tracheoesophageal fistula or esophageal atresia. Any such suspicion is reported to the physician immediately.

The infant is placed in an Isolette or under a radiant warmer, and oxygen is administered to help relieve respiratory distress. Positive pressure is contraindicated since it may add to air pressure in the stomach to compound the distress.

Preoperative care. The infant's mouth and nasopharynx are carefully suctioned, and he is placed in an advantageous position. It is common practice to place an infant who appears to have difficulty with secretions in the head-down position to facilitate drainage. Without a fistulous communication to the stomach (as in type A or B) this would be of

Summary of nursing care of the infant with esophageal atresia and tracheoesophageal fistula

Goals	Responsibilities
Preoperative	
Recognize defect early	Be alert to danger signs Excess salivation Three C's—choking, coughing, and cyanosis Acute gastric distention Assist with diagnostic procedures
Prevent aspiration pneumonia	Administer nothing by mouth Position advantageously Change position every 2 hours Aspirate secretions from oropharynx and esophageal pouch Facilitate drainage from gastrostomy
Maintain patent airway and lung expansion	Remove accumulated secretions from oropharynx Position for patent airway, lung expansion, and prevention of aspiration of saliva or stomach contents Observe for signs of respiratory distress
Postoperative	
Prevent infection at operative sites	Administer judicious care of operative site Observe for signs of inflammation, bleeding, and/or other drainage Cleanse and apply dressings as ordered
Maintain fluid and electrolyte balance	Record accurate measurement of intake and output Regulate intravenous fluids carefully Measure and record gastrostomy drainage Record weight daily Measure specific gravity of urine
Facilitate ventilation	Maintain patent airway Suction secretions as needed Maintain care of chest tubes and drainage apparatus Position for optimum ventilation Administer oxygen as indicated Prevent aspiration of feedings

benefit, but since the majority are type C anomalies, the head-down position could have adverse effects. The most desirable position for a newborn who is suspected of having a tracheoesophageal fistula is supine with the head elevated on an inclined plane of at least 30 degrees. This positioning serves to minimize the reflux of gastric secretions up the distal esophagus into the trachea and bronchi, especially when intra-abdominal pressure is elevated during episodes of crying.

It is imperative that the source of aspiration be removed at once. Until surgery the blind pouch is kept empty by intermittent or continuous suction through an indwelling nasal catheter that extends to the end of the pouch. The catheter needs attention since it has a tendency to become clogged with mucus. It is usually replaced daily by the physician. On diagnosis the gastrostomy tube is inserted and left open so that air entering the stomach through the fistula can escape, thus minimizing the danger that gastric contents will be regurgitated into the trachea. The tube empties by gravity drainage. Feedings through the gastrostomy tube and irrigations with fluid are contraindicated prior to surgery.

Often the infant must be transferred to a hospital with specialized care units. Care is exercised to maintain the position and continue suctioning during transport. Specially designed units are equipped for transporting infants to criti-

Summary of nursing care of the infant with esophageal atresia and tracheoesophageal fistula—cont'd

Goals	Responsibilities
Postoperative—cont'd	
Administer postoperative nutrition	Administer gastrostomy feedings when tolerated Progress to oral feedings as prescribed according to child's condition
Control pneumonia	Administer antibiotics as ordered Administer oxygen as needed Suction secretions Position for optimum ventilation
Administer comfort measures	Provide tactile stimulation Position comfortably postoperatively Avoid restraints where possible Administer mouth care
Educate parents in home care	Teach parents Positioning Signs of respiratory distress Signs of contracture—refusal to eat, dysphagia, increased coughing Care of gastrostomy and esophagostomy when infant has staged surgery including techniques such as suctioning, care of operative site and/or ostomies, dressing changes, and so on Assist in acquiring needed equipment and services
Administer oral feedings	Teach to take feedings orally after repair Introduce foods one at a time Provide foods with various textures and flavors Begin with slightly liquid feedings and progress to more solid food
Maintain contact with family	Refer to appropriate clinics and/or agencies for needed services Continue nursing follow-up care

cal care facilities. During transport the infant is accompanied by a physician, nurse, or a physician/nurse team (see p. 325 for transportation of high-risk infants).

Postoperative care. Postoperative care for these infants is essentially the same as for any high-risk newborn (see p. 330). The infant is returned to the warm, high-humidity atmosphere of the Isolette, and the gastrostomy tube is returned to gravity drainage until the infant can tolerate feedings, usually the second or third postoperative day. At this time the tube is elevated and secured at a point above the level of the stomach. This allows gastric secretions to pass to the duodenum, whereas swallowed air can escape through the open tube. If tolerated, gastrostomy feedings are continued until the esophagus anastomosis is healed, about the tenth to fourteenth day, after which oral feedings are initiated.

The initial attempt at oral feeding must be carefully observed to make certain that the infant is able to swallow without choking. Oral feedings are begun with glucose water followed by frequent, small feedings of formula. Until the infant is able to take a sufficient amount by mouth, oral intake may need to be supplemented by gastrostomy feedings. Ordinarily the infant is not discharged until he is taking oral fluids well and the gastrostomy tube has been removed. However, the infant who has undergone palliative surgery will be discharged with the gastrostomy tube in place. The nurse is responsible for making certain that the care giver is educated and practiced in the care of the gastrostomy (see p. 945).

Special problems. Upper respiratory complications are a threat to life in both the preoperative and postoperative period. In addition to pneumonia, there is a constant danger of respiratory embarrassment resulting from atelectasis, pneumothorax, and laryngeal edema. Any persistent respiratory difficulty after removal of secretions is reported to the surgeon immediately.

In the infant awaiting esophageal replacement surgery, the catheter is removed and the upper esophageal segment is drained by means of an artificial opening in the neck (cervical esophagostomy), which allows escape of the swallowed saliva. This is a source of annoyance as the skin may become irritated by moisture from the continual discharge of saliva. Frequent removal of drainage and application of a thin layer of protective ointment are usually sufficient treatment.

Meeting the oral needs of infants who are unable to suck on a bottle should not be overlooked. A pacifier offered periodically is an acceptable substitute until oral feedings are instituted. The child who has corrective surgery delayed until 18 to 24 months of age may have a different problem. Some children who have not been able to go through the processes of eating in the normal manner have difficulty with this new task and require patient, firm guidance in learning the techniques of taking food into the mouth and swallowing.

Discharge. Preparing parents for discharge of their infant involves teaching the techniques that will be continued in home care such as careful suctioning, gastrostomy feeding, and so on. The parents are taught child or infant behaviors that might be expected after corrective surgery, such as those that indicate that the child needs to be suctioned, signs of respiratory difficulty, and signs that indicate constricture of the esophagus. They are reminded that it is particularly important to guard against the child swallowing foreign objects. With a child in any of the stages of locomotion this is no simple problem. Parents will also need help in acquiring needed equipment, such as a suction machine, and special services, for example, crippled children's services.

See the boxed material on pp. 404 to 405 for a summary of nursing care of the infant with esophageal atresia and tracheoesophageal fistula.

ANORECTAL MALFORMATIONS

Malformations in the anorectal region of the gastrointestinal tract are manifest in several variations, all classified as *imperforate anus*. They are among the more common congenital malformations caused by abnormal development (approximately one in 5000).

The most widely used classification describing anorectal malformations is illustrated and described in Fig. 11-20. The rectum may end blindly or may have a fistulous connection to the perineum, urethra, bladder, or, in females, the vagina. In 10% of anorectal anomalies the anal aperture is small (anal stenosis) (Fig. 11-20, *A*). Incomplete obliteration of the anal membrane results in anal membrane atresia, also called imperforate anal membrane or membranous obstruction of the anus (Fig. 11-20, *B*). In anal agenesis the rectal pouch ends blindly above the perineal surface (Fig. 11-20, *C*). The pouch may end "low" near the surface or "high," 1.5 cm or more from the surface. This type of deformity occurs in 80% of anorectal anomalies, and fistulas are present in 80% to 90% of these cases (Fig. 11-20, *E* and *F*). An anal dimple may or may not be present. Rectal atresia consists of a normal anus with a blind rectal pouch and may be mistaken for a normal rectum unless a careful examination is done (Fig. 11-20, *D*).

Etiology and pathophysiology

About the seventh week of gestation the future rectum and anus develop from an expanded portion of the caudal hindgut, the *cloaca,* which is subsequently divided by downward growth of a urorectal septum into a urogenital sinus and a rectum. At about the same time, the lower urogenital portion has acquired an external opening whereas the rectum is separated from the exterior by the *anal membrane*. This membrane breaks down by the beginning of the eighth week of gestation to form a continuous patent communication between the outside and the remainder of the gut. Most anorectal malformations result from abnormal partitioning of the cloaca by the urorectal septum. A large number of infants with anorectal defects will have another serious associated congenital anomaly, the most common of which are those involving the genitourinary tract, heart, and esophagus.

Diagnostic evaluation

Checking for patency of the anus and rectum are routine parts of the newborn assessment, including observation or inquiries regarding the passage of meconium. Inspection of the perineal area reveals absence of an anal opening or the thin translucent membrane of anal membrane atresia. Digital and endoscopic examination identify constriction or the blind pouch of rectal atresia. Stenosis may not become apparent until 1 year of age or older when the child has a history of difficult defecation, abdominal distention, and ribbon-like stools. Fistulas associated with types B and C anomalies are not usually apparent at birth, but as peristalsis gradually forces the meconium through the fistula they can be identified by careful examination. A rectourinary fistula is diagnosed on the basis of meconium in the urine.

Definitive diagnosis of the extent and location of the rectal pouch is made by x-ray examination. With the infant inverted and an opaque marker at the anal dimple, air ascending into the rectum and lower bowel will outline the location of the pouch in relation to the anal depression. The infant should be thoroughly evaluated for the presence of other anomalies.

Medical management

Successful treatment for anal stenosis is generally accomplished by manual dilatations. The procedure, begun

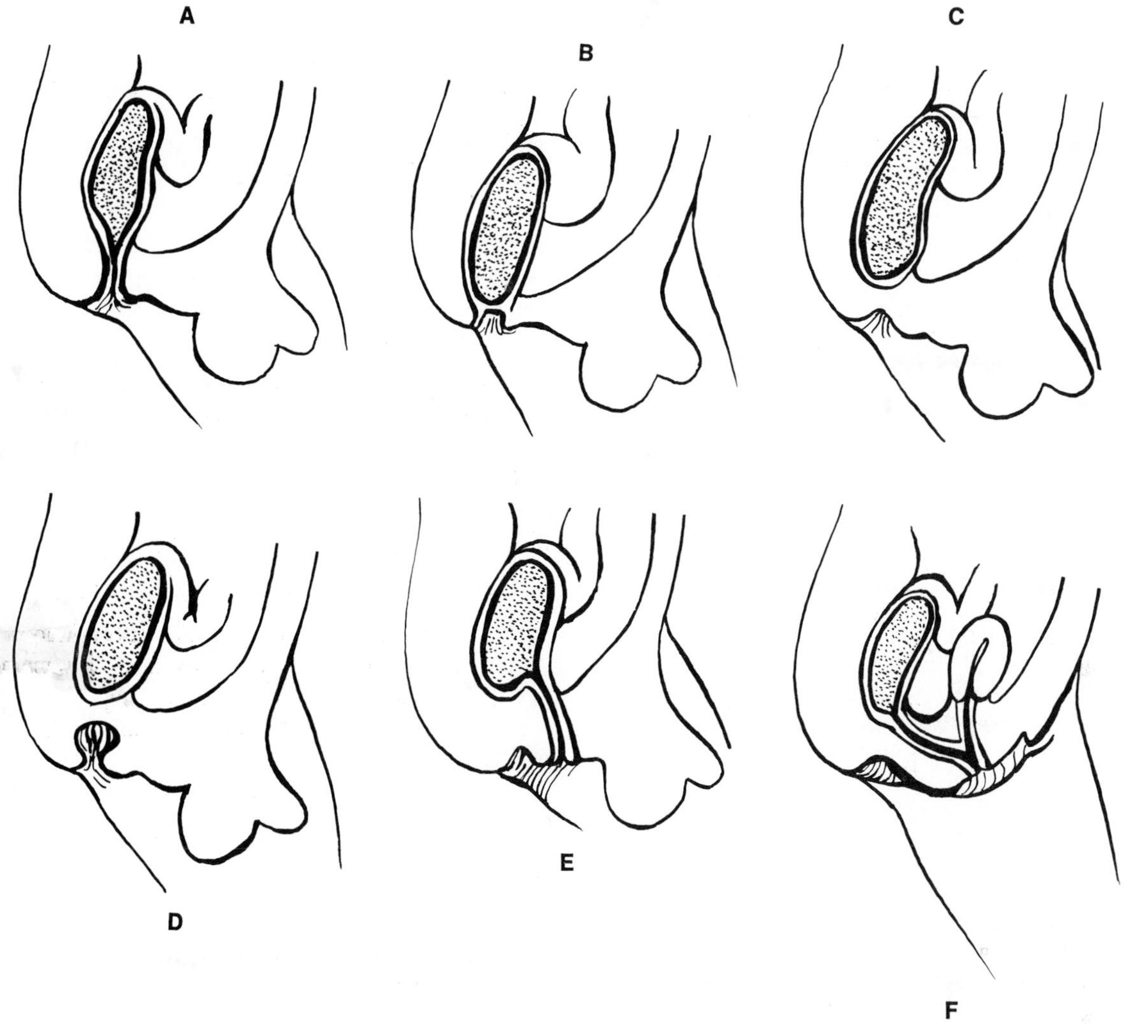

Fig. 11-20. Anorectal stenosis and imperforate anus. **A,** Congenital anal stenosis; **B,** anal membrane atresia; **C,** anal agenesis; **D,** rectal atresia; **E,** rectoperitoneal fistula; **F,** rectovaginal fistula.

by the physician, is repeated on a regular basis by the nurses in the hospital and continued at home by the parents, after they are carefully instructed in the technique. An imperforate anal membrane is excised and followed by daily anal dilatations.

Reconstruction of an anus in the proper position is the goal of surgical treatment of other anorectal malformations. The most important consideration in the probable success of reconstruction is the level at which the rectum terminates, especially in its relationship to the puborectalis sling of the levator ani muscle. Where the bowel has come through this structure, surgical correction often can be accomplished in the neonatal period by way of an abdominal-perineal pull-through procedure and/or anoplasty. Infants with higher anomalies require a divided sigmoid colostomy in the newborn period. This allows time for the infant to gain weight, a more leisurely evaluation of the anomaly, and protection of the genitourinary tract from fecal contamination from a fistula. Antibiotics are usually administered prophylactically. Final correction of higher defects is usually postponed for a year.

Nursing considerations

The first nursing responsibility is identification of undetected anorectal malformations. The undetected deformity is most often revealed when the nurse finds it impossible to insert a thermometer when taking the initial rectal temperature. A newborn who does not pass a stool within 24 hours of birth requires further assessment, and meconium that appears at an inappropriate orifice should be reported.

Postoperative nursing care ordinarily presents few problems and is primarily directed toward healing of the anoplasty without infection or other complications. Where the infant has undergone a pull-through procedure with anoplasty, special nursing care involves maintaining the anal area as clean as possible with scrupulous perineal care.

There may or may not be a temporary dressing and drain, but, when the infant is passing stool, dressings are of little value. The preferred position is a side-lying prone position with the hips elevated or a supine position with the legs suspended at a 90-degree angle to the trunk to prevent pressure on perineal sutures. Periodic application of a heat lamp facilitates healing.

The infant is administered regular infant formula as soon as peristalsis returns. In the meantime there may be a nasogastric tube for abdominal decompression and intravenous feedings. Care of the infant with a colostomy involves frequent dressing changes, meticulous skin care, and correct application of a collection device (see p. 929).

Hernias

A hernia is a protrusion of a portion of an organ or organs through an abnormal opening. The danger from herniation arises when the organ protruding through the opening is constricted to the extent that circulation is impaired or when the protruding organs encroach upon and impair the function of other structures. The herniations of concern here are those that protrude through the diaphragm, the abdominal wall, or the inguinal canal. A summary of hernias including site, diagnostic evaluation, medical and nursing management, and outcome is outlined in Table 11-5.

HERNIAS THROUGH DIAPHRAGM

The diaphragm forms between the eighth and tenth weeks of fetal life from four separate embryonic structures that fuse to form the partition that separates the thoracic and abdominal cavities. Failure of these diaphragmatic components to fuse at the proper time and place produces an abnormal opening between the two cavities. The diaphragm normally contains apertures through which the esophagus and great vessels traverse the partition. If an aperture is larger than normal, it allows other structures to protrude through the opening. The degree and timing of the clinical manifestations depend on the degree to which abdominal viscera encroach upon the thoracic structures.

Diaphragmatic hernia

In congenital herniations through a large diaphragmatic defect on the left side, it is not unusual to find most of the abdominal organs (stomach, small intestine, spleen, left lobe of liver, left kidney, and all but the descending colon) in the thorax. Ineffective motion of the leaf of the diaphragm on the affected side interferes with the normal diaphragmatic breathing of the neonate. Respiration is further compromised by atelectasis of the lung on the affected side and by the stomach and intestine (generally found within the chest), which rapidly become distended with swallowed air as the result of crying. Moreover, this increased volume in the chest cavity displaces the mediastinum to the unaffected side to produce a partial collapse of the opposite lung. The infant should be positioned on the affected side to take advantage of gravity, which facilitates expansion of the unaffected lung.

The affected infant requires immediate respiratory support, which includes administration of oxygen, nasogastric suction for decompression of the stomach, and conscientious efforts to prevent the infant from crying. Negative thoracic pressure from crying tends to pull the intestines into the chest and further distend those already there. Following these and other preparations the infant is taken to surgery or transported to a special facility for surgical repair of the defect.

When the abdominal viscera are replaced in the abdomen and the defect repaired, the infant recovers with the usual postoperative care and management. Fatalities are usually the consequence of pulmonary insufficiency caused by the compressed and often hypoplastic lung on the affected side. Contributing factors include circulatory problems secondary to a mediastinal shift, pulmonary infection, and complications associated with a high incidence of prematurity and other anomalies.

Hiatal hernia

Congenital herniations through the normal esophageal hiatus in the newborn are usually of the sliding type. Because the muscular ring of the hiatus is not snug, it permits the cardiac end of the stomach to slide above the diaphragm and back into the abdomen. This produces the symptoms seen with associated incompetent or relaxed cardiac sphincter *(chalasia),* that is, reflux of gastric contents into the esophagus with subsequent regurgitation. When conservative management such as upright posture and feeding modification is disappointing, the defect is repaired surgically.

HERNIAS THROUGH ABDOMINAL WALL

Herniations of abdominal contents through openings in the abdominal wall are usually confined to the midline or located symmetrically in the lower abdominal wall. This discussion is limited to the more common hernias that are located at sites of important embryologic activity—the umbilicus and inguinal-perineal areas.

Umbilical hernia

Ordinarily the umbilical ring, through which the umbilical blood vessels provide essential elements to the developing fetus, undergoes spontaneous, gradual closure after birth. Incomplete closure of this fascial ring results in the protrusion of portions of omentum and intestine through the opening. The size of the defect varies from less than

1 cm to 4 or 5 cm. The hernias are seen as soft swellings or protrusions covered by skin that are readily reducible with the finger, and small defects usually close spontaneously by 1 or 2 years of age. Very large hernias often persist. Those that have not disappeared by school age require surgical closure.

Because the sight of an umbilical hernia is very disconcerting to parents, they need reassurance regarding the innocuous nature of the defect. Taping or strapping appears to be of no value in expediting closure and may even cause troublesome skin irritation. Strangulation or incarceration of herniated bowel is rare but requires immediate surgical intervention.

Omphalocele

Omphalocele is a serious congenital malformation in which a variable amount of the abdominal contents protrudes into the base of the umbilical cord. As the embryonic midgut grows and elongates, it projects from the abdomen, which is too small to contain it, into the umbilical cord. This migration takes place from the sixth to the tenth week of fetal life. Normally the intestines return rapidly into the abdomen by the eleventh week of gestation; failure to return produces an omphalocele. In contrast to an umbilical hernia, the omphalocele is covered only by a translucent sac of amnion to which the umbilical cord inserts. The sac may contain only a small loop of bowel or most of the bowel, and other abdominal viscera. If the sac ruptures, the abdominal contents eviscerate through the opening in the abdominal wall. The abdomen is smaller than usual, making replacement of the bowel more difficult.

The treatment is immediate surgical repair before infection or tissue damage takes place. The omphalocele is covered immediately with moist gauze and kept moist until the infant is taken to the operating room. When the abdomen is too small to accommodate the extruded contents, a protective sac of Silastic or other synthetic material is constructed to contain the omphalocele to aid in reduction of the viscera until surgical closure is attempted. Rarely nonoperative treatment, consisting of repeated application of a cicatrizing or toughening solution to the sac, is used with excessively large omphaloceles. Complications include infection, rupture, and intestinal obstruction. The defect is often associated with other malformations. Special nursing care consists of careful positioning and handling to prevent infection or rupture of the sac.

Inguinal hernia

Inguinal hernia is derived from persistence of all or part of the processus vaginalis, the tube of peritoneum that precedes the testicle through the inguinal canal into the scrotum during the eighth month of gestation. Following descent of the testicle, the proximal portion of the processus vaginalis normally atrophies and closes whereas the distal portion forms the tunica vaginalis, which envelopes the testicle in the scrotum. When the upper portion fails to atrophy, the abdominal fluid or an abdominal structure can be forced into it, creating a palpable bulge or mass. The persistent sac may end at any point along the inguinal canal; it may stop at the inguinal ring or extend all the way into the scrotum (Fig. 11-21). The hernial sac is present at birth but does not usually become apparent until the infant is able to build up sufficient intra-abdominal pressure to open the sac, usually 2 to 3 months of age. Since the inguinal canal is short, hernias occur relatively early. Inguinal hernia occurs much more frequently in boys (90%), but it is seen in girls, also.

Diagnostic evaluation. This very common defect is asymptomatic unless the abdominal contents are forced into the patent sac. Most often it appears as a painless inguinal swelling that varies in size. It disappears during periods of rest or is reducible by gentle compression; it appears when the infant cries or strains or when the older child strains, coughs, or stands for a long period. The defect can be palpated as a thickening of the cord in the groin, and the ''silk glove'' sign can be elicited by rubbing together the sides of the empty hernial sac.

Sometimes the herniated loop of intestine becomes partially obstructed, producing variable symptoms that may include fretfulness and irritability, tenderness, anorexia, abdominal distention, and difficulty in defecating. Occasionally the loop of bowel becomes incarcerated (irreducible), with symptoms of complete intestinal obstruction that, left untreated, will progress to strangulation and gangrene. Incarceration occurs more often in infants under 10 months of age and is more common in girls.

Medical management. The treatment for hernias is prompt, elective surgical repair in healthy infants and children as soon as the defect is diagnosed. Many physicians advocate exploration of both sides since there is a high incidence of recurrence on the contralateral side. This remains controversial, however. It is preferable to attempt reduction of a recently incarcerated hernia in order that surgery can be delayed to allow the injured tissues to recover somewhat, but irreducible or strangulated hernias are treated as emergencies.

Nursing considerations. Both infants and children tolerate surgery very well. There is usually no restriction placed on their activities, and it is not uncommon for the child to be discharged from the hospital on the day of surgery. Every attempt is made to keep the wound clean and reasonably dry. With infants and small children who are not yet diaper trained, the wound is left without a dressing. Changing diapers as soon as they become damp helps reduce the chance of irritation or infection of the incision, or the child may be left undiapered. It is seldom necessary to apply a urine-collecting device, and in doing so it is often difficult or impossible to avoid the incision.

Table 11-5. Summary outline of diaphragmatic, abdominal, and inguinal hernias

Type	Site of herniation	Diagnostic evaluation
Diaphragmatic		
Through foramen of Bochdalek	Posterolateral (80% on left) or retrosternal (rare—1%)	Symptoms—mild to severe respiratory distress within a few hours after birth; tachypnea, cyanosis, dyspnea, and severe acidosis Breath sounds absent in affected area; bowel sounds may be present Rarely asymptomatic Diagnosis made by x-ray study
Through foramen of Morgagni	Anteromedial through slits in attachment of diaphragmatic muscle	Symptoms—vague, including substernal pain and indigestion Diagnosis made by x-ray study
Hiatal		
Sliding	Esophageal hiatus Esophagogastric junction, located above hiatus	Symptoms—dysphagia, failure to thrive, vomiting, neck contortions, frequent unexplained respiratory problems, bleeding, incompetent cardiac sphincter Diagnosis made by fluoroscopy
Paraesophageal	Esophagus normal to hiatus; stomach herniated into thorax through hiatus	Symptoms of esophageal stricture
Abdominal		
Omphalocele	Anterior abdominal wall at base of umbilical cord	Obvious on inspection Observation for other malformations
Umbilical	Umbilicus	Inspection and palpation of abdomen High incidence in black infants
Inguinal	Right or left inguinal canal Higher incidence in males Higher incidence on right side Often bilateral	History of intermittent appearance of mass in inguinal area History of symptoms Palpation of mass

Medical management	Nursing considerations	Outcome
Supportive treatment of respiratory distress and correction of acidosis Prophylactic antibiotic administration Surgical reduction of hernia and repair of defect	Preoperative Prevent crying Carry out distressing procedures at one time Maintain suction, oxygen, and intravenous fluids Place in semi-Fowler's position Assist with diagnostic and preoperative procedures Administer medications Postoperative Carry out routine postoperative care and observation Use comfort measures Support parents	Untreated—symptoms are progressive Treated—uneventful recovery anticipated Fatalities caused by respiratory insufficiency, circulatory problems, prematurity, and associated anomalies
Surgical repair of defect	Be alert to significant signs Carry out routine postoperative care	Usually cause no problems in newborn period High incidence of complications if untreated, including strangulation
Conservative Positioning, modified feeding, mild sedation, and sometimes anticholinergics and antacids Operative Esophageal dilatation or surgical repair of hiatus	Position in semiupright posture Give small, frequent feedings with bubbling Use comfort measures to reduce irritability and distress Teach parents	Gastroesophageal reflux with aspiration pneumonia Esophagitis followed by severe esophageal stricture
Surgical "snugging" of hiatus	Carry out routine nursing management	Satisfactory
Preoperative Prevention of drying, rupture of the sac, or eviscerated bowel Give intravenous fluids Central venous hyperalimentation in long-term care Bowel decompression Prophylactic antibiotic administration Surgical repair of defect	Keep sac or viscera moist Use Isolette for warmth Carry out routine care of intravenous line, nasogastric suction Give nothing by mouth Use comfort measures	Depends on extent of defect
No treatment of small defects Operative repair if persists to age 2 to 5 years Strangulation requires immediate attention	No special care required Reassure parents	Spontaneous closure by age 1 to 2 years
Surgical repair Bilateral exploration recommended	Carry out routine postoperative care Child can resume normal activities	High incidence of recurrence on opposite side

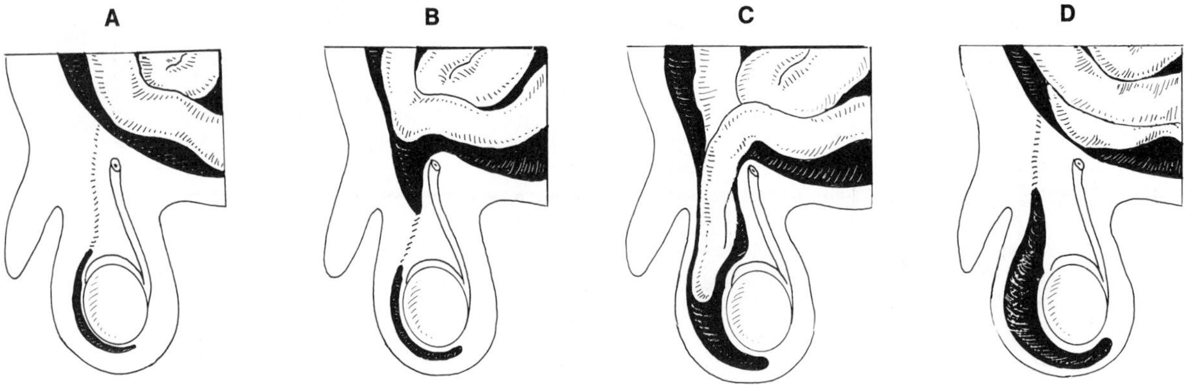

Fig. 11-21. Inguinal hernias. **A,** Normal; **B,** partially obliterated processus vaginalis; **C,** hernia; **D,** hydrocele.

Hydrocele

Hydrocele is the presence of fluid in the persistent processus vaginalis and is the result of the same developmental process as inguinal hernia (Fig. 11-21, *D*). When the upper segment of the processus vaginalis has been obliterated but the tunic vaginalis still contains peritoneal fluid, this is called a *noncommunicating hydrocele*. This type of hydrocele is common in newborns and often subsides spontaneously as fluid is gradually absorbed.

A *communicating hydrocele* is one in which the processus vaginalis remains open and into which peritoneal fluid may be forced by intra-abdominal pressure and gravity. The length of the hydrocele depends on the length of the processus vaginalis and may extend into the tunica vaginalis within the scrotum. The hydrocele is asymptomatic except for a palpable bulge in the inguinal or scrotal areas. Unlike a hernia, the hydrocele is unable to be reduced and cannot be produced by a sudden increase in intra-abdominal pressure (such as straining). The scrotum appears to be larger after an active day and smaller in the mornings. Since a hydrocele represents a patent processus vaginalis, it can predispose to herniation; therefore, surgical repair is indicated.

Defects of genitourinary tract

External defects of the genitourinary tract are usually obvious at birth. Several, such as hypospadias, epispadias, and undescended testes (cryptorchidism), do not necessitate immediate repair but may require one or more staged repairs during early childhood. Others, such as exstrophy of the bladder, require initial intervention at birth with repeated medical and surgical treatment for several years. The anatomic location of these defects frequently causes more psychologic concern to children and parents than does the actual condition or treatment.

HYPOSPADIAS

Hypospadias refers to a condition in which the urethral opening is located behind the glans penis or anywhere along the ventral surface of the penile shaft (Fig. 11-22). In very mild cases the meatus is just off center from the tip of the penis. In the most severe malformations the meatus is located on the perineum between the two halves of the scrotum. Chordee, or ventral curvature of the penis, results from the replacement of normal skin with a fibrous band of tissue, causing constriction of the penis. In addition the foreskin is usually absent ventrally and, when combined with chordee, gives the organ a hooded and crooked appearance (Fig. 11-23). The altered appearance may leave the sex in doubt at birth, since the perineal position of the meatus may be mistaken for a female urethra. Since undescended testes may also be present, the small penis may appear to be an enlarged clitoris. Occasionally a vaginal vault is also found, further complicating the sexual identity. In any case of ambiguous genitalia, further study, such as chromosomal analysis, is essential.

Surgical correction

The principal objectives in surgical correction are (1) to enable the child to void in the standing position by voluntarily directing the stream in the usual manner, (2) to improve the physical appearance of the genitalia for psychologic reasons, and (3) to produce a sexually adequate organ. The procedure involves releasing the chordee, extending the length of the urethra, and constructing a new meatal opening. Since the prepuce is valuable skin for the reconstructive surgery, circumcision should not be done on these infants. A minimal defect without chordee usually requires no

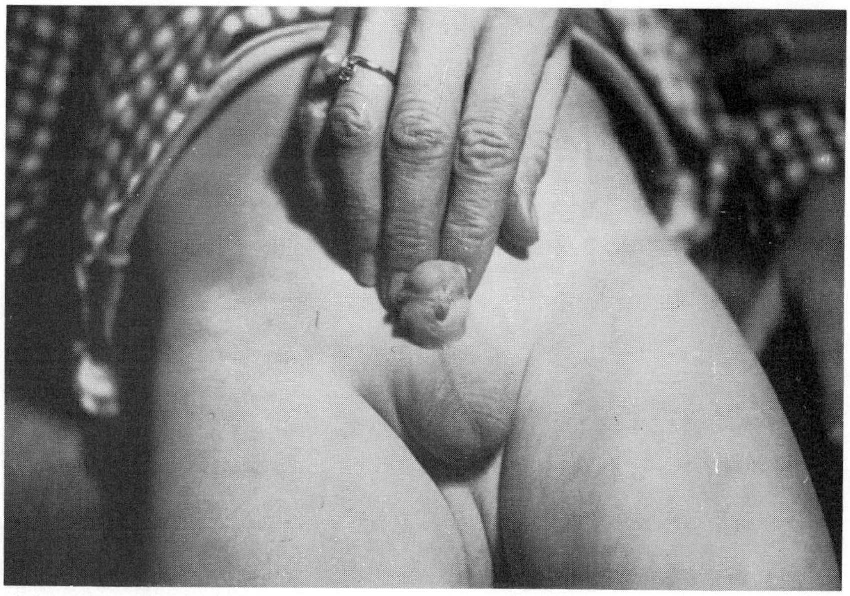

Fig. 11-22. Hypospadias. (Courtesy M. C. Gleason, M. D., San Diego, Calif. From Ingalls, A. J., and Salerno, M. C.: Maternal and child health nursing, ed. 4, St. Louis, 1979, The C. V. Mosby Co.)

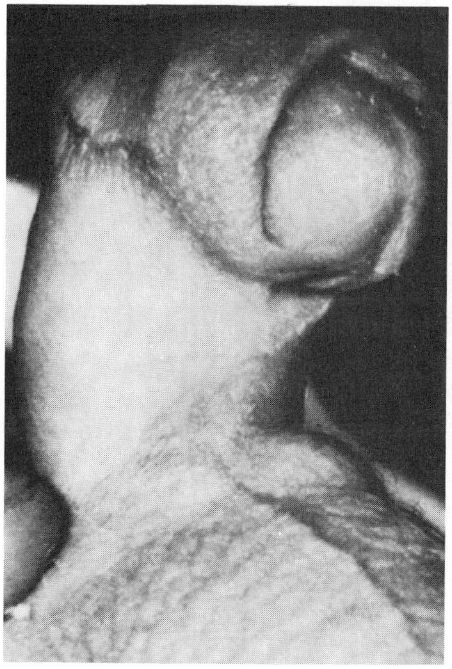

Fig. 11-23. Hypospadias with significant chordee. (From Shirkey, H. C.: Pediatric therapy, ed. 5, St. Louis, 1975, The C. V. Mosby Co., p. 1123.)

treatment except perhaps for cosmetic reasons; when the meatus is located on the glans penis, no intervention may be required except to release the chordee. When the hypospadias is more severe, the repair often requires more than one surgical procedure, progressively extending the length of the urethra. The surgery is usually performed at about 3 years of age when the phallus is of sufficient size and the child has not yet developed mutilation anxiety and is not yet attending school. Sometimes repairs for more severe cases of hypospadias may result in fistulas and strictures, necessitating additional surgical intervention.

Psychologic problems

The location of the defect and the need for repeated surgery cause these children more emotional concern than does the actual defect. Voiding usually presents no problem when diapers are used, and the infant and young child are not unduly affected by an altered body image. However, initial repairs, such as release of the chordee, are performed early, which imposes hospitalization and possible separation from parents on the child. Delaying the repair until later years increases the anxieties of castration and mutilation in preschool children. In addition parental concerns for acceptable physical appearance and adequate future sexual competency may be transmitted to the child.

Nursing considerations

Preparation of parents and child for the type of procedure to be done and the expected cosmetic result helps avert later problems. Frequently parents are informed of what is to be surgically corrected but are not advised of what to expect as a reasonable consequence. As a result they are greatly disappointed to see a physically imperfect penis. If the child is old enough to understand what is occurring, he is also prepared for the operation and the expected outcome. It is particularly important to emphasize that the operation is necessary because of a problem he was born with and is in no way a punishment for misdeeds or thought. Considering the sexual curiosity of preschoolers, the operation can be mistakenly viewed as retribution for masturbation, sex play, or erotic feelings. Correction of the deformity should be completed before entrance into school to prevent criticism and embarrassment from peers and to foster a more positive body image.

Urethroplasty usually requires some type of urinary diversion to promote optimal healing and to maintain the position and patency of the newly formed urethra. The nurse employs all measures to avoid infection of the urinary tract and operative site.

EPISPADIAS

In this congenital anomaly the urethra is located on the dorsal surface of the penis. As in hypospadias the defect can occur in differing degrees of severity. In the mildest cases the meatus is located in front of the glans penis. In the most severe instance epispadias extends to exstrophy of the bladder. The treatment is surgical and usually requires more than one procedure. The psychologic problems and nursing considerations are similar to those discussed under hypospadias.

EXSTROPHY OF BLADDER

Exstrophy of the bladder is an obvious and serious congenital defect that occurs three times more frequently in males than in females (Fig. 11-24). There is no familial tendency, although rarely it occurs in siblings. There are varying degrees of the defect, ranging from an abdominal opening (epispadias) to vestiges of the primitive cloaca, embryonic endodermal tissue from which the bladder is eventually derived. Incontinence accompanies all degrees of the anomaly.

Etiology and pathophysiology

Exstrophy results from failure of the abdominal wall and underlying structures, such as the ventral wall of the bladder, to fuse in utero. As a result the lower urinary tract is exposed. The everted bladder appears bright red through the abdominal opening. The abnormal ureteral outlets and the external urethral meatus cause a constant seepage of urine, making the area malodorous and highly susceptible to infection. The constant accumulation of urine on the surrounding skin promotes tissue ulceration and further infection. Progressive renal damage from infection and obstruction may terminate in renal failure.

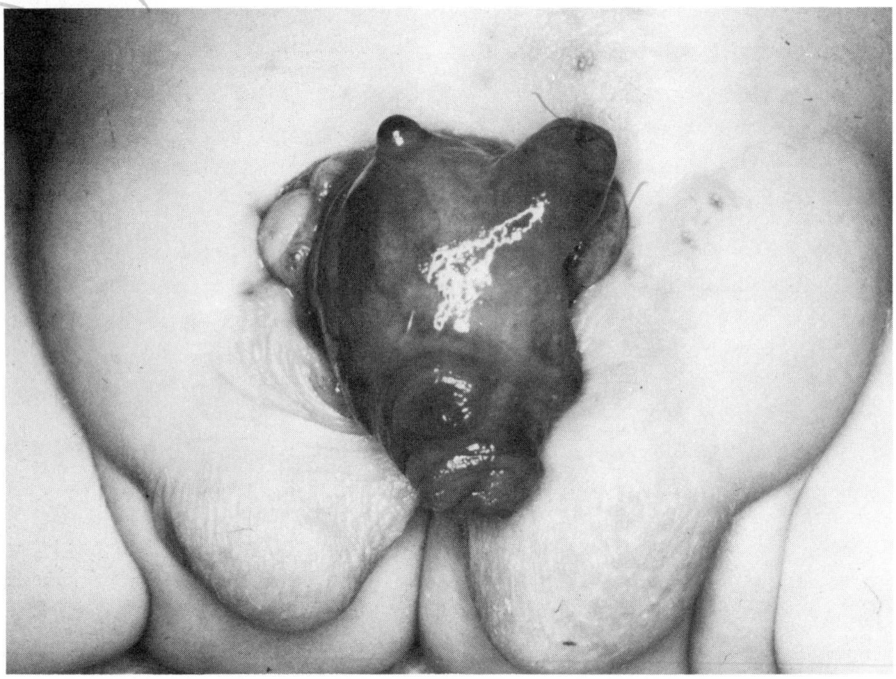

Fig. 11-24. Exstrophy of bladder. (Courtesy E. S. Tank, M. D., Division of Urology, University of Oregon Health Sciences Center, Portland, Oreg. From Jensen, M. D., Benson, R. C., and Bobak, I. M.: Maternity care: the nurse and the family, St. Louis, 1977, The C. V. Mosby Co., p. 590.)

In males the defect may be associated with other problems, such as undescended testes, a short penis, epispadias, or inguinal hernia. The sexual handicap in males may be severe because the penis protrudes inadequately. In females the genitalia may be affected, with a cleft clitoris, completely separated labia, and absent vagina. In either sex, separation of the pubic bones causes difficulty in walking, such as a waddling gait.

Medical management

The objectives of treatment include (1) preservation of renal function, (2) attainment of urinary control, (3) adequate reconstructive repair for psychologic benefit, and (4) improvement of sexual function, particularly in males. The success of each of these goals depends on the severity of the exstrophy. The exact surgical intervention is frequently a matter of preference. However, in those cases where continence is not possible, some type of urinary diversion is generally necessary, such as ureteral sigmoid implant, bilateral ureterostomy, or ileal conduit. In a *sigmoid implant* the ureters are transplanted into the sigmoid portion of the lower colon. Urine is then continually passed with stool. When the child is old enough to learn bowel control, he is taught to constrict the anal sphincter for voluntary elimination of stool and urine. However, complications from this procedure are common and serious. Chronic infection from ascending colonic bacteria and hydronephrosis from reflex and backup of urine into the pelvis of the kidneys cause progressive renal damage.

A more satisfactory procedure, and the one that is usually performed, is an *ileal conduit,* also called a ureteroileal cutaneous ureterostomy. A small section of the ileum or colon is resected, and the remaining bowel is reanastomosed. The physiologic characteristics of the colon appear to make it a more suitable conduit than the ileum, because the colon eventually becomes peristaltically inert.[15] One end of the resected bowel is sutured closed and the other end is attached to a small opening in the lower abdomen, forming a stoma. The distal ends of the ureters are severed from the bladder and attached to the ileum, which acts like a bladder, although there is no voluntary control in the regulation of voiding. The child wears an ileostomy appliance over the stoma, which collects the continuously flowing urine. In a young child diapers serve the same purpose as the collecting appliance, although the surrounding skin must be kept clean and relatively dry of urine to prevent excoriation. A complication of this type of urinary diversion is gradual dilation of the urinary tract from occasional stomal occlusion caused by constricting clothing, body posture, or the diversion appliance, which produces high pressure in the conduit and ureters.

In a cutaneous *ureterostomy* the ureters are attached directly to the abdominal wall, usually at a site proximal to the level of the kidneys. A collecting appliance may also be worn, although in exstrophy of the bladder two appliances are necessary to accommodate the bilateral openings. Infection is more common because of the short length of the ureters, and general care is more cumbersome. Usually ureterostomy is a method of choice for temporary urinary diversion to prevent renal function deterioration.

Nursing considerations

One of the most devastating aspects of exstrophy of the bladder is its gross appearance. Parents must first deal with the loss of the perfect child before being able to learn the nursing aspects of general care and to comprehend the potential lifelong handicaps imposed by a severe defect. The nurse's acceptance of the child is an important component of care in helping the parents adjust to this anomaly.

Frequently surgical intervention is delayed until the infant has attained more physiologic maturity to withstand the operation and increased body growth to allow for improved abdominal closure. As a result the newborn may be discharged from the nursery before the parents have had sufficient opportunity to adjust to the defect and learn the procedures for home care. It is advisable to prolong the hospital stay of mother and child until at least one parent feels somewhat comfortable in caring for the child and the nurse has had an opportunity to evaluate that parent's ability. Although the actual procedures are not difficult, it is not easy for parents to assume responsibility for what to them seems an enormous task because of the emotional impact of the defect. Care includes meticulous hygiene of the bladder area to prevent infection and excoriation of the surrounding tissue. Sterile petrolatum gauze is placed over the exposed bladder area to prevent infection and to keep the diaper from adhering to the mucosa. Some type of ointment may be prescribed for the surrounding skin to protect it from the constantly draining urine. Ordinarily diapers are placed over the defect in the usual manner, although extra thickness may be added with an additional cloth diaper wrapped around the lower abdomen for added absorbency. Diapers are changed frequently to prevent infection, ulceration, and odor and immediately after a bowel movement to prevent contamination of the exposed area. The presence of continually draining urine makes controlling odor a difficult and embarrassing problem, especially for older children. Rubber pants or tight, binding clothing are avoided as additional insurance against promoting infection or trauma to the exposed bladder. General infant care remains unchanged except for sponge baths rather than immersion in water. A public health referral is an important component of discharge planning, and, ideally, home visits should begin immediately after the infant's release from the hospital.

Surgical correction may require more than one procedure. Depending on the age of the child, preparation for hospitalization includes an adequate description of what can be expected postoperatively. Generally the immediate surgical concerns are closure of the opening and urinary control or diversion. Cosmetic surgery of the genitalia is deferred until later. Parents and child should be aware of this since unrealistic expectations of the cosmetic result may leave them very disappointed and discouraged. Continuous care by one nurse helps the family adjust to all aspects of recovery. Since the mother has usually established her own method and schedule of caring for the child, the nurse should encourage her to continue this in the hospital or if this is not feasible, to explain to the staff the usual home procedure. In this way the child will gain security and comfort from a continued daily routine.

As difficult as it was for parents to adjust to the defect at the time of the child's birth, it may be equally disturbing for them to accept the fact that surgical closure does not ensure normal urination and that urinary diversion is necessary. The prospect of a permanent ileal conduit or other similar procedure provokes powerful emotional responses. Parents often worry about the child's sexual adjustment, even though they may not voice such thoughts. No operation should be performed until parents (and child if old enough) are ready psychologically and emotionally. Frequently it is difficult for nurses to assess the family's degree of readiness because of a limited preoperative period. However, part of the nursing admission history is directed toward evaluating the parents' and child's expectation of the surgical repair, knowledge of the possibility of eventual ileostomy appliance for an ileal conduit or urinary control with a sigmoid implant, and feelings concerning this permanent change in body function. It is not unusual for parents to be ambivalent in their feelings, especially if they have become accustomed to the general care, which for infants differs little from diapering an unaffected child. In such situations it is well to discuss the long-range advantages of a permanent urinary diversion in contrast to the ever-present danger of infection and kidney damage and the constant inconvenience of seeping urine from incontinence. A well-fitting ileostomy bag allows the child almost unrestricted freedom in activities enjoyed by other children and results in no major alteration in toileting, except emptying the bag at periodic intervals. This is extremely important to older children and adolescents who want to be accepted as one of the group and deplore any stigma of being different.

Other aspects of preoperative care are similar to those for any major abdominal surgery. Since a routine urinalysis is part of most admission procedures, a urine specimen can be obtained by allowing urine to drip into a container by holding the child prone over a basin or by aspirating some urine directly from the bladder area into a medicine dropper or syringe. If a sterile specimen is needed for evaluation of existing infection, the former procedure is preferable, but a sterile container must be used.

Postoperative care differs little from that of any surgical patient. An abdominal dressing is placed over the closure site and is kept clean and checked for any presence of urine. If an ileal conduit or ureterostomy was performed, a separate absorbant dressing is placed over the stoma to collect the urine and prevent contamination of the other dressing. An appliance is usually fitted as soon as possible to allow the child and parents adequate time to learn its proper use and adjust to the change in body image.

Even with improved reconstructive surgery for these patients, substantial psychologic support and guidance are needed to help them adjust to their fears of inadequate penile size, ugliness of genitalia, potential inability to procreate, and rejection by peers, especially the opposite sex. Ongoing discussion groups for parents and children are particularly useful in promoting resolution of these fears and allowing for optimal psychologic adjustment, particularly during adolescence.[4]

PHIMOSIS

Phimosis is an abnormal narrowing or stenosis of the preputial opening of the foreskin over the glans penis. In an uncircumsized child the foreskin cannot be retracted over the penis, and in rare cases the narrowing obstructs the flow of urine, resulting in a dribbling stream rather than a steady flow of urine during voiding.

Etiology and pathophysiology

Phimosis can occur as a congenital anomaly or, more commonly, as a result of poor hygiene. In the latter case smegma accumulates between the prepuce and penis, infections occur, and adhesions form, preventing the easy retraction of the foreskin.

Medical management

Prevention and treatment of phimosis is circumcision. Although this procedure is performed on most male neonates, the medical indications and justifications are not well established.

Nursing considerations

True cases of congenital phimosis are rare, and proper hygiene prevents most instances of acquired phimosis. Circumcision for older children may be done to relieve the phimosis, but psychosexual factors are important to consider. For example, a 5-year-old child who had undergone circumcision for phimosis became acutely anxious and upset after surgery. He was unable to void, despite a variety of attempts to encourage micturition. The palpable bladder was proof of his need to urinate, but every suggestion to do so was met with tears. Finally the nurse asked him what he knew about this operation. He stated that his mother told him that some skin would be removed and the end of the penis stitched together. The obvious presence of the stitches was sufficient to convince him that the opening had indeed been stitched closed. The nurse clarified this misunderstanding and pointed out that the stitches were not near the opening but below the tip where the skin had been cut away. After much reassurance that the opening was still functional, the child voided with no difficulty.

Treatment of mild cases includes manual retraction of the foreskin and proper cleansing of the area. Retraction is best accomplished during the child's bath. However, caution must be exercised in instructing mothers to replace the foreskin back over the glans penis. If left retracted, the tight band of skin constricts the blood vessels, causing edema, bluish discoloration, pain, dysuria, and eventually necrosis. The resulting edema and pain further complicate attempts to replace the foreskin in its normal position. Local applications of cold compresses and use of analgesics may help, but a physician should always evaluate the condition.

CRYPTORCHIDISM

Cryptorchidism is failure of one or both testes to descend in the scrotal sac. Because the testes normally descend during the seventh to ninth month of gestation, infants born prematurely are likely to have cryptorchidism.

Etiology and pathophysiology

The cause is not known, although there is an increased chance of finding an upper urinary tract anomaly on the same side as the undescended testes. There are two types of cryptorchidism. In true, undescended testes the organ has never been in the scrotal sac but lies somewhere along the path of descent above the inguinal ring. In ectopic testes the organ has passed down the inguinal canal through the external rings but is fixed in an upward direction, such as in the perineum or proximal scrotum. Congenital hydrocele or inguinal hernias frequently accompany the defect.

Diagnostic evaluation

Diagnosis of undescended testes is complicated by the normal retraction of testes by the cremasteric reflex. This reflex is particularly sensitive to touch and cold. However, it can be obviated by placing the child in a squatting or tailor-like position or by applying firm finger pressure on the external ring before palpating the abdomen or genitalia (see Fig. 5-46). Retracted testes can be "milked" or pushed back into the scrotum, but truly undescended ones cannot. Ectopic testes may be felt along the inguinal canal, but those in the abdominal cavity usually cannot.

Medical management

In some cases hormonal therapy in the form of human chorionic gonadotropin may be initiated to help enlarge the scrotum or testes. Testes below the external ring may descend by hormonal treatment, but those lodged inside the inguinal canal or fixed in an abnormal position usually require surgical intervention (orchiopexy). Hormone treatment may be attempted during the ages of 1 to 4 years. If hormone treatment is unsuccessful, orchiopexy should be performed by the time the child is 5 years of age. If left in the abdomen any longer, the testes are likely to be damaged by the higher degree of body heat, resulting in sterility. Also, having both testes in the scrotum by school age prevents psychologic problems related to body image and peer group embarrassment, since the empty scrotum is smaller in size and altered in shape.

Adequate treatment usually results in functional testes, although infertility may be a problem if spermatic production is impaired. Undescended testes are regarded as worth saving because of their unimpaired secretion of testosterone, which is necessary for pubertal changes. Also, cancers in undescended testes are more frequent than in descended ones, although testicular cancer is rare and is not prevented by orchiopexy. Because of their increased propensity toward neoplastic changes, cryptorchid testes are better observed in the scrotal position.[15]

Nursing considerations

In the routine procedure for undescended testicles, the testes are brought down into the scrotum and secured in that position by attaching one end of a rubber band to a retraction suture in the scrotum and securing the other end to the inner thigh with adhesive tape for about 5 to 7 days. Care must be exercised to preserve this necessary tension or else the testes may reascend to an abnormal location. Infection of the operative site is prevented by careful cleansing of stool and urine. If surgery is done after the child is toilet trained, prevention of contamination is simplified.

The optimum age for treatment of cryptorchidism is influenced by several factors.[8] Many testes descend spontaneously during the first year, especially in premature infants. During the second year surgery is complicated by tissue that is still very fragile and easily traumatized. An important psychologic factor is the effect of separation on the child imposed by hospitalization.

ABERRANT SEXUAL DEVELOPMENT

The birth of a child with ambiguous genitalia is a situation that constitutes a crisis situation quite different from that of many other congenital anomalies. Uncertain sex is no threat to life in a physical sense but is a potential lifetime social tragedy for the child and family. The problem of appropriate sex must be solved quickly and accurately and requires no less speed and skill than life-threatening anomalies such as tracheoesophageal fistula. There are studies that can be carried out during the first few days of life that help guide those involved in making a correct gender choice. Even a brief delay in gender assignment can generate rumors that can be a source of distress to an infant and family for years.[3]

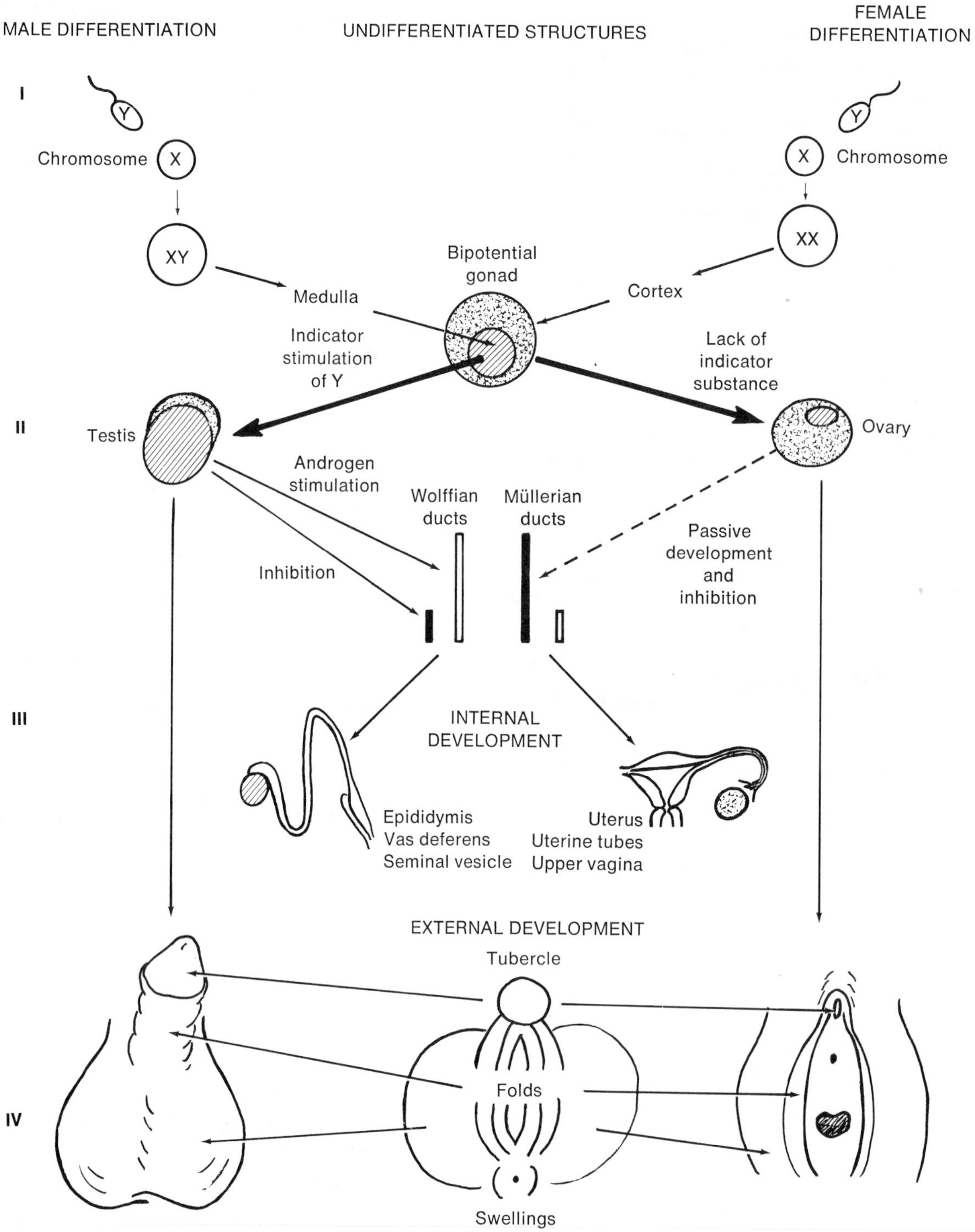

Fig. 11-25. Sex differentiation in male and female.

Etiology

Genetic sex is determined at the time of conception and depends on whether the ovum is fertilized by a sperm bearing an X chromosome or one bearing a Y chromosome. The phenotypic evidence of sex depends on whether subsequent processes proceed normally: differentiation of the primitive gonads, differentiation and development of internal duct systems, and differentiation and development of external genitalia. Disturbances in any of these processes will lead to abnormal sexual development evidenced by the presence of ambiguous genitalia at birth. The normal order of events can be altered by abnormalities of the chromosomal complement, defects of embryogenesis, or biochemical (hormonal) abnormalities.

Normal sexual development. For the first 6 weeks of life the developing embryo is morphologically neutral, neither male nor female. The primitive, bipotential (able to form either a testicle or an ovary) gonad consists of an outer layer, the cortex, and an inner medulla. Differentiation into testes and ovary takes place during the seventh and eighth weeks of gestation. At this time, in the male the medullary portion develops and the cortical zone regresses; in the female the cortex is preserved while the medulla regresses. It appears that without the presence of a masculine inductor stimulus determined by the Y chromosome the primitive gonad has an inherent tendency to feminize. The embryonic ovary develops in the absence of stimulation.

In the 7-week-old embryo the internal genital ducts of the bipotential embryo consist of both wolffian and müllerian duct systems. Differentiation of these duct systems depends on the presence or absence of locally acting male organizer substances secreted by Leydig's cells of the testes. One, an androgen, stimulates development of the wolffian duct system into epididymis, vas deferens, and seminal vesicles; another, not an androgen, actively inhibits the müllerian duct system, which subsequently regresses. In the absence of a testis the müllerian system is preserved to give rise to the uterine tubes, uterus, and upper vagina whereas the wolffian system passively regresses (Fig. 11-25).[3,20]

The final stage of sex development is differentiation of the external genitalia, which in the early embryo consists of a urogenital sinus, two lateral labioscrotal swellings, and an anteriorly situated genital tubercle. Depending on the presence or absence of male hormones, the genital tubercle differentiates into a penis or a clitoris. In response to testicular androgens, the labiosacral folds fuse to form a scrotum and ventral skin of the penis; the urethral folds form the perineal and penile urethra. Without the influence of masculinizing secretions, the urethral folds do not fuse and instead become the labia minora, the labiosacral folds remain unfused to separate into the labia majora, and the urogenital sinus differentiates into a lower vagina and the vaginal and urethral openings (see Fig. 11-25).

Abnormal sexual development. Disturbances in the normal order of events in sex determination will produce abnormal sex development with the presence of ambiguous or inappropriate external genitalia at birth. Ambiguous genitalia can be variable and often closely conform to one sex or the other. In some forms the external sexual structures represent those of a perfectly normal male or female whereas the genetic sex is the direct opposite. A situation in which the phenotypic sex differs from the chromosomal sex is often termed *intersex*.

A failure or abnormality in any of the four steps of sexual development can lead to abnormal development in subsequent stages. The mechanisms and site of defective development are summarized below.[20]

abnormal sex determination chromosomal abnormalities that result in disturbance of sexual development are discussed on p. 189 and in relation to delayed development in Chapter 20.

abnormal differentiation of gonads when induction of the bipotential gonad fails, sex differentiation proceeds in the direction of the female phenotype, regardless of the genetic sex.

abnormal differentiation of ductal systems biologic inactivity of androgenic male organizer substance or insensitivity of ductal tissue to its action results in deficient wolffian duct differentiation, whereas normal secretion of the second male organizer produces normal regression of the müllerian duct system (seen in testicular feminization syndrome). Defective function of the second male organizer substance causes persistence of the müllerian duct system, which leads to the presence of a uterus and uterine tubes, whereas the normal androgenic substance stimulates normal male differentiation (uterine hernia syndrome).

abnormal secretion of or tissue insensitivity to testicular androgen complete failure of male hormone secretion produces female external genitalia in a genetic male. Partial or incomplete failure results in incomplete masculinization with ambiguity of external genitalia. The genetic female fetus exposed to large amounts of androgenic hormone (from maternal hyperproduction, fetal adrenal hyperplasia, or maternal ingestion of androgenic steroid substances) may exhibit varying degrees of masculinization of the external genitalia (adrenal genital hyperplasia).

Types of abnormalities

Some disorders with abnormal sexual development are not characterized by ambiguous genitalia in the newborn period. For example, the most common sex chromosomal disorders do not become apparent until later childhood, adolescence, or even young adulthood when the individual seeks medical attention because of problems of delayed development or infertility. The four conditions producing ambiguous genitalia in the newborn that require prompt and accurate evaluation are: the masculinized female (female pseudohermaphrodite), the incompletely masculinized male (male pseudohermaphrodite), the true hermaphrodite, and mixed gonadal dysgenesis.

The most common condition that produces ambiguous

genitalia in the newborn is the masculinized female as the result of virilization by adrenal androgens after the time of early differentiation of gonadal tissues. The most common type, congenital adrenal hyperplasia, is caused by an inherited deficiency in the enzymes of adrenal corticoid synthesis. The resulting decrease in cortisol stimulates pituitary secretion of corticotropin (ACTH), which causes the adrenal cortex to respond with increased production of other adrenal hormones, including the androgens. Since the adrenal gland differentiates later than the gonadal duct systems but before differentiation of the external genitalia, the masculinization of the external genitalia is the predominant feature. The internal female anatomy is normal. This inherited disorder is the only intersex problem that is life-

Table 11-6. Abnormalities of sexual development

Abnormality	Genetic sex	Description	Etiology
Masculinized female (female pseudohermaphrodite)	Female XX, chromatin positive	Congenital adrenal hyperplasia	Endogenous adrenal androgens Autosomal-recessive inheritance Maternal virilizing adrenal tumor Maternal ingestion of steroids or progestinal agents
Incompletely masculinized male (male pseudohermaphrodite)	Male XY, chromatin negative	Complete testicular feminization	Inherited (autosomal dominant[?] X-linked[?])
	Male XY, chromatin negative	Incomplete testicular feminization	Inherited (autosomal dominant[?] X-linked[?])
	Male XY, chromatin negative	Pseudovaginal perineoscrotal hypospadius (PPSH)	Inherited (autosomal recessive)
Uterine hernia syndrome	Male XY, chromatin negative		Unclear
Anorchism	Male XY, chromatin negative		Unclear
True hermaphrodite	Male XY, female XX or XX/XY; chromatin variable		Unknown
Mixed gonadal dysgenesis	X/XY		Unknown
Turner's syndrome	Female X, chromatin negative		Chromosomal aberration
Klinefelter's syndrome	Male XXY, chromatin positive		Chromosomal aberration

threatening, and it should be considered in any situation where sex is doubtful. Congenital adrenal hyperplasia is discussed further in Chapter 38.

In the incompletely masculinated male the external evidence may be incompletely masculinized, ambiguous, or completely female. The complex nature of virilization offers numerous opportunities for disturbance in the process. In some disorders there is deficient production of fetal androgen, in others there is deficiency in any of the enzymes needed in the numerous steps of testosterone biosynthesis, or, more commonly, there is unresponsiveness or subresponsiveness of genital structures to testosterone. True hermaphrodites are rare and may be either genetic males or females with *both* ovarian and testicular tissues

Internal structures	External genitalia	Gender assignment	Management
Ovaries present Female duct system present Fertile at maturity if course arrested	Ambiguous with enlarged clitoris and varying degrees of labial fusion Often indistinguishable from cryptorchid male	Female	Close observation for adrenal crisis Administration of hydrocortisone for life in endogenous disorder—progressive virilization if not treated Exogenous disorder not progressive after birth Surgical correction if needed, for example, clitoral recession, vaginoplasty
Testes in abdomen, inguinal canal, or labia Duct systems present Germ cells absent or early forms	Female with blind vaginal pouch	Female	Secondary sex characteristics
Testes in abdomen, inguinal canal, or labia Duct systems present Germ cells absent or early forms	Ambiguous with blind vaginal pouch	Female	Female secondary sex characteristics (may be minimal)
Testes in labial folds, inguinal canal, or abdomen Duct systems and sperm cells (immature forms only) present	Ambiguous, severe hypospadias Blind vaginal pouch	Usually male	Masculinization at puberty
Testes in scrotum or inguinal canal Normal duct system and germ cells Hernia containing müllerian structures	Male (often cryptorchid)	Male	Normal masculinization at puberty
Absent internal genital structures and germ cells	Male (small)	Male	No secondary sex characteristics Androgen therapy at puberty
Ovary and testes or ovotestis present Germ cells present Internal structures present and correspond to adjacent gonads	Male, female, or ambiguous (majority)	Either	Sex assignment depends on predominant characteristics
Infantile uterus, vagina, and fallopian tubes present Usually a unilateral testis with streak gonad contralateral	Male, female or ambiguous	Usually female	Sex assignment depends on predominant characteristics Masculinization at puberty
Absent or mere vestiges	Female	Female	May develop varying degrees of secondary sex characteristics
Dysgenic duct system present Small testes present; germ cells absent	Male	Male	Deficient masculinization at puberty Gynecomastia common

with an ovary on one side and a testis on the other, or a combination of ovotestis. The external genitalia may be male, usually cryptorchid, or normal female, but in the majority of cases are ambiguous. The second most frequently seen disorder is mixed gonadal dysgenesis in which affected infants are sex chromosomal mosaics (see p. 190). Genitalia vary greatly, but, in those who appear predominantly female, the dysplastic testis may cause masculinization at puberty.

Some of the defects in sexual development are outlined in Table 11-6.

Diagnostic evaluation

Diagnostic tools with their corresponding significant findings that help determine gender assignment include:

history previous abortions may help identify chromosomal aberrations; ingestion of steroids; relatives with ambiguous genitalia or death in the first weeks of life.
physical examination seldom of significant value.
buccal smear detects presence or absence of sex chromatin.
chromosomal analysis detects chromosomal abnormalities and precise genetic sex.
endoscopy and x-ray contrast studies reveal presence, absence, or nature of internal genital structures.
biochemical tests urinary steroid excretion patterns help detect several of the adrenal cortical syndromes. Tests include 17-ketosteroids, 17-hydroxycorticoids, and urinary pregnanetriol.
laparotomy or **gonad biopsy** in some instances this is the only way to arrive at a definitive diagnosis.

Medical management

The assignment of a gender sex to the infant whose sex is doubtful constitutes a social emergency. The long-term implications are such that a hasty decision based on appearance alone may be disastrous, and the optimal sex of rearing may not be the same as the genetic or gonadal sex. The infant's anatomy rather than genetic sex is the primary criterion on which the choice of gender should be based. An incomplete female is better able to adjust than is an inadequate male. A functional vagina can be constructed surgically, and with appropriate administration of hormones the anatomically incomplete female can lead a relatively normal life, but it is as yet impossible to construct a satisfactory penis from an inadequate phallus for an equally satisfactory adjustment of the incomplete male.

In most instances of ambiguous genitalia it is recommended that the infant be reared as a female. Genetic males with a phallus of adequate size that will respond to testosterone at the time of puberty can be considered for male rearing. Adequate studies should be carried out early to assist in gender selection even though they may delay final sex assignment for several days or even weeks. Supportive measures, such as appropriate surgical reconstruction techniques, that provide normal-appearing internal structures are carried out. Removal of inappropriate internal structures and dysgenic gonads is recommended.

Nursing considerations

Families need a great deal of support and encouragement from nurses and other members of the health team to cope with this emotionally charged situation. Parents are confused, anxious, and overwhelmed by feelings of guilt and shame. They may pressure for immediate sex assignment because not only are they concerned about the child and the child's future but they must also face questioning relatives and friends. It requires sympathy and understanding to deal with parental anxiety during this trying period and to guide them throughout the long-term management (see also Chapter 22).

REFERENCES

1. Braney, M. L.: The child with hydrocephalus, Am. J. Nurs. **73:**828-831, 1973.
2. Brocklehurst, G.: The pathogenesis of spina bifida: a study of the relationship between observation, hypothesis, and surgical incentive, Dev. Med. Child Neurol. **13:**147, 1971.
3. Donahoe, P. K., and Hendren, W. H.: Evaluation of the newborn with ambiguous genitalia, Pediatr. Clin. North Am. **23:** 361, May 1976.
4. Feinberg, T., and associates: Questions that worry children with exstrophy, Pediatrics **53:**242-250, 1973.
5. Fraser, F. C.: The genetics of cleft lip and cleft palate, Am. J. Hum. Genet. **22:**336-352, 1970.
6. Freeman, J. M.: Quoted by Haller, J. S. In Bull, M., and associates: Myelodysplasia, Orthop. Clinics North Am. **7:**475-499, 1976.
7. Lambert, C. N., Hamilton, R. C., and Pellicore, R. J.: The juvenile amputee program: its social and economic value—a follow-up study after the age of twenty-one, J. Bone Joint Surg. **51A:**1135-1138, 1969.
8. Latimer, J., and associates: The optimum time to operate for cryptorchidism, Pediatrics **53:**96-99, 1973.
9. Lax, R. F.: Some aspects of the interaction between mother and impaired child: mother's narcissistic trauma, Int. J. Psychoanal. **53:**339-344, 1972.
10. Lorber, J.: Results of treatment of myelomeningocele, Dev. Med. Child Neurol. **13:**279-303, 1971.
11. Menkes, J. H.: Textbook of child neurology, Philadelphia, 1974, Lea & Febiger.
12. Mills, G. C.: Supporting parental needs after birth of a defective infant. In Brandt, P. A., Chinn, P. L., and Smith, M. E., editors: Current practice in pediatric nursing, vol. 1, St. Louis, 1976, The C. V. Mosby Co.
13. Passo, S. D.: Positioning infants with myelomeningocele, Am. J. Nurs. **74:**1658-1660, 1974.
14. Scott, F. B., Bradley, W. E., and Timm, G. W.: Treatment of urinary incontinence by implantable prosthetic sphincter, Urology **1:**252, 1973.
15. Scott, J.: Urinary diversion in children, Arch. Dis. Child. **48:** 199-206, 1973.
16. Seller, M. J.: Alpha-fetoprotein and the prenatal diagnosis of

neural tube defects, Dev. Med. Child Nuerol **16:**369-371, 1974.

17. Shannon, R. M.: The gastrointestinal system. In Scipien, G. M., and associates: Comprehensive pediatric nursing, New York, 1975, McGraw-Hill Book Co.
18. Solnit, A., and Stark, M.: Mourning and the birth of a defective child, Psychoanal. Study Child **16:**523-537, 1963.
19. Stark, G. D.: Neonatal assessment of the child with meningomyelocele, Arch. Dis. Child. **46:**539, 1971.
20. Summitt, R. L.: Differential diagnosis of genital ambiguity in the newborn, Clin. Obstet. Gynecol. **15:**112-139, March 1972.
21. Waechter, E.: The birth of an exceptional child, Nurs. Forum **9**(2):202, 1970.
22. Zimbler, S.: Practical considerations in the early treatment of congenital talipes equinovarus, Orthop. Clin. North Am. **3:** 251-259, 1972.

BIBLIOGRAPHY

Bergsma, D., editor: Birth defects atlas and compendium, Baltimore, 1973, The Williams & Wilkins Co.

Bleck, E. C., and Nagel, D. A., editors: Physically handicapped children, San Francisco, 1975, Grune & Stratton, Inc.

Brown, D.: Developmental handicaps in babies and young children, Springfield, Ill., 1972, Charles C Thomas, Publisher.

Conway, B. L.: Pediatric neurologic nursing, St. Louis, 1977, The C. V. Mosby Co.

Conway, B. L.: Carini and Owens' neurological and neurosurgical nursing, ed. 7, St. Louis, 1978, The C. V. Mosby Co.

Crocker, J. F. S., Brown, D. M., and Vernier, R. L.: Developmental defects of the kidneys: a review of renal development and experimental studies of maldevelopment, Pediatr. Clin. North Am. **18:**355-376, 1971.

Downey, J. A., and Low, N. L., editors: The child with disabling illness, principles of rehabilitation, Philadelphia, 1974, W. B. Saunders Co.

Freeman, J. M., editor: Neurological examination in practical management of myelomeningocele, Baltimore, 1974, University Park Press.

Galloway, K.: Early detection of congenital anomalies, J. Obstet. Gynecol. Neonatal Nurs., pp. 37-38, July/August 1973.

Gellis, S. S.: A practical approach to the child with multiple congenital anomalies, Orthop. Clin. North Am. **7:**261-264, 1976.

Grosfeld, J. L.: The youngest surgical patient, Emergency Med. **6:**93-115, 1974.

Harwood-Nash, D. C., Fit, C. R., and Reilly, B. J.: Cranial computed tomography in infants and children, Pediatr. Calif. Med. Assoc. J. **113:**546, 1975.

Holmes, J. E.: The physical therapist and team care, Nurs. Outlook **20:**182, 1972.

Janerich, D. T., Skalko, R. G., and Proter, I. H., editors: Congenital defects, new directions in research, New York, 1974, Academic Press, Inc.

Langman, J.: Medical embryology. Human development—normal and abnormal., ed. 3, Baltimore, 1975, The Williams & Wilkins Co.

Lewis, C.: Nursing care of the neonate requiring surgery for congenital defects, Nurs. Clin. North Am. **5:**387-398, 1970.

MacMahon, B.: Etiology of congenital defects, N. Engl. J. Med. **287:**487-489, 1972.

Milunsky, A., and Alpert, E.: The value of alpha-fetoprotein in the prenatal diagnosis of neural tube defects, J. Pediatr. **84:**889-893, 1974.

Milunsky, A., and associates: The prevention of genetic disease and mental retardation, Philadelphia, 1975, W. B. Saunders Co.

Moore, K. L.: The developing human: clinically oriented embryology, Philadelphia, 1973, W. B. Saunders Co.

Morison, J. E.: Perinatal pathology. In Aladjem, S., and Brown, A. K., editors: Clinical perinatology, St. Louis, 1974, The C. V. Mosby Co.

Motulsky, A. G., Lenz, W., and Ebling, F. J. G., editors: Birth defects: proceedings of the fourth international conference, New York, 1974, American Elsevier Publishing Co., Inc.

Norman, A. P., editor: Congenital abnormalities in infancy, ed. 2, Oxford, 1971, Blackwell Scientific Publications, Ltd.

Persaud, T. V. N., and Moore, K. L.: Causes and prenatal diagnosis of congenital abnormalities, J. Obstet. Gynecol. Neonatal Nurs. **3:**50-55, July/August 1974.

Roberts, F. B.: Perinatal nursing, New York, 1977, McGraw-Hill Book Co.

Schaffer, A. J., and Avery, M. E.: Diseases of the newborn, ed. 3, Philadelphia, 1971, W. B. Saunders Co.

Scipien, G. M., and associates: Comprehensive pediatric nursing, New York, 1975, McGraw-Hill Book Co.

Smith, D. W.: Recognizable patterns of human malformation: genetic, embryologic, and clinical aspects, ed. 2, Philadelphia, 1976, W. B. Saunders Co.

Steele, S.: Nursing care of the child with congenital anomalies and minimal brain dysfunction. In Steele, S., editor: Nursing care of the child with long-term illness, New York, 1971, Appleton-Century-Crofts.

Stevenson, A. C., and Davison, B. C.: Genetic counseling, Philadelphia, 1970, J. B. Lippincott Co.

Sucheston, M. E., and Cannon, M. S.: Congenital malformations: case studies in developmental anatomy, Philadelphia, 1973, F. A. Davis Co.

Tudor, M. J.: Family habilitation: a child with a birth defect. In Hymovich, D. P., and Barnard, M. U., editors: Family health care, New York, 1973, McGraw-Hill Book Co.

Vaughn, V. C., and McKay, R. J., editors: Textbook of pediatrics, ed. 10, Philadelphia, 1975, W. B. Saunders Co.

Waechter, E. H.: Developmental correlates of physical disability, Nurs. Forum **9**(1)90, 1970.

Waechter, E. H.: Developmental consequences of congenital abnormalities, Nurs. Forum **14**(2):108-129, 1975.

Waecther, E. H., and Blake, F. G.: Philadelphia, 1976, J. B. Lippincott Co.

Waranky, J.: Congenital malformations, Chicago, 1971, Year Book Medical Publishers, Inc.

Birth of a defective child

Brown, M. S.: The Gordons needed all the help they could get, Nursing '77 **7**(10):40-43, 1977.

Butnai, P.: Reactions of mothers to the birth of an anomalous infant: a review of the literature, Maternal-Child Nurs. J. **3:**59, 1974.

Choi, M. W.: Birth crisis: parental and professional responses to the birth of a child with a defect, Iss. Comp. Pediatr. Nurs. **2**(1):1-11, 1978.

Clay, C.: There is something wrong with your baby. In McNall, L. K., and Galeener, J. T., editors: Current practice in obstetric and gynecologic nursing, vol. 1, St. Louis, 1976, The C. V. Mosby Co.

Eyres, P. J.: The role of the nurse in family-centered nursing care, Nurs. Clin. North Am. **7:**27, 1972.

Freeman, J. M.: Is there a right to die—quickly? J. Pediatr. **80:** 904-905, 1972.

Gonzales, M. T.: Nursing support of the family with an abnormal infant, Hosp. Top. **15:**68-69, 1971.

Gracely, K. A.: Parental attachment to a child with a congenital defect, Pediatr. Nurs. **3**(5):15-17, 1977.

Irvin, N. A., Kennell, J. H., and Klaus, M. H.: Caring for parents of an infant with a congenital malformation. In Klaus, M. H., and Kennell, J. H.: Maternal-infant bonding: the impact of early separation or loss on family development, St. Louis, 1976, The C. V. Mosby Co.

Jackson, P. L.: Chronic grief, Am. J. Nurs. **74:**1288-1291, July 1974.

Johns, N.: Family reactions to the birth of a child with a congenital abnormality, Med. J. Aust. **6:**277, 1971.

Mercer, R. T.: Crisis: a baby born with a defect, Nursing '77, **7**(11):45-47, 1977.

Pillitteri, A.: Nursing care of the growing family, Boston, 1976, Little, Brown and Co.

Schroeder, E.: The birth of a defective child: a cause for grieving. In Hall, J. E., and Weaver, B. R., editors: Nursing of families in crisis, Philadelphia, 1974, J. B. Lippincott Co.

Waechter, E. H.: Bonding problems of infants with congenital anomalies, Nurs. Forum **16**(3,4):298-318, 1977.

Young, R. K.: Chronic sorrow: parent's response to the birth of a child with a defect, Am. J. Maternal Child Nurs. **2**(1):38-42, January/February 1977.

Malformations of the central nervous system

Ames, M. D., and Schut, L.: Results of treatment of 171 consecutive myelomeningoceles, 1963-1968, Pediatrics **50:**466, 1972.

Barden, G. A., Meyer, L. C., and Stelling, F. H.: Myelodysplastics—fate of those followed for twenty years or more, J. Bone Joint Surg. **57A:**643-647, 1975.

Bellam, G.: The nursing challenge of the child with neurological problems, Nurs. Forum **11:**397, 1972.

Bensman, A., and associates: Myelomeningocele birth defect, habilitation of the child, Minn. Med. **54:**599-604, 1971.

Bonine, G. N.: The myelodysplastic child: hospital and home care, Am. J. Nurs. **69:**541-544, 1969.

Bull, M. J., and associates: Myelodysplasia, Orthop. Clin. North Am. **7:**475-500, 1976.

Burr, C. H.: The hip in the meylomeningocele child, Clin. Orthop. **90:**11-21, 1973.

Carmel, P. W.: Spina bifida. In Downey, J. A., and Low, N. L.: The child with disabling illness, Philadelphia, 1974, W. B. Saunders Co.

Conway, B. L.: Pediatric neurologic nursing, St. Louis, 1977, The C. V. Mosby Co.

Culp, D., Bekhrad, A., and Flocks, R.: Urological management of the meningocele patient, J.A.M.A. **213:**753-758, 1970.

Farmer, T. W., editor: Pediatric neurology, ed. 2, New York, 1975, Harper & Row, Publishers.

Field, B.: The child with spina bifida: medical and social aspects of the problem of a child with multiple handicaps and his family, Med. J. Aust. **2:**1286, 1972.

Fishman, M. A.: Recent clinical advances in the treatment of dysraphic states, Pediatr. Clin. North Am. **23:**517-526, 1976.

Ford, F. R.: Diseases of the nervous system, ed. 6, Springfield, Ill., 1973, Charles C Thomas, Publisher.

Ford, H. A.: Nursing the spina bifida child in a general hospital, Nurs. Times **66:**293-295, 1970.

Freeman, J.: Practical management of meningomyelocele, Baltimore, 1974, University Park Press.

Freeston, B. M.: An enquiry into the effect of a spina bifida child upon family life, Dev. Med. Child Neurol. **13:**456-461, 1971.

Hayden, P. W., and associates: Custody of the myelodysplastic child: implications for selection for early treatment, Pediatrics **53:**253-256, 1974.

Hayden, P. W., and Shurtleff, D. B.: The medical management of hydrocephalus, Dev. Med. Child Neurol. (Suppl.) **27:**52, 1972.

Henderson, M. L., and Synhorst, D. M.: Bladder and bowel management in the child with myelomeningocele, Pediatr. Nurs. **3**(5):24-31, 1977.

Hide, D. W., and Semple, C.: Co-ordinated care of the child with spina bifida, Lancet **2:**603-604, 1970.

Hill, M. L., and associates: The myelodysplastic child: bowel and bladder control, Am. J. Nurs. **69:**545-550, 1969.

Kapke, K. A.: Spina bifida: mother-child relationship, Nurs. Forum **9**(3):310-320, 1970.

Kolin, I. S., and associates: Studies of the school-age child with meningomyelocele: social and emotional adapation, J. Pediatr. **78:**1013, 1971.

Lightowler, C.: Meningomyelocele—the price of treatment, Br. Med. J. **2:**385, 1971.

Lister, A. H.: Future for children with spina bifida, Lancet **2:**982-986, 1970.

Littlewood, J. M.: Spina bifida, Nurs. Times **66:**5-8, 1970.

Lorber, J.: Congenital malformations of the central nervous system, Br. J. Hosp. Med. **8:**37, 1972.

Lorber, J.: Spina bifida cystica, Arch. Dis. Child. **47:**854-872, 1972.

McCullough, D. C., and associates: Computerized axial tomography in clinical pediatrics, Pediatrics **59:**173-181, 1977.

Meservey, P. M.: Congential musculoskeletal abnormalities, Issues Comprehensive Pediatr. Nurs. **2**(4):15-22, 1977.

Milhorat, T. H.: Hydrocephalus and the cerebrospinal fluid, Baltimore, 1972, The Williams & Wilkins Co.

Milunsky, A., and Alpert, E.: The value of alpha-fetoprotein in the prenatal diagnosis of neural tube defects, J. Pediatr. **84:** 889, 1974.

Mrozinski, C. M.: Complications encountered in the course of shunt therapy for hydrocephalus in children, J. Neurosurg. Nurs. **2:**41-61, December 1970.

Naidich, T. P., and associates: Evaluation of pediatric hydrocephalus by computed tomography, Radiology **119:**337, 1976.

Owen, L. V.: Orthopedic management of a child with a spinal cord disorder, Pediatr. Nurs. **3**:37-40, July/August 1977.

Richards, I. D. G., and McIntosh, H. T.: Spina bifida survivors and their parents: a study of problems and services, Dev. Med. Child Neurol. **15**:292, 1973.

Salmon, J. H., Gonen, J. Y., and Brown, L.: Ventriculoatrial shunt for hydrocephalus ex-vacuo: psychological and clinical evaluation, Dis. Nerv. Syst. **32**:299-307, May 1971.

Scarff, J. E.: Treatment of nonobstructive (communicating) hydrocephalus by endoscopic cauterization of the choroid plexuses, J. Neurol. Surg. **33**:1, 1970.

Scherzer, A. L., and Garner, G.: Studies of the school-age child with myelomeningocele, Pediatrics **47**:424-430, 1971.

Shurtleff, D. B., and associates: Myelodysplasia: decision for death or disability, N. Engl. J. Med. **291**:1005-1011, 1974.

Spina bifida: hope through research, Public Health Pamphlet No. 1023, Health Information Series No. 103, Washington, D.C., 1970, U.S. Government Printing Office.

Stone, B. H.: Computerized transaxial brain scan, Am. J. Nurs. **77**:1601-1605, 1977.

Tew, B., and Lawrence, K. M.: Mothers, brothers, and sisters of patients with spina bifida, Dev. Med. Child Neurol. **15**:69, 1973.

Towbin, A.: Central nervous system damage in the human fetus and newborn infant, Am. J. Dis. Child. **119**:529, 1970.

Walker, J. H., Thomas, M., and Russell, I. T.: Spina bifida and the parents, Dev. Med. Child Neurol. **13**:462-476, 1971.

Wiley, L., editor: Spina bifida. Immediate concerns—long-term goals, Nursing '73 **3**(10):43-47, October 1973.

Zachary, R. B.: The improving prognosis in spina bifida, Clin. Pediatr. **11**:11-14, January 1972.

Skeletal defects

Asher, M. A.: Orthopedic screening, Pediatr. Clin. North Am. **24**:713-721, 1977.

Bailey, J. A., and Palmatier, J. A.: The nurse's role in detecting dwarfism at birth, Nurs. Clin. North Am. **6**:559, 1971.

Brashear, H. R., Jr., and Raney, R. B.: Shands' handbook of orthopaedic surgery, ed. 9, St. Louis, 1978, The C. V. Mosby Co.

Chuinard, E. G.: Femoral osteotomy in the treatment of congenital dysplasia of the hip, Orthop. Clin. North Am. **3**:157-174, 1972.

Chung, S.: Diseases of the developing hip joint, Pediatr. Clin. North Am. **24**:857-870, 1977.

Clarren, S. K., and Smith, D. W.: Congenital deformities, Pediatr. Clin. North Am. **24**:665-677, 1977.

Downie, G. R.: Limb deficiencies and prosthetic devices, Orthop. Clin. North Am. **7**:465-474, 1976.

Duthie, R. B., and Ferguson, A. B., Jr.: Mercer's orthopedic surgery, ed. 7, Baltimore, 1973, The Williams & Wilkins Co.

Hilt, N. E., and Schmitt, E. W., Jr.: Pediatric orthopedic nursing, St. Louis, 1975, The C. V. Mosby Co.

Kadkhoda, M., Chung, S. M. K., and Abdbonojo, F. O.: Congenital dislocation of the hip. Diagnostic screening and treatment: a comparative study of two populations of infants and children, Clin. Pediatr. **15**:159-166, 1976.

Kane, R., and Krom, W.: Deformities of the foot. In Downey, J. A., and Low, N. L.: The child with disabling illness, Philadelphia, 1974, W. B. Saunders Co.

Katz, J. F., and Challenor, Y. B.: Childhood orthopedic syndromes. In Downey, J. A., and Low, N. L.: The child with disabling illness, Philadelphia, 1974, W. B. Saunders Co.

Lane, P. A.: A mother's confession—home care of a toddler in a spica cast: What it's really like, Am. J. Nurs. **71**:2141, 1971.

Lowry, M. F.: Congenital dislocation of the hip, Nurs. Times **66**:72-74, 1970.

Mercer, R. T.: Crisis: a baby is born with a defect, Nursing '77 **7**(11):45-47, 1977.

Mital, M. A.: Limb deficiencies: classification and treatment, Orthop. Clin. North Am. **7**:457-464, 1976.

Siffert, R. S., Ehrlich, M. G., and Katz, J. F.: Management of congenital dislocation of the hip, Clin. Orthop. **86**:28-33, 1972.

Specht, E.: Congenital dislocation of the hip, Am. Fam. Physician **9**:88-89, 1974.

Speck, W. T.: Special orthopedic problems. In Behrman, R. E., editor: Neonatal-perinatal medicine: diseases of the fetus and infant, ed. 2, St. Louis, 1977, The C. V. Mosby Co.

Wynne-Davies, R.: The epidemiology of congenital dislocation of the hip, Dev. Med. Child Neurol. **14**:515, 1972.

Lacey, K. A., and Parkin, J. M.: Causes of short stature, Lancet **1**:42, 1974.

Cleft lip and/or palate

Battle, C. U., Pashayan, H., and Pruzansky, S.: Special management of cranio-facial problems. In Behrman, R. E., editor: Neonatal-perinatal medicine: diseases of the fetus and infant, St. Louis, 1977, The C. V. Mosby Co.

Bleiberg, A. H., and Leubling, H. E.: Parent's guide to cleft palate habilitation. The team approach, New York, 1971, Exposition Press.

Cosman, B.: Cosmetic surgery for the disabled child. In Downey, J. A., and Low, N. L.: The child with disabling illness, Philadelphia, 1974, W. B. Saunders Co.

Gorlin, R. J., Cervenka, J., and Pruzansky, S.: Facial clefting and its syndromes, Birth Defects **7**:3, 1971.

Huddart, A. G.: The care and management of the newborn cleft palate infant, Nurs. Mirror **140**:61, 1975.

Powers, G. R.: Cleft palate, Indianapolis, 1973, The Bobbs-Merrill Co., Inc.

Ross, R. B., and Johnston, M. C.: Cleft lip and palate, Baltimore, 1972, The Williams & Wilkins Co.

Gastrointestinal tract atresias

Ashcraft, K. W., and Holder, T. M.: Esophageal atresia and tracheoesophageal fistula malformations, Surg. Clin. North Am. **56**:299, 1976.

Bishop, W. S., and Head, J. J.: Care of the infant with a stoma, Am. J. Maternal Child Nurs. **1**:315-319, 1976.

Davidson, M.: Diseases of the gastrointestinal tract. In Behrman, R. E., editor: Neonatal-perinatal medicine: diseases of the fetus and infant, St. Louis, 1977, The C. V. Mosby Co.

Davis, A.: Billy had a tracheo-esophageal fistula, Am. J. Nurs. **70**:326, 1970.

Grosfeld, J. L.: Alimentary tract obstruction in the newborn, Curr. Probl. Pediatr. **5**(3):3-47, January 1975.

Tank, E. S.: Diagnosis and treatment of congenital anomalies of the anus and rectum, Dis. Colon Rectum **15:**135, 1972.

Stephens, F. D.: Embryologic and functional aspects of "imperforate anus," Surg. Clin. North Am. **50:**919, 1970.

Hernias

Bronsther, B.: Inguinal hernias in children, J. Am. Med. Wom. Assoc. **27:**523, 1972.

Darling, D. B., and associates: Hiatal hernia and gastroesophageal reflux in infants and children, Pediatrics **54:**450-455, 1974.

Herbst, J., and associates: Hiatal hernia and "rumination" in infants and children, J. Pediatr. **78:**261-265, 1971.

Kim, S.: Omphalocele, Surg. Clin. North Am. **56:**361, 1976.

Ravitch, M.: The non-operative treatment of surgical conditions in children, Pediatrics **51:**435, 1973.

Rohalgi, M., Shandling, B., and Stephens, C. A.: Hiatus hernia in infants and children: results of surgical treatment, Surgery **69:**456, 1971.

Defects of the genitourinary tract

Amar, A. D., and associates: The practical management of vesicoureteral reflux in children, Clin. Pediatr. **15**(6):562-569, June 1976.

Bongiovanni, M. A.: Diagnosis and treatment: the undescended testicle, Pediatrics **36**(5):786, November 1965.

Bradley, G. M.: Urinary screening tests in the infant and young child, Med. Clin. North Am. **35:**1457-1471, November 1971.

Cross, P. S.: Ureteral reimplantation: nursing care of the child, Am. J. Nurs. **76**(11):1800-1803, November 1976.

Groff, D.: Handbook of pediatric surgical emergencies, New York, 1975, Medical Examination Publishing Co., Inc.

Khan, A., and Pryles, C.: Urinary tract infection in children, Am. J. Nurs. **73**(8):1340-1343, August 1973.

Murray, B. S., and associates: The patient has an ileal conduit, Am. J. Nurs. **71**(8):1560-1565, August 1971.

Oster, J.: Clinical phenomena noted by a school physician dealing with healthy children, Clin. Pediatr. **15**(8):748-751, August 1976.

Woodard, J. R., and Holden, S.: The prognostic significance of fever in childhood urinary infections, Clin. Pediatr. **15**(11): 1051-1054, November 1976.

Aberrant sexual development

Federman, D. D.: Abnormal sexual development, Philadelphia, 1968, W. B. Saunders Co.

Hendren, W. H., and Crawford, J. D.: The child with ambiguous genitalia, Curr. Probl. Surg., pp. 1-64, November 1972.

Hill, S.: The child with ambiguous genitalia, Am. J. Nurs. **77:** 810-814, 1977.

Himathongkam, T., and associates: Incomplete testicular feminization syndrome with pubertal virilization, Am. J. Obstet. Gynecol. **118:**288, 1974.

McCoy, N. L.: Innate factors in sex differences, Nurs. Forum **15**(3):277-293, 1976.

McFarlane, J.: Congenital adrenal hyperplasia, Am. J. Nurs. **76:** 1290-1292, 1976.

Moloshok, R. E., and Kerr, J. M.: The infant with ambiguous genitalia, Pediatr. Clin. North Am. **19:**529-542, 1972.

Moore, K. L.: Sex determination: normal and abnormal sexual development, J. Obstet. Gynecol. Neonatal Nurs. **3**(1):32-35, January/February 1974.

Rosenfield, R. L., and associates: Androgens and androgen responsiveness in the feminizing testis syndrome. Comparison of complete and "incomplete" forms, J. Clin. Endocrinol. Metab. **32:**625, 1971.

Walsh, P. C., and associates: Pseudohermaphroditism type II, N. Engl. J. Med. **291:**944, 1974.

Young, H. H., II, and associates: The management of agenesis of the phallus, Pediatrics **47:**81, 1971.

UNIT FIVE

Infancy

The first 12 months of childhood is the period of most rapid gain in physical size and most dramatic achievement of developmental milestones of an individual's entire life. It is marked by an orderly progression of physical, intellectual, and social maturation. It is also a highly vulnerable period for both positive and negative influences governing optimum growth and development.

Chapter 12, *The First Year: Laying the Foundation,* investigates the infant's biologic, adaptive, and intellectual development. It is concerned with fostering optimum health through anticipatory guidance regarding nutrition, prevention of accidental injury, and promotion of parent-child attachment. Chapter 13, *Health Problems During the First Year,* deals with health problems that commonly occur during the first year, usually as a result of environmental, rather than pathologic, processes and that therefore are amenable to prevention. It is also concerned with conditions of unknown etiology, such as sudden infant death syndrome, which has profound emotional consequences on the developing family.

12

The first year: laying the foundation

The miracle of birth is surpassed only by the wonder of unfolding in the succeeding months and years. The biologic growth and developmental maturation of the infant are a study of perfection in nature. The nurse's understanding of these processes is essential to the optimal care of the child and family. In order to present relevant data for appreciation of growth and development, it is necessary to systematize and categorize the facts into various levels of maturation and age-groups. However, one must always bear in mind that no child will be represented in any one table or chart, for each child is as much as individual as the number of variables that influence his existence.

GROWTH AND DEVELOPMENT

General concepts of growth and development, such as stages and patterns of development and individual differences, have been extensively discussed in Chapter 3. This chapter is primarily concerned with the growth and development of the infant from 1 to 12 months of age.

Developmental tasks

Infants are born with the basic abilities needed for extrauterine survival, such as respiration, thermoregulation, and digestion. However, they cannot survive without a care giver to provide for their essential needs, such as food, warmth, and security. In addition to their basic needs, which must be supplied for them, infants have certain tasks that they must achieve for themselves during the first year of life. How their needs are met by others greatly determines to what degree they accomplish their tasks.

The stages of development have been studied and described by several noted psychoanalysts, one of the most accomplished of whom is Erik H. Erikson. Erikson's phases of development are based on Freudian theory, but they differ in several important aspects. Erikson emphasizes the *ego,* rather than the *id,* and, by doing so, deemphasizes many of the biosexual connotations of Freud's theory. His basic premise supporting the ego assumes that the individual has an innate ability to cope with a usual, predictable environment. He does not stress Freud's philosophy of instinctual motivation, such as the death wish. He believes that play provides the best vehicle for exploring a child's ego, in contrast to Freud, who believed that dreams were the doorway to the unconscious.

Another crucial difference between the theories of these two men is that Erikson stresses the relationship of the individual to his family, community, and world. This broader framework of interpersonal relationships replaces the Freudian mother-child-father triangle. Another difference involves the focus of each man's theory. Freud attempted to prove the existence of the unconscious and devoted his research to the study of pathologic development in man. Erikson, on the other hand, has endeavored to study the phases or stages of man's psychologic development and has stressed the solutions to the potential hazards inherent in each phase. He is one of the few theorists who has attempted to study the entire life span, although the greatest emphasis has been placed on the first and fifth stages, developing a sense of trust and a sense of identity. Table 12-1 lists a comparison of Freud's and Erikson's stages of development.

Freud's *oral stage* during infancy involves id gratification through oral satisfaction. Before the teeth erupt, usually during the first 6 months of life, the infant is in the oral-passive or oral-dependent stage. Pleasure is derived through sucking, eating, and rooting. During and after teething, the infant is in the oral-aggressive stage and can bite, as well as suck, for gratification. The erogenous zones are the mouth and lips; any object that comes in contact with this zone is potentially pleasurable. The "mouthing activity" of the infant is very evident during the first year, when everything is explored by sucking or biting. The sucking needs of infants vary, just as the "oral needs" of adults differ. Some infants are satisfied by the amount of sucking supplied through feeding, whereas others require additional opportunities for sucking pleasure, such as the use of a pacifier.

Erikson's phase I is concerned with acquiring a sense of basic *trust* while overcoming a sense of mistrust. The trust acquired in infancy is foundational for all the succeeding phases. It allows the infant a feeling of physical comfort and security, which assists him in experiencing unfamiliar,

Table 12-1. Comparison of Freud's and Erikson's stages of development

Age	Freud's psychosexual stages	Erikson's psychosocial phases
Birth-18 months	Oral	Trust vs mistrust
1½-3 years	Anal	Autonomy vs shame and doubt
3-5½ years	Phallic	Initiative vs guilt
5½-12 years	Latency	Industry vs inferiority
Adolescence	Genital	Identity vs role confusion
Young adulthood		Intimacy vs isolation
Middle age		Generativity vs self-absorption
Mature age		Integrity vs despair

unknown situations with a minimum of fear. The crucial element for the achievement of this task is the *quality* of the mother (care giver)-child relationship. The provision of food, warmth, and shelter (or Maslow's first two stages—physiologic needs and physical safety) are alone inadequate for the development of a strong ego. The infant and mother must jointly learn to satisfactorily meet their needs in order for mutual regulation of frustration to occur. When this synchrony fails to develop, mistrust is the eventual outcome.

The acquisition of trust involves the libidinal or psychologic energy of the erotic centers of the body, namely the mouth. Similar to Freud's theory, Erikson's has described particular stages in the oral phase. The first social modality is primarily *oral*. During the first 3 to 4 months, food intake is the most important social activity the infant engages in. The id processes are most evident; the newborn can tolerate little frustration or delay of gratification. Primary *narcissism* is at its height. However, as bodily processes such as vision, motor movements, and vocalization are more cortically controlled, the id processes, which operate on the *pleasure principle,* become a component of the ego structure, which operates on the *reality principle.* The infant gradually learns to accept delayed gratification and alternate methods of eliciting a positive response from the environment. Either extreme in terms of "delayed gratification" leads to mistrust. If the mother or care giver always meets the child's needs before he signals his readiness, the infant will never learn to test his ability to control the environment. If the delay is prolonged, the infant will experience constant frustration and eventually mistrust others in their efforts to satisfy him.

The next social modality involves an incorporative mode of reaching out to others through *grasping*. Initially grasping is reflexive, but it has a powerful social meaning to the parents. The reciprocal response of the infant's grasping is the parents' holding on and touching. Tactile stimulation is extremely important in the total process of acquiring trust. In fact, the degree of mothering skill, the quantity of food, or the length of sucking does not determine the quality of the experience. Rather, it is the total nature of the quality of the interpersonal relationship that regulates the infant's formulation of trust.

During the second incorporative stage, the more active and aggressive modality of *biting* occurs. The infant learns that he can hold on to what is his own and can more fully control his environment. During this stage the infant is confronted with one of his first conflicts of breast-feeding as he quickly learns that biting causes withdrawal of the nipple and anxiety in the mother. Yet biting also brings internal relief from teething discomfort and a sense of power or control. The successful resolution of this conflict strengthens the mother-child relationship at a time when the infant is recognizing her as the most significant person in his life. At about the same time (6 months of age), stranger anxiety is evident. The infant has formed strong attachments to the most significant people in his world, his parents. Separation can be devastating and, if prolonged, can affect future personality development. Although unpleasant to experience, demonstration of stranger anxiety is an important manifestation of the strength of the infant-parent attachment.

Play during infancy is representative of the various social modalities. The infant's activity is primarily narcissistic, revolving around his own body. At 2 months of age the infant will look at his extended hand as if it were an unfamiliar object. At about age 6 months the infant plays with his feet and also finds fingers excellent nipple substitutes. During this time the ability to grasp is well under self-control and everything is reached for and brought to the mouth for inquisitive exploration. When the pincer grasp is mastered, the infant is absorbed with growing independence, refusing to allow others to feed him. At the same time, locomotion skills are rapidly developing, bringing previously unattainable areas within easy access. The infant is thus facing another conflict by learning the meaning of the word "no." His new independence in gross motor skills necessitates his learning and adapting to limits within his environment. This is another important time for child and parents, since it represents the beginning of discipline and further delayed gratification. Successful resolution of the independence–limit setting conflict further strengthens the development of basic trust, building a solid foundation for progression to the second stage, acquisition of autonomy.

Biologic development

During embryonic development the head and brain have the fastest growth rate. Approximately 70% of head growth occurs before birth, and at birth the brain is about one fourth of its eventual adult size. During the first year elongation of the trunk predominates, which is evidenced by

Neurologic reflexes that appear during infancy

Reflex	*Expected behavioral response*	*Age of appearance (months)*
Landau	When infant is suspended in a horizontal prone position and the head is flexed against the trunk, the legs reflexly draw up against the body	3 until 12-24
Parachute	When infant is suspended in a horizontal prone position and suddenly thrust downward, infant's hands and fingers extend forward as if to protect himself from falling	7-9, persists indefinitely
Labyrinth-righting	When infant is in prone or supine position, he is able to raise the head	2, strongest at 10
Body-righting	A modification of the labyrinth-righting reflex that enables infant to sit and stand	7-12

a threefold increase in weight and a 50% increase in height. Each body system also undergoes specific changes during the first year.

Neurologic. Brain growth continues to be rapid during the first year. The brain of the newborn weighs 350 to 400 g (12 to 14 ounces) and by the end of the first year has increased about two and one half times, or to two thirds of its eventual adult weight. The average male brain weighs from 10% to 15% more than that of the average female by 1 year of age. Most of the nerve cells are present at birth, except for the formation of microneurons. The increasing growth is mainly a result of hyperplasia of nerve cells and growth of nonnerve cells (glia), dendritic branching, and the development of synaptic branching. Myelin formation, which is amost complete by the end of 2 years of age, is the chief source of white matter. Most of the brain growth occurs in the cortex, particularly in the parietal and frontal lobes. The sulci of the lobes deepen and increase in complexity until about 6 years of age.

At birth several reflexes are present (Table 8-7); some of these, such as the Moro, tonic neck, and grasp reflexes, fade during the next few months. Others, such as the knee jerk or blink reflex, are present for life, whereas still others appear at different times during infancy. Reflexes that can be elicited at particular developmental periods are listed in the boxed material above. Development of the pyramidal tract, which controls voluntary movement, occurs later but is completed by the end of the second year.

Organs of special sense

Vision. At birth the eye is structurally incomplete and vision is one of the newborn's poorest senses. During infancy visual acuity gradually improves and binocular fixation is established. The major developmental characteristics of vision during infancy are listed in the boxed material on p. 432.

Binocularity, or the fixation of two ocular images into one cerebral picture (fusion), begins to develop by 6 weeks of age and should be well established by age 12 months. Lack of binocular vision results in strabismus or cross-eye. When this occurs, two images are projected on different areas of the retina, causing diplopia. Uncorrected strabismus can cause blindness or suppression amblyopia, because the brain will suppress the image seen through the weaker eye. If the condition is not corrected by about 5 years of age, the lack of visual stimulation to the brain will result in permanent, irreversible visual loss. However, if the affected eye is forced to fixate on an object because the unaffected eye is covered, visual loss can be prevented. Some degree of visual loss from strabismus can occur by 1 year of age.

Depth perception (stereopsis) begins to develop by age 7 to 9 months but may exist earlier as an innate safety mechanism. For example, in one study, a visual cliff was erected. On one side of the transparent platform a checkerboard table was placed several feet below the platform, giving the illusion of depth. On the other side the checkerboard table was placed close to the underside of the platform. When infants who were 6 months old or more were placed on the transparent platform, most of them refused to crawl across the side that demonstrated an illusional cliff, but they easily crawled on the other side.[25] Other investigators found that even 2- to 3-month-old infants distinguish depth. They recorded heart rate when the infants were placed on the "deep" or "shallow" side of the visual cliff. The slower heart rate of the infants, when they were placed prone on the "deep" side, indicated a physiologic response of the ability to perceive depth.[11] Whether this is a learned or innate perception is still unsolved.

Infants also have a *visual preference.* At birth they show preference for bright, moving objects. They seem to be born with a preference for looking at the human face, which also has a developmental sequence. For example, at age 6 weeks, they show more interest in a picture of a face with eyes than without. By 10 weeks of age a picture with both eyes and eyebrows elicits more response, and by

Major developmental characteristics of vision

Age (weeks)	*Development*
Birth	Pupillary and corneal (blink) reflexes present Able to fixate on moving object in range of 45 degrees when held 8-10 inches away Cannot integrate head and eye movements well (doll's eye reflex—eyes lag behind if head is rotated to one side)
4	Can follow in range of 90 degrees Can watch parent intently as he or she speaks to infant Tear glands begin to function Visual acuity is hyperopic because of less spherical eyeball than adult
6-12	Has peripheral vision to 180 degrees Binocular vision begins at age 6 weeks, is well established by age 4 months Convergence on near objects begins by age 6 weeks, is well developed by age 3 months Doll's eye reflex disappears
12-20	Visual acuity, 20/200 Recognizes feeding bottle Able to fixate on a ½-inch block Looks at hand while sitting or lying on back Looks at mirror image Able to accommodate to near objects
20-28	Adjusts posture to see an object Able to rescue a dropped toy Develops color preference for yellow and red Able to discriminate between simple geometric forms Prefers more complex visual stimuli Develops hand-eye coordination Pats image of self in mirror
28-44	Can fixate on very small objects Depth perception begins to develop Lack of binocular vision indicates strabismus
44-52	Visual acuity, 20/100 Visual loss may develop if strabismus is present Can follow rapidly moving objects

Adapted from Illingworth, R. S.: The development of the infant and young child, New York, 1975, Churchill Livingstone; and Chinn, P., and Leitch, C.: Child health maintenance: a guide to clinical assessment, ed. 2, St. Louis, 1979, The C. V. Mosby Co.

Major developmental characteristics of hearing

Age (weeks)	*Development*
Birth	Responds to loud noise by startle reflex Responds to sound of human voice more readily than to any other sound Low-pitched sounds, such as lullaby, metronome, or heartbeat, have quieting effect
8-12	Turns head to side when sound is made at level of ear
12-16	Locates sound by turning head to side and looking in same direction
16-24	Can localize sounds made below ear, which is followed by localization of sound made above ear; will turn head to the side and then look up or down Begins to imitate sounds
24-32	Locates sounds by turning head in a curving arc Responds to own name
32-40	Localizes sounds by turning head diagonally and directly toward sound
40-52	Knows several words and their meaning, such as "no," and names of members of the family Learns to control and adjust own response to sound, such as listening for the sound to occur again

Adapted from Illingworth, R. S.: The development of the infant and young child, New York, 1975, Churchill Livingstone.

20 weeks of age the mouth is also necessary. By age 6 months infants respond to facial expressions and can distinguish between familiar and strange faces.

Hearing. With progressive myelination of the auditory pathway, the specific responses of locating sound replace the generalized response of the neonate. The major developmental characteristics of hearing are listed in the boxed material above right. (For a further discussion of hearing and the senses of smell, taste, and touch, see Chapter 8.)

Respiratory system. The most dramatic changes in the respiratory system occur at birth. These are discussed in Chapter 8. During infancy the rate slows somewhat (see Appendix A) and is relatively stable. Respiratory movements continue to be abdominal. Growth of the respiratory tract is gradual. Several factors predispose the infant to more severe and acute respiratory problems. The close proximity of the trachea to the bronchi and its branching structures rapidly transmits an infectious agent from one anatomic location to another. The short, straight eustachian tube closely communicates with the ear, allowing infection to ascend from the pharynx to the middle ear. In addition the immunologic ability of the mucosal lining provides less protection against infection in infancy than during later childhood.

Although the lumen of the trachea and bronchi enlarges during infancy, it remains small in comparison to the total size of the lung, maintaining low resistance to the volume of air inspired. Also the ability of the entire respiratory tract to produce mucus is diminished, decreasing the humidification of the large volume of inspired air. In addition the volume of dead space, that amount of air needed to fill the respiratory passages with each breath, is large, requiring the infant to breath about twice as fast as the adult to provide the body with the needed amount of oxygen.

The chest assumes a more adult contour, with the lateral diameter becoming larger than the anteroposterior diameter. The chest circumference approximately equals head circumference by the end of the first year.

Circulatory system. The immediate postnatal circulatory changes that accompany the respiratory changes have been discussed in Chapter 8. Complete anatomic closure of the fetal shunts may take several months, and innocent murmurs may be present in as many as 50% of children after the neonatal period. The heart rate slows (Appendix A), and the rhythm is frequently sinus arrhythmia, which is usually considered pathologic in later life. Sinus arrhythmia, which usually disappears with increased activity, is most obvious during sleep. The regularity of the rhythm seems to correlate with the respiratory rate: the faster the respiratory rate, the more regular the heartbeat, and the slower the respiratory rate (as in sleep), the more irregular the heartbeat.

The heart grows less rapidly than does the rest of the body. Its weight is usually doubled by 1 year of age in comparison to body weight, which triples during the same length of time. The size of the heart is still large in relation to the chest cavity; its width is about 55% of the width of the chest.

Blood pressure also changes during infancy (Appendix A). The rising systolic pressure is a result of the increasing ability of the left ventricle to pump blood into the systemic circulation. Fluctuations in blood pressure occur during varying states of activity and emotion. However, the usual increase of blood pressure toward evening and subsequent decrease during the night, which is normal in older children and adults, is absent during infancy.

Hemopoietic changes also occur during the first year (Appendix B). Fetal hemoglobin is usually present for the first 5 months, with adult hemoglobin forming at about 13 weeks of age. Maternal iron stores are usually present for the first 5 to 6 months and then gradually diminish, which partially accounts for lowered hemoglobin levels toward the end of the first 6 months. Physiologic anemia is also seen at 2 to 3 months of age because of the decreasing number of red blood cells. This phenomenon is thought to be caused by the depression of the hemopoietic system because of the high level of fetal hemoglobin, which represses the production of erythropoietin, a hormone released by the kidney. The occurrence of physiologic anemia is not affected by an adequate supply of iron. However, when erythropoiesis is stimulated, iron supplies are then necessary for formation of hemoglobin.

Fluid and electrolyte balance. At birth there is a shift in the total body fluid of the neonate, resulting in a higher level of intracellular fluid to extracellular fluid, probably because of the progressive growth of cells at the expense of extracellular fluid. This shift continues during the first year, resulting in about 35% extracellular fluid and 40% intracellular fluid, or a total body fluid of 75%. This is in contrast to an adult total body fluid value of about 59% (extracellular fluid, 22%; intracellular fluid, 37%). The proportionally higher ratio of extracellular fluid, which is composed of blood plasma, interstitial fluid, and lymph, predisposes the infant to a more rapid loss of total body fluid and, consequently, dehydration.

Thermoregulation. During infancy the ability of the skin to contract and shiver in response to cold increases. The ability of the peripheral capillaries to respond to change in ambient temperature serves to regulate heat loss. In response to cold, the capillaries constrict, conserving core body temperature and decreasing potential evaporative heat loss from the skin surface. In response to heat, the capillaries dilate, decreasing internal body temperature through evaporation, conduction, and convection. Shivering causes the muscles and muscle fibers to contract, generating metabolic heat, which is distributed throughout the body. Accumulation of adipose tissue serves to insulate the body against heat loss.

Gastrointestinal system. The digestive processes are immature at birth. Saliva is secreted in small amounts, but the majority of the digestive processes do not begin functioning until age 3 months, when drooling is common because of the poorly coordinated swallowing reflex. The enzyme ptyalin (also called amylase) is present in small amounts but usually has little effect on the foodstuff because of the small amount of time the food stays in the mouth. Gastric digestion in the stomach consists primarily of the action of hydrochloric acid and rennin, an enzyme, which acts specifically on the casein in milk to cause the formation of curds. A curd is a coagulated semisolid particle of milk. The curds cause the milk to be retained in the stomach long enough for digestion to occur. The amount of rennin decreases throughout life. In addition this enzyme functions best in a moderately acid medium. The child's stomach has less acidity than the adult's, which enhances the action of rennin. Digestion also takes place in the duodenum, where pancreatic enzymes and bile begin to break down protein and fat. Secretion of the pancreatic enzyme amylase, which is needed for digestion of complex carbohydrates, is deficient until about the third month of life. Lipase is also somewhat limited, especially for highly saturated fats. Trypsin is secreted in sufficient quantities to catabolize protein into polypeptides and some amino acids.

The immaturity of the digestive processes is evident in the appearance of stools. During infancy solid foods, such as peas, carrots, corn, and raisins, are passed incompletely broken down in the feces. Not until the second year are most fibrous foods completely digested. An excess quantity of roughage easily disposes the child to loose, bulky stools.

The liver is the most immature of all the gastrointestinal organs throughout infancy. The ability to conjugate bilirubin and to secrete bile is achieved after the first couple of weeks of life. However, the capacities for gluconeogenesis, formation of plasma protein and ketones, storage of vitamins, and deaminization of amino acids remain relatively immature for the first year of life.

The rapid peristaltic activity of the gastrointestinal tract slows down throughout infancy, and the stomach enlarges to accommodate a greater volume of food. By the end of the first year the infant is able to tolerate three meals a day and a bedtime bottle and may have one or two bowel movements daily. Bowel evacuation remains under involuntary, reflexive control until myelination of the spinal cord is complete, usually by 14 to 18 months of age.

The immunologic properties of the mucosal lining of the gastrointestinal tract are immature, which predisposes this system, like the respiratory system, to increased risk of infection and inflammation. When any type of gastric irritation occurs, the transit time is increased above its already rapid rate, making the infant vulnerable to diarrhea, vomiting, and dehydration (see Chapter 30).

Renal system. The immaturity of the renal structures continues to predispose the infant to dehydration. Complete maturity of the kidney occurs during the latter half of the second year, when the cubical epithelium of the glomeruli becomes flattened (see p. 1148).

Musculoskeletal system. Elongation of the trunk dominates skeletal growth during the first year (60% of total increase in height) and is succeeded by growth of the legs (66% of total increase in height) during the next year. Closure of the cranial sutures occurs during the first year. The posterior fontanel is usually obliterated by 6 to 8 weeks of age, and the anterior fontanel closes by 12 to 18 months of age.

Growth can be determined by bone age or centers of ossification. At birth five ossification centers are present in the majority of infants: (1) distal end of the femur, (2) proximal end of the tibia, (3) talus (the bone that articulates with the tibia and fibula to form the ankle joint), (4) calcaneus (the heel bone, which articulates with the cuboid and talus bones), and (5) cuboid (the bone between the calcaneus bone and the fourth and fifth metatarsals). Thereafter, various ossification centers appear in an orderly sequence. The first ossification centers to appear by 5 or 6 months of age are the capitate and hamate in the wrist. Bone age is usually determined by the number of ossification centers in the hand or wrist.

Muscle hypertrophy continues throughout the first year and parallels the acquisition of motor skills. For example, the gluteal muscles remain undeveloped until walking is well established.

Adipose tissue, which is laid down during the last trimester of pregnancy, continues to accumulate during the next 6 months of life. The amount of adipose tissue laid down during infancy probably influences the predisposition to fat accumulation later in life and should be an important fact to stress during nutritional counseling. Approximately 85% of overweight children will become overweight adults.

Dentition. Teeth arise as outgrowths of the oral epithelium during the sixth week of embryonic life. Tooth buds form at ten different points in each arch, which become the eventual enamel organs for the 20 primary (deciduous) teeth. The enamel organ is of ectodermal origin and determines the shape of the tooth and gives rise to the enamel covering. All the buds are present at birth, but the amount of enamel laid down varies with each set of teeth. In general, hard tissue formation occurs between 4 and 6 months of fetal life.

Teeth are divided into quadrants of the lower mandible and upper maxilla and are named for their location in each quadrant of the dental arch, such as central incisor, lateral incisor, and first and second molars. Teeth are also named after their specific function in the mastication of food. The central and lateral incisors, which have a knife-like, or scissor-like shape, cut the food. The cuspids, also called canines, tear the food. The term cuspid refers to the single point or cusp shape of the crown. The two premolars, or bicuspids because of their two-pointed crown, crush the food. The permanent molars, which have four or five cusps, grind the food.

Tooth eruption occurs in a fairly orderly sequence, but the rate may vary in different children (Fig. 3-8). The first teeth to erupt are usually the lower central incisors. One incisor will erupt, followed closely by the homologous incisor. These teeth usually are present by 6 to 7 months of age. The upper central incisors usually erupt by 7 or 8 months of age. The upper lateral incisors erupt at about ages 10 to 12 months, followed by the lower lateral incisors at ages 12 to 14 months. Primary dentition is usually complete by 2½ years of age. The deciduous teeth are shed in order of their appearance, to be replaced by thirty-two permanent teeth.

Immunologic system. There are five main classes of immunoglobulins: (1) IgG, which neutralizes microbial toxins, (2) IgM, which is important in combating serious infections and responding to artificial immunization, (3) IgA, which can easily cross cell barriers, (4) IgD, which has an unknown specific action, and (5) IgE, which responds primarily to allergic reactions. The newborn receives significant quantities of IgG from the mother and is able to synthesize his own by 1 to 3 months of age. Adult levels are reached by 1 to 2 years of age. The infant can manufacture significant amounts of IgM at birth and begins producing IgA 2 weeks after birth, with 40% to 80% of eventual adult levels reached by 1 year of age. The time of onset of IgD and IgE is uncertain.

Endocrine system. The endocrine system is adequately developed at birth, but its functions are immature. The interrelatedness of all the endocrine organs has a major effect on the function of any one gland. The lack of homeostatic control because of various functional deficiencies renders the infant especially vulnerable to imbalances in fluid and electrolytes, glucose concentration, and amino acid metabolism.

The pituitary gland, or hypophysis, produces several hormones that control growth and reproduction. The most important hormone produced by the anterior pituitary during infancy is growth hormone or somatotrophic hormone (STH). Growth hormone stimulates growth, increases protein synthesis and fat catabolism, and decreases carbohydrate metabolism. As a result of suppression of carbohydrate utilization, blood glucose increases, which then stimulates the secretion of insulin in the pancreas. Although the islets of Langerhans produce insulin and glucagon during fetal life and early infancy, blood sugar levels tend to remain labile, particularly under conditions of stress.

The anterior pituitary also secretes thyroid-stimulating hormone (TSH) or thyrotropin, which stimulates the thyroid gland. Both hormones, TSH and thyroxine, are produced in limited amounts during fetal life and continue to be produced in larger quantities during infancy. The most characteristic function of the thyroid gland is its ability to take up and concentrate iodine from the blood. This hormonal iodine controls the rate of metabolism and has an important effect on growth.

Another anterior pituitary hormone, which is produced in limited quantities during infancy, is corticotropin (ACTH), which acts on the adrenal cortices to produce their hormones, particularly the glucocorticoids and aldosterone. Because the feedback mechanism between ACTH and the adrenal cortex is immature during infancy, there is much less tolerance for stressful conditions, which affect fluid and electrolytes and the metabolism of fats, proteins, and carbohydrates.

The adrenal medulla produces two hormones, epinephrine and norepinephrine. Secretion of these hormones is limited during infancy and early childhood. Both hormones have several vital functions, particularly in response to stress. They increase cardiac output, induce release of free fatty acids, stimulate the sympathetic nervous system, increase heat production, and elevate the blood sugar level by accelerating conversion of liver glycogen to glucose (glycogenolysis).

Adaptive behaviors

As biologic maturation progresses there is a concurrent development of behaviors, which increasingly allows the infant to respond to and cope with the environment. These adaptive behaviors can be classified into various categories: (1) gross motor, (2) fine motor, (3) language, and (4) personal-social. The acquisition of skill in each area occurs in an orderly sequence, following the usual cephalocaudal-proximodistal laws. Although each 4-week period will be reviewed for the developmental process that occurs, the key ages are 4, 16, 28, 40, and 52 weeks of age, because they represent integrative periods and major shifts in focus and centers of organization.[17]

Knowledge of the developmental sequence allows the nurse to assess normal growth as well as minor or abnormal deviations. Knowledge of developmental milestones helps parents gain realistic expectations of their child's ability and provides guidelines for suitable play and stimulation. Emphasizing the child's *developmental age* rather than chronologic age strengthens the parent-child relationship by fostering trust and lessening frustration. Therefore, one cannot overemphasize the importance of a thorough understanding and appreciation of the growth and developmental process of children.

Gross motor behavior. Gross motor behavior includes developmental maturation in posture, head balance, sitting, creeping, standing, and walking (Fig. 12-1). The full-term neonate is born with some ability to hold the head erect and reflexly assumes the postural tonic neck position when supine. Several of the primitive reflexes have significance in terms of development of later gross motor skills. The righting reflexes, or those reflexes that elicit certain postural responses, particularly of flexion or extension, are responsible for certain motor activities, such as rolling over, assuming a crawl position, and maintaining normal head-trunk-limb alignment during all activities. The neck-righting reflex, which turns the body to the same side as the head, enables the child to roll over from supine to prone. Later the body-righting reflex allows the child to stand and sit. Other reflexes, such as the otolith-righting and labyrinth-righting reflexes, enable the infant to raise the head.

The asymmetric tonic neck reflex, which persists from birth to age 3 months, prevents the infant from rolling over. The symmetric tonic neck reflex, which is evoked by flexing or extending the neck, helps the infant to assume the crawl position. When the head and neck are extended, the extensor tone of the upper extremities and the flexor tone of the lower extremities increases. The child extends the arms and bends the knees. This reflex disappears when neurologic maturity allows actual crawling to occur because independent limb movement is required.

Head control. The full-term newborn can momentarily hold the head in midline and parallel when the body is suspended ventrally and can lift and turn the head from side to side when prone. However, marked head lag is evident when the infant is pulled from a lying to a sitting position. By 12 weeks of age the infant can hold his head well be-

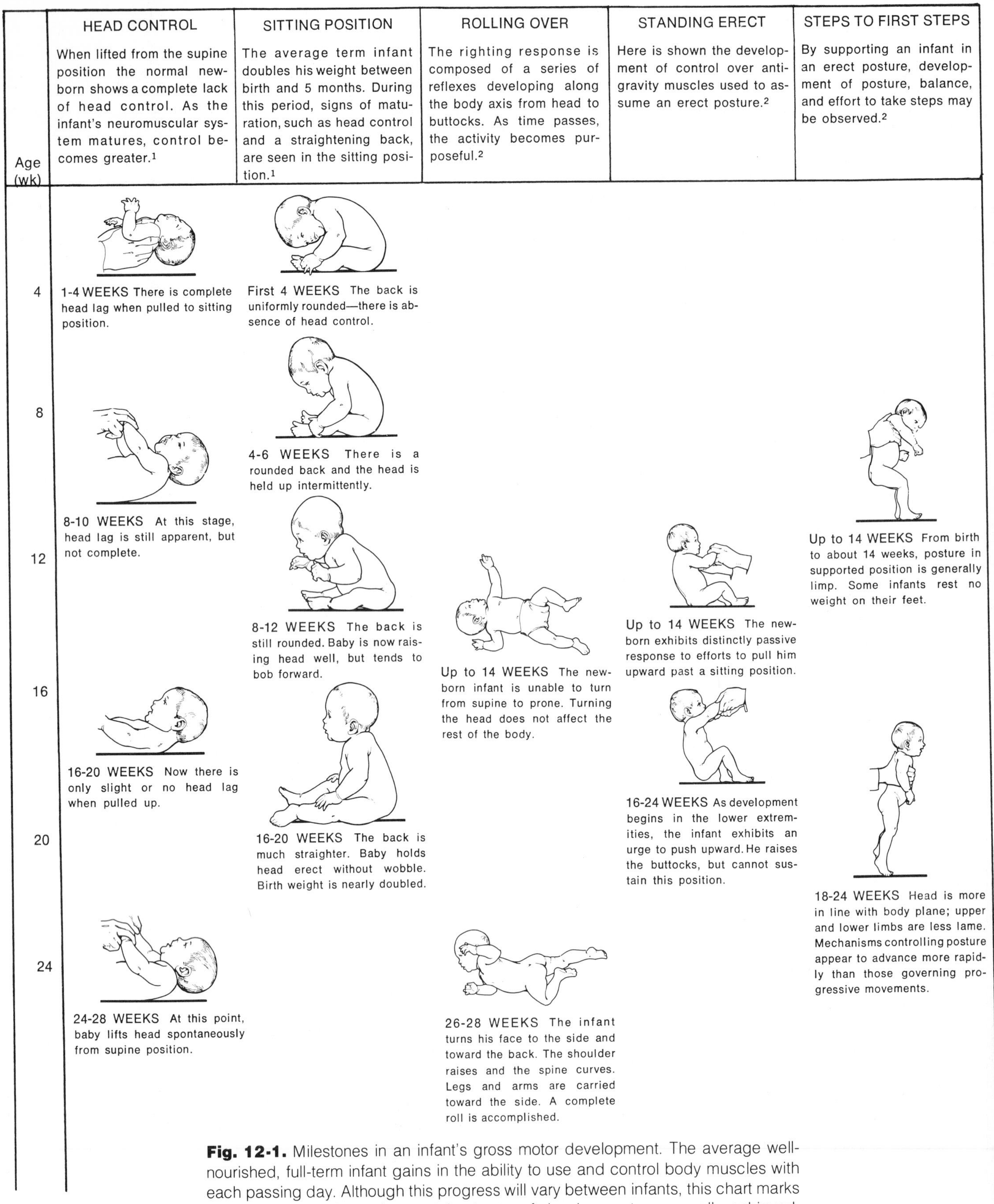
Age (wk)
HEAD CONTROL
When lifted from the supine position the normal newborn shows a complete lack of head control. As the infant's neuromuscular system matures, control becomes greater.[1]
SITTING POSITION
The average term infant doubles his weight between birth and 5 months. During this period, signs of maturation, such as head control and a straightening back, are seen in the sitting position.[1]
ROLLING OVER
The righting response is composed of a series of reflexes developing along the body axis from head to buttocks. As time passes, the activity becomes purposeful.[2]
STANDING ERECT
Here is shown the development of control over antigravity muscles used to assume an erect posture.[2]
STEPS TO FIRST STEPS
By supporting an infant in an erect posture, development of posture, balance, and effort to take steps may be observed.[2]
4
8
12
16
20
24
1-4 WEEKS There is complete head lag when pulled to sitting position.
8-10 WEEKS At this stage, head lag is still apparent, but not complete.
16-20 WEEKS Now there is only slight or no head lag when pulled up.
24-28 WEEKS At this point, baby lifts head spontaneously from supine position.
First 4 WEEKS The back is uniformly rounded—there is absence of head control.
4-6 WEEKS There is a rounded back and the head is held up intermittently.
8-12 WEEKS The back is still rounded. Baby is now raising head well, but tends to bob forward.
16-20 WEEKS The back is much straighter. Baby holds head erect without wobble. Birth weight is nearly doubled.
Up to 14 WEEKS The newborn infant is unable to turn from supine to prone. Turning the head does not affect the rest of the body.
26-28 WEEKS The infant turns his face to the side and toward the back. The shoulder raises and the spine curves. Legs and arms are carried toward the side. A complete roll is accomplished.
Up to 14 WEEKS The newborn exhibits distinctly passive response to efforts to pull him upward past a sitting position.
16-24 WEEKS As development begins in the lower extremities, the infant exhibits an urge to push upward. He raises the buttocks, but cannot sustain this position.
Up to 14 WEEKS From birth to about 14 weeks, posture in supported position is generally limp. Some infants rest no weight on their feet.
18-24 WEEKS Head is more in line with body plane; upper and lower limbs are less lame. Mechanisms controlling posture appear to advance more rapidly than those governing progressive movements.

Fig. 12-1. Milestones in an infant's gross motor development. The average well-nourished, full-term infant gains in the ability to use and control body muscles with each passing day. Although this progress will vary between infants, this chart marks the approximate times that certain stages of development are usually achieved. [1]Based on material presented by R. S. Illingworth: Development of the infant and young child, ed. 2, Baltimore, 1963, The Williams & Wilkins Co. [2]Adapted from McGraw, M.: The neuromuscular maturation of the human infant, New York, 1943, Columbia University Press, by permission of the publisher. (From Mead Johnson & Co., 1967, Evansville, Ind. Permission granted by Mead-Johnson Nutritional Division. Copyright, 1967, The Williams & Wilkins Co., Baltimore, Md.)

Age (wk)	HEAD CONTROL	SITTING POSITION	ROLLING OVER	STANDING ERECT	STEPS TO FIRST STEPS
	When lifted from the supine position the normal newborn shows a complete lack of head control. As the infant's neuromuscular system matures, control becomes greater.[1]	The average term infant doubles his weight between birth and 5 months. During this period, signs of maturation, such as head control and a straightening back, are seen in the sitting position.[1]	The righting response is composed of a series of reflexes developing along the body axis from head to buttocks. As time passes, the activity becomes purposeful.[2]	Here is shown the development of control over antigravity muscles used to assume an erect posture.[2]	By supporting an infant in an erect posture, development of posture, balance, and effort to take steps may be observed.[2]

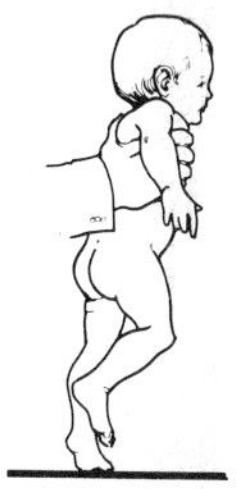

28

26-30 WEEKS Postural adjustment is much the same as in previous phase, but up and down movements and stamping may be seen. Some stepping movement may be observed.

32

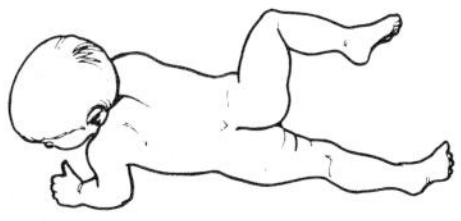

36

34-38 WEEKS Early rolling appears more involuntary than deliberate. Spinal extension is still the major initial movement. If near the edge of a bed or table, the infant shows no awareness of it. He might roll off.

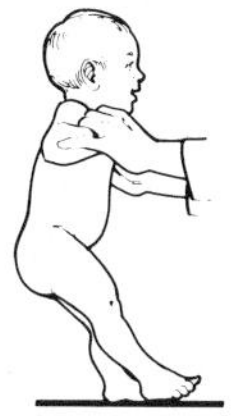

36-44 WEEKS As capacity increases, the infant extends his lower extremities and attains a somewhat erect posture. However, a vertical position usually cannot be achieved.

40

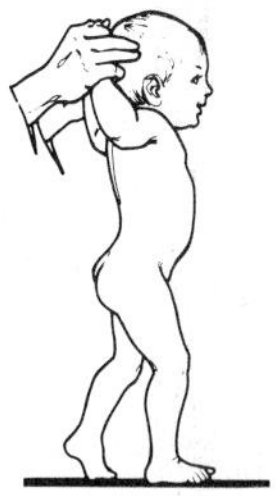

44

40-48 WEEKS Stepping and postural adjustment are more evidently deliberate at about 36 weeks. Some support is needed. Infant may begin *independent stepping* at 40-48 weeks.

48

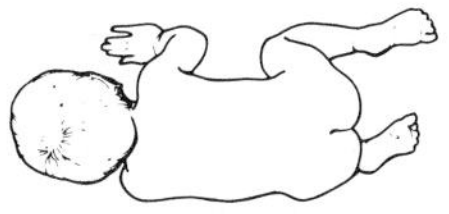

48-52 WEEKS The infant begins to use the act of rolling to complete some deliberate performance. He may flex the legs and raise the abdomen in order to creep or push into a sitting position. He shows some tendency towards adjusting to his whereabouts.

52

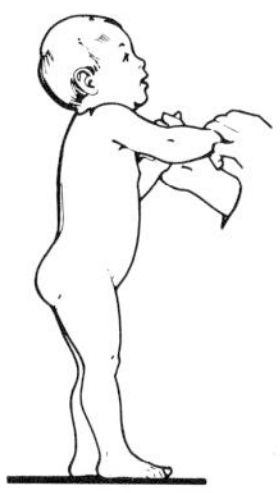

48-52 WEEKS Erect, vertical position is finally accomplished. Movements are made with effort.

Fig. 12-1. cont'd. For legend see opposite page.

yond the plane of his body, and by 16 weeks of age he can lift the head and front portion of the chest about 90 degrees above the table, bearing his weight on the forearms. Only slight head lag is evident when the infant is pulled from a lying to a sitting position. By age 24 weeks he can raise the chest and upper part of the abdomen off the table, maintaining his weight on the hands. By 28 weeks of age he can bear weight on one hand while exploring with the other.

Rolling over. The newborn may accidentally roll over because of his rounded back. The neck-righting reflex enables him to roll from back to side at age 16 weeks. The ability to willfully turn from the abdomen to the back occurs at 20 weeks of age and from the back to the abdomen at 24 weeks of age. It is noteworthy that the parachute reflex, which elicits a protective response to falling, appears at 28 weeks of age.

Sitting. The ability to sit follows progressive head control and straightening of the back. Although there is marked head lag in the sitting position at birth, the infant contracts the neck, shoulder, and arm muscles, enabling him to raise the head when half pulled to sitting. He will make attempts to lift the chin and right the head while sitting. At 12 weeks of age head lag is slight; at age 20 weeks it is absent; by 24 weeks of age the infant lifts the head when he is about to be pulled to sitting. By the next month he spontaneously raises the head in an attempt to sit up by himself.

For the first couple of months the back is uniformly rounded. The infant is born with the thoracic and pelvic curves, which are both concave, giving the vertebral column a C shape, rather than the adult double-S shape. The convex cervical curve forms about 3 to 4 months when head control is established. The convex lumbar curve appears when the child begins to sit, about age 4 months, but is usually pronounced (lordosis) for the first year or two. As the spinal column straightens, the infant is able to be propped in a sitting position. By ages 24 to 28 weeks he can sit alone, leaning forward on his hands for support. By ages 7 to 8 months he can sit well unsupported and begins to explore his surroundings in this position rather than in a lying position. By 40 weeks of age he can maneuver from a prone to a sitting position.

Locomotion. At birth the walking or dance reflex is present. It usually disappears by 3 weeks of age but can be elicited for a longer period of time if the neck is extended. If the infant is placed in a standing position, the body is usually limp at the hips and knees. By ages 24 to 28 weeks the infant is usually able to bear all his weight. By 36 weeks of age he stands holding on to furniture and can pull himself to the standing position but is unable to maneuver himself back down, except by falling. At age 44 weeks he can step with one foot, and at age 48 weeks he can cruise or walk while holding onto furniture or with both hands held. By 52 weeks of age he is able to walk with one hand held. The major gross motor milestones for the key developmental ages during infancy are listed in the box below.

Fine motor behavior. Fine motor behavior includes the use of the hands and fingers in the prehension of an object. Grasping occurs during the first 2 to 3 months as a reflex and gradually becomes voluntary. At age 4 weeks the hands are predominately closed and by age 12 weeks are mostly open. By this time the infant demonstrates a desire to grasp an object, but he "grasps" it more with the eyes than with the hands. If a rattle is placed in his hand, he will actively hold onto it. By age 16 weeks he regards a small pellet and his hands and will look from the object to his hands and back again. Hand regard is common at this age because of the limitation of symmetric positioning, which prevents the infant from exploring the periphery. Hand regard occurs in children who are blind, because it is a developmental process that occurs without visual stimulation. The fingering usually includes pulling at the blankets and clothes and sucking on the fists or fingers.

By 20 weeks the infant is able to voluntarily grasp an object, but prehension is two handed. The palmar grasp begins with grasping the object in the ulnar side of the palm (toward the fourth and fifth fingers) for the first 6 months. From ages 24 to 32 weeks, grasping occurs on the radial side (second and third fingers) and the base of the thumb. From ages 32 to 40 weeks the index, fourth, and fifth fingers form a crude pincer grasp with the lower part of the thumb (Fig. 12-2, *A*). By 40 weeks of age the index finger and thumb are used in apposition for a neat pincer grasp (Fig. 12-2, *B*).

Major gross motor developments during infancy

Key ages (weeks)	*Behavior*
4	Marked head lag, especially when pulled from lying to sitting position Holds head momentarily parallel and in midline when suspended in prone position Assumes asymmetric tonic neck reflex
16	Holds head erect in sitting position Slight head lag when pulled from lying to sitting position Lifts head in 90-degree angle from table when lying prone Assumes predominately symmetric position Rolls from back to side; rolls completely over at 20 weeks
28	Sits, leaning forward on both hands Bears full weight on feet
40	Sits alone Pulls self to standing position Creeps
52	Walks with someone holding one hand Cruises around furniture

By 6 months of age the infant has increased manipulative skill. He holds his bottle, grasps his feet and pulls them to his mouth, and feeds himself a cracker. He enjoys tearing and crumbling paper and explores it thoroughly in his mouth. If he is given two objects, he will hold one and drop the other.

By 7 months of age he transfers objects from one hand to the other, employs one hand for grasping, and holds a cube in each hand simultaneously. He enjoys banging objects and will explore movable parts in a toy. Although unidexterous prehension is dominant, handedness is not firmly established until 5 to 6 years of age, even though definite use of the dominant hand is evident at 1 to 2 years of age.

By age 40 weeks pincer grasp is established and the infant is able to pick up a raisin and other finger foods. He can deliberately let go of an object and will offer it to someone, but true casting, deliberate throwing objects one after the other, is not evident until 12 to 15 months of age. By age 44 weeks he puts objects into a container and likes to remove them. By 1 year of age the infant tries to build a tower of two blocks but fails. Deliberately releasing an object has advanced; he now releases a cube into a cup following a demonstration. The major fine motor milestones for the key developmental ages during infancy are listed in the boxed material.

Language behavior. The infant is a very social being. His first means of verbal communication is crying. He learns to signal displeasure before pleasure. Vocalizations heard during crying become the syllables and the words of the child. A classic example is the "mama" heard during vigorous crying. The infant vocalizes as early as 5 to 6 weeks of age by making small throaty sounds. By age 8 weeks he makes single vowel sounds, such as ah, eh, and uh. By 12 to 16 weeks of age the consonants n, k, g, p, and b are added and the infant coos, gurgles, and laughs aloud. By age 32 weeks he adds the consonants t, d, and w and combines syllables, such as dada, but does not ascribe meaning to the word until ages 44 to 48 weeks. He makes

Major fine motor developments during infancy

Key ages (weeks)	*Behavior*
4	Hands fisted
16	Hands open
	Searches and "grasps" with the eyes
	Reaches for object but misses, may contact a 1-inch cube
28	Palmar grasp
	Rakes at pellet
	Transfers objects from hand to hand
	Unidexterous approach to an object
	Retains one cube when second is offered
40	Pincer grasp
	Crude release beginning
52	Can release a cube into a cup following demonstration

A

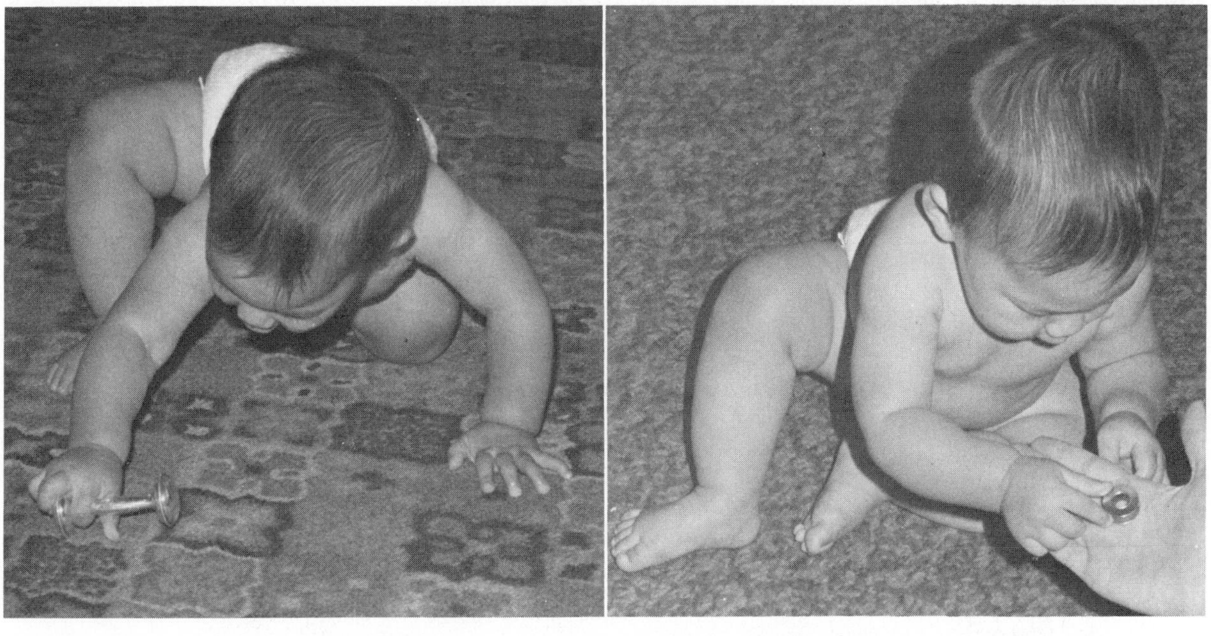

B

Fig. 12-2. A, Crude pincer grasp; **B,** neat pincer grasp.

sounds, such as coughing or snorting, to attract attention. By 36 to 40 weeks of age he can comprehend the meaning of the word "no," obey simple commands, and respond to his name. By age 1 year he can say two to three words with meaning. The major language achievements for the key developmental ages during infancy are listed in the boxed material below.

During the acquisition of new language skills it is not unlikely for the child to temporarily give up other recently learned sounds or words. This is often distressing for parents after waiting in anticipation for the words dada or mama. However, these sounds are frequently given up for other vocalizations and may not be repeated for several weeks. It is reassuring for parents to know that the child will again say these words, and probably with meaning. Not making these sounds bears no negative message from the infant.

Personal-social behavior. Personal-social behavior includes the child's personal responses to his environment. It is the area most influenced by external stimuli but, as in the other fields of behavior, follows certain developmental laws. Personal-social behavior implies communication with one's self and with others. It is foundational for the successful mastery of skills such as feeding, control of bodily functions, independence, and cooperativeness in play.

Recently research has confirmed what parents knew all along—that infants are responsive, social beings. They have the ability to shape their environment and to elicit certain responses. The newborn shows visual preference for the human face and, as early as 1 week of age, begins to watch his mother intently as she speaks to him. As he regards her face his activity diminishes, his head bobs up and down, and his mouth moves almost as if trying to say something. By ages 6 to 8 weeks a social smile in response to pleasurable stimuli is present. This has a profound effect on family members and is a tremendous stimulus for evoking continued responses from others. By age 12 weeks he shows considerable interest in the environment: excitement when a toy is presented, refusal to be left alone, recognition of mother, and demonstration of pleasure by squealing. By age 16 weeks he laughs aloud and enjoys strange, novel stimuli.

By age 6 months the infant is a very personable child. He plays games such as peekaboo when his head is hidden in a towel, he signals his desire to be picked up by extending his arms, and he shows displeasure when a toy is removed or his face is washed. There is increasing demonstration of his ability to control his environment. The acquisition of fine and gross motor skills allows him much more independence in movement.

By the second half of the first year the infant understands simple discipline, such as the meaning of the word "no" or a scolding remark. He comprehends different facial expressions and is sensitive to emotional changes in others. Imitation is developing during this time. By age 28 weeks he imitates acts and noises, by age 32 weeks, sounds, and by age 40 weeks, games such as pat-a-cake and peekaboo. From ages 44 to 52 weeks he is increasingly independent. He is learning to feed himself and use a spoon and cup and can help with dressing by putting his foot out for a shoe or pushing his arm through the sleeve. He not only comprehends the meaning of "no," but shakes his head to signal his understanding. He can follow simple directions and will gladly perform for others to attract and prolong attention. The major personal-social achievements for the key developmental ages during infancy are listed in the boxed material below.

Major language developments during infancy

Key ages (weeks)	*Behavior*
4	Small throaty sounds
16	Vowel sounds—ah, eh, uh
	Consonant sounds—n, k, g, p, b
	Coos and laughs
28	Single consonant syllables—ah goo, ba, ka, da
	Vocalizes to toys
40	Consonant sounds—t, d, w
	Combines syllables—baba, dada
	Imitates sounds
	Says one word
	Comprehends "no"
	Responds to own name
52	Says two or more words with meaning
	Recognizes objects by name
	Imitates animal sounds

Major personal-social development during infancy

Key ages (weeks)	*Behavior*
4	Regards face intently, activity diminishes
	Social smile at 6 to 8 weeks
16	Plays with hands and clothes
	Recognizes bottle; shows anticipation for feeding
	Laughs aloud
28	Stranger anxiety, preference for parents or care giver
	Plays with feet
	Regards self in mirror, pats own image
	Feeds self cracker
40	Plays simple nursery games
	Waves bye-bye, imitates pat-a-cake
52	Cooperates in dressing
	"Plays" ball
	Shakes head for "no"

Play. Play is becoming more sophisticated and interdependent. From birth to age 3 months the infant's response to the environment is global and largely undifferentiated. Play in dependent; pleasure is demonstrated by a quieting attitude (age 1 month), later by a smile (age 2 months), and then by a squeal (age 3 months). From ages 3 to 6 months the infant shows more discriminate interest in the stimuli presented to him and begins to play alone with a rattle or soft stuffed toy or to play with someone else. There is much more interaction during play. By 4 months of age he laughs aloud, will show preference for certain toys, and will be excited when food or a favorite object is brought to him. He recognizes an image in a mirror, smiles at it, and vocalizes to it.

By 6 months to 1 year of age, play is much more sophisticated and involves sensorimotor skills. Actual games are played, such as peekaboo, pat-a-cake, verbal repetition, and imitation of simple gestures in response to demonstration. Play is much more selective, not only in terms of specific toys, but also in terms of "playmates." Although play is solitary or one sided, the infant chooses with whom he will interact. At 6 to 8 months of age he usually refuses to play with strangers until he begins to know them. Parents are definite favorites, and he knows how to attract their attention. At age 24 weeks he extends his arms to be picked up, at age 28 weeks he coughs to make his presence known, at age 40 weeks he pulls the parent's clothing, and at age 52 weeks he calls them by name. This represents a tremendous advance from the newborn who signaled biologic needs by crying to express displeasure.

Stimulation is as important for developmental growth as food is for biologic growth. Knowledge of developmental milestones allows nurses to guide parents regarding proper play for infants. It is not sufficient to place a mobile over a crib and toys in a playpen for a child's optimal social, emotional, and intellectual development. Play must provide interpersonal contact, as well as recreational and educational stimulation. Infants need to be *played with,* not merely allowed *to play*. Although the type of play infants engage in is called *solitary,* this is only a figurative, not literal, term to denote one-sided play. The kind of toys given to the child is much less important than the quality of personal interaction that occurs.

Table 12-2 lists play activities that are appropriate for the developmental level of the infant in view of motor, language, and personal-social achievements. Although the activities are grouped according to the major mode of stimulation provided, there is overlap in many instances. In addition play activities suggested for one age-group may be appropriate for an older age-group but are generally inappropriate for a younger age-group.

Intellectual development

Intellectual development is concurrent with biologic, motor, language, and personal-social achievements. In fact, many of these must occur before learning can take place. For example, visual ability must be sufficient for the infant to see objects clearly before associations about the object can be made. Learning occurs when behavior changes as a result of experience or growth. Learning theories attempt to explain the acquisition and understanding of perception and knowledge. In general, learning takes place through (1) conditioning and/or reinforcement, (2) imitation, (3) insight, and (4) natural progression of one's innate capacity. Conditioning, or learning by association between a stimulus and a response, appears to be the predominant type that takes place during early infancy. As motor function progresses, learning occurs through the infant's more active participation in the environment. The theory most frequently quoted to explain cognition, or the ability to know, is by Piaget. Jean Piaget, Swiss psychologist, observed and described the unfolding of the child's inherited potentialities for intellectual growth. He has described five major phases in the development of logical thinking (Table 12-3). Subdivisions of the phases are termed stages. The phase that has been most extensively studied is the sensorimotor phase (birth to 24 months), which is composed of six stages. During this phase the infant progresses from reflex behavior to simple repetitive acts to imitative activity. Three crucial events take place during this phase. First the infant learns to separate himself from other objects in the environment. In Freudian terms, the infant progresses from the id stage to ego development. He realizes that others besides himself control the environment and that certain readjustments must take place for mutual satisfaction to occur. This coincides with Erikson's concept of the formation of trust and mutual regulation of frustration. Piaget also believes in a "conflict" during each phase. The goal during one phase is to establish a balance between the desire to function at a higher level while recognizing the limitations created by the environment. He believes that achieving a near equilibrium in a constantly changing environment is the goal of biologic, affective (emotional), and mental functions.

The second major achievement is perceiving the concept of *permanency,* or the realization that objects that leave one's visual field still exist. A typical example of the development of object permanency is the infant's ability to separate from his parents at bedtime because of his realization that they will be present when he awakens. Eventually he broadens this concept to tolerate brief periods of separation with a different care giver. The last major intellectual development of this period is the ability to use symbols or "mental representation." The use of symbols allows the infant to think of an object or situation without actually experiencing it. The recognition of symbols is the beginning of understanding of time and space.

To understand Piaget's cognitive theory, certain terms must be defined. *Adaptation* is the cognitive striving of the individual to seek an equilibrium or balance in the interaction of self with the environment. Adaptation depends on

Table 12-2. Play during infancy

Age (months)	Visual stimulation	Auditory stimulation	Tactile stimulation	Kinetic stimulation
Suggested activities				
Birth-1	Look at infant within close range Hang bright, shiny object within 8-10 inches of infant's face and in midline	Talk to infant, sing in soft voice Play music box, radio, or television Have ticking clock or metronome nearby	Hold, caress, cuddle Keep infant warm May like to be swaddled	Rock infant, place in cradle Use carriage for walks
2-3	Provide bright objects Make room bright with pictures or mirrors on wall Take infant to various rooms while doing chores Place in infant seat for vertical view of environment	Talk to infant Include in family gatherings Expose to various environmental noises other than those of home Use rattles, wind chimes	Caress while bathing, at diaper change Comb hair with a soft brush Spread soothing lotion or powder on body	Use cradle gym or swing Take in car for rides Exercise body by moving extremities in swimming motion
4-6	Place infant so that he can look in mirror Place in front of television with family Give brightly colored toys to hold (small enough to grasp)	Talk to infant, repeat sounds he makes Laugh when he laughs Call him by name Crinkle different papers by his ear Place rattle or bell in hand, show him how to shake them	Give him soft squeeze toys of various textures Allow to splash in bath Place nude on soft furry rug and move extremities	Use swing or stroller Bounce him in lap while holding him in standing position Help him roll over Support him in sitting position, let him lean forward to balance himself Put him in a box and tilt gently
6-9	Give him large toys with bright colors, movable parts, and noisemakers Enjoys mirror, pats it, talks to image (Fig. 12-3) Enjoys peekaboo, especially hiding his face in a towel Make funny faces to encourage imitation Give him paper to tear, crumble Give him ball of yarn or string to pull apart	Call him by name Repeat simple words such as dada, mama, bye-bye Speak clearly Name parts of body, people, and foods Tell him what you are doing Use word "no" only when necessary Give simple commands Show him how to clap hands, bang a drum	Let him play with various textures of fabric Have bowl with foods of different sizes and textures to feel Let him "catch" running water Encourage "swimming" in large bathtub or shallow pool Give wad of sticky tape to manipulate	Use walker Place on floor to crawl, roll over, or sit Hold upright to bear weight and bounce Pick up—say "up" Put down—say "down" Place toys out of reach; encourage him to get them Play pat-a-cake Encourage banging on pot and slapping hands on table
9-12	Show him large pictures in books Take him to places where there are animals, many people, different objects (shopping center) Play ball by rolling it to child, demonstrate "throwing" it back Demonstrate building a two-block tower	Read him simple nursery rhymes Point to body parts and name each one Imitate sounds of animals	Give finger foods of different textures Let him mess and squash food Let him feel cold (ice cube) or warm objects, say what temperature each is Let him feel a breeze (fan blowing)	Use walker Give large push-pull toys to encourage walking Place furniture in a circle to encourage cruising Encourage "roughhouse" play, turn in different positions
Suggested toys				
6-12	Various colored blocks Nested boxes or cups Books with rhymes and bright pictures Brightly colored balloons Strings of big beads and snap beads Simple take-apart toys Large ball Cup and spoon	Rattles of different sizes, shapes, tones, and bright colors Squeaky animals and dolls Records with light rhythmic music	Soft, different textured animals and dolls Sponge toys, floating toys Squeeze toys	Exercise crib toys Activity box for crib Push-pull toys Walker Swing

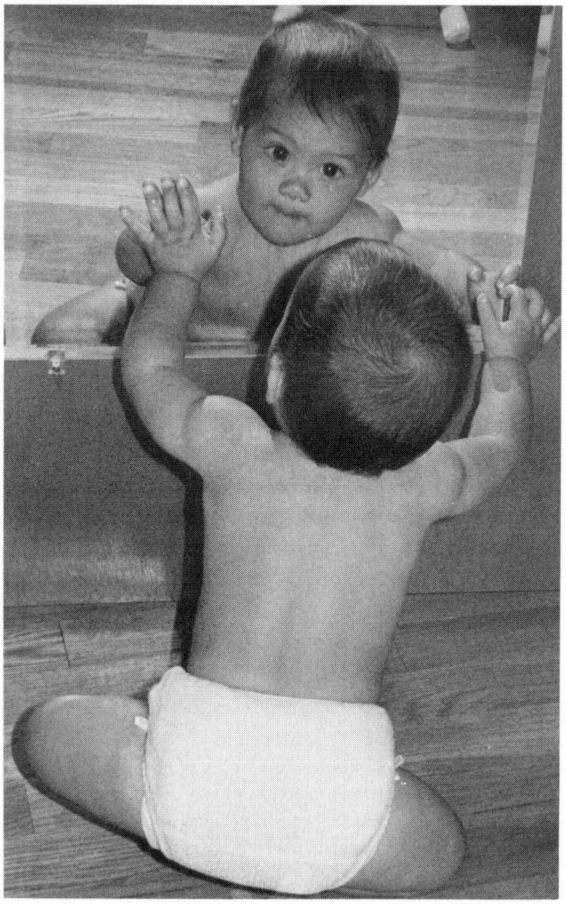

Fig. 12-3. A 9-month-old infant enjoying her image in the mirror.

Table 12-3. Piaget's phases of cognitive development

Age (years)	Phase	
Birth-2	Sensorimotor	
2-4	Preconceptual	Preoperational
4-7	Intuitive thought	
7-11	Concrete operations	
11-15	Formal operations	

two interrelated processes: assimilation and accommodation.

Assimilation is the process by which an individual incorporates knowledge about the environment as he initially perceives it. The new knowledge, skills, or insights are taken in only as far as his previous experience allows. Through *accommodation,* new knowledge is incorporated that previously was not perceived. These two processes always act together to provide an organizational pattern or *schema*. Assimilation can occur without accommodation, but accommodation must follow assimilation. When there is a balance between these two processes, adaptation occurs. Because of these two processes, it is understandable that *experience* rather than maturation is the chief determinant of intellectual development.

The period of infancy (birth to 24 months) is termed the sensorimotor phase and is composed of six stage (Tables 12-4 and 14-2). The first stage, from birth to 1 month, is identified by the *use of reflexes*. At birth the infant's individuality and temperament are expressed through the physiologic reflexes of sucking, rooting, grasping, and crying. The repetitious nature of the reflexes is the beginning of associations between an act and a sequential response. When the infant cries because he is hungry, a nipple is put in his mouth, and he sucks, feels satisfaction, and sleeps. He is assimilating this experience, while perceiving auditory, tactile, and visual cries. This experience of perceiving certain patterns or ''ordering'' is foundational for the subsequent stages.

The next stage, *primary circular reactions,* marks the beginning of the replacement of reflexive behavior with voluntary acts. During this period from 1 to 4 months, activities such as sucking or grasping become deliberate acts that elicit certain responses. The beginning of accommodation is evident. The infant incorporates and adapts his reactions to the environment and recognizes the stimulus that produced a response. Previously the infant would cry until the nipple was brought to his mouth. Now he will associate the nipple with the sound of the mother's voice. He accommodates this new piece of information and adapts by ceasing to cry when he hears her voice, before he receives the nipple. A realization of causality and a recognition of an orderly sequence of events is taking place. The environment is taken in with all the senses and with whatever motor ability is present.

The next stage, *secondary circular reactions,* is a continuation of the previous one, as its name implies. In this stage the circular primary reactions are repeated and prolonged for the response that results. Grasping and holding now become shaking, banging, and pulling. Shaking is performed to hear a noise, not solely for the pleasure of shaking. Quality and quantity of an act become evident. ''More'' or ''less' shaking produces different responses. Causality, time, deliberate intention, and one's separateness from the environment begin to develop. Three new processes of human behavior—imitation, play, and affect—occur. *Imitation* requires the differentiation of selected acts from several events. By the second half of the first year, the infant can imitate sounds and simple gestures. *Play* becomes evident as the infant takes pleasure in performing an act after he has mastered it. Much of the infant's waking hours are absorbed in sensorimotor play. *Affect* is seen as the infant begins to develop a sense of permanency. During the first 6 months the infant believes that an object exists

Table 12-4. Sensorimotor phase during early infancy*

Stage	Age (months)	Cognitive development	Behavior
I. Use of reflexes	Birth-1	Repetitious use of reflexes establishes a pattern of experiences Totally autistic (self-centered) being	Mostly reflexive (sucking, swallowing, rooting, grasping, crying) Little or no tolerance for frustration or delayed gratification
II. Primary circular reactions	1-4	Use of reflexes is gradually replaced by voluntary activity Recognition of causality occurs when repetition of events causes one stimulus to produce a consistent response Beginning notion of temporal space or time occurs as infant realizes the progression of an orderly sequence of events Beginning separation of self from others Learns from type of interaction between object or individual rather than from object itself Engages in an activity for the pleasure of the activity more than for its result	Recognizes familiar faces and objects (for example, bottle) Shows anticipation before feeding Awareness of strange surroundings indicates memory Discovers parts of own body—plays with hands, fingers, feet Becomes bored when left alone Shows no stranger anxiety unless care giver's skill differs from usual routine
III. Secondary circular reactions	4-8	Intentional activity replaces repetitious activity that did not produce a desired result Beginning of object permanency when object is beyond perceptual range Progressive idea of time, awareness of before and after in a sequence of events Able to imitate selective activity from several events Further separation of self from environment Idea of quality and quantity Beginning recognition of symbols as type of communication	Secures objects by pulling on a string Searches for objects that have fallen Shows stranger anxiety Able to tolerate some frustration and delayed gratification Imitates sounds and simple gestures Great interest in mirror image Beginning independence in self-feeding Shows displeasure if activity is inhibited Language development, attracts attention by methods other than crying Realizes that parents are present even if not in visual field
IV. Coordination of secondary schemata and their application to new situations	9-12	Concept of object permanence advances, beginning of intellectual reasoning Associates symbols with events, but classification is based on own experience Distinguishes objects from the related activity and perceives them as objects Distinguishes end products from their means, attempts to remove barriers to achieve the end	Actively searches for a hidden object Comprehends meanings of words and simple commands Knows that gestures (bye-bye, kiss) have certain meanings Is able to put objects in a container Works to get toy out of reach Ventures away from mother to explore surroundings

*For phases during later infancy and early childhood see Table 14-2.

only for as long as he can visually perceive it. In other words, out of sight—out of mind. When the object continues to be present or remembered even though it is beyond the range of perception, affect to external objects is evident. The most notable example of this is the development of stranger anxiety at 6 to 8 months of age. Another is the game of peekaboo, in which the child tests out the reality of being and not being. Some theorists postulate that this type of activity represents the beginning development of the concept of death.

During the fourth sensorimotor stage, *coordination of secondary schemata and its application to new situations,* the infant uses previous behavioral achievements primarily as the foundation for adding new intellectual skills to his expanding repertoire. This stage is largely transitional. Increasing motor skills allow for greater exploration of the environment. He begins to discover that hiding an object does not mean that it is gone but that removing an obstacle will reveal the object. This marks the beginning of intellectual reasoning. Furthermore, he can experience an event by *observing* it, and he begins to associate symbols with events, such as "bye-bye" with "Daddy goes to work," but the classification is purely his own. Unlike the second stage, where the infant learned from the type of interaction between objects or individuals, in this stage the child learns from the object itself. Intentionality is further developed in that now the infant will actively attempt to remove a barrier to his desired (or undesired) action. If something is in his way, he will attempt to climb over it or push it away. Previously an obstacle would cause him to give up any further attempt to achieve his desired goal.

The last two stages occur during the toddler period of 12 to 24 months. In the fifth stage, *tertiary circular reactions* (see Table 14-2), the child uses active experimentation to achieve previously unattainable goals. Accommodation processes are evident as he attempts to incorporate the environmental experience as it truly is. He is able to solve more complex problems through active trial-and-error experimentation. Reasoning becomes increasingly evident as the child grasps logic—that the first precedes the second, but that the second need not succeed the first. Awareness of relationships such as time and space becomes increasingly apparent. As causal relationships progress, the child is aware that events occur that are totally beyond his control and that other people are autonomous beings. This latter development is elaborated on in the sixth stage, *invention of new means through mental combinations* (see Table 14-2), during the latter half of the second year. The child has a deeper awareness of object permanence. He will now search for an object that has been displaced twice. In the previous stage the child would search for an object that was placed under one pillow. But if it was placed first under one pillow and then under a second pillow, he would not look under the second pillow. In this stage he can search under more than one location for an object. In addition he can infer what happened to something. For example, he can infer that a missing object was taken by someone else even if he did not see it being taken. Play and imitation also advance toward more sophisticated levels of intellectual functioning during the toddler years. Further discussion of cognitive development is explored in Chapter 14.

Summary of growth and development

At no other time in life are the biologic and developmental changes and achievements more dramatic than during infancy. Each month the infant learns new skills, is increasingly aware of the environment, and develops closer interpersonal attachments. Because of the complexity of the developmental process during these 12 months, Table 12-5 is presented to help organize and clarify the data that have already been presented. The material has been compiled from a variety of sources but is based primarily on the work of Arnold Gesell and Catherine Amatruda.* The age-groups have been divided into weeks rather than months for greater accuracy. For example, a 7-month-old child is really 30 weeks old. The use of 4-week divisions results in thirteen age categories rather than twelve. Although the milestones are important, some represent essential integrative aspects of development that lay the foundation for the achievement of more advanced skills. These essential milestones are designated by a bullet (•) in the chart. The table represents the *average* age at which various skills are attained. It must be remembered that although the sequence is the same, the rate will vary in different children.

*Knobloch, H., and Pasamanick, B.: Gesell and Amatruda's developmental diagnosis, New York, 1974, Harper & Row, Publishers.

HEALTH PROMOTION DURING FIRST YEAR

The infant's first year is a time of monumental change and achievement. Each month and each phase of development have implications for care of the child. Some of the general areas that are especially affected by the infant's development are feeding and safety. Physical care is fairly constant, because the infant is dependent on others for bathing and diapering, and the degree of the child's independence usually is less influential than during the toddler years, when the achievement of autonomy and tasks such as toilet training are important goals.

Health promotion also involves prevention of disease. Although nutrition and safety play a definite role in preventing illness, the most important intervention is immunizations. Immunizations are part of the routine health care of children. The recommended schedule for health supervision is monthly for the first 6 months, bimonthly for the second 6 months, every 3 months during the second year, every 6 months during the third year, and annually thereafter.

Nutrition guidance

Ideally nutrition guidance should begin prenatally with the decision to breast- or bottle-feed the infant. The choice for either is highly individual and has been discussed in Chapter 8. This section is primarily concerned with infant nutrition during the next 12 months, when growth needs and developmental milestones ready the child for introduction of solid foods. Frequently the nurse is asked when to begin feeding solid foods, how to introduce new foods, and what foods are best. A thorough understanding of each of these areas prepares the nurse to answer these questions in order to meet the nutritional needs of each child.

Infant feeding. A great deal of controversy exists regarding infant feeding and the need for solid foods. Prior to 1920 solid foods were seldom offered until 1 year of age. However, several studies were then done that demonstrated that infants tolerated solid foods well during the first year.[5] From that time on, the pendulum swung in the opposite direction, with solid foods, particularly meat, being added at an increasingly earlier age. Several claims have been advanced for the benefit of adding solid foods to the infant's diet as early as 1 or 2 weeks after birth. However, clinical studies have not offered substantial proof of superior nutritional states over breast milk, commercially prepared for-

Text continued on p. 450.

Table 12-5. Summary of growth and development during infancy*

Age (weeks)	Physical	Gross motor	Fine motor
Birth-4	Weight gain of 150 to 210 g (5 to 7 ounces) weekly for first 6 months Height gain of 2.5 cm (1 inch) monthly for first 6 months Head circumference larger than chest circumference Primitive reflexes present and strong Doll's eye reflex and dance reflex fading Obligatory nose breather	Marked head lag, especially when pulled from lying to sitting position Holds head momentarily parallel and in midline when suspended in prone position Assumes asymmetric tonic neck reflex position when supine • Assumes flexed position with pelvis high, but knees not under abdomen when prone (at birth, knees are flexed under abdomen) • Can turn head from side to side when prone, lifts head momentarily from bed Makes crawling movements when prone When held in standing position, body limp at knees and hips	Hands predominately closed Grasp reflex strong Hand clenches on contact with rattle
8	Posterior fontanel closed Crawling reflex disappears	Less head lag when pulled to sitting position Can maintain head in same plane as rest of body when held in ventral suspension When prone, can lift head almost 45 degrees off table When held in sitting position, head is held up but bobs forward Assumes asymmetric tonic neck reflex position intermittently • Assumes less flexed position when prone—hips flat, legs extended, arms flexed, head to side	Hands frequently open Grasp reflex fading
12	Primitive reflexes fading Landau reflex appears	Able to hold head more erect when sitting, but still bobs forward Only slight head lag when pulled to sitting Assumes symmetric body positioning Able to raise head and shoulders from prone position to a 45- to 90-degree angle from table; bears weight on forearms When held in standing position, able to bear slight fraction of weight on legs Regards own hand	Grasp reflex absent Hands kept loosely open • Actively holds rattle, but will not reach for it Clutches own hand, pulls at blankets and clothes
16	Drooling begins • Moro, tonic neck, rooting, extrusion, and Perez reflexes have disappeared	• Almost no head lag when pulled to sitting position • Balances head well in sitting position Able to raise head and chest off couch to angle of 90 degrees Assumes predominately symmetric position Rolls from back to side Back less rounded, curved only in lumbar area Able to sit erect if propped up	Tries to reach objects with hand but overshoots it Grasps object with both hands Plays with rattle placed in hand, shakes it, but cannot pick it up if dropped Can carry objects to mouth • Inspects and plays with hands, pulls clothing or blanket over face in play
20	Growth rate may begin to decline Beginning signs of tooth eruption Able to breathe when nose is obstructed	No head lag when pulled to sitting position When sitting, able to hold head erect and steady Able to sit for longer periods when back is well supported Back straight When prone, assumes symmetric positioning with arms extended When held in standing position, able to bear most of weight Can turn over from abdomen to back When supine, puts feet to mouth	• Able to grasp objects voluntarily Uses palmar grasp, bidexterous approach Plays with toes Takes objects directly to mouth Holds one cube while regarding a second

*Milestones that represent essential integrative aspects of development that lay the foundation for the achievement of more advanced skills are indicated

Sensory	Vocalization	Socialization
• Able to fixate on moving object Follows light to midline Quiets when hears a voice	Cries to express displeasure Makes small throaty sounds Makes comfort sounds during feeding	Watches parent's face intently as she or he talks to infant
Binocular fixation and convergence to near objects beginning When supine, follows dangling toy from side to point beyond midline Visually searches to locate sounds Turns head to side when sound is made at level of ear	• Vocalizes, distinct from crying Crying becomes differentiated Coos Vocalizes to familiar voice	• Social smile in response to various stimuli
• Follows object to periphery (180 degrees) • Locates sound by turning head to side and looking in same direction Begins to have ability to coordinate stimuli from various sense organs	Coos, babbles, and chuckles Vocalizes when smiling "Talks" a great deal when spoken to • Squeals aloud to show pleasure Less crying during periods of wakefulness	Much interest in surroundings Ceases crying when parent enters room Can recognize familiar faces and objects, such as feeding bottle Shows awareness of strange situations
Able to accommodate to near objects Binocular vision fairly well established Can focus on a ½-inch block Beginning eye-hand coordination	Makes consonant sounds n, k, g, p, b Laughs aloud Vocalization changes according to mood	Demands attention by fussing; becomes bored if left alone Enjoys social interaction with people Anticipates feeding when sees bottle Shows excitement with whole body, squeals, breathes heavy Shows interest in strange stimuli
Visually pursues a dropped object • Smiles at mirror image Able to sustain visual inspection of an object Visual acuity, 20/200 Can localize sounds made below the ear	• Squeals Vowellike cooing sounds interspersed with consonantal sounds (for example, ah-goo)	Smiles at mirror image Pats bottle with both hands More enthusiastically playful, but may have rapid mood swings Able to discriminate strangers from family Vocalizes displeasure when an object is taken away

by a bullet.

Continued.

Table 12-5. Summary of growth and development during infancy—cont'd

Age (weeks)	Physical	Gross motor	Fine motor
24	Birth weight doubled Weight gain of 90 to 150 g (3 to 5 ounces) weekly for next 6 months Height gain of 1.25 cm (½ inch) monthly for next 6 months Teething may begin with eruption of two lower central incisors • Chewing and biting occur	When prone, can lift chest and upper abdomen off table, bearing weight on hands When about to be pulled to a sitting position, lifts head Sits in high chair with back straight Rolls from back to abdomen When held in standing position, bears almost all of weight Hand regard absent	Resecures a dropped object Drops one cube when another is given Grasps and manipulates small objects Holds bottle Grasps feet and pulls to mouth
28	Eruption of upper central incisors	When prone, bears weight on one hand • Sits, leaning forward on both hands Sits erect momentarily Bears full weight on feet When held in standing position, bounces actively • When supine, spontaneously lifts head off table	• Transfers objects from one hand to the other Unidexterous approach and grasp Holds two cubes more than momentarily Bangs cube on table Rakes at a small object
32	Begins to show regular patterns in bladder and bowel elimination Parachute reflex appears Plantar reflex disappears	Sits steadily unsupported Readily bears weight on legs when supported, may stand holding on Adjusts posture to reach an object	Beginning pincer grasp using the index, fourth, and fifth fingers against the lower part of the thumb Releases objects at will Rings bell purposely Retains two cubes while regarding the third cube Secures an object by pulling on a string Reaches persistently for toys out of reach
36	Eruption of upper lateral incisor may begin	Crawls, may progress backward at first Sits steadily on floor for prolonged time (10 minutes) Recovers balance when leans forward but cannot do so when leaning sideways Stands holding onto furniture Pulls self to standing position	• Ability to use thumb and index finger in crude pincer grasp Preference for use of hand now evident Grasps third cube Compares two cubes by bringing them together
40	Neck-righting reflex disappears Labyrinth-righting reflex is strongest Body-righting reflex appears	Crawls by pulling self forward with hands Can change from prone to sitting position Pulls self to sitting position Stands while holding onto furniture, sits by falling down Recovers balance easily while sitting	Crude release of an object beginning Grasps bell by handle
44	Eruption of lower lateral incisors may begin	• Creeps with abdomen off floor While standing, lifts one foot to take a step	Can hold crayon to make a mark on paper Explores objects more thoroughly (for example, clapper inside bell)

Sensory	Vocalization	Socialization
Adjusts posture to see an object Prefers more complex visual stimuli Can localize sounds made above the ear Will turn head to the side, then look up or down	• Begins to imitate sounds Vocalizes to toys, mirror image • Babbling resembles one-syllable utterances—ma, mu, da, di, hi Laughs aloud Takes pleasure in hearing own sounds (self-reinforcement)	Recognizes parents; begins to fear strangers Holds arms out to be picked up Has definite likes and dislikes Beginning of imitation (cough, protrusion of tongue) Excites on hearing footsteps Laughs when head is hidden in a towel Briefly searches for a dropped object (object permanence beginning) Frequent mood swings—from crying to laughing with little or no provocation
• Can fixate on very small objects Responds to own name Localizes sound by turning head in a curving arch Beginning awareness of depth and space Has taste preferences	Vocalizes four distinct vowel sounds • Produces vowel sounds and chained syllables—baba, dada, kaka "Talks" when others are talking	• Increasing fear of strangers; shows signs of fretfulness when mother disappears Imitates simple acts and noises Tries to attract attention by coughing or snorting Plays peekaboo Demonstrates dislike of food by keeping lips closed Exhibits oral aggressiveness in biting and mouthing Demonstrates expectation in response to repetition of stimuli
	Makes consonant sounds t, d, and w Listens selectively to familiar words Utterances signal emphasis and emotion Combines syllables, such as dada, but does not ascribe meaning to them	Increasing anxiety over loss of parent, particularly mother, and fear of strangers Responds to word "no" Dislikes dressing, diaper change
Localizes sounds by turning head diagonally and directly toward sound Depth perception increasing	Responds to simple verbal commands Comprehends "no-no"	Parent (mother) is increasingly important for own sake Increasing interest in pleasing mother Begins to show fears of going to bed and being left alone Puts arms in front of face to avoid having it washed
	• Says dada, mama with meaning Comprehends bye-bye May say one word (for example, hi, bye, what, no)	Inhibits behavior to verbal command of "no-no" or own name Imitates facial expressions, waves bye-bye Extends toy to another person but will not release it Looks around a corner or under a pillow for an object Repeats actions that attract attention and are laughed at Pulls clothes of another to attract attention Plays interactive games such as pat-a-cake Reacts to adult anger, cries when scolded Demonstrates independence in dressing, feeding, locomotive skills, and testing of parents Looks at and follows pictures in a book
	Imitates definite speech sounds Uses jargon	Experiences joy and satisfaction when a task is mastered Reacts to restrictions with frustration

Continued.

Table 12-5. Summary of growth and development during infancy—cont'd

Age (weeks)	Physical	Gross motor	Fine motor
48		May creep with soles of feet flat on floor When sitting, pivots to reach toward back to pick up an object Cruises or walks holding onto furniture or with both hands held	• Neat pincer grasp Drops object deliberately for it to be picked up Puts one object after another into a container (sequential play) Able to manipulate an object to remove it from tight-fitting enclosure
52	Birth weight tripled Birth length increased by 50% Head and chest circumference equal (head circumference 46.5 cm [18.5 inches]) Has total of six to eight deciduous teeth Anterior fontanel almost closed Landau reflex fading Babinski's reflex disappears Lumbar curve develops, lordosis evident during walking Mouthing and drooling begin to cease	Walks with one hand held Cruises well May attempt to stand alone momentarily Can sit down from standing position without help	Releases cube in cup Attempts to build two-block tower but fails Tries to insert a pellet into a narrow-neck bottle but fails Can turn pages in a book, many at a time

mula, or modified cow's milk when solids are fed under 3 months of age. Except for the deficiency of ascorbic acid and iron in most types of infant formulas, there is little need to supplement additional foods for the first several months. There may, however, be some hazards to introducing foods too early, although nutritional research is still not complete.

The optimum caloric requirement for full-term infants is 110 to 120 kcal/kg/day. Breast milk and modified cow's milk formulas readily supply 20 kcal/ounce, and the caloric and fluid requirement (150 ml/kg) can be easily calculated. However, when solid foods are substituted or given in addition to the caloric-fluid requirement, underfeeding or overfeeding can result. In general, commercial ready-to-serve dry cereals have 8 kcal/level tbsp, strained meats have 15 kcal/tbsp, vegetables have 3.5 to 10 kcal/tbsp, fruits have 10 kcal/tbsp, and egg yolk has 30 kcal/tbsp. Since overfeeding and obesity are serious nutritional problems, this is an important consideration in the addition of solid foods. Although meat is an adequate protein substitute for milk, it is deficient in calcium. Meat supplements provide a high-protein content, accompanied by a lowered fluid intake, which places high demands on the kidneys by increasing the renal solute load. This may be particularly crucial in times of stress when the infant's system cannot meet altered fluid and electrolyte demands. The infant's immature gastrointestinal tract also is unable to handle complex carbohydrates or saturated fats early in life.

Infant nutrition and feeding are highly individualized. Human milk and properly modified cow's milk are excellent sources of nutrition for the infant for the first 3 months of life. The Committee on Nutrition of the American Academy of Pediatrics recommends the addition of 1 mg/kg/day of iron to the infant's diet.[7] Supplements of 400 U of vitamin D and 30 mg of ascorbic acid (vitamin C) should be provided, as well as fluoride, unless the local water supply is fluoridated (one part/million) and the infant consumes tap water. Supplementation of any of these minerals or vitamins is dependent on the type of formula given. Human milk contains adequate amounts of vitamin C but is deficient in vitamin D and fluoride. Although the amount of iron in human milk is low, absorption seems to be significantly higher than in cow's milk and appears to be sufficient to meet the iron requirements of the exclusively breast-fed infant until he triples his birth weight.[20] Enriched milk provides 400 U of vitamin D/liter but lacks vitamin C, iron, or fluoride. Commercially prepared formulas contain adequate amounts of vitamins C and D and may be iron enriched, but they lack fluoride. However, if any of the cow's milk prep-

Sensory	Vocalization	Socialization
		Rolls ball to another on request Aniticipates body gestures when a familiar nursery rhyme or story is being told (for example, holds toes and feet in response to "This little piggy went to market") Plays game up-down, "so-big," or peekaboo by covering face Shakes head for "no"
Visual acuity, 20/100 Discriminates simple geometric forms (for example, circle) Amblyopia may develop with lack of binocularity Can follow rapidly moving object Controls and adjusts response to sound; will listen for sound to recur	• Says two or more words besides dada, mama Comprehends meaning of several words (comprehension always precedes verbalization) Recognizes objects by name Imitates animal sounds Understands simple verbal commands (for example, "Give it to me," "Show me your eyes")	Shows emotions such as jealousy, affection (may give hug or kiss on request), anger, fear Enjoys familiar surroundings and will explore away from mother Fearful in strange situation, clings to mother May develop habit of "security blanket" or favorite toy Unceasing determination to practice locomotor skills

arations are diluted with fluoridated tap water, fluoride (usually 0.5 mg/day) does not need to be supplemented. Before recommending any food supplements, the nurse must take a thorough nutritional history regarding the earliest form of infant nutrition. The recommended daily allowance for each nutrient is listed in Appendix D.

Introduction of solid foods. There are well-documented reasons for initiating the feeding of solid foods during the first year. Probably the most important is the assurance of an adequate supply of iron. Prenatal iron stores acquired from the mother during the last trimester gradually diminish in the full-term infant by 4 to 5 months of age and by 2 to 3 months of age in premature infants. Cereal is an excellent source of iron, although the exact amount absorbed is controversial because of the phytates in the grain and the phosphates in the milk, which are binding agents that decrease iron absorption. The type of iron (ferrous sulfate) added to commercial formula is better absorbed than is the type added to enriched cereals (sodium iron pyrophosphate). Fruits and vegetables ensure an adequate supply of vitamins and minerals, particularly vitamin C.

There are also psychobiologic advantages to introducing solid foods. At about 6 months of age, when dentition begins, the infant is learning to chew and bite. Solid foods encourage this natural behavior, facilitating adequate chewing and digestion of foods later in life. Introducing various textures and tastes of foods helps the infant learn likes and dislikes and develop enjoyment and anticipation of eating. Much of the control of one's eating habits probably stems from this early introduction of food and is influenced by the sociocultural values placed on food.

Although infants seem to accept solid food best between 2½ to 3½ months of age, there should be no rigid rules regarding introduction of solids.[8] Large, rapidly growing infants may not be satisfied by drinking large quantities of milk, but they may be contented with cereal and fruit. Small infants may be quite satisfied with formula for considerably longer and be nutritionally sound, provided all the nutrients are provided. Other infants who are allergic to various foods may need a very specific schedule for introduction of each new food.

Nature seems to have provided certain cues as to how and when to feed infants. The rooting and sucking reflexes are strongest for the first 2 months, when fluids are given by breast- or bottle-feeding. The extrusion reflex, which pushes food out with the tongue, begins to fade at 3 to 4 months of age. As it fades, food placed on the tongue is carried to the back of the mouth and swallowed. Before this

Developmental milestones associated with feeding

Age (months)	*Behavior*
Birth	Sucking, rooting, and swallowing reflexes
	Feels hunger and indicates desire for food by crying; expresses satiety by falling asleep
1	Able to take food from a spoon but extrusion reflex is strong
3-4	Extrusion reflex is fading, able to take food from a spoon
	Beginning eye-hand coordination
4-5	Can approximate lips to the rim of a cup
5-6	Can use fingers to feed self a cracker
6-7	Chews and bites
	May hold own bottle, but may not drink from it (prefers for it to be held)
7-9	Refuses food by keeping lips closed; has preferences
	Holds a spoon and plays with it during feeding
	May drink from a straw
	Drinks from a cup with assistance
9-12	Picks up small morsels of food (finger foods) and feeds self
	Holds own bottle and drinks from it
	Drinks from a cup but spills some of the contents
	Uses a spoon with much spilling

time, food must be placed well back in the mouth for it to be retained and swallowed. When chewing begins at 6 months, new foods such as hard toast or crackers can be crushed against the gums and swallowed. As the pincer grasp is refined, small pieces of food can be manipulated and put into the mouth. The major developmental milestones associated with feeding are listed in the boxed material above.

Selection of foods. The choice of foods to introduce first is also variable, but it should meet the reasons for early feeding, such as supplying nutrients not found in milk. Cereal is generally introduced first because of its high-iron content (7 mg/3 tbsp of dry cereal). There are several types of commercially prepared ready-to-serve dry cereals, such as rice, barley, oatmeal, and high-protein cereals, but rice is usually suggested as an initial food because of its easy digestibility and low allergic reaction. Homemade cereal such as Cream of Farina can also be given but should be cooked longer to break down complex carbohydrates and should be mixed with milk for a thinner consistency. If the infant is breast-fed, new foods should be mixed with expressed breast milk or water, rather than with cow's milk, since the child may unknowingly be sensitive to cow's milk. Fruit is started after cereal, and any strained or blended fruit can be given. Some of the commercial dry baby cereals are combined with fruit. There is little nutritional benefit from this preparation except it is more expensive. Since all new foods should be added one at a time, mothers should avoid this type of cereal when beginning a new grain. Vegetables are added later, followed by meats, meat soup, and egg yolk. Egg white should be introduced during the second half of the first year because of difficult digestibility of the protein albumin and its high allergic response. General guideline for introducing solid foods to infants is shown in the boxed material on the opposite page.

Commercially prepared baby foods are the most commonly used types of food served to infants in the United States. They are convenient but relatively expensive and sometimes contain added salt and modified starch that may have adverse effects, although this has not been proved. The calorie content of these prepared foods varies widely, and if they are used indiscriminately they can lead to overweight and less nutrition (Table 12-6). For example, the meat dinners or combination meat and vegetable dishes contain less meat than the pure meat preparations and should be used as a vegetable dish. In addition food labels almost always list water as the first and, therefore, most abundant ingredient.

Food preparation. Preparing baby foods at home is simple and inexpensive. Fruits and vegetables can be steamed in a small amount of water and pureed in a blender or food processor. Many of them can be mashed fine with a fork, such as a ripe banana. Fruits such as apples or pears require little or no water in the cooking process. Vegetables such as carrots, potatoes, or string beans will require additional water in the cooking and blending process. It is important to stress that no water used in cooking should be discarded, since the water-soluble vitamins will be lost. Vitamin C is naturally destroyed by heat; therefore, cooked fruits or vegetables do not supply this essential nutrient. Orange juice should not be warmed for this reason. Vitamin C is also destroyed by oxidation and alkaline solutions. Containers of juice should always be kept covered and refrigerated to prevent oxidative loss.

Meats can easily be prepared by steaming, boiling, baking, or poaching but not by frying. Meat should be lean, since the infant's ability to handle saturated fats is limited. Meat can be pureed in a blender with liquid, such as leftover vegetable broth or meat broth. Baby food grinders are also available that finely grind small portions of cooked table food. Since the food is ground dry, some type of liquid or some other pureed ingredient such as mashed potatoes, squash, carrots, or other vegetable, to which the infant has already been introduced, must be added. When chewing is fairly well established, table food can be chopped finely and placed on the high-chair tray for the child to pick up and eat by himself.

Storage of commercial baby food requires a few simple rules. Unopened jars can remain on the shelf indefinitely.

Guidelines for introducing solid foods to infants

Age (months)	*Food*	*Comment*
1	Orange juice Multivitamin preparation (A, D, and C) Iron Fluoride	Orange juice is an excellent source of vitamin C but is sometimes given later if sensitivity to it is suspected Enriched apple juice is a good substitute Any vitamin or mineral supplement is added only after considering the specific formula and the infant's needs
2-3	Cereal, particularly rice Strained or blended fruits	Applesauce, bananas, and pears are fruits best tolerated
3-4	Egg yolk Vegetables	Egg yolk is usually hard boiled and sieved, later may be given soft cooked or poached May avoid early introduction of beets and spinach, especially if home processed Potatoes, rice, puddings, and other high-carbohydrate foods are are usually added after the more essential and nutritious foods are taken regularly
5-6	Meats Meat soup Cheese	Fatty meats should be avoided Should include organ meats such as liver, which has a high-iron, high–vitamin A, and high–vitamin B complex content If soup is given, be sure all ingredients in soup are familiar to child's diet Cottage cheese is an excellent meat substitute
6	Hard, chewable foods such as zwieback, cracker, dry toast, or pretzel	Introduction of finger foods should be nutritionally sound; firmly cooked vegetables (carrots or celery), slices of raw fruit (apple, banana), or raw vegetables (cucumber, pepper) are excellent additions
6-12	Fish Egg white Chopped table foods Desserts	Fish should be baked, steamed, boiled, or poached, not fried, and finely separated to remove all bones; Tuna fish packed in water is a good addition Egg white should be hard or soft cooked, mashed, and fed in *small* amounts (1 tsp) to detect any allergic manifestation Chopped table foods should be added gradually; usually by age 9 months infant has sufficient pincer grasp to feed self small morsels of food Desserts should be chosen that are nutritious, such as fruits, puddings, custards, or yogurt; concentrated sweets should be avoided or kept to a minimum to stress good food habits early and prevent overweight

Opened jars must be refrigerated and can last for a couple of days. If the infant does not finish a jar of food at one time, a portion of the food should be removed from the jar using a clean spoon. If this is not done, the salivary enzymes on the feeding spoon begin to digest unused portions of the food.

For convenience, home-prepared baby foods can be made in advance and frozen in small jars or in special plastic bags that are sealed by heat and can be reheated by placing them in boiling water. Individual portions of food can be frozen in ice cube trays, transferred to a large container, and individually defrosted as needed. With reasonable care in the preparation and storing of foods, there is little need to worry about bacterial contamination.

Generally all foods served in the home can be given to an infant. Recently there has been some question about serving fresh beets and spinach to infants because of their high-nitrate content.[6] Nitrates can be converted to nitrites, which oxidize ferrous iron in hemoglobin to the ferric state. The resulting compound, methemoglobin, which is normally found in erythrocytes in very small amounts, increases, causing methemoglobinemia. Methemoglobin is incapable of binding molecular oxygen for transfer to cells. Prolonged storage of fresh spinach increases the conversion of nitrates to nitrites and can be harmful if ingested in sufficient quantities. The processing of commercially prepared spinach inactivates this conversion system. As a precautionary measure, it is best to prepare spinach or beets quickly for use as baby food and probably to avoid feeding these vegetables uncooked to infants.

Method of introduction. When the spoon is first introduced to the infant, the likelihood is that he will push it away and appear dissatisfied. If foods are begun early, the pushing away is more a result of the extrusion reflex than the child's voluntary will. Some patience and skill is required to overcome this initial response. A small-bowled, straight, and long-handled spoon, similar to a demitasse spoon, allows a small portion of food to be placed toward the back of the tongue. If food is placed on the front of the tongue, it will be pushed out. Simply scoop it up and try again. As the child gets used to the spoon, he will more eagerly accept the food and will eventually open his mouth in anticipation (or keep it closed in dislike). Since the first introduction of food is a new experience, the spoon feeding should be attempted after ingestion of some breast milk or formula to associate this new experience with a pleasurable and satisfying experience. Trying to introduce a new food *after* the entire milk feeding is usually useless, since the infant is satiated and has no inclination to try something new.

After several spoon feedings, new food can be introduced at the beginning of a meal. It is best to introduce many new foods during the first year when the infant is more likely to eat them because of a hearty appetite resulting from a rapid growth rate. During the toddler years eating becomes less of an adventure and strong food preferences become evident.

Each new food should be introduced alone and at intervals of 4 to 7 days to allow for identification of food allergies. This is an important point to remember since elimination diets to detect a possible food allergy are difficult and frustrating to follow. Allergic manifestations to a food may be dermal, gastrointestinal, or respiratory in nature. New foods should also be introduced in small amounts, from 1 tsp to a couple of tablespoons. As the amount of solid food increases, the quantity of milk should be decreased to prevent overfeeding. Steady, even growth in height and weight is the best indicator of optimum feeding and should be regularly recorded on a growth chart.

Since feeding is a learning process as well as a means of nutrition, new foods should be given alone to allow the child to learn new tastes and textures. Sometimes it is necessary to camouflage a new food by mixing it with another favorite food to encourage the child to try it. Food should not be mixed in the bottle and fed through a nipple with a large hole. This deprives the child of the pleasure of learning new tastes and developing a discriminating palate. It can also cause problems with poor chewing of food later in life since this experience would be lacking. There are instances when diluted pureed foods are given in a bottle to minimize energy expenditure, such as in a cardiac condition, but this should be the exception rather than the rule. A summary of the principles that govern the introduction of new foods is shown in the boxed material below.

Introducing solid foods can be an exciting time for parent and child. Most infants are good eaters and enjoy eating from a spoon and, later, feeding themselves. However, the transition from "mother doing it" to "baby doing it" can be a trying experience, particularly for those who value a clean house or who view cleaning up the mess as a waste of time. The infant's first, second, and often twentieth try at self- or cup feeding is a sloppy experience. Finger foods such as soft fruits or vegetables are just as good playthings as food; they can be squeezed, smeared, squashed, and thoroughly painted on oneself, others, and the surrounding environment (Fig. 12-4). However, all of this is part of learning, and mastery follows many accidents. If parents find this experience distressing, a few suggestions may prove helpful. Designate as a feeding area a section that has a floor that can be easily wiped (not a rug) and is relatively far away from walls, upholstered furniture, or drapes. Messes will be confined to one area if the child is seated in a high chair or baby tender rather than allowed to crawl or walk around while drinking or eating. The infant should be expected to get himself covered with food; therefore, a large bib (plastic can be wiped easily) should be used and he should be dressed in washable clothes that are easily removed. Outdoor dining provides an excellent opportunity for practicing with a cup, spoon, or fingers since the accidents are simple to hose or sweep away. Children cannot be pressured into eating neatly or developing table manners before facile manipulative skill is acquired. If a young child suddenly refuses to eat, the feeding process should be investigated. It is not unusual for an 11-month-old infant to become stubborn, push the spoon away, and refuse to open his mouth. He may not be content with having his own spoon to play with while someone else feeds him; he probably wants to do it himself, even though others can do it so much

Summary of method of introducing solid foods to infants

1. Introduce solids when infant is hungry
2. Begin spoon feeding by pushing food to back of tongue because of infant's natural tendency to thrust tongue forward
3. Use small spoon with straight handle; begin with 1 or 2 tsp of food; gradually increase to a couple of tablespoons per feeding
4. Introduce one food at a time, usually at intervals of 4 to 7 days to allow for identification of food allergies
5. As the amount of solid food increases, decrease the quantity of milk to prevent overfeeding
6. Never introduce foods by mixing them with the formula in the bottle

better. Helping parents understand this may prevent many temper tantrums and power struggles later on.

Weaning. Weaning, the process of giving up one method of feeding for another, usually refers to relinguishing the breast or bottle for a cup. In Western societies this is generally regarded as a major task for infants and is frequently seen as a potentially traumatic experience. It is psychologically significant because the infant is required to give up a major source of oral pleasure and gratification. There is no one time for weaning that is best for every child, but generally most infants show signs of readiness during the second half of the first year. They have learned that good things come from a spoon. Their increasing desire for freedom of movement may lessen their desire to be held close for feedings. They are acquiring more control over their actions and can easily manipulate a cup to their lips (even if it is held upside down!). Since imitation becomes a powerful motivator by age 8 or 9 months, they enjoy using a cup or glass like others do. Since most children can approximate the rim of a cup to their lips by 4 or 5 months of age, this is not too early to introduce a cup while removing one bottle- or breast-feeding at a time. Weaning should be gradual by replacing one bottle- or breast-feeding at a time. The last feeding to be discontinued is usually the nighttime one. It is advisable to never begin allowing a child to take a bottle of milk to bed, since this is a major cause of dental caries in deciduous teeth. If breast-feeding must be terminated before 5 or 6 months of age, weaning should be to a bottle to provide for the infant's continued sucking needs. If discontinued later, weaning can be directly to a cup.

Nutritional counseling. The addition of solid foods during the first year should provide a nutritionally sound diet and teach good eating habits. Often both these objectives are controlled by the sociocultural background of the family, rather than by their knowledge of well-balanced nutrition. Since "we are what we eat," nurses have a great responsibility for teaching optimum nutrition as early as possible. Common myths such as "a fat baby is a healthy baby" are difficult to dispel. In some cultures overweight infants are regarded as a sign of good mothering, and any suggestion regarding altering the child's weight is threatening to the parent. Since obesity in infancy may predispose the individual to obesity in later life, rectifying this problem as early as possible is essential. A thorough nutritional history is a prerequisite for counseling. Asking questions such as, "Does your child drink too much milk?" yields little reliable information. Phrasing the question by saying, "Your child certainly looks well nourished (or well fed); how many bottles of milk a day does he drink?" will not cause parents to be defensive and will offer an objective number of ounces. If too much formula or milk is the problem, the solution may be to dilute the feeding to decrease the calorie content. Substituting skim milk is unacceptable since the essential fatty acids are inadequate and the solute concentration of protein is too high. Frequently the problem of overfeeding stems from the fact that as solid foods are added, milk is not decreased. Since baby foods contain different caloric contents, knowing which foods are less fattening can provide satisfactory substitutions without greatly altering feeding habits. Table 12-6 lists the calorie content of representative commercially prepared strained foods. Calculating the caloric density of the infant's diet is very

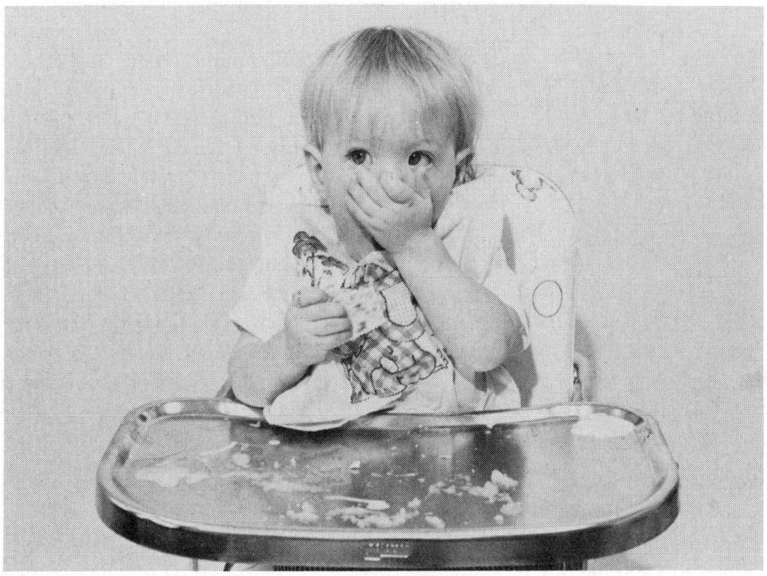

Fig. 12-4. Finger feeding at mealtime. (From Erickson, M. L.: Assessment and management of developmental changes in children, St. Louis, 1976, The C. V. Mosby Co., p. 228.)

Table 12-6. Caloric content of commercial baby food

Food	Caloric content
Juice (4.2 ounces)	
Apple	70
Orange	70
Orange-apricot	80
Apple-grape	90
Orange-apple-banana	100
Prune-orange	100
Meats (3.5 ounces)	
Veal	90
Beef	100
Lamb	100
Ham	110
Pork	120
Chicken, turkey	130
Vegetables (4.5 ounces)	
Green beans	35
Squash, carrots	40
Beets	50
Peas	60
Sweet potatoes (4.7 ounces)	90
Fruits (4.7 ounces)	
Pears	90
Applesauce	100
Peaches	110
Plums with tapioca (4.75 ounces)	140
Dairy products	
Egg yolks (3.3 ounces)	180
Creamed cottage cheese with pineapple (4.5 ounces)	160
High meat-content dinners (4.5 ounces)	
Ham or veal with vegetables	90
Chicken or beef with vegetables	100
Turkey with vegetables	120
Vegetable and meat–combination dinners	
Vegetables and turkey or chicken	50
Macaroni and cheese	80
Vegetables and bacon	100

important since commercially strained foods can yield greater or lesser concentrations of calories as compared to formula, which yields 67 kcal/100 ml. About 20% of commercial baby foods yield less than 50 kcal/100 g, whereas 20% have greater than 100 kcal/100 g. This is a considerable difference when one considers the total daily calorie consumption from formula or from solid foods. One should bear in mind that a child who is underweight or who has a congenital heart defect might benefit from the higher caloric density foods. Although government regulations regarding food labeling do not require that the caloric and nutritive content of the food be listed on the package, this information is available on request from the manufacturer.

Immunizations

One of the most dramatic advances in pediatrics has been the decline of infectious diseases over the past 30 years because of the widespread use of immunization for preventable diseases. Although many of the presently available immunizations can be given to individuals of any age, the recommended primary schedule begins during infancy and, with the exception of boosters, is completed during early childhood. Therefore, the discussion of childhood immunizations for diphtheria, tetanus, pertussis, polio, measles, mumps, and rubella is included under health promotion during the first year.

In addition to immunizations for these diseases, vaccines are also available for cholera, influenza, plague, rabies, Rocky Mountain spotted fever, smallpox, typhoid fever, typhus, yellow fever, tuberculosis (bacillus Calmette Guérin [BCG] vaccine), and strains of *Streptococcus pneumoniae* and *Neisseria meningitidis*. Although none are routinely administered in the United States, several of them are recommended for people who travel to foreign countries. Information concerning required and recommended immunizations is available in the booklets *Immunization Information for Foreign Travel* from the Superintendent of Documents, U.S. Government Printing office, Washington, D.C., and *Vaccination Certificate Requirement for International Travel* from Center for Disease Control, Atlanta, Ga.

In order to facilitate one's understanding of immunization, the following terms are defined for reference throughout the next section:

immunity an inherited or acquired status in which an individual is resistant to the occurrence or the effects of a specific disease, particularly an infectious agent.

natural immunity innate immunity or resistance to infection or toxicity.

acquired immunity immunity from exposure to the invading agent, either bacteria, virus, or toxins.

active immunity individual actively forms immune bodies against specific antigens, either *naturally* by his having had the disease clinically or subclinically or *artificially* by the introduction of an antigen (vaccine) into the individual.

passive immunity temporary immunity by transfusing plasma proteins either *artificially* from another human or an animal that has been actively immunized against an antigen or *naturally* from the mother to the fetus via the placenta.

antibody a protein found mostly in serum that is formed in response to exposure to a specific antigen.

antigen a variety of foreign substances, including bacteria, viruses, toxins, and foreign proteins that stimulate the formation of antibodies.

antitoxin antibody formed in response to a toxin (antigen).

toxin a poisonous substance usually produced by the invading microorganism.

toxoid a toxin that has been treated to destroy its toxic properties but retain its antigenic quality.

vaccine collectively a term to denote any type of active immunization, such as toxoids or attenuated live viruses; specifically a suspension of disease-causing bacteria or viruses that acts like an antigen, stimulates antibody production, and produces active acquired immunity.

attenuate reduction of the virulence (infectiousness) of a pathogenic microorganism by such measures as treating it with heat, chemicals, or cultivating it on a certain media.

Schedule for immunizations. Two organizations—The Advisory Committee on Immunization Practices (ACIP) of the U.S. Public Health Service and the Committee on Infectious Diseases of the American Academy of Pediatrics (AAP)—govern the recommendations for immunization policies and procedures. Because The Advisory Committee on Immunization Practices is concerned primarily with national health issues and the Committee on Infectious Diseases formulates its recommendations for infants and children who receive regular health care, there are occasionally different perspectives in each group's recommendations. It is important for nurses to realize the purpose of each committee and to view immunization practices in light of the needs of an individual child as well as of a community.

The policies of each committee are recommendations, not rules, and they change as a result of advances in the field of immunology. For example, the 1965 recommendation of the American Academy of Pediatrics to administer measles immunization at 12 months of age was changed in 1976 as a result of studies that demonstrated that the optimum age for measles immunization is 15 months of age. This change resulted from the findings that the antibody response increases from 80% to 85% at 12 months of age to more than 95% at 13 to 14 months of age.[4]

Another major change has been the routine discontinuation of smallpox vaccination since 1971. As a result of the vaccine's widespread use, no new cases have been reported in the United States since 1949. However, since that date, approximately 160 vaccine-associated deaths have occurred, with significant neurologic and dermal complications in an additional 8,000 people per year. The risks of vaccination greatly exceeded the risk of contracting the disease.[15]

As a result the following major recommendations have been made by The Advisory Committee on Immunization Practices and Committee on Infectious Diseases of the American Academy of Pediatrics[1,21]: (1) Routine vaccination for smallpox should be eliminated. (2) Vaccination is required of individuals at special risk, that is, for travelers to certain countries where smallpox is present, for individuals in health-related fields, and for immediate and secondary contacts in the presence of an epidemic. Health service personnel, which includes nurses, should be revaccinated every 3 years because of their susceptibility of coming in contact with a smallpox victim. (3) When smallpox vaccination is administered, contraindications to its use must be followed, such as any child under 1 year of age, individuals with eczema or individuals who would be exposed to someone with eczema, anyone with an altered immune state,

Table 12-7. Recommended schedule for active immunization of normal infants and children

Age	Immunization recommended
2 months	DTP,* TOPV†
4 months	DTP, TOPV
6 months	DTP‡
1 year	Tuberculin test§
15 months	Measles, rubella, mumps‖
18 months	DTP, TOPV
4-6 years	DTP, TOPV
14-16 years	Td¶—repeat every 10 years

Adapted from American Academy of Pediatrics: Report of the Committee on Infectious Diseases, Ill., 1977. Copyright American Academy of Pediatrics, 1977.

*DTP—diphtheria and tetanus toxoids combined with pertussis vaccine.

†TOPV—trivalent oral poliovirus vaccine. This recommendation is suitable for breast-fed as well as bottle-fed infants.

‡A third dose of TOPV is optional but may be given in areas of high endemicity of poliomyelitis.

§Frequency of tuberculin testing depends on risk of exposure of the child and on the prevalence of tuberculosis in the population group. The initial test should be at or preceding the measles vaccine.

‖May be given at 15 months as measles-rubella or measles-mumps-rubella combined vaccines.

¶Td—combined tetanus and diphtheria toxoids (adult type) for those more than 6 years of age, in contrast to diphtheria and tetanus (DT) toxoids which contain a larger amount of diphtheria antigen.

Table 12-8. Primary immunization for children not immunized in early infancy*

Time interval	Age (years): Under 6	Age (years): 6 and older
First visit	DTP, TOPV, tuberculin test	Td, TOPV, tuberculin test
1 month later	Measles,† mumps, rubella	Measles, mumps, rubella
2 months later	DTP, TOPV	Td, TOPV
4 months later	DTP, TOPV‡	
8 to 14 months later		Td, TOPV
10 to 16 months later or preschool	DTP, TOPV	
At age 14-16 years	Td—repeat every 10 years	Td—repeat every 10 years

Adapted from American Academy of Pediatrics: Report of the Committee on Infectious Diseases, Ill., 1977. Copyright American Academy of Pediatrics, 1977.

*The sequence of these schedules may be altered if specific infections are prevalent. For example, measles vaccine might be given on the first visit if an epidemic is occurring.

†Measles vaccine is not routinely given before age 15 months.

‡Optional.

Table 12-9. Contraindications to routine immunizations

Contraindication	Immunization	Rationale	Nursing considerations
Acute febrile illness or chronic debilitating diseases	All	Masks febrile reactions from the immunization, decreases body's natural defense mechanisms	Explain reason for postponing immunization to parent and reschedule it at earliest return visit For chronic diseases, check with physician before administering any immunization
Gastroenteritis	Live poliovirus vaccine	May interfere with colonization of the viruses in the intestines, which is essential for the immune response to occur	Explain reason for postponing immunization and reschedule it as soon as possible
Altered immune system Immunologic disease Generalized malignancy (leukemia, lymphoma) Immunosuppressive therapy (steroids, antimetabolites, radiation)	All live viral vaccines (measles, mumps, rubella, and polio)	Depressed immune defenses may result in extreme reactions to the immunizations	Emphasize to parents the need to prevent their children from exposure to any of these childhood diseases, since they cannot be artificially protected from them
Recently acquired passive immunity Blood transfusion or immune serum globulin within last 6 weeks Maternal antibodies during first year	Measles, mumps, and rubella vaccines	Presence of passive immunity prevents formation of antibodies to the vaccine	Inquire during the history concerning recent blood transfusions or injections of immune serum globulin; wait recommended 6 weeks before administering the immunization; follow suggested schedule for measles, mumps, and rubella (15 months)
Allergy to substances in vaccine, for example, egg protein, neomycin	Live virus vaccines grown on chick embryos, treated with neomycin	Known hypersensitivity to substance will also result in reaction to substance in vaccine	Check manufacturer's product information for specific contraindications and screen child for known allergies to potential foreign substances
History of nervous system disorders Reaction of high fever, somnolence, or convulsions following a DTP immunization	Pertussis vaccine	Danger of serious reaction to pertussis vaccination is greatly increased	Take a detailed neurologic history, including past convulsions, fainting spells, tremors, or twitching and specific reactions to DTP; report any such findings to a physician before administering the pertussis vaccine
Pregnancy	All live virus vaccines except for poliovirus	Potential risk to fetus, especially from rubella	Take a careful history of all women of childbearing age regarding the possibility of pregnancy or conception within the next 2 months

pregnant women, and patients with burns, poison ivy, impetigo, or other acute skin lesions until completely healed.*

The generally recommended age for beginning primary immunizations of normal infants is 2 months (Table 12-7). However, data from immunization surveys in the United States show declining levels of protection for these diseases. For example, although immunizations for diphtheria, pertussis, and tetanus are recommended during the first year of life, only three quarters of children between 1 and 4 years of age have been immunized. The decline in polio immunization is even more dramatic. It is estimated that only about two thirds of children under 15 years of age are immunized and that less than half the children of minority groups under 5 years of age are protected.[12] One of the dangers of such low levels of immunity is loss of the benefit of "herd immunity," which means that children who are not immunized are protected against the disease because nearly everyone in contact with them has been immunized. For herd immunity to be present, 80% of the children must be vaccinated. Recommended schedules for children not immunized during infancy are included in Table 12-8.

Contraindications and precautions. Since not all children who begin a primary immunization schedule continue with the series as recommended, it is important for the nurse to know that a delay does not interfere with the final immunity achieved and that it is unnecessary to restart any series regardless of the length of the delay. However, it is important to recognize general contraindications to immunizations (Table 12-9). Minor illnesses not associated with febrile reactions, such as the common cold, are not contraindications.

The principal precautions in administering immunizations include proper storage of the vaccine in order to protect its potency and the recommended procedure for injection. The nurse must be familiar with the manufacturer's directions for storage and reconstitution of the vaccine. Table 12-10 summarizes the recommended procedures for administration and storage of commonly used immunizations.

*In 1978 WHO declared smallpox had been eradicated, eliminating the need for immunization.

Reactions. Vaccines for routine immunizations are among the safest and most reliable drugs available. However, minor side effects do occur following many of the immunizations, and, rarely, a serious reaction may result from the vaccine. However, for the use of any vaccine to be justified, the benefit of receiving protection from the immunization must greatly outweigh the risk of contracting the disease. To illustrate the benefit of immunizations, one can look at the impressive statistics for poliomyelitis and poliovirus vaccines. Paralytic poliomyelitis declined from 18,308 cases in 1954 before the widespread use of polio vaccines to seven cases in 1975-1976.[3] With more than 25 million doses of oral poliovirus vaccine distributed annually in the United States, the current estimated risk of possible vaccine-associated paralysis in vaccines or contacts is no more than one in 10 million doses.[1]

In general with inactivated antigens, such as DTP, side effects are most likely to occur within a few hours or days of administration. However, because live attenuated virus vaccines such as measles, mumps, rubella, and oral poliovirus multiply for days or weeks, possible unfavorable reactions and "vaccine-associated" disorders can occur for a period of 30 to 60 days.[1] Table 12-11 lists the usual side effects for each immunization.

Parents and children of responsible age should be fully informed about the immunization, the reasons and benefit of its use, and its possible side effects. Since nurses frequently administer the immunization during child health visits, the responsibility for adequately informing parents is often left to them. The U.S. Department of Health, Education and Welfare, Public Health Service, Center for Disease Control publishes a pamphlet for parents entitled "Vaccines and Immunizations."* It describes the disease, vaccine, and possible side effects of each recommended childhood immunization. It also includes a card that the parents sign in order to confirm their understanding of the benefits and risks of the vaccine. In essence the card is a signed consent that the drug can be given. Although this procedure is not widely practiced, it does emphasize the need for health pro-

*Available from Center for Disease Control, Atlanta, Ga. 30333.

Table 12-10. Recommended procedures for administration and storage of routine immunization materials

Immunization	Route of administration	Storage
Diphtheria and tetanus toxoid, pertussis vaccine	Intramuscular	Store at 2°-8°C (35.6°-46.4°F)—do not freeze; loss of potency can occur if vial is left at room temperature, but during recommended storage, expiration time for vaccine is 18 months
Trivalent oral poliovirus vaccine	Oral	Store at freezing temperatures (below 0°C or 32°F); once refrigerated, must be used within 30 days; if opened, must be used within 7 days
Measles, mumps, and rubella live virus vaccines	Subcutaneous	Before reconstitution, store at 2°-8°C (35.6°-46.4°F) and protect from light; if not used immediately, store reconstituted vaccines in a dark place at the recommended temperature and discard if not used within 8 hours

Table 12-11. Possible side effects and nursing responsibilities of recommended childhood immunizations*

Immunization	Reaction	Nursing responsibilities
Diphtheria	Fever usually within 24-48 hours Soreness, redness, and swelling at site of injection	Instructions for DTP: Advise parents of possible side effects; may recommend prophylactic use of aspirin or acetaminophen if fever occurred following previous DTP immunization; recommend its use if fever occurs following present immunization; advise parents to notify physician immediately of any unusual side effects, such as those listed under pertussis
Tetanus	Same as for diphtheria but may include urticaria and malaise All may have delayed onset and last several days Lump at injection site may last for weeks, even months, but gradually disappears	
Pertussis	Same as for tetanus but may include loss of consciousness, convulsions, and thrombocytopenia	
Poliovirus (TOPV)	Essentially no side effects Vaccine-associated paralysis usually occurs within 2 months of immunization	See general comment to parents*
Measles	Anorexia, malaise, rash, and fever may occur 7 to 10 days after immunization Rarely (estimated risk 1 in 1 million doses) encephalitis may occur	Advise parents of more common side effects and use of antipyretics for fever; if a persistent high fever with other obvious signs of illness occurs, have them notify physician immediately
Mumps	Essentially no side effects other than a brief, mild fever	See general comment to parents
Rubella	Mild rash that lasts 1 or 2 days within a few days after immunization Arthralgia, arthritis, and/or paresthesia of the hands and fingers may occur about 2 weeks after vaccination and is more frequent in older children and adults	Advise parents of side effects, especially of time delay before joint swelling and pain; assure them that these symptoms will disappear; may recommend use of mild analgesics for pain

*General comment to parents regarding each immunization: The benefit of being protected by the immunization is believed to greatly outweigh the risk from the disease.

fessionals to adequately inform parents before administering immunizations both as a professional obligation and a personal legal safeguard.

Recommendations. In addition to being thoroughly familiar with the contraindications, proper administration, and reactions of childhood immunizations, the nurse must also be aware of the latest recommendations regarding their use.

Diphtheria. Diphtheria vaccine is commonly administered in three different ways: (1) in combination with tetanus and pertussis vaccines (DTP) for normal children under 6 years of age, (2) in a double vaccine with tetanus (DT) for children under 6 years of age who have some contraindication to receiving pertussis vaccine, and (3) in smaller doses (15% to 20% of that in DTP or DT) with tetanus vaccine (Td) for use in children over 6 years of age. Although the diphtheria vaccine does not produce absolute immunity, when given according to the recommended schedule, protective levels of antitoxin persist for 10 years or more.

Tetanus. Three forms of tetanus vaccine—tetanus toxoid, tetanus immune globulin (TIG) (human), and tetanus antitoxin (usually horse serum)—are available. Tetanus toxoid is generally used for routine primary immunization, usually in one of the combinations listed above, and provides long-lasting protective antitoxin levels. In response to a booster dose in persons who have had at least two previous doses of the toxoid, protective antitoxin develops rapidly.

For wound management, passive immunity is available with tetanus immune globulin or animal-source antitoxin. However, since the risk of severe reaction, such as anaphylactic shock or serum sickness, is always greater to the foreign substances of animal serum, the choice should always be tetanus immune globulin. In persons with a history of two previous doses of tetanus toxoid, a booster dose of the toxoid can be given. Table 12-12 presents a summary of the recommended procedure for tetanus prophylaxis in wound management.

Pertussis. Pertussis is recommended for all children under 6 years of age who have no neurologic contraindications to its use. It is not given to children over age 6 years because whereas the incidence, severity, and fatality of the disease decrease, the risk of receiving the vaccine increases.

Polio. The trivalent oral form of poliovirus (TOPV) (developed by Sabin) is recommended for all children under 18 years of age who have no specific contraindications, regardless of the number of administrations of inactivated poliovirus vaccine (IPV) (developed by Salk) they may al-

Table 12-12. Guide to tetanus prophylaxis in wound management

History of tetanus immunization (doses)	Clean, minor wounds		All other wounds	
	Td	TIG	Td	TIG
Uncertain	Yes	No	Yes*	Yes*
0-1	Yes	No	Yes	Yes
2	Yes	No	Yes	Not†
3 or more	No‡	No	No§	No

From Krugman, S., Ward, R., and Katz, S. L.: Infectious diseases of children, St. Louis, 1977, The C. V. Mosby Co.
*Td and TIG are given together to confer passive and active immunity.
†Unless wound more than 24 hours old.
‡Unless more than 10 years since last dose.
§Unless more than 5 years since last dose.

ready have received. For infants and children with immune deficiency diseases and for their siblings, the inactivated poliovirus vaccine is the vaccine of choice. It is also recommended for adults who have had no previous polio immunization but require it because of planned travel to an area where the disease remains endemic.[3] Inactivated poliovirus vaccine has the disadvantage of being given by subcutaneous injection but has no reported history of ever causing a case of vaccine-associated paralysis.

Measles. Because of the presence of maternal antibodies, measles virus vaccine should be delayed until 15 months of age for infants who live in communities where the disease is not prevalent. However, during the course of measles outbreaks, the vaccine can be given any time after 6 months of age, followed by a second inoculation after age 15 months.[2]

Theoretically tuberculin testing should be done before or at the same time as the measles immunization. Exacerbation of tuberculosis is known to occur with natural measles infection and, theoretically, could result from the live attenuated measles virus vaccine. In addition viral interference from the vaccine may cause a false-negative reaction. However, depression of tuberculin sensitivity is unlikely to occur within 48 hours of the immunization.[24] In actual practice, neither of these two possibilities is considered a contraindication to measles immunization, especially in the event of an epidemic.

An interval of at least 1 month is recommended between immunizations using live virus vaccines. This is based on the rationale that one vaccine may interfere with the antibody response of another vaccine. Presently there are combined live virus vaccines for primary immunization that are safe and effective, for example, mumps and rubella; measles and rubella, and measles, mumps, and rubella. However, simultaneous administration of preparations not commercially combined, such as separate injections of mumps virus vaccine and measles virus vaccine, is not recommended.

Mumps. Mumps vaccine may be given at any time to children between 15 months and 12 years of age who have not had the disease.

Rubella. Rubella immunization is recommended for (1) all susceptible children between the ages of 15 months and 12 years and (2) female adolescents and women of childbearing age who are not protected against the disease.[4] Because the live attenuated virus may cross the placenta and present a risk to the developing fetus, rubella vaccine is not given to any pregnant woman or to any whoman who may become pregnant in the 2 months following the immunization. The nurse must explain the necessity for adequate contraception for at least this 2-month period following the vaccine. There is no reported danger of giving a rubella immunization to a child if the mother is pregnant.

Safety and security

Accidents are a major cause of death during infancy, especially for children 6 to 12 months old, as well as the leading cause of mortality in children over 1 year of age until early adulthood. Constant vigilance, awareness, and supervision are essential as the child gains increased locomotor and manipulative skills, coupled with an insatiable curiosity about the environment. Accidents can be grouped into the following categories: suffocation, falls, poisoning, aspiration of foreign objects, burns, motor vehicle accidents, and bodily damage. Table 12-13 lists the major development achievement of each period during infancy and the appropriate accident prevention plan.

Suffocation. At one time suffocation was thought to be a cause of crib death or sudden infant death syndrome, but it is now known that infants can wriggle out from under small pillows or blankets. However, danger from mechanical suffocation does exist and accounts for the most frequent type of accidents in infants less than 1 year of age. An infant who is placed in a bed under blankets and sheets that are tucked in can be caught under them and be unable to wriggle free. There are potential dangers in adults' sleeping with a small infant because of the possibility of their rolling over and smothering the child. Even though this is a slight possibility, if it happens the consequent parental guilt can be devastating. Another more common cause of suffocation is plastic bags. Large plastic bags used over garments are very lightweight and can easily and quickly be wrapped around the head of an active infant. Pillows should not be covered with plastic for this reason. Older infants may play peekaboo with a plastic bag and accidently pull it over their head. Since plastic is nonporous, suffocation takes place in a matter of minutes.

Anything tied around the infant's neck potentially can cause strangulation. Bibs should be removed at bedtime, and objects such as pacifiers should never be hung on a string around the infant's neck. This is a common practice

Table 12-13. Accident prevention during infancy

Age (months)	Major developmental task	Accident prevention
Birth-4	Crawling reflex may propel infant forward May roll over Moro reflex can propel infant forward Increasing eye-hand coordination and voluntary grasp reflex	**Suffocation** Keep all plastic bags stored away from infant's reach; discard large plastic garment bags after tying in a knot Do not cover mattress or pillows with plastic Use a firm mattress, no pillows, and loose blankets Position crib away from other furniture Avoid sleeping in bed with infant Do not tie pacifier on a string around infant's neck Remove bibs at bedtime Drowning—never leave infant alone in bath **Falls** Always raise crib rails; tie them to crib if malfunctioning Never leave infant on a raised, unguarded surface When in doubt where to place child, use the floor Restrain child in the infant seat and never leave him unattended while the seat is resting on a raised surface Avoid using a high chair until child is old enough to sit well **Poisoning and aspiration** Not as great a danger to this age-group but should begin practicing safeproofing early **Burns** Check bath water and warmed formula and food Do not pour hot liquids when infant is close by, such as sitting on your lap Beware of cigarette ashes that may fall on the infant Do not leave infant in the sun for more than a few minutes Wash flame-retardant clothes according to label directions Use cool mist vaporizers Do not keep child in parked car **Motor vehicles** Transport infant (even newborn) in a specially constructed car seat with shoulder and waist restraints Do not place infant on the seat or in your lap Do not place a carriage or stroller behind a parked car **Bodily damage** Avoid sharp, jagged-edged objects Keep diaper pins closed and away from infant
4-7	Rolls over Sits momentarily Grasps and manipulates small objects Resecures a dropped object Has well-developed eye-hand coordination Can fixate and locate very small objects Mouthing very prominent	**Suffocation** May begin to teach swimming as part of water safety **Falls** Restrain in a high chair Keep crib rails raised to full height **Poisoning and aspiration** Keep buttons, beads, and other small objects out of infant's reach Use pacifier with one-piece construction and loop handle Keep floor free of any small objects Do not feed infant hard candy, nuts, or food with pits or seeds Inspect toys for removable parts Make sure that paint for furniture or toys does not contain lead Place toxic substances on a high shelf and/or locked cabinet Hang plants or place on high surface rather than on floor Avoid storing large quantities of cleaning fluid, paints, pesticides, and other toxic substances Discard used containers of poisonous substances Do not store toxic substances in food containers Know telephone number of local poison control center

Table 12-13. Accident prevention during infancy—cont'd

Age (months)	Major developmental task	Accident prevention
4-7—cont'd		**Burns** Keep faucets out of reach Place hot objects (cigarettes, candles, incense) on high surface **Motor vehicles** Transport in a specially constructed car seat with shoulder and waist restraints Do not place infant on the seat or in your lap Do not place a carriage or stroller behind a parked car **Bodily damage** Give him toys that are smooth and rounded, preferably made of wood or plastic Avoid long, pointed objects as toys
8-12	Crawls Stands, holding onto furniture Stands alone Cruises around furniture Walks Climbs Pulls on objects Throws objects Uses pincer grasp for small articles Mouthing still prominent Dislikes being restrained Explores away from mother Increasing understanding of simple commands and phrases	**Suffocation** Keep doors of ovens, dishwashers, refrigerators, and front-loading clothes washers and dryers closed at all times If storing an unused appliance, such as a refrigerator, remove the door Fence swimming pools; always supervise when near any source of water **Falls** Fence stairways at top and bottom if child has access to either end **Poisoning and aspiration** Administer medications as a drug, not as a candy Do not administer adult medications unless so prescribed by a physician Replace medications and poisons immediately after use; replace caps properly if a child protector cap is used; some insecticides have special caps that prevent short fingers from pressing the spray button Keep floor free of small objects **Burns** Place guards in front of any heating appliance, fireplace, or furnace Keep electrical wires hidden or out of reach Place plastic guards over electrical outlets Keep hanging tablecloths out of reach Do not allow infant to play with electrical appliance **Motor vehicles** Do not use adult seat or shoulder belt without infant car seat Do not allow to crawl behind a parked car If infant plays in a yard, have the yard fenced or use a playpen **Bodily damage** Do not allow infant to use a fork for self-feeding Use plastic cups or dishes Check safety of toys

in some cultures and can be remedied by pinning the string tied to a pacifier on the child's shirt.

Restraining straps, if applied too loosely or left unfastened, can be a hazard. For example, a child may slide off a high chair beneath the tray and strangle himself on the loose strap. All straps should be fastened securely or removed if not used.

Infant strangulation may occur if the infant's head becomes caught between the crib and mattress or items in close proximity to the crib.[9] Mattresses and bumper pads that fit snuggly against the slats should be purchased. The crib should be positioned away from large furniture because children who crawl out of the crib may become caught between the two objects.

Since drowning is another cause of asphyxiation, infants should never be left unsupervised in a bathtub or near a source of water, such as a swimming pool, toilet, or bucket. One way to stress water safety is to teach infants to swim. Infants under 6 months of age have two reflexes that enhance swimming. The crawl reflex causes a swimming motion strong enough to propel the infant through water for a short distance. The dive reflex inhibits breathing when the infant is submerged. Most infants, if introduced to the water *properly,* will not be afraid and can be taught to float and to swim underwater for a few feet. Not until they are 3 or 4 years old can they swim above water for longer distances because of the proportionately heavy weight of the head.[13]

Falls. Falls are most common after 4 months of age when the infant has learned to roll over, but they can occur at *any* age. Newborns are normally active, assume a flexed position, and have crawling and Moro reflexes that can propel them forward. The best advice is never to place a child unattended on a raised surface that has no type of guard rails. When in doubt, the safest place is the floor. Even though young infants cannot climb over a partially raised crib rail, it is best to form a habit of raising the side rail all the way, because one day that infant will manage to get out.

Another danger area for falling is a changing table, which is usually high and narrow. Although these tables have a restraining belt, it is unwise to leave the child unattended even when he is so restrained. The best way to avoid having to leave is to arrange the area so that all necessary articles are within easy reach so the child is always in full eyesight of the care giver. It only takes a fraction of a second for the infant to fall off. During the latter half of the first year, infants usually resist dressing and diapering and may be more of an active handful than one can always manage. If there is danger that the child is strong enough to resist restraining, he should be changed on the floor.

Infant seats, high chairs, walkers, and swings present additional opportunities for accidental falls. If the infant seat is placed on a table where the infant has an excellent panorama of his environment, he should never be left unrestrained or unattended. The same rule is essential for other baby equipment, particularly when the child has learned to crawl and stand up. Small infants can slip through a high chair if a protective harness is not used. High chairs are designed for older infants who can sit well and who are tall enough to have the tray at the level of their chest or abdomen.

Although the infant begins to develop depth perception by age 9 months, that is no guarantee of his ability to perceive danger. His curiosity may still propel him forward and over, or his immature locomotor skills may be inadequate to keep him from falling even though he is aware of the danger. Infants should not be allowed to crawl unsupervised on any raised surface, near stairs, or near any water reservoir. Gates should be used at the bottom and top of stairs, since both present dangers to the crawling and climbing infant.

Poisoning. Accidental poisoning is one of the major causes of death in children under 5 years of age. The highest incidence occurs in those in the 2-year-old age-group, with the second highest incidence in 1-year-old children. The infant who has not learned to crawl is relatively free from danger of poisonous agents by virtue of his confinement. However, once locomotion begins, danger from poisoning is present almost everywhere. There are over 500 toxic substances in the average home, and the majority of all poisonings (about 34%) occur in the kitchen. The major reason for ingestion of poisons is improper storage. For the infant, this means not placing toxic agents on a low shelf, table, or floor. Drugs that are kept in a purse pose additional dangers because if the purse is given to the infant to play with he may open it and ingest the contents. Poisoning is almost always the result of inadequate supervision, but it may not represent neglect. Children are very fast, and it takes only seconds to eat a bar of soap, an opened cleanser can, or a handful of detergent. Although infants usually do not possess the manipulative skill to open closed jars, they are amazingly persistent and inventive. For example, an ant trap placed in an out-of-the-way corner is easy for a crawling infant to find.

Plants are another source of poisoning for infants. Plants are frequently placed on the floor, where the leaves or flowers are attractive and easy to pull off. There are over 700 species of plants that are known to have caused death or illness. One leaf of a poinsettia plant can kill a child.

The only sure way to prevent poisoning is to remove toxic agents. For the infant, this means placing them high out of reach. However, since crawling infants soon become climbing toddlers, it is best to keep all toxic agents, especially drugs, in a locked cabinet. Special plastic hooks can be attached to the inside of cabinet doors to keep them securely closed. Since it requires firm thumb pressure to unlatch the hook, small children are usually unable to manipulate them. Locks are best, but for cleaning agents frequently used, such as under a kitchen sink, hooks are a practical alternative. Impractical suggestions are usually ignored, and some protection is better than none. With several hundred toxic substances in each house, locking all potentially toxic substances could present a problem; however, careful planning can help. A large surplus of cleaning agents, furniture polishes, laundry additives, paints, insecticides, and solvents should be avoided. Used poison containers should be promptly discarded and not used to store another poison without adequately marking the package. Since young children cannot read, any potentially hazardous substance should not be stored in any type of food container. A popular container that is used to store toxic liquids is soda bottles. A child who is unaware of the dangerous contents is a vulnerable victim for poisoning. Parents should know the location of the local poison control centers and call them in the event of a suspected poisoning. For children under 1 year of age, ipecac syrup is usually not administered to produce vomiting; however, a spoon or a finger stroked against the back of the pharynx will induce emesis. If a finger is used, care must be exercised to prevent damage from biting. Emergency measures for accidental poisoning are discussed in Chapter 16.

Aspiration of foreign objects. As soon as the infant has the ability to find his mouth, he is vulnerable to aspiration of a small object. The infant is subject to aspirating tiny objects that are left within his reach or removable parts of objects that may on initial inspection appear safe. Rattles, for example, have small beads in them to produce noise. A broken or cracked rattle can be dangerous since the beads can easily be swallowed while the infant has the toy in his mouth. Stuffed animals are another potentially dangerous toy if any of the parts, such as the eyes or nose, are removable buttons or plastic pieces. Sometimes no part is removable, but wire is placed inside an area to create a special shape. A typical example is wire inside a rabbit's ear to make it stand up.

All toys must be carefully inspected for potential danger. An active infant can grab a low-hanging mobile and quickly chew off a small piece. As soon as the infant crawls or plays on the floor, one must be certain that the floor is free of any small articles that can be picked up and swallowed. When new foods are given to the child, nuts, hard candies, or fruits with pits or seeds should be avoided. When infant clothes are being purchased, the type of closure used should be considered. A front button can easily be pulled off and swallowed. Safety pins for diapers should be kept closed and away from the dressing table. Even though a young infant may not search for them, practicing this good habit from the beginning prevents future accidents.

Pacifiers can also be dangerous because the entire object may be aspirated if it is small, or the nipple and shield may become detached from the handle and become lodged in the pharynx.[18] Safe pacifiers should be of one-piece construction, have a shield or flange that is large enough to prevent entry into the mouth, and have a handle that can be grasped (Fig. 12-5).

Burns. Burns are generally not thought of as a particular danger to infants, but several important hazards exist, such as scalding from water that is too hot, excessive sunburn, and burns from electrical wires, sockets, and heating elements, such as radiators, registers, and floor furnaces. The infant's skin is particularly sensitive to irritation, and the mechanisms for temperature perception are not completely developed.

The bath water should be checked before the infant is immersed. The handles of cooking utensils should be turned toward the back of the stove. When the infant is underfoot, hot liquids should not be poured from one container to another and cooking with hot oil should not be done. Hanging tablecloths should be placed out of the infant's reach.

Sunburn can be a source of a first- or second-degree burn. Exposure to direct sunlight or filtered light through a window should be gradual, about 5 minutes initially. The infant's head should be covered, since it represents a large proportion of body surface.

Electrical outlets should be covered with protective plastic caps that prevent the child from sucking on the outlet or putting objects such as hairpins into it. Live wires should be placed out of reach, since curious infants can chew on them and potentially break the rubber coating. Infants should not be allowed to play near televisions, stereo units, or other appliances, whether these units are on or off, since infants cannot determine when the appliance is safe. Any heat-producing element should have a guard placed in front of it. Fireplaces should be well screened since they are very appealing and within easy access. Small portable heaters should only be used when placed on

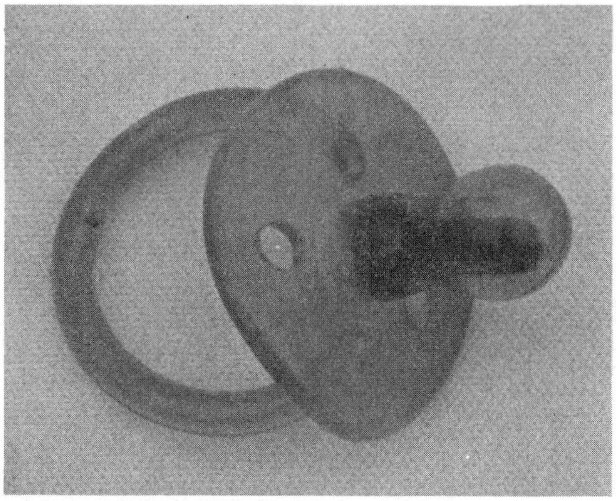

Fig. 12-5. Design of a safe pacifier.

a high surface. Burning cigarettes, candles, and incense should be kept out of reach.

Vaporizers are a hazard, particularly if they produce heated mist. Parents should be advised to purchase cool-mist vaporizers. If a heat-mist vaporizer is used, it should be placed on a high surface, away from the crib. By law, all infants' sleepwear must be flame retardant. Unfortunately this does not apply to all infants' clothes. Flame-retardant fabric must never be viewed as the ultimate protection against burns. Repeated washing reduces the flame-retardant properties, and the use of soap or bleach destroys the protection. Since only detergent should be used for washing flame-retardant clothing, infants, who are sensitive to such wash agents, are unprotected when their clothing is washed with a mild soap. If sleepwear is home sewn, mothers should be advised to look for specially treated flame-retardant fabric.

Another type of thermal injury occurs when children are exposed to excessive heat during confinement in poorly ventilated cars. The practice of leaving the windows open a couple of inches does not appear to be protective.[22] The nurse should caution parents never to leave children in parked cars, especially when the automobile is in direct sunlight.

Motor vehicle accidents. Automobile accidents are the leading cause of accidental deaths in children over 1 year of age. The major danger to the infant is improper restraint within the vehicle. It is recommended that all infants, newborns included, be secured in a special car restraint, rather than held or placed on the car seat. Child seats that hook over the back of the automobile or seats with attached gadgets, such as play steering wheels, are inadequate and may present additional hazards. A variety of car seats are available for young children. For infants the recommended type is a rearward facing molded plastic shell seat, which includes a shoulder restraint and utilizes the adult car seat belt. Children should not use the adult seat belt as their sole protection until the pelvic structures are adequately developed, which is usually between 4 and 5 years of age.[14] Use of the adult lap seat belt or shoulder belt with a child who weighs less than 40 pounds can result in severe abdominal injury or strangulation. If the portable shell seat is used, it should be strapped with the infant facing the back of the seat. If it is placed with the infant facing the front of the car, in the event of a collision the child would be propelled forward. This type of car restraint can also be used as a portable infant seat. If a car bed is preferred, it should be well padded and of strong construction. It should be placed on the seat (preferably the rear) with the child's head toward the center of the car, away from the doors. A nylon net should be stretched over the bed and tucked in. The bed must then be firmly secured to the seat with two vehicle lap seat belts.[12a]

Another potential vehicular accident is placing a carriage or stroller behind a car, particularly a car parked in a garage or driveway. It is possible that the driver may not see the small stroller and, while driving in reverse, run over the child.

Bodily damage. Accidents can occur in other ways. Sharp, jagged-edged objects can cause wounds in the skin. Long, pointed articles can be poked into the eye, causing serious visual loss. The latter is particularly important to remember because infants have less well-developed fine motor control. For this reason forks should be avoided for self-feeding until the child has mastered the spoon, usually by age 18 months.

Nursing considerations: accident prevention and discipline

When one considers the potential environmental dangers to which infants are vulnerable, the task of preventing these accidents only begins to be appreciated. Nurses must be aware of the possible causes of injury in each age-group in order for *anticipatory* preventive teaching to occur. For example, the guidelines for accident prevention during infancy presented in Table 12-13 should be discussed before the child reaches the susceptible age-group. Therefore, preventive teaching ideally occurs during pregnancy. Since two thirds of all accidents involving children occur in the home, the importance of safety cannot be overemphasized.

Accident prevention requires protection and education. For infants, this translates into protection of the child and education of the parents or care giver. Nurses in ambulatory care settings, health maintenance centers, or visiting nurse agencies are in a most favorable position for accident education. This does not exclude nurses in inpatient facilities, who could utilize visiting times as an excellent opportunity for discussing this topic. One approach to teaching accident prevention is to relate why children in various age-groups are prone to special types of accidents. Stressing the prevention is just as important as emphasizing the *why* of the accident. However, accident prevention must also be practical. For example, suggesting that *all* potentially toxic substances be locked in a cabinet or placed on a high shelf is ideal but may be so impractical that no change will occur. Asking parents for their ideas will lead to realistic suggestions that can be followed. For instance, bathroom cleaning agents, cosmetics, and personal-care items can be placed on a top shelf in the linen closet, and towels or sheets can be stored on the lower shelves and floor.

If an accident has occurred, do not be too quick to admonish the parent. Accidents do not always indicate neglect. It is a difficult task to watch children carefully without overprotecting or unnecessarily confining them. Small falls help children learn the dangers of heights. Touching a hot object once can emphasize to the child the pain of a burn. Allowing children to explore while maintaining *consistent, age-appropriate limit setting* is sound advice.

Parents need to remember that infants and young children cannot anticipate danger or understand when it is or is not present. A dead electrical wire may present no actual harm, but, if the child is allowed to play with it, a poor habit is being practiced for when the child comes across live wires. Although it is always wise to explain why something is dangerous, remember that small children will need to be physically removed from the situation.

It is not easy to teach safety, supervise closely, and refrain from saying "no" a hundred times a day. Parents become acutely aware of this triangle as soon as the infant learns to crawl. Preventing accidents is usually the first reason for discipline, because accidents not only can cause harm to children but may also damage valuable household objects. Parents are frequently caught in the dilemma of protecting their children and home from accidents caused by children by either removing potential dangers and valuable objects or by teaching rules and regulations while not removing potential dangers or special possessions. Probably neither solution is better. Small children must have dangerous objects removed or guarded, and valuable articles should be placed out of reach at least until the child has learned by breaking other things. Children, even the youngest crawling infant, will almost always test their parents and defy their commands. It is better to learn a lesson from breaking an inexpensive ashtray than a valuable crystal decanter, or by falling off a step stool rather than down a flight of stairs. In either case the lesson is similar, but the price is different.

When children are taught the meaning of "no," they should also be taught what "yes" means. Children should be praised for playing with suitable toys, their efforts at behaving or listening should be reinforced, and recreational toys that are innovative and creative should be provided for them. Infants love to tear paper and avidly pursue books, magazines, or newspapers left on the floor. Instead of always scolding them for destroying a valued book, old, discarded reading material should be kept available for them to play with. If they enjoy pots and pans, a cabinet can be arranged with safe utensils for them to explore. These actions will result in much less frustration for everyone, and in time the infants will learn to distinguish between what is theirs and what belongs to others.

One additional factor must be stressed concerning accident prevention and discipline. Children are imitators; they copy what they see and hear. Practicing safety teaches safety, which applies to parents and their children as well as to nurses and their clients. Saying one thing but doing another confuses children and can lead to discipline problems as the child grows older.

Parental concerns

For new parents, as well as for some experienced parents, there are many concerns about child rearing during the first year. How shall we feed him, why does he suck his thumb, when will he sleep through the night, why he is so irritable with each new tooth, should we discipline him so soon? These are just a sampling of questions that parents ask themselves. Although the answers are much less exciting than preparing children for surgery or assisting with complicated procedures, nurses must be aware of these concerns and provide answers that give guidance and help decrease anxiety.

Teething. One of the more difficult periods in the infant's (and parents') life is the eruption of the deciduous teeth, often referred to as teething. The exact mechanisms responsible for the eruption of teeth are not fully understood. The growth of the root, dentin, and pulp of the tooth, the pressure exerted against the peridental tissue, and the hormonal control of the pituitary growth hormone and the thyroid hormone are some of the theories under investigation.[19] Teething is a physiologic process, and as the crown of the tooth breaks through the peridental membrane considerable discomfort may be present. Some children show minimal evidence of teething, such as drooling or biting on hard objects. Others are very irritable, have difficulty in sleeping, and refuse to eat. Generally signs of illness such as fever, vomiting, or diarrhea are not symptoms of teething but of illness.

Since teething pain is a result of inflammation, cold is usually soothing. Giving the child a cold metal spoon, a frozen teething ring, or an ice cube wrapped in a washcloth helps relieve the inflammation. Analgesics, preferably nonaspirin compounds, such as acetaminophen, can be given judiciously. The use of teething powders or procedures such as cutting or rubbing the gums should be discouraged, since ingestion of the powder or infection of the tissue can occur.

Thumb-sucking. Sucking is the infant's chief pleasure, and it may not be satisfied by breast- or bottle-feeding. It is such a strong need that infants who are deprived of sucking, such as those with a cleft lip repair, will suck on their tongue. Some newborns are born with sucking pads on their fingers from in utero sucking activity. Problems arise when parents are concerned about finger- or thumb-sucking and attempt to restrain this natural tendency. Before giving advice nurses should investigate the parents' feelings and base guidance on this information. For example, some parents may see no problem with the use of a pacifier but may find the use of a finger repulsive. In general there is no need to restrain either. Malocclusion may occur if thumb-sucking persists past 4 years of age or when the permanent teeth erupt. There is probably less dental displacement with the use of pacifier than with the use of a hard, rigid finger. Pacifiers are usually relinguished earlier than thumbs because they are not so readily available. However, pacifiers can be dangerous if they are too small or improperly constructed, since in either case the entire pacifier or a part of it can be aspirated or lodged in the trachea, totally occluding the airway. A pacifier should be of a continuous, one-piece construction, and the base or perioral mouthpiece should be larger than the oral opening. Sucking pleasure can be increased by prolonging feeding time. A small-holed, firm nipple on the bottle causes stronger sucking and slower feeding.

Thumb-sucking reaches its peak at ages 18 to 20 months and is most prevalent when the child is hungry or tired. Persistent thumb-sucking in a listless, apathetic child always warrants investigation. It may be a sign of an emotional problem between parent and child or of boredom, isolation, and lack of stimulation.

Sleep. Most infants have developed a nocturnal pattern of sleep by 3 months of age. By age 6 months the majority of infants sleep through the night, with naps during the day. An 8- or 9-month-old infant may take one or two naps during the day and sleeps about 12 hours during the night. However, there is no set schedule for any child. If parents question the infant's need for sleep, it is best to investigate the reason for their concern, stressing the individual needs of each child. Infants who are active during wakeful periods and who are growing normally are sleeping a sufficient amount of time. If waking during the night persists, the diet should be investigated, since hunger will cause infants to waken. Breast-fed or small infants usually sleep less prolonged periods than do bottle-fed or larger infants because of the more rapid digestion of human milk by breast-fed infants and smaller stomach capacity of smaller infants.

PROMOTING OPTIMUM DEVELOPMENT

Although growth and development proceed in an orderly, predetermined sequence, environment does influence optimum development. No aspect of environment is more important than the quality of emotional care that the infant receives. Some of the most famous and convincing work supporting this fact has been done by Bowlby and Spitz on emotional deprivation. John Bowlby studied the effects of the infant's separation from his mother and noted severe mental and physical retardation, particularly if emotional deprivation occurred during the first 3 years of life. He observed that the progressive retardation could be arrested or reversed if no further emotional deprivation occurred after the first 2 years but that prolonged severe deprivation beginning early in the first year and lasting for 3 years led to severe permanent effects. Among these were the inability to form trusting, intimate interpersonal relationships, language impairment, and deficiency in abstract thinking.[10] He also found typical behavioral reactions of infants who were hospitalized and separated from their mothers (Chapter 25).

René Spitz studied the effects of emotional deprivation of children raised in foundling homes or institutions. The infants were cared for by one nurse who had responsibility for eight children. Although the care giver might be a loving, motherly person, she lacked the time necessary to devote individual attention and stimulation to each child. As a result, the children were retarded in physical growth, were more susceptible to disease, and demonstrated decreasing developmental quotients over a 2-year period. Spitz found that children who were given one-to-one attention by a mother substitute developed normally.[23]

The importance of human physical contact cannot be overemphasized. Parenting is not an instinctual ability but a learned acquired process. The attachment of parent and child probably begins before birth. Only recently has the importance of the first few hours of life been studied and recognized. It is the nurse's responsibility to promote parent-child bonding through each stage of development, especially during infancy when the foundation of trust is being formed.

Attachment

Parent-infant attachment has been discussed in Chapter 8, specifically in terms of the neonatal period. However, attachment behavior is not confined to the birth of the child. In fact many parents state that they felt nothing for the newborn and that feelings of motherliness or fatherliness took time to develop, usually about 3 months. The infant's behavior has a significant influence on the development of attachment or bonding. A highly responsive infant is more likely to evoke satisfaction and pleasure from a parent than is a passive, apathetic infant. However, stimulation plays an important role in enhancing the responsiveness of the infant. Since the bonding process is always a reciprocal process, any learning about each other evokes a more mutually reinforcing experience. Development and acquisition of new skills is part of the process. A parent who is aware of the child's expected level of performance promotes trust and security in the child, whereas a parent who is always pushing a child beyond his capacity for learning creates tension, frustration, and insecurity in the child.

Several components are crucial in the process of attachment. One of them, the *sensitive period,* has been discussed in Chapters 8 and 10 and relates to the importance of the first hour and days of life. Separation during this time, as in the case of the high-risk infant, has special implication for nurses. Another is the *developmental behaviors* that infants acquire during the first year. These include differential crying, smiling, and vocalization (more to mother than to anyone else), visual-motor orientation (looking more at mother even if she is not close), crying when mother leaves the room, approach through locomotion (crawling, creeping, or walking), clinging (especially in presence of a stranger), and exploring away from mother while using her as a secure base. It is important to note that the word mother does not exclusively refer to the biologic mother but to the consistent care giver with whom the child relates more than anyone else. In society's changing social climate and sex role stereotypes, this may very well be the father.

Monotropy is another component of attachment that has special meaning for health professionals. Monotropy refers to the principle that a person can become optimally attached to only one individual at a time.[16] This is very significant in the attachment process that occurs in multiple births. If a parent can form only one attachment at a time, how then can all the siblings of a multiple birth receive optimal emotional care? With increasing multiple births accompanying the more widespread use of fertility drugs, this is an area that will require additional investigation. If nurses are aware of such a component of attachment, it may be well to encourage extended family members to participate in the care of the infants.

Another aspect of monotropy is the attachment-detachment process. While mourning a loss (detachment), one may have difficulty in simultaneously forming a close attachment to someone else. This is particularly significant in cases where a child has died and another child is immediately conceived. Until mourning has been worked through (usually a minimum of 1 year), it may be best to avoid having another child. Other losses that may influence the attachment process are the birth of a sick or defective child, a difficult labor and delivery, or a serious illness of a parent or close family member. Nurses who are sensitive to the components of attachment will be able to assess disturbances in parent-child relationships, based on facts that may be altered or changed. For example, a mother who has difficulty in accepting the second twin is not an inadequate mother but one who is experiencing the difficulty of monotropy. She may need more support and help from significant others with the second twin until the time when she can devote her emotional energy to the other child.

Stranger anxiety

During the formation of attachment to a parent, usually the mother, the infant progresses through four distinct, but overlapping, stages. For the first few weeks the infant responds indiscriminately to anyone. Beginning at about 8 to 12 weeks of age, the infant cries, smiles, and vocalizes more to the mother than to anyone else but continues to respond to others, whether familiar or not. At age 6 months or so the infant shows a distinct preference for the mother. He follows her more, cries when she leaves, enjoys playing with her more, and feels most secure in her arms. As the infant demonstrates this sharp attachment to one person, he correspondingly exhibits less friendliness to others. Between ages 6 and 8 months fear of strangers and stranger anxiety become most prominent. Although interpreted by some people as a sign of undesirable, antisocial behavior, stranger anxiety really indicates a strong healthy parent-child attachment. It is a most important and sometimes difficult time for parent and child. Parents may be more confined to the home because baby-sitters are violently protested by the infant. If parents have encouraged close friends or relatives to visit often, there is usually one other person with whom the child is comfortable, who can give parents time alone. However, prolonged separation, such as hospitalization, can have severe emotional sequelae, and every effort should be employed to prevent any unnecessary separation. The effects of hospitalization and separation anxiety in children are discussed in Chapter 25.

Parents also may wonder whether they should encourage the child's clinging, dependent behavior, especially if there is pressure from others who view this as antisocial, spoiled antics. Parents need to be reassured that such behavior is healthy, desirable, and necessary for the child's optimal emotional development. If parents can reassure the infant of their presence, the infant will learn to realize that they are still there even if not physically present. In Piaget's terms this is part of learning object permanence. Talking to infants when leaving the room or allowing them to hear one's voice on the telephone reassures them of the parent's continued presence.

This is no less a trying time for infants, because parents cannot always be with the child. An excellent example of necessary separation is bedtime. Fear of going to bed or being left alone in the dark commonly occurs during the second half of the first year. Rocking, walking, prolonged nursing, or sleeping with the child may remedy the problem temporarily but does not help the child learn that separation is necessary and must be dealt with. Not giving children opportunities to deal with anxiety and frustration leaves them helpless and bewildered when the smallest crisis arises. Firmly but gently putting the child in his crib, hugging and kissing him, and then leaving the room is usually a better solution. Encouraging habits that later become nuisances, such as putting the child in the parents' bed, may eventually become greater problems to solve than initial firmness.

Care of parents

Child rearing is no easy task; it presents challenges to new parents as well as to ''seasoned'' parents. With society's changing roles and mores, combined with a highly mobile population, there is little stability for traditional role models and time-honored methods of raising children. As a result, parents look more to professionals for guidance. Nurses are in an advantageous position for rendering assistance and suggestions. Every phase of a child's life has its particular traumas, whether it is toilet training for toddlers, unexplained fears for preschoolers, or identity crises for adolescents. For parents of an infant some challenges center around dependency, discipline, increased mobility, and safety. The major areas for parental guidance during the first year are listed in the boxed material on p. 470.

At birth the major task for parents and infant is attach-

Parental guidance during infant's first year

Birth
- Understand each parent's adjustment to newborn, especially mother's postpartal emotional needs
- Teach care of infant and assist parents to understand his individual needs and that he expresses his wants through crying
- Encourage parents to establish a flexible schedule to meet needs of child and themselves

First 6 months
- Help parents understand infant's need for stimulation in environment
- Support parents' pleasure in seeing child's growing friendliness and social response, especially smiling
- Teach introduction of new foods
- Plan anticipatory guidance for safety
- Stress need for artificial immunization

Second 6 months
- Prepare parents for child's "stranger anxiety"
- Encourage parents to allow child to cling to mother or father and avoid long separation from either
- Guide parents concerning discipline because of infant's increasing mobility
- Teach accident prevention because of child's advancing motor skills and curiosity
- Encourage parents to leave child with suitable mother substitute to allow some free time
- Discuss readiness for weaning

ment. Parents, particularly mothers, expect to feel intense love and unity with their newborn and are frequently ashamed and bewildered that their feelings are so neutral. They need help in understanding that the process of parenting is learned and gradual. Mothers also have their special postpartal emotional needs. The sudden drop in hormone level may cause a temporary depression or feeling of loneliness. Stressing that this is normal and expected and encouraging her to talk about the labor and delivery experience will help relieve some anxiety, particularly if the husband or other significant person is supportive of the woman through this period.

Many new parents are unprepared for the care of the infant at home and are overwhelmed by the tasks of feeding, bathing, and changing. Rooming-in provides an excellent opportunity for nurses to teach these skills or to support the existing abilities of each parent. Fathers should be encouraged to participate and should be praised for their efforts. It is best to teach by example, rather than by lecture. Calling the infant by name, looking at him in the *en face* position, holding him closely, touching him gently, and talking to him will set an example for parents, which can enhance the attachment or bonding process. Emphasizing the individuality of their child, asking them how he differs from the other siblings when they were newborns, and describing how he behaves in the nursery help parents see their child as a unique human being. This is particularly important if the "fantasy child" differs from the "real child," which commonly happens when parents desire a child of one sex and give birth to a child of the opposite sex. The fantasy vs real child conflict is a very important component of the detachment-attachment process, which occurs with the birth of a defective or seriously ill child.

During the first 6 months there are several important areas of teaching. Parents may not realize the infant's need for stimulation or be aware of how to provide it, and suggestions for suitable toys may be needed (see Table 12-2). During the early months the infant's social responses, such as smiling, grasping, and vocalizing, should be supported. It is most important that during these first few months parent and child develop reciprocal relationships and mutually meet each other's needs. It may very well be that problems such as maternal deprivation or child abuse begin when two individuals are both relating on opposite levels. Investigating the infant's habits, sleep routine, and waking activities will yield invaluable information concerning the mother's feelings of caring for her child. This is also the time to begin discussing introduction of new foods and potential sources of accidents in the home.

During the second 6 months the child's increasing dependence on mother and increasing independence through locomotion present major challenges. Preparing parents for the child's fear of strangers and encouraging them to allow the clinging dependent behavior helps minimize potential conflicts. Stressing that such behavior indicates a strong parental attachment focuses on the *positive* aspects of stranger anxiety. Encouraging parents to find a suitable baby-sitter, particularly someone who can visit often, allows them freedom and enjoyment together, without feelings of guilt. This is not only important for the child, who learns how to adjust to a crisis, but also for the parents, who need to spend time alone with each other to communicate, to love, and to enjoy one another's company. Time for one another can easily be lost amidst the multiple responsibilities of raising a family.

As the infant achieves greater skill in all areas of development, safety becomes a major problem. Helping parents *anticipate* potential dangers in the home decreases the possibility of accidents occurring. Since discipline is part of teaching safety, establishing certain "rules" early helps children learn what is acceptable behavior. Neither a laissez-faire nor a dictator approach to discipline is advisable. A commonsense approach that incorporates understanding, firmness, and consistency by both parents usually yields the best results.

REFERENCES

1. American Academy of Pediatrics: Report of the Committee on Infectious Diseases, Evanston, Ill., 1977, The Academy.
2. American Academy of Pediatrics, Committee on Infectious Diseases: Measles immunization: new recommendations,

Am. Acad. Pediatr. News Comments **27**(12):7, December 1976.
3. American Academy of Pediatrics, Committee on Infectious Diseases: Poliovirus immunization re-examined, Am. Acad. Pediatr. News Comments **27**(12):7, December 1976.
4. American Academy of Pediatrics, Committee on Infectious Diseases: Rubella immunizations: new recommendations, Am. Acad. Pediatr. News Comments **27**(12):7, December 1976.
5. American Academy of Pediatrics, Committee on Nutrition: On the feeding of solid foods to infants, Pediatrics **21**(4): 14-21, April 1958.
6. American Academy of Pediatrics, Committee on Nutrition: Infant methemoglobinemia, Pediatrics **42**(3):475-478, September 1970.
7. American Academy of Pediatrics, Committee on Nutrition: Iron supplementation for infants, Pediatrics **58**(5):765, November 1976.
8. Beal, V. A.: On the acceptance of solid foods and other food patterns of infants and children, Pediatrics **20:**448, 1957.
9. Bergeson, P. S., Hernreid, C. S., and Sonntag, P. L.: Infant strangulation, Pediatrics **59**(6):1043-1045, June 1977.
10. Bowlby, J., and associates: Effects of mother-child separation: follow-up study, Br. J. Med. Psychol. **29:**211, 1956.
11. Campos, J., and associates: Cardiac responses on the visual cliff in prelocomotor human infants, Science **170:**196-197, 1970.
12. Diphtheria, pertussis, tetanus, and poliomyelitis in the United States, Stat. Bull. **57:**8-11, September, 1976.
12a. Don't risk your child's life, Irvington, N.J., 1977, Physicians for Auto Safety.
13. Galatioto, M.: Water babies, Baby Talk **41**(6):18, June 1976.
14. Hletko, P. J., and Hletko, J. O.: Auto safety: preventive medicine for a pediatric epidemic, Pediatr. Basics **21:**10-14, 1978.
15. Karzon, D. T.: Smallpox vaccination in the U.S.: the end of an era, J. Pediatr. **81**(3):600-608, September 1972.
16. Klaus, M., and Kennel, J.: Maternal infant bonding, St. Louis, 1976, The C. V. Mosby Co.
17. Knobloch, H., and Pasamanick, B.: Gesell and Amatruda's developmental diagnosis, New York, 1974, Harper & Row, Publishers.
18. Kravath, R. E.: A lethal pacifier, Pediatrics **58**(6):853-855, December 1976.
19. McDonald, R.: Dentistry for the child and adolescent, St. Louis, 1974, The C. V. Mosby Co.
20. McMillan, J. A., Landau, S. A., and Oski, F. A.: Iron sufficiency in breast-fed infants and the availability of iron from human milk, Pediatrics **58**(5):686-691, November 1976.
21. Public Health Service recommendation on smallpox vaccination, Morbidity Mortality **20:**339, 1971.
22. Roberts, K. B., and Roberts, E. C.: The automobile and heat stress, Pediatrics **58**(1):101-104, July 1976.
23. Spitz, R. A.: Hospitalism: an inquiry into the genesis of psychiatric conditioning in early childhood. In Fenechel, D., and associates, editors: Psychoanalytic studies of the child, vol. 1, New York, 1945, International University Press, pp. 113-117.
24. Vessal, S., and Kravis, L. P.: Immunologic mechanisms responsible for adverse reactions to routine immunizations in children, Clin. Pediatr. **15**(8):688-696, August 1976.
25. Wall, R., and Gibson, E.: A comparative and analytical study of visual depth perception, Psychol. Monogr. **75**(15):170, 1961.

BIBLIOGRAPHY

Aab, C.: Assessment of maternal behavior during early mother-infant interaction. In Brandt, P. A., and associates, editors: Current practice in pediatric nursing, St. Louis, 1976, The C. V. Mosby Co.

Barnard, K.: The acquaintance process. In Klaus, M., and associates, editors: Maternal attachment and mothering disorders, New Brunswick, N.J., 1974, Johnson & Johnson, Baby Products Co.

Barnard, K. E., and Erickson, M. L.: Teaching children with developmental problems: a family care approach, ed. 2, St. Louis, 1976, The C. V. Mosby Co.

Barness, L.: Manual of pediatric physical diagnosis, ed. 4, Chicago, 1972, Year Book Medical Publishers, Inc.

Barness, L., and associates: Calcium and fat absorption from infant formulas with different fat blends, Pediatrics **54:**217, August 1974.

Bennett, S.: Infant caretaker interactions, J. Child Psychiatry **10:** 321-335, 1971.

Bowlby, J. Separation anxiety, Int. J. Psychoanal. **41:**89-113, 1960.

Brown, M., and Murphy, M.: A child grows, Pediatr. Nurs. **1:**9, January/February 1975.

Brown, M., and Murphy, M.: A child grows: how the child grows and develops psychologically, socially, and culturally. Part II. Pediatr. Nurs. **1**(2):22-30, March/April 1975.

Brown, M., and Murphy, M.: A child grows: the child's cognitive development. Part III. Pediatr. Nurs. **1**(3):7-12, May/June 1975.

Brown, M., and Murphy, M.: A child grows: the child's perceptual and linguistic development. Part IV. Pediatr. Nurs. **9:**15, July/August 1975.

Brown, M., and Murphy, M.: Ambulatory pediatrics for nurses, New York, 1975, McGraw-Hill Book Co.

Brown, M. S.: What you should know about communicable diseases and their immunizations. Part I. The three R's, Nurs. '75 **5**(9):70-72, September 1975.

Brown, M. S.: What you should know about communicable disease and their immunizations. Part II. Diphtheria, pertussis, tetanus, and polio, Nursing '75 **5**(10):56-60, October 1975.

Brown, M. S.: What you should know about communicable diseases and their immunizations. Part III. Mumps, chickenpox, and diarrhea, Nursing '75 **5**(11):55-60, November 1975.

Chinn, P. L.: Child health maintenance: concepts in family-centered care, ed. 2, St. Louis, 1979, The C. V. Mosby Co.

Chinn, P. L., and Leitch, C.: Child health maintenance: a guide to clinical assessment, ed. 2, St. Louis, 1979, The C. V. Mosby Co.

Clark, A., and Affonso, D.: Infant behavior and maternal attachment: two sides of the coin, Am. J. Maternal Child Nurs. **1**(2): 94-99, March/April 1976.

DeAngelis, C.: Basic pediatrics for the primary health care provider, Boston, 1975, Little, Brown and Co.

Dodge, P. R., Prensky, A. L., and Feigin, R. D.: Nutrition and the developing nervous system, St. Louis, 1975, The C. V. Mosby Co.

Dreikurs, R.: Children: the challenge, New York, 1964, Hawthorn Books, Inc.

Dudgeon, J. H.: Congenital rubella, J. Pediatr. **86**(6):1078-1086, December 1975.

Ericksen, A.: Every accidental poisoning is an emergency, Point of View **11**:7, October 1974.

Erickson, E.: Childhood and society, ed. 2, New York, 1963, W. W. Norton & Co., Inc.

Erickson, M. L.: Assessment and management of developmental changes in children, St. Louis, 1976, The C. V. Mosby Co.

Essoka, G., and associates: Pediatric nursing continuing education review, New York, 1975, Medical Examination Publishing Co., Inc.

Feldman, M.: Cluster visits, Am. J. Nurs. **74**(8):1485-1488, August 1974.

Fendrick, G.: Quizzing the expert: Jay M. Arena, on saving the child who swallows poison, Hosp. Physician, November 1973, p. 44.

Filer, L. J.: The case for iron supplements in infant feeding regimens, Hosp. Pract. **6**(6):79-92, June 1971.

Filer, L. J.: Studies of taste preference in infancy and childhood, Pediatr. Basics **12**:5-9, 1975.

Fraiberg, S.: The magic years, New York, 1959, Charles Scribner's Sons.

Francis, B. J.: Current concepts in immunizations, Am. J. Nurs. **73**(4):646-649, April 1973.

Gold, E., and associates: Immune status of children one to four years of age as determined by history and antibody measurement, N. Engl. J. Med. **289**(5):231-235, August 2, 1973.

Goldstein, J. A., and associates: Smallpox vaccination reactions, prophylaxis, and therapy of complications, Pediatrics **55**(3): 342, March 1975.

Goth, A.: Medical pharmacology, ed. 9, St. Louis, 1978, The C. V. Mosby Co.

Guyton, A. C.: Textbook of medical physiology, ed. 4, Philadelphia, 1971, W. B. Saunders Co.

Hendin, D.: Save your child's life! New York, 1972, Enterprise Publications.

Hoekelman, R. A.: What constitutes adequate well baby care? Pediatrics **55**(3):313, March 1975.

Hott, J.: The crisis of expectant fatherhood, Am. J. Nurs. **76**(9): 1436-1440, September 1976.

Hughes, J. G.: Synopsis of pediatrics, ed. 4, St. Louis, 1975, The C. V. Mosby Co.

Hymovitch, D.: ABC's of pediatric safety, Am. J. Nurs. **66**(8): 1768-1770, August 1966.

Infant nutrition: feeding the infant . . . building the man, New York, 1972, Medcom Press.

Illingworth, R. S.: Development of the infant and young child, New York, 1975, Churchill Livingstone.

Krugman, S., Ward, R., and Katz, S. L.: Infectious diseases of children, ed. 6, St. Louis, 1977, The C. V. Mosby Co.

Lewis, M.: Clinical aspects of child development, Philadelphia, 1971, Lea & Febiger.

Maier, H.: Three theories of child development, ed. 2, New York, 1969, Harper & Row, Publishers.

Miller, J. R., and Pless, I. B.: Child automobile restraints: evaluation of health education, Pediatrics **59**(6):907-911, June 1977.

Miller, R., and Johnson, R.: Poison control—now and in the future, Am. J. Nurs. **66**(9):1984-1987, September 1976.

Modlin, J. F., and associates: A review of five years' experience with rubella vaccine in the U.S., Pediatrics **55**(1):20-28, January 1975.

Nysather, J. O., Katz, A. E., and Lenth, J. L.: The immune system, its development and function, Am. J. Nurs. **76**(10):1614-1616, October 1976.

Obrzut, L.: Expectant fathers' perceptions of fathering, Am. J. Nurs. **76**(9):1440-1442, September 1976.

Papalia, D., and Olds, S.: A child's world, infancy through adolescence, New York, 1975, McGraw-Hill Book Co.

Piaget, J.: The construction of reality in the child, New York, 1954, Ballantine Books, Inc.

Prival, M., and Fisher, F.: Adding fluorides to the diet, Environment **16**(5):29-33, June 1974.

Rios, E., and associates: The absorption of iron as supplements in infant cereal and infant formulas, Pediatrics **55**(5):686, May 1975.

Rudolph, A. B., editor: Pediatrics, ed. 16, New York, 1977, Appleton-Century-Crofts.

Sander, D., and Cramblett, H.: Antibody titers to poliovirus in patients ten years after immunization with Sabin vaccine, J. Pediatr. **84**(3):406-408, March 1974.

Schoenbaum, S. C., and associates: Benefit-cost analysis of rubella vaccination policy, N. Engl. J. Med. **294**(6):306-310, February 5, 1976.

Slattery, J.: Dental health in children, Am. J. Nurs. **76**(7):1159-1161, July 1976.

Smith, J.: Promoting childhood dental health, Pediatr. Nurs. **2**(3): 16-19, May/June 1976.

Sutterley, D., and Donnelly, G.: Perspectives in human development, Philadelphia, 1973, J. B. Lippincott Co.

Taylor, R. W.: Depression and recovery at 9 weeks of age, Am. Acad. J. Child Psychiatry **12**(3):506-510, 1973.

Tulkin, S., and Kagon, J.: Mother-child interaction in the first year of life, Child Dev. **43**:31-41, 1972.

Ventura, J. N.: Immunizations for foreign travel, Am. J. Nurs. **77**(6):972-973, June 1977.

Ventura, J. N.: The international traveler's health guide, Am. J. Nurs. **77**(6):969-973, June 1977.

Wachs, T. D., and associates: Cognitive development in infants of different age levels and from different environmental backgrounds: an exploratory investigation, Merrill-Palmer Quarterly of Behavior and Development **17**:283-317, 1971.

Waechter, E., and Blake, F.: Nursing care of children, New York, 1976, J. B. Lippincott Co.

Wasserman, E., and Slobody, L.: Survey of pediatrics, New York, 1974, McGraw-Hill Book Co.

Weiner, I., and Elkind, D.: Child development: a core approach, New York, 1972, John Wiley & Sons, Inc.

Wiatrowski, E., and associates: Dietary fluoride intake of infants, Pediatrics **55**(4):517-522, April 1975.

Williams, S. R.: Nutrition and diet therapy, ed. 3, St. Louis, 1977, The C. V. Mosby Co.

Wright, W.: How one poison control center works, Am. J. Nurs. **66**(9):1988, September 1966.

13

Health problems during the first year

The infant's immature physiologic system predisposes him to several potential health problems during the first year. This chapter deals primarily with health problems that are influenced by environmental factors affecting the physical or psychologic development of the child. Some of the problems, such as the nutritional disturbances, have special implications for nurses because they are preventable. Others, such as sudden infant death syndrome, are uncontrollable and unpredictable, but the intervention needed after the death of the child is crucial for the reintegration of the family. Although several of the topics discussed here can occur in other age-groups besides infancy, the greatest significance of these disorders is evident during the early months and years of life. Prompt awareness and identification of health problems hopefully will avert complications in later life. Prevention rather than treatment whenever possible should be every health professional's goal in the care of children.

NUTRITIONAL DISTURBANCES

Malnutrition is a general term that refers to poor or inadequate nutrition. Although it is generally thought of in terms of undernutrition, it also includes overnutrition, which may be manifested as obesity or hypervitaminosis. Inadequate nutrition is most commonly seen as iron-deficiency anemia or vitamin deficiencies. The most severe states of malnutrition involve protein and caloric deficiencies, such as kwashiorkor or marasmus. Each of these may occur during infancy and are related to a wide variety of factors, such as economic, sociocultural, geographic, and educational. Since all are amenable to some degree of alteration through intervention, the nutritional disturbances to be discussed could potentially be eliminated. However, adequate food supplies alone is not the answer, especially when one considers that populations with high standard of living have nutritional problems related to overeating and poor eating habits. Therefore, nutritional counseling is a complex process that must take into account all the variables influencing the physical and psychologic makeup of each individual.

Iron-deficiency anemia

Anemia caused by an inadequate supply of dietary iron is the most prevalent nutritional disorder in the United States. It most frequently occurs in children between 6 and 24 months of age and during adolescence because of the rapid growth rate of each group combined with poor eating habits of adolescents. Iron-deficiency anemia is prevalent among the lower socioeconomic groups (10% to 20% with some estimates as high as 50%) and to a lesser extent among middle class groups (3% to 6%).[8,22] Since economics is not the sole factor involved in ingesting inadequate sources of iron, any population group is at risk.

Etiology. At birth the full-term infant's supply of iron is approximately 300 mg, or 75 mg/kg. The majority of it has been transferred from the mother at the rate of 4 mg/day during the last trimester.[22] The bulk of the iron is stored in the circulating hemoglobin of the erythrocytes; the rest is deposited in the liver, spleen, and bone marrow. Maternal iron stores are adequate for the first 4 to 5 months of age in the full-term infant but are reduced considerably in premature infants or infants of multiple births. When exogenous sources of iron are not supplied to meet the infant's growth demands following depletion of fetal iron stores, iron-deficiency anemia results. Evidence of anemia prior to approximately 5 months of age is generally not caused by insufficient dietary sources of iron, but by other causes as shown in the outline below.

Causes of iron-deficiency anemia

1. Inadequate supply of iron
   - a. Deficient dietary intake
     1. Rapid growth rate
     2. Excessive milk intake, delayed addition of solid foods
     3. Poor, general eating habits
   - b. Inadequate iron stores at birth
     1. Low birth weight, premature, multiple births
     2. Severe iron deficiency in the mother (hemoglobin level below 9 g/100 ml)
     3. Fetal blood loss at or before delivery

2. Impaired absorption
   a. Presence of iron inhibitors
      1. Phytates, phosphates, or oxalates
      2. Gastric alkalinity
   b. Malabsorptive disorders
   c. Chronic diarrhea
3. Blood loss
   a. Acute or chronic hemorrhage
   b. Parasitic infestation
4. Excessive demands for iron required for growth
   a. Prematurity
   b. Adolescence
   c. Pregnancy
5. Inability to form hemoglobin
   a. Lack of vitamin B_{12} (pernicious anemia)
   b. Folic acid deficiency

Physiologic anemia, a normal process resulting from a depression of erythropoietin and hemoglobin synthesis, should not be confused with iron-deficiency anemia caused by nutritional causes. Physiologic anemia occurs at 2 to 3 months of age in the full-term infant and at approximately age 7 weeks in the premature infant.

Pathophysiology. Iron is required for the production of hemoglobin. One hemoglobin molecule consists of protein (globin) combined with four molecules of a pigmented compound (heme). Each molecule of heme contains one atom of iron. When iron stores are deficient, the production of hemoglobin is reduced. Consequently the main effect of iron deficiency is decreased hemoglobin and reduced oxygen-carrying capacity of the blood.

Clinical manifestations. The clinical manifestations are directly attributed to the reduction in the amount of oxygen available to tissues and do not differ from those seen in any type of anemia (p. 1371). Usually the signs are insidious and obscure and the severity is directly related to the duration of the dietary deficiency.

Not infrequently infants with iron-deficiency anemia are overweight because of excessive milk ingestion (so-called milk baby). These children become anemic because milk, a poor source of iron, is given almost to the exclusion of solid foods. Although chubby, these infants are pale, usually demonstrate poor muscle development, and are prone to infection. The skin color is sometimes described as porcelain-like.

Though the mechanism is unknown, iron-deficiency anemia enhances the leakage of plasma proteins in infants, causing edema, retarded growth, and decreased serum concentration of the proteins albumin, gamma globulin, and transferrin, a protein that binds iron and transports it through the plasma. The adult signs of iron deficiency, such as atrophic glossitis, dysphagia, and koilonychia (concave fingernails), are not seen in infants and only rarely in older children. The precise relationship of anemia and retarded intellectual functioning is not clear, but studies indicate a negative effect.[26]

Diagnostic evaluation. Since iron deficiency primarily affects hemoglobin synthesis, laboratory tests that measure or describe hemoglobin, the morphologic changes in the red blood cell, and iron concentration are usually performed. (For a review of the routine hematologic tests used to diagnose anemia, see Table 36-1, p. 1372.)

Red blood cell (RBC) count. Red blood cell formation is affected to a much lesser degree than hemoglobin synthesis. The red blood cell count may be normal, borderline, or moderately reduced. Typically the almost normal number of erythrocytes is strikingly out of proportion to the decreased hemoglobin concentration.

Hemoglobin. As expected, the hemoglobin level is low; diagnosis of anemia is usually defined when the hemoglobin is below 11 g/100 ml. Sometimes a hemoglobin value of 10 g/100 ml is used as the lower limit of normal.[27] However, since age affects the hemoglobin concentrations, it is more precise to set standards to meet individual needs. For example, during 6 months to 2 years of age the hemoglobin is normally between 10 and 12.5 g/100 ml; therefore, anemia is generally regarded as a hemoglobin level of 9 g/100 ml or below. However, during the preschool and school-age years, the hemoglobin level rises to about 14.5 g/100 ml; consequently, a hemoglobin value of 11 g/100 ml may be considered borderline.

Hematocrit. Although the red blood cell count may be normal, red blood cells are typically small in size. Consequently this alteration is expressed in a lowered hematocrit level (usually below 33%), since the microcytic red blood cells pack together into a smaller volume, regardless of their actual number.

Red blood cell indices. The mean corpuscular volume (MCV) is an important diagnostic measurement because it demonstrates the decreased size of a single red blood cell. As was discussed in terms of hemoglobin levels, the lower limit of normal for the mean corpuscular volume is also defined according to age. For infants around 1 year of age, a mean corpuscular volume of below 70 cuμ is considered diagnostic of microcytic anemia, whereas, in the preschool and older child, a mean corpuscular volume of 75 cuμ is usually the lower limit of normal.

Since the amount of hemoglobin in each cell is decreased, the color of the cell is hypochromic. The mean corpuscular hemoglobin (MCH) and mean corpuscular hemoglobin concentration (MCHC), which measure the average weight and concentrations of hemoglobin in a single red blood cell, respectively, are decreased. A mean corpuscular hemoglobin value of below 27 $\mu\mu$g and a mean corpuscular hemoglobin concentration below 30% are considered indicative of hypochromic anemia.

Reticulocyte count. The reticulocyte count is usually normal or reduced because of decreased stores of iron. However, in severe anemia where tissue hypoxia exerts an erythropoietic response, the reticulocyte count may be elevated to 3% or 4%.

Serum-iron concentration (SIC). The serum-iron concentration measures the amount of circulating iron and normally is about 70 μg/100 ml in infants and slightly higher in older children. In iron deficiency these values are usually below the lower limit of 30 μg/100 ml for infants.

Total iron-binding capacity (TIBC). The total iron-binding capacity measures the amount of transferrin or iron-binding globulin, which is necessary for the transport of iron in the bloodstream. When combined with transferrin, the iron is loosely bound to the globulin molecule so that it can be released easily to tissue cells anywhere in the body. In iron-deficiency anemia the total iron-binding capacity is elevated above the normal range of 250 μg/100 ml. The elevated total iron-binding capacity represents the body's compensatory mechanisms to absorb more exogenous sources of iron during states of deficiency than normally. The combination of a reduced serum-iron concentration and elevated total iron-binding capacity is of significant diagnostic value because it is not found in any other condition.[22] It is specific for differentiating between (1) hypochromic, microcrytic anemia caused by inadequate intake or absorption of iron and (2) those anemias resulting from defective utilization of iron, such as thalassemia.

In terms of differential diagnosis, a stool analysis for occult blood (guaiac test) is frequently performed to confirm or rule out the possibility of chronic fecal blood loss, especially from milk (lactose) intolerance or structural anomalies, such as diverticulitis.

Medical management. Nutritional anemia is usually treated with oral iron supplements. Ferrous iron is more readily absorbed than ferric iron, resulting in higher hemoglobin levels. Ingested iron is absorbed largely from the duodenum and is facilitated by an acid environment. Normal infants will absorb an average of 10% to 20% of oral iron supplements, but during periods of iron deficiency they will absorb an additional 5% to 10%. Dietary addition of iron-rich foods is usually inadequate as a sole treatment for iron-deficiency anemia because it provides insufficient supplemental quantities of iron. Therefore, oral iron supplements are prescribed in daily doses of 10 to 15 mg for a period of approximately 3 months to replace body stores. Ideally the iron should be given in three divided doses between meals. Side effects of oral iron therapy are minimal in infants and children but may include nausea, gastric irritation, diarrhea or constipation, and anorexia.

Parenteral iron therapy may be used if hemoglobin levels fail to rise after 1 month of oral therapy. The commonest cause of failure of oral iron therapy is unreliability of parenteral administration, which may reflect poor counseling and education by health professionals. Since parenteral iron can cause a fatal anaphylactic reaction, every attempt should be made to encourage adequate therapy with oral supplements. If iron dextran (Inferon) is ordered, it must be injected deeply into a large muscle mass using the Z-tract method to minimize skin staining and irritation. Transfusions are indicated for the severest degree of anemia (usually a hemoglobin value of 4 mg/100 ml or less), in cases of serious infection, cardiac dysfunction, or surgical emergency where anesthesia is required. Packed red cells, not whole blood, should be used to minimize the chance of circulatory overload. Supplemental oxygen is administered when tissue hypoxia is severe.

Response to oral iron therapy is reflected in a peak increase in reticulocyte count by the fifth to the tenth day of administration. Following the reticulocyte rise, the hemoglobin and hematocrit levels and red blood cell count increase. The hemoglobin level rises an average of 0.17 to 0.25 g/100 ml per day; therefore, a substantial increase should occur by the end of 1 month.[22]

Nursing considerations. The main nursing objective is prevention of nutritional anemia through parent education. The nurse discusses with parents the importance of using iron-fortified formula or the introduction of solid foods by 4 months of age in full-term infants and by 2 months of age in premature infants. The dose of supplemental iron should not exceed 1 mg/kg/day for full-term infants and 2 mg/kg/day for preterm infants, up to a maximum of 15 mg/day.[1] The source of iron varies with the family's preferences and needs. In breast-fed infants early introduction of iron-fortified cereal or oral iron drops is recommended. In infants being fed commercially prepared formula, the use of iron-fortified preparations is convenient and reliable, since ingestion of the formula ensures a constant supply of iron. Children receiving fresh cow's milk formula may be given oral iron supplements or iron-enriched solid foods (Table 13-1).[21] Heat-treated milk products, such as evaporated milk, are preferred to fresh cow's milk to decrease the possibility of iron deficiency from gastrointestinal blood loss occurring from allergy to the milk protein.

Table 13-1. Iron content of baby food

Food	Amount	Iron (mg)
Enriched cereal*	3 tbsp	7.1
Egg yolk*	1 yolk	1.0
Beef*	7 tbsp	1.82
Beef liver*	7 tbsp	4.43
Green beans*	7 tbsp	0.88
Peaches†	7 tbsp	0.40
Iron-enriched formula	1 liter	15.00
Cow's milk	1 liter	1.0-2.0
Human milk	1 liter	0.7-1.0

*Commercially prepared food.
†Home-prepared peaches contain 0.32 mg/tbsp of iron and are the highest source of iron among fruits.

One of the considerations in encouraging parents to limit the quantity of milk and introduce solid foods is dispelling the popular myth that milk is a "perfect food." Many parents believe that milk is best for the infant and equate the resultant weight gain with a "healthy child." The nurse must emphasize that, although milk is an excellent food, it is deficient in iron, vitamin C, and fluoride. Sources of each of these nutrients and the role they play in preventing deficiencies are discussed. The nurse also stresses that overweight is not synonymous with good health. If the infant has obvious signs of anemia such as pallor, listlessness, frequent infections, and muscular weakness, they are pointed out as evidence of suboptimal health. In some instances it is helpful to chart the hemoglobin or hematocrit values in order to visually impress on parents the change in iron levels. Often increased blood values correspond to improved physical status and reinforce the benefit of dietary or oral iron supplementation.

Instructing parents regarding proper administration of oral iron supplements is an essential nursing responsibility. Several factors affect the absorption of iron (Table 13-2). Ideally iron drops should be administered in three divided doses between meals when the presence of free hydrochloric acid is greatest and accompanied with a citrus fruit or juice, which helps reduce iron to its most soluble state. An adequate dietary intake of calcium helps bind and remove agents, such as phosphates and phytates, that react with iron to render it insoluble. If the iron produces vomiting and diarrhea, it should be administered with meals and in gradually increasing doses. When adequate dosage is reached, the stools usually turn a tarry green color. The nurse advises parents of this normally expected change and inquires about its occurrence on follow-up visits. Absence of the greenish black stool may be a clue to poor administration of iron, either in schedule or dosage. Liquid preparations of iron may temporarily stain the teeth. If possible the medication should be taken through a straw or given through a syringe or medicine dropper placed toward the back of the mouth. Brushing the teeth after administration of the drug lessens the discoloration.

Counseling families whose children are anemic is often a difficult and challenging task. Meal planning must be based on their financial budget, cultural pattern, and food preferences. Often this requires more than a brief discussion with the mother or usual care giver. For teaching to be effective, the nurse may need to offer recipes, assist in planning a shopping list, and investigate food prices for economy. Since the physical effects of anemia are insidious, parents may not consider their child ill and consequently may view the medication and diet changes as unnecessary. Stressing what the physical and behavioral improvements will be and what effect the improved diet will have on all family members may encourage parents to adhere to the treatment plan.

Table 13-2. Factors that affect the absorption of iron

Increase	Decrease
Acidity (low pH)—administer iron between meals (gastric hydrochloric acid)	Alkalinity (high pH)—avoid any antacid preparation
Ascorbic acid (vitamin C)—administer iron with juice, fruit, or multivitamin preparation	Phosphates—milk is unfavorable vehicle for iron administration
Calcium	Phytates—found in cereals
Tissue need	Oxalates—found in many fruits and vegetables, for example, plums, currants, green beans, spinach, sweet potatoes, and tomatoes
	Tissue saturation
	Malabsorptive disorders
	Disturbances that cause diarrhea or steatorrhea

Protein and calorie deficiencies

Hunger is one of the world's gravest and most prevalent health problems. Three fourths of the world population suffers some form of malnutrition. The mortality and morbidity rates among children support the severity of this problem in underdeveloped countries, where in the 1- to 4-year-old age-group the death rate may be twenty to fifty times higher than in the United States. Even in the United States, vitamin, iron, and protein deficiencies are not uncommon. The protein-calorie malnutrition (PCM) diseases of kwashiorkor and marasmus are reported in hospitals in the United States each year. The effects of inadequate diet are analogous to a cancer that slowly invades and destroys every living cell.

Kwashiorkor. Kwashiorkor is a deficiency of protein with an adequate supply of calories. The word comes from the Ghan language and means "the sickness the older child gets when the next baby is born." It is an appropriate name because it is a syndrome that develops in the first child, usually between 1 and 4 years of age, when he is weaned from the breast once the second child is born and fed a diet consisting mainly of starch grains or tubers. Such a diet provides adequate calories in the form of carbohydrates but an inadequate amount of high-quality proteins.

Pathophysiology. The pathophysiology of kwashiorkor results from the protein deficiency, both in quantity and quality. Since protein is essential for tissue growth and cell repair, all body systems are affected, but rapidly growing cells, such as those of mucosa, are most severely affected. The skin is scaly and dry and has areas of depigmentation. Several dermatoses may be evident, partly resulting from the vitamin deficiencies. Permanent blindness results from the severe lack of vitamin A. The hair is thin, dry, coarse, and dull. Depigmentation is common, and patchy alopecia may occur (Fig. 13-1). There is loss of weight in conjunction with edema (ascites) from the hypoalbuminemia. The edema often masks the severe muscular atrophy, making the child appear less debilitated than he actually is. Total body water increases, but total body potassium decreases with retention of sodium, causing signs of hypokalemia and hypernatremia. Diarrhea frequently occurs from the lowered resistance to infection and further complicates the electrolyte imbalance. Gastrointestinal disturbances occur, such as fatty infiltration of the liver and atrophy of the acini cells of the pancreas. Behavioral changes are evident as the child grows progressively more irritable, lethargic, withdrawn, and apathetic. Fatal deterioration may be caused by diarrhea and infection or as the result of circulatory failure.

Medical management. Treatment includes providing a diet high in quality proteins, vitamins, and minerals. Electrolyte imbalance requires immediate attention, and coexisting problems such as infection, diarrhea, parasitic infestation, and anemia necessitate prompt attention for optimum recovery.

Nursing considerations. Provision of essential physiologic needs such as rest, individually tailored activity, and protection from infection is paramount. Since the child is usually weak and withdrawn, he is dependent on others to feed him. Hygiene may be distressing because of the poor integrity of the skin, and decubiti are a constant threat. The larger problem is the prevention of this condition through education concerning the importance of high-quality protein, availability of protein-rich foods such as milk, and motivation of the people to utilize the resources provided them.

Marasmus. Marasmus is the result of general malnutrition of both calories and protein. It is most common in infants between the ages of 6 and 18 months. It is usually a syndrome of physical and emotional deprivation and is not confined to geographic areas where food supplies are inadequate. Marasmus may be seen in failure-to-thrive children, where the etiology is not solely nutritional but primarily emotional (p. 494).

Pathophysiology. Marasmus is characterized by gradual wasting and atrophy of body tissues, especially subcutaneous fat (Fig. 13-2). The child appears to be very old; his skin is flabby and wrinkled, unlike the child with kwashiorkor who appears more rounded from the edema. Fat metabolism is less impaired than in kwashiorkor, so that vitamin A deficiency is usually minimal or absent. In general the clinical manifestations of marasmus are similar to those seen in kwashiorkor with the following exceptions: no edema from hypoalbuminemia or sodium retention, contributing to a severely emaciated appearance; no dermatoses caused by vitamin deficiencies; little or no depigmentation of hair or skin; and more normal fat metabolism and lipid absorption. As in kwashiorkor, body metabolism is minimal, and maintaining body temperature is complicated by lack of subcutaneous fat. The child is fretful, apathetic, withdrawn, and so lethargic that prostration frequently oc-

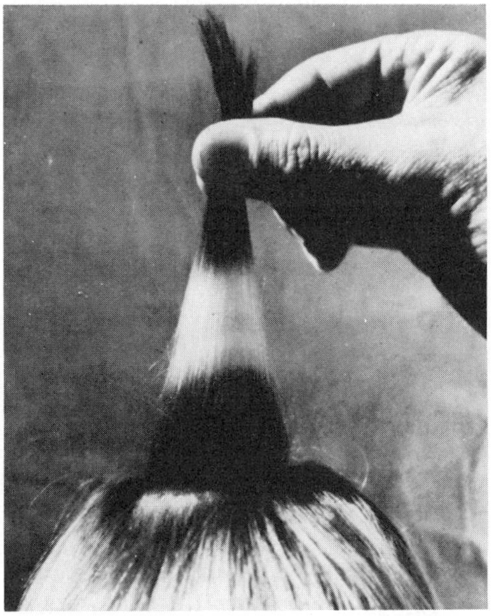

Fig. 13-1. Appearance of the hair in kwashiorkor. Pigmentation changes indicate periods of normal and abnormal growth of hair. (From Scrimshaw, N. S., and Béhar, M.: N. Engl. J. Med. **272:**137, 1965. Reprinted by permission from The New England Journal of Medicine.)

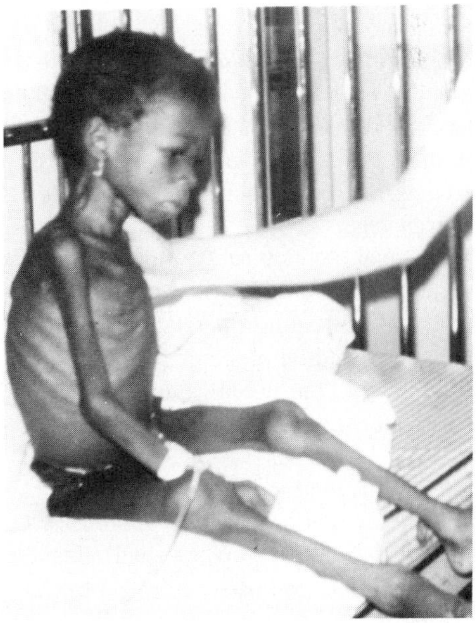

Fig. 13-2. Child with marasmus. (Courtesy Dr. Donald Anderson, Travis Air Force Base, Calif.; from Dodge, P. R., Prensky, A. L., and Feigin, R. D.: Nutrition and the developing nervous system, St. Louis, 1975, The C. V. Mosby Co.)

curs. Intercurrent infection with debilitating diseases such as tuberculosis, parasitosis, and dysentery is common.

Medical management. Treatment is similar to that of kwashiorkor. Parenteral fluid replacement is usually necessary initially to correct the dehydration and restore renal function. Occasionally oral fluids will not be tolerated, necessitating the use of hyperalimentation (p. 1091).

Nursing considerations. Since there is such a great degree of general deterioration, every nursing measure must be taken to avoid infection. Since these children frequently suffer from emotional starvation as well, care should include a consistent mother substitute and appropriate stimulation for the developmental, not chronologic, age. Nursing care of the failure-to-thrive child resulting from maternal deprivation is consistent with care of the child with marasmus (p. 494).

Vitamin disturbances

True vitamin disturbances are rare in the United States, but subclinical deficiencies are commonly seen, especially in lower socioeconomic groups, where proper dietary intake may be unbalanced. Vitamin deficiencies of the fat-soluble vitamins A and D may occur in malabsorptive disorders. With the addition of vitamins and minerals to commercially packaged foods, vitamin deficiencies have decreased, but the potential for hypervitaminosis has escalated, especially when combined with the injudicious use of vitamin supplements. Deficiencies of vitamins A, B complex, C, and D are discussed in greater detail in the following paragraphs and are summarized in Table 13-3. Other vitamin disturbances are also outlined in Table 13-3. Nursing care is discussed for each of the vitamins in the following paragraphs.

Vitamin A (retinol) deficiency. Vitamin A is a fat-soluble vitamin that is available to the body in its natural form or as carotene, a precursor. In its natural form it is found primarily in the fat of animals and in foods such as meat and dairy products. The main sources of vitamin A are the yellow and green vegetables that contain the pigment carotene. Many commercial products such as margarine and enriched cereals or breads are fortified with vitamin A. Because it is insoluble in water, vitamin A is relatively stable in cooking but may be destroyed on prolonged exposure to high temperatures. Vitamin A is stored as an ester with fatty acids in such tissues as the liver, kidney, lung, and adipose depots.

Physiologic function and deficiency. Vitamin A is necessary for the formation of the light-sensitive pigment rhodopsin (visual purple). When light hits the retina, rhodopsin is split into two parts, a protein called opsin and a vitamin A compound called retinene. When the body is deficient in this vitamin, the rods and cones of the eye become increasingly sensitive to light, causing *night blindness.*

Vitamin A is also essential for the formation and maintenance of epithelial tissue, and its deficiency causes a number of problems resulting from *keratinization,* scaling and hardening of the tissues. In the eye, the cornea and conjunctiva become hard and dry (xerophthalmia). Metaplasia of the lacrimal or tear glands leads to a loss of their secretion and their cleansing and lubricating function. Infection may follow, with corneal ulceration and scar formation. Early signs of xerophthalmia are drying, roughness, pain, wrinkling of the conjunctiva, swelling and redness of the lids, and photophobia. The cornea becomes dull, lusterless, and hazy, with a film that resembles "oil on water." At this point the process is still reversible with adequate therapy. Without treatment the cornea softens (keratomalacia), perforates, and rapidly deteriorates, resulting in total blindness.

As the epithelial cells become hard and scaly, small pustules or hardened, pigmented, papular eruptions appear around the hair follicle (follicular hyperkeratosis). The most common sites for these dermal changes, sometimes called phrynoderma or toadskin, are the thighs, upper back of the arms, abdomen, and back. Epithelial changes also occur in the mucosal lining of the respiratory, gastrointestinal, and genitourinary tracts. In the respiratory tract the cilia are lost as the lining becomes dry. The secretory cells of the salivary gland become nonfunctional and the mouth is dry and cracked, allowing invading organisms to enter, resulting in infection. The epithelial changes in the lining of the gastrointestinal tract affect the digestion and absorption of nutrients. The protective function of the mucosal lining of the genitourinary tract is diminished, increasing the chances for vaginal and urinary tract infection and the formation of renal calculi.

Vitamin A deficiency is also associated with retarded growth, although the exact mechanism is unknown. The formation and growth of bone and soft tissue are affected, probably as a result of disturbed protein synthesis, formation of mucopolysaccharides, and utilization of nitrogen. The formation of tooth enamel is also disrupted because the epithelial cells (ameloblasts) surrounding the tooth, which produce and deposit enamel, are adversely affected. Inadequate amounts of vitamin A also reduce the rate of thyroxine formation. Persons with subminimal amounts of this vitamin are more prone toward development of a goiter.

Vitamin A deficiency can occur directly as a result of decreased dietary intake or, more commonly, as a secondary result of diseases, such as celiac syndrome, sprue, or colitis, which affect its absorption. The most common age-group for its occurrence is 6 months to 4 years, especially in children mainly fed skimmed milk. A defective diet is required for several weeks for symptoms to appear. Night blindness is usually the first sign and can be detected by asking parents if the child stumbles in dim light or is especially sensitive to light in a dark room.

Medical management. Treatment is the use of vitamin A

supplements in doses determined by the severity of the symptoms. Deficiency states usually respond to oral doses of 10,000 IU/kg/day, preferably in a water-soluble form. Intensive therapy may be continued for several days, followed by a reduced daily dose of 25,000 IU, which can be supplied by 30 ml of cod liver oil. The earliest symptom of the deficiency, night blindness, may improve dramatically within 1 hour after treatment with a single large dose of vitamin A or may take several weeks to subside.

Nursing considerations. The primary nursing objective is prevention of vitamin A deficiency through dietary counseling. Adequate whole milk intake should ensure against vitamin A deficiency (one liter contains 1400 to 1500 IU). However, skimmed milk is a poor source of the vitamin. As milk intake decreases with the addition of solid foods, education should stress high-quality foods that provide vitamin A or carotene (Table 13-3). If cod liver oil is prescribed, parents need guidance in methods of introducing it. Since it is an oil, it does not mix well with liquids. One way of camouflaging its taste and consistency is to mix it with a strongly flavored gelatin, such as grape. Prepare the gelatin as directed on the package. Place a small amount (about ¼ cup) in a container. When the gelatin is soft set, mix in the cod liver oil; serve when completely jelled.

Vitamin B-complex deficiencies. Vitamins of the B complex are water soluble, mainly involved in protein, carbohydrate, or fat metabolism, and found in several food sources, especially enriched grains such as pasta, rice, bread, or cereal. For this reason, deficiencies are uncommon. However, a deficiency of one of the B vitamins usually indicates the possibility of other vitamin disturbances.

Dietary vitamin B_9 (folic acid) deficiency is rare because the body requires only minute amounts of the substance and forms endogenous sources from intestinal bacterial synthesis. However, ascorbic acid is necessary for the conversion of folic acid to folinic acid. Deficiencies can occur in cases of ascorbic acid deficiency, from prolonged antibiotic therapy, or from the use of antifolic compounds, such as aminopterin or methotrexate, antineoplastic drugs used in the treatment of many malignancies. Its absence from the body results in bone marrow depression and macrocytic anemia.

Dietary vitamin B_{12} deficiency is also rare. However, this vitamin is dependent on exposure to gastric secretions before it can be absorbed. Hydrochloric acid and intrinsic factor, a mucoprotein enzyme found in the fundus and cardia of the stomach, split the B_{12} vitamin so that it can be utilized in the ileum. In the absence of these substances, such as in the case of a complete gastrectomy, *pernicious anemia* occurs.

Medical management. In most instances treatment is large oral or intravenous doses of the B vitamin. Since deficiencies may accompany starvation, therapy may include parenteral hyperalimentation during the initial phase. In the case of pernicious anemia, vitamin B_{12} must be supplied parenterally since the oral form cannot be absorbed in the stomach.

Nursing considerations. The main nursing objective is prevention. Food sources rich in B-complex vitamins, especially foods made from enriched or natural grains, wheat germ, legumes, organ meats, and green leafy vegetables, are encouraged. The nurse stresses proper cooking techniques to avoid loss of vitamins during food preparation, such as use of minimal water to steam vegetables and avoidance of overcooking.

In this highly weight-conscious society where fad diets often advocate extreme limitations of various food groups, specific vitamin deficiencies are possible. The nurse stresses the importance of well-balanced meals with reduced calories as a sound method of weight reduction. For those individuals, especially adolescents, who experiment with various crash diets, the nurse emphasizes the necessity of oral vitamin supplements to substitute for missed dietary sources of nutrients.

Vitamin C deficiency. Vitamin C is a water-soluble vitamin that is unstable to heat, air, and alkalies. Unlike lower mammals, man is unable to synthesize vitamin C and is dependent on a constant exogenous source to prevent deficiency. Absorption takes place in the small intestine and is enhanced by hydrochloric acid. No one tissue is a major storage site for vitamin C, but small amounts circulate in the blood and greater amounts are concentrated in the metabolically active tissues such as the adrenals, kidneys, liver, and spleen. Excess is rapidly excreted in the urine. Overdose is unknown, and large amounts have controversial benefits, such as protection from infection. Vitamin C requirements are increased by needs of wound healing, fever, infection, increased growth periods, pregnancy, and reaction to stress. Excellent food sources are citrus fruits and tomatoes, as well as the other foods listed in Table 13-3. However, since vitamin C is easily destroyed by heat and oxidation and is soluble in water, one must carefully consider the preparation of the food source before evaluating its vitamin C content. For example, fresh orange juice is rich in ascorbic acid (122 mg/cup), but processing, boiling, and exposure to the air destroy the vitamin. Breast milk contains a sufficient amount of ascorbic acid (40 to 80 mg/liter) for the infant, provided the mother's diet includes adequate sources. Milk is a poor source (10 to 14 mg/liter), and, unless fortified commercial formula is used, the infant requires vitamin C supplements at some time during the first 6 months of life.

Physiologic function and deficiency. Ascorbic acid performs many functions that are essential to health. Its most important role is providing an intercellular cementing substance that is required to build supportive tissue, such as bone matrix, cartilage, collagen, dentine, and connective tissue. The capillary walls of blood vessels are particularly

Table 13-3. Vitamins and their nutritional significance

Vitamins	Physiologic function	RDA*	Sources
A (retinol)	Necessary component in formation of pigment rhodopsin (visual purple) Formation and maintenance of epithelial tissue	Infants—1400-2000 IU†; others‡—2000-5000 IU	Natural form—liver, kidney, fish oils, milk and non-skimmed milk products, egg yolk
Provitamin A (carotene)			Carrots, sweet potatoes, squash, apricots, spinach, collards, broccoli, cabbage, artichokes
B_1 (thiamine)	Coenzyme (with phosphorus) in carbohydrate metabolism	Infants—0.3-0.5 mg; others—0.7-1.5 mg (usually calculated in relation to caloric intake as 0.5 mg/1000 kcal)	Meats—pork, beef, or liver Legumes, nuts, and whole or enriched grains
B_2 (riboflavin)	Coenzyme (with phosphorus) in protein metabolism	Infants—0.4-0.6 mg; others—0.8-1.8 mg (usually calculated in relation to caloric intake as 0.6 mg/1000 kcal)	Milk and its products, eggs, organ meats (liver, kidney, and heart), enriched cereals, some green leafy vegetables, and legumes
Niacin (nicotinic acid, nicotinamide)	Coenzyme (with riboflavin) in protein and fat metabolism	Infants—5.0-8.0 mg; others—9-20 mg (tryptophan is a precursor; 60 g = 1 mg of niacin)	Meat, fish, peanuts, beans, peas, whole or enriched grains except corn and rice
B_6 (pyridoxine)	Coenzyme in protein, carbohydrate, and fat metabolism Possibly involved in metabolism of polyunsaturated fatty acids	Infants—0.3-0.4 mg; others—0.6-2.0 mg	Meats, especially liver and kidney, cereal grains (wheat and corn), yeast, soybeans, and peanuts
B_9 (folic acid) (reduced form is called folinic acid or citrovorum factor)	Coenzyme for single-carbon transfer (purines, thymine, hemoglobin)	Infants—50 μg; others—100-400 μg	Green leafy vegetables (spinach), asparagus, liver, kidney, nuts
B_{12} (cobalamin)	Coenzyme in protein synthesis, indirect effect on formation of red blood cells (particularly on formation of nucleic acids and folic acid metabolism)	Infants—0.3 μg; others—1.0-3.0 μg	Meat, liver, kidney, milk, eggs, and cheese
C (ascorbic acid)	Intercellular cement substance General metabolism Increases utilization of iron for hemoglobin formation Enhances conversion of folic to folinic acid Affects cholesterol synthesis and conversion of proline to hydroxyproline Probably a coenzyme in metabolism of tyrosine and phenylalanine May play role in hydroxylation of adrenal steroids May have stimulating effect on phagocytic activity of leukocytes and formation of antibodies	Infants—35 mg; others—40-45 mg	Citrus fruits, berries, tomatoes, melon, cabbage, green and yellow vegetables

*RDA—Recommended Dietary Allowances represent the amount of nutrients needed daily by healthy individuals, plus an excess of 30% to 50% to search Council (1974).

†One international unit (IU) is approximately equivalent to 1 milligram (mg).

‡Others—1 to 18 years of age.

Results of deficiency	Results of overdose
Night blindness Keratinization of the epithelium, xerophthalmia, conjunctivitis, phrynoderma and drying of the respiratory, gastrointestinal, and genitourinary tracts Defective tooth enamel Retarded growth Impaired bone formation Decreased thyroxine formation	Early signs—irritability, anorexia, pruritus, fissures at the corners of nose and lips Later signs—hepatomegaly, jaundice, retarded growth, poor weight gain, thickening of the cortex of long bones with pain and fragility, hard tender lumps in extremities and occiput of the skull NOTE: Overdose only results from ingestion of large quantities of the vitamin, not the provitamin; large amounts of carotene (carotenemia) cause yellow or orange discoloration of the skin (not the sclera as in jaundice), but none of the above symptoms
Beriberi Gastrointestinal—anorexia, constipation, indigestion Neurologic—apathy, fatigue, emotional instability, polyneuritis, convulsions and coma (in infants) Circulatory—cardiac failure, peripheral vasodilation, edema	None
Ariboflavinosis Lips—cheilosis, perlèche Tongue—glossitis Nose—irritation and cracks at nasal angle Eyes—burning, itching, tearing, photophobia, cornea vascularization, cataracts Skin—seborrheic dermatitis, delayed wound healing and tissue repair	None
Pellagra Oral—stomatitis, glossitis Cutaneous—scaly dermatitis on exposed areas Gastrointestinal—anorexia, weight loss, diarrhea, fatigue Neurologic—apathy, anxiety, confusion, depression, dementia	Nicotinic acid—potent vasodilator, circulatory disturbances, skin flushing, itching, and increased peristalsis
Scaly dermatitis, convulsions, peripheral neuritis, anemia, retarded growth	None
Macrocytic anemia, bone marrow depression, glossitis, intestinal malabsorption	None
Pernicious anemia General signs of severe anemia Lemon yellow tinge to skin Spinal cord degeneration	Unknown
Scurvy Skin—dry, rough, petechiae, perifollicular hyperkeratotic papules Musculoskeletal—bleeding into muscles and joints, pseudoparalysis from pain, swelling of joints, costochondral beading (scorbic rosary) Gums—spongy, friable, swollen, bleed easily, bluish red or black color, teeth loosen and fall out General disposition—irritable, anorexic, apprehensive, in pain, refuses to move Signs of anemia Decreased wound healing Increased susceptibility to infection	None, controversial reports of beneficial effects of megadoses in prevention of infection (common cold)

allow for individual variations and conditions of stress. RDA set by Food and Nutrition Board of the National Academy of Sciences—National Re-

Continued.

Table 13-3. Vitamins and their nutritional significance—cont'd

Vitamins	Physiologic function	RDA	Sources
D_2 (ergocalciferol) and D_3 (cholecalciferol)	Absorption of calcium and phosphorus and decreased renal excretion of phosphorus	400 IU	Cod liver oil, herring, mackerel, salmon, tuna, sardines, direct sunlight Enriched food sources—milk, milk products, cereals, margarine, breads, many breakfast drinks
E (tocopherol)	Production of red blood cells Muscle and liver integrity Antioxidant agent Coenzyme factor in tissue respiration Reproduction (demonstrated only in animals) Minimizes oxidation of polyunsaturated fatty acids and vitamin A in intestinal tract and tissues	Infants—4-5 IU; others—10-15 IU	Vegetable oils, wheat germ, milk, eggs, muscle meats, fish, cereal, nuts, legumes, green leafy vegetables
K	Catalyst for production of prothrombin and blood clotting factors II, VII, IX, and X by the liver	Not established	Pork, liver, green leafy vegetables (spinach, kale, cabbage), tomatoes, egg yolk, cheese

affected in cases of vitamin C deficiency. They are fragile, rupture easily, and produce symptoms such as petechiae, hemarthrosis, easy bruising, and bleeding gums. Vitamin C is also involved in general body metabolism. It enhances the formation of hemoglobin by releasing more iron into the circulation because it influences the release of iron from the protein ferritin. It affects the conversion of folic acid to its reduced form, folinic acid (citrovorum factor). It is involved with cholesterol synthesis; in states of deficiency, high cholesterolemic foods fail to exhibit their effect on blood lipid levels. It participates in the hydroxylation of proline to hydroxyproline, a compound necessary for connective tissue proliferation. Ascorbic acid may be concerned with the hydroxylation of steroid hormones in the adrenals, which may explain its role in increasing resistance to infection.

Deficiency of ascorbic acid produces scurvy, the clinical manifestations of which are directly related to the functions of vitamin C. The skin becomes dry, rough, and scaly, and raised areas develop around hair follicles (perifollicular hyperkeratotic papules), mostly on the arms, legs, buttocks, and back. Small, pinpoint hemorrhages (petechiae) develop, usually on the lower extremities, and spread upward. Purpura may be seen as areas of petechiae coalesce. Hemorrhaging into the muscle produces swelling and pain. Hemarthrosis, particularly in large joints of the lower extremities, causes local inflammation and pain, which may be so severe that the child appears paralyzed (pseudoparalysis) and maintains a fixed posture—supine with the legs and thighs partially flexed and the hips outwardly rotated (scorbutic pose). Edema from subperiosteal hemorrhage is commonly seen at all joints, but particularly directly above the knee, which may double in size.

In young children and infants, the growing bones show marked pathologic changes. The centers of ossification calcify, whereas the amount of cartilage matrix undergoing calcification is increased. At the same time the conversion of cartilage to bone is impaired. As a result the brittleness of the large masses of calcified matrix undergo microscopic fractures. Osteoblastic activity is also impaired. Subperiosteal hemorrhages are common, especially in the long bones of the arms and legs. Characteristic changes in the ribs causes sternal depression and a sharp prominence at the bony ends (costochondral beading).

The gums bleed easily with the slightest trauma, are grossly swollen, and have a characteristic bluish red or black discoloration from the hemorrhaging and thrombosis formation in the tissues. The tooth structure is damaged and weakened, and the teeth frequently self-extract. Wound healing of any kind is greatly diminished, and minor trauma may cause ulceration. Anemia is present from the hemorrhagic blood loss and the effect of deficient vitamin C on

Results of deficiency	Results of overdose
Rickets Head—craniotabes, bossing of the frontal bones, deformed shape (skull flat and depressed toward middle), delayed closure of fontanels Chest—rachitic rosary, pigeon chest, Harrison's groove Spine—kyphosis, scoliosis, lordosis Abdomen—potbelly, constipation Extremities—bowing of arms and legs, knock-knee, saber shins, instability of hip joints, pelvic deformity, enlargement of epiphysis at ends of long bones Teeth—delayed calcification, especially of permanent teeth	Acute—vomiting, dehydration, fever, abdominal cramps, bone pain, convulsions, and coma Chronic—lassitude, mental slowness, anorexia, failure to thrive, thirst, urinary urgency, polyuria, vomiting, diarrhea, abdominal cramps, bone pain, pathologic fractures Calcification of soft tissue—kidneys, lungs, adrenal glands, vessels (hypertension), heart, gastric lining Osteoporosis of long bones Elevated serum levels of calcium and phosphorus
Not well established; may involve red blood cell hemolysis, especially in premature infants, and focal necrosis of tissues Causes infertility in rats, but not in man (does *not* increase human male virility or potency)	Unknown
Hemorrhage	Hyperbilirubinemia in infants Hemolytic anemia in individuals who are deficient in glucose-6-phosphate dehydrogenase

iron and folic acid metabolism, which affects hemoglobin and erythrocyte production. In general the child is irritable, fretful, and apprehensive of pain. Tenderness in the legs is the usual presenting sign of scurvy. Vitamin C deficiency is most commonly seen in infants from 6 to 15 months of age who are fed cow's milk formula unfortified with vitamin C supplements. It is rarely seen in younger infants, because fetal supplies are usually adequate for the first few months of life.

Medical management. Treatment of scurvy is administration of vitamin C in daily amounts of 100 mg or more. Dramatic recovery is usually evident within hours of treatment. The child's disposition improves, appetite returns, and tenderness from the extremities diminishes. Hemorrhaging stops, but sites of localized hemorrhaging take longer to disappear. As the swelling of the gums recedes, a new erupting tooth may be evident. Reversal of pathologic bone changes begins immediately as new calcification of periosteal bone production resumes. Permanent skeletal deformities from scurvy have not been observed.

Nursing considerations. Nursing objectives in caring for the child with scurvy include alleviation of pain and prevention of infection. Nutritional counseling regarding natural sources of vitamin C and the effects of cooking and exposure to air on ascorbic acid is essential. For example, orange juice should not be boiled and should be stored in a covered container. Frozen orange juice is a good source of vitamin C if not thawed for a prolonged time. Fresh fruits and vegetables are better sources than if they are cooked or processed because heat and water enchance vitamin C loss. Liquid supplements should be given in one dose, rather than diluted and fed over a prolonged time. If scurvy is diagnosed, other vitamin deficiencies are also probably present, necessitating a complete nutritional assessment.

Vitamin D deficiency. Vitamin D, also called the "sunshine vitamin," is the common name for a group of steroids, the most important ones being D_2 (ergocalciferol or viosterol) and D_3 (cholecalciferol). Vitamin D_2 is formed by irradiation of the provitamin D_2 (ergosterol), which is found in ergot and yeast. Vitamin D_3 is found naturally in fish liver oils or is formed from its provitamin (7-hydrocholesterol) by the action of sunlight. All forms of vitamin D are fat soluble, heat stable, and relatively resistant to oxidation. Absorption takes place in the small intestine and requires the presence of bile since it is fat soluble. Malabsorptive disorders, such as celiac syndrome or chronic diarrhea, adversely affect its absorption. Vitamin D is stored in the liver, but in much smaller amounts than vitamin A. Food sources of vitamin D are limited; the richest source is fish liver oils and fish, such as herring, mackerel, fresh or canned salmon, tuna, or sardines. Less efficient sources are milk, egg yolk, and butter. Exposure to ultraviolet light either directly from the sun or from a lamp is an excellent source since it converts provitamin D_3 to cholecalciferol.

Physiologic function and deficiency. The primary action of vitamin D is the absorption of calcium and phosphorus from the small intestine and the conservation of phosphorus by the renal tubules. The effect on calcium absorption is more direct than on phosphorus, because it makes the cell membrane more permeable to calcium. The effect on renal excretion of phosphorus is an indirect one. As the calcium levels drop, which occurs in vitamin D deficiency, the renal threshold level for phosphorus excretion is lowered, causing increased phosphorus loss. This mechanism is necessary to preserve the calcium:phosphorus ratio in the blood and thus prevent tetany. Vitamin D also influences the metabolism of citrate, an organic acid that has a role in many metabolic functions, such as mobilizing minerals from bone tissue and removing calcium from the blood. Citrate has an anticoagulant effect on blood because when it combines with the serum calcium the calcium becomes nonionizable, which prevents coagulation from occurring.

Deficiency in vitamin D results in a decreased extracellular concentration of both calcium and phosphorus, preventing adequate mineralization and calcification of bone. A secondary effect is an overproliferation of osteoblasts, probably as a response to the poorly formed bone. As a result of the increased level of the enzyme from the osteoblasts, the serum alkaline phosphatase is elevated. The clinical manifestations of deficiency are mainly skeletal, resulting in a disease called rickets. The softened, weakened bones are deformed by the stress of weight bearing (such as bowlegs) or the pull of attached muscles (such as the rachitic rosary of the ribs). Early rickets produces cranial deformities, such as craniotabes or softening of the cranial bones, which allows one to depress the skull with a finger (similar to the response of exerting pressure on a Ping-Pong ball). Thinning is most pronounced in the posterolateral portions of the skull and should not be confused with physiologic craniotabes, which is normally found in infants less than 3 months old and is confined to the bone close to the sutures, particularly the lambdoid suture. As rickets progresses, the skull becomes thicker, with bossing or prominence of the frontal and parietal bones. Growth is retarded, resulting in open sutures past the time of expected closure (usually 12 to 18 months of age for the anterior fontanel). The head may appear large because of the thickening of the bone and deformed, particularly from the weight of lying down.

The ribs become deformed from the pull of the intercostal muscles. The costochondral junctions enlarge and form palpable nodes alongside the sternum. Since they begin close to the sternal notch and flare out as they reach the bottom of the sternum, they resemble strings of beads; hence the term "rachitic rosary." As the disease worsens the ribs are pulled in at the costal cartilage and the sternum protrudes, causing the pigeon breast deformity (pectus carinatum) (Fig. 13-3). In addition the lower portion of the rib cage flares out, but a depression is produced by pull of the diaphragm on the ribs, called Harrison's groove. From the resultant chest deformities and lax musculature, spinal deformities such as kyphosis (increased curvature of the cervical spine, called "humpback") or scoliosis (lateral curvature of the spine) occur and represent chronic, progressive rickets. Poor muscle tone results in abdominal distention, constipation, and difficulty in sitting, standing, and walking. Laxity of the ligaments causes hyperextensibility of joints. The child may assume a semiflexed froglike position (similar to that seen in scurvy) and may be unable to sit or stand.

Deformity of the extremities is common. Weight bearing causes bowing of the arms (when crawling) and the legs (when walking), knock knee (genu valgum), and instability

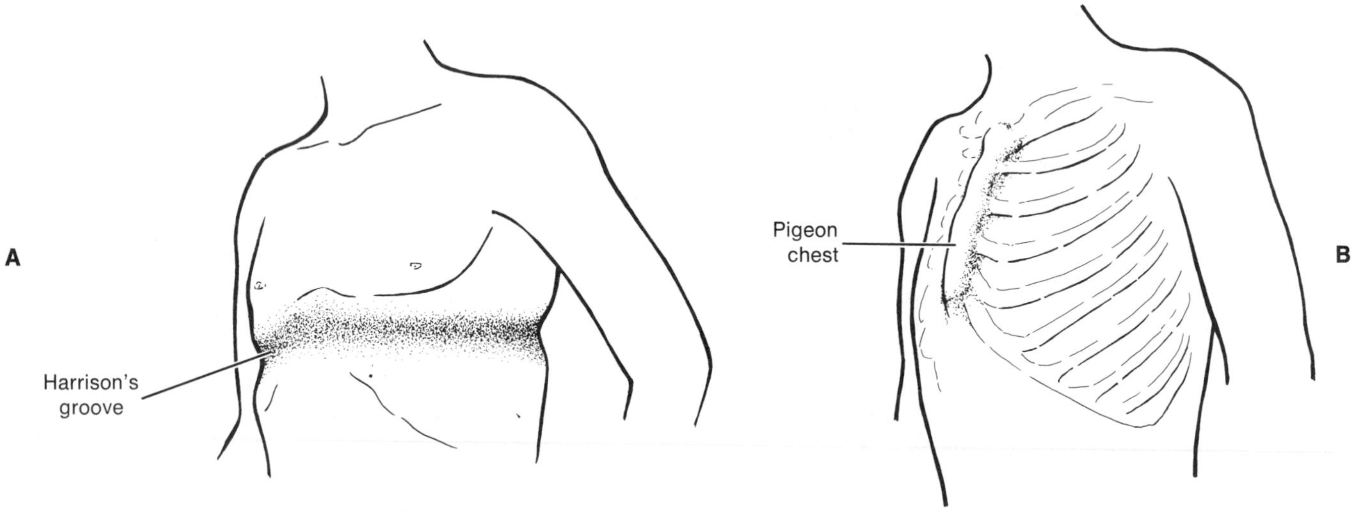

Fig. 13-3. Chest deformities in vitamin D deficiency. **A,** Harrison's groove; **B,** pigeon chest.

of the hip joints, resulting in a waddling gait. Greenstick fractures may occur in severe rickets. In addition a deformity called saber shin may result as the lower end of the tibia curves forward from the weight of the foot while the child is lying or sitting. Tooth formation is also affected from lack of calcium deposition, but usually the deciduous teeth erupt well-developed because of their formation prior to the vitamin deficiency.

Rachitic tetany may result if the serum calcium ion level drops or if the phosphate level increases, which results in situations of febrile illness or starvation. Generally the vitamin D–deficient child does not develop overt tetany because of the concurrent renal loss of phosphate. Iatrogenic tetany may occur as a result of vitamin D supplementation for treatment of tetany, probably because of decreased serum calcium levels following absorption of calcium from osteoid bone. Signs of tetany are discussed in Chapter 9, p. 304.

Rickets is most commonly seen in infants between 6 and 18 months of age, especially in premature infants who are born with inadequate calcium and phosphorus stores to accommodate the rapid growth rate. Other predisposing factors for development of rickets and vitamin D deficiency include heredity, dark-skinned individuals, who absorb less vitamin D through their skin because deeper pigmentation prevents penetration of ultraviolet light; artificially fed infants who are not receiving enriched formulas (breast milk contains inadequate amounts of vitamin D but the calcium: phosphorus ratio is more favorable); and decreased exposure to sunlight, which may occur from urban or slum living, time of the year, especially late fall, winter, and early spring, and environmental agents that filter out ultraviolet rays, such as dust, fog, smoke, clouds, and window glass.

Medical management. Treatment of rickets consists of administration of vitamin D supplements, usually 1500 to 5000 IU daily. An alternative method is to give one massive dose (600,000 IU) of vitamin D, which in cases of hypocalcemia restores the calcium serum level more rapidly than daily doses, thus preventing tetany. In all cases of treatment, 10% calcium gluconate should be available in case of convulsions. Skeletal improvement will occur, usually within 2 to 4 weeks, provided the deformity is not too severe. Orthopedic braces may be necessary to correct the long bone and joint deformities.

Nursing considerations. Nursing objectives for vitamin D deficiency are similar to those for scurvy. Prevention of infection decreases the possibility of latent tetany, which may cause convulsions. In any case seizure precautions should be planned during the treatment phase. Decubitus ulcers are a potential risk because of the rachitic posture assumed by the child as a result of weak musculature. Respiratory status may be affected in severe cases of sternal deformity and, when combined with immobility, increases the possibility of pneumonia. Since the treatment consists of high doses of vitamin D, hypervitaminosis is a potential side effect and should be observed for (Table 13-3). After treatment the child needs the usual 400 IU of vitamin D, which can be supplied by fortified milk (400 IU/liter), dairy products, and enriched foods. Parents should also know about the beneficial effects of sunlight as an additional source of vitamin D.

Vitamin E (tocopherol) deficiency. Vitamin E is fat soluble and stable to heat, oxidation, and acids but not to alkalies. Like the other fat-soluble vitamins, absorption takes place in the small intestine, after digestion by bile. Storage sites are mainly in adipose tissue, a fact that is important when considering deficiency in premature infants. Deficiency is rare because of the small amount of vitamin E required and its abundance in food. However, vitamin E deficiency may cause hemolytic anemia in premature infants or macrocytic anemia in malnourished infants.[15] Focal necrosis of skeletal muscle has been reported in individuals suffering from disorders such as cystic fibrosis or kwashiorkor, where fat metabolism and absorption is adversely affected.

Vitamin K deficiency. Vitamin K is fat soluble and sensitive to light and irradiation. Several forms exist naturally and have been synthesized, such as vitamin K_1 (phytonadione) and K_3 (menadione). A water-soluble form is available for use in individuals with altered fat metabolism. Absorption is similar to the other fat-soluble vitamins, vitamins A, D, and E. Deficiency is unusual because it is synthesized by the intestinal bacterial flora.

However, several clinical conditions may predispose to vitamin K deficiency, the commonest of which is the absence of vitamin K in the newborn because the intestine is sterile at birth. In normal neonates who are fed cow's milk shortly after birth, the level of vitamin K rises to adequate levels within 48 hours because cow's milk contains about 6 μg/100 ml of vitamin K. However, breast milk contains about one fourth of this amount; as a result hemorrhagic disease of the newborn is more likely to occur. Therefore, prophylactic administration of vitamin K is recommended for all newborns. In premature infants the effectiveness of vitamin K supplements is diminished because of the liver's immature functioning. Other indications for vitamin K supplements are intestinal disease, lack of bile, prolonged antibiotic therapy, or use of anticoagulants such as heparin or bishydroxycoumarin (dicumarol), which are vitamin K antagonists.

Hypervitaminosis. Hypervitaminosis of the fat-soluble vitamins can occur after chronic ingestion of large quantities or massive doses of vitamins A and D. The effects of excessive intake of vitamin E are unknown. Toxicity from vitamin K overdose can cause hyperbilirubinemia from hemolysis of red blood cells in premature infants. It can also occur in newborns whose mothers have received large doses of vitamin K to prevent the infant from developing hemorrhagic disease. A rare example of toxicity is in individuals who have a deficiency of the enzyme glucose-6-phosphate dehydrogenase, which is necessary for the formation of red blood cells. In susceptible individuals large doses of vitamin K may cause hemolytic anemia. Hypervitaminosis does not occur from excessive use of the water-soluble vitamins B and C because these are excreted in the urine rather than stored in the body.

The signs of vitamin A or D overdose are listed in Table 13-3. Treatment involves removing the exogenous source. In vitamin D excess, a low-calcium diet may be prescribed during the initial phase of therapy.

As a precaution against hypervitaminosis of vitamins A and D, the Food and Drug Administration has made the following classification: (1) any substance that contains less than 50% of the recommended daily allowance (RDA for vitamin A—5000 IU; RDA for vitamin D—400 IU) is a *food,* (2) any substance that contains 50% to 150% of the RDA is a *dietary supplement,* and (3) any substance that contains more than 150% of the RDA is a *drug* and can only be obtained via a physician's prescription.

Nursing considerations. Prevention involves teaching parents the correct use of vitamin supplements. In most instances adequate dietary sources of vitamin A and D contradict the use of additional exogenous supplies. The nurse should investigate the child's dietary habits to ensure that adequate but not excessive sources of vitamin A and D are ingested.

Overnutrition. Overnutrition refers to the chronic ingestion of more calories than are needed to supply the body's energy requirement. In other words, there is a positive energy balance—more is eaten than is needed. Although growth problems such as obesity may be related to hormonal imbalances, the majority of cases of overweight are caused by dietary surplus. Evaluation of overnutrition *early* in life is essential, since it has been well documented that obese infants have an 80% chance or greater of becoming obese adults. Possibly the most critical period for development of persistent, chronic obesity is during the first year of life when hyperplasia of fat cells occurs. High-caloric intake stimulates growth in the form of cellular mitosis, resulting in the formation of more fat cells (hyperplasia) rather than enlargement (hypertrophy) of existing cells. The importance of this finding is that once the new fat cells are formed, they exist for the life of the individual, undergoing hypertrophy when increased calories are consumed. It is well known that treating overweight that had its beginning in childhood is much more difficult than treating the condition if it begins later in life. Besides the physiologic component of increased numbers of fat cells, there is also the psychologic disadvantages of firmly entrenched food habits and dependency on food.

Overnutrition is usually defined as a weight gain above the ninety-seventh percentile on a growth chart. However, height and weight must always be evaluated together. A consistent gain in height and weight, even at or above the ninety-seventh percentile, is usually normal. In general overweight is defined as an increase of 10% over one's ideal or average height. Obesity is a 20% or more increase over the ideal weight. Other methods of determining obesity include measuring the skin-fold thickness or measuring the body weight by underwater weighing. Both methods attempt to calculate the amount of adipose tissue as compared to lean body mass. Regardless of the method used, obesity is an easily recognizable problem.

Less facile is the treatment for overnutrition. During infancy obesity is less the child's problem than the parents' problem, because overfeeding is more directly linked to the adult's sociocultural food habits than to the infant's increased appetite. Therefore, intervention involves helping the adult change the feeding habits of the infant. This involves much more than dietary counseling. Psychologic factors play an important role, particularly the philosophy that a fat baby is a healthy baby, or, more subconsciously, that a fat "healthy" baby is a sign of good mothering. Helping parents realize what constitutes good nutrition and health is one of the first steps toward change.

Another step in controlling overfeeding in infancy is selection of foods that provide adequate, but not excessive, calories. Whole milk contains 20 kcal/ounce and can easily supply all the calories necessary for infants (115 kcal/kg). However, when solid foods are added, the quantity of milk should be decreased to maintain the proper caloric intake. If the infant seems unsatisfied with fewer bottle feedings and refuses water, the milk or formula should be diluted to yield fewer calories per ounce. For example, diluting 1 quart of milk with 5 ounces of water yields a solution of 17.3 kcal/ounce. For a child ingesting 30 ounces of milk, this represents a saving of 81 kcal/day. Skimmed or nonfat milk contains a significant reduction in calories (10 kcal/ounce) but is not nutritionally sound for infants. Its low-fat content deprives the infant of essential fatty acids, and the significantly increased amounts of solids and electrolytes elevate the renal solute load and water demands. Half-skimmed milk is also a poor substitution unless solid foods are wisely chosen to supply the deficient fatty acids. Nonfortified skimmed milk is a very poor source of vitamin A and, unless supplemented, can lead to vitamin A deficiency. A comparison of whole, nonfat or skimmed, and lowfat or partially skimmed milk is presented in Table 13-4.

The addition of solid foods is another important aspect of controlling obesity. Approximately 20% of commercial baby foods contain less than 50 kcal/100 g, whereas another 20% contain more than 100 kcal/100 g. Choosing low-caloric foods can significantly lower the daily calorie intake without actually decreasing the total quantity of food. Table 12-6 lists calorie contents of various commerical baby foods. Another important consideration for developing nutritionally sound eating habits is keeping the introduction

Table 13-4. Nutritive values of milk (per 8 ounces)

	Whole milk	Nonfat or skim milk	Lowfat or partially skim milk
% water	87	90	87
Food energy (kcal)	160	80	135
Protein (g)	9	9	10
Fat (g)	9	Trace	5
% milk fat	3.5 minimum	0.25 (maximum)	2.0 (average)
Minimum % of solids not fat*	8.7	10.0	9.0
Fatty acids			
Linoleic (g)	Trace	—	Trace
Oleic (g)	3	—	2
Carbohydrates (g)	12	12	15
Calcium (mg)	288	296	352
Iron (mg)	0.01	0.01	0.01
Vitamin A (IU)	350	10	200
Thiamine (mg)	0.07	0.09	0.10
Riboflavin (mg)	0.41	0.44	0.52
Niacin (mg)	0.2	0.2	0.2
Vitamin C (mg)	2	2	2

Based on data from U.S. Department of Agriculture: Handbook No. 8, Washington, D.C., 1972, U.S. Government Printing Office; U.S. Department of Agriculture: Home and garden bulletin No. 72, Washington, D.C., U.S. Government Printing Office.

*Proteins, carbohydrates, minerals, and vitamins constitute solids, not fat.

of sweet foods to a minimum. Since infants seem to be born with a preference for sweet tastes, it is advisable to limit concentrated sweets. This includes not adding additional sugar to the formula or cereal and avoiding finger foods, such as cookies. Other foods rich in calories that should be restricted in serving size rather than eliminated include butter, cream, ice cream, pastries, and chocolate.

Another nutritional product that has recently been receiving much attention is the role of fiber in the diet. Fiber or roughage represents the organic but nondigestible fraction of food. Major food fiber components are cellulose, hemicellulose, lignin, and pectin. Some of the benefits of high fiber in one's diet seem to be a lowered incidence of diverticulosis, colonic cancer, hemorrhoids, diabetes, and obesity.[13] High-fiber diets reduce the intake of calories and provide a high level of satiety. In infants who are large for their age and have a voracious appetite, increasing the fiber content of their diet assists in extending the interval between feedings, as well as restricting the caloric intake. High-fiber foods that are suitable for infants include carrots, celery, cucumber, broccoli, green beans, whole-grain cereals, such as wheat and bran, whole-grain bread, and fruits.

Although children can become obese at any time, the most likely periods are the latter part of infancy, at the time of starting school, and during adolescence. It is unquestionable that the easiest time to alter food consumption and eating habits is during infancy. As the child grows older, overnutrition is not solely a result of overfeeding but of complex sociologic and psychologic factors, which are much more resistant to change. Chapter 21 presents an extended discussion of obesity during adolescence.

ALLERGIES

Allergy (or atopy as it is sometimes called) can be defined as an altered, adverse reaction to a foreign substance or antigen that usually produces no untoward effects in man. An antigen is any substance capable of stimulating the production of antibodies and, subsequently, reacting with them to initiate the allergic response. In most cases the antigenic agent is a protein, polysaccharide, or protein-polysaccharide complex. Simple substances, such as aspirin or penicillin, become antigens when they combine with body proteins to form a hapten-protein complex. Antigens enter the body through ingestion, inhalation, transepidermal penetration, or parenteral infusion. Development of the allergic state depends on the nature of the antigen, the type of exposure, and the duration of contact.

One of the most important aspects of allergies is their genetic component. Although all individuals are potentially allergic, certain people have an inherited predisposition for the development of allergies. Studies have revealed that anywhere from 40% to 80% of allergic individuals have a positive family history for allergy. Asthma seems to be more affected by heredity factors than atopic dermatitis (eczema), allergic rhinitis (hay fever), or gastrointestinal allergy. The results of one study indicated the following hereditary influence on the development of allergy: (1) individuals with asthma or eczema have a 2- to 3.5-times greater chance of developing an additional allergy. (2) First-degree relatives have a 3.3 fold increased risk of developing asthma if the individual has asthma and an additional allergy, such as eczema or hay fever. If the individual has only asthma, the risk is decreased to 1.5- to 2.0-times greater. (3) If a parent has a severe allergy, the chance of the offspring developing an allergy is about half the risk of a recessively inherited disorder (8:1).[12]

Age is another important factor in the development of allergies. During infancy, eczema (atopic dermatitis) is frequent but asthma is rare. After the third year, eczema clears spontaneously and asthma and hay fever become dominant. Sensitivity to allergens may begin even before birth via transplacental sensitization. Since foods are the most important allergens during the first 6 months of life, the diets of pregnant women who have a strong family history of allergy should contain small amounts of potentially allergenic foods, such as milk, eggs, and chocolate. Prophylaxis of allergic disease from environmental inhalants can also decrease the incidence of respiratory allergy. Suggestions for "allergy proofing" the home even before the child is born are listed in the boxed material below.

Atopic dermatitis

Atopic dermatitis, or eczema, is an allergic manifestation that is most common in children under 2 years of age. The most common allergens are foods, environmental inhalants, and pollens. During infancy foods such as cow's milk and egg albumin are the chief offenders. As the child grows older, environmental inhalants and pollen become stronger allergens. Infantile eczema usually undergoes spontaneous and permanent remission by 3 years of age. Approximately 50% of infants with eczema develop asthma as children and hay fever as adults.[14]

Pathophysiology. The cause of atopic dermatitis is unknown, although a basic factor seems to be a constitutional skin type that is hypersensitive to irritation, drying, and pruritus. Dilatation of capillaries causes erythema and edema. Papules, vesicles, and crusts form as the weeping lesions dry. There is usually intense itching associated with the rash, which results in secondary infection if the lesions are scratched. The child is usually very irritable, fretful, and unable to sleep because of the persistent pruritus. The erythematous lesions usually begin on the cheeks, spread to the rest of the face and scalp, and seem to favor the flexor surfaces of the body, such as the antecubital and popliteal areas of the arms and legs. The unaffected areas of the body are usually dry and rough. Lymphadenopathy, particularly near the affected sites, such as the cervical area, is common. Other systemic manifestations are rare. Eosinophilia is usual with 5% to 10% eosinophils in the peripheral blood smear, and positive skin tests to various allergens can be demonstrated.

Medical management. Treatment of eczema is primarily supportive. The first objective is removal of specific allergens. The onset of eczema is frequently associated with the introduction of cow's milk to breastfed infants or new foods, particularly egg white, to other infants. The child is placed on a hypoallergenic diet that restricts the following foods: milk or milk products, eggs, wheat, fish, citrus fruits, nuts, peanut butter, chocolate, strawberries, tomatoes, pork, and pineapple. A typical hypoallergenic diet for an infant would include a milk substitute such as soy formula, rice cereal, apples, apricots, carrots, string beans, beef, and aqueous multiple-vitamin supplements. The diet is followed for 10 days; if remission occurs, each food from the restricted list is added one at a time at weekly intervals to identify specific food allergens. Milk and then wheat are usually the first two foods added for suspected sensitivity. Even if all foods can be accepted, eggs are usually not permitted. If the response to the hypoallergenic diet is unsuccessful, environmental control is attempted to lessen the amount of inhalants. The boxed material lists the usual steps toward environmental adjustment.

Pruritus is the most difficult medical and nursing problem. Itching and scratching lead to infection, which in turn results in loss of the stratum corneum or lichenification. Measures that reduce skin irritation lessen pruritus. Fabrics such as wool or coarsely woven materials should be avoided. Soft, washable cottons are preferable. Long sleeves, long pants, and one-piece outfit prevent the infant from scratching exposed skin. Since heat and humidity in-

Suggestions for "allergy proofing" the home

- House dust—commonest cause of respiratory allergy in children
  - Bedroom should be for sleeping, not playing.
  - Feather pillows, which collect dust, should be avoided; if used, they should be encased in an impermeable plastic casing. Dacron pillows should be used.
  - Mattresses and box springs should also be encased in an impermeable covering.
  - Room should be dusted daily and thoroughly cleaned weekly, when the child is not present.
  - Sheets, bedspreads, and curtains should be made of washable, smooth cotton or synthetic fabirc and cleaned frequently. Window shades are preferable to curtains or venetian blinds, which collect dust.
  - Floors should be bare, with only a cotton or synthetic (not wool) "scatter rug."
  - The following should be removed from the room.
    - Stuffed animals
    - Upholstered and stuffed furniture, except those stuffed exclusively with foam rubber; in general, the less furniture, the better
    - Plants and aquariums, which can harbor molds
    - All pets (if one is already there, it should be kept outdoors at all times)
  - The closet should be kept free of stored articles, especially woolen clothing.
  - Windows and doors should be kept closed.
  - Walls should be covered with washable paint or wallpaper.
- Heating system—forced air circulates dust
  - Minimum treatment—vent or duct should be covered with cheesecloth, which is washed frequently.
  - Preferable treatment-heating ducts should be closed off in room and an electric heater (which is placed so as to prevent severe burns to the child) should be used.
  - If possible, an air cleaning machine, such as an electronic air purifier, should be used. Although expensive, small units can be rented for use in the child's room.
- Mildew exposure
  - Cellars should be avoided as play areas.
  - Showers and tile areas should be cleaned well and sprayed with an antimold agent, such as Lysol.
  - Vaporizers should be kept clean and free of mold.
  - Plants and aquariums should be kept out of child's room.

crease pruritus, proper clothing for the environmental temperature is important, especially during winter months when many people tend to overdress children. Toys, such as furry stuffed animals, should be replaced with washable, smooth, plastic or wood toys. Not infrequently the itching and irritability warrant the judicious use of medication, such as chloral hydrate, diphenhydramine (Benadryl), or cyproheptadine (Periactin).

The use of hot water and soap intensifies skin drying and irritation. Baths are either avoided or given with plain tepid water. Nonlipid, hydrophilic agents, such as Cetaphil lotion, are useful cleansing and lubricating solutions. Colloid baths, such as the addition of 2 cups of cornstarch to a tub of warm water, temporarily relieve itching and may help the child sleep if given before bedtime. Wet soaks or dressings, such as Burow's solution (aluminum subacetate solution and glacial acetic acid in water, diluted 1:20) or potassium permanganate, are soothing to the skin and provide antiseptic protection. Topical steroids in strengths of 0.01% to 1% are the most effective local treatment because of their potent anti-inflammatory effect. One important consideration to remember concerning the use of steroids is that signs of infection will be masked. In addition prolonged use of steroids must be carefully evaluated because, following discontinuation of the drug, the lesions often exacerbate in a more severe form than before treatment was begun. In cases of chronic eczema in which lichenification has occurred, tar preparations may be used to produce a mild irritation, which promotes granulation and healing. The most common tar preparations, such as ichthammol, are made by the destruction of wood or coal. Coal tars should be avoided during the summer months because of their photosensitizing effect on the skin. Coal and wood tars can have potential toxic effects on the renal system, warranting routine urinalysis of individuals treated with these preparations.

Immunizations necessitate special caution in children with eczema. These children should have their skin tested before receiving vaccines that have been cultivated in chick embryo, such as measles virus and mumps virus. Although smallpox vaccination is no longer routinely given, three groups of people should continue their artificial immunity. These include health personnel, military personnel, and travelers to foreign countries where the threat of the disease still exists. Children in these selected groups who have eczema are susceptible to developing eczema vaccinatum from contact with the persons who have been vaccinated.[11]

Nursing considerations. Long-term treatment of eczema is usually established on an outpatient basis. As a result the major burden of responsibility and physical care rests on the parents in the home. A vicious cycle of exacerbations—scratching—infection—irritability—frustration is the usual course unless the initial phase can be altered. The primary objective is to identify the allergen or allergens to which the child is sensitive. When a hypoallergenic diet is prescribed, parents need help in understanding the reason for the diet and guidelines for following it. Table 13-5 lists common sources of food that contain milk, wheat, eggs, and other hyperallergenic foods. Eliminating such foods becomes more of a problem when the child eats table food than during early infancy. Since hypoallergenic diets take time before visible effects are observed, parents need reassurance that this is not an immediate cure. Eliminating environmental allergens is another time-consuming and tedious task. Often the financial resources are not sufficient to to make optimal adjustments, and improvisation is essential. Referral to a public health nursing agency can assist the family in coping with the difficulties of following a special diet and "allergy proofing" the home.

Table 13-5. Hyperallergenic foods

Food	Sources
Milk	Ice cream, butter, margarine, cheese, pudding, baked goods, wieners, bologna, canned creamed soups, instant breakfast drinks, powdered milk drinks, or milk chocolate
Eggs	Mayonnaise, creamy salad dressing, baked goods, egg noodles, some cake icing, meringue, custard, pancakes, french toast, or root beer
Wheat	Almost all baked goods, wieners, bologna, pressed or chopped cold cuts, gravy, pasta, and some canned soups
Peanuts	Peanut butter or legumes, such as beans, peas, or lentils (peanuts are a legume, not a nut)
Nuts	Chocolate, baked goods, or cherry soda (may be flavored with a nut extract)
Fish or shellfish	Cod liver oil, pizza with anchovies, Caesar salad dressing, or any food fried in same oil as fish
Chocolate	Cola beverages, cocoa, or chocolate-flavored drinks
Buckwheat	Some cereal, pancakes
Pork, chicken	Bacon, wieners, sausage, pork fat, chicken broth
Strawberries, melon, pineapple	Gelatin, syrups
Corn	Popcorn, cereal, muffins
Citrus fruits	Orange, lemon, lime, grapefruit; any of these in drinks, gelatin, juice, or medicines
Spices	Chili, pepper, vinegar

Adapted from Rapp, D.: Sneezing, wheezing, and scratching, New York, 1974, Erie County Department of Health, Office of Public Health Information and Education.

Probably the most difficult problem of caring for the child with eczema is controlling the intense pruritus. In order to prevent infection, the child must be restricted from scratching. Aside from the use of topical or systemic medications, other measures can be taken to minimize the scratching. Fingernails and toenails are cut short, kept clean, and filed frequently to prevent sharp edges. Gloves or cotton stockings may have to be placed over the hands and pinned to shirt-sleeves. To prevent any contact with the skin, elbow restraints are sometimes necessary. One-piece outfits with long sleeves and long pants also decrease direct contact with the skin. Whether gloves or restraints are used, the child needs time when he is free from such restrictions. An excellent time to remove any protective devices is during the bath or after receiving sedative or antipruritic medication. Restraints should not be removed during sleep, because the child will scratch in his sleep and can severely traumatize the skin.

The elimination of conditions that increase itching is another approach. Woolen clothes or blankets, rough fabrics, and furry stuffed animals are irritating to the skin and should be removed. During cold months, synthetic—not wool—fabrics should be used for overcoats, hats, gloves, and snowsuits. Heat and humidity cause perspiration, which intensifies itching. Proper dress for climatic conditions lessens overheating. Since sunlight has a beneficial drying effect on weeping lesions, exposure to ultraviolet light should be encouraged but should be monitored carefully to prevent burning. Any topical beauty aid, such as perfumes, powder, or oils, must be avoided. Clothes and sheets should be laundered in a mild detergent and rinsed thoroughly. Putting the clothes through a second complete wash cycle without using detergent ensures that no residue remains.

Preventing infection is usually secondary to preventing scratching. Personal hygiene must be accomplished without the liberal use of soap. Baths should be given infrequently (unless otherwise prescribed), the water should be kept tepid, and bubble baths should be avoided as well as the use of oils or powder. Skin folds and diaper areas need frequent cleansing with plain water and without the use of any anti–diaper rash preparation. If antiseptic soaks are prescribed, they should be applied as directed. Demonstrating the technique is preferable to explaining it. For example, toddlers have great difficulty in sitting still for a 10- or 15-minute wet soak. One suggestion is to apply the wet dressing at naptime or when the child is watching television or listening to a story. If the soaking solution is to be diluted at home, demonstrate what the term "parts" means. For example, 1 part Burow's solution is mixed with 20 parts of water. For someone who is unfamiliar with this expression of measurement, it is better to express the ratio as 1 cup of Burow's solution mixed with 20 cups of water. If topical ointments are prescribed, stress to parents that one thick application is *not* equivalent to several thin applications. The same is true for oral medications, particularly systemic antibiotics for skin infections. Equally divided doses over a 24-hour time period are essential for the antibiotic to achieve continuous high blood levels.

Since adequate rest is also important for these children, who are usually fretful and irritable, planning meals, baths, medications, and treatments during awake periods is paramount. Sleepy, tired children are normally cranky, and such behavior only intensifies the urge to scratch. During periods of irritability, these children tend to be anorectic, which is worsened by restriction of their usual foods. Forcing them to eat should be avoided; it is better to be lenient about food consumption than to allow them to have a potentially allergic food. Multiple-vitamin and mineral supplements are very important during these times, particularly to prevent iron, calcium, and vitamin C deficiencies.

Perhaps it is because the physical problems seem insurmountable during periods of acute exacerbations that the emotional stress becomes so intense. Parents are told, "Don't let the child scratch," but the child scratches, the lesions worsen, infection begins, and the parents are overwhelmed with feelings of helplessness, frustration, anger, and guilt. They need time to talk about such negative feelings, and they need to be reassured that these feelings are expected, normal, acceptable, and healthy provided there is an emotional outlet to dissipate the invested energy. Supporting parents through the initial phase of identifying the specific allergens is crucial because improvement is not immediate, although dramatic recovery can occur once the sensitizing agents are completely removed. During acute phases, relieving as much anxiety as possible in both parents and child has a beneficial emotional, and physical effect, since stress tends to aggravate the severity of eczema.

When management at home becomes impossible, hospitalization is required. Since one of the risks during hospitalization is contraction of a pyogenic or viral infection, particularly herpes simplex, the child should be placed in a private room or in a room with children of similar ages who are noninfectious. Hospitalization may dramatically improve the child's condition because environmental agents are more carefully controlled and the component of constant parental frustration is lessened. Since eczema is a disease of remissions and exacerbations, frequent hospitalizations that rapidly induce remissions can be extremely discouraging to parents, who feel incompetent, helpless, and insecure in their parenting abilities. It is in these situations that follow-up care in the home by a public health nurse is mandatory, since members of the family have demonstrated their need for outside help. Not recognizing this clue for additional support can leave emotional scars long after the eczema has disappeared. (A summary of nursing care of the infant with eczema is described in the boxed material on p. 491.)

Nutritional allergies

Nutritional allergies can occur in anyone at any age, and frequently the allergic response is exhibited after the food

Summary of nursing care of the infant with eczema

Goals	Responsibilities
Prevent or minimize scratching	Keep fingernails and toenails short and clean Wrap hands in soft cotton gloves or stockings; pin to shirt cuff Dress in loose-fitting, one-piece, long-sleeve and long-pants outfit (if appropriate for weather conditions) Avoid overheating, high humidity, and perspiration Use elbow restraints when absolutely necessary, but allow supervised periods for unrestricted movement Encourage exposure to ultraviolet light, but avoid sunburn Eliminate any woolen or rough garment or furry stuffed toys; nylon garments promote sweating Launder all clothes or bedsheets in mild detergent and rinse very well
Prevent infection	Administer good personal hygiene—baths with tepid water, little or no soap (using only a mild, unperfumed product), and no bubble bath, bath oil, perfume, or powder Demonstrate proper procedure for applying wet dressings; suggest quiet times of day for applying them to child's skin Demonstrate carefully the proper dilution of soaks at home Schedule times for administering oral antibiotics that maintain continuous high blood levels of the drug
Promote rest	Plan meals, baths, medications, and treatments around nap or bedtime Make child as comfortable as possible before sleep to enhance restfulness (for example, give sedation and then give bath before bedtime) Carry out any distressing procedure when child is well rested and after he has received medication for itching
Promote nutrition	Feed child when he is well rested Do not force food or introduce a restricted food to encourage eating Stress need for vitamin and mineral supplements Allow child to feed himself if that is usual routine
Encourage play activities that are suitable to skin condition and child's developmental age	Avoid any furry, hairy stuffed toys or dolls Provide kinesthetic, moving toys, large toys, which require less fine motor skills if hands are covered, and quiet musical or visual toys Remember that there is no substitution for the stimulation and comfort of human contact
Assist parents in identifying causative allergens	Stress reason for hypoallergenic diet or removal of inhalants, especially that positive results are not immediate Give written list of foods restricted as well as those allowed Identify hidden sources of milk, wheat, and eggs Assess home environment *before* suggesting ways to eliminate inhalants Make public health referral for long-term home care follow-up
Provide emotional support for child and parents	Provide one-to-one consistent care giver for hospitalized child Encourage parents to play with child and to realize that the irritable behavior is directly related to physical discomfort Stress to parents that child still needs limit setting and discipline Be aware of overprotectiveness and restrictiveness, which can stifle child's emotional growth Allow and encourage parents, particularly the one who cares for child most of the time, to express their negative feelings, such as anger, frustration, and perhaps guilt Stress that negative feelings are normal, acceptable, and expected but that they must have an outlet in order for parents and child to remain healthy

has been ingested one or more times. Food allergies are most common during infancy, and the chief offenders are milk, eggs, wheat, vegetables, and fruits. Sensitivity to fish and nuts is also likely but is less often outgrown than allergy to the other substances. Some reactions to foods mimic allergic responses but are caused by other malfunctioning mechanisms. Classic examples of these are lactose intolerance to milk and inability to absorb the protein gluten in wheat. Nutritional allergies during infancy are common because the infant is exposed to many new food antigens. Physiologically the intestinal tract is immature and absorbs many more inadequately catabolized proteins, which, unlike the amino acids that compose them, are capable of producing an allergic response. This explains why as the child grows the food allergy may disappear.

Nutritional allergies can also be prevented. In a child who has a strong family history for allergy, certain foods should be avoided during the first year. Table 13-5 lists common foods that are potentially allergenic. In addition following careful schedules for introducing new foods can quickly identify the offending agent. Each new food should be offered one at a time for a period of 4 to 7 days. If potentially allergenic foods are introduced, they should be offered in small quantities, about ½ to 1 tsp, and served well cooked, since heat breaks down proteins. If any local inflammation occurs, such as swelling of the lip or urticaria around the mouth, the food must be avoided and is usually not reintroduced for a period of about 6 months.

Milk sensitivity. The most common nutritional allergy among infants is whole cow's milk. It is estimated that about 1% to 2% of all infants have a milk allergy and that approximately 30% of allergic children are sensitive to milk.[3] Sensitivity can be to different protein components of cow's milk. The whey fraction, which contains lactalbumin and lactoglobulin, is sensitive to heat, which means that evaporated milk or boiled homogenized milk can be substituted. The casein fraction, which is not sensitive to heat, presents additional problems for substitutions, since cow's or goat's milk cannot be utilized. The most likely alternative is soybean milk, although approximately one in five children who are allergic to cow's milk are also sensitive to soybean milk.[10] Commercially available soy formulas include Prosobee, Neo-Mull-Soy, and Isomil. Commercial formulas that are suitable cow's and soybean milk substitutes include Meat Base formula, Nutramigen, and Pregestimil. The latter two preparations are predigested synthetic milk.

Clinical manifestations of milk allergy are generally gastrointestinal disturbances, such as vomiting, diarrhea, and colic. Diagnosis of milk allergy is based on disappearance of these symptoms following elimination of all milk products. Confirmation of the diagnosis should be determined by a trial period of reintroduction of milk to ascertain if the symptoms reappear. Only after careful investigation should appropriate dietary changes occur. Milk allergy can mistakenly be diagnosed as galactosemia, which is a deficiency of the enzyme galactose-1-phosphate-uridyl transferase, or as lactose intolerance, which is an inability to digest usual levels of milk lactose.[17] Milk intolerance is more common in nonwhite groups (American Indians, blacks, and Asians) and is less prevalent in children than in adults. Most infants outgrow their sensitivity to milk, probably as a result of the maturing gastrointestinal system. Very small quantities of milk are gradually reintroduced, usually during the last half of the first year.

Nursing considerations. Management of milk allergy is elimination or modification of cow's milk. The main difficulty is identification of the exact sensitivity and selection of an acceptable substitution. This is frequently time-consuming, frustrating, and expensive. If milk allergy is suspected, the initial trial is the use of evaporated or boiled milk. If soybean milk or other substitutes must be tried, the nurse advises the parent to purchase small quantities of the formula and to ascertain if unused portions can be returned. Frequently when parents are told to try a new formula, they purchase a case, rather than a few cans. At the end of the trial period they have a large reserve of unused, costly formulas.

The nurse also stresses that all associated milk products must be avoided (Table 13-5). This requires assiduously reading all food labels for addition of milk products to the prepared food. In addition, some drugs, such as penicillin or vitamins, contain lactose as a filler or bulk agent. Parents should be advised to check with the pharmacist regarding this possibility when obtaining drugs. Since allergy to one protein may mean allergy to other proteins, particularly egg albumin and wheat, such hyperallergenic foods should be restricted from the diet for the first 9 to 12 months of life. Prevention of allergy even before the infant is born with proper antepartal counseling and emphasis on breast-feeding is preferable to treatment later on.

SEBORRHEIC DERMATITIS (CRADLE CAP)

Seborrheic dermatitis is a chronic, recurrent, inflammatory reaction of the skin. It occurs most commonly in the scalp but may involve the eyelids (blepharitis), external ear canal (otitis externa), nasolabial folds, and inguinal region. The cause is unknown, although it is more common in early infancy when sebum production is increased.

The lesions are characteristically thick, adherent, yellowish, scaly, oily patches. Occasionally areas of transient alopecia may be evident.

Although the appearance of cradle cap resembles eczematous eruptions, it differs from them in several important aspects. It is not necessarily associated with a positive family history for allergy, it is very common (approximately 50%) in infants shortly after birth, the lesions are greasy in appearance and more pink or yellow than red, and lichenification (induration and thickening of the skin from persistent irritation) does not occur. Probably the most significant distinguishing characteristic of seborrheic dermatitis is the absence of pruritus. The child's behavior is unchanged by the presence of the lesions. Diagnosis is made primarily on the appearance of the crusts and the absence of pruritus.

Medical management

Treatment is mainly directed at removing the crusts. Frequent vigorous shampooing, the use of a fine-toothed comb, and sometimes application of vegetable or mineral oil to loosen the crusts followed by thorough cleansing are usually sufficient to eliminate the condition. At other times, topical preparation may be prescribed, such as sulfur, salicylic acid, or coal tar. Topical corticosteroids are especially effective in reducing the inflammation and causing a complete remission. However, the lesions may return following discontinuation of the preparation. Occasionally the lesions become secondarily infected, requiring topical or systemic antibacterial and/or antimycotic treatments.

Nursing considerations

The initial objective is prevention of cradle cap through adequate scalp hygiene. Not infrequently parents omit shampooing the infant's hair from fear of damaging the "soft spots" or fontanels. The nurse discusses how to shampoo the infant's hair and emphasizes that the fontanel is like skin anywhere else on the body. It does not puncture or tear with mild pressure.

When seborrheic lesions are present, the nurse teaches parents the appropriate procedure to clean the scalp thoroughly. At this point, a demonstration may be necessary to ensure that the parents can institute meticulous hygiene. Shampooing should be done three to four times a week, using a mild soap or commercial shampoo, such as the no-tear preparations. If an oil is applied, it should be massaged into the scalp and allowed to penetrate the crusts for a few minutes and then thoroughly washed out. Using a fine-toothed comb after shampooing helps remove the loosened crusts from the strands of hair.

The nurse stresses prevention of secondary bacterial or fungal infection through hygiene measures and frequent changing of bed linen and clothing that comes in contact with affected sites, such as hats or diapers. Since the lesions are not puritic, measures to prevent scratching are not necessary. However, as a general precaution the infant's hands should be kept clean to prevent infecting areas such as the eyelids.

If topical preparations are used, the nurse consults with the physician regarding specific procedures for use. For example, coal tar ointments such as Pragmatar may need to be diluted with a few drops of water for use in infants. They are sometimes applied overnight and then removed with a shampoo in the morning, or they may be left on indefinitely. The nurse cautions the parents to avoid the eyes when applying any preparations. Sometimes it is helpful to use a light cotton cap to cover the infant's head to avoid accidental rubbing of the medication in the eyes.

COLIC

Colic is generally described as paroxysmal abdominal pain or cramping that is manifested by loud crying and drawing the legs up to the abdomen. It is more common in very young infants under the age of 3 months than in older infants. Despite the obvious behavioral indications of pain, the child tolerates the formula well, gains weight, and thrives. Many theories have been investigated as potential causative factors, such as too rapid feeding, overeating, swallowing excessive air, improper feeding technique, especially in positioning and/or burping, and emotional stress or tension between parent and child. Generally colic is thought to be caused by excessive fermentation and gas production in the intestines. Excessive intake of carbohydrates causes flatus, but a change in diet rarely prevents the attacks of colic. Regardless of the fact that colic is considered a minor ailment, the impact of a colicky, crying, irritable infant can have an intense emotional impact on parent-child attachment and family relationships. Mothers will often relate histories of the daily routine that are laden with feelings of frustration, anger, despair, and helplessness. A vicious cycle ensues in which the parent's own anxiety may be transferred to the infant, which further increases his tension, irritability, and crying.

Nursing considerations

The initial step in managing colic is to take a thorough, detailed history of the usual daily events. Areas that should be stressed include what time of the day the attacks occur, what the relationship of the attacks to feeding time is, which family members are present, what the activity of the mother or usual care giver is before, during, and after the crying, and which measures to relieve the crying have been tried. Of special emphasis is a careful assessment of the feeding process via *demonstration* by the mother, not solely through interviewing. The following example stresses the importance of evaluating the feeding process.

A 19-year-old mother brought her 1-month-old son to the health center for a routine visit. Her main complaint was that after feeding the child would always spit up, fall asleep for a short time, and then wake up screaming. History taking and physical assessment revealed no unusual findings. In fact the child was thriving and gaining weight more rapidly than expected. Since exact statements from the mother concerning feeding practices were vague, the nurse asked the mother to give her child a bottle of formula. The mother proceeded to feed the child a full 8-ounce bottle of formula, which he finished without interruption in about 5 minutes. As soon as the bottle was drained, the mother placed the infant in a sitting position and rather forcefully "patted" his back. As she had stated, the child promptly regurgitated about 2 ounces of undigested milk and then seemed content.

It was not necessary for the nurse to wait for the child to have abdominal cramps. The feeding procedure needed some revision. On further questioning of the mother about the method used, the nurse learned that no one had talked to the mother about infant's fluid needs and stomach capacity. She had purchased 8-ounce bottles and had assumed that they should be filled and then emptied at each feeding. Although the infant had initially resisted the large volume, she had kept the nipple in his mouth, prodding him to drink more. If she removed it to burp him, he would fall asleep before he finished the bottle. As a result he learned to meet his mother's demands and compensated by giving some back as soon as he could. Since the burping was not gentle, the mother helped the infant regurgitate. The nurse then proceeded to explain how one determines the amount of formula infants need. The mother seemed willing to try demand feedings, beginning with 4 ounces of formula, interrupted by at least one period of gentle burping. A return visit was scheduled for 1 week later.

When the mother and child returned, the mother stated that at first the infant seemed to want more than 4 ounces but that since he did not spit up or cry after the initial smaller feeding, she decided to continue following the nurse's suggestions. By the end of the first day, the infant slept well, drank 4 or 5 ounces about every 4 hours, and was beginning to sleep through the night.

All instances of colic do not respond to intervention quite so remarkably. More often than not, there is no change required in feeding practices. When no cause can be identified, it is preferable to determine the time of the onset of crying and attempt to manipulate the circumstances associated with it. For example, some infants have episodes of colic around the family's dinner time, when all household members are home and the mother is preoccupied with cooking. The overstimulating, more tense atmosphere may upset the infant. Encouraging the mother to partially prepare dinner earlier in the day and feed the infant in a more quiet area of the house may help reverse the environmental conditions that may have provoked the attack of colic.

One of the most important areas of nursing concern is the support of the mother during the colic period. Stress that despite the crying and obvious pain, the infant is doing well. Colic disappears spontaneously, usually by 3 months of age, although guarantees should never be given since it may continue for much longer. The mother should be encouraged to get out of the house and arrange for some free time. Most important, it should be emphasized that the colic is not indicative of poor or inadequate mothering. The mother's negative feelings toward the infant and her insecurities regarding her mothering abilities are normal. She should be encouraged to talk about them, since active listening may do more to relieve the colic syndrome than offering stereotyped advice, remedies, and glib statements such as, "Don't worry about it; your child will eventually outgrow the colicky spells."

Although the exact cause of colic is unknown, the abdominal cramping is painful and may be relieved by stimulating peristalsis, which can be accomplished by placing the child prone over a hot-water bottle, heated towel, or covered heating pad or by giving 1 or 2 ounces of warm dilute tea. Passage of flatus or feces can be stimulated by a glycerine suppository (child size only), stimulation by a well-lubricated little finger, or administration of a 1- or 2-ounce warm-water enema. Preventive measures include changing the infant's position frequently, burping during and after feedings using the shoulder position, smaller, frequent feedings, placing the infant in an upright seat after feedings, and maintaining a quiet, emotionally stable environment. Mild sedation may be prescribed but should be a measure of last resort.

FAILURE TO THRIVE (MATERNAL DEPRIVATION)

Failure to thrive, also referred to as maternal deprivation syndrome, is defined as children who are below the third percentile in growth but who demonstrate no organic cause. More detailed clinical criteria can be summarized as: (1) weight below the third percentile with subsequent weight gain in the presence of adequate nurturing or mothering, (2) no evidence of systemic disease or congenital abnormality that explains the growth failure, (3) developmental retardation with subsequent improvement following appropriate stimulation, (4) clinical signs of deprivation that decrease in a more nurturing environment, and (5) presence of significant environmental psychosocial interruption.[4] In summary the lack of physical growth is secondary to the lack of emotional and sensory stimulation from the mother or care giver. Besides the obvious signs of malnutrition and delayed development, the child seems to have a characteristic posture or "body language." In one extreme the child is unpliable, stiff, and rigid. He is uncomforted by and unyielding to cuddling or holding and is very slow in smiling or socially responding to others.[19] The other extreme is the floppy infant, who is like a rag doll. Neither child molds to the holder's body, maintains sustained eye-to-eye contact, or shows signs of satisfaction or contentment when any caregiving procedures are done. Frequently there is a history of difficult feeding, vomiting, sleep disturbance, and excessive irritability.

Etiology

Failure to thrive may be caused by a number of organic disorders, including congenital heart defects, neurologic lesions, urinary tract infection, renal insufficiency, malabsorption syndrome, and endocrine dysfunction. In some instances severe malnutrition, such as kwashiorkor or marasmus (see pp. 476 and 477), may underly failure to grow. However, in about 10% of cases no organic basis can be found and maternal deprivation, which really should be called parent deprivation, is thought to be the cause. But complex physical, psychosocial, and emotional variables are involved in determining the reason for why the parenting is deficient to the point of emotional and physical starvation. Although the literature almost exclusively discusses characteristics of mothers of failure-to-thrive children, it must be remembered that every child has a biologic father and that in some way he may have contributed to the parent-child disturbance either by his presence or absence. Frequently the father is not discussed because he is a covert partner, whereas the mother is visibly present and identifiable. Fathers or significant other persons, who can be helped to be more emotionally, physically, and financially supportive to the family unit, can become the emotional reservoir needed by these mothers to give nurturance to their child.

Characteristics of families of failure-to-thrive children

Many theories have been suggested to explain the etiology of maternal deprivation. One of them, role theory, proposes that the mother is unable to fulfill her role as mother because of her conflicting needs as a child herself. The role of mothering is a learning process and does not begin at the time of the child's birth or conception. Development of mothering and nurturing is influenced by the mother's life experiences since her own birth. Frequently the mother of the failure-to-thrive child has herself been maternally deprived. She may have sufficient emotional resources to nurture a family, provided no additional stresses are superimposed. It is not unusual for a mother to have reared other offspring who show no overt signs of maternal deprivation and to bear a child who is more difficult to relate to and be unable to give anymore of herself to this infant. The personalities of infants can have definite effects on the mother-child attachment process.[20] Identifying such situations of disharmony between the mother's expectations of the real child vs the fantasy child may be one approach toward prevention of maternal deprivation syndrome.*

Another explanation concerns itself with the system of reciprocity, or the mutual regulation of clues between infant and parent. Normally the infant has distinct sets of behavior whereby he controls his attention to a particular situation. In essence he can turn on and off visually and attentively to the stimulation. For example, during an attention cycle there is initiation of prolonged sensory contact with an object. This is followed by an orientation to the object, which establishes an expected set of social responses. There is acceleration to a peak of excitement, followed by deceleration of attention and physically turning away, both of which comprise the nonattention cycle.[7] An example of such activity is the simple response of an infant to a human face. As a person approaches, the infant responds to the new stimuli with decreased motor activity and initiates visual contact with the other person. In response to the infant's attention, the person begins to smile, verbalize, make faces, and move closer. The infant reacts with heightened physical activity, interest, pleasure, and satisfaction. However, he then "turns off" the interaction by withdrawing active attention and finally by turning away and directing his focus elsewhere. The individual perceives this clue and either attempts to reengage the infant's attention with some other activity or also "turns off" and respects the infant's decision to be nonattentive.

This example comprises a set of synchornous behaviors. However, in situations of disturbed parent-child relationships there is often a lack of synchrony. Whether the infant or the parent is primarily responsible for faulty clues is similar to the unanswerable question of which came first—the chicken or the egg? Is the mother insensitive to behavioral clues of attention-nonattention and consequently bombards the infant with continuous stimulation, which he eventually responds to by "turning off" altogether? Or is the infant born stiff, rigid, or excessively flaccid and unable to demonstrate appropriate pleasure or satisfaction when the attention clues are met?

Probably the answer is neither of these extremes but a combination of both, which is further complicated by a family unit laden with various stressors. Frequently these families are under stress and in multiple chronic emotional, social, and financial crises. Often there is marital discord; if fathers or husbands are present, they usually give little emotional support to their wives. The mothers tend to lead lonely, solitary lives with few outside interests or friends who can relieve them of child-rearing responsibilities in times of heightened stress. Typically these mothers have difficulty in perceiving and assessing their infants' needs. For example, they cannot distinguish "cries" of hunger, pain, or general dissatisfaction. They are unaware of what to expect developmentally from their child at a particular age and, consequently, do not know how to stimulate or play with the infant. Attempts at social interaction usually result in an acute nonsynchronous set of behaviors. The mother's reaction to the child's dissatisfied response to care-giving activities or social play is frustration and anger, resulting in a vicious, destructive cycle.

Failure-to-thrive children are not limited to lower socio-

*For additional reading about the Neonatal Perception Inventory, a useful tool for measuring the parent's perceptual difference between the average child and their child, see Broussard, E., and Hartner, M.: Further considerations regarding maternal perception of the first born. In Helmuth, J., editor: Exceptional infant studies in abnormalities, vol. 2, New York, 1972, Brunner/Mazel, Inc.

economic groups. Although financial crisis generally means "poor," families with adequate monetary resources can be in chronic financial stress if their standard of living exceeds their income. Emotional deprivation, a kind of rejection, can also occur in financially stable homes where all child-rearing responsibilities are left to others. Although this is less visible and borders more on emotionally neglected children, such families can include children who are physically and emotionally starved. It is essential for nurses to set aside stereotypes and prejudices in order to be aware of the potential for existence of maternally deprived children in *any* family situation.

Nursing considerations—families as patients

Usually the physical and developmental retardation in failure-to-thrive children is so great that hospitalization is prescribed. In order to rule out any organic etiology, a battery of diagnostic tests is generally ordered. Distinguishing failure-to-thrive from emotional starvation is usually based on negative laboratory data and on physical/psychologic improvement without major intervention. Unfortunately many of these infants are subjected to needless examinations and procedures because the emotional assessment of the family is neglected in the initial plan of care. As a result valuable time is lost in helping the parents and child meet their own needs.

Nursing care of the family with failure-to-thrive children involves a systems approach. In other words, for the entire family to become healthy, each member must be helped to change. To nurture the child back to physical, developmental, and emotional help during his hospitalization, while neglecting the emotional needs of the parents, does not solve the problem. Therefore, the nursing care plan must include at least the child and mother and, if possible, significant others such as the father or husband.

Since part of the difficulty in reciprocity between mother and child was dissatisfaction and frustration for both, altering that pattern of behavior is essential. A consistent primary nurse for all three shifts with scheduled relief for days off is a priority. Only the same nurse caring for the child over a period of time can learn to perceive the child's cues and reverse the cycle of dissatisfaction. This often takes time, patience, understanding, and a willingness to wait for positive results. The general care of the child does not differ from that given to any infant, except that more time may be necessary for each activity, such as bathing and feeding. Since these children are not ill with any physical disorder but debilitated from general malnutrition, they should be placed in a room with noninfectious children of a similar age.

Besides attending to the physical needs of the child, the nurse must plan care for *appropriate* developmental stimulation. The word "appropriate" is emphasized because it refers to the child's developmental, not chronologic, age. Assessing the developmental age should be done on admission by administering the Denver Developmental Screening Test (DDST) or other psychometric test (p. 173). The DDST will give an approximate age for the child's present achievement in gross–fine motor, social-adaptive, and language skills. Only after objective measurements are available can a plan of care for stimulation be organized. Periodic testing is an excellent tool for evaluation of the child's developmental progress.

The following example illustrates the potential errors in caring for a failure-to-thrive infant and stresses adaptive measures for promoting physical and emotional health:

A 12-month-old girl was admitted to the pediatric unit with a chief complaint of malnutrition. She weighed 5 kg (11 pounds) and was emaciated, extremely lethargic, irritable, and rigid. She showed no interest in her surroundings, had no eye contact with other people, and was grossly developmentally retarded. She was also frail, tiny, and pathetic looking and engendered a positive emotional response from others caring for her. As a result she became a "favorite" patient among the nurses, was carried most of the time, and was literally inundated with dozens of toys, mobiles, and colorful, musical stimuli. However, despite negative findings for an organic cause of failure to thrive, she continued to not gain weight or improve developmentally. When her mother came to visit, she would sit in a chair in a corner of the room and watch television. The only time the child was also in the room was during her nap. At all other times she was at the nurses' station or the playroom. Since the mother made no attempt to talk to anyone or ask about her child's condition, she was ignored by the nursing staff. After 1 month's hospitalization, a conference was called to decide the disposition of the child. A clinical nurse specialist from another pediatric unit was asked to attend the conference.

After listening to the child's history and negative progress, the clinical specialist asked about the mother's background. Silence accompanied the only answering statement, "The mother doesn't care about the child. She comes here and watches television while we care for her child." The clinical specialist briefly discussed the dynamics of maternal deprivation and failure-to-thrive children and suggested that she visit the mother in her home and then have another conference to discuss alternatives to the child's and parent's care. Although there was some resistance to this suggestion, the staff agreed since the only decision they could reach was placement in a foster home, which would take time to arrange.

At the following conference the clinical specialist described her two visits to the mother's one-room apartment. This 20-year-old, unmarried woman lived alone with her daughter. She was unemployed and received minimal welfare support. She rarely saw the child's father, occasionally visited her mother, and had no friends. When asked about a usual day's activities, she stated, "Before the baby was hospitalized, I stayed home, slept, fed her, and watched TV. Now I have a place to go because I visit her in the hospital, but I am not needed. The nurses care so well for her." When asked about her feelings toward the child, she remarked, "Well, I didn't really want her, but I had her. I thought babies slept all the time, drank their bottle, and played with people. She just cries and fusses. Sometimes I feel like I could almost strangle her." At this point she started crying. When the nurse said she would like to return in a couple of days, the mother seemed surprised but agreed. During the second visit the mother talked more openly about her childhood, expressed a desire to be a better mother, and asked if she could talk to the nurse again.

The staff's reaction to this account of the home visits was one of mixed feelings. Some members openly expressed their doubt as to the mother's concern and love for her child. Others felt guilty for avoiding her and realized that they had alienated an already insecure, lonely, depressed woman. It was agreed that the following care plan would be implemented:

I. *Care of child*

A. Assign one nurse on each shift; assign consistent weekend relief only if the nurse can be a primary nurse assistant at least 2 days before actually caring for the child
B. Limit visitors (meaning other staff) at the discretion of all three primary nurses
C. Perform an initial DDST and base stimulation on the child's present developmental age
D. Perform physical care with as much holding, rocking, and cuddling as the child responds to; encourage eye-to-eye contact, tactile stimulation, and soft vocalization
E. Assign a "foster grandmother" to the child for 2 hours everyday, who will work with the nurse; use this time for care of the mother

II. *Care of mother*

A. Welcome the mother every time she visits; talk to her about her child's progress, but do not push her into caring for the child
B. Teach the mother about the child's physical care, developmental skills, and emotional needs through example and demonstration—not through lecturing; allow the mother to proceed at her own pace; encourage the foster grandmother to participate
C. Afford the mother the opportunity to talk about her life and feelings toward her child
D. Supply emotional nurturance without encouraging dependency; promote the mother's self-respect and confidence by praising her achievements with her child

With the guidance of the clinical specialist and several conferences to deal with their feelings toward the mother and their increasing attachment to the child, a successful plan of care was implemented during the next month. The child gained 3 kg (6.6 pounds), progressed from an initial developmental age of 4 months to an age of 7 months, and had formed a close interpersonal relationship with the nurse, foster grandmother, and, especially, her mother. The latter goal was probably the staff's most difficult task. As they became closer to the child they acutely realized that they must also separate from her and encourage the mother-child relationship. Before discharge a public health referral was made, the foster grandmother agreed to continue visiting the family at home, and outpatient hospital visits were arranged at times when the clinical specialist or primary staff nurse could visit. The care of this child and mother had only begun during the 2-month hospitalization.

The prognosis for failure to thrive is uncertain. The question of whether helping the mother learn new ways of relating to and caring for her child can permanently change behavior in conflict-laden, stressful situations always remains. It is well-known that emotional starvation early in life, particularly under 3 years of age, is psychologically destructive and traumatic for the child. Many of these children remain below normal in intellectual development and fail to learn acceptable social behavior. The most common emotional scar is their lasting inability to form trusting, meaningful relationships with other individuals. Many of the mothers continue to exhibit emotional detachment from their children and are unable to cope with their chronic state of crisis.[9] However, there are those families that can change, learn, and grow, but they cannot do it alone. Sensitive, well-planned, and coordinated care by nurses and other health professionals will help fill the emotional void that led to maternal deprivation.

SUDDEN INFANT DEATH SYNDROME (SIDS)

Sudden infant death syndrome, also referred to as crib death, is a leading cause of death among infants. In fact it is the number one cause of death in children between the ages of 2 weeks and 1 year and is second only to accidents in children under age 15 years. Sudden infant death syndrome outranks deaths from all types of congenital anomalies and kills more than twice the number of children who might die from cancer. It claims the lives of 8000 to 10,000 infants each year, or about two to three in every 1000 live births.[6] Although it is defined as "the sudden death of any infant or young child, which is unexpected by history, and in which a thorough postmortem examination fails to demonstrate an adequate cause for death," it is a definite disease entity that has positive pathologic findings on autopsy.[5]

Theories of etiology

Although SIDS is always unexpected and unexplained by usual pathologic mechanisms, there is conclusive evidence that an occluded airway was the cause of death. Two characteristics of almost every death are significant factors. One, the child is asleep, and, the other, the death is silent. The fact that the child could not cry out in distress supports the conclusion that the airway was blocked at the level of the vocal cords from laryngospasm. Other consistent pathologic findings on autopsy include intrathoracic petechiae on the surface of lungs, pericardium, and thymus; the areas of the thymus outside the thoracic cavity, mainly the cervical lobes, being impressively void of these petechiae; pulmonary congestion and edema; inflammatory infiltrates in the lung and upper airway; and areas of inflammation and fibrinoid necrosis in the vocal cords. In about one third of the cases viral agents have been isolated, but this may be more significantly related to the fact that a prior upper respiratory infection was present in almost half of the victims.

Besides these internal pathologic findings, several external manifestations are consistently found and tend to support the parents' initial belief that the child died from suffocation. The child is often found in a disheveled bed, with blankets over his head, and huddled into a corner. Frothy, blood-tinged fluid fills the mouth and nostrils, and the infant may be lying facedown in the secretions, suggesting that he bled to death. The diaper is usually wet and full of stool, which is consistent with a cataclysmic type of death. The hands may be clutching the sheets as if the child were in distress before he died. The initial appearance of the child combined with the shock of such an unexpected event adds to the horror and nightmare that the parents must face.

There are a plethora of theories regarding the etiology of SIDS. Presently the exact cause is unknown. Some of the theories of causation that have been investigated include suffocation from sleeping with a parent; suffocation from blankets, sheets, or other very unlikely objects; pneumonia; laryngeal inflammation; hypersensitivity to cow's milk (breast-feeding does not prevent SIDS); immunoglobulin abnormalities; parathyroid inadequacy; electrolyte imbalance, particularly magnesium; viral infection; hyperactive "dive" reflex; and sleep pathophysiology, especially prolonged apneic periods. The last theory has received notable attention by several investigators. One of the dilemmas that has been associated with the possibility of prolonged periods of apnea as the cause of SIDS is the use of respiratory monitors in the home. Although there may be some justified use of this in special cases of research on "near-miss' infants, it presents a tremendous burden for parents who view it as a means of prevention for the subsequent child. The psychologic damage from this type of home monitoring can be more devastating than the recurrent risk of SIDS.

Some factors appear to be shared by a majority of victims of SIDS. The two most prominent, which have been termed "eligibility factors," are age and sleep. The peak age for SIDS is between 10 and 12 weeks of age, over half of the deaths occur by age 3 months, and almost 90% occur before age 6 months. This syndrome is three to four times more common in prematurely born infants. All of the deaths occur during periods of sleep. Minor viral infections of the respiratory tract and low socioeconomic status are higher-than-average associated variables. Very important to consider are the associated genetic factors. SIDS is not a genetic or inherited disorder. Although there is a slightly higher chance for it to recur within the same family, for purposes of genetic counseling the increase is *not* significant. The recurrence risk is estimated to be approximately 2%. Some of the factors that might explain the increased risk include: (1) SIDS might be influenced by polygenic factors or the concept of an "unbalanced gene," such as one that might be responsible for prolonged apneic spells, (2) some cases of SIDS may represent familial diseases that at the present time appear to be sudden, unexplained events, and (3) environmental factors that may have influenced one child's death could also be present to increase the probability of a second child's fate from SIDS.

In summary the following facts about sudden infant death syndrome are known and must be shared with parents:

SIDS is a separate disease entity, similar to any other known and recognized disorder.
SIDS cannot be predicted or prevented.
SIDS is not contagious or hereditary.
SIDS can recur within the same family, but the chances of this happening are about the same as its happening in any other family for the first time.

Nursing considerations—crisis intervention

Loss of a child from SIDS represents several additional crises for the parents to cope with. In addition to the grief and mourning for the death of their child, the parents must face a tragedy that was extremely sudden, unexpected, and unexplained. The psychologic intervention for the family must deal with these additional variables. It is the purpose of the discussion of nursing considerations to stress primarily the objectives of care for families experiencing SIDS, rather than the process of grief and mourning, which is explored in Chapter 27.

One approach toward delineating the nursing care plan for these families is to base it on the usual sequence of events that occurs after the infant is found. This approach encompasses the different areas in which nurses will be involved with the family. Usually it is the mother who finds the child dead in the crib. Frequently she is alone and must deal with her initial shock, panic, and grief, questions of the other siblings, and the decision of where to find help. The first persons to arrive may be the police and ambulance attendants. Hopefully they will handle the situation by asking few questions, giving *no* indication of wrongdoing, abuse, or neglect, making sensitive judgments concerning the resuscitation efforts for the child, and comforting the members of the family as much as possible. The trend is toward public professional education of SIDS, particularly for those who arrive on the scene first. If properly informed, police should be able to recognize signs of SIDS, particularly to distinguish them from signs of abuse, and to tell parents that their child probably died from a disease called sudden infant death syndrome, which cannot be predicted or prevented. A compassionate, sensitive approach to the family during the very first few minutes can help spare them some of the overwhelming guilt and anguish that frequently follow this type of death.

Usually the first contact that nurses have with these families is in the emergency room. The infant must be seen by a physician in order to be pronounced dead. Usually there is no attempt at resuscitation. During the time in the emergency room, several aspects warrant special consideration. Parents should be asked only factual questions, such as when they found the infant, how he looked, and who they called for help. Any remarks that may suggest responsibility, such as why didn't they go in earlier, didn't they hear him cry out, was his head buried in a blanket, or were the other siblings jealous of this child, should be avoided. The events that took place when help arrived should be inquired about. If resuscitation was attempted, the infant may have fractured ribs, internal bleeding, and traumatic bruising, which can simulate physical abuse. Also, if statements were made that were misguided, such as, "This looks like suffocation," they can be corrected before parents harbor them in their minds as indications of their guilt. Since the diagnosis of SIDS can be definitely made on postmortem findings, autopsies of all suspected cases of SIDS should be performed. The nurse is an excellent person to initiate this request. This subject should be approached positively by stating that SIDS is suspected but that it is a disease that must have an autopsy for a positive diagnosis to be made. This is not the time for a lengthy discussion of SIDS, but emphasizing that it is common in young infants and that it cannot be predicted or prevented is essential.

Another very important aspects of compassionate care toward these parents is allowing them to say good-bye to their child. Remember that a happy, beautiful, living part of themselves has suddenly been snatched from them forever. Before they go into the examining room, any blood or emesis should be removed from the child, he should be covered partially with a sheet or blanket, and the room should be straightened up, especially if instruments or equipment was used. These are the parents' last moments with their child, and they should be as quiet, meaningful, peaceful, and undisturbed as possible. The child's belongings should be packaged for the parents to take home if they wish. Nothing involved in the care of these grief-stricken people is complicated, difficult, or time-consuming. It only involves being human.

When the parents return home, they are usually not free to grieve. They have questioning neighbors staring at them, frightened siblings wondering why everyone left so suddenly, relatives to call, and funeral arrangements to make. With this type of death there is no warning, preparation, or anticipatory grieving. And if no one suggested that this is SIDS, there is also nothing to tell others that explains this sudden tragedy. In addition police may come back "just to ask a few questions" or neighbors may begin gossiping about "that family." Tragically parents have been incarcerated for erroneous charges of child abuse and homicide and SIDS families have had to move to a new community to escape the destructive rumors and remarks from others. No matter what the particular events, every family should be visited by a competent, qualified professional as soon after the death as possible. In some states there is a plan to organize SIDS information and counseling programs. Under the statewide SIDS program, there would be an organized referral system, assuring that each family would be visited by a public health nurse almost immediately after the death. Part of this program may include a direct communication from the medical examiner, who on completion of the autopsy explains the results and some information about the diagnosis. A referral should also be made to the local Foundation of Sudden Infant Death. Printed material that contains excellent information about SIDS for parents is available from the national or local chapters.*

During the initial home visit one of the nursing objectives is to assess what the parents have been told, what they think happened, and how they have explained this to the other siblings. If parents have been told about SIDS, they may answer the questions factually and seem to understand and accept the diagnosis. Although this might be so, it is unusual for parents not to have second thoughts, doubts, and feelings of guilt. It may also be intellectualization, a type of denial that can be erroneously midjudged as positive coping. Pursuing the factual answer by asking about feelings or emotions may uncover repressed thoughts that, when once said aloud, can be dealt with.

The nurse cannot deal with all the issues relating to the child's death in one visit. During the initial visit the nurse may be doing most of the talking, as the parents are helped to gain in intellectual understanding of the disease. If the visit is made within a day or two of the death, the parents are in the impact phase of crisis, in which their thinking abilities are disorganized and distracted. It is difficult for them to deal with the crisis in concrete terms, especially in exploring problem-solving approaches. During the turmoil phase, which is usually the first week following the death, there is more structure of thinking, although it is global rather than specific. During this phase the goal is to help the parents bring their feelings out into the open. This may require "precipitating" emotions by asking about crying and feeling sad, angry, or guilty. It is an attempt to provoke a display of emotion, not just an admission of a feeling. During this session the parents should be helped to explore their usual coping mechanisms and, if these are ineffectual, to investigate new approaches. It may be a time when parents are making rash decisions such as moving away to avoid questions or deciding never to have another child. This is not the time to decide these issues rationally and logically but rather to acknowledge that they are unable to deal with them. Because questions like these do arise and must be answered eventually, the number of visits and plan for intervention must be flexible. The siblings may initially appear accepting of the explanation and well-adjusted but may later refuse to go to sleep or ask questions about graves or funerals, indicating their need for further help in dealing with their sibling's death. Parents will face the question of a sub-

*Pamphlets available include *The Sudden Infant Death Syndrome,* (DHEW publication no. [HSA] 75-5137), *The Subsequent Child,* and *Facts about SIDS.*

sequent child and wonder if they could ever survive another tragedy as this. If another pregnancy occurs before both parents are ready, they are forced to deal with an additional crisis before resolution of the first. One of the dangers of having another child soon after the other's death is that this infant may become a replacement child. Sometimes this is so overt that the child is given his dead sibling's name and never allowed to express his individuality. Even when parents are well-prepared for the birth of the subsequent child, they will have doubts concerning his well-being, will be overprotective, especially near the age of the other infant's death, and will need support that these behaviors are normal.

Since the mourning process takes at least a year for completion of acceptance and social reorganization, nurses should periodically call on the family to evaluate their progress. Many families receive much solace and support from talking to other parents who have lost a child from SIDS. Parent groups have been formed throughout the United States and can be contacted through the national or local chapters of the Foundation of Sudden Infant Death.

INFANTILE AUTISM

Psychopathology is much less frequent in children than in adults. It is usually characterized by disturbances in the following areas: relationship with the social environment, use of speech for social expression and communication, developing a sense of personal identity, use of affect, and total integration and organization of personality. Autism, the earliest form of psychosis in children, occurs in about four to five children per 10,000 and is more common in males than in females, from 2:1 to 4:1.[2] It is differentiated from childhood schizophrenia in several aspects. Autistic children exhibit bizarre, deviant behavior almost from birth. Schizophrenic children develop psychotic behavior after a period of normal development. Usually the term schizophrenia is used to denote the occurrence of psychosis after 3 years of age. Also family history of schizophrenia is very common, whereas recurrence of autism among siblings or other relatives is unusual. The behavioral characteristics of both differ markedly. Autistic infants are dramatically cold, detached, and unemotional toward their parents. Schizophrenic children are typically clinging, dependent infants, who are excessively attached to their mothers. Autistic children fail to manifest the delusional and hallucinatory phenomena of schizophrenia, whereas schizophrenic children seldom demonstrate the bizarre language peculiarities and intense preoccupation with sameness that characterize autism.

Characteristics of autistic children[25]

The most prominent characteristics of infantile autism are the child's extreme interpersonal isolation and intense, abnormal concern for preservation of sameness. Autistic infants may appear undemanding, placid, and easy to care for. Their social development is retarded to the point that there is no advancement from the typical behavior of a 1-month-old child. They fail to develop a smiling response to others or the usual anticipatory movements, such as putting their arms out to be picked up, which signify their interest in their social environment. They are unyielding to cuddling and holding and fail to show any signs of satisfaction or pleasure in tactile contact. They have a blank, detached look in their eyes and do not respond to verbal stimulation, which may lead others to suspect deafness. Most notably, they fail to demonstrate the usual 6- to 8-month stranger anxiety and fear of separation from mother. In fact they have no difficulty in tolerating separation and seem unaware of the parent's absence. Autistic children are content to be left alone and provide no satisfaction or feedback to the parent or care giver for any type of nurturing.

In sharp contrast to their detachment from social interaction is their intense preoccupation with the preservation of sameness and their attachment to mechanical objects. Typically during their second year they become engrossed in odd repetitive behaviors, such as flicking a light switch on and off, passing a toy back and forth from one hand to other, or walking around a room feeling the walls. If they are interrupted while engaged in these activities or if their environment is disturbed, such as if the crib is moved even a few inches, they will react with a violent temper tantrum. Other self-stimulatory behaviors include rocking, whirling, flapping of arms, or flicking of hands and fingers before their eyes while staring at bright lights.

These behavioral disturbances may go unnoticed during the first year or two. For one thing, none of these activities is unusual for infants or toddlers when present in moderation. For example, one of the tools and tasks for infancy is autistic invention, which is defined as "a primary unsocialized state of symbol activity which makes the infant feel that he is master of all he surveys."[24] Toddlers are known to be ritualistic and negativistic. The well-known security-blanket syndrome is hardly abnormal. But for autistic children, attachment to mechanical devices or material objects is to the exclusion of social interaction or attachment. In addition they may exhibit above-average motor behavior for their age, be unusually graceful and agile in their movements, and demonstrate superior skill in visual-motor tasks, such as jigsaw puzzles. Although they may perform poorly on standard intelligence tests, many of them display superior memory, motor coordination, and spatial abilities. Certain features of autism also characterize blind, deaf, and retarded children, but autistic children rarely have sensory impairments.

Recognition of autism usually follows the appearance of the typical language and communication defects of this disorder, such as echolalia, or parrot speech—the automatic repetition of words spoken to them; pronominal reversal—the tendency to use "you" for "I" and the striking absence of the first person to refer to oneself; and literal concrete use of words, such as "in" to mean "door." Although their phonation and articulation of sounds are clear, their highly individualized and specialized speech makes communication with others almost impossible.

Origins of infantile autism

The precise origin of autism is still an unsolved question. Some authorities believe that there is a psychogenetic basis for autism, which has its pathology in the mother-child relationship. It is true that family histories may reveal an emotionally cold, detached, aloof mother who has difficulty in expressing a warm nurturing affect toward her child. But could this defective attachment be a result of the child's impersonal, unresponsive, apathetic attitude toward his social environment? Many parents of autistic children raise other well-adjusted offspring who demonstrate no emotional or psychotic disturbance. Biogenetic theorists view autism as an inborn cognitive and perceptual defect that leads to the secondary social disturbances. Recently biochemical differences that may account for the deviant behavior and for the usually poor prognosis even with intensive therapeutic intervention have been found in these children.

Another point to consider in the genesis of autism is its differences from the maternal deprivation syndrome or the failure-to-thrive child. For one thing, the failure-to-thrive child rarely exhibits the typical bizarre behaviors of the autistic child and usually demonstrates gross physical and developmental retardation. Although the social isolation and unresponsiveness may initially resemble the autistic type of interpersonal detachment, this dramatically changes under conditions of optimum physical and emotional care. Perhaps most important is that the degree of maternal deprivation that results in a child's failure to thrive is many times greater than the cold, aloof mother's reserve of affection for her child.

Nursing considerations

Therapeutic intervention for the autistic child is a specialized area of nursing. Several approaches, such as use of the therapeutic one-to-one relationship, play therapy, and behavioral modification, have been attempted and advocated.[16,23,28] In all instances the objective is to increase social awareness of others, teach verbal communication, and decrease unacceptable behavior. Unfortunately the long-range success of intervention has been disappointing. Autism, like so many other chronic conditions, becomes a "family disease." The psychogenetic theory is well-known and greatly multiplies the parents' guilt. Stressing what is known about the disorder from a biologic standpoint as well as how little is known, can help lessen guilt and shame. When one carefully questions parents about the infant's very early behavior, there is evidence of autistic tendencies before significant parental or environment factors could have negatively influenced the child.

When these children are hospitalized they usually present many management problems for nurses. Decreasing stimulation by using a private or semiprivate room, avoiding extraneous auditory and visual distraction, and encouraging parents to bring in possessions the child is attached to may lessen the disruptiveness of hospitalization. Since physical contact frequently upsets these children, minimal holding and physical care may be necessary to prevent temper tantrums. A thorough assessment of the child's usual routine and activities helps maintain an environment that is manageable and conducive to physical recovery.

REFERENCES

1. American Academy of Pediatrics, Committee on Nutrition: Iron supplementation for infants, Pediatrics **58**(5):765, November 1976.
2. Aug, R., and Ables, B.: A clinicians's guide to childhood psychosis, Pediatrics **47**(2):327-338, 1971.
3. Bachmann, K., and Dees, S. C.: Milk allergy. II. Observations on incidence and symptoms of allergy and milk in allergic children, Pediatrics **20**:400, 1957.
4. Barbero, G.: Failure to thrive. In Klaus, M., and associates: Maternal attachment and mothering disorders, New York, 1974, Johnson & Johnson, Baby Products Co.
5. Beckwith, J.: Discussion of terminology and definition of sudden infant death syndrome. In Bergman, A., and associates, editors: Proceedings of the Second International Conference on Causes of Sudden Death in Infants, Seattle, 1970, University of Washington Press.
6. Bergman, A.: Sudden infant death, Nurs. Outlook **20**(12): 777, December 1972.
7. Brazelton, T., and associates: The origins of reciprocity: the early mother-infant interaction. In Lewis, M., and Rosenblum, L., editors: The effect of the infant on its caregiver, New York, 1974, John Wiley & Sons, Inc.
8. Brigety, R., and Pearson, H.: Effects of dietary and iron supplementation on hematocrit levels of preschool children, J. Pediatr. **76**:759, 1970.
9. Elmer, E., and associates: Late results of failure-to-thrive syndrome, Clin. Pediatr. **8**:584-589, October 1969.
10. Frazier, C.: You can't always win! (a dialogue on allergy and nutrition), Pediatr. Basics **13**:12-14, March/April 1975.
11. Karzon, D.: Smallpox vaccination in the U.S.: the end of an era, J. Pediatr. **81**(3):600-608, September 1972.
12. Lubs, M.: Empiric risks for genetic counseling in families with allergy, J. Pediatr. **80**(1):26-31, January 1972.
13. Michelsen, O.: Evaluating the role of fiber in our diet, Pediatr. Basics **16**:4-7, September/October 1976.
14. Norins, A.: Atopic dermatitis, Pediatr. Clin. North Am. **18**(3):801-837, 1971.
15. Oski, F., and Barness, L.: Vitamin E deficiency: a previously unrecognized cause of hemolytic anemia in the premature infant, J. Pediatr. **70**(2):211-220, February 1967.
16. Pothier, P.: Individual therapy with a mute autistic child. In Fagin, C., editor: Readings in child and adolescent psychiatric nursing, St. Louis, 1974, The C. V. Mosby Co.

17. Protein Advisory Group of the United Nations System: PAG statement of low lactose activity and milk intake, State No. 17, February 2, 1972.
18. Rapp, D.: Sneezing, wheezing and scratching, New York, 1974, Erie County Department of Health, Office of Public Health Information and Education.
19. Rhymes, J.: Working with mothers and babies who fail to thrive, Am. J. Nurs. **66**(9):1972-1976, September 1966.
20. Robson, K., and Moss, A.: Patterns and determinants of maternal attachment, J. Pediatr. **77:**976-985, December 1970.
21. Ross Conference: Iron nutrition in infancy, sixty-second Conference on Pediatric Research, Columbus, Ohio, 1970, Ross Laboratories.
22. Smith, C.: Blood diseases of infancy and childhood, St. Louis, 1972, The C. V. Mosby Co.
23. Spurgeon, R.: Nursing the autistic child. In Fagin, C., editor: Readings in child and adolescent psychiatric nursing, St. Louis, 1974, The C. V. Mosby Co.
24. Sullivan, H.: Conceptions of modern psychiatry, New York, 1953, W. W. Norton & Co., Inc.
25. Tanguay, P.: A pediatrician's guide to the recognition and initial management of early infantile autism, Pediatrics **51**(5): 903-910, 1973.
26. Webb, T., and Oski, F.: Iron deficiency anemia and scholastics achievement in young adolescents, J. Pediatr. **82**(5):827-830, May 1973.
27. Widmann, F.: Goodale's clinical interpretation of laboratory tests, Philadelphia, 1973, F. A. Davis Co.
28. Wolf, M., editor: Application of operant conditioning procedures to the behavior problems of an autistic child. In Ulrich, R., and associates, editors: Control of human behavior, Glenview, Ill., 1966, Scott, Foresman and Co.

BIBLIOGRAPHY

Aab, C.: Assessment of maternal behavior during early mother-infant interaction. In Brandt, P. A., Chinn, P. L., and Smith, M. E., editors: practice in pediatric nursing, vol. 1, St. Louis, 1976, The C. V. Mosby Co.

Aguilera, D. C., and Messick, J. M.: Crisis intervention: theory and methodology, ed. 3, St. Louis, 1978, The C. V. Mosby Co.

Amendt, M.: Malabsorption syndromes in infancy and childhood. Part I, J. Pediatr. **81**(4):685-695, October 1972.

American Academy of Pediatrics, Committee on Infant and Preschool Child: Home monitoring for sudden infant death, Pediatrics **55:**144, 1975.

American Academy of Pediatrics, Committee on Nutrition: Childhood diet and coronary heart disease, Pediatrics **49:**305-307, 1972.

American Academy of Pediatrics, Committee to Review the Ten-State Nutrition Survey: The ten-state nutrition survey: a pediatric perspective, Pediatrics **51:**1095-1099, 1973.

Atherton, H.: Rejection . . . the deadliest poison, Pediatr. Basics **12:**11-14, 1975.

Barnard, K.: The acquaintance process. In Klaus, M., and associates, editors: Maternal attachment and mothering disorders, N.J., 1974, Johnson & Johnson, Baby Products Co.

Barnett, H. L.: Pediatrics, ed. 14, New York, 1968, Appleton-Century-Crofts.

Beale, M. G., and associates: Vitamin D.: the discovery of its metabolites and their therapeutic applications, Pediatrics **57**(5): 729, May 1976.

Bergman, A. B.: The apnea monitor business, Pediatrics **56**(1): 1-2, July 1975.

Bergman, A. B., and associates: The psychiatric toll of sudden infant death syndrome, GP **40**(6):99-105, December 1969.

Carman, D. D.: Infant and childhood obesity: guidelines for prevention and treatment, Pediatr. Nurs. **2**(6):33-40, November/December 1976.

Child nutrition programs, Dairy Council Digest **45**(1):1-5, January/February 1974.

Clark, A.: Recognizing discord between mother and child and changing it to harmony, Am. J. Maternal Child Nurs. **1**(2):100-106, March/April 1976.

Clark A., and Affonso, D.: Infant behavior and maternal attachment: two sides of the coin, Am. J. Maternal Child Nurs. **1**(2): 94-99, March/April 1976.

Cohen, D. J., and Caparulo, B.: Childhood autism, Child. Today **4**(4):2-6, July/August 1975.

Conrad, M.: A primer on iron metabolism. In Crosby, W., editor: Iron: a total clinical learning experience, New York, 1972, Medcom Press.

Crosby, W., editor: Iron: a total clinical learning experience, New York, 1972, Medcom Press.

Current concepts in infant nutrition, Dairy Council Digest **47**(2): 7-12, March/April 1976.

Dawson, A.: Survey: SIDS research and counseling, Am. J. Nurs. **76**(10):1602-1603, October 1976.

De Angelis, C.: Basic pediatrics for the primary health care provider, Boston, 1975, Little, Brown and Co.

Downing, S. E., and Cee, J. C.: Laryngeal chemosensitivity: a possible mechanism for sudden infant death, Pediatrics **55**(5): 640, May 1975.

Easson, W.: Symptomatic autism in childhood and adolescence, Pediatrics **47**(4):717-722, 1971.

Erickson, M.: Assessment and management of developmental changes in children, St. Louis, 1976, The C. V. Mosby Co.

Essoka, G., and associates: Pediatric nursing continuing education review, ed. 1, New York, 1975, Medical Examination Publishing Co., Inc.

Facts from FDA, U.S. Department of Health, Education, and Welfare, Pub. no. (FDA) 73-2042.

Fagin, C. M., editor: Nursing in child psychiatry, St. Louis, 1972, The C. V. Mosby Co.

Fasler, J., and Bryant, N.: Disturbed children under reduced auditory input: a pilot study, Except. Child. **38**(3):197-204, 1971.

Ferster, C.: The autistic child, Psychol. Today **2**(6):34, November 1968.

Filer, L. J.: The case for iron supplements in infant feeding regimens, Hosp. Pract. **6**(6):79-92, June 1971.

Fraiberg, S.: Billy: psychological intervention for a failure-to-thrive infant. In Klaus, M., and associates, editors: Maternal attachment and mothering disorders, N.J., 1974, Johnson & Johnson, Baby Products Co.

Functions and interrelationships of vitamins, Dairy Council Digest **43:**5, September/October 1972.

Goth, A.: Medical pharmacology: principles and concepts, ed. 9, St. Louis, 1978, The C. V. Mosby Co.

Gottsacker, J.: Maternal attachment in relation to failure to thrive.

In Brandt, P. A., Chinn, P. L., and Smith, M. E., editors: Current practice in pediatric nursing, vol. 1, St. Louis, 1976, The C. V. Mosby Co.

Graziano, A.: A group treatment approach to multiple problem behaviors of autistic children, Except. Child. **36**(10):765-770, 1970.

Guyton, A. C.: Textbook of medical physiology, ed. 4, Philadelphia, 1971, W. B. Saunders Co.

Hagan, J. M.: Infant death: nursing interaction and intervention with grieving families, Nurs. Forum **13**(4):372-385, 1974.

Hall, J., and Weaver, B.: Nursing of families in crisis, Philadelphia, 1974, J. B. Lippincott Co.

Hardgrove, C., and Warrick, L.: How shall we tell the children, Am. J. Nurs. **74**(3):448-450, March 1974.

Harrison, L.: Nursing intervention with the failure-to-thrive family, Am. J. Maternal Child Nurs. **1**(2):111-116, March/April 1976.

Herman, S. P., and Burgert, E. D.: Anemia and growth failure, Clin. Pediatr. **15**(10):962, October 1976.

Hughes, J. G.: Synopsis of pediatrics, ed. 4, St. Louis, 1975, The C. V. Mosby Co.

Infant nutrition: feeding the infant . . . building the man, New York, 1972, Medcom Press.

Knobloch, H., and Pasamanick, B.: Some etiologic and prognostic factors in early infantile autism and psychosis, Pediatrics **55**(2):182, February 1975.

Lewman, L.: SIDS: Oregon's model system: a statewide approach, Pediatr. Ann. **3:**11, November 1974.

Lloyd-Still, J., and associates: Intellectual development after severe malnutrition in infancy, Pediatrics **54:**306-311, 1974.

Malnutrition, learning, and behavior, Dairy Council Digest **44**(6): 31-34, November/December 1973.

Mandell, F., and Wolfe, L. C.: Sudden infant death syndrome and subsequent pregnancy, Pediatrics **56**(5):774-776, November 1975.

Marx, J.: Crib death: some promising leads but no solution yet, Science **189**(4200):367-369, August 1, 1975.

Mondale, W.: SIDS: The government's role, Pediatr. Ann. **3:**11, November 1974.

Murphy, M.: The crying infant, Pediatr. Nurs. **1:**15-17, January/February 1975.

Nakushian, J.: Restoring parents' equilibrium after sudden infant death, Am. J. Nurs. **76**(10):1600-1604, October 1976.

Patterson, K., and Pomeroy, M.: Sudden infant death syndrome, Nursing '74 **4**(5):85-88, May 1974.

Pipes, P. L.: Nutrition in infancy and childhood, St. Louis, 1977, The C. V. Mosby Co.

Purvis, G.: What nutrients do our infants really get? Nutr. Today **8**(5):28-34, September/October 1973.

Rapp, D.: Sneezing, wheezing, and scratching, New York, 1974, Erie County Department of Health, Office of Public Information and Education.

Ray, C., and associates: SIDS: an analysis of the problem, Pediatr. Ann. **3:**11, November 1974.

Reddy, V., and Pershad, J.: Lactase deficiency in Indians, Am. J. Clin. Nutr. **25:**114-119, 1972.

Ritvo, E., and Ornitz, E.: A new look at childhood autism points to CNS disease. In Roche Laboratories Report: Frontiers of hospital psychiatry, Nutley, N.J., November 1970, Roche Laboratories.

Rivlin, R.: Therapy of obesity and hormones, N. Engl. J. Med. **299:**26-29, 1975.

Roper, K., and associates: Failure to thrive: an opportunity for innovative nursing, Pediatr. Nurs. **2**(5):43-45, Sepbember/October 1976.

Rowell, P. A.: Infantile colic: reviewing the situation, Pediatr. Nurs. **4**(3):20-21, May/June 1978.

Salk, L.: Sudden infant death: impact on family and physician, Clin. Pediatr. **10**(5):248-249, May 1971.

Sampson, P.: Until crib death problem is solved, victim's parents need more help, J.A.M.A. **226**(11):1291-1300, December 10, 1973.

Sanders, H.: Allergy: a protective mechanism out of control, Chem. Engineering News **48:**20, May 11, 1970.

Shenker, I., and associates: Weight differences between foster infants of overweight and nonoverweight foster mothers, J. Pediatr. **84:**715-718, May 1974.

Stegink, L.: Current concepts of protein digestion and absorption, Pediatr. Basics **15:**9-13, July/August 1976.

Steinschneider, A.: Prolonged apnea and the sudden infant death syndrome: clinical and laboratory observations, Pediatrics **50**(4):646-653, 1972.

Steinschneider, J.: Nasopharyngitis and prolonged sleep apnea, Pediatrics **56**(6):967-971, December 1975.

Szybist, C.: SIDS: a parent's perspective, Pediatr. Ann. **3:**11, November 1974.

Tonkin, S.: Sudden infant death syndrome: hypothesis of causation, Pediatrics **55**(5):650, May 1975.

Vitamin E—miracle or myth? DHEW Pub. no. (FDA) 74-2004, FDA Consumer, July/August, 1973.

Williams, S. R.: Nutrition and diet therapy, ed. 3, St. Louis, 1977, The C. V. Mosby Co.

Wilson, P.: Iron-deficiency anemia, Am. J. Nurs. **72**(3):502-504, March 1972.

Wollerstein, R.: Iron deficiency in children. In Crosby, W., editor: Iron: a total clinical learning experience, New York, 1972, Medcom Press.

UNIT SIX
Early childhood

Early childhood comprises the period of toddlerhood and the preschool years. It is primarily a period of physical development and refinement, attainment of social skills, and achievement of independent behavior. Dramatic changes occur in the child as he leaves the dependent world of infancy and readies himself for the self-sufficient life of a school-age child. Chapters 14 and 15, *The Toddler Years* and *The Preschool Years,* are concerned with the biologic growth and psychologic development of the toddler and preschooler. Emphasis is placed on promoting optimum development during each phase of early childhood, especially through anticipatory guidance regarding nutrition, achievement of self-care activities, prevention of accidental injury, and specific parental concerns.

Chapter 16, *Health Problems of Early Childhood,* deals with health problems that commonly occur during early childhood. Although many of the disorders that occur during this period are caused by infectious processes, most of the child's care is implemented in the home, necessitating nursing guidance rather than direct intervention. The other conditions discussed are results of environmental and social factors to which toddlers and preschoolers are especially vulnerable or by which they are greatly influenced. In each of these health problems, emphasis is placed on prevention, recognition, and nursing interventions that return the child to an optimum physical and mental status following recovery.

14

The toddler years

The "terrible twos" has often been used to describe the toddler years, a period of age 12 months to the completion of 2 years of age. It is a time of intense exploration of the environment as the child attempts to find out how things work, what the word "no" means, and how to control others with temper tantrums, negativism, and obstinacy. The phrase "he gets into everything" underestimates the toddler's voracity for adventure, but the very adventure of getting into things is his means of acquisition of learning and knowledge. Although this can be a difficult time for parents and child as each learns to know the other better, it is also an extremely important period for developmental achievement and intellectual growth. Successful mastery of the tasks of this age requires a strong foundation of trust during infancy and frequently necessitates guidance from others when parent and toddler face the struggles of toilet training, limit setting and discipline, and sibling rivalry. Nurses who understand the dynamics of growth and development of the toddler can help parents deal effectively with the tasks of this age.

GROWTH AND DEVELOPMENT

Developmental tasks

The toddler is faced with the mastery of several important tasks. If the need for basic trust has been satisfied, he is ready to give up dependence for control, independence, and autonomy. Some of the specific tasks to be dealt with include differentiation of himself from others, particularly the mother; toleration of separation from mother or parent; ability to withstand delayed gratification; control over bodily functions; acquisition of socially acceptable behavior; verbal means of communication; and ability to interact with others in a less egocentric, autistic manner. Mastery of these goals is only begun during late infancy and toddler years, and such tasks as developing interpersonal relationships with others may not be completed until adolescence. However, crucial foundations for successful completion of such developmental tasks is laid during these early formative years.

Conceptually the needs and tasks of this age-group can be studied by discussing the theories of Maslow, Freud, Erikson, and Piaget to establish a continuum of developmental trends from infancy to adolescence. Chapter 12 discusses each of these theories during the developmental phase of infancy. As will be seen, the toddler period builds on previously acquired needs and completion of tasks. For example, in Maslow's hierarchy of basic human needs, the infant was most dependent on physiologic needs, physical safety, and affection. The toddler is also dependent on such levels being satisfied for him, but he now has the need for *self-esteem*—the desire to feel important, in control, competent, and, in his own way, respected. This is very closely associated with Erikson's developmental task of acquiring a sense of *autonomy* while overcoming a sense of doubt and shame. As the infant gains trust in the predictability and reliability of his parents, his environment, and his interaction with others, he begins to discover that his behavior is his own and that how he demonstrates his behavior has a predictable, reliable effect on others. However, while he realizes his will and control over others, he is confronted with the conflict of exerting his autonomy and relinquishing his much enjoyed dependence on others. Exerting his will has definite negative consequences, whereas retaining dependent, submissive behavior is generally rewarded with affection and approval. However, continued dependency creates a sense of doubt regarding his potential capacity to control his actions. This doubt is compounded by a sense of shame for feeling this urge to revolt against others' will and a fear that he will exceed his own capacity for manipulating his environment. The latter fear is a basis for instituting limit setting and consistent discipline at this age. Without appropriate limits on what is acceptable vs nonacceptable behavior, the child has no guidelines for establishing the end points of his ability to control. This is the essence of behavior modification. A set of conditioned responses is established for certain behaviors and is consistently applied to either reinforce or extinguish the behavior. A typical example of the need for limit setting during the toddler period is bedtime. Toddlers frequently resist going to bed and learn to employ various techniques to prolong the inevitable, such as asking for a drink, initiating a play activity, or crying at the initial attempt to get undressed for bed. If parents give in to these procrastination behaviors, they are reinforcing the toddler's ability to delay bedtime. This usually results in a tired, cranky child and angry, frustrated parents. However, a different set of responses to this bedtime pattern can establish reasonable limits that benefit both child and parents. For example, a schedule of quiet activity before the usual hour of retiring, dressing for bed followed by a drink, and then going to bed reinforces these behaviors and eventually extinguishes other undesirable behaviors such as crying or screaming.

The toddler's ability to control his environment is greatly enhanced by his increased gross motor skills and energy. For example, to return to the previous discussion of limit setting and bedtime ritual, the action of "being put to bed" is complicated by the toddler's ability to climb out of the crib or bed. Therefore, an additional action of locking the door may be the control necessary to reinforce the bedtime routine. As a precautionary measure in case of fire, the door should be unlocked after the child is asleep.

Just as the infant has the social modalities of grasping and biting, the toddler has the newly gained modality of holding on and letting go. To hold on and let go is evident with the use of the hands, mouth, eyes, and, eventually, the sphincters, when toilet training is begun. These social modalities are expressed constantly in the child's play activities, such as casting or throwing objects away, taking objects out of boxes, drawers, or cabinets, holding on tighter when someone says, "No, don't touch," and spitting out food as taste preferences become very strong. Control is also evident in his ability to voluntarily release objects on command. For example, by ages 12 to 14 months the child obeys the command, "Give it to me." Play also demonstrates the child's constant conflicts of expressing his autonomy while desiring dependency. The almost incessant response of "no" to commands he may want to obey is proof of his struggle to express his will. Emotions become very strongly expressed, usually in rapid mood swings. One minute the toddler can be engrossed in an activity, and the next minute he might be violently angry because he was unable to manipulate a toy or open a door. If scolded for doing something wrong, he can have a temper tantrum and almost instantaneously pull at his mother's legs to be picked up and comforted. Often these swift changes are difficult for parents to understand and cope with. Many parents find the negativism exasperating and, instead of dealing with it, give into it, which further threatens the child in his search for learning acceptable methods of interacting with others. As Erikson has stated, a parent's firmness and ability to reasonably set limits "must protect (the child) against the potential anarchy of his yet untrained sense of discrimination, his inability to hold on and to let go with circumspection."[5]

Paralleling the child's expression of his will is his increasing awareness of others' differences in tolerating those expressions. Father frequently becomes a target for the toddler's greater freedom of expressing his independence. Fathers are equally caught in a bind because they want to show more attention to the child when they are home and the child interprets this heightened attention as approval of his ability to manipulate others. If parents cannot agree on a mutual plan of managing this behavior, marital discord can become an additional problem.

The birth of a new sibling has special significance for the toddler in his quest for autonomy. In his experimentation with the degree of environmental manipulation he can control, he is suddenly faced with an intruder who totally upsets his routine, and maintenance of a ritualistic environment is as important as his manipulation of that environment. His conflict for self-assertion while retaining dependency is further complicated by his renewed desire for dependency with his mother, who is sharing her attention and affection with a second person. He resents the change in his usual pattern of events and social interactions, rather than the new infant, because other children only have significance in as far as they meet his needs.

Erikson focuses on the development of the *ego* during this phase of psychosocial development. There is a struggle as the child deals with the impulses of id and attempts to tolerate frustration and learns socially acceptable ways of interacting with the environment. The ego, which may be thought of as reason or common sense, is evident as the child is able to tolerate delayed gratification. It operates on the "reality principle," whereas the id operates on the "pleasure principle." There is also rudimentary beginning of the superego or conscience, which is the incorporation of the morals of society and the process of acculturation. With the development of the ego the child further differentiates himself from others and expands his sense of trust within himself. But as he begins to develop awareness of his own will and capacity to achieve, he also becomes aware of his ability to fail. This ever-present awareness of potential failure creates fear of doubt and shame. Successful mastery of the task of autonomy necessitates opportunities for self-mastery while withstanding the frustration of necessary limit setting and delayed gratification. Opportunities for self-mastery are present in appropriate play activities, toilet training, the crisis of sibling rivalry, and successful interactions with significant others.

Freud's *anal stage* roughly corresponds with Erikson's stage of autonomy, or the period from 18 months to 3 years of age. Within this psychosexual framework the anal zone becomes the center of the child's physical, emotional, and psychologic efforts. Pleasure comes from moving his bowels, but the child is also met with the conflict of gaining physical satisfaction from involuntary evacuation vs gaining emotional reinforcement by holding on and letting go at mother's will. The process of toilet training is regarded as the resolution of this conflict. It is theorized that difficulties with the mastery of voluntary toileting result in an "anal personality." If the cleanliness aspect of toileting is overemphasized, the child may become obsessively clean and neat or defiantly slovenly and untidy. The person may also be compulsively rigid, precise, and inflexible. If the gift-giving aspect of toileting is exaggerated, that is, the idea that the feces or urine is a gift to the parent, the child may equate love with bestowal of material objects or hoard his possessions as he retained his feces as a method of control. Evidences of "oral" or "anal" personalities are evident in most individuals, and the exact relationship of toilet training on future personality development is unclear. However, it is obvious that control of bodily functions is an important component in the acquisition of autonomy.

Biologic development

Biologic development and maturation of body systems is less dramatic during early childhood than during infancy. A brief summary of the significant changes is presented.

The physical growth and developmental achievements are not as dramatic during the toddler years as during infancy. Growth slows considerably. The usual 198 g (7 ounces) per week weight gain during early infancy is now decreased to about 198 g (7 ounces) per month, or an average weight gain of 1.8 to 2.7 kg (4 to 6 pounds) per year. The birth weight is quadrupled by 2½ years of age. The rate of increase in height also slows. During infancy the usual increase is to about one and one half times the birth length, or an increase of 25.4 cm (10 inches) for a birth length of 50.8 cm (20 inches). During the next 7 years the usual increment is an addition of 7.5 cm (3 inches) per year, then 5.0 cm (2 inches) per year until the pubertal growth spurt. Birth length generally takes 4 years to be doubled, in contrast to birth weight, which takes 6 months. In general, adult height is about twice the child's height at 2 years of age. Adult males tend to be slightly taller than this estimate and adult females slightly shorter. Accurate measurement of height and weight during the toddler years should reveal a steady growth curve but one that is more steplike in nature rather than straight. This is characteristic of the growth spurts during the early childhood years. In general, growth should be evaluated more in terms of conformity with the child's established patterns of weight and height gain during infancy than according to prescribed norms for each age period. For example, it is more important for the child to retain his usual level of growth as determined by percentiles than to gain 2 or 3 kg per year.

Head circumference slows somewhat by the end of infancy and is usually equal to the chest circumference by 1 to 2 years of age. The usual increase in head circumference during infancy is approximately 10 cm (4 inches) and during the second year is only 2.5 cm (1 inch). It continues to decrease until at age 5 years the increase is less than 1.25 cm (0.5 inch) per year. At the end of the sixth year the head has reached 90% of its eventual size. The anterior fontanel closes between the twelfth and eighteenth months of life. Chest circumference continues to increase in size and exceeds head circumference during the toddler years. Its shape also changes as the transverse or lateral diameter exceeds the anteroposterior diameter. Abdominal circumference is usually equal to or slightly larger than that of the chest and is prominent in infants. After the second year the chest circumference exceeds the abdominal measurement, which, in addition to the growth of the lower extremities, gives the child a taller, leaner appearance. However, the toddler retains a squat, "pot-bellied" appearance because of the less well-developed abdominal musculature and short legs. Bone growth is most dramatic in elongation of the legs during childhood.

Neurologic and organs of special sense. By the end of the first year, all the brain cells are present but they continue to increase in size. Myelination of the spinal cord is almost complete by 2 years of age, which parallels the completion of most of the gross motor skills associated with locomotion. Brain growth is 75% completed by the end of 2 years. Development of various areas of the brain seems to correspond with the progressive intellectual capacity of the child. Various areas of the cerebral cortex undergo specific changes as developmental progress occurs, such as Broca's area for speech and cortical areas for control of the legs, hands, feet, and sphincters. Because this neuromotor organization is so inclusive, complex, and intricate, the child is limited in his ability to attend to any one aspect of behavior for more than a few minutes. Between 2 and 3 years of age the coordination and consolidation of these voluntary functions allows the toddler to listen better, look longer, and have extended spans of attention. Although postural control is increasingly more developed as myelination of the spinal cord advances, its immaturity, combined with the child's limited experiences and lack of visual perception, makes simple acts like seating oneself in a chair or climbing down stairs difficult tasks.

The limbic system, which consists of part of the cerebral cortex and several subcortical structures, most importantly the hypothalamus, is involved with the affective nature of sensory sensations, such as pleasant or unpleasant sensations. This system is functioning in young children but is probably immature, because the adult ability of moderating the emotion even if the sensation is incongruent with the expressed behavior is less well-developed.

Visual ability is fairly well-established by 1 year of age but continues to undergo refinement until about age 6 years, when visual acuity is 20/20. Full binocular vision is well-developed by 12 months of age, and any evidence of persistent strabismus should receive professional attention before age 4 years to prevent amblyopia. By age 15 months the child is able to distinguish geometric shapes and can insert a round object into a hole without being shown. By age 24 months he can place a square cube in its respective square opening. Eye-hand coordination has developed sufficiently by age 15 months to enable him to scribble spontaneously on a piece of paper. By 24 months of age he can imitate a vertical line drawn on the paper, and by 36 months of age he can copy a circle. Depth perception continues to develop, but because of the child's lack of motor coordination, falls from heights continue to be a persistent danger.

The senses of *hearing, smell, taste,* and *touch* become increasingly well-developed, coordinated with each other, and associated with other experiences. The usual mouthing activity during infancy is replaced by exploration of the environment using all senses. The toddler will deliberately visually inspect an object by turning it over; he may taste it, smell it, and touch it several times before he is satisfied with his investigation. He will shake it to see if it makes noise and vigorously test its durability. Another example of the integrated function of the senses is the toddler's development of specific taste preferences. The child is much less likely to try a new food because of its appearance or smell, not only its taste. Nonsensory associations with objects also take on significance. Using food as the example, a parent who refuses a particular food because of his dislike will transfer this negative connotation to the child before the child has had an opportunity to taste it. The complex nature of associations of the senses with memory of previous experiences and increased comprehension of verbal statements demonstrates the child's progressive development of cognitive abilities. Awareness of these factors is important in several areas of child rearing, such as feeding, teaching socially acceptable habits, and reinforcing appropriate behavioral responses to various situations.

Touch continues to be important to the toddler. Descending development of the spinal tract is evidenced by increased sensation in the lower extremities, such as tickling the feet. Pleasant tactile sensations continue to soothe and comfort the toddler, especially in times of stress or fatigue. Particularly during periods of illness or hospitalization, regression to and dependence on tactile and kinetic sensations such as cuddling, rocking, holding, and patting become much more demanded and needed by the toddler. Painful experiences take on new significance because memory is associated with the specific event. The young infant was manageable and cooperative during physical examinations and before receiving injections, but the toddler is most uncooperative and highly suspicious of any procedure. Explanation before the procedure and play experience with equipment is much less effective with children in this age-group than with older children. The only secure base and source of comfort is the mother or father, who should be encouraged to participate in the examination or procedures as much as possible. Since the child remembers the event and circumstances associated with it, fears are likely to develop, such as resistance to people who wear white uniforms or rooms that look like the physician's office. Sometimes the child's ability to recall events is underestimated and little thought is given to his preparation for visits to a hospital or other health facility, resulting in fears that can last a lifetime. Because of the vulnerability of these early years, it is essential to prepare children for new experiences, whether it is a new baby-sitter or a visit to the dentist.

Cardiopulmonary system. Volume of the respiratory tract and growth of associated structures continues to increase during early childhood, lessening some of the factors that predisposed the child to frequent and serious infections during infancy. However, the internal structures of the ear and throat continue to be short and straight, and the lymphoid tissue of the tonsils and adenoids continues to be large. As a result, otitis media, tonsillitis, and upper respiratory infections are not uncommon.

The respiratory rate slows from approximately 40 breaths/minute at birth to 28 breaths/minute at age 1 year to 27 breaths/minute at age 2 years to 25 breaths/minute at age 3 years. Respirations continue to be abdominal during the toddler years but gradually shift to thoracic by 6 or 7 years of age.

The postnatal circulatory changes are completed by the end of infancy. The heart rate slows and the blood pressure increases. The pulse rate is approximately 100 beats/minute at age 2 years with a large standard deviation of 16 and 93 beats/minute at age 3 years with a standard deviation of 12. Blood pressure increases to a mean systolic of 99 mm Hg (plus or minus 25 mm Hg) and a mean diastolic of 64 mm Hg (plus or minus 25 mm Hg) at age 2 years and rises to 100/67 mm Hg with a continued range of 25 mm Hg for each reading at age 3 years (see Appendix A, Table A-3).

Proper evaluation of vital signs is essential because activity, anxiety, fever, or illness causes wide variations from normal. Pulse and respiration should be taken for 1 full minute since sinus arrhythmia is not uncommon during infancy and early childhood. Accurate blood pressure readings, which establish an early baseline for future evaluation, require the use of cuffs of proper size. The width of the cuff should cover two thirds of the upper arm or lower thigh. An oversized cuff results in a falsely low reading, and an undersized cuff results in a falsely high reading. Using the leg for blood pressure measurement is a reliable alternative in young children. The procedure is the same except the cuff is applied directly above the knee, with the inflatable bag against the popliteal space. The stethoscope is placed behind the angle of the knee and the reading is taken by compressing the popliteal artery.

Changes in vascular resistance continue as the lumen of vessels increases. The capillary beds enlarge and are functional at the distal portion of the extremities. They are more effective in responding to changes in temperature and contribute to the more efficient thermoregulation mechanism. Hemopoietic mechanisms are stabilized by the end of infancy. Hemoglobin levels are approximately 12 to 15 g/100 ml, and decreases are most likely a result of nutritional iron deficiency.

Fluid and electrolytes. By 2 to 3 years of age the total body fluid is similar to that of an adult. Extracellular fluid continues to decrease, whereas intracellular fluid increases because of the growth of new cells. Muscle mass accounts for an increasingly greater percentage of body weight than does adipose tissue. The approximate percentage of total body fluid is 64% in the toddler as compared to 59% in the adult male. Rapid shifts in fluid between intracellular and extracellular compartments is less likely, making the toddler somewhat less vulnerable to dehydration. The mature functioning of the renal and endocrine systems also serves to conserve fluid under times of stress, although this is still less efficient than in the older child.

Thermoregulation. Under conditions of moderate variation in temperature, the toddler rarely has the difficulties of the young infant in maintaining body temperature. The capillaries are able to conserve core body temperature by constricting in response to cold and dilating in response to heat. Shivering is much more effective as a source of thermogenesis. Shivering is an involuntary act that results in rhythmic muscle contraction, which increases cellular metabolism, producing heat. The child also learns mechanisms to control body temperature, by putting on clothing when cold or removing it when warm.

Gastrointestinal system. The digestive processes are fairly complete by the end of infancy. The salivary glands have reached mature size and functioning by the third year of life and, under the control of the autonomic nervous system, respond to associated stimuli, such as the presence of food or emotional anxiety. The acidity of the gastric contents continues to increase but does not reach adult concentrations until adolescence. The high acidity has a protective function since it is capable of destroying many types of bacteria, but this mechanism is less efficient during early childhood. Transit time decreases by the end of infancy, and stomach capacity increases to allow for the usual schedule of three meals a day. The decreased transit time also makes the toddler somewhat less vulnerable to dehydration from diarrhea.

One of the more prominent changes of the gastrointestinal system is the voluntary control of elimination. With complete myelination of the spinal cord, control of anal and urethral sphincters is gradually achieved. Urination and defecation is controlled by a visceral reflex. For example, as urine accumulates in the bladder, the proprioceptors within the muscle tissues are activated by the stretching of the walls. Impulses are sent by the visceral afferent fibers to the spinal cord to the autonomic nervous system, which in turn causes the smooth muscle of the bladder wall to contract and expel the urine. Children learn bowel and bladder control whether they are specifically taught or if left to their own discretion, which frequently occurs in other cultures. The ability to control the sphincters probably occurs somewhere between ages 18 and 24 months, although bowel training is usually accomplished before bladder training because of its regularity and decreased frequency.

Renal system. The renal system, which serves to conserve body fluid by concentrating urine, is functionally mature by the end of infancy. However, the ability to control water in times of stress is hindered by the still immature endocrine system, particularly the secretion of vasopressin or antidiuretic hormone (ADH) from the posterior pituitary gland. Bladder capacity also increases considerably. By 14 to 18 months of age the child is able to retain urine for up to 2 hours or longer. However, this usually does not indicate complete readiness for toilet training because the child may not be sufficiently aware of the sensation to urinate to communicate it to his mother.

Integumentary system. The skin becomes functionally more mature during early childhood. The epidermis and dermis are more tightly bound together, increasing their resistance to infection and irritation and creating a more effective barrier against fluid loss. Production of sebum is minimal, which contributes to the development of dry skin. The eccrine glands are functional during early childhood and react to changes in temperature, but they produce very minimal amounts of sweat. Hair grows thicker and coarser and usually darkens and loses some curliness. Fine hair is evident on the lower arms and legs. Production of adopose tissue declines as hyperplasia of muscle cells increases. With the concurrent growth of the lower extremities, the child assumes more adult-like proportions.

Musculoskeletal system. Bone growth continues to be rapid following infancy with the development of several new centers of ossification. More than twenty-five new ossification centers appear during the second year. Growth in height is primarily a result of elongation of the legs. For example, the infant's legs constitute about 30% of the total height, but by 6 years they comprise 45% of the total length. As total body length increases, the proportion of head size to total height decreases from one sixth during infancy to one eighth in adulthood. The legs retain a slightly bowed or curved appearance during the second year from the weight of the relatively large trunk. This lateral curvature disappears by 3 years of age. If it persists it may be a sign of deficient calcium utilization, which occurs in vitamin D deficiency.

Changes in the feet also occur during infancy and early childhood as locomotion and weight-bearing progress. At birth the feet are flat because the arches are protected by fat pads on the soles of the feet. As the bones in the arches develop, the pads disappear and the feet begin to assume their natural shape. A normal arch is determined by proper alignment of all the bones and development of the surrounding musculature, not by the height of the arch. When children begin walking, the shape of the shoe should conform to the anatomic shape of the foot. The shoe should be soft and flexible, with smooth interiors and few construction seams to irritate the skin. There should be firm support around the ankle, and the heel should be raised slightly, about ¼ inch. Shoes should be roomy; when bearing weight, there should be at least the space of half the width of the thumbnail between the end of the longest toe and the shoe. Socks should also be roomy and square-toed to allow for proper growth and alignment.

Growth in the muscular system is almost entirely a result of hyperplasia and is directly influenced by the degree of use. Genetic differences have more effect on muscular development than do gender differences until puberty, when hormonal changes cause increased muscle mass in males.

Dentition and dental hygiene. By 1 year of age most children have between six and eight temporary teeth—the upper and lower central and lateral incisors. During the next year and a half the cuspids and first and second molars will erupt. The usual order of appearance is listed in Fig. 3-8, *A*. By age 2½ years primary dentition is completed.

Care of the teeth becomes important during late infancy and the toddler years. Since most of the deciduous teeth are formed at birth, fluoride plays less of a role in protecting these teeth from dental caries than the developing permanent teeth. The exact protective mechanism of fluoride is not known, but it makes teeth more resistant to decay. If drinking water is not fluoridated, fluoride supplements in the dose of 0.5 to 1.0 mg should be administered daily.

Another important aspect of tooth care is prevention of "bottle-mouth syndrome," which affects children between the ages of 18 months and 3 years. Caries result when the child is allowed to take a bottle of milk or juice to bed and the liquid pools in the mouth, bathing the teeth in sugar. Although the exact cause of dental caries is not known, one theory postulates that the enzymes liberated by the bacterial flora of the mouth split carbohydrates to form lactic acid and other decay-causing acids that cause erosion and absorption of the protein matrix of the enamel and dentine.[7] The length of time the teeth are exposed to these acids seems to be a crucial factor. In bottle-mouth syndrome the teeth are bathed in these acids for several hours. The maxillary incisors tend to be affected most, since the mandibular incisors are bathed by saliva, which dilutes the acids. Prevention involves eliminating the bedtime bottle completely, feeding the last bottle before bedtime, or substituting a bottle of water for milk or juice. Juice in bottles, especially commercially available ready-to-use bottles, should be discouraged. Juice should always be offered in a cup in order to avoid prolonging the bottle-feeding habit.

Regular dental visits can be begun when the child is as young as 18 months of age, but they should be started by the time primary dentition is completed. Initial visits to the dentist (or pedodontist) should be nontraumatizing. Since toddlers react negatively to new and potentially frightening experiences, the initial visit can center around meeting the dentist, seeing the equipment, and sitting in the chair. If the child is cooperative, the dentist may just look at the teeth but reserve a more thorough examination for another visit. This type of conditioning is very important in preparing the child for future experiences.

Dental hygiene can be started when the first tooth erupts by wiping the surfaces with a clean damp cloth. Tooth brushing is not recommended before 18 months of age because the tender gingival tissue is easily damaged. Since toddlers are great imitators, introduction of a toothbrush can easily be accomplished by associating it with the parent's brushing. Since young children are inexperienced in holding any solution in their mouth, it is best to avoid toothpaste or to use a very small amount. For the time being, a random "brush anyway–everywhere" technique is satisfactory.

Defenses against infection. The defense mechanisms of the skin and blood, particularly phagocytosis, are much more efficient in the toddler than in infants. The production of antibodies is well-established. Immunoglobulin G (IgG), which neutralizes microbial toxins, reaches adult levels by the first to second year of life. Passive immunity from maternal transfer disappears by the end of infancy, necessitating the use of artificial immunizations followed by periodic booster doses during later childhood. Immunoglobulin M (IgM), which responds to artificial immunizing techniques and combats serious infection, attains adult levels during late infancy and early childhood. Immunoglobulin A (IgA) increases gradually, not reaching eventual adult levels until later childhood. Many young children demonstrate a sudden increase in colds and minor infections when entering nursery school or kindergarten because of the exposure to new antigens. Gradually resistance increases, although the body's ability to combat infections has been well-established for some time.

Endocrine system. Most of the functions of the endocrine system are functional by the end of infancy and early childhood, with the exception of the reproductive hormones. Most of the specific hormonal functions are still somewhat limited during the toddler years, especially under instances of stress. For further elaboration of these functions, refer to Chapter 12.

Adaptive behaviors

Adaptive behaviors can be classified according to developmental achievement in the following areas—gross motor, fine motor, language, and personal-social behaviors. The key developmental ages for the toddler are 18 and 24 months, although the chronologic ages of 15 and 30 months are also significant.[3] Fifteen months of age is a particularly integrative period of developmental achievement since it represents the completion or fruition of many skills that were unperfected at 1 year of age. Table 14-1 presents a summary of the major features of growth and development for the age-groups of 15, 18, 24, and 30 months.

Gross and fine motor behavior. The major gross motor skill during the toddler years is the acquisition of locomotion. By age 15 months he walks alone, by age 18 months he tries to run but falls easily, and by age 2 years he walks well and runs fairly well, using a wide stance for extra balance (Fig. 14-1). Between ages 2 and 3 years refinement of the upright, biped position is evident in improved coordination and equilibrium. By age 2 years the toddler walks up and down stairs, and by age 2½ years he jumps, using both feet, stands on one foot for a second or two, and manages a few steps on tiptoe. By the end of the second year he stands on one foot, walks on tiptoe, and climbs stairs with alternate footing.

Fine motor development is demonstrated in increasingly skillful manual dexterity. Once the pincer grasp is achieved, usually at 9 to 10 months of age, the toddler combines this skill with other developing sensory and cognitive abilities. For example, by age 12 months the child is able to grasp a very small object but is unable to release it at will. At age 15 months he is able to drop a pellet into a narrow-necked bottle. Casting, or voluntarily throwing objects, and retrieving them become almost obsessive activities around 15 months of age. By age 18 months he can throw a ball overhead without losing his balance.

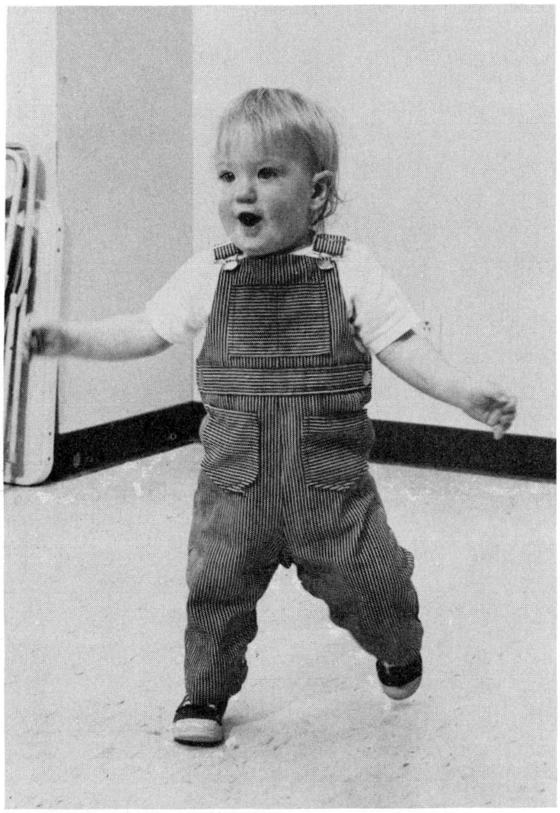

Fig. 14-1. Typical toddling gait. (From Erickson, M. L.: Assessment and management of developmental changes in children, St. Louis, 1976, The C. V. Mosby Co., p. 173.)

Visual perception of geometric shapes is also evident at this time. At age 12 months the infant selectively looks at a round hole in a special form board but is unable to insert a round object. By age 15 months he promptly places the round object in the hole, even if the board is reversed or turned upside down. Spatial relations also are evident in his ability to build a tower with blocks. By age 15 months he can build a tower of two blocks; by age 18 months, a tower of three to four blocks; by age 24 months, a tower of six to seven blocks; and by age 30 months, a tower of eight blocks or more. At 2 years of age he builds a "train" with blocks and at age 2½ years adds a chimney.

Fine motor skill and visual ability are demonstrated in the child's progressive adeptness in manipulating a pencil. Before age 12 months the child visually and orally examines a pencil but will not spontaneously use it or imitate a demonstration. By age 15 months he will scribble spontaneously and by 24 months of age will imitate a circular stroke and a vertical line. By the end of the toddler period he copies a circle and imitates a cross.

Mastery of gross and fine motor skills is evident in all phases of the child's activity, such as play, dressing, language comprehension, response to discipline, social interaction, and proneness to accidents. Activities occur less in isolation and more in conjunction with other physical and mental abilities to produce a purposeful result. For example, the infant engages in many physical activities for the sheer joy of those activities, such as crawling for crawling's sake. Now the toddler employs a skill for a purpose. He walks to reach a new location, releases a toy to pick it up or to choose a new one, and scribbles to look at the image produced. The possibilities of the exploration, investigation, and manipulation of his environment seem endless.

Language behavior. The most striking characteristic of language development during early childhood is the increasing level of comprehension. Although the number of words acquired—from about four at 1 year of age to approximately 300 at age 2 years—is notable, the ability to comprehend and understand speech is much greater than the number of words the child can say. This is particularly evident in bilingual families where the vocabulary may be delayed, but comprehension in either language is appropriate.

Regardless of cultural background, language development follows fairly well-delineated steps during early childhood. The infant progresses through the stages of undifferentiated crying, differentiated crying, cooing, babbling, lallation or imperfect imitation, and echolalia or imitation of the sounds of others. During the second year he may use ex-

Table 14-1. Summary of growth and development during the toddler years

Age (months)	Physical	Gross motor	Fine motor
15		Walks without help (usually since age 13 months) Creeps up stairs Kneels without support Cannot walk around corners or stop suddenly without losing balance Assumes standing position without support Cannot throw ball without falling	Constantly casting objects to floor Builds tower of two cubes Holds two cubes in one hand Releases a pellet into a narrow-necked bottle Scribbles spontaneously Uses cup well but rotates spoon
18	Physiologic anorexia from decreased growth needs Anterior fontanel closed Able to control sphincters	Runs clumsily, falls often Walks up stairs with one hand held Pulls and pushes toys Jumps in place with both feet Seats self on chair Throws ball overhand without falling	Builds tower of three to four cubes Release, prehension, and reach well-developed Turns pages in a book two or three at a time In drawing, makes stroke imitatively Manages spoon without rotation
24	Head circumference 49 to 50 cm (19.6 to 20 inches) Chest circumference exceeds head circumference Lateral diameter of chest exceeds anteroposterior diameter Usual weight gain of 1.8 to 2.7 kg (4 to 6 pounds) Usual gain in height of 10 to 12.5 cm (4 to 5 inches) Adult height approximately double height at 2 years of age Respiratory rate 26 to 28 breaths/minute Heart rate approximately 100 beats/minute Blood pressure: systolic, 99 mm Hg, diastolic, 64 mm Hg (plus or minus 25 mm Hg) Physiologic systems, except for endocrine and reproductive, stable and mature May have achieved readiness for beginning daytime control of bowel and bladder Primary dentition of sixteen teeth	Goes up and down stairs alone with two feet on each step Runs fairly well, with wide stance Picks up object without falling Kicks ball forward without overbalancing	Builds tower of six to seven cubes Aligns two or more cubes like a train Turns pages of book one at a time In drawing, imitates vertical and circular strokes Turns doorknob, unscrews lid
30	Birth weight quadrupled Primary dentition (twenty teeth) completed May have daytime bowel and bladder control	Jumps with both feet Jumps from chair or step Stands on one foot momentarily Takes a few steps on tiptoe	Builds tower of eight cubes Adds chimney to train of cubes Good hand-finger coordination; holds crayon with fingers rather than fist Can move fingers independently In drawing, imitates vertical and horizontal strokes, makes two or more strokes for cross

pressive jargon, a term that refers to a string of utterances that sound like sentences.[4] During most of these stages the child is acquiring a repertoire of sounds that eventually become words, phrases, and sentences. At age 1 year the child uses one-word sentences or holophrases. The word "up" can mean "pick me up" or "look up there." For the child the one word conveys the meaning of a sentence, but to others it may mean many things or nothing. During this age about 25% of the vocalizations are intelligible. By the age of 2 years the child uses multiword sentences by stringing together two or three words, such as the phrase, "mama go bye-bye" or "all gone," and approximately 66% of the speech is understandable. By age 3 years the child has a fairly extensive vocabulary of about 900 words and uses complete sentences, which include all parts of speech and major grammatical principles. However, grammatical ex-

Sensory	Vocalization	Socialization
Able to identify geometric forms; places round object into appropriate hole Binocular vision well-developed Displays an intense and prolonged interest in pictures	Uses expressive jargon Says four to six words, including names "Asks" for objects by pointing Understands simple commands May use head-shaking gesture to denote "no" Uses "no" even while agreeing to the request	Tolerates some separation from mother Less likely to fear strangers Beginning to imitate parents, such as cleaning house (sweeping, dusting, folding clothes) Feeds self using cup with little spilling May discard bottle Manages spoon but rotates it near mouth Kisses and hugs parents, may kiss pictures in a book Expressive of emotions, has temper tantrums
	Says ten or more words Points to a common object, such as shoe or ball, and to two or three body parts	Great imitator ("domestic mimicry") Manages spoon well Takes off gloves, socks, and shoes and unzips Temper tantrums may be more evident Beginning awareness of ownership ("my toy") May develop dependency on transitional objects, such as "security blanket"
Accommodation well-developed Visual acuity, 20/40 In geometric discrimination, able to insert square block into oblong space	Has vocabulary of approximately 300 words Uses two- to three-word phrases Uses pronouns I, me, you Understands directional commands Gives first name; refers to self by name Verbalizes need for toileting, food, or drink Talks incessantly	Stage of parallel play May have imaginary playmate Has sustained attention span Temper tantrums decreasing Pulls people to show them something Increased independence from mother Dresses self in simple clothing
	Gives first and last name Refers to self by appropriate pronoun Uses plurals Names one color	Separates more easily from mother In play, helps put things away, can carry breakable objects, pushes with good steering Begins to notice sex differences; knows own sex May attend to toilet needs without help except for wiping

ceptions are not well-learned or practiced, resulting in sentences such as, "Daddy goed to work today." Speech is over 90% intelligible. Hesitation or stuttering is common during this period and should be ignored.

There are several theories regarding language acquisition. Some theorists believe that humans have an innate biologic predisposition for speech. This is supported by the fact that even deaf infants coo and babble, although they lose this ability by 6 to 7 months of age. Normal children progress through the same stages of language development regardless of race and master the language somewhere between ages 4 and 6 years, regardless of its complexity. Behaviorists believe that language is a result of selective reinforcement, which shapes the various vocalizations into words, phrases, and sentences. According to this theory, the presence of a good role model is necessary for the acquisition of correct speech. Inattentiveness by the child or adult results in decreased response to the potential reinforcer. Poor language development is typically seen in failure-to-thrive infants who have received minimal parental stimulation. Delayed language is also possible in a household where too much stimulation occurs. For example, in a family where everyone talks loudly and few people listen, the child can "turn off" to cues that would reinforce specific verbalizations. The interactionist's theory views language as the result of the interaction of heredity, maturation, and environment. It is a learned process, rather than a predetermined or reinforced process. In terms of Piaget's theory, language is the use of symbols to represent objects, events, and people. It is the expected consequence of logical thought.

Which theory is correct is less important than the fact that each presents relevant facts when assessing the language behavior of the child. The ability to hear, the presence of a suitable role model, and the level of cognitive ability influence the acquisition of speech. Therefore, a nursing assessment of this area of development is much more complex than the number of words a child knows and says.

Personal-social behavior. One of the most dramatic aspects of development in the toddler is his personal-social interaction. Parents frequently wonder why their manageable, docile, lovable infant has turned into a determined, strong-willed, volatile-tempered little tyrant. In addition the tyrant of the terrible twos can swiftly and unpredictably revert back to the adorable infant. All of this is part of his "growing up" and is evident in such areas as dressing, feeding, tolerating brief periods of separation, developing fears, playing, especially with older children, and establishing self-control.

The toddler still fears strangers and is dependent on his mother for security, but he ventures away from her voluntarily to explore the environment. Verbal and visual reassurance from the parent gradually replace some of the previous need to be physically close to the parent for comfort. The toddler is more willing to meet strangers and will tolerate longer periods of separation. There is less of the extreme fear of separation that was prominent during the latter half of infancy. Persistence of this intense need to be with the parent may indicate further investigation. For example, if the infant has never been away from his mother, he is much less likely to tolerate any degree of separation. The reverse may also be true. A child who has experienced many separations from his parent may still be attempting to form trust by excessively clinging to every opportunity for attention. No fear of strangers, indiscriminate friendliness toward anyone, and no anxiety during separation from parents always warrant assessment since such behaviors are characteristic of a disturbed parent-child relationship.

Fears are common during early childhood. The ritualism of children in this age-group provides a firm base for the complexity of neuromotor, cognitive, and psychosocial development. Changes in the daily routine and environment present threats to this essential security. Hospitalization represents one of the most difficult disruptions in the life of the toddler. Any activities that simulate the home environment help to reduce the anxiety of this experience. Fears of going to sleep in the dark, hearing thunder or other loud noises, or watching leaves or shadows move are not uncommon. But the toddler responds well to comforting from the parent. For example, waking in the middle of the night and crying from fear of the dark and loneliness initially may require the parent's physical presence for reassurance. But eventually the parent's voice alone will quiet and reassure the child. Frustrating habits commonly develop when fears are unsatisfactorily dealt with. For example, picking the child up after awakening from fear of the dark reinforces this behavior and can result in more difficulties when the child refuses to go back to bed.

The toddler is also developing skills of independence, which are evident in all areas of behavior. The 15-month-old child feeds himself, drinks well from a cup, and manages a spoon, with considerable spilling. By age 18 months he uses a spoon well and may be using a fork. Between ages 2 and 3 years he eats with the family, likes to help with chores such as setting the table or removing dishes from the dishwasher, but lacks table manners and may find it difficult to sit through the family's entire meal. Dressing also demonstrates strides in independence. The 15-month-old child helps his mother by putting his arm or foot out for dressing and pulls his shoes and socks off. The 18-month-old child removes his own gloves, helps with pullover shirts, and may be able to unzip. By age 2 years he removes most of his clothing and puts on his socks, shoes, and pants without regard for right or left and back or front. By age 3 years he begins to manipulate buttons and is able to fully dress himself with supervision regarding left and right, but he cannot tie laces until age 4 or 5 years. Skills in undressing facilitate the learning of toileting, since independence helps prevent accidents.

The most dramatic social change for the toddler is his determination to express his own will. He comprehends the meaning of "no" while testing the limits of discipline and tolerance. "No" is so frequently used that he may mean "yes" but still express negativism. The best solution to this "no—I mean yes" dilemma is to make the decision for the child rather than give in or suggest additional choices. For example, when asked, "Do you want a peanut butter or cheese sandwich for lunch?" the answer frequently is "no." Rather than offering more choices, decide which one the child should have and give it to him. Toddlers like to have choices since it enhances their opportunity for independence and control, but occasionally the negativism of this age can supercede the desire for decision making.

Play. Play magnifies the toddler's physical and psychosocial development. Interaction with people becomes increasingly important. The solitary play of infancy (see Chapter 12) progresses to *parallel* play. The toddler plays alongside, not with, other children. Although sensorimotor play is still prominent, there is much less emphasis on the exclusive use of one sensory modality. The toddler inspects the toy, talks to the toy, tests its strength and durability, and invents several uses for it. Imitation is one of the most distinguishing characteristics of play and dictates the most appropriate toys for children in this age-group. With less emphasis on sex-stereotyped toys, play objects such as dolls, dollhouses, dishes, cooking utensils, child-sized furniture, trucks, and dress-up clothes are suitable for both sexes.

Increased locomotive skills make push-pull toys, stick horses, straddle trucks or cycles, a small, low gym and slide, varied size balls, and rocking horses appropriate for the energetic toddler. Finger paints, thick crayons, chalk, blackboard, paper, and puzzles with large simple pieces utilize the developing fine motor skills. Blocks in varied sizes and shapes provide hours of fun and, during later years, are useful objects for creative and imaginative play.

Because the toddler is experimenting with self-control and independence, feelings of anger and frustration are common and frequently have no suitable outlet other than screaming and temper tantrums. Toys such as drums, play nails and hammer, clay, and Play Dough provide alternative methods of dissipating psychic energy. They also begin to teach socially acceptable ways of dealing with feelings of aggression.

Talking is a form of play for the toddler, who enjoys musical toys such as play phonographs, "talking" dolls and animals, and play telephones. Appropriate children's television programs are excellent for children in this age-group, who learn to associate words with visual images. Toddlers also enjoy "reading" stories from a picture book and imitating the sounds of animals. Usually by 2 years of age they talk incessantly to everyone, including imaginary playmates. Make-believe friends provide an additional source of security and control in a somewhat complex and hectic world. Children relinguish such playmates when parallel play progresses to cooperative play, usually during the preschool years.

Tactile play is also important for the exploring toddler. Water toys, a sandbox with pail and shovel, finger paints, soap bubbles, and clay provide excellent opportunities for free creative and manipulative recreation. Parents sometimes forget the fascination of feeling slippery cream, catching airy bubbles, squeezing and reshaping clay, or smearing paints. But these kinds of unstructured activities are equally as important as educational play in order to allow children freedom of expression.

Selection of appropriate toys must involve safety factors. Although the toddler has less chance of accidently poking a pointed object into his eye because of crude fine motor skill, he is still clumsy and unaware of potential danger. Therefore, prevention involves the same principles of safety for children in this age-group as were discussed for infants (Chapter 12), although the reason may be different. For example, although mouthing activity ceases at 12 or 15 months of age, danger of swallowing harmful agents is present because of the child's insatiable curiosity, increased motor skills to reach and open containers, and unawareness of the word "danger." His increasing understanding and comprehension of the language are no guarantee to his safety, since negativism and the desire to assert his will make obeying extremely unreliable. Protection involves active measures for safeproofing the house.

Safeproofing should not be translated into total restriction. Some of the toddler's favorite toys are pots and pans, the pantry, the drawer of socks, and the laundry basket. The investigation and exploration of closed doors seem always to surpass the intrigue of the most expensive toy. Structured permissive play allows the child the opportunity to test his capacities for control, while having the reassurance that he will not overextend his limit and lose security. Play is the child's work of acquiring autonomy while overcoming a sense of doubt and shame.

Intellectual development

The toddler's increasing cognitive development parallels the infant's dramatic physical achievement. By the beginning of the second year it is quite clear that the toddler "thinks" and "reasons" things out. There is deliberate trial and error experimentation to produce certain results. The mental abstracts of time, space, and causality begin to have meaning, but the child's conception of each is different from that of the adult's. The main cognitive achievement of early childhood is the acquisition of language, which represents mental symbolism.

Piaget classifies the period of 12 to 24 months as part of infancy, which completes the six stages of the sensorimotor phase (Tables 12-4 and 14-2). In the fifth stage, *tertiary circular reactions,* the child uses active experimentation to achieve previously unattainable goals. Newly acquired physical skills are increasingly more important for the function they serve rather than for the acts themselves. The child incorporates the old learning of secondary circular reactions and applies the combined knowledge to new situations, with emphasis on the results of the experimentation. In this way there is the beginning of rational judgment and intellectual reasoning. During this stage there is further differentiation of oneself from objects. This is evident in the child's increasing ability to venture away from his mother and to tolerate longer periods of separation. Awareness of a causal relationship between two events is apparent. As the child flips a light switch, he is aware that a reciprocal response occurs. However, he is not able to transfer that knowledge to new situations. Therefore, every time he sees what ap-

Table 14-2. Sensorimotor and preconceptual phases during later infancy*

Stage	Age (months)	Cognitive development	Behavior
Sensorimotor			
V. Tertiary circular reactions	13-18	Active experimentation to achieve previously unattainable goals Increased concept of object permanence Differentiation of oneself from objects Early traces of memory Beginning awareness of spatial, causal, and temporal relationships Able to enter into an action at any point without reproducing the entire sequence	Insatiable curiosity about the environment Uses all sensory cues for exploration Ventures away from mother for longer periods Uses physical skills to achieve a particular goal Can find hidden objects, but only in first location Able to insert a round object into a hole Fits smaller objects into each other (nesting) Gestures "up" and "down" Puts objects into a container and takes them out Realizes that "out of sight" is not out of reach; opens doors and drawers to find objects Gains comfort from parent's voice even if the parent is not visually present
VI. Invention of new means through mental combinations	19-24	Awareness of object permanence regardless of the number of invisible displacements Can infer a cause while only experiencing the effect Imitation is increasingly more symbolic Beginning sense of time in terms of anticipation, memory, and ability to wait Egocentricism in thought and behavior Global organization of thought	Searches for an object through several hiding places Will infer a cause by associating two or more experiences (such as candy missing, sister smiling) Imitates words and sounds of animals Imitates adult behavior (domestic mimicry) Follows directions and understands requests Uses words "up," "down," "come," and "go" with meaning Has some sense of time; waits in response to "just a minute; may use word "now" May sit and wait for meals at the table for short period of time Refers to self by name Engages in parallel play; demonstrates awareness of ownership Very concerned with ritualistic, routinized schedule
Preconceptual	2 to 4 years†	Increased use of language as mental symbolization Egocentricism still present in thought, play, and behavior Increased sense of time, space, causality Global organization of thought Transductive reasoning Concept of animism Unable to conceptualize two aspects of one object Magical thinking	Uses two- to three-word phrases Increased vocabulary Refers to self by pronoun Possessive of own toys, uses word "mine" Begins to use past tense of verbs Uses phrases "going to, in a minute, today, all done" Uses many future-oriented words, such as "tomorrow, next day, afternoon," but poor conception of passage of time Follows directions using prepositions—up, behind, under, in back of, and so on Transfers knowledge of one object to same object in another location (for example, electrical outlet) Very traditional and ritualistic, small change in routine represents a drastic change in entire schedule Reasoning of causal relationships is directed by proximity of two or more events

*For stages during early infancy see Table 12-4.

†Cognitive development and behavior apply primarily to ages 24 to 36 months.

pears to be a light switch, he must reinvestigate its function. Such behavior demonstrates the beginning of categorizing data into distinct classes, subclasses, and so on. There are innumerable examples of this type of behavior in toddlers as they continuously explore the same object each time it appears in a new place. A classic example is their curiosity about electrical outlets. They will adamantly poke, taste, and inspect every outlet, even if they receive a shock from one of them. This inability to transfer information leaves toddlers particularly vulnerable to accidents. However, traces of memory are evident because they will usually avoid the outlet where the shock occurred.

Since classification of objects is still rudimentary, the appearance of an object denotes its function. For example, if the child's toys are stored in a paper bag or large container, that toy receptacle is no different than the garbage pail or laundry basket. If the child is allowed to turn over the toy receptable, he will just as quickly do the same to other similar objects because, for him, there is no difference. Expecting the child to judge which receptacles are permissible to explore and which are not is inappropriate for this age-group. Instead, the forbidden object such as the garbage pail should be placed out of reach.

The discovery of objects as objects leads to the awareness of their spatial relationships. The child is able to recognize different shapes and their relationship to each other. For example, he can fit slightly smaller boxes into each other (nesting) and can place a round object into a hole, even if the board is turned around, upside down, or reversed. However, not until 2 years of age can he do the same thing with a square. He is also aware of space and the relationship of his body to dimensions such as height. He will stretch, stand on a low stair or stool, and pull a string to reach an object.

Object permanence has also advanced. Although he still cannot find an object that has been invisibly displaced or moved from under one pillow to another pillow without his seeing the change, the toddler is increasingly aware of the existence of objects behind closed doors, in drawers, and under tables. Parents are usually acutely aware of this developmental achievement and find high places and locked cabinets the only places inaccessible to toddlers.

During ages 19 to 24 months the child is in the final sensorimotor stage, the *invention of new means through mental combinations*. This stage completes the more primitive, autistic thought processes of infancy and prepares the way for more complex mental operations during the phase of preoperational thought. One of the most dramatic achievements of this stage is in the area of object permanence. The child will now actively search for an object in several potential hiding places. Also, he can infer a cause when only experiencing the effect. He can infer that an object was hidden in any number of places even if he only saw the original hiding place.

Imitation displays deeper meaning and understanding. Earlier, imitation was very concrete and action oriented. For example, "bye-bye" was a behavioral response more than a conceptual gesture of departure. Now it has a broader meaning, such as Daddy is going to work, it is time for a walk, or something is no longer present. There is greater symbolization to imitation. The child is acutely aware of others' actions and attempts to copy them in gestures and in words. He can imitate his mother performing a household task both physically and verbally. Parents will often remark how they see themselves in their child. Domestic mimicry and sex-role behavior become increasingly common during this period and the second year. Identification with the parent of the same sex becomes apparent by the second year and represents the child's intellectual ability to differentiate different models of behavior and to imitate them appropriately. With less emphasis on sex-role stereotyping in child rearing, there may be less evidence of this aspect of the process of identification.

The conception of time is still embryonic, but the child has some sense of timing in terms of anticipation, memory, and the limited ability to wait. He may listen to the command, "Just a minute," and behave appropriately. However, his sense of timing is exaggerated because for him 1 minute can last an hour. The toddler's limited attention span is also indicative of his sense of immediacy and concern for the present. Egocentrism, or one's primary concern with himself, is prominent in all aspects of the child's behavior. He can play alongside, not with, other children. His whole world is for his satisfaction and benefit. However, there is advancement from the infantile form of narcissistic behavior in the child's ability to wait, increased concern with pleasing mother, and awareness of outside controls on his actions. The ecogentricity of early childhood stems from an ignorance of social perspectives and confusion of differentiating self from the external world, rather than a failure in social sensitivity.[5] For this reason it is unrealistic to expect social graces and impeccable manners from young children. By the end of early childhood there is much more concern with acquiring the sociocultural amenities because foundational physical, psychologic, and intellectual developmental achievements have been mastered.

At approximately 2 years of age the child enters the *preconceptual phase* of cognitive development, which spans the period of 2 to 4 years of age. In some of Piaget's writing, the preconceptual phase is part of a larger category, the preoperational phase, which includes the time span of ages 2 to 7 years. The period from ages 2 to 4 years is primarily one of transition, which bridges the purely self-satisfying behavior of infancy and the rudimentary socialized behavior of latency. Several of the characteristics of ages 19 to 24 months are evident here, such as egocentricity of thought, symbolic imitation, and primitive concept of time, space, and causality. The 2-year-old child is in a state of continuous investigation. The primary focus of his attention is still egocentric. He sees, experiences, and lives every event in reference to himself. For example, if a person is positioned between him and another child, the toddler will explain that both children can see the middle person's face. He is unable to view the middle person from a different perspective. Imaginary and symbolic play is rich in activities that involve total absorption with one's self. The child can be anyone, do anything, and experience everything just by thinking that it is so. Magical thinking is very prevalent during early childhood and explains the child's feelings of omnipotence and supreme authority. However, it also places him in the very vulnerable position of feeling guilty and responsible for bad thoughts, which may coincidently occur. A typical example is wishing a new sibling dead. If that sibling does die, the child thinks his wish caused the death. His inability to logically reason the cause and effect of illness or an accident makes it especially difficult for the child to understand such events.

The concept of causality is demonstrated in a phenomenon called *animism,* in which the child attributes to inanimate objects lifelike qualities. For example, if the child falls down the stairs, he blames the stairs for causing the accident and will frequently "scold" the stairs. Cause and effect is more related to the proximity of events than to anything else. In some instances this is a correct assumption, such as flicking the light switch turns the lamp on. But in other circumstances, two simultaneous events do not cause each other, such as turning the light off at bedtime and the parent leaving the room. Fears of darkness are not unlikely when, in the child's mind, darkness is the "cause" of separation. Being aware of this type of causal thinking is especially important when young children are subjected to painful or frightening procedures. For example, when lights are turned off in a radiologic room, the x-ray machine is turned on. The sudden darkness and loud noise can be frightening even though no pain is inflicted. Explaining the procedures by turning the machine and lights on with people present will help the child disassociate the two events of darkness and loud noise.

The child's reasoning is neither deductive, from the general to the specific, or inductive, from the specific to the general, but *transductive,* from the particular to the particular. For example, if he did not like one food on the table, he will not like any other food. This prelogic is often very difficult to understand and confusing for parents, who will respond to the previous example by stating, "What does this food have to do with that food?" As far as the child is concerned, his statement is logical because it is based on his own frame of reference. No amount of "reasoning" will reverse this logic.

Typical of toddlers' thinking is global organization of thought processes or, in other words, the idea that changing any part of the whole changes the entire whole. Behaviorally this is repeatedly demonstrated in the toddler's ritualistic and rigidly traditional world. Everything must remain the same for the entire event to remain constant. Changing the smallest detail disrupts the entire experience. For example, moving the crib a few inches upsets the entire room. Substituting a new dish for the usual one spoils the entire meal. Rescheduling one part of the day's activity ruins the whole day. Such preoccupation with sameness is usually not evident in every phase of the child's life. It may center around a "security blanket" or a favorite teddy bear, but the ritualism represents a secure and reassuring foundation. When one realizes the importance of tradition and routine, the great disruption that illness and hospitalization represent to toddlers can be appreciated.

Within the second year the child increasingly uses language as symbols and is concerned with the "why" and "how" of things. For example, a pencil is "something to write with," food is "something to eat," and so on. Mental symbolization is closely associated with the prelogical reasoning. For instance, a needle is "something that hurts." Through the rapid acquisition of language and the ability to associate causes, the child is able to speculate and anticipate future events. If he remembers the needle as something that hurts, he will anticipate any visit to the doctor as one that causes pain. Reminding young children about other visits that did not hurt or experiences that were pleasant will usually do little to change their frame of reference regarding such events.

PROMOTING OPTIMUM DEVELOPMENT

The toddler years can be one of the most trying and confusing periods for parents. Conceptually there are similarities between this stage of development and adolescence, because in one stage the infant becomes a child and in the other the child becomes an adult. Both stages are concerned with autonomy, self-assertion, and independence. The toddler differentiates himself from the symbiotic relationship with his mother, and the adolescent seeks identity as an individual. Children in both age-groups engage in a self-referenced type of thinking, which outwardly appears adultlike, but is often understandable only from the person's perspective. The negativism of the toddler is not unlike the stubbornness of the teenager. Both are concerned with ritualism, conformity, and sameness. It is no wonder that child rearing seems complex during both of these stages.

Developing a sense of autonomy

Behaviorally the toddler can be described as untiringly energetic, insatiably inquisitive, annoyingly negative, and obstinately ritualistic. Understanding these behaviors helps parents realize the necessity of the behaviors and allows the parents to effectively deal with the development tasks of children in this age-group. The most important psychosocial task is acquiring a sense of autonomy or self-control. Implicit in this is allowing children opportunities to assert themselves. Children who are placed in a playpen, kept on a rigid schedule, given no choices, and disciplined sternly are unable to make decisions. On the other hand, children who are given unrestricted freedom, allowed to explore anywhere, given no set schedule, and offered unlimited choices are also allowed no decision making. Therefore, appropriate limit setting and discipline are essential for children to develop self-control while learning the boundary of their abilities.

Discipline. Once infants acquire locomotion, it seems inevitable that some type of limit setting be instituted. There are as many theories regarding discipline as there are for toilet training; however, some principles are consistent for almost every approach. Firmness and consistency are essential ingredients. In the framework of behavior modification, it is well-known that intermittent negative reinforcement will greatly prolong the extinction of a behavior. For example, relenting occasionally to the child's habitual crying at bedtime will indefinitely maintain the behavior. Consistently ignoring the crying will extinguish the behavior in a few nights. Establishing rules that are reinforced by both parents and other care givers is essential.

Discipline for toddlers involves saying "no" when they perform an unpermitted act, such as touching a lamp or the television. If many objects are within reach but not allowed, toddlers can be so restrained in exploration that development is stifled. It is wiser to remove breakable, valued articles and reduce the number of "trouble spots" for children. Some restriction is almost always necessary in order to prevent accidents, such as guarding stairs and locking cabinets. Although it is a good practice to explain why such limits are imposed, it is foolish to expect toddlers to understand and abide by them. Physical punishment is not a solution to discipline, but during early childhood it may be beneficial in moderation. For example, slapping the child's hand while saying, "No, don't touch," reinforces the meaning of the statement. Another effective means of limit setting is physical restriction such as removing the child from the room or placing him in the crib or playpen. One must remember that time has less reference for young children so that 5 minutes could be hours for them. Therefore, discipline should be appropriate to the child's age and tempered judiciously.

Since the concept of causality is determined by the proximity of two events, punishment must immediately follow the wrongdoing. Telling the child "no" while talking on the telephone and then slapping his hand after he has begun to play with a toy is confusing to the child. He will interpret the slap as punishment for playing with the toy and not for touching something else earlier. Another common example of delayed punishment is telling the child, "Wait until your father comes home." Not only is this ineffectual, but it also conveys negative connotations about the other parent.

Discipline is a positive, necessary component of child rearing. It serves several useful functions as it helps children to test their limits of control, achieve in areas appropriate for mastery at their level, and channel undesirable feelings into constructive activity. Children want and need limits. Unrestricted freedom is a tremendous threat to their security and safety. Through testing the limits imposed on them, they learn how far they can manipulate their environment as well as gain reassurance from knowing that others will be there to protect them from potential harm. As they grow older, the more demonstrative forms of behavior control are replaced by subtler expressions. The following example serves as an illustration:

> Two-year-old John continuously turns the knobs on the television. He has been told repeatedly to leave the set alone and, more recently, has been spanked for not obeying. While his mother is in another room, he turns the knobs, while watching to see her reaction. She tells him to stop, and he continues, but as soon as she approaches him he leaves the television, saying, "hi, kissy John," and smiles adoringly. Mother responds by kissing him, praising him for listening, and gives him a favorite toy while moving him away from the television.

Appropriate discipline teaches socially acceptable behavior. Destructive and defiant acts may represent aggressive feelings that have no alternative outlet. Giving the child a punching bag, bean bags or balls to throw, and clay to pound helps relieve feelings of frustration and anger. Sometimes a wrong act is more the parent's fault than the child's. The child who writes on the wall may have no paper to use. Telling the child, "Walls are not for writing on; here is a coloring book," presents a positive educational approach toward discipline.

Limit setting also circumscribes areas of success and mastery for children. When allowed to play with toys that are suitable to their developmental age, children have the opportunity to master a task and feel satisfaction. When they are aware of what pleases their parents, they are certain of love and approval. Limit setting is part of establishing a routine scheduled environment for toddlers.

One of the more difficult aspects of disciplining children in this age-group is their persistent negative "no" response to every request. The negativism is not an expression of being fresh or insolent, but a necessary assertion of self-control. One method of dealing with the negativism is reducing the opportunities for a "no" answer. Asking the child, "Do you want to go to sleep now?" is an almost certain example of a question that will be answered with an emphatic "no." Instead, tell the child that it is time to go to sleep and proceed accordingly. If positively stated requests such as, "Let's get ready for bed," are met with resistance, firm but gentle discipline is required. The request should be enforced, but as soon as possible the child should be allowed to do something he enjoys. In this way he will associate compliance with positive results and approval. Children like choices such as what shirt to wear or what fruit to eat, but, if all choices are rejected, the care giver should choose one for the child. Nurses who ask a toddler which leg he prefers for the injection are asking for negativism. Choosing the site and quickly giving the injection is the best course of action.

Temper tantrums. Toddlers may assert their independence by violently objecting to discipline. They may lie down on the floor, kick their feet, and scream at the top of their lungs. Some have learned the effectiveness of holding their breath until the parent relents. The best approach toward extinguishing such attention-seeking behavior is to ignore it. Holding one's breath may cause fainting from the lack of oxygen, but the accumulation of carbon dioxide will stimulate the respiratory control center, resulting in no physical harm. When the tantrum has subsided, the child needs to feel some control and security. A different toy or a favorite activity can be substituted for the ungranted request.

A popular time for temper tantrums is before bed. Toddlers often have trouble sleeping. After so much activity and stimulation during the day, some are unable to abruptly "shut off their motors" and others may have bedtime fears, waking during the night, or nightmares. Still others may prolong the inevitable through elaborate rituals. After a careful assessment of the events surrounding the tantrum, a recommended approach involves counseling the parent about the importance of a consistent bedtime ritual and emphasis about the normalcy of this type of behavior in young children. Attention-seeking behavior is ignored, and the child is not taken into the parents' bed or allowed to stay up past a reasonable hour. If nightmares occur the child is comforted but left in his own bed. Sometimes the child's door must be locked in order to enforce the limits.[2]

Helping the child slow down before bedtime also contributes to less resistance to going to bed. Reading the child a story, playing with him in the bath, and letting him sit in the care giver's lap while listening to television or music are quieting activities. If extra stimulation such as having company arrive at bedtime is disruptive to the child's routine, it is advisable to settle the child in bed beforehand.

Some parents feel guilty when the child responds so negatively to limit setting and consequently rescind their request, which reinforces the undesirable behavior and effectively achieves control and manipulation by the child of others. It is best to investigate not only the temper tantrums but other areas of discipline, such as mealtime, bedtime, and toilet training. Stressing the positive aspects of discipline such as helping children learn the limits of their control, develop acceptable social behavior, and feel security and self-mastery within the limits imposed on them assists parents in realizing its necessity. Since parenting is a learned process that is profoundly influenced by one's own parenting, it is well to investigate the types of discipline that each parent experienced as a child.

Toilet training. Similar to discipline, there are numerous theories regarding proper toilet training, from training in less than a day to letting the child train himself. However, some principles do serve as guidelines, regardless of the particular method adopted. Voluntary elimination is a physiologic process that cannot be achieved until myelination of the spinal cord is completed. A mother who claims that her 8-month-old child is toilet trained is a mother who is trained. Infants who have regular bowel movements can be scheduled to sit on the potty-chair at the right time, but the evacuation is involuntary.

Sometime after the child is walking, voluntary control of the anal and urethral sphincters is achieved, probably between ages 18 and 24 months. However, complex psychophysiologic factors are required for readiness. The child must be able to recognize the urge to let go and hold on and be able to communicate this sensation to the mother. In addition there is probably some necessary motivation in the desire to please mother by holding on, rather than pleasing oneself by letting go. Usually, physical and psychologic readiness is not complete until the later half of the second year. By this time the child has mastered the majority of essential gross motor skills, can communicate intelligibly,

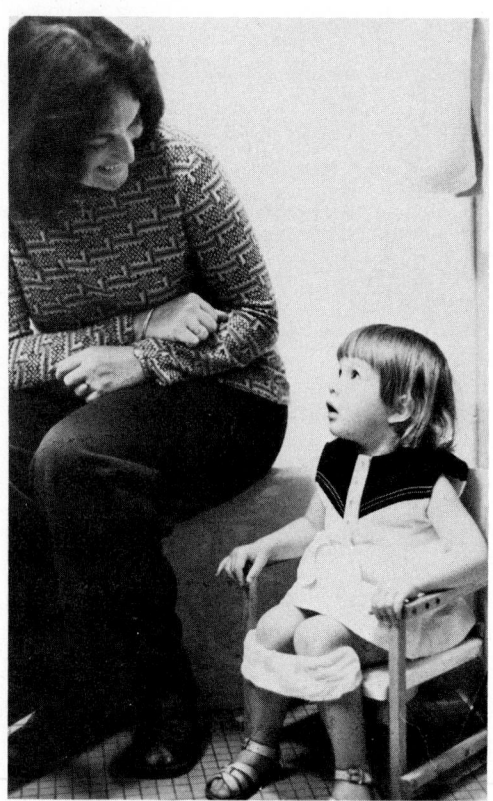

Fig. 14-2. Child is seated comfortably on a free-standing potty-chair. (From Erickson, M. L.: Assessment and management of developmental changes in children, St. Louis, 1976, The C. V. Mosby Co., p. 222.)

is less in conflict with self-assertion and negativism, and is aware of his ability to control his body and please his mother. One of the most important responsibilities of nurses is to help parents identify readiness in their child.

Child-rearing theories are also filled with various helpful techniques to encourage the child's cooperation. Some advocate the use of a freestanding potty-chair, which allows the child a feeling of security (Fig. 14-2). Others suggest a portable seat attached to the regular toilet to facilitate the transition from potty-chair to regular toilet. Using positive reinforcement through the use of training pants or fancy panties and encouraging imitation by watching others also works for some children. Forcing the child to sit on the potty for long periods of time, spanking him for having accidents, or other methods of negative control are to be avoided.

Bowel training is usually accomplished before bladder training because of its greater regularity and predictability. There is a stronger sensation for defecation than urination, which can be brought to the child's attention. Nighttime bladder training may not be completed until 4 or 5 years of age, and even later training is generally not indicative of pathology. Limiting fluid intake before the child's hour of sleep and waking him once around midnight help decrease the incidence of bed-wetting but do not teach voluntary control. Boys master the stand-up position after they have been toilet trained for some time. Imitating father during the preschool years is a powerful motivating force. Daytime accidents are also not uncommon, particularly during periods of intense activity. Preschoolers become so engrossed in play activity that if they are not reminded they will wait until it is too late to make it to the bathroom. The following example illustrates appropriate intervention:

> Three-year-old Susan had been toilet trained during the day for the last 4 months. Occasional accidents had decreased to almost zero. Now that the weather was warmer, her mother had been allowing her to play outside for a few hours each afternoon, but she noticed that Susan's pants were wet each time. She did not scold Susan for the accidents but reminded herself to bring the child into the house every hour and to show her how to open the door and call for her mother. She also brought the potty-chair downstairs where Susan could reach it quickly. After the first day of the hourly reminders, Susan called her mother and came in on her own. She still needed to be reminded, at least once during the afternoon, but the accidents were few.

For other suggestions regarding toilet training, refer to Chapter 23.

Sibling rivalry. The arrival of a new infant into the family represents a crisis for even the best prepared toddler. The toddler does not hate or resent the infant but despises the change that this additional sibling produces. Mother and father now share their love and attention with someone else, the usual routine is disrupted, and the toddler may lose his crib—all at a time when he thought he was in control of his world. It is not so difficult to understand the child's unwelcomed feelings toward this intruder when one considers the kinds of ambivalent feelings that surround the experience of parenting. Parents will ventilate feelings of jealousy concerning loss of independence and freedom. The difference between both types of jealousy is that the adult can rationalize and understand the change, but toddlers cannot.

Sibling rivalry tends to be most pronounced in the firstborn, who has experienced the wonderful position of being number one. It also seems to be most difficult for the 2-year-old child. Three- and 4-year-old children are more secure within themselves and have other interpersonal attachments besides their mother. They have achieved a greater degree of independence in dressing, feeding, toileting, and playing; therefore, they are less dependent on their mother for physical comfort and psychologic fulfillment. Five-year-old children may again have difficulty in accepting a new sibling because they are adjusting to the separation from home imposed by entering school.

Just how one prepares a child for the birth of a sibling is quite individual, but age dictates some important considerations. Time for toddlers is a vague concept. Tomorrow could be yesterday or next week, and a month from now could be never. Preparing children too soon for the birth may turn them off by the time the event occurs. Toddlers are aware of something when mother's belly gets large and changes have taken place within the house. A month or two in advance is ample time for preparing the child. Telling him that a new playmate will come home soon is foolish since it is untrue and sets up unrealistic expectations. Rather, what infants are like, how dependent they are, but also how things will stay the same should be stressed. If the toddler has had no contact with an infant, it is a good idea to introduce him to one, if that is feasible. Frequently other preparations, such as introducing the toddler to a regular bed or moving him to a different room, should be made earlier. If these changes are done well in advance, they will not be associated with the infant's arrival. Attempting to toilet train toddlers at the end of pregnancy is likely to be met with instant regression as soon as mother leaves for the hospital.

Older children need to be prepared earlier, because frequently they are aware of the expected sibling from overhearing adults' conversation. Jealousy can develop from feeling left out, and, since fantasy dictates reality, fear of the unknown can lead to fear of abandonment, separation anxiety, and insecurity.

Pregnancy is an abstraction for toddlers. They need concrete illustrations of how the baby is growing inside the mother. It is an excellent opportunity for introducing aspects of reproduction and sexuality. Showing simple pictures of the uterus and fetus, allowing the child to feel the fetus move, and involving the child in care-giving activities after the infant is born help him feel part of the experience.

How children exhibit jealousy is complex. Some will overtly hit the infant, push him off mother's lap, or pull the bottle or breast from his mouth. More often the expressions of hostility and resentment are much more subtle and covert. Toddlers may verbally express a wish that the infant "go back inside mommy," or they will revert to more infantile forms of behavior, such as demanding a bottle, soiling their diaper, clinging for attention, using baby talk, or aggressively acting out toward others. The latter is particularly common in preschoolers who may seem accepting of the new sibling at home but behave poorly in nursery school. This is a form of displacement that, says, "I can't let my parents know how I feel, so I will tell you." Encouraging parents to explore how their older child is acting with other care givers is an important aspect of intervention.

Regardless of how well-adjusted and accepting toddlers or preschoolers appear, infants must be protected by supervising the interaction between the siblings. It helps to show favoritism to the older child whenever possible, since this reinforces his acceptance and importance within the family. Visitors may initiate problems when they inadvertently shower the infant with attention and presents while neglecting the older child. Parents can minimize this by having small presents on hand for the toddler and including him in the visit as much as possible.

The first few weeks at home with a newborn and sullen toddler are difficult for parents. Assuring them that this period will pass, that the toddler will learn to accept the changes in his life-style, and that the newborn will sleep through the night is part of intervention. Allowing parents to talk about their feelings of ambivalence and frustration and suggesting ways of dealing with the jealousy help all members of the family survive this experience.

Parent-child relationships

The "terrible twos" aptly describes the parents' attitude toward this stage of child rearing. Toddlers' ceaseless activity, constant talking, lack of appreciation for danger, and preoccupation with self-assertion wear their parents' energy and patience thin. Their thinking processes, which initially appear mature but bear little resemblance to adult logic and reasoning, confuse parents. Facilitating parent-child relationships is tremendously enhanced by helping parents understand the "why's" of toddlers' behavior. Once parents realize the necessity of discipline, recognize readiness for toilet training, and deal with the negativism, they can feel more comfortable and secure in their parenting role.

Separation anxiety. A major task of the toddler period is differentiation of self from the environment. There is increased understanding and awareness of permanence and some ability to withstand delayed gratification and tolerate moderate frustration. As a result toddlers react differently to strangers than the way in which infants do, because the appearance of unfamiliar persons does not represent such a significant threat to their attachment to mother. They have learned from experience that parents exist when physically absent. Repetition of events such as going to bed without mother but waking to find her there again reinforces the reliability of such brief separations. Toddlers are also able to venture away from their parents for brief periods of time because of the security of knowing that the parent will be there when they return. Learning to tolerate and master brief periods of separation is an important developmental task of children in this age-group. In addition it is a necessary component of parenting, because brief periods of separation from toddlers allow parents to recoup their energy and patience. Without such outlets for physical and emotional relief, it is almost inevitable that their irritations and frustrations will be directed toward the children.

Prolonged separation, such as that imposed by hospitalization, represents a tremendous threat to young children's emotional stability. The stress of bodily illness alone is a major factor. However, prolonged separation can occur for other reasons, such as illness or death of the parent, particularly the mother. Children's ability to cope with a loss—and temporary separation is a loss—is influenced by many factors. The more significant the parent-child attachment, the greater the amount of anxiety produced. In addition the degree and duration of the separation, the type of preparation for the separation, the number of previous experiences with separation, the presence of additional stresses such as pain, illness, or sibling birth, and children's innate capacity for tolerance affect toddlers' reactions toward this crisis.

Although the specific reaction of young children to the separation of hospitalization is discussed in detail in Chapter 25, it is worthwhile to explore how they behave in response to separation for any reason. During the last half of the first year, infants demonstrate marked anxiety toward strangers, desperately cling to their mothers, and cry violently when their mother departs. Toddlers show less fear of strangers when their parents are present but are very fearful and angry when their parents leave. When alone, they are acutely anxious with strangers, manifest depressive behavior, such as crying and withdrawal, may become restless, hyperactive, or passive, and revert to regressive behaviors. Such reactions may be evident the first time a child is left with a baby-sitter or during the first day of nursery school. These behaviors are not pathologic or harmful if parents realize how desperately their children need them. Sensitive, perceptive parents will be aware of the child's need for increased love, affection, and attention when they are together. An attitude such as, "They will get used to the baby-sitter," will not help young children positively tolerate separation. Indeed, they will cope with the separation, but the emotional scars will also be the price for such an adjustment.

Parents often need help in realizing the necessity of preparing children for an inevitable separation. Particularly with the firstborn, parents tend to overprotect children, shield them from any anxiety-producing experience, and insulate them from less than immediate gratification. Although this is not necessarily harmful, especially if opportunities for independence are allowed later, it does not prepare children for unexpected events. A typical example is the birth of a sibling. The child is faced with the crisis of sibling rivalry as well as separation from mother. No wonder this child will not welcome the infant, because in his mind the intruder caused his mother to leave him. Allowing children to experience brief periods of separation early during infancy prepares them for such experiences later. Indeed they may still manifest the typical behaviors of protest, but they will also have learned that mother or father always returns. One can appreciate the tremendous loss that death of a parent represents for young children, because, unlike their other experiences with separation, this time the parent will not return.

Regression. Regression can be defined as the retreat from one's present pattern to past levels of behavior.[8] It usually occurs in instances of discomfort or stress, when one attempts to conserve his psychic energy by reverting to patterns of behavior that were successful in earlier stages of development. Regression is common in toddlers, because almost any additional stress lessens their ability to master present developmental tasks. Any threat to their autonomy, such as illness, hospitalization, separation, or adjustment to a sibling, represents a need to revert to earlier forms of behavior, such as increased dependency, refusal to use the potty-chair, temper tantrums, demand for the bottle, stroller, or crib, and loss of newly learned motor, language, social, and cognitive skills. At first such regression appears acceptable and comfortable for children, but on closer inspection one realizes that the loss of newly acquired achievements is frightening and threatening, because children are aware of their total helplessness in the recent past.[6] Parents, too, become frightened about regressive behavior and frequently in their efforts to deal with it force the child to cope with an additional source of stress, the pressure to live up to expected standards.

When regression does occur, the best approach is to ignore it, while praising existing patterns of appropriate behavior. Children are saying, "We can't cope with this present stress and perfect this skill as well, but we will if given patience and understanding." For this reason it is not advisable to attempt new areas of learning when an additional crisis is present or expected. An excellent example is beginning toilet training shortly before a sibling is born or attempting new areas of learning during a brief period of hospitalization.

More often than not, the regression occurs when parents can identify no unusual stress. For example, the toddler may insist on sleeping in the crib while his father is away on a business trip. It is better to let children have their request than force them to conform to one's expectations. If regressive behavior persists long after the stressful event has subsided, one should assess the present family relationships. For example, children frequently regress to using baby talk or soiling their pants when entering nursery school or day-care centers, but, once they feel comfortable in their new surroundings, such behavior disappears. If it continues, one must investigate how the child is relating to the teacher, what expectations are placed on the child, if the separation has been too long too quickly, and how parents relate to the child when he is at home. Altering any one of these variables may ease the anxiety and permit the child to return to a higher level of functioning.

HEALTH PROMOTION DURING THE TODDLER YEARS

Physical and psychosocial changes in toddlers affect two major areas of health maintenance and promotion, namely, nutrition and accident prevention. As the growth rate slows, young children require less calories and demonstrate this through increased fussiness and decreased appetite. Their negativism and awareness of food as a control mechanism pose potential problems for parents.

Gross and fine motor skills are so well-developed that toddlers seem vulnerable to almost every kind of accident. It is not difficult to appreciate the facts that accidents are the number one cause of death and that nearly half of all poisonings occur in children less than 5 years of age. Parents' ability to safeproof the environment and to reasonably set limits is the major component in preventing accidents.

Nutritional requirements

During the period from 12 to 18 months of age, the growth rate slows but the activity level increases, resulting in an adjustment from a previous caloric requirement of 110 to 120 kcal/kg (50 to 54 kcal/pound) during infancy to 100 kcal/kg (45 kcal/pound) during the next 2 years. Protein requirements also decrease slightly from 2.0 to 3.5 g/kg for infants to 2.0 to 2.5 g/kg for toddlers but are still high to meet the demands of muscle tissue growth. Fluid needs drop from an infant requirement of 150 ml/kg (2.25 ounces/pound) to a toddler requirement of 125 ml/kg (2.0 ounces/pound). The reduced fluid requirement represents a decrease in the total body water and an increase in fluid within the cells (intracellular fluid).

Vitamin requirements remain the same as those listed in Table 13-4. Need for minerals such as iron, calcium, and phosphorus is still high, particularly when one considers the poor food habits of children in this age-group and the increased mineralization within bones. Milk intake, the chief source of calcium and phosphorus, should average about 2 to 3 cups a day. More than a quart of milk consumption daily considerably limits the intake of solid foods, resulting in deficient dietary iron. Vitamin and iron supplements are generally recommended for those toddlers who have difficulty in adhering to a well-balanced diet.

At approximately 18 months of age, most toddlers manifest this decreased nutritional need in a phenomenon known as *physiologic anorexia.* They become picky, fussy eaters with strong taste preferences. They may eat voraciously one day and almost nothing the next. They are increasingly aware of the nonnutritive function of food: the pleasure of eating, the social aspect of mealtime, and the control of refusing food. They are influenced by factors other than taste when choosing food. If a family member refuses to eat something, the child is likely to imitate that response. If the plate is overfilled, he is likely to push it away, overwhelmed by its size. If food does not appear or smell appetizing, he will probably not agree to try it. In essence mealtime is more closely associated with psychologic components than nutritional ones.

Nutritional counseling

Developmentally most children by 12 months of age are eating the same food prepared for the rest of the family. Some may have mastered using a cup with occasional spilling, although most cannot adeptly use a spoon until 18 months of age or later. Some children find weaning easy and voluntarily relinquish the bottle by the first birthday. Others are unable to sacrifice that pleasure and require a bottle at nighttime or occasionally during the day. Allowing the child to give up the bottle when he is ready is preferable to forcing the issue. Just as children will achieve bowel and bladder control, they will also have no need for a bottle when they are secure enough to find pleasure in other achievements.

Some toddlers reject all solid food in preference for the bottle. This can be discouraged by gradually diluting the milk with water to make it less satisfying and introducing foods at times when the child is most likely to be hungry, such as on awakening. Occasionally it may be necessary to withhold bottle feedings for several days until the child is hungry enough to eat solid foods. This is a difficult period for child and parent and may represent the first crisis of child rearing. Reassuring parents that this temporary training period is essential for the child's present health and future eating habits helps parents feel secure during this trying time. Forcing the child to eat solid foods usually results in a battle and, in the long run, does not establish healthy eating habits. The following example illustrates one approach to changing feeding patterns:

Fifteen-month old Suzie had failed to triple her birth weight of 3.5 kg (7.7 pounds). Her present weight of 9 kg (20 pounds) was slightly above the third percentile, and her height was at the fiftieth percentile. All other physical and developmental milestones were appropriate, if not advanced, for her age. During the nurse's assessment of the child's usual routine, the mother stated that Suzie ate almost no solid foods, preferring the bottle or cup. Her usual daily milk intake averaged 900 ml (30 ounces). A "good day" of eating solid food would include ¼ slice of french toast, ¼ banana, 1 tbsp of vegetables, and a cookie or a pretzel. Any attempt at encouraging eating had been unsuccessful, and mealtime in general was unpleasant. Suzie refused to sit in the high chair, climbed onto the table if not restrained, and threw the food on the floor or played with it. Both parents were aware of the need for a change but did not know how to initiate it without force-feeding, which they were against. They had rationalized that although her caloric intake was inadequate, she was receiving all other nutrients through the milk and added vitamin, iron, and fluoride supplements.

The nurse discussed the usual appetite and behavior characteristics of toddlers as well as the need to reinforce better feeding patterns before the physiologic anorexia and negativism were greater deterrents to change in the subsequent months. Both parents agreed to try a training period. Three objectives were identified and agreed on: limiting the intake of milk, increasing the quantity of solid foods, and eliminating the disruptive behavior at mealtime. The plan involved diluting the milk by half, withholding the bottle until after meals and at bedtime, reinforcing only eating behavior through verbal attention, and ignoring all other behavior by not looking at or talking to the child. It was also decided that attempting to eliminate the disruptive behavior would be dealt with only after solid food intake had increased to at least twice its present quantity.

On the first day of the training period Suzie was not given a bottle on awakening. She was placed in the high chair and given pieces of banana and French toast. Since she refused any attempts at spoon-feeding, all food was served as finger food. Both parents sat down to breakfast. They ignored her crying and served only two pieces of food to her at a time. When she picked up the food and placed it in her mouth, they spoke to her. They did not praise her by saying, "That's a good girl for eating," and did not physically encourage her to eat, as they had done on other occasions. They showed approval for about 5 seconds, then ignored all other behavior until she ate another piece of food. A reasonable time limit of 15 minutes was predetermined for the length of the meal. At the end of this period she had finished one half slice of French toast with honey and one half of a banana. After breakfast she drank 120 ml (4 ounces) of diluted milk with vitamin supplements. Since she was accustomed to two 240-ml bottles during the morning before her usual nap at noon, she did not sleep that afternoon. Instead, at noon the same feeding routine was instituted. She ate 1 ounce of ham, ¼ cup of peas, and a few pieces of pear. She was cranky and irritable but was only offered the 120-ml bottle at midafternoon. At dinner she again ate 1 ounce of hamburger, ½ cup of corn, and 1 tbsp of baked potato. Before bedtime she was given a bottle of whole milk and allowed to drink as much as she desired. Before falling asleep she consumed 160 ml, seemed satisfied, and was put in her crib.

Although the amount consumed on the first day was still well below the suggested servings for a toddler (Table 14-3), it represented a severalfold increase in solid food consumption from any previous day.

On the second day of the training period the same plan was followed, except that intermittent, rather than continuous, positive reinforcement was practiced at each meal and the milk was not diluted. By the third day the disruptive behaviors of standing in the high chair, climbing toward the table, and playing or throwing food had almost disappeared. When feeding was well-established, positive reinforcement was given only when she was sitting in her high chair. By the end of 1 week the training period was no longer necessary.

Attention was given to the child's legitimate taste preferences and appetite patterns. For example, her appetite was never great at breakfast, but it increased after activity. During the training period she was also partially weaned from the bottle, except for one before bedtime. To compensate for the caloric deficiency, she was given homemade nutritious desserts, but they were not used as a reward or sign of approval. They were presented in the same manner as any other food. Slowly she began to gain weight, and her weight stabilized at the twenty-fifth percentile by 18 months of age.

Table 14-3. Servings per day for toddlers based on basic four food groups*

Food group	Servings per day
Milk or equivalent	4
½ cup whole milk equals:	Usual serving, ½-¾ cup
1 ounce cheese	
½ cup cottage cheese	
¼ cup evaporated milk	
½ cup yogurt	
½ cup milk pudding	
Meat, fish, poultry, or equivalent	2-3
1 ounce meat equals:	Usual serving, 1 egg or 3 tbsp meat
1 egg	
1 ounce cheese	
2 tbsp peanut butter	
¼ cup tuna fish	
½ cup legumes	
1 thin slice cold cuts	
Vegetables and fruits	4 (one citrus)
Citrus equivalents:	Usual serving, 4 ounces
1 orange or tomato	
½ cup orange or grapefruit juice	
¾ cup strawberries	
Yellow or green vegetables	
Broccoli, spinach, carrots, squash, string beans	
Other fruits and vegetables:	
Potatoes, apple, banana, legumes	
Breads and cereals	4 or more
1 slice enriched bread equals:	Usual serving, ½ cup or ½ slice bread
¾ cup dry cereal	
½ cup cooked pasta, rice, or cereal	
1 small biscuit	

Adapted from Williams, S. R.: Nutrition and diet therapy, ed. 3, St. Louis, 1977, The C. V. Mosby Co.

*Fats and carbohydrates should be served sparingly to meet caloric needs.

Eating habits established in the first 2 or 3 years of life tend to have lasting effects on subsequent years. If food is used as a reward or sign of approval, it is possible that the person may overeat for this reason. If food is forced and mealtime is consistently unpleasant, one may never develop the usual pleasure associated with eating. Mealtimes should be enjoyable rather than times for discipline or family arguments. The social aspect of mealtime may be distracting for young children; therefore, an earlier feeding hour may be appropriate. Young children are unable to sit through a long meal and become fidgety and disruptive. This is particularly common when children are brought to the table just after active play. Calling them in from play 15 minutes before mealtime allows them ample opportunity to get ready for eating while settling down their active minds and bodies.

The method of serving food also takes on more importance during this period. Toddlers need to feel control and achievement in their abilities. Giving them large, adult-size portions contributes to their feeling overwhelmed. In general what is eaten is much more significant than how much is consumed. Small amounts of meat and vegetables supply greater food value than a large consumption of bread or potato. Young children tend to like less spicy, bland food, although this is culturally determined in many instances. Substitutions should be provided for foods that they do not enjoy. The ritualism of this age also dictates certain principles in feeding practices. Toddlers like the same dish, cup, or spoon every time. They may reject a favorite food simply because it is served in a different utensil. Since toddlers are unpredictable in their table manners, it is best to use plastic dishes and cups, both for economic and safety reasons. A regular mealtime schedule also contributes to their desire and need for predictability and ritualism.

Appetite and food preferences are sporadic during these years. A child may enjoy one food for 3 days in a row and then suddenly refuse to eat it again for days. Such food fads do not ensure a well-balanced diet, but attempts to alter them are met with bitter resentment and unwavering obstinacy. It is preferable to accept such extremes and offer other foods in small portions. Generally the child will choose another "favorite food" that may adjust the nutritional inadequacy. Introducing at least three items from the basic four food groups at each meal helps develop a variety of taste preferences and well-balanced habits. The boxed material on p. 528 suggests appropriate sample menus for toddlers.

It is apparent from studying children's feeding problems that prevention rather than treatment ensures the best chance for success. When forewarned about what to expect, parents are in a much better position to deal with the erratic food demands of toddlers. Much of the dissatisfaction that parents relate about their children's nutritional habits stems from a lack of knowledge concerning normal variations in relation to age, caloric needs, energy requirements, developmental skills, and individual temperaments rather than

Sample menu for toddlers based on basic food groups

Breakfast

½ cup orange juice
1 poached egg
½ slice enriched toast with 1 tsp butter
½ cup milk

Lunch

½ cup cooked peas and carrots
2 tbsp chopped roasted chicken
½ banana or apple
½ cup milk

Dinner

½ cup baked macaroni with 1 ounce cheese*
½ cup string beans
½ slice bread
½ cup pudding
½ cup milk (after dinner or before bed)

Snack during day

½ apple
½ cup milk or juice
⅓ cup ice cream†

*Used as a meat substitute.
†Concentrated sweets and empty calories should be avoided.

pathologic deviations from normal. Each age has its special idiosyncrasies. The infant typically has a voracious appetite with few preferences or dislikes. The toddler demonstrates lack of interest in food, decreased appetite, and food fads. At age 3 years the child accepts foods well with only occasionally strong food demands. At 4 years of age the extremes in taste preference surface again. The five-year-old child is willing to accept what is offered and is strongly influenced by others' food practices. All of these demonstrate usual and expected developmental changes. Part of anticipatory guidance is preparing parents for these behavioral differences to prevent long-term problems in subsequent years.

Safety and security

The statistics concerning accidents in children 1 to 4 years old attest to the seriousness of this problem. More children in this age-group die from accidents (a death rate of 31.9 per 100,000 population) than from the combined deaths in the next seven leading causes of mortality. For example, accidents are responsible for more than three times as many deaths as from congenital anomalies, five times the number from malignant neoplasms, and over five times the number from influenza and pneumonia. In addition the accident rate has remained relatively unchanged during the past decade, whereas the corresponding rates from all other causes combined have declined by about 30%.*

Mortality from accidental causes tells only part of the story. Disability is another dominant factor. Approximately one third of the entire population under 6 hears of age suffers some injury requiring medical attention or involving 1 day's restricted activity. About two thirds of all these accidents occur in the home, and almost all accidents are preventable.* Their prominence as the leading cause of death among toddlers and preschoolers underscores the need to emphasize safety awareness among parents. Child protection and parent education are key determinants in every health professional's battle against accidents.

Growth, development, and accidents

A major factor in the critical increase of accidents during early childhood is the unrestricted freedom achieved through locomotion combined with an unawareness of danger within the environment. Specific categories of accidents and appropriate prevention are best understood by associating them with the major developmental achievements of toddlers and preschoolers (Table 14-4).

Motor vehicle accidents. Motor vehicle fatalities dominate the accident mortality of all pediatric age-groups after age 1 year. Such deaths cause more than one third of all accidental deaths among preschool boys and two fifths of those among preschool girls. Most of the deaths in children under age 3 years are caused by accidents within the car in which restraints have been improperly used. Children who are under 4 years of age or who weigh less than 40 pounds cannot use a lap belt alone. Their pelvic bone structure is not adequately developed to prevent possible internal injuries from the belt in a crash. Several types of car seats are available for children in this age-group. Car seats should be made of durable material that withstands an impact of over 30 miles/hour. Some car seats are convertible from the rear-facing type recommended for infants to the upward, forward-facing seat for older children. Regardless of the particular model, no car restraint is safe unless used properly and consistently.

Children over age 3 years are most often involved in pedestrian traffic accidents. Because of their gross motor skills of walking, running, and climbing and their fine motor skills of opening doors and fence gates they are able to leave most restricted areas when unsupervised. Unaware of danger and unable to approximate the speed of a car, they are hit by moving vehicles. Running after a ball, playing in a pile of leaves or snow or inside a cardboard box, riding a tricycle, and playing behind a parked car or near the curb are common activities that may result in a vehicular tragedy.

Preventing vehicular accidents involves protecting and

*Data from Reports of the Division of Vital Statistics, National Center for Health Statistics, 1973.

Table 14-4. Accident prevention during early childhood

Major developmental task	Accident prevention
Walks, runs, and climbs Able to open doors and gates Can ride tricycle Can throw ball and other objects	**Motor vehicles** Always use well-constructed car restraint Supervise children while playing outside Do not allow to play on curb or behind a parked car Do not permit to play in pile of leaves, snow, or large cardboard container Supervise tricycle riding Lock fences and doors if not directly supervising children Teach children to look for a car before crossing, recognize color of traffic lights, and obey traffic officers
Able to explore if left unsupervised Has great curiosity Helpless in water; unaware of its danger; depth of water has no significance	**Drowning** Supervise closely when near any source of water Have fence around swimming pool and lock gate Teach swimming and water safety
Able to reach heights by climbing, stretching, and standing on toes Pulls objects Explores any holes or opening Can open drawers and closets Unaware of potential sources of heat or fire Plays with mechanical objects	**Burns** Turn hot handles toward back of stove Place guard rails in front of radiators, fireplaces, or other heating elements Store matches and cigarette lighters in locked or inaccessible area Place burning candles, incense, hot foods, and cigarettes out of reach Do not let tablecloth hang within child's reach Do not let electric cord from iron or other appliance hang within child's reach Cover electrical outlets with protective plastic caps Keep electrical wires hidden or out of reach Do not allow child to play with electrical appliance Stress danger of open flames; teach what "hot" means Always check bathwater; adjust hot-water temperature to 52°C (125°F) or lower; do not allow to play with faucets
Explores by putting objects in mouth Can open drawers, closets, and most containers Climbs Cannot read labels	**Poisoning** Place all potentially toxic agents out of reach or in a locked cabinet Replace medications and poisons immediately; replace child-protector caps properly Administer medications as a drug, not as a candy Do not store large surplus of toxic agents Promptly discard empty poison containers; never reuse to store a food item or other poison Never remove labels from containers of toxic substances Know when and how to use emetic such as ipecac syrup Know number and location of nearest poison control center
Able to open doors and some windows Goes up and down stairs Depth perception unrefined	**Falls** Keep screen in window, nail securely, and use guard rail Place gates at top and bottom of stairs Keep doors locked when there is danger of falls (stairwells, porches)
Puts things in mouth May swallow hard or nonedible pieces of food	**Aspiration and asphyxiation** Avoid large chunks of meat Avoid fruit with pits, fish with bones, dried beans, hard candy, chewing gum, and nuts Choose large sturdy toys without sharp edges or small removeable parts Discard old refrigerators, ovens, and so on If storing an old appliance, remove the doors
Still clumsy in many skills	**Bodily damage** Avoid giving toddler sharp or pointed objects, especially when walking or running Do not let toddler have lollipops or similar objects in mouth when walking or running Teach safety precautions, for example, to carry knife or scissors with pointed end away from face Store all dangerous tools, garden equipment, and firearms in locked cabinet

educating the child about the danger from moving or parked vehicles. Although preschool children are too young to be trusted to always obey, emphasis on looking for moving vehicles before crossing the strees, recognizing the color of traffic lights for stop and go, and following traffic officers' signals is important. Most of all, practice what is preached. Children learn through imitation, and consistency reinforces learning.

Drowning. Drowning, not including drowning from water transportation, ranks second among preschool boys and third among preschool girls as a cause of accidental death. With well-developed skills of locomotion they are able to reach potentially dangerous areas, such as bathtubs, swimming pools, lakes, and so on. Their intense drive for exploration and investigation, combined with an unawareness of the danger of water and helplessness in water, makes drowning always a viable threat. It is also one category of accidents that results in death within minutes, diminishing the chance for rescue and survival. Supervising children when near any source of water and teaching swimming and water safety help eliminate this potential fatality.

Burns. Burns rank second among preschool girls and third among preschool boys. A major contributing factor to the sex difference is that girls tend to play indoors and imitate sex-related functions, such as cooking at the stove. Their ability to climb, stretch, and reach objects above their head make any hot surface a potential source of danger. Scalds from pulling pots on top of themselves are a major source of accidents. Pot handles should be turned toward the back of the stove. Ideally the knobs for controlling the range burners should be out of reach, not on the front panel where nimble fingers can turn them on and accidently touch the hot burner. Oven doors should be closed whenever the oven is turned on or when it is cooling. The outside of doors of automatic self-cleaning ovens may become hot and, if touched, could cause a burn. Other sources of heat, such as radiators, fireplaces, or accessible furnaces, should have guards placed in front of them. Portable electric heaters must be placed in a high area, well out of reach of climbing young children.

Hot objects, such as candles, incense, cigarettes, pots of tea or coffee, or irons must be placed away from children. The flame of the candle and the smoke of a cigarette invite investigation from young children. Tablecloths should not be used, or if so the edges should be placed out of reach to prevent accidents from both burns and falling objects.

Electrical burns also represent an immediate danger to children. With preschoolers' ability to manipulate small, thin objects, they are able to insert hairpins or other conducive articles into electrical sockets. Young toddlers may explore outlets and wires by mouthing them. Since water is an excellent conductor, the chance for a severe circumoral electrical burn is great. Electrical outlets should have protective guards plugged into them when not in use or made inaccessible by placing furniture in front of them when feasible. Children should not be allowed to play with electrical cords or appliances, which should be kept out of reach as much as possible.

Scald burns are the most common type of thermal injury in children. Among toddlers and preschoolers a significant type of scalding burn is caused by high-temperature tap water, either as a result of turning on the hot-water faucet, falling into a bathtub of hot water, or deliberate abuse. Besides the obvious prevention of always supervising youngsters when they are near tap water and checking bathwater temperatures, a recommended passive prevention is to limit household water temperatures to less than 52°C (125°F). At this temperature it takes 2 minutes for exposure to the water to cause a full-thickness burn. Setting the temperature only 3°C lower raises the time necessary for a third-degree burn to 10 minutes. Conversely water temperatures of 54°C (130°F), the usual setting of most water heaters, exposes household members to the risk of full-thickness burns within 30 seconds.[1] Nurses can help prevent such burns by advising parents of this common household danger and recommending that they readjust the water heater to a safe temperature of between 49° and 52°C (120 to 125°F).

Poisoning. Ingestion of toxic agents is extremely common during early childhood. The highest incidence occurs in children in the 2-year-old age-group. Although in many instances poisoning does not result in mortality, it may cause significant morbidity, such as esophageal stricture from lye ingestion. Although mouthing activity decreases after 1 year of age, exploring objects by tasting them is part of children's curious investigation. Almost every nonfood substance is potentially harmful, including many house plants, and toddlers by 2 years of age are able to climb most heights, open most drawers or closets, and unscrew most lids. By trial and error younger children also manage to undo tops of bottles, plastic containers, aerosol cans, and jars. Recent legislature has mandated the use of child-guard tops on articles such as prescription drugs, but many 4-year-old children have outwitted such "safe" caps.

The major reason for poisoning is improper storage. The guidelines suggested in Chapter 12 are applicable to children in this age-group as well. However, unlike the infant who was confined to certain heights and unable to unlatch inventive locks, preschoolers manage to find access to many high-level, tight-security places. Sometimes it is necessary to test a lock or high shelf by challenging the child to undo or reach it. Uncovering potential loopholes in one's security system now prevents tragedies later.

Although environmental hazards, developmental abilities, and insufficient parental supervision are considered causal factors in childhood poisoning, current research indicates that psychosocial variables are also significant. Abnormalities in parent-child relationships include such problems as a power struggle, misdirected anger, and prolonged and intense developmental characteristics, such as oral exploratory behavior, pica, mimicry, and negativism. Children with repeated occurrence of poisonings were found to have more behavior problems than the general population and were characterized as hyperactive, passive-anxious, and aggressive-impulsive. Risk-taking behavior and increased family stress also were present in situations of recurrent accidents. Implications for poison prevention are that concentration and emphasis on parent-child relationships may be equally as important as manipulation of environmental hazards.

By law, all poisonous agents must include an antidote on their label. This ensures that at least minimal emergency treatment can be instituted as soon as the poisoning is identified. Removing labels or reusing the empty container to store a different substance limits valuable first-aid information that may save a life. Parents should have ipecac syrup in the home and know its proper use and administration. Unfortunately some poisonings have been complicated by an overdose of ipecac syrup because parents were unaware of the proper dosage and schedule for readministration. Parents should also know the phone number and location of the nearest poison control center, which is usually a community hospital. Emergency measures for accidental poisoning are discussed in Chapter 16.

Falls. Falls are still a hazard to children in this age-group, although by the later part of early childhood, gross and fine motor skills are well-developed, decreasing the incidence of falls down stairs, from chairs, or out of windows. The climbing and running of the typical toddler is complicated by his total neglect for and lack of appreciation of danger. Gates must be placed at both ends of stairs. Accessible windows that are left open during warm weather must be screened or guarded with a rail. Falling from open windows is a major cause of accidental death in urban lower socioeconomic groups. Doors leading to stairwells or porches must be locked, since preschool children can easily open them. A convenient type of lock is a sliding bar or hook that can be attached to the door and frame at a level higher than the child can reach. One must be careful that inventive youngsters do not pull a chair over to unlatch the hook or bar.

Aspiration and asphyxiation. Usually by 1 year of age children chew well, but they may have difficulty with large pieces of food such as meat and with hard foods such as nuts or dried beans. Young children cannot discard pits from fruit or bones from fish like older children. It takes practice to learn how to chew gum without swallowing it. Play objects for toddlers must still be chosen with an awareness of danger from small parts. Large, sturdy toys without sharp edges or removable parts are safest. Coins, paper clips, thumbtacks, nails, screws, jewelry, and all type of pins are common household objects that can cause significant harm if swallowed.

Any of the objects in the preceding paragraph can accidently be aspirated, causing total obstruction or a consequent aspiration pneumonia. Emergency treatment for a *blocked* airway involves turning the child upside down, slapping him on the back, and trying to dislodge the object with the finger. Slapping the victim on the back in the upright position or if the airway is not completely obstructed is contraindicated because this may force the object further into the trachea, bronchi, or lungs. (See p. 1238 for the Heimlich maneuver.)

Suffocation is less frequent from causes seen during infancy but is an ever-present threat from old refrigerators, ovens, and other large appliances. Toddlers can climb inside these appliances and if they close the door behind them will be trapped inside. Discarding old appliances and removing all doors during storage prevent such tragic accidents.

Bodily damage. Toddlers are still clumsy in many of their skills and can seriously harm themselves when walking while holding a sharp or pointed object or having food or objects, such as spoons, in their mouth. Foreseeing such potential accidents is the best approach. For the older child, teaching safety is most important. The child should be taught that when walking with a pointed object such a knife or scissors, the pointed end is held away from the face. Dangerous garden or workshop equipment and all firearms should be stored in a locked cabinet. Safety education should include respect for firearms and their proper appropriate use.

Anticipatory guidance—care of parents

Understanding toddlers is fundamental to successful child rearing, regardless of the approach used. Nurses, particularly those in ambulatory or child health centers, are in a most favorable position to assist parents in meeting the tasks and needs of children in this age-group. It seems to be an almost universal phenomenon that prevention yields better results than treatment. Anticipatory guidance in each of the areas presented in the box on p. 532 is paramount if one wishes to prevent future problems. Advice is sometimes not the sole answer. Actual assistance, such as being available for home visiting or telephone consulting, should be part of nurses' flexible repertoire of interventions. Whether parents are experiencing the rearing dilemmas of a first or subsequent child, they benefit from sharing their feelings, frustrations, and satisfactions. They need adult companionship, freedom from child-rearing responsibilities, and periodic separations from their children. Sometimes they lose perspective of the needs of each other in the marital relationship and fail to communicate effectively. Part of nurses' responsibility is to provide opportunities for ventilation of parents' feelings and guidance in personal areas such as marital needs, career fulfillment, and peer companionship.

Parental guidance during toddler years

Age (months)	Guidance
12-18	Prepare parents for expected behavioral changes of toddler, especially negativism and ritualism
	Assess present feeding habits and encourage gradual weaning from bottle and increased intake of solid foods
	Stress expected feeding changes of physiologic anorexia, presence of food fads and strong taste preferences, need for scheduled routine at mealtimes, inability to sit through an entire meal, and lack of table manners
	Assess sleep patterns at night, particularly habit of a bedtime bottle, which is a major cause of dental caries, and procrastination behaviors that delay hour of sleep
	Prepare parents for potential dangers of the home, particularly motor vehicular, poisoning, and falling accidents; give appropriate suggestions for safeproofing the home (Table 14-4)
	Discuss need for firm but gentle discipline and ways in which to deal with negativism and temper tantrums; stress positive benefits of appropriate discipline
	Emphasize importance for both child and parents of brief, periodic separations
	Discuss new toys that utilize developing gross and fine motor, language, cognitive, and social skills
18-24	Stress importance of peer companionship in play
	Explore need for preparation for additional sibling; stress importance of preparing child for new, and potentially frightening, experiences
	Emphasize need for dental supervision, types of basic dental hygiene at home, and food habits that predispose to caries; stress importance of supplemental fluoride
	Discuss present discipline methods, their effectiveness, and parents' feelings about child's negativism; stress that negativism is important aspect of developing self-assertion and independence and is not a sign of spoiling
18-24—cont'd	Discuss signs of readiness for toilet training; emphasize importance of waiting for physical and psychologic readiness
	Discuss development of fears, such as of darkness or loud noises, and of habits, such as security blanket or thumb-sucking; stress normalcy of these transient behaviors
	Prepare parents for signs of regression in times of stress
	Assess child's ability to separate easily from parents for brief periods of separation under familiar circumstances
	Allow parents opportunity to express their feelings of weariness, frustration, and exasperation; be aware that it is often difficult to love toddlers at times when they are not asleep!
	Point out some of the expected changes of the next year, such as longer attention spans, somewhat less negativism, and increased concern for pleasing others
24-36	Discuss importance of imitation and domestic mimicry and need to include child in activities
	Discuss approaches toward toilet training, particularly realistic expectations and attitude toward accidents
	Stress uniqueness of toddlers' thought processes, especially through their use of language, poor understanding of time, causal relationships in terms of proximity of events, and inability to see events from another's perspective
	Stress that discipline still must be quite structured and concrete and that relying solely on verbal reasoning and explanation leads to accidents, confusion, and misunderstanding
	Discuss investigation of nursery school or day-care center toward completion of second year

In order to provide individualized, nonjudgmental care, nurses must explore the influences in their own lives that have shaped their attitudes toward such areas as discipline, feeding habits, toilet training, and so on. The sociocultural background of each family determines to a large extent the kind of attitudes, type of child rearing, and quality of parent-child relationship. One cannot compare two different life-styles and assess either as good or poor. Rather each must be assessed according to the results that one observes. In some highly mobile types of living, the very inconsistency of the daily schedule and uncertainty of future location may represent security, consistency, and ritualism for the young child. Parents who are not outwardly demonstrative of affection and emotion may show their strong maternal-paternal attachment in other ways to the child, such as only when alone in the privacy of their home. It is the quality of the parent-child relationship, not the particular life-style, cultural heritage, or social background of the family, that most decisively determines the child's optimum physical, psychologic, and emotional development. When stresses such as separation, illness, economic insecurity, or marital strife impair the ability of parents to relate to their children, anticipatory guidance may not be effective. Rather helping parents deal with the immediate crisis is of primary importance in one's efforts to enhance child rearing. Therefore, there are no established rules for counseling in any of the areas discussed. Nurses must assess each family's level of functioning, readiness to listen, and ability to implement suggestions in relation to their individual life-style before attempting to give anticipatory guidance. The ability to listen, observe, and silently assess is fundamental to any type of counseling and intervention.

REFERENCES

1. Feldman, K. W., and associates: Tap water scald burns in children, Pediatrics **62**(1):1-7, July 1978.
2. Inglis, S.: The nocturnal frustration of sleep disturbance, Am. J. Maternal Child Nurs. **1**(5):280-287, September/October 1976.
3. Knoblich, H., and Pasamanick, B., editors: Gesell and Amatruda's developmental diagnosis, New York, 1974, Harper & Row, Publishers.
4. Lenneberg, E.: Biological functions of language, New York, 1967, John Wiley & Sons, Inc.
5. Maier, H.: Three theories of child development, New York, 1969, Harper & Row, Publishers.
6. Oremland, E., and Oremland, J., editors: The effects of hospitalization on children: models for their care, Springfield, Ill., 1973, Charles C Thomas, Publisher.
7. Slattery, J.: Dental health in children, Am. J. Nurs. **76**(7): 1159-1161, July 1976.
8. Topalis, M., and Aguilera, D.: Psychiatric nursing, ed. 7, St. Louis, 1978, The C. V. Mosby Co.

BIBLIOGRAPHY

Accident mortality at the preschool ages, Stat. bull. Metropol. Life Ins. Co. **56:**7-9, May 1975.

American Academy of Pediatrics: Juice in ready-to-use bottles and nursing bottle caries, News and Comment **29**(1):11, January 1978.

Azrin, N. H., and Foxx, R. M.: Toilet training in less than a day, New York, 1974, Simon & Schuster, Inc.

Brown, M., and Murphy, M.: A child grows: how the child grows and develops psychologically, socially and culturally. Part II, Pediatr. Nurs. **1**(2):22-30, March/April 1975.

Brown, M., and Murphy, M.: A child grows: the child's cognitive development. Part III, Pediatr. Nurs. **1**(3):7-12, May/June 1975.

Brown, M., and Murphy, M.: A child grows: the child's perceptual and linguistic development. Part IV, Pediatr. Nurs. **1**(4): 9-15, July/August 1975.

Carlson, S., and Asnes, R.: Maternal expectations and attitudes toward toilet training: a comparison between clinic mothers and private practice mothers, J. Pediatr. **84**(1):148-151, January 1974.

Chamberlin, R. W.: Parental use of "positive contact" in child-rearing: its relationship to child behavior patterns and other variables, Pediatrics **56**(5):768-773, November 1975.

Chinn, P. L.: Child health maintenance: concepts in family centered care, ed. 2, St. Louis, 1979, The C. V. Mosby Co.

Chinn, P., and Leitch, C.: Child health maintenance: a guide to clinical assessment, ed. 2, St. Louis, 1979, The C. V. Mosby Co.

Dreikurs, R.: Children: the challenge, New York, 1964, Hawthorn Books, Inc.

Hendin, D.: Save your child's life! New York, 1972, Enterprise Publications.

Hennon, D., Stookey, G., and Muhler, J.: Prophylaxis of dental caries: relative effectiveness of chewable fluoride preparations with and without added vitamins, J. Pediatr. **80**(6):1018-1021, June 1972.

Hughes, J. G.: Synopsis of pediatrics, ed. 4, St. Louis, 1975, The C. V. Mosby Co.

Illingworth, R. S.: Development of the infant and young child, New York, 1975, Churchill Livingstone.

Jones, D.: Siblings! New Baby Talk **41**(6):16-17, 1976.

Kukuk, H. M.: Safety precautions: protecting your patients and yourself. Part 3, Nursing '76 **6**(7):45-49, July 1976.

Lewis, M.: Clinical aspects of child development, Philadelphia, 1971, Lea & Febiger.

Margolis, J.: Psychosocial study of childhood poisoning: a 5-year follow-up, Pediatrics **47**(2):439-444, 1971.

Murray, M. E.: Behavioral management in pediatrics, Clin. Pediatr. **15**(5):465-470, May 1976.

Neligan, G. A., and Prudham, D.: Family factors affecting child development, Arch. Dis. Child. **51:**853-858, 1976.

Padilla, E. R., Rohsenow, D. J., and Bergman, A. B.: Predicting accident frequency in children, Pediatrics **58**(2):223-226, August 1976.

Papalia, D., and Olds, S.: A child's world, infancy through adolescence, New York, 1975, McGraw-Hill Book Co.

Piaget, J.: The construction of reality in the child, New York, 1954, Ballantine Books, Inc.

Prival, M., and Fisher, F.: Adding fluorides to the diet, Environment **16**(5):29-33, June 1974.

Rudolph, A. M.: Pediatrics, ed. 16, New York, 1977, Appleton-Century-Crofts.

Sieben, R. L., and associates: Falls as childhood accidents: an increasing urban risk, Pediatrics **47**(5):886-892, 1971.

Simpson, J. S.: Trauma: the leading childhood killer in Canada and elsewhere, Clin. Pediatr. **15**(4):313-315, April 1976.

Smith, J.: Promoting childhood dental health, Pediatr. Nurs. **2**(3): 16-19, May/June 1976.

Snell, B., and McLellan, C.: Whetting hospitalized preschoolers' appetites, Am. J. Nurs. **76**(3):413-415, March 1976.

A source book on food practices, with special emphasis on children and adolescents, Chicago, 1974, National Dairy Council.

Sutterley, D., and Donnelly, G.: Perspectives in human development, Philadelphia, 1973, J. B. Lippincott Co.

Turbeville, D. F., and Fearnow, R. G.: Is it possible to identify the child who is a "high risk" candidate for the accidental ingestion of a poison? Comparison of oral gratification habits between 100 poison ingestors and 100 controls, Clin. Pediatr. **15**(10):918-919, October 1976.

Waechter, E., and Blake, F.: Nursing care of children, New York, 1976, J. B. Lippincott Co.

Weiner, I., and Elkind, D.: Child development: a core approach, New York, 1972, John Wiley & Sons, Inc.

Williams, S. R.: Nutrition and diet therapy, ed. 3, St. Louis, 1977, The C. V. Mosby Co.

Zarin-Ackerman, J., Lewis, M., and Driscoll, J. M.: Language development in 2-year-old normal and risk infants, Pediatrics **59**(6):982-986, June 1977.

15

The preschool years

The preschool years, a period from 3 years of age to the completion of age 5 years, comprises the end of early childhood. It is also an age of discovery, inventiveness, curiosity, and developing sociocultural patterns of behavior. In some ways it is a period of ease and comfort for parents, particularly when many of the child-rearing tasks, such as toileting, independence, and self-caring abilities, have been mastered. Preschoolers usually have less difficulty in tolerating separation, adjusting to change, behaving appropriately, and accepting compromise than toddlers. Their world is no longer confined to the home environment and the immediate family. They need and enjoy the companionship of other children. Play becomes cooperative and mirrors some of the most important tasks of this stage, such as identification of sex role, development of socially acceptable behavior, and realization of their separateness as individuals. Although their thought processes appear mature and adultlike, they are still self-referenced, which frequently leads to confusion, misunderstanding, and conflict between parents and child.

The combined physical, psychosocial, and cognitive achievements of children in this age-group prepare preschoolers for their most significant change in life-style—entrance into school. Their control of bodily systems, experience of brief and prolonged periods of separation, ability to interact cooperatively with other children and adults, use of language for mental symbolization, and increased attention span and memory ready them for the next major period—the school years. Successful mastery of previous levels of growth and development is essential for preschoolers to refine many of the tasks that were begun during the toddler years.

Many authorities believe that the period from birth to before entering school is the most critical period of emotional and psychologic development. Successful mastery of trust, autonomy, and initiative are foundational for further personality maturation, and failure to complete these stages may result in deep-seated, long-range problems in later life. It is also the period of greatest parental influence on the formation of the child. Once children enter school, their environment is only partially the home. School becomes a major contributing factor, and peers, teachers, and other authority figures, as well as selected "idols" from the mass media, greatly influence their thinking and behavior. Often parents realize the importance of others in their child's development when it is too late to exert effective parental controls, principles, or philosophies. Helping parents realize and understand the pliability and malleability of young children as early as possible is one method of preventing problems in subsequent years.

GROWTH AND DEVELOPMENT

Physical growth continues to slow and stabilize during the preschool years. Average weight gain remains about 2.3 kg (5 pounds) per year. By 6 years of age the child's weight at 1 year of age has doubled. Height also remains steady at a yearly increase of 6.75 to 7.5 cm (2.5 to 3 inches) and generally occurs in elongation of the legs rather than of the trunk. Most bodily systems are mature and stable and can adjust to moderate stress and change. Motor development consists mostly of increases in strength and refinement of previously learned skills, such as walking, running, jumping, and so on. However, muscle development and bone growth are still far from mature. Excessive activity and overexertion can injure delicate tissues. Properly fitting shoes, good posture, appropriate exercise, and adequate rest are essential for optimal development of the musculoskeletal system.

Bodily proportions no longer resemble those of the squat, potbellied toddler. The preschooler is slender but sturdy, graceful and agile, with erect posture. There is little difference in physical characteristics according to sex, except as dictated by sociocultural norms and physical activity. However, there is a great tendency to identify with the same sex and to imitate sex-related roles, such as keeping house, playing nurse or doctor, going to work, being a policeman, cowboy, and so on. In addition there is intense interest and curiosity in physical sexual differences, experimentation with one's body, and inquisitiveness regarding reproduction. For some parents this represents a problem because they are unsure of what the child is asking and how much information to supply. This is often one area where intervention is useful in solving the present dilemma, as well as in influencing healthy sexual attitudes during subsequent years (see p. 550).

Developmental tasks

If preschoolers have mastered the tasks of the toddler period, they are ready to face the developmental endeavors of this stage. As soon as children comprehend their separateness as a person, they begin to realize that there are categories of objects, such as things, people, males, females, children, adults, and so on. One of the principal goals in further differentiation of oneself from others is *learning sex differences and sexually appropriate behavior*. Child-rearing practices are tremendously sex oriented, even when parents consciously think they are avoiding stereotyped sex connotations. The way in which parents dress and talk to the child, hold, cuddle, and caress the child, and discipline him all express some aspect of sexually oriented behavior. Studies are increasingly demonstrating that gender is not solely biologic or genetic but primarily a result of complex postnatal psychologic factors and that most children are aware of their sex and the expected set of related behaviors by 1½ to 2½ years of age.[10,11] Although toddlers might be aware of their particular sex, they do not possess the language and cognitive skills to investigate sexual identity as fully as preschoolers.

Freud has long recognized this task by describing this period as the *oedipal, phallic,* or *genital* stage. The Oedipus complex is based on the Greek mythology of Oedipus, the king's son who had been raised in a foster family since infancy. When he grew to manhood he accidently killed his father, the king, and unknowingly married his mother, the queen. Conceptually this represents every small boy's wish to marry his mother and get rid of his father. Conflict arises when the child realizes that his father is much stronger and more powerful than he. Subconsciously he wishes that his father were dead. Concurrently he has noticed physical sexual differences, in specific, that boys have a penis but that girls do not. In his mind he surmises that girls have lost their penis for some wrongdoing. His guilt regarding his feelings toward his father makes him fear the same punishment of mutilation, resulting in the *castration complex*. Various authorities have negated the relevance of Freud's psychosexual theories. However, one need only observe the fear of preschool males who may need circumcision or other related surgery to realize that boys in this age-group do indeed have special fears regarding mutilation and castration.

Girls have similar wishes to marry their father and kill their mother, a phenomenon sometimes called the *Electra complex,* named after the Greek counterpart of Oedipus. Females, however, do not fear castration because they have no such anatomy to be removed, but rather they have *penis envy*. Freud has developed the female role in the phallic stage less fully than the male's part. By naming this stage phallic, he has demonstrated his sexual bias for male dominance!

The resolution of the Oedipus or Electra complex is identification with the same sex parent. Sex typing, or the process by which an individual develops the behavior, personality, attitudes, and beliefs that are appropriate for his or her culture, occurs through several mechanisms during this period.[12] Probably the most powerful are child-rearing practices and imitation. Girls are usually dressed in feminine clothes, protected from injury, and pampered more than boys. Boys are expected to be aggressive. Less restraint is placed on their activity, usually in subtle ways, such as providing more active toys. Girls are allowed more freedom of expression of emotions, especially sadness and crying. Boys are usually expected to "act grown up," "bear it like a man," and so on. Even when parents attempt to treat both sexes alike, there are other influences, such as from nursery school, relatives or friends, and mass media communication, that shape stereotyped sexual behavior. Because children recognize their biologic differences, they are adept at identifying with like expectations of behavior, attitude, dress, and so on. When ambivalent or incongruous messages concerning sex typing are received, difficulties in appropriate sexual identity arise. For example, children who are raised with emphasis on behaving like the opposite sex usually have no difficulty during preschool years but encounter tremendous conflict in social expectation and conformity when they enter school. If this conflict is not resolved, these individuals may choose alternate sexual relationships, such as homosexuality, or attempt to resolve the difference through transsexualism therapy.[1]

Development of the superego, or conscience, has its beginnings toward the end of the toddler years and is a major task for preschoolers. Learning right from wrong and good from bad is the beginning of morality. Children in this age-group are generally unable to understand the reasons for why something is acceptable or nonacceptable. They are aware of appropriate behavior mainly through punishment or reward and rely almost religiously on parental principles for developing their own moral judgment. However, verbal enforcement of limits is much more effective. For example, the toddler needed to be supervised, fenced in, and told not to run into the street to prevent accidents. The preschooler is much more aware of danger and can be relied on to listen and obey in most instances. If allowed to disagree and question, he will develop socially acceptable behavior as well as independence in thought and action.

Developing a conscience implies *learning the sociocultural mores* of the family's heritage. Depending on the type of attitudes conveyed, the child will learn not only appropriate behaviors but also tolerant, biased, or prejudiced values concerning his ethnic, religious, and social background and that of other groups. Much of this influence may remain dormant until he associates with children or adults of a different heritage. Then, depending on the particular group, he may be accepted or ostracized for his attitudes. For the school-age child this can represent a most difficult crisis, since acceptance by his peers is an important developmental need. For example, a child who is reared in a home where tolerance and respect for people of all religions and races are stressed may find it very difficult when his schoolmates disapprove of his relationship with a child of a different background.

Erikson maintains that the chief psychosocial crisis of the preschool period is acquiring a sense of *initiative*. The child is in a stage of energetic learning. He plays, works, and lives to the fullest and feels a real sense of accomplishment and satisfaction in his activities. Conflict arises when the child oversteps the limits of his ability and inquiry and experiences a sense of *guilt* for not having behaved or acted appropriately. Feelings of guilt, anxiety, and fear may also result from thoughts that differ from expected behavior. A particularly stressful thought is wishing one's parent dead. As a sense of rivalry or competition develops between the same sex child and parent, the child may think of ways to get rid of the interfering parent. In most situations this is resolved by strongly identifying with the same sex parent and peers during the school years. However, if that same sex parent dies before the identification process is completed, the preschooler can be overwhelmed with feelings of guilt for having wished, and therefore caused, the death. Clarifying for children that wishes cannot and do not make events occur is essential in helping them overcome their guilt and anxiety.

Cognitive development

One of the tasks related to the preschool period is *readiness for school and scholastic learning*. Many of the thought processes of this period are crucial for achieving such readiness. Piaget's cognitive theory actually does not include a period specifically of 3 to 5 years. The *preoperational* phase comprises the age span from 2 to 7 years and is divided into two stages, the *preconceptual* phase, ages 2 to 4 years, and the phase of *intuitive thought,* ages 4 to 7 years. One of the main transitions during each of these two phases is the shift from totally egocentric thought to social awareness and regard for others. This transition is very closely associated with the development of the superego. The child is able to think and verbalize his mental processes without having to act out his thinking. However, he can only think of one idea at a time, a concept known as *centration*. He is unable to think of all parts in terms of the whole. Outside influences or perceptions direct his understanding of a visual concept.

Piaget's concept of *conservation,* or the idea that a mass can be changed in size, shape, volume, or length without losing or adding to the original mass, is not understood by prelogical children. This is easily demonstrated by the 4- or 5-year-old child's understanding of numbers. Children in this age-group may be able to count from one to ten, but they do not have a mathematic conception. For example, if coins are placed in a straight row, the child can easily count ten of them. If they are placed in a more complex arrangement, the child is less likely to count all ten accurately. He may arrive at the number ten by recounting the same coins twice. Also, the concept of reversibility, that ten is ten no matter how the coins are arranged, is not comprehended. If the same ten coins are placed in a long row, and another shorter row of ten coins is placed alongside, the child will state that the longer row has more coins, even if he recounts each row and states that both contain the same number of coins.

Preschoolers also judge what they see by the immediate perceptual clues given them. For example, if two lines of equal length are presented in such a way that one appears longer than the other, the child will state that one line is longer, even if he measures both lines with a ruler or yardstick and finds that each has the same length. Therefore, experiences are judged by outside appearances and results, not by intrinsic, logical indicators. Understanding this prelogical thinking in young children helps other persons, such as nurses, interact with them in the most efficacious manner. One example of how manipulating matter according to the child's understanding can facilitate performing an activity concerns administration of drugs. If the child is to receive 5 ml of liquid medication, it is advisable to give it in a small medicine cup, rather than a large cup, since the child will imagine that the large vessel contains more liquid. Since he is unable to perceive the two dimensions of height and width simultaneously, the child will choose one dimension and measure the amount according to that standard. If the child refuses the medicine in the small cup, he may accept it once it is poured into a large cup because the liquid will appear less in a tall, wide container.

There are many everyday examples of how the young child's inability to conserve matter influences his behavior. Probably one of the most common situations involves eating and the amount of food placed on a dish. If the same amount of food is placed on a small and a large plate, the child may state that the large plate contains more food and may feel overwhelmed by the apparently large quantity. Parents are usually "taught" this by their children and "learn" ways to use this thinking to fool the child. Meat that is cut thin and flat appears to be more in quantity than the same amount of meat that is cut thick, and the child will generally consume more of the thicker portion. The opposite also has its advantages. Giving a child a large, flat cookie will please and satisfy him more than a small, thick one.

Children develop logical thought processes and understanding of conservation of numbers, substance, length, and so on during the school years (Chapter 17). It is no accident that learning subjects such as mathematics or science is begun at 6 years of age and later. Although some children might comprehend the meaning, reversibility, and symbolization of numbers earlier, most do not until 6 or 7 years of age.

Language continues to develop during the preschool period. Speech remains primarily a vehicle of egocentric communication. The child assumes that everyone thinks as he does and that a brief explanation of his thinking makes his entire thought understood by others. Because of this self-referenced, egocentric verbal communication, it is frequently necessary to explore and understand the young child's thinking through other nonverbal approaches. For children in this age-group, the most enlightening and effective method is *play*. Play becomes the child's work of understanding, adjusting to, and working out his life's experiences. Because of their rich imagination and unlimited ability to invent and imitate, all kinds of play hold therapeutic and communicative value. At this age the child's egocentricity dominates his interaction. Expressions about others, such as the doll, puppet, truck, dog, and so on, are actually descriptions of himself. To know what a child is really thinking demands skill, time, and patience in those willing to learn to look beyond the words and into the hearts and minds of these children.

Preschoolers afford adults, particularly parents, teachers, and nurses, the richest opportunity of comprehending the uniqueness, innocence, and genuineness of children. Children's conversation with their toys can tell more in a few minutes than many long hours of conversation between two adults, which is illustrated in the following example:

> Five-year-old Ann is playing mommy and has her family of dolls nearby. She is "talking" on her telephone, exclaiming to her doll children, "Be quiet! Can't you see that I am busy? This is an important business call. Go away and play somewhere else." She hangs up the phone and becomes the little girl at whom she had just yelled. She makes believe she is crying and says, "I always do bad things. I wish mommy wouldn't yell at me all the time."
>
> Ann's mother has overheard this play conversation and is acutely aware of the similarity between the play session and real-life experiences in the home. She had never before realized how the child must have felt when she was preoccupied with other business. She had always been irritated by her daughter's inconsiderateness. As she analyzed the example more closely, she realized that this was happening a few times a day and that, with her working part-time, she never really gave the child her undivided attention. She planned to set aside 1 hour every morning before leaving for work to play or read to Ann and to confine her business telephone calls to the evening when Ann's father was home.

This mother was perceptive to clues regarding the child's feelings. However, not all parents are this aware and frequently negate what they hear, believing it to be unimportant or irrelevant. To understand children is to listen to their spoken and nonspoken language. Communicating messages to them may also necessitate using their methods, such as play, imitation, role playing, and so on. Unlike toddlers who respond less favorably to anticipatory explanation or preparation for a potentially frightening experience, preschoolers have the ability to comprehend simple explanations, enjoy preparation such as seeing or playing with equipment, and can relate how they feel and think by using puppets or dolls.

Preschoolers increasingly use language without comprehending the meaning of words, particularly concepts of right or left, time, and causality. The child may use the concepts correctly but only in the circumstances he has learned them. For example, he may know how to put on his shoes by remembering that the buckle is always on the outside of the foot. However, if different shoes have no buckles, he cannot reason which shoe fits which foot. Any experience is judged by its end product. For example, the child who wins the race is the "fastest," even if he ran a shorter distance or started before the others. Rules of the game are only governing statements that can be changed and altered according to the specific events. To return to the preceding example, the school-age child will state that the child who ran a shorter distance or started before the others did not play fairly and, therefore, did not win and is not the fastest. This difference in thinking often complicates play activity between children in these two age-groups because each judges the situation from a different standard.

Superficially, *causality* resembles logical thought. The child explains a concept as he heard it described by others, but his understanding is limited. The concept of death illustrates this type of thinking. The adult concept of death implies inevitability and irreversibility. The preschooler may state that when a person dies it is forever. When asked what forever means, he may explain that the person has gone away, but that he may return someday. Some of the explanations offered to children about death support this idea of reversibility, such as "He has gone on a trip and will not be back for a very long time." Since *time* is still incompletely understood, the child interprets this according to his own frame of reference, such as "A long time means until Christmas." Explaining life events accurately and honestly helps children form correct concepts and leaves them with fewer self-interpreted meanings. Time is best explained in relationship to an event, such as "Your mother will visit you after you finish your lunch." Avoiding terms such as yesterday, tomorrow, next week, Tuesday, and so on to express when an event is expected to occur and associating time with usual expected daily occurrences help children learn about temporal relationships, while increasing their trust in other's predictions. Children are usually not able to tell time on a clock until 7 or 8 years of age.

Age is another concept that is judged by one set of criteria, such as size or physical appearance. A 5-year-old child's question of "Was the baby just born?" illustrates that the small 10-month-old infant could be a newborn to the preschooler. Children gradually develop the ability to judge age based on multiple factors other than size about the age of 8 years.

The preschooler's thinking is often described as *"magical."* Because of his egocentrism and his transductive reasoning (association of one event with a simultaneous event), the child believes that his thoughts are all-powerful. A classic example is the development of fears during this period (see p. 549). Because the child need not base his thinking on logical facts, any explanation that he contrives to explain an event is acceptable to him. If two events occur at the same time, his thoughts are even more strengthened. For example, if he has an injury that necessitates emergency medical attention, he may assume that the treatment is punishment for wrongdoing rather than a necessary intervention.

Preschoolers believe in the power of words and accept their meaning literally. A significant example of this type of thinking is calling the child "bad" because he did something wrong. In his mind, telling him that he is bad means that he is bad. For this reason it is better to relate such words to the act, by saying, for example, "That was a bad thing to do."

Play

Play is the young child's work and life. Play has an autotherapeutic value as the child grows and learns. Various types of play, including cooperative, associative, parallel, solitary independent, and onlooker play and unoccupied behavior, have been described as typical of preschoolers.

In *cooperative* play the child plays in a group *with* other children. There is a common interactive activity, such as a conversation, competitive game, or role playing. The group is loosely formed, but there is a marked sense of belonging or not belonging. The leader-follower relationship is definitely established, and the activity is controlled by one or two members. There is a division of labor, such as who plays what role, and the activity is organized to allow one child to supplement another's function in order to complete the goal.

The child plays with other children and engages in a common activity in *associative* play, but the rules of the group are loosely established. One child does not dictate the activity of another. There is no division of labor, leadership assignment, or mutual goal. An example of associative play is two children playing with dolls, each borrowing articles of clothing from the other, engaging in similar conversation, but neither directing the other's actions nor establishing rules regarding the limits of the play session.

In *parallel* play the child plays independently—not with, but *alongside*—other children. He may play with the same type of toys as the other children, but he plays with them as he desires and does not try to influence or modify other children's activity. There is no group association. This type of play is more common among toddlers, but it may also occur in other groups of any age. Individuals who are engaged in a creative craft with each person separately working on his own project are in parallel play.

The child plays alone and independently with toys that are different from those of other children in *solitary independent* play. He makes no effort to get close to the other children and pursues his activity without reference to what the others are doing. This differs from parallel play in that the child is *apart* from, not alongside, others.

In *onlooker* play the child watches what other children are doing but makes no attempt to enter into the play activity. There is an active interest in observing the interaction of others but no movement toward participating. Watching television is a common example of the onlooker role.

In *unoccupied behavior* the child is not playful but focuses his attention momentarily on anything that strikes his interest. He is daydreaming, fiddling with his clothes or other objects, or walking aimlessly. This differs from the onlooker, who is actively observing the activity of others.

All types of play serve some purpose for children and are normal and expected in moderation. Assessing children's activity involves investigation of how much time is spent in each type of play. A child who is mostly the onlooker or the solitary independent participant is missing the social relationships of associative or cooperative play. Excessive unoccupied behavior warrants special notice since it may indicate a troubled, unstimulated, or depressed youngster. Each type of play also benefits various aspects of development. Physical exertion is most often a part of cooperative play, particularly in games or role playing. The onlooker or the unoccupied player is in the passive role and loses the physical, social, competitive, and educational functions of play. However, passive forms of play provide needed periods of relaxation.

Imaginary playmates. Play is so much a part of the young child's life that reality and fantasy become blurred. The make-believe is reality during play and only becomes fantasy when the toys are put away or the dress-up clothes are removed. It is no wonder that imaginary playmates are so much a part of this age period. They serve many purposes—they become friends in times of loneliness, they accomplish what the child is still attempting, and they experience what the child wants to forget or remember. Parents often worry about the imaginary playmates, not realizing how normal and useful they are. Children usually give up these friends when the group process becomes much more important, usually when they enter school. Allowing children to enjoy their make-believe world and providing them with experiences with other children and community activi-

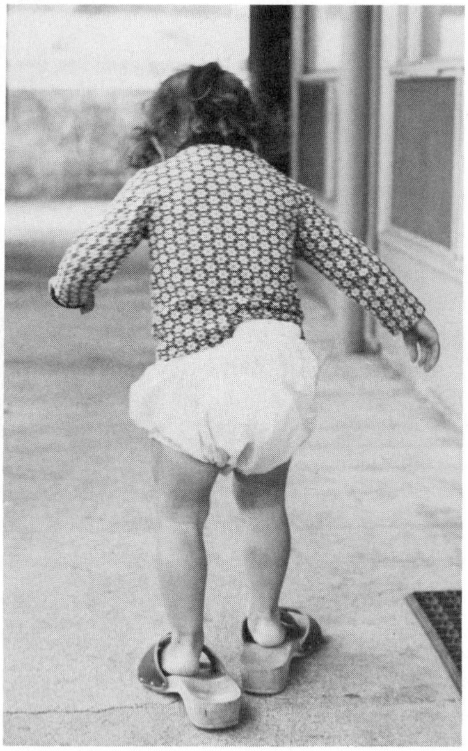

Fig. 15-1. Role playing for the preschooler. (From Erickson, M. L.: Assessment and management of developmental changes in children, St. Louis, 1976, The C. V. Mosby Co., p. 131.)

ties readies them for social interaction while giving them the security of their "special" friends.

Selection of play materials. Play activities for children in this age-group should provide for *physical growth and refinement of motor skills,* such as jumping, running, and climbing. Tricycles, trucks, wagons, gym and sports equipment, sandbox, wading pool, and winter sleds help develop muscles and coordination. Activities such as swimming, ice skating, skiing, and so on teach safety as well as muscle development and coordination.

Manipulative, constructive, creative, and educational toys provide for quiet activities, fine-motor development, and self-expression. Easy construction sets, large blocks of various sizes and shapes, a counting frame, paints, crayons, simple carpentry tools, musical toys, illustrated books, simple sewing or handicraft sets, large puzzles, and clay are suitable toys. Probably the most characteristic and pervasive preschooler activity is *imitative, imaginative, and dramatic* play. Dress-up clothes, dolls, housekeeping toys, dollhouses, play store toys, telephones, farm animals and equipment, village sets, trains, trucks, cars, planes, hand puppets, and doctor and nurse kits provide hours of self-expression (Fig. 15-1).

Television also has its place in children's play. Unfortunately, more often than not, television becomes the onlooker's paradise. Supervised selection of programs and scheduled hours of the day for quiet activity should guide how television is used. Children in this age-group enjoy and learn from educational children's programs, which are pur-

Table 15-1. The major developmental achievements of children 3, 4, and 5 years of age

Age (years)	Physical	Gross motor	Fine motor	Sensory	Language
3	Heart rate approximately 95 beats/minute Respiratory rate approximately 24 breaths/minute Blood pressure: systolic 100 mg Hg, diastolic 67 mm Hg (plus or minus 25 mm Hg) Usual weight gain of 1.8 to 2.7 kg (4 to 6 pounds) Usual gain in height of 5 to 6.25 cm (2 to 2.5 inches) May have achieved nighttime control of bowel and bladder	Rides tricycle Jumps off bottom step Stands on one foot for a few seconds Goes up stairs using alternate feet, may still come down using both feet on the step Broad jumps May try to dance, but balance may not be adequate	Builds tower of nine to ten cubes Builds bridge with three cubes Adeptly places small pellets in narrow-necked bottle In drawing, copies a circle, imitates a cross, names what he has drawn, cannot draw stickman but may make circle with facial features	Able to copy geometric figures Can place geometric forms into respective opening if form board is reversed Reading readiness may be present	Has vocabulary of about 900 words Uses primarily "telegraphic" speech Uses complete sentences of three to four words Talks incessantly regardless of whether anyone is paying attention Repeats sentence of six syllables Constantly asks questions

posely shown before dinner or after meals to provide a quiet activity. The exact influence of television on children's development and attitudes toward sex, violence, crime, and so on is a much disputed subject.[5] However, few authorities disagree on the fact that television should only be one part of children's total repertoire of social and recreational activities.

Adaptive behaviors

By 3 years of age the child has made tremendous strides from the dependency and callowness of infancy and the negativism and clumsiness of toddlerhood. The preschooler has excellent gross and fine motor control. Few physical barriers are obstacles. He is a very social and domesticated being. He cares for himself almost completely and enjoys doing simple household chores. He deliberately attempts to please others and is aware of manners and social amenities. Language use is a vehicle of communication, learning, and self-expression. The vocabulary is relatively extensive, almost completely intelligible, and fairly grammatically correct. The major developmental achievements for 3-, 4-, and 5-year-old children are summarized in Table 15-1.

Gross and fine motor behavior

Walking, running, climbing, and jumping are well established by age 36 months. Refinement in eye-hand and muscle coordination is evident in several areas. At age 3 years the preschooler rides a tricycle, walks on tiptoe, balances on one foot for a few seconds, and broad jumps. By 4 years of age he skips and hops proficiently on one foot and catches a ball reliably. By age 5 years he skips on alternate feet, jumps rope, and begins to skate and swim.

Drawing. Drawing shows several advancements in perception of shape and development of fine muscle coordination. The 3-year-old child copies a circle and imitates a cross and vertical and horizontal lines. He holds the crayon with his fingers, rather than in his fist. He scribbles or scrawls but names what he has drawn. He is not able to draw a complete stick figure but draws a round circle, later adds facial features, and, by 5 or 6 years of age, draws six parts (head, arms, legs, body, and facial features). Between ages 4 and 5 years he can trace a cross and copy a square. The triangle and diamond are usually the last geometric figures to be mastered, somewhere between 5 and 6 years of age.

Children's drawings have been studied extensively. As children progress from scribbling to picture making, they advance through four distinguishable stages.[9] In the *placement* stage the very earliest spontaneous scribblings of the 15-month-old child are placed on the paper in a specific placement pattern, such as in the center, all over, across the lower half, or across the page in a diagonal direction (Fig. 15-2). Approximately seventeen different placement patterns appear by the age of 2 years and, once developed, are never lost.

By age 3 years children are in the *shape stage*. They draw single-line outline forms such as rectangles, circles, ovals, crosses, and other odd shapes. As soon as they draw dia-

Socialization	Cognition	Family relationships
Dresses self almost completely if helped with back buttons and told which shoe is right or left Buttons and unbuttons accessible buttons Pulls on shoes Has increased attention span Feeds self completely Pours from a bottle or pitcher Can prepare simple meals, such as cold cereal and milk Can help to set table, dry dishes without breaking any Likes to "help" entertain by passing around food May have fears, especially of dark and going to bed Knows own sex and appropriate sex of others In play, parallel and associative phase; begins to learn simple games and meaning of rules, but follows them according to self-interpretation; speaks to doll, animal, truck, and so on; begins to work out social interaction through play; able to share toys, although expresses idea of "mine" frequently	Is in preconceptual phase Is egocentric in thought and behavior Has beginning understanding of time; uses many time-oriented expressions, talks about past and future as much as about present, pretends to tell time Has improved concept of space as demonstrated in understanding of prepositions and ability to follow directional command Has beginning ability to view concepts from another perspective	Attempts to please parents and conform to their expectations Is less jealous of younger sibling; may be opportune time for birth of additional sibling Is aware of family relationships and sex role functions Boys tend to identify more with father or other male figure Has increased ability to separate easily and comfortably from parents for short periods

Continued.

Table 15-1. The major developmental achievements of children 3, 4, and 5 years of age—cont'd

Age (years)	Physical	Gross motor	Fine motor	Sensory	Language
4	Pulse, respiration, and blood pressure decrease very slightly Height and weight gain remain constant Length at birth is doubled	Skips and hops on one foot Catches ball reliably Throws ball overhand Walks down stairs using alternate footing	Imitates a gate with cubes Uses scissors successfully to cut out picture following outline Can lace shoes, but may not be able to tie bow In drawing, copies a square, traces a cross and diamond, adds three parts to stick figure	Maximum potential for development of amblyopia	Has vocabulary of 1500 words or more Uses sentences of four to five words Questioning is at peak Tells exaggerated stories Knows simple songs May be mildly profane if he associates with older children Obeys four prepositional phrases, such as "under," "on top of," "beside," "in back of" or "in front of" Names one or more colors Comprehends analogies, such as, "If ice is cold, fire is ____" Repeats four digits Uses words liberally but frequently does not comprehend meaning
5	Pulse, respiration, and blood pressure decrease slightly Growth rate is similar to that of previous year Eruption of permanent dentition may begin, especially if deciduous tooth eruption was early (before age 6 months) First permanent teeth to erupt are four molars, which come in behind the last temporary teeth (often mistaken for temporary molars) Handedness is established (about 90% are right-handed)	Skips and hops on alternate feet Throws and catches ball well Jumps rope Skates with good balance Walks backward with heel to toe Jumps from height of 12 inches, lands on toes Balances on alternate feet with eyes closed	Ties shoelaces Uses scissors, simple tools, or pencil very well In drawing, copies a diamond and triangle; adds seven to nine parts to stickman; prints a few letters, numbers, or words, such as his first name	Minimum potential for development of amblyopia Visual acuity approaches 20/20 (may not be completely achieved until 8 years of age)	Has vocabulary of about 2100 words Uses sentences of six to eight words, with all parts of speech Names coins (nickel, dime, and so on) Names four or more colors Describes drawing or pictures with much comment and enumeration Asks meaning of words Asks inquisitive questions Can repeat sentence of ten syllables or more Knows names of days of week, months, and other time-associated words Defines words using action as well as description Knows composition of articles, such as, "A shoe is made of ________" Can follow three demands in succession

Socialization	Cognition	Family relationships
Very independent Tends to be selfish and impatient Aggressive physically as well as verbally Takes pride in accomplishments Has mood swings Boasts and tattles Shows off dramatically, enjoys entertaining others Tells family tales to others with no restraint Still has many fears In play, is cooperative and associative; imaginary playmates common; uses dramatic, imaginative, and imitative devices; works through unresolved conflicts, such as jealousy toward sibling, anger toward parent, or unconquered fear in himself; sexual exploration and curiosity demonstrated through play, such as being "doctor" or "nurse"	Is in phase of intuitive thought Causality still related to proximity of events Understands time better, especially in terms of sequence of daily events Unable to conserve matter Judges everything according to one dimension, such as height, width, or first Immediate perceptual clues dominate judgment Can choose longer of two lines or heavier of two objects Is beginning to develop less egocentrism and more social awareness May count correctly but has poor mathematic concept of numbers Still believes that thoughts cause events Obeys because parents have set limits, not because of understanding of reason behind right or wrong	Rebels if parents expect too much from him, such as impeccable table manners Takes aggression and frustration out on parents or siblings Do's and don'ts become important May have rivalry with older or younger siblings, may resent older's privileges and younger's invasion of privacy and possessions May run away from home Identifies strongly with parent of opposite sex Is able to run errands outside the home
Less rebellious and quarrelsome than at age 4 years More settled and eager to get down to business Not as open and accessible in thoughts and behavior as in earlier years Independent but trustworthy, not foolhardy Has fewer fears, relies on outer authority to control the world Eager to do things right and to please, tries to "live by the rules" Acts "manly" or "womanly" Takes increased responsibility for his actions Has fairly consistent and polished manners Cares for himself totally, occasionally needing supervision in dress or hygiene May complain over minor injuries but tries to be brave for major pain In play, cooperative; likes rules and tries to follow them but may cheat to avoid losing; begins to notice group conformity and sense of belonging; very industrious, tries to accomplish a goal and feels pride and satisfaction, as well as unhappiness and discontent; may demand to watch television more now that he understands programs better; not ready for concentrated close work or small print because of slight farsightedness and still unrefined eye-hand coordination; imitative play mimics the portrayed adult like a mirror image; wants to use real objects during play, such as actual ingredients to make cookies rather than sand or mud	Begins to question what parents think by comparing them to age-mates and other adults May notice prejudice and bias in outside world Is more able to view other's perspective, but tolerates differences rather than understands them Tends to be matter-of-fact about differences in others May begin to show understanding of conservation of numbers through counting objects regardless of arrangement Uses time-oriented words with increased understanding Very curious about factual information regarding his world	Gets along well with parents Doesn't run away from home May seek out mother more often than at age 4 years for reassurance and security, especially when entering school Is upset not to find parent, for example, when he comes home from school Tolerates siblings, but finds 3-year-old children a special nuisance Begins to question parents' thinking and principles Strongly identifies with parent of same sex, especially boys with their fathers Enjoys doing activities, such as sports, cooking, shopping, and so on, with parent of same sex

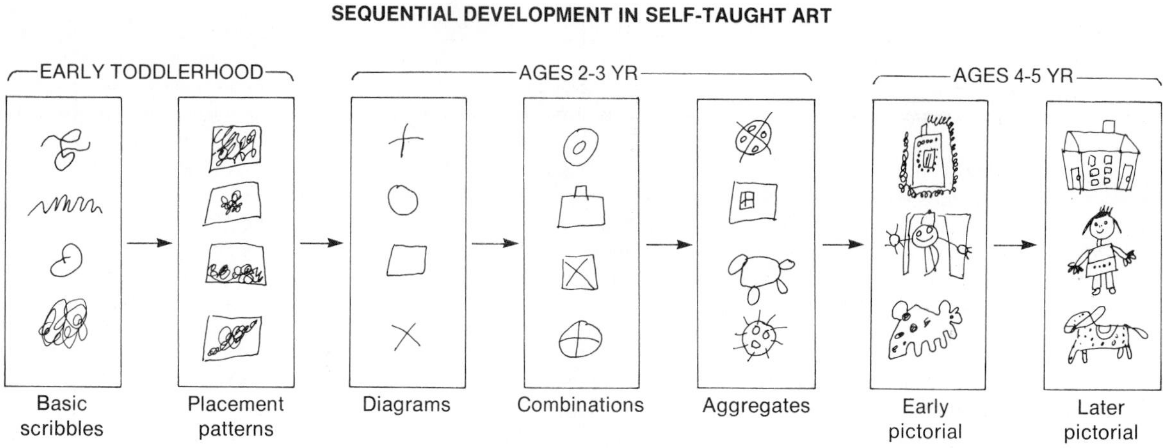

Fig. 15-2. Sequential development in self-taught art. (From Kellogg, R.: Understanding children's art. In Readings in Psychology Today, Del Mar, Calif., 1969, Communication-Research Machines, Inc.)

grams, they almost immediately progress to the *design stage,* in which simple forms are drawn together to make structured designs. When two diagrams are united, the resulting design is called a combine. Three or more united diagrams produce an aggregate (Fig. 15-2). Between the ages of 4 and 5 years most children enter the *pictorial stage,* in which the designs are recognizable as familiar objects. Early pictorial drawings are suggestive of human figures, houses, animals, trees, and so on. Later pictorial drawings are more clearly defined and recognizable. The child's pictorial drawings are not representations of the actual object, but esthetically satisfying structures that resemble familiar objects. For example, the initial human figure drawing is a circle with arms attached to the head. It is more an aggregate drawing than any attempt to copy a human figure. Drawings of animals follow the human figure drawing but are only a slight modification, such as attaching ears to the top of the head.

Children's drawings before age 6 years are strikingly similar from country to country, culture to culture, and from the past to the present. This suggests that there are some inherent neurologic mechanisms that influence the type of self-taught art forms. After age 6 years environmental influence, particularly from parents and teachers, shapes much of what children draw. It has been suggested that free scribbling and drawing are necessary for children to learn to read and that children who have been free to experiment and produce abstract forms have developed the mental set required for learning symbolic language.[9] Scribbling and drawing also help develop the fine muscle skills and eye-hand coordination eventually required for making precise letters and numbers.

Drawing is also a tool used for assessing intelligence, personality development, and psychosocial adjustment. The precise value of using drawing to measure such concepts is still an inexact science. However, children do reveal thoughts about themselves in their drawing, particularly school-age children. It is generally not necessary for one to have in-depth knowledge of children's drawings to make assumptions about their significance. One need only listen to all the clues, both verbal and nonverbal, to understand how and what children are communicating to others. For further discussion of children's drawing see Chapter 27.

Language

Language during the preschool years is quite sophisticated and complex. It also becomes a major mode of communication and social interaction. Vocabulary increases dramatically, from 300 words at age 2 years to over 2100 words at the end of 5 years of age. Sentence structure, grammatical usage, and intelligibility also advance to a nearly adult level.

Between 3 and 4 years of age children form sentences of about three to four words and include only the most essential words to convey a meaning. Such speech is often termed "telegraphic" for its brevity in length. Three-year-old children ask many questions and use plurals, correct pronouns, and the past tense of verbs. They name familiar objects, such as animals, parts of the body, and relatives or friends. They can give and follow simple commands. They talk incessantly, regardless of whether anyone is listening or answering them. They enjoy musical or talking toys or dolls and imitate new words proficiently.

From 4 to 5 years of age preschoolers use longer sentences of four to five words and more words than are used to convey a message, such as prepositions, adjectives, and a variety of verbs. They follow simple directional commands, such as "Put the ball on the chair," but can carry out only one request at a time. They answer questions, such as "What do you do when you are hungry?" by describing the appropriate action. Asking questions is at its peak, and children usually repeat the question until they receive an answer.

By the end of age 5 years children use all parts of speech grammatically correctly, except for deviations from the rule. They can define simple words by describing their use, shape, or general category of classification, not only by stating their outward appearance. For example, they define a ball as "round, something you bounce, or a toy," rather than by its color. They can give some opposites, such as, "If mommy is a woman, daddy is a man." By the time they are 6 years old, they can describe an object according to its composition, such as "a spoon is made of metal."

Not only does preschoolers' language acquisition advance, but the purpose of speaking also undergoes a radical transition. Speech can be of two types—egocentric or socialized.[13] *Egocentric* speech consists of repeating words and sounds for the pleasure of hearing oneself, either as a monologue (talking to oneself) or as collective monologue (talking *at,* not with, one or more persons). Collective monologue is an advancement over infantile speech, although no communication is intended by either. However, both forms have important functions. For one, this is pleasurable and part of one's activity and interaction with the environment, since it stimulates attention and reinforcement by others. Another is wish fulfillment. If a child cannot have something, he can wish it were so by verbalizing the desire. Since young children believe that thoughts cause events, saying the thoughts aloud reinforces this self-powerfulness. Before the age of 3 years most speech is directed at self-fulfillment or self-reference, such as "I want a drink" or "I can do it." Speech at this level is directed mostly to adults. Since children think that everyone else's world is the same as theirs, they expect others to understand their verbal messages when limited information is conveyed.

Socialized speech is for communication. At age 3 or 4 years social speech is still egocentric in that children communicate about themselves to others. They boast, tell stories of their adventures, and exaggerate their abilities. Between ages 5 and 6 years they are increasingly able to take the other's viewpoint. There is an exchange of knowledge with sharing of ideas. Conversations include much rationalization, justification, and disagreement. Without this type of communication, learning in a structured environment, such as school, would be severely hampered.

Language and sociocultural influences. Much controversy exists concerning the degree of social influence on intellectual development and academic achievement. Since within the highly verbal society of this country language is so essential a factor in learning, retardation in language development is a serious academic deterrent. Studies have repeatedly demonstrated that children from lower socioeconomic environments learn new words more slowly, retain unclear pronunciation longer, and use shorter, less complex sentences than do middle or upper class children. In addition the type of messages conveyed has been found to differ markedly.[2] Lower class families use a *restricted code* of communication. They use short sentences or phrases that include little explanation, information, and concepts. In the *elaborated code* of middle class families, messages are more complex, more individualized, and include reasons or explanations. An illustration of both types of communication occurs in the different approaches of either group toward discipline. The restricted code message dictates, "Go to bed," whereas the elaborated code suggests, "It is time to go to bed now. Tomorrow is an early day and you need your rest." The latter communication is much more personal and positive. It is an authoritative statement, whereas the other is authoritarian and dictatorial. Assessing language development from a sociologic framework yields additional information to the parent-child relationship, family interactions, and parental controls.

Personal-social behavior

The pervasive ritualism and negativism of toddlerhood gradually diminish during the preschool years. Although self-assertion is still a major theme, preschoolers demonstrate their sense of autonomy differently. They are able to verbalize their request for independence, as well as perform independently, because of their much refined physical and cognitive development. They fully care for themselves by 4 or 5 years of age, needing little, if any, assistance with dressing, eating, or toileting. They can also be trusted to obey warnings of danger, although the 3- or 4-year-old child may exceed his boundaries at times. They are also much more sociable and willing to please. They have internalized many of the standards and values of the family, and their conscience dictates many of their actions. By the end of early childhood they begin to question parental values and compare them to those of the peer group and other authority figures; as a result they may be less willing to abide by the family's code of conduct.

Preschoolers become increasingly aware of their position and role within the family. Although this is a more secure age for experiencing the addition of another sibling, relinquishing the position of first or youngest is still difficult and requires appropriate preparation (see p. 523). Sex role typing becomes a major social task and is particularly evident in the child's play. Girls imitate the female role, and boys, the male role. Even in households where there is a blurring of the traditional sex roles, children identify with certain feminine or masculine behaviors, which are demonstrated in almost all heterosexual relationships. Probably at no other time is the reproduction of the behavior of significant adults so faithful and absorbing as in 4- and 5-year-old children. Toward the end of the preschool period, children are less satisfied with make-believe or pretend objects and enjoy actually doing the activity, such as cooking, carpentry, and so on. This also explains why sexual curiosity not only involves asking questions but is also directed toward exploring and looking at the physical differences between the sexes (see p. 550).

Preschoolers have relinquished much of the stranger anxiety and fear of separation of earlier years. They relate to unfamiliar people easily and tolerate brief separations from parents with little or no protest. However, they still need parental security, reassurance, guidance, and approval, especially when entering nursery or regular school. Prolonged separation, such as that imposed by illness and hospitalization, is difficult, but preschoolers respond very well to anticipatory preparation and concrete explanation. They can cope with changes in daily routine much better than toddlers, but they may develop more imaginary fears. They gain security and comfort from familiar objects, such as toys, dolls, or photographs of family members. They are able to work through many of their unresolved fears, fantasies, and anxieties through play, especially if guided with appropriate play objects such as dolls or puppets that represent family members, medical and nursing staff, other children, and so on.

PROMOTING OPTIMUM DEVELOPMENT

In many respects the preschool years present few child-rearing problems. The preschooler is quite independent, listens and obeys most of the time, clings less to adults, and enjoys peers for playmates. To the casual observer the child's play is purely recreational. But to the more astute and perceptive observer, play is the child's work of developing into a physically, psychologically, and intellectually well-adjusted young person. Through play preschoolers channel their industrious energy toward achievement and competence or toward failure and dissatisfaction. How children feel about themselves in later life is directly influenced by how they succeed in acquiring a sense of initiative during early childhood.

Developing a sense of initiative

By the time children reach 3 years of age their gross and fine motor abilities are sufficiently developed to enable them to pursue almost limitless activities. If they have been allowed to express their independence and negativism constructively, they are ready to direct their energy toward new learning. They learn how to interact and relate to other children and adults; they learn appropriate sex role functions and socially acceptable behavior; they learn right and wrong and the types of rewards or punishment associated with each. However, learning does not necessarily imply success. Without appropriate guidance and reinforcement, children can learn unacceptable behavior and, instead of feeling accomplishment, will feel inadequacy, guilt, and inferiority.

Family relationships. Since the nuclear family is the most powerful motivating factor in the young child's life, it is logical to assume that the type of child rearing will to some degree influence the child's development. Although child rearing is a complex result of sociocultural, ethnic, religious, and economic variables in each parent's life, there are three recognizable and distinct types. *Authoritarian and dictatorial* parents try to control their children's behavior and attitudes through unquestioned mandates. They establish rules and regulations or a standard of conduct that they expect to be rigidly and unquestioningly followed. They value and reward absolute obedience, mute acceptance of their word, and unfailing respect for the family's principles and beliefs. They forcefully punish any behavior that is contrary to parental standards. Punishment need not be corporal but may be stern withdrawal of their love and approval. The familiar saying, "Children are to be seen, not heard," typifies this type of child rearing.

Permissive or laissez-faire parents are at the other extreme, exerting little or no control over their children's actions. They avoid imposing their own standards of conduct and allow their children to regulate their activity as much as possible. They consider themselves resources for the children, not role models. If rules do exist, the parents explain the underlying reason, encourage the children's opinions, and consult them in decision-making processes. They hardly ever punish the children, since most behavior is considered acceptable.

Authoritative or democratic parents combine some child-rearing practices from both extremes. They direct their children's behavior and attitudes by emphasizing the reason for rules but negatively reinforce deviations. They respect each child's individuality and allow the children to voice their objections to family standards or regulations. Parental control is firm and consistent but tempered with encouragement, understanding, and security. Control is focused on the issue, not on withdrawing love or fearing punishment. They foster "inner-directedness," the type of conscience that regulates behavior based on feelings of guilt or shame for wrongdoing, not on fear of being caught or punished.

The most successful type of child rearing seems to be the authoritative method. Parents' realistic standards and reasonable expectations result in children who are self-reliant, self-assertive, inquisitive, and content. Both the dictatorial and the noncontrol parents shield their children from the opportunity to explore their limits for self-mastery. As a result these children are uncertain, immature, less exploratory or questioning, and discontent. In order to feel a sense of mastery, accomplishment, and competence, children must be allowed reasonable freedom to test their abilities. In the authoritarian home children are concerned with meeting parental expectations and avoiding negative consequences associated with any deviation. They are not free, or willing, to judge the behavior on its own merits. If the parent states, "You are not allowed to ride a bicycle," they will not try to learn, even if mastery of the skill would eventually prove worthwhile, safe, and enjoyable. In permissive homes children are so unrestricted that they too experience little success, either because they fear to try activities above their present ability or from attempting feats that consistently exceed their competency, resulting in numerous failures. Without guidance they are always uncertain and anxious about whether their behavior is right or wrong.

Few families fit precisely into any one of the three types of child-rearing methods. There are vestiges of each in almost every home. Children quickly learn how to manipulate each parent for the most advantageous result. Problems arise when each parent adheres to different extremes, such as strict adherence to rules vs unlimited freedom. Although children are remarkably flexible in adapting to wide disparity between parents' methods of control, they need congruency in the messages they receive. Helping parents resolve some of their differences allows children much greater security and reassurance to learn acceptable behavior and achieve initiative and competency.

Father's role. Until the preschool years most of the emphasis for child development focuses on the mother's role in child rearing. Although the importance of the father's role from conception to birth and through all the child's years is now being recognized, it is well known that preschoolers, especially boys, need a male influence. In psychoanalytic theory the *negative* forces underlying the boy's resentment of his father in his attempt to possess his mother influence the child's strong identification with the male aggressor as a means of resolving the conflict. Learning theory emphasizes the *positive* forces that facilitate the father-son relationship, namely, the reward and satisfaction for acting masculine. In either case the boy must relinquish his primary attachment to his mother for stronger identification with his father. Girls, on the other hand, are spared this transition, because they continue their strong identification with the mother in the sex role typing process.

The effects of the father's absence on the development of boys and girls have been studied, but the results are far from conclusive. However, one fact emerges consistently: separation or loss of father before age 6 years, particularly during the preschool years, has a greater effect on a daughter's or son's behavior than later loss of the father.[4,7] After children enter school there are many more ways to compensate for lack of a male role model. In addition the role of the mother as single parent is important in encouraging masculine behavior in boys.[3] The effects of father loss on daughters, particularly those effects that appear during adolescence, seem to be caused by a lack of opportunity for constructive interaction with an attentive, significant male, rather than deviations in sex typing.[7]

The effects of the mother's absence on young children have not been extensively studied, except in terms of separation anxiety or institutionalized care. One reason might be that in most cases in which a mother is absent another female substitutes in her role as care giver. Also, most single-parent homes include mothers, not fathers. Loss of a father from death or divorce usually does not result in as immediate a replacement as in loss of a mother.

Nursery school. The effects of early education and stimulation on children have increasingly gained recognition and importance. These first few years are foundational for personality development, social awareness, concept formation, and language. Since social development widens to include age-mates and other significant adults, preschool provides an excellent vehicle for expanding children's experiences with others. In nursery school or day-care centers, children are exposed to opportunities for learning group cooperation, adjusting to various sociocultural differences, and coping with frustration, dissatisfaction, and anger. If activities are tailored to provide mastery and achievement, children increasingly feel success, self-confidence, and personal competence. Whether or not structured learning is imposed is less important than the social climate, type of guidance, and attitude toward the children that is fostered by the teacher or leader. With a teacher who is aware of preschoolers' developmental abilities and needs, the children will learn from any activity that is provided. Most nursery schools incorporate a similar daily schedule of quiet play, active outdoor activity, group activities such as games and projects, creative or free play, and snack and rest periods.

Nursery school is particularly beneficial for children who lack a peer group experience, such as an only child, and for children from culturally deprived homes. Nursery school provides extensive stimulation for language, physical, and social development. It also is an excellent preparation for entrance into regular school. For a child from a poor home, regular school can be so overwhelming that all learning is impeded by the sensory overload. Regular school places many more demands on children for prolonged attention, self-disciplined behavior, and demonstrated progress in performance and achievement than the less-structured atmosphere of preschool. Nursery school and kindergarten are a transitional preparation for the demands of academic learning in later years.

Children need preparation for the preschool experience, whether it is a formal nursery school, organized day-care center, or casual gathering in a neighbor's home. For young children it represents a change from their usual home environment and prolonged separation from parents. Even if the child has been cared for by a baby-sitter, preschool is still different since the individualized attention is no longer as intense or sustained. Parents should introduce their child to the teacher and school and remain for at least some part of the first day until the child is comfortable and at ease. Frequently a full day is too overwhelming and needs to be shortened to a morning or afternoon session. This is particularly important for children beginning in a day-care center. Since most day-care centers offer child-care services for the duration of a regular working day, children should be introduced slowly at first and gradually required to stay the entire day. Many parents are not aware of this and begin the day-care service the same day as they begin new employment. Both parent and child are faced with adjusting to a significant alteration in life-style and may be less able to cope successfully with the change than if the day-care center experience had been started shortly before the parent's employment.

Independent-dependent behavior. Exactly what determines the degree of dependent vs independent behavior in individuals is still an unanswered question. From birth there are obvious differences in the manageability of children. Some passively accept parental demands, show little resistance to change, and cling to parents. Others demonstrate their individuality almost as soon as they recover from the exhausting labor and birth. They demand a schedule that meets their needs, they explore away from their parents at an early age, and they tend to assume leadership roles in most group experiences. Parental practices, such as achievement behaviors, do seem to influence the development of independency in their children. Parents who reward their children's efforts to achieve and ignore or disapprove of dependent behaviors tend to have more self-reliant, independent children. These parents also reward approval-seeking behavior. When children look for approval and praise for their accomplishments, the parents respond with emotional support, reassurance, and help if needed. Precisely how parents encourage dependency is unclear. Overprotective, excessively controlling, and dominating parental practices seem to attribute to dependency in children. However, the opposite also holds true in some instances. Rejecting, punishing, emotionally cold, and nonnurturant parents encourage dependency, probably as a result of the child's continued efforts to evoke closeness and approval from them.

Personality characteristics, such as independency or dependency, are clearly evident by the preschool years. However, this may not be the critical period for future development of either attribute. It seems that the persistence of passivity during the school-age years correlates more significantly with dependency in later life. Also, a shift from dependent to independent behavior during the latency period is more evident in boys than in girls. This is probably a result of sociocultural expectations of boys from teachers and peers. Girls are less likely to be rewarded by these extrafamilial groups for independent behavior.[8]

A warm, close, nurturant parent-child relationship does not foster dependency. On the contrary such a relationship fosters trust and security that greatly helps children achieve autonomy and initiative. Children who have been rewarded with approval and affection for their accomplishments are motivated to learn and achieve in order to receive such parental reinforcement. The democratic, authoritative family encourages independent, self-reliant behavior because children are guided toward goals that are appropriate for their level of mastery. However, sometimes all children feel insecure and revert to more dependent behavior during periods of stress, such as illness, hospitalization, or sudden prolonged separation. They need help in finding ways of coping with the insecurity and frustration and activities that enhance feelings of control, self-esteem, and self-reliance. For the preschool child, play is an excellent therapeutic method for promoting independence in thought and behavior. A sensitive parent or other significant adult can help the child deal with his insecure, frightening feelings by acting out the experience with dolls or puppets. In this way the child feels powerful and in control, while releasing his anxiety through play.

HEALTH PROMOTION DURING PRESCHOOL YEARS

Nutritional guidance

Nutritional requirements for preschoolers are fairly similar to those for toddlers (Chapter 14). The requirement for calories per unit of body weight continues to decrease slightly to 90 kcal/kg (40 kcal/pound). Fluid requirements may also decrease slightly but are dependent on activity level, climatic conditions, and state of health. Protein consumption seems to be more than adequate if it comprises 15% of the total caloric intake. Although the optimal protein requirement is not known, a daily consumption of approximately 30 g is recommended.

Some preschoolers still have food habits that are typical of toddlers, such as food fads and strong taste preferences. Four years of age seems to be another period for resurgence of finicky eating, which is generally characteristic of the more rebellious and rowdy behavior of children in this age-group. By age 5 years children are greatly influenced by the food habits of others and are more agreeable to trying new foods, especially if encouraged by an adult who also experiments with a new taste or different dish. Mealtimes can become battlegrounds if parents expect impeccable table manners. Usually the 5-year-old child is ready for the "social" side of eating, but the 3- or 4-year-old child still has difficulty in sitting quietly through a long family meal.

Parents sometimes worry about the quantity of food preschoolers consume. In general the quality is much more important than the quantity, a fact that should be stressed during nutritional counseling. Young children often consume more food than parents realize. One approach toward lessening this parental concern is advising parents to keep a weekly record of everything the child eats. In particular the need for measuring the amount of food, such as setting aside ½ cup of vegetables, and serving the child from this premeasured amount should be stressed. In this way, there is a more accurate estimate of food intake at each meal. Usually, by the end of the week's food chart, parents are amazed at how much the child has consumed, even though at each meal the amount seemed so minimal. In general preschoolers consume only slightly more than toddlers, or about half of an adult's portion. (See Table 14-3 and the boxed material on p. 528 for recommended serving sizes and sample menus.)

Safety and security

Because of improved gross and fine motor skill, coordination, and balance, preschoolers are less prone to falls than toddlers. They tend to be less reckless, listen more to parental rules, and are aware of potential danger, such as hot objects, sharp instruments, dangerous heights, and so on. Putting objects in the mouth as part of exploration has all but ceased, although poisoning is still a danger. Pedestrian motor vehicle accidents increase from activities such as playing in the street, riding tricycles, running after balls, or forgetting safety regulations when crossing streets. In general the guidelines suggested for accident prevention in Table 14-4 are applicable to children in this age-group as well. However, emphasis is now on *education* for safety and potential hazards, in addition to appropriate protection. Since preschoolers are great imitators, it is especially essential that parents set a good example by "practicing what they preach." Children are very quick to observe discrepancies in what they are told to do and what they see others do. Since they faithfully and unquestioningly believe in their parent's values and rules, this is an excellent opportunity for parents to practice and teach safe, cautious habits in daily living.

Fears

Throughout life fears follow a developmental sequence. During early infancy the child startles at a loud noise or a sudden movement or jarring. Whether this is fear in a psychologic sense or purely a neurologic reflex remains to be clearly defined. By about age 6 months infants have some concept of depth and refuse to cross a visual cliff (see Chapter 12). The parachute reflex, which appears at about the same age as depth perception and persists indefinitely, also seems to indicate infants' perception of fear of falling as they place their hands in a protective position. It appears that such responses are inborn mechanisms for survival and protection.

During the first 2 years of life children are frightened by physical stimuli, such as loud noises, strange people or places, sudden movements, particularly the sensation of falling, and flashes of light. Usually by age 2 years children develop fears of the dark or of being left alone, particularly at bedtime. During ages 2 to 5 years the greatest number and variety of *real* and *imagined* fears are present. The exact cause of children's fears is unknown but can be traced to theorists such as Freud and Piaget. Freudians believe that the upsurge of fears during the preschool years results from preschoolers' anxiety of being injured or mutilated (castration complex). Piaget views fears as a product of the type of thinking of children in this age-group. Preschoolers are caught between the egocentric thinking of infants, which protects them from imagined fears, and the more logical thought processes of school-age children, which help explain and dispel potential fears. Children in the preconceptual stage still engage in egocentric thought but are now able to imagine an event without actually experiencing it. For example, seeing someone hurt is sufficient for realizing what the hurt must be like and, consequently, fearing that hurt. In medical practice this is frequently observed. If a young child witnesses another child getting an injection, he becomes very upset, almost as if he himself had gotten the injection. This is in contrast to infants or older children, who are less affected by observing such an event.

As a result of magical thinking, all kinds of fears become real and logical in the minds of young children. No amount of logical persuasion, coercion, or ridicule will send away the ghosts, boogeymen, monsters, devils, and so on. The best way to help children overcome their fears is by actively involving them in finding practical methods to deal with the frightening experience. This may be as simple as keeping a dim night-light on in the child's bedroom to assure him that no monsters lurk in the dark. Exposing children to the feared object in a safe situation also provides a type of conditioning or desensitization. For instance children who are afraid of dogs should never be forced to approach or touch one, but they may be gradually introduced to the experience by watching other children play with the animal. This type of modeling, demonstrating fearlessness in others, can be very effective if the child is allowed to progress at his own rate.

Many young children's fears seem absurd to parents, such as fear of disappearing down the bathtub drain. Adults may wonder how a child could ever fear such a preposterous event when the child's body is so much larger than the small opening in the tub. However, preschoolers have little meaningful concept of relative size; to them, if the water can be drained away, so can they. Sometimes this fear is also associated with anxiety about toilet training, specifically the experience of watching one's stools being flushed away. In the child's immature sense of body image, that product is still a part of him, which suddenly vanishes forever. In addition parents frequently express delight at seeing the stool in the toilet and do not appreciate the child's feelings of seeing it disappear. Sometimes, relaxing the pressures of toilet training may help the fear of vanishing down the drain. Another approach toward such a fear is not releasing the drain until after the child is out of the tub. Water play is also effective. Letting the child bathe a doll or play with toys in a tub of water and opening the drain with the toys still inside demonstrate that large objects cannot go down the drain. In this way the experience that created the fear in the child can be reconstructed without involving the child directly as the victim. The child is allowed alternate methods to feel in control and powerful, while overcoming his fear.

Usually by 5 or 6 years of age children relinquish these old fears. If told about a previous fear, such as disappearing down the bathtub drain, they will respond with, "That's silly. Anybody can see that I am too big to fit in that small hole." If asked about believing in ghosts or the like, they will typically remark that they do not believe in or fear them because they have never seen one. This is quite logical and very concrete and helps explain away many of the fears of younger years. However, their quest for proof and facts also makes other events, such as death, more terrifying. Before this age, death is associated with sleep and fear of separation or abandonment, but it is probably not differentiated from any other cause of temporary loss, such as illness. Since the concept of time and causality is still poorly understood, preschoolers view death as an event that is reversible, but not inevitable. One of their fears at experiencing the death of someone near to them is the realization that this could possibly happen to them. Such a fear is similar to disappearing down the drain or falling asleep and not awakening. How adults explain death to children and the opportunities provided them about loss from death, such as of a pet, affect their future attitude toward death. Young children have the right to feel. Protecting them from death or other tragic events deprives them of the opportunity to express their feelings and learn healthy outlets for sadness, grief, anger, disappointment, and so on. Very frequently adults' own fear of death hinders them from helping children understand what loss means. Fear of death, pain, and mutilation are fears that few people ever completely overcome but concerning which they continually search for explanation, reason, and meaning. Children also need assistance in finding whatever rational, logical explanation there is for death, even if that explanation is "I don't know." Honest answers allow children to express what they think, especially at a time when their thoughts and fantasies seem so real and powerful to them. (For a further discussion of children's concept of death, see Chapter 27.)

Sexual curiosity

Preschoolers have absorbed and experienced a tremendous amount of information during their short lifetimes. Although their thinking may not be adultlike, they search constantly for explanations and reasons that are logical and reasonable to them. The word "why" seems to supplant the word "no," which was common in toddlerhood. One of their major developmental achievements has been severing the psychologic "placenta" from mother as they discover their sense of self apart from others. It is only natural that as they learn about "me" they will also want to know "why me," "how me," and so on. Questions such as "Where do babies come from?" are sexual in content but informational in intent. Such inquiries are as casual as "Why is the sky blue?" "What makes it rain?" or "Who is that?" It is the *way* in which questions about procreation are answered that conditions children, even the youngest, to separate these questions from others about their world. If these questions are answered honestly and as matter-of-factly as any other inquiry, children will continue to search for answers. If they are answered with a "tall tale" or an anxious "you are too young to know about that," children will learn to keep such questions to themselves. Unfortunately, as they harbor these silent mysteries, they are formulating their own theories to explain birth. Since magical thinking need not be based on logic or fact, any fantastic, often terrifying, explanation can be substituted for the truth.

Regardless of whether children are given sex education, they will engage in games of sexual curiosity and exploration. At about 3 years of age children are aware of the anatomic differences between the sexes and are very concerned with how the other "works." This is not really "sexual" curiosity, because many children are still unaware of the reproductive function of the genitals. Their curiosity is for the eliminative function of the anatomy. Little boys wonder how girls can urinate without a penis, so they watch girls go to the bathroom. Since they cannot see anything but the stream of water coming out, they want to observe further for what makes it come out. "Doctor play" is often a game invented for just such investigation. Little girls are no less curious about boys' anatomy. It is very intriguing to have a closer inspection of this "thing" that girls do not have.

Even if children's curiosity is satisfied about the eliminative differences, once they are told about the "special place where babies come out," they are more mystified and determined to find that opening. Unfortunately investigation often yields even fewer answers and may result in anxiety and shame if they are caught and scolded for their behavior. When one thinks about the facts of reproduction and views them from the young child's thinking processes, it becomes quite clear how absurd and incredible the "facts of life" really are. Think about the "special place where the baby grows," "the seed or egg that grows when the father's seed or sperm meets it," and "the special opening" that is so small it cannot be found but through which a fairly large person emerges. And most fantastic of all is how the father's sperm meets the mother's egg! For sure, this is more preposterous than any fairy tale about witches, princesses, or monsters!

As children absorb these facts, no matter how expertly they are explained, they will form their own theories. Since the only framework they have for "special place," "growing,'' ''seed or egg,'' and ''opening'' is eating and eliminating, they fit all the new information into this understandable explanation. It is no wonder that children need the correct information repeated several times as they attempt to assimilate it as logical and reasonable. However, what framework is available for the act of intercourse? No matter how it is presented, the intrusive experience of the penis entering the vagina can only be associated with an aggressive, painful act. This explains why children who witness sexual activity or the primal scene are so upset and distraught by it. The physical motion and verbal expressions associated with coitus only intensify the children's impression that this is a violent, destructive act. Possibly they associate the explanation of penile intrusion with other painful intrusions, such as receiving an injection.

Parents' role in sex education

Preschoolers do not have the benefit of potential sex education in school or from their peer group, as older children do. They rely on parental information or misinformation in their search for ''how me.'' Although sexual mores have seen a kind of liberation movement in the past several decades, parents still may feel uncomfortable when faced with their child's probing questions. Usually overanxious parents react in one of two ways: they close communication either by giving no answers or by giving too much information. The latter approach temporarily terminates further inquiry because the child is so overwhelmed with ''illogical, incredible'' answers that he needs time to ponder them before daring to ask more questions. Probably two rules govern answering questions about sex, death, divorce, adoption, and so on. The first is to *find out what the child thinks*. By investigating the theories he has conjured in his mind as a reasonable explanation, parents can not only give correct information but also help the child understand why his explanation is inaccurate. For example, before children ever ask about where babies come from, they usually have imagined that the mother ''ate'' something, which made the baby grow in her stomach. Therefore, the baby will come out like a bowel movement. When parents give the appropriate information they can also correct this ''eating-elimination'' theory. The following example illustrates how uncorrected misconceptions can lead to unexpected problems:

> Five-year-old John knew his mother was to have a baby soon. He saw how large her abdomen was becoming and, when he asked why, was told that the baby was growing inside mother's stomach. At about the same time, John began eating excessively and became extremely constipated. He would violently object to any measures directed at relieving the constipation and if he evacuated would become very upset. During a visit to a nurse friend's home, his mother related these events. The nurse asked about John's understanding of the baby's conception and birth. Mother offered the same explanation that she had given her son. She also stated that John never asked any other questions, such as how the baby got there or how it would get out, so she assumed he understood. The nurse pointed out that based on the information of ''baby grows in the stomach,'' John probably thought he did understand. According to his logic, he was having a baby by eating a lot and didn't want it to come out in the only way he knew body products to exit. Mother saw the logic behind this theory and agreed that they should explore it with John.
>
> John related almost precisely the story as predicted by the nurse. If his mother could have a baby, so could he by eating so much that his belly would enlarge. As he saw himself grow bigger, he was sure that he was pregnant, and he greatly feared that the baby would come out ''prematurely'' (as he had overheard) if he had a bowel movement. When the nurse explained the correct facts, John was relieved, although somewhat disappointed to learn of his inability to bear children. He asked about the father's role and was given the appropriate explanation. He wondered about ''Daddy entering mommy in a special place and depositing a sperm that made the egg grow,'' and stated, ''I guess for now I won't make any babies. Can I go out and play?'' The overeating and constipation resolved without any further intervention.

Another reason for ascertaining what the child thinks before offering any information is that the ''unasked for'' answer may be given. For example, 4-year-old Sally asked her father, ''Where did I come from?'' Both parents quickly took this inquiry as a clue for offering sex education. After a lengthy miniobstetric course, Sally exclaimed, ''I don't know about all that! All I know is Mary came from New York and I want to know where I was born.''

The second rule for giving information is *honesty*. It is true that much of the correct information will be forgotten or misunderstood by the preschooler, but what is more important is that the correct information can be restated until the child absorbs and comprehends the facts. Even though the correct anatomic words may be hard to pronounce or even more difficult to remember, they become foundational content for explaining other concepts later on. They also reinforce the fact that procreation is not associated with ingestion or elimination but that it occurs in a place that is near, but not the same as, where the child urinates or defecates. Honesty also tells children that parents will be truthful in other phases of inquiry and learning. It does not establish a ''double-standard,'' whereby parents can tell ''little white lies'' but children must always be straightforward.

Honesty does not imply bombarding children with every fact of life or allowing excessive permissiveness in sexual curiosity. When children ask one question, they are looking for one answer, not the entire procreation cycle. When they are ready, they will ask about the other ''unfinished'' parts of the story. Sooner or later they will wonder how the ''sperm meets the egg'' and ''how the baby gets out,'' but it is best to wait until they ask.

The question usually arises of how much sexual curiosity should be satisfied? Developmentally children progress through different stages of sexual exploration. The infant who finds his genitals is not really masturbating, but exploring another pleasurable part of his body. The 3-year-old child who peeks into the bathroom to watch his sister urinate is not perverted, but finding out how she does it without a penis. Five-year-old children engaged in doctor play are not promiscuous, but trying to find concrete evidence to support explanations about birth. Regardless of how normal these activities are, many parents are confused and bewildered by them and do not know what to say or do when confronted with such behavior.

One positive approach is neither to condone nor condemn the sexual curiosity but to express that if the child has questions he should ask his parents, and then encourage the child to engage in some other activity. In this way children can be helped to understand that there are ways other than through playing investigative games that their sexual curiosity can be satisfied. This in no way condemns the act but stresses alternate methods to seek solutions. Allowing children unrestricted permissiveness only intensifies their anxiety and concern since exploring and searching usually yield little evidence to satisfy their sexual curiosity.

Occasionally parents are faced with a special dilemma, when children ask to see "how mommy and daddy do it." When parents are confronted with such intimate requests, they must remember that sex education is much more than textbook facts. It is part of a greater concept called "sexuality." Two people unite intimately because of the special relationship they have together. Intercourse is not a physical act apart from feeling or emotion, but a private act that two people share in caring and pleasure. Such an explanation does not deny children's right to be curious, nor does it deny them the request because their wish is bad or dangerous. On the contrary it teaches appropriate social behavior and, in particular, stresses the meaningful, intimate relationship between man and woman.

Parental concerns

Masturbation. Parents' attitudes toward masturbation closely parallel their view toward sex education for their children. Much of what has been discussed under sexual curiosity applies to masturbation as well. Masturbation, or self-stimulation of the genitals, occurs at any age for a variety of reasons and, if not excessive, is normal and healthy. For preschoolers it is a part of sexual curiosity and exploration.

Many individuals have certain beliefs about masturbation. Traditionally people have believed it to be sinful and harmful to health. A common myth was that masturbation led to insanity, probably from the observation that mentally ill people masturbate excessively. However, this behavior is a symptom—not a cause—of mental illness. Some people with strong religious beliefs think that masturbation distracts people from the true ideal of sexuality, primarily, procreation within a marital relationship. Others who think of themselves as neutral regard masturbation as a subject that requires further study, but meanwhile they do not encourage it as something positive or healthy. Finally those who take a liberal or permissive view hold that it is not only harmless but positively good, healthy, and, at times, necessary. They believe that it helps young people grow up sexually in a natural way.[15]

If parents are concerned with masturbation in their children, it is essential for nurses to assess which belief is held as doctrine for acceptable moral conduct. Individuals who view any form of masturbation as negative and unacceptable will need more help in understanding it as a natural, healthy expression of sexual development. In all cases it is advisable to investigate the circumstances associated with so-called masturbation, because all genital stimulation is not masturbation for sexual stimulation but may be an expression of anxiety, boredom, or unresolved conflicts. For example, a boy who repeatedly touches his penis all day is not masturbating for pleasure but may be reassuring himself that it is intact. This may be an expression of castration anxiety and should be investigated further. Also, children who openly and publicly masturbate are inviting a reaction, such as discipline, punishment, or criticism. They may be overwhelmed by their sexual feelings and asking others to help them channel them into more constructive outlets. Since masturbation, like other forms of sex play, is a private act, parents should emphasize this to children as part of teaching them socially acceptable behavior.

Aggression. Aggression, whether active or passive, is influenced by a complex set of sociocultural and familial variables. There is also substantial evidence that gender differences in aggressive tendencies are biologically controlled. Although it is generally accepted that the characteristics of maleness and femaleness are the result of complex environmental factors and not the product of chromosomal determination, the one exception is the increased aggressiveness in persons with male genotypes.[11] Other factors that seem to increase aggressive behavior are frustration, modeling, and reinforcement. *Frustration,* or the continual thwarting of self-satisfaction from parental disapproval, humiliation, punishment, and insults, can lead children to act out on others as a means of releasing the frustration. Especially if they fear their parents, these children will displace their anger on others, particularly peers and other authority figures. This type of aggression frequently applies to the "well-behaved child" at home who is a discipline problem at school or a "bully" among his playmates.

Modeling, or imitating behavior of significant adults, is a powerful influencing force in preschoolers. This helps explain why aggressive behavior in children from disturbed or broken homes is usually greater than in children from harmonious families. Children who see their parents fighting, both physically or verbally, are observing behavior that they come to know as acceptable. Even when children are spanked or hit as a method of discipline, parents are demonstrating a vivid example of the use of aggression at a time when they may be condemning the very act.

Another aspect of modeling is establishing a double standard for acceptable conduct. For example, in some families aggression is synonymous with masculinity and boys are encouraged to defend themselves. Although defending one's rights is to be encouraged for both sexes, at times the principle of "toughness" or "standing up for yourself" is not tempered with judgment, fairness, or equality but becomes a carte blanche excuse for ruling and dominating others. Such permissive aggression can be extremely anxiety producing for children because it makes them feel out of control, even though they outwardly may appear as the "boss" or "leader." Frequently the very aggressive behavior that is condoned when it is directed toward others is not tolerated in the home. For example, sons may be encouraged to be rough and tough yet not allowed to talk back to their parents. Sometimes children are unable to adapt to this "split" personality and sublimate the anger they feel toward their parents. This may eventually be exhibited in academic problems at school, failure to get along with peers, and inability to communicate with their parents.

Reinforcement is another shaper of aggressive behavior and is closely associated with modeling of "masculine" behavior. Sometimes the reward for aggressive behavior is negative, such as punishment or disapproval, but is reinforcing because it represents attention. For example, the child who is ignored by his parents until he hits his brother or sister is learning that such acts are forceful attention mechanisms. In addition parents who permit aggressive behavior by not interfering with it communicate silent, implicit approval of such acts.

One of the tasks of preschoolers is learning socially acceptable behavior and the ability to control and redirect the aggression toward the appropriate source. Children should not be made to feel guilty or ashamed of being angry or frustrated. When they recognize these feelings, they are better able to channel them into constructive, not destructive, outlets. One of the earliest demonstrations of aggression is temper tantrums. If parents handle them wisely by not attending to or reinforcing them and help children find control through appropriate play situations, young children will learn to acknowledge such feelings and express them in alternate ways, such as pounding on clay or hitting a punching bag. By the end of early childhood most children use verbal expressions as a method of displacing angry, frustrating feelings. This does not imply using foul language but rather intonations and expressions that direct the confrontation at the appropriate source. The following situation illustrates the developmental steps in the process of gaining control:

During the toddler years Lisa expressed anger through occasional temper tantrums. In response to this behavior her parents ignored the outbursts and interested her in another activity as soon as she was more in control of her emotions. When language comprehension was fairly advanced, by the end of 2 years of age, Lisa's parents told her that they would continue the conversation after she quieted down from yelling. They also provided her with "frustration toys" that she could pound and bang whenever she felt angry. By the time she was 4 years old, Lisa identified her feelings verbally and ventilated them with vocal expressions and physical activity. However, she was increasingly able to discuss the conflict or disagreements that led to the aggressive feelings and to explore possible alternatives or compromises for a mutually agreeable solution.

Discipline. Sometimes the root of controlling aggression lies in the type of discipline that is employed to extinguish other forms of unacceptable behavior. The basic principles for effective discipline have been discussed in Chapter 14. However, there is an additional aspect of discipline that must be emphasized in preschoolers and older children, that is, the function of teaching a lesson and developing a set of inner controls. The educational objective of punishment is to teach self-control not because one may get "caught" but because one feels guilty for displeasing or disrupting others. This principal goal explains why spanking or other forms of physical punishment fail to establish acceptable behavior patterns. When a child commits a wrongdoing, the spanking acts as a punishment that relinquishes all responsibility from the child. In other words, the child says to himself, "I disobeyed but I received my punishment; therefore, the 'slate' is clean." This is a type of external, not internal, control. Also, spanking is not a logical consequence of any wrongdoing, whereas other forms of punishment "fit the crime" and teach a lesson.

To return to the discussion of aggression, one can consider various punishments for a child who acts like a bully. If the child is spanked for the act, aggression is employed to "teach" a lesson against aggression! It is obvious that little learning takes place. However, if the child is told to come into the house and stay in his room until he believes that he can play agreeably with the other children, two things are accomplished. One, the punishment is a logical consequence of bullying the other children, and, two, the responsibility is put on the child to control his behavior. Notice that no time limit is given, which becomes another type of external control. Therefore, instead of the child stewing in his room for a prescribed sentence of so many hours, it is up to him to establish how long he needs to be punished. Since time is such an elusive concept for young children, any excessive time limit may exceed the justice of the punishment. Parents who take away a privilege for several days are negating the effectiveness of the punishment by exceeding the child's tolerance. Instead of teaching a lesson, they are encouraging hostility and resentment rather than penitence.

Speech problems. The most critical period for speech

development occurs between 2 and 4 years of age. During this period the child is using his rapidly growing vocabulary to interact with the environment. However, the rate of vocabulary acquisition does not parallel the advancing mental ability nor the degree of comprehension. This failure to master sensory-motor integrations results in the child's stuttering or stammering as he tries to say the word he is already thinking about. This hesitancy or nonfluency in speech pattern is a *normal* characteristic of language development. However, when parents or other significant care givers place undue emphasis or stress on this pattern, a real speech problem can occur. Children who are pressured into producing sounds ahead of schedule may cope by reverting to baby speech, stuttering, or dyslalia (a problem in articulation).

The best therapy for speech problems is prevention and early detection. One of the most essential factors involves anticipatory preparation of parents for the expected hesitation in speech during the preschool period and discussion of developmental achievements characteristic of children in each age-group. Each of these is discussed in Chapter 24 and should be included in the health promotion of preschoolers.

ANTICIPATORY GUIDANCE—CARE OF PARENTS

Although the preschool years present fewer child-rearing difficulties than earlier years, this stage of development is facilitated by appropriate anticipatory guidance in the areas already discussed. There is also a shift in child-rearing practices from one mainly of protection to one primarily of education. An occasional spanking during the toddler years may have been effective, but it now ceases to teach any lesson for why certain behavior is wrong or not acceptable. Likewise, accident prevention previously focused on safeguarding the immediate environment with less emphasis on reasoning. Now the protective guardrails or electrical outlet caps are substituted with verbal explanations of why danger exists and how to avoid it with appropriate judgment and understanding.

During this period an emotional transition between parent and child is also occurring. Although children are still attached to their parents and accepting of all their values and beliefs, they are nearing the period of life when they will question previous teachings and prefer the companionship of peers. Entry into school marks a separation from home for parents, as well as for children. Parents also need help in adjusting to this change, particularly if the mother has focused her daily activity primarily on home responsibilities. As preschoolers begin nursery or regular school, mothers may need to seek activities beyond the family, such as community involvement or pursuing a career. In this way all family members are adjusting to change, which is part of the process of growing and developing.

REFERENCES

1. Benjamin, H., and Ihlenfeld, C.: Transexualism, Am. J. Nurs. **73**(3):457-261, March 1973.
2. Bernstein, B.: Social class and linguistic development: a theory of social learning. In Halsey, A., and associates, editors: Education, economy, and society, New York, 1961, The Free Press.
3. Biller, H.: Father absence, maternal encouragement, and sex role development in kindergarten boys, Child Dev. **40:**539-546, 1969.
4. Biller, H., and Bahm, R.: Father absence, perceived maternal behavior, and masculinity of self-concept among junior high school boys, Dev. Psychol. **4:**178-181, 1971.
5. Brazelton, B.: TV and children: a pediatrician's advice, Am. Acad. Pediatr. News Comments **25**(9):10-11, September 1974.
6. Gustafson, S., and Coursin, D.: Childhood speech and reading disorders. In Gustafson, S., and Coursin, D., editors: The pediatric patient, Philadelphia, 1967, J. B. Lippincott Co.
7. Hetherington, E.: Girls without fathers, Psychol. Today **6**(9): 47-52, February 1973.
8. Kagan, J., and Moss, H.: The stability of passive and dependent behavior from childhood through adulthood, Child Dev. **31:**577-591, 1960.
9. Kellogg, R.: Understanding children's art. In Readings in psychology today, Del Mar, Calif., 1969, Communications/ Research/Machines/Inc.
10. Money, J.: Sex errors of the body, Baltimore, 1968, The Johns Hopkins University Press.
11. Money, J., and Ehrhardt, A.: Man and woman, boy and girl, Baltimore, 1972, The Johns Hopkins University Press.
12. Papalia, D., and Olds, S.: A child's world, infancy through adolescence, New York, 1975, McGraw-Hill Book Co.
13. Piaget, J.: The child's construction of reality, London, 1955, Routledge & Kegan Paul, Ltd.
14. Pomeroy, W.: Your child and sex: a guide for parents, New York, 1974, Delacorte Press.

BIBLIOGRAPHY

American Academy of Pediatrics, Committee on Pediatric Aspects of Physical Education, Recreation, and Sports: Fitness in the preschool child, Pediatrics **58**(1):88-89, July 1976.

Brown, M., and Murphy, M.: Ambulatory pediatrics for nurses, New York, 1975, McGraw-Hill Book Co.

Crichton, J. V., and associates: Social and environmental factors in assessing school readiness, Clin. Pediatr. **15**(6):523-526, June 1976.

Delacey, P., and associates: Effects of enrichment preschooling: an Austrailian follow-up study, Except. Child. **40**(3):171-176, 1973.

Drabman, R. S., and Thomas, M. N.: Does watching violence on television cause apathy? Pediatrics **57**(3):329-331, March 1976.

Dreikurs, R.: Children: the challenge, New York, 1964, Hawthorn Books, Inc.

Fraiberg, S.: The magic years, New York, 1959, Charles Scribner's Sons.

Ginott, H.: Between parent and child, New York, 1965, Macmillan Publishing Co., Inc.

Goldberg, S., and Lewis, M.: Play behavior in the year-old infant: early sex differences, Child Dev. **40:**21-31, 1969.

Havighurst, R.: Developmental tasks and education, New York, 1972, David McKay Co., Inc.

Heagarty, M., and associates: Sex and the preschool child, Am. J. Nurs. **74**(8):1479-1482, August 1974.

Hiles, D.: Strabismus, Am. J. Nurs. **74**(6):1082-1089, June 1974.

Illingworth, R. S.: Development of the infant and young child, New York, 1975, Churchill Livingstone.

Inglis, S.: The nocturnal frustration of sleep disturbance, Am. J. Maternal Child Nurs. **1**(5):280-287, September/October 1976.

Juenker, D.: Play as a tool of the nurse. In Steele, S.: Care of the child with long-term illness, New York, 1971, Appleton-Century-Crofts.

Knoblich, H., and Pasamanick, B., editors: Gesell and Amatruda's developmental diagnosis, New York, 1974, Harper & Row, Publishers.

Kodman, F.: Effects of preschool enrichment on intellectual performance of Appalachian children, Except. Chil. **36**(7):503-507, 1970.

Kogecshatz, J., and associates: Family styles of fatherless household, J. Child Psychiatry **11:**365-382, 1972.

Lewis, M.: Clinical aspects of child development, Philadelphia, 1971, Lea & Febiger.

Maier, H.: Three theories of child development, New York, 1969, Harper & Row, Publishers.

Matheny, A. P., Braun, A. M., and Wilson, R. S.: Assessment of children's behavioral characteristics: a tool in accident prevention, Clin. Pediatr. **11**(8):437-439, August 1972.

Millman, I., and Canter, S.: Language disturbances in normal and pathologic development, J. Child Psychiatry **11:**243-254, 1972.

Murphy, M.: When parents ask about discipline, Pediatr. Nurs. **2**(6):28-32, November/December 1976.

Osofsky, H., and Osofsky, J.: Let's be sensible about sex education, Am. J. Nurs. **71**(3):532-535, March 1971.

Penalver, M.: Helping the child handle his aggression, Am. J. Nurs. **73**(9):1554-1555, September 1973.

Piaget, J.: The construction of reality in the child, New York, 1954, Ballantine Books, Inc.

Rogers, W. B., and Rogers, R. A.: A new simplified preschool readiness experimental screening scale (PRESS), Clin. Pediatr. **11:**558-562, October 1972.

Southard, S. C., and Arena, J. M.: A comprehensive protocol for evaluating the safety of toys for preschool children, Clin. Pediatr. **15**(12):1107-1109, December 1976.

Spock, B.: Baby and child care, New York, 1968, Pocket Books.

Wilbur, C., and Aug, R.: Sex education, Am. J. Nurs. **73**(1):88-91, January 1973.

Williams, S. R.: Nutrition and diet therapy, ed. 3, St. Louis, 1977, The C. V. Mosby Co.

Wohlwill, J.: The mystery of the prelogical child. In Readings in psychology today, Calif., 1969, Communications/Research/Machines/Inc.

Your child from 1 to 6, U.S. Department of Health, Education and Welfare, Children's Bureau Publication No. 30, Washington, D.C., 1962, U.S. Government Printing Office.

Zimmerman, L., and Calvovini, G.: Toys as learning materials for preschool children, Except. Child. **37**(9):642-654, 1971.

16

Health problems of early childhood

This chapter is concerned with health problems that occur most frequently during the early childhood years, such as poisoning and child abuse, and with disease or illness that necessitates elective intervention, such as tonsillitis or communicable disease. The influence of growth and development on each health problem is of special concern, since the etiology or the treatment may be directly affected by the child's age. Optimal care includes knowledge of the pathologic, psychologic, developmental, and familial variables of the health problem in order to plan and provide care that is individualized to meet each child's particular needs.

COMMUNICABLE DISEASES

The incidence of common communicable diseases of childhood has declined tremendously since the advent of immunizations. Serious complications resulting from such infections have been further reduced with the use of antibiotics and antitoxins. For example, in 1950 there were 5796 cases of diphtheria with a mortality toll of 410. In 1974, 272 cases were reported with only five deaths.[12] Similar impressive statistics are available for tetanus, pertussis, poliomyelitis (almost nonexistent as a result of the widespread use of the vaccine introduced in 1955), measles, mumps, and rubella. Immunization against smallpox has been so successful that routine vaccination is no longer required in the United States and most parts of the world. (See p. 457 for a more detailed discussion.)

However, infectious diseases do occur and in most cases are prevalent during early childhood when resistance to infectious agents may still be low but exposure is beginning to increase as a result of social involvement outside the home. Therefore, the nurse must be familiar with the infectious agent in order to recognize the disease and institute appropriate preventative and nursing interventions (Table 16-1). Smallpox is included because, although it is not common, the nurse should be aware of its dermal manifestations in the event of contact with an isolated case.

In order to facilitate understanding of communicable diseases, the following terms are defined:

communicable disease an illness caused by a specific infectious agent or its toxic products through a direct or indirect mode of transmission of that agent from a reservoir.

epidemic a disease occurring in greater than the expected number of cases in a community.

endemic a disease occurring regularly within a geographic location.

pandemic a disease affecting large portions of the population throughout the world.

infectious agent an organism such as bacteria or virus that is capable of producing infection or infectious disease.

reservoir the environment in which an infectious agent lives and multiplies and on which it depends for survival; man is the most frequent reservoir of infections that are capable of producing disease in other humans.

source of infection the person, object, or substance from which an infectious agent passes immediately to the host; may be the reservoir (for example, man) or any one of the several modes of transmission (for example, contaminated water).

mode of transmission the mechanism by which an infectious agent is transported from the reservoir to susceptible human host. Types of transmission include the following:

- **direct contact** actual contact with infected person or other reservoir of infection.
- **indirect contact** contact with contaminated objects.
- **vehicle** any vehicle serving as an intermediate means by which an infectious agent is transported from the reservoir to the host (victim), usually water, soil, food, or biologic products such as plasma.
- **vector** arthropods or other invertebrates that transmit infection by inoculation or deposition of infectious agents on the skin, food, or other objects.
- **air-borne** dissemination and inhalation of microbial aerosols or their deposition on the skin, mucous membranes, or wounds, either by droplets or dust. (Droplet spread is considered a form of contact infection since transmission is usually over a distance of 3 feet or less.)

incubation period time interval between infection or exposure to disease and appearance of initial symptoms.

period of communicability time or times during which infectious agent may be transferred directly or indirectly from infected person to another person.

prodromal period interval of early manifestations of disease to time when overt clinical syndrome is evident.

Classification of childhood communicable diseases requiring isolation or precautions

Strict isolation (diseases—diphtheria, congenital rubella syndrome, smallpox)

Private room—necessary; door must be kept closed
Gowns—must be worn by all persons entering room
Masks—must be worn by all persons entering room
Hands—must be washed on entering and leaving room
Gloves—must be worn by all persons entering room
Articles—must be discarded or wrapped before being sent to central supply department for disinfection or sterilization

Respiratory isolation (diseases—chickenpox, measles [rubeola], mumps, pertussis [whooping cough], rubella [German measles])

Private room—necessary; door must be kept closed
Gowns—not necessary
Masks—must be worn by all persons entering room if susceptible to disease
Hands—must be washed on entering and leaving room
Gloves—not necessary
Articles—those contaminated with secretions must be disinfected
Caution—all persons susceptible to the specific disease should be excluded from patient area; if contact is necessary, susceptible persons must wear masks

Oral secretion precautions (disease—scarlet fever)

Private room—not necessary
Gowns—not necessary
Masks—not necessary
Hands—must be washed before and after patient contact
Gloves—not necessary
Articles—disposable handkerchiefs must be discarded in impervious bags, which should be sealed before being discarded in trash

Excretion precautions (disease—poliomyelitis)

Private room—not necessary
Gowns—not necessary
Masks—not necessary
Hands—careful hand washing after any patient contact and contact with secretions
Articles—no special precautions

From U.S. Public Health Service: Isolation techniques for use in hospitals (Public Health Service Pamphlet No. 2054), Washington, D.C., U.S. Government Printing Office.

control measures methods used to prevent spread of the organism; most common methods are immunizations, health education, medical treatment of infected person, and isolation or quarantine.

isolation separation of infected persons from noninfected persons for the period of communicability under conditions that will prevent the transmission of the etiologic agent (see the boxed material above).

quarantine formerly a term derived from the practice of keeping a ship suspected of carrying infection offshore for 40 days; presently used to mean limiting activity of persons who have been exposed to a communicable disease until the incubation period has expired.

Nursing considerations

Identification. Identification of the infectious agent is of primary importance in order to prevent exposure to susceptible individuals. Nurses in ambulatory care settings, such as emergency rooms, health maintenance centers, nursery or regular schools, and physicians' offices, are often the first persons to see signs of a communicable disease, such as a rash or sore throat. The nurse must operate under a high index of suspicion for common childhood diseases in order to identify potentially infectious cases and to recognize diseases that require medical intervention. An illustrative example is the common complaint of sore throat. Although most often a symptom of a minor viral infection, it can signal diphtheria or a streptococcal infection, such as scarlet fever. Each of these conditions requires appropriate medical treatment to prevent serious sequelae.

Several important factors are helpful in identifying potentially communicable diseases: (1) recent exposure to a known case, (2) history of prodromal symptoms or evidence of constitutional symptoms, such as a fever or rash (see Table 16-1), (3) history of previous immunizations, and (4) previous history of having the disease. Since immunizations are available for several of the diseases and in almost each case an attack confers lifelong immunity, one can rule out the possibility of many infectious agents based on these two criteria.

Many of the diseases require only supportive measures until the illness runs its course. Children are usually cared for at home until they are no longer communicable and feel

Text continued on p. 569.

Table 16-1. Infectious diseases that occur during early childhood

Diseases	Infectious agent	Source	Transmission	Incubation period	Period of communicability	Clinical manifestations
Chickenpox	Varicella-zoster	Primarily secretions of respiratory tract of infected person; to a lesser degree skin lesions (scabs not infectious)	Direct contact, droplet spread, and objects contaminated by contact with skin lesions and mucous membranes of infectious persons	2-3 weeks, commonly 13-17 days	Probably 1 day before eruption of lesions (prodromal period) to 6 days after first crop of vesicles when crusts have formed; most communicable in early stages of dermal eruptions	Prodromal stage: slight fever, malaise, and anorexia for first 24 hours: rash highly pruritic; begins as macule, rapidly progresses to papule and then vesicle (surrounded by erythematous base, becomes umbilicated and cloudy, breaks easily, and forms crusts); all three stages present in varying degrees at one time Distribution: centripetal, spreading to face and proximal extremities, but sparse on distal limbs Constitutional signs and symptoms: lymphadenopathy, temperature, irritability from pruritus
Diphtheria	*Corynebacterium diphtheriae*	Discharges from mucous membranes of nose and nasopharynx, from skin, and from other lesions of infected person	Direct contact with infected person, a carrier, or contaminated articles from discharge of infected person	Usually 2-5 days, possibly longer	Variable; until virulent bacilli are no longer present (identified by three negative cultures); usually 2 weeks or less, but sometimes as long as 4 weeks	Varies according to anatomic location of pseudomembrane Nasal: resembles common cold, serosanguineous mucopurulent nasal discharge without constitutional symptoms; may be frank epistaxis Tonsillar/pharyngeal: malaise; anorexia; sore throat; low-grade fever; pulse increased above expected for temperature within 24 hours; smooth, adherent, white or gray membrane; lymphadenitis possibly pronounced (bull's neck); in severe cases, toxemia, septic shock, and death within 6-10 days Laryngeal: fever, hoarseness, cough, with or without signs of above; potential airway obstruction, apprehensive, dyspneic retractions, cyanosis
Erythema infectiosum (fifth disease)	Probably virus	Infected persons	Presumably direct contact by droplet infection	6-14 days	Uncertain; most outbreaks subside in 1-2 months	Rash appears in three stages: I—erythema on face, chiefly on cheeks, "slapped face" appearance; disappears by 1-4 days II—about 1 day after rash appears on face, maculopapular red spots appear, symmetrically distributed on upper and lower extremities; rash progresses from proximal and distal surfaces and may last a week or more III—rash subsides but reappears if skin is irritated or traumatized (sun, hot, cold, friction)

Treatment	Nursing considerations	Control measures	Complications
Specific: none Supportive: benadryl or antihistamines to relieve itching; skin care to prevent secondary bacterial infection	Administer skin care: give daily bath; change clothes and linens daily; administer topical application of calamine lotion or paste of baking soda and water; keep child's fingernails short and clean; apply mittens if child must scratch Lessen pruritus; keep child occupied Remove loose crusts that rub and irritate skin Teach child to apply pressure to pruritic area rather than scratch it If older child, reason with him regarding danger of scar formation from scratching	Immunization not available Isolation of child in home until vesicles have dried (usually 1 week after onset of disease) Isolation of high-risk children (including neonates born of mothers who contract the disease 5 days or less before delivery and infants less than 1 month of age); treatment of exposed high-risk children includes administration of immune serum globulin (ISG) or zoster-immune-globulin (ZIG); one attack confers permanent immunity, although second attack of herpes zoster (shingles) can occur in susceptible children or adults	Secondary bacterial infections (abscesses, cellulitis, pneumonia, sepsis) Encephalitis Varicella pneumonia Hemorrhagic varicella (tiny hemorrhages in the vesicles and numerous petechiae in the skin)
Antitoxin (usually intravenously); preceded by skin or conjunctival test to rule out sensitivity to horse serum Antibiotics (penicillin or erythromycin) Complete bed rest (prevention of myocarditis) Tracheostomy for airway obstruction	Maintain *strict* isolation Participate in sensitivity testing; have epinephrine available Administer antibiotics; observe for signs of sensitivity to penicillin Administer *complete* care to maintain bed rest Use suctioning as needed Regulate humidity for optimal liquefaction of secretions Observe respirations for signs of obstruction	Immunization during infancy and boosters every 10 years after initial series (see Table 12-7) Strict isolation of all symptomatic persons Treatment of infected contacts (positive throat cultures and Schick test) and carriers (positive throat cultures but negative Schick test)	Myocarditis (second week) Neuritis
None necessary	Support parents regarding benign nature of condition	None specific, except isolation of child from other siblings	Self-limited arthritis and arthralgia

Continued.

Table 16-1. Infectious diseases that occur during early childhood—cont'd

Diseases	Infectious agent	Source	Transmission	Incubation period	Period of communicability	Clinical manifestations
Exanthem subitum (roseola)	Probably virus	Unknown	Unknown (limited virtually to children between 6 months and 2 years of age)	Unknown	Unknown	Persistent high fever for 3-4 days in child who appears well Precipitous drop in fever to normal with appearance of rash Rash: discrete rose-pink macules or maculopapules, appearing first on trunk, then spreading to neck, face, and extremities; nonpruritic, fades on pressure, lasts 1-2 days Associated signs and symptoms: cervical/postauriculer lymphadenopathy, injected pharynx, occasionally catarrhal otitis media
Measles (rubeola)	Virus	Respiratory tract secretions, blood, and urine of infected person	Usually by direct contact with droplets of infected person; less commonly by airborne or indirect contact with articles freshly contaminated by respiratory tract secretions	10-20 days	From 4 days befor to 5 days after rash appears, mostly during catarrhal phase	Prodromal stage: fever and malaise, followed in 24 hours by coryza, cough, conjunctivitis, Koplik spots (small irregular red spots with a minute bluish white center first seen on the buccal mucosa opposite the molars) 2 days prior to rash; symptoms gradually increase in severity until second day after rash appears, when they begin to subside Rash: appears 3-4 days after onset of prodromal stage; begins as erythematous maculopapular eruption on face and gradually spreads downward; more severe in earlier sites (appears confluent) and less intense in later sites (appears discrete); after 3-4 days, assumes brownish appearance and fine desquamation occurs over areas of extensive involvement Constitutional signs and symptoms: anorexia, malaise, generalized lymphadenopathy
Mumps	Virus	Saliva of infected persons	Direct contact with or droplet spread from an infected person	14-21 days	Most communicable immediately before and after swelling begins; virus present in saliva up to 7 days before and 9 days after parotid swelling	Prodromal stage: fever, headache, malaise, and anorexia for 24 hours, followed by "earache" that is aggravated by chewing Parotitis: by third day, parotid gland(s) (either unilateral or bilateral) enlarges and reaches maximal size in 1-3 days; accompanied by pain and tenderness Other manifestations: submaxillary and sublingual infection, orchitis, and meningoencephalitis

Treatment	Nursing considerations	Control measures	Complications
None specific Antipyretics to control fever Anticonvulsives for child with history of febrile seizures	Teach parents measures for lowering temperature (antipyretic drugs and tepid sponge baths) If child is prone to seizures, discuss appropriate precautions Reassure parents regarding benign nature of illness	None	Febrile seizures
Supportive: bed rest during febrile period Antipyretics Antibiotics to prevent secondary bacterial infection in high-risk children	Maintain bed rest during prodromal stage; provide quiet activity Fever: instruct parents to administer antipyretics and cool sponge bath; avoid chilling; if child is prone to seizures, institute appropriate precautions (fever spikes to 40°C [104°F] between fourth and fifth days) Eye care: dim lights if photophobia present; cleanse eyelids with warm saline solution to remove secretions or crusts; keep child from rubbing his eyes; examine cornea for signs of ulceration Coryza/cough: use cool mist vaporizer; protect skin around nares with layer of petrolatum; encourage fluids and soft bland foods Skin care: keep skin clean; use tepid baths as necessary	Immunization with measles virus vaccine at 15 months of age (if given earlier to provide protection during an epidemic, vaccine needs to be repeated at this age because of suppression of immunity by maternal antibodies) Gamma globulin may prevent or modify the illness and prevent complications in unimmunized and high-risk children One attack of measles confers lifelong immunity Isolation only necessary until fifth day of rash; if hospitalized, respiratory precautions are instituted	Otitis media Pneumonia Bronchiolitis Obstructive laryngitis and laryngotracheitis Encephalitis
Symptomatic and supportive: analgesics for pain and antipyretics for fever Intravenous fluid may be necessary for child who refuses to drink or vomits because of meningoencephalitis	Maintain bed rest during prodromal phase until swelling subsides Give analgesics for pain; if child is unwilling to chew medication, use elixir form Encourage fluids and soft bland foods; avoid foods requiring chewing Apply hot or cold compresses to neck, whichever is more comforting To relieve orchitis, provide warmth and local support by means of a nest of absorbent cotton in the diaper or tight-fitting underpants (stretch bathing suit works well)	Immunization of all infants at 15 months of age Passive protection with gamma globulin ineffective Confinement to the home recommended during period of communicability; respiratory isolation is required during hospitalization One attack of bilateral, unilateral, or inapparent infection usually confers permanent immunity	Sensorineural deafness Postinfectious encephalitis Myocarditis Arthritis Hepatitis Sterility (in adult males)

Continued.

Table 16-1. Infectious diseases that occur during early childhood—cont'd

Diseases	Infectious agent	Source	Transmission	Incubation period	Period of communicability	Clinical manifestations
Poliomyelitis (see also p. 1514)	Enteroviruses: type I—most frequent cause of paralysis, both epidemic and endemic; type 2—least frequently associated with paralysis; type 3—second most frequent	Feces and oropharyngeal secretions of infected persons, especially young children	Direct contact with persons with apparent or inapparent active infection; spread is via fecal-oral and pharyngeal-oropharyngeal routes	Usually 7-14 days, with range of 5-35 days	Not exactly known; virus is present in throat and feces shortly after infection and persists for about 1 week in throat and 4-6 weeks in feces	May be manifest in three different forms: Abortive or inapparent—fever, uneasiness, sore throat, headache, anorexia, vomiting, abdominal pain; lasts a few hours to a few days Nonparalytic—same manifestations as abortive but more severe, with pain and stiffness in neck, back, and legs Paralytic—initial course similar to nonparalytic type, followed by recovery and then signs of central nervous system paralysis; acute stage (about 5-7 days) characterized by headache, vomiting, fever, stiffness of back and neck (tripod sign—unable to sit up straight unless hands are used to brace self), pain in back, limbs, and neck, and finally paralysis; any muscle groups may be involved, but demonstrates predilection for large muscles; respiratory paralysis may occur from damage to nerve cells in cervicothoracic segments of spinal cord or damage to vital centers in medulla (bulbar poliomyelitis); recovery may be complete over several months or associated with residual paralysis
Pertussis (whooping cough) (see also p. 1230)	*Bordetella pertussis*	Discharge from respiratory tract of infected persons	Direct contact or droplet spread from infected person; indirect contact with freshly contaminated articles	5-21 days, usually 10	Greatest during catarrhal stage before onset of paroxysms and may extend to fourth week after onset of paroxysms	Catarrhal stage: begins with symptoms of upper respiratory infection, such as coryza, sneezing, lacrimation, cough, and low-grade fever; symptoms continue for 1-2 weeks, when dry hacking cough becomes more severe Paroxysmal stage: cough that most commonly occurs at night consists of a series of short rapid coughs, followed by a sudden inspiration that is associated with a high-pitched crowing sound or "whoop"; during paroxysms, cheek becomes flushed or cyanotic, eyes bulge, and tongue protrudes; paroxysm may continue until a thick mucus plug is dislodged; vomiting frequently follows an attack; stage generally lasts 4-6 weeks, followed by convalescent stage

Treatment	Nursing considerations	Control measures	Complications
No specific treatment, including antimicrobials or gamma globulin Supportive treatment; complete bed rest during acute phase Assisted respiratory ventilation in case of respiratory paralysis Physical therapy for muscles following acute stage	Maintain complete bed rest Administer mild sedatives as necessary to relieve anxiety and promote rest Participate in physiotherapy procedures (use of moist hot packs and range-of-motion exercise) Position child to maintain body alignment and prevent contractures or decubiti; use footboard Encourage child to move; administer analgesics for maximum comfort during physical activity Observe for respiratory paralysis (difficulty in talking, ineffective cough, inability to hold the breath, shallow and rapid respirations); report such signs and symptoms to physician; have tracheostomy tray at bedside	Immunization of all children with complete series of trivalent oral poliovirus vaccine Vaccination of close contacts who have not been adequately immunized During an epidemic, avoid visiting families with known cases, overexertion or chilling, eating unwashed fresh fruits or vegetables, surgical procedures in nose and oropharynx, and unnecessary injections, including vaccination other than for poliomyelitis	Permanent paralysis Respiratory arrest Hypertension Kidney stones from demineralization of bone during prolonged immobility
Antimicrobial therapy (such as erythromycin) Administration of pertussis-immune globulin Supportive treatment: hospitalization required for infants, children who are dehydrated, or those who have complications Bed rest Increased oxygen intake and humidity Adequate fluids Intubation possibly necessary	Maintain bed rest as long as fever is present Keep child occupied during the day (interest in play is associated with fewer paroxysms) Reassure parents during frightening episodes of whooping cough Provide restful environment and reduce factors that promote paroxysms (dust, smoke, sudden change in temperature, chilling, activity, excitement); keep room well-ventilated Encourage fluids; offer small frequent fluids; refeed child after vomiting Keep child in Croupette with high humidity; suction gently but often to *prevent* choking on secretion Observe for signs of airway obstruction (increased restlessness, apprehension, retractions, cyanosis) Involve public health nurse if child is cared for at home	Immunization during early infancy (2 months of age); no passive immunity from mother and absence of IgM antibodies (see p. 460 for precautions regarding pertussis immunization) Value of pertussis-immune globulin in preventing illness is questionable If child is hospitalized, respiratory isolation required One attack usually confers permanent immunity	Pneumonia (usual cause of death) Atelectasis Otitis media Convulsions Hemorrhage (subarachnoid, subconjunctival, epistaxis) Weight loss and dehydration Hernia Prolapsed rectum

Continued.

Table 16-1. Infectious diseases that occur during early childhood—cont'd

Diseases	Infectious agent	Source	Transmission	Incubation period	Period of communicability	Clinical manifestations
Rubella (German measles)	Virus	Primarily nasopharyngeal secretions of persons with apparent or inapparent infection; virus also present in blood, stool, and urine	Direct contact and spread via infected person; indirectly via articles freshly contaminated with nasopharyngeal secretions, feces, or urine	14-21 days	7 days before to about 5 days after appearance of rash	Prodromal phase: absent in children, present in adults and adolescents; consists of low-grade fever, headache, malaise, anorexia, mild conjunctivitis, coryza, sore throat, cough, and lymphadenopathy; lasts for 1-5 days, subsides 1 day after appearance of rash Rash: first appears in face and rapidly spreads downward to neck, arms, trunk, and legs; by end of first day, body is covered with a discrete pinkish-red maculopapular exanthema; disappears in same order as it began and is usually gone by third day Constitutional signs and symptoms: occasionally low-grade fever, headaches, malaise, and lymphadenopathy
Congenital rubella	Primarily nasopharyngeal secretions of persons with apparent or inapparent infection; virus also present in blood, stool, and urine	Direct contact and spread via infected person; indirectly via articles freshly contaminated with nasopharyngeal secretions, feces, or urine	Transplacental	Not applicable; virus is only dangerous to fetus during first trimester	Infants may be infectious for months; virus shedding from throat disappears by age 6 months in 80% to 90% of cases	Virtually any organ can be affected; classic rubella syndrome characterized by growth retardation, cerebral defects (mental retardation, microcephaly), deafness, eye defects (cataracts, strabismus, retinopathy), congenital heart disease (patent ductus arteriosus [PDA], ventricular septal defect; coarctation of the aorta, pulmonary stenosis), thrombocytopenic purpura, behavioral abnormalities—unusual pleasure in rocking, obsession with lights, lack of recognition of human relationships, little interest in food, difficulties with toilet training
Scarlet fever	Group A beta hemolytic streptococcus	Usually from nasopharyngeal secretions of infected persons and carriers	Direct contact with infected person or droplet spread; indirectly by contact with contaminated articles, ingestion of contamined milk or other food	2-4 days with range of 1-7 days	During incubation period and clinical illness, approximately 10 days; during first 2 weeks of carrier phase, although may persist for months	Prodromal stage: abrupt high fever, pulse increased out of proportion to fever, vomiting, headache, chills, malaise, abdominal pain Enanthema: tonsils enlarged, edematous, reddened, and covered with patches of exudate; in severe cases appearance resembles membrane seen in diphtheria; pharynx is edematous and briefly red; during first 1 or 2 days tongue is coated and papillae become red and swollen (white strawberry tongue); by the

Treatment	Nursing considerations	Control measures	Complications
No treatment necessary other than antipyretics for low-grade fever and analgesics for discomfort Antibiotics not indicated because secondary bacterial infection does not occur	Reassure parents of benign nature of illness Employ comfort measures as necessary Isolate child from pregnant women	Routine immunization of all children (usually at 15 months of age) and of all females before childbearing age See also measures included under congenital rubella	Complications rare (arthritis, encephalitis, or purpura); most benign of all childhood communicable diseases; greatest danger is teratogenic effect on fetus
Strict isolation of neonates with rubella until throat culture is free of virus Medical treatment as indicated by various anomalies (chief causes of death are sepsis, congestive heart failure, and general debility) Rehabilitation of children who survive infancy	Identify neonates with congenital rubella and institute *strict* isolation *immediately* Select nursing personnel to care for infant who are not at high risk for rubella infection	See also preceding discussion of rubella Do not administer rubella vaccine to pregnant women (threat of contracting disease from newly vaccinated children negligible) Immunization of women of childbearing age with low hemagglutination-inhibition (HI) titer who agree to use contraception for 2 months after receiving immunization Use of immune serum globulin in pregnant women exposed to rubella who have low HI antibodies Elective therapeutic abortion for pregnant women with known (or suspected) infection during first trimester Isolate women at risk of contracting rubella from contact with infant	Same as outlined under clinical manifestations
Treatment of choice is a full course of penicillin (or erythromycin in penicillin-sensitive children); fever should subside 24 hours after beginning therapy Supportive measures: bed rest during febrile phase, analgesics for sore throat	Ensure compliance with oral antibiotic therapy (intramuscular benzathine penicillin G [Bicillin] may be given if parents' reliability in giving oral drugs is questionable) Maintain bed rest during febrile phase; provide quiet activity during convalescent period Relieve discomfort of sore throat with analgesics, gargles, lozenges, antiseptic throat sprays (Chloraseptic), and inhalation of cool mist Encourage fluids during febrile phase; avoid irritating liquids (citrus juices) or rough foods; when child is able to eat, begin with soft diet	Respiratory isolation of children with scarlet fever until 24 hours after initiation of treatment Throat cultures of children with sore throat and penicillin therapy for those with positive group A streptococci test Antibiotic therapy for newly diagnosed carriers (nose or throat cultures positive for streptococcus) Prophylactic antibiotic therapy of household contacts, ideally those with cultures positive for streptococcus, regardless of associated symptoms, or an upper respiratory infection Proper food handling (use of pasteurized milk and exclusion of infected persons from handling food)	Otitis media Peritonsillar abscess Sinusitis Rheumatic fever Glomerulonephritis

Continued.

Table 16-1. Infectious diseases that occur during early childhood—cont'd

Diseases	Infectious agent	Source	Transmission	Incubation period	Period of communicability	Clinical manifestations
Scarlet fever —cont'd						fourth or fifth day white coat sloughs off, leaving prominent papillae (red strawberry tongue); palate is covered with erythematous punctate lesions Exanthema: rash appears within 12 hours after prodromal signs: red pinhead-sized punctate lesions rapidly become generalized but are absent on the face, which becomes flushed; rash is more intense in folds of joints; by end of the first week, desquamation begins, which may be complete by 3 weeks or longer
Smallpox (variola)	Poxvirus (variola)	Respiratory secretions and lesions of skin and mucous membranes of infected person	Prolonged direct contact with infected person; indirectly by articles freshly contaminated with crusts or secretions	12 days, with range of 7-17 days	Onset of first symptom to disappearance of all scabs, usually about 2-3 weeks	Prodromal stage: abrupt onset with chills, fever (reaches peak by end of second day), headache, backaches, and prostration; lasts 2-4 days, and symptoms begin to improve as rash develops Eruption period: painful lesions appear on mucous membranes of mouth, throat, and respiratory tract, causing symptoms of sore throat, hoarseness, and cough; macules first appear on face, forearm, trunk, (especially back), and finally lower extremities; intensity of rash is centrifugal—denser on peripheral than on central regions; within a few hours, macules become papules; by sixth day from onset of illness they become vesicles, then pustules, and finally form crusts by end of 14 days; during pustular stage constitutional signs worsen and lesions are painful; dessication of lesions is accompanied by intense pruritus and is followed by 1- to 2-week period of desquamation

Treatment	Nursing considerations	Control measures	Complications
	Advise parents to consult physician if fever persists after beginning therapy Discuss procedures for preventing spread of infection		
No specific treatment available; patients are placed under strict isolation; antibiotics are used if bacterial infection is present Supportive therapy: adequate fluids, calories, and electrolytes (may require gavage feeding because oral and intravenous routes are incapacitated by presence of lesions), analgesics, antipruritics	Ensure strict isolation procedures; maintain complete bed rest; schedule analgesics to ensure optimum comfort Cleanse eyes with sterile saline solution to remove crusts, inspect cornea for evidence of infection Observe patterns of fever (peaks on second to third day and during pustular stage but is only low grade at other times; normal by tenth to twelfth day); unusual spikes may indicate bacterial infection Although no special skin care indicated, change bedclothes and linens at least daily, especially during desquamation phase Prevent child from scratching: use mittens, keep fingernails short and clean, use elbow restraints Participate in immunization procedures of close contacts or general population if epidemic is anticipated	Routine immunization no longer recommended except for groups at risk (military, health personnel, and travelers to areas where disease is endemic) Strict isolation of infected person Vaccination or revaccination of persons presumably exposed to smallpox Use of vaccines of variola-immune globulin (VIG) may prevent or modify disease in exposed individuals	Secondary bacterial infection: impetigo, furuncles, cellulitis, pneumonia, septicemia, osteomyelitis, keratitis, scarring, laryngeal edema, encephalitis, psychoses, abortion in pregnant women

Table 16-2. Diagnostic tests used to detect communicable diseases

Test	Description	Disease detected
Culture	Organism is obtained from infected site (throat, lesion, blood, excretion) and grown in suitable medium	All diseases listed in Table 16-1 except erythema infectiosum and roseola
Complement fixation (CF)	Complement is mixture of globulins consisting of several components normally present in serum; when activated, complement produces hemolysis; complement is mixed with commercially available virus antigens and, if specific immune antibodies are present, there is binding or fixation of the complement to the antigen-antibody complex, which makes it incapable of producing hemolysis; complement fixation is usually evident 2 weeks after infection with the virus, but the reaction tends to be short lived	Measles, mumps, rubella, poliomyelitis, chickenpox, smallpox
Neutralization	When a specific immune serum is added to the corresponding virus, the virus is rendered noninfective or neutralized, as evidenced by failure to demonstrate cytoplastic changes on tissue culture cells; neutralization is usually evident a few weeks after infection with the virus and tends to be life long	Measles, mumps, rubella, poliomyelitis, chickenpox, smallpox
Hemagglutination-inhibition (HI)	Suspensions of certain viruses cause agglutination or clumping of red blood cells; if specific immune serum is added, it will inhibit the agglutination of the red blood cells in proportion to the amount of antibody present in the serum; results are expressed as a titer; for example, in rubella a titer of 1:20 or greater is indicative of immunity, whereas a titer of 1:10 or lower indicates absence of immunity; increase in a titer from early in infection to later in disease indicates that it was caused by a specific virus, such as rubella	Measles, mumps, rubella, chickenpox, smallpox
Fluorescent-antibody (FA)	A fluorescent dye is attached to selected immunoglobulin molecules and then added to a sample of serum; in the *direct test* the labeled known antigen attaches itself to the antigen present in the serum; under the microscope, this binding process is evident	Rubella, poliomyelitis, pertussis, smallpox, chickenpox
Anti-streptolysin O	Concentration of antibody formation to streptolysin O, a streptococcal extracellular product that produces lysis of red blood cells, is measured; rise in the titer indicates a recent group A streptococcal infection	Scarlet fever
Dick	Intracutaneous inoculation with 0.1 ml of group A beta hemolytic streptococcus toxin is given; a positive reaction—local erythema 1 cm or more in diameter—indicates absence of antitoxin and therefore no immunity; a negative reaction indicates neutralization of the toxin and therefore presence of immunity	Scarlet fever
Schultz-Charlton reaction (blanching test)	Intracutaneous inoculation with 0.1 ml of streptococcus antitoxin is given during the early stages of a rash; if the rash is caused by scarlet fever, there will be blanching of the injection site	Scarlet fever
Schick	Intracutaneous inoculation of a specific amount of diphtheria toxin is given; a positive reaction—an area of erythema and induration 10 mm or more in diameter—indicates absence of antitoxic immunity; a negative reaction indicates neutralization of the toxin and therefore presence of immunity	Diphtheria
Moloney	Intradermal injection of diphtheria toxoid is given; a positive reaction—erythema 10 mm or more in diameter—indicates previous exposure to the diphtheria bacillus and therefore immunity; a positive reaction contraindicates the further use of diphtheria toxoid	Diphtheria

Data from Bauer, J. D., Ackerman, P. G., and Toro, G.: Clinical laboratory methods, ed. 8, St. Louis, 1974, The C. V. Mosby Co.

well enough to resume normal activity. However, there are groups of children who are at risk for serious, even fatal, complications from communicable diseases, especially those of viral etiology. Such children include those who are on steroid or other immunosuppressive therapy, those who have a generalized malignancy, such as leukemia or lymphoma, or those who have an immunologic disorder. The nurse immediately refers children who have signs of a communicable disease to a physician. School nurses who are aware of such susceptible children have the responsibility of warning their parents of recent outbreaks of a communicable disease in order to prevent their exposure to known cases. In most instances the child is kept out of school until the outbreak is over. At the present time chickenpox is the most frequent disease requiring isolation of high-risk children, because no immunization is available.

The nurse should also be familiar with tests commonly used to confirm or rule out the diagnosis of infectious diseases (Table 16-2). Knowledge of test results allows the nurse to make appropriate decisions regarding need for treatment or isolation. For example, rubella is a benign childhood disease that requires no special intervention. Ordinarily the recommendation is to confine the child to the home until about 5 days after appearance of the rash. However, if the mother is in the first trimester of pregnancy, immediate steps need to be taken to isolate the child from her if her antibody titer is low. In addition any visitors who are pregnant should avoid close contact with the child.

Prevention. Prevention consists of the following two components: prevention of the disease and control of spread of the disease to others. Primary prevention rests almost exclusively on immunization. The tremendous success and benefit of worldwide immunization programs are clearly demonstrated in the almost complete eradication of smallpox. (The nurse's role in immunization of children is discussed in Chapter 12.) Identification of a household member with a communicable disease should alert the nurse to investigate the possibility of unimmunized contacts. Other measures available to prevent the occurrence of scarlet fever include screening for streptococcal throat infections and administration of penicillin therapy. Nurses in school systems or public health agencies are frequently involved in such programs and need to be aware of the importance of adequate follow-up of children with positive cultures.

Control measures to prevent spread of the disease include appropriate isolation and early definitive treatment when necessary. Since most children are cared for at home, the nurse is responsible for instructing parents regarding isolation techniques. The most important procedure to stress is hand washing. Persons directly caring for the child or handling contaminated articles must wash their hands before and after leaving the room. The child should be instructed to practice good hand washing technique after toileting and before eating. He should be confined to his room (preferably alone, but not necessarily so) until the period of communicability is over. The nurse stresses to parents how many days this involves. It is important to remember that many of the diseases are not infectious even if the rash is still present. For example, the scabs that form in chickenpox are not a source of the virus. The child can return to school in about 1 week and need not be confined until complete healing takes place.

With the exception of those diseases requiring strict isolation, no special precautions need to be observed in cleaning the child's room, intimate articles, or clothing. However, the child should use disposable tissues that are discarded in a plastic, sealed bag. His eating and drinking utensils should not be shared by others, unless washed thoroughly beforehand. His room should be aired out and cleaned without spraying dust in the air. Vacuuming is preferable to using a dust mop, and sheets should be collected and placed in a receptacle, not shaken in the room.

For those diseases spread by droplets, the nurse instructs parents in measures aimed at reducing airborne transmission. If the child is old enough, he should cover his face during coughing or sneezing; otherwise the parent should cover the child's mouth with a tissue and then discard it. Persons who are susceptible to the disease should not come close to the child unless special precautions are taken. Since masks are rarely available in the home, such individuals can place a paper tissue over their mouth and nose in the event that they must be in direct contact with the child. The tissue is discarded after one use.

Whenever the child is hospitalized, rigid adherence to appropriate isolation procedures is required. It is the nurse's responsibility to ensure that the correct isolation procedures are instituted and properly implemented (Table 16-3). In the case of a child who is admitted with an undiagnosed exanthema, the nurse institutes strict isolation until a diagnosis is established. To facilitate nursing care and minimize the possibility of spread of infection, nursing activities are organized to allow for the least number of trips in and out of the room.

Regardless of the type of isolation, the nurse explains to parents and older children the reason behind such procedures. Family members are more likely to practice good hand washing, toileting hygiene, and so on if they are aware of their value. If the child is hospitalized the nurse prepares him for this experience by showing him the mask, gowns, and gloves and allowing him to dress up if he desires. The nurse is introduced when entering the room and lets the child see his or her face before putting on the mask. In this way he associates the nurse with significant experiences and gains a sense of familiarity in an otherwise strange and lonely environment. When the child's condition improves, the nurse provides appropriate play activities to minimize the boredom. Rather than dwelling on the negative aspects of isolation, the child can be encouraged to view this experience as

Table 16-3. Implementation of isolation procedures

Isolation procedure	Activity
Hand washing	Wash hands immediately after contact with each patient, after handling articles that may be contaminated, and before leaving room. If a gown is worn, untie lower string when ready to remove gown, wash hands, and then untie neck string. Remove gown by grasping inside of cuffs, pull off, and discard. Rewash hands, Mask may be removed before or after hand washing, provided only the ties are handled.
Gowns	Place an adequate supply of long-sleeved gowns outside room. Before entering, put on a gown and tie it securely at the back and neck. When leaving, remove gown and discard into receptacle *before* leaving room; use correct hand washing procedure. Ideally, wear gowns only once and discard. If a gown must be worn more than once, hang it up close to the door inside the room with the *clean* side (side against nurse's clothing) folded together.
Masks	Place supply of disposable masks outside room. Apply mask before entering room and wear over nose and mouth. Discard mask in a receptacle *before* leaving room. Change masks every hour or if they become moist.
Gloves	Place supply of disposable gloves outside room for strict isolation and inside room for certain discharge precautions. Change gloves after direct contact with patient's secretion or excretions even if care is not completed. Discard gloves before leaving room and wash hands.
Disposal of contaminated articles	Use as many disposable items as possible (paper dishes, disposable needles and suction catheters, paper tissues, disposable diapers, plastic sputum cups). Place all disposable items in paper bag and then in large plastic bag and tie securely. Place disposable needles and syringe in special box marked "contaminated." Collect linen in special color-coded bag; place outside room and enclose it in second special laundry bag marked "contaminated." Send all specimens to laboratory in *closed* containers and mark "potentially infectious" (or soak in antiseptic solution). Wash and dry all instruments and equipment that are not disposable; double bag, mark "contaminated," and send for sterilization to central supply department. Supply patient with personal bedpan and urinal; room should have adjoining private bathroom, where all excretions are disposed of. If bedpan is not disposable, prepare for sterilization in central supply department.
Environmental control	Avoid creating aerosols (particles of dust dispersed in the air); dust with a damp cloth and use wet vacuuming; reduce activity in room. Keep cleaning equipment inside room. Ventilate room to outside atmosphere. Use spray disinfectant. Keep room clean. On discharge, ensure that housekeeping personnel perform terminal cleaning.

challenging and positive. For example, the nurse can help the child look at isolation as a method of keeping others out and letting only special people in. Children often think of intriguing signs for their doors, such as "Enter at your own risk" or "Many have entered but few have left." These poster-like signs also encourage people "on the outside" to enter and talk with the child about the ominous greetings.

In suggesting isolation procedures for the home, the nurse considers the family's cultural and socioeconomic background. For example, it is useless to recommend confining the child to his own room if the entire family sleeps together. A more appropriate suggestion would be to select a sleeping area, such as a couch or one end of the bed, that is not in direct contact with the other members. Ideally the best approach is to make a home visit and suggest practical measures based on the family's living situation. During a visit the nurse also questions other family members about symptoms suggestive of the disease.

In some instances prevention involves ensuring the family's compliance with antibiotic administration. In the nursing assessment a preliminary judgment is made regarding the parents' reliability and sense of responsibility. Factors supporting compliance include a history of kept appointments for health care, an up-to-date schedule of immunizations, and a past history of illnesses, such as otitis media, that were associated with no recurrences. Whenever possible, the child should receive oral medications to prevent the trauma of an injection. However, if there is serious ques-

Summary of nursing care of the child with a communicable disease

Goals	Responsibilities
Assist in identifying etiologic agent	Recognize exanthema associated with communicable diseases (Table 16-1) Operate under a high index of suspicion for children who are susceptible to infectious diseases Identify high-risk children to whom communicable disease may be fatal; in case of an outbreak, advise parents to confine child to the home Assist in performing tests used to identify the organism, such as collection of specimens for culture Be aware of significance of test results in terms of the etiologic agent and child's level of immunity (Table 16-3)
Prevent occurrence of the disease	Participate in public education regarding prophylactic immunizations, method of spread of communicable diseases, proper preparation and handling of food and water supplies, and control of animal vectors in regard to reservoirs of disease (not a factor in childhood communicable disease but in other infectious illness such as malaria) Participate in immunization programs or screening programs to identify streptococcal infections
Prevent spread of the disease	Institute appropriate isolation procedures (Table 16-3) Post isolation procedures on door to child's room Make referral to public health nurse when necessary to ensure appropriate isolation procedures in the home Work with families to ensure compliance with therapeutic regimens Identify close contacts who may require prophylactic treatment (specific immune globulin or antibiotics) Report disease to local health department
Prepare child for isolation	Explain reason for confinement and use of any special precautions Allow child to play with gloves, mask, and gown Always introduce yourself to child and allow him to see your face before donning protective clothing Provide diversionary activity Encourage parents to remain with child during hospitalization Help child view isolation experience as challenging rather than solely negative Discontinue isolation as soon as period of communicability is over; discuss this with parents if child is at home
Provide comfort measures	Schedule analgesics and antipyretics for maximum relief of discomfort Maintain bed rest; administer complete care as needed Keep mucous membranes moist with use of cool-mist vaporizer, gargles, and lozenges Apply petrolatum to chapped lips or nares Cleanse eyes with physiologic saline solution Keep skin clean (change bedclothes and linens at least daily) Administer oral hygiene
Prevent complications	Ensure compliance with therapeutic regime (bed rest, antibiotics, adequate hydration) Institute seizure precautions if febrile convulsions are a possibility Monitor temperature; unexpected elevations may signal an infection Attend to good body hygiene Prevent child from scratching the skin; keep nails short and clean; apply mittens or elbow restraints Ensure adequate hydration with small frequent sips of water or favorite drinks and soft, bland foods (gelatin, pudding, ice cream, soups); refeed after vomiting; observe for signs of dehydration
Provide emotional support	Recognize loneliness imposed by isolation; encourage contact with friends via telephone (in hospital can use intercom between room and nurse's station) Reinforce parents' effort to carry out plan of care Provide assistance when necessary, such as visiting nurse to help with home care Keep parents aware of child's progress; stress rapidity of recovery in most cases

tion regarding compliance with the full 10-day schedule, one injection of benzathine penicillin G (Bicillin) is given. As in any other situation, the nurse prepares the child beforehand for the procedure. Discomfort from the injection can be reduced if the drug is allowed to warm to room temperature before administration.

Nursing care of the child with a communicable disease is listed in the boxed material on p. 571. Since most of the diseases are associated with skin manifestations, the reader is referred to pp. 676 and 677 for a discussion of nursing care in dermatologic conditions.

TONSILLITIS

The tonsils are masses of lymphoid tissue located in the pharyngeal cavity. Their function is probably to filter and protect the respiratory and alimentary tracts from invasion by pathogenic organisms. They also may have a role in antibody formation. Although the size of tonsils varies, children generally have much larger tonsils than adolescents or adults. This difference is thought to be a protective mechanism at a time when young children are especially susceptible to upper respiratory infection.

Several pairs of tonsils encircle the pharynx, forming what is known as Waldeyer's tonsillar ring (Fig. 16-1, *B*). The *palatine* or faucial tonsils are located on either side of the oropharynx, behind and below the pillars of the fauces (opening from the mouth). A free surface of the palatine tonsils is usually visible during oral examination. The palatine tonsils are the pair of tonsils usually surgically removed during tonsillectomy. Above these are the *pharyngeal* tonsils, also known as the adenoids. They are located in the posterior wall of the nasopharynx, opposite the posterior nares. Their close proximity to the nares and eustachian tubes causes difficulties in instances of inflammation. The *lingual* tonsils are located at the base of the tongue and only rarely are removed. The *tubal* tonsils are found near the posterior nasopharyngeal opening of the eustachian tubes and are not part of Waldeyer's tonsillar ring.

Etiology, pathophysiology, and clinical manifestations

Tonsillitis usually occurs as a result of pharyngitis, inflammation of the structures of the pharynx. Because of the normally abundant amount of lymphoid tissue and the frequency of upper respiratory infection in young children,

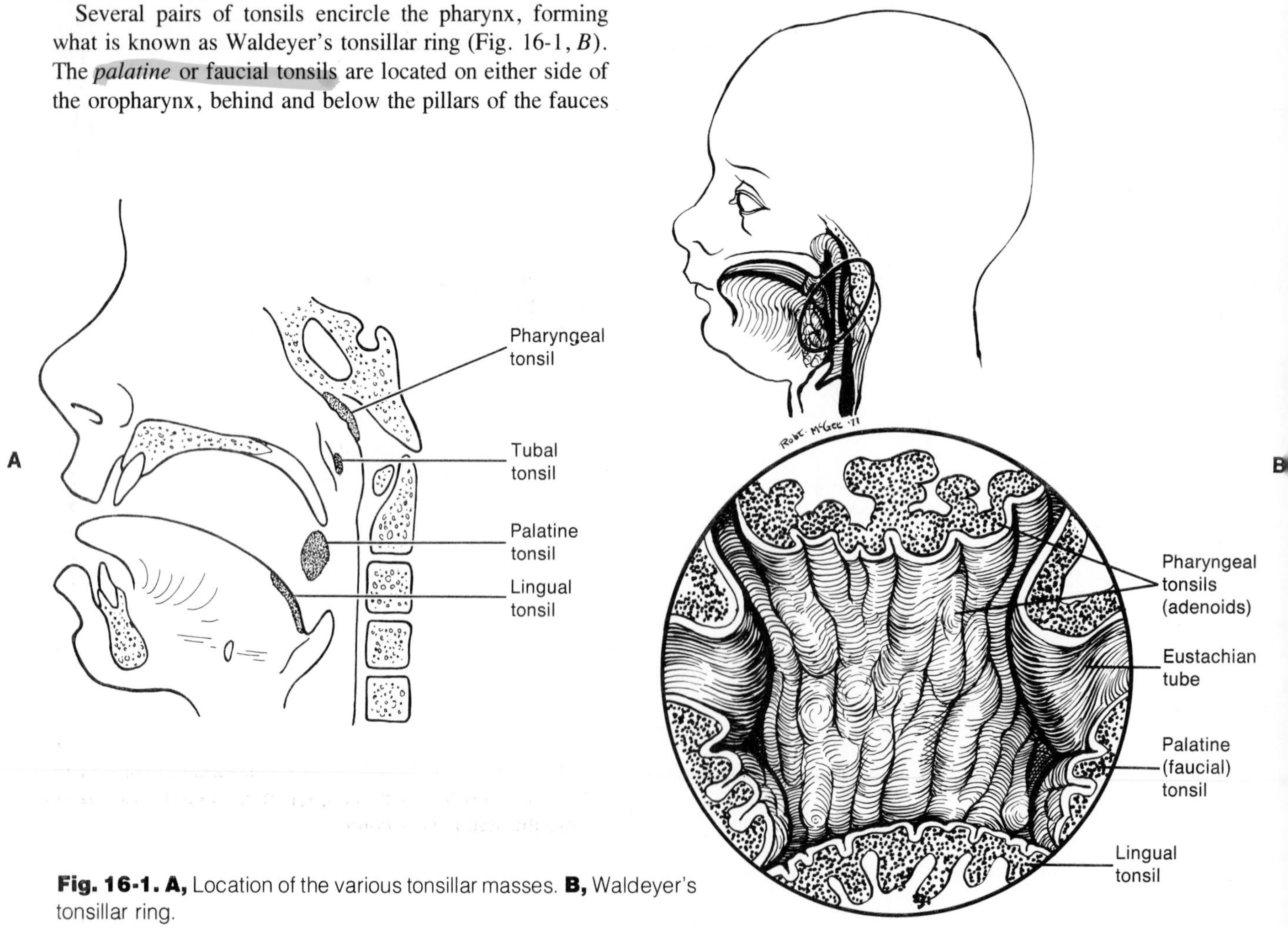

Fig. 16-1. A, Location of the various tonsillar masses. **B,** Waldeyer's tonsillar ring.

tonsillitis is a very common cause of morbidity. The causative agent may be viral or bacterial. About 15% of cases of pharyngitis are caused by group A β-hemolytic streptococci, which requires antibiotic therapy to prevent the serious potential sequelae of rheumatic fever or acute glomerulonephritis. It is often difficult to diagnose which cases are viral and which require treatment based on clinical manifestations alone. Table 16-4 contrasts some of the more typical findings characteristic of viral or bacterial pharyngitis. The only reliable method for objectively differentiating the specific cause is throat culture, which can be read within 24 hours. Because as many as 15% of children are carriers of β-hemolytic streptococci, several authorities suggest performing a throat culture on every child with a significant sore throat as a screening procedure to prevent rheumatic fever (p. 1363).[5]

The pathology and clinical manifestations of tonsillitis are chiefly caused by inflammation. As the palatine or faucial tonsils enlarge as a result of edema, they may meet in the midline (kissing tonsils), obstructing the passage of air or food. The child has difficulty in swallowing and breathing. Enlargement of the adenoids blocks the space behind the posterior nares, making it difficult or impossible for air to pass from the nose to the throat. As a result the child breathes through the mouth. If mouth breathing is continuous, the mucous membranes of the oropharynx become dry and irritated. There may be an offensive mouth odor, and the senses of taste and smell are impaired. Because air cannot be trapped for proper speech sounds, the voice has a nasal and muffled quality. A persistent, harassing cough is also common. Because of the proximity of the adenoids to the eustachian tubes, this passageway is frequently blocked in adenoiditis. As a result normal drainage is impaired and otitis media frequently occurs.

Table 16-4. Comparison of signs and symptoms of viral vs bacterial pharyngitis (tonsillitis)

Viral pharyngitis	Bacterial (streptococcal) pharyngitis
Gradual onset	More abrupt onset
Low-grade fever	Fever increased to 40°C (104°F)
Headache, rhinitis, cough, and hoarseness occur after 1 or 2 days of fever	Conjunctivitis, rhinitis, cough, or hoarseness uncommon Headache, severe sore throat, and abdominal pain more common
Slight erythema of pharynx and slight or moderate enlargement of tonsils	White exudate on posterior pharynx and tonsils; erythema and enlargement of tonsils
Firm, tender cervical lymph nodes may be present	Localized firm, tender cervical lymph nodes common
Child is moderately ill for 1-5 days	Child is acutely ill for as long as 2 weeks

Medical management

Treatment of viral pharyngitis is symptomatic, because the illness is self-limiting. If the tonsils and adenoids are enlarged the child will prefer a soft, liquid diet. A cool-mist vaporizer helps keep the mucous membranes moist during periods of mouth breathing. Warm, saltwater gargles, throat lozenges, and analgesic/antipyretic drugs such as acetaminophen (Tylenol) are useful to promote comfort.

Throat cultures that are positive for group A β-hemolytic streptococci warrant antibiotic treatment. A 10-day schedule of oral drug therapy, such as penicillin, is necessary to totally eradicate the bacilli. However, noncompliance is a major problem in the efficacy of this treatment. Several studies show that compliance with the drug regimen is significantly reduced after 3 days, when most symptoms are subsiding, and almost totally absent by the ninth day. For this reason many physicians advocate administering an intramuscular dose of parenteral benzathine penicillin G, which maintains substantial blood levels for at least 10 days. In high-risk populations where return to the health facility after 24 hours for throat culture results is questionable, an injection of benzathine penicillin G may be given for suspected streptococcal infections. Such injections are quite painful and must be administered deeply into a large muscle mass, such as the vastus lateralis or gluteus muscle in older children. Parents need to be aware of the residual tenderness, which may cause the child to limp for a day or two. Local applications of heat are helpful in relieving some of the discomfort. If the child is not seriously ill and follow-up care is reasonably certain, antibiotic therapy may be delayed for a few days to allow antibody formation against the streptococcus to occur.

Surgical treatment of chronic tonsillitis is a very controversial subject. Tonsillectomy is the most frequently performed pediatric surgical procedure. Many authorities believe that most of these surgeries are unwarranted and unnecessary. Others, who have seen children dramatically improve after tonsillectomy and adenoidectomy, continue to recommend it for selected patients. Probably the word "selective" is one key to the judicious advocacy of either procedure. Indications for tonsillectomy may include persons who have persistent chronic sore throats that result in significant morbidity, who have respiratory distress from retropharyngeal obstruction, or who are diphtheria carriers. Generally removal of the tonsils should occur after 3 or 4 years of age, because regrowth or hypertrophy of lymphoid tissue before this age is very common. The tubal and lingual tonsils often enlarge to compensate for the lost lymphoid tissue, resulting in continued pharyngeal and eustachian tube obstruction. Adenoidectomy is recommended for children with recurrent otitis media to prevent hearing loss and in those children where hypertrophied adenoids obstruct nasal breathing. Their removal may be warranted in the child under 3 years of age and should be performed without a tonsillectomy. Follow-up after adenoidectomy should include assessment of hearing, smell, and taste for expected improvement.

Nursing considerations

Since tonsillectomy/adenoidectomy is the most frequent pediatric surgery, it deserves special consideration. Since the surgery is most often an elective procedure after the infection has subsided, there is no reason why children should not be adequately prepared for hospitalization and surgery. Frequently it represents the child's first hospitalization and major separation from home or parents. Since 4 or 5 years of age is recommended for tonsillectomy, the procedure for preoperative teaching is outlined for the preschooler. (See boxed material.) No elaborate equipment is needed, although drawings, puppets, dolls, and hospital equipment such as caps, mask, gowns, and so on may be advantageous teaching aids.

Preoperative care. Care on admission and prior to surgery is similar to that for other surgical procedures. A complete history is taken with special notation of any bleeding tendencies, since the operative site is highly vascular. Bleeding and clotting times are included in the usual blood work. During physical assessment the presence of any loose teeth is noted.

Postoperative care. Postoperative nursing objectives include comfort measures to relieve the pain, proper positioning to avoid aspiration, and observation of signs of hemorrhage. The throat is very sore after surgery. An ice collar may provide relief, but many children find it bothersome and prefer not to have it. Analgesics are usually ordered but may need to be given rectally or intramuscularly to avoid the oral route. If children are very irritable, mild sedation is helpful to lessen crying, which irritates the operative site, increasing the chance of bleeding. Food and fluid are restricted until the child is fully alert and there are no signs of hemorrhage. Cool water or fruit juice is given first, although fluids with a red color are avoided to distinguish fresh blood in emesis from the ingested liquid. Citrus juice is usually poorly tolerated because of the discomfort it causes. Milk, ice cream, or pudding is generally offered after clear fluids are retained, because milk products coat the mouth and throat, causing the child to try and clear the throat more often, which may initiate bleeding. Soft foods,

Preparation of child for tonsillectomy

Objective	*Intervention*
Consistent care giver	Assign one nurse to child. Encourage parents to stay with child as much as possible and involve them in teaching and postoperative care.
Assessment of child's understanding of reason for hospitalization	Ask such questions as "Why did you come to the hospital?" or "What did your parents or doctor tell you?" If child says he doesn't know, ask him what he *thinks* is the reason. (If child refuses to offer any information, seek above answers from parents regarding what they told him beforehand.)
Determination of specific areas of information: what the child *thinks* will be done, what area of body is affected, and why operation is necessary	Ask such questions as "Where are the tonsils?" "What are they for?" and "Why must they be removed?" Using a simple diagram, pointing to the throat, or using a mirror to show the location of the tonsils is useful. Supply correct information of usual function of tonsils and reason for removal. *Reassure* child that he is not to blame for the illness and that the surgery is not a punishment for any misdeeds. Also, stress that no other body part will be operated on.
Explanation of various preoperative procedures and reason for each	Explain the following: NPO; transportation to OR; attire of OR personnel (give him mask or cap if possible); anesthesia (stress that it is *special sleep*—that unlike nighttime, he will not wake up until doctor stops the special medicine); recovery room (if used) (encourage parents to meet child in own room). Explain need for preoperative medication *last,* since anxiety over receiving an injection may block out all other information.
Explanation of various postoperative expectations and reason for each	Explain the following: position after surgery (on abdomen or side); emesis of dark blood; sore throat and measures to relieve discomfort (show him ice collar); food and fluid restrictions until fully awake, then cool juices. Stress that after surgery the child *can* talk, although it will be uncomfortable. Let him know that no one will leave him for expressing negative behavior.
Emphasis on positive aspects of experience	Besides the expected physical improvements from the surgery, stress the new things he has seen, what he can tell his friends, and any special privileges or rewards he has received.

particularly gelatin, cooked fruits, sherbert, soup, and mashed potatoes, are started on the first or second postoperative day or as the child tolerates. Eating promotes healing because it increases the blood supply to the tissues.

Before the child is fully awake he is placed on his abdomen or side to facilitate drainage of secretions. If suctioning is needed, it is carefully performed to avoid any trauma to the oropharynx. When alert the child may prefer sitting up, although he should remain in bed for the rest of the day. Some secretions are common, particularly dried blood from surgery. Dark brown blood is usually present in the emesis, as well as in the nose and between the teeth. If parents do not expect this, they may be frightened at a time when they need to be calm and reassuring for the child.

Postoperative hemorrhage is not usual but can occur. The most obvious early sign is the child's continuous swallowing of the trickling blood. The nurse observes the child when he is asleep and counts the number of swallows per minute as baseline data for subsequent postoperative assessments. The pharynx is also inspected for obvious signs of bleeding. Other signs of hemorrhage include increased pulse (above 120 beats/minute), pallor, frequent clearing of the throat, and vomiting of bright red blood. Restlessness, an indication of hemorrhage, may be difficult to differentiate from general discomfort after surgery. Decreasing blood pressure is a later sign and signals impending shock. If continuous bleeding is suspected, the nurse notifies the physician immediately since surgery may be indicated to ligate the bleeding vessel. Airway obstruction may occur as a result of edema or accumulated secretions and is indicated by progressive cyanosis. Suction equipment should always be set up at the bedside after tonsillectomy.

Discharge instructions include (1) avoiding foods that are irritating or highly seasoned, (2) avoiding the use of gargles, (3) discouraging the child from coughing or clearing the throat, (4) and using mild analgesics or an ice collar for pain. Hemorrhage may occur in 5 to 10 days after surgery, as a result of tissue sloughing from the healing process. Any sign of bleeding warrants immediate medical attention. Objectionable mouth odor and slight ear pain with a low-grade fever are common occurrences for a few days postoperatively. However, persistent severe earache, fever, or cough necessitates medical evaluation. Most children are ready to resume normal activity within 1 to 2 weeks after the operation.

OTITIS MEDIA

Middle ear infection is one of the most common early childhood diseases, particularly as a complication of upper respiratory infection, respiratory allergy, adenoiditis, or unrepaired cleft palate. It can be classified as (1) acute or chronic suppurative otitis media, in which bacterial or viral agents cause a purulent exudate to accumulate behind the eardrum in the space of the middle ear, or (2) serous otitis media, in which a nonpurulent sterile mucoid effusion collects as a result of blocked eustachian tubes.

Etiology and pathophysiology

Acute suppurative otitis media is frequently caused by *Hemophilus influenzae,* pneumococci, or streptococci. Chronic suppurative otitis media is most often a result of inadequately treated acute otitis media, recurrent adenoiditis, or unrepaired cleft palate. The etiology of the serous type is unknown, although it is a frequent result of blocked eustachian tubes from the edema of allergic rhinitis or hypertrophic adenoids.

Otitis media is primarily the result of dysfunctioning eustachian tubes. As illustrated in Fig. 16-2, the eustachian

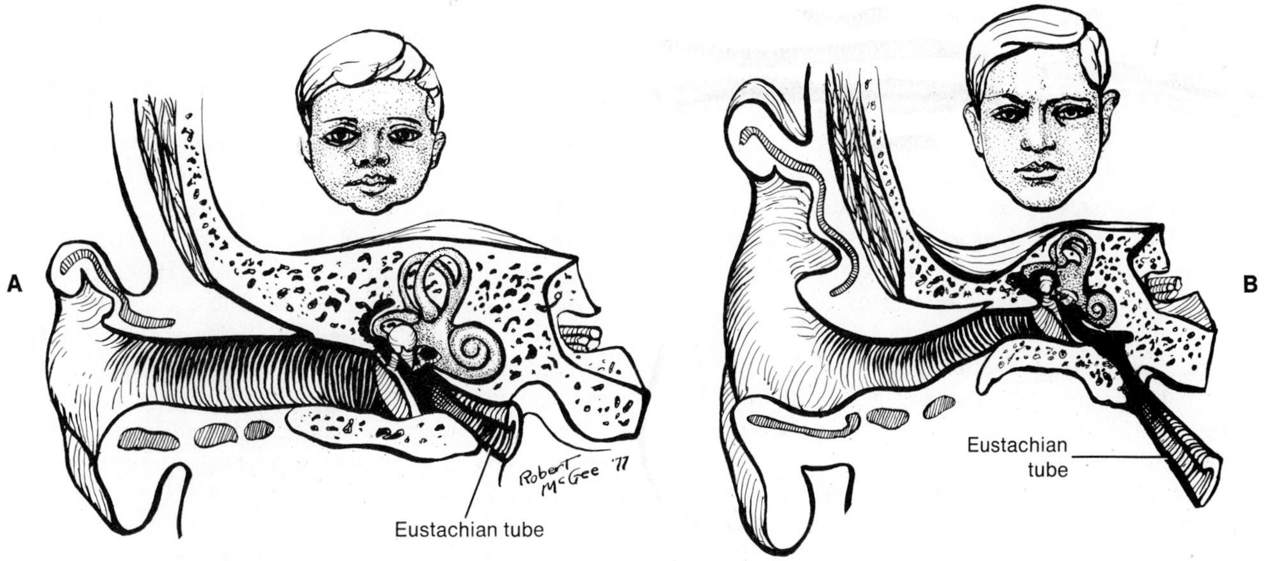

Fig. 16-2. Comparison of anatomic position of eustachian tube in child, **A,** and adult, **B.**

tube connects the middle ear to the nasopharynx. Normally it is closed and flat, preventing organisms from the pharyngeal cavity from entering the middle ear. It opens to allow drainage of secretions produced by the middle ear mucosa and to equalize air pressure between the middle ear and outside environment. If the tubes are blocked these protective functions cannot occur. With drainage impaired, the normal secretions are retained (serous type). The air that cannot escape or equalize through the blocked tube is absorbed through the vascular circulation, causing a negative pressure within the middle ear. If the tube opens, bacteria are swept up through the tube into the middle chamber as a result of this difference in pressure. Once inside the middle ear, the organisms quickly proliferate and invade the mucosa (suppurative type).

Several factors predispose infants and young children to development of otitis media: (1) the eustachian tubes are short, wide, and straight and lie in a relatively horizontal plane, (2) the cartilage lining is undeveloped, making the tubes more distensible and, therefore, more likely to open inappropriately, (3) the normally abundant amount of lymphoid tissue of the pharynx readily obstructs the eustachian tube openings in the nasopharynx, (4) the humoral defense mechanisms are still immature, and (5) the usual lying-down position of infants favors the pooling of fluid, such as formula, in the pharyngeal cavity, which hinders normal tube drainage.

Clinical manifestations

As purulent fluid accumulates in the small space of the middle ear chamber, pain results from the pressure on surrounding structures. Infants become irritable and indicate their discomfort by holding or pulling at their ears and rolling their head from side to side. Young children will usually verbally complain of the pain. A temperature as high as 40°C (104°F) is common. Postauricular and cervical lymph glands may be enlarged. Rhinorrhea, vomiting, and diarrhea as well as signs of concurrent respiratory or pharyngeal infection may also be present. Anorexia is common, and sucking or chewing tends to aggravate the pain. As the exudate accumulates and pressure increases, the tympanic membrane may rupture spontaneously. As a result there is immediate relief of pain, a gradual decrease in temperature, and the presence of purulent discharge in the external auditory canal.

Severe pain or fever is usually absent in serous otitis media, and the child may not appear ill at all. Instead there is a feeling of "fullness" in the ear, a popping sensation during swallowing, and a feeling of "motion" in the ear if air is present above the level of fluid. Since chronic serous otitis media is the most frequent cause of conductive hearing loss in young children, audiometry may reveal deficient hearing.

Diagnostic evaluation

In acute otitis media otoscopy reveals an intact membrane that appears bright red and bulging, with no visible landmarks or light reflux. The usual landmarks of the bony prominence from the long and the short process of the malleus are obscured by the outwardly bulging membrane. In the serous type of otitis media otoscopic findings may include a slightly injected, dull gray membrane, obscured landmarks, and a visible fluid level or meniscus behind the eardrum if air is present above the fluid.

Tympanometry, the objective measurement of tympanic membrane compliance (mobility), measures the change in air pressure in the external auditory canal.[20] Normally greatest membrane compliance occurs when air pressure is equal on both sides of the drum. However, when the eustachian tube is blocked, the stagnant air of the middle ear is absorbed by the blood vessels, causing negative pressure in this space. As a result, membrane mobility is decreased. Early diagnosis of eustachian tube dysfunction by tympanometry reveals a retracted, not bulging, eardrum, which, if treated, will prevent the condition of otitis media. Several authorities believe that diminished movement of the tympanic membrane is the most reliable and significant indication of suppurative otitis media or serous otitis media.[20] An inflamed eardrum alone is not sufficient evidence of either condition.

An advantage of using tympanometry is that the amount of cooperation necessary from the child is minimal. A soft rubber cuff is pressed over the external canal and, when an airtight seal is achieved, an automatic reading of air pressure registers on an attached handheld probe. Visualization of the membrane, which frequently is very difficult if cerumen is present and/or if the child is in considerable discomfort, is not necessary. Testing the drum for mobility can also be done by pneumoscopy (air blown into the canal through a pneumatic otoscope).

Medical management

Treatment of suppurative otitis media is vigorous and includes early use of antibiotics, especially penicillins such as ampicillin. Diagnosis is usually based on clinical manifestations, but if purulent discharge is present it should be cultured and a specific antibiotic chosen for that organism. The usual length of therapy is 10 to 14 days. However, compliance with the recommended schedule is a serious problem, as was discussed in the previous section under tonsillitis.

Aspiration of the fluid, surgical incision of the eardrum (myringotomy), or drainage of the middle ear with insertion of myringotomy tubes may be indicated in cases of otitis media with (1) very severe earache that does not respond to analgesics, (2) progression of symptoms in spite of adequate medical treatment, (3) suppurative complications, such as mastoiditis or meningitis, and (4) risk of progressive, significant hearing loss. Mechanical drainage promotes better healing of the membrane and prevents scar formation and loss of elasticity. Unfortunately myringotomy tubes tend to plug and often require reinsertion. In cases of chronic otitis media, they are left in place indefinitely.

Other measures include the use of a decongestant to shrink the mucous membranes and increase eustachian tube function and analgesic/antipyretic drugs such as aspirin or acetaminophen (Tylenol) to reduce the pain and fever. Although ear drops may promote comfort, they may not be used because they obscure a clear view of the tympanic membrane.

Children with suppurative otitis media should be seen at the end of antibiotic therapy to evaluate the effectiveness of the treatment and to identify potential complications, such as meningitis, mastoiditis, or hearing loss. Infants under 4 months of age are particularly susceptible to developing meningitis and should be observed for impending signs (see p. 1431). Symptoms of mastoiditis are persistent pain in the mastoid region behind the ear, high fever, and sixth nerve palsy, which is demonstrated by an inability to look toward the affected side. Hearing loss is usually not noticed by parents but should be determined by audiometric testing. (Screening tests for hearing are discussed in Chapter 5.)

Serous otitis media is treated with decongestants to improve eustachian tube function. In instances of chronic serous otitis media that do not respond to this therapy, the insertion of myringotomy tubes may be necessary to continually drain the middle ear. In any case the underlying cause should be investigated and properly treated.

Nursing considerations

Nursing objectives include relief of pain, facilitation of drainage when possible, and prevention of complications or recurrence. Analgesics are often very helpful to reduce the severe earache. Although acetaminophen is usually recommended for children, aspirin may be more effective in alleviating the pain. High fever, particularly in infants, should be reduced with antipyretic drugs and/or cool sponges to avoid febrile convulsions. The application of heat with a heating pad or hot water bottle wrapped in a towel may reduce the discomfort. Local heat should be placed over the ear with the child lying on the affected side. This position also facilitates drainage of the exudate if the eardrum has ruptured or if myringotomy was performed. An ice bag placed over the affected ear may also be beneficial since it reduces edema and pressure. If the child is cooperative either procedure can be tried to determine which offers maximum relief.

If the ear is draining the external canal may be cleansed with sterile cotton swabs or pledgets soaked in hydrogen peroxide. In order to straighten the external canal for cleansing, the ear lobe is pulled *down* and *back* for children under age 3 years and *up* and *back* for older children. If ear wicks or lightly rolled sterile gauze packs are placed in the ear after surgical treatment, they should be loose enough to allow accumulated drainage to flow out of the ear; otherwise the infection may be transferred to the mastoid process. Parents should be told to keep these wicks dry during shampoos or baths. Occasionally drainage is so perfuse that the auricle and the skin surrounding the ear become excoriated from the exudate. The nurse can prevent this by frequent cleansing and application of petrolatum or zinc oxide to the area.

Prevention of recurrence necessitates adequate parent education regarding antibiotic therapy. Antibiotics are frequently regarded as ''miracle'' drugs or as the ''one-dose'' cure for everything. Since the symptoms of pain and fever usually subside within 24 to 48 hours, the rapid outward signs of recovery support such thinking. Nurses must emphasize that, although the child looks well in a couple of days, the infection is not completely eradicated until all of the prescribed medication is taken. Although one does not want to alarm parents, it is important to stress the potential complications of otitis media, especially hearing loss, that can be prevented with adequate treatment and follow-up care. Ultimate prevention of otitis media involves eliminating the chief causes, particularly upper respiratory infections. Although an enormous task to achieve, nurses should advise parents that proper nutrition, appropriate dress, and adequate rest for all family members is one step toward preventing the ubiquitous common cold.

URINARY TRACT INFECTION

Urinary tract infection (UTI) is a significant childhood problem, probably second only to infection of the respiratory tract. Although its exact incidence is not known, studies suggest that from 1% to 2% of school-age children have urinary tract infection as demonstrated by significant bacteriuria. The peak incidence of urinary tract infection not caused by structural anomalies occurs between 2 and 6 years of age. Except for the neonatal period, females have a ten to thirty times greater risk for developing urinary tract infections than males. It has been estimated that approximately 5% of school-age females will develop bacteriuria by 18 years of age.[15] Such statistics attest to the importance of preventing, diagnosing, and treating this problem to prevent recurrent infections and possible renal damage in later years.

Factors that predispose to urinary tract infection

Anatomic and structural factors. These factors seem to account for the increased incidence of asymptomatic bacteriuria and clinical urinary tract infections in females. The short urethra, which measures about 2 cm in young females and 4 cm in mature women, provides a ready pathway for invasion of organisms. The longer male urethra (as long as 20 cm in an adult) and the antibacterial properties of prostatic secretions inhibit the entry and growth of pathogens. The cause of increased incidence of urinary tract infection in male neonates is not known, although it has been demonstrated that irrigating the preputial sac with a syringe, such as in the cleansing procedure for clean-catch urine specimens, does introduce bacteria into the bladder.[23] A similar introduction of bacteria can occur in females during tub baths. Soap or water softeners decrease the surface tension of the water, increasing the possibility of fluid entry into the short urethra. Tight clothing or diapers, poor hygiene, and local inflammation, such as from vaginitis or pinworm infestation, may also increase the risk of ascending infection.

Physical factors. Physical factors relating to the functioning of the bladder are of major importance in the occurrence and spread of infection. Ordinarily urine is sterile, but at 37°C (98.6°F) it is an excellent culture medium. Under normal conditions the act of completely and repeatedly emptying the bladder flushes away any organisms before they have an opportunity to multiply and invade surrounding tissue. However, urine that remains in the bladder allows bacteria from the urethra to rapidly become established in the rich medium.

Incomplete bladder emptying may result from reflux, anatomic abnormalities, or dysfunction of the voiding mechanism. *Vesicoureteral reflux* refers to the retrograde flow of bladder urine into the ureters. Reflux increases the chance for and perpetuates infection because with each void urine is swept up the ureters and then allowed to empty after voiding. Therefore, the residual urine in the ureters remains in the bladder until the next void (Fig. 16-3).

Primary reflux results from the congenitally abnormal insertion of the ureters into the bladder and predisposes to development of infection. Secondary reflux occurs as a result of infection. Normally the ureters enter the bladder wall in such a manner that the accumulating urine compresses the submucosal segment of the ureter, preventing reflux. However, the edema caused by bladder infection renders this mechanism at the ureterovesicular junction incompetent. Also, in infants and young children the shortness of the submucosal portion of the ureter decreases the effectiveness of this antireflux mechanism.[13] Other causes of secondary reflux are neurogenic bladder from either chronic obstruction or neural dysfunction or as an iatrogenic result from progressive dilatation of the ureters following surgical urinary diversion.[6]

Overdistension and increased pressure within the bladder may enhance the risk of infection by decreasing host resistance, probably as a result of lessened blood flow to the mucosa. This frequently occurs in neurogenic bladder or as a consequence of voluntarily holding urine back despite the urge to void. Children with neurogenic bladder can be taught nonsterile intermittent self-catheterization as an alternative to indwelling catheter or urinary diversion.[1]

Another factor that is responsible for "functional" bladder neck obstruction is chronic and intermittent constipation. The full rectum displaces the bladder and posterior urethra in the fixed and limited space of the bony pelvis, causing obstruction, incomplete micturition, and urinary stasis. Treating constipation along with antibiotic therapy for urinary tract infection reduces the recurrence of infection, whereas failure to relieve the fecal retention in spite of adequate treatment of the urinary tract infection may result in recurrence.[19]

Chemical factors. Several chemical factors of the urine

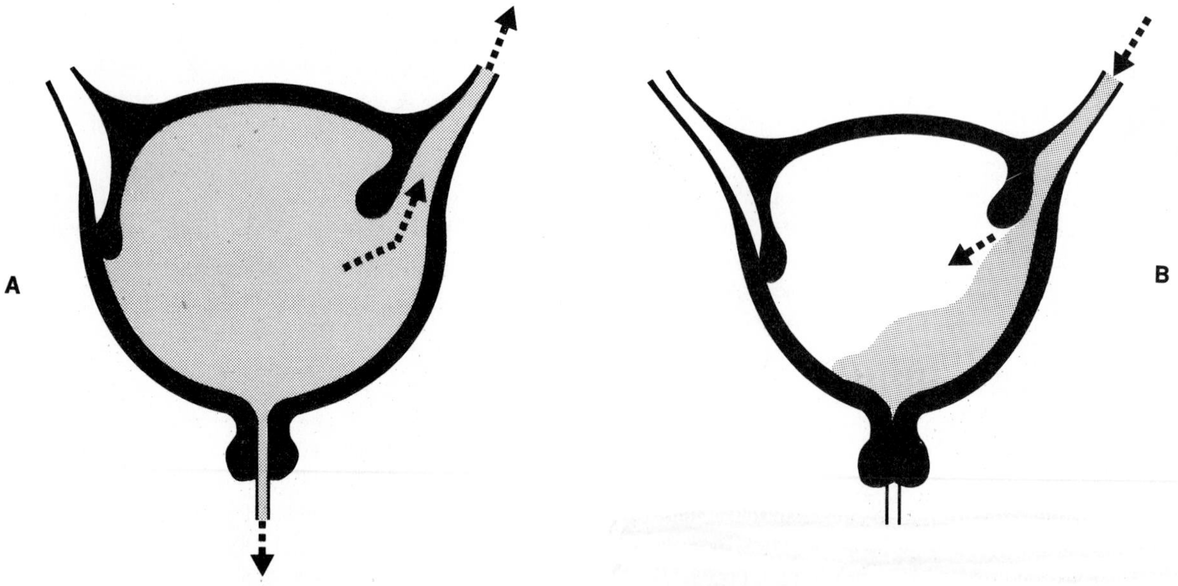

Fig. 16-3. Mechanisms of vesicoureteral reflux. **A,** During voiding, urine refluxes into ureter. **B,** After voiding, residual urine from ureter remains in the bladder.

and bladder mucosa help maintain urinary sterility. An increased fluid intake promotes flushing of the normal bladder and lowers the concentration of organisms in the infected bladder. Water diuresis also seems to enhance the antibacterial properties of the renal medulla. One effect of water diuresis is increased blood flow to the medulla (where it is normally low), thereby increasing the availability of white cells at the site of inflammation.[2]

Most pathogens favor an alkaline medium. Normally urine is slightly acidic, but it can be made more acidic by diet (apple or cranberry juices, large amounts of ascorbic acid, and animal protein) or acid-forming drugs. When the urine pH is about 5, bacterial multiplication is hampered, although the acidification rarely eliminates the bacteriuria. However, it may enhance the therapeutic effectiveness of drugs and of the natural defense mechanisms, as well as help relieve some of the symptoms. Infection by some organisms, such as *Proteus,* increases the pH by decomposing urea to ammonia, thereby increasing the favorable conditions for the continued growth of the organism.

The bladder mucosa seems to have bactericidal effectiveness by destroying the bacteria in the very thin layer of urine left on the walls after complete voiding. Since close contact of the bacteria with the mucosa is essential for lysis to occur, any residual urine prevents the mechanism from functioning.

Classification

Infection of the urinary tract may be present with or without clinical symptoms. As a result the site of infection is often difficult to pinpoint with any degree of certainty. Therefore, the term *urinary tract infection* has been used to designate instances of bacteriuria with or without signs of symptoms of inflammation in the bladder, kidneys, or both.[13] Various other terms used to denote specific locations of inflammation relating to urinary tract infection are listed below.

bacteriuria growth of bacteria in uncontaminated urine.
- **asymptomatic** bacteriuria unaccompanied by clinical symptoms.
- **symptomatic** bacteriuria accompanied by clinical symptoms such as frequency, urgency, and dysuria.

urethritis inflammation of the urethra.
cystitis inflammation of the bladder.
ureteritis inflammation of the ureters.
pyelonephritis inflammation of the kidney and upper tract (may be acute or chronic).

Acute or chronic inflammatory disease resulting from infection may involve the kidneys and upper urinary tract (pyelonephritis) or the bladder and lower tract (cystitis).

Clinical manifestations

Symptoms of bacteriuria of the lower urinary tract usually include frequency, urgency, dysuria, and lower abdominal pain. In infants any of these signs can easily be overlooked. Parents should be cautioned to observe for specific clues of urinary tract infection in suspected cases, such as frequent or infrequent voiding, constant squirming and irritability, foul-smelling urine, and abnormal stream. Checking the diaper every half hour increases the opportunity for observing the stream for such findings as straining or fretting before voiding begins, signs of discomfort before and during urinating, starting and stopping the stream intermittently, and frequent dripping of small amounts of urine. A persistent diaper rash may also be a helpful clue. Generally fever and systemic symptoms are absent.

Acute upper urinary tract infection usually is evidenced by more severe symptoms, such as fever, chills, flank pain, and vomiting. Neonates and young infants may become acutely ill with high temperature, convulsions, and gastrointestinal disturbance. Except for flank pain and tenderness, there may be no other indication on physical examination that points to pyelonephritis. However, absence of symptoms related to upper respiratory infection should lead one to suspect urinary tract infection.

Diagnostic evaluation

Bacteriuria is diagnosed by the presence of organisms in the urine. Clean-voided specimens may grow bacteria from contamination of the normal urethral flora, but growth is usually limited to a concentration less than 10,000 (10^4) organisms/ml. Significant bacteriuria is designated by a colony count of more than 100,000 (10^5) organisms/ml.[13] Colony counts between these two values may represent a contaminated specimen and should alert the nurse to the need for more careful urine collecting technique. Low counts in cases of suspected infection may be a result of diuresis before the test. Therefore, children should not be encouraged to drink large volumes of water in an attempt to obtain a specimen quickly. Urine obtained by suprapubic aspiration or from catheterization is normally sterile. Therefore, any growth of bacteria in these cases represents infection.

Urinalysis may show several variations from normal in urinary tract infection. The usual normal findings of urinalysis and those characteristic of possible infection are contrasted in Table 16-5. However, a normal urinalysis may also be present in conditions of asymptomatic bacteriuria. Other tests, such as intravenous pylogram (IVP), voiding cystourethrogram (VCUG), and cystoscopy, should be done after the initial infection subsides to identify anatomic abnormalities contributing to the development of infection and existing kidney changes from recurrent infection.

Medical management

Treatment is directed at clearing the primary infection and preventing recurrence. Antibiotic therapy should be initiated after identification of the pathogen. Antibacterial compounds used in the management of urinary tract infec-

Table 16-5. Comparison of urinalysis of normal and infected urine

Urinalysis	Normal findings	Findings indicative of infection
Color	Clear, yellow, or straw-colored	Cloudy, hazy, or thick with noticeable strands of mucus and pus
Odor	Mild if fresh Ammoniac if allowed to stand at room temperature	Fishy, unpleasant even when fresh May be ammoniac (especially with high pH)
pH	Slightly acidic (varies according to time of day and freshness of urine)	Alkaline (especially with urea-splitting organisms such as *Proteus*)
Specific gravity (concentration)	1.002-1.030	May be reduced, especially with kidney involvement
Protein	Negative	Negligible to moderate (trace to +1)
Ketones	Negative	Negative (except in diabetes mellitus)
Glucose	Negative	Negative (except in diabetes mellitus)
White blood cells and casts	Negative (may be present as a result of other systemic infection or vaginal contamination)	Present (pyuria)
Red blood cells	Absent	Generally absent
Bacteria	Absent or few	Many

Table 16-6. Drugs commonly used in the treatment of urinary tract infection

Drug	Dose (mg/kg/day)	Route	Nursing considerations
Antibiotics			
Ampicillin	50-100 25-50	IV, IM Oral	IV or IM preparation must be used within 1 hour after reconstitution; oral preparation may cause diarrhea; contraindicated in penicillin-sensitive individuals; renal excretion is rapid; dose must be repeated within 6 hours
Amoxicillin	20-40	Oral	Similar to ampicillin; better absorption allows convenience of three divided daily dosages; more expensive
Carbenicillin	200-400	IV	Expensive, suitable for *Pseudomonas* infection only
Kanamycin	5-7.5	IM	Renal and auditory complications; adequate hydration helps prevent renal irritation; local pain at site of injection
Cephalothin	50-75	IV, IM	Pain at site of injection; Side effects of neutropenia and rashes
Gentamicin	3-5	IM, IV	Renal and auditory toxicity are complications, can be minimized by slow infusion of drug (IV over 1 hour)
Chloramphenicol	50-75	IM, IV, oral	Not for prolonged use because of development of aplastic anemia; check blood count frequently, especially for decreased white blood cells and platelets
Antibacteriocides			
Sulfonamides	100-200	Oral	Observe for sensitivity (photosensitivity, drug fever, rashes); increase fluid intake to prevent crystal formation in urine (less likely to occur in alkaline urine); good for prolonged therapy; not used in newborns
Antiseptics			
Nitrofurantoin (Furadantin)	5-7	Oral	Side effects of diarrhea and vomiting may be decreased by giving drug with food or milk; increased activity in acid urine; should not be used in infants less than 3 months of age or if renal failure is present; recommended for prolonged use, since resistance develops slowly
Methenamine mandelate (Mandelamine)	50	Oral	Effective only if urine has pH of about 5 or less; acidifying agent such as high doses of ascorbic acid usually needed; should test urine daily to ensure proper pH level
Nalidixic acid (NegGram)	50-60	Oral	Many side effects; resistant organisms develop rapidly

tion include (1) systemic penicillins and sulfonamides, which are used for a short, intensive course of therapy, and (2) antiseptic preparations, which are often continued over longer periods of time to maintain urinary sterility. The drugs most commonly used in the treatment of urinary tract infection are listed in Table 16-6. If anatomic defects such as primary reflux or bladder neck obstruction are present, surgical correction of these abnormalities may be necessary to prevent recurrent infection. Medical management of constipation may be required if "functional" bladder obstruction is present.

Follow-up study is an important component of medical management, since the relapse rate is high and recurrent infection tends to occur 1 to 2 months after termination of treatment.[13] Even with recurrent infections, renal damage is rare if no anatomic abnormalities complicate the condition. The aim of therapy and careful follow-up in such cases is to prevent morbidity rather than reduce the chance of renal failure. However, the hazard of progressive renal injury is greatest when infection occurs in young children (especially under 2 years of age) and is associated with congenital renal malformations and reflux. Therefore, early diagnosis of children at risk is particularly important during infancy and toddlerhood.

Nursing considerations

Objectives of nursing care include identification of children with urinary tract infection and education of parents and child regarding prevention and treatment of infection. Identification involves isolating those children at risk for developing urinary tract infection and helping confirm the diagnosis of existing infection. Aside from the influence of renal abnormalities, females between the ages of 2 and 6 years are in general a high-risk group. Since they are not a captive population, mass screening is difficult. However, children who are receiving annual health examinations should have a routine urinalysis performed. In addition nurses should instruct parents to routinely observe for clues suggestive of urinary tract infection. Unfortunately, the signs of urinary tract infection are not as evident as those of upper respiratory infection. Therefore, many cases go undetected because no one thought to investigate this very common problem. Since infants and young children cannot complain verbally, there is no way of knowing how uncomfortable they might be because of dysuria. A careful history regarding voiding habits and episodes of unexplained irritability may well "diagnose" less obvious cases of urinary tract infection.

When infection is suspected, collecting a midstream clean-catch voided specimen is essential. Although older children can be instructed in the proper technique, the nurse performs the cleansing procedure on infants and young children. The nurses cleanses the perineum with a soap- or an antiseptic-soaked sterile pad, wiping from front to back only once with each pad. This is repeated at least two times. The area is then wiped with sterile water to prevent accidental contamination of the urine with a solution that may destroy the pathogens. To collect the urine the nurse holds the infant over a sterile container or applies a sterile plastic collecting bag (p. 929). The bag may be held in place with a tightly pinned diaper. The infant can be encouraged to void by applying pressure over the suprapubic area or by stroking the paraspinal muscles to elicit a Perez reflex. This reflex, which usually disappears by 4 to 6 months of age, results in crying, extension of the back, flexion of the arms and legs, and urination. Encouraging fluids to initiate voiding is helpful only if small amounts of liquid are given. Excessive diuresis will dilute the colony count, falsifying the results. Urine specific gravity should be at least 1.005 for sufficient concentration of bacteria.

When voiding has occurred, the nurse removes the bag immediately. Urine that has been allowed to remain at room temperature is unacceptable because the number of bacteria doubles every 20 to 30 minutes. If the urine is not tested within 30 minutes, the specimen is refrigerated. If the child has not voided within 45 minutes, the bag must be removed and the cleansing procedure repeated. Proper technique for "bagged" or clean-catch specimens yields reliable results. Routine catheterization or bladder aspiration for sterile specimens indicates poor cleansing technique and subjects children to unnecessary discomfort and trauma. It is the nurse's responsibility to take every precaution to obtain acceptable clean-voided specimens in order to avoid the use of other collecting procedures, except where absolutely indicated.

Frequently other tests are performed to detect anatomic defects. Children are prepared for these tests as appropriate for their age. Except for intravenous pyelography (IVP), voiding cystography and cystoscopy are usually done under general anesthesia. However, children still need an explanation of the procedure, its purpose, and a simple description of the urinary system. Especially for preschool children, the nurse must clarify that the urinary tract is separate from any sexual function and that the test is for a problem that they did not cause. It is not uncommon for children to associate blame for wrongdoing or unacceptable thoughts with the reason for the illness or the tests. For young children under 3 to 4 years of age, the procedure can be explained on a doll. For those who are older, a simple drawing of the bladder, urethra, ureters, and kidneys makes the explanation more understandable.[21] Children may be treated as outpatients to avoid overnight separation from home for such procedures. In such cases nurses must be careful not to overlook the need for adequate preparation, because if surgery is subsequently indicated the child will face an impending operation with facts and understanding from these procedures, which will help to decrease his fear and anxiety of more extensive medical-surgical intervention.

Since antibacterial drugs are always indicated in urinary tract infection, the nurse advices parents of proper dosage and administration. Ampicillin is frequently the drug of choice, but it must be given every 6 hours to maintain high blood levels. This generally requires waking the child during sleep for one dose. Amoxicillin, an excellent substitute, allows for 8-hour intervals, which is more convenient, but the drug is more expensive than ampicillin. When antiseptics such as nitrofurantoin are used for prolonged therapy to maintain urine sterility, parents need an explanation of their continued necessity when no signs of infection are present. Other nursing considerations in the optimal use of drugs for urinary tract infection are discussed in Table 16-6.

Prevention is certainly the most important goal in preventing both primary and secondary infection. All the suggestions included in Table 16-7 are very simple, ordinary habits that should be practiced by all females. Except for avoiding tub baths, the other measures are applicable to males as well. For sexually active adolescent females, it is also advisable for them to urinate as soon as possible after intercourse to flush out bacteria introduced during sex play.

INGESTION OF INJURIOUS AGENTS

The high incidence of poisonings in children attests to the importance of its prevention and immediate treatment. The developmental factors predisposing the vulnerable high-risk group of toddlers and preschoolers to this accident and appropriate suggestions for prevention are discussed in Chapters 14 and 15. This section is primarily concerned with the immediate emergency treatment of ingestion of common injurious household agents, especially salicylates (aspirin), and the etiology, treatment, and prevention of lead poisoning (plumbism).

Principles of emergency treatment

Identification. The first step in emergency treatment is identifying the poison. This may involve searching for an empty bottle, an opened container, or other visible evidence of the ingested substance. Any substance from the child's body such as vomitus, stool, or urine is brought to the hospital. Likewise, the partial or completely empty container is also kept for possible clues to the exact composition of the toxic substance. Since parents or baby-sitters are the most likely people to learn of the accident, they should be advised of these measures when they call the emergency squad, hospital, or Poison Control Center. When trying to determine from the responsible adult the exact quantity of poison the child may have ingested, one must remember that the estimate is likely to be inaccurate at best and, more likely, an understated amount. If an exact quantity should be given, such as "six tablets," it should be determined how this number was arrived at. If the care giver can positively state that the container was full and now "X" number of tablets are left, one can be more certain that the estimate is correct. In situations where doubt remains regarding whether a toxic dose was ingested, it is always essential to seek medical advice.

Poison Control Centers are local outreaches of the American Association of Poison Control Centers (AAPCC), a voluntary organization that has three main goals: (1) prevention of poisonings, (2) dissemination of information on potential hazards of household products and medicines, and (3) advice on the prevention, diagnosis, and treatment of acute poisonings.[17] Local Poison Control Centers are usually located in community hospitals. Every home should have the telephone number of the nearest center readily available for

Table 16-7. Prevention of urinary tract infection

Factors predisposing to development	Measures of prevention
Short female urethra in close proximity to vagina and anus	Perineal hygiene—wipe from front to back Avoid tub baths, especially with bubblebath or water softener; use showers Avoid tight clothing or diapers; wear cotton panties rather than nylon Check for vaginitis or pinworms, especially if child scratches between legs
Incomplete emptying (reflux) and overdistention of bladder	Avoid "holding" urine; encourage child to void frequently, especially before a long trip or other circumstances where toilet facilities are not available Empty bladder completely with each void Avoid straining at stool
Concentrated and alkaline urine	Encourage generous fluid intake Acidify urine with juices such as apple or cranberry and a diet high in animal protein

Methods of inducing emesis after accidental poisoning

Tickle the back of the throat with a spoon or other blunt object (not the fingers if possible) after giving a large glass of water. (This method is especially useful for children younger than 1 year of age, for whom ipecac syrup is not recommended.)

Administer large quantities of water or milk. For children between 2 and 5 years of age, administer 120 to 240 ml (1 to 2 cups); for children over 5 years of age, administer up to 1 liter (about 1 quart).

emergencies. If the local center does not have the antidote on file, it can obtain assistance from the Regional or National Clearing House for Poison Control Centers.

Removal or neutralization. The next step is removing the poison from the body. In general the immediate treatment is to induce vomiting. An effective method is to administer ipecac syrup, which probably exerts its action by direct stimulation of the vomiting center and an irritant effect on the gastric mucosa. Proper administration of this nonprescription drug is essential. The usual dose for children over 1 year of age is 10 to 15 ml (2 to 3 tsp) with one or two large glasses of water, because ipecac syrup does not work well on an empty stomach. If emesis fails to occur within 15 to 30 minutes, a second dose is given. The average period of time for emesis to occur is 17 minutes, and vomiting occurs in the vast majority (98%) of patients.[22] Overdose from ipecac syrup has occurred when multiple doses were given to induce vomiting or in those instances when fluidextract of ipecac, which is fourteen times more potent than the syrup, was mistakenly administered. Ipecac syrup is available in single-dose (15-ml) vials. However, the label information does not include directions for a second dose. Therefore, parents should be advised to always have two single-dose vials in the home, with written instructions for proper use and dose.

One of the difficulties with ipecac syrup is the need for oral administration. Toddlers often vehemently resist drinking the required amount of medication and water. Parents need to know that if "gentle persuasion" fails, they must use more directive measures for administering the liquid. A medicine dropper is helpful for instilling the ipecac syrup, and if a syringe is available it also works well. If the child resists and cries, it is important to exercise caution in giving the fluid, since aspiration may occur. Other methods of inducing emesis are listed in the box on p. 582. The important consideration is not to waste time inducing or waiting for emesis. The child should be transported to the hospital as quickly as possible, unless otherwise advised by the physician or member of the staff of a Poison Control Center. Vomiting may also be induced by subcutaneous or intramuscular injection of apomorphine, a morphine derivative that acts directly on the medulla to induce vomiting. Although its onset is more rapid than that of ipecac syrup (mean time, 4 minutes), it causes side effects of central nervous system depression, which can mask signs of toxicity from the ingested poison. Also, it is not suitable as a home remedy, which severely limits its use.

Gastric lavage may also be done to empty the stomach of the toxic agent. It is usually contraindicated for the same reasons as an emetic but is indicated if the child has ingested an antiemetic compound, methyl salicylate (wintergreen oil), or one of the tricyclic compounds, particularly imipramine (Tofranil), which is often used for treating enuresis. Some authorities also advocate lavage for petroleum-distillate poisoning, although this is controversial because of the danger of aspiration. The antiemetic compound inactivates the ipecac syrup, a cardiotoxin, which, if left in the stomach, may produce conduction disturbances, such as atrial fibrillation. The other two substances are absorbed slowly, and the tricyclics are reexcreted in the stomach, necessitating the use of repeated intermittent lavage for continuous removal of the metabolites. The potential complications of gastric lavage are impaired pulmonary function (from aspiration), gastric hemorrhage, esophageal perforation, cardiac arrest, and psychologic trauma for the child. These complications should be observed for after any use of lavage.

Inducing vomiting is contraindicated in the following in-

Table 16-8. Emergency treatment for ingestion of common household poison when vomiting is contraindicated

Poison	Signs and symptoms	Immediate treatment
Petroleum distillates—kerosene, turpentine, gasoline, lighter fluid, furniture polish, metal polish, benzene, naphtha, some insecticides, cleaning fluid	Burning sensation in mouth and throat Choking and gagging Cough Nausea/vomiting (hemoptysis) Pulmonary edema Tachypnea and tachycardia Fever Signs of central nervous system depression	Give mineral or cooking oil to reduce absorption Use activated charcoal if available If vomiting occurs, use all measures to reduce possibility of aspiration (head between knees)
Corrosives—lye (drain or oven cleaners), chlorine bleach, electric dishwasher granules, household ammonia	Severe burning pain in mouth, throat, and stomach White, swollen mucous membranes, edema of lips, tongue, and pharynx (respiratory obstruction) Violent vomiting (hemoptysis) Signs of shock Anxiety and agitation	Neutralize with 2 tbsp vinegar, lemon juice, or other weak acid in 2 glasses of water Give demulcents (milk, egg white, or oil) Keep child calm, warm, and inactive

stances: (1) if the person is comatose or is having a convulsion, (2) if the poison contains petroleum distillates, or (3) if the poison is a strong corrosive (acid or alkali). The danger in each of these instances is aspiration of the toxic substance into the lungs, causing a chemical pneumonitis. In the third situation emesis of the strong corrosive redamages the mucosa of the esophagus and pharynx. Immediate emergency treatment is aimed at reducing the rate of absorption of the substance and inactivating its harmful effect. Generally this involves as little manipulation or movement of the child as possible and administration of a suitable antidote (Table 16-8).

An antidote is any substance capable of rendering the poison harmless. There are three kinds of antidotes: (1) physical or mechanical, (2) chemical, and (3) physiologic. A *physical* antidote prevents absorption, protects the tissues, and/or aids in removal of the poison. Emollients, demulcents, emetics, or cathartics are examples. An emollient or demulcent is a softening agent used to soothe the irritated mucous membrane. Common household products used for this purpose are milk, egg white, boiled starch or flour mixture, and cooking oil.

Activated charcoal effectively absorbs most poisons, except cyanide. It also absorbs ipecac syrup; therefore, the emetic should be given and allowed to exert its effect before the charcoal is given. However, charcoal is most effective if administered within 30 minutes of the poisoning.[9] It is a black powder and is served mixed in water. Despite its appearance, most children tolerate its taste quite well. It is available as a nonprescription drug and can be used as a routine home remedy. The use of burnt toast as substitute charcoal in the universal antidote (a mixture of burnt toast, milk of magnesia, and strong tea) is considered ineffective and a waste of precious time in seeking professional help.

A *chemical* antidote is one that reacts with the poison and neutralizes it. In general, soap, baking soda, or milk of magnesia is used in poisoning caused by acids, and vinegar, orange juice, or lemon juice is administered after ingestion of alkalies. Specific antidotes are also known for a variety of other toxic agents but are not routinely carried out in a home.

A *physiologic* antidote is one that produces the opposite effect of the ingested substance. For example, naloxone (Narcan), a narcotic antagonist, reverses the respiratory depressant effects of morphine, meperidine (Demerol), and methadone. It is sometimes given to counteract the side effects of the emetic apomorphine.

Treatment of symptoms. Treating the symptoms is another important aspect in the supportive management of poisoning. Generally poisonings affect three body systems: gastrointestinal, respiratory, and central nervous systems. Knowledge of the common clinical manifestations of each system helps in initially identifying that a poisoning has occurred in the absence of other definitive evidence. The more usual symptoms in each system are listed in Table 16-9. The increased recovery from acute poisonings is largely attributable to vigorous use of supportive measures after symptoms have begun. Since shock is a complication of several types of household poisons, particularly the petroleum distillates and corrosives, measures to reduce the effects of shock, such as elevation of legs and head to level of heart to promote venous drainage and provision of warmth and rest, are important. Maintenance of respiratory function may require mouth-to-mouth resuscitation or insertion of an airway and/or mechanical ventilation. The emergency room nurse's responsibility is to be prepared for immediate intervention with any of the necessary equipment. Since time and speed are critical factors in recovery from several poisonings, anticipation of potential problems and complications may mean the difference between life and death.

See also p. 585 for a discussion of prevention of poisoning through counseling.

Salicylate poisoning

Aspirin ranks number one as the most frequently ingested poison among children, with household products and plants ranking second and third, respectively. One of the reasons for this is the readily available source of aspirin in most homes and the child's understanding of medicine as "candy." Children's aspirin is deliciously orange flavored, and parents frequently induce children to take it by referring to it as candy. Under present law, children's aspirin cannot be packaged in large quantities as a preventive measure to reduce the chance of overdose. However, no such regulation

Table 16-9. Common systemic signs of poisoning

Gastrointestinal system	Respiratory/circulatory system	Central nervous system
Abdominal pain	Depressed respirations	Convulsions
Vomiting	Labored respirations	Overstimulation
Diarrhea	Unexplained cyanosis	Sudden loss of consciousness
Anorexia	Signs of shock—increased, weak pulse; decreased blood pressure; increased, shallow respiration; pallor; cool, clammy skin	Dizziness
		Stupor, lethargy
		Coma

pertains to adult strength aspirin, and, even with child guard caps, some children are able to open the container and ingest the contents. Since the adult 5-grain tablets are four times stronger than the children's preparation, it takes much fewer adult strength aspirin to cause toxicity.

Time-released aspirin is a particularly lethal preparation for children since symptoms are delayed for several hours. In addition this type of aspirin is frequently used by people with arthritis who find the safety caps very difficult to open. As a result they may transfer the drug to an ordinary container or incorrectly replace the safety cap. Either of these possibilities increases the chance of young children gaining access to the drug and accidently ingesting it.

Etiology, pathophysiology, and clinical manifestations. Salicylate poisoning usually results from acute overdose. The toxic dose is 3.33 grains/kg. For a child who weighs 10 kg, this would represent an ingestion of approximately six adult aspirin or twenty-six baby aspirin (1.25 grains). The usual dose would be two baby aspirin (or the following rule—1 grain per year until age 5 years, then 5 grains until age 10 years or 1 grain per year until age 10 years). Aspirin exerts its peak effect in 2 to 4 hours, and its effects may last for as long as 18 hours. There is usually a delay of up to 6 hours before evidence of toxicity is noted. This delay represents a serious problem, since by the time symptoms are evident, pathophysiologic disturbances are fairly advanced.

Toxic amounts of salicylates directly affect the respiratory system by producing an increase in alveolar ventilation. Hyperventilation, the most impressive clinical manifestation of salicylate overdose, causes loss of carbon dioxide and respiratory alkalosis. Salicylates also increase metabolism, resulting in greater oxygen consumption, carbon dioxide production, and heat production, which is manifest as hyperpyrexia. The increased carbon dioxide production is compensated for by the loss of carbon dioxide during hyperventilation. However, metabolic acidosis may occur from the accumulation of ketones and other organic acids, since salicylism also interferes with the normal metabolism of carbohydrates and fats. Metabolic acidosis results in symptoms of anorexia, vomiting, and diaphoresis. Respiratory alkalosis, or loss of carbon dioxide, causes confusion, loss of consciousness, and, if not treated, coma and death from respiratory failure. Although not an acute effect of overdose, salicylates can cause bleeding tendencies since aspirin inhibits platelet aggregation and prothrombin production. In addition to the clinical manifestations, diagnosis is confirmed by determination of blood salicylate concentration.

Medical management. The immediate treatment of salicylism is to remove the drug from the stomach either by forced emesis or gastric lavage. Since an appreciable amount may have been absorbed before the stomach was emptied and because side effects are slow to develop, the child should be observed for 12 to 24 hours. Further therapy is dependent on the clinical manifestations. The acid-base disturbances are treated with appropriate electrolyte transfusions. Calories and fluids are supplied to meet the increased metabolic rate. The hyperpyrexia is controlled with cool sponges or hypothermia blankets to reduce the possibility of convulsions. Vitamin K may be administered to decrease the bleeding tendencies. In extreme cases of salicylate poisoning, external removal of the drug may be attempted through peritoneal dialysis or hemodialysis, but such intervention is usually reserved for cases of life-threatening salicylism.

Since time-released aspirin is also widely available, a major problem exists after accidental ingestion, since symptoms may not arise until 6 to 16 hours have elapsed. By this time the tablets have passed beyond the pyloric sphincter and cannot be retrieved by either induced emesis or gastric lavage. Surgical intervention is usually ineffective because the soft mass of semidigested tablets is difficult to locate and remove. Cathartics and colonic irrigations are helpful in removing the unabsorbed drug, and in severe cases dialysis may be necessary.

Nursing considerations. The major nursing objectives are removal of the poison, observation of latent effects of overdose, assistance with any medical treatments of the complications, and prevention of recurrence of the poisoning. Another aspect of care that relates to each of these goals is emotional support of the child and parents. A poisoning is more than a physical emergency for the child. It usually represents an emotional crisis for the parent, particularly in terms of guilt, self-reproach, and insecurity in the parenting role. The emergency room is no time to admonish the parent for negligence, lack of appropriate supervision, or failure to safe-proof the home. Rather it is a time to calm and support the parent, while unaccusingly exploring the circumstances of the accident. If the nurse prematurely attempts to discuss ways of preventing such an accident from recurring, the parent's anxiety will block out any suggestions or offered guidance. Instead, it is preferable to delay the discussion until the child is stabilized or, if the child is discharged immediately after emergency treatment, to make a public health referral. In either case the subject of accident prevention needs to be introduced in a nonjudgmental, nonaccusing manner for the parent to accept the information and incorporate the suggestions in the home.

One method of accomplishing effective counseling for accident prevention is first to discuss the difficulties of constantly watching and safeguarding young children. In this way the monumental task of raising children is shared as a common problem, with accident prevention as one part of the parental role, not as the central issue. This approach also incorporates other possible causes for the accident, such as inadequate discipline, parent-child disturbances, or behavior problems. A visit to the home should always be part of the follow-up care to assess the potential accidental hazards and consequently to evaluate the institution of appropriate safe-proofing measures. One method of identifying risk areas is to ask specific questions or to have the parent complete a questionnaire designed to isolate factors that predispose children to poisoning.

The box below is a sample questionnaire of items that may determine what environmental manipulation is needed to "poison-proof" homes. The box on the right is a teaching plan designed to assess the parents' preparedness in case of an accidental poisoning and to supply appropriate instruction where necessary. Tools such as these have been developed to enable nurses to systematically and efficiently counsel families in the area of accident prevention. They are not meant to supplant nurses' own creativity in a specific situation or lessen their responsibility in any situation.

Acetaminophen poisoning

Acetaminophen is increasingly used as a mild analgesic/antipyretic drug, especially as a substitute drug for aspirin. The extensive availability of this nonprescription medication increases the probability of accidental ingestion of toxic quantities by infants and children. In addition the federal safety standards regarding child-proof packaging and limited quantities of medication per container, which are imposed on children's aspirin, are not required for acetaminophen preparations. Like aspirin, acetaminophen is available in many palatable forms that are well accepted by youngsters.

Etiology, pathophysiology, and clinical manifestations. Acetaminophen poisoning usually occurs from acute

Questionnaire for poison prevention

1. Where do I store cleaning products, medicines, laundry aids, and garden supplies?
2. What do I keep under the sink in the kitchen and bathroom?
3. Do I have any medicines (aspirin, tranquilizers, birth control pills, antacids, and so on) in my purse?
4. Are all the medicines and household products clearly labeled and in their original container?
5. Do I refer to medicine as candy to encourage my child to take it?
6. Are baby aspirins or chewable vitamins left on the table or kitchen counter for handy use?
7. Do I keep drugs prescribed for previous illnesses?
8. Is my child out of sight when I take medicine?
9. When using any medicine or household product, do I put it away immediately after use, keep my eye on it at all times, or put it down where my child cannot get it?
10. Are any of my garden plants or houseplants poisonous?
11. Do all cabinets have a lock on them?
12. What is stored in the garage or basement?
13. Are paints, gasoline, solvents, insecticides, poisons, and fertilizers either on a high shelf or locked in a cabinet?
14. Do I teach my child never to touch any nonfood item without asking me first?

Teaching strategy for parent education and preparation in case of an accidental poisoning

Question	*Intervention*
If you suspected that your child had ingested (eaten) a poison, what would you do first?	If answer is correct, ask for more specifics, such as number of local Poison Control Center If answer does not include knowledge of local Poison Control Center, supply information Stress necessity of not wasting time and need to save all evidence of poisoning
Do you have ipecac syrup in your home?	If answer is yes, ask for specific directions concerning its dosage and readministration If answer is no, supply correct information Also suggest alternate methods for inducing emesis, especially for child under 1 year of age
Should you always make the child vomit?	If answer is no, ask for specific poisons that are treated differently, such as bleach, turpentine, drain cleaner, and so on If answer is yes, supply correct information Emphasize that "antidote" listed on container of household products is minimal emergency treatment; medical advice should *always* be sought before relying on that information alone
If you suspected that your child had taken a poison, but there were no signs of illness and the child denied doing so, what would you do?	Emphasize need to always seek medical advice, rather than waiting for signs or believing the child

overdose. The recommended dosage for children is as follows:

Age (years)	*Amount (mg)*
Birth-1	60
1-3	60-120
3-6	120
6-12	240
Over 12	325-650

Single doses may be repeated every 4 hours but should not exceed a total 24-hour dose of 1.2 g in children under age 12 years and 2.6 g in children over age 12 years. The precise toxic dose is uncertain, although dosages significantly above these levels can produce toxicity, especially in infants.

Hepatic damage is the lethal consequence of acute toxicity. There is usually a latent period of approximately 24 to 36 hours before signs of liver damage, especially jaundice, are evident. If the toxicity is not treated, the clinical features are those of hepatic failure and coma (see p. 1297). Signs and symptoms that occur immediately after acute toxic ingestion include gastrointestinal irritability, anorexia, nausea, vomiting, diaphoresis, and gradual drowsiness.

Medical management. Early treatment includes gastric lavage and administration of activated charcoal. If hepatic damage has occurred as evidenced by abnormal liver function tests, the treatment is similar to the child with hepatic failure.

Nursing considerations Nursing goals are essentially the same as those discussed under salicylate poisoning (p. 585). The nurse needs to be familiar with acetaminophen preparations in order to identify possible ingestion. For example, cold remedies may contain acetaminophen in excessive amounts. However, if the nurse is unaware of this the potential source of drug overdose may be missed. As with any poisoning, the primary goal is prevention. With the present emphasis on acetaminophen as a "safe" substitute for aspirin, it is important to stress that in excess this drug, like any other, is capable of toxic and lethal side effects.

The boxed material on p. 588 summarizes the principles of nursing care in an acute poisoning.

Lead poisoning (plumbism)

Heavy metal poisoning can occur as a result of acute ingestion of lead, such as from ingestion of lead salts or inhalation of lead fumes. However, the vast majority of cases are caused by chronic ingestion of lead-containing products, principally, interior or exterior lead-base paint. Since mouthing is a normal activity of young children, children in the age-group of 18 to 30 months are most at risk.

Heavy metal poisoning can also occur from a number of other substances. Two of the more common are arsenics, a common ingredient found in snail bait and rat poison, and mercury, which is most notably found in excessive quantities in seafood harvested from polluted waters. The pathologic effects are similar to those of lead poisoning, and treatment is chelation therapy.

Etiology. The exact cause of lead poisoning is unknown; however, several factors usually influence the ingestion of lead-containing substances.

Characteristics of child. The child who ingests lead often practices pica. Pica was the Latin word for magpie, a bird of voracious and indiscriminate appetite. The use of the term today denotes the habitual, purposeful, and compulsive ingestion of nonfood substances. This list of ingested substances is practically endless, but most commonly included are clay, dirt, ashes, paint chips, laundry starch, cornstarch, paper, pencils, crayons, cigarette butts, and matches. Most children have a particular craving for a few items, which is largely determined by the availability of the substance. Although several investigators have attempted to associate the practice of pica with specific nutritional deficiences, such as iron, magnesium, and so on, no evidence of nutritional inadequacy other than that caused by the exclusion of nutritious substances for the ingestion of nonfood stuffs has been found.

Developmentally children progress through various stages of oral activity. As soon as infants learn to voluntarily bring an object to their mouth, they explore the object by mouthing, chewing, sucking, or biting it. However, it is not until after 12 to 18 months of age that children also begin ingesting the object as a further extension of their curiosity and exploration. This normal mouthing activity partially accounts for the high incidence of poisoning in toddlers. Between ages 3 and 5 years this behavior tends to disappear, unless other factors, such as those discussed under parent-child relationships, persist.

Lead poisoning is not confined to the preschool child who ingests the substance. It can also occur in older children who habitually sniff leaded gasoline. The nurse must be aware of children experimenting with drugs or other psychotropic substances and the possibility of gasoline sniffing. Gasoline sniffing is believed to be especially prevalent among American Indian children on reservations.[26]

Parental characteristics. Parent-child interaction is another significant variable in the ingestion of lead. As many as 50% of mothers whose children have the pica habit also demonstrate the behavior.[8] It is postulated that a child's high level of oral activity may be reinforced by a mother with similar oral interests. Imitation alone would account for such repetition of behavior, but, in addition, oral activity is probably associated with relief of anxiety. For example, bottle-feeding after age 18 months is more common in children who develop lead poisoning. Oral gratification from sucking on a bottle may be transferred to chewing on a windowsill or eating paint chips for lack

Summary of nursing care in acute poisonings

Goals	Responsibilities
Identify that a poisoning has occurred	Call local Poison Control Center, emergency facility, or physician for immediate advice regarding treatment Save all evidence of poison (container, vomitus, urine, and so on)
Remove or counteract poison	Induce vomiting except as contraindicated Keep child as quiet as possible To save time, prepare appropriate equipment for potential medical use, such as gastric lavage
Prevent aspiration of vomitus	Keep child's head lower than chest, place head between his legs, or position him on his side
Observe for latent symptoms and complications of poisoning	Treat as appropriate, for example, institute seizure precautions, keep warm and position correctly in case of shock, reduce temperature if hyperpyrexic, and so on
Support child and parent	Keep calm; do not admonish or accuse child or parent of wrongdoing
Prevent occurrence and/or recurrence	Assess possible contributing factors in occurrence of accident, such as discipline, parent-child relationship, developmental ability, environmental factors, behavior problems, and so on Institute anticipatory guidance for possible future accidents based on child's age and maturational level Refer to visiting nurse agency to evaluate home environment and need for safe-proofing measures Provide assistance with environmental manipulation when necessary

of stimulation and attention from the mother. Times of stress, such as birth of another sibling, are frequently associated with the commencement of pica activity.

The most common maternal pattern seen in these families is dependency. Such mothers have a history of despair, passivity, and inactivity to everyday life. As a result they are usually unable to stimulate or discipline the child to more constructive forms of activity. Another frequent pattern is the parent who is unaware of the child's pica, either from ignorance that ingestion of such substances is harmful or from lack of supervision and knowledge of the child's usual behavior. The passive parent is "mentally" absent from the home, but other parents may be "physically" absent to the point of delegation of all parental responsibilities to others.

Environmental characteristics. The third necessary component in this triad of causative factors is the availability of lead in the environment. Prior to 1940, interior paint contained lead pigments. Since then, lead-based paint can only be used for exterior surfaces. However, old, dilapidated housing is a prime source of lead from old flaking paint on walls, windowsills, and floors. Other potential sources of lead are unglazed clay pottery, toys or children's furniture painted with exterior paint, discarded cans containing lead paint, newspaper with colored print, painted food wrappers, painted handles of kitchen utensils, and pet food. Common exterior sources are door frames, fences, porches, and siding. A few chips of paint the size of a thumbnail may contain 100 mg or more of lead, which is 200 times the usual safe daily ingestion (0.5 mg).[8]

Unfortunately the likelihood of all three factors being present is greatest in the lower socioeconomic population, whose members live in poor housing, depend on oral activity as one source of pleasure, and exist in a state of crisis,

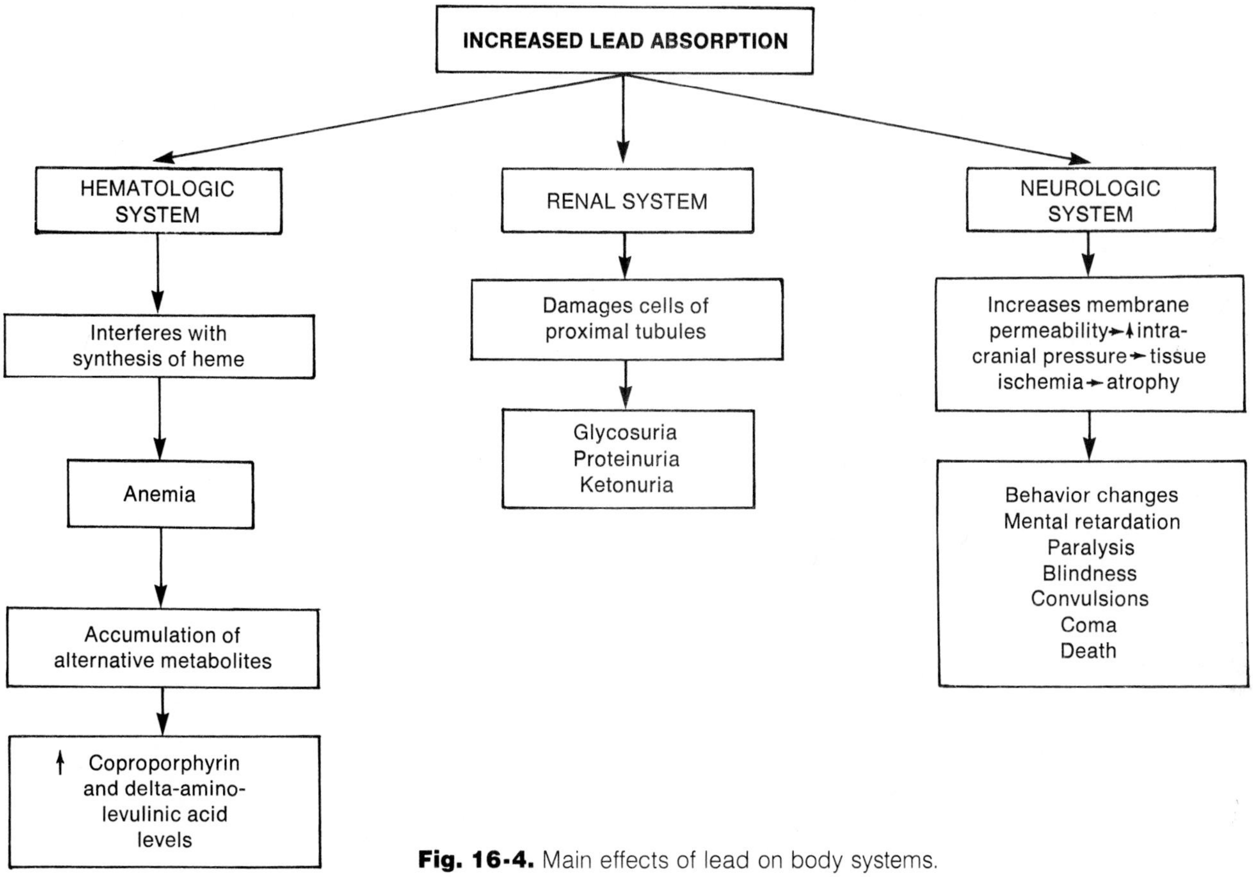

Fig. 16-4. Main effects of lead on body systems.

which leads them to dependency, passivity, and despair. Successful long-term cure and prevention of lead poisoning involves change in all three variables.

Pathophysiology and clinical manifestations. Normally lead is poorly absorbed by the body and is very slowly excreted via the kidneys, alimentary tract, and, to a small extent, sweat. Retained lead is largely stored in bone. However, under conditions of chronic ingestion, the rate of absorption exceeds the rate of excretion, and the excess lead is deposited in the tissues and circulatory system. About 90% of the lead is attached to the erythrocytes. Even when the chronic ingestion stops, it takes the body twice as long to excrete the stored lead as it did to accumulate it. As a result several body systems continue to be affected after environmental removal of the poison (Fig. 16-4).

Hematologic system. Lead is extremely toxic to the biosynthesis of heme, preventing the formation of hemoglobin and causing its precursors, especially coproporphyrin and delta-aminolevulinic acid (ALA), to increase in the body. Both of these intermediary metabolites are excreted and found in the urine in excessive amounts when the blood-lead concentration reaches 80 μg/100 ml of whole blood. Reduction of the heme molecule in the red blood cell results in anemia, one of the initial signs of the disease. The pathologic changes in the bone marrow are reversed when lead leaves the soft tissue and is excreted in urine or stored in bone.

Renal system. Lead damages the cells of the proximal tubules, resulting in abnormal excretion of glucose, protein, amino acids, and phosphate. With adequate treatment kidney damage is usually reversible. Severe irreversible lead nephropathy is probably limited to protracted childhood plumbism.

Central nervous system. The most serious and irreversible side effects of lead intoxication are on the nervous system. Initially there is an increase in membrane permeability, with a shift of fluid into the intervascular spaces of the brain. As a result increased intracranial pressure causes cortical atrophy and the sequelae of convulsions, mental retardation, paralysis, blindness, and, ultimately, coma and death. However, before acute encephalopathy occurs, behavioral changes indicate lead toxicity. Hyperactivity, aggression, impulsiveness, decreased interest in play, lethargy, irritability, delay or reversal in verbal maturation, loss of newly acquired motor skills, clumsiness, deficits in sensory perception, learning difficulties (despite adequate intelligence scores), short attention span, and distractibility are common signs of asymptomatic or borderline poisoning. Such manifestations of behavioral disturbance are important clues to the indentification of children with early poisoning.

The prominent clinical signs of gasoline sniffing are mainly those of central nervous system toxicity, namely irritability, tremor, hallucinations, confusion, lack of impulse control, depression, and sometimes delirium.[4] It may also cause signs of cerebellar dysfunction, notably chorea and ataxia.[26]

Other vague symptoms of plumbism are acute crampy abdominal pain, vomiting, constipation, anorexia, headache, and fever, which are sequelae of increasing toxicity.

Diagnostic evaluation. Several tests are available to detect the presence of toxic amounts of lead in the body (see Table 16-10). Nurses should be aware of the various tests used to establish a definitive diagnosis of the presence and severity of lead poisoning to prepare the child for the procedures and to explain to parents the necessity of several tests. The most frequently used procedure for routine screening is the blood-lead concentration and the erythrocyte-protoporphyrin level.[7] Various protocols based on the results of these two tests are available for suggesting when children should be treated. Most agree that when the blood-lead level exceeds 60 $\mu g/100$ ml, chelation therapy should be initiated. In some high-risk urban areas a blood-lead level of 50 $\mu g/100$ ml is considered indicative of treatment or careful follow-up for any rise above this level.

Nurses must be aware of the results from screening procedures in order to isolate those children at greater risk for increasing lead levels. Careful history taking is one of the most useful and valuable tools available to nurses. They should place particular emphasis on the following areas: (1) history of pica or evidence of this behavior during the interview, (2) recent change in behavior, particularly disinterest in play, (3) developmental delay or recent loss of acquired skills, especially speech, and (4) behavior problems such as aggression or hyperirritability. Maternal characteristics, such as those that are discussed in the section on etiology, are important contributing factors to high-risk situations, particularly recent crisis events, such as the birth of another child or absence of the parent. The value of a home visit to evaluate the availability of sources of lead cannot be overestimated in the overall plan for diagnosis and prevention.

Medical management. The objective of treatment is to mobilize the lead from the blood and soft tissues by enhancing its deposition in bones and its excretion in the urine. The main vehicle for accomplishing these goals is the use of chelation therapy, which involves the removal of the metal by combining it with another substance. Calcium disodium edetate (EDTA) is the principal chelating agent used. It forms a fairly stable, highly soluble compound that causes free lead to be readily excreted in the urine. It increases the urinary excretion of lead by ten to forty times, thereby relieving the symptoms of lead intoxication. It may be used singly or in combination with the chelating drug dimercaprol, also called BAL (British antilewisite). A combination of the drugs is thought to result in less saturation of each (therefore, fewer side effects) and better removal of lead from the brain. Although EDTA results in lower lead levels in general, it is less effective than BAL in the nervous system.

The exact course of therapy differs according to the severity of the child's condition and the preferred method of the physician. However, a commonly accepted regimen involves the intramuscular administration of each drug six times a day for a period of 5 days. For this treatment children are hospitalized and any supportive measures related to the child's symptoms are instituted.

Symptomatic treatment largely involves controlling seizures, which are often severe and protracted, since the anoxia that accompanies the convulsions compounds the brain damage from lead. Many of the usual drugs that are effective in managing seizures, such as the barbiturates, are not useful because repeated doses often result in medullary paralysis with respiratory and cardiac arrest. Precautionary measures for children with seizures include the use of an oxygen tent and available equipment needed in case of respiratory arrest, such as suction, endotracheal intubation set, tracheostomy set, ambu bag, and mechanical respirator.

Marked anemia is also treated. If shock is present, immediate intravenous replacement of blood is begun. If the child's clinical condition is stable, oral or intramuscular iron is used. Supplemental oxygen is helpful in situations of low-hemoglobin levels. Kidney function is carefully monitored because nephrotoxicity is a side effect of plumbism and EDTA. Decreased kidney function severely limits the effectiveness of chelation therapy. Blood calcium and phosphorus levels are measured frequently since chelation agents also remove calcium from the body, predisposing to the risk of hypocalcemia.

Various other treatments may be part of the total therapy. Vitamin D, calcium, and phosphorus may be given to enhance deposition of lead in bones. Cleansing enemas are ordered for episodes of acute lead ingestion or when lead is visible on radiologic examination in the gastrointestinal tract. Every effort is made to prevent infection and maintain adequate hydration. However, the most important aspect of treatment is prevention of recurrence. This usually involves a multidisciplinary approach of pediatrician, nurse, social worker, and social services to attack all three factors involved in lead poisoning—the child, the parent, and the environment. The role of the nurse is discussed in the following paragraphs.

Table 16-10. Diagnostic evaluation of lead poisoning

System	Pathologic change	Laboratory procedure	Result	Comments
Hematologic	Interferes with biosynthesis of heme, resulting in accumulation of alternate metabolites and hypochromic, microcytic anemia	Hematocrit	Decreased	Not specific for lead poisoning
		Hemoglobin concentration	Usually below 10 g	
		Reticulocyte count	Elevated	Helps differentiate anemia caused by lead rather than deficiency of iron
		Erythrocyte evaluation	Basophilic stippling	Indicates number of immature circulating erythrocytes by staining nuclear remnants retained in red blood cells, not reliable when done on peripheral blood samples
		Lead level	Elevated above normal (15-40 μg/100 ml of whole blood): 40-60 μg/100 ml—undue exposure 60-80 μg/100 ml—mild symptoms Above 100 μg/100 ml—great risk of encephalopathy	Highly sensitive to poor quality control; any lead contamination on skin surface (micro method) or equipment falsely elevates concentration; does not indicate if lead level is increasing, decreasing, or stabilizing
		Erythrocyte protoporphyrin (EP) level	Elevated above normal (levels between 60-189 μg/100 ml of blood are characteristic of anemia, but levels above 190 μg/100 ml are almost always caused by lead toxicity)	Less sensitive to contamination by exogenous lead Better index of potential lead toxicity; usually significantly elevated before clinical symptoms appear
Renal	Damages cells of proximal tubules, causing abnormal excretion of various substances	Urinalysis	Proteinuria, glycosuria, acetone bodies present, increased reducing substances, scattered red blood cells and casts	Not specific for lead poisoning
	Reflects paralysis of enzyme systems	Urinary coproporphyrin (UCP) level	Above 150 μg/24-hour output	Usually elevated after blood-lead level is above 80 μg/100 ml and clinical symptoms are evident; affected by state of hydration
		Urinary delta-aminolevulinic acid (ALA) level	Above 20 μg/100 ml	
		Calcium disodium edetate (EDTA) mobilization test	Increasing levels of lead in urine over 24-hour period	Inconvenient—requires collecting urine over 8- to 24-hour period; not suitable when signs of encephalopathy are present (delays treatment)
Neurologic	Increases cell membrane permeability Destroys neurons	Lumbar puncture	Spinal fluid under increased pressure, increased protein level, pleocytosis	Potentially dangerous—sudden release of pressure may result in herniation of cerebellar tonsils through foramen magnum or of temporal lobes through tentorium cerebri
Skeletal	Results in deposition of lead in bones	X-ray film	"Lead lines" in long bones	Related to *duration* of lead ingestion, not to severity of symptoms; frequently absent in children less than 2 years of age, even in presence of severe illness from plumbism
Gastrointestinal	Denotes recent ingestion of lead containing substance, such as paint chips	X-ray film	Presence of lead deposits along alimentary tract	Related to acute ingestion

Nursing considerations. The goals of nursing care are many in plumbism. The first is primary prevention of lead poisoning. However, this is an objective that cannot be accomplished by one person. It involves eliminating the environmental conditions, such as old, dilapidated housing, that contribute to the readily available source of the poison. Even further, it includes fostering the kind of parent-child relationship where pica is discouraged, the child is directed and stimulated to constructive activity, and the stresses of daily life do not overwhelm and drive the parent to despair, hopelessness, and passivity. Without such a multifaceted approach, the child will persist in the habit of pica and find substitute injurious agents to ingest, even if the source of lead is removed.

As has been discussed previously, identification of the child at risk in terms of all three causative factors is essential. Besides the laboratory screening procedures to isolate borderline or asymptomatic cases, the history is the most powerful tool available to health prefessionals. Actively looking for behavior changes, vague complaints of discomfort, signs of anemia, and situations of poor supervision or stimulation of the child can delineate potential victims who may ''pass'' the screening tests. Probably for these children the chance of preventing further lead ingestion is greater than for the child who is acutely ill.

For the child who must undergo chelation therapy, the nurse has several priority objectives. Certainly one of the most significant objectives is preparation of the child for the tremendous number of injections that he will receive. For example, if EDTA and BAL are to be administered as separate injections every 4 hours for a time period of 5 days, the child will receive a total of sixty injections. That alone is sufficient evidence of the need for anticipatory planning, but in addition the injections are very painful. The nurse can prepare the child through needle play on a doll or stuffed toy before the therapy begins and after receiving each injection. It is important to allow the child an outlet for the pain and anger he feels and to emphasize the reason for the drugs, particularly that it is not a punishment for eating lead or paint. Also, since the injections are painful, the nurse should tailor the child's activity to allow adequate rest and physical stimulation that does not aggravate the painful sites. Local application of warm soaks or insulated hot packs helps relieve the discomfort, although the pain may persist and be severe enough to limit movement. The nurse should also prepare the parents for the drug treatment and forewarn them of the child's possible psychologic and physical reactions to it.

EDTA and BAL are both viscous solutions. For adequate absorption, each must be administered deeply into a different large muscle mass. Sometimes, a local anesthetic such as procaine is injected simultaneously with the EDTA or BAL to help lessen the pain during administration. If this is done, the chelating agent is drawn into the syringe, followed by the anesthetic. In this way the anesthetic is the first medication to be injected into the tissue. It is introduced slowly in order to allow some time for it to exert its deadening effect. An air bubble at the top of the syringe flushes the needle of any remaining medication, thereby decreasing the chance of tracking the drug through the layers of the skin on withdrawal of the syringe.

Planning a rotation schedule for each series of injections is essential to prevent tissue damage and to ensure maximum tissue absorption. The preferred injection sites are the vastus lateralis muscle (anterolateral aspect of the thigh), gluteus medius muscle (upper outer quadrant of the gluteal area), and ventrogluteal site (lateral aspect of the hip). The gluteus medius muscle is composed mostly of subcutaneous tissue in children under 2 years of age or in any child who has not been using the legs for locomotion. Although the deltoid muscle is a satisfactory site in older children, it is not adequate for injection of a large volume of fluid, where a large surface area is needed for increased absorption. Since the peak incidence of lead poisoning is during the toddler years, it is likely that the vastus lateralis, ventrogluteal, and gluteal sites are satisfactory available areas for rotation of multiple injections. Table 16-11 presents one example of how these sites can be scheduled

Table 16-11. Schedule for rotation of injections* in lead poisoning†

	Day 1		Day 2		Day 3		Day 4		Day 5	
Time	EDTA	BAL	EDTA	BAL	EDTA	BAL	EDTA	BAL	EDTA	BAL
Midnight	RVL_1	LVL_1	RVL_3	LVL_3	RVL_5	LVL_5	RVL_2	LVL_2	RVL_4	LVL_4
4:00 AM	RVG_1	LVG_1	RVG_3	LVG_3	RVG_5	LVG_5	RVG_2	LVG_2	RVG_4	LVG_4
8:00 AM	RGM_1	LGM_1	RGM_3	LGM_3	RGM_5	LGM_5	RGM_2	LGM_2	RGM_4	LGM_4
Noon	LVL_2	RVL_2	LVL_4	RVL_4	LVL_1	RVL_1	LVL_3	RVL_3	LVL_5	RVL_5
4:00 PM	LVG_2	RVG_2	LVG_4	RVG_4	LVG_1	RVG_1	LVG_3	RVG_3	LVG_5	RVG_5
8:00 PM	LGM_2	RGM_2	LGM_4	RGM_4	LGM_1	RGM_1	LGM_3	RGM_3	LGM_5	RGM_5

*Abbreviations. Site: L, left; R, right; VL, vastus lateralis muscle; VG, ventrogluteal; GM, gluteus medius muscle. Rotation of injection within site: 1, upper left corner; 2, lower right corner; 3, upper right corner; 4, lower left corner; 5, center.

†Directions: cross out each site as it is used for that day and time.

Summary of nursing care of the child with lead poisoning

Goals	Responsibilities
Identify lead poisoning	Assist in screening procedures Recognize behavioral indications of asymptomatic or borderline lead poisoning Identify high-risk groups, especially "pica" child, "dependent" mother, and "lead" environment
Prevent complications from multiple injections into same site	Schedule rotation of sites, using recommended muscle areas for each individual child Palpate muscle area before preparing site to locate and avoid fibrosed tissue from previous injections
Prepare child for multiple injections	Always give reason for injection, while emphasizing that it is not a punishment for eating lead (paint) Use dramatic needle play with preschooler Involve parents in comforting child after injection
Observe for signs of encephalopathy or toxicity of chelating agents	Have seizure precautions and emergency respiratory arrest equipment at bedside; evaluate urinary functioning (intake and output record and periodic urinalysis)
Prevent occurrence and/or recurrence	Educate public about dangers of lead ingestion, signs and symptoms indicating intoxication, and need for treatment Assist in renovation of home to remove sources of lead, as well as measures to improve parenting Actively participate in social/political movement to provide suitable housing for everyone
Provide relief from pain at site of injection	Apply warm soaks or heating pad to injection site Avoid activity that places undue strain or exertion on painful muscle area, for example, use wheelchair for transportation If local anesthetic is added to syringe, inject it slowly as first drug (draw up last in syringe and do not mix)
Provide rest (depending on physical states)	Tailor activity to suit child's energy level Encourage quiet recreational activity that is stimulating and educational yet geared to present developmental level If anemia is severe, provide supplemental oxygen as needed
Educate parents	Discuss with parents dangers of lead ingestion, particularly for prevention of recurrence Inform parents of type of treatment and possible physical and psychologic reactions from child
Support parents	Suggest ways to help parents relate to their child in a more constructive manner in order to decrease pica behavior Help parents deal with additional crises in order to devote more energy to child-rearing responsibilities Locate potential child-care services to relieve some parental responsibilities, while increasing supervision of child outside the home
Acquire needed services	Refer to public health nurse, social worker, and other agencies who can assist in overall management of complex problem

to ensure that all areas are utilized to the best advantage.

A complication of multiple injections in one site is the development of hard, painful areas of fibrotic tissue. The nodules feel firm and almost circular when palpated. It is advisable practice to routinely feel the muscle mass before preparing the injection site to avoid administering additional medication into the same area. With the systematic approach used in Table 16-11, even with sixty injections, each specific location (for example, RVL_1, right vastus lateralis, upper left corner) is used only twice. If the gluteal muscle is not sufficiently developed, the alternate specific sites will each receive three injections. However, this is preferable to random selection of sites, which does not ensure that any one area will not receive multiple injections.

If the child is old enough to understand the concept of time, he can help mark off each injection as a way of helping him realize that the end of the treatment is approaching. For the toddler, little helps other than the physical presence and comfort of an adult, especially the parent. Dramatic play before and after the injection helps the preschooler feel control and mastery of the experience. All children deserve an explanation for the needle, such as "This is to take the lead (paint) out of your body so that your tummy (or other physical discomfort) feels better." Since the medication is given around the clock, the nurse must be careful to wake the child before giving the injection. Although it may seem easier to surprise the sleeping child and get it over with as quickly as possible, performing the procedure in this way can cause the child to fear going back to sleep. If he is awakened first, the child will know that nothing will be done to him unless he is forewarned.

EDTA is also a calcium-chelating agent; therefore, calcium is removed with the lead from the body. Although calcium is replaced in the calcium disodium edetate preparation, the nurse observes for signs of hypocalcemia, especially tetany and convulsions. Calcium gluconate should be readily available as the emergency antidote to calcium deficiency. Seizure precautions, such as those discussed in Chapter 37, are instituted for all children hospitalized with plumbism. If lumbar puncture is done, the nurse observes for signs of respiratory arrest from the sudden release of intracranial pressure. Signs suggestive of cerebral damage include apathy, lethargy, increased passivity and disinterest in surroundings, increased irritability, decreased alertness, difficulty in arousing the child from sleep, loss of consciousness, and coma. Each nurse should keep a detailed account of the child's behavior for the shift as a data base for comparing suspected alterations in personality and level of activity. Since chelating agents, particularly EDTA, are toxic to the kidneys, records are kept of intake and output and frequent urinalysis is performed to evaluate gross renal functioning. If the nurse suspects renal damage, a urine sample should automatically be sent for laboratory analysis.

Comprehensive management of the child with lead poisoning involves "treating" the environment to prevent recurrence after hospital discharge. However, this is not part of discharge planning, but rather a priority objective as soon as diagnosis of lead poisoning is made. When it is not possible for the family to move to better housing or expensively refurbish the present home, some simple, inexpensive measures can be utilized. As much of the old flaking paint as possible is scraped from the walls, ceilings, and floors. Since a new coating of lead-free paint does not prevent additional chips from falling away from the plaster, the walls are covered with wallpaper, contact paper, fabric, or burlap. In addition the children must be supervised and guided toward activity other than pica. Helping parents learn methods of stimulating their children, locating preschool or day-care centers, or helping parents organize a play group are methods of improving parenting and, consequently, lessening those factors that contribute to plumbism.

Health professionals have an even broader responsibility in terms of education of the public regarding the signs and symptoms of the disease. According to recent studies, subtle behavioral abnormalities may also be present in children with lead levels that are clinically borderline.[11] The most frequent behavior deviations of extreme negativism, distractibility, and constant need for attention may well be mistakenly diagnosed as other behavior problems, with labels such as learning disorder, delinquency, emotional disturbance, or hyperactivity, when in reality the child is suffering from the physical effects of a toxic substance. If such children were detected and treated earlier, the chance for optimum development would probably be greater. However, until lead poisoning is attacked as a social problem, as well as a physical problem, its high incidence, rate of recurrence, and serious irreversible sequelae may not be significantly altered.

For a summary of nursing care of the child with lead poisoning, see the boxed material on p. 593.

CHILD ABUSE

Child abuse is believed to be the result of a disturbance in parenting. Like the child with lead poisoning, the maltreated child is a victim of another triad of etiologic factors—the child's own temperament or unfortunate position in the family, the parents' background, and the compounded stresses of the environment. It is the combination of all three factors that frequently transforms corporal punishment as a form of discipline into a ruthless beating, whose purpose is no longer to control unacceptable behavior but to allow for release of pent-up frustration.

Scope of problem

Exactly how many children are maltreated is unknown, but speculations place the number above 500,000.[18] Nationwide public agencies receive over 300,000 reports of suspected child abuse each year, and annually 2000 children die from circumstances that are described as suspicious of maltreatment.[3] However, such figures probably attest to the problem of battered child syndrome, which is defined as "a clinical condition in young children who have received serious physical abuse, generally from a parent or foster parent,"[14] rather than to emotional neglect, whose definition is at best ambiguous. Emotional neglect is generally considered an omission, rather than a commission, of a direct act or behavior that has a detrimental effect on the child's psychologic development. The American Humane Association attempts to define it as follows: A child may be said to be emotionally neglected when there is failure on the part of the parents to provide him with the emotional support necessary for the development of a sound personality. This may result when the "home lacks the warmth and security essential for the development of a sound personality" or "when a child is met with overt or subtle rejection . . . and is made to feel unwanted, . . . does not belong, . . . and inferior to others."[10] When one considers the broad application of such statements, one only begins to appreciate the potential number of children who may be defined as emotionally neglected, in addition to those who are never discovered as having been physically abused.

One of the less publicized areas of maltreatment is sexual molestation. Its true incidence is highly speculative and uncertain, because, unlike physical injury or neglect, there may be no obvious signs of sexual assault. Considering the widespread reluctance to recognize or report this condition, it is likely that the available statistics grossly underestimate the frequency of this problem (see p. 597).

Etiology

The exact cause of child abuse is not known, but three major criteria—parental characteristics, characteristics of the child, and environmental characteristics—seem to be necessary in order for a child to be physically injured or neglected by his parents or guardian.

Parental characteristics. First the parents must have the potential to abuse, which is believed to be the result of specific child-rearing practices in their childhood. Although no two abusing individuals are exactly alike, there are several common factors that help identify potential abusers. One of the most significant is the type of parenting they received as a child. Most abusing parents were themselves abused as children. Therefore, the only way they know to relate to their children is through physical punishment, such as beatings or other inflictions of physical injury, or emotional neglect, such as omission of warmth, security, and affection or commission of verbal abuse, scapegoating, disapproval, and blame. When they were children they learned that no matter how hard they tried to be good or provide for their parents' needs, it was never enough. They eventually believed that they were no good and deserved to be hit. As a result they developed a poor self-image and low self-esteem. As parents they transfer this belief to their children, who they believe must also be punished in order to perform according to parental expectations.

Since their parents had little concept of what children were like or realistically could accomplish, abusing parents have little knowledge of normal developmental expectations. As a result they expect their children to nurture and parent them, in the same way as their parents demanded similar behavior. This concept of role reversal, or the parent acting as the child and expecting the child to become the parent, is an important factor in why some children escape abuse, whereas others become the victim. Understanding the concept of role reversal is also helpful in the planning of therapy for these individuals.

Developmentally when abusing parents were children they never mastered the first task of forming trust. Consequently they live in social isolation and find little pleasure and satisfaction from interpersonal relationships. With such needs unmet, they seek gratification in a marriage partner, who may be the same type of person. If this is the case, either parent may be the abuser. The marriage partner may also be a passive, dependent individual who condones the abuse by not interfering with it. If the potentially abusing individual marries a spouse who can meet his "child" needs, the likelihood of abuse occurring is diminished. However, the personality of the potential abuser usually does not attract the type of individual who compensates for the other's deficiencies, but rather, the kind of person who enhances such personality traits, to the disadvantage of the victimized child. Fig. 16-5 illustrates the cyclic pattern of the parents' rearing that perpetuates abuse.

The cumulative effect and interaction of these various factors greatly compound the task of parenting. Although these parents genuinely desire to have children, their reason for doing so is for the children to take care of them. This unrealistic expectation immediately creates crisis because the newborn demands total physical care and attention. With the parents' unsatisfied needs, there is no surplus or reserve of energy available for them to give to the infant. As the infant becomes more frustrated and irritable, the parents doubt any of their ability to provide the most minimal care and, because of their lonely, isolated lives, do not have the adequate support system, such as extended family, friends, or neighbors, that is available to other parents for periodic relief from parenting responsibilities. With no storehouse of spare emotional energy to cope with the usual tasks of child rearing, they are extremely vulnerable to additional crises of any nature and literally strike out at the child as a method of releasing their increasing frustration and anxiety. For this reason a crisis is usually the precipitating factor in isolated events of abuse, which frequently require medical intervention.

Characteristics of the child. The child also contributes to the abusing situation. In families of two or more children,

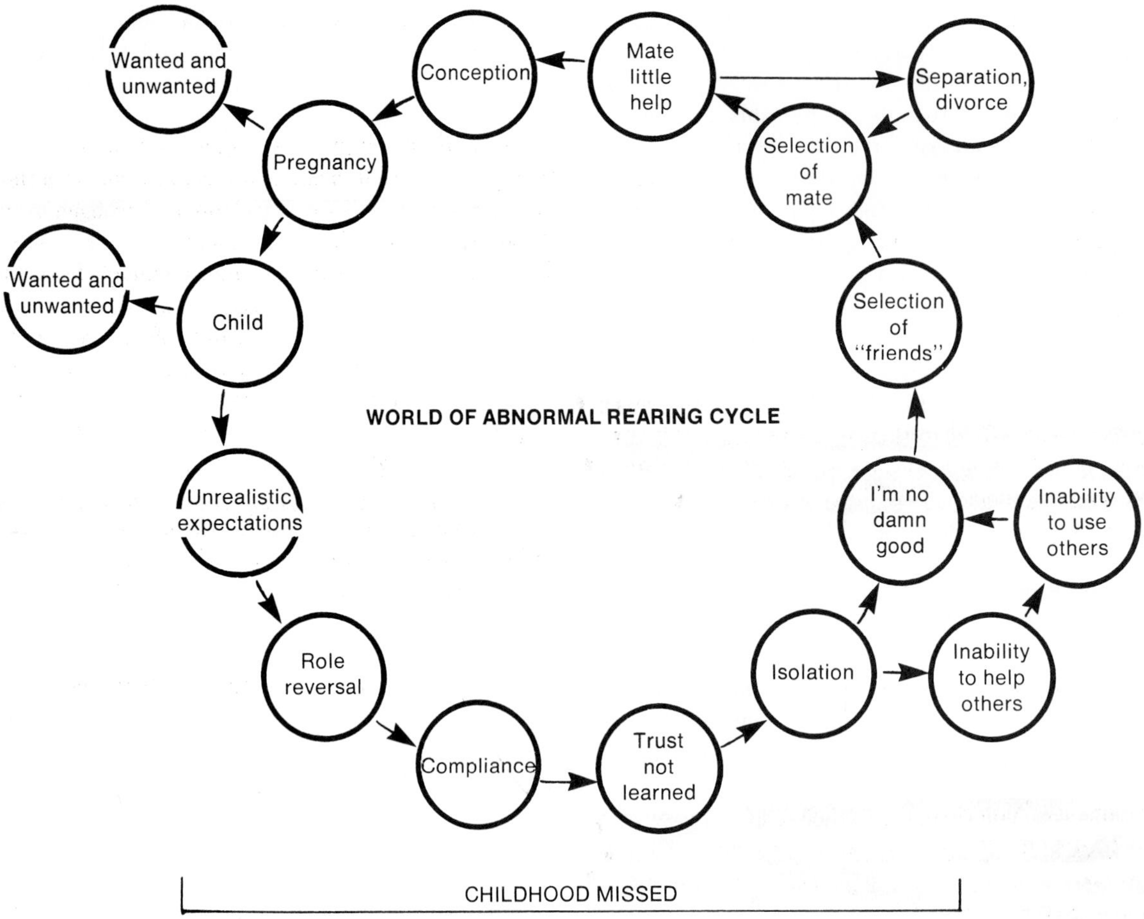

Fig. 16-5. World of abnormal rearing cycle. (From Helfer, R. E.: World of abnormal rearing cycle, Pediatr. Basics, vols. 10 and 11, 1975.)

it is usual to find only one child as the victim of abuse. This child's temperament, position in the family, additional physical needs if ill, activity level, or sensitivity to parental needs all in some way contribute to why he escapes or fosters physical abuse. For example, the firstborn may not be abused if he is the type of infant who demands little other than routine feeding and diapering. As he grows older the docile child may learn how to meet the parent's needs by being quiet, playing alone, showing the parent affection, and acting as grown up and self-sufficient as possible. However, this situation is never safe for the child. Any added stress such as illness, pregnancy, birth of a sibling, financial need, and so on can upset this precarious balance between parent-child role reversal. Often the precipitating factor for the abuse is not an identifiable stress but an ordinary task of child rearing, such as toilet training, speech development, or self-help skills. With no realistic knowledge of children's age-appropriate capabilities, the parent may expect learning to take place automatically. For example, the parent may decide that the 1-year-old child is ready for toilet training and expect that once the child is put on the potty-chair he will immediately learn to control elimination. When the child fails, the parent punishes him for not complying with the expected behavior. This partially explains why most physical injury occurs during usual child-caring activities, such as bathing, dressing, feeding, and so on, and why the majority of abused children are under school age.

Not infrequently the abused child is illegitimate, unwanted, brain damaged (especially in situations where the parents cannot accept the retardation), hyperkinetic, physically disabled, or from a broken home. Sometimes the child is abused because he reminds the parent of someone the parent dislikes, for example, a younger brother or sister who received all the attention from their own parents. Premature infants are at risk for maltreatment because of the failure of parent-child bonding during early infancy. Frequently a difficult pregnancy, labor, or delivery is a predisposing factor in abuse, especially when the infant is born prematurely or with congenital anomalies.

Although one child is usually the victim in an abusing family, if that child is removed for his own protection, the parents quickly replace him with another victim. Child abuse is not confined to one child because of a disturbed parent-child relationship but is the result of dysfunctioning parenting, which can involve any child. Therefore, no child is safe if left in the abusing environment unless the parents can be helped in some way to learn new parenting skills and to meet their needs and release their frustration through alternatives other than attacking their children.

Environmental characteristics. The environment is an integral part of the potential abusing situation. Typically it is one of chronic stress, including financial, emotional, physical, and marital crises. The social milieu of the abusive family is one devoid of adequate support systems. The environment becomes a trap from where there is no emotional exit except to direct the anger and frustration toward a helpless victim, the child.

Although most reporting of abuse has been from lower socioeconomic populations, child abuse is by no means a problem of any one societal group. It spans all educational, social, and economic levels. Certainly it is obvious that the stresses imposed by poverty, hunger, inadequate housing, and social prejudice predispose lower socioeconomic families to abusive situations. However, concealed crises can also be present in upper class families. For example, a wealthy family experiencing major life changes, such as rehousing, birth of an additional child, or marital discord, may have sufficient environmental stressors imposed on them to produce a potentially abusing situation. Nurses need to be cognizant of such factors in order to identify the hidden sources of child abuse and neglect.

Identification of abuse or neglect

Many parents favor physical punishment for disciplining their children yet do not abuse their child to the same degree of other parents. How does one differentiate between the spanking that may be severe enough to cause welts and the beating that may cause no greater physical injury but is representative of abuse? For one thing, each of the following three factors must be investigated in suspected cases of abuse: (1) Are the parents potential abusers because of their own experiences as a child and is their present behavior suggestive of foul play? (2) Is the child's behavior in any way suggestive of inducing abuse? (3) What environmental event or stressors precipitated the abuse? The answers to these questions are invaluable clues to suspected cases of abuse. A thorough physical examination and a careful, detailed history are the diagnostic tools. Nurses have a very special role because they may be the first person to see the child and parent, as well as the consistent care giver if the child is hospitalized.

Evidence of maltreatment. Physical abuse may be evident from obvious marks on the body. Some of the more common forms of physical injury include small, round burns or scars from cigarettes; localized burns on the buttocks or soles of the feet from being placed against a radiator or immersion in hot water; slap marks resembling the shape of a hand; welts from beatings with a belt, belt buckle, chains, or hangers; and circular abrasions around the ankles or wrists from tying the child down. A form of abuse that leaves no visible marks but causes severe pain from damage to the muscles and subcutaneous tissue is flogging the child with a wet towel. Another abusive act is vigorously shaking the child, which may result in a whiplash type of injury to the neck and can cause brain damage. Other evidence of abuse includes radiologic findings of healed or new fractures or dislocation of the extremities, especially the shoulder, from pulling the child or throwing him against a hard surface.

Signs of possible abuse should arouse suspicion but must be coupled with an understanding of cultural practices. For example, the Vietnamese have a practice called Cao Gio (coin rubbing) to relieve the symptoms of fever, chills, and headache. The procedure consists of applying oil to the back and chest, massaging the skin until warm, and firmly stroking the surface with the edge of a coin until petechiae or frank purpura appear. The appearance of the skin resembles that seen in a beating with a hard object. The practice is commonplace and definitely not viewed as battering by the Vietnamese people.[25]

Neglect or emotional abuse is much more difficult to recognize and document. Neglect is suspected when the child is unbathed, poorly nourished, inadequately dressed for the weather, or wearing old or torn clothing. Emotional abuse may be evident when signs of failure to thrive are seen, particularly those characteristic of the maternal deprivation syndrome (p. 494). Another clue is also the type of parent-child relationship, especially when the parent verbally abuses the child or continually belittles him in front of others.

In order to identify sexual molestation, health professionals must be willing to investigate the possibility of its existence. Besides the routine physical examination for signs of abuse or neglect, the child is carefully inspected for evidence of oral and/or anal penetration, as well as genital contact. Laboratory tests are done to detect the presence of semen and venereal disease. With the exception of congenital syphilis or gonoccocal conjunctivitis in newborns, the presence of venereal infection in children should always be an indication of possible sexual abuse.[24]

History pertaining to the incident. Besides observable evidence of abuse, the type of history revealed by the parents or other care giver, such as the baby-sitter or mother's boyfriend, is a significant diagnostic factor. Those areas of the history that should arouse suspicion of abuse include (1) conflicting stories about the "accident" from the parents or child, (2) an injury inconsistent with the history, such as a concussion and broken arm from falling off a bed, (3) a complaint other than the one associated with signs of abuse, for example, a chief complaint of a cold when the child has evidence of first- and second-degree burns on his body, (4) inappropriate parental concern for the degree of the injury, such as an exaggerated or absent emotional response; (5) refusal of the parents to sign for additional tests or agree to necessary treatment, and (6) absence of the parents for questioning.

Parental behaviors. Certain behavioral responses of the parents to their child and to the interviewer should alert the nurse to the possibility of maltreatment. Typically the parents have difficulty in showing concern toward their child. They are unable to comfort him and give no indication of realizing how the child may feel, physically or emotionally. Instead, they are critical of the child and angry with him for being injured. They maintain that the child injured himself and, if asked any question regarding their responsibility of protecting or supervising the child, become hostile and aggressive. They act as if the child's injury is an assault on them. Their entire perception of the incident is in terms of how it affects them, not the child, which is an indication of their preoccupation with their own needs and their inability to give any support to others. During the child's hospitalization they rarely become involved in the child's care and show little concern for his progress, eventual discharge, or need for follow-up care. However, if they are pressured during interrogation, they immediately demand to take the child home, regardless of the child's readiness for discharge.

If the interviewer avoids judging the parent and attempts to ask questions directed at the parents' history, the parent will usually reveal feelings about his childhood, particularly of loneliness, longing for a loving mother, and overwhelming feelings of worthlessness and dependency. As the interviewer shifts his focus from the child's "accident" to the parents' life, there is usually a marked transition in the parent's attitude, from one of distrust, suspicion, and hostility to one of attentiveness, heightened interest, and security.

Child behaviors. Battered children also exhibit behaviors that are untypical of those of well-nurtured children. They show no expectation of being comforted by their parents and, in general, are wary of physical contact by anyone else. They cry little, and, when they do so, it is in a hopeless sense, rather than as a plea for help. When admitted to the hospital unit they are less afraid of strangers than are their age-mates, and they tend to settle in quickly. They may form "friends" almost immediately, but there is little selectivity or preference in their attachments. Rather than seeking approval through verbal statements, they are always searching for satisfaction in material rewards, such as food, favors, or presents. They seem to seek safety in sizing up a situation and knowing the consequences of an act, rather than in physical contact with another person.

However, maltreated children rarely betray their parents by confessing to the abuse they received. If questioned, they will repeat the same story as the parents and try to defend their parents' actions. If the interviewer directly accuses the parents of abuse, the child will accept responsibility for the act in an attempt to vindicate his parents from the accusation. Whether the child responds in this way out of fear is uncertain, because, even when removed from the home, the child still upholds the parents' innocence. However, the child knows what he has in his parents. Even if the parent-child relationship is distorted, the child has a home, a family, and, in a sense, security. Between abusing events the child may receive some sort of attention and love from his parents, even if it is a result of his attending to their needs. If he betrays his parents, he loses all of this and is uncertain of what may be in its place. So he protects his parents because, in his thinking, a little love is better than none.

Observations of parents-to-be during prenatal care

1. Are the parents overconcerned with the baby's sex?
2. Are the parents overconcerned with the baby's performance? Do they worry that he will not meet the standard?
3. Is there an attempt to deny that there is a pregnancy (mother not willing to gain weight, no plans whatsoever, refusal to talk about the situation)?
4. Is this child going to be one child too many? Could he be the "last straw"?
5. Is there great depression over this pregnancy?
6. Is the mother alone and frightened, especially by the physical changes caused by the pregnancy? Do careful explanations fail to dissipate these fears?
7. Is support lacking from husband and/or family?
8. Where are the parents living? Do they have a listed telephone number? Are their relatives and friends nearby?
9. Did the mother and/or father formerly want an abortion but not go through with it or wait until it was too late?
10. Have the parents considered relinquishment of their child? Why did they change their minds?

From Kempe, C. N.: Approaches to preventing child abuse, Am. J. Dis. Child. **130**:941-947, September 1976. Copyright 1976, American Medical Association.

Nursing considerations

Prevention. Prevention involves identifying potential abusers and instituting supportive intervention prior to the

Observations to be made at postpartum and pediatric checkups

1. Does the mother have fun with the baby?
2. Does the mother establish eye contact (direct *en face* position) with the baby?
3. How does the mother talk to the baby? Is everything she expresses a demand?
4. Are most of her verbalizations about the child negative?
5. Does she remain disappointed over the child's sex?
6. What is the child's name? Where did it come from? When was the child named?
7. Are the mother's expectations for the child's development far beyond the child's capabilities?
8. Is the mother very bothered by the baby's crying? How does she feel about the crying?
9. Does the mother see the baby as too demanding during feedings? Is she repulsed by the messiness? Does she ignore the baby's demands to be fed?
10. What is the mother's reaction to the task of changing diapers?
11. When the baby cries, does she or can she comfort him?
12. What was/is the husband's and/or family's reaction to the baby?
13. What kind of support is the mother receiving?
14. Are there sibling rivalry problems?
15. Is the husband jealous of the baby's drain on the mother's time and affection?
16. When the mother brings the child to the physician's office, does she get involved and take control over the baby's needs and what's going to happen (during the examination and while in the waiting room) or does she relinquish control to the physician or nurse (undressing the child, holding him, allowing him to express his fears, etc.)?
17. Can attention be focused on the child in the mother's presence? Can the mother see something positive for her in that?
18. Does the mother make nonexistent complaints about the baby? Does she describe to you a child that you do not see there at all? Does she call with strange stories that the child has, for example, stopped breathing, turned color, or is doing something "on purpose" to aggravate the parent?
19. Does the mother make emergency calls for very small things, not major things?

From Kempe, C. N.: Approaches to preventing child abuse, Am. J. Dis. Child. **130:**941-947, September 1976. Copyright 1976, American Medical Association.

occurrence of an abusive act. Frequently there are clues that point to potentially abusive parents prior to the birth of a child (see the box on p. 598). Nurses in prenatal health centers need to be attuned to parents who are at risk by specifically questioning them regarding their attitude toward the pregnancy, future expectations for the child, and available support systems to help them adjust to parenthood. Of significance is information about the parents' own child rearing and incidents of physical or emotional abuse during their childhood.

As soon as the infant is born, the nurse assesses the parent-child attachment process and notes behaviors that signal lack of understanding of the infant's needs, disappointment in the child, little identification with him, lack of support from the father or other family members, and additional environment stressors (see the box above). Behaviors that signify positive adjustment to parenthood that offset the pressure of negative factors are also observed for (see the box on the right).

Once high-risk families have been identified, they need to be involved in a plan to promote the parent-child relationship. This involves helping the parents identify with the child, teaching them effective child-rearing practices, and promoting their self-esteem. Nurses in a variety of settings can implement these goals. Nurses in prenatal clinics can

Positive family characteristics

1. The parents see likable attributes in the baby and perceive him as an individual.
2. The baby is healthy and not disruptive to the parents' life-style.
3. Either parent can rescue the child or relieve one another in a crisis.
4. The parents' marriage is stable.
5. The parents have a good friend or relative to turn to, a sound "need-meeting" system.
6. The parents exhibit coping abilities, such as capacity to plan, and understand the need for adjustments because of the new baby.
7. The mother is intelligent and her health is good.
8. The parents had helpful role models when they grew up.
9. The parents can have fun together and with their personal interests and hobbies.
10. The parents practice birth control; the baby was planned or wanted.
11. The father has a steady job. The family has its own home, and living conditions are stable.
12. The father is supportive of the mother and involved in the care of the baby.

From Kempe, C. N.: Approaches to preventing child abuse, Am. J. Dis. Child. **130:**941-947, September 1976. Copyright 1976, American Medical Association.

prepare expectant families for the adjustment of parenthood. Nursery and postpartum nurses can foster the attachment process by encouraging parents to hold and look at their infant. In neonatal intensive care units nurses can minimize the effects of separation by encouraging parents to visit and help them become comfortable in the child's care. Those in ambulatory settings can teach parents appropriate methods of bathing, feeding, toileting, disciplining, and preventing accidents, while stressing the normal needs and developmental characteristics of children. Nurses need to be sensitive to the parents' needs for attention, reassurance, and reinforcement. Ideally community nurses should visit these families to ensure that adequate support and help are available.

Identification. Initially identification of cases of suspected abuse or neglect is essential. The nurse may come in contact with abused children in an emergency room, physician's office, or school. Signs that are indicative of abuse, such as the physical findings, specific parent or child behaviors, inconsistencies in the history, and contributing familial and environmental factors, must be recognized by the nurse. The priority is to remove the child from the abusive situation to prevent further injury.

All states have laws for mandatory reporting of child maltreatment. Referrals usually come to the Bureau of Child Welfare and are assigned to a caseworker in an agency such as the Child Protective Services. In most states, once a referral has been made, there is an automatic court order, which gives the agency the right to keep the child in protective custody for 72 hours. This allows the caseworker sufficient time to investigate the report in the event of intervening holidays or weekends. If the caseworker finds no justification for the charge, the child is returned to the home. If there is evidence of abuse, further action is taken against the parents.

In some states a court proceeding is necessary before the child can be placed in an institution. However, when the courts are involved, they usually require firsthand testimony by the referring parties. This may mean that nurses in the school, hospital, or public health agency are subpoenaed or that their records are introduced as evidence. In either case the nurse has a great responsibility in reporting facts, not hearsay or subjective opinion. This is particularly critical when writing nurses' notes. For example, the child's physical appearance on admission is clearly described. If possible, color photographs should be taken. Any changes in lesions, bruises, or healing wounds are noted. Behaviors are described, not interpreted, and are written down daily to establish a progress record. Conversations between the nurse and parent are written in quotes as much as possible. The nurse must bear in mind that the record of the hospital admission or home visit may be the most supporting evidence available. Nurses must be willing to take an active, responsible part in reporting and testifying to child abuse. Part of the long-term plan is help for parents, but the priority must be protection of the child.

Care of child. Frequently children suspected of abuse are hospitalized for medical management of their injuries. Their needs are the same as those of any hospitalized child but are multiplied by their situation. Even though they tend to adjust easily to their new environment and make friends quickly, they need a consistent care giver. At times the child's indiscriminate affection for any adult seems to diminish the necessity of consistency. However, such behavior is a learned response from previous relationships with others. The child wants to love and attach himself to one special person, but his efforts to do so with his parents, especially his mother, often were met with frustration and physical punishment or neglect. Therefore, he is no longer about to take the same chance, unless the effort comes from the other person. The nurse has the obligation of demonstrating acceptance of and affection for the child, while not expecting the same in return, until the child begins to trust that the nurse will not turn against him for not meeting the nurse's needs. This can be made very difficult by the child's behavior, such as his clinging for attention, which at first is flattering but later becomes very annoying and irritating. The nurse is placed in the position of showing the child acceptance while attempting to modify the negative behavior. The nurse must be careful not to use the mechanism of displacing anger on the child, which is what the child expects. Instead, a program of attention based on play, group interaction with other children, and quiet time with the child is planned beforehand. Behavior modification is also used to express disapproval of disruptive behavior. Through such modeling, alternate ways of interacting and disciplining their children can be demonstrated to parents.

Hospitalization is often extended as eventual placement is arranged. Frequently this is much longer than that necessary for recovery from the injury or neglect. The child must be guided toward physical and mental wellness during this period. He is treated as a child with the usual physical needs, developmental tasks, and play interests—not as a dramatic victim of abuse. The nurse is his advocate in this goal. Others who want to question the child without justified reason are intercepted by the nurse, who also encourages the child in his continuing relationship with his parents. The nurse does not become a substitute parent to the exclusion of the child's natural parents. Such an intent only intensifies the parents' feelings of inadequacy, worthlessness, and isolation. It in no way helps them to understand their child or to promote their trust in health professionals. The goal of the consistent nurse-child relationship is to provide a role model for the parents in helping them to relate positively and constructively to their child and to foster a therapeutic environment for the child in his reprieve from the abusing situation.

Discharge planning should begin as soon as the legal dis-

Summary of nursing care of the abused child

Goals	Responsibilities
Prevent abuse	Identify families at risk for potential abuse (see the boxed material on pp. 598 and 599) Promote parental attachment to child Emphasize child-rearing practices, especially effective methods of discipline Increase parents' feeling of adequacy and self-esteem Encourage support systems that lessen stress and total responsibility of child care on one or both parents Be available for assistance
Identify suspected cases of child abuse or neglect	Be child advocate—place protection of child above consideration for parents' rights or own wish to remain uninvolved Formulate data base of those factors that are indicative of abuse, such as signs of previous injury or neglect, inconsistencies in history, parent or child behaviors unlike those of protective parents and nurtured children, and significant familial and environmental factors Have a working knowledge of the state's child abuse laws Keep factual, objective records of the child's physical condition; behavioral response to parents, others, and environment; and interviews with family members Suspect sexual molestation in any young child with venereal infection other than congenital syphilis or ophthalmia neonatorum
Provide consistent care giver and therapeutic environment during hospitalization	Demonstrate acceptance of child while not expecting same in return Show attention while not reinforcing inappropriate behavior Plan appropriate activities for attention with nurse, other adults, and other children; use play to work through relationships Avoid displacing anger on child, such as shouting or yelling, as method of dealing with own frustration toward child's negative behavior Praise child's abilities in order to promote his self-esteem
Relieve anxiety in child	Treat child as one who has a specific physical problem for hospitalization, not as "abused" victim Avoid asking too many questions; use play, especially family or doll house activity, to investigate kind of relationships perceived by child; child should relate to one consistent person regarding events of abuse Foster healthy aspects of parent-child relationship, encourage child to talk about parents in positive sense; avoid criticizing parents' actions to child
Promote wellness in child	Besides physical needs related to injury or neglect, focus on developmental needs such as sensory stimulation and education Accept temporary regression as necessary mechanism to cope with present crisis
Promote a sense of parental adequacy during child's hospitalization	Orient parents to hospital unit and help them feel welcomed and an important part of child's care and recovery Reinforce competent child-care activities Focus on the abuse as a problem that requires therapeutic intervention, not as a behavior characteristic or deficiency of the parent Empathize with difficulties of rearing children, especially with additional life crises, while not condoning the act of abuse or neglect

Continued.

Summary of nursing care of the abused child—cont'd

Goals	Responsibilities
Plan for discharge	Prepare for discharge as soon as disposition is finalized If child is being placed in foster home, encourage family members to visit child before discharge; stress to them child's need to regress in order to complete missed stages of development If child is returning to his own home, encourage parents to visit as much as possible; plan for close supervision and counseling of family If parents' rights are being terminated permanently, help child grieve this loss, especially if it entails separation from siblings (long-term counseling is optimum goal)
Prevent recurrence	Collaborate efforts of multidisciplinary team to continually evaluate progress of child in foster home or in return to own family As public health or school nurse, actively look for signs of continued abuse or neglect Help parents identify those circumstances that precipitate an abusive act and ways in which to deal with the release of anger in ways other than attacking child
Support parents	Provide "mothering" by directing attention to parent, taking over child-care responsibilities until parent feels ready to participate, and focusing on parent's needs Refer parents to Parents Anonymous (initially may need to attend with parents as their advocate) Help identify a support group for parents, such as extended family or nearby neighbors; help these significant others understand their important role in also preventing further abuse
Teach parents	Teach realistic expectations of child's behavior and capabilities Emphasize alternate methods of discipline, such as reward and verbal disapproval Suggest methods of handling developmental problems or goals, such as toddler negativism, toilet training, independence, and so on Teach through demonstration and role modeling, rather than lecture; avoid authoritarian approach
Lessen environmental crises	Refer to social agencies who can provide assistance in financial support, adequate housing, employment, and so on

position for placement has been decided, which may be temporary foster home placement, return to the parents, or permanent termination of parental rights. The latter is the most drastic resolution, but it is necessary in situations of repeated abuse. Whenever children are remanded to a foster home or juvenile institution, they must be allowed the opportunity to ventilate their feelings. No matter how severe the abuse, they usually mourn the loss of their parents. They need help to understand why they must not return home and that this new home is in no way a punishment. Whenever possible, foster parents should be encouraged to visit, and the nurse should take an active role in helping these parents understand the child. It is unfortunate that many abused children live in hell as they are tossed from one foster home to another, sometimes enduring worse circumstances than existed in their real home. Only through constant evaluation of the placement residence and the child's adjustment to his new environment can the vicious cycle of abuse, abandonment, and neglect be stopped.

Care of parents. One of the most difficult, yet essential, components of success with abusing parents is the quality of the therapeutic relationship. It must be one of genuine concern and treatment, not one of accusation and punishment. Nurses must examine their personal feelings toward these parents, particularly when sexual abuse is present. Some see the act of abuse as disgusting and totally without justification, whereas others can identify with it, at least in the sense of realizing the exasperation and frustration occasionally felt toward their own children. In some way, such as group discussion, nurses must come to an understanding of their feelings to be effective with an abusing parent. For example, viewing the parent as the patient and the child as the victim of abuse places the emphasis on "treatment" rather than "punishment." Unless the nurse's attitude is positive, abusing parents will not be motivated to change, since they will not be working with a trusting person who demonstrates the kind of behavior that is being asked of them.

These parents cannot be fooled. Their survival as a child depended on their perception of other peoples' needs, and they are very skillful at saying what is expected of them while not making any attempts to change. Possibly it is for this reason that self-help groups, such as Parents Anonymous, are so successful, because the members cannot be deluded since they know the "game" so well. Such groups also are very accepting and nonjudgmental, because everyone has been in the same position. Group peer pressure and commitment are important motivating factors that keep parents from reverting to previous behaviors. The group also provides a release mechanism, because, when parents are angry, they can call a fellow member and ventilate their feelings over the phone rather than on the child.

Since these parents have unrealistic expectations of children's capabilities, the nurse also fosters knowledge and understanding of normal growth and development. The nurse demonstrates how to handle children, how to teach them at their age level, and what realistically to expect from them. Since these parents are very sensitive to criticism or domination and already possess a very low self-esteem, the nurse teaches through demonstration and example, rather than through lecturing. Any competent parenting abilities they demonstrate are praised in an attempt to promote their sense of parental adequacy. Abusing parents desperately need "mothering" in order to be able to mother or father their own children. The nurse attends to their needs for security, trust, release from responsibility, and so on. For home visits, the nurse may plan to visit at times when the children are at school, with a friend, or asleep. The nurse must remember that implicit in role reversal is the concept that the parent is a child and as a child will be jealous of the attention given to other children. Therefore, the nurse structures visits in the home or hospital to allow maximum attention to the parent.

The solution to child abuse is not an easy one. Success is never certain, and the penalty for failure may well be a child's life. For those children who do survive, there is the possibility of their becoming abusive parents and consequently continuing the pattern of maltreatment, the threat of institutionalization because of retardation resulting from brain damage, and the risk of becoming juvenile offenders. In fact 80% of known criminals have a history of significant abuse during their childhood. However, there are services available, such as Parents Anonymous, psychiatric or mental health intervention, and group therapy sessions, that help parents achieve major changes within themselves. Nurses have a responsibility to work individually with those families they care for in the hospital or community in terms of establishing a supportive and trusting relationship and to refer parents for additional help whenever possible.

For a summary of general nursing care of the abused child, see the boxed material on pp. 601 to 602.

REFERENCES

1. Altshuler, A., and associates: Even children can learn clean self-catheterization, Am. J. Nurs. **77**(1):97-101, January 1977.
2. Becker, E., editor: Kidney and urinary tract infections, Indiana, 1971, Eli Lilly and Co.
3. Besharov, D. J.: Building a community response to child abuse and maltreatment, Child. Today **4**(5):2-4, September/October 1975.
4. Boeckx, R. L., Postl, B., and Coodin, F. J.: Gasoline sniffing and tetraethyl lead poisoning in children, Pediatrics **60**(2): 140-145, August 1977.
5. Boyle, M., and Kaufman, A.: Strep screening to prevent rheumatic fever, Am. J. Nurs. **75**(9):1487-1488, September 1975.
6. Burko, H., and Rhamy, R.: Lower urinary tract problems related to infection: diagnosis and treatment, Pediatr. Clin. North Am. **17**(2):233-253, 1970.
7. Center for Disease Control: Increased lead absorption and lead poisoning in young children, Atlanta, March 1975, U.S. Department of Health, Education, and Welfare, Public Health Service.
8. Chisolm, J., and Kaplan, E.: Lead poisoning in childhood—comprehensive management and prevention, J. Pediatr. **73**(6):942-950, December 1968.
9. Corby, D. G., and Decker, W. J.: Management of acute poisoning with activated charcoal, Pediatrics **54:**324-328, September 1974.
10. De Francis, V.: Protecting the child victim of sex crimes committed by adults, Denver, 1969, American Humane Association.
11. de la Burde, B., and Choate, M.: Does asymptomatic lead exposure in children have latent sequelae? J. Pediatr. **81**(6): 1088-1091, December 1972.
12. Diphtheria, pertussis, tetanus, and poliomyelitis in the U.S., Stat. Bull. Metropol. Life Ins. Co. **57:**8-11, September 1976.
13. James, J. A.: Renal disease in childhood, ed. 3, St. Louis, 1976, The C. V. Mosby Co.
14. Kempe, C. H., and associates: The battered child syndrome, J.A.M.A. **181:**17-24, 1962.
15. Kunin, C.: Diagnosis, prevention, and management of urinary tract infection, Philadelphia, 1974, Lea & Febiger.
16. Lansdown, R. G., and associates: Blood-lead levels, behavior, and intelligence: a population study, Lancet **1**(7857): 538-541, 1974.

17. Mofenson, H.: The American Association of Poison Control Centers, Clin. Pediatr. **13:**305-306, April 1974.
18. Nagi, S. Z.: Child abuse and neglect programs: a national overview, Child. Today **4**(3):13-17, May/June 1975.
19. Neumann, P. Z., de Domenico, I. J., and Nogrady, M. B.: Constipation and urinary tract infection, Pediatrics **52**(2): 241-245, August 1973.
20. Northern, J., and associates: A technique for identifying ear disease in children, Pediatr. Nurs. **1**(2):32-37, March/April 1975.
21. Petrillo, M., and Sanger, S.: Emotional care of hospitalized children, Philadelphia, 1972, J. B. Lippincott Co.
22. Reid, D.: Treatment of the poisoned child, Arch. Dis. Child. **45**(241):428-433, 1970.

22a. Scott, J.: Urinary diversion in children, Arch. Dis. Child. **48**(1):199-206, 1973.

23. Thrupp, L., and associates: Transurethral reflux during cleansing procedure for clean-voided urine specimens in low-birth weight infants, J. Pediatr. **82**(6):1057-1059, June 1973.
24. U.S. Public Health Service: Gonorrhea: the latest word, Emergency Med. **7**(2):132-138, February 1975.
25. Yeatman, G. W., and associates: Pseudobattering in Vietnamese children, Pediatrics **58**(4):616-618, October 1976.
26. Young, R. S., Grzyb, S. E., and Crismon, L.: Recurrent cerebellar dysfunction as related to chronic gasoline sniffing in an adolescent girl, Clin. Pediatr. **16**(8):706-708, August 1977.

BIBLIOGRAPHY

Brown, M., and Murphy, M.: Ambulatory pediatrics for nurses, New York, 1975, McGraw-Hill Book Co.

Goth, A.: Medical pharmacology: principles and concepts, ed. 9, St. Louis, 1978, The C. V. Mosby Co.

Hamilton, W. J., editor: Textbook of human anatomy, St. Louis, 1976, The C. V. Mosby Co.

Ravel, R.: Clinical laboratory medicine, Chicago, 1973, Year Book Medical Publishers, Inc.

Rudolph, A., editor: Pediatrics, ed. 16, New York, 1977, Appleton-Century-Crofts.

Scipien, G. M., and associates: Comprehensive pediatric nursing, New York, 1975, McGraw-Hill Book Co.

Shirkey, H. C., editor: Pediatric therapy, ed. 5, St. Louis, 1975, The C. V. Mosby Co.

Waechter, E., and Blake, F.: Nursing care of children, New York, 1976, J. B. Lippincott Co.

Widmann, F.: Goodale's clinical interpretation of laboratory tests, Philadelphia, 1973, F. A. Davis Co.

Communicable diseases

Altemier, W. A., and Ayoub, E. M.: Erythromycin prophylaxis for pertussis, Pediatrics **59**(4):623-625, April 1977.

American Academy of Pediatrics: Report of the committee on infectious diseases, Evanston, Ill., 1977, The Academy.

American Hospital Association: Infection control in the hospital, ed. 2, Chicago, 1970, The Association.

Benenson, A. S., editor: Control of communicable diseases in man, ed. 11, Washington, D.C., 1970, American Public Health Association, Inc.

Brown, M. S.: What you should know about communicable diseases and their immunizations. Part I. The three R's, Nursing '75 **5**(9):70-72, September 1975.

Brown, M. S.: What you should know about communicable diseases and their immunizations. Part II. Diptheria, pertussis, tetanus, and polio, Nursing '75 **5**(10):56-60, October 1975.

Brown, M. S.: What you should know about communicable diseases and their immunizations. Part III. Mumps, chickenpox, and diarrhea, Nursing '75 **5**(11):55-60, November 1975.

Brem, J.: Koplik spots for the record, Clin. Pediatr. **11**(3):161-163, March 1972.

Dudgeon, J. A.: Congenital rubella, J. Pediatr. **87**(6):1078-1086, December 1975.

Gardner, P., Breton, S., and Carles, D. G.: Hospital isolation and precaution guidelines, Pediatrics **53**(5):663-673, May 1974.

Gardner, P., Oxman, M. N., and Breton, S.: Hospital management of patients and personnel exposed to communicable diseases, Pediatrics **56:**700-709, 1975.

Garner, J. S., and Kaiser, A. B.: How often is isolation needed, Am. J. Nurs. **72**(4):733-737, April 1972.

Judelsohn, R. G., and associates: Efficacy of zoster immune globulin, Pediatrics **53**(4):476-480, April 1974.

Karson, D. T.: Smallpox vaccination in the United States: the end of an era, J. Pediatr. **81**(3):600-608, September 1972.

Krugman, S., Ward, R., and Katz, S. L.: Infectious diseases of children, ed. 6, St. Louis, 1977, The C. V. Mosby Co.

Lentz, J.: The nurse's role in extending infection control to the community, Nurs. Clin. North Am. **5:**165, 1970.

Morrison, S., and Arnold, C.: Patients with common communicable diseases, Nurs. Clin. North Am. **5:**143, 1970.

O'Grady, R., and Dolan, T.: Whooping cough in infancy, Am. J. Nurs. **76**(1):114-117, January 1976.

Spicher, C.: Nursing care of children hospitalized with infections, Nurs. Clin. North Am. **5:**123, 1970.

U.S. Department of Health, Education and Welfare, Public Health Service: Isolation techniques used in hospitals, Washington, D.C., 1970, U.S. Government Printing Office.

Zausner, E.: Congenital rubella: pathogenesis of motor deficits, Pediatrics **47**(1):16-25, 1971.

Zoumboulakis, D., and associates: Steroids in treatment of pertussis, Arch. Dis. Child. **48**(1):51-54, 1973.

Tonsillitis and otitis media

Bluestone, C., and Shurin, P.: Middle ear disease in children, Pediatr. Clin. North Am. **21**(2):379-397, 1974.

Crawford, C., and Palm, M.: Can I take my teddy bear? Am. J. Nurs. **2**(73):286-287, February 1973.

De Angelis, C.: Basic pediatrics for the primary health care provider, Boston, 1975, Little, Brown and Co.

Dison, N.: Tonsillectomy: a mother's view, Am. J. Nurs. **69**(5): 1024-1027, May 1969.

Eavery, R. D., and associates: How to examine the ear of the neonate, Clin. Pediatr. **15**(4):338-341, April 1976.

Havener, W. H., and associates: Nursing care in eye, ear, nose, and throat disorders, ed. 3, St. Louis, 1974, The C. V. Mosby Co.

Levy, J. S., and Lovejoy, G. S.: Management of pharyngitis by pediatric nurse practitioners, Clin. Pediatr. **15**(5):415-418, May 1976.

McCurdy, J. A., and associates: Auditory screening of preschool children with impedance audiometry—a comparison with pure tone audiometry, Clin. Pediatr. **15**(5):436-441, May 1976.

Mattar, M., Markello, J., and Yaffe, S. J.: Pharmaceutic factors affecting pediatric compliance, Pediatrics **55**(1):101, January 1975.

Paradise, J.: Why T & A remains moot, Pediatrics **49**(5):648-650, 1972.

Paradise, J., and Bluestone, C.: Early treatment of universal otitis media in infants with cleft palate, Pediatrics **53**(1):48-54, 1974.

Rees, T. S.: Tympanometry as an aid in the diagnosis of middle ear disease, Clin. Pediatr. **15**(4):368-373, April 1976.

Whitson, B.: The puppet treatment in pediatrics, Am. J. Nurs. **9**(72):1612-1614, September 1972.

Wolman, I. J.: The "T and A" status in 1976. In Wolman, I. J., editor: Clinical pediatrics, Philadelphia, 1976, J. B. Lippincott Co.

Urinary tract infection

Amar, A. D., and associates: The practical management of vesicoureteral reflux in children, Clin. Pediatr. **15**(6):562-569, June 1976.

American Academy of Pediatrics, Section of Urology: Screening school children for urologic disease, Pediatrics **60**(2):239-240, August 1977.

Bradley, G. M.: Urinary screening test in the infant and young child, Med. Clin. North Am. **35:**1457-1471, November 1971.

Khan, A., and Pryles, C.: Urinary tract infection in children, Am. J. Nurs. **73**(8):1340-1343, August 1973.

Lohr, J. A., and associates: Prevention of recurrent urinary tract infections in girls, Pediatrics **59**(4):562-565, April 1977.

Ochsner, M., and associates: Assessing UTI in the infant, Nurs. Update **7:**1, January 1972.

Oster, J.: Clinical phenomena noted by a school physician dealing with healthy children, Clin. Pediatr. **15**(8):748-751, August 1976.

Slosky, D. A., and Todd, J. K.: Diagnosis of urinary tract infection: the interpretation of colony counts, Clin. Pediatr. **16**(8): 698-701, August 1977.

Woodard, J. R., and Holden, S.: The prognostic significance of fever in childhood urinary infections, Clin. Pediatr. **15**(11): 1051-1054, November 1976.

Ingestion of injurious agents

Arena, J. M.: Poisoning and its treatment. In Shirkey, H. C., editor: Pediatric therapy, ed. 5, St. Louis, 1975, The C. V. Mosby Co.

Brandt, P., and associates: IM injections in children, Am. J. Nurs. **72**(8):1402-1406, August 1972.

Chisolm, J.: Treatment of lead poisoning, Mod. Treatment **8**(3): 593-611, August 1971.

Croft, H., and Frenkel, S.: Children and lead poisoning, Am. J. Nurs. **75**(1):102-104, January 1975.

Fendrick, G.: Quizzing the expert: Jay M. Arena on saving the child who swallows poison, Hosp. Physician, pp. 44-58, November 1973.

Goulding, R.: Acetaminophen poisoning, Pediatrics **52**(6):883-884, December 1973.

Greengard, J.: Lead intoxication in children, Hosp. Med., pp. 61-82, April 1970.

Guinee, V.: Pica and lead poisoning, Nutr. Rev. **29:**267-269, December 1971.

Hankin, L., and associates: Lead poisoning from colored printing ink, Clin. Pediatr. **12:**654-655, November 1973.

Hankin, L., and associates: Lead on painted handles of kitchen utensils, Clin. Pediatr. **15**(7):635-636, July 1976.

Hendin, D.: Save your child's life! New York, 1972, Enterprise Publications.

Klein, R.: The prevention of lead poisoning in children, Pediatr. Clin. North Am. **21:**2, May 1974.

Levy, G., and Houston, J. B.: Effect of activated charcoal on acetaminophen absorption, Pediatrics **58**(3):432-435, September 1976.

Lourie, R.: Prevention of lead paint or prevention of pica? Pediatrics **48:**490-491, September 1971.

Lybarger, P. M.: Accidental poisoning in childhood: an ongoing problem, Issues Comprehensive Pediatr. Nurs. **1**(6):30-39. May 1977.

MacLean, W.: A comparison of ipecac syrup and apomorphine in the immediate treatment of ingestion of poisons, J. Pediatr. **82**(1):121-124, January 1973.

Maheffy, K. R.: Relation between quantities of lead ingested and health effects of lead in humans, Pediatrics **59**(3):448-456, March 1977.

Meadow, S., and Leeson, G.: Poisoning with delayed-release tablets, Arch. Dis. Child. **49**(4):310-312, 1974.

Mennear, J. H.: The poisoning emergency, Am. J. Nurs. **77**(5): 842-844, May 1977.

Mooty, J., Ferrand, C. F., and Harris, P.: Relationship of diet to lead poisoning in children, Pediatrics **55**(5):636, May 1975.

Perkins, K. C., and Oski, F. A.: Elevated blood lead in a 6-month-old breast fet infant: the role of newsprint logs, Pediatrics **57**(3):426-427, March 1976.

Piomelli, S., and associates: The FEP (free erythrocyte porphyrin) test: a screening micromethod for lead poisoning, Pediatrics **51**(2):254-259, February 1973.

Reed, A.: Lead poisoning: silent epidemic and social crime, Am. J. Nurs. **72**(12):2181-2184, December 1972.

Robinson, L. A., Roper, K. E., and Fischer, R. E.: Nursing considerations in the use of non-prescription analgesic-antipyretics aspirin and acetaminophen, Pediatr. Nurs. **3**(4):18-24, 1977.

Robischon, P.: Pica practice and other hand-mouth behavior and children's developmental level, Nurs. Res. **20:**4-16, January/February 1971.

Si Lin-Fu, J.: Childhood lead poisoning—an eradicable disease, Children **17:**2-7, January/February 1970.

Wright, S. P.: Usefulness of physostigmine in imipramine poisoning, Clin. Pediatr. **15**(12):1123-1127, December 1976.

Child abuse

Atherton, H. B.: Rejection: the deadliest poison, Pediatr. Basics **12:**11-14, 1975.

Barnard, M.: Early detection of child abuse. In Hymovitch, D., and Barnard, M., editors: Family health care, New York, 1973, McGraw-Hill Book Co.

Broadhurst, D. D.: Project protection: a school program to detect and prevent child abuse and neglect, Child. Today **4**(3):23-25, May/June 1975.

Davoren, E.: Working with abusive parents: a social worker's view, Child. Today **4**(3):2, May/June 1975.

Davoren, E.: Foster placement of abused children, Child. Today **4**(3):41, May/June 1975.

Ferro, F.: Combatting child abuse and neglect, Child. Today **4**(3):1, May/June 1975.

Fontana, V.: The diagnosis of the maltreatment syndrome in children, Pediatrics **51**(4):780-782, 1973.

Fontana, V. J.: The maltreated child, Springfield, Ill., 1971, Charles C Thomas, Publisher.

Fontana, V. J., and Robison, E.: A multidisciplinary approach to the treatment of child abuse, Pediatrics **57:**760-764, 1976.

Galdston, R.: Violence begins at home, J. Child Psychiatry **10:**336-350, 1971.

Geiser, R. L., and Norberta, M.: Sexual disturbance in young children, Am. J. Maternal Child Nurs. **1**(3):186-194, 1976.

Helfer, R. E., and Kempe, C. H.: The battered child, Chicago, 1968, University of Chicago Press.

Helfer, R. M.: The etiology of child abuse, Pediatrics **51**(4): 776-777, April 1973.

Isaacs, J. L.: The law and the abused and neglected child, Pediatrics **51**(4):783-788, April 1973.

Jaffe, A. C., and associates: Sexual abuse of children, Am. J. Dis Child. **129:**689-692, June 1975.

Kellogg, M.: Like the lion's tooth, New York, 1972, The New American Library, Inc.

Kempe C. H.: Pediatric implications of the battered baby syndrome, Arch Dis. Child. **46**(245):28-37, 1971.

Kempe, C. H.: A practical approach to the protection of the abused child and rehabilitation of the abusing parent, Pediatrics **51**(4):804-808, April 1973.

Kempe, C. H., and Helfer, E. E., editors: Helping the battered child and his family, Philadelphia, 1972, J. B. Lippincott Co.

Morris, M., and associates: Toward prevention of child abuse, Children, pp. 55-60, March/April 1964.

Neill, K., and Kauffman, C.: Care of the hospitalized abused child and his family: nursing implications, Am. J. Maternal Child Nurs. **1**(2):117-123, March/April 1976.

Olson, R. J.: Index of suspicion: screening for child abusers, Am. J. Nurs. **76**(1):108, January 1976.

Reed, J.: Working with abusive parents: a parent's view, Child. Today **4**(3):6-9, May/June 1975.

Rosenfeld, A. A., and Newberger, E. H.: Conceptual and practical pitfalls in the broadened definition of child abuse, J.A.M.A. **237**(19):2086-2088, May 1976.

Savino, A., and Sanders, R.: Working with abusive parents: group therapy and home visits, Am. J. Nurs. **73**(3):482-484, March 1973.

Sgroi, S. M.: Sexual molestation of children, Child. Today **4**(3): 19-21, May/June 1975.

Shydro, J., Noyes, M., and Wheeler, J.: Child abuse, Nursing '72 **2**(12):37-41, December 1972.

Steele, B. F.: Working with abusive parents: a psychiatrist's view, Child. Today **4**(3):3-5, May/June 1975.

Stone, R. K., and associates: Needle perforation of the liver in an abused infant, Clin. Pediatr. **15**(10):958-959, October 1976.

Whiting, L.: Defining emotional neglect, Child. Today **5**(1):2-5, January/February 1976.

UNIT SEVEN
Middle childhood

Children in the middle childhood years enjoy a relatively stable period of slow but steady growth and maturation with few physical or emotional stresses. It is a comfortable period of adjustment with a developmental pace sufficiently slow to meet the physical and psychologic demands placed on them. It is a period of broadening horizons when children encounter a wider sphere of influence—school, peers, and multiple opportunities for social interaction. During this period children learn the fundamental skills of their culture and develop inner resources for coping with larger social units. The emphasis during this period is on competence in physical and mental tasks and on the equally important changes in social relationships.

Chapter 17, *The School-Age Years,* provides a brief overview of the developmental changes that take place in middle childhood, including a lengthy summary of the major characteristics of each age within the period of middle childhood. Chapter 18, *Health Problems of Middle Childhood,* outlines the more common health problems encountered during these years. Few major illnesses are associated with middle childhood, although children during this time are still subject to many of the problems that characterize the earlier childhood years, such as accidents, and, with the wider social relationships, communicable diseases continue to be prevalent.

17

The school-age years

The segment of the life span that extends from age 6 years to approximately age 12 years has been tagged with a variety of labels, each of which describes an important characteristic of the period. These middle years are most often referred to as *school-age* or the *school years*. This period begins with entrance into the wider sphere of influence represented by the school environment, which has a significant impact on development and relationships. The term *gang age* describes the child's affiliation with age-mates and learning the culture of childhood. With peer groups children establish the first close relationships outside the family group. From a psychoanalytic point of view, this is the period of *latency,* which has been considered to be a time of sexual tranquility between the Oedipal phase of early childhood and the eroticism of adolescence. It is during this time that children experience the intimacy of relationships with same sex peers following the indifference of earlier years and preceding the heterosexual fascination that accompanies the changes of puberty. However, the concept of sexual latency is now being questioned in the light of early sexual exploration and the exploitation of sex in the media.

Physiologically the middle years begin with the shedding of the first deciduous tooth and end at puberty with the acquisition of the final permanent teeth (with the exception of the wisdom teeth). During the preceding 5 to 6 years, the child has progressed from a helpless infant to a sturdy, complicated individual with the capacity to communicate, conceptualize in a limited way, and become involved in complex social and motor behavior. Physical growth has been equally rapid. In contrast the period of middle childhood, between the rapid growth of early childhood and the turmoil of the prepubescent growth spurt, is a time of gradual growth and development with steadier and more even progress in both its physical and emotional aspects. Physical health is generally good, and it is a comfortable period of physical adjustment. Physiologic processes in general have attained a stage of development that permits their maintenance at stable levels under ordinary conditions and their ready adjustment to changing needs and stresses. Under normal circumstances these children are usually well able to meet the physical and psychologic demands that are placed on them.

There is a special quality about the middle childhood years. This is the period of childhood that the adult remembers with fond recollections. The school-age child likes this age period, and it is the one to which the preschooler eagerly looks ahead and for which the adolescent yearns. In the Western world the school-age child has a good deal of freedom and few responsibilities.

With a firm foundation of trust, autonomy, and initiative, the child is ready and eager for the wider world of learning and competition associated with developing a sense of industry. The child moves from the egocentricity of early childhood to the subperiod of cognitive domain described as concrete operations. Until recently middle childhood has generated the least interest and preoccupation among psychologists and others concerned with the effects of childhood experiences on later adjustments. However, it has been found that this period has an important contribution to the child's learning the fundamental skills of the culture and the development of competence and self-esteem. It is a time of intellectual growth, investment in work, and the child's first real commitment to a social unit outside of and larger than the family.

Developmental tasks of middle childhood

The major developmental tasks associated with middle childhood are predicated on the successful acquisition of earlier, simpler skills. They are accompanied by the mild but persistent expectations of the society in which the child lives, which serve as guidelines for behavior. Children who succeed in achieving the tasks of early childhood are able to move into middle childhood with the skills of locomotion, language, and control of body functions. They are now ready to undertake the tasks associated with the school experience, which are characterized by three outward thrusts. The child feels the interpersonal push from home and family into the peer group, the physical thrust into the world of active games and work that requires neuromuscular skills, and the mental thrust into the world of mature concepts, logic, symbolism, and communication. From these three developmental thrusts emerge the tasks of middle childhood[3]:

1. *Learning physical skills necessary for ordinary games.* Increasing muscular growth and neurologic maturation allow for increasingly complex and refined motor activities as childhood progresses. For most children this is a natural process facilitated by peer group rewards and cooperation.
2. *Building wholesome attitudes toward oneself as a growing organism.* Middle childhood is the most critical time for development of a positive self-concept. The child learns to care for his body, is taught the concepts of hygiene and safety, and is provided with opportunities to stimulate his mind. When he achieves success in an endeavor, the child feels competent and confident.
3. *Learning to get along with age-mates.* The social sphere of middle childhood is centered around peers whose approval and acceptance depends on the child's conformity to group standards. Through interaction with peers, children learn cooperation, social skills, and the social habits that they will retain into adulthood.
4. *Learning an appropriate masculine or feminine social role.* To gain social acceptance the child must learn the male and female roles that have been defined by his culture. Boys and girls are expected to behave in a prescribed manner, and conformity to acceptable role behavior is rewarded by family, peers, and society.
5. *Developing fundamental skills in reading, writing, and calculating.* As the nervous system matures sufficiently, the school assumes the responsibility for teaching basic skills that prepare the child to take his place in the social and economic life of the society.
6. *Developing concepts necessary for everyday living.* From a concrete basis of reality, the child, during the school years, acquires a sufficient store of concepts to allow him to think effectively about the ordinary activities of living related to occupational, civic, and social matters.
7. *Developing a conscience, morality, and a scale of values.* The child gradually learns to distinguish "good" from "bad" and "right" from "wrong" and to internalize the rules for behavior of his culture into an inner controlling force, the conscience.
8. *Achieving personal independence.* During middle childhood the child gradually becomes a person who can rely on his own store of knowledge and experience to make increasingly sound judgments. Although independence from adults comes about slowly, by the end of the middle childhood years he can assume responsibility for his personal care and safety, for use of time and a share in useful tasks, and for selection of friends and activities.
9. *Developing attitudes toward social groups and institutions.* It is during the middle years that children learn and assimilate the attitudes and values of their culture toward religious, social, political, occupational, and economic groups. Much of what is termed culture is learned during the school years.

PHYSICAL DEVELOPMENT

During middle childhood growth in height and weight assume a slower but steady pace as compared with the earlier years and the years immediately ahead. Between ages 6 and 12 years, children will grow an average of 2½ to 5 cm (1 to 2 inches) per year to gain 30 to 60 cm (1 to 2 feet) in height and will almost double in weight, increasing 1½ to 3 kg (3 to 6 pounds) per year. The average 6-year-old child is about 117 cm (46 inches) tall and weighs about 22 kg (48 pounds); the average 12-year-old child stands about 150 cm (59 inches) tall and weighs approximately 38 kg (84 pounds). During this age period girls and boys differ very little in size, although boys tend to be slightly taller and somewhat heavier than girls. Toward the end of the school-age years both boys and girls begin to increase in size, although most girls begin to surpass boys in both height and weight to the acute discomfort of both.

School-age children are more graceful than they were as preschoolers and are steadier on their feet. Their body proportions take on a slimmer look with longer legs, varying body proportion, and a lower center of gravity. Posture improves over that of the preschool period to facilitate locomotion and efficiency in using the arms and trunk. These proportions make climbing, bicycle riding, and other activities much easier. Fat gradually diminishes and its distribution patterns change, contributing to the thinner appearance of the child during the middle years. Accompanying the skeletal lengthening and fat diminution is a greater percentage increase in muscle tissue. By the end of this age period both boys and girls will double their strength and physical capabilities and their steady and relatively consistent acquisition of refined coordination will increase their poise and skill. However, this increased strength can be misleading. Although strength increases, muscles are still functionally immature when compared with those of the adolescent and are more readily damaged by muscular injury caused by overuse.

The most pronounced changes and those that seem best to indicate increasing maturity in children are a decrease in head circumference in relation to standing height, a decrease in waist circumference in relation to height, and an increase in leg length related to height. These observations often provide a clue to the child's degree of maturity that has proved useful in predicting the child's readiness for meeting the demands of school. There appears to be a correlation between physical indications of maturity and success in school.

Certain physiologic and anatomic characteristics are typical of children in the years of middle childhood. Facial proportions change as the face grows faster in relation to the remainder of the cranium. The skull and brain grow very slowly during this period and increase little in size thereafter. Since all of the primary (deciduous) teeth are lost during this age span, middle childhood is sometimes known as the *age of the loose tooth* and the early years of middle childhood as the *ugly duckling stage,* when the new secondary (permanent) teeth appear to be much too large for the smaller face.

Maturity of the gastrointestinal system is reflected in fewer stomach upsets, better maintenance of blood sugar levels, and an increased stomach capacity that permits retention of food for longer periods of time. The school-age child does not need to be fed so carefully, promptly, or as frequently as before. Caloric needs in relation to stomach size are less than they were in the preschool years and less than they will be during the coming adolescent growth spurt.

Physical maturation is evidenced in other body tissues and organs. Bladder capacity, although differing widely among individual children, is generally greater in girls than in boys. There are individual variations in frequency of urination and differences in one child under variable circumstances such as temperature, humidity, time of day, amount of fluids ingested, and emotional state.

The heart grows more slowly during the middle years and is smaller in relation to the rest of the body than at any other period of life. Consequently many believe that strongly competitive sports with prolonged, intense physical exertion may be damaging to the school-age child. The heart and respiratory rates steadily decrease and the blood pressure increases during the ages from 6 to 12 years (see Appendix A).

The shape of the eye changes during growth, and the normal farsightedness of the preschool child is gradually converted to 20/20 vision during middle childhood. There is still controversy regarding the age at which 20/20 vision is achieved, although it appears to be well established by 9 to 11 years of age. Binocular vision is well developed in most children at 6 years of age or shortly after. To aid vision throughout the school years, large print is recommended for reading matter and regular vision testing should be a part of the school health program.

Bones continue to ossify throughout childhood, but, since mineralization is not completed until maturity, bones resist pressure and muscle pull less than mature bones. Consequently care must be observed to prevent alterations in bone structure, such as providing well-fitted shoes, chairs, and desks that allow correct sitting posture with the feet able to reach the floor and the hips able to fit well back in the seat. Children should have ample opportunity to move around and should observe appropriate caution in carrying heavy loads. For example, they should shift books from one arm to the other, and newsboys who carry heavy newspapers slung from the shoulders should alternate the load from one shoulder to the other to avoid developing a low shoulder or spine curvature.

There are wider differences between children at the end of middle childhood than at the beginning, and in some individual children the difference is striking. These differences become increasingly apparent and, if extreme or unique, may create emotional problems unless the associated characteristics of height and weight relationships, rapid or slow growth, and other important features of development are recognized and explained to these children and their families. Also, physical maturity is not necessarily correlated with emotional and social maturity. The 7-year-old child who looks like a 10-year-old child will, in fact, think and act like a 7-year-old child. To expect behavior appropriate for a 10-year-old child from him is unrealistic and can be detrimental to his development of competence and self-esteem. Conversely to treat a 10-year-old as though he were 7 years old is an equal disservice to the child.

Toward the end of middle childhood the discrepancies between growth and maturation between boys and girls begin to be apparent. On the average there are approximately 2 years difference between girls and boys in the age of onset of pubescence. The average age of onset for girls is about age 10 years, whereas for boys it is about age 12 years. There are wide differences between individuals, and some girls may display characteristics or developmental changes as early as 8 years of age. Because of this discrepancy, some authors define the middle childhood or school-age years as 6 to 10 years for girls and 6 to 12 years for boys.

Relationship of body build to personality

During the school-age years children take on the characteristics of physical appearance more nearly like the adult body type they will ultimately attain; the general trend varies very little. For example, the tall, slim child will undoubtedly become a tall, slim adult. A number of classification systems have been advanced that attempt to describe specific body types. The most popular of these identifies three basic body types, and, although most persons show variations or mixtures of all three, the characteristics of one type appear to predominate in each person. The three general body types are described as *endomorphic* (persons with short, fat builds), *ectomorphic* (long, thin persons), and *mesomorphic* (muscular, athletic persons). Table 17-1 describes the three basic body types and the general temperament that appears to be associated with each. The body build of the child appears to have a subtle but significant influence on personality development. However, these observations are not conclusive since much also depends on cultural influences, health, and adequacy of nutrition.

Extremes in any one body build carry some disadvantages. Endomorphic children, for example, tend to readily become obese, whereas ectomorphic children are more likely to become underweight and to fatigue easily. During the childhood years children representing all three basic

Table 17-1. Physical and temperamental characteristics associated with the three body types

Body type	Physical characteristics	Temperament
Endomorphic	Heavy trunk, thighs, and upper arms Rounded, soft body contours Tapering forearms and legs Large amounts of subcutaneous fat Predominance of feminine physical attributes Large intestines and large amounts of other endothelial tissues	Viscerotonic—sociable, relaxed in posture and movement, loves physical comfort, slow reacting, emotionally even-tempered, tolerant, complacent
Ectomorphic	Preponderance of ectodermal tissues, that is, of skin and nervous tissues Linear build Thin bones and muscles Little fat in soft tissues	Cerebrotonic—restrained in posture movement, enjoys being alone, self-conscious, vocally restrained, tense
Mesomorphic	Heavy skeleton in body and extremities Broad, rectangular shoulders Large, strong muscles Athletic competence Predominance of masculine attributes	Somatotonic—needs activity and action, assertive, energetic, courageous, competitive, direct, generally noisy

types may be short, medium or tall; however, the general trend is for predominantly mesomorphic children to be characterized by vigorous growth in height and endomorphic children to increase in weight. Ectomorphic children are usually the smallest during school age; their development tends to be slow and late in maturing, but after the adolescent growth spurt they are usually tall adults. Frequently they grow to be physically strong with speed and endurance that permit their indulging in sports activities that do not require weight. Although not universally characteristic of these children, ectomorphic children tend to be restless and active and may have difficulty in assimilating sufficient amounts of food to meet their considerable nutritional requirements. In contrast endomorphic children tend to be relatively inactive and placid with large appetites and an interest in preparing and consuming food.

The general responses of persons in the United States to a child's physical characteristics and the physical limitations placed on the child by these characteristics are well correlated with personality development. For example, the short, fat child will seldom be selected by other children to be a member of a team in sports. As a result of this negative reinforcement, the child will turn to other interests. The well-coordinated child will be in demand for activities that involve athletic prowess and skill, and this positive reinforcement encourages his efforts in this direction. Often the child's appearance will result in his assuming a role in order to live up to the expectations that others may have determined, for example, the attractive, well-built, coordinated child will assume a leadership role and the fat, uncoordinated child will often play the clown or the "jolly fat person" to gain a place in the peer group.

Physical activity

The improved capabilities and adaptability of the school-age child permit greater speed and effort in motor activities, and larger, stronger muscles with greater efficiency and skill permit longer and increasingly strenuous play without exhaustion. During this age period children acquire the necessary coordination, timing, and concentration that are required to participate in adult-type activities, even though they may be deficient in the strength, stamina, and control of the adolescent and adult. Consequently a larger amount of physical activity should be expected and encouraged during the school years. However, it must be kept in mind that, although school-age children are large and appear to be strong, they may not be prepared yet for strenuous competitive athletics. A great deal of controversy has surrounded the trend toward earlier participation in competitive athletics and regarding the amount and type of competitive sports that are appropriate for children in the elementary grades. At present most authorities do not discourage participation in Little League baseball, soccer, swimming, and other sports for school-age children. However, it is important for those involved with children in this age-group to understand the child's physical limitations and to teach the proper techniques and safety in order to avoid injury to developing bones and muscles. Equipment should be maintained in safe condition and protective apparatus worn to prevent serious accidents.

All growing children need some regular exercise and should be afforded with opportunities of various kinds that provide satisfying experiences to meet individual likes and dislikes. Appropriate activities that promote coordination and development during the school-age years include

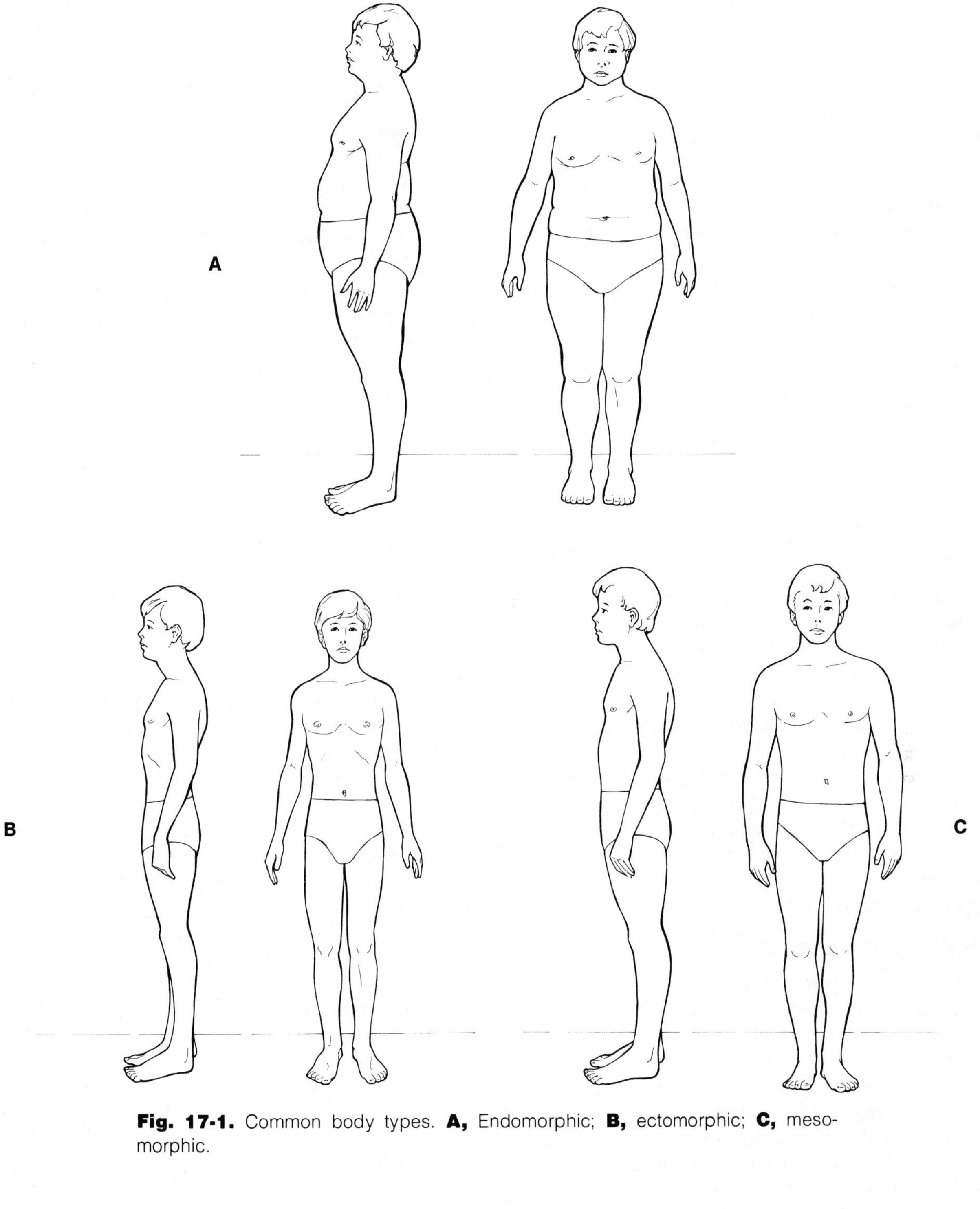

Fig. 17-1. Common body types. **A,** Endomorphic; **B,** ectomorphic; **C,** mesomorphic.

running, skipping rope, swimming, roller skating, ice skating, and bicycle riding. Positive reinforcement achieved by experiencing increasingly smooth, rhythmic, and efficient use of the body conditions the child toward regular physical activity.

Acquisition of skills

School-age children also demonstrate increasing capacities in fine muscle facility and complex artistic skills. Handedness is well established by the beginning of the school years, and the child makes great strides in writing and drawing during this age period. It is a period of energetic and vibrant creative productivity. With the tools of language and reading, children can create poems, stories, and plays. With more advanced fine motor skills, they are able to master an unlimited variety of handicrafts, such as ceramics, needlework, wood carving, and beadwork. They avidly pursue these skills in solitude, with a friend, or in programs offered through organizations such as boys' or girls' clubs, scouting, or the YWCA and YMCA, which use crafts as a means to occupy, entertain, and educate children.

Music is a favorite form of expression in middle childhood. School-age children are stimulated and invigorated by music. They can sing in harmony, play instruments in orchestras and bands, and otherwise manage music at a more complex level. They can compose original songs, learn lyrics almost effortlessly, and turn any empty moment into an occasion for singing to which any family, bus driver, or group leader can attest.

The school-age child is capable of assuming responsibility for his own needs, although his distaste for soap and water and "dress" clothes is legendary. School-age children can and want to assume their share of household tasks, which usually are related to the male and female roles that have been defined by their culture, and many assume responsibility for tasks outside the home, such as baby-sitting or paper routes.

PSYCHOLOGIC DEVELOPMENT

There is no concept more difficult to assess or more elusive than that of the personality or the "self." Most persons draw inferences regarding children's personalities from observation of their behaviors. These behaviors are based on many different innate and acquired characteristics, the way in which these characteristics are organized, and the manner in which each characteristic modifies or alters the other to contribute to the unique quality of each child. Personality is reflected in the way in which the child reacts to himself and others, the way in which others react to him, and the way in which he adjusts to his environment. Development of the personality involves a number of different aspects of development, including physical, intellectual, social, and emotional aspects, all of which are profoundly influenced by the environment in which the child grows and develops.

Cognitive development

Somewhere around the beginning of the school years, children begin to acquire the ability to relate a series of events and actions with mental representation that can be expressed both verbally and symbolically. This is the stage in development that Piaget describes as *concrete operations,* wherein the child is able to use his thought processes to experience them. Since the word "operation" implies an action that is performed on an object or set of objects, a mental operation is an alteration or transformation that is carried out in thought rather than in action. A toddler or preschool child can perform acts that involve ordering, such as correctly arranging a graduated set of circles from largest to smallest on a stick, or he can find his way to a friend's house, but he is unable to verbalize the action or actions involved in the process. The school-age child is able to articulate the process and can perform the action mentally without the need to carry out the behaviors.

As the child moves from the preschool years into the world of wider relationships, his conceptual abilities become increasingly more flexible. His rigid, egocentric outlook is replaced by thought processes that allow him to see things from the point of view of another. He becomes aware of a variety of perspectives and becomes more sensitive to the fact that others do not always perceive events exactly as he does. He is able to delay action until he has evaluated alternative responses to situations, and his steady reduction in egocentricity helps form the basis for logical thought and the development and maturation of morality.

During this stage the child develops an understanding and use for relationships between things and ideas. He progresses from making judgments based on what he sees (perceptual) to making judgments based on what he reasons (conceptual). He is increasingly able to master symbols and to use his memory store of past experiences in evaluating and interpreting the present. He gains insight into the basic components of concrete operational thought: conservation, classification, and combinational skills.[5]

Conservation. One of the major cognitive tasks of the school-age child is learning that physical matter does not appear and disappear by magic. He learns that certain properties of the environment are not changed simply by altering their disposition in space. He is able to resist perceptual cues that suggest such alterations in the physical state of an object. There appears to be a developmental sequence in the child's capacity to conserve matter. Conservation of mass usually is accomplished earliest, weight some time later, and volume last.

Conservation of mass is usually demonstrated by the use of two soft clay balls of the same size and shape. When the child has determined to his satisfaction that the balls are identical, one is flattened into a pancake-shaped mass. The child is asked to tell which has more clay or if the masses are the same. The child who is still in the preoperational phase of cognitive thought, relying on his perceptions to make the judgment, will say that the pancake-shaped mass has more clay because it is wider or larger around. The child who is able to conserve will insist that the masses still contain the same amount of clay. To explain his observation that the mass has been unaltered, the child may use one of the following three concepts[5]:

1. The concept of *identity*—since nothing has been added and nothing has been taken away, the pancake is still the same clay with nothing changed but the shape.
2. The concept of *reversibility*—the clay can be reshaped into its original form, that of a ball.
3. The concept of *reciprocity*—although the pancake appears larger in circumference, the ball is much thicker. In this instance the child demonstrates that he can deal with two dimensions at the same time and comprehend that a change in one dimension compensates for a change in another.

When the child is able to use the concepts of identity, reversibility, and reciprocity, he can conserve along any physical dimension. He no longer perceives a tall, thin glass of water as containing more volume than an equal amount in a short, wide glass; he can distinguish between the weight of items regardless of their size. He recognizes that the size is not necessarily related to the weight or volume. He can solve concrete problems that he is able to manipulate or "see" in a concrete manner. He recognizes that logical operations move in two directions, such as addition and subtraction or multiplication and division. He learns that certain properties are invariant; for example, 7 remains 7 whether it is represented by 3 + 4, 2 + 5, seven buttons, seven stars, or seven boys.

Reversibility is used by the child in selecting a course of action, thus providing greater control over himself and his environment. He has the ability to think through an action sequence, anticipate the consequences, and, if needed, return to the beginning and rethink the action in a different direction. He no longer needs to experience an action before he can anticipate the results. Reversibility allows mental action to replace physical action and provides the child with the ability to disassemble and reassemble certain kinds of things in his thoughts.

Classification. Classification skills involve the ability to group objects according to the attributes that they share in common. The school-age child now has the ability to place things in a sensible and logical order, to group and sort, and, in doing so, to hold a concept in his mind while he makes decisions based on that concept. It is characteristic of middle childhood that children derive a great deal of enjoyment from classifying and ordering their environment. They become occupied with numerous and varied collections of objects, such as wrappers, stamps, shells, dolls, cars, stones, and anything that is classifiable. They even begin to order friends and relationships, such as first best friend, second best friend, and so on.

As the child matures he progresses from collecting simply for the sake of collecting and becomes more selective and discriminating. His classification systems become more complex and based on abstract ideas rather than on perception and experience. Much of the pleasure of collections is the appraising, ordering, and reordering of the parts.

School children are able to *serialize,* that is, to arrange objects according to some ordinal scale or quantified dimension such as size, weight, or color. They develop the ability to understand relational terms and concepts, such as bigger and smaller; darker and paler; heavier and lighter; to the right of and to the left of; first, last, and intermediate relationships (fourth, second, and so on); and more than and less than. They can see family relationships in terms of reciprocal roles, for example, in order to be a brother, one must have a sibling. It is common for a preschool child to refer to the adult female in a family as "your mother" even when discussing the relationship with the woman's husband.

Combination skills. It is during the school-age years that children develop the ability to manipulate numbers and to learn the skills of addition, subtraction, multiplication, and division. They learn to apply the basic operations to any object or quantities. They learn the alphabet and the ever-widening world of symbols called words that can be arranged in terms of structure and their relationship to the alphabet. They learn to tell time, to see the relationship of events in time (history) and places in space (geography), and to combine time and space relationships (geology and astronomy).

School-age children are able to entertain a hypothesis through use of conceptual principles and perceived events and to evaluate the evidence that might support or disprove the hypothesis. These capabilities allow them to expand beyond the limits of their own experience and to consider events that happened before, will happen in the future, and are hypothesized to be happening in the present.

The most significant skill, the ability to read, is acquired during the school years and becomes the most valuable tool for independent inquiry. The child's capacity for exploration, imagination, and expansion of knowledge is enhanced with the ability to read as he progresses from the repetition and confusion of early efforts to increasing facility and comprehension.

It is through no accident that the schools are prepared to meet the essentials of intellectual capabilities at the time that the child's cognitive processes are ready to assume appropriate intellectual achievements. The increase in capacity for logical thinking during this stage of concrete operations is based on the sensorimotor schemes of infancy and the representational abilities of the preschool child.

The child is now able to move into the formal operations that characterize the period of adolescence.

Developing sense of accomplishment

Successful mastery of Erikson's first three stages of psychosocial development is probably the most important for development of a healthy personality.[2] With a foundation of trust, autonomy, and initiative, the child is fairly certain to progress through subsequent stages with relative ease. Successful completion of these stages implies a confidence in the environment of loving relationships within a stable family unit that has prepared him to engage in experiences and relationships beyond this intimate group. It is suggested that the individual's fundamental attitude toward work is established during middle childhood. It is during this time that he receives the systematic instruction prescribed by his culture and develops the skills needed to become a useful, contributing member of his social community.

The stage of industry, for which a more descriptive term is the *stage of accomplishment,* is achieved somewhere between age 6 years and adolescence. It involves an eagerness for building skills and producing meaningful and socially useful work. Interests expand in the middle years, and the child wants to engage in tasks that can be carried through to completion with a growing sense of independence. There are many attributes of industry that contribute to the child's sense of competence and mastery. Intrinsic motivation is associated with increased competence in mastering new skills and assuming new responsibilities. Children gain a great deal of satisfaction from independent behavior in exploring and manipulating their environment and from interaction with peers. Extrinsic sources of reinforcement in the form of grades, material rewards, additional privileges, and recognition provide encouragement and stimulation. Often the acquisition of skills is a means for achieving success in special activities such as athletics or social organizations such as scouting. Peer approval is a strong motivating power.

A sense of accomplishment also involves the ability to cooperate and to compete with others—to cope more effectively with people. Middle childhood is the time when children learn the value of doing things alongside and with others and the benefits derived from division of labor in the accomplishment of goals.

The danger inherent in this period of personality development is the imposition of situations that might result in a sense of inadequacy or inferiority. This may happen if the previous stages have not been successfully achieved or if the child is incapable of or unprepared for assuming the responsibilities associated with developing a sense of accomplishment. Feelings of inferiority or lack of worth can be derived from the child himself or from the social environment. The child with physical or mental limitation is at a disadvantage for acquisition of certain skills and, when the reward structure is based on evidence of mastery, the child who is incapable of developing these skills is bound to feel inadequate and inferior. Even children without chronic disabilities represent such a wide range of individual differences in capabilities and preferences that they will experience feelings of inadequacy in some areas. No child is able to do well in everything, and children must learn that they will not be able to master each skill that they attempt. All children, even children who in most instances have positive attitudes toward work and their own capabilities, will feel some degree of inferiority in regard to a specific skill that they cannot master.

To some extent, success or aptitude in one area may compensate for failure or ineptitude in another. However, the differences in reinforcement provided for success in various areas have a very significant effect on feelings of adequacy. For example, in the United States reading proficiency is more highly rewarded than mechanical aptitude such as tinkering with broken automobile engines. A higher social value is placed on success in team sports than success in operating a ham radio. To compensate for the inability to excel in more socially valued skills through mastery of other less valued skills is difficult for the child. Also, as a corollary to this, the social environment places a negative value on any kind of failure that serves to further stimulate feelings of inferiority in the less capable child. Repeated failures often generate such strong feelings in the child that eventually he is reluctant to attempt any new task in order to avoid failure or he is fearful that he will not be able to perform as well as his peers. Thus intrinsic motivation toward engaging in a task for the pleasure of the challenge conflicts with the external forces that cause feelings of doubt and inferiority. Consequently he may no longer try.

Much depends on the child's concept of success or failure. Children who aspire for more than they are capable of will usually experience failure. In contrast, children who set their aspirations lower than their level of achievement will usually experience success. Most accomplishments during the school years are very public. Success or failure in school is known to family, teachers, peers, and others. In the social environment of school and sometimes at home, feelings of inferiority may be produced through comparison with others that suggests that the child is not as good as some peer, sibling, or another subcultural group. His inadequacy becomes a source of embarrassment. He may even be shamed for his failure. The earlier conflicts of doubt and guilt are very closely associated with feelings of inferiority.

Children need and want real achievement. When they have access to tasks that need to be done, that they are able to do well despite individual differences in their innate capacities and emotional development, and for which they are suitably rewarded, children will be able to achieve a sense of industry and accomplishment.

Moral development

As children move from egocentrism to the more logical patterns of thought, they also move through stages in development of conscience and moral standards. The beginning of this development is evident during the preschool years when children have, to some extent, adopted and internalized the moral values of their parents and their standards for evaluating the behavior of themselves and others. Adopting parental standards makes children feel similar to the parents, thereby strengthening their identification with the parents.

Growth in moral thought and judgment progresses between the ages of 6 and 12 years. Young children do not believe that standards of behavior come from within themselves but that rules are established and set down by others. At first, rules are definite, cover limited situations, and require no reason or explanation. Children learn the standards for acceptable behavior, act according to these standards, and feel guilty when they violate the standards. Although children of 6 or 7 years of age know the rules and what they are supposed to do, they do not understand the reasons behind them. Young children usually judge an act by its consequences. Rewards and punishment guide their judgment; a "bad act" is one that breaks a rule or does harm. When a child and an adult conflict in judging an act, the adult is right. Children may believe that what other people tell them to do is right and that what they think of themselves is wrong. Consequently children 6 or 7 years old are more likely to interpret accidents and misfortunes as punishment for misdeeds.

Older school-age children are able to judge an act by the intentions that prompted it rather than just the consequences. Whereas a younger child can judge an act only according to whether it is right or wrong, older children will take into account a different point of view to make a judgment. They are able to understand and accept the concept of doing as one would be done by. Rules and judgments become less absolute and authoritarian and are founded more on the needs and desires of others. Rules of conduct are more readily considered in terms of mutual agreement and based on cooperation and respect for others. For older children a rule violation is apt to be viewed in relation to the total context in which it appears; reactions are influenced by the situation as well as by the morality of the rule itself. However, it is not until adolescence or beyond that children are able to view morality on an abstract basis with sound reasoning and principled thinking.

Self-evaluation

Closely associated with developing a sense of industry is developing a concept of one's value and worth. With the emphasis on skill building and broadened social relationships, children are continually occupied in the process of self-evaluation. If they regard themselves as worthwhile or satisfactory persons, they are considered to have self-esteem, self-confidence, or a positive self-image. If they view themselves as worthless, they are said to have poor or low self-esteem.

In the process of self-evaluation, children actively strive to come up to internalized goals or levels of attainment that they hope to achieve. At the same time they continually receive feedback on the quality of their performance from those whom they consider to be authorities. By the time they reach school age, children have already received messages regarding the extent to which they are able to accomplish tasks that have been delegated to them. For example, one child may have been given prestigious responsibilities at home or at school or received special commendation for an achievement. On the other hand, another child may have been sent to a special class for slow learners or may have been the last person chosen when children choose up sides for a game. These and other signs serve as clues to social evaluation that the child then incorporates as part of his self-evaluation.

Children approach the process of self-evaluation from a framework of either self-confidence or self-doubt. Children, who during the preschool years have mastered the maturational crises of autonomy and initiative, are able to face the world with feelings of pride rather than shame. At first their self-concept is formed exclusively from what they perceive to be their parents' evaluation of them. During middle childhood the opinions of peers and teachers further complicate the process. The criticisms and peer approval are sources of data for evaluation. Now parents and other adults are not the only persons who respond to their skills, talents, and abilities. Peers, also, identify the skills and capabilities, and each child soon begins to internalize these outside opinions. Childrens' self-concept is composed of their own critical self-assessment plus what they interpret as the opinions of members of their family and outside social contacts.

The difficulty that children encounter in the attempt to assess their own abilities is their inclination to rely on their own expectations or those expectations expressed by others regarding their performance. They depend almost entirely on external evidence of worth, such as school grades, teachers' comments, and parental and peer approval. Children do not yet have the capacity to develop their own, independent criteria by which they can evaluate their own accomplishments, and it is especially difficult for them to assess their achievement in abstract skills.

Nothing succeeds like success. The significant adults in a child's life can often manage, unseen, to manipulate the child's environment so that he meets with success. Each small success increases the child's self-image a little. The more positive he feels about himself, the more confident he feels in trying again for success. All children profit from a feeling that they are in some way special to a significant adult. A positive self-concept makes them feel likable, worthwhile, and someone with a valuable contribution to make in their world. Such feelings lead to self-respect, self-confidence, and a general feeling of happiness.

Preadolescence

The preadolescent years, roughly ages 10 to 13 years, are years of transition. Soon the child will leave childhood behind forever and move on to adolescence. Preadolescence is childhood at its highest form of development. It is a healthy period of childhood — the period between childhood diseases and the diseases of adulthood. Preadolescence is, for some, a period of rapid growth, especially for girls; for others, mostly boys, it is a period of steady growth in height and weight.

There is no universal age at which children assume the characteristics of preadolescence. The first physiologic signs begin to appear at about 9 years of age (particularly in girls) and are usually clearly evident in 11- to 12-year-old children. Although the preadolescent child does not want to be different, at this age the variability in physical growth and physiologic changes between children of the same sex, between the two sexes, and even within each individual child is often striking. This variability, especially in relation to the onset of secondary sex characteristics, is of utmost concern to the preadolescent. Either early or late appearance is a source of embarrassment and uneasiness to both sexes.

Preadolescence is a time when there is a good deal of overlapping of developmental characteristics with elements of both middle childhood and early adolescence. However, there are a sufficient number of unique characteristics to set it apart as an age category, even with the wide range of variability in the ages 11 and 12 years (or even 9 to 13 years in some children). The earliest age at which puberty usually begins is 10 years in girls and 12 years in boys, although there has been an increase in the number of girls reaching puberty at 9 years of age. The average age of puberty in girls is 12 years, and for boys it is 14 years. Boys do little sexual maturation during preadolescence.

Preadolescence is a time of trial for parents and teachers as well as for the child. Most of the child's behavior seems to be directed toward ego strengthening and integration. He frequently challenges authority, and, although he is highly competent, he still lacks the maturity, information, and judgment he needs to be self-sufficient, effective, and resourceful.

SOCIETY OF CHILDREN

Children at the beginning of the middle years normally enter a period of less intense emotions, secure in their dependency on their parents and family, and with self-confidence tempered by a more realistic perspective. Their energy is now available to explore the environment beyond the family, for a gradual increase in the scope of interpersonal interactions, and to invest their curiosity in a greater understanding of the world.

One of the most important socializing agents in the life of the child is members of the peer group, with whom they explore ideas and the physical environment around them. Although it has neither the traditional authority of the parents nor the legal authority of the schools for teaching information, the peer group manages to convey a substantial amount of material to its members. Children's need for the friendship of their peers brings them into an increasingly complex social system. The world of the peer group is different from the adult world. Children have a culture all their own with secrets, mores, and codes of ethics with which they promote feelings of group solidarity and detachment from adults. Through peer relationships children learn ways in which to deal with dominance and hostility and to relate with persons in positions of leadership and authority.

During their life children are exposed to value systems such as those of the family, ethnic origin, and social class. In peer group interaction children are confronted with a variety of these sets of values. The values imposed by the peer group are especially compelling because a child must accept and conform to them in order to be accepted as a member of the group. When the peer values are not too different from those of family and teachers, the mild conflict created by these small differences serves to separate children from the adults in their lives and to strengthen the feeling of belonging to the peer group. Identification with peers appears to be a strong influence in the child's gaining independence from parents. The aid and support of the group provides the child with enough security to risk the moderate parental rejection brought about by each small victory in his development of independence.

Questions of masculinity and femininity take on importance as sex-role learning assumes more prominence. Boys associate with boys and girls with girls, each pursuing their own interests with communication between the sexes confined to that which is necessary. Much of the child's concept of the appropriate sex role is acquired through relationships with peers. During the early school years there is little difference relative to sex in play experiences of children. Games and many other activities are shared by both girls and boys. However, in the later school years the differences become marked. Boys and girls grow more intolerant of each other, especially on the surface.

Social relationships and cooperation

Daily relationships with age-mates provide the most important social interactions in the life of school-age children. For the first time children are able to join in group activities with unrestrained enthusiasm and steady participation, when, formerly, interactions had been limited to short periods under considerable adult supervision. With increased skills and wider opportunities, children are able to become involved with one or several peer groups in which they can gain status as respected members.

There are valuable lessons to be learned from daily interaction with age-mates. First children learn to appreciate the numerous and varied points of view that are represented in the peer group. As they play together, children discover that there are numerous occupations for fathers and/or mothers, perhaps more than one version of the same song, different rules for the same game, and different customs for celebrating the same holiday. As the child interacts with peers who see the world somewhat differently than he does, he becomes aware of the limits of his own point of view. Because they are peers and are not forced to accept each other's ideas as they are expected to accept those of adults, other children have a significant influence on decreasing the egocentric outlook of the child. Consequently they learn to argue, persuade, bargain, cooperate, and compromise in order to maintain friendships.

Second the child becomes increasingly sensitive to the social norms and pressures of the peer group. The peer group establishes standards for acceptance and rejection, and the child may be willing to modify his behavior in order to be accepted by the group. Children are judged by the physical impression they convey, the skills they can perform, and other abilities they can demonstrate. The need for peer approval becomes a powerful influence toward conformity. The child learns to dress, talk, and otherwise behave in a manner acceptable to the group. A variety of roles, such as class joker or class hero, may be assumed by individual children in order to gain approval from the group. However, no child will be able to adapt perfectly to all the requirements made by the peer group. If the child finds that discrepancies between the values of the peer group and the values of his family are too great, he may be forced to relinquish the pleasure of interaction with the group in order to abide by the regulations established in the home. Thus, to diminish conflict within the family, the child may be forced into a position outside the peer group.

Third the interaction among peers leads to the formation of intimate friendship between two same sex peers. School-age is the time when children have "best friends" with whom they share secrets, private jokes, and adventures and come to one another's aid in times of trouble. In the course of these friendships the children also fight, threaten, break up, and reunite. These dyadic relationships, in which the child experiences love and closeness for a peer, seem to be important as a foundation for heterosexual relationships in adulthood. The conflicts encountered in the relationship are usually resolved in terms that the children are able to control. Since neither child has authority over the other, as in an adult-child relationship, the children must work through their differences within the framework of their commitment to one another.

Gangs. One of the outstanding characteristics of middle childhood is the formation of formalized groups, or gangs. Initially the child in the early middle years merely hangs around the periphery of the formalized group watching, learning, practicing various skills, and participating in the group activities whenever the members of the gang allow him to do so. In a year or two, as he advances in age, the child eventually takes his place as a full-fledged participating member. The process is facilitated if he has a buddy.

One of the prominent features of the gangs of middle childhood is the rigid rules they impose on the members. There is an exclusiveness in the selection of persons who have the privilege of joining. Acceptance in the group is often determined on a pass-fail basis that is based on social or behavioral criteria. Conformity is the core of the gang structure. There are often secret codes, shared interests, and special modes of dress, and each child must abide by a standard of behavior established by the group. An understanding of and conformity to the rules provide the child with a feeling of security and relieve him of the responsibility of making decisions. Membership in the gang provides the child with a comfortable place in society. Many of the values of the gang, such as physical strength, daring, ingenuity, and comradeship, have not been stressed in the family group, but these, too, are worthy values and contribute to the child's total personality. By merging his identity with that of his peers, the child is able to move from the family group to an outside group as a step toward seeking further independence. He substitutes conformity to a peer-group pattern for conformity to a family pattern while he is still too shaky and insecure to function independently.

During the early school years gangs are rather small, loosely organized groups with changing membership, little formal structure, and without the more prolonged cohesiveness characteristic of gangs in later school years. They do not demonstrate the elements of give-and-take, cooperation, and order that are seen in groups of older children. As a rule, girls' groups are less formalized than boys' gangs, and, although there may be a mixture of both sexes in the earlier school years, the gangs of later school years are composed predominantly of same sex groups. Common interests are a frequent basis around which a gang is structured.

Children's strong desire not to be different creates problems for children who are for various reasons unable to meet the acceptable standards of the peer group. Handicapped children or those who are in some way so deprived that they are unable to compete have a difficult time. Self-consciousness results when a child is unable to dress as the other children dress, does not have spending money like other children, or appears different from the other children, such as the child with numerous freckles, red hair, or such minor physical defects as strabismus. Any of these differences sets them apart from the group and often makes the child a target for the criticism and ridicule of the peer group.

Although peer group identification and association are essential to the child's emergence into the world, there can be dangers inherent in the strong peer-group attachment. Peer pressures may force the child into taking risks, even against his better judgment. Minor infractions and immoralities, such as stealing apples from the neighbor's tree, smoking, or sexual exposure, are disturbing to adults but seem to be a normal part of gang activity. However, acts of violence or destruction and foolhardy risks to safety are sometimes the outgrowth of overzealous gang cohesiveness.[7]

Relationships with parents

Although the peer group is highly influential and necessary to normal child development, the parents are still the primary influence in shaping the child's personality, setting standards for behavior, and establishing a value system. It is the family values that usually predominate when parental and peer value systems are in conflict. Although the child may appear to reject parental values while testing the new values of the peer group, ultimately he will retain and incorporate into his own value system the parental values he has found to be of worth. Peer associations seem to remain within the social class systems, and, not infrequently, there may be discriminate membership based on the ethnic or racial origin of the family.

As children move into the wider world of peer-group relationships, parents are faced with the task of relinquishing their hold on the child. They may find it difficult to face the rejection that is demonstrated as the child stands solidly with the peer group. The child will want to spend more time in the company of his peers and may seem anxious to leave the house; he will often prefer activities of the gang to family activities. This can be very disturbing to parents. During this time parents can best serve the interests of the child through tolerant understanding and support. The child becomes intolerant and critical of the parents and their ways when they deviate from those of the gang. In the eyes of the child the parents no longer assume the stature they previously enjoyed. Children discover that parents can be wrong, and they begin to question the knowledge and authority of the parents who previously they considered to be all-knowing and all-powerful.

Although increased independence is the goal of middle childhood, children are not yet prepared to abandon parental control. Children need and want restrictions placed on their behavior; they are not yet prepared to cope with all the problems of their expanding environment. They feel more secure knowing that there is an authority greater than themselves to implement such controls and restrictions. Children may complain loudly about the restrictions and try their best to break down parental barriers, but they are uneasy if they can succeed in doing so. Children feel secure with reasonable, consistent controls. They respect the adults on whom they can rely to prevent them from acting on each and every urge. Children sense in this behavior an expression of love and concern for their welfare.

Children also need their parents as adults, not as pals. Sometimes parents, hurt at their children's rejection, attempt to maintain their love and gratitude by assuming the role of ''pals.'' Children need the stable, secure strength provided by mature adults to whom they can turn during troubled relationships with peers or stressful changes in their world. During a disruption in their lives, such as times of failure, periods of illness, or a move that separates them from the security of friends, children need the firm, secure anchor of parental interest and concern. With a secure base in a loving family, children are able to develop the confidence in themselves and the maturity needed to break loose from the gang and stand independently.

School experience

The schools serve as agents for transmitting the values of the society to each succeeding generation of children and as the setting for much of their relationship with peers. As a socializing agent second only to the family, schools exert a profound influence on the social development of children. Until school entrance at approximately 5 or 6 years, the primary sphere of influence of the child is the family, in which his interactions are with parents and siblings. Neighborhood children provide broader relationships, but parents serve as the only continuous adult contact, those with whom he is most intimately involved and who set the pattern of his daily life. School entrance marks a sharp change in the child's experiences with others. His world at once becomes more complex, requiring adjustments to a new set of interpersonal contacts and authority figures. In addition he is separated from the parents and siblings for a substantial portion of the day.

School entrance constitutes a sharp break in the structure of the child's world. For many children it is their first experience in conforming to a group pattern imposed by an adult who is not a parent and one who has responsibility for too many children to be constantly aware of each child as an individual. Children want to go to school and usually adapt to the new conditions with little difficulty. Successful adjustment is directly related to the physical and emotional maturity of the child and the mother's readiness to accept the separation associated with school entrance. Unfortunately some mothers express their unconscious attempts to delay the child's maturity by clinging behavior, particularly with their youngest child. However, the transition from home to school is usually accomplished with little disturbance. To facilitate the process, educators select teachers, usually women, with personality characteristics that allow them to deal with potential problems of young children. Children react to the teacher on the basis of past experiences; therefore, they respond best to teachers with attributes that they would desire in a warm, loving parent. As a mother surrogate the teacher in the early grades performs many of the activities formerly assumed by the mother, such as recognizing the children's personal needs (such as a need to go to the bathroom or help with clothing) and helping to develop their social behavior (for example, manners).

Teachers, just as the parents, are concerned about the psychologic and emotional welfare of the child. Although teachers' and parents' functions differ, both place constrains on behavior and both are in a position to enforce standards of conduct. However, the teacher's primary responsibility is stimulating and guiding the child's intellectual development but not the child's physical welfare beyond the school setting. The teacher shares the parental influence in determining the child's attitudes and values. Teachers serve as models with whom children identify and whom they try to emulate. Teacher approval is sought; teacher disapproval is avoided. The teacher is a very significant person in the life of the early school child, and hero worship of a teacher may extend into late childhood and preadolescence. It is not uncommon for the first or second grader to be heartbroken and tearful at leaving a familiar teacher at the end of the school term or to be upset when faced with a substitute teacher for even a short period.

Children's interest in school and learning and much of their social interaction and self-concept are related to interactions with the teacher. The interaction between the teacher and individual pupils affects the pupil's acceptance by the other children, which in turn affects his self-concept. Behaviors praised by the teacher usually acquire a positive value, whereas those viewed negatively by the teacher are similarly devalued by the children. In this way the teacher exerts a good deal of influence in a number of areas. Teacher approval of and self-acceptance in the child are very closely related.

The teacher sets the emotional tone of the classroom. Teachers who are able to establish a positive social climate in the environment are concerned about the mental health and social dynamics of the children. Feeling a responsibility for the personality development of the pupils, they are alert and sensitive to the children's anxieties, peer-group relationships, self-concepts, and general attitudes toward school. Learner-centered behaviors, such as supportive statements that reassure or commend the child, accepting and clarifying statements that help him refine ideas and feelings to provide a sense of being understood, and constructive assistance that assists the child with his own problem solving, all contribute to the child's expansion and development of a positive self-concept.

Play

As children enter the school years, their play takes on new dimensions that reflect this new stage of development. Not only does it involve increased physical skill, intellectual skill, and fantasy, but, as they form gangs and cliques, children begin to evolve a sense of team or club. To belong to a group is of vital importance. Each individual child must abide by the rules of the group, which may be extremely rigid, and they now devote their energy to team success as well as personal success.

Rules and ritual. The need for conformity in middle childhood is strongly manifest in the activities and games that are so important in the life of school-age children. Previously children have either played games they have invented themselves or have played in the company of a friend or an adult when rules more or less evolved with the game. Now children begin to see the need for rules, and the games they play have fixed and unvarying rules that may be bizarre and extraordinarily rigid (especially those made up by the group). But part of the enjoyment of the game is to know the rules, because knowing means belonging. Once the rules are established and agreed on, the demand for conformity is vigorous. A child who does not conform to the rules is excluded because individuality is not tolerated by the group. Clubs and secret societies become part of the culture of childhood.

Conformity and ritual permeate the play of school-age children. Not only are they present in games, but they are also evident in much of the children's ritualistic behavior and language. Childhood is full of chants and taunts such as ''Eeny, meeny, miney, mo,'' ''Johnny's mad and I'm glad,'' ''Last one is a rotten egg,'' and ''Step on a crack, break your mother's back.'' Children derive a great deal of pleasure from such sayings that have been handed down with few changes through generation after generation of children. Sometimes the children elaborate on them with particular variations to meet the special attributes of their group. The undeviating ritual frequently is invested with some magical quality that serves to give the children a sense of power over the unconquerable world about them.

Team play. A more complex form of group play that evolves from the group games is team games and sports that are part of the life of the early school years. The rules of the game may even require the presence of a referee, umpire, or person of authority, in order that the rules can be followed more accurately. Team membership has three significant characteristics that are relevant to child development during the middle years.[5] First children learn to subordinate personal goals to group goals. Team membership means that each child is accountable to the other team members and carries with it the responsibility that each member's acts may affect the success or failure of the entire group. Members' behavior is open to public evaluation, and a child risks ostracism or ridicule if he contributes to a team loss. Team accomplishments reflect on all the players. Although individual skills are recognized, team successes and failures are shared by all members—the best and the poorest alike. In this way children learn the concept of interdependence, that all players must rely on one another. Unfortunately all too often instead of the better members helping the weaker members to improve, the poorer members are scorned and scapegoated, especially when the team loses.

Second children learn about division of labor as an effective strategy for the attainment of a goal. They learn that each position on a team has a specific function and that the team has a greater chance of winning if each person performs his own function instead of the work of all the other members. As children learn this concept in team play, they can transfer this knowledge to other aspects of life. Once they learn that certain goals are best accomplished by dividing tasks among several individuals, they begin to see the relationship to principles of organization of other social structures. A corollary to this is the concept that some children are best equipped to perform one part of the task, whereas other children are best suited to another aspect of the task.

Third team play helps children to learn about the nature of competition and the importance of winning—an attribute highly valued in the United States. In all team play there is a winning and losing side. Since losing is often interpreted as failure, children will go to great lengths to avoid the public embarrassment and personal shame that accompany failure. The more a child identifies himself with the team and values his membership in the team, the more distasteful losing becomes. Fear of losing and the failure it implies are strong incentives for group commitment. The importance of winning is not universally valued, however. Some cultures and subcultures place emphasis on the game and consideration for one's companions rather than on the outcome.

Team play can also contribute to children's social, intellectual, and skill growth. A child will work hard to develop the skills needed to become a member of a team, to improve his contribution to the group effort, and to anticipate the consequences of his behavior for the group. Team play helps stimulate cognitive growth as children are called on to learn many complex rules, make judgments about those rules, plan strategies, and assess the strengths and weaknesses of members of their own and the opposing team.

Quiet games and activities. Although the play of school-age children is highly active, these children also enjoy many quiet and solitary activities. The middle years are the time for collections, which constitute another ritual. The early school-age child's collections are an odd assortment of unrelated objects in messy, disorganized piles. Collections of later years are more orderly, selective, and organized neatly in scrapbooks, on shelves, or in boxes.

School-age children become fascinated with increasingly complex board or card games, such as Monopoly and rummy, that they can play with a best friend or a group. As in all games, their adherence to rules is fanatic. There is usually much discussion and argument, but the disagreement is easily resolved through reading the appropriate rule of the game.

The newly acquired skill of reading becomes increasingly satisfying as school-age children are able to expand their knowledge of the world through books. Children never tire of stories and, just as preschool children, they love to have stories read aloud. Other skills such as sewing, cooking, carpentry, gardening, or creative activities such as painting are all activities that these children enjoy. Many of these creative skills as well as athletic skills such as swimming, riding, hiking, dancing, and skating that are learned and delighted in during childhood are activities that are continued to be enjoyed into adolescence and adulthood.

Ego mastery. Play also affords children the means to acquire representational mastery over themselves, their environment, and others. Through play they can feel as big, powerful, and skillful as their imaginations will allow and they can attain vicarious mastery and power over whomever and whatever they choose. They need to feel in control in their play. School children still need the opportunity to use large muscles in exuberant outdoor play and freedom to exert their newfound autonomy and initiative. They need space in which to exercise large muscles and to work off tensions, frustrations, and hostility. Physical skills practiced and mastered in play help them develop a feeling of personal competence that contributes to a sense of accomplishment and helps provide a place of status in the peer group.

HEALTH PROMOTION DURING MIDDLE CHILDHOOD

Health supervision of children, begun in early childhood, is continued in middle childhood and includes the periodic ongoing health assessment and guidance advised for children 6 to 12 years of age. Since regular health checkups and prophylactic measures such as immunizations are a routine function of health supervision, this need not be reiterated. The regular, routine health supervision that was begun in infancy is continued throughout childhood. The frequency of checkups is usually reduced to yearly assessment of growth progress and screening for vision, hearing, posture, and general health status.

When school-age children enter school they leave the relatively protected environment of home and neighborhood and encounter broader interpersonal contacts with a larger number of children. Although the incidence of childhood disease has declined significantly in recent times, some diseases are not as yet controlled. Many can be prevented by careful health supervision. For example, most of the communicable diseases, formerly a cause of high morbidity in school children, can be prevented by immunization (see p. 456). The body's natural defenses against illness can be supported through careful attention to diet, rest, exercise, and protection from extreme mental and physical stress.

It is not uncommon for school-age children to complain of assorted physical symptoms that are particularly apparent at age 9 years and during preadolescence. The more common somatic complaints are headaches, dizziness, or sudden, unexpected pains in various part of the body, most often localized in the head or stomach but occasionally in the leg. Sometimes the discomfort can be directly related to an unpleasant situation at school or a distasteful task at home (see school phobia, p. 648), and often the desire for play overpowers the demands of the symptoms. In the preadolescent period a child may suffer periods of extreme fatigue when he is so "out of sorts" that he hates everything and everybody. At this time he may benefit from a day home from school in which to rest and recoup his resources. When school officials are aware of this need, they are ready to cooperate and allow absence when it is desirable. Children of this age do not like to miss school and usually will not take undo advantage of the situation.

Sleep and rest

The amount of sleep and rest that is required during middle childhood is a highly individual matter and unique to every child. There is no specified amount needed by a child at any given age. The amount depends, rather, on the child's age, the activity level, and other factors such as his state of health. The growth rate has slowed; therefore, less energy is expended in growth than during the preceding periods and than will be required during the adolescent growth spurt.

During the school years children usually do not require a nap, but they sleep an average of 11 to 12 hours nightly at age 6 years to 9 or 10 hours a night at 11 or 12 years of age (see p. 66). Although there are fewer bedtime problems with advancing years, there are still occasional difficulties associated with this necessary ritual. Usually there is little problem for children 6 and 7 years old, and the task of going to bed can be facilitated by encouraging quiet activity before bedtime, such as coloring and reading. For many children, bedtime is improved considerably by allowing them a small radio to which they can listen for a specified length of time.

Although most children in middle childhood must be reminded frequently to go to bed, 8- to 9-year-old and 11-year-old children are particularly resistant. Often the child is unaware that he is tired, and, if allowed to remain up later than usual, he is fatigued the following day. Sometimes the bedtime resistance can be resolved by allowing a later bedtime in deference to his advancing ages. However, it should be made clear that this privilege is dependent on compliance—going to bed without stalling and without complaints. A firm approach to bedtime is usually the most successful. Parents can help the child by giving him a little advance warning, but he should realize that when the final bedtime is announced they really mean it.

Twelve-year-old children usually offer no difficulty in relation to bedtime. Some even retire early in order to enjoy slow preparations for bed, to read, or to listen to their radio.

The cause of bedtime resistance is not always clear. For some children it is related to the normal fears of their age, such as fear of the dark, strange noises, intruders, or other imagined phenomena. Children who are subject to frightening dreams are hesitant to retire, and their sleep is more apt to be disturbed following emotional stimulation prior to bedtime. Sometimes children are loathe to give up some exciting or interesting activity in which they are involved or they are reluctant to leave the protective social circle of the family. Another factor associated with time for retirement is related to status. For example, older children are ascribed the privilege of a later bedtime than younger children. Promotion to a later bedtime is highly prestigious, and age-mates compare their bedtimes. This may explain why parental decisions are often hotly contested by a child who believes that playmates enjoy a more privileged position in this area. In some situations going to bed is used as a method of control. Where going to bed early is imposed as a punishment or staying up a little longer is a reward, the child may view bedtime as punitive or status degrading.

Nutrition

Although calorie needs are diminished in relation to body size during middle childhood, resources are being laid down for the increased growth needs of the adolescent period. It is important to impress on children and their parents the value of a diet balanced to promote growth (see Appendix D for recommended daily allowances). Influenced by the mass media and the temptation of an immense variety of "junk food," it is all too easy for children to fill up on empty calories—foods that do not promote growth, such as sugars, starches, and excess fats. They have more freedom to move without parental supervision and often have small amounts of money to spend on candy, soft drinks, and other easily accessible treats. Midafternoon snacks are common, and it is wise to encourage fruit, nuts, and other wholesome finger foods to meet this need.

Mealtime continues to be a central issue in most families. Although it should be a pleasant part of the child's day, parents' concern and emphasis on manners often make it a battleground. Likes and dislikes established at an early age continue in middle childhood, although the propensity for single food preferences is ending and children acquire a taste for an increasing variety of foods. Since the child usually eats as the family does, the quality of his diet depends to a large extent on the family's pattern of eating. Other interests and participation in outside activities often compete with mealtime. A working mother, assuming the child to be sufficiently mature, frequently leaves the responsibility for preparation of meals to him. Although most older school-age children are capable of preparing simple fare, all too often breakfast and/or lunch may be inadequate, makeshift, or nonexistent. In recognition of this problem the federal government has established the National School Lunch Program (NSLP) and, more recently, the School Breakfast Program (SBP) in many areas. These meals must meet specified nutritional requirements and furnish one third of the daily recommended dietary allowance for children in the United States. Most schools subscribe to the programs, and, although it is difficult to measure directly, it is believed that these school feeding programs positively influence the behavior and learning capacity of children.

The threat of childhood obesity is an increasingly prevalent health problem in school-age children in the United States. The easy availability of high-calorie foods combined with the tendency toward more sedentary activities such as television and the trend away from walking or cycling and toward transportation by automobile and bus have reduced the caloric expenditure. The problem of childhood obesity is discussed further in Chapter 21.

Nutrition is a joint responsibility of both the child and his family. Nutrition education can and should be integrated throughout the child's school years as part of classroom learning. In school the basic food groups and the elements of a wholesome diet are learned, as well as how food products are grown, processed, and prepared. School projects often include growing vegetables in the classroom or at home, and science projects in the more advanced grades might include some simple animal experiments. The school nurse can take an active role in nutrition education by working with teachers to plan and implement units of nutrition instruction and with parents and children to give nutritional guidance.

Exercise and activity

Exercise is essential for developmental progress in a number of areas such as the following: muscle development and tone, refinement of balance and coordination, gaining strength and endurance, and stimulating body functions and metabolic processes. Children need ample space in which to run, jump, skip, and climb and safe facilities and equipment to use both inside and outside. Most children need little encouragement to engage in physical activity. They have so much energy that they seldom know when to stop.

Children with handicapping conditions or those who hesitate to become involved in active play, such as obese children, require special assessment and help so that activities that will appeal to them, are compatible with their limitations, and, at the same time, meet their developmental needs, can be determined.

Dental health

Since it is during the school-age years that the permanent teeth erupt, good dental hygiene and regular attention to dental caries are a vital part of health supervision during this period (see p. 650). Correct brushing techniques should be taught or reinforced, and the role that fermentable carbohydrates play in production of dental caries should be emphasized. It is also important to be alert to possible malocclusion problems that may result from irregular eruption of permanent teeth and may impair function. Regular dental supervision is as essential as medical supervision and should be an integral part of the overall health maintenance program.

Sex education

Evidence indicates that many children experience some form of sex play during or prior to preadolescence as a response to normal curiosity, not from love or sexual urge. Children are experimentalists by nature, and this play is incidental and transitory. Any adverse emotional consequences or guilt feelings depend on how this behavior is managed by the parents, if discovered, or whether the child views his actions as wrong in the eyes of significant persons, particularly the parents.

Much of the child's attitude toward sex that is acquired indirectly at a very early age affects the way in which he responds to sexual information presented at a later time. With few exceptions, parents discourage sex exploration either through subtle substitution of activities that divert the child's attention from the genitalia or by expressions of anger or disgust at his behavior. These tactics set limits on his curiosity and ability to learn. In addition parents seldom teach the young child the correct terminology for sexual organs or sexual feeling; therefore, the only vocabulary available to him is the one that identifies sexual organs with excretory functions. Thus these parental attitudes influence the child's perception of the cleanliness of his genitalia in relation to their actual function.

Because parents either repress or avoid the child's sexual curiosity, the sexual information that he receives in childhood is acquired almost entirely from his peers. When peers are the primary source of sexual information, it is transmitted and exchanged in secret, clandestine conversation and contains a large amount of misinformation. The context in which these communications take place creates anxiety in the child and barriers to trust; therefore, he continues to keep sexuality a secret. These reactions inhibit spontaneous expressions to or questioning of the parents.[4]

The subject of where sex education should be taught and by whom arouses a good deal of controversy throughout the country. Many individuals and groups are unconditionally opposed to the inclusion of sex education in the schools. Others believe that sex information should not be taught separately from other information but should be presented as naturally as information about other body functions and natural phenomena such as the solar system, the changing seasons, and the migratory habits of birds. Children's questions about sex should be answered to the same extent as their questions about any other topic—honestly and at their level of understanding. During the preschool years the child will be satisfied with simple answers, but as he gains more knowledge and understanding of the world his curiosity about everything will be deeper. When sex is treated as though it is a normal part of growth and development and questions are answered matter-of-factly, parental responses are less apt to contain overtones of guilt and anxiety that in turn produce anxiety in the child.[8]

Middle childhood appears to be an ideal time for formal sex education, and many authorities believe that the topic is best presented from a life-span approach. Initial curiosity about differences in body structure between boys and girls and between children and adults has been explored in the preschool years, and the next stage, adolescence, will arouse both anxiety and excitement about sexual encounters. Information about sexual maturation and the process of reproduction presented during middle childhood helps to minimize the child's uncertainty, embarrassment, and feelings of isolation that often accompany the events of puberty.

Although sex education programs are not universally a part of the elementary school curriculum, some progressive educators have successfully incorporated sex education into a number of schools. Because of the natural social orientation of this period of development, structured group learning situations can be successfully utilized for discussion of sexuality. An ideal approach that has been advanced suggests that sexuality can best be presented in the context of its central role as a biologic mechanism for the survival of the culture. This allows children to approach the topic at a distance with sexual maturation and reproduction as each individual's contribution to the natural order of things. It then provides a natural entry into discussion of sexuality as a basis for family units, marriage, and attitudes toward children as well as into a presentation of the biologic facts of sexuality. More difficult, but equally important, is for children to view sexual intimacy as a close, personal relationship and a means of conveying love as well as a means for assuring the survival of the species.[5]

Nurse's role in sex education. No matter where nurses practice, they can provide information on human sexuality to both parents and children. Nurses can help parents by first becoming knowledgeable about human sexuality themselves, including the common myths and misconceptions associated with sex and the reproductive process. They need to know their own attitudes and feelings toward sexuality and to feel comfortable with these feelings.[4]

During encounters with parents, nurses can be open and available for questions and discussion. They can set an example by the language they use in discussing body parts and their function and by the way in which they deal with problems that have emotional overtones, such as exploratory sex play and masturbation. Parents need to be helped to understand normal behaviors and to view sexual curiosity in their children as a part of the developmental process. Assessing the parents' level of knowledge and understanding of sexuality provides cues to their need for supplemental information that will better prepare them for the increasingly complex explanations that will be needed as their children grow older. Sometimes short classes or group discussions for parents are helpful for discussing disturbing behaviors and anticipating the questions and forthcoming learning needs of the children. When possible it is wise to include both parents. Sex education in the home should be assumed by both parents so that the children will not acquire a distorted view of either the male or the female role that may alter relationships with the opposite sex in later life.

Most important of all, nurses should take an active role in encouraging, developing, and providing sex education to children at all levels as an integral part of their total education.

School health programs

Child health maintenance is ultimately the responsibility of the parents; however, the public schools and health departments in the United States have contributed to the improvement of child health by providing a healthful school environment, health services, and health education that emphasize sound health practices. Most of these constitute a major component of community health services that involves a large amount of public funds and a large number of health professionals, including nurses, on either a full- or a part-time basis. School health programs contribute to the goals of the community for the education and development of the children.

Healthful school living. A safe and healthful school environment is the first essential element of any school health program. Conditions within the school setting should make a positive contribution to the physical, mental, and social development of the children. Factors that contribute to healthful school living include the following[1]:

1. A clean, safe, and wholesome school and classroom environment. This includes a physical facility that conforms to minimum standards for safety and sanitation and that provides suitable lighting, seating, heating, ventilation, furniture, and equipment.
2. A health program that is concerned about the physical and mental health of teachers and other staff members involved in the school operation.
3. A schedule of activities that is suited to the capabilities and maturational level of each child.
4. A regular physical education program.
5. A planned food service program that provides both meal services and an example of good nutrition practices.

School health services. A school health program is also involved in ongoing health maintenance through assessment, screening, and referral activities. Routine health services provided by most schools include the following:

1. Health appraisal. Health status is determined through the modalities of observation, screening tests (vision, hearing), measurements (height, weight), and medical, dental, and psychologic examinations.
2. Emergency care and safety. Care is provided in case of accident or sudden illness, emergency treatment (first aid), notification of parents, and transportation of the ill or injured child to home or hospital.
3. Communicable disease control. Recommended immunization schedule, detection and exclusion of affected children, and policies for readmission and attendance at school are emphasized. Many state and local laws require immunizations against the common communicable diseases before the child is allowed to enter school.
4. Counseling and follow-up. Health guidance, referral, and follow-up are provided to parents and children with special health needs.
5. Adjustment is made to individual student needs.

Health education. Health education of school children is primarily directed toward providing knowledge of health and influencing habits, attitudes, and conduct in relation to health and accident prevention. Health education can be provided by means of:

1. Direct instruction. This includes regular classroom instruction that involves the teacher, a group of students, a definite time and place, and a planned sequence of learning activities.
2. Integration of health information into other school subjects. Opportunities to relate health aspects to subjects such as home economics, social studies, and biologic sciences should be taken advantage of.
3. Special activities in the school program. This may include the lunch program, assembly programs, special films, and lectures.
4. Individual health guidance. The opportunity for this may present itself at any time and under a variety of circumstances.

The variety of topics for health instruction is endless, and eager minds are ready and willing to learn.

School nursing services.[6] School nurses are in a position to assume a major role in the school health program. Working in collaboration with others in the school and community, their service consists of three interrelated aspects of child health care: health supervision, health counseling, and health education. These functions are not necessarily limited to the confines of the school environment but also extend into the community in which the students live. As a health practitioner, the school nurse is in a position to promote and evaluate health services throughout the community as they affect the children.

Traditionally school nurses have been viewed from a limited perspective that placed them in the role of disease detector, applier of Band-Aids, and official care giver in cases of illness and injury. Although these are still important functions and their importance is not to be minimized, this traditional role is acquiring much broader dimensions. School nurses are being prepared to provide primary health care on a broader scale that includes assessment of physical, psychomedical, psychoeducational, behavioral, and learning disorder problems and to provide comprehensive well-child care. The school nurse practitioner is also concerned with development, implementation, and evaluation of health care plans and programs.

The preparation, qualifications, and utilization of school nurses and school nurse practitioners vary throughout the United States. Some communities consider the school nurse an essential member of the school organization with a full-time school commitment; in other communities school health practice is merely a part of the total community health program assumed by the health department. The relative merits of the two types of services are a matter of controversy.

AGE PROFILES OF MIDDLE CHILDHOOD

The preceding stages of child development increasingly demonstrate the individuality in the patterns of development. As children grow and mature, these differences become more pronounced. Although the rate generally slows, development continues to be uneven with periods of acceleration in some areas followed by a leveling off period. At the same time, other areas progress normally. In addition each child has a unique developmental pattern; therefore, any attempt to describe the typical child of any age-group can only represent an average and should not be considered as absolute criteria for any given child.

6 years

General characteristics

Is full of surprises
Is egocentric; center of his world
Wants to be best or first
Is eager to begin a project but has difficulty in completing it
Has prodigious appetite for new experiences
Is easily distracted by environment
Is expansive; ready for anything
Is eager to try anything new
Meets new situations head-on
Has rapid mood swings
Is quarrelsome, argumentative
When all goes well, is delightful; when things go badly, resorts to tears and tantrums
Finds that backyard can no longer contain him; needs room
Dawdles much of the time

Motor behavior

Has boundless energy
Is excited by speed and motion

Runs, jumps, climbs, hops, skips
Is unable to sit still for any length of time; wriggles in chair, sits on the edge, bangs and thumps; may fall off chair
Is clumsy and awkward
Has much oral activity, that is, blowing, extending tongue, various mouthing noises
Can use scissors
Enjoys fine motor activity but becomes restless after a short time; has imprecise small-muscle coordination—a frequent cause of frustration

Personal care

Can dress and undress but may need help with dressing
Usually requires, but resists, help with bathing
Needs reminding to wash before meals
Plays exuberantly in bathtub but needs help to get clean
Leaves clothes wherever they are removed
Takes responsibility for toileting, but may have to dash; accidents are rare, but disturbing, and are usually related to overexcitement

Social behavior and manners

Experiences rapid expansion of social environment
Centers life around school
Has unpredictable behaviors—is agreeable, loving, and cooperative one minute; dislikes everything and everybody the next
Wants help but refuses to accept it
Is unaware of ethnic identity of playmates
Is demanding of others; rigid in his demands
Must have things his way; he cannot adapt—others are expected to do adapting
Does not yet know how to speak or act properly; often forgets to say "Please" or "Thank you"
Is ritualistic about food preferences
Has frequent "accidents" at mealtime: spilled milk, food on clothes
Usually has "eyes that are bigger than his stomach"

Relationships with family

Experiences sibling jealousy
Enjoys hearing about when he was a baby
Has worst relationship so far with mother; loves her one minute and hates her the next, with little provocation
Blames mother for all that goes wrong
At times is very close with parents

Relationships with peers

Rarely appears in public singly; when 6-year-old children appear, they soon move together
No longer waits for others to come to him but goes where he can find the company of others
Is found in groups that are loosely organized and flexible; there is much coming and going
Each child within group goes his own way; there is little visible cooperation
Is anxious to be with peers; fears he will lose his place in group if not there physically
Has simple group rules, for example, must not cry when hurt; must act, look, and talk like the others

Play activities

Likes rough-and-tumble play
Values wind, speed, and coordination
Loves active games
Insists on a bicycle
Is not ready for competitive sports, especially those that demand coordination; must learn to work with others before he can work against them; best suited are those with simple rules, for example, relay races
Likes group games (for example, London Bridge, tag, hide and seek) that do not demand special skills
Delights in tricks and stunts
Likes table games, for example, checkers, simple card games
Paints, colors, draws
Uses clay
Collects odds and ends
Enjoys stories, including at bedtime

Mental activity and school

Knows right from left and morning from afternoon
Can describe objects in a picture, not simply enumerate them; defines objects in terms of their use
Has not firmly established concept of "cause and effect"
Can see differences more easily than similarities
Has difficulty in making decisions
Memory: can repeat sentences of ten or twelve words; repeats four digits in order
Knows number combinations up to 10
Is in first grade
Is easily distracted at school
Loves "show and tell"
Recognizes simple words and phrases and "sounds out" words to pronounce them
Draws a man, including neck, hands, and clothes
Has somewhat clumsy pencil manipulation
Prints capital letters, some of which may be uneven or reversed
Uses every form of sentence structure
Is ready to learn to read (many children who begin school before they are ready may develop a variety of symptoms, including somatic complaints, crying, crossness, unhappiness, begging to stay home)
May find lengthy school sessions too fatiguing; half-day may be best

Tension-stress behaviors

Bites nails
Bites lower lip
Taps foot
May return to temper tantrums
Stutters
If history of thumb-sucking, may increase

Fears

Is very fearful
Fears loud noises—doorbell; telephone; ugly voice tones; animal, bird, or insect noises; static
Fears supernatural, that is, witches, ghosts, goblins
Fears large animals
Fears imagined unseen persons, that is, under bed, inside closet, in cellar
Fears elements—fire, thunder, lightning, water
Fears being lost
Fears being hurt, that is, that others will hit him
Fears that mother will not be home when he arrives; that something may happen to her; that she may die

Ethical sense and morality

Is unable to put rules of the game above need to win; therefore, may break rules—even those he made himself
Is too uncertain of himself to lose gracefully
Tattles on others who cheat

Sexuality

Has increased interest in opposite sex
Has strong interest in origin of babies; will accept idea that baby grows from seed inside mother's stomach; vague idea that babies follow marriage
Is interested to know how baby gets out and if it hurts
Giggles at sound of urine stream; name calling involves words dealing with elimination
Has marked interest in and awareness of sex differences
Mutual investigation by both sexes
Takes part in mild sex play or exhibitionism
Plays hospital
Questions

Health

Is more susceptible to diseases
Communicable diseases increased on school entry
Has frequent sore throats, colds, often with complications
Has somatic complaints related to going to school
Has hypersensitivity of face and neck to washing
Is more apt to break arm if falls

7 years

General characteristics

Is less of a problem than at 6 years of age
Is more quiet and withdrawn, introspective, pensive
Likes to be alone; wants a room of his own
At times feels that everyone is against him and picks on him
Demands much of himself; needs help to define stopping point
May lack confidence to the point of not trying
Has intense but short-lived interests
Is conscientious; tries to take responsibilities seriously, but is too young to be completely reliable
Can be reasoned with
Has good days and bad days; high-learning and "forget-everything" days
Is generally less happy and satisfied with life than younger children

Motor behavior

Has eye-hand coordination that is still not fully developed
Has cautious but not fearful gross motor actions
Is more cautious in approaches to new performances
Repeats performances to master them
Although more quiet, still displays spurts of energy and activity
Has usually learned to swim and ride a bicycle

Personal care

Needs reminding to wash hands before meals
Dawdles in bath and self-care activities
May dislike baths; can get fairly clean without help
Prefers old clothes but accepts whatever is selected for him
Still drops clothes on floor or chair
May need encouragement to go to bed; may still take favorite toy to bed with him
Can brush and comb hair acceptably without help or "going over"

Social behavior and manners

Likes to help and have a choice
Is less resistant and stubborn; is more polite, responsible and sensitive than at 6 years of age
Enjoys teasing
Is very talkative; fights verbally rather than physically
Is more cooperative
Must be called at least twice for meals
Hastens through meals so that he can return to activities
Likes to eat in front of television
Enjoys family conversation at meals

Relationships with family

Feels constantly mistreated; may threaten to run away
Complains about parents
If has vigorous imagination, may believe that he is adopted
Desires family approval
Admires older sibling

Looks after younger sibling, but fights with him a good deal; jealousy still occurs at times
Gets along better with mother
Is developing closer relationship with father

Relationships with peers

Seeks approval of peers
Sex discimination appearing in play groups
Begins to have boyfriends and girlfriends
Becomes more concerned about his place in the group and being liked
May develop "love affairs"
Is in a "for-or-against" age; an age of cliques and outsiders

Play activities

Is more careful with toys
Occupies himself alone for long periods of time
Likes to play alone, but prefers group play
Has more intense interest in some activities, fewer new ventures
Has "mania" for certain activities
Enjoys magic tricks; collecting in quantity, puzzles, "swapping"

Mental activity and school

Is more aware of consequences and cause and effect
Begins to be able to put himself in another's place; moved by sad stories
Can tell time and make small purchases
Can name day, month, and season
Has speech that is no longer egocentric but sociocentric (other-centered)
Begins to use elementary logic
Is in second grade
Can count by multiples of 2, 5, and 10
Grasps basic idea of addition and subtraction
Enjoys school and learning with others
Fears being late for school
Is more dependent on teacher as a person
Has strong emotional responses to teacher; may believe that teacher is unfair
Notices that certain parts are missing from pictures
Can copy a diamond shape

Tension-stress behaviors

Has very few tension outlets
Fidgets
Wriggles loose teeth
Blinks
Scowls
Decreases old tension-reducing habits; attempts to control those that remain

Fears

Has many fears
Fears visual things, such as the dark, attics, cellars; interprets shadows as ghosts, witches
Fears imaginary things, such as war, burglars, spies, persons hiding under the bed or in closets
Is stimulated by mass media
Worries about self—that things will be too difficult; that second grade will be too hard; that people may not like him; that something may happen to him; that he will be late for school
Fears trying something new on his own

Ethical sense and morality

Has good intentions, but may become distracted
Lies less—still concerned about other's wrongdoing
Makes alibis
Has more abstract and generalized concept of good or bad; outside influences are seen as "luck" or "fairness"
Is becoming conscious of right or wrong in self and others

Sexuality

Wants a new baby in family
Knows that having babies can be repeated
Knows that older women do not have babies
Is interested in pregnancies
Is satisfied to know that babies come from two seeds
Has less interest in sex
Takes part in some exploration, experimentation, and sex play, but less than at 6 years of age
Tends to be modest in front of opposite sex

Health

Has fewer illnesses than at 6 years of age
Is subject to communicable diseases, which are still prevalent
Is subject to frequent colds
Complains of headache with fatigue or excitement; muscular pain
Tends to have minor accidents to eyes
Becomes fatigued often

8 years

General characteristics

Is exuberant—ready for anything
Has insatiable curiosity
Is always in a hurry
Is concerned about relationships with others
Thinks that nothing is too difficult—in his estimation
Begins activities with a burst of energy and enthusiasm that may be followed by failure, discouragement, and tears

May need to be protected from trying too much and self-criticism that is too excessive
Tends to be dramatic
Enjoys taking trips and visiting new places
Is usually punctual

Motor behavior

Has increased smoothness and speed in fine motor control
Is always on the go; jumps, chases, skips
Is fluid, almost graceful, in his movements
Is apt to overdo; is often hard to quiet down after recess

Personal care

Dresses self completely
Is careless, messy, impatient
Enjoys selecting own clothes
Needs reminding to go to bed
Likes to be tucked in
Sleeps well

Social behavior and manners

Is more sociable
Is expansive, gregarious
Is constantly busy and active
Enjoys new experiences, new friends
Is better behaved
Responds to reward system
Runs useful errands
Is silly; laughs and giggles
Prefers companionship to solitude; hates to do things alone
Is alert, friendly, interested in people
Is sensitive to criticism
Is first to finish a meal
Gobbles food down
Has social manners that are generally better than at 7 years of age but that still need improvement
Verbalizes proper greetings

Relationships with family

Is easy to get along with at home
Wants a close, understanding relationship with mother—sometimes to her puzzlement and concern
Is sensitive to parental approval/disapproval
Has more to give to others; expects more in return
Competes with siblings
Is very strict when tending younger siblings
Shows preference for mother, but father gets increased share of affection

Relationships with peers

Has usually completed transition to peer culture
Shows preference in friends and groups; ready for and wants a good two-way relationship
Values best friends
Plays mostly with groups of own sex
Is interested in boy-girl relationship, but will not admit overtly
Begins to be interested in clubs and gangs, especially secret clubs
Gives allegiance to peers rather than to adults in case of conflict
Argues, plans, makes deals
Gains security through group membership

Play activities

Has variety of interests; prefers companionship in play
Likes to compete and play games
Enjoys books, comics, television, movies; may retire early in order to read
Requires supervision in play—unsupervised play frequently ends in brawl
Has collections that reflect quality as well as quantity
Likes making things
Enjoys quiet play
Loves prizes in cereal boxes, Cracker Jack
Likes to put on dramatic shows
Begins to be interested in group games

Mental activity and school

Shows interest in causal relationships
Develops through experience
Has increasing memory span
Has increased vocabulary; can give more precise definitions
Is in third grade
Finds school a source of social activity
Likes school; does not like to miss any
Is afraid of failing a grade; is ashamed of bad grades
Often finds need to communicate with his neighbor a source of difficulty
Talks about school more than previously
Evaluates his work in relation to others

Tension-stress behaviors

Cries with fatigue
May return to earlier patterns such as blinking or rubbing eyes or biting nails
Picks at fingers

Fears

Has fewer fears
Worries less
Is able to evaluate fears; has reasonable fears, for example, personal failings
Has less fear of the dark

Ethical sense and morality

Prefers to work for immediate reward (preferably cash)
Will carry out a request if it is insisted on
Considers money of utmost importance
Has more advanced concept of goodness and badness
Is essentially truthful

Sexuality

Understands growth of baby inside mother
Wants more exact information
Asks very searching questions
Has rather high interest in sex
Girls more curious than boys regarding conception, pregnancy, birth, and menstruation
Decreases exploration and play
Has interest in smutty jokes, peeping

Health

Has improving health
Has fewer illnesses; shorter duration
Has increase in allergies
Has frequent accidents—falls, automobile accidents, bicycle accidents
Is more apt to break leg if falls

9 years

General characteristics

Is more quiet and inward directed
Is independent, self-reliant, capable, and trustworthy
Is peer-oriented
Has more confidence in contacts with the world
Works hard and plays hard
Finishes jobs that he starts
Makes decisions quickly and easily
Is motivated by own interests more than by obligations
Is anxious; worries; takes things hard
Complains; often copes with an unpleasant situation with a physical complaint
Is concerned about his relationship with others
Rebels against authority—usually by complaining or passively by withdrawal

Motor behavior

Has fully developed hand-eye coordination that still needs refinement
May work hard to perfect a skill
Develops good timing and skillful control in motor activities
Has apparent individual skills

Personal care

Often rests in strange, awkward positions
Needs no help in bathing or dressing
Is unaware of dirty clothes
Girls discover an interest in clothes; are more fastidious than boys
Needs to be reminded to brush teeth
Keeps room and personal effects reasonably tidy
Is frank about food likes and dislikes
Still needs to be reminded to go to bed
Often gets up early to have time to "mess around" before school

Social behavior and manners

Is more sociable
Is easy to discipline
Has strong social feelings; shows empathy and sympathy
Begins hero worship and prejudices
Has greater refinement in behavior
Is aware of appropriate sex roles
Understands explanations and tries to do things well
Has acceptable manners when guests are present; less so when family is alone
Chews with mouth closed when reminded

Relationships with family

Resists too much bossing by parents
Considers opinions of parents less important than opinions of friends
Is less interested in relationships with parents, but enjoys going places with them
Rebels against parental oversolicitousness
Takes part in family decisions
Enjoys running errands, helping when mother is busy or ill
Willingly responds to parental demands—if he hears them
Has better relationship with siblings

Relationships with peers

Is loyal to friends
Values "special" friends
Still determines friendship on basis of sex
Enjoys chatting with groups of friends
Boys chase girls

Play activities

Develops "crazes" for certain activities
Has variety of play interests
Works hard at play
Enjoys more complicated table games
Takes part in organized play—group rewards are powerful incentives
Loves stunts of all sorts
Continues collections, some of which develop into organized hobbies
Loves making things

Participates in outdoor sports of the large-muscle, rough-and-tumble variety
Enjoys sports such as baseball, skating, and swimming
Individual differences in play become more apparent
Delights in legends; this is the age of stories
Girls enjoy dancing school; boys have little interest in dancing
Likes to hike
Loves to read
Spends much time in solitary activities
Has high interest in competitive sports

Mental activity and school

Understands explanations and tries to do things well
Has somewhat longer attention span than at 8 years of age
Is intellectually more stimulating
As a group, girls are superior to boys
Good grades are standard achievement, excellent grades less so
Is in fourth grade
Exceptionally bright children may become outcasts
Is ashamed of failure; competes for pride
Is more concerned with subjects than with teacher
Is interested in schoolwork

Tension-stress behaviors

Stamps feet
Fiddles
Picks at self
Drops and breaks things
Taps pencil
Grumbles and mutters
Feels dizzy; has other somatic complaints
Draws in lips

Fears

Has fewer fears; has reasonable fears
Worries less
Has fears that relate to personal ineptitudes
Fears failure in school
Has scary dreams, but quiets easily

Ethical sense and morality

Evaluates self and family
Recognizes his own weaknesses; often makes self-effacing remarks
Can accept blame for his actions
Is more willing to interrupt own activity in response to a request or demand from an adult—if he hears them
Is less interested in money; works for service
Is honest, fair; feels guilty when "bad"

Sexuality

Is sexually modest
Has increased awareness of sexuality
Majority know about menstruation
Has mild interest in father's part in reproduction
May discuss sex information with friends
Is interested in details of own organs and functions
Begins sex swearing; sex poems
Some 9-year-old girls begin pubertal changes
Boys hesitant to ask questions of parents

Health

Has improved health, few illnesses
Has minor complaints—usually related to a task, for example, eyes burn when studying, hands hurt when practicing piano, stomach hurts when doing dishes

10 years

General characteristics

Is relatively predictable
Is in a comfortable equilibrium; is sincere, happy, relaxed, confident, congenial
Has gradual, smooth transition from 9 to 10 years of age
Is generally content with self
Is oblivious
Is in one of the happiest ages
Is highly competitive
Has mainly superficial feelings

Motor behavior

Develops greater strength and coordination in all motor skills
Delights in physical activity—running, skating, sliding, climbing, jumping, cycling
Has greater stamina

Personal care

May wear same thing continually
Cannot be bothered with personal hygiene; needs constant reminding
Has positive antipathy for water and heroically resists bathing but in bath will play for long periods
Keeps room in constant disarray
Leaves clothes wherever they fall
Is not always aware when tired and ready for bed
Boys go to bed more easily and rapidly than girls
Has poor posture at meals

Social behavior and manners

Experiences sharp outbursts of anger; tends to be brief, explosive, and shallow
Cries when angry but does not bear a grudge or nurse hurt feelings
Experiences outbursts of happiness and demonstrations of affection
Is able to tolerate frustration
Has huge appetite
Has acceptable manners

Relationships with family

Is fond of home and loyal to it
Has closer attachment to family than at 9 years of age
Has better mother-child relationship
Respects parents and their role
Gets along well with father and enjoys his companionship
Readily participates in family activities
Gets along least well with siblings ages 6 to 9 years of age
Is nurturing to younger (preschool) children and animals

Relationships with peers

Is fond of his friends; extols their virtues to family
Is apt to be cliquey
Clubs (for example, cub scouts) have great appeal
Is serious about organized group life; avidly forms clubs, which are often short-lived
Joins informal, temporary groups as well as established gangs and organized groups
Girls prefer small, more intimate groups
Most girls have a "best friend" for an extended period
Still separate by choice into like-sex groups for group games and activities
Experiences hero worship
Wants to measure up to a challenge as defined by peer group
Can subordinate own desires for good of the group

Play activities

Enjoys just "fooling around" with neighborhood children
Loves large-muscle activity and gross motor games out-of-doors
Enjoys collections
Enjoys reading
Especially enjoys bicycle riding
Likes noise and makes a great deal of it

Mental activity and school

Manages time fairly well
Enjoys learning
Begins to handle simple fractions and numbers better
Begins to think of social problems in terms of cause and effect; still has problems combining facts and seeing relationships
May have difficulty in combining time and space to arrive at a place at a specified time
Has short interest span
Loves to memorize
Is in the fifth grade
Likes school
Likes to talk and listen rather than work, but may like to be motivated to work difficult problems
Is more aware of teacher's appearance and manner
Needs schedules—is unable to plan
Has difficulty in connecting facts

Tension-stress behaviors

May increase finger-to-mouth activity
May increase fidgeting and other motor activity at middle of tenth year; more common in girls

Fears

Has many fears, but fewer than in preadolescence to come
Fears animals, especially snakes and wild animals, high places, fires, criminals, the dark, blood, ghosts
Has fewer worries than fears
Worries about school—homework, grades, being late

Ethical sense and morality

Is concrete in matters of conscience
Is seriously opposed to cheating; wants stern codes against dishonesty
May defer to parent in solving ethical problems
Has a conscience that is still relatively immature
Is more preoccupied with wrong than right
Believes in justice and fair play

Sexuality

Expresses disinterest or disrelish of opposite sex, but not too vehemently
Most know about sexual intercourse
Is interested in smutty jokes
May begin to see discrepant growth between sexes
Girls begin to show unmistakable signs of approaching adolescence during the tenth year—slight projection of nipples, rounding of contours
No sexual maturation apparent in boys
Girls more aware of sex than boys, although less outspoken

Health

Has, on the whole, good to excellent health
Has lessening somatic complaints
Has big appetite; has more food likes than dislikes

11 years

General characteristics

Is filled with conflict, turmoil, and stormy behavior; is paradoxical
Is sulky, fidgety, restless, resentful
Is gay, kind to friends, eager, pleasant
Is relatively independent and tolerant
Assumes much responsibility for self
Has strengthened superego and greater self-control
Is full of energy and activity
Is interested in exploration and adventure

Is a clown; enjoys slap-stick humor and puns; can get silly over anything
Is unpredictable
Is interested in money—allowance or earning

Motor behavior

Has increased motor and mental activity
Is less poised
Bounces and jerks more; acts more clumsily

Personal care and responsibility

Is rebellious in relation to parental standards for mealtimes, washing, dressing
Has self-awareness in terms of grooming—especially girls
Has less resistance to bathing; still has trouble cleaning back of neck and ear
Has difficulty in keeping hair clean and combed
Is dissatisfied with earliness of bedtime; needs prodding
Has difficulty in getting up in the morning
Girls highly interested in clothes and "what to wear" but hang up only best clothes
Often has small job after school and during summer
Needs reminding and prefers to have a choice in whatever is demanded of him

Social behavior and manners

Loves conversation
Resists imposed tasks and proprieties
Strives hard for conformity
Has little interest in adults
May have increased shyness but hates to be alone
Rarely chooses to be alone; elects to be involved in family group or peer group
Is often at his best behavior away from home

Relationships with family

Is constantly present in family circle
Can be a pleasant companion
Enjoys family group activities
Has worst relationship with siblings
Is rebellious with parents
Argues about everything; is aware of parents' fallibilities and does not hesitate to point them out
Usually get along better with one parent than with the other
Boys embarrassed if mothers kiss them in front of friends
Wishes to become somewhat financially independent from parents
Family tensions may develop over parents' "nagging" to eat better, stand up straight, and so on
Is critical and resistant to mother; is more tolerant of father

Relationships with peers

Is more intense, emotional, and complicated
Chooses friends more selectively
Values membership in clubs and community activities
Girls often in friendship groups of three to five with whom they shift; boys more apt to have single "best friend"
"Detests" opposite sex, but girls enjoy being teased by boys
Is often jealous of peers
Demonstrates friendship—girls put arms around each other; boys punch each other
Boys may get into fist fights
Likes to stay overnight with a friend
May be strongly influenced by best friend

Play activities

Considers play not as important as formerly
Considers people more important than the play
Is active; team games are very popular
Has impulse to be out-of-doors
Although clumsy in the home, is agile in sports
Enjoys taking walks
Still maintains collections, especially for purpose of trading
Enjoys comic books
Loves to construct a tree house, including the problems of construction, membership, and so on
Is less interested in television; leans toward teen-age interest in popular music; has more interest in movies
Enjoys humor, puns, corny jokes

Mental activity and school

Is in sixth grade
Can define increasingly abstract terms, such as "justice"
Is still excited about learning
Often has trouble over homework
Is interested in the "why" and "how" of things
Begins to understand workings of simple machines
Is more critical in evaluating own work
Likes a teacher who provides a challenge
Takes part in a great deal of note passing
Will enjoy reading more if it was enjoyed before
Attends school primarily for peer association
Loves competition, especially, boys against girls
Works for good grades, pleased when doing well
Begins to think realistically about career and/or marriage

Tension-stress behaviors

Often expresses frustrations by withdrawal
Displays sudden, uncontrolled outbursts of anger, frequently ending in tears
May snuggle up to mother in private
Expresses anger in yelling, sometimes hitting

Uses tension outlets that involve increased motor activity, such as blinking, snuffing, and grimaces
May revert to falling down or dropping and breaking things

Fears

Is in one of the most worried and fearful ages
Is mainly afraid to be alone
Worries about school, money, parents' welfare, his own health
Girls afraid of physical pain, infection, and that something might happen to their mothers
Is afraid that no one—especially girls—likes him
Fears strange animals

Ethical sense and morality

Can extract the meaning or moral from stories
Is keenly aware of how people treat one another
Is concerned about fairness
Knows what is right but does not always *do* what is right
May not always tell the truth or accept blame; is more concerned about self-protection than truthfulness
Boys may cheat; girls may steal
Is too often influenced by feelings rather than established dogma
Has fairly good controls through conscience
Is concerned with fairness
Sometimes girls will misbehave to spite people

Sexuality

Begins to comprehend prenatal growth
Is interested to know how "seed is planted from father to mother," but has difficulty in comprehending
Is apt to consider intercourse as "nasty"
Boys are interested in smutty jokes and in observing animal copulation
Few boys are willing to discuss sex matters with parents
Frequent erections occur in many boys
Boys are becoming more aware of girls as girls
Girls have absorbed interest in their own body changes, which may be a source of pride or of embarrassment
Girls are interested in imminent onset of menstruation

Physical changes

Girls
- Have striking individual differences—some have childish form, whereas others are well advanced into adolescence
- Most have begun growth spurt in height; some have reached apex
- Average changes—some pubic hair; cone-like projections surrounding nipples are evidenced on flat chest; pelvic area developing rounded contours; 90% of mature height and 50% of adult weight achieved
- A small percentage begin menstruation in the eleventh year

Boys
- Are more uniform than girls
- Few indicate signs of sexual maturation
- Some go through a "fat period" with fat deposits around hips and nipples (transient)
- Have increase in bone size, which produces prominent skeletal structure, especially in chest area
- Average changes—80% of adult height and less than 50% of adult weight achieved
- Approximately one fourth of boys exhibit increasing genital size

Health

Has generally good health but has frequent colds
Is hypochondriacal; has many somatic complaints such as feet hurt, has a headache, is tired
Has good appetite
Understands rationale behind health and hygiene practices, such as covering mouth and nose when coughing or sneezing

12 years

General characteristics

Is more companionable, reasonable, tolerant
Is less insistent
Is even-tempered, happy, good natured
Is adjustable
Has a charming sense of humor
Is self-reliant
Is fairly satisfied with self and world
Appears to be trying to "grow up"
Becomes more calm and relaxed
Has enthusiasm as a prime characteristic (boys—enthusiasm for sports; girls—enthusiasm for child care)
Likes variety and change

Motor behavior

Takes part in intense activity; suddenly reaches saturation point and collapses
Is capable of more refined motor activities
Still enjoys gross motor activity

Personal care and responsibility

Continues to be more concerned about personal cleanliness and appearance
Bathes frequently; prefers showers
May still need help with shampoo
Has difficulty with bedtime; is more easily roused in the morning

Is concerned about wearing clothes that are in vogue, that fit well, and that match
Rapid growth often necessitates new wardrobes
Girls may try to look glamorous; want to wear lipstick for special occasions
Enjoys shopping for clothes; choice of clothes better than care of clothes
Needs reminding about care of clothes
Spends time decorating room, less on keeping it tidy
Has less interest in money, but manages money well
Is helpful with tasks but often "in a couple of minutes"
Is able to assume more complex chores
Is motivated by earning money

Social behavior and manners

Is excellent conversational company
Boys more interested in attending social gatherings, such as dancing school, parties, and so on
Enjoys group activities involving both sexes
Has better control of emotions, especially anger
Is more capable of give-and-take
Is more aware of other's feelings
Seldom gets in conflict with others
Is diplomatic in his actions
Has fairly accurate assessment of others

Relationships with family

Is less demonstrative about affection than at 11 years of age
Gets along better with parents and argues less; demands less from them
Recognizes changes of behavior with fatigue
Has less fighting with siblings near his age; young siblings may bother him, but he relates well with preschoolers
Responds especially well to sympathetic older sibling
Expects parents to respect need for privacy
Still wants limits set on his behavior

Relationships with peers

Has easy relationship with peers
May rotate among several friends; rarely at a loss for friends
Prefers smaller groups
May join larger groups for athletic activities
Most large, spontaneous clubs begin to break up
Girls are more prone to segregate into twosomes
Has interest in the opposite sex
For many, is an age of considerable boy-girl interest and activity during school
Shifts interest from one friend to another
Girls enjoy talking about boys

Play activities

Enjoys collections; new dimension—mementos such as ticket stubs, clippings, photographs
Needs bulletin board for display
Enjoys parties, but requires supervision, otherwise may get out of hand
Likes games involving close, accidental contact with opposite sex
Likes group activities but can enjoy solitude
Is seldom bored
Has wide range of interests
Segregates into athletic and nonathletic groups
Likes athletic sports in season
Likes swimming; girls like horseback riding
Enjoys some sort of organization in activities
Reads less

Mental activity and school

Has wide variety of interests in schoolwork but prefers sports
Eagerly absorbs information and accumulates ideas
Asks many questions
Is interested in scientific matters and social studies
Seeks reality in social and physical relationships
Collects facts; enjoys hearing about faraway places and distant times
Likes books about travel, biography, science, nature, home, and school; girls like books about heroines and romance; boys like stories of adventure, exploration, the wild West, mysteries, and tall tales
Tends to like teacher; wants one who knows and who demands decorum
Is concerned with schoolwork and being well liked
Competes less intensely; prefers to be even with friends
Has less interest in and time for books
Likes arithmetic
Boys excel at number manipulation; girls excel at language, rote memory, and writing skills
Likes to be involved in dramatics
Is open and uninhibited in the classroom

Tension-stress behaviors

Has nervous mannerisms that may appear when tired

Fears

Is less fearful than at 11 years of age
Is still uncomfortable in the dark; hears creaky noises at night; fears an intruder

Ethical sense and morality

Is level-headed
Makes decisions based on considered thinking, past experience, and analysis of consequences—less on feeling

Is less tempted to misbehave than at 11 years of age
Is tolerant toward self and others
Still may try to see what he can get away with
Has well-developed conscience
Is truthful about big things; may not be about little things
Believes that one can lie if there is sufficient justification, such as to protect another person
Knows when he has infringed on the rights of others
Will accept responsibility for actions
Can control cheating and stealing more easily
Expects to pay a penalty for wrongdoing or inappropriate behavior

Sexuality

Is aware that intercourse occurs apart from conception
Views sex as less "dirty"
Girls
- Are less self-conscious about development; may even flaunt their developing form
- Are usually more cognizant of sex matters in general than boys
- Are fairly comfortable in discussing sex with mother
- Few show any of the premenstrual behavior changes associated with later years

Boys
- Become more interested in sex than previously; may seek information from magazines, books, and dictionaries
- Are usually less interested in sex activity of grown-ups; are more absorbed with own sex interest
- Have frequent bull sessions about sex
- Have erections frequently
- Masturbation common

Physical changes

Girls
- Achieve greatest advancement in form and function of mature female
- Are in period of most rapid growth in height and weight (at end of twelfth year has achieved 95% of mature height)
- Experience filling out of breasts; dark areola
- Have some growth of axillary hair
- Experience menarche toward end of year; have strong interest in menstruation

Boys
- Have wide range in physical growth
- On the average, show definite indications of beginning puberty
- Many show increased growth of both penis and scrotum
- Have long, downy hair at base of penis
- Often have erections—spontaneously and under various kinds of stimulation

Health

May suffer extreme fatigue, especially after intense activity
May require a day or two of rest
Has good health but less consistent
May still have sudden, unexpected, sharp but short-lived pains, frequently in head or abdomen
Is concerned about vision

REFERENCES

1. Bryan, D. S.: School nursing in transition, St. Louis, 1973, The C. V. Mosby Co.
2. Erikson, E. H.: Childhood and society, ed. 2, New York, 1963, W. W. Norton & Co., Inc.
3. Havighurst, R. J.: Developmental tasks and education, ed. 3, New York, 1972, David McKay Co., Inc.
4. Heagerty, M., and associates: Sex and the pre-school child., Am. J. Nurs. **74:**1479-1482, 1974.
5. Newman, B. M., and Newman, P. R.: Development through life. A psychosocial approach, Homewood, Ill., 1975, Dorsey Press.
6. Oda, D.: The role of the community nurse in school systems. In Archer, S. E., and Fleshman, R.: Community health nursing: patterns and practice, North Scituate, Mass., 1975, Duxbury Press.
7. Stone, L. J., and Church, J.: Childhood and adolescence, ed. 3, New York, 1973, Random House, Inc.

BIBLIOGRAPHY

Bakwin, H., and Bakwin, R. M.: Behavior disorders in children, Philadelphia, 1972, W. B. Saunders Co.

Bigner, J. J.: The school-age child—6 to 12 years. In Scipien, G. M., and associates: Comprehensive pediatric nursing, New York, 1975, McGraw-Hill Book Co.

Blaesing, S., and Brockhaus, J.: The developing of body image in the child, Nurs. Clin. North Am. **7:**597-608, 1972.

Brozovish, R.: Characteristics associated with popularity among different social and socioeconomic groups of children, J. Educ. Res. **63:**441-444, 1970.

Chaubey, N. P.: Effect of age on expectancy of success and on risk-taking behavior, J. Pers. Soc. Psychol. **29:**774-778, 1974.

Child nutrition programs, Dairy Council Digest **45**(1):1-5, January/February 1974.

Child Study Association of America: What to tell your children about sex, New York, 1974, Pocket Books.

Chinn, P. L.: A relationship between health and school problems: a nursing assessment, J. Sch. Health **43:**85, February 1973.

Chinn, P. L.: Child health maintenance: concepts in family centered care, ed. 2, St. Louis, 1979, The C. V. Mosby Co.

Committee on Pediatric Manpower and Committee on School Health: Concepts of school health programs, Pediatrics **55:** 140, 1975.

Cornwell, G.: The differential sexual socialization of school children, Nurs. Forum **10**(4):401, 1971.

Crewe, H. J.: Fears and anxiety in childhood, Public Health **63:** 165-171, October 1973.

Czarniecki, L.: The integration of sex education in pediatric nursing practice, Pediatr. Nurs. **2**(2):12-16, 1976.

Dansky, K. H.: Assessing children's nutrition, Am. J. Nurs. **77:** 1610-1611, 1977.

Edelman, S. K.: Sex and life education in a rural school, Am. J. Maternal Child Nurs. **2**(4):233-239, 1977.

Egan, M. C.: Federal nutrition support programs for children, Pediatr. Clin. North Am. **24:**229-239, 1977.

Ehrman, M.: Sex education for the young, Nurs. Outlook **23:** 538-585, 1975.

Eisner, V., Cobb, O., and Tortosa, R.: The effectiveness of health screening in a school program for migrant children, Pediatrics **49:**128, 1972.

Elkind, D.: A sympathetic understanding of the child from six to sixteen, Boston, 1971, Allyn & Bacon, Inc.

Emmerich, W., Goldman, K. S., and Shore, R. E.: Differentiation and development of social norms, J. Pers. Soc. Psychol. **18:**323-353, 1971.

Fine, L. L., and Bellaire, J. M.: The school nurse: an obsolete professional revisited, Pediatr. Nurs. **1:**25, 1975.

Garner, G.: Modifying pupil self-concept and behavior, Today's Educ. **63:**24-28, 1974.

Gendel, E. S., and Green, P. B.: Sex education controversy—a boost to new and better programs, J. Sch. Health **41:**24, 1971.

Hawkins, N. G.: Is there a school nurse role? Am. J. Nurs. **71:** 744, 1971.

Hildebrandt, D. E., Feldman, S. E., and Detricks, R. A.: Rules, models, and self-reinforcement in children, J. Pers. Soc. Psychol. **25:**1-5, 1973.

Hilmar, N. A., and McAtte, P. A.: The school nurse practitioner and her practice: a study of traditional and expanded health care responsibilities for nurses in elementary schools, J. Sch. Health **43:**431, 1973.

Hogan, E. O., and Green, R. L.: Can teachers modify children's self-concepts? Teachers College Record **62:**423-426, 1971.

Hordin, D.: The school-age child and the school nurse, Am. J. Nurs. **74:**1476-1478, 1974.

Hoyman, H. S.: Sex education and our core values, J. Sch. Health **44:**62-69, 1974.

Husband, P., and Hinton, P. E.: Families of children with repeated accidents, Arch. Dis. Child. **47:**396, 1972.

Igoe, J. B.: The school nurse practitioner, Nurs. Outlook **23:** 381, 1975.

Jenny, J., and Grazier, P. J.: Parents' attitudes about school dental services for children, J. Sch. Health **44:**86-91, 1974.

Jersild, A. T., Telford, C. W., and Sawrey, J. M.: Child psychology, ed. 7, Englewood Cliffs, N.J., 1975, Prentice-Hall, Inc.

Johnson, R.: Sex education and the nurse, Nurs. Outlook **18:** 26-29, 1970.

Johnson, R. C., and Medinnus, G. R.: Child psychology, behavior and development, ed. 3, New York, 1974, John Wiley & Sons, Inc.

Kaluger, G., and Kaluger, M. F.: Human development: the span of life, ed. 2, St. Louis, 1979, The C. V. Mosby Co.

Kappleman, M., and associates: The school health team and school health physician: new role and operation, Am. J. Dis. Child. **129:**191, 1975.

Knifong, J. D.: Logical abilities of young children—two styles of approach, Child Dev. **45:**78-83, 1974.

Kokenes, B.: Grade level differences in factors of self-esteem, Dev. Psychol. **10:**954-958, 1974.

Kolberg, L.: Development of moral character and moral ideology. In Hoffman, L. W., and Hoffman, M. L., editors: Review of child development research, vol 1, New York, 1964, Russell Sage Foundation.

Large, J. T.: The school-age child and his family. In Hymovich, D. P., and Barnard, M. U.: Family health care, New York, 1973, McGraw-Hill Book Co.

Marks, M. B.: Recognition of the allergic child at school, visual and auditory signs, J. Sch. Health **44:**277-284, 1974.

Marlow, G.: Textbook of pediatric nursing, ed. 4, Philadelphia, 1973, W. B. Saunders Co.

Marshall, C. L., and associates: Attitudes toward health among children of different races and socioeconomic status, Pediatrics **46:**422, 1970.

McAtee, P. R.: Nurse practitioners in our public schools? An assessment of their expanded role as compared with school nurses, Clin. Pediatr. **13:**360, 1974.

Moore, G. T., and Frank, K.: Comprehensive health services for children: an exploratory study of benefit, Pediatrics **51:**17, 1973.

Murray, R., and Zentner, J.: Nursing assessment and health promotion through the life span, Englewood Cliffs, N.J., 1975, Prentice-Hall, Inc.

Mussen, P. H., Conger, J. J., and Kagan, J.: Child development and personality, ed. 4, New York, 1974, Harper & Row, Publishers.

Oda, D.: Increasing role effectiveness of school nurses, Am. J. Public Health **64:**591-595, 1974.

Osofsky, H. J., and Osofsky, J. D.: Let's be sensible about sex education, Am. J. Nurs. **71:**532, 1971.

Pasternack, S. B.: Annual well-child visits, Am. J. Nurs. **74:** 1472-1475, August 1974.

Pelizza, J. J.: A comparative study of how parents from different social classes perceive school health services, J. Sch. Health **43:**176-180, 1973.

Philips, I.: Youth permissiveness, and child development, Pediatrics **49:**1-4, 1972.

Pipes, P. L.: Nutrition in infancy and childhood, St. Louis, 1977, The C. V. Mosby Co.

Quereschi, M. Y.: Patterns of intellectual development during childhood and adolescence, Genet. Psychol. Monogr. **87**(2): 313-344, 1973.

Rybicki, L. L.: Preparing parents to teach their children about human sexuality, Am. J. Maternal Child Nurs. **1**(3):182-185, May/June 1976.

Sandstead, H. H., and associates: Nutritional deficiencies in disadvantaged preschool children: their relationship to mental development, Am. J. Dis. Child. **121:**455-463, June 1971.

Sears, R. R.: Relation of early socialization experiences to self-concept and gender role in middle childhood, Child. Dev. **44:**267-289, 1970.

Silver, H. K., Igoe, J. B., and McAtee, P. R.: The school nurse practitioner: providing improved health care to children, Pediatrics **58:**580-584, 1976.

Slattery, J.: Dental health in children, Am. J. Nurs. **76:**1159-1161, 1976.

Smart, M. S., and Smart, R. C.: Children: development and relationships, ed. 2, New York, 1972, Macmillan Publishing, Inc.

Smith, J. T.: Promoting childhood dental health, Pediatr. Nurs. **2**(3):16-19, 1976.

Southall, C.: Family life and sex education, Am. J. Nurs. **77:** 1473-1476, 1977.

Stephenson, P. S.: Working with 9- to 12-year-old children, Child. Welfare **52:**375-382, June 1973.

Sutterly, D. C., and Donnelly, G. F.: Perspectives in human development, Philadelphia, 1973, J. B. Lippincott Co.

Wany, R. M.: Streptococcal sore throat, Am. J. Nurs. **77:**1996-1998, 1973.

Weinheimer, S.: Egocentrism and social influence in children, Child Dev. **43:**567-578, 1974.

Whipple, D. V.: Dynamics of development: euthenic pediatrics, New York, 1966, McGraw-Hill Book Co.

Williams, S. R.: Nutrition and diet therapy, ed. 3, St. Louis, 1977, The C. V. Mosby Co.

Wolman, I. J.: Some prominent developments in childhood nutrition, Clin. Pediatr. **12**(2):74, 1973.

Woody, J.: Contemporary sex education: attitudes and implications for child rearing, J. Sch. Health **43:**241-246, 1973.

18

Health problems of middle childhood

As a group, school-age children are fairly healthy when compared with children in infancy and early childhood and the ages 9 to 12 years are usually the healthiest years of childhood. As would be expected, respiratory illnesses (the leading cause of morbidity) and gastrointestinal upsets are the most common illnesses. A factor contributing to this overall health state is the quantity of lymphoid tissue, at its height during this stage, which helps to fight infection and ward off disease (see p. 58). The 11-year-old child has almost twice the amount of a young adult.

Most children in this age-group have either contracted the communicable diseases of childhood or have been immunized against them. Their excellent appetites, adequate rest, and sufficient physical exercise further contribute to their general good health. Other conditions that are not uncommon in middle childhood are accidental injuries (primarily related to their normal activities), dental problems, and emotional or behavior disorders. Allergic manifestations, especially asthma (see p. 1241), may reach a peak during the middle childhood years, and a variety of other serious disorders make a significant contribution to childhood morbidity. These will be considered as appropriate in relation to the ill child.

Behavioral disorders in school-age children

A number of classification systems have been employed to outline the various problems of middle childhood that interfere with development, learning, and social relationships. Although there is no universal categorization, most authorities seem to broadly classify behavioral disorders in some manner that identifies mental subnormality, learning disabilities, neuroses, psychoses, and antisocial behavior. Many disorders have a major organic or developmental component, whereas others are seen almost exclusively in children of school-age. Still others are primarily problems of adolescence and many extend throughout the course of childhood. Very often a change in behavior is one of the manifestations of an organic disease; at other times emotional problems produce somatic symptoms of greater or lesser seriousness.

The variety and extent of emotional and behavioral disorders of childhood are much too numerous to be considered here. Some are discussed elsewhere (for example, mental retardation, Chapter 23, and sensory impairment, Chapter 24).

MINIMAL BRAIN DYSFUNCTION

A good deal of confusion surrounds the definitions and relationships of various behavior problems that in some way impair the child's capacity to profit from new experiences. Some disabilities, such as mental retardation and cultural deprivation, are very general in scope. Others are defined in more discrete terms such as hearing impairment, visual disabilities, and so on. Most of the confusion is related to the category of behaviors and special learning disabilities for which many overlapping terms have emerged—"minimal brain dysfunction," "specific learning disabilities," "neurologic handicap," "hyperkinetic syndrome," and "developmental dyslexia," to name a few. The syndrome of manifestations affects a significant number of children, persists throughout childhood, and carries with it a high rate of behavioral disturbance and academic failure.[4]

Most of the confusion involves the relationship between the terms *minimal brain dysfunction (MBD)* or *cerebral dysfunction* and *specific learning disabilities (SLD)* or simply *learning disabilities*. The definitions of these terms follow:

minimal brain dysfunction "this term as a diagnostic and descriptive category refers to children of near average, average, or above average intellectual capacity with certain learning and/or behavioral disabilities ranging from mild to severe, which are associated with deviations of function of the central nervous system. These deviations may manifest themselves by various combinations of impairment in perception, conceptualization, language, memory, and control of attention, impulse or motor function. These aberrations may arise from genetic variations, bio-chemical irregularities, perinatal brain insults, or other illnesses or injuries sustained during the years critical for the development and maturation of the central nervous system."[3]

specific learning disability "children with specific learning disabilities exhibit a disorder in one or more of the basic psychological processes involved in understanding or in using spoken or written language. These may be manifested in disorders of listening, thinking, talking, reading, writing, spelling, or arithmetic. They include conditions which have been referred to as perceptual handicaps, brain injury, minimal brain dysfunction, dyslexia, developmental aphasia, etc. They do not include learning problems which are due primarily to visual, hearing, or motor handicaps, to mental retardation, emotional disturbances, or to environmental disadvantage."[8]

Minimal brain dysfunction is the *medical* term that is applied to these children and includes the neurodevelopmental and etiologic aspects of the disorder; learning disabilities is the *educational* term that emphasizes the behavioral outcomes of impaired functioning in central processing. This dual definition has an advantage. By using the educational category learning disability, the schools can provide services for affected children without requiring a medical diagnosis.

The incidence of minimal brain dysfunction is difficult to estimate since the symptomatology and the definitions are so varied that no standard evaluation criteria is available to help identify any specific case. Unofficial estimates place the incidence at anywhere from 3% to 15% of the childhood population with boys affected more frequently than girls. However, minimal brain dysfunction is the single most important cause of school underachievement in school-age children.[11]

Etiology

The etiology of minimal brain dysfunction is uncertain, obscure, and often speculative. As the definition implies, it may be related to virtually any illness or trauma affecting the brain that occurs at any stage of development—before, during, or after birth. Multiple causes, including psychosocial factors, are probably involved.

Behavioral and learning disorders have been noted in children with some of the sex chromosomal abnormalities. For example, in girls with Turner's syndrome (see pp. 190 and 713) there is a high incidence of impaired spatial abilities and right-left directional sense, and a large number of boys with Klinefelter's syndrome (see pp. 190 and 714) have learning, behavioral, or peer problems. A sex-linked factor may be operating since the hyperkinetic syndrome is much more common in boys than in girls.

A popular theory is the concept of a developmental lag. Distractibility, short attention span, and impulsiveness are all normal characteristics of children at a much younger developmental level. Since the symptoms tend to diminish with age, it is postulated that this may have an anatomic basis, that is, a maturational lag in myelination of the prefrontal cortex that takes place through adolescence. Also, hyperactivity may be merely a normal variant of innate temperament in some children who represent the extreme end of the normal distribution curve for activity.

Support for a biochemical etiology is suggested by the way in which a majority of hyperactive children respond to central nervous system stimulant drugs. Proponents of this theory suggest that in these hyperactive children there is an absence or insufficiency of norepinephrine, a neurotransmitter that normally appears in high concentrations in areas of the brain that have much to do with activity level, mood, and awareness. Others advance the theory that there is some alteration in the reticular activating system of the midbrain, a key area for controlling consciousness and attention, that interferes with its function of filtering out extraneous stimuli. Consequently these children are unable to focus on one stimulus but are compelled to respond to every stimulus in the environment. Central nervous system stimulants that increase the level of norepinephrine and/or activate the reticular activating system cause a reduction in the undesired behavior. The fact that these children show few, if any, symptoms in a stress situation (such as the physician's or principal's office) provides additional support to this hypothesis, because stress increases the level of norepinephrine.

In recent years there has been interest in diet and hyperkinesis. There are those who believe that the observed behavioral patterns are related to an innate sensitivity to certain food items and/or food additives. Although this theory does not have wholehearted support, some children do show improvement when certain foods are eliminated from their diet, particularly those containing salicylates and those with specific additives such as artificial coloring, sweetening, and preservatives. Parents may need help with the child's diet; for example, it is the nurse's responsibility to find out what the child *can eat* and help the parents find sources for the proper foods, especially if the child is on a special metabolic diet.

Diagnostic evaluation

Early identification of affected children is needed since the characteristics of the disorder significantly interfere with the normal course of emotional and psychologic development. Many of these children, in the attempt to cope with cerebral dysfunction, develop maladaptive behavior patterns that are a deterrent to psychosocial adjustment. Their behavior evokes negative responses from others, and repeated exposure to negative feedback adversely affects the child's self-concept.

Characteristics. The behaviors exhibited by the child with minimal brain dysfunction are not unusual aspects of child behavior. The difference lies in the "intensity, persistence, and clustering of his symptoms.'' A small percentage of these children display only the hyperactivity, impulsiveness, and short attention span that characterize the *hyperkinetic syndrome*. Another group of children are not hyperactive or impulsive; in fact, most are hypoactive. The predominant features of this group are the *specific learning disabilities* such as developmental dyslexia (difficulty with reading) or dysgraphia (difficulty with writing). The largest segment of the childhood population with minimal brain dysfunction are children who have both learning disabilities and hyperactivity. This is the *mixed* group (Fig. 18-1).

The manifestations that are displayed by affected children may be numerous or few and mild or severe and will vary with the developmental level of the child. Any given child will not have every manifestation that is characteristic of a syndrome, and the degree of severity is highly variable. Mild manifestations of the symptoms may not be apparent in a good educational and family environment, whereas severe symptomatology will be recognizable even in the most healthy and accommodating environment. Every dysfunctional child is, in some respects, different from all other children with minimal brain dysfunction.

Most of the behavioral manifestations are apparent at an early age, but the learning disabilities may not become evident until the child enters school. The symptoms are more prominent prior to age 10 years, after which they become more subtle since they tend to diminish with advancing age. Although it appears that most characteristics of minimal brain dysfunction do not extend into adolescence, increasing evidence indicates that hyperactive children do not necessarily outgrow their symptoms. Concomitant emotional difficulties are frequent, and there are indications of sociopathic and psychotic behavior in a significant number of these children. It is questionable how many of these persistent behavioral problems may be caused by the cerebral dysfunction and how many by the undesirable effects of childhood experiences. The child who is unable to function normally in his home and school environment will meet with constant failure and rejection and will react with hostility or other inappropriate behaviors. His frequent recognition that he is ''bad'' or is not ''right inside'' will produce a negative self-concept and reactive hostility.

The basic characteristics described in the following segment and outlined in Table 18-1 reflect disturbances in central processing. The first five—overactivity, hyperactivity, or hyperkinesis; short attention span; distractibility; impulsiveness and inability to delay gratification; and labile emotions or excitability—are the cardinal signs of the hyperactive syndrome.

Overactivity, hyperactivity, or hyperkinesis. Hyperactivity is a central feature of the constellation of behavioral symptoms of minimal brain dysfunction. It is not certain whether the hyperactivity of minimal brain dysfunction is truly overactivity. Quantitatively the degree of activity may be no greater than in other children; however, the movements appear to be hyperactive because the activity is disorganized, nonproductive, relatively continuous, and not turned off in appropriate situations.

Severe cases are unusual, but moderate to mild degrees of hyperactivity are common. In the newborn period the hyperactive infant may be unduly sensitive to stimuli and respond in an undifferentiated, massive, averse manner. During infancy he is active in his crib, sleeps little, and cries a good deal; very early he gets out of the crib on his own and gets into everything, fingering, breaking, or demolishing objects. As he grows in mobility his sphere of activities rapidly extends to the yard and neighboring territory including the street.

Short attention span. These children are ''short samplers,'' that is, they seem unable to give their attention to any stimulus for more than a few seconds. There appears to be rapid decay of memory traces in these children. They seem able to hold only a few units of information in their minds at one time. They will explore a stimulus and then come back to it as though it were a fresh stimulus. Therefore, when confronted with a complex situation, their at-

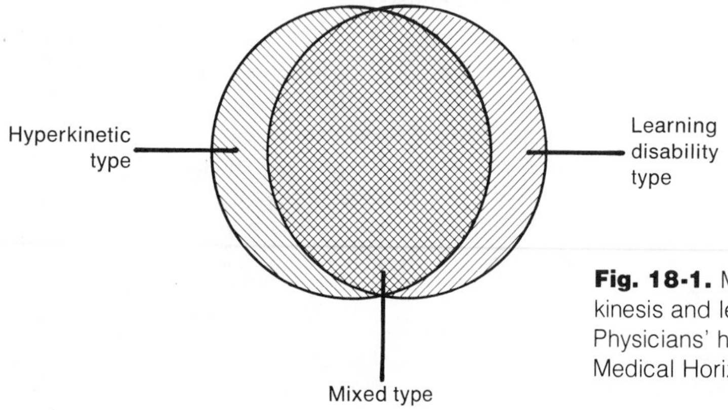

Fig. 18-1. Minimal brain dysfunction. Relationship between hyperkinesis and learning disabilities. (From Peters, J. E., and associates: Physicians' handbook; screening for MBD, Summit, N.J., 1973, Ciba Medical Horizons.)

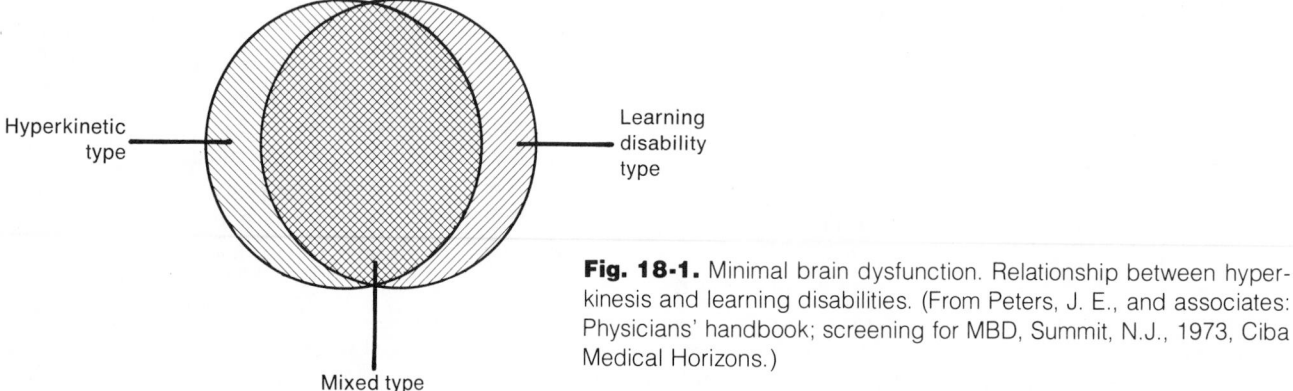

tention flits from one bit of information to another, since they are unable to integrate and synthesize the information, which results in failure.

Distractibility. Without great and conscious effort, these children are unable to inhibit their response to any stimulus, regardless of meaning or significance. Although they are able to concentrate in a quiet, isolated environment, they are highly susceptible to interruptions from any stimulus. Apparently outside stimuli (noise, movement, and so on) evoke an orienting reflex that they are unable to inhibit.

Impulsiveness and inability to delay gratification. These children have difficulty in restraining their impulses to move or speak. They appear to act or speak before they take time to reflect on it. They rush quickly into a task and are unable to wait for even a minute. They are usually overaggressive and often destructive; they tend to bully younger children and are rebellious and resentful of authority. They are accident prone.

Labile emotions or excitability. Children with minimal brain dysfunction are unable to inhibit their emotions. They may be quick to laughter or to tears. They are explosively volatile, and this irritability can be triggered by relatively minor stimuli; they recover from their emotional outburst equally fast and are easily distracted.

Poor motor integration or coordination. Integration of motor function is impaired in both fine and gross motor control. Many of these children are described as "clumsy." They also exhibit many extraneous movements and have difficulty in modulating their motions or voices. Their arms swing too fast and too hard; their voice is too loud.

Perceptual deficits. These children frequently have difficulty with perception of time, space, form, sound, and sequence. They confuse right and left; in front of and in back of; before and after; yesterday, today, and tomorrow; and so on. The concepts and names for directional movement in space and time create confusion and frustration. For example, the simple act of writing the alphabet involves a complex sequence of movements in four directions—right, left, up, and down; arithmetic processes involve the same directional movements. They may reverse letters and figures or produce mirror writing.

Impaired language or symbol development. Many children with minimal brain dysfunction are delayed in talking or in conventional word ordering. Often they have difficulty in reading (dyslexia), spelling (dysorthographia), and writing (dysgraphia).

Perseveration. Some children repeat persistently in almost every area (oral responses, movement), but this is seen more often in writing or copying when a word is involuntarily copied over and over again.

Overattention. Some children exhibit what might be termed attention fixation, in which they focus on one particular object and seem unable to break the focus.

Impaired memory. The highly complicated process of memory is often affected to the degree that a child may not be able to repeat a simple sequence of three words immediately after hearing them or remember where specific and familiar items of furniture are placed.

Hypoactivity. Although seen much less frequently than hyperactivity, a diminished activity level is not unusual in some children with learning disabilities. Since the child's behavior causes no disturbance to others, it is often overlooked as a manifestation.

Diagnosis. It is important that a diagnosis of minimal brain dysfunction be made as early as possible because of the long-term effects that may be generated by the child's behavior. The most significant and essential tool for diagnosis is a thorough history. Neurologic and psychologic examinations are useful in detecting specific defects, and observations made in a familiar environment may help confirm suspicions. However, it is the history that ultimately determines the diagnosis. The child seldom displays symptoms in the physician's office and acts reasonably normal in a one-to-one relationship.

Table 18-1. Most common behavior characteristics of children with minimal brain dysfunction

Likelihood of displaying	Hyperkinetic type	Mixed type	Learning disability type
High	Hyperactivity Short attention span Distractibility Impulsiveness Excitability	Hyperactivity Short attention span Distractibility Poor motor coordination Right-left confusion Dyslexia Dysgraphia Dysorthographia	Hypoactivity Right-left confusion Dysgraphia Dyslexia Dysorthographia
Less frequent	Clumsiness May have mild problems in writing, reading, spelling, and mathematics secondary to haste	Impulsiveness Hypoactivity Dyscalculia	Short attention span Dyscalculia

A history and description of the child's behavior should be obtained from as many observers of the child as possible, especially parents and teachers, as well as the observations of the health professionals involved. It should include descriptions of the child's behavior in home and school situations. In obtaining descriptive material the interviewer must question the observers carefully since some persons, especially parents, may be so concerned with gross behaviors that they often overlook less distressing but equally important symptoms.

The history should include both a medical and developmental history. Hyperactivity, for example, is usually evident from the onset. Parents may report a "colicky" infant, a child who began to run as soon as he walked, a toddler who was compelled to touch everything he saw, and a child who resisted sleep until exhausted. A history of delayed or atypical language development is associated with specific learning disabilities. A pregnancy and birth history may provide clues to a situation that might have produced an episode of hypoxia.

Although the history suggests the diagnosis, other neurologic tests are frequently useful. A physical examination including a detailed neurologic evaluation will help rule out any severe neurologic disorders. Psychologic testing, especially projective tests, is valuable in determining visual-perceptual difficulties, problems with spatial organization, and other phenomena that suggest cortical or diencephalic involvement and helps to identify the child's intelligence and achievement levels. Psychiatric disorders need to be ruled out. Other causes of hyperactivity that may need to be ruled out include lead poisoning, petit mal seizures, partial hearing loss, psychosis, and witnessing sexual activity (common in children in lower socioeconomic groups).

The value of the electroencephalogram as a diagnostic tool is a disputed issue. Its greatest value is probably the differentiation of other disorders, such as a temporal lobe seizure disorder or "absence spells" in a child who reacts with hyperactivity out of sheer frustration, that may show some feature of the hyperkinetic syndrome.

Management and nursing considerations

Management of the child with minimal brain dysfunction usually involves a multiple approach that includes family education and counseling, medication, remedial education, environmental manipulation, and sometimes psychotherapy for the child.

Nurses are active participants in all aspects of management of the child with minimal brain dysfunction. Nurses in the community setting work with families in the home on a long-term basis to help plan and implement therapeutic regimens and to evaluate the effectiveness of therapy. They are in the best position to coordinate services and serve as liaison between other health and education professionals directly involved in a child's therapy program. The nurse in the school who has an understanding of the child's special needs can work with teachers. The nurse in any setting (community, school, hospital, or physician's office) can provide support and guidance to children and families during the difficult tasks associated with growing up with a handicapping condition.

Family counseling and education. The management of the child with minimal brain dysfunction begins with an explanation to the parents and the child about the diagnosis, including a description of the nature of the problem and the physician's concept of the underlying central nervous system basis for the disorder. Most parents are confused and feel some measure of guilt. To some it is confirmation of the fear that the child may be "crazy" or has something irrevocably bad; to others it is a relief. They need the opportunity to ventilate their feelings and suspicions. A common complaint of parents is that health professionals have not listened to what they have to say about their child.

The parents need information about the prognosis and an understanding of the treatment plan. The greater their understanding of the disorder and its effects, the more likely they will be to carry out the recommended program of therapy. It is important that they understand that the therapy is not necessarily a panacea and that it will extend over a long period. This has particular significance for changes they need to make in environmental management.

Medication. Extensive experience with central nervous stimulants has demonstrated them to be highly effective in reducing many of the symptoms in children with minimal brain dysfunction. The most prominent of these are amphetamines, such as amphetamine sulfate (Benzedrine) and dextroamphetamine sulfate (Dexedrine), and methylphenidate (Ritalin). It is believed that these drugs produce their effect by direct action on the reticular activating system and/or by stimulating the release of norepinephrine from nerve endings in the brain stem. The effect of the medication in alleviating the signs and symptoms of minimal brain dysfunction is often so striking that it provides a diagnostic test for the condition. However, not all children benefit from medications. Those who do may respond to only one medication or to a combination of two medications, and the effective dosage varies from child to child. However, most physicians believe that any child with minimal brain dysfunction deserves a trial of medication. If no response is noted in 3 to 6 weeks, the drug is probably not effective and should be discontinued.

The child is begun on a small dosage that is gradually increased until the desired response is achieved. When evaluating the child's response to the medication, it is helpful to obtain reports from the teacher as well as from the parents, since the parents may see the child when the effects of the drug are wearing off. Observing the child's

Summary of nursing care of the child with minimal brain dysfunction

Goals	Responsibilities
Identify minimal brain dysfunction	Observe directly child's behavior Gather objective data from observers of the child Assist with screening tests Refer child with manifestations to appropriate persons or agencies for diagnosis
Provide therapeutic physical environment	Assess home and family Assist families in planning environmental manipulation program to reduce stimulation and stress Reduce or eliminate special hazards that threaten safety Help to find suitable programs that can meet child's special needs Assess school environment Assist teacher and others to reduce distracting stimuli Provide sanctuary to which child can retreat during particularly stressful times
Reduce symptoms	See that child takes medication as ordered Instruct parents in administration of medications Instruct parents in management techniques Counsel regarding diet if prescribed
Counsel family	Continue ongoing evaluation of situation Be a sympathetic listener Assist family to cope with identified problems Provide reassurance, support, and positive feedback Assist parents to improve parenting techniques Assist parents in planning activities for child Assist parents to control child's behavior with appropriate disciplinary techniques
Provide for energy outlet	Plan for periods of outdoor activity with large-muscle activity and loud vocal outlets Channel need for movement into safe, acceptable activities
Acquire needed services	Refer to appropriate persons and/or agencies Coordinate services between family, school, and agencies or persons involved in care
Participate in education of community	Seek and/or take advantage of opportunities to teach individuals and groups about minimal brain dysfunction
Evaluate effectiveness of programs	Provide ongoing observation and assessment of therapeutic regimens Report findings to appropriate persons

behavior through visits to home and school is useful for assessing his attention span, interactional patterns with others at school, and behaviors with academic tasks. The nurse can consult with the teacher about the child's behavior in general. This information provides data so that appropriate dosages can be regulated based on recorded, systematic observations of the child's behaviors in at least two settings. The optimal daily dose varies according to the child and ranges from 5 to 50 mg of amphetamine and 5 to 120 mg of methylphenidate. In time the need for medication changes and eventually becomes nonexistent. At this point if discontinuance of the drug does not bring on a return of symptoms or if, instead of reducing overactivity, symptoms of overstimulation (the usual effects of amphetamine) begin to appear, the need for medication is past.

Parents need to be informed of the possible side effects of the medication, that is, anorexia, blurred vision, and sleeplessness, which usually disappear after several weeks. A common complaint is that the child becomes quiet and very sensitive, crying at the slightest provocation. Another troublesome side effect is depressed growth probably caused by interference with the release of growth hormone; therefore, the physician may sometimes discontinue the drug on weekends or on vacations to allow for some catch-up growth. Parents may express concern that the child may become addicted to antidepressant drugs. There is always the possibility of abuse; however, usually the child is no longer interested in the drug once the need is past—particularly since the effect of the drug in these children is opposite that produced in normal individuals.

Medications that have been tried with varying success are chlorpromazine (Thorazine), chlordiazepoxide (Librium), imipramine (Tofranil), and thioridazine (Mellaril). Phenobarbital should be avoided since it may potentiate the action of some tranquilizers and antihistamines to aggravate the behavior. The therapeutic dose is very close to the toxic dose. Other treatments have been advanced by several observers but need further investigation before they achieve extensive adoption.

Environmental manipulation. The child's environment is simplified by decreasing external stimuli, reducing alternatives, encouraging desired patterns of behavior, and, sometimes, controlling his diet. The parents may need assistance to determine firm but reasonable limits and support in their efforts to provide a stable and predictable environment with regular routines of sleep, eating, working, and playing. The child needs an environment in which distractions are reduced to a minimum and that is relatively free of external stimuli. Also, the more the environment is controlled, the less medication is required.

Remedial education. Special training activities in the schools are designed to offer a direct attack on such areas of deficit as visual perception, auditory perception, and other areas involving integration and coordination. These may be accomplished in self-contained classes with a limit of six to eight children, special resource rooms with equipment and teaching teams, mobile consultants who move from room to room to provide assistance to teachers and children, and special first-grade programs in which high-risk children receive special attention to prevent or reduce the need for services as they progress. The purpose of programs for children with special learning disabilities is to assist them toward more successful achievement, personal adjustment, and eventual retention in the regular classroom.[6] However, because a true perceptual problem exists, improvement is noted by an increased attention span, allowing the child to focus on one stimulus while blocking out others; refinement of fine motor control; and advancement in other areas of disability.

Psychiatric, psychologic, and social therapies. On the whole, psychotherapy is relatively unsuccessful in the treatment of the basic characteristics of minimal brain dysfunction. However, psychotherapy is sometimes useful in the child who has experienced negative experiences to the extent that his self-image is threatened. Often children with minimal brain dysfunction describe themselves as stupid or "mentally retarded." They are different from the other children, and they know it. Although they have strengths, they do not get an opportunity to demonstrate them. Consequently they develop coping mechanisms to deal with their negative self-image. They are restless and disruptive, resort to clowning, and develop somatic symptoms. They may become apathetic, resort to daydreaming, appear "not to care," or display perfectionistic perseverence in the attempt to do well. Shy children may withdraw. The child with behavior problems is the one who will get help earlier than the quiet child. Therefore, the quiet child may not receive help until the problem is well advanced, which places him at a disadvantage since remediation takes longer when it is begun with older children. Both child and family may need help during certain periods of stress. Professionals who serve as consultants to health professionals, schools, and families include education specialists, language specialists, and behavior technologists as well as psychologists, social workers, and physician specialists. For a summary of nursing care of the child with minimal brain dysfunction see the boxed material on p. 645.

ENURESIS

Enuresis is a common and troublesome disorder that is difficult to define because of the variable ages at which children achieve bladder control. Bladder control depends on a number of factors, including the individual child's developmental tempo, the manner in which training is carried out, the personality makeup of the child, and the emotional climate of the home environment. In a broad sense enuresis can be defined as repeated involuntary urination (usually nocturnal) in children who are beyond the age when voluntary bladder control should normally have been acquired. Some authorities place 4 years as an arbitrary age by which diurnal and nocturnal bladder control is normally accomplished, although 5 years of age is probably more accurate.

Enuresis can also be defined as *primary,* wherein there has never been a long dry or symptom-free period, or *secondary* or *acquired,* in which the enuresis occurs after a dry period of at least a year, and as nightime *(nocturnal)*, daytime *(diurnal)*, or both. The incidence is approximately 5% to 17% in otherwise normal children between 3 and 15 years of age.

Etiology and pathophysiology

There is no clear-cut etiology for enuresis as a distinct entity. Some observers have established a hereditary basis in a number of instances. There appears to be a high frequency of bed-wetting in parents, siblings, and other near relatives of symptomatic children, and these observations are supported by a high concordance rate in enuretic monozygotic twins. Family studies indicate that the closer the relationship, the higher the incidence of enuresis.[2] It appears that these persons have difficulty in inhibiting the mechanisms that regulate the emptying of the bladder.

Enuresis is more common in boys than in girls, although the reason for this higher frequency is not altogether clear. Some authorities believe that it may be related to the fact that girls are usually neater and more conscious of cleanliness than boys and that they more readily respond to training procedures. There is a high frequency in children in the lower socioeconomic groups, and a higher frequency has been observed in black children than in white children. Socioeconomic differences are probably related to a number of incidental factors. Bed-wetting is less frequent in homes where cleanliness is prized, a toilet is nearby, bedtime fluid intake is regulated, the mother makes a special effort with toilet training, and the child is taken from the bed to empty his bladder during the night. Bed-wetting is more apt to be increased in children who live in homes in which poor habits of cleanliness are practiced, toilet facilities are not readily accessible, and the temperature is cold at night and in children who sleep with a bed-wetting sibling.

Organic causes that may be related to enuresis should be ruled out before psychogenic factors are considered. These include structural disorders of the urinary tract, urinary tract infection, major neurologic deficits, nocturnal epilepsy, disorders such as diabetes mellitus and diabetes insipidus that increase the normal output of urine, and disorders such as chronic renal failure or sickle cell disease that impair the concentrating ability of the kidneys. In other cases the enuresis is influenced by emotional factors, although it is doubtful that they are etiologic factors.

Enuresis is primarily a maturation problem and, as such, is benign and self-limiting. There are children who exhibit temporary regressive behavior after the birth of a sibling or who have occasional ''accidents'' when they become involved in play to such an extent that they are unaware of a full bladder, become excited, or ''forget'' to empty the bladder. In other children enuresis may be caused by problems associated with toilet training that are related to the age at which training is begun, the emotional atmosphere that surrounds the training situation, or an excessive amount of emotional dependence on the mother. In some children enuresis is one behavioral manifestation of a personality disorder. However, behavioral problems associated with enuresis are probably a result, rather than a cause, of the enuresis.

A significant number of nocturnal enuretic episodes are related to deep sleep. These children seem to sleep more soundly than others and fail to waken from either external or internal stimuli. Many of these children demonstrate increased frequency and magnitude of spontaneous bladder contractions during the non-REM stage of sleep preceding bed-wetting. Bed-wetting appears to occur as the child moves from the deeper stages of non-REM sleep into the REM stage.

Enuresis has a strong familial tendency and seems to be associated with a developmental delay that causes such intense urgency that the child is unable to inhibit bladder contraction after the bladder is distended beyond a certain volume. Such children acquire bladder control with difficulty and, even after control, are more prone to enuresis when subjected to stress than are other children. Also, most enuretic children have a borderline functional bladder capacity. The small bladder is unable to hold a full night's urine excretion.

Diagnostic evaluation

In most enuretic children nocturnal bed-wetting is a primary maturational problem and usually ceases between 6 and 8 years of age, although it sometimes continues into adolescence. The predominant symptom is urgency that is immediate and accompanied by acute discomfort, restlessness, and sometimes urinary frequency. Nocturnal enuresis is most common and is occasionally accompanied by diurnal wetting; diurnal bed-wetting without nocturnal bed-wetting is unusual.

In older children routine examinations are carried out to rule out infection and bladder capacity is determined by having the child hold off voiding until he feels urgency, at which time he voids into a measured container. A bladder volume of 300 to 350 ml is sufficient to hold a night's urine. Suspected congenital anomalies such as urethral stricture, stenosis, and valves are ruled out, and the child is tested for the presence of organic disease.

Management and nursing considerations

Enuresis not resulting from organic causes can be approached in several ways. No method is so successful as to achieve universal endorsement; however, some have proved helpful in keeping the child dry during the night. Frequently more than one technique is employed.

Emotional support. Essential to the success of any method is the supportive management of parents and child. Both need encouragement and patience. The problem is discussed with the parents and, since any treatment involves the child and requires his active participation, he should be included as well. Many parents believe that enuresis is caused by an emotional disturbance and fear that they have somehow produced the situation by imprudent child-rearing practices. They need reassurance that the bed-wetting is not a manifestation of emotional disturbance nor does it represent willful misbehavior. They should be informed about the nature of enuresis and cautioned against scolding, shaming, threatening, and punishing the child, which are useless and harmful. Communication with the child is directed toward eliminating the emotional impact of the problem by relieving him of feelings of shame, guilt, and the burden of parental disapproval and toward building up his self-confidence and motivating him toward independent control.

Conditioning devices. A number of electrical devices are available that are based on the conditioned reflex response. These consist of a wire pad attached to a bell or buzzer that wakens the child as soon as the first drops of urine create a closed circuit. The child is thus conditioned to waken at the initiation of micturition or to the stimulus of the bell or buzzer. Most have reported a substantial success rate with the device. There appear to be no undesirable emotional effects, although this is debatable.

There are disadvantages to the use of electrical devices. A practical problem is the disturbance it may create when other children sleep in the same room or in the same bed. The child may be too sleepy or forget to reset the alarm following its activation to render it ineffective for the remainder of the night. There may be a risk of ulceration and scarring caused by slow electrolysis of tissue cells when the child does not hear the alarm or turns the alarm off without waking while the current continues to flow or when the batteries have run down to a feeble point where the alarm is insufficiently loud.

Drug therapy. A number of pharmacologic agents can be used in the treatment of enuresis, either alone or in combination with other techniques. The selection depends on the interpretation of the cause. The drug used most frequently is the tricyclic antidepressant drug imipramine, which exerts an anticholinergic action on the bladder to inhibit urination. The dosage and time of administration are individualized, and the drug is given in amounts sufficient to lighten sleep but not to cause wakefulness. The suggested length of treatment is 6 to 8 weeks followed by gradual withdrawal over a period of 4 weeks. Since this drug is dangerous in overdosage, parents must be cautioned about judicious usage and keeping supplies of the drug far from the reach of younger siblings.

Bladder training. It has been known for some time that enuretic children have smaller functional bladder capacities. Bladder training is aimed at stretching the bladder to accommodate increasingly larger volumes of urine. After forcing fluids the child is instructed to postpone voiding as long as he can tolerate it before emptying his bladder. The heightened threshold for retention allows the child to remain dry throughout the night.

Withholding fluids. Restricting or eliminating fluids after the evening meal is aimed at decreasing the output of urine during the night. This method has proved to be of questionable value.

Sleep interruption. Having the child void before retiring and then wakening him and taking him to the bathroom has met with limited success. Favorable responses are probably a result of the focused concern by both parents and child and of the positive behavioral reinforcement it provides. For this to be effective the parent should be sure that the child is fully awake when he empties his bladder.

No matter what techniques are employed, the nurse can help both child and parents to understand the problem of enuresis, the treatment plan, and the probable difficulties they may encounter in the process. More important, the nurse can provide consistent support and encouragement to help sustain them through the inconsistent and unpredictable treatment process. The child needs to believe that he is helping himself and to sustain feelings of confidence and hope.

SCHOOL PHOBIA

School phobia is a term used to describe children, other than beginning students, who resist going to school because of dread of the school situation, concerns with leaving home, or both. Anxiety that frequently verges on panic is a constant manifestation, and they can develop symptoms as a protective mechanism to keep them from facing the situation that distresses them. Physical symptoms are prominent and may affect any part of the body—anorexia, nausea, vomiting, diarrhea, dizziness, headache, leg pains, or abdominal pains, to name a few. They may even develop a low-grade fever. A striking feature of school phobia is the prompt subsiding of symptoms when it is evident that the child can remain at home. Another significant observation is absence of symptoms on weekends and holidays unless they are related to other places such as Sunday school or parties. Occasional mild reluctance is not uncommon among school children, but if the fear continues for longer than a few days it must be considered as a serious problem—a warning of an important personality problem. Professional help is recommended.

Unlike most other behavior problems of children, school phobia is more common in girls than in boys, there is no relationship to socioeconomic status, ethnic origin, or other subcultural affiliation, and no particular age predominates. The onset is usually sudden and precipitated by a school-related incident, and a poor attendance record for trivial reasons can be elicited by a careful history.

Etiology

School phobia can be caused by a number of factors. Sometimes the complaints can be related to a transient, specific cause such as fear of a mismatched or overcritical teacher, fear of failing an examination or giving an oral recitation for a painfully shy child, or discrimination based on race, dress, or physical defect. Sometimes it may be related to a school bully or threatening gang. An insecure home situation in which the child fears that he may be deserted by a parent while he is gone may be the basis of anxiety, especially if the parent has previously threatened to leave for some reason.

A frequent source of fear is separation anxiety based on a strong dependent relationship between the mother and child in which the child is reluctant to leave the mother and she is equally reluctant (even though this may be unconscious) to have him leave her. The intense need for closeness between mother and child is normal in infancy, but the persistence of this type of relationship into childhood is totally inappropriate. Characteristically these children are not afraid to go to school, but rather they are afraid to leave home. The symptoms may be precipitated by any situation that intensifies the mutual dependency between the mother and child, such as illness, arrival of a new baby, move to a strange neighborhood or a new school, or parental discord.

In some instances children have an unrealistic, exaggerated view of their abilities and achievements. When they feel threatened by incidents that challenge their estimate of themselves, such as a minor episode that leads to embarrassment, return from school after an absence, transfer to another class, or even imagined social or academic failure, they become anxious and withdraw, frequently seeking close proximity to the mother.

Management and nursing considerations

The treatment for school phobia depends on the cause. The children really *want* to go to school but just cannot force themselves to do so; they are not delinquent children. They are anxious, tense, and distressed because they are unable to muster enough courage to go to school. If the cause of the problem is an examination, relationships with a bully, or a mismatch between teacher and child, it can be dealt with accordingly. When the child is helped to understand and cope with his fear, the symptoms usually disappear spontaneously.

It is important that the child not be allowed to stay home from school. The longer the child is permitted to stay out of school, the more difficult it is to reenter. For the child with severe symptoms it may be necessary to make some modifications in school attendance. If he is unable to return to the regular classes, the child may be allowed to go to school on a part-time basis, spending the time in the counselor's office or the nurse's office and getting homework from the teacher after class. It may be necessary to transport the child to and from school or even have a parent attend class with him. However, this practice is not allowed to continue for an unlimited time, and the time limit should be agreed on beforehand. The essential factor is that the child should go back to school. He should return to school right away, maintain the pattern of going, and remain there even while a solution is being worked out. The school nurse can provide both teacher and parents with support in carrying out this plan of action.

Well-meaning parents or others who permit the child to stay away from school and support his efforts with written excuses only confirm his own feelings of worthlessness and inability to cope. In severe cases when returning to school is unsuccessful, professional psychiatric consultation is usually desirable to help identify possible distorted family relationships or a personality disturbance in the child and to help both child and family to understand the sources of the problem.

CHILDHOOD SCHIZOPHRENIA

Childhood schizophrenia is a term used to describe severe deviations in ego functioning and is generally reserved for psychotic disorders that appear after the first 4 or 5 years of life. Schizophrenia in adults occurs with relative frequency, and, although childhood psychosis is not as common, it is by no means rare. Nursing of psychotic children is a highly specialized area, but since these problems are being recognized with increasing frequency, a brief outline of the disorder will be included.

The symptomatology among children shows wide variation according to each affected child's developmental level, the age of onset, the nature of early childhood experiences, and the type of defense mechanisms used. However, the basic core disturbance is a lack of contact with reality and the subsequent development of a world of the child's own. Secondary characteristics represent impairment in a wide number of areas of development including cognition, perception, emotion, language, and physical motor control. The most common manifestations involve language disturbances, impaired interpersonal relationships, and inappropriate affect (outward expression of emotion).

Etiology

There is considerable disagreement regarding the cause of schizophrenia, both adult and childhood onset. Some authorities favor a biochemical basis, whereas others support the theory of a complex combination of psychosocial and environmental stresses. There is evidence to indicate that genetic factors contribute significantly to its development. The likelihood of children born to a schizophrenic parent to develop the disorder is fifteen times greater than for children in the general population—even when they are separated from the parent at an early age. There is also a high concordance rate (40% to 60%) in monozygotic (identical) twins.

Support for an interpersonal theory of schizophrenia comes from a number of sources. The major theories point to disturbed family or parent-child relationships as an etiologic basis. The types of interpersonal relationships that are believed to contribute to the development of schizophrenia in children include (1) cold, distant, nondemonstrative, and highly impersonal and mechanistic parents who rear their children in "emotional iceboxes" and produce individuals who are unable to relate to people; (2) parents who behave inappropriately for their age and sex in regard to themselves and the child, thus preventing him from learning appropriate forms of behavior; (3) disordered patterns of family interaction, including role relationships that are too ambiguous or too rigid and an unstable home environment, which hinder the development of a stable personal identity; and (4) parents who consistently place the child in double-bind situations, producing a child who, unable to make reasonable responses to confused communications, either fails to develop or loses his hold on rational existence. Although these and other theories have been investigated, no specific etiologic factors have been identified as unique to parents and families of psychotic children.

Diagnostic evaluation

Unlike the abrupt onset of the adult disorder, childhood schizophrenia is characterized by a gradual onset of neurotic symptoms followed by any of over 100 different abnormal manifestations, including the following:

- Bizarre behavioral patterns and stereotyped movements such as robot-like walking, whirling, or graceful gyrations
- Periods of hypoactivity alternating with periods of hyperactivity
- Inappropriate affect that ranges from flatness to explosiveness
- Common occurrences of temper tantrums
- Language disturbances such as speaking in fragmented sentences, parrot-like repetition of words, development of a private language, and altered tone of voice; some schizophrenic children are mute or will only utter a single word on rare occasions
- Distorted time orientation with a blending of past, present, and future
- Distorted sense of and use of their bodies
- Apparent denial of the human quality in people, such as attempting to use a person as a step stool to reach an object
- Conveying a nonhuman identity by action, sounds, or posture, such as barking or calling himself a vacuum cleaner
- Frequent occurrences of compulsive behavior and phobias

Management and nursing considerations

Both individual and group therapy approaches have been used, and the implementation of any treatment is contingent on available resources. Home treatment, day-care facilities, and residential treatment centers are all used for management of childhood psychosis. Often a combination of these approaches is advisable, for example, short-term hospitalization followed by weeks or months of outpatient group therapy and individual psychotherapy. Since the families of affected children are so important in the ultimate outcome of treatment, they are frequently involved in the therapy either together or separately.

Some drugs have been found useful as an adjunct to other therapies. Psychoactive drugs appear to reduce anxiety, impulsiveness, and disorganized behavioral patterns and produce more harmonious interpersonal relationships. Basically the pharmacologic agents used fall into two categories—tranquilizers and antidepressants. The selection of drugs depends on the child, the philosophy of the therapist, and the environment. Convulsive therapy, because of its controversial nature, is employed less frequently than in the past.

A more recent approach to the treatment of psychotic disorders is behavior therapy, which applies the application of the principles of learning theory to the modification of behavior. Based on the principles of classical conditioning, most methods employ positive reinforcement for desired behavior responses, and, in some instances, mild punishment is used in conjunction with the positive reinforcement. Although dramatic cures are not a reality and many complain that the children are psychotic in spite of alterations in the target behaviors, most believe that the technique has produced improvement and that these gains represent substantial progress in a large number of cases.

Common health problems

DENTAL PROBLEMS

Since all of the permanent teeth (except the wisdom teeth) erupt during middle childhood, dental health is of particular importance during this stage of development. Ideally children should receive regular preventive dental care and supervision in daily hygienic care from the time the teeth begin to erupt (see p. 512). The importance of dental care is undisputed; however, limited or inadequate dental care results in the most prevalent of all childhood health problems, chiefly dental caries, malocclusion, and trauma. Although these conditions are not considered illnesses, they have harmful long-range effects on children's health.

Dental caries

Dental caries is one of the most common chronic diseases that afflict mankind at all ages; it is the principal oral problem in children and adolescents. The implications for reducing the incidence and consequences of the disorder are highly significant in childhood because dental caries, if untreated, results in total destruction of involved teeth. The ages of greatest vulnerability are ages 4 to 8 years for the primary dentition and ages 12 to 18 years for the secondary or permanent dentition (see p. 59 for sequence of tooth eruption).

Etiology and pathophysiology. Dental caries is a multifactorial disease that involves susceptible teeth, cariogenic microflora, and an appropriate oral environment. The incidence of lesions and the likelihood of progressive invasion vary considerably and depend on a number of factors in the right combination.

Teeth. The prevalence of caries is directly related to the tooth anatomy. The areas most subject to attack by bacteria are (in order of difficulty of complete cleansing) grooves and fissures, interdermal areas, gum margins, and other smooth surfaces. Newly erupted teeth that have not yet acquired sufficient surface minerals are more susceptible to decay than those that have been erupted for 2 or more years. Undoubtedly hereditary factors influence resistance and susceptibility since similar patterns and anatomic characteristics are seen in successive generations.

Bacteria. Three types of microflora that produce different effects contribute to the formation of dental caries. Acidogenic bacteria act on fermentable carbohydrates in dental plaque to produce organic acids that decalcify hard surface tooth enamel. With the inner organic matrix exposed, proteolytic organisms and acids digest and destroy the inner tooth structure. These destructive organisms are harbored and protected in a gelatinous plaque formed on the tooth surface by still another group of bacteria that are thought to play no primary role in production of decay.

Substrates. The material on which the acid-forming bacteria act consists essentially of carbohydrates. Among the fermentable carbohydrates, sucrose has been consistently implicated as the most cariogenic. Caries formation is strongly influenced by the two concurrent processes that continually operate on enamel surfaces—acid production and acid neutralization by saliva. The type and frequency of foods and fluids containing sucrose that are placed in the mouth are of particular importance. Saliva and other foods that are ingested at mealtime tend to help neutralize much of the acid formed from sucrose. Sucrose-containing substances, especially in forms that cling, such as chewy candy, or that promote prolonged contact with the teeth, such as chewing gum, hard candy, and lollipops, when ingested between meals contribute markedly to the development of dental caries.

Other factors that contribute to caries formation are hereditary factors, the amount of fluoride in drinking water, lack of or ineffectual oral hygiene, and the child's general state of health. Hereditary factors appear to influence both resistance and susceptibility to dental caries. For example, structural defects, such as deep fissures on occlusive surfaces, predispose to decay, and persons in whom acid formation exceeds neutralization are more prone to caries. The effectiveness of the buffering action of saliva is highly variable among individuals.

It has been demonstrated that children who live in communities in which drinking water contains 1.0 part per million (ppm) or more of fluoride have a significantly lower incidence of dental caries than children in areas with a fluoride content less than 0.5 ppm. It appears that fluoride incorporated into the crystallites of the surface enamel increases the resistance to acid dissolution.

Poor oral hygiene that permits the accumulation of food debris on tooth surfaces provides for proliferation of acid-forming bacteria that thrive in this environment. Removal of food particles and bacteria-laden plaque inhibits destructive acid formation.

The susceptibility to dental decay may be influenced by the general health of the child. Children who suffer from chronic debilitating disease show increased caries activity as do children with systemic conditions that alter the quality and quantity of saliva produced.

Diagnostic evaluation. As mentioned previously, caries formation is most prevalent in areas where food easily becomes impacted such as fissures, between the teeth, and at the gum line. Because the permanent teeth erupt during this time, children are more susceptible to development of dental caries during middle childhood than at any other age. Caries in the vulnerable teeth penetrate rapidly at this age as opposed to the slower, intermittent activity characteristic at later ages.

Caries on visible surfaces are easily detected by oral inspection. Large, extensive caries are apparent even to the untrained eye, but small, beginning lesions are best identified by trained professionals. Caries between the teeth may not be located without x-ray examination.

Management. Dental caries can usually be controlled by the following measures[7]:

1. Frequent, regular observation by a dentist beginning when all primary teeth have erupted but at least by 3 years of age. The recommended frequency is usually twice yearly, but this depends on the individual child.
2. Progression of a carious lesion checked by surgical removal of all affected portions of involved teeth as soon as detected, preparation of a retentive cavity, and replacement of the lost portion of the tooth with a material that is durable in the mouth environment. This restoration of involved teeth not only prevents progression of established caries but reduces the number of bacteria in the oral cavity to decrease the danger to uninvolved teeth.
3. Oral hygiene that emphasizes thorough mechanical removal of plaque and other material from tooth surfaces by brushing, rinsing, and the use of dental floss. Cleansing is most effective when carried out after meals and snacks.
4. Elimination of concentrated sugars between meals and reducing the mealtime ingestion of sweets to a minimum. This includes excessive ingestion of sweetened soft drinks and juices.
5. Sound nutrition practices that include an adequate intake of building materials, such as protein, calcium, fluoride, and vitamin D, to help form teeth that resist caries and build healthy supporting structures. Also, an adequate amount of crunchy, chewable foods in the diet, such as apples, celery, and raw carrots, provides a detergent effect and helps to cleanse tooth surfaces as the child chews.
6. Topical application of fluoride to the teeth (except in communities where fluoride is already present in large amounts) that increases the concentration of fluoride in the surface enamel is believed to be the most effective preventive mea-

sure against dental caries in young children. Many pedodontists also advocate the use of fluoridated toothpaste for dental hygiene.

Nursing considerations. Oral inspection is an integral part of the nursing assessment of the child in any setting (see p. 139). If there is any evidence of dental caries or other unhealthy state, the child is referred for dental services. The family may have a family dentist or a pedodontist who can provide needed care. However, an alarming number of children do not receive regular dental supervision and a significant number reach adulthood without having been examined or treated by a dentist.

Nurses can serve as counselors to families regarding the importance of regular dental care, oral hygiene, and dietary management. They can encourage good oral hygiene by teaching correct tooth cleaning to both children and their parents. The random brushing allowed during the early childhood years should be replaced by more careful and methodical cleansing techniques. Children are taught to brush the teeth in a vertical direction and in the direction in which the teeth grow, and the proper use of dental floss. Sometimes the greatest task for nurses is not the teaching aspect of dental care but counseling children and families for motivation to develop sound dental hygiene and nutritional practices. Nurses can be active members of preventive educational programs.

Malocclusion

When teeth of the upper and lower dental arches approximate in the proper relationships, the physiologic function of mastication is more effective and the cosmetic effect is more pleasing. Teeth that are uneven, crowded, overlapping, or otherwise interfere with their ability to meet their opponents in the opposite jaw in the appropriate relationships may predispose to dental disease in later years.

The most common cause of malocclusion is hereditary factors, but abnormal growth and habits such as thumbsucking and tongue thrusting also contribute to the disordered alignment and occlusion of the teeth. The important aspects in treatment of malocclusion are elimination of habits that aggravate the deformity and corrective therapy at the optimal time. Orthodontic treatment is usually most successful when started in the later school-age years or the early teenage years after the last primary teeth are shed and before growth ceases. However, referral should be made as soon as malocclusion is evident since some deformities can be corrected at an earlier age. Often removal of extra teeth, impacted teeth, or prosthetic replacement of missing teeth can prevent problems from developing.

Trauma

Injury to the teeth is not an uncommon occurrence in childhood. This includes fractures of varying degrees of severity, dislocation, or evulsion. All tooth injuries require prompt treatment by a competent dentist in order to prevent permanent displacement or loss. Delayed examination and diagnosis of tooth damage all too frequently result in infection or pulp involvement that can be avoided by early attention.

Evulsed teeth should be carefully placed in saline solution until they can be replanted and stabilized, preferably by a dentist. If a dentist is not available, the child, parent, or nurse should replant the tooth as soon as possible. Prognosis for retention of the tooth depends on prompt reimplantation. It is important to rinse the tooth carefully before implantation to avoid disturbing the adhering periodontal membrane, which is essential to the success of the endeavor. The tooth will usually become firmly attached, although endodontic therapy is always required and the tooth is eventually replaced by a prosthetic device. The reimplanted tooth may be retained anywhere from 6 months to 12 years and serves to facilitate normal development and occlusion, since loss of teeth during the period of permanent tooth eruption may adversely affect such development.

ACCIDENTS

Because school-age children have developed more refined muscular coordination and control and can apply their cognitive capacities to a more judicious course of action, the incidence of accidents is diminished in children in this age-group when compared with the incidence in early childhood. As previously described, the type of accidents most prevalent in children in any age-group largely reflects the child's developmental stage (see p. 79).

As in all other age-groups, the most common cause of severe accidental injury and death in school-age children is motor vehicle accidents—either as pedestrian or passenger. The school-age child's penchant for riding bicycles increases the risk of injury on streets and byways, and other serious injuries associated with moving conveyances include accidents on skateboards, roller skates, skis, and other sports equipment. The most effective means of prevention is education of the child and family regarding the hazards of risk taking and improper use of the equipment.

Physically active, school-age children are highly susceptible to cuts and abrasions, and the incidence of childhood fractures, strains, and sprains is impressive. The incidence is significantly higher in school-age boys than in school-age girls, and most occur in or near the home or school. Accidental injuries of serious nature are discussed as appropriate elsewhere in the book, that is, burns (p. 1112), eye trauma (p. 855), near drowning (p. 1239), and head injuries (p. 1421), and need not be elaborated here. There is concern regarding some accidental injuries in school children, such as poisoning, that are considered to be nonaccidental unless specifically reported otherwise. The "accident" may be a manifestation of a significant mental health problem (see suicide, p. 765). The prevalence of accidents depends on the dangers present in the environment, the protection offered by adults, and the behavior patterns of the children.

Accident proneness

Although causative factors are controversial, there is a group of children who appear to be *accident prone,* that is, they suffer significantly more accidental injuries than the overall childhood population. Certain personality characteristics seem to be typical of these children (see the box on p. 82). One type of accident-prone child is overreactive, restless, and impulsive and, in situations of stress, becomes increasingly impulsive and disorganized to the point that he is unable to recognize or heed danger signals. The resentful, hostile child and the immature child who attempts to compete with others beyond his capacity in a hazardous environment are other types of children who have many accidents. In the latter two types the quality of parent-child relationships appears to be a significant factor. These parents provide less supervision, appear more distant with their children, and are casual in their attitudes toward the injuries. It is not established to what extent these accidents may be motivated. Certainly with the first type, whose characteristics are those of the child with a minimal brain dysfunction (see p. 641), and the immature child, this is doubtful. It has also been shown that children undergoing stressful changes in their lives are more susceptible to accidents.[9]

Parasitic disorders

A parasitic relationship involves a one-sided nutritive association between two organisms of different species in which one (the parasite) derives physical protection and nourishment from the other (the host) without reciprocation. Although this relationship can be fatal to the host, it is to the advantage of the parasite that the host is not destroyed. The effect on the host may be negligible or, with heavy infections, fatal. A parasitic relationship in which the parasite lives within the body of the host *(endoparasite)* is designated as an *infection*. Parasites that are attached to the skin or temporarily invade the superficial tissues *(ectoparasites)* produce an *infestation*. Less specifically, *parasitosis* is the state of infection or infestation with an animal parasite.

There are several ways in which damage can be inflicted on the host organism. When tissue repair takes place as rapidly as tissue destruction, often without demonstrable symptoms, the host is referred to as a *carrier*. A parasite that produces considerable damage resulting in varying degrees of disease is considered to be a *pathogen*. Parasites produce damage to the host by[12]:

1. Deprivation of nutrients and essential elements for the metabolic processes of the host
2. Destruction and/or loss of blood
3. Lytic necrosis and tissue digestion that may produce extensive damage, open sores, and/or perforation of organs
4. Mechanical interference with organ function because of location, such as serious obstruction of ducts and passages
5. Production of extensive tissue reactions in the host
6. Stimulation of hypersensitivity and toxic responses

Parasitic infection or infestation may be derived from one or more of the following sources[5]:

1. Contaminated soil or water
2. Food containing the immature infective stage of the parasite
3. A blood-sucking insect
4. A domestic or wild animal harboring the parasite
5. Another person or his clothing, bedding, or immediate environment that he has contaminated
6. One's self (reinfection)

There are numerous portals of entry through which parasites invade the host organism. The most common one is by way of the mouth, either ingested in food and water or transferred to the mouth from soil or other reservoirs via the hands or other objects. Some parasites actively enter the body from soil through the skin (hookworms) or are introduced percutaneously when an arthropod punctures the skin to feed (malarial parasites). Other methods of transmission include inhalation of eggs from the air, transplacental infection (toxoplasmosis), and sexual intercourse (trichomonas vaginalis).

Parasitic diseases constitute the most frequent infections in the world, and although many are concentrated in the tropical regions, others are not. A number of these infections are encountered with relative frequency in the United States and are of importance in children in the pediatric age-groups. Of the various species capable of infecting man, the helminths (worms), arthropods (spiders, insects), and protozoa are seen most frequently. Since arthropod infestations are considered later in relation to disorders affecting the skin, only helminthic infections will be discussed here.

HELMINTHIC INFECTIONS

Biologically the structure of helminths is adapted to a parasitic existence. With a ready supply of predigested nutrients and the ability to live under conditions that are essentially anaerobic, most systems of parasitic worms are greatly reduced or absent, with the exception of the reproductive system, which is greatly elaborated. The integument or outer covering of the parasite is designed to provide protection for the organism. It may be hardened, tough or elastic, or relatively delicate, but in most cases it is highly resistant to digestion while the organism is alive. It is often equipped with spines, hooks, cutting plates, stylets, or other armature for attachment to, penetration of, or abrasion of the host's tissues. Many are provided with secretory glands near the mouth that secrete a lytic substance to digest the

Table 18-2. Common helminthic infections

Infection and organism	Life cycle and pathogenesis	Clinical manifestation
Trichuriasis—*Trichuris trichiura* (whipworm)	Adult worms live in the cecum; in heavy infections, also in the colon and rectum; passed in feces, slow development in soil (3-4 weeks); eggs swallowed, larvae hatch in small intestine, penetrate villi and mature; return to lumen and migrate to cecum	Light infections: asymptomatic Heavy infections: abdominal pain and distention; diarrhea
Hookworm disease—*Necator americanus*	Worms live in small intestine and feed on villi; process of attachment produces bleeding; ova deposited in bowel, expelled in feces; hatch in damp, shaded soil; larvae attach to skin, penetrate and enter bloodstream, migrate to lungs, exit into alveoli, migrate to upper passages to be swallowed; develop in upper intestine	Light infections in well-nourished individuals: no problems Heavier infections: mild to severe anemia, malnutrition May be itching and burning ("ground itch") followed by erythema and a papular eruption
Strongyloidiasis—*Strongyloides stercoralis* (threadworm)	Life cycle similar to that of hookworm, except that worm is not attached to intestinal mucosa and feeding larvae (not eggs) may be deposited in soil; also, sometimes penetrate colonic mucosa and enter systemic circulation, migrate to respiratory structures, and are subsequently swallowed	Light infection: asymptomatic Heavy infection: respiratory signs and symptoms; abdominal pain, distention; nausea and vomiting; diarrhea—large pale stools, often with mucus Threat to life in children with weakened immunologic defenses
Trichinosis—*Trichinella spiralis*	A true parasite in all stages; can infect any carnivorous or omnivorous homothermic animal, most commonly hogs and rats; infection initiated by ingesting flesh containing encysted larvae, larvae escape to the stomach and small intestine; at maturity, fertilized females bore through intestinal wall, deposit fully developed larvae in mucous membrane or intestinal lymph spaces; larvae carried via bloodstream to all parts of body, especially skeletal muscles and diaphragm	Nonspecific and generalized: gastroenteritis during invasive phase; later myositis, periorbital edema, dyspnea, fever, enlarged lymph nodes; eosinophilia
Ascariasis*—*Ascaris lumbricoides* (common roundworm)	Adult lays eggs in small intestine; eggs deposited in stool; incubation in soil 2-3 weeks; swallowed eggs hatch in small intestine, larvae penetrate intestinal villi, enter portal vein to liver, proceed to lungs, rupture capillaries into respiratory system, ascend to upper passages to be swallowed, proceed to small intestine, and mature into adult worms (total time 2-3 months)	Light infections: asymptomatic Heavy infections: anorexia, irritability, nervousness, enlarged abdomen, weight loss, fever, intestinal colic Severe infections: intestinal obstruction, appendicitis, perforation of intestine with peritonitis, obstructive jaundice, lung involvement—pneumonitis
Enterobiasis (oxyuriasis)*—*Enterobius vermicularis* (pinworm, scatworm)	Adult lives in rectum or colon, emerges onto perianal skin during hours of sleep to lay eggs; scratching of itching perianal area transfers eggs to hands, then to mouth to be swallowed; hatch in the upper intestine, travel to the bowel, attaches to the bowel wall and matures in about 2-3 weeks	Intense itching of perianal area; no systemic reaction In females, adult may migrate to vagina to produce perivaginal itching Rarely, appendicitis
Visceral larva migrans*—*Toxocara canis* (dogs) Intestinal toxocariasis *Toxocara cati* (cats)	In natural host (dog), larvae migrate to liver and lungs and reach maturity in intestines; when ingested by immature host (man), larvae migrate aimlessly to become encapsulated in muscles and organs such as liver, lungs, kidney, eye, and brain; most serious are those in eye and central nervous system	Depends on reactivity of infected individual May be asymptomatic except for eosinophilia Specific diagnosis difficult

*Diseases caused by nematodes (roundworms).

Special examination	Transmission and prevention	Treatment	Comments
Ova in fecal smears	Transmitted from contaminated soil, vegetables, toys, and other objects	Mebendazole (Vermox), 1 tablet twice daily for 3 days	Most frequent in warm, moist climates Occurs most often in undernourished children living in unsanitary conditions
Ova in fecal smears Positive occult blood in stools in heavier infections	Humans initiate extrinsic phase by discharging eggs on the soil and, in turn, pick up infection from direct skin contact with contaminated soil Prevention: proper sanitary disposal of human excreta	Bephenium hydroxynaphthoate (Alcopara), single dose of 2.5 g (children <20 kg), 5 g (children >20 kg), or daily Tetrachloroethylene, single dose of 0.1-0.12 mg/kg, not to exceed 5 ml Pyrantel pamoate, single dose of 10-11 mg/kg, not to exceed 1 g	Wearing shoes is helpful, although children playing in contaminated soil expose many skin surfaces
Larvae in feces and duodenal aspirate; sometimes in sputum	Same as above except autoinfection common	Thiabendazole (Mintezol), 25 mg/kg orally twice daily or 50 mg/kg once daily for 2 days	Older children and adults affected more often than young children Severe infections may lead to severe nutrition deficiency
History of eating poorly cooked pork Diagnosis by muscle biopsy	Thorough cooking of pork	Corticosteroids for symptoms Thiabendazole kills worms in intestines; no effect on larvae in muscles No treatment for muscle involvement	Seldom affects infants and young children More common in Europe and North America
Microscopic examination of stool for ova and parasites	Transferred to mouth by way of contaminated food, fingers, toys, etc. Community sanitation	Pyrantel pamoate (Antiminth), single dose of 10-11 mg/kg, not to exceed 1 g Piperazine citrate (numerous preparations), 1.0-3.5 g each day for 2 days Mebendazole (Vermox), 1 tablet twice daily for 3 days	Affects principally young children 1-4 years of age Prevalent in warm climates Reinfection is the rule
Microscopic examination of perianal swabbings Cellulose tape examinations: sticky surface of tape is firmly pressed against perianal folds, then placed, sticky side down, on a slide, which is subsequently examined under a microscope	Transferred to mouth by fingers from scratching or from soiled night clothes, underclothes, bed linens, or other contaminated objects; may breathe in and ingest airborne eggs	Pyrvinium pamoate (Povan), single dose of 5 mg/kg Piperazine citrate, 65 mg/kg/day for 8 days, not to exceed 2.5 mg/day Pyrantel pamoate (Antiminth), 10 mg/kg, not to exceed 1 g If tolerated, repeat in 2 weeks Mebendazole	Sometimes other family members are treated as well as affected child Povan stains clothing, vomitus, and stool; parents may mistake for blood
Difficult to detect in humans; organ biopsy Suspected by eosinophilia and elevated isoagglutinin titers	Transmitted by direct contamination of hands from contact with dog, cat, or objects or ingestion of soil Dogs and cats should be kept away from areas where children play; sandboxes especially important transmission areas Periodic deworming of diagnosed dogs and cats Control of dog population Continued education and laws to prevent indiscriminate canine defecation	No specific therapy known	

tissues of the host for food or enable the parasite to migrate through the host to the optimum site for maturation.

Depending on the organism, the life cycle of the parasite may or may not require an intermediate host, such as an animal, for example, dog, or insect, for example, mosquito or flea. An understanding of the life cycle of the infecting parasite, its mode of transmission, the site in the body where it becomes established, the symptomatology displayed by the host, and the habits of the host is essential in planning the eradication of the organism and/or prevention of infection. Most infections result from ingestion of parasite eggs that hatch within the environment of the host. Depending on the organism, the eggs may continue to mature within the gastrointestinal tract; the hatched larvae may burrow through the intestinal lining to the bloodstream where they are carried to the lungs (usually) or other organs; or the organisms may make their way through ducts and passages to other areas where they produce symptoms associated with the affected organs. Light infections may be asymptomatic, but all infections produce symptoms and pathology when present in large numbers. In general, parasitic worms do not multiply in the host; therefore, the number of worms in the body depends on the intensity (especially the first) and the frequency of exposure. Parasitic helminthic infections in man include those caused by nematodes (roundworms), cestodes (tapeworms), and trematodes (flukes). Tapeworm and fluke infections are rare in North America; therefore, the discussion will be limited to those caused by the more common nematodes. Table 18-2 describes the outstanding features of these parasitic infections, including treatment.

Nursing considerations

Nursing responsibilities related to parasitic worm infections are directed toward identification of the parasite, treatment of the infection, and prevention of initial infection or reinfection. Identification of the organism is accomplished by laboratory examination of substances containing the worm, its larvae, or embryonated ova. Most are identified by examining feces smears from the stools of persons suspected of harboring the parasite. Stool specimens should be large enough to get an ample sampling, not merely a fecal fragment. Fresh specimens are best for revealing parasites or larvae; therefore, collected specimens should be taken directly to the laboratory for examination. Pinworm specimens are collected in the morning before the child has a bowel movement or bathes, usually before he gets out of bed. A loop of transparent tape, sticky side out, is placed around the end of a tongue depressor, which is then firmly pressed to the child's perianal area, first one side, then the other, to attach eggs to both sides. A convenient commercially prepared tape can be given to the parents. If the parents collect the specimen, they should be instructed to place the tongue blade in a glass jar or loosely in a plastic bag so that it can be brought in for microscopic examination. For specimens collected in the hospital, physician's office, or clinic, the tape is placed smoothly on a glass slide, sticky side down, for examination.

In most worm infections examination of other family members, especially children, may be carried out to identify those who are similarly affected. (With pinworm infections, rather than performing clear tape tests on all members, the entire family is often treated.) Nurses are frequently the persons who assume the responsibility for directing and instructing the families in the collection and disposition of specimens. The treatment regimen may need further explanation and reinforcement, especially when it involves other members of the household and care of clothing and bed linen. When other members are treated, the family needs to understand the nature of transmission and that, in many cases, the medication is repeated in 2 weeks to 1 month to kill organisms that have been hatched since the initial treatment.

The child with pinworm infection is especially prone to continual reinfection, particularly via the anal-oral route. Pinworm eggs persist in the home to contaminate anything they contact, such as hands, bed linen, underwear, and food. They may float in the air. Parents are instructed to wash all bedding immediately after treatment. The child should wear a clean pair of long pajamas to sleep in each night and underclothing that fits snugly and is changed daily. All underwear and bed linen are washed in hot water to kill any adherent eggs, and pajamas are ironed with a hot iron. The child's fingernails should be cut short to minimize the chance of ova collecting under the nails. The movement of the worms on skin and mucous membrane surfaces causes intense itching that promotes scratching and contributes to reinfection and secondary infection and sometimes aids in the diagnosis. In both home and hospital, bed linen and clothing should be handled carefully to avoid scattering eggs into the air and onto the floor.

The nurse's most important function in relation to these parasites is preventive education of children and families regarding good hygiene and health habits. The importance of careful hand washing before eating or handling food, after using the toilet, or before placing fingers in the mouth should be emphasized. Children and parents need to be cautioned about washing foods that have been in or near the soil, such as raw fruits and vegetables, or food that has fallen on the floor. Children need to be discouraged from biting their nails or scratching the bare anal area. Contaminated soil can be carried long distances on feet into houses or conveyances. Children should be taught to wear shoes when they are outside.

In areas where infections are endemic or where sanitary conditions are conducive to continued infection and reinfection, nurses can, hopefully, become involved in working with public health officials for provision of better living conditions, such as reduction of overcrowding in living accommodations and provision of adequate, sanitary disposal systems for human feces.

Disorders affecting the skin

The skin, the largest organ in the body, is not merely a covering but is a complex structure that serves many functions, the most important of which is to protect the tissues that it encloses as well as protecting itself. This pliable sheath is a vital shield against the shifting physical and chemical stresses of the environment, and this role is fulfilled to the extent that outside changes are not transmitted inward to upset the body's internal equilibrium. The skin is primarily an insulator, not an organ of exchange.

Purposes of the skin

This functionally simple but morphologically complex structure serves several physical functions that are essential to life:

Protection. The skin serves as a protection against trauma, including mechanical, thermal, chemical, and radiant. Anatomically and physiologically the skin differs in different areas of the body. The intact tough outer layer is a mechanical barrier. Organisms and chemicals penetrate it with difficulty, and it is further protected by the oily and slightly acid secretions of its sebaceous glands, which limit the growth of bacteria.

Impermeability. Very few substances are able to penetrate the skin with ease. It seals the body from the environment. The outer side of the upper layer, with its low water content, is in equilibrium with the viable cells underneath. It protects against loss of essential body constituents to the environment. The effectiveness of this impermeable membrane is demonstrated by the profuse fluid loss that follows damage to the epidermis by superficial burns, injury, poison ivy, or other agents. Loss of water and some electrolytes takes place only through pores in this effective barrier.

Heat regulation. The skin also adjusts heat loss to heat production to maintain the thermal balance of the body. This is accomplished primarily through functioning of cutaneous blood vessels and sweat glands. The vascular supply to the skin, much more extensive than needed for tissue nourishment, is regulated by way of central and local neural and hormonal processes.

Touch, pain, heat, and cold. As a sensory organ, these perceptions are registered through the nerves that permeate the skin. To some extent, it is also an organ of expression that betrays strong feelings: blushing (shame or embarrassment), redness (anger), blanching (fear), and sweating (anxiety).

Structure of the skin

Anatomically and physiologically the skin differs markedly in various areas of the body, and each variation is adapted to meet special stresses. These regions, such as the soles of the feet, the eyelids, and the back, vary in thickness and looseness and in the kinds and quantities of appendages they contain, such as sweat glands and hair follicles. These variations are the basis for the localization of many disorders to specific areas and for the distribution of certain eruptions in characteristic patterns.

The basic structure of the skin consists of three layers (Fig. 18-2).

Epidermis. The epidermis, the outermost cellular membrane of relatively uniform thickness, is separated from the middle portion by a layer of specialized cells called basal cells. The cells in this layer are continually reproducing the cell population, and, as they multiply, the daughter cells are displaced outwardly by this constant stream of new cells. In their progress to the surface, these cells progressively flatten, gradually age, and are otherwise altered until they form dead cornified or horny flakes that are constantly sloughed off the surface of the body. These flattened, scalelike, adherent epidermal cells are composed of *keratin* and contain no cellular details. The epidermis is continually renewing itself, nourished by fluid from blood vessels in the dermis. In pathologic conditions these cells stick together to form flakes or scales, a sign of epidermal damage.

Elaborating this outer layer are specialized cellular invaginations of epidermal origin, the glandular appendage and hair follicles. Although they are situated mainly in the dermis, these structures are lined with epithelial cells and are derived from the epithelial skin layer. This has significance when a large area of epidermis is damaged. It is from the cells lining these structures that new epithelium is derived.

Diseases of the skin focus sharply on the epidermis, which is the site of many distinctive patterns ranging from the vesiculation of contact dermatitis to common superficial tumors. Clearly visible, these morphologic changes produce the varied patterns on which a dermatologic diagnosis is made.

Dermis. The dermis or *corium* comprises the major portion of the skin. It is a firm, fibrous, and elastic connective tissue network containing an elaborate system of blood vessels, lymphatics, and nerves and varies throughout the body from 1 to 4 mm in thickness. In addition it is invaded by the epidermal downgrowth of hair follicles and glands. Functionally the corium has a major protective role for these varied essential components of the skin.

More hidden than the epidermis, changes in the corium are more difficult to interpret on inspection. Biopsy and histologic studies are more often needed to confirm a diagnosis based on manifestations in the corium. Since it is composed predominantly of connective tissue, the dermis fre-

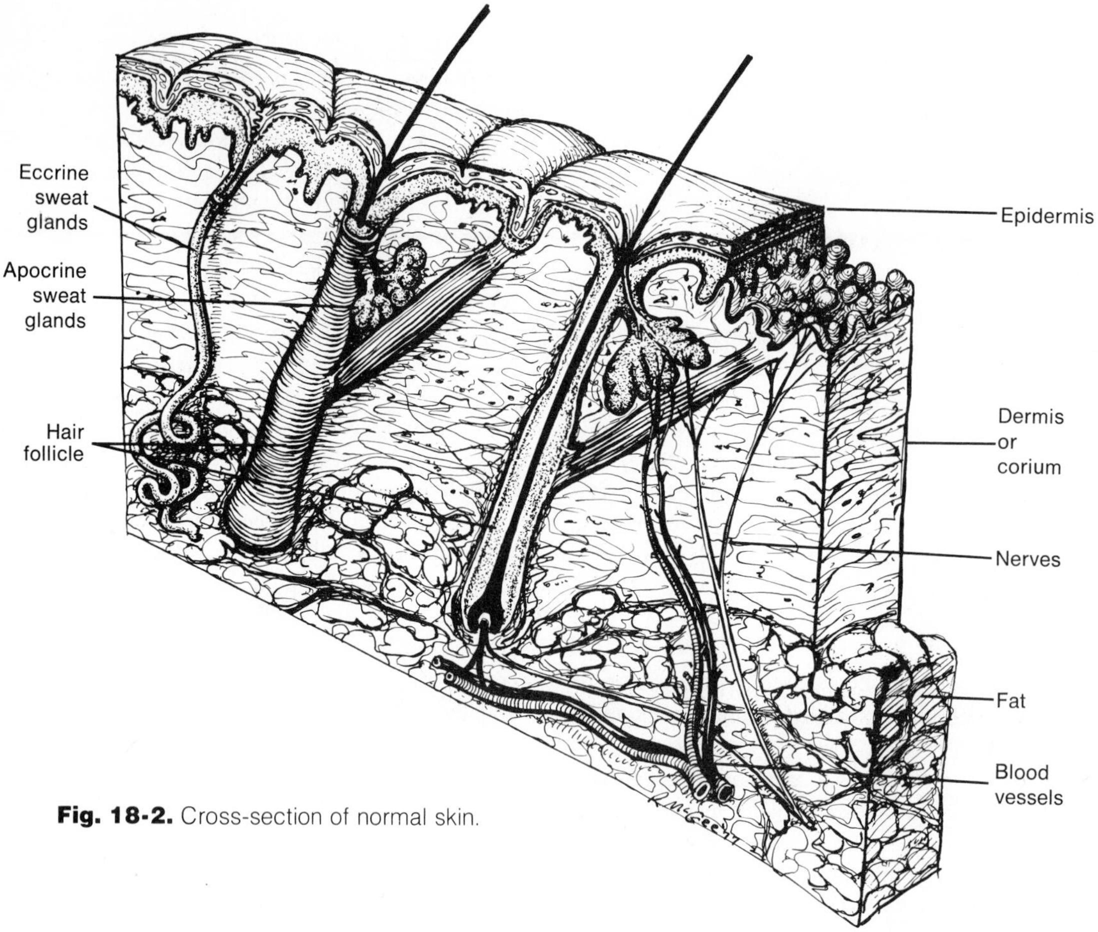

Fig. 18-2. Cross-section of normal skin.

quently permits an awareness and observation of many diffuse systemic disorders of connective tissue—the "collagen" diseases.

Subcutaneous tissue. A thick layer of *subcutaneous tissue* lies beneath the dermis and is composed of a looser type of connective tissue that varies greatly in extent in various parts of the body. In addition to larger blood vessels, lymph channels, and nerve trunks, the subcutaneous tissue serves as a depot for the storage of fat that acts as a cushion, insulates the body against cold, and largely determines its contours.

Younger children. Several characteristics influence skin responses in infants and young children. Their skin is far more susceptible to superficial bacterial infection. They are more likely to have associated systemic symptoms with some infections and are more apt to react to a primary irritant than to a sensitizing allergen. They more often show blistering (bullous) reactions caused by the poor adherence between epidermis and dermis and are frequently affected by chronic atopic dermatitis (eczema). The infant's skin is much more prone to develop a toxic erythema as a result of skin eruptions or drug reactions and is subject to maceration, infection, and the sweat retention associated with diaper rash.

Etiology and pathophysiology

Lesions of the skin or disorders with skin manifestations can be a result of a wide variety of specific etiologic factors. In general, skin lesions originate from (1) contact with injurious agents such as infective organisms, toxic chemicals, and physical trauma, (2) hereditary factors, or (3) some external factor that produces a reaction in the skin, for example, allergens. In this situation the damage is caused by the body's response to the agent rather than by the agent itself. Such responses are highly individualized. An agent that may be harmless to one individual may be damaging to another, and a single agent may produce various types of responses in different individuals.

Among other factors involved in the etiology of skin manifestations is the age of the child. For example, infants are subject to "birthmark" malformations and atopic dermatitis that appear early in life; the school-age child is susceptible to ringworm of the scalp; and acne is a characteristic skin disorder of puberty. Contact dermatitis, such as poison ivy, is seen only where the noxious agent is a feature of the area. Similarly reactions to animal bites are associated with their life cycle and seasonal activities. Although less common in children, tension and anxiety may produce, modify, or prolong many skin conditions.

The following paragraphs include the more common types of skin disorders seen in children of all ages categorized according to the major etiologic factors. Some disorders are seen with such frequency in children in other age-groups that they are discussed with the health problems of that particular period. For example, infantile dermatitis or eczema is seen so commonly in infants and young children that it is more appropriate to discuss the various forms in relation to that age-group (atopic dermatitis or eczema, p. 488; seborrheic dermatitis or "cradle cap," p. 492; and the specific contact dermatitis known as diaper rash, p. 283).

Over half of dermatologic problems are various forms of dermatitis. This implies a sequence of inflammatory changes in the skin that are grossly and microscopically similar but that are diverse in course and causation. Acute responses produce intercellular and intracellular edema, the formation of intradermal vesicles, and an initial minimal infiltration of inflammatory cells into the epidermis. In the dermis there is edema, vascular dilatation, and early perivascular cellular infiltration. The location and manner of these reactions produce the lesions that are characteristic of each disorder. The changes are reversible, and the skin ordinarily recovers without blemish, completely intact, unless complicating factors such as ulceration from the primary irritant, scratching, and infection are introduced or if underlying vascular disease develops. In chronic conditions more permanent effects are seen that vary according to the disorder, the general condition of the affected individual, and available therapy.

Diagnostic evaluation

One of the more advantageous aspects of skin disorders is that often the diagnosis is readily established after simple, careful inspection. Much can be determined by the distribution, size, and arrangement of the components of the lesions and by the morphology of individual lesions. In addition the physician must determine whether the cause is primarily extrinsic or intrinsic. Extrinsic causes usually result from physical, chemical, or allergic irritants or from an infectious agent such as bacteria, fungi, viruses, or animal parasites. Skin manifestations can be produced by such intrinsic causes as a specific infection, drug sensitization, or other allergic phenomena. Other diagnostic tools are subjective symptoms, history, and medical and laboratory studies.

Lesion. According to the nature of the pathologic process, lesions assume more or less distinct characteristics. They are usually the result of disturbance of function, inflammation, or growth. Although the names that have been applied to these lesions are of little value in themselves, they are important for descriptive purposes in the processes of record keeping and communication. To examine the various aspects of the lesion requires that the inspection take place under natural or adequate artificial light. A low-powered magnifying lens serves as a useful adjunct and, in diseases with abnormalities of pigmentation or those associated with fluorescence, a Wood's light is useful.

Several general types of skin lesions are seen in dermatologic conditions. A reddened area is usually caused by increased amounts of oxygenated blood in the dermal vasculature and is described as *erythema*. Hemorrhages into the skin produce localized red or purple discolorations such as *ecchymoses* (bruises), caused by extravasation of blood into dermis and subcutaneous tissues, and *petechiae,* pinpoint tiny and sharply circumscribed spots in the superficial layers of the epidermis. *Primary* lesions are skin changes produced by some causative factor; *secondary* lesions are changes that result from alteration in the primary lesions, such as those caused by rubbing, scratching, medication, or involution and healing. Nurses should become familiar with the more common terms used to describe skin lesions:

Distribution pattern. The pattern in which lesions are distributed over the body is a useful aid in diagnosis. Local processes are distinguished from those that are generalized. Many lesions are primarily associated with specific areas such as extensor areas in atopic dermatitis or uncovered areas that allow exposure to sun or noxious agents such as poison ivy; others are related to the location of specific cutaneous appendages, such as the unique sebaceous gland distribution of acne.

Configuration and arrangement. The size, shape, and arrangement of a lesion or groups of lesions assist in diagnosis. Discrete lesions are distinguished from clustered, diffuse, or confluent configurations. Grouped or clustered lesions are characteristic in herpes eruptions; annular (ringed) or arciform lesions are typical of ringworm and diseases resulting from vascular reactions, such as urticaria or drug reaction; linear arrangements usually represent an exogenous influence that has either caused the process or contributed to its spread, such as scratching.

History and subjective symptoms. Many cutaneous lesions are associated with local symptoms, the most common of which is itching that varies in kind and intensity. Pain or tenderness often accompanies some skin lesions, and other sensations may be described as burning, prickling, stinging, or crawling. Alterations in local feeling or sensation include absence of sensation (anesthesia), excessive sensitiveness (hyperesthesia), or diminished or lessening of sensation (hypesthesia or hypoesthesia). These symptoms may remain localized or may migrate, may be constant or intermittent, and may be aggravated by a specific activity or circumstance, such as exposure to sunlight.

It is also important to determine whether the child has had an allergic condition such as asthma or hay fever or has had previous skin disease. Atopy, often associated with allergies, frequently begins in infancy. When the lesion or symptom first became apparent should be determined, as well as if it is related to ingestion of a food or other substance, including any medication the child might be taking.

Primary lesions	Description	Example
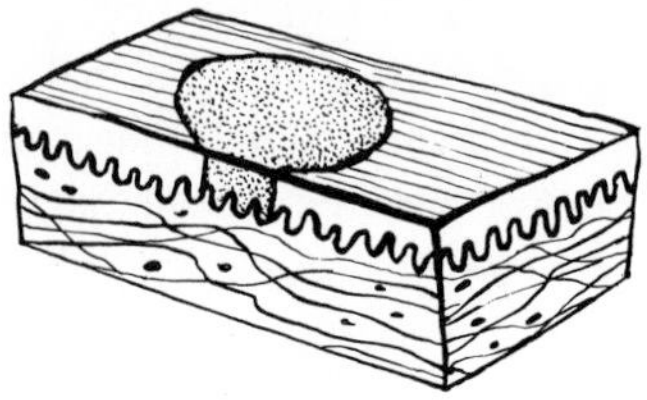 **Macule**	Flat circumscribed area of color change less than 1 cm in diameter, neither elevated nor depressed and with no alteration in skin texture.	Freckle, nevus, measles
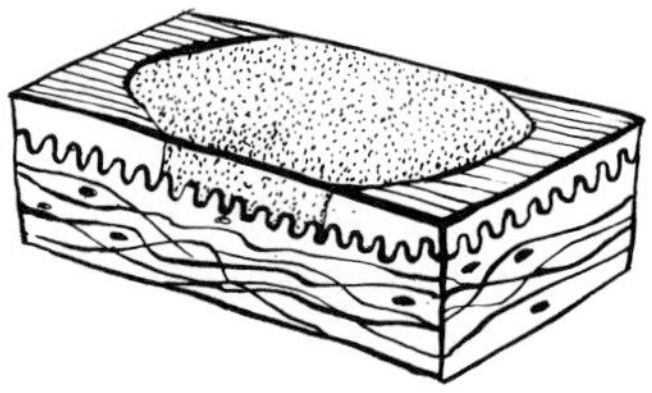 **Patch**	Flat circumscribed discoloration of skin greater than 1 cm in diameter.	Mongolian spot, vitiligo
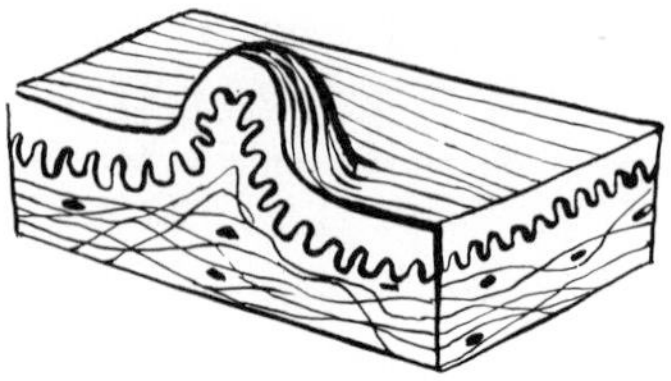 **Papule**	Small circumscribed solid elevation of the skin, less than 1 cm in diameter. It exists mostly above the plane of the skin surface, and the more superficial it is, the more distinct are the borders.	Wart, ringworm
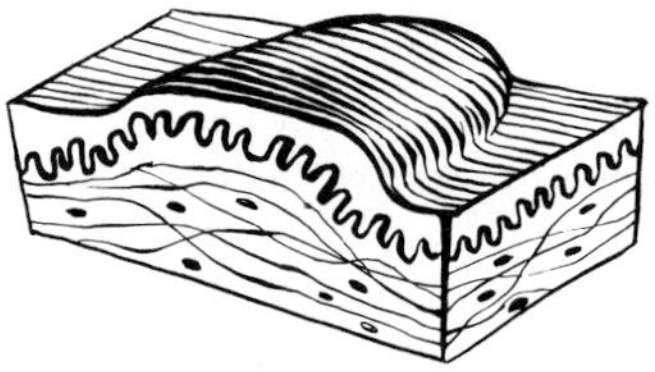 **Plaque**	Flattened, raised lesion in which the surface area involved is relatively large in relation to its height.	Psoriasis
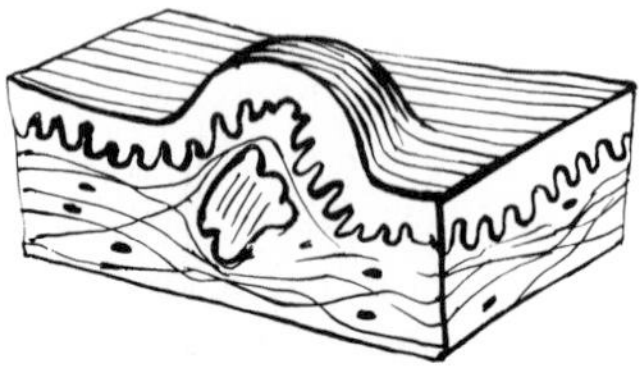 **Nodule**	Solid circumscribed elevation, round or ellipsoid, located deep in dermis or subcutaneous tissue.	Dermatofibroma
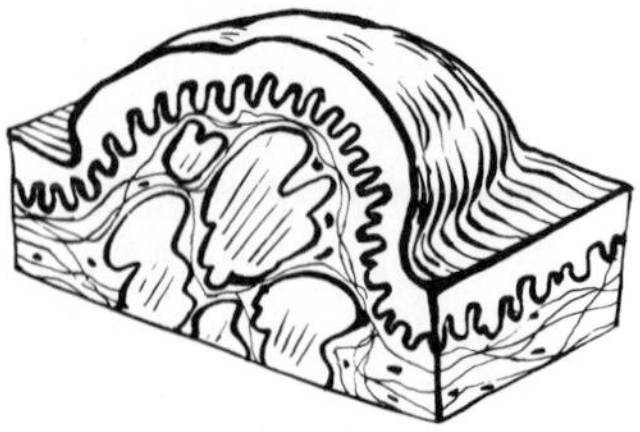 **Tumor**	Circumscribed infiltration of skin or subcutaneous tissue that is larger (greater than 1 cm in diameter) and deeper than nodule.	Cavernous hemangioma

Primary lesions	Description	Example
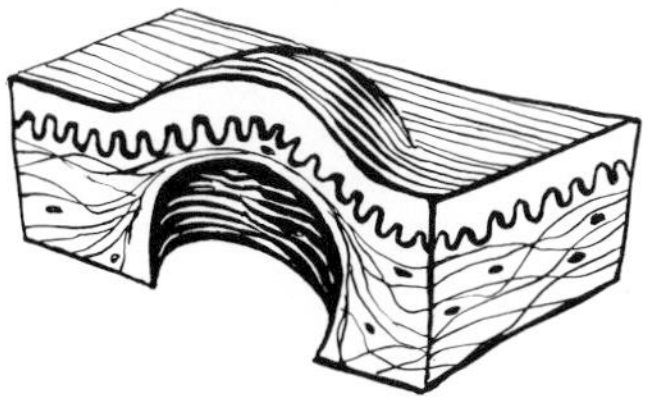 **Cyst**	Encapsulated semisolid or fluid-filled mass in dermis or subcutaneous tissue.	Epidermoid cyst
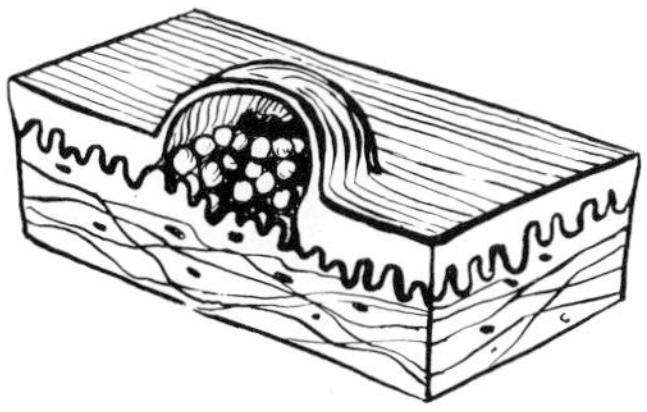 **Vesicle**	Small (less than 1 cm in diameter), superficial circumscribed elevation of the skin containing serous or blood-tinged fluid.	Chickenpox, herpes, poison ivy dermatitis
Pustule	Vesicle filled with pus that may or may not be caused by infection.	Acne, impetigo, folliculitis
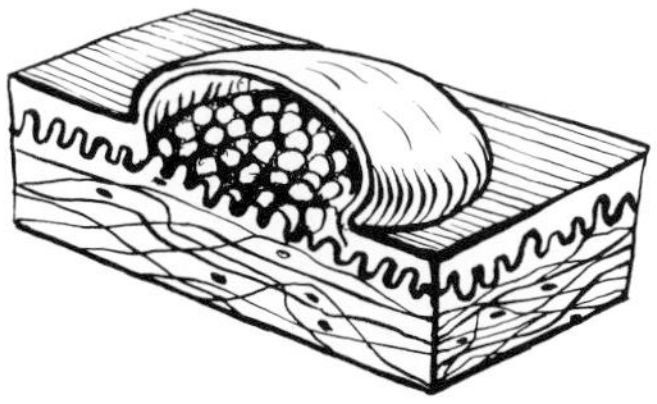 **Bulla**	Fluid-filled vesicle greater than 1 cm in diameter; a large vesicle; bleb; blister.	Second-degree burn
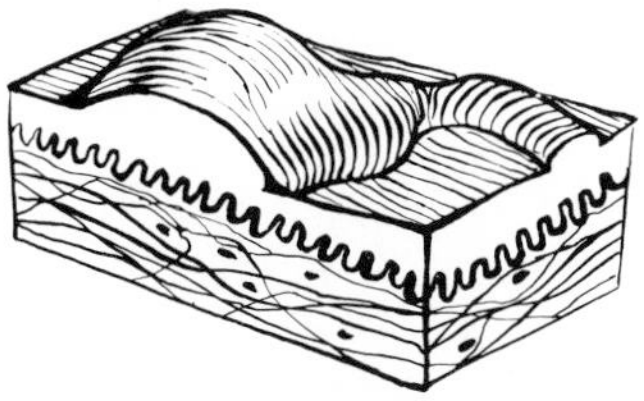 **Wheal (hives)**	Round or flat-topped and irregularly shaped, evanescent lesions resulting from acute accumulation of edema fluid in upper dermis.	Mosquito bites, urticaria

Continued.

Secondary lesions	Description	Example
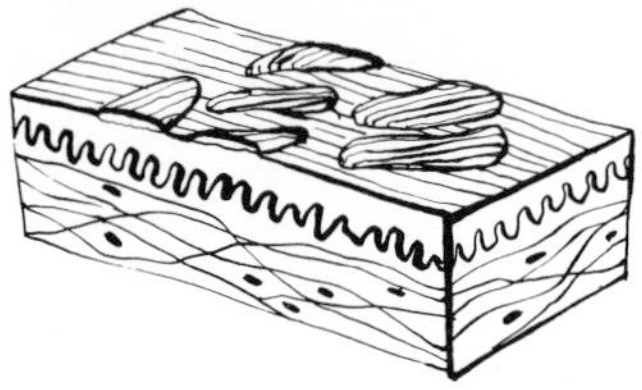 **Scales**	Flakes of dead, cornified tissue being shed from skin.	Psoriasis, ringworm
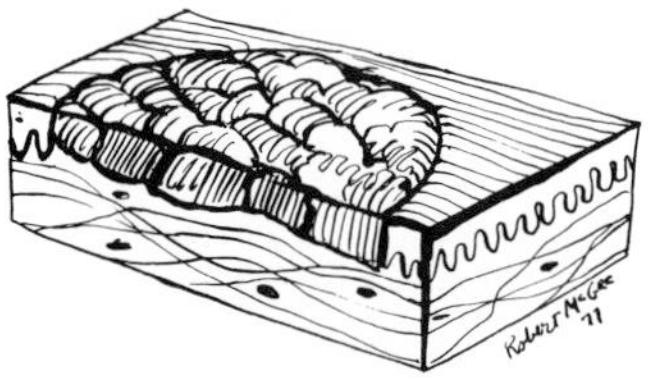 **Crusts**	Dried masses of serum, pus, dead skin, and debris that can be found surmounting any lesion.	Impetigo, other infectious dermatitis
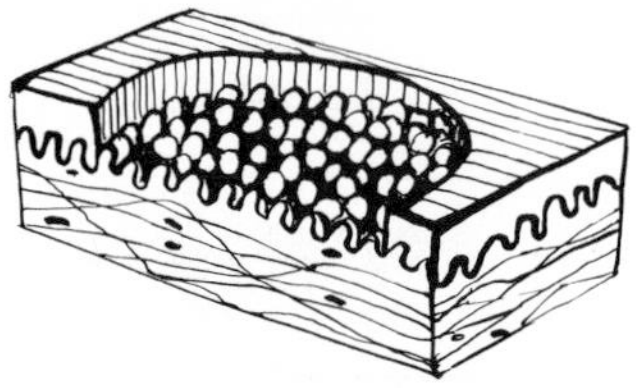 **Excoriation or erosion**	Superficial loss of skin substance that does not extend into dermis.	Superficial scratches
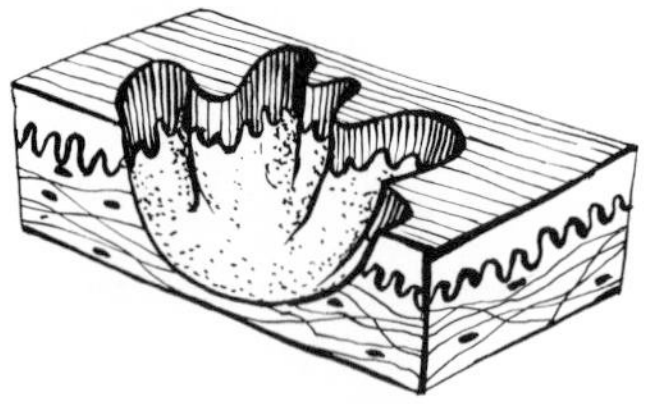 **Ulcer**	Irregularly shaped escavation caused by loss of substance with gradual disintegration and necrosis of tissue.	Decubiti
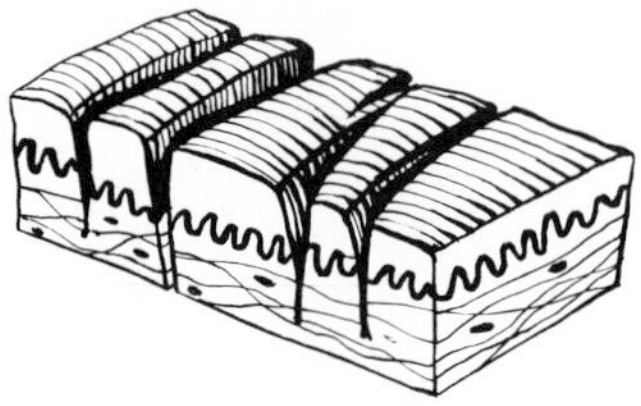 **Fissure**	Deep linear split through epidermis into dermis.	Chapping
Scars	Permanent dermal changes with production of excess collagen following damage to corium.	Vaccination, burns, deep scratches

It should be kept in mind that it may be related to an activity such as contact with plants, insects, or chemicals.

Laboratory studies. The physician who suspects that a skin problem might be related to a systemic disease, such as one of the collagen diseases or immune deficiency disease, will include studies to rule out these possibilities. Microscopic examination of a skin lesion may be essential in many chronic conditions and in pigmented nevi. Cultures in bacterial infections, scrapings for fungal infections, allergic skin testing, and various other laboratory tests (blood count, sedimentation rate) are employed when indicated.

General medical management

The living organism tends to heal; therefore, treatment is directed toward eliminating or ameliorating influences that interfere with healing so that the body can be allowed to heal itself. Some disorders may demand aggressive therapy, but, by and large, the major aim of any treatment is to prevent further damage, eliminate the cause, prevent complications, and provide relief from discomfort while tissues undergo healing. Factors that contribute to the dermatitis and may prolong the course of the disease must be eliminated where possible. The most common offenders in pediatrics are environmental factors, such as soaps, bubble baths, shampoos, rough or tight clothing, blankets, and toys, the natural elements, such as dirt, sand, heat, cold, moisture, and wind. Dermatitis can also be aggravated by home remedies and medications.

Most skin disorders will respond to topical therapy, that is, application of an active ingredient directly to the affected areas. This is applied by way of a pharmacologically inert vehicle that contributes to the therapy with physical properties that protect, soothe, or cleanse. However, there are occasions when systemic administration of therapeutic agents is employed. Since the type of medication and the active ingredient employed vary with the preference of individual practitioners, in the discussions of the various types of skin disorders only a representative example of some of the preferred therapeutic regimens are included.

Topical therapy. A variety of agents and methods are available for treatment of dermatologic problems. In selecting a therapeutic program the physician considers (1) a choice of active ingredient, (2) a proper vehicle, (3) the cosmetic effect, (4) the cost, and (5) instructions for its use.[1] In addition several basic concepts are kept in mind. Overtreatment should be avoided. For example, when the dermatitis is acute, the applications should be mild and bland to avoid further irritation. Broken or inflamed skin, especially in children, is more absorbent than intact skin, and chemicals that are nonirritating to intact skin may be quite irritating to inflamed skin. The dermatitic skin is also more apt to develop allergic contact-type sensitization to substances applied as medication or base. Infants and small children are particularly sensitive to topical antihistamines and the "caine"-type of anesthetics, both of which are potent allergic sensitizers. Phenol, often incorporated into medications as an antipruritic, should be avoided with children.

Topical applications may be applied to treat the disorder, reduce the itching associated with many diseases, decrease external stimuli, or apply external heat or cold. The emollient action of soaks, baths, and lotions provides a soothing film over the skin surface that reduces external stimuli. Application of heat tends to aggravate most conditions, and its use is usually reserved for reducing specific inflammatory processes, such as folliculitis. Ordinarily applications offer most relief when they are lukewarm, tepid, or cool.

The most frequent means for topical treatment of skin disorders are wet dressings, soaks, lotions and shake solutions, baths, creams and ointments, pastes, powders, occlusive dressings, soaps and shampoos, sunscreening agents, other topical treatments, and topical glucocorticoid therapy.

Wet dressings. Probably the mildest form of topical therapy, open wet dressings, cool the skin by evaporation, relieve itching and inflammation, and cleanse the area by loosening and removing crusts and debris. Any of a variety of ingredients, such as the time-honored Burow's solution, can be applied on kerlix gauze, plain gauze, or (preferably) soft cotton cloths such as freshly laundered handkerchiefs or strips from diaper, sheeting, or pillowcase material. Dressings immersed in the desired solution are wrung out slightly and applied to the affected area wet but not dripping. They are applied flat and smooth and in such a way that motion is not totally restricted—fingers are wrapped separately and arms and legs are wrapped so that elbows and knees can bend. Dressings are kept in place by kerlix or other cotton wrap, tubular stockinette, mittens, and socks (two pair—one to hold the dressings in place, the other to take up movement) but are left uncovered. When evaporation begins to dry them, the dressings are removed, rewet in the solution, and reapplied to the area using aseptic technique. The solution is not poured or syringed directly over the dressings. The most commonly used solutions are outlined in Table 18-3.

Fresh solution at room temperature is applied at 2-, 3-, or 4-hour intervals and is allowed to remain on anywhere from 30 minutes to 1½ hours. Wet dressings are seldom continued after about 48 hours. The child must be guarded against chilling during treatment, and no more than one third of the body should be covered at one time. After treatment the skin is dried thoroughly by patting with a towel. Application of lotion or other medication may be ordered at this time.

Soaks. When young children are uncooperative in the use of wet dressings, soaks are often employed for removal of crusts and for their mild astringent action, using the same solution employed for wet compresses. See p. 950 for play techniques to use with children who require soaks.

Lotions and shake solutions. Lotions are preparations of

powder suspended in solution. As the liquid evaporates, it not only cools but a coating of soothing, lubricating, protective, and drying powder remains on the skin. Lotions are applied evenly over the skin with gauze or an ordinary paintbrush, frequently after wet dressings or soaks. Lotions are not applied to oozing surfaces. They are not ordinarily washed off between applications but may be removed by soaking with the solution used for soaks or dressings. An emulsion can be formed by the addition of an oil and a dispersant.

Baths. Baths are especially useful in the treatment of widespread dermatitis by evenly distributing the soothing antipruritic and antiinflammatory effects of the solution. The solution is added to a tub well filled with lukewarm water. The duration of treatment is usually 15 to 30 minutes.

Creams and ointments. Creams and ointments are easily and evenly spread over the skin. Creams contain water with cold cream or oil emulsified in it; the main constituent of ointments is oil. The lipid component may consist of animal fats, such as lard or wool fat (lanolin), petrolatum, or vegetable oils. Creams tend to disappear when rubbed into the skin and are less occlusive than ointments. If ointment is not absorbed but remains on the skin, too much is being applied. Creams and ointments are used for lubrication, as a vehicle for medication, and for protection. Neither should be used in hairy, intertriginous, or macerated areas.

Pastes. Pastes are powders mixed with an ointment base. More porous and less occlusive than ointments, they absorb moisture and produce a drying effect, and medications incorporated into pastes are released more slowly than from creams and ointments. Because they are difficult to apply and must be removed from the skin with mineral oil, pastes are used less frequently than other preparations. They are most easily applied with a tongue depressor and ''buttered'' on.

Powders. Powders have a controversial use in pediatrics. They are very effective for soothing, absorbing moisture, and protecting the skin by reducing friction. Chemically inert, their chief use is prophylactic when applied to intertriginous areas. However, powder must be applied in a fine film that does not cake or form lumps when wet, and care must be exerted to prevent the child from inhaling the powder, especially those that contain talc or kaolin. To reduce the risk of inhalation, powder is sprinkled in the palm of the hand and then applied to the skin surface. Powder is never sprinkled directly onto the patient's skin.

Occlusive dressings. Used primarily in association with topical steroids, occlusive dressings are usually restricted to treatment of chronic dermatoses. A thin application of ointment or cream is covered with a thin, transparent pliable plastic film that is anchored with adhesive. Occlusive dressings promote moisture retention, nonevaporation of the vehicle, and maceration of the epidermis, all of which increase the penetration of medications. Although of value in certain situations, the dangers are bacterial and candidal infections, sweat retention, and increased likelihood of side effects from the medication used. The treatment consists of an 8- to 10-hour period, usually overnight, and covers no greater an area than 10% of the body.

Soaps and shampoos. Germicidal soaps are useful adjunctive therapy for skin infections. Bactericidal agents incorporated in soaps include hexachlorophene and the halogenated salicylanilides and carbanilides, one or more of which are found in many of the well-known soaps. Another effective topical microbicide is povidone-iodine (Betadine) skin cleanser, which contains a detergent mixture with iodine and polyvinyl pyrrolidone that assists in disinfecting the skin and is effective in eliminating common pathogens including *Staphylococcus aureus*.

Shampoos that are used in dermatologic skin conditions include tar shampoos for resistant scalp seborrhea and psoriasis and antiparasitic shampoos such as gamma benzene hexachloride (Kwell) for pediculosis capitis. Soaps containing hexachlorophene are used with caution to reduce the risk of absorption, especially on broken or denuded areas. Large amounts of the drug when absorbed can cause central nervous system symptoms.

Sunscreening agents. Some chemicals have the capacity to absorb certain wavelengths of light and thus provide protection to the cutaneous surface when applied to the skin. They are especially useful in dermatoses in which light plays an important causative role. They are applied to light-exposed areas and provide protection for about 3 to 4 hours under ordinary circumstances.

Other topical treatments. Other topical treatments include chemical cautery (especially useful for warts), cryo-

Table 18-3. Solutions most commonly used for wet dressings

Solution	Active ingredient	Preparation and use
Physiologic saline	0.9% sodium chloride	2 tsp/liter (quart) of water
Burow's	Aluminum sulfate and calcium acetate	Mildly astringent, coagulant, and bacteriostatic 1 packet or tablet, such as Domeboro or Buro-Sol, to 500 ml (1 pint) of water
Potassium permanganate		Mildly antiseptic and drying; may stain skin, clothing, and utensils, including bathtubs (remove stain with 3% hydrogen peroxide) 1:15,000 solution = one 5-grain tablet to 4½ liters (quarts) of water

surgery, electrodesiccation (chiefly used for warts, granulomas, and nevi), ultraviolet therapy (primarily used in psoriasis and acne), and special acne therapies such as dermabrasion and acne ''surgery.''

Topical glucocorticoid therapy. The glucocorticoids are the therapeutic agents used most widely for skin disorders. Their local antiinflammatory effects are merely palliative so that the medication must be applied until the disease state undergoes a remission or the causative agent is eliminated. Corticosteroids are applied directly to the affected area, and, because they are essentially nonsensitizing and have only minor side effects, they can be applied over prolonged periods with continuing effectiveness. As with the use of any steriods, in large amounts they may mask signs of infection and there may be exacerbation of symptoms following termination of the drug. Hydrocortisone preparations are available in sprays, lotions, creams, ointment, gels, suspensions, and powders.

Systemic therapy. Therapeutic agents are often used as an adjunct to topical therapy in dermatologic disorders, and those most frequently used therapeutically are the corticosteroids and the antibiotics. The corticosteroid hormones with their capacity to inhibit inflammatory and allergic reactions are valuable in the treatment of severe skin disorders. Dosage is carefully adjusted and gradually tapered to the minimum that is effective and tolerated and, in infants and children, is larger than is usually calculated from body-weight ratios. Protracted use may temporarily suppress growth, however.

Antibiotics, which interfere with the growth of microorganisms, are used in severe or widespread skin infections. The danger inherent in the use of antibiotics is their tendency to produce a hypersensitivity in the patient; therefore, they are used with caution. Antifungal agents are the only means for treating systemic fungal infections.

BACTERIAL INFECTIONS (Table 18-4)

Normally the skin harbors a variety of bacterial flora, including the major pathogenic varieties of staphylococci and streptococci. The degree of their pathogenicity depends on the specific organism's invasiveness and toxigenicity, the integrity of the skin, the barrier of the host, and the immune and cellular defenses of the host. Children with immune deficiency states are highly susceptible to bacterial invasion. This includes infants, children with congenital immune deficiency disorders, children in a debilitated condition, those on immunosuppressive therapy, and those with a generalized malignancy such as leukemia or lymphoma.

Because of the characteristic ''walling'off'' process of the inflammatory reaction, that is, abscess formation, staphylococci are more difficult to attack and the local infected area is associated with an increase in numbers of bacteria all over the skin surface that serve as a source of continuing infection. Staphylococcal infections occur most often in children in the younger age-groups, and the incidence decreases with advancing age. All of these factors emphasize the importance of careful hand washing and cleanliness when caring for infected children and their lesions to prevent spread of the infection and as an essential prophylactic measure when caring for infants and small children.

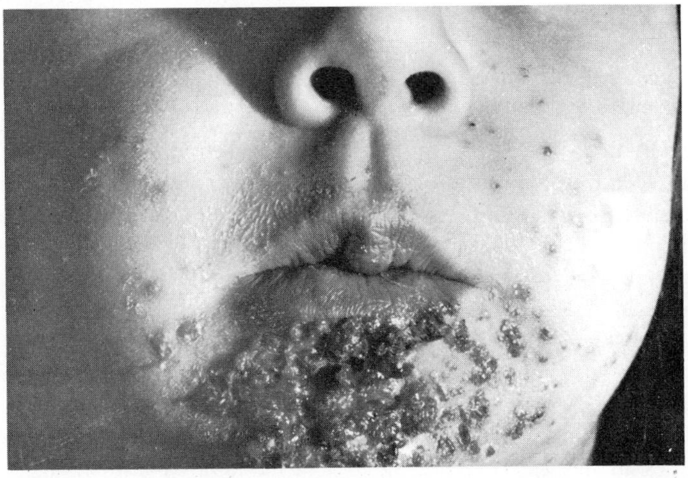

Fig. 18-3. Impetigo contagiosa. (From Stewart, W. D., Danto, J. L., and Maddin, S.: Dermatology: diagnosis and treatment of cutaneous disorders, ed. 4, St. Louis, 1978, The C. V. Mosby Co.)

Table 18-4. Bacterial infections

Disorder	Organism	Skin manifestations
Impetigo contagiosa (Fig. 18-3)	*Streptococcus* *Staphylococcus*	Begins as a reddish macule Becomes vesicular Ruptures easily, leaving a superficial, moist erosion Tends to spread peripherally in sharply marginated irregular outlines Exudate dries to form heavy, honey-colored crusts Pruritus common
Pyoderma	*Staphylococcus* *Streptococcus*	Deeper extension of infection into dermis Tissue reaction more severe
Folliculitis (pimple), furuncle (boil), carbuncle (multiple boils)	*Staphylococcus aureus*	Folliculitis: infection of hair follicle Furuncle is a larger lesion with more redness and swelling at a single follicle Carbuncle is a more extensive lesion with widespread inflammation and "pointing" at several follicular orifices
Cellulitis	*Streptococcus* *Hemophilus influenzae*	Inflammation of skin and subcutaneous tissues with intense redness, swelling, and firm infiltration Lymphangitis "streaking" frequently seen Involvement of regional lymph nodes common

VIRAL INFECTIONS (Table 18-5)

Viruses are intracellular parasites that produce their effect by using the intracellular substances of the host cells. Composed of only a DNA or RNA core enclosed in an antigenic protein shell, viruses are unable to provide for their own metabolic needs or to reproduce themselves. After a virus penetrates a cell of the host organism, it sheds the outer shell and disappears within the cell where the nucleic acid core stimulates the host cell to form more virus material from its intracellular substance. In a viral infection the epidermal cells react with inflammation and vesiculation (as in herpes simplex) or by proliferating to form growths (warts).

FUNGAL INFECTIONS (Tables 18-6 and 18-7)

Superficial infections caused by fungi live on, not in, the skin. They are confined to the dead keratin layers of the skin, hair, and nails but are unable to survive in the deeper layers. Since the keratin is being desquamated constantly, the fungus must multiply at a rate that equals the rate of keratin production to maintain itself; otherwise the infection would be shed with the discarded skin cells.

Superficial fungus infections are transmitted from one person to another or, more commonly, from infected animals to man. Of the superficial fungal infections, ringworm is the most prevalent. Diseases in this category are the tineas with further designation related to the area of the body where they are found, for example, tinea capitis or ringworm of the scalp. They exert their effect by means of an enzyme that digests and hydrolyzes the keratin of hair, nails, and the stratum corneum. Dissolved hair breaks off to produce the bald spots characteristic of tinea capitis. In the annular lesions the fungi are found principally in the edge of the inflamed border as they move outward from the inflammation. Nurses who suspect ringworm in school children are able to identify the organism by means of a Wood's light, under which the fungus is fluorescent.

When teaching families regarding the care of the child with ringworm, it is important to emphasize good health and hygiene. Because of the infectious nature of the disease, several basic hygienic measures are particularly pertinent. The affected child should not exchange any grooming items, headgear, scarves, or other articles of apparel that have been in close proximity to the infected area. The affected child should have his own towel and wear a protective cap at night to avoid transmitting the fungus to bedding, especially if he sleeps with another person. Since the infection can be acquired by animal-to-human transmission, all household pets should be examined for the presence of the disorder.

Treatment with the drug griseofulvin frequently lasts for weeks or months, and because subjective symptoms subside the child or parent may be tempted to decrease or discontinue the drug. The nurse should impress on members of the family the importance of maintaining the prescribed dosage schedule. They are also instructed regarding the possibility of side effects from the drug such as headache, gastrointestinal upset, fatigue, insomnia, and photosensi-

Systemic effects	Treatment	Comments
Minimal or asymptomatic	Careful removal of undermined skin, crusts, and debris by softening with 1:20 Burow's solution compresses Topical application of bacteriocidal ointment (Garamycin, Neo-Polycin, Neosporin) Systemic administration of oral or parenteral antibiotics (penicillin) in severe or extensive lesions	Tends to heal without scarring unless secondary infection Autoinoculable and contagious Very common in toddler, preschooler
Fever, lymphangitis	Soap and water cleansing Wet compresses (saline solution, Burow's solution, or potassium permanganate solution)	Autoinoculable and contagious May heal with or without scarring
Malaise if severe	Skin cleanliness Local warm, moist compresses (Burow's solution, saline solution, potassium permanganate) Topical application of antibiotic agents Systemic antibiotics in severe cases Incision and drainage of severe lesions, followed by wound irrigations with antibiotics or suitable drain implantation	Autoinoculable and contagious Furuncle and carbuncle tend to heal with scar formation
Fever, malaise	Oral or parenteral penicillin Rest and immobilization of both the affected area and the child	Hospitalization may be necessary for the child with systemic symptoms

tivity. For children who take the drug over a period of many months, periodic testing is required to monitor leukopenia and assess liver and renal function.

Systemic or deep fungal infections have the capacity to invade the viscera as well as the skin. The best known of these are primarily lung diseases, which are usually acquired by inhalation. They produce a variable spectrum of disease, and some are quite common in certain geographic areas. They are not transmitted from person to person but appear to reside in the soil, from which their spores are airborne. The cutaneous lesions are granulomatous and appear as ulcers, plaques, nodules, fungating mosses, and abscesses. The course of deep fungal diseases is chronic with slow progression that favors sensitization.

INSECT INFESTATIONS, BITES, AND STINGS

(Tables 18-8 and 18-9)

School children's social nature and close proximity to other children render them highly susceptible to communicable diseases, including those caused by parasites. Because they spend a great deal of time outdoors and in fields and vacant lots, children often come in contact with insects. Consequently children are frequently the victims of insects that puncture the skin for the purpose of sucking blood, injecting venom, or laying their eggs. In the process of these activities, substances foreign to the victim may create an allergic sensitivity in that individual to produce pruritus, urticaria, or systemic reactions of greater or lesser degree depending on the child's sensitivity.

Ordinarily insect bites are of little significance and cause only minor inconvenience. However, they can attain importance if[10]:

1. They cause symptoms that interfere with the child's normal activities, such as the effects of a spider bite
2. They signify the presence of a contagious skin disease, such as scabies
3. The parasite is able to transmit other diseases, for example, ticks that transmit Rocky Mountain spotted fever

Infestations with insect parasites are more prevalent in nonhygienic environmental conditions but are also encountered in scrupulously clean persons. The infestations encountered most frequently in childhood are scabies and pediculosis capitis. Body lice infestations are seen less often, and pubic lice (pediculosis pubis, or "crabs") are rare in childhood.

Persons who have become sensitized to the bites of certain insects such as bees may demonstrate a severe anaphylactic response that can be life threatening. Intramuscular administration of epinephrine provides immediate relief and must be available for emergency use. Hypersensitive children need a kit available that contains epinephrine, a hypodermic syringe, a tourniquet (to delay spread of venom from an extremity), and perhaps ephedrine and an antihistamine preparation. A child with a history of generalized reactivity to an insect sting should undertake a program of skin testing and desensitization to prevent serious or fatal reactions.

Table 18-5. Viral infections

Disease	Manifestations	Treatment	Comments
Verruca (warts)	Small benign tumors Usually well-circumscribed, gray or brown, elevated firm papules with a roughened, finely papillomatous texture Occur anywhere but usually appear on exposed areas such as fingers, hands, face, and soles	Not uniformly successful Local destructive therapy, individualized according to location, type, and number—surgical removal, electrocautery, curettage, cryotherapy (liquid nitrogen), caustic solutions (bichloracetic acid, salicylic acid plasters), x-ray treatment	Common in children Tend to disappear spontaneously Course unpredictable Most destructive techniques tend to leave scars Autoinoculable
Variants:			
Verruca vulgaris (common wart)	A skin-colored to brown, rough-surfaced epithelial growth May be single or multiple Asymptomatic Most frequent sites are dorsal and palmar surfaces of hands, fingers, and around nails	Psychotherapy often effective	Repeated irritation will cause to enlarge
Verruca plana juvenilis (juvenile wart)	Flat, skin-colored to brown, slightly raised, smooth lesion Asymptomatic Lesions multiple Commonly located on face and dorsum of hands		
Verruca plantaris (plantar wart)	Located on plantar surface of feet and, because of pressure, are practically flat; may be surrounded by a collar of hyperkeratosis		
Herpes simplex (cold sore, fever blister)	Grouped, burning, and itching vesicles on an inflammatory base, usually on or near mucocutaneous junctions (lips, nose, genitals, and buttocks) Vesicles dry, forming a crust, followed by exfoliation and spontaneous healing in 8 to 10 days May be accompanied by regional lymphadenopathy	Avoidance of secondary infection Burow's solution compresses during weeping stages Ointments (bacitracin or neomycin) when lesions are dry and crusted Aggravated by corticosteroids	Heal without scarring unless secondary infection
Herpes zoster (shingles)	Caused by same virus that causes varicella (chickenpox) Virus has affinity for posterior root ganglia, posterior horn of spinal cord, and skin; crops of vesicles usually confined to dermatome following along the course of the affected nerve Usually preceded by neuralgic pain, hyperesthesias, or itching May be accompanied by constitutional symptoms	Control of pain with salicylates or codeine Mild sedation sometimes helpful Thiamine chloride 25 to 100 mg three times daily Local moist compresses three times daily soothing Drying lotions may be helpful Ophthalmic variety: systemic ACTH and/or corticosteroids	Pain in children usually minimal Postherpetic pain does not occur in children Chickenpox may follow exposure to herpes zoster; therefore affected child should be isolated from other children in a hospital May occur in children with depressed immunity; can be fatal

Table 18-6. Superficial mycoses caused by fungi

Disease	Organism	Manifestations	Diagnosis	Treatment	Comments
Dermatophytosis (ringworm)					
Tinea capitis (see Fig. 18-4, *A*)	Usually *Microsporum*, primarily *M. audouini*, transmitted from one human being to another, or *M. canis*, usually contracted from household pets	Lesions in the scalp, but may extend to hairline or neck Scaly, circumscribed patches to patchy, scaling areas of alopecia Generally asymptomatic, but severe, deep inflammatory reaction may occur that manifests as boggy, encrusted lesions (kerions) Pruritic	Characteristic configuration Fluoresce green under Wood's lamp Direct examination of scales and culture if doubtful Check at 2-week intervals with Wood's lamp	Oral griseofulvin (Fulvicin-U/F, Grifulvin V, and Grisactin), 20 mg/kg/day for 7-10 days Effectiveness of drug is enhanced by frequent shampoos and clipping hair Sometimes local application of strong antifungal ointment such as Whitfield's ointment is advisable	Person-to-person transmission Animal-to-person transmission Rarely, permanent loss of hair
Tinea corporis (see Fig. 18-4, *B*)	Trichophyton or *Microsporum* Majority of infections in children caused by *M. canis* and *M. audouini*	Generally round or oval, erythematous scaling patch that spreads peripherally and clears centrally; may involve nails (tinea unguium)	Direct microscopic examination of scales	Oral griseofulvin, 20 mg/kg/day for 10-14 days Local application of antifungal preparation such as Whitfield's ointment or tolnaftate (Tinactin)	Usually of animal origin from infected pets
Tinea cruris ("jock itch")	*Epidermophyton floccosum* and *T. rubrum*	Skin response similar to tinea corporis Localized to medial proximal aspect of thigh and crural fold; may involve scrotum in males Pruritic	Same as tinea corporis	Local application of tolnaftate liquid Wet compresses or sitz baths may be soothing	Rare in preadolescent children Health education regarding personal hygiene
Tinea pedis (athlete's foot)	*E. floccosum* *T. rubrum* *T. interdigitale*	On intertriginous areas between toes or on plantar surface of feet Lesions vary: Maceration and fissuring between toes Patches with pinhead-sized vesicles on plantar surface Pruritic	Direct microscopic examination of scrapings	Oral griseofulvin Local applications of tolnaftate liquid and antifungal powder containing tolnaftate Acute infections: Compresses or soaks for 15 minutes twice daily followed by application of glucocorticoid cream Elimination of conditions of heat and perspiration by clean, light socks and well-ventilated shoes; avoidance of occlusive shoes	Most frequent in adolescents and adults; rare in children Transmission to other individuals is rare despite general opinion to the contrary Ointments not successful

A

B

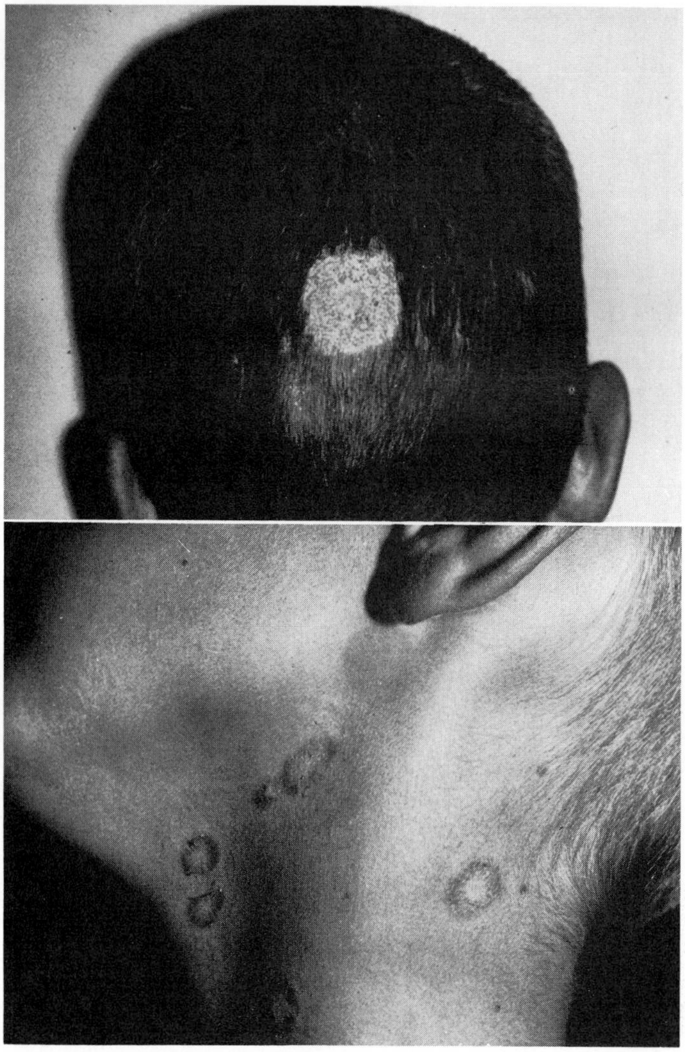

Fig. 18-4. A, Tinea capitis. **B,** Tinea corporis. Both infections caused by *Microsporum canis,* the "kitten" or "puppy" fungus. (From Stewart, W. D., Danto, J. L., and Maddin, S.: Dermatology: diagnosis and treatment of cutaneous disorders, ed. 4, St. Louis, 1978, The C. V. Mosby Co.)

MISCELLANEOUS SKIN LESIONS

There are a number of skin lesions caused by extrinsic or intrinsic factors. Table 18-10 lists some of the common manifestations.

Contact dermatitis

Contact dermatitis is an inflammatory reaction of the skin to chemical substances, natural or synthetic, that evoke a hypersensitivity response or to those agents that cause direct irritation. The initial reaction occurs in an exposed region, most commonly the face and neck, backs of the hands, forearms, male genitalia, and lower legs. There is characteristically a sharp delineation between inflamed and normal skin early in the reaction that ranges from a faint, transient erythema to massive bullae on an erythematous swollen base. Itching is a constant symptom.

The cause may be a *primary irritant* or a *sensitizing agent*. A primary irritant is one that irritates any skin; a sensitizer irritates in relatively low concentrations only persons who are allergic to it, that is, those who have met something chemically related to it, have undergone an immunologic change, and have become sensitized. Prior exposure is not a factor in the reaction. The course is relatively short (1 to 4 weeks) if the causative agent is eliminated, and it depends on the severity of the original reaction whether or not there are complications from secondary invasion or reactions to topical therapy.

Sensitizing reactions are acquired by repeated exposure

Text continued on p. 676.

Table 18-7. Systemic or deep diseases caused by fungi

Disease	Organism	Skin manifestations	Systemic manifestations	Treatment	Comments
Actinomycosis	*Actinomyces israelii*	Deep-seated granulomatous nodules, and subcutaneous abscesses that drain as chronic fistulas, especially in jaw or neck	General health not affected	Penicillin or other antibiotics Incision and wide débridement of lesions	Access frequently through a carious tooth or mucous membranes of mouth Less prevalent in children Noninfectious
North American blastomycosis	*Blastomyces dermatitidis*	Chronic granulomatous lesions and microabscesses in any part of body Initial lesion is a papule; undergoes ulceration and peripheral spread	Pulmonary symptoms such as cough, chest pain, weakness, and weight loss May have skeletal involvement, with bone destruction and formation of cutaneous abscesses	Intravenous administration of amphotericin B	Usual portal of entry is the lungs Source of infection unknown Noninfectious
Cryptococcosis	*Cryptococcus neoformans (Torula histolytica)*	Usually on face; acneiform, firm, nodular, painless eruption	Central nervous system manifestations: headache, dizziness, stiff neck, and signs of increased intracranial pressure Low-grade fever, mild cough, lung infiltration	Intravenous amphotericin B may be administered intrathecally 5-Fluorocytosine Excision and drainage of local lesions	Acquired by inhalation of dust, but may enter through skin Prognosis serious Noninfectious
Histoplasmosis	*Histoplasma capsulatum*	Not distinctive or uniform but most appear as punched-out or granulomatous ulcers	General systemic symptoms may include pallor, diarrhea, vomiting, irregular spiking temperature, hepatosplenomegaly, and pulmonary symptoms Any tissue of the body may be involved with related symptoms	Intravenous amphotericin B for severe cases Triple sulfonamides	Organism cultured from soil, especially where contaminated with fowl droppings Fungus enters through skin or mucous membranes of mouth and respiratory tract Endemic in Mississippi and Ohio river valleys Disseminated diseases most common in infants and children
Coccidioidomycosis (valley fever)	*Coccidioides immitis*	Erythema nodosum	Primary lung disease usually asymptomatic May be sign of acute febrile illness Disseminated disease is very serious	Intravenous amphotericin B	Inhalation of aerospores from soil Endemic in southwestern United States Usually resolves spontaneously

Table 18-8. Eruptions caused by bites and stings

Bite or sting	Organism	Mechanism	Manifestations
Insect bites	Flies, gnats, mosquitoes, fleas, and flies	Hypersensitivity reaction Little or no reaction in nonsensitized person Foreign protein in insects' saliva introduced when skin penetrated for a blood-sucking meal	Papular urticaria termed lichen urticatus Firm papules; may be capped by vesicles or excoriated
Hymenoptera stings	Bees, wasps, hornets, yellow jackets, and ants	Injection of venom through stinging apparatus Venom contains histamine, allergenic proteins, and often a spreading factor, hyaluronidase Some proteins are species specific; others are common to a number of species, therefore cross-reactivity is common Severe reactions caused by hypersensitivity and/or multiple stings	Local reaction: small red area, wheal, itching, and heat Systemic reactions: may be mild to severe, including generalized edema, pain, nausea and vomiting, confusion, respiratory embarrassment, and shock
Arachnid bites	Spiders	All produce venom via fangs; few are able to pierce skin or the venom is insufficiently toxic	Local tissue reaction
	Black widow spider	Venom injected through a clawlike appendage Has a neurotropic action	Mild sting at time of bite Area becomes swollen, painful, and erythematous Dizziness, weakness, and abdominal pain May produce delirium, paralysis, convulsions, and (if large amount of venom absorbed) death
	Brown recluse spider	Venom contains a powerful neurotoxin	Mild sting at time of bite Transient erythema followed by bleb or blister; mild to severe pain in 2-8 hours; purple, star-shaped area in 3-4 days; necrotic ulceration in 7-14 days Heals with scar formation Systemic reactions may include fever, malaise, restlessness, nausea and vomiting, and joint pain Generalized petechial eruption
	Scorpions	Sting by means of a hooked caudal stinger that discharges venom Venom of more venomous species contains hemolysins, endotheliolysins, and neurotoxins	Some species produce only local tissue reaction with swelling at puncture site (distinctive) Intense local pain, erythema, numbness, and burning Ascending motor paralysis with convulsions, weakness, rapid pulse, excessive salivation, thirst, and dysuria
	Ticks	Feed on blood of mammals Significant in man because of pathologic organisms they carry In the process of sucking blood, the head and mouth parts are buried in the skin	Produce firm, discrete, intensely pruritic nodules at site of attachment May cause urticaria or persistent localized edema
Animal bites	Household pets (dogs, cats, mice, hamsters, and so on) Wild animals (mice, skunks, racoon, etc.)	Puncture wounds and tears from direct penetration of skin with teeth (claws)	Puncture wound, laceration, bruise

Treatment	Comments
Antipruritic agents and baths Antihistamines Application of insect repellant when exposure is anticipated Prevention of secondary infection	Avoidance of contact Removing focus such as treating furniture, mattresses, carpets, and so on, where insects may live
Carefully scraping off stinger if present Cleansing with soap and water Application of cool compresses or ice packs Elevation of involved extremity Application of tourniquet to extremity to retard absorption of venom Antihistamines Severe reactions: epinephrine, corticosteroids; treatment for shock	Persons with known sensitivity to bites or stings should wear identifying tag to indicate allergy and therapy needed; parents should keep emergency medication and be taught its administration Child should be taught to wear shoes, to avoid wearing bright clothing or perfumed grooming products that might attract the insect, and to avoid places where the insect may be contacted
Local compresses	Most spiders are harmless, including tarantulas
Cleansing wound with antiseptic; application of ice packs Antivenin Muscle relaxant such as calcium gluconate Morphine sulfate for pain Phenobarbital	Spider is recognized by red or orange hourglass-shaped marking on underside Avoids light and bites in self-defense
Local application of cool compresses Antibiotics Corticosteroids Relief of pain	Spider is fawn to dark brown and recognized by fiddle-shaped mark on head
Delaying absorption of venom by application of tourniquets for 10-15 minutes and application of cold with ice packs or submersion in cold water Supportive measures Treatment of shock	Usual habitat is southwestern United States Symptoms subside in a few hours Deaths occur among children under 4 years of age
Careful removal of tick to avoid breaking off embedded head; heated needle applied to body will cause head to withdraw; Other items that may cause it to release its hold include kerosene, lighter fluid, and nail polish	May be vectors of various infectious diseases such as Rocky Mountain spotted fever, Q fever, tularemia, and relapsing fever
Thorough washing with soap and water Observation of animal for rabies; if animal is positive for rabies, immunization series is begun immediately	May be vectors of bacterial infections and rabies Usual habitat is very wooded area

Table 18-9. Eruptions caused by infestations

Disease	Organism	Mechanism	Manifestations
Scabies (7-year itch)	*Sarcoptes scabei*	Impregnated female burrows into superficial stratum corneum of epidermis, depositing eggs and fecal material; burrows form a minute linear, grayish-brown, threadlike lesion Transmitted by skin-to-skin contact	Characteristic minute linear lesion seen with difficulty Intense pruritus that leads to punctate discrete excoriations secondary to pruritus; maculopapular lesions characteristically distributed in intertriginous areas: interdigital surfaces, axillary-cubital area, popliteal folds, and inguinal region Alopecia in scalp involvement Diagnosis confirmed by demonstrating mite or ova from skin scrapings
Pediculosis capitis (head lice)	*Pediculus humanus capitus*	Saliva of louse on the skin produces itching	Pruritus of scalp Close examination of scalp reveals white eggs (nits) firmly attached to hair shafts; adult lice are seldom found because of brief life span and mobility Excoriations are produced from itching and may become secondarily infected
Pediculosis corporis (body lice)	*Pediculus humanus corporis*	Lice present on the skin only when feeding Diagnosis established when lice and nits identified in seams of clothing	Pruritus Erythematous macules, wheals, and excoriated papules Most often found on upper back and pressure areas caused by tight clothing

Table 18-10. Miscellaneous skin disorders

Disease	Causative agent	Local manifestations	Systemic manifestations
Intertrigo	Mechanical trauma and aggravating factors of excessive heat, moisture, and sweat retention	Red, inflamed, moist, partially denuded, marginated areas, the shape of which is determined by location Appear where opposing skin surfaces rub together, that is, intergluteal folds, groin, neck, and axilla are common sites where chafing, warmth, and moisture enable microorganisms to produce dermatitis Hyperhydrosis and obesity are often factors	None unless severe secondary infection
Urticaria	Usually allergic response	Development of wheals Vary in size and configuration and tend to appear quickly, spread irregularly, and fade within a few hours May be constant or intermittent, sparse or profuse, small or large, discrete or confluent May be acute, chronic, or recurrent in acute attacks	May be accompanied by malaise, sometimes fever and lymphadenopathy Severe cases may involve mucous membranes, internal organs, and joints Obstruction to air passages constitutes medical emergency
Psoriasis	Unknown Hereditary predisposition	Round, thick, dry, reddish patches covered with coarse, silvery scales over trunk and extremities; first lesions commonly appear in scalp; facial lesions more common in children than adults Affected cells proliferate at a much more rapid rate than normal cells	Persons are otherwise healthy individuals

Treatment	Comments
Gamma benzene hexachloride (Kwell) in vanishing cream base Benzyl benzoate emulsion Crotamiton (Eurax) After hot bath with soap and water and thorough drying, one of the above is applied over entire cutaneous surface from the neck down; is left on for 24 hours; is repeated in 10 days to kill hatched larvae Only fresh laundered linen and underclothing should be used Touch and holding contacts should be reduced until treatment is completed Soothing ointments for pruritus	All infected members of a family should be treated at the same time Previously worn clothing should be washed in very hot water and ironed Nurses caring for affected children in the hospital should wear gloves and reduce holding
Gamma benzene hexachloride (Kwell, Kwellada) shampoo One ounce is applied to wet hair to form a luxuriant lather and rubbed in for at least 4 minutes, followed by combing with a fine-tooth comb to remove any remaining nits	Children, especially those with long hair, are most frequently affected Associated with poor hair hygiene Care givers, including nurses, should protect themselves from infection during examination and treatment by wearing gloves and protective caps
All clothing should be thoroughly laundered and seams ironed	Associated with unhygienic environmental conditions

Treatment	Comments
Affected areas are kept clean and dry Cool compresses of Burow's solution provide relief Skin folds may be kept separated with a generous supply of nonmedicated powder or cornstarch Area is exposed to air and light Treat superimposed infections Remove excess clothing	A form of diaper irritation Prevent recurrence by keeping susceptible areas clean and dry Frequently associated with overheating from too much clothing
Local soothing and antipruritic applications Antihistamines Epinephrine or ephedrine Cortisone or ACTH in severe cases Severe upper respiratory involvement may require tracheostomy	Known etiologic agents should be avoided
Exposure to sunlight, ultraviolet light Children respond well to topical applications of coal tar ointments, which act synergistically with ultraviolet light Ammoniated mercury 2%-5% Trihydroxyanthracine (anthralin) Topical adrenocorticosteroid cream Systemic (used only in acute refractory cases); corticosteroids, methotrexate	Uncommon in children under age 6 years

or prolonged exposure, and the sensitizing capacity of different substances varies widely. Strong sensitizers require only one or two exposures and occur in a higher percentage of individuals; weak sensitizers require numerous exposures, and a smaller percentage of those exposed will be sensitized. The length of time from exposure to development of sensitivity varies considerably and may be as short as a week or much longer. Sometimes with repeated exposure and reactions the skin loses its capacity to return to normal or secondary factors become predominant to produce a chronic inflammatory process.

The major goal in treatment is to prevent further exposure of the skin to the offending substance. Providing there is not further irritation, the normal recuperative powers of the skin will produce satisfactory results without treatment.

The most frequent offenders are plant and animal irritants, the prototype of which is poison ivy. Contact with the dry or succulent portions of the plant produces localized, streaked or spotty, oozing and painful impetiginous lesions. The most effective management of the lesions includes administration of corticosteroids to reduce inflammation, cooling compresses, and a sedative such as diphenhydramine (Benadryl) or aspirin. Prevention of autoinoculation from the original lesions and avoidance of contact by teaching the child to recognize the plant and its removal from the environment when feasible are prophylactic measures.

The most common contact dermatitis in infants occurs on the convex surfaces of the diaper area as a result of chemical irritation from ammonia, putrefactive enzymes acting on urinary amino acids, or, less often, laundry products (see p. 283). Other agents that frequently produce dermatologic responses from contact are animal irritants such as wool, feathers, and furs, vegetable irritants such as oleoresins, oils, and turpentine, and chemicals of all kinds, including synthetic fabrics, dyes, metals, cosmetics, perfumes, and soaps. The list is endless.

Drug reactions

Adverse reactions to drugs are seen more often in the skin than in any other organ. Cutaneous manifestations can resemble almost any skin disease and can be seen in almost any degree of severity. With few exceptions, the distribution of a drug eruption is widespread since it results from a circulating agent, appears as an inflammatory response with itching, is sudden in onset, and may be associated with constitutional symptoms such as fever, malaise, gastrointestinal upsets, anemia, or liver and kidney damage.

Although any drug is capable of producing almost any form of reaction in the susceptible individual, some of them have a tendency to produce a particular reaction consistently, and some drugs are more likely than others to produce an untoward effect. Many are allergenic responses following a prior administration of the drug, even a topical application. Other factors influence a drug response in a particular individual. For example, drug eruptions occur with less frequency in children than in adults, climate may be a factor when light sensitivity produces a response on sun-exposed surfaces, and it is well known that there are genetic factors that affect the way in which some individuals are able to metabolize specific drugs.

Individual drug reactions may vary from a single lesion to extensive, generalized epidermal necrosis. Drug reactions are also related to the amount of drug administered and the route of administration. For example, larger amounts precipitate a more severe response than a small amount, and drugs taken orally are less sensitizing than those administered intravenously. Another common response is a fixed eruption, that is, a recurrent eruption at the same site with each readministration of the drug. The lesion, a purplish red round or oval plaque with a sharp border seen most frequently on the extremities, disappears slowly and the pigmentation deepens with each episode.

The most frequent offenders in drug reactions are penicillin and sulfonamides. However, even commonplace drugs including aspirin, barbiturates, and chemical agents in a number of foods, flavoring agents, and preservatives, are capable of producing an undesired response.

Treatment for cutaneous reactions consists of discontinuation of the drug. Nurses who suspect that a rash is caused by a medication should withhold any further dose and report the eruption to the attending physician. In urticarial-type eruptions antihistamines may be ordered, and, for widespread and severe lesions, corticosteroids are beneficial.

Nursing considerations

Skin disorders present nurses with some of their most challenging problems. Nurses are involved in recognizing and describing deviations from normal skin character, determining the cause, carrying out a treatment plan, and dealing with the affected child and his family.

Identification of skin disorders. To assist in establishing a diagnosis, it is important for nurses to accurately describe any deviation in the character of the skin, using both inspection and palpation. The color, shape, and distribution of the lesions are noted, including absence of pigment (vitiligo). The individual lesions are described according to the accepted terminology (p. 660) and may involve more than one type, such as a maculopapular rash.

To confirm or amplify the findings made by inspection, the skin is gently palpated to detect characteristics such as temperature, moisture, texture, elasticity, and the presence of edema in the skin. It should be indicated whether the findings are restricted to the area of the lesion(s) or are generalized.

The child's subjective symptoms provide additional information. Older children are able to describe the condition as painful, itching, tingling, or so on. However, much can

Summary of nursing care of the child with disorders of the skin

Goals	Responsibilities
Identify lesion and its cause	Describe skin lesion accurately; use descriptive terminology for type, configuration, and distribution of lesion(s) Describe any associated characteristics, such as temperature, moisture, texture, elasticity, and hardness of skin in general or in area of lesion(s) Obtain history of onset, possible precipitating events, and course of development Determine any symptoms associated with disorder, such as itching, pain, fever, and so on Participate in special tests, such as collection of specimens for laboratory examination, use of Wood's light, or elimination diet
Prevent secondary infection	Maintain careful hand washing before handling affected child; wear surgical gloves when handling or dressing affected parts if indicated by nature of lesion Teach child and family hygienic care and medical asepsis Devise methods to prevent secondary infection of lesion in small or uncooperative children
Protect healthy skin surface	Teach and impress on child importance of keeping hands away from lesion(s) Assist child to determine ways of preventing autoinoculation Devise means for keeping small or uncooperative children from spreading infection to other areas Protect healthy skin from maceration by keeping it dry
Prevent spread of infection to self and others	Isolate affected child from susceptible individuals Maintain careful hand washing after caring for child Avoid unnecessary close contact with affected child during infective stage of disease Use correct technique for disposal of dressings, solutions, and other fomites in contact with lesion(s)
Prevent occurrence and/or recurrence	Avoid or reduce contact with agents or circumstances known to precipitate skin reaction Teach child to recognize agents or circumstances that produce reaction
Promote healing	Carry out therapeutic regimen as prescribed or support and assist parents to carry out treatment plan Prevent secondary infection and autoinoculation Encourage rest Reduce external stimuli that aggravate condition Encourage well-balanced diet
Relieve discomfort	Avoid or reduce external stimuli that aggravate discomfort, such as rough clothing and bed linen Apply soothing treatments and topical applications as ordered Administer medications to relieve discomfort and/or restlessness and irritability
Support child	Teach self-care where appropriate Involve child in planning treatment schedules Support and encourage child in his efforts to deal with the multiple problems that may be associated with disorder, including discomfort, rejection, discouragement, and feelings of self-revulsion Encourage child to maintain usual activities

Continued.

Summary of nursing care of the child with disorders of the skin—cont'd

Goals	Responsibilities
Promote habits of hygiene	Teach and reinforce positive habits of hygienic care
Teach parents	Teach parents skills needed to carry out therapeutic program Inform parents of expected and unexpected results of therapy and a course of action to follow Help devise special techniques to carry out therapy
Support parents	Encourage parents in their efforts to carry out plan of care Provide assistance when appropriate Refer to agencies and services that assist with social, financial, and medical problems

be determined by observation of the child's behavior and the parents' account of his reactions. Does he scratch? Is he restless or irritable? Does he favor or avoid using a part? A careful history may provide enlightenment. Has the child had access to chemicals? Has he been in the woods or around a woodpile? Has he eaten a new food? Is he taking medication? Has he any known allergy? Do any of his playmates have a similar lesion? A doubtful diagnosis is frequently confirmed on the basis of history.

Nurse's role in therapy. Since only a few skin diseases are contagious, it is usually not necessary to isolate the affected child unless there is a danger that he may acquire a secondary infection. This is usually the child who is receiving large doses of corticosteroids or other immunosuppressant drugs or the child with an immunologic deficiency disorder. If the skin manifestation is caused by a viral exanthem, such as measles or chickenpox, the child should be prevented from exposing other susceptible children (see also impetigo contagiosa, p. 311).

Autoinoculation is a constant hazard in some disorders such as impetigo, poison ivy, or (to a lesser extent) warts. The cooperation of older children can be obtained, although they may need reminding to stop scratching or rubbing, but smaller and uncooperative children require the implementation of techniques and devices such as mittens, restraints, or special coverings. These methods, along with general cleanliness and hygiene, also serve to reduce the likelihood of secondary infection of a primary lesion.

Therapeutic programs are usually designed to provide general measures such as rest, protection, and relief of discomfort and specific treatments such as a definitive medication or physical technique. They usually involve some type of topical treatment, and the mode of application depends on the nature and location of the lesion being treated. For example, soothing lotions, creams, and intermittent wet dressings or soaks help cool and dry; ointments, lotions, and creams soften and lubricate dry, scaling areas. Most of the therapeutic regimens are directed toward relief of pruritus, the most common subjective complaint. Cooling applications that reduce external stimuli to the part are highly beneficial along with maintenance of cleanliness and good aeration. Clothing and bed linen should be soft and lightweight to decrease the irritation from friction and stimulation. During any type of treatment, both affected and unaffected skin is protected from damage and secondary infection.

Child and parental support. Childhood dermatologic conditions always involve the parents. Since few situations require hospitalization and children who do require hospitalization will complete a therapy program at home, the parents are the persons who must carry out the treatment plan; therefore, their cooperation is essential. Child and parents are more apt to be motivated if they are told why something is being done in a certain way. Success of treatment depends on the correct interpretation of instructions, and it is often the nurse's responsibility to teach the parent how to carry out the physician's instructions and offer encouragement, support, and assistance with problem solving.

Regimens that are simple to accomplish in the hospital or office situation may be frustrating and baffling at home. Parents often need assistance in adapting equipment available in the home to the therapy, for example, dressings from scraps and rags and the use of utensils for soaks. One of the most difficult areas to deal with is the child's irritability and tendency to disturb dressings and scratch or pick at lesions. Here nurses can help parents devise protective restraining devices and distracting activities for the child. Treatments at home, in the clinics, or in the physician's office that are scheduled and arranged to accommodate the child's schooling and parent's affairs are more apt to be carried out.

It is important that parents and child are given as much explanation as possible about both the expected and the unexpected results of treatments, including any ill effects that might occur. Although a treatment plan is chosen for its probability of being beneficial without doing harm using medications that contain the fewest and safest ingredients, persons with skin disorders are highly susceptible to irritation. They are directed to discontinue treatment and report any unexpected reactions to the appropriate person(s). Skin changes bother people so that they often try anything, including home remedies and patent medicines. The use of patent medicines is discouraged unless this has first been discussed with the attending physician and has received approval.

Since the skin is the most visible portion of the body, defects in its surface that alter its appearance are sometimes an additional source of distress to the affected child and his family. Unsightly lesions or medicinal preparations applied to the skin are often sources of revulsion and rejection by others. Other children will proffer derogatory comments and may even reject the affected child. Parents of other children may fear that their children will "catch" the disorder. Occasionally the affected child's own family will reduce their interaction with him, especially close physical contact, or otherwise demonstrate a distaste for his condition that he may interpret as rejection. This is seldom a difficulty with dermatitis of short duration, but chronic conditions can create problems in development of a positive self-concept. (For a summary of nursing care of the child with disorders of the skin see the boxed material on pp. 677 to 678.)

REFERENCES

1. Adams, R. M.: Principles and practice of topical therapy, Pediatr. Clin. North Am. **18:**685-712, 1971.
2. Bakwin, H., and Bakwin, R. M.: Behavior disorders in children, ed. 4, Philadelphia, 1972, W. B. Saunders Co.
3. Clements, C. K.: Minimal brain dysfunction in children: terminology and identification, Public Health Service pamphlet No. 3, Washington, D.C., 1966, U.S. Department of Health, Education and Welfare.
4. Eisenberg, L.: The clinical use of stimulant drugs in children, Pediatrics **49:**709-715, 1972.
5. Faust, E. C., Russell, P. F., and Jung, R. C.: Craig and Faust's clinical parasitology, ed. 8, Philadelphia, 1970, Lea & Febiger.
6. Gearheart, B. R.: Learning disabilities: educational strategies, ed. 2, St. Louis, 1977, The C. V. Mosby Co.
7. Jacobson, O. H.: Teeth. In Kempe, C. H., Silver, H. K., and O'Brien, D.: Current pediatric diagnosis and treatment, ed. 3, Los Altos, Calif., 1974, Lange Medical Publications.
8. The National Advisory Committee on Handicapped Children, Washington, D.C., 1967, U.S. Office of Education.
9. Padilla, E. R., and associates: Predicting accident frequency in children, Pediatrics **58:**223-226, 1976.
10. Stewart, W. D., Danto, J. L., and Maddin, S.: Dermatology: diagnosis and treatment of cutaneous disorders, ed. 4, St. Louis, 1977, The C. V. Mosby Co.
11. Wender, P.: Minimal brain dysfunction in children: diagnosis and management, Pediatr. Clin. North Am. **20:**187-202, 1973.
12. Ziai, M., and Wasti, S. M. K.: Parasitic infections. In Ziai, M., editor: Pediatrics, Boston, 1975, Little, Brown and Co.

BIBLIOGRAPHY

Bain, H. W.: Chronic vague abdominal pain in children, Pediatr. Clin. North Am. **21:**991-1000, 1974.

Boder, E.: School failure—evaluation and treatment, Pediatrics **58:**394-403, 1976.

Caldwell, P. D., and Smith, D. W.: The XXY (Klinefelter's) syndrome in childhood: detection and treatment, J. Pediatr. **80:** 250, 1972.

Crowdes, N. E.: Group therapy for preadolescent boys, Am. J. Nurs. **75:**92-95, 1975.

Cullinan, T. R.: Children at risk of accident, Community Health **2**(4):175-178, January/February 1971.

Galli, P.: Nursing in a pediatric multiphasic program, Am. J. Nurs. **74:**892, 1974.

Izant, R. J., and associates: Bicycle spoke injuries of foot and ankle in children: an underestimated minor injury, J. Pediatr. Surg. **4:**654, 1969.

Kinsbourne, M.: School problems, Pediatrics **52:**697, 1973.

Kruter, J. S.: A comprehensive nursing approach to pediatric facial injuries, Issues Comprehensive Pediatr. Nurs., pp. 1-17, May 1977.

Metz, J. R., and associates: A pediatric screening examination for psychosocial problems, Pediatrics **58:**595-606, 1976.

Rance, C. P., and associates: Persistent systemic hypertension in infants and children, Pediatr. Clin. North Am. **21:**801, November, 1974.

Rodstein, M.: Accident proneness, J.A.M.A. **229:**1495, September 4, 1974.

Rommel, J.: Referral of children with speech problems, Pediatr. Nurs. **2:**28, 1976.

Shirkey, H. C., editor: Pediatric therapy, ed. 5, St. Louis, 1975, The C. V. Mosby Co.

Tredgold, R. F.: Emotional factors and accident causation, Community Health **2**(1):7-11, July/August 1970.

Waller, J.: Bicycle ownership use, and injury patterns among elementary school children, Pediatrics **47:**1042, 1971.

Minimal brain dysfunction

Adams, J.: Clinical neuropsychology and the study of learning disorders, Pediatr. Clin. North Am. **20:**587-598, 1973.

Allmond, B. W.: Psychological testing in children, Pediatr. Clin. North Am. **21:**184-196, 1976.

Arnold, L. E.: The art of medicating hyperkinetic children: a number of practical suggestions, Clin. Pediatr. **12:**35, 1973.

Berlin, L. N.: Minimal brain dysfunction: management of family distress, J.A.M.A. **229:**1454-1456, 1974.

Bierbauer, E.: Tips for parents of a neurologically handicapped child, Am. J. Nurs. **72:**1972-1974, 1972.

Bowers, J. E.: Can you recognize childhood learning disorders? Nursing '77 **7**(11):26-29, 1977.

Box, M. C.: The assessment of the child at school entry, Pediatrics **58:**403-407, 1976.

Bruere, H.: The dyslexic child, Pediatr. Ann. **6:**129, February 1977.

Cochran, A.: Recognizing MBD in the problem child, RN **35:**35-39, May 1972.

Connors, C. K., and associates: Food additives and hyperkinesis: a controlled double-blind experiment, Pediatrics **58:**154-166, 1976.

Drabman, R. S., and Jarvie, G.: Counseling parents of children with behavior problems: the use of extinction and time-out technique, Pediatrics **59:**78-85, 1977.

Erenberg, G.: Drug therapy in minimal brain dysfunction: a commentary, J. Pediatr. **81:**359-365, 1972.

Feingold, B.: Food additives and child development, Hosp. Pract. **8:**11, 1973.

Feingold, B. F.: Hyperkinesis and learning disabilities linked to artificial food flavors and colors, Am. J. Nurs. **75:**797-803, 1975.

Freeman, R. D.: The drug treatment of learning disorders: continuing confusion, J. Pediatr. **81:**112-115, 1972.

Gofman, H. F., and Allmond, B. W., Jr.: Learning and language disorders in children, Curr. Probl. Pediatr. **1**(11):entire issue, September 1971.

Gross, M. D.: Growth of hyperkinetic children taking methylphenidate, dextroamphetamine, or imipramine/desipramine, Pediatrics **58:**423-431, 1976.

Hart, E. J., and Carter, S.: Minimal brain dysfunction. In Downey, J. A., and Low, N. L., editors: The child with disabling illness, Philadelphia, 1974, W. B. Saunders Co.

Holmberg, N. J.: Serving the child with MBD and his family in a health maintenance organization, Nurs. Clin. North Am. **10:** 381-392, June 1975.

Johnson, C. F., and Prinz, R.: Hyperactivity is in the eyes of the beholder, Clin. Pediatr. **15**(3):222-237, 1976.

Kenny, T. J., and associates: Characteristics of children referred because of hyperactivity, J. Pediatr. **79:**618, 1971.

Kenny, T. J., and associates: The medical evaluation of children with reading problems (dyslexia), Pediatrics **49:**438-442, 1972.

Keogh, B. K.: Hyperactivity and learning disorders: review and speculation, Except. Child. **30:**2, 101-109, 1971.

Lerner, J. W.: Children with learning disabilities: theories, diagnosis, and teaching strategies, Boston, 1971, Houghton Mifflin Co.

Marwit, S. J., and Stenner, A. J.: Hyperkinesis: delineation of two patterns, Except. Child. **38:**5, 401-406, 1972.

Nichamin, S. J.: Recognizing minimal cerebral dysfunction in the infant and toddler, Clin. Pediatr. **11:**255-257, May 1972.

O'Leary, K. D., and associates: Behavioral treatment of hyperkinetic children, Clin. Pediatr. **15:**510-515, 1976.

Page-El, E., and Grossman, H. J.: Neurological appraisal in learning disorders, Pediatr. Clin. North Am. **20:**599, 1973.

Palmer, S., Rapoport, J. L., and Quinn, P. O.: Food additives and hyperactivity, Clin. Pediatr. **14:**956-959, 1975.

Pearson, G. A.: Nutrition in the middle years of childhood, Am. J. Maternal Child Nurs. **2**(6):378-382, 1977.

Peters, J. E., and associates: Physician's handbook, screening for MBD, Summit, N.J., 1973, Ciba Medical Horizons.

Rogers, M.: Early identification and intervention of children with learning problems, Pediatr. Nurs. **2:**21-26, January/February 1976.

Schain, R. J.: Minimal brain dysfunction, Curr. Probl. Pediatr. **5**(10):1-30, August 1975.

Senf, G. M.: Learning disabilities, Pediatr. Clin. North Am. **20:** 607-640, 1973.

Silver, L. B.: Acceptable and controversial approaches to treating the child with learning disabilities, Pediatrics **55:**406-415, 1975.

Spring, C., and Sandoval, J.: Food additives and hyperkinesis: a critical evaluation of the evidence, J. Learning Disabilities **9**(9): 28-37, November 1976.

Sroufe, L. A., and Stewart, M. A.: Treating problem children with stimulant drugs, N. Engl. J. Med. **289:**407, 1973.

Stein, M. T.: Minimal brain dysfunction: a note of caution in management, Clin. Pediatr. **14:**840-841, 1975.

Stewart, M. A.: Hyperactive children, Sci. Am. **222:**94, 1970.

Towbin, A.: Organic causes of minimal brain dysfunction, J.A. M.A. **217:**1207, 1971.

Tredgold, R. F.: Emotional factors and accident causation, Community Health **2**(1):7-11, July/August 1970.

Warren, S. A.: Adult expectations and learning disorders, Pediatr. Clin. North Am. **20:**705-718, 1973.

Woodward, P. B., and Brodie, B.: The hyperactive child: who is he? Nurs. Clin. North Am. **9:**727-746, 1974.

Enuresis

Ballar, W. R.: Bed wetting: origins and treatment, Elmsford, N.Y., 1975, Pergamon Press, Inc.

Cohen, M. W.: Enuresis, Pediatr. Clin. North Am. **22:**545-560, 1975.

McKendry, J. B. J., and Stewart, D. A.: Enuresis, Pediatr. Clin. North Am. **21:**1019-1028, 1974.

Palmisano, P. A.: Enuresis. In Shirkey, H. C., editor: Pediatric therapy, ed. 5, St. Louis, 1975, The C. V. Mosby Co.

Pierce, C. M.: Enuresis and encopresis. In Freedman, A. M., Kaplan, H. I., and Sadock, B. J.: Comprehensive textbook of psychiatry II, vol. 2, ed. 2, Baltimore, 1975, The Williams & Wilkins Co.

Simonds, J. F.: Enuresis, Clin. Pediatr. **16:**79-82, 1977.

Starfield, B.: Enuresis: its pathogenesis and management, Clin. Pediatr. **11:**343, 1972.

Stewart, M. A.: Treatment of bedwetting, J.A.M.A. **232:**281, 1975.

School phobia and childhood schizophrenia

Fagin, C. M., editor: Readings in child and adolescent psychiatric nursing, St. Louis, 1974, The C. V. Mosby Co.

Freedman, A. M., Kaplan, H. I., and Sadock, B. J.: Comprehensive textbook of psychiatry II, vol. 2, ed. 2, Baltimore, 1975, The Williams & Wilkins Co.

Goldfarb, W., and Yahres, H.: The causes and treatment of childhood schizophrenia. In Segal, I.: The mental health of the child, Public Health Service pamphlet No. 1268, Washington, D.C., 1971, U.S. Government Printing Office.

Herbert, M.: Emotional problems in development of children, New York, 1974, Academic Press, Inc.

Lidz, T., and Yahraes, H.: Parental behavior and the origins of schizophrenia. In Segal, J., editor: The mental health of the child, Public Health Service pamphlet No. 2168, Washington, D.C., 1971, U.S. Government Printing Office.

Moughton, M. L.: Systems and childhood psychosis, Nurs. Clin. North Am. **6:**425-434, 1971.

Nader, P. R., Bullock, D., and Caldwell, B.: School phobia, Pediatr. Clin. North Am. **22:**605-617, 1975.
Schmitt, B. D.: School phobia—the great imitator: a pediatrician's viewpoint, Pediatrics **11:**195, April 1972.

Dental problems

Bernick, S. M.: What the pediatrician should know about children's teeth, Clin. Pediatr. **10:**243, 1974.
DePaola, D. P., and Alfano, M. C.: Diet and oral health, Nutr. Today **12**(3):6-11, 29-32, May/June 1977.
McBean, L. D., and Speckmann, E. W.: A review: the importance of nutrition in oral health, J. Am. Dent. Assoc. **89:**109-114, July 1974.
McDonald, R. E.: Dentistry of the child and adolescent, ed. 2, St. Louis, 1974, The C. V. Mosby Co.
Nizel, A. E.: Preventing dental caries: the nutritional factors, Pediatr. Clin. North Am. **24:**141-155, 1977.
Pillsbury, D. M.: A manual of dermatology, Philadelphia, 1971, W. B. Saunders Co.
Rowe, N. H., and associates: The effect of age, sex, race and economic status on dental caries experience of the permanent teeth, Pediatrics **55:**457-461, 1976.
Shaw, J. H.: Nutritional guidance in the prevention of oral disease, Dent. Clin. North Am. **16:**733, 1975.
Slattery, J.: Dental health in children, Am. J. Nurs. **76:**1159-1161, 1976.
Smith, J. T.: Promoting childhood dental health, Pediatr. Nurs. **2**(3):161-191, 1976.

Helminthic infections

Abadie, S. H., Blumenthal, D. S., and Wang, C. C.: When the name of the game is worms, Patient Care **9**(10):96-101, May 15, 1975.
Katz, M.: Parasitic infections, J. Pediatr. **87:**165, 1975.
Knight, R., and associates: Progress report: intestinal parasites, Gut **14:**145, 1973.
Most, H.: Treatment of common parasitic infections of man encountered in the United States. Part I, N. Engl. J. Med. **287:**495-498, 1972.
Roy, C. C., Silverman, A., and Cozzeto, F. J.: Pediatric clinical gastroenterology, ed. 2, St. Louis, 1975, The C. V. Mosby Co.
Simon, R. D.: Pinworm infestation and urinary tract infection in young girls, Am. J. Dis. Child. **128:**21-22, 1974.

Disorders affecting the skin

Alexander, M. M., and Brown, M. S.: Pediatric physical diagnosis for nurses, New York, 1974, McGraw-Hill Book Co.
Burson, I. J.: Drug reactions, insect bites, and fungal infections, Issues Comprehensive Pediatr. Nurs., pp. 12-21, 1976.
Derbes, V. J.: Rashes: recognition and management, Nursing '73 **3:**44-49, March 1973.
Derbes, V. J., and associates: Treating severe reaction to bee sting, Patient Care **10**(11):66-77, June 1, 1976.
Dufour, H. B.: Disorders of the skin. In Moidel, G. H., and associates: Nursing care of the patient with medical-surgical disorders, New York, 1971, McGraw-Hill Book Co.
Dufour, H. B.: Dermatology outline, Unpublished data.
Epstein, E.: Contact dermatitis in children, Pediatr. Clin. North Am. **18:**839-852, 1971.
Epstein, E., and Orkin, M.: Could that "maddening itch" be lice or mites? Patient care **7:**44-111, 1973.
Fisher, A. A., and Maibach, H.: Cooling poison-plant dermatitis, Patient Care **10**(11):60-65, June 1, 1976.
Forbes, M., and Scipien, G.: Communicable diseases and some infections of the skin, Issues Comprehensive Pediatr. Nurs., pp. 1-11, 1976.
Frazier, C. A.: Those deadly insects, RN **34**(4):49-55, 1971.
Freedberg, I. M.: The skin. In Ziai, M., editor: Pediatrics, ed. 2, Boston, 1975, Little, Brown and Co.
Hall, V. A., Shaw, P. K., and Smith, E. B.: Exterminating the scabies mite, Patient Care **10**(9):102, May 1976.
Hall, V. A., Shaw, P. K., and Smith, E. B.: Could that itching be scabies? Nurs. Update **7**(8):1, 13-16, 1976.
Huchinson, R.: What to do and what to worry about when treating stings and bites, Nursing '77 **7**(6):69-71, 1977.
Juranek, D. D.: The nuisance diseases: pediculosis and scabies, Assoc. Pract. Inf. Cond. Newslett. **4**(1):entire issue, February 1976.
Krugman, S., Ward, R., and Katz, S. L.: Infectious diseases of children, ed. 6, St. Louis, 1977, The C. V. Mosby Co.
Leider, M.: Some principles of dermatologic nursing, RN **35**(5): 48-53, 1972.
Matus, N. R.: Topical therapy: choosing and using the proper vehicle, Nursing '77 **7**(11):8-10, 1977.
Moschella, S. L., Pillsbury, D. M., and Hurley, H. J.: Dermatology, Philadelphia, 1975, W. B. Saunders Co.
Nahmias, A. J., and Tomkh, M. O.: Herpes simplex virus infection, Curr. Probl. Pediatr. **4**(4):3-36, February 1974.
North, C., and Weinstein, G. D.: Treatment of psoriasis, Am. J. Nurs. **76:**410-412, 1976.
Orkin, M.: Today's scabies, J.A.M.A. **233:**882-885, August 25, 1975.
Prior, J. A., and Silberstein, J. S.: Physical diagnosis: the history and examination of the patient, ed. 5, St. Louis, 1977, The C. V. Mosby Co.
Rice, A. K.: Common skin infections in school children, Am. J. Nurs. **73:**1905-1909, 1973.
Rogers, R. S., and Tindall, J. P.: Herpes zoster in children, Arch. Dermatol. **106:**204, 1972.
Sutton, R. L., Jr., and Waisman, M.: The practitioners' dermatology, New York, 1975, Yorke Medical Books.
Vaughan, V. C., and McKay, R. J.: Textbook of pediatrics, ed. 10, Philadelphia, 1975, W. B. Saunders Co.
Watson, W., and Farber, E. M.: Psoriasis in childhood, Pediatr. Clin. North Am. **18:**875-895, 1971.

UNIT EIGHT
Later childhood

Adolescence is a period of transition that is based on childhood experiences and accomplishments and has a goal of mature, independent, and responsible functioning. This transition is a biologic, emotional, and social process, a preparatory period requiring the accomplishment of defined developmental tasks in order to attain satisfactory adjustment to adulthood. The early years of adolescence are concerned with individuation from previous dependency roles and a gradual movement toward peer-group identity. The peer group is the focus of the adolescent's world—the persons in his life who are going through the same transition and who understand the problems and frustrations he is experiencing. Later years of adolescence are centered around acquiring a personal identity, completing the separation process from family, and career-directed activity.

The physiologic changes that take place during puberty have both psychologic and social significance for adolescent boys and girls, and the rate and degree of equanimity with which adolescents grow and mature vary widely among individuals. Although it is a relatively healthy period of life, most of the health and emotional problems of teenagers are directly related to the biologic alterations and the emotional responses associated with this tumultuous period in the life span.

Chapter 19, *The Adolescent Years,* provides an overview of the transitional adolescent period during which youth must adjust to rapid body changes, establish a personal identity, gain emotional and (for some) economic freedom from their parents, and evolve a set of values uniquely their own. Chapters 20 and 21 are concerned with some of the health problems associated with adolescence as a result of either the changes related to biologic maturation or the psychologic adjustments imposed by these changes and the expectations of society. Chapter 20, *Health Problems of Adolescence,* is devoted primarily to physical problems with psychologic implications; Chapter 21, *Problems of Psychologic Adjustment to Adolescence,* is focused on health problems that are induced principally by the psychologic responses to adolescence but that impose a serious threat to health and well-being.

19

The adolescent years

Adolescence begins at puberty and, accompanying the pubertal changes, there are corresponding changes in the personality. There is considerable variation in the time of onset of puberty and in the manner in which different individuals cope with the multiple developmental events associated with pubertal changes. Adolescence is a period of transition and a time of physical, social, and emotional maturing as the boy prepares for manhood and the girl for womanhood. It is during this period of development that the individual makes the most significant progress in learning to live effectively in society.

The precise boundaries of adolescence are difficult to define, but this period is customarily viewed as beginning with the gradual appearance of secondary sex characteristics at about 11 or 12 years of age and ending with cessation of somatic growth at 18 to 20 years of age. However, there are such wide individual and cultural variations that, more than any other age category, no sharp age delineation can be made. Adolescence tends to begin and end earlier in girls than in boys.

There are several terms that are commonly used in reference to this particular stage of growth and development. Puberty primarily refers to the maturational, hormonal, and growth process when the reproductive organs begin to function and the secondary sex characteristics develop. Puberty is sometimes further delineated as *pubescence,* that period of about 2 years immediately prior to puberty when the child is developing preliminary physical changes that herald sexual maturity and is characterized by the prepubertal growth spurt; *puberty,* the point at which sexual maturity is achieved, marked by the first menstrual flow in girls but by less obvious indications in boys; and *postpubescence,* a 1- to 2-year period following puberty during which skeletal growth is completed and reproductive functions become fairly well established. Puberty ends with the ability to reproduce, which in girls is soon after the onset of menstruation with the establishment of regular ovulation and in boys is soon after the first nocturnal emission when spermatogenesis is established. *Adolescence,* less firmly fixed, literally means "to grow into maturity" and is generally regarded as the psychologic, social, and maturational process initiated by the pubertal changes. The term *teenage years* is used synonymously with adolescence to describe ages 13 through 19 years.

Although the changes that take place during adolescence are primarily those of body and personality, children in this period are highly influenced by the culture in which they grow and develop. In some of the more primitive societies the transition to adulthood is recognized soon after or simultaneous with puberty. The event is solemnized by some type of ritual, ceremony, or other "rite of passage." The child from that point assumes the privileges, responsibilities, and status accorded an adult in the society. Decisions are made early, and the psychologic stage is relatively brief. The child knows from early childhood what is expected and, prepared for his role in adult activities, slips easily into the new position accepted by parents, the society, and himself.

In more complex societies this transition is less clearly delineated, and society is equally vague about attainment of adult status. School years are legally over at 16 to 18 years of age but for many young people may continue to age 25 years or beyond. Adolescents are legally permitted to drive as young as 14 years of age in some states and at a later age in others, but adult insurance premiums are not granted until age 25 years. In many states adolescents are not allowed to gamble or purchase liquor until age 21 years. Many activities in which young people are allowed to participate are considered to be those of adults, such as wars, voting, marriage, and childbearing, whereas, at the same time, they are considered as youngsters in relation to social status and control of resources in the adult community. This ambiguity of society and parents contributes to the adolescents' own confusion and ambiguity about themselves.

In addition to this prolonged period of cultural maturation, adolescents' ultimate goals and adult roles are less defined and clear-cut in advanced societies than they are in primitive societies. In advanced cultures there are choices to be made regarding occupation, marriage, and even social and religious values. Although adolescents want to achieve adult status and privileges, they are faced with so many possibilities and choices that they are often reluctant to assume the associated responsibilities. They are eager to grow up yet fearful of the implications. It is no wonder that adolescence is a time of confusion and turmoil.

Developmental tasks of adolescence

Adolescence, that transitional stage between childhood and adulthood, is a period of life that presents special problems of adjustment. With the impetus of their internal changes and the pressures of society, children must progress to emotional independence from their parents, consider prospects of economic independence, and learn the meaning of a more intimate heterosexual companionship. They learn to work with age-mates on common interests and to subordinate personal differences as they pursue a common goal. Achievement of these maturational goals to become responsible persons in control of their lives and possessing a knowledge of who they are in relation to the world are accomplished through the developmental tasks of adolescence. These tasks as defined by Havighurst are[9]:

1. *Achieving new and more mature relations with age-mates of both sexes.* A satisfactory social adjustment is achieved through social activities and experimentation with the increasingly influential peer group. Here adolescents learn to behave as adults among adults as they create, on a small scale, the society of their elders.
2. *Achieving a masculine or feminine social role.* Sex is biologically determined, but masculinity and femininity are culturally established behaviors that must be learned.
3. *Accepting one's physique and using the body effectively.* The body image is established most firmly during adolescence. The adolescent must cope with normal but rapid changes in physical appearance and concomitant alterations in functional capacity. Any deviation from the "norm" is a source of stress and may or may not be incorporated into the adolescent's body image.
4. *Achieving emotional independence of parents and other adults.* The movement away from dependence on parents that was begun during the school years is completed in this period of development. Successful accomplishment results in affection and respect for the parents without a childish dependence on them.
5. *Preparing for marriage and family life.* Sexual maturation and a strong attraction for the opposite sex serve as an impetus for examining the implications of a future life-style. Young people show varied attitudes toward marriage and having children.
6. *Preparing for an economic career.* With adulthood approaching rapidly, children must begin planning for economic independence and organizing their energies toward realistic goals and career opportunities that complement rather than conflict with their capabilities and temperament.
7. *Acquiring a set of values and an ethical system as a guide to behavior–developing an ideology.* Assuming a place in society requires the individual to make value choices on his own in a number of complex situations. During adolescence the child develops an increased interest in philosophic, political, and religious matters and incorporates the values learned in his childhood in developing his own philosophy of life.
8. *Desiring and achieving socially responsible behavior.* Throughout childhood the child learns to be a participating member of a group. First in the family group, then in the peer group, he gradually learns to subordinate his personal pleasures for the welfare of the group and to assume social obligations.

PHYSICAL DEVELOPMENT

The physical changes of puberty are primarily the result of hormonal activity under the influence of the central nervous system, although all aspects of physiologic functioning are mutually interacting. Growth and change are more dramatically and visibly demonstrated at this time than at any other period in the life span. The very obvious physical changes are noted in increased physical growth and the appearance and development of secondary sex characteristics; less obvious are physiologic alterations and neurogonadal maturity, accompanied by the ability to procreate. Physical distinction between the sexes is determined on the basis of distinguishing characteristics: *primary sex characteristics* are the external and internal organs that carry on the reproductive functions; *secondary sex characteristics* are those that distinguish the sexes from each other but play no direct part in reproduction.

Physical growth

A constant phenomenon associated with sexual maturation is a dramatic increase in growth. The final 20% to 25% of linear growth is achieved during puberty, the majority of which occurs during a 24- to 36-month period—the adolescent growth spurt. This accelerated growth occurs in all children but, as in other areas of development, is highly variable in age of onset, duration, and extent. The growth spurt begins earlier in girls, usually between ages 10 and 14 years; on the average it begins between ages 12 and 16 years in boys. During this period the average boy will gain 10 to 30 cm (4 to 12 inches) in height and 7 to 30 kg (15 to 65 pounds) in weight; the average girl, in whom the growth spurt is slower and less extensive, will gain 5 to 20 cm (2 to 7.9 inches) in height and 7 to 25 kg (15 to 55 pounds) in weight. Growth in height commonly ceases at 16 or 17 years in girls and 18 to 20 years in boys[1] (see Figs. 19-1 and 19-2).

This increase in size is acquired in a characteristic sequence of changes. Growth in length of extremities and neck precedes other areas, and, since these parts are first to reach adult length, the hands and feet appear larger than normal during adolescence. Increase in hip and chest breadth takes place in a few months followed several months later by an increase in shoulder width. These changes are followed by an increase in length of the trunk and depth of the chest. It is this sequence of changes that is

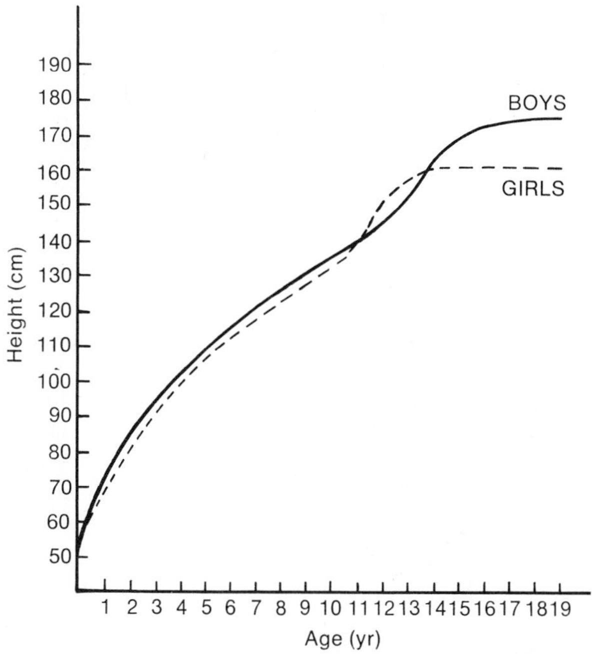

Fig. 19-1. Linear growth throughout childhood. (From Tanner, J. M., Whitehouse, R. H., and Takaishi, M.: Arch. Dis. Child. **41:**454-471, 1966.)

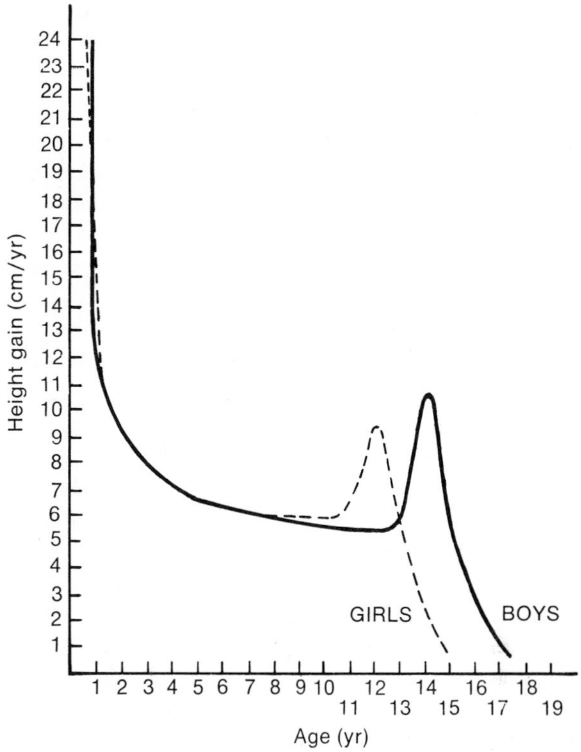

Fig. 19-2. Linear growth in centimeters per year. (From Tanner, J. M., Whitehouse, R. H., and Takaishi, M.: Arch. Dis. Child. **41:**454-471, 1966.)

responsible for the characteristic long-legged, gawky appearance of the early adolescent child.

Although the brain has achieved the major portion of its growth prior to adolescence, there are proportional changes in the skull as the face lengthens coincident with other body alterations. A disproportion is noted in the facial features as the forehead becomes higher and wider and the nose appears large since it lengthens before puberty. Later the mouth and lips become fuller and, last, the jaw reaches adult size (see also p. 54).

Sex differences in general growth patterns. Sex differences in general growth and distribution patterns are apparent in skeletal growth, muscle mass, adipose tissue, and skin. Although many of the individual variations are influenced by hereditary traits other than sex, the sex-related characteristics are under the regulation and control of sex hormones.

Skeletal growth differences between boys and girls are primarily reflected in limb length and are apparently a function of hormonal effects at puberty. The earlier cessation of growth in girls is caused by epiphyseal unity under the potent effect of estrogen secretion, and the hormonal effect on female bone growth is much stronger than the similar effect of testosterone in males. The prolonged growth period prior to puberty in boys and the less rapid epiphyseal closure is reflected in their greater overall height and longer arms and legs. Other skeletal differences are increased shoulder width in boys and broader hip development in girls (see p. 53).

Hypertrophy of the laryngeal mucosa and enlargement of the larynx and vocal cords occur in both boys and girls to produce voice changes. Girls' voices become slightly deeper and considerably fuller, but the effect in boys is striking. The "change of voice" in adolescent boys is one of the most noticeable traits of puberty as the voice shifts uncontrollably from deep to high tones in the middle of a sentence.

Growth of lean body mass, principally muscle, that tends to occur after the bone growth spurt increases steadily during adolescence and is both quantitatively and qualitatively greater in males than in females at comparable stages of pubertal development. Muscle development, under the influence of androgenic hormones, increases steadily and is remarkably well developed in boys, whereas in girls muscle mass increase is proportionate to general tissue growth.

Nonlean mass, primarily fat, is also increased but follows a less orderly pattern. There may be a transient increase in subcutaneous fat just prior to the skeletal growth spurt, especially noted in boys, that is followed 1 to 2 years later by a modest to marked decrease, again more marked in boys. Later on, variable amounts of fat are deposited to fill out and contour the mature physique in patterns characteristic of the adult of the appropriate sex. In both sexes fat on the trunk increases at a fairly steady rate, but, under the influence of ovarian hormones, the overall fatty tissue deposition in girls is more pronounced. Adipose tissue is distributed over the entire body, particularly in the regions over the thighs, hips, buttocks, and around the breast tissue, altering the angular childhood figure to the smoother, rounded body contours of the mature female.

Skin changes. Hormonal influences during puberty cause an acceleration in growth and maturation of the skin and its structural appendages. Secretion of estrogen causes the skin of the female to develop a soft, smooth, but thicker texture with increased vascularity; androgenic hormones produce increased thickness and some darkening of the skin. Sebaceous glands become extremely active at this time, especially on the genitals and in the "flush areas" of the body, that is, the face, neck, shoulders, and upper back and chest. This increased activity and the structural nature of the glands are extremely important in the pathogenesis of a common problem of puberty, acne (p. 720).

Eccrine sweat glands, present almost everywhere on the human skin, become fully functional during puberty. Under sympathetic control these glands produce sweat over the entire body, where evaporation helps eliminate body heat. The eccrine glands respond to emotional as well as thermal stimulation, and heavy sweating appears to be more pronounced in boys than in girls. The palms and soles ordinarily produce sweat on emotional stimulation but may cause sweating with more intense thermal heating. This also applies to the forehead and axillae.

Apocrine sweat glands, larger than eccrine glands and nonfunctional in childhood, reach secretory capacity during puberty. Unlike the eccrine sweat glands, the apocrine glands are limited in distribution and grow in relation to hair follicles in the axillae, around the areola of the breast, around the umbilicus, on the external auditory canal, and in the genital and anal regions. Apocrine glands secrete a thick secretion as a result of emotional stimulation that, when acted on by surface bacteria, becomes highly odoriferous. The pH of the axillae, acid during childhood, shows a progressive rise to a distinctly alkaline level during adolescence when the apocrine glands begin to function.

Body hair assumes very characteristic distribution patterns and texture changes during puberty. Some are common to both boys and girls; others appear to be related entirely to male androgen secretion. Estrogens seem to produce no consistent effect. Under the influence of gonadal and adrenal androgens, hair coarsens, darkens, and lengthens at sites related to secondary sex characteristics. Pubic and axillary hair appears in both sexes, although pubic hair is more extensive in males than in females. Beard and mustache hair is normally dependent on testicular androgens but can be increased in hirsute women. Body hair that usually appears on the chest, upward along the linea alba, and sometimes on other regions (such as the back and shoulder) is male sexual and androgen dependent. Extremity hair appears in varying amounts in both males and females but is also more prolific in the male. There is a strong genetic influence on the degree of extremity hirsutism in both sexes.

Physiologic changes

A number of physiologic functions are altered in response to some of the pubertal changes. The size and strength of the heart, blood volume, and systolic blood pressure increase, whereas the pulse rate and basal heat production decrease (see Appendix A). Consistent with the general developmental timetable, these changes appear earlier in girls and girls establish a slightly higher pulse rate and a slightly lower systolic blood pressure than boys. Blood volume that has increased steadily during childhood reaches a higher value in boys than in girls, which may be related to the increased muscle mass in pubertal boys. Adult values are reached for all formed elements of the blood, but the hematocrit levels are higher in boys, platelet count and sedimentation rate are increased in girls, and white blood cell numbers are decreased in both boys and girls.[20]

Respiratory rate, decreasing steadily throughout childhood, reaches the adult rate in adolescence. However, respiratory volume, vital capacity, and other physiologic properties related to respiratory function are increased, and to a far greater extent in males than in females. The sex differences are a result of the greater lung growth associated with the increased shoulder and chest size in boys.

Other changes relative to the attainment of mature physiologic capacity are reflected in body fluid volume and composition (see p. 1061) and in basal metabolic rate that, declining throughout life, reach adult levels during the adolescent years. The slightly higher metabolic rate in boys is thought to be a function of androgenic hormones.

Through progressive maturation of the body as it reaches adult size, the adolescent develops the ability to respond to physical stresses and strains equal to or in excess of adult competence. During this period physiologic responses to exercise change drastically—performance improves, especially in boys, and the body is able to make the physiologic adjustments needed for normal function after exercise is completed. These capabilities are a result of the increased size and strength of muscles and the increased cardiac, respiratory, and metabolic functions. Adolescents enjoy physical activity, and there appears to be a positive relationship between regular exercise and physical conditioning activities and improved general health, endurance, and appearance.

Reproductive endocrine system

It is generally accepted that the events of puberty are caused by hormonal influences and are controlled by the anterior pituitary (adenohypophysis) in response to a stimulus from the hypothalamus. Probably in some way related to brain maturation, hypothalamic stimulation causes the anterior pituitary to release gonadotropins that in turn stimulate the gonads. Stimulation to the gonads results in fulfillment of a dual function: (1) production and release of gametes—production of sperm in the male and maturation and release of ova in the female, and (2) secretion of sex-appropriate hormones—estrogen and progesterone from the female ovaries and testosterone from the male testes.

Table 19-1. Functions of pituitary gonadotropins

Hormone	Sex	Effect in gonads
Follicle-stimulating hormone (FSH)	Male	Stimulates development of seminiferous tubules Initiates spermatogenesis
	Female	Stimulates graafian follicles to mature and secrete estrogen
Luteinizing hormone (LH)*	Male	Stimulates differentiation of Leydig cells, which secrete androgens, principally testosterone
	Female	Produces rupture of follicle with discharge of mature ova Stimulates secretion of progesterone by corpus luteum

*In the male, LH is sometimes known as interstitial cell–stimulating hormone (ICSH).

Hormonal stimulation of gonadal function. The dynamics of the reproductive hormone system include both neural and endocrine functions involving principally the hypothalamus, the adenohypophysis, and the gonads. The chain of reactions that cause ripening of the ovum in the female and production of sperm in the male begins in the region of the hypothalamus. Neurosecretory hormones, the *gonadotropin-releasing factors (GnRF),* synthesized and discharged by the hypothalamus, are carried via the hypophyseal portal vessels to the adenohypophysis where they trigger the release of the gonadotropins *follicle-stimulating hormone (FSH)* and *luteinizing hormone (LH),* also known in the male as *interstitial cell–stimulating hormone (ICSH).* Increasing blood levels of these gonadotropic hormones stimulate the appropriate responses in the gonads. The pituitary gonadotropins and the effects on their target glands are listed in Table 19-1.

Inhibition, or negative feedback, in the reproductive endocrine system refers to the diminished gonadotropin secretion as a result of increasing serum levels of sex hormones. When sex hormone levels increase, GnRF secretion is diminished; when sex hormone levels decrease, the hypothalamus is stimulated to release GnRF, again initiating the sequence that produces the appropriate gonadal responses[19] (Fig. 19-3). For a more detailed review of these mechanisms the reader is referred to Chapter 38 and physiology textbooks.

Initiation of puberty. The mechanism for gonadal stimulation and the capacity for reproduction are present throughout childhood. Children are born with the hypothalamic-pituitary complex, the gonads, and the corresponding external genitalia appropriate to their sex. Although sexual function normally remains quiescent during childhood, animal experiments and abnormalities of the neuroendocrine system indicate that appropriate stimulation can produce mature responses in both the adenohypophysis and the gonads. For example, a lesion in the area of the hypothalamus can cause precocious puberty in the young child.

The precise mechanism that institutes the changes at puberty is not completely understood. Evidence suggests that the hypothalamic-pituitary-gonadal system is maintained in a dormant state throughout prepubescent childhood by some

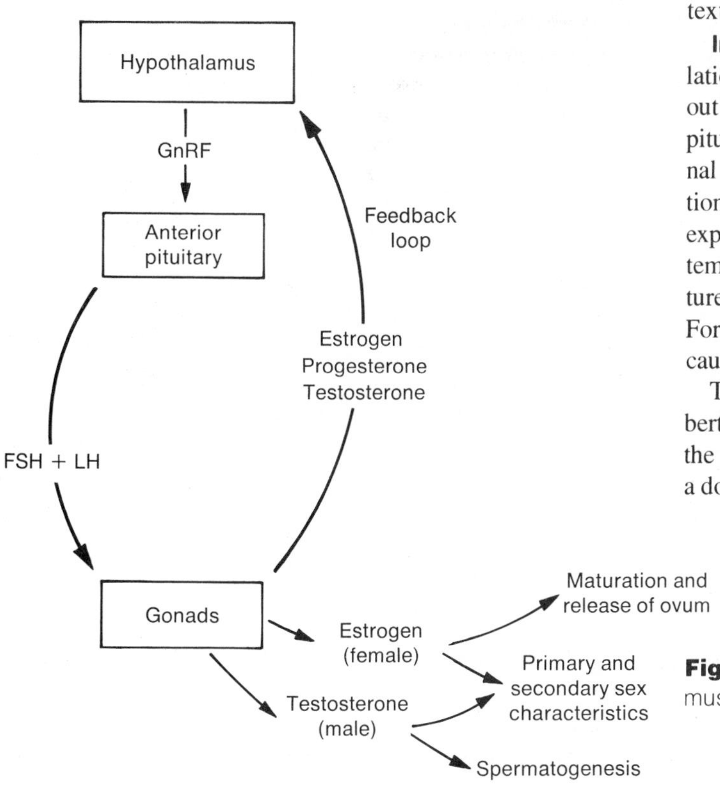

Fig. 19-3. Hormonal interaction between hypothalamus, pituitary, and gonads.

central nervous system inhibitory factor in the region of the hypothalamus and that, with maturation of the brain, it is an increased amount of GnRF that is responsible for initiating puberty. It appears that although the pituitary and gonads are capable of mature function and can be made responsive to stimuli at any age, some factor or factors operate to inhibit their function until the time of puberty. It is believed that the receptor sites in the hypothalamus are so highly sensitive that the most minute quantities of androgens and estrogens are sufficient to inhibit the secretion of GnRF during childhood. For reasons yet unknown but somehow related to brain maturation, the hypothalamus loses this extreme sensitivity at puberty and thus allows the hypothalmic-pituitary-gonadal mechanism to attain full secretory function. The sex hormones secreted in sufficient quantity produce the anatomic and physiologic effects that characterize the developmental phase known as puberty.[20]

Sex hormones. Sex hormones are secreted by the ovaries, testes, and adrenals and are produced in varying amounts by both sexes throughout the life span. The adrenal cortex is responsible for the small amounts secreted during the prepubescent years, but the sex hormone production that accompanies maturation of the gonads is responsible for the variety of biologic changes observed during pubescence and puberty. Table 19-2 summarizes the major somatic effects of the sex hormones.

Estrogen, the feminizing hormone, is found in low quantities during childhood and is secreted in slowly increasing amounts until about age 11 years. In males this continues through maturation. In females the onset of estrogen production in the ovary causes a pronounced increase that continues until about 3 years after the onset of menstruation, at which time it reaches a maximum level that continues throughout the reproductive life of the female.

Androgens, the masculinizing hormones, are also secreted in small and gradually increasing amounts up to about 7 or 9 years of age, at which time there is a more rapid increase in both sexes, especially boys, until about age 15 years. These hormones appear to be responsible for most of the rapid growth changes of early adolescence. With the onset of testicular function, the level of androgens (principally testosterone) in males increases over that in females and continues to increase until a maximum is attained at maturity.

Development of reproductive function in females. Approximately 1 to 2 years before the onset of menstruation in the female, the secretion of estrogen assumes a cyclic pattern. Under the influence of follicle-stimulating hormone, a graafian follicle containing the ovum begins to mature and secrete estrogen. Increased estrogen levels stimulate the release of luteinizing hormone from the anterior pituitary that in turn causes the follicle to rupture and discharge the ma-

Table 19-2. Sex hormones and their somatic effects

Hormone	Source	Both sexes	Female	Male
Estrogen	Female: ovaries and adrenal glands Male: testes and adrenal glands	Pubescent fat distribution	Distinctly feminine fat distribution on breasts, hips, and thighs Development of nipple and ductal structures of breast Development of labia minora, vulva, vagina, and fallopian tubes Epiphyseal unity and cessation of linear growth	Transient mammary tissue development (in some boys) Functions in mature male are unknown
Progesterone	Corpus luteum in ovaries Testes Adrenal glands		Secretory changes in uterine endometrium Lobular-acinar development in breasts	Unknown, if any
Androgens	Female: adrenal glands Male: testes and adrenal glands	Growth spurt (probably acting synergistically with growth hormone) Increased muscular development Pubic, body, and axillary hair growth Development of sweat and sebaceous glands	Development of labia majora and clitoris	Increased vascularity, circumference, and length of penis Growth and pigmentation of scrotal skin Growth of prostate gland, testes, and seminal vesicles Development of facial hair and larynx

Developmental stages of secondary sex characteristics and genital development

Genital development in boys—average age span, 12 to 16 years

Stage 1 (prepubertal)	Essentially the same as during childhood
Stage 2 (pubertal)	Initial enlargement of scrotum and testes; reddening and textural changes of scrotal skin
Stage 3	Initial enlargement of penis, mainly in length; further growth of testes and scrotum
Stage 4	Increased size of penis with growth in diameter and development of glands
Stage 5	Adult in size and shape

Development of the breast in girls—average age span, 11 to 13½ years

Stage 1 (prepubertal)	Elevation of papilla only
Stage 2 (pubertal)	Breast bud stage—small area of elevation around papilla; enlargement of areolar diameter
Stage 3	Further enlargement of breast and areola with no separation of their contours
Stage 4	Projection of areola and papilla to form a secondary mound (may not occur in all girls)
Stage 5	Mature configuration; projection of papilla only caused by recession of areola into general contour

Growth of pubic hair—average age spans for stages 2 through 5, 11 to 14 years in girls, 12 to 16 years in boys

Stage 1 (preadolescent)	No distinction between hair on penis and over the abdomen
Stage 2	Sparse growth of long, straight, downy, and slightly pigmented hair at base of penis or along labia
Stage 3	Hair darker, coarser, and curly; spread sparsely over entire pubis
Stage 4	Adult in type but restricted to pubic area
Stage 5	Adult in quantity and type with spread to inner surface of thighs

Adapted from Marshall, W. A., and Tanner, J. M.: Variations in the pattern of pubertal changes in girls, Arch. Dis. Child. **44:**291, 1969; and Marshall, W. A., and Tanner, J. M.: Variations in the pattern of pubertal changes in boys, Arch. Dis. Child. **45:**13, 1970.

ture ovum. The graafian follicle, without the ovum, rapidly becomes the *corpus luteum,* which begins to secrete progesterone. The levels of both estrogen and progesterone remain elevated for approximately 12 days and then gradually decrease. The large amounts of estrogen and progesterone secreted during the early phase cause a feedback decrease in follicle-stimulating and luteinizing hormones. When they diminish, the lack of feedback suppression again stimulates

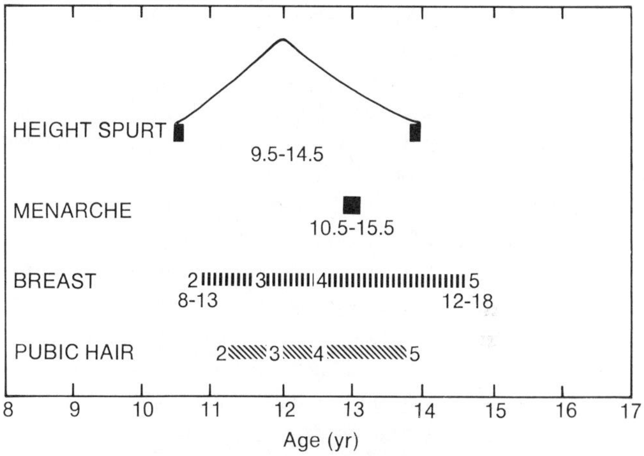

Fig. 19-4. Approximate timing of developmental changes in girls. The numbers indicate stages of development. See the boxed material for explanation. (From Marshall, W. A., and Tanner, J. M.: Variations in the pattern of pubertal changes in girls, Arch. Dis. Child. **44:**291, 1969.)

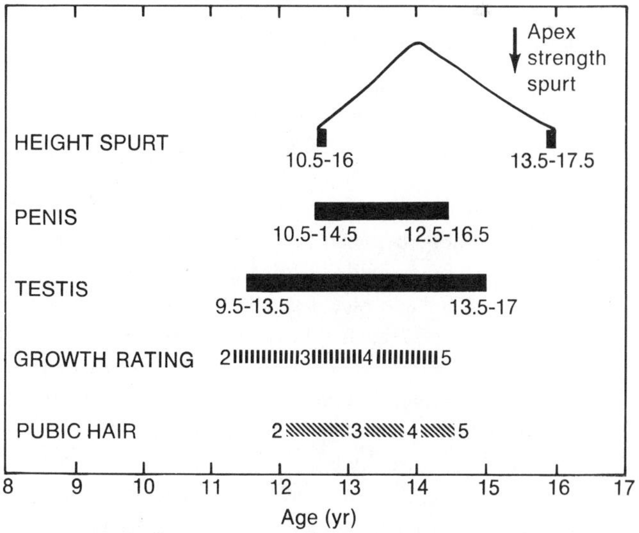

Fig. 19-5. Approximate timing of developmental changes in boys. The numbers indicate stages of development. See the boxed material for explanation. (From Marshall, W. A., and Tanner, J. M.: Variations in the pattern of pubertal changes in boys, Arch. Dis. Child. **45:**13, 1970.)

the pituitary to secrete gonadotropins and the cycle is repeated.

Coincident with and in response to these hormonal fluctuations, there are changes in the endometrium, the most conspicuous being the periodic bleeding that occurs with the shedding of the uterine mucosa or menstruation caused by diminished levels of estrogen and progesterone. The initial appearance of menstruation *(menarche)* occurs about 2 years after the first appearance of pubescent changes. The normal age range of menarche is usually considered to be 10 to 15 years, with the average age being 12.5 years for North American girls. Menarche has been related to a critical point in body weight (48 kg or 106 pounds) but may show variation with race. During the establishment of the ovarian cycle, the menstrual periods are usually scanty and irregular and may not be accompanied by ovulation. Ovulation usually occurs 12 to 24 months after menarche.

Development of reproductive function in males. The maturation of male sexual function is also under the stimulation and control of pituitary gonadotropins. Unlike the cyclic germ cell production in the female, spermatogenesis is a continuous process that is usually well established by 17 years of age. There is no sudden physical change to indicate puberty such as the menarche in girls. The overt signal in boys is the beginning of nocturnal emissions of seminal fluid that occur spontaneously during sleep at periodic intervals of approximately 2 weeks. Nocturnal emissions will persist into adulthood and will occur whenever there is a buildup of semen in the genital ducts. As with girls, mature germ cells may not be produced for several months. The average age range at which boys attain puberty is 12.5 to 16.5 years, with a mean of 14.5 years.

Determination of sexual maturity

The visible evidence of sexual maturation is achieved in orderly sequence, and the state of maturity can be estimated on the basis of the appearance of these external manifestations. The age at which these changes are observed and the time required to progress from one stage to another may vary considerably between individual children. From the appearance of breast buds to full maturity may range from 1½ to 6 years for adolescent girls; male genitalia may take from 2 to 5 years to reach adult size. The usual sequence of appearance of maturational changes in girls is rapid increase in height and weight, breast changes, increase in pelvic girth, growth of pubic hair, appearance of axillary hair, menstruation that usually begins 2 years after first signs and an abrupt deceleration of linear growth (Fig. 19-4). The usual sequence of appearance of maturational changes in boys is increase in weight, enlargement of testicles, rapid increase in height, growth of pubic hair, axillary hair, hair on upper lip, hair on face and elsewhere on body (facial hair usually appears about 2 years after appearance of pubic hair), changes in the larynx and, consequently, the voice, which usually develops concurrently with growth of the penis, nocturnal emissions, and an abrupt deceleration of linear growth (Fig. 19-5).[10]

The developmental stages of secondary sex characteristics and genital development have been defined as a guide for estimating sexual maturity.[13,14] (See the boxed material on p. 691.)

ADOLESCENT'S REACTION TO PUBERTY

Physical growth and maturation during adolescence occur so rapidly that these young people have difficulty in adjusting to a changing body image. While many of the changes of puberty have features common to both girls and boys, the implications and responses are quite different in the two sexes and many of these adjustments are influenced by the values and prohibitions of the culture. Very often the body changes per se may be less significant than the meaning and importance that these changes have for adolescents and other persons in their lives.

Adolescence is the time when young persons' self-awareness reaches a peak and, with sexual awareness, when much of their thought and concern is turned inward. The sudden growth that takes place in early adolescence creates feelings of confusion about their bodies. Typically they tend to deny changes until they are suddenly aware of the difference. They have lost the security of a familiar body and feel a strangeness about their changed bodies. Consequently they may try either to hide them or to advertise them, or they may alternate between the two extremes. Teenagers are acutely aware of their appearance as they begin to acquire an image of themselves as adults, but they see discrepancies between their ideal and actual skills and abilities.

Strange and unfamiliar feelings press on them as inner urges announce a sexual awakening. These feelings must also be integrated into the self-image. Sexuality is not the same for boys as it is for girls, and it has different psychic overtones that influence their behavior and adaptation. Although it appears that the intensity of the sexual drive is different in adolescent boys and girls, this has not been conclusively demonstrated. Current findings indicate that the difference may be related to the physiologic nature of the sex drive rather than to its intensity. Sexual arousal in males is very direct and centered in the genitals, whereas in females it is more vague, diffuse, and closely linked to their total personality.

Boys' responses to puberty

The early adolescent increases in height and muscle mass are welcomed by the adolescent boy, whose growth, for several months, has lagged significantly behind that of his female age-mates. Although his more mature physique brings highly valued increase in strength and more mature athletic skills, this rapid growth is uneven so that he has some trouble adjusting. When bones grow faster than muscles, muscles are taut and respond with quick, jerky movements; when muscles grow faster than bones, they become somewhat loose and sluggish. For a period of time he is awkward and uncoordinated. Often his size outstrips his strength and he tires more easily. Fatigue, lack of coordination, and appearing "funny" and "out of shape" are sources of embarrassment, self-consciousness, and feelings of inadequacy. He has difficulty in accepting his new body image at first, and accusations of clumsiness, laziness, or stupidity do little to strengthen his self-concept during a time that offers such strong challenges to his self-esteem.

The development of secondary sex characterisitcs, especially the growth of facial and body hair, has psychologic and social meaning to the adolescent boy. This, more than any other secondary characteristic, is associated with the masculine sex role, and the ritual act of shaving at the slightest evidence of growth is a means for the young boy to validate his identification with this role. Shaving also provides a legitimate excuse to gaze at and admire the broadening shoulders and altered features of his changing body image. Unfortunately, with many adolescent boys, the appearance of acne and an awkward appearance when assuming adult poses often interfere with the pleasure of this experience.[16]

The growth of the penis and testes creates some important problems for the adolescent male. Unlike the reproductive organs in the female, the male reproductive organs are readily visible and provide the boy with concrete evidence of his masculine character. He knows by the sensations localized within these organs that he is now a man. His reproductive organs become very sensitive to sexual stimulation. Sexual feelings are directly related to the genitals, desire is urgent, and he seeks rapid relief from pressure and tension through ejaculation. Sexual needs in the pubertal boy are a highly specific physical phenomenon, centered around the sex act itself, and are initially quite separated from ideas of love. These sexual cravings appear to reach a peak in the 1 or 2 years after puberty.

Adolescent boys are generally not well prepared for the maturation of the reproductive organs. Spontaneous ejaculations are frequently puzzling, troublesome, and embarrassing events. Unless he has been prepared in advance for this eventuality, the boy often finds it difficult to seek an explanation from his parents; therefore, he turns to friends or reading material to gain information or he may puzzle about the meaning in his own mind.

The opportunity for gratification of these genital urges through heterosexual expression is denied to the adolescent by Western cultural standards. Premarital sexual involvement is fraught with many problems and conflicts, and homosexual activities are generally condemned by society. As a consequence, the teenage boy resorts to masturbation, the manipulation of the genitals for the purpose of ejaculation, to relieve him of the accumulated pressures in his genital organs. It is essentially a normal activity, and almost every boy masturbates alone or in relation to sexual experimentation with others of the same sex. However, this too is often associated with guilt and anxiety. Misconceptions still dominate the feelings of many people who believe masturbation to be evil, unmanly, or "not nice" and who attribute a wide assortment of ills to the practice. Current enlightenment accepts that to engage in the practice from time to time is normal and temporarily helps provide the young man with important information about how his body works and how adult physical sexuality and reproduction are accomplished. He learns that organ responses to sexual excitement can be initiated at will and that orgasmic climax with a predictable release of tension, or repeatedly deferred at will, contributes to a developing sense of mastery over sexual impulses and new sexual capacities. Without guilt and worry, the adolescent boy can incorporate this aspect of his masculinity into a more positive self-concept.[7,16]

Girls' response to puberty

As girls begin the pubertal changes, they, too, become very body conscious. Because the onset in girls is almost 2 years in advance of boys, their initial reaction to increased height may be embarrassment as they find themselves towering above their male classmates. They worry about becoming too tall. Adolescent girls often slouch or adopt a hunched posture in an attempt to minimize this increased height, especially early-maturing girls who are normally of above-average height. The increase in weight and the normal plumping of features with fat deposition are predominant concerns of the pubescent girl. They perceive this to be evidence of a tendency toward obesity that many attempt to avoid by strict and rather faddish dieting. This ill-timed strategy can deprive their bodies of essential nutrients during a period of rapid body development.

The young girl is interested in her changing form and feminine curves. The average girl looks on her budding breasts with pleasure as a sign of approaching maturity and evidence of her femininity. She observes and may even measure the progress of her developing breasts and continually compares her own progress with that of her friends and classmates. She begins to wear a brassiere. Some girls are sensitive about their breast development and attempt to hide their breast development, whereas others are delighted with their new figures and wear tight sweaters and clothes that accentuate their curves.

Development of some of the secondary sex characteristics may be less pleasing to girls than they are to boys, particularly the growth of body hair. A culture in which smooth-skinned females are preferred makes it necessary for the girl to shave her underarms and legs regularly to meet the cultural standards for feminine appearance. Whereas this practice is another indication of maturity, it does not have the same sex-role significance as face shaving for the adolescent boy. The girl becomes increasingly conscious of the feminine ideal and, in an effort to approach this standard, experiments with a variety of cosmetics and hair styles. Alone and together, she and her friends spend endless hours before the mirror posing, applying cosmetics, and combing their hair. This practice provides the same narcissistic outlet for the girl that is available to the boy through shaving.[16]

The advent of menstruation, that exclusive feature of female puberty, provides the greatest impetus toward full realization and acceptance of female sexuality. Menstruation is positive evidence of womanhood and the potential for pregnancy and childbearing. Most girls are adequately prepared for the event and take this new function in stride, looking forward to menstruation, feeling satisfaction at its onset, and seeing it as the symbol of their passage from childhood to womanhood. Others find it distressing, are frightened by it, and find it difficult to accept. In some it reawakens old fears of body injury and castration. Still others accept it matter-of-factly. Because of its sudden onset, the first menstruation can be a traumatic experience for the girl who has not been taught what to expect. As a rule, if the young girl has established a positive gender role during childhood, the transition to womanhood, with all its ramifications, is accepted as the normal phenomenon that it is.[4]

Unlike the adolescent boy, strong sexual feelings in the adolescent girl are not usually centered in the genital region but are more generalized and ill defined. Her reproductive apparatus, less obvious than in the boy, contributes in only a vague way to sexual awareness. The girl in early adolescence may experience pleasant sensations and even tingling in the genital area, but these feelings are diffuse and difficult to separate from other body sensations. Her sexual feelings are centered less on the genitals and erotic gratification with release of tension than on manipulating a pleasant state with romatic feelings about love. Sexual impulses tend to be secondary rather than primary as they are in the boy. However, with the more open, liberal views regarding female sexual responses, it is being revealed that much of the nature of the adolescent girl's sexual arousal may have more of a cultural than biologic basis.

The urge for self-stimulation in the adolescent girl is not as strong as it is in the male. Although many girls handle the genitals for the pleasant sensation this evokes, not all carry the activity to a climax. Masturbation is frequently combined with fantasy.

A difficulty faced by the pubescent girl is related to the discrepancy in the onset of puberty in girls and in boys. She is often placed in the position where she must explain or hide the fact of her own body changes from her male peers. The dissemination of information to boys about these changes lags significantly behind; therefore, the girl finds it difficult to accept the changes she is experiencing while attempting to hide or mask them from the boys whose attention and approval she is seeking.

Disturbances of body image

Adolescents are continually comparing themselves with their peers and making judgments of their own normality based on these observations. Pubertal children feel most comfortable when they are just like their friends and age-mates. Deviations from the group average or perceived defects are threatening to their idealized image. Any blemish is apt to be magnified out of proportion, and any delay of the visible evidence of maturity is cause for worry. Unfortunately this is also the time when the hormonal effect of the sebaceous glands produces the acne that creates problems for many youngsters. To the adolescent, even the most insignificant pimple may be viewed as a colossal disfigurement; every blemish is a major catastrophe. The advent of chronic disease or a permanent physical disability has very special significance during adolescence and creates additional problems for both the affected youngster and health workers.

Both early- and late-maturing children feel out of place among their classmates, but the slow-maturing children appear to suffer the most pronounced inner turmoil as their age-mates are progressing through puberty. Late-maturing children find themselves being left out of private discussions about body changes experienced by the group—some to the point of ostracism or, especially in boys, an object of scorn and ridicule. They feel cheated and may well believe that they are doomed to a permanent position outside the group. Such fears and failures only serve to accentuate the normal doubts and concerns about the self that are part of this critical age period. Early-maturing boys are less at a disadvantage than early-maturing girls or late-maturing boys. Late-maturing boys usually suffer most.[5]

PSYCHOLOGIC AND EMOTIONAL DEVELOPMENT

While adolescents are adjusting to physical changes that may contribute to or detract from their feelings of self-worth, they are learning how to use their developing mental capacities. Their ability to reason, to assess and evaluate, and to use divergent thinking to come up with new ideas increases during this period of life. The adolescent begins to think beyond the present into the future. However, these capacities and the ability to make good judgments are still limited by inexperience and as yet inadequate knowledge from which to gain an adequate perspective for problem solving.

Cognitive development[17,18]

Progression in the realm of cognitive thinking culminates with the capacity for abstract thinking. The preceding stages have been outlined and discussed in general (p. 68) and as they apply to the appropriate developmental period. This stage, the period of formal operations, is Piaget's fourth and last stage and is attained at different ages, depending on the individual child's motivation, practice, opportunities, and cultural differences.

Young people now are able to begin thinking about the world in new ways. Living in the nonpresent as well as the present, they are no longer concerned with and restricted to the real and actual, which was typical of the period of concrete thought, but they are also concerned with the possible. They now think beyond the present. At this time their thoughts can be influenced by more logical principles than by their own perceptions and experiences. They now become capable of scientific reasoning and formal logic. Without having to center attention on the immediate situation, they can imagine the possible—a sequence of events that might occur, such as college and occupational possibilities; how things might change in the future, such as relationships with parents; and the consequences of their actions, such as dropping out of school.

They are capable of mentally manipulating more than two categories of variables at the same time. For example, they can consider the relationship between speed, distance, and time in planning a trip. They are now able to detect logical consistency or inconsistency in a set of statements and to evaluate a system or set of values in a more analytic manner. For instance, they question the parent who insists on honesty in the youngster but, at the same time, cheats on an income tax report or expense account.

Young people are now able to think about their own thinking and the thinking of others. They wonder what opinion others have of them, and they are increasingly able to imagine the thoughts of others. With this capacity comes the ability to differentiate between others' thoughts and their own and to interpret those of others more accurately. Thus they are able to see themselves and the world in a more relativistic way. As they come to know that other cultures and communities have different norms and standards from their own, it becomes easier to accept members of these other cultures and the decision to behave in their own culture in an accepted manner becomes a more conscious commitment to that culture.

Moral development[12,21]

As children move through the stages of cognition and logical thought, they also progress through sequential stages of moral development. Kohlberg's theory of development of moral judgment and thought proposes three levels of reasoning—preconventional, conventional, and postconventional. During the preconventional level, which encompasses the ages from 4 to 10 years, children have been concerned with the external consequences of their acts and the power exerted by those who represent authority. At the conventional level, which includes youngsters of preadolescence and adolescence, ages 10 to 16 years, the major concern is to act or behave in such a way that will gain or maintain the approval of others. There is obedience to rules and respect for authority.

The change from conventional to postconventional morality that takes place during late adolescence involves a serious questioning of existing moral values and their relevance to society and the individual. Adolescents can easily take the role of another. They understand duty and obligation based on reciprocal rights of others as well as the concept of justice that is founded on making amends for misdeeds and repairing or replacing what has been spoiled by wrongdoing. However, they seriously question established moral codes, often as a result of observing that adults verbally ascribe to a code but do not adhere to it. Their advanced cognitive development renders adolescents more aware of moral questions and values and closely parallels the general process of identity formation. Coincident with these advancements are rapidly changing social demands that require continual reappraisal of these values and beliefs. They are aware of the contradictions in the existing social and value structures in which they participate.

Adolescent boys and girls must make choices. They are changing, and their social world is also changing. They find that there are many ways to live their lives, their behavioral domain is expanded, and they encounter situations that they have never before faced that require decisions about action to be taken and decisions based on moral evaluation and judgment. Whereas the younger child merely accepts the decisions or point of view of adults, the adolescent, to gain autonomy from adults, must substitute his own set of morals and values. When old principles are challenged but new and independent values have not yet emerged to take their place, young people search for a moral code that preserves their personal integrity and guides their behavior, especially in the face of strong pressure to violate these moral beliefs. Their decisions involving moral dilemmas must be based on an internalized set of moral principles that provides them with the resources to evaluate the demands of the situation and to plan a course of action that is consistent with their ideals.

Idealism

With the capacity for abstract thinking and the use of deductive reasoning, youth become concerned about gaining a clear understanding of life and its purpose. They often become disillusioned with the world they see and search for an ideal and decent world to which their ideal and decent selves can respond. This part of the self is hidden from view and may not be revealed to any but closest friends. Adolescents are continually discarding old illusions and constructing new ones to take their place. Consequently they may embrace idealistic movements and causes. Many turn to religion—their own or a new one—as a source of comfort and reassurance.

Most adolescents accept society as it exists and attempt to adjust as best they can to things as they are. Some devote themselves to a life of pleasure and seek to extend this existence as long as they possibly can. Others, convinced that injustice and repression have reached an intolerable point, become revolutionaries or radical reformers in an attempt to create a better place in which to live. A highly visible few resort to psychopathic behavior as they seek gratification by an exploitive and sometimes brutal approach to others.

As a whole, adolescents are able to maintain the conviction that virtue and decency are possible, and they are seldom totally disillusioned. They are able to discern in others the idealism that they feel. They are prone to setbacks with feelings of helplessness and depression, and few are able to carry their idealism beyond adolescence in careers and organizational activities. By late adolescence most have come to terms with things as they are. They have evaluated their capabilities in relation to their ambitions and economic realities and have either entered the work force or the armed forces or embarked on the pursuit of an educational goal. Very few are able to hold fast to their ideals in the face of the pressures and stress associated with the turbulent transition to adulthood.

Search for identity

Whereas the changes that take place during the middle childhood years are relatively gradual and regular, during early adolescence the changes are rapid. Adolescents experience rapid body changes; a shift from the homogeneous uniformity of grade school to the heterogeneous world of classmates, teachers, and classes in high schools; and expanding relationships and expectations for behavior. These rapid changes undoubtedly are responsible for much of the inner turmoil that finds external expression in the adolescent.

The traditional psychosocial theory identifies the developmental crisis of adolescence as developing a sense of identity.[2] Throughout childhood individuals have been going through the process of identification as they concentrate on various parts of the body at specific times. During infancy the child identifies himself as separate from the mother, during early childhood he establishes a gender role identification with the appropriate sex parent, and in later childhood he establishes who he is in relation to others. In adolescence he comes to see himself as a distinct individual, somehow unique and separate from every other individual. In the light of their observations, some authorities see the central conflict of identity vs role diffusion of adolescence as accomplished in two stages[16]: The early period of adolescence begins with the onset of puberty and extends to relative physical and emotional stability at or near graduation from high school. It is characterized by the rapid physical changes and conceptual maturation already discussed and a heightened sensitivity to peer approval. During this time the adolescent is faced with the crisis of *group identity* vs alienation. In the period that follows, the individual hopes to attain autonomy from the family and develop a sense of *personal identity* as opposed to role diffusion. A sense of group identity appears to be essential as a prelude to a sense of personal identity. Young adolescents must resolve questions concerning relationships with a peer group before they are able to resolve questions about who they are in relation to family and society.

Group identity. During the early stage of adolescence the pressure to belong to a group is intensified. Teenagers find it essential to find a group to which they feel that they can belong and that provides them with status. Belonging to a crowd helps adolescents to define the differences between themselves and their parents. They dress as the group dresses and wear makeup and hairstyles according to group criteria—all of which are different from those of the parental generation. Language, music, and dancing reflect a culture that is exclusive to the adolescent. When adults begin to emulate these fashions and interests, the style changes immediately. The evidence of adolescent conformity to the peer group and nonconformity to the adult group provides teenagers with a frame of reference in which they can display their own self-assertion while they reject their identity with their parents' generation.

The group offers an identity to the young adolescent in terms of acceptance and of the roles it defines. Within the group the young person can try out and experiment with a variety of roles while remaining in the security and warmth of those who face the same problems, feel the same way, behave the same way, and wear the same symbols of belonging. There is comfort in standing together against those who do not understand—to giggle, shout, and act silly in the company of those with whom they share an emotional attachment. To be different is to be unaccepted and alienated from the group.

Individual identity. The quest for personal identity is part of the ongoing identification process. As the child establishes identity within a group, he or she is also attempting to incorporate multiple body changes into a concept of the self. Body awareness is part of self-awareness, and for some time the adolescent will engage in assimilating the self represented by this dimension. It has been determined that the body image established during adolescence is the one that the individual retains throughout life. Much of the adolescent's search for identity takes place before a mirror as he tries to read from the reflected features just who he is and what he looks like to other people. The adolescent practices facial expressions and postures, tries out hair arrangements, worries about a pimple, and in other ways attempts to assess the best means to achieve a maximum effect—to reveal the "true self."

In this search for identity, adolescents take into consideration the relationships that have developed between themselves and others in the past as well as the directions they hope to be able to take in the future. Significant others hold certain expectations for the behavior of the adolescent. Often these expectations or demands are persistent enough to induce certain decisions that might be made differently or not at all if the individual could be solely responsible for identity formation. It is all too easy to slip into the roles that are expected by these external influences without incorporating personal goals or questioning these decisions in relation to the developing personality. Thus the individual becomes what parents or others wish him to be based on these premature decisions. Also, a young person might form a negative identity when society or the culture provides him with a self-image that is contrary to the values of the community. Labels such as "juvenile delinquent," "hood," or "failure" are applied to certain adolescents, who then accept and then live up to these labels with behaviors that validate and strengthen them.

The process of evolving a personal identity is time-consuming and fraught with periods of confusion, depression, and discouragement. To determine an identity and a place in the world is a critical and perilous feature of adolescence. However, as the pieces are gradually shifted and settled into place, an eventual positive identity will emerge from the confusion. Role diffusion results when the individual is unable to formulate a satisfactory identity from the multiplicity of aspirations, roles, and identifications.

Sex-role identity. Adolescence is the time for consolidation of a sex-role identity. In the preschool and early school years children learned to apply an appropriate gender label to themselves, they acquired information about sex-linked expectations, and they developed a sex-role preference. The establishment of close relationships with same-sex peers, which began in later childhood, is intensified during early adolescence. Through these relationships children learn about the possibility of intimacy between equals and are exposed to peer standards for appropriate sex-role behavior. During early adolescence the peer group begins to communicate some expectations regarding heterosexual relationships, and, as development progresses, adolescents encounter expectations for mature sex-role behavior from both peers and adults. Expectations such as these vary from culture to culture, between geographic areas, and between socioeconomic groups. Boys may find that they will be expected to be competitive, hold a steady job, and be able to provide for a family. Adult expectations for girls may include maternal, nurturant behaviors and being a good homemaker. Adolescents are urged to make a career choice, and the decision about an occupation has important implications for their sex-role identity. Many jobs or careers are viewed and categorized in terms of how they relate to sex-role expression, and if the choice is considered "sex appropriate," the work environment will support the sex-role identity. To enter a career that is not generally selected by one's own sex may lead to constant tension as a result of challenges directed toward the individual's competence and sex-role identity. The trend toward equalizing career opportunities and minimizing the sex-role connotations of many occupations hopefully will eliminate much of this source of tension.

Emotionality and adolescent behavior

The pubertal changes in physical appearance are accompanied by changes in emotional control and response. The stability of the prepubescent period is replaced by the turmoil precipitated by the physical and psychologic alterations that teenagers experience. They are deluged with new sensations and feelings that they cannot understand. The behavior of adolescents is bewildering to others and often to the adolescents themselves. They are frequently labeled as unstable and always as inconsistent and unpredictable. The behaviors they exhibit have even been described as pseudopathologic or as representing a normal psychosis. It is true that many of the transient symptoms that are relatively common in adolescence resemble pathologic syndromes in the adult, such as mood swings, depression, periodic regression to childhood, and mild antisocial behavior.

Most feelings in early adolescence seem to originate from within the individual rather than from the environment. Adolescents characteristically exhibit alternating and recurrent episodes of disturbed behavior with periods of relative tranquility. There is an increase in moods and sentiments. They vacillate up and down and between considerable maturity and childlike behavior. One minute they are exuberant and enthusiastic; the next minute they are depressed and withdrawn. Unpredictable, but essentially normal, outbursts of primitive behavior appear as the teenager loses control over instinctual drives. Little things can cause an emotional upheaval and, depending on the teenager's interpretation, can mean a great deal. As the tension is relieved, emotion is brought under control and the individual retreats in order to work over what has happened, to attempt to master his anger, and in the overall process to grow in his ability to control his emotions and gain from the new experience. These emotional outbursts and ensuing periods of calm may last only a few minutes or hours or may extend over a period of weeks. Adolescents are given to extensive daydreaming that may be so intense that they do not hear another person speaking to them. On the other hand, they may become hostile or ready to fight, complain, or resist everything.

The cyclic pattern that has been apparent throughout childhood continues in adolescence (p. 51). The outgoing, balanced child is replaced by the withdrawn, pensive, and moody early adolescent child who is often most unhappy and humorless. Adolescents again shift to a more vigorous, expansive state during the middle teens. They are less apt to get their feelings hurt and are less inclined to cry at the least provocation as was evident earlier. Teenagers again retreat into a phase of withdrawal, moodiness, and introspection. They often feel excessively tired. For many it is a troubled time. Adolescents begin to take hold of themselves in later adolescence; their emotions are better controlled. They can approach problems more calmly and rationally, and, although they are still subject to periods of depression, their feelings are less vulnerable and they are beginning to demonstrate the more mature emotions of later adolescence.

In later adolescence the source of emotion is more apt to come from the external environment than from within. Anger is the most disruptive emotion, most often as a consequence of interruption or restriction of activities. However, whereas early adolescents react immediately and emotionally, older adolescents can control their emotions until a socially acceptable time and place for expression. They are still subject to heightened emotion, and, when it is expressed, their behavior reflects feelings of insecurity, tension, and indecision.

Interests and activities. During early adolescence the interests and activities of girls and boys are in rather sharp contrast. Boys spend a great deal of time in active outdoor sports or "just going out with the guys." They enjoy hobbies and clubs, and television takes up a good bit of their time. Girls and mixed-sex activities occupy their interest and concern but less prominently until their development more nearly approaches that of the more rapidly maturing girls. As their bodies gain strength and size, "making the team" is a major concern for many youths, and a boy may spend an excessive amount of time in attempting to perfect athletic skills. The essential bicycle of middle childhood is replaced by the automobile, the symbol of status to the adolescent. If a car cannot be acquired, a motorcycle or motor bike is preferable to walking, riding the bus, or the humiliation of being chauffered by a parent or sibling. Most avidly seek part-time employment, many because of economic necessity.

Although girls' leisure interests involve many outdoor activities, an increased interest in parties and social activities is evident. They are interested in hobbies, volunteer activities, and many part-time jobs through necessity or in order to purchase more clothes and other teenage "necessities." They are avid conversationalists and spend much of their time in the company of other girls talking, listening to records, and experimenting with makeup, hairstyles, and clothes. They enjoy shopping for clothes, but there is seldom agreement between mother and daughter regarding types and styles of clothing. Many of their thoughts and feelings are confessed in a diary. Daydreaming is a prominent characteristic of the adolescent.

Both sexes enjoy movies, rock concerts, disco dancing, and other communal activities and entertainment. Girls seem to prefer sentimental, romantic-type films when they are available, whereas boys would rather see sports, mystery, or action films. The x-rated movies are crowded with adolescents. They both begin to appreciate and enjoy the theater and to share in the experience of audience reaction to the performance. They increasingly progress toward enjoyment of more adult activities and interests, and their developing social competence makes them more willing to accompany adults on occasion to share in the fun and activity.

Reading is still a favorite occupation with teenagers and may serve to satisfy some of their needs for vicarious experiences. Reading is more purposeful at this stage than at earlier ages, and most adolescents prefer to read magazines rather than books. Boys read magazines of a scientific or technical nature, and girls prefer women's magazines. The avid interest in collections that was so prominent in middle childhood declines during adolescence to be replaced by individual hobbies in the areas of the arts and sciences.

Television viewing declines in adolescence, and many teenagers have a decided preference for the radio and are avidly addicted to the transistor radio that accompanies many of their other activities, such as studying, walking, and so on. Closely associated with the radio is the stereo, which assumes an important part in teenagers' life. Much of their money is spent on records and tapes that are collected in much the same way as books. Often a favorite recording is regarded with the feeling accorded a well-loved book and is played over and over again.

When they are not engaged in other activities, they are probably talking in "rap sessions" or in endless telephone conversations. The telephone serves that essential link to peers when they are physically removed from one another. It is a means for fulfilling the need for flight from parents to the peers without leaving the home. The conversations may consist of gossip, plans, experiences, or an account of the activities of the day. The topics vary greatly, but the amount of time so engaged is often measured in hours. For boy-girl conversations, the telephone provides a means for closeness without fear of complications that physical proximity may engender.

Teenage interests and activities are subject to rapid change, and each succeeding "generation" of teenagers has its own peculiar characteristics that are evidenced by their behavior, vocabulary, dress, and other external manifestations that reflect and establish a clear line of separateness, although superficial, between the peer and the adult cultures. The rapidity with which these external trappings change is often astonishing.

It is apparent from the preceding that the adolescent age-group is a major force in the economic marketplace. Today's adolescents have more money to spend than any previous generation of teenagers, and the advent of television and movies for some ethnic groups has made them a much more visible and identifiable group. Symbols of their identity are brought to their attention through the media by advertisers of cosmetics, radios, records, fad clothing, and so on. Members of this easily exploitable group are readily persuaded to part with money in their ever-present quest for acceptance and popularity, even though based on very superficial values.[15]

INTERPERSONAL RELATIONSHIPS

To achieve full maturity, adolescents must free themselves from family domination and define an identity independent of parental authority. However, this process is fraught with ambivalence on the part of both teenagers and their parents. Adolescents want to grow up and to be free of parental restraints, yet they are fearful as they try to comprehend the responsibilities that are linked with independence. Part of this emancipation involves developing social relationships outside the family that help the teenagers identify their role in society. Increasing absence from home through frequent contacts with peers is essential to this socialization process. Adolescence is a time of intense sociability and often a time of equally intense loneliness. Acceptance by peers, a few close friends, and the secure love of a supportive family are requisites for the interpersonal maturation process.

Adolescents and their parents

During adolescence the parent-child relationship changes from one of protection-dependency to mutual affectionate equality. The process of achieving independence often involves turmoil and ambiguity as both parent and adolescent learn to play new roles and work toward this end while, at the same time, resolving the often painful series of rifts essential to establishing the ultimate relationships.

Most of the behavior observed in the adolescent is related to the struggle for independence and the external restrictions and checks that are placed on this spontaneous maturation process. On the one hand, adolescents are accepted as maturing preadults. They are allowed privileges heretofore denied and are provided with increasing responsibilities. On the other hand, because of their unpredictability and insecurity in evaluating situations and making sound judgments, they must conform to regulations and restrictions set by adults. This is particularly exemplified by the struggle between parents and adolescents concerning the hour at which they are to come in at night.

As teenagers assert their rights for grown-up privileges, they frequently create tensions within the home. They resist parental control and resent being treated like a child. Conflicts can arise from almost any situation or any subject. Some of the favorite topics of dispute include use of the telephone, manners, dress, chores and duties, homework, disrespectful behavior, friendships, dating, money, automobiles, and time schedules. Present in these areas of conflict are the overriding argument that "Everyone else has one" or is allowed the desired item or privilege and the ever-present assertion that "You don't understand me" and "You always treat me like a baby." Parents' reactions, spoken or unspoken, consist of, "Is this all the thanks I get for what I have done, or am doing, for you?"

The teenager's earliest attempts to achieve emancipation from parental controls are manifest in a period of rejection of the parents. Adolescents are critical, argumentative, and generally remote with both parents. They absent themselves from home and family activities and spend an increasing amount of time with the peer group. They are less close and confiding in relationships with parents. This rejection is not consistent, however, and varies with mood changes. At times the young teenager feels highly competent and demands his "rights"; at other times, after being hurt in battles with the world, he may accept the parental guidance and security.

With advancing adolescence, teenagers become more competent, and with this competence comes a need for more autonomy. However, although they are psychologically better prepared for independence, they are often thwarted in their efforts by lack of money or other parental barriers. Much conflict arises from the teenager's outside activities and the elements of privacy and trust. Too many parents believe that they must know all of the adolescent's activities and feelings; they may go through the teenager's belongings in an attempt to find out what he is doing. To gain the respect and trust of their adolescent, parents must respect his privacy and show an honest and sincere interest in what he believes and feels. Teenagers need not only guidance and support from their parents but also enough leeway to establish their own individuality.

Sometimes teenagers prove to be a source of pleasure and fulfillment beyond the parents' expectations. The adolescent may be one who is of a particularly happy disposition or one whose talents and abilities in areas such as music, art, scholastic achievement, or athletics provide the parents with pleasure and gratification. Most parental disappointments in their adolescent children are related to their expectations for success or failure.

The recent trends in society in terms of equality and relaxation of previous moral standards have made the adjustments of teenagers and parents increasingly difficult. The so-called generation gap is widening in relation to a number of attitudes, values, and beliefs. Parents can no longer find guidance from their own experiences in understanding the needs of today's teenager. Consequently, in their frustration, bewilderment, and disappointment, they are forced to undertake a painful reevaluation of a number of their previously held attitudes and beliefs.[8]

Autonomy from parents requires a great deal of energy during the adolescent struggle for independence. It is difficult for the teenager to continue to be a son or daughter and meet the obligations imposed by this role while, at the same time, abandoning the role of the dependent child and gradually assuming the position of independent, autonomous adult. Although the individual is continually involved throughout childhood in some phase of self-differentiation and separation from parents, it is during later adolescence that the real and final liberation from parental domination takes place.

Peer relationships and influence

Although parents remain the primary influence in their lives, for the majority of adolescents peers assume a more significant role in adolescence than they did during childhood. The peer group serves as a strong support to teenagers, individually and collectively, providing them with a sense of belonging and a feeling of strength and power. It forms that transitional world between dependence and autonomy. As adolescents spend increasing amounts of time among their peers and have less contact with their parents, the peer group becomes an important socializing agent. The group is a support for conformity and for questioning and challenging adult values and societal institutions—a new frame of reference from which to reject the old.

Peer group. Adolescents have always been social, gregarious, and group minded. Although there are a few who remain outside either from preference or rejection, the majority seek the safety, companionship, and reciprocal reinforcement of a group. The peer group now has an intense influence on the adolescent's self-evaluation and behavior. In order to gain acceptance by a group, the early teenager tends to conform completely in modes of dress, hairstyle, taste in music, vocabulary, and so on, often at the expense of individuality and self-assertion. The teenager's entire being is measured by the reaction of his peers. Since most teenagers are still insecure and lacking in confidence, they are unable to tolerate differences between themselves and their peers; therefore, conformity is the rule within primary friendship groups. To belong is of utmost importance; therefore, the adolescent behaves in a way that will ensure his establishment in a group. Adolescents are highly susceptible to social approval, acceptance, and demands. To be ignored or criticized by peers creates feelings of inferiority, inadequacy, and incompetence.

Except in a few small, homogeneous high schools, teenagers distribute themselves into a relatively predictable social hierarchy. The largest social division is the set. Both boys and girls are members of the crowd, but for some occasions and activities they separate into like-sex crowds. The adolescents know to which set they and others belong, although in large schools they may not all know each other. Thus the circle of acquaintances is broadened and within this set the adolescent develops the adult social skill of exchanging breezy, pert greetings with people he knows only slightly.

Within the set are smaller, distinct, and rather exclusive crowds or cliques of selected close friends, based on common tastes, interests, and background, who are emotionally attached to each other. Although they may become formalized, most cliques remain informal and small but each has an identifying feature that proclaims its difference from others and its solidarity within itself in much the same manner as the adolescent generation as a whole sets itself apart from the adult generation. Although the criteria for membership may not be publically voiced, the groups tend to include or exclude persons according to consistent standards. Cliques are usually made up of one sex, and girls tend to be more cliquish than boys and to have a greater need for close friendships. Groups congregate at lunch, at a favorite hangout, or in the intimacy of someone's bedroom to talk about things that are of utmost concern to teenage girls, such as clothes, makeup, and, especially, boys. Boy's groups tend to revolve around sports, hobby activities, and rough games, although they, too, gossip and discuss the opposite sex. Within the intimacy of the group adolescents gain support in learning about themselves, consideration for the feelings of others, and increased ego development and self-reliance.

The school is psychologically important to adolescents as a focus of social life, a setting in which to define and elaborate relationships with peers. In addition most teenagers have a selected gathering place or hangout to which they can go alone or, preferably, with others of the same sex for the purpose of mingling with a group of persons from the opposite sex without the formalities or financial obligations of a date.

Best friends. Personal friendships of the one-to-one variety usually develop between like-sex adolescents. This relationship is closer and more stable than in middle childhood and is important in the quest for identity. A best friend is the best audience on whom to try out possible roles and identities that each wants to test. Best friends may try a role together, each providing support for the other. Each cares about what the other thinks and feels. Since a sense of intimacy grows within a permanent relationship, the stability of this like-sex friendship is an important link in the progress toward an intimate heterosexual relationship in young adulthood.

Heterosexual relationships. During adolescence relationships with members of the opposite sex take on new importance. The increased interest in heterosexual relationships is a natural outgrowth of the physical maturation of the reproductive organs that is taking place at this time. The interaction between body development and cultural expectations helps adolescents incorporate ideas about mature sexuality. As they begin to assimilate and integrate the changes of puberty, adolescents turn increasingly toward the opposite sex, not motivated by a need to find a permanent partner, but rather, as a means to enhance their own sex-role identity. Early dating is usually closely related to peer-group membership and social status and, like other phases of development, follows a rather predictable, sequential pattern. However, the time and rapidity of progress is influenced by many cultural factors, such as the philosophy of the community, traditions, parents' wishes, and the teenagers themselves.

Typically 12-year-old children still maintain same-sex friendships, although there are increasing opportunities for mixed-group activities. Although there seems to be a trend toward earlier dating, on the *average,* dating activities begin in the seventh and eighth grades and are usually "crowd" dates at organized school functions. For example, a group of girls just happens to be around a certain group of boys at most activities. There is seldom pairing off within the group, although a few boys and girls may see each other on a paired-off basis. By the ninth grade crowd dates are still popular, but now there is more pairing off of couples. In the tenth grade paired crowd dates, in which some boys and girls come as a couple and join the crowd consisting of several couples and perhaps a few unattached friends, are the rule. Double-dating follows group dating and is the more common practice in the eleventh grade, and both doubledating and single-pair dating are common by the twelfth grade. Most adolescents are dating to some degree by the time they leave high school. The group dating patterns provide a means whereby the potential stress and anxiety associated with heterosexual relationships are buffered by the peer group. When the focus is on group activities rather than on diadic contacts, heterosexual friendships are less threatening.[11]

The type and degree of seriousness of heterosexual relationships vary. The initial stage is usually noncommittal, extremely mobile, and seldom with any deep romantic attachments. Crushes, those strong feelings of attachment to an important or well-liked adult in the youngster's life who embodies the qualities considered most valuable by the adolescent, are common in early adolescence and are one of the earliest "love" attachments. During early midadolescence, as their sexual capacity is evolving, young boys frequently feel the need to test out the power of their sexuality by numerous exploits and conquests. It may be a response to inner sexual pressures or a need to conform to group expectations. With advancing adolescence and a more firm sexual identity, steady dating and boy-girl love relationships with deeper commitment become more numerous among teenage youngsters. Steady dating is evidence of adolescent insecurity and uncertainty—an escape from loneliness, of being left out—and provides a sense of belonging. The relationship continues until misunderstanding or boredom ends the association, and the process is often repeated with another partner. During this time the relationship between love and sexuality is brought into focus. Boys and girls in the middle teens find it hard to believe that sex can exist without love; therefore, each boy-girl attachment is viewed as real love. Parental attempts to break up these early heterosexual relationships may only cause the youngsters to prolong the attachments as a further expression of defiance. Hasty marriages based on such rebellion are, therefore, usually doomed to failure.

Authorities disagree regarding the value of early opposite sex relationships in the development of a sexual identity. Some believe that longer like-sex relationships are necessary to fully develop the characteristics of their own sex, whereas others believe that dating provides adolescents with experience in human relationships, promotes social skills, and enhances their ability to choose a mate wisely. A variety of dating partners and experiences undoubtedly promote a wiser mate selection and favor earlier and longer dating practices; however, early dating can involve an adolescent pair in a close sexual relationship before they are ready for intimacy. The sense of intimacy, the developmental crisis of early adulthood, is built on a firm sense of identity.

Sexual codes. Attitudes toward heterosexual codes among teenage youngsters have undergone a notable change in recent years. The extent to which adolescents engage in intimate sexual relationships is not known precisely. Studies indicate that casual sexual relationships are generally not acceptable. Some degree of permanent commitment is needed before sexual intimacy is considered appropriate. Most adolescents have indulged in petting, including transient, exploratory homosexual petting, and petting is generally more acceptable than intercourse as a form of sexual expression. However, available information indicates that at least 40% of girls and 80% to 95% of boys experience coitus by the end of adolescence. The prevalence increases with advancing age so that the largest numbers of sexually active youngsters are college students. In general whereas males have experienced sexual relationships with a number of females, most girls restrict their experiences to steady boyfriends, most often their future mates. For girls such intimacy is closely allied to an affectionate commitment. The overall major sexual codes in adolescence appears to be (1) petting with affection, in which the couple stops short of full sexual intercourse; (2) permissiveness with affection, which permits coitus in a stable relationship, usually between a steady-dating pair of older adolescents; and (3) the double standard of male sexual behavior, in which the majority of boys feel justified to engage in coitus with other girls to demonstrate and enhance their virility while expecting abstinence from the girl to whom they become romantically committed.

Adolescents engage in sexual relationships for pleasurable sensations, to satisfy sexual drives, to satisfy curiosity, as a conquest, as an expression of some degree of affection, or from inability to withstand pressures to conform. Often the urge to belong and gain reassurance and the wish to really belong to someone provoke a series of increasing intimate physical contacts with a favored boyfriend or girlfriend, each contact more sexually provocative than the last. Eventually sexual intercourse becomes established as a behavior pattern and a method for ensuring social participation—or even as an end in itself.

Society places the responsibility on the girl for inhibiting the boy's sexual advances; therefore, if she concedes through a need to conform or for acceptance she is faced with fears of disease, pregnancy, and/or being labeled "fast" or "bad." Often the experience can be psychologically harmful, especially when it produces a conflict of values, resulting in feelings of guilt and worthlessness. The increasing incidence of sexual activity among teenagers has important implications for health professionals because of the associated health-related problems.

The current trend toward greater permissiveness regarding adolescent sexual behavior will undoubtedly have an effect on the adolescent developmental experience. It is quite likely that young people will be accorded progressively more decision making concerning and control over their bodies. These alterations in the attitudes and value systems toward sex will have important implications for health professionals. It has been predicted that attitudes toward sex will shift from a moral context to a predominantly health context within a few years.[22]

HEALTH PROMOTION DURING ADOLESCENCE

Adolescents are, on the whole, healthy individuals. The disease level is low during this age period, but there is heightened concern about the body. Most of the health problems and the more common illnesses are in some way related to the body changes of puberty. The more common disorders associated with adolescent development are discussed in Chapter 20; health promotion in persons in this age-group is primarily one of health teaching and guidance.

Adolescents as a group are eager to learn about themselves, and nurses who are truly interested in them, respect them as persons, and are willing to listen to them will be able to gain their confidence and trust. During this period of gaining independence from families and the strong peer-group influences, teenagers are vulnerable to practices that may be hazardous to their health and well-being. They need someone to whom they can turn for guidance, with whom they can test out ideas, and with whom they feel free to express their fears and feelings. Nurses as health professionals and respected adults have the opportunity to provide adolescents with factual information about what is taking place in their bodies and to clarify misconceptions about menstruation, nocturnal emissions, and other physical changes of puberty. Both individual and group conferences with teenagers provide excellent opportunities to discuss actual or potential health problems, such as pregnancy, venereal disease, and the hazards of smoking and experimenting with drugs, including alcohol. Adolescents are often confused about the information they receive from parents, friends, and written material to which they have access. Very often teenagers feel more comfortable in the group situation. With peer support they are better able to explore ideas that they may not be able to express individually. Individual counseling provides adolescents with a knowledgeable adult in whom they can confide without the threat of an intimate relationship.

Personal care

The body-conscious teenager is highly amenable to discussion and counseling about personal care and hygiene. Body changes associated with puberty bring with them special needs for cleanliness. The hyperactive sebaceous glands and newly functioning apocrine glands make the daily bath imperative, and underarm deodorants assume an important place in personal care. The adolescent will find that hair requires more frequent shampooing, and girls will have questions about hair removal, use of cosmetics, and menstrual hygiene. Many group discussions center around the virtues of particular products or methods. Adolescents are continually bombarded with messages from the media regarding the best means to enhance their popularity and appeal to the opposite sex. Nurses are in a position to help them evaluate the relative merits of commercial products.

Teenagers vary in their need for sleep and rest. The rapid physical growth, the tendency toward overexertion, and overall increased activity of this age contribute to the fatigue in adolescents. They find it very difficult to get out of bed in the mornings and sleep late at every opportunity. Adequate sleep and rest at this time are important to a total health regimen.

Ear piercing. The currently popular trend of ear piercing may sometimes create a health problem in the uninformed teenager. It is a nursing responsibility to caution girls or boys against the practice of having their ears pierced by friends, mothers, or themselves. Although in most cases there are few if any serious side effects, there is always a danger of complications such as infection, cyst or keloid formation, bleeding, dermatitis, or metal allergy. Therefore, the procedure should be performed by a physician or qualified nurse using proper sterile technique. This is especially important if the youngster has a history of diabetes, allergies, or skin disorders. Teenagers are prone to develop keloids, particularly if there is a history of keloid formation.

Vision. Regular vision testing is an important part of health care and supervision during adolescence. The incidence of visual refractive difficulties reaches a peak at this time that is not exceeded until the fifth decade. Adolescents may not have poorer vision than children or adults, but the increased demands of schoolwork make good vision important for academic success. Consequently teenagers are more likely to be referred for visual evaluation at this time. The need for corrective lenses can create psychologic problems for teenagers if they believe that glasses spoil their appearance or do not fit their body image. For those who are able to tolerate and afford them, contact lenses are a happy solution. For some, the impact of a visual defect, no matter how slight, may prove to be a great personal concern.

Smoking. The problem of smoking among teenagers is becoming an increasingly serious one. The habit appears to be spreading among teenagers even as the evidence of the relationship between smoking and health and other harmful effects reaches greater proportions. The latest statistics indicate that the incidence of smoking among teenagers 12 to 18 years of age has not only increased but that the proportion of girls who smoke regularly almost equals that of male smokers. Consequently the ways of dealing with the problem become more important.

There are a variety of reasons for teenage smoking. Normal pressures to smoke include imitation of parents and other adults, the association of smoking with maturity or as representing a ''mature habit,'' pressures from peers who look on smoking as the popular, ''in,'' or ''cool'' thing to do, and the use of smoking as an outlet for real or imagined school, social, or home pressures. Other pressures come from advertisers who aim directly at members of this vulnerable age-group.

Obviously getting to the children before they begin smoking regularly is most effective in prevention. The problem is at what age should those involved start warning children against the hazards of smoking. The most successful programs begin such education in grade school and junior high school and continue it throughout the school years.

A variety of methods have been employed to deal with the problem. Communication through posters, charts, displays, statistics, and the use of examples of actual damaged lungs all have their supporters and doubters. While some believe that these are a waste of time, others give evidence that many children are influenced by these ''scare tactics.'' Presentation of films and demonstrations in science classes have proved relatively successful in some schools.

The economic aspects are sometimes effective. That is, calculating the amount of money spent on cigarettes over a period of time and demonstrating what the accumulated money can buy has an impact on some. Anything that will make the habit distasteful to the young people offers hope. If a significant number of influential peers can ''sell'' their classmates on the idea that the habit is not popular, the followers will imitate their behavior. Another ploy that seems to be meeting some success is emphasizing the effect of smoking on personal appearance, such as the unattractive stains on teeth and hands and the unpleasant odor that smoking gives to the breath. Nurses in schools and other agencies of the community are in a position to implement and reinforce teaching, to serve as consultants and counselors to student, teacher, and parent groups, and to be advocates in all areas where antismoking campaigns might be effective.

Nutrition

The rapid and extensive increase in height, weight, muscle mass, and sexual maturity of adolescence is accompanied by new and greater nutritional requirements. Since nutritional needs are closely related to the increase in body mass, the peak requirements occur in the year of maximum growth, during which time the body mass almost doubles. This takes place between the tenth and twelfth years in girls and about 2 years later in boys. The calorie and protein requirements during this year are higher than at almost any other time of life. As a result of this increased anabolic need, the adolescent is highly sensitive to caloric restrictions. Adolescents want food, their appetities soar, and their capacity to consume food is often awe-inspiring, as any parent of a teenage boy can attest. A fast-growing boy may never get filled up. His stomach may be too small to accommodate the amount of food he requires to meet his growth needs unless he eats at very frequent intervals. Not only do teenagers eat at every pause in the day's activities, but they enjoy food and the pleasures related to its consumption. Food is part of the attraction of ''hangouts'' and gathering places that teenagers frequent. For example, the corner drugstore or fast-food diner provides such favored items as hamburgers, ice cream, soft drinks, and the company of their equally starved peers. Large bags of assorted munchables are an essential part of beach gatherings, rock concerts, or other outdoor gatherings.

The nutritional needs of adolescents are difficult to determine because of meager nutritional information on members of this age-group. This is further complicated by the influence of emotional and other stress factors affecting nutrient utilization and the psychologic factors that influence their eating habits. In addition the wide variations in growth rates during adolescence and the equally wide variations in ages at which these changes take place complicate any attempt to set minimum dietary standards for this age-group. Consequently the Recommended Dietary Allowances for teenagers (Appendix D) include a safety factor that attempts to allow for these differences.[3] There is an additional need for iron during adolescence because of the increased muscle and soft tissue growth in both sexes and the rapid growth demands of an expanding red cell mass. Girls may be especially susceptible to iron deficiency at menarche.

Eating habits and behavior. Eating and behavior towards food are primarily family centered during early and middle childhood, and food habits are largely related to cultural and individual family preferences and patterns. With adolescence and the move toward independence, family influences on the child change. Children's interests, attitudes, and routines are altered as an increasing number of meals are eaten away from home. These changes are largely a result of the high value that teenagers place on peer acceptability and sociability; therefore, their eating habits are easily influenced by their associates. Also, family criticism about food habits tends to have a negative effect on wise selection of an adequate diet.

Omitting breakfast or eating breakfast nutritionally poor in quality is frequently a problem. Often adolescent youngsters are so sleepy in the morning, hate to get up, and delay getting up as long as possible that they have no time to eat. Many do not like breakfast food items. Other reasons for skipping breakfast are that they are not hungry, there is no one with whom to eat, or no breakfast is prepared for them. The youngster who dislikes traditional breakfast fare may react favorably to a peanut butter sandwich or a hamburger, both of which are nutritionally good and often more acceptable to the teenager. The goal of an adequate, good-tasting breakfast requires that someone prepare it and that the youngster arrange the time to eat it.

Pressure for time and their commitments to activities adversely affect the teenager's eating habits. Snacks, usually selected on the basis of accessibility rather than nutritional merit, become more and more a part of the habitual eating pattern during adolescence. Adolescents characteristically reject or only infrequently eat a sufficient amount of fresh fruits and vegetables, especially those that are rich in ascorbic acid. Milk is usually passed over in favor of soft drinks, the appropriate social drink of the peer culture.

Overeating or undereating during adolescence presents special problems. As they experience the normal increase in weight and fat deposition of the growth spurt, teenage girls often resort to dieting. The desire for the admired slim figure and a fear of becoming "fat" prompt teenage girls to embark on nutritionally inadequate reducing regimens that sap their energy and deprive their growing bodies of essential nutrients. They resort to diets on their own or with peers in an effort to conform. Many adopt the current fad diets and are victims of food misinformation. Boys are less inclined to undereat. They are more concerned about gaining in size and strength. However, they tend to eat foods high in calories but low in other essential nutrients.

Iron-deficiency anemia (p. 473) is relatively common in undernourished teenage girls, and the severe form of malnutrition, anorexia nervosa, occurs most frequently in adolescence when the girl becomes obsessed with self-denial of eating pleasures (p. 753). Obesity from either overeating or underactivity is another form of inadequate nutrition often seen in adolescence (p. 754).

Nursing considerations. Nothing can make adolescents eat wisely. Since their food habits reflect many influences and conditions, these must be considered when planning nutritional education and guidance. Food habits begun in early childhood are difficult to break. Failure to develop the habits of eating nutritious foods and a habitual lack of variety in a family's diet contribute to a lack of adequate nutrition. The quality of a diet is related to the number of different food items eaten in a day, and consistently skipped meals are associated with a poor diet.

In helping teenagers select a nutritious diet, it is best to begin where they are and actively involve them in the process. In helping teenagers analyze their nutritional intake, it is well to remember that there are many ways in which to achieve an adequate diet and that no pattern should be prejudged as inadequate until it is determined that it is indeed deficient in essential nutrients. Adolescents do not respond well to judgmental attitudes. It is not unusual to discover that their diet patterns, although unusual by adult standards, are actually satisfactory. Teenagers dislike being talked down to or preached at, but they do respond when their independence is respected and they are given the opportunity to make their own decisions regarding food choices.

In general, adolescents are body-conscious and concerned about their appearance. When diet is associated with clear skin, firm flesh, and glossy hair, the teenager is more likely to be receptive to nutritional education. However, helping young persons arrive at a decision for change is more difficult than providing information. They respond best when the counselor provides straightforward information, talks with them and not at them, and listens to what they have to say. Listening objectively to their ideas, clarifying misconceptions without ridicule, and involving them in diet planning are necessary if essential knowledge is to be translated into action. It is best to begin where the individual is. A current food fad may be a good point from which to build a nutritious diet, taking into consideration other factors, such as, cultural, social, and economic factors, without prohibitions or declaring any food to be "bad."

As snacks become more and more a part of the adolescents' eating pattern, it is important that they contribute something other than calories to their diet. More often than not, what the adolescent eats is determined by what is available. Items such as fruits, vegetables, and dairy products, when made readily available, are excellent and nutritious snack foods. A refrigerator shelf stocked by the mother with good-tasting snack items specially for the youngster can contribute significantly to improving an adolescent's diet and giving him a feeling that he is an important and worthwhile person. Similarly schools should provide nutritious snack foods in cafeterias and on-campus vending machines to encourage the purchase of these items by the teenage population.

It is often necessary to work with parents to help them understand the dietary needs and eating behavior of their teenagers. Many are conscious of their responsibility for the nutrition of their children, whereas others are indifferent. Family influence on adolescents is likely to change as they move toward independence and the peer group exerts a greater influence. Poorer food practices appear to result when status, sociability, independence, and enjoyment are predominant influences. Diets tend to be better when adolescents consider health to be an important factor. Good family relationships, emotional stability, and adjustment to reality are also characteristics associated with better food habits.

Posture

The process of normal development during adolescence does little to promote good posture in the teenage girl or boy. The rapid skeletal growth that is usually associated with a significant lag in muscular growth leads to weakness, easy fatigability, and awkwardness. This predisposes youngsters to slumping and makes them less inclined to stand or sit erectly. A relative reduction in physical activity that often accompanies this aggravates the situation, especially in teenage girls. The adolescent who is routinely engaged in vigorous physical activity appears to have fewer problems with posture.

Many adolescents, especially those early-maturing few who gain additional height in advance of their peers, feel conspicuous and attempt to disguise their height by adopting a slouching posture. Early pubescent breast development may cause the shy girl to hunch forward and drop her head. This is usually a transient phase that disappears as she develops confidence and maturity. Most of these postural problems resolve as the adolescent matures.

A few preexisting musculoskeletal problems, such as lateral spine deviation, or scoliosis, are likely to become exaggerated during the growth spurt and require treatment. However, most postural problems do not require special attention and treatment, and poor posture is not a source of pain. Actually the teenager's posture is primarily of concern to the parents, who continually admonish the youngster to "sit up" or "stand up" straight. The teenager, unaware of any postural defect, fails to see or understand the problem. Consequently the parental nagging only creates additional hostility and resistance on the part of the adolescent.

The best approach to counseling teenagers about posture is to show, not tell, them and to serve as a proper model. Good posture can be demonstrated best when standing before a full-length mirror. Postural defects and desired alterations can be pointed out in full view of both the young person and the nurse. A sunken chest, winged scapulas, swayback, protruberant abdomen, and drooping head and shoulders are clearly visible, and the nurse is able to demonstrate the simple corrections that can transform the youngster into a more attractive and, ultimately, healthier person. Adolescents will need reassurance that the fatigue they feel when attempting to maintain correct posture is a transient effect caused by weaker muscles, especially those of the back, and that they will soon acquire the strength and endurance to maintain the desired posture. If they concentrate on assuming correct positioning several times each day, with regular practice it will eventually become a permanent aspect of their person.

Serious postural defects, detected in the process of a physical assessment, will require early medical intervention. Scoliosis (p. 1528) is usually intensified during adolescence, and tight muscles often produce postural problems that need special attention. Nurses can refer the youngster to the appropriate source, such as the family physician, pediatrician, or health clinic, for evaluation and implementation of corrective therapy. Nurses are important sources of support and reassurance to the teenager and the parents throughout lengthy bracing, casting, and/or exercise programs.

Dental health

Dental health should not be neglected during adolescence, although the rate of caries formation is not as great as it was in childhood. Early adolescence is usually the time when corrective orthodontic appliances are worn, and these are frequently a source of embarrassment and concern to the youngster. Reassurance regarding the temporary nature of the annoyance and anticipation of an improved appearance help to make the inconvenience tolerable. It is also important to reinforce the orthodontist's directions regarding use and care of the appliances and to emphasize careful attention to brushing during this time.

Slow maturation

A group of adolescents who are under a great deal of stress and who may be hesitant to voice their concerns are slow-maturing youngsters. The rate of maturation is important during the school years, but at puberty it assumes gigantic proportions to these children and often to their parents. Girls or boys who lag behind their peers in physical maturation are painfully aware of their shortcomings. The girl feels out of place among her companions, whose hips and bosoms are developing, feels cheated because she has not yet menstruated, and feels that she is not a part of the giggling and boy-talk of her friends. The boy feels weak and small compared with his muscular companions with whom he can no longer compete, and his high voice sounds childish compared to the deep tones around him. Slow-maturing youngsters need much support and reassurance that they are not abnormal and need only hold on until the time comes when they, too, will develop the characteristics for which they yearn. The child with endocrine or genetic disorders that interfere with the maturation process needs special help, which will be discussed in Chapter 20.

Sex education and guidance

Contemporary adolescents are constantly exposed to sex symbolism and erotic stimulation from the mass media. At the same time the development of primary and secondary sex characteristics and the increased sensitivity of these body parts generate thoughts and fantasies about heterosexual relationships. In addition the culture expects that adolescents will date, flirt, and experience tender feelings. As a result teenagers are often confused and ambivalent about sexuality and heterosexual relationships. Although many adolescents have received sex education from parents and school throughout childhood, this does not always prepare them adequately for the impact of puberty. A large portion of their knowledge is acquired from peers, provocative illustrations, and inscriptions on the walls of public restrooms. Consequently much of the sex information they accumulate is incomplete, often inaccurate, riddled with cultural values and morality, and usually not very helpful.

Sex education should be education concerning a normal body function and presented in a straightforward manner using correct terminology. However, the questions of who is responsible for teaching and how the teaching can be best accomplished must be considered. Sex education is, and has been, assumed by parents, schools, churches, community agencies such as Planned Parenthood–World Population, and health professionals. Among this last group, nurses should be, and many are, taking an active role in talking to young people about their sexuality. To be able to discuss the topic with teenagers adequately, nurses must have not only an understanding of the physiologic aspects of sexuality and a knowledge of cultural and societal values but also an awareness of their own attitudes, feelings, and biases about sexuality. One cannot give information without simultaneously conveying attitudes. These attitudes in turn influence the behavior of young people.

The most comprehensive approach to sex education is offered by the Sex Information and Education Council of the United States (SIECUS), an interdisciplinary organization founded to establish sexuality as a health entity and to dignify it by openness of approach, study, and scientific research. SIECUS maintains that every sex program should present the topic from six aspects: biologic, social, health, personal adjustments and attitudes, interpersonal associations, and the establishment of values.

Whether nurses counsel young people on an individual basis, in mixed groups, or in groups segregated by sex makes little difference. Some nurses and teenagers are uneasy in mixed groups for discussions of sexuality, and no hard-and-fast rule prevails. Ideally boys and girls should be able to discuss sex objectively with one another and in groups, but this is not always possible. The difference in the rate of maturation between boys and girls and between different members of the same sex often makes it desirable to discuss certain aspects of sexuality in segregated groups. Sometimes individuals or small groups will deliberately seek the opportunity to talk over some subjects in the security of unmixed company. As a general rule, the need for separate discussion groups diminishes as the young person progresses toward maturity.

When discussing sex and sexual activities, it is best to use simple but correct language—not street language, highly scientific terminology, or evasive jargon. For example, the term sexual intercourse is usually understood by teenagers, whereas few are familiar with the terms coitus or copulation, the term sexual relationships is too vague, and the four-letter street terms are inappropriate. Once the meaning of biologic terms such as uterus, testicles, vagina, and so on is understood, teenagers prefer to use them in their discussions.

Both boys and girls need to know more about what is going on in their bodies than they are able to see. Although most girls are adequately prepared for menstruation, they do not always understand its relationship to the total process of reproduction. Many are under the impression that the "safe" time for sexual intercourse is midway between menstrual periods. Whether they are sexually active or not, adolescents should receive accurate information about pregnancy, when and how it occurs, and ways by which it can be avoided. They need to know about venereal diseases, the manner in which they are transmitted, symptoms, and how to get treatment if one becomes infected.

Teenagers as a whole are limited in their knowledge and understanding of sexuality in the opposite sex. Unless they are taught differently, each assumes that members of the other sex feel as they do. When girls understand the directness of the drive for sexual release that is experienced by young boys, they are better able to conduct themselves appropriately. This same knowledge will help boys to understand that girls do not feel the same urges as they do. Both need to recognize that they have a responsibility for their own behavior.

It is also important for teenagers to know that the thoughts and fantasies that may be disturbing to them are a normal part of the developmental process and should not be a source of guilt feelings. Adolescents, girls in particular, will want answers to questions, such as, "What is it like?" "Does it hurt?" "What happens when . . . ?" and "Is it all right if you . . . ?" Boys are often concerned about the fallacy that there is a relationship between penis size and sexual function. They need reassurance that masturbation is a normal and common practice, that pornography is not harmful, that some degree of homosexuality is not unusual in early adolescence, and that some "perversions," such as oral genital relations, are normal substitutes for intercourse in certain situations.[6]

Young people are at the stage of life when the sexual aspects of interpersonal relationships become particularly important. Societal expectations push them toward dating, and their own inner sex drive urges them toward exploration. Teenagers' curiosity and desire for information extend beyond the need for anatomic and physiologic knowledge. They need to know more than the mechanics of conception, gestation, and birth. They need to know about sexuality in the opposite sex and to be helped to view the nature of sex as a powerful life force—a force to be utilized as an intense, vital human experience that is earned by maturity and not a childhood game at which to play.

REFERENCES

1. Cooper, H. E.: Adolescence. In Kempe, C. H., Silver, H. K., and O'Brien, D.: Current pediatric diagnosis and treatment, ed. 3, Los Altos, 1974, Lange Medical Publications.
2. Erikson, E. H.: Childhood and society, ed. 2, New York, 1963, W. W. Norton & Co., Inc.
3. Food and Nutrition Board, National Research Council: Recommended dietary allowances, ed. 8, Washington, D.C., 1974, National Academy of Sciences.
4. Frisch, R. E., and Revelle, R.: Height and weight at menarche and a hypothesis of menarche, Arch. Dis. Child. **46:**695, 1971.
5. Gold, M., and Donovan, E.: Adolescent development: readings in research and theory, Boston, 1969, Allyn & Bacon, Inc.
6. Gordon, S.: What adolescents want to know, Am. J. Nurs. **71:**535-536, 1971.
7. Group for the Advancement of Psychiatry: Normal adolescence, New York, 1968, Charles Scribner's Sons.
8. Group for the Advancement of Psychiatry: The joys and sorrows of parenthood, New York, 1973, Charles Scribner's Sons.
9. Havighurst, R. J.: Developmental tasks and education, ed. 3, New York, 1972, David McKay Co., Inc.
10. Illingworth, R. S., and Ziai, M.: Physical growth and development. In Ziai, M., editor: Pediatrics, ed. 2, Boston, 1975, Little, Brown and Co.
11. Kaluger, G., and Kaluger, M. F.: Human development: the span of life, ed. 2, St. Louis, 1979, The C. V. Mosby Co.
12. Kohlberg, L., and Gilligan, C.: The adolescent as a philosopher: the discovery of the self in a post conventional world. In Kagan, J., and Coles, R., editors: 12 to 16: Early adolescence, New York, 1972, W. W. Norton & Co., Inc.
13. Marshall, W. A., and Tanner, J. M.: Variations in the pattern of pubertal changes in girls, Arch. Dis. Child. **44:**291, 1969.
14. Marshall, W. A., and Tanner, J. M.: Variations in the pattern of pubertal changes in boys, Arch. Dis. Child. **45:**13, 1970.
15. Muhich, D. F., and Johnson, B. J.: Youth and society: changing value and roles, Pediatr. Clin. North Am. **20:**771-778, 1973.
16. Newman, B. M., and Newman, P. R.: Development through life, a psychosocial approach, Homewood, Ill., 1975, Dorsey Press.
17. Phillips, J. L.: The origins of intellect: Piaget's theory, San Francisco, 1969, W. H. Freeman and Co. Publishers.
18. Piaget, J.: The theory of stages in cognitive development, New York, 1969, McGraw-Hill Book Co.
19. Tichy, A. M., and Malasanos, L. J.: The physiological role of hormones in puberty, Am. J. Maternal Child Nurs. **1:**384-388, 1976.
20. Timeras, P. S.: Developmental physiology and aging, New York, 1972, Macmillan Publishing, Inc.
21. Turiel, E.: Conflict and transition in adolescent moral development, Child Dev. **45:**14-29, 1974.
22. Vincent, C. E.: A historical perspective for the growth and developmental tasks of today's adolescents. In American Medical Association First National Congress on the Quality of Life: The early years, Acton, Mass., 1974, Publishing Sciences Group Inc.

BIBLIOGRAPHY

Adams, G.: The sexual history as an integral part of the patient history, Am. J. Maternal Child Nurs. **1**(3):170-175, May/June 1976.

Alissi, A. S.: Bridging the concept gap in work with youth, Children **18:**13, January/February 1971.

Amenta, M. M.: Free clinics change the scene, Am. J. Nurs. **74:** 284, 1974.

Anderson, F. J.: The developmental experience of adolescence, Issues Comprehensive Pediatr. Nurs., 1976.

Barnes, H. V.: Physical growth and development during puberty, Med. Clin. North Am. **59:**1305-1318, 1975.

Bellaire, J.: Teenagers learn to care about themselves, Nurs. Outlook **19:**792, December 1971.

Brown, F.: Sexual problems of the adolescent girl, Pediatr. Clin. North Am. **19:**759-764, 1972.

Bryt, A.: Adolescent sex crises, Hum. Sexuality, pp. 8-34, October 1976.

Caghan, S. B.: The adolescent process and the problem of nutrition, Am. J. Nurs. **75:**1728-1731, 1975.

Cassidy, J. T.: Teenagers in a family planning clinic, Nurs. Outlook **18:**30-31, November 1970.

Chard, M.: An approach to examining the adolescent male, Am. J. Maternal Child Nurs. **1**(1):41-43, January/February 1976.

Children are different, Columbus, Ohio, 1970, Ross Laboratories.

Chinn, P. L.: Child health maintenance: concepts in family centered care, ed. 2, St. Louis, 1979, The C. V. Mosby Co.

Conger, J. J.: Adolescence and youth, New York, 1973, Harper & Row, Publishers.

Daniel, W. A., Jr.: The adolescent patient, St. Louis, 1970, The C. V. Mosby Co.

Davis, R. C.: The adolescent and his family. In Hymovich, D. P., and Barnard, M. U., editors: Family health care, New York, 1973, McGraw-Hill Cook Co.

DeGrave, G., Riordan, B., and Mathias, R.: Sex education for delinquent boys—unveiling the taboo, Nursing '76 **6**(22, 25, June 1976.

Dempsey, M. O.: The development of body image in the adolescent, Nurs. Clin. North Am. **7:**609-616, 1972.

Duffy, T. P.: Anemia in adolescence, Med. Clin. North Am. **59:** 1481-1488, 1975.

Duran, M. T.: Family-centered care and the adolescent's quest for self-identity, Nurs. Clin. North Am. **7:**65-73, 1972.

Dylag, H.: How difficult the "I." The adolescent maturation of critical identity. In Hall, J. E., and Weaver, B. R.: Nursing of families in crisis, Philadelphia, 1974, J. B. Lippincott Co.

Elder, M. S.: The unmet challenge—nurse counseling on sexuality, Nurs. Outlook **18:**38-40, November 1970.

Erikson, E. H.: Identity: youth and crisis, New York, 1968, W. W. Norton & Co., Inc.

Erikson, E. H.: Dimensions of a new identity, New York, 1974, W. W. Norton & Co., Inc.

Fielding, J. E., and Nelson, S. H.: Health care for the economically disadvantaged adolescent, Pediatr. Clin. North Am. **20:**975-988, 1973.

Fine, L. L.: What's a normal adolescent? Clin. Pediatr. **12:**1-5, 1973.

Frankle, R. T., and Heussanstamm, F. K.: Food zealotry and youth, Am. J. Public Health **64:**11-17, 1974.

Frisch, R. E., and Revelle, R.: Height and weight at menarche and a hypothesis of critical body weight and adolescent events, Science **169:**377-399, 1970.

Gadpaille, W. J.: Adolescent sexuality and the struggle over authority, J. Sch. Health **40:**479-483, 1970.

Gallagher, J. R., Heald, F. P., and Garell, D. C.: Medical care of the adolescent, ed. 3, New York, 1976, Appleton-Century-Crofts.

Gallagher, U.: Changing focus on services to teen-agers, Child. Today **2:**24-27, 1973.

Gecas, V., Thomas, D. L., and Weigert, A. J.: Social identities in Anglo and Latin adolescents, Soc. Forces **51:**477-484, 1973.

Gendel, E. S., and Green, P. B.: Sex education controversy—a boost to new and better programs, J. Sch. Health **41:**24, January 1971.

Giuffra, M. J.: Demystifying adolescent behavior, Am. J. Nurs. **75:**1724-1727, 1975.

Graf, C. M.: Sex and the adolescent, Issues Comprehensive Pediatr. Nurs., pp. 31-41, 1976.

Guyton, A. C.: Textbook of medical physiology, ed. 5, Philadelphia, 1976, W. B. Saunders Co.

Hammar, S. L.: The approach to the adolescent patient, Pediatr. Clin. North Am. **20:**779-788, 1973.

Heald, F. P.: Adolescent nutrition, Med. Clin. North Am. **59:** 1329-1336, 1975.

Hill, J. P., and Shelton, J., editors: Readings in adolescent development and behavior, Englewood Cliffs, N.J., 1971, Prentice-Hall, Inc.

Horrocks, J. E., and Weinberg, S. A.: Psychological needs and their development during adolescence, J. Psychol. **74:**51-69, 1970.

House, E.: Medical services for sexually active teenagers, Am. J. Public Health **63:**285-287, 1973.

Johnston, F. E., Molina, R. M., and Galbraith, M. A.: Height, weight and age of menarche and the "critical weight" hypothesis, Science **174:**1148, 1971.

Josselyn, I. M.: The adolescent and his world, New York, 1972, Family Service Association of America.

Keniston, K.: Youth: a "new" stage of life, Am. Scholar **39:**631-654, 1970.

Kogut, M. D.: Growth and development in adolescence, Pediatr. Clin. North Am. **20:**789-806, 1973.

Konapka, F.: Formation of values in the developing person, Am. J. Orthopsychiatry **43:**86, 1973.

Krizinofski, M. T.: Human sexuality and nursing practice, Nurs. Clin. North Am. **8:**673-681, 1973.

Kulin, H. E., and Reiter, E. O.: Gonadotropins during childhood and adolescence; a review, Pediatrics **51:**260, 1973.

Landbaum, J., and Willis, R.: Conformity in early and later adolescence, Dev. Psychol. **4:**334, 1971.

Long, W. A.: Adolescent maturation—a clinical observation, Postgrad. Med. **57:**54, 1975.

Lowery, G. H.: Growth and development of children, Chicago, 1973, Year Book Medical Publishers, Inc.

Maddox, J.: Sex in adolescence, Adolescence **8:**325, 1973.

Malina, R. M.: Adolescent changes in size, build, composition and performance, Hum. Biol. **46:**117-131, February 1974.

Mandetta, A. F., and Woods, N. F.: Learning about human sexuality—a course model, Nurs. Outlook **22:**525-527, 1974.

Monge, R. H.: Developmental trends in factors of adolescent self-concept, Dev. Psychol. **8:**382-393, 1973.

Mussen, P. H., Conger, J. J., and Kagan, J.: Child development and personality, ed. 4, New York, 1974, Harper & Row, Publishers.

Osofsky, H. J., and Osofsky, J. D.: Let's be sensible about sex education, Am. J. Nurs. **71:**532-535, 1971.

Osokby, H. J.: Adolescent sexual behavior: current status and anticipated trends for the future, Clin. Obstet. Gynecol. **14:**405, 1971.

Quereshi, M. Y.: Patterns of intellectual development during childhood and adolescence, Genet. Psychol. Monogr. **87**(2): 313-344, 1973.

Rajokovich, M. J.: High schools need nurse counselors, too, Nurs. Outlook **18:**60, May 1970.

Rauh, J. L., Johnson, L. B., and Burket, R. L.: The reproductive adolescent, Pediatr. Clin. North Am. **20:**1005-1020, 1973.

Reiter, E. O., and Kulin, H. E.: Sexual maturation in the female, Pediatr. Clin. North Am. **19:**581, 1972.

Reiter, E. O., and Root, A. W.: Hormonal changes in adolescence, Med. Clin. North Am. **59:**1289-1304, 1975.

Root, A. W.: Endocrinology of puberty. Part I. Normal sexual maturation, J. Pediatr. **83:**1-19, 1973.

Rosendorf, F.: Youth has its say in the Rockies, Children **18:**122, July/August 1971.

Ross, D. C., Sr., and Ross, D. C., Jr.: Youthful alienation and social mobility, Clin. Pediatr. **12**(1):22-27, January 1973.

Schorr, B. C., SanJur, D., and Erickson, E. D.: Teenage food habits, J. Am. Diet. Assoc. **61:**415-420, 1972.

Semmens, J. P., and Semmons, J. H.: Sex education of the adolescent female, Pediatr. Clin. North Am. **19:**765, 1972.

Sinclair, D.: Human growth after birth, New York, 1969, Oxford University Press, Inc.

Sternlieb, J. J., and Munan, L.: A survey of health problems, practices, and needs of youth, Pediatrics **49:**177-186, 1972.

Stone, L. J., and Church, J.: Childhood and adolescence, ed. 3, New York, 1973, Random House, Inc.

Sutterly, D. C., and Donnelly, G. F.: Perspectives in human development, Philadelphia, 1973, J. B. Lippincott Co.

Trott, A. W.: Disorders of bone and muscle. In Gallagher, J. R., Heald, F. P., and Garell, D. C., editors: Medical care of the adolescent, ed. 3, New York, 1976, Appleton-Century-Crofts.

U.S. Department of Health, Education and Welfare: How children grow, Washington, D.C., 1972, U.S. Government Printing Office.

Waechter, E. H., and Blake, F. G.: Nursing care of children, ed. 9, Philadelphia, 1976, J. B. Lippincott Co.

Wagner, H.: Increasing impact of the peer group during adolescence, Adolescence **2:**52-53, 1971.

Wattenberg, W. W.: The adolescent years, New York, 1973, Harcourt Brace Jovanovich, Inc.

Webb, T., and Oski, F.: Iron deficiency anemia and scholastic achievement in young adolescents, J. Pediatr. **82:**827-830, 1973.

Westman, J. C.: Understanding teen-agers, Minn. Med. **56:**94-98, 1973.

Whipple, D. V.: Dynamics of development: euthenic pediatrics, New York, 1966, McGraw-Hill Book Co.

Wilbur, C., and Aug, R.: Sex education, Am. J. Nurs. **73:**88-91, 1973.

Williams, S. R.: Nutrition and diet therapy, ed. 3, St. Louis, 1977, The C. V. Mosby Co.

Wingerd, J., Solomon, I. L., and Schoen, E. J.: Parent-specific height standards for pre-adolescent children of three racial groups, with method for rapid determination, Pediatrics **52:**555, 1973.

Wolfish, M. G.: Adolescent sexuality, Clin. Pediatr. **12**(4):244-247, 1973.

Wolfish, M. G.: A clinic for the ambulatory adolescent, Clin. Pediatr. **12:**13-15, 1973.

Woods, N. F.: Human sexuality in health and illness, ed. 2, St. Louis, 1979, The C. V. Mosby Co.

Yacenda, J. A.: Smoking behavior and young people. The need for new directions, Clin. Pediatr. **12:**13A, January 1973.

Yaros, P. S.: The adolescent. In Scipien, G., and associates, editors: Comprehensive pediatric nursing, New York, 1975, McGraw-Hill Book Co.

Young, C. M.: Adolescents and their nutrition. In Gallagher, J. R., Heald, F. P., and Garell, D. C.: Medical care of the adolescent, New York, 1976, Appleton-Century-Crofts.

Zacharias, L., Wurtman, R. J., and Schatzoff, M.: Sexual maturation in contemporary American girls, Am. J. Obstet. Gynecol. **108:**833, 1970.

20

Health problems of adolescence

In many ways the health problems of adolescents are very different from those of either children or adults. Teenagers are relatively healthy individuals on the whole, as the health status of the preadolescent period continues into pubescence. However, the multiple aspects of adolescence, both physiologic and psychologic, influence the evaluation and care of members of this age-group. It is characteristic of adolescents that the very nature of their health problems is a deterrent to seeking health care. Most health problems are related to the physical changes taking place in their bodies and the crucial psychosocial crisis of identity formation. Major diseases are at a relatively low incidence but, when they do occur, have unusual significance for the adolescent.

Delayed growth and/or maturation

The absence of sexual maturation at a time when other children are experiencing positive evidence of sexual development and its associated spurt in growth and physical strength is a matter of concern to both the parents and their affected child. Fortunately in most instances the delay in development is a simple physiologic or constitutional delay that merely represents one end of the normal genetically influenced variation of pubertal growth. These children will go through a delayed but normal puberty to finally catch up, in their late teens, with their more rapidly developing age-mates. However, this becomes a psychosocial problem for some young people. Less benign causes of delayed development may be of endocrine origin or caused by chromosomal aberrations. In other situations delayed development may be a result of chronic diseases such as malabsorption, chronic asthma, and poorly controlled diabetes mellitus that are serious enough to retard the developmental process.

CONSTITUTIONAL DELAY

Delayed development, manifested by short stature and other indications, is often the reason the adolescent is brought to the attention of health professionals and is the more common presenting complaint in endocrine clinics. Although it occurs with equal frequency in both girls and boys, the problem seems to be more serious in boys than in girls. Therefore, it is boys who more often seek assistance. Since the psychosocial factors are of importance and there are rare situations in which delayed development is caused by a pathogenic condition, it is important to determine the reason for developmental delay.

Diagnostic evaluation

Clinical diagnosis of delayed development can usually be determined with relative ease on the basis of some simple criteria:

Family history. Parents and/or other relatives often have a history of a similar type of delayed growth and maturation. Height and weight of siblings at comparable ages and their present measurements are helpful.

Child's history. Prenatal and birth history will reveal whether or not the child's height and weight were appropriate for gestational age, and a pregnancy history might reveal factors that could have influenced a deviation from normal. Concurrent chronic diseases influence growth, and past illnesses such as head injuries and gastrointestinal, renal, or neurologic disorders may provide clues for the examiner.

History of the child's dietary habits, strength, stamina, and susceptibility to infection are investigated as well as attainment of developmental milestones and school progress. Any emotional problems or problems of social adjustment are considered, especially those that may indicate past family instability. It is well known that prolonged emotional upset has a significant influence on growth.

Previous growth pattern. If the growth rate is known, it is often found that it has decreased during the second year of life or just prior to puberty or that the child has remained relatively small throughout the growth period with a growth curve that is parallel or slightly below the third percentile. If records are not available, information can be obtained regarding when it was first noticed that the child was small compared to other children.

Physical examination. An accurate measurement of

height and weight is taken with the child stripped to underclothing. This may also include measurements of body proportions from crown to pubis and pubis to heel to detect any abnormality of body proportion. Signs of sexual development are noted using standard criteria (p. 691). The first evidence of puberty is breast budding in girls and testicular enlargement (testicular volume greater than 2 ml) in boys. If these signs are present, normal sexual development can be expected to follow in 1 to 2 years.

Bone age. Bone age, assessed from wrist x-ray films, is always delayed in these children.

Endocrine studies. Hormonal investigations reveal essentially normal results. Growth hormone (GH) responses, gonadotropin levels, and responses to gonadotropin-releasing factor (GnRF) are usually low for the child's chronologic age but consistent with his bone age. The same is true for the plasma levels of testosterone and estrogen and urinary excretion of 17-ketosteroids. In addition, as these children mature, they have a corresponding change in endocrine response consistent with normal pubertal changes.

Summary. The child with constitutional delay in development usually displays the following[2]:

A positive family history
A growth pattern in the lower range of normal
Delayed bone age
Evidence of early sexual development on careful examination
Normal physical and mental health

Outcome and treatment

The untreated child will proceed through normal changes as expected on the basis of bone age. These changes, although occurring later than in the average child, will appear in normal sequence and manner, and treatment is not usually indicated. The management consists of continued medical observation, attention to general health and nutrition, and psychologic support. Further assurance can be provided by predicting the youngster's adult height from available tables and other criteria devised from comprehensive studies of child development. Very often the longer an individual takes to pass through puberty, the better are his prospects for achieving an acceptable adult height, since epiphyseal fusion is more advanced in youngsters who mature earlier. Where the psychosocial situation is such that the young boy is 14 years of age or older and miserable as a result of peer ridicule and indignities, hormonal therapy has proved to be advantageous, and many authorities recommend treatment in these instances. However, hormonal therapy is undertaken with caution. Thyroid hormone is of no value unless hypothyroidism is present; anabolic steroids increase protein synthesis and stimulate growth but often have undesirable androgenic effects that may persist after administration; and human growth hormone, although capable of increasing height, is in short supply and is, at present, confined to the treatment of hypopituitary dwarfism.[22]

DELAYED DEVELOPMENT CAUSED BY PATHOLOGIC CONDITIONS

A small group of children suffer delay of growth or onset of adolescence because of disorders that may or may not be amenable to treatment. From a worldwide point of view, the most common cause of short stature and/or delayed development is probably inadequate nutrition; however, the major disorders that produce delayed development can be classified into three groups: (1) chronic diseases, (2) endocrine dysfunction, and (3) syndromes of primary gonadal failure.

Chronic diseases

Chronic diseases can interfere with growth, but, unless the illness is unduly prolonged, catch-up growth will occur. There are a number of chronic illnesses that fit in this category, and these will be discussed at the appropriate time. Those encountered most frequently are respiratory disorders such as asthma, cystic fibrosis, and recurrent upper respiratory infection; illnesses caused by defective organ or disturbed immune mechanisms; gastrointestinal diseases such as parasitic infestations, cystic fibrosis, and other malabsorption syndromes; cardiac anomalies and blood dyscrasias such as sickle cell anemia; and chronic renal disturbances, especially renal tubular acidosis. It appears that the duration of the illness is more significant than the intensity in its effect on growth, although the precise length of time necessary to affect growth permanently has not been determined precisely.

Skeletal disorders that affect growth in stature are principally those described as dwarfism. Most are caused by a variety of congenital defects and disorders, such as achondroplasia, and some of the inborn errors of metabolism, such as Hurler's or Hunter's syndrome. Whereas some are readily apparent at or shortly after birth, milder cases may not be recognized until later in life and are diagnosed on x-ray and biochemical examinations.

Endocrine dysfunction

The major hormones that promote physical growth are thyroid hormone, growth hormone, and sex hormones. Insulin can be said to promote growth by its effect on carbohydrate metabolism, whereas cortisol inhibits growth. Therefore, deficiencies of growth-promoting hormones or an excess of cortisol can cause growth retardation in children. Endocrine deficiencies can be the result of abnormal secretory function in the glands responsible for their production, the pituitary hormones that stimulate their secretion, or the releasing factors from the hypothalamus. In some instances growth retardation may be the result of increased production of factors that inhibit hormone secretion (Table 20-1). The complex relationships of endocrine function and their disturbances are discussed in Chapter 38; therefore, the reader is directed there for further elabora-

Table 20-1. Effects of endocrine deficiency on growth and maturation

Hormone	Source	Action	Effects of deficiency on growth and/or maturation
Thyroid hormone	Thyroid gland	Controls rate of chemical reactions in the body Is essential for normal growth and reproduction	General growth is greatly reduced; extent depends on age at which deficiency occurs Early epiphyseal closure Disproportional linear growth
Thyroid-stimulating hormone (TSH)*	Pituitary gland	Stimulates thyroid to produce thyroid hormone	Marked delay of puberty
Growth hormone (GH) or somatotropic hormone (SH)*	Pituitary gland	Increases rate of protein synthesis; conserves carbohydrate utilization and fat mobilization	Generalized growth retardation Proportional diminished growth Eventual spontaneous puberty
Gonadotropin*	Pituitary gland	Stimulates gonads to mature and produce sex hormones and germ cells	Absent or incomplete spontaneous puberty
Sex hormones Testosterone Estrogen Progesterone	Gonads Testes Ovaries	Produces sex cells and secondary sex characteristics	Absence of secondary sex characteristics Infertility

*For each anterior pituitary hormone there is a corresponding hypothalamic releasing factor. A deficiency in these factors caused by inhibiting anterior pituitary hormone synthesis produces the same effects (see Chapter 38 for more detailed information).

tion. This segment is limited to a summary of those factors that affect growth.

Thyroid hormone deficiency. Thyroid hormone deficiency is always associated with poor growth and delayed bone maturation. Hypothyroidism that is present from birth causes severe stunting of linear growth, which is evident early in life. When the deficiency begins before the skeletal age of 9 or 10 years, the child maintains infantile proportions with short legs compared to the length of the spine; he tends to be pale, sluggish, inactive, and obese; and intellectual achievement at school deteriorates. Acquired hypothyroidism varies with the degree and duration of the deficiency, but skeletal age is delayed if the condition has been present more than 12 months (see p. 1465 for diagnosis and treatments).

Growth hormone deficiency. Growth hormone deficiency, associated with hypopituitarism, inhibits somatic growth in all cells of the body. Although children with hypopituitarism are normal at birth, they show growth patterns that progressively deviate from the normal growth rate, often beginning in infancy. The chief complaint in most instances is short stature. Of those who seek help, boys outnumber girls three to one. Skeletal proportions are normal for the age, but these children appear younger than their chronologic age, tend to be relatively inactive, and are less apt to participate in aggressive, sporting-type activities. Bone age is nearly always retarded but is closely related to height age; the degree of retardation depends on the duration and extent of the hormonal deficiency. Diminished function of recent onset may show little retardation in skeletal age, whereas children with a long-standing deficiency may evidence a skeletal age only 40% to 50% of their chronologic age. In children with a partial growth hormone deficiency, the growth retardation is less marked than in children with a growth hormone deficiency.

Growth hormone deficiency may be attributed to an *idiopathic* or *organic* etiology. The extent of idiopathic growth hormone deficiency may be complete or partial, but the cause is unknown. It is frequently associated with other pituitary hormone deficiencies, such as deficiencies of thyroid-stimulating hormone and ACTH; thus it is theorized that the disorder is probably secondary to hypothalamic deficiency. It has also been observed that there is a higher than average frequency in some families, which indicates a possible genetic etiology in a number of instances.

The most common organic causes of growth hormone deficiency are tumors of the pituitary or hypothalamic region, in which case the child may evidence growth retardation for quite some time before developing any symptoms or signs of increased intracranial pressure, local compression, or destructive effects of the tumor. Other causes sometimes include encephalitis, head trauma (rarely), and congenital hypoplasia of the hypothalamic area.

Sex hormone deficiency. Sex hormone deficiency that causes delayed puberty can occur as a result either of pituitary dysfunction or of hypogonadism. A hypofunctioning pituitary gland as briefly discussed in the preceding segment on endocrine dysfunction, can produce a deficiency in either the gonadotropic hormones, which retards maturation of the gonads, or growth hormone, which will diminish total growth during childhood. In addition there are a large variety of disorders that cause absence or deficiency of sex hormone secretion by their effect on the gonads directly. These may be genital abnormalities that are related to defective gonadal differentiation or those that are associated with functional abnormalities of the already differentiated fetal gonad (see p. 419 for abnormal sexual development). The largest group of disorders in which deficient gonadal development is a prominent feature includes the sex chromosomal aberrations. Two of these, Klinefelter's and Turner's syndromes, will be elaborated later in this chapter.

Cortisol excess. Cortisol excess as a result of organic causes or of prolonged cortisone therapy also has an adverse effect on growth in children. This effect is produced by direct action on growing cartilage, interference with production of growth hormone, or interference with the response to or production of somatomedin, a substance that mediates the action of growth hormone on tissues. Because of the growth-suppressing effect of cortisone in excess of minimal requirements, therapy is limited to short-term administration whenever possible.

Syndromes of primary gonadal failure

The most frequently seen disorders associated with primary gonadal failure are the sex chromosomal defects categorized collectively as gonadal dysgenesis, principally Turner's syndrome. Chromosomal impairment of male sexual function is most commonly caused by Klinefelter's syndrome. The general concepts and mechanisms responsible for sex chromosomal anomalies have been discussed in Chapter 6 (see p. 190), and disorders associated with aberrant sexual development were outlined in Chapter 11 (see p. 418). Derangements that become apparent at puberty are more common. Clinical presentation in the female may be masculinization, sexual infantilism or hypoplasia, primary absence of menstruation *(amenorrhea),* or abnormally scanty or infrequent menstruation *(oligomenorrhea* or *hypomenorrhea).*

Turner's syndrome. Although this disorder is often recognized at birth, it is diagnosed most frequently at puberty because of three outstanding features: short stature, sexual infantilism, and amenorrhea. The incidence of the condition in the population has been variously estimated at 1 in 1500, 1 in 3000, to 1 in 10,000 live female births.

Etiology. Turner's syndrome is caused by absence of one of the X chromosomes; as a result the number of chromosomes in these girls is forty-five—forty-four pairs of autosomes and one X chromosome (45,X), sometimes referred to as *monosomy X*. The disorder is caused by nondisjunction during germ cell formation and, unlike most disjunction phenomena, is related to paternal meiotic error.

Diagnostic evaluation. A tentative diagnosis can be made

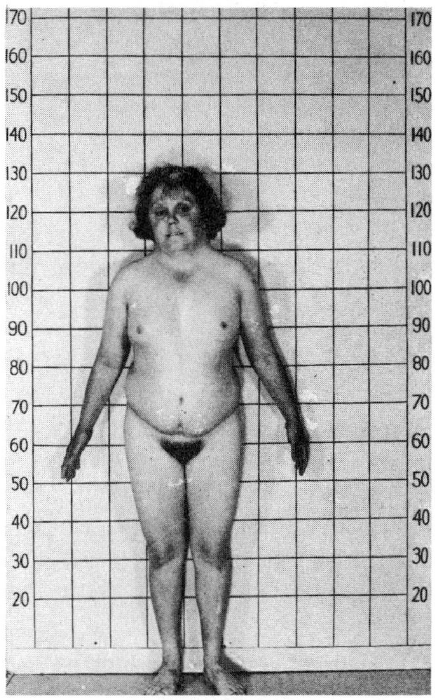

Fig. 20-1. Turner's syndrome. (From McKusick, V. A.: Medical genetics, 1959, J. Chron. Dis. **12:**1-202, 1960.)

on the physical appearance in most instances. Only a few persons with this syndrome manifest all of the possible clinical features, which include the following[15] (Fig. 20-1):

- Significant short stature, which is common to all (many adults are less than 5 feet tall)
- Redundant skin folds on the neck (webbed neck) with low posterior hairline (present in 40% to 50% of cases)
- Rather "old" facial appearance with micrognathia and low-set and sometimes malformed ears
- Shield-shaped chest with widely spaced hypoplastic nipples
- Increased carrying angle at the elbow (cubitus valgus)
- Cardiac anomalies, principally coarctation of the aorta or aortic valvular stenosis
- Moderate degrees of learning difficulty
- Abnormal growth patterns; absence of normal growth spurts and sexual development at puberty with primary amenorrhea and sterility; sparse pubic and axillary hair; gonads replaced by fibrous streaks
- In infancy, congenital lymphedema of hands and feet

Definitive diagnosis is confirmed on the basis of a negative sex chromatin test (see p. 189); chromosomal analysis is rarely necessary.

Medical management. Therapy is always individualized for these girls and consists primarily of hormone treatment and psychologic counseling for both child and parents. Linear growth often can be increased by the administration of anabolic steroids (chiefly synthetic androgenic hormone) continuously or intermittently over a period of 2 to 3 years. The length of treatment depends on the response to and side effects of therapy, which are usually minimal. Androgenic therapy is followed by estrogen therapy to promote the development of secondary sex characteristics. Responses to estrogen therapy vary from girl to girl, but gradual feminization is accomplished to some degree in most individuals accompanied by a positive effect on the young girl's self-image. Cardiac anomalies, if present, require treatment, and surgical correction of the webbed neck may be undertaken if the defect is disfiguring. Psychologic counseling is such an important aspect of management that it will be discussed in relation to nursing considerations of all problems of pubertal development (see p. 716).

Klinefelter's syndrome. Young boys with this disorder are seldom seen before puberty, at which time varying degrees of failure of adolescent virilization occur. Some males are not detected until they appear for evaluation for infertility. All have absence of sperm in the semen (azoospermia), small testes, and defective development of secondary sex characteristics. The incidence of Klinefelter's syndrome is estimated to be approximately 1 in 500 live male births.

Etiology. The most common of all chromosomal abnormalities, Klinefelter's syndrome is caused by the presence of one or more additional X chromosomes, probably as a result of meiotic nondisjunction (see p. 185). The majority of males with this syndrome have a chromosomal complement of 47,XXY, but there are numerous variants in the number of extra sex chromosomes, and the clinical features are essentially the same in all.

Diagnostic evaluation. There are no physical characteristics that are helpful in detecting Klinefelter's syndrome before the advent of puberty, with the possible exception of mental retardation. Mental impairment of varying degrees is a frequent finding and appears to have a direct relationship to the number of X chromosomes in the cells. The severity of retardation increases with the number of X chromosomes. Characteristic features of the disorder include (Fig. 20-2):

- Tall, eunuchoid figure with legs disproportionately long in relation to the trunk
- Sparse facial and pubic hair, often with a female distribution pattern
- Gynecomastia of some degree (seen in half the cases and often the reason for seeking medical advice)
- Small, firm, and insensitive testes; small penis and prostate
- Aspermia or oligospermia

In 80% of these boys there is a chromatin-positive buccal smear and the extra chromosome is apparent on chromosomal analysis.

It has also been observed that Klinefelter's syndrome is associated with learning and/or behavioral problems in school-age boys. Therefore, it has been suggested that buccal smears be part of the assessment of school boys with behavior problems and other signs such as slender, long legs and small testes and penis.

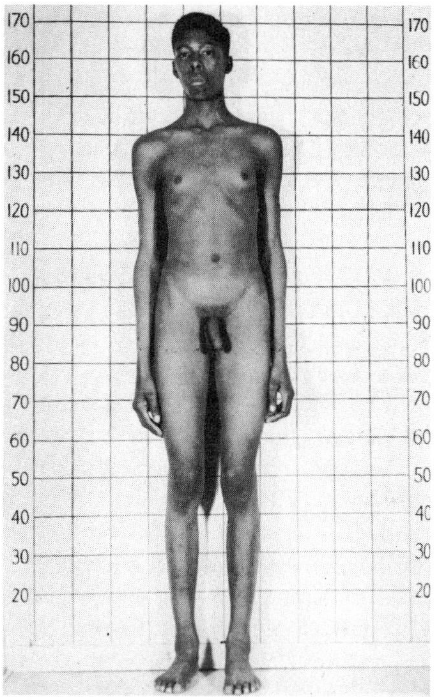

Fig. 20-2. Klinefelter's syndrome. (From McKusick, V. A.: Medical genetics, 1959, J. Chron. Dis. **12:**1-202, 1960.)

Medical management. The major effort in medical treatment is directed toward enhancing the masculine characteristics through the administration of male hormones, principally testosterone. Cosmetic surgery will eliminate embarrassment for the boy with gynecomastia. As with other pubertal development, psychologic counseling and support are considered in the segment on psychologic problems associated with developmental difficulties (p. 716).

Psychosocial dwarfism[13]

Psychosocial or deprivation dwarfism is a term applied to children who are significantly retarded in growth because of environmental circumstances. Children from homes in which they receive little, if any, psychosocial stimulation display markedly delayed skeletal development, and various tests in these children for growth hormone release are consistent with those that indicate a pituitary dysfunction. When these children are removed from the deprived environment, their growth proceeds at a normal or increased rate. This has been repeatedly demonstrated in infants and very young children. Some investigations attribute the growth retardation to malnutrition. Although this may be a factor in infants, it may also be a contributing factor in adolescents with short stature and delayed puberty secondary to psychosocial factors, particularly in the loss of appetite related to the disorder anorexia nervosa (p. 753).

Although the mechanism is not entirely clear, it is hypothesized that deprivation dwarfism occurs as a response to increased cortisol secretion in response to the prolonged stress of a disturbed environment or to unsettled patterns of sleep. Evidence indicates that deprivation dwarfism is often associated with sleep abnormalities. Since growth hormone is secreted in largest amounts during sleep, it follows that anything interfering with normal sleep patterns will interfere with the hormone secretion.

OTHER PROBLEMS OF PUBERTAL DEVELOPMENT

Delayed sexual development and short stature are manifestations of only one end of the developmental spectrum. On the other end are conditions that can be equally distressing to the developing child.

Precocious puberty

Precocious puberty is the manifestation of pubertal development that appears prior to the expected age of onset. Although puberty is gradually appearing earlier in most societies, manifestations of sexual development before age 10 years in boys or age 8½ years in girls are considered precocious and should be investigated. Early sexual development can be a result of a number of causes and may result from a disorder of the gonad, the adrenal gland, or the hypothalamic-pituitary mechanism (see p. 689). Precocious sexual development can be divided into two types: true, or complete, precocious puberty and pseudoprecocious, or incomplete puberty (also called precocious pseudopuberty or pseudosexual precocious puberty).

True (complete) precocious puberty. True precocious puberty is always isosexual and results from premature activation of the hypothalamic-pituitary-gonadal axis, which produces early maturation and development of the gonads with secretion of sex hormones, development of secondary sex characteristics, and (sometimes) production of mature sperm or ova. True precocious puberty may be caused by a variety of organic brain lesions, such as tumors, congenital lesions, or postinflammatory disorders, but in most instances no cause can be found. Cases in which the cause cannot be identified are termed *functional idiopathic* or *constitutional precocious puberty,* which may occur at any time during childhood and can be explained only as an unusually early activation of the maturation process that is regarded as a normal course of events at a later age. This is believed to be the cause of precocious puberty in 90% of girls and 50% of boys with the disorder and is nine times more common in girls than in boys. A familial incidence of male sexual precocity has been observed in some families, but sexual precocity occurs as an isolated event in girls. In sexual precocity there is early acceleration of linear growth with early epiphyseal fusion and ultimate height less than would have been anticipated with later pubertal onset.

Psychologic management and guidance of the child and family constitute the most important aspects of treatment. Parents need a detailed explanation and reassurance of the benign nature of the condition. Dress and activities for the physically precocious child should be appropriate to the age. Heterosexual interest is not usually advanced beyond the child's chronologic age, and parents need to understand that the child's mental age is congruent with the chronologic age and that the child's normal, overt manifestations of affection are age appropriate and do not represent sexual advances. In a few instances a tumor can be removed, and medroxyprogesterone acetate has been used to inhibit the production of gonadotropin in some cases. However, undesirable consequences limit the drug's usefulness as a routine measure.

Precocious pseudopuberty. Precocious pseudopuberty differs from true sexual precocity in that there is no early secretion of gonadotropin. Most cases result from early overproduction of sex hormone, usually as a result of a tumor of the ovary or testis, a tumor or hyperplasia of the adrenal gland, or exogenous sources of androgens or estrogens. There is no maturation of the gonads, but there is appearance of secondary sex characteristics. Unlike true sexual precocity, precocious pseudopuberty may be heterosexual. For example, a tumor of the adrenal gland in a girl can cause early and inappropriate female development, including clitoral enlargement and masculinization.

Isolated manifestations that are usually associated with puberty may be seen as variations in normal sexual development. They appear without other signs of pubescence and are probably caused by unusual end organ sensitivity to prepubertal levels of estrogen or androgen. Included are the following:

premature thelarch development of breasts in prepubertal females.

premature pubarche (premature adrenarche) early development of sexual hair.

Tall stature

Tallness is rarely a problem to boys, but, to the girl who is or is likely to be much taller than her age-mates, it can be a source of acute distress. Despite the fact that the average height of both boys and girls is steadily increasing, there is still a small group of children who, because of some organic disorder or a familial tendency, are excessively tall when compared with their contemporaries. Many girls like the idea of being tall and manage to cope effectively with any height-related problems that may arise. For others, it can be a source of intense anxiety and a severe social handicap.

When the rate of height change prior to puberty suggests the probability of excessive adult height, treatment with hormones may be considered. Cyclic administration of estrogens has proved effective in controlling height when therapy is initiated prior to menarche and before the end of the adolescent growth spurt that normally precedes menarche. Estrogen therapy is continued over several years until the epiphyses are fused, as determined by periodic wrist x-ray films. If treatment is stopped before that time, growth will continue. Although estrogen treatment has reduced the height from that estimated on prediction tables in a number of cases, there is still a good deal of controversy regarding its use for this purpose.[3,12,27]

Before therapy is instituted a number of factors such as the following must be considered: the prediction of future height based on present height and bone age; determination of whether predicted height is really an excessive one, that is, over 178 cm (70 inches); assessment of the child's and parents' attitudes toward the predicted height; and evaluation of the child's capacity to cope with day-to-day problems associated with such height. If hormone therapy is elected, the parents and the young girl will need to know the anticipated length of treatment, the probability of success, the side effects associated with estrogen administration, such as menorrhagia (progesterone is usually added on the last 7 days of the ovarian cycle to assure sloughing of endometrium), dark pigmentation of areola, nipples, and labia, and in some cases moderate obesity. Both parents and child will need continued support and encouragement during the extent of therapy.

Hormonal therapy has also been shown to be effective in reducing the ultimate height of excessively tall teenage boys. Long-acting testosterone esters administered periodically over the period of 1 year have proved effective in a limited sample. The testosterone has the effect of accelerating bone maturation and growth with more rapid epiphyseal closure. As with girls, the selection of children is made on the basis of careful evaluation of physical, psychologic, and social factors.[29]

Gynecomastia

Some degree of bilateral or unilateral breast enlargement frequently occurs in young boys during puberty. In most instances it is a transient phenomenon that subsides spontaneously with achievement of male development. Occasionally, however, it is associated with abnormalities such as Klinefelter's syndrome or endocrine dysfunction; therefore, these possibilities are ruled out by appropriate diagnostic examination.

Treatment usually consists of assurance to the boy and his parents that this is a benign and temporary situation. If the condition persists or is extensive enough to cause acute embarrassment or to produce doubts about gender identity in the young boy, plastic surgery is indicated for cosmetic and psychologic considerations. Administration of testosterone has no effect on breast development or regression and may even aggravate the condition. Since the boy is distressed about his physical integrity and masculinity, he will need reassurance regarding this apparently incongruous development.

Nursing considerations

Deviation from the normal course of puberty is always of concern to the affected adolescent, and, to some, it assumes monumental proportions. This distress is often so intense that the youngster hesitates to voice his concerns for fear that his worries and doubts will be confirmed. Nurses, especially school nurses, working with adolescents encounter young people who are delayed in development or who are destined to be shorter in stature than their average agemates. Most of the problems of delayed development are those caused by simple constitutional delay of puberty, and in this situation the child can be assured that the normal course of events will eventually take place. This is not always reassuring to them. They are impatient to grow and are not easily convinced. Even after direct and thorough discussion of growth and the normal variations in rate and timing of maturation, they often doubt that they will grow. It is important to maintain contact with these children, convey to them a concern about their feelings, and let them know that they are accepted as they are.

Those young people who cannot be assured that they will eventually achieve more than a minimal height will need even more acceptance and support. The suffering is especially acute in young boys who may have hoped for success in athletics or those who may have been hurt by thoughtless remarks of their more fortunate associates. They need to know that they have a sympathetic listener who understands the importance of their anguish and who can help them develop their potential in areas that do not demand size in order that they will find recognition and acceptance and acquire self-confidence and self-esteem.

One of the difficulties related to a size that is incongruent with chronologic and mental age is the manner in which others, especially adults, relate to the child. People quite naturally respond to children with short stature as though they are younger than their age. Consequently these children often react with babyish or juvenile behavior, thus setting in motion a circular pattern of behavior and response. Conversely children who are tall or physically advanced for their age are treated as though they are more advanced than their years. They are often considered to be retarded or behaviorally immature when they actually perform according to the normal behavioral expectations for their age.

Listening to distressed adolescents and conveying to them genuine interest and concern are prerequisite to any successful intervention. Counseling and therapy are individualized to meet the needs of each youngster and his problems. Encouraging these children to accentuate the positive aspects of their body and personality with sound health practices and good grooming helps foster a more positive self-image. Helpful devices include a padded brassiere for girls, hairstyling, and selection of clothing that adds the illusion of height (or diminishes it in the tall girl). In many areas there are special clothing and footwear stores that cater to persons with atypical sizes, in which the youngster can find age-appropriate clothing. They can be taught to make their own clothing.

Cosmetic surgery is often advisable when deviation from normal threatens the self-image. Breast surgery for boys with gynecomastia or for girls with oversize breasts, implantation of prosthetic testes for boys whose own are missing, and reduction of deformities, such as the webbed neck of Turner's syndrome, can often avert the development of a negative body image or self-concept.

These youngsters also need help to redirect their goals from aspirations that are unattainable to those commensurate with their capabilities. Adjustments may be accompanied by psychophysiologic or behavioral manifestations, and health workers need to be alert for signs and prepare the parents for this possibility with anticipatory guidance. Some disorders, such as Turner's or Klinefelter's syndrome, in which sterility is a fact or a decided probability, may present a need for special sex education during adolescence, particularly in relation to fertility and alternative routes to parenthood.

Common problems of adolescence

There are a number of health problems that have their onset in adolescence or are more prominent at this stage of development than at earlier or subsequent ages. Most are not life threatening but may create psychologic problems that influence the establishment of a positive identity.

MENSTRUAL DISORDERS

A menstrual history and gynecologic examination should be a routine part of the assessment of the adolescent girl. Menstrual delay, irregularities, or discomfort is a frequent concern and is worthy of consideration and understanding from health professionals.

Amenorrhea

It is not unusual for an adolescent to skip a menstrual period or two when establishing normal menstrual and ovulatory cycles. Delay in initiation of menstruation is ordinarily a temporary problem resulting from late onset of puberty and requires no intervention. This is of little concern unless it creates undo anxiety on the part of the girl and her parents, which can ordinarily be allayed by explanation and reassurance. Careful examination will reveal any congenital defects of the genital tract (a rare cause).

Amenorrhea is considered to be *primary* when menarche is delayed beyond age 17 years. *Secondary* amenorrhea is prolonged absence of menstruation for 12 months or more between periods in the first 2 years following menarche or when more than three periods have been missed after menses have become established. The most common cause of secondary amenorrhea are emotional disturbances and pregnancy, which is accompanied by the signs and symptoms associated with this state.[9,26]

Primary amenorrhea may be the result of absence or malformation of the female genital structures or the inability of normal structures to respond to hormonal stimulation. This can be of hypothalamic, pituitary, ovarian, or uterine origin and can include hypopituitarism, Turner's syndrome, tumors, and infections. Pseudoamenorrhea, resulting from imperforate hymen or transverse vaginal septum, is an unusual cause of absent menses in a girl who exhibits all the evidences of estrogen production and sexual maturation and who complains of periodic (usually monthly) lower abdominal pain. The treatment is simple surgical perforation and drainage.

A group of systemic disorders that may affect the functions of the reproductive tract are thyroid hypofunction or hyperfunction, prolonged or severe infections, adrenal hyperplasias, diabetes mellitus, or other chronic diseases. Obesity, malnutrition (including protein, vitamin, or iron deficiencies), or any rapid change in weight either up or down can produce amenorrhea. Management involves determining and treating the cause.

Dysfunctional uterine bleeding

Irregularities in the timing, length, or amount of menstrual flow are common conditions in adolescent girls and are caused primarily by either imbalance in the secretion of hormones that control menstrual function or variability in responsiveness of the target organs in adolescence. Anovulatory menstruation is characteristic of the early menstrual periods following menarche and is self-limited for the majority of teenage girls. Occasionally chronic diseases and thyroid dysfunction are causative factors, and abnormal bleeding is associated with systemic diseases that cause bleeding from a variety of mucosal surfaces, such as purpura, scurvy, and leukemia.

Treatment. Ordinarily only reassurance and attention to general health status are needed, with emphasis on a well-balanced diet, adequate rest, and moderate exercise. Anticipatory supportive therapy often includes a high-protein diet with vitamin and iron supplements. In persistent cases hormonal therapy has proved beneficial. Dilatation and curettage may be necessary to control hemorrhage in severe cases or in those that do not respond to more conservative management.

Dysmenorrhea

A certain amount of discomfort during the first day or two of the menstrual flow is extremely common. Most girls experience cramping, abdominal pain, backache, and leg ache, but in a few the pain is intolerable and incapacitating. The term *primary dysmenorrhea* is applied to these symptoms when there is no pelvic pathology to account for the cramping discomfort that is severe enough to interfere with normal activity. When the discomfort can be attributed to endometriosis, infection, adhesions from peritonitis, or other pelvic disease, the complaint is described as *secondary dysmenorrhea*.

No specific etiology of primary dysmenorrhea is known; however, some contributory factors are recognized. The first factor present in all instances of primary dysmenorrhea is the occurrence of prior ovulation. Although it is not invariable, the symptoms do not occur during the first few postmenarchal months or months of irregular anovulatory menses. Estrogen production alone does not appear to be related to uterine discomfort; however, progesterone secretion that follows ovulation is apparently responsible for the symptoms. Whereas estrogen produces fine, regular uterine contractions, progesterone causes the uterus to contract in large, irregular waves. Local discomfort is related to vascular changes in the endometrial bed during menstruation caused by alternating vasoconstriction and vasodilatation of endometrial vessels that induce local ischemia, edema, necrosis, and slough. In some girls the discomfort may be a result of low pain tolerance.

The second factor is psychologic—the reaction of the young girl to this normal female function or an emotional reaction to slight pain. It is not uncommon for girls to outgrow the severity of the symptoms once they have overcome their resentment toward menstruation or resolved the conflict between an unconscious wish to remain a little girl and a conscious drive to gain maturity. These psychic factors, tension, and anxiety can accentuate the local symptoms and produce the associated autonomic nervous system symptoms such as nausea, vomiting, pallor, diaphoresis, and fainting.

Treatment. A thorough gynecologic examination is carried out to exclude any pelvic abnormalities, and a careful history is taken regarding the type and duration of pain, its relationship to menstrual flow, and any associated symptoms. These questions not only provide information to the examiner but also serve to provide the girl with evidence that her problem is being taken seriously. An explanation of the physiology of menstruation helps to give reassurance.

Treatment consists of mild analgesics, with precautions to use them with discretion, and simple exercises similar to those recommended for relief of prenatal discomfort, such as pelvic rocking, assuming the knee-chest position, and breathing exercises. The girl is encouraged to practice good hygiene and participate in regular activities. Sometimes cyclic estrogen therapy to prevent ovulation provides dramatic and predictable relief from pain.

Premenstrual tension. Some adolescents will complain of associated symptoms such as headache, weight gain, irritability, depression, bloating, and breast congestion prior to their flow. These symptoms are grouped under the general term premenstrual tension. The cause is not agreed on but appears to be a result primarily of water and sodium retention as a result of progesterone production following ovulation. Characteristically these symptoms are relieved at the onset of the menstrual flow. Premenstrual tension does not seem to occur before ovulatory cycles begin and is not ordinarily a problem in adolescence.

Nursing considerations

The nurse is most frequently the person to whom a young girl turns for advice regarding menstrual problems. Usually all the youngster needs is reassurance about this normal function, but this also provides an opportunity for the nurse to listen to what the adolescent is saying and to engage in health teaching concerning menstrual physiology and hygiene and the importance of a well-balanced diet, exercise, and general health maintenance. It is a time to dispel any myths the girl may have in relation to menstruation and her femininity. When assessment indicates a potential problem and need for further evaluation, the girl is referred to a physician, health service, or clinic.

One of the most difficult experiences facing the adolescent girl is the gynecologic examination. Whether it is her first experience or not, she is most likely filled with apprehension. Almost all adolescents are extremely self-conscious about their bodies and the changes taking place. She will need continuing support in the form of anticipatory guidance regarding what she can expect and suggestions of what she can do to help herself relax during the procedure. It is essential for the nurse to remain with her during the examination to offer support and guidance.

ACCIDENTS

Accidents are the greatest single cause of death in the adolescent age-group and claim more lives than all other causes combined. The most vulnerable ages are the years 15 to 24, when accidents account for 61% of deaths in boys and 39% of deaths in girls. The tragedy of this is that the figures remain fairly constant from year to year and almost all fatal accidents are preventable. The most frequent causes of death are automobile accidents, drowning, falls, and accidents caused by firearms.

As in all age-groups, accidental injury is closely related to the developmental characteristics associated with normal growth and maturation. During adolescence, peak physical, sensory, and psychomotor function gives teenagers a feeling of strength and confidence that they have never experienced before and the physiologic changes of puberty give impetus to many basic instinctual forces. One manifestation of this is an increase in energy that simply must be discharged through action, often at the expense of logical thinking and other control mechanisms. Because of this need for action, adolescents are prone to act impulsively. Their propensity for risk-taking behavior plus a feeling of indestructibility make adolescents especially prone to accidents.[7]

The care and management of specific types of accidental injuries are discussed where appropriate throughout the book and will not be considered here. These include head injuries (p. 1421), spinal cord injuries (p. 1579), burns (p. 1112), near drowning (p. 1239), and fractures (p. 1558).

Motor-vehicle accidents

Almost half the accidents in the adolescent age-group are motor-vehicle accidents. The adolescent's newly acquired ability to drive and the normal developmental need for independence and freedom make the automobile an attractive, if not necessary, part of adolescents' life. They love to be propelled through space at a rapid pace. A significant number of fatal teenage accidents involved vehicles that are driven too fast for the existing conditions. Almost all are related to the actions of the driver and are disproportionately high among young drivers—often caused by ignorance of or disregard for sound, defensive driving principles. Most fatal accidents involving adolescent drivers occur because of improper driving or poor judgment on the part of the driver. These young people, delighted with the freedom that a driver's licence affords them, are less concerned about the new responsibilities associated with this freedom. They have yet to learn behavioral patterns that are gained with experience and maturity.

The recent upsurge in the use of drugs, including alcohol, by adolescents has further compounded the problem of motor-vehicle accidents involving youth. Overindulgence in alcohol is known to impair the ability of the best driver. The combination of inexperience, lack of defensive driving skills, and inexperience with drinking is a lethal one, and the unfortunate consequences are predictable.

Accidents are preventable, but, although the implications for prevention are obvious, the preventive measures are not always easy to implement, especially when behavioral characteristics such as poor impulse control, recklessness, and hostility are also operating.

The role that nurses can play in prevention of motor-vehicle accidents is to become active proponents of driver education and safety programs in the school and community that emphasize the use of good driving habits and judgment. They can encourage teenagers to obtain such instruction and encourage parents to determine the quality of this instruction and to take measures to improve the quality if it is found lacking.

Sports injuries

Adolescents probably spend more time and energy practicing and participating in sports activities than members of any other age-group. The practice of sports and games contributes significantly to growth and development, to the education process, and to better health. It provides exercise for growing muscles, interactions with peers, and a socially acceptable means to enjoy stimulation and conflict. In addition competitive activities help the teenager in the process of self-appraisal, development of self-respect, and concern for others.

Every sport has some potential for injury—whether one participates in serious competition or is actively engaged in the activity for pure enjoyment. Serious injury is not limited to the athlete who competes in rough contact sports. In fact, a large number of severe or fatal injuries occur to persons who are not physically prepared for the activity. For example, their body build may not be suited to the sport, their muscles and support systems (respiratory and cardiovascular) have not been sufficiently conditioned to withstand the rigors of the physical stress, or they do not possess insight and judgment to recognize when an activity is beyond their capabilities. Rapidly growing bones, muscles, joints, and tendons are especially vulnerable to unusual strain. The awkward and inexperienced youngster suffers more injury than the more skilled and experienced one, strong muscles are less easily damaged than weak ones and will provide better protection to the joints they cross, and fatigue significantly impairs muscle function and judgment. The increase in strength and vigor in adolescence may tempt youngsters to overextend themselves, especially boys who are egged on by teammates or are stimulated by the admiration of female observers.

Not only does the activity itself pose a hazard of greater or lesser degree, but the environment and the sports or recreational equipment provide additional risks. Adolescents participate in physical activity in a variety of environments, both indoors and outdoors, on floors, on the ground, on snow, on or beneath water surfaces, and sometimes in free air space. These activities frequently involve equipment that intensifies the risk factor. Some of the sports that contribute to adolescent accident injuries by their activity and equipment are those related to bicycles, football, basketball, baseball, snow skiing, hockey, trampoline jumping, and water activities such as swimming and fishing.

The range of injuries sustained in sports or recreational activities can involve any part of the body and extend from relatively minor cuts, bruises, and abrasions to totally incapacitating central nervous system injuries or death.

The role of health professionals in relation to sports injuries is directed toward prevention, treatment, and rehabilitation. Of these, the area of prevention is perhaps the most important. To this end, those youth who are actively involved in athletic programs need medical evaluation as a prerequisite to participation; education in sports skills with correct training and conditioning methods; omission of those tactics that are dangerous beyond the ordinary risk associated with the specific sport; use of appropriate protective equipment, properly maintained and suited to the individual; and an environment with maximal provision for safety and availability of first-aid and medical services. These same protective principles apply to noncompetitive sports enthusiasts. They need the same education in basic safety precautions, encouragement to acquire proper instruction in the skills required for performance of the activity (for example, instruction in water safety, skiing techniques, and so on), and proper maintenance of equipment.

Firearms

Injury and death from improper use of firearms continue to be one of the leading causes of accidental death in the adolescent age-group—most of which occur in or on home premises. The natural interest in gun-related activities is accelerated at this time, when almost half the victims of firearm fatalities are between the ages of 15 and 24 years. Instruction in the use of firearms should be taught at an appropriate age by parents and is probably best accomplished in cooperation with a youth organization or professional association. Most accidental injuries can be prevented when proper safety precautions are taken in the use and storage of firearms. For example, loaded guns should never be permitted in or around the home, and they must be stored where only appropriate adults have access to them.

Nursing considerations

Accident prevention is an ongoing part of nursing responsibility throughout the childhood years. Anticipatory guidance to parents regarding the expected problems and hazards related to growth and development does not end as the child nears maturity. However, at adolescence, health and safety education and guidance are more effective when the young people are involved directly. They can emphasize the importance of safety in the execution of activities and skills and the proper use of equipment. They can encourage the proper conditioning and preparation for sports, including rest, nutrition, and the activity that is best suited to the individual child's physical and emotional capabilities.

School nurses, in cooperation with other persons involved with youth, such as teachers, activity leaders, and parent groups, can help to evaluate sports and athletic programs, to assess environmental conditions, and to institute changes that emphasize prevention of injury. They can help to assess the needs for emergency services, to institute such services, and to provide care and guidance when needed.

ACNE

Adolescents are subject to the same skin conditions that affect the school-age child, such as bacterial, viral, and fungal infection, contact dermatitis, and drug reactions. However, there is one skin disorder that, although not limited to the adolescent age-group, appears predominantly at this time—*acne vulgaris*. The skin undergoes many alterations during a lifetime, but perhaps the most difficult period of adaptation occurs during adolescence, at which time the final transition to adult skin takes place. Acne is an almost universal occurrence during these years and involves anatomic, physiologic, biochemical, genetic, immunologic, and psychologic factors of significant import.

It is estimated that over 90% of all teenage boys and 80% of all teenage girls suffer from acne. The degree to which they are affected may range from nothing more than a few isolated comedones to a severe inflammatory reaction. The greatest incidence is in late adolescence, from about ages 16 to 20 years, after which it usually slackens off, but it may persist well into adulthood. Although the disease is self-limited and is not life threatening, its significance to the affected adolescent is great, and it is a mistake to underestimate the impact that it can have on young persons.

Etiology and pathophysiology

Acne is usually classified as a disorder of the sebaceous glands. However, there is no abnormality of the gland; rather, it is the glandular secretion, sebum, initiated by androgenic hormones, that is involved in the pathogenesis of this disease. The etiology of acne is still unclear, although a number of factors appear to be related to its development. Its distribution in families and a high degree of concordance in identical twins suggest that hereditary factors predispose to susceptibility to acne. Androgens are implicated since observations indicate a diminished effect on acne during pregnancy, its virtual absence in castrated males and young children, and its higher incidence in adolescent males. The disease seems to be aggravated by emotional stress, winter weather, some stimulant drugs, and the premenstrual period. There is no positive evidence that any specific foods are factors, except perhaps with individual youngsters. Corticosteroids administered systemically over a period of weeks may produce a form of acne with typical lesions that does not appear to be associated with sebaceous hyperplasia and that slowly subsides after the steroids are discontinued.

Pathophysiology. Acne is a disease that involves the pilosebaceous follicles (the hair follicle and sebaceous gland complex) of the face, neck, shoulders, back, and upper chest—the so-called "flush areas" of the skin. There are two basic types of lesions seen in acne: (1) *noninflamed* lesions called *comedones,* consisting of compact masses of keratin, lipids, fatty acids, and bacteria that dilate the follicular duct, which may be plugged (closed comedones, or whiteheads with no visible opening) or open (blackheads, with visible dilated openings that are discolored as fatty acids are oxidated by air), and (2) *inflamed* lesions that result when the follicular wall ruptures to produce papules, pustules, nodules, and cysts (Fig. 20-3). The inflammatory acne is responsible for the destructiveness and propensity for scarring.

The maturation of the sebaceous glands begins as an early pubertal occurrence, and the development of acne as adolescence progresses appears to be the result of a sequence of events. Under the influence of the accelerated androgen secretion from the adrenal glands and gonads, the gland in-

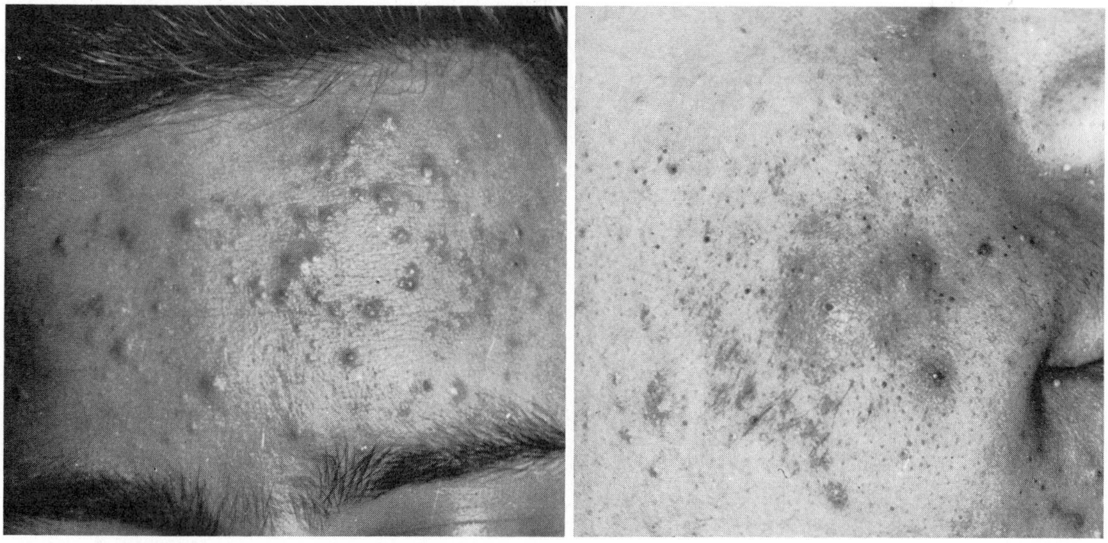

Fig. 20-3. Acne vulgaris. Papular pustules and comedones. (From Stewart, W. D., Danto, J. L., and Maddin, S.: Dermatology: diagnosis and treatment of cutaneous disorders, ed. 4, St. Louis, 1978, The C. V. Mosby Co.)

creases in size, secretory productivity, and turnover of the follicular epithelium. These changes are accompanied by an alteration in the follicular lining that allows the accumulation and stagnation of sebum and keratinized material derived from the lining cells. Normally the growing hair shaft prevents this accumulation by functioning as a "pipe cleaner" and moving the material out of the follicle. In acne the small, fine, vellus hairs occupying sebaceous follicles are unable to move the fixed material and the acne lesion develops. The noninflammatory comedones may resolve or become infected pustules. A normally harmless bacteria, *Corynebacterium acnes,* is attracted to the sebum, which it hydrolyzes into fatty acids. These fatty acids are the major tissue irritants in the sebum and initiate the inflammatory response. Inflammation is preceded by rupture of the distended follicles, which allows the follicular contents to leak into the dermis. The resultant damage causes a further wall-rupturing effect from leukocytes that invade the dermis. Those that become cystic are likely to form scars when they heal.

Secondary invasion by *Staphylococcus albus* can complicate the acne lesion, and adolescents' concern about their appearance tempts them to pick, finger, squeeze, and otherwise manipulate the lesions, which plays an important role in the perpetuation of acne. In addition to the precipitating factors mentioned previously, the application of creams, oils, and some cosmetics that add to the plugging of the follicles may aggravate acne; therefore, cosmetic agents should be selected to avoid those with greasy or occlusive bases. Also, it has been shown that iodides markedly increase the cellular phase of inflammation.

Exposure to oily substances, chlorinated hydrocarbons, and coal tar distillates profoundly exaggerate acne, which may influence the choice of occupation among adolescents. Exposure to excessive warmth and humidity may cause marked exacerbations in adolescents with more severe types of acne, which may necessitate discontinuing some active sports, such as football or wrestling, or employment in a hot, humid environment, such as working as a cook. Local increases in heat produced by occlusive clothing or mechanical irritation by wool and other rough textures may also produce exacerbations.

Medical management

There is little evidence that treatment shortens the duration of the entire course of the disease. However, much can be done to control acne, reduce the inflammatory process and scarring, and improve the appearance. All too often parents and health professionals have a tendency to dismiss acne as a normal part of "growing up." In addition there is no uniform treatment that can be applied to every case; therefore, in many instances, inadequate or inappropriate treatment may result in damaging consequences to the emotional health of the affected youngster.

Self-treatment is extremely common and associated with the many myths related to the cause and treatment of acne. Teenagers are subject to the influence of commercial advertising in many media concerning acne care and have ready access to a variety of over-the-counter preparations. Therefore, it is important that affected adolescents receive an explanation of the disease so that they have some knowledge of its causes and the rationale underlying the prescribed treatment. They need to understand the lengthy course of the disease so that they will not have unrealistic expectations and disappointments concerning the progress of therapy and will be more apt to comply with instructions for personal hygiene.

The management of acne is directed toward removal of the comedo, preventing its formation, controlling excessive sebaceous gland activity, controlling infection, and preventing scar formation. The treatment consists of some general measures of care and specific treatments largely determined by the type of lesions involved.

General measures. A general explanation of the disease process and the plan of care is given to the youngster with emphasis on his responsibility to faithfully carry out the program for as long as the process persists. It is also important to obtain the cooperation and understanding of the parents; therefore, they should be present at the initial discussion.

Improvement of the adolescent's overall health status is part of the general management. Adequate rest, moderate exercise, a well-balanced diet, reduction of emotional stress, elimination of any foci of infection, and correction of constipation (if it exists) are all part of general health promotion. There is no convincing evidence to implicate any single dietary item or combination of foods in the exacerbation of acne with the possible exception of iodides and bromide in therapeutic amounts. Occasionally a youngster will demonstrate an aggravation of symptoms after each ingestion of a given food. In such instances the food is eliminated for a period of time to assess its influence on the disease.

Dermatologists do not uniformly agree on the efficacy of various therapeutic agents and treatment modalities. For convenience the therapies are discussed in relation to the disease process in the two types of acne.

Treatment of noninflammatory acne. Noninflammatory acne is predominantly an obstructive disease characterized by open and closed comedones. Therefore, the treatment consists of the removal of these comedones and the prevention or reduction of the formation of new lesions. This is usually accomplished by surgical therapy and peeling agents. Recent findings indicate that zinc sulphate administered orally after meals has a controlling effect on acne. It appears to decrease the number of comedones in some adolescent patients. However, its efficacy is questioned by many dermatologists.

Expression of comedones. The nontraumatic removal of comedones serves two purposes. It reduces the risk of possible future inflammatory lesions and scarring and produces a prompt improvement in the youngster's appearance. Blackheads, with open communication with the skin surface, can be effectively expressed by direct pressure with a comedo extractor, a small metal scoop with a hole in the center. The hole is placed directly over the blackhead and pressure applied against the skin with a slight sliding movement across the skin. Removal of whiteheads, which do not have open communication with the skin surface, cannot be removed easily with the extractor alone. The epidermal covering of the whitehead must be gently and superficially nicked with a Bard-Parker No. 11 blade before extrusion with the comedo extractor.

Initially the procedures are carried out in the physician's office by the physician or nurse, but a parent or other family member often can be taught to use the extractor. The face should be washed with soap and water before and after extraction, and the instrument should be cleaned and cared for in the manner directed by the individual physician, which usually consists of cleaning it with soap and water and then either storing it in alcohol or wiping it with alcohol and storing in a clean receptacle such as a clean, dry envelope. The parent is cautioned against excessive pressure that might bruise the skin. The blackhead that cannot be removed readily should be left until another time. Some dermatologists limit home treatment to removal of blackheads only. Satisfactory results can be obtained by the removal of a limited number (five or ten) each day on a regular basis, thus avoiding any family friction. Although the comedones tend to recur in the same follicle, periodic removal properly carried out by this procedure will produce no scarring and will reduce the likelihood of follicular rupture and subsequent inflammation with possible scar formation.

Peeling agents. A number of therapeutic modalities appear to function in the same way, that is, to produce erythema and desquamation. The effectiveness of this treatment is probably the result of an increased rate of turnover of the superficial epithelium that lines the follicular duct, thereby preventing or reducing the compaction that produces the comedo. This helps to diminish the development of new lesions and contributes to the loosening of the comedo within the duct, which facilitates its mechanical removal or spontaneous shedding.

Peeling agents and modalities include: (1) cleansing agents; (2) astringents, (3) creams, lotions, gels, and so on, (4) Cryoslush therapy, (5) ultraviolet light, and (6) topical applications of vitamin A acid. Not all dermatologists subscribe to all of these methods, but the majority prescribe some form of peeling agent. Table 20-2 lists the most commonly used peeling modalities and some important aspects of each. Treatment may involve the use of a single agent or one or more of these in combination. When more than one modality is prescribed, they are usually added gradually since they tend to be additive in their effect and the goal is minimal, not gross, erythema and desquamation. Some dermatologists prescribe frequent shampooing as part of the regimen.

Treatment of inflammatory acne. The measures used for the management of noninflammatory acne are not of great value in treatment of inflammatory acne, except in the mildest forms. The modalities employed in therapy of the pustu-

Table 20-2. Peeling modalities used in acne therapy

Modality	Effect	Agent	Method of application	Comments
Cleansing agents	Redness and peeling	Ordinary soaps and detergents Medicated soaps (Actaveen, Acne-aid, Acne-Dome, Brasivol, Fostex Cake, Neutrogena, Pernox, and so on)	Wash affected areas in lukewarm water with prescribed cleansing agent, with or without washcloth; if washcloth is used, it should be used gently, not as an abrasive tool Lather thoroughly and gently into skin for approximately 1 minute, rinse with lukewarm water; repeat Dry gently	No arbitrary number of washings prescribed Frequency adjusted to individual Gross chapping should be avoided Ritualistic washing should be avoided Some areas of the face, such as the nose and forehead, may require more frequent washing than others, such as the cheeks
Astringents	Removal of surface film	Numerous preparations in liquid or saturated pads containing substances such as alcohol or acetone; Seba-nil (liquid) and Therapads (towelettes)	Use as skin cleansers	No evidence that they are effective in control of acne
Topical preparations	Peeling and drying Keratolytic Cosmetically acceptable covering agents	A variety of preparations available, tinted and colorless Active ingredients: sulfur, resorcinol, salicylic acid, and benzoyl peroxide, in various combinations May also contain alcohol, zinc oxide, and glycerin	Applied in lotions, creams, powders, and cakes	Persons with dry, fair skin respond more strongly to these preparations
	Increased epidermal turnover and desquamation	Retinoic or vitamin A acid (Retin-A)	Daily applications for 6 weeks, followed by intermittent applications as needed	Very effective but requires careful use Primarily useful in obstructive type of acne Greater sensitivity to sun and tendency to burn because of thinning of stratum corneum; may enhance cancer-causing effects of sun on skin; should avoid or minimize exposure of treated areas to sun
	Desquamation Reduces level of free fatty acids Bacteriostatic	Benzoyl peroxide (Benoxyl, Loroxide)	Apply daily or every other day Apply alternatively with retinoic acid	Very effective but requires careful use Should not be used in same application as retinoic acid
Cryoslush therapy	Freezes skin to produce erythema and desquamation	Carbon dioxide mixed with small amount of acetone to a slushlike consistency	Brushed lightly on skin with gauze held in a clamp Frequency of application and length of contact time between slush and skin determines the degree of injury and thus the redness and peeling	Initial applications should be a very few seconds until patient's skin reactivity is determined
Ultraviolet light	Redness and peeling	Natural—sunlight Artificial—hot or cold quartz lamp	Adequate protection to eyes—goggles or glasses Reliable means for timing exposure (not unusual for user to fall asleep under lamp) Exposure should be sufficient to produce mild to moderate erythema 24 hours after exposure Important to maintain same distance from lamp at each exposure	Home use should be confined to small, relatively weak floodlight-type screw-in bulb As tanning develops the dose may need to gradually increased to produce desired erythema and desquamation Acne often improves during summer months; may be associated with relaxed, vacation-like atmosphere in which sun exposure is likely to occur

lar and cystic forms include surgical techniques, chemotherapeutic agents (systemic and intralesional), and x-ray therapy.

Acne surgery. Minor surgery such as incision and drainage of cystic or pustular lesions is performed occasionally, although it is seldom necessary in any but the most severe suppurative cysts and nodules. The preferred methods in most cases are treatment with intralesional corticosteroids or prevention with systemic antibacterial therapy.

Chemotherapy. The most effective means for managing pustular and cystic lesions that may result in scarring is long-term administration of chemotherapeutic agents, particularly the broad-spectrum antibiotics, the safest of which appear to be the tetracyclines.[1] Corticosteroids have been valuable for short-term therapy in selected cases, and intralesional injections have proved helpful for the more severe nodular and cystic forms. Estrogen-progestin therapy in a cyclic routine, has produced good responses in carefully selected females. Table 20-3 outlines the various forms of chemotherapeutic agents used in treatment of inflammatory acne.

X-ray therapy. Ionizing radiation is rarely used since newer and more effective methods have been developed and is usually reserved for cases refractory to other forms of treatment. The inescapable hazards of the multiple biologic effects associated with its use make it undesirable. If it is employed, x-ray therapy requires a specialist highly skilled in its use.

Other. In some adolescents hygiene of the hair and scalp appears to be related to the clinical activity of acne. In these persons acne of the forehead can be improved by brushing the hair away from the forehead. Frequent shampooing seems to be beneficial in these cases. Also, there is often acne associated with seborrheic dermatitis (dandruff), but its control seems to have little influence on the course of acne.

Dermabrasion. Despite the best modes of therapy, it is not always possible to prevent the disfiguring scars that result from the more severe forms of the disease. With the passage of time much of the scarring is filled in, but the final result often leaves a great deal to be desired. In selected individuals a plastic corrective procedure sometimes provides some improvement in appearance. The procedure has decreased in popularity in recent years because of some untoward results, including hyperpigmentation at the margins of the treated areas and extreme resentment of psychologically unstable adolescents who had unrealistic expectations of improvement.

The procedure consists of abrading the skin with a high-speed rotating wire brush or steel abrasive wheel after the skin has been hardened and anesthetized with a refrigerant. Dermabrasion cannot be performed during the course of the disease and is usually not considered until late adolescence or adulthood. It should not be attempted by anyone but an experienced physician, usually a dermatologist or plastic surgeon. In addition the selection of patients is carried out very carefully from the viewpoint of the stage of the disease, the skin type, the character of the scarring, and, perhaps most importantly, the personality and stability of the individual. It is not recommended for young persons who are likely to react unfavorably to the procedure and to a result less desirable than anticipated.

Nursing considerations

As in many long-term problems of adolescence, nurses are involved in the assessment and therapy of the teenager with acne on a sustained basis. Often it is the nurse who established the initial contact with the affected adolescent and is instrumental in the youngster's seeking medical advice and embarking on a course of treatment. Teenagers do not always seek advice on their own; therefore, the nurse will need to ferret out their concerns about facial blemishes. During professional contact with an adolescent, such as a routine physical assessment or incidental visit for another problem, nurses can ask the youngster if he or she would like them to do something about "those few pimples (or 'zits')." It is not uncommon for troubled teenagers to deliberately seek advice on another matter in hopes that they may get the opportunity to discuss the skin condition without revealing the extent of their concern. To the adolescent even a minor facial blemish can assume monumental proportions. In addition adolescents may have unspoken concerns about the relationship of acne to sexual feelings, sexual intercourse or lack of it, masturbation, venereal disease, contagion, being unclean, and a myriad of myths that surround acne. Voluntary reassurance can do much to relieve these unspoken fears.[23]

The adolescent should be encouraged to seek medical treatment for the skin lesions from a sympathetic and understanding dermatologist; however, the extent of physician involvement varies. Simple over-the-counter acne remedies are available, and most adolescents do not see a physician, but they need education regarding the many factors associated with the disorder and a supportive, caring individual to help them maintain the persistence required to deal with the disorder over such an extended period of time. It is essential that the youngster with inflammatory lesions obtain medical treatment in order to control the process and reduce the incidence of scarring.

The adolescent needs education regarding the disease process and instruction in the prescribed therapy. Instruction should be definite and as specific as practical for each individual youngster. A written instruction sheet that describes the etiology and therapeutic regimen is often helpful, and parents should be cautioned against nagging. Adolescents should assume responsibility for following through on the instructions. They need to be cautioned against damaging the skin through too vigorous scrubbing and the im-

Table 20-3. Chemotherapeutic agents for treatment of inflammatory acne

Chemotherapeutic agent	Method of administration	Therapeutic action	Precautions and adverse reactions
Antibiotics			
Tetracycline	Orally Initial dose of 500 mg/day, then reduced as improvement occurs Maintained on small doses for many months	Appears to be excreted through sebaceous glands Reduces the normal follicular population of *Corynebacterium acnes,* thus preventing lipolysis of sebum and liberation of free fatty acids Appears to be most effective and safest antibiotic for long-term use	Inexpensive Relatively free from toxicity Allergic reactions rare Gastrointestinal irritation with nausea, vomiting, and superinfections with yeast (especially vaginal candidiasis) relatively uncommon May cause temporary or permanent discoloration of teeth in children younger than 12 years of age Contraindicated during pregnancy and in persons with renal disease Impaired absorption from gastrointestinal tract by food, iron supplements, milk, and aluminum hydroxide gels; should be taken on an empty stomach Outdated drug may cause severe toxicity
Erythromycin Clindamycin	Oral administration Topically as 2% lotion	Used in persons sensitive to tetracycline Topical administration effective in milder forms; not effective in severe forms	Intense photosensitivity from clindamycin
Hormones			
Corticosteroids	Intralesional injection	Antiinflammatory Causes rapid regression of nodules and cysts—reduces scarring Helpful in softening and flattening keloid scarring that occurs in some persons	Care must be taken to avoid intravascular injection May cause local and persistent atrophy of skin and adjacent tissues (pseudoatrophy, since process is spontaneously reversible after a time)
	Systemic oral administration (Prednisone)	Effective in reducing inflammatory component of severe nodulocystic acne Used for control of acute exacerbations not responsive to other therapy	May produce papulopustular follicular acneiform eruption Reserved for carefully selected patients
Estrogen-progestins	Cyclic oral administration	Suppresses sebum production	Acne may flare up in first few months Improvement usually not apparent until 3 to 5 months after treatment is begun May cause menstrual abnormalities Emboli and other adverse effects associated with its use

portance of using only those preparations and appliances (such as the ultraviolet light) prescribed for their particular needs and carrying out associated directions such as hairstyling and shampooing and, for girls, not leaving cosmetics on the face overnight should be emphasized. Nurses can help girls select proper cosmetic preparations. The nurse is often the person who teaches a family member in the use of a comedo extractor.

During conversations with teenagers, the nurse can dispel the common myths often associated with acne and allow them to discuss any feelings related to the disorder, such as self-consciousness and anxieties regarding relationships with others, and, sometimes, help them explore job or other after-school interests. The acne lesions need not become an excuse to avoid social contacts and activities after school.

INFECTIOUS MONONUCLEOSIS

Infectious monomucleosis is an acute, self-limiting infectious disease presumed to be of viral etiology that is most common among young persons between 12 and 25 years of age. The disease is characterized by an increase in the mononuclear elements of the blood and general symptoms of an infectious process. The course is usually mild but occasionally can be severe or, rarely, accompanied by serious complications.

Etiology and pathophysiology

Recent evidence implicates the herpes-like EB (Epstein-Barr) virus as the probable cause of infectious mononucleosis. It appears in both sporadic and epidemic forms, the sporadic cases being most common. The mechanism of spread has not been proved, although it is believed to be transmitted by direct intimate contact. It also appears to be only mildly contagious, and the period of communicability is unknown. The incubation period following exposure is 2 to 6 weeks. There is enlargement of lymph nodes from mononuclear infiltration and variable infiltration of most of the body tissues.

Diagnostic evaluation

The onset of symptoms appears anywhere from 10 days to as much as 6 weeks following exposure and may be acute or insidious.

Clinical manifestations. The common presenting symptoms of infectious mononucleosis vary greatly in type, severity, and duration. The characteristics of the disease are malaise, sore throat, and fever with generalized lymphadenopathy and splenomegaly that may persist for several months. Most often the symptoms appear insidiously with fatigue, lack of energy, and sore throat that may not become prominent. The youngster's chief complaint is often difficulty in maintaining his usual level of activity. This is often attributed to lack of sleep, an upper respiratory infection, or both. In many instances the manifestations never arouse enough concern to bring the affected individual to medical attention. Many cases of infectious mononucleosis are no doubt never recognized as such.

A skin rash is present in a few cases, most often a discrete macular eruption most prominent over the trunk. Other symptoms may include headache, epistaxis, and abdominal pain. The tonsils may be enlarged, reddened, and sometimes covered with a diphtheria-like membrane. Hepatic involvement to some degree is almost always present, often associated with jaundice, which may cause the disease to be confused with infectious hepatitis. The extensive mononuclear infiltration produces symptoms related to any body tissue so that the clinical picture can resemble that of many conditions, including neurologic manifestations and cardiac involvement.

Laboratory diagnosis. The diagnosis is established on the basis of clinical manifestations, absolute increase in atypical leukocytes in a peripheral blood smear, and a positive heterophil agglutination test. Differential diagnosis depends on the clinical symptoms present. For example, the pharyngitis may simulate symptoms of other diseases such as diphtheria and streptococcal pharyngitis. Lymphadenopathy, fever, and malaise are all characteristic of numerous disorders. Jaundice, nervous system manifestations, and skin eruptions are each similarly indicative of a variety of conditions.

The leukocyte count may be normal or low, but usually lymphocyte leukocytosis develops; of these, approximately 10% are atypical lymphocytes.

The heterophil antibody test determines the extent to which the patient's serum will agglutinate sheep red blood cells. In infectious mononucleosis, a titer of 1:160 is considered diagnostic, although a rising titer during the earlier stages is the best indicator.

The more recent "spot test" (Monospot), a slide test of high specificity, has been developed for the diagnosis of infectious mononucleosis. It is rapid, sensitive, inexpensive, easy to perform, and has the advantage that it can detect significant agglutinins at lower levels, thus enabling earlier diagnosis.

Patients may have a falsely positive complement fixation reaction for syphilis at about the second week, which usually becomes negative within 2 or 3 weeks.

Nursing considerations related to medical management

The course of infectious mononucleosis is self-limiting and usually uncomplicated. Contrary to popular belief, mononucleosis is not necessarily a difficult, prolonged, disabling disease, and the prognosis is generally good. Acute symptoms usually disappear within 7 to 10 days, and the persistent fatigue subsides within 2 to 4 weeks. A number of affected youngsters may need to restrict activities for 2 or 3 months; rarely the disease extends for longer periods.

There is no specific treatment for infectious mononucleosis. Common symptoms are ordinarily relieved by simple remedies. Aspirin is usually sufficient to relieve the bothersome symptoms of headache, fever, and malaise. Bed rest is encouraged for fatigue but is not imposed for any specified period of time. Affected youngsters are instructed to regulate activities according to their own tolerance, unless complicating factors are present. If the spleen is enlarged, for example, activities in which they might receive a blow to the abdomen or chest should be avoided.

A short course of oral penicillin is sometimes prescribed for sore throat, especially if β-hemolytic streptococci are present. Administration of ampicillin frequently precipitates a maculopapular rash in affected persons; therefore, its use is contraindicated. Sore throat can be relieved by gargles, hot drinks, analgesic troches, or aspirin. Some physicians favor the use of corticosteroids for suppression of high fever and/or severe sore throat but usually limit its use to the period of more intense symptoms or if the youngster is severely ill. Complications are uncommon but can be serious and require appropriate management. Liver involvement is present to some degree in almost all cases and may become chronic. Neurologic complications are seen in some outbreaks and vary in severity and outcome. Other complications include pneumonitis, myocarditis, hemolytic anemia, thrombocytopenia, and ruptured spleen. There is also some evidence to indicate a depressed cellular immune reactivity during the course of the disease and for some time afterward so that live vaccines are best avoided until several months following recovery.

Nursing responsibilities are directed toward comfort measures to relieve the symptoms and helping the affected youngster and his family determine appropriate activities according to the stage of the disease and his interests. They may need diet counseling to select foods that contain sufficient calories to meet growth and energy needs and yet are easy to swallow. Every effort should be made to prevent a secondary infection; therefore, the adolescent is counseled to limit exposure to persons outside the family, especially during the acute phase of illness.

The protracted nature of the illness and its associated weakness and fatigue frequently cause depression and resentment on the part of the usually vigorous, active teenager. It is important to spend time with the youngster to listen to his concerns and to allow him to express his feelings and vent his anger. The adolescent needs to be reassured that the limitations are only temporary and that social activities, so essential at this stage of development, can be resumed after the acute phase and that he will have sufficient autonomy to determine the extent of his capabilities and the rate of resumption of activities.

SYSTEMIC HYPERTENSION

Hypertension occurs in a variety of acute and chronic illnesses of childhood and adolescence. Secondary hypertension of a sustained nature accompanies renal, cardiovascular, adrenal, and some neurologic disorders as well as such miscellaneous conditions as lead and other poisoning and ingestion of excessive amounts of licorice. Until recently, primary hypertension has been considered to be a disease of middle-aged or older persons. However, in recent years there has been increasing interest in this disorder as it occurs in adolescents and children. Routine blood pressure measurements of children in the pediatric age-group have detected hypertension similar to essential hypertension in adults with surprising frequency in asymptomatic children, especially teenagers. A conservative estimate suggests at least a 1% to 2% incidence of sustained hypertension in the age-groups under 20 years. The prevalence of the condition in adolescents is difficult to evaluate since no firm criteria have been established to determine what constitutes hypertension in the pediatric age-groups or which of the three blood pressure levels (supine, sitting, or standing) provides the most significant prognostic information. However, evidence is accumulating to indicate that the essential hypertension of adulthood may have its origin in childhood; therefore, its early detection has significance for prevention and treatment.

Definitions

hypertension blood pressure elevated above that considered to be normal.

primary, essential, or **idiopathic hypertension** hypertension that develops without apparent cause.

benign hypertension hypertension that develops slowly over a period of time. It may progress to the same conclusion as malignant hypertension but at a slower rate.

malignant hypertension hypertension that develops and progresses rapidly, often to a fatal conclusion if untreated.

Blood pressure levels vary widely within a normal range in children of the same age and in the same child on any given day. In addition, the pressures are subject to false readings because of the stress associated with the examination, use of improper size blood pressure cuffs, or mechanical factors. Most of the confusion regarding hypertension is related to a cutoff point to differentiate normal from abnormal blood pressure in children, especially in borderline cases. It is generally agreed, however, that any child or adolescent who has a diastolic blood pressure repeatedly in the range of 90 to 95 mm Hg in the supine position should be considered hypertensive. Recent studies suggest that children or teenagers whose systolic and/or diastolic pressures are repeatedly in the ninetieth percentile for age or occasionally above the ninetieth percentile constitute a borderline group who are probably at high risk to develop hypertension at a later age. This takes into account the age and sex factors, since blood pressure measurements rise steadily with age; thus a blood pressure reading of 140/90 mm Hg, which is considered to be the upper limit of normal in adults, would be clearly abnormal in the pediatric age-group.[18,20]

Etiology

The causes of primary hypertension are undetermined, but there is evidence to indicate that both genetic and environmental factors play a role. Hypertension has been shown to be increased in parents whose children are considered to be hypertensive. American blacks have a higher incidence of hypertension that whites, and in these persons it develops earlier, is frequently more severe, and results in mortality at an earlier age. In fact, hypertension among American blacks is more prevalent and more fatal than sickle cell disease. In such susceptible persons emotional and mental stresses, excessive salt ingestion (often associated with "soul foods"), and obesity are significant environmental factors.

Diagnostic evaluation

It is clear from the increasing numbers of hypertensive or potentially hypertensive children and adolescents being identified that a blood pressure determination should be a routine part of a child assessment in children over 3 years of age. The blood pressure of a child at *any* age should be measured if they are diagnosed or suspected of (1) coarctation of the aorta, (2) unexplained heart failure, (3) unexplained heart murmurs, (4) unexplained seizures or other neurologic signs, (5) an abdominal mass or masses, (6) edema, ascites, and/or evidence of renal failure, (7) hypernatremia, (8) failure to thrive, (9) raised intracranial pressure, (10) tumors of the orbit, or (11) respiratory distress. Black teenagers of both sexes are at greater risk to develop primary hypertension than the teenage population as a whole. White male adolescents are more likely to be hypertensive than white females, in whom elevated blood pressure is more often secondary than primary. The conditions associated with secondary hypertension in children and adolescents are listed in the boxed material.

Conditions associated with secondary hypertension in children and adolescents

- Renal disorders
  - Congenital malformations
    - Polycystic kidney, ectopic kidney, horseshoe kidney, and so on
    - Obstructive anomalies
    - Hydronephrosis
  - Renal tumor
    - Wilms' tumor
  - Acquired disorders
    - Glomerulonephritis—acute or chronic
    - Pyelonephritis
    - Nephritis associated with collagen disease
- Metabolic and endocrine diseases
  - Adrenal tumors
    - Adenoma
    - Pheochromocytoma
    - Neuroblastoma
  - Cushing's syndrome
  - Adrenogenital syndrome
  - Hyperthyroidism
  - Aldosteronism
  - Hypercalcemia
  - Diabetes mellitus
- Cardiovascular disease
  - Coarctation of the aorta
  - Abnormalities of the renal arteries
  - Renal vein thrombosis
- Neurologic disorders
  - Space-occupying lesions of the cranium
    - Tumors, cysts, hematoma
    - Cerebral edema
    - Encephalitis (including Guillain-Barré and Reye's syndromes)
- Iatrogenic causes
  - Administration of corticosteroids (including oral contraceptives)
  - Administration of pressor agents
  - Following genitourinary surgery
  - Intravascular overload (blood fluid)
- Miscellaneous causes
  - Toxemia of pregnancy
  - Poisoning
    - Lead
    - Mercury
  - Amphetamine overdosage

Although clinical manifestations associated with hypertension depend largely on the underlying cause, there are some observarions that can provide clues to the examiner that an elevated blood pressure may be a factor. Adolescents and older children with hypertension complain of frequent headaches, dizziness, and/or changes in vision. In infants or young children who cannot communicate symptoms, observation of behavior provides clues, although gross behavioral changes may not be apparent until complications are present. Parents of infants and small children who have been treated for hypertension report that their child had previously been irritable, often indulged in an abnormal degree of head banging or rubbing, and may have wakened screaming in the night (when blood pressure tends to be highest).

To obtain an accurate reading, care should be taken to quiet the child or relax the adolescent while the measurement is recorded to avoid false readings caused by excitement. The chief cause of falsely elevated blood pressure readings is the use of improperly fitting, narrow cuffs. Sphygmomanometer cuffs must be selected according to the individual's build and weight (see p. 116 for selection of blood pressure cuff and method of measurement). Measurements on obese adolescents may require the use of specially designed cuffs that are longer and wider than an average

Table 20-4. Drugs most frequently used in treatment of hypertension in children and adolescents

Drug	Mode of action	Average oral dosage and administration	Side effects
Reserpine (variety of trade names, including Serpasil, Sandril, Serfin, Reserpoid, Rau-Sed)	Acts on sympathetic nervous system Reduces norepinephrine levels in sympathetic nerves by altering ability of nerve cells to bind norepinephrine, which inhibits stimulation of vascular smooth muscle	Initial dose—children less than 25 kg: 0.2-0.5 mg/day in one to two doses; children more than 25 kg: 0.25-0.5 mg/day in one to two doses	Flushing (parenteral administration), drowsiness, irritability, depression, nasal stuffiness, bradycardia, weight gain, and diarrhea Occasionally parkinsonian state, tremors, dryness of mouth, itching, and skin eruptions
Hydralazine (Apresoline)	Acts on vascular smooth muscle Thought to produce its effect by direct action on the blood vessels to cause arterial vasodilatation	0.75 mg/kg/day in four to six doses	Tachycardia, headache, anorexia, nausea, vomiting, flushing, and symptoms of rheumatic arthritis or lupus erythematosis Occasionally severe depression or other psychic symptoms and peripheral neuropathy
Methyldopa (Aldomet)	Acts on vascular smooth muscle Reduces blood pressure by lowering peripheral vascular resistance; also lowers norepinephrine levels; sodium and water retention may occur if a diuretic is not given with the drug	10 mg/kg/day in three to four doses	Drowsiness, irritability, emotional lability, bradycardia, dry mouth, and gastrointestinal symptoms such as abdominal distention, flatus, and diarrhea Occasionally fever, abnormal liver function tests, and paradoxical pressor effect
Guanethidine (Ismelin)	Acts on sympathetic nervous system Causes release and subsequent depletion of norepinephrine from adrenergic nerve endings to produce dilatation of both arterial and venous vessels; sodium and water retention if not given with a diuretic	0.2 mg/kg/day in a single dose	Postural hypotension, postexercise syncope, diarrhea, bradycardia, fatigue, nausea, nasal stuffiness, weight gain, and impotence and failure of ejaculation

adult cuff, or sometimes an adult thigh cuff is needed.

Detection of elevated blood pressure calls for a full diagnostic evaluation to determine the etiology. When there is a strongly positive family history of hypertension, and in the absence of other signs or symptoms, the youngster with borderline readings is not usually submitted to an intensive barrage of diagnostic tests. The blood pressure is monitored for a period of time to rule out possible transient hypertension, after which the tests are more likely limited to renal function tests and intravenous pyelography. In adolescents with more severe hypertension, a full diagnostic evaluation is indicated.

Medical management

Therapy for secondary hypertension involves diagnosis and treatment of the underlying cause. In those cases amenable to surgical repair, the nature of the condition, the type of surgery, and the age of the child are all essential considerations. For example, vascular repair in a child with renovascular hypertension is usually delayed when possible to allow for sufficient growth of both the child and his blood vessels. Most surgeons prefer that the child be kept on a medical regimen until he weighs at least 18 kg (40 pounds). On the other hand, coarctation of the aorta is frequently repaired at an early age to avoid prolonged preoperative hypertension and its associated sequelae (see p. 1318). Pheochromocytoma, a rare benign tumor of the hypertensive catecholamines (norepinephrine and epinephrine), is usually removed as soon as a diagnosis is confirmed.

Children or adolescents who have consistently elevated blood pressure readings with no known etiology or those in whom secondary hypertension is not amenable to surgical correction are placed on hypotensive drug therapy. Antihypertensive drugs most frequently prescribed for adolescents and children are listed in Table 20-4. The drug is tailored to meet the needs of individual children and is determined by the hypotensive effect produced and the appearance of any side effects. The aim is to achieve a normotensive state throughout the day without any accompanying side effects. The drug regimen is kept simple, preferably with a single antihypertensive agent in combination with a suitable diuretic. If the teenager is unreliable in taking a drug pharmocologically best suited to his particular form of hypertension several times a day, the physician may prescribe a less optimal drug that can be taken only once a day if it produces an adequate lowering of the pressure. Also, a drug such as guanethidine that has a tendency to cause post-exercise syncope is not advised for the athletic youngster. The choice of agent may need to be changed if it is found to produce depression, for example, reserpine. Although it is definitely established that therapy should begin immediately in persons definitely diagnosed as hypertensive, it is less clear in borderline cases.

Since there is a close association between overweight and subsequent weight gain in persons with hypertension, a weight-reduction program is recommended for overweight youngsters. It has also been confirmed that high-salt intake increases the risk of hypertension in genetically predisposed persons and aggravates existing hypertension unless salt intake is limited. This is not uniformly seen in children, however.

The role of exercise in hypertension has not been fully evaluated, and at the present time there is no good evidence to indicate that hypotensive children should be restricted in their activities. However, it is well known that blood pressure rises to high levels in hypertensive adults after exercise, and some preliminary evidence indicates that this also occurs in adolescents; however the ultimate effects have not been adequately evaluated. Until more substantial evidence is available, restriction of physical exercise in the teenager is kept to a minimum to avoid psychologic trauma, except in specific circumstances. Adolescents who are on drugs that might produce dizziness or syncope are cautioned not to engage in physical activities in which these symptoms could be a hazard during exertion.

Nursing considerations

The nurse is a valuable link in the health-care delivery system in relation to hypertension in the pediatric age-group. Active in detection, diagnosis, and therapy in any setting—hospital, school, clinic, private office, public health services, and private practice—nurses are frequently the persons who operate screening and follow-up units and are usually the primary contact between health services and the child and his family.

A blood pressure measurement should always be a part of the routine assessment of infants and children. In carrying out the procedure it is most important to make certain that the cuff used is suited to the individual child and that any questionable reading is repeated, using different instruments if doubtful. When an elevated pressure is detected the procedure should be carried out in the standing, sitting, and supine positions and comparison readings made between both upper extremities to ascertain if they are equal.

Nursing counseling and guidance of the hypertensive teenager pose a number of problems. In the hospital situation diet and medication regimens can be carefully regulated. Home management necessitates motivating youngsters in the adolescent age-group and their parents to cooperate in carrying out a treatment plan. The major problem in hypertensive adolescents is compliance in relation to maintaining contact with the physician or clinic for follow-up care, taking antihypertensive drugs as prescribed, and allowing home blood pressures to be taken. An important aspect of nursing care is to convince these youngsters that their disorder is probably a lifelong concern and that management must include drug therapy, perhaps some modification in diet and activity, and regular follow-up care.[19]

Home blood pressure measurements greatly facilitate surveillance in youngsters with chronic hypertension. Someone in the hypertensive child's family, such as a parent, sibling, or other responsible person, must be assisted in securing proper equipment and instructed in its use. He or she needs to know about fluctuations in readings that can be expected in relation to the time of day, posture (sitting, lying, or standing), activity, and stress. He or she needs to be told at what levels to seek advice. The nurse can help this person set up a system for recording the measurements, usually using a graphic record.

The drug therapy program, including the need for taking the drug, how the drug works and its duration of action, any side effects that may be expected, and what to do if such effects are experienced, must be explained to the youngster and his family. It is important to impress on the youngster the importance of taking the drug continuously as prescribed and the fact that it is effective only during the time it is taken regularly. The adolescent who has no symptoms and feels no ill effects may discontinue taking the medication, having his blood pressure checked, or visiting the office or clinic for checkups. For these youngsters nursing follow-up and guidance are extremely important. Young hypertensive women should avoid the use of oral contraceptives because of their pressor effects, which may have broader implications in relation to compliance to a regimen, that is, in regard to the sexually active teenager.

Unfortunately not all adolescents and their families are able to accept the responsibility and the stress of continuous management. In such cases the school nurse may need to assume the responsibility for taking blood pressure measurements regularly or making arrangements for another individual to do so. It is simple to stress the importance of weight control or reduction and suggest restricting salt intake to teenagers, but it is another matter to see that they follow through on these instructions. The family may be reluctant to impose necessary modifications to the usual family diet, and the youngster who enjoys food-related activities with friends is less likely to comply. Both the teenager and the mother will need guidance in the preparation and selection of palatable, low-salt foods. For example, the adolescent can select unsalted peanuts or popcorn instead of the salted variety and substitute unsalted French fries for potato chips.

The learning needs vary greatly among affected adolescents. Some require a great deal of support, education, and guidance; others need only education and periodic follow-up. Scolding the noncompliant adolescent is useless and may serve only to alienate him from the nurse and continued health care. Exploring with him the reasons for difficulty in following the prescribed regimen will assist both nurse and teenager in problem solving. Continued reinforcement for positive behavior is a major nursing responsibility, and a good nurse-patient relationship is essential to the continued compliance. The adolescent needs education and guidance as well as support and reassurance.

Sexually active adolescents

The biologic maturity that results from the pubertal changes and the emotional responses that accompany these changes provide the impetus for sexual experimentation and expression. The increase in numbers of teenagers, their earlier maturation, plus a more mobile, permissive, and contraceptive-conscious society allow more adolescents the opportunity to become sexually active at an increasingly younger age. Sexual involvement has attendant problems; consequently health professionals are seeing more and more health problems related to adolescent sexuality. Those of major importance are sexually acquired diseases and teenage pregnancies.

SEXUALLY TRANSMITTED DISEASES

Traditionally known as venereal diseases (a term derived from Venus, the goddess of love), newer terminology designates them as sexually transmitted diseases (STD). They are among the most prevalent and dangerous of the communicable diseases and are now epidemic in the United States, with a disproportionate number occurring in adolescents and young adults. Of the reportable diseases, gonorrhea ranks first and syphilis fourth in numbers of cases with an alarming increase in the adolescent age-group (Fig. 20-4). Although they constitute only about 20% of the total population in the United States, adolescents experience one of the highest attack rates for sexually transmitted diseases. Even with the large number of cases that are reported, this is considered to be a conservative estimate of the true incidence because of underreporting of cases and failure to diagnose all cases as they occur. Sexually active adolescents are particularly at risk because they are often late in seeking medical attention. Traditional sexually transmitted diseases and those that are now also designated as such in the adolescent age-group are listed in the box on p. 732. It is important that when a patient has one of these conditions, the history and examination should encompass the others. The more serious diseases, gonorrhea and syphilis, are discussed further.

Gonorrhea

The most common of the traditional sexually transmitted diseases is gonorrhea, also known by such common names

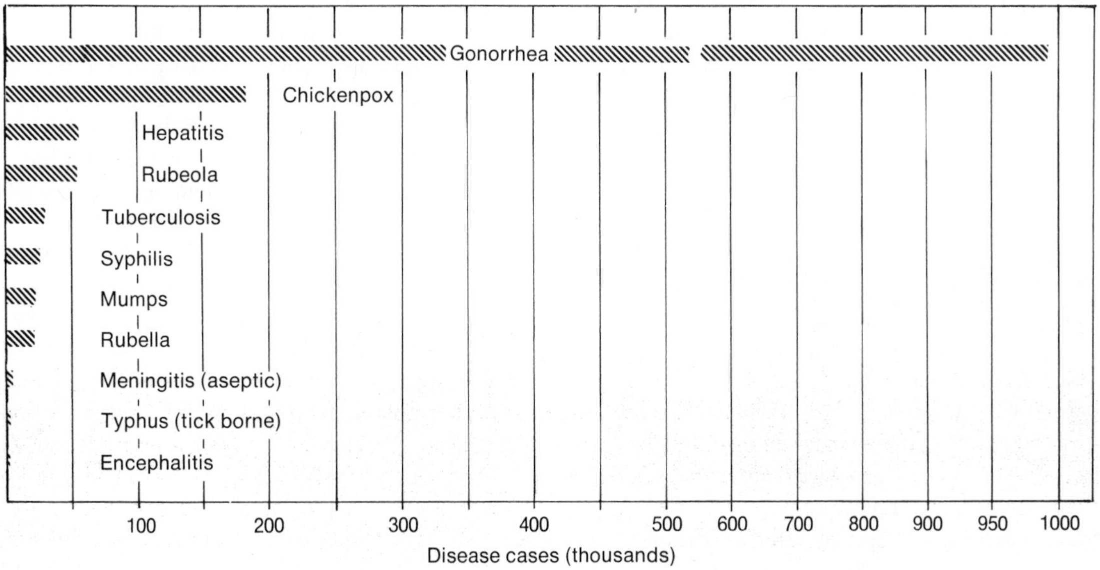

Fig. 20-4. Communicable diseases. Number of reported cases, United States, calendar year, 1977. (Data from Center for Disease Control: Morbidity and Mortality Weekly Report **27**(1):10, January 6, 1978.)

as the whites, clap, the drips, and the dose. It is a disease that primarily occurs in larger metropolitan areas where the rate of infection is higher than in more rural areas. There are three times as many males affected as females, and it is more prevalent in nonwhite than in white populations. The highest incidence is in young adults aged 20 to 24 years, but adolescents 15 to 19 years of age are the next group most frequently affected.

Gonorrhea is a disease that appears to be everywhere, and an attack confers no immunity to subsequent reinfections. In fact, subsequent infections are often caused by the same untreated partner, and a potentially vicious cycle is created until the infected partner is identified and treated. Gonorrhea is almost always sexually contracted, except when it appears as conjunctivitis. Other manifestations such as pharyngitis and proctitis reflect variant modes of sexual contact.

Etiology and pathophysiology. The causative organism is *Neisseria gonorrhoeae,* a gram-positive diplococcus. The organisms, commonly known as gonococci, have been divided into four types; types 1 and 2 are pathogenic, and types 3 and 4 are considered nonpathogenic. The difference in pathogenicity appears to be the presence of hairlike projections on types 1 and 2 that cause them to adhere to the mucosa where they remain attached for 36 to 48 hours, the incubation period of the organism. The organisms have very specific survival requirements. They prefer a moist, alkaline environment (pH, 7.2 to 7.6) and a temperature of 35 to 36° C (95 to 96.8° F). They quickly die on drying, exposure to the weakest acids, and an increase or decrease of 3° C in temperature. The gonococcus organism survives only on the columnar and transitional epithelium of man; stratified epithelium is resistant to its onslaught. The organisms spread along the mucosa from the point of entry. They penetrate between the epithelial cells and, when they die, liberate an irritant that produces the inflammatory response characterized by localized capillary dilatation, edema, and leukocytosis. This process accounts for the purulent discharge and erosive balanitis and cervicitis observed in affected persons.

Clinical manifestations. Symptoms can appear as early as 1 day or as late as 2 weeks after sexual contact. Gonococcal infection can occur in many diverse ways with four basic presentations: asymptomatic, uncomplicated symptomatic, complicated symptomatic, and disseminated disease. Table 20-5 illustrates the diverse manifestations of these four clinical forms as they are seen in males and females. The pelvic inflammatory disease (PID) in females simulates the inflammatory process caused by other bacterial infections, and differential diagnosis is made for more definitive medical treatment. Since a large percentage of affected persons are asymptomatic, gonorrhea should be considered in the evaluation of all sexually active adolescents. Lack of clinical symptoms is especially true of the rectal and pharyngeal infections.[17]

There is a difference in the way the disease affects children. Whereas uncomplicated urogenital infection in postpubescent girls involves the cervix, in prepubescent girls it is seen as vulvovaginitis. Early complaints of vulvovaginitis include dysuria and perineal or vulvar discomfort, often associated with perianal soreness that is increased during defecation. Examination reveals edematous vaginal mucosa, and a greenish-yellow discharge may be present; the perianal area often appears inflamed and edematous with some discharge from anal crypts.

Sexually transmitted diseases

Traditional	*Newer inclusions*
Syphilis	Scabies
Gonorrhea	Pediculosis
Chancroid	Herpes progenitalis
Lymphogranuloma venereum	Condyloma acuminata (genital warts)
	Hemophilus vaginalis
Granuloma inguinale	*Trichomonas* infestation
	Cytomegalovirus
	Monilial vaginitis
	Molluscum contagiosum of the genitalia
	Nongonococcal urethritis

Diagnosis. The diagnosis is established on identification of the organism from direct smear or culture techniques. In males the diagnosis is relatively easy. Since gram-negative diplococci are not normally present in the male genitourinary tract, their intracellular presence in smears is diagnostic. A false-negative result may be seen in the very early course of the disease, in old, untreated cases, and in persons who have taken penicillin or a wide-spectrum antibiotic within a few hours of the examination.

The diagnosis is more difficult in females, which has been a significant obstacle in effective control programs. Although cervical and urethral smears are fairly reliable in the acute phase of the disease, with less acute or asymptomatic cases there is a high yield of both false-positive and false-negative results. Specimens of pus from the urethra or cervix (not the vagina) should be cultured immediately on special media (Thayer-Martin VCN or Transglow) designed for these discriminating organisms. Because of their adverse effects on organisms, surgical jelly or any fatty substance (including some types of swabs) should not be used in securing the specimen. Presence of menses is not a contraindication. Actually the menstrual secretions provide an optimum environment for growth of the organism.

Recently blood tests for gonorrhea have become available that are proving effective for screening females and can be performed in a physician's office or clinic in 2 minutes.

Medical management. Effective treatment of both males and females with uncomplicated gonorrhea is administration of penicillin (preferably) or other antibiotic therapy (Table 20-6). Most desirable is an effective single-dose ap-

Table 20-5. Clinical forms of gonococcal infections

Type	Male		Female	
	Infection	**Observations**	**Infection**	**Observations**
Asymptomatic	Urethral, rectal, pharyngeal	Asymptomatic in up to 68% of affected males	Cervical, rectal, pharyngeal	Asymptomatic in up to 80% of affected females
Uncomplicated	Urethritis	Symptoms: dysuria with associated profuse yellow discharge, frequency, urgency, and nocturia	Cervicitis	Usually limited to cervix in postpubertal females; vagina not involved
	Proctitis	Always result of homosexual contact		May be associated with purulent cervical discharge, dysuria, and dyspareunia
			Proctitis	From genitorectal exposure or spread from vaginal discharge
			Bartholin's abcess	Caused by inflammatory process with edema and obstruction of duct
	Pharyngitis	Erythema and edema of pharynx with or without superficial erosion		
	Ophthalmitis	Acute and severe purulent conjunctivitis Usually spread from genitals to eyes by hands or (rarely) fomites, such as a damp towel		
Complicated	Direct spread through genital tract		Direct spread through genital tract	
	Prostatitis	Fever Urinary symptoms associated with pain in suprapubic or inguinal regions; same with seminal vesicle involvement	Endometritis	Sometimes confused with menstrual cramps Shed with menses
			Salpingitis	May appear acutely ill with fever, chills, and abdominal pain Bilateral adnexal pain on examination and pain on gentle movement of cervix
	Epididymitis	Pain and swelling of scrotum		
			Peritonitis, perihepatitis	Pain and other symptoms associated with infection of these areas
Disseminated	Arthritis	Occurs in approximately 3% of untreated patients May be accompanied by tenosynovitis, especially in wrists and dorsa of hands Two types: (1) painful, swollen joint(s) from pressure of purulent exudate in synovial capsule; aspirated fluid contains diplococci; causes rapid destruction of articular cartilage and underlying bone; usually accompanied by other symptoms of gonorrheal infection; (2) painful joint(s) with little or no swelling or heat; aspirated fluid culture negative for diplococci		
	Dermatitis	Visible as vestibular and pustular eruptions on extremities followed by petechial and purpuric eruptions (similar to meningococcemia)		
	Endocarditis, meningitis	Rarely seen but may occur when gonococci invade bloodstream		

Table 20-6. Antibiotic therapy in gonorrhea

Drug	Dosage		Method	Administration
	Adolescents	**Children**		
Procaine penicillin G	4.8 million U	75,000 U/kg	IM	Administered at two sites during single visit
Probenecid	1 g	25 mg/kg	PO	Administered simultaneously or 20-30 minutes prior to IM penicillin as initial dose to delay excretion of penicillin by kidneys
	500 mg	10 mg/kg	PO	Given every 6 hours for 24 hours
Ampicillin	3.5 g	100 mg/kg	PO	Single dose preceded 30 minutes earlier by probenecid
Amoxicillin	Same as ampicillin		PO	Can be given without probenecid
Spectinomycin dihydrochloride (Trobicin)	2 g	—	IM	For patients allergic to penicillin Single-dose drug, therefore useful only in treatment of uncomplicated disease Not used in children who weigh less than 50 kg (110 pounds)
Tetracycline	1.5 g 500 mg	25 mg/kg 10-15 mg/kg	PO	Initial dose Given 4 times per day for total dosage of 9.5 g (adolescents) Given every 6 hours for 5 days (children)

proach in order to avoid problems of follow-up and patient cooperation. Adequate penicillin therapy achieves a 95% success rate in acute genital gonorrhea, but follow-up is essential since an acute infection may convert to the asymptomatic carrier state and the incidence of reinfection is high. Relief of symptoms cannot be equated with cure. All affected youngsters should have a serologic test for syphilis, and all their sexual contacts should be traced and treated.

Complicated and disseminated infections may require longer antibiotic therapy, and complications are treated appropriately. In all cases of gonorrhea the long-term genitourinary problems in the male and possible occlusion of the fallopian tubes or tubo-ovarian abscesses in the female from untreated or repeated infections can lead to severe debilitation in later life or even death. Therefore, case finding and early treatment are imperative.

Preventive aspects. A genuine prophylaxis against gonorrheal infections is not yet available. There is a protective vaccine in the process of development, but when it becomes available the decision must be made concerning who should be vaccinated and when they should be vaccinated. Until such time as such protection is in common use, preventive efforts must be directed toward finding and treating affected persons, locating and examining contacts of affected persons, educating young people regarding the facts of the disease and its spread, and encouraging the use of barriers in sexually active young people.

The increasing incidence of gonorrhea in young people is influenced to a great extent by the larger numbers of teenagers who engage in sexual activity more casually, at younger ages, and with more partners. In addition the changing pattern of contraceptive use is a contributing factor to more promiscuous sexual activity and the concomitant rise in gonorrhea. The newer contraceptive methods, oral contraceptive and intrauterine devices, appear to provide no protection against sexually transmitted diseases, and barrier devices, such as the condom, that offer some protection are not well accepted by teenagers. Unfortunately many girls who take oral contraceptive pills mistakenly believe that they are also effective in preventing sexually transmitted diseases. Actually evidence indicates that the pill alters the vaginal pH sufficiently to facilitate growth of the gonococcal organisms. Since the gonococcus is a very fragile organism, any device that interferes with its environmental needs and nutrition will help eradicate the organism and prevent its becoming established in the genital tract. To decrease the likelihood of infection, sexually active youngsters should be encouraged to use a mechanical barrier (condom) and/or some substance that alters the environment. Vaginal sprays, lubricants, or douches that lower the vaginal pH are fairly effective, for example, a vinegar douche *soon* after intercourse. Interest has been generated regarding copper-coated intrauterine devices that seem to have an adverse effect on the gonococcus. Copper that leeches out over a period of time appears to be sufficient to eradicate the organism.

Essential measures for control of the disease are treating the disease, reporting it *promptly,* and tracing and treating contacts. The obstacle of the youngster's fear of parental wrath or shame has been overcome in most areas by permitting physicians to treat affected minors without requiring the consent of the parent. In many areas medical clinics and practitioners specializing in members of this age-group have gained the trust of the adolescent, who may readily seek their services in such an emergency. However, there is a dirty connotation to sexually transmitted diseases, which must be overcome before many teenagers will cooperate. Most teenagers have intercourse with someone they are fond of, and they do not like to think of the partner with this implication. Even when youngsters trust the health workers, they may hesitate being seen entering a venereal disease clinic.

Syphilis

Less a health hazard in adolescence than gonorrhea, syphilis is nevertheless a serious disease with destructive long-term consequences in untreated cases. The disease constitutes only 0.5% of all sexually transmitted diseases in the adolescent age-group. About forty cases of gonorrhea occur to one case of syphilis. The incidence of syphilis is higher in males than in females (2.5 to 1), and the largest number of reported cases (about 70%) are in the nonwhite population.

Etiology. The causative organism in syphilis is *Treponema pallidum,* a fragile spirochete found naturally only in the tissues of infected humans. Viability outside the body is short. The organism is rapidly killed by oxygen, soap, common bacterial agents, and drying. The disease is spread by sexual exposure, kissing (moist kissing, not dry "pecks"), prenatal transmission from infected mother to unborn child, and (rarely) needle punctures, significant breaks in the skin, and blood transfusions. About 95% is transmitted sexually, and the affected person is most infectious during the first year of the disease, after which the communicability diminishes.

Clinical manifestations. Syphilis appears in the following stages: the primary stage, characterized by a chancre; a secondary stage, characterized by systemic symptoms and a generalized rash; a latent stage, with no clinical signs or symptoms; and a later stage, a destructive stage that can involve one or more body systems.

Primary syphilis. Following an incubation period of approximately 3 weeks, a characteristic lesion, the hard chancre, appears at the point of inoculation, usually the penis, vulva, or cervix. Extragenital chancres may occur on other areas of the body. The chancre is a hard, painless, red, sharply defined lesion with an indurated base, raised border, eroded surface, and scanty yellow serous discharge.

Secondary syphilis. The second stage frequently, but not invariably, develops 1 to 3 months (average, 3 weeks) after spontaneous healing of the primary lesion. It is characterized by a variety of signs and symptoms that may be grouped into three syndromes: (1) influenza-like symptoms of headache, lacrimation, nasal discharge, sore throat, and generalized arthralgia with a slight temperature elevation and loss of weight; (2) generalized lymphadenopathy, in which the lymph nodes are enlarged and have a hard, rubbery feeling but are not usually painful; and (3) a generalized skin eruption that may mimic a variety of skin diseases. This eruption involves skin and mucous membranes and, except for the follicular type, is painless and nonpruritic. The lesions are discrete, sharply demarcated, and coppery-colored, with the color intensifying toward the center. There may be hard, indurated papules on the soles and palms. The distribution is bilateral, symmetric, and tends to be more profuse on the upper extremities. It may persist for a few weeks or as long as 12 months.

Latent syphilis. The latent, or quiescent, phase commences with the spontaneous resolution of secondary syphilis and may persist from 1 to 20 years or even longer. It is asymptomatic but is characterized by positive blood tests.

Late (tertiary) syphilis. Late effects of syphilis infection do not usually occur in the pediatric age-group. The cardiac and neurologic manifestations of severe destructive disease appear 10 to 20 years after the initial infection.

Congenital syphilis. The special situation in which the unborn child contracts the disease transplacentally from an infected mother is again increasing in incidence, along with the other forms of the disease. Not all infants of women with syphilis will have the disease, although most will be stillborn or will eventually display clinical evidence of infection or its sequelae (see p. 232).

Diagnostic evaluation. Positive identification of the treponema organism is made by examination of the exudate from primary or secondary lesions under a darkfield microscope. Although less reliable than microscopy, serologic tests are valuable for screening purposes. Serologic tests are of two basic types: nontreponemal or nonspecific reagin antigen tests and treponemal or specific antibody tests.

Nontreponemal tests are the least expensive. The most frequently used tests are the Kahn, Kolmer's, and VDRL (Venereal Disease Research Laboratories) tests, all of which are laboratory tests. Newer tests that do not require laboratory equipment are the Rapid Plasma Reagin (RPR) and plasmacrit (PCT) tests, which can be performed in the clinic or physician's office. They are mainly screening tests to be confirmed by more specific studies in doubtful cases. Acute infectious diseases and collagen disorders may produce false-positive results, and some false-negative results are obtained in syphilitic infections. A positive VDRL reaction develops in 10 to 90 days. Approximately 50% of infected persons have a positive reaction within the first 3 weeks, 90% are positive at 6 weeks, and the remainder are positive by 13 weeks. It is important to note that a biologic false-positive VDRL reaction secondary to heroin abuse is a possibility in adolescents, a population at risk for both drug abuse and sexually transmitted disease.[25]

Treponemal tests such as the *Treponema pallidum* immobilization (TPI) and the fluorescent treponemal antibody absorption (FTA-ABS) tests are specific for antigens and more accurate than reagin tests. However, they require elaborate equipment (especially the TPI test), and are more expensive than screening tests.

Medical management. The drug of choice for the treatment of syphilis is penicillin in doses sufficient to maintain an adequate blood level for a minimum of 10 to 14 days. This is attained with 2.4 million U of benzathine penicillin G administered at two sites at a single visit. Alternative drugs for allergic individuals are tetracycline and erythromycin.

At the time of therapy the patient should be warned of the possibility of the Jarisch-Herxheimer reaction, or therapeutic shock, that occurs in 50% to 90% of persons with primary or secondary syphilis. Characteristically within 12 hours of treatment the patient will experience a flu-like syndrome consisting of fever, chills, lethargy, headache, joint and muscular pain, and reappearance of the rash. The reaction is over in a matter of 1 or 2 hours, sometimes up to 48 hours, and can be controlled by mild sedation.

Follow-up VDRL tests are performed at 3-month intervals for a year and biannually the second year. As with gonorrhea, sexual contacts are sought and examined, and the same general preventive and educational concepts apply.

Nursing considerations in sexually transmitted diseases

Nursing responsibilities encompass all aspects of sexually transmissible disease education, prevention, and treatment. Part of the sex education of young people should include information about these diseases, such as their symptoms and treatment, and dispelling the myths associated with their mode of transmission. These diseases are not contracted from toilet seats, drinking glasses, bath towels, and so on. It is true that most persons in the vulnerable teenage population are uninformed or misinformed about these diseases. Helping to promote the inclusion of venereal disease information in schools is an important function of the nurse.

No matter what their area of practice, nurses are in a position to disseminate information, identify probable cases, and refer these cases for treatment. In the hospital, school, clinic, or private practice, nurses who recognize the signs and symptoms of disease can call these to the attention of the attending physician. This includes not only nurses working in pediatric practice but those in prenatal and obstetric services as well. A characteristic rash on a pregnant woman may be evidence of disease and a threat to the unborn child. It is nurses who are most successful in persuading pregnant women to receive early and regular prenatal care. The earlier the mother is treated, the less the hazard to the unborn child, especially in the case of syphilis, which does not affect the fetus during the first 4 months of gestation. Gonorrheal infection is most dangerous to the child during delivery and in the postpartum period.

Nurses, too, should not overlook the need for care in handling infected infants and children to prevent cross-contaminating others or contracting the disease themselves. Gloves should be worn when handling secretions and areas most likely to contain the organisms, and any breaks in the skin should receive special protective covering.

Nurses in all areas must make certain that all cases of sexually transmitted disease are reported to the public health authorities. Public health nurses play a vital role in epidemiologic investigations, including interviewing, tracking down contacts (including homosexual contacts) of reported cases, and frequently follow-up of treated cases.

Very often teenagers who suspect they have a sexually transmitted disease will seek a trusted nurse for help rather than their parents. It is probably best to try to persuade the youngsters to tell their parents, but, if they are reluctant, the alternative is to refer them to some source where they can receive medical help. Although not all states permit private physicians to treat minors, most public health departments are prepared to accept them for treatment without parental consent since they are legally allowed to treat persons of all ages for communicable diseases.

When dealing with adolescents, nurses need highly developed interviewing skills to elicit a history of sexual contacts. The connotation that the diseases are "dirty," the belief that "nice" people from "nice" families do not contract the disease, and the fear of parental displeasure and of "squealing" on friends can be deterrents to getting needed information. To gain youngsters' cooperation the nurse conveys acceptance, helps them feel at ease, and assures them that the information they give will be used to help those persons whom they name as contacts. They can be reassured that their identity and the identity of the persons they name as contacts will be kept confidential. The purpose is not to embarrass or punish but to trace and treat affected persons. This is the most effective means presently available for controlling these diseases.

ADOLESCENT PREGNANCY

The biologic maturation that forms the foundation of adolescent development and the transition to adulthood is accompanied by conflicting feelings, attitudes, and social practices related to the developing sexuality. Sexual enticements by the mass media to enhance physical attractiveness conflict with traditional religious and societal expectations for chastity. Easy access to cars, unsupervised after-school activities, removal of other safeguards, and decline of social and religious controls have left youth defenseless against the environmental forces to which they are exposed. The importance of having "popular" daughters frequently causes parents to push young girls into situations they are not mature enough to handle. One of the consequences of experimentation, acting-out, the need to conform, impulsivity, and the search for a sexual identity is pregnancy. Factors that contribute to the increasing number of adolescent pregnancies include:

Increase in the number of teenagers in the population
Earlier age at which girls reach sexual maturity
Adolescent age-specific fertility
Earlier age at marriage and younger age at first pregnancy
Greater degree of sexual freedom and permissiveness

Although the incidence of adolescent pregnancy is influenced by the availability of contraception and abortion, pregnant teenagers present a population at risk—medically, socially, economically, and educationally.

Medical aspects

With better facilities available for care, the mortality rates for teenage pregnancies are decreasing, but the morbidity still remains high. Teenage girls and their unborn infants are at greater risk for complications of both pregnancy and delivery. The most frequent complications are premature labor and infants of low birth weight, high neonatal mortality, toxemia of pregnancy, iron-deficiency anemia, fetopelvic disproportion, and prolonged labor. There may be a greater incidence of weight gain in young mothers and, in younger girls, a competition in the nutritional needs for growth between the fetus and the teenage girl.

Developmental aspects. Particularly at risk are early-maturing girls who have not completed their adolescent growth (especially girls age 10 to 13 years). If they become pregnant while still in the active anabolic phase of growth, the additional anabolic demands of the pregnancy may have an adverse effect on their ultimate adult stature. For the girl whose adolescent growth has ceased and who has achieved physical and reproductive maturity, a pregnancy is no longer as biologically hazardous.

It does not necessarily follow that early biologic development is accompanied by early emotional and psychologic development. The young teenager is still a teenager who must cope with the developmental tasks of adolescence. When the tasks of motherhood or impending motherhood are superimposed on adolescent needs, the girl is ill prepared to deal appropriately with either.

Complications of pregnancy. The most serious complication of teenage pregnancy is toxemia. Girls less than 16 years of age have five times the chance of developing preeclampsia than older girls and young women, and, since there is greater likelihood of repeat pregnancy at an earlier age, the threat is not eliminated with the termination of one pregnancy. Younger women are statistically destined to have more than the average number of additional pregnancies, and these earlier and repeated episodes of toxemia are detrimental to the cardiovascular-renal system. Consequently each subsequent pregnancy bears the risk of increased severity of toxemia, and the resulting renal damage can produce chronic renal disease in the young woman by age 30 years or so.

A number of authorities have cited a relatively high prevalence of iron-deficiency anemia among pregnant teenage girls, and the incidence increases sharply when there are repeated pregnancies during the adolescent years. Anemia is not an unusual finding in nonpregnant adolescent girls, but during pregnancy the deficit is increased because of the normal hemodilution associated with pregnancy and the growth demands of the fetus.

There appears to be little difference in the incidence of placental accidents and antepartal and postpartum hemorrhage in teenagers compared to older-aged women, although the findings vary with the observers. Lacerations of the genital tract are more frequent in younger, smaller patients.

Structural aspects. Labor may be prolonged in younger teenagers and is directly related to fetopelvic incompatibility, a reflection of teenagers' smaller stature and incomplete growth process. This is particularly true regarding girls age 12 to 16 years and is highest in girls less than 14 years of age. Girls 12 and 13 years old have the highest rate of cesarean sections, primarily necessary because of cephalopelvic disproportion. However, older adolescents, 15 to 21 years of age, often have labors that are shorter than average, especially those girls who have previously delivered a baby. The critical point between pelvic disproportion and adequacy appears to occur around 15 years of age in the average adolescent.

Nutritional aspects. Caloric requirements during adolescence closely parallel the growth curve, and the need for protein, calcium, and iron is increased concomitantly. Young adolescents tolerate caloric restriction poorly, and the anabolic need for calories during pregnancy places an added burden on their bodies. The nutritional status at the time of pregnancy is a reflection of lifetime nutritional practices. Unfortunately, because of an attempt to attain fashionably slim figures, denial of the pregnancy, and zealous restriction of diet to control pregnancy weight gain, many teenagers have been placed at risk.

There is a high correlation between adequacy of diet and successful pregnancy outcome. It has been found that adequate diet is more significant in determining the weight of the infant at birth and a trouble-free pregnancy than either maternal size or age. Since there is marked variation in the dietary needs of individual teenagers, no hard and fast rule can be laid down to describe the adequate diet for all pregnant girls. It must provide sufficient nutrients to meet growth needs of both the prospective mother and the unborn child without the threat of obesity and other evidences of malnutrition. Adolescent girls often adopt unusual dietary patterns that can seriously compromise the health of themselves and their infants.

Infants. There is a higher incidence of prematurity and low birth weight and a slight increase in congenital defects (especially some neural tube anomalies) in infants of young mothers. It is difficult to determine if this is a result of the developmental stage of the mother or a reflection of multiple factors associated with teenage pregnancies, including first pregnancy, poor nutrition, lower socioeconomic status, concomitant disease and deleterious habits, and deficiency of or lack of prenatal care. Several factors that demonstrate a high degree of association with prematurity, such as first birth, preeclampsia, immaturity, illegitimacy, and the young age of the mother, can create an accumulative effect that places the pregnant teenager in a perilously high-risk situation.

Psychologic and emotional aspects

Becoming pregnant is not something that merely happens to a girl. Although she may not be aware of it, she has arrived at the pregnant state through her own actions—conscious or unconscious. She is usually not promiscuous, that is, engaging in sexual intercourse with a variety of partners. Often the pregnancy is planned; however, an unwanted or ill-advised pregnancy can be disruptive and, in the adolescent, catastrophic.

The motivation and meanings for pregnancy during the teen years are multiple. The pregnant teenager may be a girl who has been submitted to at home and uses the same submissive treatment on herself that her parents have given her. She acts on her impulses with little control over her desires. It is difficult for her to say "no." She may be a girl from a home where the parents are critically demanding, distrustful, and punitive who chooses pregnancy as an expression of hostility toward the parents. She may be a girl from a home in which something has prevented her from receiving the care and interest that would enable her to think well of herself as a person. When parents are absent, too busy, or preoccupied with their own problems, the girl feels (and often is) neglected. Consequently she turns to another, frequently a boy in similar circumstances, for comfort and love.

Motivation for pregnancy may also reflect maladaptive attempts to solve psychologic conflicts peculiar to the stage of the girl's development. The early adolescent girl has little or distorted information about sexuality, conception, and contraception. Her motivation appears to reflect a complex relationship with her own mother, in which she wishes to break away from her mother and, at the same time, become dependent on her. Another motivation seems to be a testing of her new and mysterious body functions. She tends to disavow any responsibility for her pregnancy and blames it on a little-known boy or on her mother for failing to provide adequate sex education. This is the type of girl who often denies her pregnancy.

The girl in middle adolescence appears to have sufficient

understanding of her sexuality to avoid pregnancy but does nothing to protect herself. She too invariably places the blame on someone else for her predicament. At this time sexual activity and pregnancy may reflect a resurgence of the Oedipal feelings, in which she indulges in competitive fantasy with her mother and becomes pregnant through a wish to have a baby for her father. It may be a way to express independence from her parents and to break away from them in a less rebellious manner while she is still dependent on them. She is very conscious of her pregnant state and often takes a romantic view of maternity. This is also the type of girl who identifies with an older, married sister or another young mother and becomes pregnant to emulate these models.

Girls in late adolescence seem to have a good understanding of conception and contraception and are aware that the pregnancy is their responsibility—the result of a conscious or unconscious slip, such as forgetting to take the pill. They are rarely surprised at finding themselves pregnant and may even admit that the conception was manipulated in an attempt to force a reluctant boyfriend into a more permanent commitment to them. The late adolescent, unlike the early or middle adolescent girl, views pregnancy as a happy event under the right circumstances, and the motivation to obtain love and commitment from the boyfriend contrasts sharply with the younger girl, to whom the boy is irrelevant and whose pregnancy generally ends their relationship. The older girl shows the beginnings of a genuine wish to love and care for a child.

A teenage pregnancy frequently compels the young girl to cope with several developmental tasks at once—adolescence, pregnancy, marriage, and motherhood. The need for dependency during pregnancy conflicts with the adolescent need for independence. Instead of the independent person breaking away from her family, she is forced to become more dependent on them for physical, emotional, and financial support. The father of her child, usually a teenager himself and faced with many of the same conflicts, is seldom able to provide the support she needs.

Social and economic aspects

The teenage girl who finds herself pregnant and unmarried will frequently become the victim of a forced early marriage that, in most cases, fails. Statistically teen marriages are notoriously unstable. The highest divorce rate occurs in couples who are married between ages 15 and 19 years and is three to four times higher than that among those married at a later age. Teenagers find themselves still dependent on parents for support or, unskilled and inexperienced, in an unfavorable position to earn enough to adequately support a family. A high percentage of young people, especially unmarried mothers, are forced to go on welfare. In addition the late teen years are considered to be the most fertile; therefore, without appropriate intervention, these young mothers tend to fall into a pattern of repeated pregnancies and bearing more children at risk.

Teenage pregnancy is one of the greatest causes of school dropout in young female students. Previously the stigma attached to teenage out-of-wedlock pregnancies was such that the girls were not allowed to remain in school. They were considered to be bad influences and publicly condemned for their misconduct. Such punitive behavior was not successful in reducing the number of pregnancies; however, it may have contributed to damaging numerous young lives.

Another significant aspect of school dropout and accelerated maturity is the girl's alienation and isolation from her peers during a stage of development when identity formation is so closely allied with peer identification. She is deprived of the interrelationship with the adolescent social system that is so essential to the development of a sense of identity. The girl believes that she no longer "belongs" to the peer group and does not qualify for membership in the older peer group normally associated with marriage and motherhood.[28]

Today most communities have some arrangement for continuation of the girl's education by allowing her to remain in regular classes or providing a curriculum to meet her special needs either within the school system or through programs associated with other community agencies. Most community programs designed for the assistance of pregnant teenagers involve the cooperative efforts of several organizations. The major service components of the programs include[28]:

1. Early and consistent prenatal care
2. Continuing education on a classroom basis
3. Counseling on an individual or group basis

Infants. Infants of the teenage mother are at risk medically because of the higher incidence of prematurity and low birth weight, but they are also at risk in other aspects of their existence. Although many adolescent mothers want their babies and are prepared to care for them in a mature manner, many others have unrealistic expectations for the child. The young mother often sees the infant as a plaything or a love object for herself. These infants are also at risk for child abuse, neglect, retarded development, and various maladaptive behaviors in childhood. Many are raised by grandparents, a situation that can be fraught with problems and confused identities for the child.[28]

Teenage fathers.[21] In the past the role of the father of an unwed teenage mother has been almost completely ignored by health professionals. Contrary to prevalent attitudes, the boy is often concerned about the girl he impregnates and wants to act in a responsible way in supporting the girl and helping her share the burden of decisions regarding the new life. With help, the couple can explore all the alternatives available regarding the future of the child, including marriage, adoption, or either the mother or father assuming responsibility to care for and rear the child. Most teenage fathers are willing to accept their obligations and demonstrate strong paternal feelings for the newborn child. They also need to be made aware of their legal right in relation to the child.

Health care during the course of pregnancy

The girl who does not choose to marry is faced with a sequence of problems. She must first decide whether to terminate or continue the pregnancy—a difficult decision for a mature woman but even more so for an immature teenager. Liberalized abortion laws have provided a means for terminating an unwanted pregnancy, and a significant number of girls choose this alternative when it is readily accessible to them and the pregnancy is not too far advanced. However, the procedure is not without risk, both physically and psychologically, and those who select this route will require abortion counseling from supportive, nonjudgmental professionals. The girl will have feelings about the therapy, and termination of the pregnancy does not always solve the underlying problem.

The girl who elects to maintain the pregnancy throughout the normal period of gestation is confronted with the decision of whether to keep the infant and attempt to provide a home, either alone or in some type of family arrangement; to relinquish the child and pursue her educational and career goals; or to provide for the child and pursue her personal goals. The girl who chooses to place her child for adoption, often a difficult and painful decision, will require guidance in selecting a suitable agency to provide this service and support during the trauma of separation from the infant. The girl who decides to keep her child is often faced with loneliness, the burden of responsibility, a new role, and the task of rebuilding a new life. She will need assistance and support in providing care for herself and the child. Factors that appear to be crucial to making a satisfactory adjustment to the pregnancy and to creating a healthy environment for the child include[28]:

1. The presence of a care-taking person who will provide the necessary emotional and financial security until the adolescent is self-sufficient
2. A realistic view of the maternal role as well as the needs of the infant
3. The motivation for pregnancy being for positive and healthy reasons rather than for self-destructive or neurotic ones

Health care. Medical management of the pregnancy or its alternative, abortion, does not vary significantly in teenage mothers from that of more mature women, with the exception of the special nutritional needs of young teenagers. For routine medical and nursing management throughout the maternity cycle, the reader is referred to an obstetric nursing textbook (see Bibliography). However, pregnant teenagers *do* require a broader range of health and auxiliary services for care. This is best accomplished by a team approach toward quality care for the teenager that includes the parents, the school, the father of the child, and, where feasible, social services and (sometimes) legal council in addition to medical and nursing care.

Nursing considerations

It is evident from the preceding that nurses play a central role in meeting the needs of pregnant teenagers. It is frequently the nurse to whom the young girl turns for help and guidance in her dilemma and on whom she relies for support and reassurance.

The most important goal in nursing care of the pregnant teenager is to obtain medical care for her if she has not already done so. Typically girls in this age-group are reluctant to seek medical help in part because of anxiety but more often because of a tendency to deny the pregnancy (especially in younger girls) or in an attempt to conceal their condition as long as possible to avoid being dropped from school (older girls). The importance of early prenatal care is well known for the welfare of both mother and infant when the girl chooses to continue the pregnancy and to facilitate a safe abortion when she elects this option. For guidelines, teaching, and general support measures during pregnancy, the reader is directed to the excellent textbooks available on nursing care throughout the maternity cycle.

Basic to the implementation of any program of care is communication and the establishment of a trusting relationship. Initially the adolescent girl frequently appears apathetic and displays little interest in discussing her pregnancy. She may be abrupt, impatient, defensive, hostile, or indifferent. It is important for the nurse to make every effort to put the youngster at ease and avoid undo pressure until a rapport can be developed so that the girl is comfortable in sharing her feelings and concerns. Conveying a nonjudgmental and genuine caring acceptance of the girl and her goals will assist the nurse to gain her confidence and trust, although this may take a good deal of time and several visits to accomplish. The girl may have encountered rejection and open criticism from authority figures and peers depending on the social and cultural attitudes of the school, the community, and her own family structure.

Communication takes time and patience. Asking open-ended questions and listening for cues will help identify physical, emotional, social, and cultural influences that might affect the adolescent's progress through the maternity cycle. For example, various cultural groups have different attitudes toward unsanctioned pregnancies, and it is important to determine other sources of support, such as the family. Factors that might affect her physical status, such as smoking, drug use, and nutritional state and habits, need to be explored and confronted. Each teenager presents a unique situation in relation to background, life-style, support structure, and coping mechanisms.

Summary of nursing care of the pregnant teenager

Goals	Responsibilities

Assist in attaining good health for mother and infant	Facilitate early diagnosis and intervention (case finding)
	Encourage early and active participation in suitable health-care program
	Provide special nutritional guidance
	Maintain surveillance for complications related to pregnancy
	Prepare mother for delivery
	Provide and encourage follow-up health services after delivery
	  Maintaining contact with mother
	  Referral to health agency
	  Coordination of services
	  Family planning services

Aid in stable family life during pregnancy and following delivery	Help with decisions regarding marriage, living with parents Assess adequacy of home Facilitate placement into home for pregnant teenagers when other alternatives not feasible Support family
Help mother to relinquish infant at birth if desired	Secure services of official adoption agency Support girl through separation process
Help mother to develop competence as a mother	Conduct or arrange for preparation for mothering activities (acquiring layette) Provide instruction in infant care (introduction to child development and child care) Help to establish positive mother-child relationship Reinforce positive behavior toward infant Provide referral services where needed
Aid mother in integration back into her community	Help secure day-care services for infant Help secure vocational or special education services
Help mother develop maturity and independence	Help mother develop her own resources for coping and problem solving

Aid mother in accomplishing developmental tasks of adolescence	Help mother develop positive self-image
	  Positive reinforcement
	  Helping to achieve successes and a sense of accomplishment
	Give individual support
	Provide for group identification (group discussions)

Aid mother in meeting educational needs	Arrange for continuing education during pregnancy
	  Reentry into regular school
	  Enrollment in special classes for pregnant teenagers
	  Tutoring where other services are not available

The young girl needs to know what is happening to her, what is expected of her, and how she can help in developing a plan of care. Adolescents have their own ideas of the type of help they need and support that would be beneficial. They should be consulted and provided with the opportunity to share their ideas and to feel that they make an important contribution to planning their care.[24]

Maternity care for the teenager involves physical, emotional, social, and educational goals. The nurse interprets and explains to the girl what is happening to her and what will happen to her and provides her with simple, clear directions. Explanations may have to be repeated again and again. Working with social agencies, the school, and the family are all part of nursing care of the pregnant teenager.

The girl will need help to improve her altered self-image, a crucial factor in adolescence. Giving her as much individual attention as possible, being a sympathetic listener, providing the opportunity for her to know, support, and be supported by other girls in the same situation, and helping her to experience success at every opportunity will facilitate progress toward achieving this goal. Individual or group discussions of clothes, hairstyles, makeup, and involvement in creative and self-improvement activities help to enhance her self-concept.

The nurse also involves the family whenever possible. The parents of the girl and the father of the child need to express feelings and attitudes about the situation. Often they must deal with their own feelings before they are able to provide support and help in problem solving for the pregnant girl. The girl may or may not wish to have these persons involved in her decisions and care. The nurse must attempt to determine the teenager's true feelings regarding these relationships. The pregnant adolescent, although still ostensibly under parental control, has legal authority over the conduct of her pregnancy and the disposition of the child. Adolescents who are clearly no longer under parental control, for example, those who are living alone, are married, are economically self-sufficient, or otherwise demonstrate the capacity to give informed consent are considered "emancipated" or "mature" minors and, as such, are responsible for their actions in seeking and accepting medical care. For a summary of nursing care of the pregnant teenager see the boxed material on the opposite page.

CONTRACEPTION

Family planning services in general have developed and expanded during recent years, and, with the increase in sexual activity among the teenage population, there is also an increased awareness of the need for contraceptive services as a part of the health care of adolescents. It is well known that the morbidity and mortality risks of pregnancy exceed those for use of contraceptive measures. Although all teenagers need sex education, not all of them are candidates for contraception. Among the large adolescent population there are those youngsters whose voluntary sexual restraint eliminates the need for control measures and those who are married and wish to have a child. For others, fertility control is advisable. This includes premarital counseling, postpartum counseling for both married and unmarried mothers, and counseling for the sexually active unmarried teenager.

Since contraceptive advice and management of premarital and married teenagers differ little from fertility control offered to older women, little need be added regarding this group of teenagers. The group that represents the greatest difficulty is the unmarried, dependent, sexually active girl, whether she has been pregnant or not. Although there is still resistance from parents, physicians, lawyers, and legislators in regard to treatment of legal minors without parental consent, a liberalized trend throughout the country makes it possible in most areas to provide such medical services to minors without parental consent. The predominant feeling is that the "parents' rights" view is not necessarily sensitive to the health needs and basic rights of youth. There is no evidence to substantiate the belief that providing contraceptive guidance contributes to sexual irresponsibility and promiscuity. Actually a request for contraceptive information indicates a responsible effort on the part of the teenager to avoid an undesirable pregnancy.

Contraceptive methods

The choice of a contraceptive method, to be safe and effective, must be suited to the individual. The choice is based on the youngster's preference and the physician's judgment. Although a girl may prefer to use the pill, if her menstrual pattern suggests that she is not ovulating normally, she will be guided to another method. Also, the girl must be motivated to use whatever method is recommended or prescribed. No matter what method is selected, the provision of a birth control device is only part of a comprehensive sex education program.

The advantages and disadvantages of various contraceptive methods recommended for use in adolescents are outlined in Table 20-7.

Simple methods. Sometimes, despite the effectiveness of prescription methods, teenagers persist in using less effective methods because of the necessity for medical screening and supervision inherent in the use of superior devices. Commonplace methods such as withdrawal, douches, and reliance on hopefully "safe" periods are often reported in teenage obstetric histories. Factual knowledge about more effective methods such as the condom and chemicals and clarifying some of the myths regarding safe times in the menstrual cycle help to reduce the incidence of unwanted pregnancy. Although they may have a limited use for infrequent or short-term exposure to pregnancy, the simple methods are generally unpopular with teenagers. Their use requires unusual consistency and care in following directions and inhibits the spontaneity of the activity.

Table 20-7. Advantages and disadvantages of contraceptive methods in the adolescent

Method	Characteristics	Advantages	Disadvantages
Oral contraceptives	Estrogen and progesterone-like compounds Inhibit ovulation by blocking release of gonadotropins from anterior pituitary gland	Theoretically 100% effective Some gynecologists consider pregnancy significant index of maturity to justify administration	Higher failure rate in adolescents than in older women Need to follow precise instructions; require continued motivation Should not be given to immediate postmenarchal females because of critical period in physiologic maturation of hormone system Should not be used until well-established menstrual cycle is present (2 years) Serious side effects have been reported, especially thrombophlebitis and hypertension
Combined	Estrogen and progesterones in set dosage Taken daily for 20-21 days or for 28 days, with twenty-one active tablets and seven inert or iron-containing tablets	Combined are slightly more effective than sequentials	
Sequential	Estrogen for 14-15 days, followed by progesterone for 5-6 days	Some gynecologists consider pregnancy significant index of maturity to justify administration	
Intrauterine devices (IUDs)	Plastic or metal devices worn inside the uterine cavity Local foreign body effect prevents implantation Copper IUD continually releases minute amounts of copper that has an adverse effect on implantation	During menses cervical dilation allows easier insertion Especially suited for long-term contraception Requires short period of time to insert More effective than oral contraceptives in teenagers Suitable for nulliparous or parous girls No significant side effects or interference with ovulation Eliminates need for motivation or compliance	Perforated uterus possible but infrequent when device is in competent hands Contraindicated in acute pelvic infections, some forms of heart disease (source of septic foci), cervical stenosis, polyps, or congenital anomalies of uterus Significantly increases blood loss in patients with iron-deficiency or sickle cell anemias Expulsion of IUD may be a problem Side effects include cramps, pelvic discomfort, and excessive bleeding for one to three menstrual cycles
Abstinence	Medically ideal contraceptive	100% effective if carried out	Peer pressure to conform Relatively high failure rate Crisis services, for example, morning-after estrogen therapy, should be made available
Condom	Penal covering to trap sperm	Simple to use Available without prescription Provides some protection from venereal disease	High failure rate Requires consistent use Requires premeditated intent for sexual union
Diaphragm	Cervical covering to prevent sperm from reaching egg For maximum effectiveness, must be used in conjunction with spermicide	Virgins can be fitted May be inserted up to 6 hours before intercourse and left in place as long as convenient (varies according to authorities)	Low failure rate when used correctly High failure rate in adolescents because of inconvenience of use Requires consistent use Requires fitting and instruction by medical personnel If inserted early, should be checked for placement before coitus Requires premeditated intent for sexual union

Table 20-7. Advantages and disadvantages of contraceptive methods in the adolescent—cont'd

Method	Characteristics	Advantages	Disadvantages
Chemicals—spermicidal foam, jelly, cream, etc.	Substance injected into vagina to kill sperm	Available without prescription	High failure rate unless combined with mechanical barrier Possible for sperm to be ejaculated directly into uterine os, bypassing spermicide in vagina Must be used shortly before coitus, therefore requires interruption of sexual experience Repeated sexual union requires repeated application Requires premeditated intent for sexual union
Sterilization	Usually tubal ligation Most often limited to girls with chronic medical problems (diabetes, sickle-cell anemia, rheumatic heart disease) in whom one or more pregnancies have occurred Hysterectomy Vasectomy	100% effective	Likely to be associated with repercussions on reaching adulthood Almost universally irreversible

Prescription methods. Birth control methods that require a medical prescription are considered by many teenagers to be too premeditated; as a result they are less popular among teenagers. However, prescription methods are now being used by greater numbers as attitudes are changing in a more open and permissive atmosphere. Oral contraceptives appear to be the preferred method and are usually prescribed unless there are contraindications.

Oral contraceptives consist of estrogen and progestogen in varying ratios. The administration of estrogen for 20 to 21 days inhibits the secretion of follicle-stimulating hormone by the anterior pituitary and thus prevents ovulation; progestogen helps endometrial buildup, thereby more nearly simulating a normal menstrual cycle. Discontinuance of the drug at the end of 21 days allows the endometrial involution to take place.

As with any medication, oral contraceptives are tailored to the individual. The same screening is carried out for teenagers as for women in any other age-group; thus steroid contraception is contraindicated where there is history of thromboembolic disorder, diabetes, liver impairment, severe migraine, or seizure disorder. Since many girls in this age-group are still establishing ovulatory regulation, care must be exercised in introducing hormonal control so that future fertility is not jeopardized. Oral contraceptives are potent hypothalamic-pituitary suppressors and should not be prescribed for postpubescent girls until they demonstrate a well-established menstrual cycle of at least 2 years. This also prevents masking of abnormalities of the reproductive system that are manifest by irregular or absent menses. Also, failure to develop withdrawal bleeding (bleeding that occurs during the days when the pill is not taken) in girls who were regular prior to the use of oral contraceptives is cause to discontinue the drug and change to a nonhormonal method of fertility control. Young females usually require higher levels of estrogen than older women, especially those with a tendency toward acne or hirsutism.

Intrauterine devices (IUDs), plastic or metal devices placed inside the uterus, probably prevent implantation through a local foreign body effect. They are easily inserted during menses by a trained professional and appear to be suitable for long-term contraception. The intrauterine device requires no motivation once it is already in place and has proved particularly useful in teenage girls.

Use of contraception

Although teenagers frequently seek contraceptive advice and do not wish for a pregnancy, they are inconsistent users of contraception. Studies indicate that a large number had used no contraceptive at the preceding act of intercourse and that only a small number of sexually active youngsters use contraception with regularity. There are several reasons why teenagers are not making better use of contraception.[21]

Lack of information. Sometimes health professionals have a tendency to confuse a teenager's sophistication with knowledge. Although youngsters are acutely aware of their sexuality, their understanding of reproductive anatomy and physiology is incomplete. If they are using contraception, they often do so with little or no instruction and with only vague understanding. Misinformation is commonplace. Lacking a fundamental understanding of fertility, they often believe that they are too young or have sex too infrequently to become pregnant. A majority of girls mistakenly believe that maximum fertility begins with menses and that the safe period occurs midway between menstrual periods.

Anxiety regarding contraception. Teenagers often express the fear of arguments or threats if they seek assistance via health services. Some are concerned that parents will be notified. Many have exaggerated ideas about the hazards of oral contraceptions or intrauterine devices.

Conflict about sexual activity. Many teenagers feel ambiguous regarding their sexual activity and avoid contraceptives (especially the pill or intrauterine device) because their use seems too premeditated. This implies that sex is planned rather than a spontaneous activity. Most of these girls believe that sex is alright if one is "swept away" (after all, what can one do about it?) but that planning to do something to prevent pregnancy is wrong.

Desire for pregnancy. There are a few teenagers who deliberately expose themselves to the risk of a pregnancy as a conscious or unconscious act of hostility, response to entrapment, or expression of self-assertion. Even though the youngster has an effective contraceptive, she may fail to use it, use it improperly (conveniently forgetting to take a pill), or use a method not suited to her needs. The girl may know how a contraceptive works but fail to put her knowledge to use.

Nursing considerations

Much of contraceptive education and service is assumed by nurses as part of sex education programs, family planning services, or postpartum health services. The initial introduction should, ideally, be associated with ongoing sex education. When included as a part of this education process, the sexually active school-age adolescent will consider contraceptives as a natural and logical part of sex life. It is important that youngsters learn about sexuality, conception, and contraception from someone who can provide them with accurate information in a straightforward, nonjudgmental manner. In birth control and family planning clinics, nurses take the leadership in conducting group discussions and most of the individual counseling and guidance. They instruct the girls in correct use of their contraceptive. Establishing rapport and open communication with teenagers, nurses provide youngsters with a person in whom they can confide.

An essential part of contraceptive services to teenagers is follow-up. The recipient is expected to return frequently for a checkup on the effectiveness of the method and her general health and welfare. Prescriptions are usually dispensed for 1 or, sometimes, 2 months only so that the girl must return at regular intervals to maintain her contraceptive. Intrauterine devices are checked after the first menstrual flow and periodically to ascertain that they are maintained in proper placement and to evaluate any persistent side effects such as excess flow, cramps, and so on.

Nurses are continually on the alert for clues that indicate physical, mental, or emotional problems. Discussions about contraception may provide some insight into disturbed interpersonal relationships and other problems related to the health and well-being of the sexually active adolescent. Participation in regularly scheduled "rap sessions" has proved to be a most important means for exchange between nurses and both male and female adolescents.

SEXUAL TRAUMA*

Sexual trauma, sexual abuse, and sexual assault involve situations in which children or adolescents "are pressured into sexual activity by a person who stands in a power position over them as through age, authority, or some other way."[5] Sexual assault can consist of manual, genital, or oral contact with the genitalia of the victim without consent, usually perpetrated by force, drugs, fraud, or threats of retaliation. The actual incidence of sexual assault is unknown since many instances (probably 10% to 30%) are never reported because the victim, female or male, is afraid, feels guilty or ashamed, thinks he or she will not be believed, or fears the loss of love from someone such as a boyfriend. The adolescent girl is particularly vulnerable to sexual assault, and it is estimated that more than 50% of such victims are between 10 and 19 years of age.[16] Definitions of several types of sexual assault follow:

rape sexual assault in which the penis is forced into the genitalia of the victim. Fitting the penis between the labia without disruption of the hymen or evidence of ejaculation is also considered sufficient penetration to constitute rape.

statutory rape this may be charged when the victim is unable to give consent legally by virtue of age (age varies from state to state, but is usually less than 16 years of age), mental deficiency, psychosis, or an altered state of consciousness caused by sleep, drugs (including alcohol), or illness.

molestation sexual assault without intercourse.

incest sexual intercourse between persons too closely related to contract a marriage legally and/or culturally.

Assault

Adolescent females are the victims in approximately half of the reported rapes. They are frequently selected at random because they are apparently helpless and are usually in a vulnerable situation, such as the teenage runaway, the unsuspecting hitchhiker, and the braless youngster in a T-shirt walking alone in an unprotected neighborhood. The assailant may be someone who knows the victim and has waited

*The material in this section has been drawn extensively from the writings of Burgess and Holmstrom.

for an opportunity when the victim is defenseless, such as the teenager at home alone with an uncle or cousin or the baby-sitter being driven home.

In the case of younger adolescents and children, the offender is known to the victims or their families in the majority of instances and is often a friend, relative, neighbor, or someone in a position of authority. In a significant number of cases concerning young victims, the sexual abuse has taken place repeatedly over a period of weeks or months. Families are often ambivalent about reporting abuse to avoid disgrace, or they may not believe the victim. Abuse that involves family members creates additional problems that will be discussed later.[6,11,16]

Most rapists are men in their late teens or early twenties, and a large number of rapes involve more than one assailant. The time of the assault is most often between 9 PM and 2 AM and rarely takes place between 6 and 11 AM. There is a slightly higher incidence in warm weather. Most rapes are intraracial, with the rapist and victim of the same race. Most studies suggest a high proportion of rape among black assailants and black victims, but the significance of this is unclear. It may reflect biased reporting and apprehension of assailants.[14,16] Physical force, including roughness, nonbrutal beating (slapping), brutal beating (slugging, kicking, beating repeatedly with fists), and choking or gagging, is present in a large number of cases. The predominant reaction of the victim is fear—of the rape and of injury. Thus the victim is faced with the dilemma of submission or resistance. Resistance increases the victim's chances of escape but also increases the likelihood of violence against her.[11]

Young victims.[5] In contrast to adult victims, young children and many adolescents are largely "accessories to sex." The nature of the sexual activity ranges from molestation to rape, and the victim often remains silent for an extended period of time—often a period of years. Most offenders are family members or friends who stand in a relationship of dominance over the victim and who pressure the victim into being an accessory to the sexual activity through various means. The methods of pressure are such that the child may be totally unaware that sexual activity is part of the offer. Frequently used methods include (1) The child is offered material goods, such as candy or money, for example, "I'll give you some candy if you take down your pants." (2) The adult misrepresents moral standards by telling the child that it is "okay to do." Children grow up believing that if an adult tells them to do something they should do it. (3) In a small percentage of cases extremely isolated and emotionally and socially impoverished children are enticed by adult males who meet their needs for warmth and human contact.

The successful sex offender also employs means to pressure the victim into secrecy regarding the activity. In cases in which the sexual activity is pleasurable to the youngster, the activity is described as a "secret between us." The offender also plays on the child's fears, including fear of punishment by the offender, fear of repercussions if the child tells, and fear of abandonment or rejection by the family. It is not uncommon for the child to reveal the fear that their parents would not believe them if they told—especially if the offender is a trusted member of the family. Some fear they will be blamed for the situation, and many young children with limited vocabulary have difficulty in describing the activity when they do have the courage or opportunity to complain.

Children usually describe the experience in terms of whether it was unpleasant or hurt, or was pleasurable (usually a response to hand-genital contact); some indicate no reaction. The disclosure of the secret comes about in a variety of ways—the act is observed by others, resulting in a direct confrontation; the child tells someone, such as a parent of a friend; visible clues are observed, such as an accumulation of coins, gifts, or candy; or more obvious clues are seen, such as a child coming home without clothes or becoming pregnant; and physical or behavioral signs and symptoms are observed, such as complaints of a stomachache, the child staying inside more, refusal to go to school, an excessive number of baths, unprovoked crying, or sudden onset of bed-wetting.

Medical management

Adolescents who have been raped arrive at the emergency room or physician's office under a variety of circumstances. They are usually brought in by parents, friends, or police, but some girls may seek medical help on their own. It is advisable to obtain parental consent for examination, but the examination may be performed without consent if the adolescent is mature and the parents are unavailable. A nurse should be present during the history and examination. Since rape is a legal matter to be determined by the courts, medical examination merely provides evidence of penetration, ejaculation, and, when possible, use of force. The latter is difficult to determine since many young women are left unmarked when forced to comply at the point of a gun or other weapon.

History. The history should be as complete as possible and must be taken and presented in the patient's own words, including any account of force or threats. Some youngsters are able to provide detailed descriptions of the event; others are afraid, stammer, cry, and have difficulty in selecting words or are unable to speak at all. The presence of a parent and/or policemen in the room often inhibits the child's ability to describe the incident.

Information includes date, time, location, and an accurate description of all types of sexual contact. All related activities are included. For example, evidence can be altered if the victim has bathed, urinated, defecated, douched, or changed clothing; therefore, these activities should be recorded. Use of a condom by the alleged assailant can alter evidence. For adequate care, other important data include date of last menstrual period, date of last intercourse (where applicable), use of contraception, and any possibility of a preexisting pregnancy or venereal disease. Behavior and emotional state should be recorded also, since responses range from outward calm and controlled behavior and affect to excessive agitation or hysteria. Some girls are inappropriately giddy or nonchalant.[10,16]

Examination. The physical examination is carried out as soon as possible, since physical evidence deteriorates rapidly. The victim is examined thoroughly, including nongenital areas for evidence of injury that might substantiate the use of force. Sometimes the stress of the incident makes the girl unaware of physical trauma or even serious injury. Physical injury varies greatly in victims of rape. A few are murdered, many suffer physical injury, and practically all are disturbed emotionally.[10] Photographs are taken of bruises, lacerations, or scratches for evidence, and rips or tears in clothing and the presence of dirt or grass stains are noted and recorded. Perineal or rectal lacerations are suggestive of rape.

Specimens are obtained from the vaginal cul-de-sac, and a hang-drop preparation is examined immediately to assess sperm mobility. A Papanicolaou (Pap) smear is prepared and sent to the laboratory. Vaginal secretions are also tested for acid phosphatase, since this enzyme is not normally present in the female genital tract but is found in high concentrations in semen. This is especially important if the assailant has had a vasectomy or is infertile. It is the most accurate test up to 14 hours after the alleged assault; the Papanicolaou smear is the most reliable test for documentation of sexual intercourse from 14 to 26 hours after the event.[16]

A baseline serology is drawn, and a gonococcal culture is obtained to prove that the victim did not have any preexisting infection. The child is reexamined at appropriate intervals (4 to 6 weeks for syphilis; 2 to 3 days for gonorrhea) to determine if the child acquired disease from the assailant.

Treatment. Any injuries sustained by the victim that require surgical treatment are repaired. Lacerations of the vagina are not uncommon. Most physicians prescribe, and many of the victims and/or their parents prefer the girl to receive, prophylactic administration of penicillin at the time of initial examination. Pregnancy prophylaxis, usually diethylstilbestrol, is offered to the victim who is not using oral contraceptives, pregnant, or menstruating.

Psychologic aspects of sexual assault in children and adolescents

The literature concerning sexual abuse in children is singularly scarce, and most reports are concerned with the medical and legal aspects. Burgess and Holstrom through their observations have identified what they describe as the *rape trauma syndrome*. The rape trauma syndrome involves two phases (1) the acute phase of disorganization of lifestyle and (2) a long-term process of reorganization. These phases encompass behavioral, somatic, and psychologic reactions to the stressful event.[6]

Acute phase of disorganization. During the acute phase victims exhibit either an expressed style or a controlled style of demonstrating emotional reactions. Those with the expressed style are able to express their feelings of fear, anger, and/or anxiety. Those with the controlled style hide or mask their feelings and do not express their feelings openly but display a calm, subdued affect. Since a common emotional response to sexual assault is terror, the psychologic mechanisms evoked in an attempt to cope with the stress are equally powerful. Often the emotional shock creates an exaggerated sense of unreality and dissociation, giving the victim the appearance of indifference to an untrained observer. The controlled victim is equally as upset as the victim who expresses her feelings.

Other acute reactions include physical reactions such as body soreness, disturbances in sleep patterns, and alterations in eating patterns. In addition to fear responses, the victims demonstrate other emotional responses, including anger, self-blame, guilt, shame, and/or feelings of degradation. Feelings of embarrassment are prominent, particularly in adolescents. Mood swings, enhanced mood lability, and increased irritability with others are often observed. Almost all victims spend a good deal of time thinking about how the assault might have been avoided. Many concerns of children focus on how the event will affect them at school.

Long-term reorganization process. Changes in lifestyle are often observed during the reorganization phase. Victims may continue previous activities such as attending school but achieve only a minimal level of functioning. A teenager may attend school but be apprehensive that other students know about the incident and are talking about her. Frequently an adolescent girl is raped by a male student or gang of boys from the school; as a result she is afraid to return to school and may beg to move to a different neighborhood. It is not unusual for the attacker to telephone and taunt the victim or for the girl to receive anonymous obscene calls. Most children experience nightmares, phobias about being left alone, and panic reactions on seeing the assailant, the scene of the crime, or a symbolic reminder of the assault. Sexual fears are prominent and difficult for the victim to discuss.[5,14,16]

Feelings of helplessness and powerlessness are experienced as the victim feels that events are totally beyond her control. Many demonstrate a marked degree of self-blame because of society's impression that women provoke sexual attacks. Victims are concerned about the potential effects that the assault will have on their relationships with others, particularly regarding the extent to which persons close to them will blame them for the assault. There are concerns about who to tell about the event and how to go about telling them. Sexual assault produces varied and profound long-term effects on the victims.

Families. Families respond to sexual assault with a wide variety of emotional responses that may be as intense and disruptive as they are for the victim, regardless of the type of assault. The immediate reactions range from emotional shock to near hysteria on the part of one or both of the parents, which may interfere with care of the victim. There may be surprising inability on the part of the parents to provide adequate emotional support to the child at this time, even when their attitude toward the child has been supportive in the past. Parents and other family members may display the same type of emotional responses as the victim, such as inability to eat or sleep and somatic complaints of headache or backache. In the acute emotional phase, parents have a need to blame someone. Burgess and Holstrom have identified three targets for this blame: the assailant, the child, and themselves.[6] The parents not uncommonly express anger at the child for "stupid" behavior and may even restrict the child's privileges as punishment. When the victim is an adolescent, the parents may question her sexual provocation of the event. Self-blaming parents assume full responsibility, believing that they have been inadequate parents or should not have allowed the child to go out. When a baby-sitter or trusted relative is involved in the assault and the child's complaint has not been believed until gross evidence is presented, the parents are often devastated by guilt.

Incestuous relationships. Incest takes place in all levels of society but is more apt to be detected and reported in the lower socioeconomic groups. The incidence is unknown but is probably much more common than is generally suspected. By far the most prevalent relationship in reported cases is father-daughter incest; brother-sister incest is less common, multiple relationships comprise a small percent, and mother-son incest is relatively uncommon. Whereas sexual play or experimentation is common among young siblings, it is usually transient and stops as the children become older and it has less disturbing emotional consequences for them. Therefore, these cases are less likely to come to the attention of authorities.

Incestuous relationships between father and daughter are generally prolonged, and the victims are usually reluctant to report the situation through fear of retaliation and fear that they will not be believed. Most relationships are directly related to sexual maladjustment and estrangement between husband and wife and begin following the cessation of sexual relationships with the usual partner. Most fathers experience little guilt, and the wives almost invariably are aware of the incestuous affair. The wife reacts by tolerating the situation or resorts to the obvious use of denial.

Incest between father and daughter is not always damaging and may be a satisfying relationship. A few girls see nothing wrong with it and state that they intend to continue the relationship. In some isolated populations it is a common practice and is generally accepted, particularly in the event that the mother dies. However, in general the incestuous relationship is the source of emotional damage and the daughters attempt to avoid contact with the father, moving away from home as soon as possible. Many avoid any relationship with a sexual connotation; others become promiscuous. Frequently emotional problems continue into adulthood.[10]

Nursing considerations

In no other area of nursing practice is there greater need for understanding and compassion toward patients and their families. When a child is seen initially it is extremely important for the health personnel to take time with the child and attempt to help her through this crisis. Many girls feel uncomfortable with a male physician or nurse and are unwilling to have them examine them after a sexual assault. A female nurse should remain with the child during the examination, and she is frequently the person who is able to elicit the necessary information from the child.

Although many children are able to talk spontaneously about the incident, others find it difficult. The child is encouraged to talk not only to provide needed information but also because talking makes people feel better, and children are no exception. It is often easiest to begin the interview with neutral questions dealing with such things as the child's reaction to the hospital and then to proceed to a discussion of the incident in general terms. Burgess and Holstrom[6] suggest that interviews might include such questions as, "Do you know why you were brought to the hospital?" "Do you know what will happen here?" or "How do you feel about being here?" Later the question, "Can you tell me what happened?" and other questions hopefully will elicit an account of the incident. Sometimes the parents are able to help the child to describe the incident, and questions can become directed to the circumstances of the assault. Questions should progress chronologically and proceed from the nonsexual to the more sexual content. If the child shows evidence of becoming too upset, the focus can be redirected to more neutral and less emotionally charged areas. It is usually difficult for young people to express feelings verbally. Talking in physical rather than sexual terms helps to facilitate discussion.

It is extremely important in this instance that the nurse and the physician take time to explain exactly what is to be done to the child clearly, thoroughly, and in language the child can understand. The physical examination is quite upsetting to the child, and she will be frightened of physical contact, especially in the genital area and other painful areas. Often young girls will cry before, during, and after the examination. The roles of the nurse and the physician should be explained to the child as well as the procedures to be performed. Ambiguity and uncertainty provoke anxiety, and simple explanations reduce a significant source of stress for the child.

After the questioning, physical examination, and any medical or surgical treatment required, it is important to discuss the situation with the parents and elicit their feelings and reaction to the assault. The family's need to discuss the incident and their feelings are essential in order that they can provide the support needed by the child. They are the strongest support system available to the child, and their ability to cope with the situation determines the degree to which they can be supportive. In most families a major concern is the physical injury sustained by the child rather than the psychologic trauma.

Members of the family are advised to encourage the child to resume normal activities and to observe the child for signs of distress. Children and adolescents express their feelings primarily through behavior. Parents should be alert for changes in behavior that indicate distress resulting from the rape trauma syndrome, such as remaining in the house, refusing to go to school, changes in sleeping patterns, and frequency of dreams and nightmares. The child should be encouraged to talk about these feelings and nightmares, since the more the child can talk about the experience, the more she will be able to gain control over it. Contrary to popular belief, children remember more than they are given credit for and thus have need for expression.

Follow-up contact with the child and family helps to assess the state of reorganization, to help mobilize family and friends to be supportive, and to provide positive reinforcement for progress. It also offers the family the opportunity to take advantage of the nurse as a source of support and guidance.

REFERENCES

1. Ad Hoc Committee on the Use of Antibiotics in Dermatology: Systemic antibiotics for treating acne vulgaris: efficacy and safety, Arch. Dermatol. **111:**1630, 1975.
2. Bailey, J. D.: Management of the teenager with retardation of physical growth or sexual maturation, Pediatr. Clin. North Am. **21:**1029-1042, 1974.
3. Bayley, N., and Pinneau, S. R.: Tables for predicting adult height from skeletal age: revised for use with the Greulich-Pyle Hand Standards, J. Pediatr. **40:**423, 1952. (Corrected in erratum for J. Pediatr. **41:**371, 1952.)
4. Blount, J. H., Darrow, W. W., and Johnson, R. E.: Venereal disease in adolescents, Pediatr. Clin. North Am. **20:**1021-1031, 1973.
5. Burgess, A. W., and Holmstrom, L. L.: Sexual trauma of children and adolescents, Nurs. Clin. North Am. **10:**551-563, 1975.
6. Burgess, A. W., Holmstrom, L. L., and McCausland, M. P.: Counseling the child rape victim, Issues Comprehensive Pediatr. Nurs., pp. 45-57, 1976.
7. Committee on Adolescence, Group for the Advancement of Psychiatry: Normal adolescence, New York, 1968, Charles Scribner's Sons.
8. Cook, C.: Contraceptive usage among teenagers, J. Am. Med. Wom. Assoc. **28:**639-642, 1973.
9. Cooper, H. E.: Adolescence. In Kempe, C. H., Silver, H. K., and O'Brien, D., editors: Current pediatric diagnosis and treatment, ed. 3, Los Altos, Calif., 1974, Lange Medical Publications.
10. Daniel, W. A., Jr.: Adolescents in health and disease, St. Louis, 1977, The C. V. Mosby Co.
11. De Francis, V.: Protecting the child victim of sex crimes committed by adults, Fed. Probation **35:**15, 1971.
12. Frisch, R. E., and Nagel, J. S.: Prediction of adult height of girls from ages of menarche and height at menarche, J. Pediatr. **85:**838-841, 1974.
13. Gardner, L. I.: Deprivation dwarfism, Sci. Am. **229:**76-82, July 1972.
14. Hilberman, E.: The rape victim, New York, 1976, Basic Books, Inc., Publishers.
15. Hughes, J. G.: Synopsis of pediatrics, ed. 4, St. Louis, 1975, The C. V. Mosby Co.
16. Kreutner, A. K., and associates: The adolescent rape victim. In Kreutner, A. K., and Hollingsworth, D. R., editors: Adolescent obstetrics and gynecology, Chicago, 1978, Year Book Medical Publishers, Inc.
17. Litt, I. F., Edberg, S. C., and Finberg, L.: Gonorrhea in children and adolescents: a current review, J. Pediatr. **85:**595-607, 1974.
18. Loggie, J. M. H.: Hypertension in children and adolescents, Hosp. Pract. **10:**81-92, 1975.
19. Loggie, J. M. H., and Rauh, L. W.: Persistent systemic hypertension in the adolescent, Med. Clin. North Am. **59:**1371-1384, 1975.
20. Londe, S., and Goldring, D.: Hypertension in children, Am. Heart. J. **84:**1, 1972.
21. Pannor, R.: The teen-age unwed father, Clin. Obstet. Gynecol. **14:**466-472, 1971.
22. Prader, A.: Delayed adolescence, Clin. Endocrinol. Metab. **4:**143-155, 1975.
23. Reisner, R. M.: Acne vulgaris, Pediatr. Clin. North Am. **20:** 851-864, 1973.
24. Schroeder, E.: The teenage unwed mother. In Kalafatich, A. J.: Approaches to the care of adolescents, New York, 1975, Appleton-Century-Crofts.
25. Stern, M. S., and MacKenzie, R. G.: Venereal disease in adolescents, Med. Clin. North Am. **59:**1395-1407, 1975.
26. Sturgis, S. H.: Menstrual disorders. In Gallagher, J. R., Heald, F. P., and Garell, D. C., editors: Medical care of the adolescent, ed. 3, New York, 1976, Appleton-Century-Crofts.
27. Tanner, J. M., and associates: Prediction of adult height from height, bone age, and occurrence of menarche, at ages 4 to 16 with allowance for midparent height, Arch. Dis. Child. **50:** 14-26, 1975.
28. Youngs, D. D., and Niebyl, J. R.: Adolescent pregnancy and abortion, Med. Clin. North Am. **59:**1419-1428, 1975.
29. Zachmann, M., and associates: Testosterone treatment of excessively tall boys, Pediatrics **88:**116-123, 1976.

BIBLIOGRAPHY

Bailey, E. N., and associates: Screening in pediatric practice, Pediatr. Clin. North Am. **21:**123-165, 1974.

Bellam, G.: The postsurgical experiences of a preadolescent girl. In Brandt, P. A., Chinn, P. L., and Smith, M. L.: Current practice in pediatric nursing, vol. I, St. Louis, 1976, The C. V. Mosby Co.

Burgess, A. W., and Holmstrom, L. L.: Sexual trauma of children and adolescents: pressure, sex, and secrecy, Nurs. Clin. North Am. **10:**551-564, 1975.

Copperman, S. M.: "Alice in wonderland" syndrome as a presenting symptom of infectious mononucleosis in children, Clin. Pediatr. **16:**143-146, 1977.

Daniel, W. A.: An approach to the adolescent patient, Med. Clin. North Am. **59:**1281-1288, 1975.

Drucker, E.: Hidden values and health care, Med. Care **7:**266, 1974.

Duffy, T. P.: Anemia in adolescence, Med. Clin. North Am. **59:** 1481-1488, 1975.

Fernbach, D. J., and Starling, K. A.: Infectious mononucleosis, Pediatr. Clin. North Am. **19:**957, 1972.

Fiedler, D. E., and associates: Pathology in the "healthy" female teenager, Am. J. Public Health **63:**962-965, 1973.

Gallagher, J. R., Heald, F. P., and Garell, D. C., editors: Medical care of the adolescent, ed. 3, New York, 1976, Appleton-Century-Crofts.

Garrell, D., editor: Symposium on adolescent medicine, Pediatr. Clin. North Am. **20**(4):entire issue, 1973.

Hofmann, A. D., and Pilpel, H. F.: The legal rights of minors, Pediatr. Clin. North Am. **20:**989-1004, 1973.

Hughes, J. G.: Synopsis of pediatrics, ed. 4, St. Louis, 1975, The C. V. Mosby Co.

Jelneck, L. J.: The special needs of the adolescent with chronic illness, Am. J. Maternal Child Nurs. **2**(1):57-61, 1977.

Kalafatich, A. J.: Approaches to the care of adolescents, New York, 1975, Appleton-Century-Crofts.

Kempe, C. H., Silver, H. K., and O'Brien, D.: Current pediatric diagnosis and treatment, ed. 5, Los Altos, Calif., 1978, Lange Medical Publications.

Leese, S. M.: Sexual urges in adolescents, Nurs. Times **70:**475, September 1974.

Leichtman, S. R., and Friedman, S. B.: Social and psychological development of adolescents and the relationship to chronic illness, Med. Clin. North Am. **59:**1319-1328, 1975.

Levine, M. S., and associates: Adolescents with developmental disabilities. A survey of their problems and management, Clin. Pediatr. **14:**25-32, January 1975.

Lore, A.: Adolescents: people, not problems, Am. J. Nurs. **73:** 1232, 1973.

Rudolph, A. M., Barnett, H. L., and Einhorn, A. H., editors: Pediatrics, ed. 16, New York, 1977, Appleton-Century-Crofts.

Shirkey, H. C., editor: Pediatric therapy, ed. 5, St. Louis, 1975, The C. V. Mosby Co.

Sorensen, R. C.: Adolescent sexuality in contemporary America, New York, 1973, World Publishing Co.

Stein, R. F.: The hospitalized adolescent's dilemma. In Reinhardt, A. M., and Quinn, M. D., editors: Current practice in family-centered community nursing, vol. I, St. Louis, 1977, The C. V. Mosby Co.

Sternlieb, J. J., and Munan, L.: A survey of health problems, practices, and needs of youth, Pediatrics **49:**177-186, 1972.

Tiedt, E.: The adolescent in the hospital: an identity-resolution approach, Nurs. Forum **11:**120-140, 1974.

Torre, C. T.: Nutritional needs of adolescents, Am. J. Maternal Child Nurs. **2:**118-127, March/April 1977.

Vaughan, V. C., and McKay, R. J.: Textbook of pediatrics, ed. 10, Philadelphia, 1975, W. B. Saunders Co.

Webb, T. E., and Oski, F. A.: Iron deficiency anemia and scholastic achievement in young adolescence, J. Pediatr. **82:**827, 1973.

Wolfish, M. G.: A clinic for the ambulatory adolescent, Clin. Pediatr. **12:**13, 1973.

Wolfish, M. G., and McLean, J. A.: Chronic illness in adolescents, Pediatr. Clin. North Am. **21:**1043, November 1974.

Delayed growth and/or maturation

Bailey, J. D.: Management of the teenager with retardation of physical growth or sexual maturation, Pediatr. Clin. North Am. **21:**1029-1041, 1974.

Barnes, H. V.: The problem of delayed puberty, Med. Clin. North Am. **59:**1337-1348, 1975.

Blunck, W.: Sexual precocity, Pediatr. Ann. **3**(7):30-46, 1974.

Brown, G. M., and Reichlin, S.: Psychological and neural regulation of growth hormone secretion, Psychosom. Med. **34:**45-60, 1972.

Ehrhardt, A. A., and Meyer-Bahlburg, H. F. L.: Psychological correlates of abnormal pubertal development, Clin. Endocrinol. Metab. **4:**207-222, 1975.

Gardner, L. I.: The child with "excessive" height prediction: clinical dilemma, Am. J. Dis. Child. **129:**17, 1975.

Gotlin, R. W., and Silver, H. K.: Endocrine disorders. In Kempe, C. H., Silver, H. K., and O'Brien, D., editors: Current pediatric diagnosis and treatment, ed. 3, Los Altos, Calif., 1974, Lange Medical Publications.

Illig, R.: Delayed adolescence, Pediatr. Ann. **3**(7):17-29, 1974.

Kaplan, J. G., and associates: Constitutional delay of growth and development: effects of treatment with androgens, J. Pediatr. **82:**38-44, 1973.

Marshall, W. A.: Interrelationships of skeletal maturation, sexual development and somatic growth in man, Ann. Hum. Biol. **1:** 29-40, 1974.

McDonough, P. G.: Gonadal dysgenesis and its variants, Pediatr. Clin. North Am. **19:**631-653, 1972.

Patton, R. G., and Gardner, L. I.: Deprivation dwarfism (psychosocial deprivation): disordered family environment as a cause of so-called idiopathic hypopituitarism. In Gardner, L. I., editor: Endocrine and genetic diseases of childhood and adolescence, ed. 2, Philadelphia, 1975, W. B. Saunders Co.

Root, A. W.: Endocrinology of puberty. II. Aberrations of sexual maturation, J. Pediatr. **83:**187, 1973.

Wolff, G., and Money, J.: Relationship between sleep and growth in patients with reversible somatotropin deficiency (psychosocial dwarfism), Psychol. Med. **3:**18, 1973.

Menstrual disorders

Altcheck, A.: Dysfunctional menstrual disorders in adolescence, Clin. Obstet. Gynecol. **14:**975, 1971.

Gilson, M. D.: Primary amenorrhea: a simplified approach to diagnosis, Am. J. Obstet. Gynecol. **117:**400, 1973.

Sloan, D.: Pelvic pain and dysmenorrhea, Pediatr. Clin. North Am. **19:**669-676, 1972.

Wentz, A. C.: Oligomenorrhea and secondary menorrhea in the adolescent, Med. Clin. North Am. **59:**1385-1394, 1975.

Accidents

Drain, C. B.: The athletic knee injury, Am. J. Nurs. **71:**536-537, 1971.

Heldreth, H. E., and Griffin, P.: Accidents and adolescents. In Gallagher, J. R., Heald, F. P., and Garell, D. C., editors: Medical care of the adolescent, ed. 3, New York, 1976, Appleton-Century-Crofts.

O'Boyle, C. M.: Sports injuries in adolescents: emergency care, Am. J. Nurs. **75:**732-1739, 1975.

Ostaszewski, T. M., and Marshall, J. L.: Prevention and treatment of sports injuries, Am. J. Nurs. **75:**1737, 1975.

Shaffer, T. E.: The adolescent athlete, Pediatr. Clin. North Am. **20:**837-850, 1973.

Acne

Akers, W. A., and Maibach, H. I.: Relative safety of long-term administration of tetracycline in acne vulgaris, Cutis **17:**531-534, 1976.

Arundell, F. D.: Acne vulgaris, Pediatr. Clin. North Am. **18:**853-874, August 1971.

Bart, B. J.: Dermatoses of adolescence, Minn. Med. **1:**121, 1973.

Brookman, R. R.: Adolescents on the surface: common dermatologic problems, Med. Clin. North Am. **59:**1473-1480, 1975.

Committee on Drugs: The treatment of acne with antibiotics, Pediatrics **48:**4, 663-665, 1971.

Cunliff, W. J., and Cotterill, J. A.: The acnes, Philadelphia, 1975, W. B. Saunders Co.

Evans, J. C., and Singleton, C. E.: Acne: the scourge of adolescence, Issues Comprehensive Pediatr. Nurs., pp. 60-68, 1976.

Fulton, J. E., and Pablo, G.: Topical antibacterial therapy for acne, Arch. Dermatol. **110:**83, 1974.

Marvin, J. A., Teefy, I. L. K., and Johnson, J. M.: The integumentary system. In Scipien, G. M., and associates: Comprehensive pediatric nursing, New York, 1975, McGraw-Hill Book Co.

Montagna, W., Bell, M., and Straus, J., editors: Advances in biology of the skin, vol. XIV, J. Invest. Dermatol. **62:**118, 1974.

Orentreich, N., and Durr, N. P.: The natural evolution of comedones into inflammatory papules and pustules, J. Invest. Dermatol. **62:**316, 1974.

Pochi, P. E., and Strauss, J. S.: Endocrinological control of the development and activity of the human sebaceous gland, J. Invest. Dermatol. **62:**191, 1974.

Reisner, R. M.: The rational therapy of acne, Cutis **17:**527-530, 1976.

Stewart, W. D., Danto, J. L., and Maddin, S.: Dermatology, ed. 4, St. Louis, 1978, The C. V. Mosby Co.

Strauss, J. S., and Pochi, P. E.: Acne and some other common skin disorders. In Gallagher, J. R., Heald, R. P., and Garell, D. C., editors: Medical care of the adolescent, ed. 3, New York, 1976, Appleton-Century-Crofts.

Strauss, J. S., Pochi, P. E., and Downing, D. T.: The role of skin lipids in acne, Cutis **17:**485-487, 1976.

Tolman, E. L.: Acne and acneiform dermatoses. In Moschella, S. L., Pillsbury, D. M., and Hurley, H. J., editors: Dermatology, Philadelphia, 1975, W. B. Saunders Co.

Systemic hypertension

Aagaard, G. N.: Treatment of hypertension, Am. J. Nurs. **73:**621-623, 1973.

Berman, E.: Children with hypertension, Am. Fam. Physician **12:** 99-103, 1975.

Botwin, E. D.: Should children be screened for hypertension? Am. J. Maternal Child Nurs. **1**(3):152-158, May/June 1976.

deCastro, F. J., and associates: Hypertension in adolescents, Clin. Pediatr. **15**(1):24, 1976.

Finnerty, F. A., Jr.: Hypertension is different in blacks, J.A.M.A. **216:**1634, 1971.

Freis, E. D.: Age, race, sex and other idices of risk in hypertension, Am. J. Med. **55:**275, 1973.

Greenfield, D., Grant, R., and Lieberman, E.: Children can have high blood pressure, too, Am. J. Nurs. **76:**770-772, 1976.

Griffith, E. W., and Madero, B.: Primary hypertension. Patient's learning needs, Am. J. Nurs. **73:**624, 1973.

Gruskin, A. B.: Clinical evaluation of hypertension in children, Primary Care **1:**233-292, 1974.

Hussar, D. A.: Antihypertensive agents, Nursing '74 **4:**37-42, March 1974.

Kilcoyne, M. M., Richter, R. W., and Alsup, P. A.: Adolescent hypertension. I. Detection and prevalence, Circulation **50:**758, 1974.

Kilcoyne, M. M.: Adolescent hypertension. II. Characteristics and response to treatment, Circulation **50:**1014, 1974.

Kotchen, J. M., and associates: Blood pressure distributions of urban adolescents, Am. J. Epidemiol. **99:**315, 1974.

Lancour, J.: How to avoid pitfalls in measuring blood pressure, Am. J. Nurs. **76:**773-775, 1976.

Loggie, J. M. H.: Systemic hypertension. In Gallager, J. R., Heald, F. P., and Garell, D. C., editors: Medical care of the adolescent, ed. 3, New York, 1976, Appleton-Century-Crofts.

Londe, S., and associates: Hypertension in apparently normal children, J. Pediatr. **78:**569, 1971.

Long, M. L., and associates: Hypertension. What patients need to know, Am. J. Nurs. **75:**765-770, 1976.

Maill, W. E.: Heredity and hypertension, Practitioner **207:**20, 1971.

Mitchell, E. S.: Protocol for teaching hypertensive patients, Am. J. Nurs. **77:**808-809, 1977.

Mitchell, S. C., and associates: Commentary: the pediatrician and hypertension, Pediatrics **56:**3-5, 1975.

Ooi, B. S.: Causes of hypertension in the young, Br. Med. J. **3:** 744, 1970.

Rance, C. P., and associates: Persistent systemic hypertension in infants and children, Pediatr. Clin. North Am. **21:**810, 1974.

Silverberg, D. S., and associates: Screening for hypertension in a high school population, Can. Med. Assoc. J. **113:**103-108, 1975.

Sexually transmitted diseases

Ahern, C.: "I think I have VD," Nurs. Clin. North Am. **8:**77-90, 1973.

Altcher, A.: Adolescent vulvovaginitis, Pediatr. Clin. North Am. **19:**735, 1972.

Atwater, J. B.: Adapting the venereal disease clinic to today's problem, Am. J. Public Health **64:**433-437, 1974.

Blount, J. H., Darrow, W. W., and Johnson, R. E.: Venereal disease in adolescents, Pediatr. Clin. North Am. **20:**1021, 1973.

Briody, B. A.: Venereal infections. In Briody, B. A., and Gillis, R. E.: Microbiology and infectious disease, New York, 1974, McGraw-Hill Book Co.

Brown, M. A.: Adolescents and VD, Nurs. Outlook **21:**99, 1973.

Brown, M. S.: Syphilis and gonorrhea: an update for nurses in ambulatory settings, Nursing '76 **6:**71-74, January 1976.

Brown, W. J.: Acquired syphilis, drugs, and blood tests, Am. J. Nurs. **71:**713, 1973.

Chang, T., and associates: Genital herpes; some clinical and laboratory observations, J.A.M.A. **229:**544-545, 1974.

Drusin, L. M., and associates: An epidemiologic study of sexually transmitted disease on a university campus, Am. J. Epidemiol. **100:**8, 1974.

Eberly, F. W.: Venereal disease in the adolescent. In Kalafatich, A. J., editor: Approaches to the care of adolescents, New York, 1975, Appleton-Century-Crofts.

Faulkner, W. L., and Ory, H. W.: Intrauterine devices and acute pelvic inflammatory disease, J.A.M.A. **235:**1851-1853, 1976.

Fiscina, B., and associates: Gonococcicidal action of copper in vitro, Am. J. Obstet. Gynecol. **116:**86, 1973.

Fiumara, N. J.: Venereal disease. In Gallagher, J. R., Heald, F. P., and Garell, D. C., editors: Medical care of the adolescent, ed. 3, New York, 1976, Appleton-Century-Crofts.

Gedden, J. O.: International symposium on gonorrhea, Can. Med. Assoc. J. **109:**1043-1050, 1973.

Golub, S.: VD—The unconquered menace, RN **33:**38, 1970.

Hein, K., Marks, A., and Cohen, M. I.: Asymptomatic gonorrhea: prevalence in the population of urban adolescents, J. Pediatr. **90:**634-635, 1977.

Jerome, E., and associates: Gonorrhea at a teenage medical service, Minn. Med. **57:**245, 1974.

Kraus, S. J.: Complications of gonococcal infection, Med. Clin. North Am. **56:**1115-1124, 1972.

Lenz, P. E.: Women, the unwitting carriers of gonorrhea, Am. J. Nurs. **71:**717, 1971.

Mathews, R.: TLC with the penicillin, Am. J. Nurs. **71:**720, 1971.

Minkowski, W., and associates: A view of health education for venereal disease control, Clin. Pediatr. **11:**613, 1972.

Tunnessen, W. W., and Jastremaki, M.: Prepubescent gonococcal vulvovaginitis, Clin. Pediatr. **13:**675-676, 1974.

Vandermeer, D. C.: Meet the VD epidemiologist, Am. J. Nurs. **71:**722-724, 1971.

Venereal Disease Control Advisory Committee: Gonorrhea—Communicable Disease Center recommended treatment schedules, Morbid. Mortal. **23:**341-348, 1974.

Wallace, H. M.: Venereal disease in teen-agers, Clin. Obstet. Gynecol. **14:**432-441, 1971.

Adolescent pregnancy

Abernathy, V.: Illegitimate conception among teenagers, Am. J. Public Health **64:**662, 1974.

Anderson, C.: Adolescent pregnancy, Issues Comprehensive Pediatr. Nurs., pp. 1-16, 1976.

Anonymous: Does anybody care? Am. J. Nurs. **73:**1563, 1973.

Arnold, C. B., and Cogswell, B. E.: A condom distribution program for adolescents: the findings of a feasibility study, Am. J. Public Health **61:**739, 1971.

Bacon, L.: Early motherhood accelerated role transition and social pathologies, Soc. Forces **52:**333-341, 1974.

Ballared, W. M., and Gold, E. M.: Medical and health aspects of reproduction in the adolescent, Clin. Obstet. Gynecol. **14:**338-366, 1971.

Bancroft, A. V.: Pregnancy and the counterculture, Nurs. Clin. North Am. **8:**67-76, 1973.

Brown, F.: Sexual problems of the adolescent girl, Pediatr. Clin. North Am. **19:**759, 1972.

Brown, J. T., and Clancy, B. J.: Meeting the needs of teens regarding their sexuality, Issues Comprehensive Pediatr. Nurs., pp. 29-44, November/December, 1976.

Bryan-Logan, B. N., and Dancy, B. L.: Unwed pregnant adolescents, their mother's dilemma, Nurs. Clin. North Am. **9:**57-68, 1974.

Clancy, B.: The nurse and the abortion patient, Nurs. Clin. North Am. **8:**469-478, 1973.

Clausen, J. P., and associates: Maternity nursing today, New York, 1973, McGraw-Hill Book Co.

Cobliner, W. G., Schulman, H., and Romney, S. L.: The termination of adolescent out-of-wedlock pregnancies and the prospects for their primary prevention, Am. J. Obstet. Gynecol. **115:**432-444, 1973.

Connell, E. B., and Jacobson, L.: Pregnancy, the teenager and sex education, Am. J. Public Health **61:**1840, 1971.

Curtis, F. L.: The pregnant adolescent, Nursing '74 **4:**77, 1974.

Curtis, F. L. S.: Observations of unwed pregnant adolescents, Am. J. Nurs. **74:**100-102, 1974.

Davis, L., and Grace, H.: Anticipatory counseling of unwed pregnant adolescents, Nurs. Clin. North Am. **6:**581-590, 1971.

Dickens, H. O., and associates: One hundred pregnant adolescents: treatment approaches in a university hospital, Am. J. Public Health **63:**794-800, 1973.

Duenhoelter, J. H., and associates: Pregnancy performance of patients under fifteen years of age, Obstet. Gynecol. **46:**49-52, 1975.

Dwyer, J. F.: Teenage pregnancy, Am. J. Obstet. Gynecol. **113:** 373-376, 1974.

Fischman, S. H.: The pregnancy resolution decision of unwed adolescents, Nurs. Clin. North Am. **10:**217-228, 1975.

Frye, B. A., and Barham, B.: Reaching out to pregnant adolescents, Am. J. Nurs. **75:**1502-1504, 1975.

Glasser, M., and associates: The unwanted pregnancy in adolescence, J. Fam. Pract. **2:**91-94, April 1975.

Grant, J., and Heald, F. P.: Complications of adolescent pregnancy. Survey of the literature on fetal outcome in adolescence, Clin. Pediatr. **11:**567-570, 1972.

Harvey, K.: Caring perceptively for the relinquishing mother, Am. J. Maternal Child Nurs. **2:**24-28, January/February 1977.

Howard, M.: Comprehensive community programs for the pregnant teenager, Clin. Obstet. Gynecol. **14:**473-487, 1971.

Jacobson, H. N.: Pregnancy in school age girls. Part I, Food Nutr. News **41**(8):1, 1970.

Jacobson, H. N.: Pregnancy in school age girls. Part II, Food Nutr. News **41**(9):1, 1970.

Jensen, M. D., Bensen, R. C., and Bobak, I. M.: Maternity care:

the nurse and the family, St. Louis, 1977, C. V. Mosby Co.

Jones, P. H., and associates: Pregnancy among high school students, Health Serv. Res. **88:**187-192, 1973.

Juhasz, A. C.: The unmarried adolescent parent, Adolescence **9:** 262-271, 1974.

Kaminetzky, H. A., and associates: The effect of nutrition in teenage gravidas on pregnancy and the status of the neonate. A nutritional profile, Am. J. Obstet. Gynecol. **115:**639, 1971.

Kappelman, M., and associates: A unique school health program in a school for pregnant teenagers, J. Sch. Health **44:**303, 1974.

Klein, L.: Early teenage pregnancy, contraception and repeat pregnancy, Am. J. Obstet. Gynecol. **120:**249-255, 1974.

LaBarre, M.: Emotional crisis of school-age girls during pregnancy and early motherhood, J. Child Psychol. Psychiatry **11:**537-555, 1972.

Malo-Juvera, D.: What pregnant teenagers know about sex, Nurs. Outlook **18:**32-35, November 1970.

Mardosa, S. A.: Rebecca was a primipara—unmarried, retarded, 14 years old and hostile, Nursing '74, pp. 35-36, March 1974.

Marinoff, S. C., and Schonholz, D. H.: Adolescent pregnancy, Pediatr. Clin. North Am. **19:**795, 1972.

McAnarney, E. R.: Adolescent pregnant—a pediatric concern? Clin. Pediatr. **14:**19-22, January 1975.

Menken, J.: The health and social consequences of teenage childbearing, Fam. Plann. Perspect. **4:**45, 1972.

Mercer, R.: Becoming a mother at sixteen, Am. J. Maternal Child Nurs. **1:**44-52, January/February 1976.

Nadelson, C.: Abortion counselling: focus on adolescent pregnancy, Pediatrics **54:**768, 1974.

Naugle, E. H.: Nurse, make it well, Nurs. Outlook **18:**41, 1970.

Nelson, S. A.: School age parents, Child. Today **2:**31-33, 1973.

Osofsky, H. J.: Adolescent out-of-wedlock pregnancy: an overview, Clin. Obstet. Gynecol. **14:**442-456, 1971.

Osofsky, H. J.: The pregnant teen-ager: a medical, educational, and social analysis, Springfield, Ill., 1972, Charles C Thomas, Publisher.

Osofsky, H. J., and Kendall, N.: Poverty as a criterion of risk, Clin. Obstet. Gynecol. **16:**103-109, March 1973.

Pannor, R.: The forgotten man, Nurs. Outlook **18:**36-37, 1970.

Papademetriou, M.: Use of a group technique with unwed mothers and their families, Soc. Work **16:**85-90, October 1971.

Poole, C. J.: Adolescent mothers: can they be helped? Pediatr. Nurs. **2:**7-11, March/April 1976.

Singleton, N., Lewis, H., and Praker, J.: The diet of pregnant teenagers, J. Home Econ. **68**(4):42, 1976.

Smith, E. W., and associates: Adolescent maternity services: a team approach, Children **18**(6):208-213, 1971.

Stickle, G.: Pregnancy in adolescents: scope of the problem, Contemp. Obstet. Gynecol. **5:**85-91, June 1975.

Wallace, H. M., and associates: A study of services and needs of teenage pregnant girls in the large cities of the United States, Am. J. Public Health **63:**28, November 1973.

Walters, J.: Birth defects and adolescent pregnancies, J. Home Econ. **67**(6):23, 1975.

Contraception

Cassidy, J. T.: Teenagers in a family planning clinic, Nurs. Outlook **18**(11):30-31, November 1970.

Connell, E. B.: The pill and its problems, Am. J. Nurs. **71:**326-332, 1971.

Cowart, M., and Newton, D. W.: Oral contraceptives: how best to explain their effects to patients, Nursing '76 **6:**44-48, 1976.

Gedan, S.: Abortion counseling with adolescents, Am. J. Nurs. **74:**1856-1858, 1974.

Goldsmith, S., and associates: Teenagers, sex and contraception, Fam. Plann. Perspect. **4:**32-38, January 1972.

Gordis, L., and associates: Evaluation of a program for preventing adolescent pregnancy, N. Engl. J. Med. **282:**1078-1081, 1970.

Hubbard, C. W.: Family planning education, ed. 2, St. Louis, 1977, The C. V. Mosby Co.

Johnson, C. J.: Attitudes toward premarital sex and family planning for single never pregnant teenage girls, Adolescence **9:** 254-261, 1974.

Johnson, L. B., Burket, R. L., and Rauh, J. L.: Problems with contraception in adolescents: the successful use of an intrauterine device, Clin. Pediatr. **10:**315, 1971.

Manisoff, M. T.: Intrauterine devices, Am. J. Nurs. **73:**1188-1192, 1973.

Miller, W. B.: Sexuality, contraception and pregnancy in a high school population, Calif. Med. **119**(2):14-21, 1973.

Morris, L.: Estimating the need for family planning services among unwed teenagers, Fam. Plann. Perspect. **1:**91-97, 1974.

Oster, O., and Salgi, M.: The copper intrauterine device and its mode of action, N. Engl. J. Med. **293:**432-437, 1975.

Pion, R. J.: Family planning education, Clin. Obstet. Gynecol. **14:**409-419, 1971.

Pomeroy, R., and Landman, L. C.: Public opinion trends: elective abortion and birth control services to teenagers, Fam. Plann. Perspect. **4:**44, 1972.

Rauh, J. L., Burket, R. L., and Brookman, R. R.: Contraception for the teenager, Med. Clin. North Am. **59:**1407-1418, 1975.

Rauh, J. L., Johnson, L. B., and Burket, R. L.: The reproductive adolescent, Pediatr. Clin. North Am. **20:**1005-1020, 1973.

Reichelt, P. A., and Werley, H. H.: Contraception, abortion, and venereal disease; teenager's knowledge and the effect of education, Fam. Plann. Perspect. **7:**83-88, 1975.

Taylor, D.: A new way to teach teens about contraceptives, Am. J. Maternal Child Nurs. **1**(6):378-383, 1976.

Wilcox, A. J., and McAnarney, E. R.: The pediatrician and the prevention of adolescent pregnancy, Clin. Pediatr. **14:**266, 1975.

Sexual assault

Brant, R. S. T., and Tisza, V. B.: The sexually misused child, Am. J. Orthopsychiatr. **47:**80-90, 1977.

Burgess, A. W., and Holmstrom, L. L.: Rape: victims of crisis, Bowie, Md., 1974, Robert J. Brady Co.

Katan, A.: Children who were raped, Psychoanal. Stud. Child. **28:**208, 1973.

Leaman, K.: The sexually abused child, Nursing '77 **7**(5):68, 1977.

Sgroi, S. M.: Sexual molestation of children, Child. Today **4:**18, 1975.

Weitzel, W. D., and associates: Clinical management of father-daughter incest, Am. J. Dis. Child. **132:**127, 1978.

21

Problems of psychologic adjustment to adolescence

Adolescence is a time of transition, maturational crisis, and adjustment. It involves an increasingly larger segment of the population with a larger peer group. In addition adolescence is becoming more prolonged and intense. The transition to adulthood with its prescribed developmental tasks is characterized by change, growth, and stress. Ineffective and unsuccessful accomplishment of these developmental tasks produces a sense of diffuse discomfort within some adolescents who respond with faulty problem solving in their search for relief from the discomfort and stress of this transitional period of life.

Psychophysiologic disorders

The term psychophysiologic disorders is applied to physical disturbances in which psychologic factors play a prominent role. They involve those organ systems that are regulated by the autonomic nervous system, including the skin, the respiratory system, the gastrointestinal system, the cardiovascular system, and the nervous system itself. There are probably innate biologic factors that predispose to these disorders with psychologic and social factors that act as additional predisposing, precipitating, or perpetuating influences. Some of these diseases are discussed elsewhere, such as asthma (p. 1241), eczema (p. 488), peptic ulcer (p. 1285), ulcerative colitis (p. 1281), and recurrent abdominal pain as related to school phobia (p. 648). Other disorders with a strong psychologic component that are seen with increased frequency in late childhood and adolescence are the so-called disorders of eating—anorexia nervosa and obesity. Emotional difficulties appear to be associated with both undereating and overeating.

ANOREXIA NERVOSA

Anorexia nervosa (AN) is the term applied to a long-recognized disorder characterized by severe weight loss in the absence of obvious physical cause. The term anorexia nervosa inaccurately describes the disorder in which emaciation occurs as a result of self-inflicted starvation. Anorexia nervosa occurs predominantly in adolescent females, and the incidence appears to be increasing significantly.

Etiology and characteristics

The onset of anorexia nervosa generally takes place at or near menarche, but it may begin in preadolescence or in adulthood. The peak ages are 12 and 13 years, with another peak occuring around ages 19 to 20 years or in the mid-twenties. Anorexia nervosa is relatively rare in males. Young women who have this disorder are most often from the upper or middle classes, are often described as "good children," are academically high achievers, are conforming, are conscientious, and have a high energy level, even with marked emaciation. These girls are usually strongly dependent on their parents, and frequently an ambivalent mother-daughter relationship is present. There is often a history of family strife with the anorexia nervosa being a symptom of the family pathology. However, the etiology of the disorder remains unclear. There is a distinct psychologic component, and the diagnosis is based primarily on psychologic and behavioral criteria. Nevertheless, the physical manifestations of anorexia nervosa lend support to possible organic factors in the etiology.

In the wake of the severe weight loss, these young girls exhibit signs of altered metabolic activity. They develop secondary amenorrhea, bradycardia, lowered body temperature, decreased blood pressure, and cold intolerance. They have dry skin and brittle nails and develop lanugo hair. The changes are usually reversible with adequate weight gain and improved nutritional status.

Psychologic aspects. Dominating the psychologic aspects of anorexia nervosa are a relentless pursuit of thinness and a fear of fatness, usually preceded by a period of a year or two of mood disturbances and behavior changes. The weight loss is usually triggered by a typical adolescent crisis such as the onset of menstruation or traumatic interpersonal incidents that precipitate serious dieting that continues out of control. Frequently there is an exaggerated misinterpretation of the normal fat deposition characteristic of the early adolescent period, or someone may comment that the adolescent girl is putting on weight. The weight loss may be a response to teasing, some change in her life (such as changing schools or going off to college), or an incident that requires an independent decision that she is unprepared to make (such as a career choice).

The syndrome of anorexia nervosa consists of three major areas of disordered psychologic functioning[7]:

1. *Disturbed body image and body concept of delusional proportions.* The young girl identifies with her emaciation, defending the skeletonlike appearance as normal, actively maintains it, and denies that it is abnormal. She indicates that it is rewarding to achieve and maintain this emaciated state. She is increasingly fearful of weight gain and interprets the concern of others as attempts to make her fat.
2. *Inaccurate and confused perception and interpretation of inner stimuli.* Inaccurate hunger awareness is pronounced. The adolescent does not recognize signs of nutritional need in herself and is unable to assess the amounts of food taken. She may feel "full" after only a few bites and derives pleasure from the refusal of food. She may even resort to induced vomiting after eating and use of laxatives to speed passage of food. Associated with this eating behavior, a preoccupation and tremendous involvement with food and related activities are demonstrated, as she frequently assumes all meal planning and preparation for others. Also, girls with anorexia nervosa often increase their activity to help counteract the possibility of weight gain. This hyperactivity may continue until emaciation is far advanced.
3. *Paralyzing sense of ineffectiveness that pervades all aspects of daily life.* Contrary to the defiant and rebellious attitude displayed by anorectic children, they are overwhelmed by a deep sense of ineffectiveness. They are convinced that they only function in response to demands and wishes of others rather than doing as they want or choose to do. They have always been compliant children, but careful analysis reveals this to be mechanical obedience and overconformity that is not recognized as a reflection of a serious problem—a self-doubt regarding their ability to stand up for themselves or even the right for self-assertion.

Organic etiology. Evidence of organic etiology has been accumulated that may implicate abnormalities of hypothalamic-pituitary and end-organ function in individuals with anorexia nervosa. This is based on the observation that secondary amenorrhea is a common finding and that appetite and satiety are hypothalamic functions. Associated symptoms manifest in anorexia nervosa that relate to hypothalamic dysfunction include abnormalities of thermoregulation and water conservation. There is evidence that supports the possible involvement of the hypothalamus in the pathogenesis of the abnormalities of anorexia nervosa in the following ways[32]:

1. The severe starvation may directly damage the hypothalamus.
2. The hypothalamic dysfunction may be secondary to primary psychologic abnormalities.
3. Anorexia nervosa may be a primary hypothalamic disorder that produces secondary psychologic changes.

Nursing considerations related to medical management

The treatment and management of anorexia nervosa are directed toward correction of the severe state of malnutrition and resolution of the psychologic disorganization. Because of the psychogenic nature of the disorder, treatment is difficult and requires long-term management. All of those involved in therapy must keep in mind the adolescent's distorted sense of body image and self-awareness and her feelings of self-doubt, ineffectiveness, and helplessness that prompt such bizarre behavior in order to feel in control of her own body functions.

The initial goal is to treat the life-threatening malnutrition with strict adherence to dietary requirements, which sometimes necessitates intravenous and tube feedings. The most successful approach uses simple operant conditioning that emphasizes positive reinforcement for weight gain. A clearly defined behavior modification plan is communicated to the child and maintained through a unified team approach by all persons involved in her care. Children whose pathology can be clearly related to a dysfunctional family situation respond to therapy best when separated from the family. Many of those whose therapy plan is implemented in the hospital need a continued behavior modification program after discharge in order to maintain the desired weight.

Psychotherapy is aimed at helping the child resolve the adolescent identity crisis, particularly as it relates to a distorted body image. Nurses need to adopt and maintain a kind, supporting, yet firm, manner in managing the care of an anorectic child without creating a passive-dependency attitude in the child. The child requires the sustained support and reassurance as she copes with ambivalent feelings related to her own body concept and the desire to see herself as cooperative, reliable, and worthy of the kindness she receives. Encouraging the child with education and activities that strengthen her self-esteem facilitates her resocialization process and social acceptance among her peers.

OBESITY

There is probably no problem related to adolescence that is so obvious to others, is so difficult to treat, and has such long-term effects on psychologic and physical health status as obesity. It is the most common nutritional disturbance of children and one of the most challenging contemporary health problems at all ages. The incidence of obesity has been conservatively estimated to be 10% to 12% of prepubertal children and anywhere from 10% or 15% to 30% of adolescents. Fully 80% to 85% of obese children perpetuate their obesity into adulthood; 50% of grossly obese adults were obese as children. Since adult obesity is associated with increased mortality and morbidity from a variety of complications, both physical and psychologic, the presence of adolescent obesity is a serious condition that deserves the interest and attention of health professionals.

The definition of obesity has always led to some confusion and, at best, is very imprecise. Because there is such variability in height and weight among normal healthy children, it is often difficult to determine the presence or extent of obesity from comparing a set of numbers with a standardized table of weights and heights. This is especially true in adolescence, when there is normally a period of rapid weight gain and linear growth together with varying rates of muscular development. The greatest amount of confusion is related to the distinction between the terms "overweight" and "obesity." *Obesity* is an increase in body weight resulting from an excessive accumulation of fat or simply the state of being too fat. *Overweight* refers to the state of weighing more than average for one's height and body build, which may or may not include an increased amount of fat. It is possible for two children to have the same height and weight and for one to be obese whereas the other is not. This is particularly evident during early adolescence when there are considerable differences in the rates of muscular development. Obesity is easily recognized, although it is difficult to assess its severity, especially in children who are overweight to a lesser degree.

Etiology and pathophysiology

Obesity results from a caloric intake that consistently exceeds caloric requirements and expenditure. The causes that produce this disequilibrium are complex and may involve a variety of influences including metabolic, hypothalamic, hereditary, social, cultural, and psychologic factors. Evidence indicates that obese children and adults were not obese at birth. Birth weight offers no clue in detection and prediction of childhood obesity; obese children do not have higher birth weights than nonobese children. However, there is a high correlation between adolescent obesity and a significantly increased weight at 1 year of age.

The various etiologies attributed to childhood obesity have been classified in a number of ways, such as endogenous and/or exogenous, and regulatory and metabolic. Many factors are involved and often are so closely interrelated that it is usually impossible to isolate any cause.

Genetic factors.[25] Heredity has been demonstrated to be an important factor in the development of obesity in some cases. It has been repeatedly illustrated that the incidence of obese children born to obese parents is significantly higher than those born to parents of normal weight: 3% to 7% of children born to parents of normal weight are obese, 40% of obese children have one parent who is obese, and 80% of obese children have both parents who are obese. Comparison of natural and adopted children shows a positive correlation for weight between children and their natural parents. Also, studies of identical and fraternal twins reveal an extremely high correlation between identical twins but not fraternal twins—even identical twins who were reared in different environments. The tendency to obesity is manifest whenever environmental conditions are favorable, such as an abundance of food and reduced or minimal physical activity (such as ready availability of automobiles).

General body build seems to have some effect on obesity. Observations of obese adolescent girls indicate that they tend to be more endomorphic (see p. 611), somewhat mesomorphic, but considerably less ectomorphic than nonobese children of comparable ages. Endomorphy is, then, an established inherited characteristic that predisposes to the accumulation of fat, unless there is insufficient diet, greater activity, disease, or other intervening factors. There is also evidence from animal experiments to indicate that some humans may inherit a metabolic defect that interferes with the breakdown of fat once it has been stored in adipose tissue. For these persons maintaining an ideal weight is much more difficult than it is for others. There are some inherited diseases in which obesity develops as one of the features of a symptom complex. In these instances obesity may be caused by endocrine or hypothalamic dysfunction or inactivity.

In any situation in which heredity is suspected as a predisposing cause of obesity, there are also environmental implications. It is almost impossible to distinguish between hereditary and environmental factors, since both may be operative in any situation, especially when other family members are also obese. Family eating patterns, ethnic diet, and psychologic factors play an important role; to many persons, fat is still considered to be an indication of good health.

Metabolic and endocrine factors.[3,16,25] The complex interrelationships between hunger, satiety, the central nervous system, and the metabolism of carbohydrates, fats, and protein continue to be investigated in relation to their role in obesity. The primary source of energy storage is adipose tissue, with its high-caloric density and mass. The status of this stored energy is constantly changing, and its volume depends on the equilibrium between deposition and release of triglycerides, the storage form of fat. Experiments with laboratory animals have led to a number of theories regarding fat utilization and obesity. It appears that the obese are able to store fat easily but are either unable to release this stored fat or to burn it for energy. In obesity there is a diminished capacity to mobilize fat stores, but it is unclear whether the obese state causes this alteration in metabolism. There is some indication that human beings and animals may possess a mechanism that prevents the development of obesity. A malfunction of this theorized mechanism, which normally converts excess calories into heat, would lead, instead, to conversion of calories into triglycerides that are then deposited in the fat cell.

It is known that the metabolism of glucose plays an important role in the regulation of fat deposition, since excess calories from carbohydrates are stored as fat and a lack of glucose prompts the release of fat as a source of energy. It also appears that glucose is the prime substance to which the satiety center responds and that there is a relationship between hyperinsulinism and the promotion of fat storage. Insulin enhances glucose entry into the adipose cell, stimulates the synthesis of triglycerides, and inhibits triglyceride lipolysis. Therefore, it is a potent lipogenic agent that favors the maintenance of the obese state and complicates treatment.

Defects in any one or a combination of these processes may alter the rate of fat storage. Although none of these mechanisms has been conclusively demonstrated in man, it has been observed that many obese persons do not eat a greater amount than normal persons—often they consume even less. Whereas the metabolism of carbohydrates and fats is known to be impaired in obesity, neither is actually considered to be a primary cause of obesity, but, rather, they are secondary to the obese state.

Work with experimental animals has also provided support to possible physiologic regulatory and metabolic mechanisms in the etiology of obesity, although the implication for humans is still speculative. Dysfunction of the central regulatory mechanism involving hunger and satiety causes an increased intake of food, possibly by interfering with transmission of signals to the satiety center or by altering the threshold of the center to such signals. The individual, unaware when satiety is reached, continues to eat. The relationship of hypothalamic dysfunction and obesity is substantiated in observations of obese persons who have been demonstrated to have suffered discrete or diffuse hypothalamic injury, for example, following tumors or trauma.

Malfunction of various endocrine glands has sometimes been associated with the development of obesity. These include abnormal responses of the pancreatic secretions insulin and glucagon, hypothyroidism (p. 1465), and hyperactivity of the adrenal cortex (p. 1472). Abnormalities in both metabolic and endocrine function have been observed in obese individuals, but the relationships remain unclear.

It has also been observed that on the whole obese children tend to be taller than average with somewhat larger lean body mass. There is some evidence to indicate that growth is accelerated by overnutrition much the same as it is retarded by undernutrition. Consequently children who are obese in infancy seem to attain relatively greater height than those with later-onset obesity.

Caloric equilibrium and obesity. As stated previously, obesity develops when caloric intake consistently exceeds caloric output and may arise from either an excessive intake of calories or a reduced expenditure of calories. It is consistently observed that obese children are less active than lean children, but it is uncertain whether the inactivity creates the obesity or if the obesity is responsible for the inactivity. However, it appears that in childhood overeating is the dominant feature, whereas in adult life reduced physical activity with normal intake is more likely to be the rule.

Although the intake of obese persons who are inactive is lower than that of leaner persons, obese persons eat more at a given sitting and eat more rapidly than nonobese persons. It appears characteristic that obese persons not only exhibit an overwhelming appetite but often overeat when they are not hungry or have no appetite. They apparently respond to other cues as well as to the hunger stimulus. It has also been shown that feeding habits and frequency of food ingestion may produce alterations in enzyme activities in both adipose cells and muscle cells. Comparison of individuals who consume similar amounts of calories ingested either as one meal (gorging) or intermittently over a period of time (nibbling) results in an increase of body fat in the "gorgers." It appears that lipogenesis is accelerated following "gorging" patterns of food intake when compared with "nibbling" patterns.[5,20] Obese adolescents are characteristically night eaters and often skip meals, particularly breakfast.

There are some children and adolescents who, from early infancy, demonstrate a significantly lower level of activity. In fact, there is no correlation between the total calories consumed and weight, but there is an inverse relationship between the amounts of subcutaneous fat and calorie intake of extremely thin and extremely fat infants. Fat children often consume fewer calories than thinner ones; however, there is a striking correlation between food intake and activity level of infants. Extremely thin infants move more and eat more than normal infants, and extremely fat infants move less and eat less.[11] This same relationship is often observed in older obese children and adolescents. For example, obese adolescents expend much less energy during exercise activities than their nonobese counterparts.

Cellular structure. Two distinct types of obesity have been identified based on the cellular character of the adipose tissue: hyperplastic (10%), in which there is a small to moderate increase in adipose cell size but an increase in cell number, hypertrophic (20%), in which there is a large increase in cell size alone, and combined hyperplastic and hypertrophic (70%). It is also recognized that there is a decided relationship between the age of onset of obesity and the cell type: hyperplastic obesity is associated with early-onset obesity and a marked increase in obesity at the time of puberty and hypertrophic obesity with later-onset obesity at mid to late adolescence. The onset of the combined form is usually in early childhood with a dramatic increase during puberty, and adiposity is relatively greater in the combined form than in the other two types.[3]

At the time of birth the infant has about one fourth to one fifth the total number of adipocytes when compared with an adult, although the total amount of lipid is about one fourth that of the adult. Therefore, between birth and adulthood both the size and number of adipose cells increase four to five times. One of the last specific tissues to develop, the adipose tissue cells begin forming at many sites during the third to fourth months of gestation and begin to accumulate fat. The major portion is deposited during the latter part of the prenatal period until, at birth, adipose tissue accounts for approximately 28% of total body weight. Development of adipose tissue continues to increase steadily during the first 9 months after birth and then reaches a plateau, after which there is a slight increment until 7 to 9 years of age, when fat again increases. The final spurt occurs during early adolescence.

Expansion of fat deposits in obese persons is a result principally of an increase in cell number, which consists of a twofold to threefold increase in most obese subjects. Some also have an increase in cell size as well, but many possess normal-size cells. Persons who become obese very early are those who have most nearly normal cell size but the greatest increase in cell number. In extremely obese persons cell numbers increase threefold and cell size increases by 50%. This hypercellular state persists into adulthood, unchanged by diet manipulation. The most sensitive periods of development that have major consequences for adult adiposity appears to be during the rapid cell proliferation and growth phases of the years between birth and 5 years of age. The two peak periods of onset of juvenile obesity are from birth to 4 years of age and the ages between about 7 and 9 to 11 or 13 years.[6]

Although the relationship between infantile and later-onset obesity has been reported by a number of authorities, not all overweight infants are doomed to become obese adults. The genetic predisposition, family eating patterns, activity level, and other factors also play an important role in ultimate size. It may be that overfeeding establishes a lifetime eating pattern, but it can be equally true that some infants are more easily programmed into a pattern of overeating.[30]

Psychologic, social, and cultural factors. Patterns of eating are culturally and socially based in most instances, and, in some, the food preferences of the culture contribute to the development of obesity. Many cultures consider plump children to be a sign of health, and some look on obesity as evidence of well-being and foster weight gain as a desirable feature. In others obesity is a status symbol or an indication of affluence. It is not uncommon for obese children to be a product of families in which eating patterns of large meals are emphasized or in which children are taught to eat everything on their plates and are admonished for leaving any food. Parents often have an exaggerated concept of the amount of food children should eat and expect them to eat more than they need.

It has also been observed that in the developed countries such as the United States and countries in Western Europe there is a marked difference in the prevalence of obesity between upper and lower class children and that these differences are frequently apparent before 6 years of age. Lower socioeconomic groups have a greater prevalence of obesity, especially in girls, and this obese state is established earlier and increases at a more rapid rate.[29]

Psychologic factors may provide a basis for eating patterns in childhood. In infancy the child first experiences relief from discomfort through feeding and learns to associate eating with feelings of well-being, security, and the comforting presence of the mothering person. Soon eating is deeply associated with the feeling of being loved. To the infant, to be fed is to be loved; satiety is security. In addition the pleasurable oral sensation of sucking provides an additional connection between emotions and early eating behavior. Many parents use food, such as candy and other "treats," as a positive reinforcer for desired behavior or as a way to compensate for their own feelings of guilt, especially if the child was unwanted or overvalued because of loss of a previous child. This practice soon acquires symbolic significance to the extent that the child continues to use food as a reward, a comfort, and a means by which to deal with feelings of depression or hostility.

In some children overweight may be the normal state and may simply represent the upper end of the normal distribution curve. These children are most comfortable when they are well filled out, and they may or may not have emotional problems. Others may begin overeating and reducing activity in response to a traumatic or upsetting event in their lives, such as the death of a parent or sibling, separation from parents, or social or scholastic failure, or as a response to illness or surgery.[7]

Obesity may be one manifestation of a disturbed way of life. Typically families of obese children are markedly socially introverted and rely on family members for socialization. Television viewing is the primary source of entertainment. Frequently the family is composed of a domineering, ambitious mother and a passive, docile father. Marital disharmony is common. There are usually only one or two children in the family. The obese child assumes the role of active participant with dependent, submissive, and generally immature behavior. The child follows the family's social pattern of isolation and tends to react to frustration with withdrawal or hostility. On school entrance the child is totally unprepared for experiences outside the shelter of the family group. Consequently he turns to food for solace, which has become the child's manner of coping with traumatic experiences, failure, and disappointment. Once obesity has developed, the family patterns of personal and social interaction tend to perpetuate it.[2]

Obesity in adolescence

Obesity in adolescence may appear simultaneously with the onset of adolescence, or it may have existed prior to puberty. Although there may be differences in the psychophysiologic dynamics in its development, the effect of the obese condition on the teenager is the same. A great deal has been hypothesized about the psychogenic factors in obesity; however, the psychologic *effects* of being obese are undoubtedly underestimated. Obesity is a serious handicap to the social life of a child and, to an even greater extent, to the life of a teenager. The common emotional sequelae of obesity in adolescence are defective body image, low self-esteem, social isolation, and feelings of rejection and depression.[15]

Adolescent-onset obesity appears to be closely related to the child's inability to master the developmental tasks of adolescence; as a result he regresses to the self-satisfying tactic of overeating to compensate. Unfortunately this mechanism only creates an additional obstacle to achieving the desired goal. The obesity, however, serves to ward off the pressures engendered by the internal changes of puberty and the outside world. The obesity becomes the safeguard. As long as the child remains fat, he does not have to deal with this repressed emotional material. He may come to view his obesity as a handicap responsible for all his disappointments. He thus avoids making the adaptations necessary to growth and maturation. Eating is his means of coping with the normal drives of adolescence and more closely binds him to the family, especially the mother, who provides the food. Thus he becomes increasingly dependent on food as a means of gratification. This impedes the normal processes of separation and individuation, since he tends to shy away from his peers and become more closely bound to the family.

Vulnerable personality. Obesity is most often a symptom in passive-dependent, compliant youngsters who are easily controlled by guilt and shame. They are easily influenced by outside forces, such as parents, peers, and school, that they consider to be more powerful than themselves. When faced with an internal or external stress, these youngsters react with helplessness, ambivalence, and a tendency to seek support from someone they see as stronger than themselves, either adult or peer.[18]

There are many psychologic implications in the development and perpetuation of obesity. It may represent aggression directed at the self, an attempt (in younger children) to grow bigger in order to physically deal with a hated person, or a means to bring shame and embarrassment to another (often the mother). Many overweight adolescents use obesity as a means of revenge. However, they easily become a scapegoat for the frustrations and anger of parents and others as a source of embarrassment and shame. A common problem is the ambivalence of mothers who like to see their daughters eat but, at the same time, desire them to have slender figures.

Self-concept and obesity. Obese adolescents score higher on depression-measurement tests than thinner teenagers and significantly lower on body-image tests, indicating a less positive or a more impaired body concept. Unlike many disorders, the fact of the youngster's obesity is a matter of general knowledge, continually on display for others to see. Some of the personality characteristics reflecting the psychologic effects of obesity have been likened to those experienced by ethnic and racial minorities who have been subjected to intense discrimination. These include passivity, obsessive concern with the self-image, expectation of rejection, and progressive withdrawal. This sets into motion a cyclic pattern wherein the youngsters expect rejection, feel awkward and out of place in the social situation, isolate themselves from social contacts, and then experience actual rejection. The decreased opportunity for activity outside the home provides increased exposure to food that leads to an increase in the obesity.[15]

Obese adolescents, particularly obese girls, consider obesity undesirable and intensely dislike their figures and physical characterisitcs. They are concerned about their obesity, are extremely self-deprecating, and judge other people in terms of degree of adiposity. They express contempt for fat persons and admiration for thin ones. They consider their bodies to be grotesque and are certain that others, too, are contemptuous of them. Stylish, age-appropriate clothing is difficult to find and, when available, is restricted to special shops or departments with labels that further emphasize the negative aspects of appearance. Sexual attractiveness is severely impaired or nonexistent; obese youngsters rarely date.

There are three major factors that contribute to the development of a disturbed body image: (1) the age of onset of the obesity—body-image disturbances are primarily found in persons who were obese as children and adolescents or as adolescents alone; (2) presence of emotional disturbances or neuroses—a stable personality and a secure childhood appear to prevent body-image distortion, whereas emotional disturbances caused by the effects of a disturbed family will invite the development of a distorted body image; and (3) a negative evaluation of the obesity by others—the child internalizes the attitudes conveyed by significant others. It appears that there is a critical period for development of a distorted body image that is characteristic of persons who were obese during adolescence. Those who become obese as adults rarely demonstrate this disturbance. During adolescence and when the youngster is establishing a sense of identity, derogatory views by peers and parents are incorporated into enduring views of the self.[28] Fig. 21-1 illustrates the interrelated factors that contribute to adolescent obesity.

Diagnostic evaluation

The presence of obesity is obvious from appearance alone, and a gross determination can be made by a rough comparison of height and weight with standard growth charts. Children who are 20% over the normal for their height and weight should be further evaluated. Evaluation

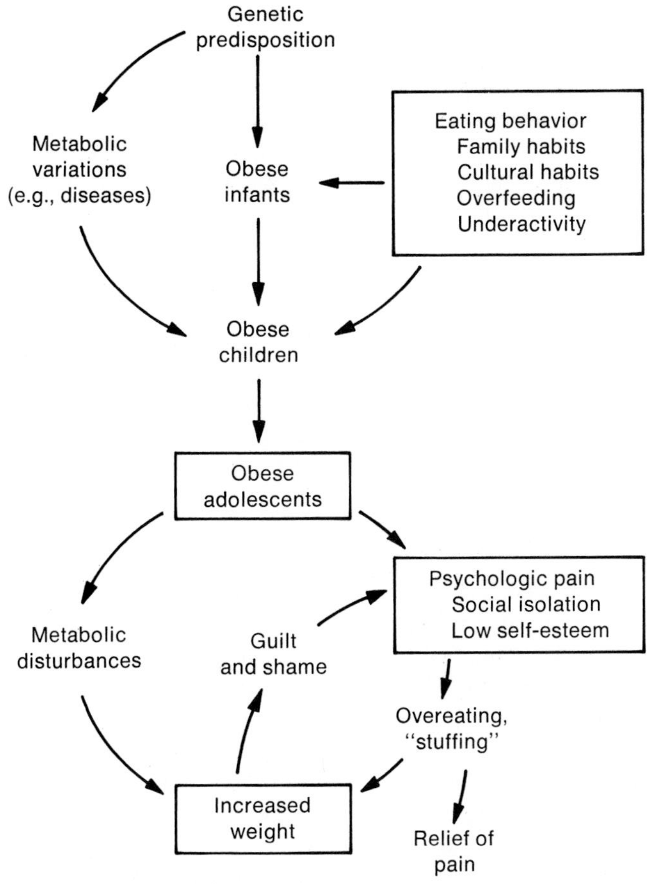

Fig. 21-1. Complex relationships in adolescent obesity.

includes a height and weight history of the child, parents, and siblings as well as eating habits, appetite and hunger patterns, and physical activities engaged in. A careful history is taken regarding the development of the obesity, and a physical examination is carried out to help differentiate simple obesity from increased fat resulting from organic causes. Psychologic assessment, accomplished via interviews with the child and standardized personality tests, provides insight into personality and emotional problems that contribute to obesity and that might interfere with therapy. Appropriate diagnostic tests rule out suspected metabolic and endocrine disorders.

It is useful to have an estimation of the degree of fatness in order to have some idea of the component of body weight that can be modified. Several tests, both scientific and unscientific, can be employed to assess obesity. Simple screening tests for use in older children and adolescents include weight tables, observation, ruler test, belt-line test, pinch test, and anthropometric measurements.

Weight tables. Comparison with weight charts is an initial screening device that does not take into consideration the body build. The tables vary according to the source of data.

Observation. The child *looks* fat.

Ruler test. Normally the slope of the abdomen between the ribs and the pelvis is flat or slightly concave when the individual is lying on the back. If a ruler that is placed on the midline of the body touches both the ribs and the pelvis, the individual is not too fat.

Belt-line test (older boys). The circumference of the chest at the level of the nipples normally exceeds that of the abdomen at the level of the umbilicus. If the abdominal girth is greater, the abdominal fat is excessive.

Pinch test. At least half the body fat is found directly beneath the skin. At many locations on the body, a fold of skin and subcutaneous fat can be lifted free, between thumb and forefinger, from underlying tissues. These areas include the midtriceps area of the upper arm, the side of the lower chest, the subscapular region of the back, the back of the calf, and the abdomen. Ordinarily this subcutaneous layer should be from 6 to 12 mm (0.25 to 0.5 inch) thick, and, since a fold of skin is double thickness, a skinfold should be between 12 and 25 mm (0.5 to 1 inch) thick. The normal range in adolescents is somewhat less, about 12 to 15 mm (0.5 to 0.6 inch). A fold significantly greater than 18 to 20 mm or approximately 1 inch (an "inch to the pinch") indicates an excess of subcutaneous fat. A practical and more accurate means for determining obesity from skin-fold thickness is by the use of special skin-fold calipers. This device, calibrated in millimeters, allows the operator to control the pressure on the skin fold and provides a more precise measurement of its thickness. The Committee on Nutritional Anthropometry of the National Research Council recommends use of the triceps and subscapular areas for skin-fold measurements.

More rigorous but more refined methods for assessing body fat involve a variety of indirect techniques. The only direct method, chemical analysis, cannot be conducted on living human beings.

Anthropometric measurements. A series of assessments of body fat are carried out by a number of measurements: caliper measurement of skin-fold thickness; circumferences and diameters of chest, abdomen, and limbs; and x-ray determination of soft-tissue, muscle, and bone mass.

More sophisticated techniques include the *densimetric* method of determining body fat from measures of body density (fat has a low specific gravity); *hydrometry,* which estimates body fat from measurement of total body water; and *radiopotassium,* which evaluates the extent of fat from whole-body potassium content (fat cells contain almost no potassium).

Complications of childhood obesity

The most prevalent complication of childhood obesity is its persistence into adulthood, with its remarkable resistance to treatment. With few exceptions, clearly identifiable hazards are rarely present in childhood, but the dangers of obesity increase with its duration. The adult with long-standing obesity is subject to the development of associated medical complications that include diabetes and cardiovascular disease.[15]

The most serious physical effect of severe obesity encountered in childhood is the Pickwickian syndrome, named after the Charles Dickens' character "Fat Boy Joe," who was continually falling asleep. Although the mechanism is unknown, narcolepsy associated with this obese state is thought to be caused by carbon dioxide narcosis from a decreased ventilatory capacity. There is an increased incidence of certain orthopedic problems in obese children, especially Legg-Perthes disease (p. 1525) and genu valgum (knock knee). Probably the most destructive complications are the psychosocial problems that affect obese youngsters as a result of teasing, ridicule, and rejection by peers and family.

Nursing considerations in medical management

Because of the self-perpetuating nature of obesity, efforts to treat the condition have been universally disappointing. A high proportion of obese children become obese adults. Because most of the nonsurgical approaches to weight reduction and maintenance suffer from a lack of lasting success, a more effective and sustained approach is a preventive one—early recognition and establishment of control measures before the child arrives at an obese state. However, varying degrees of success have been achieved in some highly motivated individuals through weight-reduction techniques, including diet and exercise, drugs, behavior modification, and psychologic support.

Medical and nursing management care are considered together since nearly all successful weight-reduction programs involve professional nurses. Few physicians are able or inclined to devote the time to the long-term supportive care needed to maintain the motivation of obese youngsters. Although therapy involves a team approach that includes the physician, dietitian, family, and the child himself, nurses play a dominant role in any regulated and promising program of weight reduction. Interested nurse practitioners are able to evaluate, treat, and follow the overweight adolescent. They also assume an important position in recognizing potential weight problems and assisting parents and their children in programs of prevention.

Guidelines for treatment. There are several factors related to the adolescent that health professionals must keep in mind when planning and implementing treatment for youngsters in this age-group. First weight gain and anabolism are normal and necessary to healthy development during adolescent years and any weight-reduction program must protect the teenager from prolonged catabolism that may permanently impair growth. Second the energy-absorbing developmental tasks of adolescence are sufficiently stressful in themselves that the psychologic stress of food deprivation may be more than the adolescent can handle.[16]

Motivation to lose weight is the key to success. The reasons behind the teenager's desire to lose weight need to be explored with him, but success is rarely achieved unless the youngster is motivated to lose weight and takes personal responsibility for his dietary habits and exercise program. Teenagers who are forced by parents to seek help are seldom sufficiently motivated, become rebellious of parental nagging, and are unwilling to control dietary intake. A rigid approach and one that is based on parental enforcement of the regimen is usually doomed from the start. The strained relationships between parents and teenager are intensified by parental coercion, and, because adolescents get food outside the home, adults simply cannot control their food intake. The result is an angry, sullen, and rebellious youngster who gains rather than loses weight.[3,16]

Diet. Planning caloric restriction for the adolescent during the rapid growth period requires a careful design. Adolescents are unusually sensitive to caloric restriction, both physically and psychologically. It is extremely difficult to achieve the ideal reduction in body fat without concurrent loss in lean body mass. The nature of energy metabolism is such that protein and carbohydrate are the preferred substrate for metabolism and are, therefore, utilized before fats. Even a moderate reduction in calories can, and often does, produce a negative nitrogen balance in adolescent youth. Sharp restriction in calories may result in relatively large losses of lean body mass and is not recommended for children or adolescents. Consequently the diet must be calculated carefully with the assistance of someone, usually a dietitian, who has a thorough understanding of diet and metabolism. Sometimes the most realistic approach during the rapid growth period is simply to prevent an increase in body fat. Children in early adolescence are usually less motivated than older adolescents and are more easily subject to a negative nitrogen balance. In middle or late adolescence, after the peak spurt in height and weight, the goal might be a relatively constant loss of weight to achieve an approximate ideal weight over a period of several months. Adipose tissue and any gains or losses are easily monitored by measuring triceps skin folds.

Since obesity is usually a lifelong problem, it is best to provide the individual with a diet that can be maintained throughout life with the emphasis on restricting calories. The most successful diets are those that use ordinary foods in controlled portions rather than diets that require the avoidance of any specific food. The youngster is taught how to incorporate favorite foods into the diet and how to select substitutes that are also satisfying. The dieting youngster should eat what the rest of the family eats, but less of it, and should not be deprived of favorite foods. These can be allowed—in small amounts. There are a multitude of restricted calorie diets available from a number of sources, such as the American Dietetic Association, and the caloric values for a wide variety of commercial foods are available to facilitate meal planning.[9]

Adolescents must be cautioned about the risk of dieting without the guidance of a health professional. They are easy prey to current fads and the influence of friends and well-meaning adults. Unfortunately many teenagers resort to complete abstinence, a liquid protein diet, and other diet methods that may reflect the current mode. Such severe restrictions are particularly hazardous to the teenager.

Snacking, for the teenager, is an integral part of the daily routine, which makes dieting especially difficult for the obese adolescent. Consequently the youngster who is serious about dieting should be helped in elimination or judicious selection of snack foods. For example, getting rid of high-calorie junk foods and placing snack foods out of sight help divert attention away from eating. Also, when snacking, several of a particular item are usually eaten; therefore, substituting several items with lower caloric value for one item higher in calories is more satisfying. For example, three vanilla wafers should be substituted for one Oreo cream sandwich or several small stick pretzels at 1 kcal each for one large pretzel with 58 kcal.

No adolescent should be encouraged to initiate a reduction diet without a health assessment, evaluation, and counseling. It is also important to emphasize the undesirable nature of the fad diets and crash programs that continually appear in various publications. Although some success has been achieved with low-carbohydrate, high-fat diets, their unpalatability and dietary boredom contribute to a high failure rate. Exotic diets have not been successful, and their unbalanced nature makes them potentially dangerous for growing children or adolescents. To be successful from all aspects, a dietary program should be nutritionally sound with sufficient satiety value, produce the desired weight loss, and be accompanied by nutrition education and continued support.[8]

Exercise. Since weight loss will occur only when caloric expenditure is greater than caloric intake, physical activity in the form of regularly scheduled exercise, progressively increased over the child's usual activity, is an integral part of a weight-reduction program. Activities should be those that stress self-improvement rather than competition, and teenagers need continued psychologic support and encouragement to prevent the beginning of the destructive cycle of passivity, withdrawal, and rejection.

Drugs. A variety of preparations have been introduced as a means for achieving weight loss, ostensibly to decrease appetite to help the individual follow a reduction diet or to utilize energy more effectively and to a greater degree. Most authorities agree that drugs have limited value in achieving permanent weight loss and are transient in action, useless, or actually harmful. They are used occasionally as a matter of convenience or as a supportive measure for a short period during the initial phase of therapy. Some drugs that may be prescribed include anorectics, thyroid preparations, fat-mobilizing substances (FMS), hydrophilic substances, human chorionic gonadotropin (HCG), laxatives, and diuretics.

Anorectics, or appetite depressants. These are usually the amphetamines. They have relatively short-lived effectiveness and can produce tolerance, habituation, addiction, and, sometimes, psychoses. Because of their potential for dependence and abuse, they are usually contraindicated.

Thyroid preparations. Drugs that stimulate the thyroid are potentially dangerous to growing children since they accelerate the already increased tissue metabolism, which may have deleterious effects on the functioning of vital organs.

Fat-mobilizing substances (FMS). Since obese persons have been shown to demonstrate diminished levels of fat-mobilizing substances, injections of these substances have produced weight loss in some patients by mobilizing the fat. However, further evaluation is needed in relation to their use in children.

Hydrophilic substances. Indigestible bulk preparations such as methylcellulose have been prescribed to produce anorexia by expanding the stomach and thus producing a feeling of satiety. Their value is questionable.

Human chorionic gonadotropin (HCG). Injections of human chorionic gonadotropin have become popular in weight control clinics, ostensibly to increase metabolism fat. There is no evidence to support its effectiveness in treatment of obesity, and its potential harmful effects, especially on the ovary, contraindicate its use in children and adolescents.

Laxatives and diuretics. Laxatives and diuretics, used without a prescription, are often tried by the individual to induce a temporary loss of weight. Undesirable effects in the form of metabolic inbalances and nutritional deficiencies make this practice potentially harmful as well as ineffective.

Surgical techniques. Surgical techniques are available that bypass substantial portions of the intestine or occlude a large segment of the stomach to produce a marked diet restriction and, hence, weight loss. These shunting techniques are hazardous surgical procedures with many metabolic complications, including severe water and electrolyte depletion, persistent diarrhea, vitamin deficiency, internal herniation, and fatty infiltration and degeneration of the liver. Use of such a drastic measure in children and adolescents is still controversial. Most authorities believe that the complex metabolic effects need clarification and that certainly this procedure should be restricted to those massively obese youngsters in whom other therapies have failed and whose obesity is life threatening in disease states that demand weight loss for effective management. It

Summary of nursing care in assessment and modification of eating habits

Goals	Responsibilities
Identify eating patterns and behaviors	Keep a record of everything eaten, including Time eaten Amount eaten Where food was consumed, for example, table, chair, in front of television, and so on Activity engaged in while eating With whom the food was eaten or if it was eaten alone Feelings at the time food was eaten, for example, angry, depressed, lonely, elated, and so on Analyze preceding data for patterns of eating and relationships of other factors as a basis for making adjustments
Control eating patterns	Eat only at specific times Eat only in a specific place (selected according to the family's eating pattern) Do nothing else while eating, such as watching television, reading, talking, talking on the telephone (it is easy to consume more than intended when distracted from eating) Prepare low-calorie foods in an attractive, inviting way Get rid of junk foods Put snacks out of sight and put away remaining food after meal or snack preparation (such as sandwich makings) before beginning to eat Avoid purchase of problem foods
Change the act of eating	Slow pace of eating Use smaller plates to make amount of food seem larger Leave a small amount of food on the plate Serve food from stove or other place out of reach of the established eating place to make seconds more difficult
Use methods other than eating to deal with emotional stress, boredom, and fatigue	Substitute other activities for eating in response to these feelings: activities help divert attention from food, for example, sewing, working at a hobby, taking a short walk, straightening up the room, and so on Become involved in activities out of the house and away from food
Give positive reinforcement for accomplishments	Provide a system of rewards for changes in eating behavior, exercise, and weight loss Point system Tangible rewards such as a trip, a new record, a concert Think positively (overweight individuals are negative thinkers) Have a family member serve as a monitor at home to help in progress toward goals and to encourage youngster with positive statements daily

should not be considered as a cosmetic procedure that is available on request.[4]

Behavioral therapy. Probably the most successful method for treating obesity is diet combined with behavioral modification, which emphasizes identification and elimination of inappropriate eating habits. Although the long-term effects of this method are still in need of evaluation, it appears to hold promise for the treatment of obesity in adolescents. Some of the techniques used in this approach are listed in the boxed material above.[1,3,8,21]

Group involvement. Some persons on weight-reduction programs find that the support and mutual reinforcement provided by a group of persons with a similar problem help them to adjust to the changes needed for successful accomplishment of their goals, including weight loss. Commercial groups such as Weight Watchers, TOPS, or diet workshops composed primarily of adults may be helpful to a few, but, for teenagers, a group composed of persons their own age is more acceptable. Some types of teenage groups include summer camps designed for obese youngsters and conducted by health professionals, school groups organized and led by the school nurse, and groups associated with special clinics.

The group is concerned not only with weight loss but also emphasizes the development of a positive self-image. Nutrition education and diet planning are essential elements of the group function, but equally important are discussions centered around better grooming and improvement of social skills. Improvement is measured by positive changes in all aspects of endeavor. Group support and reinforcement are basic to success.

Nurses' role in prevention and management of obesity

Unfortunately the results of most weight-reduction regimens are disappointing. Few obese adolescents attain successful long-term weight loss. Any weight loss that is achieved is usually brief, and relapses are frequent. Early-acquired obesity is remarkably resistant to therapy. Any regimen requires extraordinary motivation, perseverance, and self-discipline, all of which are extremely difficult for children and adolescents. Once a child has become obese, attempts at weight reduction are fraught with frustration, consistent failure, and potential physical and psychologic harm as a result of desperate measures. Therefore, a more effective, safe, and sustaining approach is one directed toward prevention and control during the stages of early development.

Preventive measures during infancy. Nurses are key persons who can identify infants at risk and practices that may lead to obesity in vulnerable infants. They are in a position to work with mothers to assist them in developing feeding habits that will help control the tendency toward adiposity. A family history for obesity provides a clue as to which infant might be at risk for acquiring obesity. These mothers or expectant mothers should be encouraged to breast-feed if they are at all disposed to do so and to continue breast-feeding for at least 3 months whenever possible. Breast-feeding allows the infant a sufficient amount of sucking without the risk of overnutrition. Mothers who choose to bottle-feed their infants are counseled not to force the infant to empty the bottle at each feeding. It is also important to be certain that the mother understands how to mix the formula correctly so that her infant is not receiving a more concentrated, higher-calorie formula than is prescribed.

Early feeding of solid food may contribute to increased weight gain in early months; therefore, it is wise to discourage the addition of solid foods to the diet until 4 to 5 months of age, provided the infant receives an iron supplement.[30] When solid foods are added to the diet, the mother should be advised and encouraged to prepare her own baby foods in a blender (preferably) or to select plain vegetables and meats rather than the mixed vegetable and meat varieties, which contain a higher percentage of carbohydrate. It is advisable to periodically assess the infant's diet, including the type and amount of milk consumed and the nature and amount of solid foods. To estimate the caloric intake and eating pattern of the infant, the mother is asked to keep a careful record of the infant's daily feedings. Sweet desserts are discouraged for infants at risk of obesity, and the mother should be counseled in proper use of other foods in the diet.

Periodic assessment of the child's height and weight attainment, plotted on a growth chart, helps to identify a rapid weight gain or an increase in weight percentile that forewarns of a potential problem. It is also important to evaluate the quality of mothering, especially in relation to feeding behaviors. Overfeeding is not uncommon in mothers who associate feeding with being a "good mother," and overfeeding is often related to the mother's inability to interpret the child's needs from his behavior. These mothers respond to all of the infant's cries with an offering of food. Nurses are able to help these mothers learn to distinguish between their infants' needs for food and other infantile needs and to provide more tactile stimulation to relieve the infant's stress. Parents should also be encouraged to allow their infants free movement of body and extremities because physical activity is an important aspect of both development and weight control, even in infancy. For further discussion of obesity in infancy, see p. 486.

Management in childhood. Beginning in the infancy period, mothers of obese or potentially obese children need nutrition counseling to help them select proper foods for optimal development of their children. This is often difficult in the lower socioeconomic class where families rely on starchy, filling foods and frequent use of quick-energy foods with concentrated calories that substitute for more expensive protein-containing foods. Even the children of more affluent families are highly influenced by the promotion of economically and nutritionally unsound foods by commercial television advertisers. Empty-calorie foods should be discouraged and replaced by more nutritious snack foods, such as fresh fruits, cheese, Vienna sausages, and fruit juices.

Mothers need to be prepared for changes in children's appetite at various stages in their development, for example, the reduced appetite that accompanies the onset of toddlerhood. They should be encouraged to serve appropriate portions to their children and to limit second portions and desserts. The mother's attitudes toward foods and philosophy about feeding are influential in developing eating habits. These include forcing the child to join the "clean plate'' club, withholding food as a punishment, and using sweets as a bribe or a reward for good behavior. The nurse can help the mother or family to explore the reasons for these practices, to look at them in the light of consequences, and to encourage them to substitute other rewards and punishments. The family may need education regarding their concept of what constitutes a healthy child—in many families large size is considered a sign of good health.

Continued encouragement of physical activity for children and helping families and children find facilities where this can be attained are also important. In many depressed areas children do not have access to safe recreational facilities or adequate physical education programs. For large numbers of children in all socioeconomic levels, especially girls, the television set is a substitute for activity.

In assessing the obese child's environment, nurses should be alert to family relationships, particularly the mother-child relationship. For example, evidence of maternal overprotectiveness and the degree of dependency and maturity that are displayed by the child provide clues to environmental factors that may influence the approach to therapy. School nurses are able to observe the child's interaction with peers. Any dietary, exercise, and supportive regimen must involve the family, since it is the parents who control the food that is available to the young child and the family as a whole that creates and maintains the eating and emotional environment.

Adolescent obesity. The role of the nurse in helping obese adolescents is to provide them with the information they need to help them lose weight and improve their diets, to serve as a consultant and guide, and to help them to develop a positive attitude toward themselves. Since weight reduction is a long-term process that requires sustained self-motivation, nurses who work with obese teenagers must be willing and able to maintain a continuous supportive relationship with these youngsters and their families. Adolescents want to actively participate in the solution of their own problems, but the support of others is an important factor for the achievement of success. Most successful results are achieved in girls with later onset of obesity, good academic performance, and family support.[14] Weight loss requires the combined efforts of the nurse, physician, nutritionist, family, and obese youngster.

In helping adolescents establish realistic goals and a plan for their attainment, nurses need to keep in mind that any approach must be tailored to the individual youngster and must take into consideration the child's pubertal stage, the duration and degree of obesity, eating and activity patterns, and psychosocial aspects, such as the degree of maturity and dependency, motivation, depression, socialization, and the child's self-concept. Some youngsters will be able to benefit from group involvement and reinforcement from the onset; others will require intensive counseling before initiating a therapeutic program and group association.

Above all, obese youngsters need to be treated with respect as worthwhile human beings. The goal is not to point out the adolescents' faults or subject them to criticism but rather to emphasize their attributes and achievements. They must be convinced that there is hope for controlling their weight and that they can count on support and encouragement but that they must be willing to take the major responsibility of a regimen themselves. To this end, health professionals attempt to shape a reduction program that incorporates individual youngsters' preferences in diet and exercise plans. The closer a regimen conforms to their tastes and interests, the more success can be expected in getting obese youngsters to adhere to a weight-reduction program. Although a team effort is required, it is almost always the nurse who plays the central role by providing the sustained professional contact with obese adolescents and their families.

Adolescents in distress

The teen years are the most unstable stage of life—a period of considerable normative stress. There are many anxieties, crises, and pains associated with the search for identity, independence, and a meaningful social role. It is a particularly lonely, difficult period of biologic upheaval and social change. With internal pressures, social turmoil, expectations from parents and friends, and rigid standards for achievement and acceptance, adolescents' coping mechanisms are stretched to the utmost. Consequently youngsters in this age-group are vulnerable to additional stresses that may result in maladaptive behavior, particularly those children who have no family support. Some of the expressions of this inner turmoil and distress are juvenile delinquency, drug abuse, and suicide or attempted suicide.

JUVENILE DELINQUENCY

Technically a delinquent can be defined as one whose behavior is brought to the attention of law enforcement agencies because it endangers the juvenile, other individuals, or the community. Juvenile delinquency refers to persons who are younger than the statutory age limit in the individual state and community. This definition helps to identify behaviors or delinquent acts in social terms and in relation to consequences but fails to take into consideration the psychologic sources within the individual. Psychologic origins of delinquency are described as[27]:

normal delinquency or **casual delinquent behavior** this is a normal part of the developmental process, is not serious, and is usually outgrown. For example, a 6- to 7-year-old child will attempt experimental stealing; gangs indulge in a certain amount of prankishness with a superficial delinquent character; and young boys engage in street fighting to ''prove'' themselves.

subcultural or **socialized delinquency** this is characteristic of the child in the lower socioeconomic classes who is reared in a delinquent culture. Primarily a gang delinquency, the individual members behave in culturally sanctioned ways, feeling no guilt, and the delinquency is considered as such only in terms of middle class mores. However, it may be a breeding ground for individual criminality.

neurotic delinquency this is an indirect expression of an unformulated wish or need. It is manifest as stealing from parents (or a teacher) by a child who feels isolated. In stealing money and other objects from the parents, the child is symbolically stealing the love he believes the parents do not give him, or this may represent a way of punishing the parents for not loving him. The child may even use the stolen money to buy favor with his peers.

acting-out delinquency in this the child engages in deliberate, often malicious indulgence of impulse, mainly as a form of revolt. Usually aggressive in nature, this form of delinquency is more an individual matter than group sanctioned and represents hostility against the adult world in general or the individual's parents in particular.

psychopathic delinquency this begins very early in life and represents a failure of the basic identification process that normally takes place in the first 5 years of life. The individual becomes incapable of true feelings for others. He has an intact personality but is lacking a conscience and can never see his responsibility for anything that goes wrong. He lies, steals, or commits physical harm casually and unthinkingly. He seems indifferent to the consequences for others of what he does and does not seem concerned about unfortunate consequences for himself. He steals when he is sure to be caught and lies without reason. Because of his lack of strong feeling, punishment does not alter his behavior.

It appears that the single most predictive indicator of adolescent delinquency is the youngsters' relationship with their parents. Family studies indicate that delinquency in children is associated with personal and marital inadequacy in the parents. The better adolescents get along with their parents, the less delinquent their behavior. Relationships between delinquents and their parents are more likely to be characterized by mutual hostility and lack of family cohesiveness than relationships between nondelinquents and their parents. Parental disciplinary methods are apt to be lax, erratic, or overly strict and involve physical punishment rather than reasoning. Parental rejection, indifference, and apathy are common observations.[26]

Recently it has been observed that there is a major link between delinquency and learning disabilities. As many as 80% of institutionalized delinquents show some form of educational handicap. This emphasizes the importance of early detection of learning disability. Management of present delinquents with these problems must include remediation of their learning disabilities and rebuilding their shattered self-images.

Prevention and treatment of delinquency have been less than encouraging. Numerous approaches, such as foster home placement, recreational programs, "street corner" youth workers, work-study programs, and various forms of family casework, have been tried with limited success. Correctional institutions and other traditional forms of punishment only serve to aggravate the situation. The prevalence of juvenile delinquency is a reflection of numerous fundamental problems of society—social, psychotic, economic, educational, vocational, physical, and even philosophic. Therefore, efforts to deal with the problem of delinquency must necessarily be aimed at the broader problems of society to improve the social conditions that foster delinquency.

SUICIDE

The problem of suicide is worldwide and increasing in many countries. A striking feature is the rise among persons in the younger age-groups. The true incidence of suicide in children and adolescents is not known because of general underreporting. Frequently deaths by suicide are reported as accidental because of pressures exerted by family and society to avoid the cultural and religious stigma associated with self-destruction. Also, there appears to be some degree of certainty that the high accident rate in persons in this age-group reflects suicides masked by accidental death or homicide.

Suicidal behavior

Suicide is defined as the deliberate act of self-injury with the intent that the injury should kill. Suicidal gestures in children and adolescents differ from those in adults in several aspects. Motivation and methodology are often related to sex and age and determine to some extent whether suicides are attempted, committed, threatened, "partial," or probable.[12]

Persons who attempt suicide are predominantly female, are younger, and no more than 10% of those who attempt suicide later kill themselves; the majority of those who are successful succeed on the first try. It is significant that 12% of all suicide attempts are made by adolescents and that 90% of these are made by adolescent girls. There are approximately seven to eight times more attempts than completed suicides at all ages, and in children and adolescents attempts are estimated to be fifty to 100 times more frequent.[12]

The outcome of suicidal behavior is influenced to some extent by the method used. Violent methods of destruction, such as jumping from heights or in front of trains, which are used by adults, are less frequently employed by younger persons. Overdose of drugs is the method of choice for most adolescents who attempt suicide, and these are usually medications prescribed for parents, such as barbiturates and antidepressants, or those intended for household use, such as aspirin.

Of successful suicides in children of both sexes, aged

10 to 14 years, firearms and hanging account for the largest number of deaths. The predominant method at ages 15 to 19 years is the use of firearms by males and poisons by females. The less lethal methods selected by girls contribute to the preponderance of suicide attempts in adolescent females.

Sometimes an adolescent will threaten suicide in order to manipulate the environment. Unfortunately, with no self-destructive intent, a youngster may make a halfhearted attempt that leads to death. A "partial" or chronic suicide is illustrated by the adolescent with a chronic illness, such as a diabetic youngster who refuses to comply with the prescribed medical regimen, the accident-prone adolescent, and the drug-abusing youngster.

The high incidence of accidental death in the adolescent age-group has led some to speculate that many of these young people intentionally or unintentionally invite injury or become victims of homicide. For example, when does the propensity for risk-taking behavior in the normal adolescent male become a deliberate courting of death? It is suggested that a significant number of teenage accident victims are probable suicides and that since the incidence of adolescent homicide is twice that of suicides troubled youngsters have allowed others to kill them.

Epidemiology

In observation of suicide, both completed and attempted, some epidemiologic information has been accumulated regarding predisposing and related factors, although no single factor or group of factors fits all adolescent suicides.

Age. In the pediatric population there is a direct relationship between the rate of suicide and advancing age. Suicide is nonexistent in children less than 5 years of age and most unusual, or not reported, in children aged 5 to 9 years, although a large number (about 10%) of those who do attempt to kill themselves are successful. The rate of suicide increases in ages 9 to 14 years, and the rate and number have been rising steadily each year. At age 14 years there is a sharp rise, and in ages 15 to 19 years the rate increases eightfold to tenfold and doubles again at ages 20 to 24 years. The greatest increase in suicides is among young men 15 to 24 years of age, where it ranks as one of the leading causes of death. In college students suicide is second only to accidents as a cause of death.[12]

Sex. In all age-groups three times as many males commit suicide as females and the males are generally successful in the first try. The rate is reversed for attempted suicides, where females outnumber males three to one. The reason for this is not entirely clear; however, males tend to use more violent means and those that are more likely to succeed, such as firearms, hanging, and explosives. Females, on the other hand, use less violent methods that allow time for rescue, such as ingesting pills or poisons.

Race and ethnic origin. The incidence of suicide varies in different countries. The suicide rates reported in Hungary, Austria, Germany, Japan, and the Scandinavian countries, with the exception of Norway, are two to three times higher than those reported in the United States and Canada. Catholic and Moslem countries report the lowest incidence, but it is uncertain whether this is a reflection of underreporting because of religious stigma attached to the act or the influence of religion on the population as a whole.[2]

Generally the suicide rates for nonwhites are below those for whites. There are, however, two exceptions: in females age 15 to 19 years, nonwhites have slightly higher rates than white females of the same age, and recently there has been a substantial increase in suicides among young nonwhite males between ages 15 and 20 years. This increase in suicides in nonwhite males may be caused by the stresses related to urban migration and tensions of unemployment and ghetto living. Other racial differences have been noted. American Indian youths living on reservations have been considered to be at risk for suicide, but the rate varies among tribes—some have very high rates, whereas others have lower rates. Orientals as a whole and Jews tend to have a lower rate of suicide than the population as a whole, possibly as a reflection of the more cohesive family units.

Religious affiliation. Observations indicate that youth of the Protestant faith have the highest rate of suicide, Catholic youth have the second highest rate, and there is a lower incidence in those of the Buddhist and Jewish faith. The lower incidence among Catholics is thought to be a result of either the church's strong opposition to suicide or the degree to which individual members are integrated into the church.

Time of day and year. The largest number of adolescent and childhood suicides occur between 3:00 PM and midnight, whereas the highest incidence in adults is between midnight and dawn. Adolescent and childhood suicides take place more often in spring and summer, with the highest incidence in May and the lowest in December. Most occur at home.

Family determinants. Suicidal adolescents are usually from homes experiencing some disruption. Broken homes, divorce, separation, abandonment, alcoholism, and death are highly significant factors and are frequently noted in the histories of suicidal youth. In instances in which the family is intact, the disorganization is manifest by marital discord, lack of or disturbed communication, abnormal patterns of interaction, physical aggression, and general lack of unity and solidarity within the family system. There is often a lack of supportive response to the children's problems. Younger children who are treated badly at home react with rebellious behavior and may commit suicide for fear of punishment. It is not uncommon to find a family history of suicide.

Developmental determinants. The increase in suicides at 14 years of age is a reflection of the changes and turmoil associated with the developmental process. During the ages 12 to 14 years youngsters are concerned with final resolution of the Oedipal situation, which has a resurgence at puberty. Adolescents begin to relinquish the emotional attachment to their parents and shift their affection to peers and other significant persons in their interpersonal environment. With limited capacities for problem solving and with fewer and less sophisticated resources for resolving difficulties, they may resort to methods of handling problems that were acquired at an earlier age. It often appears to adults that adolescents "overreact" to situations. Actually they experience emotions and react to events more intensely than adults.

Immature adolescents with poor ego development tend to react impulsively to situations much as they did at a younger age. Turning aggression inward in stressful situations, they seek to avoid discomfort, join a lost object, or gain love; in the process they may attempt or commit suicide.

Motivation

Suicidal behavior is generally divided into (1) primarily "acting-out" behavior, representing a cry for help, and (2) a true death wish.

Suicidal gestures are not uncommon among adolescents, and most are impulsive acts committed to force parents or other significant persons in their lives to pay attention to their need for help. The attempt usually is the culmination of a behavioral pattern. These youngsters often have a history of attention-getting behaviors that range from minor acts to increasingly dramatic ones. With the ultimate act of attempted suicide, the teenager finally makes himself heard. He seldom actually plans a suicidal act because he really wants to die; successful suicides are committed either impulsively or accidentally.

A frequent motive for suicide in children and younger adolescents is the desire to punish others who will be grieved by their death. Angry children who are unable to punish directly those who have injured or insulted them will take revenge on those who love them through self-destruction ("They'll be sorry when they find me dead"; "They'll be sorry they were mean to me"). This motive is more common in girls and more likely to persist longer.[2]

Occasionally there are adolescents who are so severely depressed that suicide appears to them to be the only means of release from their despair. These youngsters rarely give evidence of their intent, concealing their suicidal thoughts for fear of outside intervention. Sometimes this self-destructive behavior on the part of adolescents is a desire to punish themselves for guilt-filled actions, such as masturbation, or, more often, thoughts. Peer pressure, too, has convinced many young persons that there is something wrong with them if they feel lonely or depressed; therefore, they direct these feelings inward to avoid the risk of rejection.

Adolescents often respond to feelings of anger, failure, or loss with overt flight reactions. Some of these adaptive techniques are rebellion, withdrawal into the self with silence, physical withdrawal, such as running away from home, or, the most drastic of all, suicide. Social isolation is seen in many suicidal adolescents, but it appears to be the most significant factor in distinguishing those who will kill themselves from those who will not. It is more characteristic of completed suicides than attempts or threats.

Although suicide is often linked to a trivial event, such as a family fight, an important school examination, death of a teen idol, or the breakup of a youthful romance, that produced an impulsive response in the child, careful analysis will usually reveal an ongoing depressive process that has been expressed periodically and behaviorally. Teachers often report changes in the behavior of a child who previously has not been a behavior problem. He may become easily irritated, demonstrate a low frustration point, or exhibit clowning and active, restless behavior. Older children may begin using drugs and alcohol.[24]

Suicidal threats should be taken very seriously. It has often been a general tendency to dismiss a suicide attempt as an impulsive act resulting from a temporary crisis or depression. If this drastic move to gain attention fails to draw attention to their problems or makes them worse, adolescents may conclude that taking their lives is their only means to solve these escalating, unsolvable, and unbearable problems.

Depression

Depression is a symptom common to all human beings. It is a normal part of life, and even adolescents who are healthy and happy experience alternating periods of depression and elation as a part of the growth process. Depression is part of the breaking away process. When adolescents break away from their parents, they need something or someone to belong to. Belonging to a peer group is a way of coping. However, this and other coping mechanisms are often stretched to the utmost, and adolescents' heightened vulnerability to added stresses sometimes precipitates maladaptive behavior. The ego is under pressure to adapt to the physical changes and instinctual drives of puberty, whereas at the same time the expectations of family and the environment for mature, independent, and responsible behavior must be met. Although some suicides occur in conjunction with a psychotic process, most frequently they are a part of the general picture of depression. When depression appears as a predominant mood, persists for an undue length of time, or is so disabling that the adolescent is unable to fulfill the normal tasks of this period of life, then the condition is serious and warrants special attention and intervention.

Depression is recognized by both subjective symptoms and objective signs that reflect adolescents' grief (see grief process, p. 970). Depressed persons describe feelings of sadness, despair, helplessness, hopelessness, boredom, loss of interest, and isolation. They may also feel self-reproach, self-depreciation, and guilt. These subjective symptoms are accompanied by objective signs, such as sighing respirations, weakness, fatigue, somatic complaints such as digestive disturbances and headaches, difficulty in concentrating, disturbances in sleep pattern, and general physical retardation (slow speech and movements).

Although the evidence of depression in older adolescents is similar to that observed in adults, depression in early adolescence and childhood is frequently masked by a variety of behaviors. Child psychiatrists describe depression in terms of "depressive equivalents," the symptoms of feeling sad that are expressed as boredom, restlessness, fatigue, difficulty in concentrating, and various behavioral problems. Children express feelings in actions rather than words. Much of the behavior that represents hidden depression has been labeled "acting-out" and is manifest as delinquency, aggression, truancy, bullying younger children, promiscuity, running away from home, school failure, and accident proneness.

Reaction to a loss. Depression is always a reaction to a loss, and since adolescents experience many losses during the process of attaining adulthood, periods of depression occur more frequently in adolescence. The way in which youngsters deal with these losses and the coping mechanisms that can be brought into play determine their ability to make a healthy adaptation. Some losses are experienced normally in the course of development, whereas others are superimposed on these developmental separations.

Developmentally the young person progresses through several stages of separations in the process of detachment, individuation, and autonomy. At each stage of development the reality of these separations forces the individual to make certain psychologic adjustments to further develop and enhance the sense of self. Inability to adapt to these separations and other losses associated with growing up often cause the child to react in maladaptive ways.

The *psychologic loss of parents* is a loss common to all adolescents. As they distance themselves from these first love objects, adolescents experience a feeling of emptiness, go through a mourning process, and tend to withdraw into themselves. *Loss of childhood identity* is another cause for depression when the secure identity of childhood is lost and the adolescent looks ahead to the uncertain promise of the future. *Loss of self-esteem* is probably the most destructive loss experienced by adolescents through repeated defeats without meaningful relationships to help them tolerate failures. Finally, the actual *loss of a significant love object*—parent, friend, pet, and so on—must be worked through in the normal grief process. The loss of the state of well-being associated with these relationships is probably what is really lost, however. Studies indicate that a high percentage of adolescents who commit suicide have experienced the loss of a parent, either from death or divorce, at some point in their life. A large number are victims of a broken home. The timing is also significant. Suicidal adolescents have parents who were divorced, separated, or remarried after the onset of adolescence—resulting in additional stresses imposed on a particularly stressful period in the life span.[13]

There appears to be a sequence leading to isolation from the important people in the lives of suicidal adolescents. First, these teenagers all have a long-standing history of multiple problems deriving from childhood and extending into adolescence. Second, problems related to identity and emancipation seem to mount and expand, usually at the beginning of adolescence, and seem to exceed those of peers and friends. There is difficulty with intrafamily communications, and tensions accelerate. The young person believes that the parents no longer understand him and that they impose excessive punishment. The youngster withdraws and exhibits further rebellious behavior. Third, the isolation occurs in the days or weeks preceding the suicide attempt and is characterized by "chain reaction dissolution of any remaining meaningful social relationships." For example, many of these adolescents had formed a possessive and exclusive romatic attachment in which they concentrate so intensely on the other that they tend to cut themselves off from friends, which isolates them further.[31] When the romance breaks up, they feel hopeless, lost, and despairing. It is often at the point when the relationship breaks up that suicide is attempted. Other factors that correlate with the suicide attempt are a real or feared pregnancy, profound school problems, loss of relationships from school dropout, loss of a family member through death, a major family row, and the feeling that there is no one to turn to for help.[17]

Nursing considerations

Care of the suicidal adolescent includes early recognition, management, and prevention. Probably the most important aspect of management is the recognition of prodromal signs that indicate that a youngster is troubled and might attempt to take his life. Health professionals need to be alert to the signs of adolescent depression, and any youngster who exhibits such behavior, subtle or overt, should be referred for thorough psychologic assessment. Depression can be manifest in two ways: youngsters who feel depressed may talk about suicide and feelings of worthlessness or they may build themselves a solid defense against such intolerable feelings of depression with behavioral or psychosomatic disturbances.

Too often suicidal threats or minor attempts are confused with bids for attention. No threat of suicide should be ignored or challenged in any way. It is a symptom that must be taken seriously. The child needs to know that someone cares and must be provided with swift and efficient crisis intervention. Most larger communities have 24-hour service in the form of "hot lines"—telephone communication that is within reach of troubled youngsters or their families where they can make ready contact with someone to listen to them. The function of the hot line is to help them through the immediate crisis. Through skillful questioning, but without imposing a solution on the caller, the listener helps the caller arrive at a course of action that will contribute to a solution for his problem.

The child should be given no false reassurance, but it is essential to make clear to him that his life is considered of great importance and that he will be protected from doing himself harm. Hospitalization, if only briefly, is usually recommended. The youngster needs to be removed from the acute situation that troubles him and given the structure and security he needs during the crisis period. Hospitalization also provides the surveillance that is impossible to accomplish in the home. It is especially valuable if he can be placed in a unit where other adolescents can offer warmth, support, and understanding.[24]

As soon as the youngster who attempts suicide is out of danger from medical problems resulting from the attempt, the data-gathering process should begin and should include information from several sources to help evaluate the extent to which the child is suffering, direction for therapy, and the probability of a repeated attempt. Some guidelines have been suggested to help evaluate the seriousness of an attempt to commit suicide, which include the following areas for exploration[12]:

1. *Social set*—determine what steps were taken to prevent rescue, if another person was present in the room or the house during the attempt, and if others were aware of the attempt either before or immediately after.
2. *Intent*—if a suicide note or letter was written, determine how detailed the suicidal plans were. Such communication often expresses the true depth of the youngster's despair.
3. *Method*—examine the means that the child selected to destroy himself and his understanding of the method, for example, the kind, number, and action of the pills taken.
4. *History*—determine if the attempt was an isolated event and, if not, the number and nature of previous attempts or gestures. A family history of suicide is significant.
5. *Stress*—determine the nature of the precipitating event, the alternative courses of action available to the child, and his previous methods of coping with stress.
6. *Mental status*—assess the present mental status of the child and compare it with pre-attempt status as described by others.
7. *Support*—evaluate the type of support that could be expected from his family, friends, peers, teachers, and others.

Not only is it important to treat the suicidal adolescent, but, since the suicide attempt is an outgrowth of family distress, it is essential to deal with the family as well. Ideally the most effective approach would be recognition of susceptible youngsters during the earlier stages of intrafamily distress so that family counseling can be instigated. This emphasizes again the importance of parent-child relationships and the role of the nurse in assessing family interactions and the early recognition of disturbed relationships. Prevention efforts must be directed toward improving child-rearing practices through support and education of parents and changing societal conditions that generate defeat, despair, and maladaptive behavior.

DRUG ABUSE

The use of drugs by children and adolescents to produce an altered state of consciousness is widespread and is believed to reflect the variety of changes taking place in their life and the stresses engendered by these changes. The discomfort associated with the growth and changes of this prolonged and intense transitional process encourages the adolescent to search for relief or for escape or even facilitates exploration of the self. To relieve this discomfort, young people often turn to the exhilarating, mind-easing, euphorigenic qualities of drugs.

Most drugs to which young people turn induce changes in perception, a feeling of well-being, and a sense of closeness. To most, they provide a feeling of happiness. With the exception of some stimulant drugs used for practical purposes, such as working better, studying, or increasing cognitive effectiveness, the drugs used are simply pleasure-promoting chemicals used in the hope for altered consciousness or the attainment of a different level of functioning. Most of these drugs have some hallucinogenic properties.

Definitions

The greatest area of misinformation and confusion is related to the terms applied to drug use. Previously drug abuse was defined in terms of *addiction* and *habituation*. Because of the confusion and controversy related to these two terms, the World Health Organization's Expert Committee on Addiction-Producing Drugs suggests the use of the term *drug dependence* to indicate the high degree of involvement with drugs that occurs when they are taken repeatedly. Drug dependence implies the need or desire to take a drug despite untoward consequences and the psychologic inability to give up the drug. *Physical dependence* is an adaptive physiologic state that occurs when the drug is taken in increasing amounts and is manifest by the development of physiologic symptoms when the drug is withdrawn. These symptoms can be relieved only by the administration of the drug or a pharmacologically similar drug. *Psychologic dependence* refers to the emotional reliance on the effects of the drug, even though a particular drug does not produce physical symptoms when discontinued. However, its psychologic and medical disturbances may be just as severe and long-lasting as the effects of those that produce physical dependence.

Drug abuse is the regular use of drugs for other than the

accepted medical purposes and to the extent that it results in physical or psychologic harm to the user and/or is used in a way that is detrimental to society. *Misuse* is the overzealous use of drugs or the exercise of bad judgment in their use. Closely related to drug dependence is *tolerance,* the clinical need to increase the dosage of a drug in order to attain the same desired effect. Drug tolerance is caused by an increased capacity to metabolize and eliminate the drug or the ability of the individual's tissues to adapt to the drug.

The broad term "drug abuse," which is often applied to all forms of drug misuse, can be a confusing term and does not necessarily define the problem related to drug use. Many of the substances are controlled by law and accompanied by severe penalties for their illegal use; others are sanctioned from a legal, social, and medical standpoint. Problems concerning drug use, therefore, can be defined as legal, social, medical, and individual.

Legal. Drug use can become a legal problem when the drug being taken is strictly controlled by law and is accompanied by severe penalties for its use or possession. Some youngsters in the pursuit for peer approval merely carry a supply of such drugs in order to impress their peers and achieve acceptance by the group, although they have no intention of actually taking the drug.[23] This is primarily a legal problem.

Social. When the use of a substance by the adolescent leads to disruptive or bizarre behavior that alienates the user from the rest of society, this results in a social problem. The deviant behavior may lead to rejection by family, school, employer, and even the peer group. Such behavior also increases the risk of confrontation with legal authorities and a forced change in life-style.

Medical. When the current or continued use of a substance may adversely affect the physical or mental health of the youngster, it becomes a medical problem. This includes life-threatening situations such as an overdose or withdrawal in which medical intervention is mandatory or the demonstration of aberrant behavior patterns that represent acute mental stress, such as panic, toxic psychosis, or acute brain syndrome.

Individual. An individual problem is one that focuses on the person. It requires continued assessment and intervention related to the role that drug use plays in the individual's life and the factors that contribute to his need for the drug.

Patterns of drug use

Many factors influence the extent to which drugs are used by teenagers. The type of drug used, the mode of administration, duration of use, frequency of use, and whether or not the drugs are used singly or in combination must be considered in determining the severity of the individual drug problem. Most drug use begins with experimentation. The individual may try a drug only once, it may be used occasionally, or it may become an integral part of a drug-centered life-style. Identification of the pattern of drug use in an individual facilitates the formulation of an approach to the problem. Patterns have been observed based on dose and frequency of use.

There are two broad categories of adolescents who use drugs: the *experimenters* and the *compulsive users*. There is a wide range of use between these groups that represents two ends of a continuum in terms of degree of use. With the exception of a "bad trip" or accidental overdose, the experimenters present few medical problems, although they probably represent the bulk of adolescent drug users. Some of these youngsters with a predisposition to heavy drug use proceed to compulsive use after a time, but, by and large, they are in the minority. However, the experimenters are frequently equated with compulsive users and consume a great deal of medical and legal energies that might be better utilized to deal with the more serious, compulsive users.[33]

Between the experimenters and compulsive users are a broad range of *recreational* users of drugs, principally drugs such as marihuana and alcohol. For many, the goal is merely relaxation, and these fit more closely with the experimenting, intermittent users. For others the goal is intoxication, and these are more nearly like the compulsive users. The group of greatest concern to health workers are those whose patterns of use involve high doses with the danger of overdose and those compulsive users with all the threat of dependence, withdrawal syndromes, and altered life-style.

A more definitive description of experimental, intermittent and compulsive use of drugs follows.[23]

Low-dose intermittent use (taster). The substance is experimental, used in low dosage, and taken without regularity. Time intervals between use are erratic. More often the drug is limited to social use from curiosity, to see what it is like, or in response to nonverbalized peer pressure. Its use is a response to expected behavior in the setting, perhaps as need to be accepted or to avoid rejection by the peer group.

High-dose intermittent use (chipper). This is an episodic more daredevil or spree use. The use may begin with an initial pleasurable or beneficial experience that is repeated periodically—usually in social gatherings. This type of use is often based on ignorance or inexperience; as a result the outcome may prove to be a life-threatening overdose. It may be associated with intense mood swings, and the drug may be used as an attempt to cope with the emotional distress being experienced at the time.

Low-dose compulsive use (head). In this pattern there is a decided regularity in time intervals with active drug-seeking behavior. The user may or may not be physically dependent on the drug, and the use is often accompanied by a great deal of denial regarding the need to continue to drug. The individual may use more than one drug.

High-dose compulsive use (freak). This pattern of drug use represents psychologic and/or physical dependence with the presence of definite time intervals of administration. Drug-seeking behavior is overwhelming, including stealing, trafficking in drugs, and prostitution, the individual accepts the dependence, and the need for the drug markedly influences his life-style—socially, emotionally, and economically.

Motivation

There are several common motives for drug use. Adolescents try drugs out of curiosity, for kicks. Drugs produce for some persons a dreamy state of altered consciousness and a feeling of power, excitement, heightened acuity, or confidence. Others seek visual hallucinatory experiences and sexual sensation. Many youngsters use drugs not only for the perceptual and sensory experiences but also for the social aspects. They use drugs because others use them and because they want to "turn on" or "tune in" to the drug culture. Teenagers are highly influenced by fads and fashions within their society, and they are, developmentally, sensation-hungry risk takers. It is characteristic that they are eager to test their mental and physical capabilities to the utmost. Also, adolescents are forever trying to find a means to cope with their disenchantment with the adult world and its social and technologic concerns and with their powerlessness to change it. They seek escape from reality and want to achieve a sense of closeness and intimacy with other people, to escape from distress or decision making, and to feel a sense of insight into the mysteries of God, death, and rebirth.

During early and mid-teenage years, drug use seems to fall into rather distinct groups in relation to motivation[10]:

Social group. These youngsters are members of the giggly social group who indulge in occasional use as a social act of sharing. They pass around a bottle so that each youngster can take a drink or a marihuana cigarette so that each member can have a puff. The pleasant act of sharing reinforces membership in the group, sets them apart from adults, and provides them with an atmosphere of doing something against the rules—something that is fun to get away with. With most youth drug use is a passing fancy and, after a few times, is dispensed with and forgotten.

Escapist group. The majority of youth who experiment with drugs are seeking escape from feelings of anger and depression when they are unable to communicate effectively with their parents concerning their problems or to cope with their emotions. Getting drunk or "freaking out" seems to work for them. Unfortunately this flight not only leaves the problems unsolved but also interferes with the satisfactory resolution of the problems. Consequently the retreat into use of drugs tends to be repeated.

Punitive group. This smaller group of adolescents seem determined to punish the world for making them angry, depressed, or frustrated. Although they use, sell, and/or push drugs, they do so in the hope that they will be discovered and arrested so that their families will suffer the anguish that the youngsters themselves feel.

Self-destructive group. A few youth are openly self-destructive individuals who internalize their anger to the extent that death seems to provide the only relief from their anger. These youngsters often give evidence of suicidal thoughts or demonstrate suicidal behavior.

Types of drugs abused

Any drug can be abused, and most are potentially harmful to adolescents still going through formative life experiences. Although rarely conceived as drugs by society, the chemically active substances most frequently abused are the xanthines and theobromines contained in chocolate and in common beverages such as tea, coffee, and colas. Common analgesics such as aspirin, Darvon compound, and fiorinal; ethyl alcohol; and nicotine are others that, although recognized as drugs, are sanctioned by society. Any of these can produce mild to moderate euphoric and/or stimulant effects and can lead to physical and psychic dependence.

A great many factors determine personal preferences for gratification. Many drugs are not harmful for all teenagers, and some, used intermittently, will probably not produce ill effects or result in dependence. Reactions vary according to the drug used and its purity, the expectations of the user, and the context in which the drug is used. These factors determine to a great extent whether the experience is viewed as pleasant or unpleasant. The type of drugs used varies according to sections of the country, socioeconomic status, urban as opposed to suburban areas, and various times. A drug that is popular with one "generation" of adolescents may not be attractive to another, and changing trends are influenced by the adolescent's constant search for new and different experiences.[22]

Drugs with mind-altering capacity that are available on the black market and that are of medical and legal concern are the hallucinogenic, narcotic, hypnotic, and stimulant drugs. In addition those of concern to the health professionals are alcohol and various volatile substances, such as antifreeze, plastic model airplane cement, and organic solvents, that are inhaled to achieve altered sensation in the user. Drugs available on the street are often mixed with other compounds and fillers so that the purity of the drug, its strength, and the nature of additives are highly variable. Many of the hazards associated with drug use are related to driving a car or operating equipment that may be harmful when carelessly used while under the influence of the drug.

Table 21-1 lists the drugs that are most often associated with drug abuse, and the following discussion identifies the more common characteristics of each group.

Narcotics. Narcotic drugs include opiates such as heroin, morphine, hydromorphone (Dilaudid), and hydrocodone (Dicodid). Codeine, although closely related to these drugs, rarely produces a physical dependency. Chemically differ-

Table 21-1. Major drugs abused by adolescents

Chemical agent	Slang terms*	Route	Physical signs	Behavior	Complications
Opiates					
Heroin	H, horse, junk, smack, scrag, stuff	Injected subcutaneously or IV	Constricted pupils, respiratory depression, cyanosis	Initial euphoria, tranquilization, lethargy, coma	Overdose: coma, respiratory arrest, death
Morphine	M, morph, white, stuff	Intranasal (sniffing)	Needle marks		Injection site infection, hepatitis, abcesses, septicemia, tetanus, pulmonary complications
Methadone (Dolophine)	Dolly	Oral			Withdrawal: muscle cramps, stomach cramps, diarrhea, runny nose and eyes, restlessness, convulsions, death Dental caries
Depressants					
Barbiturates—secobarbital, amobarbital, pentobarbital, amobarbital/secobarbital	Downers, goofers, reds, red devels, blue heaven, blues, yellow jackets, yellows, tooies, rainbows, Christmas trees	Oral, IV	Slurred speech, ataxia, slowed reflexes, constricted pupils (barbiturates); dilated pupils (glutethimide)	Short attention span, impaired judgment, combativeness, violence	Overdose: respiratory depression, coma, death Injection site infection, hepatitis, septicemia Withdrawal: hyperreflexia, irritability, convulsions, death
Alcohol—ethanol	Sauce, hootch, booze, juice	Oral	Incoordination	Impaired judgment and perception, loss of inhibitions, emotional lability, quarrelsomeness, aggressiveness, hostility Lethargy	Hazards related to impaired judgment, for example, automobile accidents, fights Nutritional deficiencies Gastritis Overdose: coma, death, especially when used in combination with barbiturates Withdrawal: anxiety, tremors, hallucinations, hyperreflexia, convulsions, death
Minor tranquilizers					
Chlordiazepoxide (Librium), diazepam (Valium), meprobamate	Tranks	Oral	Nonspecific	Decreased anxiety and tension Occasional disinhibition	Similar to barbiturates but with reduced intensity

Organic solvents					
Hydrocarbons & fluorocarbons—glue, cleaning fluid, lighter fluid, aerosol sprays, nail polish, gasoline		Sniffed	Nonspecific	Euphoria, dysphoria, confusion, impaired perception and coordination Loss of consciousness	Secondary trauma, asphyxia from plastic bags used to inhale fumes Lead poisoning Possible irreversible damage to central nervous system, kidneys, liver, and bone marrow
Stimulants					
Amphetamines—amphetamine sulfate (Benzedrine), dextroamphetamine, methamphetamines	Uppers, leapers, speed, bennies, dexies, pep pills, crystal, whites	Oral, subcutaneous, IV	Hypertension, weight loss, dilated pupils Sweating (injected)	Psychologic and motor stimulation Hyperactivity, false bravado, euphoria, increased alertness, insomnia, anorexia, irritability, personality change	Injection site infection Paranoia, severe depression with suicidal tendency when drug stopped
Cocaine	Coke, Coca Cola, snow	Intranasal, IV	Hypertension, tachycardia, hyperreflexia	Restlessness, hyperactivity, intense euphoria	Nausea and vomiting, inflammation or perforation of nasal septum
Hallucinogens					
Cannabis—marihuana, hashish	Stick, joint, grass, pot, weed, hash, reefers, Mary Janes	Smoke, oral	Occasionally tachycardia, delayed response time, poor coordination	Simple euphoria, mild intoxication, heightened sensory awareness, drowsiness	Occasionally depressive or anxiety reactions
LSD, PCP, DMT, STP, THC, mescaline	Acid, sugar, pearly gates, cubes, big D, mushrooms, peace pill	Oral	Dilated pupils, reddened eyes, occasionally hypertension, hyperthermia, piloerection	Euphoria, heightened sensory awareness, increased appetite, hallucinations, confusion, paranoia	Primarily psychiatric: may intensify latent psychotic tendencies, panic, suicide possible, flashbacks

*Street names are colloquial and vary according to geographic region.

ent and somewhat less addictive are meperidine (Demerol) and methadone (Dolophine). The direct effect of narcotic substances is to alleviate pain and suffering. They produce a state of euphoria by removing painful feelings and creating a pleasurable experience of specific quality and a sense of success. These feelings are accompanied by clouding of consciousness and a dreamlike state.

Although they produce psychologic and physical dependence, heroin and related narcotics do not cause detectable tissue damage and do not impair coordination and judgment when taken in average doses. However, following dependence and withdrawal, physiologic functions may remain unchanged for quite some time. Perhaps more important are the indirect consequences related to the illegal states of narcotic use and the problems associated with securing the drug—time-consuming searches and methods used to meet the high cost. Health problems result from self-neglect of physical needs (nutrition, cleanliness, and dental care), overdose, contamination, and infection. Withdrawal from opiates is extremely unpleasant unless controlled with supervised substitution of methadone.

Central nervous system depressants. A variety of hypnotic drugs that produce physical dependence and withdrawal symptoms on abrupt discontinuance may be used by adolescents. They create a feeling of relaxation and sleepiness, and they impair general functioning. Barbiturates combined with alcohol produce a profound depressant effect.

Also classified as a depressant and socially accepted, acute or chronic abuse of ethanol is responsible for many acts of violence, suicide, and accidental injury and death. It reduces inhibitions against aggressive and sexual acting-out. Abrupt withdrawal is accompanied by severe physical and psychologic symptoms, and long-term use leads to slow tissue destruction, especially of the brain and liver cells.

Central nervous system stimulants. Amphetamines (Benzedrine), methamphetamine (Methedrine), dextroamphetamine (Dexedrine), and cocaine do not produce strong physical dependence and can be withdrawn without much danger. However, psychologic dependence is strong and acute intoxication can lead to violent aggressive behavior or psychotic episodes manifest by paranoia, uncontrollable agitation, and restlessness. Physical deterioration may occur from loss of appetite and sleep during the time the drug is being taken, and severe suicidal depression is often experienced while ''coming down'' off the drug. Combined with barbiturates (''goofballs''), the stimulant effect is canceled out by the depressants. However, the euphoric effects of both are synergistic, cumulative, and particularly addictive. Cocaine is the most potent antifatigue agent known and, although it is not a narcotic, is legally categorized as such.

Mind-altering drugs. Hallucinogens, also known as psychedelic, psychotomimetic, psychotropic, or illusionogenic drugs, consist of a wide variety of agents that produce vivid hallucinations and euphoria. The substance induces a dreamlike state in which the user experiences a whirl of images and strong emotion accompanied by a feeling of boundless union with the environment, not uncommonly associated with feelings of self-disintegration. These drugs do not produce physical dependence since they can be abruptly withdrawn without ill effect. However, acute and long-term effects are variable. In some individuals the dissociative behavior may be unduly protracted. Drugs included in this category are cannabis (marihuana, hashish), mescaline (peyote), lysergic acid diethylamide (LSD), psilocybin (PCP), 2,5-dimethoxy-4-methylamphetamine (DOM or ''STP,'' which stands for ''serenity, tranquility, peace''), and tetrahydrocannabinol (THC), the active ingredient of cannabis. Street drugs sold as mescaline, psilocybin, or tetrahydrocannabinol rarely contain the stated drug. They more often contain LSD or a combination of two or more chemical agents.

Hydrocarbons and fluorocarbons. Glue ''sniffing,'' the inhalation of plastic cement, and inhalation of other volatile substances that youngsters breathe and rebreathe in paper or plastic bags produce euphoria and altered consciousness. They are extremely hazardous to the individual since they cause rapid loss of consciousness and respiratory arrest. Many persons taking these drugs do not have time to remove the bag from their heads and quickly become asphyxiated.

Sequence of drug use[23,33]

All drugs may be abused by teenagers, and most adult users are introduced to the habit at this critical stage of development. However, the type of drugs and the sequence in which they are used follow a fairly typical pattern. The earliest drug use involves easily accessible materials, such as the inhalant or ''sniffing'' substances. They are popular in late childhood and early adolescence (ages 8 to 13 years) because children in this age-group are involved in making models with airplane glue and have more difficulty in acquiring other drugs.

At ages 13 to 14 years and sometimes earlier, alcohol is abused; most adolescents have ''tasted'' alcohol by the time they are 14 years of age. Although most are infrequent drinkers, an alarming number drink regularly. Some drinking takes place at home sanctioned by parents who shudder at the prospect of their children becoming dope users. However, most alcohol is consumed away from home in cars, in alleys, at unchaperoned parties, and openly on the street. Teenagers as a whole have substituted alcohol for dope as the ''lesser of two evils'' with characteristic disregard for its devastating effects. Teenage alcoholism is rising and beginning at earlier ages. Simultaneous use of other drugs compounds the seriousness of alcohol intoxication. For example, barbiturates decrease the rate of alcohol detoxification by live enzymes, thus intensifying the effect.

Amphetamines are popular with young people and are apt

to be one of the first drugs ingested by adolescents, probably obtained from the parents' medicine cabinet and used at first for studying and then later for kicks. Many are able to take them without ill effects, but tolerance quickly develops. From ages 14 to 16 years these and a variety of other drugs including hypnotics, tranquilizers, and cannibis (marihuana), the most popular drug of youth, may be taken. The onset of regular use of the most risky drugs usually does not take place until somewhere between 16 and 18 years of age. These include the narcotics and mind-altering drugs such as LSD, 2,5-dimethoxy-4-methylamphetamine, psilocybin, and marihuana.

Nursing considerations related to medical management

Nurses in almost every setting are increasingly likely to have contact with youthful drug abusers or to be in a position to serve as educator and patient advocate. They are often in a position to serve as listener, confidant, and counselor to troubled youngsters. Nurses are essential members of health teams whose efforts are directed toward short-term and long-term therapy for drug abusers.

The nurse most often encounters youthful drug abusers when they are (1) experiencing overdose symptoms, (2) experiencing withdrawal symptoms, (3) manifesting bizarre behavior or confusion secondary to drug ingestion, or (4) worried that they are becoming or will become addicted.

Many youngsters (or their parents) first seek help when they fear that they are addicted. Most of the young teenagers who claim to be addicted are badly frightened by some contact with drugs or believe that they are addicted because they are drawn to a drug and want to take it again despite the knowledge that they should not. Some adolescents, after an initial exposure to a drug, proudly announce to their parents that they are addicted simply for the shock value of the statement. For many, the legal implications are the primary concern. Therefore, it is important to determine what these youngsters mean when they claim to be addicted, why they are saying this, and what they mean by "addicted." Such claims, as well as actual use, are often a cry for help—a means of drawing attention to them and their needs. It is extremely important to determine if the youngsters are really using drugs and to determine which agent (or agents) is being used. In this way the problems associated with dependence, withdrawal, tolerance, and related health hazards can be anticipated.[10]

Nurses may encounter drug use in relation to other health problems. Nurses caring for adolescents in the hospital or under treatment for other illnesses need to know if the youngsters use drugs compulsively, since withdrawal phenomena can seriously complicate the illness. They should be able to recognize physical or behavioral clues that indicate the onset of withdrawal or the effects of drugs that might have been brought to the youngster secretly by well-meaning relatives or friends. An unwary nurse could administer a prescribed medication that might constitute an overdose in a drugged patient.

Obstetric and nursery personnel sometimes encounter the problem of drug dependence and withdrawal in newborn infants or in a compulsive drug-using mother. These infants are at risk and require special surveillance for complications of withdrawal; therefore, the nursing staff should be aware of the drug dependence in those mothers who come to the hospital for delivery (see p. 353).

Acute care. Adolescents experiencing toxic drug effects or withdrawal symptoms are frequently seen as emergencies. Experienced emergency room personnel are familiar with the management of acute drug toxicosis; the signs, symptoms, and behavioral characteristics of a variety of substances; and differences and similarities among them. When the drug is questionable or unknown, knowledge of these factors facilitates handling of the youngster and implementation of a treatment regimen. Often observation of or description of the behavior is of more value than a report by patients or their friends as to the chemical agent taken. For example, aggressive behavior and disorientation are often seen in barbiturate, alcohol, stimulant, or hallucinogen intoxication but not in opiate intoxication.[22] Overdose from either barbiturates or opiates can result in respiratory failure and coma. Pinpoint pupils are seen only in opiate toxicity. Nurses must be alert for life-threatening consequences of drug toxicity; therefore, equipment and personnel should be available or the patient should be transferred to facilities that are prepared to provide supportive measures for physiologic depression and psychogenic phenomena.

The treatment for drug toxicity or withdrawal varies according to the drug and the method used. Every effort should be made to determine the type and amount of drug taken, the time it was taken, the mode of administration, and factors related to the onset of presenting symptoms. It is helpful to know the patient's pattern of use. For example, if two types of drugs are involved they may require different treatments. Gastric lavage may be employed when the drug has been ingested recently and the cough reflex is intact but would be of little value when the drug has been administered by the intravenous ("mainlined") or intranasal ("sniffed") route. Since the actual content of most street drugs is highly questionable, other pharmaceutical agents are administered with caution, except perhaps the narcotic antagonists in cases of suspected opiate overdose. It is necessary to assess for possible trauma that might have been sustained while under the influence of the drug.

Stimulation should be kept to a minimum for agitated, frightened youngsters. Treatment or tests that are not required immediately are best postponed. Primarily these youngsters need psychologic support in a nonthreatening environment and close contact with a sympathetic person who can stay with them and help them maintain contact with reality.

Long-term management. A major factor in the treatment

and rehabilitation of the young drug user is careful assessment, in the nonacute stage, to determine the function that the drug plays in the youngster's life. The adolescent needs help to identify the problem that motivated him to resort to drugs and to recognize his own role in self-destructive, inappropriate drug-abuse behavior before he can embark on a rehabilitation program.

The motivated phase of treatment is directed toward exploring the factors that influence drug use and establishing in the youngster a feeling of self-worth and a commitment to self-help. It requires a trust relationship between the youngster and the health team and involves a thorough physical examination and assessment of physical, psychologic, educational, and vocational status. A realistic appraisal of the adolescent's potential and efforts aimed at short-term goal satisfaction with building of self-esteem lay the groundwork for a successful rehabilitation program. It may require withdrawing the youngster from his environment as well as from the chemical agent. Programs must be suited to the individual and may involve foster home placement or residential treatment setting, although many are handled in an ambulatory setting. Programs often include group sessions with other troubled youth.

Many drug-abusing adolescents have histories of maladaptive behavior, including family conflicts, school failure, and/or delinquency. Drug use is often a manifestation of a faulty problem-solving process and maladaptive stress-coping mechanisms. A number of teenagers blame their parents, peers, or society for their predicament and need help to understand that they made the choice to use drugs and must assume the responsibility for a course of action—to continue or to select an alternative.[19]

Rehabilitation begins when a youngster has decided that, with the help of concerned and supportive adults, he can and is willing to change. Rehabilitation implies not only environmental manipulation and involvement therapy but also commitment on the part of the patient to substitute dependency on people for his dependency on drugs and to explore alternative mechanisms for problem solving and coping with stress. Persons working with troubled youth must be prepared for recidivism, or the tendency to relapse, and maintain a plan for reentry into the treatment process.

Prevention. Drug abuse in adolescence is both an individual and a community problem, and nurses play an important role in education and legislation as well as in individual observation, assessment, and therapy. In this drug-oriented society, patterns of drug use may be established through parental models and the influence of the media as an effective means to make the user "feel better." Impressionable youth need to be educated regarding appropriate use of chemicals. More important, those associated with adolescents should listen to what they are saying, determine what is bothering them, and try to help them meet these needs through alternative methods before they resort to drugs.

REFERENCES

1. Asher, W. L.: Bariatric medicine and obese teenagers, In Collipp, P. J., editor: Childhood obesity, Acton, Mass., 1975, Publishing Sciences Group, Inc.
2. Bakwin, H., and Bakwin, R. M.: Behavior disorders in children, ed. 4, Philadelphia, 1972, W. B. Saunders Co.
3. Barnes, H. V., and Berger, R.: An approach to the obese adolescent, Med. Clin. North Am. **59:**1507-1516, 1975.
4. Blackburn, G. L., and Bristrain, B. R.: Surgical techniques in the treatment of adolescent obesity. In Collipp, P. J., editor: Childhood obesity, Acton, Mass., 1975, Publishing Sciences Group, Inc.
5. Bray, G. A.: Lipogenesis in human adipose tissue: some effects of nibbling and gorging, J. Clin. Invest. **51:**537, 1972.
6. Brooks, C. G. D.: Evidence for a sensitive period in adipose cell replication in man, Lancet **2:**624, September 23, 1972.
7. Bruch, H.: Anorexia nervosa in adolescence. In Gallagher, J. P., Heald, F. P., and Garell, D. C., editors: Medical care of the adolescent, ed. 3, New York, 1976, Appleton-Century-Crofts.
8. Carman, D. D.: Infant and childhood obesity. Guidelines for prevention and treatment, Pediatr. Nurs. **2**(6):33-38, November/December 1976.
9. Church, C. F., and Church, H. N.: Food values of portions commonly used, ed. 12, Philadelphia, 1975, J. B. Lippincott Co.
10. Faigel, H. C.: Teenage drug abuse. What should you do when one of your adolescent patients says he is a drug addict? Clin. Pediatr. **8**(3):123-125, March 1969.
11. Fisch, R. O., Bilek, M., and Ulstrom, R.: Obesity and leanness at birth and their relationship to body habitus in later childhood, Pediatrics **56:**521-527, 1975.
12. Garfinkel, B. D., and Golombek, H.: Suicide and depression in childhood and adolescence, Can. Med. Assoc. J. **110:** 1278-1281, 1974.
13. Godenne, G. D.: The masked signs of adolescent depression, Med. Insight, pp. 9-11, March 1974.
14. Gross, I., Wheeler, M., and Hess, K.: The treatment of obesity in adolescents using behavioral self-control, Clin. Pediatr. **15:**920-924, 1976.
15. Hammar, S. L., and associates: An interdisciplinary study of adolescent obesity, J. Pediatr. **80:**373-383, 1972.
16. Heald, F. P., and Khan, M. A.: Teenage obesity, Pediatr. Clin. North Am. **20:**807-818, 1973.
17. Hofman, A. D.: Adolescents in distress: suicide and out-of-control behaviors, Med. Clin. North Am. **59:**1429-1438, 1975.
18. Kornhaber, A., and Kornhaber, E.: Obesity in adolescents: contributing psychopathological factors and their treatment. In Collipp, P. J., editor: Childhood obesity, Acton, Mass., 1975, Publishing Sciences Group, Inc.
19. Kramer, R. A.: Drug abuse by adolescents. In Vaught, V. C., and McKay, R. J., editors: Textbook of pediatrics, ed. 10, Philadelphia, 1975, W. B. Saunders Co.
20. Leveille, G. A., and Romsos, D. R.: Meal eating and obesity, Nutr. Today **9**(6):4-9, 1974.
21. Levitz, L. S., and Stunkard, A. J.: A therapeutic coalition for obesity: behavior modification and patient self-help, Am. J. Psychiatry **131:**4, 1974.

22. Long, B. L., and Krepick, D. S.: New perspectives on drug abuse, Nurs. Clin. North Am. **8:**25-40, 1973.
23. MacKenzie, R. G.: A practical approach to the drug-using adolescent and young adult, Pediatr. Clin. North Am. **20:** 1035-1046, 1973.
24. Marthas-Sampson, M.: Adolescents who commit suicidal acts: suicidogenic factors, Issues Comprehensive Pediatr. Nurs., 1976.
25. Mayer, J.: Overweight. Causes, cost, and control, Englewood Cliffs, N.J., 1968, Prentice-Hall, Inc.
26. Mussen, P. H., Conger, J. J., and Kagan, J.: Child development and personality, ed. 4, New York, 1974, Harper & Row, Publishers.
27. Stone, L. J., and Church, J.: Childhood and adolescence, ed. 3, New York, 1973, Random House, Inc.
28. Stunkard, A. J.: Body image disturbance in obesity, Feelings and their Medical Significance **10**(1):1-4, January/February 1968.
29. Stunkard, A. J., and associates: Influences of social class on obesity and thinness in children, J.A.M.A. **221:**579-584, 1972.
30. Taitz, L. S.: Obesity in pediatric practice: infantile obesity, Pediatr. Clin. North Am. **24:**107-115, 1977.
31. Teicher, J. D., and Luce, G.: Why adolescents kill themselves. In Segal, I., editor: The mental health of the child, Public Health pamphlet No. 2168, Washington, D.C., 1971, U.S. Government Printing Office.
32. Vigersky, R. A., and associates: Anorexia nervosa: behavioral and hypothalamic aspects, Clin. Endocrinol. Metabol. **5:** 517:535, 1976.
33. Wurmser, L.: Drug use and abuse in adolescence. In Gallagher, J. R., Heald, F. P., and Garell, D. C., editors: Medical care of the adolescent, ed. 3, New York, 1976, Appleton-Century-Crofts.

BIBLIOGRAPHY

Aguilera, D. C., and Messick, J. M.: Crisis intervention: implications for community nursing with the "now" generation. In Reinhardt, A. M., and Quinn, M. D., editors: Current practice in family-centered community nursing, vol. I, St. Louis, 1977, The C. V. Mosby Co.

Amenta, M. M.: Free clinics change the scene, Am. J. Nurs. **74:** 284, 1974.

Bernard, B. H.: When a child's distress is a family affair, Nurs. Clin. North Am. **5:**677, 1970.

Blackford, G. S.: The professional and the contemporary youth scene. The design of a course, Nurs. Clin. North Am. **5:**261-268, 1970.

Emmert, J.: Youth clinic: A nurse's challenge, Nursing '72 **2:**13, September 1972.

Fagin, C. M., editor: Readings in child and adolescent psychiatric nursing, St. Louis, 1974, The C. V. Mosby Co.

Feighner, J. P., and associates: Diagnostic criteria for use in psychiatric research, Arch. Gen. Psychiatry **26:**57-63, 1972.

Fredlund, D.: Juvenile delinquency and school nursing, Nurs. Outlook **18:**57, 1970.

Gallagher, J. R., Heald, F. P., and Garell, D. C., editors: Medical care of the adolescent, ed. 3, New York, 1976, Appleton-Century-Crofts.

Guthrie, A. D., and Howell, M. C.: Mobile medical care for alienated youths, J. Pediatr. **81:**1025, 1972.

Kalafatich, A. J., editor: Approaches to the care of adolescents, New York, 1975, Appleton-Century-Crofts.

Quinn, D. C.: No room at the inn: gaps in services for troubled youth and the role of the community health nurse. In Reinhardt, A. M., and Quinn, M. D., editors: Current practice in family-centered community nursing, St. Louis, 1977, The C. V. Mosby Co.

Rudolph, A. M., Barnett, H. L., and Einhorn, A. H., editors: Pediatrics, ed. 16, New York, 1977, Appleton-Century-Crofts.

Vaughn, V. C., and McKay, R. J.: Textbook of pediatrics, ed. 10, Philadelphia, 1975, W. B. Saunders Co.

Weiner, I. B.: Juvenile delinquency, Pediatr. Clin. North Am. **72:** 673-684, 1975.

Anorexia nervosa

Bruch, H.: Psychosomatic aspects of malnutrition during adolescence, Postgrad. Med. **47:**99, May 1970.

Combrinich-Graham, L.: Structural family therapy in psychosomatic illness, Clin. Pediatr. **13:**827, 1974.

Crisp, A. H.: Primary anorexia nervosa or adolescent weight phobia, Practitioner **211:**525, 1974.

Halmi, K. A., and associates: Treatment of anorexia nervosa with behavior modification, Arch. Gen. Psychiatry **32:**93-96, 1975.

Hext, M., and Murchland, A.: Adolescent anorexia nervosa: the patient; an approach, J. Psychiatr. Nurs. **10:**23, November/December 1972.

Melton, J. H.: A boy with anorexia nervosa, Am. J. Nurs. **74:** 1649-1651, 1974.

Schmidt, M. P. W., and Duncan, B. A. B.: Modifying eating behavior in anorexia nervosa, Am. J. Nurs. **74:**1646-1648, 1974.

Silverman, J. A.: Anorexia nervosa: clinical observations in a successful plan, J. Pediatr. **84:**68-73, 1974.

Tolstrup, K.: The treatment of anorexia nervosa in childhood and adolescence, J. Child. Psychol. Psychiatry **14:**76, January 1975.

Warren, M. P., and VandeWiele, R. L.: Clinical and metabolic features of anorexia nervosa, Am. J. Obstet. Gynecol. **117:**435, 1973.

Watson, W. C.: On psychological factors and disease states, Gastroenterology **59:**646-647, 1970.

Obesity

Adebonojo, F. O.: Primary exogenous obesity: a conceptual classification, Clin. Pediatr. **13:**715, 1974.

Brook, C. G. D., Lloyd, J. K., and Wolff, O. H.: Relation between age of onset of obesity and size and number of adipose cells. Br. Med. J. **2:**25-27, 1972.

Bruch, H.: Treatment of eating disorders, Mayo Clin. Proc. **51:** 266-272, 1976.

Charney, E., and associates: Childhood antecedents of adult obesity, N. Engl. J. Med. **295:**6, 1976.

Collip, P. J.: Obesity in children. In Asher, W. L., editor: Treatment of the obese, New York, 1974, Medcom Press.

Collip, P. J., editor: Childhood obesity, Acton, Mass., 1975, Publishing Sciences Group, Inc.

Craft, C. A.: Body image and obesity, Nurs. Clin. North Am. **7:** 677-685, 1972.

Davis, B., and Stuart, R. B.: Slim chance in a fat world: behavioral control of obesity, Champaign, Ill., 1974, Research Press.

Dobbing, J.: Fat cells in childhood obesity, Lancet **1**:224, 1975.

Eden, A. N.: Growing up thin, New York, 1975, David McKay Co., Inc.

Fineberg, M. D.: Diet: the realities of obesity and fad diets, Nutr. Today **7**(4):23, 1972.

Fisch, R. O., Bilek, M., and Ulstrom, R.: Obesity and leanness at birth and their relationship to body habitus in later childhood, Pediatrics **56**:521-527, 1975.

Garn, S. M., and Clark, D. C.: Trends in fatness and the origins of obesity, Pediatrics **57**:443, 1976.

Green, R. S., and Rau, H. N.: Treatment of compulsive eating disturbances, Am. J. Psychiatry **131**:428, 431, 1974.

Grollman, A.: Drug therapy of obesity in children, Pediatr. Ann. **4**:266, 1975.

Hammar, F.: Adolescent obesity, J. Pediatr. **80**:373, 1972.

Hammar, S. L.: Obesity: early identification and treatment, Pediatr. Ann. **4**:250, 1975.

Hicks, C. B.: "Eat" says fat little Johnny's mother, Today's Health **48**:48-52, 86, February 1970.

Jones, Y. H., and Jenkins, L. A.: A nurse-directed outpatient obesity clinic, Hospitals **47**:74-78, 1973.

Kaufmann, N. A., and associates: Eating habits and opinions of teenagers on nutrition and obesity, J. Am. Diet. Assoc. **66**:264-268, March 1975.

Knittle, J. L.: Obesity in childhood: a problem in adipose tissue cellular development, J. Pediatr. **81**:1048-1059, 1972.

Kopelke, C. E.: Group education to reduce overweight . . . in a blue collar community, Am. J. Nurs. **75**:1993-1995, 1975.

Lenitz, L. S.: Behavior therapy in treating obesity, J. Am. Diet. Assoc. **62**:22, 1973.

Lepkovsky, S.: Newer concepts in the regulation of food intake, Am. J. Clin. Nutr. **26**:271-284, 1973.

Mann, G. V.: The influence of obesity on health, N. Engl. J. Med. **291**:178-185, 226-231, 1974.

Martin, M. M., and associates: Obesity, hyperinsulinism, and diabetes mellitus in childhood, J. Pediatr. **82**:192-201, 1973.

Mayer, J.: Obesity, Postgrad. Med. **51**:66, 1972.

Meyer, E. E., and Neumann, C. G.: Management of the obese adolescent, Pediatr. Clin. North Am. **24**:123-132, 1977.

Peckos, P.: The treatment of adolescent obesity, Issues Comprehensive Pediatr. Nurs., pp. 17-30, 1976.

Pipes, P. L.: Nutrition in infancy and childhood, St. Louis, 1977, The C. V. Mosby Co.

Reiter, E. D., and Wright, E.: Endocrine causes and treatment of obesity. In Barness, L., editor: Report of second Wyeth nutrition symposium, Philadelphia, 1976, Wyeth Laboratories.

Salams, L., Cushman, S., and Weismann, R. E.: Studies of human adipose tissue: adipose cell size and number in non-obese and obese patients, J. Clin. Invest. **52**:929, 1973.

Stanley, E. J., and associates: Overcoming obesity in adolescents. A description of a promising endeavor to improve management, Clin. Pediatr. **9**:29-36, 1970.

Steiner, M. M.: Childhood obesity, Pediatr. Digest **18**:9, 1976.

VanItallie, T. B., and Campbell, R. C.: Multidisciplinary approach to the problem of obesity, J. Am. Diet. Assoc. **61**:385, 1972.

Winick, M.: Childhood obesity, Nutr. Today **9**(3):6-12, May/June 1974.

Zakus, M.: The family situation of obese adolescent girls, Adolescence **8**:33, 1973.

Suicide

Bakwin, R. M.: Suicide in children and adolescents, J. Am. Med. Wom. Assoc. **28**:643, 1973.

Barnett, H. R.: Suicide in children and adolescents, Pediatrics **49**:290, 1972.

Bell, K. K.: The nursing consultant in a suicide prevention center, Nurs. Clin. North Am. **5**:687-697, 1970.

Blomquist, K. B.: Nurse, I need help: the school nurse's role in suicide prevention, J. Psychiatr. Nurs. Ment. Health Serv. **12**:22-26, 1974.

Fenton, K. F.: Adolescent suicide and the suicidal adolescent. In Kalafatich, A. J., editor: Approaches to the care of adolescents, New York, 1975, Appleton-Century-Crofts.

Hofmann, A. D.: Adolescents in distress: suicide and out-of-control behaviors, Med. Clin. North Am. **59**:1429-1438, 1975.

Holland, J., and Plumb, M.: Management of the serious suicide attempt: a special ICU nursing problem, Heart Lung **2**:378, May/June 1973.

Jacobziner, H.: Attempted suicides in adolescence, J.A.M.A. **191**:101-105, 1975.

Lordi, W. M.: Suicide in children and adolescents, Va. Med. **98**:209, 1971.

Malmquist, C. P.: Depressions in childhood and adolescence, N. Engl. J. Med. **284**:887-893, 1971.

McAnarney, E. R.: Suicidal behavior in children and youth, Pediatr. Clin. North Am. **22**:595-604, 1975.

Mitchell, M. L.: Suicide is a family nursing problem. In Hymovich, D. P., and Barnard, M. V., editors: Family health care, New York, 1973, McGraw-Hill Book Co.

Musgrave, L. C.: Hot line takes the heat off, Am. J. Nurs. **71**:756-759, 1971.

Rohn, R. D., and associates: Adolescents who commit suicide, Pediatrics **90**:636-638, 1977.

Schowalter, J.: Adolescent patient's decision to die, Pediatrics **51**:97, 1973.

Shore, J. H.: American Indian suicide—fact or fantasy, Psychiatry **38**:86-92, 1975.

Stanley, E. J., and Barter, J. T.: Adolescent suicide behavior, Am. J. Orthopsychiatry **40**:87: 1970.

Strutzel, E. A.: A disturbed adolescent. The nursing process in a collaborative treatment, Nurs. Clin. North Am. **6**:727-744, 1971.

Teicher, J. D.: Children and adolescents who attempt suicide, Pediatr. Clin. North Am. **17**:687, 1970.

Toolan, J. M.: Suicide in children and adolescents, Am. J. Psychother. **29**:334-339, 1975.

Weinberg, S.: Suicidal intent in adolescence: a hypothesis about the role of physical illness, J. Pediatr. **77**:579-586, 1970.

Westercamp, T. M.: Suicide, Am. J. Nurs. **75**:260-262, 1975.

Yusin, A.: Attempted suicide in an adolescent, Adolescence **8**:18, 1973.

Drug abuse

Bergersen, B. S., and Goth, A.: Pharmacology in nursing, ed. 14, St. Louis, 1979, The C. V. Mosby Co.

Blades, S.: Clinical notes on adolescent drug abuse, Issues Comprehensive Pediatr. Nurs., pp. 59-64, 1976.

Bosma, W. G. A.: Adolescents and alcohol. In Gallagher, J. R., Heald, F. P., and Garell, D. C., editors: Medical care of the adolescent, ed. 3, New York, 1976, Appleton-Century-Crofts.

Bourne, P. G.: Is drug abuse a fading fad? J. Am. Coll. Health Assoc. **21:**198-200, 1973.

Boyer, C. M.: Caring for a young addict with tetanus, Am. J. Nurs. **74:**265, 1974.

Caskey, K. K., Blaylock, E. V., and Wauson, B. M.: The school nurse and drug abusers, Nurs. Outlook **18:**27-30, 1970.

Charalampous, K. D.: Drug culture in the seventies, Am. J. Public Health **61:**1225-1228, 1971.

Choi, S. Y.: Death in young alcoholics, J. Stud. Alcohol **36:**1224-1229, 1975.

Faigel, H. C.: Commentary: why our children drink, Clin. Pediatr. **16:**509, 1976.

Flynn, W. R.: Drug abuse as a defense in adolescence—a follow-up, Adolescence **8:**363, 1973.

Foreman, N., and Zerwekh, J.: Drug crisis intervention, Am. J. Nurs. **71:**1736, 1971.

Fort, J.: Youth: drugs, sex and life, Curr. Probl. Pediatr. **6**(11): 1-68, September 1976.

Geist, R. A.: Some observations on adolescent drug use, J. Am. Acad. Child Psychiatry **13:**54-71, 1974.

Herzog, E., and associates: Drug use among the young, as teenagers see it, Children **17:**207, 1970.

Kandell, D.: Adolescent marijuana use: role of parents and peers, Science **181:**1067, 1973.

Korobkin, R., and associates: Glue-sniffing neuropathy, Arch. Nuerol. **32:**158-162, 1975.

Krepick, D. S., and Long, B. L.: Heroin addiction: a treatable disease, Nurs. Clin. North Am. **8:**41-52, 1973.

Lieber, C.: Alcohol and nutrition, Nutr. News **39**(3):9, 1976.

Litt, I. F., and Schonberg, S. K.: Medical complications of drug abuse in adolescents, Med. Clin. North Am. **59:**1445-1452, 1975.

MacKenzie, R. G.: Caring for the adolescent drug user, Med. Clin. North Am. **59:**1439-1444, 1975.

Musgrave, L. C.: Hot line takes the heat off, Am. J. Nurs. **71:**756-759, 1971.

Nelson, K.: The nurse in a methadone maintenance program, Am. J. Nurs. **73:**870, 1973.

Notaro, C.: Adolescents and alcohol, Issues Comprehensive Pediatr. Nurs., 1976.

Petit, J. M., and Biggs, J. T.: Tricyclic antidepressant overdoses in adolescent patients, Pediatrics **59:**283-287, 1977.

Stephenson, J. N.: Drug abuse in adolescence. In Kalafatich, A. J., editor: Approaches to the care of adolescents, New York, 1975, Appleton-Century-Crofts.

Thornburg, H.: The adolescent and drugs: an overview, J. Sch. Health **43:**640-644, 1973.

Yancy, W. S., Nader, P. R., and Burnham, K. L.: Drug use and attitudes of high school students, Pediatrics **50:**739-745, 1972.

Yankelovich, D.: Drug users vs. drug abusers: how students control their drug crisis, Psychol. Today **9:**39-42, October 1975.

UNIT NINE
The child with developmental problems

Units Four through Eight have focused on the growth and development of the well child. Most of the health problems discussed for each age-group were those that temporarily incapacitated the child. Unit Nine is concerned with the child who has a permanent or chronic physical and/or developmental handicap. Unlike the child who is well, these children need to master the same developmental achievements in accordance with their potential abilities despite the handicapping condition. Families of these children, likewise, are faced with exceptional challenges for which there is little guidance or few role models to emulate. As a result the entire family unit is highly vulnerable to psychologic and sometimes physical problems that arise from unsuccessful attempts to deal with the primary condition.

Chapter 22, *The Handicapped Child,* is an overview of the child's and family's reactions to a handicap and nursing interventions that assist each member in adjusting to the condition and developing to their fullest despite the disability. This chapter serves as a basis for understanding the stresses and needs of families when the child is chronically ill, physically disabled, mentally retarded, or sensory impaired. Chapter 23, *The Child with Mental Retardation,* is primarily concerned with the retarded child and discusses the classification of mental retardation, its causes, and the nursing interventions required to help the child become independent. Chapter 24, *The Child with a Sensory or Communication Disorder,* deals with the child who has a sensory loss or a communication disorder. Emphasis is placed on the effect of the impairment on development, detection of the disorder, and nursing interventions that promote rehabilitation.

22

The handicapped child

The term "handicapped" is one that almost defies definition, because in a complex society there are innumerable abilities necessary for functioning. Loss of any physical or mental power immediately poses an obstacle to one's ability to meet societal expectations. Because nurses are intimately involved in every type of health deviation, it is inevitable that they will be responsible for some phase of care with handicapped children. This discussion focuses on handicapping conditions in general, including (1) chronic illness—any illness with a protracted course that can be progressive and fatal or one that is associated with a relatively normal life span despite impaired physical or mental functioning[15]; (2) permanent loss of a physical or sensory ability; (3) developmental disability—any disability that is attributable to mental retardation, cerebral palsy, epilepsy, autism, dyslexia, or any other condition related to mental retardation; that originates before age 18 years and has continued to be or can be expected to continue indefinitely; and that constitutes a substantial handicap to the ability to function normally in society[13]; and (4) multiple handicaps—the presence of more than one handicapping condition. Although many congenital conditions are handicapping, the response of parents to a defective newborn has been discussed in Chapter 11.

SCOPE OF PROBLEM

Statistics regarding handicapping conditions are formidable. It is estimated that as many as 10% to 15% of all children under 18 years of age have some type of chronic illness, including sensory impairments.[18] The most frequent chronic childhood conditions are caused by diseases of the respiratory system, chiefly asthma and bronchitis, neurologic diseases, and a variety of musculoskeletal disorders. Significantly the majority of chronically ill children suffer from a disorder that primarily or indirectly affects motor activity. In addition to this group, 3% of the population has some form of mental retardation,[7] and each year approximately 250,000 infants are born who survive with significant birth defects. Broadly expanding chronic conditions to include speech, learning, and behavioral disorders yields an estimated 30% to 40% of children who are suffering from a significant long-term disorder.[15] If one considers that the average American family has between three and four members, the numbers of individuals intimately affected by the handicapped child are staggering.

The numbers alone suggest that comprehensive nursing approaches are needed to meet the vast problems of children, youth, and families. Clearly nurses have a more crucial role than ever before in early screening, case finding, assessment, and diagnostic studies. Another major responsibility is preventing further handicapping conditions by eliminating their known causes. Nurses are responsible for assuring immunization programs, identifying infants and mothers who may be at risk prenatally or postnatally, identifying the disability early, and implementing innovative health education programs. Table 22-1 lists conditions of high risk for causing handicaps in infants.

CHANGING TRENDS IN CARE

American society has passed through three stages in providing services to handicapped children,[4] the first stage of which is *forget and hide*. The parents and family were encouraged to place the handicapped child in an institution or send him away to relatives. Persons were oriented to an "out of sight–out of mind" philosophy in order to cope with differences. Negative attitudes prevailed, and handicapped persons were neglected. Many constitutional rights were abused or violated.

The second phase is described as *screen and segregate*. During the years following World War II, special classes for handicapped children were offered by specially trained personnel. Many believe that this was a subtle way of segregating handicapped children from regular teachers and classrooms.

The present stage is referred to as *identify and help* and is characterized by finding children in need of services at the earliest possible age and beginning treatment. Different trends in care of handicapped persons are listed in the boxed material on p. 784.

Table 22-1. At-risk conditions for handicaps in infants

Maternal factors	Infant factors
History of infertility History of abortions (3 times) Previous delivery stillborn or suffered neonatal death Previous premature delivery Previous delivery of infant with congenital defects Weight gain during pregnancy less than 4.5 kg (10 pounds) Threatened abortion in first or second trimester Premature labor Prolonged rupture of membranes (more than 20 hours) Cesarean section Abruptio placentae Cord prolapse Fetal distress (decreasing fetal heart tones) Multiple birth Breech birth Preeclampsia-eclampsia	Fetal distress, meconium-stained ileus Prematurity or postmaturity Low gestational weight Congenital defects Apgar score of 6 or below at 1 or 5 minutes Addiction withdrawal symptoms Hypoglycemia requiring treatment Seizures Use of oxygen at greater than 40% concentration for more than 24 hours Recognized viral syndromes Recognized bacterial, protozoan, or fungal infections Bilirubin level 15 mg/100 ml or above in premature or low gestational weight infants Bilirubin level 20 mg/100 ml or above in full-term infants Metabolic disease Drug depression Resuscitation needed for more than 2 minutes Chromosomal anomaly Placenta/infant weight ratio indicating a small placenta

Adapted from criteria used by the Nursing Child Assessment Project, University of Washington; from Barnard, K. E., and Erickson, M. L.: Teaching children with developmental problems: a family care approach, ed. 2, St. Louis, 1976, The C. V. Mosby Co.

PRINCIPLES OF WORKING WITH HANDICAPPED CHILDREN

The concept of individual differences, the need to treat persons with dignity, and the need to reject stereotypes have been manifest and appreciated only recently. Nurses working with a handicapped child need to have a comprehensive knowledge of the individual needs of these children. They must know each child and be able to assess his strengths, deficits, and unique characteristics. Nurses should be sensitive to his capabilities, his progress, the need for an individualized program, and the efficacy of the care and services received.

Changing trends in care

Outmoded concepts of care	*Emerging trends in care*
Use of pediatric pathologic medical model	Use of developmental and educational model
Waiting for gross clinical manifestations before making a diagnosis	Beginning to observe infants early
Generalizing, stereotyping, and labeling of children	Observation for individual differences
Looking for negative features or traits	Emphasizing assets and positive features of infant, child, or parent
Guessing about how well a child is doing	Collecting objective data in decision-making process
Gathering data only once	Gathering data on serial basis
Omitting parents in assessment and care process	Eliciting parent's perceptions of child's development and behaviors
Failure to share assessment and care progress data with parents	Use of mutual participation model for problem solving
Lack of standardized assessment tools	Use of recent standardized screening and assessment tools
Instant advice given	Thinking of ways to collect data and solve problems
Use of trial and error approach	Documentation of behavioral change and evaluation of it
Focusing on one symptom	Looking for clusters of minor anomalies that may signal presence of major defect
Focusing on child alone	Consideration of needs of siblings and parent
Screening at school entrance	Early case finding during newborn period—periodic screening
Physician responsible for diagnosis and treatment	Use of interdisciplinary approach
Planning short-term goals	Consideration of lifetime goals
Intervention during crisis	Anticipation of guidance before stress and crisis
Physical evaluation	Developmental screening
Yearly checkups	Ongoing, repeated assessments
Telling parents what to do	Asking parents what their concerns are and what they want to do
Emphasizing abnormalities in child	Looking for similarities child has with others
Viewing handicap first	Seeing child as individual first and emphasizing handicap(s) second

Nurses' understanding needs to be thorough enough to communicate the child's strengths and weaknesses to him, his parents, care givers, or personnel who work with him at home, in schools, in special remedial programs, in rehabilitation centers, or in job placement training programs. The professional nurse must be able to view the child in relationship to his handicap and not have perceptions clouded by the handicap. *The nurse must be sensitive to the child first and to his handicap second.* Thus the nurse can respond to the handicapped child with a spontaneous and genuine interest, rather than with misplaced sympathy.

The nurse's manner similarly conveys an attitude to the child's parents and teachers. A dislike, rejection, or nonacceptance of a child cannot be disguised. A nurse having difficulty in liking or accepting a child may need to examine personal feelings about differences in others, stigma, and difficulty in accepting and interacting with persons who display unattractive features or behaviors. All child-care professionals at one time or another need to permit themselves to work through their feelings. Sometimes this is difficult and painful. The first step is awareness of uncomfortable feelings. The nurse needs to know that the feelings that first emerge may be fear, anger, or grief. As these feelings are dealt with appropriately, there is a greater chance that more positive feelings can emerge, and, as they are gradually worked through, there is a greater sense of acceptance of one's feelings, appreciation for self and others, more tolerance and flexibility, and the gratification of learning and discovering something new about one's self.

As nurses become more attuned to their personal feelings, they may be in a better position to help others get in touch with their feelings. The handicapped person can interact better with the professional person who has developed healthy, nurturing attitudes rather than stereotyped, primitive, inappropriate, and unhealthy ones. The person with a handicapping condition needs to interact with persons who are intact, sensitive, and responsive to new growth on their own part. There has been less emphasis in the past on assisting the handicapped person to discover and appreciate his own strengths. A sensitive nurse can encourage and foster the handicapped person's self-acceptance. A handicapped person who continually receives negative, subtly disguised cues that he is different and unaccepted learns to perceive himself in a less than healthy way. The nurse should serve as a role model for parents, teachers, and others who work with persons who are handicapped, demonstrating that the person is acceptable, is unique, does have strengths, can change, and can contribute in his own way.

The nurse must be sensitive to parents' reactions to handicapped persons and help them express and clarify their feelings. Parents should be taught that their feelings are normal and that expressing fear, hurt, grief, or anxiety is both healthy and helpful. The nurse needs to orient the mother and father to the child's emotional needs as well as seek their permission to allow the child to express feelings he has about himself, his handicap, and what it means to him now and in the future. A skilled nurse can use many supportive techniques in communicating with a child. Developing a sense of trust is essential to allow the child to feel safe in expressing himself. This requires a long-term relationship with the child through his stages of development and changing feelings.

The nurse needs skills in collaborating, sharing, and exchanging roles with other members of the child-care disciplines. Nurses need to understand that comprehensive management begins with systematic, objective observations and assessments. Comprehensive care means ongoing surveillance, not episodic care planning. They have to be aware of appropriate screening tools, systematic observational methods, and newer trends in assessment and management. They should be able to recognize and reject outmoded concepts of care and help parents do so. They need to listen to parents' thoughts and hear the child's point of view. The child should be included in planning and decision making that affects him.

Nurses need to be willing to plan care with other health care workers and to seek additional expertise when needed. The nurse must be oriented to anticipatory care and prevention rather than emergency intervention. Nurses need to be willing to keep systematic records of the following behaviors: (1) sleep, eating, toileting, and dressing; (2) limit-setting responses; (3) interactions with peers, interactions with adults, play, and preacademic behaviors; (4) behaviors during illness and before and after hospitalization; (5) behaviors indicating independence or dependence and maladaptive and adaptive, desirable and undesirable, and compliant and noncompliant behaviors; and (6) behaviors that show traits of being a leader or a follower. Objectivity is necessary in documenting the kind of behavior. The parents are encouraged to be objective also. The nurse must observe and record adult behaviors as well and use the data to encourage change when appropriate.

Nurses' actions need to be based on scientific knowledge of growth and development, biochemistry, and theories from the social and behavioral sciences. Interventions should be founded on sound, theoretic frameworks and well-defined behavioral objectives that can be documented and measured. Nurses must be flexible and willing to revise plans of care appropriately. They should encourage the child and family to set realistic goals and maintain an outlook of success rather than failure. Using instruments such as the Home Observation for Measurement of the Environment (HOME) birth to three and HOME three to six, the nurse ensures that the home and the school environments meet the needs of the child and his family (see p. 793). Community resources and their standards of care, advantages, and disadvantages should be discussed and evaluated with parents.

FAMILIES OF HANDICAPPED CHILDREN

Impact of diagnosis

Many of the reactions of parents to the birth of a defective child are observed when the diagnosis of a handicapping condition is made later in life. The parents have, in a sense, lost the perfect child they had and now have to adjust to a child with a disability. The parents need the opportunity to mourn the loss of the perfect child before they can adjust to and fully accept a child who is handicapped. This period varies with each parent but usually proceeds through the following stages (Fig. 22-1).

Shock. The initial stage is one of shock and a period of intense emotion. It may be accompanied by denial, especially if the handicap is not obvious, such as in chronic illness. If the defect is highly obvious and overwhelming, such as the loss of eyesight or a limb, this period may be characterized by disintegration, because the emotional demands for dealing with the diagnosis leave no reserve for dealing with realistic problems.

The period of shock is usually short-lived because of the necessity of making decisions regarding treatment. However, the denial may be protracted. Denial as a defense mechanism is not always abnormal; in fact, it may be the necessary cushion to prevent disintegration. Probably all parents experience various degrees of adaptive denial as they learn of the impact that the diagnosis has on their lives. Denial becomes maladaptive when it prevents recognition of treatment rehabilitative goals necessary for the child's optimal survival. For example, denial of diabetes mellitus that results in failure to administer insulin has life-threatening consequences. However, this is not infrequently seen in diabetic children who forget to give themselves the drug or eat excessive quantities of carbohydrates. Other common examples of parental denial are physician shopping for additional opinions and the frequently heard expression, "No one tells us anything about our child's condition."

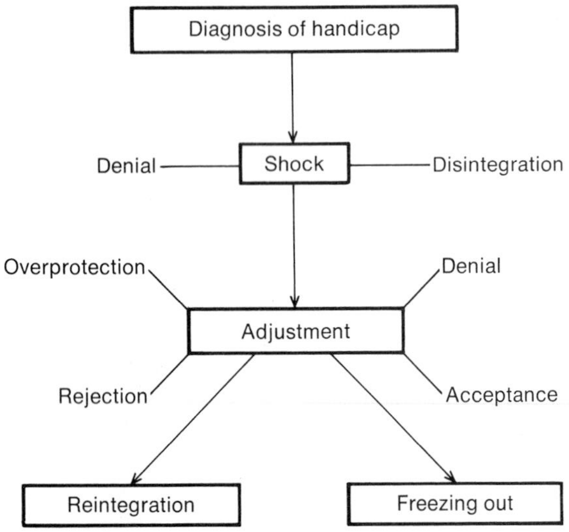

Fig. 22-1. Reactions to diagnosis.

The response of a family to mental retardation may differ from those discussed in the preceding paragraphs, because as long as the family can maintain a fiction of normality and handle the deviance within the present familial roles and values, there may exist no recognition of the diagnosis.[22] Instead the problem is explained as slow maturation or an easily remedied disorder. The denial may be enforced by the child's social development, which belies the degree of motor and speech retardation. Not infrequently this ability to rationalize delayed development is successful until the child enters school, when his differences are compared to other children and become blatantly evident. At this point the family may begin to recognize the diagnosis as a crisis and react with shock and disbelief.

Adjustment. Adjustment soon follows shock and is usually characterized by an open admission that the handicap exists. This stage is one of "chronic sorrow" and only partial acceptance.[17] This period is manifest by several responses, probably the most universal of which are *guilt* and *self-accusation*. Guilt arises from a human need to find rational causes for events. The concept of cause and effect implies an ability to change future events. It is often greatest when the cause of the handicap is directly traceable to the parent, such as in genetic diseases or from accidental injury. However, it occurs even without any scientific or realistic basis for parental responsibility. Frequently the guilt stems from a fallacious assumption that the handicap is a result of personal failing or wrongdoing. The ability to master resentful and self-accusatory feelings of having "caused" the child's disorder is a crucial factor in determining the parents' acceptance of their handicapped child.[15]

Other common reactions are *bitterness* or *anger* because the child is an obstacle interfering with parental goals and *envy* toward those who are not burdened with a handicapped child. Because the real reason for such feelings are usually unacceptable to parents, the emotions may be redirected toward others, such as health professionals, for not "curing" their child.

Parents who have a retarded child are faced with major psychologic stress, and, even though they may be generally well adjusted, they are likely to manifest responses that interfere at least temporarily with optimum coping. Typical parental reactions include[19]: (1) *loss of self esteem,* in which parents perceive a defect in their child as a defect in themselves; their life goals may be abruptly and dramatically altered, and they lose the fantasy of immortality through their child; (2) *shame,* in which parents anticipate social rejection, pity, or ridicule and related loss of social prestige and may experience social withdrawal; (3) *ambivalence,* in which the simultaneous experience of love and hatred normally experienced by parents toward their children is likely to be greatly intensified in parents of a retarded child; (4) *depression,* in which parents experience chronic feelings of sorrow as a nonneurotic reaction to having a retarded child; to some parents mental retardation symbolizes the child's death and therefore precipitates a grief reaction; (5) *self-sacrifice,* in which parents adopt a "martyr" attitude and focus their total interest on the child with mental retardation, often to the detriment of other family members; and (6) *defensiveness,* in which parents become acutely sensitive to implied criticism of their retarded child and may react with resentment and belligerence, or they may deny the existence of mental retardation and seek professional opinions to substantiate their own belief that "there is really nothing wrong with him." Although these reactions have been noted specifically in parents of retarded children, they are frequently observed in other handicapping situations as well.

During the period of readjustment, there are four types of parental reactions to the child[16]: (1) *overprotection* or the benevolent overreaction,[2] in which the parents fear letting the child achieve any new skill, avoid all discipline, and cater to every desire to prevent frustration; (2) *rejection,* in which the parents detach themselves emotionally from the child but usually provide adequate physical care or constantly nag and scold the child; (3) *denial,* in which parents act as if the handicap does not exist or attempt to have the child overcompensate for it, and (4) *gradual acceptance,* in which parents place necessary and realistic restrictions on the child, encourage self-care activities, and promote reasonable physical and social abilities.

The most common initial response, especially among mothers, is the benevolent overreaction. It is usually a consequence of unresolved guilt or fear, such as ambivalent feelings of not wanting the child during pregnancy, feeling responsible for the handicap, believing that the child would die at the time of birth or diagnosis, or reactivated feelings about a previous death of a loved one.[15] It results in a vicious cycle of overprotective, permissive parent and dependent, demanding child (Fig. 22-2). It prevents the child from developing self-control, independence, initiative, and self-esteem. Fortunately it is a reaction that responds to early intervention and prevention.

Reintegration and acceptance. The last stage is characterized by realistic expectations for the child and reintegration of family life with the handicap in proper perspective. Since a large portion of the adjustment phase is one of grief for a loss, total resolution is not possible until the child dies. Therefore, one can regard adjustment to chronic sorrow as "increased comfortableness" with everyday living.[17]

It is also one of social reintegration in which the family broadens its activities to include relationships outside of the home with the handicapped child as an acceptable and participating member of the group. This last criterion often differentiates the reaction of gradual acceptance during the adjustment period from total acceptance.

Freezing-out phase.[8] Not all families reach the stage of

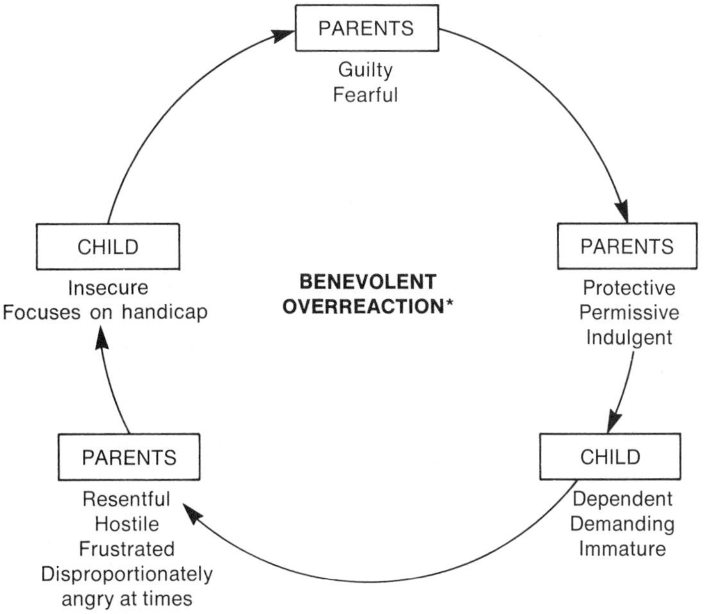

Fig. 22-2. Common cyclical response between parents and handicapped child.
*(From Boone, D. R., and Hartman, B. H.: The benevolent over-reaction, Clin. Pediatr. **11**(5):268-271, May 1972.)

acceptance and reintegration. Many maintain the patterns of overprotection, rejection, or denial. However, if strategies of coping cannot be employed to minimize the stress and disorganization of maintaining the child within the home to tolerable levels, the handicapped child may be permanently eliminated by placing him outside the home in some type of residential setting, usually institutionalization. The evolvement of this phase is directly related to the degree of physical and mental handicap.

This phase is not necessarily one of maladjustment. Placement may be the only strategy that will preserve the integrity of the family. Aging parents may be forced to accept this alternative from progressive inability to meet the demands of a severely retarded or multihandicapped offspring. Relinquishing the role of primary care giver is followed by an initial sense of loss, relief, guilt, and ambivalence.[12] The pattern of reactions is not unlike that seen following the death of a terminally-ill child (see p. 984).

Effects on family members

Each family who has a child with a handicap comprises a "handicapped family." No one member remains uninvolved or unaffected by the experience. The child's and siblings' reactions are usually direct consequences of the parents' responses.

Parents. Besides grieving for the loss of a perfect child, parents of a handicapped child are less likely than most parents to receive positive feedback from transactions with their child. Parenting such children may be a series of unrewarding experiences, which continually support the parents' feelings of inadequacy and failure. These responses may be most evident in mothers who are responsible for the child's care. For example, they may become preoccupied with their ability to carry out certain procedures, overlooking the child's personal comfort and satisfaction or failing to praise him for anything less than perfect cooperation or performance. They often pursue a frustrating activity until they achieve "success" long after the child has become irritable and uncooperative. They may unrealistically withhold privileges until the child completes a certain task or exercise. As a result the mother becomes caught in a pattern of interaction that is mutually unrewarding and minimally productive. For these mothers it may be beneficial to reduce the quantity of time spent with the child to increase the quality of the relationship.[14]

Parents may have excessive demands placed on their time, energy, and financial resources. Depending on the roles assumed by each spouse, the wife often receives the brunt of the time and energy demands and the husband the financial responsibilities. However, with changing sex roles these responsibilities may be shared or shifted more heavily to one member. For example, the working mother may feel the need to continue employment to help defray the expenses, but this also incurs the added burden of additional child/home responsibilities. The result can eventually be marital conflicts as one partner views his or her share as unequal. In addition the partner who is not included in the care-giving activities may feel neglected since all the attention is directed toward the handicapped child. Without active participation in the care of the child, the parent has little appreciation of the time and energy involved in performing those activities. Whereas one parent feels neglected, the other feels resentful for the responsibility and the other's uninvolvement.

Each partner may displace feelings of resentment, anger, and bitterness on the other for having their life-style disrupted by the child's handicap, unaware of the true reason for such feelings. For example, a mother who is forced to terminate a career in order to assume full-time child care may express her feelings of resentment and bitterness as anger toward her husband for not sharing more in the household chores. Even if he participates more, she may continue to be angry with him because of her need to express the other unresolved feelings. He, in turn, may refuse to participate since nothing he does can satisfy her. As a result communication breaks down and neither is able to support the other.

Reports indicate that divorce and suicide rates are higher in families with a handicapped child than in the general population. Problems contributing to marital disintegration aside from those already discussed include avoidance of sex for fear of conceiving another handicapped child, financial stress, and disagreement regarding expectations from the affected offspring.[20] Each of these potential problems guides the nurse to preventive counseling measures that can preserve the marital relationship.

Although a great deal of emphasis has been placed on the mother's reaction to a handicapped child, little research has focused on the father's response. The available findings indicate that fathers of chronically ill children feel less competent and inferior as parents. They have been found to lack gratifying relationships with their children and to experience significant stress even though they may have other healthy children. Fathers, compared to mothers, generally have fewer opportunities to do something directly helpful for their handicapped child, such as taking the child to the physician, the drugstore, the physical therapist, the special school, or other special health services. Organizations for parents of handicapped children seem to offer fewer services to fathers. Fathers are less adequately provided for than are mothers by supportive mental health services for parents of handicapped children. As a result they have fewer opportunities available to them to mourn the loss of the perfect child and to deal with lowered self-esteem associated with fathering a handicapped child.[6] Their needs to adjust to the loss of a perfect male child may be even greater than the mother's when the expectations of immortality through a son can no longer be realized.

Siblings. Siblings are deeply affected by the handicapped child's membership in the family. Many of the reactions discussed under the terminally-ill child (see p. 977), namely anger and resentment over added responsibility and loss of attention, apply here. Frequently the developmentally disabled child causes a revision of age and sex roles within the family. For example, if the retarded child is firstborn, he becomes the "youngest" by virtue of his developmental age. Conversely the second-born becomes the oldest, often shouldering adult-like responsibilities and achieving parental expectations that would have been reserved for the eldest. Therefore, it is not uncommon for the siblings to express the same feelings of depression, envy, bitterness, and so on that were described earlier for parents.

Reactions of siblings to a mentally retarded child differ. In one study about half the siblings reported that they benefited from the experience, about half believed that they were harmed, and a minority felt unaffected. In the investigator's opinions those siblings who had benefited had a greater understanding of people, showed more compassion, were more sensitive about prejudice and its consequences, and had more appreciation of their own good health and intelligence than many of their peers who had not had the experience of growing up with a mentally retarded sibling. They also viewed the experience as having drawn the family closer together. In contrast the siblings who were judged to be harmed exhibited shame about their handicapped sibling and guilt about their feelings, conveyed a sense of being defective themselves, experienced a sense of guilt about their own good health, felt neglected by their parents, and believed that the handicapped child had negatively affected the rest of the family.[11]

Another study found that boys who interacted daily with their retarded siblings placed a greater emphasis than noninteractors on the following goals: success in business, devotion to a worthwhile cause, making a contribution to mankind, and learning not to take life too seriously. These same boys showed less interest in having many close friends, focusing life around marriage and the family, and being a respected community leader. The girls who interacted daily with their retarded siblings gave a higher rank than noninteractors to learning to accept hardships, devotion to a worthwhile cause, and making a contribution to mankind. In summary frequent interactors wanted to turn their life career toward the improvement of mankind, whereas noninteractors were more concerned with goals involving interpersonal relationships.[9]

Such findings emphasize the positive, maturing attitudes that can form in siblings of handicapped children and stress the responsibility of health professionals to involve the entire family unit in the adjustment process.

Handicapped child. The child's reaction to his handicap depends to a great extent on the reactions of significant others to him and to his disability, the child's developmental level and his available coping mechanisms, and, to a lesser extent, the handicap itself. Four patterns of behavior are evident that directly relate to parental responses to child rearing: (1) marked dependency, especially on the mother, fearfulness, inactivity, and lack of outside interests; (2) overactivity, defiance, risk-taking behavior; (3) resentment and hostility, especially to normal individuals; and (4) dependence/independence appropriate for age and responsibility and achievement commensurate with limitation, pride, confidence, and self-esteem.[15]

Because it is often easier to recognize the child who adjusts poorly to his handicap, it is worthwhile to delineate those behaviors that describe the well-adjusted child. The well-adapted child slowly learns to accept his physical limitations but finds achievement in a variety of compensatory motor and intellectual pursuits. He functions well at home, at school, and with peers. He has an understanding of his disorder that allows him to accept his limitations, assume responsibility for care, and assist in treatment and rehabilitation regimens.

He expresses appropriate emotions, such as sadness, anxiety, and anger at times of exacerbations but confidence and guarded optimism during periods of clinical stability. He is able to identify with other similarly affected individuals, promoting positive self-images. The well-adjusted handicapped person displays pride and self-confidence in his ability to master a productive, successful life despite the disability.

When a child experiences a serious disability, he proceeds through three predictable stages. The first is immediate *withdrawal,* in which the child becomes depressed and nonresponsive. The second is *preoccupation with self,* in which the child focuses on his disability and loss of previous abilities. The third is a *gradual return to reality,* which is closely linked to the parents' ability to adjust to the handicap. Response to loss of a body function and/or part is manifest in grief responses, "No, not me" (denial), "Why me?" (anger), and "Yes me" (depression). (See Chapter 27 for a more detailed discussion of the grief process.)

The onset of a crippling condition generates a state of confusion for the child who may have trouble differentiating between his actual body functions and his image of his body. He may also experience problems in identifying himself and that extension of himself in the form of wheelchairs, braces, crutches, or other mechanical or prosthetic devices and may have tremendous difficulty in accepting functional aids.

For example, one 8-year-old child partially paralyzed from the waist down drew a picture of herself without legs. When asked if she had forgotten anything, the child responded, "No, that's me." When asked if she should draw legs with braces on, she again replied, "No, the braces are not part of me. You said to draw a picture of me." From the drawing and her comments it was obvious that she had dissociated nonfunctional parts of her body from having any meaning in terms of body image. It helped explain why the child refused to wear her braces for ambulation, preferring to be wheeled everywhere by others. Gradually through therapeutic play sessions the child was able to talk about her paralysis and consequently took a more active role in learning to walk with the orthopedic appliance.

The type of handicap also influences the emotional response. Considering children's cognitive ability and their delay in achieving abstract thinking until adolescence, it is likely that an obvious handicap is easier to accept because its limitations are concrete.[16] For example, the blind or crippled child is constantly reminded of his inability to run. However, the hemophiliac child must not only live by rules he does not understand, but he also only vaguely and occasionally senses his illness, such as when he runs and accidently initiates a bleeding episode. Therefore, some chronic illnesses pose special threats to the child. The following is an overview of some disorders that have special significance.[15]

Children with serious respiratory disorders commonly harbor fears of suffocation, drowning, or dying while asleep. Children with convulsive disorders frequently fear loss of consciousness or uncontrollable strange behavior. They may resist obtaining a driver's license for fear of a seizure, which prolongs their dependency on their parents. Children with bleeding disorders may fear hemorrhaging to death and may resist medical procedures, such as injections, for fear of initiating such an episode.

Children with chronic renal disease often have frightening fantasies about hemodialysis, such as fears of bleeding to death or of the machine assuming control of them. After kidney transplant parents may overprotect them and use possible graft rejection as a means of controlling their activity. If an actual rejection occurs, the child may respond with depression, withdrawal, and self-blame for having destroyed the kidney.

Chronically ill children also experience emotional stress associated with long-term illness. Pain in young children is often perceived as punishment for some real or imagined transgression. Children may believe that they became ill because their parents failed to protect them. Diseases transmitted by hereditary factors may cause strain in the parent-child relationship once children discover the etiology of the disorder. During frequent and lengthy hospitalizations that result in separations from family, school, and friends, which can temporarily terminate needed sources of support, children may resent the need to be helped with bathing, feeding, or toileting. Painful procedures such as injections and surgery often reactivate fears of bodily mutilation and fantasties of punishment.

Although handicapped children frequently learn to use aspects of their illness or disability to control members of the family, they also may feel responsible for much of the stress created by their condition, such as marital discord, financial problems, additional responsibilities on other members, interruption of previous life-style, and interference with future goals. They may also feel insecure in terms of their true worth to the family. For example, it is not unusual for the handicapped child to wonder if the concern and attention focused on him is because of his handicap. He may question his real worth as a person, especially if his disability has received more emphasis than his abilities.

Extended members. Extended members include two groups of people who experience the effects of a handicapped child: (1) the significant nonnuclear family members or friends, and (2) society as a whole. Although extended family relationships are often helpful to parents in rearing a handicapped child, they may also be sources of stress. Grandparents may have far more difficulty in accepting the diagnosis than the parents themselves do, and parents may have concerns about the best way in which to respond to the grandparents' anger over the diagnosis or criticism regarding parental care. For example, grandparents or other well-meaning relatives may attempt to reassure the parents that the child "will grow out of" his slowness at a time when parents are struggling to accept reality.

Although society's views of handicapped individuals are changing toward a more accepting, unjudgmental, and open attitude, parents, siblings, and the child himself frequently are victims of prejudice, ostracism, or criticism. A great deal of this stems from public ignorance and fear and remains a crucial area for intervention by the health professional.

Factors affecting the family's adjustment

Those factors that are discussed in terms of affecting the family's adjustment to loss of a child (Chapter 27) are similarly applicable to accepting a seriously handicapped child. In addition there are other influences that may have special significance in the latter situation. One is sex of the child. Although the initial impact is sex-linked, that is, the mother experiences greater trauma if the child is a female and vice versa for the father, the effects shift as the child grows older. Parents are more adversely affected by a handicapped son, especially if he is the firstborn. Conversely it has been noted that the impact is least if the child is the last born, probably because the other offspring have shared in fulfilling the parents' expectations.

Socioeconomic status has an effect based on parental expectations. Families of higher socioeconomic standards usually have high ideals and experience greater stress. Religion is also a contributing factor. It has been found that parents who are Catholic seem to make a more rapid adjustment to having a handicapped child, viewing this as a responsibility given to them from God. Although few studies have focused on ethnic differences, one study found that Puerto Rican parents were less traumatized than white parents by the diagnosis of mental retardation in their child.[3] This may be related to socioeconomic and religious factors, as well as ethnic differences.

The obviousness of the child's defect also influences parents' adjustment in much the same way as it does the child's. The more visible the defect, the more difficult it is to deny or minimize its existence. This is often one of the key elements that hinders adjustment to mental retardation, since the behaviors can so easily be missed or shrouded in excuses. Likewise families of multihandicapped children often adjust sooner, not because the problems are easier, but because they are more readily apparent.

Another highly significant factor is the parents' lack of models on which to base child-rearing methods. Unlike normal children who can be reared by asking the advice of relatives or friends or by reading books on the subject, parents of handicapped children often feel inadequate and helpless in their role as parents. The benefits of professional guidance and parent support groups directly relate to providing usable, practical models for child rearing.

NURSING INTERVENTIONS WITH HANDICAPPED CHILDREN

The major goal of the nurse is to help the family remain intact and functioning at maximum levels throughout the child's life. This involves not merely supporting the child and his parents during the critical period of the newborn phase when the infant is being diagnosed or when the parents encounter problems in the child of preschool or school age. It involves using the mutual participation model to facilitate better communication and alleviate feelings of parental inadequacy and child inferiority. This model invites the parents' early input, encourages them to be more accountable and responsible for the child's care, and does not reinforce the dangerous attitude that the professional will "fix" the child and give him back to the parents. It also reinforces the fact that it is not so much the handicap itself that affects the child's progress and developmental outcomes, but the family's ability to cope successfully with the child's problems. Thus long-term, comprehensive, systematic, family-centered approaches must be applied.

Basic concepts of rehabilitation

In the past, health professionals have looked at handicapped persons within a pathologic framework, probing for weaknesses and negative features. Much attention has been given to the technologic aspects of the child's care and health needs, whereas less attention has been paid to the child's individuality, personality, or strengths, the family's needs, and the overall concerns of those who interact with handicapped children. Under the developmental model, attention is directed to the child's functional development, changes, and adaptation to the environment. Nurses often are in vital positions to redirect attention from the pathologic to the developmental model to meet the unique needs of the child and his family. The following are basic principles underlying rehabilitation efforts:

1. The child and family are the primary rehabilitators; professional health team members only assist the family in the process of rehabilitation.
2. The focus of rehabilitation is the treat the *effect* of the handicap on the child, not merely the disorder.
3. The goal is to promote optimum development, independence, and emotional adjustment within all family members.
4. The child's developmental age, not chronologic age, is the criteria for beginning rehabilitation efforts.
5. Health professionals' role is in preventing the disorder, the treatment regimen, and those working with the child (specifically, health team members) from interfering with the development of the child and disrupting the family unit.

These principles underly each of the following nursing objectives. Since the handicapped child involves several different categories of conditions, general guidelines are discussed as well as specific interventions where appropriate. However, the reader is also encouraged to refer elsewhere in the text for more detailed nursing considerations related to the child's diagnosis.

Assessing family's strengths and level of adjustment

Since the nurse may meet a family during any phase of the rehabilitation process, it is essential that the family members' individual strengths, coping mechanisms, and reaction to the handicap be assessed. The preceding discussion delineated the major factors involved in each of these areas. Table 22-2 is a rating scale for detecting families at risk for adapting poorly to chronic illness. Such a scale can be used to assess a family's adjustment to any type of handicap. Although such a tool does not provide exact measurements or negative or positive adaptation, it does provide an initial assessment plan for devising strategies of care. The assessment of coping behaviors in the boxed material on p. 987 is also applicable to the handicapped child, with the exception of those behaviors dealing directly with death.

The nurse also assesses the parents' reaction to the child, using as a guideline the four categories of child rearing—overprotection, rejection, denial, and acceptance. Questions that may be helpful in revealing child-rearing practices and attitudes toward the handicapped child include, "How is this child different from his siblings?" "Do you find yourself being a little more cautious with this child than your other children?" "How has your life-style changed since you learned of the diagnosis?" "When you think of your child's future, what thoughts do you have?" and "Describe your child's personality."

The parents' and child's understanding of the handicap is another significant assessment area. Although this may be apparent in discussions with the family, often it is not,

Table 22-2. Scale for detecting family at risk for adapting poorly to chronic illness

Factors	Rating 4	3	2	1	0	Score*
Age	<20	20-25	26-30	31-35	>35	
Income	<5000	5000-7500	7501-10,000	10,001-15,000	>15,000	
Race	Black		Other		White	
Years married	<2	2-4	5-7	8-10	>10	
Strength of marriage	Weak		Average		Strong	
Number of children	1	2	3	4	>4	
Education level	<High school	High school	1-2 years college	3-4 years college	>4 years college	
Religious conviction	None		Average		Strong	
Community involvement	None	One group	Two groups	Three groups	>Three groups	
Support from maternal grandmother	None		Average		Strong	
Husband/wife experiences with and feelings about chronic illness	Negative		Neutral		Positive	
					TOTAL	

From Lawson, B. A. Copyright January/February 1977, The American Journal of Nursing Company. Reproduced with permission from MCN, The American Journal of Maternal Child Nursing **2**(1):49-56, 1977.
*The higher the total score, the higher the risk factor.

necessitating direct inquiry. One way of eliciting information is to ask the person how he would explain the child's condition to a stranger. This approach frequently eliminates the use of medical jargon that the family has learned to conveniently cover up their true feelings. For example, if a parent explains that mental retardation means an IQ (intelligence quotient) of 75, the nurse can respond that the stranger is unfamiliar with such numbers and needs to know what it means to have an IQ of 75.

While inquiring about the parents' level of understanding, the nurse also focuses on the child's and siblings' knowledge of the condition. It is not unusual for parents who appear well adjusted and knowledgeable to state that they have never told the children the truth. Although this is less of a problem when the handicap is visible, it may occur when the disability can be cloaked in terms such as "a little behind" or "slow learner." Conflict arises when the child or siblings learn of the diagnosis from nonparental sources. Although this issue is similar to the "to tell or not to tell dilemma" when a child has a terminal illness, it has greater ramifications here because the disability may be lifelong, may require assistance from the siblings later in life, and influences the entire family's social reintegration as a final phase to acceptance.

Children present special challenges in assessing their feelings regarding having a handicap or living with a handicapped child. Chapter 27 focuses on several approaches to encourage a child to discuss feelings about his diagnosis and future. These same approaches can be used with the handicapped child, provided they are appropriate for his developmental age. For example, using drawing and play as a method of communication is usually more appropriate in the developmentally disabled child, who may be retarded in verbal skills.

Assessment is a continuous process that includes each member of the family. Traditionally the mother and handicapped child have been active participants and receivers of professional care, whereas fathers and siblings have been excluded. However, for one to realize the goal of optimum development for the family unit, each member must be included. This involves scheduling office and/or home visits at times when other family members can be present. Although occasionally this necessitates appointments during evenings or weekends, it can also be done late in the afternoon or early morning. It is surprising how often fathers will change their work schedule to meet with a health professional once an invitation is extended.

The nurse positively approaches the task of including other family members in a visit. If they have not been included previously, they may interpret such an invitation as a portent of more bad news or an indication of their own difficulties. One way of welcoming others to join in a visit is to state that the nurse hears so often about the other siblings and the father that he or she wishes to meet them. This informal, casual approach is nonthreatening and implies only friendly intonations.

Ideally a thorough assessment includes observing the child and family in a variety of settings. Undoubtedly the

Home observation for measurement of the environment

Birth to three

Date of interview________

Child designee____
Name — Age — Sex — Ethnicity

Child's birthday ____________________ Birth order ____________________

Mother's name ____________________ Father's name ____________________

Address ____

Categories	**Raw scores**	**Percentile scores**
I. Emotional and verbal responsivity of mother	______	______
II. Avoidance of restriction and punishment	______	______
III. Organization of physical and temporal environment	______	______
IV. Provision of appropriate play materials	______	______
V. Maternal involvement with child	______	______
VI. Opportunities for variety in daily stimulation	______	______
TOTALS	______	______

I. Emotional and verbal responsivity of mother	**Yes**	**No**
1. Mother spontaneously vocalizes to child at least twice during visit (excluding scolding).		
2. Mother responds to child's vocalizations with a verbal response.		
3. Mother tells child the name of some object during visit or says name of person or object in a "teaching" style.		
4. Mother's speech is distinct, clear, and audible.		
5. Mother initiates verbal interchanges with observer—asks questions and makes spontaneous comments.		
6. Mother expresses ideas freely and easily and uses statements of appropriate length for conversation (e.g., gives more than brief answers).		
*7. Mother permits child occasionally to engage in "messy" type of play.		
8. Mother spontaneously praises child's qualities or behavior twice during visit.		
9. When speaking of or to the child, mother's voice conveys positive feeling.		
10. Mother caresses or kisses child at least once during visit.		
11. Mother shows some positive emotional responses to praise of child offered by visitor.		
SUBSCORE		

From Caldwell, Bettye M.: Home Observation for Measurement of the Environment (birth to three), 1970.
*Items that may require direct questions.

Continued.

richest environment for observing a child's development and interactions with family members is the home. One tool that can be used to systematically assess subtle aspects of the home environment is the Home Observation for Management of the Environment (HOME)[5] (see the box above), which is divided into two age-groups—birth to 3 years of age and 3 to 6 years of age. However, for developmentally disabled children, the tool is applicable for a wider chronologic age range, since it should be used based on the child's developmental or functional age. Some of the items require direct observation, whereas others necessitate questioning of the parents. Each item receives a "yes" or "no" response. The number of "yes" scores correlates with the amount of appropriate environmental stimulation. Any "no" scores indicate possible areas for intervention and counseling.

The following is a summary of the objectives that the nurse should accomplish during home visits:

1. Monitor progress of the child's development.
2. Gather records of the child's discrete behaviors.
3. Assess and measure the environment in which the child is growing and developing.
4. Gather diagnostic data on the child before a diagnosis is made.

Text continued on p. 798.

Home observation for measurement of the environment—cont'd

Birth to three—cont'd

II. Avoidance of restriction and punishment	Yes	No
12. Mother does not shout at child during visit.		
13. Mother does not express overt annoyance with or hostility toward child.		
14. Mother neither slaps nor spanks child during visit.		
*15. Mother reports that no more than one instance of physical punishment occurred during the past week.		
16. Mother does not scold or derogate child during visit.		
17. Mother does not interfere with child's actions or restrict child's movements more than three times during visit.		
18. At least ten books are present and visible.		
*19. Family has a pet.		
SUBSCORE		

III. Organization of physical and temporal environment	Yes	No
20. When mother is away, care is provided by one of three regular substitutes.		
21. Someone takes child into grocery store at least once a week.		
22. Child gets out of house at least four times a week.		
23. Child is taken regularly to doctor's office or clinic.		
*24. Child has a special place in which to keep his toys and "treasures."		
25. Child's play environment appears safe and free of hazards.		
SUBSCORE		

IV. Provision of appropriate play materials	Yes	No
26. Child has some muscle activity toys or equipment.		
27. Child has a push or pull toy.		
28. Child has stroller or walker, kiddie car, scooter or tricycle.		
29. Mother provides toys or interesting activities for child during interview.		
30. Provides learning equipment appropriate to age—cuddly toy or role-playing toys.		
31. Provides learning equipment appropriate to age—mobile, table and chairs, high chair, play pen.		
32. Provides eye-hand coordination toys—items to go in and out of receptacle, fit together toys, beads.		
33. Provides eye-hand coordination toys that permit combinations—stacking or nesting toys, blocks or building toys.		
34. Provides toys for literature and music.		
SUBSCORE		

V. Maternal involvement with child	Yes	No
35. Mother tends to keep child within visual range and to look at him often.		
36. Mother talks to child while doing her work.		
37. Mother consciously encourages developmental advance.		
38. Mother invests "maturing" toys with value via her attention.		
39. Mother structures child's play periods.		
40. Mother provides toys that challenge child to develop new skills.		
SUBSCORE		

VI. Opportunities for variety in daily stimulation	Yes	No
41. Father provides some caretaking every day.		
42. Mother reads stories at least three times weekly.		
43. Child eats at least one meal per day with mother and father.		
44. Family visits or receives visits from relatives.		
45. Child has three or more books of his own.		
SUBSCORE		

*Items that may require direct questions.

Home observation for measurement of the environment—cont'd

Three to six

Date of interview ________

Child designee ________________________________
Name ______ Age ______ Sex ______ Ethnicity ______

Child's birthday ______________ Birth order ______________

Mother's name ______________ Father's name ______________

Address ________________________________

Categories	Raw scores	Percentile scores
I. Provision of stimulation through equipment, toys, and experiences	______	______
II. Stimulation of mature behavior	______	______
III. Provision of stimulating physical and language environment	______	______
IV. Avoidance of restriction and punishment	______	______
V. Pride, affection, and thoughtfulness	______	______
VI. Masculine stimulation	______	______
VII. Independence from parental control	______	______
TOTALS	______	______

I. Provision of stimulation through equipment, toys, and experiences	Yes	No
1-12 The following are present in home and either belong to child subject or he is allowed to play with them:		
1. Toys to learn colors, sizes, shapes—typewriter, pressouts, play school, peg boards, etc.		
2. Toy or game facilitating learning letters (e.g., blocks with letters, toy typewriter, letter sticks, books about letters, etc.).		
3. Three or more puzzles.		
4. Two toys necessitating some finger and whole hand movements (crayons and coloring books, paper dolls, etc.).		
5. Record player and at least five children's records.		
6. Real or toy musical instrument (piano, drum, toy xylophone or guitar, etc.).		
7. Toy or game permitting free expression (finger paints, play dough, crayons or paint and paper, etc.).		
8. Toys or game necessitating refined movements (paint by number, dot book, paper dolls, crayons and coloring books).		
9. Toys to learn animals—books about animals, circus games, animal puzzles, etc.		
10. Toy or game facilitating learning numbers (e.g., blocks with numbers, books about numbers, games with numbers, etc.).		
11. Building toys (blocks, tinker toys, Lincoln logs, etc.).		
12. Ten children's books.		
13. At least ten books are present and visible in the apartment.		
14. Family buys a newspaper daily and reads it.		
15. Family subscribes to at least one magazine.		
16. Family member has taken child on one outing (picnic, shopping excursion) at least every other week.		
17. Child has been taken out to eat in some kind of restaurant three-four times in the past year.		
18-20 Child has been taken by a family member to the following within the past year:		
18. Airport		
19. A trip more than 50 miles from his home (50 miles radial distance, not total distance).		
20. A scientific, historical, or art museum.		
21. Child is taken to grocery store at least once a week.		
SUBSCORE		

From Caldwell, Bettye M.: Home Observation for Measurement of the Environment (three to six), 1976.

Continued.

Home observation for measurement of the environment—cont'd

Three to six—cont'd

II. Stimulation of mature behavior	**Yes**	**No**
22-29 Child is encouraged to learn the following:		
22. Colors		
23. Shapes		
24. Patterned speech (nursery rhymes, prayers, songs, TV commercials, etc.)		
25. The alphabet		
26. To tell time		
27. Spatial relationships (up, down, under, big, little, etc.)		
28. Numbers		
29. To read a few words		
30. Tries to get child to pick up and put away toys after play session—without help.		
31. Child is taught rules of social behavior which involve recognition of rights of others.		
32. Parent teaches child some simple manners—to say, "Please," "Thank you," "I'm sorry."		
33. Some delay of food gratification is demanded of the child, e.g., not to whine or demand food unless within ½ hour of meal time.		
SUBSCORE		

III. Provision of a stimulating physical and language environment (observation items, except **45)	**Yes**	**No**
34. Building has no potentially dangerous structural or health defect (e.g., plaster coming down from ceiling, stairway with boards missing, rodents, etc.).		
35. Child's outside play environment appears safe and free of hazards (no outside play area requires an automatic "No").		
36. The interior of the apartment is not dark or perceptibly monotonous.		
37. House is not overly noisy—television, shouts of children, radio, etc.		
38. Neighborhood has trees, grass, birds—is esthetically pleasing.		
39. There is at least 100 square feet of living space per person in the house.		
40. In terms of available floor space, the rooms are not overcrowded with furniture.		
41. All visible rooms of the house are reasonably clean and minimally cluttered.		
42. *Mother uses complex sentence structure and some long words in conversing.		
43. Mother uses correct grammar and pronunciation.		
44. Mother's speech is distinct, clear, and audible.		
**45. Family has TV and it is used judiciously, not left on continuously (no TV requires an automatic "No"—any scheduling scores "Yes").		
SUBSCORE		

IV. Avoidance of restriction and punishment (observation items, except **51 and **52)	**Yes**	**No**
46. Mother does not scold or derogate child more than once during visit.		
47. Mother does not use physical restraint, shake, grab, pinch child during visit.		
48. Mother neither slaps nor spanks child during visit.		
49. Mother does not express over-annoyance with or hostility toward child—complain, say child is "bad" or won't mind.		
50. Child is not punished or ridiculed for speech.		
**51. No more than one instance of physical punishment occurred during the past week (accept parental report).		
**52. Child does not get slapped or spanked for spilling food or drink.		
SUBSCORE		

*Throughout interview this refers to *mother* OR other *caregiver* who is present for interview.

Home observation for measurement of the environment—cont'd

Three to six—cont'd

V. Pride, affection, and thoughtfulness (observation items, except **53, **54, **55, **56, **57, **58, **59)	Yes	No
**53. Parent turns on special TV program regarded as "good" for children (*Captain Kangaroo, Magic Toy Shop,* Walt Disney, *Flipper, Lassie,* educational TV, etc.).		
**54. Someone reads stories to child or shows and comments on pictures in magazines five times weekly.		
**55. Parent encourages child to relate experiences or takes time to listen to him relate experiences.		
**56. Parent holds child close ten to fifteen minutes per day, e.g., during TV, story time, visiting.		
**57. Parent occasionally sings to child, or sings in presence of child.		
**58. Child has a special place in which to keep his toys and "treasures."		
**59. Child's art work is displayed some place in house (anything that child makes).		
60. Mother introduces interviewer to child.		
61. Mother converses with child at least twice during visit (scolding and suspicious comments not counted).		
62. Mother answers child's questions or requests verbally.		
63. Mother usually responds verbally to child's talking.		
64. Mother provides toys or interesting activities or in other ways structures situation for child during visit when her attention will be elsewhere. (To score "Yes" mother must make an active guiding gesture or suggestion to structure child's play.)		
65. Mother spontaneously praises child's qualities or behavior twice during visit.		
66. When speaking of or to child, mother's voice conveys positive feeling.		
67. Mother caresses, kisses, or cuddles child at least once during visit.		
68. Mother sets up situation that allows child to show off during visit.		
SUBSCORE		

VI. Masculine stimulation	Yes	No
69. Child sees and spends some time with father or father figure four days a week.		
70. Child eats at least one meal per day, on most days, with mother (or mother figure) and father (or father figure). (One-parent families get an automatic "No.")		
71-73 The following are present in home and either belong to child subject or he is allowed to play with them:		
71. Ride toy (tricycle, scooter, wagon, bike with or without training wheels).		
72. Medium wheel toys—trucks, trains, doll carriage, etc.		
73. Large muscle toy (jump rope, swing, ball, climbing object, etc.).		
SUBSCORE		

VII. Independence from parental control	Yes	No
74. Child is encouraged to try to dress himself.		
75. Child is permitted to choose some of his clothing to be worn except on very special occasions.		
76. Child is permitted some choice in lunch or breakfast menu.		
77. Parent lets child choose certain favorite food products or brands at grocery store.		
78. Child is permitted to go to another house to play without having the caregiver accompany him.		
79. Child can express negative feelings without harsh reprisal.		
80. Child is permitted to hit parent without harsh reprisal.		
SUBSCORE		
TOTAL SCORE		

5. Determine the functional levels of development of the child within his home.
6. Make direct observations of the child's behaviors in activities of daily living.
7. Observe parent-child interactions.
8. Collect records on behavioral frequencies and duration.
9. Solve problems with parents in the home setting.
10. Administer standardized screening tools in the child's natural setting.
11. Observe mothers teaching their child tasks such as drinking from a cup, eating with a spoon, undressing, dressing, language, discipline, or toilet training.
12. Acknowledge parents' progress in teaching their children developmental tasks.
13. Assist in the implementation of behavioral management strategies.
14. Encourage the child.
15. Explore the child's feelings about his handicapping condition.
16. Reinforce continuation of planned programs.
17. Observe the child at play.
18. Observe the effects of medication on the child's behavior.
19. Answer questions about the child's progress or lack of it.
20. Assist family members with programs in which they play a part.
21. Acknowledge parents' efforts at record keeping.
22. Support and encourage the parents.

Probably the second most important environment for a child is school. Besides his parents, teachers exert a tremendous influence on the child's developmental progress, feelings of self-esteem, learning capacity, and formation of social relationships. Whenever feasible the nurse should visit the school to observe directly the child's behavior and interaction among teachers and classmates. The following is a summary of objectives for school visits:

1. Observe the child's classroom behaviors, such as the ability to sit, follow directions, and comply with requests, determine appropriate responses to teachers questions and determine the child's independence in functioning.
2. Gather data on reported behavioral problems such as "hyperactivity," "noncompliance" or "stubbornness."
3. Observe the child's interactions with peers in class and at play.
4. Observe the child's behaviors in structured and nonstructured activities.
5. Observe the teacher's appropriate and nonappropriate interactions with the child.
6. Observe the teacher's teaching strategies with the child. (Are the strategies consistent with home teaching?)
7. Determine the teacher's concerns for the child.
8. Determine the teacher's expectations of the child.
9. Administer standardized screening tools with the teacher.
10. Observe the child's behavior before, during, and following a medication regimen.
11. Observe the child's eating patterns at school.
12. Collaborate with the teacher in future planning for the child.
13. Determine the effectiveness of programs of care for the child.
14. Offer support to the teacher in her efforts to assist the child.
15. Coordinate parents, teachers, and others' plans for the child.

Revealing diagnosis

The impact of the crisis usually occurs at the time of diagnosis, which may be at the time of birth, following a long period of physical and/or psychologic testing, or immediately after a tragic accident. It is a critical time for parents. Although they may not hear or remember all that is said to them, they frequently sense a certain attitude of acceptance, rejection, hope, or despair from the informant. As was mentioned earlier, the informant must honestly convey information without pronouncing himself or herself the "omnipotent curer." Rather the informant must stress the role of the parents and child as primary rehabilitators, with health team members as facilitators of the process.

The nurse is increasingly responsible for conducting the informing interview with parents, explaining the handicap, giving follow-up information, and coordinating services with other agencies. With increased awareness of the need for a reality approach rather than a therapy approach, there has also arisen the recognition of a primary care giver. Whether nurses assume the role of primary or secondary care giver, they must have guidelines to follow during the informing interview. (Refer to the discussion of Down's syndrome [p. 816] for other recommendations regarding revealing the diagnosis.)

The nurse should encourage parents to be together when they are informed of their child's condition, thus avoiding the problem of one parent having to interpret complex findings and deal with the initial emotional reaction of the other. It also gives the nurse an opportunity to observe the interaction between the parents as they are confronted with the tragedy of discovering a handicap in their child. The nurse should remember that because of its social and emotional implications, the concepts of handicaps such as mental retardation are very difficult to convey to parents and require tremendous patience and increased sensitivity on the nurse's part. For example, the nurse must be both realistic and cautious, stressing that mental retardation refers to a description of the individual's level of functioning in intellectual and adaptive skills at a given time.

Nurses must keep in mind that although they have their agenda for presenting information, the parents also have their agenda in terms of receiving the information and asking questions. It is important that the nurse answer questions as they arise, rather than focus on revealing information.

It is the responsibility of the nurse to make certain that the parents understand the information. One way to assure understanding is to ask simple questions, such as, "Do you see what I mean?" The nurse should then check further with the parents and have them repeat to the nurse what they have just been told and to interpret it in their own way if they understood the information. It is at this point that if clarification needs to be made, it is done by the nurse.

For example, if the diagnosis is one of developmental disability, the nurse can intersperse the information with, "Do you agree with these observations?" "Have you made similar observations of your own?" "Is this the kind of behavior you have seen at home or at school?" "Are these the observations that you were hoping we would make about your child?" "Has this been your experience?" "Is this information making sense to you?" and "Do you have any questions?" The nurse should then wait, even though it may appear that a long silence is occurring, for the parents to think about and to comment on what they have just heard. Technical terms are used with constant clarification. If the parents are unaware of the term, the nurse gives them written literature or, at least, a written summary of the diagnosis.

The nurse also observes the parents' behavior to determine their reaction to the diagnosis, especially if they seem overwhelmed by the seriousness of the child's condition. Expressions on their faces, the times they look down, their ability to maintain eye contact with the nurse, their behaviors that show they are avoiding what the nurse is saying, such as turning their heads, looking around, looking away, or any other activity that shows that they are indeed dealing with a very difficult subject, is observed. When the nurse does perceive different changes in the expression of the parents' faces, these observations are checked by asking questions, such as, "I can see that this is very difficult for you, am I right?" or "This seems to be pretty overwhelming to you, am I right?"

If the observations are confirmed, the nurse offers to terminate the conference and continue it at another time, while providing them with an opportunity to ask questions. For example, the nurse may state, "I know that the diagnosis is serious and a great deal to accept at one time. We can talk again at another time unless there are questions you would like to ask now." Their emotional needs are acknowledged by expressing acceptance of crying, sadness, anger, disappointment, and so on. The nurse can offer emotional support by having Kleenexes ready for when one of the parents cries. The nurse can reach out and touch the parents, show support, and demonstrate through facial and bodily language an understanding that indeed this is a difficult and painful period.

The nurse should be prepared to assess and respond to the variety of reactions displayed by the parents, who are being told for the first time that their child is handicapped. For example, some respond realistically to the diagnosis of a developmental disability, whereas others respond defensively. The most common initial defense is that of denial. Parents may openly reject the diagnosis of mental retardation even in the light of overwhelming evidence, or they may superficially accept the diagnosis but secretly cling to the belief that nothing is wrong. Other parental reactions include guilt, depression, loss of self-esteem, projection of blame to others, including health professionals, and feelings of ambivalence. The atmosphere of the informing session should be one in which parents feel free to express their own emotion. If their feelings can be expressed and acknowledged, the parents can be helped to deal openly with them and their need for further counseling can be determined.

Lastly the informing conference should not end with presentation of devastating news. Instead the nurse stresses the strengths of the child, his appealing behaviors, his potential for development, and available rehabilitation efforts or treatment. Although it may not be the time to discuss orthopedic appliances, special schools, or corrective surgical procedures in depth, it is appropriate to stress the positive future expectations for the child. The nurse also communicates to parents that life with their child who is handicapped is very similar to life with other children. Their experiences should be thought of as a series of problem-solving processes that they are capable of handling, particularly with available professional feedback. The parents are assured that the nurse will be available to answer questions and to provide further assistance as it is needed in the future.

The preceding discussion relates primarily to the initial informing interview. However, because of the need for long-term follow-up, it is only one in a series of continuing discussions. Although it is not possible to detail every issue that should be discussed with parents throughout the course of the rehabilitation process, the following points deserve further mention.[10]

1. Be certain that parents clearly understand that there is no such thing as an unchanging diagnosis and that if a label has to be used, it is merely a way of communicating about a child; it really tells very little about the child's *current* and *future* capabilities.

2. Remember that parents must understand their child's abilities and assets, not only his negative traits, deficits, disabilities, and dysfunction. Assist the parents in learning to observe even the slightest changes in their child and in being honest with him. Parents need to know that one of their most important contributions to the child's life will be the manner in which they show respect for his appropriate behaviors and help him "feel good about himself." Parents should teach the child as early as possible that his disability cannot be blamed on anyone and is not his fault.

3. Tell parents that some people may dwell on the negatives of their child; this is to be expected. Help them to discover how to reverse this trend by thinking and acting in positive ways so that others can learn from them. Parents need to present their child in positive ways rather than emphasizing his negative traits.

4. Teach parents that they are important and vital contributors to the decision making that is done for their child's welfare and well-being. They should insist that no decisions be made about their child without their input and final approval. Their legal right to all services should be stressed.

5. Encourage parents to become as well informed as possible about their child, his programs, progress, and the ways in which others are treating him. Parents need to learn to interact effectively with other people who help their child and to present their own ideas with tact and confidence.

6. Be supportive of parents as they establish growth-producing and appropriate relationships with various professionals who will work with them on a longitudinal basis.

7. Stress the value of parents keeping their own records, including names, addresses, phone numbers, dates of visits, persons present during visits, and as much as they can remember of what was said.

8. Before giving advice about a problem, remember to ask about what the parent was told by another professional.

9. Encourage parents to speak up and ask professionals when they do not understand what is being said to them. Urge parents to gain confidence in talking openly and honestly with professionals, stating exactly what they want.

10. Guide the parents to appropriate sources of literature and remind them that some literature is out of date and presents only partial descriptions or answers.

11. Help parents get into the habit of seeking out and talking with other parents, to help them evaluate the advantages and disadvantages of all available programs. Point out to them that their child is an individual and that just because a program worked for another child does not mean that it will necessarily provide the same benefits for their child. Encourage them to visit each facility and to ask the nurse to go with them to help them be objective whenever possible.

12. Encourage parents not to discount what their own child is saying to them, just because he is a child, because only the child can tell the parents how he perceives what is happening to him.

13. Remind parents that they are their child's best example of people working together in a mutually supportive, honest, and cooperative manner. Give parents credit for all the strengths they have shown and all the successful interactions they have had. Caution them not to dwell on their weaknesses and fears, but not to discount them either. Convey to parents that they are the primary and best resource for their child and that they should treat themselves with respect because of their many strengths and their powers.

The preceding paragraphs encompass guidelines for discussing a handicap in general. However, some situations present special problems. The following is a brief discussion of special considerations based on the diagnosis.

Mental retardation. Unless mental retardation is associated with other physical handicaps, it is often easy for parents to miss clues to its presence or to make defensive excuses regarding diagnosis. Since the impact of a diagnosis is associated with the reactions of shock and denial, it is important for the nurse to help parents develop self-awareness of the handicap. The best approach lies not so much in careful preparation of how to tell, but in planning situations that help them become aware of the problem.[1] This may deliberately involve a prolonged period of evaluation to help the parents gain an appreciation of the child's strengths and weaknesses.

The nurse can encourage parents to discuss their observations of the child without offering diagnostic opinions. For example, the parents may be asked how this child's development compares with that of other siblings or peers, how he is doing in school, if the parents have any concerns about his progress, or what they have been told by others. By focusing on what the child can do and appropriate interventions to help him progress, such as infant-stimulation programs, the nurse can involve parents in their child's care while helping them gain an awareness of his disability.

Physical disability. Loss of a motor or sensory ability offers little difficulty in revealing the diagnosis because it is readily apparent. The challenge lies in helping the child and parents over the period of shock and grief toward the phase of acceptance and reintegration. One of the most helpful interventions is to institute early rehabilitation, such as using a prosthetic limb, learning to read braille, learning to read lips, and so on. However, physical rehabilitation usually precedes psychologic adjustment. Therefore, persons working with crippled or sensory-impaired children must bear in mind that even though the child is proficient in compensatory skills, he may still be grieving for his loss and in great need of emotional support.

A special dilemma exists when the cause of the disability is accidental, since parental and child guilt can be overwhelming. It is imperative at the time of diagnosis to avoid implying that the parents or child was responsible for the injury. However, at the same time the nurse should allow the parents and the child the opportunity to discuss feelings of blame. The third-person technique, which involves expressing a feeling in terms of a third person, can be used. This technique is less threatening than directly asking a person how he feels, because it gives him the opportunities to agree or disagree without being defensive. For example, the nurse can encourage parents to express their feelings by stating, "Sometimes it is so difficult for a parent to anticipate hidden dangers in a child's life," or "Parents often feel responsible for things that happen to their child even if there was no way they could have prevented it." Statements directed at eliciting the child's feelings are, "Sometimes when tragic things happen, people often wonder what they did to deserve them," or "When people tell others not to do things, it is easy to forget their warnings because they may not realize the actual dangers, but then when something happens, they wish they had listened." The nurse can either wait for a response with silence or encourage a reply with a statement such as, "Did you ever feel that way?"

Chronic illness. Realization of the true impact of a diagnosis of chronic illness may take months or years. Conflict over parents' vs child's concerns may result in serious problems. For example, whereas parents worry about preventing bleeding episodes and joint deformity, the hemophiliac child may only focus on the activity restriction. Unless each member is able to gain an appreciation of the other's concerns, it is likely that no one's needs will be met.

A special dilemma arises when the illness is inherited, since parents may blame themselves, and/or the child may blame the parents. This aspect should be discussed with parents at the time of diagnosis to lessen guilt and accusatory feelings on any person's part. The child should be allowed to express his feelings. Using the third-person technique helps open discussion in this area. For example, the nurse may comment, "Sometimes when a person has an illness that was passed on by the parents that person feels angry or bitter toward them." This approach allows the child three choices: to disagree, to agree and hopefully express how he feels, or to not reply, in which case he probably has such feelings but is unable to express them.

Multiple handicaps. The multihandicapped child may present special challenges because the child or parent may require additional time for the shock phase. The child or parent may only be able to attend to one diagnosis before hearing significant information regarding the other handicap. This serves as a clue to the nurse to tailor the informing conference to prevent overwhelming the family.

When an obvious and a more hidden handicap coexist, such as cerebral palsy and mental retardation, the nurse must be careful to acknowledge parents' understanding and acceptance of both diagnoses. Not infrequently the parents intellectualize that any retarded development is the result of the physical impairment and resist in accepting the intellectual deficit.

The nurse must also appreciate the devastating consequences of two handicaps to a child, especially if they interfere with expressive-receptive abilities. The overwhelming example is the blind-deaf child. Although both these defects may be present at birth, they may also have different onsets, such as partial deafness at birth with progressive loss of vision. In this situation the child's experiences with the outside world are severely limited. The nurse must rely heavily on the ability to observe facial/bodily expressions as cues to the child's feelings and to use touch as a method of communication.

Helping the family prosper

In order for the family to meet the stresses of optimally adjusting to the child's handicap, each member must be individually supported so that each part of the family system is strong. Although the family unit can indefinitely support a member who is in need of assistance, its greatest strength lies in every member supporting each other. The nurse should bear in mind that the "member in need" is not necessarily the handicapped child but may be a parent or sibling who is dealing with stresses that require intervention.

Parents. The nurse can provide support by being attentive to the family's responses to the child. Mothers and fathers need to experience success, joy, and pride in their child to give him the support he needs from them. The child, too, requires support for his interactions, adjustments, and efforts. He must be reinforced for attempts to get to know his care providers and to communicate his needs to them.

Since mothers and fathers of handicapped children have few role models to imitate, they need support from the nurse to help them adjust. Above all, the nurse should ensure that the parents and siblings learn to perceive the handicapped child as a child first with unique and individual needs. The nurse needs to convey a humanistic, accepting approach of the child, so that the parents can observe this acceptance. The way the nurse interacts with, approaches, touches, or holds the child makes this obvious. Any signs of rejection of the child, though subtle in nature, are readily interpreted by parents. This attitude of liking, concern for, and acceptance of the child should begin in early infancy and continue throughout the handicapped child's life.

The nurse should ask the parents for suggestions on care planning, implementation, and evaluation, using the mutual participation model. The nurse can play a valuable role in ensuring that the child learns about his handicap. The nurse can foster communication between the child and his parents so that he shares his concerns with them. The parents can be helped to realize the child's level of maturity and understanding. The nurse needs to determine if the parents agree on what and when to tell the child about his condition. The nurse should emphasize that the parents must stress to the child the hopeful aspects of his condition, as well as the problems. The nurse should help the parents stress hopeful aspects to themselves before beginning to discuss them with the child. Careful consideration should be given to avoid overwhelming him and to supporting him as he reacts to information about himself. The nurse again needs to stress and to impress on the family that the child is normal—his handicap is not.

Most families can be helped to feel adequate about their roles and responsibilities. They should understand from the beginning that they can shape their child's outcome. At the same time, the lack of stable cultural practices on which they can rely may make parents feel insecure in their roles, inadequate, burdened, and anxious. The nurse's role is to help alleviate these feelings by pointing out the parents' and child's strengths. For example, a handicapped infant may be more demanding if he has difficulty in eating and needs more feedings. The child might be less responsive than the parents thought he would be. Therefore, the parent-infant relationship is vulnerable from the beginning. The nurse can support the parents in these concerns and supply information about what to expect from the infant in different phases of development.

The nurse encourages communication among all family members. Although some families do this automatically, many do not and need help in learning how to converse as a group within an atmosphere of freedom that fosters honesty and openness. Parent group sessions are helpful in assisting parents to verablize thoughts and feelings to each other but often do not take into account siblings' or the handicapped child's viewpoint. Therefore, the nurse may need to set up a family session, such as during a home or clinic visit. Although the ideal situation is to have all the members present at once, this is often not possible within the confines of traditional nursing practice. However, inviting members to participate at various visits is an appropriate alternative.

The nurse encourages parents to discuss their feelings toward the handicapped child, the impact of this event on their marriage, and associated stresses, such as financial burdens. It is important for the nurse to listen nonjudgmentally, avoiding any urge to align herself with one parent's feelings. Rather both parents are provided an equal opportunity to discuss their perceptions of events and relationships in the family.

The nurse makes every effort to include the father in visits, such as to the nursery, clinic, special school, stimulation programs, and so on. His relationship with the child is observed, noting verbal interactions, tendency to assist the child, ability to give praise or set limits, and sensitivity to the child's needs. He is included in the assessment process with specific emphasis on having him describe the child's strengths and difficulties. It is not unusual to find two parents who have found opposing views of the child's abilities, especially in the area of developmental disabilities. The nurse encourages the father to express his expectation for the child now and in the future. Because fathers tend to repress their feelings and feel less competent, the nurse acknowledges their difficulties and strengths, such as parenting skills and problem-solving abilities.

The nurse investigates community resources for the family. For example, State Crippled Children's Programs fund many handicapping conditions and can greatly relieve financial stresses. Several official and volunteer agencies offer special services for the handicapped child. Many of these are discussed elsewhere in the text under the diagnosis. Parents' organizations are especially helpful because they provide information and mutual support among the members. The nurse who is aware of similarly affected families can be instrumental in organizing a self-help parent group. Sometimes all the effort this entails is identifying one or two parents as leaders, sharing with them the names, telephone numbers, and addresses of other families, and guiding them in how to initiate a first meeting. Although the nurse may not participate in the actual meeting, he or she should be available to the parents as a resource person or as an intermediary to locate professional guidance when necessary. It is just as important for the nurse to recognize personal limitations as abilities in working with a group.

Siblings. As pointed out previously, the presence of a handicapped child in a family may result in parents paying less attention to the other children or expecting older siblings to take on greater responsibility for the care of the child. The siblings may respond by developing negative attitudes toward the child or by expressing anger in different forms. The nurse can help by using "anticipatory guidance," questioning the parents about what they believe is the best way to have siblings respond to the handicapped child and about whether they have any concerns about the way in which they are assigning responsibility to older siblings. This questioning should take place before serious negative effects occur.

In cases in which neglect and increased responsibility on the part of other siblings are kept within normal limits, siblings may experience embarrassment associated with the stigma of a handicap such as mental retardation. Parents are then faced with the difficulty of responding to this embarrassment in an understanding and appropriate manner without punishing the siblings for feeling the way they do. The nurse should encourage parents to talk with the siblings about how they view their handicapped sibling. For example, siblings of a retarded child may express fears about their ability to bear normal children. Adolescents in particular may not be able to discuss these vital issues with their parents and may prefer to consult with the nurse. The nurse should emphasize to parents that such questioning is natural for adolescents and should not be misconstrued as rebelliousness or rejection.

Many parents express concern about when and how to inform the other children in the family about the birth or the presence of a child who is handicapped. The answer depends on each child's level of sophistication and understanding. However, it is usually best to inform the siblings before a neighbor or other nonfamily member does so. Nurses can show by their behavior that they see the parents as being capable in their own unique style of imparting information about the condition. However, they should make it clear that if the parents postpone informing the siblings they run the risk of hindering the siblings' ability to develop a realistic understanding of the problem. Uninformed siblings may fantasize or develop apprehensions that are out of proportion to the child's actual condition. Furthermore, if parents choose to be silent or deceptive about the issue, they are setting a negative precedent for the siblings to follow, rather than encouraging the siblings to cope with the experience in a healthy and nurturing way.

The nurse must be sensitive to the reactions of siblings and whenever possible intervene to promote more positive adjustments. For example, siblings often mention that they are expected to take on additional responsibilities to help the parents care for the handicapped child. It is not unusual for them to express a positive reaction to assuming the extra duties but a negative response to feeling unappreciated for doing so. Such feelings can often be remedied by encouraging the siblings to discuss this with the parents and by suggesting to parents ways of showing gratitude, such as an increase in allowance, special privileges, and, most significantly, verbal praise.

Handicapped child. Through ongoing contacts with the child, the nurse can observe the child's responses to his handicap, ability to function, and adaptive behaviors within the environment and with significant others. The nurse can explore the child's own understanding of the nature of his illness or condition and support him while he learns to cope with his feelings. The nurse can ask how the child views himself and his condition. He should be supported and encouraged to express his concerns rather than allowing the nurse to express them for him, since open discussions may reduce anxiety.

Parents sometimes convey concern because the child cannot express the anxieties *he feels*. If the child cannot or will not talk, the nurse may have the child play out his feelings. He can be provided with toys to allow him to express threatening or stressful emotions. The nurse may find that the child responds best to drawing pictures or telling stories. Puppets can also be used to help him express himself. By demonstrating to parents how useful these techniques are, the nurse also helps them learn new ways of communicating with him.

Since school and peer relationships are so meaningful to the child, a chronically ill or handicapped child who must be hospitalized or stay at home should have some means of maintaining contact with his peers. The nurse and school teacher can plan care to create and maintain an environment that meets this need. Besides periodic visits, peer contact can be fostered through telephone calls, letter writing, special cards, or the use of tape recordings.

The nurse also helps the child and parents express frustrations about restrictions imposed on his movements and activities. They can be helped to plan appropriate activities for when he is immobilized. The nurse and child need to discuss what he wants and is able to do. The nurse needs to check with him repeatedly to see how he is responding to restrictions of his movement and help find creative ways in which he can entertain himself. Although the point seems obvious, parents and health professionals often fail to include the child in his care planning.

Extended members. The nurse must also be sensitive to family's cues regarding sources of stress from extended members, such as grandparents. For example, the nurse may want to encourage the parents to invite the grandparents to be present during one of the child's visits to a clinic, during the diagnostic workup, or to a parent conference. Including grandparents in a discussion in which they can discuss their concerns may help them deal with their feelings, thus reducing stress on the entire family. Grandparents' feelings of blame and anger as well as any "cure fantasies" they harbor can be brought out in the open and discussed if such discussions seem necessary. The nurse can help the grandparents understand the effects of their behavior on the family with an appropriate statement, such as, "Your daughter is currently experiencing a great deal of pain and anguish. We realize that this is difficult for you as well as your daughter; however, you can be of tremendous help by being supportive toward her."

Considerable stress can also arise from nonfamilial sources, such as friends, neighbors, or strangers. Inability to cope with comments about the disorder or curious stares by others may foster the tendency to isolate and protect the child within the home. The family needs guidance in preparing for these inevitable experiences. One approach is encouraging parents to dress the child as much as possible like other children. Good grooming is very important in minimizing differences in appearance. Through role playing, parents can practice responses to comments, such as, "Is your child retarded?" or "Has he always been crippled?" Through parent groups, family members can share experiences and learn from each other how they successfully deal with probing questions or unkind remarks. Such interventions must include the siblings and handicapped child, who also must face and deal with these events.

Fostering reality adjustment

Fostering a reality adjustment primarily involves education of the parents regarding the handicap, developmental needs of the child, and realistic goal setting. Ideally education should be aimed at preventing problems, rather than at relearning to change existing dilemmas. Like the interventions previously discussed, this goal requires an ongoing process that is part of assessment and emotional support of the family.

Knowledge of handicap. Educating the family about the handicap is actually an extension of revealing the diagnosis, especially those points listed on p. 799. Education involves not only supplying technical information but also discussing how the handicap will affect the child. For example, it is of little benefit to discuss mental retardation in terms of numbers. Rather parents need to understand what the moderately retarded child can do in terms of self-help, academic learning, and independence. Similarly the child who has lost a limb needs more than an explanation of the prosthetic leg. He must know the limitations it places on his activity as well as the opportunities available for him.

Parents also need guidance in how the handicap may interfere or alter activities of daily living, such as eating, dressing, sleeping, toileting, and so on. One area frequently affected by handicaps such as chronic illness or developmental disability is nutrition. The most common problems are undernutrition as a result of food being inappropriately restricted, loss of appetite, or motor deficits that interfere with feeding and overnutrition usually caused by a caloric intake in excess of energy expenditure or from boredom and lack of stimulation in other areas.

Although a handicapped child requires the same basic nutrients as other children, the daily requirements may differ. For example, the child who has a handicap may have a different body composition. A child with cerebral palsy grows more slowly than a normal child yet needs additional calories because of constant muscular activity. Feeding the child with cerebral palsy is usually very difficult because of spasticity or rigidity, and the nurse and nutritionist need to monitor height and weight to assure optimum nutrition. The hypermetabolic child requires more calories. Thus it is important to individually define the calorie level for each child. The nurse must consider that anticonvulsant drugs, such as diphenylhydantoin (Dilantin) and phenobarbital, increase the need for vitamin D and alter folic acid metabolism. Therefore, the child who is being given anticonvulsant drugs must be monitored carefully for evidence of calcium or phosphorus depletion. He should receive an adequate supply of milk as a source of vitamin D and important minerals.

Unfortunately few reliable standards exist regarding nutritional requirements for handicapped children. To ensure optimum nutrition, the nurse should record the child's diet for a 7-day period to determine if deficiencies exist. The nurse can collaborate with the nutritionist to select a diet that best meets the child's nutritional needs.

In addition to educating the family about the effect of the handicap on the child, it is also advisable to discuss the prognosis for parental feelings and actions. Once parents realize that the response of overcompensating for their feelings of guilt and inadequacy through overprotection is normal but potentially destructive, they can then begin to consider other ways of relating to the child. Obviously the goal is for the parents to realistically accept the child's handicap, promote his optimum development, and grow together as a family unit.

Insight into normal development. Aside from knowledge of the handicap and its effect on the child's abilities, the family must be guided toward fostering appropriate development in their child. Although each stage may take longer to achieve, parents must be guided to helping the child fully realize his potential in preparation for the next phase of development.

For example, during infancy the normal child is achieving basic *trust* through a satisfying, intimate, consistent relationship with his parents. However, the handicapped child's early existence may be stressful, chaotic, and unsatisfying. Consequently he may need more parental support and expressions of affection to achieve trust.[21] Likewise the parents require assistance in ways of meeting the infant's needs, such as how to hold a rigid or flaccid infant, how to feed a child with tongue thrust or episodes of dyspnea, and how to stimulate a child who seems incapable of achieving any skills.

During early childhood the goal is to achieve separation from mother, autonomy, and initiative. For the child who is hospitalized, the ability to separate may be extremely difficult and realistically may have to be delayed. However, the natural parental response to this continued dependence is overprotection. Parents need help in realizing the importance of brief separations from the child, including others in the child's care, and providing social experiences outside the home whenever possible.

Another consequence of overprotection is decreased independence on the part of the child. Frequently the child is able to learn self-help skills, such as holding the bottle, finger-feeding, removing simple articles of clothing, and so on, but the parent continues to perform the act. The nurse, therefore, must guide parents to the usual milestones expected from the child. Initially this requires developmental assessment of functional age, such as using the Denver Developmental Screening Test (Appendix F) or the Washington Guide to Promoting Development in the Young Child (Appendix G). The latter tool is especially helpful in providing suggestions regarding common functional activities in a young child's daily life, namely motor skills, feeding, sleep, play, language, discipline, and toilet training.

Once the child's developmental level is obtained, the nurse systematically reviews with parents what the child should be achieving and ways of accomplishing this goal. The parent is also encouraged in any present pursuits, such as giving the child a spoon during mealtime. Instructions should be written, not only verbal. If presented similarly to those of the Washington Guide to Promoting Development in the Young Child (Appendix G), written instructions can be individualized for each child by selecting the specific age-group for each activity and compiling it into one form. The nurse should avoid presenting the entire guide to the parents to prevent them from becoming overwhelmed by the number of future skills still to be learned. (Tables 23-4, 23-6, and 23-7 list stimulation programs for developing independent behavior.)

At each visit the nurse evaluates the child's developmental process. Since each child develops at his own rate, there are no rigid guidelines for expecting when a handicapped child will achieve a particular skill. However, the nurse inquires about lack of progress in any one area. For example, sometimes a delay in self-feeding is not caused by lack of motor skill but by the parents' impatience in waiting for the skill to develop. Cleaning up the spilled food may seem like one more unnecessary task unless the nurse stresses the importance of using a cup or spoon. All that may be necessary to encourage parent participation are suggestions to avoid large accidents, such as pouring only a small amount of juice in a cup or having the child feed himself mashed potatoes (a sticky food) rather than gelatin (a slippery food).

Not all handicapped children are capable of achieving normal developmental milestones. For example, the mentally retarded child may never achieve cognitive skills above a preschool level. The child who is deaf may achieve only rudimentary verbal language. In these situations adjustments must be made to compensate for the lack of or severely delayed achievement in one area. However, such adjustments must be based on an understanding of normal development. Since motoric handicaps are present in a majority of handicapping conditions, this disability is used as an example to illustrate psychologic implications in making developmental changes.

During early childhood the basic innate drive for movement is dominant. During toddlerhood there is rapid development of motor skills, which eventually becomes the basis for learning and coping with the complex world. Psychologically this period is critical for developing a desire for independence. Language development, bowel control, locomotion, and fine-motor control all converge to produce a feeling of competency. Gradually during the early school years this basic motor urge shifts to a more goal-directed, symbolic expression in which words and thoughts replace actions as a way of problem solving.[16]

When the young child has a handicap that interferes with motor development, there is the potential hazard of shifting to development of compensatory intellectual pursuits before the child is ready. If this occurs, achievement of autonomy and initiative may be severely compromised, setting the stage for permanent emotional problems. Therefore, intervention must be based on providing activities that allow maximum motor development. For example, if a child has paraplegia, it is not sufficient to strengthen the upper extremities to compensate for the lower ones. Rather the activity must take into account the child's need for social interaction, sense of control over his body, feeling of competence and achievement, and an outlet for aggression. Suitable activities may include ball throwing, swimming, building blocks, or pounding with a hammer. In this way the child's developmental needs based on motor activity are met within the limitations of his physical handicap.

Another critical component for normal child development is discipline. Unfortunately this is one of the earliest child-rearing practices eliminated when parents react with "overbenevolence." Not only does lack of discipline destroy the child's security because he has no boundaries on which to test out his behavior, it also fails to teach the child socially acceptable behavior and creates resentment and hostility among the siblings if different standards are applied to each child. One of the most effective approaches to discipline, especially with developmentally disabled children, is the use of behavior modification.

The nurse's responsibility is to help parents learn successful methods of controlling behavior before they become a problem. Simple limit-setting measures that should be applied to the handicapped child include a regular bedtime or nap hour, routine feeding schedule, preferably with the family, dressing in the morning, and scheduled play time, such as outdoor activity or limited watching of television. Such measures not only enforce certain expectations from the child but also encourage "normalization" of the handicapped child. (See Chapter 23 for a more detailed discussion of this concept.)

The next major development is entry into school and achieving a sense of industry. Both should be easily accomplished by the handicapped child who has experienced peer relationships and achieved some developmental skills. The nurse encourages parents of handicapped children to provide appropriate nursery school experiences, to encourage peer play within the home, and to foster as many independent behaviors as possible. For example, handicapped children who are able to attend regular nursery schools are excluded unless they are toilet trained.

The adolescent is achieving a sense of identity. Even under the best circumstances, this period is often difficult because of the pressure of group conformity and acceptance. For the handicapped child it may be a time of insurmountable obstacles, especially if he has not accepted his disability. Parents need to offer a great deal of support. While demonstrating their love and acceptance of the child, they must be careful to encourage independence and not shelter the adolescent from the necessary conflicts of his age-group. For example, they should encourage the child to learn to drive, since the mobility offered by that skill greatly increases independence and social opportunity.

Setting realistic goals. One of the most difficult adjustments is setting realistic future goals for the handicapped child and for those who must assume his continued care. Sometimes the impact of this decision does not surface until the child finishes school or the parents near retirement. At that time another crisis can arise because all the family roles and relationship that maintained stability are now disrupted.

Planning for the future should be a gradual process. All along the parents should cultivate realistic vocations for the child. For example, if the child has a physical handicap, he should be directed to intellectual, artistic, or musical pursuits. If the child is developmentally disabled, he should be taught a manual skill that can be done in a special workshop. In this way the child's development proceeds in the direction of self-support through gainful employment.

Unfortunately vocational pursuits are not realistic for every handicapped person. Multiple or severely handicapped persons may require lifelong care and assistance. In these situations parents must look to the future when they will no longer be able to care for their child. Residential placement may be very difficult unless the family mutually participates in the decision-making and planning process. Institutionalization should not be viewed as abandonment. Not infrequently it is the only way to preserve the family unit. The nurse should help the family investigate suitable placements, discuss their feelings regarding this discussion, and explore measures to maintain meaningful communication with the handicapped member. Alternatives to home care are described on p. 833.

NURSING INTERVENTION WITH MULTIHANDICAPPED CHILDREN

It is estimated that the largest group of multiply handicapped children are those with mental retardation and physical disabilities, such as epilepsy or cerebral palsy. Although these children need a great deal of consideration and care, there is little knowledge and research about them and few programs designed to meet their needs. Nursing interventions may not only seem insurmountable but also hopeless at the same time. The following report of a nurse's involvement with a multihandicapped child is presented to illustrate specific interventions used in this situation and to emphasize previously discussed principles in caring for handicapped families.

A 12-month-old infant was referred to a multidisciplinary setting for a comprehensive evaluation. Her parents suspected that she could not see objects but that she did respond to light. She could not lift her head, and she rarely moved about or played. She did respond to voices. Her legs made scissor-like movements, and her body stiffened when her mother held her. She had no difficulty in swallowing or sucking. She was referred for a physical examination, a speech and hearing examination, and neurologic, nutritional, and psychologic tests. She was also scheduled to see the nurse.

The nurse did not understand how to contribute to the child's assessment, since the child could not pass any items on standardized screening tests as the Denver Developmental Screening Test, except for lifting her head slightly off the surface of a table.

In thinking further, however, the nurse realized that some very valuable data about the infant could be collected so that this information could be applied to an intervention program.

First the nurse decided that it was important to find the child's strengths, using the Denver Developmental Screening Test. Her deficiencies were glaringly obvious. The infant could not accomplish 90% of the developmental tasks that are expected of a 1-year-old child. Instead of concluding that nothing could be done for the child, the nurse formulated objectives to facilitate a plan of care that could be shared with the professional team members.

During the diagnostic process it was vital that the nurse properly assess the infant's ability to suck and swallow food, her sleep patterns, and mother-infant interactions. It was also clear that someone who made home visits, namely the nurse, assess the child's home environment. The nurse chose the Home Observation for Measurement of the Environment (HOME) and discovered that the infant was failing to thrive because she lacked stimulation. It was also observed that the infant blinked when a flashlight was flashed before her eyes. The nurse discovered that the infant could hold her head up for 2 to 3 seconds when she was placed on her abdomen. Her breathing rate changed when she was given a rattle and when rattling noises were made. She could place and hold a rattle in each hand when it was presented. Still, she could not hold her head up when sitting, her head lagged severely when she was pulled to a sitting position, and she did not respond differentially to sounds. During the assessment process the nurse realized that it was important to assess the child's functional status, adaptive behaviors, levels of independence, and responsiveness to her environment. It also became clear that it would be valuable to learn how the mother perceived her infant. The nurse realized that it was imperative that the mother describe whether the infant responded to sounds, voices, movement, light and its different intensities, and persons. The nurse had to discover what stimulation the child enjoyed—touch, movement, or voices, how the infant showed interest in animate and inanimate stimuli, what maintained her interest longest, and what decreased her interest. No matter how insignificant they seemed, it was important that the mother learn of her infant's interests, strengths, and behaviors.

The nurse also had to know what strengths the mother perceived in the infant, what her main concerns were, and what worried her the most. The nurse discovered that the mother did not respond with interest when the different professionals told her what her child *could not do*. When the nurse asked the mother what the child did when she was placed in the living room, the mother said that the child blinked when the sun shone in the room. It was discovered that the mother felt inadequate in her ability to help her own infant. Through home visits and systematic observations of the parent-infant interaction, the nurse learned that the mother talked continuously and automatically to the infant, who did not show signs of visual tracking. By using the Home Observation for Measurement of the Environment, the nurse was able to convince the mother that she indeed offered the child appropriate auditory stimuli. It also became evident that the child responded to sounds and voices.

The nurse acknowledged the mother's persistent efforts to get the child to respond to something in her environment.

The nurse explained to the mother that she was doing the right thing by placing the infant in different environments throughout the day. In determining the infant's strengths, the nurse made a point of asking the parents what they thought the infant's capabilities were. Could she, for instance hold her head steady while sitting, or did she turn to different sounds? The nurse asked the mother and father to describe the infant's feeding patterns. Both parents reported that she was able to suck and swallow without choking. The nurse praised them for their ability to make observations of their infant.

In the period when the infant was being tested by various professionals, the nurse made several home visits and watched how the mother and father interacted with the infant at home, rather than in a clinical setting. The parents and nurse had observed that the 1-year-old child was consistently startled by loud noises, a reflex that should have disappeared months before. The nurse then realized the need to find whether the infant was startled by other stimuli. It was also important to learn how the infant was approached, touched, and held, because she was startled so easily. The nurse observed that the parents approached her gently and held her firmly and securely. This was important because it appeared that the infant could not see and needed a secure feeling and a sense of trust about her environment. The nurse realized that it would be important to help the mother first observe the infant and then plan different places in which to place the infant and help her experience different postures, so that she could become oriented to her environment through many different stimuli, motions, and movement.

The nurse was concerned by the mother-infant patterns of interaction. It was obvious that it was difficult for the mother to interpret and respond to the infant's need for play, to be picked up, to go to sleep, or to have new stimuli. On the other hand, it was impossible for the infant to read or interpret the mother's facial cues of pleasure or displeasure. Both were experiencing difficulty in interpreting each other's cues of expectations, needs, approval, gratifications, and disappointments or disapproval. The nurse subsequently played a vital role in reducing the mother's confusion about what the infant needed and wanted. Simultaneously the nurse supported the mother for her ability to reinforce the infant when the infant made attempts to make her own unique needs known. The nurse began by asking the mother to describe the infant's behaviors when eating and sleeping. The mother was able to distinguish cries of hunger from cries of boredom and signs of fatigue from behavior indicating lack of interest. As the weeks passed, the nurse screened the infant on a number of important developmental items. The nurse learned what interested the infant as well as that the infant could hold her head steady and that she could turn to voices. She enjoyed her bath and liked her hands in the water. She responded when a breeze blew across her face when she sat on the front porch. The nurse and parents continued to search for activities or stimuli that would generate more exploratory activity by the infant.

Remembering that the ultimate goal was to help this child become as *independent as possible,* despite her lack of vision and mobility, the nurse and parents watched as she drank from her bottle. They observed that, for the most part, her environment was brought to her, that is, food and toys were brought to her and people came to her. *Nothing* was expected of the infant. In keeping with realistic present goals it was determined that she would have to turn her head when her bottle was brought to her. The infant reacted to the bottle when it was being prepared and when it was presented to her. Before eating she would cry, fuss, and scream, and she would immediately become quiet when given food. It was also observed that she could move her tongue forward and backward. Gradually she was fed small pieces of food so that she could become accustomed to different textures and consistencies and could practice moving her lips, mouth, and tongue to receive food.

Because the nurse was concerned that the child was not receiving adequate stimulation, she asked the parents to keep records of how often the infant was picked up, held, or positioned elsewhere. The nurse wanted to teach the parents that the infant, although she appeared not to respond, needed more stimuli to learn from her environment. The parents thus learned that the child was left alone for long periods of time without any animate or inanimate stimulation. The parents learned from their own records that she needed to be picked up, talked to, held, and touched more often.

The nurse was also concerned that the mother considered the infant "very irritable." The mother agreed to keep records of when the infant cried and when she was happy. As a result the nurse could acknowledge the mother's concerns about the infant's irritable cry. The nurse supported the mother by saying, "It must be difficult and frustrating, and it must really drain you when she cries so often throughout the day." The nurse was particularly sensitive to the need for supporting these parents, since the infant could not respond by smiling when they came near or showing pleasure when she was held. The mother needed to discuss her frustration, her fear, her sense of helplessness, and her potential loss of hope. The mother's greatest fear was that the child would be totally blind, would have cerebral palsy and be paralyzed, and would not profit from any learning experiences or whatever the parents might offer.

The mother needed support from the nurse, too, that feeding was a very demanding activity. Simply giving her a bottle took 40 minutes three times a day. The mother needed to know that she was doing a good job as a mother and was trying her best under overwhelming circumstances.

The nurse realized the importance of observing appropriate interactions between the mother and infant and mentioning them to the mother. For example, when the mother held the infant gently and protectively and talked to the infant, even though the infant did not respond, the nurse would comment, "That's nice the way you talk with her. It's good you keep on trying even though she doesn't let you know she understands." Clearly the mother needed to hear of her own resources and efforts, especially when the infant gave no conspicuous signs that she perceived what the mother intended. During the time the infant was being assessed by a multidisciplinary group, the nurse realized how important it was for the mother to use specific descriptions of the child's behavior. The nurse encouraged her to say, for example, that she cries about ten times in the morning for about 20 minutes, it takes 40 minutes to give her her bottle, and she is fussy 2 hours every night instead of that she cries all the time, it takes forever to feed her, and she is fussy every minute. The nurse encouraged the mother to be assertive in questioning child-care professionals when she did not understand their answers. The nurse emphasized to the mother that she had a right to such answers without feeling guilty, stupid, or inadequate. When the mother and father were invited to the informing parent conference, the nurse encouraged them to ask questions when the information was unclear. The nurse took on the responsibility of follow-up care and attempted to determine how much of the shocking information the parents had assimilated. Little had actually been remembered. The parents recalled with grief that they were told that the child was totally blind. The nurse added to, corrected, or offered alternative explanations.

Throughout the diagnostic workup the mother continuously expressed fear of what she would find out and of how she had caused the infant's problems. In subsequent visits to the home, the nurse made every effort to help alleviate the mother's guilt. Over time, the mother cried and grieved, moving through periods of mourning, grief, and despair. The nurse kept in mind the mother's needs throughout the evaluation period when most of the other professionals were intent on diagnosing the child. Throughout this time the nurse focused on the mother's need to talk about the constant supervision required of her infant, the fact that the infant was irritable and screamed, and that she responded barely or not at all to everyone's effort to elicit a response. The nurse also gently supported the mother through her fears about the child's future.

It is especially important that throughout the time when other professionals were testing the infant for developmental delays, the *nurse* emphasized the infant's strengths. One important reason for this focus was to encourage the attachment process between infant and mother. The mother had repeatedly stressed that her infant was not cuddly. Her comments were valid on observation. The infant had extensor thrust of the legs and arms. By helping the mother hold the infant and move her head into the midline, the nurse was able to facilitate an improved posture. The mother no longer felt that the infant was "rejecting" her. The nurse continued to allow the mother to talk about her infant's lack of being cuddly. The mother was asked to describe the infant's ability to cuddle, what she thought a cuddly infant was, and if there were times the infant did cuddle. Interestingly enough, the mother described times when the infant would relax and mold into her arms and snuggle against her shoulder and neck. The nurse sympathized with the mother's disappointments and lack of gratification in holding her infant. The nurse asked the mother to describe what was gratifying about her infant and what activities were mutally satisfying. Of greatest importance was the mother's ability to express her deep feelings of sorrow, her disappointments, her struggles, and what *she* rather than the child-care professional thought.

Summary of nurses' role in assessment and management of multihandicapped children

The nurse realized that personal significant contributions to the family were: (1) The parents were helped to consider and provide the appropriate stimuli that would elicit and maintain the infant's attention. (2) The infant's frustration was reduced and the parents were helped to interpret the infant's cues. (3) The infant was helped to learn to use her own resources to adapt or cope with stress, conflict, or frustration, and the parents were helped in refraining from aiding the infant too soon. (4) The parents were helped to promote the infant's independent behaviors in language, head raising, cooperating with undressing, holding her bottle, and experiencing sitting up so that she could practice head control. The nurse also helped the parents see the need for the infant to turn her head in search of food when it was presented to her. (5) The mother's needs were met, which included giving credit to the mother for her strengths, goals, and child-rearing methods; acknowledging the mother's observational skills; letting the mother express her views of her infant's behaviors and what these meant; allowing the mother to express her feelings about the infant's serious sensorimotor deficits; encouraging the mother to talk about what she liked about the infant; discovering what the mother and father's goals were for the infant; learning of the mother's and father's concerns about the infant's development; and encouraging problem-solving and decision-making skills of the mother and the father.

REFERENCES

1. Barnard, K. E., and Erickson, M. L.: Teaching children with developmental problems: a family care approach, ed. 2, 1976, The C. V. Mosby Co.
2. Boone, D. R., and Hartman, B. H.: The benevolent over-reaction, Clin. Pediatr. **11**(5):268-271, May 1972.
3. Budner, S., Goodman, L., and Aponte, R.: The minority re-

tardate: a paradox and a problem in definition, Soc. Serv. Rev. **43:**174-183, 1969.

4. Caldwell, B. M.: The importance of beginning early. In Karnes, M., editor: Not all little wagons are red, Reston, Va., 1973, Council for Exceptional Children.
5. Caldwell, B. M.: Instruction manual inventory for infants (Home Observation for Measurement of the Environment), Little Rock, Ark., 1970.
6. Cummings, S. T.: The impact of the child's deficiency on the father: a study of fathers of mentally retarded and of chronically ill children, Am. J. Orthopsychiatry **46**(2):246-255, April 1975.
7. Ehlers, W. H., Krishef, C. H., and Prothero, J. C.: An introduction to mental retardation: a program text, Columbus, Ohio, 1973, Charles E. Merrill Publishing Co.
8. Farber, B.: Family organization and interaction, San Francisco, 1964, Chandler Publishing Co.
9. Farber, B., and Jenne, W. C.: Interactions with retarded siblings and life goals of children, Marriage Fam. Liv. **25:**96-98, 1963.
10. Gorham, K. A., and associates: Effects on Parents. In Hobbs, N., editor: Issues in the classification of children, San Francisco, 1975, Jossey-Bass, Inc., Publishers.
11. Grossman, F. K.: Brothers and sisters of retarded children: an exploratory study, New York, 1972, Syracuse University Press.
12. Hersh, A.: Changes in family functioning following placement of a retarded child, Soc. Casework **15:**93-102, 1970.
13. Hobbs, N.: The futures of children, San Francisco, 1975, Jossey-Bass, Inc., Publishers.
14. Kogan, K. L., and Tyler, N. B.: Mother-child transactions in cerebral palsy therapy, Seattle, 1975, Child Development and Mental Retardation Center, University of Seattle.
15. Mattsson, A.: Long-term physical illness in childhood: a challenge to psychosocial adaptation, Pediatrics **50**(5):801-811, November 1972.
16. McDermott, J. F., and Akina, E.: Understanding and improving the personality development of children with physical handicaps, Clin. Pediatr. **11**(3):130-134, March 1972.
17. Olshansky, S.: Parent responses to a mentally defective child, Ment. Retard. **4:**20-25, 1966.
18. Pless, I. B., and Douglas, J. W. B.: Chronic illness in childhood. Part I. Epidemiological and clinical characteristics, Pediatrics **47**(2):405-414, February 1971.
19. Roos, P.: Parents and families of the mentally retarded. In Kauffman, J. M., and Payne, J. S.: Mental retardation: introduction and personal perspective, Columbus, Ohio, 1975, Charles E. Merrill Publishing Co.
20. Sultz, H. A., and associates: Long-term childhood illness, Pittsburgh, 1972, University of Pittsburgh Press.
21. Yancy, W. S.: Approaches to emotional management of the child with a chronic illness, Clin. Pediatr. **11**(2):64-67, February 1972.
22. Zelle, R. S.: The family with a mentally retarded child. In Hymovitch, D. P., and Barnard, M. U.: Family health care, New York, 1973, McGraw-Hill Book Co.

BIBLIOGRAPHY

Battle, C. V.: Chronic physical disease: behavioral aspects, Pediatr. Clin. North Am. **22:**525, 1975.

Gould, R. K., and Rothenberg, M. B.: The chronically ill child facing death—how can the pediatrician help? Clin. Pediatr. **12**(7):447-449, July 1973.

Guralnick, M. J.: A language development program for severely handicapped children, Except. Chil. **39**(1):45-49, 1972.

Holdaway, D.: Educating the handicapped child and his parents, Clin. Pediatr. **11**(2):63-64, February 1972.

Jones, R.: The hierarchical structure of attitudes toward the exceptional, Except. Child. **40**(6):430-435, 1974.

Kogan, K. L., and Tyler, N.: Mother-child interaction in young physically handicapped children, Am. J. Ment. Defic. **77:**492-497, 1973.

Lepler, M.: Having a handicapped child, Am. J. Maternal Child Nurs. **3**(1):32-33, January/February 1978.

Love, H. D.: Parental attitudes toward exceptional children, Springfield, Ill., 1970, Charles C Thomas, Publisher.

Mackeith, R.: The feelings and behavior of parents of handicapped children, Dev. Med. Child. Neurol. **15:**524, 1973.

Meadow, K. P., and Meadow, L.: Changing role perceptions for parents of handicapped children, Except. Child. **38**(1):21-27, 1971.

Pless, I. B., and Satterwhite, B.: Chronic illness in childhood: selection, activities, and evaluation of non-professional family counselors, Clin. Pediatr. **11**(7):403-410, July 1972.

Poznanski, E.: Psychiatric difficulties in siblings of handicapped children, Clin. Pediatr. **8:**232-234, April 1969.

Poznanski, E.: Emotional issues in raising handicapped children, Rehabil. Lit. **34:**322, 1973.

Schulman, J. L.: Coping with tragedy: successfully facing the problem of a seriously ill child, Chicago, 1976, Follett Publishing Co.

Shepherd, C. W.: Childhood chronic illness and visual motor perceptual development, Except. Child. **36**(1):39-42, 1969.

23

The child with mental retardation

Mental retardation is one of the most prevalent handicapping conditions in the United States. An estimated 6.5 million persons, or 3% of the entire population, are afflicted with mental retardation and fall into the following categories: mildly retarded (5.3 million individuals), moderately retarded (360,000 individuals), severely retarded (210,000 persons), and profoundly retarded (90,000 persons).[2] Most mentally retarded individuals live at home, and their condition intimately affects other family members. Therefore, mental retardation touches the lives of at least 20 million persons in the United States.

Since mentally retarded children are no longer automatically admitted into institutional settings, but often remain at home to learn basic self-care skills, parents need role models and adequate preparation to effectively teach the child to function optimally within his environment. Nurses are in a strategic position to assume a vital role in assisting these parents with observation, problem solving, and decision making. With expanded roles in nursing, it is not unlikely that nurses will assume additional responsibility for the care of mentally retarded children in schools, sheltered workshops, residential settings, and ambulatory care centers, as well as in hospitals.

DEFINITION

The most commonly accepted definition of mental retardation by the American Association on Mental Deficiency (AAMD) states that "mental retardation refers to significantly sub-average general intellectual functioning existing concurrently with deficits in adaptive behavior and manifested during the developmental period."[10] An important aspect of this definition is that it emphasizes both intelligence and behavior as criteria for mental retardation. Generally intelligence is measured by a standard test, such as the Stanford Binet test or Wechsler Intelligence Scale for Children. Subaverage intellectual functioning is usually defined as an intelligence quotient (IQ) that is 2 standard deviations or more below the mean (generally an IQ of 70 or lower). However, according to the AAMD definition, subaverage intelligence is defined as 1 standard deviation below the mean, or a score of 83 or 84, depending on the scale used. According to this one criterion, nearly 16% of the population can be classified as mentally retarded, which provides educational opportunities for a group of children who are usually neglected such as those defined as "slow learners" or "borderline intelligent."

Adaptive behavior is usually considered in terms of academic performance. Low academic performance is a score on an achievement test that is more than 1½ years below grade level.[6] Therefore, in terms of this definition, a child with a subaverage IQ who manages to succeed in a regular classroom is not strictly classified as mentally retarded, because the child's adaptive behavior reflects a higher level of intellect than is demonstrated by the usual intelligence tests. Conversely a child who fails in academic learning but whose intelligence is within normal limits cannot be defined as mentally deficient.[6] These dual criteria for classification of mental retardation attempt to balance other factors that may influence poor intellectual performance, such as emotional or environmental deprivation.

Another implication of this definition is that a child's classification may change with improvements in adaptive behavior. For example, a child with low intelligence will probably also do poorly in academic work. However, with good vocational preparation he may be able to support himself after graduation from high school; therefore, he no longer fulfills the requirement of poor adaptive behavior. This is particularly relevant to mildly retarded individuals who can learn to function independently within society by the early adult years. It is also significant in terms of children who because of sensory impairment may be erroneously classified as retarded. However, once they receive appropriate rehabilitation that allows them to learn and adapt using compensatory skills, it is obvious that such labeling is incorrect.

Another implication of the definition is its focus on subaverage intelligence or poor adaptive behavior originating within childhood development or from birth to adolescence. By these criteria adults who through disease or injury lose such functions are not classified as retarded.

Classification

Mentally retarded children can be classified according to several criteria. The most useful is classification based on educational potential or symptom severity (Table 23-1). The approximate range of IQ for each category is given to familiarize the nurse with scoring standards usually used to diagnose subaverage intelligence. However, the nurse should refrain from using numbers as the criteria for assessing or evaluating the child's abilities, since they provide little value in counseling parents or training retarded children.

Borderline. Borderline mentally retarded children are usually called slow learners. Although they often exhibit no abnormal delays in development, they tend to achieve marginal success in the regular classroom. Many are found in classes for the educationally handicapped or learning disabled. They usually require special educational assistance within the regular classroom to achieve academic success. They are capable of graduating from high school, learning gainful skilled or semi-skilled labor, and adjusting to social relationships, including marriage and child rearing. However, they may need additional support during major stressful periods during their life.

Mildly retarded. Mildly mentally retarded children are also referred to as educable, because they are able to benefit from educational programs. Although they may develop slowly, they have the potential to be assimilated into their community economically and socially. They require educational programs directed toward their adjustment to accepted social interaction patterns and realistic occupational goals, as well as supportive guidance in selecting and holding suitable jobs. On occasion they may require special

Table 23-1. Classification of mental retardation*

Level (IQ)†	Preschool (0-5 years)—maturation and development	School age (6-21 years)—training and education	Adult (21 years and over)—social and vocational adequacy
Borderline—68-83	Usually has few if any lags in development; often not detected until demonstrates marginal success in school	Can achieve in a regular classroom with additional help; achievements close to normal mental age	Capable of competitive employment, although vocational choices may be limited to skilled labor; self-supporting; can adjust to marriage and child rearing; may need additional support when experiencing unusual stress
Mild—52-67	Often not noticed as retarded by casual observer but is slower to walk, feed self, and talk than most children; follows same sequence in development as normal children	Can acquire practical skills and useful reading and arithmetic to a third to sixth grade level with special education; can be guided toward social conformity; achieves mental age of 8 to 12 years	Can usually achieve social and vocational skills adequate to self-maintenance; may need occasional guidance and support when under unusual social or economic stress; can adjust to marriage but not child rearing
Moderate—36-51	Noticeable delays in motor development, especially in speech; responds to training in various self-help activities	Can learn simple communication, elementary health and safety habits, and simple manual skills; does not progress in functional reading or arithmetic; achieves mental age of 3 to 7 years	Can perform simple tasks under sheltered condition; participates in simple recreation; travels alone in familiar places; usually incapable of self-maintenance
Severe—20-35	Marked delay in motor development; little or no communication skills; may respond to training in elementary self-help, for example, self-feeding	Usually walks, barring specific disability; has some understanding of speech and some response; can profit from systematic habit training; achieves mental age of toddler	Can conform to daily routines and repetitive activities; needs continuing direction and supervision in protective environment
Profound—0-19	Gross retardation; minimal capacity for functioning in sensorimotor areas; needs nursing care	Obvious delays in all areas of development; shows basic emotional responses; may respond to skillful training in use of legs, hands, and jaws; needs close supervision; achieves mental age of young infant	May walk, needs complete custodial care, has primitive speech; usually benefits from regular physical activity

*Based on classification from American Association on Mental Deficiency.
†According to Stanford-Binet scale.

assistance and guidance to cope with major life crises, but generally they are capable of working in competitive situations and living independent lives. They function well in compatible marital relationships but are usually unable to cope with the responsibilities of child rearing.

Moderately retarded. Moderately retarded individuals are referred to as trainable, because they can be taught to independently care for their own needs. Although they may require supervision and support throughout life, they can learn to do meaningful tasks at home and work at appropriate simple jobs such as those in sheltered workshops maintained by community agencies for special work training. Some of these persons may live in special residential care centers, which are available to them when no responsible relative or significant others can be responsible for them.

Severely retarded. Children with severe retardation are limited in their language, social skills, motor capabilities, and communication abilities and may have associated physical handicaps. They may have impaired judgment and require help in making important life decisions for themselves. They are certainly capable of learning selected self-care skills and learning to protect themselves within their environment. Although they may need to be placed in residential facilities for various reasons, many of them can live at home under the supervision of their parents.

Profoundly retarded. Children who are profoundly retarded generally need complete custodial care or supervision. They exhibit major impairments in physical coordination and in sensorimotor development. They generally require supervised living whether they live at home or in a specially designed residential facility. They may acquire minimal speech development, but their chances for achieving self-sufficiency are extremely limited.

No matter which set of criteria characterize a retarded child, it is crucial that both nurses and parents capitalize on the child's unique capabilities, strengths, and abilities and carefully evaluate those areas in which he requires help.

CAUSES OF MENTAL RETARDATION

Estimates suggest that less than 6% of the cases of mental retardation have actual recognized causes; in the other 94% the causes are either unknown or are not classified.[2] Generally the etiologic classifications of mental retardation can be divided into the following nine broad categories[16]:

1. Infection and intoxication, including any agent associated with abnormalities or malformations, such as rubella, syphilis, thalidomide or other maternal drug consumption, exposure to industrial chemicals, increased blood levels of lead, Rh incompatibility resulting in kernicterus, or maternal disorders, such as toxemia
2. Trauma or physical agent, namely injury to the brain suffered during the prenatal, perinatal, or postnatal period, including physical injury or lack of oxygen or exposure to radiation
3. Metabolism or nutrition, including imbalances in fat, carbohydrates, and amino acids, inadequate nutrition, and metabolic disorders, such as phenylketonuria
4. Gross postnatal brain disease, including diseases characterized by skin eruptions, lesions, and tumors, such as, neurofibromatosis and tuberous sclerosis
5. Unknown prenatal influence, including cerebral and cranial malformations such as microencephaly and hydrocephaly
6. Gestational disorders, including prematurity, low birth weight, and postmaturity
7. Psychiatric disorders that have their onset during the child's developmental period up to age 18 years
8. Environmental influences, including evidence of a deprived environment associated with a history of mental retardation among parents and siblings; an estimated 80% to 90% of all persons with mental retardation are characterized as being psychosocially disadvantaged
9. Chromosomal abnormalities, including chromosomal aberrations resulting from radiation, viruses, chemicals, parental age, and genetic mutations, such as Down's and cri du chat syndromes

Down's syndrome

Down's syndrome is the most common chromosomal abnormality of a generalized syndrome, occurring once in every 600 to 650 live births. It was first described by Dr. John Langdon Haydon Down in 1866 and owes its more common yet increasingly unacceptable name, mongolism, to the particular facial characteristics, which resemble those of the Mongol race.

About 95% of all cases of Down's syndrome are attributable to an extra chromosome 21 (group G), hence the name *trisomy 21*. About 4% of the cases may be caused by *translocation* of chromosomes 15 and 21 or 22. A small percentage of persons with this disorder are called *mosaics,* because their cells show both normal and abnormal chromosomes on analysis.

Origin of chromosomal defect. Trisomy 21 is associated with advanced maternal age, particularly over 35 years of age (Table 23-2). Several investigators have reported that early biologic aging may be more important than chronologic age. This hypothesis has been supported by the finding of increased incidence of gray hair and earlier onset of menarche in younger women who had given birth to an infant with Down's syndrome. The number of pregnancies and paternal age were not significant.[3]

Aging is important in the female because the germ cells in the adult ovary, which were formed during intrauterine development, remain in the stage of early meiotic division until one completes its division to form an ovum during the ovulation cycle once every month. Besides aging of the ova, exogenous influences such as radiation or drugs can adversely affect the genetic makeup. In the male fresh sperm are continuously formed.

Trisomy is the result of nondisjunction during meiotic or mitotic division. Failure of the chromosome to split results in one gamete receiving the entire pair and the other gamete receiving none, a condition that is nonviable. Nondisjunction can also occur after fertilization during mitosis. The earlier the nondisjunction occurs, the greater the number of cells affected. If it occurs later, then both normal and trisomic cells will be present, resulting in *mosaicism*. The degree of mosaicism will determine the extent of physical characteristics and the severity of mental retardation. As a rule mosaicism is associated with significantly higher intellectual potential, better verbal facility, and fewer visual perceptual difficulties than trisomy 21.[5]

Table 23-2. Maternal age related to incidence of Down's syndrome

Maternal age (years)	Incidence of Down's syndrome/ 1000 live births
20-29	0.5-1.0
30-34	1.5-2.0
35-39	3.0-4.0
40-44	9.0-10.0
45+	15.0-17.5

Data from Hughes, J. G.: Synopsis of pediatrics, ed. 4, St. Louis, 1975, The C. V. Mosby Co.

Translocation is a defect in chromosomal structure rather than in cell division. It involves the transfer of genetic material from one chromosome to another chromosome of a different pair or group. In Down's syndrome, translocation most frequently involves the chromosomes of groups D and G (group D contains chromosomes 13 to 15, group G contains chromosomes 21 to 22). This type of genetic aberration is usually hereditary and is not associated with maternal age. The translocation carrier, who has forty-five chromosomes but is phenotypically normal, mated to a normal individual can produce four categories of outcome: normal individuals, viable children with Down's syndrome, normal translocation carriers, and nonviable monosomies. Since the latter category is aborted early, the chance of producing an affected child is theoretically 1 in three (33⅓%) but actually 1 in five if the mother is the carrier and 1 in twenty if the father is the carrier. (For a further discussion of the genetics involved in Down's syndrome, see Chapter 6.)

Clinical manifestations. Down's syndrome can usually be diagnosed by the clinical manifestations alone (see boxed material below), but a chromosomal analysis should

Observable physical characteristics (stigmata) associated with Down's syndrome

- Head
  - Brachycephalic
  - Skull rounded and small
  - Flat occiput
  - Sparse hair (variable)
- Face
  - Flat profile
- Eyes
  - Inner epicanthal folds
  - Oblique palpebral fissures (upward, outward slant)
  - Speckling of iris (Brushfield's spots)
  - Short, sparse eyelashes
  - Blepharitis
- Nose
  - Small
  - Depressed nasal bridge (saddle nose)
- Ears
  - Small
  - Short pinna (vertical ear length)
  - Overlapping upper helices
  - Sometimes low set
- Mouth
  - Small osseous orbit
  - Protruding tongue, may be fissured at lip and furrowed on on the surface
  - Hypoplastic mandible
  - Downward curve (especially noted when crying)
  - High-arched palate
- Teeth
  - Delayed eruption
  - Alignment abnormalities common
- Neck
  - Short and broad
  - Skin laxity, lateral aspects
- Abdomen
  - Protruding
  - Muscles lax and flabby
    - Diastasis recti
    - Umbilical hernia
- Genitalia
  - Small penis
    - Cryptorchidism
  - Bulbous vulva
- Hands
  - Broad, short
  - Stubby fingers
  - Incurved little finger (clinodactyly)
  - Transverse palmar crease (simian line)
  - Characteristic dermal ridge patterns
    - Distally located axial triradius
    - Increased ulnar loops on fingers
- Feet
  - Broad, stubby
  - Wide space between big and second toes
  - Plantar crease
- Muscles
  - Hypotonic
  - Hyperextensible and lax joints
- Skin
  - Dry, cracked, and frequent fissuring
  - Cutis marmorata (mottling)

always be done to confirm the genetic abnormality (Fig. 23-1). Trisomy 21 is a sporadic event, associated with a low risk of recurrence (0.5% to 1.0%), whereas translocation has a much greater incidence of occurring within the same family more than once (theoretically, 33%). In addition some infants may have characteristics of Down's syndrome, usually epicanthal folds, narrow palate, short, broad hands, and a simian crease, but be cytologically normal.[14]

Intellectual and social characteristics. The most outstanding and significant feature of Down's syndrome is mental retardation. The brain is smaller in size than normal, especially the brainstem and cerebellum. Degrees of mental retardation differ, but the IQ is generally within the trainable range. In the past this disorder has accounted for approximately 10% of institutionalized mentally defective people.

Children with Down's syndrome do not appear abnormal in their mental development in the beginning, even though they may be hypotonic and have physical stigmata that are present at birth. They are reported to have a nearly normal developmental course during early infancy, followed by a relative decline during the next 2 years of life and then a slower decline in developmental quotient to age 4 years, at which time the decline tends to plateau and level off.

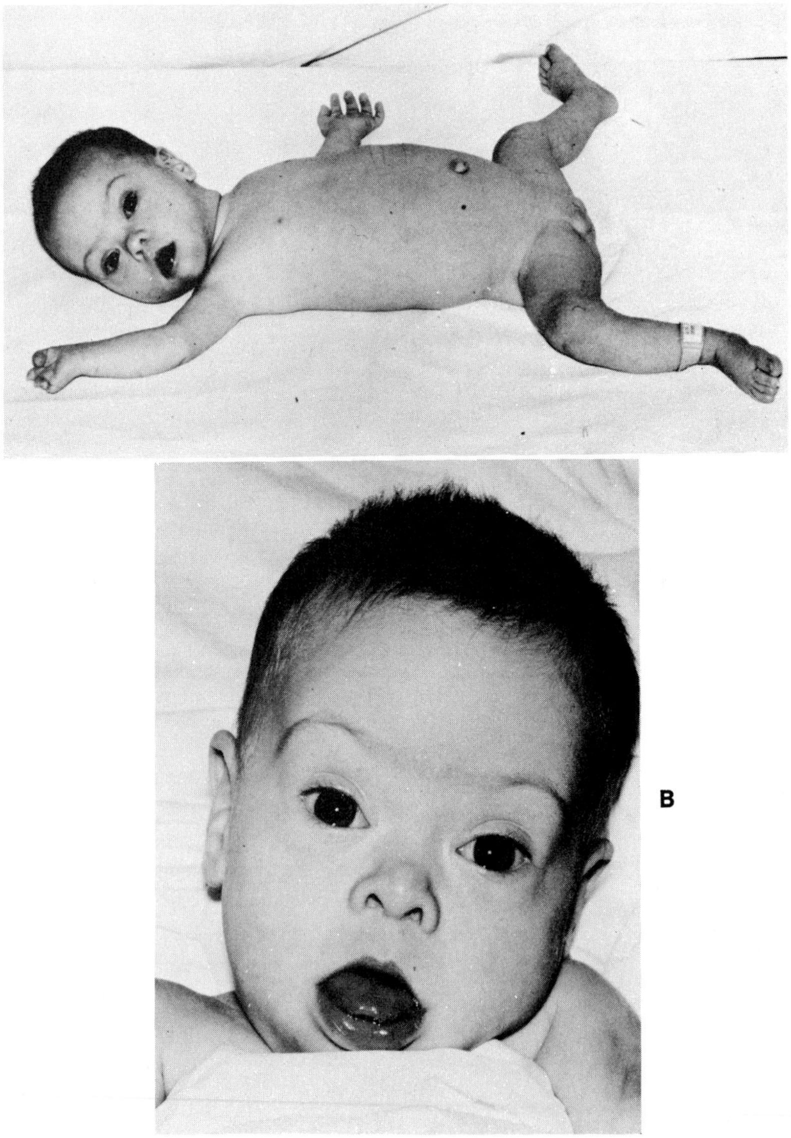

A

B

Fig. 23-1. Down's syndrome in newborn. **A,** Floppy, hypotonic newborn. **B,** Small, square head with mongoloid slant to the eyes, flat nasal bridge, and protruding tongue. (From Reisman, L. E., and Matheny, A. P.: Genetics and counseling in medical practice, St. Louis, 1969, The C. V. Mosby Co., p. 71.)

Much of what is known about children with Down's syndrome has been documented from observations or reports of children who were institutionalized in the past. Longitudinal systematic observations and data of social and intellectual development about children reared at home are incomplete at this point in time. There is evidence of overall deficits in intellectual competence and limitations with higher-level integrative abilities, such as concept formation, abstraction, and expressive language skills.[18] Table 23-3 lists ages of achieving motor and speech milestones in children with Down's syndrome who were reared at home. It is obvious from this data that there is great variability within each aspect of development as demonstrated by the range and standard deviation. It also appears that females develop earlier than males in skills such as sitting, standing, walking, and speaking first words.

Congenital anomalies and physical disorders. Several physical problems are associated with Down's syndrome. About 40% of these children have congenital heart disease, the most common being septal defects. Structural defects such as renal agenesis, duodenal atresia, aganglionic megacolon (Hirschsprung's disease), and tracheoesophageal fistula are common. Respiratory infections are very prevalent and account for the high morbidity in these children. When combined with cardiac anomalies, it is the chief cause of death, particularly during the first year of life. Hypotonicity of chest and abdominal muscles probably predisposes to the development of respiratory infection. Visual defects such as strabismus, myopia, nystagmus, or cataracts are common. Inflammation of the conjunctiva and lids occurs frequently. The incidence of different types of leukemia is about fifteen times more frequent in children with Down's syndrome. The increased incidence has been attributed to the imbalance of genes on the trisomic chromosome 21. This imbalance probably upsets the humoral control of tissue growth during embryonic development, affecting the regulation of the leukopoietic mechanism later in life.

Table 23-3. Motor and speech development in children with Down's syndrome

Attribute	Range*	Average*	Standard deviation
Motor			
Holds head up when held vertically	1-18 weeks	3.95 weeks	3.12
Rolls over	1-60	6.38	5.85
Sits up unsupported (boy)	5-72	12.52	7.77
Sits up unsupported (girl)	5-36	11.14	5.04
Creeps on hands and knees	4-24	12.19	4.55
Stands up (boy)	8-84	22.17	11.62
Stands up (girl)	7-72	18.97	9.36
Walks unassisted (boy)	7-74	26.09	11.40
Walks unassisted (girl)	8-72	22.72	8.89
Is toilet trained	8-108	34.78	20.32
Speech			
Speaks first word (boy)	6-72	26.59	15.70
Speaks first word (girl)	6-84	21.82	13.33
Speaks first phrase	12-96	41.82	17.15
Speaks first sentence	17-132	52.05	19.81

From Melyn, M. A., and White, D. T.: Pediatrics **52**(4):542-545, October 1973. Copyright American Academy of Pediatrics 1973.
*In months, except where otherwise indicated.

Height and weight. Children with Down's syndrome tend to be shorter than average and seem to be stocky in build because their legs and arms are shorter in relationship to the trunk of the body. Birth length may be within the normal range, and linear growth up to age 4 years is usually slightly below the normal range. After age 4 years, and with each successive year, the rate of growth begins to fall beneath the normal range. The average final height for men with Down's syndrome is about 5 feet, and for women it is about 4 feet, 7 inches.

Weight measurements tend to be in the range of low normal at birth. As children grow older, weight, although low for chronologic age, corresponds to their shorter height. Children with Down's syndrome are manifesting different and larger growth trends than in the past, because of better nutrition, fewer serious infections, availability of antibiotics, and improved developmental environments.

General health. About 20% to 40% of infants with Down's syndrome do not survive the first few years. If the child does not suffer from some of the more serious physical problems such as pneumonia, gastroenteritis, major heart defects, and incomplete development of the gastrointestinal tract, such as intestinal blockage, the prospect for survival to adulthood is enhanced. If the child does not experience serious physical problems, it is probable that he will be healthy and will not present unusual difficulties in general care. He may be susceptible to the usual childhood illnesses and may experience a few minor problems that other children do not experience as often. He may have a tendency, for example, to be prone to minor infections of the ear or eye or respiratory tract and may have more frequent colds than his siblings. Children with Down's syndrome may have runny noses that are a persistent problem even though they do not have colds. Because of the problems associated with the ear, it is important that the child be screened yearly for hearing and any deficits in hearing loss.

Adolescent and sexual development. Sexual development may be delayed or incomplete or both. The genitalia of the male may be underdeveloped because males tend to produce less male hormone. Secondary sex characteristics such as facial hair are also underdeveloped. The breast development of females is mild to moderate. Menstruation usually occurs at the average age and follows the usual course.

The sexual drive in persons with Down's syndrome is reported as being diminished. Only a few affected women have had babies; of their offspring, half have had Down's syndrome and half have been normal. It is presumed that men with Down's syndrome are infertile. There is no documentation available that a man with Down's syndrome has ever fathered a child.

Aging. Those who survive the first few years have the same mortality rate as for normal persons up to about age 40 years, at which time the mortality rate begins to increase. Persons affected with Down's syndrome seem to age more rapidly than normal. Aging is evident by a drying of the skin and a gradual coarseness in appearance. The gums begin to recede more rapidly than normal and usually result in premature loss of the teeth. Adults with Down's syndrome are jeopardized with respiratory infections, pneumonia, and lung disease, which can be problematic and a potential cause of death.

Nursing considerations. Caring for the child with Down's syndrome involves several short- and long-term goals. Support for parents from health professionals, especially nurses, is increasingly more important with the present trend to rear these children at home. This discussion focuses on supporting parents at the time of diagnosis and preventing physical problems in the child. Long-term interventions for the child with mental retardation are discussed later in this chapter.

Informing parents of diagnosis. Because of the characteristic facies and other stigmata, the infant with Down's syndrome is usually diagnosed at birth. However, parents are not always informed of the diagnosis at this time. This presents special difficulties for those caring for the postpartal mother, since she or the father may notice differences in the child and question others about their concern. Therefore, the nurse needs some guidelines to help in assessing when, how, and what parents should be told.

Generally parents wish to know the diagnosis as soon as possible. This approach prevents such dilemmas as telling others that the child has Down's syndrome after indicating that he was fine and experiencing unconfirmed doubt over the child's development. Most parents prefer that both of them be present during the informing interview because it is a problem that both of them will have to face, they can emotionally support each other, and it eliminates the difficult task of revealing the diagnosis to the other partner. They appreciate receiving reading material about the syndrome* and being referred to others for help or advice, such as parent groups or professional counseling.[7]

Once parents are aware of the diagnosis, they are confronted with the crisis of losing a perfect or dream child and grieving for and accepting their reality child. For the nurse to support parents during this period, variables surrounding the birth must be assessed in order to understand parental reactions. For example, it is not uncommon for the advanced maternal age at the time of the child's birth to be the result of inability to conceive for many years. Consequently the birth of this child is a most anticipated and desired event. On the other hand, this pregnancy may have been unplanned, unwanted, and resented. When the infant is born, the parents may feel extremely guilty concerning their previous thoughts, equating this event with punishment for their rejection of the child.

The parents' responses to the child may greatly influence decisions regarding future care. Whereas some families willingly wish to take the child home, others consider immediate institutionalization. The nurse must carefully answer questions regarding developmental potential and institutionalization, since the responses may influence the parents' decision. It is obvious from ranges such as those in Table 23-3 that the child's ability for developmental achievement varies greatly. Therefore, it would be inaccurate and unfair to predict the child's intellectual capacity at birth. However, the nurse emphasizes the potential abilities of a retarded child to learn self-help skills, communication, social behavior, and a semiskilled vocation with or without supervision.

It is also not possible to predict which child will present few problems for child rearing. Although most children with Down's syndrome adjust extremely well to the home environment and thrive with appropriate stimulation, a few do have severe handicaps or aggressive tendencies that cannot be dealt with in the home. It is important to stress to parents that a decision regarding placement will affect all of their lives and need not be made at the time of diagnosis. The nurse should emphasize every available source of assistance, such as parent groups,[15] professional guidance, literature, and so on, to help them learn to live with the child and deal with child-rearing problems.

Assisting parents in preventing physical problems. Many of the physical characteristics of Down's syndrome present nursing problems. The hypotonicity of muscles and hyperextensibility of joints complicate positioning. The limp, flaccid extremities resemble the posture of a rag doll; as a result holding the infant is difficult and cumbersome. Some-

*Several books are available. One that is written very positively in terms of home care and includes a list of other references is: Pitt, D.: Your Down's syndrome child, available from the National Association for Retarded Citizens, 2709 Avenue E East, P.O. Box 6109, Arlington, Texas 76011.

times parents perceive this lack of molding to their bodies as evidence of inadequate mothering or fathering. The extended body position promotes heat loss because more surface area is exposed to the environment. The nurse teaches the parents to swaddle or wrap the infant tightly in a blanket before picking him up to provide security and warmth. The nurse also discusses with parents their feelings concerning attachment to the child, emphasizing that the child's lack of clinging or molding is a physical characteristic, not a sign of detachment or rejection.

Decreased muscle tone compromises respiratory expansion. In addition the underdeveloped nasal bone causes a chronic problem of inadequate drainage of mucus. The constant stuffy nose forces the child to breathe by mouth, which dries the oropharyngeal membranes, increasing the susceptibility to upper respiratory infections. The nurse teaches parents to clear the nose with a bulb-type syringe, rinse the mouth with water after feedings, use a cool-mist vaporizer to keep the mucous membranes moist and the secretions liquified, change the child's position frequently, and perform postural drainage and percussion. If antibiotics are ordered, the nurse stresses the importance of completing the full course of therapy for successful eradication of the infection and prevention of growth of resistant organisms.

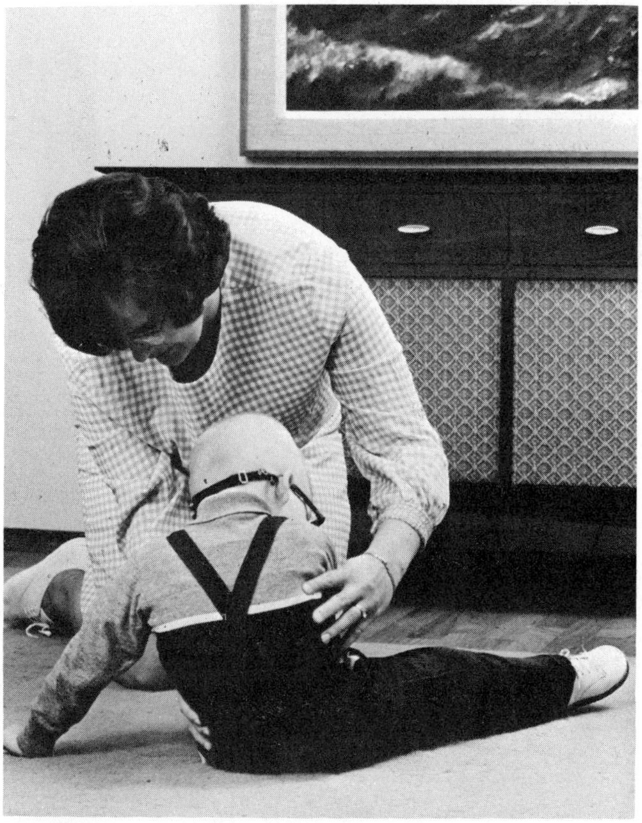

Fig. 23-2. Encouraging child to learn balance while sitting up. (From Barnard, K. E., and Erickson, M. L.: Teaching children with developmental problems: a family care approach, ed. 2, St. Louis, 1976, The C. V. Mosby Co., p. 114.)

Inadequate drainage and pooling of mucus in the nose also interfere with feeding. Because the child breathes by mouth, he is unable to suck for any length of time as a result of his need for air. When eating solids, he may gag on the food because of mucus in the oropharynx. The nurse advises parents to clear the nose before each feeding, give small, frequent feedings, and allow opportunities for rest at mealtime.

The large, protruding tongue also interferes with feeding, especially of solid foods. The nurse discusses with parents the fact that the tongue thrust is not an indication of refusal to feed, but a physiologic response. Parents are advised to use a small but long, straight-handled spoon to push the food toward the back and side of the mouth. If food is thrust out, it should be refed.

Dietary intake needs supervision. Decreased muscle tone affects gastric motility, predisposing the child to constipation. Dietary measures such as increased residue and fluid promote evacuation. The child's eating habits may need careful scrutiny to prevent obesity. Height and weight measurements should be obtained on a serial basis, especially during infancy, since excessive weight gain can impede motor development. The child should receive calories in accordance with his height and weight, not his chronologic age.

During infancy the child's skin is pliable and soft. However, it gradually becomes rough and dry and is prone to cracking and infection. Skin care involves the use of minimal soap and application of lubricants such as creams or bath oil. Lip balm should be applied to the lips, especially when the child is outdoors, to prevent excessive chapping.

Promoting children's developmental progress. The hypotonicity also affects muscular development. Supporting skills such as rolling over, sitting up, standing, or pulling oneself to a sitting or standing position may be delayed. Since it has been found that the child's developmental potential seems greatest during infancy, it is imperative that parents be involved in an infant stimulation program. If a formally organized program is not available, the nurse can individualize one by assessing the infant's present abilities and selecting appropriate activities that he should be learning. Table 23-4 lists several exercises to help a child learn gross motor skills. Suggestions for teaching independent self-help behaviors are discussed later in this chapter and are summarized in Tables 23-5 to 23-7.

After the nurse plans a stimulation program based on the child's developmental abilities, the parents are given detailed written instructions regarding each exercise and how often it should be performed. The nurse requests a return demonstration of each activity to ensure the parents' understanding. The importance of verbally repeating the instructions to the child to enhance his comprehensive and, later,

Table 23-4. Infant stimulation program for gross motor development

Normal age of achievement (months)	Behavior	Activity*
Birth	Assumes flexed position, kicks, has dance reflex	Exercise limbs several times each day Place child in flexed position, encourage movement such as kicking Hold child upright with feet touching a flat surface to stimulate dance reflex
3-4	Holds head erect	Hold child prone, encourage him to raise head Place child supine and pull up by arms; encourage him to raise head forward Place child in sitting position, hold head erect, gradually release support on sides of head for him to learn muscle control If child holds head erect, tilt him to one side to learn balance Support child in sitting position with head erect; if head falls forward, attract child's attention to encourage him to look up
4-5	Rolls over—prone to supine	Place child prone but slightly lying on one side; place hand on hip and push down as you are pulling up on the ipsilateral arm; encourage child to push with arm underneath him; gradually encourage child to use free arm to push himself over completely
5-6	Rolls over—supine to prone	Place child supine, cross one leg over the other and gently push him to one side; reduce assistance as he learns to roll by himself Roll him over and over
8	Sits up unsupported	Place child in sitting position but supported several times each day Support child in sitting position; gently tilt him to one side to learn balance (see Fig. 23-2) Place child in sitting position with his back against a wall; kneel in front of him and encourage him to lean away from the wall to learn balance Sit child on floor with knees in an Indian position; place his hands on floor so he can balance himself Use same Indian position, kneel down in front of him, and gently push him to one side so that he practices righting himself Sit child on large beach ball with his feet flat on the floor; sway him from side to side to regain balance
9-10	Goes from sitting to standing position	Sit child on a low stool or chair with feet firmly placed on floor; place a towel around his chest and gently pull him up to standing position, help him sit down again, gradually reduce assistance Place child in crib or playpen and in sitting position; encourage him to get up to reach an object

Adapted from Gregory, P.: Pediatr. Nurs. **1**(4):23-29, July/August 1975.
*With each activity the parent continues the actual behavior with a verbal command and praises the child for each increment in motor development, as well as for cooperation and/or signs of enjoyment.

speech development, gradually reducing assistance as the child gains strength and coordination, and praising the child for success and cooperation are emphasized. At regular intervals the nurse assesses the child's developmental progress to ensure compliance with the program. Screening tools such as the Denver Developmental Screening Test are not sufficiently detailed to evaluate indices of progress such as increased strength, balance, coordination, or muscle tone. Therefore, the nurse must keep detailed written records of the child's motor abilities in order to distinguish subtle changes in functioning.

With the present trend toward home care, the parents should be encouraged to investigate special day-care programs for the child as soon as possible, since frequently there are long waiting lists. They should also investigate the public school system for special educational classes. In essence the same child-rearing goals that are established for normal children are pursued for these children.

Prevention. There is no cure for Down's syndrome. However, through amniocentesis, chromosomal analysis of fetal cells can detect the presence of trisomy or translocation. The nurse has a role in genetic counseling of those women of advanced maternal age or who have a family history of the disorder to discuss the possibility of amniocentesis. If the fetus is affected, the nurse must allow the parents to express their feelings concerning elective abortion and support their decision either to terminate or proceed with the pregnancy.

For long- and short-term nursing care of the child with Down's syndrome, see the boxed material on pp. 820 to 821.

Table 23-4. Infant stimulation program for gross motor development—cont'd

Normal age of achievement (months)	Behavior	Activity*
10	Crawls	Place child on abdomen, encourage him to come forward by moving an object away from him Place child over a large rolled towel that is high enough to allow him to rest his hands on the floor; encourage him to bear weight on his hands; straighten his arms to increase weight bearing Use same position but with small towel so that elbows and lower arms rest on floor; encourage him to lift up or come forward slightly; press down on his shoulders to stimulate his effort at maintaining this position When bearing weight on hands, place rolled towel or beach ball under his chest to stimulate getting on all fours; gently support him around the waist and pull him up, release assistance as he bears more weight Lay child across beach ball; roll him forward, backward, and to each side to stimulate balance in either direction Play wheelbarrow; hold him at his hips and let him walk forward on his hands; as he bears more weight, hold him by his feet and let him go forward Encourage "walking like a bear" (last step before walking); stand him upright, support him at the hips, and have him lean forward or gently push him over to bear weight on his hands; encourage him to walk in this position and to straighten up
	Stands with support	If child resists standing, place him upright with his back against the wall, grasp his knees, and manually straighten the legs; as he controls his legs, reduce the amount of assistance While child is in crib or playpen, place him in standing position and holding onto railing While child is in standing position, have him hold your hands; encourage him to bear weight and "jump" up and down Place him in jumper seat to encourage standing and jumping
10-12	Stands alone for short periods	With child in standing position, release supports for a moment to encourage standing alone Place him in a walker and encourage him to stand up and release holding onto it by placing an object in front of him to grasp
12-14	Walks with support	Place him in a walker several times each day Hold his two hands in front of you and guide him in walking, gradually hold only one hand Encourage him to cruise around furniture and push a chair or carriage
14	Walks alone	Place child in standing position in front of you; reach out to child but do not actually support him; encourage him to walk forward Hold child by one hand; release your grasp while he is walking

CHANGING TRENDS IN CARE

Common myths about mental retardation

In the past, professional orientation to interacting with and planning care for persons with mental retardation was affected by some very archaic, destructive models and concepts. Four particular kinds of stereotyping that have led to subhuman treatment are[20]:

1. *Menace*. Mental retardation was equated with criminal tendencies or reproduction of defective children; therefore, prisonlike institutions were necessary to protect society.
2. *Object of pity*. Mental retardation was viewed as suffering; therefore, overprotection was necessary.
3. *Eternal child*. Mental retardation was equated with childhood; individuals were not allowed to make choices and were not held accountable for their behaviors.
4. *Diseased organism*. Mental retardation was perceived as a sickness; therefore, medical services and custodial care were necessary.

Shattering the myths

In view of such stereotypes it is extremely important for nurses to examine their own attitudes in order to feel more comfortable with the individual with mental retardation and to convey to him the feeling that he is acceptable. Such self-examination requires energy, time, and thoughtfulness but also enables nurses to deal more constructively with the mentally retarded person and his family. Nurses need to treat persons who are different with dignity and respect and to use the developmental model rather than the pathologic model to look for change and strength rather than seeing only a person's deficits and weaknesses.

Summary of nursing care of the child with Down's syndrome

Goals	Responsibilities
Support parents at time of diagnosis	Inform parents as soon as possible after birth Have both parents present at informing conference Give parents written information about syndrome Discuss with parents benefits of home care vs institutionalization; allow them opportunities to investigate all residential alternatives before making a decision Encourage parents to meet other families with Down's children Refrain from giving definitive answers about the degree of retardation; stress the potential learning abilities of retarded children, especially with early stimulation Demonstrate acceptance of infant through own example Emphasize normal characteristics of child
Prevent physical problems associated with syndrome	
Respiratory infections	Teach parents postural drainage and percussion Stress importance of changing child's position frequently, especially use of a sitting posture Encourage use of cool-mist vaporizer Teach suctioning of nares Stress importance of good mouth care (follow feedings with clear water)
Feeding difficulties	Suction nares before each feeding Schedule small frequent feedings; allow child to rest during feedings Feed solid food by pushing it to back and side of mouth; use long, straight-handled infant spoon Point out to parents that tongue thrust does not indicate refusal of food Calculate caloric needs to meet energy requirements; base intake on height and weight, not chronologic age Monitor height and weight at regular intervals Provide sufficient bulk and fluids to prevent constipation
Skin breakdown	Keep skin well lubricated with topical creams or lotions Use soap sparingly Apply lip balm when child is outdoors
Promote optimum development	Involve child and parents in an early infant stimulation program (Table 23-4) Assess child's developmental progress at regular intervals; keep detailed records to distinguish subtle changes in functioning Help parents set realistic goals for child Encourage learning of self-care skills as soon as child achieves readiness (Tables 23-5 to 23-7) Encourage parents to investigate special day-care programs and educational classes as soon as possible; point out that toilet training may be a prerequisite to eligibility Emphasize that child has same needs as other children* Play Discipline Social interaction Prior to adolescence, counsel child and parents regarding physical maturation, sexual behavior, marriage, and family* Encourage optimal vocational training
Help family prepare for future care of child*	As child grows older, discuss with parents options to home care, especially as parents near retirement or old age Help family investigate residential settings other than institutionalization Encourage family to include retarded member in planning and to continue meaningful relationships with him after placement

*These interventions are discussed in greater depth later in this chapter.

Summary of nursing care of the child with Down's syndrome—cont'd

Goals	Responsibilities
Prevent Down's syndrome	Discuss with high-risk women risks of giving birth to child with Down's syndrome Encourage all pregnant women at risk (age over 35 years, family history of Down's syndrome, or previous birth of child with Down's syndrome), to consider amniocentesis during twelfth to sixteenth week of pregnancy to rule out Down's syndrome in fetus Discuss option of elective abortion with women who are carrying an affected fetus Discuss with parents of adolescent children with Down's syndrome the probability of conception in a female and the need for contraceptive methods

It is also important to consider the attitudes of parents and to encourage them to discuss what mental retardation means to them and what they expect of their child. Parents should be aware that the mentally retarded child is capable of adapting to his environment, independently performing some or all of the functions of daily living, having and expressing feelings, and changing, no matter how slightly. He has the same needs as a normal person for approval, attention, and love. Depending on the degree of retardation, he may be able to marry, have gainful employment, and be a successful care provider for his family.

Applying developmental model

The developmental model implies that the child's present strengths and abilities guide the goals for education and training. Therefore, the nurse's primary responsibility is in assessing the child's functional or mental age by using screening tools such as the Denver Developmental Screening Test (Appendix F) or the Washington Guide to Promoting Development in the Young Child (Appendix G). If the child has already undergone extensive psychologic testing, it is possible to estimate the mental age from the intelligence score by using the following formula:

$$\frac{\text{Mental age (MA)}}{\text{Chronologic age (CA)}} \times 100 = \text{IQ}$$

For example, if the child's chronologic age is 10 years and his IQ is 50, his mental age is approximately 5 years.

Although this method of estimating functional age is less exact and useful than appropriate screening tests, it is helpful in determining at what level to begin an assessment. It also guides the nurse to an understanding of the child's eventual capabilities within the categories of mental retardation.

One assessment tool, the Progress Assessment Chart of Social and Personal Development (PAC), is designed specifically to help assess mentally retarded individuals. It gives information about a child's or adult's level of functioning in self-help, communication, socialization, and occupational skills. The primary usefulness of the PAC is that it gives hope to parents and other care givers because it allows the examiner to break down skills into many component parts so that people are able to teach the child additional skills.

The Home Observation for Measurement of the Environment (p. 793) in conjunction with developmental assessment tools results in the most comprehensive composite of the child's level of development and quality of his environment in enhancing or hindering his development. Using the Home Observation for Measurement of the Environment, the nurse can provide objective feedback to parents about ways in which to regulate the environment to best facilitate their child's optimal functioning.

The box on p. 822 is an example of a written report to parents using the developmental model to assess the child's functional ability.

Applying principles of normalization

Normalization refers to establishing a normal pattern to activities of daily living.[20] Traditionally the mentally retarded person performed all his activities in one room, unlike normal individuals who conducted various activities in specified places. However, by applying the principles of normalization, the environment for the retarded child is "normalized" and "humanized."

One example of applying the principles of normalization concerns sleeping. The mentally retarded child should not be put to bed earlier than his siblings or peers simply because he is retarded. He should sleep in a regular bed, not unnecessarily restrained in a crib. He should not have a light burning all night just for him. He should engage in daily

Dear Mr. and Mrs. Brown,

For the past 2 months I have been visiting your home and accompanying you to clinic visits at the child development center. My objectives have been to become acquainted with you and your family; to establish a relationship with a mutual exchange of questions, observations, and concerns; to observe Susan as she grows and develops in her home environment; and to increase my own skills in the assessment of children. The tools I used were the Denver Developmental Screening Test, the Developmental Profile, and the Home Observation for Measurement of the Environment. I also had the opportunity to videotape Susan at mealtime with you present. As a result of these interactions I have identified the following areas of strength as well as some areas of concern for the near future:

Susan's functional areas of strength

1. *Personal-social*
   She is spontaneously friendly; initiates interactions with others; reaches out to others with her eyes, hands, and expressions; plays games with others (pat-a-cake, peekaboo); is curious and attempts to solve problems, such as how to open or turn over a toy; looks for objects out of sight; moves towards objects out of reach; is able to entertain herself for at least 15 minutes; and is beginning to imitate speech sounds.
2. *Fine-motor*
   She is increasing her self-feeding skills with finger foods and with a cup; has a neat pincer grasp; and is increasing her skill in transferring objects from hand to hand.
3. *Gross-motor*
   She sits, rolls over, crawls, pulls herself up to a standing position, and is able to bear weight and alternate weight. Her ability is increasing in balancing, shifting weight, and protecting herself when falling.

Parental areas of strength

Both parents are warm, affectionate, and gentle with Susan and are interested in her optimal growth and development. In particular Mary (mother) spontaneously offers praise and encouragement to her and frequently initiates interactions with her and responds to her cues, particularly during mealtime. Mary is sensitive to Susan's needs; is able to identify and anticipate Susan's development and encourage mastery of new skills; maintains interests away from home; is able to find and to use support systems in times of crisis (relatives, friends, professionals); is able to express questions and concerns in an appropriate manner about Susan's development; and is able to express frustration and appropriate anger about complications associated with previous hospital, clinical, and personal experiences.

Appropriateness of home environment

Both parents provide a variety of learning and developmental experiences for Susan, such as frequent trips away from home, to a day-care center, and to relatives' homes. At mealtime a variety of foods with different textures are offered. Toys are provided that promote problems solving, exploration, eye-hand coordination, and the development of new skills. All members of the family consistently spend appropriate time playing with Susan.

Areas of concern for near future

For Susan, areas of concern for the near future include reinforcement and encouragement of speech development and continuing encouragement of self-feeding (using a cup and finger foods—offering one item at a time and allowing Susan to choose).

My concern for you, Mary, is that amid all the time and the effort you are taking to provide such an excellent environment for Susan, you take some time for yourself. I am concerned that you spend time apart from Susan, that you relax at times in some of your efforts, and that you continue to give yourself permission to express feelings of fatigue or worry or discouragement as they come.

Hopefully you will also share your joys and successes. My concern for your relaxing from your persistent efforts for Susan does not at all suggest a weakness on your part, but more of a genuine concern I have felt for you as I have observed you and Susan interact together. For example, one day when you were allowing Susan to finger-feed herself, I noticed that you initiated a verbal interchange with her ninety-one times. Your initiation of verbal exchange with her was very commendable; however, I think that at times it may be disappointing when she does not react or initiate interchanges with you.

I do want you to know that it has been a privilege to have become acquainted with you and Susan. Your love, your interest, and your ongoing concerns for her and for other members of the family are obvious indeed, and you are promoting and providing an optimum environment for Susan. She is a very fortunate child to have both of you as parents.

Sincerely,
Kathy Phillips, R.N.

activities appropriate for his developmental age and not be forced to take daytime naps.

The principle of normalization is discussed in detail in terms of teaching the child independence in activities of daily living.

NURSING INTERVENTIONS WITH MENTALLY RETARDED CHILDREN

The goal of caring for a retarded child is to promote his optimum development as an individual within a family and community. The nurse is in a vital position to teach parents how to foster learning in their child. The following discussion focuses on principles involved in educating these children, specific interventions to teach self-care skills, guidelines for promoting optimal development, helping families adjust to future care, and caring for the hospitalized retarded child.

Educating mentally retarded children

In order to learn how to teach mentally retarded children, it is necessary to investigate their learning abilities and deficits. Research indicates that retarded children have a marked deficit in their ability to discriminate between two or more stimuli because of difficulty in paying attention to relevant cues.[6] Unfortunately the ability to discriminate between symbols is essential in learning the alphabet for reading or numbers for arithmetic. However, these children can learn to discriminate if the cues are presented in an exaggerated concrete form and all extraneous stimuli are eliminated. For example, the use of colors to exaggerate visual cues or music for auditory cues can help them learn. The latter is particularly effective for teaching speech by singing the same word rather than only saying it.

Their deficit in discrimination also implies that concrete ideas are learned much more effectively than abstraction. Therefore, demonstration is preferable to verbal explanation, and learning should be directed toward mastering a skill rather than understanding scientific principles underlying the procedure.

Another deficit of retarded children is in short-term memory.[6] Whereas normal children can remember several words, numbers, or directions at one time, these children are unable to do so. Therefore, they need simple one-step directions. They respond to learning how to remember, such as by "clustering" pairs or triads together. This approach is helpful when trying to teach them their telephone number. Rather than having them memorize the entire seven-digit number, the set is broken into pairs. After the pairs are memorized the child puts them all back together.

Learning through a step-by-step process requires the teacher to break down each task into its necessary components. For example, if the child is learning to tie a shoe, the teacher must practice the skill, divide it into steps, and teach each step completely before proceeding to the next activity.

One critical area of learning that has had a tremendous impact on education for the retarded is motivation. Programs based on the motivation principles of positive reinforcement for specific tasks or behaviors have demonstrated marked improvement in retarded children's ability to learn. Such principles can easily be implemented in the home in learning self-help skills. Maintaining feelings of success in accomplishing specified goals also promotes a feeling of self-esteem in the child.

Another consideration that has relevance to any learning situation is the concept of teacher expectancy. Research has demonstrated that children who were labeled as "brighter" by their teachers actually gained points on an IQ score as compared to a control group who had initially the same measured intelligence but who were not labeled "brighter."[17] The implication is that mentally retarded children may also learn according to parent-teacher expectation. If parents are negatively informed about their child's potential, they may gear their expectations below the child's actual potential. This point emphasizes the need for an individualized stimulation program that continuously monitors the child's developmental progress.

Promoting independent self-help skills

When a defective child is born, there is frequently little or no transference of normal child-rearing practices to the child without special guidance or instruction from nonfamily members.[8] Parents need assistance in promoting normal developmental skills that are almost automatically learned by other children. For the nurse to be successful in meeting this goal, the parents must be supported, included as the primary rehabilitators with the child, and provided with written detailed descriptions of the stimulation program.

Feeding. Self-feeding is recognized as the first major self-help skill that children learn.[4] It actually involves the integration of fine motor skills, visual perception, and gross motor skills. Most mothers take for granted that they will be successful in teaching their children to feed themselves. Therefore, the nurse must also be especially sensitive to the needs of the parent as well as of the child when assistance is offered.

Before beginning a self-feeding program the nurse should do a task analysis, breaking the process of feeding into its smallest component parts. For example, the tasks in self-feeding with a spoon include: the child (1) orients to the food by looking at, (2) looks at the spoon, (3) reaches for it, (4) touches it, (5) grasps it, (6) lifts it, (7) delivers the spoon to the bowl, (8) lowers it into the food, (9) scoops food onto the spoon, (10) lifts it, (11) delivers the spoon to his mouth, (12) opens his mouth, (13) inserts the spoon into his mouth, (14) moves his tongue and mouth to receive the food, (15) closes his lips, (16) swallows the food, and (17) returns the spoon to the bowl. It is important that the nurse observe the child in an eating situation to determine whether he has mastered any of these small steps that make up the entire task of self-feeding. If he has, the nurse should comment about them positively to the mother.

In addition to doing a task analysis, the nurse assesses a number of other factors. The shape of the child's mouth and his control of mouth, lips, and tongue movements (whether the tongue moves forward and backward, from side to side, and whether there are rotary movements) are examined. The nurse looks for the presence of teeth, which determines the textures and the consistencies of food that may be offered to the child. The child's developmental readiness for self-feeding, such as his ability to maintain head and trunk support, to sit without support, eye-hand coordination, the firmness of his grasp, and his ability to reach for an object, hold it, and release it, are examined. If the child has any physical handicaps that interfere with holding

A

B

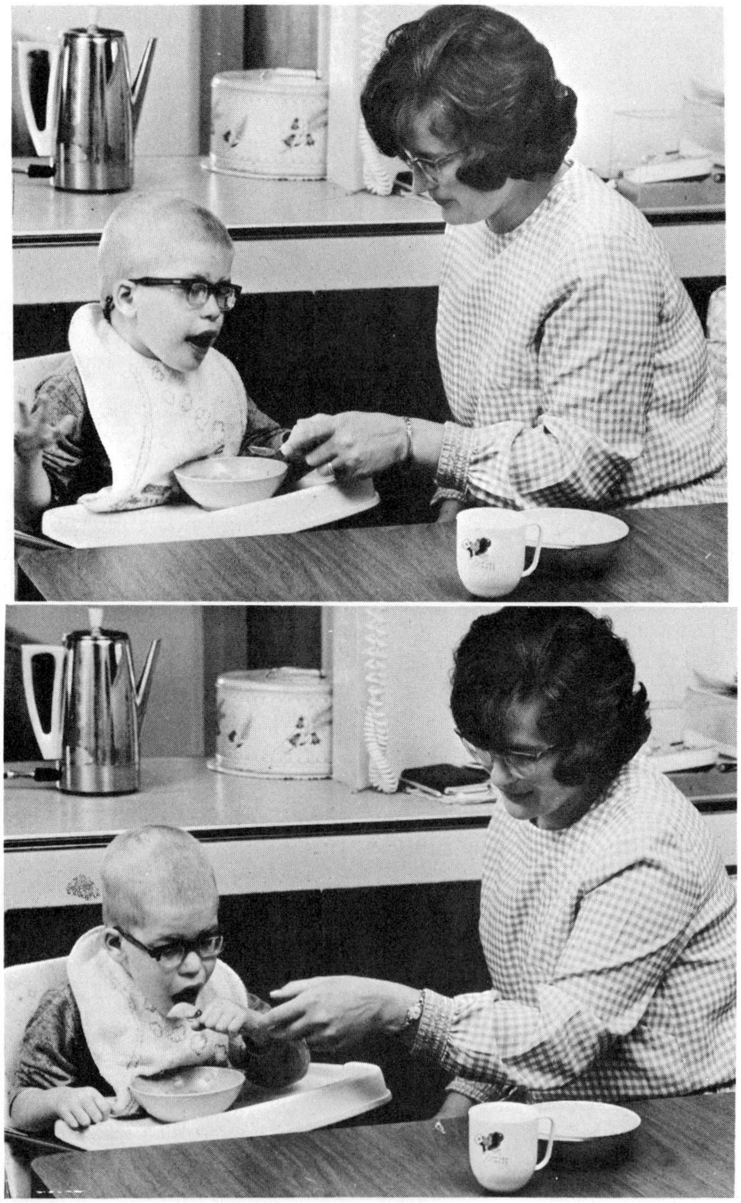

Fig. 23-3. The technique of fading. **A,** Mother's hand guides child's hands through the motions in learning self-feeding. **B,** Mother decreases her guidance of actual hand movement. **C,** Expectations for independence are scaled to the child's performance. Getting food into the mouth is often the first successful independent achievement. (From Barnard, K. E., and Erickson, M. L.: Teaching children with developmental problems: a family care approach, ed. 2, St. Louis, 1976, The C. V. Mosby Co., pp. 130-131.)

or grasping the utensil, the nurse improvises handles that are easier to grasp, such as by building the handle up with a sponge or piece of wood or by bending it so that it accommodates arm movement.

The nurse determines whether the child has any dietary deficiencies as revealed by a 7-day dietary history kept by the mother, whether there have been any changes in the child's eating habits, or if he is on a metabolic diet. The nurse also assesses neurologic factors, such as if the child has seizures, is on medications to control seizures, chokes often, or has difficulty in swallowing or a history of such difficulties.

The nurse obtains further data from the mother by interviewing her specifically about the family's approach to teaching. For example, who feeds the child regularly? Does the child eat at regularly scheduled times? Is the child fed when he is hungry or according to a prescribed schedule? What are the child's appetite patterns? Does the mother know when the child is full? What foods does the child like? How long does feeding take? A short length of feeding time, such as 10 or 20 minutes, might indicate that the child is being deprived of sensory experiences or appropriate interactions; a long time might indicate frustration and fatigue on the mother's part. Does the mother describe the feeding environment as quiet and nondistracting? What is the best time for the mother to begin teaching this new task? If the family is going on vacation, if someone is visiting, or if there has been a major stress in the family, this may not be the ideal time to begin a teaching program. The nurse also determines whether the mother is really asking for help by the questions she asks, the comments she makes, and her ability to keep records.

The nurse discusses various principles of learning with the mother before beginning a feeding program. The mother needs to know that the behavior she reinforces is the behavior that will be repeated and that it is vitally important to attract and maintain the child's attention and to give him specific cues regarding what is expected of him. The mother must understand the technique of *fading,* physically taking the child through each sequence of feeding and gradually fading out her physical assistance to the child so that the child becomes more independent (Fig. 23-3). She should also be familiar with the technique of *shaping,* waiting for the child to give a response that approximates the desired behavior, then reinforcing the child by social approval, such as touching or talking to him.[1]

The mother should understand that it is crucial not only to continuously reinforce desirable behavior but also to consistently ignore undesirable behavior. Ignoring the child is particularly difficult for many mothers, because they may equate ignoring their child with being a "bad mother." Therefore, the nurse must be especially supportive as the mother attempts negative reinforcement. The mother should realize that repetition plays an important part in her child's learning. As the child gains mastery, the mother will be encouraged to thin out the social reinforcement or physical reinforcement she has been offering her child. She should understand that if the feeding program does not move forward successfully she and the nurse will reevaluate the last sequence the child mastered to determine if she is expecting too much too soon.

The nurse also discusses preparation for the feeding activity, such as proper placement of the child at the table, protection of the area against spills, and so on. The principle of normalization is employed to make feeding a family activity. For example, the child should be fed in the

C

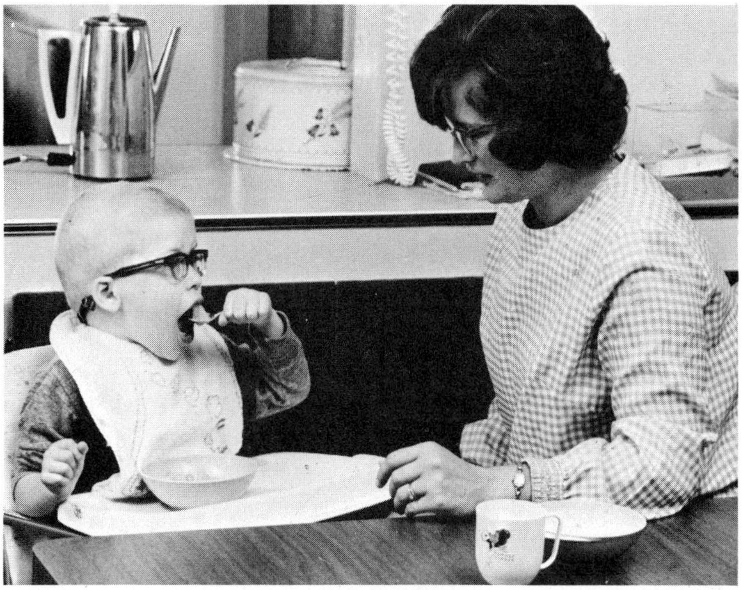

Fig. 23-3, cont'd. For legend see opposite page.

kitchen, at the table, or in a highchair in a sitting position, and with other family members whenever possible. Food should be served in attractive utensils, offered singly—not pureed or mixed together, served at the appropriate temperature—not routinely lukewarm, and of sufficient variety and texture from each of the basic four food groups.

Once the feeding program is begun the nurse is in an important position to give parents supportive feedback. The nurse calls attention to the mother's observational skills and ability to share observations as well as her ability to keep records of the child's progress. The nurse comments on the mother's ability to establish a goal that is appropriate and realistic for both the child and the mother. The mother is supported and encouraged by the nurse for her willingness to try a feeding program *now* rather than waiting. The nurse also acknowledges the mother's creativity and resourcefulness, the appropriate speed or the frequency with which the mother gives reinforcement to the child, her beginning success, her continued efforts when behavioral change seems slow, and her ability to withhold reinforcement (that is, ignore the child, remove the food, and wait until the child is exhibiting desirable behaviors before proceeding). By acknowledging all of these aspects of the mother's continued efforts, the nurse promotes mastery of a task that is extremely important to the child who is mentally retarded.

Table 23-5 lists activities to help the child learn self-feeding.

Toileting. Independent toileting is another major self-help skill that can be taught using behavioral modification principles. It should be started after self-feeding, since this is the normal sequence of development. It is an important achievement because the child may be denied enrollment in educational programs unless he is trained, whereas self-feeding or dressing skills may not be prerequisites.

The nurse begins by assessing the child's physical readiness for a toilet-training program: Can he sit by himself? Can he stand alone? Does he balance well, walk backward and forward, and climb onto a chair? Can he retain urine for at least 2 hours? All of these skills require coordinated movement, posture, and balance and suggest that the child is physically and neurologically ready for toilet training. Children with physical handicaps that prevent walking are not able to meet each of these criteria. However, if they are able to sit and stand with good balance, training can be attempted.

If the child is physically ready for toilet training, the nurse also assesses if he is exhibiting behavioral signs of readiness. The parents are asked to describe differences in his behaviors that signal his need to urinate or defecate or the fact that he has wet or soiled clothing. For example, does he become quieter or verbally seek attention? Does he shift his weight? Does the color of his face change? Does he cry? Does he fuss or become more dependent and clinging? Has he developed a word, gesture, or symbol indicating that he needs to eliminate? Does he associate the bathroom with eliminating?

The nurse interviews parents regarding their readiness to pursue a toilet-training program that is characterized by a positive, consistent, individualized, nonpunitive, nonpressured style of teaching. It is important to explore the parents' willingness to participate, the time they have to invest in the program, the advantages they see, the inconveniences that toilet training may cause them, the reason they wish to start, and whether this is the best time for both the parents and the child to begin. As was mentioned earlier, any major stress or change may be a contraindication to training at that time.

The nurse should ask the parents about any past attempts at toilet training the child: When and why did the parents start training? What methods did they use? Did they experience feelings of frustration, indifference, or discomfort? How long did they attempt training and what were their reasons for discontinuing training efforts? Looking back, how did they view the experience for themselves and the child? Were their efforts consistent? What did they do most consistently? Do they think that it is important to try again? If the parents admit to using punishment in any form, including spanking, scolding, withholding privileges, using suppositories, withholding fluid, getting the child up in middle of the night, or making the child wash his sheets or clothes, the nurse appeals to them to discontinue these unnecessary, ineffective methods.

As part of the procedure for determining the readiness of both parents and child to become involved in a successful toilet-training program, the nurse asks parents to keep detailed records for a period of 7 days. They should be cautioned to discontinue record keeping if the child becomes ill or if fluid intake is changed. Parents must record the exact time that the following events occur: (1) The child ate or drank, no matter how little he consumed. (2) The child's behavior was suddenly distinctly different, for example, when the child was noticeably quiet or louder, started fussing or tugging at his clothes, pointed toward the bathroom, cried, or squirmed. (3) Parents gave the child positive attention related to toileting behaviors only, in the form of praise, concrete rewards, affection, or approval. (4) Parents gave attention in the form of scolding, threatening, or spanking if the child had wet or soiled his underclothes or did not tell them before eliminating. (5) The child indicated his need to go to the toilet either by gestures or words. (6) The child was noted to have dry underclothes. (7) The child was noted to have wet underclothes.

It is crucial to refrain from beginning any toilet-training program until such records are completed, because they show how parents are responding to the child's behaviors and at what times the child is most likely to eliminate. After the records are completed to the parents' express satisfaction, the nurse should acknowledge their efforts to

Table 23-5. Infant stimulation program for self-feeding from birth to age 15 months*

Normal age of achievement (months)	Behavior	Activity
Birth	Has sucking, rooting, and swallowing reflexes	If sucking is weak, gently stroke around child's lips and mouth to stimulate puckering in order to strengthen lip muscles†
1	Is able to take food from a spoon	Press spoon on the tongue to stimulate jaw closure; press gently above the thyroid cartilage to stimulate swallowing; after spoon is withdrawn, close the mouth by pushing up on the mandible; wipe excess food from the lips in one stroke to prevent disrupting the normal closing and swallowing sequence† Introduce pureed foods of different tastes and textures
4-5	Can approximate cup to lips	Offer small amounts of milk or juice from a cup
5-6	Can use fingers to bring food to mouth	Give child dry toast, zwieback, pretzel, or cracker Dip fingers into food and bring hand to his lips If child is not used to voluntarily grasping objects, place food in his hand; gradually make him reach for it
6-7	Is able to chew solids	Introduce soft foods that require some chewing (soft cooked carrots, baked meats, baked potato, cheese, and so on) To stimulate chewing, place a small piece of food on the back molar area†
8-9	Holds a spoon and plays with it during feeding	Give child a small spoon at feeding time Reinforce any attempts at self-feeding (putting spoon in mouth, in food, and so on) If child has difficulty in holding spoon, improvise appropriate utensil
9	Holds his own bottle	Place the bottle in child's hands and bring it to his mouth; gradually release your hand If it is too heavy, fill it only part way with milk or use a small (4-ounce) bottle If child is unable to tilt the bottle, purchase a special nipple with a straw attached that draws milk from the bottom of the bottle
12	Drinks from a cup with much spilling	Give child a cup, beginning with the same procedure as for a bottle
15	Drinks well from a cup	Use a wide unbreakable cup with two handles If child is unable to lift a cup, introduce a straw; to initiate sucking liquid up the straw, fill the straw with juice, cover the top end with your finger, place the bottom end in child's mouth, and gradually release your finger to let the fluid in when child makes sucking movements Gradually wean child from one bottle at a time, eliminating the nighttime one last
	Uses a spoon with much spilling	Give child a spoon, a bowl, and "sticky" food (applesauce or mashed potatoes) If child is unwilling to feed himself, guide his hand toward the bowl and then into his mouth; gradually fade out the assistance If child has poor motor coordination, anchor the bowl to the table

*Use of a fork and, lastly, use of a knife are introduced after all the preceding steps are mastered. Table manners are usually learned after the second year and, most successfully, from imitation of role models.
†Data from Godfrey, A.: Am. J. Nurs. **75**(1):56-59, January 1975.

keep accurate records, their diligence in making observations, and their ability to follow through.

The goal of any toilet-training program is to help the child achieve small goals and experience comfort and success and to help the parents simultaneously experience feelings of adequacy, minimal tension, and success. Parents should understand that they will be capitalizing on the times the child is most likely to eliminate and that they should respond immediately to any cues indicating his need to eliminate. They must be cautioned to ignore accidents.

A task analysis of toileting reveals the following steps, which parents must systematically reinforce in positive, natural, spontaneous ways: (1) sitting on the toilet or potty-chair and playing there without fussing, crying, or attempting to get off, (2) eliminating into the toilet on a regular basis when sitting on it, (3) waiting to eliminate before being placed on the toilet, (4) indicating the need to eliminate before going into the bathroom, (5) asking to go to the toilet or just going to it, (6) remaining dry for longer periods of time, (7) climbing onto the toilet independently, (8) helping undress himself before getting on the toilet, (9) independently undressing himself before getting onto the toilet, (10) wiping independently, (11) flushing the toilet, (12) dressing, (13) washing his hands with soap in a correct manner, and (14) drying his hands with a towel.

A positive and relaxed attitude toward toilet training is important. The parents should begin by leading the child gently into the bathroom, staying with him, and showing approval for each aspect of his cooperative behavior. If a potty-chair is used, it should be kept in the bathroom, not in the kitchen, bedroom, or living room. If the child has not had any success after 5 minutes, he should be wiped, praised for sitting quietly and appropriately, and asked to get off the potty-chair. Children associate diapers with their old habits of elimination; therefore, parents should begin substituting training pants during the toilet-training program. To facilitate independence in undressing, the child should be dressed in pants with elastic waistbands for easy removal or in a dress that can be pulled up. Ideally parents should place the child on the potty-chair for voiding when he first gets up in the morning, just before breakfast, at midmorning, after snacks, after lunch, at midafternoon, before and after dinner, and again before bedtime. They cannot expect the child to have a regular pattern of elimination unless they feed him at approximately the same times each day. Parents should also remember to help the child only when he needs it. Although this may take longer, it is the best way for a child to learn complete independence.

Dressing. Dressing skills develop without special training in normal children, usually as a consequence of autonomy and imitation. For children who are retarded, special training is necessary to promote this skill. Factors that interfere with spontaneous learning include immature motor skills, lack of motivation, physical handicaps, or lack of opportunity.[13] The last variable should always be considered when assessing delayed development of independent dressing.

The level of independence in dressing varies according to the degree of retardation. Mildly and moderately retarded children without physical handicaps can become independent in all dressing skills, except for more complex tasks such as color coordination. Severely retarded children can achieve most dressing skills, except the ability to fasten complicated closures, such as buttons or ties. Profoundly retarded children are usually able to assist in undressing and dressing but achieve no independent skills.

Prior to instituting a self-dressing program, the nurse assesses the child's physical readiness by doing a task analysis of the following gross and fine motor skills: (1) can stand alone, (2) can balance in a chair or on the floor without support, (3) can lean free from the chair when seated, (4) can raise one knee up toward the chest when seated, (5) can place either hand on the opposite shoulder, (6) can place one or both hands on top of head, (7) has apposition with one or both hands, (8) can grasp and hold slim objects with one or both hands, (9) can pick up a 1-inch button using thumb and forefinger, (10) can push with one or both hands with all fingers grasped around an object, and (11) can pull with one or both hands with all fingers grasped around an object.[12]

The child is considered to be mentally ready for dressing training if he can sit quietly for 3 to 5 minutes while working on a task, can watch what he is doing while working on a task, can follow physical gestures or cues, can follow verbal commands, and can relate clothing to the appropriate body part, such as socks with feet. As with other self-help skills, the child may not be able to master every task but should be evaluated for evidence of willingness to participate at his level of readiness.

After assessing the child's readiness, the nurse requests the parents to keep a detailed record of what the child can do in dressing, what is being taught, and how well the child is progressing with the new skill. The program for self-dressing follows the same sequence as normal development: dressing is done for the child but with demonstration of the procedure, the child undresses and then dresses with assistance, the child undresses completely without supervision, the child dresses with little assistance but with supervision, and the child assumes all responsibility for dressing. It also follows the guidelines used for other programs: namely, the skill is first broken down into step-by-step process; each procedure is demonstrated and the child's performance is guided; after one step is completely learned, a new step is introduced; and the child is praised for success. Table 23-6 suggests activities for promoting independent dressing. Since normal children do not master fastening back closures or tying shoelaces until age 6 years or older, it is unrealistic to expect such skills until after this age in retarded children.

Choice of clothing is an important aspect of the training program. Clothes should be clean, up-to-date, and well fitted. Minimizing the appearance of a "retarded" child is a major goal in promoting acceptance from others and self-esteem in the child. The following is suggested clothing for use in a training program: undershirts with large neck openings, brassieres that have elastic straps and front fasteners, half-slips, underpants with elastic waists, boxer shorts for boys, slip-on polo shirts with large armholes (tight turtleneck sweaters should be avoided), front-buttoning shirts or dresses, pants with elastic waistbands or side large hook fasteners, wool or cotton ankle socks (tight nylon knee socks should be avoided), panty hose with sewn-in panty for girls, and slip-on shoes. If the child cannot manage but-

Table 23-6. Infant stimulation program for self-dressing

Normal age of achievement (months)	Behavior	Activity
15	Cooperates by extending arm or leg	Give child verbal direction ("put your hands over your head") and assist child in procedure; gradually give only verbal command
18	Takes off mittens, hat, or socks	Demonstrate taking off article of clothing; then give only verbal command. Use loose-fitting socks
	Unzips	Place child's finger on zipper head; pull it down with him; gradually reduce assistance until he can do it on verbal command
	Tries to put on shoes	Begin with having child extend foot, put open shoe or slipper in child's hand, and demonstrate getting it over toes; show him how to push foot into shoe and hit the sole with his hand to make sure heel is inside; demonstrate "stepping into" shoes Use oversized shoes at first
21	Undresses	Demonstrate step-by-step procedure, for example, pants: pull down pants to child's ankles, have him pull them off, then pull down to knees, then hips, and lastly, have child pull them from waist For shirt: unbutton shirt, pull off shoulders and one arm, have child pull off other arm, then pull off shoulders only and have child do both arms
24	Removes shoes	Loosen shoes completely; demonstrate taking them off by pushing from heel; take them off part way, have child do rest; gradually have child do it himself Demonstrate untying shoe by placing two beads or bells at the ends of the laces, grasping each, and pulling the bow out; have child first pull one string with parent, until gradually he can do both unaided
	Helps in dressing	Use same technique as for learning to cooperate with undressing (15 months) and self-undressing (21 months) Use simple articles of clothing Concentrate on putting the clothes on first and fastening them later Sew tabs or colorful appliques on shirts and pants to indicate front or back Practice buttoning with large buttons; use front-fastening clothes

tons, hooks, or straps, Velcro fasteners are excellent substitutes.

Grooming. Learning self-grooming is usually part of other independent skills, such as washing hands during toilet training. The same principles are followed in teaching grooming measures as have already been discussed: assess the child's readiness and present level of competency, proceed with skills in the normal sequence of development, analyze the task into its component parts, and set up an individualized teaching program. As with self-dressing, a major factor in learning independent grooming is the opportunity to practice the skills. Table 23-7 suggests activities for promoting self-grooming. Complete independence for bathing and hair washing are learned during the school years and, therefore, are late skills for the retarded child.

Special mention must be made of dental hygiene. An odor-free mouth and a white set of teeth are essential in promoting a positive image. In addition sound teeth are necessary for proper functioning of the mouth in terms of mastication and speech. Diseased teeth and gums increase drooling and prevent proper preparation of food for subsequent digestion. Missing teeth interfere with proper tongue positioning for clear speech.[9]

Not all causes of dental problems in handicapped or retarded children are a result of physical abnormalities. On the contrary, most are the result of neglected dental hygiene and excessive quantities of carbohydrates. Most dental problems are preventable with proper brushing at home, avoidance of cariogenic foods, especially sugars that remain in the mouth (lollipops, sucking candies, chewing candies, and gum), frequent ingestion of detergent foods (uncooked fruits and vegetables), periodic dental examinations (at least every 6 months, but more often for children who demonstrate a predisposition to decay), and use of fluoride, either in the drinking water, in toothpaste, as a mineral supplement, or applied topically by the dentist. Care of the teeth begins as soon as they erupt with attention to diet and frequent wiping of the tooth surface with a cloth.

If the child has physical handicaps that limit his ability to brush, special devices may be necessary, such as a larger handle or a curved toothbrush, to reach all surfaces of the teeth. Electric toothbrushes may be a worthwhile investment for some children. The use of dental disclosing tablets is an excellent aid in visually showing the child the thoroughness (or lack of) in his toothbrushing technique. Any devices that help to motivate the child to brush should be

Table 23-7. Infant stimulation program for self-grooming

Normal age of achievement (months)	Behavior	Activity
14	Brushes teeth with help	Establish a routine (after each meal and before bedtime) Demonstrate toothbrushing to child on yourself Use small toothbrush with pleasant-tasting toothpaste (preferably containing fluoride) Use a mirror for child to observe procedure Place toothbrush in child's hand and assist in brushing Teach child how to rinse toothbrush and mouth
18	Helps with bath	Explain to child what you are doing ("I am washing my face") Give child washcloth and soap, guide his hand to imitate your action; gradually reduce assistance
24	Washes hands with help	Demonstrate procedure Place child by sink with a stool so he can easily reach bowl Regulate water, give him soap, help him rub soap on hands, rinse, and dry; gradually reduce assistance
	Helps with washing hair	Place child's hands in hair while lathering scalp; show him the bubbles on his hands and use a mirror for him to observe shampooing; as he learns to rub scalp, gradually reduce assistance During rinse, give him towel to hold over his eyes Give him a large-toothed comb for his hair; guide his hand in learning to comb his hair
30-36	Brushes teeth alone	Demonstrate placing paste on toothbrush Encourage child to brush his own teeth using "any direction" method Reinforce any previously learned skills Remind child to brush according to set routine Begin visits to the dentist
36	Washes hands alone	Place all utensils within easy reach Regulate water for child (safety measure against burning) Teach child to turn off faucets Reinforce all previously learned skills When child has sense of responsibility concerning danger (hot), teach him how to regulate water and check the temperature each time

used. For example, the parent can place a special "tooth calendar" on the wall and mark each date with stars to represent the number of brushings per day. At the end of so many accumulated stars, the child can receive a special reward.

Routinely the child should be taken to a dentist. To accustom him to this experience, he should go for visits with other members of the family *before* the dentist examines or looks at his teeth. It is important to attend to the child's preparation for such visits, since it is much more difficult to reason with the retarded child concerning the necessity of dental examinations than it is with a normal child. Therefore, once he is traumatized by the experience, parents may be less inclined to take the child back for fear of temper tantrums or other resisting behavior. The nurse can assist in this area by locating dentists who are familiar with treating retarded children[9] and discussing with parents preparatory procedures for the visit.

Promoting optimum development in children

Optimum development involves more than achieving independence. It requires appropriate guidance for establishing acceptable social behavior and personal feeling of self-esteem, worth, and security. These attributes are not simply learned through a stimulation program. Rather they must arise from the genuine love and caring that exists among family members. However, parents need guidance in providing an environment that fosters optimal development. Often it is the nurse who can provide continuing assistance in these areas of child rearing.

Play. The retarded child has the same needs for play as any other child. However, because of his slower development, parents may be less aware of the need to continue appropriate stimulation. They may also feel inadequate in how to play with the child, since the usual reciprocal satisfaction between child and parent may be slower in developing. Therefore, the nurse guides parents toward selection of suitable toys and interactive activities. Since play has been discussed for children in each age-group in earlier chapters and is also outlined in the Washington Guide to Promoting Development in the Young Child (Appendix G), only the exceptions for the retarded child are discussed.

Play is based on the child's developmental age. For the retarded child, the need for sensorimotor play may be prolonged for several years. Parents should use every opportunity to expose the child to as many different sounds, sights, and sensations as possible. Appropriate play includes musical mobiles, stuffed toys, water play, floating toys, rocking chair or horse, baby swing, bells, and rattles. The child should be taken on outings, such as trips to the grocery store or shopping center, other people should be encouraged to visit in the home, and the child should be related to directly, such as cuddling, holding, rocking, talking to him in the *en face* position, giving him rides on the parents' shoulders, and so on.

Toys should also be selected for their educational value. For example, a large inflatable beach ball is a good water toy, encourages interactive play, and can be used to learn motor skills, such as balance, rocking, kicking, and throwing. A doll with removeable clothes and different types of closures can help the child learn dressing skills. Musical toys that mimic animal sounds or respond with social phrases are excellent ways of encouraging speech. Toys should be simple in design so that the child can learn to manipulate them without help. Toys that are suitable in terms of teaching skill but that are too complicated to work are frustrating to the child.

Safety is a major consideration in selection of toys. Toys that may be appropriate developmentally may present dangers to a child who is strong enough to break them. Even if more advanced toys are suitable for the child's developmental skills, the parent must keep in mind the child's level of responsibility in using them properly. For example, the child may be physically able to use a bow and arrow but may lack the judgment in properly using it to only shoot at a target.

Retarded children often lack the motivation to institute appropriate play activities on their own. As a result of boredom, they resort to self-stimulatory behavior such as rocking, head hitting, twirling, masturbating, or finger-sucking. Such behaviors are destructive in that they limit developmental progress and impede social acceptance. If the nurse is aware of such behavior in a child, appropriate play activities, especially as a method of distraction from self-stimulation, are discussed with the parents. Behavior techniques, such as ignoring the child when he engages in such behavior and attending to him when he is behaving acceptably, should also be used.

Communication. Verbal skills are often delayed more than other physical skills. Since suggestions for promoting speech development are discussed in Chapter 24, only brief comments are included here.

Speech requires hearing and interpretation (receptive skills) and facial muscle coordination (expressive skills). Both may be impaired in mentally retarded children. For example, in children with Down's syndrome the large protruding tongue often interferes with speech. These children may need tongue exercises to correct the tongue thrust or gentle reminders to keep the lips closed. Deficits in discrimination impede learning of different sounds. Often it helps to exaggerate the word's pronunciation or associate it with another stimuli, such as singing. Singing attracts the child's attention so that he attends to the cue longer. Parents also must remember that since learning is slower, their teaching must continue longer. The nurse encourages them not to give up or believe that speech is hopeless.

Shaping techniques are useful in fostering meaningful vocalization. Every time the child vocalizes a sound that either represents a letter of the alphabet or an intelligible syllable, the parent reinforces him with praise and social approval. The nurse instructs parents to record all meaningful vocalizations the child has learned in the past in order to continue reinforcing them. A written record also helps parents monitor evidence of progress in this area.

Discipline. As was discussed in Chapter 22, one of the earliest child-rearing practices eliminated when the parents have a handicapped child is discipline. This not only can result in serious behavior problems, but it also interferes with the child's developing a sense of security and self-control. It may also foster resentment from siblings who are forced to abide by a double standard.

Discipline must begin early. For the retarded child, limit-setting measures must be simple, consistent, and appropriate for his age. Control measures are based on teaching a specific behavior—not on understanding the reasons behind it. Stressing moral lessons are of little value to a child who cannot learn from self-criticism or from a lesson based on previous wrongdoing.

Behavior modification is an excellent technique for limit setting. For example, to teach the child to stay in the yard and not run in the street, the parent makes a simple rule, such as "You must stay behind this gate." If the child breaks the rule, the parent immediately shows disapproval, such as confining him to his room or taking away a special privilege. It does little good to give him a speech about the dangers of traffic as the sole method of disapproval, since this is an abstraction that has little meaning. Such types of discipline are appropriate regardless of the child's age. As he grows older, it is important to stress the reason why a certain act is forbidden, provided the explanation is simple, but only as a secondary measure to a more concrete approach.

The nurse stresses supervision during play and other activities, since these children are slow to learn inherent dangers. Parents may need to place reminders around the house to prevent accidents, such as signs to keep the doors closed or the gate locked. They should also be taught first-aid measures for minor injuries.

Socialization. Parents should be encouraged early to teach their child socially acceptable behavior, such as waving good-bye, saying hello, thank you, and so on, responding to his name, greeting visitors but not being overly affectionate, sitting modestly, and so on. The greatest teaching method is being a role model combined with gentle, consistent reminders to perform the behavior. Parents also need to expose the child to strangers so that he can practice manners. Although it is well to teach social amenities in the home, the child may not transfer the learning to other situations unless the parent provides the opportunity.

Prior to preschool age the parents should contact the nearest day-training center or special school. Not only do these centers provide appropriate education and training, they also offer an opportunity for social experiences among the children. As the child grows older, he should have peer experiences similar to those of normal children, including group outings, sports, and organized activity, such as Boy Scouts or Girl Scouts for retarded children. He should be encouraged to form a close relationship with a best friend. Often parents neglect this aspect of the child's life, believing that once he leaves school he should be sheltered in the home. On the contrary he needs to feel companionship and belonging by being able to invite friends home, talk to them on the telephone, and plan and participate in special events.

Adolescence may be a particularly difficult time for parents, especially in terms of the child's sexual behavior, future plans to marry, and ability to be independent. Frequently little anticipatory guidance has been offered parents to prepare the child for physical and sexual maturation. The nurse can help in this area by providing parents with information about sex education that is geared to the child's developmental level. For example, the adolescent female needs a *simple* explanation of menstruation and instructions on personal hygiene during the menstrual cycle.*

Parents often express a great deal of concern about sexual drives and interest in their retarded child, especially fear of pregnancy in a girl. Generally the moderately and more severely retarded adolescents exhibit limited sexual drives. Their interest is mainly exploratory and characteristic of young preschool children. The behavior of most concern to parents is masturbation. If this occurs the nurse should investigate the situation for evidence of boredom in the child or excessive provocative sexual behavior among family members. Parents should be cautioned against nudity, teasing, and sexually stimulating material as a source of promoting sexual behavior in the child.

Mildly retarded adolescents often have normal sexual drives, including the wish to marry and have children. Because they are more socially acceptable and have greater access to peers, they are more vulnerable to heterosexual or homosexual experiences. These adolescents need practical sexual information regarding anatomy, physical development, conception, and personal hygiene. Because of their easy persuasion and lack of judgment, they need a well-defined, concrete code of conduct. The subtleties of social sexual behavior are less beneficial than specific instructions for handling certain situations. For example, a girl should be firmly told never to go alone anywhere with any man she does not know well. A boy should be warned of intimate advances from other males. To protect their children from abusive sexual activities, parents must closely observe their teenager's activities and associates.[11]

Retarded adolescents need social outlets for heterosexual experiences. Unfortunately few schools or communities provide for this recreational need. The nurse can be instrumental in indirectly initiating such activities by encouraging parents to discuss these unmet social needs with educational staff. Clubs, sports, hobby projects, and dances can be organized for the teenagers to provide experience that teaches acceptable social behavior.

Parents of retarded adolescents are often very concerned about the advisability of marriage between two retarded individuals. There is no conclusive answer; rather each situation must be judged individually. In many instances marriage would help the couple achieve a mutually satisfying and supportive relationship, meaningful companionship, and a more normal social sexual adjustment. However, parenthood is usually not desirable because the retarded couple may not be able to cope with the dependency needs of offspring for several years. In addition pregnancy presents the problem of perpetuating mental deficiency, since the offspring of one or two retarded parents is on the average below normal intelligence.[11] The nurse should discuss this topic with parents and with the retarded couple, stressing suitable living accommodations and contraceptive methods to prevent pregnancy.

The question of contraceptive protection for female retarded adolescents is often a parental concern. Of the available methods, the intrauterine device or birth control pills are the most satisfactory. The effectiveness of birth control pills can be maximized by devising reminder charts or by using dated pill dispensers. Their use should be investigated for girls at risk for pregnancy, for example, those in lower socioeconomic levels who have poor parental supervision/ or for females contemplating marriage. Sterilization is a special dilemma because of moral and ethical questions as well as psychologic effects on the adolescent.

In summary the nurse has the following three major areas of guidance, counseling, and intervention in assisting retarded adolescents to adjust to adulthood: (1) helping them achieve a significant degree of independence, particularly mastery of self-help skills; (2) guiding them toward appropriate vocational training; and (3) counseling them and their parents regarding physical maturity, sexual behavior, marriage, and family planning. Assisting families in each of these goals must begin early if the crises of this difficult period are to be prevented.

Helping families adjust to future care

Not all families are able to cope with home care of a retarded child, especially one who is severely or profoundly

*A helpful book on this subject is Pattulio, A.: Puberty in the girl who is retarded, available from the National Association of Retarded Citizens.

retarded and/or multihandicapped. Older parents may be able to assume care responsibilities until they reach retirement or old age. Unfortunately some parents view institutionalization as the only alternative to coping with problems of adolescent retarded children. For these parents, the decision regarding residential placement is a difficult one. The nurse's role is to assist parents in exploring the reasons regarding placement, especially of retarded adolescents, investigating alternatives to home care prior to their necessity, and establishing ways in which to maintain contact and communication with the retarded member of the family.

The following are alternatives to living at home that are compatible with the national trend toward returning institutionalized mentally retarded persons to their community[19]:

Children under 18 years. For children under age 18 years, alternatives to living at home include: (1) foster homes (private homes with a full-time family-type care program for less than five children); (2) group foster homes (full-time family-type homes for five to eight children); (3) child-welfare institutions (possibly temporary facilities within the community for four or more mentally disabled children who cannot remain in their own or foster homes and who require specialized training, care, and services); (4) boarding home (homes for one to four children who need a place to live while attending a specialized school program—especially rural children; the children go home on weekends and for vacations); and (5) temporary-care homes (short-term care for one to four children to relieve the family or to provide emergency housing while plans are made for more permanent living arrangements).

Adults age 18 years and older. For adults age 18 years and older, alternatives to living at home include: (1) foster homes (private homes with a family-type care program for less than five adults who can tend to their personal needs and who do not need continuing medical nursing services; they may be working and paying a part of their expenses or being trained for employment); (2) group foster homes (family-type homes for up to eight retarded adults who need supervision and personalized living; may offer short-term or long-term care); and (3) boarding homes (homes for up to eight retarded adults who are capable of independent living for total self-care; most pay their room and board from earnings; sometimes placement agencies supplement the cost; little supervision required).

Residential care institutions for adults. This includes (1) long-term care for a maximum of fifty semidependent individuals, most of whom will be able to care for themselves with minimal supervision but require special social and vocational help; emphasis on training by specialists in nonmedical fields; and (2) short-term care in a program resembling a hostel or halfway house for nine to thirty residents living semi-independently, with social, minimal nursing, and community living needs met in the home; some work or go to training programs in the community.

Nursing home care for adults who require specialized attention. This includes (1) *skilled,* for persons requiring services of a registered nurse because of severe handicaps, (2) *limited,* for semiambulatory persons with some self-help skills, and (3) *personal,* for ambulatory handicapped persons who require minimal medications and are capable of supervised community activities.

Nurses working with a family may wish to visit each facility directly to evaluate its suitability for the child or may guide parents on how to assess the facility's adequacy. The following are objectives to assist in assessment of visits to residential institutions, foster or group homes, and special programs:

1. Clarify the facility's philosophy of care.
2. Assess the environment for adequacy of inanimate and animate stimuli available to children.
3. Determine the appropriateness of amounts of stimuli in the child's environment.
4. Observe care provider–to-child ratios.
5. Observe care personnel interacting with children in a variety of teaching and learning experiences.
6. Determine the appropriateness of the setting for a child being considered for placement.
7. Observe the quality of physical care administered to children.
8. See if children are attended to regularly and consistently, instead of when inappropriate behaviors occur.
9. Determine if activities are child oriented.
10. Determine the existence of structured and nonstructured activities.
11. Determine if individual plans of care are available.
12. Determine if individual plans of care are evaluated.
13. Determine the functional levels of children who reside in settings, for example, are they ambulatory and is speech encouraged?
14. Determine if speech, physical, and occupational therapies are available.
15. Determine if each child is perceived as unique and distinct and if care is given to each child according to his needs.
16. Determine the advantages and disadvantages of the setting for a child.
17. Determine the criteria for meeting standards of care.
18. Determine if and to what degree official standards of care are met.
19. Meet with parents of children who reside in special settings to hear their comments, both positive and negative.

Caring for hospitalized retarded children

Caring for retarded children during hospitalization is a special challenge to nurses. Frequently nurses are unfamiliar with retarded children and cope with their feelings of insecurity and fear by ignoring or isolating the retarded child. Not only is this approach nonsupportive, it may also be destructive for the child's sense of self-esteem and optimum development and in terms of the parents' ability to cope with the stress of the experience. One method of successfully avoiding this nontherapeutic approach is to use the mutual participation model in planning the child's care. Parents should be encouraged to room with their child but should not be made to feel as if the responsibility is totally theirs.

When the child is admitted, the nurse takes a detailed history (see p. 892), especially in terms of all self-help activity. During the interview the nurse simultaneously assesses the child's developmental age. It is best to avoid directly asking about IQ levels, since this may make the parents uncomfortable and often tells little about the child's actual abilities. Questions are approached positively. For example, rather than asking, "Is he toilet trained yet?" the nurse may state, "Tell me about his toileting habits." The assessment should also focus on any special devices the child uses, effective measures of limit setting, unusual or favorite routines, and any behaviors that may require intervention. For example, if the patient states that the child engages in self-stimulatory activities, the nurse inquires about events that precipitate them and techniques that the parents use to manage them.

The nurse also assesses the child's functional level of eating and playing, his ability to verbally express his needs, his progress in toilet training, and his relationship with objects, toys, and other children. He is encouraged to be as independent as possible, even though he is in a hospital setting. If the child has already accomplished self-help skills in eating, the nurse encourages the child to continue to eat with a spoon or a fork. He is also encouraged to be independent in his toileting functions and to make his needs known.

The nurse ensures that the child has toys and other activities to entertain him. Realizing that he may be lonely in the hospital, the nurse makes certain that he is included in group activities on the ward and sets time aside each day to talk to or play with him. He is placed in a room with other children of approximate developmental age, preferably an area with two beds, to avoid overstimulation. The nurse discusses with the other parents the retarded child's abilities and introduces the parents and children to each other. By the nurse's example of treating the retarded child with dignity and respect, others who may be fearful of what they do not understand are encouraged to accept deviation.

The nurse explains procedures to the child using methods of communication that are at his cognitive level. Generally explanations should be simple, short, and concrete, emphasizing what the child will *physically* experience. Demonstration either through actual practice or with visual aids is always preferable to verbal explanation. The nurse repeats instructions often and evaluates the child's understanding by asking questions, such as, "What did I say it will feel like?" "What will the doctor look like?" "Show me how you must lie." "Where will the dressing be?" and so on. Parents are included in preprocedural teaching for their own learning and to help the nurse learn effective methods of communicating with the child.

During hospitalization the nurse should also focus on growth-promoting experiences for the child. For example, hospitalization may be an excellent opportunity to emphasize to parents abilities that the child does have but has not had the opportunity to practice, such as self-dressing. It may also be an opportunity for social experiences with peers, group play, or new educational/recreational activities. For example, one child who had had the habit of screaming and kicking demonstrated a definite decrease in those behaviors after he learned to pound pegs and use a punching bag. Through social services the parents may become aware of specialized programs for the child. Nutritional counseling is available if the child is overweight or has evidence of specific deficiencies, such as iron deficiency. Hospitalization may also offer parents a respite from everyday care responsibilities and an opportunity to discuss their feelings with a concerned professional.

REFERENCES

1. Barnard, K. E., and Erickson, M. L.: Teaching children with developmental problems: a family-care approach, ed. 2, St. Louis, 1976, The C. V. Mosby Co.
2. Ehlers, W. H., Krishef, C. H., and Prothero, J. C.: An introduction to mental retardation: a program text, Columbus, 1973, Charles E. Merrill Publishing Co.
3. Emanuel, I., and associates: Accelerated aging in young mothers of children with Down's syndrome, Lancet **2**:361-363, August 19, 1972.
4. Erickson, M. L.: Assessment and management of developmental changes in children, St. Louis, 1976, The C. V. Mosby Co.
5. Fishler, K., Koch, R., and Donnell, G. N.: Comparison of mental development in individuals with mosaic and trisomy 21 Down's syndrome, Pediatrics **58**(5):744-748, November 1976.
6. Forness, S. R.: Education of retarded children, Am. J. Dis. Child **127**:237-242, February 1974.
7. Gayton, W. F., and Walker, L.: Down syndrome: informing the parents, Am. J. Dis. Child. **127**:510-512, April 1974.
8. Godfrey, A.: Sensory-motor stimulation for slow-to-develop children, Am. J. Nurs. **75**(1):56-59, January 1975.
9. Green, A.: A preventive care guide for multihandicapped children: dental care begins at home, Rehabil. Lit. **31**(1):10-12, January 1970.
10. Grossman, H. J.: Manual on terminology and classification in mental retardation, American Association on Mental Deficiency, Special Publication Series, No. 2, Baltimore, 1973, Garamond Pridemark Press.
11. Hammar, S. L., and Barnard, K. E.: The mentally retarded adolescent: a review of the characteristics and problems of 44 non-institutionalized adolescent retardates, Pediatrics **38**(5): 845-857, November 1966.
12. Henderson, S., and McDonald, M.: Step-by-step dressing, Ill., 1973, Suburban Publications.
13. Kluss, K.: Training the mentally retarded child in self-help

skills. In Brandt, P. A., Chinn, P. L., and Smith, M. E.: Current practice in pediatric nursing, vol. 1, St. Louis, 1976, The C. V. Mosby Co.
14. Lee, L. G., and Jackson, J. F.: Diagnosis of Down's syndrome: clinical vs. laboratory, Clin. Pediatr. **11**(6):353-356, June 1972.
15. Mori, W.: "My child has Down's syndrome," Am. J. Nurs. **73**(8):1386-1387, August 1973.
16. Payne, J. S., and Mercer, C. D.: Biological and environmental causes. In Mental retardation: introduction and personal perspective, Columbus, 1975, Charles E. Merrill Publishing Co.
17. Rosenthal, R., and Jacobsen, L.: Pygmalion in the classroom, New York, 1968, Holt, Rinehart and Winston, Inc.
18. Smith, D. W., and Wilson, A. A.: The child with Down's syndrome, Philadelphia, 1973, W. B. Saunders Co.
19. Weinberger, C. W.: Islands of excellence, Reports of the President's Committee on Mental Retardation, Washington, D.C., 1972, U.S. Government Printing Office.
20. Wolfensberger, W.: The principle of normalization in human services, Toronto, 1972, National Institute on Mental Retardation.

BIBLIOGRAPHY

Aase, J., and associates: Small ears in Down's syndrome: a helpful diagnostic aid, J. Pediatr. **82**(5):845-847, May 1973.

Barnard, K. E.: Developmental disabilities, Am. J. Nurs. **74**(10): 1700-1704, October 1975.

Bartel, N. R., and associates: Language comprehension in the moderately retarded child, Except. Child. **39**(5):375-382, 1973.

Bean, N. R., and Bell, B. J.: Nursing intervention in the care of the physically handicapped, severely retarded child, Nurs. Clin. North Am. **10**(2):353-359, June 1975.

Blackwell, M. W., and Roy, S. A.: Surgical "routines" for profoundly retarded patients, Am. J. Nurs. **78**(3):402-404, March 1978.

Christiansen, T.: Visual imagery as a factor in teaching elaborative language to mentally retarded children, Except. Child. **35**(7):539-541, 1969.

Cohen, H., and associates: Some considerations for evaluating the Doman-Delacata "Patterning" method, Pediatrics **45**(2):302-313, 1970.

Dunham, P.: Teaching motor skills to the mentally retarded, Except. Child. **35**(9):739-744, 1969.

Dybwad, G.: Who are the mentally retarded? Children **15**(2):43-48, March/April 1968.

Eddington, C., and Lee, T.: Sensory-motor stimulation for slow-to-develop children: a home-centered program for parents, Am. J. Nurs. **75**(1):59-62, January 1975.

Erickson, M.: Talking with fathers of young children with Down's syndrome, Child. Today **3**(6):22-25, November/December 1974.

Erickson, M.: Developmental assessment. In Curry, J. B., and Peppe, K. K., editors: Mental retardation: nursing approaches to care, St. Louis, 1978, The C. V. Mosby Co.

Fackler, E.: The crisis of institutionalizing a retarded child, Am. J. Nurs. **68**:1508-1512, July 1968.

Gibson, B. S., and Reed, J. C.: Training nurses in mental retardation, Ment. Retard. **12**(6):19-22, December 8, 1974.

Golden, D., and Davis, J.: Counseling parents after the birth of an infant with Down's syndrome, Child. Today **3**:2, March/April 1974.

Gorham, K. A.: A lost generation of parents, Except. Child. **41**: 521-525, May 1975.

Gregory, D.: Family assessment and intervention plan, Pediatr. Nurs. **1**(4):23-29, July/August 1975.

Haring, N. G., Hayden, A. H., and Beck, R.: General principles and guidelines in programming for severely handicapped children and young adults, Focus Except. Child. **8**:1-14, 1976.

Johnson, C., and Opitz, E.: The single palmar crease and its clinical significance in child development, Clin. Pediatr. **10**:392-403, July 1971.

Kauffman, M., and Payne, J. S.: Mental retardation: introduction and personal perspectives, Columbus, 1975, Bell and Howell Co.

Krajicek, M. J., and Tearney, A. I., editors: Detection of developmental problems in children, Baltimore, 1977, University Park Press.

Kugel, R.: Combating retardation in infants with Down's syndrome, Children **17**:188-192, September/October 1970.

Lappalainen, J., and Kouvalainen, K.: High hematocrits in newborns with Down's syndrome, Clin. Pediatr. **11**:472-474, August 1972.

Lawrence, E. A., and Winschel, J. F.: Self concept and the retarded: research and issues, Except. Child. **39**(4):310-317, 1973.

Lawson, L. J., and Schoofs, G.: A technique for visual appraisal of mentally retarded children, Am. J. Ophthalmol. **72**(3):622-624, September 1971.

Lepler, M.: Having a handicapped child, Am. J. Maternal Child Nurs. **3**(1):32-33, January/February 1978.

Maddock, J.: Sex education for the exceptional person: a rationale, Except. Child. **40**(4):273-278, 1974.

Melym, M. A., and White, D. T.: Mental and developmental milestones of noninstitutionalized Down's syndrome children, Pediatrics **52**(4):542-545, October 1973.

Myers, P. A., and Warkany, S. F.: Working with parents of children with profound developmental retardation: a group approach, Clin. Pediatr. **16**(4):367-370, April 1977.

Neman, R., and associates: Experimental evaluation of sensorimotor patterning used with mentally retarded children, Am. J. Ment. Def. **79**(4):372-384, 1974.

Norris, G. J.: National concerns for children with handicaps, Nurs. Clin. North Am. **10**(2):309-318, June 1975.

Pipes, P. L.: Nutrition and feeding of children with developmental delays and related problems. In Pipes, P. L.: Nutrition in infancy and childhood, St. Louis, 1977, The C. V. Mosby Co.

Quick, A. D., and associates: Early childhood education for exceptional foster children and training of foster parents, Except. Child. **40**(3):206-208, 1973.

Robinson, N. M., and Robinson, H.: The mentally retarded child, New York, 1976, McGraw-Hill Book Co.

Russell, F.: Interdisciplinary early intervention program, Phys. Ther. **56**:155-158, 1976.

Schein, J. D., and Salvia, J. A.: Color blindness in mentally retarded children, Except. Child. **35**(8):609-612, 1969.

Seidel, M.: Nursing care of children with mental retardation and other developmental disabilities: career development in the health professions, Bureau of Community Health Services, Title V Maternal and Child Health, U.S. Public Health Service, Department of Health, Education and Welfare, 1976.

Tudor, M.: Nursing intervention with developmentally disabled children, Am. J. Maternal Child Nurs. **3**(1):25-31, January/February 1978.

Wolfensberger, W., and Kurtz, R. A.: Measurements of parents' perceptions of their children's development, Genet. Psychol. Monogr. **83**:3, 1971.

24

The child with a sensory or communication disorder

Sensory impairments pose special threats to a child's developmental potential. Deprived of visual or auditory cues, the child must rely more heavily on other sensory experiences to learn about and relate to his environment. The child with a communication disorder may function well during early childhood but be unable to achieve in an academic setting. Without assistance and rehabilitation, these children are vulnerable to the lifelong disadvantages of being a handicapped individual.

Parents are the major rehabilitors of the child. However, they need guidance and support from specially trained professionals to help the child learn. The nurse is often in a strategic position to prevent and identify sensory or communication disorders, support the family in adjusting to the handicap, and assist them in learning methods of overcoming or compensating for the impairment.

HEARING IMPAIRMENT

Scope of the problem

Hearing loss is the most frequent handicap in the United States. It is estimated that 3 million children and 13 million adults have some degree of hearing loss.[12] The number of children with subnormal hearing is approximately 4% of the school-age population.[20] The Bureau of Education for the Handicapped reports that there are 52,000 deaf children and 350,000 hard-of-hearing children from birth to 19 years of age.[13] The prevalence of profound congenital deafness is about 1:1500 live births.[1]

Classification of hearing defects

Hearing defects may be classified according to etiology, pathology, or symptom severity. Each is important in terms of treatment, possible prevention, and rehabilitation.

Etiology. The precise etiology is not known in about 30% of hearing impaired children; however, many of these children demonstrate histories of conditions in which the risk of deafness is greatly increased (see the box on p. 838). With environmental noise levels increasingly exceeding normal limits, the significance of this potential causative influencing factor must receive special consideration. Evidence is accumulating that hearing levels in young people under 21 years of age are following an awesome trend toward loss of high-frequency acuity.[19] In addition high-risk neonates who are surviving formerly fatal prenatal or perinatal conditions may be susceptible to hearing loss from the disorder or its treatment. For example, sensorineural hearing loss may be the result of continuous humming noises or high noise levels associated with incubators, oxygen hoods, or intensive care units.[8,30] Continuous exposure to excessive noise levels in the premature infant may represent an even greater risk when combined with the use of potentially ototoxic antibiotics.

Pathology. Disorders of hearing are divided according to location of the defect. *Conductive* or middle-ear hearing loss results from interference of transmission of sound to the middle ear. It is the most common of all types of hearing loss and most commonly involves the external auditory canal, tympanic membrane, middle-ear chamber, the ossicles (incus, stapes, and malleus), or the eustachian tube. It may be the result of developmental anomalies, such as atresia of the external canal, or mesenchymal changes, most frequently as a result of recurrent otitis media.

Conductive hearing impairment mainly involves interference with loudness of sound. Although air conduction is impaired, bone conduction is intact. Many conductive defects are amenable to medical or surgical treatment. Hearing is improved with the use of a hearing aid to amplify sound.

Sensorineural hearing loss, also called perceptive or nerve deafness, involves damage to the inner ear structures and/or the auditory nerve. In almost half the cases the etiology of sensorineural loss is unknown. The most common causes are congenital defects of inner ear structures or consequences of acquired conditions, such as infection, hyperbilirubinemia, administration of ototoxic drugs, or exposure to excessive noise.

Sensorineural hearing loss results in distortion of sound and problems in discrimination. The hearing loss is often selective for various frequencies, especially those in the high range. Loss of discrimination of high frequencies makes perception of consonants, such as "s," "z," "ch,"

Conditions associated with hearing loss

Familial/genetic factors
- Skeletal defects (Treacher Collins and Klippel-Feil syndromes)
- Retinitis pigmentosa
- Cerebral palsy
- Mental retardation
- Visual handicaps
- Pigment abnormalities (Waardenburg's syndrome, albinism)
- Congenital abnormalities, especially those involving the ear, eye, mouth (cleft palate), central nervous system, heart, or kidney
- Chromosomal abnormalities, such as D and E trisomies
- Connective tissue disorders (osteogenesis imperfecta, Hurler's syndrome)
- Family history of congenital deafness

Prenatal/intrauterine factors
- Rubella during first trimester
- Diabetes mellitus, syphilis, alcoholism
- Drugs such as quinine, salicylates, and certain ototoxic antibiotics
- Maternal anoxia
- Preeclampsia/eclampsia

Perinatal factors
- Premature birth
- Prolonged or difficult birth
- Kernicterus, especially from hemolytic disease

Postnatal factors
- Ear infection (chronic otitis media)
- Acute infection (mumps, rubella, measles, encephalitis, meningitis)
- Respiratory conditions (hypertrophied adenoids, allergy)
- Ototoxic drugs, including topical applications to the ear (kanamycin, streptomycin, gentamycin, neomycin, vancomycin, viomycin)
- Trauma (burns, frostbite, lacerations, perforations, bone fracture)
- Exposure to excessive noise (urban living, loud rock music, model airplanes, snowmobiles, sport shooting, motorcycle and sport racing, heavy machinery)

or "th" impossible; loss in the middle range eliminates hearing vowels, semivowels, and most consonants. Although the child hears some of everything going on around him, the sounds are distorted, resulting in discrimination and comprehension being severely affected. Medical/surgical intervention is rarely of any benefit. Since the defect is not one of intensity of sound, hearing aids are of little value in improving discrimination, since they merely amplify distorted sounds.

Mixed conductive-sensorineural hearing loss results from interference with transmission of sound in the middle ear and along neural pathways. It frequently results from recurrent otitis media, which causes damage to middle- and inner-ear structures. The conductive loss is more amenable to treatment and improvement with a hearing aid than the sensorineural component.

Table 24-1. Intensity of sounds expressed in decibels

Decibels (db)	Representative sound
0	Softest sound normal ear can hear
10	Heartbeat
20	Whisper at 5 feet
30-45	Normal conversation
70-80	Street noises
90-100	Train
120	Thunder
140	Jet airplane during departure

Central auditory imperception includes all hearing losses that do not demonstrate defects in the conductive or sensorineural structures. They are usually divided into organic or functional losses. In the organic type of central auditory imperception, the defect involves the reception of auditory stimuli along the central pathways and the expression of the message into meaningful communication. Terms used to describe such receptive-expressive disorders are *aphasia,* an inability to express ideas in any form, either written or verbally, *agnosia,* the inability to interpret sound correctly, and *dysacusis,* difficulty in processing details or discrimination among sounds. In each of these conditions the difficulty is in processing, patterning, and interpreting the information within the brain, not in hearing the sound. Perception of sound eventually becomes so confusing and distressing that it results in complete inhibition of response to all auditory stimuli. Consequently the aphasic child acts as if he were deaf.

In the functional type of central auditory imperception, there is no organic lesion to support a central auditory loss. Examples of functional hearing loss are conversion hysteria (an unconscious withdrawal from hearing to block remembrance of a traumatic event), infantile autism, and childhood schizophrenia. Another common type is psychogenic selective hearing loss, in which the child who is continually bombarded with auditory stimuli tunes out extraneous sounds. This is in contrast to selective sensorineural loss, in which the child has normal hearing for some frequencies and a substantial loss for others.

Symptom severity. Hearing loss is often expressed in decibels (db), a unit of loudness (Table 24-1). Hearing impairment is divided into two groups: those children who are hard of hearing and those who are deaf (Table 24-2). A child is considered legally deaf when hearing is depressed 80 db in the better ear (from 500 to 2000 cycles per second, the range of speech frequencies).[1]

Most deaf children have some perception of loud sounds

Table 24-2. Classification of hearing loss based on symptom severity

Hearing loss (db)	Effect
Slight—<30	Has difficulty in hearing faint or distant speech Usually is unaware of hearing difficulty Likely to achieve in school but may have problems No speech defects
Mild—30-45	Understands conversational speech at 3 to 5 feet but has difficulty if speech is faint or speaker is not in *en face* position May have speech difficulties
Moderate—45-60	Unable to understand conversational speech unless it is loud Considerable difficulty with group or classroom discussion May not be able to hear telephone conversation Requires special speech training
Severe—60-80	May hear a loud voice if nearby May be able to identify loud environmental noises Can distinguish vowels but not consonants of high frequency (s, z, ch, th) Requires speech training
Profound—<80	May hear only loud sounds Requires speech training

but no usable hearing. Their primary mode of communication is visual (lipreading or sign language). Children who are hard of hearing use auditory cues in conjunction with visual cues to communicate.

Detection of hearing impairment

Discovery of a hearing impairment within the first 6 to 12 months of life is essential to prevent social, physical, and psychologic damage to the child. Detection involves isolating those children who by virtue of their history are at risk, observing for behaviors that indicate a hearing loss, and screening all children for auditory function. This discussion focuses on developmental/behavioral indices associated with hearing impairment. Tests for assessing hearing are included in Chapter 5.

Infancy. At birth the nurse can observe the neonate's response to auditory stimuli as evidenced by the startle reflex, head turning, eye blinking, and cessation of body movement. The Brazelton Neonatal Behavioral Assessment Scale evaluates the infant's orientation response to the sound of a voice. Scoring is based on the following: (1) no reaction; (2) respiratory change or blink only; (3) general quieting as well as blink and respiratory changes; (4) stills, brightens, no attempt to locate source; (5) shifting of eyes to sound, as well as stills and brightens; (6) alerting and shifting of eyes and head turned to source; (7) alerting, head turned to stimulus, and searching with eyes; (8) alerting prolonged, head and eyes turned to stimulus repeatedly; and (9) turning and alerting to stimulus presented on both sides on every presentation of stimulus.[3] The infant may vary in the intensity of his response, depending on his state of alertness. However, a consistent score of "no reaction," especially with absence of the startle reflex, should lead the nurse to suspect hearing loss.

During infancy children demonstrate developmental changes in response to localizing a source of sound (see Chapter 12, p. 432.) Failure to orient to a sound and to attempt to localize it by age 6 months is an important clue to auditory loss. Other danger signals suggesting hearing problems in the developing infant include (1) persistence of the Moro reflex beyond age 4 months, (2) failure to be awakened or disturbed by loud environmental sounds during the first 4 months, (3) absence of babbling or voice inflection by age 7 months, (4) inability to understand words or short phrases by age 12 months, and (5) the consistent use of gestures rather than verbalization to indicate wants after age 15 months.

Childhood. The profoundly deaf child is much more likely to be diagnosed during infancy than the less severely affected one. If the defect is not detected during early childhood, the likelihood is that it will surface during entry to school, when the child has difficulty in learning. Unfortunately some of these children are erroneously placed in special classes for the learning disabled or the mentally retarded. Therefore, it is essential that the nurse suspect a hearing impairment in any child who demonstrates the following behaviors: (1) shows less interest than his peers in casual conversation; (2) is often inattentive unless the environment is quiet and the speaker is close to the child; (3) is more responsive to movement than to sound; (4) intently observes the speaker's face, responding more to facial expression than verbalization; (5) often asks to have statements repeated; (6) may not follow directions exactly; (7) tends to be shy, withdrawn, timid, and dreamy; and (8) tends to avoid social interaction with other children.[22] In response to the frustration of not being able to make others understand him, the child may develop temper tantrums, yelling, head banging, or other behavioral patterns.

Of primary importance is the effect of hearing impairment on speech development. A child with a mild conductive hearing loss may speak fairly clearly but in a loud voice. A child with a sensorineural or selective hearing loss usually has difficulty in articulation. Depending on the degree of loss, sounds of certain frequencies may not be audible. For example, inability to hear higher frequencies renders the child unable to perceive or to imitate some consonants, especially sounds such as "s," "z," "ch," and

Signs suggestive of hearing impairment in infants and young children

Orientation response
- Lack of startle or blink reflex to a loud sound
- Persistence of Moro reflex beyond 4 months of age (associated with mental retardation)
- Failure to be awakened by loud environmental noises during early infancy
- Failure to localize a source of sound by 6 months of age
- General indifference to sound
- Lack of response to the spoken word; failure to follow verbal directions
- Response to loud noises as opposed to the voice

Vocalizations and sound production
- Monotone quality, unintelligible speech, lessened laughter
- Normal quality in central auditory loss
- Lessened experimental sound play and squealing
- Normal use of jargon during early infancy in central auditory loss, with persistent use later on
- Absence of babble or inflections in voice by age 7 months
- Failure to develop intelligible speech by age 24 months
- Vocal play, head banging, or foot stamping for vibratory sensation
- Yelling or screeching to express pleasure, annoyance, or need
- Asking to have statements repeated or answering them incorrectly

Visual attention
- Augmented visual alertness and attentiveness
- Responding more to facial expression than verbal explanation
- Being alert to gestures and movement
- Use of gestures rather than verbalization to express desires, especially after age 15 months
- Marked imitativeness in play

Social rapport and adaptations
- Less interest and involvement in vocal nursery games
- Intense preoccupation with things rather than persons
- Avoidance of social interaction; often puzzled and unhappy in such situations
- Inquiring, sometimes confused facial expression
- Suspicious alertness, sometimes interpreted as paranoia, alternating with cooperation
- Marked reactivity to praise, attention, and physical affection

Emotional behavior
- Use of tantrums to call attention to self or his needs
- Frequently stubborn because of lack of comprehension
- Irritable at not making himself understood
- Shy, timid, and withdrawn
- Often appears "dreamy," "in a world of his own," or markedly inattentive

Adapted from Knobloch, H., and Pasamanick, B., editors: Gesell and Amatruda's developmental diagnosis, New York, 1974, Harper & Row, Publishers.

"th." Therefore, to the child who is unable to discriminate all sounds, the word "spoon" acoustically sounds like "poon." Consequently the child's speech will be a reflection of the distortion of sound.

A child with a central auditory hearing loss presents a special dilemma for diagnosis. During early infancy there is little or no evidence that the child has a hearing impairment because he responds normally to sounds. It is often impossible to ascertain that the child cannot interpret what is heard until 18 months of age or older, at which time associated behavioral characteristics become apparent.[15] At this age the child behaves as if he is deaf because he inhibits all response to sounds that are confusing and have little meaning for him.

Communication deficits are important clues to a central auditory hearing loss. The child with a mild loss learns language and can easily give stereotyped responses, such as his name, sex, address, or age. In other words, he can answer questions for which he has learned a patterned response. He can also make appropriate spontaneous remarks or comments. However, when asked a question, such as, "What's this?" (pointing to a shoe), he is unable to answer. He may continually repeat the question or answer it incorrectly. Parents frequently become irritated with the monotonous repetition or interpret the wrong response as evidence of stupidity.

He may also experience an inordinate amount of difficulty in learning the correct use of pronouns, especially "you" and "I." Although he may learn usable language, he is unable to manipulate it to express wants, answer questions, or engage in social conversation of any complexity. His speech is not as monotonous as that of a child with conductive or sensorineural loss, but it may be so limited that it seems inarticulate. Loud sounds (about 90 db) are irritating and even painful to the child; as a result he may inhibit such sounds as a banging door or a dropped plate but attend to sounds such as rustling paper or a verbal comment. Obviously such behaviors can lead one to seriously question the existence of a hearing deficit unless he has a high index of suspicion for each type of loss. The best rule to follow is that if the child *acts* as though he were deaf to the human voice, he should be treated as though he has a hearing impairment.[15]

Signs suggestive of hearing impairment in children are outlined in the boxed material. Of primary significance is the nurse's willingness to *listen* to parents' reports of suspicion regarding hearing loss.

Effects of hearing impairment

Loss of hearing affects speech, language, and social development. The severity of the handicap depends not only on the extent of the defect but on the age of occurrence, interval until diagnosis, and adequacy of rehabilitation. To understand the tremendous effect loss of hearing has on a young child, it is necessary to explore the role of hearing in normal childhood development.

The full-term infant is born with auditory sensitivity to all ranges of sound frequencies heard by human beings. From birth, and possibly before, sound acquaints the infant with events in the physical world. Significantly the sound of the mother's voice becomes an important component of maternal-infant bonding. Long before he understands the words, he learns the emotional intonations of what is said to him. Likewise, his vocal response, such as small throaty sounds or squeals, gives reciprocal satisfaction and meaning to the parents.

He learns from sounds in the environment what is expected of him. For example, when he cries and hears footsteps or his parents' voice, he associates them with anticipated meeting of his needs. He learns that quiet sounds, such as singing when he falls asleep, are soothing. He judges the emotional behavior of others by the way in which they inflect their voices in anger, praise, disapproval, sadness, or joy. From these cues he learns to relate in a complimentary manner.

Sounds associated with objects give them additional meaning. For example, a ride in the car is much more stimulating when one hears the myriad of sounds than if one hears only silence or distorted, confusing noise. Much of the child's initial knowledge about objects is related to the sound they make, such as animal sounds, the sound of a clock, and so on.

The infant learns speech from the pleasure derived from hearing his own voice, the reinforcement each vocalization evokes, and the usefulness of substituting words for gestures in expressing desires. By the end of the first year he listens to and discriminately behaves according to auditory cues. A primary example is his ability to stop an activity in response to the word "no." Although this may appear to be an insignificant act, it marks the beginning of deliberate socially acceptable behavior, ability to accept frustration, and recognition of a less egocentric existence.

Audition also has a motor component. Although less obvious than the effect of vision on motor development, hearing encourages the child to move rhythmically and later to run, jump, or rock in time with music and use facial muscles for singing. Sounds, such as banging for the resultant noise, striking piano keys for the different notes, or splashing water for the slapping sound, often encourage motor activity. Audition also alerts the child to potential danger, such as a car coming down the street, and to the need for various responses, such as answering the door and coming home when called.

The effect of hearing on academic learning is profound. Most learning is done through auditory cues, primarily verbal language. Even if other media are used, such as visual aids, the child must understand verbal directions concerning their use and meaning. If the child has some hearing and has learned compensatory visual skills, he may function well in a one-to-one relationship. However, he may have difficulty in school because of his placement distant to the teacher, the teacher's continuous movement while talking (walking back and forth, turning to a blackboard, looking down to a book), group discussions, and extraneous noise.

Socialization is dependent on communication. Although the infant relies heavily on nonauditory cues, such as vision and tactile sensations, for social interaction, language becomes increasingly important to social development during early childhood. Verbal symbols gradually replace gestures and by school age are a prerequisite for social relationships. The hearing-impaired child is at a great disadvantage. He is often unable to proceed past parallel play within a group because of his inability to follow directions during cooperative play. Even if he has speech, in a group setting his hearing deficit may not allow him to interpret enough of the conversation to join in. His inability to quickly grasp the meaning of a discussion often labels him by his peers as "slow," "square," or "dumb." As a result he learns to stay on the periphery or to avoid social interaction altogether. His self-concept becomes severely damaged, which may result in permanent emotional problems.

Nursing interventions with hearing-impaired children

Prevention. The primary nursing role is prevention of hearing loss. Since the most common cause of impaired hearing is chronic otitis media, it is essential that appropriate measures be instituted to treat existing infections and prevent recurrences. Since acute otitis media is usually treated with a 10-day course of oral antibiotics, the nurse's role is in ensuring parent compliance with the treatment regimen (see p. 577). Children with histories of ear or respiratory infections or any other condition known to increase the risk of hearing impairment should receive periodic auditory testing. Many conductive hearing losses benefit from medical/surgical therapy, such as the use of decongestants for eustachian tube blockage or tympanoplasty for a perforated drum. Allergic otitis can be managed by hyposensitization, avoidance of the allergens, and antihistamines.

Routine immunization eliminates the possibility of acquired sensorineural loss from rubella, mumps, and measles (encephalitis). Drugs used to treat infections should be used cautiously with avoidance of ototoxic agents. If such drugs are used, the nurse evaluates changes in the child's hearing for prompt recognition and discontinuation of therapy. Groups at special risk for receiving ototoxic antibiotics are premature or sick neonates and children with chronic illnesses, such as cystic fibrosis, immune-deficiency diseases, and conditions requiring immunosuppressant therapy, such as leukemia or nephrosis.

The nurse counsels pregnant women regarding the ne-

Assessment of child for impaired hearing

Family history
- Genetic disorders associated with hearing impairment
- Family members, especially siblings, with hearing disorders

Prenatal history
- Miscarriages
- Illnesses during pregnancy (rubella, syphilis, diabetes)
- Drugs taken
- Exposure to childhood diseases
- Toxemia

Delivery
- Duration of labor, type of delivery
- Fetal distress
- Presentation (especially breech)
- Drugs used
- Blood incompatibility

Birth history
- Apgar score
- Weight
- Associated anomalies
- Cyanosis, oxygen therapy
- Jaundice
- Transfusions

Past health history
- Immunizations
- Serious illnesses, childhood illnesses
- Convulsions
- High unexplained fevers
- Ototoxic drugs
- No history (adopted child)
- Frequency of colds, ear infections, allergies
- Surgical/medical treatment of ear problems
- Visual difficulties

Hearing and testing
- Parental concerns regarding hearing loss (what cues, at what age)
- Response to name calling, loud noises, sounds of different frequencies (crinkling paper, whisper, bell, rattle)
- Audiometric testing in several frequencies
- Use of screening tests (five-toy test, tuning fork, galvanic skin resistance, or EEG)

Motor development
- Age of sitting, standing, walking
- Level of independence in self-care, feeding, toileting, grooming

Speech development
- Age of babbling, first meaningful words, phrases
- Intelligibility of speech
- Present vocabulary

Adaptive behavior
- Play activities
- Socialization with other children
- Behaviors: temper tantrums, stubbornness, self-vexation, vibratory stimulus
- Educational achievement
- Recent behavioral/personality changes

cessity of early prenatal care, including genetic counseling for known familial disorders, avoidance of all ototoxic drugs, especially during the first trimester, tests to rule out syphilis, rubella, or blood incompatibility, medical management of maternal diabetes, control of alcoholism whenever possible, and adequate dietary intake. Since maternal rubella is the single most common cause of congenital sensorineural deafness, the nurse discusses the possibility of elective abortion in affected mothers.

Exposure to excessive noise pollution is a well-established cause of sensorineural hearing loss. In individuals who are exposed to loud noise, there are fewer sensory hairs lining the organ of Corti than in unaffected persons. These hairs are the direct pathways to cranial nerve VIII. Although exact criteria for damaging noise levels in infants and children are not firmly established, in adults the maximum sound intensity that does not produce sensorineural hearing loss is approximately 80 db. Depending on duration of exposure to sounds louder than 80 db, hearing loss may result.[5]

Children are exposed to a wide variety of high-intensity sounds, one of the most common of which is loud rock music. The greatest danger seems to be at dances, concerts, or discotheques where the noise levels reach between 120 and 140 db and persist for 3 or more hours.[27] The nurse should routinely assess the possibility of environmental noise pollution and advise children and parents of the potential danger. Signals suggesting exposure to excessive noise are ringing or buzzing in the ears and/or perceiving sounds as muffled or dull after leaving the source of the noise. It is recommended that when individuals engage in activities associated with high-intensity noise, such as flying model airplanes, target shooting, or snowmobiling, they wear ear protection such as earmuffs or earplugs (not ordinary dry cotton).[2]

Detection. Aside from prevention, the most important nursing responsibility is detection. Both prenatally and postnatally, the nurse must have a high index of suspicion for children who may have congenital hearing loss, as well as those who may be at risk for acquired auditory impairment (see the boxed material). In the nursery nurses routinely assess newborns' hearing by observing orientation responses to sound (startle reflex and detailed responses in the Brazelton Neonatal Behavioral Assessment Scale). During infancy and early childhood, simple orientation tests to grossly assess hearing are used. (Tests for screening auditory function are discussed in Chapter 5.) Any child suspected of a hearing loss because of either the history or a screening test is referred for specialized audiometric testing.

The value of a thorough history cannot be overemphasized. Parents' concerns about hearing deficits or behavior problems must be taken seriously. The nurse evaluates information from the history with the observations of the child. For example, many of the signs of central auditory imperception resemble those seen in autism. However, there are some notable differences, namely that the autistic child completely lacks normal social relationships, may have exceptional verbal skills that are rarely used for communicative purposes, and visually orients to objects but not to people. Likewise a deaf child may appear retarded but usually demonstrates nonverbal development appropriate for his age. An observant, knowledgeable nurse will be aware of these differences and make an appropriate referral. At the same time the nurse reassures parents that their concerns are valid, realizing that selective sensorineural or central auditory loss may be seen as confusing, often conflicting, evidence of hearing ability.

The nurse assesses speech development, response to hearing, past history of ear infections, and behavioral patterns (see p. 842). Since speech is a direct consequence of hearing sounds, the nurse evaluates the quality of speech as well as the quantity of vocabulary. Children with hearing impairment often have a monotone, flat type of speech. A deaf infant babbles and vocalizes the same sounds as a normal infant until age 6 to 8 months, when the sounds decrease and are of a different pitch and phonetic content. The deaf child also vocalizes a primitive sound, "amah," which parents may mistake for "mama."[6] The nurse carefully evaluates the pronunciation of words to ensure that meaningful speech has been learned. Articulation, especially loss of high or low frequencies, is noted. Loud speech may be a sign of conductive hearing loss, although it may also represent a learned behavior. The child's ability to use language in conversation that does not rely on stereotyped answers is assessed.

The nurse may need to specifically question parents about the child's response to hearing. Some children become so adept at learning visual cues that even a severe loss may go undetected. In particular the nurse inquires about response to vibratory sound, such as music, and to the human voice. Profoundly deaf children enjoy music and may be skillful dancers, not because they hear the sound, but because they sense the rhythm of the vibrations. Such behavior may be mistaken as evidence of hearing. Other clues to vibratory stimulus may be persistent banging activity, such as hammering pegs, playing musical instruments, placing hands against a radio to feel vibrations, or sudden attentiveness to loud noises, such as a door slamming.

Past history of ear disorders may lead to suspicion regarding conductive hearing loss. In addition to inquiry about ear or throat infection, respiratory allergies, colds, and tonsillitis, the nurse asks about treatment for each disorder and associated complications, such as a "draining" ear or sudden relief of pain (perforation of the membrane). Otoscopic examination may reveal areas of tympanic scarring, perforation, or obstruction. A foreign body or packed cerumen in the external canal is a common temporary cause of conductive hearing loss. If an obstruction is seen, the nurse refers the child to a physician for removal of the impaction. Return of normal hearing is frequently confirmed by the child's complaint that "everything is so loud."

The nurse listens for descriptions of behavior that parallel those seen in children with hearing impairment. Of special significance is the child's social interaction with peers. Although the child may have no difficulty in a one-to-one relationship, he often is unable to cope with a group situation because of few visual cues to supplement his comprehension. A child who does poorly in nursery or regular school, who has temper tantrums alternating with cooperative behavior, and who frequently seems frustrated in attempts to follow directions or make himself understood, may be a child who hears little of what is going on around him.

Since the deaf child's primary mode of learning is based on visual cues, the nurse also assesses him for visual problems, such as refractive errors, strabismus, and color blindness. It has been found that the incidence of eye defects is twice as common in hearing-impaired children as in normal children.[9,17] Although the precise nature of the association between visual and auditory deficiencies is unclear, it follows the frequent biologic adage that one physical defect is often accompanied by others. Correction of visual impairment when possible is essential to reduce additional handicaps to learning. When color blindness is present, teaching aids may need revision to eliminate the influence of color in learning situations.

Rehabilitation. Once the diagnosis of hearing impairment is made, parents may need extensive support to adjust to the shock of learning about their child's disability. This may be the first time they learn that the child's poor speech development and behavior problems are the result of a hearing deficit, not because of difficulty with his tongue, refusal to talk, or disobedience and naughtiness. Parents may need time to deal with guilt feelings over previous attempts to teach the child to talk or punishment for misbehavior.

Parents also need an opportunity to realize the extent of the hearing loss. Sometimes parents benefit from a demonstration of what it is like to be deaf or hard of hearing. For example, showing them a moving film without sound helps them appreciate the profound effect of living in a world devoid of hearing and the great difficulty in comprehending the spoken word. If the child has a selective hearing loss, the parents can better understand the distortion of sound and difficulty with discrimination if they are placed in a soundproof room and allowed to hear only the frequencies the child hears. Central auditory imperception is similar to hearing a foreign language with no understanding of the meaning of the words.

The nurse also explains the benefit of amplifying devices in different types of hearing impairment. Hearing aids are of value in conductive hearing losses, although all ambient noise is also amplified, often making conversational speech difficult to hear. However, if it is a sensorineural or central auditory loss, hearing aids are of little benefit and constitute only a minor part of rehabilitation, since they amplify distorted sound and are unable to conduct sounds the way the nerves do.

The parents will gradually need to adjust to the idea that the child's major obstacle will be in his development and use of language. The parents may benefit from being told that with appropriate teaching the child can learn receptive language skills. This step will precede his attempts to use expressive language, because he needs to know and understand what is being communicated to him before he can be expected to communicate expressively to others.

After the parents have been able to assimilate the magnitude of the burden of their child's loss, they may benefit from encouragement and support to set realistic goals for themselves and for their child. A deaf child's education cannot wait until he is 6 years old and is ready for school. It must begin as early as possible and be continued in the home, where the parents play a significant role in teaching and reinforcing language skills.

The nurse also discusses with parents how impaired hearing affects a child's normal development. For example, the infant with a hearing loss, especially in the moderate or greater range, is unaware of parental verbal cues. Consequently he is less likely to demonstrate the same degree of reciprocity in relating to his parents as a hearing child. However, he does attend to significant others by looking at them, nestling in their arms during holding, or quieting when his needs are met. The nurse stresses these behaviors to parents to help them in establishing meaningful contact with the infant. Although the child is unable to hear, the nurse encourages the parents to talk to him as they would a normal child, supplement his stimulation needs with visual and tactile cues, and relate to him in the *en face* position to help him learn facial expressions.

Rehabilitation training consists of learning lipreading (speech reading), sign language, and verbal communication. Since even profoundly deaf individuals have some residual hearing, a hearing aid is used to maximize this ability. Approaches to education depend on the severity of the hearing loss. Children with a slight loss usually do well with lipreading and favorable positioning to the speaker. Children with mild or greater losses require lipreading, hearing aid and auditory training, speech therapy, and sign language. Most of them are able to function in regular classroom settings, provided they have no additional handicaps.

The nurse's initial role in rehabilitation is to help the family accept the defect and participate in an auditory training program.* The parents are assisted in their ability to help the child understand the spoken word by waiting for the child's attention before they speak, speaking clearly and distinctly at eye level and in good lighting, facing the child directly, carrying on a conversation with the child in the same room and close to the speaker, and helping him focus on all sounds in his environment and talking to the child about them. The nurse encourages the parents to learn role modeling by attending the auditory clinic. It is important that the father be included in the educational process so that he learns to communicate with his child.

Hearing aids. The nurse should be familiar with the types of hearing aids (Table 24-3).* Basically the system consists

*A list of approved programs are available from the Alexander Graham Bell Association for the Deaf, 3417 Volta Place, Washington, D.C. 20007. Home training correspondence programs are sponsored by the John T. Tracy Clinic, 806 West Adams Blvd., Los Angeles, Calif.

*A booklet, *Facts about hearing and hearing aids: a consumer's guide*, is available from the United States Department of Commerce, National Bureau of Standards, Washington, D.C. 20234.

Table 24-3. Types of hearing aids

Type	Description
In the ear	Aid fits directly in the ear canal, supported by the ear shell Has volume control but may have no tone control Very light in weight Useful if hearing loss is mild
Behind the ear	Aid is housed in a small curved case that fits behind the ear Microphone, amplifier, and receiver are housed in the case and connected to the ear mold by a plastic tubing Useful with hearing losses in the mild to severe range More comfortable, less conspicuous, and eliminates sound of fabric rubbing on aid that is common with on-the-body type
On the body or pocket	Microphone, amplifier, and power supply are enclosed in a case worn in a pocket or attached to clothing External receiver is attached directly to ear mold and is powered through a flexible wire from the amplifier Powerful aids for severe hearing losses Controls are easy to adjust Some models have variable tone control to selectively strengthen or diminish sounds Sturdier than in-the-ear or behind-the-ear type aids Fabric rubbing against case produces excessive annoying noise
Eyeglass model	Similar to behind-the-ear models except that the aid is built into the eyeglass frame Convenient for binaural (two-ear) hearing aids

of a tiny *microphone,* which picks up sound waves and converts them into electrical signals, an *amplifier,* which increases the strength of the electrical signals, a *receiver* or loudspeaker, which converts the amplified signals back into sound waves and directs them into the ear via a specially fitted *ear mold,* and a *battery* source, which provides electrical current for operation of the device.

Hearing aids are expensive and require care to maintain optimum functioning. The nurse should be familiar with basic care and handling of the device, especially when the child is hospitalized (Table 24-4). One of the most common problems with the device is an annoying whistling sound, usually caused by improper fit of the ear mold. If this occurs it may be remedied by reinserting it, making certain that no hair is caught between the ear mold and canal, cleaning the ear mold or ear, or lowering the volume of the aid. Sometimes the whistling may be at a frequency that the child cannot hear but that is annoying to others. The child should be told of the noise and asked to readjust the aid.

Table 24-4. Care of hearing aids

Part	Instructions for care
Hearing aid casing	Store it away from high heat or excessive cold Keep it dry; remove during hair washing, showering, or swimming Avoid dropping or bumping it Remove it when using hair spray or a hair dryer Turn switch to off *before* removing aid to prevent accidental drain on the batteries
Ear mold	Keep it clean, detach it from receiver, and wash in soap and water; dry thoroughly If opening becomes clogged with wax, clean it gently with a pipe cleaner Do not use alcohol or other cleaning solutions
Batteries	Store extra batteries in a cool, dry place If stored in refrigerator, allow them to warm to room temperature before using If carried in a pocketbook, wrap them in plastic to avoid accidental contact with a metal object Remove batteries from the aid when it is not worn Keep battery contacts clean (remove residue with a pencil eraser) Insert batteries correctly (proper negative and positive charges to contacts)
Tubing and cord	Avoid twisting the cord or bending the tubing Replace worn-out tubing or too short cord (on-the-body model)
Microphone	Check microphone openings; if clogged, wipe off particles with a *dry* cloth Do not use damp cloth or pipe cleaner to open holes; consult hearing aid dealer for advice

As the child grows older, he may be self-conscious of the device. Every effort should be made to make the aid inconspicuous, such as an appropriate hairstyle to cover behind-the-ear or in-the-ear models, attractive frames for glasses, and placement of the on-the-body type where it is not seen, such as under a blouse or sweater. The child should be given responsibility for the care of his device as soon as he is able, since fostering independence is a primary goal of rehabilitation.

Lipreading. Even though the child may become expert at lipreading, only about 40% of the spoken word is understood, and less if the speaker has a mustache or a beard. Exaggerating pronunciation or speaking in an altered rhythm (too slow or too fast) further lessens comprehension. The child learns to supplement the spoken word with sensitivity to visual cues, primarily body language and facial expression (tightening the lips, muscle tension, eye contact, and so on).

Sign language. The child who is severely or profoundly deaf is usually taught sign language and is encouraged to supplement talking with his mouth with "talking" using his hands. Unfortunately this method of communication is useful only when the other person understands the symbols. Family members are encouraged to learn sign language because hands require much less concentration to watch than lipreading. Sign language also enables some deaf children to learn more and to learn faster.

Speech therapy. The most formidable task in the education of a deaf child is learning to speak. Speech is learned through a multisensory approach, using visual, tactile, kinesthetic, and auditory stimulation. Since the usual mechanism for learning language is not available to the deaf child, namely, through imitation and reinforcement, systematic formal education is required. Parents should be encouraged to participate fully in the learning process. For example, language that serves a useful purpose is taught. Teaching is related to significant and meaningful experiences. The home environment fosters an atmosphere in which language is used and books are read. While spontaneous language is encouraged, poor articulation, rhythm, and voice quality are corrected.

As the deaf child learns to compensate for his lack of hearing, he becomes extremely perceptive to visual and vibratory changes. He often knows when another person wishes to talk to him because the person will walk close by him but not pass. He learns to be alert to other people approaching him by seeing their shadows or feeling the vibrations of their footsteps. He is acutely aware of facial expressions and may comprehend the unspoken word more quickly than the spoken word. However, this constant alertness and sensitivity to all environmental cues is exhausting. These children often need extra sleep or rest periods when they are alone and able to relax.

Everyday activities present problems to the older child. For example, he may not be able to hear the telephone, doorbell, or alarm clock. Several commercial devices are available to help the deaf person adjust to these dilemmas. Flashing lights can be attached to a telephone or doorbell to signal its ringing. Recently, trained hearing ear dogs have provided great assistance to deaf individuals because they alert the person to sounds, such as someone approaching, a moving car, a signal to wake up, a child's cry, and so on. Special teletypewriters help deaf people communicate with each other over the telephone because the typed message is conveyed via the telephone lines.

Since socialization is extremely important to the child's development, the nurse discusses with the family methods of fostering social contact. If the child attends a special school for the deaf, he is able to socialize with peers in that setting. Many programs specifically focus on the ability to relate to peers in a group situation by providing classroom and recreational activities. Classmates become a potential source of close friendships since they communicate more easily among themselves. Parents should be encouraged to promote these relationships whenever possible.

The child with a hearing impairment may need special help in school or social activities. Since lipreading is the main mode of receptive communication, the environment should facilitate visualization of the speaker's face, such as good lighting, favorable seating close to the speaker, and as much eye contact as possible. Since many of these children are able to attend regular classes, the teacher may need assistance in adapting methods of teaching for the child's benefit. The school nurse is often in an optimum position to emphasize methods of facilitated communication, such as speaking while facing the class, standing still rather than walking back and forth, and refraining from speaking when turning away from the group. Since group projects and audiovisual teaching aids may hinder the deaf child's learning, these educational methods should be carefully evaluated.

When the child is in a group setting, it is helpful for the other members to sit in a semicircle in front of him so that he can see their faces. Since one of the difficulties in following a group discussion is that the deaf child is unaware of who speaks next, it helps to have someone point out each speaker. This can inconspicuously be accomplished by giving each speaker a number or using his name and marking this down as that person talks. If one person writes down the main topic of the discussion, the child is able to follow lipreading more closely. Such suggestions can increase the child's ability to participate in sports, clubs such as Boy Scouts or Girl Scouts, and group projects.

If the child and family are to be followed on a longitudinal basis, the nurse will have to learn the teaching techniques being employed, whether they are sign language, lipreading, or enhancing speaking through extrasensory modalities. The nurse should be aware of the educational objectives of the school curriculum so that he or she can check with the parents on their perceptions of the educational goals and determine if these are perceived as compatible with the parents' goals. The nurse should be aware of subject matter being taught at school and know if a plan of continuity has been made for carry-over and consistency into the child's home setting.

The nurse must learn and become knowledgeable about diagnostic reports (medical, audiologic, and psychologic) so that their meaning can be interpreted and explained to parents when they ask questions or seem perplexed by the meaning of the diagnosis or treatment. It is very important that the nurse know what the parents have been told and what this information means to them. In addition the nurse must be astute and acutely aware of available community agencies and special programs (and their standards) so that parents can be referred when they have needs for information about medical, psychiatric, educational, or vocational programs. A summary of nursing care of the hearing-impaired child is listed in the box on pp. 847 to 848.

Caring for hospitalized deaf children

The needs of the hospitalized deaf child are the same as those of any other child, but his disability presents special challenges to the nurse. For example, the nurse must supplement verbal explanations as the primary method of preparation for admission or procedures with tactile and visual aids, such as books or actual demonstration and practice. The nurse needs to constantly reassess the child's understanding of the explanation. If the child's verbal skills are poorly developed, he can answer questions through drawing, writing, or gesturing. For example, if the nurse is attempting to clarify where a spinal tap is done, the child should be asked to point to where the doctor will insert the needle. Since deaf children often need more time to grasp the full meaning of an explanation, the nurse is careful not to judge the slowness as a sign of retardation.

When communicating with the child, the nurse uses the same principles as those that are outlined for facilitating lipreading. The nurse also makes certain that the child's hearing aid is working properly. If it is necessary to awaken the child at night, the nurse gently shakes him to signal his or her presence or turns on the hearing aid before arousing the child. The nurse always makes sure that the child can see him or her before any procedures, even routine ones such as changing a diaper or regulating an infusion, are per-

Summary of nursing care of the hearing-impaired child

Goals	Responsibilities
Prevention	Identify pregnant women at risk Counsel pregnant women regarding risk of ingesting ototoxic medications Isolate pregnant women from exposure to rubella if their immune titers are low Encourage immunization of all females against rubella Participate in immunization programs for children Assess hearing ability of children who are receiving ototoxic antibiotics Promote compliance with treatment regimens for otitis media Discuss with parents measures to prevent otitis media (see p. 577) Evaluate auditory ability of children prone to chronic ear or respiratory problems Assess sources of excessive noise in child's environment; institute appropriate measures to decrease sound levels (turn music lower, use ear protection)
Detection	At birth assess neonate's response to a loud noise; observe for signs associated with congenital deafness At each well-baby visit assess orientation responses; as early as possible administer hearing tests and refer for audiometry Listen carefully to parents' concerns regarding hearing loss Take a thorough history regarding factors that support an auditory impairment (see p. 840); carefully evaluate speech development Observe for behaviors that may suggest a hearing impairment Test child for visual problems that may interfere with learning to lip-read or use sign language
Rehabilitation	
Assist the family in adjusting to child's loss of hearing	Anticipate the usual grief reaction to loss Help parents deal with any guilt feelings regarding previous responses to child when true nature of the problem was unknown Help parents realize extent of child's disability and its tremendous influence on speech and language development Discuss advantages and limitations of amplifying devices with different types of hearing loss Encourage formal rehabilitation as soon as possible
Promote parent-child attachment	Help parents identify clues other than verbal ones that signify infant's communication with them Encourage parents to stimulate child with visual and tactile cues; stress importance of continuing to talk to child even though he may not hear their voice Encourage parents to discuss their feelings regarding attachment process
Promote communication process	Encourage both parents to attend the rehabilitation program in order to continue learning in the home; encourage them to learn sign language Teach language that serves a useful purpose Encourage use of language and books in the home Encourage spontaneous language but correct speech impairments
Facilitate lipreading	Attract the child's attention before speaking Speak clearly and distinctly; do not exaggerate pronunciation or rhythm of words Stand at eye level with child Face child directly; do not turn away to show him something while talking or move back and forth Ensure that speaker's face is well illuminated Stand close to child while speaking, but do not shout

Continued.

Summary of nursing care of the hearing-impaired child—cont'd

Goals	Responsibilities
Rehabilitation—cont'd	
Maximize residual hearing	Help family investigate reliable hearing aid dealers Discuss types of hearing aids and their proper care (Tables 24-3 and 24-4) Teach child how to regulate hearing aid for maximum benefit Help child focus on all sounds in his environment and talk to him about them For older child, discuss methods of camouflaging the aid to make it less conspicuous
Promote independence and development	Help family transfer normal child-rearing practices to this child Emphasize importance of attaining independence in self-care Provide child with devices that foster independence (hearing ear dog, special signaling aids for telephone or door bell) Discuss importance of discipline and limit setting Stress child's need for additional rest to meet the demands of his environment
Provide opportunities for play and socialization	Guide parents in selection of toys that maximize visual and tactile senses, as well as residual hearing Encourage child to participate in group activities; help him follow group discussion by pointing out the speaker and arranging the group in a semicircle Help him develop friendships among hearing and deaf peers Help him achieve a sense of security in his ability to compete with his peers
Encourage education within a regular classroom	Discuss with teacher ways of communicating effectively with child (such as through facilitating lipreading) Promote socialization with his classmates
Provide emotional support	Be available to the family for assistance Encourage family members to discuss their feelings regarding the disability Stress child's abilities rather than disability If following the family on a longitudinal basis, become familiar with techniques used for communication Refer family to appropriate community agencies for medical, psychiatric, educational, vocational, or financial assistance Involve parents in local parent groups for deaf children

formed. It is important to remember that the child may not be aware of one's presence until alerted through visual or tactile cues.

Ideally the nurse encourages parents to room with the child. However, it must be conveyed to them that this is not to serve as a convenience to the nurse but as a benefit to the child. Although the parents' aid can be enlisted in familiarizing the child with the hospital and explaining procedures, the nurse also talks directly to him, encouraging expression of his feelings about the experience. If the nurse has difficulty in understanding the child's speech, an effort is made to become familiar with his pronunciation of words. Parents often can be helpful by explaining the child's usual speech habits.

The nurse should honestly admit if the child cannot be understood, and he should be encouraged to write his statements. However, at no time does the nurse imply that the child's speech is inferior. Rather the nurse lets the child know that it will take some time to become familiar with his words and that in the meantime he can help by using gestures or written messages. Expressing an interest in learning sign language, especially useful words, such as yes, no, water, toilet, and so on, not only improves communication efforts but greatly strengthens the nurse-child-parent relationship.

The nurse has a special role as child advocate with the deaf. The nurse is in a strategic position to alert other health team members and other patients to the child's special needs regarding communication. For example, the nurse should accompany the physician on visits to the child's room to ensure that the physician speaks to the child and that the child understands what was said. Not infrequently care givers forget that the child has the abilities to perceive and learn despite a hearing loss and consequently communicate only with the parents. As a result, the child's needs and feelings remain unrecognized and unmet.

Since deaf children often have difficulty in forming social relationships with other children, the nurse introduces the child to his roommates and encourages them to engage in play activities. The hospital setting can provide growth-promoting opportunities for social relationships. With the assistance of a play therapist, the child can learn new recreational activities, experiment with group games, and engage in therapeutic play. The use of puppets, dollhouses, role playing with dress-up clothes, building with a hammer and nails, finger painting, needle play, and water play can help the deaf child express feelings that previously were suppressed.

VISION IMPAIRMENT

Scope of the problem

Serious visual impairments occur in approximately one of every 1000 school-age children. There are nearly 70,000 visually impaired children aged birth to 19 years, and about 24,000 of whom are enrolled in special education programs.[13] These figures do not take into account the number of children with refractory errors that require corrective lenses. It is estimated that about 7½ million school children have some type of visual difficulty, yet only one fourth will demonstrate symptoms.[18] The other three fourths require specific testing to identify the problem. The nurse's role is clearly one of detection, referral, and in some instances rehabilitation.

Classification of visual defects

Visual defects are legally classified as *blind,* a corrected vision of 20/200 or less or peripheral vision (tunnel vision) of less than 20 degrees in the better eye, and *partially seeing,* corrected vision between 20/200 and 20/70. Visual defects are also divided into congenital and acquired types. Any child who suffers a loss of vision before the age of 5 or 6 years is classified for educational purposes as a child with a congenital visual defect. Children who lose their sight before the age of 6 years are unable to retain much visual imagery and memory of color as they get older. The impact of a loss of vision after the age of 5 years has different implications, both emotionally for the child as well as for the provision of educational services. The child who is newly blinded may retain the basic process of reading and transfer this to new learning of the braille system.[28]

Causes of visual impairment

The etiology of visual impairment can be classified according to the following divisions: (1) familial factors, including genetic diseases associated with visual defects, such as Tay-Sachs disease or inborn errors of metabolism; (2) prenatal/intrauterine factors, especially maternal infections such as rubella, syphilis, or toxoplasmosis; (3) perinatal factors, including prematurity and oxygen toxicity (retrolental fibroplasia); and (4) postnatal factors, primarily trauma, infections (mumps, measles, rubella, poliomyelitis and chickenpox), and disorders such as juvenile rheumatoid arthritis, leukemia, and myasthenia gravis. The following discussion focuses on the most common types of visual disorders in children.

Refractive errors. The term refraction means "bending" and refers to the bending of light rays as they pass through the lens of the eye. Normally light rays enter the lens and fall directly on the retina, usually at the fovea centralis (center of the macula), the region of greatest visual acuity. However, in refractive disorders the light rays either fall in front of the retina (myopia) or beyond it (hyperopia) (Fig. 24-1). Children are normally hyperopic until 5 to 6 years of age, at which time their visual acuity approaches 20/20. This is an important fact to remember when screening children for refractive errors, since hyperopia in children in this age-group does not require correction. (See p. 432 for a summary of the development of vision in young children.)

Three reflexes—accommodation, convergence, and pupillary constriction—are necessary to bring the image into clear focus. The *accommodation reflex* focuses the image sharply on the retina. It causes an increase in the curvature of the lens, constriction of the pupils, and convergence of two eyes. The reflex depends on contraction of the ciliary muscle to change the lens to a more convex shape, thus increasing refractive power. As an object is brought to close range, the pupils constrict (pupillary contraction), and, as the object is moved farther away, the pupils dilate (pupillary relaxation).

The *convergency reflex* permits the object seen through each eye to focus on corresponding areas on the retina (binocularity). Convergence refers to the movement of the eyeballs inward as an object is brought closer to the face. The nearer the object, the greater the degree of convergence. When the eyes do not converge, two images are produced (diplopia).

For an object to be seen there must exist adequate illumination. The amount of light entering the retina is controlled by the *pupillary reflex.* In bright light the pupils constrict; in dim light the pupils dilate. If a bright light is shown into one eye, both eyes constrict (consensual light reflex). Changes in pupillary size are a function of the iris and are controlled by the smooth muscles that surround this pigmented structure.

Refractive errors are evaluated by testing visual acuity (see Chapter 5). They are best assessed by eliminating the accommodative powers of the eye with the use of a cycloplegic drug, such as atropine, that paralyzes the ciliary muscles (Table 24-5).

Myopia. Myopia or nearsightedness refers to the ability

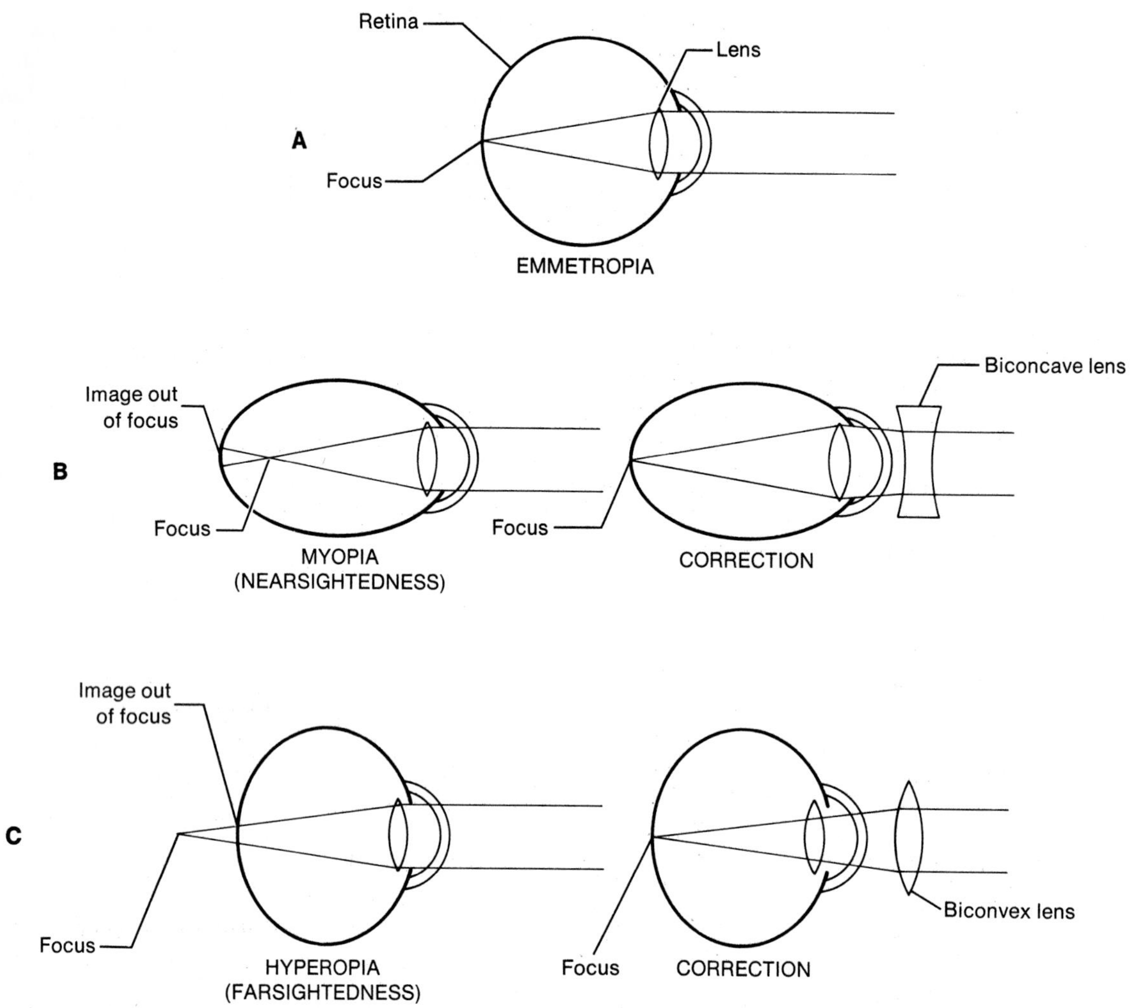

Fig. 24-1. Comparison of normal vision and refractive errors. **A,** Emmetropia (normal vision). **B,** Myopia (nearsightedness). **C,** Hyperopia (farsightedness).

to see objects clearly at close range but not at a distance. In most instances it results from an eyeball that is too long, resulting in the focal point falling in front of the retina. The eye possesses no ability to accommodate itself to this condition. Only when objects are brought close to the eye so that the image falls on the retina is vision clear. The child often squints in an attempt to try and correct the defect.

Correction involves the use of biconcave lenses, which cause the parallel rays to diverge, thus permitting the lens of the myopic eye to focus the two rays on the retina (see Fig. 24-1). Unfortunately myopia tends to increase in severity until adulthood. There is evidence to suggest that the use of hard contact lenses retards myopia by preventing further changes in the curvature of the eyeball.

Some children have congenital myopia. Unlike the acquired type, vision tends to improve with age and approaches normal acuity by adolescence. However, very young children may need to wear corrective lenses if the defect is severe.

Hyperopia (hypermetropia). Hyperopia or farsightedness is the reverse of myopia. The eyeball is too short in length; as a result rays of light are theoretically focused behind the retina. These children can see objects clearly at a distance and, because of their accommodative ability, can usually see objects in close range. However, the continual muscular effort produces eyestrain and may result in strabismus from overexertion of the ciliary muscles.

Correction involves the use of convex lenses that bend the light rays so that the lens of the eye can focus them on the retina (Fig. 24-1). Controversy exists over whether hyperopic children should wear corrective lenses; however, if close work is impaired or causes excessive eyestrain, corrective lenses are recommended.

Astigmatism. The refractive surfaces of the eye are rarely

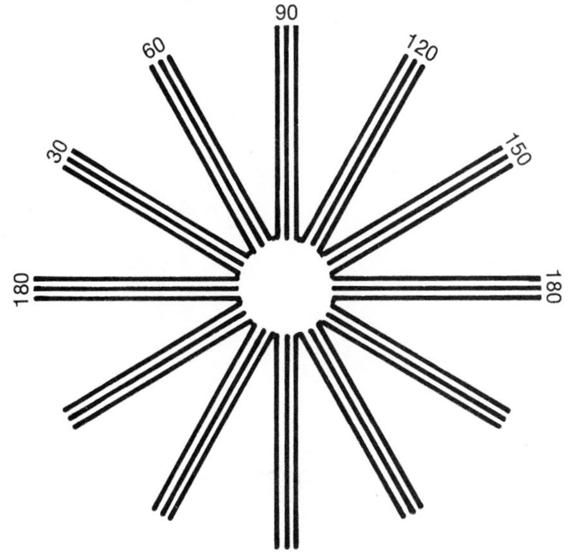

Fig. 24-2. Chart for astigmatism.

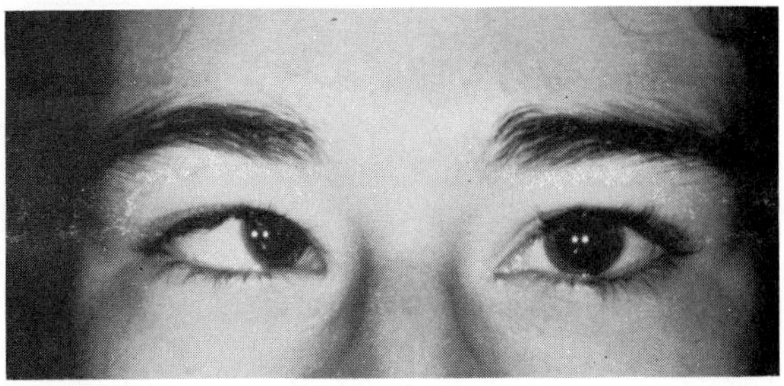

Fig. 24-3. Strabismus. Note the obvious malalignment of the eyes. The light reflections are centered in the left cornea and to the side of the right cornea. (From Havener, W. H., Saunders, W. H., Keith, C. F., and Prescott, A. W.: Nursing care in eye, ear, nose, and throat disorders, ed. 3, St. Louis, 1974, The C. V. Mosby Co., p. 99.)

perfectly spherical. Normally the imperfection is so slight that it does not interfere with refraction or vision. In astigmatism there are unequal curvatures in the cornea or lens so that light rays are bent into different directions, producing a blurred image. Although the eye attempts to accommodate for the distortion, it is unsuccessful, causing eyestrain.

Correction involves the use of specially ground lenses that compensate for the errors in refraction. A special chart is used for astigmatism in order to isolate the exact location of deviation in curvatures along the meridians (Fig. 24-2). Astigmatism may occur with or without other refractive disorders.

Amblyopia. Amblyopia is a reduced visual acuity in one eye that is not related to obvious structural or pathologic anomalies, such as cataract, scarred cornea, or retrolental fibroplasia.[21] It is diagnosed by at least a two-line difference in Snellen testing between two eyes, such as 20/20 in the right eye and 20/30 in the left eye.[25] Although amblyopia ex anopsia (dimness of vision from nonuse) is usually the result of strabismus, it also occurs with unequal refractive errors in each eye (anisometropia). In the latter instance the child has straight eyes. If visual testing is not done with one eye occluded, the child will use his better eye and the amblyopia will be undetected.

Normally the two eyes work as a unit (binocular vision). Images of an object are focused on the retina of each eye and passed to the brain so that the images are seen as one (fusion). When fusion is disrupted, each retina receives two different images, resulting in diplopia (double vision). The brain accommodates for the visual confusion by suppressing the less intense image (those light rays that fall adjacent to but not directly on the macula). If the defect is not corrected, the macular suppression scotoma (visual blind spot) becomes permanent, resulting in loss of vision in the weaker eye.

The optimal time for correction of amblyopia is during early childhood. The treatment consists of patching the good eye so that the child will be forced to use the weaker eye. If refractive errors are present, corrective lenses are worn. It is more difficult to encourage school-age children to wear the occlusive patch because the poor visual acuity of the uncovered weaker eye interferes with schoolwork and the patch sets them apart from their peers.

Strabismus. Strabismus, which literally means squinting, refers to malalignment of the eyes (Fig. 24-3). The types of, and screening tests for, strabismus have been discussed in Chapter 5. The esodeviations are divided into two groups: accommodative and nonaccommodative. In the *accommodative* type the visual axis for distance seeing is parallel and binocular. However, when the object is brought to close range and accommodation is necessary for fixation, fusion is disrupted and an esotropia or esophoria is evident. The child attempts to produce clearer vision by squinting, which forces convergence through increased muscle strength. Accommodative strabismus is believed to be the result of a defect in the innervation of the medial rectus and ciliary muscles. It may or may not be present with excessive hyperopia.

The diagnostic features of this type of strabismus include (1) onset between 2 to 3 years of age, at which time the child begins to use accommodation to see small objects closely; (2) orthophoric eyes when seeing distant objects and malaligned eyes when viewing close objects; (3) disappearance of the squint when accommodation is removed, such as with the use of cycloplegic drugs; (4) a tendency for the esophoria to become constant (esotropia), with the risk of amblyopia ex anopsia developing; and (5) often a family history of a positive esophoria that developed after 1 year of age.[31]

Table 24-5. Classification of ophthalmic drugs

Classification	Action	Uses	Side effects	Comments
Cholinergic Pilocarpine Carbachol (Carcholin) Acetylcholine chloride (Miochol)	Chemically related to acetylcholine, the neurohormone that mediates nerve impulse transmission at all cholinergic or parasympathetic nerve sites Miosis—contraction of the sphincter muscle of the iris, resulting in pupillary constriction Decreased accommodation for near vision—causes spasms of the ciliary muscle and deepening of the anterior chamber Decreased intraocular pressure—causes vasodilatation of vessels where intraocular fluids exit from the eye	Antidote for short-acting anticholinergic drugs During ocular surgery to reduce risk of imprisoning iris tissue at limbus during wound closure Strabismus Glaucoma	Visual blurring Headaches Difficulty in adjusting to changes in light, especially at nighttime Spasm of the wink reflex Irritation of external structure of the eye Cysts of iris or synechiae Retinal detachment Obstruction to tear drainage Cataracts Systemic effects Decreased blood pressure Sweating Salivation Flushing Diarrhea Abdominal cramps Enuresis May precipitate asthmatic attack (bronchospasm)	Apply pressure to lacrimal duct, and wipe excess fluid away promptly to prevent its flow into the lacrimal system and systemic circulation Advise individual of possible difficulty of seeing in the dark and temporary blurring of vision Administer cautiously to anyone with asthma or low blood pressure Warn parents of possibility of bed-wetting Shorter acting than anticholinesterase drugs In chronic glaucoma, drug of choice over anticholinesterase agents because side effects are less frequent and less severe
Anticholinesterase Isoflurophate Fluorophosphate (Floropryl) Physostigmine salicylate (Eserine salicylate) Neostigmine bromide (Prostigmin) Demecarium bromide (Humorsol) Echothiopate iodide (Phospholine iodide)	Inhibits the enzymatic (cholinesterase) destruction of acetylcholine Action is similar to cholinergic drugs, but longer acting	Same as above	Same as above	Same as above Prolonged use lowers blood cholinesterase activity; instruct parents to inform surgeon of the fact that the child is receiving miotics, since they may interfere with certain anesthetic agents (succinylcholine) and result in muscle paralysis and apnea

Anticholinergic Atropine Scopolamine Homatropine Cyclopentolate hydrochloride (Cyclogyl) Tropicamide (Mydriacyl)	Blocks the actions of acetylcholine Mydriasis—blocks innervation of the circular smooth muscles of the iris, which normally constrict the pupil Cycloplegia—paralyzes the ciliary muscle, preventing accommodation	Atropine—antidote to cholinergic drugs Relieves pain in inflammatory conditions such as uveitis and keratitis; places eye at rest Ophthalmic (fundoscopic) examination Postoperatively to prevent synechiae and pupillary occlusion During examination for refractive errors Strabismus	Ocular effects—pupillary dilatation can cause sharp rise in intraocular pressure, aggravating glaucoma Systemic effects Dryness of the mouth Flushing Tachycardia Fever Inhibition of sweating Delirium Coma	Mydriatics produce less response in persons with deeply pigmented irides than in persons with lightly pigmented irides Advise individual of impairment of close vision as a result of loss of accommodation Dilated eyes are sensitive to light; encourage use of tinted glasses Instruct parents to omit next dose if systemic side effects occur (dryness of mouth, flushing, and so on) *Contraindicated in glaucoma*
Adrenergic Epinephrine Hydroxyamphetamine hydrobromide (Paredrine) Phenylephrine hydrochloride (Neo-Synephrine)	Acts on the sympathetic nervous system Mydriasis—causes contraction of the radial or dilator muscle of the eye Decreased intraocular pressure—decreases formation of aqueous humor and increases outflow Decreased congestion—constricts conjunctival blood vessels Slight relaxation of ciliary muscle	Ocular examination Wide-angle glaucoma Ocular congestion and hyperemia	Eye pain Ocular irritation Tearing Systemic effects—tachycardia and elevated blood pressure	Give cautiously to individuals with cardiovascular disease Do not administer to individuals with narrow-angle glaucoma (mydriasis restricts ocular fluid outflow)
Carbonic anhydrase inhibitors Acetazolamide (Diamox) Ethoxzolamide (Cardrase) Methazolamide (Neptazane) Dichlorphenamide (Daranide)	Inhibits the enzyme carbonic anhydrase, one of the substances necessary for the production of aqueous humor	Glaucoma	Lethargy Anorexia Numbness Tingling of face and extremities Diuresis, loss of potassium	Given as oral preparation Teratogenic—avoid use during first trimester of pregnancy Encourage foods rich in potassium Stress importance of regular administration of drug

Treatment involves the use of eye patching, corrective lens for excessive hyperopia or the use of anticholinesterase agents to reduce accommodation, and adjunctive orthoptic exercises to improve muscular coordination. The latter measure is controversial and usually reserved for mild cases. Anticholinesterase agents (see Table 24-5) are used instead of eyeglasses in very young children or in older children who refuse to wear them. A particular advantage to the use of these drugs over optical correction is that when the accommodative defect is combined with excessive hyperopia, appropriate accommodation is controlled for all distances. When bifocal lenses are used (a system of two lenses to decrease accommodation), they only provide correction for seeing close and distant objects but not for intermediate ranges.

Nonaccommodative esodeviation includes selected cases of accommodative squint in which muscular dysfunction develops from constant overconvergence and congenital types, usually caused by abnormal muscles, abnormal attachments to the globe, or imbalance between the medial and lateral rectus muscles. In either case treatment is surgical either to weaken the muscles (myectomy or myotomy) or tendonous attachment (tenectomy or tenotomy) or to strengthen them.

Another important cause of strabismus is any lesion that impairs vision in one eye, such as cataracts, corneal opacities, chorioretinitis, and retinal detachment. Acquired strabismus is one of the earliest signs of optic atrophy from brain tumors and retinoblastoma (see Chapter 28). Therefore, early recognition of squint cannot be overemphasized to prevent amblyopia or detect associated disorders.

The goal in treating strabismus is preservation of vision, binocularity, and improvement in cosmetic appearance. However, all of these goals may not be achieved. Fortunately lack of binocularity is not a serious handicap for most children. However, it does result in failure to develop stereopsis or depth perception, the ability to locate an object in spatial relationship to another object. The individual has difficulty in judging distances, such as when driving a car or reaching for a close object, and when using binocular instruments, such as a microscope or field glasses.

Cosmetic effects can be difficult for older children. Peers may taunt them with remarks such as "cross-eyed." Other children often have difficulty in looking directly at them because the wandering eye is distracting. This may force the speaker to look away, making the person with strabismus feel insecure. If this occurs the best advice is to look directly at the focusing or straight eye and avoid contact with the deviated eye, since the person then receives a clear, direct image.

Cataracts. A cataract is an opacity of the crystalline lens. Since the lens is normally transparent to allow light rays to enter the eye and refract them for a clear image on the retina, a cataract interferes with both of these functions. Cataracts may be congenital, such as those caused by maternal rubella during the first trimester, or acquired, most commonly as a result of penetrating injuries or, less frequently, as a secondary complication to diseases such as galactosemia.

Congenital cataracts are removed as early as possible (usually between 6 months to 3 years of age) to preserve useful vision, since the early childhood years are critical for development of visual reflexes. If monocular congenital cataracts are not removed early, permanent blindness from amblyopia results. Removal at an early age results in useful vision because the eyes have had an opportunity to develop fixation reflexes. Lens are worn or implanted surgically to compensate for the lost refractive power of the lens.

Several surgical techniques are available for removal of the lens. One of the most widely used procedures is phacoemulsification, which entails the use of high-frequency ultrasonic vibrations combined with controlled irrigation to maintain normal ocular pressure in the anterior chamber and aspiration of the lens fragments through a needle. It requires only a minute 2- to 3-mm incision at the limbus (corneal-scleral junction).[23]

Postoperative recovery with this procedure is short (2 to 3 days), involves no eye patching, requires only limited activity restriction, and is associated with little pain. Mydriatics (Table 24-5) are used to keep the pupil dilated to prevent posterior synechiae formation (adhesion of the iris to the lens capsule or face of the vitreous) and occlusion of the pupil, which can lead to glaucoma. Steroid drops are administered to reduce postsurgical inflammation.

Glaucoma. Glaucoma refers to a condition in which intraocular pressure is increased, causing pressure on the optic nerve and, eventually, atrophy and blindness. Intraocular pressure is the result of pressure exerted by aqueous humor in the anterior cavity of the eye (the space posterior to the cornea and anterior to the lens). Aqueous humor is believed to be produced by the ciliary body and normally passes from the anterior chamber through the pupil, canal of Schlemm, and finally into the anterior ciliary veins.

Congenital glaucoma results from defective development of the structures of the eye in the region of the anterior chamber angle (outflow tracts for aqueous humor). Consequently there is obstruction to the flow of fluid resulting in increased intraocular pressure. Because of the distensibility of the infant's eye, the increased pressure pushes the anterior structures forward, causing thinning of the ocular layers until rupture of the globe may occur.

The earliest symptoms of this rare condition are tearing (epiphora), photophobia, and redness. As the glaucoma progresses, the cornea becomes cloudy from edema. Corneal haziness is the most significant objective sign and in the early stages is reversible once the ocular pressure is reduced.

Surgical treatment (goniotomy) is required to open the outflow tracts (canal of Schlemm) sufficiently to facilitate the flow of aqueous humor. Occasionally more than one operation is necessary to produce an anterior chamber angle that is wide enough.

Acquired glaucoma is rare in children (as opposed to adults, in whom it is the second most common cause of blindness in the United States). It is usually the result of some superimposed obstacle to the flow of aqueous humor. The most common causes are retrolental fibroplasia or retinoblastoma, which result in a narrowing of the anterior angle from forward displacement of the fibrous tissue or tumor, respectively, and trauma or inflammation that results in the formation of synechiae and scarring in the angle. Treatment is aimed at eliminating the cause and is frequently surgical.

Trauma. Trauma is the most common cause of blindness in children over 2 years of age. Injuries to the eyeball and adnexa (supporting or accessory structures, such as eyelids, conjunctiva, lacrimal glands, and so on) can be classified as penetrating or nonpenetrating. Penetrating wounds are most often the result of sharp instruments, such as knives or scissors, propulsive objects, such as firecrackers, guns, bows and arrows, or slingshots, and a powerful contusion by a blunt object, which may occur during a fight or from a serious car accident. Nonpenetrating injuries may be the result of foreign objects in the eyes, lacerations, a blow from a blunt object such as a fist, and thermal or chemical burns.

Visual impairment is caused by a number of possible posttraumatic events. These include (1) corneal ulceration and scarring; (2) herniation of the intraorbital contents through a fracture of the orbital floor (blow-out fracture); (3) complications from a hyphema (hemorrhage into the anterior chamber), such as secondary bleeding, blood staining of the cornea, glaucoma, or sympathetic ophthalmia (autoimmune disease of the uveal tract often occurring in the uninjured eye); (4) damage to the lens and cataract formation; (5) symblepharon (adhesions between the bulbar and palpebral conjunctiva) usually from scarring caused by burns; (6) rupture of the choroid, resulting in scar formation of the retina; (7) damage to the ciliary body; (8) infections of any structures of the eye, including panophthalmitis (Table 24-6); (9) retinal detachment from retraction of scar tissue formed along the path of a penetrating wound; and (10) therapeutic enucleation.[31]

Treatment is aimed at preventing further ocular damage and is primarily the responsibility of the ophthalmologist. It involves adequate examination of the injured eye (with the child sedated or anesthetized in severe injuries), appropriate immediate intervention such as removal of the foreign body or suturing of the laceration, and prevention of complications, such as administration of antibiotics or steroids and complete bed rest to allow the eye to heal and blood to reabsorb. Prognosis varies according to the type of injury. It is usually guarded in all cases of penetrating wounds because of the high risk of serious complications, especially retinal detachment, panophthalmitis, and sympathetic ophthalmia.

Infections. Infections of the adnexa and the structures of the eyeball or globe are not infrequent in children. The most common eye disease is conjunctivitis. Table 24-6 lists the

Table 24-6. Types of ocular infections

Structure	Infection	Common causes
Orbit	Orbital cellulitis	Paranasal sinusitis meningitis Penetrating injury
Lids	Blepharitis	Bacteria (hordeolum [stye], chalazion, pyodermas) Virus (herpes zoster, herpes simplex)
Conjunctiva	Conjunctivitis (often called pinkeye)	Bacteria (ophthalmia neonatorum) Virus
Cornea	Keratitis	Bacteria (congenital syphilis) Virus (herpes simplex, chickenpox)
Uvea (choroid, iris, and ciliary body) Ciliary body Anterior segment of uvea Posterior segment of the uvea (with secondary involvement of retina)	Uveitis, panuveitis Cyclitis Iritis, iridocyclitis Choroiditis Choroidoretinitis	Bacteria (tuberculosis, congenital syphilis) Virus (herpes simplex, herpes zoster, cytomegalic inclusion disease) Fungus Parasite Protozoa (toxoplasmosis) Rheumatoid arthritis Trauma
Uvea, retina, and vitreous body (with involvement of sclera)	Endophthalmitis Panophthalmitis	Bacteria Fungi Parasite Penetrating wound Intraocular surgery

various types of ocular infections. Treatment is usually ophthalmic antibiotics. Severe infections may require systemic antibiotic therapy. Steroids are used cautiously because they exacerbate viral infections such as herpes simplex, increasing the risk of damage to the involved structures.

Effects of visual impairment

Vision is the most sophisticated and objective of all the senses.[15] It is intimately involved with motor development because through sight the child learns spatial relationships, form, size, position, and distance. Without sight the child's mental constructs regarding these visual-motor perceptions are confined to the sense of touch and are limited to the periphery of his reach. Although the child hears, this sense cannot compensate fully for vision, because sounds are a subjective experience. The child can hear a dog bark but does not have the visual image to attach deeper meaning to the sound. Although sounds imply spatial distances, it is difficult for the blind child to associate the concepts of "near" or "far" with respective sounds.

To comprehend the impact of visual impairment on a child, it is helpful to review the role of sight in childhood development. At birth the newborn is able to distinguish forms at close range. The importance of the first hour of life (sensitive period) to parent-infant bonding has been partly attributed to the neonate's visual alertness. He is able to maintain eye contact with his parents, which evokes a powerful reciprocal response from them. Throughout the attachment process visual responsiveness is extremely influential in assisting parent and child in learning about each other, identifying the parent as a significant care giver, and perceiving emotional responses and physical needs in the child.

Vision is so essential to learning about one's environment that "seeing" or "not seeing" is the criteria for wakefulness and sleep. Visual stimulation is intense with the presentation of color, motion, size, and shape. Many blind or partially seeing children develop self-stimulatory habits called *blindisms,* such as eye rubbing, body rocking, finger flicking before the eyes, sniffing and smelling, arm twirling, or repetitive vocal tics, as substitutes for inadequate sensorimotor stimulation. The infant gradually separates himself from his surroundings by learning that blankets, garments, toys, furniture, and so on are not a part of his body. His body image is heavily dependent on the visual cues he receives, as well as on tactile sensations.

Visual-motor perception is believed to be a dependent ability. Retinal images supply the data that guide motor function for prehension, manipulation, and locomotion. For example, an infant learns to voluntarily grasp an object by seeing it first and reaching out to prehend it. If he does not see the object, he will have no self-stimulus to reach for it. The stimulus must be provided through another sense, usually touch. For example, the object is taken away and the infant's hand is guided to search for it through touch.

When the infant learns to crawl, he is guided in his locomotion through sight. Likewise as he becomes more mobile he uses his depth perception to learn how to go up and down steps and climb off or onto furniture. For the blind child these visual perceptions are learned through experimentation. For example, blind infants will substitute crawling on all fours with hitching (using legs to propel themselves while in a sitting position) to feel for obstacles with their hands rather than their heads. If the environment is not made reasonably safe for experimentation, they may be thwarted in their efforts toward locomotion by repeated accidental bumps and bruises.

The four visual motor perceptions basic to the establishment of body image and spatial perception are (1) balance and posture, (2) contact activities (reach, grasp, and release), (3) locomotion, and (4) receipt and propulsion (receipt relates to an object moving toward a child and propulsion relates to an object moving away from the child).[34] Each of these activities becomes the foundation for helping blind children develop motor skills.

During the preschool years imitation is a primary form of cognition. The child learns appropriate roles by watching and imitating the activities of significant others. Much of social behavior is learned by observing how others relate to one another. It is extremely difficult for a blind child to play cooperatively with peers because he cannot see what they are doing. Although he can hear and follow verbal commands, he may not be able to participate because of limitations in his motor ability. For example, a blind child who is able to walk well may refrain from running for fear of accidental collision with obstacles.

Academic learning is highly dependent on visual intactness. The normal child learns the meaning of words, letters, and numbers by associating the sound with the visual image of the object or symbol. The blind child hears only the word but has no concept of the object other than through touch. He is deprived of the richness of learning provided by pictorial books, photographs, movies, and television. Blind children often have misinformation, fragmented concepts, and a limited use of differentiation of information. This deprivation in learning is not sufficiently compensated by giving them auditory and tactile information.[14] However, despite these handicaps blind or partially seeing children are able to learn with sighted children, provided they have no additional disabilities.

The preceding discussion has focused primarily on the child with severe visual impairment. However, children with a mild loss of visual acuity may experience difficulties. One of the most common problems is borderline academic performance from inability to see distant objects, such as projected visual aids, or difficulty in reading small print. Manual skills may be retarded, especially if the child is hyperopic or severely myopic. Personality problems result from failure to achieve and loss of self-esteem. Social interaction may be retarded because the child is unable to compete with his peers in activities that require visual accuracy, such as catching a ball. The parent-child relationship may be disturbed when the parents mistakenly contribute poor academic achievement and psychosocial adjustment to causes such as lack of concentration, disinterest, passivity, and so on.

Since the visually impaired child, like the deaf or hard of hearing child, has no knowledge of his sensory handicap, he is totally unaware that he is missing important visual (or auditory) cues in his environment. Consequently he begins to believe that his difficulties are the result of behavioral problems, thus creating a vicious destructive cycle of interactions. Only through early detection of sensory problems and appropriate rehabilitation can the sensory-impaired child adjust and develop optimally despite his handicap.

Nursing interventions with visually impaired children

Prevention. The primary nursing objective is to prevent visual impairment. This involves many of the same interventions discussed under hearing impairments, namely (1) prenatal screening for pregnant women at risk, such as those with rubella or syphilis infection and family histories of genetic disorders associated with visual loss; (2) adequate prenatal and perinatal care to prevent prematurity and iatrogenic damage from excessive administration of oxygen; (3) periodic screening of all children, especially newborns through preschoolers, for congenital blindness and visual impairments caused by refractive errors, strabismus, and so on; (4) adequate immunization of all children; and (5) safety counseling regarding the common causes of ocular trauma (Table 24-7).

Following detection of eye problems, the nurse has a responsibility to prevent further ocular damage by ensuring that corrective treatment is employed. For the child with strabismus, this often necessitates occlusion patching of the stronger eye. Compliance with the procedure is greatest during the early preschool years and increasingly more difficult after school entry. If an older child requires occlusive patching, the nurse discusses the importance of the patch in preserving eyesight, allows the child an opportunity to discuss his feelings regarding the obvious dressing, and attempts to overcome difficulties imposed by the patch. For example, sole use of the weaker eye may make schoolwork more difficult unless the child is positioned favorably (closer to the blackboard) and allowed extra time to read or complete an assignment.

For the child with refractive errors, the nurse helps the child adjust to wearing glasses. Young children who often pull glasses off benefit from temporal pieces that wrap around the ears or an elastic strap attached to the frames and around the back of the head to hold them on securely. Once a child appreciates the value of clear vision, he is more likely to wear the corrective lenses.

Older children may refuse to wear glasses because of cosmetic reasons. Although this can be a traumatic experience for some children, with support and encouragement, combined with the benefit of improved vision, most children agree to wear them when necessary. The nurse helps parents understand the psychologic implications of altered body

Table 24-7. Anticipatory guidance for prevention of eye injuries

Age-group	Recommendations
Infants and toddlers	Avoid any toys with long pointed handles, such as a pinwheel on a stick Keep pointed instruments and tools out of reach (scissors, knives, screwdrivers, rulers, pencils, sticks, and so on) Do not allow child to *walk* or *run* with any pointed object in his hand (spoon, lollipop, toothbrush) Keep child away from play of older children and adults that involves projectile activities (throwing a ball, golf, target shooting, swings) Stress importance of fire safety and poison protection in preventing thermal/chemical burns to the eye Shield child's eyes when in direct sunlight
Preschoolers	Supervise use of sharp or pointed objects, especially scissors Teach proper use of pointed objects, such as toy guns or scissors, namely, to always point them *away* from their face or from anyone else at close range Teach child to walk carefully (never run) while carrying any sharp or pointed object Keep child away from projectile activities Begin teaching respect for firearms
School-age children and adolescents	Teach proper use and respect for potentially dangerous equipment such as power tools (flying objects from them), firearms, and firecrackers where legally permitted Stress use of eye protection when riding motorcycles or using equipment such as power saws or chemistry sets Advise them of danger of excessive sunlight (ultraviolet burns) If child wears contact lens, monitor duration of wear to prevent corneal scratching and possible scarring

image, especially in the adolescent. The nurse discusses the importance of including the child in the selection of frames, since they become a significant article of wearing apparel. Frames need not be changed each time further correction is needed. Therefore, it is sometimes a worthwhile investment to purchase more expensive, attractive frames since this may induce the child to wear them. Of course, such decisions must be made in light of the child's age, physical activity, and family's financial resources. All corrective lenses should be made from safety glass, which is shatterproof.

Depending on the reason for corrective lenses, some children may be required to wear them continuously whereas others may need them only for close work or distance seeing. If they are to be worn continuously, the nurse discusses with the physician the feasibility of short periods of disuse for special occasions, such as parties or other social activities. Children are usually much more cooperative when they know that there is flexibility in the wearing schedule that permits them to appear at their best with peers.

Glasses should not interfere with any activity. Special protective guards are available during contact sports to prevent accidental injury. Often corrective lenses improve visual acuity so dramatically that children are able to compete more effectively in sports. This in itself is a tremendous inducement to continue wearing glasses.

Contact lenses have been gaining in popularity and usage during the past several years. The two main types are hard or soft lenses. There is a third type called scleral lenses, which are rarely used because the wearing time is limited to about 4 hours. Contact lenses offer several advantages over conventional spectacles, namely, greater visual acuity, total corrected field of vision, and optimum cosmetic benefit. Unfortunately they are quite costly, require much more care than glasses, and involve considerable practice in learning techniques for insertion and removal. If they are prescribed the nurse can be very helpful in teaching parents or older children how to care for the lenses. Nurses should be aware of basic techniques for care and removal, especially during emergency situations when they may be responsible for such procedures (Table 24-8). Prolonged wearing of contact lenses, especially during sleep, damages the cornea because it deprives the corneal layers of their oxygen supply, which is received via exchange of gases in the atmosphere and tears. Normally when the eyes are closed the metabolic

Table 24-8. Care and removal of contact lenses

Type of lenses	Description	Removal	Care
Hard	Inflexible Always smaller than the cornea Visible against the iris (often appears an an "eyelash") Tinted or clear May wander from center or dislodge completely from eyeball	Manual technique—place thumb or finger of one hand on upper lid directly at the margin and thumb or finger of other hand on the lower lid; separate the lids; slowly push the lower lid upward until the lens is trapped between the lids; the lower lid ejects the lens by breaking the suction Suction method—use same procedure to separate the lids, but use a suction cup to lift off the lens NOTE: if lens has wandered from center (positioned on sclera, usually under top lid), manipulate lens back onto cornea by gently pushing on lid; if lens does not move freely, instill sterile saline solution	Store in sterile saline solution or distilled water May be rinsed in sterile saline solution and stored dry to prevent bacterial contamination of soaking solution Label each lens container as right or left during storage Can be worn again after cleaning and moistening with special wetting solution or sterile saline solution
Soft	Flexible; bends in half Slightly larger than cornea (extends to limbus) Almost invisible Clear Rarely wanders from center or falls out	Separate lids as for hard lenses; have child look up, slide lens toward bottom lid onto sclera; pinch lens between fingers of hand used to separate bottom lid If lens adheres to cornea, moisten with saline solution, then remove Do not use suction cup	Store in sterile distilled saline solution (never dry) Label each lens container as right or left Before lenses are worn again, they should be sterilized Do not use tap water in caring for lenses (causes chemical deposits on surface)

Data from Gould, H.: Am. J. Nurs. **76**(9):1483-1485, September 1976.

rate of the cornea decreases so that the oxygen supply via the circulation is sufficient. However, when lenses are worn, the metabolic rate remains high and oxygen via the blood is inadequate to maintain tissue metabolism.[10]

Treatment of several eye disorders (infection, strabismus, glaucoma, and so on) requires instillation of ophthalmic medication. The nurse teaches parents the correct procedure. With the child lying supine or sitting with the head hyperextended, the parent uses one hand to pull the upper lid upward and the other hand to pull the lower lid downward. The child is asked to look up. As the lower lid is manipulated, a small conjunctival sac is formed; the solution or ointment is applied to this area, never directly on the eyeball (see Fig. 26-23). The lids are gently closed to prevent expression of the medication, and the child is asked to look in all directions to enhance even distribution of the preparation. Excess medication is wiped from the inner canthus outward to prevent contamination to the contralateral eye.

If the child is not cooperative it may be necessary to have two people perform the procedure: one to properly position the lids and the other to instill the drug. If the child is cooperative the parent administers the medication with the same hand that separates the upper lid. A convenient method is to use the third finger to pull the lid upward and the thumb and index finger to manipulate the dropper.

Since trauma is the leading cause of blindness, the nurse has the major responsibility of preventing further eye injury until the physician orders specific treatment. The major principles to follow when caring for eye emergencies are: (1) reassure the child and parents—everyone with an eye injury fears blindness; (2) test visual acuity; (3) never apply a patch on a penetrated eye (an eye patch will exert more pressure, causing further structural damage); instead, use a Fox shield (a small metal shield shaped like an eye that has tiny perforations); (4) never try to remove a foreign body that has penetrated the eye; (5) never use anesthetic *ointment* unless ordered by a physician (the ointment, not the solution, may cause a corneal ulcer and masks signs of painful injury); and (6) never use steroids unless specifically ordered.[7] Table 24-9 summarizes basic emergency nursing care procedures for eye injuries.

Preservation of sight is such an essential goal that the nurse incorporates the following preventive health teachings concerning care of the eyes regardless of the presence or absence of deviations: (1) avoidance of excessive eyestrain;

Table 24-9. Emergency nursing care for eye injuries

Type of trauma	Nursing responsibility
Foreign object	Examine eye for presence of a foreign body (evert upper lid to examine upper eye) If a freely movable object is seen, it may be removed with the pointed corner of a gauze pad lightly moistened with sterile saline solution Do not irrigate eye or attempt to remove a penetrating object If fluorescein dye is used to detect corneal abrasions, be careful to use aseptic technique because fluorescein drops are highly susceptible to contamination and growth of *Pseudomonas* (sterile fluorescein strips are preferred)
Chemical burns	Irrigate eye copiously with normal saline solution or tap water; evert upper lid to flush thoroughly; hold child's head and eye under tap of running lukewarm water Check pH if possible; continue irrigating until pH is normal (15-20 minutes) Do not administer any ointments (may interfere with ophthalmic examination) If child is in severe pain, may be necessary to administer anesthetic drops Allow child to rest with eyes closed
Ultraviolet burns	If child is in severe pain, instill anesthetic drops; test visual acuity Patch both eyes (make sure lids are completely closed); if skin is burned, secure dressing with Kling bandages wrapped around the head rather than tape
Hematoma ("black eye")	Test visual acuity With a flashlight, check for gross hyphema (visible fluid meniscus across iris; more easily seen in light-colored than in brown eyes) If no hyphema is present, apply ice for first 24 hours to reduce swelling, followed by heat to absorb extravasated blood If hyphema is present, have child examined by an ophthalmologist
Penetrating injuries	*Never remove an object that has penetrated eye* Follow strict aseptic technique in examining eye; observe for aqueous or vitreous leaks (fluid leaking from point of penetration), hyphema, shape and equality of pupils, prolapsed iris (not perfectly circular), and pupillary reaction to light If leaks are present, apply a Fox shield and maintain bed rest with child in 30-degree Fowler's position Caution child against rubbing eye

when doing close work, periodically looking into the distance to relax the muscles of accommodation; (2) use of proper lighting; light should not be glaring or cast shadows on reading material (light source should come from behind the left shoulder in a right-handed individual and vice versa); watching television with a light in a dark room to decrease contrast; (3) getting the proper amount of rest; and (4) having the eyes checked at least yearly by a licensed optometrist or ophthalmologist.

Detection. Equally important as prevention is early detection of eye problems. As has already been pointed out, detection and treatment of many ocular defects, such as strabismus, often prevent any permanent visual impairment. Every child from birth onward should receive periodic visual screening. Chapter 5 includes tests for visual acuity in children in various age-groups. Table 24-10 summarizes the usual signs and symptoms associated with ocular disorders.

Infancy. At birth most infants demonstrate specific orientation responses to visual stimuli, such as a bright or shiny object held in their line of vision. According to the Brazelton Neonatal Behavioral Assessment Scale, the infant may exhibit the following responses (scores): (1) does not focus on or follow stimulus; (2) stills with stimulus and brightens; (3) stills, focuses on stimulus when presented, little spontaneous interest, no following; (4) stills, focuses on stimulus, follows for 30-degree arc, jerky movements; (5) focuses and follows with eyes horizontally for at least 30-degree arc, smooth movement, loses stimulus but finds it again; (6) follows for 30-degree arc with eyes and head, eye movements are smooth; (7) follows with eyes and head at least 60 degrees horizontally, maybe briefly vertically, partly continuous movement, loses stimulus occasionally, head turns to follow; (8) follows with eyes and head 60 degrees horizontally and 30 degrees vertically; and (9) focuses on stimulus and follows with smooth, continuous head movement horizontally, vertically, and in a circle; follows for 120-degree arc.[3] The nurse refers any infant with a score of

Table 24-10. Detection of visual impairment

Cause	Behavior	Signs/symptoms
Congenital blindness	Does not follow a moving light; no orientation response to visual stimuli Does not initiate eye-to-eye contact with care giver	Constant nystagmus Fixed pupils Marked strabismus Slow lateral movements
Refractive errors	Rubs eyes excessively Tilts head or thrusts head forward Has difficulty in reading or other close work Holds books close to eyes Writes or colors with head close to table Clumsy; walks into objects Blinks more than usual or is irritable when doing close work Is unable to see objects clearly Does poorly in school, especially in subjects that require demonstration, such as arithmetic	Dizziness Headache Nausea following close work
Strabismus	Squints eyelids together or frowns Has difficulty in focusing from one distance to another Inaccurate judgment in picking up objects Unable to see print or moving objects clearly Closes one eye to see Tilts head to one side If combined with refractive errors, may see any of the above	Diplopia Photophobia Dizziness Headache Cross-eye
Glaucoma	Mostly seen in acquired types—loses peripheral vision; may bump into objects that are not directly in front of him; sees halos around objects; may complain of mild pain or discomfort (severe pain, nausea, and vomiting if sudden rise in pressure)	Redness Excessive tearing (epiphora) Photophobia Spasmatic winking (blepharospasm) Corneal haziness Enlargement of the eyeball (buphthalmos)
Cataract	Gradually less able to see objects clearly May lose peripheral vision	Nystagmus (with complete blindness) Gray opacities of lens Strabismus

1 or the signs listed in Table 24-10, which are early clues to congenital blindness.

Of special importance in detecting visual impairment during infancy are the parents' concerns regarding visual responsiveness in their child. Their concerns must be taken seriously. The nurse encourages parents to document the objects, faces, persons, or toys that the infant actually looks at during a 1-week period of time. Such information helps the nurse plan for specific testing and appropriate ophthalmologic referral.

During infancy the child should be tested for strabismus. Lack of binocularity after 4 months of age is considered abnormal. Although strabismus is most common between the ages of 2 and 3 years when the child uses accommodation for near vision, accommodative esotropia can occur as early as age 4 months and requires immediate intervention to prevent amblyopia.[24] Tests for strabismus are discussed in Chapter 5.

Childhood. Since the most common visual impairment during childhood is refractive errors, testing for visual acuity is essential. Besides the testing methods discussed in Chapter 5, a Home Eye Test for Preschoolers is available from the National Society for the Prevention of Blindness,* a voluntary organization devoted to preservation of sight through public education and research. This test is designed for use by parents for children 3 years or older and employs the letter "E." It explains how to interpret the results and when to refer the child to an ophthalmologist. It also lists the following major signs of visual difficulties in children and suggests that if any of them are present, the child should receive professional eye examination:

BEHAVIOR. Behaviors that should be checked for include (1) rubbing eyes excessively; (2) shutting or covering one eye, or tilting head or thrusting head forward; (3) having difficulty in reading or in other work requiring close use of the eyes; (4) blinking more than usual or becoming irritable when doing close work; (5) holding books close to eyes; (6) inability to see objects clearly; and (7) squinting eyelids together or frowning.

APPEARANCE. Appearance of the child with visual difficulties includes (1) crossed eyes; (2) red-rimmed, encrusted, or swollen eyelids; (3) inflammed or watery eyes; (4) recurring styes.

COMPLAINTS. Complaints include (1) eyes that itch, burn, or feel scratchy; (2) not being able to see well; (3) dizziness, headaches, or nausea following close eye work; and (4) blurred or double vision.

The school nurse usually assumes major responsibility for vision testing in school-age children and adolescents. Besides refractive errors, the nurse should be aware of signs and symptoms indicative of other ocular problems. If a referral is made to the family requesting further eye testing, the nurse is responsible for follow-up concerning the recommendation. Often parents do not willingly neglect their child's care out of disinterest, but rather because of contributing factors, such as financial difficulty. The school nurse can be instrumental in seeking financial assistance for the family, such as through health centers that provide care on a sliding-fee basis.

It is also important for the nurse to stress that children continue to need periodic eye examination. Myopia commonly continues to worsen throughout childhood, necessitating stronger corrective lenses. Conversely a hyperopic child may outgrow his need for glasses by 7 or 8 years of age. One pair of glasses frequently affords only temporary visual correction.

Rehabilitation

Adjusting to diagnosis. The shock of learning that their child is blind or partially sighted is an immense crisis for parents. Of all types of disabilities, many people fear loss of sight the most. Certainly it is one of the senses that is involved in almost every activity of daily living. Parents need support during the initial phase of learning about the diagnosis. The nurse can help them understand that their grief reaction to the loss is normal and that adjustment requires considerable time and emotional working through. The nurse also helps parents gain a realistic understanding of their child's abilities. Although it is impossible to predict the future for the blind child, it is reasonably safe to assume that a blind child without other severe handicaps can live a productive, independent life provided he is afforded the opportunity to learn and develop.

Parents should know from the beginning that rearing a blind child is a difficult task for which there are few role models and even fewer ready-made solutions. The nurse discusses with them that the usual reaction is to overprotect the child in an attempt to make the environment as safe as possible for him. However, the destructive effects of the "benevolent overreaction" (see p. 787), especially to a child who needs encouragement and structured stimulation to learn about his world and venture forth where he cannot see, are emphasized. The family is encouraged to investigate appropriate stimulation and educational programs for their child as soon as possible.*

When blindness is not congenital but acquired, the newly blind child needs a great deal of support to help him adjust to the handicap. He is usually frightened and confused by the sudden or progressive loss of sight and benefits from an environment that provides security and familiarity. This is especially important for the nurse to remember when he is hospitalized. The child needs careful orientation to his immediate surroundings, elimination of as many extraneous stimuli, such as strange noises, as possible, and provision of

*79 Madison Avenue, New York, N.Y. 10016.

*Information about services for the blind is available from American Foundation for the Blind, 15 W. 16th Street, New York, N.Y. 10011.

safety measures to prevent accidents and encourage ambulation. (Interventions for meeting these needs are discussed on p. 866.) He should be encouraged to continue as many independent behaviors as possible and be taught methods to help him compensate for the loss of vision, such as localization of objects through sound or touch, organization of personal belongings to facilitate identification of clothes, grooming aids, and so on, and learning braille.

Parent-child attachment. A crucial time in the life of the blind infant is when he and his parents are getting acquainted with each other. Pleasurable patterns of interaction between the infant and his parents may be lacking if there is not enough reciprocity. For example, if the parent gazes fondly at the infant's face and seeks eye contact but the infant fails to respond because he cannot see the parent, a troubled cycle of responses may occur. The nurse can help parents learn to look for other cues that indicate the infant's responding to them, such as if his eyelids blink, whether his activity level accelerates or slows, if respiratory patterns change, such as if he breathes faster or slower when they come near, and whether the infant makes throaty sounds when they speak to him. In time parents learn that the infant has his own unique way of relating to them even though he cannot return a smiling gaze of the eyes.

Parents need opportunities to discuss this emotionally laden topic because of the importance of attachment with the infant. Both the infant and parents are vulnerable to having this bonding interrupted if they perceive a lack of reciprocity. It is crucial that the parents do not feel that their infant dislikes or is rejecting them. It is also important for them to have support for the feelings they have and to understand how they affect their interactions with an infant who cannot see them. Sometimes it is appropriate for the nurse to serve as the interpreter of the blind infant's communication.

Parents also need advocates for their blind child. The nurse demonstrates by personal example acceptance of the child as a unique and special person. The child's positive aspects, such as physical appearance, cooperative behavior, developmental progress, and so on, are emphasized. The parents are supported in any of their attempts to foster the child's development. Through this approach the nurse indirectly encourages attachment by influencing and strengthening the parents' acceptance of their child.

Development and independence. Motor development is almost as dependent on sight as verbal communication is on hearing. From earliest infancy the nurse encourages parents to expose the infant to as many visual-motor experiences as possible, such as sitting supported in an infant seat or swing and given opportunities for holding up his head, sitting unsupported, reaching for objects, crawling, and so on. Ideally the child should be enrolled in an educational stimulation program for blind infants to develop age-appropriate motor skills. (Many of the activities suggested in Table 23-4 for motor stimulation are applicable for a home program, with modification of those exercises that depend on sight.) The nurse stresses to parents that the blind child who receives formal instruction in movement can learn and master balance, coordination, and mobility within his environment.

Even after accomplishing the major motor developments, many blind children are restricted in their participation in activities that require large-muscle coordination. Parents may prohibit the child from engaging in active play, such as riding a tricycle or bicycle, swimming, active sports, running, and so on. Sometimes the child himself fears these activities. Parents and child both need support to work through their fears and misconceptions about the dangers of active play. It is helpful to ask parents questions, such as, "What is the worst thing that can happen if your child rides a tricycle?" and "What opportunities and benefits are available to him once he learns to master the skill?" The nurse can also suggest safe ways of introducing active play, such as learning to ride a tricycle in a confined area with few obstacles or counting the number of rotations for pedaling before reaching a wall.

Blind children often lack experiences that help develop fine motor coordination. For example, young sighted children pick up pieces of paper and fine objects from a table or floor surface because they see them. The child who cannot see small objects misses the opportunities for such practice and may have poor fine motor coordinated skills. The nurse suggests to parents that they provide the child with a variety of experiences that include touching small toys and other objects. He should also be introduced to a variety of textures such as silk, satin, coarse burlap, soft cotton, wooly-fuzzy materials, sand, slippery objects, water, hard surfaces, soft toys, and cold and warm temperatures. Such experiences will increase his sensitivity as well as enable him to master braille reading and writing skills more readily.[28]

Despite visual impairment the child can become independent in all aspects of self-care. (See Chapter 23 for a discussion of helping slow-to-develop children learn self-care.) He may need help in dressing, such as special arrangement of clothing for style coordination and various tags or identifying marks to distinguish colors, prints, and so on. He should be encouraged to take pride in his appearance, with attention to good grooming and dress, since these assets greatly increase his social acceptance within society.

The child learns self-feeding as a normal child would. If he is given a deep bowl and a lightweight spoon, he is able to scoop food more easily and can determine the quantity by the increased weight of the utensil. Securing the dish to the table surface makes locating it easier and eliminates accidents. Food and fluids should be arranged in the same position at each meal so that the child can choose what to eat and when. Once the child is old enough to tell time or understand the numerical positions on a clock, food can be arranged in a circle and its location designated by a number, such as the meat being placed at the 12 o'clock position. During the preschool years the child is encouraged to develop table manners. Parents need to realize that without the assistance of imitation they must verbally explain the importance of manners and gently remind the child to practice them.

Toilet training should proceed according to the usual physical and psychologic signs of readiness. Since the child cannot see the toilet or imitate other's toilet habits, he must be verbally instructed regarding its purpose. Using the step-by-step approach outlined in Chapter 23 is often helpful for the blind child to learn independent toileting. Toilet training is an important achievement because it is usually a prerequisite for entry into nursery schools or special programs.

Play/socialization. The blind child does not automatically learn to play. Because he cannot imitate others or actively explore his environment as sighted children do, he is much more dependent on others to stimulate him and to teach him how to play. (For negative environmental influences, see Chapter 23.) Parents also need help in selecting appropriate play material. Toys should encourage fine and gross motor development and stimulate the senses of hearing, touch, and smell. (See Table 12-2 for toys appropriate during infancy.) The nurse stresses to parents that the blind child will usually need more time and help in learning how to use toys but that this is not an indication of his slowness or inability to learn. It represents the loss of one sense in the learning process and the compensatory effort required from the other senses.

The blind child has the same needs for socialization as normal children. Since he has little difficulty in learning verbal skills, he is able to communicate with age-mates and participate in suitable activities. Contact with peers often enables blind children to participate much more easily in activities that require running, jumping, and falling. Parents should take an active part in the socialization process, especially during the phase of parallel play when the blind child may be totally unaware of what the other children are doing, unless someone tells him about the activity. Parents should encourage group activities that are appropriate for the young blind child, such as "ring-around-the-rosy," singing nursery rhymes, playing tag, and so on. The nurse discusses with parents opportunities for socialization outside of the home, especially regular nursery schools. The trend is to include these children with other normal children to help them adjust to the outside world for eventual independence.

Blindisms are usually an indication of inadequate compensatory stimulation for the child. Since such habits retard socially acceptable behavior, the nurse assesses the child's environment for clues to when they occur and how parents manage them. Suitable substitute stimulation within an appropriate social context, such as a play group of peers or within the family setting, is suggested. Providing the blind child with appropriate tactile and musical toys alone in his room is inadequate stimulation. He needs the social contact to sustain his interest.

Education. The early education of the blind child must avoid unnecessary confusion. There should be fixed orientation to familiar environments. Each room in the house should be arranged to allow the child maximum mobility and safety. If the child has partial vision, special identifying markers can be used to emphasize certain locations, such as a bright light in the bathroom or a ticking clock near the stairway. When the child is in unfamiliar surroundings, parents should orient him to the room. This point is especially relevant during hospitalization when the nurse may have to repeat directions regarding room arrangement, location of the bathroom, and so on.

Since strange sounds have no meaning without visual orientation, these are explained whenever necessary. Sighted people often selectively inhibit extraneous sounds because of the more compelling visual cues. However, the blind child is acutely aware of auditory stimuli and can be easily confused or frightened by them unless he is aware of their source. This is similar to deaf children's preoccupation with visual cues, such as facial expressions, which can be upsetting to them if they are not sure of their meaning.

The main obstacle to learning is the child's total dependence on nonvisual cues. Although the child can learn via verbal lecturing, he is unable to read the written word or to write without special education. Therefore, he must rely on braille, a system that uses raised symbols to represent letters and numbers. The child can then read the braille with his fingers and can "write" a message using a braille typewriter. The partially sighted child may learn this system but also benefits from large-print books.

Touch is also a principle media for learning concepts, such as comparison in size, weight, and so on. Touch becomes extremely important in gaining some idea of "appearance." For example, using the fingers to touch someone's face helps the child learn distinguishing marks for each individual. Blind children are frequently able to decipher a person's emotional mood from facial muscle tenseness, positioning of the lips, cheeks, and eyes, and other subtle body language.

The blind child also must learn to become independent in navigational skills. The two main techniques are the tapping method (use of a cane to survey the environment for direction and avoidance of obstacles) and guides, such as a human sighted guide or a Seeing Eye dog. Both afford the blind person sufficient mobility to travel in unfamiliar surroundings using public transportation.

Blind children are exposed to stresses that sighted people rarely experience. Because the environment beyond the fingertips is almost always a source of unknown dangers, the blind person constantly experiences tension when moving about. Such tension combined with constant alert-

Summary of nursing care of the visually impaired child

Goals	Responsibilities
Prevention	
Prior to occurrence of ocular problems	Identify pregnant women at risk Encourage adequate prenatal care to decrease likelihood of premature delivery or low birth weight infant Administer oxygen cautiously to neonate Periodically screen all children from birth through adolescence for visual impairment Participate in immunization programs for children Teach safety regarding common accidental causes of eye injuries (Table 24-7) Stress importance of good eye care—use of proper lighting, avoidance of excessive close work, proper rest and nutrition, and yearly eye examinations
Following detection/or diagnosis of eye disorders	Encourage compliance with corrective therapies
Strabismus	Discuss with school-age child necessity of patch in preserving vision; allow him to verbalize feelings regarding altered facial appearance; help him overcome visual difficulties imposed by seeing with weaker eye (favorable seating in school, large-print books, and additional time to complete assignments) Teach parents correct procedures for instilling anticholinesterase drugs
Refractive errors	For secure fit of glasses, use ones with rounded temporal pieces or attach elastic strap to handles and around back of head Include older child in selection of frames Encourage parents to compare value of more expensive attractive frames and inducement for wearing them against cost If glasses are recommended for continuous wearing, discuss possibility of temporary removal for special occasions Encourage use of protective shields during contact sports Stress improvement in visual acuity as reason for wearing glasses Discuss feasibility of contact lenses with selected families Know procedures for care, insertion, and removal of lens; teach these to parents and older children (Table 24-8)
Infections	Teach parent correct procedure for instilling ophthalmic preparations (always in conjunctival cul-de-sac) Ensure proper dosage by holding dropper vertically, slowly closing the lids, and having child rotate the eyeball for even distribution Wipe excess medication from inner canthus outward to prevent contamination of contralateral eye Emphasize regular administration of drug for entire term of therapy to completely eradicate infection
Trauma	Prevent further injury by instituting appropriate emergency care (Table 24-9) Obtain history of incident; avoid any implication of guilt Reassure parent and child; avoid giving false reassurance; appraise them of each step of treatment, especially if therapy interferes with vision (patching eyes)
Detection	
Infancy	At birth assess neonate's response to a bright, shiny object; observe for signs associated with congenital blindness (Table 24-10) After 4 months of age, check for strabismus (lack of binocularity); refer to ophthalmologist for evaluation Listen to parents' concerns regarding visual loss

Summary of nursing care of the visually impaired child—cont'd

Goals	Responsibilities
Detection—cont'd	
Childhood	Test for visual acuity as soon as child is cooperative (sometimes by age 2 years) Advise parents of Home Eye Test for Preschoolers, which is available from National Society for the Prevention of Blindness Observe for signs or behaviors indicative of eye problems (Table 24-10); specifically include questions regarding behavioral indications of vision impairment in health histories As school nurse, assume responsibility for follow-up care of children who require corrective lenses or other types of treatments, such as patching Stress to parents importance of continued periodic eye examinations, since the child's eyesight may change significantly in a short period of time
Rehabilitation	
Assist family in adjusting to child's loss of sight	Anticipate the usual grief reactions to loss Stress to parents (and older child) that such feelings are normal and that grief takes time to resolve Help parents gain a realistic concept of child's handicap and abilities Encourage formal rehabilitation as soon as realistically feasible Assist parents in orienting newly blind child to his environment and in making immediate surroundings safe to encourage ambulation
Promote parent-child attachment	Help parents identify clues other than eye contact from the infant that signify his communication with them Encourage parents to discuss their feeling regarding lack of visual contact or smiling from the child Stress that lack of such responses is not an indication of child's rejection or dislike of his parents Demonstrate by own example acceptance of the child; emphasize positive abilities or attributes; encourage parents in their attempts to promote child's development
Promote development and independence	Provide visual-motor activities for infant (sitting in chair or swing, holding head up, standing, crawling, grasping for objects, and so on) Provide an environment that fosters familiarity and security, arrange furniture to allow safe ambulation; place identifying markers to denote steps or other dangerous areas Enroll child in special programs for the blind as soon as possible to learn independent skills, braille reading and writing, and navigational skills (cane method, sighted guide, or Seeing Eye dog) Encourage participation in active play Discuss need for experimenting with active play in safe environment and with other children
Provide opportunities for play/socialization	Always talk to child about his environment Guide parents to selection of play material that encourages motor development and stimulates the senses of hearing and touch Discuss with parents how play for blind children differs from that of sighted children Encourage parents to initiate play activities and teach child how to use toys If blindisms are present, assess adequacy of environmental stimulation Discuss importance of consistent limit setting in helping child learn acceptable behavior and tolerate frustration

Continued.

Summary of nursing care of the visually impaired child—cont'd

Goals	Responsibilities
Rehabilitation—cont'd	
Provide emotional support	Be available to family for assistance Encourage parents, child, and siblings to discuss their feelings regarding the disability Stress child's abilities rather than disability Refer families to appropriate community agencies for medical, psychiatric, vocational, or financial assistance Encourage child to discuss his feelings regarding constant tension and alertness needed to cope with a strange environment Stress that such tension is natural for all blind people Help him find ways of relieving tension, such as relaxing while moving about and resting at frequent intervals throughout the day

ness to nonvisual cues is exhausting. These children often require additional rest. They may also benefit from expressing how they feel and discovering that such tension is natural for blind persons. Attention should be directed at finding ways of helping them cope more securely and successfully with potential dangers. They should be encouraged to relax while moving about and to plan their day to allow for rest periods. (For nursing care of the visually impaired child, see the boxed material on pp. 864 to 866.)

Caring for hospitalized children with temporary loss of vision

Children may be hospitalized for ocular surgery that requires temporary patching, such as strabismus or some types of cataract removal, or because of trauma and temporary loss of vision resulting from the injury or treatment. The nursing care objectives in either situation are to (1) reassure the child and family throughout every phase of treatment, (2) orient the child to his surroundings, (3) provide a safe environment, and (4) encourage independence. Whenever possible the same nurse should care for the child to assure consistency in the approach. These same principles also apply to a blind child who requires hospitalization.

When a sighted child temporarily loses his vision, almost every aspect of his environment becomes bewildering and frightening. He is forced to rely on nonvisual senses for help in adjusting to the blindness without the benefit of any special training. Nurses have a major role in minimizing the effects of temporary loss of vision. They talk to the child about everything they are doing, emphasizing aspects of procedures that are felt or heard. They approach the child by always identifying themselves as soon as they enter the room. Since unfamiliar sounds are especially frightening to the child, the nurse is alert to them and explains what they are. Parents are encouraged to room with him and participate in his care. Familiar objects, such as a teddy bear or doll, should be brought from home to help temper the strangeness of the hospital. As soon as the child is able to be out of bed, the nurse orients him to his immediate surroundings. If the child is able to see on admission, this opportunity is taken to point out significant aspects of his room and he is encouraged to practice ambulating with his eyes closed to accustom him to this experience.

The room should be arranged with safety in mind. For example, a stool or chair is placed next to the bed to help the child climb in and out of bed. The furniture is always placed in the same position to prevent accidental collisions. The nurse should remind cleaning personnel of the necessity of putting the room back in order. When the child is in bed (even if not asleep), side rails must be up. If the child has difficulty in navigating on his own, a rope can be attached from the bed to the point of destination, such as the bathroom. The child follows the rope for direction. Attention to details such as well-fitting slippers or robes that do not hang on the floor is important in preventing tripping.

The nurse encourages the child to be independent in self-care activities, especially if the visual loss may be prolonged or potentially permanent. For example, during bathing the nurse sets up all the equipment and encourages the child to participate. At mealtime the nurse explains where each food item is on the tray, opens any special containers, prepares cereal or toast, but encourages the child to feed himself. Since manipulating utensils may be difficult, favorite finger foods, such as sandwiches, hamburgers, hot dogs, or pizza, are selected. The child is encouraged to use a straw to drink soups or fluids, rather than feeding him. If he has accidental spills, the nurse quickly cleans them up, with no emphasis on his clumsiness. Instead he is praised for efforts at being cooperative and independent, and the importance of any improvements he makes in self-care, no matter how small, is stressed.

The nurse provides appropriate recreational activities for the child. If a play therapist is available, such planning should be done jointly. Since the child with temporary blindness has a wide variety of play experiences to draw on, he should be encouraged to select activities. For example, if he liked to read, he may enjoy being read to. If he preferred manual activity, he may appreciate playing with clay or building blocks or feeling different textures and trying to guess what they are. If he needs an outlet for aggression, activities such as pounding or banging on a drum can be helpful. However, guessing games should be avoided because they increase frustration. He should have familiar toys from home to play with, since they are more easily manipulated than new ones. If parents wish to bring him presents, they should be things that stimulate hearing and touch, such as a radio, music box, or stuffed animal.

Occasionally children who are blind come to the hospital for procedures to restore their vision. Although this is an extremely happy time, it also requires intervention to help the child adjust to sight. The child needs an opportunity to take in all that he sees. He should not be bombarded with visual stimuli. He may need to concentrate on people's faces or his own to accustom himself to this experience. He often has the need to talk about what he sees and to compare the visual image with his mental one. The child may also go through a period of depression as he begins to realize all that he had lost. This depression must be respected and supported. The nurse or parents should refrain from statements, such as, "How can you be so sad when you can see again?" Instead the child should be encouraged to discuss how it feels to see, especially in terms of seeing himself.

The child also needs time in adjusting to his ability to engage in activities that were impossible before. For example, he may prefer to use braille to read, rather than learning a new "visual approach" because of his familiarity with the touch system. Eventually, as he learns to recognize letters and numbers, he will integrate these new skills into reading and writing. However, parents and teachers must be careful not to push the child before he is ready. This applies to social relationships and physical activities as well as learning situations.

DEAF-BLIND CHILDREN

The most traumatic sensory impairment is loss of sight and hearing. Causes of deaf blindness include the following: (1) congenital blindness, acquired deafness (meningitis); (2) congenital deafness, acquired blindness (eye trauma); (3) congenital deaf blindness (congenital rubella); and (4) acquired deaf blindness (accidents).[11] In most instances deaf-blind children have some residual hearing and vision to supplement the senses of touch, smell, and taste.

Obviously, auditory and visual handicaps have profound effects on the child's development. They interfere with the normal sequence of physical, intellectual, and psychosocial growth. Although the child often achieves the usual motor milestones, they are more slowly developed. Children only learn communication with specialized training. The following communication systems are used with deaf-blind children[11]:

1. *Vibration (Tadoma method).* The sense of touch is used for receptive language. The child puts his hand on the face of the person to whom he is talking. The thumb covers the mouth and feels the movement of the lips, jaws, and tongue. The four other fingers are spread over the cheek and jaw to pick up vibrations.
2. *Finger spelling.* In this system each letter in the alphabet has a specific finger position. The letters are spelled into the hand of the deaf-blind person, and the deaf-blind person spells out his ideas to the person with whom he is talking.
3. *Gesture.* The normal young child finds movement and language inseparable. Spontaneous gesturing is rare in the congenitally deaf-blind child, and he must be taught to use gestures as one of the first steps in learning language. Natural gestures are necessary but are not the final goal.
4. *Sign language:* Each word has as its symbol a movement of hands and arms. Movements are combined to form a language used mainly by deaf students. Deaf-blind children can use this system, but speech and finger spelling are more often preferred. The movements of sign language are difficult for the deaf-blind child to pick up through touch or residual sight.
5. *Communication using a machine.* One machine consists of a typewriter keyboard and a braille cell. The deaf person puts his finger on the braille cell, and the person talking to him uses the keyboard. For example, pressing "A" on the keyboard makes the braille "A" appear.

Some deaf-blind children, especially those with residual hearing or sight, can learn to speak. Whenever possible, speech is encouraged, since it allows communication with individuals not familiar with the preceding list of approaches. The principles discussed under hearing (p. 843) are utilized to help the deaf-blind child learn language.

Programs for these children vary. The four types of programs recommended include[32]:

1. An early management program emphasizing psychoeducational management conjointly with medical care, which is designed to identify and train the child who is nonambulatory, delayed in self-care skills, and whose potential for learning has not been determined
2. Day programs for ambulatory deaf-blind children who have basic self-care skills and a determined potential for learning
3. Residential programs for children described in the preceding

category who would benefit from concentrated residential learning
4. Custodial programs for severely involved children who do not demonstrate any learning potential

Nursing interventions with deaf-blind children[4]

One of the major concerns of families with deaf-blind children is helping them establish communication. The nurse is in a vital position to help parents with this goal. Since the infant cannot coo, laugh, or make eye movements, he is limited in the cues he can send and in those he can receive. Therefore, initiating and maintaining communication is the responsibility of the care giver. The nurse discusses with parents behaviors that signal the infant's recognition of them, such as quieting behavior, blinking, change in respiration, and so on. The parents are encouraged to find ways of increasing stimulation for the child, especially cues that help the child identify each parent. For example, each person involved with the child should choose something that he, and only he, does, such as a kiss on the forehead or a stroke on the cheek. In this way the infant learns to discriminate among people in his environment.

The infant should be held close to the adult with his hands placed on the face while the person talks or changes facial expression. Eventually this technique becomes structured to associate a certain facial vibration with a word. However, such associations take time, patience, and effort on the part of both the child and the parents.

Much of the same stimulation for motor and sensory development that was discussed for the blind child is instituted here. He should be placed in as many different positions as possible throughout the day in relation to light and provided variation in stimuli so that he will be motivated to move toward, reach, touch, and explore his own environment. Sounds should be brought near and made interesting to the child. For example, he can participate in hearing by placing his hand on a radio or on a person's throat. The child's position should be altered frequently to orient him to space and to encourage muscle development and movement patterns. Consistent tactile cues should be associated with a change of position and activities so that the movement is experienced as a positive nonthreatening experience. The nurse should encourage family members to urge the child to participate in games that require repositioning and body action, such as peekaboo and pat-a-cake.

The nurse encourages parents to provide secure, safe experiences while the child is learning to walk and gaining confidence. Once ambulatory, the child needs help in exploring the environment on a gradual *planned* basis. The environment should not be haphazard, for the child may become fearful and avoid growth-producing experiences. After the child succeeds in becoming well oriented to his environment and can overcome any abnormal movement patterns, he is ready for a plan of locomotion. Sighted guide, trailing (movement directed by touching objects, such as the wall), and cane walking are three methods. An individually planned mobility program should be based on the child's age, needs, and functional status and shared with the child's therapist, teachers, parents, and siblings.

The nurse points out to parents the necessity for fostering independence as early as possible in all self-help tasks. The deaf-blind child's success in learning and his parents' success in teaching self-care will be determined to a great extent by the obvious cues that can be built into any teaching task. All activities must be kept as simple as possible. Care providers must remain sensitive to the child's last step mastered before introducing new steps in the learning process. (The guidelines for stimulating independent self-care activities in Chapter 23 can be modified for application here.)

The nurse can help the parents with specific child-rearing problems. One of the most frequent is sleep. Parents often complain that the child refuses to go to sleep, wakes up for extended intervals, has irregular sleeping habits, or wants to sleep in the parents' bed. The nurse discusses with parents the value of a behavior modification program to change these habits. The nurse helps the parents keep a detailed record of undesirable behaviors, formulates a plan for positive and negative reinforcement, and supports them during the modification period. Assisting parents with one child-rearing problem in this fashion often allows them to deal with other undesirable or socially unacceptable behaviors. Parents for the first time may sense a feeling of control and order that was lacking previously because of the overwhelming implications of this handicap.

The future prospects for deaf-blind children are at best unpredictable. Not infrequently congenital blindness or/and deafness is accompanied by other physical or neurologic handicaps, which further lessen the child's learning potential. The most favorable prognosis is often for children who have acquired deaf blindness and have few, if any, associated disabilities. Their learning capacity is greatly potentiated by their previous developmental progress prior to the sensory impairments. Although total independence, including gainful vocational training, is the goal, some deaf-blind children are unable to develop to this level. They may require lifelong parental or residential care. The nurse working with such families helps them deal with future goals for the child, including possible alternatives to home care during the parents' advancing years. In this respect much of the nurse's role is similar to that discussed in Chapter 23 for the mentally retarded or severely handicapped child.

COMMUNICATION DISORDERS

One of the most outstanding differences between man and lower animals is the human ability to communicate by using verbal language. The profound effect of hearing loss on speech development, discussed on p. 840, laid a foundation for understanding how inability to communicate hinders every aspect of a child's life. However, hearing impairment is only one of several reasons for communication disorders. Often the child has language and speech but is still unable to communicate effectively. This discussion focuses on types of communication disorders, guidelines for detecting children who require referral, and techniques to promote language/speech development and prevent problems.

Types of communication disorders

Communication disorders can be classified into language disabilities and speech impairments. *Language* is the arbitrary symbol system whereby a person relates thoughts or feeling to others.[26] The two major types are *receptive* language, or comprehension of the spoken word, and *expressive* language, or formulation of verbal symbols. *Speech* is the oral production of language, including articulation of sounds, rhythm, and tone. Difficulties can occur in either one or both components of communication.

Language disabilities. Language disorders may be characterized by an inability to (1) assign meaning to words (vocabulary), (2) organize words into sentences, (3) alter word forms to indicate tense, possession, and plurality, and (4) produce speech sounds comprising the words of language (frequently a form of an articulation disorder). Articulation patterns in language disorders differ from those seen in speech impairment. In the latter instance the child tends to distort or substitute a few consonants, especially those that are learned last—"s," "l," "r," and "th". As a result speech is fairly intelligible. In the former instance the child omits many consonants, usually at the end of words, and frequently substitutes the letters "t," "d," "k," or "y" for them. Consequently speech is almost unintelligible.[29]

Speech impairment. Speech impairments include differences from the normal in articulation, voice production, and fluency. *Articulation* errors refer to those sounds that a child makes incorrectly or inappropriately. *Voice disorders* are defined as differences in terms of pitch, loudness, and quality. *Dysfluency* or rhythm disorders usually consist of repetitions of sounds, words, or phrases. One of the most common and serious dysfluencies is stuttering.

Causes of communication disorders

The most common cause of communication disorders is mental retardation; the next most common is hearing impairment. Other causes include central nervous system dysfunction, which tends to result in central auditory imperception or language disability; poor role models for developing language and speech; severe emotional disturbance, such as autism and schizophrenia; and organic problems, such as cleft palate, vocal cord injury, and paralysis or foreshortening of the soft palate or uvula. In some instances, such as in stuttering, the cause is unknown or speculative.

Nursing interventions

Detection. Communication disorders can occur at any age but are most commonly found during childhood. The preschool period is considered critical to language development and therefore is a prime age for detection and intervention. Failure to detect communication disorders during early childhood affects the development of social relationships and emotional interactions, increases difficulty in developing academic skills, and lessens the chances for successful correction of deficit skills. Since nurses are frequently involved in preventive health maintenance of well preschool children and care of ill or hospitalized youngsters, they are in an optimum position to assess children for adequate communication development and to detect deviations.

The first step toward detection of abnormalities is knowledge of normal language and speech development. Unless nurses are aware of when children achieve such milestones, they will not be able to distinguish when specific communication characteristics are expected and when they are considered deviations (Table 24-11). Nurses must also be aware of clues indicative of language disorders and speech impairment (Table 24-12).

The nurse investigates known causes of communication disorders, most notably mental retardation and hearing loss. The Denver Developmental Screening Test (Appendix F) is a reliable, easy tool for assessing developmental or functional age. A child who performs near his chronologic age in all areas except language should be further evaluated by a speech therapist for communication disorders.

The nurse has three methods available for assessing speech and language development: (1) direct observation of the child's verbal skills, (2) questioning of the parents, and (3) testing. Direct observation necessitates spontaneous language interaction between the child and nurse. Suggestions for initiating conversation include showing the child an object and asking him to describe it (asking him to name it often results in one-word responses that are too limited for evaluation of speech, although appropriate for evaluation of language), or posing questions, such as, "If you could have three wishes, what would you want?" The nurse may also use the word-imitative procedure by having the child repeat sentences or words. It is believed that children are not able to reproduce statements using correct grammatical forms that they have not previously learned to use.[29] Whenever possible, the nurse should tape-record the child's conversation for serial documentation of his progressive language/speech development and further evaluation by or consultation with a language or speech therapist.

Indirect assessment relies on parental information obtained through a history. Key questions that reflect problems in language or speech are listed in the boxed material on p. 871. Information obtained from the history must be viewed cautiously. Not infrequently parents are less aware of the child's difficulties because of lack of comparison with normal language development. They may not realize the degree of unintelligible speech because of familiarity with the child's approximation of words. Conversely parents may have unrealistic expectations regarding verbal develop-

Table 24-11. Normal language and speech development during early childhood

Normal language development		Normal speech development		
Age (years)	**Speech**	**Age (years)**	**Speech**	**Intelligibility**
1	Says two to three words with meaning Imitates sounds of animals	1-2	Omits most final and some initial consonants Substitutes consonants "m," "w," "p," "b," "k," "g," "n," "t," "d," and "h" for more difficult sounds Height of unintelligible jargon at age 18 months	Usually no more than 25% intelligible to unfamiliar listener Almost 100% unintelligible
2	Uses two- to three-word phrases Has vocabulary of about 300 words Uses "I," "me," "you"	2-3	Uses above consonants with vowels, but inconsistently and with much substitution Omission of final consonants Articulation lags behind vocabulary	At age 2 years, 65% intelligible in context At age 3 years, 70%-80% intelligible
3	Says four- to five-word sentences Has vocabulary of about 900 words Uses "who," "what," and "where" in asking questions Uses plurals, pronouns, and prepositions	3-4	Masters "b," "t," "d," "k," and "g"; sounds "r" and "l" may still be unclear; omits or substitutes "w" Repetitions and hesitations common	90%-100% intelligible
4-5	Has vocabulary of 1500 to 2100 words Able to use most grammatic forms correctly such as past tense of verb with "yesterday" Uses complete sentences with nouns, verbs, prepositions, adjectives, adverbs, and conjunctions	4-5	Masters "f" and "v"; may still distort "r," "l," "s," "z," "sh," "ch," "y," and "th" Little or no omission of initial or last consonant	Speech is totally intelligible, although some sounds are still imperfect
		5-6	Masters "r," "l," and "th"; may still distort "s," "z," "sh," "ch," and "j" (usually mastered by age 7½ to 8 years)	

Table 24-12. Cues for detecting communication disorders

Disorder	Characteristics
Language disability*	
Assigning meaning to words	First words not uttered before second birthday Vocabulary size reduced for age Difficulty in describing characteristics of objects, although may be able to name them Infrequent use of modifier words (adjectives or adverbs)
Organizing words into sentences	First sentences not uttered before third birthday Short and incomplete sentences Tendency to omit words (articles, prepositions) Misuse of the "be," "do," and "can" verb forms Difficulty understanding and producing questions Plateaus at an early developmental level
Altering word forms	Omission of endings for plurals and tenses Inappropriate use of plurals and tense endings Inaccurate use of possession words
Articulation patterns	Intelligibility of conversational speech reduced for age Omission of consonants at end of words Substitution of "t," "d," "k," and "g" for most other consonants Slowed or plateaued progress in the acquisition of new sounds
Speech impairment†	
Dysfluency (stuttering)	Repetition of sounds, words, or phrases Obvious frustration when attempts to communicate Demonstration of struggling behavior while talking (head jerks, eye blinks, retrials, or circumlocution)
Articulation deficiency	Omission of a sound where one should occur Distortion of a sound Substitution of an incorrect sound for a correct one
Voice disorders	Deviations in pitch (too high or too low, especially for age and sex) Deviations in loudness Deviations in quality (hypernasality or hyponasality)

*Data from Schwartz, A. H., and Murphy, M. W.: Pediatrics **55**(5):717-722, May 1975.
†Data from Van Hattum, R. J.: Nursing '75 **5**(3):12-15, March 1975.

Assessment of communication disorders

*Key questions for language disorders**

1. How old was your child when he began to speak his first words?
2. How old was your child when he began to put words into sentences?
3. Does your child have difficulty in learning new vocabulary words?
4. Does your child omit words from sentences (that is, do his sentences sound telegraphic?)
5. Does your child speak in short or incomplete sentences?
6. Does your child have trouble with verbs such as "is," "am," "are," "was," and "were"?
7. Does your child have difficulty in following directions?
8. Does your child seem to have difficulty in understanding you if you use long sentences?
9. Does your child respond appropriately to questions?
10. Does your child ask questions beginning with "who," "what," "where," and "why?"
11. Does your child use present and past tense verbs correctly?
12. Does it seem that your child has made little or no progress in speech and language in the last 6 to 12 months?
13. Does your child omit sounds from his words?
14. Do you believe that your child's speech is more difficult to understand than it should be in view of his age?
15. Does it seem like your child uses "t," "d," "k," or "g" in place of most other consonants when he speaks?

Key questions for speech impairment

1. Does your child ever stammer or repeat sounds or words?
2. Does your child seem anxious or frustrated when trying to express an idea?
3. Have you noticed behavior in your child such as blinking his eyes, jerking his head, or attempting to rephrase his thought with different words when he stammers?
4. What do you do when any of these occur?
5. Does your child omit sounds from his words or substitute the correct consonant with another one (such as "rabbit" with "wabbit")?
6. Do you have any difficulty in understanding his speech?
7. Has anyone else ever remarked about having difficulty in understanding him?
8. Do you believe that his speech is appropriate for his age (for example, as intelligible as that of his peers)?
9. Has there been any recent change in the sound of his voice?

*From Schwartz, A. H., and Murphy, M. W.: Cues for screening language disorders in preschool children, Pediatrics **55**(5):717-722, May 1975. Copyright American Academy of Pediatrics 1975.

ment and may exaggerate the degree of dysfluency, misarticulation, or word usage.

To obtain more objective data, the nurse administers language/speech tests. One test, which employs the word-imitative procedure, is the Denver Articulation Screening Examination (DASE) (see Appendix F). The child repeats twenty-two words but pronounces thirty different sound elements. The raw score, or the number of correctly pronounced sounds, is then compared to the percentile rank for children in that age-group. The examiner must be careful to evaluate the specific sound, rather than the quality of the entire word. For beginning examiners it is helpful to validate the final score by comparing the results with a different examiner, ideally a speech therapist. The child is also scored on intelligibility, by selection of one of four possible categories: (1) easy to understand, (2) understandable half of the time, (3) not understandable, or (4) cannot evaluate. The Denver Articulation Screening Examination is a reliable, effective screening tool for nurses because it requires only 10 minutes to perform and it is designed to discriminate between significant delay and normal variations in the acquisition of speech sounds. It also detects common abnormal conditions such as hyponasality, hypernasality, tongue thrust, and lateral lisp.

Development of language and speech is influenced by many variables, making evaluation of assessment findings difficult, especially when communication patterns are normal but delayed. The nurse can better formulate a decision regarding referral based on knowledge of the following environmental factors—bilingualism, multiple birth, socioeconomic level, and gender—that are known to hinder or promote language/speech development.

Bilingualism may have a deleterious effect on both articulation and acquisition of vocabulary when parents pressure children to use both languages skillfully and interchangeably. However, if parents are encouraged to allow children to proceed at their own pace and to use either language when it is easiest for them, the effect of learning two languages simultaneously can advance the learning above the norms for that age level.

There is also some evidence that multiple birth, such as twins or triplets, results in delayed speech development in these children as compared to children of single birth. In this case nurses should assess and evaluate the level of twins' or triplets' communication with a broader range of expected language development than other children. They also should caution parents against comparing each twin's development to that of the other and expecting both to develop at the same rate.

Socioeconomic level has a measurable and significant effect on acquisition of verbal skills. Children from higher socioeconomic families surpass children from lower socioeconomic homes in all criteria of language development. Since an adequate role model and appropriate reinforcement are part of the reason for this difference, nurses can help parents and others from less advantageous backgrounds carry out adequate role modeling for the child and can discuss ways of positively reinforcing proper speech sounds. They can explain to parents that a suitable role model with appropriate reinforcement, such as parental approval, is essential for children to acquire speech.

Gender is also a significant variable in assessing speech problems. There is some evidence that preschool girls surpass boys in vocabulary, comprehension, and length of response. However, by school age, boys generally equal or excel the opposite sex, especially in vocabulary acquisition. Despite this fact, the predominance of males to females in problems of stuttering has been found to be from 3:1 to 5:1 as school years advance. Therefore, a male child who persists in speech difficulties, such as the pattern of normal hesitancy, is probably a vulnerable candidate for serious speech problems later on. This is an important fact to remember when deciding which child may need closer evaluation of present speech difficulties.

Following assessment and detection of language or speech problems, the nurse must make a decision regarding appropriate referral. The all too frequent advice of "wait and let's see what happens" or "he will grow out of it" is often to the detriment of the child's future development. Since children normally vary greatly in their development of verbal skills, the nurse needs some guidelines for determining which child's development is abnormal. Table 24-13 lists general recommendations for referring children for specialized audiologic and language evaluations. Information regarding available services for language, speech, and hearing can be obtained from the American Speech and Hearing Association.*

Prevention and education. The primary intervention for communication disorders is prevention. Much of prevention directly relates to factors that predispose to causes of language/speech impairment, namely, mental retardation and hearing loss. Infants at risk for either condition (see pp. 784 and 838) should be referred for audiologic evaluation prior to 6 months of age so that audiologic and speech therapy can be initiated immediately, when required.

Prevention also involves early recognition of children at risk for language delays, such as those exposed to inadequate role models, or children at risk for speech impairment, such as those who are expected to communicate above their present developmental level. In either case prevention necessitates parental education to foster the child's communication development.

Language delay.[16] The nurse can emphasize to parents that when a child is delayed in his language development it becomes very important to try and structure what the parents do so that when they are with their child he has the op-

*9030 Old Georgetown Road, Washington, D.C. 20014.

Table 24-13. Guidelines for referral regarding communication disorders

Age	Assessment findings
2 years	Failure to speak any meaningful words spontaneously Consistent use of gestures rather than vocalizations Difficulty in following verbal directions Failure to respond consistently to sound
3 years	Speech is largely unintelligible Failure to use sentences of three or more words Frequent omission of initial consonants Use of vowels rather than consonants
5 years	Stutters, stammers, or has any other type of dysfluency Sentence structure noticeably impaired Substitutes easily produced sounds for more difficult ones Omits word endings (plurals, tenses of verbs, and so on)
School age	Poor voice quality (monotonous, loud, or barely audible) Vocal pitch inappropriate for age Any distortions, omissions, or substitutions of sounds after age 7 years Connected speech characterized by use of unusual confusions or reversals
General	Any child with signs suggestive of a hearing impairment Any child who is embarrassed or disturbed by his speech Parents who are excessively concerned or who pressure the child to speak at a level above that appropriate for his age

Adapted from Marlowe, N. B.: Clin. Pediatr. **12**(12):675-677, December 1973.

portunity to learn. The underlying principle is not to bombard the child with words so that he will learn more language but to plan what will be said to him, how he will be observed, what responses will be expected of him, and how he will be reinforced.

COMPREHENSIVE INTERACTION. No matter what the child's age or level of development, it is important for the parents to try and respond to him by talking to him, praising him, or taking time to listen when he does the following: (1) comes to the parents and tries to tell them something; (2) attempts to follow through with a question the parents have asked or a direction they have given; (3) brings the parents toys or books; (4) tries to imitate what the parents are saying or doing; and (5) seems to enjoy playing near the parents.

COMPREHENSION. It is important to remember that children usually understand many more words than they can say. Also a child usually has to understand a word before he can produce it. Many language-delayed children are somewhat more delayed in comprehension of specific words, questions, directions, and so on, than in other areas of development. Therefore, it is important to concentrate on teaching the meaning of new words to the child, giving him verbal information, and providing listening activities for him as well as helping him produce speech. The nurse can suggest that parents select a small group of words to use each time they are involved in different activities with the child. For example, each time the parent opens a door or a box the parent should say, "Open." After doing this many times, the parent only says, "Open" and waits to see if the child starts carrying through with the motion. The parent praises the child after he has attempted to respond to a word.

If the parents give the child a specific word to respond to, such as, "Find the dog," and he does not attempt to do so, they should gently shake his hand and place it on the picture of a dog in the book and then praise him for finding it. After doing this many times the child should be able to locate the picture after hearing the word. The parents should try to give short verbal descriptions of whatever the child is attending to at the time he is involved in a particular activity. For example, if he is emptying a drawer, the parents should say, "Pots out—you're taking all the pots out." If the child points to a picture, the parents talk about the particular thing he is looking at. The parents should try to expand his comprehension vocabulary by talking about what is happening, such as "Timmy's running," where things are (up, high), how things feel ("grass is wet"), how things compare (big ball), and less familiar words (empty, sunny).

PRODUCTION OF WORDS. By studying the first words that children use and how they begin to put words together, it is interesting to note that what is actually happening is that children are telling parents how they see the world around them and what is happening to them at the time. Although initially some children do learn the names of common items or people in their environment, such as "mama," "doggie," and "bottle," most of the first meaningful words that they will use indicate egocentric desires, such as "more," "mine," "no," "I do," and so on.

In choosing vocabulary parents should consider the following: the *usefulness* of the word to the child, such as the word "more," which can denote more food, another ride in the car, or the desire to be read another story; ease of pronunciation, especially use of vowels and the consonants "b," "d," "m," "k," "t," "p," or "d"; and words the meaning of which the child comprehends. Children normally learn monosyllabic words, such as "mama," "bye," and so on. When learning to pronounce polysyllabic words, they frequently only pronounce the initial sound, such as "ba" for "bottle." Any approximation of words that the child uses should be repeated back to him with a clearer model. At the same time parents should praise him for his attempts to pronounce the word.

Parents can also encourage vocabulary by having the child say a word before some request is fulfilled. For example, each time he wants to go outside the parent should try to have him say part of the word "out," or each time he wants more cookies, the parent should expect him to try to say part of the word "more." As he progresses and can imitate more easily, the parents can expect him to do more, such as imitating more single words or two-word combinations. If the parents think that he can at least vocalize or make any kind of sound before he gets something, they should be sure to expect this rather than giving in to any kind of whining, grunting, or gesturing.

TALKING AND RESPONDING TO THE CHILD. It will help the child if the parents plan ahead in regard to the specific things they will say and how they will respond to him. The child needs the parents to point things out to him. For example, as the child is attending to or is involved in a particular activity, the parents should try to describe what the child is doing. If he is looking at what the parents are doing, the parents should describe what they are doing. *They should reduce the length of what they are saying to approximately one level above the level at which the child is talking.* If he is just beginning to use single-word approximations, they should describe his activities in one or two words. For example, as he points to the "duck," they should say, "Duck" or "Quack-quack." If the child is using single words, the parents could add two- or three-word models, such as, "Duck swimming," "Duck in water," "Big duck," or "Duck says quack-quack." If the child is using two-word combinations, the parents could describe what he is doing or looking at in three to four words, such as, "See duck swimming," or "Lots of big ducks."

Sometimes parents ask many questions of the child who has a language delay. The usual reaction from the child is silence. If there is a high frequency of questions, the parents should try to reduce this by making statements about what the child is doing rather than asking questions about it. For example, instead of saying, "What's this?" they should say, "Look, here's a cow." To help the child answer questions, parents should present the question while the child is listening, wait for him to try to answer, praise him if he does so, and, if he has difficulty, give him the answer. For example, if the parent states, "What does the cow say?" and the child has no response, the parent replies, "The cow says moo moo."

TEACHING GRAMMATICAL FORMS. Children will begin to use adult-like forms of words only after they are using two-word combinations for an extended period of time. Parents should remember that when they are using single words and beginning to combine these single words into two-word relationships, the child is talking about ideas and how the world appears to them. For example, when the child says, "Ducky water," he is telling the parent that he sees the duck and the duck is in the water. At that point of development, if he used the word "is" it would not add any meaning for him, because it is the underlying idea that is important rather than the grammatical rules.

When the child is ready, he will begin to apply the "rules of grammar," usually by imitating what he hears around him. He will understand that when "s" is added to the word "dog," it means more than one dog. Or if "ed" is added to a word, that means that something has already happened. Children, however, benefit from having these specific word endings emphasized and exaggerated. Therefore, if the child has been using two-word combinations for some time, it helps if the parents stress different parts of grammar that he has omitted or the order of words in a sentence. For example, if the child says, "Push ball," the parent could respond with a subject-verb model, such as, "Boy push ball." If the child says, "Kitty eat," the parent could exaggerate the parts of speech he left out, by saying, "Yes, a kitty is eating."

REINFORCEMENT. Whenever possible, parents want to respond to the child with what he is trying to say. As mentioned previously, it helps to give him a hug, praise him directly, or comment on what he is saying. However, in order to know what he is trying to say, it is essential that the parents watch and listen to him as carefully as possible. Parents should try to develop a habit of looking at what the child is doing when he is talking. Some attempts on his part to talk will be rather obvious, for example, if he struggles to get out of the parent's arms and says, "Dou," it will be easy for the parent to understand his meaning and imitate him by saying, "Down, good boy, you said down," as he is put down. However, if he points to a dog and says, "Oo," the parent needs to try to think about what he is referring to. Perhaps he is saying to himself that this is a four-legged animal and that all four-legged animals go "moo" or look like a cow.

It is not always easy to understand what a child is trying to say. Sometimes parents choose the wrong word to stress and the child becomes frustrated in his attempts to make himself understood. However, success in guessing at the correct meaning of the child's word approximation is greatly reinforcing to him because it symbolizes the usefulness and efficiency of language. The nurse needs to bear this fact in mind, especially when the child is hospitalized and dependent on others to understand him. In these instances it is beneficial to have the parent write a list of the child's vocalizations and related meanings, particularly those that refer to his needs regarding toileting, dressing, bathing, eating, sleep, and play.

Speech impairment. One of the most serious speech problems is stuttering. This hesitancy or dysfluency in speech pattern is a *normal* characteristic of language development

Suggestions for parents regarding stuttering in children

To be encouraged	*To be avoided*
Viewing the hesitancy and dysfluency as a normal part of speech development	The natural tendency to "help" the child by supplying the word when he is having a block
Giving the child plenty of time and the impression that you are not rushed or in a hurry	Telling him to stop and start over, to think before he speaks, or to take it easy and go slowly
Looking directly at the child while he is talking; being patient and never ridiculing or criticizing	Showing great concern, embarrassment, or disapproval for the hesitancy
Speaking clearly and articulating well but not stressing that all sounds must be perfected too early	*Anything* that emphasizes the stuttering and calls the child's attention to his speech skills
Identifying situations when stuttering increases and avoiding them or ignoring the hesitancy	
Capitalizing on periods of fluent speech with positive reinforcement	

during the preschool years. It occurs because the child's advancing mental ability and level of comprehension exceed his vocabulary acquisition. The child knows what he wants to say but hesitates or repeats words or sounds as he tries to find the vocabulary to express himself. Eventually his language skills parallel the other abilities and speech becomes fluent.

However, when parents or other significant persons place undue emphasis or stress on this pattern of dysfluency, an abnormal speech pattern may result. Chances for reversal of stuttering are good until about 7 years of age. Therefore, prevention must begin early. The nurse discusses with parents the normal dysfluencies in children's speech. When stuttering does occur, parents are advised to use the suggestions listed above in the boxed material in order to prevent inadvertently reinforcing this pattern. If excessive concern on the part of the parent or frustration and struggling behavior from the child are noted, they are referred for language and speech evaluation. The critical point to remember is that the dysfluency must be arrested before the child develops an awareness or anticipation of the difficulty and begins to mistrust his speech skills.

Children who are pressured into producing sounds ahead of their developmental level may develop dyslalia (articulation problems) or revert to using infantile speech. Prevention involves discussing with parents the usual achievement of speech production during childhood. The Denver Articulation Screening Examination is an excellent tool to assess articulation skills in the child and to explain to parents the expected progression of sounds. Since the consonants "s," "l," "r," and "th" are mastered at about 7 to 8 years of age, true articulation problems are usually seen during the school years.

Voice disorders are tolerated by society more than other types of speech impairment. However, recognition of voice disorders is important because this can lead to prevention or identification of other problems. For example, continued vocal abuse may result in permanent damage to the vocal cords, hoarseness may be an early sign of carcinoma, and nasality may indicate an undiagnosed palatal problem or paralysis of the velum following adenoidectomy.[33] The nurse encourages parents to seek further evaluation by a physician and speech therapist to rule out any of these disorders.

REFERENCES

1. American Academy of Pediatrics, Committee on Children with Handicaps: The physician and the deaf child, Pediatrics **51**(6):1100-1110, June 1973.
2. Bess, F. N., and Powell, R. L.: Hearing hazard from model airplanes; a study on their potential damaging effects on the auditory mechanism, Clin. Pediatr. **11**(11):621-624, November 1972.
3. Brazelton, T. B.: Neonatal Behavioral Assessment Scale, Philadelphia, 1973, J. B. Lippincott Co., and London, 1973, William Heinemann, Ltd.
4. Bumbalo, J., and Seidel, M.: Identifying and serving a multiple handicapped population, Nurs. Clin. North Am. **10**(2): 341-352, June 1975.
5. Davis, H., and Silverman, S. R.: Hearing and deafness, New York, 1970, Holt, Rinehart and Winston, Inc.
6. Downs, M. P., and Silver, H. K.: The "A.B.C.D." to "HEAR," Clin. Pediatr. **11**(10):563-565, October 1972.
7. Dupont, J.: What to do for common eye emergencies, Nursing '76 **6**(5):17-19, May 1976.
8. Falk, S. A., and Farmer, J. C.: Incubator noise and possible deafness, Arch. Otolaryngol. **97:**385-387, May 1973.
9. Frey, R. M., and Krause, I. B.: The incidence of color blindness among deaf children, Except. Child. **37**(5):393-394, 1971.

10. Gould, H.: How to remove contact lens from comatose patients, Am. J. Nurs. **76**(9):1483-1485, September 1976.
11. Guldager, L.: The deaf blind: their education and their needs, Except. Child. **36**(3):203-206, 1969.
12. Hearing alert, Washington, D.C., Alexander Graham Bell Association for the Deaf.
13. Hobbs, N.: The futures of children, San Francisco, 1975, Jossey-Bass, Inc., Publishers.
14. Kephart, J. G., and associates: A journey into the world of the blind child, Except. Child. **40**(6):421-427, 1974.
15. Knobloch, H., and Pasamanick, B., editor: Gesell and Amatruda's developmental diagnosis, New York, 1974, Harper & Row, Publishers.
16. Kriegsman, E.: A guide for the language delayed child, unpublished manuscript, University of Washington, 1977.
17. Lawson, L. J., and associates: Ophthalmological deficiencies in deaf children, Except. Child. **37**(1):17-20, 1970.
18. Lippman, O.: Vision screening of young children, Am. J. Public Health **61**(8):1598-1601, August 1971.
19. Lipscomb, D. M.: Environmental noise is growing—is it damaging our hearing? Clin. Pediatr. **11**(7):374-375, July 1972.
20. Lipscomb, D. M.: How frequent are ear lesions and hearing defects among U.S. children? Clin. Pediatr. **12**(3):125-126, March 1973.
21. Moody, E. A.: Amblyopia. In Harvey, R. D., editor: Pediatric ophthalmology, Philadelphia, 1975, W. B. Saunders Co.
22. Payne, P. D., and Payne, R. L.: Behavior manifestations of children with hearing loss, Am. J. Nurs. **70**(8):1718, August 1970.
23. Pilgrim, M., and Sigler, B.: Phaco-emulsification for cataracts, Am. J. Nurs. **75**(6):976-977, June 1975.
24. Pollard, Z. F.: Accommodative esotropia during the first year of life, Arch. Ophthalmol. **94:**1912-1913, November 1976.
25. Pollard, Z. F.: Are we missing amblyopia? The answer is preschool screening, Pediatrics **60**(4):603-605, October 1977.
26. Rommel, J.: Referral of children with speech problems, Pediatr. Nurs. **2**(2):28-32, March/April 1976.
27. Rupp, R., and Koch, C.: Effects of too-loud music on human ears, Clin. Pediatr. **8**(2):60-62, February 1969.
28. Scholl, G. T.: The education of children with visual impairments. In Cruickshank, W. M., and Johnson, G. O., editors: Education of exceptional children and youth, Englewood Cliffs, N.J., 1975, Prentice-Hall, Inc.
29. Schwartz, A. H., and Murphy, M. W.: Cues for screening language disorders in preschool children, Pediatrics **55**(5): 717-722, May 1975.
30. Seleny, F. L., and Streczyn, M.: Noise characteristics in the baby compartment of incubators, Am. J. Dis. Child. **117:** 445-450, April 1969.
31. Shirkey, H. C., editor: Pediatric therapy, ed. 5, St. Louis, 1975, The C. V. Mosby Co.
32. Stein, L. K., and Green, M. B.: Problems in managing the young deaf blind child, Except. Child. **38**(6):481-484, 1972.
33. Van Hattum, R. J.: Communication disorders in children: a guide for detection and referral, Nursing '75 **5**(3):12-15, March 1975.
34. Whitcraft, C. J.: Motor engramming for sensory deprivation or disability, Except. Child. **38**(6):475-478, 1972.

BIBLIOGRAPHY

Hearing impairment

Auxter, D.: Learning disabilities among deaf population, Except. Child. **37**(8):573-577, 1971.

Gustafson, S. R., and Coursin, D. B., editors: The child with a hearing problem. In The pediatric patient, Philadelphia, 1966, J. B. Lippincott Co.

Herth, K.: Beyond the curtain of silence, Am. J. Nurs. **74**(6): 1060-1061, June 1974.

Holm, V. A., and Thompson, G.: Selective hearing loss: clues to early identification, Pediatrics **47**(2):447-451, February 1971.

Keaster, J., Hyman, C. B., and Harris, I.: Hearing problems subsequent to neonatal hemolytic disease or hyperbilirubinemia, Am. J. Dis. Child. **117:**406-410, April 1969.

Kennedy, P., and Bruininks, R. H.: Social status of hearing impaired children in regular classrooms, Except. Child. **40**(5):336-342, 1974.

Lesser, S. R., and Easser, B. R.: Personality differences in the perceptually handicapped, J. Child Psychol. Psychiatry **11:**458-466, 1972.

Martin, V.: What it means to the parent of a deaf child, Otolaryngol. Clin. North Am. **5:**59, 1975.

McConnell, F.: A new approach to the management of childhood deafness, Pediatr. Clin. North Am. **17**(2):347-362, 1970.

Moores, D. F., and associates: Receptive abilities of deaf children across five modes of communication, Except. Child. **40**(1):22-28, 1973.

Northern, J., and Downs, M.: Hearing in children, Baltimore, 1974, The Williams & Wilkins Co.

Roach, R. E., and Rosecrans, C. J.: Verbal deficit in children with hearing loss, Except. Child. **38**(5):395-399, 1972.

Schlesinger, H. S., and Meadow, K. P.: Development of maturity in deaf children, Except. Child. **38**(6):461-467, 1972.

Schwartzberg, J.: When a hearing impaired child must go to the hospital, Volta Review **74:**30, 1972.

Stark, E. W., and Borton, T. E.: Klippel-Feil syndrome and associated hearing loss, Arch. Otolaryngol. **97:**415-419, May 1973.

Wright, J.: Deaf but not mute, Am. J. Nurs. **76**(5):795-799, May 1976.

Visual impairment

Breinin, G. M.: Accommodative strabismus and the AC/A ratio, Am. J. Ophthalmol. **71**(1):303-311, January 1971.

Burns, R. P.: Effect of silicone contact lenses on corneal epithelial metabolism, Am. J. Ophthalmol. **71**(2):486-489, February 1971.

Calvert, D. R., and associates: Experiences with preschool deaf-blind children, Except. Child. **38**(5):415-421, 1972.

Catford, G. V., and Oliver, A.: Development of visual acuity, Arch. Dis. Child. **48**(1):47-50, 1973.

Corn, A. L., and Martinez, I.: When you have a visually handicapped child in your classroom: suggestions for teachers, New York, 1977, American Foundation for the Blind.

Hiles, D. A.: Strabismus, Am. J. Nurs. **4**(6):1082-1089, June 1974.

Hulsey, S.: Liberating the blind student, Am. Educ., pp. 19-22, July 1973.

Is your child blind? New York, 1975, American Foundation for the Blind.

Kahn, H.: Visual dysfunctions, Nursing '74 **4**(10):26-27, October 1974.

Moor, P. M.: Toilet habits: suggestions for training a child who is blind, New York, American Foundation for the Blind.

Murphy, J. A.: How does a blind person get around? New York, 1977, American Foundation for the Blind.

Ryan, S. J., and Von Noorden, G. K.: Further observations in the aspiration technique in cataract surgery, Am. J. Ophthalmol. **71**(3):626-630, March 1971.

Thurrell, R. J., and Rice, D. G.: Eye rubbing in blind children: application of a sensory deprivation model, Except. Child. **36**(5): 325-330, 1970.

Tweedie, D.: Demonstrating behavioral change of deaf-blind children, Except. Child. **40**(7):510-512, 1974.

Vaughan, D.: Common ocular disorders, Hosp. Med. **8**:22, 1972.

Von Noorden, G. K.: Diagnosis and management of eye muscle problems in childhood, Surg. Clin. North Am. **50**(4):885-894, August 1970.

Language and speech impairment

Berry, M.: Language disorders in children, New York, 1969, Appleton-Century-Crofts.

Brown, M. S.: Testing of a young child for articulation skills, Clin. Pediatr. **15**(7):639-644, July 1976.

Dickson, S.: Communication disorders: remedial principles and procedures, Chicago, 1974, Scott, Foresman and Co.

Gonzalez, G.: Language, culture, and exceptional children, Except. Child. **40**(8):565-570, 1974.

Kirk, S. A.: Ethnic differences in psycholinguistics abilities, Except. Child. **39**(2):112-118, 1972.

Kulig, S. G., and Baker, K. A.: Preliminary field-testing of the physician's developmental quick screen for speech disorders ("PDQ"), Clin. Pediatr. **15**(12):1146-1150, December 1976.

Marlowe, W. B.: The pediatrician and the child with a communication disorder, Clin. Pediatr. **12**(12):675-677, December 1973.

Travis, L. E.: Handbook of speech pathology, New York, 1972, Appleton-Century-Crofts.

Van Riper, C.: The treatment of stuttering, Englewood Cliffs, N.J., 1973, Prentice-Hall, Inc.

UNIT TEN
The hospitalized child

When illness requires hospitalization, it creates a crisis for the child. Depending on his age, the child must deal with separation from familiar care givers and environment, exposure to painful experiences, loss of independence, and disruption of nearly every aspect of his usual life-style. Often the reason necessitating hospitalization is of much less concern to the child than the consequences of confinement. Emergency admissions pose an even greater threat because of the lack of time to prepare the child for this event.

Chapter 25, *The Child's Reaction to Illness and Hospitalization,* is concerned with the child's age-related reactions to illness and hospitalization and interventions that lessen the psychologic trauma of the experience, particularly parent participation and preparation for admission to the hospital and prior to medical procedures. It also discusses general principles of preoperative and postoperative nursing care. Chapter 26, *Pediatric Variations of Nursing Intervention,* deals with pediatric variations of nursing procedures. It is not designed to present a detailed description of how to perform specific procedures but rather how to safely implement them with children.

25

The child's reaction to illness and hospitalization

For children illness and hospitalization constitute a major life crisis. It is the purpose of this chapter to acquaint nurses with the various aspects of illness and hospitalization in children in order to assist them in providing the kind of care that promotes optimum resolution of the crisis and positive growth from the experience.

ILLNESS AND HOSPITALIZATION AS A CRISIS

The word "crisis" has many definitions, such as "upset in steady state," "any sharp or decisive change for which old patterns are inadequate," "situations which block the usual patterns of action and call for new ones," or "a turning point."[14] All of these definitions have two things in common: (1) an event occurs that is perceived as stressful, and (2) the usual coping mechanisms are inadequate to solve the problem. The latter characteristic implies a growth potential because three outcomes are possible: (1) the person solves the problem at a lower precrisis level of coping, (2) the person maintains the precrisis level of functioning, or (3) the person attains a higher level of problem solving. The second and third outcomes are the minimal and optimal therapeutic goals, respectively.

Children are particularly vulnerable to the crises of illness and hospitalization because (1) either stress represents a change from the usual state of health and environmental routine, and (2) children have a limited number of coping mechanisms to solve the stressful events. Children's reactions to these crisis are influenced by their developmental age, previous experience with illness, separation, or hospitalization, available support system, and the seriousness of the illness and threat of hospitalization.

Stressors and reactions related to developmental stage

Children's understanding of, reaction to, and method of coping with illness or hospitalization are influenced by the significance of individual stressors (those events that produce stress) during each developmental phase. Although the major stressors of separation, loss of control, and bodily injury and the behavioral reactions are discussed in the following section, a review of the previous chapters on normal growth and development will facilitate a more thorough understanding of children's physical, psychosocial, and cognitive abilities and limitations. In addition Chapter 27 presents an in-depth discussion of children's and family members' reactions to a life-threatening illness. Table 25-1 summarizes the principal behavior responses to each stressor during the developmental periods of childhood.

Separation anxiety. The major stress from middle infancy throughout the preschool years is separation anxiety. Three distinct phases are evident in the crisis of separation. During the phase of *protest,* the child cries loudly, screams for his mother, refuses the attention of anyone else, and is inconsolable in his grief. The child may continue this behavior for a few hours to several days. Some children may protest continuously, ceasing only from physical exhaustion. If a stranger approaches the child, he will initially protest even louder.

During the phase of *despair,* the crying stops. The child is much less active, is disinterested in play or food, and withdraws from others. The child looks sad, lonely, isolated, and apathetic. The major behavior characteristic is depression, a result of increasing hopelessness, grief, and mourning.

The third stage is *detachment,* which is sometimes also called *denial.* Superficially it appears that the child has finally adjusted to the loss. He becomes more interested in his surroundings, plays with others, and seems to form new relationships. However, this behavior is the result of resignation and is not a sign of contentment. He detaches from his mother in an effort to escape the emotional pain of desiring her presence. The child copes by forming shallow relationships with others, becoming increasingly self-centered, and attaching primary importance to material objects. One dominant characteristic of these children is their future inability to form intimate, trusting interpersonal attachments to significant others.

Without an understanding of the meaning of each stage of behavior, hospital personnel may erroneously label the behaviors as positive or negative. In the stage of protest, hos-

Table 25-1. Children's reactions to stress

Age	Development achievement and major fears	Behavior reactions
Infants	Trust vs mistrust	
	Separation	Protest—cries, screams; searches for parent with eyes; clings to parent; avoids and rejects contact with strangers Despair—inactive, withdrawn, depressed, disinterested in environment Detachment—resignation; superficial "adjustment," that is, appears interested in surroundings, happy, friendly
	Pain	Neonate—total body reaction, easily distracted Later infancy—localized reaction, uncooperative, offers physical resistance
Toddlers	Antonomy vs shame and doubt	
	Separation	Protest—verbal cries for parent; verbal attack on others; physical fighting, that is, kicks, bites, hits, pinches; tries to escape to find parent, clings to parent and physically tries to force parent to stay Despair—passive, depressed, disinterested in environment, uncommunicative; loss of newly learned skills Detachment—similar to infants, less regressive behaviors
	Loss of control—physical striction, loss of routine and rituals, dependency Bodily injury and pain	Resistance Physical aggression Verbal uncooperativeness Regression Negativism Temper tantrums
Preschoolers	Initiative vs guilt	
	Separation	Protest—less direct and aggressive than toddlers, may displace feelings on others Despair, Detachment } similar to toddlers
	Loss of control—sense of own power Bodily injury and pain—intrusive procedures, mutilation	Aggression—physical and verbal Regression—dependency; withdrawal; feelings of fear, anxiety, guilt, shame; physiologic responses
School-age children	Industry vs inferiority	
	Separation (parents as well as peers) Loss of control—enforced dependency, altered family roles	Usually do not see stage behavior of protest, despair, or detachment Any of following may indicate separation as well as other fears—loneliness, boredom, isolation, withdrawal, depression, displaced anger, hostility, frustration
	Bodily injury and pain—fear of illness itself, disability, and death; intrusion in procedures of a sexual nature	Seeks information Passively accepts pain Groans or whines Holds rigidly still Tries to act brave Communicates about pain May try to postpone an event
Adolescents	Identity vs role diffusion	
	Loss of control—loss of identity, enforced dependency	Rejection Uncooperativeness Withdrawal Self-assertion
	Bodily injury and pain—mutilation, sexual changes	Self-control Cooperativeness Fear, anxiety Overconfidence May capitalize on gains from pain
	Separation (especially peer group)	Depression Loneliness Withdrawal Boredom

pital personnel may view the loud crying as bad behavior. Since the protesting increases if a stranger approaches, they may interpret the reaction as evidence of their need to stay away. During the quiet, withdrawn phase of despair, they regard the child as finally "settling in" to his new surroundings. The detachment behaviors are proof of a "good adjustment." The faster a child reaches this stage, the more likely he will be regarded as the "ideal patient."

Since children seem to react "negatively" to visits by their parents, uninformed observers feel justified in restricting parental visiting privileges. For example, during the protest stage, children outwardly do not appear happy to see their parents. Instead, they may cry louder than before their visit. If they are depressed, they may reject their parents or begin to protest once more. Often they cling to their parents in an effort to assure their continued presence. Hospital personnel may view such behavior reactions as disturbing the child's adjustment to his surroundings. If the separation has progressed to the phase of detachment, children will respond no differently to their parents than to any other strange or familiar person.

Such reactions are equally distressing to parents, who are unaware of their meaning. If hospital personnel regard parents as intruders, parents will view their absence as "beneficial" to the child's adjustment and recovery. They may respond to the child's behavior by staying for short periods of time, decreasing the frequency of visits, or lying to the child when it is time to leave. Consequently a destructive cycle of misunderstanding and unmet needs results.

Infants. Although infancy is generally regarded as the period from birth to the completion of 1 year of age, to understand the reactions of infants to illness and hospitalization it is more relevant to divide this age span into preattachment to the significant care giver and postattachment. Prior to the recognition and attachment of young children to their parents, the major reaction of infants to illness or hospitalization is bodily sensations of pain, immobilization, and change in the usual caring activities of bathing, dressing, and feeding. The seriousness of the illness, the events of hospitalization, and separation from parents have meaning only in terms of disruption of infants' comfort and established routine.

Separation. Somewhere by the end of the first 6 months of life, infants selectively recognize their mothers, are strongly attached to them, and protest furiously if separated from them. The fear of strangers or so-called eighth-month anxiety, which was originally thought to occur in the third quarter of the first year, is now believed to begin as early as 4 months of age.[17] Reactions to the stress of pain, illness, or hospitalization occur mostly from separation of child and mother. If separation is avoided, infants seem to have a tremendous capacity for withstanding any type of stress.

Pain. Behavioral reactions to pain also correlate with age. Neonates' degree of perception of pain is still controversial. The observed general reaction is total body movement associated with brief loud crying that ceases on distraction.[16] Because of the effectiveness of distraction, medical personnel may perform painful procedures without the use of local anesthetics, as in the case of circumcision. However, there is presently no way of knowing what future psychologic effect such exposure to pain may cause. This is particularly significant in high-risk neonates, who are subjected to multiple, continuous painful procedures.

By the end of the first month, there is a noticeable decrease in the diffuse body response to pain. Somewhere between 3 and 10 months of age, infants localize the pain. For example, they react to an injection by withdrawing the leg. Since all their cognitive and sensory abilities are advancing, they also begin to associate environmental factors with painful events. By 4 months of age infants no longer react solely to the painful stimulation, but to a complex range of perceptual cues from their environment. Individual differences in temperament are marked. Some infants may cry loudly following the procedure, whereas others are easily calmed by a gentle hug. It is important to recognize and respect such early signs of individuality and intervene accordingly.

Infants less than 6 months of age seem to have no memory of previous painful experiences and react to a potentially stressful situation with less apprehension and fear than older children. However, after this time, children's response to pain is influenced by their recall of prior painful experiences and the emotional contagion of parents during the procedure.[20] Infants react intensely with physical resistance and uncooperativeness. They may refuse to lie still, attempt to push the person away, or try to escape with whatever motor activity they have achieved. Distraction does little to lessen their immediate reaction to pain, and anticipatory preparation, such as showing them the equipment, tends to increase their fear and resistance. The most supportive intervention is to perform the procedure as quickly as possible and maintain parent-child contact.

Since emotional contagion is a factor in the child's response to pain, it may be necessary to prepare parents for the event. Decreasing their fear of the procedure will increase their effective support of the child during the experience.

The most common indication of pain in children, but particularly in preverbal youngsters, is behavioral changes such as irritability, lethargy, loss of appetite, or disturbed sleep patterns. Specific reactions often indicate discomfort in localized body regions, such as rolling the head from side to side or pulling the ears from an earache, lying on the side with legs flexed on the abdomen for abdominal pain, or favoring a body part during usual activity.

Toddlers

Separation. Toddlers' main reaction to stress is also caused by separation. Although toddlers are friendlier and more tolerant of strangers and tend to stray away from parents for brief periods of time, they are still very attached and dependent on them for continued emotional growth. The stages of separation are the same as those observed during infancy, but the behaviors may be more goal directed. Toddlers verbally plea for their parents to stay and physically attempt to secure or find them. They may demonstrate displeasure on their return or departure by having temper tantrums, refusing to comply to the usual routines of mealtime, bedtime, or toileting, or regressing to more primitive levels of development.

Toddlers' reactions to stress are compounded by their developmental striving for autonomy. In addition to separation, the main threats to the achievement of this goal are (1) loss of control from physical restriction, altered routine or rituals, and dependency and (2) bodily injury and pain. Their principal responses to these stressors are physical resistance, aggression, negativism, and regression.

Loss of control. Any restriction or limitation on toddlers' newly gained motor skills results in an immediate threat to their sense of security and is met with physical resistance. Toddlers' needs for freedom of movement are so essential that the simple act of lying toddlers on their back can cause forceful resistance and noncompliance. Although pain is a component of many similar reactions from toddlers, painless procedures such as taking rectal temperatures, monitoring blood pressures, or administering oral drugs can produce considerable anxiety.

Nurses who appreciate toddlers' reactions to physical restrictions can alter many of the usual hospital routines to allow maximum movement and independence. Physical examinations should be done in a sitting or partially reclining position and preferably in the parent's lap. Gaining toddlers' cooperation for painless procedures by showing them the equipment, performing the skill on a doll, or letting them imitate the nurse's role lessens the need for physical restriction. When painful procedures are performed, it is best to avoid lengthy anticipatory preparation, discussions, or choices and to complete the task as quickly as possible. Since toddlers still require the presence of their parents for maximum support and comfort, preparing parents for such procedures may take priority.

The physical environment of the hospital should also be conducive to toddlers' motor skills. Chairs, tables, beds, sinks, and toilets should be low and stable enough to facilitate and encourage their independence. Since toddlers persist in using all their motor skills, sometimes beyond the limits of acquired proficiency, their hospital area should be within view of the nurses' station. Glass walls with curtains for privacy and nighttime darkness facilitate preventive supervision for safety.

Loss of control also results from altered routines and rituals. Toddlers rely on the consistency and familiarity of daily rituals to provide a measure of stability and control in their complex world of growing and developing. The experience of hospitalization or illness severely limits their sense of expectation and predictability, because practically every detail of the hospital environment differs from that of the home. Table 25-2 presents some of the major differences between these two environments. It is obvious from this comparison that an alteration in usual sensory stimulation also exists and exerts an effect over the child's reaction to stress. Although the usual sensory stimulations are lacking, the additional hospital stimuli of sight, sound, and smell may be bombarding and overwhelming. Without an insight into the type of environment conducive to children's optimum growth, the hospital experience can at best tem-

Table 25-2. Differences between the hospital and home environments

Variable	Home	Hospital
Environment	Own room and bed and familiar occupants	Strange room, bed, or crib and unfamiliar occupants
Mealtimes	At table with family, feeds self, usual schedule, favorite foods	In bed or crib, isolated, fed by strangers, new schedule, new foods, preparation, and packaging
Toileting	Own potty or toilet	Diapers, bedpan, strange adult toilet
Dressing and bathing	Routine of separate clothes for night and day, bath in tub	Pajamas all the time, bedbath or strange tub
Bedtime	Established rituals	Loss of rituals, strange environment, separation from parents
Parents and siblings	Usual roles, established hours of contact	Altered role (loss of parenting function, absence of siblings), limited contact
Recreation	Own toys, games, television, books; individualized attention; safe, pleasurable activities	Strange or limited toys, limited personal attention, exposure to *painful* experiences

porarily slow development and at worst permanently retard it.

Toddlers' main areas for rituals include eating, sleeping, bathing, toileting, and play. When the routines are disrupted, one can expect to see difficulties in any or all of these areas. The principal reaction to such change is regression. For example, when mealtime and food choices differ from those at home, toddlers often refuse to eat, demand a bottle, or request others to feed them. Although regression to earlier forms of behavior may seem to increase toddlers' security and comfort, in reality it is very threatening for them to relinquish their most recently acquired achievements.

Toddlers' striving for autonomy is evident in most of their behaviors. Play, interpersonal relationships, activities of daily living, and communication focus on their desires and needs. When their egocentric pleasures are met with obstacles, toddlers react with negativism, especially temper tantrums. Enforced dependency seems to be a chief characteristic of the sick role and of the hospital patient and accounts for the numerous instances of toddler negativism. For example, rigid schedules, altered care-giving activities, unfamiliar surroundings, separation from parents, and medical procedures usurp toddlers' control over their world. Although most toddlers initially react negatively and aggressively to such dependency, prolonged loss of autonomy may result in passive withdrawal from interpersonal relationships and regression in all areas of development. Therefore, the effects of the sick role are most severe in instances of chronic, long-term illnesses or in those families in which the sick role is fostered despite the child's improved state of health.

Bodily injury and pain. Toddlers' concept of body image, particularly the definition of body boundaries, is poorly developed. Intrusive experiences, such as examining the ears or mouth or taking a rectal temperature, are very anxiety producing. Toddlers may react to such painless procedures as intensely as they do to painful ones.

Toddler's reactions to pain are similar to those seen during late infancy, except that the number of variables influencing the individual response is highly complex and varied. Memory, physical restraint, parent separation, emotional reactions of others, and lack of preparation partially determine the intensity of the behavioral response. In general, children in this age-group continue to react with intense emotional upset and physical resistance to any actual or perceived painful experience. Cultural expectations, fears of mutilation, or psychosomatic disorders are not evident until later.

By the end of this age period toddlers usually are able to verbally communicate about their pain. Although they have not developed the ability to describe the type or intensity of the pain, they usually are able to localize it. For example, they may tell their parents that their ear or belly hurts. Such complaints should be taken seriously because children in this age-group rarely imagine or fake discomfort.

Although toddlers are primarily concerned with the pain related to illness or medical procedures, they are aware of the seriousness of their condition from the emotional reactions of others, especially their parents. They sense feelings of fear, confusion, anger, or sadness from those around them, but they are in the difficult position of not being able to understand the reason for the reactions unless others are perceptive of toddlers' needs. Since these children only comprehend concrete explanations, particularly those based on facts they can see, it is often most supportive to help parents work through their reactions to the child's illness before approaching him. In this way the child is spared some of the more volatile parental emotions that prevent them from meeting his needs. In addition toddlers should be given honest but appropriate explanations of their illness and reason for hospitalization in order for them to have some base for understanding the responses of significant others. Telling toddlers all the positive aspects about a hospital, such as the playroom, while avoiding any of the negative ones confuses children and weakens their trust in others.

Preschoolers. Preschoolers have advanced dramatically since infancy. Most of their fine and gross motor skills endow them with practically limitless freedom. They appear quite mature and self-sufficient in usual activities of daily living. They can tolerate brief periods of separation without difficulty. They begin to assume increasing responsibility, and their cognitive powers seem almost adultlike. However, these descriptions of preschoolers are deceptively shallow because much of the displayed independence rests on a fragile surface of ego strength. Under the stress of illness and hospitalization, preschoolers exhibit many of the same needs as toddlers.

Separation. Preschoolers are much more secure interpersonally than their predecessors. Not only can they tolerate brief periods of separation from their parents, but they also are able to develop substitute trust in other significant adults. However, the stress of illness usually renders them less able to cope with separation; as a result they manifest many of the stage behaviors of separation anxiety. In general, however, the protest behaviors are more subtle and passive than those seen in children in earlier age-groups. Preschoolers may demonstrate separation anxiety through refusing to eat, difficulty in sleeping, crying quietly for their parents, continually asking when they will visit, or withdrawing from others. They may express anger indirectly by breaking their toys, hitting other children, or refusing to cooperate during usual self-care activities. Nurses need to be sensitive to these less obvious signs of separation anxiety in order to intervene appropriately.

Fathers are increasingly more important to preschoolers,

especially in view of the psychosexual changes in relationships during this period. Boys may desire the presence of their father during a hospital stay to support them during procedures or to engage in usual play activities. Girls may demonstrate difficulty in relating to their mothers and find more comfort in their fathers. Often mothers sense such preferences and are disturbed by them. It is important for nurses to assess the significance of each parent to the ill child and to encourage both to visit. It is equally essential to include fathers in care-giving activities as much as possible. At the same time, it may be necessary to help mothers understand their son's or daughter's shifting preference for the father.

Loss of control. Preschoolers also suffer from loss of control caused by physical restriction, altered routines, and enforced dependency. However, their specific cognitive abilities, which make them feel omnipotent and all-powerful, also have the effect of making them feel out of control. This loss of control as a result of their sense of self-power is a critical influencing factor in their perception of and reaction to separation, pain, illness, and hospitalization.

Preschoolers' egocentric and magical thinking limit their ability to understand events because they view all experiences from their own self-referenced perspective. Without adequate preparation for unfamiliar settings or experiences, preschoolers' fantasy explanation for such events are usually more exaggerated, bizarre, and frightening than the actual facts. One typical fantasy to explain the reason for illness or hospitalization is that either event represents punishment for real or imagined misdeeds. The response to such thinking is usually feelings of shame, guilt, and fear.

Preschoolers' cognitive ability is also concrete. Explanations are understood only in terms of real events. Purely verbal instructions are often inadequate for them because of their inability to abstract and synthesize beyond what their senses tell them. When combined with their egocentric and magical powers, they can interpret any message according to their particular past experiences. Even with the best preparation for a procedure, they may misconstrue the details.

Transductive reasoning implies that preschoolers deduct from the particular to the particular, rather than from the specific to general or vice versa. For example, if preschoolers' concept of visiting a physician's office is receiving an injection, they will think that every visit results in this procedure, regardless of the reason for the visit.

Because of these three characteristics of preschoolers' cognitive development, it is important that an event be explained in terms of how they may perceive it. It is always necessary to clarify and emphasize the concrete facts in order to lessen the powers of magical thinking and, therefore, increase their sense of control. Since fear of the unknown is greater than fear of the known, the value of anticipatory preparation for the stress of pain, illness, or hospitalization cannot be overstated.

Bodily injury and pain. The psychosexual conflicts of children in this age-group make them very vulnerable to threats of bodily injury. Intrusive procedures, whether painful or painless, are threatening to preschoolers, whose concept of body integrity is still poorly developed. It is not uncommon for preschoolers to react to an injection with as much concern for withdrawal of the needle as for the actual pain. They fear that the intrusion or puncture will not reclose and that their "insides" will leak out. For this reason, bandages are very important to children in this age-group. A small Band-Aid on a pricked finger renders immediate comfort. Conversely removing any size skin covering can be a traumatic experience because of the child's perception of his vulnerability to exposure.

Concerns of mutilation are paramount during this age period. Loss of any body part is threatening, but preschoolers' fears of castration complicate their understanding of surgical or medical procedures associated with the genital area, such as circumcision, repair of hypospadias or epispadias, cystoscopy, or catheterization. Their limited comprehension of body functioning also increases their difficulty in understanding how or why body parts are "fixed." For example, telling preschoolers that their tonsils are to be removed may be interpreted as "taking out their voice," or having the penis "fixed" may be understood as cutting it off. Although in general it is best to use the term "fixed" rather than removed, it is also important to explain what will be done to them as concretely as possible. In addition their perception of the procedure is much more relevant than the actual degree of risk or seriousness.

Reactions to pain also change during this age period. By the end of the fourth year, many preschoolers exhibit an increasing degree of self-control while experiencing pain.[20] Anticipatory preparation, such as explaining the reason for the procedure and giving them an opportunity to explore and use the equipment, assists them in coping with the potential stress. Likewise, lack of such preparation and information may increase the reactions of physical resistance and uncooperativeness, since children in this age-group often supply their own reasons, such as punishment, abandonment, or disapproval, to explain events. The child who is docile, cooperative, and passive may well be a victim of such thinking.

Cultural expectations are also evident in these children. The stereotyped sex role of "brave men don't cry" is often seen in young boys who attempt to be courageous and, if they fail, feel guilty and ashamed. Telling these children that the procedure will hurt but that it is all right to say "ouch," scream, or cry allows them to express their feelings in an atmosphere of support and acceptance.

The potential gains from the sick role also become obvious to preschoolers, and psychosomatic pain may surface at this time. Recurrent abdominal pain is the most common somatic complaint in children and may first occur in preschoolers who are facing the crisis of entering kindergarten.[16] Therefore, it becomes important during this age period to evaluate complaints of pain on both a soma (body) and a psyche (mind) framework.

Preschoolers' reactions to the stress of pain and fear are aggression, verbal expression, dependency, and physiologic responses.[19] *Aggression* in preschoolers is more specific and goal directed than in younger children and is geared toward fight or flight. Instead of total body resistance, preschoolers may push the person away, try to secure the equipment, or attempt to lock themselves in a safe place. Much more thought is evident in their plan of attack or escape.

Verbal expression in particular demonstrates their advanced development in response to stress. They may verbally abuse the attacker by stating, "Get out of here" or "I hate you." They may also use a more cunning approach of trying to persuade the person to give up the intended activity. A common plea expressed by preschoolers is, "Please don't give me that shot; I'll be good." Some statements are not only attempts to avoid the event but also evidence of children's perceptions about the experience.

Besides verbal expression serving as a form of nonphysical aggressiveness, it is also used to communicate pain, fear, anxiety, confusion, power, or dependency. Although language helps them communicate more fully, their ability to use concrete thinking rather than abstraction makes it necessary for others to interpret the words in light of the behavior. For example, the child who exclaims, "I hate you," may really be expressing his fear of strange, unfamiliar sights and sounds. The nurse who interprets that statement as personal rejection cannot meet the underlying need expressed by the child.

Dependency very often represents regression to more stable and comforting modes of behavior. Anxiety related to uncertainty, fear, pain, or separation may be expressed through behaviors such as clinging to a parent, refusing to play with other children, reverting to nonverbal means of communication, wanting to be held, or refusing to be left alone. A common expression denoting the need for dependency is, "Help me." Children, who are adept at self-help skills, such as dressing, bathing, or feeding, suddenly request assistance with these activities. It is important to recognize such requests as the need for support from others during a time of stress. Admonishing children to act grown-up or encouraging them to do things by stating, "I know you can do it yourself," deprives them of the support they are requesting and increases their own feelings of guilt and shame.

Preschoolers also react to the stress of pain with observable *physiologic responses,* such as flushing of the skin, vomiting, increase in pulse and respiration, restlessness, and dilatation of the pupils. Since emotions such as fear, anxiety, or anger may produce similar physiologic reactions, it is important for nurses to differentiate the cause of the response. This is particularly significant for preschoolers who develop fears easily during the phase of magical thinking. Their very exposure to a potentially frightening environment such as the hospital can produce acute physiologic signs of stress, which are the result of fear, not pain.

School-age children. The period of school-age includes children from 6 years of age to the end of preadolescence. Since this is a fairly large age span, it is more relevant to view this period as three separate, but overlapping groups: (1) late preschool—early school-age, (2) middle school-age, and (3) late school-age—preadolescence. Many of the fears and reactions of children in this age-group are carried over from the preschool years, whereas others commence during preadolescence. For a more complete understanding of school-age children's reactions to stress, nurses must consider their specific chronologic and developmental age, not merely their classification as "school-age" or "latent childhood."

Separation. School-age children are increasingly better able to cope with the stress of pain, illness, or hospitalization. Because of their gradual separation from their parents through school entry and social peer attachment, the separation imposed by hospitalization is much less of a threat to their security. With broader support systems in other adults, siblings, and age-mates, they are able to adjust to the strange hospital environment while maintaining stability in usual interpersonal relationships. At times the hospital stay provides a maturing opportunity for them to challenge their decision-making ability and growing sense of independence.

Although school-age children are better able to cope with separation in general, the stress imposed by illness or hospitalization may increase their need for parental security and guidance. This is particularly true for young school-age children who have only recently left the safety of the home and are struggling with the crisis of school adjustment. These youngsters may still require the presence of their parents during hospitalization because the usual response of regression to stress may leave them with the same needs as preschoolers.

Middle and late school-age children may react more to the separation from their usual activities and social attachments than to absence of their parents. Their high level of physical and mental activity frequently finds no suitable outlets in the hospital environment. Even when they dislike school, they admit to missing its routine and associated activities. Since children in this age-group are also very involved in group recreation, such as sports, Boy Scouts or Girl Scouts, or youth groups, temporary absence may increase their feelings of loneliness, boredom, isolation, and depression. It is important to recognize that such reactions may occur more as a result of separation than from concern over the illness, treatment, or hospital setting. Helping school-age children to maintain their usual nonhome contacts by continuing school lessons during the period of illness and confinement, visiting with friends either directly or through letter writing, telephone calls, and so on, and participating in extracurricular projects whenever possible minimize the effects of separation imposed by hospitalization.

School-age children may need and desire parental guidance or support from other adult figures but be unable or unwilling to ask for it. Because the goal of attaining independence is so important to them, they are reluctant to seek help directly for fear that they will appear weak, childish, or dependent. Cultural expectations to "act like a man" or to "be brave and strong" bear heavily on these children, especially males, who tend to react to stress with stoicism, withdrawal, or passive acceptance. Often the need to express hostile, angry, or other negative feelings finds outlets in alternate ways, such as irritability and aggression toward parents, withdrawal from hospital personnel, inability to relate to peers, rejection of siblings, or subsequent behavioral problems in school. Because nurses spend more time with children than any other health team member, it is important to note deviations in one particular area of behavior. For example, the children who appear to be very accepting of the separation from parents and school may be the same children who cannot relate to hospitalized age-mates because their repressed resentment toward the change imposed by the illness and confinement is directed against these children. Helping them express their repressed feelings of anger may also assist them in finding companionship and support from their peers.

Middle school-age children and preadolescents may welcome the temporary separation from home. Encouraging parents to stay may increase these youngsters' reactions to hospitalization because they are denied needed privacy, independence, and control in making decisions and choices. Frequently they appreciate the opportunity to room with an age-mate, to meet new friends, to explore a strange environment, and to learn about their bodies and themselves. For the hospital experience to have maximum beneficial effects, nurses must assess the individual needs of each child for the continued presence of their parents or for the need to have privacy and independence. Unless this objective is met, older school-age children may regress to primitive levels of behavior to meet the imposed dependency needs or reject all efforts directed at their physical well-being. In either case illness and hospitalization will exert greater than usual stress and may result in maladaptive coping mechanisms. Since a crisis is a time for change, the minimum nursing goal of preserving the precrisis level of functioning may not be met.

Loss of control. Because of their striving for independence and productivity, school-age children are particularly vulnerable to events that may lessen their feeling of control and power. In particular, altered family roles, physical disability, fears of death, abandonment, or permanent injury, loss of peer acceptance, lack of productivity, and inability to cope with stress according to perceived cultural expectation may result in loss of control.

Because of the nature of the patient role, many routine hospital activities usurp individual power and identity. For these children, dependent activities such as enforced bed rest, use of a bedpan, inability to choose a menu, lack of privacy, help with a bed bath, or transport by use of a wheelchair or stretcher can be a direct threat to their security. Although all of these usual hospital procedures seem routine and inconsequential, nurses must remember that to children who want to "act grown-up," these activities allow no freedom of choice. However, when children are allowed to exert a measure of control, regardless of how limited it may be, they generally respond very well to any procedure. For example, some of the most cooperative, satisfied, and contented patients are those school-age children who help make their beds, choose their schedule of activities, assist in procedures, and help the nurses care for the younger children. An increased sense of control is usually an outcome of a feeling of usefulness and productivity.

Besides the hospital environment, illness may also cause a feeling of loss of control. One of the most significant problems of children in this age-group centers on boredom. When physical or enforced limitations curtail their usual abilities to care for themselves or to engage in favorite activities, school-age children generally respond with depression, hostility, or frustration. Keeping a normally active child on bed rest is no small challenge. However, emphasizing areas of control and capitalizing on quiet activities, particularly hobbies such as building models or collecting specific objects, promote their adjustment to physical restriction. Nursing judgment regarding selection of a roommate is one of the most important contributing factors to their overall adjustment to illness and hospitalization.

Even under the most optimal hospital conditions, loss of control can result from actual or perceived changes in the roles of family members. If hospitalized school-age children think that they are being displaced from their usual position in the family, they may feel extremely threatened. Although some shift in family roles is almost always necessary, it is important for parents to discuss them with the hospitalized child. For example, during his absence the next-oldest sibling may be granted the temporary use of the vacant bedroom. To an ill child this does not represent a better use of space but an unforgivable invasion of his territory. It is best to advise parents of the impact such changes can have on the hospitalized child and the importance of continuing his contact with all family members. There can be little substitute for the advantages of sibling visitation privileges, but telephone calls and letter writing are alternate means of keeping the family together during this time of stress. In addition the beneficial effects are multidimensional because the siblings feel included in the other child's experiences and the parents are spared some, if not all, of the possible emotional aftereffects of the crisis on their children.

Bodily injury and pain. Fears of the physical nature of the illness surface at this time. There may be less concern with actual pain than there is for disability, uncertain recovery, or possible death. Because of their developing cognitive abilities, school-age children are aware of the significance of different illnesses, the indispensability of certain body parts, the potential hazards in treatments, the lifelong consequences of permanent injury or loss of function, and the meaning of death. They generally take a very active interest in their health or illness. Even those children who rarely ask questions usually reveal detailed knowledge of their condition by attentively listening to all that is said around them. They request factual information and quickly perceive lies or half-truths. Seeking information tends to be one way of their maintaining a sense of control despite the stress and uncertainty of illness.

School-age children begin to show concern for the potential beneficial and hazardous effects of procedures. Besides wanting to know if a procedure will hurt, they want to know what it is for, how it will make them better, and what injury or harm could result. For example, these children fear the actual procedure of anesthesia. Unlike preschoolers who fear the mask and the strange surroundings, school-age children fear what may happen while they are asleep, if they will wake up, and if they may die. Preadolescents also worry about the operation itself, particularly one that will result in visible changes in body image.

Intrusive procedures of a nonsexual nature, such as routine physical examination of the ears, nose, mouth, and throat, are generally well tolerated. However, concerns for privacy become evident and increasingly significant. Although school-age children may be cooperative during examination of, or procedures that are performed on, the genital area, it is usually very stressful for them, especially for preadolescents who are beginning pubertal changes. Nurses who respect children's need for privacy provide them with much assurance and support. Since the parents' presence may or may not be wanted by children during such procedures, nurses should also assess the child's individual preference. It may also be necessary to explain to parents why children prefer to be alone. Many parents forget the special needs of children in this age-group and believe that concerns for privacy surface only during adolescence.

By the age of 9 or 10 years most school-age children show little fright or overt resistance to pain. They generally have learned passive methods of dealing with discomfort, such as holding rigidly still, clenching their fists or teeth, or trying to act brave by the "grin and bear it" routine. If they do display signs of overt resistance, such as biting, kicking, pulling away, trying to escape, crying, or plea bargaining, they tend to deny such reactions later, especially to their peers for fear of losing status within the group.

School-age children verbally communicate about their pain in respect to its location, intensity, and description. They may also use words as a means of controlling their reactions to pain. For example, these children may ask the nurse to talk to them during a procedure. Some prefer to participate in a procedure, whereas others choose to distance themselves by not looking at what is happening. Most appreciate an explanation of the procedure and seem less fearful when they know what to expect. Others try to gain control by attempting to postpone the event. A typical request is, "Give me the shot when I am finished with this." Although the ability to make decisions does increase their sense of control, unlimited procrastination results in heightened anxiety. When choices are allowed, such as selection of the injection site, it is best to structure the number of possible sites and to limit the number of "procrastination" techniques.

Similar to their more passive acceptance of pain is their nondirective request for support or help. School-age children will rarely initiate a conversation about their feelings or request someone to stay with them during a lonely or stressful period. In fact, their visible composure, calmness, and acceptance often belie their inner longing for support. It is especially important to be aware of nonverbal clues, such as a serious facial expression, a halfhearted reply of, "I am fine," silence, lack of activity, or social isolation, as signs of the need for help. Usually when someone identifies the unspoken messages and offers support, they readily accept it.

Adolescents. Of all periods during childhood, adolescents have the most well-developed coping mechanisms to deal with stress. They have a widely developed support system, the ability to think abstractly as well as concretely, the communication powers to make all their needs known, the physical stability to withstand bodily injury and stress, and previous life experiences to guide them through the present and future. Yet, with all these strengths, they are one of the most vulnerable groups to succumb to the stress of illness and hospitalization.

Although their support system has expanded to include new significant adults and peers, they may be very reluctant to rely on their parents and may be suspicious of strange adults. Even though they have well-developed cognitive abilities, they are also struggling with the definitions of right and wrong, moral and ethical, and so on. Such issues often cloud their perspective of relevant issues. For example, in their investigations of different religious beliefs, they may feel strongly about agreeing to certain forms of medical treatment. Their decision to refuse such procedures may be related to peer conformity rather than to devoted adherence to the underlying religious principle.

Their well-developed means of verbal and nonverbal communication is often hampered by their equally extensive jargon. The words and expressions used by adolescents may be as unintelligible to outsiders as a foreign language. Also, because of their increasingly expert use of adult camouflages to distort their true feelings, communication may be totally blocked between adolescents and their potential sources of support.

Although their body systems are more mature to withstand physical stress, their developmental needs for group conformity and acceptance greatly influence their response to body injury. For example, the potential scar from an appendectomy may cause exaggerated concern in the female adolescent who wants to wear a bikini in order to be like her friends. Adolescents' concern with body image is often greater than the actual seriousness of the illness.

Adolescents have acquired a fairly large reserve of previous experiences to help them cope with present crises. In general, if their coping mechanisms have been successful for past crises, they will be beneficial for future ones. However, adolescents are expected to behave more like adults than children. If their previous coping behaviors reflect more childlike defenses, such as regression, physical aggression, or dependency, adults may be less tolerant and supportive of such behaviors than in younger children. Therefore, while facing new crises with additional developmental handicaps, adolescents are also forced to give up previous coping mechanisms and to form more mature and sophisticated ones.

The sum total of the comparison of adolescents' advantages and disadvantages toward dealing with stress is an obvious potential for excessive negative forces against adaptive coping. The main threats to persons in this age-group are loss of control, especially in terms of loss of identity, fear of altered body image, and separation, primarily from members of their peer group.

Loss of control. Adolescents' struggle for independence, self-assertion, and liberation centers on the quest for personal identity. They seek answers in the home, from peers, in other authority figures, from "idols," and within themselves. Anything that interferes with these associations poses a threat to their sense of identity and results in a loss of control. Illness, which limits their physical abilities, and hospitalization, which separates them from usual support systems, constitute major situational crises.

The patient role fosters dependency and depersonalization. Adolescents may react to dependency with rejection, uncooperativeness, or withdrawal. They may respond to depersonalization with self-assertion, anger, or frustration. Regardless of which response they manifest, hospital personnel generally tend to regard them as difficult, unmanageable patients. Parents may not be a source of help because these behaviors serve to further isolate them from understanding the adolescent. Although peers may visit, they may not be able to offer the kind of support and guidance needed. Sick adolescents often voluntarily isolate themselves from age-mates until they feel they can compete on equal bases and meet group expectations. As a result ill adolescents are left with virtually no support systems.

Loss of control also occurs for many of the reasons discussed under school-age children. However, adolescents are more sensitive to potential instances of loss of control and dependency than younger children. For example, both groups seek information about their physical status and rely heavily on anticipatory preparation to decrease fear and anxiety. However, adolescents react not only to the kinds of information supplied them but also to the means by which it is conveyed. They may feel very threatened by others who relate facts in a derogatory manner. Adolescents want to know that others can relate to them on their own level. This necessitates a careful assessment of their intellectual abilities, previous knowledge, and present needs. It may also require a willingness on the part of the information giver to learn the language of the adolescent.

Bodily injury and pain. Although body image, or the conscious and unconscious perceptions and feelings about one's body, begins at birth, its relevance is paramount during adolescence. Injury, pain, disability, and death are viewed primarily in terms of how each affects the adolescent's view of himself in the present. Any change that differentiates the adolescent from his peers is regarded as a major tragedy. For example, diseases such as diabetes mellitus often present a more difficult adjustment period for children in this age-group than for younger children because of the necessary changes in the adolescent's life-style. Conversely, serious, even life-threatening illnesses that entail no visible body changes or physical restrictions may have less immediate significance for the adolescent. Therefore, the nature of bodily injury may be more important in terms of adolescents' perception of the illness than its actual degree of severity.

Adolescents' rapidly changing body image during pubertal development often makes them feel insecure about their bodies. Illness, medical or surgical intervention, and hospitalization increase their existing concerns for normalcy. They may respond to such events by asking numerous questions, withdrawing, rejecting others, or questioning the adequacy of care. Frequently their fear for loss of control and body image change is demonstrated as overconfidence, conceit, or a "know-it-all" attitude.

Because of the sexual changes, adolescents are very concerned about privacy. Lack of respect for this need can cause greater stress than physical pain. In addition adolescents look for signs that indicate that they are developing normally and according to acceptable standards. When illness occurs, they fear that growth may be retarded, leaving them behind their peers. Although they may not voice this concern, they may demonstrate it by carefully observing others' reactions during physical examinations or procedures.

Illness may also have significance in terms of perceived punishment, guilt, or shame. Since sexual impulses are strong, adolescents may misinterpret the cause of illness. For example, they may regard masturbation, homosexual acts, or heterosexual experimentation as causes of specific disorders. Although they have higher-level cognition than preschoolers, much magical thinking occurs during this time. It is particularly important to assess imagined cause and effect associations, because the related guilt may interfere with adaptive coping.

Adolescents react to pain with much self-control. Physical resistance and aggression are unusual at this age, unless the adolescents are totally unprepared for a procedure. However, the social gains from playing the sick role are clearly evident. Psychosomatic complaints are frequent and most often disclose an underlying psychosocial problem. Complaints of fatigue, abdominal pain, headache, or backache may indicate problems in the home, school, or peer group. Effective intervention involves a careful assessment of adolescents' environment, not only an investigation of organic problems. Inquiring about sexual activity is an area of prime significance. Psychosomatic complaints may follow initial sexual relationships because of associated guilt, shame, or confusion.

Since pain is a complex psychobiologic event, assessment of pain must include several factors. Unlike younger children who may refuse to admit that pain exists for fear of receiving injectable medications, adolescents may use this excuse to continue a source of drugs. In a drug-using society it would be naive of nurses to fail to consider the secondary gains from pain medication. In addition use of narcotics during hospitalization may be an adolescent's first experience with euphoric drugs. The judicious use of such medications is part of the prevention of future drug abuse. Emphasizing to adolescents the curative and supportive benefits of medicine is no different than stressing to young children that medicine is not candy.

Separation. Separation from home and parents may be a welcomed and appreciated event. However, loss of peer-group contact may be a severe emotional threat because of loss of group status, inability to exert group control or leadership, and loss of group acceptance. Deviations within peer groups are poorly tolerated, and, although members may express concern for the adolescent's illness or need for hospitalization, they continue their group activities, quickly filling the gap of the absent member. During the temporary separation from their usual group, ill adolescents may benefit from group associations of other hospitalized age-mates. A formal or informal gathering of this nature may provide a substitute supportive peer system.

The potential benefits of hospitalization for emotional growth are great for children in this age-group because of their ability to temporarily separate from home, provided their needs for control, independence, and bodily concern are met. The challenge of nursing is to realize the stressors of each age period, to accept the behavioral reactions, and to provide the support and assistance needed to overcome the obstacles of successful coping.

Nurses' role: minimizing stress of illness and hospitalization

Although children in each developmental age-group respond differently to the stressors of separation, loss of control, and bodily injury and pain, it is evident that intervention in each of these areas is essential for optimum adjustment to illness and/or hospitalization. In addition supportive nursing approaches to the principal behavioral reactions of separation anxiety, aggression, regression, depression, and fear are necessary in order to lessen the possible deleterious effects of either stressor.

Separation. The primary nursing goal is preventing or minimizing the effects of separation, particularly in children under 5 years of age. Prevention of separation requires rooming-in facilities in pediatric hospital settings. Although some health facilities provide special accommodations for parents, the concept of rooming-in can be instituted anywhere. The first requirement is the staff's positive attitude toward parents. When hospital personnel genuinely appreciate the importance of continued parent-child attachment, they foster an environment that encourages parents to stay. When parents are included in the care planning and made to feel as if they are a contributing factor to the child's recovery, they are more inclined to remain with their child and have more emotional reserves to support themselves and the child through the crisis.

Since the mother tends to be the usual family care giver, she usually spends more time in the hospital than the father. However, not all mothers feel equally comfortable in assuming responsibility for their child's care. Some may be under such great emotional stress that they need a temporary reprieve from total participation in care-giving activities. Others may feel insecure in participating in specialized areas of care, such as bathing the child after surgery. Individual assessment of each parent's preferred involvement is necessary in order to prevent the effects of separation while supporting the parent in her or his needs as well.

All too often nurses' response to parent participation is abandonment of their patient responsibilities. Nurses need to restructure their roles to complement and augment the care-giving functions of parents. It seems that members of the staff who view their primary nursing functions as similar to those of the parents have the most difficulty in redefining their roles, whereas others who value "family-centered care" and place emphasis on the supportive roles of nursing have the least difficulty in adjusting to parental involvement.[18] With many of the usual tasks of feeding, bathing, dressing, and making beds performed by parents, nurses should be more available to the parents and children for greater emotional support and preparatory teaching.

Although most of the research on separation has focused on the mother-child relationship, the role of fathers in the emotional development of children is increasingly being recognized. With life-styles and sexual roles changing, it is conceivable that some fathers may assume all or some of the usual mothering roles in the household. In this case it may be the father-child relationship that requires preservation. Since the majority of nurses are women, it is necessary for them to include fathers in the plan of care and respect the sexual role of that person. It is equally important to support the mother's role as family provider or part-time housekeeper in order to meet the needs of each parent. In single-parent families the care giver may not be a parent but an extended family member, such as a grandparent or aunt.

Although prevention of separation is the ideal goal, often this is not possible. Therefore, minimization of the effects of separation becomes the substitute objective. This necessitates a consistent nurse to meet the child's needs. Becoming a surrogate mother requires a thorough, detailed nursing history that specifically identifies the child's established daily routine. Usual daily activities such as food preparation and method of feeding help establish a complementary schedule of care-giving practices. It also helps the parent feel as if he or she is participating in the child's care but through another person. A nursing admission history for children is outlined in the boxed material below.

The nurse caring for the child must have an appreciation

Nursing admission history for activities of daily living

Eating

Usual mealtimes (with other family members or alone)
Favorite foods, snacks, and beverages; average amounts
Way in which food is served (warmed, cold, one item at a time)
Food and beverage dislikes
Feeding habits (cup, spoon, bottle, eats by self, needs assistance)
Description of usual appetite
Any problems (spitting up, ruminating)
Remedies for problems

Sleeping

Usual hour of sleep and awakening
Schedule for naps
Routine before sleeping (bottle, drink of water, bedtime story, night-light, favorite blanket or toy, prayers)
Type of bed
Sleeps alone or with others (siblings, parents, or other relatives)
Favorite sleeping position
Any problems (waking during night, nightmares, sleep walking)
Remedies for problems

Elimination

Toilet trained (day and/or night, use of word to communicate urination or defecating, potty-chair, diapers, other routines)
Usual pattern of elimination (bowel movements)
Any problems (bed-wetting, constipation, diarrhea)
Remedies for problems

Hygiene

Usual habits for bathing (daily bath in tub or shower, sponge bath, usual schedule for shampoo)
Dental habits
Dressing
Degree of assistance needed for above
Any problems (refusal to wash or brush teeth, disliking having hair washed)
Remedies for problems
Care of special prostheses (glasses, contact lenses, hearing aid, orthodontic appliances, dentures, artificial elimination appliances, orthopedic devices)

Play

Schedule during day (nursery, day-care center, regular school [grade in school], extracurricular activities)
Preferred play companions (peer groups, alone, adults, younger or older children)
Favorite activities or toys (both active and quiet interests)
"Security" objects (pacifier, bottle, blanket, thumb, doll)
Any favorite objects with him in hospital
Any television restrictions, favorite programs
Interest in or fear of animals (if playroom has live animals)

Family data

Child's favorite name or nickname
Other members of immediate family, others who live in home (relatives, pets)
Usual care giver (other than parent), baby-sitter, relative
Experiences with and reactions to temporary separation or absence of parent
Parents' occupations
Special considerations (adoption, foster child, stepparent or siblings, divorce, single parent)

of the child's separation behaviors. As was discussed on p. 881, the phase of protest and despair is normal. The nurse allows the child to cry. Even if he rejects strangers, the nurse provides support through physical presence in the room. Saying to the child, "I know you are unhappy because you miss your mommy and daddy. It's all right to cry. I will sit here for awhile so you are not alone," reinforces to the child the nurse's awareness of his feelings without abandoning him. If the behaviors of detachment are evident, the nurse maintains the child's contact with his parents by frequently talking about them, encouraging him to remember them, and stressing the significance of their visits, telephone calls, or letters.

Besides similar routines, familiar surroundings also increase the child's adjustment to separation. If parents cannot room-in, they should leave favorite home articles, such as a blanket, toy, bottle, feeding utensil, or article of clothing, with the child. Since young children associate such inanimate objects with significant people, they gain comfort and reassurance from such possessions. They make the association that if the parent left this, the parent will surely return. A tape recording of the parent's voice, such as reading a story, singing a song, or relating events at home can help the child feel closer to his loved ones.

Older children also appreciate familiar articles from home, particularly photographs, a radio, a favorite toy or game, and usual pajamas. The use of the telephone and letter writing is advantageous in maintaining contact with family members and friends. For extended hospitalizations they usually enjoy personalizing the hospital room to make it "home." Decorating the walls with posters and cards, placing growing plants in the room, rearranging the furniture (when possible), and displaying a collection or hobby are all means of defining their territory.

Some children resist such activities, because in anticipating a prolonged admission they fear that they will never leave. Nurses who are perceptive of their hesitancy can help them overcome their fear by suggesting "personalizing ideas," while emphasizing a departure date. Making a calendar and crossing off each passing day helps some children gain a perspective of time.

Probably of all hospital facilities no room does more to alleviate the stressors of hospitalization than the playroom. In this room children temporarily distance themselves from the fears of separation, loss of control, and bodily injury. They can work through their feelings in an unthreatening, comfortable atmosphere and in the manner that is most natural for them.

Play provides them with a sense of control because they can become whomever they want to be. They also know that the boundaries of this room are safe from intrusive or painful procedures, strange faces, and probing questions. The playroom becomes a sanctuary of peace and safety in an otherwise frightening environment.

Although play is every child's natural medium of expression, children in various age-groups require different types of play facilities. Infants and toddlers need maximum safety, whereas school-age children and adolescents benefit most from group recreation. Providing space for special needs of children in each age-group can be difficult in overcrowded institutions, but innovational solutions can assure practical answers. Playroom schedules can accommodate children in one age-group at one session and another group at a later time, for example, adolescents can utilize the facility in the evening when younger children are asleep. Older children can also congregate in one patient's room and listen to music, play games, or just talk about their experiences. If the location of the recreational session is rotated each evening, older children can look forward to arranging or setting up for the activities.

Separation may be equally as difficult for parents, especially when they do not understand the behaviors of separation anxiety. To avoid the immediate protest, parents may sneak out or lie to the child about leaving. As a result the child does not learn that absence is associated with a guaranteed return but that absence means loss of parents, possibly forever. Helping parents realize the necessity and value of telling their children when they will leave assists children in adjusting to the temporary separation. Although infants do not understand the reason for the departure or the expected time of return, when parents openly admit their good-byes, infants learn that such behavior is eventually met with a "hello."

Toddlers and preschoolers have a very limited concept of time. The young child's question of, "Will my mommy come yesterday?" symbolizes a lack of understanding for usual measurements of time, such as days, hours, weeks, and so on. Time is measured in associations, such as, "Eating dinner when daddy comes home." Therefore, when helping parents with their fears of separation, nurses need to suggest ways of explaining leaving and returning. For example, if parents must leave to go to work or to make meals for the other family members, they should tell the hospitalized child the reason for leaving. They also need to convey the expected time of return in terms of anticipated events. For example, if the parents return in the morning, they can tell the child that they will see him "After the sun comes up," or "When a favorite program is on television." When such promises are made, parents must be fairly certain that they will be able to be present at that time. Otherwise the child will have little trust in relying on his parents' word. If parents do not know when they can return, they should tell the child so, rather than stating a definite time and failing to adhere to it. Because hours may seem endless to waiting children, nurses can encourage parents to call when they know their expected time of arrival. If a child's room has a telephone, the parent can communicate this directly.

For older children who know how to tell time, it is helpful to give them a clock or watch. However, these children have the same needs for honesty from their parents regarding visiting schedules. Because peer groups are also important, adolescents often appreciate planning visiting hours with their parents to provide them with some private time for friends.

One of the ways of supporting parents through their separation anxieties is to assure them that a nurse will be with their child. Parents who room-in often remark that they rarely see a nurse and that if they were to leave they fear that no one would care for their child. When nurses redefine their roles away from technical tasks toward supportive intervention, more time should be available to spend with parents. The very presence and interest of the nurse in the care of the child assures parents of continued care during their absence.

Explaining to parents how the child reacts after they leave may also be helpful. Many parents imagine that the child cries for hours after they leave, whereas in reality he may cry for a few minutes but settle down when comforted by someone else. Since parents who leave on false pretenses may be unaware of negative reactions in the child, nurses may also help them see the value of honesty by explaining this response.

Supporting parents through their own feelings of separation, concern for the child's recovery, and anxiety over the hospital experience allows them to effectively support the child and avoids major disruptions in family life and in parenting roles. Accepting parents' inability to stay with their child helps them deal with their feelings of guilt. Encouraging parents to participate in their child's care emphasizes the importance of the parenting role in the child's recovery. Preparing parents for anticipated, potentially frightening procedures allows them to calmly and constructively support the child through the experience.

Loss of control. Feelings of loss of control result from separation, physical restriction, altered routines, enforced dependency, magical thinking, and changed status within the family or peer group. Although some of these, such as separation from parents, can be prevented, most of them can be minimized through individualized planning of nursing care.

Physical restriction. Younger children react most strenuously to any type of physical restriction or immobilization. Although some restraint, such as immobilizing an extremity for maintenance of an intravenous line, is frequently necessary, much physical restriction can be prevented if the nurse gains the child's cooperation.

For young children, particularly infants and toddlers, preserving parent-child contact is the best means of decreasing the need for or stress of restraint. For example, almost the entire physical examination can be done in a parent's lap, with the parent hugging the child for procedures such as otoscopy or rectal temperatures. For painful procedures parents may not wish to participate in restraining the child either because of their own fear or because they do not want the child to associate them with the event. In this case the parents can be readily available to console the child immediately following the procedure.

Although involving the parents in performing stressful procedures is believed to be supportive for the child, it does present dilemmas. If parents directly assist in the event, young children may believe that their parents are punishing them. If they are not involved but remain in the background, children wonder why their parents do not rescue them and prevent the procedure. In either case it is essential that the nurse repeatedly clarify to the child the reason for the procedure and assess the parents' preferences for assisting, observing, or waiting outside the room, since emotional contagion can also be a stress-provoking factor.

Older children may or may not wish their parents' presence, particularly if privacy is a concern. Most children feel more in control when they know what to expect because the element of fear is reduced. Anticipatory preparation and information giving is a significant method of lessening stress and often results in little need for physical restraint.

Environmental factors also influence the need for physical restraint. Keeping children in cribs or playpens may not represent immobilization in a concrete sense, but it certainly limits sensory stimulation. Increasing mobility by transporting children in carriages, wheelchairs, carts, wagons, or on stretchers or beds provides them with mechanical freedom.

The choice of a transporting conveyance should be guided by the child's age, physical condition, and destination. In general the sitting position is preferred to the horizontal position, regardless of age. However, sometimes a stretcher or bed is required, such as when the child is in traction or has a spica cast. Young children feel more secure in proportionately smaller conveyances, such as wagons, carriages, or narrow wheelchairs. Older children prefer wheelchairs because they can move and guide them without assistance, thus increasing their independence. Safety is also a prime factor, especially when children are left in group-supervised areas. For example, toddlers may satisfactorily be transported in any sitting-type conveyance, but a carriage with a restraining belt may provide the most protection.

In some cases physical restraint is necessary for promotion of recovery, such as using elbow restraints on children with eczema. Whenever possible, restraints should be removed to allow the child some period of supervised freedom, such as during the bath or when parents visit. In those instances when restraints cannot be moved, such as in severe burns, nurses can manipulate the environment to increase sensory freedom. For example, moving the bed toward the door or window, providing musical, visual, or tactile toys, and increasing interpersonal contact can substitute mental mobility for the limitations of physical movement.

Altered routines. Altered daily schedules and loss of rituals are particularly stressful for toddlers and early preschoolers and may increase the stress of separation. As has been discussed previously, the nursing admission history provides a baseline for planning care around the child's usual home activities.

Children's response to loss of routine and ritualism is often demonstrated in problems with activities such as feeding, sleeping, dressing, bathing, toileting, and social interaction. Although some regression is to be expected in all of these areas, sensitivity to the special needs of children can minimize the negative effects. For example, loss of appetite and marked food preferences are common in ill or hospitalized children. In addition the food selections on hospital menus may differ greatly from preferred cultural or ethnic food preparation. In general, hotdogs, hamburgers, peanut butter and jelly sandwiches, spaghetti, and pizza are favorite foods of most children. Although alone they may not typify well-balanced diets, they can be adjusted to include sufficient amounts from the basic four food groups. It is better to work with preferred food choices than with selections that children rarely eat. Encouraging parents to stay with their children during mealtime, serving meals group style, planning box lunches or "picnics" in a special area of the hospital, celebrating special occasions such as birthdays, and using feeding utensils and dining furniture appropriate for the child's age often improve the appetite.

An understanding of children's feeding habits can also increase food consumption. For example, if children are given all of their food at one time, they will generally eat the dessert first. Likewise, if they are presented with large portions, they often push the food away because the amount overwhelms them. If young children are not supervised during mealtime, they tend to play with the food rather than eat it. Therefore, nurses should present food in the usual order, such as soup first, followed by small portions of meat, potatoes, and vegetables, and finally, ending with dessert. The principles of conservation that were discussed in Chapter 15 (p. 537) can also be used to increase food consumption.

After each meal nurses should record the amount and type of food eaten. Statements, such as "Ate poorly," "Ate well," or "Left most of meal" yield little objective data regarding food consumption and give no indication of the quality of nutritional intake. A dietary record should be specific and detailed. For example, a tally of breakfast might be stated: "4 ounces of orange juice, one pancake, no bacon, and 8 ounces of milk." A comparison of the intake at each meal can isolate food deficiencies, such as insufficient intake of meat or vegetables. Behaviors associated with mealtime also identify possible factors influencing appetite. For example, the observation that, "Child eats well when with other children but plays with food if left alone in room," helps the nurse plan mealtime activities that stimulate the appetite.

Because most children cope with the stress of illness and/or hospitalization by regressing to a more dependent and secure level of functioning, hospitalization is generally regarded as a poor time to introduce children to new skills. For example, young children who do not feed themselves should continue to be fed during this time. Expecting them to use a spoon "because they are old enough" does not respect their present level of functioning or their need for increased or maintained dependency.

Although regression is expected and normal, nurses also have the responsibility of fostering children's optimum growth and development. There are instances during which hospitalization becomes a significant opportunity for learning and advancing. For example, extended hospitalization for long-term chronic illness or situations of failure to thrive, abuse, or neglect represent instances in which regression must be seen as one adjustment period, to be followed by plans for promoting appropriate developmental skills.

Helping parents understand and accept the meaning and importance of regression is necessary for them to tolerate and support the behavior. Besides the regression observed during hospitalization, nurses should also forewarn parents of the usual continuance of such reactions following discharge. Young children who have been separated from their mothers during hospitalization may continue to show regressive behavior, such as emotional dependence, food finickiness, resistance to going to bed, and regression in self-toileting, for a month or longer. Older children may express posthospitalization behaviors such as anger, jealousy, and emotional coldness, followed by intense, demanding dependence on the mother. Other negative behaviors include new fears, nightmares, insomnia, withdrawal and shyness, hyperactivity, temper tantrums, attachment to blanket or toy, and tics or other nervous mannerisms. Younger children tend to exhibit more of these behaviors for longer periods of time.[6] Parents who do not expect such reactions may misinterpret them as evidence of the child's "being spoiled" and demand perfect behavior at a time when he is still reacting to the stress of illness and hospitalization. If the regressive behaviors, especially the demand for attention, are dealt with in a supportive manner, accompanied with reasonable limits on and expectations for acceptable behavior, most children are able to relinquish the more primitive behaviors and assume precrisis levels of functioning.

Enforced dependency. The dependent role of the hospitalized patient imposes tremendous feelings of loss on older children. The principal interventions focus on respect for individuality and the opportunity for decision making. Although these sound simple, their efficacy lies with nurses who are flexible, tolerant, and personally secure. The latter is particularly important because when decision making is geared toward the patient, nurses can feel threatened by their own sense of lessened control.

Promoting children's control involves maintaining independence through activities such as jointly planning care, wearing street clothes, making choices in food selections, bedtime, and so on, continuing school activities, and rooming with an appropriate age-mate. For example, although school-age children may enjoy the responsibility of caring for a toddler or preschooler in their room, adolescents generally prefer quarters that are separate from the pediatric unit. Because their self-concept is so dependent on outside influences, they are sensitive to even slight associations with childish "stigma," such as cartoons painted on their walls. They need surroundings and significant individuals who enhance their identity as adolescents. Nurses who call them by name, take an interest in them personally, and talk to them on their level usually are most supportive of adolescents' needs for control and self-identity.

Magical thinking. Loss of control can occur from feelings of too little influence on one's destiny as well as from a sense of overwhelming control over fate. Although the cognitive abilities of preschoolers predispose them most significantly to magical thinking and self-power, all children are vulnerable to misinterpreted causes for stresses such as illness and hospitalization. As has already been pointed out, the principal felt reason for either crisis is punishment, which results in feelings of guilt, shame, self-reproach, and depression.

Maintaining a feeling of realistic control involves removing the magic from egocentric, magical thinking. This is best accomplished through age-appropriate preparation for hospitalization and related procedures, which is discussed on p. 909. It also involves repeatedly clarifying that illness occurs because of germs, accidents, inborn problems, or unknown causes.

Because children perceive the reactions of their parents to illness or hospitalization, nurses must assess parental remnants of magical thinking. Although this is discussed more in detail in Chapter 27, asking parents why they think their child is ill uncovers relevant hidden explanations. Superstition, religion, or cultural beliefs play particular roles in such fantasy thinking. Not uncommonly statements, such as, "Ever since you became sick nothing but trouble has come into this home," greatly burden children with feelings of guilt. Assisting parents in realizing the significance of such statements can be helpful in alleviating children's feelings of responsibility for "creating all the family's difficulties."

Altered family and social roles. Besides the effects of separation on family roles, loss of the parenting, sibling, and offspring roles may affect each family member differently. One of the most common reactions of parents is specialized and intensified attention toward the sick child. The other siblings usually regard this as unfair and interpret the parents' attitude toward them as rejection. Although such responses are usually unconscious and unintended, they place unique burdens on ill children. For example, the ill child may feel obligated to play the sick role in order to meet his parents' expectations. This is especially frequent in children who have had limited physical ability and regain normal health status, such as following corrective heart surgery. Parents may be unable to perceive the child as well and, therefore, need to continue the pattern of overprotection and indulgent attention.

Ill children may also feel the jealousy and resentment from other siblings. Because of their singular position in the family, they may be denied the companionship of their brothers and sisters. Rivalry between siblings tends to be greatest in the sibling who is nearest the ill child's age.[3] Without an understanding of the interpersonal dynamics between siblings, parents are likely to blame the well children for antisocial behavior.

Illness may also result in children's loss of status within either their family or social group. For example, illness in the oldest child may temporarily terminate his special privileges as "big" brother or sister. The hospitalized adolescent loses his rank within the peer group. The effects of such losses have already been discussed.

The nurse's role is to counsel parents regarding the effects of altered roles. In specific, parents should keep the family well informed and communicating as much as possible. They should treat all the children as equally and as normally as before the illness occurred. Discipline, which initially may be lessened for the ill child, should be continued to provide a measure of security and predictability. When ill children know that their parents expect certain standards of conduct from them, they feel certain that they will recover. Conversely when all limits are removed, they fear that something catastrophic will happen.

Nurses should also forewarn parents of the reactions of siblings to the ill child, particularly anger, jealousy, and resentment. Older siblings may deny such reactions because they provoke feelings of guilt. However, everyone needs outlets for emotions, and the repressed feelings may surface as problems in school, with age-mates, as psychosomatic illnesses, or in delinquent behavior.

Parents also need help in accepting their own feelings toward the ill child. If given the opportunity, parents often disclose their feelings of loss of control, particularly with decreased tolerance and understanding of all offspring. The anger-depression-guilt syndrome of normal parenthood becomes intensified during periods of crisis, such as childhood illness.[11] Parents often resist admitting to such feelings because they expect others to disapprove of behavior that is less than perfect. Unfortunately health personnel, including nurses, sometimes do exercise little tolerance for deviation from the expected norm. This only increases the psychologic impact of a child's illness on family members. Helping parents identify the specific reason for each behavior and emphasizing that each is a normal, expected, and healthy response to stress provides them with an opportunity to unburden their emotional toll.

Bodily injury and pain. Beyond early infancy, all children fear bodily injury either from fears of mutilation, bodily intrusion, body image change, disability, or death. In general, preparation of children for painful procedures decreases their fears (see p. 909). Manipulating procedural techniques for children in each age-group also minimizes fear of bodily injury. For example, since toddlers and young preschoolers are traumatized by insertion of a rectal thermometer, axillary temperatures or electronic temperature probes can effectively be substituted. Gaining the child's cooperation for examining the throat prevents the need for a tongue blade.

Because of young children's poorly defined body boundaries, the use of bandages may be particularly significant. For example, telling them that the bleeding will stop after the needle is removed does little to relieve their fears, whereas applying a small Band-Aid usually provides much reassurance. The size of bandages is also significant to children in this age-group. The larger the bandage, the more importance is attached to the wound. Using successively smaller surgical dressings is one way of their measuring healing and improvement. Prematurely removing a dressing may cause them considerable concern for their well-being. Such reactions may be erroneously interpreted as their fear of looking at the wound. In contrast it is an expression of their need for assistance in defining body image.

In children who fear mutilation of body parts, repeatedly stressing the reason for a procedure and evaluating their understanding is essential in order to minimize fear. For example, explaining cast removal to preschoolers may seem simple enough, but the child's comprehension of the details may vary considerably from the explanation. Asking them to draw a picture of what they think will happen presents substantial evidence of the perceived events. For example, one child who was to have a leg cast removed drew a picture of the doctor using a large saw to cut through the cast. When the nurse asked him how the doctor would know when to stop, the child answered, "I don't know. I guess he could cut off my leg." The nurse again clarified that the special saw blade was only long enough to go through the hard cast and automatically stopped if it touched soft material, such as the cotton lining of the cast. To evaluate this teaching the nurse had the child draw a second picture, which depicted the doctor using a tiny saw. The child in this picture had a happy smile on his face, in contrast to the first one, in which the face was expressionless. From this drawing the nurse judged that the child was more aware of and confident about the actual events of cast removal.

Children may fear bodily injury from a great variety of sources. X-ray machines, use of strange equipment for examination, unfamiliar rooms, or awkward positions can be perceived as potentially hazardous. In addition thoughts and actions can be imagined sources of bodily damage. For older children, masturbation or sex play may be perceived as powerful weapons of potential destruction. Therefore, it is important that nurses investigate imagined reasons for illness, particularly of a sexual nature. Since children may fear revealing such thoughts, using projective techniques such as drawing or doll play may provide previously undisclosed misconceptions.

Older children fear bodily injury of both internal and external origins. For example, school-age children are aware of the significance of the heart and may fear the actual operation, as well as the pain, the stitches, and the possible scar. Adolescents may express concern for the actual procedure but be much more anxious over the resulting scar. An appreciation of each child's special concerns helps nurses focus on critical areas during preparation for procedures or explanations of disease processes.

Assessment of pain. Assessment of pain is a critical component of the nursing process. Knowledge of children's response to pain yields valuable data for an assessment plan. Several basic assumptions regarding pain perception and expression are foundational: (1) pain is subjective, personal, and not directly communicable; (2) pain is integrally interwoven with emotions such as fear, anxiety, anger, loneliness, or depression, and the emotion itself may increase the perception and expression of pain; (3) the expression of pain varies with age; and (4) nonverbal communication, specifically a change in behavior, precedes verbal communication of pain.[19]

Recognition of the existence and evaluation of the severity of pain is facilitated by an understanding of the response to pain of children in each age-group, as well as the influence of factors such as cultural or ethnic background, previous experience with pain, and response from others to the pain. Although this has been discussed in the previous section, the major responses are summarized as follows: *Preverbal children* express pain through behaviors such as tense body posture, irritability, inability to be comforted by usual measures, rolling of the head, flexing extremities on the body, rubbing or pulling a body part, lethargy, and overreaction to usual stimuli. Reaction to induced pain is primarily physical resistance. *Preschoolers* also exhibit pain primarily through behavior but begin to verbally communicate its location. Psychosomatic pain and cultural expressions become evident, as well as an increased ability to control pain responses. *Older children* explicitly describe their pain but are also more sophisticated in hiding or exaggerating it for personal gain. However, subtle behaviors such as a strained facial expression, rigid positioning of a body part, or unusual quietness are clues to the presence of pain. The absence of these behaviors may also disclose an exaggerated or feigned expression of pain.

It is obvious that the most important tool in assessing pain is observation. For a more systematic approach, nurses can observe for signs of pain in the following areas: verbal indications, behavioral changes, and physiologic responses. Fig. 25-1 presents an inventory of pain indicants. Such a tool can be used to familiarize oneself with developmental expressions of pain, to learn how each child communicates his pain, and to nonjudgmentally evaluate the degree of pain by observing actual behaviors.

The child's response to medication is another valuable indicator of actual or imagined pain. For example, in preverbal children who communicate a wide variety of emotions through behavior, obvious change in behavior following administration of analgesics is suggestive of existing pain. In older children psychologic gains from pain may be evident in their punctual request for pain medication. The use of a placebo and resultant relief of pain symptoms may

I. Time observation began:_______
Time observation ended:_______

II. Time observation began:_______
Time observation ended:_______

	I	II
A. VERBAL INTROVERTED		
1. Asks to be left alone		
B. NONVERBAL INTROVERTED		
2. Draws knees up to abdomen		
3. Turns away from people		
4. Covers face		
5. Sucks thumb or bottle		
6. Hides under bed covers		
7. Pushes helping person away		
8. Tightly holds favorite toy		
9. Sleeps		
10. Touches painful area		
C. VERBAL EXTROVERTED		
11. Asks to be held		
12. Asks someone to stay with him		
13. Calls for mother		
14. Asks for nurse or doctor		
15. Asks to have little things done		
16. Asks to go home		
17. Asks for medication		
18. Asks not to be moved		
19. Refuses food or drink		
D. NONVERBAL EXTROVERTED		
20. Holds another person's hand		
21. Reaches out to another person		
22. Pulls another person toward him		
23. Strikes out at those around him		
24. Bites		
25. Tears falling		
E. DESCRIPTION OF PAIN EXPERIENCE		
26. Tells you where it hurts		
27. States he is in pain		
28. Tells how it hurts		
29. States he doesn't have pain		
30. Says not to look at him		
31. Points to where it hurts		

	I	II
F. SYMPATHETIC		
32. Change in skin color		
33. Changes position frequently		
34. Changes in pulse		
35. Changes in body temperature		
36. Changes in BP		
37. Changes in respirations		
38. Perspiration		
39. Hands trembling or shaking		
40. Sighing		
G. RESPONSE TO FOOD		
41. Pushes food and drink away		
42. Plays with food but doesn't eat		
43. Reluctant to swallow		
H. VERBAL		
44. Cries		
45. Screams		
46. Groans, moans, or grunts		
47. Whines		
I. MOTOR		
48. Winces, grimaces, or frowns		
49. Paces floor		
50. Stands up in bed		
51. Jumps up and down on bed		
52. Holds body rigid		
53. Lies quietly in bed		
54. Flings arms and legs, kicks		
55. Lies with eyes open		
56. Lies in one position		
57. Clenches jaw		
58. Grits teeth		
59. Walks hunched over		
60. Fidgets		

J. COMMENTS

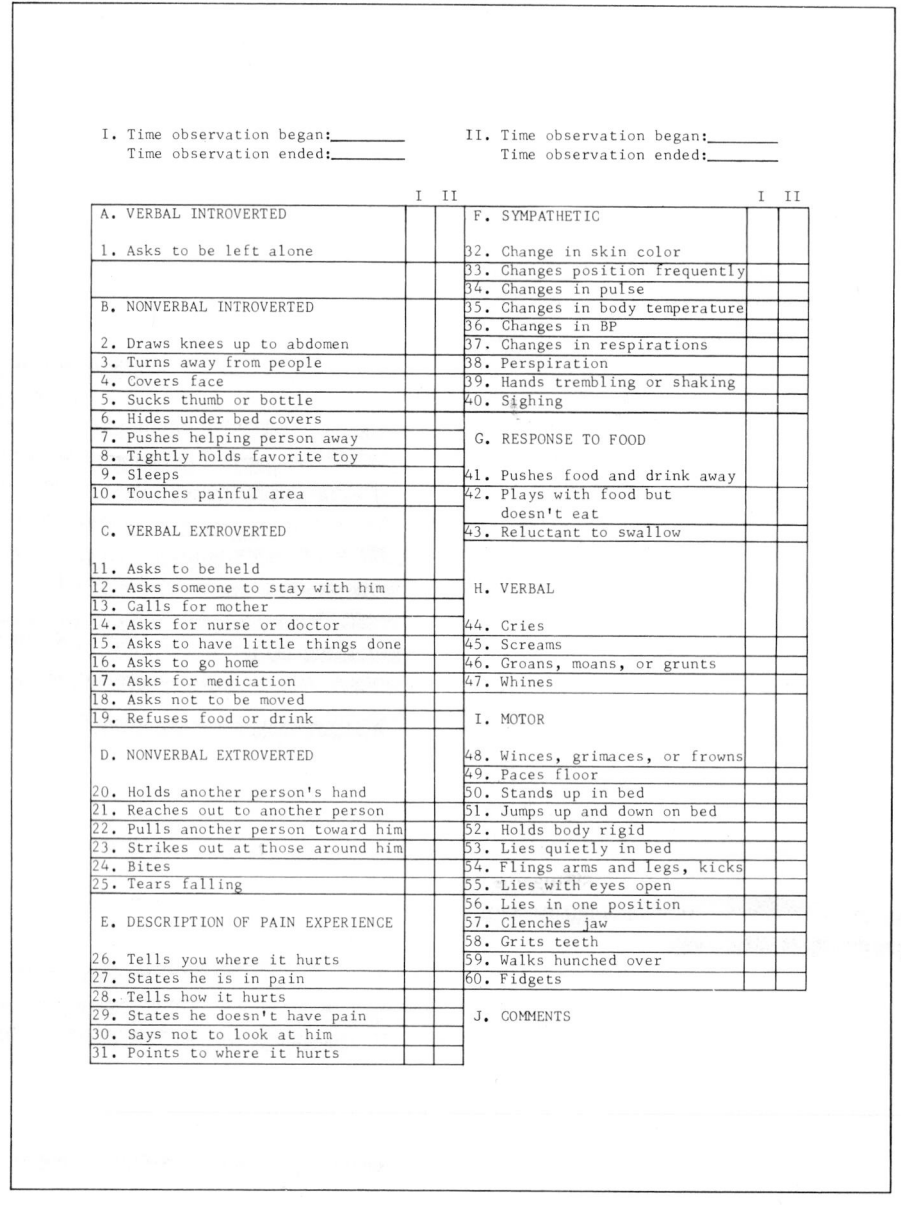

Fig. 25-1. Inventory of pain indicants. (From Smith, M. E.: The preschooler and pain. In Brandt, P. A., Chinn, P. L., and Smith, M. E.: Current practice in pediatric nursing, vol. 1, St. Louis, 1976, The C. V. Mosby Co., p. 206.)

be indicative of nonorganic causes. It is important in such situations to refrain from labeling the child a "faker," because fear can often mimic pain. The personal attention from the nurse administering the medication may be sufficient to reduce the fear and, thereby, alleviate the responses indicative of pain.

Nurses' role: maximizing growth potential of illness and hospitalization

Thus far the stressors of illness and hospitalization have been viewed as crisis situations that are capable of producing negative adjustments in children. However, since the theory of crisis includes the potential for growth, it follows that the experience of illness and hospitalization can lead to positive changes. Therefore, nurses' role must focus on both minimizing the stress and maximizing the growth potential of either experience.

Support in parent-child relationships. The crisis of illness and/or hospitalization can mobilize parents into more acute awareness of the needs of their children. For example, one school-age child who was diagnosed with a serious physical condition commented to the nurse that he "enjoyed" the hospital because it was the first time that he had seen so much of his parents. He expressed concern over discharge because he anticipated the loss of the intensified love and attention. The nurse was able to discuss these feelings with the parents and to increase their awareness of their child's need for them.

Hospitalization provides opportunities for parents to learn more about their children's growth and development. When nurses help parents understand children's usual reactions to stress, such as regression or aggression, parents are not only better able to support the child through the hospital experience but also may extend their insights into child-rearing practices following discharge.

Difficulties in parent-child relationships that may result in feeding problems, negative behavior, enuresis, and so on may decrease during hospitalization. The temporary cessation of such problems sometimes alerts parents to the role they may play in propagating the negative behavior. With assistance from health professionals, parents can restructure ways of relating to their children to foster more positive behavior.

Hospitalization may also represent a temporary reprieve or refuge from a disturbed home. Typically, abused or neglected children's dramatic physical and social improvement during hospitalization is proof of the growth potential of this experience. Hospitalized children temporarily are able to seek support, reassurance, and security from new relationships, particularly with nurses, hospitalized peers, and others.

For older children who have contemplated leaving home, hospitalization can provide them with an opportunity to think through the benefits and dangers of such a move. For example, an adolescent who was hospitalized unexpectedly for emergency surgery confided to the nurse his plans for running away from home. His fantasies concerning this decision were heavily influenced and glorified by stories from friends who had run away. However, he had given little thought to the practicalities of self-support and the prevalent street dangers to runaways. Although the nurse did not attempt to dissuade him from his plans, she concentrated on directing his thoughts to the more serious consequences of this move and introduced possible other alternatives. His parents were included in some of the discussions and were made aware of the influences their marital problems had on the other children. During his admission the nurse and social service department were able to find the adolescent a temporary home in a supervised group setting for troubled youths. The parents agreed to this arrangement and began to participate in family counseling sessions.

Educational opportunity. Illness and hospitalization represent excellent opportunities for children and other family members to learn more about their bodies, each other, and the health professions. For example, during a hospital admission for a diabetic crisis, the child may learn about his disease, the parents may learn about the child's needs for independence, normalcy, and appropriate limits, and each of them may find a new support system in the hospital staff.

Since nurses are in an optimum position to institute health teaching, they often can help people of different cultures understand the goals and philosophy of modern medicine and, thereby, help them adhere to prescribed treatment plans. For example, Chinese medicine relies heavily on the use of herbs. When a Chinese person is ill, he receives one dose of a preparation from the herbalist, who tells him to return if he does not improve. Therefore, many Chinese persons have difficulty in comprehending treatment that requires continuous use of medication, such as in diabetes.[2] Nurses who are aware of such cultural variations can use the hospital experience as an extended opportunity for health teaching.

Illness or hospitalization can also help older children in choosing a vocational career. Frequently children have impressions of physicians or nurses that are disproportionately glorified or horrified. However, actual experience with different health professionals can influence their decision for or against a health career. For example, an adolescent who was hospitalized for an orthopedic problem related to the nurse that she had no idea of what she would like to do following graduation. She was steadily dating a young man, who had asked her to marry him. She admitted that she liked, but did not love, him. However, she saw marriage and child bearing as a substitute role for a career. She also confided that she was sexually active with him but did not fear a pregnancy, since that would "make up her mind" about marriage. The nurse recognized the adolescent's superficial motives for marriage and focused her discussions on possible careers. The girl stated that she had always wanted to become a nurse but that she did not like ''hurting people.'' She had never seen nurses ''supporting'' people by talking with them. As a result of her several-week hospital stay and her trusting relationship with her nurse, she made definite plans with her school guidance counselor to begin nursing education, began birth control measures, and continued to see her boyfriend, but with marriage as a possible long-range goal.

Self-mastery. The experience of facing a crisis such as illness or hospitalization, coping successively with it, and maturing as a result of it constitutes an opportunity for self-mastery. Younger children have the chance to test out fantasy vs reality fears. They realize that they were not abandoned, mutilated, castrated, or punished. In fact, they were loved, cared for, and treated with respect for their individual concerns. It is not unusual to hear children who have undergone hospitalization or surgery tell others of how ''it was nothing,'' or proudly display their scars or bandages.

For older children hospitalization may represent an opportunity for decision making, independence, and self-reliance. They are proud of having survived the experience and may expect their parents to treat them as more ''grown-up'' following discharge. School nurses can capitalize on the school-age child's hospital experience by encouraging the child to discuss it with his classmates. In this way the child feels important as a result of having faced the crisis, and the other children vicariously learn about hospitalization.

Socialization. Hospitalization may offer to children a special opportunity for social acceptance. Lonely, asocial, sometimes delinquent children find a sympathetic environment in the hospital. Children who are physically deformed or in some other way ''different'' from their age-mates may find an accepting social peer group. Although this does not always spontaneously occur, nurses can structure the environment to foster a supportive child group.

For example, on a preadolescent unit, the children derided a new patient who was a paraplegic as a result of accidental gunshot wounds. They made fun of his confinement to a wheelchair and deliberately provoked incidents in which he could not compete. The nurse was disturbed by these events and decided to have a group session in which all the children discussed why they were hospitalized. As each related his health problem, it became obvious that they too had defects that could be criticized. Following the discussion, some of the children asked the paraplegic child to join them in a game. When he was able to compete on an equal basis, the children accepted him and no longer taunted him with his limitations.

Parents may also encounter a new social group in other parents who have similar problems. The waiting room or corridor ''self-help'' groups are inherent to every institution. Nurses can capitalize on this informal gathering by encouraging parents to collectively discuss their concerns and feelings. They can also refer parents to organized parent groups or can utilize the help and support of recovered hospitalized patients. The ''ostomy club'' is a well-known organization of osteotomy patients who help other new osteotomy victims adjust to the change in body image and function.

FAMILIES OF ILL CHILDREN

The crisis of childhood illness and hospitalization affects every member of the nuclear family and, to various degrees, members of the extended family. Because a family is a system of interdependent parts, a change in any one member of the system causes a corresponding change in every other member. Schematically the family system can be viewed as a set of gears or cogwheels; movement in any one gear causes a reciprocal movement in every other gear. Under normal circumstances the parents are the dominant force in the family or the major directional gears of the system. However, when illness occurs, the child often becomes the principal directional force and, as such, causes major responses in each of the other family members.

Parents' reactions and ability to cope

Parents' reactions to illness in their child depend on a variety of influencing factors, such as (1) the seriousness of the threat to their child, (2) previous experience with illness or hospitalization, (3) medical procedures involved in diagnosis and treatment, (4) available support systems, (5) personal ego strengths, (6) previous coping abilities, (7) additional stresses on the family system, (8) cultural and religious beliefs, and (9) communication patterns among family members. Assessment of each of these variables gives nurses baseline data on which to evaluate the degree of risk each family faces in trying to cope with illness.

Denial and disbelief. Although a life-threatening illness presents the greatest stress to parents (see Chapter 27), many of the reactions demonstrated in response to terminal illness are also seen in less serious conditions. Initially parents may react with *denial* and *disbelief*. For example, if a child complains of severe abdominal pain, parents initially may ascribe it little meaning. Even when the diagnosis of appendicitis is confirmed, parents may question the immediate need for surgery.

Anger and guilt. Following the realization of illness, parents react with *anger*, *guilt*, or both. To return to the example in the preceding paragraph, parents may direct the anger at the child for not having complained sooner or at themselves for not having realized the severity of the condition. Guilt is almost a universal response to such situations. Even in the mildest of illnesses, parents question their adequacy as care givers and review any actions or omissions that could have prevented or caused the illness. When hospitalization is indicated, parental guilt is intensified because they feel helpless in alleviating the child's physical and emotional pain. Nurses who realize the impact of childhood illness can reduce the burden of guilt by including parents in the care of their child, keeping them informed of the child's progress, and providing emotional support to all family members.

The child's reactions of anger, regression, negativism, and resistance often intensify parents' feelings of guilt because they think that these behaviors are directed toward them. The child who withdraws is a special dilemma because parents interpret the reaction as rejection at a time when they wish to console and comfort. However, children who cope in this manner may fear losing control if they express emotion. Therefore, they protect themselves through social isolation. Helping parents understand the child's possible need or reason for withdrawal assists them in accepting it without feeling rejected.

Although parents may feel guilty when confronted with such behaviors, they also tend to counteract them with overt anger. Children, in turn, interpret the anger as evidence of parental rejection. Consequently a destructive cycle of misunderstood reactions occurs. Intervention involves preventing the nonsupportive parent-child interactions by preparing parents for the usual reactions of children to illness and hospitalization.

Fear, anxiety, and frustration. *Fear, anxiety,* and *frustration* are common feelings expressed by parents. Fear and anxiety may be related to the seriousness of the illness and the type of medical procedures involved. Often a great deal of anxiety is related to the trauma and pain inflicted on the child because of the various procedures. Since the perception of an event is more significant than the actual circumstances, it is necessary to assess parents' degree of comfort and familiarity with hospital routines. For example, seeing a young child restrained to a bed with intravenous equipment connected to his arm or foot can be extremely frightening. Nurses, who work with such equipment daily, may have difficulty in perceiving this event from a stranger's viewpoint. Putting oneself in the parents' and child's place often yields the best guidelines for intervention.

Parents' anxieties regarding their child's hospitalization also fuel their feelings of frustration. Mothers who were questioned about their reactions to the child's hospital stay reported that lack of information about procedures and treatment caused them the greatest concern.[6] Frustration and a feeling of loss of control also occur as a result of unfamiliarity with hospital rules and regulations, a sense of unwelcomeness from the staff, or fear of asking questions. It is obvious that much frustration can be alleviated in a pediatric unit in which parents participate in their child's care and are regarded as the most significant contributors to the child's total health.

Depression. From the culmination of all the previous reactions, parents eventually react with some degree of *depression*. Contrary to common belief, the depression usually occurs when the acute crisis is over, such as following hospital discharge or complete recovery. Prior to this, depression would result in a lowered level of activity and would negatively affect one's ability to cope with stress. Mothers often comment on their feeling of physical and mental exhaustion after all the other family members have adapted to the crisis. Both parents may express concern for the financial burden incurred from the hospitalization.

To understand this delayed reaction, one can relate the response to the system of gears. The mother senses her responsibility as a prime care-giving force and is unable to relinquish some of the roles until the system is ready to respond on its own. In an emotionally healthy family the other members support the mother's needs by reciprocally assuming some of her roles. In the moderately or severely disturbed family the other members are not able to change roles interdependently. Therefore, at some point the system fails.

Coping mechanisms

Since illness or hospitalization becomes a crisis when the family does not have adequate coping mechanisms to deal with it, there is benefit in elucidating parents' usual coping mechanisms to stress. The major defense mechanisms can be classified as denial, intellectualization, projection, displacement, regression, and introjection. These mechanisms are psychologic processes that temporarily protect individuals from anxiety by providing a measure of security or relief from stress. These defenses are normal and healthy; they may become pathologic when they prevent the person from successfully resolving the crisis situation.

Denial. *Denial* is rejection of reality. It is an almost universal response to stress. It helps parents distance themselves from the emotional onslaught of the crisis until they have summoned sufficient alternate defenses to help them cope. It becomes pathologic and destructive when it prevents movement or action toward decision making. For example, continued denial of a child's serious illness may fatally delay medical care. Denial of children's usual reactions to the stressors of illness may prevent parents from offering them any emotional support.

Intellectualization. *Intellectualization* is the use of knowledge to control the intense emotional impact of the illness's meaning. Parents intellectualize when they attempt to find out all the information available on their child's illness but fail to face the issues of that disorder. Medical and nursing personnel are frequently caught in this trap because they feel more comfortable in supplying the facts than in helping the family deal with more critical problems. Although gaining knowledge about the child's condition is an important component of eventual acceptance, in its extreme it can represent a form of denial.

Projection. *Projection* is resolving conflicts by placing the responsibility outside oneself. For example, parents may project their blame and anger onto the child, other spouse, or hospital staff. Consequently they accept little or no responsibility for the illness. In this way the parent's own self-esteem can be maintained. Projection can be destructive when it alienates the parent from all potential sources of support.

Displacement. *Displacement* is the transference of emotion or concern from one object or event to another, less threatening one. For example, parents may transfer their fear of the child's recovery into concern for a specific symptom, such as the pain from surgery. A common displacement of anger is toward the well siblings. Parents who have tried to be patient and tolerant of the ill child's negative behavior may literally explode with anger at the slightest provocation from other siblings. Siblings interpret such reactions as parental rejection.

Regression. *Regression,* or the return to a less stressful level of functioning, is evident in parents, as well as children, although the behaviors may be more subtle. Fears, "temper tantrums" or sudden outbursts of anger, and demanding behavior toward others, such as the spouse or hospital staff, are characteristic patterns of regressive behavior.

Introjection. *Introjection,* in which parents turn all their blame, anger, and guilt inward, expecting punishment for their misdeeds, is the opposite of projection. The ultimate result of introjection is self-punishment by suicide. Less severe and more common examples of self-blame are verbally downgrading one's parenting abilities, searching for evidence of one's responsibility in causing the illness, and neglecting one's physical health. Introjection of this nature is often a component of depression.

How parents cope with the stress of illness and how they resolve the feelings of guilt and self-blame often determine how the family system will be affected. Those who can successfully accept the illness and deal with self-accusatory feelings are generally able to allow the child a return to normal life. Those who are guilt ridden, overpermissive, and overprotective usually cause the child to be dependent, fearful, and demanding. The repressed hostility toward the child often results in outbursts of anger, usually directed toward all other family members.

Nurses' role

Because dealing with a crisis involves a feeling of loss of control when previous coping mechanisms fail, parents' principal need is a reestablishment of control. Nurses' main mode of intervention is supportive, which involves (1) acting as a support system, (2) referring to available support resources, and (3) providing information. Since each individual copes differently, it is apparent that the type of support and depth of information vary. For example, parents who cope with stress through active involvement benefit most from the support provided through parent-participation programs. Parents who deal with stress by problem solving require frequent and detailed information about the child's progress.

Support. The term "family-centered care" defines the focus of pediatric care because nursing of children cannot be optimally performed unless each family member is designated the "patient" or "client." Support involves the willingness to stay and listen to parents' verbal and nonverbal messages. Sometimes the support is not given directly by the nurse. For example, the nurse may offer to stay with the child to allow the parents time alone. In this way the nurse provides support through each spouse. The nurse may discuss with other family members the parents' need for extra relief. Often, extended relatives and friends want to help but do not know how. Suggesting ways such as baby-sitting, preparing meals, tending the garden or home, doing laundry, or transporting the siblings to school lessens the responsibilities that burden parents.

Nurses may also provide support through the clergy. Parents with deep religious beliefs may appreciate the counsel of a clergy member, but because of their stress may not have sufficient energy to initiate the contact. Nurses can also be supportive by upholding parents' religious beliefs and respecting their individual meaning and significance. For example, during a child's hospitalization for elective surgery, the mother prayed constantly but did not participate in any of the child's care, even though the staff encouraged parent involvement. The nurses were initially critical of her behavior, until one of them asked her if she would like to help with the child's bath. The mother responded, "No, I appreciate if you do it, because I can pray, but you cannot." The mother was conveying her priority of needs.

Support also involves an acceptance of cultural, socioeconomic, and ethnic values. Although it is not the intent to stereotype, each group defines health and illness differently. For example, Mexican-Americans perceive illness as a state of physical discomfort. Health is determined by a sturdy body, high level of physical activity, and absence of persistent pain. Therefore, disorders that have no outward manifestation of illness, such as diabetes, hypertension, or cardiac problems, are not viewed as "illness." In addition causes of diseases, such as germs, are not strongly believed. Instead the common idea that God decides when a person is to be ill as a sign of his displeasure is upheld as the reason for illness.[1] Medical treatments are often seen as an interference with God's will.

The culture of poverty also dictates attitudes toward illness. The effects of economic deprivation are expressed in four life themes: fatalism, authoritarianism, concreteness, and present orientation.[8] Poor persons' fatalistic impression of life and orientation to the present hinder them from taking an active role in treatment or prevention of disease. Authoritarianism and concreteness direct their trust in the validity of strength and observable results. Therefore, decisions regarding health care are often made on the basis of authority and power rather than reason or understanding.

How individuals respond to stress such as illness is also culturally influenced. For example, Oriental parents are often judged as cold, distant, aloof, and uncaring because of their limited outward display of emotion. However, when one realizes that self-discipline and emotional restraint are valued attributes in their culture, one will also realize that lack of overt emotion is no measure of the depth of feeling and involvement.

Nurses must also exercise awareness of cultural and individual patterns of relating. For example, although direct eye contact is generally regarded as a sign of interest and attention, the American Indian regards direct visual contact as a sign of impoliteness and invasion of one's privacy.[5] Therefore, downcast eyes may have very different meanings for this group of parents than for those of other ethnic backgrounds.

Information. The term "information" involves much more than relaying facts. It is guidance through (1) knowledge of the disease, its treatment, and prognosis; (2) awareness of the child's emotional, as well as physical, reaction to illness and hospitalization; and (3) anticipation of the probable emotional reactions of the parents and siblings to the crisis.

Conveying knowledge about the child's illness involves assessing the parents' present level of understanding and desire for additional information. Often this prerequisite for effective intervention is ignored, resulting in overloading them with information or leaving them unaware of significant facts.

Because parental anxiety selectively decreases their perception of information and leads to misinterpretation, nurses need to repeatedly assess the level of understanding. Although the degree of anxiety is directly related to the seriousness of the disease, parents' perception of potential threats may vary from the actual risk. For example, although a child may be undergoing routine elective surgery, to the parents he may be facing a critical and hazardous experience. Their level of anxiety may not only necessitate repeated explanations but may also prevent them from being able to prepare the child for the event.

Communicating effectively requires (1) an understanding of parents' reactions to stress, particularly those responses that may block communication, such as guilt, fear, denial, or anxiety; (2) relating to parents on their intellectual level; (3) repeatedly clarifying and evaluating their level of understanding; and (4) being aware of the blocks to communication, such as stereotyping, information overload, and the use of generalizations. Specific interventions include providing parents with written information, defining and clarifying all medical terms, suggesting the use of a written list of questions for obtaining information from other members of the health team, acting as liaison and interpreter for parents in their relationship with other disciplines, and offering repeated explanations while supporting their self-esteem.

Siblings' reactions and ability to cope

Siblings' reactions to a sister's or brother's illness or hospitalization have briefly been discussed in this chapter and are elaborated on in Chapter 27. Their main reactions are anger, resentment, jealousy, and guilt. Guilt is usually a result of repressing the other feelings and occurs more commonly in older children.

Siblings' ability to cope is determined primarily by their developmental age but is also influenced by the strength of the family system, previous or concurrent experiences with stress, and usual coping mechanisms. For example, young children may have more difficulty in adjusting to the stress imposed by the parents' separation. Older children who use verbal communication as a coping mechanism may have less difficulty in adjusting, provided they are given adequate information. Children who are experiencing concurrent stresses, such as entry into school, may have increased difficulty in coping, regardless of their age.

Nurses' role. One of the dilemmas in helping siblings deal with the stress of illness or hospitalization is the lack of nursing contact. Traditionally preparation programs for hospitalization or related procedures involve the child (patient) and parents. Limited visiting hours and rigid age requirements further decrease nurses' opportunities to meet with siblings. In addition unawareness of the effects of a child's illness and hospitalization on other siblings usually results in a total lack of concern with this group.

Nursing approaches with siblings can be direct or indirect. Direct services might include (1) incorporating siblings into hospital admission programs; (2) liberalizing visiting regulations; (3) extending parent participation programs to include sibling involvement, such as through family dining or group play sessions; and (4) developing programs designed specifically for siblings, such as group sessions to discuss their concerns or posthospital discharge visits to evaluate the siblings' adjustment.

Indirect services, which are amenable to any existing nursing role, involve helping parents understand, cope with, and support the siblings' reactions to the experience. Parents who are unaware of the effect of a child's illness on siblings are likely to expect behavioral patterns that are beyond the siblings' ability. For example, parents may expect older siblings to assume too much responsibility or to comfort them in their parental needs. When the siblings express resentment for the parents' absence, the parents respond with anger and resentment. If each party realized the other's needs, there would be less likelihood of a destructive, nonsupportive cycle of relating.

Probably one of the most neglected areas regarding siblings involves information giving. Frequently age becomes the only factor that leads to an awareness of this problem, because older children may begin to ask questions or request explanations. However, even in this situation the information may be seriously inadequate. Children in every age-group deserve some explanation for the child's illness or hospitalization. Although the exact wording may differ, the answer should focus on the following concerns: (1) "Will I get sick and have to go to the hospital?" (2) "Did I cause the illness?" (for actual or imagined reasons), and (3) "Will my parents abandon me if my brother or sister doesn't recover?" If parents or nurses address the explanations to these three questions, the siblings' own fears of illness, guilt, and adandonment are minimized.

Nurses also provide indirect care when they prepare parents for some of the behaviors siblings may exhibit as evidence of their stress. Regression, demand for parental attention, difficulty in school, social withdrawal, and psychosomatic complaints may be indicative of the siblings' emotional needs. When parents anticipate such reactions, they can cope more effectively, either by seeking additional professional help or by supporting the child through the difficult readjustment period.

PREPARING FOR HOSPITAL EXPERIENCE

The rationale for preparing children for the hospital experience and related procedures is based on the theorem that fear of the unknown (fantasy) exceeds fear of the known. Therefore, decreasing the elements of the unknown results in less fear. When children do not have paralyzing fear to cope with, they are then able to direct their energies toward dealing with the other unavoidable stresses of hospitalization and to benefit optimally from the growth potential of the experience.

Ideally preparatory procedures should be (1) planned by the nursing staff prior to any child's admission to the hospital, (2) appropriately designed for each child's developmental age, and (3) sufficiently individualized to account for different children's previous experience with hospitalization, present reason for admission, and available support system. Although the following discussion will address each of these ideal requirements, for practical reasons each institution may implement them differently. For example, some hospital admission programs focus on group preparation prior to actual admission, whereas others prepare each child either prior to or on the day of admission. Regardless of which method is used, whether it be formalized or spontaneous, the value of a consistent primary nurse during the child's entire hospitalization is of paramount importance. Primary nursing allows individualized care based on age, family constellation, and previous experience with illness. It also offers a substitute support system when stressors such as separation cannot be prevented. It ensures a continuity of assessment, implementation, and evaluation of care that facilitates the minimization of negative effects and maximization of beneficial effects from the hospital experience for all family members.

Although the preparation procedures presented are most effective when the hospital experience is expected, special considerations for emergency admission are also discussed. Emergency hospitalization presents special dilemmas and challenges because time is usually insufficient to lessen the fear of the unknown until after many of the events have occurred. However, the concept of *postvention,* or preventive counseling after the fact, is considered as the basis for decreasing stress as much as possible for this experience and for subsequent ones as well.

Prehospital counseling

For children past the years of infancy and early toddlerhood, preparation prior to hospital admission is recommended. Even when children are too young to benefit from this procedure, parents need prehospital counseling to lessen their fears and, thereby, increase their ability to psychologically support the child. Prehospital counseling has two major goals: (1) to make the hospital less strange and frightening to parents and children, and (2) to establish a positive atmosphere regarding hospitalization for all family members. Although the specific details of each program may vary, the following principles serve as guidelines for accomplishing these goals: (1) the tour, literature, "show," or discussion should be designed to be as nonfrightening as is possible; (2) the entire family should be included in the program; (3) time should be allowed for each family member to ask questions or to express individual needs; (4) the program should be scheduled for the most optimum time for retention of information and prevention of fantasy reproduction; and (5) the interpersonal needs of parents and children should be focused on by including significant members of the hospital staff in the program. The following example of a hypothetical prehospital admission program illustrates how each principle is implemented.

Prehospital counseling by professionals. Children between the ages of 2 and 18 years who are electively scheduled for hospital admission are invited to attend a regularly planned prehospital admission program. The entire family is invited to the program either by letter or telephone. Some hospitals have found that inner city families respond better to direct telephone contact than to written invitations.[9] When the family arrives at the hospital, they are greeted by a nurse or other person who groups the families according to specific ages: older toddlers and preschoolers, school-age children, and adolescents.

Because most scheduled admissions are for elective surgery, the family watches a puppet show reenacting the basic steps of this hospitalization: admission procedures; preparation for surgery in the "slumber" room, the operating room, and the recovery room; and postsurgical treatment. The main focus of each scene is the use of concrete actions and props to familiarize the family members for what will actually occur. The puppets talk about children's common fears, such as pain, anesthesia, parent separation, and so on. Although the sophistication of the materials varies, the basic characters include a puppet family (mother, father, and child) and hospital staff (physician and nurse), that are racially representative of the patient and hospital population. For example, both black and white dolls are required in many urban areas. Hospital equipment includes mask, cap, gloves, gown, intravenous bottle, stand, tubing, syringes, thermometer, blood pressure machine, stethoscope, scale, oxygen mask, suture removal set, bandages, bed, and sheets. If children are routinely admitted for diagnostic evaluations, miniature replicas of machinery, such as x-ray equipment, or the use of slides as visual aides may be used. The use of scaled down models is especially beneficial for young children who may be frightened by the actual proportions of some equipment. However, it is the intent of what is conveyed that greatly surpasses the sophistication of the materials used.

Following the show there is a question and answer period, monitored by a nurse. Sometimes the group is reticent about asking questions. In this case the nurse can stimulate discussion by posing a question to the audience or inviting the children to see and touch the puppets and equipment.

The children in each age-group with their family members are taken on a tour of the hospital facilities, specifically the pediatric unit, a typical inpatient room, the playroom (a highlight of the tour) the parents' waiting room, the x-ray department and laboratory area, the slumber or induction room, and the recovery room. Different hospitals may tailor this tour to include special rooms, such as the "OR playroom," where children and parents first go before any induction is administered.[9] Children who are undergoing serious surgery requiring special postoperative care may be taken to visit the intensive care unit. Children scheduled for special tests, such as cardiac catheterization or cystoscopy, are sometimes shown these areas. Young children may respond better to shorter tours that concentrate on the areas of most concern, such as the pediatric unit, playroom, and recovery room.

During the tour the nurse encourages family members to ask questions and to familiarize themselves with the environment by sitting on a bed, using the electric bed controls, riding in a wheelchair, or handling the equipment in the special rooms. Ideally the tour should also be an opportunity for meeting the child's primary nurse. Although this is not always possible because of staffing schedules, the nursing staff should be introduced to the children by name. Introducing the parents to one specific nurse, such as the head nurse or clinical specialist, helps them feel more comfortable in knowing who is available for questions or concerns during the hospital stay.

Following the tour the groups reconvene for a final discussion. Serving refreshments helps people relax to ask a last-minute question. By informally visiting each table, the nurse has an excellent opportunity to discuss individual concerns. At this time the nurse can also invite the parents to call the pediatric unit for any reason prior to admission, since questions may arise during this interval.

Prehospital admission programs should be scheduled for the time of day when nursing staff are most available and the majority of medical procedures are completed. They should take place before actual admission occurs. For children 4 to 7 years of age, informing them of anticipated hospitalization about 1 week in advance is ample time for them to assimilate the information and ask questions. For older children, the time may be longer. However, for young children, who may begin to fantasize about what they observed, 1 or 2 days prior to admission is sufficient time for anticipatory preparation.[15] This is an important consideration for hospitals in which group programs are planned at widely spaced times, such as once a month. In these situations it may be best to include only children who are of school age or older and either individualize prehospital counseling for younger children or prepare them on the day of admission. Home preparation of young children is another option and can be a valuable experience for nursing students.

Often it is difficult to decide whether a child who has had previous experiences with hospitalization should attend these admission programs. As a general rule, children who adjusted well to a previous hospitalization may not need to attend. However, children who were frightened by the experience, exhibited prolonged regressive behaviors following discharge, or express fear regarding the next admission will probably benefit from such programs. Since age influences each child's reaction to hospitalization, a child who was admitted during an earlier period of development may gain new insights and perspectives from prehospital counseling.

Prehospital counseling by parents. In many situations the preparation of children for the hospital experience is left up to parents. Parents may abdicate this responsibility for a variety of reasons. For example, they sometimes think the child is too young to understand or is better off not knowing beforehand; often they are unable to prepare the child because of their own lack of knowledge and understanding.

Professionals can help parents prepare their children by adequately informing them of the specific details of hospitalization and related procedures, through both direct discussion and written material. Responsibility for such guidance often rests with office and clinic nurses. Although the elaborate preparation described in the preceding paragraphs in a hospital program is usually not possible for parents to perform, the principles outlined on p. 904 are guidelines for home preparation. For example, the use of a picture book about going to the hospital can substitute for an actual tour. A selection of references follows:

Chase, F., and Coleman, L.: A visit to the hospital, New York, 1974, Grosset & Dunlap, Inc.

Clark, B.: Pop-up going to the hospital, New York, 1970, Random House, Inc.

Collier, J.: Danny goes to the hospital, 1970, W. W. Norton & Co., Inc.

Rey, M., and Rey, H.: Curious George goes to the hospital, New York, 1966, Houghton Mifflin Co.

Stein, S.: A hospital story, New York, 1974, Walker & Co.

Weber, A.: Elizabeth gets well, New York, 1970, Thomas Y. Crowell Co.

Hospital admission

The preparation that children require on the day of admission depends on the kind of prehospital counseling they have received. If they have been prepared in a program similar to the one described on p. 904, they will usually know what to expect in terms of initial medical procedures, inpatient facilities, and nursing staff. However, prehospital counseling does not preclude the need for support during procedures such as drawing blood, x-ray tests, or physical examination. For example, undressing young children before they feel comfortable in their new surroundings can be very upsetting. Causing needless anxiety and fear during admission may adversely affect the nurse's establishment of trust with these children. Therefore, nursing assistance during the admission procedure is vital, regardless of how well prepared any child is for the experience of hospitalization. In addition spending this time with the child gives the nurse an opportunity to evaluate his understanding of subsequent procedures, such as surgery. The usual admission procedures for children are outlined in the boxed material below, left.

Nursing admission history. In those cases in which children have not had the benefit of prehospital counseling, the day of admission is a critical time for preparation for hospitalization and related procedures. However, before beginning any preparation, nurses must assess the needs of the child. Performing an admission history elicits such baseline data and should be a routine part of every hospital admission. Sample questions that nurses can use to plan their care for further hospital preparation are listed in the box below, right. As with any history form (see also the boxed material on p. 892) the questions are only guidelines; for maximum communication nurses should ask these questions as a part of conversation, not as a direct ques-

Outline of admission procedures

Preadmission

1. Assign a room based on developmental age, seriousness of diagnosis, and projected length of stay.
2. Prepare roommate or roommates for the arrival of a new patient (where children are too young to benefit from this consideration, prepare parents).
3. Have the room ready for child, with admission forms and equipment nearby to eliminate need to leave child.

Admission

1. Introduce primary nurse to child and parents.
2. Orient family to inpatient facilities, especially own room (call light, emergency bell, lights, bed controls, bathroom, telephone, and television [where applicable]). Emphasize positive areas of pediatric unit such as playroom, dining room, or other.
3. Introduce family to roommate and his or her parents.
4. Apply identification band to child's wrist, ankle, or both.
5. Explain hospital regulations for visiting hours (give written information if available).
6. Perform nursing history.
7. Take vital signs, blood pressure, height, and weight. Obtain urine sample.
8. Support child and assist physician with physical examination (for purposes of nursing assessment).

Nursing admission history for preparation for hospitalization

1. What does child know about this hospitalization?
   a. Ask child what he came to the hospital for.
   b. If answer is, "For an operation," ask child to tell you about what will happen before, during, and after the operation.
   c. Is there anything the parents do not want child to know? If so, inquire as to the reason.
2. Has child ever been in the hospital before?
   a. Did anything unpleasant or traumatic occur in earlier hospitalization that could have been avoided?
   b. Has anyone close to child died in a hospital?
3. Are there any current illnesses or disabilities other than those for which child is now admitted that limit his activity or require special care?
4. Have any major changes in the family occurred lately (death, divorce, separation, birth of a sibling, loss of a job, financial strain, mother beginning a career)? If so, explain child's reaction.
5. How does child act when he is upset or annoyed? What do the parents usually do?
6. Does child have any fears (places, objects, animals, people, situations)? If so, what do the parents do?

tionnaire. Answers to questions, such as, "What does your child know about this hospitalization?" that are broad and nonspecific, such as, "We told him everything," tell the nurse nothing. Rephrasing the question to, "Tell me what you told him," focuses on concrete details that assist nurses in evaluating the adequacy of the explanation. For example, children may respond to questions regarding their knowledge of hospitalization with statements, such as, "I don't know why I am here." Although this may be correct, frequently they have been given some explanation concerning the reason for hospitalization. Such an answer may mean that the explanation was inadequate, their anxiety blocked the recall, or they are testing out the explanation by prompting the nurse to supply additional information.

The admission history leads to the formulation of nursing diagnoses. A *nursing diagnosis* is defined as "a *conclusion* based on scientific determination of an individual's nursing needs, resulting from critical analysis of his behavior, the nature of his illness, and numerous other factors which affect his condition."[10] Although there are established classifications of nursing diagnoses, nurses' primary role is to make a judgment regarding the child's needs. To return to the discussion of hospital preparation, the nursing admission history may reveal that (1) the child is well prepared, (2) the child has had some preparation but needs additional information and support, or (3) the child has minimal knowledge of the hospital experience and requires thorough preparation.

Physical assessment. Although physical examinations by physicians are a required part of the admission procedure, nurses should also utilize the valuable information gained from physical assessments in their planning of care (Chapter 5). Subjecting children to two separate examinations is unnecessary if the nurse and physician cooperate during the procedure. For example, when the nurse is present to psychologically support the child, the opportunity can also be used to observe the child's body for any bruises, rash, signs of neglect, deformities, or physical limitations. The nurse should also listen to the heart and lungs with the physician to assess overall physical status. For example, it is impossible for a nurse to evaluate improvement in respiratory function in a child admitted with pulmonary disease unless there is baseline data with which to compare subsequent findings.

Placing child. Room assignments are usually made before the child is admitted to the pediatric unit. The minimum considerations for room assignment are age and nature of the illness. Ideally, however, room selection should be based on a variety of developmental and psychobiologic needs. Determining compatible roommates, both for the children and rooming-in parents, greatly influences the growth potential from the hospital experience.

Although there are no absolute rules to govern room selection, in general, placing children of the same age-group and with similar types of illness in the same room is both psychologically and medically advantageous. However, there are many exceptions. For example, a school-age child may thrive on the responsibility of caring for a younger child. A child in traction may be very therapeutic for another child confined to bed because of a serious illness, such as rheumatic fever. An adolescent may find social acceptance from a peer of the opposite sex who is in a neighboring room. A child who is very independent despite handicaps may help another child with similar or different physical limitations and his parents achieve deeper insight and acceptance of the disability.

Preventing information overload. Frequently children who are admitted for elective surgery or diagnostic evaluation are scheduled for these procedures the day after admission. In ambulatory surgical units children are admitted the day of surgery. This leaves nurses little time to prepare children for procedures. However, nurses must be cognizant of the effect of information overload. Following the admission procedures outlined in the box on p. 906, when possible it is advisable to delay further preparation until the child has had some time to settle in. When procedures are scheduled for the following day, early evening is an opportune time to begin explaining the event. In ambulatory or daytime units, prehospital counseling is indispensable. However, when it is not possible, surgery should be scheduled to allow some time for children to get acquainted with their surroundings and nurses to assess, plan, and complement appropriate teaching.

Emergency admission

Lengthy preparatory admission procedures are frequently inappropriate for emergency situations. In such instances nurses must focus their nursing interventions toward the most essential components of admission counseling. Since the objective of prehospital counseling is to decrease the fear and anxiety of a potentially stressful experience, planning emergency admission care based on the stressors of separation, loss of control, and bodily injury can result in prevention or minimization of negative effects. The following steps, although not necessarily applicable to every emergency situation, can serve as a general outline for nurses to use during emergency admissions.

Defining emergency. There is a wide discrepancy between what constitutes a medically defined emergency and a client-defined emergency. Studies show that acute life-threatening emergencies account for less than 1% of all emergency visits and that acute nonlife-threatening emergencies account for approximately 6%. In pediatric populations the majority of visits are for respiratory infections, whereas skin conditions, gastrointestinal disorders, and trauma such as poisoning account for the remainder of the cases. The most common reason parents give for bringing the child to the emergency room is concern for the illness worsening. However, physicians generally do not consider the progressive symptoms as necessitating emergency care.[12] Therefore, it is obvious that "emergency" is a term that is perceived differently by various people. One of nursing's primary goals is to assess the parents' perception of the events and their reason for considering it serious or life threatening.

Admission history. As soon as the child enters an emergency room, the strange, unfamiliar surroundings coupled with the parents' emotional state and the child's physical condition constitute a stressful situation. The nurse should introduce himself or herself to the family and begin an admission history. In medically defined emergencies a lengthy admission interview may not be feasible. However, several items are essential: (1) the child's name should be asked and he should be called by that name—terms such as "honey" or "dear" often confuse children; (2) the child's age should be determined and some judgment made about developmental age (if the child is of school age, asking about his grade level will offer some evidence for concurrent intellectual ability); (3) the child's general state of health, any problems that may interfere with medical treatment, such as sensitivity to medication, and previous experience with hospital facilities should be ascertained; and (4) the chief complaint should be focused on, both from the parents' and child's viewpoints.

The latter area is particularly important in decreasing stress, because children frequently supply their own reasons for why an event occurred. Most often the child's perception of the events increases his feelings of guilt, blame, and punishment. Although this occurs more frequently in accidental injuries, it can also happen when a physical illness worsens. For example, a preschooler who was brought to the emergency unit with severe respiratory distress told the nurse that she had difficulty in breathing because she cried too much. The mother realized that the reason the child thought this was that during the night the mother had asked the child to try and be quiet in order for the other children to remain asleep. The nurse and mother emphasized to the child that her crying had not made her cough worse and that if she needed to cry it was certainly all right. Such immediate intervention was extremely beneficial because the child's condition was diagnosed as epiglottitis, and an emergency tracheotomy was later performed. During the child's hospitalization, the nurses on the pediatric unit who were aware of the emergency history reinforced to the child that the temporary loss of speech was caused by the tracheotomy, not her crying.

Preventing separation. Nurses should also maintain parent-child contact during emergency admissions. Although the effects of separation are well documented for young children, older children, including adolescents, may need the support of their parents during stressful periods. Since many emergencies do not occur in the home, it is likely that parents may be unaware of the problem. In notifying parents nurses should factually and calmly state the emergency situation, refraining from emotional overtones that may increase the parents' anxiety. Supporting the parents will foster their ability to support the child.

Maintaining control. Unless an emergency is life threatening, children need to participate in their care in order to maintain a sense of control. Because emergency units are frequently hectic, there is a tendency to rush through procedures in order to save time. However, the extra few minutes needed to allow children to undress themselves may save many more minutes of useless resistance and uncooperativeness during subsequent procedures.

Maintaining control also involves assuring privacy, accepting various emotional responses to fear, pain, and so on, preserving parent-child contact, explaining all events prior to when or as they occur, and personally remaining calm. Nurses' ability to make judgments under stress, to collaborate and coordinate effectively with other disciplines, and to keep the patient's total welfare as their priority of care are probably the most essential elements in preparing children for emergency admissions.

Decreasing fear of bodily injury and pain. During emergency procedures nurses need to remember the special concerns of children in each age-group about bodily injury. Explaining each procedure, altering it whenever possible to decrease the child's fears, and supporting the child during the procedure are essential. Since many emergency visits do not require hospital admission, giving children an object that symbolizes their courage, such as a "hero badge," helps them face their fears and anxiety. It is a positive momento of an otherwise stressful experience. Giving them a choice in choosing which color or design of the badge they prefer also provides them with an opportunity for control in decision making.[13]

Postvention. There are occasions when, because of the child's physical condition, little or no preparatory counseling for emergency hospitalization can be done. In such situations the implementation of postvention, or counseling subsequent to the event, has therapeutic value. The process of postvention involves evaluating children's thoughts regarding emergency hospital admission and related procedures. It is similar to precounseling techniques; however, instead of supplying information, the nurse listens to the explanations offered by the child. Projective techniques such as drawing, doll play, or storytelling are especially effective. The nurse then bases additional information on what has already been revealed.

For example, a child who was admitted to the hospital for an emergency appendectomy described the usual admission and preoperative procedures correctly but had no understanding of why they were done. His most prominent recollection focused on all the "shots" he had received (blood tests, intravenous fluid, and sedation). When the nurse asked him why he had received so many (he had stated "millions of shots"), he responded *too* appropriately, "To make me better." Because the nurse sensed that he had been programmed or taught to view injections in this way, he was asked, "Why wouldn't one shot have been enough?" He thought for a moment, then replied, "I guess because I didn't tell my mommy about my stomachache soon enough." Based on this statement, which supports self-blame, guilt, and punishment, the nurse described the entire admission and preoperative procedure, stressing the reason for each shot. The child was also asked to confirm the details and to count the number of injections to lessen the enormity of "millions" of shots.

PREPARING FOR HOSPITAL PROCEDURES

The principles governing preparation for hospital procedures, such as surgery, diagnostic tests, medical treatments, physical therapy, and so on, follow those already described for hospitalization. In summary the following are the major guidelines: (1) determine the details of the exact procedure to be performed; (2) review the parents' and child's present level of understanding; (3) plan the actual teaching based on the child's developmental age and existing level of knowledge; (4) incorporate parents in the teaching if they desire, but especially if they plan to participate in the care; and (5) while preparing the child, allow for ample discussion to prevent information overload and ensure adequate feedback.

Psychologic preparation

Although the precise words used to describe a procedure will vary for children in each age-group and for each specific event, several important considerations apply to any situation:

1. Use concrete, not abstract, terms and visual aides to describe the procedure. For example, use a simple line drawing of a boy or girl (Fig. 25-2) and mark what body part will be involved in the procedure.
2. Emphasize that no other body part will be involved.
3. Use neutral words to describe the procedure, such as "fixed" instead of "cut out" or "taken out" and "discomfort" rather than "pain."
4. Clarify all words, such as "anesthesia is a *special* sleep."
5. Use medical terminology for body parts when teaching school-age children or adolescents.
6. Allow child to practice those procedures that will require his cooperation, such as turning, coughing, deep breathing, using a blow bottle or mask, or breathing on an intermittent positive pressure (IPPB) machine.
7. If body part is associated with a specific function, stress the change or noninvolvement of that ability, for example, following tonsillectomy, the child can still speak.
8. Introduce anxiety-laden information last, such as the preoperative injection or postoperative discomfort.
9. Plan teaching sessions at times most conducive to learning, for example, after a rest period, and for the child's usual span of attention.
10. Use drawing, doll play, or storytelling to evaluate the

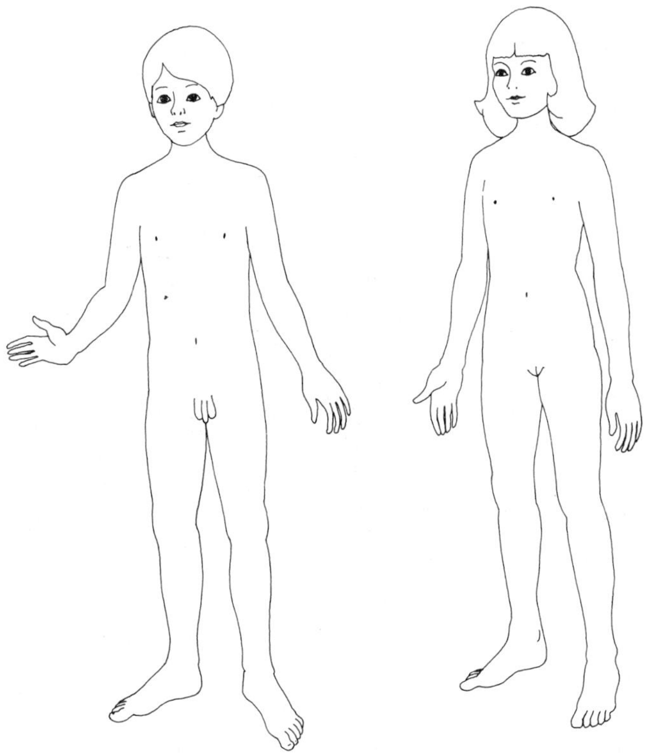

Fig. 25-2. Use of line drawings in preparing child for procedures.

teaching session, both before and after the procedure is performed.

11. Stress the positive benefits of the procedure, for example, "After your tonsils are fixed, you won't have as many sore throats."

For a more detailed description of preparing a child for surgery, specifically a tonsillectomy, refer to the boxed material on p. 574.

Fear of anesthesia. One special concern in preparing children for surgery is explaining about anesthesia. Just as children have age-related fears about bodily injury, they have similar fears of anesthesia. Children under 5 years of age primarily worry about what will happen when they wake up, such as where they will be and who will be with them. Showing youngsters the recovery room whenever possible, telling them where their parents will visit them after surgery, and encouraging the parents to be with the children as soon as possible after surgery decreases these fears. School-age children fear the anesthesia itself. Seeing the mask and learning how the "gas" or "medicine" works helps minimize their concerns. Children about age 9 years and older fear the anesthesia, the operation itself, and possi-

Preoperative preparation

Intervention	*Significance*
Check that admission laboratory tests, such as urinalysis and complete blood count, are on chart (other diagnostic tests may be pertinent, such as x-ray examination).	Laboratory values are checked for any sign of systemic abnormality, such as infection (increased white blood cells), anemia (decreased hemoglobin and/or hematocrit), or bleeding tendencies (reduced platelets or prolonged bleeding or clotting time)
Check that surgical consent form is signed.	For legal purposes an informed consent must be obtained from the child's legal guardian
Maintain child NPO (nothing by mouth) usually 12 hours prior to surgery. If oral medication is ordinarily given, consult with physician for appropriate change in schedule or route of administration.	To prevent aspiration from vomiting during anesthesia (gag reflex is depressed); child should be hydrated well before NPO begins
Monitor temperature, pulse, respiration, and blood pressure.	Any deviations from admission readings, especially elevated temperature, which may indicate infection, are reported
Cleanse site according to prescribed method.	Special cleansing and shave may not be done in children, but operative area should be cleansed during regular bath
Have child void before surgery.	To prevent bladder distention or incontinence during anesthesia
Properly attire child.	Special operating room gown may be needed; privacy may be a concern; if possible, allow child to wear underwear or pajama bottoms; mark personal articles of clothing with name
Administer preoperative sedation 20 minutes prior to surgery.	To achieve optimum relaxation and sedation prior to arriving in operating room
Fasten side rails of bed or crib.	To ensure safety
Check that identification band is securely fastened.	To ensure safety
Check for loose teeth and remove prostheses or jewelry.	To ensure safety Some cultures wear objects for religious or other reasons; to respect these traditions, these objects should be fastened securely to gown or body part
Remove any makeup or nail polish.	To observe for cyanosis
Complete nurses' notes.	All preoperative procedures, including child's emotional status prior to surgery (for example, asleep, drowsy, anxious, crying, or other), are recorded
Encourage parents to accompany child as far as possible to operating area.	To increase child's sense of security
Use restraints during transport by use of stretcher (or other conveyance).	To ensure safety
Do not leave child unattended. Explain what is happening, unless child is asleep.	To ensure safety To orient child to strange surroundings and decrease anxiety

ble death. They may ask, "Will I wake up?" or "What happens if I don't wake up?" Adolescents share these concerns with a special anxiety for change in body image. They fear the loss of control while under anesthesia, both in terms of their behavior and for their body integrity. Reassuring them that only what is supposed to be done will be performed is essential.

Because anesthesia is a type of sleep, children often supply their own definitions to this concept. Children worry about whether they will awaken during the procedure and how the doctor knows when to awaken them. Stressing that anesthesia is a "special sleep," caused by the mask, gas, and so on, that is controlled by a special person, called the anesthesiologist, is important in minimizing children's fear-provoking fantasies.

Because children are often restless when coming out of anesthesia, it is best to have the parents with them or, if this is not possible, to have a favorite possession or person, such as the primary nurse, greet them on gaining consciousness. This helps decrease the disorienting effect of anesthesia.

Physical preparation

Besides psychologic preparation, children usually require various types of physical preparation for procedures. Because these differ, the physical care usually instituted prior to surgical procedures is outlined in the box on the opposite page. Although these preparations are routine, nurses should keep in mind that they can be anxiety provoking for children and parents. For example, seeing their infant's scalp shaved for a craniotomy can intensify parents' fears of the actual surgical procedure. For preschoolers, having to wear a loose-fitting hospital gown without the security

Postoperative procedures

Intervention	*Significance*
Monitor vital signs every 15 minutes for 1 hour, every 30 minutes for 1 hour, then every hour until stable.	Recorded more frequently if any value fluctuates; blood pressure cuff kept in place but deflated in order to lessen amount of disturbance to child
Evaluate vital signs for signs of shock. Increased weak, thready pulse Increased weak, shallow respirations Decreased temperature Decreased blood pressure Cool, clammy, pale skin	Reported immediately; child kept warm, calm, and supine with lower extremities raised and head slightly elevated
Evaluate for effects of postanesthesia. Hyperthermia Decreased blood pressure Respiratory depression	Hyperthermia during immediate postoperative period not a sign of infection Decreasing blood pressure evaluated as possible sign of shock Signs of respiratory depression reported immediately; oxygen and suction equipment placed at bedside
Check dressing.	Presence of dark or fresh blood noted immediately after surgery; area circled with pen and time marked Areas below surgical site observed for blood that may have drained toward bed If dressing is loose, it should be reinforced but not removed Physician should be notified of signs of continuous bleeding, especially if accompanied by signs of shock
Maintain child NPO until fully awake; start with small sips of water. Avoid red-colored fluids.	To prevent aspiration To distinguish fresh blood from red oral fluids (NOTE: for gastrointestinal procedures, bowel sounds are listened for before and after beginning fluids; nasogastric tube usually inserted to prevent abdominal distention and removed after oral fluids are retained)
Monitor intravenous infusion at prescribed rate; check that infusion solution corresponds to physician's order; observe for signs of infiltration.	To ensure accuracy and patency of infusion
Encourage to turn, cough, and deep breathe.	Operative site splinted with hand or pillow if possible before coughing or deep breathing; pain medication administered prior to activity when necessary

of underpants or pajama bottoms can be traumatic. Explaining the reason for each preoperative procedure and altering it whenever possible to meet the needs of various children and parents combines physical care with effective psychologic support.

Postprocedural care

After medical/surgical procedures, various physical interventions and observations are required to prevent or minimize possible untoward effects. The usual postoperative care for surgical procedures is outlined in the boxed material on p. 911. Although most of these interventions are prescribed by physicians, it is the nurse's responsibility to exercise judgment in their implementation. For example, vital signs should be taken as frequently as necessary until they are stable. Simply recording temperature, pulse, respiration, and blood pressure without comparing the present readings to previous ones is a useless technical function. Each value should be evaluated in terms of side effects from anesthesia and signs of impending shock.

The procedures outlined in the boxed material on p. 911 represent the minimal nursing responsibilities for postsurgical care. However, they are applicable to most procedures that require general anesthesia and, if accurately implemented, are the basis for evaluating the child's physical status after surgery.

Minimizing effect of elective hospital procedures

Regardless of the quality of physical and psychologic care, medical and surgical procedures are difficult for children. Therefore, when procedures are elective, the following guidelines can help minimize the stress[7]:

1. Elective surgery should be postponed during the vulnerable years of infancy through preschool. The best time seems to be when major psychosexual conflicts have been resolved and ego strengths have developed, roughly between the ages of 6 and 10 years (latency period).
2. Surgery should be avoided during times of preexisting stress, such as following the death of a family member.
3. Hospitalization should be planned for the optimal length of time. For children younger than 4 or 5 years of age in whom separation anxiety is a major threat, admission, operation, and discharge on the same day is advantageous. For prolonged admissions, preservation of parent-child contact is critical. For older children a period of adjustment of about 24 hours prior to surgery helps allay their fears and allows for preoperative preparation.
4. The hospital experience should avoid as many strange and frightening events prior to surgery as possible to decrease the anxiety associated with the procedure.

PREPARING FOR DISCHARGE AND HOME CARE

Assessment

Ideally preparation for hospital discharge and home care begins during the admission assessment. Specifically the establishment of short- and long-term goals determines discharge planning. Frequently only short-term goals are identified. For example, following a tonsillectomy, discharge planning focuses on home care of the child until complete healing of the surgical site takes place. However, general extended or long-term goals for tonsillectomy patients can be summarized as: (1) evaluating improvement in physical status, (2) assessing possible improvement in hearing if an adenoidectomy was performed, and (3) evaluating the child's subsequent psychologic adjustment to the hospital experience. It is important for nurses to consider the obvious short-term goals and the more subtle, but equally significant, long-range objectives.

Discharge planning also focuses on those procedures that parents or children are expected to continue at home. In planning for such goals, nurses need to assess (1) the actual and perceived complexity of the skill, (2) the parents' or child's willingness to assume the responsibility, and (3) the parents' or child's previous or present experience with such procedures. To illustrate each point, the very common expectation of continuing antibiotic medication following discharge should be examined. Although a relatively simple task for older children, administering liquid medication to young children can be difficult. Parents may agree to continue the procedure, but if they have not been helped to carry it out or fully convinced of its necessity, the probability exists that they will fail to comply.

Nurses' responsibility is to prepare parents for the specifics of the task. For example, telling them that the child needs 1 tsp of medicine four times a day is not necessarily adequate, since parents may routinely schedule the doses at incorrect times. Instead, a preplanned schedule based on 6-hour intervals should be set up with the number of days required for therapeutic dosage listed, as in the following:

Schedule for home administration of antibiotic medication

General instructions: Give child 1 tsp ampicillin four times a day.

Specific instructions

1. Use medicine dropper and fill with liquid to 5-ml mark.
2. Give *1 hour* before meals.
3. Avoid giving acidic fruit juices with drug.
4. Refrigerate bottle and *shake well* before using.
5. Use for each day listed below, then discard remaining medicine.
6. Cross off appropriate time and date each time child is given medicine.

Date*	Times†			
5/21	Discharge	12:00 PM	5:00 PM	11:00 PM
5/22	6:30 AM	12:00 PM	5:00 PM	11:00 PM
5/23	6:30 AM	12:00 PM	5:00 PM	11:00 PM
5/24	6:30 AM	12:00 PM	Discard remaining drug	

*Based on number of days for administration of drug after discharge.

†Optimum administration schedule is approximately every 6 hours but is altered to conform with most convenient family routine to increase compliance.

Also, how to give medication to young children should be demonstrated. For example, using a syringe, mixing the drug with a small amount of juice or food, or using a small cup may increase the child's willingness to take the preparation. One mother shared her success in inducing her toddler to cooperatively drink the liquid. She gave the child a medicine dropper filled with juice. The child fed herself the juice and asked for more. The mother then filled the dropper with the medicine. The child willingly consumed the contents of that dropper. By making it a game, the mother eliminated the need to force the child to take her medicine.

Rooming-in automatically facilitates preparing parents for home procedures, because they are available to observe and participate in the child's care. However, even though multiple opportunities exist for teaching, nurses should establish a specific plan that incorporates levels of learning, such as observing, participating with assistance, and, finally, acting without help or guidance. In those situations in which parents visit during scheduled times, such plans must be carefully determined to allow sufficient time for observation, participation, and evaluation.

It is also advisable to include more than one family member in discharge planning. Although the most consistent care giver is the prime student, at least one other member should be prepared, in order to allow the other person freedom from the responsibility. For example, a mother had learned to give the injectable medication to her child at home. However, because of the frequency of administration, she was never able to leave the house for more than a few hours. Although this presented no problem during the initial discharge period, it added to the mother's continued stress. As a result the visiting nurse taught the father the procedure. This not only freed the mother from the home, but it also enhanced the father's feelings of inclusion and importance in his child's recovery.

Referral

Establishing appropriate referrals also stems from short- or long-term goals. This may be formal, such as referring to the visiting nursing service, or informal, such as introducing parents to another family with similar experiences. It may be initiated by the nurse or by the family. Regardless of which method is used, nurses need to assess the specific needs of the family and their probable reactions to the referral. The latter is particularly significant, because, although the needs may be quite evident, the family may reject the offered help. Preparing the family for the referral is as important as informing the referral service of the family's needs.

Some of the more usual referrals following hospital discharge include visiting nurse agency, private nurse practitioner, private physician, school tutor, physical therapist, mental health counselor, social worker, or other specialist. Sharing the important issues surrounding the child's hospitalization is essential. However, sharing opinions can also be detrimental. Referral summaries should be concise, specific, and factual. For example, if part of the referral to the visiting nurse focuses on the parent-child relationship, it is more effective to state observations supporting the reason for the referral, rather than judgmental statements. In this way visiting nurses have actual areas designated to help them form a plan of care.

Long-term follow-up

Initiating a referral is only one step in providing post-hospitalization care. Coordinating and sharing the results of other health team members' efforts is also important. For example, in many situations, more than one referral is necessary following discharge, such as to the visiting nurse, the outpatient clinic, and the school tutor. The referral should not only be unidirectional, but multidirectional as well (Fig. 25-3). This allows for comprehensive follow-up care that treats the family and child.

Although Fig. 25-3 illustrates the hospital nurse as the

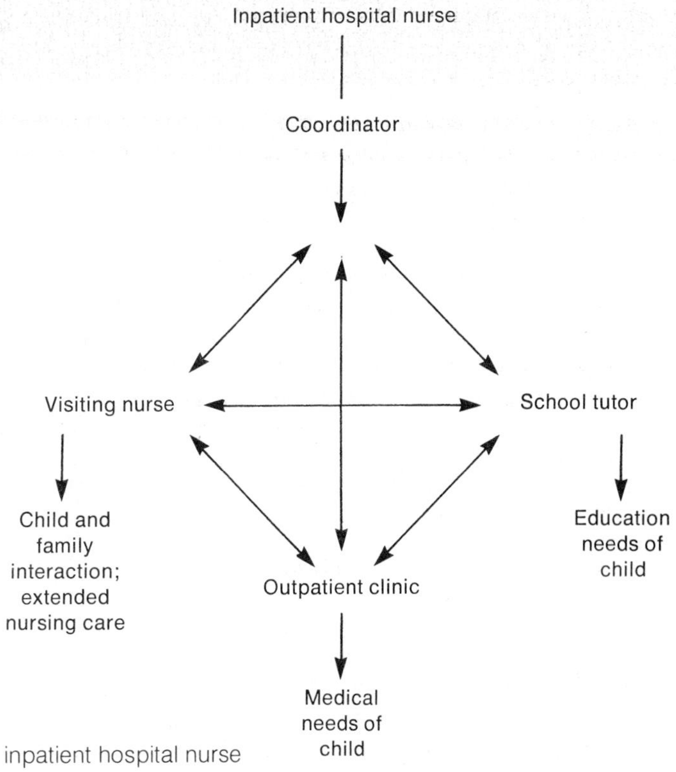

Fig. 25-3. Multidirectional referring system that designates inpatient hospital nurse as system's liaison and coordinator.

central focus of the referral system, this may vary according to the specific requirement of each situation. For those children who repeatedly return to the hospital for subsequent care, this person is a strategic liaison. For children who primarily require the services of outpatient facilities, the visiting nurse may play a more vital role as coordinator. However, the essential ingredient for successful referral and follow-up is the designation of a particular person to assume leadership and coordination of all services.

REFERENCES

1. Abril, I. F.: Mexican-American folk beliefs: how they affect health care, Am. J. Maternal Child Nurs. **2**(3):168-173, May/June 1977.
2. Campbell, T., and Chang, B.: Health care of the Chinese in America, Nurs. Outlook **21**(4):245-249, April 1973.
3. Everson, S.: Sibling counseling, Am. J. Nurs. **77**(4):644-646, April 1977.
4. Fagin, C.: The effects of maternal attendance during hospitalization on the post hospital behavior of young children: a comparative study, Philadelphia, 1966, F. A. Davis Co.
5. Farris, L. S.: Approaches to caring for the American Indian maternity patient, Am. J. Maternal Child Nurs. **1**(2):82-87, March/April 1976.
6. Freiberg, K. H.: How parents react when their child is hospitalized, Am. J. Nurs. **72**(7):1270-1272, July 1972.
7. Hoch, S.: Problems associated with surgical emergencies and brief elective procedures. In Oremland, E., and Oremland, J., editors: The effects of hospitalization on children, Springfield, Ill., 1973, Charles C Thomas, Publisher.
8. Irelan, L., editor: Low-income life styles (No. 14), Washington, D.C., 1968, U.S. Department of Health, Education and Welfare.
9. Johnson, B. H.: Hospitalization: a preparation program for the child and his family, Child. Today **3**(6):18-21, November/December 1974.
10. Komorita, N.: Nursing diagnoses, Am. J. Nurs. **63**(12):83-86, December 1963.
11. McBride, A. B.: The anger-depression-guilt go around, Am. J. Nurs. **73**(6):1045-1049, June 1973.
12. McFarlane, J. M.: Pediatric care in the emergency room, Pediatr. Nurs. **2**(2):22-25, March/April 1976.
13. McLellan, C. L.: Hero badges mean more than courage, Pediatr. Nurs. **2**(3):7, May/June 1976.
14. Parad, H. J.: Crisis intervention: selected readings, New York, 1965, Family Service Association of America.
15. Petrillo, M., and Sanger, S.: Emotional care of hospitalized children, Philadelphia, 1972, J. B. Lippincott Co.
16. Poznanski, E. O.: Children's reaction to pain: a psychiatrist's perspective, Clin. Pediatr. **15**(12):1114-1119, December 1976.
17. Robson, K. S.: Development of object relations during the first year of life. In Schwartz, J. L., and Schwartz, L. H., editors: Vulnerable infants: a psychosocial dilemma, New York, 1977, McGraw-Hill Book Co.
18. Seidl, F. W.: Pediatric nursing personnel and parent participation, Nurs. Res. **18**(1):40-44, January/February 1969.
19. Smith, M. E.: The preschooler and pain. In Brandt, P. A., Chinn, P. L., and Smith, M. E.: Current practice in pediatric nursing, St. Louis, 1976, The C. V. Mosby Co.
20. Watson, J.: Research and literature on children's responses to injections: some general nursing implications, Pediatr. Nurs. **2**(1):7-8, January/February 1976.

BIBLIOGRAPHY

American Academy of Pediatrics, Section on Urology with the co-operation of the Section on Child Development: The timing of elective surgery on the genitalia of male children with particular reference to undescended testes and hypospadias, Pediatrics **56**(3):479-483, September 1975.

Barrell, L. M.: Crisis intervention: partnership in problem-solving, Nurs. Clin. North Am. **9**(1):5-16, March 1974.

Barton, P.: Play as a tool of nursing, Nurs. Outlook **10**:162, March 1962.

Baxter, P.: Frustration felt by a mother and her child during the child's hospitalization, Am. J. Maternal Child Nurs. **1**(3):159-161, May/June 1976.

Bell, J. G., and associates: Family participation in hospital care for children, Children **17**(4):154-157, July/August 1970.

Bellack, J. P.: Helping a child cope with the stress of injury, Am. J. Nurs. **74**(8):1491-1494, August 1974.

Bergman, T., and Freud, A.: Children in hospitals, New York, 1966, International Universities Press.

Berner, C.: Assessing the child's ability to cope with stresses of hospitalization. In Brandt, P. A., Chinn, P. L., and Smith, M. E., editors: Current practice in pediatric nursing, St. Louis, 1976, The C. V. Mosby Co.

Blake, F.: The child, his parents, and the nurse, Philadelphia, 1954, J. B. Lippincott Co.

Bothe, A., and Goldstein, R.: The child's loss of consciousness: a psychiatric view of pediatric anesthesia, Pediatrics **50**(2):252-263, August 1972.

Bowlby, J., and associates: Maternal care and mental health, New York, 1966, Schocken Books Inc.

Brooks, M. M.: Why play in the hospital? Nurs. Clin. North Am. **5**(3):431-444, September 1970.

Canright, P., and Campbell, M. J.: Nursing care of the child and his family in the emergency department, Pediatr. Nurs. **3**(4):43-45, July/August 1977.

Colainni, J. A.: Parents care in intensive care, Pediatr. Nurs. **1**(2):16-19, March/April 1975.

Condon, S.: Day-time hospital for children, Am. J. Nurs. **72**(8):1431-1433, August 1972.

Crawford, C. F., and Palm, M. C.: Can I take my teddy bear? Am. J. Nurs. **73**(2):286-287, February 1973.

Di Fabio, S.: Crisis: a complex process, Nurs. Clin. North Am. **9**(1):47-56, March 1974.

Dombro, R. H.: The surgically ill child and his family, Surg. Clin. North Am. **50**:759-769, August 1970.

Farrell, S. E., and Kiernan, B.: A positive approach to nutrition for hospitalized children, Am. J. Maternal Child Nurs. **2**(2):113-117, March/April 1977.

Faulkner, B. L.: From first base to home plate, Am. J. Nurs. **71**(12):2331-2333, December 1971.

Gardner, G. G., and Simkins, R. A.: Does it really matter what nurses wear in the intensive care unit? Am. J. Maternal Child Nurs. **1**(4):239-242, July/August 1976.

Green, C. S.: Understanding children's needs through therapeutic play, Nursing '74 **4**(10):30-31, October 1974.

Green, C. S.: Larry thought puppet-play "childish," but it helped him face his fears, Nursing '75 **5**(3):30-33, March 1975.

Griffin, C., and Aufhauser, T.: Don't let them hurt me, Am. OR Nurs. J. **17:**59-65, May 1973.

Guerin, L. S.: Hospitalization as a positive experience for poverty children, Clin. Pediatr. **16**(6):509-513, June 1977.

Haka-Ikse, K., and Van Leeuwen, J.: Care of the long-term hospitalized infant: a developmental approach, Clin. Pediatr. **15**(7): 585-588, July 1976.

Hardgrove, C. B., and Dawson, R. B.: Parents and children in the hospital: the family's role in pediatrics, Boston, 1972, Little, Brown and Co.

Hardgrove, C. B., and Rutledge, A.: Parenting during hospitalization, Am. J. Nurs. **75**(5):836-838, May 1975.

Hilt, N. E.: Pride, prejudice, and parents, Pediatr. Nurs. **2**(3):32-35, May/June 1976.

Issner, N.: The family of the hospitalized child, Nurs. Clin. North Am. **7**(1):5-12, March 1972.

Jelneck, L. J.: The special needs of the adolescent with chronic illness, Am. J. Maternal Child Nurs. **2**(1):57-61, January/February 1977.

Johnson, J. E., Kirchhoff, K. T., and Endress, M. P.: Easing children's fright during health care procedures, Am. J. Maternal Child Nurs. **1**(4):206-210, July/August 1976.

Juenker, D.: Child's perception of his illness. In Steele, S., editor: Nursing care of the child with long-term illness, New York, 1971, Appleton-Century-Crofts.

Juenker, D.: Play as a tool of the nurse. In Steele, S., editor: Nursing care of the child with long-term illness, New York, 1971, Appleton-Century-Crofts.

Klinzing, D., and Klinzing, G.: The hospitalized child: communication techniques for health personnel, Englewood Cliffs, N.J., 1977, Prentice-Hall, Inc.

Knudsen, K.: Play therapy: preparing the young child for surgery, Nurs. Clin. North Am. **10**(4):679, December 1975.

Kunzman, L.: Some factors influencing a young child's mastery of hospitalization, Nurs. Clin. North Am. **7**(1):13-26, March 1972.

Lawson, B. A.: Chronic illness in the school-aged child: effects on the total family, Am. J. Maternal Child Nurs. **2**(1):49-56, January/February 1977.

Lee, J. S., and Greene, N. M.: Parental presence and the emotional state of children prior to surgery, Clin. Pediatr. **8:**126-130, March 1969.

Lore, A.: Adolescents: people, not problems, Am. J. Nurs. **73**(7): 1232-1234, July 1973.

Luciano, K., and Shumsky, C. J.: Pediatric procedures: the explanation should always come first, Nursing '75 **5**(1):49-52, January 1975.

Luckmann, J., and Sorenson, K.: What patients' actions tell you about their feelings, fears, and needs, Nursing '75 **5**(2):54-61, February 1975.

Lyons, M.: What priority do you give preop teaching? Nursing '77 **7**(1):12-14, January 1977.

Mandelco, B. H.: Monitoring children's reactions when they are hospitalized for percutaneous renal biopsy, Am. J. Maternal Child Nurs. **1**(5):288-292, September/October 1976.

Millar, T. P.: The hospital and the preschool child, Children **17:**171-176, September/October 1970.

Mioduszewski, D.: Preparing a child for hospitalization. In Brandt, P. A., Chinn, P. L., and Smith, M. E.: Current practice in pediatric nursing, St. Louis, 1976, The C. V. Mosby Co.

Norberta, S.: Caring for children with the help of puppets, Am. J. Maternal Child Nurs. **1**(1):22-26, January/February 1976.

Norris, C. M.: The professional nurse and body image. In Carlson, C. E., editor: Behavioral concepts and nursing intervention, Philadelphia, 1970, J. B. Lippincott Co.

Oremland, E., and Oremland, J., editor: The effects of hospitalization on children, Springfield, Ill., 1973, Charles C Thomas, Publisher.

Ormond, E. A., and Caulfield, E.: A practical guide to giving oral medications to young children, Am. J. Maternal Child Nurs. **1**(5):320-325, September/October 1976.

Penalver, M.: Helping the child handle his aggression, Am. J. Nurs. **73**(9):1554-1555, September 1973.

Pillitteri, A.: Nursing care of the growing family, Boston, 1977, Little, Brown and Co.

Plank, E. N.: Working with children in hospitals, Chicago, 1971, The Press of Case Western Reserve University.

Robertson, J.: Young children in hospitals, New York, 1958, Basic Books, Inc., Publishers.

Robischon, P., and Scott, D.: Role theory and its application in family nursing, Nurs. Outlook **17**(7):52-57, July 1969.

Schultz, N. V.: How children perceive pain, Nurs. Outlook **19:** 670-672, October 1971.

Seidl, F. W., and Pillitteri, A.: Development of the attitude scale on parent participation, Nurs. Res. **16**(1):71-73, 1967.

Smith, J. C.: Spending time with the hospitalized child, Am. J. Maternal Child Nurs. **1**(3):164, May/June 1976.

Snyder, J. C., and Wilson, M. F.: Elements of a psychological assessment, Am. J. Nurs. **77**(2):235-239, February 1977.

Stein, R.: The hospitalized adolescent's dilemma. In Reinhardt, A. M., and Quinn, M. D.: Current practice in family-centered community nursing, St. Louis, 1977, The C. V. Mosby Co.

Stephens, K. S.: A toddler's separation anxiety, Am. J. Nurs. **73**(9):1553-1555, September 1973.

Visintainer, M. A., and Wolfer, J. A.: Psychological preparation for surgical pediatric patients: the effect of children's and parents' stress responses and adjustment, Pediatrics **56**(2):187-202, August 1975.

Whitson, B. J.: The puppet treatment in pediatrics, Am. J. Nurs. **72**(9):1612-1614, September 1972.

Williams, F.: The crisis of hospitalization, Nurs. Clin. North Am. **9**(1):37-45, March 1974.

Zweig, I. K.: A new way to get acquainted with the hospital—pediatric open house for well children, Am. J. Maternal Child Nurs. **1**(4):217-219, July/August 1976.

26

Pediatric variations of nursing intervention

Children are not simply small adults. They differ from their older counterparts in the areas of biologic, cognitive, and emotional function and response. Consequently many of the standard techniques employed in nursing practice must be altered to meet the special needs of this small but important group of patients. After this chapter is read, it is hoped that the reader will be able to apply principles of growth and development in planning, implementing, and evaluating nursing care of infants and children.

CONSENT

Parents have always been considered to have full responsibility for the care and rearing of their children, including legal control over their minor children. Therefore, as long as a child remains classified as a minor, the parent or the person designated as legal guardian for the child is required to give consent before medical treatment is implemented or any procedure is performed on the child. In most situations this creates little difficulty. The parent or guardian accompanies the child and is willing to give blanket permission or consent for specific procedures. Problems may arise in situations in which parents are not available to give consent, the child is a borderline or emancipated minor, or the parents neglect or refuse care for their minor children. Although it is the physician's duty to explain the procedure or treatment to the parents or guardian, the nurse is often the person responsible for making certain that such consent is a part of the child's record.

Common law has considered an individual to be a minor and legally unable to enter into a contractual agreement before reaching the age of 21 years. Since the voting age has been lowered to 18 years of age, an increasing number of states have lowered the age of majority for all purposes. In addition there have been a number of changes based on legislation and court decisions that differ from the traditional legal view of parental responsibility and control. Because the age of majority and other changes vary within jurisdictions, nurses should become acquainted with the way in which the law functions in their state regarding medical care to children.

When consent is required

Written consent of the parent or guardian is usually required for medical or surgical treatment, including many diagnostic procedures. One blanket consent is not usually sufficient. Separate permission must be obtained for each surgical or diagnostic procedure, including:

1. Major surgery
2. Minor surgery, for example, cutdown, biopsy, dental extraction, suturing a laceration (especially one that may have a cosmetic effect), removal of a cyst, and closed reduction of a fracture
3. Diagnostic tests with an element of risk, for example, bronchoscopy, needle biopsy, angiography, electroencephalogram, lumbar puncture, cardiac catheterization, ventriculography, and bone-marrow aspiration
4. Medical treatments with an element of risk, for example, blood transfusion, thoracentesis or paracentesis, radiation therapy, and shock therapies

In addition there are certain situations such as the following that are not directly related to medical treatment but that require parental consent:

1. Taking photographs for medical, educational, or other public use
2. Removal of the child from the hospital against the advice of the physician
3. Postmortem examinations
4. Examination of medical records by unauthorized persons, such as attorneys, insurance representatives, and so on

Consent of persons other than parents or guardian. Although a parent or guardian is ordinarily the source of consent, in the absence of the parents a person in charge of the child is usually allowed to give consent for treatment. This person, *in loco parentis,* may be a relative or other person who is caring for the child while the parents are away.

Oral consent. When the parent is not immediately available to sign a consent form, oral consent, for example, a telephone consent or an oral consent from a parent who is for some reason unable to sign, such as because of an injury following an accident, may be obtained. When verbal consent is being secured, it is wise to have a witness, such as another nurse, on a telephone extension. Both nurses can record that consent was given and the name, address, and relationship of the person giving consent, together with their signatures indicating that they witnessed the consent.

Mature and emancipated minors

One of the areas in which modifications have been made in the usual view of parental obligation is in regard to borderline minors, that is, youngsters who are legally minors but who are considered to possess the maturity to give consent for their own medical care.[1] Although not legally emancipated, they understand and appreciate the consequences of treatment. There are a number of situations in which this is highly desirable from the standpoint of health care, for example, the youngster who seeks medical care for a venereal disease without the knowledge of the parents as well as the unmarried pregnant minor.

A number of states have enacted legislation that permits emancipated and married minors to give consent for their medical and surgical treatment. An emancipated minor is one who is legally underage but is recognized as having the legal capacity of an adult. This may be the youngster who is married or who lives apart from the parents and is self-supporting. Some states do not recognize emancipation, and others vary in their interpretation of what constitutes an emancipated minor. Nurses need to be aware of the statutes regarding the attainment of majority and all its variables in the state in which they practice.[2]

Treatment without parental consent

An exception to the general rule that parental consent is obtained prior to medical treatment of minor children occurs in situations in which children need prompt medical or surgical treatment and a parent is not readily available to give consent. Many states recognize this exception and permit treatment if the life or health of such a minor is in jeopardy or if delayed treatment would create a risk to the health of the minor. When surgical intervention is indicated in such situations, the procedure is usually begun only after consultation with another physician.[2]

Parental negligence

The state is able to intervene in situations that jeopardize the health and welfare of children. Children may need protection from their parents in cases in which parents neglect or impose excessive or improper punishment on a child (see p. 594). Neglect includes failure to provide protection for the child, for example, failure to provide or permit needed or required medical attention. This may include situations in which the parent, for religious or other reasons, refuses treatment such as a blood transfusion or immunization. In most communities there are procedures by which custody of the child can be transferred to a governmental or a private agency when parental neglect can be proved. Sometimes the parental refusal is in direct violation of the law, for example, concerning immunizations and examinations that are required for school attendance and compulsory prophylaxis against ophthalmia neonatorum in the newborn. In many cases the state interferes with the parental rights in the interest and protection of minor children.

GENERAL CARE AND HYGIENE

Hygienic care is continued throughout the child's hospital stay and is essentially no different from that provided to persons of any age. The primary differences are those related to the size of the patient. Grooming aids and attractive attire are important adjuncts to hygienic care. Children are delighted with anything that makes them feel more attractive.

Bathing

Unless contraindicated, most infants and children can be bathed in a tub at the bedside, on the bed, or in a standard bathtub located on the unit, which is often conveniently adapted for pediatric use.

Infants and small children are *never* left unattended in a bathtub, and infants who are unable to sit alone are securely held with one hand during the bath. The infant's head is supported securely with one hand or the farthest arm is firmly grasped in the nurse's hand while the head rests comfortably on the wrist. This provides secure control of the infant while the other hand is free to wash the infant's body (Fig. 26-1). Infants or children who are able to sit without assistance need only close supervision and a pad placed in the bottom of the tub to prevent slipping and loss of balance, which could result in a bumped head or submersion of the face.

Older children may enjoy a shower if it is available. School-age children may be reluctant to bathe, and many are not accustomed to a daily bath. However, most children who feel well require little encouragement to participate in their daily care. Nurses will need to use judgment regarding the amount of supervision the child requires. Some can be trusted to assume this responsibility unaided, whereas others will need someone in constant attendance. Retarded children, those with physical limitations such as severe anemia or leg deformities, and suicidal or psychotic children (who may commit bodily harm) require close supervision.

Areas that require special attention from the nurse during bed baths and for children performing their own care are the ears, between skin folds, the neck, the back, and the genital area. The genital area should be carefully cleansed and dried with particular care to skin folds, and, in uncircumcised boys, the foreskin should be gently retracted and the exposed surfaces cleansed and then the foreskin replaced. Older children have the tendency to avoid these areas; there-

A 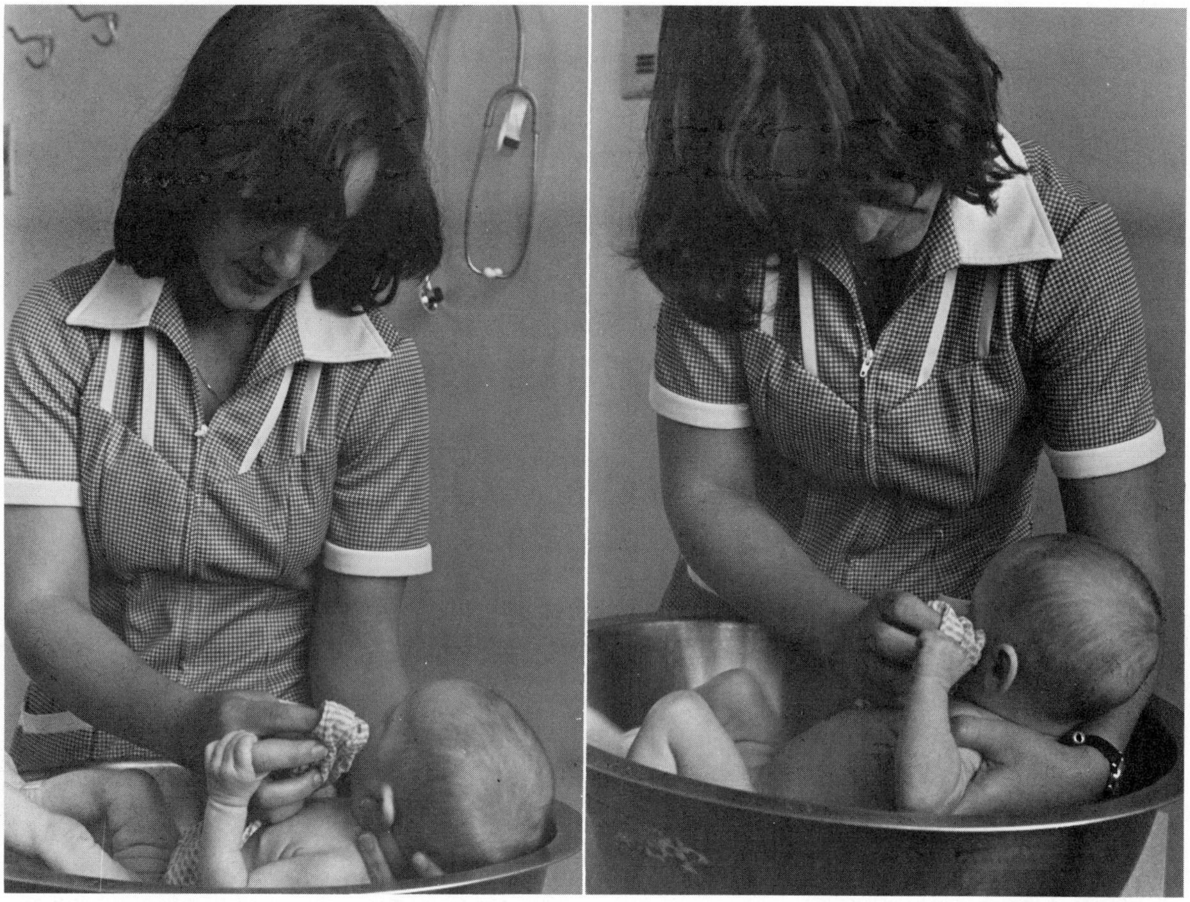 B

Fig. 26-1. Proper method for holding infant for tub bath. **A,** Supporting neck; **B,** neck supported on wrist.

fore, they may need a gentle reminder from the nurse.

Children who are ill or debilitated will need more extensive assistance with bathing and other aspects of hygienic care, but they should be encouraged to perform as much as they are capable without overtaxing their energies. Increasing involvement can be expected with improved strength and endurance. Children who are limited in the capacity for self-help and who have no other contraindications benefit a great deal from tub baths. They can be transported to the tub and, with the aid of lifting devices and/or an appropriate number of persons to assist, gain the advantages of a tub bath.

Cooling baths. Cool, moist applications to the skin help to reduce the core temperature. Cooled blood from the skin surface is conducted to inner organs and tissues, and warm blood is circulated to the surface where it is cooled and recirculated. The surface blood vessels dilate as the body attempts to dissipate heat to the environment and facilitate this cooling process.

Baths to reduce a fever can be given in a tub, or the bed or crib. Tepid tub baths are fast, simple, and effective for reducing an elevated temperature in a child. When using the tub, it is usually best to start with warm water and gradually add cool water until the desired water temperature is reached. In this way the child becomes more easily accustomed to the lower water temperature. The child is placed directly into the tub of tepid water for 20 to 30 minutes while water is gently squeezed from a washcloth over his back and chest or gently sprayed over his body from a sprayer. The bath is even more effective if the child can tolerate lying down in the water with his head supported on the nurse's arm or a padded support. This is more easily accomplished with a small infant or an older child. Small children dislike lying down and often resist any efforts to force them into the horizontal position. For conscious children a floating toy or other distraction can be employed during the bath. The child's temperature is retaken 30 minutes to 1 hour after removal from the tub (the length of time may vary according to circumstances). The child is never left alone in the tub.

The cooling bath can also be given in the bed or crib. The child is completely undressed and placed on an absorbent blanket or towel spread over the bed. He is covered with a large towel or lightweight, absorbent cotton blanket. A cool washcloth or ice pack is placed on the child's forehead and changed as it warms. One area of the body is exposed at a time and sponged with a washcloth soaked in tepid water. Special care is taken where two body surfaces touch. The sponge bath is continued for approximately 30 minutes.

A safe, easy, and effective alternate method, and the one most often employed, is the towel method. The child is undressed and placed on an absorbent towel or blanket, and a cool cloth or ice bag is applied to the forehead. Each extremity is wrapped in a towel moistened in tepid water, one is placed under the back, and another covers the neck and torso. Special care is taken to make certain that opposing body surfaces, such as the groin and lateral torso between the arms and chest, are covered. The towels are changed as they warm. This is continued for approximately 30 minutes.

After the tub or sponge bath, the child is dried and dressed in lightweight pajamas, nightgown, or diaper and placed in a dry bed. The temperature is retaken 30 minutes after the tub bath or sponge bath and repeated as often as indicated. The child should be observed carefully during any of these procedures, and if he shows signs of chilling the cool treatment is discontinued immediately. The child is dried by gently rubbing the skin surface with a towel to stimulate circulation. The bath or sponge should not be continued or restarted until the skin surface is warm. Chilling causes vasoconstriction, which defeats the purpose of the cool applications. In this condition little blood is carried to the skin surface but remains primarily in the viscera to become heated. Also, the process of shivering generates additional heat. Therefore, cool tub or sponge baths should never be continued if the child shows evidence of chilling.

Mouth care

Mouth care is an integral part of daily hygiene and should be continued in the hospital. Infants and debilitated children will require the nurse to perform mouth care. Although small children can manage a toothbrush and should be encouraged to use it, most will need assistance to perform a satisfactory job. Older children, although capable of brushing without assistance, sometimes need to be reminded that this is a part of their hygienic care. Most hospitals have equipment available for those children who do not have toothbrush or toothpaste of their own. Brushing with a soft toothbrush should begin as soon as teeth emerge. (See Chapter 28 for mouth care of children with oral ulcers.)

Hair care

Brushing and combing hair are a part of the daily care for all persons in the hospital, including infants and children. If the child does not have a brush or comb, many hospitals provide one as part of the usual admission kit. If not, the parents should be asked to bring hair care equipment for the child's use. Both boys and girls should be helped to comb and/or brush their hair, or it should be done for them, at least once daily. There is no special hairstyle that is prescribed for hospitalized children. The hair should be styled for comfort and in a manner pleasing to the child and parents. The hair should not be cut without parental permission, although shaving hair to provide access to a scalp vein for intravenous needle insertion is frequently carried out without permission.

Infants require little extra attention. The hair is washed daily as part of the bath in the newborn period and less often in later infancy. It is usually sufficient for most children to wash the hair and scalp once or twice weekly, but if there is any indication otherwise in children of any age, it is washed more frequently. Some hospitals have shampoo basins, but almost any child can be conveniently transported by a gurney to an accessible sink or washbasin for shampooing. Those who are unable to be transported can receive a shampoo in their beds with adequate protection and/or specially adapted equipment or positioning.

Teenagers, with their normally increased oily sebaceous secretions, are particularly in need of frequent hair care and usually require more frequent shampoos. Commercial "dry shampoo" products also may prove useful on a short-term basis. If a commercial variety is not available, talcum powder placed on the hair will absorb oils and can be removed by vigorous brushing.

Black children require special hair care, and this need is frequently neglected or inadequately managed. For the black child with kinky hair, most standard combs are inadequate and may cause hair breakage and discomfort to the child. If a special comb with widely spaced teeth is not available on the unit, the parent can be reminded to bring a comb, if possible, for the child's use. This type of hair also requires a special hair dressing or pomade, which usually has a coconut oil base. The preparation is rubbed on the hands and then transferred to the hair to make it more pliable and manageable. The child's parents should be consulted regarding the preparation they wish to be used on their child's hair and asked if they can provide some for use during the child's hospitalization. Vaseline or petroleum jelly should *not* be used. For boys and girls with short hair, a simple combing is sufficient. The most satisfactory style for girls with longer hair is the French braid, which is created by starting with three equal portions of hair from the top of one side of the scalp; as the hair is braided, segments of hair are added at successive intervals until all the hair has been incorporated into one neat, head-hugging braid on each side of the head. The ends are firmly anchored with a malleable holder or barrette.

Health teaching

Nurses have a unique opportunity for teaching and reinforcing good hygienic care while the child is hospitalized. Although most children have learned self-care and hygiene in the home or at school, many have not. For some young children this is their first introduction to the use of a toothbrush. A great deal of health teaching can be accomplished even when the child is hospitalized for only a short time. The daily bath, hand washing before meals and after bowel and bladder evacuation, and conscientious dental hygiene are taught by example during routine care. Clean hair, nails, and clothing as well as good grooming are emphasized as essential to a pleasing appearance. Positive reinforcement of good hygiene practices helps to create a positive body image, promote the development of self-esteem, and prevent health problems, for example, teaching girls to wipe the genital area from front to back after toileting.

SAFETY

Since small children are separated from their usual environment and do not possess the capacity for abstract thinking and reasoning, it is the responsibility of everyone who comes in contact with them to maintain protective measures throughout their hospital stay. Nurses need a good understanding of the age level at which each child is operating and plan for safety accordingly.

Name bands, a part of hospital safety practices, are particularly important for children in the pediatric age-group. Infants and unconscious patients are unable to tell or respond to their names. Toddlers may answer to any name or to a nickname only. It is not uncommon for older children to exchange places, give an erroneous name, or choose not to respond to their own names as a form of joke, unaware of the hazards of such practices.

Environmental factors

All the environmental safety measures in operation for the protection of adults apply to children as well, such as good illumination, floors clear of fluid or other objects that might contribute to falls, and nonskid surfaces in showers and tubs; electrical equipment that is maintained in good working order, is used only by personnel familiar with its use, and is not in contact with moisture or near tubs where it could prove to be a shock hazard; beds of ambulatory patients locked in place and at a height that allows easy access to the floor; proper care and disposal of small breakable items such as thermometers, bottles, and so on; and a well-organized fire plan known to all staff members. Medical asepsis and isolation techniques differ very little from those in any other hospital unit and should be strictly adhered to by personnel, since infants and small children are highly susceptible to cross-infection.

All windows should be securely screened and elevators and stairways made safe. Ideally electrical outlets should be provided with covers to prevent burns in small children whose exploratory activities may extend to inserting objects into the small openings. Bath water should be carefully checked by the nurse before placing the child in the bath, and children must never be left alone in a bathtub. Infants are helpless in water, and small children (and some older ones) may turn on the hot water faucet and be severely burned.

Furniture is safest when scaled to the child's proportions, sturdy, and well-balanced to prevent its being easily tipped over. Infants and small children must be securely strapped into infant seats, feeding chairs, and strollers. Infants and small, agitated, or mentally retarded children should not be left unattended on treatment tables, on scales, or in treatment areas. Even tiny premature infants are capable of surprising mobility; therefore, portholes in Isolettes must be securely fastened when not in use.

Crib sides should be kept up and fastened securely unless an adult is at bedside. It is safer to leave crib sides up even when the crib is unoccupied, to remove the temptation to climb in. Anyone attending an infant or small child in a crib with the sides down should never turn away without maintaining hand contact with the child, that is, one hand should be kept on the child's back or abdomen to protect him from rolling, crawling, or jumping from the open crib (Fig. 26-2). The crib bars should be spaced close enough together not to allow a child's head to be caught between them. A child who is apt to or has demonstrated the inclination to

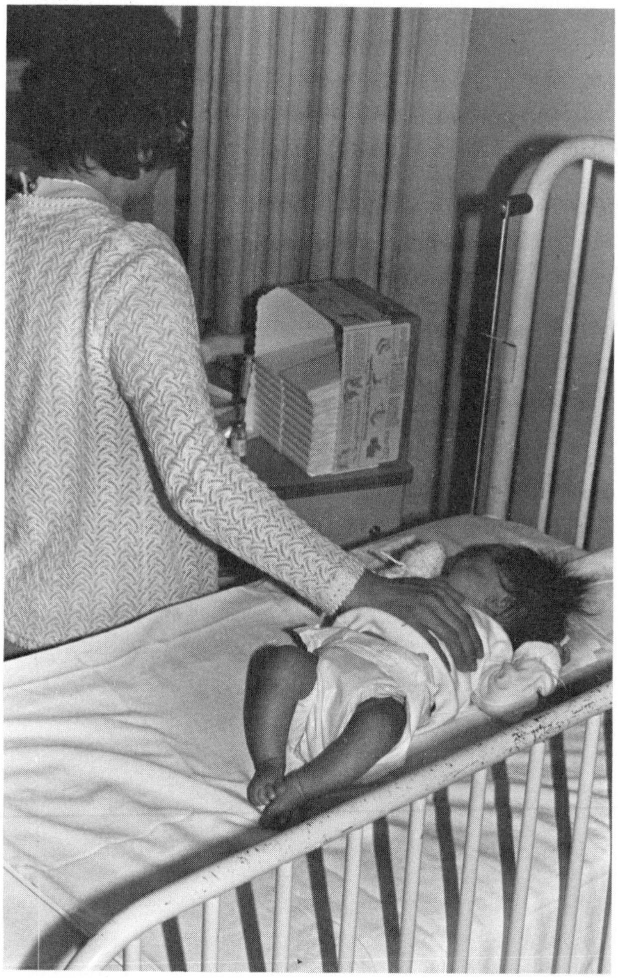

Fig. 26-2. Nurse maintains hand contact when back is turned.

climb over the sides of the crib is safest when placed in a specially constructed crib with a cover or one that has a safety net placed over the top. If the net is used it must be tied to the frame in such a manner that there is ready access to the child in case of emergency. Nets are never tied to the movable crib sides, and the knots should be tied in a manner that permits quick release. Cribs should not be placed within reach of heating units, appliances, dangling cords, or other objects that can be reached by curious hands.

Toys. Toys play a vital role in the everyday life of children, and they are no less important in the hospital setting. However, it is up to nurses to assess the safety of toys brought to the hospital by well-meaning parents and friends. Toys should be appropriate to the child's age and condition and inspected to make certain that they are allergyfree, washable, and unbreakable and that they have no small, removable parts that can be aspirated or swallowed or that can in other ways inflict injury to a child.

Limit setting

Setting limits is essential to a child's safety. Children must understand where they are permitted to go and what they are permitted to do in the hospital. These limitations should be made clear to them, consistently enforced, and repeated as frequently as necessary to make certain that they are understood. The nurse is responsible for where children are at all times. Children can easily wander off unnoticed.

Normal active, older children often become restless when their activity is restricted and may resort to pillow fights, water fights, and other rough play that might endanger the safety of the involved children or of bystanders (other children, staff, and visitors). Children in the hospital require surveillance, and appropriate tension-reducing activities can be planned and supervised by nurses and/or by the play therapist.

Transporting children

In the course of a hospital stay, infants and children usually need to be transported within the unit and to areas outside the pediatric unit. It is ordinarily safe to carry infants and small children for short distances within the unit, but for more extended trips the child should be securely transported in a suitable conveyance.

Transporting infants. Small infants can be held or carried in the horizontal position with the back supported and the thigh grasped firmly by the carrying arm (Fig. 26-3, *A*). In the football hold the infant is supported on the nurse's arm with the head supported by the hand and the body held securely between the nurse's body and her elbow (Fig. 26-3, *B*). Both of these holds leave the nurse's other arm free for activity. The infant can be held in the upright position with buttocks on the nurse's forearm and resting against the nurse's chest. The infant's head and shoulders are supported by the nurse's other arm to allow for any sudden movement by the infant (Fig. 26-3, *C*). Older infants are able to hold their heads erect but are still subject to sudden movements.

Infants can be transported to other areas, such as the x-ray department, in their bassinet or crib. Baby buggies are sometimes used for infants who are not likely to stand up. Strollers and wheeled feeding chairs or tables are also convenient transporters in some situations, such as trips to the playroom, nurse's station, or sun porch.

Transporting children. The method of transporting children is determined by their age, condition, and destination. Most older children are safe in wheelchairs or in gurneys. Younger children can be transported in their crib, on a gurney, or in a wheelchair with a safety belt. Gurneys should be equipped with high sides and a safety belt, both of which are kept in place during transport.

Restraints

Frequently some method of restraint is needed for a child's safety or comfort, to facilitate examination, or to carry out diagnostic and therapeutic procedures. Restraint can be accomplished with the hand or with physical devices. Restraining the child with the hand provides an element of human contact that is lacking in restraint by mechanical means. For example, a large infant or small child can be effectively restrained by having him sit astride the lap facing an assistant. The assistant hugs him close against the body to provide both comfort and restraint while the nurse safely carries out the necessary procedure (Fig. 26-4).

Mechanical restraints are never used as a punishment or as a substitute for observation. When a child must be restrained, he and his parents need a simple explanation, and, if the restraint is applied for an extended period of time, the explanation must be repeated often to gain his cooperation and to help him understand that it is not a punishment. Restraining devices are not without risk and must be checked frequently to make certain that they are accomplishing the purpose for which they are intended, that they are applied correctly, and that they do not impair circulation.

Parents need to know the purpose of restraints, how to remove and reapply them, and the signs of complications from their use. Parents are sometimes upset when their child must be restrained and need to understand how they can help to assure the maximum benefit and minimize the stress related to their use. Children, too, should be prepared for both the procedure or the circumstance for which the restraint is required. (See p. 909 for preparation of children for procedures.)

Jacket restraint. A jacket restraint is sometimes used as an alternative to the crib net to prevent the child from climbing out of the crib or to keep the child safe in various kinds of chairs. The jacket is put on the child with the ties in back so that the child is unable to manipulate them, and the long tapes, secured to the understructure of the crib,

A B C

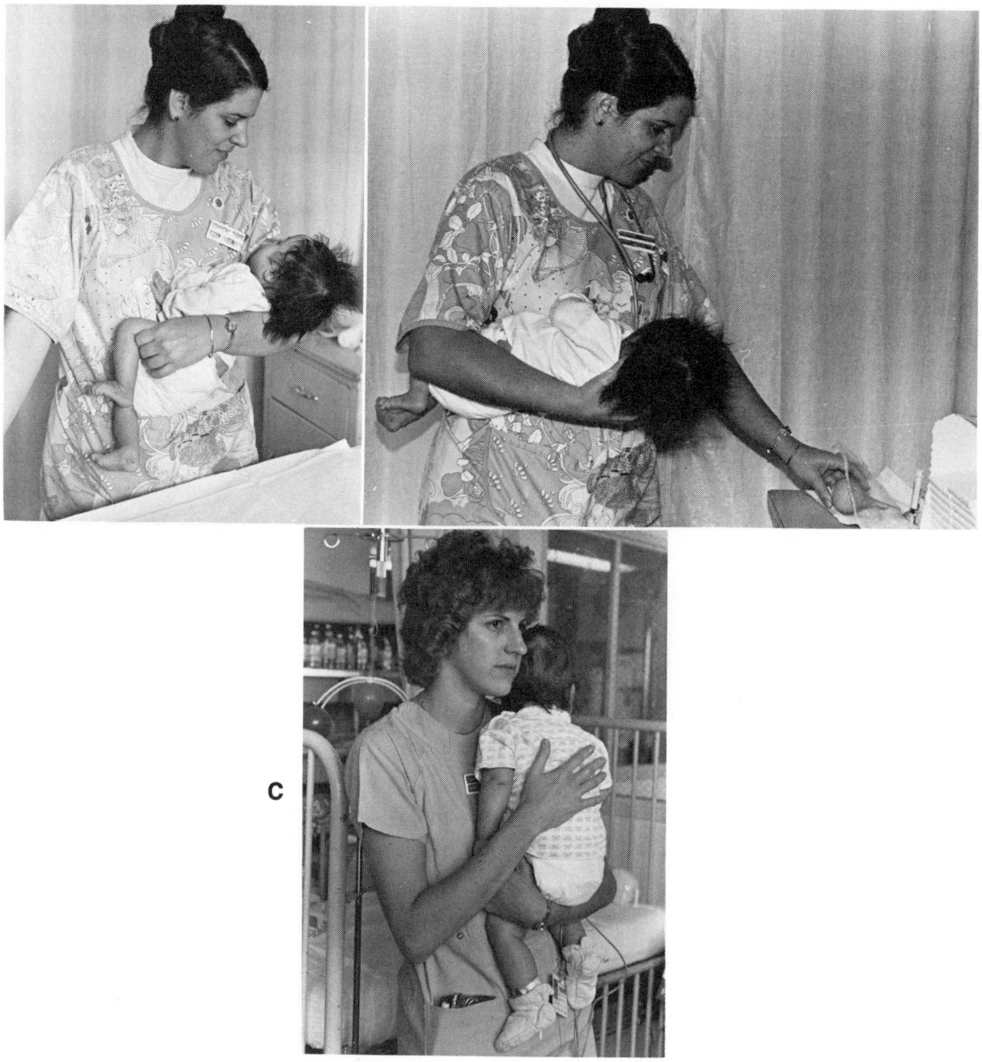

Fig. 26-3. Transporting infants. **A,** Infant's thigh firmly grasped in nurse's hand; **B,** football hold; **C,** back supported.

keep the child inside the crib (Fig. 26-5). The jacket restraint is also useful as a means to maintain the child in a desired horizontal position. A Posey belt scaled to fit the child is an alternative device.

Mummy restraint. When an infant or small child requires short-term restraint for examination or treatment that involves the head and neck, such as venipuncture, throat examination, gavage feeding, and so on, the mummy device effectively controls the child's movements. A blanket or sheet is opened on the bed or crib with one corner folded to the center. The infant is placed on the blanket with his shoulders at the fold and his feet toward the opposite corner (Fig. 26-6, *A*). With the infant's right arm straight down against his body, the right side of the blanket is pulled firmly across the infant's right shoulder and chest and secured beneath the left side of his body (Fig. 26-6, *B*). The left arm is placed straight against his side, and the left side of the blanket is brought across the shoulder and chest and locked beneath the child's body on the right side (Fig. 26-6, *C*). The lower corner is folded and brought over the body and tucked or fastened securely with safety pins. Safety pins can be used to fasten the blanket in place at any step in the process.

To modify the mummy restraint for chest examination, the folded edge of the blanket is brought over each arm and under the back, after which the loose edge is folded over and secured at a point below the chest to allow visualization and access to the chest (Fig. 26-7).

Arm and leg restraints. Occasionally one or more extremities must be restrained or limited in motion. A number

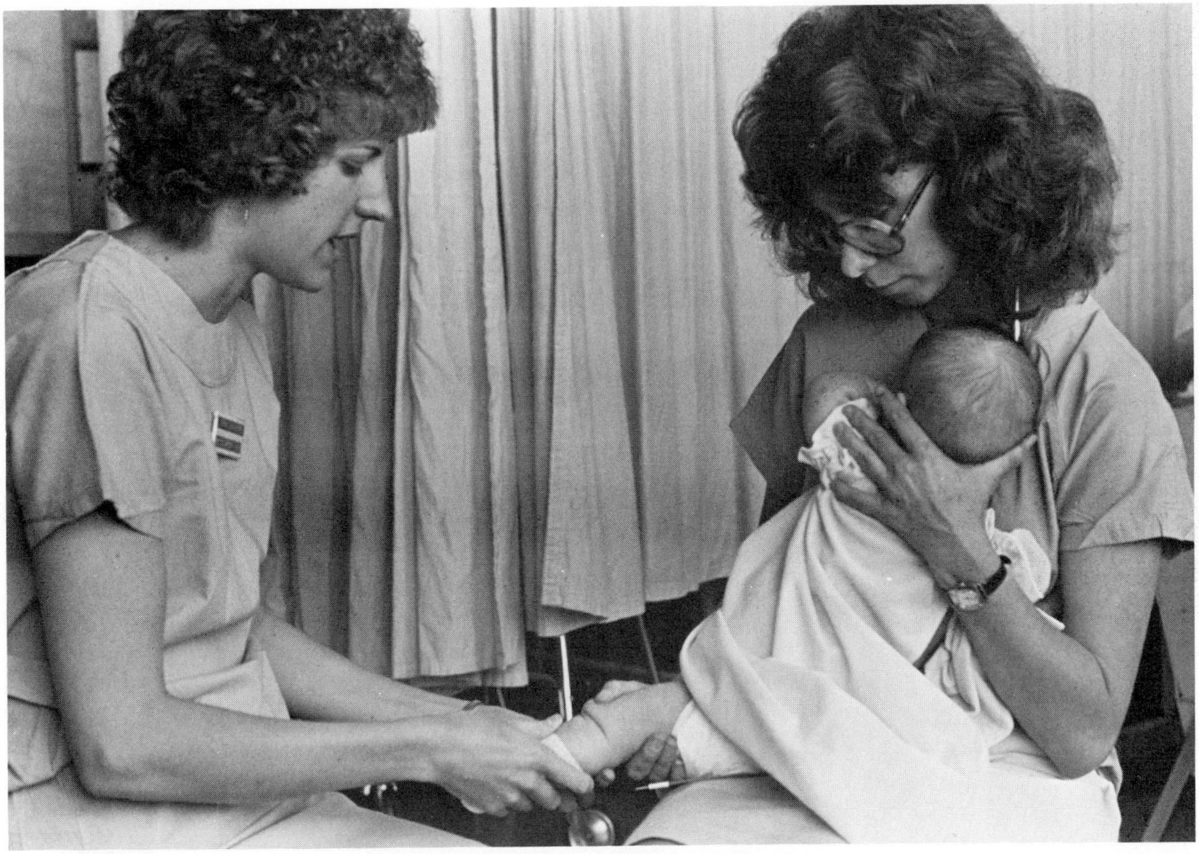

Fig. 26-4. Assistant supplies comfort and security while nurse carries out procedure.

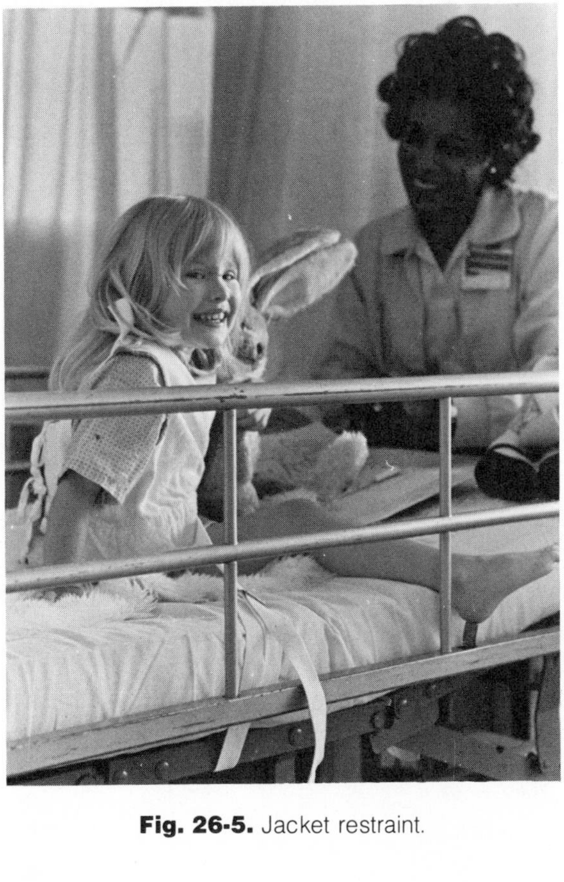

Fig. 26-5. Jacket restraint.

A B

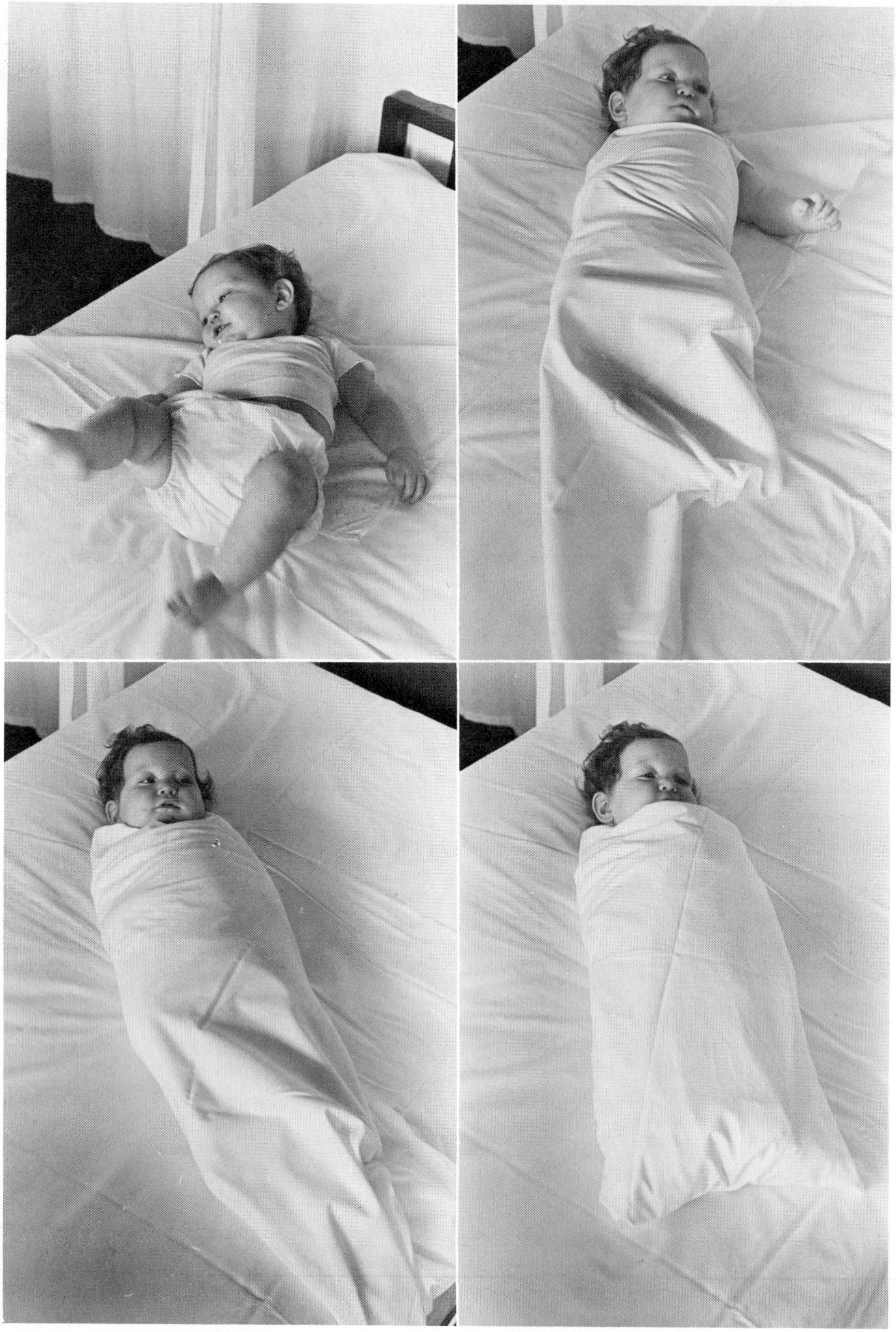

C D

Fig. 26-6. Application of mummy restraint. **A,** Infant placed on folded corner of blanket; **B,** one corner of blanket brought across infant and secured beneath body; **C,** second corner brought across body and secured; **D,** lower corner folded and tucked or pinned in place.

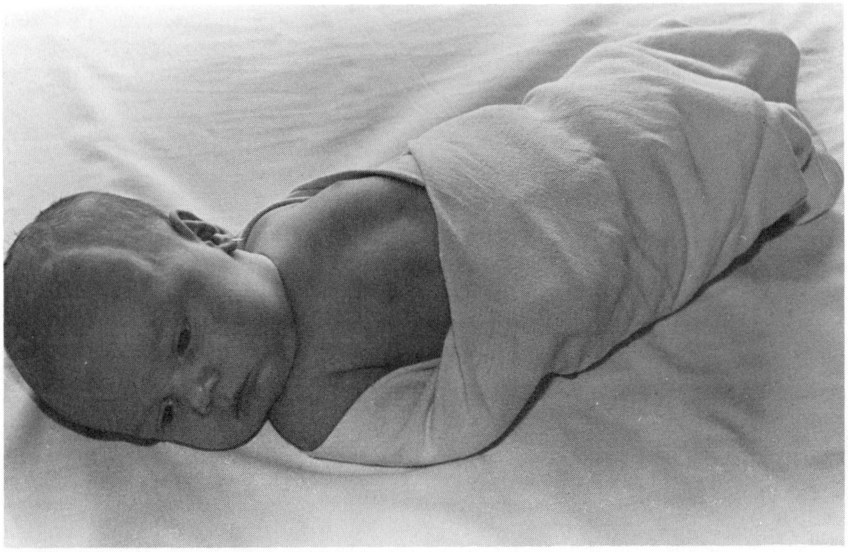

Fig. 26-7. Modified mummy restraint with chest uncovered.

of commercial restraining devices are available, or a restraint can be fashioned from gauze tape, muslin strips, or a length of narrow stockinette. When this type of restraint is used, it must be appropriate to the size of the child, it must be padded to prevent undo pressure, constriction, or tissue injury, and the extremity must be observed frequently for signs of irritation and/or impairment of circulation.

The *clove hitch* restraint is fashioned from a length of gauze or muslin tape. When properly applied, the restraint should provide a snug fit with minimum danger of pulling too tightly. See Fig. 26-8 for the method of tying and applying a clove hitch restraint.

The ends of the restraints are never tied to the crib rails, since lowering of the rail will disturb the extremity, frequently with a jerk, that may hurt or injure the child. Restraints can and should be released periodically to allow the child to move the restrained extremities. The child can remain unrestrained when someone can be with him to achieve the desired restraints on his movements.

Elbow restraint. Sometimes it is important to prevent the child from reaching his head or face, for example, after lip surgery, when a scalp vein infusion is in place, or to prevent scratching in skin disorders. For this purpose, elbow restraints fashioned from a variety of materials function very well. The most common form of elbow restraint consists of a piece of muslin long enough to reach comfortably from just below the axilla to the wrist with a number of vertical pockets into which tongue depressors are inserted (Fig. 26-9). The restraint is wrapped around the arm and secured with tapes or pins. Sometimes it is necessary to pin the tops to the child's undershirt to prevent the restraint from slipping (see also Fig. 11-18, p. 398).

Similar restraints can be made from padded large-diame-

1

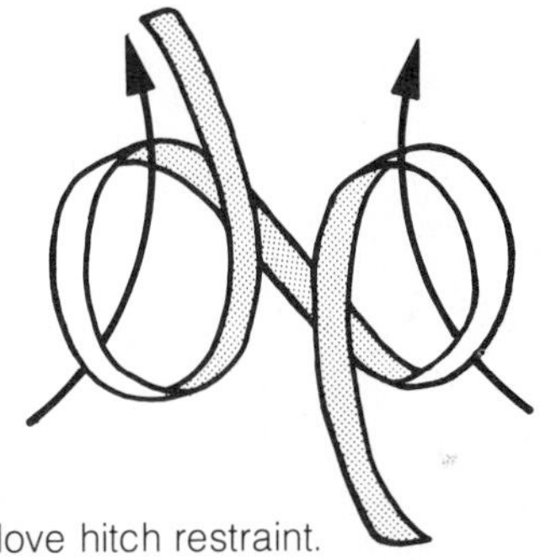

Fig. 26-8. Clove hitch restraint.

2

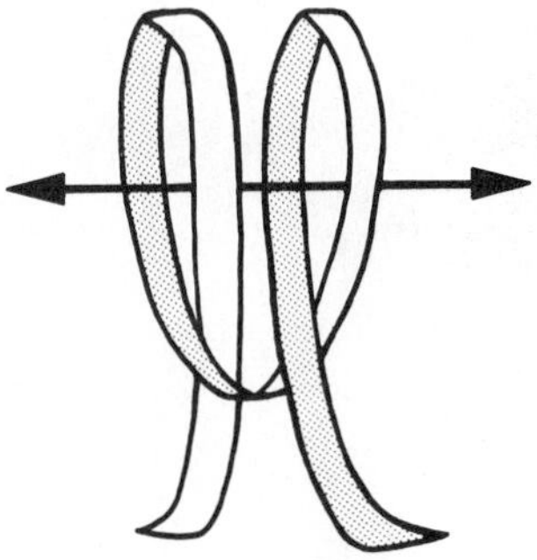

3

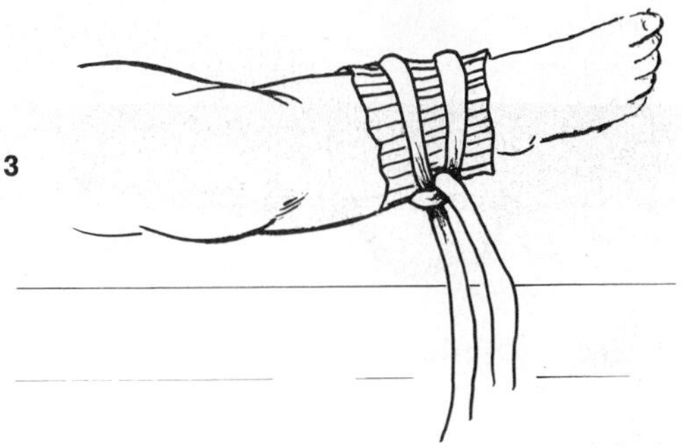

ter towel rollers or appropriately sized plastic containers from which the tops and bottoms have been removed. Both types need to be padded and to have some means to prevent the restraint from slipping from the extremity.

Positioning for procedures

Infants and small children are unable to cooperate for many procedures; therefore, the nurse is responsible for minimizing their movement and discomfort with proper positioning. Older children usually need only minimal, if any, restraint. Careful explanation and preparation beforehand and support and simple guidance during the procedure are ordinarily adequate.

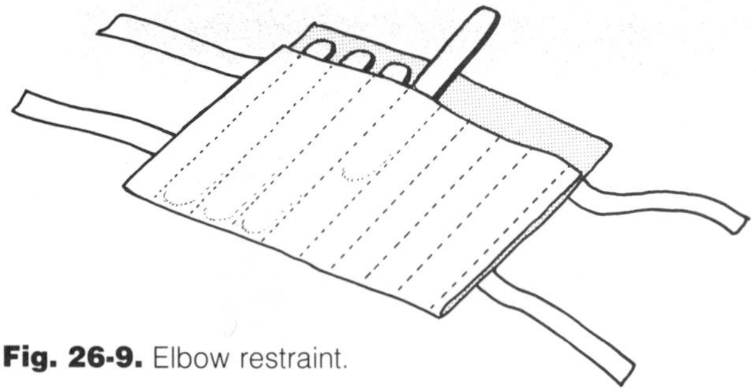

Fig. 26-9. Elbow restraint.

Jugular venipuncture. The large, superficial external jugular vein is frequently used to obtain blood specimens from infants and young children. For easy access to the vein, the child is first placed in a mummy restraint in which the top edge of the restraint is low enough to allow sufficient exposure to permit access to the vein. The child is placed so that his head and shoulders extend over the edge of a table or a small pillow with his neck extended and his head turned sharply to the side (Fig. 26-10). One alternate method for restraining arms and legs is with the nurse restraining the child's arms and legs with his or her arms at the same time as the head is restrained and positioned. It is important for the nurse holding the infant to maintain control of the infant's head without interfering with the operator's approach to the vein. The infant's crying during the procedure increases intravenous pressure, which facilitates visualization of the vein. Following venipuncture, digital pressure is applied to the site with a dry gauze square for 3 to 5 minutes or until bleeding has been stopped. Care must be taken not to apply excessive pressure that might compromise circulation or breathing during or following the procedure.

Femoral venipuncture. Other commonly used sites for venipuncture are the large femoral veins. The nurse restrains the infant by placing him supine with his legs in a frog position to provide extensive exposure of the groin

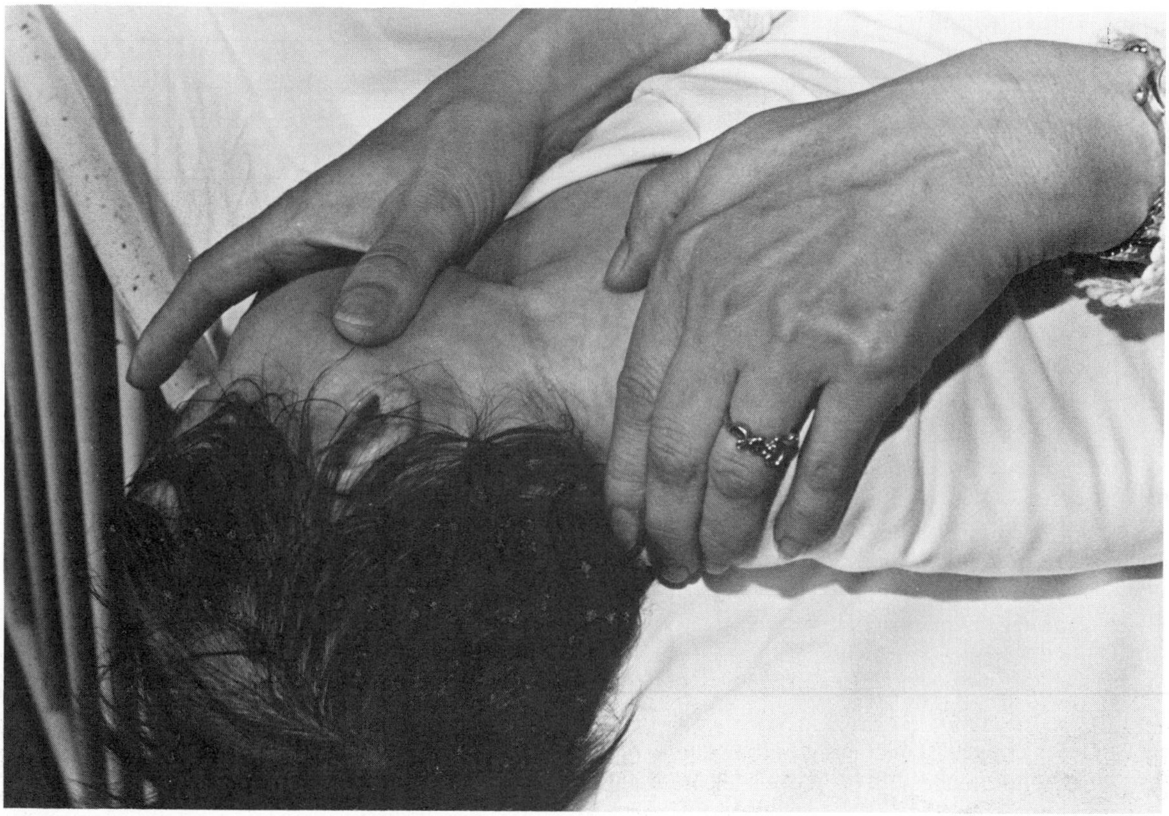

Fig. 26-10. Restraining child for jugular vein puncture.

area. Both the arms and legs of the infant can be effectively controlled by the nurse's forearms and hands (Fig. 26-11). Only the side used for the venipuncture should be uncovered so that the operator is protected if the child should urinate during the procedure. Pressure should be applied to the site after the withdrawal of blood to prevent oozing from the site.

Lumbar puncture. The technique for lumbar puncture in infants and children is similar to that in the adult. Pediatric lumbar puncture sets contain smaller spinal needles, but sometimes the operator will specify a particular size or type of needle that the nurse should make certain is placed on the tray.

Children are usually controlled best in the side-lying position, with the head flexed and the knees drawn up toward the chest. Even cooperative children need to be restrained to prevent possible trauma from unexpected, involuntary movement. They can be reassured that, although they are trusted, the restraint will serve as a reminder to maintain the desired position. It also provides a measure of support and reassurance to them.

The child is placed on the side with the back close to the edge of the examining table on the side from which the operator is working. The nurse maintains the child's spine in a flexed position by holding the child with one arm behind his neck and the other behind his thighs. The position can be effectively stabilized if the nurse's hands are clasped in front of the child's abdomen (Fig. 26-12, *A*). The flexed position enlarges the spaces between the lumbar vertebral spines, which facilitates access to the spinal fluid space. It is helpful to wrap the legs prior to positioning to decrease leg movement. An alternate position used with small infants and some older children is the sitting position. The child is placed with the buttocks at the edge of the table and with the neck flexed so that the chin rests on the chest. The infant's arms and legs are immobilized by the nurse's hands (Fig. 26-12, *B*). Since this position may interfere with chest expansion and diaphragm excursion, the child is observed for difficulty in breathing. Also, the soft, pliable trachea of the infant is subject to collapse. Specimens and spinal fluid pressure are obtained, measured, and sent for analysis in the same manner as for the adult patient. It is advisable for the child to lie quietly for an hour following the procedure to decrease the likelihood of headache, and he is offered fluids to drink. Vital signs are taken as ordered, and the child is observed for any changes in level of consciousness, motor activity, or other neurologic signs.

Other. For subdural puncture through a fontanel or burr hole, the infant is wrapped in a mummy restraint and placed in the supine position with the head accessible to the exam-

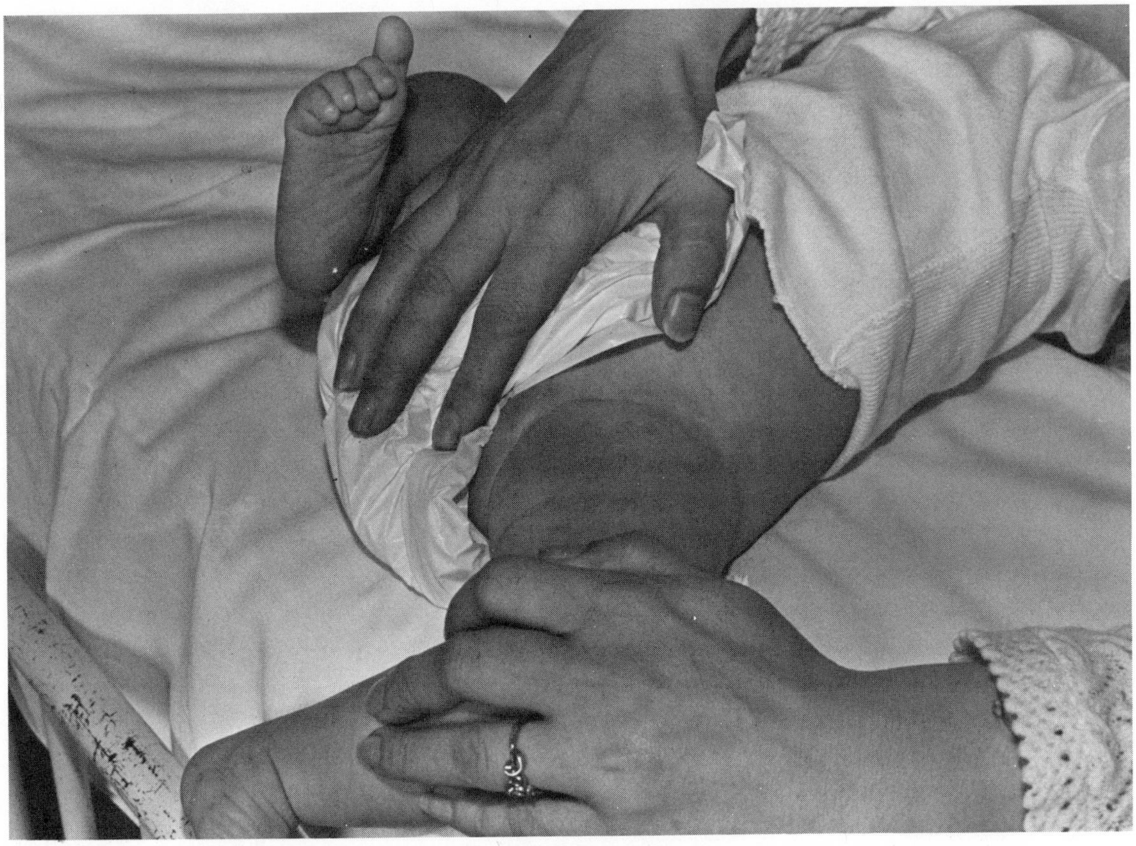

Fig. 26-11. Restraining child for femoral vein puncture.

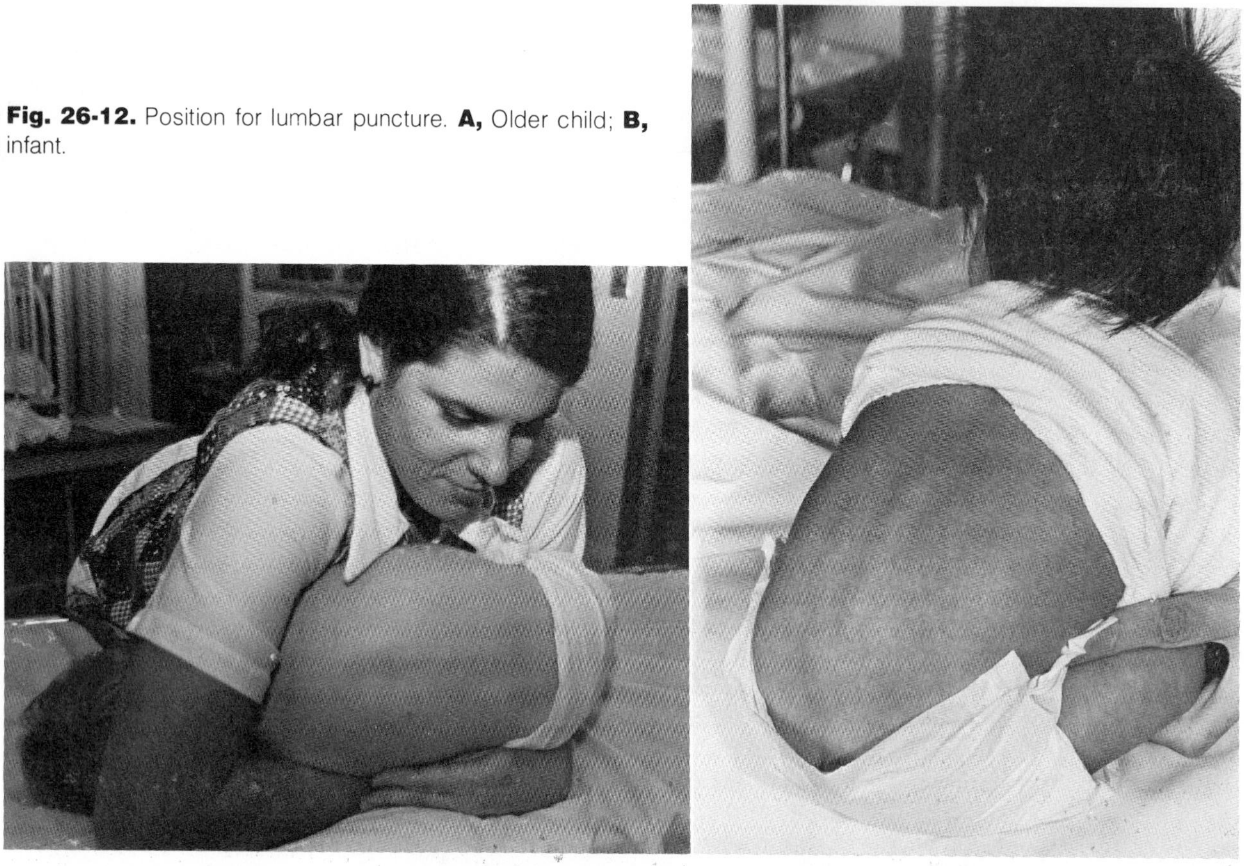

A B

Fig. 26-12. Position for lumbar puncture. **A,** Older child; **B,** infant.

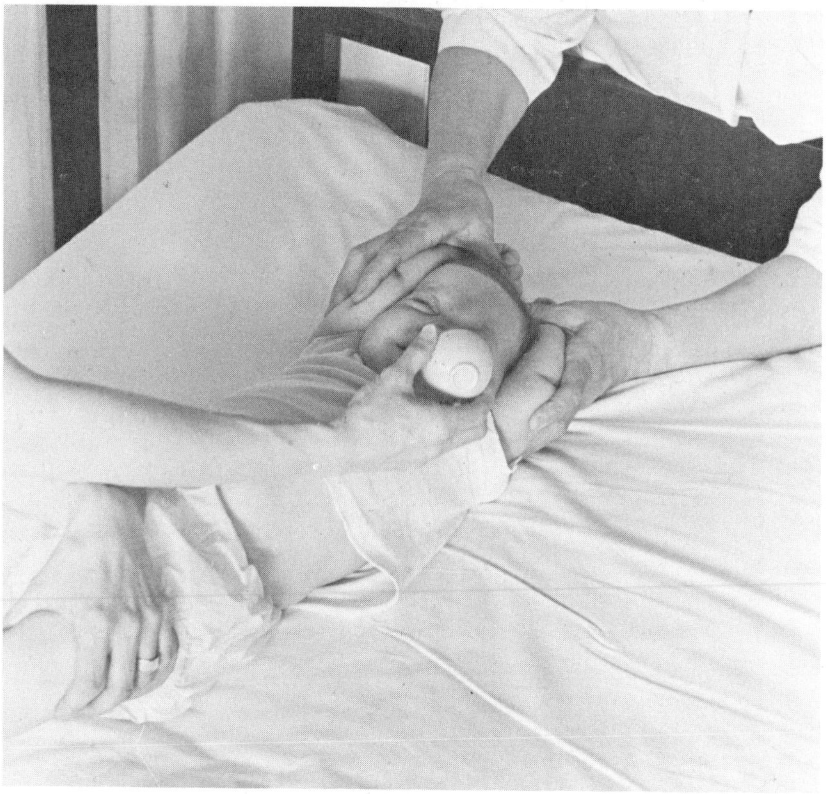

Fig. 26-13. Child's head immobilized with arms extended.

iner. The head is controlled with a firm hold on each side by the nurse. For access to the nose or throat, an alternate means for controlling head movement is immobilization of the head with the child's arms held extended above the head. This prevents movement of both arms and head (Fig. 26-13). Ears are examined with the child positioned as for jugular venipuncture but without the neck extension. (See p. 132 for other approaches for examining the ear.)

COLLECTION OF SPECIMENS

Many of the specimens needed for diagnostic examination of children are collected in much the same way as they are for adults, and older children are able to cooperate if given proper instruction regarding what is expected from them. Infants and small children, however, are unable to follow directions or control body functions sufficiently to help in collecting some specimens.

Urine specimens

All children admitted to the hospital and most clinic or office visits require a urine specimen as a routine diagnostic procedure. Older children and adolescents will readily use the bedpan or urinal or can be trusted to follow directions for collection in the bathroom. Self-conscious adolescents who may be reluctant to carry a specimen bottle through a hallway or waiting room can be provided with a paper bag or other means for disguising the container. The presence of menses is sometimes an embarrassment to teenage girls; therefore, it is a good idea to ask them if it might be that particular time of the month and make adjustments as necessary. The specimen can be delayed or a notation made on the laboratory slip to explain the presence of red blood cells.

School-age children are cooperative but curious. They are concerned about the reasons behind things and are likely to ask questions regarding the disposition of their specimen and what one expects to find out from it.

Preschoolers and toddlers are less cooperative primarily because they are usually unable to void on request. It is often best to offer them water or other liquids that they enjoy and wait 30 minutes or so until they are ready to void voluntarily. The child will better understand what is expected if the nurse uses his terms for the function, such as "pee-pee" or "tinkle." Some will have difficulty voiding in an unfamiliar receptacle. Potty-chairs or a bedpan placed on the toilet will ordinarily prove satisfactory. Toddlers who have recently acquired bladder control may be especially reluctant, since they undoubtedly have been admonished for "going" in places other than those approved by parents. A useful approach is to enlist the help of a parent; the parent is likely to be successful, and this helps them to feel a part of the child's care.

For infants and toddlers who are not toilet trained, special urine collection devices are used. These devices are clear plastic single-use bags with self-adhering material around the opening at the point of attachment. To prepare the infant, the genitalia, perineum, and surrounding skin are washed and dried thoroughly, since the adhesive will not adhere to a moist, powdered, or oily skin surface. The collection bag is easiest to apply if attached first to the perineum, progressing to the symphysis (Fig. 26-14). With little girls the perineum is stretched taut during application to that area to assure a leak-proof fit. With small boys the penis and scrotum are placed inside the bag. The adhesive portion of the bag must be firmly adhered to the skin all around the genital area to avoid possible leakage. The diaper is carefully replaced. The bag should be checked frequently and removed as soon as the specimen is available, since the moist bag may become loosened on an active child. (See p. 581 for collecting a clean-catch specimen.)

Twenty four–hour collection. Infants and children who are on accurate output measurements or are bagged for 24-hour urine collection will require a special collection bag, because frequent removal and replacement of adhesive collection devices can produce skin irritation. A thin coating of tincture of benzoine applied to the skin helps to protect it and aids adhesion. Plastic collection bags with collection tubes attached are ideal when the container must be left in place for a length of time. These can be connected to a collecting device or emptied periodically by aspiration with a syringe. When such devices are not available, a regular bag with a feeding tube inserted through a puncture hole at the top of the bag serves as a satisfactory substitute. However, care must be taken to empty the bag as soon as the infant urinates to prevent leakage and loss of contents.

Older children and adolescents will share the responsibility for long-term urine collection or measurement if they are given instructions and provided with the equipment. They can keep output records and transfer each voiding to the 24-hour collection container if this is permitted.

Blood specimens

Most blood specimens are obtained by the laboratory staff or physicians. However, nurses are often responsible for making certain that specimens, such as serial examinations, fasting specimens, and so on, are collected on time and that the proper equipment, such as correct collection tubes and ice for blood gas samples, is available. However, in some areas such as intensive care units, nurses routinely collect specimens that are needed frequently.

Venous blood samples can be obtained by venipuncture or by aspiration from an intravenous infusion site. When using an intravenous infusion site for specimen collection, it is important to consider the type of fluid being infused. For example, a specimen collected for glucose determination would be inaccurate if removed from a catheter through which glucose-containing solution is being administered.

No matter how or by whom the specimen is collected, nurses should be aware that children, even some older

A

B

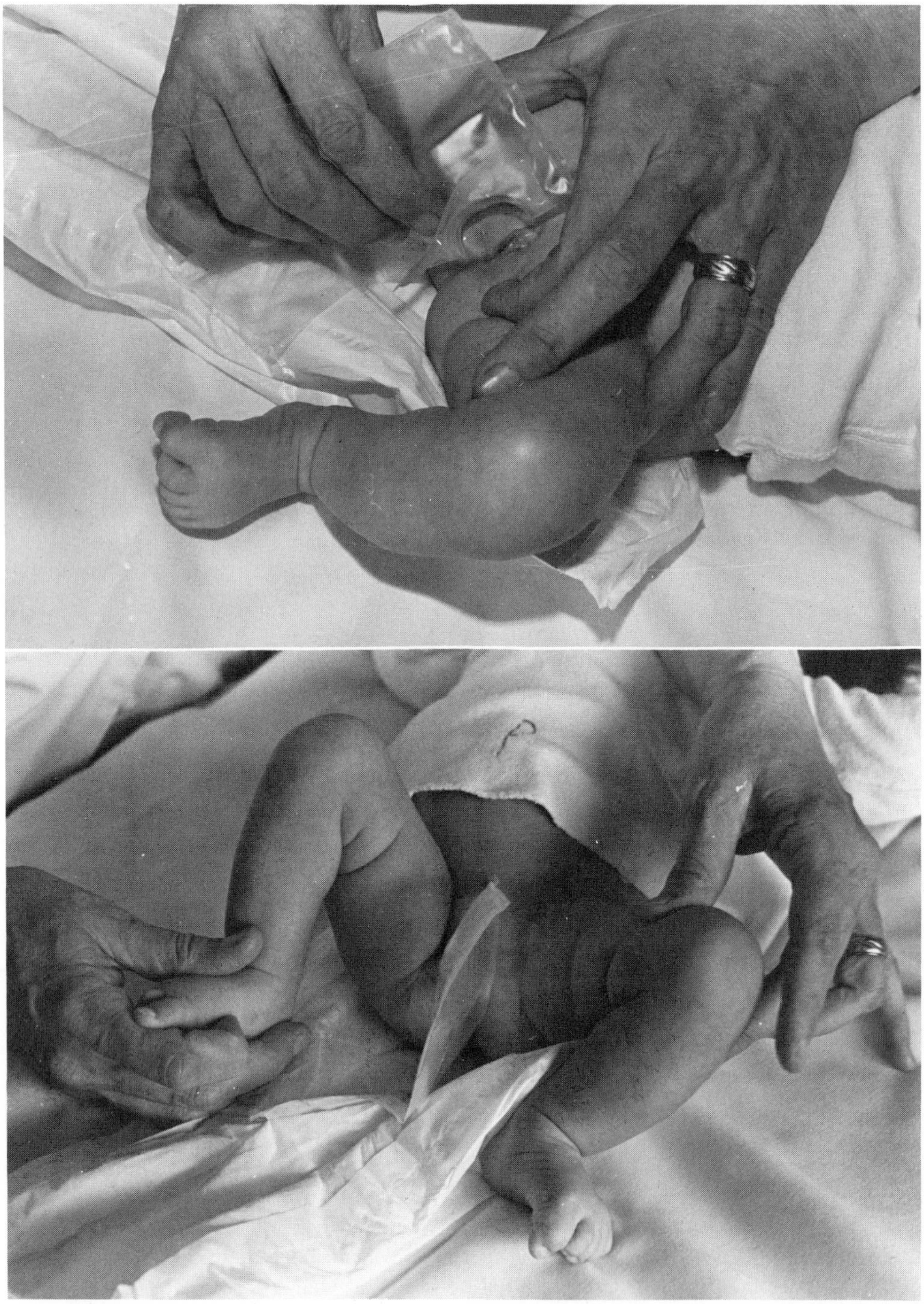

Fig. 26-14. Application of urine collection bag. **A,** On little girls the adhesive portion is applied to the exposed and dried perineum first. **B,** The bag adheres firmly around the perineal area to prevent urine leakage.

ones, fear the loss of their blood. This is particularly true for children whose condition requires frequent blood specimens. Ignorant about the process of hemopoiesis, they mistakenly believe that blood removed from their bodies is a threat to their lives. Explaining to them that their blood is continually being produced by their bodies provides them with a measure of reassurance regarding this aspect of the stress-provoking procedure. When the blood is drawn, a simple comment, such as, "Just look how red it is. You're really making a lot of nice red blood," confirms this information and affords them an opportunity to express their concern. A Band-Aid gives them added assurance that the vital fluids will not leak out through the puncture site.

Capillary blood samples from children are taken by finger or earlobe stick methods, just as in the adult patient. The best method for taking peripheral blood samples from infants is by a heel stick. Prior to taking the blood sample, the heel is warmed with warm, moist compresses for 5 to 10 minutes in order to dilate the vessels in the area. The area is cleansed with alcohol, and, with the infant's foot firmly restrained with the free hand, the heel is punctured with a Bard-Parker No. 11 or Redi-Lance blade deep enough to get a free flow of blood. Punctures should be made at the outer aspects of the heel in order to avoid the medial plantar artery. Also, repeated trauma to the walking surface of the heel can cause fibrosis and scarring that may interfere with locomotion. Frequent heel punctures have also been associated with development of plantar warts at a later age. The needed specimens are quickly collected and pressure applied to the puncture site with a dry gauze square until bleeding stops. The site is then covered with a Band-Aid. Applying warm compresses to ecchymotic areas to increase circulation helps remove extravasated blood and decreases pain.

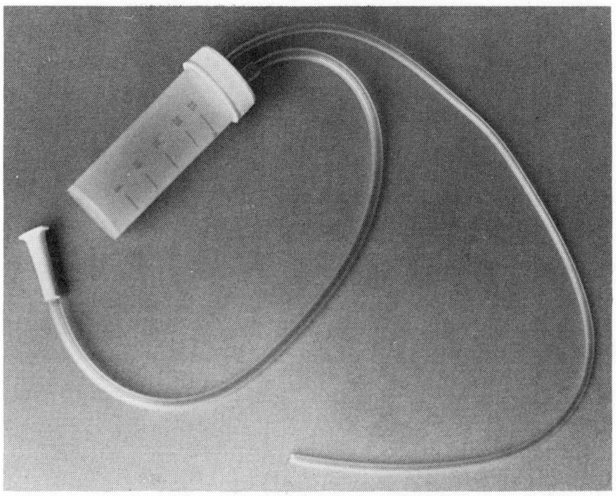

Fig. 26-15. Devices for collecting sputum specimens.

Sputum specimens

Older children and adolescents are able to cough as directed and supply sputum specimens when given proper directions. It must be made clear to them that a coughed specimen, not what is cleared from the throat, is needed. It is helpful to demonstrate a deep cough so that communication is clear. Infants and small children are unable to follow directions to cough and will swallow any sputum produced when they do. Sometimes it is possible to get a satisfactory specimen by using a suction device such as a mucous trap if the catheter is inserted into the trachea and the cough reflex elicited. A catheter that is inserted into the back of the throat is not sufficient. For children with a tracheostomy, a specimen is easily aspirated from the trachea or major bronchi by attaching a collecting device to the suction apparatus (Fig. 26-15).

ADMINISTRATION OF MEDICATIONS

The administration of medications to children presents a number of problems that are not encountered with giving medication to adult patients. Children vary widely in age, weight, surface area, and the ability to absorb, metabolize, and excrete medications. Nurses must be particularly alert when computing and administering drugs to infants and children.

Determining drug dosage

It is the physician's responsibility to prescribe drugs in the correct dosage to achieve the desired effect without endangering the health of the child. However, nurses must have an understanding of the safe dosage of medications they administer to children as well as the expected action, possible side effects, and signs of toxicity. Unlike adult medications, there are no standardized dosage ranges for children in the pediatric age-groups, and, with a few exceptions, drugs are prepared and packaged in average adult-dosage strengths.

Factors related to growth and maturation significantly alter the capacity of an individual to metabolize and excrete drugs, and deficiencies associated with immaturity become more important with decreasing age. Immaturity or defects in any or all of the important processes of absorption, distribution, biotransformation, or excretion can significantly alter the effects of a drug. Newborn and premature infants with immature enzyme systems in the liver where most drugs are broken down and detoxified, lower plasma concentrations of protein for binding with drugs, and immaturely functioning kidneys where most drugs are excreted are particularly vulnerable to the harmful effects of drugs. However, there are some drugs, such as epinephrine and the barbiturates, to which small children show surprising tolerance. For instance, a 2- to 4-year-old child can tolerate a dose equivalent to roughly half the adult dose of pentobarbital, and infants and young children are more resistant than adults to the effects of digitalis preparations.

Other factors that create problems in drug dosages in children include the difficulty in evaluation of drug response. For example, how does one assess in an infant a toxic manifestation such as ringing in the ears? In disease states, particularly in children, water losses and water requirements are both increased, whereas the fluid intake decreases. Since water is required to excrete the drug, dehydration poses the danger of toxic accumulation. For example, aspirin, which is commonly prescribed for fever, is excreted in the kidney, and its excretion is decreased with diminished urine pH and renal blood flow, both of which are associated with fever states.

Various formulas involving age, weight, and body surface area (BSA) as the basis for calculations have been devised to determine children's drug dosage from a standard adult dose. Since the administration of medication is a nursing responsibility, nurses need not only a knowledge of drug action and patient responses but some resources for estimating safe dosages for children. The methods most

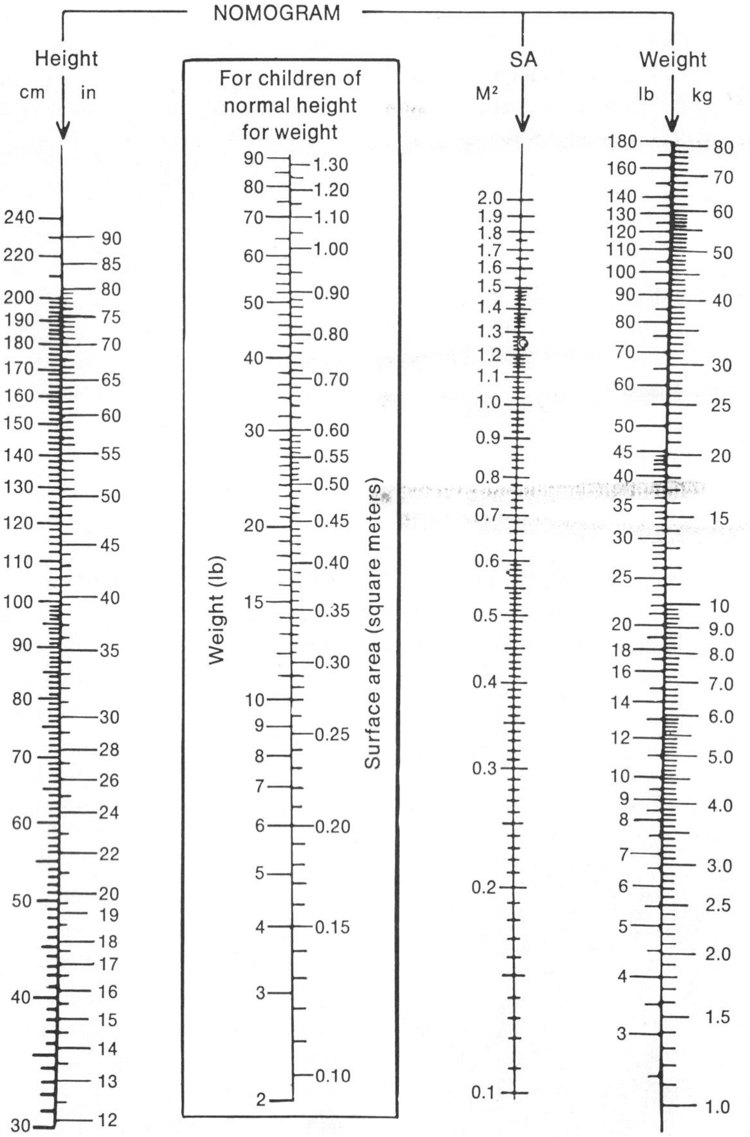

Fig. 26-16. West nomogram (for estimation of surface areas). The surface area is indicated where a straight line connecting the height and weight intersects the surface area (SA) column or, if the patient is roughly of normal proportion, from the weight alone (enclosed area). (Nomogram modified from data of E. Boyd by C. D. West; from Shirkey, H. C.: Drug therapy. In Vaughan, V. C., III, and McKay, R. J., editors: Nelson's textbook of pediatrics, ed. 10, Philadelphia, 1975, W. B. Saunders Co.)

often used to determine children's dosage are based on weight or surface area.

Weight as a basis. A method for quick calculation of dosage for children 2 years of age or older is Clark's rule, which uses the child's weight in pounds, the average adult weight in pounds, and the average adult dose.

$$\frac{\text{Weight of child in pounds}}{150} \times \text{Average adult dose} = \text{Estimated child's dose}$$

Since the average adult weight has increased over a number of decades, the "150" figure no longer represents the average. However, even with its limitations, this method continues to be favored by many physicians for calculating pediatric dosage.

Body surface area as a basis. The most reliable method for determining children's dosage is to calculate the proportional amount of body surface area to body weight. The ratio of body surface area to weight varies inversely to length; therefore, the infant who is shorter and weighs less than an older child or adult has relatively more surface area than would be expected from his weight.

The usual determination of surface area requires the use of a nomogram, such as that devised by West (Fig. 26-16). Body surface area is estimated from height and weight of the child, and then this information is applied to a formula for dosage. One formula that will obtain the appropriate fraction of the adult dose is:

$$\frac{\text{Body surface area of child}}{\text{Body surface area of adult}} \times \text{Adult dose} = \text{Estimated child's dose}$$

Another formula expresses the child's dose without relationship to the adult dose but requires knowledge of average dose per square meter (m^2) of surface area:

$$\text{Surface area of child } (m^2) \times \text{Dose}/m^2 = \text{Estimated child's dose}$$

Preparation for administering medications

Unit dose packaging, which is gaining wide usage in hospital pharmacies, does not usually extend to pediatric medications. Therefore, the ability to calculate fractional doses from larger dosages is absolutely essential. In addition, measuring doses, identifying patients, and gaining their cooperation create problems not usually encountered in giving medications to adults.

Checking dosage. Administering the correct dosage of a drug is a shared responsibility between the physician who orders the drug and the nurse who carries out that order. Children react with unexpected severity to some drugs, and ill children are especially sensitive to drugs. Therefore, checking the dose if there is any doubt about the accuracy of the dose ordered is a valuable habit to acquire. When a dose is ordered that is outside the usual range or if there is some question regarding the preparation ordered or the route of administration, this should always be checked with the physician before proceeding with the administration, since the nurse is legally liable for any drug administered.

Administering some medications requires added safeguards. Even when it has been determined that the dosage is correct for a particular child, there are many drugs that are potentially hazardous or lethal. Most hospital units or other facilities where medications are given to children have regulations requiring that specified drugs be double-checked by another nurse before they are given to the child. Among those drugs that require such safeguards are digoxin, heparin, and insulin. Others that are frequently included are epinephrine, narcotics, and sedatives. Even if this precaution is not mandatory, nurses would be wise to take such precautions for their own sense of security.

Identification. No matter what route is used to administer a medication, the child must be correctly identified. As mentioned previously, children are not totally reliable in giving correct names on request. An infant is unable to give his name, a toddler or preschooler may admit to any name, and a school-age child may deny his identity in an attempt to avoid the medication. Children sometimes exchange beds for awhile. Parents may be present to identify their child, but the only safe method for identifying children is to check their hospital identification bands with the medication card.

Parents. Parents can be useful sources of information regarding the child and his capabilities. Nearly all parents have given some kind of medication to their child and can describe the approaches that they have found to be successful. They can also provide information regarding the child's reaction to similar experiences if the child has been hospitalized before or if he has been given medication in a physician's office or clinic. In some cases it is less traumatic for the child if a parent gives the medication to the child, provided the nurse prepares the medication and supervises its administration and the practice is consistent with hospital or ward policy. Children being given daily medications at home are accustomed to the parent functioning in this capacity and are less apt to fuss than they would if the medication is administered by a stranger. It is not advisable to involve a parent in giving a painful or distressful medication such as a shot. The child is apt to view the parent's participation as complicity, and he will then blame the parent for allowing such indignities or pain to be inflicted on him. Children normally associate parents with a comforting, "make it better" role; therefore, parents should be a source of comfort and security to the child.

Patient approach

Even nurses who are experienced and who are skilled in administration of drugs to adults find that giving medications to children is challenging but, often, time-consuming and frustrating. A child's responses are strongly influenced by developmental characteristics such as physical abilities and cognitive capabilities, environmental influences, including past experiences with hospitalization, medications, and medical personnel, and his perception of the present situation. The child's general disposition and behavior patterns should be assessed as well as his condition and the degree of regression he has experienced as a result of his illness. All of these are considered in planning an approach best suited to the child as an individual. Also, nurses need to know how to communicate with children.

The nurse who has spent time with a child and established a positive relationship with him will usually find it easier to gain his cooperation in taking medications. If the relationship is based on trust, the child will associate the nurse with care-giving activities that give him comfort and pleasure most of the time and not as someone who brings discomfort and stress. There are a few guidelines that nurses working with children find useful in giving medication to children.

Expect success. Nurses who approach children with confidence and convey the impression that they expect to be successful are less likely to encounter difficulty. It is best to approach a child as though he is expected to cooperate without a fuss. Children sense anxiety in another and will respond to a perceived threat by striking out or with active resistance. Although it is not possible to eliminate such behavior in every child, a firm approach with a positive attitude on the part of the nurse tends to convey a feeling of security to most children. It is not always possible to estimate the extent to which a child will cooperate. Many very small children readily comply, whereas some older children or adolescents will offer unexpected resistance.

Provide an explanation. Children need an explanation for anything that involves them directly. Before giving a medication, the nurse should explain to the child what is to be done and what is expected of him. A short, simple explanation appropriate to the child's level of comprehension, for example, "It's time to drink your medicine now," is all that is required. This can be qualified with, "Swallow it and then you can have a drink of water." Long explanations are not necessary and may only increase anxiety in a small child. This is especially true regarding painful or unpleasant medications. Very small children understand simple instructions and are entitled to an explanation. Also, an accepting or a rejecting attitude is readily apparent to a child.

Allow choices. A choice should be given to the child only in situations in which one is available to him. To ask a child, "Do you want to take your medicine now?" or "I'm going to give you a shot now, okay?" leads him to believe that there is an option and provides him with the opportunity legitimately to refuse or delay the medication. This places the nurse in an awkward, if not impossible, position. It is much better to state firmly, "It's time to drink your medicine now." Children usually like to make choices, but the choice must be one that they do indeed have, for example, "It's time for your medicine. Do you want to drink it plain or with a little water?" "Do you want to hold the cup or shall I hold it for you?" or "Do you want a little drink of water or juice to swallow after it?" An older child can be permitted to state a preferred injection site.

Be honest. Honesty is essential to effective communication with children. For example, a child should be informed that a shot will hurt but that the hurt will not last very long. It may be helpful to try to describe how the injection will feel, but analogies should be carefully selected. A mosquito bite may be an adequate example for an intradermal skin test but is not descriptive of a painful injection of iron. Nurses who lie to a child will risk destroying any trust relationship that they have established or hope to establish with the child. Also, it is unwise to refer to medicine as candy. A child can innocently swallow fatal amounts by helping himself to medication unobserved.

The nurse should taste a minute amount of an oral preparation to ascertain if it is palatable or bitter. In this way legitimate signs of dislike from the child can be accepted and the taste camouflaged whenever possible.

Involve the child. As in any other aspect of care, involving children helps to gain their cooperation. Permitting them to make choices gives them some measure of control. Many children respond to tactics that appeal to their maturity or courage. This also gives them a sense of achievement. For example, preschool children will be proud that they can hold their own medicine cup or take their own pills from the container without assistance. Involving children generates a sense of participation. The same is true for the school-age child who submits to an injection with a minimum of resistance.

Provide distraction. When a child is occupied with some activity that interests him, he is less likely to focus on the medication. For example, a child at play will often accept the medication if he knows that he can return to his activity immediately afterward. When an injection is being given, it is helpful to give the child something to do or something on which to focus his attention. For example, asking the child to point the toes inward and wiggle them not only helps to relax the gluteal muscles but provides a diversion. Other strategies for diverting attention are to have the child tightly squeeze the hands of a parent or an assistant, count aloud, or verbally express his discomfort.

Allow expression of feelings. The child should be allowed to express without judgment feelings of anger, anxiety, fear, frustration, or any emotion he feels. It is natural for children to strike out in frustration or try to avoid stress-provoking situations. The child needs to know that it is all right to cry. Whatever the response, it is important that the nurse accept the behavior for what it is. Telling a child with limited verbal skills, such as a toddler, to stop kicking, biting, or otherwise expressing his frustration conveys to him that he is not being understood. Behavior is his primary means of communication.

Some planned activity is helpful in encouraging expression of feelings in a constructive way. For example, even older children are able to vent their anger and frustration in acceptable pounding or throwing activities. Play Dough is a remarkably versatile medium for pounding and shaping. One of the most effective activities for reducing the stress of injections is to permit the child to give a "shot" to a doll or stuffed toy. Dramatic play such as this provides an outlet for his anger and places the child in a position of control, in contrast to his position of helplessness in the real situation.

Praise the child. The child needs to hear from others that they know that he did the best he could in the situation—no matter how he behaved. It is important for the child to know that his worth is not being judged on the basis of his behavior in a stressful situation. Although bribes are seldom effective over an extended period, some reward systems, for example, saving the empty medicine cup as evidence of achievement, are often helpful. Children who require distasteful medications or shots over a period of time can look with pride on a series of stars or check marks on a calendar, especially if an accumulated number of marks represents a special privilege or reward.

Relate to the child. Returning to the child a short while after the medication has been given helps the nurse to strengthen a relationship with the child. This is an ideal time to engage him in hospital play such as giving a shot or other stress-provoking procedures to a doll. Relating with the child in a relaxed and nonstressful period allows him to see the nurse not only as someone associated with stressful situations but as someone with whom to share pleasurable experiences as well.

Accept the child. Most children are able to tolerate any number of insults and indignities if they know that both they and their reactions are accepted. Children need to know that they will not be rejected because of their methods of coping.

Oral medications

The oral route is preferred for administering medications to children whenever possible and, because of the ease of administration of oral medications, most are dissolved or suspended in liquid preparations. Although some children are able to swallow or chew solid medications at an early age, solid preparations are not recommended for children under 5 years of age. There is danger of aspiration in any oral preparation, but solid forms (pills, tablets, and capsules) are especially hazardous if their administration causes marked resistance or crying.

Most pediatric medications come in palatable and colorful preparations for added ease of administration. Some have a slightly unpleasant aftertaste, but the majority of children will swallow these liquids with little if any resistance. Many oral medications are more readily swallowed if they are diluted with a small amount of water and followed by a "chaser" of water, juice, a soft drink, or a Popsicle or frozen juice bar. Carbonated beverages poured over finely crushed ice given prior to or immediately after a medication are an excellent means to prevent or allay nausea. If large quantities of water are used, the child may refuse to drink the entire amount and, thus, receive only a partial dose of the medication. Disagreeably tasting medications should be disguised if possible, and most pediatric units have preparations available for this purpose. Sweet-tasting substances that are suitable include honey, flavored syrups, jam, and some fruit purees. Syrups are ideal for mixing with medicines that do not dissolve in water and for powdered drugs or pulverized tablets. Nurses cannot describe the taste of a medication to a child unless they have tasted the drug themselves. When selecting a substance to mix with a medication, *essential food items*, such as milk, cereal, and orange juice, should be avoided. If they are used, children may become conditioned against them and refuse these foods in their diet.

Preparation. Selecting a vehicle to measure and administer a medication requires careful consideration. The devices available to measure medicines are not always sufficiently accurate for measuring the small amounts needed in pediatric nursing practice (Fig. 26-17). Standard medicine glasses have been replaced by disposable plastic or paper cups. Although the carefully molded plastic cups offer reasonable accuracy in measuring moderate or large doses of liquids, the paper cups are likely to have irregularly shaped or crumpled bottoms. Calibrations on the cups

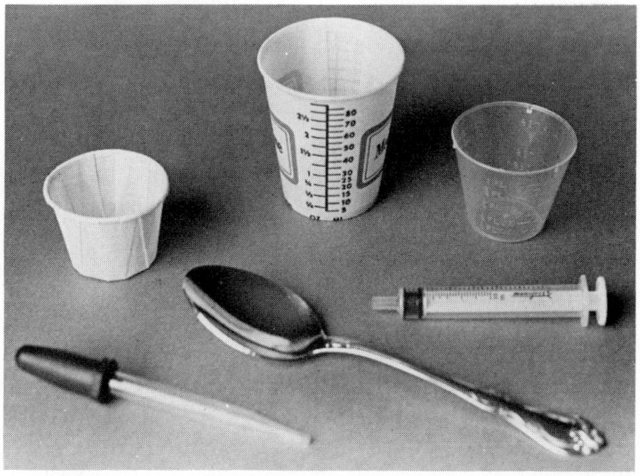

Fig. 26-17. Devices for administration of medications to pediatric patients.

(especially the teaspoon mark) and the personal equation or interpretation of a given measure are highly variable. Measures less than a teaspoon are impossible to determine accurately with a cup.

Many liquid preparations are prescribed in measurements of teaspoons. However, the teaspoon (and other household measures) is an inaccurate measuring device and is subject to error from a number of variables. For example, household teaspoons vary greatly in capacity, and different persons using the same spoon will pour different amounts. This variability is also influenced by the adequacy of available light, the color of the liquid, and the size of the bottle from which it is poured. Therefore, a drug ordered in teaspoons should be measured in milliliters. The American Standards Institute has established 5 ml as the standard teaspoon measurement; this is also the volume accepted by the United States Pharmacopeia (U.S.P.).

Another device that is not reliable for measuring liquids is the drop, which varies to a greater extent than the teaspoon or measuring cup. Droppers are available in numerous sizes but, even with the standard U.S.P. dropper, the volume of a drop will vary according to the viscosity of the liquid measured. Viscid fluids produce much larger drops than thin liquids. Many medications are supplied with caps or droppers designed for measuring each specific preparation. These are accurate when used to measure that specific medication but are not reliable for measuring other liquids. Emptying dropper contents into a medicine cup invites additional error. Since some of the liquid clings to the sides of the cup, a significant amount of the drug can be lost.

The most accurate means for measuring small amounts of medication is the syringe, and, for volumes less than 1 ml, the tuberculin syringe offers even greater accuracy. Not only does the syringe provide a reliable measure, but it also serves as a convenient means for transporting and administering the medication. The medication can be placed directly into the child's mouth from the syringe. However, only the disposable plastic syringes are safe for placing in children's mouths to avoid the possibility that they may be cut by broken glass if they should clench their teeth on the syringe. For added safety, a short length of flexible tubing can be placed on the tip of the syringe to prevent injury to the mouth.

Small children and some older children as well have difficulty in swallowing tablets or pills. Since a surprising number of drugs are not available in pediatric preparations, the tablet will need to be crushed before it can be given to these children. To minimize loss of the drug, the tablet can be crushed between two spoons or placed between

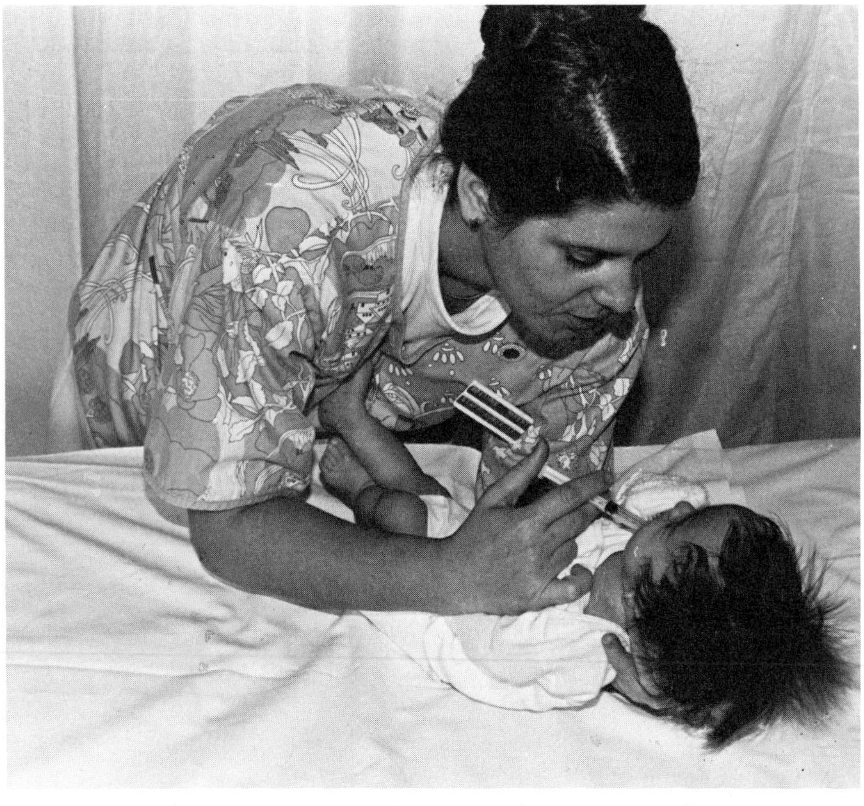

Fig. 26-18. Administering medication.

two small paper soufflé cups and crushed in a mortar and then mixed with syrup or juice for the child to swallow. The nurse must make certain that the bits of pulverized medication that tend to cling to the sides of the medicine cup or spoon are not lost.

Preparing dosage. Since pediatric doses often require dividing adult preparations of medication, the nurse may be faced with the dilemma of accurate dosage. With tablets, only those that are scored can be halved or quartered. If the medication is soluble, the tablet or contents of a capsule can be mixed in a small premeasured amount of liquid and the appropriate portion given. For example, if half a dose is required, the tablet is dissolved in 5 ml of water and 2.5 ml is administered.

Medications that are not scored cannot be divided accurately. For example, suppositories cannot be divided into two equal halves. In addition the manufacturer does not guarantee that the drug is evenly dispersed throughout the petrolatum base.

Administration. Administering liquids to infants is relatively easy, but care must be observed to prevent aspiration. With the infant held in a semireclining position (Fig. 26-18), the medication is placed in his mouth from a spoon, plastic cup, plastic dropper, or plastic syringe (without needle). The dropper or syringe is best placed along the side of the infant's tongue and administered slowly to avoid causing him to choke. Medicine cups can be used effectively for older infants who are able to drink from a cup. Because of the natural outward tongue thrust in infancy, medications may need to be retrieved and refed from lips or chin. Allowing the infant to suck the medication that has been placed in any empty nipple is another convenient method for giving liquid medications to infants. Medication is never added to the infant's formula feeding.

The small child who refuses to cooperate or resists consistently despite explanation and encouragement may require mild physical coercion. If so, it is carried out quickly and carefully. Every effort should be made to determine why the child resists, and the reasons for this alternative should be explained to the child in such a way that he will know that it is being carried out for his well-being and is not a form of punishment. There is always a risk in using even mild forceful techniques. A crying child can aspirate a medication, particularly when he is lying on his back. If the nurse holds the child in the lap with the child's right arm behind the nurse, the left hand firmly grasped by the nurse's left hand, and the head securely restrained between the nurse's arm and body, the medication can be slowly poured into the mouth (Fig. 26-19).

Intramuscular injections

Injections constitute some of the most traumatic health-related experiences for children. No one likes a "shot," especially those children in the age-groups when the procedure may be associated with other meanings such as fear of body mutilation, punishment, and so on (p. 886). At times it can be no less stressful to the nurse who must inflict the distress. Because of this characteristic of children, injections are given only when the drug cannot be given by the oral route.

Determining site. Factors that are considered when selecting a site for an intramuscular injection on an infant or child include the amount and character of the medication to be injected, the amount and general condition of the muscle mass, the frequency or number of injections to be given during the course of treatment, the type of medication being given, factors that may impede access to or cause contamination of the site, and the ability of the child to assume the required position safely. Ordinarily older children and adolescents pose few problems in selecting a suitable site for intramuscular injections, but infants with their small and underdeveloped muscles have fewer available sites. It is sometimes difficult to assess the amount of fluid that can be safely injected into a single site. Usually 1 ml is the maximum volume that should be administered in a single site to small children and older infants. The muscles of small infants may not tolerate more than 0.5

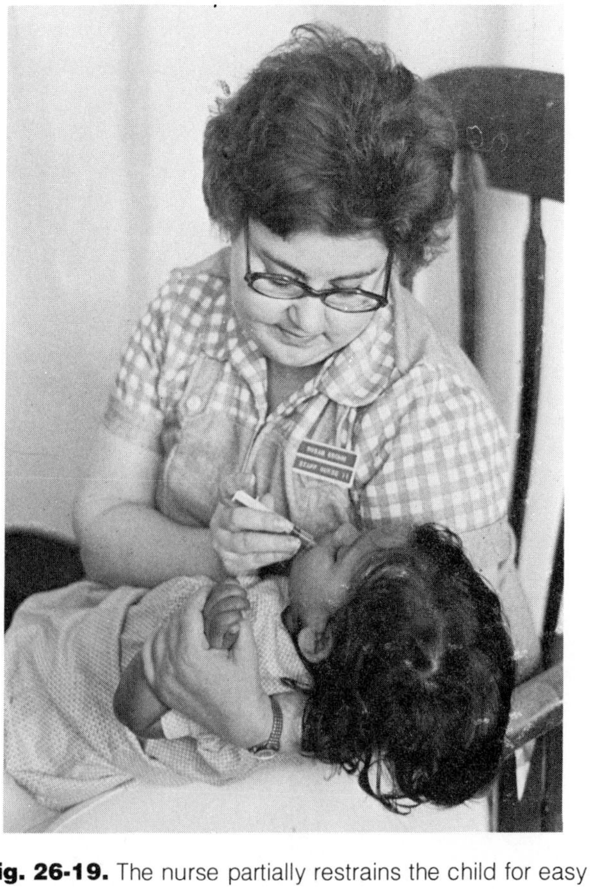

Fig. 26-19. The nurse partially restrains the child for easy and comfortable administration of medication.

ml. As the child approaches adult size, volumes approaching those given to adults may be used. However, the larger the amount of solution, the larger must be the muscle into which it is injected.

Injections must be placed in muscles large enough to accommodate the medication, yet major nerves and blood vessels must be avoided. There is no universal agreement regarding the best intramuscular injection site for children, and in older children and adolescents the preferred sites are much the same as in the adult: the posterior gluteal, ventrogluteal, quadriceps femoris (especially vastus lateralis), and deltoid muscles. In infants, however, there is less latitude. The preferred sites for infants are the vastus lateralis and ventrogluteal muscles, although the rectus femoris muscle can be used also. These are free of important nerves and blood vessels, with the exception of the femoral artery on the medial aspect of the thigh. The vastus lateralis muscle is the largest of the three and is well developed in the infant, and the ventrogluteal muscle is larger than the posterior gluteal muscle and has less subcutaneous tissue. On the other hand, the posterior gluteal muscle is very small, poorly developed, and dangerously close to the sciatic nerve, which occupies a larger proportion of space in infants than in older children. Therefore, it is not recommended as an injection site until the child has been walking for at least a year. The gluteal musculature develops with locomotion. Fig. 26-20 illustrates the location of the preferred intramuscular injection sites for children.

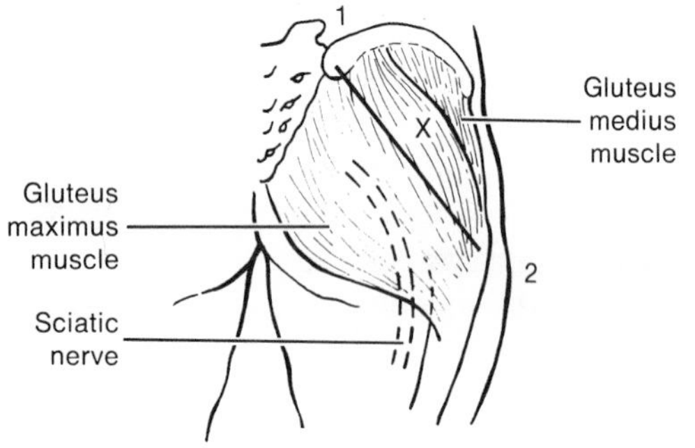

POSTERIOR GLUTEAL MUSCLE
LANDMARKS
1 Posterior superior iliac spine
2 Greater trochanter
INJECTION SITE: superior and lateral to imaginary line connecting landmarks; inject perpendicular to surface on which the child is lying

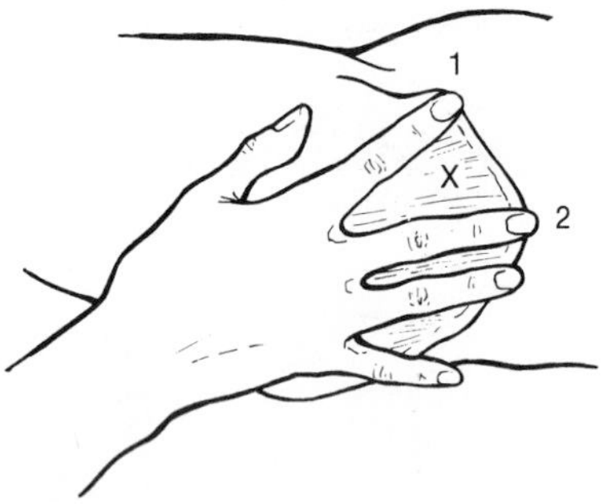

VENTROGLUTEAL
LANDMARKS
1 Anterior superior iliac spine
2 Iliac crest
INJECTION SITE: within V formed between index finger on anterior superior iliac spine and second finger at iliac crest; inject perpendicular to surface on which child is lying

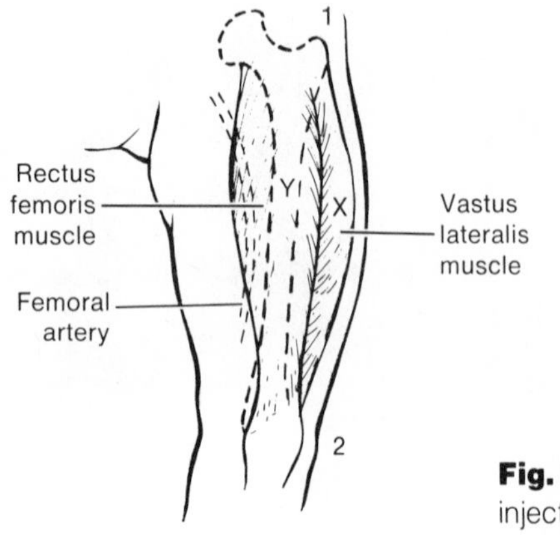

VASTUS LATERALIS MUSCLE
LANDMARKS
1 Greater trochanter
2 Knee
INJECTION SITE: lateral aspect of muscle mass in middle third of distance between landmarks; injected at 45 degree angle in direction of knee

Fig. 26-20. Acceptable intramuscular sites for children. *X*, Injection site; *Y*, alternate injection site.

Although injections that are executed with care seldom produce trauma to the child, there have been reports of serious disability related to intramuscular injections in children. Rotating sites is a safety factor well known in nursing practice when multiple injections are to be administered. Repeated use of a single site has been associated with fibrosis of the muscle with subsequent muscle contracture, and injections in the neighborhood of large nerves, such as the sciatic nerve, have been responsible for permanent disability, especially when potentially neurotoxic drugs are administered. Therefore, careful attention to detail is essential. The injection area should be well exposed to permit an unobstructed view of the injection site for identification of landmarks. The needle should be selected so that the medication is deposited well within the body of the muscle, and the drug should be injected slowly to allow the muscle to distend and accommodate the medication. Injections given too rapidly may cause the medication to be displaced into surrounding tissues, where it can produce irritation and discomfort.

Administration. Most children are unpredictable and few are totally cooperative when receiving an injection. Even children who appear to be relaxed and constrained can lose control under the stress of the procedure. It is advisable to have someone available to help restrain the child if needed. Since children often jerk or pull away unexpectedly, it is a good idea to carry an extra needle to exchange for a contaminated one so that there is a minimum of delay. The child, even a small one, should be told that he is getting an injection, and then the procedure should be carried out as quickly and skillfully as possible to avoid prolonging the stressful experience. Delay caused by lengthy explanations, attempts to hide the syringe from sight, or efforts to soothe the child will only serve to increase his anxiety. It must be kept in mind that intrusive procedures such as injections and rectal temperatures are especially anxiety provoking in preschool children and that small children usually associate any assault to the ''behind'' area with punishment.

It is also a good idea to carry a small Band-Aid to place on the puncture site. Most children associate this simple device with injury and derive comfort from its presence. Decorated Band-Aids are enjoyed by children of all ages. Drawing a smiling face on the surface of a plain Band-Aid reflects the nurse's reaction to the child's behavior during the procedure and serves as a positive reinforcement.

Small infants offer little, if any, resistance to injections. Although they squirm and may be difficult to hold in position, they can usually be restrained without assistance. The muscle mass of the thigh to be injected is firmly grasped in one hand to stabilize the limb and compress the muscle mass for injection with the other hand (Fig. 26-21). The body of a larger infant can be securely restrained between

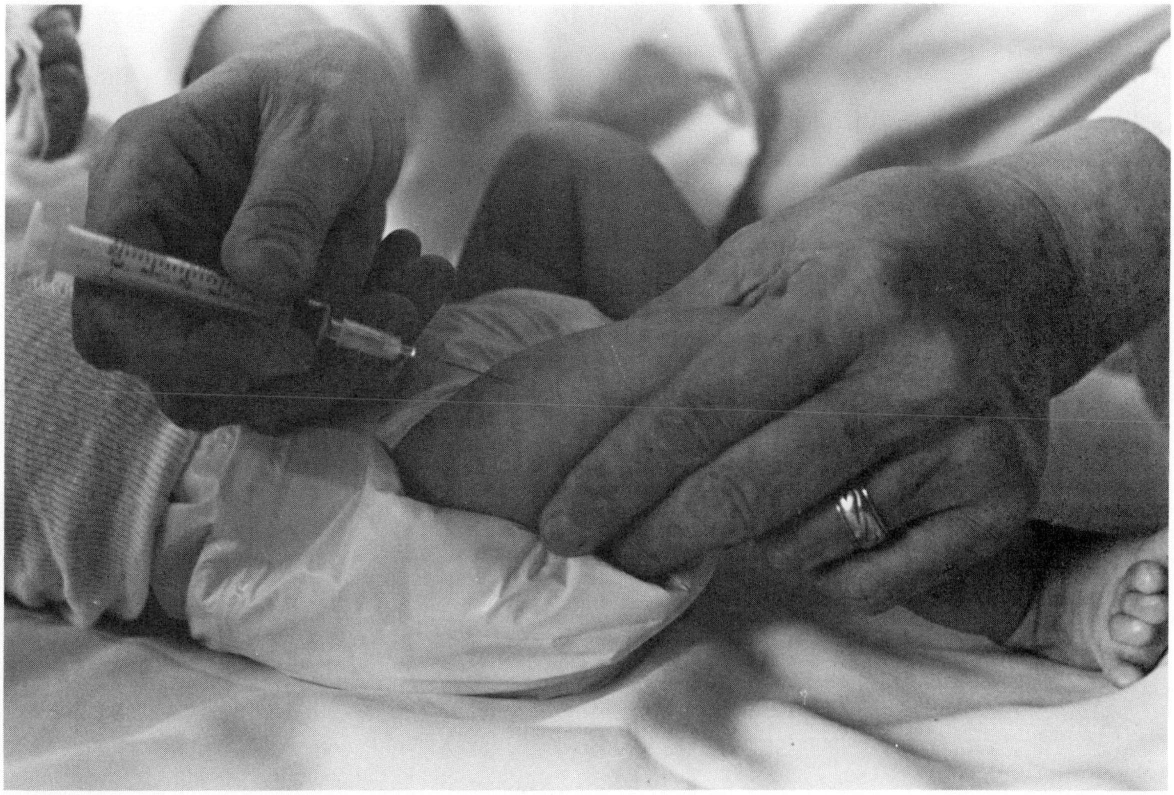

Fig. 26-21. Infant's leg stabilized for intramuscular injection.

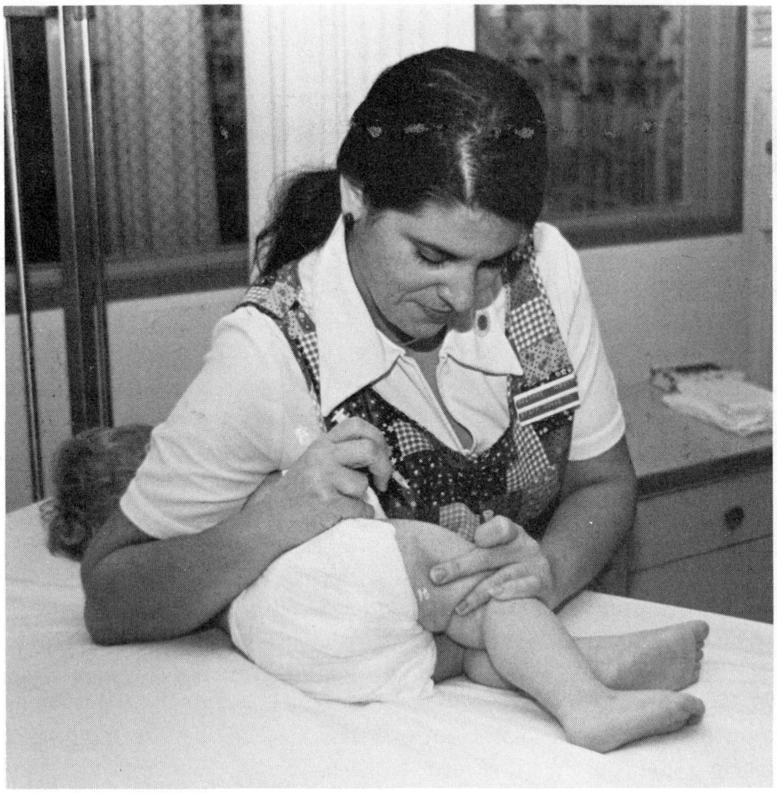

Fig. 26-22. Small child restrained for intramuscular injection.

the nurse's elbow and body (Fig. 26-22). After the procedure the child needs to be held and comforted. If parents are present, they usually require little encouragement to cuddle and comfort their child.

It is helpful to give an older child something on which to concentrate while the injection is being given. Squeezing a hand or bed rail, "toeing in," pinching his own nose, or humming are some of the devices. Children appreciate being permitted to say "ouch" as an approved outlet for feelings and to know that the nurse accepts whatever behavior they may display. They also need recognition of their fortitude. One small boy was heard to comment between sobs that "Kisses would make it better."

Rectal medications

The rectal route for administration is less reliable but sometimes used when the oral route is difficult or contraindicated. Some of the drugs available in suppository form are aspirin, sedatives, and antiemetics. The difficulty in using the rectal route is that, unless the rectal ampulla is empty at the time of insertion, the absorption of the drug may be delayed, diminished, or prevented by the presence of feces. Sometimes the drug is later evacuated, securely surrounded by stool. However, the rectal route is used most frequently in children who are unable to take anything by mouth and are unlikely to have large amounts of stool. It is also used when oral preparations are unsuitable to control vomiting.

Using a glove or finger cot, the suppository is quickly but gently inserted into the rectum, making certain that it is placed beyond both of the rectal sphincters. The buttocks are then held or taped together firmly to relieve pressure on the anal sphincter until the urge to expel the suppository has passed—5 to 10 minutes. Sometimes the amount of drug ordered is less than the dosage available. The irregular shape of most suppositories makes the process of dividing them into a desired dose difficult if not dangerous.

The same procedure is used to administer medication in a retention enema. Drugs given by enema are diluted in the smallest amount of solution possible to minimize the likelihood of being evacuated.

Nose, ear, and eye drops

There are few differences in administering nose, ear, and eye drops to children than to adults. The major difficulty is in gaining their cooperation or employing restraining techniques. Older children need only explanation and direction. When the drops are being instilled, the hand that holds the dropper should rest on the head of the child

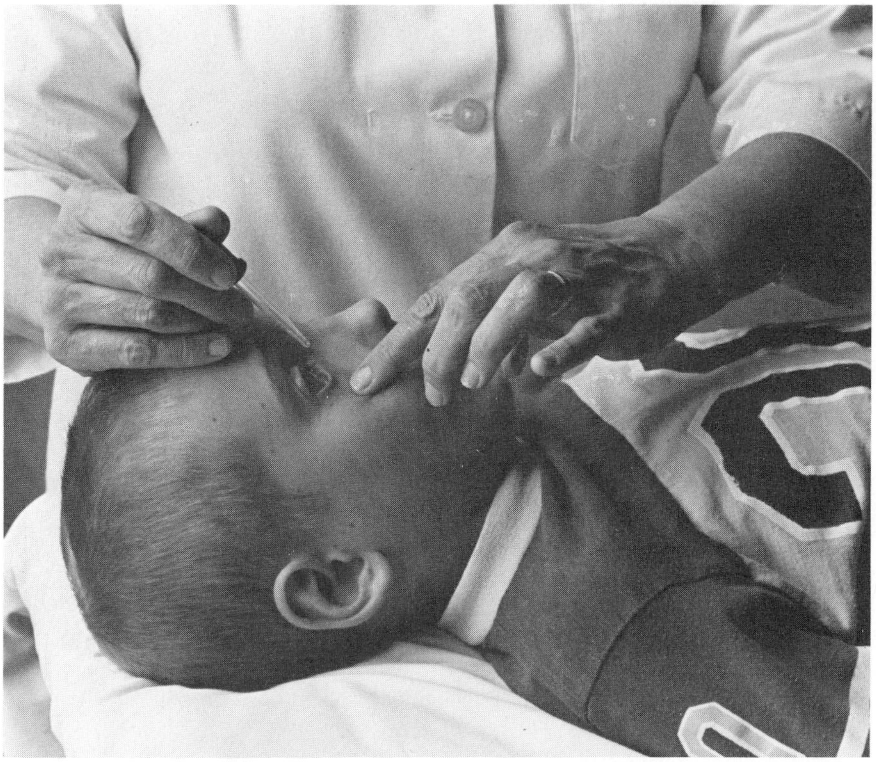

Fig. 26-23. Administering eye drops.

(Fig. 26-23). In this way the hand moves synchronously with the child's head and reduces the possibility of trauma to a struggling child or dropping medication on the face. The head of the infant or small child is immobilized in the same manner as described for obtaining specimens or assisting with procedures. Medications stored in the refrigerator should be warmed to room temperature before instillation.

For administering eye drops, the eyelids are gently separated with the thumb and index fingers and the prescribed number of drops instilled onto the conjunctiva of the lower lid. Another effective technique is to pull the lower lid down and out to form a cup effect, into which the medication is dropped (Fig. 26-23).

Ear drops are instilled with the child restrained in the supine position and the head turned to the appropriate side. For children younger than 3 years of age, the external auditory canal is straightened by gently pulling the pinna downward and straight back. The pinna is pulled upward and back in children older than 3 years of age (see Fig. 5-27). After instillation, the child should remain lying on the unaffected side for a few minutes. Gentle massage of the area immediately anterior to the ear facilitates the entry of drops into the ear canal. The use of cotton pledgets prevents medication from flowing out of the external canal. However, they should be loose enough to allow any discharge to exit from the ear. Ear drops are warmed to near body temperature, since cold solutions striking the tympanic membrane may produce pain or vertigo.

Nose drops are instilled in the same manner as in the adult patient. Unpleasant sensations associated with medicated nose drops are minimized when care is taken to position the child with the head extended well over the edge of the bed or a pillow (Fig. 26-24). Strangling sensations are caused by medication trickling into the throat rather than up into the nasal passages. Following instillation of the drops, the child should remain in position for 1 minute to allow the drops to come in contact with the nasal surfaces.

Plain saline or vasoconstricting nose drops are frequently prescribed for infants with ''stuffy noses'' caused by upper respiratory infections. Since these children naturally breathe by nose, nasal congestion interferes with feeding; therefore, drops are instilled prior to feedings to clear nasal passages and reduce congestion. Depending on the size of the infant, he can be positioned in the football hold (p. 922), in the nurse's arm with the head extended and stabilized between the nurse's body and elbow and the arms and hands immobilized with the nurse's hands, or with the head extended over the edge of the bed or a pillow.

Intravenous administration

Use of the intravenous route for administering medications has gained widespread use in pediatric therapy. For some important drugs it is the only effective route of ad-

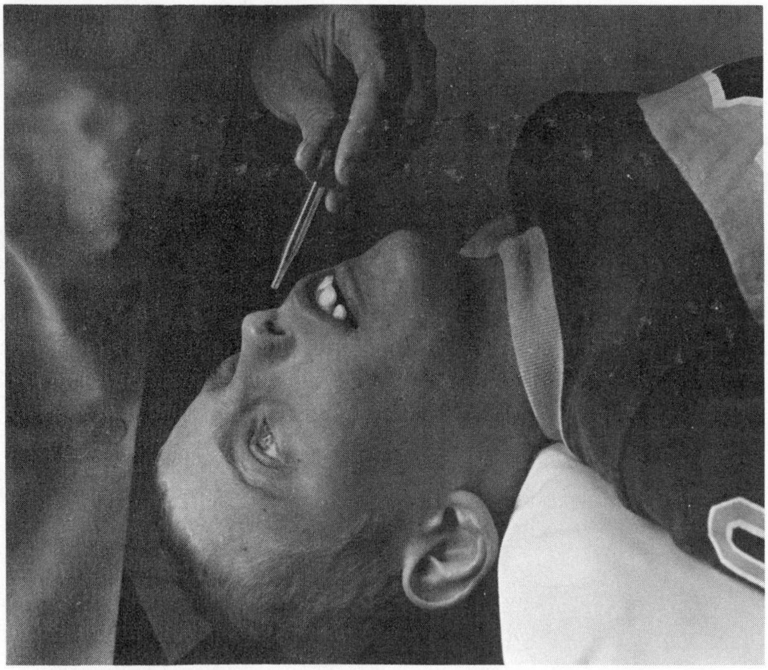

Fig. 26-24. Proper position for instilling nose drops.

ministration. This method is used for giving drugs to children who have poor absorption as a result of diarrhea, dehydration, or peripheral vascular collapse; children who need a high-serum concentration of a drug; and those with resistant infections that require parenteral medication over an extended period of time.

Insertion sites and observation of the intravenous infusion are discussed in Chapter 29. However, there are a number of factors to be considered and nursing responsibilities related to intravenous medication. When a drug is administered intravenously, the effect is almost instantaneous and further control is limited. Most drugs for intravenous administration require a specified minimum dilution and/or rate of flow, and many are highly irritating or toxic to tissues outside the vascular system. In addition to the precautions and nursing observations related to intravenous therapy, factors that are considered when preparing and administering drugs to infants and children by way of the intravenous route include:

Amount of drug to be administered
Minimum dilution of drug
Type of solution in which drug can be diluted
Length of time over which drug can be safely administered
Rate of infusion that child and his vessels can tolerate safely
Time that this or another drug is to be administered
Compatibility of all drugs that child is receiving intravenously

Prior to any intravenous infusion, the site of insertion is checked for patency. Medications are never administered by way of blood products.

When a drug with poor stability, such as ampicillin, is being administered, it should be kept in mind that not only must the Volutrol (or similar container) be emptied of the drug-containing solution but also that the tubing from the Volutrol to the insertion site contains the drug as well. The child does not receive the full dose of the drug until the 10 ml or more of solution within the tubing has also been infused. This is a significant consideration when drugs are given in small amounts of fluid. For example, if a drug is added to 10 ml of fluid in the Volutrol, it does not reach the bloodstream until all of the fluid in the tubing is absorbed.

Teaching parents

It is usually the nurse who assumes the responsibility for preparing parents to administer medications at home. The parent should have an understanding of why the child is receiving the medication and the effects that might be expected, as well as the amount, frequency, and length of time the drug is to be administered. Instruction should be carried out in an unhurried, relaxed manner, preferably in an area away from busy ward of office routine.

The parent or other care giver is carefully instructed regarding the correct dosage. Some persons have difficulty in understanding or interpreting terminology from the pharmacy, and just because they nod or otherwise indicate an understanding it cannot be assumed that the message is clear. It is important to ascertain their interpretation of, for example, a teaspoon—is it rounded, level, or scant? If the drug is packaged with a dropper in the cap, the nurse should show the point on the dropper that indicates the prescribed dose and demonstrate how the dose is drawn up and measured and the bubbles eliminated. If the nurse has any doubts about the parent's ability to administer the correct dose, it is wise to have him or her give a return demonstration. This is especially important when the drug has potentially serious consequences from incorrect dosage, such as insulin or digitalis. The nurse should demonstrate and receive a return demonstration of administration of eye, ear, or nose drops. Teaching a parent to give an injection usually requires instruction and practice over a period of 2 or 3 days.

The time that the drug is to be administered should be clarified with the parent. For instance, when a drug is prescribed in association with meals, the number of meals that the family is accustomed to eat influences the amount of drug the child receives. Do they have meals twice a day or five times a day? When a drug is to be given several times during the day, together the nurse and parents can work out a schedule that fits around the family routine. This is particularly significant if the drug must be given at equal intervals throughout a 24-hour period (see p. 912).

ALTERNATIVE FEEDING TECHNIQUES

Children who are unable to take nourishment by mouth because of anomalies of the throat or esophagus, impaired swallowing capacity, severe debilitation, respiratory distress, or unconsciousness are frequently fed by way of a tube inserted directly into the stomach (gastrostomy) or by gavage. Premature infants who are either unable to suck or who become exhausted from bottle-feeding are fed by gavage.

Gavage feeding

Infants and children can be fed simply and safely by a tube passed into the stomach through either the nares or the mouth. The tube can be left in place or inserted and removed with each feeding. In older children it has usually been found to be less traumatic to tape the tube securely in place between feedings. When this alternative is used, the tube should be removed and replaced with a new tube once every 24 to 72 hours, depending on hospital policy or specific orders.

Preparation. The equipment needed for gavage feeding includes:

A rubber, polyethylene, or polyvinyl feeding tube selected according to the size of the child and the viscosity of the solution being fed; for infants a 15-inch French catheter or feeding tube size 5 to 8 is appropriate. In larger children longer catheters with a larger diameter, usually sizes 10 to 14 French, are needed.

A receptacle for the fluid; for small amounts a 10- to 30-ml syringe barrel or Asepto syringe is satisfactory; for larger amounts a 50-ml syringe with a catheter tip is more convenient.

A syringe to aspirate stomach contents and/or to inject air after the tube has been placed

Water to lubricate the tube; sterile water is used for infants

Paper or nonallergenic tape to mark the tube and to attach the tube to the infant's or child's face

A stethoscope to determine the correct placement in the stomach

The solution for feeding

Procedure. Infants will be easier to control if they are first wrapped in a mummy restraint (p. 924). Even tiny infants with random movements can grasp and remove the tube. Premature infants do not ordinarily require restraint, but, if they do, a small towel folded across the chest and secured beneath the shoulders is usually sufficient. Care must be taken so that breathing is not compromised.

Gavage feeding is usually carried out with the infant or child lying on the back or toward the right side and the head and chest elevated slightly. A folded blanket under the head and shoulders is satisfactory for infants, and a pillow is useful for small children. The head of the bed is raised for larger children. The feeding tube can be passed through either the nose or the mouth. Since young infants breathe by mouth, insertion through the mouth causes less distress to the infant and helps to stimulate sucking. A tube passed through one of the nares in older infants and children seems quite satisfactory once the tube is in place. An indwelling tube is almost always placed through the nose; the nares are rotated with each insertion to minimize irritation, chance of infection, and possible breakdown of mucous membranes from pressure that occurs over a period of time.

The procedure for gavage feeding is carried out as follows:

1. Measure the tube for correct length of insertion and mark the point with a small piece of tape. Correct length can be determined by one of two methods: (1) measuring from the bridge of the nose to the umbilicus, or (2) measuring from the tip of the nose to the earlobe (or vice versa) and then to the tip of the xiphoid process (ensiform cartilage) of the sternum (Fig. 26-25). However, new information indicates that this may not be a sufficient distance.[4] The tube may need to be advanced a few centimeters farther for correct placement as verified by aspiration of stomach contents in step 3.

2. Insert the tube that has been lubricated with sterile water or water-soluble lubricant through either the mouth or one of the nares to the predetermined mark. Since the esophagus is situated behind the trachea, the tube is more easily inserted when the child's head is hyperflexed. This reduces the chance of the tube entering the trachea. When using the nose, the tube is slipped along the base of the nose and directed straight back toward the occiput; when entering through the mouth the tube is directed toward the back of the throat. The tube is passed quickly and, if the child is able to swallow, synchronized with swallowing.

3. Check the position of the tube by using one or both

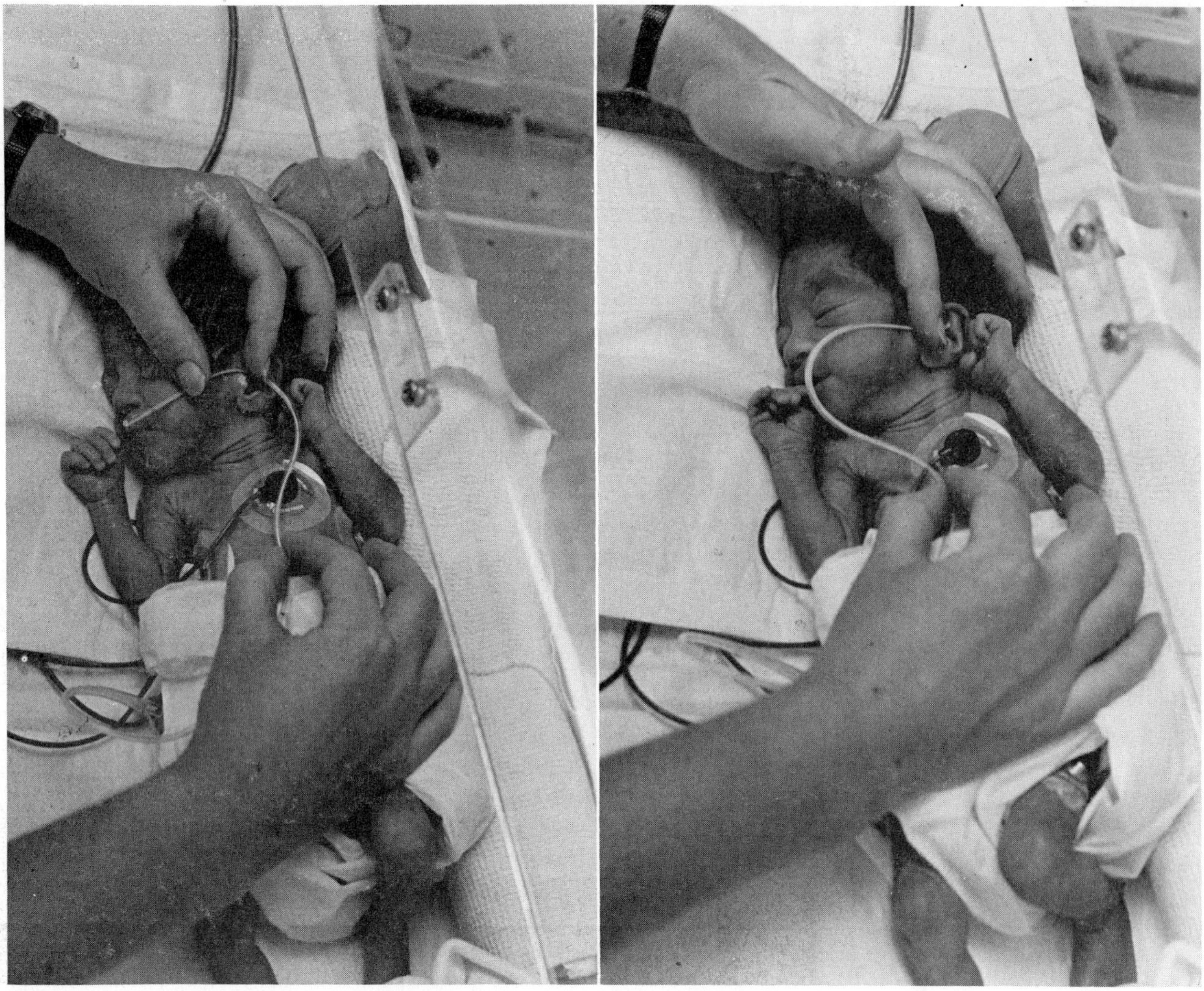
A B

Fig. 26-25. Measuring tube for gavage feeding. **A,** From tip of nose to earlobe and to tip of sternum. **B,** From earlobe to tip of nose and to tip of sternum.

of the following: (1) The syringe is attached to the feeding tube and gentle negative pressure applied. Aspiration of stomach contents indicates proper placement. The amount and character of any fluid aspirated is noted and returned to the stomach. Absence of fluid is not necessarily evidence of improper placement. The stomach may be empty or the tube may not be in contact with stomach contents. (2) With the syringe, inject a small amount of air into the tube while simultaneously listening with a stethoscope over the stomach area. Sounds of gurgling or growling will be heard if the tube is properly situated in the stomach. The air is then withdrawn. The amount of air injected is determined by the size of the child: 0.5 to 1 ml in premature or very small infants to 5 ml in larger children.

4. Stabilize the tube by holding or taping it in place with tape to maintain correct placement. When taped, the tube is secured to the cheek, not to the forehead because of possible damage to the nostril.

5. Feed the formula, which has been warmed to room temperature. Formula is poured into the barrel of the syringe attached to the feeding tube (Fig. 26-26, *B*). To start the flow a gentle push with the plunger may be required, but the plunger should then be removed and the fluid allowed to flow into the stomach by gravity. The rate of flow should not exceed 5 ml per 5 to 10 minutes in premature and very small infants and 10 ml/minute in older infants and children to prevent nausea and regurgitation. The rate is determined by the diameter of the tubing and the height of the reservoir containing the feeding and is regulated by adjusting the height of the syringe. A usual feeding requires 15 to 20 minutes to complete.

6. Flush the tube with sterile water (1 or 2 ml for small

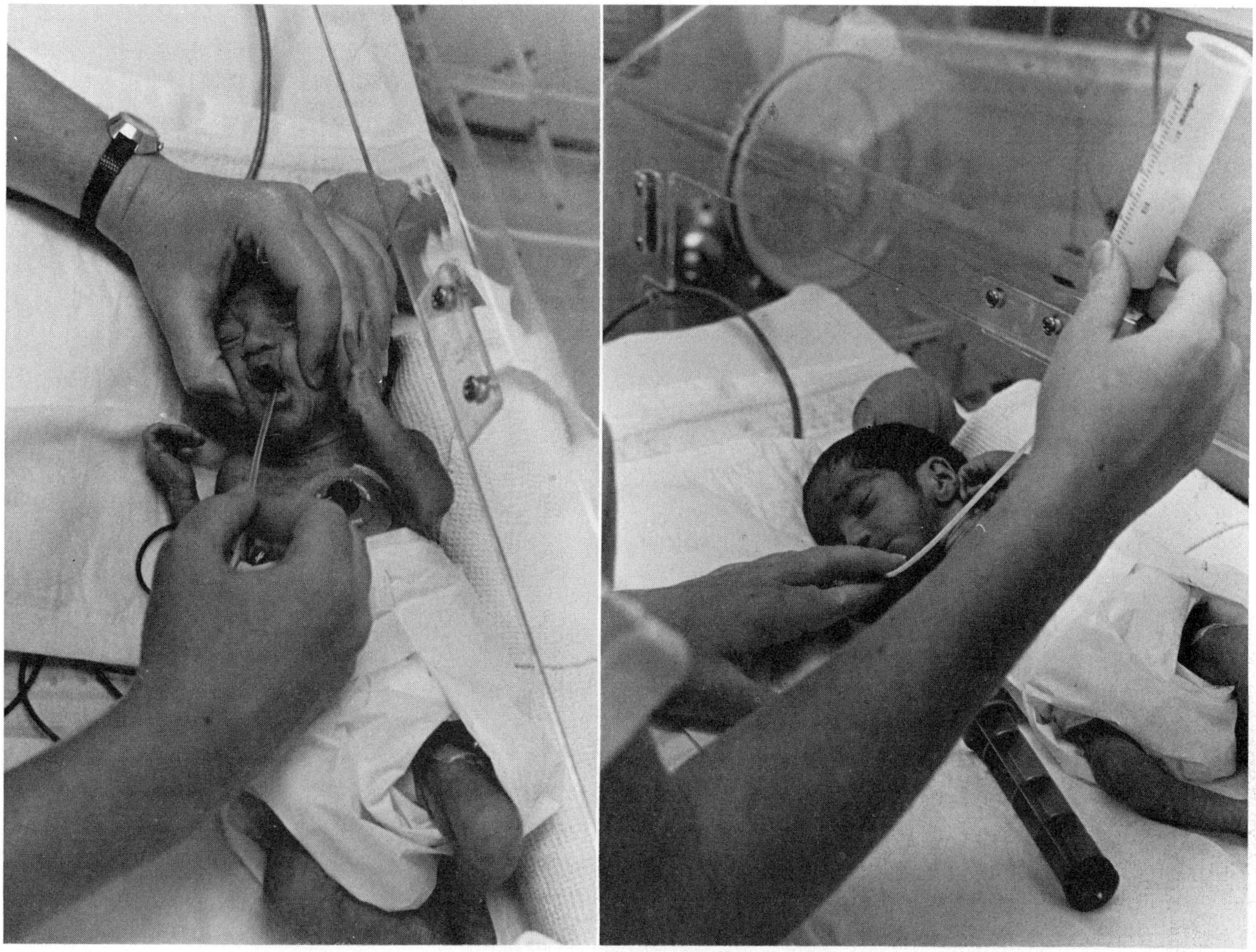

A B

Fig. 26-26. Gavage feeding. **A,** Insertion of tube. **B,** Formula flowing into tube by gravity.

tubes to 5 ml for large ones) to clear it of formula. Indwelling catheters are capped or clamped to prevent loss of feeding and entry of air into the stomach.

7. Remove the tube by first pinching it firmly to prevent escape of fluid as the tube is withdrawn. Withdraw the tube quickly.

8. Position the child on the right side or abdomen for at least 1 hour in the same manner as following any infant feeding to minimize the possibility of regurgitation and aspiration. If the child's condition permits, he can be bubbled after the feeding.

9. Record the feeding, including the type and amount of residual, the type and amount of formula, and the manner in which it was tolerated. For most infant feedings any amount of residual fluid aspirated from the stomach is refed and the amount subtracted from the prescribed amount of feeding. For example, if the infant is to receive 30 ml and 3 ml is aspirated from the stomach before the feeding, the 3 ml of aspirated stomach contents is refed plus 27 ml of feeding.

Gastrostomy feeding

Feeding by way of gastrostomy tube is a variation of tube feeding that is often used for children in whom passage of a tube through the mouth, pharynx, esophagus, and cardiac sphincter of the stomach is contraindicated or impossible or to avoid the constant irritation of a nasogastric tube in children who require tube feeding over an extended period of time. Placement of a gastrostomy tube is an operative procedure performed under general anesthesia. The tube is inserted through the abdominal wall into the stomach about midway along the greater curvature and secured by a purse-string suture. The stomach is anchored to the peritoneum at the operative site. The tube used can be a plain, Foley, or mushroom catheter with the tip removed. Immediately after surgery the catheter is usually left open and attached to gravity drainage for approximately 24 hours. Postoperative care of the wound site is directed toward prevention of infection and irritation. The area is cleansed and covered with a sterile dressing daily or as often as needed to keep the area dry. After healing takes place a dressing is usually not required, but meticulous care is needed to keep the area surrounding the tube clean and dry to prevent excoriation and infection. Daily applications of ointment, karaya powder, or other preparations may be prescribed to aid in healing and prevention of irritation. Care is exercised to prevent excessive pull on the catheter that might cause widening of the opening and subsequent leakage of highly irritating gastric juices.

Positioning and feeding of water, formula, or pureed foods are carried out in the same manner and rate as gavage feeding. After feedings the infant or child is positioned on the right side or in Fowler's position, and the tube may be left open and suspended or clamped between feedings, depending on the child's condition (Fig. 26-27). Sometimes a Y tube is used to allow for simultaneous decompression during feeding. The tube is usually left open for the first few days after insertion, but a clamped tube allows more mobility. If a Foley catheter is used as the gastrostomy tube, very slight tension should be applied after feeding to ascertain that the balloon is at the gastrostomy opening. The tube is then securely taped into place to prevent the possibility that the balloon might make its way to the pyloric sphincter and occlude the stomach outlet.

When the gastrostomy is no longer needed, the skin opening ordinarily closes spontaneously by contracture after removal.

PROCEDURES RELATED TO ELIMINATION

Children seldom have problems with elimination, but in cases of severe constipation or when an empty rectum is needed prior to surgery or diagnostic procedures, an enema may be administered to stimulate rectal emptying. A number of conditions in the newborn and childhood period also require formation of an ostomy for purposes of elimination. Ostomy care and management are discussed in relation to gastrointestinal problems on p. 1274.

Enema

The procedure for giving an enema to an infant or child does not differ essentially from that for an adult. Infants and small children do not have sensory control in the rectum and are unable to retain the fluid; therefore, the enema is administered and expelled while the child is lying with the buttocks over the bedpan and his head and back supported with pillows. A french catheter size 10 to 12 is inserted approximately 2 to 4 inches into the ampulla of the rectum. An isotonic solution is used in children; if prepared saline

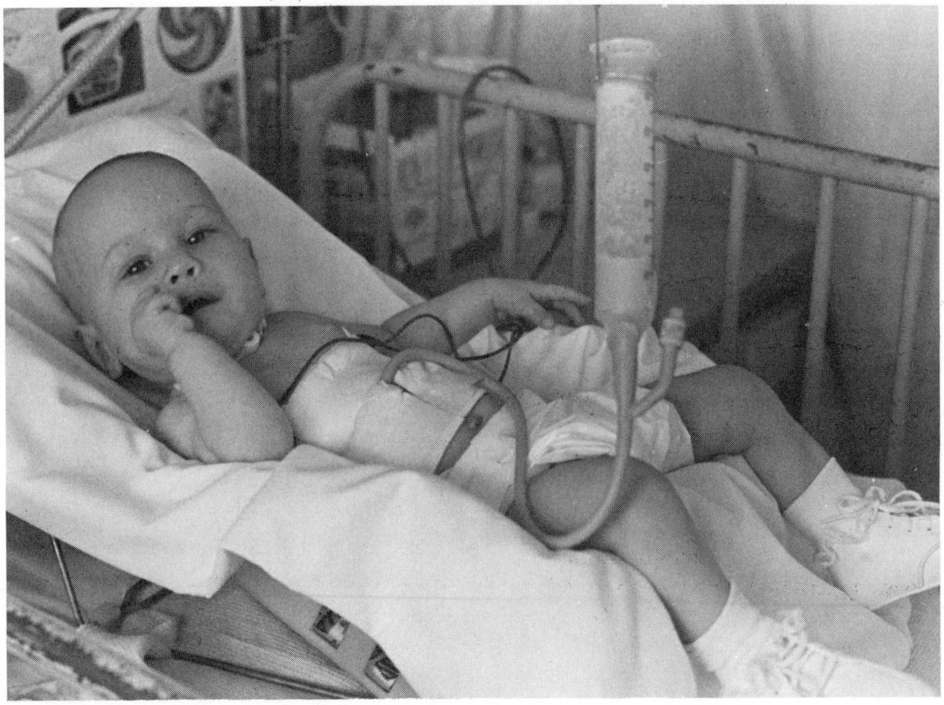

Fig. 26-27. Gastrostomy feeding. Syringe barrel suspended to allow thick formula to enter stomach by gravity.

is not available, it can be made from 1 tsp table salt in 500 ml (1 pint) of tap water. Plain water is rarely used in children because, being hypotonic, it can cause rapid fluid shift and fluid overload. The Fleet enema is not advised for children because of the harsh action of its ingredients (sodium biphosphate and sodium phosphate). Commercial enemas can be dangerous to patients with megacolon and to dehydrated or azotemic children.

The amount of solution to be administered varies with the size of the child. Suggested amounts are:

Age	*Amount (ml)*
Infant	150-250
Small child	250-350
Larger child	300-500
Adolescent	500-750

Infants and small children are unable to retain the solution after it is administered; therefore, the buttocks must be held together for a short time if fluid is to be retained. Older children are ordinarily able to hold the solution if they understand what to do and if they are not expected to hold it for too long a period of time. It is well to have the bedpan handy or, for the ambulatory child, to make certain that the bathroom is clear and available before beginning the procedure. An enema is an intrusive procedure and thus threatening to the preschool child; therefore, a careful explanation is especially important.

USE OF PLAY AS NURSING INTERVENTION

Play is one of the most important aspects of a child's life. It is children's natural means of expression and a major way in which they learn about the world around them. It can be one of the most effective tools for managing stress. Since illness and hospitalization constitute crises in the life of a child and these situations are often fraught with overwhelming stresses, to play out their fears and anxieties affords a means by which children can cope with these stresses in any setting—home, clinic, and hospital.

Play is the "work" of children. It is essential to their mental, emotional, and social well-being, and, like their developmental needs, the need for play does not stop when children are ill or when they enter the hospital. Through play children learn to deal with other children. Play also provides a medium for understanding some of the adult roles and activities that are puzzling and frustrating to them. Play, although primarily imaginative, is related to reality and, thus, leads to learning. Children in the hospital have the same basic needs as children in other settings; therefore, their medical needs should be supplemented by those activities that maintain their identity, make them feel secure in the foreign environment, and build self-esteem while they cope with new and difficult experiences. Play in the hospital relieves tension and anxiety, lessens the stress of separation and feelings of homesickness, and helps the child to relax, achieve a sense of security, understand procedures and therapies, express fears and fantasies, learn, and build social relationships.

Diversional activities

Almost any form of play can be used for diversion and recreation, but the activity should be selected on the basis of the child's age, interests, and limitations. Children do not necessarily need special direction for using play materials. All they require is the raw materials with which to work, adult approval, and supervision to help keep their natural enthusiasm or expression of feelings from getting out of control. Small children enjoy a variety of small colorful toys that they can play with in bed or in their room or more elaborate play equipment, such as playhouses, sandboxes, rhythm instruments, and large boxes and blocks, that may be a part of the hospital playroom.

Games that can be played alone or with another child or an adult are popular with older children, as are puzzles; reading material; quiet individual activities such as sewing, stringing beads, and weaving; and Tinker-Toys, Lincoln logs, and other building materials. Assembling models is an excellent pastime, but it is a good idea to make certain that all pieces and necessary materials are included in the package. It is disappointing to the child to be ready to begin a project only to find that an essential item, such as glue, is missing from the set.

Well-selected books are of infinite value to the child. Children never tire of stories. To have someone read aloud provides endless hours of pleasure and is of special value to the child who has limited energy to expend in play (Fig. 26-28). A radio and/or television set, a part of most hospital room equipment, is a useful tool for entertaining a child, but parents and nurses should monitor program selection and it should not be used as a substitute for social interaction or therapeutic play.

When supervising play for ill or convalescent children, it is best to select activities that are simpler than normally would be chosen according to the specific developmental level of the child. These children usually do not have the energy to cope with more challenging activities. Other limitations also influence the type of activities. Special consideration must be given to the child who is confined in terms of movement, has an extremity restricted, or is isolated. Toys for isolated children must be capable of being disposed of or disinfected after use.

Toys. Parents of hospitalized children often ask nurses about the types of toys that would be best to bring for their child who is hospitalized. Most want to bring new ones to cheer and comfort the child and assuage their own guilt feelings regarding the child's need for hospitalization. It is wise to assure the parents that, although it is natural to want to provide these things for their child, it is often better to wait awhile to bring new things, especially in the case

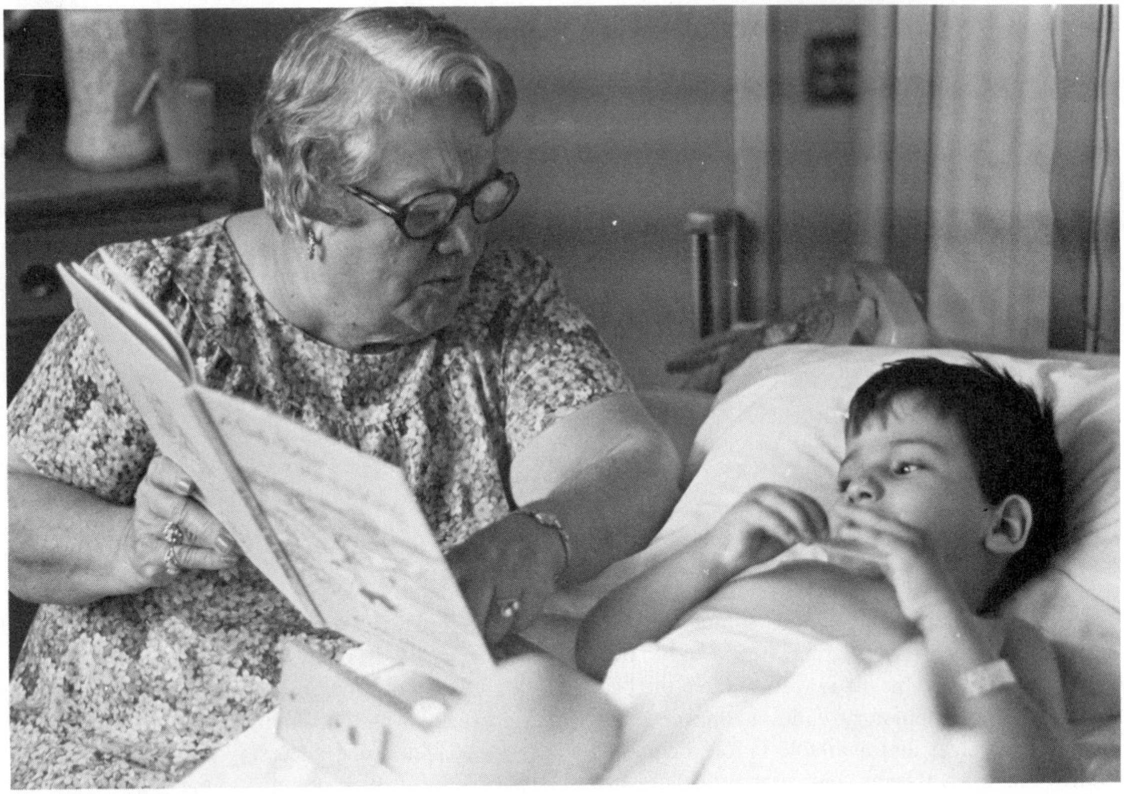

Fig. 26-28. Children never tire of listening to stories. A ward "grandmother" reads to a bedfast boy.

of younger children. Small children need the comfort and reassurance of familiar things, such as the stuffed animal the child hugs for comfort and takes with him to bed at night. These are a link with home and the world outside the hospital.

Large numbers of toys often confuse and frustrate a small child. A few small, well-chosen toys are usually preferred to one large expensive one. Children who are hospitalized for a period of time benefit from changes. Rather than a confusing accumulation of toys, older toys are replaced periodically as interest wanes. A helpful suggestion is to have parents provide the child with a shoe box, a child's small suitcase, or a knapsack to attach to the bed for an easy storage receptacle to prevent small items from becoming lost in the sheets or under the bed. Children love putting things in and taking things out of a larger container. Many simple items, such as a small magnifying glass, a magnet, grooming aids, a small mirror, crayons and coloring books, colorful paper with scissors and paste, a magic slate, small dolls or toy soldiers, small cars, and beads to string, afford endless hours of amusement. It is the responsibility of the nurse to assess the safety of the toys brought to the child.

A highly successful diversion for a child who is hospitalized for a length of time and whose parents are unable to visit frequently is for them to bring a box with seven small, inexpensive, and brightly wrapped items with a different day of the week printed on the outside. The child will eagerly anticipate the time for opening each one. When the parents know when their next visit will be, they can provide the number of packages that corresponds to the days between visits. In this way the child knows that the diminishing packages also represent the anticipated visit from the parent.

Use of play in nursing activities

The use of play is an integral part of relationships with children, and, as such, its value in specific situations is discussed throughout this book. Many institutions have very elaborate and well-organized play areas and programs under the direction of specially trained occupational therapists, whereas some have limited facilities and others have no designated play area. No matter what the institution provides for the children, nurses can still include play activities as part of nursing care. Play is an effective means of diversion or a means of occupying long, lonely hours. It can be used to teach, for expression of feelings, or as a method to achieve a therapeutic goal.

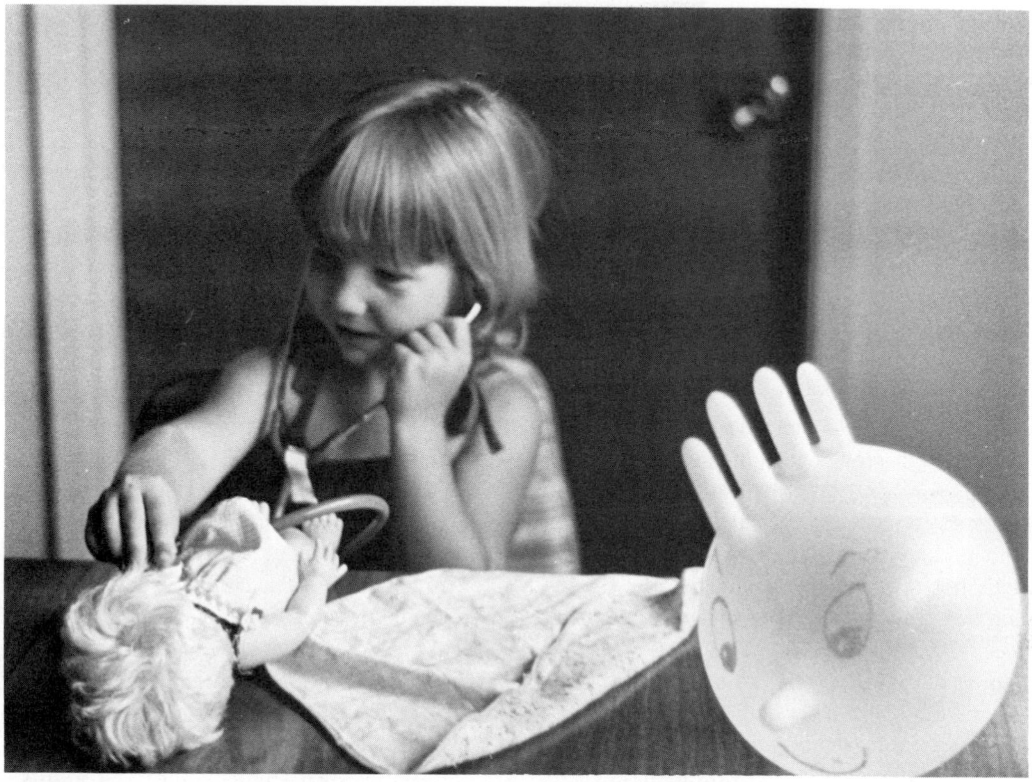

Fig. 26-29. Balloon fashioned from surgical glove.

Fluid intake. Sometimes it is difficult to persuade children to drink an adequate amount of fluid. They may not feel well, their throat or mouth may hurt, or the unfamiliar hospital environment and the strangers who inhabit it may be deterrents. When a child refuses to drink or drinks an insufficient amount of fluid, whether or not the reason can be determined from careful assessment, a variety of techniques can be employed to encourage an intake of fluid. Appealing forms of fluids are Popsicles, frozen juice bars, and Slurpies or Snowcones made by pouring flavored syrup over crushed ice. Vegetable coloring added to water or milk makes the liquid more interesting, and Jell-O is always a favorite with children. When circumstances permit, the child can help make the Jell-O and pour it into small, interesting containers (such as a medicine cup) to set.

Children are more likely to take fluid if drinking is part of a game or other fun activity. Incorporating the drinking into a story is a useful ploy, for example, taking a drink each time the page is turned. A drink can be part of the child's "turn" in a game, and children love to drink from interesting containers such as small decorated cups, glasses, or other containers. Colorful or unusually shaped drinking straws add appeal. A child may enjoy filling a syringe with water and squirting it directly into his mouth or using it to fill a small cup. A medicine cup is a convenient size for this purpose, but it should be decorated or otherwise modified so that the intake of fluid is not associated with taking medicine. Children will often drink a great deal when fluid is served at a tea party at which they can pour drinks from a toy teapot, pitcher, or coffeepot into toy cups or glasses. This is especially appealing when the child can include others and sit on a chair at a small table.

Deep breathing. There are a number of devices and activities that can be used effectively to encourage a child to breathe deeply. There are several devices manufactured specifically for this purpose; however, when these are unavailable, a number of play activities serve as practical substitutes or supplemental exercises. Blowing soap bubbles appeals to many children, and blowing up balloons is an excellent measure for increasing end-expiratory pressure. Interesting balloons can be fashioned from surgical gloves (Fig. 26-29), which the child can also decorate with felt pens. Blow bottles designed to force liquid from one container to another can be constructed with discarded bottles, stoppers, and tubing and are more enticing when the water is colored with food coloring. Other activities that stimulate lung expansion are blowing feathers, whistle toys (such as those used for parties), musical instruments (ocharina, harmonica) where the environment permits, and blowing cotton balls around the table through a straw.

Range of motion and use of extremities. There are a variety of ways to provide range of motion exercises for children that combine fun with therapy. Any kind of throwing activity provides movement for the shoulder, elbow, and wrist. Wadded-up paper or bean bags can be thrown into a wastebasket, a box, or a target such as a hole cut into a large box. Toys attached to the end of a pulley are fun to manipulate. Activities that involve imaginative movement encourage exercising the extremities, for example, pretending to be a bird, a butterfly, or a wild horse. A tricycle, where permitted, requires knee, hip, and ankle movement. Positioning the bed so that the child must turn to view the television or the doorway encourages him to assume different positions.

Soaks. To gain young children's cooperation for hand or foot soaks is difficult unless the procedure is made attractive to them through play. Older infants and toddlers delight in playing with brightly colored marbles scattered over the bottom of the receptacle, and preschoolers can be challenged to hold a floating item beneath the water surface. These activities require supervision, because infants and small children will often place items in their mouths and children can easily lose control with water play. Washing dishes, cars, dolls, or doll clothes will occupy many children for quite some time. The older child is able to cooperate but may need something to do while confined during the procedure. Therapeutic baths are always more interesting when the child is accompanied by toy boats or other items for water play.

Expression

Play provides one of the best opportunities for encouraging emotional expression, including the safe release of anger and hostility. Nondirective play that allows children freedom for expression can be tremendously therapeutic. Therapeutic play, however, should not be confused with the psychologic technique of play therapy. *Play therapy* is reserved for use by trained and qualified therapists who use the technique as an interpretative method with emotionally disturbed children. *Therapeutic play,* on the other hand, is a very effective nondirective modality for helping children deal with their concerns and fears, whereas, at the same time, it often helps the nurse to gain insights into their needs and feelings.

Tension release can be facilitated through almost any activity and, with younger ambulatory children, large-muscle activity such as use of tricycles, wagons, and so on is especially beneficial. A great deal of aggression can be safely directed into pounding and throwing games and activities. Bean bags are often thrown at a target or open receptacle with surprising vigor and hostility. A pounding board is employed with enthusiasm by young children; clay and Play Dough are marvelous media for use at any age. It is not uncommon to see an angry child of 9 or 10 years of age attacking a mound of clay with the same intensity that is observed in his 3- or 4-year-old counterpart.

Creative expression. Drawing and painting are excellent media for expression. The child need only be supplied with the raw materials, such as crayons and paper; pots of bright poster color, large brushes, and an ample supply of newsprint supported on easels; or materials for finger painting. Children usually require little direction for self-expression; however, older children may be given some direction in what to paint or draw. For example, they may be asked to draw the hospital room, draw what they like about the hospital, or draw what they do not like about the hospital. Groups of children can enjoy this creative activity either working individually or, with older children, collaborating on a group project such as a mural painted on a long piece of butcher paper. For children confined to bed, an old sheet (acquired from the laundry) spread over the bed and a large gown that extends down over the bedclothes to cover their own gown provide protection to clean linen.

Holidays provide stimulus and direction for unlimited creative projects. The children can participate in decorating the pediatric unit, and making pictures and decorations for their rooms gives the children a sense of pride and accomplishment. This is especially beneficial for immobilized and isolated children. Making gifts for someone at home helps to maintain interpersonal ties.

Dramatic play. Dramatic play is a well-recognized technique for emotional release, as children reenact frightening or puzzling hospital experiences. Through use of puppets, replicas of hospital equipment, or some actual hospital equipment, children can play out the situations that are a part of their hospital experience. Dramatic play enables children to learn about procedures and events that will concern them and to assume the roles of the adults in the hospital environment (Fig. 26-30). Miniature versions of hospital properties such as gurneys and x-ray and intravenous equipment can be used to explain what the children can expect and permit them to experience vicariously the situations that are unfamiliar and potentially frightening. Allowing children to handle actual items that will be used in their care, such as a stethoscope, sphygmomanometer, or oxygen mask, helps them to develop familiarity with these items and to reduce the threat often associated with their use. Children delight in listening to their own or another's heartbeat and to act out both commonplace and unusual events that take place in the course of their hospitalization.

Puppets are universally effective for communicating with children. Most children view them as peers and readily communicate with them. Children will relate to the puppet feelings that they hesitate to express to adults. Puppets can share children's own experiences and help them to find solutions to their problems. Puppets dressed to represent figures in the child's environment, for example, a physician, nurse, or therapist and members of the child's own family, are especially useful. Small, appropriately attired

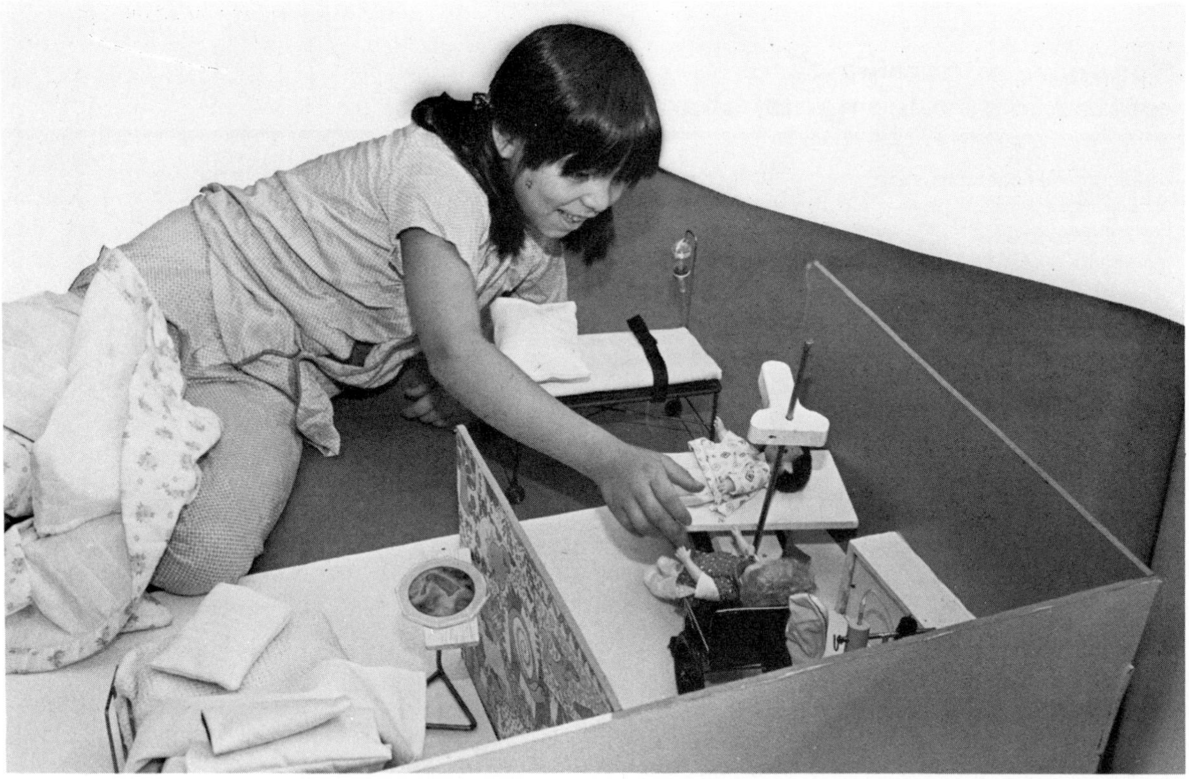

Fig. 26-30. Child playing with miniature hospital furniture.

dolls are equally effective in encouraging the child to play out situations, although puppets are usually best for direct conversation.

Injections One of the most threatening procedures and a familiar one to all children is the hypodermic injection. Hospital play involving this stress-provoking equipment can be very revealing as well as therapeutic. Children respond in various ways to play with syringes. Usually children approach the syringe with respect and caution as though it were a dangerous weapon. Many hesitate to handle the equipment and require some time to muster the courage to touch the feared object. Once the initial hesitancy is overcome, however, children cannot resist handling the syringe and are willing to "give a shot" to a doll or stuffed animal. Some handle the syringe gingerly and carefully imitate the ritual they have observed in their role models, that is, wiping the area with an alcohol sponge before and after injecting the solution and placing a Band-Aid over the puncture site. Others repeatedly ram the needle into the doll with surprising vigor and expression of hostility.

It has been found repeatedly that children who are exposed to needle play and who are able to act out the unpleasant experience are then able to tolerate the procedure with less apparent distress. Although they still protest when they must receive an injection, the overt manifestations are less violent and last for a shorter period of time.

Hospitalized children

In planning any play activities for the hospitalized child, the nurse must not lose sight of the fact that the reason for the child's hospitalization always takes precedence over other considerations, including the need for play. Play must be scheduled around medical needs and any limitations imposed by the child's condition. For example, it is not uncommon for small children to eat paste and other creative media; therefore, a child who is allergic to wheat should not be given finger paint made from wallpaper paste or play dough made with flour. A child on a restricted salt intake should not play with modeling dough, since salt is one of its major constituents. Treatment schedules and the rules and policies of the institution must be considered, also. At home the play program should be planned around the therapy regimen. However, play can be satisfactorily incorporated into the child's care if the nurse and others involved allow some flexibility and use creativity in planning for play.

SUMMARY OF DEVELOPMENTAL CHARACTERISTICS AND NURSING INTERVENTIONS

The task of providing care to children is facilitated by the understanding and application of developmental concepts. The boxed material on pp. 952 to 955 relies heavily

Text continued on p. 956.

Summary of nursing care related to developmental characteristics

Developmental characteristics	Responsibilities
Early infancy: developing a sense of basic trust	
Diffuse, global response to stimuli	Control head for administration of medications to prevent spilling
Random limb movements; reflex withdrawal of limb	Restrain limbs for injection, dressing, or intravenous therapy
Strong grasp reflex	Keep harmful objects out of reach of hands Keep in mind that infant may grasp and pull at tubing, for example, intravenous or gavage tubes
Strong sucking reflex	Administer medications through nipple; control rate of flow from dropper or syringe to prevent possible choking from administration that is too rapid
Crying in response to noxious stimuli	Increase likelihood of aspiration if distressed by solutions placed in mouth
Satiety center fully functioning; when full, child falls asleep	Administer medications and perform procedures prior to feeding
Tongue thrust, which is used for sucking, may eject substance from mouth	Place food well back in mouth Refeed medication and food if necessary Place medications at side of mouth between tongue and cheek
Relaxed cardiac sphincter	Perform procedures prior to feeding to avoid stimulating vomiting
Later infancy: establishing basic trust	
Able to sit with support; stands holding onto crib sides	Employ adequate safety measures
Increasing mobility	Keep in mind that child who does not wish to cooperate is able to resist with entire body Request assistance to immobilize child if necessary
Developing fine motor hand control	Keep medicines and harmful objects out of reach
Beginning active cortical control	Restrain adequately for unpleasant procedures
Active lip and tongue movements	Retrieve and refeed food and medications
Eating well with fingers	Provide finger foods
Swallowing and tongue movements better syncronized	Give fluids and medications in a cup
Relaxed cardiac sphincter	Perform procedures prior to feeding to reduce likelihood of vomiting
Recognition of family and association of care givers with comfort and security	Enlist care giver as ally for giving medications that are not unpleasant Encourage care giver to be involved in care Use care giver as comforter after unpleasant experiences

Summary of nursing care related to developmental characteristics—cont'd

Developmental characteristics	Responsibilities
Later infancy: establishing basic trust—cont'd	
Stranger anxiety	Make advances slowly and in nonthreatening manner
Memory for pleasant and unpleasant experiences	Keep in mind that infant associates objects or persons with prior painful experiences Keep in mind that infant will cry and resist at sight of persons or objects that inflict pain or discomfort
Imitation of gestures	Model desired behavior, for example, opening mouth
Toddlerhood: developing a sense of autonomy	
Increasingly able and prefers to do things for himself	Allow to drink liquids, including medicine, from a cup Help with medicine to prevent spills if needed Involve in own care whenever possible
Resistive behavior; dominant "no" stage	Use firm, direct approach Allow choices whenever possible Expect treatments to be resisted Be prepared in case food or medication is spit out Be prepared in case mouth is tightly clamped shut Use distraction techniques
Increased mobility	Keep harmful items out of reach Restrain for procedures Be prepared in case child attempts to run away Be prepared for child to throw items
Responses to simple commands	Use few and simple terms in giving directions Use words familiar to child
Increased control of muscles	Expect child to spit out distasteful substances Expect child to resist vigorously Restrain adequately for procedures and treatments
Recalling impressionable experiences	Keep in mind that previous experiences will affect current responses Disguise unpleasant tastes, such as medications and crushed tablets, in syrup
Little understanding of time	Use immediate concrete rewards Avoid having child wait when possible Have preparations for activities made before involving the child, for example, bath water in tub, tray at table, and so on
Conflict between "hanging on" and "letting go"; therefore, tendency to dawdle	Use firm, positive approach with simple direct commands Make choices simple
Poor frustration tolerance; tantrums common	Ignore temper tantrums Be consistent in expectations and demands Realize that bargaining is usually ineffectual

Continued.

Summary of nursing care related to developmental characteristics—cont'd

Developmental characteristics	Responsibilities
Toddlerhood: developing a sense of autonomy—cont'd	
More comfortable with the familiar; ritualistic	Determine child's way of doing things and words he uses Use familiar terms for objects and behaviors, for example, toileting Involve care giver when possible Use items familiar to child Allow child to handle unfamiliar items to become familiar and more apt to cooperate
Participating in routines of daily living	Allow to participate in care
Imitativeness	Demonstrate behaviors expected Use small replicas of adult equipment, such as dishes and cups Use games to gain cooperation
Limited language	Communicate with behaviors
Close attachment to parents	Encourage frequent visiting Encourage family to bring items that child relates with home and loved ones, for example, photographs, favorite toy, transitional items (blanket) Involve parents in care Encourage child to talk about home and family
Seeing parents as protectors	Use parents as comforting persons Do not involve parents in painful procedures
Preschool period: developing a sense of initiative	
Concrete thought; egocentric	Explain procedures in simple terms and in relationship to how activity will affect child personally
Increased fine motor coordination	Realize that preschool child is better able to participate in his own care Realize that preschool child is able to take pills and tablets Allow to participate in more complex activities
Refined senses of taste and smell	Realize that disguising tastes is usually less effective Determine child's preferences when planning for diet needs
Increasing use of initiative	Include child in decision making Request assistance in evaluating alternatives Set clear definitions of limitations for behavior and activity
Little concept of conservation	Use the size of container or serving that gives child the impression that the amount or volume is smaller
Increased language capabilities	Encourage to verbalize feelings and ideas Realize that preschool child is able to understand simple explanations
Better concept of time; better able to delay gratification	Use rewards that are not immediate Use social interaction as effective motivating force
Frustration tolerance still limited but better developed	Take time for short explanation Do not prolong explanations or argue, which will increase anxiety Realize that preschool child has poor ability to cooperate in unpleasant treatments and procedures
Able to retain information for longer periods of time	Spend time on health teaching, which can have long-term benefits
May view illness and hospitalization as punishment	Elicit child's concept of situation Give careful explanations, which are beneficial Allow control when possible Encourage positive relationships with significant persons Allow expression of hostile feelings in acceptable activities

Summary of nursing care related to developmental characteristics—cont'd

Developmental characteristics	Responsibilities
Preschool period: developing a sense of initiative—cont'd	
Fear of body mutilation dominant	Explain procedures carefully Explain relationship between cause of illness and therapy Realize that preschool child is likely to resist intrusive procedures
Dramatic play predominates	Use hospital play, which can be very effective in reducing anxiety Use role playing for tension release, understanding experiences, and teaching Use dramatic play, which is an excellent mechanism for teaching and explaining
Fear of unknown and dark—especially when alone	Make certain that call bell or other means for communicating is at hand Allow night-light Explain unfamiliar situations
School-age period: developing a sense of industry	
Can assume responsibility for actions	Allow responsibility for simple tasks, such as collecting specimens Include in decision making
Industrious; enjoys helping	Allow active involvement in care Involve in ward activities where possible—collating charts, playing with small children, and so on
Interested in acquisition of knowledge	Explain procedures Explain functioning and mechanisms of equipment in simple terms Allow child to manipulate equipment when possible Provide materials for child to "play hospital" Arrange to continue with schoolwork
Competitiveness	Expect school-age child to respond to challenges and rewards Arrange to keep up with schoolwork so child will not fall behind classmates
Beginning to see relationships	Reason with child
Increased self-control	Attempt to gain child's cooperation Request assistance to maintain control in stressful situations as needed
Peer relationships important	Place with children of similar age Allow visits from peers (where hospital policy allows)
Developing self-esteem	Provide positive feedback Accept loss of control without reprimand
Adolescence: developing sense of identity	
Importance of peer group	Allow visiting from peers Provide telephone for maintaining contact outside Allow adolescent to continue activities that are important to him, for example, playing records and tapes
Increasingly capable of abstract thought	Realize that adolescent is able to see long-term consequences of actions Realize that adolescent is able to understand explanations of condition and therapy program
Striving for independence	Involve adolescent in decision making and planning activities Impose as few restrictions as feasible Realize that adolescent may have difficulty in adjusting to new authority figures—resistance to therapy not uncommon Expect noncompliance
Acutely conscious of body and appearance	Provide for some privacy Encourage grooming activities and wearing attractive attire Relate health teaching to appearance

on work developed and compiled by Ormond and Caulfield[3] and presents the major developmental characteristics that have implications for nursing interventions.

REFERENCES

1. Creighton, H.: Law every nurse should know, ed. 3, Philadelphia, 1975, W. B. Saunders Co., Chapter 3.
2. Hershey, N.: Minors and consent, Am. J. Nurs. **68:**2396-2398, 1968.
3. Ormond, E. A. R., and Caulfield, C.: A practical guide to giving oral medications to young children, Am. J. Maternal Child Nurs. **1:**320-325, 1976.
4. Ziemer, M., and Carroll, J. S.: Infant gavage feeding, Am. J. Nurs. **78:**1543-1544, 1978.

BIBLIOGRAPHY

Asnes, R. S., Grebin, B., and Maqboll, S.: The inaccuracy of paper medicine cups; a warning, J. Pediatr. **83:**848, 1973.

Bergersen, B. S., and Goth, A.: Pharmacology in nursing, ed. 13, St. Louis, 1976, The C. V. Mosby Co.

Bishop, B.: How to cool a feverish child, Pediatr. Nurs. **4**(1): 19-20, 1978.

Bishop, W. S., and Head, J. J.: Care of the infant with a stoma, Am. J. Maternal Child Nurs. **1:**315-319, 1976.

Braddom, J.: Intramuscular injections, J.A.M.A. **214:**466-467, 1970.

Brandt, P. A., and associates: IM injections in children, Am. J. Nurs. **72:**1402-1406, 1972.

Bromberg, M. J.: Legal problems and safeguards in the ED, RN **49:**66-76, May 1973.

Campbell, A. G. M.: Infants, children, and informed consent, Br. Med. J. **39:**334-448, 1974.

Chinn, P. L.: Infant gavage feeding, Am. J. Nurs. **71:**1964-1967, 1971.

Chudzik, G. M., and Yaffee, S. J.: Introduction to the special problems of pediatric drug therapy, Drug Ther. Bull. p. 17, July 1973.

Conway, B., Mandelco, B., Trufant, J., and Scoblic, M.: The seventh right, Am. J. Nurs. **70:**1040-1043, 1970.

Dowd, E. L., Novak, J. C., and Ray, E. J.: Releasing the hospitalized child from restraints, Am. J. Maternal Child Nurs. **2:**370-373, 1977.

Duff, R. S., and Campbell, A. G. M.: Moral and ethical dilemmas in the special-care nursery, N. Engl. J. Med. **289:**890-894, 1973.

Erickson, R., and Storlie, F.: Taking temperatures: oral or rectal, and when? Nursing '73 **3:**51-53, April 1973.

Greenfield, D., Grant, R., and Lieberman, R.: Children can have high blood pressure, too, Am. J. Nurs. **76:**770-772, 1976.

Grier, M. E.: Hair care for the black patient, Am. J. Nurs. **76:** 1781, 1976.

Holder, A. R.: Minors and contraception, J.A.M.A. **216:**2059, 1971.

Johnson, J. E., Kerchhoff, K. T., and Endress, M. P.: Easing children's fright during health care procedures, Am. J. Maternal Child Nurs. **1**(4):206-210, 1976.

Littman, D.: Stethoscopes and auscultation, Am. J. Nurs. **72:** 1239-1241, 1972.

Lowenthal, W.: Factors affecting drug absorption, Am. J. Nurs. **73:**1391, 1973.

Luciano, K., and Shumsky, C. J.: Pediatric procedures, Nursing '75 **5:**49-52, January 1975.

Mason, G.: Bottle type restraints, Am. J. Nurs. **76:**1258, 1976.

McCaffery, M.: Children's responses to rectal temperature: an exploratory study, Nurs. Res. **20:**32, 1971.

McCloskey, J. R., Stanley, M. K., and Chung, M. K.: Quadriceps contracture as a result of multiple intramuscular injection, Am. J. Dis. Child **131:**416-417, 1977.

McLaughlin, G. W., and associates: Indirect measurement of blood pressure in infants utilizing Doppler ultrasound, J. Pediatr. **79:**300-302, 1971.

McLellan, C. L.: Hero badges mean more than courage, Pediatr. Nurs. **2**(3):7, 1976.

Norman, M. G., and associates: Infantile quadriceps femoris contracture resulting from intramuscular injections, N. Engl. J. Med. **282:**964-966, 1970.

Petrillo, M., and Sanger, S.: Emotional care of hospitalized children, Philadelphia, 1972, J. B. Lippincott Co.

Pitel, M.: The subcutaneous injection, Am. J. Nurs. **71:**76-79, 1971.

Plank, E. N.: Working with children in hospitals, ed. 2, Chicago, 1971, The Press of Case Western Reserve University.

Rowland, M.: Influence of route of administration on drug availability, J. Pharm. Sci. **61:**70, 1972.

Shaw, A.: Dilemmas of informed consent in children, N. Engl. J. Med. **289:**885-890, 1973.

Shirkey, H. C.: Dosage forms for administration—factors of importance for infants and children, Chapter 4; Dosage, Chapter 6; and Drug administration, Chapter 12. In Shirkey, H. C.: Pediatric therapy, ed. 5, St. Louis, 1975, The C. V. Mosby Co.

Snell, B., and McClellan, C.: Whetting hospitalized preschooler's appetites, Am. J. Nurs. **76:**413-415, 1976.

Soparkar, B. A. P.: Trickery, white lies, and deception in pediatrics, Nursing '74 **4:**11-13, 1944.

Virnig, N. L., and Reynolds, J. W.: Reliability of flush blood pressure measurements in the sick newborn infant, J. Pediatr. **84:**594-598, 1974.

Warren, F. M.: Blood pressure readings: getting them quickly on an infant, Nursing '75 **5**(4):5, 1975.

Use of play as nursing intervention

Azarnoff, P., and Flegal, S.: A pediatric play program: developing a therapeutic play program for children in medical settings, Springfield, Ill., 1975, Charles C Thomas, Publisher.

Brooks, M. M.: Why play in the hospital? Nurs. Clin. North Am. **5:**431-442, 1970.

Byers, M. L.: Play interviews with a five-year-old boy, Maternal Child Nurs. J. **1:**133-141, Summer 1972.

Caplan, F., and Caplan, T.: The power of play, New York, 1973, Anchor Press.

Gerbing, D. D.: Putting play to work in pediatrics, Am. J. Maternal Child Nurs. **2**(6):387, 1977.

Gibbons, M. B.: When parents ask about play, Pediatr. Nurs. **3**(6):19-22, 1977.

Gnus, M.: A therapeutic play session in a health center, Am. J. Maternal Child Nurs. **2:**193, Fall 1973.

Green, C. S.: Understanding children's needs through therapeutic play, Nursing '74 **4**(10):31-32, 1974.

Green, C. S.: Larry thought puppet-play "childish," but it helped him face his fears, Nursing '75 **5**(3):30-33, 1975.

Hames, C. C., and Ingham, M.: The colorful creatures of continuous care, Am. J. Maternal Child Nurs. **2**(6):385-386, 1977.

Hott, J.: Rx: play PRN in pediatric nursing, Nurs. Forum **9**(3): 288, 1970.

Juenker, D.: Play as a tool of the nurse. In Steele, S., editor: Nursing care of the child with long-term illness, New York, 1971, Appleton-Century-Crofts.

Knudsen, K.: Play therapy: preparing the young child for surgery, Nurs. Clin. North Am. **10:**679-686, 1975.

Murphy, D. C.: The therapeutic value of children's literature, Nurs. Forum **11**(2):142-164, 1972.

Norberta, Sr.: Caring for children with the help of puppets, Am. J. Maternal Child Nurs. **1**(1):22-25, 1976.

Piers, M. W., editor: Play and development, New York, 1972, W. W. Norton & Co., Inc.

Porter, C. S.: Grade school children's perceptions of internal body parts, Nurs. Res. **23:**384-391, 1974.

Shufer, S.: Teaching via the play-discussion group, Am. J. Nurs. **77:**1960-1962, 1977.

Smith, E. C.: Are you really communicating? Am. J. Nurs. **77:** 1966-1968, 1977.

Smith, L. F.: An experiment with play therapy, Am. J. Nurs. **77:**1963-1965, 1977.

Wheeler, A. C.: The magic cart, Am. J. Nurs. **71:**2172-2174, 1971.

Whitson, B. J.: The puppet treatment in pediatrics, Am. J. Nurs. **72:**1612-1614, 1972.

UNIT ELEVEN
The child with a terminal illness

Although most childhood illnesses respond favorably to appropriate medical/surgical intervention, some do not. However, with advances in treatment, many invariably fatal illnesses are now amenable to a prolonged period of remission and possibly cure. Despite this fact, families constantly live under the threat of potential loss of their child. As a result health professionals are faced with the challenges of providing the best medical and nursing care for the physical problem and meeting the family's psychologic and emotional needs as well.

Chapter 27, *The Child Who is Potentially Terminally Ill,* is an overview of each family member's reaction to a life-threatening illness, the grieving process before and after death, and nursing interventions to assist the family through each phase of the illness. Because of the chronic nature of many terminal illnesses, the intent of this chapter is to detail the family's responses and needs from the time of diagnosis to the resolution phase after death.

Chapter 28, *The Child With a Life-Threatening Disorder,* discusses those disorders that at present are life threatening despite advances in treatment that indefinitely prolong life. They have been grouped together and placed in Chapter 28 to reinforce the psychologic and physical nursing activities necessary for comprehensive care of the child and family.

27

The child who is potentially terminally ill

The finality of life is a fact that most people effectively deny until they are faced with their own impending death or the loss of a loved one. As a famous philosopher stated, "One can no more look steadily at death than at the sun." However, many nurses are forced to cope with dying and death, regardless of their preparation and readiness to shed the denial and deal directly with this experience.

There is probably no more difficult death to face than that of a child, because the end of life is premature and without purpose or fulfillment. It is the purpose of this chapter to establish some theoretic and practical guidelines for helping families cope with the loss of a child. There are no absolute, definitive answers, only the personal willingness to become involved, to feel with the child and family, and to find one's own answers through individual experiences and dedicated learning.

CHILDREN'S UNDERSTANDING AND REACTIONS TO DYING AND DEATH

The concept of death is acquired through the sequential development of cognitive abilities. Although throughout childhood death is greatly influenced by the child's personal experiences with it and the explanations and attitudes offered by others, the abstract adult meaning of death as irreversible, inevitable, and universal is not understood by most children until preadolescence. Unless nurses understand how children perceive death, their fears associated with death in each age-group, and the personal meanings of death and bereavement during various stages of development, they cannot effectively counsel parents and children through the multiple crises associated with expected or unexpected death.

Infants and toddlers

Concept of death. Death has the least significance to infants younger than 6 months of age. Before the recognition of familiar persons, attachment to the consistent care giver, usually the mother, and demonstration of stranger anxiety, death, loss, or separation has little meaning for the infant. However, once parent-child attachment and the development of trust are well established, the loss, even temporarily, of that significant person elicits profound resistance from the child. Prolonged separation during the first several years is thought to be more significant in terms of future physical, social, and emotional growth than at any subsequent age.

Exactly how preverbal children view death is a mystery, although there are various developmental characteristics that support the beginning development of "predeath" or being vs nonbeing.[6] The favorite game of peekaboo amuses infants as young as 4 months of age and is based on the idea of visually being present or absent. The very nature of wakefulness and sleep establishes a cycle of being and nonbeing. The toddler and preschool years are prime periods for nightmares or fears of the dark.

Casting, the practice of throwing objects away, is a high-level activity for infants about 15 months old. Adults who persist in retrieving the cast objects will entertain the child for a prolonged time. From these games come phrases such as "all gone," another example of the beginning awareness of absence.

During the period of ages 1 year to 18 months, the ability to find hidden objects, even if the hiding place is not readily apparent, is increasingly expert. The child knows that "out of sight" does not mean "absent." Seeing an object hidden, hearing voices or footsteps, and watching someone walk behind a door may no longer indicate the physical absence of that object or person. Indeed toddlers unceasingly pursue finding objects regardless of the obstacles.

It is likely that such awareness is a precursor of the ability to perceive death on a more concrete and abstract level later in life. Also, how toddlers tolerate brief periods of separation may be an important determinant in their eventual acceptance of permanent separation—death.

Toddlers' egocentricity (self-centeredness) and vague separation of fact and fantasy make it impossible for them to comprehend absence of life. Although they may repeat what initially sounds like a correct definition of death, such as, "Grandpa is dead; he went to heaven," they may later refer to this person as if he still exists. They can only think about events in terms of their own frame of reference—living.

Reactions to death. To the amazement and dismay of adults, toddlers may persist in wanting to visit the dead person, request that all that person's possessions and living quarters remain unchanged, and talk about the deceased as if nothing has happened. Dealing honestly and openly with such reactions is preferable to admonishing the child or trying to prove to him what dead means. For example, the parent can restate that the person cannot visit because he is dead and in a special place (cemetery, heaven, or other explanation) and can offer to bring the child to visit the burial plot if possible.

Since ritualism is extremely important to toddlers, any change in the home following the death can be anxiety producing. There is no harm in allowing the ritualism, such as setting an extra place at the table for the deceased person, because, for the child, imagining the person to be present is almost as real as life. What is important is to stress that although the place is set at the table the dead person will return only in thoughts and memories. As the child grows older, forms new attachments, and develops stronger ego defenses, he will be increasingly able and willing to let go of this fantasy person.

Reactions to dying. Infants and toddlers react more to the pain and discomfort of a serious illness than to the probable fatal prognosis. Immobilization, regression to less independent levels of behavior, separation, intrusive procedures, and alteration in ritualistic routine represent the greatest threats to children in this age-group. However, they may perceive the seriousness of the illness from the parents' reactions of anxiety, sadness, depression, or anger. Although the children are unaware of the reason for such emotions, they are disturbed and upset by their parents' behavior. Helping parents deal with their feelings allows them more emotional reserve to meet the needs of their children. Encouraging them to stay in the hospital as much as possible and to participate in the child's care promotes the parents' and child's adjustment to a serious, potentially fatal illness.

Preschool children

Concept of death. Children between 3 and 5 years of age have usually heard the word "death" and have some connotation of its meaning. They see death as a departure, possibly as a kind of sleep. They may recognize the fact of physical death but do not separate it from living abilities. The dead person in the coffin still breathes, eats, sleeps, and so on. Death is temporary and gradual; life and death can change places with one another. Because of their immature concept of time, there is no real understanding of the universality and inevitability of death. Words such as "forever" and "everyone" have meaning only in the child's egocentric thinking. Waiting until Christmas may be "forever," and anybody the child denotes is "everyone."

Several characteristics of the preschoolers' cognitive and psychologic development affect their conception of death. Because of their sense of precausality, they are unable to differentiate physical cause from logical or psychologic motivation. Also, their egocentricity implies a tremendous sense of self-power and omnipotence. Therefore, they believe that their thought is sufficient to cause events. The consequence of such magical thinking is the burden of guilt, shame, and punishment.

Preschoolers' psychosexual development heavily influences their understanding of death. They strongly identify with the parent of the opposite sex and wish to replace the same-sex parent. Casual expressions such as a daughter's desire to marry her father are evidence of this attachment to the opposite-sex parent. Usually this Oedipus or Electra complex is resolved by eventually identifying with the same-sex parent in terms of role functions. However, if the same-sex parent should die during this time, preschoolers feel responsible for the death because of their wishes to rid themselves of the competition. If the opposite-sex parent dies, they may be troubled because the desired object is taken from them.

Reactions to dying. If preschoolers become seriously ill during this time, they conceive of the illness as a punishment for their thoughts against the competitor parent. The usual diagnostic and treatment procedures, combined with enforced hospitalization, only confirm their belief that they are being punished. If the parents do not stay with them during hospitalization or prevent the traumatic procedures, they are convinced that the parents are retaliating for the child's previous misdeeds or bad thoughts.

The same principles of magical thinking and omnipotence affect preschoolers when a sibling becomes critically ill or dies. One of the most significant types of death is sudden infant death syndrome (SIDS). Because it occurs unexpectedly to a healthy infant, who may have been rejected and unwanted by a jealous sibling, preschoolers find no evidence to support a physical cause of death. Indeed the parents are frequently unaware of the reason for the fatality and may question any possible cause. If preschoolers are in any way accused or suspected of having harmed the infant, they may feel extremely guilty and responsible for the tragedy. On observing their parent's acute grief, they may interpret the anger or depression as a rejection of them.

When a sibling becomes ill, the well siblings experience the loss of routine and parental attention. It is natural for them to resent such disruptions and to blame the changes on the ill child. However, preschoolers have less ability to understand the reasons for the parents' prolonged absence from the home than older children. Even though parents may explain how ill the sibling is, what the hospital is like, and why they must be there, preschoolers only see the special attention and the material rewards that the ill sister or brother receives. Since they are also unable to differentiate causes for separation of the parents and ill child, they fear that the parents may never return. If they should learn that the ill child may not get well or come home, they interpret this to mean that the parents will also never return. Their greatest fear concerning death is separation from parents.

Reactions to death. In relation to death, preschoolers may engage in activities that seem strange or abnormal to adults. For example, if a pet dies, preschoolers usually request a "funeral" or some ceremony to symbolize their loss. Perceptive parents realize that the function of such rites of passage is as important to the preschooler for the loss of a pet as to an adult for the loss of a significant person. After the "funeral" and "burial," preschoolers may dig up the remains. Many parents are confused by this behavior and label it as morbid. However, these children have no concept of the irreversible nature of death and must continually reassure themselves that the animal has not returned or gone somewhere else. If left alone to satisfy their curiosity, they will see that the dead animal is still in the ground.

Because young children accept the literal meaning of words, it is important for others to examine the implications of possible explanations for death. Those with a religious affiliation may equate death with an afterlife and explain that dead animals or people go to heaven. The act of digging up the dead pet may be a result of trying to ascertain if the animal did go to heaven. Parents who are aware of the reason for this behavior can explain that the "soul" goes to heaven but the body remains in the earth. If parents dismiss this activity without some clarification, the child may interpret the religious message as a lie.

Another common euphemism for death is "gone to sleep." Again preschoolers attach the literal meaning of sleep to death and may fear going to sleep for fear of dying or never waking up. One 5-year-old child who had been told that her aunt died because she was very tired refused to engage in any strenuous activity and took naps frequently. Her parents became concerned about her sudden lassitude and finally asked her why she was always tired. The child exclaimed that she *was not* tired; she took naps to avoid fatigue because she did not want to die like her aunt. When the parents explained that her aunt was tired from old age and sickness, not from playing too much or sleeping too little, the child immediately resumed her usual behaviors.

Because of their fewer defense mechanisms to deal with loss, young children may react to a less significant loss with more outward grief than to the loss of a very significant person. This can be extremely disconcerting to parents who view their child's undisturbed behavior as evidence of his lack of interest or response to the tragedy. However, the reverse is most likely true. The loss is so deep, painful, and threatening that the child must deny it for the present in order to survive its overwhelming impact. Behavioral reactions such as giggling, joking, attracting attention, or regressing to earlier developmental skills indicate the child's need to distance himself from the tremendous loss. Understanding the function of such behaviors and supporting the child through the reactions until such time as he feels enough self-control to grieve will help him gradually resolve the loss.

School-age children

Concept of death. Much of what pertains to the preschool period regarding the understanding of death also relates to school-age children, particularly those near 6 or 7 years of age. However, these children have a deeper understanding of death in the concrete sense. They attempt to ascribe a more comprehensible meaning to the event by personifying death as a devil, God, ghost, "bogeyman," and so on. As some of these names imply, there is a destructive connotation to death. These children particularly fear the mutilation and punishment they associate with death.

Although school-age children have a better understanding of causality, less egocentricity, and advanced perception of time, they still associate misdeeds or bad thoughts with causing death and feel intense guilt and responsibility for the event. However, because of their higher cognitive abilities, they respond well to logical explanation and comprehend the figurative meaning of words more than children in younger age-groups. Although they are less likely to interpret explanations in a purely literal sense, they are still prone to self-referenced definitions. It is important for adults to clarify the meanings of statements and to repeatedly ask them what they think.

By 9 or 10 years of age most children have an adult concept of death. They realize that it is inevitable, universal, and irreversible. Their attitudes toward death are greatly influenced by the reactions and attitudes of others, particularly their parents. Some investigators have found that those children with a religious orientation that stresses a benevolent God and reunion after death have less anxiety and fear of death than those children who equate death with sin, punishment, and hell.[1,11]

Reactions to dying. School-age children's increased ability to comprehend and reason places additional risks on them. They may fear the reason for the illness, communicability of the disease to themselves or others, consequences of the disease on their functioning and relationships with others, and the process of dying and death itself. They tend to fear the expectation of the event more than its realization. Their fear of the unknown is greater than the known, because, like preschoolers, their fantasy explanations for the unexpected or unknown are usually much more frightening and extreme than the actual situation. For this reason anticipatory preparation is very necessary and effective. These children respond well to explanations of the disease, names of drugs, and so on. Since the developmental task of this age is industry, helping children maintain control over their bodies by understanding what is happening to them and participating in what is done to them allow these youngsters to achieve independence, self-worth, and self-esteem and to avoid a sense of inferiority.

Because dying is a loss of control over every aspect of living, the realization of impending death or failing to recover is a tremendous threat to their sense of security and ego strength. These children are likely to exhibit their fear more through verbal uncooperativeness than actual physical aggression. Health professionals may erroneously interpret this behavior as rude, impolite, insolent, or stubborn. In reality the words are conveying the same meaning as physical attempts to run away or to fight others off. This verbal ''flight or fight'' reaction to stress is a plea for some control and power. Encouraging children to talk about their feelings and providing aggression outlets through play are means of dealing with this type of uncooperativeness.

Reactions to death. School-age children are very interested in postdeath services, such as wakes, funerals, and burials. They may be inquisitive about what happens to the body, such as who dresses it, what happens in an autopsy, and so on. Adults sometimes find these questions distressing, particularly when they are about a death of a significant person. However, such inquiries are children's way of assimilating all the facts about death into a concrete, logical framework. Avoiding such questions or fabricating euphemistic stories only confuses and frustrates children's attempts at understanding what may happen *to them* if they should die.

Parents usually question whether or not school-age children should attend funeral or burial services. Sharing moments of deep significance with parents helps children understand the experience and deal with their own feelings of shock, sorrow, and grief. However, children need preparation for postdeath services. They should be told what to expect, particularly how the deceased person will look if the coffin is open. Ideally the parent should explain the details to the child, but if the parent's grief prevents this communication a significant family member or friend should substitute.

It is often helpful to bring the child to the funeral service before many visitors arrive. The child is allowed his private time to say good-bye but is spared some of the unpredictable emotional reactions of others, which can be very distressing to him. Allowing the child to stay as long as he wishes but respecting his need to leave provide maximum control for the child over his ability to grieve comfortably.

Adolescents

Concept of death and reactions to dying. By far, adolescents have the most difficulty in coping with death. Although they have reached the level of adult comprehension of the concept of death, they are least likely to accept cessation of life, particularly if it is their own. Developmentally one can understand the rejection of death because the adolescent's task is to establish an identity by finding out who he is, what his purpose is, and where he belongs. Any suggestion of being different or nonbeing is a tremendous threat to the answers to such questions. Adolescents' concern is for the present much more than the past or future.

Adolescents strive for group acceptance and independence from parental constraints. As a result they rely on peer rules and beliefs for personal direction and reject opposing parental demands. However, when they are faced with the crisis of serious illness, they may consider themselves alienated from peer associations and unable to communicate with their parents for emotional support. Therefore, they may be virtually alone in their struggle for survival.

Healthy adolescents must deal with several maturational crises, such as acceptance of bodily changes and socialization of intensifying sexual impulses. Any threat to either task increases the vulnerability of adolescents to the stress of coping with such crises. The ravages of a terminal illness and the deleterious effects of chemotherapy may be greater concerns than the prospect of dying. Adolescents' orientation to the present compels them to worry about physical changes even more than the prognosis for future recovery. Sometimes parents fail to understand the emotional impact on the adolescent of side effects from chemotherapy, such as hair loss, weight gain, fatigue, or skin eruptions. They wonder why the adolescent cannot accept the temporary altered body image for the possible benefit of the treatment. Intellectually adolescents can understand the necessity of treatment, but emotionally they have great difficulty in overcoming the feelings of being different, unable to equal others, and physically compromised because of the illness.

Although older children have a mature understanding of death, they are still very much influenced by ''remnants'' of magical thinking and are subject to the feelings of guilt and shame. Since adolescents are exploring many new areas of interpersonal relationships, they are likely to see deviations from accepted behavior as reasons for their illness. It is important to clarify that thoughts and deeds do not cause leukemia, Hodgkin's disease, and so on. Focusing on the normalcy of sexual or aggressive experimentation as part of adolescent development rather than as isolated acts of deviant behavior helps adolescents rationally deal with possible misconceptions of causality.

One of the difficulties in working with adolescents is their tendency to reject adult authority for peer-group direction. Anyone who has been successful in forming trusting relationships with adolescents is acutely aware of the need to accept them as individuals and to wait for them to test out the potential risks in establishing a friendship. They want guidance, answers, and emotional support, but they also need to retain independence, control, and decision-making power.

Nurses are in a most advantageous position, because in the hospital setting they spend the greatest amount of time with the child. They can structure the hospital admission to allow for maximum self-control and independence, while allowing the adolescent the opportunity to learn to know the nurse. Answering adolescents' questions honestly, treating them as mature individuals, and respecting their needs for privacy, solitude, and personal expressions of emotions such as anger, sadness, or fear convey to adolescents the adult's true concern for their physical and emotional welfare. Nurses can help parents to communicate with their adolescent children by acting as a role model, avoiding alliances with either parent or child, and allowing parents the opportunity to ventilate their feelings of frustration, incompetence, or failure in an atmosphere of acceptance and nonjudgment.

AWARENESS OF DYING IN FATALLY ILL CHILDREN

One of the initial reactions of parents (and many health professionals) to the discovery of a potentially fatal illness is to protect the child from the impact of the diagnosis. This usually results in the "to tell or not to tell" dilemma. One of the choices is not informing the child about his illness and fabricating a plausible story to explain the treatments without implying the seriousness of the actual condition. The other choice is including the child in what is happening by explaining simply and honestly the disease process, the treatments, and the chances of recovery. Although the options seem well defined and absolute, in reality the decision is influenced by the child's level of understanding, the parents' ability to communicate with the child, and the support systems available to both.

Observations of fatally ill children

The question of whether children realize how ill they are frequently arises in discussions with parents and seems to be an important influencing factor in the final parental decision of whether or not to tell children about their disease. Several authors have studied the behaviors of terminally ill children and conclude that there is some level of comprehension, even in those situations in which children are protected from the truth. Anxiety may not be attributable to fear of death but may be demonstrated in relationship to separation, pain, intrusive procedures, bodily change or mutilation, loneliness, immobilization, and punishment. Children as young as 2 or 3 years of age perceive their parents' emotions and react accordingly.

A study by Waechter, which attempted to measure the difference in anxiety level, found that children with a fatal illness told stories of loneliness, separation, and death much more frequently than children who were well, briefly ill, or chronically ill.[13] Their stories contained a significantly greater number of references to negative affect, such as fear, sadness, and so on. Many of their stories described facts about death that related the make-believe character to themselves. One of the most significant findings indicated that the children who had an opportunity to discuss their illness, treatment, and prognosis expressed less anxiety than did the other terminally ill children who had been denied this opportunity.

Morrissey attempted to identify the specific type of anxiety in children of various ages who were fatally ill.[9] Of the three types of anxiety that were defined, he found that the majority of children 5 years of age or younger demonstrated separation anxiety and that the majority of children older than 10 years of age exhibited death anxiety (apprehensive responses related to the child's concerns with his existence or identity, as he perceives it). Very few children showed overt signs of castration anxiety. The drawings of most of the children contained many symbols of death, particularly the use of dark colors, such as black or brown. The author also found that the way in which children expressed their death anxiety was significant. Younger children tended to express it symbolically and physiologically, whereas older boys acted out and older girls became depressed and withdrawn.

Symbolic language

One of the difficulties in attempting to answer the question of whether or not children are aware of their potentially fatal prognosis is that children frequently speak in symbolic or nonverbal language. Even when asked direct questions and given the opportunity to discuss their thoughts, children may answer in a way that must be interpreted and understood by others in view of the child's age and cognitive abilities. One family who had tried to convey openness and honesty to their 9-year-old son were uncertain of his present level of understanding. After several years of remission he had relapsed and chemotherapy was no longer effective. His parents told him that the physician planned to try new drugs but that the leukemic cells had returned and had not responded to the usual treatment. He seemed to accept this information very casually. However, one day as he and his mother returned home from an outpatient visit, he began asking about funerals. He had never attended any wakes or burial ceremonies, but he wanted detailed information regarding disposal of the body. His main concern was, "Who dresses the person—does a man dress a man and a woman dress a woman?" The mother answered as honestly as she could but was disturbed by this question because he exhibited many needs for privacy and usually refused to allow female nurses to dress or bathe him. During her next session with the nurse counselor, she related this conversation and wondered if her son was inquiring about his death. The nurse felt certain that the questions were not random curiosity but were an indication of his awareness of the seriousness of the relapse.

When children convey thoughts using symbolic language, intervention must also be expressed symbolically. In the above example, the mother realized the importance of assuring him that a man dresses a man. She also understood that he could only ask these questions about someone else. Therefore, she avoided directly confronting him with his own fears concerning postdeath rituals and answered his questions in the same way he presented them.

Children may also symbolically communicate their thoughts through writing or telling stories. Several techniques employ this type of expressive nonverbal and verbal communication. The nurse can show the child a picture of a particular event, such as a child in a hospital with other people in the room, and ask the child to describe the picture. Comic strips cut from a newspaper with the words removed are excellent vehicles when the child ascribes his own statements to each comic scene.[3] If the child draws a family or hospital scene, he can fill in short verbal communication above each person, similar to a comic strip theme. Asking older children to write a short story or a letter to someone about what it is like to be ill or hospitalized also evokes powerful evidence of their hidden thoughts or fears.

Art and play

Children also communicate through drawing and play. Both mediums of self-expression are much less altered by learned defense mechanisms than verbal communication. True fears can be uncovered by asking children to draw a person in the hospital or to engage in dramatic play, such as a "hospital setting." For example, one preadolescent drew a picture of a small girl in a large bed, with the sheet pulled up to her chin and only the head and small hands exposed. The child was very careful to point out that the girl in the bed was not herself. In reality, however, the small, scared, helpless patient greatly resembled the fatally ill child.

Through play, children reveal their perceptions of interpersonal relationships with their family, friends, or hospital personnel. Children may also reveal the wide scope of knowledge they have acquired from listening to others around them. For example, through needle play children may disclose how carefully they have watched each procedure by precisely duplicating the technical skills. They may also reveal how well they remember those who performed procedures. One child who painstakingly reenacted every detail of a lymphangiogram also played the role of the physician who had continually shouted at her to be still for the entire 5-hour ordeal. Her anger at him was extremely evident during the play session and revealed the cause for her abrupt withdrawal and passive hostility toward the medical and nursing staff following this test.

Drawings and play sessions serve not only as assessment tools for determining children's awareness and perception of their illness but also as methods of intervention and evaluation. In the adolescent's drawing described previously, the nurse conveyed an understanding of the child's fear and loss of control by drawing a person sitting on the bed touching the patient's hand. Also, in the preceding example, when the child revealed anger toward the doctor, the nurse acted the part of the patient but this time did not accept the physician's harsh commands to stay still. Instead the nurse said to the physician all the things the child had wished she could say.

Subsequent drawings or play sessions can also be used for evaluation of the child's progress. A change in the type of drawing or the theme of the play may indicate progression toward or away from ability to deal with anxiety. For example, the preadolescent's later drawing of a larger girl in a smaller bed, with outstretched arms on top of the covers, demonstrated her feeling of more control and power in the hospital setting.

Dreams

Dreams often reveal unconscious and repressed thoughts and feelings. Although interpretation of dreams is a specialized area of psychotherapy, asking a child or parent to talk about a dream may uncover areas that were previously unknown to the nurse. For example, one father who appeared physically and emotionally strong described a recurrent dream of being trapped by vicious dogs against a high wall. The color of his dream was always red and black. It was obvious that such a nightmare revealed his feelings of entrapment, loss of control, fear of mutilation, and death.

Because the material revealed in dreams may be too threatening for the person to deal with, it is often advisable to view the dream as an assessment tool. In this case the nurse helped the father explore ways in which he could maintain control in his grief. His fantasies of his son's anticipated death from gross hemorrhage were also investigated, and the usual ways in which children with leukemia die were discussed. Although the dream was never directly analyzed, these interventions were sufficient to lessen the frequency and intensity of the nightmare.

"To tell or not to tell" dilemma

The initial reaction of parents following discovery of the potentially terminal diagnosis is shock and disbelief. Probably one way of further shielding themselves from the overwhelming reality of the situation is to deny its existence to the child and siblings. Another reason for their inability to deal with the question of preparing the child may be their total concern with the present crisis and a lack of emotional reserve to cope with one more stress. As a result most parents seem to fabricate an alternate excuse as the reason for the child's hospitalization. Frequently many health professionals support such improvised explanations because of their own unresolved fears and insecurity in dealing with the truth. With no direction or help in deciding whether to protect the child or openly discuss with him the facts of his illness, many parents persist in fostering this conspiracy.

The decision not to tell. Initially the decision not to tell the child the truth has its superficial advantages. For one, it avoids the entire issue of what and how to explain the illness. Also, it solves the problem of the child asking his parents or staff any difficult, probing questions. After induction therapy most children attain a remission and are physically well and ready to resume prehospital activities. For parents it seems easier to return to normalcy with the diagnosis hidden.

However, the disadvantages of this decision are soon readily apparent. Following the course of remission therapy, there are future courses of treatment and evaluatory procedures, such as lumbar punctures, bone marrow aspirations, and blood tests. There is always the threat of relapse or recurrence of the illness, as well as intermittent problems with infection, hemorrhage, drug toxicity, and so on. What plausible explanation is available for these future problems? The answer is more lies, more excuses, and more flimsy explanations.

Effects on terminally ill children. Children are perceptively aware of conspiracies. They can detect the poorly hidden tears, the look of hopelessness after a conference with the physician, the vague telephone conversations that end abruptly if the child is present, or the whispers in the hallway and the overuse of big words. Children realize from the reactions of others that something is very wrong. But they also know that no one wants to talk about it with them, so they tacitly agree to the "don't tell him game" and protect others by not asking questions. However, such a conspiracy denies these children any opportunity to discuss their fears, questions, or thoughts. They are deprived of the truth and forced to supply their own answers or interpretations to events, which frequently are more extreme, frightening, and bizarre than the truth.

For example, in a family where the adolescent son had metastatic cancer, the father refused to allow anyone to talk openly to the boy. Although the mother felt strongly that her son knew and needed to discuss his feelings with someone, she also respected the established code of behavior in the Mexican culture of abiding by the patriarch's commands. Members of the medical and nursing staff agreed to the conspiracy, which was facilitated by the adolescent's passive, outwardly accepting behavior. However, one night he had a severe central nervous system reaction to an antiemetic medication. He became extremely upset and panic-stricken. The nurse understood that he misinterpreted the reaction as a terminal stage of his disease and spoke softly to him, explaining that the symptoms were caused by a drug, not the illness. He immediately relaxed. The look of relief in his eyes was the clearest message to everyone present that he had feared dying. Although the nurse later tried to discuss with him his behavioral reactions during this episode, he again refused to talk about his illness. As the nurse began to leave, he asked her to stay with him until he fell asleep. She held his hand and reassured him that he was not alone. They communicated in this way for the next several nights until he died.

Effects on siblings. The "to tell or not to tell" dilemma also involves the siblings and the support system that may be available to the family. During the initial hospitalization admission, many parents elect to room-in or stay with their child as much as possible. This is understandable and probably necessary to help them work through their initial grief reactions of denial, disbelief, or anger. If there are other children in the family, they are usually cared for temporarily by a relative, friend, or "part-time" parent. Unless parents give them a reasonable explanation for their continued absence from the home, the siblings will regard the sick child as responsible for the disruption and inconvenience.

To the well children, the brother or sister in the hospital receives the undivided attention of one or both parents and is showed with gifts, cards, and other visitors. Consequently the "neglected and forgotten" siblings feel resentful, angry, and jealous of such special treatment. Even when parents do attempt to convey a realistic picture of the hospitalized child's ordeal, few children are able to cast aside their negative feelings for genuine reactions of sympathy and concern. Being truthful with the siblings, including them in family discussions, and encouraging them to visit during the hospital stay help them realize the seriousness of the situation while allowing them the opportunity to be a contributing (not neglected) part of the family.

Many subsequent behavioral problems in well siblings, such as aggressiveness, regression, acting out, separation anxiety, and so on, can be prevented or resolved by including these children in the discussion, decision making, and care of the ill child. Preparing them for expected changes in the child, such as hair loss, physical deterioration, loss of function, and so on also helps them cope with questions or remarks from other children or adults and facilitates their adjustment to such alterations.

Effects on parents. The conspiracy of hiding or camouflaging the truth also places additional burdens on parents in their social milieu because it robs them of potential support from relatives or friends. It is true that not telling anyone about the child's diagnosis preserves the protective fortress constructed for the ill child and siblings and avoids sometimes distressing questions from others. However, a successful conspiracy is rarely, if ever, possible, and as a result the established code of silence alienates the family from others who are aware of the situation and might wish to help. The more families isolate and close themselves off from their world, the less likely they are to regain emotional strength to help them successfully resolve this crisis. This is particularly significant after the death, when parents wish to reenter their social environment and find their previous relationships and interests affected by their absence.

"Cruel" truth vs "gentle" truth. One of the strongest arguments for protecting the child from knowledge of the disease is that truth dispels hope, unnecessarily increases anxiety, and destroys the will to survive. Many people cite examples of individuals who stopped fighting and died shortly after learning of their terminal illness. Although there is some justification to this because some people do will themselves to die, one must also distinguish between "cruel" truth and "gentle" truth. To tell someone that he has an incurable illness and that he is going to die does dispel hope and possibly life. On the other hand, to tell someone the name of his illness, its effect on body functioning, and the reason for the treatment instills hope, allows for support from others, and serves as a basic foundation for explaining and understanding future crises.

Even when parents agree that their child should be told the truth, they encounter difficulty in using the words cancer, leukemia, tumor, and so on. They believe that such highly emotional words will upset the child by implying hopelessness, disability, or death. However, often these terms have little meaning for children, other than the connotations conveyed by others. The emotional impact of the word cancer is a learned response. If a cure were suddenly found for all malignancies, the fear, anxiety, and hopelessness presently associated with such diseases would diminish.

Once children know the name of the disease, the treatments, the required laboratory tests, and expected outcomes from each, they are able to deal with what is happening to them by seeking support and understanding from others. The following examples compare the different responses from children who were protected from the truth and those who were exposed to it.

Example A:

Eight-year-old Ann was recently diagnosed as having leukemia. Her parents explained to her that "something was wrong with her blood," which they called anemia. After the initial hospitalization Ann went into remission and returned to school. After 2 days at school, a classmate exclaimed, "You have leukemia. You are going to die." Ann was so upset by this that she told the teacher she was sick and consequently was sent home. The following day Ann refused to return to school and was very depressed. She offered no explanation to her parents, except that she was not feeling well. Her parents allowed her to remain at home for several weeks, which greatly intensified the child's fear of returning to school. It was not until the family sought professional help that the child was able to disclose the reason for her fear and to understand the actual illness and related facts.

Example B:

Nine-year-old Tom also was recently diagnosed with leukemia, but his parents had decided to be honest and open with their son. They had explained what effect the disease had on the blood, the reason for the treatments, and the chances for recovery. They agreed to tell their son that there was no cure for leukemia, that it was a serious illness, but that there were drugs that could kill the leukemia cells indefinitely, possibly forever. They emphasized that at one time such drugs were not available and people died shortly after the diagnosis was made. During the course of the induction therapy Tom went into remission and, following hospital discharge, returned to school. During his first day back at school, a classmate said to him, "I heard you had leukemia. I thought you were dead." Tom calmly responded, "I did have leukemia. I don't anymore. Do I look dead?" The other boy shrugged his shoulders and replied, "Come on, let's play." Tom immediately agreed.

Explaining death to children

Many adults attempt to shield children from any tragedy, especially death. They argue that children are too young, too fragile, or too vulnerable to cope with grief, sadness, unhappiness, or disappointment. What such individuals fail to understand is that life never shields anyone from eventual tragedy and that allowing children to feel emotions, particularly for less significant or important losses, prepares them for more traumatic events later. For example, a mother of a 5-year-old child decided to spare her son the grief of learning that his cat had been killed by a car. She planned to replace the animal with a substitute before the child returned home that day. However, in the interim she discussed her intended plans with a nurse friend, who emphasized the importance of telling the child the truth, because he would realize that the new animal was a replacement and resent its immediate presence. The mother agreed but asked the nurse to be there when she told her son about the accident. The nurse provided the support the parent needed and attended the "burial services" for the animal.

A year later the child's father also died in an accident. The mother used the example of the cat's death to explain this event to her son. She later told her nurse friend that had she shielded her child from the animal's death by substituting a replacement, she did not know how she could have explained the husband's sudden death.

Children need to feel, to express their emotions, and to learn appropriate outlets for anger, sadness, anxiety, or resentment. If others protect them from unhappy truths, children may respond to future stresses with few resources for how to handle their emotions. For example, inappropriate behavior, regression, problems with learning or relating to others, passivity, denial, dependence on drugs, development of psychosomatic symptoms, and withdrawal are a few of the alternative responses children may use to deal with stress.

Exactly how and what to tell children about events such as serious illness, dying, and death is a very individual matter. There is as much danger in telling children too much as there is in telling them too little. However, there are guidelines that can help in determining how to present facts in a way that fosters trust, enhances meaningful communication, and offers emotional support to the child and parents.

Developmental age. A primary concern in any relationship with children is their age, because the level of comprehension is a function of children's cognitive development. As has been discussed earlier in this chapter, children at various ages have different understandings and fears of death. The younger child fears separation, which can be imposed by any number of circumstances, only one of which is death or illness. The older child fears the results of illness, particularly pain or bodily injury, as well as death itself. Anyone working with children must be aware of such developmental variations and be sensitive to their verbal, nonverbal, and symbolic language.

Previous knowledge. Besides age, another essential principle is first to find out what the child is thinking. Before any explanations (true or false) are offered to children, they have invented their own. Asking such questions as, "What do you think is wrong with you?" or "What have you heard others say?" provides information on which to structure further explanations. Very often a child will respond with an answer of such detailed, accurate information that the only element lacking is the name of the disease. Other answers may reveal possible areas of misconception, which can then be clarified or refocused.

Sometimes parents and other adults hear the child's words but fail to comprehend their meaning. They erroneously assume that because the child recites all the facts he also understands their implications or has dealt with all his fears. This may not be so, because intellectualizing about one's condition can be a powerful defense mechanism. For example, an adolescent who was undergoing serious open-heart surgery knew precisely every detail of the operation, preoperative and postoperative care, involved risks, and so on. The medical and nursing staff considered her exceptionally well prepared. However, everyone had failed to ask her about how she felt. When the clinical nurse specialist asked her this before her surgery, the child answered, "I fear that I may die." Once this was verbalized, the child, her parents, and the nurse focused on her fears instead of on the facts of her illness.

Honesty. The last principle in explaining events such as death to children is honesty. Although the truth is usually the most difficult answer to give, in the long run it lessens many of the conflicts or problems that arise from lies, half-truths, or conspiracies. The truth provides answers for future questions. It also fosters trust. Children adeptly perceive the maxim: Do as I say, not as I do. It is very difficult to encourage children to be honest, to confide in others, and to openly discuss their fears if parents refuse to do the same.

Honesty is certainly not the easiest solution, because the truth may prompt children to ask other distressing questions. The question many parents and health professionals dread the most is, "Am I going to die?" because what honest answer also implies hope? One possible response is to use the principle of first ascertaining why they are asking questions *now*. Are they asking about dying today, in the future, from the disease, from the treatments, during the relapse, or from the infection? The following conversation between the nurse and a terminally ill child who was undergoing reinduction therapy following a recurrence of the disease illustrates a possible intervention.

CHILD: What is happening to me?
NURSE: What do you mean?
CHILD: I feel so awful. Sometimes I think I may die.
NURSE: What do you think about dying?
CHILD: I get very scared. I don't know how it will be or if anyone will be there to help me. [Starts to cry, nurse comforts child in her arms.] Am I going to die?
NURSE: I don't know. We hope these new medicines work. But you won't be alone. No matter what happens, we will be here.
CHILD: I'm glad. That's what I fear the most. [Nurse remains silent but continues to physically comfort the child to reinforce the promise that he won't be left alone.]

The truth can be very overwhelming to children. In the preceding example the nurse could have focused on the child's question of, "How will it [dying] be?" and have missed that the real concerns were loneliness, isolation, and abandonment. Had the nurse begun to explain about dying, this probably would have added to the child's fears and not met his expressed needs.

If given the opportunity, children will tell others how much they want to know. Asking questions, such as, "If the disease came back, would you want to know?" "Do you want others to tell you everything, even if the news isn't good?" or "If someone were not getting better [or more directly, "were dying"], do you think they would want to know?" helps children set the limits for how much truth they can accept and cope with. Children need time to proceed through the stages of denial, shock, anger, and so on before they can assimilate and hopefully accept the inevitable fact of mortality.

The way in which children ask questions is also indicative of the answer they are seeking. Few children seem to ask such direct questions as, "Am I going to die?" Instead they may ask, "Have the bad cells gone away?" or "Will this medicine make me better?" They tend to avoid final questions, such as, "What happens *if* the bad cells don't go away?" or "What happens *if* there are no more medicines?" In this way they always leave the opportunity for hope to be present. In a leukemic ward where all the children 9 years and older were routinely told about their illness and the chemotherapy, no child ever questioned the possibility of no more drugs being available. As the authors conclude: "The fatally ill child is sustained by hope and avoids any confrontation by the physician which could lead to its denial."[5]

GRIEF PROCESS IN EXPECTED AND UNEXPECTED DEATH

Lindemann has defined grief work as the behavioral reactions that result in the resolution of the loss.[8] *Acute grief* is a normal reaction to a distressing situation and has the following characteristics: (1) it is a definite syndrome with psychologic somatic symptomatology; (2) the syndrome may appear immediately after a crisis, be delayed, be exaggerated, or apparently be absent; (3) in place of the normal syndrome there may appear distorted reactions that represent one special aspect of the syndrome; and (4) through intervention, distorted reactions can be transformed into normal grief work with successful resolution.

Investigators such as Erich Lindemann, George Engel, and Elisabeth Kübler-Ross have contributed greatly to the present understanding of grief and bereavement. In expected death one must involve the identified patient and his family in the plan for intervention both before and after the death. In unexpected death the survivors face the tremendous task of integrating the loss into their lives, with no opportunity for anticipatory grief. However, in either situation nurses can facilitate the grief process by being aware of expected psychologic and somatic reactions and supporting the grievers through each stage.

Lindemann: symptomatology of grief

Lindemann analyzed and described the reactions of people who had survived the loss of significant others and found that several symptoms, both somatic and psychologic, characterized each individual's response to awareness of the loss. Table 27-1 summarizes the five characteristics of the normal grief syndrome.

Lindemann also identified several distortions of normal grief, which he termed morbid grief reactions (Table 27-2). Through appropriate intervention he found it possible to transform these morbid or potentially pathologic responses into normal reactions that resulted in successful resolution of the acute grief.

Intervention. The importance of such work is that health professionals such as nurses can use this theoretic framework to support those individuals who demonstrate adaptive behaviors (approach toward resolution of the crisis) and to intervene in those who exhibit maladaptive behaviors (avoidance or movement away from resolution of the crisis).

One example of emotional support toward the bereaved is to emphasize that reactions such as hearing the dead person's voice, feeling distant from others who want to help, or seeking reassurance that they did everything possible for the lost person are normal, necessary, and expected responses. They in no way signify insanity or approaching mental breakdown. On the contrary such behaviors following the loss signify that the survivor is working through the acute grief and will probably satisfactorily resolve the loss and resume or restructure a meaningful role in his social environment.

Table 27-1. Symptomatology of normal grief

Normal reaction	Symptoms
Sensations of somatic distress	Feeling of tightness in the throat Choking, with shortness of breath Marked tendency toward sighing Empty feeling in abdomen Lack of muscular power Intense subjective distress described as tension or mental pain
Preoccupation with image of the deceased	Hears, sees, or imagines that the dead person is present Slight sense of unreality Feeling of emotional distance from others May believe that he is approaching insanity
Feelings of guilt	Searches for evidence of failure in preventing the death Accuses himself of negligence or exaggerates minor omissions
Feelings of hostility	Loss of warmth toward others Tendency toward irritability and anger Wish not to be bothered by friends or relatives
Loss of usual pattern of conduct	Restless, inability to sit still, aimless moving about Continual searching for something to do or what he thinks he ought to do Lack of capacity to initiate and maintain organized patterns of activity

Adapted from Lindemann, E. In Parad, N. J., editor: Crisis intervention: selected readings, New York, 1965, Family Service Association of America.

Another significant finding in Lindemann's work is that most acute grief reactions are resolved within a period of 4 to 6 weeks. This is especially pertinent to the discussion of the child with a potentially terminal illness because for leukemia (the number one cause of death other than accidents in children above infancy), this same time span corresponds to the phase of discovery of the diagnosis and induction therapy. Nurses, therefore, have an excellent opportunity to work with the family during this initial crisis period. Although most crises are resolved regardless of intervention, the individual may return to a level of func-

Table 27-2. Symptomatology of morbid grief

Morbid reactions	Characteristics
Delay in or postponement of grief	None of the expected psychosomatic reactions of grief for the loss of the significant person immediately after death
	May see grief for an unresolved earlier loss
	Grief reaction may begin as "anniversary reaction"
	Acute grief may be postponed because of other immediate tasks, such as sustaining morale of others
Distorted reactions	Overactivity without a sense of loss
	Acquisition of symptoms belonging to the last illness of the deceased
	Acquisition of a recognized psychosomatic illness, such as ulcers, asthma, or rheumatoid arthritis
	Conspicuous alteration in relationship to friends and relatives, usually social isolation
	Furious hostility against specific persons
	Repression of hostility, resulting in altered affect and conduct, similar to schizophrenic symptoms
	Lasting loss of patterns of social interaction, especially lack of decision and initiative
	Altered behavior that is detrimental to his own social and economic existence, such as unjustified generosity
	Agitated depression, with danger signs of suicide

Adapted from Lindemann, E. In Parad, N. J., editor: Crisis intervention: selected readings, New York, 1965, Family Service Association of America.

tioning that is below or equal to the precrisis level. However, the minimal therapeutic goal is to assume the return to at least the precrisis level, and the maximum goal is improvement in functioning above the precrisis level, with increased problem-solving skills.

If one views a crisis as a transitional period, representing both the risk of increased vulnerability and an opportunity for personality growth, one can also focus on the discovery of a potentially fatal illness as a time for increased strength and maturity, rather than solely as a time to prepare for death. It may be that such a perspective will help health professionals and family members deal with their own feelings of fear and insecurity in working with dying patients, because the positive, hopeful aspects of the crisis situation are emphasized rather than the negative, hopeless aspects.

Kübler-Ross: stages of dying

Unlike Lindemann, who concentrated his investigation on the reaction of survivors, Elisabeth Kübler-Ross has identified five stages that people experience in terms of expected death.[7] In some ways one can conceptualize the stages of dying as behavioral reactions of anticipatory grief. One important point to remember when discussing each stage is that it pertains to the dying person and to those experiencing this person's expected death. With children, the "patient" is the ill child, the parents, and the siblings.

Denial. In the first stage, *denial,* the person responds with shock and disbelief. The "no, not me" reaction occurs regardless of whether or not the person is explicitly told his diagnosis. The duration of the denial is dependent on the coping mechanisms used by the person in previous crises, the support systems available to the person to help him give up the denial, and the reactions of others, especially physicians and nurses, to the resistance that is demonstrated. Unfortunately the need of others to deny the reality of the situation may be so great that it supports and fosters the patient's own denial and retards his progression toward other stages.

Examples of denial may include any of the following: physician shopping, attributing the symptoms of the actual illness to a minor condition, refusal to believe the diagnostic tests, delay in agreeing to treatment, acting very happy and optimistic despite the revealed diagnosis, refusing to tell or talk to anyone about the condition, insisting that no one is telling the truth regardless of others' attempts to do so, denying the reason for admission, and asking no questions about the diagnosis, treatment, or prognosis. Each of these mechanisms allows individuals to distance themselves from the onslaught of a tremendous emotional impact and to collect and mobilize their energies toward goal-directed, problem-solving behaviors. Partial denial, such as seeking additional professional consultations or occasionally acting as if nothing were wrong, is used by most people throughout the dying process. Without such a temporary protective mechanism, few people could survive the constant emotional drain of anticipating their own death or the death of a family member. Particularly with parents, anticipating the death of child is the same as losing part of one's personal hope for achievement, prestige, and accomplishment. There is no comfort or justice in the loss of youth, because death occurs before self-fulfillment.

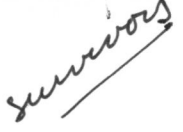

Nurses' response to denial is a critical component of the individual's need for sustaining this defense mechanism. Dr. Kübler-Ross maintains that the helping person's role in all stages of dying is to support the person (where he is at), not to maneuver him from one stage to another. If support is truly therapeutic the strength gained from this active intervention will help the person proceed on his own to another stage. The ultimate goal is for the dying person, and hopefully all family members or significant others, to reach the final stage of acceptance. However, persistence of denial prevents the person from even minimally accepting death. Therefore, it is important for others to support denial in such a way that neither reinforces nor rejects it.

Intervention. The most effective method of support is active listening. Silence neither reinforces nor rejects denial (or any other stage of dying) but implies a willingness and acceptance of the person's need for this behavior. However, silence alone can be misinterpreted. For example, if the person demonstrates denial, such as by saying, "I am sure the doctors made a mistake," and the nurse responds silently and leaves, the person may infer disapproval, agreement, avoidance, or rejection from this behavior. To be effective, silence and listening must be accompanied by physical and mental concentration and use of body language to communicate interest and concern. Direct eye contact, touch, physical geographic closeness, and body posture, such as sitting and leaning slightly forward, demonstrate silent but effective communication. Sometimes this type of support is sufficient to give the patient or family members enough strength to relinquish the denial and deal with the impact of reality.

The following example illustrates effective therapeutic use of active support:

> The pediatric clinical specialist was asked to see the mother of a 5-year-old boy who had been recently diagnosed with acute lymphocytic leukemia. The nursing staff expressed concern that the mother was not aware of the seriousness of the child's condition. They identified the following behaviors as signs of denial: asking few questions, never crying, seeming composed, calm (almost flighty), and never upset, and engaging in casual conversation with members of the staff and other parents without focusing on the child's problem.
>
> The nurse, who had never met the mother except through report, made an appointment with her at a specified time. When the nurse arrived, the mother was waiting in the hallway for her. The nurse introduced herself by saying, "You're Mrs. ________? I'm ________. Let's find a quiet place to sit and talk about what's been happening." She looked directly at the mother and touched her arm to convey where they would sit. Before the nurse closed the office door, the mother broke into tears, sobbing almost uncontrollably. The nurse moved a chair close to the mother, touched her knee, and encouraged her to cry. Then she remained silent. After a few minutes the mother stated through her tears, "It's almost as if I waited for you to come. I have kept these tears inside for several days, afraid that if I started to cry, I would never stop." The nurse responded, "Cry, it sometimes helps. I'm here for as long as you want." The woman replied, "Thank you. I feel better now. I'd like to talk about what's been happening since my son was admitted."
>
> As the mother spoke, it became very clear that the observed behaviors of denial were the mother's attempt to remain in control. She felt that she had to boost the morale of her relatives and had seen the nurses' and physicians' roles as task oriented, with little time for meaningful conversation. This was unfortunate, because in reality the nurses desperately wanted to support her but did not know how to channel the casual conversation into therapeutic communication. Through staff conferences with the clinical specialist, they were able to clarify their impressions of denial, analyze how their responses had supported it, and utilize new behaviors that encouraged the mother to feel accepted enough to let down her protective defenses.

Anger. The second stage in the dying process is *anger*. Although it usually follows denial, it may occur and recur at any time during the dying process. It is important to always remember that these stages represent a set of static, ever-changing behaviors that surface as the need for them arises within individuals' attempts to cope with expected loss.

When the denial fails and the reality of the situation penetrates consciousness, the person's reaction is, "Why me?" The anger, rage, hostility, envy, or resentment may be directed at oneself or at others, notably members of the medical and nursing staff. However, unlike denial, anger is not socially approved or condoned. The tacit reinforcement of denial gives way to overt rejection of anger. As a result the person is harshly judged for his angry refusal to accept mortality and is further isolated in his struggle for life, as well as death.

When one thinks about why the dying person or the parents of a dying child become enraged and resentful, one only begins to imagine the tremendous consequences of loss. Everything of life that the person dreamed of, hoped for, and expected to achieve is now only painful memories. He is angry toward those who are physically strong, who can make the dreams reality, and who live without pain or suffering. He is not angry at these people but at the things they represent, which for the dying person are no longer possible.

Intervention. The angry person needs to express these feelings but without feeling guilty or being judged by others. Sometimes the freedom to express angry thoughts is in itself therapeutic. One adolescent who had continually been verbally uncooperative with the hospital staff was labeled a "problem." Most people responded to the child's angry outbursts with admonishments or other direct signs of disapproval. For example, as soon as a procedure was finished, they would quickly leave the room. However, during a lumbar puncture, one nurse attempted to support the child by asking what she could do for him. He snapped back with, "Nothing. I hate you." The nurse said nothing and continued to assist in the procedure.

After the test was completed the nurse remained in the room, sat down next to the bed, and quietly said, "Lots of painful things are done to you, aren't they?'' He looked directly at her, and retorted, ''Yes, what would you know?'' She met his stare and reached out to touch his hand. He pulled it away but almost immediately began to cry, expressing his fear of pain, doubt for eventual recovery, and wish for another way to handle the anger. The nurse supported his need for the anger and later conveyed the experience to members of the nursing staff. Once they understood that the anger was not personally directed against them, which had increased their own feelings of helplessness, insecurity, and fear, they were better able to nonjudgmentally accept it. They also allowed the adolescent as much control and decision-making power over his hospital admission as possible to help him cope with his loss of independence and personal identity.

Bargaining. The next stage, and one that is often difficult to identify, is *bargaining*. It is the dying person's attempt to postpone the inevitable. The bargaining for additional time may be with God, with oneself, or with the most significant other person. One way of exploring a person's silent bargaining is to ask, ''If you could do one more thing, what would that be?'' Frequently the answer will reveal a hidden desire.

Intervention. Because bargaining may be associated with guilt, it is always important to explore the reasons behind the expressed wish. One mother who prayed that God would make her daughter live a little longer later revealed that this child was illegitimate. The mother was certain that if the child died, God was punishing her for the out-of-wedlock pregnancy. All the other half siblings, who might have been bone-marrow donors for this child, were not compatible. If the child continued to survive, the mother fantasized that a suitable random donor might eventually be found.

Unfortunately this child died shortly after the diagnosis was discovered. The mother was convinced that this was a sign of God's revenge. Following the death she exhibited several signs of morbid grief reactions. She refused to accept the child's death and acted as if she were still alive. Although members of the nursing staff had been aware of the implications of this child's failure to recover, they were powerless in helping the mother, who isolated herself from everyone.

Bargaining also occurs in children. The dying child may wish for additional time for himself, or the child who is facing the loss of a parent may hope for a delay of that person's death. One must listen very carefully to children in order to understand their symbolic language. One child who had recently been told that he had relapsed with leukemia, casually said to his mother, ''Do you know what I wished for on my last birthday? Another birthday.'' The mother was shocked by this statement and thought that it meant nothing. However, at a later time she asked a nurse, with whom the family had a trusting, working relationship, if this wish could mean that her son anticipated the consequences of the relapse. The nurse was certain that this was the child's way of bargaining for more time against the odds that he knew existed.

Depression. Without the denial to protect the person from realizing the seriousness of his condition, the anger to displace the emotional anxiety, and the bargaining to postpone the inevitable, the person eventually experiences *depression*. Generally there are two types of depression: the one experienced for past losses and the one experienced for anticipated or impending losses.

In a chronic terminal illness there are many reasons for the first kind of depression, such as loss of hair from therapy, loss of a body part or function, restricted physical ability, and change in life-style. The second kind of depression signals the person's preparation for the impending loss of all love objects. It is a difficult time for the dying person because he realizes the enormity of his loss. Unlike the survivors who are saying good-bye to one person, the dying person is saying good-bye to everyone and everything he ever loved.

Intervention. Dealing with each loss in a constructive, positive manner can greatly relieve the first type of depression. For example, purchasing an attractive wig, emphasizing the person's ability, rather than disability, and manipulating the individual's life-style to accommodate his physical changes help him deal with the depression of each crisis.

Since this type of depression is frequently associated with guilt, shame, or self-punishment, it is necessary to investigate less obvious reasons for the behavior. For example, one mother became very depressed after a neighbor told her that the child's malignant tumor was probably inherited. Since kidney disease had been present on the maternal side of the family, the mother was certain that she had transmitted the defect to her child. It was not until she discussed this fear that she was able to deal with her depression.

During the next period of preparatory grief or depression, there is little need for verbal reassurances. Attempts to ''lighten the mood'' or ''cheer up the person'' are not only ineffective but may also burden the griever with additional expectations to appear happy in order to meet the needs of those around him. It is a time of listening and of being physically present with the dying person. Toward the terminal stage the person may request the company of only one or two significant people. Children usually desire the presence of their parents more than anyone else.

Acceptance. The final stage of dying is *acceptance*. The person is no longer angry or depressed. If bargaining occurs, it is usually for a peaceful, painless death rather than for prolongation of life. It is not a happy time but rather one of inner peace and resolution that death is a certainty. The person may signal his acceptance by being disinterested in present or future events and preoccupied with past events, preferring few visitors, and wanting quiet and solitude.

Intervention. Such behavior may be very upsetting to others close to him, including health personnel who have not reached the same level of acceptance. One critical objective is to recognize the behaviors of acceptance in the patient and help others understand its relevance. Often the medical plan for continued treatment does not allow the patient the opportunity to accept the inevitable end. Nurses can be instrumental in planning care with all members of the health team with the goal of the patient's and family's wishes as the priority. This may involve the willingness to terminate extraordinary or lifesaving measures when death is imminent.

For example, one family whose teenage son was dying requested that all chemotherapy be terminated except those measures directed at keeping the child comfortable. When the child's respirations became labored, the nurse administered oxygen by way of nasal cannula, but the adolescent resisted. The father calmly told the nurse, "Take it away. We are ready for our son to die in peace and with dignity." The nurse respected the parents' acceptance of death, removed the tube, and summoned the other members of the nursing staff to say their last good-byes to the child. In a few minutes the child's breathing stopped. Everyone cried, but it was the parents who consoled the nurses.

Expected death

Although the stages of dying are described in terms of the ill person, the survivors also progress through several or all of them. When death is expected there is time for anticipatory grieving. This does not mean that the actual loss hurts less, but that the length of acute grief and work of mourning following the loss is probably shortened. Many parents reflect that the physical absence of the child is the most difficult aspect of the death to bear. Although there is preoccupation with the image of the deceased, parents are able to resume daily activities much more quickly than parents who experienced a sudden loss. This hastened mourning process is frequently very difficult for others to understand who are experiencing the child's death as an unexpected event. Helping parents anticipate the various reactions of other individuals lessens any guilt they may feel.

For example, one mother who had cared for her child at home before his death remarked at the wake services, "I wonder if I should be more upset." The visitors cried and were unable to offer any solace to the parents, who frequently reacted to this behavior by stating, "We will be all right. Our son is now in peace." After the funeral services the parents needed to discuss these feelings in order to validate that their more calm acceptance of their son's death was a positive reaction.

In long-term, potentially fatal illnesses, the grief for anticipated loss becomes chronic. The parents mourn the loss of their child long before he dies. Unlike parents who experience a sudden loss, these family members are unable to resolve their grief until the child is considered cured or dead. Each time they see the pain the child must endure or anticipate the sudden loss of hope from a relapse, they are reminded of their child's uncertain future.

However, the prolonged period of chronic grief provides families with the precious opportunity to complete all "unfinished business," such as helping the child and siblings understand and cope with a fatal prognosis. Many families reflect on their changed perspective of time after learning of the diagnosis, particularly their heightened awareness of the value and worth of each day. As one father stated, "I used to plan ahead for a better job, more money, and more prestige. But now I find myself wanting to stay home to be with my family. I never before realized how important time really is. Now I only wish we had more of it."

Unexpected death

In sudden, unexpected death the family is deprived of any of the advantages of anticipatory grief. There is no opportunity to prepare oneself or others for the death, only the cruel reality that nothing remains of their child except memories. Because of this lack of time to prepare, many families feel great guilt and remorse for not having done something additional or different with the child. For example, they may berate themselves for not having prevented the accident or for depriving the child of some desired material object or privilege. It is important to assess how parents feel about the events just prior to the tragedy to help them work through their feelings so that they may progress through the resolution of grief. Specific reactions to unexpected death are discussed in Chapter 13, p. 498.

REACTIONS OF FAMILIES TO A FATAL ILLNESS

Because of the many advances in the treatment of previously short-term fatal illnesses, diseases such as leukemia are now chronic disorders with a potentially fatal prognosis. As a result the family's adjustment to the diagnosis is extended over an indefinite period of time with several phases: discovery of the diagnosis, induction and remission, maintenance, recovery, relapse, terminal stage, post-death. Fig. 27-1 describes the cycle of reactions during each phase. Because the priorities of intervention change, the nurses' role will be discussed for each stage.

Phase I—discovery of diagnosis

Shock and disbelief. When parents learn of the life-threatening diagnosis, they usually react with numb disbelief. Many parents relate that after they heard the physician confirm the diagnosis, they were deaf to everything else he related. As one mother described, "All I heard the doctor say was the word leukemia. I didn't hear anything else. All

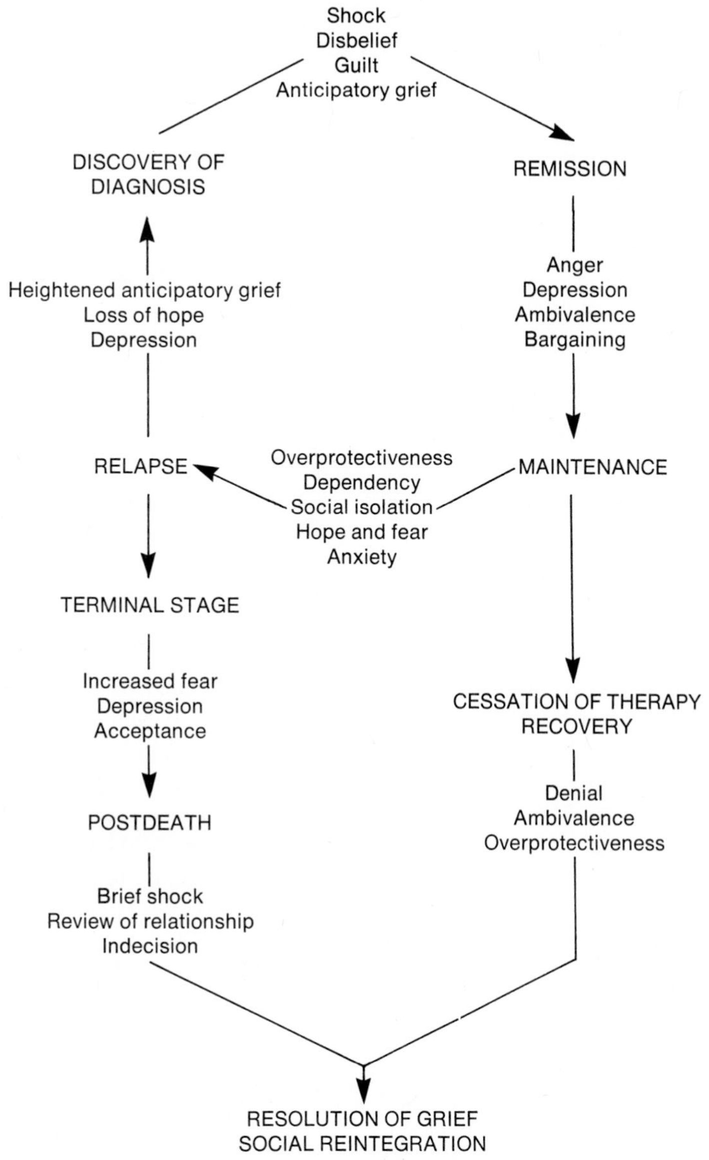

Fig. 27-1. A family's reaction to a fatal illness in a child.

I could think of was that leukemia was fatal. I was certain my child was going to die. My husband heard the doctor say it was curable, but I didn't. I won't believe that until I see it. Even if my child is 50 years old, I will worry about it coming back.'' The pessimistic response of this mother is typical of many parents who are afraid to believe that their child will recover despite the obvious odds. If parents are not helped to understand the improved prognosis of these diseases, they may react by psychologically burying the child.

It usually takes parents a few days to overcome the shock and denial. During this time many behaviors are characteristic of their attempt to assimilate the facts of this serious diagnosis. For example, they have an insatiable quest for knowledge and information about the illness, they may actively seek out those people who support an optimistic outlook, they may attempt to validate the diagnosis by questioning the ability of the physicians and members of the hospital staff, or they may withdraw in order to shield themselves from additional alarming news. It is important to recognize and accept such reactions as necessary protective defenses in the initial stage of the diagnosis. For example, some parents react to the news by staying with their child and participating in his care as much as possible. Others may need to distance themselves from the entire hospital situation by visiting for short periods each day. Accepting each parent's individual method of coping with the crisis is essential in the overall support of the family.

Guilt. Almost a universal reaction to the discovery of a catastrophic illness is guilt. Parents review every detail of the child's prodromal symptoms, searching for some clue that they missed or overlooked. There is also questioning, either voiced or silent, regarding the genetic influence on the disease. Many parents are greatly concerned about their role in transmitting the condition and the chances of it occurring in other siblings, particularly subsequent children. For example, one father was extremely interested in recent research on the investigation of chromosomal defects in children with leukemia. During this discussion he made no reference to the implication of heredity, but later he asked about the danger of having another offspring develop the disease. These clues led the nurse to question why he thought his child had leukemia. The father admitted his concern over whether or not he or his wife may have transmitted some genetic defect to their son.

Guilt may also be associated with religious beliefs. Some parents are convinced that they are being punished for some previous misdeed. Others may see the illness as a sacrifice sent by God to test their religious strength and faith. It is always advisable to pursue the meaning of each person's religious background to identify hidden sources of guilt and punishment.

Children, too, may interpret their serious illness as retribution for past misbehavior. The nurse should be particularly sensitive to the child who passively accepts all painful procedures. This child may believe that such acts are inflicted as punishment that he deserves. It is always vital to assure children that what happens to them in the hospital is to make them well.

Some parents displace their own feelings of guilt onto another person whom they regard as responsible for some aspect of the disease. A common target for the transferred guilt is the other spouse, particularly in marriages in which there is less communication between the partners. For example, in a session with one mother the nurse learned that she had taken the child to the physician despite the father's decision to wait a little longer. When the nurse spoke to the father, he stated that it was his decision to seek medical help, not his wife's. Although neither expressed overt anger toward the other party or guilt for having waited as long as they did, the nurse concluded that there were unspoken messages in these opposing statements. It was not until the nurse talked with them together that the parents were able to openly discuss their true feelings.

Anticipatory grieving. Almost immediately after learning of the diagnosis, most parents begin grieving for the loss of a perfect healthy child. Much of this acute grief remains until there are signs of physical improvement in the child. During the impact phase parents have great difficulty in making decisions, such as what to tell the ill child, how to prepare the siblings, and so on. Unfortunately despite their decreased ability to solve problems, they are forced to make a great many decisions. Nurses can be very helpful in supplying direction in areas in which alternatives are possible. For example, one family decided to move to a new location as soon as they heard that their child had cancer. This sudden uprooting would have been extremely disruptive to the entire family and would have introduced multiple new crises into the already critical stress situation. The nurse was able to intervene by listening to the parents' reasons for wanting to relocate and then discussing with them some of the disadvantages of doing so at the present time. It was stressed that if they still felt inclined to move, they could more effectively plan a change after the child's discharge. The parents realized the tremendous implications of such a decision and decided to wait. Following the hospitalization the mother remarked to the nurse, "When I heard the diagnosis, I was in such a state of mental upset that I could have done anything foolish. I am so glad we didn't make any decisions at that time."

Nurses' role. The time of diagnosis is a critical period for the development of therapeutic relationships. Ideally a consistent nurse should be present with both parents when the physician reveals the diagnosis. In single-parent families the nurse can become a substitute support system for the parent. The nurse can also assess how much of what the physician related the parent actually heard and understood. The nurse can clarify, refocus, or supply additional information at the parent's request.

In many instances the nurse becomes the only consistent, available person to the family. For example, in the case of a child with Wilms' tumor, a family physician, pediatrician, urologist, surgeon, radiologist, and hematologist/oncologist participate in the medical/surgical care of the child. Even under the best of circumstances, parents receive opposing messages from many physicians and are confused about who can answer their questions. The nurse is in an advantageous position to interpret those messages and to direct the parents to the most appropriate source of information.

Many parents elect to stay with their child and to participate as much as possible in his care. Because the possibility of death in a child is a highly emotional experience, nurses may unknowingly usurp parents' roles or relinquish nursing responsibilities. They need to be aware of their approach toward parents in order to support them in the way most comfortable for the parents. Planning the child's care *with* family members is a most effective way of communicating genuine concern and avoiding either hazard.

Phase II—induction and remission

Almost immediately after the diagnosis is confirmed, induction therapy aimed at a total remission of the disease begins. During this period families commonly react with anger, depression, ambivalence, and bargaining. Much of the psychic energy is directed at waiting for the confirmation of a remission. If that does not occur, one can expect to see all the initial reactions repeated again, with increased anticipatory grieving.

Parents' anger. Anger, closely associated with guilt, may be directed at oneself, the other spouse, the child, or members of the staff. Anger directed inward may be evident as self-reproaching or punitive behavior, such as neglecting one's health and verbally degrading oneself. Anger directed at the spouse may be manifest in open arguments or withdrawal from communication. Since quarreling in public is not socially acceptable, the other type of anger is substituted. Nurses need to be aware of parents who each ask them the same question at different times, which may be a clue to their lack of communication. Passive anger toward the ill child may be evident in decreased visiting, refusal to believe how sick he is, or inability to comfort him.

One of the most common targets for parental anger is members of the staff. Parents, mothers in particular, complain about the nursing care, the insufficient time physicians spend with them, or the lack of skill of those who draw blood or start intravenous infusions. Parents frequently question the physician's skill in making a diagnosis, choosing the correct treatment, and so on.

One particularly difficult situation is when parents express anger at the physician for not diagnosing the condition sooner. Since it is quite common knowledge that the prognosis for cancer is related to the time of discovery, parents understandably wonder if their child's illness was diagnosed as early as possible. In retrospect parents frequently recall signs or symptoms that they now regard as early clues to the disease. Nurses need to be aware of the implications of their responses to parents during such discussions. For example, agreeing that the physician missed an early diagnosis may actually increase the parents' guilt and decrease their trust in the present treatment program. Conversely defending the physician's medical judgment may weaken the parents' trust in the nurse. Listening to the parents' views and refraining from choosing sides helps them ventilate their anger, while maintaining confidence in their child's care.

However, there are times when parents' anger at medical or nursing personnel is justified. In such cases it may be therapeutic for the nurse to encourage parents to confront the specific person with their feelings. For example, one mother was so consumed with rage toward the physician for neglecting the seriousness of the child's condition that she was unable to deal with some of the other issues surrounding the hospitalization. The nurse helped the mother identify the specific reasons for the anger and encouraged her to discuss them with the physician. Even though the pediatrician was intolerant of her comments, the mother felt much more calm and personally satisfied for having directed her anger at the appropriate source.

Child's anger. Children also feel angry, particularly because of all the traumatic procedures done to them. Once they begin to feel better, they frequently express their anger through uncooperativeness. Parents receive the brunt of much of the child's anger and often find coping with it extremely difficult. A common reaction is to ignore it and try to pacify the child by giving in to his requests whenever possible. Since overprotectiveness and permissiveness are typical reactions during the maintenance phase of the illness, helping parents deal with the child's anger constructively during the hospitalization also prevents some of the potential future problems.

Children of various ages manifest anger differently. Young children may demonstrate their uncooperativeness by yelling, screaming, and physically fighting off the adversary. Older children may verbally express anger through abusive language. Passive anger, expressed in statements, such as, "I don't know" or "I don't care," usually evokes aggressive anger in others. Such passive anger may be misinterpreted as sullen, obnoxious, or hostile reactions. As a result these statements are effective in keeping people at a distance, when the hidden message of such statements really is, "I need to talk. Please help me understand what is happening."

Siblings' anger. Siblings also feel anger and resentment toward the ill child and parents for their temporary loss of routine and parental attention. Although they are forced to cope with a disrupted family life, they are usually given no rewards and, sometimes, inadequate explanations. It is difficult for older children and almost impossible for younger children to comprehend the plight of the ill child. Their perception is of a brother or sister who has the undivided attention of their parents, is showered with cards and gifts, and is the focus of everyone's concern. Although siblings seem to adjust to the required changes during the period of hospitalization, many of them demonstrate the effects of the emotional strain during the maintenance phase. Helping siblings understand the reason for the abrupt change in family life and continuing as much contact as possible with the hospitalized child and absent parents through visiting, telephone contact, letter writing, cards, or photographs fosters the siblings' adjustment to the crisis situation.

Depression and ambivalence. The shock of discovering the diagnosis is followed by depression, which usually lasts until there is physical evidence of improvement. Since in many cases the chemical and/or surgical intervention results in further deterioration of the child's physical status, many parents are ambivalent in their decision to agree to treatment. Although this is rarely voiced, parents may infer their ambivalence in such statements as, "Will the medicine always make him so sick?" "Is surgery really necessary?" "Wouldn't one drug do just as well as so many?" or "Is radiation just an extra measure in case the drugs don't work?" Supplying an automatic answer is less effective than encouraging parents to discuss their thoughts about the treatments. Many parents verbalize that when they consented to the interventions they were not aware of the significance of the side effects, regardless of how well they were informed.

Reactions to altered body image. One side effect of chemotherapy and/or cranial irradiation that has particular psychologic significance for children in different age-groups and for parents is hair loss.

Infants, toddlers, and preschoolers. For young children baldness has little significance. Preschoolers may attach superficial concern to the hair loss, particularly if it affects their sex-role image. For example, one 4-year-old girl was disturbed about her baldness because she thought she looked like a boy. Once her parents emphasized her femaleness in dress, she was unconcerned about the temporary change.

Parents of young children usually have the most difficult adjustment. However, they may be unwilling to admit their concern and lack of acceptance. For example, the mother of a 3-year-old boy refused to openly discuss the hair loss in front of her son. She had decided to hide the change from him until new hair grew in. She had formulated a fantastic conspiracy to maintain the secret. For example, she planned to remove all mirrors in the house, to isolate him from children, to keep his head always covered with hats, and to buy a soft brush and groom the hair as if it were still present. She explained that this was necessary because he was very vain. When asked what she would do if he discovered the baldness, she calmly said, "I'll just tell him what happened." It was not possible for her to see the pitfalls of such a scheme until she verbalized her personal feelings about the hair loss.

School-age children. The reactions of school-age children depend on their preparation for the loss and the type of parental adjustment. Much of their anxiety relates to the anticipation of the loss, rather than the actual baldness. Telling children about the change before it occurs, stressing that it is temporary, and suggesting ways of camouflaging it, such as with a wig, hat, or scarf, fosters better adjustment to the altered body image.

Adolescents. Adolescents have the most difficulty in accepting and adjusting to the hair loss, because it occurs at a time when peer acceptance and group conformity are essential. They need the opportunity to express their anger and fears of rejection without being judged or reproached. Sometimes parents try to reason with their adolescent child that the hair loss is a small sacrifice for a possible future recovery. Although that fact is true, it does little to comfort the adolescent in his present struggle.

Involving adolescents in selecting a wig *before* the hair falls out provides them with a feeling of participation and allows them to secure a wig that is most similar to their own hair. For example, a 13-year-old girl, whose wig was styled exactly like her hair, commented, "I think I like my wig even better than my own hair." Before she began to lose her hair, she wore the wig to school to see if anyone could detect the difference. Because no one could, she felt very comfortable about wearing it when it was necessary.

Bargaining. During the initial phase of induction therapy, most of the concern is focused on the child's recovery from the actual disease. Once physical improvement is evident, attention centers on the prospect of a remission. Parents constantly look for signs of a remission, which to them may be indicated by increased appetite, less irritable behavior, more energy, better color, and so on. However, the clinical confirmation of a remission usually takes several weeks or more. During this waiting period, parents bargain for a postponement of any pessimistic reports. Parents frequently make comments, such as, "If we can make it through this hospitalization, I think everything will be all right." The significance of the child's attaining a remission cannot be overestimated. For many, it represents a second chance.

Nurses' role. Anger is one of the more difficult reactions to accept and deal with therapeutically. The responses to anger may be reciprocal anger, fear, acceptance, and/or encouragement. The first two reactions close off communication and express disapproval and rejection of the person. They most commonly occur when the listener views the anger as a personal assault. The latter responses allow the individual to ventilate his feelings in an atmosphere of nonjudgmental acceptance. The following steps encourage expression of emotions[3]:

1. Describe the behavior: "You seem angry at everyone."
2. Give evidence of understanding: "Being angry is only natural."
3. Give evidence of caring: "It must be difficult to endure so many painful procedures."
4. Help focus on feelings: "Maybe you wonder what you've done to deserve all this misery."

One essential element to the successful implementation of this process is to wait for the person to respond to a statement before proceeding to the next step. Since the objective of each statement is for the person to speak freely, the responses should avoid "yes" or "no" type of answers. For example, one can describe the behavior as in the list above or ask, "Are you angry?" The latter question hinders further expressive communication and places the burden of subsequent conversation on the nurse, who should be the listener.

During the remission phase, parents, ill children, and siblings need reassurance that their reactions are normal and expected. Helping parents understand the children's reason and need for anger promotes adjustment to the present situation and may avoid additional problems. For example, one mother thought that the child's aggressive, uncooperative behavior was a reaction to the drug therapy. She verbalized her concern over coping with such behavior following discharge. The nurse discussed with her possible causes of the child's anger, such as loss of control, pain, and fear, and suggested various interventions. One especially effective outlet for the behavior involved hanging a large punching balloon over the bed. The child hit it furiously *after* he drew the physician's face on the balloon. Other aggression outlets include needle play, dramatic physician-nurse-patient play, and action toys, such as dart sets, water guns, drums, or hammering tools.

Parents and children need thorough, detailed, and repeated explanations of the plan of therapy. They need reassurance that a change in the child's condition is most likely a result of chemotherapy, not the disease. Decreasing the chance for the unexpected to occur lessens the opportunities for increased anxiety. For example, forewarning the family about the side effects of therapy, such as alopecia, weight gain, constipation, stomatitis, and nausea and vomiting, and the necessary laboratory procedures prepares them for these expected events and increases their sense of security and control.

As the ill child improves toward the end of the induction phase, the nurse should encourage parents to refocus their priorities and areas of responsibility. There may be less need for the parents to stay continuously with the hospitalized child and more need for them to prepare the siblings for his homecoming. It is also time for the nurse to begin discharge planning, particularly in those areas discussed in the maintenance phase.

Phase III—maintenance

Once the child is in remission, there is a long period of hope for an eventual recovery and fear of a possible relapse. Parents commonly react to these feelings by overprotecting the child, encouraging dependency, and liberalizing discipline. All of these reactions support the child's sick role and hinder his optimal physical and emotional development. Family members may attempt to escape or avoid the problems of this period through social isolation.

Overprotectiveness. Although many children return home in relatively stable and much improved physical health, parents frequently treat them as invalids. One of the most common manifestations of overprotectiveness is parents' inability to set appropriate limits. It is understandable that under the stress of potential loss parents might respond by overindulging the child in his every desire and wish. Although this is probably part of the grieving process during the initial phase of the illness, persistence of this reaction culminates in special problems during the often long period of remission.

For ill children, overprotection and "special" treatment increase their fears of serious illness and failure to recover. Without structure, they are unable to do what they desire most—live a normal life like other children. Each time they are granted extra favors they are reminded that they cannot compete or measure up to usual expectations. It is not unusual for these children to deliberately misbehave in order to force their parents into disciplinary action. With few limits or controls, these children are high-risk candidates for the development of emotional and behavioral problems. If they are given everything during periods of wellness, they will become very frustrated, unhappy, and demanding children during the terminal phase, when it will be impossible to meet all their requests.

Within the family system, parents may regulate discipline among the child and his siblings by setting up double standards. This results in the added problem of siblings' resentment and anger toward their sister or brother. With the visible effects of the illness no longer evident, the siblings are much less tolerant of special treatment or favors granted to the other child. They may express their disapproval through sibling fights, arguments, bouts of jealousy, and uncooperativeness.

Dependency. Closely associated with the overprotectiveness is increased dependency between parents and child. Parents may be unwilling to send their child to school because of their inability to let go of the perceived "sick child." If not helped toward reintegration of usual activities, they may use the hair loss, frequent visits to the physician, or continued treatment as excuses for keeping the child home.

For school-age children a special area of concern is resumption of school attendance. Having a tutor resume school lessons in the hospital as soon as the child is able helps him readjust to the classroom following discharge. The longer the child is protected within the safety and security of his home, the more difficult it is for him to reintegrate his usual social attachments and responsibilities.

Preparation for resumption of school is best accomplished through a team approach with the parents, child, school teacher, school nurse, and the primary nurse in the hospital. Ideally this planning should begin before hospital discharge, provided the child is well enough to resume usual activities. The plan should also include the special needs of the parents, the child, and the school personnel.

Parents' needs. Parents need support in understanding the necessity of encouraging a normal life for the child. It is difficult for them, especially the mother, to relinquish the intensive parenting role, particularly if many of their other social attachments have weakened. A successful approach is to plan school attendance concurrently with the parents' recommencement of prehospital activities. In this way the nurse also intervenes to prevent some of the destructive social isolation that can occur during the maintenance phase.

Children's needs. Children also need preparation before resuming school. They need to investigate possible answers to the many questions others will ask. One method of anticipatory preparation is to role play, with the child as the "returned pupil" and the nurse as "other schoolmates." The nurse asks questions about the reason for the child's absence, the name of the disease, and so on. The child is thus provided with a safe opportunity to explore possible answers and to experience some of the possible reactions of others. If the child returns to school with some obvious physical change, such as hair loss, amputation, or visible scar, the nurse might also ask questions about these alterations to prompt preparatory responses from the child.

Plans for return to school must be based on the individual child's ability to resume usual activity. Initially the child may find it easier to attend half-day sessions or to participate in a limited number of activities. It is preferable to plan the school program with as much participation and leadership from the child as possible. For example, during the planning stage of a preadolescent's return to school, the mother had talked to the physical education teacher concerning her daughter's need for limited activity. However, a problem occurred when a substitute teacher taught the class. Since no one had informed her of the child's condition, she expected the child to participate as fully as the others. The child tried to comply, but physically was unable to do so. Instead of explaining the situation to the teacher, she became depressed and withdrawn. Because she had not been included in the planning discussions, she assumed this confusion was her mother's fault. However, none of this was disclosed until the child described the events to the nurse. During the next session with the teacher, she and her mother explained the physical limitations imposed by the illness. All agreed at that time that if there were any further changes in teachers, it would be the child's responsibility to clarify the situation.

School personnel's needs. The nurse can also be instrumental in explaining to the school nurse and teacher the effects of therapy, the physical limitations of the disease, and the expected future prognosis. A common, often unvoiced fear of school personnel is that the child will become fatally ill while in the classroom. During the discussion of the disease, the nurse should include the usual course of the illness and its specific implications, such as the child's increased susceptibility to common childhood diseases or unexpected epidemics, such as chickenpox. In this case the school nurse should report the instance of prevalent illness to the mother.

Several issues should also be approached with the school teacher and nurse, particularly other parents' questions about the disease, such as the chance of communicability, preparation of the class for expected physical changes, and possible future absences. During the terminal phase the parents should also discuss the likelihood of the child's death and the need for discussing this with the other students. In the case of siblings who attend the same school, their teachers should also be included in the discussions. For example, the siblings may be demonstrating in school their difficulties in adjusting to the child's illness. Such behavior may erroneously be interpreted as learning disabilities, behavioral or emotional problems, delinquency, and so on. Unless the teachers are aware of the extenuating circumstances, these children can be saddled with negative labels for the rest of their academic life.

Social isolation. The critical nature of the crisis frequently closes off communication with those people not integrally involved in the child's care. Consequently when the child returns home, the parents may find it easier to keep their secret behind closed doors. Although the community is usually aware of the child's diagnosis, many individuals avoid the family. If parents are helped to understand the reactions of others and are guided to answer questions, they will be less likely to need protective isolation.

Although friends and relatives may be a significant support system to the family, frequently they are not. For example, casual remarks can burden the family with increased guilt. One mother who had returned home with her child after a lengthy hospital stay had gained weight. The neighbors expressed surprise at "how good the mother looked." During the next hospital admission, the mother deliberately limited her caloric intake. She commented to the nurse, "I can't gain weight this time. They will never understand how difficult this is if I look healthy." It took many discussions before the nurse was able to help the mother realize that what others thought was less important than her physical well-being.

Another reason for parents' social isolation is their intolerance of other families' comparatively insignificant problems. Many parents voice their frustration about others who complain of petty problems and who seem so out of touch with real tragedy or disaster. It is for this reason that parent groups of children with similar life-threatening diagnosis seem to band together automatically. There is a special camaraderie between these parents that seems to sustain them through the long ordeal. Many professionals have utilized the informal group process and have worked with the members to reach more long-range, identifiable goals. National organizations, such as the Candlelighters and the American Cancer Society, may be aware of local self-help groups in various areas. The primary nurse or the public health nurse should make these resources available to the parents.

Hope and fear. Throughout the transition period from discovery of the diagnosis to recovery or death, there is a constant mixing of hope and fear. Parents are continually investigating new avenues to potential cure. For example, one mother whose child remained in remission much longer than expected literally toured the globe in hope of finding a cure. She investigated occult rituals, religious crusades, unapproved drugs, and a multitude of unorthodox remedies. It was an extremely difficult time for her, other family members, and the treating physicians. Fortunately the mother was supported in the emotional need for such a search and gradually came to the opinion that the present therapy was the most valid. However, she stated that the search was necessary in order for her to feel that she had done everything possible.

Accompanying hope is the ever-present fear of return of the disease. Any intervening physical crisis, such as infection, drug toxicity, or depressed bone marrow, causes marked parental concern and anxiety. There is a constant need for reevaluation of the child's progress, reassurance that the child is in remission, and reconfirmation that some children do recover.

If the child is hospitalized during a remission for almost any reason, the parents may respond with what appears to be exaggerated fear and concern. However, health professionals need to understand that any complication magnifies the seriousness of the underlying illness. Nurses should encourage families to express their feelings while emphasizing to them signs of improvement in the child's condition.

Many parents find that the best times are the most difficult, because in the light of hope lurk the shadows of fear. As one parent explained, "I never can enjoy the good times too much because the fear of leukemia recurring is always there. If I have too much hope and allow my spirits to get too high, I am afraid that if something goes wrong, I will have too far to fall. If that would happen, I worry that I will never be able to pick myself up again. So I protect myself by staying on a cautious level of optimism."

Anxiety. Besides the concerns discussed in the preceding paragraphs, parents are anxious over many additional stresses. The financial strain of a long chronic illness is a constant worry. Job security is always a necessary consideration, since unemployment may jeopardize insurance coverage. There are also additional costs besides the actual medical care, such as transportation to the hospital, meals while away from home, baby-sitting cost for other siblings, or temporary housing for distant medical care. The nurse can provide assistance by referring the family to available organizations, such as the Leukemia Society of America or the American Cancer Society, who may be able to provide financial help.

Nutrition is also a continuing concern. Many of the drugs cause severe nausea and vomiting, thereby decreasing the child's appetite. The illness usually results in marked weight loss. Mealtime can become a battleground for family members. The nurse can prevent some of the problems by forewarning parents of the expected change in appetite and by suggesting ways of encouraging children to eat without causing a power struggle. For example, during the course of steroid therapy, appetite improves dramatically. Parents should be told that the increased hunger is a result of medication, not a change in the child's behavior or attitude. During periods of chemotherapy when the appetite is decreased, providing small, frequent meals of favorite foods often encourages some cooperation. Growth may also be slowed during the treatment phase from the various drugs and use of radiation. If parents are aware of some of these expected changes, they may be more accepting of the child's fluctuating appetite.

Nurses' role. In many health systems the role of the nurse during the maintenance phase is limited by confinement to a specific agency. There may not be one primary nurse who can act as liaison and coordinator among the nurses in the hospital, school, clinic, physician's office, and community. Often this results in a lack of preventive intervention. The problems caused by overprotection, dependency, and social isolation are identified after a crisis exists. One group of nurses who are in a particularly advantageous position to become a primary link with the family are public health nurses. They can counsel the family regarding resumption of usual activities, such as school, the need for discipline, the hazards of protective isolation, and the availability of various supports, such as parent groups.

Nurses who work closely with many families of potentially fatally ill children can be instrumental in forming self-help groups or participating as the professional leader of the group. Parent-founded organizations often provide many services that health professionals are less able to institute, such as temporary housing, child-care services for siblings, meals, transportation, resources for wigs, blood donors, and so on. Nurses who work with such groups can often help the group meet needs of individual members. One special instance is the support of those parents who have lost a child. The group may be extremely uncomfortable with the problems of these members and unable to mutually solve the dilemma.

Phase IV—recovery

The maintenance period may be followed by cessation of therapy in the hope of a permanent recovery. Although this is a very happy time, it is mixed with feelings of grief and ambivalence.

Denial and ambivalence. At the time the decision is made to terminate therapy, many parents deny the fact that treatment is no longer warranted. They may express ambivalence through such questions as, "Are you sure that a longer period of drugs wouldn't guarantee a better chance for a cure?" There is great difficulty in giving up the security of the rituals of medication, radiation therapy, and frequent examinations. Occasionally health professionals erroneously label the ambivalence or denial as a psychologic need for the child's sick role. Although this may be true in isolated instances, in general this reaction is characteristic of the grieving for the loss of security afforded by medical intervention and adjustment to the hazards of "waiting it out'' again. Parents need almost as much support during this phase as they did when they were told of the diagnosis.

Overprotectiveness. Parents also relate a resurgence of the need to overprotect and isolate their child from any potential physical harm. As one mother stated, ''I became fanatical about examining my child for signs of recurring illness when the drugs were stopped. If he had a runny nose or sore throat, I immediately took him to the doctor, requesting a blood count. I was so sure those leukemic cells had returned.'' She later compared this reaction to the ways in which she treated the child following his first remission. She added, ''You would think that after 3 years of living with drugs, side effects, blood tests, and doctors, I would be thrilled to give it all up, but here I am, as shaky and nervous as if I had just found out he had the disease.''

Nurses' role. Probably the most important component of care is acceptance of the parents' need to regress to earlier forms of coping, such as denial or overprotection. Parents need to feel comfortable in calling the physician or clinic about any concern or problem. They also should be encouraged to verbalize their feelings and thoughts of cessation of therapy. It may be helpful for the nurse to acquaint them with another family who had progressed through this transition period.

Phase V—relapse

Heightened anticipatory grieving. Once the remission has ended, there is an exacerbation of all the previous stages of grieving. Denial may be present in various degrees, from minimal disbelief on discovery of the relapse to complete refusal to accept the diagnosis. However, most families tend to practice partial denial. For example, one parent explained that although the leukemic cells were present in the spinal fluid, the physician was not certain ''If this is a relapse or a 'slight failure' of the drugs to kill these cells.'' Children also seem to defend themselves against the complications of a relapse. For example, one adolescent emphasized that Hodgkin's disease had not returned. The physician had just found a node that was ''missed'' during radiation therapy.

During a relapse any of the stages of dying may be exaggerated. Children in particular may become very angry or depressed, especially if they have not been told the truth or if the truth has been distorted to imply that the treatment is a cure. For example, children who may have been very accepting and cooperative during the initial hospitalization may respond to subsequent hospital admissions with hostility and rage. Parents and staff members frequently do not comprehend the reason for the altered behavioral reaction and, instead of trying to understand and deal with it, scold or admonish the child. However, for the child, this hospitalization may be more difficult and frightening than the initial one, because the severity and uncertainty of the disease have become a reality.

Loss of hope and depression. One of the most difficult realizations for parents is the knowledge that with each relapse the chances for eventual recovery diminish. The reality of possible death looms before them, particularly during the reinduction phase when a recurrent remission may or may not be feasible. Once another remission is attained, reason for hope is again present.

However, many parents relate that after termination of the primary remission they never again felt as hopeful or optimistic. Some also discussed their silent preparation and grieving for the child's eventual death. Nurses need to be sensitive to such thoughts and aware of the possible beneficial aspect of this reaction, since repeated relapses are associated with poorer prognoses.

The usual reaction to loss of hope is depression. This may be the type of depression for past losses but most often is anticipatory grieving for impending losses. Nurses need to carefully assess the reason for the depression and to realistically plan intervention. For example, if another remission is likely, the nurse would plan to help the parents work through their depression. If this is not done, the parents may psychologically bury the child and end his living prematurely. However, if this relapse is actually the commencement of the terminal stage, the nurse would plan to support the parents in their depression, since it is a necessary precursor of acceptance.

Nurses' role. Relapse is a difficult phase for nurses because it often initiates a loss of hope and their own grieving process. One of the dangers during the phase of relapse is that nurses may transfer their feelings of either pessimism or optimism to the parents. It is extremely important to assess one's own personal response to the relapse and to plan the intervention according to the person's needs. This seems to be particularly critical at the time the final relapse occurs. Nurses can help parents and children formulate realistic short-term goals and establish reasonable priorities of care. It is also the time to discuss with parents their wishes and expectations for the terminal phase. For some families the alternative of home care rather than hospitalization is a very significant and fulfilling means of sharing their child's last days.

Phase VI—terminal stage

The terminal stage is actually a continuation of the final relapse. The families' reactions are influenced by their previous acceptance or denial of the child's illness. It is a period of intense anticipatory grieving, characterized by the relapse reactions of depression, loss of hope, and, hopefully, acceptance. As the child's condition worsens, there is an intensification of numerous fears. These fears may be particularly worrisome for those parents who have chosen home care because they must assume primary responsibility for the child. The nurse's role in preparing them to deal with each fear and in providing assistance through home visits, telephone counseling, and the alternative of hospital admission at any time assumes great significance for these families.

Fear of death. The most prevalent fear is of death itself. Parents frequently ask about death through questions, such as, "What will he die from?" "How will we know he is dying?" and "What will happen when he dies?" It is important to listen sensitively to such questions, because the real concern may be hidden behind the question. For example, when parents ask, "What will he die from?" they are less concerned with the medical cause of death, such as hemorrhage or infection. What they may really be asking is, "What is hemorrhage like?" Most people have a fantasy idea of how death will occur that is much more horrifying than the actual events. For example, parents will relate that their idea of hemorrhage is uncontrollable gushing of blood from every orifice. In reality is is usually internal bleeding with oozing of blood from the nose. When nurses are aware of the imagined events, they can clarify the misconceptions and supply the correct information.

Fear of pain. The fear of uncontrollable pain is almost universal. Whatever bargaining occurs during the dying stage is for a peaceful, quiet, and quick death. Often parents will relate that the child has pain even when it appears that he is comfortable. It is important for nurses to understand that pain is much more than physical. Watching one's child die is a pain that must certainly be immeasurable and that subjectively shadows one's perception of surrounding events.

Fear of loss of control. A fear that is shared by the dying and the survivors is losing emotional and physical control as death approaches. Some parents attempt to cope with this fear by requesting that their child be heavily sedated during the terminal stage. However, the loss of control imposed by medication may make the child very distraught. Since nurses usually regulate the administration of drugs, it is important for them to carefully assess the needs of both the child and parents. Supporting parents at the time of impending death by being physically present, making the child as comfortable as possible, and talking to the awake child help parents feel in control without the need for sedating the child.

Fear of isolation and loneliness. Parents fear that their child will die when they are not with him. Dying children often request that their parents stay by their bedside. Although everyone dies alone, no one need die in lonely isolation. Nurses should encourage family members to be present. If death approaches sooner than expected, nurses should recognize the physical signs of death and summon the parents to the child's bedside. They should also prepare the family members for expected death. For example, if the child's condition worsens, the parents should be told that he may die. Sometimes health professionals' need to deny death is so strong that parents are continually given messages of false hope that prevent them from preparing themselves for the worst news. Although others may think such false hope is helpful, in reality it may be extremely painful for family members to live in uncertainty.

Nurses' role. During the terminal stage the fears of parents and children form the foundation for nursing care. Assessment of such fears guides nurses toward therapeutic intervention. Keeping the family informed as much as possible about the child's condition helps them feel more in control. One essential aspect of intervention is awareness of approaching death and concurrent physical needs.[4]

Loss of sensation and movement. An initial sign of impending death is loss of sensation and motion in the lower extremities, progressing toward the upper body. At this time the child may complain that the bedsheets or pajamas annoy him. Loose clothing, untucked bedsheets or use of a bedcradle and frequent, gentle change of positioning make the patient feel much more comfortable and may decrease the need for analgesics.

Loss of senses. As death nears, tactile sensation decreases, although touch may become annoying. Usually at this point the less manipulation of the child's body, the greater his degree of comfort. This may entail abandoning the usual hygienic measures of bed bath, clothing change, and bed making. However, it is important to allow the child as much decision-making power as possible, since prematurely enforced dependency can also be upsetting. For example, some children want to use the bathroom until the very end, whereas others prefer to void in the bed. However, when the child requests that no one touch or bother him, it is important for others to respect this request.

Vision also fails, and the dying child will usually turn toward a light source. Although bright, direct light is annoying, drawing the shades and dimming the light too much can also be disturbing. Those who are with the child should be seated near the head of the bed in direct line with the child's vision.

Hearing is the last sense to fail. Even those who appear asleep or comatose may hear all that is said around them. Parents should talk to their children in a clear, distinct voice, never in whispers. If others must converse, it should be done outside the room, where the child normally would not hear them. Nurses should encourage family members to continue talking to the child until he dies. In one family, where the child died at home, the parents spent the last few hours telling their son they loved him, reassuring him that he was not alone, and encouraging him not to be afraid. He died peacefully, calmly, and with a smile on his face.

Sensation of heat. Most dying patients are not aware of cold, regardless of how cool their skin feels, because internal body temperature rises. At this point light clothing and fresh circulating air increases their comfort. Nurses should explain the reason for this change in environmental conditions to parents who may interpret their child's external coolness as a need for increased warmth.

Minimal need for pain medication. If all the preceding needs are met, the child is usually comfortable with little or no pain medication. This may be in contrast to his previous need for high doses of analgesics. If sedating drugs are administered only as required, most children are conscious until the very end. It is striking to observe that they die as they lived. For example, one preadolescent who had maintained his independence and individuality through the several weeks of pain and failing strength was conscious, alert, and behaving as characteristically as he always had until the last moments of his life.

Heightened spiritual needs. If the child has had a strong spiritual orientation, he may desire a priest, minister, or rabbi at the time of death. Parents who sense that death is near may also have this request. Nurses who are aware of spiritual needs can summon the clergy to be with the family at the time of death. In those cases in which it may not be possible to reach a clergyman, the nurse may have to provide the spiritual needs by praying with the family, reading from the Bible, or listening to the review of their life. It does not matter what nurses' religious beliefs are, provided they accept others' faith without judgment or criticism.

Peace before death. Those patients who are conscious until the very end experience a period of peace and calm before death. Frequently this follows a period of restlessness that is unaltered by drugs or other physical comfort measures. It is important to recognize the period of restlessness as a sign of approaching death and avoid oversedating the person, since the loss of control from excessive medication may prolong the restlessness and shorten the period of calm. Nurses should forewarn parents of both behavioral reactions and stay with them as much as possible.

The terminal stage is also a period of preparing for postdeath. It may be a time when the focus on the dying child and mother needs to shift to the father and siblings. Often these family members are the silent, forgotten mourners. Siblings need to be prepared for the fact of the child's death and, according to their age, to be included in the burial services. Fathers may need encouragement to express their emotions. At the time of death, family members may benefit more from a "screaming room," where they can ventilate their anger and deep sorrow, than a quiet room, where they must hold back their intense emotions.

Phase VII—postdeath

The crisis of loss does not end with the child's death. In many ways, it only begins. Families can prepare themselves for the expected loss, but when it occurs there is a period of acute grief, followed by an extended phase of mourning.

Brief shock. When death occurs there is a brief period of shock. As one parent described, "We were as prepared for our son's death as anyone could be, but it was a shock when in a moment his life was finished. I just can't get over the rapidity with which life ends." Following the death, there is a period of time that family members still need to say good-bye to the child. The body should be left in the room. If there is any reason to clean the body or remove medical equipment, the nurse should do so before the parents reenter the room. It is important for family members to remember the child in quiet, peaceful, pleasant surroundings.

Review of relationship. During the immediate postdeath period, there is a tendency to review the events of the child's life during his illness and to evaluate the effectiveness of the parents' efforts to care for him. Parents will frequently look for validation of their efforts from the nurses who were with the child during his final hospitalization. It is important to support all parental actions and to listen for any feelings of guilt, which may delay the resolution of grief.

Indecision. Intervention is necessary after the child's death because new conflicts, such as the decision to have additional children, may arise. Many parents fear the recurrence of the illness in the subsequent child. Although nurses cannot make such a decision for parents, they can assess their readiness for another pregnancy. The successful resolution of mourning is characterized by decreased preoccupation and realistic memory of the deceased, establishment of new interests, and resumption of self-enjoyment and pleasure.[2] If such behaviors are evident, the parents are probably ready for the additional responsibilities of another child. However, signs of unresolved grief, such as continued preoccupation with and idealization of the dead child, may indicate that the subsequent offspring will become a "replacement child."[10]

Social reintegration. The final resolution of grief is not only reintegration within the immediate family but also resumption of social attachments. Families demonstrate this response in a variety of ways. Some desire to become involved in helping other families cope with a similar crisis. Others attempt to distance themselves as much as possible from the past loss. It is important to accept either adjustment as positive and adaptive.

Sometimes social reintegration follows a period of postdeath dissolution of remaining family relationships. The divorce rate is high among the parents of fatally ill children. In these situations siblings and parents need additional help to resolve their grief and reestablish their social attachments and societal roles. Public health nurses can assist these parents by locating temporary housing, child-care services, and so on. In addition they can serve as a substitute support system while resolution of the divorce crisis occurs.

FAMILIES AT RISK

Death of a family member is a major situational crisis that tremendously affects the entire family system. One nursing goal is to assess which families are at greater or lesser risk for succumbing to the effects of the crisis. Three categories—available support system, perception of the event, and coping mechanisms—influence the resolution of a crisis.

Available support system

The significant others who are available to individuals for emotional strength during periods of crisis comprise their support system. Support systems may be available through a variety of relationships and may consist of one significant other, such as a marital partner, or a group of significant others, such as the extended family or members of the health team. Although a support system exists, it may not be effective unless the individual is able to utilize the system through mutual channels of communication.

Status of the marital relationship. The marital relationship is a prime source of potential support. When the spouses can openly discuss their feelings there tends to be much less guilt, anger, blame, and indecision. Each crisis during the long period of potential fatal illness is successfully resolved, lessening the accumulation and overlapping of multiple stresses.

Unlike the emotionally healthy family, there are other family styles that have less available support. For example, the single-parent family is frequently devoid of immediate support. The single or sole parent bears all the responsibility for decision making that ordinarily would be shared by two people. In the moderately adjusted family there are no major difficulties between the marital partners until a crisis occurs. Without open communication and mutual sharing of ideas, the spouses react to the crisis with opposing opinions, blame, bitterness, and anger. In the poorly adjusted family the marital relationship is precarious under the least stressful circumstances. The spouses have few common interests, do not share responsibilities, and communicate ineffectively. During a crisis they react by blaming each other, emphasizing past misdeeds, and searching for reasons to instill guilt in the other partner. Unable to cope constructively with the crisis, they may seek destructive coping mechanisms, such as excessive drinking, drug abuse, promiscuous behavior, or physical aggression.

Alternate support systems. Support systems may be available with significant others outside the marital relationship. For example, the single-parent family may have the support of extended family, such as that of the parent's own parents. Occasionally parents may be able to communicate with each other but are unable to talk with the child. This is particularly evident with very young children, who communicate least through verbalization, and with adolescents, who may be unwilling to discuss or listen to adults. In this case the child is left without an available support system.

Ability to communicate. Besides the availability of significant others, family members must have the ability to utilize the support system. Almost all methods of psychologic intervention, such as support through active listening, counseling, crisis intervention, or psychotherapy, require verbal communication between two individuals. The ability to verbalize about feelings, such as anger, fear, guilt, or anxiety, helps individuals cope with the particular emotion. Verbalization allows for validation of feelings and thoughts. For example, one mother secretly believed that she had caused her son's illness because prior to the discovery of the diagnosis she had had recurrent dreams of his dying. Through discussions about this fear and the realistic impact of dreams on future events, the mother was able to resolve her guilt.

Not all individuals are able to communicate verbally. Some rely on religious faith and silent prayers for support. Others, such as children, communicate best through nonverbal methods, such as play, drawing, movement, and so on. Some individuals may not be able to communicate with anyone because of their interpersonal withdrawal and social isolation. These individuals are most at risk because, even if a support system is available, they may be unable to share their problems with others.

Perception of event

Although death is a crisis to everyone, its meaning and significance are influenced by the individual's perception of that event. In particular the association of guilt may complicate one's ability to realistically view the death and ultimately resolve his grief. Guilt implies a degree of control over one's actions. The more guilt an individual has, the more control that person perceives in the prevention or alteration of the event. Assessment of specific perceptions concerning the illness aids in evaluating the individual's ability to cope with various aspects of the event and identifies possible areas for intervention.

Knowledge of disease. Although family members may be shocked to learn that their child has a serious illness, they usually have some knowledge about the disorder from previous associations. It is important to explore the extent of that information, since there is a great tendency to compare the recently disclosed facts with the other knowledge. One very prevalent discrepancy is parents' past awareness that diseases, such as leukemia, are inevitably fatal. If nurses identify the specific source of that information, they can effectively begin to clarify the reasons for a more favorable prognosis.

Parents' reactions to the discovery of the diagnosis may also be influenced by past knowledge of the disorder. For example, a mother who initially refused to agree to chemotherapy was labeled "hostile and dumb." Instead of trying to discover the reason for her resistance, the physicians continued to coerce her into signing the consent forms by threatening her. During a conversation with the nurse, the mother disclosed that her best friend's daughter had recently died from the same illness. The mother knew of this child's suffering from the drugs and eventual fatal outcome.

She was understandably hesitant in agreeing to a serious treatment that carried no guarantee of success. However, as the nurse discussed with the mother her thoughts of refusing treatment, the mother stated that she knew she could not deny her child any chance for recovery. With the opportunity to talk about the events of the other child's illness, the mother was able to deal with her feelings of ambivalence and to agree to treatment with a more positive attitude.

Past experiences with death. Most individuals are able to relate some previous experience with death. Their perceptions of that event influence their ability to cope with and prepare others for dying and death. In particular, instances of unresolved grief over a previous loss may interfere with or delay resolution of the anticipated loss. For example, a young mother who was dying of cancer refused to allow anyone to tell her 8-year-old daughter of the seriousness of the illness. Instead, she continued to tell the child that she was improving. She felt that this approach was necessary because her brother's death during her childhood was so traumatic that afterward she was not able to talk about death or attend any other funeral services. The mother imagined that if her daughter learned of the serious illness, she would react similarly. It was only after the family had been helped to see the differences in the two situations that they could agree to a more honest, open approach toward preparing the child for the impending loss of her mother.

Influence of religion. Religious beliefs and faith have various meanings for different people. For some, religion comprises the foundation of their support system. For others, it may intensify feelings of guilt, shame, bitterness, or punishment. For example, some individuals may interpret the illness as a punishment from God. They may exclaim, "What have I done to deserve this?" or "God, why are you punishing me in this way?" It is important to take such statements seriously and to explore reasons for why the person believes that this is a punishment. For example, after a father learned of his son's failure to respond to the therapy, he stated, "It took me 5 years to get used to the fact that my child has Down's syndrome. It seems like God is punishing me for rejecting my child by taking him away after I began accepting him." When the child died, the father expressed his guilt for not having wanted this child.

Imagined cause of disease. Although the etiology of many disorders is unknown, parents and children usually supply their own answers. Sometimes this is associated with religious beliefs, but it may also be influenced by previous events. For example, children may interpret the reason for the illness as a punishment for not obeying others. Parents may be convinced that the disease was inherited. Sometimes there is a strong belief in curses, occult witchcraft, or devils as perpetrators of the disorder. Once the fantasied cause is revealed, the person can be helped to deal with the irrationalities of that thinking and, hopefully, will be relieved of feelings of guilt, blame, or anger.

Effects of illness on family. How the child's illness affects the family reveals how its members perceive the event. For example, the following statements could be representative of a particular reaction: (1) denial—"everything is the same as it always was," (2) inability to express feelings—"we have more *things* to do," (3) anger, blame, or bitterness—"we never should have had children," (4) resentment and hostility—"my sister gets everything because she is sick," and (5) acceptance and ability to express feelings—"the perspective of time has changed because we realize how precious and limited it is."

Coping mechanisms

Coping mechanisms are those behaviors that are aimed at reducing the tension caused by a crisis. Approach behaviors are those coping mechanisms that result in movement toward adjustment and resolution of the crisis. Avoidance behaviors result in movement away from adjustment or maladaptation to the crisis. Several approach and avoidance behaviors used in the crisis of a fatal illness are listed in the box at the top of p. 987. None of the indices can be used singly to assess the possible success or failure in resolving the crisis. Each behavior must be viewed in the context of all the variables affecting the family. For example, the observation of several avoidance behaviors in an emotionally healthy family may denote significantly less risk to the successful resolution of the crisis than an equal number of avoidance behaviors in a poorly adjusted family or in an individual who has few available supports.

Reactions to previous crises. Exploring the way in which a family dealt with a previous crisis identifies their possible reactions to the present stressful event. The type of family structure frequently offers valuable clues to the general approach the family may use to solve the crisis.

In the authoritarian family one or both parents decide what is best for all its members. In such a family structure there is little chance for the children to exercise their own rights or desires. As a result the type of coping behavior demonstrated is usually chosen by a specific individual, regardless of others' needs. In the laissez-faire family the excessive freedom or permissive attitude may result in important issues being undecided, because no one member takes responsibility for the decision making. Often children are uncertain of what is acceptable behavior and may test out both desirable and undesirable approaches toward problem solving. Although new coping mechanisms may be explored, family members offer little direction, approval, or validation of the effectiveness of the behavior. In the authoritative or democratic family there is flexibility and respect for each other's opinions, although the adults exercise direction and guidance for decision making. This type of family usually demonstrates the most ability in

Assessment of coping behaviors

Approach behavior (directed toward acceptance and successful resolution of the crisis)

Asks for information regarding diagnosis and child's present condition
Seeks help and support from others
Anticipates future problems; actively seeks guidance and answers
Talks about the process of dying and death, either of own child's or others'
Plans realistically for the future
Acknowledges and accepts child's awareness of diagnosis and prognosis
Expresses feelings, such as sorrow, depression, and anger, and realizes reason for the emotional reaction
Realistically perceives the child's condition, adjusts to changes (such as remission to relapse)
Recognizes own growth through passage of time, such as earlier denial and nonacceptance of diagnosis
Expresses feelings openly
Experiences somatic distress when fear of loss or actual loss is greatest

Avoidance behaviors (directed toward denial and avoidance of the crisis)

Fails to recognize the seriousness of the child's condition despite physical evidence
Refuses to agree to treatment
Intellectualizes about the illness, but in areas unrelated to the child's condition
Is angry and hostile to members of the staff, regardless of their attitude or behavior
Avoids staff, family members, or child
Entertains unrealistic future plans for child, with little emphasis on the present
Is unable to adjust to or accept a change in progression of disease
Continually looks for new cures with no perspective toward possible benefit
Refuses to acknowledge child's understanding of disease and prognosis
Uses magical thinking and fantasy, may seek ''occult'' help
Places complete faith in religion to point of relinguishing own responsibility
Withdraws from outside world
Punishes self because of guilt and blame
Makes no change in life-style to meet needs of other family members
Is unable to discuss death on any level, such as previous experiences with loss

exploring new coping mechanisms that are aimed at successful resolution of the crisis for the ultimate benefit of the entire family.

Nurses' role

The value of identifying possible methods for assessing the potential risk factor in families in crisis is to isolate those families who need more intense intervention in order to prevent future problems. Ideally assessment of risk factors should begin as soon as the family learns of the diagnosis. Sample questions that are designed to elicit information for evaluating the degree of risk are listed in the boxed material to the right. Assessment must be a continuous process because approach behaviors during one phase of the illness do not ensure reciprocal coping mechanisms in subsequent phases. Since support systems may change and perception of events may be altered at any point during the illness, nurses must continually evaluate the effectiveness of their interventions.

After assessment of the family's strengths or weaknesses in coping with the crisis, nurses can intervene in any or all of the preceding categories. If a support system is lacking, they can substitute as a significant person and can locate potential sources of support, such as other parents, extended family members, specific service agencies, religious clergy, or community members. If parents are hav-

Questions for assessing degree of risk in families of terminally ill children

1. ''Who do you talk to when you have something on your mind?'' If answer is not the spouse, ask for reason.
2. ''When something is worrying you, what do you do?''
3. ''Does talking seem to help when you feel upset?''
4. ''Have you ever heard the word [name of diagnosis] before?'' If answer is ''yes,'' say, ''Tell me about it.''
5. ''Have you known anyone who died?'' If answer is ''yes,'' say, ''Tell me about it.'' Alternate question, ''Are all your family members living?'' Ask for further description of those who died.
6. ''Has your religion or faith been of help to you?'' If answer is ''yes,'' say, ''Tell me how.'' If person has a religious orientation, ask, ''Have you ever wondered why God sent you this illness?''
7. ''I know the physicians said that there is no known cause of this disease, but what do you think *really* caused it?''
8. ''How has your child's illness affected you and your family?''
9. ''Tell me about a time that you have had another crisis (problem, bad time) in your family. How did you solve that problem?''
10. ''Who usually makes the decisions in your family?''

ing difficulty in relating to their children, nurses can intervene by serving as interpreters, role models, or temporary supports for the child. When perception of the illness interferes with successful resolution of the crisis, nurses can clarify misconceptions, encourage family members to discuss their feelings, help other professionals to understand the family's reactions, and refer to other specialists for additional assistance in dealing with specific problems. Nurses can help families explore new coping mechanisms or alter old ones to successfully meet the present crisis. Since a period of crisis is a time for exceptional growth and change, nurses can guide individuals toward seeking original coping behaviors that may affect their overall functioning as well as adjustment to the crisis. An example of the positive benefits of stressful events is the observation that potentially fatally ill children mature earlier, cope better, and adjust easier to normal life changes than healthy children.

NURSES' REACTIONS TO FATALLY ILL CHILDREN

Nurses experience reactions that are very similar to the responses of family members to a fatal illness. Some of these help nurses provide care by protecting them from the emotional impact of the event. Others interfere with the establishment of a therapeutic relationship with family members. An analysis and understanding of these reactions are as important in providing effective care to the dying child as is the recognition of specific responses in the family.

Denial

When children are admitted to a pediatric unit with a suspected diagnosis of a serious illness, the initial response from nurses is shock and denial. However, their behavioral reaction may be withdrawal from the child and family. They choose the "cure" philosophy over the "care" philosophy as a method of distancing themselves from the implications of emotional involvement. Since there usually is a favorable prognosis for induction of remission, nurses attempt to focus on the medical treatment of the disease. They may avoid family members' questions or answer them in terms of a medical orientation. As a result they may not understand the reason or hidden meanings behind the family's reactions to discovery of the diagnosis. For example, they may interpret a family member's anger as a personal affront to their adequacy as nurses rather than as a necessary component of eventual acceptance of the diagnosis.

Because of their own dependency on denial, nurses may support denial in parents. There are several methods of conveying this message, such as emphasizing only the optimistic "survival statistics," negating the seriousness of the illness, focusing on "cheering up" the family, and engaging in casual conversation to avoid meaningful dialogue. Although this increases nurses' comfort in caring for the dying child, it does little to provide family members with an opportunity to progress beyond denial and begin anticipatory grieving.

Some denial is as important for nurses as it is for the child or parents, because it protects them from the overwhelming reality of death. It would be extremely difficult to participate in the medical treatment plan without some expectation of a cure. Denial is also necessary to prevent feelings of failure. The nursing and medical goal is curing illness and saving lives, not allowing patients to die. However, denial loses its beneficial functions when nurses refuse to admit failure and adhere to the "curing" regimen, regardless of its effectiveness or value. Consequently nurses and other members of the health team do not allow children to die with dignity and focus on the quantity of life, rather than its quality. One of the reasons for this is that health professionals may not progress past the point of denial in the grieving process and, therefore, are unable to let go of the child even when death is imminent. As a result of this continued denial, the family members are isolated and often hindered in their own efforts to prepare for death.

Anger and depression

Some nurses may be angry for having been assigned to the "leukemic case," because the very exposure to potential failure in a fatal illness is extremely threatening. Others may feel angry for having to subject the child to painful procedures or for being unable to relieve his physical and emotional suffering. Still others may identify with the parents and share the cultural belief that children should not die before their chance for fulfillment. Instead of anger, some nurses may feel depression for any of the preceding reasons.

However, without an understanding behind the reason for the emotion, nurses may project the anger onto others, particularly family members. They may be unable to tolerate the child's uncooperative behavior or the parents' continual request for information. Since anger instigates more anger, parents react with hostility and think that the members of the nursing staff are rejecting them. Consequently a vicious cycle of resentment, mistrust, and frustration results.

Depression also has adverse effects on a therapeutic relationship, because nurses may withdraw from the child and parents as a method of controlling their sadness. Unaware of the reason for the avoidance, family members interpret this behavior as evidence of inadequate care. This reaction also fosters a nonsupportive cycle of avoidance, withdrawal, resentment, and frustration. However, the messages are usually more covert than when the nurses' reaction is anger and may prevent a climax that could result in a solution to the problem.

Guilt

A reaction to one's inability to deal with a fatally ill child is often guilt. Nurses who become angry or depressed when caring for a dying child often reveal that they are very uncomfortable with this response but are unable to choose a more direct, constructive approach. They express guilt for having been intolerant of the child's or parents' behavior and, even more importantly, realize the missed opportunity in providing these individuals with professional support and guidance.

Nursing staff may experience guilt even when they can deal effectively with the family. For example, when a young adolescent with leukemia died unexpectedly from a rare complication, the primary nurse, who had had an excellent, supportive relationship with him, felt guilt and remorse for not having predicted or prevented the fatality. Even though everyone assured the nurse that responsible nursing judgment had been exercised, the nurse was convinced that impending signs of the complication had been missed. It was several weeks before the nurse was able to realize that guilt was a typical reaction and part of the resolution of grief.

Nurses may also experience guilt for having failed the expectation that they are supposed to save lives, not let people die. Unfortunately nursing education has often been negligent in its preparation of nurses to help people die. Guilt is particularly intense when one fails to do something for the child or misses clues from parents for help. For example, a nurse who had been working with a family whose son was dying procrastinated in seeing them because of her difficulty in relating to the nonverbal parents. The seriousness of the child's illness was denied as a defense for not visiting. After he died, the nurse felt extremely guilty for meeting personal needs by staying away.

The one important difference between a dying child and an ill child is that there may be no second chance to meet the needs of the dying child. This finality is difficult to comprehend but can be a catalyst toward better understanding of one's own responses to dying. For example, when guilt makes one uncomfortable enough to seek alternate behavior patterns, there is an opportunity for change to occur, provided the individual is given some assistance and support.

Ambivalence

One of the most universal reactions of nurses is ambivalence in their feelings toward a dying child. There is the fluctuating adherence to hope and fear or the continuous bargaining for oneself, the child, and other family members. There is also frustration as one confronts many conflicts in the care and cure philosophies.

Hope and fear. Nurses hope for an eventual cure for the child and fear a relapse. Sometimes the motivations for either are more for personal comfort than genuine concern for others. For example, they may hope that the child recovers so that he does not return to the hospital. Or they may wish for a remission so that his discharge is assured. Such thoughts are certainly understandable in light of the emotional toll of nursing a fatally ill child. Although nurses often feel guilty for having such selfish thoughts, it is important to recognize the human need each individual has for personal comfort and security. If one can accept the ambivalence, especially the fear, then the challenge of facing a child's death becomes easier because nurses can share in the strength and support of the family.

Bargaining. Ambivalence may be demonstrated in a particular type of bargaining. Rather than bargaining for extra time, nurses may hope that their colleagues are assigned the patient or that a death may occur on a shift other than their own. Occasionally the bargaining may progress to the extreme that nurses refuse to care for the child. Although this overt reaction is uncommon, nurses may demonstrate such feelings by avoiding the child and family whenever possible.

Bargaining for a temporary absence from the dying child is a healthy response, because it denotes nurses' awareness of their own emotional limits. Nurses who continually work in any high-stress environment must have time to recoup their own emotional reserves. This may occur through various support systems, such as one's own family, colleagues, clinical supervision, and so on. Nurses who are unable to recognize their personal emotional limits are in danger of seeking from the professional relationship their own needs for gratification, achievements, and fulfillment. This results in the loss of an objective evaluation of therapeutic interventions and the increased potential for subjective overinvolvement with the family.

Frustration

Caring for the terminally ill child creates dilemmas of conflict, such as what to tell the child, the responsibility of carrying out medical orders, the risks of emotional involvement, and the potential need for extraordinary medical treatment. Some nurses react to the conflict by staunchly supporting the medical orders. For example, if the physician decides not to tell the child the truth or plans to use lifesaving measures in the face of impending death, the nurse may avoid the potential conflicts by following the physician's mandates. However, the risk in such an approach is that the physician's needs will be met at the expense of those of the child and family.

The opposite approach is to become the child's advocate despite the opinions of other health team members and, sometimes, despite the desires of parents. As the child's advocate the nurse may demonstrate control through possession of the child. When this occurs, nurses usurp the usual parental responsibilities and privileges and create an atmosphere that keeps parents from participating in their child's care. Typical ways of exercising this power are by restricting visiting hours, providing no privacy for the child and parents, and informing parents of the child's ''cooperative, good behavior'' when they are not visiting. Often this tacit ''no welcome'' approach is sufficient to keep parents away from an already threatening, frightening environment. However, once the parents do limit their visiting time, nurses seize the opportunity to label them as uncaring, aloof, or uninvolved. What nurses fail to realize is that their position as the child's advocate has limited the child's most important support system, his family.

A more desirable approach to the conflicts of caring for a potentially fatally ill child is to become the child's advocate while respecting the wishes of others. Rather than choosing sides, it is beneficial to listen to each person's decisions and attempt to mediate a mutually agreeable solution. Since individuals achieve different degrees of acceptance during the course of a fatal illness, supporting one person's reaction may reject another's. Often, effective communication requires involving all significant members in a group discussion. A team approach ensures a more equitable and agreeable plan of care for all family members and avoids much of the frustration caused by conflicts.

Nurses' role

Nursing approaches to the care of potentially terminally ill children and their families, particularly for each phase of the illness, have been discussed throughout this chapter. The roles nurses assume can be summarized as (1) support system for the child and family throughout the course of the illness; (2) educator of family members regarding knowledge of the disease, its treatment, and the psychologic reactions of others; and (3) coordinator, liaison, and advocate of the family with each other and among the members of the health team.

However, there are other nursing responsibilities that do not directly relate to the recipient of care. These goals are personal and individual. They involve understanding, insight, and awareness of one's own reactions to death and loss. Becoming a nurse who can cope effectively and therapeutically with children who are dying requires deliberate and concerted effort on the part of the nurse, an opportunity to acquire and translate theory into practice, and the availability of personal and professional support systems.[12]

Self-awareness and consciousness raising. The initial step in effectively caring for a dying child is making a deliberate choice to become involved. Many nurses react negatively to the word ''involvement'' because they believe that professionals must remain uninvolved in order to maintain objectivity. Involvement does not displace objectivity. On the contrary, allowing oneself to feel with the other person expands one's ability to comprehend the meaning and depth of that emotion. Involvement does have the potential risk of clouding objectivity, but awareness of one's reactions and investments in the care of a dying child prevents such possible hazards.

Developing awareness requires the willingness to investigate one's motivations for choosing to work in such an area, to review one's resolution of past losses, and to contemplate one's own fears of death. Often nurses realize that their cold, impersonal, detached reaction to dying patients stems from previous unresolved conflicts or losses. Once they are able to talk about such experiences, they are usually able to gain insight into their behavior and begin to form alternate methods of reacting.

Knowledge and practice. Intervening therapeutically with terminally ill children and their families requires more than self-awareness. It also necessitates basing one's practice on sound theoretic formulations. Although many of the discussions in this chapter may resemble stereotyping, they are meant to serve as a general, concise analysis of the typical reactions of families. Every individual is different and responds to events or crises in a way that is influenced by all his previous life's experiences. However, there must be some beginning point for understanding the more typical responses of individuals and for making some decision as to their importance in the eventual resolution of the crisis. In this way nurses can plan care that meets the needs of each family member in terms of prevention as well as intervention of problems.

Nurses also must explore ethical issues surrounding the definition of death, the use of extraordinary, lifesaving measures vs passive or active euthanasia, and patients' rights to know and choose their own destiny. Once they have soundly formulated principles by which to practice, they need opportunities for decision making. When a team approach is used, nurses can be valuable members of the group, provided that their own values are clarified and that they have critically assessed the family's responses.

Support systems. The value of an available support system in the overall adaptation of family members to the crisis of anticipated death has already been explored. The same importance and necessity exist for a support system that allows nurses to effectively investigate their attitudes toward death and translate theory into practice. Social supports may be personal family members such as parents or spouses, extended relatives, and friends. Professional supports are usually colleagues, consultants, teachers, or supervisors. Professional persons may be of their own field or may be from related disciplines.

Although professional supports may include social relationships, it is best if the roles remain separate. For example, it may be very difficult to discuss a personal experience of a previous loss if the individual believes that the revelation of such an event would alter the friendship. In a professional relationship the responsibilities of a social attachment are absent. The individual can disclose personal feelings without the hazards of judgment or criticism. It is for this reason that regular sessions with a preceptor or clinical supervisor are probably most constructive and conducive to professional growth. Consultants or counselors who are not involved in the actual work situation are better able to objectively evaluate the effectiveness of nurses' roles. They provide the necessary insurance against professional overinvolvement with the dying child and family.

Although personal awareness of one's feelings about death, an understanding of children's and other family's reactions to death, and a functional support system are prerequisites toward effective care of the dying child, approaches toward effective nursing care of the dying child are determined by each nurse's willingness to bear the pain of trial and error, to seek answers by facing challenges, and to reap the rewards from dedicated efforts.

REFERENCES

1. Caprio, F.: A study of some psychological reactions during pre-adolescence to the idea of death, Psychiatr. Q. **24:**495-505, 1955.
2. Engel, G. L.: Psychological development in health and disease, Philadelphia, 1962, W. B. Saunders Co.
3. Epstein, C.: Nursing the dying patient, Reston, Va., 1975, Reston Publishing Co.
4. Gray, V. R.: Some physiological needs. In Dealing with death and dying, Philadelphia, 1977, Intermed Communications Inc.
5. Karon, M., and Vernick, J.: An approach to the emotional support of fatally ill children, Clin. Pediatr. **7:**274-280, 1968.
6. Kastenbaum, R.: The child's understanding of death: how does it develop? In Grollman, E., editor: Explaining death to children, Boston, 1967, Beacon Press.
7. Kübler-Ross, E.: On death and dying, New York, 1969, Macmillan, Inc.
8. Lindemann, E.: Symptomatology and management of acute grief. In Parad, H. J., editor: Crisis intervention: selected readings, New York, 1965, Family Service Association of America.
9. Morrissey, J.: Death anxiety in children with a fatal illness. In Parad, H. J., editor: Crisis intervention: selected readings, New York, 1965, Family Service Association of America.
10. Poznanski, E.: The "replacement child"-a sign of unresolved parental grief, J. Pediatr. **81**(6):1190-1193, December 1972.
11. Schowalter, J. E.: The child's reaction to his own terminal illness. In Schoenberg, B., and associates, editors: Psychosocial aspects of terminal care, New York, 1972, Columbia University Press.
12. Suarez, M., and Benoliel, J.: Coping with failure: the case of death in childhood. In Scipien, G., and associates, editors: Issues in comprehensive pediatric nursing, New York, 1976, McGraw-Hill, Inc.
13. Waechter, E.: Children's awareness of fatal illness, Am. J. Nurs. **71**(6):1168-1172, June 1971.

BIBLIOGRAPHY

Aguilera, D. C., and Messick, J. M.: Crisis intervention: theory and methodology, ed. 3, St. Louis, 1978, The C. V. Mosby Co.

Aradine, C. R.: Books for children about death, Pediatrics **57**(3): 372-378, March 1976.

Binger, C. M., and associates: Childhood leukemia—emotional impact on patient and family, N. Engl. J. Med. **280:**414-418, 1969.

Bivalec, L. M., and Berkman, J.: Care by parent, Nurs. Clin. North Am. **11**(1):109-113, March 1976.

Bowlby, J.: Grief and mourning in infancy and early childhood: psychoanalytic study of the child, vol. 15, New York, 1960, International Universities Press.

Bozeman, M. F., and associates: The adaptation of mothers to the threatened loss of their children through leukemia, Parts I and II. Psychological impact of cancer and its treatment, Part III, Cancer **8**(1):1-33, January/February 1955.

Bright, F., and France, M.: The nurse and the terminally ill child, Nurs. Outlook **15:**39-42, September 1967.

Buschman, P.: The child with leukemia: group support for parents, Am. J. Nurs. **76**(7):1121, July 1976.

Cain, A. C., and associates: Children's disturbed reactions to the death of a sibling, Am. J. Orthopsychiatry **34:**741-752, 1964.

Chodoff, P., Friedman, S., and Hamburg, D.: Stress, defenses, and coping behaviors: observations in parents of children with malignant disease, Am. J. Orthopsychiatry **120:**174-194, 1964.

Clapp, M. J.: Psychosocial reactions of children with cancer, Nurs. Clin. North Am. **11**(1):73-82, March 1976.

Cobb, B.: Psychological impact of long illness and death of a child on the family circle, J. Pediatr. **49:**746-751, 1956.

Craven, J., and Wald, F.: Hospice care for dying patients, Am. J. Nurs. **75:**1816, October 1975.

Easson, W.: The dying child, Illinois, 1970, Charles C Thomas, Publisher.

Engel, G. L.: Psychological development in health and disease, Philadelphia, 1972, W. B. Saunders Co.

Evans, A.: If a child must die . . . , N. Engl. J. Med. **278:**138-142, 1968.

Everson, S.: Sibling counseling, Am. J. Nurs. **77**(4):644-646, April 1977.

Fergusson, J. H.: Late psychologic effects of a serious illness in childhood, Nurs. Clin. North Am. **11**(1):83-93, March 1976.

Fond, K. I.: Dealing with death and dying through family-centered care, Nurs. Clin. North Am. **7**(1):53-64, March 1972.

Friedman, S.: Care of the family of the child with cancer, Pediatrics **40:**498-504, 1967.

Friedman, S., and associates: Behavioral observations on parents anticipating the death of a child, Pediatrics **32:**610-625, 1963.

Furman, E.: A child's parent dies, New Haven, 1975, Yale University Press.

Green, M.: Care of the dying child, Pediatrics **40:**492-498, 1967.

Green, M., and Solnit, A. J.: Reactions to the threatened loss of a child: a vulnerable child syndrome: pediatric management of the dying child, Part III. In Schwartz, J. L., and Schwartz, L. H., editors: Vulnerable infants: a psychosocial dilemma, New York, 1977, McGraw-Hill, Inc.

Greene, P.: The child with leukemia in the classroom, Am. J. Nurs. **75**(1):86-87, January 1975.

Grollman, E., editor: Explaining death to children, Boston, 1967, Beacon Press.

Guimond, J.: We knew our child was dying, Am. J. Nurs. **74**(2): 248-249, February 1974.

Gyulay, J. E.: The forgotten grievers, Am. J. Nurs. **75**(9):1476-1479, September 1975.

Gyulay, J. E.: Care of the dying child, Nurs. Clin. North Am. **11**(1):95-107, March 1976.

Gyulay, J. E.: Dealing with the family of a dying child. In Scipien, G. M., and Barnard, M. U., editors: Issues in comprehensive pediatric nursing, New York, 1976, McGraw-Hill, Inc.

Gyulay, J. E., and Miles, M. S.: The family with a terminally ill child. In Hymovitch, D., and Barnard, M., editor: Family health care, New York, 1973, McGraw-Hill, Inc.

Hardgrove, C., and Warrick, L.: How shall we tell the siblings? Am. J. Nurs. **74**(3):448-450, March 1974.

Heffron, W. A.: Group therapy sessions as part of treatment of children with cancer, Pediatr. Ann. **3**:102-112, February 1975.

Hopkins, L. J.: A basis for nursing care of the terminally ill child and his family, Am. J. Maternal Child Nurs. **2**(2):93-99, 1973.

Jackson, P. L.: Chronic grief, Am. J. Nurs. **74**(7):1289-1291, July 1974.

Karon, M., and Vernick, J.: Who's afraid of death on a leukemia ward? Am. J. Dis. Child. **109**:393-397, 1965.

Kartha, M., and Inta, J.: Short-term group therapy for mothers of leukemic children, Clin. Pediatr. **15**(9):803-806, September 1976.

Kavannaugh, R. E.: Children's "special needs." In Chaney, P. S., editor: Dealing with death and dying, Philadelphia, 1976, Intermed Communications Inc.

Keleman, S.: Living your dying, New York, 1974, Random House, Inc.

Kübler-Ross, E.: Death: the final stage of growth, Englewood Cliffs, N.J., 1975, Prentice-Hall, Inc.

Lowenberg, J.: The coping behaviors of fatally ill adolescents and their parents, Nurs. Forum **9**(3):270-272, March 1970.

Mann, S. A.: Coping with a child's fatal illness, Nurs. Clin. North Am. **9**(1):81-87, March 1974.

Martinson, I. M.: Home care for the dying child: professional and family perspectives, New York, 1976, Appleton-Century-Crofts.

Martinson, I. M.: Parents help each other, Am. J. Nurs. **76**(7): 1120-1122, July 1976.

Morrissey, J.: Children's adaptation to fatal illness, Social Work **8**:81-88, October 1963.

Nagy, M.: The child's view of death, J. Genet. Psychol. **73**:3-27, 1948.

Natterson, J., and Knudsen, A.: Observations concerning fear of death in fatally ill children and their mothers, Psychosom. Med. **22**:456-465, 1969.

Northrup, F. C.: The dying child, Am. J. Nurs. **74**(6):1066-1068, June 1974.

Popoff, D.: What are your feelings about death and dying? Part I, Nursing '75 **5**(8):15-24, August 1975.

Pothier, P.: Mental health counseling with children, Boston, 1976, Little, Brown and Co.

Puff, R. S., and Campbell, A. G.: In deciding the care of severely handicapped or dying persons: with particular reference to infants, Pediatrics **57**(4):487-493, April 1976.

Schowalter, J. E., Ferholt, J. B., and Mann, N. M.: The adolescent patient's decision to die, Pediatrics **51**(1):97-103, January 1973.

Schowalter, J. E.: Children's reactions to terminal illness, Pediatr. Ann. **3**:93-100, November 1974.

Schulman, J. L.: Coping with tragedy: successfully facing the problem of a seriously ill child, Chicago, 1976, Follett Publishing Co.

Schulz, R., and Aderman, D.: Clinical research and the stages of dying, Omega **5**:137-143, 1974.

Solnit, A., and Green, M.: The pediatric management of the dying child: the child's reaction to fear of dying, Mod. Perspect. Child Dev. **8**:217-228, 1963.

Spinetta, J. J., Rigler, D., and Karon, M.: Anxiety in the dying child, Pediatrics **52**(6):841-845, December 1973.

Surveyer, J. A.: Coma in children: how it affects parents, Am. J. Maternal Child Nurs. **1**(1):17-21, January/February 1976.

Wentzel, K. B.: The dying are the living, Am. J. Nurs. **76**(6): 956-957, June 1976.

Wiener, J. M.: Children and dying, Pediatr. Ann. **3**:83-92, November 1974.

Wolf, A.: Helping your child to understand death, New York, 1973, The Child Study Press.

28

The child with a life-threatening disorder

There are few situations in nursing that exceed the challenges of caring for a child with a life-threatening illness. The general psychologic needs of these children and families, which have been discussed in Chapter 27, are tremendous and mesh inextricably with their physical needs. This chapter is concerned with the physical and specific emotional problems associated with several disorders that have potentially fatal prognoses.

The purpose of isolating these conditions from other areas of the text is to present a comprehensive model of the nursing care that applies to such disorders. For example, most of the emphasis focuses on the discussion of leukemia because it is the most frequent form of cancer and because it serves as a prototype for problems and needs encountered in other conditions. In addition, since many of the medical therapies differ little from one type of cancer to another, discussing them in unison allows for a detailed exploration without undue repetition.

Although these conditions are all life threatening because of an uncertain, and often unfavorable, prognosis, this chapter should be viewed with hope and optimism rather than despair or pessimism. Newer trends in therapy are briefly discussed to alert the nurse to those advances that may herald a new future for these children. In the last decade significant advances have resulted in improved survival rates for several disorders. However, the emphasis focuses on those problems that demand nursing expertise for the child undergoing current modes of treatment.

CANCER IN CHILDREN

Incidence

Cancer is the leading cause of death from disease in children ages 1 through 14 years and accounts for 1 out of twenty-seven of all childhood deaths, exceeded only by accidents. The incidence of cancer in children in this age-group is approximately 10 per 100,000 children yearly. The mortality rate annually is 5.3 per 100,000. If the present rates continue, the projected number of new cases will be about 6400, with about 2800 deaths per year.[6]

The difference between yearly mortality rates and incidence reflects the longer survival time of children with cancer. For example, children who are diagnosed before age 15 years are included in the incidence figures, but if they survive past 15 years they obviously cannot be included as a mortality statistic. This is an important consideration when investigating the incidence of cancer, because mortality tables do not accurately reflect the total number of children who actually have the disease and survive.

There is considerable disparity in the statistics available for childhood cancer. A great deal of this is because of the innumerable variables in statistical surveys that are not readily apparent when investigating the data. For example, in most epidemiology studies mortality rates are tabulated from death certificates. Incidence data are derived from diagnosis and are believed to be more correct. However, recent advances in diagnosis also account for possible "false trends." Two examples of this include leukemia and Wilms' tumor.

Prior to 1940, bone marrow examination was not mandatory for confirming the diagnosis of leukemia. Following this period there was an increase in incidence, which may actually represent more reliable diagnostic criteria. In the case of Wilms' tumor the reclassification of many reported cases of the nephroblastoma to nonmalignant mesoblastic nephroma has cast doubt on the validity of the dramatic improvement in survival rates.[17]

Despite statistical inconsistencies, most investigators believe that the incidence of cancer in children has been increasing over the past half century. This is partly a result of better diagnostic procedures for detecting cancer and partly a result of decreased mortality caused by infectious diseases. However, the rising number of cases of childhood cancer above expected population growth probably reflects a significant increase in carcinogenic agents or an increased exposure to such agents.[17] For instance, some types of cancer have increased dramatically after exposure to carcinogens such as radiation or drugs. The rise in thyroid carcinoma, normally a rare type of cancer in children, during the early 1950s as a result of low-dose therapeutic irradiation, is a classic example of the relationship between exposure to carcinogens and changes in incidence rates.[18]

Table 28-1. Incidence of cancer in United States among children under 15 years of age

Type of cancer	% of cases	
	White	Black
Leukemia	42.1	24.3
Central nervous system	23.9	23.9
Lymphoma	13.2	13.9
Neuroblastoma and other sympathetic nervous system tumors	9.6	7.0
Rhabdomyosarcoma and other soft tissue sarcomas	8.4	3.9
Wilms' tumor and other kidney tumors	7.8	7.8
Bone tumors	5.6	4.8
Retinoblastoma	3.4	3.0
Other	10.5	9.1

From Young, J. L., and Miller, R. W.: J. Pediatr. **86**(2):254-258, February 1975.

During childhood there are changing incidences for various types of cancer. For children in all pediatric age-groups, leukemia is the most frequent type of cancer (Table 28-1). The second most common type includes tumors of the central nervous system and brain. However, for children in the age-group between 15 and 29 years, the lymphomas are the second most common form, followed by the sarcomas. There is a striking absence of neoplastic disease during the age period from 8 to 14 years.[7] It has been suggested that this lag is caused by a quiescent period of growth prior to puberty.[11]

There are also peak incidences for various types of cancer. The age period from 2 to 4 years is a peak for acute lymphocytic leukemia, Wilms' tumor (nephroblastoma), neuroblastoma, retinoblastoma, and rhabdomyosarcoma. The high frequency of the blastomas in young children suggests an intrauterine origin for these types of cancer.

Race and sex also influence incidence rates. For example, the usual peak for leukemia seen in white children is absent in nonwhite groups. In general, leukemia incidence is lower for the American black than for the country's entire population, and American Indians have less leukemia than either group. The frequency of death from leukemia is almost twice as high among the Jewish as among the non-Jewish population. Whether these differences are the result of genetic or socioeconomic factors is still unclear. For example, the high incidence among Jews may be related to their increased likelihood to seek medical care than to any genetic factor.[17]

For many types of cancer there is a preponderance of males, although this changes with age. For example, during infancy more leukemia is observed in females than males, but in later childhood the incidence is greater in males. Likewise, in bone sarcomas the incidence is virtually identical until 13 years of age, when the rate for boys exceeds that for girls. This change suggests a pattern that may be an important clue to etiology, because the occurrence of this neoplasm is closely related to bone growth. Other specific differences in incidence are discussed under the individual cancers.

Since 1950 mortality rates for all types of childhood cancer have decreased. This is primarily the result of improved survival rates for Wilms' tumor, retinoblastoma, rhabdomyosarcoma, and leukemia. For all forms of cancer occurring in children under age 15 years, the 5-year survival rate age-adjusted (a rate that mathematically removes the effect of age to allow more accurate comparison for different groups) for normal life expectancy is 39%. For the ten most frequent types of cancer, the range is as low as 15% for some leukemias to a high of 84% for cancer of the eye tumors.

Etiologic factors

The cause of many types of cancer is not known, and even less is known about the etiology of childhood than adult forms of the disease. In recent years the discovery of *carcinogens* (cancer-producing substances) has led to increased knowledge about the causes and high-risk factors for some types of cancer. The leading single known cause of cancer is cigarette smoking, which causes about 80% of all lung cancers and has been associated with cancers of the mouth, larynx, esophagus, kidney, bladder, and perhaps pancreas. However, cigarette smoking as a carcinogen is directly related to *exposure* to the substance and, therefore, is extremely rare in young children.

The following discussion is a brief overview of some of the etiologic factors implicated in childhood cancer.

Environmental agents. A gamut of environment agents that are carcinogenic in humans have been described, but only one of these—ionizing radiation—has been implicated in children. Low doses of radiation have been known to cause thyroid cancer and leukemia. There is some evidence that exposing pregnant women to diagnostic x-ray procedures increases the occurrence of leukemia and other forms of cancer among their children.

Although drugs, particularly those containing radioisotopes and immunosuppressive agents, can increase the risk of developing childhood cancer, the one drug most notably recognized for its carcinogenic effect is diethylstilbestrol. Large doses of this hormone given to pregnant women to prevent abortion cause adenocarcinoma of the vagina in a significant proportion of the female offspring when they reach adolescence and early adulthood.

Viruses. The role of viruses in causing cancer, particularly leukemia, has received much attention. Various cancers have been induced in laboratory animals by inoculation with viruses extracted from cancer sites in other animals. However, there is no direct proof for the virus-cancer relationship in humans. To date, one of the few conclusive findings for the viral theory has been the discovery of the Epstein-Barr (EB) virus, a type of herpes virus, in Burkitt's lymphoma. The high clustering of this type of cancer in Africa in contrast to its rarity in other parts of the world suggests an infectious mode of transmission. However, the Epstein-Barr virus is found in other conditions, particularly in mononucleosis, in which there is no associated cancer.

The fact that viruses are implicated in the etiology of cancer is highly probable, even though a causal relationship is still unsupported. It is likely that the type of cellular reaction produced by the virus depends on the degree to which the host can resist viral invasion or, in other words, on the development of an antibody response. Such a conclusion is already supported by the success of immunotherapy in treating certain types of human cancer and by the increased susceptibility to cancer in individuals with immune deficiencies or following immunosuppressive therapy for transplants. It is also probable that the latent virus is triggered by a variety of environmental carcinogens. For example, it has been found that exposure to x-rays could only produce leukemia in mice who were carriers of the leukemia virus.

One of the implications of a viral etiology for cancer involves its communicability. Until more evidence is available, it must be assumed that cancer is not contagious. There is no scientific evidence that anyone with cancer can transmit the disease to another person by any known mode of transmission. Likewise, there is even less proof to support any transmission between man and animal.

Familial/genetic factors. Whether childhood cancers are genetically determined is uncertain. Considerable evidence exists that retinoblastoma is a genetically inherited disorder. Its transmission is autosomal dominant, although the gene has reduced penetrance; therefore, about 10% of children with the gene do not develop tumors. For this reason a family history of the disorder may not be readily apparent. In many of the cases, particularly if the retinoblastoma is unilateral, the occurrence of the disorder represents a fresh mutation.

Leukemia occurs excessively in children with chromosomal aberrations. For example, in children with Down's syndrome, of all three forms the probability of developing leukemia is about 1 in 200, or fifteen times the normal rate for whites.[21] In addition unaffected siblings of children with Down's syndrome also have an increased risk of developing leukemia. A consistent feature of leukemia in children with Down's syndrome is that the age of onset is 2 to 3 years earlier than it is in children generally. Leukemia is also associated with some disorders with mendelian modes of transmission, such as Fanconi's syndrome (a deficiency of all cellular elements of the blood) and Bloom's syndrome (dwarfism and skin changes).

The high incidence of leukemia in children exposed to radiation is possibly caused by long-lasting chromosomal aberrations from the agent. An abnormal chromosome in the G group, commonly known as the Philadelphia chromosome, has been found in chronic myelogenous leukemia and is considered diagnostic of that condition.

Wilms' tumor is associated with several congenital anomalies. One of them, aniridia (bilateral absence of the iris), occurs 1000 times more often in children with Wilms' tumor. Ordinarily this condition is caused by an autosomal-dominant gene, which suggests some genetic influence on Wilms' tumor.

The high frequency of embryonal tumors (the blastomas) in very young children has led to the belief that they are present at birth. The theory of a misplaced embryonal rest suggests that a group of cells or fetal tissue has become misplaced and under certain conditions begins renewed growth as a neoplasm. Exactly what triggers the proliferation and unrestricted growth of these cells is still unknown.

A familial tendency or clustering of cancer also occurs. For example, there are some families who have a higher than expected incidence of cancer, although no environmental or host factor can explain the event. Likewise, there are clustering of cases of cancer within a geographic location that exceeds the incidence expected by chance. However, even in these situations one common denominator cannot be found to explain the phenomenon. Unfortunately such situations can cause considerable concern and even panic in the community.

Some forms of cancer have occurred with greater than random frequency among siblings, although, besides retinoblastoma, these occurrences are rare. However, leukemia carries an extraordinary risk of twin concordance with ratios approximately 1:5 for monozygotic twins, 1:80 for dizygotic twins, and 1:500 for ordinary siblings.[9] The risk is greatest for identical twins during the first year of life. In most instances twins with concordant leukemia have their onset of illness within weeks or months of each other. These events suggest a similar inciting factor responsible for the leukemia, particularly one that was transferred or shared during fetal life.

Host factors. Although carcinogens are defined as agents capable of producing cancer, an exact cause-effect relationship is not present. Rather there are a variety of complex environmental and genetic factors that influence the probability that certain events will occur. An example of this is the relationship between lung cancer and smoking. Although smoking is considered a "cause," it is really a "high-risk factor," because not all people who smoke develop lung cancer and some individuals who never smoked do. In childhood cancers, with so few "causes" identified, there is even less knowledge about the host factors that predispose a child to cancer.

However, there exist what are known as "cancer-susceptibles"—children who have a greater risk than average for developing the disorder. As has already been discussed, children born with some congential anomalies or chromosomal aberrations are more prone to develop a specific type of cancer.

Another host factor implicated in increasing the risk of cancer is immune deficiency. Children with cell-mediated deficiencies, such as Wiskott-Aldrich syndrome, are at a greater risk for developing lymphoma. Similarly children whose immune system has been suppressed, such as following transplant procedures, develop various cancers more often than average. The theory behind this is that in the body somatic mutations occur that result in cells with cancer properties. Normally the altered cells contain antigens that stimulate the immune system to destroy these cells. If the immune system fails to respond, the altered cells are free to proliferate. Recently this theory has received clinical application by artificially stimulating the body's immune system to develop antibodies that may recognize the cancer cells as foreign and, therefore, destroy them. (See p. 1004 for a more detailed discussion.)

Properties of tumors

Broadly a *tumor* means a "swelling" or a "mass." Some tumors are *benign* in that they demonstrate slow, controlled, and noninvasive growth. Others are *malignant neoplasms* because they demonstrate uncontrollable growth and dissemination (metastasis).

Tumors can arise from any tissue of the body and are classified according to tissue and cell type. The major classifications are (1) *carcinoma,* derived from epithelial tissue such as skin and lining of the body cavities; (2) *adenocarcinoma,* a carcinoma of glandular tissue, such as the breast or prostate; (3) *sarcoma,* derived from connective and supporting tissue, such as bone, cartilage, nerve, and fat; (4) *embryonal* tumor, arising from embryonic tissue, such as the blastomas; (5) *lymphomas* of the lymphatic system; and (6) *leukemias* of the blood-forming organs.

Malignant neoplasms are considered "cancer," a word that actually comprises a large group of diseases. Although many cancers are "tumors" or masses, some types, such as the leukemias, are not masses but widely disseminated cells with characteristics of malignant neoplasms. The following discussion details the biology of malignant growth and will be referred to later in the chapter under the discussion of chemotherapeutic agents.

Growth rate. The cell growth rate of tumors is usually very rapid, in contrast to other cells of the body, which divide slowly. However, there are groups of tissue, namely, the bone marrow, gastrointestinal mucosa, and hair follicles, that normally divide at a rate comparable to malignant cells. It is for this reason that therapeutic agents that are toxic to cancer cells also affect these normal cells.

Generation and doubling time. The growth rate and eventual size of a tumor is dependent on generation time and cell death rate. *Generation time* is the time it takes a cell to complete one cycle of growth and division (mitosis). *Doubling time* is the time it takes for the tumor to double in size. Rapid tumor growth occurs when generation time is short and cell death rate is low. Slow tumor growth can occur with a short generation time but a high cell death rate. Large tumors usually expand more slowly than small ones because their cells are increasingly removed from the core blood supply.

Autonomy. Besides a rapid growth rate, cancer cells exhibit varying degrees of independent behavior. The usual growth regulatory mechanisms of the body do not exert a homeostatic effect on these cells. Therefore, the usual differentiation and organization of cells to perform a specific function is absent. This loss of orderly orientation and structure is called *anaplasia*. As a result rapidly proliferating, nonfunctional cells compete with normal cells for essential nutrients, until eventually the normal cells die and are replaced by cancer cells.

Expansion and invasion. The abnormal, unrestricted growth of cancer cells produces organ damage by *expansion,* resulting in adjacent tissues being compressed and their normal functions altered. This characteristic is typical of space-occupying benign tumors, such as those occurring in the brain. Most malignant tumors also exert injury by *invading* adjacent tissues. In this process the host tissues may be totally replaced by cancer cells that are incapable of the original cells' functions.

Metastasis. A unique property of several cancer cells is their ability to spread to distant sites within the body and establish secondary colonies of malignant growth. Although not all cancer cells exhibit this characteristic, in general they demonstrate an exceptional degree of flexibility in adjusting to adverse conditions elsewhere in the host.

This property is significant for several reasons. It has been demonstrated that the transplantation of a single cell is capable of producing cancer. For example, in leukemia, failure to destroy every leukemic cell may result in a relapse. Transplantation of tumor cells may also occur by implantation during surgery or needle biopsy. For instance, in removing a malignant tumor, there is the risk of allowing cancer cells to break off and implant (metastasize) elsewhere in the body.

Characteristics of neoplastic disease in children[7]

Malignancies in children exhibit the same tumor properties as discussed in the preceding paragraphs but also demonstrate some striking differences. For example, many of the types of cancer seen in children, especially embryonal tumors, are rarely seen in adults. Similarly many of the

Table 28-2. Comparison of incidence for types of cancer in children and adults

Type of cancer	% of cases: Children ages 1-14 years	% of cases: All ages
Leukemia/lymphoma	41	6.5
Sarcomas	27	3
Embryonal tumors	16	1
Neural tumors	6	1.5
Carcinomas and adenocarcinomas	5	85.5
Others	5	2.5

From Sutow, W., Vietti, T., and Fernbach, D., editors: Clinical pediatric oncology, ed. 2, St. Louis, 1977, The C. V. Mosby Co.

adult tumors of the lung, breast, genitalia, and gastrointestinal tract are rarely seen in children (Table 28-2). One of the possible theories explaining the marked difference in cancer sites involves growth rate of cell types and length of exposure to environmental agents. Childhood cancers occur most frequently in rapidly growing tissue, especially the bone marrow. Adult cancers result in tissues that have been in prolonged contact with various carcinogens, such as excessive sunlight on the skin.

Metastasis of cancer cells seems to occur more readily in children than adults. For example, the dissemination of cancer cells during surgery, nonsurgical manipulation, or biopsy results more frequently in children than is generally expected.

However, spontaneous regression of even widely metastasized malignancy occassionally occurs in children. Although the reason is not known, one theory suggests that embryonal tumors undergo maturation to become benign masses.

Cancer cells, particularly of embryonal tumors, exhibit an extremely malignant appearance, which often makes classification of cell types very difficult. Frequently, encapsulated tumors in adults are benign, but in children any tumor should be regarded as malignant until histologically identified.

Prevention

Some cancers can be prevented by avoiding their cause. However, in children the known carcinogens are limited to radiation and a few drugs given to the mother during pregnancy. Therefore, at the present time there is really no known prevention.

Health professionals do have two roles, however. One is aimed at preventing adult-type cancers by educating parents and children about the hazards of known carcinogens, particularly the effects of cigarette smoking and excessive exposure to sunlight in fair-skinned individuals.

Table 28-3. Cancer's seven warning signals

Adults	Children
Change in bowel or bladder habit	Marked change in bowel or bladder habits; nausea and vomiting for no apparent cause
Unusual bleeding or discharge	Bloody discharge of any sort: blood in urine, spontaneous nosebleed or other type hemorrhage, failure to stop bleeding in the usual time
Thickening or lump in breast or elsewhere	Swellings, lumps, or masses anywhere in the body
Obvious change in wart or mole	Any change in the size or appearance of outward growths, such as moles or birthmarks
Nagging cough or hoarseness	Unexplained stumbling in a child
A sore that does not heal	A generally run-down condition
Indigestion or difficulty in swallowing	Pains or the persistent crying of a baby or child, for which no reason can be found

From Cancer in children, New York, 1964, American Cancer Society, Inc.

For example, the death rate for lung cancer among men has increased more than twenty five times over the past 45 years, and 5-year survival rates are low for all stages in both sexes. Female adolescents should be taught the method of self-breast examination and be encouraged to seek periodic health examinations, including a Papanicolaou (Pap) smear. Breast cancer occurs mainly in women over age 35 years and is the leading cause of death among women 40 to 44 years old. It is one of the earliest forms of the adult cancers.

Second, health professionals should teach parents the warning signals of childhood cancer. A comparison of the warning signals for children and adults illustrates the differences in the most common types of cancer seen in each group (Table 28-3). Although cancer occurs less frequently in children (1:27) than in adults (1:5), it is still a leading cause of death. If parents suspect an abnormality, they must be encouraged to seek professional advice. The greatest weapons against all forms of cancer are early detection and treatment.

MODES OF THERAPY

Several advances in the understanding of cancer and improvements in technical processes have greatly influenced present modes of therapy. At the present time, treatment regimens include (1) surgery, (2) chemotherapy, (3) irradiation, (4) immunotherapy, and (5) bone marrow trans-

Text continued on p. 1003.

Table 28-4. Summary of chemotherapeutic agents used in the treatment of childhood cancers*

Type	Agent	Administration	Indication	Side effects and toxicity	Comments and specific nursing considerations
Alkylating agents	Mechlorethamine (nitrogen mustard, Mustargen)	IV, IT†	Hodgkin's disease and other lymphomas Neuroblastoma Retinoblastoma	N/V‡ (½-8 hours later) BMD§ (2-3 weeks later) Alopecia Local phlebitis	Use caution in mixing drug—wear eyeglasses or goggles to avoid vapors in eyes; if solution comes in contact with skin, rinse copiously with water; unstable once mixed, use immediately Infuse through free-flowing infusion; extravasation causes necrosis and sloughing of skin
	Cyclophosphamide (Cytoxan, CTX, Endoxan)	PO, IV, IM	Leukemias Hodgkin's and other lymphomas Neuroblastoma Retinoblastoma Sarcomas	N/V (3-4 hours later) BMD (7-14 days later) Alopecia Hemorrhagic cystitis Severe immunosuppression Mucosal ulceration Hyperpigmentation Transverse ridging of nails Infertility	BMD has platelet-sparing effect Force fluids before administering and for 2 days after drug to prevent chemical cystitis; encourage frequent voiding, even during night Warn parents to report signs of burning on urination or hematuria to physician
	Chlorambucil (Leukeran)	PO	Hodgkin's disease Chronic lymphocytic leukemia	N/V BMD Diarrhea Dermatitis Less commonly may be hepatotoxicity	Usually slow onset; side effects related to high doses
Antimetabolites	Cytosine arabinoside (Ara-C, Cytosar, Cytarabine, arabinosyl cytosine)	IV, IM, SC, IT	Leukemia (AML) Lymphoma Brain tumor	N/V BMD (7-14 days later) Mucosal ulceration Immunosuppression Hepatitis (usually subclinical)	Crosses blood-brain barrier Use with caution in patients with hepatic dysfunction
	5-Azacytidine (5-AzaC)	IV	Leukemia (AML)	N/V BMD Diarrhea	Infuse slowly to decrease severity of N/V
	Mercaptopurine (6-MP, Purinethol)	PO	Leukemia	N/V Diarrhea Abdominal pain Anorexia Stomatitis BMD (4-6 weeks later) Immunosuppression Dermatitis Less commonly may be hepatic dysfunction	Abdominal pain usually relieved by defecation 6-MP is an analog of xanthine; therefore allopurinol (Zyloprim) delays its metabolism and increases it potency

	Methotrexate (MTX, Amethopterin)	PO, IV, IM, IT	Leukemia Sarcomas Brain tumors	N/V Diarrhea Mucosal ulcerations (2-5 days later) BMD (10 days later) Immunosuppression Dermatitis and sensitivity to sun Photosensitivity Alopecia (uncommon) Toxic effects include Hepatitis (fibrosis) Osteoporosis Nephropathy Pneumonitis (fibrosis) Hemorrhagic enteritis	Potency and toxicity increased by salicylates, sulfonamides, and aminobenzoic acid; avoid use of aspirin Citrovorum factor (folinic acid or leucovorin) decreases cytotoxic action of MTX; used as an antidote for overdose and to enhance normal cell recovery following intense therapy; avoid use of vitamins during drug administration unless prescribed by physician Increased toxicity with IT use—pain at injection site, meningismus (signs of meningitis without actual inflammation), especially fever and headache; potential sequelae—transient or permanent hemiparesis, convulsions, dementia, and death Meningeal irritation can be minimized by (1) using a preservative-free diluent, (2) allowing it to warm to room temperature, and (3) filtering it through a Millipore filter prior to administration; use of an Ommaya reservoir also decreases side effects
	6-Thioguanine (6-TG, Thioguan)	PO	Leukemia (AML)	N/V BMD Stomatitis Rarely Dermatitis Photosensitivity Liver dysfunction	Side effects are unusual
Plant alkaloids	Vincristine (Oncovin)	IV	Leukemia Hodgkin's and other lymphomas Wilms' tumor Neuroblastoma Sarcoma Brain tumor	BMD (especially anemia) Alopecia Neurotoxicity—paresthesia (numbness), ataxia, weakness, footdrop, hyporeflexia, constipation (adynamic ileus), hoarseness (vocal cord paralysis), abdominal, chest, and jaw pain, mental depression	Extravasation causes cellulitis; administer through free-flowing infusion Individuals with underlying neurologic problems may be more prone to neurotoxicity Institute safety precautions when ambulation is impaired (side rails, wheelchair, assistance when walking) Monitor stool patterns closely Report signs of neurotoxicity because may necessitate cessation of drug Excreted primarily by liver into biliary system; administer cautiously to anyone with biliary disease
	Vinblastine (Velban)	IV	Hodgkin's and other lymphomas	N/V BMD (especially neutropenia) Alopecia Neurotoxicity (same as above but less severe)	Same as for vincristine

*A general discussion of side effects common to many drugs is discussed on pp. 1014 to 1018.
†IT, intrathecal.
‡N/V, nausea and vomiting.
§BMD, bone marrow depression.

Continued.

Table 28-4. Summary of chemotherapeutic agents used in the treatment of childhood cancers—cont'd

Type	Agent	Administration	Indication	Side effects and toxicity	Comments and specific nursing considerations
Antibiotics	Actinomycin-D (Dactinomycin, Osmegen, ACT-D)	IV	Wilms' tumor Neuroblastoma Sarcomas	N/V (2-5 hours later) BMD (especially platelet) Immunosuppression Mucosal ulceration Abdominal cramps Diarrhea Anorexia (may last few weeks) Alopecia Acne Erythema or hyperpigmentation of previously irradiated skin Fever Malaise	Extravasation causes skin necrosis and pain; administer through free-flowing infusion Enhances cytotoxic effects of radiation therapy but increases toxic effects May cause serious desquamation of irradiated tissue
	Doxorubicin, adriamycin (Doxyrubicin)	IV	Leukemia Lymphomas Sarcomas Neuroblastoma	N/V Stomatitis BMD Fever Local phlebitis Alopecia High-dose toxicity includes Cardiac abnormalities ECG changes Heart failure	Administer through free-flowing infusion to minimize vascular irritation Observe for any changes in heart rate or rhythm and signs of failure Cumulative dose must not exceed 550 mg/m² Warns parents that drug causes urine to turn red (for up to 12 days after administration); this is normal, not hematuria
	Daunorubicin (Daunomycin, Rubidomycin)	IV	Leukemia (AML)	Similar to adriamycin	Similar to adriamycin
	Bleomycin (Blenoxane)	IV, IM, SC	Hodgkin's lymphoma	Allergic reaction—fever, chills, hypotension, anaphylaxis N/V Stomatis Cumulative dose effects include Skin—rash, hyperpigmentation, thickening, ulceration, peeling, nail changes, alopecia Lungs— Pneumonitis with infiltrate that can progress to fatal fibrosis	Should have test dose before therapeutic dose administered Have Benadryl and epinephrine at bedtime Hypersensitivity occurs with first one to two doses Concentration of drug in skin and lungs accounts for toxic effects

Hormones	Corticosteroids (prednisone most frequently used; many proprietary names such as Meticorten, Deltasone, Paracort)	PO; also IM or IV but rarely used	Leukemia Hodgkin's and other lymphomas	For short-term use, no acute toxicity Usual side effects are mild BMD, moon face, fluid retention, weight gain, euphoria, increased appetite, gastric irritation, susceptibility to infection	Explain expected effects, especially in terms of body image, increased appetite, and personality changes Monitor weight gain, evaluate true weight (muscle mass) from water retention May recommend moderate salt restriction Administer with an antacid and early in the morning (sometimes given every other day to minimize side effects) Observe for potential infection sites; usual inflammatory response and fever are absent
				Long-term effects of chronic steroid administration are mood changes, hirsutism, trunk obesity (buffalo hump), thin extremities, muscle wasting and weakness, osteoporosis, poor wound healing, bruising, potassium loss, gastric bleeding, hypertension, diabetes mellitus	All of above; in addition, encourage foods high in potassium (bananas, raisins, prunes, coffee, chocolate) Test stools for occult blood Monitor blood pressure Test urine for sugar and acetone
Enzymes	L-Asparaginase (Elspar)	IV, IM	Leukemia	Allergic reactions (including anaphylactic shock) Fever N/V Anorexia Weight loss Toxicity— Liver dysfunction Hyperglycemia Renal failure	Have epinephrine (1 : 1000) at bedside (usual dose 0.01 ml/kg) Record signs of allergic reaction, such as urticaria, facial edema, hypotension, or abdominal cramps Check weight daily Normally, BUN and ammonia levels rise as a result of drug—not evidence of liver damage Check urine for sugar
Nitrosoureas	Carmustine (BCNU)‖ Lomustine (CCNU)	IV PO	Hodgkin's and other lymphomas Brain tumors Neuroblastoma	N/V (2-6 hours later) BMD (4-6 weeks later) Burning pain along IV infusion BCNU—flushing and facial burning on infusion	Should be used cautiously if BMD already present Avoid extravasation; contact with skin causes brown spots Oral form—give 4 hours after meals when stomach is empty Crosses blood-brain barrier

‖Abbreviations stand for chemical compound.

Continued.

Table 28-4. Summary of chemotherapeutic agents used in the treatment of childhood cancers—cont'd

Type	Agent	Administration	Indication	Side effects and toxicity	Comments and specific nursing considerations
Other miscellaneous agents	Hydroxyurea (Hydrea)	PO	Sarcomas	N/V Anorexia Less commonly Diarrhea BMD Mucosal ulceration Alopecia Dermatitis	Must be given cautiously in patients with renal dysfunction
	Procarbazine (Matulane)	PO	Hodgkin's and other lymphomas Neuroblastoma Embryonal cell carcinoma	Severe N/V BMD (3-4 weeks) Lethargy Dermatitis Myalgia Arthralgia Less commonly Stomatitis Neuropathy Alopecia Diarrhea	Central nervious system depressants (phenothiazines, barbiturates) enhance central nervous system symptoms Monoamine oxidase (MAO) inhibition sometimes occurs; therefore sympathomimetic drugs and natural foods such as aged cheese, yogurt, and bananas should be avoided
	Dacarbazine (DTIC-Dome)	IV	Hodgkin's lymphoma	N/V (especially after first dose) BMD Flulike syndrome	Must be given cautiously in patients with renal dysfunction

plant. The following is an overview of each of these procedures. In addition they are also discussed later in the chapter when applicable to the specific type of cancer.

Surgery

The main goal of surgery is to remove all traces of tumor and restore normal body functioning. Surgery is most successful when the tumor is encapsulated and localized (confined to the site of origin). It may only be palliative when the cancer is regional (metasized to an area adjacent to the original site) or advanced (widespread throughout the body). Obviously the best prognosis is directly related to early detection of the tumor.

The recent trend is toward more conservative surgical excision. For example, in some types of bone cancer such as Ewing's sarcoma, patients are successfully treated with resection of the diseased portion of the bone rather than amputation. There is an increasingly greater emphasis on the use of combination drug and irradiation therapy after limited surgical intervention.

Chemotherapy

One of the greatest advances in the treatment of widely disseminating cancers, such as the leukemias and lymphomas, has been the discovery and effective use of neoplastic agents. Basically these drugs fall into two classifications: cycle-dependent agents (also called cell-cycle phase specific agents) and cycle-independent agents (also called cell-cycle phase nonspecific agents).

To understand how these agents work, it is necessary to review the phases of the cell life cycle. The G_0 phase (''G'' stands for gap) is the period of rest or out-of-cycle phase, during which the cell retains the ability to enter cell division at any time. Undividing stem cells of the hemopoietic system are an example of G_0. G_1, the presynaptic phase, is the phase of cell growth, differentiation, and function. During G_1, RNA and protein are synthesized. When this activity is high, the G_1 interval is short. Usually the major portion of the cell's life is spent in this phase.

The DNA-synthetic or ''S'' phase is the time for replication of chromosomal complement from 46 to 92 and transcription of its genetic information to the RNAs, which then contain the instructions for the correct amino acid sequence for cell functioning and renewal.

The interval after DNA synthesis but preceding mitosis is G_2, or postsynthetic gap phase, during which cells undergo a sequence of biochemical events, such as RNA synthesis, which prepares them for division. Mitosis (M) is the phase of cytoplasmic and nuclear division (prophase, metaphase, anaphase, and telophase), which results in two identical daughter cells. (For a discussion of cell division, see p. 182.)

Cycle-dependent agents destroy cells when they are in a specific phase of division. They are most effective for rapidly growing cells and produce the least toxic effects to normal cells when given for a short period of time. Examples of these types of agents are cytosine arabinoside and methotrexate, which interfere with DNA synthesis; vincristine, which inhibits mitosis; and L-asparaginase, which inhibits the movement of cells from the G_1 to the S phase.

Cycle-independent agents destroy proliferating cells regardless of their cell phase and, therefore, are most effective for slow-growing, bulky tumors, Although generally they are more effective against proliferating cells, they also may destroy cells during the stationary phase G_0 or G_1. Examples of this type are the alkylating agents and the antibiotics.

Although several agents have been found effective in treating different forms of cancer, the remarkable survival rates have been the result of improved combination drug regimens. Combining drugs allows for optimal cell-cycle destruction with minimal toxic effects and decreased resistance by the cancer cells to the agent. For example, the combination MOPP (mechlorethamine [Mustargen], vincristine [Oncovin], procarbazine, and prednisone) combines complimentary cytotoxic effects with nonsimilar side effects. Mechlorethamine and procarbazine are myelosuppressive, vincristine is neurotoxic, and prednisone produces mild bone marrow depression with beneficial effects of improved appetite and a feeling of well-being.

Another example relating to drug resistance involves the single use of corticosteroids. When used only to induce a remission, there is a 40% to 50% chance that steroids alone will induce a second remission. However, when used as maintenance therapy until a relapse occurs, this drug alone will no longer be effective in achieving a successful remission.[21]

Chemotherapeutic agents are classified according to their cytotoxic action. The agents are discussed below, and the principal drugs used in treatment of childhood cancer are summarized in Table 28-4. An understanding of drugs' actions and side effects is essential to nursing care of children with cancer. Frequently the problems requiring nursing care are drug related rather than a consequence of the disease.

Alkylating agents. Alkylation is the replacement of a hydrogen atom of a molecule by an alkyl group. The irreversible combination of alkyl groups with nucleotide chains, particularly DNA, causes unbalanced growth of unaffected cell constituents so that the cell eventually dies. They are radiomimetic, in that their action is similar to irradiation.

Antimetabolities. These agents resemble essential metabolic elements needed for cell growth but are sufficiently altered in molecular structure to inhibit further synthesis of DNA and/or RNA.

Plant alkaloids. These agents from the periwinkle plant

Vinca rosea arrest cells in metaphase (a phase of mitosis) by binding to microtubular protein needed for spindle formation. These two agents, vincristine and vinblastine, differ structurally by only one oxygen atom but are markedly different from each other with regard to dose, toxicity, and antitumor activity. Although both are neurotoxic, vincristine causes more severe side effects than vinblastine.

Antitumor antibiotics. These agents are natural products that interfere with cell division by reacting with DNA in such a way as to prevent further replication of DNA and transcription of RNA.

Hormones. Both adrenal and gonadal hormones have antineoplastic properties. The precise mechanism of action is still unclear. Adrenocorticosteroids greatly depress the production of lymphoid cells by inhibiting mitosis. Although there are a number of cortisone preparations, prednisone is most frequently used.

Androgens and estrogens are effective against certain cancers, such as of the prostate and breast, probably because the hormones exert a growth-regulating rather than a cytotoxic effect on the cells.

Miscellaneous agents. A number of agents do not fall into any of the preceding classifications. The most commonly used ones are described in the following paragraphs.

L-Asparaginase is unique because it is selectively cytotoxic only for certain cancer cells. L-Asparagine, an enzyme necessary for cellular growth, is synthesized by normal cells but must be exogenously supplied to certain leukemic and lymphoma cells. Administration of the enzyme L-asparaginase destroys the essential exogenous supply while sparing normal cells of untoward effects.

Unfortunately this drug is associated with a high incidence of allergic reactions because of the impurities present in its commercially prepared form. The enzyme is harvested from large vats of *Escherichia coli;* as a result complete purification of endotoxin contaminants is difficult. However, for patients allergic to this drug, another L-asparaginase derived from a different bacterium can be used instead.

Hydroxyurea, a cell-cycle dependent agent, inhibits ribonucleotide reduction to deoxyribonucleotide. DNA synthesis is impaired, but protein and RNA synthesis are less affected; therefore, the unbalanced growth results in eventual cellular death.

Nitrosoureas, of which a number of compounds are available, act similarly to alkylating agents and are sometimes classified as such because they replace an essential DNA molecule, thus inhibiting DNA, RNA, and protein synthesis. One of their unique properties is the ability to cross the blood-brain barrier.

Procarbazine is a weak monoamine oxidase (MAO) inhibitor. (MAO is an enzyme that destroys the neurohormones epinephrine, norepinephrine, and serotonin. MAO inhibitors act as psychic energizers.) Its exact cytotoxic action is not known, although it inhibits DNA, RNA, and protein synthesis.

Dacarbazine is an analog of aminoimidazole carboxamide. It interferes with purine synthesis and also exhibits alkylating properties in DNA synthesis. It has shown significant antitumor activity when combined with other drugs, especially doxorubicin.

Irradiation

Irradiation is frequency used in the treatment of childhood cancer, usually in conjunction with chemotherapy and/or surgery. It can be used for curative purposes and is often employed for palliation to relieve symptoms by shrinking the size of the tumor. Recent advances in radiation therapy have optimized its beneficial effects and minimized many of the undesirable side effects. One of these has been the development of high-speed, high-energy machines, such as the linear accelerator, which deliver a concentrated electron or x-ray beam to a precise area of the body. The elimination of extraneous scatter doses of radiation decreases the reactions in adjacent sites.

Cytotoxic effect. Ionizing radiation is cytotoxic in at least three different ways: (1) damaging the pyrimidine bases cytosine, thymine, and uracil needed for the synthesis of nucleic acids, (2) causing single-strand breaks in the DNA or RNA molecule, or (3) causing double helical–strand breaks in these molecules.[21] The effect of disturbing cellular metabolic and reproductive function is either sublethal or lethal damage.

Lethal damage refers to the death of the cell. *Sublethal* damage refers to injured cells that may subsequently be repaired. Many of the acute side effects are the result of lethal damage to radiosensitive tissue, particularly proliferating cells such as those of the bone marrow, gastrointestinal tract, and hair follicles. Late effects may be the result of cell death, such as in infertility, or the consequence of sublethal damage, such as premature aging from a shortened cell life span.

Side effects. The acute untoward reactions from radiation therapy are primarily dependent on the area to be irradiated. Although many factors influence the development of late effects, some of the more important ones include the total dose given, the age of the child (the younger the child, the more radiosensitive his body organs), and the location of the tumor. Total-body irradiation (TBI) is associated with the most severe reactions. It is a necessary preparatory procedure for bone marrow transplants. Table 28-5 summarizes the acute and late effects of radiation therapy and nursing interventions that may he helpful in lessening or preventing them.

Immunotherapy

One of the most exciting research discoveries in the treatment of certain cancers has been the stimulation of

Table 28-5. Side effects of radiotherapy

Site	Early effects	Nursing interventions	Late effects
Gastrointestinal tract	Nausea/vomiting	Give antiemetic on a regular schedule Measure amount of emesis to prevent dehydration	Potential effects: Small bowel or gastric ulceration, perforation Esophageal stricture Radiation hepatitis Gastrointestinal cancer
	Anorexia	Encourage fluids and foods best tolerated, usually light, soft diet Monitor weight loss	
	Mucosal ulceration	Use frequent mouthwashes and oral hygiene to prevent mucositis	
	Diarrhea	Can be controlled with antispasmodics and kaolin pectin preparations Observe for signs of dehydration	
	Potential effects: Pancreatitis Parotitis Loss of taste	May need analgesics to relieve the discomfort Combat severe dryness of mouth with oral hygiene and liquid diet	
Skin	Alopecia (within 2 weeks, begins to regrow by 3-6 months) Dry or moist desquamation	Introduce idea of wig Stress necessitity of scalp hygiene and need for head covering in cold weather Do not refer to skin change as a "burn" (implies use of too much radiation) Keep skin clean Wash daily, using soap sparingly; avoid removing skin markings for radiation fields Avoid exposure to sun For dryness, apply lubricant For desquamation, consult physician for skin hygiene and care	Hyperpigmentation Potential effects: Scarring from moist desquamation Skin cancer Permanent hair loss
Head	Nausea/vomiting (from stimulation of emetic control center) Alopecia Potential effects (area to neck): Parotitis Loss of taste	Same as for gastrointestinal tract	Rarely brain necrosis
Eyes	None	Encourage regular eye examinations	Cataracts
Ears	Potential effect: Radiation-induced otitis media	Encourage regular auditory tests	Potential effect: Hearing loss
Lungs	Potential effect: Pneumonitis	Lung involvement evidenced by coughing and mild chest pains Encourage rest	Potential effect: Fibrotic changes
Heart	Potential effect: Pericarditis	Pericarditis evidenced by friction rub, pain, and ECG changes Encourage rest	Potential effects: Endocardial or myocardial fibrosis Myocardial infarctions
Kidneys	Potential effect: Acute nephritis	Nephritis evidenced by lassitude, headache, vomiting, nocturia, edema of legs, shortness of breath, and sometimes hypertension	Potential effect: Chronic nephritis
Urinary bladder	Rarely cystitis	More likely to occur with concomittant use of cyclophosphamide Encourage liberal fluid intake and frequent voiding	Rarely fibrosis

Continued.

Table 28-5. Side effects of radiotherapy—cont'd

Site	Early effects	Nursing Interventions	Late effects
Bones	None	Inform parents of eventual bone changes; examples—with spinal radiation, retarded height; with Wilms' tumor, scoliosis	Potential effects (depending on site and age): Linear growth retardation Spinal deformities Asymmetric growth Pathologic fractures Benign tumors Sarcomas
Bone marrow	Myelosuppression	Institute bleeding and infection precautions Observe for signs of anemia	Potential effects: Protracted anemia Leukemia
Endocrine glands	None	Encourage anyone who has been exposed to radiotherapy of the neck and thorax to to seek yearly thyroid examinations	Potential effect: Thyroid carcinoma
Testes	None Secretion of testosterone is not affected (normal appearance of secondary sexual characteristics)	Advise family of possibility of sterility	Sterility Testicular hypertrophy
Ovaries	Secondary sexual characteristics may be delayed or absent	Advise family of possibility of delayed secondary sexual characteristics, sterility, and chromosomal damage	Potential effects: Sterility Menopause In presence of fertility, chromosomal damage to germ cells may result in defective product of conception (less likely in sperm because of constant spermatogenesis)

the body's natural immune defenses to combat malignant cells. One of the theories behind the development of immunotherapy is that since cancer cells are constantly developing in everyone's body, there must be a natural immunity that prevents the cells from proliferating to cause disease. Based on this premise and several documented reports linking cancer to the immune system, such as the increased incidence of cancer in immunosuppressed individuals, immunotherapy has become an important component of cancer control.

Immunotherapy may be divided into three classifications: (1) *active,* which uses specific cancer antigens, either those prepared from the patient's own tumor cells or from a similar type tumor, to stimulate a specific host-immune response; (2) *passive,* which involves using antibodies or other immunologically active lymphocytes; and (3) *adaptive,* which involves the transfer of the mechanism for a prolonged nonspecific immune response to the recipient's own immune system.

The latter form of nonspecific immunotherapy is most frequently used in treating childhood cancer. Although several products are under investigational use, the most popular is the Calmette-Guerin bacillus (BCG), an attenuated tuberculin bacillus. Calmette-Guerin bacillus has been used for many years as an immunization for tuberculosis in countries in which the disease is endemic. As an immunologic adjuvant, it stimulates the body's immune system to react by producing antitumor antibodies as well as nontumor antibodies.

Calmette-Guerin bacillus may be administered directly into the tumor or given systemically by intradermal injection (tine technique, multiple puncture, scarification, or Heaf Gun method). Within a few hours a local inflammatory reaction occurs, which indicates an immunologic response. In addition the patient may also experience low-grade fever, malaise, and regional lymphadenopathy within 24 hours of receiving the preparation. With subsequent injections a more severe local reaction can occur from increasing sensitivity to the bacillus. Possible side effects are a disseminated tubercular infection, hypersensitivity reactions, and local skin sloughing at the injection site.

Results with immunotherapy have been promising in leukemic patients. However, this form of therapy only controls cancer growth and, therefore, must be used with other cytotoxic regimens such as chemotherapy.

Bone marrow transplant

Another dramatic approach to the treatment of some forms of cancer, particularly the leukemias, is bone marrow transplant. Unlike immunotherapy, the goal of this procedure is complete cure. Bone marrow transplant involves the matching of a histocompatible donor recipient and complete eradication of all cancer cells from the recipient's body prior to transplantation. The principle behind this procedure is that once the patient is totally aleukemic and immunosuppressed, the donor's marrow cells will begin to produce functioning blood cells without transplant rejection. In essence a new blood-forming organ will be accepted by the recipient.

Although the actual transplant procedure is simple (see p. 1400), the preoperative and postoperative care are complex. The first stage is identifying a compatible donor. The second phase is producing a totally aleukemic immunosuppressed state, which involves intense chemotherapy (usually administration of high-dose cyclophosphamide) and total-body irradiation. The third phase is preventing complications. During the preoperative aplastic phase and for the 10- to 20-day period after transplantation, the patient is extremely susceptible to infection and hemorrhage, as well as to toxic effects from chemotherapy and total-body irradiation. After the procedure there is the grave complication of graft-vs-host reaction (see p. 1400). Unfortunately a high percentage of patients who receive nonidentical donor cells develop this reaction, for which there is no known antidote. Another depressing finding is that in some of the successful transplant patients there is a recurrence of the leukemia.

However, despite these drawbacks, bone marrow transplantation has heralded new hope for patients with poor prognostic characteristics and/or terminal leukemia. With advances in controlling graft-vs-host reaction, deeper understanding of the cancer process, and methods of using nonidentical donors, the prospect for this procedure in treating other forms of cancer and various blood disorders is promising.

Nurses' role

Nurses working with cancer patients have a significant supportive role in helping the family understand the various therapies and prevent or manage expected side effects or toxicities. They also must be cognizant of those treatments, such as diets, devices, and drugs, that are not sanctioned by the medical profession. Cancer quackery is a threat to every cancer family, because it may produce unnecessary harm by itself or render injury because other proved modes of therapy are avoided. In many instances it causes financial burden and emotional strife among family members.

Nurses can be instrumental in working against cancer quackery by identifying those individuals most likely to become victims, such as the miracle seekers, the impatient, and the straw-graspers, communicating effectively with families about the diagnosis and forms of therapy, and providing all possible support and reassurance during treatment.[4] Nurses must be fortified with knowledge to substantiate present treatment protocols and to discredit unauthorized methods. The American Cancer Society and local and state medical societies are reliable sources of information concerning research on investigational vs quack methods of cancer therapy.

LEUKEMIAS

Leukemia, cancer of the blood-forming tissues, is the most common form of childhood cancer. The annual incidence in children under 15 years of age is approximately 4 per 100,000, although the risk is greater in white children in the United States (1 in 2880).[21] It occurs more frequently in males than females after age 1 year, and the peak onset is between 2 and 5 years of age. It is one of the forms of cancer that has demonstrated dramatic improvements in survival rates. Before the use of antileukemic agents in 1948, a child with acute lymphocytic leukemia (ALL) lived only a few weeks or months. Today 5-year survival rates for children with ALL exceed 50% in major research centers, and a proportion of these children may be cured.

However, even for the child with the most favorable prognosis, leukemia presents innumerable physical, emotional, financial, and familial stresses. Nurses in the hospital, clinic, physician's office, and community can do much to prevent some problems and lessen others.

Classification

Site of origin. The leukemias are classified according to site of origin of the white blood cell (leukocyte) within the lymphomyeloid complex. (For a review of the origin of the formed elements of the blood, see Chapter 36 and Fig. 36-1.) Traditionally, acute leukemia has been divided into three groups: (1) lymphatic, (2) myelocytic, and (3) monocytic. Each implies the specific cell of origin. Subdivision into further cell types has resulted in much confusion regarding exact classification. In addition in the majority of children with acute leukemia there is such poor differentiation of immature cells that the general term "stem cell" or "blast cell" leukemia is used.

Presently two forms are generally recognized: *acute lymphoid leukemia (ALL)* and *acute nonlymphoid leukemia*. Synonyms for ALL include lymphatic, lymphocytic, lymphoblastic, and lymphoblastoid leukemia. Usually the term stem cell or blast cell leukemia also refers to the lymphoid type of leukemia. Synonyms for the acute nonlymphoid type include granulocytic, myelocytic, monocytic, myelogenous, monoblastic, and monomyeloblastic. More simply, the nonlymphoid type is termed AML for the monocytic or myelocytic series. Unless a specific cell type is definitively classified, these various synonyms are used interchangeably for either ALL or AML. There are also much rarer forms of leukemia that are named for the specific cell involved, such as basophilic or eosinophilic leukemia.

A second classification of leukemia has been used to differentiate between acute and chronic types. These terms have traditionally referred to the maturity of the leukemic cells and, before the advent of chemotherapeutic agents, also indicated the expected course of the illness. For example, "acute" refers to immature, undifferentiated leukemic cells, which without treatment herald a rapidly fatal course. "Chronic" suggests the presence of mature or maturing leukocytes, which, although produced in excess quantities, still retain some functional ability and, therefore, represent a chronic, long-term disease process. Although these terms are still used, particularly in regard to childhood (acute) and adult (chronic) forms of leukemia, they are no longer truly correct regarding prognosis because of long-term remissions from present therapy.

Because of the confusion and inconsistency in classifying the leukemias, some researchers suggest that other factors, such as morphologic and immunologic cell surface characteristics, be used to identify the cell type. For example, the enzyme muramidase is present only in cytoplasmic granules. Because there are no granules in lymphoblasts, muramidase levels are low. However, in the myelocytic forms of leukemia, levels of this enzyme are markedly elevated.

Recently the type of lymphocyte has been classified into T-lymphocytes (T cells), B-lymphocytes (B cells), or "null" cells, those cells that lack T or B cell characteristics. This further classification of lymphocytic leukemia appears to have prognostic importance in that persons with leukemias of the "null" category (about 85% of ALL) demonstrate better survival rates.

Predominant type. The predominant type of leukemia is lymphoid. Since classification systems vary according to different investigators, it is difficult to precisely state how many cases constitute each type of leukemia. An average estimate seems to range between 80% and 85% for ALL and 15% and 20% for AML. Some investigators include a third group called chronic myeloid or lymphocytic leukemia (4%), which is very rare in children.

Anticipated course. Although the clinical manifestations are similar regardless of the cell involved, classifying leukemia as ALL or AML is extremely important in terms of response to therapy and prognosis. The dramatic improvements seen in children with leukemia almost exclusively occur in ALL. For example, over 90% of children with ALL can be expected to attain an initial remission, and about half of these children will survive for 5 years. With AML the chances of attaining an initial remission are about 70% with considerably shorter duration of remissions and higher mortality rates than ALL.

In addition to the predominant cell type, several other characteristics at diagnosis have prognostic importance. Characteristics associated with the most favorable prognosis (low-risk group) are ages between 3 and 6 years inclusive and a white blood count below $10,000/mm^3$. The average-risk group includes children younger than age 3 years or older than age 7 years with a white blood count above $50,000/mm^3$ or ages 3 to 6 years with a count between $10,000/mm^3$ and $50,000/mm^3$. The high-risk group includes all ages with an initial white blood count above $50,000/mm^3$.

Therefore, from the time of establishment of the diagnosis, the nurse has some idea of the expected course the child will follow. However, in some instances, because of the variety of cell types observed and the marked undifferentiation of immature cells, a definitive classification cannot be made or the diagnosis may be changed. The nurse should be aware of the importance of such events in counseling and supporting family members.

Pathology and related manifestations

Leukemia is an unrestricted proliferation of immature white blood cells in the blood-forming tissues of the body. Although not a "tumor" as such, the leukemic cells demonstrate the same neoplastic properties of solid cancers. Therefore, the resultant pathology and clinical manifestations of the disease are caused by infiltration and replacement of any tissue of the body with nonfunctional leukemic cells. Highly vascular organs of the reticuloendothelial system are most severely affected.

In order to understand the pathophysiology of the leukemic process, it is important to clarify two common misconceptions. First although leukemia is an overproduction of white blood cells, most often in the acute form the leukocyte count is low (hence, the term "leukemia"). Instead, the peripheral blood smear and, more definitively, the bone marrow examination reveal greatly elevated counts of immature cells or "blasts." Second these immature cells do not deliberately attack and destory the normal blood cells or vascular tissues. Cellular destruction is by the process of infiltration and subsequent competition for metabolic elements. The following discussion elaborates the pathologic process and related clinical manifestations in the most susceptible organs of the body (Fig. 28-1).

Bone marrow dysfunction. In all types of leukemia the proliferating cells depress bone marrow production

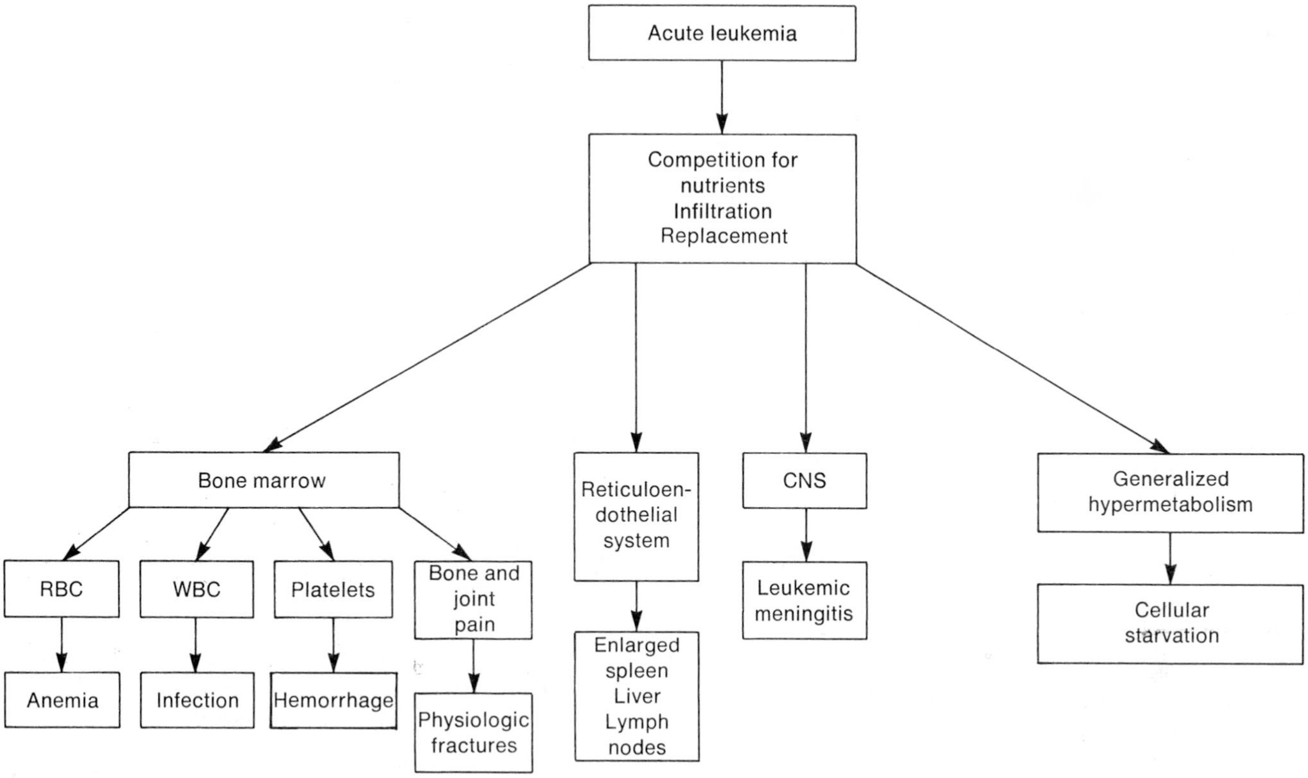

Fig. 28-1. Principal sites of tissue involvement in leukemia.

of the formed elements of the blood by competing for and depriving the normal cells of the essential nutrients for metabolism. The three main consequences are (1) *anemia* from decreased erythrocytes; (2) *infection* from neutropenia; and (3) *bleeding tendencies* from decreased platelet production.

The invasion of the bone marrow with leukemic cells gradually causes a weakening of the bone and a tendency toward physiologic fractures. As leukemic cells invade the periosteum, increasing pressure causes severe pain.

The most frequent presenting signs and symptoms of leukemia are a result of infiltration of the bone marrow. These include fever, pallor, fatigue, anorexia, hemorrhage (usually petechiae), and bone and joint pain. In the presence of neutropenia the body's normal bacterial flora can become aggressive pathogens. Any break in the skin is a potential site of infection. Frequently, vague abdominal pain is caused by areas of inflammation from normal flora within the intestinal tract.

Disturbance of involved organs. The organs of the reticuloendothelial system, namely, the spleen, liver, and lymph glands, demonstrate marked infiltration, enlargement, and eventually fibrosis. Hepatosplenomegaly is typically more severe than lymphadenopathy. Toxic chemotherapeutic agents seem to account for more liver and spleen damage than the disease process.

The next most important site of involvement is the central nervous system. Initially at the time of diagnosis leukemic cells do not tend to invade this area, probably as a result of the protective blood-brain barrier. However, this normal protective mechanism also prevents the antileukemic drugs, with the exception of steroids, from entering the brain in sufficient therapeutic doses to be effective. Prior to the prophylactic use of cranial irradiation and intrathecal methotrexate, central nervous system involvement was frequent in children who survived 6 months or more. However, newer modes of therapy have significantly changed the course of the disease, although central nervous system complications still occur, even during bone marrow remission.

The usual effect of leukemic infiltration of the meninges is increased intracranial pressure. The pathogenesis is presumably attributable to invasion of the arachnoid with proliferating cells, which then interferes with the flow of cerebrospinal fluid in the subarachoid space and at the base of the brain. The increased fluid pressure causes dilation of all four ventricles and, consequently, the signs and symptoms normally associated with this condition, such as severe headache, vomiting, papilledema, irritability, lethargy, and eventually coma. Irritation of the meninges also causes pain and stiffness in the neck and back.

Additional sites of involvement may be the cranial

nerves, most often cranial nerve VII, or the facial nerve, and spinal nerves, particularly of the lumbar sacral plexus, hypothalamus, and cerebellum. Clinical manifestations for these sites are directly related to the area involved. For example, with lumbar-sacral invasion, there is weakness in the lower extremities, pain radiating down the legs to the feet, and difficulty in voiding. Although such signs may be suggestive of a brain tumor, the absence of localized signs often leads to the discovery of central nervous system involvement in leukemia.

Other long-term sites of involvement include the kidneys, testes, prostate, ovaries, gastrointestinal tract, and lungs. With long-term survivors becoming increasingly more common, it is likely that such extramedullary sites of leukemic invasion will become more important clinically. For example, the development of renal masses not only impairs kidney function until uremia may result but also seriously affects the chemotherapeutic regimen of those agents normally excreted in the urine.

Hypermetabolism. The immense metabolic needs of proliferating leukemic cells eventually deprive all body cells of nutrients necessary for survival. Muscle wasting, weight loss, anorexia, and fatigue are natural consequences. Obviously, in addition to the risk of death from infection and hemorrhage, uncontrolled growth of leukemic cells can also terminate in metabolic starvation.

Onset

The precise onset of leukemia is unknown. Its clinical appearance varies markedly from acute to insidious. In most instances the child displays remarkably few symptoms. For example, it is quite typical for leukemia to be diagnosed when a minor infection, such as a cold, fails to completely disappear. The child continues to be pale, listless, irritable, febrile, and anorexic. Parents often suspect some underlying problem when they observe the weight loss, petechiae, bruising without cause, and continued complaints of bone and joint pain.

At other times leukemia is diagnosed after an extended history of signs and symptoms mimicking such conditions as rheumatoid arthritis or mononucleosis. There are also occasions when the diagnosis of leukemia accompanies some totally unrelated event, such as a routine physical examination or accidental injury.

The history not only yields valuable medical information regarding the subsequent course of the illness but also bears heavily on the parents' emotional reaction to the discovery of the diagnosis. In most instances the diagnosis is an unexpected revelation of catastrophic proportion.

Diagnostic evaluation

Leukemia is usually suspected by the history, physical manifestations, and a peripheral blood smear that contains immature forms of leukocytes, frequently combined with low blood counts. Definitive diagnosis is based on bone marrow aspiration or biopsy. Typically the bone marrow is hypercellular with greatly elevated numbers of blast cells. Normally the bone marrow contains between 1% and 5% blast cells. Although the criteria for leukemia are more than 25% blast cells, in almost all cases the number of immature cells exceeds this value.

Once the diagnosis is confirmed, a lumbar puncture is performed to determine if there is any central nervous system involvement. Only about 10% of children demonstrate the presence of leukemic cells in the spinal fluid at the time of diagnosis.

Although several tests may be performed to evaluate the child's general physical condition, those that are usually included are an intravenous pyelogram and biochemical studies to assess liver and kidney function. Since almost all of the chemotherapeutic agents are dependent on these two systems for detoxification and excretion, evaluation of normal functioning is imperative prior to beginning therapy.

Medical management

Treatment of leukemia involves the use of chemotherapeutic agents and irradiation in three phases: (1) induction, which achieves a complete remission or disappearance of all leukemic cells; (2) sanctuary therapy, which prevents leukemic cells from invading or destroys leukemic cells in those areas of the body normally protected from cytotoxic drug levels; and (3) maintenance, which serves to maintain the remission phase. Although the combination of drugs and radiation may vary according to institutions, the prognostic or risk characteristics of the patient, and the type of leukemia being treated, the following general principles for each phase are quite consistently employed.

Remission induction. Almost immediately after confirmation of the diagnosis, induction therapy is begun. Because of the various side effects of the drugs and the possibility of complications from leukemia, especially infection and hemorrhage, the child is usually hospitalized for part or all of the 4- to 6-week induction regimen.

The main drugs used for induction in ALL are the corticosteroids (especially prednisone), vincristine, and L-asparaginase (Table 28-4). Since the use of combination-drug therapy has been more successful in inducing remissions than single-agent schedules, these two drugs are used simultaneously. Oral steroids are administered daily in three divided doses to maintain consistently high blood levels. Vincristine is given by intravenous infusion once a week for a total of four to six doses. L-Asparaginase is given intramuscularly three times a week for a total of nine doses.

Another drug included as part of therapy that is not an antineoplastic agent is allopurinol, a xanthine-oxidase inhibitor, which prevents the metabolic breakdown of xanthine to uric acid. Uric acid, a chemical released during cell breakdown, can accumulate and precipitate in the renal tubules. Eventually tubular obstruction results in uremia. Since the chemotherapeutic agents cause massive cellular destruction, allopurinol is administered to inhibit uric acid production. Diuresis is also helpful in ensuring adequate excretion of the metabolites.

A complete remission is determined by the absence of leukemic cells in the bone marrow and disappearance of all signs and symptoms of the disease. Since the bone marrow normally contains less than 5% blast cells, a remission may also be achieved with some cells remaining. However, since research indicates that one remaining leukemic cell is capable of producing disease, the aim of therapy is usually total destruction of all blast cells. Some treatment regimens include a week of *consolidation* or *intensification therapy* with one or more of the usual remission drugs to achieve an aleukemic state.

Since many of the drugs also cause myelosuppression of normal blood elements, the period immediately following a remission can be critical, because the body is defenseless against invading organisms (including normal bacterial flora) and highly susceptible to spontaneous hemorrhage. Those children who die during the induction phase frequently succumb at this point in treatment.

Ninety percent to 95% of children with ALL can be expected to attain an initial remission based on a combination of these drugs. Only about 75% as many children with AML will achieve a remission, and the drug therapies will differ from those used for lymphoid leukemia. The principal drugs used for induction therapy are 6-thioguanine, daunomycin, cytosine arabinoside, 5-azacytidine, vincristine, and prednisone.

Sanctuary therapy. The second phase involves prophylactic treatment of the central nervous system with cranial irradiation and/or intrathecal administration of methotrexate. Therapy is usually begun during the first 6 to 8 weeks after diagnosis and consists of daily high-dose radiation treatments for about 2 weeks and weekly or twice weekly doses of methotrexate for a total of five to six injections.

Most often irradiation for prophylactic treatment of central nervous system involvement is limited to the cranium, although some institutions advocate craniospinal radiation. However, exposing the spine of a young child to irradiation results in markedly retarded linear growth.

Maintenance. Maintenance or continuation therapy is begun after completion of successful induction and sanctuary therapy to preserve the remission and further lessen the number of leukemic cells. It most often begins after the child is discharged from the hospital and when blood values begin to approach normal levels. As with induction therapy, combined drug regimens have been more successful in maintaining remissions and preventing drug resistance. Although a variety of combinations are used, a frequent schedule includes daily doses of oral 6-mercaptopurine and weekly doses of oral methotrexate. Intermittently short-term intensified therapy with prednisone and vincristine may be included. Similarly, periodic doses of intrathecal methotrexate are given to maintain central nervous system prophylaxis. Depending on the type of leukemia and the risk factors of the child, several other drugs may be added to the intensification protocol.

During maintenance therapy weekly or monthly complete blood counts are taken to evaluate the marrow's response to the drugs. If myelosuppression becomes severe (usually indicated by a white blood cell count below 2000/mm^3) or toxic side effects occur, therapy is temporarily stopped or the dose decreased. If the initial remission is maintained, all therapy is terminated after a period of about 3 years, although this varies according to different institutions.

Cessation of therapy is based on clinical experience that demonstrates that continuing therapy for longer than 2 to 3 years does not increase survival time. Since the effects of prolonged therapy are not completely known, current recommendations include that all drugs be stopped. After cessation some children will continue in a permanent remission, but about 20% will relapse within the first year.[1]

Reinduction. For many children a fourth phase of therapy becomes necessary when a relapse occurs, as evidenced by the presence of leukemic cells within the bone marrow. Usually reinduction includes the use of prednisone and vincristine with a combination of other drugs not previously used. Sanctuary and maintenance therapy follow as outlined above if a remission is induced.

In children who have responded to the induction regimen of prednisone-vincristine and who have not been on these drugs for maintenance therapy, the chances of attaining a second remission are better than 80% to 90%, the chance of a third remission are between 60% and 70%, and the chances of a fourth remission are between 50% and 60%.[21] Obviously each relapse heralds an increasingly poorer prognosis, since with each additional induction phase the effectiveness of previously used drugs and availability of new chemotherapeutic agents decrease.

Immunotherapy and bone marrow transplant. Recently newer modes of therapy have been used in treating leukemia. Immunotherapy with Calmette-Guerin bacillus is sometimes combined with the usual agents of maintenance therapy. Although not effective in inducing a remission, it has had some success in prolonging a remission, even after all chemotherapy has been stopped.

Bone marrow transplant has provided hopeful treatment for children who have AML or terminal ALL. Although usually limited to those individuals with a compatible donor, it has been successful in producing long-term remissions in about 10% to 20% of cases. Unfortunately it involves many hazardous procedures and complications to which some parents may not be willing to subject their child. It is a procedure that involves total team support to assist the parents and child through their tremendous physical and emotional needs.

Nursing considerations

Nursing care of the child with leukemia is directly related to the regimen of therapy. Secondary complications that necessitate supportive physical care are caused by myelosuppression, drug toxicity, and leukemic infiltration. Although this discussion is primarily concerned with the physical problems requiring nursing care, it also focuses on the specific emotional needs during diagnosis, treatment, and relapse. The general psychologic interventions during each phase of therapy are discussed in Chapter 27.

Preparation of family for diagnostic and therapeutic procedures. From the time before diagnosis to cessation of therapy, children must undergo several tests, the most traumatic of which are bone marrow aspiration or biopsy and lumbar punctures. Multiple fingersticks and venipunctures for blood analysis and drug infusion are common occurrences for several years after the diagnosis. Therefore, the child needs an explanation of why each procedure is done and what can be expected.

Depending on the age of the child, one way of beginning such preparation is to explain the basic elements of the blood. Using a drawing or letting the child look at a drop of blood under a microscope not only teaches but also encourages trust between the nurse and child. It also allows the nurse to assess the child's level of understanding. One error many health professionals make is to overestimate children's knowledge about their bodies. For example, a bone marrow aspiration only makes sense when one clarifies that the center of a bone is hollow and contains the cells that later become ''working'' blood cells or leukemic cells.

Bone marrow aspiration. There are three types of bone marrow tests: (1) aspiration, which consists of aspirating marrow through a large-bore needle; (2) biopsy, which consists of aspirating a piece of bone through a special type needle; and (3) trephine, which is a surgical biopsy of a section of bone. Aspiration is the method of choice, unless the cells are so tightly packed that suction is inadequate to remove a sample. In that case a biopsy is done. In children the posterior iliac crest is most frequently used. The sternum is avoided because the bone is more fragile and adjacent to vital organs.

When preparing the child for the test, it is best to describe each step as it occurs, stressing what will be done and what it will feel like. When the posterior iliac crest is used, everything is done behind the child's line of vision. Although this is often less traumatic than actually viewing the procedure, such as occurs when the sternum or anterior iliac crest is used, it also increases the fear of the unknown. If each step is explained beforehand, having the child recall the next step during the procedure can be a distraction mechanism. The sequence of events during a bone marrow aspiration or biopsy is outlined in the boxed material on the opposite page.

A bone marrow aspiration is routinely done at the time of diagnosis, during and/or after induction therapy, and whenever a relapse is suspected. Since it is a traumatic test, it is important to stress the few times it is needed. Sometimes children fear that a bone marrow aspiration will be necessary every time they visit the physician.

Lumbar puncture. A lumbar puncture (LP) is usually done at the time of diagnosis to evaluate central nervous system involvement and at scheduled intervals for the administration of intrathecal methotrexate. It is usually a less traumatic procedure than the bone marrow aspiration because the only pain is from the injection of lidocaine (Xylocaine). The steps outlined in the boxed material on the opposite page are modified for a lumbar puncture.

Before explaining any test, the nurse should know the exact routine employed by the institution. For example, some physicians recommend that the child remain flat for 1 or more hours after the lumbar puncture to minimize the chance of a headache. Others prefer that the child be placed in a slight Trendelenburg's position for 30 minutes to facilitate circulation of the medicated spinal fluid. Others recommend no special positioning, advocating that the child resume normal activity at once. To eliminate the power of suggestion, it may be best to avoid telling the child about the possibility of a headache after the lumbar puncture, regardless of the position or activity he assumes afterward.

Much of the anxiety and discomfort children experience for either procedure is caused by the subcutaneous injection of an anesthetic. A noninvasive technique for numbing the skin has been developed, which uses a patch impregnated with lidocaine cream.[15] The patch is kept in place over the involved area for 3 hours prior to the procedure. The subcutaneous layers of tissue become sufficiently numbed for the procedure to be performed without additional anesthetic or for a painless injection of lidocaine to be administered. The anesthetic patch is useful not only for bone marrow aspiration or lumbar puncture but also for intravenous infusions and skin testing (such as in immunotherapy).

Another advance in the intrathecal administration of methotrexate is the Ommaya reservoir, which eliminates repeated lumbar punctures. In this procedure a silicon rubber tube is surgically inserted into one of the ventricles and connected to a reservoir placed beneath the scalp. To instill medication the area of scalp covering the reservoir is cleansed with an antiseptic and a small needle is inserted through the skin into the reservoir. The drug is then in-

Explanation of a bone marrow aspiration or biopsy and lumbar puncture

Bone marrow aspiration or biopsy	*Lumbar puncture**
Step 1. You will be lying on your *stomach.*	Side with your knees bent so that they touch your chest. The nurse (parent) will "hug" you to help you maintain this curled up position (see Fig. 26-12, p. 928).
Step 2. Your pants or pajamas will be pulled down a little so that this part of your back *(point to posterior iliac crest)* will be visible.	Point to the lumbar area of the spine.
Step 3. The physician will have a tray with the equipment for the test. He or she will put on rubber gloves and then clean your back with a special antiseptic solution. It will probably feel cold. Then the physician will place sterile towels on your back so that only a small section of skin is visible.	Same.
Step 4. Next the nurse will hold a bottle of numbing medicine (called lidocaine) so that the physician can fill the syringe. He or she needs help because the gloves must remain sterile.	Same.
Step 5. After the syringe is filled with the lidocaine, the physician will give you a shot in the spot where the *bone marrow aspiration* will be done. It will hurt, but only for a few seconds until the area is numb or asleep.	Lumbar puncture.
Step 6. Next the physician will use a special needle that is hollow with a solid plug inside. The plug makes the needle strong. You will feel the physician touching your skin with the fingers. Because the area is asleep, you will only feel pressure *(demonstrate pushing)* as the needle is put in.	Do not demonstrate pushing.
Step 7. The physician will remove the solid plug and attach a syringe to the hollow needle so that some *cells* can be taken out. *This may hurt for a few seconds, but it tells you that the test is almost over.*	Fluid. Eliminate last sentence and add: The physician may attach a long tube that looks like a thermometer to measure the pressure of the fluid, after which an exact amount of fluid will be removed and replaced with medicine.
Step 8. If the sample of cells is sufficient, the physician will pull out the needle, place a bandage over the spot to stop the bleeding, and then put on a Band-Aid. The physician will then look at the cells under a microscope.	Same.
Step 9 (possible). Sometimes the cells are packed so tightly that the physician cannot get enough of them into the syringe. In this case he or she has to try again. Because your back is still asleep, you will feel some pushing.	Eliminate entire step.
Step 10. After the test your back may feel a little sore and the Band-Aid must stay on, *but there is no reason that you cannot do whatever you feel like.*	Some physicians recommend that the child be flat for a period of time to lessen the chance of a headache.

*The explanation of the lumbar puncture is the same except for the modifications of italics in the left column.

jected into the reservoir and by gently compressing the skin over this site is pumped into the ventricles.

Venipuncture. Multiple venipunctures are performed for blood tests and intravenous infusions. The child needs the same preparation for this as for the more traumatic procedures. A recent development that eliminates the need for multiple venipunctures or continuous infusion when fluid replacement is not required is the heparin lock. It employs the standard venipuncture technique, but with a special adaptor attached to allow for a completely closed system. A commercial product frequently used is the Butterfly-21, INT,* which consists of a 21-gauge scalp vein needle attached to a piece of 3½-inch tubing that ends in a resealing rubber diaphragm.

The infusion line is kept patent by instilling a heparin solution into the tubing. Ordinarily 1 ml of the solution is

*Manufactured by Abbott Laboratories, Chicago, Ill.

administered prior to and after instillation of medication. Routine heparin flushing is performed every 8 hours to maintain patency. No adverse systemic alterations in blood clotting have been observed.[12]

The heparin lock is advantageous for children who require daily doses of chemotherapeutic agents. It allows them maximum mobility while in the hospital, minimizes the trauma of repeated injections, and on occasion may allow them to remain at home, provided the parent can be instructed in administration of the heparin. The venipuncture site requires no special care other than a sterile bandage to keep it securely in place.

Prevention of complications of myelosuppression. The leukemic process and most of the chemotherapeutic agents cause myelosuppression. The reduced numbers of blood cells result in secondary problems of infection, bleeding tendencies, and anemia. Supportive care involves both medical and nursing management. Because they are so closely linked, they are discussed in unison rather than separately.

Infection. The most frequent cause of death from leukemia is overwhelming infection. The leukemic child is most susceptible to overwhelming infection during three phases of his disease: (1) at the time of diagnosis and relapse when the leukemic process has replaced normal leukocytes; (2) during immunosuppressive therapy; and (3) after prolonged antibiotic therapy that predisposes to the growth of resistant organisms.

The organisms most lethal to these children are (1) viruses, particularly varicella (chickenpox), herpes zoster, herpes simplex, measles, rubella, mumps, and poliomyelitis; (2) *Pneumocystis carinii* (a parasite); (3) fungi, especially *Candida albicans;* (4) gram-negative bacteria, such as *Pseudomonas aeruginosa, Escherichia coli, Proteus,* and *Klebsiella;* and (5) gram-positive bacteria, especially *Staphylococcus aureus, S. epidermidis,* and group A β-hemolytic streptococcus. Because the usual viral infections of childhood are particularly dangerous, immunizations against these diseases are not given until the child's immune system is capable of responding appropriately to the vaccine. If given when the immune system is depressed, the attenuated virus can result in an overwhelming infection. (Salk vaccine for poliomyelitis is recommended in lieu of Sabin's oral vaccine.)

The first defense against infection is prevention. When the child is hospitalized, the nurse employs all measures to control transfer of infection. This may include strict reverse isolation or, more frequently, the use of a private room, restriction of all visitors and health personnel with active infection, and strict hand-washing technique with an antiseptic solution. In some research centers special germ-free environments are available during complete myelosuppression from intensive chemotherapy or for bone marrow transplant.

The nurse evaluates the child for any potential sites of infection, such as from a needle puncture, mucosal ulceration, or minor abrasion. Any elevation of temperature is considered a sign of infection, even in the absence of symptoms. To identify the source of infection, blood, stool, urine, and nasopharyngeal cultures and chest x-ray films are taken. Broad-spectrum intravenous antibiotic therapy is begun before the organism is identified and continued for the usual 7- to 10-day period, regardless of whether a specific agent is isolated.

Continuous intravenous therapy can be difficult for the child because it usually means numerous venipunctures to restart the infusion, limited activity because of the immobilized body part, and a prolonged hospital admission. The nurse can help the child adjust to these problems by choosing the intravenous site that least hinders mobility, such as in the nondominant hand, and by taking every precaution to preserve a patient infusion, such as an arm board for site immobilization, a protective shield over the needle to prevent accidental dislodgement, and instructing the child in moving the body part cautiously.

Boredom can be minimized by attention to appropriate recreational activity, such as reading, watching television, listening to music, talking on the telephone, needlepoint or other crafts, and so on. Since induction hospitalization is fairly long (4 to 6 weeks without complications), it may be helpful to "personalize" the child's room by hanging get-well cards on the wall, placing plants in the room, and bringing photographs in from home. Many families seem to develop their own "hospital projects," such as group jigsaw puzzles, hooked rugs, model cars, and so on. It is important to encourage such activities for the child as well as the family members.

If an infection does not respond to antibiotics, transfusions of concentrated leukocytes (granulocytes) can be given. Preparation of leukocyte transfusions requires compatible blood donors and the use of a special machine called a blood-cell separator (leukophoresis), which removes only the white cells from the donor's blood, allowing the rest of the blood to be reinfused. By using this continuous-flow centrifuge it is possible to obtain as many granulocytes from one normal donor at one time as are contained in 30 to 40 units of blood collected by standard methods. Since the other blood components are returned, the donor is able to give blood as frequently as twice a week for up to 3 months.

Febrile reactions from leukocyte antigens are common, especially from repeated transfusions. Although the patient may experience moderate to severe chills and an elevated temperature, this is not an indication to stop the transfusion. The nurse should record and report these reactions and explain their significance to the child and family. Also, if the child's blood type is rare, the nurse should encourage parents to locate suitable donors in case leukocytes or platelets are needed. Often this anticipatory guidance is neglected and parents are forced to meet this need when an emergency arises.

Prevention of infection continues as a priority after discharge from the hospital. However, rigid social restriction must be tempered with the child's need for resuming normal activity. Ordinarily the child can return to school when the white blood cell count (WBC) is about 2000/mm^3. If the level falls below this value, cautious isolation from crowded areas, such as shopping centers or subways, is advisable. Family members should be encouraged to practice good hand washing to avoid introducing pathogens into the home.

A very important indication for isolation is an outbreak of childhood diseases, especially chickenpox. The child is confined from all known sources of the infection, such as schoolmates, until the epidemic is over. Ideally the school nurse should work with the treating physician to decide the optimum time for school reattendance. If the child has been exposed to the varicella virus, zoster immune globulin (ZIG) given within 72 hours may favorably alter the course of the disease. Death from disseminated varicella (about 7%) is usually caused by pneumonia; however, other serious although nonfatal complications include hepatitis, pancreatitis, meningitis, and bacterial skin infections.[20]

Nutrition is another important component of infection prevention. An adequate protein-calorie intake provides the child with better host defenses against infection and increased tolerance to chemotherapy and irradiation. However, providing optimum nutrition during periods of anorexia is a tremendous challenge. Measures to encourage eating are discussed on p. 1016.

Hemorrhage. Prior to the use of transfused platelets, hemorrhage was a leading cause of death in leukemia. Now most bleeding episodes can be prevented or controlled with judicious administration of platelet concentrates or platelet-rich plasma. Spontaneous hemorrhage usually does not occur until the platelet count is below 20,000/mm^3. Some children can tolerate extremely low levels, probably because of a combination of inherent factors such as decreased capillary fragility.

Since infection increases the tendency toward hemorrhage, and bleeding sites become more easily infected, a combined effort at controlling and preventing infection and hemorrhage has cumulative beneficial effects. The nurse takes special care in cleaning all puncture sites such as fingersticks, venipunctures, intramuscular injections, and so on. Meticulous mouth care is essential since gingival bleeding with resultant mucositis is a frequent problem. (Oral hygiene measures are discussed on p. 1017.) The nurse also attends to skin care. Since the rectal area is prone to ulceration from various drugs, feces and urine are removed immediately and the perineal area washed. Frequent turning, the use of a flotation or alternating-pressure mattress, and sheepskin under bony prominences prevent pressure areas and decubital ulcers.

Platelet transfusions are generally reserved for active bleeding episodes that do not respond to local treatment. Epistaxis and gingival bleeding are the most common. The nurse teaches parents and older children measures to control bleeding. Pressure at the site without disturbing clot formation is the general rule. Two measures employed for hemostasis are salt pork packs for epistaxis and dry tea bags for gingival bleeding.[20] For epistaxis a piece of salt pork is cut to the size of the nostril to fit securely as packing, which serves as an astringent and pressure pack. Removal of the salt pork is less traumatic than conventional gauze or tissue because it remains moist and does not adhere to the clot formation. (See p. 1398 for other measures to control epistaxis.) For gingival bleeding, a dry tea bag placed against the mucosa promotes hemostasis. Both of these articles are inexpensive, easily available, and convenient first-aid devices for use in the home.

Platelet counts may be low during chemotherapy when the child is at home. Although there may be no visible evidence of bleeding, the nurse should encourage the parents to restrict sports that may result in accidental injury, such as football, soccer, bicycle riding, tree climbing, skateboard riding, and so on. Such restriction may be more difficult for boys than girls. However, one way of avoiding a battle is to discuss with the child the meaning of blood values. For example, by telling the child that the platelet count is below 50,000/mm^3, which means that the cells needed for blood clotting are low, the child can assume responsibility for tailoring his activity. It also allows him the opportunity to resume normal sports when he learns that the platelet count has risen.

Two of the problems with multiple platelet transfusions are the risk of febrile reactions and decreased life span of the platelets. Platelet concentrates normally do not have to be crossmatched for blood group or type. However, because platelets contain specific antigen components similar to blood group factors, children receiving multiple transfusions may become immunized to a platelet group other than their own. Therefore, it is advisable to crossmatch platelets with the donor's blood components whenever possible.

Transfused platelets generally survive in the body for 1 to 3 days. The peak effect is reached in about 2 hours and decreased by half in 24 hours. Therefore, after a transfusion the nurse observes and records the approximate time when hemostasis of bleeding sites occurs. Delayed effect of hemostasis is evidence of platelet destruction. For long-term leukemic patients, multiple transfusion therapy becomes progressively less effective.

During bleeding episodes the parents and child need much emotional support. The sight of oozing blood is very upsetting. Often parents will request a platelet transfusion, unaware of the necessity of trying local measures first. The nurse can be instrumental in allaying anxiety by explaining the reason for delaying a platelet transfusion until absolutely necessary. Since compatible donors decrease the risk of antigen formation in the recipient, the nurse should encourage parents to locate suitable donors for eventual blood use.

Anemia. Initially anemia may be profound from complete replacement of the bone marrow by leukemic cells. During induction therapy, blood transfusions with whole blood or packed red cells may be necessary to raise hemoglobin to levels approaching 10 g. The nurse institutes usual precautions in caring for the anemic child (see p. 1374).

Anemia is also a consequence of drug-induced myelosuppression. Although not as severely affected as the white blood cells, erythrocyte production may be delayed. Since children have an amazing capacity to withstand low hemoglobin levels, the best approach is to allow the child to regulate his activity with reasonable adult supervision. It may be necessary for the parents to alert the schoolteacher to the child's physical limitations, particularly in terms of strenuous activity. At home, parents should encourage quiet periods during the day, such as before dinner and bedtime, to avoid exhaustion. A well-rested child is more likely to resist infection than one who is continually fatigued.

Management of problems of irradiation and drug toxicity. Tables 28-4 and 28-5 list the major side effects associated with chemotherapy and irradiation. The following is a discussion of each of these reactions and appropriate interventions.

Nausea and vomiting. The nausea and vomiting that occur shortly after administration of several of the drugs and as a result of cranial radiation can be profound. They can be controlled with antiemetics such as prochlorperazine (Compazine) or trimethobenzamide (Tigan), which are available in oral, injectable, or suppository form. The injectable and rectal forms relieve nausea and vomiting within several minutes, but the oral preparation may require 20 minutes or more to become effective. They are most beneficial if given prior to the onset of nausea and vomiting.

To calculate the optimum time for administration, the nurse should administer the first dose immediately after nausea begins. The subsequent dose is given 20 minutes before the nausea is expected. For example, with cyclophosphamide (Cytoxan), nausea and vomiting may not begin until 3 to 4 hours after administration. Therefore, if the antiemetic were given with the drug, it would lose its maximum effectiveness when needed. However, if it were given 2½ hours later (based on symptoms of nausea at 3 hours) it would exert its maximum benefit during the onset of symptoms. For children, the oral or suppository form is recommended. However, if rectal ulcers are a problem, the suppository is not advisable because of increased tissue trauma.

Anorexia. Loss of appetite is a direct consequence of the chemotherapy, irradiation, and nausea and vomiting. It is a major problem for parents because it is the one area they feel responsible for, particularly when so many other facets of care are outside their control. There are no panaceas for encouraging a sick child to eat. However, there are some guidelines that can be helpful during the anorexic period and can prevent additional problems during the remission.

The most important measure is to encourage parents to relax. Forcing a child to eat only meets with rebellion and negativism. In turn, refusing to eat becomes a controlling mechanism for the child. Second, it should be impressed on parents that during the period of intense therapy the child legitimately does not feel like eating. This is a time for the parents to concentrate on giving the child anything he wants to eat. Although it is best to encourage high-quality nutritious foods, the child may desire foods and liquids that contain mostly calories. Allow him what he wants whenever he desires and plan to encourage a more balanced diet when he is physically improved. Some well-tolerated foods include gelatin, clear soups, carbonated drinks, popsicles, dry toast, crackers, and hard candy. Even though these substances are not nutritious, they can provide necessary fluid and calories.

Once the child is feeling better, his appetite usually begins to improve, especially if he is being administered steroids. It is best to take advantage of any hungry period by serving high-quality foods. For example, the nurse can advise parents to fortify soups with extra pieces of meat or vegetables, to prepare pudding, mashed potatoes, cooked cereal, or "shakes" with added powdered milk, to serve nutritious desserts such as frozen yogurt, ice cream, pudding, and oatmeal or peanut butter cookies, and to have handy snacks available, such as cheese "kisses," raw pieces of vegetable, or dried fruits. If the child still refuses to eat, nutritious fluids, such as prepared breakfast drinks, should be encouraged.

The results of successful approaches to encouraging the child to eat are cumulative. However, they require a willingness to let the child proceed at his own pace. Sometimes it is helpful to encourage the child to participate in noneating activities, such as grocery shopping, menu planning, and food preparation. For young children, making food appealing by providing decorative accessories in the form of paper plates, fancy cups, or straws, decorating food with a "face" on a hamburger or a cookie-cutter shaped sandwich, and eating a "picnic lunch" in another room or eating a meal on a tray in front of the television may encourage eating because their interest in different aspects of food is increased.

Some children still do not eat despite these approaches. The following theories have been postulated to explain persistent anorexia: (1) a physical cause related to the cancer that is nonspecific; (2) a conditioned aversion to food from nausea and vomiting during treatment; (3) stress in the environment, either related to eating and or to the child's condition; (4) depression; (5) a control mechanism when so much else has been imposed on him; and (6) an opportunity to express anger and punishment at his parents for "allowing" him to become sick.[19] When loss of appetite and weight continue to persist, the nurse should investigate the family situation to identify if any of these variables are contributing to the problem. Often it is possible to improve eating habits by using the approaches listed on p. 1016 once the real problem has been dealt with.

Mucosal ulceration. One of the most distressing side effects of several drugs is gastrointestinal mucosal cell damage, which results in ulcers anywhere along the alimentary tract. Oral ulcers (stomatitis) are red, eroded, painful areas in the mouth and/or pharynx. They may extend along the esophagus and frequently occur in the rectal area. They greatly compound anorexia because eating is extremely uncomfortable. When oral ulcers develop; the following interventions are helpful: (1) a bland, moist, soft diet, (2) use of a soft sponge toothbrush (Toothettes)* or cotton-tipped applicator, (3) frequent mouthwashes with diluted hydrogen peroxide (1 part hydrogen peroxide and 4 parts normal saline), and (4) local anesthetics such as Chloroseptic spray or viscous lidocaine. Other oral hygiene agents frequently used include lemon glycerin swabs or milk of magnesia. However, glycerin, a trihydric alcohol, absorbs water and is drying to the membranes, whereas lemon may be irritating to eroded tissue. Milk of magnesia is also thought to have a drying effect because unabsorbed magnesium salts exert an osmotic pressure on tissue fluids.[5] Many children also find the chalky taste unpleasant.

Administering mouth care is particularly difficult in infants and toddlers. A satisfactory method of cleaning the gums is to wrap a piece of gauze around a finger, soak it in diluted hydrogen peroxide, and swab the gums, palate, and inner cheek surfaces with the finger. Mouthwashes are best accomplished with plain water since the child cannot gargle or spit out excess fluid. Mouth care should be done routinely before and after any feeding and at least every 4 hours. The main objective is to rid the mucosal surfaces of debris that become an excellent medium for bacterial and fungal growth.

Although local anesthetics are effective in temporarily relieving the pain, many children dislike the taste and numbing feeling they produce. Viscous lidocaine is not recommended for young children, because, if applied to the pharynx, it may depress the gag reflex, increasing the risk of aspiration.

Difficulty in eating is a major problem with stomatitis and may warrant hospitalization if the child refuses fluids. The child will usually choose the foods that are best tolerated. Surprisingly some children prefer salty foods to more bland ones. Drinking can usually be encouraged if a straw is used, since the fluid bypasses the ulcerated oral mucosa. The nurse should encourage parents to relax any eating pressures because the anorexia accompanying stomatitis is well justified. Also, since it is a temporary condition, once the ulcers heal the child can resume good food habits. Ordinarily severe mucosal ulceration indicates a need for decreased medication and complete healing takes place within a week.

*Manufactured by Halbrand, Inc., Willoughby, Ohio.

Dental hygiene can become a serious problem if the child wears an orthodontic appliance. The accumulated debris on braces is difficult to remove without vigorous brushing, and the appliance itself traumatizes the gums. In some situations braces may have to be removed to allow chemotherapy to continue.

If rectal ulcers develop, meticulous toilet hygiene, warm sitz baths after each bowel movement, and periodic exposure of the ulcerated area to warm heat promote healing. Sometimes a rectal ulcer can be so uncomfortable that the child prefers to spend as much time as possible in the bathtub. Applying A and D Ointment helps in some situations, particularly when the child must pass stool. Parents should be advised to record bowel movements since the child may voluntarily avoid defecation to prevent discomfort. Rectal temperatures are not taken since they may further traumatize the area.

Peripheral neuropathy. Vincristine and to a lesser extent vinblastine can cause various neurotoxic effects, one of the more common of which is severe constipation from decreased bowel innervation. The nurse advises parents to record bowel movements and to notify the physician of a change in stool habits. Stool softeners may be helpful in preventing the problem, but laxatives or enemas are often necessary to stimulate evacuation.

Footdrop and weakness and numbing of the extremities may cause difficulty in walking or fine hand movement. The nurse should warn parents of these side effects, which are reversible once the drug is stopped. If the child is on bed rest, a footboard should be used to preserve proper alignment. If weakness occurs while the child is attending school, a temporary alteration of activity may be necessary. The teacher should be apprised of the situation so that unrealistic expectations of the child's ability are not made.

Another side effect that can be severe is jaw pain. Analgesics may be necessary to relieve the discomfort. Avoiding movement by not talking or chewing is usually self-imposed. Since the pain is temporary, usually for a day or two, the child can be given fluids through a straw.

A neurologic syndrome may develop 5 to 8 weeks after central nervous system irradiation and may last for 3 to 15 days.[20] It is characterized by somnolence with or without fever, anorexia, and nausea and vomiting. Although of no apparent clinical significance, parents should be warned of the possibility of such symptoms and encouraged to allow the child a period of needed rest.

Hemorrhagic cystitis. Sterile hemorrhagic cystitis is a side effect of chemical irritation to the bladder from cyclophosphamide. It can be prevented by a liberal fluid intake (at least one and one half times the recommended daily fluid requirement) and frequent voiding, including nighttime voiding. If signs of cystitis, such as burning on urination, occur, fluids are increased with more frequent voiding. The physician is notified of these symptoms immediately. Hemorrhagic cystitis warrants cessation of the drug and is more frequently a complication of oral cyclophosphamide than from intravenous administration. In the latter instance intravenous fluids are given before, during, and after the drug to ensure adequate hydration, thereby eliminating the need for the child's drinking large amounts of fluid.

Alopecia. Hair loss is a side effect of several chemotherapeutic drugs and cranial irradiation. Although nothing can prevent alopecia from cranial irradiation, the use of a scalp tourniquet may prevent hair loss from drugs during the maintenance phase. A scalp tourniquet is a wide rubber band that is placed around the head near the hairline during drug infusion and kept in place for 5 minutes after administration of the drug. It is not recommended for induction therapy, since leukemic cells may be missed. However, it is used by some physicians when the child is in remission, since it may prevent complete hair loss.

Not all children lose their hair during drug therapy; however, this is the exception rather than the rule. It is better to warn children and parents of this side effect than to allow them to think that it is only a remote possibility. Encouraging a child to choose a wig similar to his own hairstyle and color before the hair falls out is helpful in fostering later adjustment to hair loss. The nurse should also inform the family that hair regrows in 3 to 6 months and may be of a different color and texture. Frequently, the hair is darker, thicker, and curlier than before.

If the child chooses not to wear a wig, attention to some type of head covering is important, especially in cold climates. Scalp hygiene is also important. The scalp should be washed like any other body part to prevent sebum accumulation or cradle cap (see p. 492).

Many children demonstrate increased tolerance to hair loss on reinduction therapy. Rather than complete baldness, the hair may thin out. If the hair is cut short, kept clean, and blow dried with an electric hair drier, it usually can look full enough to make a wig unnecessary. This can be a tremendous psychologic boost to the child who is already depressed about learning of a relapse and the need for additional chemotherapy.

Moon face. Short-term steroid therapy produces no acute toxicities and results in two beneficial reactions—increased appetite and a sense of well-being. However, it does produce alterations in body image, which, although not clinically significant, can be extremely distressing to older children. One of these is moon face. The child's face becomes rounded and puffy. Unlike hair loss, little can be done to camouflage this obvious change. It is not unusual for other children to make fun of the child with such remarks as "porky-pig" or "fat face." For the child who experiences such name-calling, it is helpful to reassure him that after cessation of the drug the facial changes will return to normal. If the child resumes activity early in the course of treatment, the change may be less noticeable to peers than after a long absence.

In contrast, parents may appreciate the full-rounded appearance because it simulates the look of a well-nourished healthy child. Because of their own needs, they may be less able to understand the child's misery over his altered body image. The nurse can foster a better understanding between the parents and child if both parties are encouraged to openly discuss their feelings.

Children on steroid therapy do look healthy. The moon face, red cheeks, supraclavicular fat pads, protuberant abdomen, and fluid retention indicate weight gain. However, the actual weight gain resulting from increased muscle mass and subcutaneous tissue may be small. Therefore, the nurse should evaluate weight gain carefully during steroid therapy to make certain that some of it is a result of increased dietary intake by observing the extremities and measuring the size of muscle bulk and power.

Mood changes. Shortly after beginning steroid therapy, children experience a feeling of well-being. This change in behavior may be striking after a period of depression following hospitalization, discovery of the diagnosis, and induction therapy. Once the drug is discontinued, the loss of the euphoric effect may also be noticeable. If parents are unaware of these drug-induced changes, they may interpret the mood swings erroneously. Therefore, the nurse should warn them of the reactions and encourage them to discuss the behavioral changes with each other and the child.

Relief of pain. Toward the terminal stages of the disease there are two complications—central nervous system meningitis and bone pain—that may require nursing intervention. The main objective in each is relief of discomfort with analgesics, environmental manipulation, and positioning.

Environmental manipulation. Depending on the type of pain, manipulating the environment to avoid unnecessary exertion or altering sensory input may be beneficial. For example, headaches are common from central nervous system involvement of leukemia. Dimming the lights and diminishing ambient noise may be helpful. If bone pain is a problem, arranging the room for easy access to the commode, telephone, or television is important. Lightweight sheets and pajamas to avoid pressure on painful areas, minimal handling, and application of warmth can also be beneficial. Although none of these measures alone may eliminate the discomfort, combined they are frequently effective enough to foster maximum pain control with minimal medication.

Positioning. Good body alignment is important when bone pain is present. However, pressure against these tender sites produces more pain. Some devices that may be helpful are reclining chairs, a water bed, or a bean-bag chair. The latter is relatively inexpensive and may be worth the investment if the child remains at home.

Once the child assumes a position of comfort, he is usually reluctant to move. However, frequent turning and repositioning are necessary to prevent pressure sores. To facilitate movement, it is advisable to coordinate position changes with pain medication schedules. Also, moving the television to the opposite side of the bed may be enough incentive to encourage the child to assume a new position.

Analgesics. Because aspirin enhances the effects of methotrexate and promotes bleeding tendencies, nonsalicylate analgesics are used. For home use, acetaminophen is recommended. However, it is only effective for mild to moderate pain. Management for more severe pain demands experimenting with various analgesics, such as oxycodone (Percodan), levorphanol tartrate (Levo-Dromoran), methadone, codeine, meperidine (Demerol), or morphine. Whenever possible the oral form of the least addicting drug is used. Although the physician must prescribe these drugs, the nurse should be familiar with each. For example, the effective use of oral nonnarcotic analgesics may eliminate the need for injectable narcotics or allow their use during the terminal stage when maximum pain relief is desired.

Besides the choice of an analgesic, the schedule of administration is important. For maximum benefit the drug should be given before the pain is severe. If pain is continuous, which may occur in the terminal stage, the goal should be relief of pain with minimum medication and maximum mental functioning. Administration of medications as needed is not conducive to meeting this goal. Rather, scheduled medication times that are individualized for each child are necessary. The nurse plans such a schedule by recording for at least one 24-hour period the times of day when the child needs pain medication. Based on this chart, a preventive schedule of drug administration is plotted. For example, if the child complains of pain at 4- to 6-hour intervals, the nurse would plan to give pain medication prior to the times the child would ask for it. Although for the first day the child may be taking a larger cumulative dose, as pain is controlled the dosage required is progressively smaller. To evaluate a continued need for this regular schedule, the nurse gradually widens the interval between doses until the same amount of pain relief is maintained.

Provide continued emotional support. The preceding discussion of nursing care of the leukemic child is based on typical problems with which the family is confronted during the treatment phases. It is not unlikely for a child who discontinues therapy after 2 or 3 years and maintains a permanent remission to experience many of these side effects. Therefore, the nurse's role is continually one of support, guidance, clarification, and judgment. Parents need to know how to recognize symptoms that demand medical attention. Although some of the reactions discussed are expected, parents still should report them to their physician. Warning parents of their possible occurrence beforehand, however, allows parents the opportunity to prepare for them. At the same time it reassures them that these reactions are not caused by a return of leukemic cells.

The nurse must also use judgment in recognizing which side effects are normal reactions and which indicate toxicity. Frequently it is the office or clinic nurse who screens such telephone calls and gives advice when appropriate. Usually, nausea and vomiting are not indications for drug cessation. However, severe vomiting may require immediate intervention to prevent dehydration. Signs of infection, mucosal ulceration, hemorrhagic cystitis, peripheral neuropathy, and obstipation require medical supervision.

Another aspect of continued emotional support involves prognosis. Certainly leukemia can no longer be defined as invariably fatal. However, present statistics must also be correctly interpreted. The fact that 90% of the children with ALL will achieve an initial remission and 50% of them will live 5 years or longer is applicable to those children treated with the latest protocols since diagnosis. Of the 50% who do survive 5 years after diagnosis, only a portion of them will remain in remission. Therefore, at the present time there is no definitive finding and criteria to positively identify which child is ultimately "cured" of the disease.

The nurse must be familiar with these statistics in order to interpret them correctly to parents. At the same time the nurse must realize that a realistic understanding of the chances for survival requires an adjustment period. For example, it is not unusual for parents to interpret the "90% remission" as the probability for a cure. When a relapse occurs, parents may for the first time be able to "hear" the correct facts.

Parents may interpret the fifty-fifty odds in a very practical way. For example, they may believe that if another child dies of the disease, then one must live, and that one could be their child. Indeed, their thinking is correct, but it may also create guilt and stifle communication with other families. The nurse who works with groups of parents may find it helpful to discuss this aspect of survival statistics in order to focus on the normalcy of such thinking.

Comprehensive emotional support for the family through all phases of the illness is discussed in Chapter 27.

Statistics are numbers. Sometimes they bring hope and, at other times, despair. Although very important in terms of research, better treatment, identification of high- or low-risk populations, and so on, they present a general picture of what to expect. The nurse who is working with family

Summary of nursing care of the child with leukemia

Goals	Responsibilities
Prepare family for diagnostic/therapeutic procedures	Explain reason for each test (fingersticks, venipunctures, bone marrow aspirations, lumbar punctures, x-ray treatments) Explain basic elements of blood to provide foundational information for tests and therapies Encourage older children and parents to learn the meaning of various blood values Explain bone marrow aspiration and lumbar puncture with a step-by-step approach and point out those few procedures that are painful Use the recall of each step as a method of distraction Whenever possible, make use of newer procedures that minimize discomfort, such as the anesthetic patch, heparin lock, or Ommaya reservoir
Prevent complications of myelosuppression	Be aware of which drugs cause bone marrow depression Interpret current peripheral blood counts to guide implementation of specific infection/bleeding precautions
Infection	Institute reverse isolation: private room, restriction of visitors/personnel with active infection, and strict hand washing; the use of gown and mask is optional Evaluate child for any potential sites of infection (needle punctures, mucosal ulceration, minor abrasions, dental problems, and so on) Monitor temperature elevations closely, although steroids may depress this symptom Administer meticulous skin care, especially in the mouth and perianal regions Prevent skin breakdown with frequent change of position Encourage adequate calorie-protein intake Avoid exertion or fatigue Teach preventive measures at discharge (hand washing and isolation from crowds) Stress importance of isolating child from any known cases of chickenpox or other childhood communicable diseases; work with school nurse and physician to determine optimum time for school reattendance
Hemorrhage	Use all measure to prevent infection, especially in ecchymotic areas Use local measures to stop bleeding Restrict strenuous activity that could result in accidental injury Involve child in responsibility for limiting activity when platelet count drops
Anemia	Allow the child to monitor his activity tolerance Encourage rest periods throughout the day and at least 8 to 10 hours of sleep at night For severe anemia, see the box on p. 1374 for nursing interventions
Support child during treatment for myelosuppression	Explain reason for antibiotics and/or transfusions, particularly why platelets are reserved for acute, uncontrolled bleeding episodes Anticipate need for crossmatched platelets and white blood cell count; encourage parents to locate potential donors Observe for signs of transfusion reaction (Table 36-2); a febrile reaction is common with leukocyte transfusion and is *not* a contraindication for its use Record approximate time for hemostasis to occur after administration of platelets

Summary of nursing care of the child with leukemia—cont'd

Goals	Responsibilities
Support child during treatment for myelosuppression—cont'd	Minimize limited activity and boredom imposed by continuous intravenous infusion Encourage appropriate quiet activities Choose site for intravenous infusion that allows maximum mobility Protect intravenous infusion from dislodgement during movement (armboard, protective shield over needle)
Manage problems of radiotherapy and drug toxicity Nausea and vomiting	Be aware of treatment protocols and expected reactions/toxicities resulting from each (see Tables 28-4 and 28-5) Give antiemetic prior to onset of nausea and vomiting; calculate optimum time by establishing when nausea and vomiting occur after the first dose; then administer about 20 minutes before the expected reaction during subsequent doses Whenever possible, give drug before bedtime and/or on an empty stomach Stress that this side effect is only temporary; with some drugs (such as dacarbazine [DTIC]) the nausea and vomiting lessen after the first dose If dehydration occurs, notify physician
Anorexia	Encourage parents to relax; stress legitimate nature of loss of appetite Allow child *any* food he tolerates; plan to improve quality of food selections when appetite increases Stress expected increase in appetite from steroids Take advantage of any hungry period; serve small "snacks" Fortify foods with nutritious supplements, such as powdered milk in custards, puddings, and so on; use nutritious drinks, such as prepared breakfast drinks Allow child to be involved in food preparation and selection (grocery shopping, trying new recipes, eating "picnic" lunch) Make food appealing (for example, "face" on hamburger) Remember usual food practices of children in each age-group, such as food jags of toddlers or normal occurrence of physiologic anorexia If anorexia persists despite improved physical status, assess family for additional problems (for example, use of food by child as a control mechanism)
Oral ulcers	Inspect mouth daily for oral ulcers Institute meticulous oral hygiene as soon as a drug is used that causes oral ulcers Use a soft-sponge toothbrush, cotton-tipped applicator, or gauze-wrapped finger Administer frequent (at least every 4 hours and after meals) mouthwashes (1 part hydrogen peroxide to 4 parts normal saline) Report evidence of ulcers to physician Apply local anesthetics to ulcerated areas before meals and as needed Serve bland, moist, soft diet Encourage fluids, drinking through a straw may help bypass painful areas
Rectal ulcers	Wash perineal area after each bowel movement Use warm sitz baths or tub baths as frequently as necessary for comfort Expose ulcerated area to warm heat to hasten healing Apply A and D Ointment or other nonporous lubricant, especially before a bowel movement

Continued.

Summary of nursing care of the child with leukemia—cont'd

Goals	Responsibilities
Rectal ulcers—cont'd	Observe for constipation resulting from child's voluntary refusal to defecate Avoid rectal temperatures or suppositories
Peripheral neuropathy	Advise parents of possible reactions Record bowel movements; may use stool softener to prevent constipation; may need stimulants for evacuation If weakness occurs, alter activity to prevent accidents (including school attendance) Use footboard if footdrop occurs Administer analgesics (not aspirin) for jaw pain; give fluids rather than solid foods to lessen chewing movements Advise parents of neurologic syndrome from central nervous system irradiation (5 to 8 weeks after treatment); allow child to rest
Hemorrhagic cystitis	Observe for signs (burning and pain on urination) Give liberal (3000 ml/m^2/day) fluid intake Encourage frequent voiding, including during nighttime
Alopecia	May be lessened with use of scalp tourniquet; discuss this procedure with physician Introduce idea of a wig prior to hair loss Administer good scalp hygiene Provide adequate covering during sunlight, wind, or cold If hair thins, keeping it clean, short, and fluffy may camouflage partial baldness Stress that hair begins to regrow in 3 to 6 months and may be a slightly different color or texture Stress that alopecia during a second treatment with the same drug may be much less severe
Moon face	Understand often conflicting reactions of child (negative) and parents (positive) to moon face Encourage rapid reintegration with peers to lessen contrast of changed facial appearance Stress that this reaction is temporary Evaluate weight gain carefully (in weight gain resulting from administration of steroids, extremities remain thin)
Mood changes	Prepare family for expected euphoric effect from steroids Interpret mood changes based on drugs or reactions to disease/treatment
Relieve pain	Carefully assess pain to determine its true cause—may be a manifestation of fear, loneliness, or depression During terminal stage, appreciate that pain control is necessary component of physical and emotional care
Environmental manipulation	Avoid excess noise or light Place all commodities within easy reach Use gentle, minimal physical manipulation Avoid pressure (bedclothes, sheets) on painful areas Experiment with using heat or cold on painful areas (use cautiously because of easy skin breakdown)

Summary of nursing care of the child with leukemia—cont'd

Goals	Responsibilities
Positioning	Change position frequently; if difficult for child, coordinate with pain relief from analgesics Avoid pressure on bony prominences or painful sites (water bed, bean bag chair, flotation mattress); ensure good body alignment
Analgesics	Administer analgesics as needed; never use aspirin or any of its compounds Select narcotic drugs carefully to use them when most needed When pain is severe, administer drugs before the pain becomes severe (administration as needed for severe pain is inadequate to provide optimal relief) Evaluate effectiveness of pain relief with degree of alertness vs sedation; excessive sedation and somnolence indicate a need for decreased analgesics
Provide continued emotional support	Always advise parents of expected therapy side effects vs toxicities; clarify which demand medical evaluation (mucosal ulceration, hemorrhagic cystitis, peripheral neuropathy, evidence of infection or dehydration) Reassure parents that such reactions are not caused by return of leukemic cells Interpret prognostic statistics carefully, realizing parents' temporary need to interpret them as they see necessary (For additional interventions, refer to Chapter 27)

members must individualize the "numbers" to relate to the people. An understanding of each member's emotional needs, as well as competent care of physical ones, is essential to the positive, growth-promoting support of the family.

Nursing care of the child with leukemia is summarized in the boxed material on pp. 1020 to 1023.

BRAIN TUMORS

Next to leukemia, tumors of the central nervous system cause more deaths in children than any other type of cancer. Although they may occur at any age, their peak incidence in childhood is between 5 and 10 years of age. Males are affected more than females.

The majority of tumors (about 60%) are *infratentorial,* which means that they occur in the posterior third of the brain, primarily in the cerebellum or brain stem. This anatomic distribution accounts for the frequency of symptoms resulting from increased intracranial pressure. A smaller number are *supratentorial,* or within the anterior two thirds of the brain, mainly the cerebrum. In adults the majority of tumors are of the latter type, which accounts for the more common clinical manifestations of behavioral change, loss of speech, mental impairment, and motor dysfunction in the adult age-group.

Classification

Because the neoplasms can arise from any cell within the cranium, it is possible to have tumors originating from the nerve cells, neuroepithelium, glia, cranial nerves, blood vessels, pineal gland, and hypophysis. Glimoas, arising from glial cells, the supporting structures of the brain, are the most common brain tumors in children.

Within each of these structures, specific cells may be involved, which histologically results in a classification of tumor types. Since the list is long, only the major tumors found in children are discussed.

Cerebellar astrocytomas. These tumors, so named because the cells resemble astrocytes, are the most common type of brain tumor. They are benign, cystic, and slow growing but may gradually replace the cerebellar hemisphere. Surgical excision is associated with a high rate of cure (80% to 90%).

Medulloblastomas. These tumors, whose cells resemble those of the primitive medullary tube, are fast-growing, highly malignant neoplasms that are most commonly found in the cerebellum. Rapid invasion of neural tissue makes surgical excision difficult, decreasing the chances of long-term survival. Radiation and chemotherapy are resulting in somewhat longer survivals.

Brain stem gliomas. These slow-growing tumors are usually astrocytomas or glioblastomas. However, their anatomic placement within vital control centers of the body, namely of respiration and heat rate, make surgical excision impossible, thus lowering chances for survival. Radiation is used palliatively to shrink the size of the tumor and thus prolong survival. However, few children with brain stem gliomas live past 12 months of age. These tumors frequently involve cranial nerves V through X.

Ependymomas. These tumors are derived from the ependyma, the membrane lining the central canal of the spinal cord and the cerebral ventricles. They most frequently arise on the floor of the fourth ventricle, causing cerebrospinal fluid obstruction. They grow with varying speed and, because of their anatomic position, can invade the cardiorespiratory center, the cerebellum and the spinal cord. Only partial surgical removal is possible because resection from the floor of the fourth ventricle could damage vital control centers. Because of the invasiveness of the tumor, the entire craniospinal axis is irradiated postoperatively.

Craniopharyngiomas. These tumors are the most common nongliomatous neoplasm of childhood and are located near the sella turcica, a saddle-like prominence of the sphenoid bone that houses the pituitary gland. Because of the anatomic location, they compress the foramen of Monro, blocking the flow of cerebrospinal fluid; cause disturbance of pituitary function; compress the optic chiasm, causing visual problems; and depress functioning of the hypothalamus.

Total surgical extirpation may not be possible with this tumor because of its insidious optic growth. However, children with this tumor have an excellent chance for survival, since radiation therapy and repeated surgical intervention are successful in reducing the size of the tumor. Unfortunately residual visual, endocrine, and hypothalamic defects are not uncommon. These children usually require hormone replacement at puberty, antidiuretic hormone to prevent diabetes insipidus, and corticosteroids to control fluid and electrolyte balance (see Chapter 38).

Cerebral tumors. The most common cerebral neoplasms are astrocytomas and ependymomas. Astrocytomas grow rapidly and invade adjacent structures, such as the basal ganglia, and thalamus. Ependymomas most often occur in the lateral ventricles, although they tend to metastasize anywhere along the cerebral hemisphere. Surgical excision is often difficult because of their location within the cerebrum.

Optic nerve gliomas. Almost all tumors of the optic nerve and chiasm (junction of the optic nerves) are astrocytomas. Tumors confined to one orbit produce moderate, straightforward exophthalmos and decreased visual acuity in the involved eye. Tumors affecting the chiasm usually result in symptoms affecting both eyes, as well as signs of increased intracranial pressure caused by obstruction of the foramen of Monro. Strabismus is a common finding because of defective fixation of a poorly seeing eye. Optic nerve atrophy is an invariable consequence from tumor compression.

Treatment is surgical extirpation. If the glioma is confined to one orbit, total resection may be possible. Since the optic nerve is also removed, vision is lost in the affected eye. However, the globe (eyeball) can usually be preserved, allowing for a natural prothesis.

If the tumor is chiasmal, it usually cannot be totally removed, although partial resection may eliminate the obstruction to the flow of spinal fluid. At other times a ventricular shunt may be necessary to bypass the tumor. Radiotherapy may be successful in reducing the size of the tumor and improving visual acuity. Because of the proximity of chiasmal gliomas to the pituitary gland, hormone imbalance, especially diabetes insipidus, after surgery may be a problem.

Clinical manifestations

The signs and symptoms of brain tumors are directly related to their anatomic location and size. In children infratentorial tumors most often cause signs of cerebellar dysfunction and increased intracranial pressure.

Ataxia. Ataxia is the most frequent sign of cerebellar involvement. Any of the tests for muscular coordination discussed in Chapter 5 are helpful in assessing loss of functioning. Early signs of ataxia may be missed because parents or teachers regard the incoordination as clumsiness. Loss of balance may only be evident when the child is asked to turn quickly and has to resort to a wide-based stance to maintain an upright position. Later, falling, tripping, banging into objects, and poor fine motor control become more obvious signs of a cerebellar insult.

Weakness. Hypotonia and hyporeflexia are frequent signs of cerebellar involvement. Neoplasms of the cerebrum, brain stem, or spinal cord may also produce lower-extremity weakness with hyperreflexia, positive Babinski's sign, spasticity, and paralysis. Early signs that may be missed include subtle changes of handedness, posture, and dexterity.

Head tilt. Abnormal posturing of the head is an important sign of a possible brain tumor, particularly of the posterior fossa. Head tilt may be the result of extraocular muscle paresis, particularly with cranial nerve IV involvement. It is frequently the first sign of decreased visual acuity. *Nuchal rigidity* may also be present with head tilt and can be the result of traction on the dura by the tumor.

Visual defects. Several visual defects may be present with infratentorial neoplasms, the most common of which are nystagmus, diplopia, strabismus, decreased visual acuity, and visual field defects. *Nystagmus* (rhythmical oscillation of the eyeball) is best elicited by having the child gaze at an object to the side. If there are coarse movements of the eye as the child looks to one side but either fine or absent movement on the other side, the lesion is usually on the side of the obvious movement.

Diplopia and *strabismus* are most often the result of sixth nerve (abducens) palsy, either caused specifically by a brain stem glioma or generally by increased intracranial pressure. Frequently the child may not verbalize double vision but characteristically tilts his head to one side to view objects near the central field of vision or closes one eye to allow unilateral fixation. Parents may observe diplopia when the child reaches for an object but misses it because he sees a different one in front of him or states that there are "two" of everything. However, since children quickly accommodate for either defect, the early signs may be missed.

Decreased visual acuity is difficult to judge, especially in young children, but it may be evident in behavior, such as banging into objects, looking closely at objects, rubbing the eyes, or failing in school.

Visual field defects may be seen with any lesion involving the optic pathways behind the optic chiasm, particularly craniopharyngiomas. It is often difficult to identify decreased peripheral vision in children until other symptoms are present from advanced tumor growth. However, parents may suspect difficulty when the child is unaware of activity until it is directly in front of him.

Cranial neuropathy. Any of the cranial nerves can be involved, depending on tumor location and severity of intracranial pressure. Of all the tumors, brain stem gliomas characteristically cause cranial nerve damage because of infiltration and compression. The nerves most commonly involved in order of frequency are VII (facial), IX (glossopharyngeal), X (vagus), V (trigeminal, sensory roots), and VI (abducens). In general, cranial neuropathy is bilateral, mixed, and incomplete. (For a discussion of the cranial nerves, see Table 5-12, p. 172.)

Vital sign disturbance. Tumors invading the brain stem most commonly cause regulatory disturbance in the cardiorespiratory center. This is usually manifest by decreased pulse and respiration, increased blood pressure, and decreased pulse pressure (difference between systolic and diastolic blood pressure). Hypothermia or hyperthermia is also related to involvement of the hypothalamus from craniopharyngiomas.

Headache. Recurrent and progressive headaches in the frontal or occipital areas may indicate a brain tumor. Characteristically these headaches are worse on arising, lessen during the day, are affected by position (intensified by lowering the head), and increase during straining, such as during a bowel movement, coughing, or sneezing. In infants persistent irritability, crying, and head rolling often indicate a headache.

Vomiting. Vomiting not preceded by nausea or associated with feeding and progressively becoming projectile is an early clue to increased intracranial pressure or direct tumor compression of the emetic control center. Like headaches, vomiting is usually more severe in the morning but relieved by moving about and changing position.

Cranial enlargement. Widening of the sutures may appear before complete closure has occurred, usually by age 18 months. However, it is not noticeable once the skull has no flexible openings. Exophthalmos may be present, especially with optic nerve tumors, but is regarded as a late sign of tumor involvement.

Papilledema. Papilledema (edema of the optic nerve) is ordinarily a late sign of increased intracranial pressure but may be the only sign of a posterior fossa neoplasm. Papilledema is visible under ophthalmoscopy as a swelling of the optic disc, blurring of the disc margins, and dilatation of disc capillaries and veins.

Behavioral changes. Behavioral changes such as irritability, lethargy, and coma may result from the tumor but more likely are caused by increased pressure. Obvious personality changes are more related to cerebral tumors than the types of tumors most commonly seen in children.

Seizures. Seizures are most often a sign of cerebral neoplasms and generally cause electroencephalogram (EEG) changes. When accompanied by changes in vital signs, the seizures may indicate a herniation of a cerebellar tumor through the foramen magnum into the brain stem.

Diagnostic evaluation

Diagnosis of a brain tumor is based subjectively on presenting clinical signs and objectively on a battery of neurologic tests. Table 11-2 summarizes the major tests used in neurologic evaluation. One recently developed procedure, computerized transverse axial tomography (CAT), has major advantages over the other tests because it is a noninvasive test that provides an exact estimation of the tumor's location. It can also provide valuable information about the tumor's properties, such as whether it is solid, semisolid, or cystic. Besides locating intracranial abnormalities, it is also advantageous in assessing tumors in the lungs and orbit.

Although there are virtually no complications from the test, with children there are special considerations, such as the need for sedation to achieve absolute immobility, the inability of an abnormally large head size (hydrocephalus) to fit into the machine, vomiting and the danger of aspiration from the injection of dye, and a worsening of pulmonary edema or intracranial pressure from the supine position.[2]

Medical/surgical management

The treatment of choice is total extirpation of the tumor without residual neurologic damage. With the exception of brain stem gliomas, surgery is usually attempted in order to determine the type of tumor, the extent of invasiveness, and potential for removal. In those cases in which surgical resection is limited, radiation and/or chemotherapy are begun. The drugs most commonly used are nitrosoureas, vincristine, methotrexate, and cytosine arabinoside. With the exception of the nitrosoureas, the other drugs must be introduced intrathecally either by lumbar puncture or the Ommaya reservoir to bypass the blood-brain barrier.

One major postoperative medical problem that may require intervention is brain edema. Parenteral administration of adrenocorticosteroids and hypertonic solutions, such as mannitol and urea, are beneficial in decreasing cerebral edema. Fluids are also monitored closely to allow for hydration without circulatory overload.

Nursing considerations

Nursing care of the child with a brain tumor involves (1) observing for signs and symptoms related to the tumor, (2) preparing the child and parents for the diagnostic tests and operative procedure, (3) preventing postoperative complications, and (4) planning for discharge. The principles of care are similar regardless of the type of intracranial lesion. However, knowledge of the specific tumor location allows the nurse to more definitively tailor the observations. Since a brain tumor is a potentially fatal diagnosis, the reader is urged to incorporate the psychologic interventions discussed in Chapter 27 with those elaborated on in the following paragraphs.

Observation for signs and symptoms. A child admitted to the hospital with neurologic dysfunction is often suspected of having a brain tumor, although the actual diagnosis is as yet unconfirmed. Establishing a baseline of data on which to compare preoperative and postoperative changes is essential toward planning physical care and preventing complications. It also allows the nurse to assess the degree of physical incapacity and the family's emotional reaction to the diagnosis. For example, children with cerebellar astrocytoma may have displayed vague cerebellar symptoms for several years before a tumor is suspected. For these parents the revelation of a neoplasm may be more of a shock than for those who have witnessed a rapid deterioration in their child's ability.

Vital signs. Vital signs are taken routinely and more often when any change is noted. They are monitored for 1 full minute to note subtle changes in rate or rhythm and recorded along with the child's activity. The nurse should also chart pulse pressure. Any sudden variations are reported immediately to the physician. Hyperthermia must be evaluated carefully since it may represent dysfunction of the hypothalamus or brain stem rather than an infectious process. Measures to lower temperature, such as tepid sponge baths, electric cooling blanket, or antipyretic medications, should be employed to avoid seizures.

Signs of increasing intracranial pressure are slowly falling pulse and respiratory rates with a rising blood pressure. It is essential to note a change in vital signs after diagnostic procedures, especially after a lumbar puncture, in which sudden release of spinal fluid may precipitate herniation of the brain stem and cardiorespiratory arrest.

Ocular signs. Ocular signs are taken routinely with vital signs. The procedures for pupil size, equality, reaction to light, and accommodation are described on p. 129. If the nurse is skilled in the funduscopic examination, papilledema is also routinely checked for. Other visual tests include evaluation of nystagmus, by having the child gaze at lateral objects; diplopia, by asking the child to count one or two fingers held before his eyes; visual acuity, by having the child read a book or describe some object held at a distance; peripheral vision, by moving a finger from the side of the head to the midline; and strabismus, using the corneal light reflex test or alternate cover test (see p. 127).

These tests, which can be presented as games, should be done in the morning and evening. Consistency in testing is important to yield reliable results. For example, the same book or distant object is used, and peripheral distance is measured in approximate degrees. Ideally the same day and evening nurses should perform the tests to eliminate judgment discrepancies. Each finding should be charted sequentially to allow instant identification of a change.

Level of consciousness. Level of consciousness is recorded with vital signs. For an older child the nurse can assess alertness and mental functioning by asking him simple questions, such as his name, where he is, how to work an addition problem, or what program is on television. An alert child may question why the nurse asks these "silly" questions. It is important to answer this wisely, since the child may deliberately attempt to fool the nurse. The nurse can reply, "I want to make sure that you are as smart today as you were yesterday."

For younger children the nurse assesses level of consciousness by recording intervals of sleep and wakefulness, noting the activity level when awake. Progressively longer sleep periods with decreased activity and a change in behavior from contentment to irritability are signs of altered consciousness.

Function. Muscle strength, coordination, and cranial nerve function, which are discussed in detail in Chapter 5, are routinely assessed. Simple muscle tests include handgrip and moving the extremities against resistance applied by the nurse. Coordination can be tested by observing for tremors, having the child write his name each day, and having him balance on one foot. The nurse observes the child's gait at least once daily. Head tilt, as well as any other change in posturing, is always recorded. Cranial nerves V through X, the nerves most often involved, are tested daily.

Unless otherwise ordered, the child is allowed out of bed with no restrictions. However, the nurse must be aware of muscle weakness or ataxia, which may necessitate special safety precautions. The child may need assistance and supervision when ambulating to prevent accidental injury. Side rails are always raised when the child is in bed.

Headache. Headache indicates increasing intracranial pressure. The nurse notes location, severity, and duration. If the child is unable to verbalize these characteristics, the nurse relies on observations of behavior. The child with a headache may assume a characteristic position, such as lying flat and facing away from light. He is often irritable but lethargic, refusing to engage in play. If the headache subsides or if analgesia is relieving the discomfort, the nurse will note a dramatic change in behavior.

Although aspirin or acetaminophen may be given for pain or fever, depressant analgesics are avoided because they obscure state of consciousness. If sedation is required for extreme irritability, the nurse carefully assesses level of alertness and orientation to surroundings, even it if requires waking the child periodically.

Since straining at stool increases intracranial pressure and headache, the nurse records daily bowel movements to prevent constipation. Stool softeners may be necessary to prevent straining, especially postoperatively. Enemas are avoided since they can dangerously increase pressure, causing compression of the brain stem.

Vomiting. Vomiting is charted for time, amount, and relationship to feeding and nausea. If the child vomits soon after waking in the morning, breakfast should be delayed until after vomiting has occurred. If the child vomits after feedings, he should be refed whenever possible. The quantity of emesis is measured since fluid replacement may be strictly calculated to prevent increased intracranial pressure.

To assure adequate hydration, the nurse records intake and output, tests urine for specific gravity, and observes for other signs of dehydration, such as dry skin and mucous membranes. In a child with open sutures, the fontanel will normally bulge from increased pressure. Therefore, observing for a depressed fontanel as a sign of dehydration is not reliable in this situation.

Cranial enlargement. Cranial enlargement occurs in children whose fontanels are not completely closed. Head circumference is measured daily. Since a progressive change is significant, the head should be measured in centimeters with the cranial landmarks clearly identified (directly over the eyes and around the occiput). The fontanels are measured using a calibrated instrument, such as a ruler.

In children over age 2 years the eyes are observed for obvious protrusion. For a more objective evaluation, the nurse can rely on observing the normal placement of the lower and upper lids on the iris or sclera (setting-sun sign).

Seizures. Seizures are recorded as described on p. 1447. They may be caused by increased intracranial pressure, hyperthermia, or a cerebral lesion. Accurate description of a convulsive episode can help the physician locate the possible site of the tumor. All children suspected of a brain tumor should have seizure precautions at their bedside. After seizure activity the nurse closely monitors vital signs and blood pressure. Normally pulse and respiration are elevated after a convulsion. However, a depressed pulse and respiration are reported immediately since they may indicate brain stem involvement.

Preparation of family for diagnostic and operative procedures. The suspected diagnosis of a brain tumor is always a crisis event. Despite the fact that some tumors are removed with excellent results, the physician can rarely give definitive answers regarding prognosis until after surgery. Therefore, parents and older children require much emotional support to face the diagnostic procedures and a craniotomy.

Preparing the child for the diagnostic tests depends on his age and previous experience. Since most of the tests involve x-ray equipment, the child may be familiar with the procedure. School-age children usually appreciate a more detailed description of why dye or air is injected. The importance of lying still for tests, particularly tomography, should be stressed. Children unfamiliar with the machines should be shown a picture beforehand. Although x-ray examinations are not painful, the machinery is often so frightening in appearance that the child protests because of anxiety. This is especially true of tomography, which requires that the child's head be placed within a special immobilizing chamber for 20 minutes or more (Fig. 28-2). To maintain a secure position, the head is placed in a rubber cap and surrounded by water pressure. Chin and cheek pads are sometimes used to prevent the slightest movement. Straps are applied to the body to prevent a slight change in position. The nurse can explain these events to a frightened child by comparing them to an astronaut's preparation for a space flight. It is emphasized to the child that at no time is the procedure painful.

A lumbar puncture is usually done to analyze spinal fluid for tumor cells, increased protein content, and increased pressure or to inject air (pneumoencephalography) into the ventricular system. The explanation summarized on p. 1013 can be modified according to the specific purpose of the lumbar puncture. Some of the other diagnostic procedures, such as ventriculography and arteriography, are usually done under general anesthesia. An older child needs a brief explanation of the procedure, particularly the reason for dressings on the scalp (burr hole) or neck (carotid artery), respectively.

Once surgery is scheduled, the child needs an explanation of what will be done. By the time most children are late preschoolers, they know that the head and brain are important parts of their body. It may be helpful to have a child draw his concept of the brain in order to clarify misconceptions and base the explanation on his level of understanding.

Although the temptation is to justify the need for surgery by stating that removing the tumor will take away various

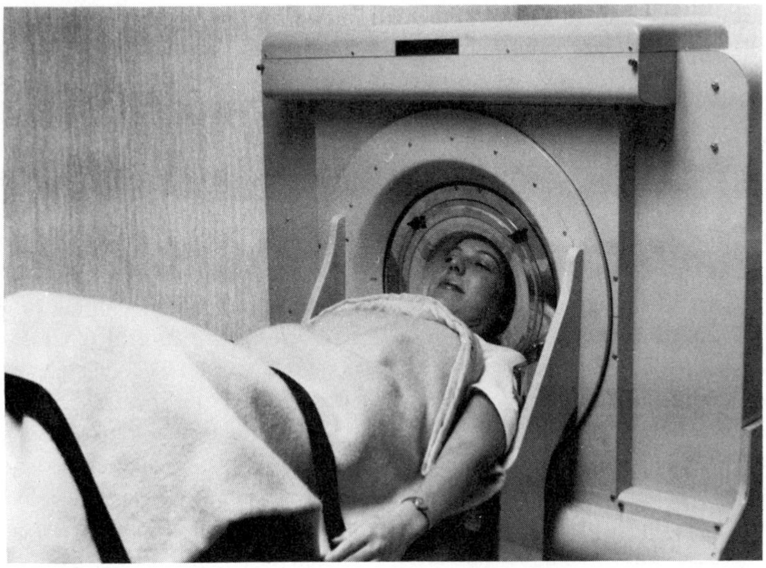

Fig. 28-2. Patient under CAT scanner (tomography). (From Conway, B. L.: Carini and Owens' neurological and neurosurgical nursing, ed. 7, St. Louis, 1978, The C. V. Mosby Co., p. 179.)

symptoms, the nurse should refrain from emphasizing this point too strenuously. Postsurgery headaches and cerebellar symptoms, such as ataxia, may be aggravated rather than improved. Surgery may not improve vision. With optic gliomas the child will be blind in one eye. Finally surgical removal of the mass may be impossible, and, after surgery, there will be deterioration of functioning. Being honest before surgery most often makes honesty after the operation easier because no false hopes were created.

Honesty does not negate instilling hope. A truthful explanation regarding the operation is: ''The physician will see exactly where the tumor is. If it is small and in one place, it will be removed. If it is large, as much of it as possible will be removed so that some of your symptoms will go away.'' It is best to deliver information in small amounts to let the child pursue additional answers. For example, some children will ask about what happens when part of the tumor is left in. An honest reply is that, after surgery, the physician will try to shrink the tumor altogether with a special radiation machine and/or drugs. A further explanation of radiation or drug side effects is unwarranted since the child will be bombarded with information before it is relevant.

Two aspects of preoperative preparation need emphasis. Usually the night before surgery the child's head is shaved. This can be traumatic to the child and parents. However, it can be approached in a sensitive, positive way. If the child's hair is long, it should be braided so that the long swatch can be saved. Showing the child how he looks at different stages of the process helps him prepare for the final appearance.

Once the hair is clipped very short or shaved, the child can be given a cap or scarf to wear in order to camouflage the baldness. The nurse takes every precaution to protect the child from teasing or ridicule by other children prior to surgery. It is also emphasized that the hair will regrow shortly after the operation. Depending on the child's immediate adjustment to the hair loss, the nurse may introduce the idea of wearing a wig until the hair is grown in, particularly if additional irradiation or chemotherapy is anticipated.

Although the shaving procedure varies, in some hospitals a special technician shaves the scalp to minimize the risk of skin cuts. The scalp is shampooed prior to surgery. During these procedures the child is afforded maximum privacy.

The nurse also tells the child about the size of the dressing. Usually the entire scalp is covered to maintain a tight wound closure, even if a small incision is made. Infratentorial head dressings may be attached to the upper back and around toward the neck in order to maintain slight extension and alignment as a precaution against wound rupture. Applying a similar dressing or ''special hat'' to a doll is often a less traumatic way of demonstrating the physical appearance.

The child also needs a brief explanation of how he will feel after surgery and where he will be. Ordinarily he will return to a special intensive care unit, which he may visit beforehand. Unlike other postsurgical instructions, which include frequent moving and coughing, the nurse stresses that he will sleep for awhile, sometimes even a couple of days, and that when he wakens he will need to lie still. He should be forewarned about the headache, but it should be stressed that it will go away after a few days.

Parents need similar explanations prior to surgery, especially in terms of special equipment used in the intensive care unit, dressings, and their child's behavior. For example, they should know that it is not unusual for the child to be comatose or lethargic for a few days after surgery. The nurse may wish to encourage less frequent visiting during this period so that parents can rest and be able to support their child when he awakens.

It is also advisable for the nurse to participate in preoperative conferences with the physician and parents. The nurse needs to know what information the parents have been informed of in order to be able to give further explanations or emotional support when necessary.

Preventing postoperative complications. Usually the surgeon will prescribe specific orders for vital signs, positioning, fluid regulation, and medication. These vary somewhat, depending on the location of the craniotomy. The following are general principles of care for infratentorial or supratentorial surgery.

Observation. Vital signs are taken as frequently as every 15 to 30 minutes until stable. Temperatures taken rectally are particularly important because of hyperthermia resulting from surgical intervention in the hypothalamus or brain stem and from some types of general anesthesia. To prepare for this reaction, a cooling blanket should be placed on the bed *before* the child returns to the unit so that it is ready for use when needed. Since the temperature control centers are affected, the nurse monitors body temperature often when any cooling measures are employed, because hypothermia can occur suddenly.

When the temperature is elevated, an infectious process must always be suspected, particularly if the febrile state occurs 1 to 2 days after surgery. The most likely types of infection are meningitis and respiratory infection. The probable cause of meningitis is wound contamination. Signs of meningitis, such as opisthotonos, Kernig's and Brudzinski's signs (p. 170), and nuchal rigidity (see also Chapter 37), are very similar to those of increased intracranial pressure and must be carefully evaluated to distinguish whether they are indications of an infection.

There is an especially high risk of respiratory infections because of the imposed immobility, danger of aspiration, and possible depression from the brain stem. The nurse auscultates the lungs to identify adventitious sounds or any areas of diminished or absent breath sounds. Early signs of respiratory involvement are abnormal rate and shallow depth. These findings are reported immediately. Usually chest x-ray films are taken to objectively evaluate pulmonary dysfunction. To prevent hypostatic pneumonia, respiratory excursion can be encouraged with blow bottles, blowing a pencil across a flat surface or on the chest, or having the child "raise" his chest by inspiring. If these measures are presented as games, the child is more likely to comply.

Blood pressure is also taken at frequent intervals. The deflated cuff should be left on the arm between readings to allow for the least movement and disturbance to the child. Ocular signs are recorded at least every hour. Sluggish, dilated, or unequal pupils are reported to the physician, since they may indicate increased pressure.

Observations for function are not instituted until the child regains consciousness. However, as soon as possible the nurse should begin testing reflexes, handgrip, and functioning of the cranial nerves. Muscle strength is usually less after surgery from general weakness but should improve daily. Ataxia may be significantly worse with cerebellar intervention, but it will slowly improve. Edema near the cranial nerves may depress important functions such as the gag, blink, or swallowing reflex.

The nurse records behavior at regular intervals, noting sleep patterns, response to stimuli, and level of consciousness. Although a child may be comatose for a few days, once he regains consciousness there should be a steady increase in alertness. Regression to a lethargic, irritable state indicates increasing pressure, possibly caused by meningitis. Seizure precautions are kept at the bedside for emergency use.

Dressings are observed for evidence of drainage. If a drain is in place the physician specifies this, since drainage frequently soaks through the dressing. If soiled, the dressing is not removed but reinforced with dry sterile gauze. The approximate amount of drainage is estimated and recorded. To keep an accurate account of drainage the nurse can circle the soiled area with a pen every hour or so. In this way continuous bleeding is easily recognized. If a colorless drainage is noted, the nurse reports this immediately, since it most likely is cerebrospinal fluid from the incisional area. A foul odor from the dressing may indicate an infection. The nurse reports such a finding, and a culture is taken.

Once the child is alert, his arms may need to be restrained to prevent him from removing the dressing. Even a child who has been cooperative before surgery must be closely supervised during the initial stages of regaining consciousness, when disorientation and restlessness are common. Elbow restraints are satisfactory to prevent the hands from reaching the head, although additional restraint may be necessary to preserve an infusion line and maintain a side-lying position.

Positioning. The child with an infratentorial operation is usually positioned flat and on either side. He is kept off his back to prevent pressure against the operative site and to avoid the danger of aspiration. He should be positioned with pillows placed against his back, not his head, to maintain the desired position. If a large tumor was removed, the child is not placed on the operative site, since the brain may suddenly shift to that cavity, causing trauma to the blood vessels, linings, and the brain itself.

The nurse confers with the surgeon to assess the allowable flexibility of the neck. Ordinarily the head and neck are kept in midline with the body and slightly extended. When the child is turned this alignment must be preserved to prevent undue strain on the sutures. Two nurses, one supporting the head and the other the body, are needed. The use of a turning sheet may facilitate turning of a heavy child.

In a supratentorial craniotomy the head is usually elevated above the heart to facilitate cerebrospinal fluid drainage and decrease excessive blood flow to the brain to prevent hemorrhage. Trendelenburg's position is contraindicated in both types of surgeries because it increases intracranial pressure and the risk of hemorrhage. If shock is impending the physician is notified immediately before the head is lowered.

The first 24 to 48 hours after brain surgery are critical. If position is restricted notice of this is posted above the head of the bed. When the child is turned every precaution is used to prevent jarring or malalignment. Brain edema may severely depress the gag reflex, necessitating suctioning of oral secretions. Facial edema may also be present, necessitating eye care if the lids remain partially open. Ice compresses applied to the eyes for short periods help in relieving the edema. A depressed blink reflex also predisposes to corneal ulceration. Irrigating the eyes with saline drops and covering them with eye dressings are important in preventing this complication.

Fluid regulation. With an infratentorial craniotomy, the child is allowed nothing by mouth for at least 24 hours and longer if the gag and swallowing reflexes are depressed or he is comatose. With a supratentorial operation, feeding may be resumed soon after the child is alert, sometimes within 24 hours.Clear water is always started first, because of the possible danger of aspiration. If the child vomits, oral liquids are stopped. Vomiting not only predisposes to aspiration but also increases intracranial pressure and incisional rupture.

Intravenous fluids are continued until fluids are well tolerated. Because of the cerebral edema postoperatively and the danger of increased intracranial pressure, fluids are very carefully monitored. If drugs, such as prophylactic antibiotics, are given intravenously, the amount of the medication is calculated as part of the intravenous fluid. For example, if the child is to receive 20 ml/hour and the diluted drug is 5 ml, the child will receive 15 ml of solution that hour. When small amounts are infused the intravenous drip should be electronically monitored for greater accuracy.

A hypertonic solution such as mannitol or dextrose may be necessary to remove cerebrospinal fluid. These drugs cause rapid diuresis. After surgery the child may have a Foley catheter. The nurse monitors urine output after administration of these drugs to evaluate their effectiveness.

When the child is able to take fluids, he should be fed by the nurse to conserve strength and minimize movement. If there is any sign of facial paralysis, the nurse feeds the child slowly to prevent choking or aspiration. Scrupulous mouth care is essential to prevent oral infection. Sometimes gavage feeding is necessary when bodily functions are too depressed to permit safe oral feedings or the child refuses to eat or drink. In the latter instance the nurse should employ every measure to encourage acceptance of fluids or solids. (See p. 1016 for nursing interventions.)

Pain relief. Unlike most other types of surgery, postoperative analgesics are not routinely prescribed. In fact, every attempt is made to avoid using any type of drug, since it can mask signs of altered consciousness or body functioning. In particular, narcotics, especially morphine, are contraindicated because of their depressant effect on the respiratory center. The one exception is the use of antipyretics, namely acetaminophen or aspirin, to control hyperthermia. Since these drugs also have moderate analgesic benefits, they help relieve the discomfort of headache pain. When oral intake is limited, the suppository forms are used.

Headache, usually severe, is the expected consequence of a craniotomy, particularly as a result of cerebral edema. Measures to relieve some of the discomfort include providing a quiet, dimly lit environment, restricting visitors to a minimum, avoiding any sudden jarring movement, such as banging into the bed, and preventing an increase in intracranial pressure. The latter is most effectively achieved by proper positioning and prevention of straining, such as during coughing, vomiting, or defecating. Bowel movements are monitored to prevent constipation. Stool softeners may be given as soon as liquids are tolerated to facilitate easy passage of stool. Placing an ice bag on the forehead may also provide some headache relief, especially if facial edema is severe.

Plan for discharge. Discharge planning depends on many variables, such as the extent of surgery, any neurologic deficits, expected prognosis, and additional therapy. The entire postoperative period, which is actually one of discharge planning, involves a great deal of emotional support for parents. Since few definitive answers can be given prior to surgery, the surgeon's report is a significant finding and can vary from a completely benign, resected neoplasm to a highly malignant, invasive, and only partially removed tumor. Although parents try to prepare themselves for a potentially fatal diagnosis, it is a shock for them. In some ways it is fortunate that the child is unconscious for a brief period of time, because this allows parents to deal with their acute grief.

This is an opportune time for the nurse and physician to discuss with parents the expected prognosis and plan of therapy. Although parents may hear only a fraction of what they are told, they can begin to put the future into perspective. For example, with most brain tumors, except those of the brain stem and a metastasized medulloblastoma, sur-

Summary of nursing care of the child with a brain tumor

Goals	Responsibilities
Observe for signs and symptoms	Keep daily records of signs and symptoms to help locate site and extent of tumor, to assess child's physical capabilities, and to assist parents in adjusting to insidious or acute deterioration
Vital signs and blood pressure	Record more frequently whenever a change occurs Monitor vital signs for 1 full minute to note subtle difference in rate or rhythm Record values with child's activity Report changes immediately (signs of increasing intracranial pressure are decreased pulse and respiratory rates and rising blood pressure) Institute measures to lower temperature
Ocular signs	Check pupils for size, equality, reaction to light and accommodation (PERRLA) Evaluate nystagmus, strabismus, diplopia, visual acuity, and peripheral vision Perform funduscopic examination for papilledema Each test should be performed by same nurses and charted sequentially with vital signs
Level of consciousness	Record intervals of sleep and wakefulness; observe level of activity when awake Assess mental functioning by asking simple questions (name, age, residence, and so on) If child sleeps for a long interval, assess ease of arousal
Function	Test cranial nerves, especially cranial nerves V through X Assess muscle strength (extremities) Assess coordination Observe gait and changes in posture, especially head tilt For safety, keep side rails up and assist child during ambulation if weakness is present
Headache	Assess location, severity, duration, and relationship to time of day and position
Vomiting	Chart time, amount, and relationship to feeding and nausea If child characteristically vomits in morning, delay breakfast until after emesis Refeed after vomiting whenever possible Observe for signs of dehydration (*sunken* fontanel is not a sign, since it usually remains bulging because of increased intracranial pressure)
Cranial enlargement	In child with open sutures, measure head circumference daily In older child, note evidence of setting-sun sign
Seizures	Have seizure precautions at bedside Record seizures accurately (see p. 1447) Record vital signs and blood pressure; depressed pulse and respiratory rates may indicate brain stem involvement

Prepare family for diagnostic/operative procedures	Explain reason for each test; if tomography (CAT) is done, emphasize need to remain motionless (younger child often needs sedation)
	Explain operative procedure honestly, being careful not to overemphasize positive benefits, which may not be evident for several days postoperatively
	Allow child to visit special intensive care unit that he will be in postoperatively
	Prepare child and parents for head shaving
	  Provide absolute privacy
	  Save long hair by braiding it first
	  Allow child to look into mirror at different stages to lessen shock of total baldness
	  Provide an attractive scalp covering (lacy nightcap or baseball cap)
	When shaving the head, be careful of skin cuts, which can become infected; shampoo scalp as prescribed
	Prepare child and parents for the large dressing; may help to show a picture or wrap gauze around a doll's head

Continued.

Summary of nursing care of the child with a brain tumor—cont'd

Goals	Responsibilities
Prepare family for diagnostic/operative procedures—cont'd	Explain to child what it will be like after surgery, for example, he may be very sleepy, have a headache, and must remain quiet May advise parents to visit less frequently during immediate postoperative period because of child's decreased state of consciousness
Prevent postoperative complications	Take vital signs, blood pressure, and ocular signs every 15 to 30 minutes until stable Place hypothermia blanket on bed prior to child's return to room View any temperature elevation as potential sign of infection Auscultate respiratory status, especially for evidence of decreased breath sounds Institute breathing exercises (use of blow bottle) when child is awake Institute tests for function after child is alert Observe level of consciousness, noting sleep pattern and response to stimuli Observe dressings for drainage; reinforce with sterile gauze pads but do not remove bandage; circle area of drainage to note further seepage; report evidence of clear fluid (cerebrospinal fluid) immediately; restrain child's hands as necessary to preserve intact dressing
Positioning	Always check with surgeon for specific orders, which may differ from the following Infratentorial—position child flat and on either side, not on back; neck is usually slightly extended to prevent strain on sutures Supratentorial—elevate head, usually above level of heart; do not lower head unless ordered by physician Post sign above bed noting exact position of head Turn child cautiously to maintain proper position
Eye care	Apply ice compresses to eyes for short intervals to relieve edema Keep eyes closed or apply eye dressings May need to instill normal saline eye drops to prevent corneal ulceration if blink reflex is depressed
Fluid regulation	Before beginning clear water, check gag and swallowing reflexes If vomiting occurs, stop fluids Calculate all fluids very carefully to prevent overload Measure urinary output, especially if hypertonic solutions for brain edema are given Feed child to conserve energy
Pain relief	Most analgesics/sedatives are contraindicated because they mask level of consciousness and/or depress respiratory center Provide pain relief with environmental manipulation (dimly lit room, no noise, no sudden movement) Prevent increasing intracranial pressure (no straining at stool, coughing, or sneezing)
Plan for discharge	Once parents learn of diagnosis, help them plan for future, especially toward helping child live a normal life Encourage parents to discuss their feelings regarding child's course prior to diagnosis and his prospects for survival Discuss with parents how they will tell the child about the outcome of surgery and need for additional treatment Help parents plan a realistic activity schedule, including resumption of school; child may need limited physical activity (for example, may have to wear a helmet to protect the skull until it is completely healed) but should be encouraged to pursue academic goals Help child prepare for questions from peers regarding "brain surgery," hair loss, or any residual neurologic deficit Provide continuing support for family through comprehensive oncology clinic and/or community nursing service (For interventions regarding emotional care, see Chapter 27)

vival time may be several years. Although the parents are in acute grief, their thinking must be directed toward helping the child recover and regain a normal life to his fullest potential, not toward preparing for imminent death.

It is also a time to encourage parents to verbalize their feelings about the diagnosis. Often they express tremendous guilt for attributing the insidious onset of symptoms, such as ataxia, visual difficulty, or headache, to minor "complaints" by the child. Parents may have punished their child for clumsiness, thinking he was being careless. The nurse listens to such statements, emphasizing the normalcy of the parents' reactions. Sometimes it may be helpful to precipitate such a discussion with a statement, such as, "It is difficult to know when a child's complaints are significant because so often they are caused by minor ailments." The nurse avoids any comments that insinuate that the parents should have sought medical advice sooner, since such remarks only add to the parents' guilt feelings.

During this period the nurse should also discuss with parents what they plan to tell the child when he regains consciousness. It he was prepared honestly as described previously, the diagnosis can be expressed in a similar manner, such as, "The physician removed most of the tumor and the rest will be treated with special drugs and x-ray treatments." As the child improves he will need additional explanation about the treatment (similar to that discussed for leukemia) as well as the reason for residual neurologic effects, such as ataxia or blindness. Since the hair was shaved before surgery, hair loss is less of a concern from treatment, although its regrowth will be delayed by 3 to 6 months, depending on the length of therapy. At this point it is well to reinforce the idea of a wig.

At the time of discharge the nurse discusses with parents the child's activity schedule, especially the need for resumption of normal activity such as returning to school. Until the skull is completely healed, the child may need to wear a helmet if he engages in any physical sport. The school nurse and teacher should confer with the parents to discuss activity restrictions, such as physical education, and the reactions of schoolmates to the child's appearance. Since children often equate "brain surgery" with "going crazy," it is important to prepare the child for possible remarks to this effect. As one child told a classmate, "It's *your* head they should have fixed because you're crazy. Can't you see that I'm all better?"

After discharge the family needs continuing medical and emotional support from health personnel. Even with children who are long-term survivors after treatment for a brain tumor, residual disabilities, such as growth retardation, cranial nerve palsies, sensory defects, motor abnormalities, especially ataxia, intellectual deficits, and emotional/social problems, are not common.[3] It is difficult to assess the exact cause of the nonphysical handicaps, since numerous variables influence the total rehabilitation of the child. However, the high frequency of emotional/social problems, such as aggressive behavior, solitude, emotional liability, insecurity, and depression, attest to the tremendous need for follow-up care despite successful treatment of the tumor.

The realm of possible consequences following the diagnosis of a brain tumor is numerous. Rather than discussing each, the reader is urged to refer to other sections of the text that deal with possible outcomes such as the handicapped, paralyzed, visually impaired, or unconscious child or the care of a child with a ventricular shunt, seizure disorder, or meningitis. Nursing care of the child with a brain tumor is summarized in the box on pp. 1031 to 1032.

LYMPHOMAS

The lymphomas are a group of neoplastic diseases that arise from the lymphoid and reticuloendothelial system. They are usually divided into the Hodgkin's and non-Hodgkin's lymphomas (NHL) and further subdivided according to tissue type and extent of disease (staging). In children non-Hodgkin's lymphomas, which have also been called lymphosarcoma, reticulum cell sarcoma, and giant follicular lymphoma, are three to four times more common than Hodgkin's disease. Although Hodgkin's disease is extremely rare before 5 years of age, there is a striking increase during adolescence and until 30 years of age. In children in the 15- to 19-year-old age-group, Hodgkin's disease occurs with almost equal frequency as leukemia. All the lymphomas are more common in males than females.

Hodgkin's disease

Hodgkin's disease originates in the lymphoid system and primarily involves the lymph nodes. It predictably metastasizes to nonnodal or extralymphatic sites, especially the spleen, liver, bone marrow, and lungs, although no tissue is exempt from involvement (Fig. 28-3). It is usually classified according to four histologic types: (1) lymphocytic predominance, (2) nodular sclerosis, (3) mixed cellularity, and (4) lymphocytic depletion. Histologic pattern and staging of the extent of disease have significant prognostic implication. The first two types and stages are most likely to result in a 90% chance of cure.

Clinical staging. Accurate staging of the extent of disease is the basis for treatment protocols and expected prognoses. The specific classification for each patient is derived from the history, physical examination, x-ray and isotope studies, urine and blood tests, and biopsy findings from diagnostic laparotomy.

Stage I Lesions are limited to one lymph node area or only one additional extralymphatic site (I_E), such as the liver, lungs, kidney, or intestines.

Stage II Two or more lymph node regions on the *same* side of the diaphragm or one additional extralymphatic site or organ (II_E) on the same side of the diaphragm is involved.

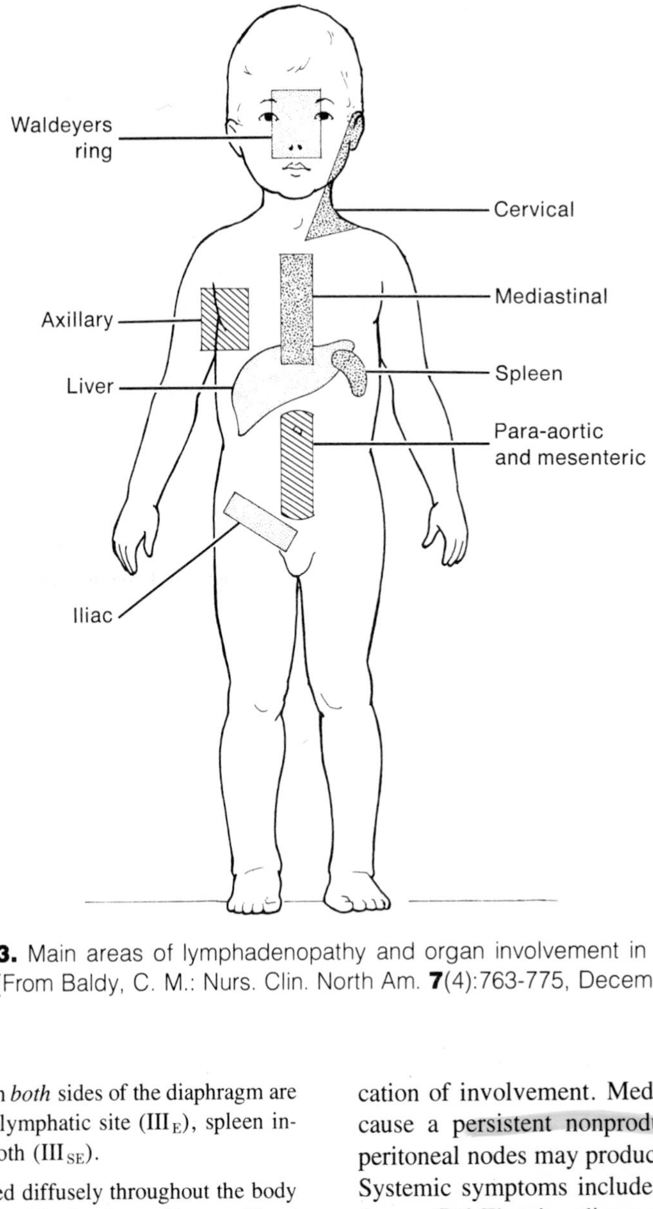

Fig. 28-3. Main areas of lymphadenopathy and organ involvement in Hodgkin's disease. (From Baldy, C. M.: Nurs. Clin. North Am. **7**(4):763-775, December 1972.)

Stage III Lymph node regions on *both* sides of the diaphragm are involved, or one extralymphatic site (III_E), spleen involvement (III_S), or both (III_{SE}).

Stage IV Cancer has metastasized diffusely throughout the body to one or more extralymphatic sites with or without involvement of associated lymph nodes.

Each stage is further subdivided into *A* or *B*. *A* denotes absence of associated general symptoms. *B* indicates presence of symptoms such as night sweats, fever, or weight loss of 10% or more during the preceding 6 months. *A* or *B* does not influence prognosis.

Clinical manifestations. Hodgkin's disease is characterized by painless enlargement of lymph nodes. The most common finding is enlarged, firm, nontender, movable nodes in the cervical area. In children the ''sentinel'' node located near the left clavicle may be the first enlarged node. Enlargement of axillary and inguinal lymph nodes is less frequent.

Other signs and symptoms depend on the extent and location of involvement. Mediastinal lymphadenopathy may cause a persistent nonproductive cough. Enlarged retroperitoneal nodes may produce unexplained abdominal pain. Systemic symptoms include low-grade and/or intermittent fever (Pel-Ebstein disease), anorexia, nausea, weight loss, night sweats, or pruritus. Generally such symptoms indicate advanced lymph node and extralymphatic involvement.

Diagnostic evaluation. Because of the multiple organs that can become involved, diagnosis consists of several tests to confirm the presence of Hodgkin's disease and to assess the extent of involvement for accurate staging. The history and physical include a thorough assessment of constitutional symptoms and palpation of enlarged lymph nodes, spleen, or liver. Routine laboratory tests include complete blood count, uric acid levels, liver function tests, urinalysis, and erythrocyte sedimentation rate.

Radiologic studies. Chest x-ray examinations and/or tomograms and liver, spleen, and bone scans are done to detect metastasis. An intravenous pyelogram may be done if renal involvement is suspected. The most diagnostic radiologic procedure is a lymphangiogram, in which a dye (usually alphazurine) is injected intradermally in the first interdigital space of each foot. Within a few seconds the lymphatic vessels are visualized. One or more vessels are chosen for catherization, and a radiopague medium, usually ethiodized oil (Ethiodol), is injected under pressure to visualize the entire lymphatic chain in the lower extremities, groin, iliopelvic and abdominal-aortic regions, and the thoracic duct. If the axillary, periclavicular, and supraclavicular lymph nodes must be examined, the same procedure is performed in the hands. X-ray films are taken during the procedure, 24 hours later, and sometimes after therapy to chart the progression of treatment or disease, since the contrast material remains in the vessels for up to 1 year.

Another test that may be performed 24 or 48 hours after the lymphangiogram is inferior venacavography. In this procedure a radiopague dye is infused through a catheter in the right femoral vein. X-ray films are taken immediately and 10 and 30 minutes later. The right iliac vein, inferior vena cava, and ureters are visualized against a background of contrast-filled retroperitoneal nodes.

Biopsy is essential to diagnosis and staging. Biopsy is usually done in two stages. First the enlarged lymph node is excised and analyzed for histologic type and evidence of the Sternberg-Reed cell, a giant cell with a dark-staining nucleolus. Although the cell is considered diagnostic of Hodgkin's disease because it is absent in the other lymphomas, it may occur in infectious mononucleosis. At the present time laparotomy is recommended for definitive staging purposes. During this procedure the entire abdomen is examined for evidence of disease, samples of organs are taken for microscopic study, any involved lymph nodes are biopsied, and the spleen is usually removed, although the exact value of splenectomy is still controversial. During surgery metal clips are placed to outline margins of involved sites for irradiation and monitor any disease progression. The ovaries may be moved out of the radiation field to potentially protect them from irradiation damage.

Bone marrow aspiration is done in selected patients when hematologic involvement is expected, usually only in stage III or IV. Occasionally the diagnostic Sternberg-Reed cell may be present in the marrow.

Medical treatment. The mode of therapy is based on the clinical stage. For stages I, II, and IIIA, tumoricidal doses of radiotherapy that are delivered by megavoltage machines such as cobalt 60 units or linear accelerators for maximum deep-tissue concentration are the treatment of choice. Patients with stage I disease may only receive local irradiation to the involved site. Those with stage II or IIIA Hodgkin's disease usually are candidates for extended field irradiation (above and below the diaphragm) and/or total nodal irradiation (to all lymph node regions from the mastoid to the groin). Intensive radiotherapy is usually given daily (except weekends) for a 4- to 5-week period.

The primary form of therapy for stages IIIB and IV is combination chemotherapy. The most widely used drug regimens are MOPP (mechlorethamine [Mustargen], vincristine [Oncovin], prednisone, and procarbazine) or COPP (the substitution of cyclophosphamide [Cytoxan] for mechlorethamine). Other drugs that are cytotoxic for Hodgkin's disease include the nitrosoureas (CCNU, BCNU), doxorubicin (Adriamycin), bleomycin, chlorambucil, and dimethyl-triazeno-imidazole-carboxamide (DTIC or dacarbazine). Present research is investigating the effects of combined radiotherapy and chemotherapeutic agents for stages IIIA, IIIB, and IV. Currently the best results have occurred in stage IIIA. Length of chemotherapy depends on individual response to the drugs but usually lasts at least 6 months. Some centers are advocating continuing therapy for 18 months.

Prognosis. Prognosis for patients with Hodgkin's disease has improved dramatically in the past few years, largely a result of the systematic staging procedure and treatment protocols. The overall 5-year survival rate for any type or stage of disease is 60%; 10-year survival rates decrease to 50%. Stage I patients have a 90% chance of 10-year survival, and patients in stage II, an 80% chance. Stage IIIA patients have a somewhat less favorable prognosis. In Stage IV the chances decrease to about a 25% chance for 5-year survival. Those patients who do relapse usually do so within 2 years after diagnosis and treatment. Since relapse after 4 or 5 years is rare, a 10-year disease-free period is considered a cure.

Nursing considerations. Nursing care involves the same objectives as for patient with other types of cancer, namely, (1) preparation for diagnostic and operative procedures, and (2) explanation of treatment side effects. The nurse bases the specific care plan on the clinical stage of the disease. Since this is most often a disease of adolescents and young adults, the nurse must have an appreciation of their psychologic needs and reactions during the diagnostic and treatment phases.

Preparation of family for diagnostic and operative procedures. Once the child is hospitalized for suspected Hodgkin's disease, a battery of diagnostic tests is ordered. The family needs an explanation of why each test is performed, since many of them, such as a bone marrow aspiration (see p. 1013), are not routine. The one test that deserves special mention is lymphography. Prior to the test the nurse informs the child of the length of the procedure, which is anywhere from 2 to 10 hours and frequently averages 4 to 5 hours. Although the feet are anesthesized, the initial injections are painful. Immobilization of feet during lymphatic vessel catheterization may be uncomfortable and tiresome, especially since the child must remain still for long periods. The nurse and/or technician attending during the procedure should talk to the child to help pass the time. Whenever possible the child is encouraged to sleep. Ideally a family member should be allowed to accompany the child. Fluids and food are not necessarily restricted. If allowed, provisions are made for the child to have a favorite drink or snack.

The procedure is not without complications, the most serious of which is pulmonary embolism from the oil-based dye ethiodized oil (Ethiodol). Fine pulmonary emboli produce symptoms of slight fever, chills, pleuritic pain, mild dyspnea, and a dry cough. Aspirin is helpful to reduce the fever and relieve the pain. The symptoms usually subside within 24 to 48 hours.

Severe oil embolism may occur after dye has been infused too rapidly. Signs alerting the nurse to this complication include cyanosis, distended neck veins, hypotension, liver tenderness, and edema in the lower extremities from increased venous resistance. Emergency medical treatment usually involves supplemental oxygen and antihypotensive drugs. The child may become very apprehensive and need considerable reassurance. Usually sedation is avoided, because it may depress the respiratory center.

Normal reactions to the dye include abnormal taste sensations, retrosternal burning, headache, sleeplessness, diarrhea, and elevated temperature. The alphazurine turns the urine and skin of the feet and/or hands bluish green. Although the urine clears rapidly, the discoloration of skin may last as long as 1 year. Adolescents may be very self-conscious of the staining, especially in the hands.

Since a cutdown procedure is done for vessel catheterization, a pressure bandage may be in place. The nurse observes the area or areas for signs of bleeding and subsequent infection. Sutures are usually removed in 7 to 10 days. Ordinarily the child has no restrictions on activity after the test. However, he is cautioned to keep the wound clean and to avoid excess irritation from shoes.

Preparation for a laparotomy is similar to any other surgery. One special area of concern for families is the effects of the splenectomy on bodily functions. They are informed of the benefits and potential risks. Since the spleen is usually the first organ of extralymphatic involvement, its removal and microscopic investigation are believed to be important in terms of staging. Although not a vital organ, it does have an important role in resisting infection, particularly in young children. Adolescents and adults are at less risk for developing a fulminant infection, probably because of their increased antibody production from continuous exposure to infectious agents. For prophylactic purposes, oral penicillin is usually given daily for the first 1 to 2 years after the splenectomy.

Explanation of treatments and side effects. Limited field radiation for localized disease results in few side effects, sometimes consisting only of a mild skin reaction. With extended field radiation to the chest and abdomen, nausea and vomiting, weight loss, and mucosal ulceration (esophagitis and gastric ulcers) are common side effects. The usual measures for providing relief have been discussed on p. 1017 and are outlined in Table 28-5. More serious reactions are pneumonitis and pericarditis. The nurse observes for signs indicative of either condition (see Table 28-5).

The most common side effect is malaise, which may last for a year after surgery. This is particularly difficult for active, outgoing adolescents, because it prevents them from keeping up with their peers. Sometimes the adolescent will push himself to the point of physical exhaustion rather than admit and succumb to the decreased activity tolerance. The nurse cautions parents to observe for such behavior, such as extreme fatigue at the end of the day, falling asleep at the dinner table, inability to concentrate on homework, or an increased susceptibility to infection. Regular bedtimes and periodic rest times are important for these children, especially during chemotherapy when myelosuppression increases the risk of infection and debilitation. Prior to discharge the nurse should discuss a feasible school schedule with the parents and child. If alterations are necessary, such as elimination of strenuous physical education, they are discussed with the teacher, nurse, and principal.

The nurse can be instrumental in helping the child adjust to activity restrictions by introducing new hobbies or sports. For example, one young adolescent who had hoped to be a cheerleader prior to the diagnosis of Hodgkin's disease found much joy in beginning guitar and painting lessons, joining a youth group, and learning needlework crafts. During periods of rehospitalization for complications from radiation, these projects helped prevent much of the boredom and depression that accompanied her absence from school and friends.

An area of concern for female adolescents is the possibility of sterility from irradiation. Even though the ovaries may be moved out of the field of radiation during the laparotomy, the scatter effect is likely to cause sterility and/or genetic mutations. Sexual function is not altered, although the appearance of secondary sexual characteristics and menstruation may be delayed in the pubescent child. Adolescents should be informed of these side effects early in the course of the diagnosis and treatment. Delayed sexual maturation may be an extremely sensitive and painful area for children (see Chapter 20). It is important for the nurse to respect their concern and refrain from casually placating them with expressions, such as, "You'll catch up someday."

Sexually active adolescents who may want to become pregnant or wish to avoid pregnancy should discuss their plans with the physician. However, the nurse may need to initiate this discussion if the adolescent feels embarrassed or hesitant. Although pregnancy does not alter the course of the disease, treatment generally causes a spontaneous abortion or stillborn child. Pregnancy is usually delayed until the patient has had no therapy for at least 1 year, preferably after a prolonged period of remission. The nurse's role may be to discuss birth control methods with the adolescent.

Explanations of chemotherapeutic reactions are dependent on the specific drug regimen. Drugs commonly used are outlined in Table 28-4, and the most common side effects, such as nausea and vomiting, body image changes, peripheral neuropathy, and mucosal ulcerations, are discussed on pp. 1014 to 1018.

Non-Hodgkin's lymphoma

Non-Hodgkin's lymphoma in children is strikingly different from Hodgkin's disease and adult types of non-Hodgkin's lymphoma in several aspects: (1) the disease is usually diffuse rather than nodular; (2) the cell type is either undifferentiated or poorly differentiated; (3) dissemination occurs early, more often, and rapidly; (4) control of the primary tumor, especially mediastinal presentation, is difficult; (5) current methods of treatment are less effective; and (6) consequently prognosis is much poorer.

Non-Hodgkin's lymphoma is classified according to the predominant malignant cell type—(1) undifferentiated, including Burkitt's lymphoma; (2) lymphocytic, poorly or well differentiated; (3) histiocytic; and (4) mixed lymphocytic and histiocytic. Each classification is further subdivided into the pattern of histologic presentation, namely nodular (circumscribed) or diffuse (spread out). Immunologically these cells are also classified as derived from T-lymphocytes (T cells), B-lymphocytes (B cells), an example of which is Burkitt's lymphoma, or null cells, which lack specific immunologic properties (most commonly found in childhood lymphomas). The intended purpose of the classification system is to allow more direct comparison among treatment protocols for reliable research findings that result in improved prognoses.

Since nursing care of the child with non-Hodgkin's lymphoma is very similar to that for Hodgkin's disease or leukemia, only a brief overview of the medical aspects are presented.

Clinical staging. The same staging used for Hodgkin's disease is employed for non-Hodgkin's lymphoma. However, the staging has little prognostic value, since most newly diagnosed cases are widely disseminated and stage I disease confined to the mediastinum heralds a poor prognosis. Treatment is not based on the staging, and exploratory laparotomy is not essential for staging, although it may be necessary for diagnosis.

Clinical manifestations. Clinical manifestations depend on the anatomic site and extent of involvement. Many of those seen in Hodgkin's disease may be present in non-Hodgkin's lymphoma, although rarely does a single symptom give rise to the diagnosis. Rather metastasis to the bone marrow or central nervous system may produce signs and symptoms typical of leukemia. Lymphoid tumors compressing various organs may cause intestinal or airway obstruction, cranial nerve palsies, or spinal paralysis.

The exception to the usual presentation of non-Hodgkin's lymphoma is Burkitt's lymphoma, a type of cancer that is rare in the United States but endemic in parts of Africa. It is the most rapidly growing human neoplasm, with a doubling time of 24 hours.[22] Therefore, it most commonly is seen as a mass in the jaw, abdomen, or orbit. However, no anatomic site appears exempt from involvement. Peripheral lymphadenopathy, hepatosplenomegaly, or signs of conversion to leukemia are rarely seen.

Diagnostic evaluation. All of the tests normally performed in Hodgkin's disease are included in the diagnostic workup for non-Hodgkin's lymphoma, although the order varies. For example, bone marrow biopsy is routine in non-Hodgkin's lymphoma because of diffuse myeloid involvement. Often the differentiation between leukemia and non-Hodgkin's lymphoma is difficult. The lymphangiogram is another test of diagnostic importance in assessing the extent of lymphatic involvement. Definitive diagnosis rests on histologic typing of biopsy from the primary tumor mass or regional nodes. Whether laparotomy should be routinely done is controversial, since many other tests are capable of reliably assessing disseminated disease.

Treatment. The present treatment protocols for non-Hodgkin's lymphoma, regardless of stage, include combination high-dose, extended-field, or total nodal irradiation with chemotherapy. In some centers the value of total-body irradiation is being investigated. The drug regimens vary and include cyclophosphamide, methotrexate, vincristine, and prednisone (COMP) and other combinations of daunomycin, 6-thioguanine, cytosine arabinoside, and L-asparaginase. Generally 6 to 9 weeks of chemotherapy are required to induce a remission. If relapse does not occur, treatment is usually continued for 18 to 24 months.

Prognosis. Because of the lack of uniformity in applying the staging procedures, reports on remissions and survival rates vary. However, intensive multimodal therapy is improving prognosis. Children with stage I disease, except if localized in the mediastinum, have a 75% chance of a cure. Those with stage II disease have a 50% or less chance. Children with extensive involvement have only a 10% to 20% probability of survival. Relapse most often occurs within 6 months and represents a grave prognostic sign. With relapse, conversion to leukemia with central nervous system involvement is common. Relapse after 12 months is rare, and a 24-month survival rate essentially equals the cure rate.

NEUROBLASTOMA

Neuroblastoma is probably the most common malignant solid tumor in children. It occurs in about 1 per 10,000 live births, with a slightly higher incidence in males. About half the cases occur in children under 2 years of age, and the other fourth occur in children under age 4 years. Because these tumors develop from embryonic neural crest tissue, they may arise anywhere along the craniospinal axis. The majority of the tumors arise from the adrenal gland or from the retroperitoneal symphathetic chain. Therefore, the primary site is within the abdomen. Other primary sites may be within the head, neck, chest, or pelvis.

Staging

In recent years there has been an attempt to classify tumors according to stages for improved criteria for treatment and prognosis at the time of diagnosis and surgery. Neuroblastoma has been classified into five different stages:

Stage I The tumor is confined to the organ or structure of origin.

Stage II The tumor extends in continuity beyond the primary site but does not cross the midline; regional lymph node involvement on the same side may be present.

Stage III The tumor extends in continuity beyond the midline; bilateral regional lymph node involvement may be present.

Stage IV There is remote disease involving the skeleton, parenchymal organs, soft tissue, or distant lymph nodes.

Stage IV-S Stage I or II with remote disease confined to only one or more sites, either the liver, skin, or bone marrow, without x-ray evidence of skeletal metastasis.

Prognosis

Neuroblastoma is a ''silent'' tumor. In over 70% of cases, diagnosis is made after metastasis occurs, the first signs caused by involvement in the nonprimary site, usually the lymph nodes, bone marrow, skeletal system, skin, and liver. Metastasis to bone usually heralds a fatal outcome, whereas metastasis to the liver, unlike in other types of cancer, may still represent a curable stage. Because of the frequency of invasiveness, prognosis for neuroblastoma is poor. The age of the child and the stage of the disease at diagnosis are important prognostic factors. The younger the child, usually under age 1 year, and the earlier the stage (I, II, or IV-S) with a primary site of the neck, pelvis, or thorax, the better the chances for long-term survival (about 90%). The overall survival rate is about 30% to 35%. The child who remains free of disease for 2 years after treatment is considered cured. Unfortunately some children demonstrate a recurrence of the tumor 8 to 10 years later.

Neuroblastoma is one of the few tumors that demonstrates spontaneous regression, possibly a result of maturity of the embryonic cell. Autopsies of many young infants without gross evidence of neuroblastoma demonstrate tumor cells within the adrenal gland. This has led to the belief that inherent control mechanisms are present that prevent the proliferation of these cells. Newer methods of treatment, such as immunotherapy, may improve survival rates for these children.

Clinical manifestations

The signs and symptoms of neuroblastoma depend on the location and stage of the disease. Most presenting signs are caused by compression of adjacent structures. With abdominal tumors the most common presenting sign is a firm, nontender, irregular mass in the abdomen that crosses the midline (in contrast to Wilms' tumor, which is usually confined to one side). Compression of the kidney, ureter, or bladder may cause urinary frequency or retention.

Distant metastasis frequently causes supraorbital ecchymosis, periorbital edema, and proptosis (exophthalmos) from invasion of retrobulbar soft tissue (Fig. 28-4). Lymphadenopathy, especially in the cervical and supraclavicular areas, may also be an early presenting sign. Bone pain may or may not be present with skeletal involvement. Vague symptoms of widespread metastasis include pallor, weakness, irritability, anorexia, and weight loss.

Other primary tumors may cause significant clinical effects, such as neurologic impairment from an intracranial lesion, respiratory obstruction from a thoracic mass, or varying degrees of paralysis from compression of the spinal cord. Infrequently a child may have symptoms of increased catecholamine excretion, such as flushing, hypertension, tachycardia, and diaphoresis.

Diagnostic evaluation

Diagnostic evaluation is aimed at locating the primary site and areas of metastasis.

Radiologic studies. Skull, neck, chest, and abdominal x-ray examinations are done to locate a tumor mass. With an adrenal neuroblastoma an intravenous pyelogram often demonstrates a downward displacement of the affected kidney but normal renal function. Complete bone surveys and liver scan are done to detect metastasis to those sites.

Hematologic studies. A bone marrow aspiration is performed to rule out metastasis. Although it is often difficult to distinguish neuroblastoma cells from other cancer cells, such as leukemia, the neuroblasts frequently clump or form ''pseudorosettes.'' Peripheral blood smears demonstrate signs of generalized malignancy, especially anemia and thrombocytopenia.

Catecholamine excretion. Neuroblastomas, particularly

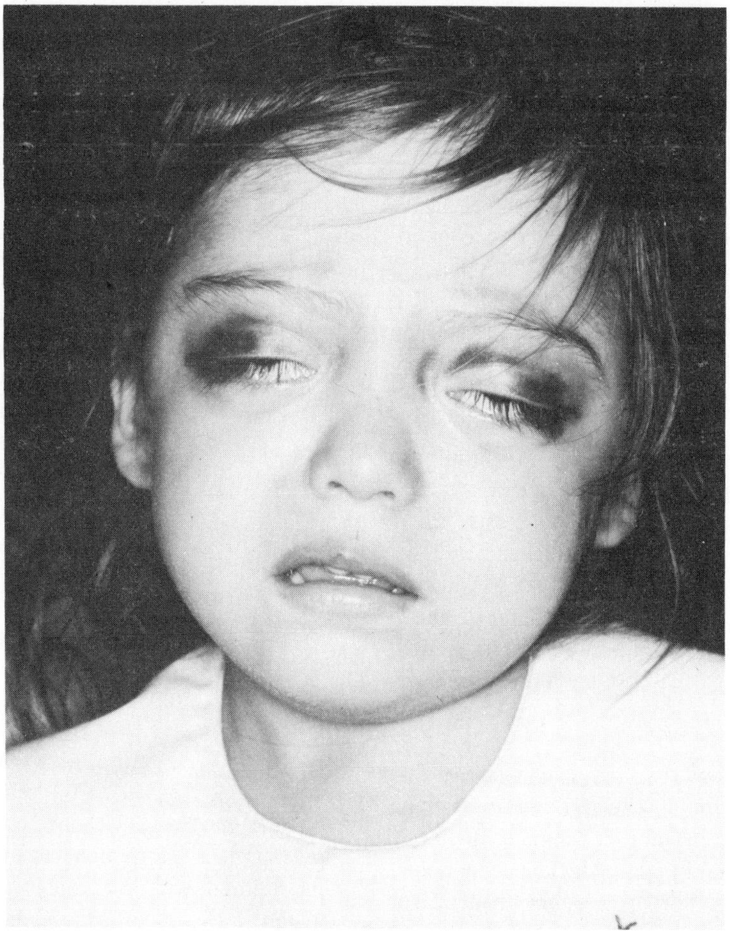

Fig. 28-4. Supraorbital ecchymoses associated with periorbital metastases. (Courtesy Howard A. Britton.) (From Sutow, W. W., Vietti, T. J., and Fernbach, D. J., editors: Clinical pediatric oncology, ed. 2, St. Louis, 1977, The C. V. Mosby Co., p. 511.)

those arising on the adrenal glands or from a sympathetic chain, excrete the catecholamines epinephrine and norepinephrine. By analyzing the breakdown products that are normally excreted in the urine, namely vanillylmandelic acid (VMA), homovanillic acid (HVA), dopamine, and norepinephrine, the physician can detect the presence of a possible tumor both before and after medical/surgical intervention.

The most commonly used test is excretion of vanillylmandelic acid. Since vanillylmandelic acid demonstrates a diurnal pattern with decreased excretion at night, a 24-hour specimen is required. It must also be kept at a pH below 3 and refrigerated (a type of hydrochloric acid is usually added to the container before collection). For accurate test results, the child must be placed on a special diet eliminating vanilla, chocolate, banana, and nuts for 3 days prior to urine collection.

Carcinoembryonic antigen (CEA). Some cancer cells, including neuroblastoma, produce a specific antigen—carcinoembryonic antigen—that can be detected and measured from the blood of a person suspected of having a malignancy. Although not a definitive test for diagnosing cancer, it is of clinical value in monitoring the effects of surgery, radiotherapy, and chemotherapy.

Medical/surgical management

The ideal treatment is complete extirpation of the tumor. However, because of the high frequency of metastasis at the time of diagnosis, total removal is often impossible. Fortunately this tumor is very radiosensitive and even incomplete removal may result in favorable results after irradiation.

Unlike other types of cancer, there is considerable controversy concerning the exact mode of treatment. Some physicians prefer to stage the tumor by performing a surgical biopsy and then use irradiation to shrink it before attempting removal. If localized disease is present, chemotherapy is used by some physicians in the hope of preventing metastasis. The drugs of choice are vincristine, dacarbazine, and cyclophosphamide, because of their different mechanisms of cytotoxicity and side effects. One of the arguments against using chemotherapy is the immunosuppressive effect of the drugs, since the host's immune defenses seem to play a role in this disease.

Nursing considerations

Nursing considerations are similar to those discussed previously for leukemia or brain tumors, such as psychologic and physical preparation for diagnostic and operative procedures, prevention of postoperative complications for abdominal, thoracic, or cranial surgery, and explanation of radiotherapy and drug actions and side effects (see Tables 28-4 and 28-5).

Since this tumor carries a poor prognosis for many children, every consideration must be given the family in terms of coping with a fatal illness. Because of the high percentage of metastasis at the time of diagnosis, many parents suffer much guilt for not having recognized signs earlier. Often the guilt is expressed as anger toward the physician for not diagnosing it sooner. Parents need much support in dealing with these feelings and expressing them to the appropriate people, particularly the physician.

WILMS' TUMOR

Wilms' tumor or nephroblastoma is the most frequent intra-abdominal tumor of childhood and the most common type of renal cancer. Its frequency is estimated to be 1: 10,000 live births with a slightly higher incidence in males. The peak incidence is in the third year of life. It is one of childhood cancers that shows an increased incidence (about 20%) among siblings and identical twins, reflecting evidence of genetic inheritance. It is also associated with several congenital anomalies, particularly aniridia, hemihypertrophy, and, less frequently, hypospadias, cryptorchidism, microcephaly, pigmented and vascular nevi, pinna deformities, mental and growth retardation, and pseudohermaphroditism. Although the exact mechanism that results in tumor formation and anomaly development is unknown, it does allow for identification of high-risk children.

Staging

Wilms' tumor probably arises from a malignant, undifferentiated metanephrogenic blastema (a cluster of primordial cells capable of initiating the regeneration of an abnormal structure). Its occurrence slightly favors the left kidney, which is advantageous because surgically this kidney is easier to manipulate and remove. In about 10% of cases both kidneys are involved. Although the tumor may become quite large, it remains encapsulated for an extended period of time. During surgery the tumor is staged to maximize treatment protocols. The following criteria for staging are most commonly used[8]:

Stage I Tumor is limited to kidney and completely resected. The surface of the renal capsule is intact. The tumor is not ruptured before or during removal. There is no residual tumor apparent beyond the margins of resection.

Stage II Tumor extends beyond the kidney but is completely resected. There is local extension of the tumor, that is, penetration beyond the pseudocapsule into the perirenal soft tissues, or periaortic lymph node involvement. The renal vessels outside the kidney substance are infiltrated or contain tumor thrombi. There is no residual tumor apparent beyond the margins of resection.

Stage III Residual nonhematogenous tumor is confined to abdomen. Any one or more of the following occur: (1) the tumor has been biopsied or ruptured before or during surgery; (2) there are implants on peritoneal surfaces; (3) there are involved lymph nodes beyond the abdominal periaortic chains; and (4) the tumor is not completely resectable because of local infiltration into vital structures.

Stage IV Hematogenous metastases; deposits beyond stage III, namely to lung, liver, bone and brain.

Stage V Bilateral renal involvement either initially or subsequently.

Prognosis

Survival rates for Wilms' tumor are the highest among all childhood cancers. Children with localized tumor (stages I and II) have a 90% chance of cure with multimodal therapy (surgical extirpation, irradiation, and chemotherapy). In children with metastasis, survival rates are approximately 50%. Metastasis is most commonly to the lungs, followed by the liver, bone, and brain.

Clinical manifestations

The most common presenting sign is a swelling or mass within the abdomen. The mass is characteristically firm, nontender, confined to the midline, and deep within the flank. If it is on the right side it may be difficult to distinguish from the liver, although, unlike that organ, it does not move with respiration. Parents usually first discover the mass during routine bathing or dressing of the child.

Other clinical manifestations are the result of compression from the tumor mass, metabolic alterations secondary to the tumor, or metastasis. Hematuria occurs in less than one fourth of children with Wilms' tumor. Anemia, usually secondary to hemorrhage within the tumor, results in pallor, anorexia, and lethargy. Hypertension probably caused by secretion of excess amounts of renin by the tumor occurs occasionally. Other effects of malignancy include weight loss and fever. If metastasis has occurred, symptoms of lung involvement, such as dyspnea, cough, shortness of breath, and pain in the chest, may be evident.

Diagnostic evaluation

In a child suspected of having Wilms' tumor, special emphasis is placed on the history and physical examination for presence of congenital anomalies, family history of cancer, and signs of malignancy, such as weight loss, size of liver and spleen, indications of anemia, and lymphadenopathy. Specific tests include radiographic studies, hematologic studies, biochemical studies, and urinalysis.

Radiographic studies. The usual tests include abdominal and chest x-ray examinations, an intravenous pyelogram, and organ and skeletal surveys. An abdominal x-ray examination usually shows a soft tissue density that displaces the intestines toward the opposite side. An intravenous pyelogram is done to demonstrate the relationship of the tumor to the ipsilateral kidney and the presence of a normal functioning kidney on the contralateral side. A normal unaffected kidney is essential, since a nephrectomy is part of the surgical tumor resection. If a large tumor is present, an inferior venacavagram is necessary to demonstrate possible tumor involvement adjacent to the vena cava. Radioisotope scans and tomography to rule out bone, liver, or lung metastasis may be performed after surgery to expedite the preoperative phase.

Hematologic studies. A complete blood count and peripheral smear are done preoperatively to evaluate the degree of anemia, especially in terms of increasing surgical risks. Polycythemia is sometimes associated with Wilms' tumor because the tumor secretes excess erythropoietin, a hormone that stimulates bone marrow production. A bone marrow aspiration is electively performed to rule out metastasis.

Biochemical studies. Liver function tests, including measurement of levels of bilirubin, serum glutamic-oxaloacetic transaminase (SGOT), serum glutamic-pyruvic transaminase (SGPT), lactic dehydrogenase (LDH), alkaline phosphatase, total protein, and albumin, are performed to assess liver dysfunction from metastasis or any preexisting abnormality that may alter antineoplastic drug metabolism and excretion. (See Table 34-3 for a discussion of these tests.) Renal function tests such as blood urea nitrogen (BUN), creatinine, and creatinine clearance determine function of the unaffected kidney. Uric acid levels are measured in anticipation of cellular catabolism after radiotherapy and chemotherapy. The level of serum electrolytes is measured, since high levels of renin cause marked imbalance with loss of sodium and potassium.

Urinalysis. A complete urinalysis is done, particularly for microscopic examination of sediment, such as white or red blood cells, epithelial cells, casts, and bacteria. An Addis count for quantitation of sediment may be done on urine collected over a 12-hour period.

Medical/surgical management

The principal modes of treatment are surgery, irradiation, and chemotherapy. Although in some institutions the exact sequence of treatment varies, with the administration of chemotherapy prior to surgery preferred in some institutions, the following is the usual approach.

Surgery. Surgery is scheduled as soon as possible after confirmation of a renal mass, usually within 24 to 48 hours after admission. A large midline incision is performed for optimal visualization of the abdominal cavity. The tumor, affected kidney, and adjacent adrenal gland are removed. Great care is taken to keep the encapsulated tumor intact, since rupture can seed cancer cells throughout the abdomen, lymph channel, and bloodstream. The contralateral kidney is carefully inspected for evidence of disease or dysfunction. Regional lymph nodes are inspected and biopsed when indicated. Any involved structures, such as part of the colon, diaphragm, or vena cava, are removed. Metal clips are placed around the tumor site for exact marking during radiotherapy.

If both kidneys are involved, several approaches are advocated. When the tumor is well encapsulated on one side, a partial nephrectomy is done on that side with a total nephrectomy on the opposite side. If both tumors are diffuse, the more involved kidney is removed and the remaining kidney is treated with radiotherapy and chemotherapy. When a transplant is feasible, such as from a twin, sibling, or parent, bilateral nephrectomy is considered. At present the value of each of these procedures is still uncertain because of the few comparative cases of bilateral Wilms' tumor.

Radiotherapy. Postoperative radiotherapy is usually indicated for all children with Wilms' tumor except those under 18 months of age with stage I disease. The normal tissues of infants are extremely radiosensitive, resulting in devastating skeletal and soft-tissue deformities. Irradiation of the tumor site and metastasized areas may be begun within 1 to 3 days postoperatively if the child's condition is stable.

Chemotherapy. The most effective agents for treating Wilms' tumor are actinomycin D and vincristine. Although treatment protocols vary, the commonly advocated approach is a 5-day course of actinomycin D immediately postoperatively, followed by courses 6 weeks and 3 months after surgery. Vincristine is given once weekly for a total of eight injections and thereafter every 3 months on the first and fifth days of actinomycin therapy. This is continued at regular 3-month intervals until a total of seven courses over 15 months have been completed. Present studies are investigating the feasibility of discontinuing therapy as early as 6 months.

Treatment of metastasis. The most common site for metastasis is the lungs. If pulmonary involvement occurs, additional treatment consists of surgical excision of the nodule when feasible, chemotherapy, and irradiation to the involved site. Although metastasis to the brain is considered a grave prognostic sign, treatment of cranial involvement with drugs and radiotherapy has resulted in some long-term survivors. With present modalities for treatment, the prospects of a cure are hopeful despite residual metastasis.

Nursing considerations

The nursing care of the child with Wilms' tumor is similar to that of other cancers treated with surgery, irradiation, and chemotherapy. However, there are some significant differences that are discussed for each phase of nursing intervention.

Preoperative care. Like many of the other cancers, the diagnosis of Wilms' tumor is an unexpected shock. Frequently the child has no physical indication of the seriousness of the disorder other than a palpable abdominal mass. Since in the majority of instances it is the parents who discover the mass, the nurse needs to take into account their feelings regarding the diagnosis. While some parents are grateful for their detection of the tumor, others feel guilt for not finding it sooner or anger toward the physician for missing it on earlier examinations.

The preoperative period is one of swift diagnosis. Typically surgery is scheduled within 24 to 48 hours of admission. The nurse is faced with the challenge of preparing the child and parent for all laboratory and operative procedures. Because of the little time available, explanations should be kept simple and repeated often.

There are several special preoperative concerns, the most important of which is that the tumor should not be palpated unless absolutely necessary because manipulation of the mass may cause dissemination of cancer cells to adjacent and distant sites. In teaching hospitals in which many medical and nursing students are assigned to one patient, it may be necessary to post a sign on the bed, such as "DO NOT PALPATE ABDOMEN." This same precaution is extended to parents as soon as Wilms' tumor is suspected. Careful bathing and handling are also important in preventing trauma to the tumor site.

Children and parents need preparation for the size of the incision and dressing. An extensive abdominal incision is required to adequately view the internal organs. Postoperatively a large dressing and retention sutures are in place. If the child is unprepared, he may become upset and angry on viewing the surgical area.

Besides the usual preoperative observations, the nurse carefully monitors blood pressure, since hypertension from excess renin production is a possibility. This is particularly important in young children in whom improperly sized blood pressure cuffs can yield inaccurate readings (see p. 116).

Since radiotherapy and chemotherapy are usually begun immediately after surgery, parents need an explanation of what to expect. Although they should be told the major benefits and side effects from each, they should not be overwhelmed with negative information. For example, scoliosis and retarded height are common long-term effects from irradiation, but their present importance is minor compared with the favorable prognostic statistics associated with such treatment. Ideally the nurse should be present during physician-parent conferences in order to place such information into proper perspective.

Parents should be aware of the usual side effects from the chemotherapeutic agents, such as nausea and vomiting, hair loss, peripheral neuropathy, and so on, to differentiate these expected reactions from surgical complications. It is usually better to reserve telling the child about these side effects until after surgery. Alopecia, usually of most concern to older children, does not occur until 2 weeks after the initial treatment regimen. Therefore, the child can be prepared for the hair loss a few days postoperatively.

Postoperative care. Despite the extensive surgical intervention necessary in many children with Wilms' tumor, the recovery period is usually rapid. The major nursing responsibilities are those following any abdominal surgery (see the boxed material on p. 1282). Since these children are at risk for intestinal obstruction from vincristine-induced adynamic ileus, radiation-induced edema, and postsurgical adhesion formation, the nurse carefully monitors gastrointestinal activity, such as bowel movements, bowel sounds, distention, vomiting, and pain.

The nurse also monitors a fall in blood pressure after removal of the tumor, urinary output to assess functioning of the remaining kidney, and signs of infection, especially during chemotherapy. Because of the myelosuppression from the drugs, the nurse institutes pulmonary hygiene measures in the immediate postoperative period to prevent lung involvement.

The postoperative period is frequently difficult for parents. The shock of seeing their child immediately after surgery may be the first realization of the seriousness of the diagnosis. It also marks the confirmation of the stage of the tumor. Again, during this period, the nurse should be with parents to assure them of the child's recovery after surgery and to assess the parents' understanding of the operative report. One mother who had been told by the pediatric hematologist that the child probably had Wilms' tumor realized only after the surgeon spoke to her that the tumor was cancer. The two physicians who had examined her child had broached the subject so differently that the mother was not aware of the actual diagnosis until the surgeon straightforwardly told her that he had found localized cancer. As a result the mother began to doubt the competency of both physicians. If the nurse had assessed the parent's understanding prior to surgery, this could have been avoided.

Older children need an opportunity to deal with their feelings concerning the many procedures that have been done to them in rapid succession. Play therapy with dolls, puppets, or drawing can be extremely beneficial in helping them adjust to the surgery and hair loss. It is not unusual for children to feel betrayed because they were not adequately prepared for the extent of surgery, the need for additional therapy, or the seriousness of the disorder.

One child who had been told very little about the proposed surgery became withdrawn, noncommunicative, and depressed after surgery. She refused to look at her stitches or talk about the operation. During a play session with the child, the nurse placed a dressing on a doll and stated, "Her operation is closed with a red, white, and blue zipper [referring to the large retention sutures]." The child reported, "No, they're green." She subsequently disclosed that one day she had peeked inside the dressing and once she had seen "those metal things" (retention sutures) she told herself that they were so ugly that she would never look again. Through continued doll play the child was gradually able to express her angry feelings and look at her incision. Instead of dreading its ugly appearance, she began to focus on signs of healing with eventual acceptance of the change in body image. For this child the permanent scar was more important in terms of self-image than hair loss.

Discharge planning. The overall objective in discharge planning is returning the child to his normal preoperative life-style. The nurse emphasizes the usual needs for discipline, moderate protection from infection, and so on. Treatment schedules are planned to allow uninterrupted school attendance.

Because the length of therapy is relatively short (15 months), these families seem to adjust to the inconvenience imposed by treatment quite well. They may, however, experience feelings of ambivalence and insecurity when the therapy is ended. Some parents remark that they fear the child's having a cold because of the knowledge of potential lung metastasis. The nurse who has been working on a long-term basis with the family needs to understand such feelings and reemphasize their normalcy. Fortunately with such favorable survival rates even with metastasis the nurse can offer families much hope and reassurance throughout the disease.

RHABDOMYOSARCOMA

Soft-tissue sarcomas are those malignant neoplasms that originate from undifferentiated mesenchymal cells in muscle, tendons, bursae, and fascia or fibrous, connective, lymphatic, or vascular tissue. They derive their name from the specific tissue(s) of origin, such as myosarcoma (*myo*—muscle). Rhabdomyosarcoma (*rhabdo*—striated) is the most common soft-tissue sarcoma in children. Because striated (skeletal) muscle is found almost anywhere in the body, these tumors occur in many sites, the most common of which are the head and neck, especially the orbit.

Rhabdomyosarcoma occurs in children in all age-groups but most commonly in children between 2 and 6 years of age or younger than 1 year of age. Its early appearance suggests an origin during prenatal life. It occurs fairly equally in both sexes, with the exception of sarcoma botryoides (*botryoid*—grapelike) of the vagina.

Classification and prognosis

Rhabdomyosarcoma has not been staged like many other tumors but is divided into four categories—embryonal, alveolar, pleomorphic, and mixed—according to cell type.

Embryonal rhabdomyosarcoma. This is the most common type in children (50% to 96%) and is most frequently found in the head, neck, abdomen, and genitourinary tract. *Sarcoma botryoids,* which appears as multiple grapelike clusters or polyps, is usually found in cavities, such as the vagina, urinary bladder, larynx, ear, biliary tree, and nasopharynx. It is associated with the best prognosis. Other types of embryonal rhabdomyosarcoma have varying survival statistics.

Alveolar rhabdomyosarcoma. This is the second most frequent type found in children and is most often seen in the extremities. It has the poorest prognosis because it is usually more extensive at the time of diagnosis and tends to metastasize earlier than the embryonic type.

Pleomorphic rhabdomyosarcoma. This type of tumor is rare in children. It has a tendency toward hemorrhage and is associated with a poor survival rate.

Mixed rhabdomyosarcoma. As the term implies, this type is a variety of any of the preceding types.

In general, prognosis for these children is guarded. The most favorable survival statistics are attributable to: (1) early age at diagnosis, specifically under 7 years of age; (2) localized disease; (3) histologic type, especially sarcoma botryoides or embryonal type; and (4) site of tumor, especially orbital. Cure is most likely when the child has remained free of disease for 2 years after diagnosis. The majority of recurrences (about 90%) occur by the end of the second year, although late local recurrence or metastasis is possible. The most common sites of metastasis are the lungs, lymph nodes, bone, bone marrow, liver, brain, and breast.

Clinical manifestations

The initial signs and symptoms are related to the site of the tumor and compression of adjacent organs (Table 28-6). Some tumor locations, particularly the orbit, produce symptoms early in the course of the illness and contribute to rapid diagnosis and improved prognosis. Other tumors, such as those of the retroperitoneal area, produce no symptoms until they are large, invasive, and widely metastasized. In some instances a primary tumor site is never identified.

Diagnostic evaluation

Unfortunately many of the signs and symptoms attributable to rhabdomyosarcoma are vague and frequently suggest a common childhood illness, such as "earache" or "runny nose." However, diagnosis begins with a careful examination of the head and neck area, particularly palpation of a nontender, firm hard mass. The nasopharynx

Table 28-6. Clinical manifestations of rhabdomyosarcoma according to tumor site

Location	Signs and symptoms
Orbit	Rapidly developing unilateral proptosis Ecchymosis of conjunctiva Loss of extraocular movements (strabismus)
Nasopharynx	Stuffy nose (earliest sign) Nasal obstruction—dysphagia, nasal voice (obstruction of posterior nasal chonchae), serous otitis media (obstruction of eustachian tube) Pain (sore throat and ear) Epistaxis Palpable neck nodes Visible mass in oropharynx (late sign)
Paranasal sinuses	Nasal obstruction Local pain Discharge Sinusitis Swelling
Middle ear	Signs of chronic serous otitis media Pain Sanguinopurulent drainage Facial nerve palsy
Retroperitoneal area (usually a "silent" tumor)	Abdominal mass Pain Signs of intestinal or genitourinary obstruction
Perineum	Visible superficial mass Bowel or bladder dysfunction (from tumor compression)

and oropharynx are inspected for any evidence of a visible mass. Several techniques, such as mirror nasopharyngoscopy, anterior rhinoscopy, or fiberoptic transnasal nasopharyngoscopy, are available for indirect examination.

Radiographic studies to isolate a tumor site are performed, accompanied by chest x-ray examinations, lung tomograms, bone surveys, and bone marrow aspiration to rule out metastasis. Any number of tests may be indicated to differentiate this tumor from others, such as Wilms' tumor or metastatic neuroblastoma. Whenever possible, an excisional biopsy is done to confirm histologic type.

Medical/surgical management

Since this tumor is highly malignant, with metastasis occurring in more than one third of the patients at time of diagnosis, aggressive multimodal therapy is recomended.

Surgery. Radical surgical removal of tumors in accessible anatomic sites is the treatment of choice. This may involve enucleation of the affected eye for orbital tumors or amputation of a limb for tumors on an extremity.

Radiotherapy. Embryonal rhabdomyosarcomas, and to a lesser extent, the alveolar type, are extremely radiosensitive. Irradiation is sometimes used preoperatively to reduce the size of the tumor for more accessible surgical extirpation, after removal to prevent metastasis, or in place of surgery with or without chemotherapy.

Chemotherapy. Several drugs including actinomycin D, methotrexate, vincristine, cyclophosphamide, and daunorubicin, have demonstrated antitumor activity for rhabdomyosarcoma. At the present time various combined drug regimens are under investigation in the hope of improving long-term survival rates.

Nursing considerations

The specific nursing responsibility, aside from general considerations in terms of any potentially fatal cancer, is related to tumor site. Radical surgery may involve removal of an eye or limb or disfiguring surgery, such as radical neck dissection. Children, even young ones, must be prepared for this potential loss prior to surgery. Helping the child adjust to an amputation is discussed on p. 1049 and in Chapter 40.

RETINOBLASTOMA

Retinoblastoma is a congenital malignant tumor arising from the retina. It is a relatively rare tumor in the United States, occurring in 1 per 14,000 to 34,000 live births. The incidence is increasing, probably as a result of increased exposure to radiation sources and improved survival among affected children, who in future matings will increase the number of abnormal genes in the gene pool.

Retinoblastoma may be present at birth or may arise in the retina during the first 2 years of life. The average age of the child at the time of diagnosis is 17 months; it is usually diagnosed earlier in hereditary cases and later in nonhereditary types. Twenty-five per cent to 30% of all retinoblastomas are bilateral and almost always represent independent tumor origins in each eye, rather than extension of the tumor from one eye to the other.

Heredity

Retinoblastoma may be caused by (1) a somatic mutation, (2) a germinal mutation, or (3) a chromosomal aberration. *Somatic mutations* (those occurring in the general body cells, as opposed to the germ cells or gametes) are nonhereditary and account for 55% to 65% of all retinoblastomas. They are always unilateral, but not all unilateral retinoblastomas are nonhereditary. In fact, about 10% to 15% of all unilateral cases are caused by germinal mutations.

Germinal mutations take place in the gametes or parent cells and consequently are passed to future generations. One third of the resulting retinoblastomas are unilateral, and the remaining two thirds are bilateral. Hereditary retinoblastomas are transmitted as an *autosomal-dominant trait*. The penetrance of the gene is from 75% to 95%. Con-

Table 28-7. Empiric risks of recurrence in families without a history of retinoblastoma

Type of tumor in proband	Risk to subsequent sibling	Risk to offspring
Unilateral	3%*	7%-10%
Bilateral	10%	50%

From Sutow, W. W., Vietti, T. J., and Fernbach, D. J.: Clinical pediatric oncology, St. Louis, 1977, The C. V. Mosby Co.
*Some sources report the risk to be as low as 1% for subsequent siblings with a 5% chance that an affected child will be born somewhere in the ensuing family line. (From Ellsworth, R. M.: retinoblastoma. In Duane, T., editor: Clinical ophthalmology, vol. 3, New York, 1976, Harper & Row, Publishers.)

sequently about 5% to 25% of gene carriers remain unaffected.

Retinoblastoma has also been associated with *partial deletion* of the long arm of a group D chromosome (number 13) and chromosomal polyploidy (excess numbers of chromosomes), such as trisomy 21. In children who have chromosomal aberrations and retinoblastoma, there is often an increased incidence of mental retardation and congenital malformations. The vast majority of children with retinoblastomas apparently have normal chromosomes, but it is possible that they have a slight aberration that at the present time is undetectable by current chromosomal analysis. However, possibly in the future advances in genetic testing will allow for screening of such individuals.

Affected children with bilateral retinoblastoma or a positive family history of the disorder have nearly a 50% chance of passing the disease to their offspring, provided the mate has normal genes. Affected offspring have a 70% chance of developing bilateral tumors. In addition all patients with the hereditary form of the disease demonstrate an increased risk of developing a secondary carcinoma, especially osteogenic sarcoma, particularly if they received irradiation as part of the treatment protocol.

Children with unilateral retinoblastomas have much less chance of transmitting the disease to their offspring. Unilateral retinoblastomas caused by somatic mutations cannot be transmitted; however, those that are a result of germinal mutations can. Unfortunately at the present time there is no way of detecting gene carriers. Empiric risks for subsequent siblings and offpsring of affected children in families without a history of the disorder are listed in Table 28-7. It is recommended that all subsequent offspring of unaffected parents and survivors undergo regular periodic indirect ophthalmoscopy under anesthesia to detect retinoblastoma at its earliest stage.

Staging and prognosis

Staging of retinoblastomas has been done to allow for more direct comparison of treatment results. The classification refers entirely to the prognosis for survival of the eye under treatment with preservation of useful vision, not to prognosis for life in general. Staging is done under indirect ophthalmoscopy before surgery to accurately determine tumor size (measured in disc diameters—DD) and location (according to an imaginary line called the equator drawn on the midplane of the eye) (Fig. 28-5). The following classification is currently used:

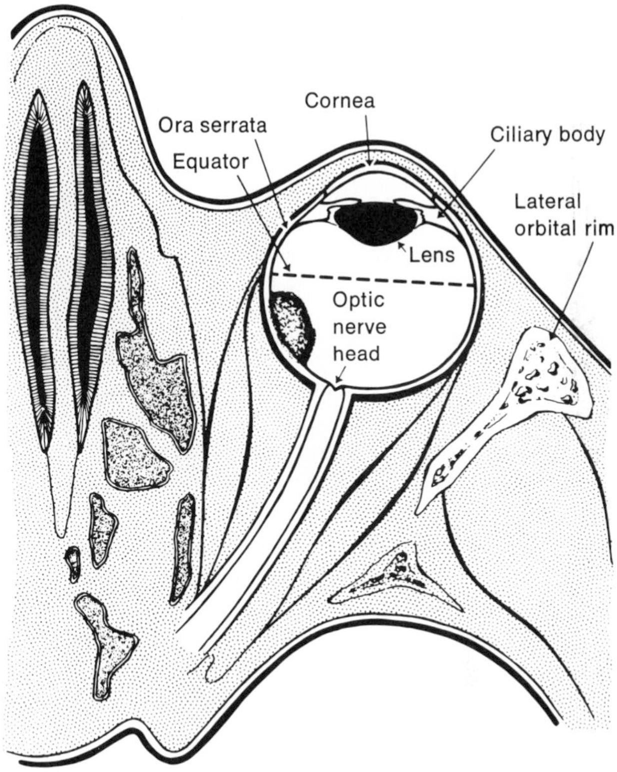

Fig. 28-5. Horizontal section through an eye that contains a single tumor. The equator, the midplane of the eye, is used as a reference line in staging the extent of disease for prognosis. (From Sutow, W. W., Vietti, T. J., and Fernbach, D. J., editors: Clinical pediatric oncology, ed. 2, St. Louis, 1977, The C. V. Mosby Co., p. 665.)

Group I
(very favorable)
1. Solitary tumor, less than 4 DD in size, at or behind equator
2. Multiple tumors, none over 4 DD in size, all at or behind equator

Group II
(favorable)
1. Solitary tumor, 4 to 10 DD in size, at or behind the equator
2. Multiple tumors, 4 to 10 DD in size, behind equator

Group III
(doubtful)
1. Any lesion anterior to equator
2. Solitary tumors larger than 10 DD in size, behind equator

Group IV
(unfavorable)
1. Multiple tumors, some larger than 10 DD in size
2. Any lesion extending anteriorly to the ora serrata

Group V
(very unfavorable)
1. Massive tumors involving over half the retina
2. Vitreous seeding

The overall prognosis for retinoblastoma is very favorable, with a mortality rate of approximately 18%. The highest rate of cures occurs in groups I and II. Unfortunately the largest numbers of patients are diagnosed when the disease has progressed to stage V, but even these children demonstrate good survival rates. Mortality is most often caused by intracranial spread and/or distant metastasis. Because of the location of the tumor, growth along the optic nerve through the lamina cribrosa can cause dissemination of tumor cells to the cerebrospinal fluid and seeding along the meninges, base of the brain, and the ventricles.

Tumor cells may invade the blood vessels, especially after metastasis to the choroid, the highly vascular middle coat of the eyeball. Once the tumor has extended outside the globe or eyeball into the orbit (bony socket encasing the globe), spread by way of the lymphatic glands can also occur. Common distant metastatic sites include the bone marrow, skeleton, lymph nodes, and liver. Unlike other childhood tumors, the lungs are rarely involved.

Clinical manifestations

Retinoblastoma has few grossly obvious signs. Typically it is the parent who first observes a whitish "glow" in the pupil. The white reflex known as the *cat's eye reflex* represents visualization of the tumor as the light momentarily falls on the mass (Fig. 28-6). When a tumor arises in the macular region, it will present a white reflex in the pupil when the tumor is still quite small. It is seen when the child looks straight ahead at the observer. When the tumor arises in the periphery of the retina, it must grow quite large before the reflex is obvious. It is usually seen only when the child looks in certain directions or if the observer stands at an oblique angle to the child's face. The fleeting nature of the reflex often leads to a delayed diagnosis because health professionals fail to appreciate the ominous significance of the parents' findings.

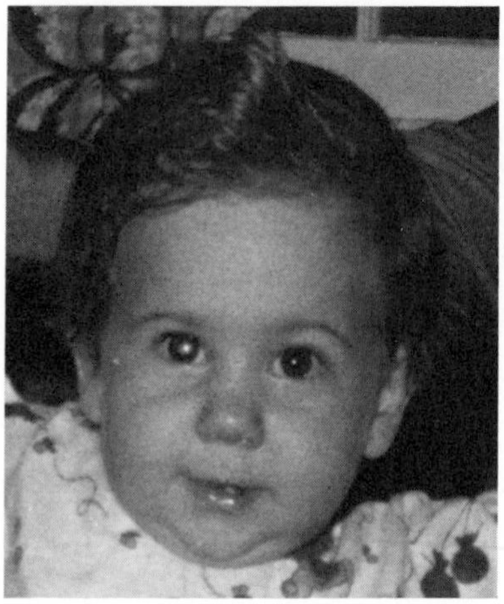

Fig. 28-6. Cat's eye reflex. Whitish appearance of lens is produced as light falls on tumor mass in right eye.

The next most common sign is strabismus resulting from poor fixation of the visually impaired eye, particularly if the tumor develops in the macula, the area of sharpest visual acuity. Blindness is usually a late sign, but it frequently is not obvious unless the parent consciously observes for behaviors indicative of loss of sight, such as bumping into objects, slowed motor development, or turning of the head to see objects lateral to the affected eye.

Another common presenting sign is a red, painful eye, often accompanied with glaucoma. Other uncommon clinical manifestations include orbital cellulitis, unilateral mydriasis, a change in the color of the iris, hyphema, white spots on the iris, nystagmus, and complaints indicative of systemic metastasis, such as weight loss, poor appetite, or fatigue.

Diagnostic evaluation

The first step in diagnosis is carefully listening to and recognizing the significance of reports from family members regarding suspected abnormalities within the eye. Since the cat's eye reflex is a momentary sign visualized only under specific conditions, the physician or nurse must attempt to duplicate those conditions necessary to observe the tumor. Children suspected of having this disorder are referred to an ophthalmologist. Definitive diagnosis is usually based on indirect ophthalmoscopy employing scleral indentation, which is done under general anesthesia with maximum dilatation of the pupils.

Two features are almost pathognomonic of retinoblastoma. The first is *calcification* of the surface of the tumor, which is sharply demarcated and glistening white and resembles "cottage cheese." This finding seen through the ophthalmoscope can be verified in the majority of cases by an x-ray examination. The second finding is *vitreous seeding,* peripheral portions that break away from the tumor mass and float freely in the vitreous. They are considered a poor prognostic sign because they remain viable for a long period of time, may establish reimplantation growths in the retina, and are not affected by chemotherapeutic agents which penetrate the vitreous poorly.

A potentially useful test is catecholamine excretion by measuring vanillylmandelic or homovanillic acid in the urine. These substances are excreted by some retinoblastomas as well as by neuroblastomas. Increased carcinoembryonic antigen levels have been found in some children with retinoblastoma and in family members who had neither the disease nor a history of the disorder. Testing carcinoembryonic antigen levels may prove to be a useful method of locating individuals with inherited premalignant disease.[10] However, this is of limited use in very young children because of normally high levels of the antigen. Other tests that may be done to confirm the diagnosis in unusual circumstances include transillumination of the retina, fluorescein angiography, ^{32}P (radiophosphate) uptake, or ultrasonography. If distant metastasis is suspected, a bone marrow aspiration, bone survey, and lumbar puncture may be done.

Medical/surgical management

Treatment of retinoblastoma depends chiefly on the stage of the tumor at diagnosis. In general, unilateral retinoblastomas in stages I, II, and III are treated with irradiation. The aim of radiotherapy is to preserve useful vision in the affected eye and eradicate the tumor. A megavoltage photon beam that supplies maximum irradiation with minimal scatter effect is employed, since the dose delivered to the lens is minimal, thus decreasing the danger of subsequent cataract formation. During this procedure it is imperative that the child lie perfectly still. For infants and young children, this often necessitates heavy sedation and a special cast to hold the head in perfect alignment (Fig. 28-7). Other approaches toward treating small localized tumors involve (1) cobalt plaque applicators (surgical implantation of a cobalt 60 applicator on the sclera until the maximum radiation dose has been delivered to the tumor), (2) light coagulation (use of a laser beam to destroy retinal blood vessels that supply nutrition to the tumor), and (3) cryotherapy (freezing of the tumor, which destroys the microcirculation to the tumor and the cells themselves through microcrystal formation).

With advanced tumor growth, especially optic nerve involvement, enucleation of the affected eye is the treatment of choice. Chemotherapy, particularly the use of vincristine and cyclophosphamide, has been beneficial in treating or preventing distant metastasis. When confirmed clinical metastastic disease is present, chemotherapy can provide palliation (not cure) for a period of 1 to 2 years.

With bilateral disease, every attempt is made to preserve useful vision in the least affected eye with enucleation of the severely diseased eye. Irradiation of the preserved eye, sometimes combined with chemotherapy, is used to eradicate the tumor and prevent metastatic spread.

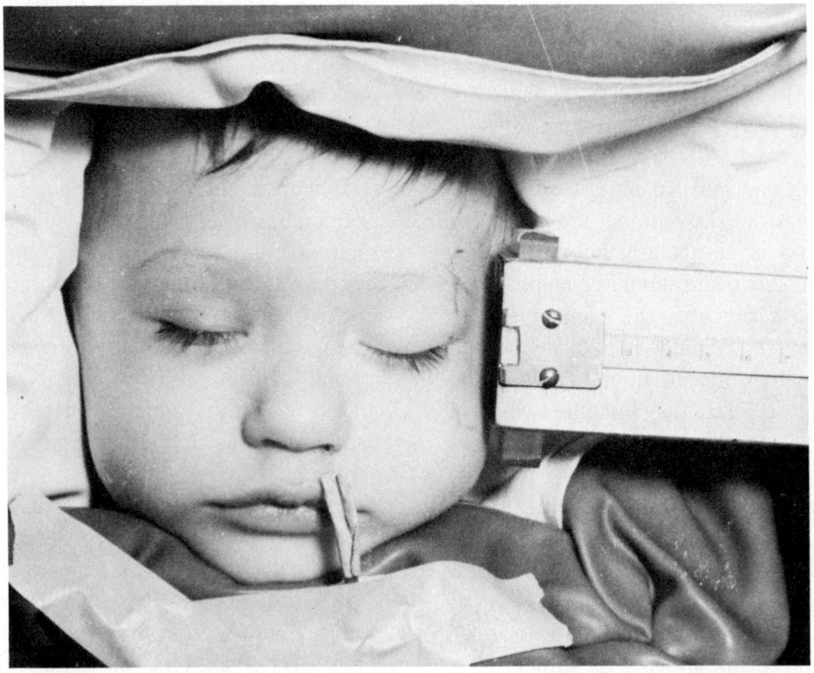

Fig. 28-7. Patient has been sedated and is asleep. He is firmly swaddled and his head is held in treatment position by a Flexicast (Picker X-Ray Corp., White Plains, N.Y.). A Thermistor wire is placed at the child's nostril to monitor breathing during treatment, since swaddling and restraining coverings make it difficult to observe respiratory movements. (From Sutow, W. W., Vietti, T. J., and Fernbach, D. J., editors: Clinical pediatric oncology, ed. 2, St. Louis, 1977, The C. V. Mosby Co., p. 673.)

Nursing considerations

The care of the child with retinoblastoma involves much attention to individual aspects of diagnosis, possible hereditary factors, and treatment protocols. Families with a history of the disorder may feel great guilt for transmitting the defect to their offspring. However, when the defect is suspected, early treatment results in such favorable outcomes that parental adjustment may be rapid. In families with no history of retinoblastoma, the discovery of the diagnosis is a shock, frequently complicated by guilt for not having found it sooner. Since parents frequently are the first to observe the cat's eye reflex, they may feel angry at themselves or others, especially physicians, for delaying a more thorough examination. The nurse assesses each of these variables in planning care based on understanding the parents' emotional reactions and adjustment.

Since the tumor is usually diagnosed in infants or very young children, most of the preparation for diagnostic tests and treatment involves parents. After indirect ophthalmoscopy, the child may not see very clearly or his eyes may be sensitive to light because of pupillary dilatation. Parents are made aware of these normal reactions prior to the procedure. They also are informed that a battery of screening tests, such as bone surveys, bone marrow aspiration, and so on, may be performed to detect metastasis.

Once the disease is staged, the physician confers with the parents regarding treatment. Unless the diagnosis is made very early, an enucleation is performed. Parents are told about the procedure as well as about the positive benefits of a prosthesis. Showing them pictures of another child with an artificial eye may be very helpful in their adjusting to the thought of disfigurement. Although the idea of blindness is a very distressing one, most parents seem to realize that there is no alternative. The fact that the unaffected eye retains normal vision is particularly helpful in their accepting the imposed handicap and should be emphasized.

After surgery the nurse prepares the parents for the child's facial appearance. An eye patch is in place, and the child's face may be edematous or ecchymotic. Parents often fear seeing the surgical site because they imagine a cavity in the skull. On the contrary, the lids are usually closed and the area does not appear sunken because a surgically implanted sphere maintains the shape of the eyeball. The implant is covered with conjunctiva, and when the lids are open the exposed area resembles the mucosal lining of the mouth. Once the child is fitted for a prosthesis, usually within 3 weeks, the facial appearance returns to normal. Parents are taught the care of the prosthesis, namely techniques for removal, insertion, and cleansing.

A long-term consideration is the survior's ability to transmit the defective gene to his offspring. Parents are encouraged to seek genetic counseling after the diagnosis in terms of subsequent childbearing and to continue counseling when the child reaches puberty. With improving prognosis for these children, the necessity of genetic counseling to prevent transmission of the disease will assume greater proportions.

BONE TUMORS

Malignant bone tumors represent less than 1% of all malignant neoplasms but are more frequent in children than adults. The peak ages during childhood are 15 to 19 years. The sexes are affected equally until puberty, at which time the ratio approaches 2:1 in favor of males. This propensity for males with a peak incidence during adolescence is thought to be because of the accelerated growth rate of osseous tissue.

Neoplastic disease can arise from any tissues involved in bone growth, such as osteoid matrix, bone marrow elements, fat, blood and lymph vessels, nerve sheath, and cartilage. The basic classifications are spindle-cell sarcoma (osteogenic sarcoma) and small-cell sarcoma (Ewing's sarcoma). In children these two types account for 85% of all primary malignant bone tumors.

Clinical manifestations

Most malignant bone tumors produce localized pain in the affected site, which may be severe or dull and in most cases is attributable to trauma or the vague complaint of "growing pains." It is often relieved by a flexed position, which relaxes the muscles overlying the stretched periosteum. Frequently it draws attention when the child limps, curtails his own physical activity, or is unable to hold heavy objects.

Diagnostic evaluation

Diagnosis begins with a thorough history and physical examination. A primary objective is to rule out causes such as trauma or infection. Careful questioning regarding pain is essential in attempting to determine the duration and rate of tumor growth. Physical assessment focuses on functional status of the affected area, signs of inflammation, size of the mass, involvement of regional lymph nodes, and any systemic indication of generalized malignancy, such as anemia, weight loss, frequent infection, and so on.

Definitive diagnosis is based on radiologic studies, particularly tomography, to determine the extent of the lesion, radioisotope bone scans to evaluate metastasis, and bone biopsy. Bone marrow aspiration is helpful in diagnosing Ewing's sarcoma. Radiologic findings are characteristic for each type of tumor. In osteogenic sarcoma needlelike new bone formation growing at right angles to the diaphysis produces a "sun burst" appearance. In Ewing's sarcoma the deposits of new bone in layers under the periosteum produce an "onionskin" appearance. In both types soft-tissue infiltration may be apparent.

At the present time there is no reliable biochemical test

for bone cancers. Elevated alkaline phosphatase levels may occur in osteoid tumors. Several tests may be done for differential diagnosis in terms of secondary bone metastasis from Wilms' tumor, neuroblastoma, retinoblastoma, rhabdomyosarcoma, lymphoma, or leukemia. Lung tomography is usually a standard procedure, since pulmonary metastasis is the most common complication of primary bone tumors.

Treatment and prognosis

A better understanding of the biology of neoplastic growth has resulted in more aggressive treatment and improved prognosis. The natural history of osteogenic sarcoma and Ewing's sarcoma suggests that multiple submicroscopic foci of metastatic disease are present at the time of diagnosis despite clinical evidence of localized involvement. Prior to the use of aggressive multimodal therapy, pulmonary metastasis invariably appeared in 6 to 9 months in patients with osteogenic sarcoma who were treated with surgical excision of the tumor. Now, with radical surgery for osteosarcoma or intensive radiotherapy for Ewing's sarcoma combined with chemotherapy, survival statistics are improving for both types of bone cancer.

Generally the survival statistics for Ewing's sarcoma are more favorable than for osteogenic sarcoma. Children with nonmetastastic Ewing's sarcoma at the time of diagnosis who are given intensive radiotherapy and chemotherapy have an 80% chance of cure. Those with osteosarcoma arising from the small bones of the hands and feet, where radical amputation is most easily accomplished, have a better than 50% chance of 5-year survival.[14] However, tumors closer to the trunk carry poorer prognoses, especially if metastasis occurs.

Osteogenic sarcoma

Osteogenic sarcoma (osteosarcoma) is the most frequently encountered malignant bone cancer in children. Its peak incidence is between 10 and 25 years of age. It presumably arises from bone-forming mesenchyme, which gives rise to malignant osteoid tissue. Most primary tumor sites are in the diaphysis (shaft) of long bones, especially in the lower extremities. Over half occur in the femur, particularly the distal portion, with the rest involving the humerus, tibia, pelvis, jaw, and phalanges.

Medical/surgical treatment. Aggressive treatment involves radical surgical ablation followed by intensive chemotherapy. Depending on the tumor site, surgery includes amputation of the affected extremity at least 7.5 cm (3 inches) above the proximal tumor margin or above the joint proximal to the involved bone. With tumors of the distal femur, preservation of the hip joint may be possible. Other procedures include an above-the-knee amputation for tumors of the tibia or fibula, a hemipelvectomy for tumors of the innominate (hip) bone, and a forequarter amputation (removal of arm, scapula, and portion of the clavicle on the affected side) for tumors of the upper humerus.

After surgery chemotherapy with high-dose methotrexate followed by citrovorum factor (citrovorum "rescue") is advocated. Other drugs commonly administered in combination with methotrexate include vincristine, adriamycin, cyclophosphamide, and derivatives of nitrogen mustard. Although the period of treatment varies according to institutions, many centers advocate adjuvant chemotherapy for 2 years in nonmetastatic osteogenic sarcoma and for 3 years when metastasis is present.

Another approach to treatment is the preoperative use of intensive chemotherapy followed by an en bloc resection of the primary tumor with prosthetic replacement of the involved bone. For example, with osteosarcoma of the distal femur, a total femur and joint replacement is done. After surgery adjuvant chemotherapy is continued for approximately 1 year. At present, long-term survival rates to determine limb function and disease-free status are still incomplete.

Nursing considerations. The main nursing consideration is preparation of the child and family for an amputation. Straightforward honesty is essential in gaining the cooperation and trust of the child. The diagnosis of cancer should not be disguised with falsehoods such as "infection." For the child to gradually accept the need for an amputation, he must be aware of the lack of alternatives to treatment. Conservative surgery offers virtually no hope for a cure. He should also know if the operation will immediately follow the biopsy procedure. Informing him that only a biopsy will be done in the hope of sparing him anxiety over the operation only weakens his trust once he is aware of the deception.

Most often the responsibility of telling the child about the surgery is left to the physician. Ideally the nurse should be present at the discussion or be aware of exactly what is said to the child. The child should be told a few days before surgery to allow him time to think about the diagnosis and consequent treatment and to ask questions.

Sometimes children have many questions about the prosthesis, limitations on physical ability, and prognosis in terms of cure. At other times they react with silence or with a calm disposition that belies their concern and fear. Either response must be accepted, because it is part of the grieving process of a loss. For those who wish information, it may be helpful to introduce them to another amputee prior to surgery or to show them pictures of the prosthesis. However, the nurse must be careful not to overwhelm them with information. A sound approach is to answer their questions without offering additional information. For those who do not pursue additional information, the nurse expresses a willingness to talk, with such expressions as, "Anytime you would like to talk or ask questions about the surgery, tell me." The nurse should not push the topic unless the child initiates the conversation. Silence does not always mean nonacceptance.

The child is also informed of the need for chemotherapy. Although it is well to introduce this subject prior to surgery, since treatment begins as soon as possible postoperatively, caution must be exercised in offering too much information at one time. It is well to discuss hair loss with emphasis on positive aspects, such as wearing a wig. Since bone tumors affect adolescents and young adults, it is not unusual for them to become angry over all the radical body alterations. One child remarked, "By the time you are done with me I will be more false than real." Sensing a feeling of powerlessness, the nurse encouraged the child to discuss his thoughts about surgery and chemotherapy, focusing on what alternatives there were available to him. The child finally stated, "I know there is no other way, but I don't have to like it." The nurse agreed, supporting the child's legitimate right to such feelings.

In most instances the child is fitted with a temporary prosthesis immediately after surgery. For a leg amputation the prosthesis consists of a rigid dressing pylon and a foot-ankle assembly, which permits early ambulation and fosters psychologic adjustment to a lost limb. A permanent prosthesis is usually fitted within 6 to 8 weeks. During hospitalization the child begins physical therapy to become proficient in the use and care of the device.

Discharge planning must begin early during the postoperative period. Once the child has begun physical therapy, the nurse consults with the therapist and physician to evaluate the child's physical and emotional readiness to reenter school. It is an opportune time to involve a community nurse in the home care of the child. Every effort is made to promote normalcy and gradual resumption of realistic preamputation activities. Environmental handicaps, such as stairs, are assessed in terms of the accessibility of the school and/or home, especially since the child may need to use crutches or a wheelchair before complete healing and prosthetic competency are achieved.

If the child needs to remain at home for any length of time, a tutor is arranged. Parents should encourage friends to visit to prepare the child for the reactions and questions of others. The longer the child remains absent from his peers, the more estranged he may feel. Role playing in anticipation of such experiences is very beneficial in preparing the child for the inevitable confrontation by others.

The nurse encourages the child to select clothing that best camouflages the prosthesis, such as pants or long-sleeved shirts. Well-fitted prostheses are so natural looking that girls can usually wear sheer stocking without revealing the device. Emphasizing feminine or masculine apparel helps the child regain his feeling of self-identity. Even during the postoperative period, encouraging the child to wear blue jeans and a shirt may distract his attention from the deformity and focus it on familiar aspects of personal appearance.

One note of caution concerning the adjustment phase is realizing the child's need for time in accepting the diagnosis and surgery. Loss of a limb constitutes a grieving process. Before the child can realistically accept the altered body image, he must go through the usual reactions of anger, depression, intellectualization, and so on. Health professionals who are aware of the normalcy of such stages can help parents understand the child's emotional reactions. Often parents view the anger as a direct affront to them for allowing the amputation to occur, or they see the depression as rejection. On the contrary these are not interpersonal attacks but self-attempts to cope with a loss.

Ewing's sarcoma

Ewing's sarcoma arises in the marrow spaces of the bone rather than from osseous tissue. The tumor originates in the shaft of long and trunk bones, most often affecting the femur, tibia, fibula, humerus, ulna, vertebra, scapula, ribs, pelvic bones, and skull. It occurs almost exclusively in individuals under age 30 years, with the majority between 4 and 25 years of age.

Medical treatment. Surgical tumor excision and/or amputation have not demonstrated improved survival rates. The treatment of choice is intensive irradiation of the involved bone, usually for a period of 6 to 8 weeks, combined with chemotherapy for a period of 2 years. A widely used drug regimen includes vincristine, actinomycin D, and cyclophosphamide (often referred to as VAC).

Investigational approaches toward treatment include total-body irradiation to destroy widespread foci of disease and immunotherapy to control and/or metastasis. However, at the present time these techniques represent ancillary, not primary, modes of therapy.

Nursing considerations. The psychologic adjustment to Ewing's sarcoma is typically less traumatic than to osteogenic sarcoma because of the preservation of the affected limb. Many families accept the diagnosis with a sense of relief in knowing that this type of bone cancer does not necessitate amputation. However, they still need preparation for the various diagnostic tests, including bone marrow aspiration and surgical biopsy, and adequate explanation of the treatment regimen. High-dose radiotherapy often causes a skin reaction of dry or moist desquamation followed by hyperpigmentation. The nurse advises the child to wear loose-fitting clothes over the irradiated area to decrease additional skin irritation. Because of increased sensitivity, the area is protected from sunlight and sudden changes in temperature, such as from heating pads or ice packs. The child is encouraged to use the extremity as tolerated. Occasionally an active exercise program may be planned by the physical therapist to preserve maximum function.

The child needs the same considerations for adjusting to the effects of chemotherapy as any other cancer patient. The regimen consisting of vincristine, actinomycin D, and cyclophosphamide usually results in hair loss, severe nausea and vomiting, peripheral neuropathy, and possibly cardiotoxicity. Every effort should be made to outline a treatment plan that allows the child maximal resumption of a normal life-style and activities.

APLASTIC ANEMIA

Aplastic anemia refers to a condition in which all formed elements of the blood are simultaneously depressed. The peripheral blood smear demonstrates pancytopenia or the triad of profound anemia, leukopenia, and thombocytopenia. *Hypoplastic anemia* is characterized by a profound depression of erythrocytes but normal or slightly decreased white blood cells and platelets.

A type of hypoplastic anemia is pure red cell anemia, a congenital condition marked by complete or almost complete absence of all cells of the erythroid series with normal production of the other myeloid cells. Its treatment, which consists of transfusions, splenectomy, and administration of corticosteroids, is similar to that of other diseases, such as the thalassemias, that result in profound anemia. Prognosis varies, although long-term survival is possible. The principal causes of death are cardiac failure, hepatitis from transfusion therapy, and sepsis. Hemosiderosis and hemochromatosis (p. 1384) also play a role in affecting vital tissues necessary for survival.

Acquired hypoplastic anemia can result from several factors, including suppressed erythropoiesis from multiple transfusion therapy, hemolytic syndromes, such as sickle cell anemia, infections, toxic substances, drugs, and autoimmune or allergic states. The following discussion, however, focuses on aplastic anemia, which carries a much poorer prognosis and follows a more rapidly fatal course.

Causes

Aplastic anemia can be primary (congenital) or secondary (acquired). Of the congenital variety, one of the best known disorders of which aplastic anemia is an outstanding feature is *Fanconi's syndrome*. Besides pancytopenia, the condition is associated with a large number of congenital anomalies, including microcephaly; dwarfism; mental retardation; anomalies of ears, skeleton, kidney, and heart; strabismus; ptosis; nystagmus; deafness; and excess deposits of melanin in areas of the skin. The syndrome appears to be inherited as autosomal-recessive trait with varying penetrance; therefore, affected siblings may demonstrate several different combinations of defects. The treatment is the same as for other causes of aplastic anemia. Prognosis is variable but is better than for acquired types.

The most common causes of acquired aplastic anemia are (1) irradiation; (2) drugs, such as the chemotherapeutic agents and several antibiotics, one of the most notable being chloramphenicol; (3) industrial and household chemicals, including benzene and its derivatives, which are found in petroleum products, dyes, paint remover, shellac, and lacquers; (4) infections, especially hepatitis or overwhelming infection; and (5) infiltration and replacement of myeloid elements, such as in leukemia or the lymphomas. A sixth category, idiopathic, is included, because no identifiable precipitating cause can be found. Prognosis is worst for children in this group.

Clinical manifestations and diagnosis

The clinical manifestations, which include anemia, leukopenia, and decreased platelet count, are usually insidious. The onset is not unlike that seen in leukemia. Definitive confirmation is bone marrow aspiration, which demonstrates the conversion of red bone marrow to yellow, fatty bone marrow.

Treatment

The objectives of treatment are (1) to remove the causative agent whenever possible, (2) to provide supportive therapy with transfusions, and (3) to stimulate erythropoiesis. In a selected number of patients splenectomy may be beneficial if a hemolytic reaction (as in hypersplenism) can be demonstrated. A potential curative approach is bone marrow transplant when a compatible tissue donor is available.

Adrenocorticosteroid therapy. The vanguard of treatment to stimulate erythropoiesis is the use of testosterone and prednisone. Although the exact mechanism of erythropoietic action is unclear, testosterone increases production of erythroid elements, converting the fatty, hypocellular bone marrow to one of erythroid hyperplasia. Several testosterone preparations are available. Those most commonly used and their methods of administration are oxymetholone (dihydrotestosterone; oral), methyltestosterone (Metandren, Oreton-M; oral or sublingual), and testosterone enanthate (Delatestryl; intramuscular).

Corticosteroids used in combination with androgens have the following important effects: (1) an increase in capillary resistance to prevent bleeding tendencies, (2) a decrease in the rate of erythrocyte destruction, and (3) opposition of the anabolic action of testosterone, thus preventing increased bone maturation and premature closure of the epiphyses.[17]

Prognosis

Response to drug therapy is usually gradual. Elevations in hemoglobin and red blood cells may take as long as 3 to 6 months. During this period the child must be protected from infection and hemorrhage and treated for the anemia with transfusions. Unfortunately the prognosis is poor. The mortality rate is about 70% for acquired aplastic anemia. Almost 50% of these children die within 4 to 6 months after diagnosis. Prospects for improved survival lie in preventing the condition and researching better approaches to treatment, such as bone marrow transplants.

Nursing considerations

The care of the child with aplastic anemia is similar to that of the leukemic child, namely, preparing the family for the diagnostic and therapeutic procedures, preventing complications from the severe pancytopenia, and emotionally supporting them in terms of a potentially fatal outcome. Since each of these has already been discussed, only the exceptions are presented.

Explanation of therapeutic procedures. Testosterone produces several undesirable effects that, when combined with the effects of steroid therapy, such as moon face, result in dramatic body image alterations. The virilizing effects of testosterone include deepening of the voice, hirsutism, growth of pubic hair, enlargement of the penis in males, flushing of the skin, and acne. Potentially testosterone can cause muscular and skeletal maturation, resulting in severely retarded height in a young child. Not only are these changes difficult to accept, they are especially difficult to explain to children not approaching puberty. Parents may feel embarrassed because they are unprepared for the sexual changes.

The nurse can help by deemphasizing the sexual nature of the effects and matter-of-factly explaining each in the same tone as moon face, truncal obesity, and so on. Expressing embarrassment or surprise to the child at observing mature sexual characteristics must be avoided. New members of the staff who may be assigned to care for the child, such as nursing students, need to be prepared for the experience of seeing a sexually mature "6-year-old male with a slight beard and a deep masculine voice."

Since chemotherapeutic agents are not used, many of the reactions, such as nausea and vomiting, alopecia, mucosal ulceration, and so on, are encountered. However, extensive ecchymotic areas of the oral mucosa from thrombocytopenia require meticulous mouth care to prevent breakdown, bleeding, and infection. Fortunately these lesions are not painful, although their appearance may lead one to expect discomfort. Local anesthetics are not necessary, but anorexia is still a consequence because of the edematous nature of the lesions. Liquid, bland, and soft diets are usually tolerated best.

SYSTEMIC LUPUS ERYTHEMATOSUS (SLE)

Lupus erythematosus, which literally means "red wolf" because of the characteristic butterfly rash on the face of some affected individuals, is a chronic inflammatory disease of the collagen or supporting tissues of the body. It characteristically follows a course of remissions and exacerbations. Because connective tissue is found practically everywhere, almost any organ or structure can be affected.

Although it is usually classified as one of the collagen diseases, such as rheumatic fever or rheumatoid arthritis, it is included here because it is potentially a life-threatening illness. The gravest prognostic sign in lupus is renal involvement and consequent kidney failure. Although supportive approaches, such as hemodialysis and kidney transplant, have improved the outlook for these patients, tissue damage in other vital organs, especially the heart and lungs, may foreshorten the benefits derived from life-supporting techniques.

Systemic lupus erythematosus affects approximately 1 in 100,000 people. The majority of cases are diagnosed between the ages of 16 and 30 years. It is seven times more frequent in females and more common in blacks than whites. It is estimated that there 4000 to 5000 new cases each year, second only to rheumatoid arthritis among the connective tissue diseases.

Etiology

The cause of lupus erythematosus is not known. The theory generally accepted, which is based on response to steroids and immunosuppressant agents, is autoimmunity. It is believed that some inciting event such as stress, infection, extreme fatigue, or exposure to various chemicals, drugs, or excessive sunburn triggers a reaction that alters the body's immune response to its own tissues. The supporting evidence for this finding is that (1) many individuals report such events prior to onset of symptoms and (2) such events enhance an exacerbation of known lupus disease.

Technically lupus erythematosus is not an inherited disease, although it demonstrates a tendency to occur within families. In addition family members without actual disease may have findings suggestive of lupus, such as LE cells, abnormal sensitivity to sun, a history of arthritis or allergies, or unusual drug reactions. It is well-documented that some individuals develop a lupus-like reaction to drugs such as isoniazid, penicillin, tetracycline, sulfa preparations, phenothiazines, and phenytoin (Dilantin).

Classification

Lupus erythematosus is classified according to the types of tissue involved and the extensiveness of the disease. The first major classification is discoid lupus erythematosus, which describes its sharply demarcated skin lesions on the face, neck, and upper chest. When the lesions are more extensive, the term "disseminated lupus erythematosus" is used.

The other classification refers to systemic involvement with or without skin lesions. The following discussion focuses on systemic lupus erythematosus.

Clinical manifestations

Because systemic lupus erythematosus can affect almost any tissue, the clinical manifestations are variable. The onset is usually insidious, with vague signs such as low-grade fever, chills, weakness, generalized aching, and malaise. However, rapid involvement of vital organs, primarily the kidney, can herald an accelerated course with minimal or absent involvement of other sites. Although the variety and severity of symptoms vary tremendously, the following is a discussion of potential clinical manifestations.

Skin. The most typical skin involvement, although seen in only a few patients, is a type of ''butterfly rash'' over the bridge of the nose and symmetrically extending to each cheek. It is described as ''fleeting, faint to pink, pink to red, flat to slightly raised, and mild to severe.''[13] These same types of lesions can occur anywhere on the body. Sometimes they are pruritic, look like severe sunburn or hives, or may become bullous. They have a tendency to scar and are aggravated by exposure to ultraviolet rays.

Some patients experience sensitivity to cold (Raynaud's phenomenon), especially in the hands and feet. Cyanosis may be present and skin ulcers often develop if the skin is allowed to dry and crack. Patchy areas of alopecia may occur, although during remission the hair usually regrows.

Musculoskeletal system. The most common symptom is generalized weakness, usually accompanied by arthritis, myalgia, joint swelling, and stiffness. Usually the joint involvement is not severe enough to cause deformity, although it may result in temporary disability because of pain.

Central nervous system. Evidence of neurologic involvement varies from forgetfulness, excitability, and headache to seizures and frank psychosis. Idiopathic epileptic seizures may be an early sign of beginning, yet undiagnosed, systemic lupus erythematosus. Any of the cranial nerves may be affected, and paralysis from spinal cord involvement may occur.

Heart and lungs. The serous linings of the lungs and heart may become inflamed, resulting in pleurisy or pericarditis, respectively. Both complications are usually reversible with rest. However, renal involvement within a few weeks or months may follow an attack of pleurisy.

Kidneys. The glomerulus is the usual site of destruction. Presumably antigen-antibody complexes are despoted primarily in the glomerular basement membrane, initiating an inflammatory response that resulsts in tissue damage. An early sign of renal involvement is proteinuria. (For other signs and symptoms of progressive renal failure, see p. 1179).

Blood. Anemia from decreased erythrocytes is common, although the exact reason is unclear. In females amenorrhea may be secondary to the anemia. The platelets and plasma proteins may also be affected.

Lymphoid system. Sometimes the spleen and often the cervical, axillary, and inguinal lymph nodes are enlarged. A type of lupus erythematosus hepatitis may develop during the course of the disease.

Gastrointestinal tract. Nausea and vomiting, diarrhea, and abdominal pain may be present and at times may falsely suggest conditions such as appendicitis.

Diagnostic evaluation

Systems lupus erythematosus has been called the ''great imitator,'' since its clinical manifestations may point to a variety of unrelated conditions. Definitive diagnosis is essential, particularly among the other collagen diseases, because treatment and prognosis vary. History is an important part of the diagnosis, since it may reveal prelupus erythematosus signs such as chronic weakness and fatigue, unexplained anemia or seizures, a false-positive syphilis test, and so on.

Several laboratory tests are performed to confirm the diagnosis, including (1) complete blood count for evidence of anemia; (2) blood chemistry for elevated blood urea nitrogen, blood sugar, abnormal plasma proteins, and electrolyte imbalances; (3) erythrocyte sedimentation rate, a nonspecific test demonstrating evidence of inflammation; (4) serologic tests for syphilis, which may be false positive; (5) complete urinalysis, particularly for proteinuria, and occult hematuria, urine sedimentation (Addis count), and renal function tests, including urea and creatinine clearance; and (6) specific tests for the LE cell.

The test for the LE (lupus erythematosus) cell is considered most diagnostic. Although there is no circulating LE cell, it can be artificially created by adding a source of nucleoprotein to a sample of the patient's leukocytes, which contain the LE factor. The LE phenomenon, a demonstration of autoimmunity, will result in phagocytosis of the nucleoprotein by the white blood cell. Other antinuclear antibodies can be qualitatively measured by immunofluorescence (fluorescent antinuclear antibody [FANA] test).

Other tests that may be used to confirm the diagnosis and/or evaluate the degree of renal damage include skin and kidney biopsies. However, they are not the routine diagnostic procedures in a suspected case of lupus erythematosus.

A neurologic examination should be done to provide baseline data for evaluatng subtle changes in behavior and function. Sometimes a psychiatric evaluation may also be warranted, since personality alterations caused by steroids and renal damage are difficult to distinguish from those resulting from central nervous system involvement of the disease.

Medical management

The objectives of medical treatment are (1) to reverse the autoimmune and inflammatory process and (2) to prevent exacerbations and complications. Therapy involves the use of specific and supportive medications and regulation of activity and diet.

Medications. The principal drugs used to control inflammation are the corticosteroids. Another group of drugs effective in relieving the dermatologic, arthritic, and renal symptoms of the disease are antimalarial preparations, such as hydroxychloroquine (Plaquenil) and chloroquine (Aralen). Although the exact action of these drugs on lupus erythematosus is not known, often they permit a continued remission with a lowered dose of steroids.

Recently another group of drugs, the immunosuppressants, have been used with varying degrees of success. The drugs most commonly employed are cyclophosphamide, azathioprine (Imuran), and nitrogen mustard derivatives (mechlorethamine and chlorambucil [Leukeran]). Although the steroids are potent anti-inflammatory agents, they have not been successful in preventing progressive renal damage. The immunosuppressants, which interfere with the formation of antigen-antibody complexes, have been able to halt the resultant interstitial cell infiltrate in the kidneys, which ordinarily leads to tissue destruction.

Aspirin has played an important role by relieving muscle and joint pains and reducing tissue inflammation. Drugs used to control various complications include anticonvulsants, antihypertensives, and antibiotics. The selection of appropriate medication in each of these categories is essential, since many of them greatly aggravate the disease process.

Regulation of activity and diet. The goal of restricted activity is to prevent a recurrence of the disease. Although the exact relationship is unclear, fatigue, stress, or sudden exertion brings about a relapse of symptoms. An effective schedule must provide for gradual resumption of pre–lupus erythematosus activity and maximal rest periods, usually 8 to 10 hours of sleep a night and one or two rest times during the day.

Diet may be restricted depending on weight gain and/or fluid retention from steroids and renal damage. The most frequently prescribed diet modification is moderate or low salt. Low-protein diets may be necessary to prevent elevated nitrogen levels. Weight reduction may help preserve maximal joint function and conserve energy.

Nursing considerations

The principal nursing goal is to help the child and family adjust to the limitations and treatments of the disease and to prevent exacerbations and complications. Since older female adolescents are the most likely group to be affected, the nurse must have an awareness of their special needs, such as body image changes, present and future vocational activities, and social relationships. Although this is a potentially fatal disorder, the reader is encouraged to apply those principles of adjusting to a chronic illness that are discussed in Chapter 22.

Assisting family in adjusting to disease and its treatment. Systemic lupus erythematosus is a complex disease. Although much is known about its effect on connective tissues and appropriate types of treatment, few concrete facts are available. However, family members need an understanding of the disease process to gain an appreciation of the necessity of regular, uninterrupted drug administration, moderate activity, and dietary modifications. Usually diagnostic tests are performed during hospitalization, which allows the nurse an opportunity to help the child and parents learn about the disease. Several booklets are available, and local lupus erythematosus organizations* have been formed to help victims learn about and adjust to the disease. The nurse should be aware of what information the family is receiving, because learning about joint deformity, sudden bouts of pain and disability, a disfiguring rash, and the possibility of renal failure can be overwhelming. Nurses should also be aware of advertised nonmedical approaches to treatment, since quackery abounds when no known cure exists.

The nurse has the responsibility of helping the adolescent adjust to drug therapy. The side effects of steroids and immunosuppressant drugs have already been discussed under leukemia and outlined in Table 28-4. Most of the antimalarial drugs have few side effects. However, hydroxychloroquine and chloroquine can cause irreversible retinal damage; as a result frequent ophthalmic examinations are necessary. Also, after exposure to the sun, the skin may tan less and become more erythematous and the hair may lighten.

Body image changes from both the disease and drugs are a major concern. Each of these should be approached in a positive manner by discussing the use of cosmetics and wigs. Sometimes health professionals fail to adequately assess the child's adjustment reactions and regard the depression and withdrawal as effects of the disease rather than a response to body image changes.

For example, during hospitalization for a relapse, a 17-year-old adolescent became very withdrawn, a distinct change in behavior from her previous admission. Because of her rapidly deteriorating physical and renal condition, the physicians and nurses assumed the personality changes to be physiologically based. However, two nursing students who had been working with her learned that since she had lost most of her hair and had "become fat," she stayed at home more and more. They concluded that her depression could be stemming from these events. They began to talk to her about wigs, makeup, and fashionable clothes that were slenderizing. As soon as she showed interest in these topics, the students brought in makeup, a wig, and fashion magazines. Although the physician advised against using any creams on her face, the application of lipstick, eye makeup, a wig, and street clothes made a dramatic difference in her appearance. Consequently she willingly left her room to socialize with other patients and only infrequently seemed depressed, and the times of de-

*Addresses of local lupus erythematosus societies are usually listed in community telephone directories.

pression corresponded to physical symptoms, such as joint pain or weakness.

Restricted activity imposes many hardships for these children. Unlike other diseases that may require a long convalescent period with ultimate resumption of normal activity, this disease warrants lifelong activity restrictions. The adolescent may need to continue school on a part-time basis to avoid fatigue. Frequently vocational choices must be changed. The inability to keep up with peers is exceptionally difficult to accept. The nurse can help these children by realistically discussing with them what alternatives are available. Although a threatening approach is to be deplored, the nurse should place the complications of uncontrolled disease, especially renal failure, in perspective.

Many adolescents are concerned about childbearing. There is no definite answer to this question. For some people pregnancy causes a complete remission, whereas for others it may result in a relapse. In general, women with the discoid type of lupus erythematosus have few difficulties during pregnancy. Those with systemic lupus erythematosus need individual counseling by the physician. Usually, progressive kidney damage is a contraindication to pregnancy.

Whenever dietary restrictions are necessary, the nurse works with the child and parents, focusing on the family member who regularly prepares meals. Several commercial cookbooks are available for salt-restricted recipes. The booklet "Primer on L.E."* also contains recipes for low-salt food preparation. Since there are so many hidden sources of sodium, besides what is added at the table, families need a written list of restricted and allowed foods.

The nurse also takes into account "adolescent" snacks outside the home that are high in sodium, such as pizza, hamburgers, frankfurters, and most baked goods. Unfortunately there are few well-accepted "fast-food" substitutions. However, compromising by eating a hamburger without cheese, ketchup, or pickles and French fried potatoes without added salt may be acceptable. The adolescent can always disguise her real motives by stating that she is "watching her figure."

Prevention of exacerbations and complications. The list of "don'ts" for these individuals is long. The importance of adequate rest has already been stressed. The necessity of adhering to the medication schedule is paramount. Some adolescents, in an attempt to lessen the side effects of steroids, may elect to skip a few doses. The nurse emphasizes that steroids not only are essential to maintaining a remission but must be taken daily (or as prescribed) to prevent sudden withdrawal from the drug, which may precipitate a serious physiologic crisis. They are also advised to seek medical attention during periods of stress, illness, or prior to elective surgical procedures, such as dental extraction, because the body may require larger amounts of the drug. They should carry an identification card or Medic Alert tag emphasizing their dependence on steroids.

As was mentioned previously, many drugs can precipitate a flare-up of the disease and must be avoided. The patient should keep a drug record in order to identify any prescription that may be contraindicated. For example, a physician unfamiliar with the patient may prescribe penicillin by using one of its trade names and the patient may unknowingly develop a reaction. If the family frequents one pharmacist, this person should be aware of restricted drugs.

Skin care is important. In those individuals who are sensitive to the sun, exposure to it must be avoided. It is important to stress that reflected sun through clouds, on snow, on water, or on white cement can cause a severe reaction. Although clothes can protect most areas of the body, special sunscreening agents are necessary for the face. An ingredient that effectively blocks ultraviolet rays is para-aminobenzoic acid (PABA), which is available in over-the-counter creams, lotions, and lip balms. A large-brimmed hat helps in partially shading the face.

Another source of ultraviolet rays is fluorescent lighting. Such lighting is used extensively in commercial buildings, including hospitals, and in homes, especially in the bathroom and kitchen, and for desk lamps. Because it is impossible to totally avoid this type of light, the person uses the same precautions as for the sun.

If the skin is hypersensitive to cold, the person should wear gloves or warm socks to maintain body heat. To prevent ulcers, lubricant creams should be applied to any dry, cracked areas of skin. Wearing rubber gloves while doing housework may be necessary to prevent excessive skin irritation.

Sometimes patients are requested to routinely check their urine for protein by using a reagent strip that changes color when protein is present. Just as in diabetic testing, the nurse assesses the adolescent's understanding of the test. The patient immediately reports any evidence of proteinuria or of advanced renal diseases, such as fluid retention, azotemia (for example, ammonia odor on breath), irritability, and exhaustion.

Long-term care of the patient with systemic lupus erythematosus may entail hemodialysis and/or kidney transplant. Nursing considerations for each procedure are discussed in Chapter 31.

*Hasererick, J., and Kellum, R.: Primer for patients with lupus erythematosus, available from Pinehurst Dermatology, Pinehurst, N.C.

REFERENCES

1. Aur, R. J., and associates: Cessation of therapy during complete remission of childhood acute lymphocytic leukemia, N. Engl. J. Med. **291:**1230-1234, December 5, 1974.
2. Bachman, D. S., Hodges, F. J., and Freeman, J. M.: Computerized axial tomography in neurologic disorders of children, Pediatrics **59**(3):352-363, March 1977.
3. Bamford, F. N., and associates: Residual disabilities in chil-

dren treated for intracranial space-occupying lesions, Cancer **37:**1149-1151, February 1976.
4. Brown, H.: Cancer quackery: what you can do about it? Nursing '75 **5**(5):24-26, May 1975.
5. Bruya, M., and Madeira, N.: Stomatitis after chemotherapy, Am. J. Nurs. **75**(8):1349-1352, August 1975.
6. Cancer facts and figures, 1977, New York, 1976, American Cancer Society.
7. Cook, R. E., editor: The biologic basis of pediatric practice, New York, 1968, McGraw-Hill, Inc.
8. D'Angio, G. J.: Management of children with Wilms' tumor, Cancer **30:**1528-1533, 1972.
9. Falletta, J. M., Starling, K. A., and Fernbach, D. J.: Leukemia in twins, Pediatrics **52**(6):846-849, December 1973.
10. Felberg, N. T., Michelson, J. B., and Shields, J. A.: CEA family syndrome, Cancer **37:**1397-1402, March 1976.
11. Finkelstein, J. Z., and associates: Acute leukemia during the first year of life, Clin. Pediatr. **11**(4):236-240, April 1972.
12. Hanson, R. L.: Heparin-lock or keep-open I.V.? Am. J. Nurs. **76**(7):1102-1103, July 1976.
13. Haserick, J. R., and Kellum, R. E.: Primer for patients with lupus erythematosus, Southern Pines, N.C., 1973, The Pilot, Inc.
14. Jaffe, N.: Malignant bone tumors, Pediatr. Ann. **4**(2):10, February 1975.
15. Lubens, H. M., and associates: Anesthetic patch for painful procedures such as minor operations, Am. J. Dis. Child. **128:**192-194, August 1974.
16. Porvars, D.: Wilms' tumor: recent advances and unresolved problems, Pediatr. Ann. **3**(5):55-70, 1974.
17. Miller, D. R., and Pearson, H. A.: Smith's blood diseases of infancy and childhood, ed. 4, St. Louis, 1978, The C. V. Mosby Co.
18. Scott, M. D., and Crawford, J. D.: Solitary thyroid nodules in childhood: is the incidence of thyroid carcinoma declining? Pediatrics **58**(4):521-525, October 1976.
19. Sherman, M.: Feeding the sick child, DHEW Publication No. 76-795, Washington, D.C., 1976, Department of Health, Education and Welfare, National Cancer Institute.
20. Stagner, S. A., and Wood, A.: The child with cancer on immunosuppressive therapy, Nurs. Clin. North Am. **11**(1):21-34, March 1976.
21. Sutow, W. W., Vietti, T. J., Fernbach, D. J.: Clinical pediatric oncology, ed. 2, St. Louis, 1977, The C. V. Mosby Co.
22. Ziegler, J. L.: Management of Burkitt's lymphoma, Pediatr. Ann. **4**(2):60, February 1975.

BIBLIOGRAPHY

Cancer in children

Burchenal, J.: Advances in the treatment of childhood cancer 1944-1974, Pediatr. Ann. **3**(4):9-12, 1974.

Conway, B. L.: Pediatric neurologic nursing, St. Louis, 1977, The C. V. Mosby Co.

Conway, B. L.: Carini and Owens' neurological and neurosurgical nursing, ed. 7, St. Louis, 1978, The C. V. Mosby Co.

Koos, W. T., and Miller, M. H.: Intracranial tumors of infants and children, St. Louis, 1971, The C. V. Mosby Co.

Lascari, A.: Leukemia in childhood, Springfield, Ill., 1973, Charles C Thomas Publisher.

Levin, D., and associates: Cancer rates and risks, Washington, D.C., 1974, U.S. Department of Health, Education and Welfare, Public Health Service, National Institutes of Health.

Ravel, R.: Clinical laboratory medicine, Chicago, 1973, Year Book Medical Publishers, Inc.

Rudolph, A. M., editor: Pediatrics, New York, 1977, Appleton-Century-Crofts.

Widmann, F. K.: Goodales' clinical interpretation of laboratory tests, Philadelphia, 1973, F. A. Davis Co.

Modes of cancer therapy

Aisner, J.: Platelet transfusion therapy, Med. Clin. North Am. **61**(5):1133-1145, September 1977.

Bergersen, B. S., and Goth, A.: Pharmacology in nursing, ed. 13, St. Louis, 1976, The C. V. Mosby Co.

Blount, M., and Kinney, A. B.: Chronic steroid therapy, Am. J. Nurs. **74**(9):1626-1629, August 1974.

Bochow, A. J.: Cancer immunotherapy: what promise does it hold? Nursing '76 **6**(10):50-56, October 1976.

Burkhalter, P. K.: Cancer quackery, Am. J. Nurs. **77**(3):451-453, March 1977.

Drugs vs. cancer, DHEW Publication No. (NIH) 76-786, Washington, D.C., 1976, U.S. Department of Health, Education and Welfare, National Institutes of Health.

Elliot, C.: Radiation therapy: how you can help, Nursing '76 **6**(9):34-41, September 1976.

Gardner, G. G., August, C. S., and Githens, J.: Psychological issues in bone marrow transplantation, Pediatrics **60**(4):625-631, October 1977.

Gilladoga, A. C., and associates: The cardiotoxicity of adriamycin and daunomycin in children, Cancer **37:**1070-1078, February 1976.

Greene, T.: Current therapy for acute leukemia in childhood, Nurs. Clin. North Am. **11**(1):3-19, March 1976.

Herbst, S. F.: A new approach to parenteral drug administration, Am. J. Nurs. **75**(8):1345, August 1975.

Hubbard, S., and DeVita, V.: Chemotherapy research nurse, Am. J. Nurs. **76**(4):561-565, April 1976.

Livingston, B. M., and Krakoff, I. H.: L-Asparaginase, Am. J. Nurs. **70**(9):28-33, September 1970.

Marino, E., and LeBlanc, D.: Cancer chemotherapy, Nursing '75 **5:**22-33, November 1975.

Marsh, J. C., and Mitchell, M. S.: Chemotherapy of cancer, Parts II and III. Drugs in current use, Drug Ther. (hospital edition) **1:**43-47, October/November 1976.

McCaffery, M.: Pain relief for the child: problem areas and selected nonpharmacological methods, Pediatr. Nurs. **3**(4):11-16, July/August 1977.

McCalla, J. L.: Immunotherapy: concepts and nursing implications, Nurs. Clin. North Am. **11**(1):59-71, March 1976.

Nirenberg, A.: High-dose methotrexate, Am. J. Nurs. **76**(11): 1176-1780, November 1976.

Powles, R. L.: Immunologic maneuvers in the management of acute leukemia, Med. Clin. North Am. **60**(3):463-472, May 1976.

Rossman, M., Slavin, R., and Taft, E.: Pheresis therapy: patient care, Am. J. Nurs. **77**(7):1135-1141, July 1977.

Schiffer, C. A.: Principles of granulocyte transfusion therapy, Med. Clin. North Am. **61**(5):1119-1131, September 1977.

Schwitter, G., and Beach, J.: Bone marrow transplantation in children, Nurs. Clin. North Am. **11**(1):49-57, March 1976.

Silverstein, M. J., and Morton, D. L.: Cancer immunotherapy, Am. J. Nurs. **73**(7):1178-1181, July 1973.

Sontesgard, L., and associates: A way to minimize side effects from radiation therapy, Am. J. Maternal Child Nurs. **1**(1):27-31, January/February 1976.

Sparks, F. C.: Hazards and complications of BCG immunotherapy, Med. Clin. North Am. **60**(3):499-509, May 1976.

Stern, R. C., and associates: Use of a "heparin-lock" in the intermittent administration of intravenous drugs, Clin. Pediatr. **11** (9):521-523, September 1972.

Tealey, A. R.: Getting children to keep still during radiotherapy, Am. J. Maternal Child Nurs. **2**(3):178-181, May/June 1977.

Tenczynski, J.: Leukapheresis: the process, Am. J. Nurs. **77**(7): 1133-1134, July 1977.

Vaeth, J. M.: Radiation therapy—a double-edged sword? Pediatr. Ann. **4**(2):72-73, February 1975.

Varicchio, C. G.: Nursing care during total body irradiation, Am. J. Nurs. **77**(8):1314-1317, August 1977.

Vietti, T., and Edelstein, M.: Pediatric chemotherapy, Pediatr. Ann **4**(2):76-100, February 1975.

Walker, P.: Bone marrow transplant: a second chance for life, Nursing '77 **7**(1):24-25, January 1977.

Wiley, F. M., and Rhein, M.: Challenges of pain management: one terminally ill adolescent, Pediatr. Nurs. **3**(4):26-27, July/August 1977.

Zimmerman, S., and associates: Bone marrow transplantation, Am. J. Nurs. **77**(8):1311-1315, August 1977.

The leukemias

Baker, L. S.: You and leukemia: a day at a time, Philadelphia, 1978, W. B. Saunders Co.

Desotell, S.: A brighter future for leukemia patients, Nursing '77 **7**(1):19-24, January 1977.

Esterhay, R. J., and associates: Cost analysis of leukemia treatment, Cancer **37:**646-652, February 1976.

Fernbach, D., and Starling, K.: Acute leukemia in children, Pediatr. Ann. **3**(5):13-26, 1974.

Fochtman, D.: Leukemia in children, Pediatr. Nurs. **2**(3):8-13, May/June 1976.

Foley, G., and McCarthy, A.: The child with leukemia: the disease and its treatment, Am. J. Nurs. **76**(7):1108-1114, July 1976.

Foley, G., and McCarthy, A.: The child with leukemia: in a special hematology clinic, Am. J. Nurs. **76**(7):1115-1119, July 1976.

Greene, P.: The child with leukemia in the classroom, Am. J. Nurs. **75**(1):86-87, January 1975.

Greene, P.: Acute leukemia in children, Am. J. Nurs. **75**(10): 1709-1714, October 1975.

Leventhal, B. L., and Hersh, S.: Modern treatment of childhood leukemia: the patient and his family, Child. Today **3**(3):2-6, May/June 1974.

Martinson, I.: The child with leukemia: parents help each other, Am. J. Nurs. **76**(7):1120-1122, July 1976.

McIntosh, S., and associates: Chronic neurologic disturbance in childhood leukemia, Cancer **37:**853-857, February 1976.

Morgan, S. K., Grooms, A. M., and Loadholt, C. B.: Is the bone marrow uniformly reactive in pediatric hematologic conditions? Clin. Pediatr. **11**(10):471-572, October 1972.

Rivera, G., and associates: Recurrent childhood lymphocytic leukemia following cessation of therapy, Cancer **37:**1679-1686, April 1976.

Shalet, S. M., and associates: Growth hormone deficiency after treatment of acute leukemia in children, Arch. Dis. Child. **5:**489-493, 1976.

Stimone, J. V., and associates: Combined modality therapy of acute lymphocytic leukemia, Cancer **35:**25-35, January 1975.

Wellnik, L.: Management of the child with cancer on an outpatient basis, Nurs. Clin. North Am. **11**(1):35-48, March 1976.

Brain tumors

Dyment, P. G., and associates: Computerized tomography in the detection of intracranial metastasis in children, Pediatrics **58** (1):72-77, July 1976.

Petito, C. K., De Girolami, U., and Earle, K. M.: Craniopharyngiomas, Cancer **37:**1944-1952, April 1976.

Stone, B. H.: Computerized transaxial brain scan, Am. J. Nurs. **77**(10):1601-1604, October 1977.

Wheeler, P.: Care of patient with a cerebellar tumor, Am. J. Nurs. **77**(2):263-266, February 1977.

Lymphomas

Baldy, C. M.: The lymphomas: concepts and current therapies, Nurs. Clin. North Am. **7**(4):763-775, December 1972.

Bolin, R. H., and Auld, M. E.: Hodgkin's disease, Am. J. Nurs. **74**(11):1982-1986, November 1974.

Keaveny, M., and Wiley, L.: Hodgkin's disease. Part I: the curable cancer, Nursing '75 **5**(3):48-54, March 1975.

Nebe, D. E., and Gavaghan, M.: Lymphography and patients' reactions, Am. J. Nurs. **73**(8):1366-1368, August 1973.

Non-Hodgkin's lumphomas: a brief introduction to their evaluation and management, Delaware, 1977, Adria Laboraties, Inc.

Qazi, R., and associates: The natural history of nodular lymphoma, Cancer **37:**1923-1927, April 1976.

Rogers, T. M.: Hodgkin's disease. Part II; hope is the key to nursing care, Nursing '75 **5**(3):55-58, March 1975.

Showfety, M. P.: The ordeal of Hodgkin's disease, Am. J. Nurs. **74**(11):1987-1991, November 1974.

Stein, R. S., and associates: Bone marrow involvement in non-Hodgkin's lymphoma, Cancer **37:**629-636, February 1976.

Walker, M. D.: Treatment of brain tumors, Med. Clin. North Am. **61**(5):1045-1051, September 1977.

Wollman, I. J.: Staging in childhood Hodgkin's disease, Clin. Pediatr. **11**(8):441-442, August 1972.

Wollner, N., and associates: Non-Hodgkin's lymphoma in children, Cancer **37:**123-124, January 1976.

Blastomas

Arneil, G. C., and associates: Nephritis in two children after irradiation and chemotherapy for nephroblastoma, Lancet **1** (7864):960-963, 1974.

Bedford, M. A.: Management of retinoblastoma, Mod. Probl. Ophthalmol. **18:**101-105, 1977.

CEA-ROCHE, carcinoembryonic antigen assay, Nutley, N.J., 1974, Hoffman-LaRoche, Inc.

Ellsworth, R. M.: Retinoblastoma. In Duane, T. D., editor: Clinical ophthalmology, New York, 1976, Harper & Row, Publishers.

Evans, A. E., D'Angio, G. J., and Koop, C. E.: Diagnosis and treatment of neuroblastoma, Pediatr. Clin. North Am. **23**(1): 161, February 1976.

Fochtman, D.: Malignant solid tumors in children, Pediatr. Nurs. **2**(6):11-17, November/December 1976.

Francois, J.: Genetics of retinoblastoma, Mod. Probl. Ophthalmol. **18:**165-172, 1977.

Grosfeld, J. L., Ballantine, T. V., and Baehner, R. L.: Current management of childhood solid tumors, Surg. Clin. North Am. **56**(2):513-553, April 1976.

Helson, L.: Neuroblastoma: early diagnosis a key to successful treatment, Pediatr. Ann. **3**(5):46-54, 1974.

Jaffe, B. F., and Jaffe, N.: Head and neck tumors in children, Pediatrics **51**(4):731-740, April 1973.

Jensen, R. D., and Miller, R. W.: Retinoblastoma: epidemiologic characteristics, N. Engl. J. Med. **285**(6):307-311, August 5, 1971.

Knudson, A. G.: Mutation and cancer: statistical study of retinoblastoma, Proc. Natl. Acad. Sci. USA **68**(4):820-823, April 1971.

Knudson, A. G.: Mutation and human cancer, Adv. Cancer Res. **17:**317-350, 1973.

Knudson, A. G., and associates: Chromosomal deletion and retinoblastoma, N. Engl. J. Med. **295**(20):1120-1123, November 11, 1976.

Martin, E. W., and associates: Carcinoembryonic antigen: clinical and historical aspects, Cancer **37:**62-81, January 1976.

Merten, D. F., Yang, S. S., and Bernstein, J.: Wilms' tumor in adolescence, Cancer **37:**1532-1538, March 1976.

Michelson, J. F., Felberg, N. T., and Shields, J. A.: Fetal antigens in retinoblastoma, Cancer **37:**719-723, February 1976.

Morgan, S. K., and Busse, M. B.: Survival following brain metastases in Wilms' tumor, Pediatrics **58**(1):130-132, July 1976.

Reynoso, G., and associates: Carcinoembryonic antigens in patients with different cancers, J.A.M.A. **220:**361-365, 1972.

Schwartz, A. D.: Neuroblastoma and Wilms' tumor, Med. Clin. North Am. **61**(5):1053-1071, September 1977.

Wilbur, J. R.: Treatment of soft tissue sarcomas, Pediatr. Clin. North Am. **23**(1):171, February 1976.

Wilson, M. G., and associates: Chromosomal anomalies in patients with retinoblastoma, Clin. Genet. **12:**1-8, 1977.

Bone tumors

Chang, P.: Progress in the treatment of osteogenic sarcoma, Med. Clin. North Am. **61**(5):1027-1038, September 1977.

Rosen, G.: Management of malignant bone tumors in children and adolescents, Pediatr. Clin. North Am. **23**(1):183, February 1976.

Rosen, G., and associates: Chemotherapy, en bloc resection, and prosthetic bone replacement in the treatment of osteogenic sarcoma, Cancer **37:**1-11, January 1976.

Staudt, A. R.: Femur replacement in osteogenic sarcoma, Am. J. Nurs. **75**(8):1346-1348, August 1975.

Aplastic anemia

Pochedly, C.: Fanconi's anemia: clues to early recognition, Clin. Pediatr. **11**(1):20-24, January 1972.

Systemic lupus erythematosus

Epstein, W. V.: Laboratory tests in rheumatic diseases, Med. Clin. North Am. **61**(2):377-387, March 1977.

Fries, J. F.: The clinical aspects of systemic lupus erythematosus, Med. Clin. North Am. **61:**229-239, March 1977.

Roe, R. L.: Drug therapy in rheumatic diseases, Med. Clin. North Am. **61**(2):405-437, March 1977.

Sato, F. F.: Trials with cyclophosphamide in SLE, Am. J. Nurs. **72**(6):1077-1079, June 1972.

Torbett, M. P., and Ervin, J. C.: The patient with systemic lupus erythematosus, Am. J. Nurs. **77**(8):1299-1302, August 1977.

UNIT TWELVE

The child with a disturbance of fluid and electrolytes

Some of the most common problems associated with the care of infants and children are related to the assessment and maintenance of fluid balance. The physiologic characteristics of young children render them more susceptible to fluid imbalances, and almost any early childhood illness is complicated by fluid disturbances. These differences are particularly noted in the infant, whose proportion of total body water is considerably greater than that of the adult or older child. Also, the usual childhood responses to illness, such as fever and anorexia, further contribute to water depletion and dehydration.

It is essential that nurses who work with children have an understanding of the basic principles underlying the pathologic processes that produce fluid and electrolyte disturbances, the rationale behind fluid therapy, and the nurse's role in maintaining or restoring fluid balance. Chapter 29, *Balance and Imbalance of Body Fluids,* provides a brief review of the basic concepts of fluid and electrolyte balance and imbalance and the nurse's role in fluid administration. Chapter 30, *Conditions that Produce Fluid and Electrolyte Imbalance,* discusses some of the major causes of fluid disturbance, and Chapter 31, *The Child with a Disturbance of Renal Function,* deals with the more specific fluid problems of renal dysfunction.

29

Balance and imbalance of body fluids

The basic elements related to fluid and electrolyte balance—body water, electrolytes, and pH—are so closely interrelated that they rarely can be separated in clinical disorders; however, for simplicity, they will be reviewed separately. An understanding of the basic principles of fluid dynamics and acid-base balance is essential for the nurse to be able to interpret observations, correlate these findings with the course of the disease process, and comprehend the rationale behind therapy in order to participate intelligently in a treatment regimen.

To facilitate a discussion of fluids and electrolytes, a few of the terms will be briefly defined. For more detailed explanation of these terms and fluid and electrolyte physiology, the reader is referred to basic physiology or chemistry textbooks.

electrolyte a substance that, when dissolved in water, is capable of conducting an electric current. This capacity is a result of its ability to dissociate into charged particles called *ions*. In their natural state, molecules are held together by an electric force. When molecules are dissolved, the electric bond is broken and the electrically charged atoms or radicals (groups of atoms) wander about in the solution. In a solution the number of positively charged ions *(cations)* must equal the number of negatively charged ions *(anions)*. The chief cations in body fluids are sodium (Na^+), potassium (K^+), calcium (Ca^{++}), and magnesium (Mg^{++}). The major anions are chloride (Cl^-), bicarbonate (HCO_3^-), phosphate (HPO_4^{--}), and sulfate (SO_4^{--}).

milliequivalent (mEq) the measure of the chemical activity or chemical combining power of an ion. It expresses the capacity of cations to combine with anions to form molecules and describes the amount of each ion that is needed for the combining process. One milliequivalent is equal to the chemical combining power of 1 ml of hydrogen. The weight of a substance has no relationship to its chemical combining power, much the same as the weight of various coins have no relationship to their buying power. Two nickels are heavier than one dime, but the purchasing power is the same.

milliosmole a measure of the number of dissolved particles in a liter of solution, regardless of their electric charge.

dynamic equilibrium a balance between continually varying, shifting, and opposing forces that is characteristic of living processes.

COMPOSITION AND DISTRIBUTION OF BODY FLUIDS

Water is the major constituent of body tissues, and the total body water (TBW) in an individual ranges from 45% to 75% of total body weight.[10] Its importance to body function is related not only to its abundance but also to the fact that it is the medium in which body solutes are dissolved and all metabolic reactions take place. Since these metabolic processes are affected by even small alterations in fluid composition, precise regulation of the volume and composition of the fluid is essential. In healthy individuals body water remains singularly constant, but marked alterations in either its volume or distribution that occur in many disease states can produce severely damaging physiologic consequences.

The percentage of total body water varies among individuals and, in adults and older children, is related primarily to the amount of body fat. Consequently females, who have significantly more body fat than males, and obese persons have less water content in relation to weight. Total body water content also varies with age. The difference is marked in the newborn infant, whose total body water is 20% greater than that of the adult. The total body water content diminishes rapidly in the neonatal period and continues to decrease steadily until the approximate adult percentage is reached at about age 2 years (Fig. 29-1). The sex differences become apparent at puberty.

Body fluid compartments

The composition and volume of body fluid are not static but remain relatively constant through a state of dynamic equilibrium. There is a continual movement of water, and, to a lesser extent, of solutes, between the individual and the external environment and between the various fluid compartments within the internal environment. The fluids are composed principally of water, in which a variety of substances are either dissolved or suspended. These substances consist of both electrolytes and nonelectrolyte particulate matter, the presence or absence of which in any fluid compartment influences the concentration and movement of water from other compartments.

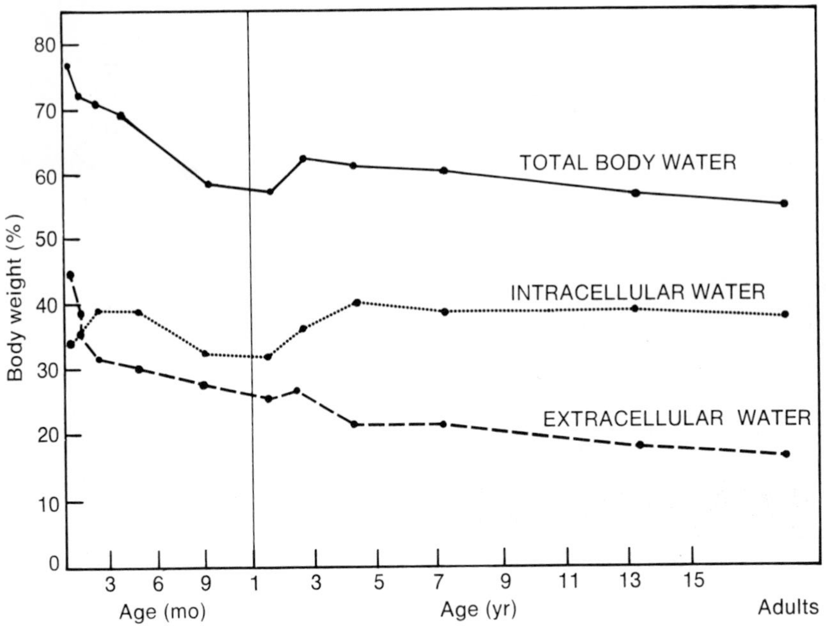

Fig. 29-1. Changes in total body water, extracellular water, and intracellular water in percentages of body weight. (After Friis-Hansen, B.: Body water compartments in children, Pediatrics **28:**169, 1961.)

Body water is distributed chiefly between two large compartments that differ markedly in composition—the *intracellular* and the *extracellular* fluid compartments. The amount and composition of these compartments are maintained by the boundary organs through regulatory mechanisms within the internal environment. The volume of body water is arbitrarily described, for illustrative purposes, as 60% of total body weight—intracellular fluid is 40% of total body weight and extracellular fluid is 20% of total body weight. Of the extracellular fluid, 5% is found in the intravascular space and 15% in the extravascular spaces (Fig. 29-2).

Extracellular fluid. The extracellular fluid (ECF) is defined as the body fluid external to the cells. This consists of[10,13]:

1. Intravascular fluid. Circulating plasma exclusive of the cellular components
2. Interstitial or intercellular fluid. That portion of the extracellular fluid that is extravascular, sometimes described as an ultrafiltrate of plasma, since its electrolyte composition closely resembles that of plasma; it is this fluid that perfuses body cells
3. Dense connective tissue, cartilage, and bone. Fluid contained in these tissues in negligible and has little, if any, significance in fluid balance
4. Transcellular fluids. Those fluids that are directly elaborated from cells, including cerebrospinal fluid, aqueous humors, sweat, and gastrointestinal fluids, including secretions from the pancreas, liver, and biliary tree; cavities within the body that ordinarily contain minimal amounts of fluid but have the potential to fill with large amounts of fluid are the peritoneal, pleural, pericardial, and synovial spaces; many authorities consider urine a transcellular fluid

The major electrolyte components of extracellular fluid are sodium, chloride, bicarbonate, and, to a lesser extent, potassium, calcium, organic acids, and phosphate. Of these, the chief cation is sodium and the most abundant anion is chloride. In addition the plasma contains proteins that, although they normally do not move freely between compartments, usually carry a negative charge and, as anions, contribute significantly to regulation of volume between compartments (Fig. 29-3).

Intracellular fluid. The largest proportion of body water is contained in the intracellular fluid (ICF) compartment. The amount is difficult to measure, but it is estimated that almost two thirds of the total body water is contained within the cells (including circulating blood cells). The major cations in the intracellular fluid are potassium and magnesium, and the chief anions are proteins and the organic phosphates (see Fig. 29-3).

The differences between the extracellular and intracellular fluid are primarily related to the amount of potassium and sodium in the two compartments. Whereas sodium is the chief cation in the extracellular fluid, its concentration is relatively low in the intracellular fluid. Chloride, the major cation of extracellular fluid, is in much smaller concentrations in the intracellular fluid and is believed to be

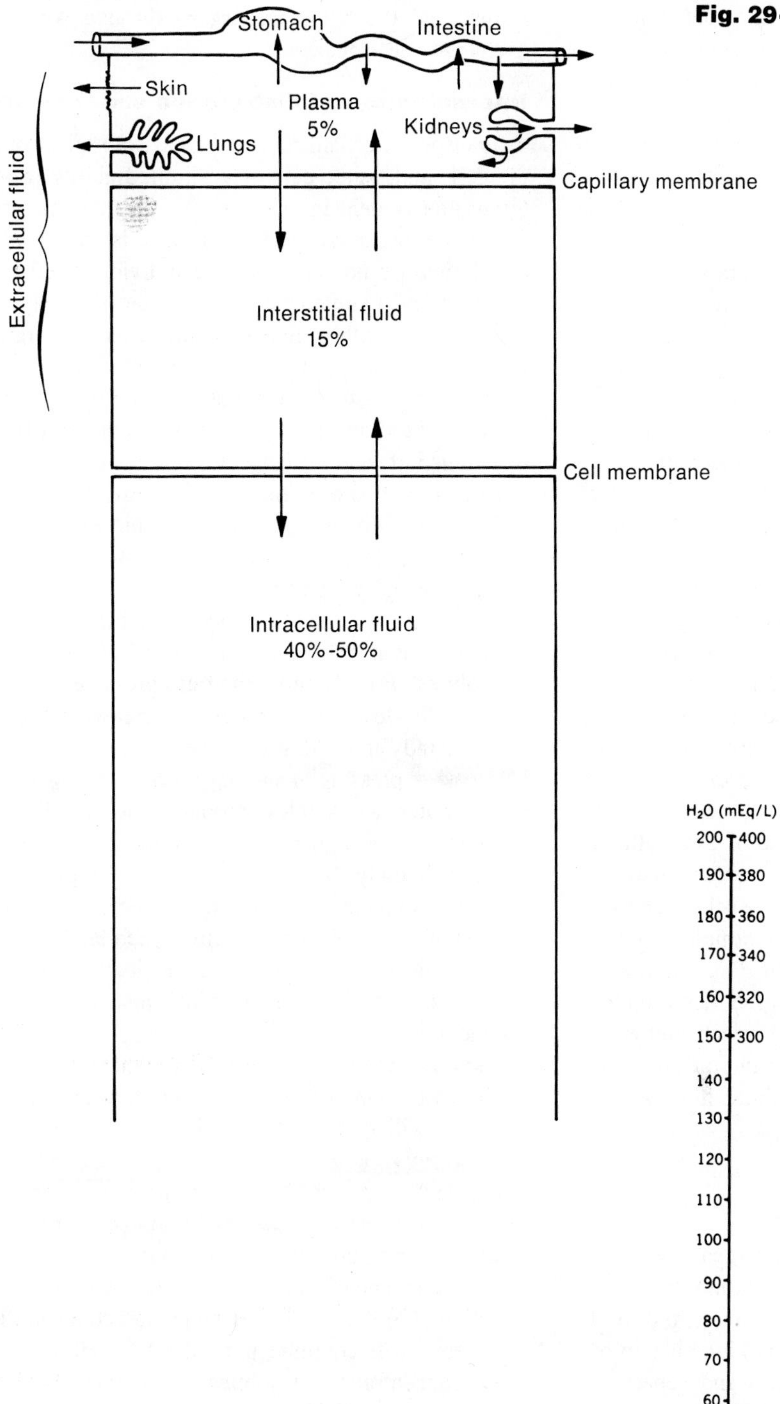

Fig. 29-2. Major fluid compartments in the body.

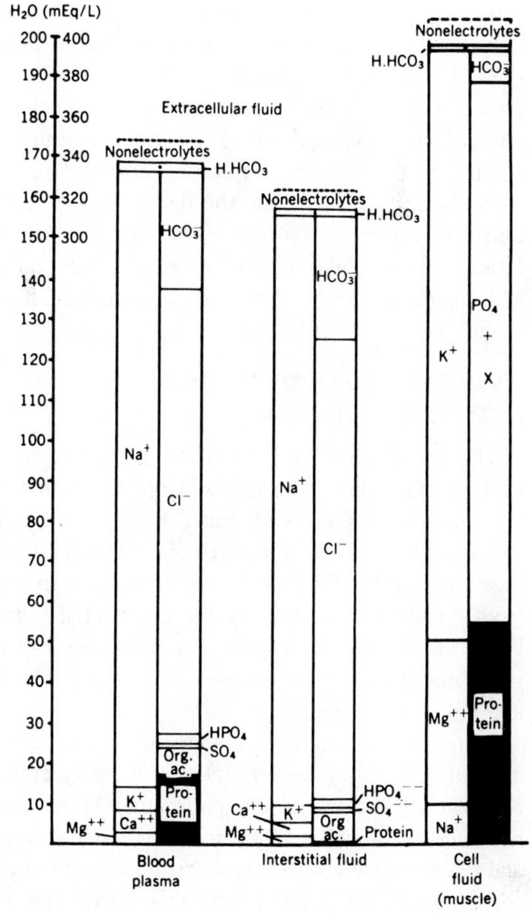

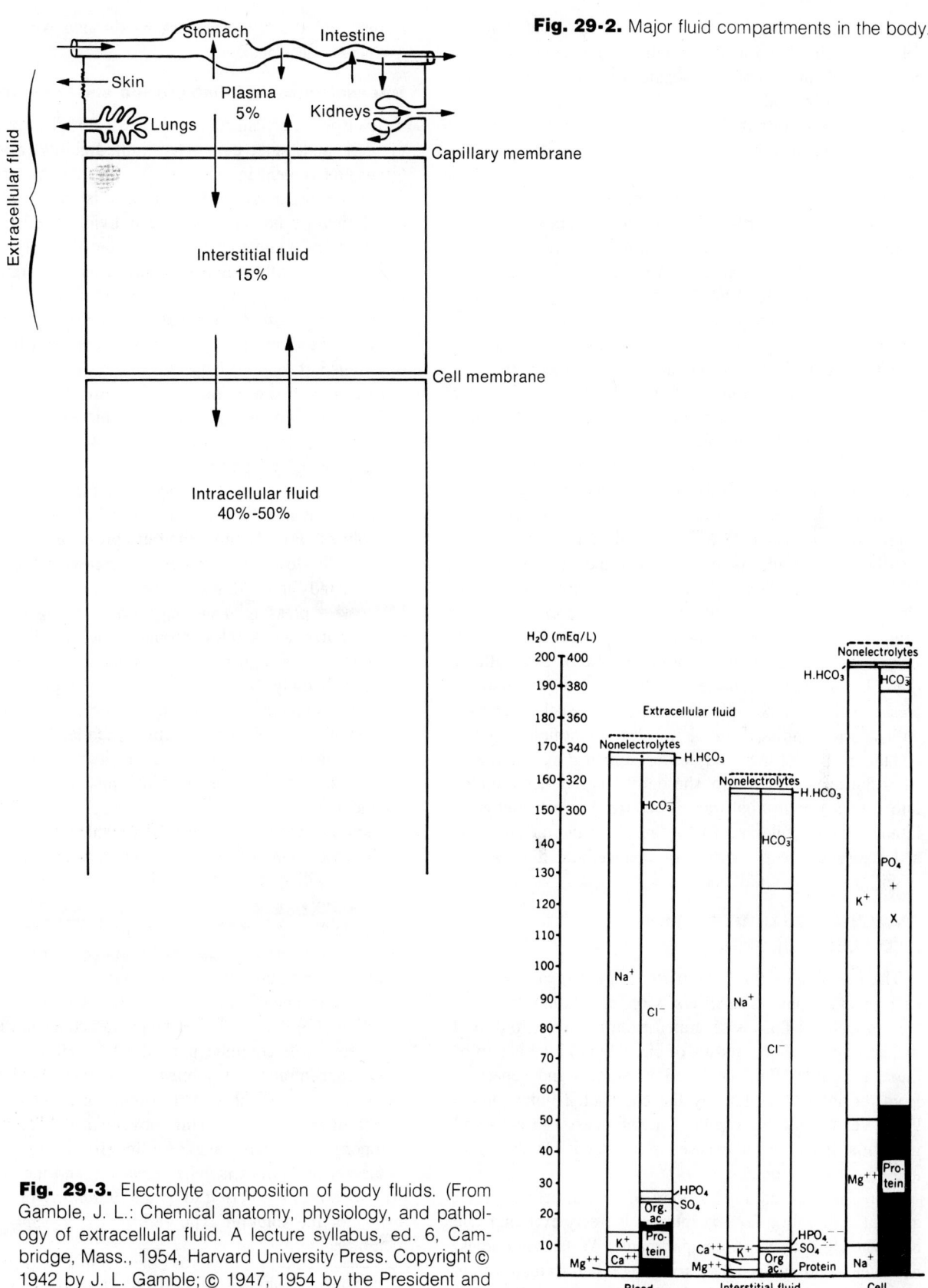

Fig. 29-3. Electrolyte composition of body fluids. (From Gamble, J. L.: Chemical anatomy, physiology, and pathology of extracellular fluid. A lecture syllabus, ed. 6, Cambridge, Mass., 1954, Harvard University Press. Copyright © 1942 by J. L. Gamble; © 1947, 1954 by the President and Fellows of Harvard College.)

virtually nonexistent in some cells (for example, muscle cells). Proteins have a higher intracellular concentration, but the concentration of bicarbonate is much lower in intracellular than in extracellular fluid.

Difference in infants.[1,6] The fluid compartments in the infant vary significantly from those in the adult primarily because of an expanded extracellular compartment. The extracellular fluid compartment comprises over half of the total body water at birth and, accompanying this, a greater relative content of extracellular sodium and chloride. This neonatal ''excess'' extracellular fluid is largely lost in the first 10 days of life through insensible perspiration that amounts to up to 10% of the infant's birth weight. The infant maintains a larger amount of extracellular fluid than the adult until about 2 years of age, and this, together with other anatomic and physiologic differences (to be discussed later), contributes to greater and more rapid water loss and poorer adjustment during this age period.

During the first year there is a sharp decrease in total body water when expressed as a percentage of body weight. The percentage of extracellular fluid also decreases from approximately 45% to 27%. The gradual alteration in water distribution that accompanies growth and maturation is a result of several changes from infancy to childhood. Muscle growth associated with increasing size of individual cells increases the actual and relative intracellular fluid volume and decreases the relative volume of extracellular fluid. In addition to muscle growth, other organs also increase in size; for example, the size of nerve cells increases with a corresponding decrease in extracellular fluid volume, and the fraction of total body water contained in skin diminishes during growth. Also, the daily volume of secretions into the gastrointestinal tract is relatively much higher in infants than in children. The net result of these changes is a decrease in the proportion of extracellular fluid as the infant grows into childhood.

DYNAMICS OF BODY WATER AND ELECTROLYTES

The major body fluid compartments are separated from each other by physical barriers. Confined within the cells, the intracellular fluid is separated from the interstitial fluid that surrounds it. The plasma of circulating blood is part of the extracellular fluid enclosed in vessels and separated from the interstitial fluid by the endothelial lining of the blood vessels and the capillary membranes. The cells and interstitial spaces are all encased in a protective layer of skin and mucous membranes.

Water is retained in the body in a relatively constant amount and, with a few exceptions, is freely exchangeable between all body fluid compartments. Water volume is, however, continually subject to change, and its distribution and maintenance are largely determined by the solutes dissolved in the body water, physical forces that act at the site of the partitioning membranes, internal control mechanisms, and the boundary organs through which external exchanges take place.

Internal forces of distribution and transport

Transport mechanisms are the basis for all activity within the cell, and, since cells have limited ability to store materials, movement in and out of them must be very rapid. Therefore, the transportation distance is very small and the capillaries are not far from the individual cells. The distribution and maintenance of fluid and electrolyte balance between and within fluid compartments are largely determined by physical forces, the most important of which are hydrostatic pressure and osmotic pressure. Other forces that influence fluid and electrolyte movement are diffusion, active transport, and vesicular transport.

Hydrostatic pressure. Fluids at rest, when enclosed in a container, produce pressure by their weight. The pressure of fluids increases toward the bottom of the container because of the weight of the water and is directly related to the height of the container—the higher a column of fluid, the greater the pressure exerted at the lower end of the column. For example, the fluid pressure of blood in the veins of the lower extremities is increased when the individual stands and is diminished when the feet are elevated. Hydrostatic pressure is the force behind filtration, the transfer of water and solutes through a permeable membrane from an area of high pressure to one of lower pressure. In the human body the force created by the pumping action of the heart increases the hydrostatic pressure in the arterial portion of the circulatory system, which tends to force fluid through the capillary wall into the interstitial spaces and from the glomerular capillaries into the collecting tubules of the kidneys.

Osmotic pressure. When two aqueous solutions are separated by a membrane permeable to water, an exchange of water will occur between the two solutions. A selectively permeable membrane allows free movement of water molecules but partially or completely prevents passage of particles dissolved or suspended in the water. When the solute concentration of the two solutions differs, the principal movement of water across the membrane is in the direction of the solution with the greater concentration. This movement will continue until the two solutions have an equal concentration of solutes and allows for rapid reestablishment of equilibrium if volume or pressure in either compartment is altered. This movement of water across a semipermeable membrane resulting from a difference in solute concentrations is called *osmosis,* and the concentration of solutes is referred to as the *osmolality* or the *osmolarity** of the solution. The cell wall is a semipermeable membrane.

*The terms osmolality and osmolarity are often used interchangeably. Osmolality refers to the concentration of the solution as expressed in osmoles/kg of water; osmolarity is the concentration of the solution expressed as osmoles/liter of solution.[8]

The degree of osmotic pressure exerted by a solution is determined by the *number* of osmotically active particles dissolved or suspended in the solution, regardless of their weight or electric charge. For example, although it is larger, one molecule of glucose has only half the osmolality of one molecule of sodium chloride, since the sodium chloride ionizes in solution into two particles, the sodium and the chloride ions. Thus one molecule of sodium chloride exerts twice the osmotic pressure of one molecule of glucose.

Osmolality can also be expressed as *tonicity* and relates to the osmolality of body fluids. A solution that is *isotonic* has the same osmolality, or tonicity, as body fluids such as plasma. A *hypertonic* solution is one that has a greater concentration of solutes than plasma; a *hypotonic* solution has a lower concentration. Examples of isotonic solutions are 0.9% saline solution and 5% dextrose in water; 10% glucose in water is a hypertonic solution; plain water and 0.2% sodium are hypotonic solutions.

The cell membrane is the selectively permeable membrane that separates the intracellular from the extracellular fluid compartments; normally the two are maintained in a state of equilibrium. The effect of osmotic pressure can be illustrated by placing a cell in solutions with greater or lesser osmolality (Fig. 29-4, *A*). There is no movement of fluid when the cell, such as a red blood cell, is placed in an isotonic solution (Fig. 29-4, *B*). To establish osmotic equilibrium when the concentration of solutes is greater or less than that of the cell, water moves to the area of greater density. A hypertonic solution causes crenation, or shriveling, as water leaves the cell (Fig. 29-4, *A*). The cell will swell, sometimes to the point of bursting (hemolysis), as water diffuses into the cell from a hypotonic solution (water intoxication) (Fig. 29-4, *C*). This is a risk in situations such as rapid intravenous infusions, blood transfusions, and tap water enemas.

An important solute that is significant in producing osmotic pressure, especially at the capillary membrane, is protein. Protein molecules ordinarily do not diffuse readily through a semipermeable membrane, and, since it is only those particles that fail to pass through the pores of a selectively permeable membrane that exert osmotic pressure, the proteins in the plasma and interstitial fluids are responsible for osmotic pressure at the capillary level. The osmotic pressure created by protein is termed *colloidal osmotic pressure (COP)* or *oncotic pressure (OP)*. The major effect is that as hydrostatic pressure tends to force fluids out of the capillaries, the opposing force of the plasma proteins tends to pull them back into the intravascular compartment. The difference between these forces is the major factor in edema formation.

Diffusion. Diffusion is the random movement of molecules from a region of greater concentration to regions of lesser concentration. When a substance of high concentration is added to a solution of low concentration, the molecules will diffuse through the solution until the concentration of the solution is uniform. Factors that influence the rate of diffusion include (1) size of the particle (smaller molecules move more rapidly than larger ones), (2) temperature (heat increases the molecular activity rate of diffusion), and (3) agitation (stirring hastens diffusion). Diffusion is the means of transfer of oxygen and carbon dioxide in the alveoli, nutrients through the intestinal membrane, and water across the cell membrane in osmosis.

Some substances, although unable to diffuse through a cell membrane in their natural states, can do so when chemically combined with a *carrier* substance within the membrane. This process is called *facilitated diffusion,* and the rate with which the substance is able to pass through a membrane depends on the concentration of the substance on each side of the membrane, the amount of carrier available, and the rapidity with which the substance can combine with the carrier. For example, glucose requires a carrier for transport across a cell membrane, but the rate of transport is greatly increased by the presence of the pan-

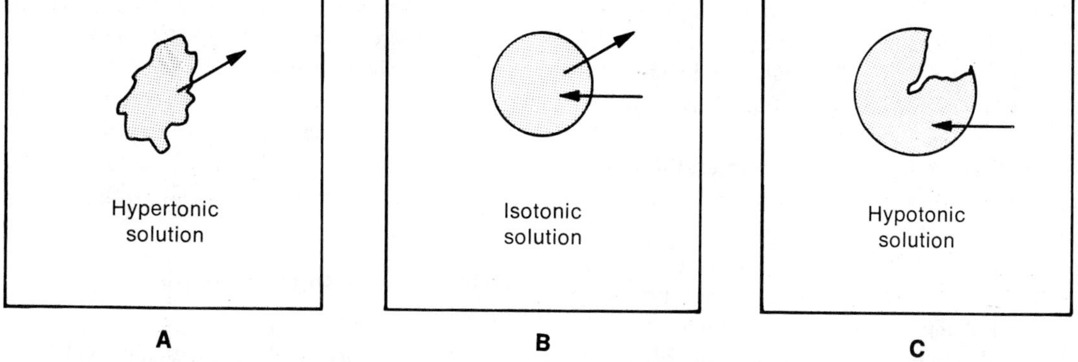

Fig. 29-4. Osmotic pressure. **A,** Hypertonic solution; **B,** isotonic solution; **C,** hypotonic solution.

creatic hormone insulin and is diminished in its absence.

Active transport. The movement of molecules across the cell membrane in osmosis and filtration is referred to as a *passive transport* mechanism, because only the random molecular motion is needed and no metabolic energy is required. Some solutes move across biologic membranes in a direction opposite to that which would be predicted from the concentrations on each side of the membrane. Since no substance can diffuse against a concentration gradient (that is, move from a region of lesser concentration to one of high concentration) without the expenditure of energy, the energy for such movement must be supplied by the cell. The mechanism of active transport is believed to depend on a carrier substance much the same as that required in facilitated diffusion. The difference lies in the fact that active transport enables the substance to be transported *against* the pressure gradient, and, to accomplish this, high energy (principally adenosine triphosphate [ATP]) is imparted to the system. The major electrolytes sodium, potassium, chloride, hydrogen, calcium, and iron, amino acids, urea, and many sugars traverse the cell membrane by way of active transport.

Vesicular transport. Larger molecular substances that are unable to move across cell membranes do so by *vesicular transport*. They move into cells by the process of *pinocytosis* and out of cells by the process of *exocytosis*. When the substance makes contact with the membrane, a segment of the cell membrane invaginates and engulfs a small amount of the substance, pinches off from the remainder of the membrane, and releases the membrane-encased substance into the interior of the cell. To move out, the membrane around the substance fuses with the membrane, the point of fusion breaks down, and the molecule is released on the outside of the membrane. This is the only means by which some larger molecules, such as protein, can enter and leave the cell.

Internal exchanges of water and electrolytes

The distribution and maintenance of water and solutes between the body fluid compartments take place by way of osmosis, diffusion, active transport, and vesicular transport. Movement is determined by the concentration of particles in the solution, the electric potential of the particles, and the pressure exerted on the fluid. The major exchanges take place between the intracellular and extracellular fluid and between the extracellular fluid and the plasma.

Exchange between intracellular and interstitial fluid. Although there is no difference in osmolality between the extracellular and intracellular fluid compartments, the ionic composition differs markedly (see Fig. 29-3). The way in which the body maintains the differences in cations and anions is not completely understood. Through an active transport mechanism the cell retains or pumps in potassium ions and repels or eliminates sodium ions. Hydrostatic pressure gradients at the cellular level are not appreciable, but cell membranes are relatively freely permeable to water; therefore, osmotic pressure is maintained primarily by the movement of water between the two compartments. Because the osmotically active solutes in the cells are not ordinarily subject to rapid alteration, it is the concentration of solutes in the extracellular fluid that usually controls the transfer of water between the intracellular and extracellular fluid compartments.

Exchange between plasma and interstitial fluid. The distribution of extracellular fluid between the vascular and interstitial compartments is determined primarily by the balance between two opposing forces—hydrostatic pressure and colloidal osmotic pressure—at the level of the capillaries. Most ions and small molecules diffuse across the capillary wall to a greater or lesser extent so that the solute composition of interstitial fluid closely resembles that of the plasma. Therefore, these substances contribute little to the osmotic pressure of plasma. However, capillaries are relatively impermeable to protein, and, whereas the protein content of interstitial fluid is usually quite low, almost the entire colloidal osmotic pressure of plasma proteins is effective. Likewise, tissue hydrostatic pressure is a small, but variable, force in maintaining fluid balance at the capillary membrane. Blood enters the capillaries at the arterial end with a hydrostatic pressure significantly greater than the colloidal osmotic fluid, causing fluid to filter from the plasma into the tissue spaces. As blood flows through the capillaries, the hydrostatic pressure diminishes and the colloidal osmotic fluid increases as a result of the loss of fluid to the interstitial space. Following this, the blood colloidal osmotic pressure causes reabsorption of fluid, and balance is restored.

Although capillaries are relatively impermeable to protein, small amounts are able to leak out. If this protein is not returned to the plasma, as occurs in pathologic conditions that increase capillary permeability, such as burns, the colloidal osmotic pressure of tissue would soon equal or surpass that of the plasma. However, protein that leaks into interstitial spaces gains access to the lymphatic channels and is then eventually returned to the plasma, facilitated by muscle contraction and tissue tone. Also, tissue hydrostatic pressure is ordinarily of little consequence. However, it plays a significant role in determining distribution of edema fluid in certain pathologic conditions. Loose tissues allow a greater amount of fluid accumulation than tissues that are tightly bound by dense fibrous bands, in which tissue pressure rapidly increases to limit further extravasation of fluid.

External exchanges of water and electrolytes

The day-to-day consistency of the total body fluid balance is the result of the dynamic equilibrium maintained between intake and output. The major routes through which water is gained or lost from the body are the boundary organs of the body—the gastrointestinal tract, lungs, kidneys, and skin. More specifically, water and electrolytes are gained through ingested water, ingested foods, oxidation of food substrates, and oxidation of body tissues. Water is normally lost through urine, feces, lungs, sweat, and insensible perspiration. Under normal conditions the amount of water ingested closely approximates the amount of urine excreted in a 24-hour period, and the water in food and from oxidation balances that lost in feces and through evaporation. Under normal conditions the balance is maintained.

Water intake. The amount of water ingested is highly variable among individuals and under various circumstances. Approximately half is acquired from drinking water and other fluids. The remainder is gained from the water content of ingested food and as a product of food oxidation. The water content of solid food is surprisingly high, varying from less than 50% to as high as 95% in some vegetables and fruits. Ordinarily only small amounts are derived from catabolism of body tissues and, are, therefore, negligible in health.[1,10]

The amount of water formed in the process of food metabolism depends on the nature of the food substances being oxidized, since the three basic nutrients vary in the amount of water produced. For example, complete oxidation of 100 g of fat yields 100 ml of water, 100 g of carbohydrate produces 60 ml of water, and 100 g of protein produces 45 ml of water.[10] Not only do these three nutrients differ in the amount of water they produce, they also differ in the manner in which the end products of metabolism are eliminated from the body. Whereas the chief end product of fat and carbohydrate is carbon dioxide, which is readily eliminated by the lungs without the need for additional water, the products of protein metabolism, for example, urea, require water for their excretion in the urine. Therefore, persons on a high-protein diet must ingest larger volumes of water.

Gastrointestinal tract. Although the net amount of fluid loss through the gastrointestinal tract is small, the exchanges of water and electrolytes throughout the length of the gastrointestinal tract are large. The numerous secretions of the gastrointestinal tract are produced in large amounts, but, under ordinary conditions, most of the fluid is reabsorbed in the lower bowel. With the exception of saliva, which is hypotonic, the total solute concentration in most of the gastrointestinal secretions is similar to that of interstitial fluid, but there are marked differences among the secretions in electrolyte composition. Therefore, the consequences of fluid lost from the gastrointestinal tract depend a great deal on the composition of the fluid that is lost. Fluid losses from the gastrointestinal tract in vomiting, diarrhea, or other routes (fistula, nasogastric tube) not only produce rapid and profound depletion of extracellular volume but can cause marked distortion of the electrolyte composition as well. Replacement requires careful attention to both volume and solute composition.

Insensible loss. A significant amount of solute-free fluid is lost by way of the lungs and respiratory passages and evaporative loss through the skin. This continuous and obligatory loss of water is a function of temperature regulation and, therefore, is subject to the influences of environmental conditions and body metabolism. Water lost in expired air from the lungs depends on the temperature and humidity of inspired air, the body temperature, and the volume of respiratory exchange. It is also closely related to the metabolic rate. Any factor that increases the metabolic rate, such as exercise, fever, respiratory distress, or metabolic acidosis, will increase the respiratory loss of fluid. Moreover, infants and children have a more rapid rate of metabolism normally.

The rate of losses from both of these routes is a function of the vapor pressure of the extracellular fluid. This pressure increases when body temperature is increased and is decreased when the extracellular fluid osmolality increases, as occurs in a state of dehydration. Insensible water loss through the skin is relatively constant in relation to metabolic activity but tends to be greater in infants and young children because of their larger ratio of surface area to body volume. Less water is lost by either route when the body is surrounded by an atmosphere of high vapor pressure, such as that found in a mist tent.

Sweat. Unlike the insensible pulmonary and cutaneous water loss, which is constant and obligatory, water lost in the sweat through sensible perspiration contains significant quantities of electrolytes and urea. Losses are negligible when the body is at rest and in an environment of controlled ambient temperature and humidity, but losses of fluid in sweat increase with increased environmental temperature, fever, or vigorous exercise. In general, sweating increases by approximately 30 ml per degree Centigrade rise in environmental temperature.[15] Since sweat is hypotonic, adequate fluid and electrolyte replacement is necessary to prevent a hypertonicity of extracellular fluid, but water replacement without replacement of electrolytes will result in a hypotonic extracellular fluid followed by a diffusion of water to the intracellular fluid (edema).

Renal excretion. The principal organs of water volume and solute regulation are the kidneys. Although there are limitations imposed by what is ingested, it has been said that "the composition of the blood [and the internal environment] is determined not by what the mouth ingests but by what the kidneys keep."[14] Under normal conditions the kidneys are able to adjust the urine and solute excretion in response to the requirements for body water and electrolyte balance. They are able to excrete or conserve both water and most electrolytes in addition to excreting end products of protein metabolism, principally urea. The volume of urine excreted by the kidneys in a given period of time depends on the water balance (including intravascular filtration pressure), the quantity of solutes presented to the kidneys, and the capacity of the kidneys to dilute or concentrate the filtrate. The immaturely functioning kidneys of the neonate do not concentrate solutes well; therefore neonates are more apt to become dehydrated when given concentrated formulas.

The ability of the kidneys to conserve or excrete depends to some extent on other forces in the body. Blood enters the nephron, the basic unit of the kidney, at a substantial pressure. This hydrostatic pressure forces plasma fluid and solutes through the capillary membrane into the collecting apparatus of the unit. As this filtrate travels through the renal tubules, water and solutes are selectively reabsorbed back into the vascular compartment. That which is not reabsorbed is excreted as urine. In a state of dehydration, more water is reabsorbed; when water intake is increased, more is excreted as urine. Conditions that produce osmotic diuresis (that is, when large solutes, such as glucose, are filtered through the capillaries in such excessive amounts that they cannot be reabsorbed), the osmotic attraction of the solute causes less water to be reabsorbed, resulting in water being excreted in the urine with the solute. Renal function and malfunction are discussed in Chapter 31.

Regulation of fluid balance

A number of mechanisms in the body play an important role in the control of extracellular fluid volume. Important among these are thirst and antidiuretic hormone; less important are aldosterone and the renin-angiotension system.

Thirst. The conscious desire to ingest water is the principal regulator of water intake. The mechanism of thirst is complex and not completely understood but is a subjective sensory impression. Although thirst can be induced in several ways, the outstanding feature is a decreased output of saliva with a resulting dryness of the mouth and throat that causes the thirst sensation and serves as a stimulus to drink. Ordinarily an individual who has free access to water will drink sufficient quantities to maintain fluid balance.

Thirst is related to the concentration of solutes in body fluids resulting from an increase in osmolality of the extracellular fluid, which may reflect an absolute or a relative deficit of water. It can be produced by either a water deficit or administration of a hypertonic solution of sodium chloride, both of which cause cellular dehydration and a sensation of thirst. Thirst is also stimulated by diminished intravascular volume, such as occurs in acute hemorrhage and in sodium depletion, which causes fluids to shift to the intracellular fluid compartment, thus reducing the extracellular fluid volume.

Antidiuretic hormone (ADH). The pituitary hormone antidiuretic hormone has the major responsibility for maintaining body fluid balance. Its primary effect is to increase the retention of water by the kidneys, and the principal physiologic stimuli for its secretion are increased plasma osmolality and decreased vascular volume. Lesser stimuli are emotional stress, exercise, and some drugs. The result of antidiuretic hormone stimulation is a decreased urine output.

Antidiuretic hormone is synthesized in the hypothalamus and stored in the posterior pituitary. In response to an increase in extracellular fluid, sodium concentration osmoreceptors, believed to be located in the supraoptic nuclei of the hypothalamus, send impulses to the posterior pituitary, from which stored antidiuretic hormone is released. Antidiuretic hormone promotes water retention in the renal system, in which it causes reabsorption of water by increasing the permeability of the renal tubules to water. In the absence of antidiuretic hormone the distal tubules are impermeable to water, which is consequently excreted. Antidiuretic hormone has no effect on solute reabsorption.

Antidiuretic hormone is also released in response to decreased plasma volume. Although the location of volume receptors is not know with certainty, it is believed that they are situated in the vascular system, probably in the veins of the chest. Any small reduction in blood volume to this area, regardless of the total volume, is monitored by these receptors. For example, antidiuretic hormone is released when blood is shifted from the chest to other areas, such as occurs when the position is changed from supine to sitting or standing, during positive-pressure respiration, or even as a result of an increased blood flow to the skin from an increase in ambient temperature. Thus this mechanism appears to provide a more sensitive minute-to-minute regulation of blood volume.[10]

Aldosterone. Aldosterone secreted by the adrenal cortex plays a role in water conservation by enhancing sodium reabsorption in the renal tubules, which promotes osmotic reabsorption of water. Consequently urine volume is diminished and the extracellular fluid volume is increased. Aldosterone is secreted in response to decreased plasma sodium, but the mechanisms that respond to diminished blood volume are more sensitive.

Renin-angiotensin system. Diminished blood flow to the kidneys stimulates receptor sites in the glomeruli to secrete renin into the bloodstream. There it reacts with plasma globulin to generate angiotensin, a powerful vasoconstrictor. In addition to increased blood flow, angiotensin stimulates aldosterone release, which promotes sodium retention in the kidneys while allowing normal excretion of metabolic waste products.

Water balance in infants

Because of several characteristics, infants and young children have a greater need for water and are more vulnerable to alterations in fluid and electrolyte balance. Compared to older children and adults, they have a greater fluid intake and output relative to size, water and electrolyte disturbances occur more frequently and more rapidly, and they adjust less promptly to these alterations. As mentioned previously, the infant's proportionately greater extracellular fluid volume is subject to rapid and profound water depletion in dehydration states as a result of intake restriction or excessive losses from disease. Likewise, overhydration from excessive intake, especially in intravenous fluid administration, is also more serious in infants. Other physiologic factors that contribute to disturbed water and electrolyte balance are mainly the infant's larger surface area, higher metabolism, and immature renal function.

Surface area. The infant's relatively greater surface area allows larger quantities of fluid to be lost in insensible perspiration through the skin. It is estimated that the body surface area of the premature infant is five times as great, and that of the newborn is two to three times as great, as that of the older child or adult. The gastrointestinal tract, sometimes considered to be an extension of the body surface area, is also proportionately larger in infancy and is a source of relatively greater loss in infancy, especially from diarrhea. The larger surface area is an important factor in metabolism and heat production, which influences fluid loss.[1,12]

Metabolic rate. The rate of metabolism in infancy is significantly higher because of the larger surface area in relation to the mass of active tissue. Consequently there is a greater production of metabolic wastes that must be excreted by the kidneys. Any condition that increases metabolism causes greater heat production, with its concomitant insensible fluid loss and an increased need for water for excretion.

Kidney function. The kidneys of the infant are functionally immature at birth and are, therefore, inefficient in excreting waste products of metabolism. Of particular importance for fluid balance is the inability of the infant's kidneys to concentrate or dilute urine, to conserve or excrete sodium, and to acidify urine. Therefore, the infant is less able to handle large quantities of solute-free water than the older child.[15]

Fluid requirements. As a result of these characteristics, infants ingest and excrete a greater amount of fluid per kilogram of body weight than older children. Since electrolytes are excreted with water and the infant has limited ability for conservation, maintenance requirements include both water and electrolytes. The daily exchange of extracellular fluid in the infant is greatly increased over that of older children, which leaves them little fluid volume reserve in dehydration states.

Water requirements for infants and children at various ages are listed in Table 29-1.

Electrolytes

All electrolytes in body fluids contribute to body function and are essential to the maintenance of life and equilibrium. Since water moves freely between fluid compartments and responds to changes in osmolality, it is the solutes that regulate water movement and fluid composition. The sodium ion is the key to extracellular fluid movement, whereas the major ion in intracellular fluid is potassium, which is essential to cellular metabolism. Serum sodium can be measured as a reflection of the relationship of sodium to water in the extracellular fluid; it is not a measure of body sodium. The intracellular fluid potassium content is impossible to measure. For normal serum concentration of electrolytes, see Fig. 29-3 and Appendix B, p. 1602. The importance of the major electrolytes is outlined briefly as follows:

Table 29-1. Ranges of daily water requirements of infants and children at different ages under normal conditions

Age	Average body weight (kg)	Total water requirements per 24 hours (ml)	Water requirements per kg per 24 hours (ml)
3 days	3.0	250-300	80-100
10 days	3.2	400-500	125-150
3 months	5.4	750-850	140-160
6 months	7.3	950-1100	130-135
9 months	8.6	1100-1250	125-145
1 year	9.5	1150-1300	120-135
2 years	11.8	1350-1500	115-125
4 years	16.2	1600-1800	100-110
6 years	20.0	1800-2000	90-100
10 years	28.7	2000-2500	70-85
14 years	45.0	2200-2700	50-60
18 years	54.0	2200-2700	40-50

From Vaughn, V. C., and McKay, R. J.: Nelson's textbook of pediatrics, ed. 10, Philadelphia, 1975, W. B. Saunders Co.

sodium (Na^+) the most abundant cation in extracellular fluid; largely responsible for osmotic pressure of extracellular fluid, stimulates reactions with nerve and muscle tissues; a component of sodium bicarbonate ($NaHCO_3$); important in maintaining acid and base balance in body fluid; contained in gastrointestinal secretions in varying amounts; concentration controlled by osmoreceptors and aldosterone; excreted in urine, sweat, and feces.

potassium (K^+) the most abundant cation of intracellular fluid; helps maintain intracellular fluid water and electrolyte balance; essential for chemical activity of cells; required for transmission of nervous impulses in skeletal, smooth, and cardiac muscles; large quantities contained in gastrointestinal secretion; body has no mechanism for conserving potassium; excreted in urine and feces.

calcium (Ca^{++}) the most abundant cation in the body and mostly concentrated in bones and teeth in association with phosphorus; important to cell membrane integrity; helps maintain normal transmission of nerve impulses—important in initiation of muscle contraction; essential for blood coagulation; important in chemical activity of cells.

magnesium (Mg^{++}) activates numerous reactions; important to normal neuromuscular activity, especially skeletal and heart.

chloride (Cl^-) most abundant anion of extracellular fluid; important for maintaining osmotic pressure.

bicarbonate (HCO_3^-) see p. 1071.

phosphate (PO_3^{--}) see p. 1071.

hydrogen (H^+) see below.

ACID-BASE BALANCE

The ability of the body to regulate the acid-base status is one of its most crucial physiologic processes. Many disease states, such as diarrhea, vomiting, or febrile states, are complicated by disturbances in the acid-base balance that are often more hazardous to the child's survival than the primary disease process. Sometimes simply providing adequate hydration, replacing electrolytes, and correcting acid-base disturbances are all that is needed to sustain an infant or child until the primary disorder has run its course.

Hydrogen ion: pH, acidity, and alkalinity

In body fluids, as in other solutions, the concentration of hydrogen ion determines the degree of neutrality, acidity, or alkalinity of the solution and is a reflection of the body's production, neutralization, and elimination of acids. The higher the hydrogen ion concentration, the more acid the fluid; the lower the concentration, the more alkaline. The mechanisms regulating the hydrogen ion concentration in extracellular fluid are very important, since body cells are especially sensitive to changes in hydrogen ion concentration and because the intracellular fluid, although slightly different in hydrogen ion concentration, depends on the composition of the extracellular fluid. This is especially true regarding enzyme systems and nervous tissue.

pH. The pH notation represents the power of hydrogen, or the concentration of hydrogen ions, and the acidity of a solution is expressed as its pH. The pH scale (derived from the logarithm of the reciprocal of the hydrogen ion concentration) ranges from 1 to 14. A pH of 7 is neutral, less than 7 is acid, and greater than 7 is alkaline. The pH of arterial plasma is normally 7.4, and that of venous plasma is slightly lower because of acid by-products of cellular metabolism. Technically *acidemia* or *acidosis* is present whenever the pH is less than 7.4, and *alkalemia* or *alkalosis* is present when the pH is above 7.4. Ordinarily the plasma pH is maintained in the narrow range of 7.35 to 7.45. At a pH outside this range cellular function is impaired, and this is indicative of profound and life-threatening physiologic disturbances. Although authorities differ regarding the outside limits compatible with life, the upper and lower limits at which an individual can sustain life for more than a few hours are 7.7 and 7.0.[7,8]

Acids. Acids are substances that are *proton donors,* that is, capable of releasing hydrogen ions when they are in solution. Strong acids are those that readily dissociate into their component atoms. For example, hydrochloric acid is considered to be a powerful acid because it dissociates almost completely in solution and, in doing so, releases large numbers of hydrogen ions and produces a strongly acid solution. Carbonic acid (H_2CO_3), on the other hand, is considered a weak acid because it does not dissociate readily and surrenders fewer hydrogen ions in solution.

The most abundant of the acid metabolites is carbonic acid, since carbon dioxide, generated from tissue metabolism of carbohydrates and fats, is largely hydrated to carbonic acid. This is a *volatile* acid; the carbonic acid dissociates to form water and carbon dioxide gas that is excreted by way of the lungs. Other acids, derived from the sulfate and phosphates of protein metabolism, remain in the extracellular fluid as sulfuric acid (H_2SO_4) and phosphoric acid (H_2PO_4), both of which are *nonvolatile* acids (sometimes called *fixed acids*), which are buffered in the blood and excreted by the kidneys. Other physiologic sources of nonvolatile acid are lactic acid from strenuous exercise and keto acids from oxidation of fatty acids.

Bases. Bases are *proton acceptors,* that is, substances that do not have hydrogen ions but are able to accept them. The dissociated hydrogen ions of an acid added to a base solution will bind with the base to form a weak acid, thereby decreasing the number of hydrogen ions and elevating the pH. In this way the base acts as a buffer to diminish the potential acidity of a solution. In the body the major cations that combine with the anion bicarbonate are sodium, potassium, calcium, and magnesium. A decrease in hydrogen ion concentration is less frequently a problem than an increase.

Acid-base regulation

Very simply, the problem of acid-base balance is the maintenance of the hydrogen ion concentration of the extracellular fluid.[7] The continuous metabolism of various foodstuffs produces acid by-products that must be excreted if pH is to be maintained. The ability of the body to maintain a relatively constant pH despite the continuous production of acids is possible because of (1) the action of the chemical buffer systems that act immediately to alter the hydrogen ion concentration and (2) the slower physiologic responses involving primarily respiratory and renal adjustments of the buffer mechanisms.

Buffer systems. A buffer is a device that lessens or absorbs the forces of impact. In the body fluids a chemical buffer is a substance that has the ability to produce a change in pH by binding or releasing hydrogen ions in solution. Buffers exist in the body in pairs that consist of a weak acid and a salt of that acid, and the pH is determined by a *ratio* of the constituents of these buffer pairs. It is the *relative* quantities of the acid and the base that are significant, not the *absolute* quantity of either constituent. An increase or decrease in the amount of one will not disturb the acid-base balance as long as there is a relative increase or decrease in the other to maintain the desired ratio. For example, the major buffer, the carbonic acid–base bicarbonate system, is maintained at an acid-base ratio of 1:20. When these acids and their salts are present in the proper proportion, there is maximum resistance to changes in hydrogen ion concentration and the pH remains within normal limits. The buffers exert their effects by converting a strong acid to a weak one and, in doing so, decreasing the hydrogen ion concentration and elevating the pH.

Chemical buffers in the body fluids can be classified as (1) bicarbonate buffers and (2) nonbicarbonate buffers. Bicarbonate buffers are widespread throughout the plasma, throughout the interstitial fluid, and in red blood cells. Nonbicarbonate buffers, which operate primarily within the cells to absorb or release hydrogen ions, include hemoglobin (Hb) and oxyhemoglobin (HbO_2), organic and inorganic phosphates, plasma proteins and intracellular proteins, and solid body constituents such as bone and collagen tissues. Within the body all the buffer systems maintain equilibrium with each other, that is, a change in one buffer system is buffered by the other buffer systems. The principal buffer in the plasma is the bicarbonate system, with lesser contributions from plasma proteins and inorganic phosphate. In erythrocytes the major buffers are hemoglobin and oxyhemoglobin, with smaller contributions from the organic phosphate and the bicarbonate systems. Over half of the whole blood buffering is caused by the bicarbonate system and half by the nonbicarbonate buffers, principally hemoglobin in the erythrocytes. The principal bicarbonate buffer, the carbonic acid–bicarbonate buffer, is probably the most important buffer in the extracellular fluid and serves as a prototype for all buffer systems.

Bicarbonate. The bicarbonate–carbonic acid buffer pair consists of the buffer acid carbonic acid and a base bicarbonate such as sodium bicarbonate ($NaHCO_3$). Carbonic acid is a weak acid because it dissociates into hydrogen ions and bicarbonate ions poorly when compared with many other acids; however, it dissocaites readily into water and carbon dioxide. Because of this property, end products of the bicarbonate buffer system are excreted readily by the body: carbon dioxide and water from carbonic acid ($H_2CO_3 \rightarrow H_2 + CO_2$) are excreted through the lungs; hydrogen ions and bicarbonate ($H_2CO_3 \rightarrow H^+ + HCO_3^-$) are excreted by the kidneys.

When a strong, nonvolatile acid, such as lactic acid, is buffered by a base bicarbonate, such as sodium bicarbonate, the products are sodium lactate and the weaker carbonic acid:

$$\underset{\text{(strong acid)}}{H^+\ \text{lactate}} + \underset{\text{(buffer base)}}{NaHCO_3} \rightarrow \underset{\text{(salt)}}{\text{Na lactate}} + \underset{\text{(weak acid)}}{H_2CO_3}$$

The carbonic acid then dissociates to be excreted through the respiratory and renal mechanisms.

In like manner, a strong base, such as sodium hydroxide (NaOH), is neutralized by carbonic acid to form the weak base sodium bicarbonate and water:

$$\underset{\text{(strong alkali)}}{NaOH} + \underset{\text{(buffer acid)}}{H_2CO_3} \rightarrow \underset{\text{(weak base)}}{NaHCO_3} + \underset{\text{(water)}}{H_2O}$$

Buffer systems function rapidly, within seconds, to form the first adjustment to deviation in pH. However, more definitive adjustments take place in the lungs and kidneys.

Hemoglobin. The same type of reaction takes place within the red blood cells as the potassium salt of hemoglobin (KHb) combines with carbonic acid to form a weaker acid to reduce the hydrogen ion concentration in the cell. In the red blood cell the enzyme carbonic anhydrase allows the carbon dioxide generated by metabolic processes and diffused into the cell to combine rapidly with water to form bicarbonate and hydrogen ions. The hemoglobin salt, which has a strong affinity for hydrogen ions, absorbs the hydrogen ions to form $KHCO_3$ + HHb. The HHB dissociates as H + Hb, but, since it is a weak acid, fewer hydrogen ions are released to remain in the blood. As the blood circulates to the lungs, hemoglobin picks up oxygen and the action is reversed, resulting in carbon dioxide and water being formed and eliminated through the lungs.

Lungs. Less rapid than the chemical buffers, the respiratory mechanism begins to act within 1 to 3 minutes to make adjustments in pH by eliminating or retaining carbon dioxide. When the levels of carbon dioxide are altered sufficiently, the respiratory centers in the brain respond by either increasing or decreasing the rate and depth of respirations. For example, when the pH of the blood drops, as from increased exercise, there is a compensatory increase in respirations to rid the body of carbon dioxide derived from carbonic acid formed from buffered acid metabolites. Carbon dioxide buildup from breath holding will produce the same response, again reducing the carbonic acid and, thus, the serum pH. The lungs, then, are the compensatory organs in metabolic disturbances and relatively prompt in their response.

Kidneys. The kidneys serve as a final regulating mechanism for both bicarbonate and hydrogen ions and are especially important when acid-base alterations extend over a long period of time. The renal mechanism requires from several hours to days to make adjustments in acid or base concentrations. When the serum carbonic acid level is lowered for some reason, the kidneys respond by increasing the excretion of bicarbonate (alkaline urine); when the bicarbonate ion level drops, the kidney conserve bicarbonate and, at the same time, excretes hydrogen ions (acid urine):

$$\underset{}{H_2CO_3} \rightarrow \underset{\text{Excreted}}{H^+} + \underset{\text{Conserved}}{HCO_3^-}$$

More important quantitatively, the kidneys also excrete hydrogen combined with ammonia (NH_3) as ammonium (NH_4). Therefore, the kidneys are the compensatory organs in respiratory disturbances.

Three important reactions take place in the kidneys that remove free hydrogen ions from the extracellular fluid. Two of these—the bicarbonate ($NaHCO_3$) and the phosphate (Na_2HPO_3) systems—involve reactions with the major sodium buffers. The other is the reaction of hydrogen ions with ammonia to form ammonium. The formation of ammonium depends on the amount of ammonia secreted by kidney tubules. The bicarbonate buffer system operates in the kidneys as it does in other areas of the body. Hydrogen ions are secreted by the kidney tubules, where they react with bicarbonate ions to form carbonic acid, which breaks down to form water and carbon dioxide. The carbon dioxide is readily reabsorbed to combine with hydrogen ions to form bicarbonate ions. Secreted hydrogen ions also react with dibasic phosphate ($2NaHPO_4^=$) to form monobasic phosphate ($NaHPO_4^=$), which is excreted in the urine, and base bicarbonate ($NaHCO_3$), which is reabsorbed.

The major functions of the respiratory and renal mechanisms maintaining acid-base balance are (1) to conserve or exhale carbon dioxide in the lungs and (2) to conserve or excrete bicarbonate through the kidneys.

DISTURBANCES OF ACID-BASE BALANCE

A disturbance of acid-base equilibrium in the direction of acidosis or alkalosis may come about in a variety of ways. However, very simply stated; acidosis (acidemia) results from either accumulation of acid or loss of base, and alkalosis (alkalemia) results from either accumulation of base or loss of acid.

When the fundamental acid-base ratio is altered for any reason, the body attempts to correct the deviation. In a simple disturbance there is a single *primary* factor that affects one component of the acid-base pair and is usually accompanied by a *compensatory* or *secondary* change in the component that is not primarily affected. For example, increased formation of metabolic acid rapidly reduces the base bicarbonate in the formation of carbonic acid. The respiratory mechanism immediately attempts to compensate for the imbalance by eliminating the carbonic acid through exhaled carbon dioxide and water. The imbalance is corrected when the kidneys excrete hydrogen and ammonium ions in exchange for reabsorbed sodium bicarbonate.

When the secondary changes (the hyperventilation and urine acidification in the preceding example) succeed in preventing a distortion of the acid-base ratio and the pH is restored to normal, the disturbance is described as *compensated*. A *partially compensated* state is one in which the serum pH is not within normal limits but in which there is no discernible compensatory effect. The *uncompensated* state exists when there is no compensatory effect and the pH remains uncorrected. The imbalance is said to be *corrected* when physiologic mechanisms fully correct the primary abnormality.[16]

Laboratory measurements

Several laboratory tests are employed to assess the nature and extent of acid-base disturbances. The importance of this data is readily apparent when a clinical observation such as hyperventilation can represent either the primary factor in respiratory alkalosis or a secondary or compensatory factor in metabolic acidosis. The laboratory tests of value in the assessment of acid-base status are outlined in Table 29-2. To determine the acid-base status, three variables—the respiratory component (PCO_2), the metabolic component (base, bicarbonate, or carbon dioxide), and the serum pH—must be determined. Measurement of any two will allow computation of the third. A summary of relationships between these three variables is outlined in Table 29-3.

Table 29-2. Laboratory tests employed in assessment of acid-base status

Abbreviation	Test	Normal values*	Description
pH	Partial pressure of hydrogen	Newborn: 7.25-7.47 Child: 7.35-7.45	Expression of hydrogen ion concentration
Pco_2	Partial pressure of carbon dioxide or carbon dioxide tension	Arterial blood: 35-45 mm Hg Venous blood: 40-50 mm Hg	Measure of carbon dioxide tension; reflects carbonic acid concentration of plasma
CO_2	Carbon dioxide content or carbon dioxide combining power	Newborn: 19-27 mEq/liter Infant: 20-28 mEq/liter Young child: 18-27 mEq/liter Older child: 23-29 mEq/liter	Concentration of base bicarbonate
BE	Base excess	Newborn: +4 to −4 Child: +2 to −2	Used to express extent of deviation from normal buffer base concentration; indicates quantity of blood buffers remaining after hydrogen ion is buffered

*Data from Vaughan, V. C., and McKay, R. J., editors: Textbook of pediatrics, ed. 10, Philadelphia, 1975, W. B. Saunders Co.

Table 29-3. Summary of simple acid-base disturbances (partially compensated)

Disturbance	Plasma pH	Plasma Pco_2	Plasma HCO_3
Respiratory acidosis	↓	↑	↑
Respiratory alkalosis	↑	↓	↓
Metabolic acidosis	↓	↓	↓
Metabolic alkalosis	↑	↑	N or ↑

Acid-base imbalance

The pH, representing the concentration of hydrogen ions, indicates only whether the imbalance is acidosis or alkalosis. It does not reflect the nature of the imbalance, that is, whether it is of metabolic or respiratory origin. Body metabolism affects primarily the base bicarbonate; therefore, alterations in the concentration of base bicarbonate are termed *metabolic* disturbances of acid-base balance, and, since the amount of carbon dioxide exhaled through the lungs affects the carbonic acid, changes in the carbonic acid concentration are referred to as *respiratory* disturbances. Consequently the simple disturbances, that is, those with a single primary cause, are categorized as metabolic acidosis or alkalosis and respiratory acidosis or alkalosis.[12]

It is also significant that the major signs and symptoms of hydrogen ion imbalances, acidosis and alkalosis, are reflections of central nervous system involvement. Depression of the central nervous system, manifest by lethargy, diminished mental capacity, delirium, stupor, and coma, is observed in acidosis of either metabolic or respiratory origin. Alkalosis, on the other hand, produces clinical manifestations of nervous system stimulation and excitement, including overexcitability, nervousness, tingling sensations, and tetany that may progress to convulsions. Persons with epilepsy are particularly susceptible to seizures, which can be precipitated by hyperventilation. The extent and severity of signs and symptoms depend on the length of time the imbalance has existed and the magnitude or degree of the deviation from normal. A rapid, severe imbalance will seriously compromise the compensatory mechanisms to the point where it is incompatible with life, whereas the body will be able to compensate adequately for a mild, gradual distortion and produce few, if any, observable signs or symptoms.[11]

Respiratory acidosis. Respiratory acidosis results from diminished or inadequate pulmonary ventilation that causes an elevated plasma Pco_2 with an increased concentration of dissolved carbon dioxide, which leads to elevated carbonic acid and hydrogen ion concentration. Conditions that produce respiratory acidosis can originate at three levels in the respiratory system and result in inadequate gas exchange. These are[16]:

1. Factors that depress the respiratory center, such as head injury, depressant or narcotizing drugs, and infections of the central nervous system
2. Factors that affect the lung proper, such as obstructive pulmonary disease, pneumonia, cystic fibrosis, acute pulmonary edema, atelectasis, and occlusion of respiratory passages
3. Factors that interfere with the bellows action of the chest wall, including trauma to the chest wall, skeletal diseases or deformities, and diseases of the thoracic muscles or their innervation (such as muscular dystrophy or muscular atrophy)

Compensation is mediated through the kidneys, which are stimulated to conserve and thus increase the plasma bicarbonate concentration and to excrete hydrogen ions. Laboratory findings in respiratory acidosis include lowered urine pH (less than 7.35), elevated plasma bicarbonate concentration (over 29 mEq/liter in older children, over 25 mEq/liter in young children), and elevated Pco_2 (above 38 mm Hg, arterial).

The treatment of respiratory acidosis is aimed at correcting the primary defect, improving gas exchange at the alveolar level to provide more efficient removal of carbon dioxide, and administration of buffers such as bicarbonate or the organic buffer tromethamine (THAM) to reduce hydrogen ion concentration during critical periods.

Respiratory alkalosis. Conversely respiratory alkalosis is caused by a primary increase in the rate and depth of pulmonary ventilation, resulting in unusually large amounts of carbon dioxide being exhaled or "blown off." This reduces the plasma Pco_2, carbonic acid, and hydrogen ion concentration and leaves an excess of base bicarbonate. Conditions that cause stimulation of the respiratory center to produce hyperventilation include[16]:

1. Primary central nervous system stimulation resulting from emotions, including hysteria, fear, or apprehension; central nervous system infection (encephalitis); and certain drug reactions, such as early salicylate intoxication (a primary respiratory stimulant)
2. Reflex central nervous system stimulation from peripheral chemoreceptors as a result of hypoxia, which provides the stimulus for hyperventilation at high altitudes, fever or high environmental temperatures, and cardiac conditions
3. Reflex central nervous system stimulation from intrathoracic stretch receptors, which is believed to be the cause of hyperventilation in localized pulmonary disease

A frequent cause of hyperventilation in children is voluntary hyperventilation prior to underwater swimming. It is also a consideration in the care of persons on assisted ventilation. Incorrectly set mechanical ventilators can cause respiratory rates and tidal volumes in excess of physiologic needs.

Compensation of respiratory alkalosis takes place in the kidneys and consists of excretion of bicarbonate in association with sodium and potassium ions to conserve hydrogen ions. Laboratory findings include elevated urine pH (over 7), elevated plasma pH (over 7.45), depressed plasma bicarbonate concentration (less than 25 mEq/liter in older children, less than 20 mEq/liter in young children), and lowered Pco_2.[12]

Treatment of respiratory alkalosis consists of correction of the primary defect and prevention of lost anions and the associated potassium deficit. Carbon dioxide administered by mask slows respirations and provides rapid relief.

Metabolic acidosis. Metabolic acidosis is a lowered plasma pH caused by any process that reduces the base bicarbonate concentration. Metabolic acidosis can be produced by the gain of nonvolatile acids or the loss of base bicarbonate. Strong acid is gained by several specific mechanisms, including the following[16]:

1. Gain of exogenous acid (such as ammonium chloride) by ingestion or infusion
2. Incomplete oxidation of fatty acids, which occurs in conditions such as diabetic acidosis, starvation (including patients receiving nothing by mouth for therapeutic purposes), and salicylate poisoning
3. Incomplete oxidation of carbohydrate that produces large amounts of lactic acid as a result of primary lactic acidosis (rare) or secondary to tissue hypoxia from excessive exercise, severe trauma, and severe infections
4. Inability of the renal system to excrete the normal, ongoing production of inorganic acid metabolites resulting from the azotemic acidosis of advanced renal failure

Base bicarbonate is lost from the extracellular fluid by the following two general routes:

1. Losses from the gastrointestinal tract—secretions distal to the pyloric sphincter contain large amounts of bicarbonate, which may be lost during conditions that produce diarrhea or vomiting, including fistula drainage and suction.
2. Losses as a result of inappropriate bicarbonate excretion in the kidneys as a result of renal tubular acidosis

Compensation of metabolic acidosis is respiratory. Strong acids are immediately buffered to generate the weaker carbonic acid, which the respiratory system attempts to eliminate through increased alveolar ventilation. In this respiratory effort the breathing is deep and rapid—the Kussmaul or air hunger type of respirations. Bicarbonate conservation and excretion by the kidneys is a slower mechanism. Laboratory findings of uncompensated metabolic acidosis include lowered urine pH (less than 6), lowered plasma pH (below 7.35), diminished plasma bicarbonate concentration (below 25 mEq/liter in older children, below 20 mEq/liter in young children), and carbon dioxide combining power that is lowered and approximately equivalent to the plasma bicarbonate in concentration.[12]

Treatment is directed toward correction of the basic defect and replacement of the excessive losses of bicarbonate with sodium or potassium bicarbonate or sodium lactate.

Metabolic alkalosis. Metabolic alkalosis is an elevated plasma pH that occurs when there is a reduction of hydrogen ion concentration and an excess of base bicarbonate. This can be caused by a gain in base or a loss of acid, which is almost the same as base gain. Loss of acid can result from the following:

1. In children the most common cause of hydrogen ion depletion is loss of hydrochloric acid (HCl) incident to hypertrophic pyloric stenosis. The infant produces large

amounts of hydrochloric acid, which is vomited with repeated feedings
2. Less often, hydrogen ions are lost through the kidney in diuretic therapy, potassium depletion, or administration of adrenocortical hormones

A gain in base is usually iatrogenic and relatively uncommon in children but can result from the following:

1. Gain of exogenous bicarbonate from ingestion or infusion
2. Oxidation of the salts or organic acid from infusion or ingestion of lactate, citrate, or acetate

Compensation in metabolic alkalosis theoretically should be respiratory; however, such compensation is irregular and unpredictable. Also, renal correction is complicated by losses of sodium, potassium, and chloride ions, which accompany vomiting in pyloric stenosis. The kidneys will attempt to conserve the sodium and potassium ion concentration at the expense of hydrogen ion concentration and acid-base balance. Laboratory findings include elevated urine pH (often above 7; may be lowered if associated with potassium ion depletion), elevated plasma pH (above 7.45), elevated plasma bicarbonate concentration (above 27 mEq/liter in older children, above 25 mEq/liter in young children), and, if associated with chloride deficit, reduced chloride ion concentration (below 98 mEq/liter).[12]

Treatment of metabolic alkalosis is aimed at preventing further losses of acid and replacement of lost electrolytes.

Associated disturbances in acidosis and alkalosis

Physiologic functions of the body take place optimally when the pH is maintained within a normal range. The disequilibrium created by moderately altered pH can produce disordered function of physiologic and enzyme systems, but great divergences are incompatible with life. Also, electrolyte shifts that take place in response to changes in pH alter the electrolyte concentration in the fluid compartments to disturb the normal concentrations. For example, cell membrane permeability is affected by changes in pH. A lowered pH allows potassium to move from the intracellular to the extracellular fluid. Serum potassium levels increase with acidosis and decrease with alkalosis.

One of the disturbances that complicates both fluid losses and acid-base imbalance is an alteration in potassium levels. During dehydration, fluid moves out of the intracellular fluid compartment into the extracellular fluid compartment in an attempt to balance the fluid losses. In doing so, potassium also moves out, creating a total body potassium depletion. Since renal function is drastically reduced in dehydration, normal excretion of potassium does not take place. This causes elevated serum levels that can produce all the signs and symptoms of hyperkalemia. During rapid rehydration therapy for gastrointestinal losses and diabetic ketoacidosis, the extracellular fluid potassium moves back into the intracellular fluid compartment, thereby creating the risk of hypokalemia unless there is anticipated replacement. However, potassium is not replaced until the intravascular fluid is sufficient to restore adequate renal function.

Disturbed extracellular fluid calcium levels may occur in various types of dehydration. Usually the disturbance is in the form of reduced serum calcium levels, especially where there is a concomitant potassium loss. Although the hypocalcemia is a common finding, it rarely reaches a point of tetany in current practice that includes adequate replacement of potassium losses. Immediate effects of calcium imbalance associated with acidosis or alkalosis are seen in the tetany of metabolic alkalosis and long-term effects related to bone resorption in chronic acidosis from renal disturbances (p. 1178).

The capacity of oxygen to combine with hemoglobin is also affected by changes in pH. The affinity of hemoglobin for oxygen decreases with a decrease in pH so that, in a state of acidosis, less oxygen will be picked up by the hemoglobin as blood travels through the lungs. However, the oxygen is more easily released to the tissues when the pH is lowered. The opposite effects operate during an increase in pH.

Blood flow in various areas is altered by changes in pH. Pulmonary circulation constricts in acidosis, whereas a decreased pH causes vasodilatation in systemic vessels.

DISTURBANCES OF FLUID AND ELECTROLYTE BALANCE

Disturbances of fluids and their solute concentration are closely interrelated. Alterations in fluid volume affect the electrolyte component, and changes in electrolyte concentration influence fluid movement. Intracellular water and electrolytes depend on diffusion and transport to and from the extracellular fluid compartment so that any imbalance in the intracellular fluid is a reflection of an imbalance in the extracellular fluid. Disturbances in the extracellular fluid involve either an excess or a deficit of fluid and/or electrolytes; of these, fluid loss occurs more frequently. Depletion of extracellular fluid, usually caused by gastroenteritis, is one of the most common problems encountered in infants and children. Until modern techniques for fluid replacement were perfected, it was one of the chief causes of infant mortality. Fluid and electrolyte problems related to specific diseases and their management are discussed throughout the book where appropriate. The major fluid and electrolyte disturbances, their most frequent causes, and clinical manifestations are outlined in Table 29-4, and the most common disturbances — dehydration and edema — will be elaborated further. Problems of fluid and electrolyte disturbance always involve both water and electrolytes; therefore, replacement always includes administration of

Text continued on p. 1080.

Table 29-4. Disturbances of fluid and electrolyte balance

Primary disturbance	Mechanisms	Clinical situations	Clinical manifestations	Laboratory findings	Comments
Water depletion	Complete sudden cessation of water intake Prolonged diminished intake Failure to absorb or reabsorb water Loss from gastrointestinal tract Excessive renal excretion Extrarenal causes	Neglect of intake by self or care giver—confused, psychotic, unconscious, or helpless (infant, handicapped) Diarrhea or other intestinal disorders such as obstruction Vomiting, diarrhea, fistula, nasogastric suction Disturbed body fluid chemistry Inappropriate antidiuretic hormone secretion (head injury, diabetes insipidus) Glycosuria of diabetes mellitus	General symptoms: Thirst Variable temperature—can be increased (infection) or decreased (shock states) Dry skin and mucous membranes Poor skin turgor Longitudinal wrinkles in tongue Weight loss Fatigue	High specific gravity of urine (except in inappropriate antidiuretic hormone secretion) Increased blood urea nitrogen Serum sodium concentration variable Potassium levels normal or increased Increased hematocrit	Symptoms depend to some extent on proportion of electrolytes lost with water
	Renal causes Iatrogenic	Renal disease Overzealous use of diuretics Improper postoperative fluid replacement	Oliguria Depressed fontanel (infant) Irritability and lethargy		
	Loss through skin or lungs Excessive perspiration or vaporization	Hyperventilation Febrile states Increase in ambient temperature such as by use of an overheated warmer Heat prostration	Sunken eyeballs Severe symptoms Signs of shock Soft eyeballs Rapid pulse and respirations Low blood pressure		
	Impaired integrity of skin	Transudate from burns, wounds, and so on Hemorrhage			
Interstitial fluid–to–plasma shift	Recovery from plasma–to–interstitial fluid shift (remobilization of edema fluid)	Recovery from burns	Signs of hypervolemia—bounding pulse, peripheral vein engorgement, moist rales in lungs, weakness, pallor, hyperpnea	Decreased red blood cell count, packed cell volume, hemoglobin concentration	
	Volume replacement after hypovolemia	Hemorrhage Administration of excessive amounts of blood, plasma, blood expanders, or hypertonic solutions			
Water excess	Water intake in excess of output	Excessive oral intake Overloading with hypotonic solutions or glucose and water Plain water enemas	Edema: Generalized Pulmonary (moist rales) Intracutaneous, particularly noted in loose areolar tissue of eyelids and scrotum	Low specific gravity of urine Dilution of electrolytes Decreased hematocrit Variable urine volume	
	Failure to excrete water in presence of normal intake	Kidney disease Congestive heart failure Malnutrition	Elevated venous pressure Bradycardia Weight gain		

			Lethargy Increased spinal fluid pressure Cerebral manifestations such as convulsions, coma		
Plasma-to-interstitial fluid shift	Portal hypertension Decreased oncotic pressure with increased capillary permeability: Cutaneous Renal Vasodilatation Decreased venous return	Chronic liver disease Malnutrition Starvation edema Burns Massive crushing injury Nephrotic syndrome Shock	Ascites Peripheral edema Signs of hypovolemia—pallor, tachycardia, low blood pressure, weak pulse, cold extremities, disorientation	Elevated hematocrit, red blood cell count, packed cell volume	
Sodium depletion (hyponatremia)	Inadequate sodium intake Loss through perspiration Loss through nonintact skin Loss through gastrointestinal tract Excessive renal excretion	Prolonged low-sodium diet Fever Excess sweating Cystic fibrosis Burns and wounds Vomiting, diarrhea Nasogastric suction, fistulas Adrenal insufficiency Renal disease Diabetic acidosis	Associated with water loss: Same as with water loss—dehydration, weakness, dizziness, nausea, abdominal cramps, apprehension Mild—apathy, weakness, nausea, soft pulse Moderate—decreased blood pressure	N = 140 mEq/liter; Sodium concentration may be high, low, or normal Specific gravity depends on water deficit or excess	May be associated with water deficit or excess
Sodium excess (hypernatremia)	Increased intake without increase in output Decreased output (renal disease)	High-salt intake—nasogastric or intravenous Renal disease	Intense thirst Dry, sticky mucous membranes Flushed skin Temperature may be increased Hoarseness Oliguria Nausea and vomiting Firm tissue turgor Irritability and possible progression to disorientation, convulsions	Serum sodium concentration increased or normal High plasma volume Alkalosis	
Potassium depletion (hypokalemia)	Inadequate intake of potassium Loss from gastrointestinal tract	Starvation Clinical conditions associated with poor food intake Intravenous fluid without added potassium Diarrhea, vomiting, fistulas, nasogastric suction	Muscle weakness, stiffness, paralysis, hyporeflexia Hypotension Cardiac arrhythmias, gallop rhythm Tachycardia or bradycardia	N = 4.1-5.6 mEq/liter Decreased serum potassium concentration Abnormal ECG:—flat T waves, prolonged ST segment	

Continued.

Table 29-4. Disturbances of fluid and electrolyte balance—cont'd

Primary disturbance	Mechanisms	Clinical situations	Clinical manifestations	Laboratory findings	Comments
Potassium depletion (hypokalemia)—cont'd	Excessive renal excretion	Diuresis Administration of diuretics Administration of corticosteroids Diuretic phase of nephrotic syndrome Healing stage of burns Potassium-losing nephritis Hyperglycemic diuresis Familial periodic paralysis	Ileus Apathy, drowsiness Irritability Fatigue		
	Movement from extracellular to intracellular fluid	Intravenous administration of insulin in ketoacidosis Alkalosis			
Potassium excess (hyperkalemia)	Inadequate excretion	Renal disease Renal shutdown Adrenal insufficiency (Addison's disease) Associated with metabolic acidosis	Muscle weakness, flaccid paralysis Twitching Hyperreflexia Bradycardia Ventricular fibrillation and cardiac arrest Oliguria	High serum potassium concentration Variable urine volume Flat P wave on ECG	
	Increased intake	Too rapid administration of intravenous potassium chloride Transfusion with old donor blood			
	Movement from intracellular to extracellular fluid	Severe dehydration Crushing injuries Burns Hemolysis from sudden massive water intake	Apnea—respiratory arrest		
	Hemoconcentration	Dehydration			

Chloride depletion (hypochloremia)	Inadequate intake	Starvation Inadequate replacement of losses	Symptoms associated with alkalosis—lethargy, muscle hypertonicity Depressed respirations Metabolic alkalosis	N = 100 mEq/liter High carbon dioxide combining power Low plasma chloride concentration
	Excessive excretion	Vomiting Pyloric obstruction Nasogastric suction		
Chloride excess (hyperchloremia)	Excessive ingestion	Treatment with ammonium chloride	Tachypnea Weakness Symptoms associated with acidosis	Low carbon dioxide combining power High plasma chloride concentration
	Decreased output	Renal disease		
Calcium depletion (hypocalcemia)	Inadequate intake Malabsorption from gastrointestinal tract	Inadequate dietary calcium Vitamin D deficiency Rapid transit through gastrointestinal tract	Neuromuscular irritability Tingling of nose, ears, fingertips, toes Tetany Laryngospasm Generalized convulsions May be changes in clotting Positive Chvostek's sign Cardiac arrest	N = 4-5 mEq/liter Decreased serum calcium concentration
	Excessive losses of calcium Decreased bone resorption Unavailable for use as ionized calcium	Advanced renal insufficiency Hypoparathyroidism Alkalosis Trapped in diseased tissues Cow's milk formula—tetany of the newborn Exchange transfusion with titrated blood		
Calcium excess (hypercalcemia)	Converted from nonionized to ionized form	Acidosis Prolonged immobilization Conditions associated with increased bone catabolism	Few problems Constipation Anorexia Dryness of mouth Muscle hypotonicity	Increased calcium concentration in urine—may cause formation of kidney stones
	Inadequate elimination Increased absorption of calcium from gastrointestinal tract	Kidney disease Hypervitaminosis D		
	Increased resorption of calcium by kidney	Hyperparathyroidism		

both, calculated on the basis of ongoing processes and laboratory serum electrolyte values.

In problems that involve alterations in the amount and composition of body fluid compartments, the following five areas are considered when planning management[6]:

1. Volume of the body fluids, that is, the water content of the patient
2. Osmolality of the body fluids, a factor that has an effect on the distribution of body water among the various compartments
3. Hydrogen ion status, that is, whether or not there has been a disturbance in the pH of body fluids or a disturbance in the homeostatic mechanisms that maintain the pH
4. Electrolyte deficits from cells as well as extracellular water
5. Disturbances in the equilibrium between the mineral skeleton and body fluids

Dehydration

Dehydration is one of the most common body fluid disturbances encountered in nursing of infants and children and occurs whenever the total output of fluid exceeds the total intake, regardless of the underlying cause. Although dehydration can result from lack of oral intake, more often it is a result of abnormal losses, such as those that occur in vomiting or diarrhea, when oral intake only partially compensates for the abnormal losses.

In early dehydration (the first 2 days), fluid loss is derived from both the extracellular and the intracellular fluid as the increased osmolality of the diminished extracellular fluid volume causes fluid from the intracellular compartment to move into the extracellular fluid compartment. As dehydration becomes chronic, the cellular losses become predominant. Dehydration can be classified as three general types according to the compositional changes in the plasma: (1) isotonic or iso-osmotic, (2) hypotonic or hypo-osmotic, and (3) hypertonic or hyperosmotic.

Isotonic dehydration. Isotonic (iso-osmotic) dehydration occurs in conditions in which the electrolyte and water deficits are present in approximately balanced proportion. The observable fluid losses are not necessarily isotonic, but losses from other avenues make adjustments so that the sum of all losses, or the net loss, is isotonic. Since there is no osmotic force present to cause a redistribution of water between the intracellular and extracellular fluid, the major loss is sustained from the extracellular compartments. This significantly reduces the plasma volume and, hence, the circulating blood volume with its effect on skin, muscle, and kidneys. Shock is the greatest threat to life in isotonic dehydration, and the child with isotonic dehydration displays the symptoms characteristic of hypovolemic shock. Plasma sodium remains within normal limits, between 130 and 150 mEq/liter.

Hypotonic dehydration. Hypotonic (hypo-osmotic) dehydration occurs when the electrolyte deficit exceeds the water deficit. Since intracellular fluid is more concentrated than extracellular fluid in hypotonic dehydration, water moves from the extracellular to the intracellular fluid to establish osmotic equilibrium. Therefore, this further increases the extracellular fluid volume loss, and shock is a frequent finding. Since there is a greater proportional loss of extracellular fluid in hypotonic dehydration, the physical signs tend to be more severe with smaller fluid losses than isotonic or hypertonic dehydration. Plasma sodium concentration is less than 130 mEq/liter.

Hypertonic dehydration. Hypertonic (hyperosmotic) dehydration results from water loss in excess of electrolyte loss and is usually caused by either a proportionately larger loss of water and/or a larger intake of electrolytes. This sometimes occurs in infants with diarrhea who are given fluids by mouth that contain large amounts of solute or in children receiving high-protein nasogastric tube feedings that place an excessive solute load on the kidneys. In hypertonic dehydration fluid shifts from the lesser concentration of the intracellular to the extracellular fluid. Plasma

Table 29-5. Physical signs of dehydration

	Isotonic (loss of water and salt)	Hypotonic (loss of salt in excess of water)	Hypertonic (loss of water in excess of salt)
Skin			
Color	Gray	Gray	Gray
Temperature	Cold	Cold	Cold or hot
Turgor	Poor	Very poor	Fair
Feel	Dry	Clammy	Thickened
Mucous membranes	Dry	Slightly moist	Parched
Tearing and salivation	Absent	Absent	Absent
Eyeball	Sunken and soft	Sunken and soft	Sunken
Fontanel	Sunken	Sunken	Sunken
Body temperature	Subnormal or elevated	Subnormal	Subnormal or elevated
Pulse	Rapid	Very rapid	Moderately rapid
Respirations	Rapid	Rapid	Rapid
Behavior	Irritable to lethargic	Lethargic to comatose; convulsions	Marked lethargy with extreme hyperirritability on stimulation

sodium concentration is greater than 150 mEq/liter. Since the extracellular fluid volume is proportionately larger, hypertonic dehydration has a larger degree of water loss for the same intensity of physical signs. Shock is less apparent in hypertonic dehydration. However, neurologic disturbances, such as seizures, are more likely to occur. Cerebral changes are serious and may result in permanent damage. Table 29-5 outlines the general physical signs of dehydration.

Degree of dehydration. The magnitude of fluid loss is best ascertained by a comparison of preillness weight with the current weight, since any weight loss is substantially equivalent to the amount of water lost. If preillness weight is unknown, the degree of dehydration is estimated by assessing the intensity of clinical signs. In infants, who are most vulnerable to rapid and extensive fluid losses, isotonic dehydration is usually described as 5% (mild), 10% (moderate), and 15% (severe). Older children and adolescents, with proportionately less total body water, display smaller proportional losses; therefore, the estimates of 3%, 6% and 9% values more nearly describe mild, moderate, and severe dehydration in these age-groups.[15]

Shock is a common feature of severe depletion of extracellular fluid volume with tachycardia and low blood pressure. Peripheral circulation is poor as a result of reduced blood volume; therefore, the skin is cool and mottled, with poor capillary filling after blanching. Impaired kidney circulation often leads to oliguria and prerenal azotemia (see p. 1171). Skin and mucous membranes are dry, skin turgor is poor, and, in infants, the anterior fontanel is depressed. At the opposite extreme, a mild degree of dehydration is associated with barely discernible physical signs and absence of shock (Table 29-6).

Medical management. Medical management is directed toward correcting the fluid imbalance and treating the underlying cause. To initiate a therapeutic plan, there are several factors that must be determined[3]: the degree of dehydration based on physical assessment; the type of dehydration based on the pathophysiology of the specific illness responsible for the dehydrated state, specific physical signs other than general signs, and initial plasma sodium concentrations; and associated electrolyte (especially serum potassium) and acid-base imbalances. Initial and regular, ongoing evaluations are carried out to assess the patient's progress toward equilbrium and the effectiveness of therapy. Assessment makes use of two major types of information:

1. Clinical observation—accurate body weights, circulatory status, urinary output, and the presence and intensity of signs of dehydration
2. Chemical analysis—blood plasma electrolyte (sodium, potassium, and chloride ion) concentrations, blood urea nitrogen (BUN), acid-base status, hemoglobin, and plasma protein concentrations; urine specific gravity; pH; and the presence or absence of sugar and ketone bodies

Most dehydration is of the mild form and can be managed at home with oral administration of fluids. Full diet is usually withheld until the child is well hydrated and the basic problem is under control. Parenteral fluid therapy is instigated whenever the child is unable to ingest sufficient amounts of fluid and electrolytes to (1) meet ongoing daily physiologic losses, (2) replace previous deficits, and (3) replace ongoing abnormal losses.

In moderate and severe dehydration, replacement of body fluid deficits includes three phases. Since it constitutes the greatest threat to life, the first priority is restoration of circulation by rapid expansion of the extracellular fluid volume, either to treat shock or to prevent its occurrence. Intravenous administration of fluid is begun immediately, even though the exact nature of the dehydration and the serum electrolyte values are not known. The solution selected is based on what is known regarding the probable type and cause of the dehydration—usually a saline solution. Sodium bicarbonate may be added, since acidosis is usually associated with severe dehydration, but potassium is not administered until kidney function is restored, unless the child is known to be hypokalemic. As the circulation improves, the glomerular filtration pressure increases to improve renal function, which is essential to electrolyte readjustments.

The goal of the next phase is the restoration of extracellular fluid volume. With improved circulation, water and

Table 29-6. Intensity of clinical signs associated with varying degrees of isotonic dehydration in infants

	Degree of dehydration		
	Mild	**Moderate**	**Severe**
Body weight	Up to 5%	5%-9%	10%-15%
Skin color	Pale	Gray	Mottled
Skin turgor	Decreased	Poor	Very poor
Mucous membranes	Dry	Very dry	Parched
Urine output	Decreased	Oliguria	Marked oliguria and azotemia
Blood pressure	Normal	Normal or lowered	Lowered
Pulse	Normal or increased	Increased	Rapid and thready

electrolyte deficits can be evaluated and acid-base status corrected either directly through fluids administered or indirectly through improved renal function. Next, potassium lost in intracellular fluid must be replaced slowly by way of the extracellular fluid. Finally, the body fat and protein stores are replaced through diet. If the child is unable to eat or if feeding aggravates the condition (such as diarrhea), intravenous alimentation is provided to prevent serious malnourishment. Table 29-7 outlines the goals of therapy and expected outcome in the management of dehydration.

While the initial phase of fluid replacement is rapid in both isotonic and hypotonic dehydration, it is contraindicated in hypertonic dehydration because of the risk of water intoxication, especially of the brain cells. There is an apparent physiologic difference in the manner and length of time for diffusion of sodium into and out of brain cells. There is a significant time lag for sodium to reach a steady state in these cells, whereas water diffuses almost instantaneously. Consequently rapid administration of fluid will cause equally rapid diffusion of water into the dehydrated brain cells, causing marked cerebral edema. Since extracellular fluid volume is maintained relatively well in hypertonic as opposed to the other types of dehydration, shock is not a usual manifestation.

Edema

Edema is the presence of excess fluid in the interstitial spaces as a result of some defect in the normal circulation of body fluids that causes increased pressure in the interstitial spaces. Fluid removal from the interstitial spaces depends on the following:

1. Venous hydrostatic pressure
2. Colloidal osmotic pressure of both the intravascular and interstitial spaces
3. Intact semipermeable capillary wall
4. Tissue tension
5. Lymphatic flow

A defect in any of these factors can cause fluid accumulation of interstitial fluid and disease results from anything that (1) alters the retention of sodium, such as renal disease or hormonal influences; (2) affects the formation or destruction of plasma proteins, such as starvation or liver disease; and (3) alters membrane permeability, such as nephrotic syndrome or trauma. Edema may be localized to a small or large area, as seen in urticaria, infection, and pulmonary congestion, or it can be generalized, as in the hypoproteinemia of the nephrotic syndrome and starvation. A severe, generalized accumulation of great amounts of fluid in all body tissues is termed *anasarca*.

Increased venous pressure. The colloidal osmotic pressure of the plasma proteins draws fluid back into the vascular system as long as this force is greater than the venous hydrostatic pressure. However, when the venous pressure is increased, fluid tends to be retained in the interstitial spaces. This occurs when an individual remains in the

Table 29-7. Principles of therapy and expected outcomes for dehydration

Phase	Goal	Method	Expected outcome
I	Restore circulation (0-24 hours)	Intravenous administration of fluid containing appropriate Na^+ and anion composition, usually both Cl^- and HCO_3^-; 20-30 ml/kg at 10 ml/kg/hour	Improved circulation as evidenced by increased blood pressure, stronger pulse, and peripheral circulation Increase in urine output Improved level of consciousness
II	Restore extracellular fluid and more completely correct deficits and acid-base status 2-4 to 18-24 hours	Continuation of therapy in phase I at slower rate of infusion	Weight gain Sustained adequate urine output Stable adequate circulation Diminished intensity in physical signs of dehydration Partial or complete restoration of abnormal Na^+ Decreased blood urea nitrogen Partial adjustment of acid-base disequilibrium
III	Repair body potassium in status (18-24 to 2-4 days)	Carefully calculated intravenous and/or oral electrolyte solutions based on laboratory findings; 125-150 ml/kg/day Na^+-K^+ maintenance solution	Sustained gain in body weight Normal or decreased blood urea nitrogen; normal Na^+, K^+, and acid-base balance
IV	Restore caloric and protein deficiencies (2-4 days to 1-3 weeks)	Gradually resume normal diet; nature of diet depends on basic pathologic condition	Slow steady weight gain Normal plasma constituents

Data from Dell, R. B.: In Winters, R. W., editor: The body fluids in pediatrics, Boston, 1973, Little, Brown and Co.

same position for a long period of time, such as swollen ankles and feet after standing or sitting for long periods. Constrictive dressings or restraints applied too tightly to extremities will obstruct venous return, increase venous and capillary pressure, and cause edema. The most graphic pathologic illustrations are pulmonary edema caused by pulmonary circulation overload in cardiac defects with a left-to-right shunt (p. 1342) and ascites caused by portal hypertension (p. 1293). Edema from any cause is increased in dependent areas because of this added factor of increased venous hydrostatic pressure and the gravitational effects in these areas.

Capillary permeability. Damage to capillary walls or alteration in their permeability will permit exudation of plasma protein into the interstitial space. Most commonly this occurs as local edema, such as seen in inflammatory and hypersensitivity reactions. Capillary damage from burns allows extensive exudation of protein-rich fluid into the interstitial spaces to compound edema formation.

Diminished plasma proteins. A fall in plasma protein levels hampers the osmotic pull back into the vessels. Consequently fluid remains in the interstitial spaces. Although other factors play a role, such as hydrostatic pressure of both the arterial vascular system and the tissues and sodium ion concentration, significantly low protein levels (below 4.5 mg%) are associated with edema. Examples of this are the massive albumin losses of the nephrotic syndrome (p. 1153), diminished serum protein from insufficient dietary protein, and (sometimes) hemodilution of plasma proteins from intravenous fluid administration in chronic dehydration.

Lymphatic obstruction. Obstruction of lymph flow creates edema high in protein content. This is uncommon in childhood but can result from trauma to the lymphatic glands or removal of lymph nodes.

Tissue tension. As mentioned earlier, edema appears earlier and more readily in loose structures such as those in the periorbital and genital tissues. The areolar structure of tissue is probably a contributing factor in pulmonary edema as well as in increased hydrostatic pressure in the pulmonary vessels.

Other factors in edema formation. Any factor that causes sodium retention by the kidneys will produce or augment edema formation. This includes stimulation of the renin-angiotensin-aldosterone mechanisms for sodium reabsorption created by the diminished plasma volume in edema resulting from primary causes. The salt-retaining property of steroids is responsible for the edema associated with their administration.

A particularly threatening form of edema is cerebral edema caused by trauma, infection, or other etiologic factors, including vascular overload or injudicious intravenous administration of hypotonic solutions. The problems and assessment of cerebral edema, discussed on p. 1424, are always nursing considerations in fluid administration.

Medical management. The primary goal in management of edema is treatment of the basic pathology, which will be discussed in relation to the specific disorders. However, an essential aspect in management of any fluid overload is early recognition, in which nurses play a vital role.

NURSING RESPONSIBILITIES IN FLUID AND ELECTROLYTE DISTURBANCES

Nursing observation and intervention are essential to the detection and therapeutic management of disturbances in fluid and electrolyte balance. There are a wide variety of circumstances in which imbalances may be precipitated, and the balance is so precarious, especially in infants, that changes can take place in a very short time. Therefore, an important nursing responsibility is perceptive observation for any signs of imbalance, particularly in those situations and conditions in which imbalance is likely to occur. Conditions in which changes can occur with surprising rapidity in young children include diarrhea, vomiting; sweating; fever; disorders such as diabetes, renal disease, and cardiac anomalies; administration of certain drugs such as diuretics and steroids; and trauma, such as major surgery, burns, and other extensive injury.

Nurses need to be comfortable with equipment used to deliver fluids to infants and children and the knowledge and techniques for assessment. An understanding of normal serum values provides additional data on which to base assessments and interventions and to validate observations. Data that are helpful in assessment related to fluid and electrolyte balance are the medical diagnosis, the treatment that the child is receiving (especially medications and fluid therapies), laboratory reports, history, and records of intake and output. An important nursing role in child care is teaching parents to recognize early signs of dehydration.

Assessment

Whether the child is at home, in the physician's office or clinic, or in the hospital, nursing assessment is an essential part of the nursing care plan.

General appearance and behavior. The nursing assessment of infants and children with suspected or potential fluid and electrolyte disturbance begins with observation of general appearance. Ill children usually have drawn, flaccid expressions, and their eyes lack luster. Anorexia is one of the first behaviors observed in the majority of childhood illnesses, and the infant's or child's activity level is diminished. The cry of an ill infant is less vigorous, often whining, and higher pitched than usual. The child is irritable, seeks the comfort and attention of the mother, and displays purposeless movements and inappropriate responses to people and familiar things. As the child's illness becomes more severe, the irritability progresses to lethargy and even unconsciousness. Much of this information can be elicited from the parent, along with a history of excessive fluid losses, diminished output, and other clues to body fluid disturbance, for example, the number and consistency of stools the child has passed in the past 24 hours, the number of times voided, and the type and amount of food and fluid ingested, or vomited. Parents frequently omit this information. They tell how much has been taken but not how much is excreted. Information about the hospitalized child is acquired from persons who care for the child and from the chart and other records.

Objective observation. Observation of the status or changes in status of infants and children is vital in assessment of fluid and electrolyte status. A variety of parameters, as outlined in Table 29-8, are utilized to arrive at a meaningful assessment. Vital signs are assessed as often as every 15 to 30 minutes, and weight is recorded frequently during the initial phase of therapy. It is important to use the same scale each time the child is weighed and to predetermine the weight of any equipment and/or device that must remain attached during the weighing process, such as arm boards, sandbags, and so on. Routine weights should be taken at the same time each day.

Intake and output (I & O) measurement

One of the most important roles of the nurse in fluid and electrolyte disturbance is related to intake and output. Accurate measurements are essential to the assessment of fluid balance. This concerns measurements from all sources and includes both gastrointestinal and parenteral intake and output from urine, stools, vomitus, fistulas, nasogastric suction, sweat, and drainage from wounds. Although the physician usually indicates when intake and output are to be recorded, it is a nursing responsibility to keep an accurate intake and output record on patients in the following situations[12]:

Receiving intravenous therapy
After major surgery
Severe thermal burns or injuries
Renal disease or damage
Congestive heart failure
Dehydration
Diabetes mellitus
Oliguria
Diuretic therapy
Corticosteroid therapy

Infants or small children who are unable to use a bedpan or those who have bowel movements with every voiding will require the application of a collecting device (p. 929). If collecting bags are not used, wet diapers or pads are carefully weighed to ascertain the amount of fluid lost. This includes liquid stool, vomitus, and other losses. The volume of fluid in milliliters is equivalent to the weight of the fluid measured in grams. The specific gravity as a measure of osmolality is determined with a urinometer or a refractometer and assists in assessing the degree of hydration.

It is important to measure and record all intake, oral and parenteral, and output from all sources, including urine, stool, emesis, drainage tubes, fistulas, and wounds from which appreciable amounts of fluid are lost.

Nasogastric tubes

Special problems are encountered with infants and children who must be fed through a nasogastric or gastrostomy tube and those who require nasogastric suction. Nasogastric suction removes important electrolytes along with fluid from the stomach and intestine, which must be replaced by the parenteral route. If replacement is omitted or inadequate, imbalance is likely to occur; therefore, an accurate record of the amount and type of fluid entering and leaving the tube is crucial. When the tube requires irrigation to maintain patency, an electrolyte solution, usually saline, is used to prevent further depletion of electrolytes, since plain water irrigation stimulates electrolyte secretion and removal.

Tube-fed children are vulnerable to imbalances, principally in relation to solute load, with the ever-present threat of fluid deficit. This is especially true when tube feedings contain a large concentration of protein and the water intake is limited. An osmotic diuresis associated with the solute load can cause water to be drawn from tissues to supply a deceptively adequate urine output. Eventually hypernatremic dehydration and accumulation of nitrogenous waste products will occur. It is the nurse's responsibility to assure an adequate water intake, since most of these children, such as infants and unconscious, confused, or mentally retarded children, are unable either to perceive or respond to the stimulus of thirst. These children are not able to communicate the need for fluid. They must rely on the competence of the nurse to recognize signs of fluid deficit or hyperelectrolytemia and to take appropriate action.

Parenteral fluid therapy

Since most hospitalized infants and children with serious disturbance of fluid and electrolyte balance are almost always maintained on intravenous fluids, monitoring intravenous fluid replacement is a major nursing responsibility. Most of the general principles of intravenous therapy apply to infants and children, but with a number of important variations.

The site. The site selected for intravenous infusion depends on accessibility and convenience. In older children any accessible vein may be used. In small infants a scalp vein or a superficial vein of the wrist, hand, foot, or arm is usually most convenient and most easily stabilized (Fig. 29-5). Since superficial veins of the scalp have no valves, they can be infused in either direction and are used frequently for intravenous therapy in infants.[9]

Equipment. There are several modifications in equipment used for intravenous infusion for children. A gravity

Table 29-8. Significance of observations and probable problem

Observation	Significant variation	Probable imbalance	Comments
Temperature	Elevated	Early water depletion Sodium excess	Elevated temperature will increase rate of water loss
	Lowered	Fluid volume deficit	Caused by reduced energy output Shock is outcome of severe fluid deficit
Pulse	Rapid, weak, thready, easily obliterated	Circulatory collapse may result from fluid deficit, hemorrhage, plasma-to-interstitial fluid shift	Pulse rate should include assessment of volume and quality as well as rate
	Bounding, easily obliterated	Impending circulatory collapse Sodium deficit	Pulse may be influenced by activity or emotions
	Bounding, not easily obliterated	Fluid volume excess Interstitial fluid-to-plasma shift	
	Weak, irregular, rapid	Severe potassium deficit	
	Weak, irregular, slowing	Severe potassium excess	
	Increased	Sodium excess Magnesium deficit	
	Decreased	Magnesium excess	
Respiration	Slow, shallow	Respiratory alkalosis	Rapid respirations increase water loss
	Rapid, deep	Metabolic acidosis Respiratory alkalosis	Not a reliable sign of respiratory alkalosis in infants
	Dyspnea	Fluid volume excess either general or pulmonary	
	Moist rales	Fluid volume excess Pulmonary edema	
	Shallow	Potassium excess or deficit	Secondary to paralysis of respiratory muscles
	Stridor	Severe calcium deficit	
Blood pressure	Increased	Fluid volume excess	Blood pressure not a reliable sign in young children Elasticity of blood vessels may keep blood pressure stable
	Decreased	Sodium deficit Diminished vascular volume (loss or plasma-to-interstitial fluid shift) Severe potassium excess or deficit	
Skin			
Color	Pallor	Protein deficit Fluid deficit Fluid compartment shifts	
	Flushed	Sodium excess	
Temperature	Cold extremities	Severe fluid volume deficit, even with fever Severe sodium depletion	Caused by decreased peripheral blood flow
Feel	Dry	Fluid depletion Sodium excess	
	Clammy, cold	Sodium deficit Plasma-to-interstitial fluid shift Hypotonic dehydration	
	Poor capillary filling	Fluid volume deficit	
Turgor	Poor to very poor	Fluid depletion	Pinch of skin from abdomen or inner thigh is lifted and remains raised for several seconds
Pitting edema	Slight to severe	Fluid volume excess Plasma-to-interstitial fluid shift	Obese infants may appear normal

Compiled from Kee, J. L., and Gregory, A. P.: Nursing '74 **4:**28-36, 1974; Metheny, N. M., and Snively, W. D.: Nurses' handbook of fluid balance, Philadelphia, 1974, J. B. Lippincott Co.; and Burgess, A.: The nurses' guide to fluid and electrolyte balance, New York, 1970, McGraw-Hill Book Co.

Continued.

Table 29-8. Significance of observations and probable problem—cont'd

Observation	Significant variation	Probable imbalance	Comments
Mucous membranes	Dry Longitudinal wrinkles on tongue	Fluid volume depletion	
	Sticky; rough, red, dry tongue	Sodium excess Hypertonic dehydration	
Salivation and tearing	Absent	Fluid volume deficit	
Fontanel	Sunken	Fluid volume deficit	
Eyeballs	Sunken Soft	Fluid volume deficit	
Sensory alterations	Tingling in fingers and toes	Calcium deficit Alkalosis	Sensory alterations unreliable in infants and young children who are unable to communicate symptoms
	Abdominal cramps	Sodium deficit Potassium excess	
	Muscle cramps	Calcium deficit Potassium deficit	
	Lightheadedness	Respiratory alkalosis	
	Nausea	Calcium excess Potassium excess Potassium deficit	
	Thirst	Fluid deficit Sodium excess Calcium excess	May be difficult to assess in infants May be masked by nausea Any conditions that reduces intravascular volume will stimulate thirst receptors
Neurologic signs	Hypotonia	Potassium deficit Calcium excess	
	Flaccid paralysis	Severe potassium deficit Severe potassium excess	
	Weakness	Metabolic acidosis	
	Hypertonia		
	Positive Chvostek's sign	Calcium deficit	Children may suffer calcium deficit easily, since growing bones do not readily relinquish calcium to circulation
	Tremors, cramps, tetany	Alkalosis with diminished calcium ionization	
	Twitching	Calcium deficit Magnesium deficit	
Behavior	Lethargy	Fluid volume deficit	Behavioral changes among the first indication of dehydration as reported by parents
	Irritability	Fluid volume deficit	
	Comatose condition	Hypotonic fluid deficit Profound acidosis or alkalosis	
	Lethargy with hyperirritability on stimulation	Hypertonic fluid deficit	
	Extreme restlessness	Potassium excess	
Weight	Loss	Fluid deficit	
	Up to 5%	Mild	
	5% to 9%	Moderate	
	10% or above	Severe	
		Protein or calorie deficiency	
	Gain	Edema—general or pulmonary Ascites	
Urine	Increased (polyuria)	Interstitial fluid–to–plasma shift Increased renal solute load	Normal range* Newborn: 1.5-12.5 ml/hour Neonatal period: 11-18 ml/hour Infant: 17-25 ml/hour Child: 20-40 ml/hour Adolescent: 20-62 ml/hour
	Diminished	Mild fluid deficit	
	Oliguria	Moderate to severe fluid deficit Plasma–to–interstitial fluid shift Sodium deficit Potassium excess Severe sodium excess Renal insufficiency	

*Data from Vaughn, V. C., and McKay, R. J.: Textbook of pediatrics, ed. 10, Philadelphia, 1975, W. B. Saunders Co.

Table 29-8. Significance of observations and probable problem—cont'd

Observation	Significant variation	Probable imbalance	Comments
Urine—cont'd	Specific gravity		
	Low (1.010 or less)	Adequate hydration Fluid excess Renal disease Sodium deficit	Used to monitor hydration status in infants Fixed low reading seen in renal disease
	High (1.030 or above)	Fluid deficit Sodium excess Glycosuria Proteinuria	
	pH		
	Acid	Acidosis—metabolic or respiratory Alkalosis accompanied by severe potassium deficit	
	Alkaline	Alkalosis—metabolic or respiratory Hyperaldosteronism Acidosis accompanied by chronic renal infection and renal tubular dysfunction Diuretic therapy with carbonic anhydrase inhibitors	

drainage apparatus used for children is much the same as that for adults except that it is designed to deliver a reduced drop size (60 drops/ml) and contains a calibrated volume control chamber that limits the maximum amount of fluid that can be infused. A microdropper greatly facilitates calculation of flow rate because a prescribed number of milliliters per hour equals the number of drops per minute. For example, if the solution is to infuse at a rate of 30 ml/hour, the nurse regulates the infusion to deliver 30 drops per minute. A variety of types are available, but all have a limited capacity, refillable from the bottle above, to minimize the possibility of overloading the circulation (Fig. 29-6). When using this device it is important that the tubing between the bottle and the chamber is firmly clamped to prevent additional fluid from dripping into the chamber. When sets with collapsible chambers and rigid cylinders with an automatic shutoff valve are employed, the infusion stops automatically when the chamber is empty. It is an important nursing responsibility to calculate the amount to be infused in a given length of time, set the infusion rate, and monitor the apparatus frequently to make certain that the desired rate is maintained and the infusion does not stop.

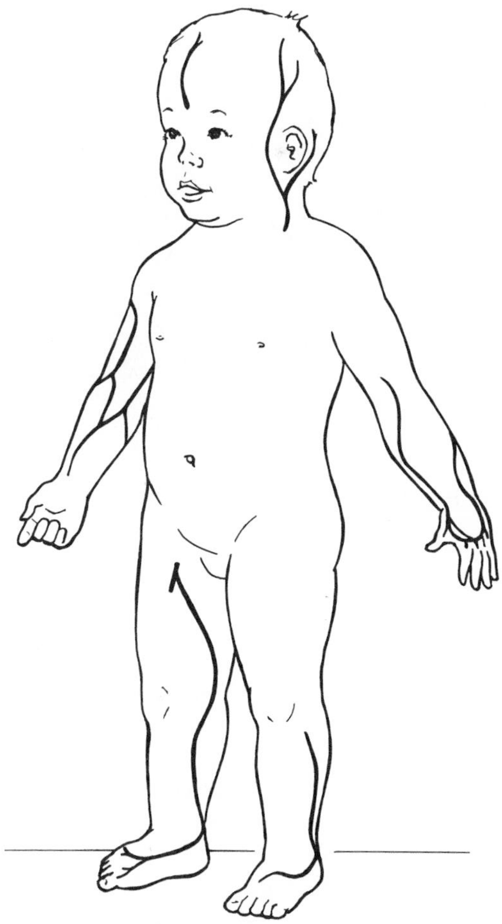

Fig. 29-5. Superficial veins used most often for intravenous infusion. (From Kempe, C. H., Silver, H. K., and O'Brien, D.: Current pediatric diagnosis and treatment, ed. 5, Los Altos, Calif., 1978, Lange Medical Publications.)

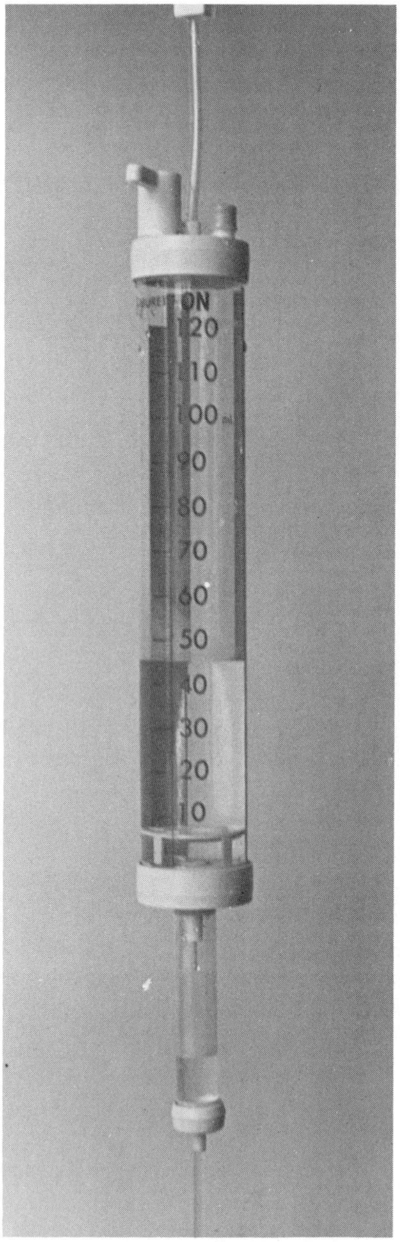

Fig. 29-6. Gravity drainage apparatus.

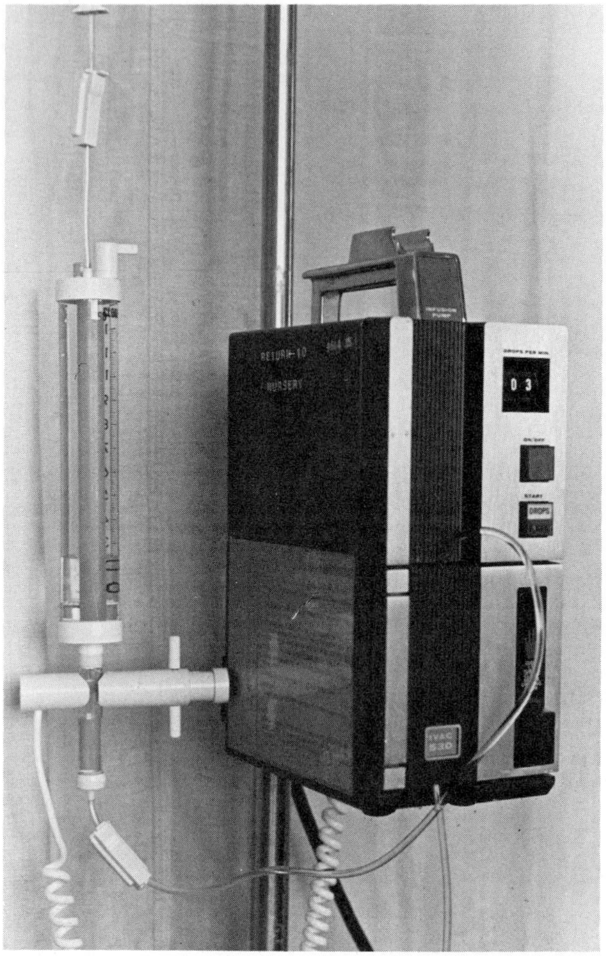

Fig. 29-7. Infusion pump for administration of intravenous fluids (IVAC Corp.).

To facilitate a more precise flow rate, a number of mechanical infusion pumps are now available and are used increasingly for pediatric intravenous fluid administration (Fig. 29-7). Most of these devices pump a given amount of fluid by peristaltic action on the tubing, governed by a flow rate setting, and regulated by a drop sensor that activates an alarm when no drops are formed. For administering a very small amount of fluid over a specific period of time, precision-controlled syringe pumps may be preferable (Fig. 29-8). These devices, although convenient and efficient, are not without attendant risks. Overreliance on the accuracy of the machine can cause either too much or too little fluid to be infused; therefore, its use does not obviate careful periodic assessment by the nurse. Excess pressure can build up if the machine is set at a rate faster than the vein is able to accommodate (or continues to pump when the needle is out of the lumen). This is especially true in very small infants and when circumstances necessitate the use of a capillary. No matter what device is used, a thorough understanding of the apparatus is essential for safe fluid administration.

For most intravenous infusions in children, a scalp-vein needle size 21 or 23 is used with flexible winged tabs that are easily secured to the skin (Fig. 29-9). For long-term therapy a flexible plastic catheter is often used, and, in situations in which fluids are urgently needed and there is difficulty in entering a vein, a polyethylene tube inserted by the surgical cutdown procedure may be necessary. The vein of choice for this alternative is the internal saphenous

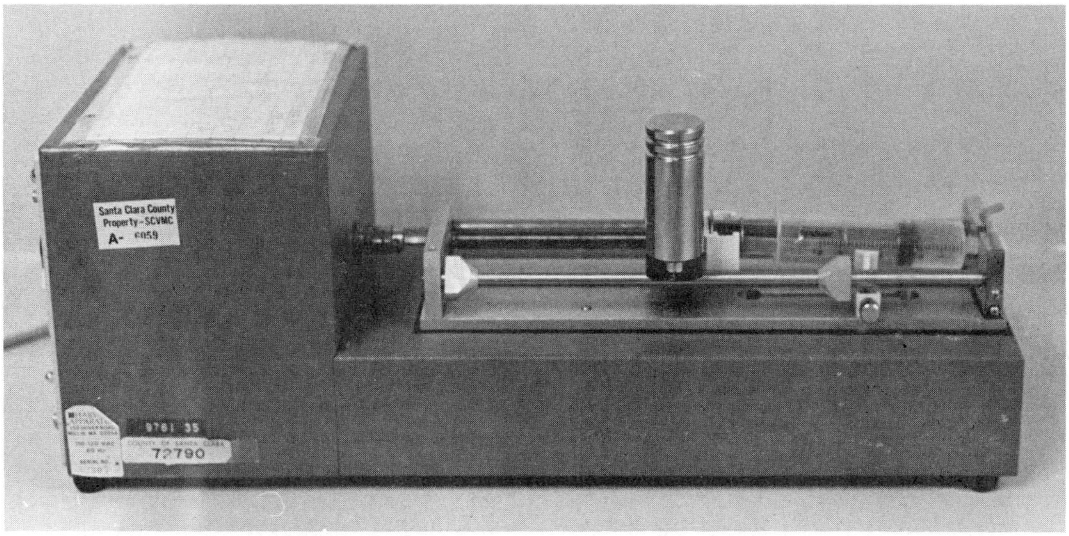

Fig. 29-8. Syringe (Harvard) pump for infusion of a very small amount of fluid over a specified period of time.

vein located just anterior to the medial malleolus of the tibia.

Selection of a scalp vein as the venipuncture site requires shaving the area around the site to better visualize the vein and provide a smooth surface on which to tape the tubing (Fig. 29-10). A rubber band slipped onto the head from brow to occiput will usually suffice as a tourniquet. Shaving off a portion of the infant's hair is very upsetting to parents; therefore, they should be told what to expect and reassured that the hair will grow in again rapidly.

Special precautions. To maintain the integrity of the intravenous site, the child will require adequate restraint. The needle is secured firmly at the puncture site with non-allergenic tape and protected from becoming dislodged by immobilization of the extremity. A plastic or wax paper cup that is applied directly over the needle site will further protect the infusion. The head can be immobilized with covered sandbags. A sandbag or a small board, well padded with plastic foam and a cloth or stockinette cover, provides a suitable means for immobilization (Fig. 29-11). Some form of resilient padding is required to prevent areas of pressure necrosis over bony prominences, such as the ankle. To prevent trauma to the skin from removal of tape, gauze can be placed between the skin and the adhesive.

Older children who are alert and cooperative can usually be trusted to protect the intravenous site. Infants, small children, and uncooperative children require restraint. The board is secured to the bed, and the remaining extremities that might be used to dislodge the needle are restrained as described previously (p. 922). This includes feet as well as hands, since most infants will attempt to brush away the offending attachment by rubbing it against another extremity or body part. Range of motion exercises are employed on infants and children who are too ill or unable to move their extremities, but others should be encouraged to move their arms and legs in response to a natural stimulus. Most infants or small children will instinctively move their extremities when released. If not, a toy or other stimulus can be provided for an incentive.

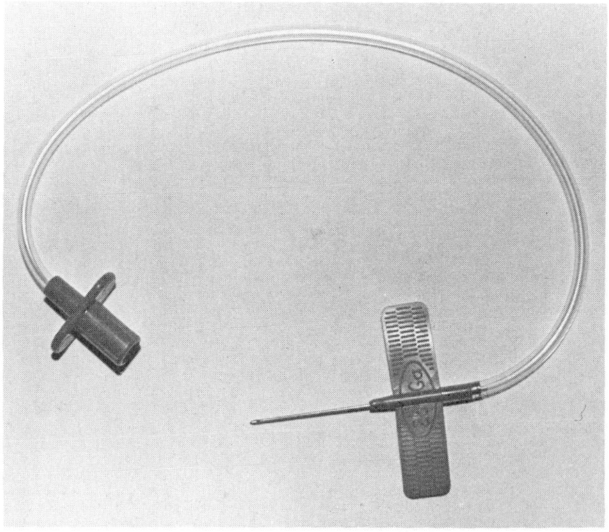

Fig. 29-9. Scalp vein needle.

The same precautions regarding maintenance of asepsis, prevention of infection, and observation for infiltration are carried out with patients of any age. However, infiltration is more difficult to detect in infants and small children than

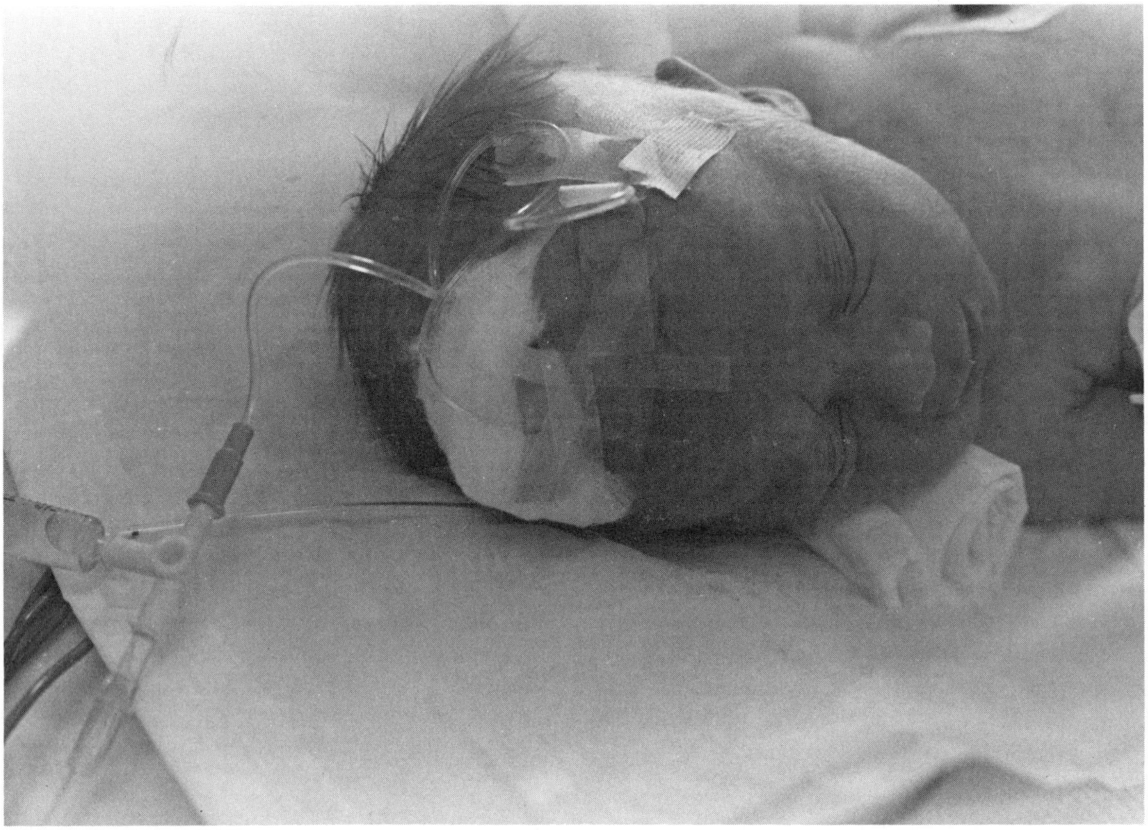

Fig. 29-10. Scalp vein infusion.

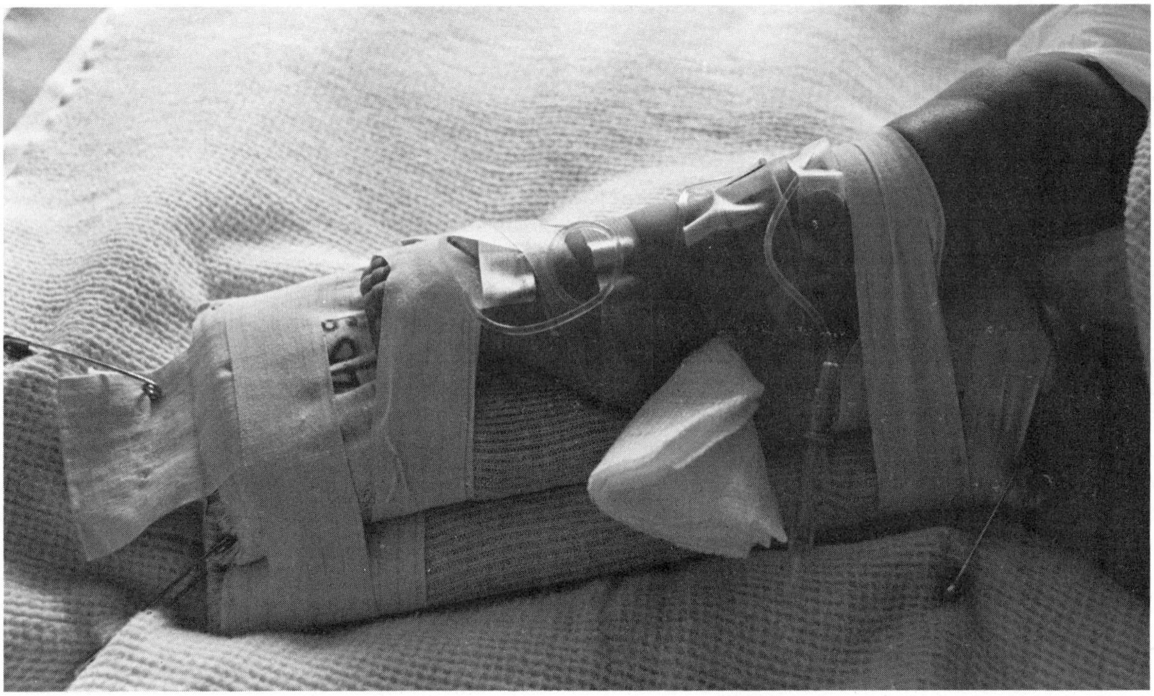

Fig. 29-11. Extremity immobilized with board and firmly secured to bedding with pins.

it is in adults. The increased amount of subcutaneous fat and the amount of tape used to secure the needle often obscure the signs of early infiltration. When the fluid appears to be infusing too slowly or ceases, the usual assessment for obstruction within the apparatus, that is, kinks, screw clamps, shutoff valve, and positioning interference (a bent elbow, for example), often locates the difficulty. When these actions fail to detect the problem, it may be necessary to remove carefully some of the tape and other material that obscures a clear view of the venipuncture site. Dependent areas, such as the palm and undersides of the extremity or the occiput and behind the ears, with a scalp vein infusion, are examined. To check for return blood flow through the needle, the bottle is lowered below the level of the infusion site. If the tubing is connected to an infusion pump, it must be removed from the pump prior to lowering.

Prevention of infection is a major nursing function. The infusion site is protected from trauma and entry of bacteria. When an intravenous infusion continues for several days or longer, the tubing and bottle are changed every 24 hours; however, this may vary according to the institution. To ensure that the equipment is changed regularly it is labeled with the date and time that the new bottle and tubing are attached. Any signs of inflammation such as redness or pain should be reported immediately. This usually requires removal of the infusion and restarting it at another site.

Application of basic scientific principles is employed to increase the flow rate when the needle is ascertained to be in place and no obstructive mechanism is detected. The rate of flow is influenced by the physical factors related to fluids in motion, some of which include pressure gradient, length of tubing, diameter of tubing and orifice, friction, and viscosity of the fluid (Table 29-9).

Intravenous alimentation

A relatively recent advance in intravenous therapy is total parenteral nutrition (TPN), also known as intravenous alimentation, which provides for the total nutritional needs of infants or children whose lives are threatened because feeding by way of the gastrointestinal tract is impossible, inadequate, or hazardous. Common conditions for which total parenteral nutrition is used therapeutically include chronic intestinal obstruction from peritoneal sepsis or adhesions, bowel fistulas, inadequate intestinal length, chronic nonremitting severe diarrhea, extensive body burns, and abdominal tumors treated by surgery, irradiation, and chemotherapy.[4] It may also be initiated prophylactically in situations in which prolonged starvation is expected.

Hyperalimentation therapy involves intravenous infusion of highly concentrated solutions of protein, glucose, and other nutrients. The hyperalimentation solution is infused through conventional tubing with a Millipore filter attached to remove particulate matter or microorganisms that may have contaminated the solution. The highly concentrated

Table 29-9. Physical factors that influence the rate of intravenous infusion

Factor	Principle	Nursing action
Pressure gradient	Force of attraction between two objects causes fluids to flow from a region of higher pressure to one of lower pressure; rate of flow varies directly with pressure difference	Increase height of the fluid column to increase rate of flow Care must be exercised not to increase pressure to a point that can cause injury to the patient
Length of tubing	Fluid flow rate is affected inversely by length of tubing, that is, the longer the tube, the slower the flow	When one or more extension tubes are added to intravenous tubing, pressure may need to be increased to compensate
Diameter of tubing or orifice	The larger the diameter of the tubing, needle, and/or blood vessel, the greater the fluid flow	Larger vein and/or needle will allow greater amount of fluid to infuse Greater pressure will be required to propel a given amount of fluid through a small needle than through a large needle
Friction	Friction produced by the interaction between the molecules in the fluid and the surface of the inner wall of the tubing decreases rate of flow; thus the smoother the inner wall, the faster the flow	Change tubing every 24 hours (necessary for prevention of infection as well) When physician's order permits, heparinized solution allowed to run through tubing and/or needle will eliminate cells attached to wall of lumen Wider-diameter needle and/or tubing will reduce amount of friction
Viscosity of fluid	Inverse relationship exists between degree of viscosity and rate of flow	It requires a larger needle and more pressure to infuse blood than it does to infuse saline solution Viscous liquid forms larger drops

solutions require infusion into a vessel with sufficient volume and turbulence to allow for rapid dilution. The wide-diameter vessels selected are the superior vena cava and innominate or intrathoracic subclavian veins approached by way of the external or internal jugular veins. In some situations the inferior vena cava from a femoral vein serves as an alternative route. The highly irritating nature of concentrated glucose precludes the use of the small peripheral veins in most instances. However, dilute glucose-protein hydrolysates that are appropriate for infusing into peripheral veins are sometimes used in patients who are able to tolerate the fluid load. Also, the recently developed emulsified fat can be administered through peripheral veins in selected cases. Since this fat solution cannot be mixed with the glucose solutions, it requires administration through a separate bottle and tubing that enters the circuit near the venous entry site through a Y type of injection adaptor. There is controversy regarding whether this secondary route should be used for intravenous administration of drugs, open central venous pressure monitoring, and blood withdrawal. Most authorities believe that the risk of infection is great enough to warrant an additional intravenous infusion site for purposes other than total parenteral nutrition.

For central venous hyperalimentation, the special Silastic catheter is placed with meticulous aseptic technique under local or general anesthetic. The jugular vein is entered through a small cutdown site and threaded to the central venous location, confirmed by fluoroscopic dye injection and then sutured in place. To stabilize the catheter, the remainder is tunneled to a previously shaved and surgically prepared exit site behind the ear (Fig. 29-12).[2] The cutdown site is surgically closed, and the catheter is sutured to the scalp at the exit site and a sterile dressing applied. An alternative method eliminates the second site by simply introducing the catheter into the central venous location through a single cutdown or percutaneous puncture site into the vein of choice, usually the subclavian vein.

Nursing responsibilities. The major nursing responsi-

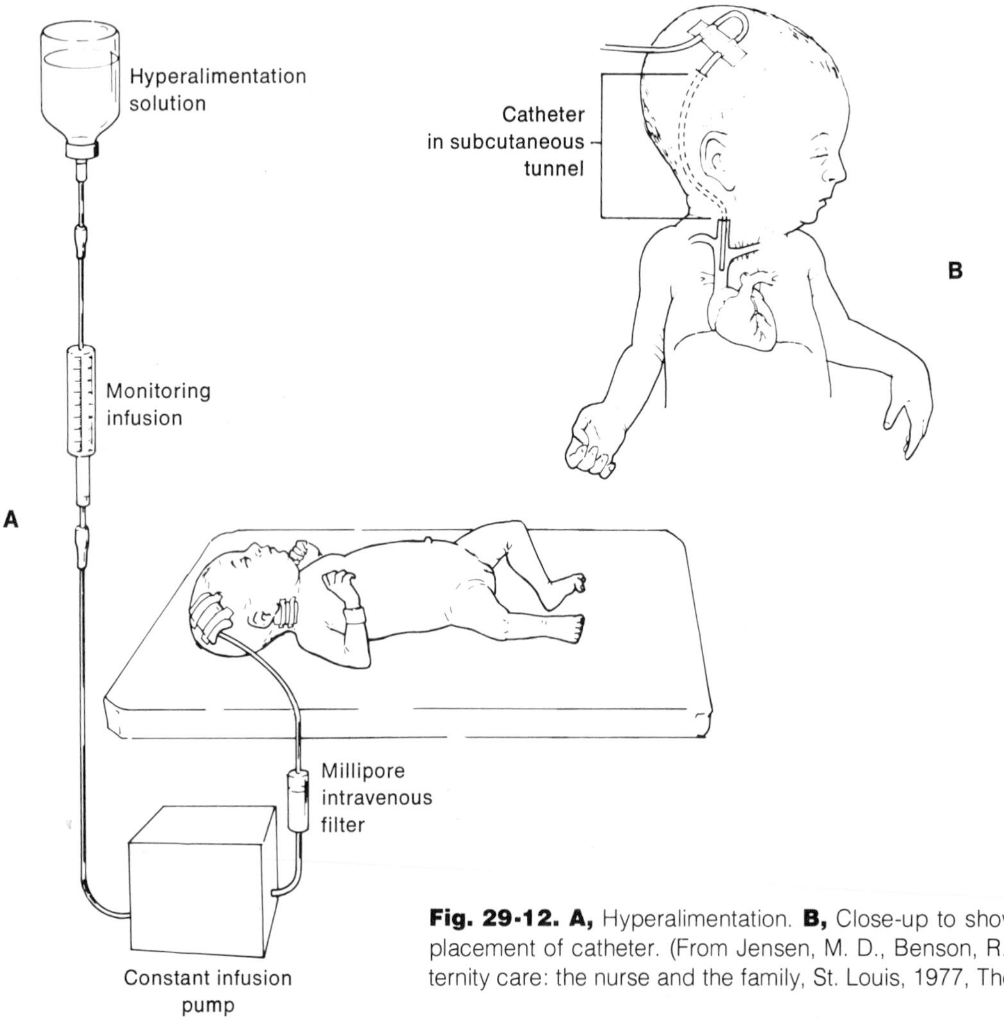

Fig. 29-12. A, Hyperalimentation. **B,** Close-up to show infusion site and internal placement of catheter. (From Jensen, M. D., Benson, R. C., and Bobak, I. M.: Maternity care: the nurse and the family, St. Louis, 1977, The C. V. Mosby Co., p. 623.)

bilities are the same as for any intravenous therapy: control of sepsis, monitoring of infusion rate, and continuous observations.

The total parenteral nutrition solutions must be prepared under rigid aseptic conditions best accomplished in the pharmacy under a Laminar Air Flow hood by specially trained technicians. The solution and tubing are changed and the infusion site redressed by the specially trained intravenous team every 24 hours, using meticulous aseptic precautions. In some institutions this may be a nursing responsibility. The infusion site is carefully exposed and examined for kinks, catheter displacement, loose sutures, and signs of inflammation, such as redness, edema, or observable sediment in the line (an indication of possible infection). The area around the infusion site is first defatted with acetone, followed by application of povidone-iodine (Betadine) solution and covered with a sterile occlusive dressing. An antibiotic ointment (such as bacitracin) is often applied to the infusion site.

The tubing is changed with rapid transfer of insertion ends to reduce the likelihood of microorganism entry and to avoid air embolism. If an air bubble is detected in the tubing, it should be removed by milking the bubble back toward the bottle or removed by aspirating the bubble with an empty, sterile syringe inserted into the special rubber diaphragm on the tubing. The tubing should not be disconnected. A hemostat with padded prongs is used to clamp off the central venous line during the change. Air can easily be drawn into the open end of the line with negative pressure during the inspiratory phase of respiration.

The infusion is maintained at a slow uniform rate to ensure proper utilization of glucose and amino acids, usually by means of a constant infusion pump. This requires accurate calculation of the rate required to deliver a measured amount in a given length of time. Since alterations in flow rate are relatively common, the drip should be checked frequently to ensure an even, continuous infusion. If for some reason the infusion rate slows, the rate should not be increased to compensate for the uninfused amount.

General assessments such as vital signs, intake and output measurements, and checking results of laboratory tests facilitate early detection of infection or fluid and electrolyte imbalance. Additional amounts of potassium and sodium chloride are often required in hyperalimentation; therefore, observation for signs of potassium or sodium deficit or excess is part of nursing care. This is rarely a problem except in children with reduced renal function or metabolic defects. Another problem may occur during the first day or two, as the child adapts to the high-glucose load of the hyperalimentation solution. The addition of insulin may be required to assist the body's adjustment to the hyperglycemia. Nursing responsibilities include testing urine for the presence of glucose and, thus, the effectiveness of the insulin therapy. To prevent hypoglycemia at the time the hyperalimentation is disconnected, the rate of the infusion and the amount of insulin are decreased gradually. The high concentration of glucose may produce an osmotic diuresis with the risk of hypertonic dehydration. Whereas more dilute solutions are often prescribed for this period of time, the nurse must be alert for this possibility.

Special needs

Infants or children who are unable to take fluids by mouth will require special mouth care. Oral hygiene, a part of routine hygienic care, is especially important when fluids are restricted or withheld. Glycerin and lemon swabs help reduce the feeling of dryness but tend to have a dehydrating effect on tissues. To meet the need to suck, infants should be provided with a pacifier, either a commercial variety or one constructed from a nipple stuffed with a gauze or cotton pledget.

To prevent imbalances resulting from the inadvertent substitution of salt for sugar in infant or nasogastric formulas, great care should be exerted in their preparation. Children, especially infants, are quickly subject to life-threatening hypernatremic dehydration from this rare but conceivable accident. It is important to stress to parents and others responsible for mixing formula feedings the harm that excessive sodium intake can cause and the simple modes of prevention. The hazard is not limited to infants. A teenager who had recently undergone surgery for an esophageal stricture with nasogastric tube feedings was given formula in which salt had been substituted for sugar during preparation. He developed a fever, physical signs of dehydration, and extreme lethargy before the cause was detected by serum electrolyte examination. Laboratory electrolyte values were hematocrit, 44 vol%; sodium, 187 mEq/liter; chloride, 169 mEq/liter; carbon dioxide, 18 mEq/liter; and potassium, 3.4 mEq/liter. Intravenous fluid therapy produced a gradual reduction of sodium and chloride to normal levels over a period of 48 hours, cleared his sensorium, and relieved other signs of dehydration. In this instance it was the nurse who persistently pointed out the significant observations that resulted in the correct diagnosis.

Emotional care of children with intravenous therapy, either short- or long-term, requires varying degrees of immobilization. Infants and very young children must be completely immobilized to prevent removal of the intravenous infusion or rubbing the site on another limb or the bed. This is intolerable to the naturally active child, and every effort should be extended to relieve the stress of immobilization (see p. 1542). Frequent removal of the restraints provides the child with the opportunity to move the extremities. Whenever possible, the infant or child should be held and cuddled to help meet his emotional needs during this trying time.

REFERENCES

1. Brooks, S. M.: Basic facts of body water and ions, ed. 3, New York, 1977, Springer Publishing Co., Inc.
2. Colley, R., and Phillips, K.: Helping with hyperalimentation, Nursing '73 **3:**6-17, July 1973.
3. Dell, R. B.: Pathophysiology of dehydration. In Winters, R. W., editor: The body fluids in pediatrics, Boston, 1973, Little, Brown and Co.
4. Filler, R., and Eraklis, A.: Care of the critically ill child: intravenous alimentation, Pediatrics **46:**456-460, 1970.
5. Fineberg, L.: Diarrheal dehydration. In Winters, R. W., editor: The body fluids in pediatrics, Boston, 1973, Little, Brown and Co.
6. Fineberg, L.: Metabolic disorders. In Ziai, M., editor: Pediatrics, ed. 2, Boston, 1975, Little, Brown and Co.
7. Ganong, W. F.: Review of medical physiology, ed. 8, Los Altos, Calif., 1977, Lange Medical Publications.
8. Guyton, A. C.: Textbook of medical physiology, ed. 5, Philadelphia, 1976, W. B. Saunders Co.
9. Kempe, C. H., Silver, H. K., and O'Brien, D.: Current pediatric diagnosis and treatment, Los Altos, Calif., 1974, Lange Medical Publications.
10. Lassiter, W. E., and Gottschalk, C. W.: Volume and composition of the body fluids. In Mountcastle, V. B., editor: Medical physiology, ed. 13, St. Louis, 1974, The C. V. Mosby Co.
11. Luckman, J. L., and Sorensen, K. C.: Medical-surgical nursing, Philadelphia, 1974, W. B. Saunders Co.
12. Metheny, N. M., and Snively, W. D.: Nurses' handbook of fluid balance, Philadelphia, 1974, J. B. Lippincott Co.
13. Moon, J. B., and O'Brien, D.: Fluid and electrolyte therapy. In Kempe, C. H., Silver, H. K., and O'Brien, D.: Current pediatric diagnosis and treatment, ed. 5, Los Altos, Calif., 1978, Lange Medical Publications.
14. Smith, H. W.: Lectures on the kidney, Lawrence, Kan., 1943, University of Kansas.
15. Winters, R. W.: Maintenance of fluid therapy. In Winters, R. W., editor: The body fluids in pediatrics, Boston, 1973, Little, Brown and Co.
16. Winters, R. W.: Physiology of acid-base disorders. In Winters, R. W., editor: The body fluids in pediatrics, Boston, 1973, Little, Brown and Co.

BIBLIOGRAPHY

Burch, G. E., Cade, J. R., and Tintinalli, J.: Sorting out the heat syndromes, Patient Care **10**(11):23-36, June 1, 1976.

Burgess, A.: The nurse's guide to fluid and electrolyte balance, New York, 1970, McGraw-Hill Book Co.

Dell, R. B.: Normal acid-base regulation. In Winters, R. W., editor: The body fluids in pediatrics, Boston, 1973, Little, Brown and Co.

Dreszer, M.: Fluid and electrolyte requirements in the newborn infant, Pediatr. Clin. North Am. **24:**537-546, 1977.

Fenton, M.: What to do about thirst, Am. J. Nurs. **69:**1014-1017, 1969.

Flitter, H. H.: An introduction to physics in nursing, ed. 7, St. Louis, 1976, The C. V. Mosby Co.

Grant, M. M., and Kubo, W. M.: Assessing a patient's hydration status, Am. J. Nurs. **75:**1306-1311, 1975.

Heath, J. K.: A conceptual basis for assessing body water status, Nurs. Clin. North Am. **6:**189-198, 1971.

Jung, R. C.: Analysis and interpretation of acid-base balance, Crit. Care Update **3**(11):5-17, November 1976.

Kee, J. L., and Gregory, A. P.: The ABC's (and mEq's) of fluid balance in children, Nursing '74 **4:**28-36, June 1974.

Keyes, J. L.: Basic mechanisms involved in acid-base homeostasis, Heart Lung **5:**239, 1976.

Kubo, W., and associates: Fluid and electrolyte problems of tube-fed patients, Am. J. Nurs. **76:**912-916, 1976.

Lee, C. A., Stroot, V. R., and Schaper, C. A.: What to do when volume imbalance, Am. J. Nurs. **74:**888-891, 1974.

Lee, C. A., Stroot, V. R., and Schaper, C. A.: What to do when acid-base problems hang in the balance, Nursing '75 **5:**32-37, August 1975.

Lee, J. L., and Gregory, A. P.: The ABC's of fluid balance (and mEq's) in children, Nursing '74 **4:**28-36, June 1974.

Lorch, V., and Lay, S. A.: Parenteral alimentation in the neonate, Pediatr. Clin. North Am. **24**(3):547-556, 1977.

Reed, G. M.: Confused about potassium? Nursing '74 **4:**20-27, March 1974.

Robinson, J. R.: Water, the indispensable nutrient, Nutr. Today **5:**16-23, 28-29, Spring 1970.

Sharer, J. E.: Reviewing acid-base balance, Am. J. Nurs. **75:**980-983, 1975.

Snively, W. D., and Roberts, K. T.: The clinical picture as an aid to understanding body fluid balances, Nurs. Forum **12**(2):132-159, 1973.

Stiehm, E. R., and Rich, K.: Recognition and management of shock in pediatric patients, Curr. Probl. Pediatr. **3:**3-29, 1973.

Stroot, V. R., Lee, C. A., and Schaper, C. A.: Fluids and electrolytes: a practical approach, ed. 2, Philadelphia, 1977, F. A. Davis Co.

Tripp, A.: Hyper and hypo calcemia, Am. J. Nurs. **76:**1142-1145, 1976.

Vaughn, V. C., and McKay, R. J.: Textbook of pediatrics, ed. 10, Philadelphia, 1975, W. B. Saunders Co.

Vaziri, N. D., and Mirahmadi, K.: New concepts in disorders of fluids and electrolytes, Crit. Care Update **4**(6):5-15, June 1977.

Voda, A. M.: Body water dynamics, Am. J. Nurs. **70:**2594-2601, 1970.

West, C. D.: Parenteral fluid therapy. In Shirkey, H. C., editor: Pediatric therapy, ed. 5, St. Louis, 1975, The C. V. Mosby Co.

Winters, R. W., editor: The body fluids in pediatrics, Boston, 1973, Little, Brown and Co.

Intravenous therapy

Beaumont, E.: The new infusion pumps, Nursing '77 **7:**31-35, July 1977.

Colley, R., Wilson, J. M., and Wilhem, M. P.: Intravenous nutrition—nursing considerations, Issues Comprehensive Pediatr. Nurs. **1**(5):50-83, 1977.

Crossley, K., and Matsen, J. M.: Scalp-vein needle: a prospective study of complications, J.A.M.A. **220:**985-987, 1972.

Donn, R.: Intravenous admixture incompatibility, Am. J. Nurs. **71:**325, 1971.

Egan, A.: Perfecting piggy-back techniques, Nursing '74 **4:**28-33, January 1974.

Hanson, R. L.: Heparin-lock or keep-open I.V.? Am. J. Nurs. **76:**1102-1103, 1976.

Heird, W. C., and Winters, R. W.: Fluid therapy for the pediatric surgical patient. In Winters, R. W., editor: The body fluids in pediatrics, Boston, 1973, Little, Brown and Co.

Heird, W. C., and associates: Intravenous alimentation in pediatric patients, J. Pediatr. **80:**351, 1972.

I.V. sets. Product survey, Nursing '72 **2:**28-34, October 1972.

Johnson, N. E.: Coping with complications of intravenous therapy, Nursing '72 **2:**5-8, February 1972.

Kee, J. L.: The critically ill patient and possible fluid and electrolyte imbalances, Nursing '72 **2:**6-11, March 1972.

Kubo, W., and associates: Fluid and electrolyte problems of tube-fed patients, Am. J. Nurs. **76:**912-916, 1976.

Kurdi, W. J.: Refining your I.V. therapy techniques, Nursing '75 **5:**41-47, November 1975.

Liebert, P. S.: Central venous catheters in children—their placement and care, Clin. Pediatr. **10:**218-222, 1971.

McGill, D.: Giving I.V. push, Nursing '73 **3:**15-18, June 1973.

Monahan, J. J., and Webb, J. W.: Intravenous infusion pumps—an added dimension to parenteral therapy, Am. J. Hosp. Pharm. **29:**54, 1972.

Moore, V. B.: I.V. fluids. Product survey, Nursing '73 **3:**32-38, June 1973.

Parsa, M. H., Thornton, B. H., and Ferrer, J. M.: Central venous alimentation, Am. J. Nurs. **72:**2042-2047, 1972.

Payne, J. E., and Kaplan, H. M.: Alternative techniques for venipuncture, Am. J. Nurs. **72:**702-703, 1972.

Plumer, A. L.: Principles and practice of intravenous therapy, ed. 2, Boston, 1975, Little, Brown and Co.

Robinson, L. A., and Whitacre, N. F.: Intravenous administration of antibiotics in children, Pediatr. Nurs. **3**(3):21-25, 1977.

Tashima, C.: Temperature of intravenous infusions, N. Engl. J. Med. **289:**922, 1973.

Ungvarski, P. J.: Parenteral therapy, Am. J. Nurs. **76:**1974-1977, 1976.

Vinnars, E.: Recent advances in parenteral nutrition, Crit. Care Med. **2:**143, 1974.

Wilmore, D. W.: The future of intravenous therapy, Am. J. Nurs. **71:**2334-2338, 1971.

Wilson, J. A.: Infection control in intravenous therapy, Heart Lung **5:**430-436, 1976.

Winters, R. W.: Total parenteral nutrition in pediatrics, Pediatrics **56:**17, 1975.

Hyperalimentation

Colley, R., Wilson, J. M., and Wilhem, M. P.: Intravenous nutrition—nursing considerations, Issues Comprehensive Pediatr. Nurs. **1**(5):50-83, April 1977.

Filler, R. M., and Coran, A. G.: Total parenteral nutrition in infants and children: central and peripheral approaches, Surg. Clin. North Am. **56:**395, 1976.

Grant, J. A. N.: Patient care in parenteral hyperalimentation, Nurs. Clin. North Am. **8:**165-181, 1973.

Grant, J. A. N.: The nurse's role in parenteral hyperalimentation, RN **36:**28-33, July 1973.

Heid, W. C., and associates: Intravenous alimentation in pediatric patients, J. Pediatr. **80:**351, 1972.

Humphrey, N. M., Wright, P., and Swanson, A.: Parenteral hyperalimentation for children, Am. J. Nurs. **72:**286-288, 1972.

Michener, W. M., and Law, D.: Parenteral nutrition: the age of the catheter, Pediatr. Clin North Am. **17:**373, 1970.

Nelson, R.: Minimizing systemic infection during complete parenteral alimentation of small infants, Arch. Dis. Child. **49:**16-19, 1974.

Nursing grand rounds: hyperalimentation, its help and risk, Nursing '72 **2:**26-31, April 1972.

Parsa, M., and associates: Central venous alimentation, Am. J. Nurs. **72:**2042-2047, 1972.

Vinnars, E.: Recent advances in parenteral nutrition, Crit. Care Med. **2:**143, 1974.

30

Conditions that produce fluid and electrolyte imbalance

Fluid and electrolyte disturbances are common in the pediatric age-group. Acute attacks of vomiting and diarrhea are so common in this group that they can almost be regarded as part of the normal way of life. However, the nature of the anatomic and physiologic structure of the infant and small child renders them particularly vulnerable to imbalances when pathologic changes affect the fluid compartments. Most illnesses create some disturbance in body fluids and/or electrolytes, and, in many, these disturbances are more threatening than the primary pathology.

DIARRHEA

Diarrhea is defined as an increase in the number of stools or a decrease in their consistency as a major clinical manifestation of alterations of water and electrolyte transport by the alimentary tract.[20] It is a symptom of diverse origin and results from disorders involving digestive, absorptive, and secretory functions. However, a precise definition and identification of what constitutes diarrhea pose a problem in terms of number or consistency of stools, since there are wide variations in colonic function between individuals. For example, one infant may have one firm stool every second or third day, whereas another normally passes from five to eight small, soft stools daily. Therefore, more important are (1) a noticeable or sudden increase in number of stools, (2) a reduction in their consistency with an increase in fluid content, and (3) a tendency for the stools to be greenish in color.

Diarrhea is one of the symptoms encountered most frequently in infants and children and was, at one time, one of the chief causes of death in infancy. With improved public health measures, the incidence has been dramatically reduced during the past century, and, although it still remains a major health problem in many areas of the world, a greater understanding of the pathophysiology of diarrhea and more effective management of the disorder have also reduced the death rate from the consequences of diarrhea. Severe cases, however, continue to present serious problems, especially with more widespread adoption of bottle-feeding throughout the world.

Diarrhea may be acute or chronic, and the physiologic consequences vary considerably in relation to its severity, duration, associated symptoms, the age of the child, and the child's nutritional status prior to the onset of diarrhea.

Etiology and pathophysiology

Diarrhea can be attributed to a large number of specific causes, mechanisms, and predisposing factors. Factors that predispose a child to diarrhea and its physiologic consequences include[14]:

1. *Age.* As a rule, the younger the child, the more susceptible he is to diarrhea and the more severe the diarrhea is likely to be. Diarrhea occurs more frequently in infancy, is a lesser threat in early childhood, and usually constitutes only a minor problem in older children.
2. *Impaired health.* Children who are malnourished or debilitated from disease are more susceptible to diarrhea, and it tends to be more severe in these children.
3. *Climate.* In areas in which sanitation and refrigeration are a problem, saprophytic organisms (organisms that grow more readily in the warmer weather) are more apt to proliferate. Most organisms that cause diarrhea are more prevalent in warmer weather. Also, the dehydration that accompanies diarrhea is aggravated by hot weather.
4. *Environment.* Diarrhea occurs with greater frequency in circumstances in which living conditions are inadequate. Crowding, substandard sanitation, poor facilities for preparation and refrigeration of food, and generally inadequate health care and education all tend to increase the likelihood for spread of pathogens. The frequency of diarrhea in infancy is closely related to the ingestion of contaminated milk. Significantly there is a lower incidence of diarrhea in breast-fed infants even where formula preparation is satisfactory.

Specific etiologic mechanisms. There are several major mechanisms that produce diarrhea in the infant or child who is susceptible and/or is exposed to a causative agent. In some cases more than one mechanism may be operating. There are numerous agents that are responsible for causing diarrhea by way of these mechanisms. Some agents create their effect by direct invasion of the intestinal tract, whereas others exert their effect through parenteral means, that is,

Table 30-1. Common causes of acute diarrhea

Factors	Condition or circumstance
Dietary	Overfeeding Introduction of new foods Unripe fruit Reinstituting milk too soon after diarrheal episode Osmotic diarrhea from excess sugar or fat in formula
Toxic	Ingestion of Heavy metals (arsenic, lead, mercury) Organic phosphates Ferrous sulfate Antibiotics
Parenteral infection	Communicable diseases Upper respiratory tract infections Urinary tract infections Otitis media
Emotional	Episodes of nervous excitement Periods of emotional tension Fatigue Psychogenic "irritable colon syndrome" in hyperactive children

not by way of the intestinal tract. Following are mechanisms known to produce diarrhea[22]:

1. *Osmotic factors*. Water is passively absorbed as a function of solute transport and normally accompanies solute movement in isotonic proportions across the intestinal mucosa in response to osmotic gradients. The presence of unabsorbed solutes creates an osmotic gradient, causing movement of sodium and water in the intestinal lumen, for example, ingestion of nonabsorbable solutes and malabsorption of water-soluble nutrients.
2. *Diminished absorption or increased secretion of water and electrolytes*. Diminished absorption of solutes will also cause decreased absorption of water and electrolytes, for example, mucosal disease. Increased secretion can be either passive secretion secondary to inflammation or active secretion secondary to stimulation of mucosal cells, for example, toxin-producing bacteria.
3. *Reduction in anatomic or functional surface area*. There is reduced absorptive surface to absorb all ingested substances in the anatomically short bowel. Both hypermotility and hypomotility reduce the amount of substance absorbed by the intestinal mucosa.

Specific causes. A variety of factors can produce diarrhea in the infant or child either as the presenting symptom or as an associated symptom. Often a specific etiologic diagnosis is lacking. *Acute* diarrhea, a sudden change in frequency and consistency of stools, is more often caused by an inflammatory process of infectious origin but may also be the result of a toxic reaction to ingestion of poisons, dietary indiscretions, or associated with infection outside the alimentary tract (Table 30-1). Most are self-limited and will ultimately subside without specific treatment if consequent dehydration does not create a serious complication. *Chronic* diarrhea, the passage of loose stools with increased frequency of more than 2 weeks' duration, is more apt to be associated with disorders of malabsorption, anatomic defects, abnormal bowel motility, hypersensitivity (allergic) reaction, or an inflammatory response (Table 30-2).

Table 30-2. Causes of chronic diarrhea*

Type of disorder	Examples of disease or condition
Anatomic or mechanical	Small bowel syndrome Hirschsprung's disease Partial small bowel obstruction (stenosis) Malrotation
Malabsorption	Cystic fibrosis Celiac disease Specific carbohydrate or fat malabsorption syndromes caused by enzyme deficiencies such as lactase deficiency, bile-salt deficiency
Food allergy	Milk colitis Allergic gastroenteropathy
Inflammatory bowel disease	Ulcerative colitis Regional enteritis Nonspecific enterocolitis of infancy
Parenteral causes	Neoplastic disease (lymphoma, neuroblastoma, polyposis, and so on) Immune deficiency diseases (Wiskott-Aldrich syndrome, agammaglobulinemia, and so on) Endocrinopathies (hyperthyroidism, congenital adrenal hyperplasia, and so on)
Malnutrition	Protein malnutrition (kwashiorkor) Protein-calorie malnutrition (marasmus)

*See Chapter 34 for discussion of chronic gastrointestinal disorders.

Diarrheal disturbances can involve the stomach and intestine *(gastroenteritis)*, the small intestine *(enteritis)*, the colon *(colitis)*, or the colon and intestine *(enterocolitis)*. *Dysentery* is a term that describes intestinal inflammation, especially of the colon, that is accompanied by cramping abdominal pain, tenesmus, and watery stools containing blood and mucus.

Enteropathologic organisms. There are many organisms that can cause diarrheal disturbances in children, especially in infants. These can be enteric pathogens primarily, such as the *Shigella* and *Salmonella* groups of bacteria, or other organisms that have the potential to produce diarrhea under favorable circumstances, such as *Staphylococcus aureus*. Most infectious organisms are transmitted

Table 30-3. Enteropathologic causes of bacterial diarrhea

Organism	Incubation	Pathology	Characteristics	Comments
Pathogenic *Escherichia coli*		Enterotoxin production (small bowel) Invasion of epithelium (small bowel and colon) Secretion of fluids and electrolytes	Variable clinical manifestations Most—green, watery diarrhea with mucus Afebrile Symptoms generally subside in 3-7 days Relapse rate approximately 20%	Usually interpersonal transmission but may transmit via inanimate objects A cause of nursery epidemics
Salmonella groups (nontyphoidal)—gram-negative, nonencapsulated, nonsporulating	6-72 hours for intraluminal; 7-21 days for extraluminal Communicable as long as organisms are excreted	Penetration of lamina propria (small bowel and colon) Local inflammation Stimulation of intestinal fluid excretion Systemic invasion of other sites	Variable symptoms—mild to severe Nausea, vomiting, and colicky abdominal pain followed by diarrhea, occasionally with blood and mucus Chills not uncommon Hyperactive peristalsis and mild abdominal tenderness Symptoms usually subside within 5 days May have high fever, headache, and cerebral manifestations, for example, drowsiness, confusion, meningismus, or seizures	Two thirds of patients are less than 20 years of age; highest incidence in children under age 9 years, especially infants Highest incidence occurs July through October, lowest from January through April Transmission primarily via contaminated food and drink—most from animal sources, including fowl, mammals, reptiles, and insects Most common sources are poultry and eggs In children—pets, especially pet turtles
S. typhi	Same	Rapid invasion of bloodstream from minor sites of inflammation Septicemia develops and is cleared by reticuloendothelial system organs where organisms multiply, and produce local inflammation Organisms reenter bloodstream to cause secondary infection Marked inflammation and necrosis of intestinal mucosa and lymphatics	Variable in infants Older children—irregular fever, headache, malaise, lethargy Diarrhea occurs in 50% at early stage Cough is common In a few days, fever rises and is consistent; fatigue, cough, abdominal pain, anorexia, and weight loss develop; diarrhea begins	
Shigella groups—gram-negative, nonmotile, anaerobic bacilli	1-7 days Communicable for 1-4 weeks	Enterotoxin Stimulates loss of fluids and electrolytes Invasion of epithelium with superficial mucosal ulcerations *S. dysenteriae* forms exotoxin	Onset variable but usually abrupt Fever and cramping abdominal pain initially Fever—may reach 40.5°C (105°F) Convulsions in about 10%—usually associated with fever Patient appears sick Headache, nuchal rigidity, delirium Watery diarrhea with mucus and pus starts about 12-48 hours after onset Stools preceded by abdominal cramps; tenesmus and straining follow Symptoms usually subside in 5-10 days	Approximately 60% of cases in children under age 9 years with more than one third between ages 1 and 4 years Peak incidence late summer Transmitted directly or indirectly from infected persons
Vibrio cholerae (cholera) groups		Enterotoxin causes increased secretion of chloride and possibly bicarbonate Intestinal mucosa congested with enlarged lymph follicles Intact mucosal surface	Sudden onset of profuse, watery diarrhea without cramping, tenesmus, or anal irritation, although children may complain of cramping Stools are intermittent at first then almost continuous Stools are whitish, almost clear, with flecks of mucus—"rice water stools"	Rare in infants less than 1 year old Mortality rate high in both treated and untreated infants and small children Transmitted via contaminated food and water Endemic in Bengal Attack confers immunity

through contaminated feedings or by infected "carriers," including animal reservoirs.

Bacterial invasion of the gastrointestinal tract produces diarrhea and related symptoms in three ways[22]:

1. *Enterotoxin production.* The organisms do not invade the mucosal epithelium. They produce their effect by multiplication in the gastrointestinal tract followed by adhesion to the mucosa, where they release an exotoxin that binds to the small bowel villi. Interaction of this toxin and the mucosa stimulates the profuse secretion of water and electrolytes. Examples include *Shigella, Escherichia coli,* and *Vibrio cholerae.*
2. *Invasion and destruction.* The organisms directly invade and destroy the cells of the intestinal epithelium. The infection proceeds from the upper to the lower intestines in a descending manner, producing bloody mucoid stools. They also produce a powerful endotoxin that promotes loss of fluids and electrolytes into the intestine. Within the epithelium the organisms multiply and cause superficial ulcerations of the mucosa. Examples include *Shigella* and *E. coli.*
3. *Penetration and systemic invasion.* There is stimulation and excretion of intestinal fluids. Local inflammation is produced as organisms invade the thin layer of connective tissue (lamina propria) lying immediately beneath the epithelium of the mucous membrane in the distal small bowel and colon. The mucosa becomes hyperemic and edematous. From this point the organism has access to the systemic circulation, in which it can produce foci of infection elsewhere in the body. An example is *Salmonella.*

Organisms that are considered "normal flora" in most situations are enteropathic under certain conditions and in susceptible children, particularly newborns and young infants. These include certain strains of *E. coli* and *Staphylococcus aureus.* Some strains of *E. coli* produce diarrhea by invasion of the intestinal mucosa and others by elaboration of enterotoxins. *S. aureus* can cause diarrhea by (1) food poisoning from contamination (especially milk or egg products) with exotoxin production, (2) enteritis as a result of prolonged broad-spectrum antibiotic therapy that destroys and eliminates enteric organisms that normally control staphylococcal invasion, (3) enteritis as a complication of staphylococcal infection elsewhere (skin or lungs), and (4) primary staphylococcal infection in newborn infants who have not yet established competing enteric flora. Other bacteria may cause diarrhea but are less likely to do so. The enteropathic bacteria are briefly outlined in Table 30-3.

Viral diarrheas are probably quite common, but, with the possible implication of the enteroviruses and adenoviruses, no specific etiologic agents have been identified. Other agents such as *Pseudomonas, Klebsiella,* and *Proteus* organisms may cause diarrhea but do not ordinarily have a tendency to do so. Amebic dysentery seldom occurs in infants.

Consequences of severe diarrheal disease. The most serious and immediate physiologic disturbances associated with severe diarrheal disease are (1) dehydration, (2) acid-base derangements with acidosis, and (3) shock that occurs when dehydration progresses to the point that circulatory status is seriously disturbed.

Dehydration, which can be isotonic (70%), hypotonic (15%), or hypertonic (5%), is the result of:

- Voluminous losses of fluid and electrolytes in frequent watery stools
- Losses when there is frequent vomiting
- Reduced fluid intake resulting from nausea and/or anorexia
- Increased insensible losses from fever, hyperpnea, and, sometimes, high environmental temperature
- Continued (although diminished) obligatory renal losses

All of these losses contribute to the rapid deterioration in diarrheal disease in infancy, and, although the fluid deficit cannot be stated precisely, it can be estimated from changes in body weight and objective clinical signs. The losses are customarily referred to in terms of percentage of body weight and estimated in the general ranges of 5%, 10%, or 15%, as described previously (p. 1081). At each of these levels, in addition to weight, certain manifestations provide clues to the extent of dehydration. The first of these appear when about 5% of the weight has been lost; the child is nearly moribund when water loss approaches 15%. Initial and ongoing losses can be determined from body weight loss with a high degree of reliability. Compensatory mechanisms attempt to maintain fluid volume by adjusting to these losses. Interstitial fluid moves into the vascular compartment to defend the blood volume in response to hemoconcentration and hypovolemia, whereas vasoconstriction of peripheral arterioles helps maintain pumping pressure. When fluid losses exceed the body's ability to sustain blood volume and blood pressure, circulation is seriously compromised and the blood pressure falls. This results in tissue hypoxia with accumulation of lactic acid, pyruvate, and other acid metabolites, which contributes to the development of acidosis.

Renal compensation is impaired by reduced blood flow through the kidneys, and little urine is formed. If dehydration increases in severity, urine formation is markedly diminished and metabolites and hydrogen ions that are normally excreted by this route are retained. The metabolic acidosis of severe diarrhea is the result of several factors[14]:

- Losses of bicarbonate, sodium, and potassium in diarrheal stools
- Impaired renal function
- Accumulation of lactic acid from tissue hypoxia
- Ketosis from fat metabolism when glycogen stores are depleted in untreated diarrheal dehydration or inadequate carbohydrate intake

In association with both fluid losses and acidosis, there are alterations in body potassium. Potassium is continually lost in stools, cellular potassium leaves the cells in exchange for sodium and hydrogen ions entering the cells, and potassium is lost from cells damaged by hypoxia. Thus the cellular potassium is seriously depleted. However, since renal excretion is impaired as a result of the circulatory adjustments, the serum levels of potassium are normal or even elevated. When circulatory volume and renal function are restored, potassium redistribution and excretion may produce a potassium deficit unless adequate amounts are restored at this time.

Intractable diarrhea of infancy. The term intractable diarrhea has been used only recently to describe infants whose diarrhea is not caused by recognized pathogens and is refractory to treatment. It is classified as either primary, which is identified as nonspecific enterocolitis, or secondary, associated with disease entities such as allergy, bowel anomalies, or a variety of congenital diseases included in Table 30-2. The age of onset ranges from 4 days to 3 months of age. Dehydration is always present, and a prominent feature is malnutrition with hypoproteinemia and hypoalbuminemia.[22]

The primary form, although the triggering factor is not well defined, may be secondary to such trivial causes as an infection or feeding difficulties. The diarrhea rapidly becomes self-perpetuating through a combination of secondary consequences—malnutrition deprives the infant of the elements protein, vitamins, calcium, and magnesium needed for mucosal regeneration; the villi of the small intestine atrophy; the bowel wall becomes inflamed and irritated by undigested foodstuffs or microorganisms; and secondary digestive and absorptive disorders develop as a result of malnutrition, various patterns of motility, and overgrowth of bacteria caused by the infant's debilitated state (Fig. 30-1).

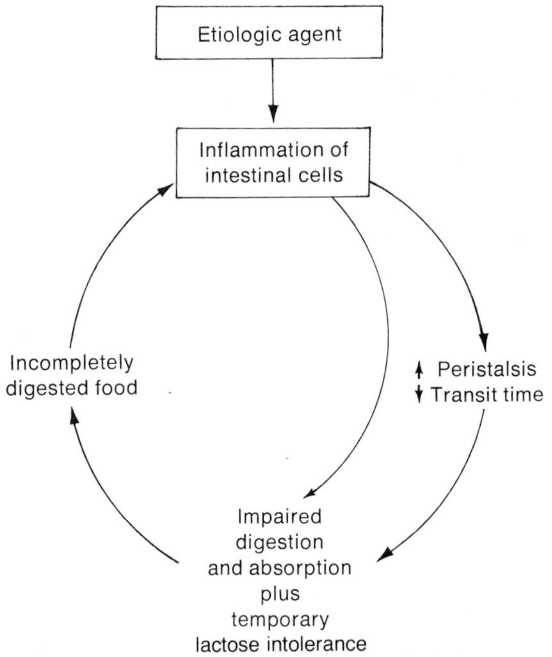

Fig. 30-1. Vicious pathologic cycle in diarrhea plus temporary lactose intolerance.

Diagnostic evaluation

The history provides valuable information regarding exposure to infectious agents, personal contact, travel, or probable contact with contaminated foods. Allergic and dietary history may indicate food allergies.

The age of the child provides clues to the eitology of diarrheal disturbances. For example, with the exception of nursery epidemics, infectious enteritis is uncommon during the first days of life. *E. coli* disease is the usual agent after the first week of life, with a peak incidence from 1 to 3 months of age in bottle-fed infants; it is uncommon after 1 year of age. In breast-fed infants the time sequence is later. Shigellosis is most common from ages 2 to 4 years, but the most severe form is more apt to occur in children over 5 years of age. Although *Salmonella* infection is encountered in children in any age-group, it appears to be most prevalent in children under age 2 years, as are the so-called viral diarrheas of unknown etiology. It is characteristic that multiple cases in a household are usually shigellosis, whereas a single case is more typical of enteropathogenic *E. coli*. Likewise, milk allergy or intolerance of other formula constituents is suspected in early infancy. In later infancy new foods added to the diet are frequent offenders. Parenteral infections are very common causes of diarrhea in infancy.

Most acute, inflammatory diarrheas are infectious, and the type of stools and symptoms associated with diarrhea provide clues to the organism. Fever is not a symptom of *E. coli* disease until late, whereas it is a common early feature even in mild cases of shigellosis. Abdominal cramps are common in shigellosis. Explosive onset of diarrhea accompanied by or preceded by vomiting suggests food poisoning. Although vomiting may occur in all infectious diarrheas, it is not a major feature.

Laboratory examination. Peripheral blood leukocyte count is of little value in differentiating organisms, but the presence of many band forms in the differential white blood count is characteristic of shigellosis but not of most other infectious diarrheas.

Examination of the stool for leukocytes often differentiates between some bacteria. No leukocytes appear in normal stools or in diarrheal disease of viral or enterotoxin-producing bacteria, but many leukocytes or clumps of pus cells are seen in infections caused by enteroinvasive organisms. The stool specimen is obtained from evacuated stool and should include mucus or tissue shreds, if present. The specimen is also examined for the presence of red blood cells. Rectal swabs for culture are indicated whenever a bacterial agent is suspected.

Stool examination with indicator paper for pH and a Clinitest tablet will detect the acid stool containing sugar that is characteristic of disaccharide intolerance. Bulky stools containing fat suggest malabsorption diarrhea.

Serum electrolyte values are obtained in the young infant who is hospitalized with diarrhea because of the likelihood of complicating dehydration and associated electrolyte imbalances, particularly in relation to sodium and potassium alterations. Dehydrated infants will have an elevated hematocrit as a result of volume loss, and an elevated blood urea nitrogen will be found in the presence of reduced renal circulation.

Medical management

Mild or moderate diarrhea is usually managed by simple measures and seldom requires hospitalization. Mild diarrhea is described as a few loose stools each day without other evidence of illness that terminates in a few days. With moderate diarrhea, the child is sicker, may have a fever, vomits, appears fretful and irritable, and passes several loose or watery stools daily. Although the child may not gain weight or may even show a slight loss, signs of dehydration are usually absent.

The extent to which the child should be examined and observed by a nurse or a physician depends a great deal on the intelligence and cooperation of the care giver in following instructions and assessing the progress of treatment. When the competency of the care giver is questionable in regard to estimating the child's condition, the child should be seen daily by a health worker. If the diarrhea persists, if the child loses weight, if there is blood in the stools, or if the child develops associated signs such as deep breathing, listlessness, or reduced urinary output that may signal complications, the child should be seen by the physician. When the moderate diarrhea becomes worse or does not respond to simple measures, hospitalization is indicated. This provides the opportunity for closer observation and examination and for a brief course of parenteral fluid therapy, which usually results in rapid improvement.

Home treatment. Home treatment consists of reducing the child's activities. Infants and young children are usually placed on bed rest and closely observed. Most authorities recommend withholding food for a brief period of time (12 to 24 hours), especially if there is vomiting. It is believed that this helps to slow down the increased intestinal activity and allows the bowel to rest, thus reducing the number and volume of stools. During this time the child is permitted clear fluids to replace fluid loss. Clear liquids are offered, and, although it is not uniformly accepted, most physicians prescribe small amounts of fluids, with electrolytes and calories, at frequent intervals. The amount of fluids is gradually increased and the intervals are lengthened as tolerated. The thirst mechanism is the most sensitive guide to fluid needs, and ad lib. administration of a glucose-electrolyte solution to an alert child will restore water and electrolytes satisfactorily. It is important to include carbohydrate to spare body protein and since there is a tendency for ketosis resulting from exhaustion of glycogen reserves to develop. Once vomiting has abated, more liberal amounts can be offered, followed by bland solids. Some physicians believe that small, frequent feedings actually induce further losses through activation of the gastrocolic reflex and prescribe large volumes, initially, at less frequent intervals. Care must be exercised in the use of electrolytes to avoid the possibility of hyperelectrolytemia.

In many children a secondary lactase deficiency may cause a temporary intolerance to milk and exacerbation of diarrhea; therefore, reintroduction of lactose is attempted progressively. Milk is usually withheld until at least a week after the disappearance of symptoms and consists of a hydrolyzed lactose-free formula.

Antimicrobial therapy is instituted in some types of diarrhea. It significantly shortens the course of shigellosis and appears to be beneficial in *E. coli* infections but does not affect the course of *Salmonella* disease. It is always indicated in bacteremia, and parenteral infections are treated with appropriate drugs. Absorbents, such as kaolin-pectin, increase stool consistency and decrease the frequency of evacuation but do not reduce the amount of fluid loss and may actually mask the volume lost. Antidiarrheal agents are not administered to infants but may be of limited value in older children. Some physicians prescribe low doses of sedatives to control abdominal pain and cramps, but routine use of opium derivatives, such as paregoric or opium tincture, are not advised since they tend to cause somnolence and mask pain that may signal complications such as intussusception in infants. However, they may be prescribed for older children with tenesmus. Diphenoxylate with atropine (Lomotil) may be given to older children but is contraindicated in children under 2 years of age because of its narrow margin of safety.[20]

Severe diarrhea. Severe diarrhea is largely a problem of infants and very young children, and, regardless of the etiology, successful management relies primarily on appropriate treatment of physiologic disturbances and is only secondarily concerned with specific treatment of the etiologic agent. Severe diarrhea warrants hospitalization, comprehensive evaluation, and parenteral fluid therapy. Fluid therapy is directed toward replacement of (1) the fluid deficit, (2) ongoing normal losses, and (3) abnormal ongoing losses. The magnitude of the deficit is determined from loss of body weight and ongoing losses by calculating the energy requirements of the child. The energy requirements include not only predicted caloric expenditure for age and size but other factors that increase the use of energy, such as elevated temperature (metabolism increases by about 12% for each 1° C) and hyperventilation. Additional replacement covers abnormal losses as determined by output measurement, weight, and electrolyte determinations.

The therapeutic plan for severe diarrhea closely parallels that described for dehydration in general (p. 1081). It is conducted in four phases—emergency, repletion, early recovery, and late recovery—with the goal of replacement of the initial losses in a period of 12 to 24 hours from admission to the hospital with follow-up maintenance fluids.[8]

Emergency phase. The *emergency phase* is designed to restore circulation rapidly. In isotonic deficit a solution of dextrose in water is administered with addition of suitable electrolytes—sodium as the cation and chloride and bicarbonate as anions. For this purpose, numerous commercially prepared solutions are available that meet the desired electrolyte concentration. In many instances, and especially in hypertonic dehydration with shock, protein-containing solutions, principally plasma substitutes such as a 5% albumin solution, are administered. Because of concern about hepatitis and problems of availability, blood and plasma are used less frequently. Glucose water without added sodium is contraindicated because of the danger of cerebral edema. The length of this phase is usually from 20 or 30 minutes to 3 or 4 hours. Other therapies that are often indicated are measures to control fever and administration of oxygen.

Repletion phase. The *repletion phase* aims to restore body fluids to a volume that will permit adequate circulation and good renal function. Once the emergency phase is past, the replacement solution of dextrose and electrolytes is administered more slowly, and potassium is added when renal function is established. The repletion phase takes approximately 6 to 8 hours in isotonic deficit but is more gradual in hypertonic dehydration. Shock is seldom a problem in hypertonic dehydration, but the risk of cerebral changes is greater.

Early recovery phase. In the *early recovery phase,* which lasts from 6 to 8 hours to 24 hours, oral feedings of a glucose-electrolyte solution are begun unless anorexia, vomiting, or nervous system disturbances prevent the use of this route. In this event, parenteral feedings are continued. A number of commercially prepared fluids are available, or a solution can be made with simple ingredients. Milk feedings are not resumed until at least the end of 24 hours. At the end of the early recovery phase, the effects of therapy are reassessed to evaluate the extent of fluid replacement and appropriate adjustments made if needed.

Late recovery phase. The *late recovery phase* is concerned with realimentation. Reintroduction of milk feedings is conducted slowly. Ordinarily about one fifth the usual daily intake of milk is recommended for the initial reintroduction, with the remainder provided by the glucose-electrolyte solution already employed. The amount of milk is gradually increased each day until the former diet is resumed. As mentioned in relation to moderate diarrhea, the possibility of a secondary lactase deficiency (especially in severely affected infants) makes a nonlactose-containing formula the feeding of choice. A normal nutritional regimen is usually resumed by the end of the fourth or fifth day.

Once the severe effects of dehydration are under control, specific diagnostic and therapeutic measures are instigated to detect and treat the cause of the diarrhea. This includes mild sedation, antimicrobial therapy where indicated, and treatment of secondary effects of the illness or its therapy. For example, secondary bacterial growth may be countered with a short course of nonabsorbable antibiotics and/or the oral administration of lactobacilli to recolonize the normal flora of the gastrointestinal tract.

Nursing considerations

The infant or child admitted to the hospital with diarrhea is always isolated from other children, and appropriate precautions are implemented to prevent possible spread to other children and personnel. Each hospital has a policy regarding isolation and enteric precautions.

The child is weighed on admission and frequently during the emergency phase of rapid hydration. Accurate intake and output measurement is imperative, and a urine collection bag is placed to determine the volume of output, to measure specific gravity, and as an indication that renal blood flow is sufficient to permit administration of potassium. Unless urine is separated from stool, this essential information cannot be obtained.

Children who are sufficiently ill to require hospitalization are almost always placed on parenteral fluid therapy with nothing by mouth for 12 to 24 hours. Monitoring the intravenous infusion is a primary nursing function, with careful attention to ascertain that the correct fluid and electrolyte concentration is infused, the flow rate is adjusted to deliver the desired volume in a given period of time, and the intravenous site is maintained. Restraint of some type is needed with infants and small children, whose purposeful or random movements might disturb the needle placement (pp. 922 and 1089). Frequent assessment of the intravenous site for infiltration and of the restrained limbs for circulation and pressure areas is necessary. Restraints should be released as frequently as possible to allow the child to move the extremities. Children are sufficiently active that range of motion exercises are seldom necessary when they are unconstrained and not in severe pain.

The nurse is responsible for examination of stools and the collection of specimens for laboratory examination. Care is exerted in obtaining and transporting stools to prevent possible spread of infection. Containers are manipulated and transported to the laboratory in appropriate media and containers and in accordance with hospital policy. Tests for pH, blood, and sugar can be done without removing the stool from the diaper. A clean tongue depressor can be used to obtain specimens for laboratory examination when a larger volume is needed or as an applicator for transfer to a culture medium.

Since diarrheal stools are highly irritating to the skin, extra care is needed to protect the skin of the diaper region from becoming excoriated. Exposing the reddened areas to heat and light is an effective method to facilitate healing. An excellent way to provide dry heat to the area is by means of a goose-necked lamp, but the lamp must be placed at a distance sufficient that the child is unable to reach any part of it. The heat source should be no closer than 18 inches. The child will require close observation during treatment, and the length of each application should not exceed 20 minutes. Active children will require restraint to maintain proper exposure, prevent any possibility of injury, and minimize possible spread of any feces that may be expelled. Contamination is especially likely in children with bowel movements of explosive character. Holding an infant or small child in the lap, protected with blankets and/or diapers, during the heat application serves as an excellent means for observing and restraining the child as well as providing tactile stimulation.

Oral feedings are begun according to the physician's orders. Although the amount and frequency vary according to individual philosophy, the initial oral fluids are water, usually with some added electrolytes. The electrolytes most frequently used are the commercial electrolyte solutions Pedialyte or Lytren, which contain a balanced electrolyte content. When the diet is advanced to clear liquids, diluted fruit juice, liquid or solid Jell-O, sweetened tea, Popsicles, and decarbonated cola or ginger ale are well tolerated. Broth or other high-sodium liquids are used with caution to avoid the possibility of hypernatremia. Soft foods are gradually added when liquids are well tolerated, as evidenced by no vomiting and an increased consistency and decrease in number of stools. Appropriate soft foods include gelatin desserts, soups (not creamed), bananas, applesauce, strained carrots, crackers (including pretzels), rice, and toast with jelly. Milk and lactose-containing formulas are usually withheld for at least a week in children with severe diarrhea. Hydrolyzed protein formulas with nonlactose sugar, such as Nutramagin or Pregestin, are substituted until the gastrointestinal tract is again able to tolerate milk and milk products.

Mild diarrhea. The observation and assessment of children who are treated at home, which are often the responsibility of a nurse who is under the supervision of the physician, involve assessment, therapy, and education. The status of the child must be evaluated to determine the extent of disease—the nature and frequency of stools, associated signs such as tenesmus, cramping, vomiting, or fever, and assessment of the state of hydration. When the diarrhea consists of a few loose stools each day without evidence of illness, the physician usually elects to treat the child with continued observation and diet management.

The mother is usually allowed to give fluids to the child. The length of time before initial feedings and the amount and type of fluids suggested depend on the philosophy of the physician. Acceptable fluids found in the home include those described for hospitalized children. If an electrolyte formula is prescribed, it is advisable to have the mother demonstrate her ability to prepare it, since a mistake or misunderstanding of measurements, for example, substitution of a tablespoon for the teaspoon measure, using heaping rather than level measurements, or adding other ingredients, such as milk, can significantly alter the electrolyte concentration.

Most often fluids are first offered in very small amounts, such as a teaspoon, and the amount is gradually increased at 15-minute intervals. If there is no vomiting, more liberal amounts can be fed. Fluids are usually tolerated best at room temperature, and the parent should be cautioned against giving solutions containing large amounts of sodium, since this can lead to hypernatremia. Undiluted fruit juices are hypertonic and contain a high concentration of carbohydrates, which may produce an osmotic diarrhea; therefore, these should be diluted until the diarrhea is controlled (Table 30-4).

Milk is added to the diet cautiously, usually 1 part skim milk diluted in 1 to 2 parts water with 5% carbohydrate added. If 30 to 60 ml of this solution every 2 to 3 hours in addition to an electrolyte fluid is tolerated, the ratio of milk should be gradually increased until the usual formula is tolerated. Simple foods are then reintroduced, and the customary diet is gradually resumed.

Table 30-4. General outline of dietary management of mild diarrhea

Time	Diet
First 8-12 hours	Small amounts (15 to 30 ml every ½ to 1 hour) of sweetened dilute tea, dilute cola, ginger ale, sugar water, or dilute Jell-O water
12-24 hours (if number of stools has lessened or not increased in frequency)	Increase clear fluids to 60 to 90 ml every 2 hours
24 hours (if definite improvement)	Plain solids such as Jell-O, bananas, applesauce, or salt crackers
36 to 48 hours	Gradual return to regular diet (dry toast, baked potato without butter, infant cereals mixed with water, fruits)
3 to 5 days	Gradual addition of milk and milk products; begin with half-strength skim, then full-strength skim, half-strength whole milk, and finally undiluted whole milk

Part of the home assessment includes taking a history to help elicit probable etiologic agents, such as introduction of a new food, travel to an area of high susceptibility, contact with foods that might be contaminated, and contact with pets that are known to be sources of enteric infections. Unrefrigerated milk and egg products provide an excellent media for growth of *Staphylococcus,* and fowl, both wild and domestic, is a well-known source of *Salmonella*. Animals of all varieties can be infected by other animals and birds. Recent evidence has implicated pet chickens, mammals (dogs, cats, mice, and so on), and reptiles, especially turtles, as sources of infection in children. Home assessment should include detection of such sources of contamination as well as observation of general cleanliness and sanitation in preparation and storage of food. (For a summary of nursing care of acute diarrheal disturbances, see the boxed material on pp. 1105 and 1106.)

It may be necessary to obtain stool specimens from the child and other family members who are affected or suspected to be carriers of infectious organisms. The parents are provided with specimen containers and instructed in collection and disposition of stool samples.

VOMITING

Vomiting, a very common symptom in childhood, is usually of little concern. Often it is of a minor and temporary nature, but when vomiting is persistent and prolonged the consequences to the infant or child can be rapid and serious. An associated hazard is the risk of aspiration, especially in very young and debilitated infants and children, with the possibility of asphyxiation, atelectasis, or pneumonia.

The amount and character of the vomiting are important observations, and nurses should be able to distinguish between and describe the various forms this behavior takes. Correct description is a valuable aid to diagnosis in a number of disorders. The following are terms used to describe vomiting:

spitting up dribbling of unswallowed formula from the infant's mouth immediately after a feeding.

regurgitation the return of undigested food from the stomach, usually accompanied by burping.

vomiting the forcible ejection of stomach contents, usually accompanied by nausea.

projectile vomiting vomitus ejected with such force that it projects as far as 2 to 4 feet from the child. The vomiting is not associated with nausea.

Etiology and pathophysiology

The etiology of vomiting is varied and is often one of the first symptoms of a variety of common infections as well as a manifestation of more serious conditions. Vomiting is a relatively frequent symptom during the neonatal period, usually simple regurgitation from overfeeding or insufficient bubbling, and has little clinical significance. However, it can indicate the presence of gastrointestinal tract disorders or increased intracranial pressure.

Vomiting in childhood can be caused by numerous intrinsic and extrinsic factors but is usually caused by readily detected infections or psychologic causes. Vomiting and diarrhea are common manifestations of a variety of infectious disorders, responses to an allergen or ingestion of drugs or other toxic substances, and symptoms associated with appendicitis or gastrointestinal obstruction. Recurrent, prolonged, or persistent vomiting is also associated with encephalographic variations and results from increased intracranial pressure caused by space-occupying lesions.

Pathophysiology. Vomiting, one of the most primitive protective functions with which animals are endowed, is controlled through the vomiting center located in the reticular core of the medulla. The vomiting center receives stimuli from three sources:

1. Higher cortical centers—either deep-seated or superficial psychologic disturbances. Stimuli include those associated with unpleasant sights, repugnant odors, and fright.
2. A chemosensitive trigger zone located on the floor of the fourth ventricle posterior to the medullary surface, which transmits impulses to the center. Stimuli include chemical stimulation by drugs such as apomorphine, morphine, ipecac, and some digitalis derivatives and toxins such as metabolic substances that result from uremia, infections, or radiation; cerebral hypoxia from decreased cerebral blood supply; the direct effect of increased intracranial pressure; and disturbances of the semicircular canals of the inner ear.
3. Reflex excitement from vagal and sympathetic afferent nerves resulting from disturbed gastrointestinal and other viscera. Stimuli include irritation, inflammation, or mechanical disturbance at any level of the gastrointestinal tract, such as distention or obstruction; irritation of other viscera, such as the heart, renal pelvis, and bladder; and pain of many sources.

Vomiting involves a complex reflex that is associated with widespread autonomic discharge that causes salivation, pallor, sweating, and tachycardia. Motor reaction, transmitted to the upper gastrointestinal tract, causes the vomiting act. The stomach antrum and duodenum contract; the remainder of the stomach, the esophagus, and its sphincters relax; the glottis closes to occlude the pulmonary airway; and the soft palate closes the nasopharynx. Then the diaphragm and abdominal muscles contract sharply, raising the intra-abdominal pressure, which compresses the abdominal contents and propels them into the esophagus and out through the mouth. Actual vomiting is usually preceded by severe cycles of reflux into the esophagus.[16]

Diagnostic evaluation

When vomiting is persistent and cannot be attributed to an obvious and temporary condition, a more comprehen-

Summary of nursing care of acute diarrheal disturbances

Goals	Responsibilities

Prevent spread of hospital infection	Isolate affected child from contact with others
	Implement protective techniques as dictated by hospital policy, including
	  Disposal of excreta and laundry
	  Appropriate handling of specimens
	Maintain careful hand washing
	Apply diaper snugly to reduce likelihood of fecal spread
	Instruct others (parents, members of staff) in protective procedures
	Teach affected children protective methods to prevent spread of infection, for example, remaining in restricted area, hand washing, handling genital area, care after using bedpan or toilet, and so on
	Endeavor to keep infants and small children from placing hand and objects in contaminated areas
	Assess home situation and implement protective measures as feasible in individual circumstances

Observe for signs of complications	Assess frequently
	  Vital signs—temperature, pulse, respiration, and blood pressure
	  Skin characteristics
	  Sensory response
	  Neurologic signs
	  Behavior

Prevent skin breakdown	Change diaper after each soiling; disposable diapers absorb poorly, cloth diapers are preferred May need to apply rubber pants or thick cotton panties to keep stool contained in diaper Cleanse buttocks and genital area well Apply protective lotion or ointment Expose reddened area to heat and air where feasible (risk of contamination great in explosive diarrhea)
Prevent dehydration	Administer fluids as prescribed and as tolerated
Prevent interference with therapeutic regimen	Apply appropriate restraining methods where indicated
Prevent complications from restraining devices	Remove restraints from extremities as often as possible Change position at least every 2 hours Observe frequently circulation, position, and pressure points

Rehydrate child	Administer fluids as ordered
	  Intravenous
	    Administer correct fluid
	    Maintain desired drip rate
	    Add appropriate electrolytes as prescribed
	    Maintain integrity of infusion site
	  Oral
	    Feed electrolyte-containing solutions as prescribed
	    Observe response to feedings
	    Describe feeding behavior
	Maintain accurate record of intake

Assess progress of hydration	Weigh child daily or as ordered Assess all parameters, for example, vital signs, skin characteristics Apply urine collection device when indicated Measure urine volume and specific gravity Collect specimens as needed

Continued.

Summary of nursing care of acute diarrheal disturbances—cont'd

Goals	Responsibilities

Assess status of diarrhea	Record fecal output
	  Number
	  Volume
	  Characteristics
	Observe and record presence of associated signs
	  Tenesmus
	  Cramping
	  Vomiting
	Collect specimens as needed
	Assist with specimen collection when indicated
	Make appropriate diagnostic tests
	  Stools
	    pH
	    Blood
	    Sugar
	  Urine
	    pH
	    Specific gravity

Provide comfort measures	Administer special mouth care while fluids by mouth are restricted Provide pacifier for infants who are receiving nothing by mouth Bubble child periodically to help expel swallowed air Hold infant or child when this does not interfere with therapy Touch, talk, and otherwise comfort child who is unable to be held Provide sensory stimulation and diversion appropriate to child's level of development Encourage parents to visit and allow them to comfort and care for child to the extent possible
Eradicate infectious agent	Administer antimicrobial medications as prescribed Administer other medications as prescribed
Reestablish diet appropriate for age	Gradually reintroduce foods as prescribed
Detect source of infection	Examine other members of household and refer for treatment where indicated Collect stool specimens from household members where indicated

Support parents	Reassure parents, especially mother
	Explain therapeutic measures that may be distressing to parents
	  Nothing by mouth
	  Parenteral fluids
	  Restraints necessary
	  Shaving of infant's head for intravenous therapy
	  Isolation from other children
	  Need for precautions that parents must observe
	Help parents provide comfort and support for child

Educate parents	Instruct parents in diet planning Help care giver plan diet to meet needs of affected child in relation to family diet pattern Instruct in preparation and storage of food, based on assessment of individual family needs and facilities Instruct in care and disposal of waste materials Teach and emphasize importance of good hygiene and sanitation
Arrange for follow-up care	Emphasize importance of posthospitalization health assessment Refer to community health agency for care and instruction when indicated

sive evaluation is warranted. It may be the only symptom the child presents; however, more often it is only one clinical feature of any one of a variety of disorders. The importance of vomiting in relation to the associated disease is also variable. It may be a minor manifestation of a serious illness or the dominant clinical feature. The following nursing observations can provide valuable information for evaluating the nature and importance of vomiting.

Character of vomitus. Vomitus that contains unchanged food and no gastric juice is esophageal. A relaxed cardiac sphincter (chalasia) or rumination (habitual regurgitation) will produce frequent small amounts of vomitus emitted with little force. The presence of sour milk curds with no green or brown color indicates vomitus from the stomach and eliminates an esophageal cause. Uncurdled milk may also be vomited during or shortly after feedings. Vomitus containing greenish-colored material indicating the presence of bile pigment is most likely to occur when an obstruction is situated below the ampulla of Vater; bile in the vomitus almost excludes pyloric stenosis. Vomitus with a fecal odor suggests a lower intestinal obstruction or peritonitis.

Blood in the vomitus may appear as bright red, bloody streaks, or brown coffee-ground emesis and may be insignificant or of major importance. Hematemesis is sometimes observed in the immediate neonatal period in infants who have swallowed maternal blood during delivery or, occasionally, from a cracked nipple. Maternal blood can be distinguished from the infant's blood by the alkaline denaturation test, which is based on the presence or absence of fetal hemoglobin. Other causes of hematemesis in early infancy include hemorrhagic disease of the newborn or other defects of coagulation and early esophageal erosion associated with regurgitation of gastric juice in diaphragmatic hernia. Trauma from nasogastric tubes or tracheal catheters may cause bleeding followed by vomiting of swallowed blood.

In older children hematemesis may be caused by swallowed blood from epistaxis or after nose or throat surgery. Rupture of esophageal varices and peptic ulcer can cause profuse hematemesis. Coagulation defects or vascular damage may cause bloody vomiting in many diseases.

Frequency and persistence. Frequent and/or persistent vomiting indicates that the causative factor is still operating. The primary danger is loss of fluids and electrolytes, which increases with the frequency and duration of vomiting. In early infancy the most frequent causes are pylorospasm, pyloric stenosis, adrenocortical insufficiency, and urinary tract infections. Recurrent vomiting suggests gastrointestinal allergy, an epileptic equivalent ("abdominal epilepsy"), a childhood form of migraine, or inconsistent intestinal obstruction, as might occur with malrotation of the colon. It is frequently associated with the onset of a febrile illness or a period of increased emotional tension.[24]

Amount. The amount of the emesis should be measured and recorded since it often furnishes information regarding the amount of fluid lost in relation to intake. This provides a clue to the extent of dehydration. Overfeeding or too rapid feeding may cause the child to vomit part of the feeding.

Force of vomiting. Repeated regurgitation is most often related to rumination or a relaxed cardiac sphincter. Forceful vomiting during or after a meal is usually caused by overdistention with milk and air. Repeated forceful vomiting of the projectile nature is one of the cardinal signs of pyloric stenosis in early infancy and can be a result of a brain tumor at any age. When combined with abdominal distention, it suggests intestinal obstruction.

Relationship to feeding. Emesis in infants may be related to the nature of their formula. Highly diluted formula may cause hungry infants to consume so much that they vomit from overdistention. High-fat or acidified formulas may cause others to vomit. Food that is contaminated by bacteria or food that is inappropriate to the child, such as unripe fruits or rich, highly seasoned foods may cause a child to vomit.

Vomiting soon after eating may be the result of food allergy or a symptom of an acute, febrile illness. More often it is caused by gastric distention associated with improper feeding techniques. Overdistention by milk and air initiates vomiting, which is caused by such feeding practices as failure to bubble the infant during and immediately after feedings, feeding formula through nipples with holes so small that the infant takes in air while sucking for milk, improper positioning of the bottle so that air instead of milk enters the nipple, feeding too rapidly, swallowing air from prolonged sucking on an empty breast, and underfeeding, which leads to hunger and causes the infant to swallow air while sucking on fingers or fists. Unwarmed formula may cause a few infants to vomit, and hurried eating at any age may precipitate vomiting, particularly when the child is excited or overly tired.

History. Sometimes the cause of vomiting is readily apparent from the history. Vomiting associated with diarrhea is usually caused by gastroenteritis; vomiting that occurs suddenly in a previously healthy child suggests the early stages of an infection. When several children or members of a family who have eaten together vomit, food poisoning is the most likely possibility. Vomiting accompanied by fever and abdominal pain and tenderness is a frequent symptom of appendicitis or other surgical conditions of the abdomen. Vomiting is not an uncommon reaction to toxins and to drugs taken as prescribed or ingested accidentally.

Many children are prone to motion sickness when riding in an automobile or airplane or even swinging in a swing. Some children, especially overly dependent children, maladjusted children, or children who react to environmental stress (such as a high-anxiety home environment), with somatic symptoms, respond to tension or stress with stomach upset and vomiting.

Diagnostic tests. Physical examination and routine tests of blood and urine are performed, but special laboratory tests are seldom employed. X-ray studies can detect anomalies of the alimentary tract. If vomiting has persisted to the degree that dehydration and electrolyte imbalance is present, the weight and serum electrolyte, blood urea nitrogen, and carbon dioxide content of the blood are determined to assess the state of hydration and to serve as the basis for therapy.

Medical management

Medical management is directed toward detection and treatment of the cause of the vomiting and prevention of complications of the vomiting. Vomiting that results in fluid loss of considerable degree may require parenteral fluid therapy. Fluids are administered in the same manner and in a similar electrolyte composition to those administered in diarrhea (p. 1101). This includes both parenteral and oral fluids.

Sometimes children will require a barbiturate, usually given by rectal suppository, or a tranquilizer, such as chlorpromazine (Thorazine) rectally or intramuscularly. For children who are prone to motion sickness, it is often helpful to administer an appropriate dose of dimenhydrinate (Dramamine) prior to a journey.

Nursing considerations

The major emphasis of nursing care of the vomiting infant or child is on observation and reporting of vomiting behavior and associated symptoms and the implementation of measures to reduce the vomiting. Accurate assessment of the type of vomiting, the appearance of the vomitus, and the child's behavior associated with the vomiting greatly aids in establishing a diagnosis of disorders that have vomiting as a clinical manifestation.

Nursing interventions will be determined by the cause of the vomiting. When the vomiting is identified as a manifestation of improper feeding methods, establishing proper techniques through teaching and example will usually correct the situation. If the vomiting is assessed as a probable manifestation of a gastrointestinal obstruction, food is usually withheld or special feeding techniques are implemented. In situations in which vomiting is related to concurrent infection, dietary indiscretion, or emotional factors, efforts are directed toward maintaining hydration or preventing dehydration by offering small amounts of palatable fluids such as ice chips, ginger ale, or diluted fruit juices, much the same as the oral intake described for diarrhea. If the child is able to retain the fluids, the diet can be expanded to include simple foods such as gelatin, crackers, clear broth, and buttered toast in small amounts, when the child desires, followed by gradual resumption of the regular diet.

HYPERTROPHIC PYLORIC STENOSIS

Obstruction at the pyloric sphincter by hypertrophy of the circular muscle of the pylorus is one of the most common surgical disorders of early infancy. This functional anomaly is seen soon after birth with vomiting that becomes progressively more severe and projectile. It is five times more common in male than female infants, affecting approximately 5 of every 1000 males and only 1 of every 1000 females. It is seen less frequently in black and Oriental than in white infants. It is more likely to affect a full-term than a premature infant.

Etiology and pathophysiology

The cause of the increased size of the pyloric musculature is unknown. A higher incidence in first-degree relatives and in monozygotic as opposed to dizygotic twins implicates heredity in the etiology, although the nature of the hereditary factors is only speculative.

Pathophysiology. The circular muscle of the pylorus is grossly enlarged as a result of both hypertrophy and hyperplasia. This produces severe narrowing of the pyloric canal between the stomach and duodenum. Consequently the lumen at this point is partially obstructed. Over a period of time inflammation and edema further reduce the size of the opening until the partial obstruction may progress to complete obstruction. The muscle is thickened to as much as twice its usual size—2 to 3 cm long—and is almost cartilaginous in consistency. The distal portion ends abruptly and is externally distinct and easily palpated, but the proximal end merges into the gastric antrum. The stomach is usually dilated (Fig. 30-2, *A*).

Diagnostic evaluation

Clinical manifestations. The age of onset and pattern of vomiting are variable. Typically infants with pyloric hypertrophy are well during the first weeks of life. Initially there is only regurgitation or occasional nonprojectile vomiting that begins about the second to the fourth week after birth, although in a few infants symptoms begin at birth. Others do well for the first few weeks and then suddenly develop projectile vomiting that rapidly leads to dehydration. The vomiting becomes projectile in nature, usually within a week, and may lead to complete obstruction by 4 to 6 weeks. The vomiting is forceful, and vomitus may be ejected 3 to 4 feet from the child in a side-lying position and 1 foot or more when the infant is lying on the back. Vomiting occurs most often shortly after a feeding, although it may occur as long as several hours later. In some instances the vomiting may follow each feeding; in others it appears intermittently. The infant is hungry and an avid nurser who eagerly accepts a second feeding after a vomiting episode. The vomitus is nonbilious, containing only gastric contents, but may be blood-tinged. The infant does not appear to be in pain other than the discomfort of chronic hunger.

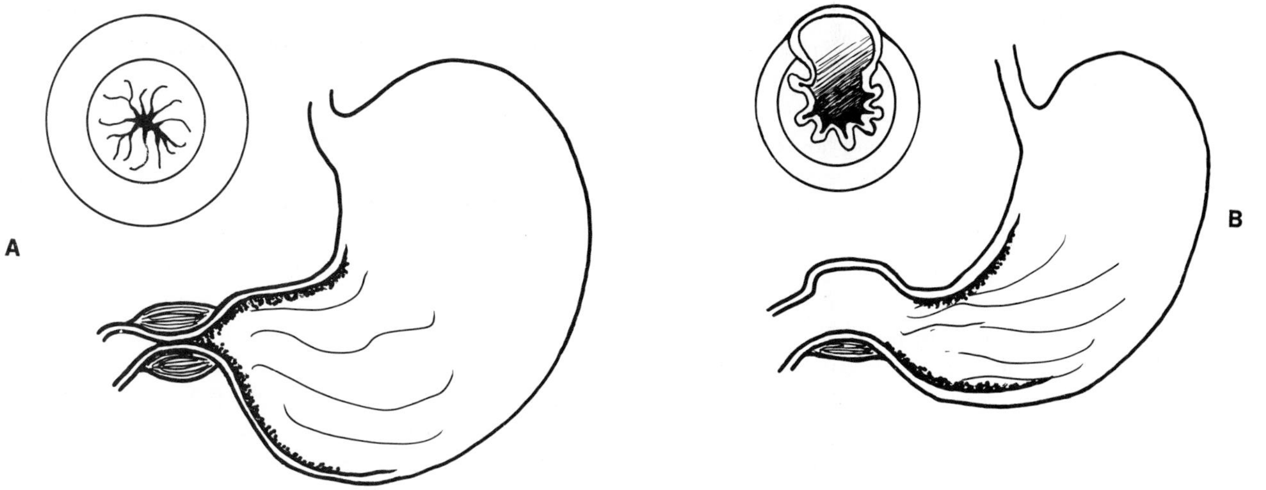

Fig. 30-2. Hypertrophic pyloric stenosis. **A,** Enlarged muscular tumor nearly obliterates pyloric channel. **B,** Longitudinal surgical division of muscle down to submucosa establishes adequate passageway.

The infant fails to gain weight or may lose weight, the stools diminish in number and size from the reduced intake, and evidence of dehydration becomes increasingly obvious. There is decreased elasticity of the skin, loss of subcutaneous tissue, and sunken eyeballs. The upper abdomen is distended, and diagnosis can be established on the basis of (1) a readily palpable olive-shaped tumor in the epigastrium just to the right of the umbilicus and (2) visible gastric peristaltic waves that move from left to right across the epigastrium. The pyloric tumor is most easily felt when the abdominal muscles are relaxed during a feeding or immediately after vomiting. Positive identification of these physical signs is sufficient evidence to establish a diagnosis (usually corroborated by a second physician).

Difficulty in diagnosis is related to children with feeding difficulties associated with disturbed mother-child relationships or hyperkinetic infants who are exceptionally reactive to external stimuli and vomit more frequently than usual in the early weeks of life.

Diagnostic tests. If diagnosis is inconclusive from the history and physical signs, upper gastrointestinal x-ray studies will reveal delayed gastric emptying and an elongated, thread-like pyloric channel. Laboratory findings reflect the metabolic alterations created by severe depletion of both water and electrolytes from extensive and prolonged vomiting. There are decreased serum levels of both sodium and potassium, although these may be masked by the hemoconcentration from extracellular fluid depletion. Of greater diagnostic value are a decrease in serum chloride levels and increases in pH and bicarbonate (carbon dioxide content) characteristic of metabolic alkalosis. Hemoconcentration is evidenced by elevated hematocrit and hemoglobin values.

Medical management

Surgical relief of the pyloric obstruction by pyloromyotomy is simple, safe, and effective and is, with very few exceptions, the standard treatment for this disorder. Nonoperative management is possible but seldom employed today since the treatment is lengthy and the results uncertain.

Surgical treatment. Since the surgery is not an emergency procedure, the initial efforts are directed toward rehydration of the infant, replenishment of body potassium stores, and correction of alkalosis with parenteral fluid and electrolyte administration. The type of fluids administered depends on the degree of dehydration and associated metabolic alterations. In well-hydrated infants with no evidence of electrolyte imbalance, surgery is performed without delay. Replacement fluid therapy usually delays surgery for 24 to 48 hours. Some surgeons prefer the stomach to be empty during surgery to diminish postoperative vomiting from gastric irritation. For these infants, gastric lavage with isotonic saline solution is part of preoperative preparation. The lavage tube is often left in place during the surgical procedure to keep the stomach empty of fluid, air, or barium from x-ray procedures.

The surgical procedure is performed through a right upper quadrant muscle-splitting incision and consists of a longitudinal incision through the circular muscle fibers of the pylorus down to, but not including, the submucosa (Fredet-Ramstedt operation), Fig. 30-2, *B*. The procedure has a very high success rate when infants receive careful preoperative preparation to correct fluid and electrolyte imbalances.

Feedings are usually begun 4 to 6 hours postoperatively, beginning with small, frequent feedings of glucose in water or electrolyte solutions. If clear fluids are retained, about 24 hours after surgery formula is started in the same stepwise increments, gradually increasing the amount and the interval between feedings until a full feeding schedule is reinstated, which usually takes about 48 hours. The infant is ready to be discharged from the hospital by about the fourth postoperative day. The prognosis is excellent, and the mortality rate is low.

Nonsurgical treatment. Medical treatment of pyloric stenosis is not widely used, since there is such a high success rate with surgical management. However, it may be employed when the diagnosis is uncertain, symptoms are mild, or surgery is contraindicated for other reasons. Nonsurgical treatment consists of a long-term regimen of small, frequent feedings of formula thickened with cereal, maintaining an upright position after feedings, refeeding, sedation, and administration of a cholinergic blocking agent. Parenteral fluids are administered as needed, and stomach lavage for epigastric distention reduces the likelihood of vomiting. Sometimes the treatment is successful in a short period of time; more often it requires prolonged hospitalization, which further complicates normal growth and development, especially in the area of maternal-child relationships.

Nursing considerations

Nursing care of the infant with hypertrophic pyloric stenosis involves primarily observation for physical signs and behaviors that help establish the diagnosis, careful regulation of fluid therapy, and reestablishment of normal feeding behaviors. Nurses are in a position to recognize signs of the disorder in infants and to refer them for medical evaluation. Hypertrophic pyloric stenosis should be considered as a possibility in the very young infant who appears alert but fails to gain weight and has a history of vomiting after meals.

Preoperative care. Preoperatively the emphasis is placed on restoring hydration and electrolyte balance and beginning replacement of depleted body fat and protein stores. These infants are usually given no oral feedings and placed on intravenous fluids with glucose and electrolyte replacement based on laboratory serum electrolyte values, usually sodium chloride solution with added potassium (when there is adequate urine output). Depleted calcium must also be replaced. Careful monitoring of the intravenous infusion and assiduous attention to intake, output, and urine specific gravity measurements are important to the success of fluid replacement. Accurate description of any vomiting, as well as the number and character of stools, is observed and recorded.

If the infant is fed either thickened or unthickened feedings, special techniques are needed to minimize the likelihood of vomiting. Feedings are given slowly with the infant held in a semiupright position. Because these infants tend to suck their fingers and hands, they swallow a good deal of air; therefore, bubbling before and frequently during feedings will lessen gastric distention. After a feeding the infant is turned slightly on the right side in high-Fowler's position in an infant seat or propped in the crib to facilitate gastric emptying. Minimal handling, especially after a feeding, helps prevent vomiting. If vomiting occurs, the type, amount, character, and its relationship to the feeding are observed and recorded. Refeeding of formula is usually ordered in an amount equivalent to the volume lost.

Observations include assessment of vital signs, particularly those that might indicate fluid or electrolyte imbalances. These infants are especially prone to metabolic alkalosis from loss of hydrogen ions and to potassium, sodium, and chloride depletion, all of which are contained in gastric secretions (see p. 1074 for signs of deficits). The skin and mucous membranes are assessed for alterations in hydration status, and daily weight provides added clues to water gain or loss (see p. 1081).

When stomach decompression and gastric lavage are part of preoperative management, it is the responsibility of the nurse to ensure that the tube is patent and functioning properly and to measure and record the type and amount of drainage. The infant is usually positioned flat or with the head slightly elevated. The infant who is receiving intravenous fluids and/or has a nasogastric tube to continuous drainage must be adequately restrained to prevent the needle and/or tube from becoming dislodged.

General hygienic care, with particular attention to skin and mouth in dehydrated infants, is an important part of care. Protection from infection is also important, since infants with impaired nutritional status are even more susceptible than normal newborn infants. Sensory stimulation is incorporated into nursing care, and parental involvement is encouraged and promoted.

Postoperative care. Postoperative vomiting is not uncommon, and most infants, even with successful surgery, exhibit some vomiting during the first 24 to 48 hours. Intravenous fluids are administered until the infant is taking and retaining adequate amounts by mouth. Therefore, much of the same care that was instituted prior to surgery is continued postoperatively, that is, observation of physical signs, monitoring intravenous fluids, and careful observation and recording of intake and output. In addition the infant is observed for responses to the stress of surgery. The nasogastric tube may be maintained after surgery for a variable length of time. Feedings are usually instituted relatively soon, beginning with clear liquids containing glucose and electrolytes. They are offered slowly and at frequent intervals as ordered by the physician. If the infant has been breast fed, breast milk, expressed by the mother, is given by bottle when the infant is able to tolerate feedings, and breast-feeding is resumed as soon as feasible. Observation and recording of feedings and the infant's responses to feed-

Summary of nursing care of the child with pyloric stenosis

Goals	Responsibilities

Help establish diagnosis	Recognize signs of pyloric stenosis and refer for medical evaluation
	Obtain specimens and assist with diagnostic tests and procedures
	Observe and record:
	  Physical signs of upper gastrointestinal obstruction, hyperperistalsis
	  Amount, type, and character of vomiting
	  Amount, type, and character of stools
	Observe oral behaviors, including eating, hand-sucking, and so on

Prevent vomiting	Give small, frequent feedings; feed slowly Bubble before and frequently during feedings Position in high-Fowler's position and slightly on right side after feeding Handle minimally and gently after feeding
Promote gastric decompression	Give nothing by mouth Carry out lavage as ordered Maintain patency of nasogastric tube Measure and record amount and type of drainage

Recognize signs of complications	Observe, report, and record any signs of upper gastrointestinal fluid loss:
	  Alkalosis
	  Hypokalemia
	  Hypochloremia
	  Dehydration
	  Altered neurologic signs
	  Shock
	Postoperatively, check incision site

Prevent removal of intravenous or nasogastric tube	Apply and maintain adequate restraining devices

Prevent infection	Continue general protective measures, including
	  Avoidance of contact with infected persons
	  Good hand washing before handling infant
	  Only clean or sterile supplies in contact with infant

Provide nutrition	Administer feedings as ordered Administer and monitor parenteral fluids as ordered at desired rate of flow
Maintain warmth	Place infant in Isolette or warmer or provide adequate covering

Assess adequacy of intake	Weigh daily or as ordered
	Assess status of skin and mucous membranes
	Measure carefully
	  Intake—oral and/or parenteral
	  Output—vomitus, nasogastric tube drainage, stools, and urine
	  Urine specific gravity

Maintain general hygiene	Administer good skin care Change diapers immediately when wet or soiled Administer special care to reddened or excoriated areas Administer mouth care

Continued.

Summary of nursing care of the child with pyloric stenosis—cont'd

Goals	Responsibilities
Provide comfort	Provide pacifier to meet oral needs Provide sensory stimulation Encourage parents' visitation and involvement in care Whenever possible, arrange to hold, or have others hold, infant
Support parents	Keep parents informed regarding infant's progress Assure mother or other care giver that the problem is organic and is in no way a reflection of inadequate mothering skills Allow parents to express concerns and anxieties
Teach parents	Instruct parent in feeding and positioning techniques Instruct in care of incision Instruct regarding signs of Expected behavior Behaviors and signs that should be reported
Administer follow-up care	Instruct parents regarding posthospitalization evaluation Refer to public health agency if needed

ings and feeding techniques are a vital part of postoperative care. Positioning with the head elevated is usually continued postoperatively. Care of the operative site consists of observation for any drainage or signs of inflammation and care of the incision as directed by the surgeon.

As with any child in the hospital, parents are encouraged to visit and become involved in the child's care. Vomiting of a projectile nature is frightening to parents, and they often believe that they may have done something wrong. Most mothers need support and reassurance that the condition is caused by a structural problem and is in no way a reflection on their mothering skills and capacities. (For a summary of nursing care of the child with pyloric stenosis, see the boxed material on pp. 1111 and 1112.)

BURNS

Minor burn injuries are experienced by everyone in day-to-day living and are relatively commonplace in nursing practice. Extensive burns, on the other hand, are relatively uncommon; however, they account for some of the most difficult nursing problems encountered in the pediatric age-group. The third most important cause of accidental death in childhood, burns are outranked only by automobile casualties and drownings. In addition serious burn injury accounts for a very large number of children who must undergo prolonged, painful, and restrictive hospitalization. These children frequently emerge from the experience with scars to both body and personality, which profoundly affect their social and emotional development. It is tragic, too, that the great majority of burn injuries (75%) are preventable.[5,26]

Although severe burns are manifest primarily in damage to the skin, they produce a complex illness that requires the utmost in nursing skill and care. Every organ system becomes involved, and sometimes even the treatment creates additional problems. Nursing care of patients with extensive burns involves an understanding of a variety of specialized areas, including surgical principles and techniques, respiratory physiology, fluid and electrolyte physiology, nutrition, bacteriology, growth and development, occupational therapy, physical therapy, and principles of psychiatric nursing.[6,15]

Epidemiology

It is estimated that 150,000 children are badly burned each year—one every 4 minutes—and that 30% of the approximately 7800 deaths from burn injury are persons under 15 years of age.[26] Figures contributed from major burn centers that specialize in the care of children reveal that the largest percentage of burns in the pediatric age-group occurs in children under 5 years of age. Until age 9 years there is no sex difference in the incidence of burns, but after age 9 years boys outnumber girls three to one.[21] Table 30-5 describes the types of burn that are most often associated with children at different developmental levels.

Children under 5 years of age constitute 70% of burn

Table 30-5. Burn hazards of children

Age-group	Type of burn	Hazard	Time/place
Toddlers (6-24 months)	Scalds	Playing underfoot in kitchen, overturning cups, pulling electric cords off coffee-pots or frying pans; bath water too hot; parental neglect/abuse	Daytime/home
	Electric burns	Chewing extension cords	
Young children (2-6 years)	Flame burns	Playing with matches, climbing on stove, warming with heating source	Early morning/kitchen, bedroom, and so on
6- to 14-year-old children	Scalds	Water too hot	
Boys	Flame burns	Playing/working with gasoline, campfires, barbecues, chemistry sets, firecrackers, rockets, matches, and so on	After school, holidays/outdoors, indoors
	Electric burns	Climbing around high-tension wires	
Girls	Flame burns	Reaching over stove, candles, making candles, "innocent bystander" (observing others play with fire or gasoline)	Morning, evening/kitchen; after school/yard
All children	Flame burns	House fires; gas tank explosion during automobile accident	Usually night, anytime

Courtesy Northern California Burn Council, San Francisco, and Elizabeth McLoughlin, Director of Burn Injury Project, Shriners Burns Institute, Boston, Mass.

injuries, and the incidence is closely related to the quality and quantity of adult supervision. The most hazardous periods are the early morning hours when parents are still in bed and the interval between the time school is out and the evening meal. Burns in children in this age-group occur more often in large than in small families.[12] Whereas young children are more apt to receive scalds, older children are more likely to be burned severely by flaming clothing from open flames, heaters, and explosions—very often in an unsupervised play situation in which combustible materials, such as gasoline and matches or cigarette lighters, are present. A significant number of burns occur in garages and basements in which there is an open-gas heating unit or pilot light. Many children die or are seriously injured in burning buildings, especially when left unattended.[13]

Electric burns of the mouth from chewing on an electric cord are more typical of children in the crawling or toddler stage of development. Younger children are more likely to be burned by poking metal objects into electric outlets, whereas burns from tension wires occur in older children.

Burns also have a seasonal incidence. Since furnaces and other heating devices are used most extensively during cold weather, burns from heaters and house fires are more frequent in the winter months. Flash burns from explosive ignition of outdoor barbecues with volatile liquids increase in summer months. Burns caused by clothing catching fire from campfires occur in summer and from burning leaves in autumn. In all seasons young girls sustain burn injuries to the chest and arms when loose, frilly clothes (especially nightwear) are ignited from an open fire, gas ranges or heaters, and candelabra.

Psychologic factors are often related to burn injury in children. For example, burns that are inflicted as punishment are a common form of child abuse, and it is the unwanted or least desirable child who is the last to be rescued from a burning building. The frequency of burn injury, as well as other accidental injuries, is increased in families in which there is emotional disturbance, such as marital discord, a disturbed parent, or a disturbed or retarded child. Setting fires by small boys and burns of either boys or girls can often be interpreted as a signal of distress related to loss of a parent to whom the child had a strong attachment. In many children difficult behavior for varying periods of time precedes the burn injury. Not only do these psychologic and behavioral problems contribute to the injury, but they also influence the child's hospitalization and convalescence.[12]

Etiology of burns

Burns can be caused by thermal, chemical, electric, or radioactive agents. Most burn injuries are caused by thermal agents, principally flame and hot water (including steam), and, to a lesser extent, friction and frostbite. Chemical burns can be caused by either acids or alkalis and radiation burns by either x-rays or ultraviolet radiation. The extent

A

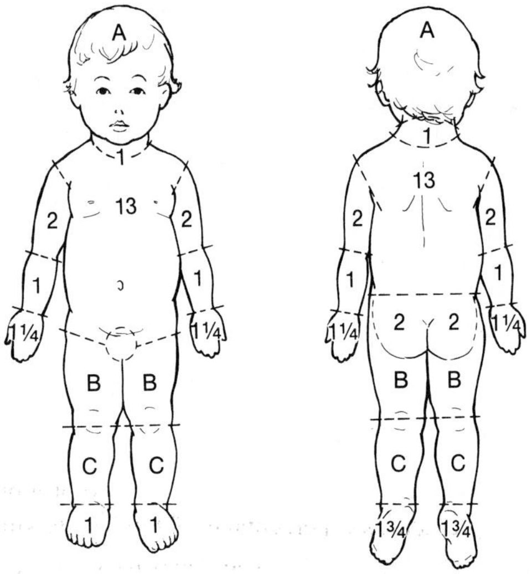

RELATIVE PERCENTAGES OF AREAS AFFECTED BY GROWTH

AREA	BIRTH	AGE 1 YR	AGE 5 YR
A = ½ of head	9½	8½	6½
B = ½ of one thigh	2¾	3¼	4
C = ½ of one leg	2½	2½	2¾

B

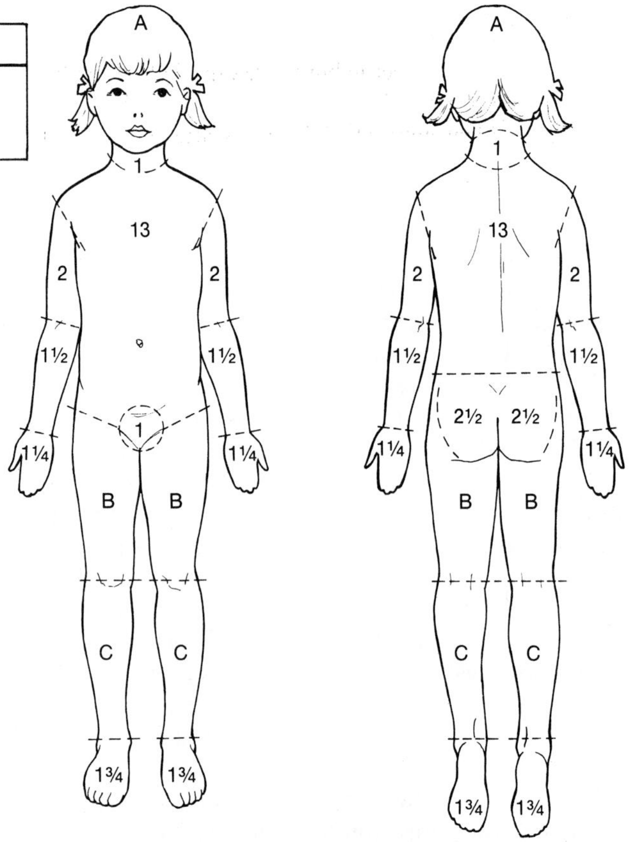

Fig. 30-3. Estimation of distribution of burns in children. **A,** Children from birth to age 5 years; **B,** older children.

RELATIVE PERCENTAGES OF AREAS AFFECTED BY GROWTH

AREA	AGE 10 YR	AGE 15 YR	ADULT
A = ½ of head	5½	4½	3½
B = ½ of one thigh	4½	4½	4¾
C = ½ of one leg	3	3¼	3½

of tissue destruction is determined by the intensity of the heat source, the duration of contact or exposure, and the speed with which the heat energy is dissipated by the burned surface. For example, a brief exposure to high-intensity heat, such as a flame, or a longer exposure to a low-intensity heat, such as hot water, can produce similar burn injuries. Burns caused by boiling oil or liquid fat tend to cause deep partial-thickness burns. Prolonged exposure to the sun's rays or to a heated object, such as a sidewalk, is also capable of producing burns of significant extent.

Full-thickness destruction frequently occurs when clothing is ignited. Cotton and nylon clothing burns most easily whereas clothing made from wool or other animal fibers burns less readily. Synthetic fabrics melt and stick to the skin surface. Contact burns from heated metal or liquids (such as tar) at extreme temperatures, prolonged immersion in hot water, chemical burns without rinsing with water, and electric burns are all significant in the etiology of severe burn trauma. Chemical agents continue to cauterize the tissues until the injurious agent is chemically united with tissue elements, neutralized, or removed by washing with running water. Electric burns are especially deceptive, since they are characterized by more extensive thrombosis that is not evident until 24 to 36 hours after injury. Their extensive destruction has been described as resembling a crush injury.

Assessment of burn wound

The physiologic responses, therapy, prognosis, and disposition of the injured child are all directly related to the *amount of tissue destroyed;* therefore, the severity of the burn injury is assessed on the basis of:

Percentage of body surface burned
Depth of the burn
Location of the burn(s)

Also important in determining the seriousness of the injury are:

Age of the child
Etiologic agent
Extent of respiratory involvement
General health of the child
Presence of any associated injury or condition

Percentage of body surface. The size of a burn is usually expressed as a percentage of total body surface area, which is most accurately estimated by using specially designed age-related charts (Fig. 30-3). Because of the body proportions, especially the head and lower extremities, the standard "rule of nines" charts used for adults are not applicable to small children.

Depth of injury. A thermal injury is a three-dimensional wound and, therefore, is also assessed in relation to depth of injury. Traditionally the terms first-, second-, and third-

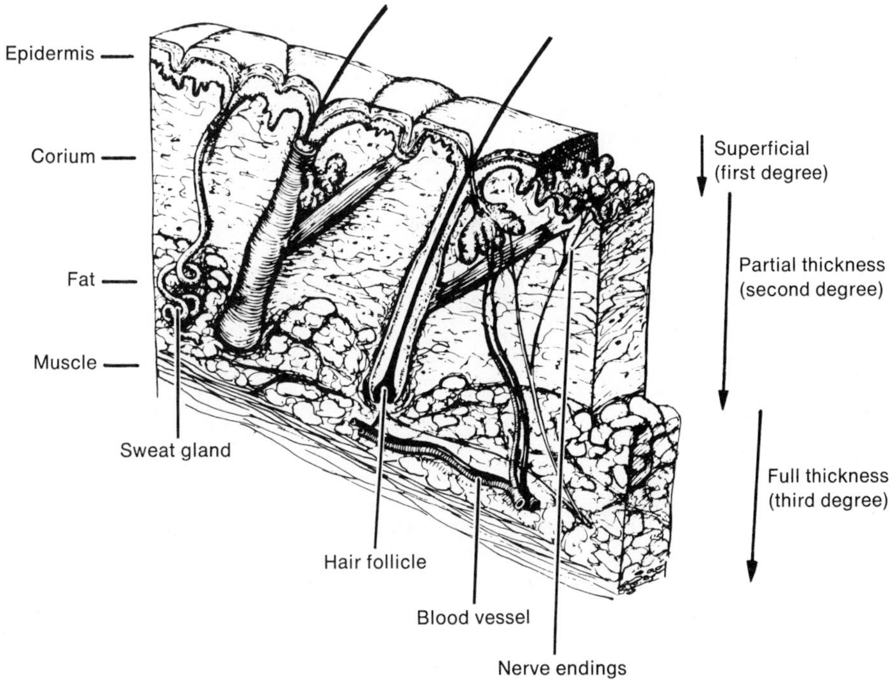

Fig. 30-4. Cross section of skin illustrating depth of tissue destruction in first-, second-, and third-degree burns.

degree have been used to describe the depth of tissue injury. However, with the current emphasis on burn healing, these are gradually being replaced by more descriptive terms based on the extent of destruction to the epithelializing elements of the skin. Partial-thickness burns heal in time; full-thickness burns require skin grafting for closure. Partial-thickness injury is further categorized, by many, as superficial or deep-dermal burns, depending on how rapidly they heal. Since both terminologies are used, often interchangeably, both are presented in describing the characteristics of burn wounds (Fig. 30-4 and Table 30-6).

First-degree burns are usually of minor significance. There is frequently a latent period followed by erythema. Tissue damage is minimal, protective functions remain intact, and systemic effects are rare. Pain is the predominant symptom.

Second-degree, or partial-thickness, burns are deeper and involve not only the epithelium but a minimal to substantial portion of the corium. The severity of the injury and the rate of healing are directly related to the amount of undamaged corium from which new tissue can regenerate. Superficial burns are often classified with first-degree burns and heal uneventfully. Deep-dermal burns, although classified as second-degree or partial-thickness burns, in many respects resemble third-degree burns. There is hyperemia in areas with less heat and leakage of protein in areas with the most heat. Systemic effects are similar to those that occur with deeper burns. Whereas first-degree and superficial partial-thickness burns are painful, deep, dermal burns are often anesthetic for the first 1 or 2 days after injury.

Third-degree, or full-thickness, burns are serious injuries in which all layers of the skin are destroyed, may involve underlying tissues as well, and are usually combined with extensive partial-thickness damage. Systemic effects can be life threatening and involve every organ system in the body.

Severity of burn injury.[3,15] Burns are also appraised on the basis of their severity. This is useful in determining the disposition of the patient for treatment. Burned patients can usually be distinguished as (1) those with a critical burn who require the services and equipment of a special burn facility; (2) those with moderate burns who may be treated in any hospital unit; and (3) those with minor burns who are able to be treated on an outpatient basis. Although each burn unit and specialist in the field of burn management has criteria for admission to special units, there are a number of factors that influence the effects of the injury, the probability of recovery, and response to therapy.

Initial assessment to estimate the extent of skin destruction is made on the basis of observation and simple diagnostic techniques. The extent of surface involvement is readily calculated, and the surface appearance of the wound

Table 30-6. Characteristics of burn wounds

Degree	Depth	Tissues	Type of burn	Appearance	Sensation
First degree	Epidermal (partial thickness)	Epidermis May include stratum germinativum	Overexposure to sun Brief flash Brief scald	Dry surface Erythematous Blanches readily on pressure; refills quickly on release	Painful (hyperesthetic)
Second degree	Partial thickness Superficial	All epidermal layers and much of the corium or dermis	Intense flash heat Immersion in hot liquids Contact with hot objects	Blistered, moist, mottled pink or red Blanches on pressure and refills	Very painful (hyperesthetic) Sensitive to air
	Deep dermal	Extends deep into corium		Mottled, red, dull white, or tan Reddened areas blanch on pressure and refill Blistered, moist, or dry	Deep dermal burns may be anesthetic for 1 or 2 days after injury
Third degree	Full thickness	Entire skin and all its structures	Scalds from live steam, open flame, chemicals, or electric current Long-term contact with milder heat	Tough, leathery surface Brown, tan, black, pearly white, or even red No blistering—may develop vesicles that represent necrosis Does not blanch and refill on pressure Area may be depressed Dull and dry	Little pain (hypesthetic to anesthetic)

provides clues to whether the injury involves the full thickness of the skin or only a portion of the skin layers. The extent to which the wound is capable of regeneration depends on the areas destroyed. Epithelial regeneration can take place from residual basilar cells and from the epithelial lining of sweat glands and hair follicles.

Blisters do not occur in full-thickness burns, but with superficial burns in general, the deeper the burn, the more common is blister formation. Blisters increase in size in the hours immediately after the burn occurs, and, usually, the larger the blister, the deeper the burn. Touching injured surfaces gives more additional information. Testing for capillary filling by blanching and refilling indicates whether circulation in the area is intact. Since the sensory end organs are concentrated in the deep dermal areas, presence of sensation indicates tissue viability; absence of sensation suggests full skin thickness destruction. This is easily determined by pricking the skin with a sterile needle.[17]

The burn source can help to estimate and classify the extent of the injury. Hot liquids may result in partial-thickness injury, whereas full-thickness injury is associated with flame burns. This can vary with the age of the child, however. Because infants' skin is so thin, it is readily destroyed by thermal agents. This makes estimation of depth difficult in children in this age-group, especially in scalds. Electric burns appear to be less serious than they actually are, since they often involve deep structures. The electric current will follow nerves and blood vessels, and it may cause thrombosis with subsequent severe tissue destruction.[26] Children with facial burns, those with burns acquired in an enclosed area, or those in whom inhalation is suspected for other reasons are at risk for developing airway obstruction or severe hypoxia during the hours after inhalation.

In calculating the risk related to thermal injuries, children less than 2 years of age have a significantly higher mortality rate than older children with burns of similar magnitude. They are subject to rapid fluid shifts, which places them in jeopardy in the early hours, and their immune competence is not well developed; therefore, sepsis is a frequent complication.

According to severity, burns are classified as follows:

Minor burns
- Partial-thickness burns of less than 15% of body surface
- Full-thickness burns of less than 2% of body surface

Moderate burns
- Partial-thickness burns of 15% to 30% of body surface
- Full-thickness burns of less than 10% of body area, except in small children and when the burns involve critical areas

Major or *critical* burns
- Burns complicated by respiratory tract injury
- Partial-thickness burns of 30% total area or greater
- Burns of face, hands, feet, or genitalia, even if they appear to be partial thickness
- Full-thickness burns of 10% of body surface or greater
- Any child under 2 years of age, unless the burn is very small and very superficial
- Electric burns
- Deep chemical burns
- Burns complicated by fractures or soft tissue injury
- Burns complicated by concurrent illness, such as obesity, diabetes, epilepsy, and cardiac and renal diseases

Pathophysiology: local responses

Local changes at the site of the burn injury begin to occur at approximately 45°C (113°F); tissues die at 65°C (149°F) and over because of coagulation necrosis. The tissue coagulates, desiccates, or becomes carbonized, depending on the extent of exposure to the source of heat. At the same time, changes in the intercellular cement that binds the epidermis to the dermis cause the epidermis to detach and either peel away or form a blister between the two layers.[15] In infants and young children the skin is so thin and contains such shallow dermal appendages that full-thickness loss occurs easily on exposure to heat. There are also fewer skin appendages in prepubescent children than in adolescents.

The burn wound consists basically of three distinct layers (Fig. 30-5)[26,27]:

1. *Zone of coagulation.* In this zone, beneath the obviously destroyed tissue, capillary flow has ceased and tissue destruction is irreversible. The tissue is dead.
2. *Zone of stasis.* Beneath and surrounding the zone of coagulation there is a zone with markedly reduced capillary flow. The tissue is severely damaged from heat but is not coagulated. The tissue in this zone can be saved with prevention of further injury and adequate perfusion.
3. *Zone of hyperemia.* An area metabolically active and displaying the usual response to tissue injury.

It is the two outer zones in which significant changes take place and that are involved in the pathophysiology of the burn wound and the systemic responses to the initial burn injury.

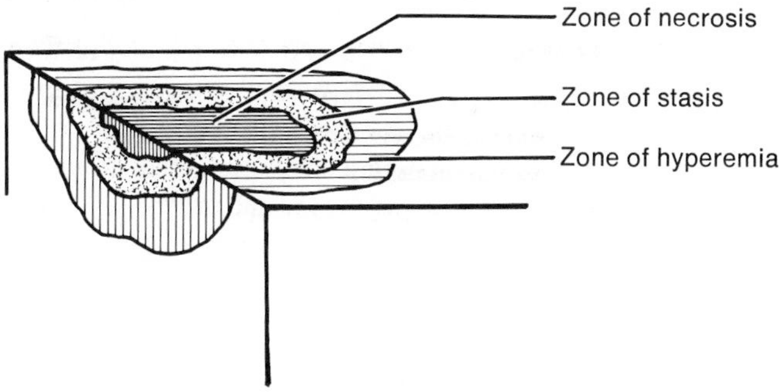

Fig. 30-5. Zones of injury in burns. (After Zawacki, B.: Reversal of capillary stasis and prevention of necrosis in burns, Ann. Surg. **180:**98-102, 1974.)

Edema formation. Increased capillary permeability in these two outer zones is due to thermal injury to the vessels. At the same time, vasodilatation causes an increase in hydrostatic pressure within the capillaries. The increased hydrostatic pressure plus the increased capillary permeability cause loss of water, protein, and electrolytes from the intravascular compartment into the interstitial spaces. This shift is further enhanced by a diminishing intravascular oncotic pressure, as protein and sodium are lost to the interstitial spaces. Although the edema involves both burned and nonburned areas, at the site of injury the accumulation of edema fluid beneath and around the burn can reach tremendous proportions until the extravasation of fluid is limited by tissue tension.

In addition there are also changes in the permeability of tissue cells in and around the burned area that allow an abnormal exchange of electrolytes between the cells and the interstitial fluid, that is, sodium enters the cells in exchange for potassium, causing further depletion of intravascular sodium.

Fluid loss. Without the protective skin, fluid loss at the air-wound interface can be extremely high. These losses reach a maximum about the fourth day after the burn occurred but continue to pose problems until the denuded surfaces are debrided and grafted.

Circulatory stasis. Significant circulatory alterations take place in the zone of stasis located around the coagulated dead tissue. When red blood cells are heated, they become spherical in shape. These heat-damaged cells, together with hemoconcentration from fluid loss, depressed cardiac output, and tissue edema, reduce the blood flow in the burn area, causing capillary stasis. Thrombi develop that further impede circulation, producing tissue ischemia and eventual necrosis. This may also prolong the edema phase. Further hyperviscosity and impaired blood flow are attributed to the release of substances from damaged cells, such as thromboplastin and clot-activating factors, that cause the production of microthrombi, platelet adhesiveness and aggregation, and increased pain and swelling.[3,4,9,15]

In partial-thickness burns circulation around the burn area ceases immediately after injury but is rapidly restored within 24 to 48 hours. In full-thickness burns, however, the vascular supply is completely occluded and no appreciable circulation is reestablished until granulation takes place at the interface between burned and unburned tissue.[19]

Burn wound. In first-degree destruction of the vascular epithelium, tissue damage is minimal. Protein loss is insignificant and edema barely perceptible. The burning sensation and pain resolve in 48 to 72 hours and, in 5 to 10 days, the damaged epithelium peels off in small scales or sheets, leaving no scarring.

In second-degree, partial-thickness burns there is considerable edema and more severe capillary damage. In 3 to 5 days a crust of dried exudate and injured tissue covers the wound to form a protective seal while healing takes place from underneath. With reasonable care, superficial burns heal spontaneously and uneventfully through the generative capacity of the stratum germinativum and epithelial cells of appendageal linings. The crust separates in 10 to 14 days with minimal or no scarring.

Deep-dermal burns heal more slowly by regeneration from the epithelial lining of skin appendages, sweat glands, and hair follicles. A thin epithelial covering develops in 25 to 35 days, but this type of burn may require several months to heal. Scarring is common, and trauma or infection can easily convert a partial-thickness burn to a full-thickness injury, especially in young children with their normally thinner skin. Fluid loss and metabolic effects may be considerable.

In third-degree, full-thickness burns there is cell destruction by coagulation necrosis. The dead tissue and exudate convert to a thick leathery eschar in 48 to 72 hours, which liquifies and begins to separate in 12 to 21 days as a result of autolysis, leukemic digestion, and disintegration of collagen fibers. New granulation tissue will form on the wound bed, which, if not grafted, will heal by slow proliferation from the edges with severe scarring. In full-thickness burns there is severe edema with fluid and electrolyte shifts and extensive metabolic changes.

Pathophysiology: systemic response

Along with and subsequent to the pathophysiologic response at the site of thermal injury, a number of systemic responses occur.

Circulatory. The immediate postburn period is marked by dramatic alterations in circulation, known as *burn shock*. There is a precipitous drop in cardiac output (about 50% of normal resting values) that precedes any changes in circulating blood or plasma volume. With the large fluid losses through denuded skin, vasodilatation, and edema formation, the blood volume decreases rapidly and cardiac output is reduced even further, usually leveling off at 20% of normal resting values. Cardiact output returns to normal spontaneously in 24 to 36 hours, although the plasma volume lags far behind.[19]

The initial decrease in cardiac output is attributed to a circulating myocardial-depressant factor, associated with severe burn injury, that affects the contractility of heart muscle directly. The blood volume deficit, although slower in onset, can be profound and appears to be directly proportional to the extent and depth of the burn.[4]

Capillary permeability with leakage of fluid takes place in noninjured areas as well as in the outer zones of the burn wound. The edema fluid accumulates rapidly in the first 18 hours after injury to reach a maximum in about 48 hours. Capillary permeability returns to normal and the fluid is reabsorbed, chiefly by way of the lymphatics. Reabsorption usually proceeds at the rate of fluid accumulation, although it may persist longer. Redistribution of fluid is often complex and unpredictable. After a time the lymphatics become incompetent and inapparent lymph accumulation may take place in compartments within the trunk or extremities.

In most children the cardiovascular system is able to withstand the demands placed on it, although shock is a prominent feature of large thermal injuries and many children are prone to develop congestive heart failure and pulmonary edema. Also, peripheral circulation in the infant is less efficient and more labile, which complicates burn response and therapy in children in this age-group.

Anemia. Loss of circulating red cell mass is significantly reduced and is associated predominantly with deep burns. The anemia characteristic of thermal injury is attributed to several factors—red blood cells are destroyed by heat; circulating red blood cells are lost in the zone of stasis; red blood cells are damaged by heat; hemolysis from circulating plasma and from *Pseudomonas* invasion occurs; direct bleeding from the wound occurs; bone marrow is depressed as a result of sepsis; and (later) loss from bleeding during repeated debridement of the wound surface occurs.

Renal responses. The loss of fluid from the intravascular compartment causes renal vasoconstriction that in turn leads to reduced renal plasma flow and depressed glomerular filtration. When adequate fluids are provided, the glomerular filtration rate returns to normal, and, by the third or fourth day of fluid therapy, urine output increases as edema fluid is mobilized and eliminated. In the first few days oliguria is more commonly the result of inadequate fluid replacement than of acute renal failure. If the patient does not respond to treatment or if there is inadequate fluid resuscitation, acute renal failure may develop with permanent kidney damage. Children with a history of a prior kidney disorder are at increased risk.

Blood urea nitrogen and creatinine levels are elevated from tissue breakdown and oliguria. Hematuria may also be evident from hemolysis of red blood cells, and oliguria may develop as a consequence of the increased pigment load the kidneys must handle, especially myoglobin from extensive electric burn destruction, which blocks the kidney tubules. Renal failure is uncommon in burns involving less than 20% of the body surface. It occurs more frequently following flame burns sustained indoors than after scalds.

Metabolic responses. The metabolic rate of burned patients is greatly accelerated, and the nitrogen losses are far in excess of those seen in other types of injuries. The magnitude of energy requirements of a burned child frequently exceeds the requirements of a normal active child and, when the burned area is extensive, may approach twice the normal requirements.

The response to the stress of injury places high demands on the body. The stress-invoked glycogen breakdown depletes the energy stores in 12 to 24 hours, after which the body resorts to glyconeogenesis for high energy needs. Blood glucose levels are elevated and, since insulin resistance is evident, remain elevated for some time. Protein breakdown is rapid, as reflected in blood urea nitrogen and urine urea nitrogen levels. Each gram of urinary urea nitrogen represents a loss of 30 g of lean body mass.

Many of the metabolic consequences of extensive burn injuries are attributed to the amount of energy needed for the energy-consuming process of evaporation of water from the damaged skin surface. The infant or young child is especially vulnerable because of the large surface area relative to metabolically active tissue. Burning destroys a lipid layer and converts skin that is normally virtually impermeable to water to a freely water-permeable state that transmits water vapor at least four times as rapidly as normal skin. In partial-thickness burns this loss is greatest the day of injury; in full-thickness areas it rises slowly at first and then rapidly increases to reach a peak about the fourth day after the burn occurred. Evaporative losses are maintained until partial-thickness burns are healed and full-thickness injuries are grafted. Thus body stores of energy are rapidly depleted unless sufficient replacement is provided or losses are reduced.[7,19]

Neuroendocrine responses. As occurs in response to any stress, the hypothalamic-hypophyseal mechanism restores equilibrium by secreting tropic hormones, which stimulate various target organs of the neuroendocrine system. Adrenal activity is stimulated maximally. The medulla responds by secreting increased amounts of the catecholamines epinephrine and norepinephrine, which appear to have a sustained elevation. Adrenocortical hormones are elevated and reach a peak immediately after injury but remain high for some time. Aldosterone secretion is elevated and sustained at a high level throughout hospitalization, and there is release of antidiuretic hormone. Despite this increased adrenal activity, adrenal insufficiency is a rare complication.

Acidosis. Most burned patients exhibit some degree of metabolic acidosis. Reduced blood volume and cardiac output result in diminished tissue perfusion with resultant tissue hypoxia, which causes a shift to anaerobic metabolism with formation of metabolic acids. However, this is usually sufficiently compensated by increased ventilation as a result of pulmonary irritation or an independent respiratory alkalosis. Renal compensatory mechanisms are impaired by the decreased blood flow.[9]

Growth changes. Changes in the growth pattern are frequently observed, particularly in older children who have burns covering large areas of their body. As in any severely burned individual, nail and hair growth essentially cease during the catabolic phase of burn response. It is believed that bone growth is also affected; weight loss is marked. During convalescence following full recovery, there is a catch-up spurt in bone growth and weight recovery. In prepubertal children who suffer thermal injury, there is frequently a rapid acceleration of pubertal changes with development of secondary sex characteristics, which may occur 2 to 3 years prior to the usual time. It is believed that these changes are probably caused by a prolonged and heavy production of growth hormone.[3]

Complications of burn injury

Thermally injured persons are subject to a number of serious complications, both from the wound and from systemic alterations resulting from the wound. The immediate threat to life is asphyxia resulting from irritation and edema of the lungs and respiratory passages. In the first 48 to 72 hours the greatest hazard is unremitting shock, followed by possible renal shutdown and potassium excess during the first week. During healing, infection—both local and generalized sepsis—is the primary complication. Mortality associated with thermal injury in children decreases with the age of the child and increases with the extent of the burn. In children over the age of 3 years the fatality rate is similar to adults, but below this age resistance to the burn or its complications is considerably lessened. Although the cause for this is unknown, it may be a function of physiologic immaturity.[3,19]

Pulmonary problems. Pulmonary problems persist as the major cause of fatality in patients with thermal burns or a result of injury to or complications in the respiratory tract. A full range of respiratory insufficiency can occur, including inhalation injury, aspiration in unconscious patients, bacterial pneumonia, pulmonary edema, pulmonary embolus, and posttraumatic pulmonary insufficiency.[1]

Inhalation injury may be caused by heat injury to the tissues of the airway or inhalation of carbon monoxide or other noxious gases. Although direct thermal injury to the upper airway may occur, heat damage below the vocal cords is rare. Above the glottis the damage is thermal (laryngeal edema); below the glottis damage is chemical.[26] The inspired heated air is cooled in the upper airway before reaching the trachea, and reflex closure of the cords and laryngeal spasm prevent full inhalation. Evidence of direct thermal injury to the upper airway includes burns of the face, lips, and nasal hairs and signs of pharyngeal swelling or necrosis. Acute edema formation may lead to airway obstruction and asphyxiation. Symptoms may not develop for as long as 24 hours. Wheezing, prolonged expiratory phase, wet rales, and copious secretions are signs of respiratory involvement. In such situations tracheal intubation or tracheostomy with gentle suction to clear the bronchial tree is indicated.

Inhalation of carbon monoxide is suspected when the injury occurs in a closed space. Carbon monoxide combines with hemoglobin to form carboxyhemoglobin (HbCO). Hemoglobin clings to carbon monoxide with 200 times the affinity of oxygen, thereby displacing oxygen. As a result the patient's color remains good despite marked tissue hypoxia. Since the carotid body is not stimulated, respirations are characteristically shallow. Mild carbon-monoxide saturation causes headache, slight dyspnea, diminished visual acuity, and some confusion. Moderate poisoning produces irritability, dim vision, nausea, and fatigability. In severe carbon monoxide poisoning, hallucinations, confusion, ataxia, collapse, and coma occur. When carbon monoxide poisoning is suspected, 100% humidified oxygen should be administered, since the half-life of carboxyhemoglobin is approximately 4 hours when breathing room air but only 1 hour on 100% oxygen.[18,26]

Inhalation of other by-products of combustion, that is, smoke and toxic chemicals, can produce varying degrees of lung damage, depending on the type of burning material. Burning wood smoke is extremely irritating, and smoke from burning plastic material, especially polyvinyl chloride, is the most irritating. Poisonous gases such as chlorine, sulfuric acid, or cyanide can be lethal if absorbed into the bloodstream. Pathology of respiratory injury is manifest as severe mucosal edema followed by sloughing of the mucosa and replacement by a mucopurulent membrane. This purulent material together with edema seriously compromise respiration. Acute bronchitis and bronchopneumonia commonly develop within a few days of injury.

The most common etiologic factor in respiratory failure in the pediatric age-group is bacterial pneumonia, which may be secondary to airway injury or contamination from a tracheostomy or acquired through hematogenous spread of bacteria, usually from the burn wound. However, the largest percentage (65%) is caused by airborne infection, which occurs early in the postburn period and is associated with poor mentation, abdominal distention, and immobilization. The hematogenous variety occurs later from either the septic burn wound or other foci, such as phlebitis at an old cutdown site.[19]

Less common pulmonary complications are pulmonary emboli and pulmonary edema resulting from fluid overload during early fluid replacement. Sometimes deep burns of the chest may cause restriction of chest movement secondary to the effect of the binding, inelastic eschar formation. This is relieved by longitudinal incision of the eschar to prevent fatal hypoxia. Posttraumatic pulmonary insufficiency, which is difficult to distinguish from bacterial pneumonia, is sometimes a consequence of severe burns and is associated with sepsis and intravascular coagulation. It is the result of pulmonary capillary damage and leaking of fluid and protein into interstitial spaces of the lung, which causes loss of compliance and interference with oxygenation.

Wound sepsis. Sepsis is the most critical problem in treatment of burns and is an ever-present threat after the shock phase. Initially burns are relatively pathogen free, unless the wound is contaminated with potentially infectious material (dirt, polluted water, and so on). However, dead tissue and exudate provide a fertile field for bacterial growth. Early colonization of the wound surface by a preponderance of gram-positive organisms (primarily staphylococci) changes, on about the third postburn day, to predominantly gram-negative organisms, particularly *Pseudomonas aeruginosa* organisms. By the fifth postburn day the bacterial invasion is well underway beneath the surface of the wound.

Characteristics of the burn wound contribute to the proliferation of pathogenic organisms. The vascular supply to full-thickness burns is occluded immediately, and there is no appreciable blood supply to the area for approximately 3 weeks after the injury. In partial-thickness burns the circulation to the burn area stops immediately but returns in about 24 to 48 hours, unless infection supervenes. Thrombosis from bacterial invasion will impair circulation sufficiently to convert the partial-thickness injury to full-thickness destruction. These large amounts of nonviable tissue provide an excellent medium for the growth of microorganisms.[19]

Occlusion of the local blood supply is believed to impair the delivery of both humoral and cellular defense mechanisms to the burn area. Initially there is a decrease in inflammatory and phagocytic cells to the area, but the number of phagocytes gradually increases until they are present in abundance by the third postburn week, when good granulation tissue is forming. Granulating tissue, with its rich blood supply, affords increasing resistance to infection. Since organisms are normally a part of skin flora, cultures that reveal an organism concentration of 10^5/g of tissue have been arbitrarily set as the level at which burn wound invasion occurs.

Normally there is a cyclic variation in the ability of phagocytes to kill ingested bacteria, and it appears that burn injury accentuates this process markedly. Burn-wound sepsis occurs only during the periods when this phagocytic killing power is depressed. Although the amount of complement, the system plasma enzymes that mediate the antigen-antibody response, is also depressed, it is still present in sufficient quantities. This has led to development of a specific antibody against *P. aeruginosa,* the primary organism involved in burn wound sepsis.[2] The success of this approach is presently being evaluated.

Disorientation in the patient is one of the first signs of overwhelming sepsis. A spiking fever and, usually, paralytic ileus develop and progressively increase in severity over a period of 2 to 3 days, after which the temperature falls to below normal. At this time the wound deteriorates, the white count is depressed, and septic shock becomes manifest.[26]

Curling's ulcer. Recurrent or intermittent bleeding resulting from Curling's, or stress, ulceration is a major noninfectious complication of burns. Routine antacid administration has reduced the incidence of this complication in recent years, but these superficial erosive lesions still occur in a number of burn injuries. The cause is obscure, and, although gastric ulcers are more common in the total burn population, duodenal ulcers occur twice as frequently in children as in adults. Whereas gastric ulcers are observed in persons in all age-groups during the first postburn month, the peak occurrence of duodenal lesions is in the first week in adults but not until the third or fourth week in children.[19]

Children with burns covering more than 20% of body surface usually develop a partial paralytic ileus in the early postburn period that lasts for 2 to 3 days. Gastric decompression and parenteral nutrition are needed until bowel motility is reestablished and oral feedings are started.

Central nervous system complications. In children a frequent complication of both large and small burn injuries is central nervous system dysfunction. The manifestations range from hallucinations, personality change, and delirium to seizures and coma. Postburn seizures seem to be unique to children. In most cases the etiology of this burn encephalopathy can be attributed to hypoxemia, electrolyte imbalance (hyponatremia), hypovolemia, septicemia, and drug administration.[12] When the cause is determined, appropriate treatment can be initiated. Although the cause is unknown in one third of the cases, full neurologic recovery is usual, even with prolonged and serious manifestations.

Hypertension.[12,15,26] Approximately one third of children with severe thermal injuries develop arterial hypertension. The etiology is unclear but may be related to the increased secretion of catecholamines or high plasma renin levels. Hypercalcemia secondary to immobilization is occasionally a factor. It may appear at any time during the burn course and may persist for a few days or several months. Control is achieved by administration of diuretic and antihypertensive drugs.

First aid for burn injury[3,10,17]

The aims of immediate treatment of thermal injury are stopping the burning process, covering the burn, transporting the child to medical aid, and providing reassurance.

Stopping burning process. In flame burns the chief aim in rescue is to smother the fire, not to fan it. Children tend to panic and run, which only serves to fan the flames and make assistance more difficult. The victim should not run and should not remain standing. The injured child should be placed in a horizontal position and rolled in a blanket, rug, or similar article, being careful not to cover the child's head and face because of the danger of the child's inhaling the toxic fumes. If none is available, he should be made to lie down and roll over slowly. If the victim remains in a vertical position, the hair may be ignited or it may cause him to inhale flames, heat, or smoke. Spontaneous cooling of burns by slow immersion in cold water or any nonflammable liquid helps to relieve the pain, inhibit edema formation, and slow the process of heat damage, especially in the zone of stasis. Ice water or ice packs are contraindicated because the resulting vasoconstriction interferes with capillary perfusion and carries the risk of further damage from cold burn. Unless there is nothing else available, no dirt or sand should be thrown on the burn. In chemical burns it is particularly important to wash the burn with copious amounts of cool running water.

Burned clothing is removed to prevent further damage from smoldering fabric or hot beads of melted synthetic material. This also provides better access to the wound and precludes more painful removal later on.

Covering burn. The burn wound should be covered with a clean cloth to prevent contamination and to alleviate pain by avoiding air contact. Application of topical ointments, oils, or other home remedies should be avoided.

Transporting child to medical aid. The child with an extensive burn should not be given anything by mouth because of the risk of aspiration and water intoxication. The child is transported to the nearest place where medical aid is available. If this cannot be accomplished within a relatively short time and if facilities for intravenous fluid therapy and oxygen administration are available, they should be instigated to prevent burn shock.

Providing reassurance. Providing reassurance and psychologic support to both the parents and the child helps immeasurably during postinjury crisis. Reducing anxiety helps to conserve energy needed to cope with the physiologic and emotional stress of a traumatic injury.

Medical management of minor burns

Treatment of burns classified as minor usually can be managed adequately on an outpatient basis when it is determined that the parents can be relied on to carry out instructions for care and observation. Children with burns of the hands and most children with burns of the feet are admitted to the hospital so that they can receive careful local wound care and proper splinting to prevent deformity. Also, burns of the face should be observed for airway obstruction.

The wound is cleansed and debrided (all foreign material and devitalized tissue removed) with a tepid or cool dilute, nonirritating soap solution and rinsed with sterile saline solution. Coolness reduces pain and probably reduces edema that can interfere with capillary flow in the zone of stasis. Blisters may or may not be debrided. Whereas removal of the dead skin makes a cleaner wound and reduces the chance of infection in the blister fluid, it is more painful and the intact blister skin provides a biologic dressing.

Most physicians favor covering the wound with a dry dressing or fine-mesh gauze lightly lubricated with water-soluble antiseptic or antimicrobial cream and then wrapping it with bulky dry gauze dressings. Some physicians prefer that an occlusive dressing be left in place for 7 to 10 days if the dressing remains clean and the child afebrile. The parents are instructed to cleanse the wound with mild soap and tepid water, change the dressings once or twice daily, and return to the office or clinic as directed for wound observation. If there is a high probability of infection or other complications or if there is doubt about their ability to carry out the directions, the parents may be directed to return daily for dressing change and inspection or a nurse may be assigned to make a home visit for that purpose. Frequent removal of dressings is an effective mode of debridement. Soaking the dressing in tepid water prior to removal will help loosen the dressings and debris and reduce the discomfort. Burns about the face are usually treated by exposure, since a protective crust will form in 24 to 36 hours provided the atmosphere is cool and dry.

A tetanus history is obtained on admission and tetanus toxoid administered if the child has not received a booster within the previous year. When there is no history of immunization, human tetanus antitoxin should be administered. Administration of antibiotics for minor burns is controversial.

Most mild burns heal with little difficulty, but if the wound margin becomes erythematous, gross purulence is noted, or the child develops evidence of systemic reaction, such as fever or tachycardia, hospitalization is indicated.

Medical management of major burns

When a child with serious burns is admitted to the hospital for treatment, a variety of assessments are made and therapies initiated. Of these, the priority concerns are (1) to establish and maintain an adequate airway, (2) to establish a lifeline for fluid resuscitation, and (3) to care for the burn wound. Although the order of implementation may vary from institution to institution and from patient to patient, there are a number of procedures and activities generally initiated on admission. Some are carried out simultaneously.[12,15,25]

- Ascertain the adequacy of the airway and provide oxygen, intubation, and ventilatory assistance as indicated
- Provide intravenous sedation only if necessary
- Remove clothes and examine for trauma to head, skeleton, or nervous system
- Insert an intravenous line to deliver fluids at a rapid rate and, in patients with extensive injury, to accommodate a central venous pressure line
- Weigh the child
- Insert an indwelling Foley catheter to obtain specimens and measure hourly output
- Empty stomach through nasogastric tube
- Obtain blood sample for baseline laboratory studies
- Examine the burn wound and evaluate the extent and depth of injury

Carry out an escorotomy (incision through the eschar) for constricting circumferential eschar of chest or extremities
Cover flame or contact burns and apply topical medication and gauze dressings
Calculate fluid requirements and establish appropriate regimen
Administer appropriate protection against tetanus
Initiate low-dosage penicillin prophylaxis
Obtain history regarding the injury and other pertinent data

Other needs and therapies, including nutritional support, splinting to prevent contractures, treatment of anemia and hypoproteinemia, and the rehabilitative aspects of burn management, are initiated as appropriate throughout the course of treatment.

Establishment of adequate airway. The first priority of care is airway maintenance. Thermal injuries to the face, nares, or upper torso, history of fire in an enclosed area, or examination of the oral and nasal membranes that reveals edema of these membranes, hyperemia, burns of mucous membranes, or evidence of trauma to upper respiratory passages all suggest inhalation of noxious agents or presence of respiratory burn. Oxygen is administered and blood gases, including carbon monoxide, are quickly determined. If the child exhibits air hunger or otherwise appears in critical condition, an endotracheal tube is inserted to maintain the airway. The usual practice is to intubate if there is any question regarding the possibility of respiratory problems. Pharyngeal edema may make delayed intubation difficult, and the child will become restless from hypoxia.

The trend in recent years has been to avoid the use of tracheostomy because of the serious complications with significant mortality associated with this therapy in childhood burn injuries, such as a high incidence of infection, tracheobronchitis, delayed hemorrhage, and cannula obstruction from secretions and granulations. Since early edema subsides within 24 to 48 hours and many have been managed successfully for longer periods of time without significant damage, nasotracheal intubation is the safer and preferred approach. It allows for delivery of humidified air with oxygen, easy removal of secretions from respiratory passages, and the use of a pressure ventilator if needed.

Frequently placing the child in a Croupette or under an oxygen hood with a high flow of oxygen and maximum humidity is sufficient to reduce reflex bronchospasm produced by trauma to the bronchial mucosa. To combat continued respiratory distress, frequently a large dose of an anti-inflammatory corticosteroid compound is given rapidly by the intravenous route to augment the already elevated blood level of circulating steroids. This therapy still remains somewhat controversial, however.

Fluid replacement therapy. The objectives of fluid therapy are to (1) compensate for water and sodium lost to traumatized areas and interstitial spaces, (2) replenish sodium deficits, (3) restore plasma volume, (4) obtain adequate perfusion, (5) correct acidosis, and (6) improve renal function.[9]

Fluid and electrolyte therapy for children in the first 24 hours postburn is still controversial. This controversy is centered primarily around whether or not colloid solution, usually albumin, dextran, Plasmanate, or plasma, should be part of the resuscitation phase of fluid therapy. Those who favor crystalloid solutions believe that during this time the altered capillary membrane is unable to provide a structural barrier and that, therefore, colloidal solutions are of questionable value in restoring the plasma oncotic pressure. Instead, the colloid crosses the membrane and becomes trapped in the interstitial spaces as capillary permeability is restored during the next 24 hours, augmenting the extravascular fluid retention. This has serious implications for fluid accumulation in the lungs and brain.

The predominant therapy at the present time is the use of crystalloid rather than colloid solutions in resuscitation of burn shock. The composition of the fluid selected varies with the philosophy of the physician and may consist of isotonic saline solution, a near-isotonic solution (such as Ringer's lactate), or even a hypertonic saline solution. Needs are determined by several parameters, such as vital signs, including blood pressure, urine volume and character, central venous pressure and other evidence of fluid overload, peripheral flow, and clinical signs of hydration and level of consciousness. These criteria, based on individual needs, are more effective for fluid resuscitation. Periodic monitoring of serum sodium, potassium, chloride, carbon dioxide, blood urea nitrogen, and osmolality help determine the adequacy of fluid therapy.[9,26]

After diuresis, in 48 to 72 hours, when capillary permeability is restored, colloid solutions such as albumin or plasma are useful in maintaining plasma volume. During this phase interstitial fluid is returning rapidly to the vascular compartment, and increasing intake to match urine output may cause circulatory overload. Oral fluids are usually withheld in the early resuscitative phase but may be administered in 24 to 48 hours.

Fluid balance may continue to be a problem throughout the course of treatment, especially during the periods in which there may be considerable evaporative loss from the wound.

Nutrition. The high metabolic requirements and catabolism in severe burns make nutritional needs of paramount importance and often difficult to provide. The diet must provide sufficient protein to avoid protein breakdown and extra calories to utilize the proteins, sustain the adaptive hypermetabolism, and spare protein breakdown. Extra calories should be derived from carbohydrates, since fat, although higher in total calories, will not spare protein. The normal energy stores of glycogen are depleted; therefore, exogenous glucose must be provided early. Intravenous 5% glucose can supply minimal requirements, but these are inadequate to meet added needs.

Most burn patients are able to eat, and the child is given

oral feedings as soon as possible. Since burned children are often anorexic, whereas the caloric requirements may be as much as two to three times their usual requirements for size and age, the diet for burned children is high calorie and high protein, supplemented with high doses of vitamins B and C and iron. An adequate anabolic state is reached when the blood urea nitrogen level begins to fall.

Nasogastric feedings may be needed to supplement oral intake, and intravenous hyperalimentation has been used to provide a large amount of concentrated glucose and amino acids, especially in infants. The anorexia, delayed gastric emptying, and osmotic diarrhea secondary to high-solute tube feedings lead to this mode of nutrition despite difficulties encountered in placement of the catheter and the increased risk of sepsis.

Medication. Controversy also exists regarding the use of antibiotics during the first few days after injury. Some authorities believe that low doses of penicillin should be given prophylactically to all children with serious burns because of (1) their susceptibility to rapidly spreading cellulitis as a result of β-hemolytic streptococci and (2) lowered immunoglobulin levels. Others prefer to treat the streptococcus only when it becomes a problem. Broad-spectrum antibiotics are avoided to prevent the possibility of a superimposed infection. Also, impaired circulation in the wound area prevents their access to the site.

Use of heparin is also controversial. Proponents argue that its administration prevents (1) thrombosis in the microcirculation, (2) thromboemboli from prolonged immobilization, and (3) disseminated intravascular coagulation, which is common after burn injury.

To facilitate growth and proliferation of epithelial cells, administration of vitamin A is begun early in the postburn period. Zinc sulfate is also administered by some physicians, since zinc stores are depleted during catabolism and since it, too, appears to facilitate wound healing and epithelialization.

Care of burn wound

After the initial period of shock and restoration of fluid balance, the primary concern is the burn wound. The objectives of management for epidermal and superficial (first- and second-degree) burns is to prevent infection by providing as aseptic an environment as possible. Occlusive dressings help to reduce pain by minimizing exposure to air. The objectives for management of full-thickness wounds are prevention of invasive infection, removal of dead tissue, and closure of the wound.[26]

Methods of burn care. There are essentially three methods of therapy for the burn wound, each of which has its place in the treatment of children. All meet the objectives of preparation for permanent wound coverage (Table 30-7). The occlusive dressings are used more frequently, although primary excision is gaining popularity as a major modality of burn care. Both the exposure and occlusive methods employ topical antibacterial applications and daily hydrotherapy or tubbing to remove loose tissue and debris and to allow inspection of the wound.

Soaking in the Hubbard tank for 20 to 30 minutes once or twice daily facilitates the loosening and removal of sloughing tissue, eschar, exudate, and topical medications. The mesh gauze serves to entrap exudative slough

Table 30-7. Methods of burn care

Method	Description	Advantages	Disadvantages
Exposure therapy	After cleansing, wound remains exposed to air and allowed to dry Natural protective barrier formed by hard coagulum from exudate of partial-thickness burns and dry eschar of full-thickness burns	Patient not immobilized with bulky dressings Allows frequent inspection Dry crust is poor culture medium Fluid loss less in initial phases Less odor	Risk of cross contamination greater Requires strict isolation technique Requires maintenance of optimal environmental temperature Often requires restraints on extremities to prevent picking at crust Presents unsightly appearance
Occlusive dressings	Wound surface covered with nonadherent, water-permeable fine-mesh gauze Inner layer covered with even layer of absorptive, resilient fluffed gauze held in place by nonconstricting stretch gauze bandages	Protection from cross contamination Protection from injury Better immobilization, if desired Aids in positioning and putting injured part at rest Less pain initially	Requires skilled nursing care Higher incidence of hyperpyrexia Warm, moist environment more conducive to bacterial growth Often requires pain medication for uncomfortable dressing changes
Primary excision	Immediate surgical excision of devitalized tissue and grafting	Immediate removal of necrotic eschar Permanent coverage of damaged skin Reduces exposure to infection	Difficult to distinguish between full-thickness and deep partial-thickness injury Associated with significant blood loss

and is readily removed during the tubbing procedure (Fig. 30-7). Any loose tissue or eschar is carefully trimmed away before redressing (Fig. 30-8). Debridement can be painful and usually requires premedication with a light dose of meperidine or codeine (Fig. 30-6). The use of hydrotherapy has reduced the need for surgical debridement under general anesthetic.

Topical antimicrobials. Prior to the development of effective topical agents for reducing the incidence of invasive organisms, wound sepsis was the major cause of mortality from thermal injury. Systemic administration cannot reach the area because of thrombosed vessels. Although wound sepsis remains a problem, the incidence is now lower and mortality has declined. Topical agents do not eliminate organisms from the burn wound, but they can effectively inhibit or delay bacterial growth. Successful burn therapy relies on both topical antibacterial applications and thorough cleansing and debridement to reduce the amounts of necrotic material on which the bacteria grow. To be effective, a topical application must be nontoxic, capable of diffusing through eschar, harmless to viable tissue, nonallergenic, one that does not cause an increase in resistant strains, inexpensive, and easy to apply.[3]

A number of topical agents are employed, but those used most frequently are 0.5% silver nitrate solution, 10% mafenide acetate (Sulfamylon) and 1% silver sulfadiazine (Silvadene). All three are effective bacteriostatic agents, but each has advantages and disadvantages. Less frequently used are 0.1% gentamicin sulfate (Garamycin) and povidone-iodine (Betadine) ointment. The significant aspects of each are summarized in Table 30-8.

Ointments are applied directly to the burn wound surface with sterile tongue blades or the hand with a sterile glove. The layer of cream or ointment should be applied thick enough so that the wound cannot be seen. It can be left uncovered or covered with a layer of fine-mesh gauze and secured with stretch gauze or elastic tubular netting. For areas that are small or difficult to cover, strips of fine-mesh gauze are impregnated with the medication and then applied to the wound (Fig. 30-9).

Wound closure and resurfacing. Temporary or permanent coverage of full-thickness wounds is accomplished with grafts. Temporary grafts are those that provide bio-

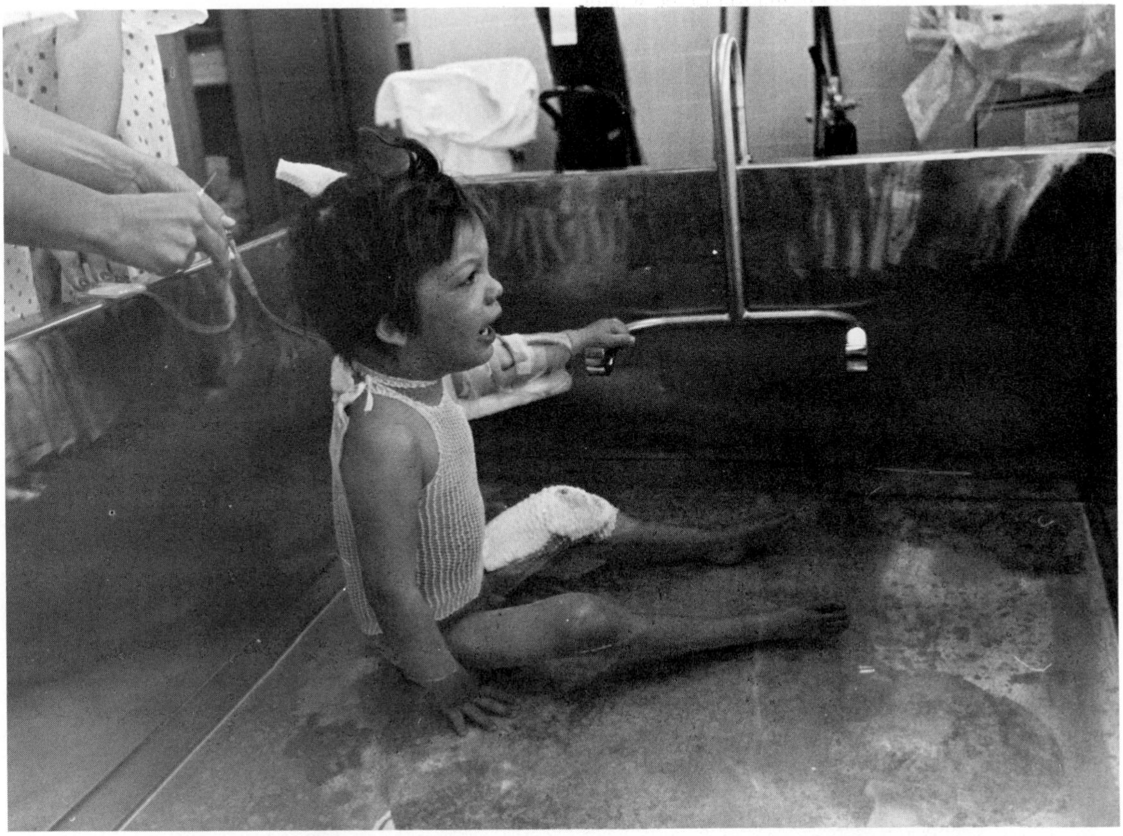

Fig. 30-6. An analgesic is administered prior to removal of dressings and débridement. In this instance the analgesic is injected directly into the intravenous line at the time of tubbing.

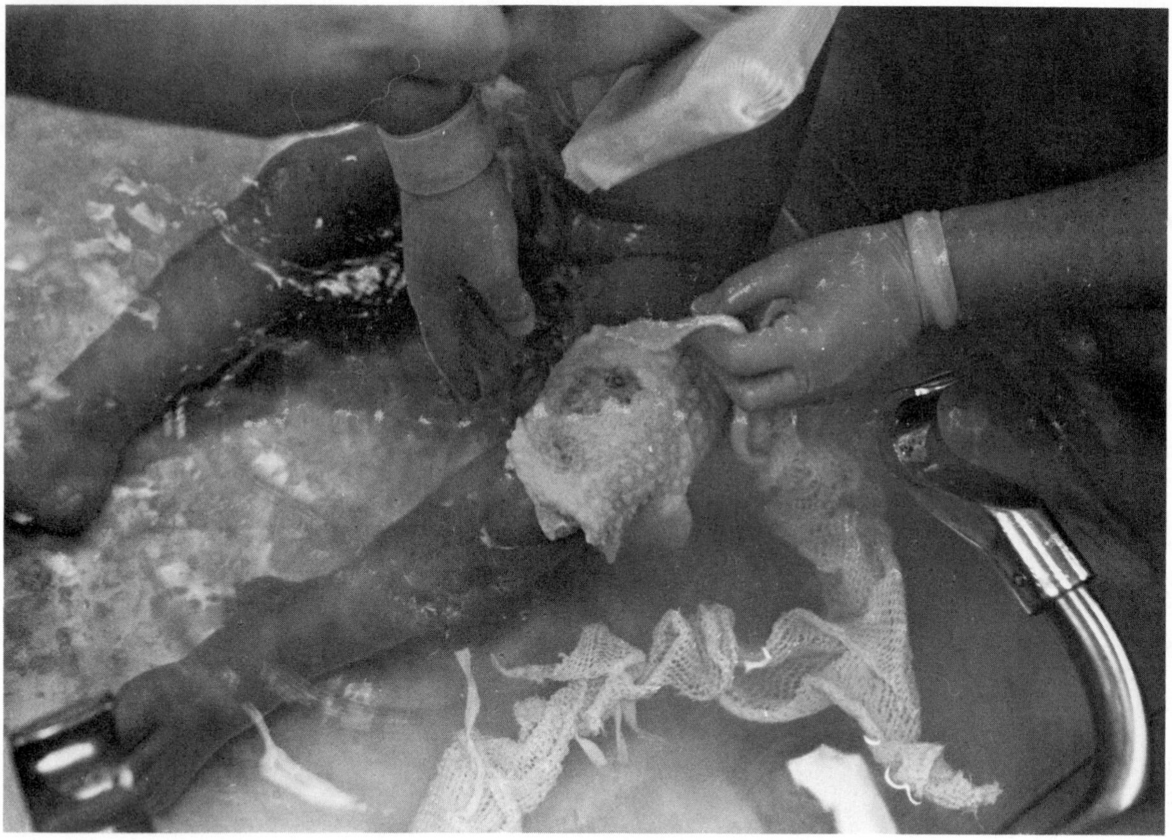

Fig. 30-7. Removal of dressings during tubbing.

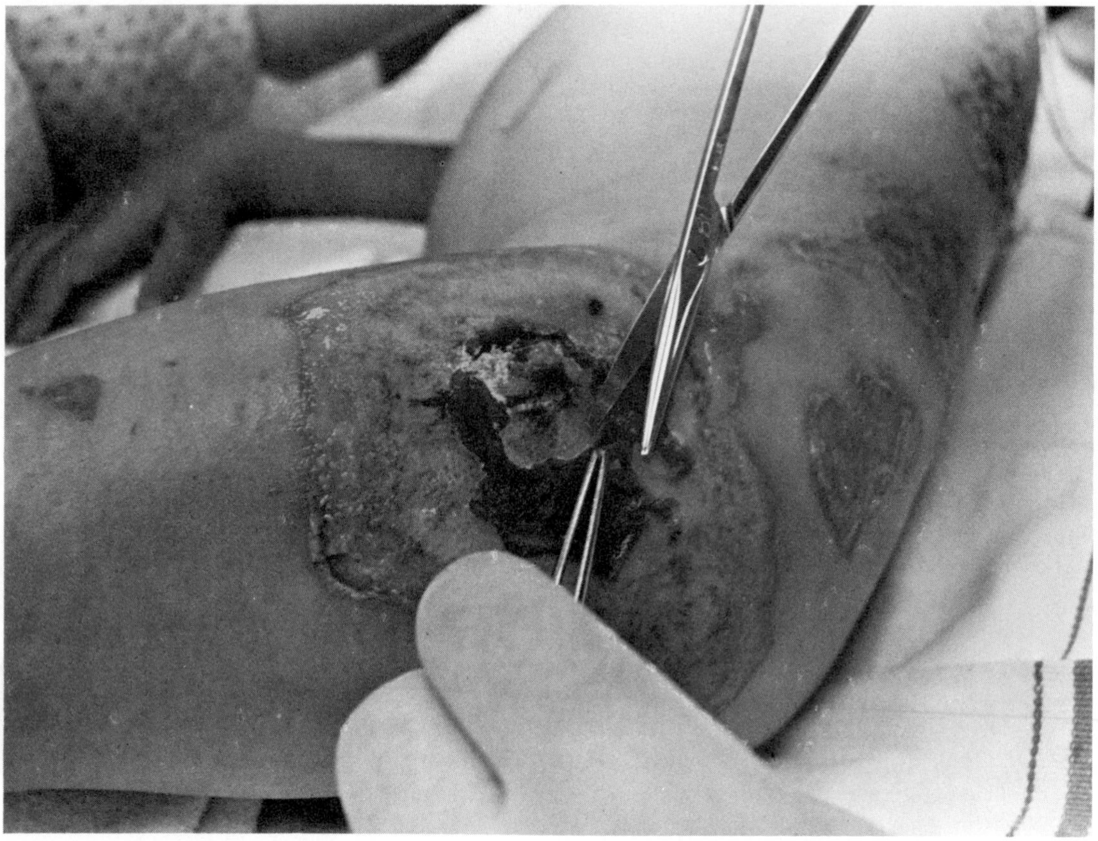

Fig. 30-8. Dead skin and debris are carefully trimmed away before dressing is applied.

A

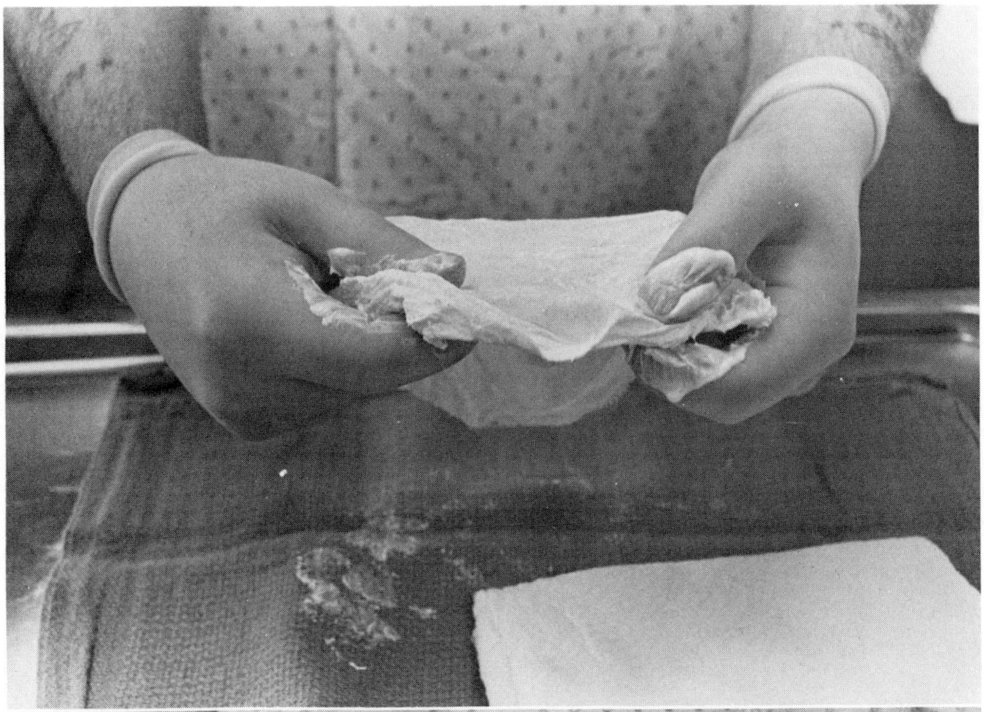

B

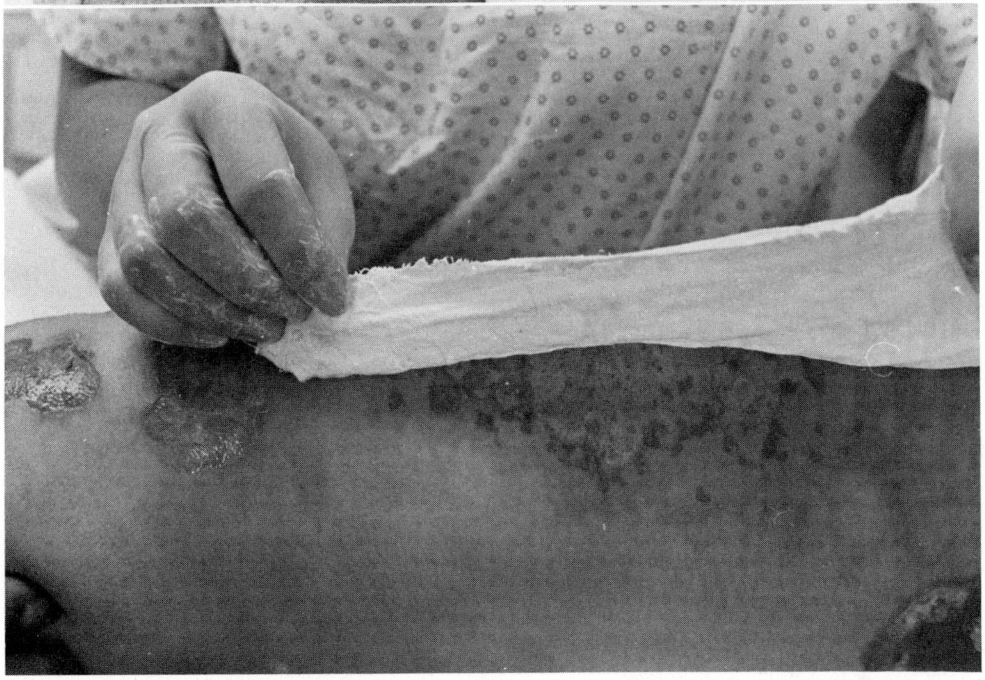

Fig. 30-9. Application of burn dressing. **A,** Gauze impregnated with ointment; **B,** ointment and gauze applied to burn wound.

Continued.

C

D

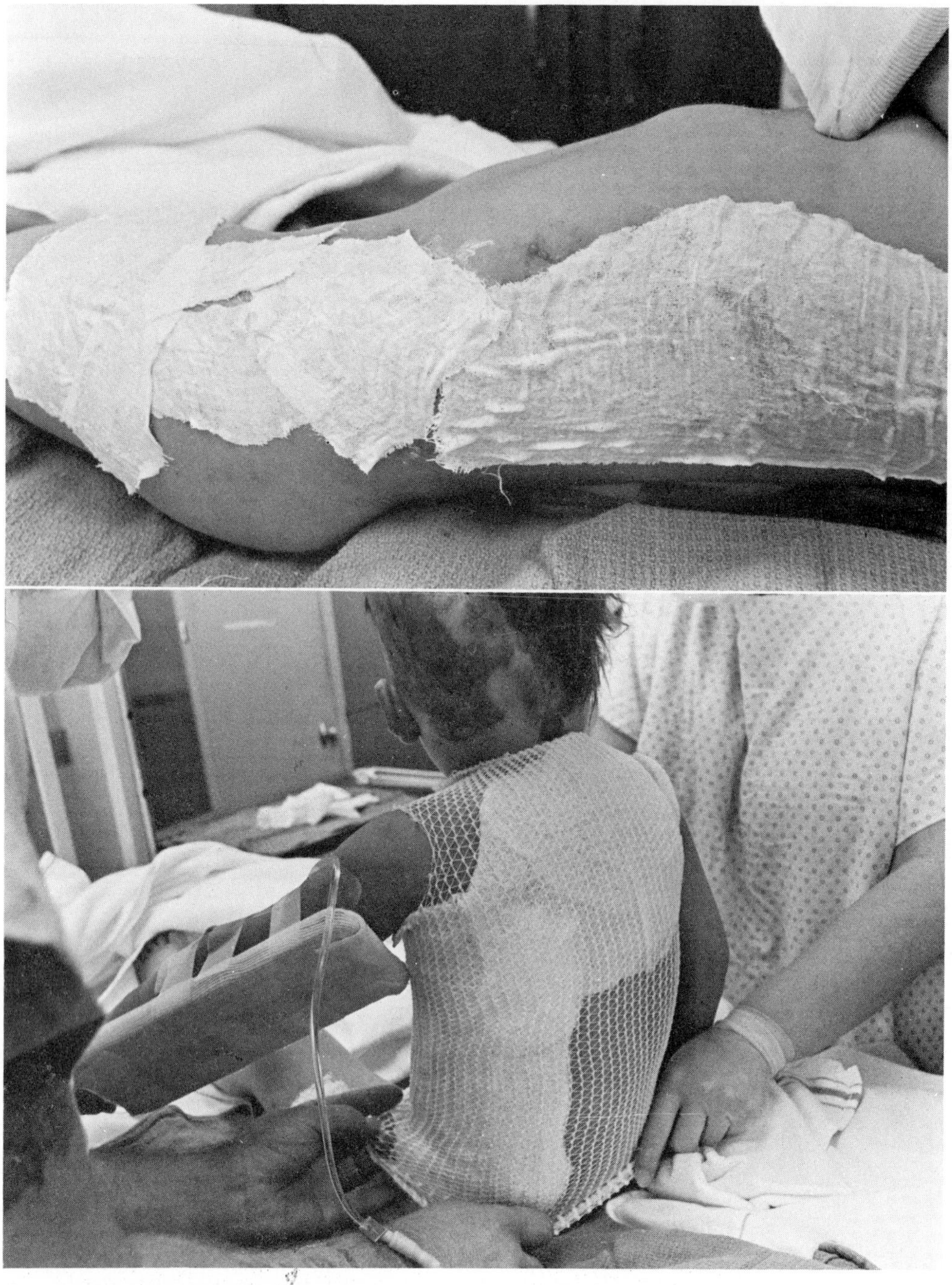

Fig. 30-9, cont'd. C, Burn wound covered with gauze dressings; **D,** dressings secured with tubular elastic netting.

E

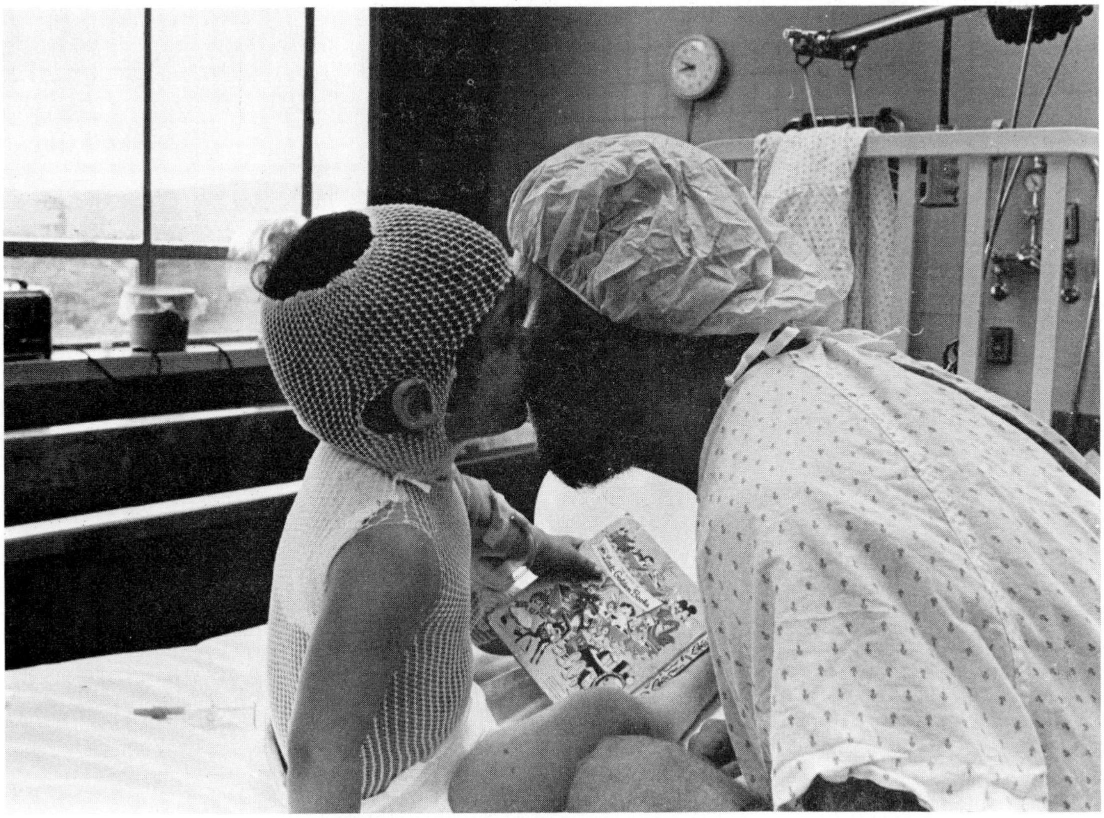

Fig. 30-9, cont'd. E, Back in bed ready to visit with Daddy.

logic dressings during the acute phase of therapy to protect the wound from bacterial invasion and to minimize fluid loss. Permanent grafting is part of the rehabilitative stage to restore cosmetic appearance and to achieve maximum functional capacity. In recent years the early application of temporary biologic dressings to partial-thickness burns, especially in children, has significantly improved burn management and is gaining in popularity.[15]

Grafts are derived from several sources. Permanent grafts are obtained from only two sources:

autografts tissues obtained from undamaged areas of the patient's own body.

isografts histocompatible tissue obtained from genetically identical individuals, that is, the patient's identical twin.

Temporary grafts include:

allografts (homografts) tissues obtained from genetically different members of the same species, living or dead—usually cadavers—that are free from disease.

xenografts (heterografts) tissues obtained from members of a different species. At present most grafts are derived primarily from pigskin, either fresh or frozen.

The type of graft particularly suitable and used most frequently for temporary covering in children is the porcine xenograft (Fig. 30-10). The split-thickness pigskin is available commercially and is an effective agent after eschar separation. Changed regularly, it reduces evaporative loss, protects the wound bed, and is believed to protect the wound from infection and trauma. The grafts usually adhere within a few hours, and dressings are not needed. They are particularly effective in children with second-degree scald burns of hands and face, since they allow relatively pain-free movement, which reduces contracture and has the added benefit of improved appetite and morale. The pigskin dressings are replaced daily or at least every 3 to 4 days; as a result acceptance of the graft is minimal. When left in place for longer periods of time, antibody development causes increasingly rapid rejection.

Permanent grafting of full-thickness burns is usually accomplished with a split-thickness skin graft. This consists of the epidermis and part of the dermis being removed from an undamaged area by a special instrument, the dermatome, which is designed to excise split-thickness skin. The priority areas for coverage are the face, neck, and areas around joints, especially the hands. With extensive burns it is often difficult to find enough viable skin to cover the wounds; therefore, available donor sites are used to the best advantage by special techniques.

Table 30-8. Comparison of common topical preparations

Agent	Antibacterial efficacy	Dressings	Advantages	Disadvantages
Silver nitrate, 0.5% ($AgNO_3$)	Gram negative	Thick occlusive dressings Impedes joint movement Dressings changed twice daily	Greatly reduces evaporative losses; thus lower metabolic rate and lower weight loss Effective in controlling *Pseudomonas* Does not interfere with wound healing Nonallergenic Inexpensive Effective against major burn flora, including *Pseudomonas* and *Staphylococcus*	Cannot allow dressings to become dry; requires frequent wetting (at least every 2 hours) Difficult to use Ineffective on established burn wound infections Does not penetrate eschar; therefore, should be applied before bacterial growth established Hypotonicity pulls electrolytes from wound, causing depletion of sodium, chloride, potassium, and magnesium that necessitates continuous monitoring and replacement Little effect on *Klebsiella* and *Aerobacter* groups
Mafenide acetate (Sulfamylon), 10%	Gram negative and positive	Usually exposure Occasionally with dressings Reapplied twice daily	Diffuses rapidly into burn wound and underlying tissues Rapidly excreted Easily applied Penetrates through eschar and deeply into burn wound; therefore, effective in deep flame, electric, and older wounds Effective against many gram-positive and gram-negative organisms, including *Pseudomonas* and *Clostridium*	Mild acidosis caused by inhibition of carbonic anhydrase in kidney Hypersensitivity reaction in many children Causes discomfort after application Inhibits wound healing
Silver sulfadiazine (Silvadene), 1% (AgSD)	Gram negative *(Candida)*	Exposure or dressings Motion of joints maintained Applied once or twice daily	Nontoxic Combines advantages of silver nitrate and mafenide acetate Painless Easy to apply Absorbs slowly Bacteriocidal for up to 48 hours Effective against gram-positive and gram-negative bacteria and *Candida albicans*	Does not penetrate eschar as well as mafenide acetate or gentamicin sulfate
Gentamicin sulfate (Garamycin), 0.1%	Gram positive and negative	Exposure or occlusive dressings	No pain associated with use Relatively nontoxic Penetrates burn wound quickly Especially effective against *Klebsiella* and *Enterobacter*	40% of pseudomonal organisms have become resistant Occasionally nephrotoxicity and ototoxicity
Povidone-iodine (Betadine) ointment	Gram positive and negative Fungicide	Usually dressings Impedes joint movement	Apparently nontoxic Effective against broad spectrum of organisms	Elevation of protein-bound iodine (PBI) Use associated with mild degree of pain Causes eschar to "tan" and become very stiff, making debridement difficult

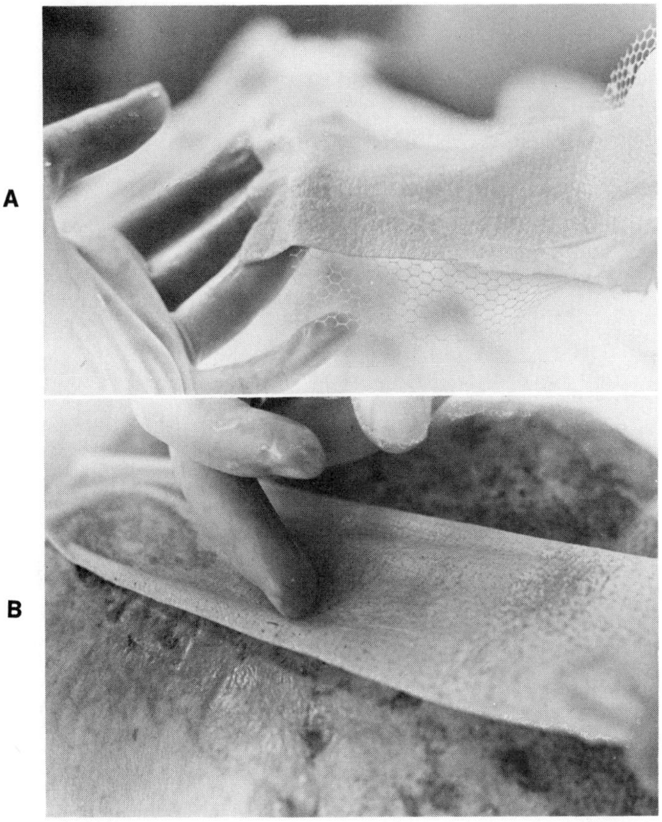

Fig. 30-10. Porcine dressing. **A,** Removed from net backing; **B,** applied to wound.

The various methods of applying split-thickness grafts are:

full-cover graft a sheet of skin, removed from the donor site, is placed intact over the recipient site. It may be sutured or maintained in place by pressure dressings.

postage-stamp graft a sheet of skin from the donor site is cut into postage-stamp sizes and placed on the recipient bed. Spaces between grafts allow for drainage. These may be covered with a dressing or, when possible, left exposed for inspection and for rolling serum from beneath the graft to aid contact between surfaces. These are not removed from the site as readily as large sheet grafts.

mesh, lace, or slit graft a sheet of skin, removed from the donor site, is run through a special instrument to make multiple slits so that, when stretched, the skin expands to cover from one and one half to nine times (usually three times) the area of a full-cover graft. This type of graft requires suturing to maintain tension. The openings allow drainage of serum and bacteria, thus allowing earlier closure of the burn. The graft may be exposed or covered with an occlusive dressing for about 48 hours. Mesh grafts are an effective method of covering large areas with a small amount of donor skin (Fig. 30-11).

Full-sheet grafts are used in areas in which a cosmetic effect is desired. Patch and mesh grafts result in a less desirable appearance. Requirements for a successful ''take,'' regardless of graft type, are:

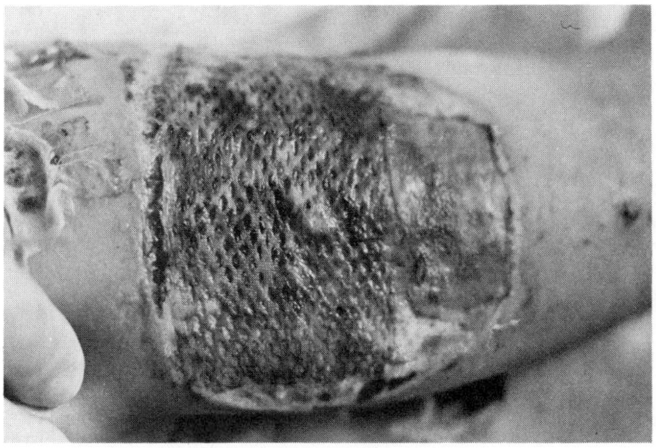

Fig. 30-11. Mesh graft.

- Sufficient nourishment until new blood supply grows in from the base of the recipient bed
- Primary tissue contact, that is, actual contact between cut surface of the graft and the recipient bed
- Avoidance of bleeding; the possibility of even the slightest bleeding must be controlled with light pressure
- Prevention of infection, especially in full-cover grafts; postage-stamp grafts will often ''take'' in contaminated areas

Until blood supply is established, the grafted skin is nourished by osmotic interchange with the recipient bed. Wound healing takes place as the recipient area throws out fibrin that attaches the graft to the new bed. The fibrin is infiltrated by leukocytes and fibroblasts, and the capillary buds of the granulation tissue spread through the fibrin. Within 3 days there is vascularization of the graft; after 2 weeks the graft is attached to the base by connective tissue.

The donor site is dressed with either a xenograft or fine-mesh gauze and left exposed until the graft falls off in about 10 to 14 days. Dressings are not changed on donor sites to prevent tearing the new, delicate epithelium.

Nursing considerations

Nursing care is the most important aspect of burn therapy. Because the care of the severely burned child encompasses such a broad range of skills and foci, this discussion is divided into segments that correspond with the major phases of burn treatment: the *acute phase* (also referred to as the resuscitative, emergent, or metabolic phase), which involves the first 24 to 48 hours; the *management phase,* which extends from the time the child has been adequately resuscitated until the major rehabilitative aspects of care are initiated; and the *rehabilitative phase,* which begins with permanent grafting. This phase continues until all full-thickness injuries are covered and reconstructive proce-

Summary of nursing care in the acute or resuscitative phase of burn care

Goals	Responsibilities
Implement care	Have respiratory resuscitation equipment ready Remove all clothing, jewelry, and so on Evaluate level of consciousness Summon medical assistance if not present Ascertain religious affiliation Get parental consent for treatment or notify parents if not present Begin "critical care" record keeping according to unit policy Give analgesia if ordered Insert Foley catheter Insert nasogastric tube
Obtain baseline information	Take vital signs Weigh child Help evaluate extent and depth of burn wound Help assess condition Request laboratory studies as ordered—hematocrit, sodium, chloride, potassium, carbon dioxide, blood urea nitrogen, creatinine, and serum protein levels
Prevent shock	Help establish intravenous line Administer fluids as ordered Monitor vital signs (including central venous pressure, if employed) Monitor intravenous infusion closely Monitor urinary output, specific gravity, and pH (sometimes protein) every ½ to 1 hour Obtain needed specimens for examination or perform needed studies
Treat burn wound	Shave hair from wound and area immediately surrounding burn Thoroughly cleanse wound and surrounding skin; debride of devitalized tissues Apply topical medication as ordered Dress or leave exposed as ordered Check eyes; if indicated, irrigate with saline and apply protective ointment
Control bacterial growth on wound	Implement and maintain reverse isolation precautions Maintain careful hand washing by members of staff and visitors Wear clean or sterilized gown, cap, mask, and sterile gloves when handling wound area Avoid injury to crust and eschar Avoid patient contact with persons who have upper respiratory or skin infection Cover wound and/or patient according to protocol of unit Administer tetanus prophylaxis Administer penicillin prophylaxis, if ordered Obtain cultures of wound, nose, throat, and stool as ordered Administer mouth care
Relieve pain	Administer analgesics as indicated
Prevent complications	
Acute respiratory distress	Administer humidified oxygen Observe for signs of respiratory distress Obtain blood for blood gas determination, if indicated Have respiratory resuscitation equipment available Have tracheostomy tray available Check for constricting eschar of chest Observe nasopharynx for edema or redness Obtain chest x-ray film

Summary of nursing care in the acute or resuscitative phase of burn care—cont'd

Goals	Responsibilities
Fluid overload	Monitor vital signs frequently Observe for signs of impending overhydration Be alert for altered behavior or sensorium Perform or request laboratory studies
Abdominal distention, nausea and vomiting	Insert nasogastric tube and attach to low Gomco suction Administer nothing by mouth
Impaired circulation in extremities	Check circulation in extremities or other areas peripheral to burns—color, capillary filling, pulses, sensation Check for constricting eschar
Cardiac failure	Check vital signs Order electrocardiogram if indicated Give digitalis as ordered
Renal failure	Check hourly urine for amount, color (dark brown indicates blood or products of hemoglobin breakdown)
Seizures	Monitor serum electrolytes and blood gases
Hypothermia	Maintain warm, humid environment Monitor temperature at least every 2 hours; in severe burns keep continuous record with direct-reading probe
Obtain history of burn injury	Ascertain information concerning burn Time of occurrence (needed for assessment of fluid shifts) Nature of burning agent Length of contact with agent (to help assess depth) If occurred in enclosed area (clue to possible respiratory involvement) Pain—severe, mild (can affect blood pressure) Any medications given Preburn weight Preexisting illnesses Any known allergies
Prevent heat loss	Adjust ambient temperature according to child's temperature Use direct-probe thermometer when feasible Avoid drafts
Support child psychologically	Reassure child and parents Allow parents to visit child Facilitate parent-child interaction Do not allow isolation technique to unduly separate parent and child Allow child to express anger and distress Answer questions as honestly as possible
Support parents	Reinforce factual information Answer questions regarding therapy Allow for expression of feelings Help alleviate feelings of guilt Instruct in techniques required for visiting child Isolation procedures Help to devise means for providing tactile contact with child Help parents deal with anxiety regarding pain to child

dures and corrective measures have been accomplished. This often extends over a period of months or years.

Nursing care during resuscitative phase

The primary emphasis during the initial phases of burn care is prevention of burn shock. Checking vital signs, monitoring the intravenous infusion, and measuring urinary output are ongoing nursing activities in the hours immediately after injury. The intravenous infusion is started immediately by intracatheter or cutdown and is regulated according to urine output and specific gravity, laboratory data, and objective signs of adequate hydration. Urine volume, measured at least every hour, should be:

20 to 30 ml/hour in a child over 2 years of age
10 to 20 ml/hour in a child less than 2 years of age[15]

The child is observed for all parameters outlined in the summary of nursing care (see the box on pp. 1132 and 1133). The child requires constant observation and assessment with special attention to signs of complications. Respiratory, cardiac, and renal complications may appear early in the postburn period.

Care of the burn wound is secondary to the more critical problems of circulatory and/or respiratory failure. When a special burn facility is available, the child is wrapped in a sterile sheet and covered with a blanket to keep him warm during transfer and the burn wound is attended to after arrival at the unit. If no burn unit is available, the wound is cleansed and dressed in the emergency department. Many units take photographs of the burn wound initially and periodically as a record of wound progress and for legal purposes, if needed—especially in cases of suspected child abuse. Evaluation of the wound is more accurately accomplished during or after cleansing. Ideally the cleansing should take place in a hydrotherapy tub. Water is maintained at body temperature (about 37.2°C or 99°F) and is disinfected with chlorine (pool chlorine or Clorox).

The burn wound is treated according to the protocol of the specific burn facility. Extensive wounds may require the use of special beds and other equipment, such as Circoelectric beds, flotation beds, alternating pressure mattresses, and many other devices, depending on the extent and location of the wound.

Throughout the acute phase of care the child's emotional needs should not be overlooked. The child is frightened, uncomfortable, and often confused. He is isolated from familiar persons and surroundings, and the often overwhelming physical needs at this time are the primary focus of staff and parents. The child needs to be reassured that he is all right and that he will get better.

Nursing care during management phase*

After the patient's condition is stabilized, the long management phase begins. The major goals for this period are (1) care of the wound to facilitate healing and prepare for permanent closure; (2) prevention and minimization of infection, both local and generalized; (3) provision of adequate nutrition and reduction of metabolic losses; and (4) meeting the emotional and developmental needs of the child.

One of the most difficult aspects of burn care, especially in children, is the impact it has on nurses. The appearance and smell of the burn and the necessary discomfort that must be inflicted on the child as a part of the therapy are often beyond the nurse's ability to cope and remain therapeutic. Throughout the entire process of burn management, nurses must deal with their own feelings and anxieties regarding their therapeutic role in burn care. It is always difficult to deal with a child in pain, and to inflict pain on a helpless child is contrary to the empathetic nature of nursing. It is a temptation to sedate the child and disturb him as little as possible, although to do so can significantly impede his progress or produce deformities that may require months of additional pain and stress for the child.

The child should begin early to do as much for himself as possible and to be an active participant in his care. It takes a great deal of warm firmness and fortitude on the part of the nurse to force the child to do this. Moving hurts. Many children are able to move and help themselves. Others need considerable help and encouragement. If the child is unable to move, he should be told firmly but gently that it must be done, that the nurses will help him, and that it will be done as quickly as possible. He should be told how he can help to make it easier.

It is difficult to handle a child with extensive burns. It is almost impossible to move and turn the child without touching a burned area. Fortunately the discomfort lasts only for the short time the child is being handled; once repositioned it hurts no longer. The child may cry, but he usually stops once the procedure is over. Some children cry in anticipation of the move and may continue to cry afterward, but even small children learn that the hurt stops when the moving is over. Special frames and beds can be used to facilitate the process and to keep the child positioned in an attitude that prevents contracture deformity. Fowler's position is comfortable but may produce hip and knee contracture that take months to correct.

The child should be encouraged to participate in as many aspects of his care as possible. With illness, children always regress to the developmental level that allows them to deal with the stress. However, there are limits to the length of time a child should be permitted to remain at a lower level of functioning. To lie passively while others tend to his needs is not "normal" and may be detrimental to the child. As their condition permits, children can be expected to do things that they were capable of doing for themselves before they were burned, such as oral hygiene, face washing, feeding themselves, and playing. Allowing the child to make choices and to help make decisions about

*Drawn extensively from Rubin.[23]

the time of his care and recreational activities makes him feel a part of the team and provides him a small measure of control. The child will probably require assistance; however, as the child sees himself contributing to his care, he gains confidence and self-esteem. Fears and anxieties diminish with accomplishment and self-confidence.

Activities are selected and encouraged according to the child's level of development and interest, but, as with any ill child, they should be somewhat simpler and less challenging than would be expected in a state of health. Otherwise, his already taxed energies may be further depleted and his self-esteem threatened. Quiet games and activities such as reading, coloring, drawing, games, puzzles, and so on are always appropriate. Television is a satisfactory diversion but should not replace active participation and should not substitute for contacts with others. Play that encourages the expression of feelings of guilt, frustration, and anger is especially therapeutic. During the acute, resuscitative phase, the child is frequently isolated but should be moved where he has contact with others, especially other children, as soon as his condition allows. School-age children should continue with schoolwork.

Children need to be bolstered in other ways. They like to look and smell nice, and the unattractive burns, dressings and assorted paraphernalia do little to foster a positive self-image. They know how they appear to others, and small things such as careful hair combing and a bright ribbon, colorful nightgown or pajamas (when possible), slippers, or any decoration (a flower, pin, necklace, badge) will help make them feel that they look better and are worthwhile to others.

All hospitalized children, especially those who must undergo painful procedures, must be allowed to express their anger and frustration appropriately through verbalization and/or play. They need to know that their injury and the treatments are not punishment for specific, general, real, or imagined transgressions and to know that nurses understand their fears, anger, and discomfort. They also need body contact. This is often difficult to arrange for the child with massive injury. The discomfort associated with moving, the bulky, messy dressings, or the bare open wound are deterrents and frequently provide a justification for the nurse to avoid such action because of her own fear or repulsion. Even older children enjoy sitting on the nurse's lap and being cuddled and hugged. This can be a comfort in times of stress or used as a reward, but, most of all, it should be kept in mind that it is a natural part of childhood.

Care of burn wound. The nurse has the major responsibility for cleansing, debriding, and applying topical medication and dressings to the burn wound. Because dressing removal is a painful procedure, the child should receive light analgesia about 30 minutes prior to the scheduled tubbing. Both nurse and child must recognize it for exactly what it is—a dreadful but absolutely necessary procedure. Because it is painful, the child should know that it is all right to cry when the treatment hurts, but only *when it hurts*. Since it is easy for the child to give way to emotional excesses he cannot control, he needs the firm control of a caring adult. This includes both actual and anticipated hurt. The child needs help to gain and maintain control of his emotions. He needs to know why things are being done to him, how they will help him get better, and how he can contribute. New procedures or changes in routine need to be explained. When possible, there should be consistency in members of the staff who care for the child and the routine for procedures and activities. Providing some order in his world reduces the anxieties related to apprehension about the unknown. Children feel comfortable with the known, the routine.

Outer dressings (if any) are removed before placing the child in the tub, but adherent dressings are more easily removed after soaking in the water. It is helpful to involve the child in the process. Whereas a child will cry and protest vigorously when others remove the dressings, he will remove adherent gauze with a minimum of fuss. In this way he maintains some control of the situation. Loose or easily detached tissue is also removed during hydrotherapy, and the child is encouraged to move about as much as possible to exercise muscles and reduce contracture formation. He needs encouragement and every little bit of healing pointed out as evidence that he is getting better. Merely saying that he is better is insufficient as he gazes at an unsightly wound. Providing something constructive for the child to do during dressing application, such as holding a package of dressings or a roll of kerlix or simply holding someone's hand helps him to focus on something other than the procedure. In dressing the wound, it is important that all areas are clean, that medication is amply applied, and that no two burned surfaces touch, such as fingers or toes.

There are some psychologic implications that may influence the child's reaction to the tubbing and application of medication. Children who acquired the burn from hot water are particularly fearful, especially if the injury was inflicted as a punishment (battered child). Application of the medication can be a painful experience also, when mafenide (Sulfamylon) cream is the agent employed. Both the nurse and the child must understand that there is a painful sensation often described as "burning" that may have special significance for burned children. They must be reassured that the medication is not inflicting further injury.

When occlusive dressings are applied, elastic bandages are worn over dressings to prevent epithelial breakdown, stimulate circulation, and make mobility easier. This is especially important when the child is ambulatory.

Nutrition. After the initial phase of care, children are usually allowed oral feedings (unless paralytic ileus persists). If they will not eat, tube feeding is necessary, but every effort should be made to encourage oral intake. Serving regular meals even though the child may take only a small amount helps to maintain the habit of eating by

Summary of nursing care in the management phase of burn care

Goals	Responsibilities
Control bacterial growth on wound	Maintain clean environment Maintain careful hand washing Wear sterile gown, mask, and gloves when handling burn wound Carefully cleanse wound and remove devitalized tissue and eschar Apply prescribed topical antimicrobial preparation and dressings (if ordered) to wound Administer good oral hygiene Avoid injury to crusts and eschar Avoid contact with infected persons Obtain wound cultures three times per week to ascertain any increase in wound flora
Facilitate wound healing	Keep child from scratching and picking at wound Maintain care in handling wound to avoid damaging epithelializing and granulating tissues Administer supplementary vitamins and minerals—vitamins A, B, and C and zinc sulfate Offer high-calorie, high-protein meals and snacks Prevent infection
Prevent evaporative heat loss	Maintain critical environmental temperature at wound and air interface Prevent drafts
Maintain adequate nutrition and prevent nitrogen loss	Provide high-calorie, high-protein meals and snacks Encourage oral feeding by Providing foods child likes Allowing self-help Providing meals when child is most apt to eat well Providing attractive meals and surroundings Providing companionship at meals Employing "contract" with older children
Recognize signs of complications	Take vital signs (temperature, pulse, respirations, blood pressure) as ordered Observe, record, and report deviations from expected vital signs Record intake and output
Wound infection	Assess wound for signs of invasive infection, including redness, purulent drainage, unpleasant odor
Generalized sepsis	Recognize signs of septicemia Marked temperature elevation (104°-107°F, rectally) Chills Rapid, irregular pulse Hypotension Diminished urine output Paralytic ileus (distention, vomiting, absent bowel sounds) Alterations in sensorium Obtain blood culture of child with temperature of 39.5°C or over
Pneumonia	Observe for signs of respiratory distress, elevated temperature, presence of rales, lethargy
Ear and eye infection	Carefully cleanse and observe for signs of infection

Summary of nursing care in the management phase of burn care—cont'd

Goals	Responsibilities
Curling's ulcer	Assess for abdominal discomfort Check for recurrent or intermittent bleeding Determine hematocrit Administer antacids as ordered
Fecal impaction	Record regular bowel movements If fecal impaction present, administer enema or remove impacted feces
Hypertension	Check blood pressure regularly
Renal	Observe amount, color, specific gravity, and reaction of urine daily or as ordered Periodically send specimens for laboratory examination
Cerebral disorders	Observe for seizures Alterations in sensorium Behavioral changes
Prevent pressure necrosis	Turn frequently Stimulate circulation
Preserve body function	Encourage mobility Carry out range of motion exercises if child is unable to move extremities Splint joints to prevent contracture deformity Position for minimum deformity and optimum function
Meet emotional needs	Convey positive attitude toward child Encourage parents to visit Encourage as much independence as condition allows Help child build self-esteem and a positive self-image Provide recreational and diversional activities Promote constructive thinking in child Point out evidence of healing Arrange for continued schooling Promote peer contact where possible

mouth. For older children, forming a contract with them that regulates the need for supplemental tube feeding based on the amount of oral food consumed often encourages them to eat solids in order to avoid tube feedings.

Because children are frequently anorexic, whereas their caloric needs and protein needs are markedly increased, a great deal of encouragement, help, and patience are required on the part of the nursing staff. Consultation with the parents and the dietitian is arranged to determine the best way to provide needed nutrients in foods the child will be more likely to eat. Children who are old enough to participate should be included in the planning. Nourishing snacks are provided between regular scheduled mealtimes, and, if a child eats better at a time other than a scheduled mealtime, that is the time he should be fed. Most important, meals should not be scheduled immediately after a dressing change. Most children are too physically exhausted and too emotionally upset to eat at this time.

Many children eat better when they can feed themselves and when they can eat in an atmosphere more nearly like what they are accustomed to at home. Even if they are unable to feed themselves (for example, if their arms are bandaged), they do better if they can sit up or at least see the tray of food so that they can instruct the person feeding them how they prefer their food and what they want to be fed next. When their conditions allows, children enjoy sitting at a table for their meals. Parents are encouraged to bring a child's favorite dish from home.

To reduce caloric expenditure as much as possible, the ambient temperature in the environment is usually maintained at a temperature above the temperature of the burn surface (30 to 34 °C or 86 to 93.2°F).[19] Although evaporative heat loss is unchanged, this reduces the conductive, convective, and radiant heat losses from the denuded areas. The heat is often provided by means of a heat cradle over the child, but, if employed, the heat source should be situated well away from the child's body. Other methods include electric heaters, which if used should be situated 4 to 5 feet away to avoid overheating, and maintaining room temperature sufficiently elevated to reduce evaporative loss. This can be extremely uncomfortable for persons attending the child, however.

Prevention of complications. The chief danger in this phase of burn care is infection—wound infection, generalized sepsis, and bacterial pneumonia. It is important to make accurate ongoing assessments of all parameters that provide clues for diagnosis. For example, wound cultures are done at least three times weekly and a blood culture is indicated in any child with a rectal temperature of 39.5°C (103°F) or above.

Antacids are usually administered prophylactically to prevent or minimize the effect of Curling's ulcer, but nurses must be alert for any signs of bleeding.

Continued observations are made to detect any indication of other complications associated with burns and their management. Rashes are not uncommon in children and may be of viral origin or a reaction to medications. They should be evaluated. The nurse must be alert to the possibility of any of the complications described previously—hypertension, renal disorders, and convulsion disorders.

Because the child is reluctant to move since doing so causes pain or discomfort, stiffness and joint contracture develop easily. In an effort to prevent this complication, he is encouraged to move whenever feasible and active physiotherapy is included as an essential aspect of burn care. When the child is resting or sleeping, contracture is prevented by proper splinting. The child's natural tendency is to be active, and he will usually move spontaneously unless the pain is severe. (For a summary of nursing care in the management phase of burn care, see the boxed material on pp. 1136 and 1137.)

Nursing care during rehabilitative phase

The rehabilitative phase of burn care begins when permanent closure of the wound is implemented. The primary focus of this phase is to obtain functional use of burned areas and cosmetic results as nearly normal as possible.

Effort in the care of children with skin grafts is directed toward facilitating a "take." Trauma, infection, and bleeding must be avoided for a successful transplantation to occur. When the grafted area is left exposed, the child must be immobilized to prevent the graft from becoming dislodged. Flat surfaces usually pose few problems, but grafts over irregular or mobile areas may require special techniques such as splints or skeletal traction. Small children may need to be restrained. Sedation may be needed for very restless and/or uncooperative children for the first 2 or 3 days after surgery.

The exposed method allows for easier inspection of the grafts, and collection of fluid under the graft can be removed by gently rolling the fluid out with a sterile applicator. This should be attempted with collections of fluid ½ inch or less from the edge of the graft. For those further toward the middle, a tiny slit is made in the graft tissue through which the fluid can be rolled. The less disturbance to any fibrous attachments, the better.[15]

Some plastic surgeons prefer to use occlusive pressure dressings over the grafted tissue or secured with sutures attached to normal surrounding skin and tied over the grafted skin to hold it in place. Wet dressings are occasionally applied over lace grafts and kept moist with antimicrobial agents, silver nitrate, or normal saline. Moist dressings are covered with dry absorbent gauze. Plastic wraps are contraindicated, since they cause buildup of heat and moisture that may cause maceration of the graft.

Wound contraction and scar tissue formation are normal parts of wound healing. Scar tissue is metabolically active tissue that continually rearranges itself; as a result disabling contractures, deformity, and disfigurement are ever-present possibilities. Physical therapy, splints, and other methods are employed to minimize these long-term effects. Pressure splints and elastic bandages or elasticized garments help reduce scar hypertrophy and are sometimes worn for months after hospitalization. Often severely burned children must return to the hospital periodically for additional skin grafts and scar revisions, especially to release contractures over joint spaces and for cosmetic considerations. Often achievement of optimum results requires years. In the meantime, burn scars are unsightly and, although *improvements* can be made, hope should not be extended to the parents and child for total resolution.

The psychologic pain and sequelae of severe burn trauma are as intense as the physical trauma. Each burned child goes through a tremendous amount of pain, often continuous for varying periods, and separation from families for extended periods. During the painful ordeal of hospitalization, children develop coping mechanisms for dealing with the acute and ever-present pain. Self-induced hypnosis is not uncommon. In addition there is a continual barrage of painful therapeutic and diagnostic procedures that are inflicted by others. This pain, however, is usually psychologically repressed, as the child attempts to forget these painful incidents.

Life becomes a struggle for the child after burn trauma. He is puzzled, confused, and bombarded by a new way of life in a frightening world of strange people, things, and language. He wonders why this has happened to *him*—what he has done that he should be punished so. Past experiences cannot serve him in this crisis. He does not understand the "ugliness" and disfigurement he sees as his body. He wonders, "Am I going to die?"

Preparation for facing friends and classmates may be more than he is able to cope with. Some severely burned children are ashamed to show their bodies in the hospital. It is not difficult to imagine how the child dreads facing a world of stares or imagined stares. Undressing at school can be a painful experience. It is not surprising that many children withdraw from contacts with others, even at a very early age. In time, as understanding and acceptance increase, they may feel more comfortable with themselves, and the emotional scars fade somewhat.

The impact of such severe injury taxes the capabilities of children at all ages, but the young child, who suffers acutely from separation anxiety, and the adolescent, who is developing an identity, are probably most affected psychologically. The toddler cannot begin to comprehend why the parents whom he loves and who have protected him from hurt can leave him in such a dreadful place and allow others to inflict such painful indignities on him.

The adolescent, in the process of achieving independence from families and seeking to find out who he is in the world, finds himself in a dependent position with a damaged body. Being different from others at a time when conformity and being like his peers are so important is difficult to accept. These children need understanding adults to help them deal with the struggles concerning resentment and other feelings generated by such a catastrophe. A psychiatric nurse is often an integral member of the burn team and is invaluable to the total management of the child and his family. (For a summary of nursing in the rehabilitative phase of burn care, see the boxed material on p. 1140.)

Family of burned child

Members of the family as well as the child feel the impact of severe burn injury. They are concerned about the child's survival, recovery, and future appearance. Because they, too, have overwhelming anxieties, fears, frustrations, and feelings of guilt, their needs must be met in order that they, in turn, can provide the support and encouragement so desperately needed by the child. It is the family, particularly the parents, who are the most significant persons in the child's life.

As in any emergency situation, all attention is focused on the child and the parents are forced to abandon their child to others. Often they do not know what is happening, how the child is doing, or if he is even alive. They feel powerless and ineffectual. Nurses can do much to alleviate parents' anxiety simply by acknowledging that they appreciate their concern, explain what is being done, explain why the child is crying, and offer whatever small physical comfort is available.

Most parents feel overwhelming guilt about the child's illness. Whether justified or not, they feel responsible for the accident or injury—as if in some way they should have been able to prevent it. These feelings sometimes impede the child's rehabilitation. Parents may indulge the child and give in to his each and every whim. Some are unable to look at or touch the child as they see him grow edematous, lethargic, and covered with unsightly eschar. Parents need to be told what to expect in the child, concerning both appearance and behavior. The burn wound will look worse before it looks better, and the child may exhibit unpredictable behavior when the parents are present. Ill children often cry when the parents are around, almost certainly when they prepare to leave; at other times they may reject the parents.

Nurses are in the most opportune position to assist parents to cope with the stresses of the child's illness and their own feelings of guilt and helplessness. The parents need to be informed of the child's progress and helped in their efforts to cope with their feelings while providing support to the child. The nurse is the person who can help them understand that it is not selfish to look after themselves and their own needs in order that they can better meet the needs of the child. For parents whose response to the illness is too severe or whose response to stress is manifest in destructive behavior, professional help may be needed.

Prevention of burn injury

Nurses have an obligation to be active in educating parents, children, and others in prevention of burn injuries. Children can be taught the hazards of flame and what to do in case of fire. They should be taught respect for matches, lighters, and other items, such as firecrackers, torches, and so on, that might cause fires or catch clothing afire. Any heating unit, flame heater, or fire is a potentially lethal device, and children must learn to maintain a safe distance from the heat source. They can learn to be "fire marshals" and inspect their homes and neighborhood for fire hazards.

Children can also be taught how to behave in case of fire. Every family should practice fire drills and designate specific responsibilities for the child in getting himself to safety from any location. Special decals are available that can be placed in windows to help firemen identify children's rooms in burning buildings. Older children should know how to report a fire and the location of the nearest fire-alarm box. All children should be taught to crawl to safety. Children have a tendency to crawl under beds or into cupboards, where they are difficult to locate. They should also be taught how to behave if their clothing becomes ignited. For example, a child who calmly walked to the kitchen where her mother was working and reported that her nightgown was afire received much less severe burns than a child in a similar situation who ran around in a panic.

Summary of nursing care in the rehabilitative phase of burn care

Goals	Responsibilities
Facilitate wound healing	Protect graft from trauma Protect from infection (as in summaries on pp. 1132 and 1136) Provide high-protein foods as a major part of the diet Administer vitamins and other medications as prescribed
Protect graft area	Position for minimal disturbance of graft site Restrain if necessary Apply topical treatment and dressings as ordered Observe for signs of infection
Promote optimal functioning (physical)	Carry out range of motion exercises Encourage mobility Ambulate as soon as feasible Splint involved joints at night and rest periods Encourage and promote self-help activities
Minimize scar formation	Position in functional attitude Apply splints as ordered and designed Wrap healing tissue with elastic bandage or dress in elastic garments as ordered Carry out physical therapy
Prepare child for discharge	Begin early in hospitalization to discuss "going home" Accept regressive behavior where appropriate Help child develop independence and self-help capabilities Explore feelings about returning to home and family, school, and friends Explore feelings concerning physical appearance Provide reinforcement of positive aspects of appearance and capabilities Discuss aids that camouflage disfigurement Wigs Clothing, for example, turtleneck sweaters Makeup
Prepare family for discharge	Teach wound care to care giver Discuss diet, rest, and activity Explore attitudes toward child's reentry into the family Explore parents' concept regarding child's capabilities and the possible restrictions and freedom they will allow Help parents set realistic goals for themselves, child, and other family members Help parents acquire needed equipment and supplies
Participate in follow-up care	Coordinate team management of child and family Arrange for return visits Assess needs of family Arrange for referral to agencies based on need assessment Collaborate with school nurse to help with child's reintegration into school and the world of peers

Parent education should be aimed at prevention and emergency care for burns. Parents can be taught commonsense safety precautions. Many persons are not aware that simple acts such as turning pot handles over the stove rather than extended over the edge where they can be reached by small hands, covering exposed hot water pipes, placing protective barriers around heating units, avoiding letting appliance cords hang below the tabletop, and covering electric outlets can prevent tragedy. Small or helpless children should not be left alone in the kitchen or bathroom. The child can turn on a gas range, especially where the knobs are situated at the front of the stove, run hot water, and pull hot items onto himself. It is also characteristic of small children in a bathtub of hot water to remain still or even to squat down rather than to climb out. Crawling infants or toddlers should be kept away from electric cords on which they might chew. Parents should recognize that children's thin skin is sensitive to direct sunlight and limit the time the child is exposed to the sun. Other preventive measures regarding burns are discussed in Chapters 12, 14, and 17.

Instruction in emergency first-aid measures should be part of parent education. Most lay persons still treat burns with application of butter or Vaseline. They need to be aware that current treatment is cooling the area with cool water. It is important that they have some criteria for determining when the injury can be treated with a simple dressing and when to seek medical aid.

Public education through community groups, the communication media, and offices, clinics, and homes is part of nurses' responsibility in preventive care. Information regarding safety devices for the home, such as smoke detectors and fire extinguishers, can be disseminated to a large audience. Nurses can be effective campaigners for safety legislation, such as fire-proofing children's clothing and for improvement of substandard housing. As health professionals, their voices can and should be heard.

REFERENCES

1. Achauer, B. M., and associates: Pulmonary complications of burns: the major threat to the burn patient, Ann. Surg. **177:** 311, 1973.
2. Alexander, J. W., Dionigi, R., and Meakins, J. L.: Periodic variations in the antibacterial function of human neutrophils and its relationship to sepsis, Ann. Surg. **173:**206-213, 1971.
3. Artz, C. P., and Moncrief, J. A.: The treatment of burns, ed. 3, Philadelphia, 1974, W. B. Saunders Co.
4. Baxter, C. R.: Crystalloid resuscitation of burn shock. In Polk, H. C., Jr., and Stone, H. H., editors: Contemporary burn management, Boston, 1971, Little, Brown and Co.
5. Berman, W., Jr., and associates: Childhood burn injuries and deaths, Pediatrics **51:**1069, 1973.
6. Bernstein, N. R.: Emotional care of the facially burned and disfigured, Boston, 1976, Little, Brown and Co.
7. Davies, J. W. L., and Liljedahl, S. O.: Metabolic consequences of an extensive burn. In Polk, H. C., Jr., and Stone, H. H.: Contemporary burn management, Boston, 1971, Little, Brown and Co.
8. Finberg, L.: Diarrheal dehydration. In Winters, R. W., editor: The body fluids in pediatrics, Boston, 1973, Little, Brown and Co.
9. Fox, C. L., Jr.: Fluid therapy and control of infection in burns. In Winters, R. W., editor: The body fluids in pediatrics, Boston, 1973, Little, Brown and Co.
10. Frye, S., and Lander, J.: The initial management of the acutely burned child, Issues Comprehensive Pediatr. Nurs., pp. 39-59, 1976.
11. Hamilton, J. R., and associates: Recent developments in viral gastroenteritis, Pediatr. Clin. North Am. **22:**747-755, 1975.
12. Herrin, J. T., and Crawford, J. D.: The seriously burned child. In Smith, C. A., editor: The critically ill child, ed. 2, Philadelphia, 1977, W. B. Saunders Co.
13. Holter, J. C., and Friedman, S. B.: Etiology and management of severely burned children, Am. J. Dis. Child. **118:**680-686, 1969.
14. Hughes, J. G.: Synopsis of pediatrics, ed. 4, St. Louis, 1975, The C. V. Mosby Co.
15. Jacoby, F. G.: Nursing care of the patient with burns, ed. 2, St. Louis, 1976, The C. V. Mosby Co.
16. Lumsden, K., and Holden, W. S.: The act of vomiting in man, Gut **10:**173, 1969.
17. MacMillan, B. G.: Management of burns in children. In Shirkey, H. C., editor: Pediatric therapy, ed. 5, St. Louis, 1975, The C. V. Mosby Co.
18. Mellins, R. B., and Parks, S.: Respiratory complications of smoke inhalation in victims of fires, J. Pediatr. **87:**1, 1975.
19. Moncrief, J. A.: Burns, N. Engl. J. Med. **288:**444-454, 1973.
20. Nelson, J. D., and Haltalin, K. C.: Acute diarrheal diseases of infectious origin. In Shirkey, H. C., editor: Pediatric therapy, ed. 5, 1975, The C. V. Mosby Co.
21. Reports on the epidemiology and surveillance of injuries, No. F.Y. 71-R3, September, 1970, U.S. Department of Health, Education, and Welfare, Public Health Service, Division of Planning and Standards, Environmental Epidemiology Branch.
22. Roy, C. C., Silverman, A., and Cozzetto, F. J.: Pediatric clinical gastroenterology, ed. 2, St. Louis, 1975, The C. V. Mosby Co.
23. Rubin, M.: Balm for burned children, Am. J. Nurs. **66:**296-302, 1966.
24. Silverberg, M., and Davidson, M.: Vomiting. In Shirkey, H. C., editor: Pediatric therapy, ed. 5, St. Louis, 1975, The C. V. Mosby Co.
25. Song, I., and Bromberg, B. E.: Burns. In Shefton, G. W., and Gardner, B., editors: Quick reference to surgical emergencies, Philadelphia, 1974, J. B. Lippincott Co.
26. Trunkey, D., and Parks, S.: Burns in children, Curr. Probl. Pediatr. **6**(3):3-51, January 1976.
27. Zawacki, B.: Reversal of capillary stasis and prevention of necrosis in burns, Ann. Surg. **180:**98-102, 1974.

BIBLIOGRAPHY
Diarrhea

Briody, B. A., and Gillis, R. E.: Microbiology and infectious disease, New York, 1974, McGraw-Hill Book Co.

Castle, M.: Isolation. Precise procedures for better protection, Nursing '75 **5:**50-57, May 1975.

Copeland, L.: Chronic diarrhea in infancy, Am. J. Nurs. **77:**461-463, 1977.

Davidson, G. P., and associates: Importance of a new virus in acute sporadic enteritis in children, Lancet **1:**242, 1975.

Davidson, M., and Silverberg, M.: Acute and chronic diarrhea. In Shirkey, H. C., editor: Pediatric therapy, St. Louis, 1975, The C. V. Mosby Co.

Diarrhea as caused by *Salmonella* and *Shigella,* Nursing '75 **5:**59-60, November 1975.

Drachman, R. H.: Acute infectious gastroenteritis, Pediatr. Clin. North Am. **21:**711, 1974.

Dupont, H. L., and Hornick, R. B.: Clinical approach to infectious diarrheas, Medicine **52:**265-270, 1973.

Finberg, L.: Diarrheal dehydration. In Winters, R. W., editor: The body fluids in pediatrics, Boston, 1973, Little, Brown and Co.

Gall, D. G., and Hamilton, J. R.: Chronic diarrhea in childhood: a new look at an old problem, Pediatr. Clin. North Am. **21:** 1001, November 1974.

Grady, G. F., and Keusch, G. T.: Pathogenesis of bacterial diarrheas, N. Engl. J. Med. **285:**831-841, 891-900, 1971.

Hamilton, J. R.: Diarrhea in infants, Mod. Med. **38:**131-139, 1970.

Ironside, A. G.: Gastroenteritis of infancy, Br. Med. J. **1:**284-286, 1973.

Keusch, G.: Bacterial diarrheas, Am. J. Nurs. **73:**1028-1032, 1973.

Rudoy, R. C., and Nelson, J. D.: Enteroinvasive and enterotoxigenic *Escherichia coli:* occurrence in acute diarrhea of infants and children, Am. J. Dis. Child. **129:**688, 1975.

Spicher, C.: Nursing care of children hospitalized with infections, Nurs. Clin. North Am. **5:**123-129, 1970.

Top, F. H., and Wehrle, P. F., editors: Communicable and infectious diseases, ed. 8, St. Louis, 1976, The C. V. Mosby Co.

Vaughn, V. C., and McKay, R. J., editors: Textbook of pediatrics, ed. 10, Philadelphia, 1975, W. B. Saunders Co.

Hypertrophic pyloric stenosis

Benson, C. D.: Infantile pyloric stenosis, Progr. Pediatr. Surg. **1:**63-88, 1970.

Huguenard, J. R., and Sharples, G. E.: Incidence of congenital pyloric stenosis within sibships, J. Pediatr. **81:**45-49, 1972.

Martin, L. W.: Pediatric surgery—general. In Shirkey, H. C., editor: Pediatric therapy, ed. 5, St. Louis, 1975, The C. V. Mosby Co.

Thompson, J. S., and Thompson, M. W.: Genetics in medicine, Philadelphia, 1973, W. B. Saunders Co.

Whaley, L. F.: Understanding inherited disorders, St. Louis, 1974, The C. V. Mosby Co.

Winters, R. W.: Metabolic alkalosis of pyloric stenosis. In Winters, R. W., editor: The body fluids in pediatrics, Boston, 1973, Little, Brown and Co.

Burns

Allyn, P., and Bartlett, R.: Management of the burn patient. In Zschoche, D. A., editor: Mosby's comprehensive review of critical care, St. Louis, 1976, The C. V. Mosby Co.

Arnoff, M., Fleishman, P., and Simon, D. L.: Experience in the application of porcine xenograft donor sites, J. Trauma **16:**280-283, 1976.

Baxter, C. R., Marvin, J., and Curreri, P. W.: Fluid and electrolyte therapy of burn shock, Heart Lung **2:**708, 1973.

Baxter, C. R., Marvin, J. A., and Curreri, P. W.: Early management of thermal burns, Postgrad. Med. **55:**131, 1974.

Bell, J. G.: Bitsy was so little . . . and her problems so big, Nursing '77 **7**(6):35-37, 1977.

Bellock, J. P.: Helping a child cope with the stress of injury, Am. J. Nurs. **74:**1491, 1974.

Berman, W., Jr., and associates: Childhood burn injuries and deaths, Pediatrics **51:**1069, 1973.

Bernstein, N. R.: Emotional care of the facially burned and disfigured, Boston, 1976, Little, Brown and Co.

Bezzeg, E. D., and associates: The role of the child care worker in the treatment of severely burned children, Pediatrics **50:**617-624, 1972.

Birch, J. R.: Flammable fabrics and human burns, Can. J. Surg. **14:**177-178, 1971.

Boswick, J. A., and Pandya, N. S.: Emergency care of the burned patient, Surg. Clin. North Am. **52:**115-123, 1972.

Bowden, M. L., and Feller, I.: Family reaction to a severe burn, Am. J. Nurs. **73:**317-319, 1973.

Burke, J. F., Quinby, W. C., and Bondoc, C. C.: Primary excision and prompt grafting as routine therapy for the treatment of thermal burns in children, Surg. Clin. North Am. **56:**477, 1976.

Burrell, Z. L., and Burrell, L. O.: Critical care, ed. 3, St. Louis, 1977, The C. V. Mosby Co.

Calleia, P., and Boswick, J. A.: A home care nursing program for patients with burns, Am. J. Nurs. **72:**1442-1444, 1972.

Campbell, L.: Special behavioral problems of the burned child, Am. J. Nurs. **76:**220-224, 1976.

Caudle, R. R. K., and Potter, J.: Characteristics of burned children and the after effects of the injury, Br. J. Plast. Surg. **23:** 63, 1970.

Claudea, M.: TLC and Sulfamylon for burned children, Am. J. Nurs. **69:**755-757, 1969.

Corliss, S.: Improving care of severe burn wounds, Nursing '72 **2**(4):6-12, 1972.

Cosman, B.: The burned child. In Downey, J. A., and Low, N. L., editors: The child with disabling illness, Philadelphia, 1974, W. B. Saunders Co.

Crikelair, G. F.: Burn prevention, J. Trauma **12:**363-364, 1972.

Davidson, S. P., and Noyes, R.: Psychiatric nursing consultation on a burn unit, Am. J. Nurs. **73:**1715-1718, 1973.

Davies, J. W. L., and Liljedahl, S. O.: Metabolic consequences of an extensive burn. In Polk, N. C., Jr., and Stone, H. H.: Contemporary burn management, Boston, 1971, Little, Brown and Co.

Eckauser, F., and associates: Tracheostomy complicating massive burn injury; a plea for conservatism, Am. J. Surg. **127:**418, 1974.

Epstein, M. F., and Crawford, J. D.: Cooling in the emergency treatment of burns, Pediatrics **52:**430, 1973.

Fagerhaugh, S. Y.: Pain expression and control on a burn care unit, Nurs. Outlook **22:**645-650, 1974.

Feller, I., and Crane, K. H.: National burn information exchange, Surg. Clin. North Am. **50:**1425, 1970.

Fujita, M. T.: The impact of illness or surgery on the body image of the child, Nurs. Clin. North Am. **7**:641, 649, 1972.

Gentry, W. C., and Pathak, M. A.: Help for your sunburn-prone patients, Patient Care **10**(11):40-45, June 1, 1976.

Gifford, G. H., Jr., and associates: The management of electrical burns in children, Pediatrics **47**:113, 1971.

Gruber, R. P., Vistnes, L., and Pardoe, R.: The effect of commonly used antiseptics on wound healing, Plast. Reconstr. Surg. **55**:472-476, 1974.

Hartford, C. E.: The early treatment of burns, Nurs. Clin. North Am. **8**:447-456, 1973.

Herrin, J., and Crawford, J.: Care of the critically ill child: major burns, Pediatrics **45**:449-458, 1970.

Hunter, G. R., and Chang, F. C.: Outpatient burns: a prospective study, J. Trauma **16**:191-195, 1976.

Jacoby, F. G.: Individualized burn wound dressings, Nursing 77 **7**(6):62-63, 1977.

Jones, C. A., and Feller, I.: Burns, what to do during the first crucial hours, Nursing '77 **7**(3):23-31, 1977.

Kavanagh, C.: A portrait of need and of giving, Am. J. Maternal Child Nurs. **2**(4):229, 1977.

Klonoff, H.: Head injuries in children: predisposing factors, accident proneness, and sequelae, Am. J. Public Health **61**:2405, 1971.

Kunsman, J.: Nursing the acutely burned child: nursing after primary excision, RN **37**:25, August 1974.

Larsen, D. L., and associates: Zinc deficiency in burned children, Plast. Reconstr. Surg. **46**:13, 1970.

Lilly, J. R., and Peck, C. A.: Immediate porcine heterografting of burns in children, J. Pediatr. Surg. **9**:335-340, 1974.

MacArthur, J. D., and Moore, F.: Epidemiology of burns—the burn prone patient, J.A.M.A. **231**:259-263, 1975.

MacMillan, B. G.: The use of mesh grafting in treating burns, Surg. Clin. North Am. **50**:1347, 1970.

Margolius, F.: Burned children, infection and nursing care, Nurs. Clin. North Am. **5**:131-142, 1970.

Martin, H. L.: Antecedents of burns and scalds in children, Br. J. Med. Psychol. **43**:39-47, 1970.

Martin, H. L.: Parents and children's reaction to burns and scalds in children, Br. J. Med. Psychol. **43**:183-191, 1970.

McDonnell, C., Kramer, M., and Leak, A.: What would you do? Am. J. Nurs. **72**:296-301, 1972.

McGranahan, B. G.: Nursing care of burn patient, A.O.R.N. **20**: 787-793, 1974.

McLoughlin, E., and associates: One pediatric burn unit's experience with sleepwear related injuries, Pediatrics **60**:405-409, 1977.

Metheny, N. M., and Snively, W. D.: Nurse's handbook of fluid balance, ed. 2, Philadelphia, 1974, J. P. Lippincott Co.

Minckley, B. B.: Expert nursing care for burned patients, Am. J. Nurs. **70**:1888-1893, 1970.

Ninman, C., and Shoemaker, P.: Human amniotic membranes for burns, Am. J. Nurs. **75**:1468-1469, 1975.

O'Neill, J. A., Jr.: Continuing care of the acutely burned child, RN **37**:93-106, September 1974.

Pascoe, D. J., and Grossman, M.: Quick reference to pediatric emergencies, Philadelphia, 1973, J. B. Lippincott Co.

Polk, H. C., and Stone, H. H., editors: Contemporary burn management, Boston, 1971, Little, Brown and Co.

Quinby, S. V., and Bernstein, N. R.: How children live after disfiguring burns, Psychiatry Med. **2**:146-159, 1971.

Quinby, S. V., and Bernstein, N. R.: Identity problems and the adaptation of nurses to severely burned children, Am. J. Psychiatry **128**:58-63, 1971.

Rinear, C. E., and Rinear, E. E.: Emergency! Part 3. On-the-spot care for aspiration, burns, and poisoning, Nursing '75 **5**(4):40, 1975.

Rogenes, P. R., and Moylaw, J. A.: Restoring fluid balance in the patient with severe burns, Am. J. Nurs. **76**:1953-1957, 1976.

Royce, J.: Shock—emergency nursing implications, Nurs. Clin. North Am. **8**:377, 1973.

Rubin, M.: Balm for burned children, Am. J. Nurs. **66**:296-302, 1966.

Savedra, M. K.: The child and his family at home: what then? Am. J. Maternal Child Nurs. **2**(4):224-227, 1977.

Savedra, M. K.: Moving from hospital to home, Am. J. Maternal Child Nurs. **2**(4):220-222, 1977.

Seligman, R., Carroll, S., and MacMillan, B. G.: Emotional responses of burned children in a pediatric intensive care unit, Psychiatry Med. **3**:59, 1972.

Seligman, R., MacMillan, B. G., and Carrol, S. X.: The burned child: a neglected area of psychiatry, Am. J. Psychiatry **128**: 52, 1971.

Sevitt, S.: Reactions to injury and burns and their clinical importance, Philadelphia, 1974, J. B. Lippincott Co.

Shaw, B. L.: Current therapy for burns, RN **34**:33-41, March 1971.

Sheehy, E.: Primary excision. Innovation in pediatric burn care, RN **37**:21-26, August 1974.

Siner, E., and Allyn, P.: Emergency burn care, Crit. Care Update **4**(3):24-27, 1977.

Smith, E. C., and associates: Reestablishing a child's body image, Am. J. Nurs. **77**:445-447, 1977.

Smith, E. I.: The epidemiology of burns, the cause and control of burns in children, Pediatrics **44**:821, 1969.

Smith, E. I.: Acute management of thermal burns in children, Surg. Clin. North Am. **50**:807, 1970.

Stinson, V.: Porcine skin dressings for burns, Am. J. Nurs. **74**: 111-112, 1974.

Stone, N. H., and associates: Child abuse by burning, Surg. Clin. North Am. **50**:1419-1424, 1970.

Talabere, L., and Graves, P.: A tool for assessing families of burned children, Am. J. Nurs. **76**:225-227, 1976.

Wagner, M. M.: Emergency care of the burned patient, Am. J. Nurs. **77**:1788-1795, 1977.

Wiley, L.: Burn care, Nursing '72 **2**(7):32-37, 1972.

Wilkinson, A. W.: Burns, Community Health **2**(1):23-28, 1970.

Willis, B. A., Larson, D. L., and Abston, S.: Positioning and splinting the burned patient, Heart Lung **2**:697, 1973.

Wright, L., and Fulwiler, R.: Long range emotional sequelae of burns; effects on children and their mothers, Pediatr. Res. **8**: 931-934, 1974.

Zitomer, M. M.: Protecting children from the tragedy of burns, Am. J. Maternal Child Nurs. **2**(2):129-130, March/April 1977.

Zschoche, D. A.: The burn patient—a challenge in critical care, Heart Lung **2**:686-689, 1973.

31

The child with a disturbance of renal function

Diseases involving the kidneys are relatively common in childhood and are caused by a variety of etiologic factors. To better understand the way in which the pathologic processes produce an effect, the basic kidney structure and function are briefly reviewed and the most frequently used tests of renal function are outlined to help the reader understand the relationship of these studies to renal physiology and pathology. Discussion of the more common disorders of renal function is followed by the critical therapies of dialysis and renal transplant.

REVIEW OF RENAL FUNCTION

The primary responsibility of the kidney is to maintain the composition and volume of the body fluids constant. To maintain this constant internal environment, the kidney must respond appropriately to alterations in the internal environment caused by variations in dietary intake and extrarenal losses of water and solutes. This is accomplished by the formation of an ultrafiltration of plasma, with subsequent reabsorption of most of the water and electrolytes by the renal tubules and the secretion of certain other substances into the tubular urine. *Reabsorption* is the transport of a substance from the tubular lumen to the blood in surrounding vessels. *Secretion* is transport in the opposite direction, that is, from the blood to the lumen. These processes can be active or passive. *Excretion* is the elimination of a substance from the body, in this case urine.

A secondary function of the kidney is the production of certain humoral substances. One such substance is an enzyme *erythropoietic stimulating factor* (*ESF* or *erythrogenin*), which acts on a plasma globulin to form erythropoietin, which in turn stimulates erythropoiesis in the bone marrow. Its production is increased in the presence of hypoxia and androgens. Few red blood cells are formed in the absence of erythropoietin, which accounts in some measure for the anemia associated with advanced renal disease. Another enzyme, *renin,* is also secreted by the kidney, probably from the juxtaglomerular cells located at the point at which the afferent arteriole enters the glomerulus. Renin secretion is produced in response to reduced blood volume, decreased blood pressure, or increased secretion of catecholamines. Renin stimulates the production of the angiotensins, which produce arteriolar constriction and an elevation in blood pressure and stimulate the production of aldosterone by the adrenal cortex.

Renal physiology and formation of urine

The structural and functional unit of the kidney is the nephron. Approximately 1 million nephrons collectively form the bulk of each kidney proper. The kidneys themselves are bean-shaped organs normally situated behind the parietal peritoneum against the posterior wall at the level of the last thoracic and first three lumbar vertebrae and held in place by a heavy cushion of fat and anchoring connective tissue. The kidney itself is almost totally lacking in connective tissue, except for the tough fibrous capsule that surrounds it. This arrangement of connective tissue is able to support a high buildup of pressure within the kidney.

The appearance of a kidney in a longitudinal section is illustrated in Fig. 31-1. The principal features are an outer *cortex* and an inner *medulla,* within which are wedge-shaped *pyramids* separated by extensions of the cortex, the *renal columns.* The tips of the pyramids form the renal *papillae,* each of which opens into a smaller or *minor calyx.* A number of calyces empty into one of several *major calyces* that converge into the *renal pelvis.* The renal pelvis narrows after it leaves the kidney and forms what then becomes a *ureter,* through which urine drains into the *urinary bladder.* The renal artery and nerves enter and the ureter and renal vein exit through a medial depression in the kidney, the *hilum.*

The nephron. The nephron, the functional unit of the kidney, is a complex system of tubules, arterioles, venules, and capillaries (Fig. 31-2). The nephron itself consists of *Bowman's capsule,* enclosing the capillary tuft of the *glomerulus,* which is joined successively to the *proximal convoluted tubule, Henle's loop,* the *distal convoluted tubule,* and the straight or *collecting duct.* Collecting tubules join larger ducts, and all the larger collecting ducts of one renal pyramid join to form a single duct that opens into

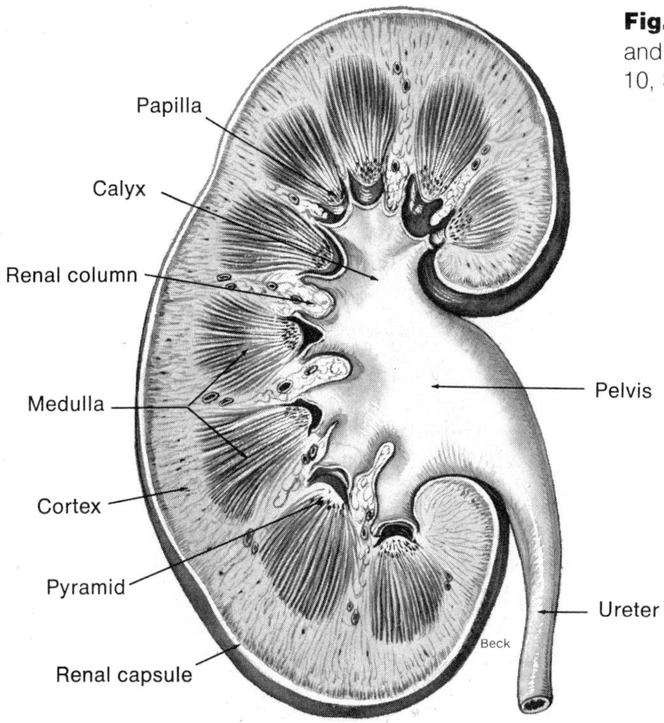

Fig. 31-1. Longitudinal section of kidney. (From Anthony, C. P., and Thibodeau, G. A.: Textbook of anatomy and physiology, ed. 10, St. Louis, 1979, The C. V. Mosby Co.)

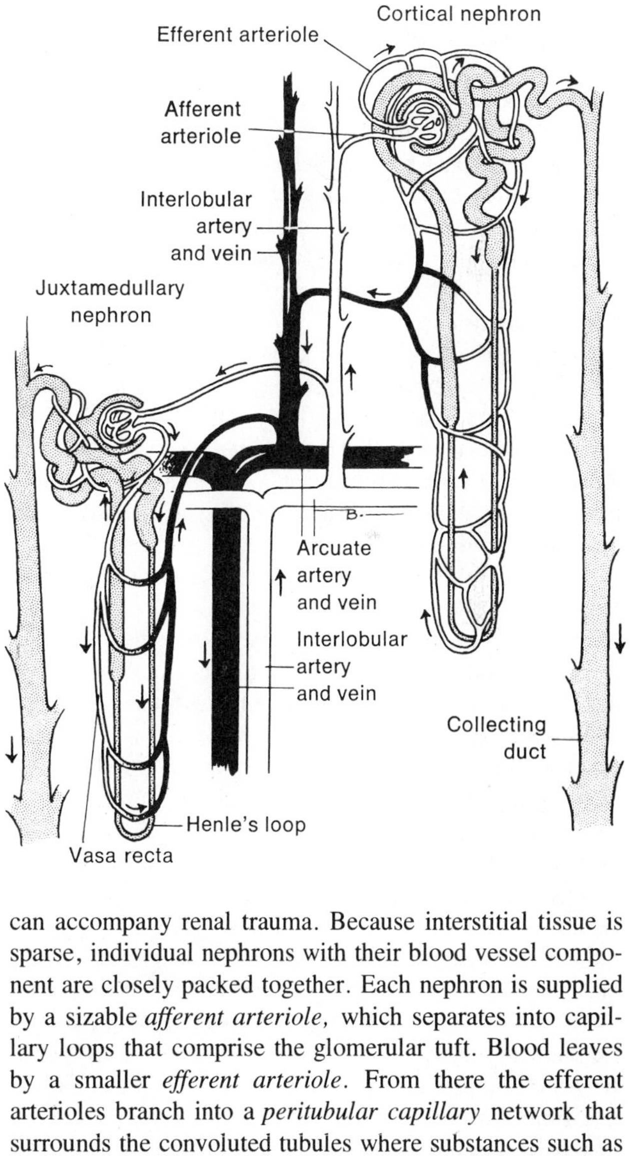

Fig. 31-2. Basic structure of a nephron. (From Brundage, D. J.: Nursing management of renal problems, St. Louis, 1976, The C. V. Mosby Co., p. 7.)

a minor calyx. Although structurally similar, two types of nephrons are recognized: those situated superficially in the cortical region of the kidney (cortical nephrons) and those that lie deeper in the cortex (juxtamedullary nephrons). All the glomeruli, the proximal and distal tubules, and most of Henle's loops lie in the renal cortex and renal columns. However, Henle's loops of the juxtamedullary nephrons are longer and extend well into the renal medulla; therefore, they have the greatest concentrating ability. Cortical nephrons outnumber juxtamedullary nephrons by a factor of seven to one.

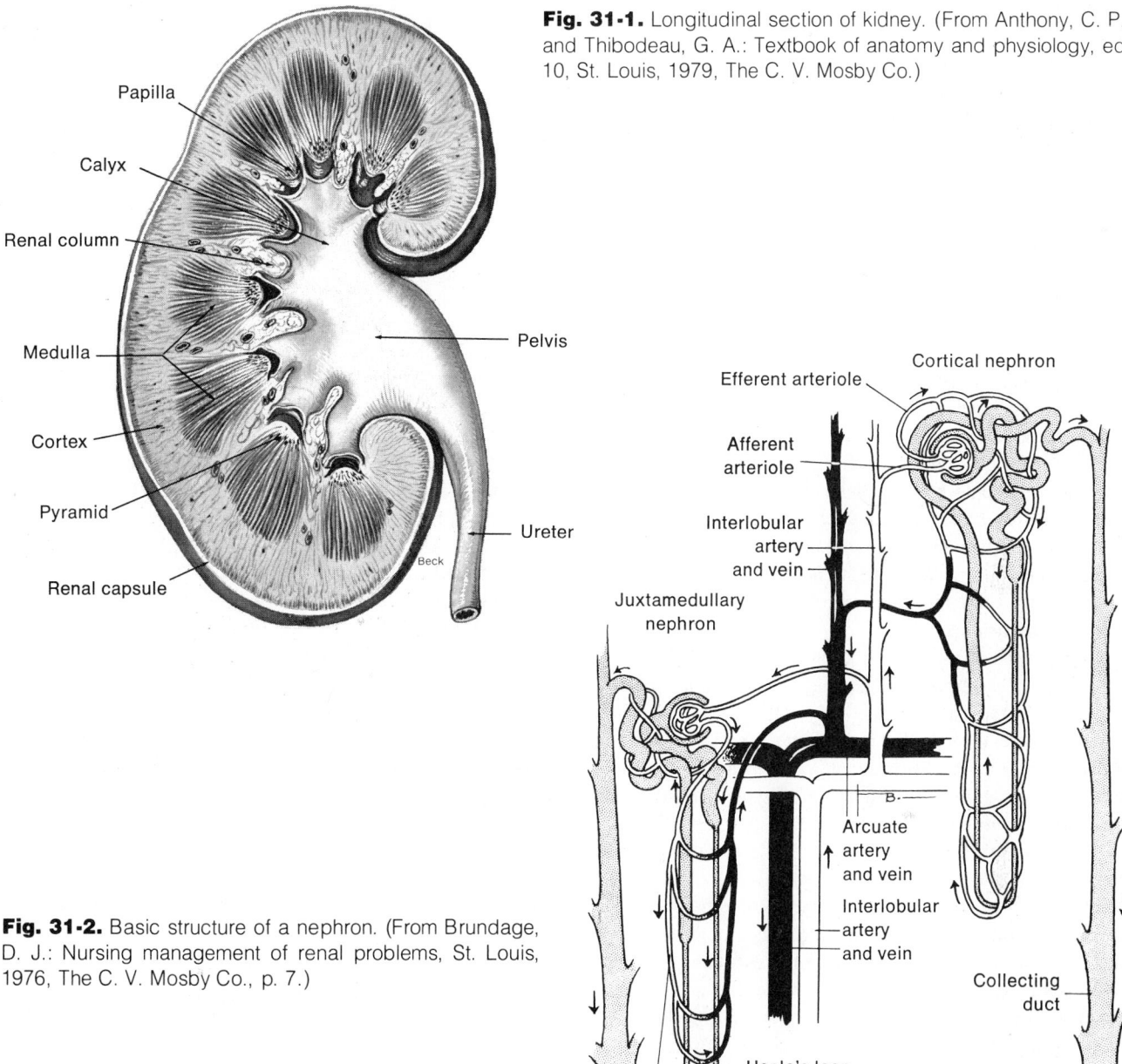

The blood supply to the kidneys constitutes about one fifth of the total cardiac output; therefore, profuse bleeding can accompany renal trauma. Because interstitial tissue is sparse, individual nephrons with their blood vessel component are closely packed together. Each nephron is supplied by a sizable *afferent arteriole,* which separates into capillary loops that comprise the glomerular tuft. Blood leaves by a smaller *efferent arteriole.* From there the efferent arterioles branch into a *peritubular capillary* network that surrounds the convoluted tubules where substances such as glucose are quickly reabsorbed into the circulation. In the longer juxtamedullary nephrons the efferent arteriole separates. One branch breaks up to form a peritubular plexus of capillaries, whereas the other branches into hairpin loops called the *vasa recta,* which parallel the Henle's loops and the collecting ducts. The total surface area of the renal capillaries is approximately equal to the total surface of the tubules.

In Bowman's capsule the *glomerular capsule* is composed of two cellular layers that separate the blood from the glomerular filtrate: the capillary endothelium and a layer of tubular epithelial lining cells. Situated between these layers is the basal lamina or basement membrane. The permeability of this glomerular membrane is a result of its structure; the capillary endothelium is fenestrated with pores or *fenestrae,* and the outer surface of the glomerular epithelium consists of fingerlike projections (*pseudopodia* or *podocytes*), which cover the entire surface to form slits called *slit pores*. The basement membrane has no visible openings but behaves as if it contains pores or channels. Consequently the glomerular filtrate, which has essentially the same composition as plasma except for the large protein molecules and cellular elements, passes through these three layers and does so at a very rapid rate. The structure of these layers becomes altered in kidney disease. The walls of the remaining portions of the nephron are composed of single cell layers, the structure of which differs with the function of each segment.

Glomerular filtration. Filtration through the glomerular capillaries is governed by the same mechanism as filtration across other capillaries in the body, that is, the size of the capillary bed, the permeability of the capillaries, and the hydrostatic and osmotic pressure gradients across the capillaries. Water and solutes filter from glomerular capillaries faster than from other capillaries because of a significantly higher intracapillary pressure, and capillary walls are more freely permeable to these substances. Also, the smaller efferent arteriole causes higher resistance to outflow of blood from the glomerulus. The filtration capacity of the glomerulus is the product of three pressure forces—the glomerular hydrostatic pressure, the colloidal osmotic (oncotic) pressure, and the intracapsular pressure—and the permeability of the glomerular capillaries.[9] The main determinant of net filtration pressure is glomerular hydrostatic pressure. The volume of filtrate formed per unit of time, usually expressed as ml/minute, is termed the glomerular filtration rate (GFR). This can be measured by determining the rate at which certain materials leave the circulation and enter the filtrate (see Table 31-1, p. 1151). Filtration takes place as long as hydrostatic pressure within the glomerular capillaries exceeds the opposing colloidal osmotic pressure (COP) of the plasma proteins. Isotonic protein-free fluid is lost from the plasma as it moves through the capillaries, thereby increasing the colloidal osmotic pressure within the capillaries at the efferent end of the glomerulus. If the pressure becomes equal through decreased hydrostatic pressure or decreased colloidal osmotic pressure, no further filtration takes place.

Factors that affect glomerular filtration include[9]:

1. Alterations in renal blood flow caused by hemorrhage, fluid overload, and increased cardiac output.
2. Changes in glomerular hydrostatic pressure caused by alteration in systemic blood pressure and afferent or efferent arteriole constriction.
3. Changes in hydrostatic pressure within Bowman's capsule caused by obstruction in kidney edema and collecting system, for example, renal pelvis or ureters.
4. Changes in plasma protein concentration caused by dehydration and hypoproteinemia.
5. Increased glomerular capillary permeability caused by glomerular disease.
6. Decrease in total area of glomerular capillary bed caused by destructive disease and nephrectomy.

Autoregulation of blood flow through glomerular capillaries can alter vascular resistance and stabilize filtration to some extent, but constriction of either arteriole decreases tubular blood flow. Diseases that alter capillary permeability permit proteins to escape into the urine to produce proteinemia. Any disease or condition that causes destruction to large numbers of nephrons and/or glomeruli reduces the functioning capacity of the kidneys.

Tubular function. The function of the renal tubules is to modify the glomerular filtrate. Tubular cells may add more of a substance to the filtrate (tubular secretion), remove some or all of a substance from the filtrate (tubular reabsorption), or both. Approximately 98% of the filtrate is reabsorbed from the tubules—about four fifths from the proximal tubules. The reabsorption is selective and discriminating for substances essential to body processes and equilibrium, whereas nonessential substances are eliminated as waste. The substances are secreted or reabsorbed in the tubules by osmosis, passive diffusion down a chemical or electric gradient, or actively transported against these gradients. These processes operate throughout the length of the tubules, but there are variations in the types, amounts, and mechanisms by which substances are secreted or reabsorbed in the different tubular segments, caused in large part by the cellular characteristics of each segment (Fig. 31-3).

Active transport mechanisms move vital substances both inward and outward from the tubular filtrate. For example, glucose molecules and sodium ions are reabsorbed and potassium and hydrogen ions are secreted by active transport mechanisms, but water is reabsorbed by osmosis and ammonia is secreted by diffusion. Active transport requires the expenditure of energy and is often one of the first powers affected by kidney disease. Essential items such as glucose, amino acids, and sodium ions are reabsorbed in the proximal tubule and returned directly to the blood. Active transport mechanisms, as elsewhere, have a limited capacity, or threshold, for moving the solute. When the maximum of the transport mechanism is reached, no more of the substance is reabsorbed and the remainder is excreted in the urine. For example, the transport mechanism for glucose

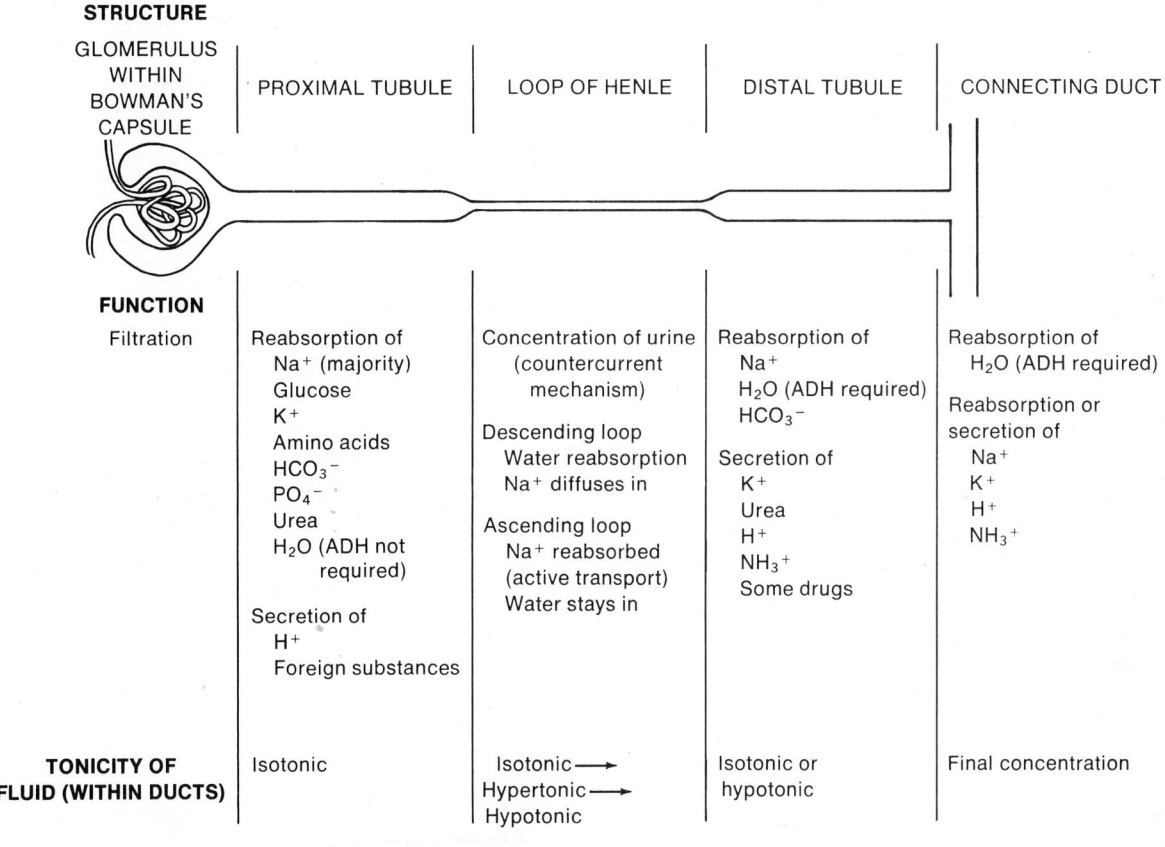

STRUCTURE	GLOMERULUS WITHIN BOWMAN'S CAPSULE	PROXIMAL TUBULE	LOOP OF HENLE	DISTAL TUBULE	CONNECTING DUCT
FUNCTION	Filtration	Reabsorption of Na^+ (majority) Glucose K^+ Amino acids HCO_3^- PO_4^- Urea H_2O (ADH not required) Secretion of H^+ Foreign substances	Concentration of urine (countercurrent mechanism) Descending loop Water reabsorption Na^+ diffuses in Ascending loop Na^+ reabsorbed (active transport) Water stays in	Reabsorption of Na^+ H_2O (ADH required) HCO_3^- Secretion of K^+ Urea H^+ NH_3^+ Some drugs	Reabsorption of H_2O (ADH required) Reabsorption or secretion of Na^+ K^+ H^+ NH_3^+
TONICITY OF FLUID (WITHIN DUCTS)		Isotonic	Isotonic → Hypertonic → Hypotonic	Isotonic or hypotonic	Final concentration

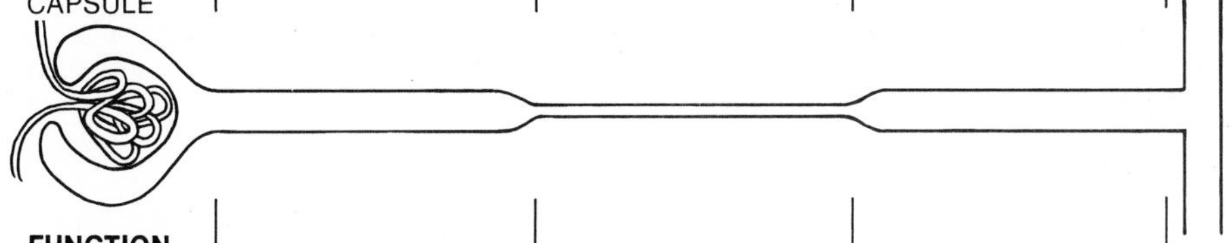

Fig. 31-3. Major functions of nephron components.

has a maximum threshold of about 180 mg/100 ml of blood; therefore, when blood glucose concentrations exceed this capacity, the surplus remains in the filtrate to be excreted in the urine (glycosuria). Active transport mechanisms are sometimes shared by two or more substances. When two substances share a common transport mechanism, the first substance may be blocked by the addition of a second substance (selective inhibition). The effect of many therapeutic agents, for example, diuretics, depends on this process.

Electrolytes are moved by both active transport and diffusion, and the transport of some, particularly sodium, has important effects on other substances. For example, sodium is actively transported from all parts of the nephron. The movement of sodium ions produces both an electric and an osmotic gradient, which causes chloride ions and water to diffuse from the tubules in an effort to establish equilibrium. This is the obligatory water reabsorption in the kidneys.

In some segments of the nephron the tubes are either impermeable to water (the ascending limb of Henle's loop) or the permeability is regulated by antidiuretic hormone (antidiuretic hormone distal tubules and collecting tube). The descending Henle's loop is highly permeable to water but not to solutes; as a result there is a movement of water out, increasing the sodium ion concentration within the tube. The ascending limb is relatively impermeable to water but is permeable to sodium ions and urea. Consequently sodium ions move outward along a concentration gradient, whereas water, which is unable to follow, remains in the filtrate, which becomes increasingly hypotonic as it reaches the distal tubule (the countercurrent mechanism). The distal tubule and collecting tube are impermeable to urea, but the pressure of antidiuretic hormone increases the permeability of the tubes to water. Consequently as sodium is transported out, water diffuses out and a concentrated urine is excreted. Thus antidiuretic hormone controls the excretion or retention of water in the distal tubule and collecting duct. The amount of sodium reabsorbed is, in turn, regulated by aldosterone. The presence of aldosterone stimulates the cells of the distal tubule to increase reabsorption of sodium ions from the filtrate into the blood. The presence of aldosterone is relatively constant under normal circumstances, but the concentration of antidiuretic hormone varies according to the osmolality of the blood and is, therefore, the major force controlling urine volume. However, the presence of an abnormal amount of unabsorbed solutes (for example, glucose or mannitol) in the tubules exerts an osmotic effect, which produces an increase in urine volume called osmotic diuresis. There is also a limit to the concentration gradient against which sodium can be transported out; therefore, when larger than normal amounts of sodium ions remain in the tubules, water is obliged to remain with the sodium.

Acidification of urine. The amount of acid secreted by the kidney depends on tubular activity, and the pH of urine ranges from 4.5 to 8.3. The kidney eliminates hydrogen ions in three ways: (1) neutralization with ammonia (60% to 75%), (2) excretion in the form of titratable acid (25% to 40%), and (3) excretion is free, dissociated hydrogen ions (small amounts). The maximum capacity for elimination of hydrogen ions corresponds to a limiting pH of 4.5. It is these three processes that constitute the renal contribution to maintenance of hydrogen ion concentration in extracellular fluids.[2]

Hydrogen ions are secreted by both the proximal and distal tubules. The bicarbonate buffer operates in the proximal tubule, the only cells of the tubule system that contain carbonic anhydrase, to break down carbonic acid to carbon dioxide and water. The hydrogen ion is exchanged for the sodium ion in sodium bicarbonate, and the resulting carbonic acid is broken down into carbon dioxide, which is readily reabsorbed to form bicarbonate and water, which is excreted. The hydrogen ions exchange with one of the sodium ions of the phosphate buffer in the distal tubules and collecting ducts to form the titratable acid NaH_2PO_4. Ammonia (NH_3) is secreted from cells of all segments, and the amount of hydrogen ions that react with ammonia to form ammonium (NH_4) depends on the pH of tubular fluid and the rate of ammonia production. Ammonia is secreted by ionic diffusion.

The renal tubules are able to excrete either hydrogen or potassium in exchange for the sodium they absorb. Consequently the more hydrogen ions they excrete, the fewer potassium ions can be excreted. Thus in acidosis there is a corresponding increase in the serum potassium levels, since their excretion is reduced.

Renal blood flow. The preservation of a relatively constant rate of flow and filtration rate, even within a wide range of systemic pressures, is achieved by alterations in the diameter of the afferent glomerular arterioles. The precise nature of this self-regulation, or *autoregulation,* is only speculative. The ascending Henle's loop reaches the glomerulus of its nephron and passes close to the afferent arteriole. At this point the wall of the arteriole contains the renin-secreting *juxtaglomerular cells* and the epithelium of the tubule is modified with specialized cells, the *macula densa*. These groups of cells, together with a few granulated cells between, are known collectively as the *juxtaglomerular apparatus*. It is this structure that is believed to contain sensor devices that respond to changes in intraarteriole pressure, sodium ion concentration, and circulating catecholamines to inhibit or stimulate the secretion of renin. Decreased blood volume or sodium ion concentration stimulates its secretion, as does sympathetic nerve activity, circulating catecholamines, and probably one of the prostaglandins. Renin secretion at any given time is apparently the result of the combined activity of these regulators.

Renal function in early infancy

Kidney function in early infancy is less efficient than at later ages. Glomerular filtration rate is low and does not reach adult values until the child is between 1 and 2 years of age. This appears to be related to a barrier imposed by more cuboidal-shaped glomerular epithelial cells and a higher afferent arteriole resistance. There is a large variation in the tubular length between nephrons, although glomerular size is less variable. The juxtaglomerular nephrons show more advanced development than cortical nephrons.[11]

The concentrating ability of the newborn kidney does not reach adult levels until about the third month of life. Although adequate amounts of antidiuretic hormone are secreted by the newborn pituitary gland, other factors appear to interfere with water reabsorption. The Henle's loop essential to concentrating ability is incompletely developed in the newborn, and urea synthesis and excretion are slower during this time. Also, the newborn retains large quantities of nitrogen and essential electrolytes in order to meet needs for growth in the first weeks of life. Consequently the excretory burden is minimized. The lower concentration of urea, the principal end product of nitrogen metabolism, reduces concentrating capacity, since it also contributes to the concentration mechanism.

Other characteristics of the newborn kidneys create differences in renal function from that of older children and adults. Because of some as yet undetermined cause, newborn infants are unable to excrete a water load at the rates of older persons. Hydrogen ion excretion is reduced, acid secretion is lower for the first year of life, and plasma bicarbonate levels are low. As a result of these inadequacies of the kidney and less efficient blood buffers, the newborn is more liable to develop severe acidosis. Sodium excretion is reduced in the immediate newborn period, and the kidneys are less able to adapt to deficiencies and excesses of sodium. For example, an isotonic saline infusion may produce edema because the ability to eliminate excess sodium is impaired. Conversely inadequate reabsorption of sodium from tubules may compound sodium losses in disorders such as vomiting or diarrhea. In addition infants have a diminished capacity to reabsorb glucose and, during the first few days, to produce ammonium ions.

ASSESSMENT OF RENAL INTEGRITY

Assessment of kidney and urinary tract integrity and the diagnosis of renal or urinary tract disease is based on several evaluative tools. Physical examination, history, and observation of symptoms are the initial procedures. In suspected urinary tract disorders, further assessment by laboratory, radiologic, and other evaluative methods is carried out.

Clinical manifestations

As in most disorders of childhood, the incidence and type of kidney or urinary tract dysfunction changes with the age and maturation of the child. Also, the presenting complaints and the significance of these complaints varies with maturation. For example, a complaint of enuresis has greater significance at age 8 years than at age 4 years. In the newborn, urinary tract disorders are associated with a number of obvious malformations of other body systems, including the curious and unexplained association between malformed or low-set ears and urinary tract anomalies.

Important signs and symptoms that suggest possible renal or urinary tract disease in children at different ages include[11]:

Neonatal period (birth to 1 month)

- Poor feeding
- Vomiting
- Failure to gain weight
- Rapid respiration (acidosis)
- Frequent urination
- Screaming on urination
- Poor urinary stream
- Jaundice
- Convulsions
- Dehydration
- Other anomalies or stigmata
- Enlarged kidneys or bladder

Infancy (1 to 24 months)

- Poor feeding
- Vomiting
- Failure to gain weight
- Excessive thirst
- Frequent urination
- Straining or screaming on urination
- Foul-smelling urine
- Pallor
- Fever
- Persistent diaper rash
- Convulsions (with or without fever)
- Dehydration
- Enlarged kidney or bladder

Childhood (2 to 14 years)

- Poor appetite
- Vomiting
- Growth failure
- Excessive thirst
- Enuresis, incontinence, frequent urination
- Painful urination
- Swelling of the face
- Convulsions
- Pallor
- Fatigue
- Blood in urine
- Abdominal or back pain
- Edema
- Hypertension
- Tetany

Many of the clinical manifestations are common to a variety of childhood disorders, but their presence is an indication to obtain further information from past history, family history, and laboratory studies as part of a complete physical examination. Suspected renal disease can be further evaluated by means of radiographic studies and renal biopsy.

Laboratory tests of renal function

Both urine and blood studies contribute vital information for detection of renal problems. The single most important test is probably the routine urinalysis. Specific urine and blood tests provide additional information. Since nurses are usually the persons who collect the specimens for examination and who often perform many of the screening tests, they should be familiar with the test, its function, and factors that can alter or distort the results of the test.

Collecting specimens. Collection of specimens varies with the purpose of laboratory study. Proper collection and use of clean procedures and containers ensure minimal contamination. For routine urine analysis, a fresh, early-morning specimen of urine collected in the bladder overnight is usually best. The urine is more concentrated at this time; therefore, formed elements in the sediment are better visualized. Since this is difficult to accomplish in infants, a random sample is satisfactory. A specimen obtained from an infant or child who is urged to drink large volumes of water in an effort to obtain a specimen quickly is too dilute and yields misleading results (see p. 929 for collection of specimens). Most specimens are clean-catch and/or midstream specimens to minimize contamination with urethral or skin bacteria.

Collection of urine voided over a 24-hour period creates some special problems in infants and children. Collection bags and, sometimes, restraining methods are required to collect specimens from infants and small children. Older children require special instruction about notifying someone when they need to void or have a bowel movement so that urine can be collected separately and not discarded. Some older school-age children and adolescents can be trusted to take responsibility for collection of their own 24-hour specimens. As in any 24-hour urine collection, the collection period always starts and ends with an empty bladder. At the time the collection begins the child is instructed to void and the specimen is discarded. All urine voided in the subsequent 24 hours is saved in a refrigerated container. Twen-

Table 31-1. Urine tests of renal function

Test	Normal range	Deviations	Significance of deviations
Physical tests			
Volume	Age related (see p. 1613)	Polyuria	Osmotic factors (urinary glucose level in diabetes mellitus)
		Oliguria	Retention caused by obstructive disease Inadequate bladder emptying caused by neurogenic bladder or obstructive disorder
Specific gravity	With normal fluid intake: 1.016-1.022 Newborn: 1.001-1.020 Others: 1.001-1.030	High	Dehydration Presence of protein or glucose Presence of radiopaque contrast medium after radiologic examinations
		Low	Excessive fluid intake Distal tubular dysfunction Insufficient antidiuretic hormone Diuresis
		Fixed at 1.010	Chronic glomerular disease
Osmolality	Newborn: 100-600 mOsm/liter Thereafter: 50-1400 mOsm/liter	High or low	Same as for specific gravity More sensitive index than specific gravity
Appearance	Clear pale yellow to deep gold	Cloudy	Contains sediment
		Cloudy reddish pink to reddish brown	Blood from trauma or disease Myoglobin following severe muscle destruction
		Light	Dilute
		Dark	Concentrated
Chemical tests			
pH	Newborn: 5-7 Thereafter: 4.5-8.0 Average: 6	Weak acid or neutral	If associated with metabolic acidosis, suggests tubular acidosis If associated with metabolic alkalosis, suggests potassium deficiency Urinary infection
		Alkaline	Metabolic alkalosis
Protein level	Absent	Present	Abnormal glomerular permeability, for example, glomerular disease, changes in blood pressure Most kidney disease Orthostatic in some individuals
Glucose level	Absent	Present	Diabetes mellitus Infusion of glucose-containing fluids Impaired tubular reabsorption
Ketone levels	Absent	Present	Conditions of acute metabolic demand (stress)
Microscopic tests			
White blood cell count	Less than 1 or 2	More than 5 polymorphonuclear leukocytes/field	Urinary tract inflammatory process
		Lymphocytes	Allograft rejection Malignancy
Red blood cell count	Less than 1 or 2	4-6/field in centrifuged specimen	Trauma Stones Infection Neoplasms

Table 31-1. Urine tests of renal function—cont'd

Test	Normal range	Deviations	Significance of deviations
Presence of bacteria	Absent to a few	More than 100,000 organisms/ml in centrifuged specimen	Urinary tract infection
Presence of casts	Occasional	Protein casts	Pronounced renal malfunction Tubular or glomerular disorders
		White blood cell casts	Pyelonephritis
		Red blood cell casts	Glomerulonephritis
		Epithelial casts	Glomerulonephritis
		Hyaline casts	Usually temporary; must be correlated with other findings

Table 31-2. Blood tests of renal function

Test	Normal range (mg/dl)	Deviations	Significance of deviations
Blood urea nitrogen (BUN)	Newborn: 5-15 Thereafter: 10-20	Elevated	Renal disease—acute or chronic (the higher the BUN, the more severe the disease) Increased protein catabolism Dehydration Hemorrhage High protein intake Corticosteroid therapy
Uric acid	Child: 2.0-5.5	Increased	Severe renal disease
Creatinine	0.3-1.1	Increased	Severe, long-standing renal impairment

ty-four hours from the time the precollection specimen was discarded, the child is again instructed to void, the specimen is added to the container, and the entire collection is taken to the laboratory for examination.

Catheterized or suprapublic aspiration is employed when a specimen is urgently needed or when the child is unable to void or otherwise provide an adequate specimen. Catheterization is most often used when urethral obstruction or anuria caused by renal failure is believed to be the cause of the child's failure to void. Suprapubic aspiration is useful in clarifying the diagnosis of suspected urinary tract infection in acutely ill infants.

Catheterizing a child requires aseptic technique and good light, gentle, thorough cleansing of the vulva or glans penis. Most children, including female infants, accommodate a size 8 or 10 French catheter, but in male infants or when the larger catheters cannot be passed, a smaller, soft plastic feeding tube may be needed. Most children are frightened of this procedure, and few small children are entirely cooperative; therefore, even when the procedure is adequately explained, the presence of an assistant is needed to help restrain and reassure the child.

Suprapubic aspiration, which is performed by the physician, involves aspirating bladder contents by inserting a 20- or 21-gauge needle in the midline approximately 1 cm above the symphysis and directed vertically downward. The skin is prepared as for any needle insertion, but the bladder should contain an adequate volume of urine. This can be assumed if the infant has not voided for at least 1 hour, or the bladder can be palpated above the symphysis. This technique is especially useful for obtaining clean specimens from young infants. The bladder is an abdominal organ at this time and is easily accessible.

Specific tests. Glomerular filtration rate is a measure of the amount of plasma from which a given substance is totally cleared in 1 minute. Clearance is calculated from the ratio of substance excreted to the concentration of that substance in the plasma. A number of substances can be used, but the most useful clinical estimation of glomerular filtration is the clearance of creatinine, an end-product of protein metabolism in muscle and a substance that is freely filtered by the glomerulus and secreted by renal tubular cells. The production and secretion of creatinine remain relatively constant from day to day, and its appearance in the urine is determined by the serum level. When the collection is complete and accurately timed, the results are fairly reliable and compare favorably with clearance of other substances, such as inulin, that require special equipment and long

Table 31-3. Radiologic and other tests of renal function

Test	Procedure	Purpose	Comments and nursing responsibilities
Radiologic tests			
Intravenous pyelography (IVP) (intravenous urogram; excretory urogram)	Intravenous injection of a contrast medium Medium secreted and concentrated by tubules X-ray films made 5, 10, and 15 minutes after injection	Defines urinary tract Provides information about integrity of kidneys, ureters, and bladder Retroperitoneal masses visualized when they shift position of ureters	Preparation for test: Infants less than 2 years of age—no solid food, omit one bottle on morning of examination, studies should be done early to avoid withholding of fluids Children aged 2-14 years—administer cathartic evening before examination, nothing is given orally after midnight, enema (Fleet or soapsuds) is given morning of examination Support during procedure
Time-sequence IVP	Modification of above Films made every 5 minutes after injection of contrast media	More accurately distinguishes differences between kidneys Differences in times of excretion indicate unilateral disease	Normal kidneys show dye before abnormal ones
Retrograde pyelography	Contrast medium injected through catheter inserted into kidney pelvis via urethra, bladder, and ureter	Visualizes pelvic calyces, ureters, and bladder	Used less frequently than in the past
Renal angiography	Contrast medium injected directly into renal artery via catheter placed in femoral or umbilical artery in newborn and advanced to renal artery	Visualizes renal vascular system, especially for renal arterial stenosis	Give cathartic if ordered Give preoperative medication if ordered Observe for reaction to contrast medium
Radioisotope renography and renal scanning	Radioisotopes injected intravenously and recorded with special camera and computer analysis	Records appearance and disappearance of radioactivity in each kidney Gives detailed picture of excretory performance Helps define intrarenal masses	Give sedation as ordered Insert or assist insertion of intravenous infusion Monitor intravenous infusion
Cystoscopy	Direct visualization of bladder and lower urinary tract through small scope inserted via urethra	Investigation of bladder and lower tract lesions; visualizes urethral openings, bladder wall, trigone, and urethra	Give nothing orally after midnight Carry out preoperative preparations
Voiding cystourethrography	Contrast medium injected into bladder through urethral catheter until bladder is full; films taken before, during, and after voiding	Visualizes bladder outline and urethra, reveals reflux of urine into ureters, and shows complications of bladder emptying	

immobilization of the child. The glomerular filtration rate is calculated by the following formula:

$$GFR = \frac{U \times V}{P}$$

U, concentration of substance in urine
V, volume of urine excreted in selected time
P, concentration of substance in plasma

Any significant degree of renal disease can diminish the glomerular filtration rate, but diseases of the glomerulus and renal vascular disease have the most immediate effect. The nurse's responsibility in this test is collection of urine, usually a 12- or 24-hour specimen.

The major blood and urine tests are outlined in Tables 31-1 and 31-2. Special tests and nursing responsibilities are briefly described in Table 31-3.

Table 31-3. Radiologic and other tests of renal function—cont'd

Test	Procedure	Purpose	Comments and nursing responsibilities
Radiologic tests—cont'd			
Scout film (KUB)	Flat plate roentgenogram of abdomen and pelvis	Detects and establishes renal outlines, presence of calculi, or opaque foreign bodies in bladder	Prepare as for routine x-ray film
Miscellaneous tests			
Renal biopsy	Removal of kidney tissue by open or percutaneous technique for study by light, electron, or immunofluorescent microscopy	Yields histologic and microscopic information about glomeruli and tubules; helps to distinguish between types of nephrotic syndromes Distinguishes other renal pathologies	Obtain parental permission Give nothing orally 4-6 hours prior to test Premedicate as ordered Prepare setup for procedure Assist with procedure Take vital signs Apply pressure to area with pressure dressing and, if feasible, a sandbag Bed rest for 24 hours Observe for abdominal pain, tenderness Monitor input and output; surgical incision may be required in infants
Nephrosonography	Transmission of ultrasonic sound waves through kidney areas to outline kidney mass	Distinguishes between cystic and solid masses and renal and nonrenal masses, localizes kidneys, and delineates nonfunctional kidney	Administer sedation if needed
Urine culture and sensitivity	Collection of sterile specimen	Determines presence of pathogens and the drugs to which they are sensitive	Does not require specific parental permission Send specimen to laboratory immediately after collection Catheterization, clean-catch, or suprapubic specimen

Glomerular disorders

Kidneys react to tissue injury in the same manner as all other body tissues. Acute inflammation evokes a pattern of exudation, white blood cell accumulation, and tissue damage; chronic longstanding inflammation results in scarring and permanent destruction of tissue elements. Several renal diseases affect the renal glomeruli, causing alterations in renal function that subsequently produce a variety of generalized symptoms. Conversly glomerular dysfunction represents only one feature of a diffuse systemic disease. This discussion is directed toward those nonsuppurative disorders collectively described as *nephritis*. The majority of causes of glomerular kidney dysfunction in childhood are caused by acute poststreptococcal glomerulonephritis and idiopathic nephrotic syndrome. Since the clinical features of nephrotic syndrome are associated with a number of renal disorders, it will be discussed first.

NEPHROTIC SYNDROME

Nephrotic syndrome is a clinical state that may develop during the course of several different renal disorders in which increased glomerular permeability to plasma protein results in massive urinary protein loss. Loss of protein leads to marked hypoproteinemia, hypovolemia, and variable degrees of edema. Hyperlipemia is usually present, and, occasionally, systemic hypertension and azotemia are seen. Nephrotic syndrome can be roughly categorized into three groups—congenital, secondary, and idiopathic.

Congenital nephrotic syndrome

The hereditary form of nephrotic syndrome is caused by a recessive gene on an autosome (see p. 191 for autosomal inheritance). Infants who have nephrotic syndrome are small for gestational age, and proteinuria and edema are manifest early. The disease does not respond to the usual therapy, and death in the first year or two of life is the rule. Renal transplant in the newborn periods has been attempted with a few successes.

Secondary nephrotic syndrome

Nephrotic syndrome may occur after or in association with glomerular damage of known or presumed etiology. Prominent among causes of glomerular damage is acute or chronic glomerulonephritis. Less commonly secondary nephrotic syndrome occurs during the course of collagen diseases (such as disseminated lupus erythematosus and anaphylactoid purpura) or as the result of toxicity to drugs (such as trimethadione and heavy metals), stings, or venom. Diverse, rare causes are sickle cell disease, malaria, cyanotic heart disease, diabetes mellitus, amyloidosis, tuberculosis, infected ventriculojugular shunts, or after renal vein thrombosis.

Idiopathic nephrotic syndrome

Approximately 80% of cases of nephrotic syndrome in children occur in the absence of recognizable systemic disease or preexisting renal disease and are categorized as idiopathic. Idiopathic nephrotic syndrome is predominantly a disease of the preschool child, with a peak age of onset between 2 and 3 years of age. The incidence is rare in children younger than 6 months of age, uncommon in infants younger than 1 year of age, and rare after the age of 8 years. The incidence varies in areas and countries reporting. The estimate in children in the United States varies from 2 to 3 per 100,000 white children. Of affected children, 60% are males.[1,30] The focus of the remainder of the discussion is on idiopathic nephrotic syndrome.

Etiology and pathophysiology

The cause of idiopathic nephrotic syndrome (also known as "minimal lesion" nephrosis, childhood nephrosis, lipoid nephrosis, or uncomplicated nephrosis) remains obscure. Often a nonspecific illness, usually a viral upper respiratory infection, precedes the manifestations by 4 to 8 days but is considered to be a precipitating factor rather than a cause. It is doubtful that there is a single cause of idiopathic nephrotic syndrome; rather, the disease probably represents several different pathologic processes affecting the glomerular membranes.

Pathophysiology. The pathogenesis of this disorder is not understood. There may be a metabolic, biochemical, or physiochemical disturbance in the basement membrane of the glomeruli that leads to increased permeability to protein, but the causes and mechanisms are only speculative.

The glomerular membrane, which is normally impermeable to albumin and other large proteins, becomes permeable to proteins, especially albumin, which leak through the membrane and are lost in urine (hyperalbuminuria). This reduces the serum albumin level (hypoalbuminemia), which decreases the colloidal osmotic pressure in the capillaries. As a result the hydrostatic pressure exceeds the pull of the colloidal osmotic pressure and fluid accumulates in the interstitial spaces and body cavities, particularly the abdominal cavity (ascites). The shift of fluid from the plasma to the interstitial spaces reduces the vascular fluid

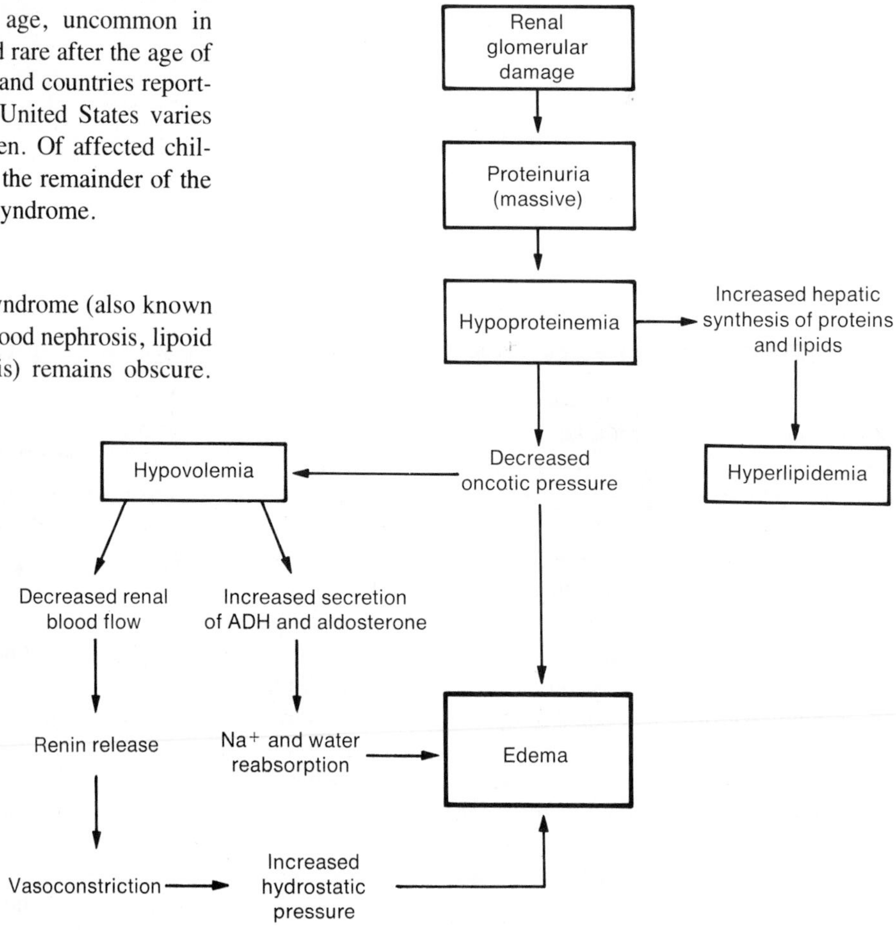

Fig. 31-4. Sequence of events in nephrotic syndrome.

volume (hypovolemia), which in turn stimulates the renin-angiotensin system and the secretion of antidiuretic hormone and aldosterone. Tubular reabsorption of sodium and water are increased in an attempt to increase intravascular volume. The elevation of serum cholesterol, phospholipids, and triglycerides is unexplained. The sequence of events in nephrotic syndrome is diagrammed in Fig. 31-4.

Diagnostic evaluation

The diagnosis is made on the basis of remarkably consistent history, typical clinical manifestations, and proteinemia. A previously well child begins to gain weight, which progresses insidiously over a period of days or weeks. Puffiness of the face, especially around the eyes, is apparent on arising in the morning but subsides during the day, when swelling of the abdomen and lower extremities is more prominent. The generalized edema develops so slowly that parents may consider it to be a sign of healthy growth. Although an acute infection may precipitate severe generalized edema (anasarca), the usual course is one of progressive weight gain until either rapid or gradual increase in edema prompts the family to seek medical evaluation. Usually present are abdominal swelling from ascites, respiratory difficulty from pleural effusion, and labial or scrotal swelling (Fig. 31-5). Edema of the intestinal mucosa may cause diarrhea, anorexia, and poor intestinal absorption. The volume of urine is decreased, and it appears darkly opalescent and frothy. Neurologic examinations are negative, and the sensorium is clear.

Extreme skin pallor is often present, and the child has a tendency toward skin breakdown during periods of edema. The child is irritable and may be easily fatigued or lethargic but does not appear seriously ill. Malnutrition from poor appetite and loss of protein is not uncommon, although it is frequently obscured by edema. However, changes in the quality of the hair give evidence of the malnourished state. The blood pressure is usually normal or slightly decreased. The child is more susceptible to infection, especially cellulitis, pneumonia, peritonitis, or septicemia.

In children with idiopathic nephrotic syndrome, there is absence of significant or persistent hypertension, gross or persistent hematuria, significant or persistent azotemia (presence of increased nitrogenous products in the blood), and depression of serum $B1_c$ globulin.

Diagnostic tests. Massive proteinuria is reflected in urine excretion of protein that frequently reaches levels in excess of 2 $g/m^2/day$ of body surface with relatively greater clearance of low molecular weight proteins. Hyaline casts from high protein and sluggish flow and oval fat bodies, as well as a few red blood cells, can be found in the urine of most affected children, although there is seldom gross hematuria. Specific gravity is high and proportionate to the amount of protein concentration. If hypovolemia is not significant and the child is well hydrated, the glomerular filtration rate is usually normal.

Total serum protein concentrations are reduced, with the albumin fractions significantly reduced (less than 2 g/100 ml) and elevation of $alpha_2$ globulins and plasma lipids. Serum cholesterol may be as high as 450 to 1500 mg/100 ml. Hemoglobin and hematocrit are usually normal or even elevated as a result of hemoconcentration. Serum sodium concentration is usually low, about 130 to 135 mEq/liter.[6]

Renal biopsy and the appearance of renal tissue under the light and electron microscope provide information regarding the glomerular status and type of nephrotic syndrome, response to drugs, and probable course of the disease. Under the microscope the foot processes of the basement membrane appear fused.

Differential diagnosis. The major focuses in differential diagnosis are to establish the edema as renal in origin and to

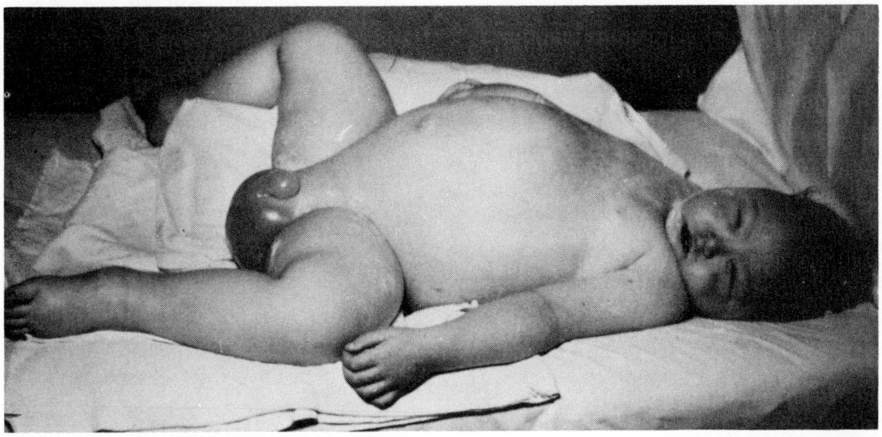

Fig. 31-5. Two-year-old child with nephrosis. (From Shirkey, H. C.: Pediatric therapy, ed. 5, St. Louis, 1975, The C. V. Mosby Co., p. 792.)

distinguish idiopathic nephrotic syndrome from other glomerulopathies with nephrotic syndrome as a manifestation.

Medical management

The medical management consists of both general and specific measures. The primary objective is to reduce the excretion of urinary protein and maintain a protein-free urine. Additional objectives include prevention or treatment of acute infection, control of edema, establishment of good nutrition, and readjustment of any disturbed metabolic processes. Children with severe symptoms or whose disease is newly recognized are hospitalized for assessment and observation for evidence of infection and response to therapy.

General measures. General treatment is principally supportive. During the edema phase the child is often placed on bed rest, but activity is not restricted during remission. Acute and intercurrent infections are treated with appropriate antibiotics, and efforts are made to eliminate possible infection.

Diet. The child who is in remission is allowed a regular diet; however, during periods of massive edema, salt is restricted, which is usually tolerated by the child for a time. Although edema cannot be removed by a low-sodium diet, its rate of increase may be reduced. Water is seldom restricted. A diet generous in protein is logical and beneficial and especially important in growing children but is not well accepted by most children. The presence of azotemia and renal failure is a contraindication for high-protein intake.

Corticosteroid therapy. The response of most affected children to corticosteroids has established these drugs as prime therapeutic agents in management of nephrotic syndrome. Corticosteroid therapy is begun as soon as the diagnosis has been determined and administered orally in a dosage of 2 mg/kg or 60 mg/m^2/day in evenly divided doses. Prednisone, the safest and least expensive drug, is the steroid of choice. The drug is continued until the urine is free from protein and remains normal for 10 days to 2 weeks.[28]

The course of the disease is fairly predictable. There is little change during the first few days of therapy. In most patients diuresis occurs, urine protein excretion disappears within 7 to 21 days, and other clinical manifestations stabilize or return to normal. In 90% of patients urine returns to normal within 4 weeks; in many this occurs as early as 3 or 4 days. If the child has not responded to therapy in 28 days of daily administration, the likelihood of subsequent response diminishes rapidly. When the child is free of proteinuria and edema, the daily dose is usually increased one and one half to two times and the medication is given as a single dose every 48 hours for a time. It is then gradually tapered to discontinuance over a variable period of time, from several days to weeks or months, depending on the philosophy of the physician. When the larger single dose is given intermittently, it is less likely to depress the pituitary-adrenal function and fewer side effects are produced during prolonged therapy. If a tendency to relapse is demonstrated, the number of relapses can be reduced by an interrupted schedule of prednisone therapy that continues for 6 months to 1 year following the initial daily dose.

Children with nephrotic syndrome are often described according to their response to corticosteroid therapy: (1) 20% to 40% of children are "steroid-sensitive" and have little tendency to recurrence after a single course of therapy; (2) 60% to 80% are "steroid-dependent" and respond well to steroid therapy, but their course is dominated by intermittent exacerbations and remissions over a period of several years before they clear completely and lose the tendency to active disease; and (3) 5% to 10% are "steroid-resistant," or are resistant to steroids at some stage and eventually go on to chronic renal failure.

The prognosis depends on the child's response to therapy. With early detection and prompt implementation of therapy to eradicate proteinuria, progressive basement membrane damage is minimized so that when the tendency to exacerbations is past, renal function is usually normal or near normal. It is estimated that approximately 80% of nephrotic children have this favorable prognosis.

Children who require frequent courses of steroid therapy are highly susceptible to complications of steroids, such as growth retardation, hypertension, gastrointestinal bleeding, Cushing's syndrome, bone demineralization, infections, and diabetes mellitus. Children who do not respond to steroid therapy, frequently relapsing children, and those in whom the side effects threaten their growth and general health are considered for a course of immunosuppressant drug therapy.

Immunosuppressant therapy. It is often possible to reduce the relapse rate and induce long-term remission with administration of an oral alkalyzing agent, usually cyclophosphamide (Cytoxan) 1 to 2.5 mg/kg/day, alternating with prednisone. Both drugs are administered for up to 2 months, after which cyclophosphamide is discontinued abruptly and the prednisone is decreased by decrements.

There are significant side effects of cyclophosphamide that must be considered and discussed with parents of children for whom this drug is contemplated. Leukopenia and alopecia, although uncommon in the recommended dosage, must be anticipated, and evidence suggests that cyclophosphamide may cause azoospermia with sterility in males treated for more than 2 to 3 months and variable effects on gonadal function in females.

Diuretics. One characteristic of the edema of nephrotic syndrome is its usual lack of responsiveness to diuretic agents. However, in cases in which edema is unresponsive to other measures, diuretics that decrease sodium retention are sometimes useful, usually spironolactone in combination with hydrochlorothiazide. Also, plasma expanders such as salt-poor human albumin may be administered; however, they must be administered frequently since the glomeruli are readily permeable to albumin in the acute stage.

Antimicrobials. The increased susceptibility to infection during the edematous phase of the disease and the lowered resistance associated with corticosteroid therapy are a constant hazard of nephrotic syndrome. Therefore, a broad-spectrum antimicrobial agent is often administered in an effort to reduce the risk of infection until the initial phase of treatment is completed and the child is receiving reduced dosages of corticosteroids.

Other therapies. When ascites or pulmonary effusion is severe and interferes with respiratory efforts, abdominal or thoracic paracentesis may be required.

Nursing considerations

Children hospitalized with nephrotic syndrome are placed on bed rest during the edema phase of the disease. They seldom offer resistance, since they are usually lethargic and easily fatigued and since their cumbersome edematous bulk is not conducive to movement. Most are content to lie in the prone position. These children must be encouraged and helped to turn regularly to prevent tissue breakdown. Areas that are particularly edematous, such as the scrotum, abdomen, and legs, may require support, and skin surfaces should be cleaned and separated with clothing, cotton, or antiseptic powder or cornstarch to prevent intertrigo.

Infection is a constant source of danger to edematous children and those on corticosteroid therapy. These children are particularly vulnerable to upper respiratory infection; therefore, they must be kept warm and dry, turned frequently, and protected from contact with infected roommates, visitors, and personnel. Vital signs are monitored to detect any early signs of an infective process.

Continuous monitoring of fluid retention or excretion is an important nursing function. Strictly accurate records of intake and output are essential but may be difficult in very young children. Application of collection bags is highly irritating to sensitive skin readily subject to breakdown. Application of diapers or weighing wet pads may be necessary, or, sometimes, estimating the size of the wet area may be allowed. If so, it is wise to pour a measured amount of water on a similar pad as a comparison. Other methods of monitoring progress include urine examination for specific gravity and albumin, daily weight, and measurement of abdominal girth. Assessment of edema such as increased or decreased swelling around eyes and dependent areas, degree of pitting (if noted), and color and texture of skin are part of nursing care.

The anorexia that accompanies active nephrosis creates a perplexing problem for nurses. During this time the combined efforts of nurse, dietitian, parents, and the child himself are needed to formulate a nutritionally adequate and attractive diet. Salt is usually restricted, but not eliminated, during the edema phase. A generous protein intake is highly desirable to minimize negative nitrogen balance but is poorly accepted by most children. Fluid restriction is limited to short-term use during massive edema. Every effort should be made to serve attractive meals with a minimum of fuss, but it usually requires a considerable amount of ingenuity and enticement to get the child to eat. Games, rewards, and special treats often help, but each child is unique, and it may require considerable trial and error to arrive at a successful strategy. Also, the same strategy may not work consistently.

As the edema subsides, children are allowed increased activity, which is desirable in order to prevent bone demineralization from immobilization and corticosteroid administration. Although they are easily fatigued, they are usually able to adjust their activities according to their tolerance, but they may require guidance in selection of play activities. Suitable recreational and diversional activities are an important part of their care. Once edema fluid has been lost, children are allowed to resume their usual activities with discretion. Irritability and mood swings accompanying the inactivity, disease process, and steroid therapy are not unusual manifestations in these children, which create an additional challenge to the nurse and the family.

Home care

Many children are treated at home during exacerbations. Parents are taught to detect signs of relapse and to bring the child for treatment at the earliest indications. Unless the edema and proteinuria are severe or the parents, for some reason, are unable to care for the ill child, home care is preferred. Parents are instructed in testing urine for albumin, administration of medications, and general care. Salt is restricted during relapse, but a regular diet is suitable for the child in remission. Parents are instructed regarding avoiding contact with infected playmates, but the child is permitted to attend school. It is important for parents of children on corticosteroid therapy to be aware of the common side effects of steroid therapy, such as rounding of the face, increased appetite, abdominal distention, and hirsutism, and to distinguish some of these from the edema formation of the disease. They should be reassured that the symptoms will disappear gradually after discontinuation of the drug. The child should receive close medical and/or nursing observation to detect unusual but more serious side effects.

Support of child and family

The prolonged course of the relapsing form of nephrotic syndrome is taxing to both the child and the family. The up-

Summary of nursing care of the child with nephrotic syndrome

Goals	Responsibilities
Prevent and control acute infection	Avoid contact with infected persons Observe medical asepsis Administer antibiotics if ordered Keep child dry and warm Monitor vital signs for early signs of infectious processes Collect specimens, such as urine for culture, blood
Prevent skin breakdown	Provide meticulous skin care Cleanse and powder opposing skin surfaces several times daily Separate skin surfaces with soft cotton Support edematous organs, such as scrotum Cleanse edematous eyelids with warm saline wipes Change position frequently; maintain good body alignment
Prevent further edema formation	Provide salt-restricted diet Administer steroids and diuretics, if ordered Administer salt-poor albumin intravenous infusion if ordered
Prevent hypovolemia	Monitor vital signs to detect physical signs Assess pulse quality and rate Take blood pressure Report deviations
Conserve energy	Maintain bed rest initially Balance rest and activity when ambulatory Plan and provide quiet activities Instruct child to rest when he begins to feel tired
Control edema	Administer corticosteroids as ordered Administer diuretics, if ordered Limit intake, if ordered
Assess changes in edema	Weigh daily (or more often if ordered) Measure abdominal girth at umbilicus Measure accurately intake and output Test urine for specific gravity, albumin Collect specimens for laboratory examination
Establish good nutrition	Administer high-protein, high-carbohydrate diet (restrict sodium during edema) Administer supplementary vitamins and iron as ordered
Stimulate appetite	Enlist aid of child, parents, and dietitian in formulation of diet Provide cheerful, clean, relaxed atmosphere during meals Serve small quantities intially to stimulate appetite; encourage seconds Provide special and preferred foods Serve foods in an attractive manner
Establish good mental hygiene	Encourage activity within limits of tolerance Encourage socialization with persons without active infection Provide positive feedback Explore areas of interest and encourage their pursuit

Summary of nursing care of the child with nephrotic syndrome—cont'd

Goals	Responsibilities
Prepare for home care	Instruct parents Testing urine for albumin daily Administration of medications Initial signs of relapse Side effects of drugs Prevention of infection Impress on parents importance of following prescribed regimen
Support parents	Listen to parents Assist parents with problem solving Provide education when indicated Provide positive feedback Refer to parent groups
Continue follow-up care	Maintain contact with family Refer to appropriate persons or agencies for assistance

and-down course of remissions and exacerbations with periodic disruption of family life by hospitalization places a severe strain on the child and the family, both psychologically and financially. Parents and children over 5 or 6 years of age need reassurance regarding this characteristic of the course of the disease so that they will not become discouraged with the frequent relapses. At the same time it is important to impress on them the importance of long-term care to gain their cooperation. A satisfactory response is more likely when relapses are detected and therapy instituted early, and remissions are prolonged when instructions are carried out faithfully. For example, one child went into an exacerbation when his mother reduced the dosage of his drug because it was so expensive.

Social isolation is a concomitant problem for these children. Isolation is related to frequent hospitalization or confinement during relapse, the risk of infection that may precipitate an exacerbation, lack of energy, and the child's reluctance to face friends at home or school because of the changes in his appearance resulting from the disease or the medication. Both parents and child need someone to listen to their complaints, to assist them to cope with both short-term and long-term problems associated with the disease, and to find solutions to their problems. Continuous support to the child and his family is one of the major nursing considerations. (For a summary of nursing care of the child with nephrotic syndrome, see the boxed material.)

ACUTE GLOMERULONEPHRITIS (POSTSTREPTOCOCCAL)

Acute glomerulonephritis (AGN) is the most common of the noninfectious renal diseases in childhood and the one for which an etiology can be established in the majority of cases. Acute nephritis occurs most frequently in children 2 to 12 years of age, with a peak incidence at about age 6 years. It is decidedly uncommon in children younger than 2 years of age, and males outnumber females two to one in most series studied. The disease frequently occurs in siblings, but, in these instances, there are often variations in the degree of severity of the disease. Although the true incidence in the population is unknown, acute glomerulonephritis accounts for 0.5% of children admitted to hospitals.[16]

Etiology and pathophysiology

Etiology. It is now generally accepted that acute glomerulonephritis is an immune-complex disease, that is, a reaction that occurs as a by-product of an antecedent streptococcal infection with certain strains of the group A β-hemolytic *Streptococcus*. Most streptococcal infections do not cause acute glomerulonephritis. The development of acute glomerulonephritis follows a limited number of subtypes, principally types 4, 12, and 49, and the clinical pattern of the disease is the same whether the disease is associated with type 12 or type 49 pharyngitis, which produces the skin disease impetigo. There is a latent period of 10 to 14 days between the streptococcal infection and the onset of clinical manifestations. The peak incidence of disease, which is in the school-age years, corresponds to the incidence of streptococcal infections. Disease secondary to streptococcal pharyngitis is more common in the winter or spring, but, when associated with pyoderma (principally impetigo), it may be more prevalent in later summer or early fall, especially in warmer climates.

Pathophysiology. The mechanism by which the reaction takes place is still speculative. The most popular proposal to explain the pathologic process is that the streptococcal infection is followed by the release of a membrane-like material from the specific organism into the circulation. Because it is antigenic, antibody is formed, and, after the appropriate period of time, an immune-complex reaction occurs. These immune complexes become trapped in the glomerular capillary loop, much the same as experimental serum sickness.[35]

The kidney itself appears normal or moderately enlarged, but microscopic examination reveals a diffuse proliferative and exudative process. Glomerular capillary loops are almost obliterated by swelling, and infiltration with polymorphonuclear leukocytes adds to the appearance of increased cellularity. Consequently the glomeruli appear dense and bloodless. Further examination reveals discrete nodules or "humps" on the basement membrane, which are identified as deposits of immune complexes. These deposits are not evident after about 6 weeks.[22]

Endothelial cell proliferation and edema occlude the capillary lumen of affected glomeruli, and the afferent arteriole is probably constricted by vasospasm, both of which significantly reduce the glomerular filtration rate. This occurs without a proportional decrease in renal blood flow and results in a reduced capacity to form filtrate from the glomerular plasma flow. Vascular and tubular changes are mild and nonspecific; therefore, tubular function is less severely impaired.

The decreased filtration of plasma results in an excessive accumulation of water and an avid retention of sodium. These cause expanded plasma and interstitial fluid volumes that lead to circulatory congestion and edema. It is unclear whether the decreased glomerular filtration rate, increased capillary permeability, or vascular spasm is responsible for these various manifestations. The cause of the hypertension associated with acute glomerulonephritis is also unexplained. Plasma renin activity is low during the acute phase, but the hypervolemia may be a factor.

Diagnostic evaluation

Typically, affected children are in good health until they experience the antecedent infection. In some instances there is no history of an infection, or it is only described as a mild cold. The onset of nephritis appears after an average latent period of about 10 days. Since the child appears well during this time, the association is not recognized by parents.

Clinical manifestations. Initial signs of nephrotic reaction include puffiness of the face, especially around the eyes (periorbital edema), anorexia, and passage of dark-colored urine. The edema is more prominent in the face in the morning but spreads during the day to involve the extremities and abdomen. The edema is only moderate and may not be appreciated by someone unfamiliar with the child's normal appearance. The urine is cloudy, smoky brown, or what parents describe as resembling tea or cola, and severely reduced in volume.

The child is pale, irritable, and lethargic. He appears unwell but seldom expresses specific complaints. Older children may complain of headaches, abdominal discomfort, and dysuria. Vomiting is not uncommon. On examination there is usually a mild-to-moderate elevation in blood pressure (diastolic, 80 to 120 mm Hg; systolic, 120 to 180 mm Hg). Occasionally a child will have an atypical mode of onset with severe symptoms such as convulsions (secondary to cerebral ischemia and/or hypertension), pulmonary and circulatory congestion, minimal urine findings, or hematuria in the absence of hypertension and edema.[11]

Laboratory tests. *Urinalysis* during the acute phase characteristically shows hematuria, proteinuria, and increased specific gravity. The specific gravity is moderately elevated and seldom exceeds 1.020. Proteinuria generally parallels the hematuria, and the content usually shows 3+ of 4+ but is not the massive proteinuria seen in nephrotic syndrome. Gross discoloration of urine reflects its red blood cell and hemoglobin content. Microscopic examination of the sediment shows many red blood cells, leukocytes, epithelial cells, and casts, primarily composed of epithelial and red blood cells. Bacteria are not seen, and urine cultures are negative.

Blood examination reveals normal electrolytes (sodium, potassium, and chloride ions) and carbon dioxide levels, unless the disease has progressed to renal failure. Azotemia resulting from impaired glomerular filtration is reflected in elevated blood urea nitrogen and creatinine levels in at least 50% of cases. When proteinuria is heavy, there may be changes associated with nephrotic syndrome, that is, transient hypoproteinemia and hyperlipidemia.

Cultures of the pharynx are positive for streptococci in only a few cases, and the numbers are not significantly greater than the normal carrier incidence in many communities. Positive cultures help to establish a diagnosis. Cultures should be obtained from other household members, and persons positive for group A streptococci should receive a course of antistreptococcal therapy.

Some *serologic tests* may help in diagnosis. The antistreptolysin O (ASO) titer is the most familiar and readily available test for streptococcal infection and is used to detect the presence of antibodies, which documents a recent infection. Antistreptolysin O appears in the serum about

10 days after the initial infection and persists for 4 to 6 weeks; however, there is no correlation between the degree of elevation and its duration and the severity or prognosis of the glomerulonephritis. It is a useful diagnostic tool when nephritis follows a pharyngeal infection but is of less value after pyoderma. An antistreptolysin O titer of 250 Todd units or higher is of diagnostic significance, as is a rising titer in two samples taken a week apart. (This is also a significant laboratory finding in rheumatic fever. See p. 1360.) More consistent and reliable antibody tests following streptococcal skin infections are elevated antihyaluronidase and antideoxyribonuclease B titers.

Nonspecific acute-phase reactants that reflect acute inflammatory processes, such as the erythrocyte sedimentation rate (ESR), C-reactive protein (CRP), and serum mucoprotein tests are elevated during the early stages of acute disease and then gradually return to normal as healing takes place. The erythrocyte sedimentation rate is sometimes used as a guide to the progress of the nephritis.

Since glomerulonephritis is an immune-complex disease, there is reduced total serum complement activity in the early stages of acute disease. The simpler measurements of the C3 complement component (beta$_1$ C globulin) is used as an index of total complement activity. The test is most useful in children with no edema or minimal urine findings.

Other studies that are employed include a chest x-ray examination, which shows characteristic generalized cardiac enlargement, pulmonary congestion, and pleural effusion during the edematous phase of acute disease. Electrocardiography reveals elevation or depression of the ST segment, prolonged QRS and ST segments, lengthening of the P-R interval, and flattened or inverted T waves. Renal biopsy for diagnostic purposes is seldom required but may be useful in the diagnosis of atypical cases.

Correlations between laboratory and morphologic findings indicate a significant relationship between creatinine clearance and severity of glomerular damage. Greater damage is reflected in a reduced creatinine clearance and is also associated with a higher blood urea nitrogen level. An increased excretion of cellular protein is associated with increasing glomerular capillary obliteration. There appears to be no correlation between the extent of glomerular damage and antistreptolysin O titer, oliguria, or blood pressure.[16,34]

Differential diagnosis. Diagnosis can generally be established on the basis of the following clinical and laboratory criteria[11]:

Acute onset
Edema
Hypertension
Hematuria with red blood cell casts in the sediment
Evidence of antecedent streptococcal infection

Table 31-4. Childhood glomerulonephritis: some clinical forms and characteristics*

Type	Etiology	Microscopic changes	Major clinical manifestations
Acute poststreptococcal	Antecedent group A hemolytic streptococcal infection	Diffuse, proliferative neutrophil exudation	Edema Hypertension Hematuria Proteinuria
Rapidly progressive	Unknown	Diffuse Glomerular necrosis Epithelial crescents in over 80% of glomeruli	Oliguria and/or anuria Azotemia Acute nephrotic syndrome or progressive renal failure
Proliferative	Unknown; occasional streptococcal infection	Diffuse, proliferative Hypercellularity	Variable manifestations
Membranoproliferative	Unknown; sometimes with lipodystrophy	Diffuse Glomerular enlargement Basement membrane thickening Histologically, three clinical groups: types I, II, and III	Nephrotic syndrome Occasional hypertension
Focal segmented	Unknown	Focal or segmented glomerulosclerosis Hypercellularity	Nephrotic syndrome Hematuria
Focal segmented proliferative	Unknown	Focal, proliferative	Hematuria
Childhood nephrosis; idiopathic nephrotic syndrome, minimal change disease	Unknown	Foot process fusion	Nephrotic syndrome

*See Table 31-5 for those associated with systemic disease processes.

Table 31-5. Renal involvement associated with a systemic disease process

Disease	Mechanism	Renal manifestation	Comments
Systemic lupus erythematosus (SLE)	Deposition of autoantibody-antigen complexes in kidney	Variable degrees of hematuria and proteinuria More severe—nephrotic syndrome, hypertension renal insufficiency	Responds to corticosteroid and antimetabolite therapy Renal failure is most common cause of death from SLE Rare prior to adolescence but may occur in school-age children
Anaphylactoid (Schönlein-Henoch purpura)	Unknown	Hematuria (gross or microscopic) Less common—edema, hypertension Nephrotic syndrome with oliguria and hypertension indicates severe involvement Rarely—acute renal failure	Incidence varies from 20% to 70% of cases Renal involvement is most serious manifestation of the disease More common in children over age 6 years Responds to corticosteroid therapy Management similar to that for persistent glomerulonephritis
Sickle cell disease	Infarction of renal vessels by sickled cells (especially medullary) Results in decreased circulation in vasa recta and impaired sodium and chloride ion reabsorption in collecting ducts	Hematuria Nephrotic syndrome Defective urine collection Progressive glomerulonephritis	Becomes irreversible with increasing age Severe urinary tract infections with bacteremia not uncommon
Polyarteritis nodosa	Fibroid necrosis of arterial walls Large vessels—patchy renal infarction Microscopic vessels—necrotizing glomerulitis	Proteinuria Hematuria Severe hypertension	Kidney involvement of secondary importance in infancy Variable course Long-term prognosis guarded
Bacterial endocarditis	Focal of diffuse, immune-complex deposition related to chronic bacteremia Some embolization of glomeruli by bacteria and fibrin from endocardial vegetations	Proteinuria Hematuria	Seen in about 50% of cases Renal involvement seldom of major significance
Prolonged bacteremia (infected atrioventricular shunts)	Immune-complex deposition with exudation and cellular proliferation	Variable degrees of persistent nephrotic syndrome	Requires vigorous antibiotic therapy and/or removal of infected shunt

Lowered serum beta$_1$ C globulin concentration
Spontaneous improvement in a few days or weeks

However, problems in diagnosis are sometimes presented by other glomerulopathies that simulate poststreptococcal disease. Some of these are outlined in Tables 31-4 and 31-5. Table 31-6 compares the manifestations of acute glomerulonephritis and nephrotic syndrome.

Clinical course. The acute edematous phase of glomerulonephritis usually persists from 5 to 10 days but may persist for 2 or 3 weeks, during which time the child remains listless, anorexic, and apathetic. The weight fluctuates, the urine remains thick and smoky brown in color, and the blood pressure may suddenly reach dangerously high levels at any time during this phase.[11]

The first sign of improvement is a small increase in urine output with a corresponding decrease in body weight, followed in 1 or 2 days by copious diuresis. With diuresis the child begins to feel better, the appetite improves, and the blood pressure decreases to normal within the reduction of edema. Gross hematuria diminishes, in part because of dilution of the red blood cells in the more dilute urine, but microscopic hematuria may persist for weeks or months. The blood urea nitrogen level decreases during diuresis, but it, along with a slight to moderate proteinuria, may persist for several weeks.

Almost all children correctly diagnosed as having acute poststreptococcal glomerulonephritis recover completely, and specific immunity is conferred so that subsequent recurrences are uncommon. Deaths from complications still

Table 31-6. Comparison of symptomatology in acute poststreptococcal glomerulonephritis and idiopathic nephrotic syndrome

Manifestations	Acute poststreptococcal glomerulonephritis	Idiopathic nephrotic syndrome
Streptococcal antibody titers	Present	Absent
Blood pressure	Elevated	Normal
Edema	Primarily periorbital and peripheral	Generalized, severe
Proteinuria	Present	Massive
Hematuria	Gross	Microscopic
Casts	Present	Present
Azotemia	Present	Absent
Serum potassium levels	Increased	Normal
Serum protein levels	Minimal reduction	Markedly decreased
Serum lipid levels	Normal	Elevated
Anorexia	Present	Present
Fatigue	Present	Present
Age at onset (years)	2-5	2-3

occur but are, fortunately, rare. A few of these children may develop chronic disease, but many of these cases are believed to be probably different glomerular diseases misdiagnosed as poststreptococcal disease.

Complications. The major complications that may develop during the acute phase of glomerulonephritis are hypertensive encephalopathy, acute cardiac decompensation, and acute renal failure. Normally cerebral blood flow responds to acute arterial hypertension by vasoconstriction. However, acute and severe hypertension may cause this protective autoregulation of cerebral blood flow to fail, leading to hyperperfusion of the brain and cerebral edema.[8] The premonitory signs of encephalopathy are headache, dizziness, abdominal discomfort, and vomiting. If the condition progresses there may be transient loss of vision and/or hemiparesis, disorientation, and generalized convulsions of the grand mal type.

Cardiac decompensation during the acute edematous phase of nephritis is caused by hypervolemia and not by cardiac failure. Signs of circulatory congestion are evident, however. The heart is enlarged, and increased pulmonary vascular markings are evident on x-ray examination. Increased pulmonary capillary permeability is also believed to be an important factor in the development of pulmonary edema.

Acute renal failure with persistent oliguria or anuria is an uncommon complication but one that requires an appropriate treatment regimen (see p. 1171).

Medical management

There is no specific treatment for acute glomerulonephritis, and recovery is spontaneous and uneventful in most cases. Management consists of general supportive measures and early recognition and treatment of complications. Children who have normal blood pressure and a satisfactory urine output can generally be treated at home. Those with substantial edema, hypertension, and/or oliguria should be hospitalized because of the unpredictability of complications. Short hospitalization is the rule in uncomplicated cases; prolonged hospitalization is required only for children with severely impaired renal function.

General measures. Bed rest is recommended during the acute phase, but ambulation does not seem to have an adverse effect on the course of the disease once the gross hematuria, edema, hypertension, and azotemia have abated.[16] Since they are generally listless and experience fatigue and malaise, most children voluntarily restrict their activities during the most active phase of the disease. After diuresis has occured, ambulation is allowed for those children without hypertension and gross urine abnormalities. Occasionally a rebound phenomenon, characterized by a transient increase in blood urea nitrogen level, hematuria, and/or proteinuria, may appear after ambulation but does not require resumption of bed rest.[30]

Fluid balance. Regular measurement of vital signs, body weight, and intake and output is essential in order to monitor the progress of the disease and to detect complications that may appear at any time during the course of the disease. A record of daily weight is the most useful means to assess fluid balance and should be kept for children treated at home as well as for those who are hospitalized. Water restriction is seldom necessary unless the output is significantly reduced (less than 200 to 300 ml/24 hours). In these children the water allowed is equivalent to the calculated insensible loss plus the volume of urine excreted. Children on restricted fluids, especially those who are not severely edematous or those who have lost weight, should be observed for signs of dehydration.

Diet. Dietary restrictions depend on the severity of edema. Regular diet is permitted in uncomplicated cases, but the intake of sodium is usually limited (no salt is added to foods). Moderate sodium restriction is usually instituted for children with hypertension or edema. Severe sodium restriction is not well tolerated by children and may interfere with caloric intake in these already anorexic children. Foods with substantial amounts of potassium are generally restricted during the period of oliguria. Protein restriction is reserved only for children with severe azotemia resulting from prolonged oliguria. The anorexia associated with the disease usually limits the protein intake sufficiently.

Drugs. Antibiotic therapy is indicated only for those children with evidence of persistent streptococcal infections. Authorities are divided in their use of prophylactic antimicrobials for other family members. Hypertension is controlled with hydralazine (Apresoline), usually in conjunction with reserpine. Some authorities recommend hydralazine with furosemide (Lasix). A mild sedative may help to control mild hypertension. Seizure activity associated with hypertensive encephalopathy requires anticonvulsant therapy as well as antihypertensive agents. However, the child must be closely observed for cumulative effects of drugs, such as phenobarbital, that are eliminated by the kidneys.

Diuretics are usually of limited value, since very little sodium reaches the distal tubules as a result of the reduced filtration rate. However, furosemide has been used with some success in severe cases. Digitalis may be employed sometimes, although there is question regarding its effectiveness in acute nephritis.

Rarely children with acute glomerulonephritis develop acute renal failure with oliguria that significantly alters the fluid and electrolyte balance. These children require careful management that may include peritoneal dialysis or hemodialysis.

Nursing considerations

Nursing care of the child with glomerulonephritis involves careful assessment of the disease status, with regular monitoring of vital signs, fluid balance, and behavior. Vital signs provide clues to the severity of the disease and early signs of complications. They are carefully measured and any abnormalities reported and recorded. The volume and character of urine are noted, and the child is weighed daily. Assessment of the child's appearance for signs of cerebral complications is an important nursing function, since the severity of the acute phase is variable and unpredictable. The child with edema, hypertension, and gross hematuria may be subject to complications, and anticipatory preparations such as seizure precautions and intravenous equipment are included in the nursing care plan.

For most children a regular diet is allowed, but it should contain no added salt. Foods high in sodium and salted treats are eliminated, and parents and friends should be advised not to bring items such as potato chips or pretzels. However, the total amount of salt ingested is usually less than prescribed because of poor appetite. Fluid restriction, if prescribed, is more difficult, and the amount permitted should be evenly divided throughout the waking hours and served in small cups to give the illusion of larger servings. Meal preparation and service requires special attention, since the child is anorexic and indifferent to meals during the acute phase. Again, collaboration with parents and the dietitian and special consideration for food preferences facilitate meal planning.

During the acute phase children are generally quite content to lie in bed, but activities should be those that require little expenditure of energy. As they begin to feel better and their symptoms subside, activities should be planned to allow for frequent rest periods and avoidance of fatigue.

Children with mild edema and no hypertension as well as convalescent children being treated at home need follow-up care. Parents are instructed regarding general measures, including activity, diet, and prevention of infection. The children are permitted to be ambulatory but should not attend school or participate in outside games and sports until the risk of complications has passed. Strenuous activity is usually restricted until there is no microscopic evidence of proteinuria or hematuria, which may persist for months. No diet restrictions are imposed, but many parents continue to limit salt intake "just in case."

Health supervision is continued with weekly, followed by monthly, visits for evaluation and urinalysis. Parent education and support in preparation for discharge and home care include education in home management and the need for follow-up care and health supervision. (For a summary of nursing care of the child with acute glomerulonephritis, see the boxed material on the opposite page.)

CHRONIC OR PROGRESSIVE GLOMERULONEPHRITIS

The majority of cases of renal glomerular disease are acute glomerulonephritis, idiopathic nephrotic syndrome, and glomerulonephritis associated with systemic diseases. These pose relatively few problems of diagnosis, and their natural course is fairly predictable. A few cases present a prolonged course and poor ultimate prognosis. They are a rather heterogenous group that is defined by correlating the clinical manifestations, pathology, and natural course of the individual diseases. *Persistent glomerulonephritis* is a term used to describe those cases of glomerulonephritis that have no specific histologic picture but that fail to show the rapid recovery expected in acute nephritis. *Chronic glomerulonephritis* (CGN) describes advanced glomerular disease, which includes a variety of different disease processes (see Table 31-4). *Rapidly progressive glomerulonephritis* is a term used to describe an acute illness with severe, acute onset resembling acute poststreptococcal glomerulonephritis but that causes rapidly progressive deterioration of renal function in 6 to 12 months.[11]

Etiology and pathophysiology

In most cases of chronic glomerulonephritis immunologic mechanisms can be implicated either through direct attack on the kidney or secondary to the accumulation of immune complexes in the glomerular filter or fibrin deposition from previously damaged glomeruli. Either can contribute to further glomerular damage and can initiate chronic changes in the glomerular structure. In many cases there is no history of an attack of acute glomerular disease. In other cases it may represent one of a succession of exacerbations of a preexisting disease. Chronic glomerulonephritis that is

Summary of nursing care of the child with acute glomerulonephritis

Goals	Responsibilities
Prevent infection	Avoid contact with infected persons Administer antibiotics if ordered Keep warm and dry
Prevent or control progress of edema	Help plan and serve restricted or low-sodium diet Limit fluids if ordered
Prevent hyperkalemia	Restrict foods high in potassium during oliguria Monitor laboratory findings Observe for incipient signs of hyperkalemia
Assess progress of edema	Assess objectively general appearance and behavior Weigh daily Measure intake and output
Reduce blood pressure	Institute bed rest Administer antihypertensive agents Administer diuretics if ordered
Observe for signs of complications	Report significant deviations of Vital signs—blood pressure, pulse, respiration, temperature Appearance and volume of urine Weight gain relative to size of child Report any dyspnea Report unusual symptoms Vomiting Visual disturbances Motor disturbances Seizure activity Severe headache Abdominal pain Changes in behavior and/or activity level, for example, lethargy, restlessness
Provide nourishment	Administer high-carbohydrate diet Allow sodium and protein as prescribed
Stimulate appetite	Serve attractive meals in small portions Serve preferred foods Arrange meals with other children or family
Provide comfort	Encourage parents to visit Spend time with child Provide opportunity to socialize with noninfectious children Provide appropriate play activities
Educate parents for home care	Teach urine testing for blood and protein Teach early signs of complications
Continue follow-up care	Arrange for regular checkups Provide for public health nurse if needed Refer to proper agency for home tutoring if needed
Promote growth and development	Encourage normal activity within limitations imposed by state of disease process Allow for regression when appropriate

not associated with other diseases may go undetected for years and be relatively asymptomatic until kidney destruction produces marked reduction in renal function. Consequently the disease is more common in adolescents than in younger children. Renal insufficiency with all its manifestations occurs as the ultimate event.

Diagnostic evaluation

The varied clinical manifestations and laboratory findings generally reflect deteriorating renal function. Nephrotic syndrome, with its usual manifestations, frequently develops. Hypertension, edema, proteinuria, cardiac failure, dyspnea, osteodystrophy, and anemia are common manifestations of progressive disease.

Laboratory findings may include proteinuria, with casts and red and white blood cells. Failing renal function is evidenced by elevated blood urea nitrogen, creatinine, and uric acid levels. Electrolyte alterations include metabolic acidosis, decreased sodium from the chronic salt-losing state, elevated potassium, elevated phosphorus, and decreased calcium levels. As the disease progresses, urine specific gravity eventually stabilizes at an isotonic state (about 1.012) as a result of the inability of the kidney to reabsorb solutes or respond to antidiuretic hormone. The renal insufficiency may extend from 5 to 15 years and even longer, or rapid deterioration may cause death in 1 to 2 years.[23]

Medical management

Early in the course of the disease, treatment is appropriate to the underlying disease and is largely symptomatic in most cases. Efforts are directed toward providing optimal conditions for the child's physical, psychologic, and social development. As few restrictions as feasible are imposed, and the child is allowed to live as normal a life as possible for as long as possible.[11] Drug treatment offers little lasting benefit, although diuretic therapy may be helpful occasionally for edema or hypertension. Marked hypertension is controlled with antihypertensive agents, and anemia may require periodic transfusion with fresh packed cells. Salt is only moderately restricted. Ultimately dialysis and transplantation may restore relatively good health; however, these are usually not available alternatives until renal failure is far advanced. (See chronic renal failure [p. 1177] for more detailed management of specific problems.) Children with rapidly progressive glomerulonephritis are usually referred to a center specializing in renal disease.[33]

Nursing considerations

The problems of chronic glomerular nephritis and those encountered in chronic renal insufficiency from any cause will be discussed in association with chronic renal failure (p. 1177).

Renal tubular disorders

Disorders of renal tubular function include a variety of conditions in which there are one or more abnormalities in specific mechanisms of tubular transport or reabsorption, whereas, initially, glomerular function is normal or comparatively less impaired. Eventually there may be more widespread kidney destruction with renal failure. In some cases the dysfunction has little, if any, effect on renal function. These disorders may be permanent or transient and may originate as primary defects or arise as a secondary effect of metabolic disease or exogenous toxins. Renal tubular disorders may be congenital (usually displaying characteristic patterns of genetic transmission), appear without evidence of hereditary transmission, or be acquired as a result of known or unknown causes.

Unlike the classic manifestations of glomerular diseases, edema and hypertension are absent and the blood urea nitrogen level and routine urinalysis are usually normal. Proteinuria may be demonstrated but only by elaborate tests. Manifestations of tubular disorders are primarily metabolic disturbances or deficiencies, such as failure to thrive, metabolic bone disease, or persistent acidosis. Because the variety of these disorders is extensive and the incidence rare, only a brief discussion of a few is included. For convenience, renal tubular dysfunction is divided into those affecting proximal and distal tubules, although some may affect both.

DISORDERS OF PROXIMAL TUBULAR DYSFUNCTION

The function of the proximal tubules is the reabsorption of substances from the glomerular filtrate, including sodium, potassium, chloride, bicarbonate, glucose, phosphate, and amino acids. A number of disorders feature impairment of reabsorption of one or more filtrate constituents, and most involve defects in the transport mechanisms for these substances. Impaired tubular reabsorption of any specific substance will cause that substance to appear in the urine, usually with reduced levels in the blood.

Disorders of amino acid transport

Normally amino acids filtered by the glomerulus are almost completely reabsorbed by the proximal tubules by way of transport mechanisms specific for those amino acids. In the following situations abnormal amounts of amino acids appear in the urine (aminoaciduria). In the first two there is no impairment of renal function, but the plasma concentrations of amino acids are significantly elevated to produce symptoms related to defective metabolism of the amino acid. The last two are principally renal in origin, and in these disorders the plasma concentration of the amino acids is normal. The loss of amino acids in the urine is seldom sufficient to cause a deficiency state.

1. *Overflow aminoaciduria,* in which the concentration of a specific amino acid in the plasma and filtrate is greatly increased so that the specific transport mechanism is exceeded. This includes, largely, the inborn errors of metabolism, such as phenylketonuria, tyrosinosis, and maple syrup urine disease.
2. *Combined aminoaciduria,* in which amino acids that share a common transport mechanism both appear in the urine when the plasma level of one is increased. For example, the amino acids ornithine, arginine, and lysine have similar chemical structures and share a common transport mechanism.
3. *Specific renal aminoaciduria,* in which there is a defect in the transport mechanism for a single amino acid or group of amino acids.
4. *Nonspecific renal aminoaciduria,* in which there is generalized dysfunction of renal transport with no specificity of amino acids excreted. These are generally the result of toxic injury to the transport mechanism, for example, nephrotoxic substances, such as heavy metal salts, toxic metabolites from metabolic diseases, or drugs.

Medical management is directed toward diagnosis of the basic cause of the aminoaciduria and implementation of appropriate therapy.

Disorders of glucose transport

Essentially all glucose in the glomerular filtrate is reabsorbed in the proximal tubules by a specific transport mechanism. Glucose begins to appear in the urine when:

Plasma concentration exceeds the renal threshold (180 to 200 mg/100 ml)
Renal threshold is reduced below normal
Maximum tubular transport capacity for glucose (TmG) is diminished

Most glycosuria is caused by increased plasma concentrations associated with diabetes mellitus (p. 1478). Renal causes may include a hereditary disorder that appears in two forms—type A, in which both glucose threshold and the tubular transport (Tm) are reduced, and type B, in which only the renal plasma threshold is reduced. Neither requires specific treatment. Glycosuria is also seen in some cases of renal insufficiency in which the amount of glucose filtered by remaining functional glomeruli exceeds the tubular capacity for reabsorption.

Disorders of phosphate transport

Normally 85% to 95% of filtered phosphate is reabsorbed in the proximal tubules, but this depends on numerous factors. Both hyperphosphatemia and hypophosphatemia may be encountered in renal disease. Hyperphosphatemia is most commonly associated with reduced filtration rate in chronic renal failure. It is also seen in the newborn period when the excessive phosphate intake in cow's milk and the characteristic low filtration rate of the newborn infant contribute to the development of neonatal tetany (p. 285).[30]

Hypophosphatemia with hyperphosphaturia may be secondary to endocrine disturbance, such as hyperparathyroidism or pseudohyperparathyroidism, a hereditary disorder in which the proximal tubule is unresponsive to parathyroid hormone; caused by deficiency of vitamin D (p. 483) or a disturbance in its metabolism, such as the hereditary disorder vitamin D–resistant rickets; or a result of other renal tubular dysfunction associated with phosphate wasting, such as Fanconi's syndrome, proximal renal tubular acidosis, and so on.[32] Treatment for disorders of phosphate transport is determined by the cause.

Disorders of bicarbonate reabsorption

These disorders, known as proximal tubular acidosis, are discussed with distal tubular acidosis.

Fanconi's syndrome

A variety of complex forms of tubular insufficiency with a common pathogenesis are designated as Fanconi's syndrome (de Toni-Fanconi syndrome). The principal features of this syndrome are glycosuria, aminoaciduria, and phosphaturia. Frequently, toxic and metabolic disorders that impair the ability of the tubules to transport one of these substances affect the transport of the others. The primary causes of Fanconi's syndrome are[11,30,31]:

1. Metabolic diseases in which the transport mechanisms are damaged by the accumulation of toxic metabolites, for example, cystinosis, galactosemia, and Wilson's disease.
2. Exogenous poisons, especially drugs and heavy metals such as lead or arsenic.

DISORDERS OF DISTAL TUBULAR FUNCTION

The primary functions of the distal renal tubules are acidification of urine, potassium secretion, and the selective and differential reabsorption of sodium, chloride, and water, which determines the final urinary concentration. Since the contribution of the distal tubule to urine composition depends in part on the volume and composition of the filtrate from the proximal tubule, the net contribution of the distal tubule is related to proximal tubular function and glomerular filtration.[30]

Renal tubular acidosis

Renal tubular acidosis (RTA) is a syndrome of metabolic acidosis in which there is impaired reabsorption of bicarbonate and/or excretion of net hydrogen ion, whereas glomerular function is normal or comparatively less impaired. On the basis of underlying pathophysiology, renal tubular acidosis is divided into *proximal renal tubular acidosis,* which results from a defect in absorption of bicarbonate, and *distal renal tubular acidosis,* which results from an inability to establish an adequate gradient of pH between blood and tubular fluid.[29]

Proximal, bicarbonate-wasting, or rate-type renal tubular acidosis. Proximal tubular acidosis is caused by impaired bicarbonate reabsorption in the proximal tubule. It may occur as an isolated defect (primary); however, more often it appears in association with other proximal tubular disorders (secondary). As a result of a depressed renal threshold, bicarbonate reabsorption in the proximal tubule is incomplete, causing the plasma concentration of bicarbonate to stabilize at a lower level than normal. This results in a hyperchloremic metabolic acidosis. There is no impairment of distal tubular integrity or, in most cases, of the distal acidifying mechanism.

The cause of the primary disorder is unknown, but it appears to be almost entirely restricted to male infants. The major clinical manifestation and presenting symptom is growth failure. Complications are rare. Therapy usually involves administration of large volumes of bicarbonate to compensate for large urinary losses and maintaining bicarbonate within a normal range. The disorder appears to be transient and resolves spontaneously in time.

Distal or gradient-type renal tubular acidosis. Distal tubular acidosis is caused by the inability of the kidney to establish a normal pH gradient between tubular cells and tubular contents. Its most characteristic feature is the inability to produce a urinary pH below 6.0 despite the presence of severe metabolic acidosis.[11,29,31]

Distal renal tubular acidosis may occur as a primary, isolated defect or in association with other diseases or disorders. Most secondary causes are rare. The primary disorder is usually considered to be a hereditary defect with a variable degree of expression and a greater penetrance in females. After the age of 2 years the child usually has growth failure, although there is often a history of vomiting, polyuria, dehydration, anorexia, and failure to thrive. Evidence of bone demineralization (rickets or osteomalacia) may be present along with, occasionally, the formation of urinary calculi (urolithiasis) in older children.

The inability to secrete hydrogen ion causes an accumulation of the ion in the body, which soon depletes the available hydrogen buffer, producing a sustained acidosis. Acidosis retards normal somatic growth, and demineralization of bone occurs as bone salts are mobilized to buffer the excessive hydrogen ions. Increased serum levels of both calcium and phosphorus contribute to the development of stones within the renal system. Both sodium and potassium are secreted in larger amounts. Serum potassium levels are depleted as the distal tubules excrete large amounts of potassium ions in an attempt to conserve sodium, since hydrogen ions are unable to participate in the exchange. Hyponatremia stimulates increased aldosterone secretion, which further aggravates the hypokalemia. With the depletion of bicarbonate ions, more chloride is reabsorbed in the proximal tubule to create a hyperchloremia.

Treatment consists of administration of sufficient bicarbonate or citrate to balance metabolically produced hydrogen ions. Most authorities favor a mixture of sodium and potassium bicarbonate (or citrate) in order to prevent deficiencies of either cation. Although the primary disorder is permanent, with early diagnosis and therapy secondary effects on growth and stone formation can be avoided.

Disorders of concentrating mechanisms

The major disorder associated with a defect in the ability to concentrate urine is *nephrogenic diabetes insipidus (NDI),* in which the distal tubules and collecting ducts are insensitive to the action of antidiuretic hormone or its exogenous counterpart vasopressin. The nature of the defect is unknown, but it is usually inherited as an X-linked recessive trait that affects males primarily, although female carriers of the defective gene may exhibit a mild defect in urine-concentrating ability. Sometimes nephrogenic diabetes insipidus may result from chronic obstructive renal disorders, sickle cell disease, renal tuberculosis, and other renal disorders.[6,23,26]

The disease is manifest in the newborn period by vomiting, unexplained fever, failure to thrive, and severe recurrent dehydration with hypernatremia. The passage of copious amounts of dilute urine, which produces severe dehydration and hypoelectrolytemia, is a serious threat to life during this period and may be responsible for the high incidence of mental and motor retardation associated with affected persons. Growth retardation is probably related to diminished food intake and general poor health because of uncontrolled polydipsia. Diagnosis is suspected on the basis of patient and family history and confirmed by a urine osmolality value consistently below that of plasma. Lack of response to vasopressin administration rules out other causes.[25]

Therapy involves provision of adequate volumes of water to compensate for urinary losses. As a result of this insatiable thirst, most of the child's time is spent drinking and voiding, with little time for activity and stimulation. These children may go to great lengths to satisfy their thirst. A low-sodium/low-solute diet and the use of thiazide diuretics to increase the reabsorption of sodium and water in the proximal tubule help to reduce the amount of tubular fluid delivered to the distal tubules and diminish the volume of water excreted. Supplemental potassium may be required to prevent hypokalemia as a result of thiazide therapy. If the disease is recognized early and treatment instituted and maintained, normal growth can be expected and a normal life span anticipated.[11]

Miscellaneous renal disorders

Renal damage occurs as a major or minor complication in many systemic diseases and with varying degrees of severity. In some the renal complications may be the principal cause of death or one of several complications with fatal consequences. In others it may be only a source of discomfort but no direct threat to life. Sometimes renal complications provide a clue to diagnosis of the underlying disease; at other times renal involvement confuses the diagnosis. Some of the disorders in which renal dysfunction is acquired as a manifestation of a systemic disease have been outlined previously (see Table 31-5).

The importance of urinary tract infections and congenital defects has been discussed elsewhere (pp. 412 and 577). There are a wide variety of hereditary disorders of renal function, some of which have been mentioned. It is estimated that 15% of renal diseases are genetically determined. These may be disorders of glomerular function, tubular defects, metabolic disorders that may lead to renal damage, disorders involving more than one system, or structural abnormalities and tumors. In addition there are miscellaneous renal conditions for which an etiology is unknown.

Obstructive uropathy

Structural or functional abnormalities of the urinary system that obstruct the normal flow of urine can produce renal pathology. When there is interference with urine flow, the collecting system above the obstruction causes hydronephrosis (the collection of urine in the renal pelvis to the extent of cyst formation from the distention) with eventual pressure destruction to renal parenchyma, although the dilating ureters form a reservoir that reduces the effect on the kidneys for a long time. Obstruction may be unilateral or bilateral and complete or incomplete and can occur at any level of the upper or lower urinary tract (Fig. 31-6). Partial obstruction may not be symptomatic unless there is a water or solute diuresis.

With hydronephrosis, glomerular filtration ceases when intrapelvic pressure equals the filtration pressure in glomerular capillaries. However, a pressure gradient usually is established because of some flow beyond the obstruction as a result of periodic relaxation of ureteral wall musculature. There is also an exchange of solutes and water between the pooled urine in the renal pelvis and the adjoining tissues and fluid compartments (such as interstitial fluid in the pelvic wall and inner kidney medulla), and an intrarenal vascular adjustment caused by a corresponding increase in peritubular capillary pressure. Partial obstruction results in progressive loss of renal function as a result of irreversible damage to the nephrons. Pooled urine serves as a medium for bacterial growth; therefore, urinary tract infection further increases the extent of renal damage. Early diagnosis and surgical correction or amelioration are essential in order to prevent progressive renal damage.

Hemolytic-uremic syndrome

Hemolytic-uremic syndrome is an uncommon acute renal disease that occurs primarily in infants and small children

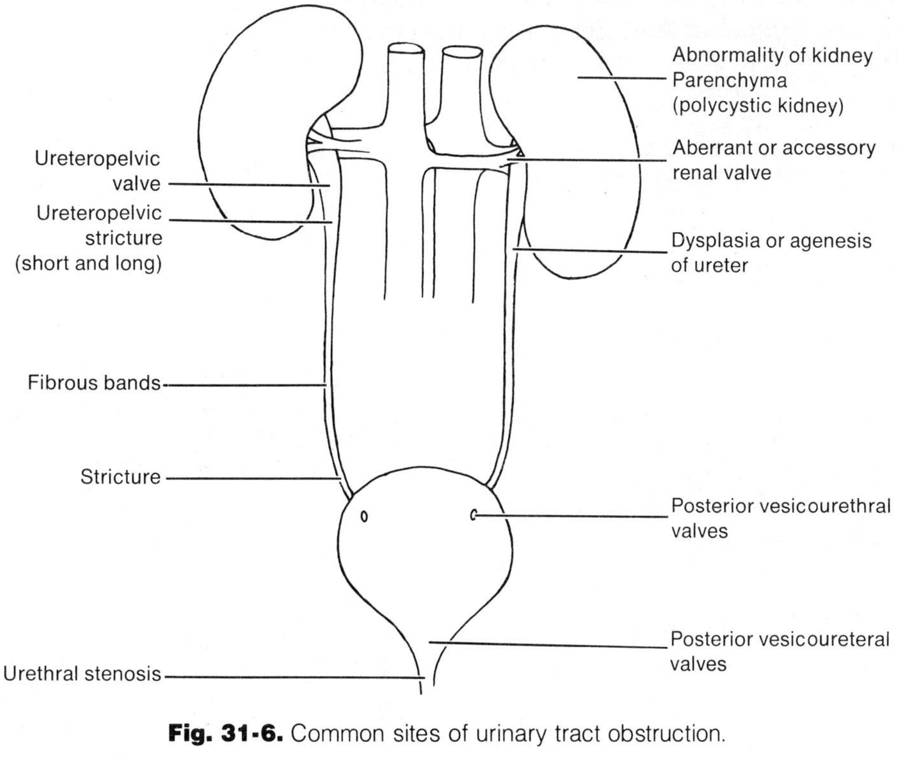

Fig. 31-6. Common sites of urinary tract obstruction.

between the ages of 6 months and 3 years. It has been recognized predominantly in whites and, whereas it occurs worldwide, is more prevalent in South Africa, Argentina, and the West coasts of North and South America. Although uncommon, hemolytic-uremic syndrome represents one of the most frequent causes of acute renal failure in children.[14,39]

Etiology and pathophysiology. In the majority of cases no causative agents have been identified; however, many possible agents or precipitating events have been suggested. The appearance of the disease has been correlated with both rickettsial and viral agents and may represent an unusual response to these infections. The disease usually follows an acute gastrointestinal or upper respiratory infection and tends to occur in scattered outbreaks in small geographic areas. The primary site of injury appears to be the endothelial lining of the small glomerular arterioles, which become swollen and occluded with deposition of platelets and fibrin clots (intravascular coagulation). Red blood cells are damaged as they move through the damaged, partially occluded blood vessels. These fragmented red blood cells are removed by the spleen, causing acute hemolytic anemia. Fibrinolytic action on the precipitated fibrin causes these fibrin-split products to appear in the serum and urine. The platelet aggregation within damaged blood vessels or the damage and removal of platelets produce the characteristic thrombocytopenia. In adults a similar condition is associated with thrombocytopenic purpura, which has led to the speculation that it may be the adult version of the hemolytic-uremic syndrome of infancy and early childhood.[36]

Diagnostic evaluation. The hemolytic process persists for several days to 2 weeks. During this time the child is anorectic, irritable, and lethargic. There is marked and rapid onset of pallor, accompanied by hemorrhagic manifestations such as bruising, purpura, or rectal bleeding. Renal involvement is evidenced by proteinuria, hematuria, and presence of urinary casts; blood urea nitrogen and serum creatinine levels are elevated. Usually there is oliguria or anuria, although nonoliguric acute renal failure may be manifest. Convulsions and stupor suggest central nervous system involvement, and there may be signs of acute heart failure.[6,11,23]

Medical management. In general, treatment is directed toward the control of the complications and hematologic manifestations of renal failure. The most consistently effective treatment is peritoneal dialysis, which is instituted in any child who has been anuric for 24 hours or who demonstrates oliguria with hypertension and seizures. Blood transfusions with fresh, washed packed cells are administered for severe anemia but are used with caution to prevent circulatory overload from added volume.

There is no substantial evidence that heparin, corticosteroids, or fibrinolytic agents are beneficial, and in some instances they may aggravate the condition. With prompt treatment the recovery rate is about 95%, but residual renal impairment ranges from 10% to 50% in various areas. Death is usually caused by residual renal impairment or central nervous system injury.[13,14]

Nursing considerations. Nursing care is the same as that provided in acute renal failure and, for children with continued impairment, includes management of chronic disease.

Benign recurrent hematuria

Benign recurrent hematuria is characterized by recurrent episodes of gross hematuria in the absence of systemic disease. The etiology is unknown, but the episodes of hematuria are frequently precipitated by viral respiratory infections, other mild febrile illnesses, or strenuous exercise.

The disorder may be confused with other forms of renal disease; therefore, renal biopsy is indicated to confirm the diagnosis and rule out more serious renal disease. There is no loss of renal function, and treatment is seldom indicated.

Familial glomerulopathy (Alport's syndrome)

The syndrome of chronic hereditary nephritis consists of hematuria, nerve deafness, ocular disorders, and chronic renal failure. The disease appears to be inherited as an autosomal-dominant trait, although rare male-to-male transmission occurs, which suggests a possible X-linked dominant trait. The disease is uncommon but not rare and accounts for a significant percentage of persistant glomerular disease in childhood.

The clinical manifestations are indistinguishable from mild acute nephritis. Initial symptoms include hematuria, proteinuria, malaise, and mild edema. The symptoms are often associated with an acute respiratory infection. The condition begins in infancy and slowly progresses until uncontrollable renal failure develops in adolescence or early adulthood. There is a positive family history. Most untreated boys develop severe symptoms, whereas affected girls generally have a milder disease and a normal life expectancy.

Treatment is symptomatic and supportive, and every effort should be made to restrict the activities of affected children as little as possible. Dialysis and renal transplantation are ultimate therapeutic measures for renal involvement. Hearing loss and ocular disorders should receive appropriate attention, and families should be counseled regarding the genetic implications of the disease.

Unexplained proteinuria

Often apparently healthy children with no suggestion of renal disease will demonstrate proteinuria on routine urinalysis. The percentage of children with unexplained proteinuria ranges from 1% at 6 years of age to 11% at puberty, reaching a maximum prevalence at 13 years of age in girls and 16 years of age in boys.[11]

Unexplained proteinuria can be categorized as (1) *transient* (inconstant), (2) *persistent,* or (3) *orthostatic* or *postural.* Transient proteinuria is a common finding with no known cause, but it sometimes increases with febrile illness, exercise, cold, or emotions.

Persistent proteinuria usually signifies renal disease but may occur consistently in children with no impairment of renal function. Orthostatic proteinuria is seen in 3% to 5% of adolescents and young adults, and, although proteinuria is evident in the recumbent as well as the erect position, it is readily detected by qualitative tests. Reactions of 2+ or 3+ are frequently encountered. The cause is unknown, although there are minor glomerular changes in many instances. The condition is benign and generally resolves over a period of time.[11]

In cases of unexplained proteinuria it is important to confirm or exclude renal disease with appropriate diagnostic tests. Repeated examination for proteinuria, an orthostatic test, and, if proteinuria is persistent, more definitive tests, including 24-hour protein excretion, intravenous pyelogram, and urine culture, are indicated.

Renal trauma

The kidneys are among the organs most often injured in children, despite their relatively protected location. However, the outer borders are less well protected and are separated from the skin surface by only 2 to 3 cm in young children. Most injuries are of the nonpenetrating or "blunt" type, usually involving falls, athletic injuries, and motor vehicle accidents. In many children (10%) preexisting renal abnormalities, particularly congenital anomalies associated with mild to moderate hydronephrosis, are found that were unrecognized prior to the accident. In approximately 40% of childhood cases, other injuries are found, most commonly those involving the brain and spleen.[11,24]

Renal injury can be suspected in children who complain of flank pain, and frequently there are abrasions or contusions on the overlying skin. Hematuria is consistently present, but the amount of blood in the urine is not a reliable indicator of the seriousness of the injury. Many relatively insignificant injuries are associated with grossly bloody urine, whereas some of the severest injuries are found in children with only microscopic hematuria.

Renal injury can be divided into two types—contusions and ruptures. In renal contusion the capsule, parenchyma, and collecting system are usually intact but subcapsular bleeding occurs into the parenchyma and appears in the urine. Renal contusion is an important cause of gross hematuria in active children. Renal rupture involves the actual splitting open of the kidney capsule, causing extravasation of blood or a mixture of blood and urine into the surrounding retroperitoneal space. Renal vascular injury, although unusual, requires immediate recognition and surgical intervention.

In active children there may or may not be history of unusual trauma. Abdominal or flank pain and tenderness are caused by bleeding around the kidney and may or may not be associated with fever. Clots passing down the ureter may cause pain similar to that of renal colic, and dysuria is common. Diagnosis is made on the basis of intravenous pyelography, angiography, and/or retrograde pyelography. Unsuspected hydronephrosis often is first detected as a result of traumatic injury.

Severe injury requires close observation in the hospital intensive care unit as well as blood replacement if there is severe internal or external bleeding. In most cases bleeding subsides spontaneously. Surgical exploration is indicated in multiple injuries, extravasation of blood around the kidneys, or disruption of the major vessels or the collecting system. Children with less severe injury, such as contusions only, are placed on bed rest. They should remain on bed rest for 3 days after cessation of gross bleeding, since the substance released from injured renal tissue (urinary urokinase) has strongly fibrinolytic properties that may precipitate serious bleeding.

ACUTE RENAL FAILURE

Acute renal failure (ARF) is said to exist when the kidneys suddenly are unable to regulate the volume and composition of urine appropriately in response to food and fluid intake and the needs of the organism. The principal feature is oligoanuria* associated with azotemia, acidosis, and diverse electrolyte disturbances. Acute renal failure is not common in childhood, but the outcome depends on the cause, associated findings, and prompt recognition and treatment.[19,26,38]

The terms azotemia and uremia are often used in relation to renal failure. *Azotemia* is the accumulation of nitrogenous waste within the blood. *Uremia* is a more advanced condition in which retention of nitrogenous products produces toxic symptoms. Azotemia is not life threatening, whereas uremia is a serious condition that often involves other body systems.[12]

Etiology

Acute renal failure can develop as a result of a large number of related or unrelated clinical conditions—poor renal perfusion, acute renal injury, or the final expression of chronic, irreversible renal disease. The most common cause in children is transient renal failure resulting from dehydration or other causes of poor perfusion that responds to restoration of fluid volume. Causes of acute renal failure

*The definition of oligoanuria varies extensively, from 180 to 400 ml/m²/24 hours, in the literature.

are usually classified according to *prerenal, renal,* and *post-renal* causes (see the box below). This implies that only renal causes are characterized by damage to the renal parenchyma while prerenal and postrenal causes can be more easily remedied. However, severe or long-standing prerenal or postrenal etiologies can produce severe secondary renal damage.[38]

Prerenal. Prerenal causes of acute renal failure are most common in children and are always related to reduction of renal perfusion to an anatomically and physiologically normal kidney and collecting system. Dehydration secondary to diarrheal disease or persistent vomiting is the most frequent cause of prerenal failure in infants and children. Surgical shock and trauma (including burns) are also common causes. Hypovolemia and decreased renal perfusion cause a decreased glomerular filtration rate and stimulate the secretion of renin, aldosterone, and antidiuretic hormone, which further diminish urine flow. Extended and severe hypoperfusion can produce cortical or tubular necrosis; however, where medical care is available, this is seldom allowed to occur. Azotemia that accompanies this type of renal failure generally is rapidly reversible with prompt attention to expansion of the extracellular fluid volume. Prerenal failure is often difficult to distinguish from tubular or cortical necrosis.

Postrenal. Acute renal failure resulting from obstructive uropathy is uncommon in children except in the first year of life. However, renal function can be restored by relief of the obstruction. The degree of recovery depends on the duration of the renal failure. When the obstruction persists for more than 3 weeks, complete recovery is unlikely.[11]

Renal. Renal causes of acute renal failure comprise the largest group that requires extended management. These include diseases and nephrotoxic agents that damage the glomeruli, tubules, or renal vasculature. Glomerular disease is the most common cause of glomerular damage, whereas tubular destruction is more often caused by ischemia or nephrotoxins. Vascular damage is an uncommon cause of renal failure in childhood. The type and extent of damage determine the degree and duration of renal insufficiency, and it is difficult to predict in any given case whether or not acute necrosis will develop.

Etiology of acute renal failure in infants and children

Prerenal (decreased perfusion)

- Hypovolemia
  - Hemorrhage (within or outside kidney)
  - Gastrointestinal losses (vomiting, diarrhea, nasogastric tubes)
  - Sequestered or isolated accumulation (local injury, trauma, or disease)
  - Burns
  - Hypoproteinemia
  - Diabetic acidosis
- Circulatory insufficiency
  - Congestive heart failure
  - Cardiac defects
  - Shock
  - Acute anemia (hemolytic crises, including sickle cell crisis)
- Peripheral vasodilatation
  - Sepsis
  - Drug-induced (antihypertensives, anesthesia)
- Increased vascular resistance
  - Anesthesia
  - Surgery
- Renal arterial occlusion
  - Renal vein thrombosis or embolus
  - Narrowing of arteries (congenital stricture)
  - External compression (tumor)

Renal

- Diseases of kidney
  - Glomerulopathies
  - Pyelonephritis
  - Cortical or medullary necrosis
  - Diseases associated with systemic disease
  - Hemolytic-uremic syndrome
  - Tumors
  - Intravascular coagulation
- Tubular distruction
  - Nephrotoxins (drugs, chemicals, dyes)
  - Intravascular hemolysis (hemoglobinuria)
  - Crush injury (myoglobinuria)
  - Transfusion reaction
- Vascular
  - Thrombosis
  - Polyarteritis or systemic vasculitis
  - Acute and/or chronic rejection
- Hypoxic ischemia
  - Near drowning
  - Shock

Postrenal

- Upper tract obstruction
  - Stones
  - Tumors
  - Uric acid or sulfonamide crystals
  - Ureterocele
  - Stricture
- Bladder neck obstruction

Pathophysiology

Acute renal failure is usually reversible, but the deviations of physiologic function can be extreme and the mortality rate in the pediatric age-group is still high. There is severe reduction in glomerular filtration rate, an elevated blood urea nitrogen level, and decreased tubular reabsorption of sodium from the proximal tubule. Consequently there is increased concentration of sodium in the distal tubule, which causes stimulation of the renin mechanism. The local action of angiotensin causes vasoconstriction of the afferent arteriole, which further reduces glomerular filtration and prevents urinary losses of sodium. There is a significant reduction in renal blood flow.[10]

The pathology that produces acute renal failure caused by glomerulonephritis, hemolytic-uremic syndrome, and other renal disorders has been discussed in relation to those disease processes. The necrotic processes within the nephron can be cortical, tubular, or both.

Cortical necrosis. Complete cortical necrosis usually results from severe ischemia, infection, or intravascular coagulation and represents a severe irreversible cause of acute renal failure. In the pediatric age-group this occurs as a fatal event most frequently during the neonatal period as a result of hypoxia and shock. When cortical destruction is incomplete, some recovery of renal function may occur. Intravascular coagulation is believed to play a significant role as an intermediate factor in the development of acute renal failure, especially in cases related to sepsis.

Tubular necrosis. Damage to the renal tubules can be broadly classified as (1) secondary to renal ischemia and (2) associated with the ingestion or inhalation of substances toxic to the kidneys. Renal tubules are particularly vulnerable to a wide variety of toxic agents that produce vasoconstriction and to focal patches of ischemia that cause a uniform necrosis of the tubular epithelium down to, but not including, the basement membrane. The lesion produced by sustained reduction in renal blood flow involves the basement membrane as well, which may become fragmented and ruptured to the extent that the continuity of tubular structure is disrupted. The lesions may affect any segment of the tubules, appearing at irregular intervals along with normal segments throughout the kidney.[11,38]

Healing of tubular lesions is accomplished by reepithelialization in the areas with intact basement membrane. In those areas in which the basement membrane has been disrupted, such healing is unable to take place and connective tissue grows through the ruptured membrane, thus preventing reestablishment of tubular integrity. Individual cells within the nephron are capable of regeneration, but the entire nephron is not capable of this.[38]

Clinical course. The clinical course of the child with acute renal failure is variable and depends on the cause. In reversible acute renal failure there is a period of severe oliguria, or the low-output phase, followed by an abrupt onset of diuresis, or a high-output phase, followed by a gradual return to, or toward, normal urine volumes. The length of the oliguric phase in older children and adolescents is 10 to 14 days, although it is highly variable at all ages. It tends to be shorter (3 to 5 days) in infants, children, and milder cases. The onset of the diuretic phase appears unexpectedly and, over a period of several days, proceeds in stepwise fashion from very low to supernormal urine volumes. During the oliguric phase, manifestations of uremia are present but may also be accompanied by other clinical disorders that make assessment difficult, such as infection, anoxia, and shock.[11,12]

The published data indicate a recovery rate from acute renal failure of 75% in children with competent care and management. The outcome is least favorable in children with rapidly progressive nephritis and cortical necrosis. Children in whom acute renal failure is a result of hemolytic-uremic syndrome or acute glomerulitis may recover completely, but residual renal impairment or hypertension is more often the rule. Complete recovery is usually expected in children whose renal failure is a result of dehydration, nephrotoxins, or ischemia. Acute renal failure following cardiac surgery is less favorable. It is often impossible to assess the extent of recovery for several months.[11]

Diagnostic evaluation

In many instances of acute renal failure the infant or child is already critically ill with the precipitating disorder and the explanation for development of oliguria is readily apparent. When a previously well child develops acute renal failure without obvious cause, a careful history is taken to reveal symptoms that may be related to glomerulonephritis, to obstructive uropathy, or regarding exposure to nephrotoxic chemicals, such as ingestion of heavy metals or inhalation of carbon tetrachloride or other organic solvents, or drugs, such as methicillin, sulfonamides, neomycin, polymyxin, and kanamycin.

The prime manifestation of acute renal failure is oliguria, generally a urine output less than 50 ml in 24 hours. Anuria is uncommon except in obstructive disorders. No other symptoms are specific to acute renal failure, although nausea and vomiting and drowsiness may develop. Some nonspecific physical findings, such as edema or hypertension, may serve to identify the underlying cause. With continued oliguria, biochemical abnormalities can develop rapidly and circulatory and central nervous system manifestations appear. Laboratory data reflect the kidney dysfunction—hyperkalemia, hyponatremia, metabolic acidosis, hypocalcemia, anemia, or azotemia (Table 31-7).

Medical management

The most effective management of acute renal failure is prevention. The development of acute renal failure is a known risk in certain situations. This should be anticipated, recognized, and adequate therapy implemented, for example, fluid therapy for children with hypovolemia in such

Table 31-7. Laboratory findings associated with acute renal failure

Clinical problem	Mechanism	Clinical considerations
Azotemia		
Elevated BUN levels	Ongoing protein catabolism Significantly decreased excretion	Lower rate of production in neonates and persons with depleted protein stores Increased in situations involving large amounts of necrotic tissue or extravasated blood
Elevated plasma creatinine levels	Continued production Significantly decreased excretion	Production less affected by other factors More sensitive measure of intensity of azotemia Low in neonate because of small muscle mass relative to size
Metabolic acidosis	Continued endogenous acid production Significantly decreased excretion Depletion of extracellular and intracellular fluid buffers	Compensatory hyperventilation Opisthotonus Major threat to life
Hyponatremia	Dilution of extracellular fluid Decreased excretion of water	May develop cerebral signs
Hyperkalemia	Ongoing protein catabolism Decreased excretion compounded by metabolic acidosis	Most important electrolyte to be considered in acute renal failure May contribute to cardiac arrhythmia With ECG changes, major threat to life May be lost from gastrointentinal tract
Hypocalcemia	Associated with metabolic acidosis and hyperphosphatemia	During alkali therapy, may cause tetany

conditions as dehydration, burns, and hemorrhage, carried out in these situations. Nephrotoxic drugs should be used with caution or avoided in children with renal disease, and all personnel should be knowledgeable in the precautions related to their administration. For example, a generous fluid intake is needed for children receiving antimetabolite drugs and after radiotherapy.

The treatment of acute renal failure is directed toward (1) treatment of the underlying cause, (2) management of the complications of renal failure, and (3) provision of supportive therapy within the constraints imposed by the renal failure.[7,19,26]

Treatment of poor perfusion resulting from dehydration consists of volume restoration as described previously in treatment of dehydration. If oliguria persists after restoration of fluid volume or the renal failure is caused by intrinsic renal damage, the physiologic and biochemical abnormalities that have resulted from kidney dysfunction must be corrected or controlled.

Initially a Foley catheter is inserted to rule out urine retention, to collect available urine for analysis, and to monitor results of mannitol or furosemide administration. The catheter may or may not be removed. Many authorities who believe that it serves little purpose during the oliguric phase and predisposes to bladder infection prefer collection bags for measuring urine output. Others maintain a catheter for hourly urine measurements.

Oliguria. When there is persistent oliguria in the presence of adequate hydration and no lower tract obstruction, mannitol, furosemide, or both are administered rapidly as a test to provoke a flow of urine. When glomerular function is intact, the administration of these substances will behave as nonreabsorbable solute in the tubular fluid to evoke an osmotic diuresis. The presence of mannitol in tubular fluid and the obligatory water that follows it also serve to dilute the concentration of any nephrotoxin that may be present in the tubules below toxic levels. The furosemide blocks reabsorption of tubular filtrate. If urine flow is generated to the extent of 6 to 10 ml/kg in 1 to 3 hours, the initial dosage is reduced and continued, if needed, to sustain the flow. If no urine is produced within 2 hours after the single dose, the drugs are not repeated and an oliguric regimen is instituted to control water balance and other abnormalities.[19,26]

Fluid and calories. The amount of exogenous water provided should not exceed the amount needed to maintain zero water balance. It is calculated on the basis of estimated endogenous water formation and losses from sensible (primarily gastrointestinal) and insensible sources. No allotment is calculated for urine as long as oliguria persists.

The child with acute renal failure has a tendency to develop water intoxication and hyponatremia, which make it difficult to provide calories in sufficient amounts to meet the needs of the child and reduce the tissue catabolism, metabolic acidosis, hyperkalemia, and uremia. If the child is able to tolerate oral foods, concentrated food sources high in carbohydrate and fat but low in protein, potassium, and sodium may be provided. However, many children have functional disturbances of the gastrointestinal tract, such as nausea and vomiting; therefore, the intravenous route is generally preferred and usually consists of highly concentrated carbohydrate solutions in small volumes of water administered by the central venous route (see total parenteral nutrition, p. 1091).

Control of water balance in these patients requires careful monitoring of feedback information, such as accurate intake and output, body weight, and electrolyte measurements. In general during the oliguric phase no sodium, chloride, or potassium is given unless there are other large ongoing losses. Regular measurement of plasma electrolyte, pH, blood urea nitrogen, and creatinine levels is required to assess the adequacy of fluid therapy and to anticipate complications that require specific treatment.[11,23,38]

Hyperkalemia. Elevated serum potassium is the most immediate threat to the life of the child with acute renal failure. Potassium ions are not being excreted, whereas at the same time release of potassium from cells is accelerated by acidosis, stress, and tissue breakdown in cases associated with internal bleeding or trauma. Since cardiac arrhythmia and cardiac arrest may result, electrocardiograms as well as serum potassium ion level are monitored regularly. Hyperkalemia can be minimized and sometimes avoided by eliminating potassium from all food and fluid, by reducing tissue catabolism, and by correcting acidosis. Serum potassium concentrations in excess of 7 mEq/liter or the presence of ECG abnormalities, such as prolonged QRS complex, depressed ST segment, high peaked T waves, bradycardia, or heart block, constitute an emergency situation.

Several measures are available to reduce the serum potassium concentration, and the priority of implementation is usually based on the rapidity with which the measures are effective. Temporary measures that produce a rapid but transient effect are[26,38]:

1. Calcium gluconate, 0.5 ml/kg, administered intravenously over a period of 2 to 4 minutes, with continuous ECG monitoring, exerts a protective effect on cardiac conduction.
2. Sodium bicarbonate, 2 to 3 mEq/kg, administered intravenously over a period of 30 to 60 minutes, elevates the serum pH to cause a transient shift of extracellular fluid potassium into the intracellular fluid. However, there is risk of hypocalcemia, tetany, and fluid overload.
3. Glucose, 50%, and insulin, 1 U/kg, administered intravenously, accelerate glycogen synthesis, causing glucose and potassium to move into the cells. Insulin facilitates the entry of glucose into cells.

These effects produce only transient protection by redistributing of existing potassium stores; they do not remove potassium from the body. However, they provide relief while more definitive but slower-acting measures are being implemented. Potassium can be removed by:

1. Administration of an ion-exchange resin such as polystyrene sodium sulfonate (Kayexalate), 1 g/kg, administered orally or rectally, to bind potassium and remove it from the body. This requires time to be effective, and a sodium ion is exchanged for each potassium ion. This increased sodium concentration adds to the body fluids, which may potentially contribute to fluid overload, hypertension, and cardiac failure.
2. Dialysis (discussed on p. 1181). Hemodialysis is efficient but requires specialized facilities. Peritoneal dialysis is simpler and can be carried out in almost any hospital setting. Indications for dialysis in acute renal failure are continued oliguria associated with any of the following[11]:
   - Severe, persistent acidosis
   - Inability to reduce serum potassium levels to a safe range with other methods
   - Clinical uremic syndrome, consisting of nausea and vomiting, drowsiness, and progression to coma
   - Circulatory overload, hypertension, and evidence of cardiac failure

   A popular philosophy is to institute dialysis after 24 to 48 hours of oliguria, regardless of other symptoms. Supporters of this approach believe that early and frequent dialysis is associated with reduced morbidity and mortality and that it permits improved nutrition with relaxed diet restrictions. The combination of dialysis and nutrition tends to reduce the complications of acute renal failure.

Other complications. Other complications that may occur with acute renal failure are hypertension, anemia, convulsions and coma, cardiac failure, and pulmonary edema. The most common cause of *hypertension* in acute renal failure is hypervolemia, or overexpansion of the extracellular fluid and plasma volume, together with hypersecretion of renin. Treatment is controlled by limiting water and sodium, but antihypertensive drugs are often used with caution. The most useful drug for treating moderate hypertension is hydralazine, administered intravenously or intramuscularly. If this is ineffective, administration of methyldopa (Aldomet) may be effective.

Anemia is frequently associated with acute renal failure, but transfusion is not recommended unless the hemoglobin drops below 6 g/100 ml. Transfusions, if used, consist of fresh, packed red blood cells given slowly to reduce the likelihood of increasing blood volume, hypertension, and hyperkalemia.

Seizures occur rather often when renal failure progresses to uremia and are also related to hypertension, hyponatremia, and hypocalcemia. Treatment is directed to the specific cause when known. More obscure etiologies are managed with anticonvulsant drugs.

Cardiac failure with pulmonary edema is almost always associated with hypervolemia. Treatment is directed toward reduction of fluid volume, with water and sodium restric-

Summary of nursing care of the child with acute renal failure

Goals	Responsibilities
Prevent or correct dehydration	See summary of nursing care in dehydration (p. 1083)
Distinguish between urine retention and diminished urine formation	Insert Foley catheter Measure output Send urine obtained (if any) for laboratory analysis
Help establish diagnosis and extent of renal function	Assist with diagnostic procedures Collect specimens for laboratory examinations Perform tests as ordered Observe, record, and report clinical manifestations

Monitor fluid balance	Weigh child daily or as ordered
	Measure intake and output accurately
	Measure urine specific gravity
	Monitor vital signs
	  Blood pressure
	  Heart rate
	  Respiratory status
	  Central venous pressure, if indicated
	Replace fluid losses as ordered (gastrointestinal, perspiration, and so on)
	Observe for signs of dehydration or fluid overload

Prevent complications Infection	 Observe medical asepsis Avoid contact with infected persons Keep skin clean and dry Change position at least every 2 hours Administer aseptic care of intravenous, hyperalimentation, or dialysis sites Administer antibiotics if ordered
Hypertension	Administer antihypertensives if ordered Carefully regulate fluid administration Observe for signs of fluid overload Monitor blood pressure and central venous pressure Administer diuretics as ordered
Minimize catabolism	Provide nutrition as ordered Reduce energy expenditure

Reduce elevated levels of electrolyte and nitrogenous waste	Oral
	  Become well acquainted with protein, potassium, and sodium content of common foods and beverages
	  Provide low-protein, low-sodium, and low-potassium diet
	Parenteral
	  Administer hyperalimentation formula as ordered
	Prevent catabolism
	Assist with peritoneal dialysis
	  Gather necessary equipment
	  Warm dialysate solution
	  Assist with catheter insertion
	  Carry out procedure as ordered
	  Observe response to treatment
	  Monitor vital signs frequently
	  Collect specimens as ordered
	Hemodialysis
	  Transport to specialized unit as ordered

Summary of nursing care of the child with acute renal failure—cont'd

Goals	Responsibilities
Support child	Remain with child Provide as much comfort as possible within limitations imposed by treatment regimen Provide means for child to express feelings
Support parents	Allow parents to visit child Explain or reinforce explanations of treatments Keep parents informed of child's progress Allow parents to express feelings and concerns Provide reassurance where possible Refer to agencies for social service and financial aid

tion and administration of diuretics. Digitalis is ineffective and can be hazardous.

Diuretic or high-output phase. When the output begins to increase, either spontaneously or in response to diuretic therapy, the intake of fluid, potassium, and sodium must be monitored and adequate replacement provided to prevent depletion and its consequences. In some cases the high-output phase is mild and lasts only a few days; in others enormous amounts of electrolyte-rich urine are passed.

Nursing considerations

Nursing care of the infant or child with acute renal failure involves care of the underlying cause plus careful observation and management of the renal status. The major goal is reestablishment of renal function, with emphasis on providing an adequate caloric intake to minimize reduction of protein stores, prevention of complications, and monitoring of fluid balance, laboratory data, and physical manifestations. The probability of dialysis must be considered and the necessary equipment made available in anticipation of such an eventuality. Because the child requires intensive observation and, often, specialized equipment, he is usually admitted to an intensive care unit in which needed equipment and personnel trained in its use are available.

Meticulous attention to the fluid intake and output is mandatory, including all the physical measurements discussed previously in relation to problems of fluid balance. Monitoring of fluid balance is a continuous process, and nursing measures, such as maintaining an optimal thermal environment, reducing any elevation of body temperature, and reducing restlessness and anxiety, are employed to decrease the rate of tissue catabolism. Although these children are usually quite ill and voluntarily diminish their activity, infants may become restless and irritable and children are often anxious and frightened. There are frequent painful and stress-producing treatments and tests that must be performed. The presence of a supportive, empathetic nurse can provide comfort and stability in a threatening and unnatural environment.

The nurse must be continually alert for changes in behavior that indicate the onset of complications. Infection from reduced resistance, anemia, and general morbidity is a constant threat. Fluid overload and electrolyte disturbances can precipitate cardiovascular complications such as hypertension and cardiac failure. Fluid and electrolyte imbalances, acidosis, and accumulation of nitrogenous waste products can produce neurologic involvement manifest by coma, convulsions, or alterations in sensorium.

Parental support and reassurance are among the major nursing responsibilities. The seriousness and emergency nature of acute renal failure are stressful to parents, and most parents feel some degree of guilt regarding the child's condition, especially when the illness is the result of ingestion of a toxic substance, dehydration, or genetic disease. They need reassurance and a sympathetic listener. They also need to be kept informed of the child's progress and provided explanations regarding the therapeutic regimen. The equipment and the child's behavior are sometimes frightening and anxiety provoking. Nurses can do much to help them comprehend and deal with the stresses of the situation. (For a summary of nursing care of the child with acute renal failure, see the boxed material.)

CHRONIC RENAL FAILURE

The kidneys are able to maintain the chemical composition of fluids within normal limits until more than 50% of functional renal capacity is destroyed by disease or injury. Chronic renal insufficiency or failure begins when the diseased kidneys can no longer maintain normal chemical structure of body fluids under normal conditions. Progressive deterioration over a period of months or years produces a variety of clinical and biochemical disturbances that eventually culminate in the clinical syndrome known as uremia. The pattern of renal dysfunction is remarkably uniform no matter what disease process initiates the advanced disease.

Etiology

A variety of diseases and disorders can result in chronic renal failure (CRF). The most frequent causes of chronic renal failure before age 5 years are congenital renal and urinary tract malformations (particularly renal hypoplasia and dysplasia) and vesicoureteral reflux (p. 578). Glomerular and hereditary renal disease predominate in children 5 to 15 years of age. Glomerular diseases that most frequently lead to chronic renal failure are chronic pyelonephritis, chronic glomerulonephritis, and glomerulonephropathy associated with systemic diseases such as anaphylactoid purpura and lupus erythematosus. Hereditary nephritis, congenital nephrotic syndrome, Alport's syndrome, polycystic kidney, and several other hereditary disorders result in renal failure in childhood. Renal vascular disorders such as hemolytic-uremic syndrome, vascular thrombosis, or cortical necrosis are less frequent causes.[6,17,23]

Pathophysiology

Early in the course of progressive nephron destruction, the child remains asymptomatic with only minimal biochemical abnormalities. Unless its presence is detected in the process of routine assessment, signs and symptoms that indicate advanced renal damage frequently emerge only late in the course of the disease. Midway in the disease process, as increasing numbers of nephrons are totally destroyed and most others are damaged in varying degree, the few that remain intact are hypertrophied but functional. These few normal nephrons are able to make sufficient adjustments to stresses to maintain reasonable degrees of fluid and electrolyte balance. Definitive biochemical examination at this time will reveal restricted tolerance to excesses or restrictions. As the disease progresses to the terminal stage, because of severe reduction in the number of functioning nephrons the kidneys are no longer able to maintain fluid and electrolyte balance and the features of the uremic syndrome appear.

The pathophysiology of specific biochemical abnormalities is briefly summarized in the following paragraphs:

Retention of waste products. Moderate decrease in renal function is not associated with a rise in fasting blood urea nitrogen concentration. With progressive nephron destruction and diminished function, the serum level of these end products of protein metabolism is elevated increasingly. However, the blood urea nitrogen level is affected by protein intake, whereas the creatinine concentration is not; therefore, creatinine is a more reliable index of renal failure.

Water and sodium. The damaged kidneys are able to maintain sodium and water balance under normal circumstances, although the few remaining functional nephrons are required to increase their rate of filtration and reabsorption in proportion to their numbers. The limitations of this capacity become apparent under stress. The nature of abnormalities in adjustment depend on the underlying renal disease: infants and small children with kidney dysplasia or urinary obstructive disease tend to excrete large volumes of dilute urine low in sodium content; children with glomerular disease tend to retain both sodium and water as a result of a greater reduction in glomerular filtration than of tubular reabsorption; and children with defective sodium reabsorption from tubular disease tend to lose sodium with a corresponding osmotic water loss. Consequently sodium excesses may cause edema and hypertension, whereas sodium deprivation can result in hypovolemia and circulatory failure. Only in end-stage renal disease is markedly reduced glomerular filtration inadequate to handle normal amounts of sodium and water. Retention of these substances then leads to edema and vascular congestion.[7,11,17]

Potassium. Dangerous hyperkalemia is an infrequent occurrence in chronic renal failure until the terminal stages. However, the kidneys are unable to adjust readily to increased ingestion of potassium, and they require a longer period to time to rid the body of this excess.

Acidosis. A sustained metabolic acidosis is characteristic of chronic renal failure resulting from the inability of the damaged kidney to excrete the normal acid load of metabolic acids generated by normal metabolic processes. There is reduced capacity of the distal tubules to produce ammonia and impaired reabsorption of bicarbonate. Although there is continual hydrogen ion retention and bicarbonate loss, the plasma pH is maintained at a level compatible with life by other buffering mechanisms, particularly the bone salts (see following paragraphs).

Calcium and phosphorus. One of the distressing features of chronic renal failure is its effect on calcium and phosphorus homeostasis. Profound and complex disturbances in the metabolism of these substances result in significant bone demineralization and impaired growth. This appears to be related to several factors:

1. In a state of acidosis there is dissolution of the alkaline salts of bone to serve as buffers and the release of phosphorus and calcium into the bloodstream
2. Reduced glomerular filtration and excretion of inorganic phosphate lead to an elevation of plasma phosphate with a concomitant decrease in serum calcium
3. Decreased serum calcium concentration stimulates the se-

cretion of parathyroid hormone (PTH), which results in resorption of calcium from bones. Under normal circumstances parathyroid hormone inhibits the tubular reabsorption of phosphates
4. Diseased kidneys are unable to complete the synthesis of vitamin D to its most active form, 1,25-dihydrocholecalciferol, which is necessary for the absorption of calcium from the gastrointestinal tract and deposition of calcium in bone. This acquired resistance to vitamin D decreases calcium absorption, permits retention of phosphorus, and contributes to secondary hyperparathyroidism.

In chronic renal failure the result of these complex disturbances in calcium, phosphorus, and bone metabolism produces growth arrest or retardation, bone pain, and deformities known as *renal osteodystrophy,* sometimes called *renal rickets* since the disorganization of bone growth and demineralization is similar to that caused by vitamin D–resistant rickets.[3,6,11]

Hematologic disturbances. A consistent feature of chronic renal insufficiency is anemia that appears to result from:

1. Shortened life span of red blood cells caused by some extracorpuscular factor associated with the uremic state
2. Impaired red blood cell production resulting from decreased production of erythropoietin
3. Increased tendency to bleed, associated with a prolonged bleeding time probably related to impaired platelet function
4. Superimposed nutritional anemia

Growth disturbance. Most children with chronic renal disease fail to grow. The cause is poorly understood but may be related to[4,11,16]:

1. Renal osteodystrophy
2. Poor nutrition associated with dietary restrictions (especially protein) and anorexia
3. Biochemical abnormalities associated with renal failure, such as sustained acidosis

Sexual maturation may be delayed or may not occur in children with chronic renal failure, and secondary amenorrhea frequently develops in girls past puberty.

Miscellaneous disturbances. Children with chronic renal failure seem to be more than usually susceptible to infection, especially pneumonia, urinary tract infection, and septicemia, although the reason for this is not entirely clear. Hyperventilation, a manifestation of the respiratory compensatory mechanism for metabolic acidosis, and pulmonary edema may contribute to upper respiratory infection. These children become extraordinarily sensitive to changes in vascular volume that may cause, in addition to pulmonary overload, cerebral symptoms and circulatory manifestations such as hypertension and cardiac failure.

Numerous neurologic manifestations appear with advanced renal failure, although no specific toxin or biochemical defect has been identified. However, disturbances in enzyme function, disturbances in water and electrolyte balance, altered calcium ion concentration, hypertension, and accumulation of various "uremic toxins" have been implicated.

Diagnostic evaluation

The diagnosis of chronic renal failure is usually suspected on the basis of any of a number of manifestations, history of prior renal disease, and/or biochemical findings. The onset is usually gradual and the initial signs and symptoms vague and nonspecific.

Clinical manifestations. The first evidence of difficulty is usually loss of normal energy and increased fatigue on exertion. For example, the child may prefer quiet, passive activities rather than participation in more active games and outdoor play. The child is usually somewhat pale, but it is often so inconspicuous that the change may not be evident to parents or others. Sometimes the blood pressure is elevated. As the disease progresses, other manifestations may appear. The child eats less well (especially breakfast), shows less interest in normal activities, such as schoolwork or play, and has an increased urinary output and a compensatory intake of fluid. For example, a previously dry child may wet the bed at night. Pallor becomes more evident as the skin develops a characteristic sallow, muddy appearance as the result of anemia and deposition of urochrome pigment in the skin. The child may complain of headache, muscle cramps, and nausea. Other signs and symptoms include weight loss, facial puffiness, malaise, bone or joint pain, growth retardation, dryness or itching of the skin, bruised skin, and sometimes sensory or motor loss. Amenorrhea is common in adolescent girls.

The therapy is generally instigated prior to the appearance of the *uremic syndrome,* although there are occasions in which the symptoms may be observed. Manifestations of untreated uremia reflect the progressive nature of the homeostatic disturbances and general toxicity. Gastrointestinal symptoms include anorexia and nausea and vomiting. Bleeding tendencies are apparent in bruises, bloody diarrheal stools, stomatitis, and bleeding from lips and mouth. There is intractable itching, probably related to hyperparathyroidism, and deposits of urea crystals appear on the skin as "uremic frost." There may be an unpleasant "uremic" odor to the breath. Respirations become deeper as a result of metabolic acidosis, and circulatory overload is manifest by hypertension, congestive heart failure, and pulmonary edema. Neurologic involvement is reflected by progressive confusion, dulling of sensorium, and, ultimately, coma. Other signs may include tremors, muscular twitching, and seizures.

Laboratory data. Laboratory and other diagnostic tools and tests are of value in assessing the extent of renal damage, biochemical disturbances, and related physical dysfunction. Often they can help establish the nature of the underlying disease and differentiate between other disease processes and the pathologic consequences of renal dysfunction.

Medical management

In irreversible renal failure the goals of medical management are to promote effective renal function, to maintain body fluid and electrolyte balance within acceptable limits, to treat systemic complications, and to promote as active and normal a life as possible for the child for as long as possible.[11] This becomes increasingly difficult as the disease progresses toward its inevitable end. Even therapeutic measures designed to relieve one manifestation may prove detrimental to another. For example, antihypertensive agents may further impair renal function, and sodium bicarbonate given to correct acidosis may precipitate tetany.

Activity. The child is allowed unrestricted activity and to set his own limits regarding rest and extent of exertion. He is encouraged to attend school as long as he is able. When the effort is too great, home tutoring is arranged.

Diet. Regulation of diet is the most effective means, short of dialysis, for reducing the quantity of materials that require renal excretion. The goal of the diet in renal failure is to provide sufficient calories and protein for growth while limiting the excretory demands made on the kidney, to minimize metabolic bone disease (osteodystrophy), and to minimize fluid and electrolyte disturbances. Dietary phosphorus, principally the intake of cow's milk, is restricted. This reduces the excretory load on the kidneys, the phosphorus content in the diet, and one of the principal sources of metabolic acids. The limited protein should include foods high in essential amino acids; those foods with protein of lesser value can be omitted from the diet. Bottle-fed infants are placed on a low-protein, low-electrolyte formula with additional caloric supplements. When given with meals, substances that bind phosphorus in the intestines prevent its absorption and allow a more liberal intake of phosphorus-containing protein. Sodium and water are not usually limited, unless there is evidence of edema or hypertension, and potassium is not restricted. Restrictions of any or all three may be imposed in later stages or at any time at which factors cause abnormal serum concentrations.[6,11,17]

Osteodystrophy. Measures directed at prevention or correction of the calcium/phosphorus imbalance are reduction of dietary phosphorus, administration of a phosphorus-binding agent, provision of supplemental calcium, control of acidosis, and administration of vitamin D.

Dietary phosphorus is controlled by the reduction of protein and milk. Phosphorus levels can be further reduced by the oral administration of aluminum hydroxide gel (Amphojel) or tablets that combine with the phosphorus to decrease gastrointestinal absorption and, thus, the serum levels of phosphate. At the same time, serum calcium levels are increased with supplementary calcium preparations, calcium gluconate, calcium carbonate, or calcium lactate.

In addition to reducing the formation of metabolic acids by decreasing the dietary intake of protein, acidosis is alleviated by alkalizing agents such as sodium bicarbonate or a combination of sodium and potassium citrate (Shohl's solution*).[38] Correction of acidosis is best attempted after calcium levels are elevated, since rapid correction may precipitate tetany in a hypocalcemic child. When serum phosphate levels are within a normal range, vitamin D in increasing doses or the recently available and biologically more active dehydrotachysterol is administered to increase the absorption of calcium through the gastrointestinal tract.

Osseous deformities that result from renal osteodystrophy, especially those related to ambulation, are troublesome and require correction as soon as feasible. However, until the osteodystrophy is healed and under control, the deformities will recur.

Miscellaneous complications. Because the anemia associated with renal failure is related to decreased production of erythropoietin, it usually cannot be successfully managed with hematinic agents. However, sufficient sources of folic acid and iron should be provided in the diet, and iron losses that may occur should be replaced. Blood transfusions carry the risk of aggravating or precipitating cardiovascular disturbances and also tend to inhibit erythropoiesis. If needed for symptomatic anemia, packed red blood cells are given slowly over several hours.[11,30]

Hypertension of advanced renal disease may be managed initially by cautious use of a low-sodium diet, fluid restriction, and perhaps diuretics such as hydrochlorothiazide or furosemide. Severe hypertension requires the use of antihypertensive agents, usually reserpine, hydralazine, and methyldopa, singly or in combinations.

Intercurrent infections are treated with appropriate antimicrobials at the first sign of infection. Most of these drugs are excreted through the kidneys; therefore, the dosage is usually reduced in proportion to the decrease in renal function and the interval between doses extended in these children to avoid possible toxic effects from accumulation. Any drug eliminated through the kidneys is administered with caution. Other complications are treated symptomatically, for example, chlorpromazine (Thorazine) or prochlorperazine (Compazine) for nausea, anticonvulsants for seizures, and diphenhydramine (Benadryl) for pruritus.

Once symptoms of uremia appear in a child, the disease runs its relentless course and terminates in death in a few weeks, unless waste products and toxins are removed from

*Each milliliter of Shohl's solution contains 1 mEq of citrate ion, which metabolizes to yield 1 mEq of bicarbonate. Citric acid exerts no effect on acid-base balance but enhances the palatability of the mixture.

body fluids by dialysis and/or kidney transplantation. Since these techniques have been adapted for infants and small children, these alternatives are implemented in most cases of renal failure once palliative management is no longer effective.

Dialysis

Two methods of dialysis are currently available for clinical management of renal failure:

1. Peritoneal dialysis, wherein the abdominal cavity acts as a semipermeable membrane through which water and solutes of small molecular size move by osmosis and diffusion according to their respective concentrations on either side of the membrane
2. Hemodialysis, in which blood is circulated outside the body through artificial cellophane membranes that permit a similar passage of water and solutes

As a rule, hemodialysis is reserved for children who are in end-stage renal disease (ESRD), since it requires creation of a vascular access and special equipment. Peritoneal dialysis is preferred for children in acute renal failure, because it is usually a temporary therapy, is generally an emergency procedure, and, therefore, is more readily available, requires less expertise, and does not require specialized facilities.

Peritoneal dialysis. Peritoneal dialysis is used in children to treat a number of acute disorders as well as acute and chronic renal failure. Examples include such acute conditions as severe metabolic acidosis, accidental poisoning, intractable heart failure, hypernatremia, hyperkalemia, and hepatic coma. Although each child is assessed on an individual basis, indications for instituting dialysis in chronic renal failure are biochemical abnormalities such as blood urea nitrogen level greater than 150 mg/100 ml, serum bicarbonate concentration less than 12 mEq/liter, serum potassium concentration greater than 6 mEq/liter, and a falling hematocrit less than 20 ml/100 ml requiring transfusion in the face of the attendant hazards of hypertension and hyperkalemia.[5,11] Evidence of deteriorating central nervous system function and congestive heart failure that is unresponsive to other therapy is an indication for dialysis. Growth failure, severe osteodystrophy, insufficient caloric intake, and inability to carry out normal activities are sometimes criteria for dialysis. The only contraindication for use of peritoneal dialysis is intra-abdominal bleeding from a coagulation disorder.

After administration of an analgesic and local anesthetic, the abdomen is surgically prepared and a trochar and catheter are inserted through the anterior abdominal wall. The trochar is removed and the catheter maneuvered into the desired position. Any abdominal fluid is aspirated, after which commercially prepared dialysis solution is allowed to flow by gravity into the abdominal cavity where it remains while equilibration between plasma and the dialysis fluid takes place. The fluid then flows out by gravity drainage, and fresh dialysate is again instilled. Each pass generally takes about 1 hour: 15 minutes for the fluid to flow into the peritoneal cavity, 30 minutes for equilibration, and 15 minutes for removal. The procedure is usually continued for 48 hours, although a shorter time may suffice if it is being used to reduce hyperkalemia. After a period of 48 hours, the risk of peritoneal infection increases considerably. The catheter is removed and a sterile dressing applied. The procedure is repeated as needed until renal function is restored, poisons are reduced, or, in prolonged need, treatment is converted to hemodialysis.

The length of the dialysis period requires the child to remain relatively quiet for long periods of time, and the attendant risk of peritonitis makes peritoneal dialysis relatively unsuited to the long-term dialysis of chronic renal failure. Accidental perforation of bowel or bladder during trochar insertion is an added hazard.

Hemodialysis. Hemodialysis is better suited to long-term therapy, although, when facilities are available, it is sometimes used for prolonged episodes of acute renal failure to allow better dietary intake and minimize symptoms. Dialysis is absolutely essential in children with bilateral nephrectomies performed for intractable hypertension or bilateral neoplastic disease. Many children are being successfully managed on hemodialysis either as a maintenance procedure while awaiting kidney transplant or as a means in itself.[21]

Hemodialysis requires the use of special dialysis equipment—the hemodialyzer, or so-called artificial kidney. Hemodialyzers are available in three forms—coil, parallel flow (plate) and hollow fiber—but not all are suited to pediatric patients, especially those that require relatively large priming volumes. Experience has demonstrated that pediatric dialysis can be safely carried out when the fluid volume required to fill both hemodialyzer and blood tubing does not exceed 10% of the child's calculated blood volume. The parallel-flow hemodialyzer is most often preferred for children.

Hemodialysis also requires blood access by the establishment of an external or internal arteriovenous shunt created by implantation of a Teflon cannula in an artery and adjacent vein connected by an external loop of Silastic tubing. Recently special pediatric cannulas have been developed that allow an access route even in infants. The most common sites for cannula placement are the radial artery and a forearm vein (older children), brachial artery and cephalic vein (younger children), and the superficial femoral artery and the saphenous vein (very small children). Sometimes the posterior tibial artery and the long saphenous vein are used, especially for home dialysis. An alternative to the external Teflon shunt is the creation of a subcutaneous (internal) arteriovenous fistula by anastomosing a segment of a saphenous vein autograft or a bovine arterial xenograft to the brachial artery and brachiocephalic vein, which produces dilatation and thickening of the superficial vessels of the forearm to provide easy access for repeated venipuncture. There appear to be fewer complications and less restriction of activity with this approach; however, it requires needle insertion at each dialysis. Various hemodialysis schedules are employed, but most centers recommend dailysis three times a week for periods of 4 to 6 hours, depending on the size of the child.[11,21,27] For complete description of the highly specialized process of hemodialysis, the reader is directed to the numerous references available on this topic.

Dietary limitations are necessary in chronic dialysis in order to avoid biochemical complications and to facilitate adequate dialysis. Fluid and sodium are restricted in order to prevent fluid overload with its associated symptoms of hypertension, cerebral manifestations, and congestive heart failure. Potassium is restricted to prevent complications related to hyperkalemia, and phosphorus restriction helps to prevent parathyroid hyperactivity and its attendent risk of abnormal calcification deposits in soft tissues. Limited intake of protein reduces high levels of blood urea nitrogen. Fluid is usually limited to 500 $ml/m^2/day$ plus an amount equal to daily urine output.

Response to dialysis. Most children show rapid clinical improvement with the implementation of dialysis, although it is directly related to the duration of uremia prior to dialysis and the extent to which dietary regulations are adhered to. Growth rate and skeletal maturation usually improve, but recovery of normal growth is infrequent. In many cases sexual development, although delayed, has progressed to completion.[27]

Seizures during or after hemodialysis are not uncommon. The cause is uncertain, but they probably result from cerebral edema caused by alterations in osmolality in the brain when the blood urea nitrogen level is lowered rapidly. Hyponatremia may be a factor, also. Seizures are most likely to occur at the time dialysis is first initiated, when large changes in serum osmolality may occur.[11]

Home dialysis. With appropriate cannulization and proper training and education of both the child and the parents, hemodialysis can be performed at home. Time spent in transportation is eliminated, the environment is more pleasant and secure, and the child is able to assume a more active role in the treatment program. Home dialysis is especially advantageous for children who live a great distance from the dialysis center or who have had one or more kidney transplant failures.

Transplantation

Renal transplantation is now an acceptable and effective means of therapy in the pediatric age-group. The criteria for selection are quite liberal, but uniform criteria have not been established among the various centers that specialize in the procedure. Children who are excluded from most transplant programs are those with (1) significant mental retardation that would require continuous custodial care; (2) malignant disease that has metastasized, (3) active systemic fungal infection, and (4) coexistence of systemic disease with multisystem involvement. Many children with systemic disease and tumors have had successful transplants. On the other hand, there is a high incidence of recurrent disease in the donor kidney in children who receive a transplant for rapidly progressive glomerulonephritis with irreversible renal failure.[11,27]

Procedure. The kidney graft is placed in the extraperitoneal space, usually the anterior iliac fossa, and the renal artery is anastomosed to the internal iliac or hypogastric artery, the renal vein is anastomosed to the hypogastric vein, and the ureter is implanted into the bladder or anastomosed to the recipient's ureter. Small children receiving a large donor kidney may require placement within the abdomen with vessel anastomoses to the aorta and inferior vena cava. Unless there is medical contraindication, the recipient's failed kidneys are left in place. Severe hypertension, neoplasm, or immunologic glomerulonephritis with antibody formation against the recipient's kidney tissue are the usual causes for nephrectomy.

The primary goal in transplantation is the long-term survival of the grafted tissue. The means by which this is attempted is (1) securing tissues that are antigenically similar to that of the recipient and (2) suppressing the recipient's immune mechanism.

Selection of donor tissue. The source of a donor kidney is either a live person or a cadaver soon after death. The closer the genetic relationship between the donor and recipient, the better the possibility of long-term survival. The only truly compatible tissue match is that between identical twin siblings. The next best possible match is a sibling, then a parent, and finally an uncle or aunt. Use of siblings is impossible, however, until the possible donor is of age to give consent for removal of a kidney. Unrelated donors are least likely to be compatible. Careful studies are carried out to determine the donor whose kidney is least likely to be rejected by the recipient.

Suppression of the immune response. After the best possible tissue match is obtained for a transplant, the survival time can be significantly lengthened by suppressing the immune response of the recipient. The immunosuppressant therapy of choice in kidney transplantation includes azathioprine (Imuran) and prednisone. To a lesser extent cyclophosphamide and antilymphocyte globulin have been used in some centers.

The administration of these drugs is not without hazard. The major problem encountered with nonspecific immunosuppression is that it not only suppresses the immune response to the grafted tissue but also suppresses the body's capacity to respond to other antigenic stimuli. Consequently the child is vulnerable to overwhelming infections. The problem related to the toxic effect of azathioprine is mainly hepatic dysfunction, which is managed by reduced dosage or by substituting cyclophosphamide. A number of complications that are directly attributable to corticosteroid therapy are cause for concern in children on steroid therapy. Retardation of linear growth is always a problem, and in some centers alternate-day administration is being used in an effort to improve growth rates. Other corticosteroid-induced side effects may include the characteristic fat distribution of Cushing's syndrome, cataracts, and gastric ulcer. (See pp. 997 and 1016 for discussion of immunosuppressant therapy and related nursing care.)

Rejection. Rejection of a transplanted kidney is the most frequent cause of transplant failure. The rejection can be one of three types—hyperacute, acute, or chronic. Hyperacute rejection is irreversible, develops immediately or within a few hours after revascularization, and is related to circulating antibodies preformed in the recipient against the donor tissue antigens. These are seen in second transplants or in persons sensitized from blood transfusions.

Acute rejection usually occurs between the first few days and 6 months after transplantation but may occur as late as 1 or 2 years later. Rejection is evidenced by both biochemical and clinical abnormalities. The most frequent finding is fever, which is usually accompanied by swelling and tenderness over the graft, hypertension, and diminished urine output. A severe reaction may cause oliguria. Increases in serum blood urea nitrogen and creatinine levels are laboratory evidence of decreased transplant function. Most acute rejection episodes respond to intravenous administration of methyl-prednisolone sodium succinate (Solu-Medrol).

Chronic rejection is characterized by slow gradual deterioration of renal function that typically begins 6 months or more after transplantation. Evidence of rejection may be heralded by proteinuria and/or hematuria, and the rejection may have symptomatology indistinguishable from the original kidney disease. No present therapy can halt the progressive process, which inevitably leads to loss of the implanted kidney.

Nursing considerations

The child with chronic renal failure is a prime example of an individual whose life is maintained by drugs and artificial means, and the multiple stresses placed on these children and their families are often overwhelming. The unrelenting course of the disease process is one of progressive deterioration. There is no means to prevent the irreversible progress of renal insufficiency, nor is there any known cure. As the affected child progresses from renal insufficiency to uremia and then to hemodialysis and transplantation with a need for intensity of therapy, the need for supportive nursing care is also intensified. Team effort is more important than ever and involves coordination of personnel from medicine, nursing, social services, dietetics, and psychologic or psychiatric specialties.

Progressive disease places a number of stresses on the child and his family. There is continuing need for repeated examinations that often entail painful procedures, side effects, and frequent hospitalizations. Diet therapy becomes progressively more restricted and intense, and the child is required to take a variety of medications. Ever present in all aspects of the treatment regimen is the agonizing realization that without treatment death is the inevitable outcome.

End-stage renal disease presents the same nonspecific stresses on child and family as any other potentially fatal illness (see Chapter 27). The reactions and adaptation of the child and family depend on the age and developmental stage of the child, the cultural and socioeconomic background of the family, the quality of the interpersonal relationships of family members, and communication patterns within the family. In general the problems observed and emotional responses to the stress of the illness are influenced less by the nature of the illness than by the characteristics of the family relationships and the personalities of its members. In some families illness and stressful experiences act as a unifying force; in others stress aggravates preexisting problems and contributes to family disharmony.[20] Some specific stresses related to end-stage renal disease and its treatment are predictable. When it first becomes apparent that kidney failure is inevitable, both parents and child experience great depression and anxiety. Acceptance is particularly difficult if renal failure progresses rapidly after diagnosis. Denial and disbelief are usually pronounced, especially among parents. Once the kidney failure is established and symptoms become progressively more distressing, the initiation of hemodialysis is usually perceived as a positive experience, and, after the initial concerns of implementing the treatment, the child begins to feel better and parental anxiety is relieved for a time.[11]

Hemodialysis. Initiating a hemodialysis regimen is a traumatic and anxiety-provoking experience for most children. It involves surgery for implantation of the shunt or fistula, and the initial experience with the hemodialysis machine and its implication is frightening to most children. They need reassurance about the nature of the preparations for dialysis and conduct of the treatment. They are anxious concerning repeated venipunctures (with implanted shunts and for blood chemistries) and the sight of their blood leaving their body and entering the machine (see also p. 790. Once the initial fear of the machine has been resolved, younger children adjust fairly well to maintenance hemodialysis.

Adolescents, with their increased need for independence

and their urge for rebellion, usually adapt less well. They resent the control and enforced dependence imposed by the rigorous and unrelenting therapy program. They resent being dependent on a machine, parents, and professional staff. Depression, hostility, or both are common in adolescents undergoing hemodialysis. The adverse effects of the disease include diet restrictions, limitations to physical activity (resulting from lack of energy, frequent illnesses, and specific restrictions related to the shunt, such as forbidden swimming with an external shunt), and simply the sense of being different from other children. Withdrawal from peers and social isolation are the rule. Depression, hostility, and noncompliance are not uncommon in the adolescent.[15]

Body changes related to the disease process, such as growth retardation, skin color, and lack of sexual maturation, are stress provoking. Dietary restrictions are particularly burdensome for both children and parents. Children feel deprived when unable to eat foods previously enjoyed and unrestricted for other family members. Consequently failure to cooperate is not uncommon. Diet restrictions are interpreted as punishment and, since they may not be able to fully understand the purpose of restrictions, some will sneak forbidden food items at every opportunity. Allowing children, especially adolescents, maximum participation in and responsibility for their own treatment program is helpful. The extent of compliance and adjustment depend on the personalities of the involved persons, the quality of the relationships, and their coping mechanisms.

After weeks or months of hemodialysis, parents and child feel anxiety associated with the prognosis and continued pressures of the treatment. The relentless need for treatment interferes with family plans. Transportation to and from the dialysis unit and the time spend on the machine cut into time for outside activities, including school. Shunt and fistula problems are not uncommon and present a common source of aggravation. Shunts and fistulas are prone to infection and are easily subject to clogging, which may necessitate further surgery. The occurrence of seizures during dialysis is highly stressful to both child and family. Eventually most severely affected children face nephrectomy, which predictably causes depression in both child and family. Most families have maintained some hope throughout dialysis, but imminent nephrectomy necesitates final acceptance of the diagnosis.[15]

Transplantation. The possibility of renal transplantation often comes as a hope for relief from the rigors of hemodialysis and the hated diet restrictions. Except for children with preexisting personality problems or residual physical disabilities, most children and families respond well to kidney transplant and the majority return to normal life within a year after surgery.[11] The dynamics related to accepting and donating kidneys are fraught with emotional overtones, caused in part by the issues related to the child's receiving an organ from another person. A variety of serious emotional and psychologic conflicts may arise as a consequence of donor selection, including ambivalence of donors faced with surgery and relinquishing a kidney, feelings of guilt if one should prove to be unacceptable as a donor, and the emotional impact of having a live-relative donated kidney rejected by the recipient. This is especially guilt producing when a parent is the donor.

The child recipient responds in various ways to kidney transplant. The concept of having a foreign body, especially a cadaver kidney, inside their own body is sometimes disturbing to children. They often speculate about the age, sex, personality, and physical characteristics of the donor. They may fear that the kidney will wear out if it came from an older person. Corticosteroid therapy, necessary in kidney transplants, creates undesirable side effects, for example, growth failure, obesity, characteristics of Cushing's syndrome, acne, and hirsutism, that are frequently a source of emotional and social problems for older children. The cosmetic implications of these side effects can be overwhelming, especially to adolescent girls. Deliberate discontinuation of the drugs is most commonly observed in teen-age girls.[20]

Working with children and their families during the various stages of renal failure, dialysis, and transplantation is a difficult and challenging experience. Nurses must become familiar with the family, assess their strengths, weaknesses, and coping mechanisms, and be prepared to provide intensive support and guidance during the prolonged experience. The child and family need help in accepting what is happening to them, anticipating guidance regarding predictable stresses, and dealing constructively with the physical, emotional, and financial burdens that are an ongoing part of this prolonged disability.

REFERENCES

1. Arneil, G. C.: Management of the nephrotic syndrome in the child. In Lieberman, E.: Clinical pediatric nephrology, Philadelphia, 1976, J. B. Lippincott Co.
2. Bauman, J. W., Jr., and Chinard, F. P.: Renal function. Physiologic and medical aspects, St. Louis, 1975, The C. V. Mosby Co.
3. Beale, M. G., and associates: Renal osteodystrophy, Pediatr. Clin. North Am. **23:**873-884, 1976.
4. Betts, P. R., and Magrath, G.: Growth pattern and dietary intake of children with chronic renal insufficiency, Br. Med. J. **2:**189, 1974.
5. Chan, J. C. M., and Campbell, R. A.: Peritoneal dialysis in children: a survey of its indication and applications, Clin. Pediatr. **12:**131, 1974.
6. Drummond, K. N.: The urinary system. In Vaughn, V. C., and McKay, R. J., editors: Nelson's textbook of pediatrics, ed. 10, Philadelphia, 1975, W. B. Saunders Co.
7. Edelmann, C. M., Jr.: Pathophysiology of chronic renal failure. In Winters, R. W., editor: The body fluids in pediatrics, Boston, 1973, Little, Brown and Co.

8. Finnerty, F. A.: Hypertensive encephalopathy, Am. J. Med. **52:**672, 1972.

9. Ganong, W. F.: Review of medical physiology, ed. 8, Los Altos, Calif., 1977, Lange Medical Publications.

10. Gordillo-Paniagua, G., and Velasquez-Jones, L.: Acute renal failure, Pediatr. Clin. North Am. **23:**817-828, 1976.

11. James, J. A.: Renal disease in childhood, ed. 3, St. Louis, 1976, The C. V. Mosby Co.

12. Johnson, H. K., and associates: Nursing care of the patient with acute renal failure, Nurs. Clin. North Am. **10:**421-430, 1975.

13. Kaplan, B. S., Chesney, R. W., and Drummond, K. N.: Hemolytic uremic syndrome in families, N. Engl. J. Med. **292:**1090, 1975.

14. Kaplan, B. S., Thomson, P. D., and de Chadarevian, J.: The hemolytic uremic syndrome, Pediatr. Clin. North Am. **23:** 761-776, 1976.

15. Korsch, B., and associates: Experiences with children and their families during extended hemodialysis and kidney transplantation, Pediatr. Clin. North Am. **18:**625-637, 1971.

16. Lewy, J. E.: Acute poststreptococcal glomerulonephritis, Pediatr. Clin. North Am. **23:**751-760, 1976.

17. Lewy, P. R., and Hurley, J. K.: Chronic renal failure, Pediatr. Clin. North Am. **23:**829-842, 1976.

18. Lewy, J. E., and New, M. I.: Growth in children with renal failure, Am. J. Med. **58:**65, 1975.

19. Lieberman, E.: Acute renal failure. In Lieberman, E., editor: Clinical pediatric nephrology, Philadelphia, 1976, J. B. Lippincott Co.

20. Malekzadeh, M. H., and associates: Current issues in pediatric renal transplantation, Pediatr. Clin. North Am. **23:**857-872, 1976.

21. Mauer, S. M., and Lynch, R. E.: Hemodialysis techniques for infants and children, Pediatr. Clin. North Am. **23:**843-856, 1976.

22. McDonald, B. M., and McEnery, P. T.: Glomerulonephritis in children: clinical and morphologic characteristics and mechanisms of glomerular injury, Pediatr. Clin. North Am. **23:**691-706, 1976.

23. McIntosh, R. M., Moon, J. B., and O'Brien, D.: Kidney and urinary tract. In Kempe, C. H., Silver, H. K., and O'Brien, D.: Current pediatric diagnosis and treatment, ed. 5, Los Altos, Calif., 1978, Lange Medical Publications.

24. Morse, T. M.: Renal injuries, Pediatr. Clin. North Am. **22:** 379-392, 1975.

25. Orloff, J., and Burg, M. B.: Vasopressin-resistant diabetes insipidus. In Stanbury, J. B., Wyngaarden, J. B., and Fredrickson, D. S., editors: The metabolic bases of inherited disease, ed. 3, New York, 1972, McGraw-Hill Book Co.

26. Orloff, S., Potter, D. E., and Holliday, M. A.: Acute renal failure. In Smith, C. A., editor: The critically ill child, ed. 2, Philadelphia, 1977, W. B. Saunders Co.

27. Potter, D.: Management of the child on chronic dialysis. In Lieberman, E., editor: Clinical pediatric nephrology, Philadelphia, 1976, J. B. Lippincott Co.

28. Rance, C. P., Arbus, G. S., and Balfe, J. W.: Management of the nephrotic syndrome in children, Pediatr. Clin. North Am. **23:**735-750, 1976.

29. Rodriguez-Soriano, J.: The renal regulation of acid-base balance and the disturbances noted in renal tubular acidosis, Pediatr. Clin. North Am. **18:**529-545, 1971.

30. Roy, S., III, and Arant, B. S.: Nephrology. In Hughes, J. G.: Synopsis of pediatrics, ed. 4, St. Louis, 1975, The C. V. Mosby Co.

31. Schulman, J. D., and Schneider, J. A.: Cystinosis and the Fanconi syndrome, Pediatr. Clin. North Am. **23:**779-795, 1976.

32. Scriver, C. R.: Rickets and the pathogenesis of impaired tubular transport of phosphate and other solutes, Am. J. Med. **57:**43, 1974.

33. Travis, L. B., Dodge, W. F., and Dalschner, C. W., Jr.: Nephritis. In Ziai, M., editor: Pediatrics, ed. 2, Boston, 1975, Little, Brown and Co.

34. Travis, L. B., and associates: Acute glomerulonephritis in children: a review of the natural history with emphasis on prognosis, Clin. Nephrol. **1:**169, 1973.

35. Treser, G., and associates: Partial characterization of antigenic streptococcal plasma membrane components in acute glomerulonephritis, J. Clin. Invest. **49:**762, 1970.

36. Tune, B. M., Leavitt, T. J., and Gribble, T. J.: The hemolytic-uremic syndrome in California: a review of 28 nonheparinized cases with long-term follow-up, J. Pediatr. **82:** 304, 1973.

37. Van Wierigen, P. M. V., Monnens, L. A. H., and Schretlen, E. D. A. M.: Hemolytic uremic syndrome, epidemiological and clinical study, Arch. Dis. Child. **49:**432, 1974.

38. Williams, G. S., Klenk, E. L., and Winters, R. W.: Acute renal failure in pediatrics. In Winters, R. W., editor: The body fluids in pediatrics, Boston, 1973, Little, Brown and Co.

BIBLIOGRAPHY

Brundage, D. J.: Nursing management of renal problems, St. Louis, 1976, The C. V. Mosby Co.

Burton, B. T.: Current concepts of nutrition and diet in disease of the kidney, J. Am. Diet. Assoc. **65:**623-633, 1974.

Cannon, P. J.: Diuretic therapy in patients with renal disease. In Winter, R. W., editor: The body fluids in pediatrics, Boston, 1973, Little Brown and Co.

Chan, J. C. M., editor: Symposium on pediatric nephrology, Pediatr. Clin. North Am. **23**(4), November 1976.

Edelmann, C. M., editor: Symposium on pediatric nephrology, Pediatr. Clin. North Am. **18**(2), May 1971.

Fennell, S. E.: Percutaneous renal biopsy, Am. J. Nurs. **75:**1292-1294, 1975.

Goldman, H. S., and Freeman, L. M.: Radiographic and radioisotopic methods of evaluation of the kidneys and urinary tract, Pediatr. Clin. North Am. **18:**409-434, 1971.

Gottschalk, C. W., and Lassiter, W. E.: Mechanisms of urine formation. In Mountcastle, V. B., editor: Medical physiology, ed. 13, St. Louis, 1974, The C. V. Mosby Co.

Gottschalk, C. W., and Lassiter, W. E.: Urine formation in the diseased kidney. In Mountcastle, V. B., editor: Medical physiology, ed. 13, St. Louis, 1974, The C. V. Mosby Co.

Guyton, A. C.: Textbook of medical physiology, ed. 5., Philadelphia, 1976, W. B. Saunders Co.

Haughey, E. J., and Sica, F. M.: Diuretics. How safe can you make them? Nursing '77 **7**(2):33-39, 1977.

Leonard, M.: Health issues and primary nursing in nephrology care, Nurs. Clin. North Am. **10:**413-420, 1975.

Lieberman, E., editor: Clinical pediatric nephrology, Philadelphia, 1976, J. B. Lippincott Co.

Loggie, J. M. H., Kleinman, L. I., and Van Maanen, E. F.: Renal function and diuretic therapy in infants and children, J. Pediatr. **86:**485, 657, 1975.

McCrory, W. W., and associates: Studies of renal function in children with chronic hydronephrosis, Pediatr. Clin. North Am. **18:** 445-465, 1971.

Northway, J. D.: Hematuria in children, J. Pediatr. **78:**381, 1971.

Rubin, M. J., and Barratt, T. M., editors: Pediatric nephrology, Baltimore, 1975, The Williams & Wilkins Co.

Rudolph, A. M., Barnett, H. L., and Einhorn, A. H., editors: Pediatrics, ed. 16, New York, 1977, Appleton-Century-Crofts.

Schumann, D.: Tips for improving urine testing techniques, Nursing '76 **6:**23, 1976.

Steele, S.: Nursing care of the child with kidney problems. In Steele, S., editor: Nursing care of the child with long-term illness, New York, 1971, Appleton-Century-Crofts.

Strauss, J.: Pediatric nephrology, New York, 1974, Stratton Inter-Continental Medical Book Corporation.

Strauss, M. B., and Welt, L. G., editors: Diseases of the kidney, ed. 2, Boston, 1971, Little, Brown and Co.

Tilkian, S. M., and Conover, M. H.: Clinical implications of laboratory tests, St. Louis, 1975, The C. V. Mosby Co.

Widmann, F. K.: Goodale's clinical interpretation of laboratory tests, ed. 7, Philadelphia, 1973, F. A. Davis Co.

Winter, C. C., and Morel, A.: Nursing care of patients with urologic diseases, ed. 4, St. Louis, 1977, The C. V. Mosby Co.

Ziai, M., editor: Pediatrics, ed. 2, Boston, 1975, Little, Brown and Co.

Ziegler, E., and Foman, S.: Fluid intake renal solute load, water balance in infancy, J. Pediatr. **78:**561, 1971.

Renal diseases

Arneil, G.: The nephrotic syndrome, Pediatr. Clin. North Am. **18:**547-559, 1971.

Balsan, S.: Renal osteodystrophy. In Lieberman, E.: Clinical pediatric nephrology, Philadelphia, 1976, J. B. Lippincott Co.

Bernstein, J.: Heritable cystic disorders of the kidney: the mythology of polycystic disease, Pediatr. Clin. North Am. **18:**435-444, 1971.

Blount, M., and Kinney, A.: Chronic steroid therapy, Am. J. Nurs. **74:**1626, 1974.

Dillon, H. C., and Reeves, M. S.: Streptococcal immune responses in nephritis after skin infection, Am. J. Med. **56:**333, 1974.

Dobrin, R. S., and associates: The critically ill child: acute renal failure, Pediatrics **48:**286-291, 1971.

Dodge, W. F., and associates: Poststreptococcal glomerulonephritis—a prospective study in children, N. Engl. J. Med. **286:** 273, 1972.

Edelmann, C. M., Jr.: Renal tubular acidosis. In Winter, R. W., editor: The body fluids in pediatrics, Boston, 1973, Little, Brown and Co.

Etteldorf, J. N., and Shane, R., III: Noninfectious disorder of the urinary system. In Shirkey, H. C., editor: Pediatric therapy, ed. 5, St. Louis, 1975, The C. V. Mosby Co.

Hekelman, F. P., and Ostendarp, C. A.: Nursing approaches to conservative management of renal disease, Nurs. Clin. North Am. **10:**431-434, 1975.

Lewis, E. J., and Couser, W. G.: The immunologic basis of human renal disease, Pediatr. Clin. North Am. **18:**467-507, 1971.

Lewy, J. E.: Treatment of acute glomerulonephritis in children. In Lieberman, E.: Clinical pediatric nephrology, Philadelphia, 1976, J. B. Lippincott Co.

Lieberman, E.: Hemolytic-uremic syndrome, J. Pediatr. **80:**1, 1972.

Morse, T. S., and Harris, B. H.: Nonpenetrating renal vascular injuries, J. Trauma **13:**497, 1973.

Nash, M. A., and associates: Renal tubular acidosis in infants and children: clinical course, response to treatment and prognosis, J. Pediatr. **80:**738, 1972.

Riley, C. M.: Nephrosis. In Shirkey, H. C., editor: Pediatric therapy, ed. 5, St. Louis, 1975, The C. V. Mosby Co.

Rodriguez-Soriano, J., and associates: Distal renal tubular acidosis in infancy: a bicarbonate-wasting state, J. Pediatr. **86:**524, 1975.

Siegel, N. J., and associates: Long-term follow-up of children with steroid-responsive nephrotic syndrome, J. Pediatr. **81:** 251, 1972.

Smith, F. G., Jr., and associates: The nephrotic syndrome: current concepts, Ann. Intern. Med. **76:**463, 1972.

Spitzer, A.: Renal physiology. Impact of recent developments on clinical nephrology, Pediatr. Clin. North Am. **18:**377-393, 1971.

Stickler, G. B.: Growth failure in renal disease, Pediatr. Clin. North Am. **23:**885-894, 1976.

Trygstad, C. W., and Anand, S. K.: Glomerulonephritis in childhood, Curr. Probl. Pediatr. **2:**3, 1972.

Tune, B. M.: The hemolytic-uremic syndrome. In Lieberman, E.: Clinical pediatric nephrology, Philadelphia, 1976, J. B. Lippincott Co.

Renal failure

Bricker, N. S., and associates: The pathophysiology of renal insufficiency, Pediatr. Clin. North Am. **18:**595-611, 1971.

Chan, J. C. M.: Acute renal failure in children: principles of management, Clin. Pediatr. **13:**686, 1974.

Chesney, R. W., and associates: Acute renal failure: an important complication of caridac surgery in infants, J. Pediatr. **87:**381, 1975.

Fearing, M. O.: Osteodystrophy in patients with chronic renal failure, Nurs. Clin. North Am. **10:**461-468, 1975.

Flamenbaum, W.: Pathophysiology of acute renal failure, Arch. Intern. Med. **131:**911, 1973.

Gentile, D. E.: Management of renal failure. In Zschoche, D. A., editor: Mosby's comprehensive review of critical care, St. Louis, 1976, The C. V. Mosby Co.

Holliday, M. A.: Calorie deficiency in children with uremia; effect upon growth, Pediatrics **50:**71, 1972.

Holliday, M. A., Potter, D. E., and Dobrin, R. S.: Treatment of renal failure in children, Pediatr. Clin. North Am. **18:**613-624, 1971.

Jain, R.: Acute renal failure in the neonate, Pediatr. Clin. North Am **24:**605-618, 1977.

Schrier, R. W.: Acute renal failure, diagnosis, management, and pathogenesis, Calif. Med. **115:**28-37, 1971.

Dialysis and transplantation

Bernstein, D. M.: After transplantation—the child's emotional reactions, Am. J. Psychiatry **127:**1189, 1971.

Cummings, J. W.: The pressure and how patients respond, Am. J. Nurs. **70:**70-76, 1970.

Dolan, P. O., and Greene, H. L., Jr.: Renal failure and peritoneal dialysis, Nursing '75 **5**(7):41-49, 1975.

Donley, D. L.: Nursing the patient who is immuno-suppressed, Am. J. Nurs. **76:**1619-1625, 1976.

Fine, R. N., and associates: Renal homotransplantation in children, J. Pediatr. **76:**356, 1970.

Fine, R. N., and associates: Renal transplantation in young children, Am. J. Surg. **125:**559, 1973.

Hassett, M.: Teaching hemodialysis to the family unit, Nurs. Clin. North Am. **7:**349, 1972.

Juliani, L., and Reamer, B.: Kidney transplant: your role in aftercare, Nursing '77 **7**(10):46-53, 1977.

Khan, A. V., and associates: Social and emotional adaptations of children with transplanted kidneys and chronic hemodialysis, Am. J. Psychiatry **127:**1197, 1971.

Kobrzycki, P.: Renal transplant complications, Am. J. Nurs. **77:**641-643, 1977.

Korsch, B. M., and associates: Kidney transplantation in children: psychosocial follow-up study on child and family, J. Pediatr. **83:**399, 1973.

Kossoris, P.: Family therapy. An adjunct to hemodialysis and transplantation, Am. J. Nurs. **70:**1730-1733, 1970.

Melber, S., Leonard, M., and Primack, W.: Hemodialysis at camp, Am. J. Nurs. **76:**935-938, 1976.

Mofenson, H. C., and Greensher, J.: Peritoneal dialysis. An outline of the procedure, Clin. Pediatr. **11:**534, 1972.

Potter, D., and associates: Treatment of chronic uremia in childhood. I. Transplantation, Pediatrics **45:**432, 1970.

Potter, D., and associates: Treatment of chronic uremia in childhood. II. Hemodialysis, Pediatrics **46:**678, 1970.

Read, M., and Mallison, M.: External arteriovenous shunts, Am. J. Nurs. **72:**81-85, 1972.

Schlotter, L.: What do you teach the dialysis patient? Am. J. Nurs. **70:**82-83, 1970.

Schumann, D.: The renal donor, Am. J. Nurs. **74:**105-110, 1974.

Smith, L. J.: Large surface area dialysis, Nurs. Clin. North Am. **10:**481-490, 1975.

Topor, M. A.: Kidney transplantation especially in pediatric patients, Nurs. Clin. North Am. **10:**503-516, 1975.

Wheeler, D.: Teaching home-dialysis for an eight-year-old boy, Am. J. Nurs. **77:**273-274, 1977.

Wiley, M.: Care of the patient with a kidney transplant, Nurs. Clin. North Am. **8:**127, 1973.

Wilson, C. J., Potter, D. E., and Holliday, M. A.: Treatment of the uremic child. In Winters, R. W., editor: The body fluids in pediatrics, Boston, 1973, Little, Brown and Co.

Wolf, Z. R.: What patients awaiting kidney transplant want to know, Am. J. Nurs. **76:**92-94, 1976.

UNIT THIRTEEN

The child with problems related to the transfer of oxygen and nutrients

The survival of an individual depends on a continuous supply of energy for maintaining the function of all the cells in the body. This energy is obtained through oxygen and nutrients incorporated by the body and converted to energy by the process of oxygenation-reduction. Any circumstance or condition that requires an increase in energy requires a concomitant increase in the materials that the body converts into energy.

The need for oxygen is most acute and, without this vital substance, the body is unable to survive more than a few minutes without permanent damage to vital structures or death. Therefore, oxygen must be supplied constantly. Nutrients and water, on the other hand, can be stored within the body for use at times of increased need or diminished supply.

Alterations in the ability to supply oxygen or nutrients are some of the most common health problems of childhood. Interference with respiratory and gastrointestinal function is encountered at all ages, but very young children are especially vulnerable to dysfunctions in these systems. Respiratory and gastrointestinal disorders are encountered most frequently and the effects are more serious in children in the younger age-groups. Chapters 32, *The Child with a Disturbance of Oxygen and Carbon Dioxide Exchange,* and 33, *Conditions with Disturbed Respiratory Function,* describe the more common conditions that impair the exchange of oxygen and carbon dioxide. Chapter 34, *The Child with a Gastrointestinal Disorder,* is concerned with factors that interfere with digestion or absorption of body nutrients. There are other situations in which there are disturbances in the availability of oxygen and nutrients for energy, for example, diabetes mellitus and disorders of fluid and electrolyte balance, but these are more appropriately discussed elsewhere.

32

The child with a disturbance of oxygen and carbon dioxide exchange

Disorders involving the respiratory tract, many of which can be life-threatening, are very common in infancy and childhood. A number of factors influence the development of respiratory disease in infancy and childhood. To better understand the way in which pathologic processes produce an effect, the basic anatomy and physiology of the respiratory tract are reviewed. The physiologic responses are no different in the child than in the adult, for example, gas exchange, oxygen and carbon dioxide tension, and the activity of chemoreceptors are very much the same in children and in adults. Anatomically, however, there are a number of differences that influence the way in which children respond to respiratory disturbances. Some have been mentioned relative to overall childhood growth and development (p. 63), whereas others have been discussed in relation to the normal newborn (p. 256).

REVIEW OF RESPIRATORY FUNCTION

The primary responsibility of the respiratory system is to distribute air and exchange gases so that cells are supplied with oxygen for body metabolism and the volatile product of the metabolism (carbon dioxide) is removed. The organs of the respiratory system—nose, pharynx, larynx, trachea, bronchi, and lungs—provide the means whereby gases enter the body; the circulatory system distributes gases to and from the millions of cells throughout the body. All the structures of the respiratory system, except the minute air sacs (alveoli) of the lung tissue, function in air distribution. It is within the alveoli that the gas exchange takes place.

Structure

The thoracic cavity, which is encased in the bony framework provided by the ribs, vertebrae, and sternum, consists of three major partitions: the three-lobed lung on the right, the two-lobed lung on the left, and the space between them—the mediastinum, which contains the esophagus, trachea, large blood vessels, and heart. The entire thoracic cavity is lined by the smooth parietal pleura, which adheres to the ribs and superior surface of the diaphragm. Each lung is encased in a separate visceral pleural sac that, when inflated, lies against the parietal pleura. Normally the two pleural membranes are separated by only enough fluid to lubricate the surfaces for painless movement during filling and emptying of the lungs. In disease states this space may contain air (pneumothorax), fluid (hydrothorax), or pleural effusion of blood (hemothorax). Inflammation of the pleura causes the painful friction of pleurisy.

The shape of the chest changes gradually from a relatively round configuration at birth to one that is more or less flattened in the anteroposterior diameter in adulthood (Fig. 32-1). In severe obstructive lung disease the anteroposterior measurement approaches the transverse measurement. Periodic measurements provide clues to the course of lung disease or the efficacy of therapy.

The elliptic shape of the ribs and the angle at which they are attached to the spine allow the thorax to change size during respiration. Contraction of the intercostal muscles lifts the ribs from a downward angle to a more horizontal angle, which increases both the anteroposterior and lateral dimensions of the chest. This also changes the diameter of the bronchi. The diameter increases during inspiration and decreases during expiration—an important factor when the bronchi are narrowed as a result of obstruction or inflammation. Contraction and relaxation of the diaphragm cause the chest cavity to lengthen and shorten, which also increases the volume of the chest cavity during inspiration. Normal expiration is passive, although contraction of the internal intercostal muscles pulls the rib cage downward and contraction of the abdominal muscles forces the diaphragm upward to decrease the chest size actively. The ribs of the newborn infant articulate with the spine at a horizontal rather than a downward slope, preventing the "bucket-handle" type of respiratory motion seen at a later age. Therefore, the chest size is altered little during inspiration (see p. 256) and breathing in the newborn is diaphragmatic.

Also facilitating respiration are (1) the elastic properties of lung tissue, which allow them to expand with increasing volume (compliance) and to collapse away from the

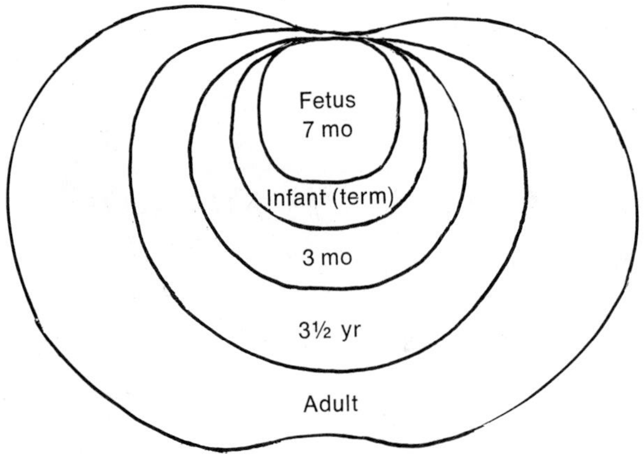

Fig. 32-1. Changes in chest shape with age.

pleural wall with decreased volume (elastic recoil), and (2) the presence of a lipoprotein (surfactant) layer at the air-fluid interface, which allows even alveolar expansion and prevents alveolar collapse. Compliance also changes with age. It is very high in the newborn, facilitated in part by a more pliant rib cage. Factors that interefere with compliance and recoil increase the work of respiration, for example, a deficiency of surfactant in respiratory distress syndrome (see p. 343) or reduced compliance from fibrotic changes as a result of chronic lung disorders such as cystic fibrosis (p. 1252) and chronic asthma (p. 1241).

Airways. The rigid nasal structures, which are lined with ciliated mucous membranes, serve as passageways for air, warming and moistening air and filtering it of impurities. In infancy the nasal passages are narrow, and infants are obligatory nose-breathers, which substantially increases airway resistance. Any factor that decreases the size of the passages and further increases airway resistance, such as nasal mucosal swelling and mucous accumulation, hampers the breathing and feeding of infants. The *pharynx* is also a passageway for the entry and exit of air, but in addition it plays a role in phonation by helping produce vowel sounds. The pharynx contains the palantine and lingual tonsils (see p. 572), which play an important role in infection control.

The *larynx,* situated at the upper end of the trachea, is constructed of a rigid circular framework of cartilage and contains the epiglottis and the glottis (vocal cords). These structures prevent solids or liquids from entering the airway during swallowing, and the vibrations of the vocal cords produce voice sounds. In infancy the glottis is located more cephalad than in later childhood and the laryngeal reflexes are very active. The epiglottis is longer and projects further posteriorly.[5] The narrowest portion of the larynx is at the level of the cricoid cartilage. In the infant and young child the ciliated columnar epithelium below the vocal cords is loosely bound with areolar tissue and is, therefore, more susceptible to edema formation.[9] Swelling of the glottis and epiglottis produces hoarseness and, often, life-threatening obstruction of this narrow portion of the airway (croup).

The *trachea,* which is composed of smooth muscle supported by C-shaped rings of cartilage, ensures an open airway to the bronchi and lungs. The trachea divides into two *primary bronchi,* the right one situated slightly more vertical than the left, which causes aspirated objects to lodge more frequently in the right bronchus. Each bronchus enters the lung on its respective side where it divides into *secondary bronchi* that continue to branch and divide into progressively smaller *bronchioles.* The entire bronchial tree is lined with mucous membrane and is composed of spiral smooth muscle supported by rings of cartilage. As the bronchioles become smaller the cartilaginous rings become increasingly irregular and then disappear completely in the smallest bronchioles, the walls of which consist of only a single layer of cells.

The airways of the newborn have very little smooth muscle, but in children 4 to 5 months of age they contain sufficient muscle to cause narrowing in response to irritating stimuli. Smooth muscle development and reactivity are comparable to that in the adult by 1 year of age.[5] Growth of the respiratory system follows the general growth curve during the early weeks of life, but the airways grow faster than the thoracic and cervical portions of the vertebral column. Consequently the larynx and trachea descend in relation to the upper spine. For example, the bifurcation of the trachea that lies opposite the third thoracic vertebra in the infant descends to a position opposite the fourth in adulthood. Likewise, the cricoid cartilage descends from a position opposite the fourth cervical vertebra in the infant to opposite the sixth cervical vertebra in the adult. The function of the tracheobronchial tree is to distribute air to the alveoli of the lung. A variety of diseases and conditions, such as mucosal swelling, muscular contraction, and mechanical obstruction by mucus or a foreign body, can cause localized or generalized airway occlusion.

Respiratory units.[7,8,9] The two cone-shaped structures, the *lungs,* consist of the bronchi, bronchioles, and innumerable small air sacs, or *alveoli.* It is through these thin-walled structures that gas exchange takes place between the inspired air and the bloodstream. The amount of gas exchanged depends on many factors, for example, the amount and composition of air inhaled, the thickness of the alveolar wall, adequacy of circulation to the alveoli, and substances within the alveoli that either prevent their inflation (the surface-active substance surfactant) or prevent gas exchange, such as fluids.

The major changes that take place in the respiratory system with age are in the number and size of alveoli and in the increased branching of terminal bronchioles. Whereas the number of conducting airways is complete early in fetal life, the air sacs are shallow and wide necked but have few septa at birth. This promotes patency but limits surface area for gas exchange. As the child grows, the peripheral bronchioles continue to branch and the alveoli grow in size. They also develop septa that partition and divide existing alveoli to increase their number. It is unclear when septal division ceases and an increase in size begins. It appears to occur sometime during middle childhood, although there is evidence to indicate that an increase in number of alveoli for each terminal airway takes place at puberty. Also, collateral pathways of ventilation develop, including pores through alveolar walls and, possibly, pathways between bronchioles. All of these factors have significance for respiratory disorders in young children; infants and young children have less alveolar surface area for gas exchange, the narrow branching peripheral airways become easily obstructed, and lack of collateral pathways inhibits ventilation beyond obstructed units. Consequently young children are more readily subject to obstruction and atelectasis, especially as a result of repeated infection.

Ventilation

Ventilation takes place as air moves in and out of the lungs as the result of changes in pressure gradients created by changes in the size of the thoracic cavity. Contraction of the diaphragm and external intercostal muscles increases the size of the thorax and decreases the intrathoracic pressure. As a result, air moves from the atmosphere, which has a higher pressure, into the lungs, which have a lower pressure. The principles of artificial ventilation are based on this concept. Artificial respiratory devices increase the pressure entering the air passages (positive-pressure breathing devices), lower the pressure around the body (iron lung, negative-pressure ventilator), or increase the negative pressure within the thoracic cavity (rocking bed). The shorter abdominal length of infants makes this latter method ineffectual for them.

The alveoli are surrounded by pulmonary capillaries, and, in most areas of the lung, the membranes that separate these structures are exceedingly thin. The gas exchange takes place by simple diffusion in the alveoli; gas in other parts of the respiratory tract is unavailable for exchange with capillary blood.

The diameter of the airways and, thus, the air flow are determined by the balance of forces that tend to widen or narrow the airways. One of these is neural regulation of bronchial smooth muscles mediated through autonomic nerves. Sympathetic impulses relax the airways; parasympathetic impulses constrict them. Reflex constriction occurs in response to irritating inhalants such as dust, smoke, or sulfur dioxide; arterial hypoxemia and hypercapnea; cold air; and some drugs, such as acetylcholine and histamine.[4] These factors are discussed further in relation to bronchial asthma (p. 1241). Other factors that alter airway size are peribronchial pressure, which tends to narrow the airways, and intraluminal pressure, which tends to keep airways open. For example, forced expiration causes increased peribronchial pressure and, hence, narrowing of the airways; positive pressure breathing apparatus increases intraluminal pressure, keeping airways open.

Gas exchange. The exchange of gases in the lungs takes place between the alveolar air and the capillary blood. The amount of alveolar ventilation must be adequate to keep the Po_2 and Pco_2 at values that promote the escape of carbon dioxide from pulmonary capillaries and uptake of oxygen from the alveoli. Each gas moves in both directions through the alveolar-capillary membrane by diffusion in accordance with the pressure gradient for each gas. The pressure gradients of the gases between alveolar air and pulmonary blood cause outward diffusion of carbon dioxide from lung capillary blood and inward diffusion of oxygen from alveolar air. This exchange lowers the Pco_2 and raises the Po_2, converting the blood from its venous to its arterial saturation. In health arterial Po_2 is approximately 95 to 100 mm Hg and arterial Pco_2 is 40 mm Hg.

Since carbon dioxide diffuses twenty-one times faster than oxygen, there is no impairment of diffusion for carbon dioxide from the blood to the alveoli. The amount of oxygen that diffuses into the blood depends on several factors, including (1) the pressure gradient between alveolar air and capillary blood—when the oxygen content of alveolar air is increased with administration of oxygen, more oxygen enters the blood; when concentration of inspired alveolar Po_2 is reduced by large amounts of air trapped in the alveoli (as in asthma), the amount that enters the blood is decreased; (2) the total functional surface area of the alveolar-capillary membrane—when the surface area is decreased in conditions such as emphysema or pneumonia, the amount that can cross the membrane is also reduced; (3) the minute volume (the amount of air inhaled with each breath times the number of respirations per minute)—conditions that reduce the respiratory rate, such as depressant drugs, or reduce the capacity, such as paralysis, will significantly alter the amount of oxygen; and (4) alveolar ventilation, or the amount of air that reaches the alveoli—obstruction of air flow in the bronchi prevents air from reaching the respiratory unit.

Oxygen transport. Once oxygen has diffused from the alveolus to the pulmonary capillary, it is transported throughout the body in two ways. A small amount (Po_2) is transported as a solute dissolved in the plasma and the water of the red blood cells. A larger portion (forty to seventy times as much) is carried by the hemoglobin as oxyhemoglobin. Since each gram of hemoglobin can combine with 1.34 ml of oxygen, the transport capacity is largely determined by the amount of hemoglobin present. Children with severe anemia tend to be fatigued, be somewhat cyanotic, and breathe more rapidly. Also, increasing the amount of oxygen delivered to the alveoli can increase the amount carried by the blood only in relation to the amount of hemoglobin present, for example, at a Po_2 of 100 mm Hg, hemoglobin is 97.5% saturated.

The oxygen, in order to combine with hemoglobin molecules, must diffuse from the plasma into the red blood cells. The degree to which oxygen combines with hemoglobin is affected by several factors. An increasing Po_2 and a decreasing Pco_2 both accelerate the hemoglobin association with oxygen to form oxyhemoglobin, and a decreasing Po_2 and an increasing Pco_2 accelerate the dissociation from oxyhemoglobin. A decrease in pH or an increase in temperature also increases the dissociation of oxygen from oxyhemoglobin. Therefore, the percent saturation of Po_2 is less under conditions of acidosis or hyperpyrexia.

Carbon dioxide is carried in the blood in a number of ways. A small amount (Pco_2) is transported dissolved in the plasma and the water of red blood cells; a large amount, over half, hydrates to form carbonic acid, which dissociates and is carried as bicarbonate and hydrogen ions; and the remainder combines with certain plasma proteins and hemoglobin. The association of carbon dioxide with hemoglobin is accelerated by an increasing Pco_2 and a decreasing Po_2 and is decreased by the opposite conditions. The diffusion of carbon dioxide into the alveoli is very rapid, thus the equilibrium between the Pco_2 of the pulmonary capillaries and the alveoli is achieved promptly.

Transport between blood and tissue cells is accomplished down a diffusion gradient just as it is between the blood and the alveoli.

Regulation of respiration. The mechanisms that control respirations can be divided into two large categories: (1) a neural system that maintains a coordinated, rhythmic respiratory cycle and regulates the depth of respiration and (2) a chemical (neurohumoral) system that regulates alveolar ventilation and maintains normal blood gas tensions.

Neural control in the respiratory center consists of three areas: (1) a *pneumotaxic center,* which modulates respiratory frequency and depth; (2) an *apneustic center,* which produces an inspiratory spasm and is modulated by the pneumotaxic and medullary centers and by vagal afferent impulses; and (3) *medullary respiratory centers,* both inspiratory and expiratory, which regulate the rhythmicity of respirations.

Impulses from other areas also affect the respiratory centers. *Proprioceptive vagal* impulses in the lung parenchyma are sensitive to stretch. When lungs become stretched, impulses are transmitted by the vagus nerve to the respiratory center, which inhibits further inflation and prevents overdistention—the *Hering-Breuer reflex.* The *cerebral cortex* also helps to control respirations by voluntary inhibition or acceleration of rate and depth of respirations. Reflex apnea can result from sudden painful stimulation, sudden cold stimulation, and stimulation to the larynx or pharynx (the choking reflex, which serves to prevent aspiration).

Chemical, or neurohumoral, control is mediated by specialized structures that respond to changes in pH, Pco_2, and Po_2—central chemoreceptors, probably located in the medulla, and peripheral chemoreceptors located in the great vessels. Peripheral chemoreceptors of greatest physiologic importance are the carotid bodies located at the division of the common carotid artery into its external and internal branches and the aortic bodies that lie between the ascending aorta and the pulmonary artery. Carbon dioxide and hydrogen ions control respiration by acting directly on the respiratory center; the peripheral chemoreceptors respond to changes in oxygen tension. Thus an increase in ventilation can result from either (1) stimulation of the respiratory center by increased Pco_2 or hydrogen ion concentration or (2) a decreased Po_2 that stimulates the carotid and aortic bodies, which, in turn, transmit signals to the brain to excite the respiratory center.

DIAGNOSTIC TOOLS

A variety of diagnostic tools are available for assessing respiratory function and diagnosing respiratory disease. For nurses caring for the child with respiratory disorders, understanding how the test is carried out helps them to devise the best strategies for preparing children for the tests, gaining their cooperation, and supporting them during the procedure. Moreover, this knowledge provides nurses with information on which to base nursing interventions, such as positioning, use of supplemental oxygen, and need for coughing or deep breathing.

Physical examination

A great deal can be determined about the child's respiratory status from simple observations of physical signs and behavior. However, to make a useful assessment, the nurse needs to know what to look for, and what is observed must have meaning (see physical assessment of the chest, p. 141). To assess deviations from the usual, the observer must know the normal type and rate of respiration in relation to the size and age of the child (see Appendix A), which is best observed when the child is sleeping or quietly awake. Much can be determined from the configuration of the chest and the pattern of respiratory movement, including rate, regularity, symmetry of movements, amplitude (deep or shallow), effort expended in respiration, and use of accessory muscles of respiration. Increased respiratory rate is observed with anxiety, with elevated temperature, with severe anemia, as the result of metabolic acidosis, and sometimes associated with respiratory alkalosis caused by psychoneurosis, salicylate ingestion, and some central nervous system disturbances.[15] The progress of disorders that contribute to low compliance, such as the pneumonias, pulmonary edema, and pleural effusion, can be followed and evaluated by observing changes in respiratory rate.

Alterations in the depth of respirations—too deep *(hyperpnea)* or too shallow *(hypopnea)*—are recognized as abnormal only in the extremes. Hyperpnea is noted with fever, severe anemia, respiratory alkalosis associated with psychosis, salicylate ingestion, central nervous system disturbances, and respiratory acidosis that accompanies disorders such as diabetes mellitus or diarrhea. Hypoventilation is less easily detected but occurs with metabolic alkalosis in conditions such as pyloric stenosis and respiratory acidosis that accompanies diaphragmatic paralysis or central nervous system depression.

Retractions, or a sinking in of soft tissues relative to the cartilaginous and bony thorax, may be noted in some pulmonary disorders. Although slight intercostal retractions are normal, in disease states (particularly in severe airway obstruction) retraction becomes extreme. Subcostal retraction, observed anteriorly at the lower costal margins, indicates a flattened diaphragm as it not only lowers the floor of the thorax but also pulls on the rib cage in response to a greater than normal decrease in intrathroacic pressure. In severe obstruction retractions extend to the supraclavicular areas and the jugular notch. Palpation and percussion provide information regarding areas of pain and tissue density, and auscultation is essential to determine the patency of airways. The type of sounds heard helps to identify specific areas of obstruction to air flow. For example, wheezing usually indicates small bronchiolar narrowing, rhonchi are more characteristic of obstruction to large airways, and rales are related to secretions in the respiratory unit.[5] However, in infants wheezing often originates in the larger airways because of their smaller diameter. Auscultation is more difficult in the young patient because of insufficiently deep breaths. Older children can cooperate after instruction; the use of games, such as pretending to blow out the candles on a birthday cake or "panting like a dog," can be successfully applied to young children. In infants often the deep breaths just before and after crying may be the means for assessing deep breath sounds.[16]

Associated observations contribute to assessment. For example, *head bobbing* in a sleeping or exhausted infant is a sign of dyspnea. The head, supported on the mother's arm only at the suboccipital area, will bob forward with each inspiration. This is caused by neck flexion resulting from contraction of the scalene and sternocleidomastoid muscles. Noisy breathing, such as *"snoring"* is frequently associated with hypertrophied adenoidal tissue, choanal obstruction, polyps, or a foreign body in the nasal passages. *Stridor,* a harsh inspiratory sound, is usually caused by laryngeal or tracheal obstruction. Audible wheezes are heard in children with bronchial asthma and foreign bodies in the trachea or bronchi. *Grunting* is frequently a sign of chest pain, suggesting acute pneumonia or pleural involvement. It is also observed in pulmonary edema and is a characteristic feature of the respiratory distress syndrome.

Color changes of the skin, specifically the distribution, degree, and duration of *cyanosis,* are noted. Except for the peripheral bluish discoloration resulting from circulatory stasis in the newborn, cyanosis is significant and usually indicates cardiopulmonary disease. The most common causes of cyanosis in children are[16]:

1. Acute or chronic alveolar hypoventilation as seen in airway obstruction, weakness of the respiratory muscles, or a depressed respiratory center
2. Uneven distribution of gas and blood throughout the lungs, as might occur in bronchopneumonia
3. Anatomic right-to-left shunts of blood that occur in some forms of congenital heart disease or congenital arteriovenous aneurysms of the lung
4. Disturbances of alveolocapillary diffusion, a rare cause of cyanosis as a result of interstitial pneumonia or pulmonary fibrosis

Chest pain may be a complaint of older children and may be a result of a variety of causes both pulmonary and nonpulmonary. It may be caused by disease of any of the chest structures—esophagus, pericardium, diaphragm, pleura, or chest wall. Parietal pleural pain is usually localized over the affected area and is aggravated by respiratory movements. It is not uncommon for the pain of diaphragmatic pleural irritation to be referred to the base of the neck posteriorly and anteriorly or to the abdomen. Most pleural pain is related to respiration; therefore, respiratory movements are shallow and rapid.

Clubbing, or proliferation of tissue about the terminal phalanges, accompanies a variety of conditions, frequently those associated with chronic hypoxia, primarily cardiac defects and chronic pulmonary disease. The degree of clubbing reflects the severity of the hypoxia, and serial measurements provide clues to the progress of the disease. For example, increased clubbing correlates with worsening of the condition and indicates a poor prognosis in cystic fibrosis. On the other hand, diminished clubbing often occurs with intensive pulmonary therapy. The degree of clubbing is determined by the extent to which the nail base is lifted on the dorsal surface of the phalanx by the tissue proliferation. The greater the angle formed above the finger at the skin-nail junction, the more pronounced the clubbing, especially when there is a decided curvature to the nail.

Pulmonary function tests

Pulmonary function tests are used less frequently in children than in adults, since most tests require understanding and the active participation of the child. In those children who are able to cooperate, the tests provide valuable information that assists in the diagnosis and management of many types of pulmonary disease. Most children over

Table 32-1. Pulmonary function tests used in children

Test	Definition	Significance
Vital capacity	Maximal amount of air that can be expelled from the lungs after maximal inspiration	Reduced in obesity Reduced in obstructive airway disease Normal in restrictive disease
Forced expiratory volume in 1 (FEV_1) or 3 (FEV_3) seconds	Amount of air that can be forced from the lungs after maximal inspiration in 1 and 3 seconds	Normally 80% of vital capacity is exhaled in 1 second Reduced in obstructive disease
Tidal volume (TV or V_T)	Amount of air inhaled and exhaled during any respiratory cycle	Multiplied by respiratory rate provides minute volume Information needed to determine rate and depth of artificial ventilation
Functional residual volume (FRV); functional residual capacity (FRC)	Volume of air remaining in the lungs after passive expiration	Allows for aeration of alveoli Increased in hyperinflated lungs of obstructive lung disease

5 years of age can be taught to perform the more simple tests when personnel involved are trained in the use of the equipment and know how to relate to children. Children need to know what is expected of them and to have time to practice the expected maneuver in a pleasant laboratory environment free from distractions. The most useful tests and their use are outlined in Table 32-1.

Radiology

X-radiation is used frequently in diagnostic evaluation of children. Although there is no definitive information on the effects of low-dose radiation, measures are carried out to protect vulnerable areas from possible damage. When possible, technicians and others try to avoid unnecessary exposure of the child (and personnel), and the more radiosensitive areas should be protected. Careful protection of the immature gonads of the infant or child is essential. Other sensitive areas are the thyroid gland, ocular lens, and the bone marrow.

Although nurses have limited control over the length, frequency, and correct application of the x-ray beam, they can make certain that the infant or child receives proper protection from possible hazards. Lead shields, correctly placed and consistently applied to areas not needed for diagnostic purposes, are essential. Special radiologic examinations used in respiratory diagnosis are outlined in Table 32-2.

Diagnostic procedures

Several diagnostic procedures are employed to assist in diagnosis of lung disorders (Table 32-3). Most require specialized equipment and skills. All require some type of preparation of the child.

Blood gas determination

Blood gas measurements are sensitive indicators of change in respiratory status in acutely ill patients. They provide valuable information regarding lung function, lung adequacy, and tissue perfusion. They are invaluable for monitoring conditions involving hypoxemia, carbon dioxide retention, or both. For the nurse who cares for the acutely ill respiratory patient, this information provides cues for decision making regarding therapeutic interventions, such as adjusting the respirator, increasing percussion and vibrating, use of oxygen, or positioning the child for maximal ventilation.

Blood gases measurements include the Po_2 and Pco_2 in association with the pH. Often the oxygen saturation and base excess values are also included. The P represents the partial pressure of the gas being measured, and the figures following indicate the pressure in millimeters of mercury. The pH indicates the hydrogen ion concentration (see acid-base balance, p. 1070). Arterial blood samples are used and are expressed as Pao_2 or $Paco_2$. Venous blood does not indicate the true values and is not used for blood gas determination.

There is some controversy regarding the collection of ''arterialized'' capillary blood for blood gas measurements; however, many believe it to be a safe, convenient, and relatively accurate method. The blood samples are obtained by taking a deep heel stick following dilatation of the vascular bed by warming (see p. 931). The first drop of blood is discarded, and subsequent blood is collected directly into heparinized capillary tubes held in a horizontal position. The filled tube is sealed on one end with wax or clay, a small piece of iron wire is placed inside, and the other end is sealed. The blood is thoroughly mixed by passing a magnet back and forth along the length of the tube, then the tube is placed in a basin of cracked ice and delivered to the laboratory as soon as possible.

Samples are obtained through an indwelling catheter or by way of arteriopuncture. The artery most frequently used is the radial artery, since there are no nearby veins. The temporal and umbilical arteries can be used effectively in the newborn. Other arteries that may be used are the femoral or brachial arteries. The normal values are much

Table 32-2. Radiologic examinations

Test	Description	Purpose	Comment
Fluoroscopy	Electronically intensified image to allow its projection on a viewing screen	Used primarily to study diaphragmatic excursion and respiratory motion of the lungs Examination of barium-filled esophagus to outline mediastinal abnormalities	
Bronchography	Contrast medium is instilled directly into bronchial tree through opaque catheter inserted via orotracheal tube	Most valuable to demonstrate and inspect bronchiectasis Detects distal bronchial obstruction Detects malformations	Carried out under general anesthesia Used less frequently than other examinations
Esophagram	Esophagus is outlined when barium solution or colloid is swallowed	Esophageal displacement defines mediastinal masses Detects swallowing disorders and malformations, for example, tracheoesophageal fistula	Valuable adjunct for diagnosis Usually performed under fluoroscope
Angiography	Injection of dye to visualize pulmonary vasculature	Investigation of pulmonary vascular anomalies and pulmonary hypertension	Seldom used in children
Tomography	Sequence of x-rays, each representing a cross section or "cut" through the lung tissue at a different depth	Useful in identifying the presence of calcium or a cavity within a lesion, hilar adenopathy, mediastinal masses, or abnormalities	Usually reserved for children old enough to be able to suspend respiration voluntarily
Isotope study	Intravenous injection of albumin labeled with radioisotopes or inhalation of radioactive aerosols or xenon gas followed by radiation scanning	Delineates defects in pulmonary arterial perfusion and diseased areas of lung Detects location of aspirated foreign body	Requires cooperation of child

Table 32-3. Diagnostic procedures used in respiratory disorders

Procedures	Description	Purpose
Tracheal aspiration	Sputum is obtained by direct aspiration from trachea	Obtains secretions for culture
Bronchoscopy	Direct observation of tracheobronchial tree via bronchoscope	Localizes abnormalities in major airways Provides access to (1) remove aspirated foreign bodies from major airways, (2) remove obstructive mucous plugs, and (3) perform bronchial lavage
Lung puncture	Needle aspiration of lung fluid via syringe and needle through intercostal space	Obtains lung aspirate for histologic study or culture
Lung biopsy	Removal of lung tissue via open thoracotomy or closed needle procedures	Diagnosis of protracted pulmonary disease unexplained by other means
Brush biopsy	Material for biopsy obtained with a nylon brush on the end of a wire passed through a tube placed via the nose, pharynx, trachea, and airways (via fluoroscope) to the involved lung segment	Obtains material for culture and histologic examination
Diagnostic pneumoperitoneum	Injection of air into peritoneal cavity sharply outlines the diaphragm on radiography	Visualizes position of diaphragm Differentiates eventration of diaphragm from extralobular sequestration

the same for all ages and depend on the concentration of the gases in the ambient air the child is breathing. The normal values for ambient oxygen concentration are less at high altitudes than at sea level and the arterial Po_2 should rise in proportion to the oxygen concentration being inhaled. Therefore, when assessing the significance of blood gas values, the data should include the percentage of oxygen administered (if any), the child's body temperature, since as little as 1°F can alter the blood gas values 5% to 8%, and the presence of anxiety, which causes many children to hyperventilate and blow off extra carbon dioxide.[1,3]

Unclotted blood is required; therefore, a syringe rinsed with heparinized solution is used to draw blood samples, and no air bubbles should enter the syringe to alter the blood gas concentration. The amount collected depends on the size of the child. Ideally, 2.5 ml of blood is drawn for blood gas analysis, but, depending on the laboratory facilities, as little as 0.1 ml may be sufficient in small infants. The normal arterial blood gas and pH measurements in patients breathing room air (21% oxygen) at sea level are:

Pao_2	92-100 mm Hg
$Paco_2$	35-39 mm Hg
pH	7.35-7.45

The significance of blood gas determinations is related primarily to the relationships between these three determinations. Much of this has been discussed in relation to acid-base imbalance in Chapter 29. Any change in a blood gas value must be compared to the other values and to previous readings as well as to the child's clinical appearance and behavior, his medical history, and associated physiologic factors. It is essential to understand the relationship between pH and Pco_2 readings.

The nurse has the following responsibilities in monitoring blood gases. The first is to determine when a blood gas sample should be taken. Sometimes a specified schedule is ordered; at other times the sample is to be drawn as indicated by clinical observations. In this situation the nurse must understand the factors influencing blood gas levels and be able to recognize the need for a blood gas examination. Factors that influence blood gas levels include the amount and method of oxygen administration, the position of the child, and nature of the respiratory disorder. Signs that indicate the need for blood gas examination include a change in color, depth or rate of respirations, behavior or sensorium, and sometimes other vital signs. The nurse may or may not be able to obtain the blood sample by arteriopuncture, depending on the policies of the institution. Nurses are usually able to withdraw the sample from an arterial catheter, and they should become skilled in the techniques of drawing blood and flushing the line. No matter who obtains the sample, the nurse is responsible for its speedy transport to the technician for analysis.

The results of the gas analysis provide the nurse with information on which to base further nursing action. Nurses must be able to understand the significance of the report and to implement nursing activities, for example, adjusting the concentration of oxygen the patient is receiving, changing the position, administering suction, administering prescribed drugs, or notifying the attending physician, according to the interpretation of the gas analysis.

THERAPEUTIC PROCEDURES

Procedures to improve ventilation are employed with increasing frequency in the prevention and management of pulmonary dysfunction. Most of these involve the nurse in the hospital or the home situation.

Inhalation therapy

The term inhalation therapy is an all-inclusive term that encompasses a variety of therapies that involve changing the composition, volume, or pressure of inspired gases. This includes primarily increasing the oxygen concentration of inspired gas (oxygen therapy), increasing the water vapor content of inspired gas (humidification), addition of airborne particles with beneficial properties (aerosol therapy), and various means for controlling or assisting respiration (artificial ventilation, intermittent positive pressure breathing).[15]

Oxygen therapy. The indication for administration of oxygen is hypoxemia as evidenced by reduced arterial oxygen tension and cyanosis. Cyanosis is a late sign but remains the single best criterion for supplemental oxygen. Dyspnea, on the other hand, is not necessarily relieved by oxygen. Oxygen is administered by mask, hood, nasal cannula, face tent, intermittent positive pressure breathing apparatus, or oxygen tent. The mode of delivery is selected on the basis of the concentration needed in the inspired air and the ability of the child to cooperate in its use. The concentration of oxygen delivered should be regulated according to the needs of the individual child. For most conditions an ambient oxygen concentration of 40% to 50% is satisfactory and should be analyzed periodically for percent concentration. There are hazards related to its use; therefore, oxygen should not be continued after the indication for its use (such as cyanosis) is no longer present. Since oxygen is dry, it is always humidified in some manner.

Oxygen therapy is almost always carried out in the hospital. Oxygen delivered to the infant Isolette is satisfactory when lower levels are adequate to prevent cyanosis, but the highest concentration (almost 100%) is supplied by way of a plastic hood (Fig. 32-2). The gas should not be allowed to blow directly into the infant's face, and the hood should not rub against the infant's neck, chin, or shoulder. Older cooperative children can use a nasal cannula or prongs, which can supply a concentration of about 50%. A nasal catheter or a mask is not well tolerated by children.

For most children beyond early infancy the oxygen tent,

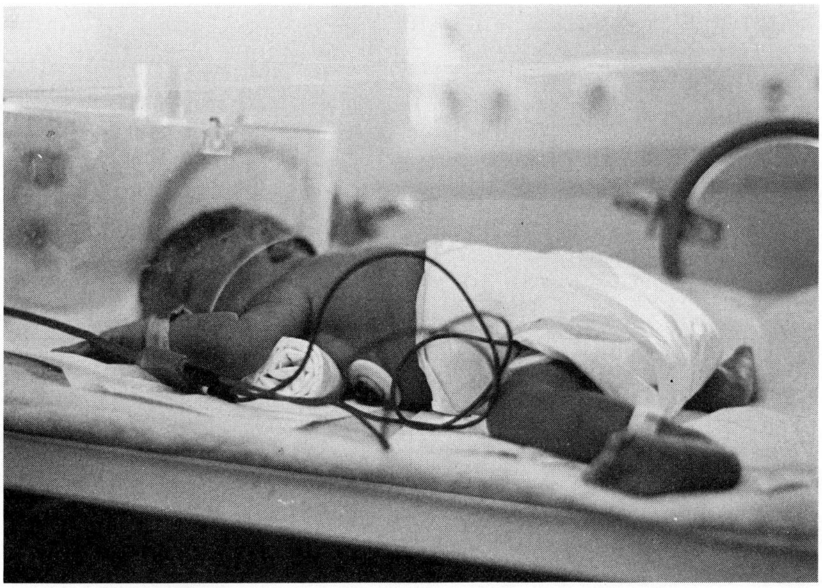

Fig. 32-2. Oxygen administered to infant by plastic hood.

or canopy, is the most satisfactory means for administration of oxygen (Fig. 32-3).[2] A tent does not require any device to come into direct contact with the face, but the concentration of oxygen within the tent is difficult to control and to maintain above about 40%. The comfort to the child makes it the method of choice except in cases of marked respiratory distress. A major difficulty with the use of the tent is keeping the tent closed so that oxygen concentration is maintained. To reduce oxygen loss, nursing care should be planned carefully so that the tent is opened as little as possible. Since oxygen is heavier than air, loss will be greater at the bottom of the tent; therefore, the tent should be tucked in snugly without open edges. The bottom of the tent should be examined more often when the child is restless and fussy and liable to pull the covers loose. Some tents are even open at the top. Because of the rapid diffusing qualities of carbon dioxide, the levels of the gas do not build up within these enclosures.

The enclosed tent becomes very warm; therefore, some type of cooling mechanism, such as an ice chamber or a refrigeration unit, is provided. The temperature inside the tent must be checked periodically to be certain that it is maintained at the desired temperature. If the coolant is an ice chamber, this is not allowed to become empty. It is important to make certain that the child is kept warm and dry. Mist is usually prescribed in conjunction with oxygen therapy, and the moisture condenses on the tent walls. The child's bedding and clothing are examined periodically and changed as needed to prevent chilling.

The reactions of children to the oxygen tent are variable. Some, especially older children, feel comfortable in and like the cozy, close privacy the tent affords. Others, more often younger children, may be frightened by the forced enclosure. The plastic walls distort their view of the world and constitute a barrier between them and their source of comfort, the mother. Their distress can be minimized if they are able to see someone nearby and are reassured that they will not be left alone. A favorite toy or object can accompany the child inside the tent. However, all toys should be inspected for safety and suitability. The high oxygen environment makes any source of sparks (such as some mechanical toys) a potential fire hazard. Other familiar items can be placed at the foot of the bed or otherwise in view.

No matter what method is used to administer the oxygen, the child's color and respiratory status are monitored frequently and evaluated in terms of efficacy of treatment. The oxygen content within the device is analyzed periodically (always at a point near the child's head) to determine the rate of flow needed to maintain the desired concentration. The equipment is changed and/or cleaned at regular intervals (at least once weekly) to prevent bacterial growth when the child requires oxygen over an extended period.

In most instances the child can be removed from the oxygen tent for activities such as feeding and bathing, whereas in other cases the child is placed in the tent only during periods of rest. Still others may require oxygen continuously and can be removed from the tent or Isolette only if an oxygen source is held close to the child's face. Any change in color, increased respiratory effort, or restlessness is an indication to return the child to the oxygen tent.

Oxygen toxicity. Oxygen is essential to life and a valu-

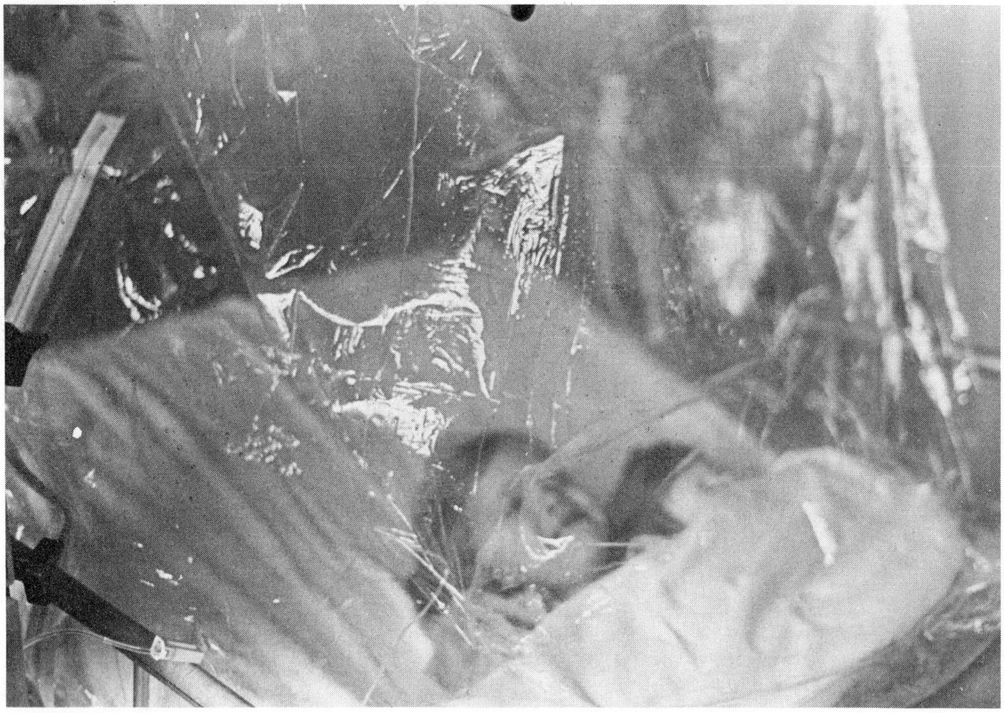

Fig. 32-3. The tent provides a comfortable method for oxygen administration but may be frightening to a small child even when shared by a familiar "friend."

able therapeutic aid. However, prolonged exposure to high oxygen tensions can be damaging to some body tissues and functions. The organs most vulnerable to the adverse effects of excessive oxygenation are the retina of the premature infant and the lungs of persons at any age. Although the exact pathogenesis of the pulmonary changes is unclear, there is evidence to indicate damage to lung capillaries, which causes diffuse microhemorrhagic changes, diminished mucous flow, and inactivation of surfactant. The total effect appears to be the direct result of "lung burn" and is, therefore, a result of the alveolar oxygen (PA_{O_2}) and not the arterial oxygen tension (Pa_{O_2}). The result of these changes is a gradual impairment of alveolar ventilation.[2,13]

Retrolental fibroplasia, once a major cause of blindness in premature infants treated with high concentrations of oxygen, is a function of elevated Pa_{O_2} rather than alveolar oxygen concentration (PA_{O_2}). The effect on the retina appears to be due to vasoconstriction of the incompletely vascularized retina of the prematurely born child. Continued hyperoxia leads to endothelial damage and ultimate obliteration of the retinal vessels. There is some speculation regarding the possibility of a similar vasospastic effect on other blood vessels of cerebral origin with resultant diminished blood flow to various areas of the brain.

Atelectasis may occur as the result of the "washing out" of nitrogen from the alveoli by the high concentrations of oxygen. This is more apt to occur in persons with low tidal volume and retention of mucus or other secretions.[14]

Oxygen-induced carbon dioxide narcosis is a physiologic hazard of oxygen therapy that may occur in persons with chronic pulmonary disease. It is seldom encountered in children except those with cystic fibrosis. These children have chronic alveolar hypoventilation with a concomitant chronic carbon dioxide retention and hypoxemia. In these patients the respiratory center has adapted to the continuously higher P_{CO_2} levels, and, therefore, hypoxia becomes the more powerful stimulus to respiration. When the P_{O_2} is elevated during oxygen administration, the hypoxic drive is removed, causing increasing hypoventilation and increased P_{CO_2} levels, and the child rapidly becomes unconscious. Carbon dioxide narcosis can also be induced by the administration of sedation in these patients.[4,14]

Other toxic effects of oxygen that are suspected include changes in the renal tubules, sympathoadrenal medullary stimulation precipitating neurogenic seizures, and an increased rate of destruction of red blood cells.[4]

Aerosol therapy. The inhalation and subsequent deposition of airborne water particles within the airway is the function of aerosol therapy. This may be merely saline to help moisten the airway and help liquify secretions, or the particles may contain mucolytic, bronchodilating, decongestant, or antimicrobial agents. The particles can vary in size, depending on the mode of delivery, and may be administered intermittently and briefly or continuously and prolonged. In all forms of aerosol therapy the nebulized substance is distributed according to the gas flow. Large droplets are usually deposited in larger airways, and any unventilated areas receive none of the aerosol. The smaller the droplets formed, the more widely they are distributed.

For continuous aerosol therapy a misting device is attached to or incorporated into the mist tent. Distilled water is used most commonly, although propylene glycol in aqueous solution is often employed, especially in jet-type nebulizers. For intermittent administration of small quantities of an agent with specific pharmacologic action, a small nebulizer can be used powered by a small electric motor or in association with a positive pressure breathing apparatus.

Aerosol therapy is widely used in treatment of both upper and lower respiratory tract disease, including croup, bronchitis, pneumonia, asthma, cystic fibrosis, and conditions in which there is weakness of the muscles of respiration. In some instances aerosol therapy is employed prophylactically (for example, cystic fibrosis) to prevent complicating pulmonary problems. There is a decided relationship between aerosol therapy and bronchial drainage. Drainage is much more effective immediately after aerosol therapy.

Aerosol therapy is usually performed under the guidance of a respiratory therapist, although nurses may assume this responsibility in the home or in association with the therapist. Nebulizers attached to mist tents are monitored to be certain that the fluid is maintained within the desired level and that the nebulization takes place. When mist cannot be observed, the apparatus is checked for interruption of patency or other malfunction. Children using nebulization by mask or other device are taught how to use the aerosol effectively and are supervised in its operation. Nurses need to know how the apparatus works and to recognize when it is functioning properly. Because of the danger of bacterial growth, the equipment is thoroughly cleaned daily.

Bronchial (postural) drainage

Bronchial drainage is indicated whenever excessive fluid or mucus in the bronchi is not being removed by normal ciliary activity and cough. The techniques of segmental drainage, percussion, and vibration assist the normal cleansing mechanisms of the lung. Positioning the child to take maximum advantage of gravity further facilitates removal of secretions. The effect is sometimes dramatic in children with chronic lung disease characterized by thick mucous secretions, such as asthma and cystic fibrosis.

Postural drainage is carried out three to four times daily and is more effective when it follows other respiratory therapy, such as bronchodilator and/or nebulization medication. Bronchial drainage is generally performed before meals (or 1 to 1½ hours after meals) to minimize the chance of vomiting and at bedtime. The length and duration of treatment depend on the child's condition and tolerance level—usually 20 to 30 minutes. There are positions to facilitate drainage from all major lung segments (Fig. 32-4), but all positions are not employed at each session. The child will usually cooperate for four to six positions, but more than six tend to exceed their limits of tolerance. In older children longer periods can be reasonably expected. In the hospital an older child can be positioned over the elevated knee rest. Small children and infants can be positioned with pillows (Fig. 32-5) or on the therapist's lap and legs (Fig. 32-6). Special modifications of the techniques are required in children whose conditions contraindicate the standard positioning, such as head injuries, some types of surgical incisions or burns, and casts or traction. At home small children can be positioned on a padded ironing board. Children who require postural drainage over a period of months or years may benefit from specially constructed tables padded and adjusted to their individual needs.

The position used and the frequency and duration of treatment are individualized. The simile used to illustrate this concept is that of a freshly opened catsup bottle. Even inverted, the catsup will not flow until it is loosened and ejected by repeated blows to the bottom of the bottle. Since viscid secretions may not drain by gravity alone, various maneuvers, including deep breathing, reinforced cough, thoracic "squeezing," "cupping," or "clapping," and vibration, are performed in association with drainage to assist in their removal.

Deep breathing. When the child is relaxed in the desired position for drainage, he is directed to take several deep breaths, using diaphragmatic breathing. The use of deep breathing enlarges the tracheobronchial tree, enabling air to circulate around and through secretions that are not affected by usual tidal volumes. Expirations after these deep breaths often carry secretions and may stimulate a cough. Other methods that can be employed to stimulate deep breathing are blow bottles of various types and incorporation of play with items such as balloons (see also p. 949).

Cough. With or without stimulation, the child is encouraged to cough. He is taught not to suppress a cough and not to waste strength and energy with repeated weak and ineffective coughs. One or two hard coughs after a deep breath are more efficient. The therapist can reinforce the child's efforts by encircling the chest with the therapist's hands, which compress the sides of the lower chest in synchrony with the cough. This is less fatiguing and increases the effectiveness of the cough efforts. Since many children have difficulty in coughing when in a dependent position, they should be allowed to sit up while they cough.

"Squeezing." A squeeze is sometimes a useful maneuver while the child is in the drainage position. He is directed to take a deep breath and then to exhale through the mouth rapidly and as completely as possible. The depth of the expiratory effort is increased by brief, firm pressure from

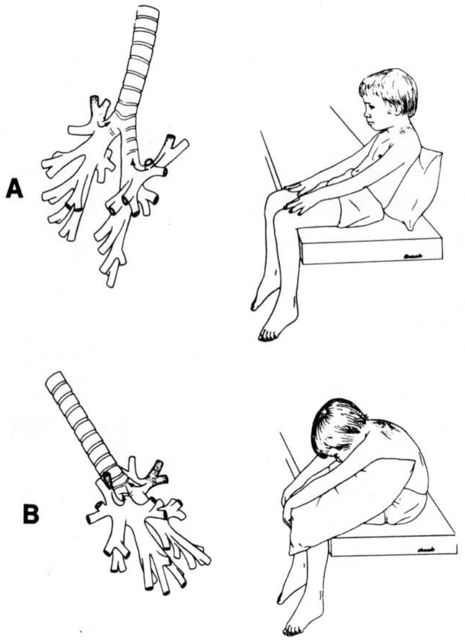

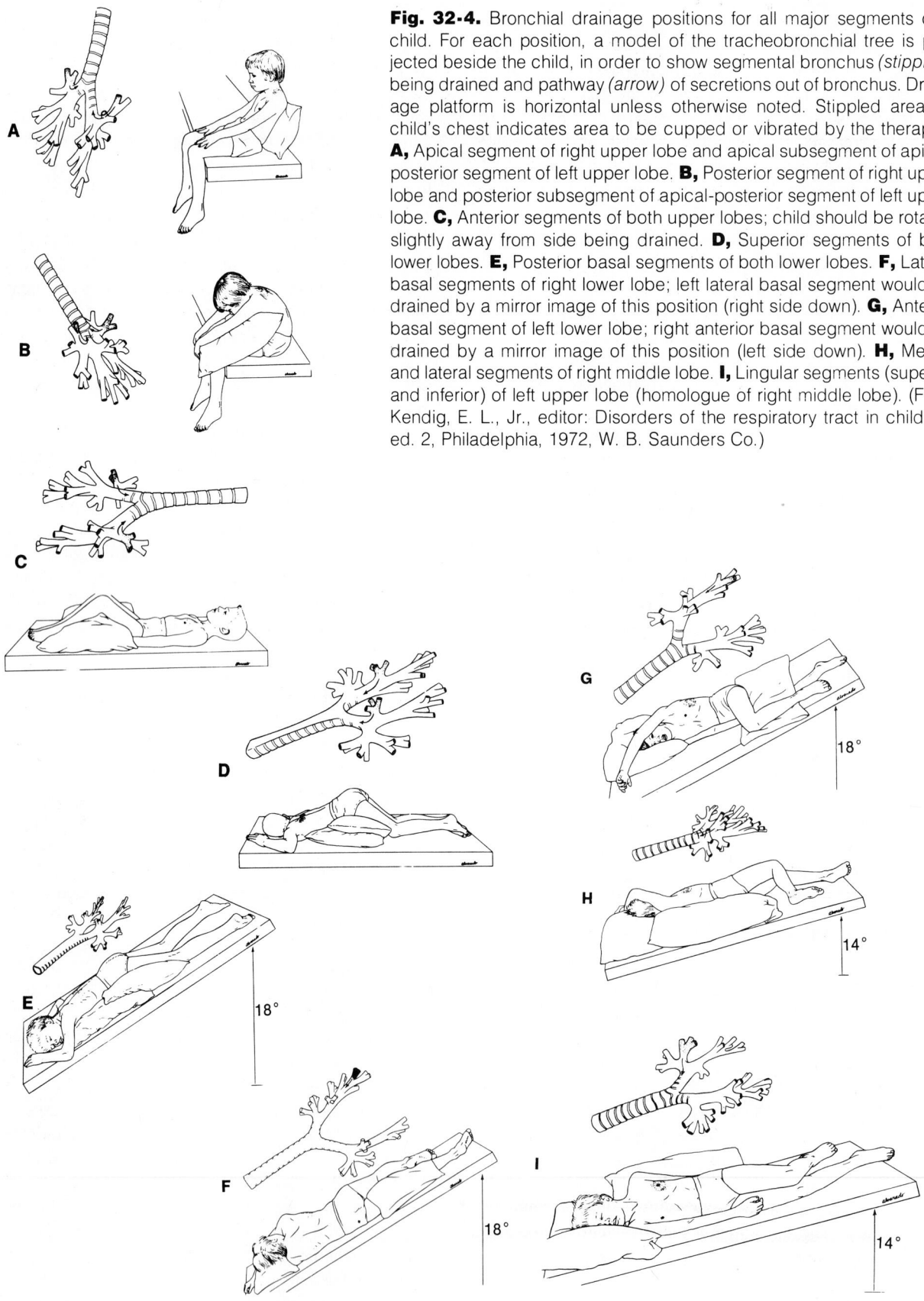

Fig. 32-4. Bronchial drainage positions for all major segments of a child. For each position, a model of the tracheobronchial tree is projected beside the child, in order to show segmental bronchus *(stippled)* being drained and pathway *(arrow)* of secretions out of bronchus. Drainage platform is horizontal unless otherwise noted. Stippled area on child's chest indicates area to be cupped or vibrated by the therapist. **A,** Apical segment of right upper lobe and apical subsegment of apical-posterior segment of left upper lobe. **B,** Posterior segment of right upper lobe and posterior subsegment of apical-posterior segment of left upper lobe. **C,** Anterior segments of both upper lobes; child should be rotated slightly away from side being drained. **D,** Superior segments of both lower lobes. **E,** Posterior basal segments of both lower lobes. **F,** Lateral basal segments of right lower lobe; left lateral basal segment would be drained by a mirror image of this position (right side down). **G,** Anterior basal segment of left lower lobe; right anterior basal segment would be drained by a mirror image of this position (left side down). **H,** Medial and lateral segments of right middle lobe. **I,** Lingular segments (superior and inferior) of left upper lobe (homologue of right middle lobe). (From Kendig, E. L., Jr., editor: Disorders of the respiratory tract in children, ed. 2, Philadelphia, 1972, W. B. Saunders Co.)

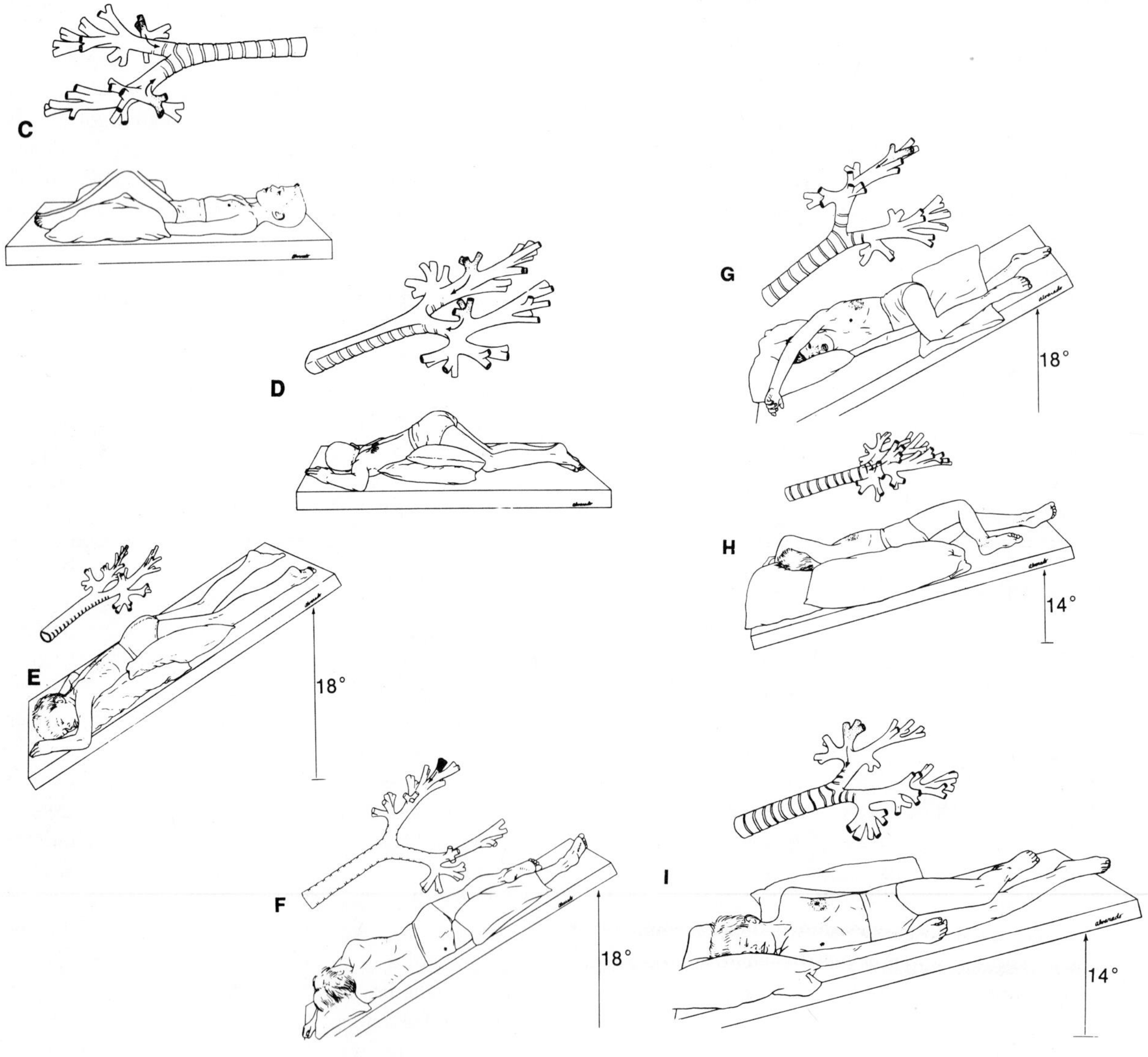

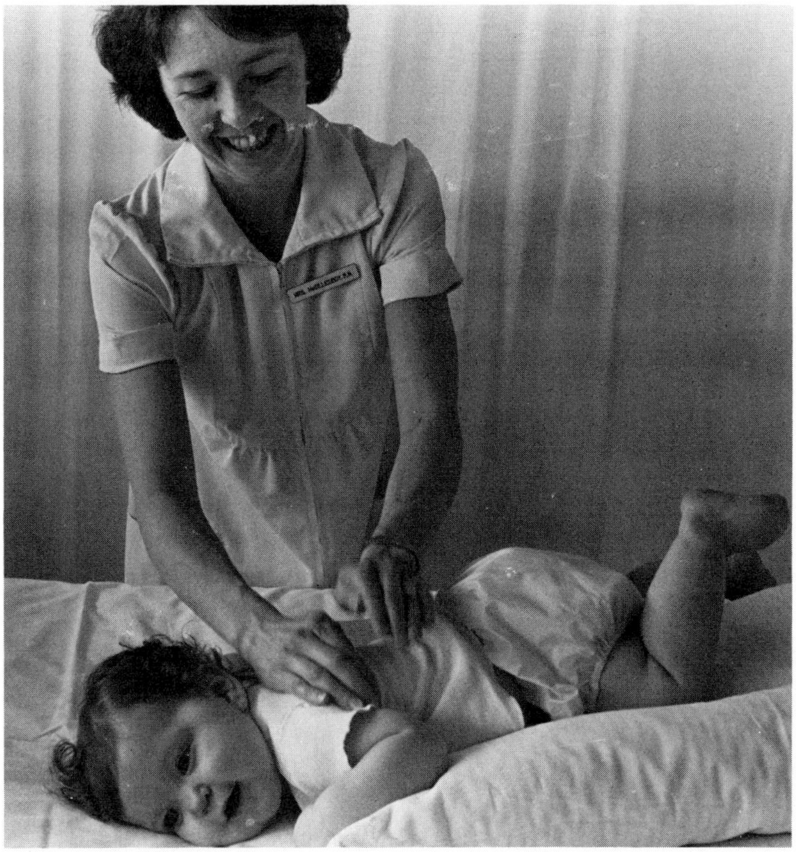

Fig. 32-5. Child positioned for postural drainage.

the therapist's hands compressing the sides of the chest. This decreases the volume of the tracheobronchial tree and facilitates the expression of secretions. The inspiration after the activity often stimulates a deep, productive cough (reinforced by the operator).

Percussion. Percussion—clapping or cupping—is performed intermittently during postural drainage. The operator's hands are held in the cupped position (Fig. 32-7) and vigorously and repeatedly strike the chest wall under which the specific lung segment to be drained is situated. Performed properly, percussion is painless. The operator's hand should not strike the bare skin. A light cotton undershirt or gown is an appropriate covering to protect the skin from possible irritation. The hand does not slap but conforms to the contour of the chest wall, the entire circumference of the cupped hand touching the chest wall at the same instant. When correctly applied the clapping emits a loud, hollow sound. Care is exerted to clap over the *rib cage only*.

For infants who chest is too small for conventional hand percussion, a small face mask is substituted for the operator's hand (see Fig. 10-13).

Vibration. Vibration, a more difficult procedure, is performed only during the exhalation phase of breathing. The child is instructed to take a deep breath and exhale slowly through pursed lips. The operator places one hand on top of the other over the target lung segment and, as the child exhales, transmits a rapid vibratory impulse through the chest wall by a tensing contraction of the forearm flexor and extensor muscles. After full expiration, pressure is released.

Breathing exercises

Breathing and postural exercises have not been widely applied to children but are useful techniques with older, motivated children. They are especially of value to children with kyphoscoliosis, cystic fibrosis, asthma, and bronchiectasis. Breathing exercises are employed as part of a total therapy program and are more convenient when performed in association with bronchial drainage.

The goals of breathing exercises are to (1) develop more effective diaphragmatic and lower intercostal breathing, (2) relax all muscles, especially those of the upper chest, shoulder girdle, and neck, and (3) attain a good, easy posture. The number and type of exercises depend on the age, moti-

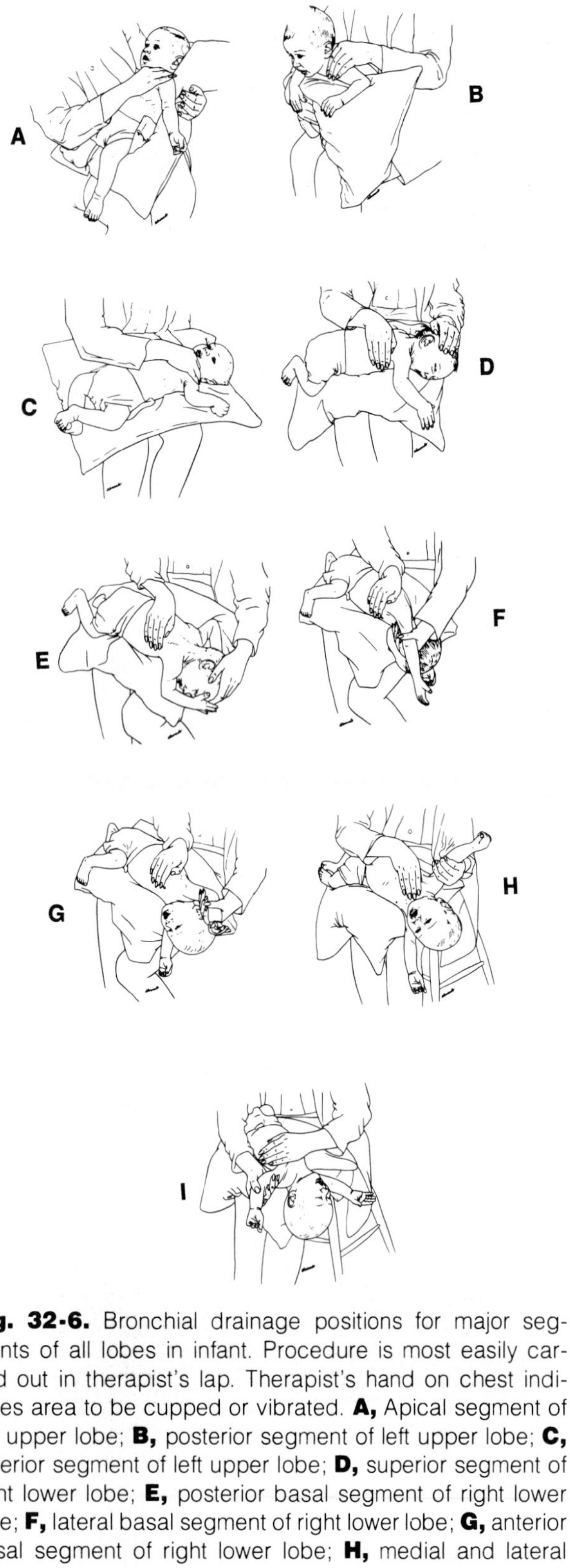

Fig. 32-6. Bronchial drainage positions for major segments of all lobes in infant. Procedure is most easily carried out in therapist's lap. Therapist's hand on chest indicates area to be cupped or vibrated. **A,** Apical segment of left upper lobe; **B,** posterior segment of left upper lobe; **C,** anterior segment of left upper lobe; **D,** superior segment of right lower lobe; **E,** posterior basal segment of right lower lobe; **F,** lateral basal segment of right lower lobe; **G,** anterior basal segment of right lower lobe; **H,** medial and lateral segments of right middle lobe; **I,** lingular segments (superior and inferior) of left upper lobe. (From Kendig, E. L., Jr., editor: Disorders of the respiratory tract in children, ed. 2, Philadelphia, 1972, W. B. Saunders Co.)

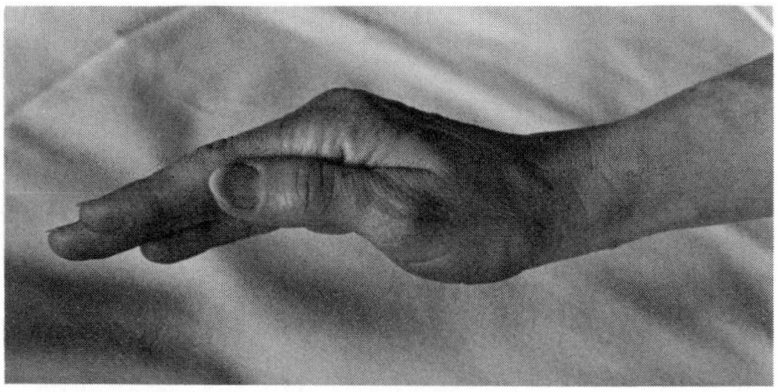

Fig. 32-7. Cupped hand position for percussion.

vation, and strength of the child as well as the type and extent of the physiologic disturbance.[15]

A variety of exercises are employed, but any individual child is unable to tolerate all of them; therefore, they are either selected to meet the needs of the specific child or alternated in their use. The most important exercises are diaphragmatic breathing and side bending, concentrating on both abdominal expansion and lateral expansion.

Diaphragmatic breathing. This exercise is performed lying down on the floor or mat after a short period of rest in the supine position, which stretches the pectoral, chest, and upper back muscles in preparation for the exercise. For abdominal expansion the child lies on the back with knees flexed, with one hand placed on upper chest and one on the abdomen. He breathes out *slowly* while compressing the lower rib cage and upper abdomen and then inhales, relaxing and expanding the upper abdomen. There should be no movement in chest or neck. The exercise is also carried out in the sitting position with the back supported.

To concentrate on lateral expansion the child lies on the back with knees flexed and palms of hands on the sides of the lower rib cage. The child is instructed to breathe out *slowly* while compressing the lower ribs and upper abdomen and squeeze the ribs at the end of expiration to get rid of as much air as possible from the bases of the lung. He then inhales, expanding the lower ribs outward against a small amount of pressure from the hands. Again there should be no movement of chest or neck. After back lying the exercise is repeated in the sitting position with the back supported.

Side bending. The child sits comfortably in a chair with the feet apart. To stretch the rib cage on the left, the left hand is placed on the right lower ribs and the right arm is allowed to hang relaxed at the right side. The child is instructed to breathe out slowly while bending the head and shoulders to the right and pressing the left hand against the ribs. Pressure from the left hand together with the torso bending permits more air to be expelled from the right lung. The child then sits upright and inhales with the head and shoulders turned slightly to the left, thus expanding the right lower ribs to the right as much as possible. This allows the lung segments on the right to expand. Bending takes place at the waist and trunk while the hips remain level. The exercise is repeated on the opposite side.

Special techniques

Several techniques can be employed to aid relaxation, especially during periods of exertion or stress. Accelerated diaphragmatic breathing, or panting, is often useful for "catching the breath" during or after episodes of dyspnea. Breathing is rapid and panting for approximately 30 seconds to 1 minute and is then decelerated slowly to the normal rate. Breathing remains diaphragmatic.

Positioning during periods of stress promotes relaxation and diaphragmatic breathing for easier and more efficient respiratory effort. These include[12]:

Squatting and leaning forward with elbows on knees
Sitting on a chair backward with forearms on chair back and leaning forward with head on forearms
Sitting on a chair and leaning forward with elbows on knees and forearms relaxed
Leaning forward against a wall or railing
Lying on side with top shoulder and side leaning over pillows placed as follows—one between knees, one under head and upper trunk, and one between arms and under head

When engaged in activity such as climbing stairs, the child should be taught to regulate breathing with the activity. For example, when climbing stairs the child inhales while taking two steps and exhales while taking six steps. The expiratory phase should be extended as long as possible; however, the expiration should be three times the length of the inspiration.

RESPIRATORY FAILURE

Disorders of respiratory structure and function that may result in ventilatory failure are a significant cause of childhood illness. They may be caused by a variety of causes, both pulmonary and nonpulmonary, and the pulmonary dysfunction can result in disturbances in other organs and systems. The primary function of the lungs is to provide sufficient oxygen for metabolic needs and to remove the carbon dioxide therapy produced. Inadequacy of the oxygen-supplying role results in hypoxemia and tissue hypoxia; inadequate carbon dioxide removal causes hypercapnia. Often both gases may be insufficiently exchanged.

In general the term *respiratory insufficiency* is applied to two conditions[10]: (1) children with increased work of breathing while preserving gas exchange function near normal—ventilatory insufficiency, and (2) children who are unable to maintain normal blood gas tensions and develop hypoxemia and acidosis secondary to carbon dioxide retention.

Respiratory failure is defined as the inability of the respiratory apparatus to maintain adequate oxygenation of the blood, with or without carbon dioxide retention.[14]

Respiratory arrest is the cessation of respiration.

Effective pulmonary gas exchange requires clear airways, normal lungs and chest wall, and adequate pulmonary circulation. This functional pulmonary unit plus normal respiratory control mechanisms ensure adequate total alveolar ventilation and perfusion, which are reflected in oxygen and carbon dioxide tensions in arterial blood leaving the lung. Anything that affects these functions or their relationships can compromise the respiration.

Respiratory dysfunction may have an abrupt or an insidious onset. Respiratory failure, therefore, can occur as an emergency situation or may be preceded by gradual and progressive deterioration of respiratory function.[11] Physical examination does not reveal the presence of either hypoxemia or hypercapnia. Most clinical manifestations are nonspecific and are affected by variations among individual patients and differences in the severity and duration of inadequate gas exchange.

The diagnosis of respiratory failure is determined by the combined application of three sources of information[14]:

1. Presence or history of a condition that might predispose to respiratory failure
2. Observation of respiratory failure
3. Measurement of arterial blood gases and pH

Conditions that predispose to respiratory failure

Respiratory disorders are more conveniently classified according to three dominant functional abnormalities, although all three types may be present in the disease. The three primary types of functional disorders and examples of each are:

1. *Obstructive lung disease,* in which there is increased resistance to airflow in either the upper or lower respiratory tract. Examples include airways obstructed by foreign body, mucus or vomitus, stenosis, bronchial constriction, laryngospasm, and tumors.
2. *Restrictive lung disease,* in which there is impaired lung expansion resulting from loss of lung volume, decreased distensibility, or chest wall disturbance. Examples include muscular paralysis, tuberculosis, pulmonary edema, kyphoscoliosis, atelectasis, pneumonia, and severe obesity.
3. *Inefficient gas transfer,* in which there is insufficient alveolar ventilation for carbon dioxide removal or impaired oxygenation of pulmonary capillary blood as a result of dysfunction of the respiratory control mechanism or a diffusion defect. Examples include (1) control mechanism dysfunction caused by cerebral trauma, central nervous system infections, intracranial tumors, and depressant drugs, and (2) diffusion defect caused by pulmonary edema, hyaline membrane disease, pulmonary fibrosis, anemia, and pulmonary hypertension.

Recognition of respiratory failure

Respiratory failure that occurs as the result of acute obstruction of a major airway or cardiac arrest is sudden and readily apparent. Gradual and more covert development of signs and symptoms is less easily recognized. Insufficient alveolar ventilation from any cause ultimately leads to hypoxemia and hypercapnia. However, there are situations in which severe respiratory distress may be present without significant carbon dioxide retention, and hypoxemia may occur without clinically detectable cyanosis. Therefore, evaluation of respiratory adequacy is based on both clinical assessment and laboratory studies. Nursing observation and judgment are vital to successful management of respiratory failure. Nurses must be able to assess a situation and initiate appropriate action within moments.

Unless respiratory arrest occurs suddenly, signs of hypoxemia and hypercapnia are usually subtle in their development and become more obvious as respiratory failure progresses. The early signs can be detected by the alert observer. These include:

- Mood changes, such as euphoria or depression
- Headache
- Altered depth and pattern of respirations (deep, shallow, apnea, irregular)
- Tachypnea
- Hypertension
- Exertional dyspnea
- Anorexia
- Increased cardiac output and renal output
- Cyanosis, peripheral or central (may or may not be evident until later)
- Central nervous system symptoms, such as decreased efficiency, impaired judgment, anxiety, confusion, restlessness, and irritability
- Flaring nares
- Chest wall retractions
- Expiratory grunt
- Wheezing and/or prolonged expiration
- Signs of more severe hypoxia, including hypotension or hypertension, dimness of vision, cyanosis, somnolence, stupor, coma, dyspnea, depressed respirations, and bradycardia

In clinical situations in which impaired ventilation can be anticipated or clinical manifestations indicate impending hypoxemia, serial measurements of blood gases should be obtained and monitored in order to detect impending respiratory failure and implement therapy before respiratory acidosis becomes extreme.

Management of respiratory failure

The interventions used in the management of respiratory failure are often dramatic, requiring special skills, and are often emergency procedures. Some of the techniques employed to assist ventilation include artificial ventilation, artificial airway, and cardiopulmonary resuscitation.

Artificial ventilation. There are a variety of methods for controlling or assisting ventilation. Temporary assistance can be provided by a hand-operated self-inflating ventilation bag with mask and a nonreturnable valve to prevent rebreathing (AMBU bag). With the mask placed on the nose and mouth (an open airway is established by correct positioning with the chin forward and the neck extended to the ''sniffing'' position), the bag is rhythmically compressed, forcing the gas from the bag into the patient's lungs.

For more prolonged assistance, mechanical ventilation is employed to replace the bellows function of the diaphragm and thoracic wall muscles. The lungs are inflated by the application of either positive or negative pressure. The positive-pressure machine inflates the lung by increasing airway pressure above atmospheric pressure, and a negative-pressure ventilator creates a subatmospheric pressure around the chest wall, whereas airway pressure remains atmospheric. Application of positive pressure by mechanical means usually improves the distribution of gas within the lung and often reinflates partially collapsed lung segments. The overall effect is the improvement of gas exchange.

Ventilators, or respirators, are characterized by the way in which gas is generated (constant pressure or constant flow) and by the way in which the gas is cycled to change from the respiratory to the expiratory phase of respiration. They are classified as *pressure cycled, volume cycled,* and *time cycled.* The pressure-cycled ventilator produces a preset pressure and ceases to deliver gas once this pressure is reached. With this type, changes in compliance allow changes in volume of gas delivered. Volume-cycled ventilators deliver a fixed volume of gas and are more effective in maintaining alveolar ventilation when compliance is severely diminished, as in asthma or pulmonary edema (Fig. 32-8). Time-cycled ventilators terminate inspiration and expiration by a preset cycle duration and gas flow rate. Most negative-pressure ventilators are time cycled.

Pressure ventilators can be regulated to either assist or substitute for the patient's respiratory effort. When used to assist ventilation, the ventilator transmits the prescribed volume of gas in response to the patient's own respiratory effort. In controlled ventilation the machine automatically controls both the rate and depth of ventilation at fixed settings. Ventilators are attached to the patient by mask, endotracheal tube, or tracheostomy.

The regulation and maintenance of mechanical ventilators are the responsibility of respiratory therapists. However, nurses should understand the function of the ventilator in use and be able to detect signs of malfunction and deviations from the desired settings. The nurse also promotes the effectiveness of ventilation by suctioning, positioning, and providing support and reassurance to the child receiving mechanical respiration. See p. 346 for assisted and controlled respiration in the neonate.

Artificial airways. An artificial airway is usually used in association with artificial ventilation and in children with upper airway obstruction. Endotracheal intubation can be accomplished by the nasal (nasotracheal), oral (orotracheal), or direct tracheal (tracheostomy) routes. Although it is

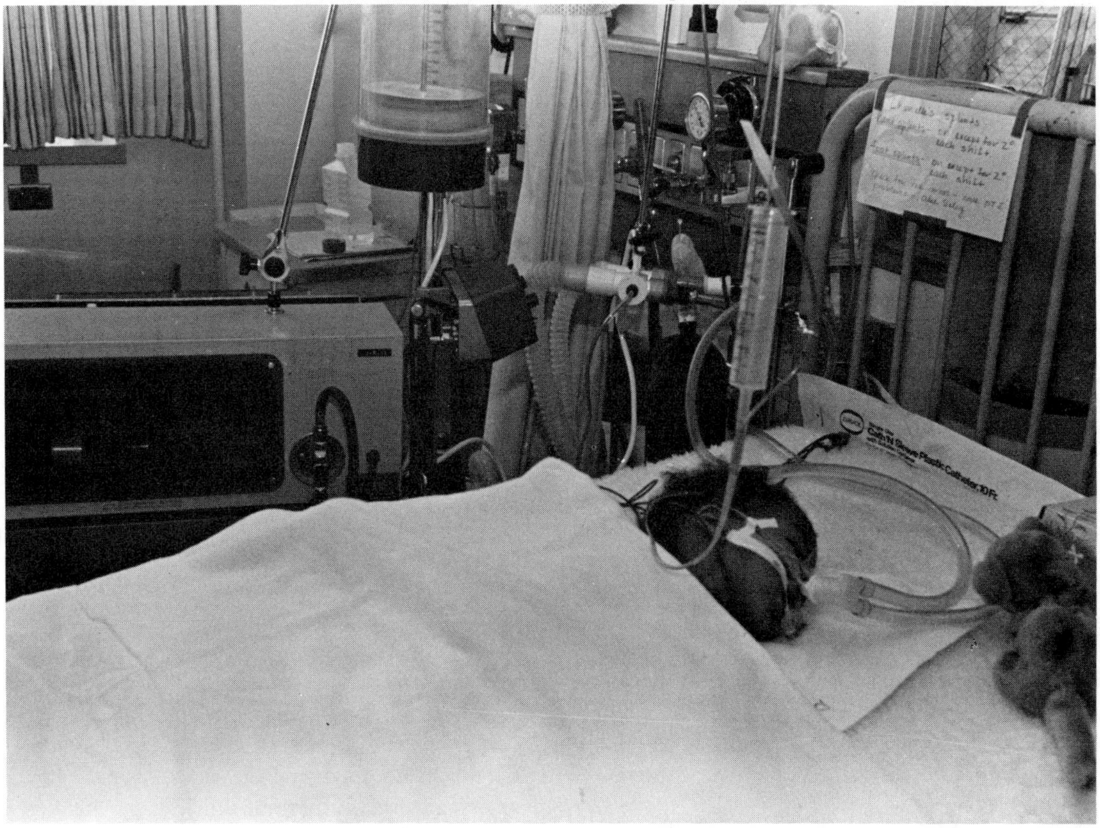

Fig. 32-8. Child receiving artificial ventilation from volume-cycled respirator through orotracheal tube. Open syringe suspended in foreground is for nasogastric feedings by gravity.

more difficult to place technically, nasotracheal intubation is preferred to orotracheal intubation because it facilitates oral hygiene and provides more stable fixation, which reduces the complication of tracheal erosion and the danger of accidental extubation. Endotracheal tubes may be cuffed to provide an airtight seal or uncuffed. Cuffed tubes are used when high-inflation pressures are needed, they are inflated to the minimum volume, and the pressure cuff must be deflated hourly for 2 to 5 minutes to minimize the possibility of pressure necrosis. However, pressure cuffs are rarely used in children younger than 10 years of age. Air or gas delivered directly to the trachea must be humidified as in tracheostomy. Although newborn infants have been successfully maintained on nasotracheal tubes for longer periods, in older children who require intubation beyond a week, a tracheostomy is usually performed.

Tracheostomy. Tracheostomy can be a lifesaving procedure. It is performed as an emergency or an elective procedure and may be combined with mechanical ventilation. The usual indications for tracheostomy are[15]:

1. Mechanical obstruction of the upper airway, for example, croup, foreign body, and laryngeal paralysis
2. Disease of the central nervous system, for example, head injury, craniotomy, and drug depression
3. Neuromuscular disease, for example, poliomyelitis, tetanus, myasthenia gravis, amyotonia congenita, and Guillain-Barré syndrome
4. Secretional obstruction, such as debility with weak cough, severe thoracic or chest pain (from incision or injury)
5. Conditions with disturbances of gas diffusion or distribution, such as blunt chest injuries, smoke inhalation, and widespread pneumonia
6. Prophylaxis for radical neck or head surgery—an unusual need in children

Plastic and Silastic have largely replaced silver as the preferred material for tracheostomy tubes, especially for pediatric use (Fig. 32-9). These materials can be constructed with a more acute angle and, since they soften at room temperature, are better able to conform to the contours of the airway. The flexibility of the material resists kinking, and the smooth surface reduces crust formation; therefore, most tubes are constructed without an inner cannula. The tube is held in place by appropriate length of sturdy cloth tape around the child's neck. Umbilical cord tape is ideal. A better fit can be achieved if the child's head is flexed, rather than extended, while the tape is fixed. If the cord is too loose the tube may be coughed out. The ties should fit snugly enough that one finger can be inserted with difficulty between the tape and the child's neck. The obturator is kept in a sterile package taped to the head of the bed.

Since the normal warming, wetting, and filtering functions of the upper airway are inoperative, air entering the tracheostomy opening is humidified by placing the child in a mist tent, by attaching a special tracheostomy mask or "collar" to deliver humidified gas directly to the tracheostomy opening, or by direct attachment to a mechanical ventilator. The humid gas helps to loosen mucus and reduce the chances of crust formation and a mucous plug. Moisture from the humidified gas tends to accumulate on the inner surface of the flexible plastic tubing and must be eliminated periodically to prevent occlusion of the tube and/or accidental aspiration. The tubing is disconnected at the collar or tracheostomy tube and drained into a container. It is not allowed to flow back into the humidifying receptacle.

The airway must remain patent and requires frequent suctioning during the first few hours posttracheostomy to remove mucous plugs and excess secretions. A small amount of sterile isotonic saline injected into the tube helps to loosen the secretions and crusts for easier aspiration. The amount of saline used (0.5 to 2 ml) depends on the size of the child. The suction catheter is one with a side hole or Y connector so that the catheter can be introduced without suction and removed while simultaneously applying intermittent suction. This reduces the likelihood of mucosal damage from the catheter. The entire process should take no longer than 15 to 30 seconds. A convenient method used by many nurses to estimate the length of time the tube is occluded is to hold their own breath during the procedure. Suctioning is carried out at frequent intervals to avoid buildup of crusts and as often as needed for signs of mucus in the airway, such as bubbling, noisy breathing, or coughing. The cough, although noisy, is ineffectual because the glottis, which normally closes and releases suddenly to effect a cough, is bypassed by the tracheostomy. The child is allowed to rest after each aspiration, then the process is repeated until the trachea is clear.

Aseptic technique is essential during care of the tracheostomy. Secondary infection is a major concern, since the air entering the lower airway bypasses the natural defenses of the upper airway. If the suction tubes are not the type that comes equipped with a plastic sleeve, a sterile glove is worn during the aspiration procedure and both suction tubes are discarded after suction. A fresh tube and glove are used each time. Aseptic technique is used to clean and dress the site. Sterile saline solution used to moisten and clean the tube should be discarded after each use. A container of saline for multiple use is discouraged since it serves as a reservoir for organisms from secretions aspirated through the tube. A duplicate tracheostomy tube and equipment needed for its insertion are kept at the bedside in the event that the tube becomes dislodged and needs to be replaced. If the tube inadvertently becomes dislodged, the attending nurse should maintain the patency of the incision by spreading the edges with a sterile clamp until the tube can be replaced. Children with tracheostomies that must remain in place for months or years require a weekly tube change.

A child with a tracheostomy requires continuous nursing attendance. Vital signs are monitored regularly, and the patency of the tube is maintained. The child is observed close-

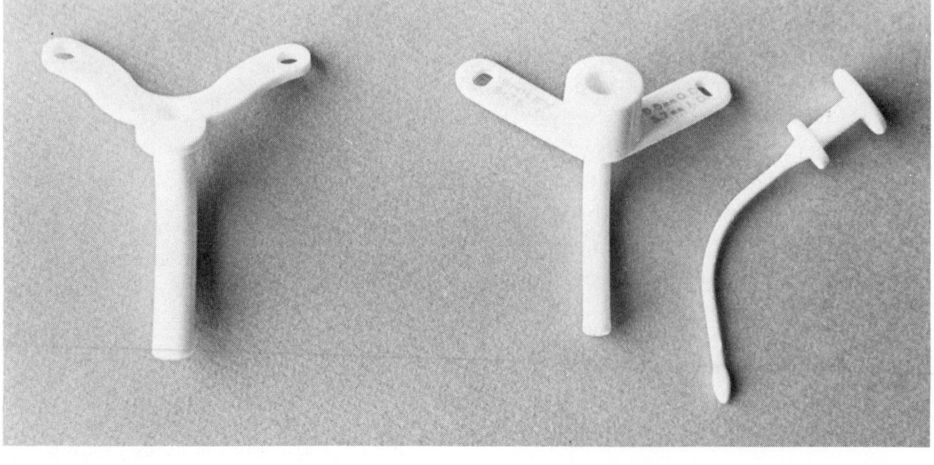

Fig. 32-9. Silastic pediatric tracheostomy tube. *Left,* tube without obturator; *right,* tube with obturator.

ly for any signs of distress or complications. Complications of tracheostomy include infection, atelectasis, cannula occlusion, tracheal bleeding, expulsion of the tube, tracheal ulceration and granulation, tracheal stenosis, air swallowing, and delayed healing of the stoma. Nursing observation is vital to the child who is unable to signal for help. Signs of impending difficulty include restlessness, dyspnea, pallor or cyanosis, changes in pulse or blood pressure, overt bleeding from the trachea or around the incision site, retractions, and noisy respirations.

If the child is fatigued and in distress prior to the procedure, he will probably fall into a restful sleep after establishment of the airway. However, unless he remains unconscious or semiconscious, he will probably be anxious and frightened when he is unable to communicate. It is often a terrifying experience for a young child to discover that he is unable to make vocal sounds, including crying. It is also stressful to parents to watch their child plead with frightened eyes and cry noiselessly. It is important to talk to the child and to reassure him that his voice will return when he is able to breathe again. Children whose tracheostomies are more or less permanent but needed to facilitate pulmonary toilet are taught to occlude the opening with a clean finger so that they can use the vocal cords to communicate.

Parents have numerous concerns relative to the procedure. If time allows prior to the procedure, the reasons for the decision to perform the tracheostomy, the expected results, and the approximate length of time it will remain in place should be discussed with them. Parental concern is centered around the (often) life-threatening implications generated by the need for the procedure and the possible long-term effects on the child, both physiologic and psychologic. They are concerned about the visible wound and the scar that will remain. Parents who must face the possibility of caring for the child with a tracheostomy at home have additional worries regarding their ability to assume this responsibility.

The tracheostomy tube is removed as soon as it is no longer needed. Diseases of short duration, such as croup, usually allow early removal, but some conditions, such as tracheomalacia, tracheal stenosis, or paralysis, may require the tube to remain in place indefinitely. Opinions differ regarding the best means for removing a tube, especially after it has been in place for an appreciable length of time. More commonly the diameter of the tube is reduced daily by inserting tubes of decreasing size. When a tube several sizes smaller than the original is tolerated without difficulty, the tube is plugged. If the child has no problems after 24 hours, the plugged tube is removed. Any air leaks through the wound nearly always cease within 72 hours.

Some children may be discharged from the hospital with tracheostomy tubes. Prior to discharge the parents will need careful instruction and practice in the care and management of the tracheostomy. During hospitalization the parents should be involved in the child's care as soon as possible in anticipation of this eventuality. The more comfortable they are with all the aspects of tracheostomy care, the more confident and less anxious they will be when faced with total care of the child at home. It sometimes requires weeks before they feel comfortable with suctioning, cleaning, and changing the tube. Instructions should be detailed and explicit. To facilitate their adjustment, supplies identical to the ones they are accustomed to should be available to the parents. Parents often become anxious when they encounter even small differences from the familiar. In the event of substitution, they need to be reassured that the unfamiliar equipment is safe to use on their child.[6]

A nurse from the public health department or other service should be available to the family and should periodically assess the family's ability to carry out the activities needed in care of the child.[8a] The parents may find it helpful to talk to other parents of children with tracheostomies. They also need to know whom to call and where they can get help and support in times of uncertainty or in an emergency.

They should be encouraged to provide as normal a life as possible for their child and other family members. The child can usually be allowed to engage in most activities that are appropriate for his age. He may even play outdoors with a scarf or other protection to cover the tracheostomy stoma. Both child and parents must be cautioned regarding play near any collection of water, such as a swimming pool or stream, and informed about safety precautions in the bathtub. Young children who may spill food in the direction of the stoma should wear a bib or other device to prevent dribbled food or crumbs from being aspirated.

Other siblings should not be neglected because of the needs of the tracheostomized child, and the care of the child should not be left to only one of the parents. Both should become involved in his care, and the presence of both should be encouraged at follow-up conferences. Most parents are eager to share the responsibilities but need the continued support and reassurance of the nurse and other health-care providers.

Pharmacologic agents. Several drugs may be used in the treatment of respiratory failure, and an intravenous route for administration is started after the initial establishment of an airway (unless it was already in existence prior to the respiratory failure). To correct metabolic acidosis, sodium bicarbonate is usually the drug of choice, although tromethamine (THAM) has been employed successfully in some instances. Cardiac stimulants are given in cardiac arrest or severe bradycardia, and bronchodilators are essential in cases of status asthmaticus. Narcotic antagonists are administered in cases of depression caused by drugs, most often in the newborn after placental transfer during labor and delivery. Nurses should anticipate the need for drugs during respiratory failure, maintain an adequate emergency supply,

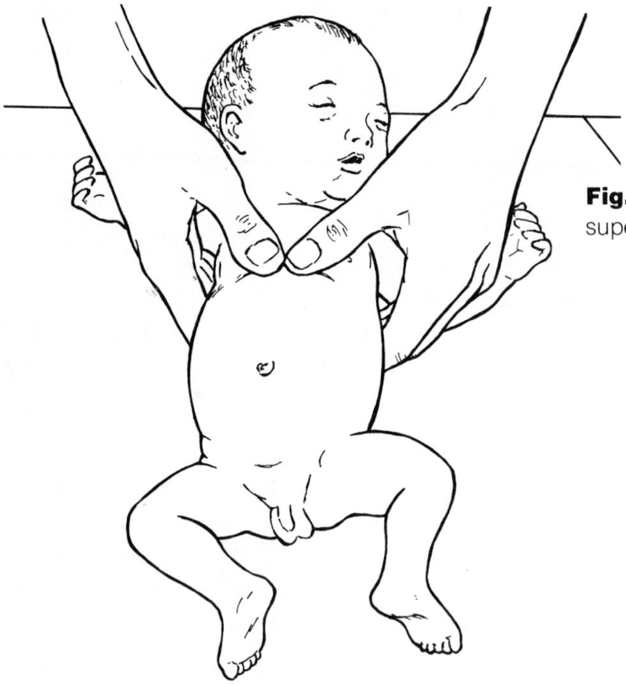

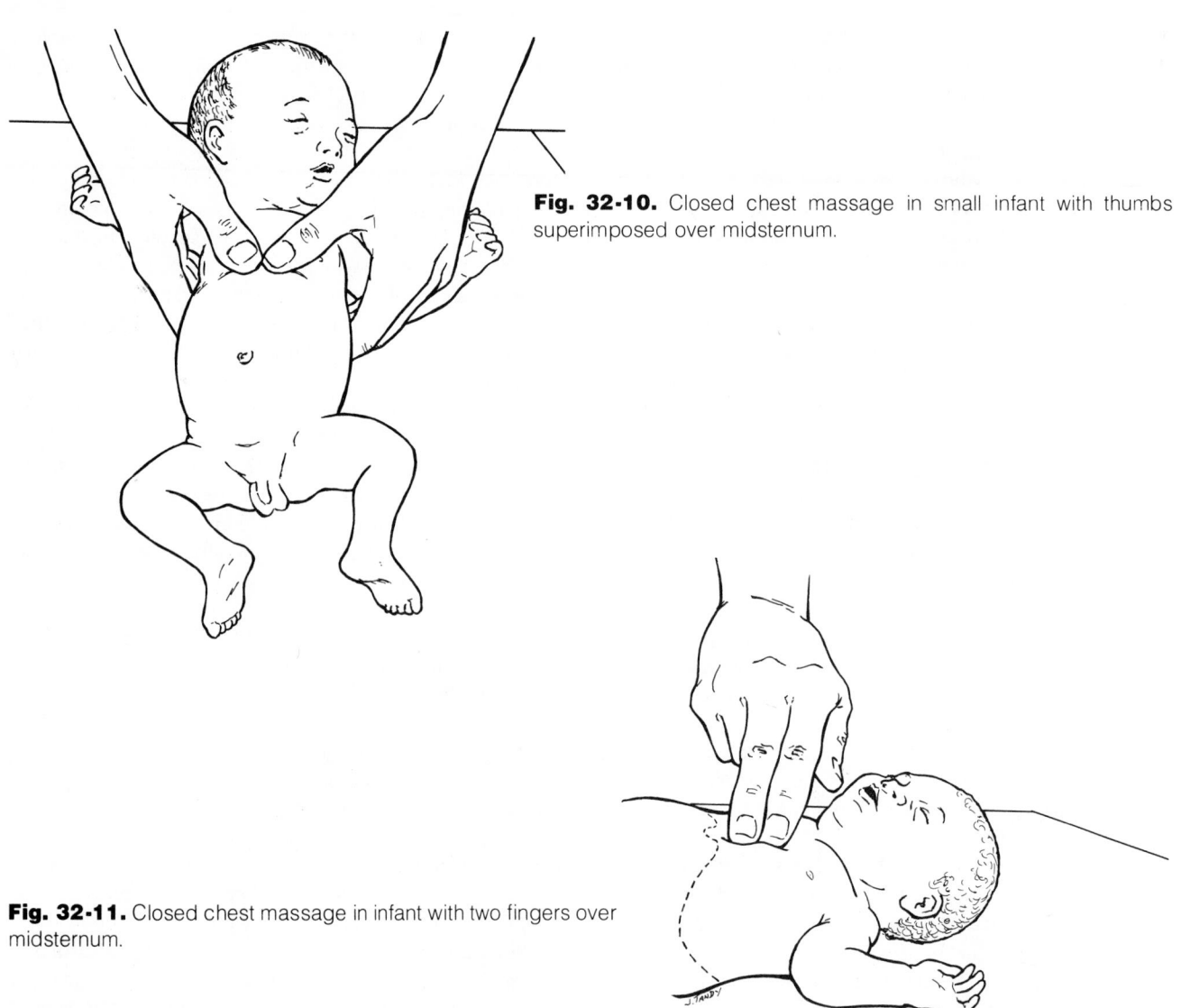

Fig. 32-10. Closed chest massage in small infant with thumbs superimposed over midsternum.

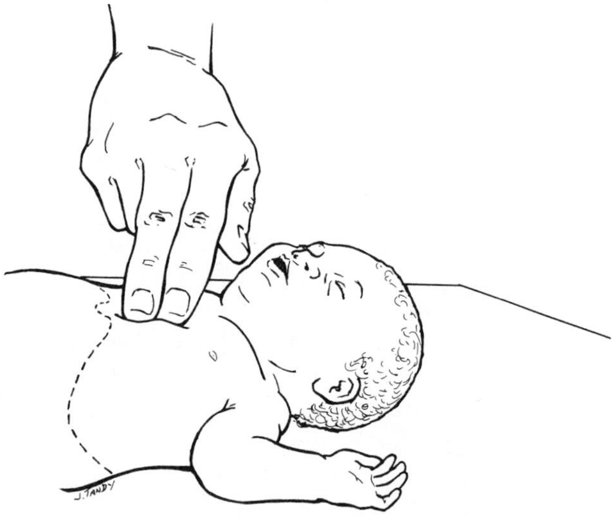

Fig. 32-11. Closed chest massage in infant with two fingers over midsternum.

and be familiar with their administration and the nursing responsibilities related to their use.

Cardiopulmonary resuscitation

Complete apnea signals the need for rapid and vigorous action to prevent cardiac arrest. In such situations nurses must be prepared to initiate action immediately. In anticipation, emergency equipment should be readily available in areas in which respiratory arrest might take place, and the status of this resuscitation equipment should be checked regularly (at least once daily). Regardless of the cause of the arrest, some very basic procedures are carried out, modified somewhat according to the size of the child.

The initial step after cessation of respiration is to palpate peripheral pulses and quickly check the heartbeat. Absence of carotid or temporal pulse is considered sufficient indication to begin external cardiac massage.[11] However, two essential elements determine the safety and efficacy of external cardiac massage: (1) the patient's spine must be supported during compression of the sternum, and (2) sternal pressure must be forceful but not traumatic.

After rapid ascertainment and restoration of a patent airway by removal of foreign material and secretions (if indicated), cardiac massage is initiated. Sternal compression is applied to small infants with both thumbs on the midsternum while joining the fingers of both hands behind the infant's back (Fig. 32-10).[11] It is best applied from the superior direction with the operator at the infant's head to minimize the chance of damage that might occur to the liver and/or spleen if applied from an inferior position. For an older infant a firm board is placed beneath the spine and pressure is applied with two fingers on the midsternum exerting a sharp downward thrust (Fig. 32-11). For children over age 5 years pressure is applied with the heel of one or both hands at the junction of the middle and lower two-thirds of the sternum. The depth of compression is also adapted to the size of the child—infants, 0.5 to 0.75 inch; young children, 0.75 to 1 inch; and older children, 1.5 to 2 inches. The location, rate, and depth for adolescents is the same as for adults.

External massage is administered at a rate of 100 to 120 times/minute in the newborn and 60 to 80 times/minute in older children. Cardiac compression should be interspersed with ventilation, administered by the mouth-to-mouth method or artificial ventilator, at a ratio of one breath for five to eight compressions. Massage is continued until there are signs of recovery as evidenced by palpable peripheral pulses, return of pupils to normal size, and the disappearance of mottling and cyanosis.

REFERENCES

1. Are you underusing blood gas analysis? Patient Care **10**(7): 120-129, 1976.
2. Avery, M. E., and Stern, L.: Oxygen therapy. In Shirkey, H. C., editor: Pediatric therapy, ed. 5, St. Louis, 1975, The C. V. Mosby Co.
3. Betson, C.: The nurse's role in blood gas monitoring, Cardiovasc. Nurs. **7**(6), November/December 1971.
4. Chernick, V., and Avery, M. E.: The functional basis of respiratory pathology. In Kendig, E. L., and Chernick, V., editors: Disorders of the respiratory tract in children, ed. 2, Philadelphia, 1977, W. B. Saunders Co.
5. Cotton, E. K., and Parry, W. H.: Respiratory tract and mediastinum. In Kempe, C. H., Silver, H. K., and O'Brien, D.: Current pediatric therapy, ed. 3, Los Altos, Calif., 1974, Lange Medical Publications.
6. Eigen, H., and Warning, W. W.: Tracheostomy care. In Shirkey, H. C., editor: Pediatric therapy, ed. 5, St. Louis, 1975, The C. V. Mosby Co.
7. Hislop, A., and Reid, L.: Development of the acinus of the human lung, Thorax **29:**90, 1974.
8. Hogg, J. C.: Age as a factor in respiratory disease. In Kendig, E. L., and Chernick, V., editors: Disorders of the respiratory tract in children, ed. 2, Philadelphia, 1977, W. B. Saunders Co.

8a. Kaler, J., and Kaler, H.: Michael has a tracheostomy, Am. J. Nurs. **74:**852-855, 1974.

9. Levin, R. M.: Pediatric respiratory intensive care handbook, Flushing, N.Y., 1976, Medical Examination Publishing Co., Inc.
10. Mellins, R. B.: Cardiorespiratory disorders in children. In Winters, R. W., editor: The body fluids in pediatrics, Boston, 1973, Little, Brown and Co.
11. Pagtakhan, R. D., and Chernick, V.: Intensive care of respiratory disorders. In Kendig, E. L., and Chernick, V., editors: Disorders of the respiratory tract in children, ed. 2, Philadelphia, 1977, W. B. Saunders Co.
12. Respiratory Therapy Department, Children's Hospital Medical Center of Northern California, Oakland, Calif.
13. Stern, L.: The use and misuse of oxygen in the newborn infant, Pediatr. Clin. North Am. **20:**447-463, 1973.
14. Wade, J. F.: Respiratory nursing care: physiology and technique, St. Louis, 1977, The C. V. Mosby Co.
15. Waring, W. W.: Diagnostic and therapeutic procedures. In Kendig, E. L., and Chernick, V., editors: Disorders of the respiratory tract in children, ed. 2, Philadelphia, 1977, W. B. Saunders Co.
16. Waring, W. W.: The history and physical examination. In Kendig, E. L., and Chernick, V., editors: Disorders of the respiratory tract in children, ed. 2, Philadelphia, 1977, W. B. Saunders Co.

Bibliography

Affonso, D., and Harris, T.: Continuous positive airway pressure, Am. J. Nurs. **76:**570-573, 1976.

Connor, G. H., and associates: Tracheostomy, Am. J. Nurs. **72:** 68-77, 1972.

Dyer, E. D., and Peterson, D. E.: Safe care of IPPB machines, Am. J. Nurs. **71:**2163-2166, 1971.

Foss, G.: Postural drainage, Am. J. Nurs. **73:**666-669, 1973.

Gale, R., Redner-Garmi, R., and Gale, J.: Accumulation of carbon dioxide in oxygen hood, infant cots, and incubators, Pediatrics **60:**453-456, 1977.

Imbruce, R. P., Nair, S., and Weg, J. G.: Are you understanding blood gas analysis? Patient Care **10**(7):120-129, April 1, 1976.

Indyk, L.: Po_2 in the seventies, Pediatrics **55:**153, 1975.

Jacquette, G.: To reduce hazards of tracheal suctioning, Am. J. Nurs. **71:**2362-2364, 1971.

Johnson, M.: Outcome criteria to evaluate postoperative respiratory status, Am. J. Nurs. **75:**1474-1475, 1975.

Kearns, B.: Tracheostomy suctioning technique, Can. Nurs **66:**44, 1970.

Kendig, E. L., and Chernick, V., editors: Disorders of the respiratory tract in children, ed. 3, Philadelphia, 1977, W. B. Saunders Co.

Laycock, J.: Nursing the patient on the ventilator, Nurs. Clin. North Am. **10:**17-26, 1975.

Libman, R. H., and Keithley, J.: Relieving airway obstruction in the recovery room, Am. J. Nurs. **75:**603-605, 1975.

Moody, L. E.: Primer for pulmonary hygiene, Am. J. Nurs. **77:** 104-106, 1977.

Nett, L., and Petty, T. I.: Oxygen toxicity, Am. J. Nurs. **73:**1556-1558, 1973.

Oaks, A., and Morrow, H.: Understanding blood gases, Nursing '73 **3**(9):15-21, 1973.

Pinney, M.: Postural drainage for infants, Nursing '72 **2**(10):45-48, 1972.

Sandham, G., and Reid, B.: Some Q's and A's about suctioning, Nursing '77 **7**(10):60-65, 1977.

Segal, S.: Oxygen: too much, too little, Nurs. Clin. North Am. **6:** 39, March 1971.

Stern, L.: The use and misuse of oxygen in the newborn infant, Pediatr. Clin. North Am. **20:**447, 1971.

Tinker, J. H.: Understanding chest x-rays, Am. J. Nurs. **76:**54-58, 1976.

Tinker, J. H., and Wehner, R.: The nurse and the ventilator, Am. J. Nurs. **74:**1276-1278, 1974.

Unquarski, P.: Mechanical stimulation of coughing, Am. J. Nurs. **71:**2358-2361, 1971.

Weber, B.: Eating with a trach, Am. J. Nurs. **74:**1439, 1974.

33

Conditions with disturbed respiratory function

Some of the most common problems in the pediatric age-group are related to disturbed respiratory function, and respiratory failure is the chief cause of morbidity in the newborn period. Respiratory illness can be caused by disease, trauma, or physical anomalies or can be seen as a manifestation of a disturbance in another organ or system, such as neurologic disorders involving the respiratory center or innervation to the respiratory musculature. Most communicable diseases have respiratory symptoms. The type and pattern of respiratory disturbances also vary tremendously according to the age of the child. There are differences in susceptibility to infections and in response to various organisms and conditions at various ages. Moreover, manifestations of illness vary according to the age of the child and may involve different organ systems. For example, diarrhea is often the manifestation of a viral infection in infancy that produces a pharyngoconjunctivitis in the older child.

This chapter is primarily concerned with infectious, allergic, and mechanical disturbances.

Defenses of respiratory tract

The respiratory tract has several anatomic and biochemical characteristics that provide natural defenses against the multitude of both biologic and inanimate agents that can damage respiratory tissues. Intact defenses help to repel and resist the impact of deleterious agents; factors that reduce the integrity of these mechanisms increase the vulnerability of these tissues to invasion and disease.

lymphoid tissues faucial, lingual, pharyngeal tonsils (adenoids) and other pharyngeal lymphoid tissues, which form a protective circle around the entrance to the respiratory tract, help to localize and contain invading organisms where they can be destroyed by the body's humoral defense mechanisms.

viscid secretions the epithelium of the respiratory tract secretes a sticky mucus to which airborne organisms adhere.

ciliary action the mucus secreted by the columnar epithelium of the respiratory tract is kept flowing, carrying microorganisms and other hostile agents away from the lungs to be coughed or swallowed.

epiglottis the epiglottis and the epiglottis reflex protect the respiratory tract from invading material, including infectious exudate from the upper tract, from being aspirated into the lower tract.

cough the expulsive force of the cough reflex propels foreign material out of the lower tract.

tracheobronchial dynamics the tracheobronchial tree elongates and dilates on inspiration and shortens and narrows on expiration.

position changes changes in body position encourage drainage of tracheobronchial passages.

lymphatics lymphatics draining the terminal bronchi and bronchioles remove invading organisms to be filtered and destroyed in the regional lymph nodes.

humoral defenses organisms and other foreign material are removed and/or destroyed by the action of phagocytes, enzymes, and immune globulins, especially immunoglobulin A (IgA).

Effective as these natural barriers are, they are frequently breached. For example, there are children who have conditions that predispose to infection resulting from interference with the efficiency of these mechanisms, such as chronic asthma, cystic fibrosis, and the various immune-deficiency disorders. Frequent intense exposure to organisms that accompanies conditions of crowding or continual exposure to irritating substances in the air results in breakdown of healthy defenses. Concurrent illness, malnutrition, or fatigue reduces the efficiency of natural defenses.

ACUTE RESPIRATORY INFECTION

Acute infection of the respiratory tract is the most common cause of illness in infancy and childhood. Young children ordinarily have four or five such infections each year that manifest a wide range of severity from trivial to severe or even fatal illness. The type of illness and the physical response are also related to a variety of factors, including the type of infectious agent, the age of the child, and the integrity of the child's defense mechanisms. Despite the effectiveness of the natural defense mechanisms in the respiratory tract, circumstances alter their ability to repel invading organisms.

The various areas of the respiratory tract will be discussed according to the general areas of involvement in the more common infections: the upper respiratory tract or upper airway, which consists primarily of the nose and pharynx; the lower respiratory tract, consisting of the structurally stable or nonreactive portion of the airway, which includes the epiglottis, larynx, and trachea; the bronchi and bronchioles, which constitute the reactive portion of the airway because of their smooth muscle content and ability to constrict; and the primary respiratory unit, the lungs.

Etiology

The etiology and course of respiratory tract infections are influenced by a number of factors. They are seldom localized to a single anatomic structure or area but tend to spread to a variable extent as a result of the continuous nature of the mucous membrane lining the respiratory tract. Consequently infections of the respiratory tract generally involve several areas rather than a single structure, although the effect on one may predominate in any given illness.

Numerous factors, including the nature of the agent, the age of the child, and the resistance offered by natural defenses, influence the incidence and severity of respiratory infections.

Infectious agents. The respiratory tract is subject to a wide variety of infective organisms, but the largest percentage of infections are caused by viruses, particularly in the upper respiratory passages. Other organisms that may be involved in primary or secondary invasion are group A β-hemolytic *Streptococcus, Streptococcus aureus, Hemophilus influenzae,* and *pneumococci*. Of special significance is the β-hemolytic *Streptococcus* because of the relationship between respiratory infection with this organism and the incidence of subsequent nephritis (p. 1159) or rheumatic fever (p. 1356).

Size and frequency of dose. The larger the dose of an infectious agent, the greater the likelihood of a significant infection. Pathogenic bacteria are natural inhabitants of the oropharynx, as evidenced by positive throat cultures from healthy persons. These organisms increase in number when the local defenses are lowered by damage to the mucous membranes from viral infections or concurrent respiratory, debilitating, or immunologic disorders.[22]

Age. The pattern of respiratory infection varies considerably with the age of the child. Infants with few outside contacts acquire fewer infections than children entering nursery school or grade school with frequent exposure to a wider circle of contacts. The susceptibility to specific organisms varies with age also, for example, there is a lower incidence of infection in infants exposed to group A β-hemolytic *Streptococcus* than in children in older age-groups. The incidence of influenza is lower in infants. The older child, on the other hand, has an advantage over the infant. Some of the viral agents produce a mild illness in older children but cause severe lower respiratory tract illness and croup in infants. The amount of lymphoid tissue increases throughout middle childhood, and repeated exposure to organisms confers increasing immunity as the child grows older; thus older children have a greater resistance to most organisms. Whooping cough is a relatively harmless tracheobronchitis in childhood but a serious disease in infancy.

Size. In the young child the diameter of the respiratory tract is relatively smaller than in older children and is, therefore, subject to considerable narrowing from edematous mucous membranes and increased production of secretions. Also, the distance between structures within the tract is shorter anatomically in the young child; therefore, organisms move more rapidly down the respiratory tract for more extensive involvement.

Resistance. The ability to resist invading organisms depends on several factors. Deficiencies of the immune system place the child at risk for any infectious process. The general conditions that appear to decrease resistance to infection are malnutrition, anemia, fatigue, and chilling of the body. Conditions affecting the respiratory tract that weaken its defenses and predispose to infection include allergies such as allergic rhinitis and asthma, cardiac anomalies that have the tendency to pulmonary congestion, and cystic fibrosis of the pancreas.

General manifestations of acute respiratory tract infections in children

Infants and young children react more severely to acute respiratory tract infection than older children, and they appear to be much more ill than their local manifestations would indicate. This is especially true regarding children between 6 months and 3 years of age. Young children display a number of generalized signs and symptoms as well as local manifestations that differ from those seen in older children and adults. An infant or child may display any or all of the following signs and symptoms as described by Hughes.[22]

Fever. A characteristic of illness in newborn infants is the presence of sepsis without an elevation of temperature. Even severe infections in newborns can occur without fever. The temperature may even be subnormal. However, the infant tends to develop fever more readily with advancing age. This capacity is greatest at ages 6 months to 3 years. Even with mild infections the temperature may reach 39.5° to 40.5°C (103° to 105°F). Children may have a fever before any other sign of infection is evident; therefore, any child with a fever should be observed for development of symptoms.

Although an elevated temperature usually makes children listless and irritable, they may become somewhat euphoric and more active than normal, temporarily. Some children talk with unaccustomed rapidity when they have a fever, and parents learn to recognize this as a sign of illness. The tendency to develop high temperatures with infection seems to occur in certain families.

Febrile convulsions. In some small children a sudden temperature rise to 40°C (104°F) or higher will precipitate febrile convulsions of a tonic-clonic character (see p. 1439). A more gradual temperature rise will not elicit a seizure. Approximately one third of these children have a family history of febrile convulsions that appear to be unrelated to epilepsy in most cases. Febrile convulsions are uncommon after 3 or 4 years of age.

Meningismus. Meningeal signs without infection of meninges may be present in small children who have an abrupt onset of fever. The signs of fever, which may include headache, pain and stiffness in the back and neck, and presence of Kernig's and Brudzinski's signs (see p. 170), subside as the temperature drops. Cerebrospinal fluid is normal but may be under slightly elevated pressure.

Anorexia. Loss of appetite is a symptom common to most childhood illnesses, and it almost invariably accompanies acute infections in small children. It is frequently the initial evidence of illness, preceding fever and other overt signs of infection. When a child who usually has a good appetite develops a distaste for food, he should be observed for impending infection. The loss of appetite persists to a greater or lesser degree throughout the febrile stage of illness and often into convalescence. Return of appetite is a well-recognized sign that the peak of illness has passed.

Vomiting. Small children vomit readily with illness, and vomiting occurs so frequently at the onset of infection that its appearance for no obvious reason is a clue to the advent of infection. It often precedes other signs, such as fever, by several hours. Although usually short lived, vomiting may persist during the illness to become the dominant feature with the associated risk of dehydration and electrolyte imbalance.

Diarrhea. Mild transient diarrhea often accompanies respiratory infections in small children, particularly viral infections. However, it may be severe, creating a greater problem than the respiratory aspects of the illness.

Abdominal pain. Abdominal pain, sometimes indistinguishable from the pain of appendicitis, is a common complaint in small children with acute respiratory infections. Mesenteric lymphadenitis that accompanies throat infection may be a cause of acute symptoms. Muscle spasms from vomiting may be a factor or a manifestation in a nervous, tense child.

Nasal blockage. The small nasal passages of the infant are easily blocked by mucosal swelling and exudation. Infants have difficulty in breathing through their mouth; therefore, this occlusion can interfere with respiration and feeding. The infant becomes restless, feeding is difficult, and fluid intake is compromised. It also contributes to the development of complications such as otitis media and sinusitis.

Absence of sore throat. Young children who are able to describe symptoms often do not complain of sore throat, even when the throat is highly inflamed. It may be that the elastic nature of the tissues in young children causes less pressure on sensitive nerve endings.

Complications. There is a higher incidence of complications with acute respiratory infection in young children, probably because of decreased resistance to infection and because of local circumstances such as a greater degree of nasal and paranasal blockage, large adenoid tissue, and shorter distance between structures (shorter and straighter eustachian tube). Complications that are common include otitis media, cervical adenitis, retropharyngeal abscess, and downward extension of infection to lower respiratory structures. Septicemia and meningitis also occur more frequently after respiratory infections in children.

ACUTE INFECTIONS OF UPPER RESPIRATORY TRACT

Acute pharyngitis and nasopharyngitis (the equivalent of the "common cold" in adults) are extremely common in the pediatric age-groups. These disorders can be merely a part of a generalized upper respiratory infection, or they may be the dominant feature of an infection. The usual organisms responsible are the viruses, but those of bacterial origin are caused predominantly by group A β-hemolytic *Streptococcus*. In general, viral infections have a relatively gradual onset as contrasted with an abrupt onset in bacterial infection, they produce a shorter and milder illness with less intense inflammation, and they cause fewer complications. Differentiation on the basis of symptoms is often difficult. Diagnosis is confirmed by throat culture, although many children harbor streptococci as part of their normal flora. See Table 33-1 for comparison of common upper respiratory infections.

Medical management of upper respiratory infection

Children with upper respiratory infections are treated at home unless there are serious complications. Treatment is important, however, to prevent or minimize complications. The usual recommendations are rest in bed until the child is free of fever for at least 1 day, encouraging liquids, and control of fever.

Most physicians prescribe antipyretic drugs for temperatures exceeding 38°C (100°F) taken orally or 38.4°C (101°F) rectally, usually acetylsalicylic acid (aspirin) or acetaminophen (Tylenol). The aspirin dosage is generally calculated at 65 mg (1 grain) per year of age up to a maximum dose of 650 mg (10 grains), administered once every 4 hours, for a child 10 years of age or older.[39] The peak effect is reached in 2 to 3 hours; however, since the average half-life of aspirin is 6 hours, too frequent administration carries the risk of aspirin toxicity. Infants younger than 6

Table 33-1. Comparison of common upper respiratory infections*

	Nasopharyngitis	Pharyngitis
Anatomic site	Nose and pharynx	Principal involvement is throat, including tonsils
Etiology	Viral, principally rhinoviruses	Viral, group A β-hemolytic *Streptococcus*
Epidemiology	Occurs throughout the year Most common respiratory infection	Uncommon in children under age 1 year Peak incidence between ages 4 and 7 years Prevalent throughout childhood
Manifestations	Younger child Fever Irritability, restlessness Sneezing Vomiting and/or diarrhea, sometimes	Fever General malaise Anorexia Moderate sore throat Headache
	Older child Dryness and irritation of nose and throat Sneezing, chilly sensation Muscular aches Cough, sometimes	Fever (may reach 40°C) Headache Anorexia Dysphagia Abdominal pain Vomiting
Pathology	Edema and vasodilatation of mucosa	Younger child Mild to moderate hyperemia May or may not exhibit follicular exudate; if so, limited to posterior wall Cervical lymph nodes not enlarged or only slightly enlarged Older child Mild to fiery red, edematous Hyperemia of tonsils and pharynx; may extend to soft palate and uvula Often abundant follicular exudate that spreads and coalesces to form pseudomembrane on tonsils Cervical glands enlarged and tender Polymorphonuclear leukocytosis
Complications	Infant Otitis media Lower tract infection	Usually causes no complications Otitis media, sometimes
	Older child Sinusitis	May cause otitis media Acute cervical adenitis Retropharyngeal abscess Downward invasion of respiratory tract May be followed by nephritis or rheumatic fever

*Tonsillitis and otitis media are discussed on pp. 572 and 575.

months of age should not receive more than 30 mg (½ grain). Aspirin is usually contraindicated in infants younger than 3 months of age because of the immaturity of renal function that impairs the child's ability to excrete the drug, thus increasing the risk of salicylate poisoning.

Local measures may be advised, including nose drops to shrink congested membranes, local irrigations (in older cooperative children), hot or cold applications, and carefully managed moist air administration. Nose drops are helpful in relieving nasal stuffiness. Plain saline drops may be all that is necessary to clear secretions in small infants, and vasoconstrictive nose drops, isotonic with nasal secretions, are useful for older infants and children (see p. 940 for administration of nose drops). Saline nose drops can be prepared at home by dissolving one tsp of salt in 1 pint of warm water. Phenylephrine (Neo-Synephrine), 0.25%, is the usual choice of decongestant nose drops, although others such as ephedrine, 1%, may be prescribed. Nasal sprays may be employed effectively in older cooperative children. Medication instilled into the nose should not be continued beyond 4 to 5 days. Beyond this time the medication may cause a chemical irritation that produces nasal congestion indistinguishable from that of the original illness.

Oral decongestants are sometimes prescribed to reduce the swelling of nasal mucosa, but there is little evidence that they are effective in the majority of cases. Potent antitussives to depress the cough reflex are contraindicated where nasal discharge is profuse because of the increased risk of aspirating the secretions.

Although 80% to 90% of all cases of acute pharyngitis are viral, a throat culture should be done to rule out group A β-hemolytic *Streptococcus* infection. If streptococcal sore throat infection is present, penicillin is administered in dosage sufficient to control the acute local manifestations and to maintain an adequate level for at least 10 days to eliminate any organisms that might remain to initiate kidney or rheumatic symptoms. Intramuscular injection of a long-acting preparation of penicillin such as benzathine penicillin G (Bicillin, Permapen) guarantees a satisfactory level for the length of time advised. Oral penicillin such as penicillin V potassium (phenoxymethylpenicillin potassium) may be prescribed for the necessary length of time, provided the parent and/or the child complies with the therapy. Erythromycin is the alternative medication most often used for children who are sensitive to penicillin.[14,22]

Nursing considerations

Since the majority of children with upper respiratory tract infections are treated at home, most of the nursing care is directed toward education and guidance of parents in caring for their child and serving as resources for problem solving. If the physician has given the parents written instructions, these can be explained and reinforced as appropriate. If written instructions have not been furnished, the nurse should provide the parents with written guidelines and, in some cases, outlines of procedures to be employed.

Rest. Any child who has an acute febrile illness should be placed on bed rest. This is usually not difficult while the temperature is elevated but may be difficult when the child feels fairly well, particularly in young children. When parents take the advice seriously and consistently keep the child in bed, most children learn to cooperate during illness. Often the child is more apt to comply if he is allowed to lie quietly on the couch where he can watch television or participate in an alternative quiet activity. If he is unreasoning and expends an inordinate amount of energy in protest, playing quietly on the floor serves the purpose of rest better than crying excessively in bed. A number of entertainment devices can be employed to keep the child quiet, based on the child's individual interests.[22]

Every endeavor should be made to remove the child from contact with other children. Ideally the ill child should be isolated in a separate bedroom at the first sign of illness. This is seldom a problem with an only child but is often difficult when living arrangements are crowded and there are several children in the family. If the child has no bedroom of his own, sometimes another child can sleep on a couch, cot, or with relatives or friends. Well children can be taught to stay away from the ill child if the living conditions allow for segregation and the rule is rigidly enforced.

Nutrition. Anorexia is characteristic of acute infections in children, and, in most cases, the child can be permitted to determine his own need for food. Many children show no decrease in appetite, and others respond well to certain foods such as Jell-O, soup, and puddings. Since the illness is relatively short, the nutritional state is seldom compromised. In fact, urging foods on the anorexic child may precipitate nausea and vomiting and, in some cases, even cause an aversion to the feeding situation that can extend into the convalescent period and beyond. Sometimes reducing the milk intake of formula-fed infants is helpful during the initial phase of an acute respiratory infection.[22]

Dehydration is always a hazard when children are febrile or anorexic, especially when accompanied by vomiting or diarrhea. An adequate fluid intake should be encouraged by offering small amounts of favored fluids at frequent intervals. High-calorie liquids such as colas, fruit juices, water flavored and sweetened with corn syrup, or similar drinks help prevent catabolism and dehydration. Fluids should not be forced, and the child should not be wakened from his rest to take fluids. Forcing fluids may create the same difficulties as urging unwanted food. Gentle persuasion with preferred beverages will usually meet with success. The mother should be advised to observe the number of times and how much the child voids. Infants younger than 1 year of age normally void every 1 to 2 hours; toddlers usually urinate approximately every 3 hours. The older the child, the less frequently he voids. The mother is instructed to notify the nurse or physician if the child appears to be voiding an insufficient amount or if he vomits persistently.

Control of fever. If the child has a significantly elevated temperature, controlling the fever becomes a major nursing task. The parent should know how to take the child's temperature and read the thermometer accurately. Most parents are able to do this, but nurses cannot make this assumption. Those who cannot will require instruction in use of the thermometer.

If the physician has prescribed aspirin or acetaminophen for the child, the parents may need help in administering the drug (see p. 935). Most parents can read the label and calculate the desired dosage, but some have difficulty and will require careful instruction or precise direction. It is important to emphasize accuracy in both the amount of drug given and the time intervals at which the drug is administered in order to avoid accumulation effects. The parents are advised to observe for signs and symptoms of salicylate toxicity (p. 584). The usual method of administration is oral in either tablet or liquid preparations. Older children are able to swallow the tablet; younger ones chew the flavored variety or can be given the tablet crushed and mixed in syrup or jelly. The tablet must be well crushed in order to avoid chunks that might be aspirated into the larynx or trachea. Sometimes the rectal route, using aspirin or acetaminophen suppositories, is easier, especially with infants or children with sore, swollen throats. However, it is almost impossible to divide a suppository accurately; therefore, unless the suppository contains the exact dose, the oral route should be encouraged. Some children will respond well to aspirin incorporated into a chewing gum (Aspergum).

Mothers should be cautioned about administration of aspirin, since there is risk of toxic effects from accumulation if given too often. Every 6 hours is recommended, and it should not be given more often than every 4 hours. If given as often as every 4 hours, the total doses for 24 hours should be kept to a minimum. In most cases the temperature decreases at night; therefore, three to four doses are usually sufficient to control most fevers and the discomfort associated with upper respiratory tract infection.[39] Sometimes aspirin and acetaminophen are given alternately for fevers that do not respond to a single drug. For example, aspirin might be given at 2, 6, and 10 PM and acetaminophen at 4 and 8 PM and 12 AM. This regimen is implemented with the approval of the physician and continued only until the fever is controlled with less frequent administration.

Temperature reduction from the skin is also promoted by evaporation, radiation, or conduction. The feverish child should wear light clothing and have minimal or no bedclothes. Blankets should not be used until the temperature returns to normal. The room should be well ventilated with good circulation of air. A small fan is sometimes helpful to keep the air moving to help dissipate heat by convection but with care to avoid chilling.

Tepid water baths or sponge baths are usually effective for reducing fevers in children (see p. 918 for procedure). Younger children usually tolerate a tepid bath very well. It is seldom wise to delay cooling procedures, since the temperature can rise very rapidly with the attendant risk of febrile convulsions. The parent can be reassured that the cooling procedure is desirable and will not cause the child to "catch more cold." However, if the parent is administering the cooling bath, he or she should be cautioned about making certain that the temperature of the water is not too cold or too warm and to stop the procedure if the child begins to show signs of chilling.

Cool liquids are encouraged to help reduce the temperature and to minimize the chances of dehydration.

Local measures. Older children are usually able to manage nasal secretions with little difficulty. They should be taught to use a tissue when they cough or sneeze and to dispose of the tissues properly. The parents are instructed concerning the correct administration of nose drops and throat irrigations, if ordered. For very young infants, who normally breathe through their noses, an infant nasal aspirator or a rubber ear syringe is helpful in removing nasal secretions prior to feeding. This, followed by instillation of saline nose drops, often clears nasal passages and promotes feeding.

For older infants and children who can better tolerate decongestants, phenylephrine nose drops may be administered 15 to 20 minutes prior to feeding and at bedtime. Two drops are instilled, and, since this shrinks only the anterior mucous membranes, 2 more drops are instilled 5 to 10 minutes later. Older cooperative children often prefer nasal sprays. They are taught to compress the plastic container at the moment of inspiration to gain relief. Spray bottles and bottles of nose drops should be used for one child only and only for one illness, since they become easily contaminated with bacteria.

Hot or cold applications sometimes provide relief to older children with painful cervical adenitis. An ice bag or heating pad applied to the neck may decrease the discomfort, but safety precautions must be observed in order to prevent burns. The ice bag or heating device must be covered, and the heating pad should not be set at the high ranges.

Vaporizers offer both heat and moisture to soothe inflamed membranes. They are especially beneficial when there is hoarseness or any laryngeal involvement. However, the hazards related to their use require that they be carefully evaluated and supervised. A vaporizer is never placed where it can be reached by a small child or accidentally tipped over. It should not be allowed to boil dry. An improvised "croup tent," which consists of a sheet placed to form a hood over the child or a tent over the crib, helps to localize the vapor near the child rather than dissipating it throughout the room. An opened umbrella can also serve as a support for a tent canopy. The parent should be cautioned against adding salt to the liquid in the vaporizer, since this increases the boiling temperature of the fluid, which might easily result in breakage. One method of producing steam is the shower. Running the shower of hot water into the empty bathtub or open shower stall with the bathroom door closed produces a quick source of steam. Ten to 15 minutes in this environment offers the same advantages as the croup tent without the fear and restraint often associated with the confines of a tent. A small child can be held on the lap of a parent or other adult. Older children can sit in the bathroom under the supervision of an adult.

Medication. In addition to antipyretics and nose drops, the child may require antibiotic therapy if the infection is caused by group A β-hemolytic *Streptococcus*. The nurse is often the one who collects the throat-culture specimens, administers medication, and instructs the parents regarding continuing the medication. Parents of children who are sent home with oral antibiotics need to understand the importance of regular administration and to continue the drug for

Summary of nursing care of the child with an acute infection of the upper respiratory tract

Goals	Responsibilities
Provide rest	Keep child in bed until free of fever for 1 full day Provide entertainment and quiet diversional activities appropriate to age and interest of child
Reduce fever	Reduce environmental temperature Place in lightweight clothing and bedclothes Administer antipyretic drugs (aspirin, acetaminophen) in prescribed dosage Administer tepid sponges or baths Encourage cool liquids
Prevent spread of infection	Isolate child from other family members as much as possible Separate bedroom if possible Avoidance of close contact between well persons and ill child Discouraging parents and others from lying down with ill child Keep others from using child's eating and drinking utensils Use separate washcloth and towel for ill child Teach child proper behavior when coughing or sneezing and proper disposal of tissues
Facilitate respirations and promote comfort	Provide moist air Shower "Croup tent" Vaporizer Humidifier Administer nose drops as prescribed Remove secretions with suction apparatus, nasal aspirator, or ear syringe Administer throat irrigations (older children) Administer hot or cold compresses
Prevent dehydration	Offer high-calorie liquids Encourage fluid intake Keep track of number of times and amount of voiding Observe child for signs of dehydration
Rule out streptococcal sore throat	Assess nature of throat manifestation Obtain throat culture
If bacterial infection, eradicate organisms	Administer antibiotics as ordered

the prescribed length of time, regardless of whether the child appears to be ill or not.

For a summary of nursing care of the child with an acute infection of the upper respiratory tract, see the boxed material above.

ACUTE INFECTIONS OF LOWER RESPIRATORY TRACT (NONREACTIVE)

The general term "croup" is applied to a symptom complex characterized by hoarseness, a resonant cough described as "barking" or "brassy" (croupy), inspiratory stridor, and varying degrees of respiratory distress resulting from swelling of the larynx. Acute infections of the larynx are of greater importance in infants and small children than they are in older children in part because of the increased incidence in children in this age-group and partly because of the smaller diameter of the airway, which renders it subject to significantly greater narrowing with the same degree of inflammation.

The infection is seldom restricted to a single area of the

respiratory tract but affects to varying degrees the larynx, trachea, and bronchi. However, the laryngeal involvement often dominates the clinical picture because of the severe effects on the voice and breathing. The syndrome appears more often in males, commonly between the ages of 3 months and 3 years. It is more prevalent in the winter months and tends to recur in the same child.

Although acute lower respiratory infections of the non-reactive airway, or croup, involve all areas to some extent, they are usually described according to the primary anatomic area affected, that is, acute epiglottitis, acute infectious laryngitis, acute laryngotracheobronchitis, and acute spasmodic laryngitis. In general, laryngotracheobronchitis tends to occur in very young children, whereas epiglottitis is more characteristic of older children. Table 33-2 compares and contrasts the major types of croup.

The principal etiologic agents in croup are viruses, except those cases associated with diphtheria, pertussis, and acute epiglottitis in which the usual organism is *Hemophilus influenzae*. The viral croup is more common in children in the younger age-group, 3 months to 3 years of age, whereas croup caused by *H. influenzae* and *Corynebacterium diphtheriae* is more often seen in children ages 3 to 7 years. There often appears to be a positive family history for croup.

In most children the disease is relatively mild with cough, stridor, and mild retractions and gradual improvement to recovery in 3 to 7 days. However, complications of viral croup occur in a number of children, the most common of which are extensions of the infection to other areas of the respiratory tract to cause otitis media, bronchiolitis, and pneumonia. The most serious complication, and the one responsible for most deaths from croup, is laryngeal obstruction. Complications of tracheostomy are another hazard related to these disorders.

Medical management

The major objective in medical management of infectious croup is maintaining an airway and providing for adequate respiratory exchange. Afebrile children with mild laryngitis and a croupy cough are usually managed at home with symptomatic treatment. Rest in bed and humidified air during sleep may be helpful.

Children with spasmodic croup are also managed at home. Steam inhalation as described for upper respiratory infection, especially the quick vaporization that is afforded by steam from hot running water in a closed bathroom, if a shower is available, is recommended. This quick and easy treatment usually provides almost immediate relief of acute laryngeal spasm and respiratory distress. Sometimes the spasm is relieved by sudden exposure to cold air (as when the child is taken out into the night air to see the physician). Parents are usually advised to have the child sleep with either warm or cool humidified air until the cough has subsided so that, hopefully, subsequent episodes will be prevented.

Although many children with croup and significantly elevated temperatures above 39°C (102.2°F) can be managed at home, hospitalization is often advised. Those for whom hospitalization is indicated are children with:

- Presence or suspicion of epiglottitis, progressive stridor and respiratory distress (especially during the daytime)
- Presence of hypoxia, restlessness, cyanosis, pallor, and/or depressed sensorium
- A high temperature and appear to be toxic

Facilities and equipment for tracheostomy, as well as reliable observation, are readily available in the hospital setting. If the hospital does not provide close, skilled observation, the child may be safer at home where the parents can maintain vigilance. Immediate tracheostomy is usually considered for *H. influenzae* epiglottitis with severe respiratory distress. Endotracheal intubation is a satisfactory alternative. In cases of suspected epiglottitis, attempts to visualize the epiglottis directly with a tongue depressor may precipitate sudden laryngospasm, complete obstruction, and death. Therefore, the nurse does not attempt examination of the throat. Examination is made by a physician with intubation or tracheostomy equipment at hand.

Children with croup, whether treated at home or in the hospital, require close observation for signs of respiratory obstruction. They are placed in high humidity, preferably in a mist tent or Croupette with cool mist vapor. Since a rapidly rising heart rate is an early signal of hypoxia and impending airway obstruction, regular monitoring of cardiac rate is instituted, preferably using a cardiac monitor. Oxygen therapy is also indicated.

Fluid by the intravenous route is indicated to lessen physical exertion and to reduce the likelihood of vomiting with the attendant risk of aspiration. Infants with rapid respirations may aspirate feedings.

Medications. Children with suspected bacterial epiglottitis are given ampicillin intravenously (150 mg/kg/day). The use of corticosteroids for reducing edema has not been determined to be of benefit. Expectorants, bronchodilators, and antihistamines are rarely helpful in croup, and sedatives are contraindicated because of their depressant effect on the respiratory center. Dramatic relief of laryngeal stridor has been achieved in treatment of croup with the use of racemic epinephrine (Vaponefrin) in nebulized mist or intermittent positive-pressure breathing.

Nursing considerations

The most important nursing function in the care of children with croup is vigilant observation for signs of respiratory embarrassment and relief of laryngeal obstruction. The child is placed in a cool high-humidity environment with oxygen, usually administered by way of a mist tent or Croupette (p. 1198) and with skilled nursing personnel in attendance to observe for any indications of respiratory distress. Vital signs are monitored frequently, and the child's

Table 33-2. Comparison of common infections of the nonreactive portion of the lower respiratory tract

	Acute epiglottitis	Acute infectious laryngitis	Acute laryngotracheobronchitis	Acute spasmodic laryngitis (spasmodic croup)
Description	Severe, rapidly progressive infection of the epiglottis and surrounding area	Common infectious condition; may be localized or one manifestation of a variety of conditions	Most common form of croup	Distinct clinical entity characterized by paroxysmal attacks of laryngeal obstruction that occur chiefly at night
Age-group affected	Chiefly ages 3 to 7 years May occur in younger children	Most common at ages 3 months to 3 years	Infants and small children primarily	Usually affects small children ages 1 to 3 years
Etiologic agent	Generally *Hemophilus influenzae*, type B	Viral agents, especially parainfluenza viruses	Viruses	Viral agents In some cases, allergy and psychogenic factors have been implicated Certain children appear to be predisposed
Manifestations	May be preceded by upper respiratory tract infection Abrupt onset; rapidly progressive Sore throat Difficulty or inability to swallow Drooling of saliva Retching Difficulty in breathing progressing to severe respiratory distress in minutes or hours Child will sit upright, leaning forward, with chin thrust out and mouth open—tripod position Thick, muffled voice Croaking, "froglike" sound on inspiration Anxious and frightened expression Suprasternal and substernal retractions may be visible Seldom struggle to breathe; breathing slowly and quietly provides better air exchange Sallow color of mild hypoxia to frank cyanosis Throat red, inflamed Distinctive large, cherry-red, edematous epiglottis	Preceded by upper respiratory tract infection Wide range of manifestations from few symptoms to severe obstructive laryngitis Hoarseness to loss of voice Brassy cough Generally mild but may be severe with marked hoarseness, inspiratory stridor, retractions, dyspnea, and restlessness May be slight temperature elevation	Begins with what appears to be simple upper respiratory tract infection for several days Infection rapidly descends, with first laryngeal symptoms—hoarseness, brassy cough, stridor, respiratory distress Fever and prostration increase Respiratory distress, especially inspiratory dyspnea with substernal and suprasternal retractions Bronchi involvement becomes evident with increased dyspnea Expiratory difficulty with labored and prolonged expirations Scattered rales of various types; rhonchi Diminished breath sounds bilaterally Pallor or cyanosis Irritability and restlessness	Usually preceded by mild to moderate nasopharyngitis or slight laryngitis Child suddenly wakens with characteristic barking, metallic cough, hoarseness, noisy inspirations, and restlessness; child appears anxious, frightened, and prostrated Accessory muscles of respiration used and inspiratory retractions sometimes evident Dyspnea aggravated by excitement May be some cyanosis Attack wears off in a few hours and child appears well the following day except for some hoarseness and cough May be repeated 1 or 2 nights in succession
Treatment	Establishment of an airway is urgent—endotracheal tube or tracheostomy Mist tent with oxygen Vigorous antibiotic therapy intravenously Nasopharyngeal culture Blood culture Rest	High-humidity atmosphere If mild, treated at home If severe, hospitalized Rest; disturb as little as possible; reduce need to talk or cry Intravenous fluids to save strength and decrease possibility of vomiting	Hospitalization Tracheostomy set at bedside High-humidity therapy with high-oxygen concentration Nasopharyngeal and blood cultures and sensitivity tests Tracheostomy if indicated Adequate fluid intake, usually intravenous Less severely affected—oral fluids	Vaporization Induction of expectoration with single dose of ipecac (1 drop per month of age up to 2 years; 2-5 ml for older children) Mild sedation with phenobarbital, 4-6 mg/kg/24 hours divided into three doses

Summary of nursing care of the child hospitalized with lower respiratory tract infection (croup)

Goals	Responsibilities
Assess respiratory status and detect impending airway obstruction	Monitor respirations Rate Depth Pattern Presence of retractions, flaring nares Auscultate lungs Evaluation of breath sounds Detection of presence of rales or rhonchi Observe color of skin and mucous membranes Pallor Cyanosis Observe for presence of Hoarseness Stridor Cough Monitor heart rate and regularity Observe behavior Restlessness Irritability Apprehension Report and record significant observations
Ease respiratory efforts	Provide high-humidity environment Place in mist tent or Croupette with cool vapor Promote rest Implement measures to reduce anxiety and apprehension Provide oxygen as prescribed Give nothing by mouth to prevent aspiration of fluids
Conserve energy	Promote rest Implement measures to reduce apprehension Disturb as little as possible
Prevent dehydration	Administer fluids as prescribed Monitor intravenous infusion during acute phase Administer oral fluids when tolerated Keep accurate records of intake and output Measure urine specific gravity to assess state of hydration
Be prepared to assist with tracheostomy	Have tracheostomy equipment at bedside Obtain parental permission for procedure
Reduce apprehension	Remain in constant attendance Hold and cuddle child whenever possible—preferably by parent or familiar person Provide comforting devices such as familiar toy, blanket, and so on Encourage parental attendance and, when possible, involvement in child's care
Provide nutrition	Administer intravenous glucose during acute phase Encourage high-calorie liquids when no longer danger of aspiration Progress to regular diet as condition improves
Reduce parental anxiety	Recognize parental concern and need for information and support Explain therapy and child's behavior Provide support as needed Encourage to become involved in child's care
Educate parents	Prepare parents for child's discharge Refer to appropriate health agency as indicated

appearance and behavior are observed to detect early signs of impending airway obstruction, such as increased pulse and respiratory rate, substernal, suprasternal, and intercostal retractions, flaring nares, and increased restlessness. Equipment for performing a tracheostomy or endotracheal intubation should be at hand in case an artificial airway must be supplied immediately and is left there until respiratory difficulty has subsided completely. Any child with laryngeal stridor requires constant surveillance. Laryngeal stridor is a shrill, harsh respiratory sound, often described as a ''crowing'' sound, that is particularly marked during inspiration.

As distress increases, the child becomes increasingly restless and anxious. He dozes, wakens startled, and makes visible efforts to draw in air. Tracheostomy is usually performed at this stage of distress. If not, the inspiratory stridor and retractions progress until he becomes markedly pale or ashen, his skin is cold and clammy, and all his attention and effort are focused on fighting for air. He becomes increasingly agitated, thrashes about, and tries to climb the sides of the Croupette in his efforts to breathe. His status is critical. An artificial airway is manditory for survival. The child may or may not be cyanotic. Cyanosis is often a late sign.

Fortunately only a small percentage of children with croup require a tracheostomy. Immediately after the procedure the child becomes more relaxed as a result of the relief from laryngeal obstruction, breathing becomes regular, and he usually falls asleep from exhaustion. Later he may become frightened to discover that he is unable to speak or to cry. One of the greatest fears is that he will be unable to call someone to his side. He will need continued emotional support as well as physical vigilance required in tracheostomy care (see p. 1207). The tracheostomy is usually left in place only as long as needed to relieve respiratory distress.

To conserve energy, the child is given every opportunity to rest. Fluids are administered intravenously during the acute phase of illness, and other measures are implemented to promote rest and to reduce anxiety. An infant or small child finds that being enclosed within the mist tent, coughing, laryngeal spasms, and restraint for intravenous therapy are additional sources of distress. He needs the security of the parent's or the nurse's presence. When his condition allows, a small child can be removed for short periods for comfort and reassurance, especially to reduce apprehension during coughing spells.

As the crisis subsides and the child responds to therapy, his breathing becomes easier and recovery is generally prompt. Home care after discharge includes continued humidity, adequate hydration, and nourishment. Parents are encouraged to ask questions about home care and preparation for discharge. Referral to a public health agency for follow-up care may be advisable. (For a summary of nursing of the child hospitalized with lower respiratory tract infection [croup], see the boxed material on p. 1221.)

ACUTE INFECTIONS OF LOWER RESPIRATORY TRACT (REACTIVE)

The reactive portion of the lower respiratory tract includes the bronchi and bronchioles in children. Cartilaginous support of the large airway is not fully developed until adolescence. Consequently the smooth muscle in these structures represents a major factor in the constriction of the airway, particularly in the bronchioles, that portion that extends from the bronchi to the alveoli.[9]

The infectious disorders involving the reactive portion of the airway are diverse in nature and etiology. Inflammation of the bronchi (bronchitis) as an isolated clinical entity is uncommon in childhood if it exists at all. Bronchial inflammation is usually seen as tracheobronchitis or laryngotracheobronchitis. Infection of the bronchioles (bronchiolitis, or capillary bronchitis) is an entirely different illness that is more closely related to interstitial pneumonia. Asthmatic bronchitis is often confused with bronchiolitis and represents a peculiar response to a variety of upper respiratory tract infections.

Asthmatic bronchitis. In *asthmatic bronchitis* the predominant pathology is bronchospasm with increased mucus production. The affected children are seldom ill, but wheezing, productive cough, and signs of moderate emphysema are apparent. There is usually a history of attacks associated with upper respiratory infections.

Bronchitis. *Bronchitis,* although an isolated condition and unusual in childhood, may be associated with either upper or lower respiratory tract conditions. A variety of etiologic agents may initiate the dry, hacking, and nonproductive cough. Noxious chemicals in urban air pollution are becoming an important cause.

Bronchiolitis. *Bronchiolitis* is represented by severe infectious and mechanical changes in the bronchioles. Bronchiole mucosa is swollen, and lumina are filled with mucus and exudate, the walls of the bronchi and bronchioles are infiltrated with inflammatory cells, and peribronchiolar interstitial pneumonitis is usually present. The variable degrees of obstruction produced in small air passages by these changes lead to hyperinflation, obstructive emphysema resulting from partial obstruction, and patchy areas of atelectasis. Dilatation of bronchial passages on inspiration allows sufficient space for intake of air, but narrowing of the passages on expiration prevents air from leaving the lungs. Thus air is trapped distal to the obstruction and causes progressive overinflation (emphysema). The chest appears barrel shaped from overinflation, and respiratory excursions are usually shallow and rapid with suprasternal and subcostal retractions. This in turn causes increased alveolar oxygen tension (PAO_2). Severe disease may be followed by a rise in arterial carbon dioxide tension (hypercapnia), leading to respiratory acidosis. Hypoxemia may persist for 4 to 6 weeks after the peak of the illness.

Table 33-3 compares the major characteristics of bronchial and bronchiolar infections.

Table 33-3. Comparison of acute infections of the reactive portion of the lower respiratory tract

	Asthmatic bronchitis	Bronchitis	Bronchiolitis
Description	Exaggerated response of bronchi to upper respiratory tract infection, with spasm and exudation similar to those of older children with asthma	Seldom occurs as an isolated entity in childhood Acute tracheobronchitis commonly found in association with upper respiratory tract infection	One of more common infectious diseases of lower respiratory tract, with maximal obstructive impact at bronchiolar level; consists of hypersecretion, edema, and inflammatory reaction confined to smaller bronchioles
Age-group affected	Late infancy and early childhood	Affects children in first 4 years of life Highest incidence in September and October	Usually children between ages 2 and 12 months; number 3 cause of death in children in this age-group Rare after age 2 years Peak incidence at approximately age 6 months of age Increased incidence in children born prematurely
Etiologic agent	Response to variety of infections, most commonly viral infections of upper respiratory tract	Usually viral agents—same as those responsible for croup syndrome; other agents, such as bacteria, fungus, allergic disorders, and airborne irritants, may trigger symptoms	Viral; predominantly respiratory syncytial (RS) virus; also, adenoviruses, parainfluenza viruses, and *Mycoplasma pneumoniae*
Manifestations	Previous upper respiratory tract infection Wheezing Productive cough Moderate signs of emphysema	Abrupt onset with upper respiratory tract infection Persistent dry, hacking, nonproductive cough that is worse at night and becomes productive in 2-3 days Audible and palpable rhonchi May be low-grade fever	Begins as simple upper respiratory tract infection with serous nasal discharge May be accompanied by moderate temperature elevation Gradually develops increasing respiratory distress, paroxysmal cough, dyspnea, and irritability Tachypnea with flaring nares and intercostal and subcostal retractions Emphysema with barrel chest and palpable liver and spleen from depressed diaphragm Shallow respiratory excursion Fine rales and prolonged expiratory phase; diminished breath sounds, hyperresonance, and scattered consolidation May be wheezing
Treatment	Bronchodilators, such as epinephrine, ephedrine Sedatives, such as phenobarbital Expectorants, principally saturated solution of potassium iodide (SSKI) High-humidity atmosphere	No specific therapy Symptomatic and supportive therapy	Rest High-humidity atmosphere Oxygen in moderate to severe cases Adequate hydration

Medical management

Asthmatic bronchitis is effectively treated with sympathomimetic bronchodilators and expectorants. Immediate relief of dyspnea and wheezing is obtained by subcutaneous administration of epinephrine, and the effect is maintained with oral administration of an ephedrine preparation (pseudoephedrine [Sudafed], triprolidine [Actifed]). The stimulant effect of these drugs is offset or counterbalanced by small doses of phenobarbital. An expectorant, usually saturated solution of potassium iodide (SSKI), is given to help liquify and remove bronchial secretions in addition to providing a high-humidity atmosphere. Since the majority of attacks are triggered by viral infections, antimicrobials are rarely indicated.[17]

There is no specific treatment for viral bronchitis, and the treatment is, therefore, symptomatic. Expectorants are sometimes used, but their value is questioned, and cough suppressants are contraindicated since coughing is necessary to bring up secretions. High humidity or mist helps liquify secretions and provides symptomatic relief, and percussion and postural drainage promote the mobilization of secretions.

Bronchiolitis is treated with an atmosphere of high humidity, an adequate fluid intake, and rest. Hospitalization is usually recommended, and the child is placed in a mist tent or Croupette to help loosen tenacious secretions and minimize fluid loss from the lungs. Mist therapy is generally combined with oxygen in concentrations sufficient to alleviate dyspnea and hypoxia, after which mist alone is continued for mild dyspnea. Fluids by mouth may be contraindicated because of tachypnea, weakness, and fatigue; therefore, intravenous fluids are preferred until the crisis of the disease has passed.

Most authorities use the conservative approach regarding medications. Antibiotics are not routinely employed, bronchodilators are ineffectual since bronchospasm is not part of the pathology, corticosteroids have not been proved to be of universal value, cough suppressants and expectorants have not been found to be useful, and sedatives are contraindicated. Digitalization is indicated in the presence of cardiac decompensation from cor pulmonale (heart failure secondary to pulmonary disease).[17]

Arterial blood gas analysis and pH determination to detect impending respiratory failure are carried out. Acute respiratory failure and threatened asphyxia require endotracheal intubation and positive-pressure ventilation, often accompanied by administration of a skeletal muscle relaxant such as curare, which is given in order that the ventilation can be slowed and the expiratory phase extended. This serves to more effectively empty the hyperexpanded lungs.

The disease lasts about 7 to 10 days, and the prognosis is generally good. The disorder is most often confused with infantile asthma and asthmatic bronchitis. Diagnosis of asthma is favored in repeat attacks, where there is a family history of asthma, and if the child responds favorably to administration of epinephrine, which is frequently used to differentiate between viral bronchiolitis and asthmatic conditions.[9] Other disorders that may be confused with bronchiolitis are congestive heart failure (p. 1342), cystic fibrosis (p. 1252), foreign body in the trachea (p. 1236), pertussis (p. 1230), and the bronchopneumonias.

Nursing care of the child with lower respiratory tract infections is considered on p. 1229.

ACUTE INFLAMMATION OF LUNGS (PNEUMONIA)

Pneumonia, inflammation of the pulmonary parenchyma, is common in childhood but occurs more frequently in infancy and early childhood. Pneumonias can be classified according to morphology, etiology, and clinical forms. Clinically pneumonia may occur as either a primary disease or as a complication of some other illness. Morphologically pneumonias are recognized as:

1. *Lobar pneumonia,* in which all or a large segment of one or more pulmonary lobes is involved. When both lungs are affected it is known as bilaterial or "double" pneumonia.
2. *Bronchopneumonia,* which begins in the terminal bronchioles that become clogged with mucopurulent exudate to form consolidated patches in nearby lobules, also called lobular pneumonia.
3. *Interstitial pneumonia,* in which the inflammatory process is more or less confined within the alveolar walls (interstitium) and the peribronchial and interlobular tissues.

Other terms that describe pneumonias are hemorrhagic, fibrinous, and necrotizing. *Pneumonitis* is a localized acute inflammation of the lung without the toxemia associated with lobar pneumonia.[24]

The most useful classification of pneumonia is based on the etiologic agent. In general, pneumonia is caused by four etiologic processes: viruses, bacteria, mycoplasmas, and pneumonia associated with aspiration of foreign substances. Less often pneumonia may be caused by histomycosis, coccidioidomycosis, and other fungi. The clinical manifestations of pneumonia vary greatly depending on the etiologic agent, the age of the child, the child's systemic reaction to the infections, the extent of the lesions, and the degree of bronchial and bronchiolar obstruction. The etiologic agent is identified largely from the clinical history, the child's age, his general health history, the physical examination, radiographs, and the laboratory examination.

Viral pneumonia

Viral pneumonias occur more frequently than bacterial pneumonia and are seen in children in all age-groups. They are often associated with viral upper respiratory infections, and the pathologic changes involve interstitial pneumonitis with inflammation of the mucosa and the walls of bronchi and bronchioles. Of the many viruses that produce pneumonia in children, the respiratory syncytial (RS) virus accounts for the largest percentage. Others are the influenza virus, parainfluenza virus, psittacosis, rhinovirus, and adenovirus. There are few clinical symptoms to distinguish between the responsible organisms, and differentiations between viruses can be made only by laboratory examination.

The onset may be acute or insidious, and symptoms are variable, ranging from mild fever, slight cough, and malaise to high fever, severe cough, and prostration. Early in the course of the illness the cough is likely to be unproductive or productive of small amounts of whitish sputum. There is often evidence of obstructive emphysema as bronchi become plugged by necrotic material from ulceration and necrosis of tracheal and bronchial mucosa. The alveoli are generally free of fluid. Chest physical signs are noncontributory but may include a few rhonchi or fine crepitant rales. Radiographs reveal diffuse or patchy infiltration with a peribronchial distribution.

The prognosis is generally good, although viral infections of the respiratory tract render the affected child more susceptible to secondary bacterial invasion, especially when there is denuded bronchial mucosa. Treatment is usually given symptomatically. Although some recommend antimicrobial therapy in hope of reducing or preventing secondary bacterial infection, it is usually reserved for cases in which the presence of such infection is demonstrated by appropriate cultures.

Primary atypical pneumonia

Approximately 10% to 20% of hospital admissions of children with pneumonia are caused by *Mycoplasma pneumoniae*. It occurs principally in the fall and winter months and is more prevalent where there are crowded living conditions. The onset may be sudden or insidious and is usually manifest first by general systemic symptoms including fever, chills (in older children), headache, malaise, anorexia, and muscle pain (myalgia). These are followed by rhinitis, sore throat, and a dry, hacking cough. The cough, initially nonproductive, becomes productive of seromucoid sputum that later becomes mucopurulent or blood streaked. The duration and degree of fever vary widely and may last from several days to 2 weeks. Dyspnea is uncommon.

Radiographic examination reveals evidence of pneumonia before physical signs are apparent. There may be fine crepitant rales over various areas of the lung fields, but consolidation is usually not demonstrated. The pathologic process consists of interstitial round cell infiltration and edema of alveolar septa and varying distribution of areas of inflammation, necrosis, and ulceration of the mucosal lining of bronchi and bronchioles. Areas of consolidation and emphysema are present.

Most affected persons recover from acute illness in 7 to 10 days with symptomatic treatment followed by a week of convalescence. Hospitalization is rarely necessary.

Bacterial pneumonia

In children beyond the neonatal period, bacterial pneumonias display distinct clinical patterns that facilitate their differentiation from other etiologies, and each individual microorganism produces a distinctive clinical picture. In very small infants (younger than 3 to 4 months of age), however, bacterial pneumonias appear as a diffuse process indistinguishable from viral pneumonia. The largest percentage of bacterial pneumonias in childhood are caused by the pneumococcus. Onset is abrupt and is generally preceded by a viral infection that disturbs the natural defense mechanisms of the upper respiratory tract and allows the pathogenic bacteria normally harbored in the upper passages to increase in number.[18]

Children with bacterial pneumonia appear ill and exhibit both general and localized physical findings. Symptoms and signs include fever, malaise, rapid and shallow respirations, cough, and chest pain that is often exaggerated by deep breathing. The pain may be referred to the abdomen and confused with appendicitis. Chills frequently occur, and meningeal symptoms (meningism) are also common. Pleural reactions and effusions often accompany the disease, and the consolidation process usually proceeds rapidly.[18]

The three major organisms causing pneumonia are the pneumococcus, *Streptococcus,* and *Staphylococcus.* Pneumonia caused by *H. influenzae* is seldom responsible for pneumonia in children. Since the availability of antimicrobial agents, the incidence of pneumococcal and streptococcal pneumonia has dropped sharply, although pneumococcal pneumonia is still the most common form encountered in childhood. Staphylococcal pneumonia has not shown a similar decline but remains a serious disease and is seen more frequently in infants than in children. The major bacterial pneumonias are compared and contrasted in Table 33-4.

Medical management. Antimicrobial therapy has significantly reduced the morbidity and mortality from bacterial pneumonia. Penicillin G, administered parenterally, is effective in treatment of pneumococcal and streptococcal pneumonia and is implemented as soon as the diagnosis is suspected. Because staphylococcal infections are caused by penicillinase-producing (penicillin G–resistant) staphylococci, semisynthetic penicillins, principally methicillin, nafcillin, or oxacillin, are employed. Medications are given parenterally for rapid action and maximum effect. Sometimes a single daily dose of procaine penicillin G or administration of oral penicillin every 6 to 8 hours for a period of 7 to 10 days may be given for pneumococcal pneumonia.

The majority of older children with pneumococcal pneumonia can be treated at home, especially if the condition is recognized and treatment initiated early. Antibiotic therapy, bed rest, liberal oral intake of fluid, and administration of aspirin for fever constitute the principal therapeutic measures. Hospitalization is indicated when pleural effusion or empyema accompanies the disease and is mandatory for children with staphylococcal pneumonia. Pneumonia in the infant or young child is best treated in the hospital since the course of illness is more variable and complications are more common in very young patients. Also, fluids usually are given intravenously, and oxygen administration greatly reduces the restlessness associated with respiratory distress.

At the present time the classic features and clinical course of pneumonia are rarely seen because of early and vigorous antibiotic and supportive therapy. However, a large number of children, especially infants, with staphylococcal pneumonia develop empyema, pyopneumothorax, or tension pneumothorax. Pleural effusion is not uncommon in children with lobar (pneumococcal) pneumonia. A diagnostic thoracocentesis is performed if there is suspected fluid in the pleural cavity. Nonpurulent effusions, such as occur in pneumococcal pneumonia, do not require surgical drainage.

Table 33-4. Comparison of the three major bacterial pneumonias

	Pneumococcal pneumonia	Staphylococcal pneumonia	Streptococcal pneumonia
Etiology and epidemiology	Most common agent in lobar pneumonia (approximately 90% of all pneumonias) Occurs most often in late winter and early spring Organisms transmitted by droplet infection Highest attack rate during the first 4 years and declines with increasing age Uncommon in infants less than age 1 year	Most common agent in bronchopneumonia Greatest incidence in first 2 years of life; 30% of all cases occur in children less than 3 months of age; 70% before 1 year of age Occurs most often in winter months Usually contracted as primary infection Cross contamination common in hospitals	Usually lobular Less common than other bacterial pneumonias Usually occurs as complication of influenza or measles
Pathology	Usually lobar but may be lobular Progresses through four stages: (1) engorgement—lobe is congested, heavy, and dark with effusion of blood and serum into alveoli; (2) red heparinization—lobe is solid, dark red, and airless; alveoli contain fibrin, serum red blood cells, neutrophils, and pneumococci; (3) gray heparinization—lobe is larger than normal, firm, gray, and pleural surface appears dull; fibrin present in alveoli but decreased cellular elements and bacteria; (4) resolution	Localized abcesses in older children; more diffuse in infants Exotoxin causes necrosis and sloughing of bronchial mucous membranes Formation of peribronchial abcesses Pneumatocele formation—frequently, abscesses erode bronchial wall, abscess material is discharged into lumen; air enters abscess cavity and becomes trapped to form pneumatoceles visible on radiographs (pathognomonic of staphylococcus pneumonia), which usually develop during the first 10 days of illness; most disappear within a few weeks	Interstitial pneumonia Spreads via lymphatics Although usually lobular, areas of consolidation may coalesce to become lobar
Radiographic findings	Areas of consolidation, usually patchy in children in one or more lobes; may involve entire lung	Patchy clouding in one or more lobes Pneumatoceles of varying sizes appear as thin-walled translucencies	Disseminated infiltration
Laboratory findings	Elevated white blood cell count—15,000-40,000/mm³ Positive sputum culture Positive blood culture in 30% of cases	Leukocytosis of 20,000/mm³ or more in older children; may be normal in infants Positive sputum culture Bacteremia in 10% of cases	Polymorphonuclear leukocytosis Blood cultures positive Elevated antistreptolysin O titer
Complications	Fibrinous pleurisy Pleural effusion Empyema Occasionally postpneumatic pneumatocele formation	Empyema Tension pneumothorax Pyopneumothorax	Pleural effusion Empyemia in approximately 20% Streptococcal foci may appear in other areas, for example, bones
Clinical manifestations	Infants: Usually preceded by upper respiratory tract infection Fretfulness and diminished appetite followed by abrupt onset of fever, 39°-40.5°C (102°-105°F) May be accompanied by convulsions Restlessness Apprehension Respiratory distress Appears acutely ill	Usually in infants less than age 1 year, often with history of staphylococcal skin lesion and preceded by upper respiratory tract manifestations Abrupt onset of fever, listlessness and lethargy when undisturbed, irritability on arousal, anorexia, nasal discharge, cough, grunting respirations, progressively severe dyspnea that may include subcostal and sternal retractions and cyanosis	May appear without evidence of illness May follow streptococcal infection of upper respiratory tract or as complication of contagious disease Symptoms similar to those of pneumococcal pneumonia Onset sudden High temperature Chills Signs of respiratory distress At times, extreme prostration

Table 33-4. Comparison of the three major bacterial pneumonias—cont'd

	Pneumococcal pneumonia	Staphylococcal pneumonia	Streptococcal pneumonia
Clinical manifestations—cont'd	Infants:—cont'd Moderate to severe air hunger Flushed cheeks Circumoral cyanosis Physical—may be decreased breath sounds and crackling rales; exaggerated breath sounds on opposite side; pleural friction rub may be heard Older children: Usually follows an upper respiratory tract infection Shaking chill followed by high fever, 40°-40.5°C (104°-105°F) Chest pain Drowsiness with intermittent periods of restlessness Tachypnea Hacking, unproductive cough (initially) Anxiety Occasionally, delerium Circumoral cyanosis Splinting of side caused by pleurisy pain Physical—dullness; diminished breath sounds, tactile and vocal fremitus; consolidation on second or third day evidenced by dullness, increased fremitus, tubular breath sounds, and disappearance of rales With resolution—moist rales; productive cough with large amounts of blood-tinged mucus	Shocklike state may be present Symptoms of complications, for example, pneumothorax, empyema, septicemia, and so on Some infants have gastrointestinal disturbances, for example, vomiting, diarrhea, and sometimes abdominal distention Rapid progression of symptoms characteristic Physical findings—early, diminished breath sounds, rales, and rhonchi with effusion or pneumothorax; dullness on percussion; breath sounds diminished; respiratory lag on affected side; exaggerated excursion on opposite side; tubular breathing above fluid level and on unaffected side	Occasionally, only mild symptoms Tachypnea usually mild Rales generally unilateral and exaggerated by deep inspiration
Antibiotic therapy	Pneumococcus highly susceptible to penicillin G and therefore the preferred drug Administered IV or IM, 25,000-50,000 U/kg/day or 300,000-400,000 U orally every 6-8 hours Continued 4-5 days after temperature returns to normal Alternate drugs—ampicillin, tetracycline, chloramphenicol, erythromycin, and sulfonamides Resolution begins about 24 hours after initiation of therapy	Methicillin, 250-300 mg/kg/day parenterally Equally effective are oxacillin, cloxacillin, dicloxacillin, or nafcillin For penicillin-sensitive organisms, penicillin G, 100,000-200,000 U/kg/day, may be given Duration of treatment usually 3 weeks If empyema—aspiration of empyema fluid and instillation of penicillin May require closed chest drainage for a while	Penicillin G (IV or IM) is highly effective—30,000-50,000 U/kg/day for infants; 500,000-1 million U/kg/day for children
Prognosis	Good when recognized and treated early Mortality less than 1%; higher in debilitated children Rapid recovery with treatment	Prognosis ranges from 5% to 40% mortality and varies with length of illness prior to treatment Course is usually prolonged, often 6-10 weeks Early recognition and treatment usually effective	Variable in duration Radiographic findings may be seen for 3 or 4 weeks, with spontaneous resolution

Summary of nursing care of the child with a lower respiratory tract infection

Goals	Responsibilities
Promote rest	Maintain rest in bed Organize nursing care to disturb as little as possible Remove or minimize sources of anxiety Administer sedatives as indicated if ordered for restlessness and pain Avoid stimulating excessive coughing
Maintain patent airway	Administer nothing by mouth during acute stage of dyspnea Promote drainage of secretions from airway Suction secretions as needed Carry out percussion, vibration, and drainage and/or suctioning Prevent aspiration of secretions
Ease respiratory efforts	Promote rest Maintain patent airway Provide high-humidity atmosphere Position for comfort Administer oxygen as needed Reduce anxiety Organize activities to allow for minimal expenditure of energy
Control fever	Provide cool environment Administer antipyretics as indicated Monitor temperature to detect status of temperature

Prevent dehydration	Administer intravenous fluid as prescribed
	  Monitor intravenous infusion for patency
	  Regulate intravenous infusion rate
	Observe for signs of dehydration
	Monitor intake, output, urine specific gravity, and daily weight
	Encourage fluids when tolerated

Determine causative organisms	Collect specimens, as needed
	Assist with diagnostic procedures
	  Radiographs
	  Thoracentesis
	  Venipuncture

Control causative organisms	Administer antimicrobial medications if prescribed Support body's natural defenses
Provide nutrition	Encourage high-calorie fluids when tolerated, then progress to diet as tolerated

Monitor respiratory status	Observe respiratory rate and pattern
	Auscultate to determine
	  Breath sounds
	  Presence of rales, rhonchi, wheezing
	  Areas of consolidation
	Assess
	  Skin color
	  Presence or absence of retractions, nasal flaring

Summary of nursing care of the child with a lower respiratory tract infection—cont'd

Goals	Responsibilities
Reduce anxiety and apprehension	Provide constant attendance during acute phase of illness Encourage presence of parents Provide comfort and cuddling when possible Remove restraining devices when and as often as possible Provide quiet diversion appropriate to child's age and condition

Detect complications early	Carry out periodic assessment of respiratory status
	Change position every 2 hours
	Observe for signs of
	  Chest pain
	  Abdominal pain
	  Dyspnea
	  Pallor or cyanosis

Continuous closed chest drainage is instituted when purulent fluid is aspirated, a frequent finding in staphylococcal infections. If a large amount of purulent drainage is obtained, an appropriate antibiotic is instilled into the cavity and the suction is discontinued for approximately 1 hour after the instillation. Closed drainage is continued until drainage fluid is free of pathogens—rarely more than 5 to 7 days. Sometimes repeated pleural taps are sufficient to remove fluid; however, the purulent drainage accumulates so rapidly and is so highly viscous that continuous drainage is preferred. Also, continuous drainage is less traumatic to the child than repeated thoracocentesis.

A newly developed vaccine for pneumococcal pneumonia is promising but is not available for widespread use. It is recommended for children over age 2 years who are debilitated and children with diseases that predispose to pneumonia, such as cystic fibrosis.

Nursing considerations in acute lower respiratory tract infections

Nursing care of the child with a lower respiratory tract infection is primarily supportive and symptomatic to meet each child's needs. The child is assigned a bed away from others, frequently in a small, segregated ward used only for children who have respiratory infections. Children with staphylococcal infections are isolated to prevent cross-contamination. Rest and conservation of energy are encouraged by relief of physical and psychologic stresses. The child is disturbed as little as possible. Since rapid improvement is the rule in most types of pneumonia, feedings may be omitted, especially when the respiration is rapid, in order to prevent possible aspiration. To prevent dehydration, fluids are frequently administered intravenously during the acute phase. Oral fluids, if allowed, are given cautiously to avoid aspiration and to decrease the possibility of aggravating a fatiguing cough.

The child is placed in a mist tent with oxygen. Cool mist moistens the airways, helps mobilize secretions, reduces bronchial edema, and provides a cool atmosphere that aids in temperature reduction. The child often requires frequent clothing and linen changes to prevent chilling in the damp atmosphere. He is usually more comfortable in a semierect position but should be allowed to determine his position of comfort. Lying on the affected side (if pneumonia is unilateral) splints the chest on that side and reduces the pleural rubbing that often causes discomfort.

Fever is usually controlled by the cool environment and administration of antipyretic drugs as prescribed. Temperature is monitored regularly to detect a rapid rise that might trigger a febrile seizure.

Vital signs and chest sounds are monitored to assess the progress of the disease and to detect early signs of complications. Children with ineffectual cough or those with difficulty in handling secretions, especially infants, will require suctioning to maintain a patent airway. A simple bulb syringe is usually sufficient for clearing the nares and nasopharynx of infants, but a suction machine should be readily available if needed. Older children can usually handle secretions without assistance. Percussion, vibration, and suctioning or drainage are generally prescribed every 4 hours or more often, depending on the child's condition.

The child in the hospital is apprehensive, and many of

the treatments and tests are frightening and stress producing. Reducing anxiety and apprehension not only reduces psychologic distress in the child but, when the child is more relaxed, the respiratory efforts are lessened. Easing respiratory efforts makes the child less apprehensive, and encouraging the presence of the care giver provides the child with his customary source of comfort and support.

For a summary of nursing care of the child with a lower respiratory tract infection, see the box on pp. 1228 to 1229.

Thoracocentesis. Dyspnea resulting from pressure from fluid accumulation in the pleural cavity requires removal by thoracocentesis. Thoracocentesis is also performed in order to obtain fluid for culture or to instill antibiotics directly into the pleural cavity. Equipment and preparation for the procedure are the same as for an adult. Nursing responsibilities include obtaining and setting up equipment, preparing the child physically and psychologically, and assisting the physician with the procedure. If continuous closed chest drainage is anticipated, this equipment should also be available. Thoracocentesis is performed with the child in a sitting position, preferably with arms and trunk bent forward over pillows or over an overbed table with a pillow. Infants are positioned in a semirecumbent position on the unaffected side. The child will need to be physically restrained in the desired position by the nurse. The nurse provides explanation, offers emotional support during the procedure, and observes the child for any changes in color, respiration, and pulse, and any alterations in behavior (such as coughing) and sensorium.

After the procedure the child is made comfortable and observations and recording of physical and emotional responses are continued. The amount and description of the fluid obtained and any medication instilled are recorded, and specimens are sent to the laboratory for culture. Continuous closed chest drainage is managed according to the same protocol as for the child with a thoracotomy (p. 1335).

Other infections of respiratory tract

Although less common than the previous illness, several infectious disorders are capable of causing significant morbidity, especially in the infant and very young child.

PERTUSSIS (WHOOPING COUGH)

Pertussis, or whooping cough, is an acute respiratory infection caused by *Brodetella pertussis* that occurs chiefly in children younger than 4 years of age who have not been immunized. It is highly contagious and is particularly threatening in young infants, in whom there is a higher morbidity and mortality rate. In many developing countries where widespread immunization is not available, the disease presents a major health problem. The incidence is highest in spring and summer months. A single attack confers lifetime immunity. Pertussis vaccine is effective, but the immunity diminishes after several years. Since the common practice is to discontinue pertussis vaccination at about 6 years of age, there is imperfect immunity in the older population. Consequently unrecognized disease in adults may be a source of infection in infants.

Pathophysiology

Infection is acquired by inhalation of infectious particles. Inflammatory changes are seen as the organism proliferates in the mucosa throughout the respiratory tract, especially in the bronchi and bronchioles. The mucosa is congested and infiltrated with neutrophils, and there is an accumulation of sticky mucus and leukocytes in bronchial lumina. Clumps of bacilli are seen enmeshed in the cilia of tracheal and bronchial epithelium, underneath which there is necrosis of the basilar epithelium. Patchy areas of atelectasis and emphysema often appear secondary to obstruction or partial obstruction by mucous plugs in the bronchi.

Diagnostic evaluation

After an incubation period of about 7 days, the clinical course of the disease extends over a period of 6 to 8 weeks and is characterized by three stages—catarrhal, paroxysmal, and convalescent.[20,25]

Catarrhal stage. The *catarrhal stage,* which lasts approximately 1 to 3 weeks, begins with upper respiratory symptoms including coryza, sneezing, cough, mild fever, listlessness, and irritability. After a week the cough, instead of improving, becomes more severe and is especially troublesome at night.

Paroxysmal stage. The *paroxysmal stage* lasts for about 4 to 6 weeks and consists of a severe, strangling cough that comes in explosive bursts on expiration and is associated with marked facial redness or cyanosis, bulging eyes, protruding tongue, and a characteristic high-pitched crowing sound or whoop on inspiration. The child's facial expression conveys anxiety and distress. A number of paroxysms may be grouped together until, with the final one, the child succeeds in dislodging and bringing up thick, tenacious mucus. After an attack vomiting frequently occurs and the child is exhausted and appears listless, dazed, or out of touch. Profuse perspiration often accompanies an attack. The number of paroxysms varies from four or five a day in mild cases to dozens in severe cases. The characteristic whoop may not be present, especially in infants younger than 6 months of age. The attacks increase in frequency and severity during the first 1 or 2 weeks, then gradually decline until whooping and vomiting disappear.

Convalescent stage. The whooping and vomiting cease and the number and severity of paroxysms diminish. A simple cough may persist for a while but usually fades away in 2 to 3 weeks. The child may develop recurrent paroxysmal coughing attacks, including whoop, during subsequent respiratory infections for months or even 1 or 2 years after an attack of pertussis.

Diagnosis is made on the basis of the characteristic cough of the paroxysmal phase, history of contact with a known case, and isolation of the pertussis bacillus from nasopharyngeal cultures. Leukocytosis at the end of the catarrhal phase may be contributory.

Complications. Complications of pertussis may occur in the respiratory, nervous, and digestive systems. The most common and most severe complication is pneumonia, primarily interstitial bronchopneumonia. Atelectasis, emphysema, and otitis media are frequent complications. A serious nervous system complication is convulsions, probably caused by anoxia secondary to paroxysms. Also associated with paroxysms are intracranial hemorrhages that result from increased venous pressure and congestion during coughing attacks. Cerebral edema may occur, and subconjunctival hemorrhages and skin petechiae are common. Loss of weight, dehydration, and nutritional disturbance may follow excessive vomiting.

Medical management

The aims of medical care are prevention of asphyxia by skilled observation and management during paroxysms, maintenance of nutrition, control of organisms to prevent the spread of infection, and reduction of the risk of secondary bacterial invasion.[35]

Most cases of pertussis are mild, but young infants and children of any age who have prolonged paroxysms (especially when associated with cyanosis) are best treated in the hospital, primarily so that skilled observation will be available during attacks. Oxygen by mask is administered for relief of dyspnea and cyanosis, and intravenous therapy may be needed in cases in which vomiting interferes with adequate intake. Intubation is rarely needed but may be lifesaving when asphyxia is unrelieved by suctioning upper airway mucus.

The administration of hyperimmune serum (pertussis immune globulin) is available, but its efficacy in established pertussis is questionable. However, since it may exert a beneficial effect, it is sometimes recommended for patients younger than 2 years of age. The use of vaccines after onset of illness has not been shown to be effective and is not recommended.[25]

Antibiotics have not been demonstrated to be effective in shortening the course or modifying the effects of the disease but are often administered to eliminate the organism and reduce the contagiousness of the affected child.

Nursing considerations

Nurses may be involved in both home and hospital management of the infant or child with pertussis. The hospitalized child should be isolated from others who might contract the disease, and, since the primary purpose of hospitalization is attention during paroxysms, the child should be located where he can be seen and coughing can be heard easily. Suction apparatus, oxygen, and intubation equipment are made available at the bedside. Nurse attendance during paroxysms is the focus of nursing care in the hospital, and someone should attend the child immediately when coughing is heard. A calm, reassuring manner helps to allay the asphyxiation anxiety that accompanies such spells, and the nurse should be prepared to implement suctioning and oxygen administration as indicated for relief of symptoms. Respiratory distress, especially if associated with cyanosis, that extends beyond 60 seconds is an indication for suctioning. Suctioning should be gentle and not overlong. Frequently, prolonged suctioning can be traumatic and may even provoke further paroxysms. When cyanosis is not relieved by brief suctioning, the nurse should give the child oxygen by mask and notify the physician.

Adequate nutrition and hydration may be difficult to maintain when vomiting and poor intake extend over several weeks. Frequent small feedings of oral liquids and soft, highly nutritious and favorite foods are usually accepted best. Feedings offered after a paroxysmal attack are more apt to be retained for a longer period of time.

Most children with pertussis can be managed satisfactorily at home. The mother is given careful instructions, and, if indicated, the nurse can make a home visit to assess the environment and assist the mother to equip the child's room with needed equipment (emesis basin and bulb aspirator) and to reduce external stimuli such as noises, smoke, and dust. The mother needs to know how to manage the child during a paroxysm. The best way is to hold the child on the lap with a basin at hand and to provide assurance and comfort. The mother should be taught how to aspirate mucus gently but needs to be cautioned against too frequent and vigorous suctioning. As long as respirations are regular and the color is good, a small rattling sound is of little concern. An excited, anxious mother only serves to increase anxiety in the child. The mother needs to know how to recognize when symptoms require professional help and how to contact such assistance.

As in any communicable disease, the most important aspect of care is prevention. Active immunization by routine administration of pertussis vaccine is recommended in combination with diphtheria and tetanus toxoids (p. 456). An affected child should be separated from contact with susceptible children. Since the disease is extremely contagious, children younger than 2 years of age should not be brought into a household where they might be exposed to a case.

TUBERCULOSIS

Tuberculosis, although controlled in most developed countries, still remains a health problem and a leading cause of death throughout many parts of the world. Tuberculosis in children is still a problem.

Etiology and pathophysiology

Tuberculosis is caused by *Mycobacterium tuberculosis,* an acid-fact bacillus, that is, the organism is not readily decolorized by acids after staining. The main types of tubercle bacilli that cause disease in man are the human *(M. tuberculosis)* and the bovine *(M. bovine)*. Children are susceptible to both varieties, and, in parts of the world where tuberculosis in cattle is not controlled or pasteurization of milk is not practiced, the bovine type is a common source of infection in children.

Although the causative agent is the tubercle bacillus, other factors influence the degree to which the organism is able to produce an altered state in the host. Resistance to the bacillus can be modified by several factors:

1. *Heredity*. There is no positive evidence to indicate a hereditary tendency to tuberculosis infection, but there is evidence that resistance to the infection may be genetically transmitted. For example, there is a higher disease rate in the nonwhite population, particularly in the American indian. However, this may be related to environmental factors, including circumstances that are not hygienic, poor housing conditions, and crowded conditions that result in more frequent contact between infected and noninfected persons.
2. *Sex*. There are not sex differences in the incidence of the disease in early years, but, in later childhood and adolescence, the morbidity and mortality rates are higher in girls than in boys.
3. *Age*. The age of the child has a decided influence on resistance to tuberculosis infection. Infants have a diminished resistance to infection, and during puberty and adolescence there is an increased tendency to develop the disease. In infancy this may be ascribed to a delay in development of acquired immunity. Infants also have a diminished capacity to resist extension of the infective process. The heightened tendency to acquire the disease during adolescence may be caused by a new infection superimposed on an old one associated with increased contacts or as a result of indigenous reinfection stimulated by metabolic changes or suboptimal diets during a period of rapid growth. There are also age differences in the type of lesion initiated, which are discussed later.
4. *Stress states*. Temporary circumstances that produce a state of stress, such as injury or illness, undernutrition, and emotional distress or chronic fatigue, may increase susceptibility to infection. Increased secretion of adrenal steroids that occurs during stress suppresses the protective inflammatory response, which permits the infection to spread. Therapeutic administration of corticosteroids causes a similar effect; therefore, they are reserved for cases with meningitis and complications such as pleural effusion.

Pathophysiology. The source of infection in children is usually an infected adult. The tubercle bacillus from a lung lesion is expelled in microdroplets from the respiratory tract during a cough or a sneeze where they disperse into the air; therefore, the lung is the most frequent portal of entry in human beings. Less often the organism gains entrance to the body by ingestion. Because droplet transmission accounts for most initial infections, almost all primary lesions are in the lungs. At the focal site there is first an inflammatory reaction with accumulation of polymorphonuclear leukocytes, followed by a localized acute bronchopneumonia. There is a proliferation of epithelial cells that surround and encapsulate the multiplying bacilli in an attempt to wall off the invading organisms, thus forming the typical tubercle. During the inflammatory process some of the bacilli leave the focal area and are carried to the regional lymph nodes that drain the anatomic area of the organism; as a result the child develops a fever. X-ray examinations may be positive if such tests are made, as in cases in which the child is known to have been exposed. The tuberculin test is positive. In children (usually infants) who are unable to contain the spread of infection, the fever persists, the generalized symptoms are manifest, and they develop pallor, anemia, weakness, and weight loss. As increasing amounts of lung tissue become involved, the respiratory rate increases, the lung on the affected side does not expand as well as the other, auscultation reveals diminished breath sounds and rales, and there is dullness to percussion. Cough may or may not be present.[24]

The outcomes of pulmonary tuberculosis are outlined in Table 33-5.

Diagnostic evaluation

Several tests and procedures are employed to establish a diagnosis. In addition it must be determined whether or not the lesion is in active, quiescent, or healed stage. A definitive diagnosis is made by demonstrating the presence of the organisms, but in the absence of this positive evidence diagnosis is based on information derived from physical examination, history, reaction to tuberculin tests, and x-ray examinations.

History. Symptoms generally do not contribute significantly to a diagnosis. History of possible contact with a person known to be infected or subsequently found to be infected is helpful. All contacts of an affected child are examined for the disease.

Various factors can affect the response to the test and produce false reactions. A negative reaction will usually mean that the child has never been infected with the organism. However, circumstances that may produce a false-negative reaction include[22]:

1. *Intercurrent diseases,* especially viral diseases such as measles, rubella, influenza, mumps, varicella, and probably others which suppress the tuberculin reaction for about 4 weeks
2. *Viral vaccines,* such as measles, mumps, and rubella suppress the reaction for about 4 weeks

Table 33-5. Possible outcomes of pulmonary tuberculosis

Outcome	Description	Comments
Hilar lymphadenitis	Enlarged lymph nodes of hilus and mediastinum May cause compression on adjacent trachea and bronchi or partial or complete occlusion of bronchi	Signs of infection variable Cough caused by compression Obstruction relieved when infection brought under control
Intraluminal or endobronchial lesions	Extension of adjacent lesions (usually adherent lymph nodes) through bronchial wall, creating ulcerous or granulomatous lesion	Often resistant to therapy because organism is difficult to reach
Extraluminal lesions	Complete or partial occlusion of bronchi by adjacent enlarged lymph nodes	Obstruction results in emphysema, absorption, atelectasis, and pneumonitis
Caseous bronchiopneumonia	Widespread pneumonia develops from discharge of material from foci in lung parenchyma or lymph nodes	Children are quite ill Bacilli can be recovered from sputum Requires prompt, intensive therapy
Progressive primary disease	Extension of primary lesion at original site causes progressive tissue destruction May become so marked as to create cavities (cavitational)	May or may not be accompanied by signs of systemic illness Cavitation tuberculosis has more prolonged course
Tuberculous pleuritis	Fluid or fibrinous exudate forms and collects in pleural space Usually unilateral	Affected children seldom exhibit signs of pleural involvement May be severe enough to cause respiratory embarrassment Symptoms relieved by thoracocentesis
Miliary tuberculosis	Erosion of blood vessels by primary lesion causes widespread dissemination of tubercle bacillus to near and distant sites	Child becomes acutely ill with fever and prostration Tiny foci of infection in lungs visible on radiographs similar to bronchiolitis Spleen enlarged Uniformly fatal if untreated
Tuberculous meningitis	Bacilli gain access to meninges from distant focus; consists of three stages: (1) prodromal stage—invasion of organisms; (2) meningeal stage—definite, clear-cut meningeal manifestations; (3) terminal stage—paralysis, coma, and death	Dread complication General illness with indefinite complications Signs of meningeal irritation and increased intracranial pressure Lasts about 7-10 days (untreated) Stupor progresses to coma Fatal if untreated
Tuberculous adenitis	Term usually reserved for disease of superficial glands Cervical gland involvement most common Glands enlarge, adhere to each other, and form irregular nodular masses May rupture to form a draining sinus	Several glands usually involved Differentiate from pyogenic adenitis, lymphosarcoma, leukemia, tularemia, and other causes of lymph node enlargement
Osseous involvement	See p. 1534	

3. *Corticosteroids* and other *immunosuppressive agents* suppress the reaction
4. *Cellular immune deficiency disease*
5. *Severe malnutrition*
6. *Too early testing* before the body develops a sensitivity to the protein fraction of the tubercle bacillus
7. *Use of impotent, outdated testing material,* as a result of a mixture that has been prepared for too long or has been exposed to sunlight
8. *Faulty technique,* such as too deep injection, no wheal formed, improper measurement of solution, or leaking of solution from a defective or loosely fitting syringe
9. *Overwhelming tuberculosis infections,* such as end-stage and terminal miliary disease, which may cause the allergy to disappear

Bacteriologic examination. The organism can be isolated by several bacteriologic examinations: (1) microscopic examination of properly prepared and stained smears from a lesion, sputum, gastric washings, spinal fluid, draining lymph nodes, and so on; (2) guinea pig inoculations with any of these materials, which produce the disease in the animal; and (3) culture, the most effective method.

Radiographic studies. Radiographic examinations are usually carried out, but numerous chronic intrathoracic diseases may simulate tuberculous lesions; therefore, the use of x-ray examinations is chiefly supplementary to other diagnostic methods.

Biopsy. Biopsy of lung tissue or scalene nodes is seldom required for diagnosis.

Medical management

Medical management of tuberculous lesions in children consists of chemotherapy, general supportive measures, prevention of reinfection, and, sometimes, surgical procedures. The child is placed on bed rest to conserve energy, avoid fatigue, and decrease metabolic demands. Bed rest is continued until the child is free of fever, exhibits evidence of returning strength, has no manifestations that limit ambulation, and desires to be up and about. Since metabolic deficits, particularly negative calcium and nitrogen, occur easily in infected children, special attention is given to planning an adequate intake of the necessary nutritional elements.[22]

Physical examination. The child should have a complete examination, but physical signs in children tend to be disproportionately few in relation to the pulmonary involvement.

Tuberculin test. This is the single most important test to determine whether a child has been infected with the tubercle bacillus. A primary infection initiates a hypersensitivity reaction to the protein fraction of the tubercle bacillus. This can be detected 2 to 10 weeks after the infection. Two types of tuberculin preparations are used for skin tests: Old tuberculin (OT) and purified protein derivative (PPD) of tuberculin. The PPD is used most widely, and the standard dose is 5 tuberculin units (TU) in 0.1 ml of solution, injected intracutaneously. The techniques for injection are (1) the Mantoux test, in which 0.1 ml of PPD is injected directly into the dermis, (2) the multiple-puncture test (tine, Heaf, Sterneedle, Mono-Vac), and (3) tests using a jet injector. The Mantoux test is the most definitive and the one recommended in suspected cases. The others are useful tests for screening purposes.

A positive reaction indicates that the person has been infected and developed a sensitivity to the protein of the tubercle bacillus. It does not indicate the length of time elapsed since infection or the extent of the lesion. Once the individual reacts positively, he will continue to react positively. If a child who previously has reacted negatively shows a positive reaction, this indicates that he has been infected since the last test. Tests are read according to instructions provided by the manufacturer.

Surgical procedures. Surgical procedures may be required to remove the source of infection in tissues that are inaccessible to chemotherapy or that are destroyed by the disease, orthopedic operations for correction of bone deformities, bronchoscopy for removal of a tuberculous granulomatous polyp, or resection of a portion of a diseased lung.

Chemotherapy. Chemotherapy is the single most important therapeutic modality available for management of tuberculosis. A variety of chemical agents can be employed, and a regimen involving two or more drugs simultaneously has been found to be effective and is usually the mode of choice. The most commonly used combinations of drugs are isoniazid (INH) and rifampin (RMP) or isoniazid and ethambutol (EMB). For severe, life-threatening disease the triple combination of isoniazid, rifampin, and either ethambutol or streptomycin (STM) is used.[43] Drugs used to treat tuberculosis are listed in Table 33-6. The optimal duration of therapy is unknown, but the usual course of treatment is no less than 12 months of an initial treatment or 18 to 24 months for more serious forms of the disease. The most valuable drug, isoniazid, is rapidly conjugated to an inactive form by approximately 25% of the population. In these persons the drug must be tailored to the individual's needs. The only serious side effect of the drug is peripheral neuritis, which seems to be related to a deficiency of pyridoxine. Supplementary administration of pyridoxine is advisable in children in whom dietary meat and milk do not provide sufficient amounts of pyridoxine, such as adolescents, preadolescents, and malnourished children.

Prognosis. Most children recover from primary tuberculosis infection and are often unaware of its presence. However, very young children have a higher incidence of disseminated disease. It is a serious disease during the first 2 years of life and during adolescence. Except for tuberculosis meningitis, death seldom occurs in treated children. Antibiotic therapy has decreased the death rate and the hematogenous spread from primary lesions.

Prevention. The only certain means to prevent tuberculosis is to avoid contact with the tubercle bacillus. Maintaining an optimal state of health with adequate nutrition and avoidance of fatigue and debilitating infections promote natural resistance but do not prevent infection. There is no means to induce reliable immunity.

Pasteurization of milk and routine testing and elimination of diseased cattle have helped reduce the incidence of bovine tuberculosis. Infants and children should be given only pasteurized milk from tuberculosis-free cattle.

Limited immunity can be produced by administration of the only successful vaccine to date, BCG (bacillus Calmette-Guerin) vaccine containing bovine bacilli with reduced virulence. The freshly prepared vaccine, injected intradermally, produces a definite although incomplete protection against tuberculosis. In most instances positive tuberculin reactions develop after inoculation. The distribu-

Table 33-6. Drug therapy in pulmonary tuberculosis

Drugs	Dosage (per 24 hours)	Duration of treatment (months)	Side effects	Comments
Isoniazid (INH)	Minimal 5 mg/kg Average dose 10-30 mg/kg	12-18	Peripheral neuropathy	Most universally used drug About 25% of population rapidly inactivate INH Administer oral, IM, or IV Few neurotoxic symptoms if pyridoxine administered in conjunction with INH
Para-amino-salicylic acid (PAS)	200-300 mg/; single dose initially then three or four times daily	6-18	Gastric irritation, fever, rash, jaundice	Give *after* meals Given as sodium (NaPAS), potassium (KPAS), or calcium (CaPAS) salt Can be given orally or IM Used with decreasing frequency since newer drugs available
Streptomycin (STM)	20 mg/kg; single daily dose; then three times weekly	2-4	Ototoxic—vestibular damage Nephrotoxic	Must be given IM Reserved for serious cases Frequent testing of auditory function
Rifampin (RMP)	10-20 mg/kg	12-18	Hepatotoxic	Administer orally Used in conjunction with INH May cause reddish color to urine and other body secretions Used with increasing frequency
Ethambutol (EMB)	15-20 mg/kg	12-18	Optic neuritis	Not recommended for children less than age 5 years because of difficulty in testing visual fields in young children Replacing use of PAS in older persons
Ethionamide (ETA)	12-15 mg/kg	12-18	Gastric irritation	Used in conjunction with INH Used in treatment of bacilli resistant to more usual drugs

tion of BCG vaccine is controlled by local or state health departments but is not used extensively, even in areas with a high prevalence of disease. Greater protection is afforced by daily prophylactic administration of isoniazid. The drug is given to children with a high probability of exposure to tuberculosis despite the disadvantage of the need for continuous therapy. The drug has no effect on the child's reaction to tuberculin; therefore, the test continues to be useful in detecting acquired infection.

Nursing considerations

Most children with pulmonary tuberculosis are almost always noninfectious; therefore, they seldom need to be isolated. There are few bacilli in the sputum, the amount of sputum produced is quite small, and it is swallowed rather than expectorated. Exceptions are children with draining fistulas from cervical adenitis or other infectious lesions and the rare child with cavitating tuberculosis.

Hospitalization is seldom necessary except for needed diagnostic tests. Only those children with the more serious forms are placed in the hospital for therapy; others are managed satisfactorily at home. Therefore, the major nursing care of children with tuberculosis involves nurses in ambulatory settings—outpatient departments, schools, and, especially, public health agencies.

Asymptomatic children are able to lead an essentially unrestricted life. They can, and should, attend school (or nursery school), but older children are restricted from vigorous activities such as competitive games and contact sports during the active stage of primary tuberculosis. They should be protected from stresses, including parental anxieties, overprotection, and pressures regarding nutritional intake. The regular immunization schedule should be continued. Care should be exerted to maintain an optimum health status with proper diet, adequate rest, and avoidance of infection.

Diagnosis. Nurses assume several important roles in management of the disease, including assisting with x-ray examinations, performing skin tests, and obtaining specimens for laboratory examination. Skin tests, whether used as screening tools or diagnostic aids, must be carried out correctly in order for the results to be accurate. For the Mantoux intradermal injection 0.1 ml of solution is measured into a tuberculin syringe with a small, sharp 27 or 26 gauge needle. After cleansing and drying the skin site, preferably the flexor surface of the forearm, the needle is inserted into the skin. To facilitate this and to avoid injecting the solution subcutaneously, the syringe is held in a position horizontal to the skin surface with the bevel of the needle directed upward so that the solution will be more apt to enter the upper layer of the skin. The needle need only be inserted enough to obliterate the bevel. A wheal 6 to 10 mm in diameter is formed in the skin when the solution is injected. If a wheal is not formed, the procedure is repeated. The injection site is circled with a ball-point pen for easy identification, and the date, time, and site are recorded. The results are read at 24, 48, and 72 hours, and any induration or redness is measured and evaluated. A transverse measurement of 10 mm or more of induration constitutes a positive reaction; 5 to 9 mm is a doubtful reaction and may indicate the presence of atypical mycobacteria; and 0 to 4 mm is a negative reaction. Multiple-puncture tests, such as the tine and Mono-Vac tests, are less standardized, but usually 5 mm or more of induration is considered a positive reaction, 2 to 4 mm a doubtful reaction, and less than 2 mm a negative reaction.[42]

Sputum specimens are difficult or impossible to obtain in an infant or young child, since they swallow any mucus coughed from the lower respiratory tract. Therefore, the best means for obtaining material for smears of culture is by gastric washing, that is, aspiration of lavaged contents from the fasting stomach. The procedure is carried out and the specimen obtained early in the morning before the customary breakfast time (see p. 931).

Ambulatory care. Nursing supervision of the child at home involves teaching parents and child about the disease and its ramifications. Since children usually acquire the disease from an adult in the home, parents often feel guilty. Historically the disease has been regarded with fear, and numerous misconceptions need to be clarified. Reducing parental anxieties helps them to deal with the illness more constructively and to collaborate more effectively in planning for the child's continued care. The success of therapy depends on the acceptance and cooperation of the family. The nurse can help the family to understand the rationale of diagnostic procedures, therapy, and the importance of maintaining the therapeutic plan over the extended period of time needed for recovery. Promoting optimum general health and prevention of intercurrent infections and reinfections with the tubercle bacillus are also of primary importance.

Case finding. Case finding and follow-up of known contacts are important nursing responsibilities. Every case of tuberculosis identified in the community involves nurses in follow-up of known contacts—contacts from which the affected person may have acquired the disease and persons who may have been exposed to the diseased individual. Early diagnosis affords a means for early protection or treatment and prevents further spread of the disease.

Periodic skin testing of all school children and adults could serve to identify positive reactors, particularly in areas in which there is a high incidence of the disease. Annual skin tests are recommended for preschool children and every 2 to 3 years thereafter through adolescence. Exposed tuberculin-negative children should have a skin test done every 2 months for about 6 months after contact has been terminated.[19]

PULMONARY DISTURBANCE CAUSED BY NONINFECTIOUS IRRITANTS

Inflammation of lung tissue can occur occasionally as the result of irritation from foreign material. Aspiration of food, oral secretions, or other substances by otherwise normal infants or children can set up an inflammatory response or chemical pneumonia. Young children are especially prone to aspiration of foreign substances, and weak and debilitated children are subject to aspiration of food or secretions. The major problems associated with aspiration in children are asphyxia or respiratory tract inflammation as the result of inhaling foreign material. Medical and nursing care of a subsequent pneumonitis and/or bronchitis are similar to that for lower respiratory treact inflammation resulting from infectious agents.

Foreign body aspiration

Small children characteristically explore matter with their mouths and are, therefore, particularly prone to aspirate foreign bodies into the air passages. Aspiration of foreign bodies can occur at any age but is most commonly seen in children aged 1 to 3 years. The signs and changes produced depend on the degree of obstruction and the nature of the foreign body. For example, dry vegetable matter, such as a seed, nut, or piece of carrot or popcorn, that may swell when wet creates a particularly difficult problem. A sharp or irritating object produces irritation and edema. A small object may cause little if any pathologic changes, whereas an object of sufficient size to obstruct a passage can produce various changes, including atelectasis, emphysema, inflammation, and abscess.

General manifestations. Initially a foreign body in the air passages produces choking, gagging, wheezing, or cough. After the initial period there is often an interval of hours, days, or even weeks without symptoms. Secondary symptoms are related to the anatomic area in which the foreign body is lodged and are usually caused by a persistent respiratory infection focused distally to the obstruction. Often, by the time secondary symptoms appear, the parents have forgotten the initial episode of coughing and gagging.[36]

Foreign bodies in specific segments of air passages

Larynx. A foreign body in the larynx produces hoarseness, cough that rapidly becomes croupy with inspiratory stridor, and inability to speak. There may be hemoptysis, dyspnea with wheezing, and cyanosis. Obstruction of the airway from the foreign body alone or in combination with the local inflammatory reaction constitutes an emergency that requires prompt recognition and relief of the obstruction. The foreign body is located and removed by direct laryngoscopy.

Trachea. A foreign body in the trachea may produce cough, hoarseness, dyspnea, and cyanosis, but, characteristically, there is an asthmatic wheeze, an audible slap, and a palpable thud as air becomes trapped at the subglottic level.

Bronchi. Initial symptoms are similar to those described previously—cough, blood-tinged sputum, and dyspnea. The symptoms are largely determined by the degree of obstruction created by the foreign body and the stage at which the child is seen. A nonobstructive, nonirritating object may cause few symptoms; an obstructive object quickly produces signs of pathologic changes; and a slight obstruction may only be evidenced by a wheeze. A foreign body is always a possibility in acute or chronic pulmonary lesions. Symptoms may include limited expansion (unilateral), decreased vocal fremitus, and diminished breath sounds distal to the obstruction. Percussion may reveal hyperresonance (caused by emphysema) or impaired sounds (resulting from atelectasis).

Signs that are characteristic of obstruction caused by a foreign body in a bronchi can be explained by the same mechanisms that control the flow of fluids in pipes (Fig. 33-1). During normal respiration the caliber of bronchi and bronchioles becomes larger during inspiration and smaller during expiration. When a small object partially obstructs a passage, air passes around the obstruction during both inspiration and expiration (bypass valve). In this type of obstruction a wheeze is heard. A somewhat larger obstruction will allow air to enter the distal portion when bronchioles enlarge during inspiration, but, when they diminish in caliber during expiration, the lumen becomes occluded and air becomes trapped distal to the obstruction (check valve). This type of obstruction produces obstructive emphysema. When there is complete blockage of the bronchus by a foreign body or by the foreign body and swollen mucosa, air is unable to move in either direction (stop valve) and the air distal to the obstruction is soon absorbed, leaving an area of obstruction atelectasis.

On fluoroscopy, a check-valve obstructed lung will remain expanded, the diaphragm will remain low and fixed on the obstructed side, and the heart and mediastinum will shift to the unobstructed side during expiration. In a stop-valve obstruction the heart and mediastinum are drawn to the obstructed side and remain there during both inspiration and expiration. The diaphragm on the obstructed side remains high, whereas that on the unobstructed side moves normally.

Diagnostic evaluation. The diagnosis of a foreign body is usually suspected on the basis of history and physical signs. X-ray examination reveals opaque foreign bodies but may be of limited use in localizing vegetable matter. Bronchoscopy is usually required for a definitive diagnosis of foreign bodies in the larynx and trachea. Fluoroscopic examination is a valuable aid in detecting and localizing foreign bodies in the bronchi (see previous paragraph).

Treatment. Foreign bodies rarely are coughed up spon-

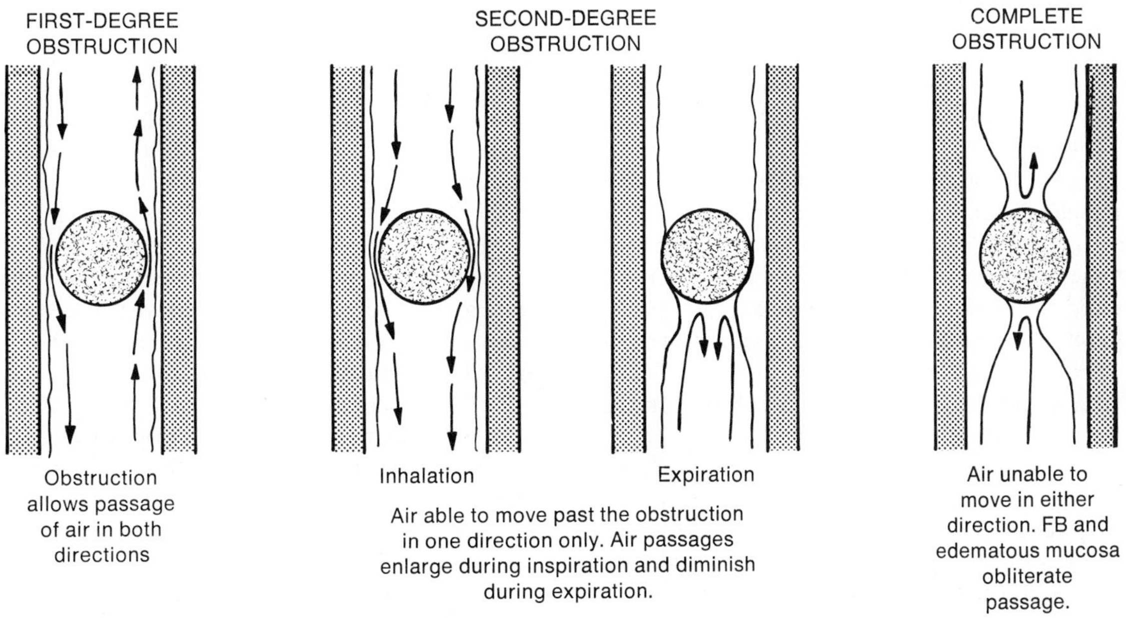
FIRST-DEGREE OBSTRUCTION
SECOND-DEGREE OBSTRUCTION
COMPLETE OBSTRUCTION
Obstruction allows passage of air in both directions
Inhalation
Expiration
Air able to move past the obstruction in one direction only. Air passages enlarge during inspiration and diminish during expiration.
Air unable to move in either direction. FB and edematous mucosa obliterate passage.

Fig. 33-1. Mechanisms of airway obstruction by foreign body (FB).

taneously; therefore, they must be removed instrumentally by direct laryngoscopy or bronchoscopy. This should be carried out as soon as possible, since the progressive local inflammatory process triggered by the foreign material hampers removal, a chemical pneumonia soon develops, and vegetable matter begins to macerate within a few days, causing it to be even more difficult to remove. After removal of the foreign body, the child is placed in a high-humidity atmosphere and any secondary infection is treated with appropriate antibiotics.

Heimlich maneuver

All persons working with children should be prepared to deal effectively with a choking emergency. Choking on food or other material should not be fatal. A very simple procedure, the Heimlich maneuver, which can be used by both health professionals and lay persons, saves children's lives. It is the obligation of nurses to learn the technique and to teach it to parents and other groups.

To aid a child who is choking, nurses need to recognize when he is indeed in distress. Not every child who gags or coughs while eating is truly choking. The child in distress *cannot speak*, *becomes cyanotic*, and *collapses*. These three signs indicate that the child is truly choking and requires immediate and quick action to save his life. He can die within 4 minutes.

When a child is obviously choking, the initial step is to open his mouth and reach in and try to remove the obstruction *without forcing it farther down*. If this fails the next step is the Heimlich maneuver, which is carried out the same in children as in adults[8]:

1. The fisted hand is placed, thumb side in, against the child's abdomen at a point just below the rib cage and slightly above the navel. The fist is firmly grasped with the other hand.
2. The fist is pressed into the abdomen with a quick upward thrust.
3. The thrust is repeated if needed.

The operator stands or kneels behind the child, with arms around the child's waist and hands correctly placed, and carries out the procedure as described above. If the child is sitting, the operator's arms are wrapped around both chair and child. For a child who is lying on his back, the operator takes a position facing the child from above, places the *heel* of the bottom hand at the proper location on the abdomen, and administers the quick inward and upward thrust.

It is neither necessary nor desirable to squeeze or compress the arms during the procedure. It is not a punch or a bear hug. The child may vomit after relief of the obstruction and should be positioned to prevent aspiration. After breathing is restored, the child should receive medical attention so that he can be assessed for complications.[8]

The success of the technique is primarily a result of the fact that obstruction takes place at the end of a maximum respiration. The victim is most likely to choke on food during inspiraton; therefore, the tidal volume plus expiratory reserve volume are present in the lungs. When pressure is exerted on the diaphragm by the maneuver, the food bolus is ejected with considerable force by this trapped air.

Aspiration pneumonia

Aspiration of fluid or food substances is a particular hazard in the child who has difficulty with or is unable to swallow because of paralysis, weakness, debility, congenital anomalies, such as cleft palate or tracheoesophageal fistula, or absent cough reflex (unconscious) or who is force fed, especially while crying or breathing rapidly. It also occurs after the ingestion of hydrocarbons. The newborn may develop a severe pneumonia from aspirating amniotic fluid and debris during the process of birth. Rarely aspiration causes immediate death from asphyxia; more often the irritated mucous membrane becomes a site for secondary bacterial infection. In addition to fluids, food, vomitus, and nasopharyngeal secretions, other substances that cause pneumonia are aspiration of hydrocarbons, lipids, or powder (rare).[18]

Hydrocarbon pneumonia. Children frequently develop pneumonia secondary to the ingestion of various forms of hydrocarbons, such as kerosine, gasoline, solvents, and lighter fluid. The pathogenesis of the pulmonary involvement is the subject of conflicting interpretations, but the most generally accepted explanation is irritation from aspiration during swallowing, vomiting, or gastric lavage. Pathologic changes (based on animal studies) consist of edema, inflammation, and hemorrhage. Coughing and vomiting occur almost immediately after ingestion and probably contribute to aspiration. Central nervous system symptoms may consist of agitation and restlessness, confusion, drowsiness, or coma. The temperature is elevated (37.8° to 40°C or 100° to 104°F).

Inducing the child to vomit is contraindicated because of the renewed danger of aspiration. Hydrocarbons are readily absorbed by the gastrointestinal tract and excreted by the lungs. Bronchitis or pneumonia usually develops early (within the first 24 hours) but may be delayed. Recovery from pulmonary involvement occurs in most instances despite a severe clinical course. Death, if it occurs, is generally the result of hepatic failure complicated by pulmonary factors. Treatment is the same as for any lower respiratory tract inflammation and consists of high humidity, oxygen, hydration, and treatment of any secondary infection.

Lipoid pneumonia. Oily substances aspirated into the respiratory passages cause progressive changes to take place in the lung tissues. First an interstitial proliferative inflammation occurs that may include an exudative pneumonia. The next stage involves a diffuse, chronic, proliferative fibrosis that is often complicated by acute bronchopneumonia. The final stage features multiple localized nodules or tumor-like paraffinomas. There are no characteristic manifestations. Cough is usually present, and dyspnea is seen in severe cases. Secondary bronchopneumonia infections are common. The outcome depends on the extent of pulmonary damage, the general condition of the infant, and discontinuance of the oily inhalation. There is no specific treatment.

Powder. Since the use of powder has been discouraged for infants, aspiration pneumonia from inhalation of zinc stearate is now rare. Formerly is was fairly common in infants. Severe respiratory distress occurs immediately as a result of an inflammatory reaction in small bronchioles initiated by deep inhalation of the extremely light powder. Treatment is symptomatic.

Prevention

The primary treatment for aspiration of foreign substances is prevention. Small children should not be allowed access to enticing small objects that they might place in their mouth. Children younger than 2½ years of age should not be allowed nuts, popcorn, or whole-kernel corn. Proper feeding techniques should be carried out for weak, debilitated, and uncooperative children and preventive measures used to prevent aspiration of any material that might enter the nasopharynx. Solid foods are not introduced until the child is old enough to handle them and has teeth for proper chewing. Thorough chewing, not talking while chewing, and cutting solid food into bite-size pieces should be emphasized. Children should not be permitted to eat or place small items in their mouths while lying on the floor or while they are overactive. Oily nose drops and oil-based vitamin preparations are not appropriate for infants and small children. Solvents, lighter fluid, and other hydrocarbon substances should be kept away from older infants and small children who are apt to put anything in their mouths and who may be attracted by their slightly sweet taste.

Nurses, as child advocates, are in a position to teach prevention in a variety of settings. They can educate parents, singly or in groups, about hazards of aspiration in relation to the developmental level of their children and encourage them to teach their children safety. Parents teach by example; therefore, they should be cautioned about behaviors that their children might imitate, for example, holding foreign objects, such as pins, nails, toothpicks, and so on, in their lips or mouth. Infants and debilitated children should be positioned on the abdomen or the right side after feedings to minimize the possibility of aspirating vomitus or regurgitated feeding. Nurses are major forces in education for accident prevention (pp. 79, 465, and 528).

Near drowning[6,21]

Drowning is not an uncommon accident in childhood. Of accidental deaths from drowning, the majority are children between ages 10 and 19 years but a significant number are infants under 3 years of age. Most are accidental, usually involving children who are helpless in water, such as inadequately attended children in or near swimming pools or infants in bathtubs; small children who fall into ponds, streams, and flooded excavations, usually near home; occupants of pleasure boats who fail to wear life preservers; and children who are able to swim but overestimate their endurance. With expeditious treatment many children can and are being saved. To clarify this discussion, several terms need clarification[33]:

drowning death from asphyxia while submerged, regardless of whether fluid has entered the lungs.
near drowning survival after submersion.

These can be further described as:

drowning without aspiration death from respiratory obstruction and asphyxia while submerged, usually as a result of prolonged laryngospasm. This is also called *dry drowning* (approximately 10% of drownings).
drowning with aspiration death from the combined effects of asphyxia and changes secondary to fluid aspiration while submerged.
near drowning without aspiration survival, at least temporarily, following asphyxia after submission in a liquid medium.
near drowning with aspiration survival, at least temporarily, following aspiration of fluid while submerged.
delayed death caused by drowning death as the result of complications subsequent to successful resuscitation following submersion.

Pathophysiology. The major changes that occur in drowning are directly related to the length of submersion, regardless of the type and amount of fluid aspirated. The major difficulty is acute respiratory insufficiency with primary *hypoxia, hypercapnia,* and *acidosis,* which terminate in cardiopulmonary arrest. Electrolyte imbalances are contributing factors but are not the major causes of morbidity and mortality, as has been previously thought. The pathologic events are directly related to the duration of submersion. The major difficulty is acute ventilatory insufficiency. Approximately 10% of drowning victims die without aspirating fluid but succumb from acute asphyxia as a result of prolonged reflex laryngospasm. Simple asphyxia is the primary cause of death when fluid is aspirated.

In persons who survive submersion, regardless of the amount and type of water aspirated, the major problems are arterial hypoxemia and metabolic acidosis as a result of atelectasis with shunting of blood through the nonventilated alveoli. Although these major problems are present, the related pathology is different after near drowning in fresh as opposed to salt water because of the differences in the osmolality of the fluid aspirated.

When fresh water is aspirated, the hypotonic fluid within the alveoli is rapidly absorbed through the alveolar membrane into the vascular compartment and interstitial spaces, producing a hemodilution and hypervolemia proportionate to the amount of water aspirated. Massive hemodilution may cause severe hyponatremia and red blood cell destruction with release of potassium in quantities sufficient to cause ventricular fibrillation (Fig. 33-2, *A*). This has been demonstrated in laboratory experiments but has not been consistently demonstrated in victims who survive. However, alveolar collapse and pulmonary edema follow the reduced surface tension of alveoli caused by destruction of surfactant.

Aspiration of salt water causes the shift of large amounts of water with protein from the circulation into the alveoli, producing massive pulmonary edema or "secondary drowning" (Fig. 33-2, *B*).

The different mechanisms causing pulmonary edema can be summarized by the following: in salt-water aspiration the osmotic pressure of the hypertonic fluid draws water into the alveoli; in fresh-water aspiration loss of surfactant results in negative intra-alveolar hydrostatic pressure. In both cases the alveolar-capillary membrane is impaired, that is, there is shunting of blood through the nonventilated alveoli. In fresh-water aspiration this is a result of collapsed alveoli and caused by fluid-filled alveoli in salt-water aspiration.[6,21]

In both types of aspiration there is decreased lung compliance and an increased airway resistance. The acidosis accompanying fluid aspiration is a combined respiratory acidosis resulting from retained carbon dioxide and metabolic acidosis caused by buildup of acid metabolites as a result of anaerobic metabolism.

Older children are sometimes victims of hypoxia prior to aspiration of fluid as a result of shallow-water blackout or breath holding while diving. Male teenagers are typical victims of shallow-water blackout when they attempt to swim long distances (several lengths of the pool) underwater. Prior to entering the water, the youngster hyperventilates, which reduces respiratory stimulation from carbon dioxide accumulation and stretch receptors in the lung. Consequently the Po_2 reaches a dangerous level before the respiratory center is stimulated. Also, breath holding with hyperinflated lungs (Valsalva's maneuver) causes further decrease in oxygen to the brain. The cerebral hypoxia causes the youngster to lose consciousness before he has the desire to surface for air. Often these youngsters are found dead at the bottom of a lake or pool. Similarly persons who engage in breath holding while diving in deep water suffer hypoxia as a result of decreasing Po_2 as they ascend from the depths. These are usually older (and experienced) divers.

Treatment. At the scene of a drowning resuscitative

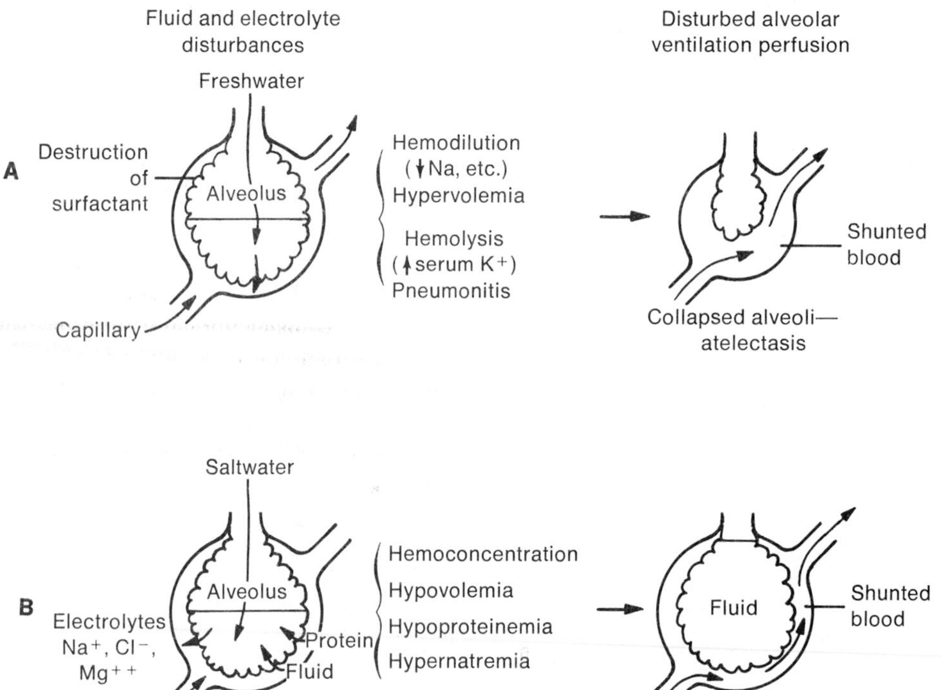

Fig. 33-2. Disturbances as a result of near drowning. **A,** Freshwater; **B,** saltwater.

measures should begin at once, and any near-drowning victim should be transported with maximum ventilatory and circulatory support to the hospital. Many need care for some time after aspiration of fluid. In the hospital intensive pulmonary care is implemented and continued according to the needs of the patient. A spontaneously breathing child will do well in an oxygen-enriched atmosphere, whereas the more severely affected child will require endotracheal intubation and mechanical ventilation. Blood gases and pH are monitored frequently as a guide to oxygen, fluid, and electrolyte therapies. In severe cases central venous pressure provides additional information regarding the status of blood volume. Acidosis is corrected by intravenous administration of sodium bicarbonate. Electrolyte imbalances are corrected in a short time. Isoproterenol may be administered to decrease bronchospasm.

Because of the frequency of complications after near drowning, the patient should be hospitalized for 48 hours for observation. If the victim is one of the 10% who do not aspirate water, is rescued and resuscitated prior to circulatory arrest, and does not suffer damage to the central nervous system, recovery should be complete. Aspiration pneumonia is a frequent complication that occurs about 48 to 72 hours after the episode. Bronchospasm, alveolar-capillary membrane damage, atelectasis, abscess formation, and hyaline membrane disease are other complications that occur after aspiration of fluid. The child who suffers from prolonged hypoxia is in danger of irreversible central nervous system damage, which then becomes a neurologic problem after recovery from pulmonary disturbances.

Prevention. Every child should be taught to swim. Even very young children can learn to handle themselves in the water sufficiently to avoid panic and propel themselves to safety until they can be removed from the water. Water safety and survival training should be required for all school-age children, and nurses can be active advocates in their communities. Nurses are also in a position to emphasize the importance of adequate adult supervision when children are in the water. Young children should never be left unattended when in the water.

BRONCHIAL ASTHMA

Bronchial asthma is a reversible obstructive process characterized by an increased responsiveness of the airway, especially the lower respiratory tract. It is manifest by labored breathing, bilateral wheezing, prolonged expiration, and an irritative tight cough caused by a reduction in the diameter of the airway. The symptoms can vary from a mild cough to severe respiratory distress with hypoxemia, retention of carbon dioxide, and respiratory acidosis that may result in prostration and even fatal asphyxia.[13,27,37]

Asthma is a common disorder and one of the leading causes of chronic illness in childhood. It is believed by many to be the single most important cause of morbidity in childhood. Prior to puberty it occurs twice as often in boys as in girls; during adolescence boys and girls are affected equally; and in adulthood women outnumber men slightly.[13] Onset is rare in the first year of life but not uncommon in the second, and the majority of childhood cases have their onset before the seventh year. Socioeconomic level appears to have no effect on the incidence, but urban dwellers appear to be more prone to asthma than persons who live in the country.[37]

Etiology

The usual cause of the asthmatic manifestations is an allergic hypersensitivity to foreign substances, usually those carried in the air, such as plant pollens. However, in some instances no allergic process can be detected. It is a complex disorder in which biochemical, immunologic, infectious, endocrine, and psychologic factors are involved to varying degrees in different persons. Consequently asthma is classified variously as *allergic* (reaginic) and *nonallergic* (nonreaginic). Most asthma in children is caused by an allergic reaction in the bronchi, but there may be nonallergic etiologies such as bronchial compression from external pressure, a foreign body in the airway, a diffuse endobronchial inflammation, or postexercise bronchial constriction. Asthma is also described as *extrinsic asthma,* caused by allergens or other external factors, and *intrinsic asthma,* caused by nonallergic factors such as bacterial infection or emotional stimuli.

Asthma is further described as:

spasmodic attacks occur intermittently with long symptom-free intervals.

continuous daily wheezing is present.

intractable symptoms are constant and unrelieved by bronchodilators.

status asthmaticus there is little or no response to bronchodilators, and respiratory metabolism is unbalanced.

There is a heritable tendency in asthma. In approximately 75% of children with asthma there is a positive family history with an immediate family member manifesting some form of allergy. Usually the child has other manifestations of allergy such as nasal allergy (hay fever), eczema, or urticaria. Frequently there is a history of eczema in early childhood.[38]

Pathophysiology

There is general agreement that heightened airway reactivity is characteristic of children with asthma. The reasons for this are less clear, and most theories do not explain all types and causes of asthma. Some of the theories attribute the hyperreactivity to (1) an exaggeration of the normal defenses of the respiratory tract, (2) abnormal tissue reactions in the bronchioles, possibly immunologically induced, or (3) an imbalance of normally balanced responses. However, the mechanisms responsible for the obstructive symptoms of asthma are (Fig. 33-3):

1. Edema of the mucous membranes
2. Accumulation of tenacious secretions from mucous glands
3. Spasm of the smooth muscle of the bronchi and bronchioles, which decreases the caliber of the bronchioles

The role that each of these mechanisms play varies from patient to patient and during the course of the disease. In some patients, smooth muscle contraction is the major factor early in the episode, followed by mucosal edema and increased mucous secretion, which are predominant in contributing to the obstruction. In others the sequence of the responses is reversed.[13]

Associated factors. Many of the stimuli that provoke asthmatic episodes may do so by being directly toxic or irritative, such as smoke, fumes, odors, or infection, by eliciting the immune response, or by a combination of mechanisms. Other factors that contribute to the responses are rapid changes in environmental temperature (especially cold), physical stress (fatigue, exertion), psychologic stress (tension, fear, anxiety), or infections in the respiratory tract or nearby structures (such as the ears or sinuses).[10,13]

Immunologic factors. In the majority of cases of childhood asthma there is a very strong allergic component. A vast number of substances in the environment are capable of inducing an asthmatic response, but the most significant are those that are antigenic, that is, that evoke the immune response. The antigen (or foreign substance) is deposited on the respiratory mucosa, where lysozymes immediately digest its outer coating, releasing fragments of foreign protein that initiate the immune sequence. The antibodies (immunoglobulins) most active in the allergic disorders, including asthma, are immunoglobulin E (IgE), located primarily in skin and mucous membranes, and immunoglobulin A (IgA), found in mucosal secretions. IgA acts on foreign antigens trapped in secretions of the bronchial tree. IgE mediates the immediate hypersensitive reaction in the bronchial mucosa that leads to *specific tissue binding*. Both immunoglobulins attach themselves to surfaces of mast cells and basophils, where they react with the specific antigen to which they have developed a bonding capacity.

Chemical mediators. Antigenic substances, as they encounter the antibodies (IgA or IgE) fixed to the lung tissue of sensitized individuals, trigger an immediate hypersensitivity reaction, with the subsequent release of chemical mediators from mast cells and basophils—histamine, slow-reacting substance of anaphylaxis (SRS-A), eosinophil chemotactic factor of anaphylaxis (ECF-A), and other substances including prostaglandins, serotonin, and various kinins (Fig. 33-4). Histamine, with its major effect on central nervous system receptors, causes capillary dilatation, increased permeability of the blood vessels, contraction of smooth muscle, and stimulation of mucous gland secretion. SRS-A, although its effects are less well defined, produces contraction of bronchial muscles with a delayed and more prolonged action than histamine.

Vagal stimulation. Normally the balance of vagal and sympathetic nerve influences maintains the tone of bronchial smooth muscle. Irritant receptors on the bronchial mucosa stimulated by various antigenic (pollens, dust) or nonantigenic (smoke, fumes, cold) stimuli trigger a reflex bronchospasm that narrows the airway. This normal reflex mechanism is designed to protect the alveoli from harmful stimuli in the bronchi; however, in the asthmatic person the bronchial constriction is abnormally severe. Acetyl-

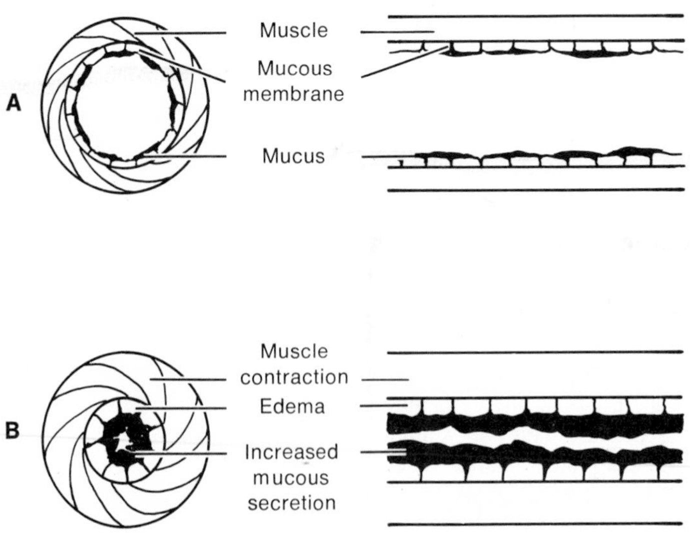

Fig. 33-3. Mechanisms of obstruction in asthma. **A,** Normal bronchus; **B,** asthmatic bronchus.

choline, a neurotransmitter, mediates the vagal response.

β-Adrenergic system. The two basic adrenergic receptors, alpha and beta, are located in the smooth muscle of the bronchi. Normally the physiologic tone of the bronchial airway represents a balance between bronchorelaxation, induced by sympathetic (β-adrenergic) stimulation, and bronchoconstriction, caused by vagal (cholinergic) stimulation and, to some extent, by α-adrenergic stimulation. Beta receptors are located in the glands, smooth muscle, and blood vessels of the bronchi. Stimulation of β-adrenergic receptors activates the enzyme *adenyl cyclase*, which catalyzes the synthesis of another essential intracellular substance, *cyclic adenosine monophosphate (cyclic 3'-5'-AMP* or *cyclic AMP)*. Cyclic AMP inhibits the release of mediator substances from mast cells and also activates the mechanism that either prevents contraction or induces relaxation of bronchial smooth muscle. Cyclic AMP is degraded by the enzyme *phosphodiesterase*. The tissue level of cyclic AMP is modulated by these two enzymes, and drug therapy for bronchial asthma is based on the intracellular activities of these substances[34] (Fig. 33-5).

In persons with asthma, bronchial reactions may be caused by diminished responsiveness of beta receptors or by blockage of these receptors, which allows the cholinergic effects to dominate, causing unopposed bronchoconstriction. Blockage of the beta receptors is thought to be the result of a deficiency or malfunction of adenyl cyclase. A deficiency of adenyl cyclase may be acquired as a result of infection, the presence of certain metabolites or certain drugs, such as propranolol, or a genetic defect.

Ventilation. Bronchilar constriction is a normal reaction to foreign stimuli, but in the asthmatic child it is abnormally severe, producing impaired respiratory function. The rigid cartilaginous rings of the upper airways act to modify the constrictive forces, but, in the smaller bronchi and the bronchioles, the cartilage has been replaced by membranous tissue. The smooth muscle, arranged in spiral bundles around the airway, causes narrowing and shortening of the airway, which significantly increases airway resistance to airflow. Since the bronchi normally dilate and elongate during inspiration and contract and shorten on expiration, the respiratory difficulty is more pronounced during the expiratory phase of respiration.

Increased resistance in the airway causes forced expiration through the narrowed lumen. The volume of air trapped in the lungs increases as airways are functionally closed at a point between the alveoli and the lobar bonchi by the combined mechanisms just described. As the severity of the asthma increases, the airways close at higher residual volume. This gas trapping is the central physiologic feature in the clinical manifestations of asthma, as it forces the individual to breathe at a higher and higher lung volume. This in turn increases the elastic work of breathing and decreases the mechanical efficiency of respiratory muscles. Consequently the person with asthma fights to inspire sufficient air, and there is hyperinflation of alveoli, which increases the diameter of the airways by exerting lateral traction on bronchiolar walls. This helps gas exchange but requires more energy during inspiration to overcome the tension of already stretched elastic lung tissues. This expenditure of effort for breathing causes fatigue, decreased respiratory effectiveness, and increased oxygen consumption and car-

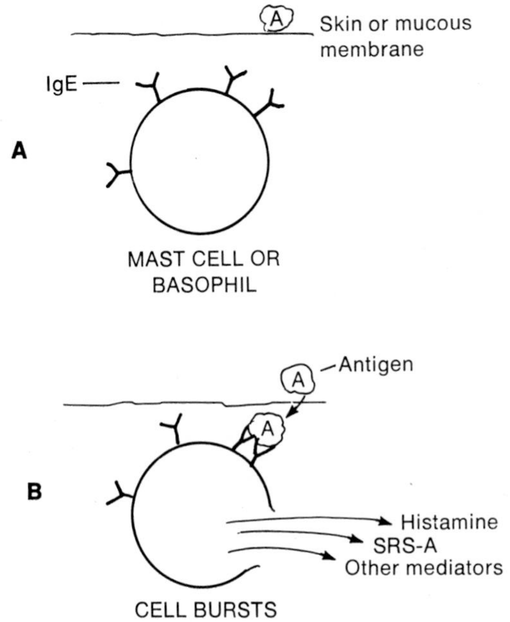

Fig. 33-4. Local response to an allergen. **A,** Antigen in contact with skin surface; **B,** release of chemical mediators.

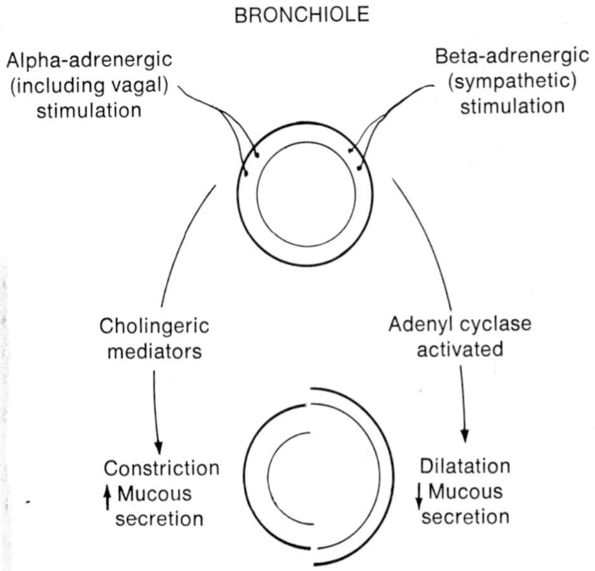

Fig. 33-5. Effect of beta-adrenergic system on the bronchiole.

diac output at a time when the gas exchange and cardiac output are already compromised. Also, the inspiration occurring at higher lung volumes reduces the effectiveness of the cough. The child becomes progressively dyspenic, cyanotic, and tachypneic.[38]

Gas exchange. The degree to which impaired respiration interferes with gas exchange depends to a large measure on the ratio of poorly ventilated and hyperextended alveoli to well-ventilated alveoli. Other factors that reduce the ventilatory efficiency include atelectasis and pneumonia. When the number of poorly ventilated alveoli increases, the degree of arterial hypoxemia also increases; in cases of complete airway obstruction there is a right-to-left pulmonary shunt with total absence of ventilation.

Whereas there are a sufficient number of well-ventilated alveolar-capillary units, perfusion remains adequate and carbon dioxide elimination is not impaired. As the severity of obstruction increases, there is a reduced alveolar ventilation with carbon dioxide retention, hypoxemia, respiratory acidosis, and, eventually, respiratory failure.

Diagnostic evaluation

Bronchial asthma in children is sometimes confused with acute middle and lower respiratory tract infections, congenital stridor, upper airway edema resulting from multiple causes, a foreign body in the bronchi or trachea, bronchial or tracheal compression, and cystic fibrosis. There is often a history of atopic dermatitis or allergic rhinitis in the child and/or a history of familial allergic disease. The age of the child is often a significant factor, since the onset of most cases occurs between ages 3 and 8 years. In infancy an attack usually follows a respiratory infection. If the child has a history of asthma, the diagnosis is almost assured.

Clinical manifestation. Children with bronchial asthma may show signs and experience symptoms that range from discrete, acute episodes of shortness of breath, wheezing, and cough followed by a quiescent period to a relatively continuous pattern of chronic symptoms that fluctuate in severity. The onset of an attack may develop gradually or appear abruptly and may be preceded by an upper respiratory infection. As a rule, episodes associated with infections are insidious in onset and prolonged; those caused by a specific allergen are acute and short lived if the causative agent is removed. An asthmatic episode usually begins with a hacking, paroxysmal, irritative, and nonproductive cough caused by bronchial edema. Accumulated secretions, acting as a foreign body, stimulate the cough. As the secretions become more profuse, the cough becomes rattling and productive of frothy, clear, gelatinous sputum. Bronchial spasm and mucosal edema reduce the size of the bronchial lumen, which is, as a result, more easily occluded by mucous plugs.

The child appears short of breath, he tries to breathe more deeply, and the expiratory phase becomes prolonged and is accompanied by an audible wheezing. He often appears pale but may have a malar flush and red ears. His lips assume a deep, dark red color that may progress to cyanosis observed in the nail beds and skin, especially around the mouth. The child is restless and apprehensive, and his facial expression is anxious. Sweating may be prominent as the attack progresses. Older children have a tendency to sit upright with shoulders in a hunched-over position, hands on the bed or chair, and arms braced to facilitate the use of accessory muscles of respiration. The child speaks with short, panting, broken phrases. Infants and small children are restless, irritable, and difficult to make comfortable.[10,13]

The prolonged expiratory phase is less apparent in infants and young children because of a more pliable chest and the normal rapid respiratory rate. Therefore, expiratory and inspiratory dyspnea are more difficult to differentiate. Infants may display intercostal and suprasternal retractions.

Examination of the chest reveals hyperresonance on percussion. Breath sounds are course and loud, with sonorous rales throughout the lung fields. Expiration is prolonged. Coarse rhonchi, as well as generalized inspiratory and expiratory wheezing that becomes more high pitched as obstruction progresses, can be heard. With minimal obstruction, wheezing may be only slight or even absent, but it can be accentuated by rapid, deep breathing.

With severe spasm or obstruction, breath sounds and rales may become almost audible. Cough is ineffective despite repeated, hacking maneuvers. This represents lack of air movement and may be misinterpreted as improvement by unknowing examiners. Shallow or irregular respirations and a sudden rise in the rate of respiration are ominous signs indicating ventilatory failure and imminent asphyxia.

Children with chronic asthma develop generalized vascularization, mucosal thickening, and hypertrophy of the mucous glands and fibers of the bronchial musculature. With repeated episodes the thoracic cavity becomes fixed in a hyperventilated state (barrel chest) with depressed diaphragm, elevated shoulders, and use of accessory muscles of respiration. The child's face takes on a typical appearance with flattened malar bones, circles beneath the eyes, narrow nose, and prominent upper teeth.

Diagnostic tests. The diagnosis is determined on the basis of clinical manifestations, history, physical examination, and, to a lesser extent, laboratory tests. X-ray examinations are used primarily to rule out other diseases and to evaluate coexisting disease. Sputum examination shows large numbers of eosinophils and colorless crystalloid fragments representing degenerations of eosinophils—Charcot-Leyden crystals, a unique feature of asthma.

There may be leukocytosis resulting from stress, dehydration, or infection. Most asthmatic children tend to have above-average hematocrit values and hemoglobin concentration, which are probably related to chronic hypoxemia with dehydration as a contributing factor. The eosinophil count is frequently over 5% and may reach 30% to 40% in long-standing, severe disease. There is no conclusive proof concerning significant alterations in gamma globulin levels.

Complications. The most prominent complications associated with asthma are:

Infection resulting from diminished efficiency of defenses and mucous growth media
Atelectasis—partial, recurrent, or chronic
Emphysema caused by chronic hyperinflation
Pneumothorax
Collapsed lung
Status asthmaticus
Cor pulmonale with right-sided heart failure
Misuse of medications (sedatives, aerosols, tranquilizers, theophylline)
Emotional and behavioral problems

Prognosis. So many variables are involved in the pathogenesis and severity of asthma that control of symptoms or eventual disappearance of symptoms will differ markedly. Overall evidence indicates that symptom-free control in childhood asthma is generally good. An impressive number of asthmatic children lose their symptoms at puberty, but there is no factor that can predict which children will "outgrow" their asthma. Some develop other forms of allergy in adulthood. It has been postulated that, just as the skin manifestations of infancy (eczema) shift to the bronchi in childhood, there may be another shift in the susceptible tissues (shock organ) at adulthood—most frequently to the nose.

Medical management

The general management of childhood asthma follows the same principles of therapy as for any allergic disorder:

1. Elimination or avoidance of the offending allergen
2. Symptomatic treatment
3. Hyposensitization, where possible

Therapy specific to asthma involves (1) treatment of acute attacks with nonspecific measures, including drugs, fluids, and supportive therapy and (2) treatment aimed at the specific etiologic agent in a given case.

Medical management: acute. Acute attacks of asthma are a medical emergency. The goal is to control the acute attack; therefore, early recognition and treatment at the onset are most important. Rapid relief of the bronchospasm reduces the need for drastic measures and increases the likelihood that relief will be complete. Objectives of therapy for an acute asthmatic attack are to relieve bronchial obstruction by dilating the bronchi, reducing the mucosal edema, and removing excess bronchial secretions. Supportive measures include maintenance of adequate hydration, prevention and relief of fatigue, and treatment of coexisting bacterial infection.[10,13]

Drugs. Rapid-acting bronchodilators are the major therapeutic tools for the relief of bronchospasm. These are the sympathomimetics (β-adrenergic) and the methylxanthines. Following are the major drugs used to relieve bronchospasm.

β-Adrenergics. Epinephrine (Adrenalin) is probably the most important drug in treatment of an acute severe attack by direct stimulation of adenyl cyclase. Subcutaneously administering 0.1 to 0.3 ml (0.01 ml/kg/dose) of 1:1000 aqueous solution rapidly relieves most cases of acute bronchospasm.[13] Duration of action is short; therefore, if there is not relief, the dose is repeated in 20 minutes two or four times. If there is no relief after three to four doses, the drug is discontinued. Since the drug is readily destroyed by light, only preparations that are stored in dark glass vials should be used. Brownish discoloration or the formation of sediment is an indication of deterioration. Sus-Phrine, also given subcutaneously, is composed of 50% epinephrine for immediate effect and 80% crystalline epinephrine, which is released slowly over 4 to 8 hours to prolong the immediate effect. The dose is 0.05 to 0.3 ml of 1:200 solution. The side effects of epinephrine are tachycardia, elevated blood pressure, pallor, weakness, tremors, and nausea. An aerosol form is available for use in nebulizers but is not generally recommended for children because of the overdependency it produces.

Isoproterenol (Isuprel), also a β-adrenergic, gives rapid relief when administered by intermittent positive-pressure breathing to relieve severe asthma in the hospital. Although the drug is available in Freon-propelled aerosol units, like epinephrine, this route is not recommended for use in children. Isoproterenol, because it acts on beta receptors in the heart as well as those in the bronchi, potentiates the side effects of epinephrine and should not be given within 1 hour after administration of epinephrine or Sus-Phrine. Isoproterenol also increases the velocity of mucous transport in the trachea to facilitate expectoration of mucus.

Ephedrine is an effective, but less potent, sympathomimetic bronchodilator with a more prolonged action than epinephrine; therefore, it is better suited to preventing a mild episode from progressing to a severe attack. It is also thought to act as a direct stimulation of beta receptors. It is usually administered orally, often combined with phenobarbital to minimize the side effects. It is also combined with theophylline.

Isoetharine (Bronkosol-2) is used for administration by intermittent positive-pressure breathing, 0.5 ml in 2 ml normal saline every 4 hours. Other drugs that are effective beta-stimulating drugs are *metaproterenol (Metaprel, Alupent),* which can be administered by inhaler or orally; *terbutaline (Bricanyl, Brethine),* a potent bronchodilator that has been approved for older children only, which provides prolonged effects up to 6 hours with minimal side effects; and *salbutamol (Albuterol),* a widely acclaimed beta stimulator without side effects, which is not available in the United States.

Methylxanthines. The methylxanthine drugs, principally theophylline, are probably the most effective and versatile asthmatic drugs. They are prepared for intravenous, intramuscular, oral, or rectal administration. The xanthines block the effect of phosphodiesterase to prevent the breakdown and thus prolong the action of adenyl cyclase, the adrenergic activator. *Theophylline* is given in doses of 5 mg/kg every 6 hours and then increased slowly, if needed, to maximum tolerance. *Aminophylline* is 85% theophylline and is given in corresponding doses. There is wide individual variation in the rapidity with which persons metabolize the drug, and children metabolize it 60% more rapidly than adults. Use of the intravenous route is recommended for hospitalized children only, and they must be carefully monitored during administration for signs of toxicity, which include fever, restlessness, nausea, vomiting of coffee-ground emesis, hypotension, and abdominal discomfort that may progress to convulsions and coma. Some of the signs of toxicity are easily confused with worsening of the asthma.

Corticosteroids. The administration of a corticosteroid preparation may provide significant relief of an attack when symptoms are not controlled by other therapies. The drugs can be given intravenously, orally, or topically by aerosol. The corticosteroids are not actually drugs but act by their hormonal effect; therefore, results are delayed for up to 6 hours. The anti-inflammatory effect diminishes the inflammatory component of asthma and thereby reduces the airway obstruction. The hormonal effects are less clear. There is evidence to indicate that they in some way increase β-adrenergic sensitivity and induce a decreased phosphodiesterase activity in tissues, thus allowing accumulation of cyclic AMP.

Corticosteroids are lifesaving in status asthmaticus, but detracting from their uses are dangers of steroid dependency and undesirable side effects, including cushingoid changes, increased susceptibility to infection, and growth suppression. When steroids are used over a long period of time, they are gradually reduced to the smallest possible maintenance dose, then discontinued as soon as possible. *Hydrocortisone (Solu-Cortef)* and *methylprednisolone (Solu-Medrol)* are the preferred intravenous preparations, and prednisone, which is short acting in terms of suppression of adrenal function, is the preferred oral preparation. Longer-acting varieties are *triamcinolone, betamethasone,* and *dexamethasone.* An inhaled insoluble corticosteroid, beclomethosone dipropionate, is now available in the United States. The drug is deactivated the first time through the liver; therefore, it produces relief without the usual steroid effects. When steroid-dependent children are changed to beclomethosone, adequate supportive therapy will be needed with gradual weaning and additional systemic steroids for periods of stress to prevent adrenal insufficiency. Beclomethosone is not usually recommended for children under 6 years of age.

Expectorants. An important part of asthma therapy is the use of expectorants. Oral administration of *saturated solution of potassium iodide,* 1 drop per year of age in water or juice, three times a day; *guaifensin (glyceryl guaiacolate)* usually given in syrup form *(Robitussin),* 5 ml, three times a day; or *ipecac syrup* in subemetic dosage is frequently helpful for mobilizing mucous secretions. Mucolytic agents such as acetylcysteine (Mucomyst) may be administered in conjunction with nebulization.

Antibiotics. Infection is frequently the triggering mechanism in cases of bronchial asthma in children; therefore, antibiotic therapy is an important part of overall management. The choice of the antibiotic agent is determined by physical findings, cultures, and other evidence that identifies the causative organism.

Sedation. Sedation is often needed to relieve the severe anxiety associated with severe asthma. Mild sedatives such as *phenobarbital* and *chloral hydrate* orally or rectally or the tranquilizer *hydroxyzine (Vistaril, Atarax)* is frequently employed to reduce anxiety and provide relaxation. Morphine and its derivatives are contraindicated because of their depressant effect on both respirations and the cough reflex.

Combination drugs. Preparations containing several drugs such as pseudoephedrine (Sudafed) or Tedral (a combination of theophylline, ephedrine, and phenobarbital), are convenient but are not generally advantageous. They are less effective than specific drugs given individually and adjusted to the needs of each child.

Other drugs. Atropine has been found to be useful in interrupting the vagal afferent or efferent limbs of the vagal reflex. This is most useful in persons with "irritable bronchi." New compounds are being developed that selectively stimulate beta receptors; others inhibit the release of chemical mediators. The role of the prostaglandins in human asthma may be important. For example, PGE_1 and PGE_2 are known to be powerful bronchodilators that act directly on smooth muscle and may prove to be of value; however, other prostaglandins potentiate the tissue injury induced by other chemical mediators. Further investigation will determine whether or not they are of value in treatment of asthma.

Status asthmaticus. Children who continue to display respiratory distress despite vigorous therapeutic measures, especially injections of epinephrine, are considered to be in status asthmaticus. The condition may develop gradually or rapidly, often coincident with complicating conditions such as pneumonia that can influence the duration and treatment of the attack. These children are acutely ill and require hospitalization, preferably where intensive care is available. They need continuous nursing attendance with frequent monitoring and observation.

Persistent hypoventilation leads to accumulation of carbon dioxide, with decrease in arterial pH and respiratory acidosis. As a result compensatory buffering mechanisms become overtaxed and the pH may drop to dangerous levels. Vomiting and dehydration cause further reduction of arterial pH by promoting retention of metabolic acids. Therapy of status asthmaticus is directed toward correction of dehydration and acidosis, improvement of ventilation, and treatment of any concurrent infection.

The child is given intravenous fluids and nothing by mouth except liquids if his condition permits. The intravenous infusion provides a means for hydration, liquifying secretions, and administering medications. The correction of dehydration, acidosis, hypoxia, and electrolyte derangements is guided by frequent determination of arterial pH, Po_2, Pco_2, and serum electrolytes. Acidosis is corrected by administration of sodium bicarbonate or the organic hydrogen-ion acceptor tromethamine (THAM Tris [hydroxymethyl] aminomethane) in sufficient amounts to maintain pH at acceptable levels. Tromethamine is usually given in association with assisted ventilation because of its tendency to depress respirations.

Humidified oxygen is administered by tent, face mask, or cannula. Care is exercised in the use of oxygen, and high concentrations are given with assisted ventilation to avoid the danger of oxygen narcosis. Since oxygen is a stimulus for respiration, high levels may significantly depress respirations. When assisted ventilation is used, volume respirators are usually more satisfactory than pressure-cycled respirators for children. Volume-type respirators ensure proper alveolar ventilation without overinflation and prevent high pressure caused by sudden obstruction.

Corticosteroids such as hydrocortisone and aminophylline are given intravenously to reduce bronchospasm, and frequently isoproterenol is administered by intermittent positive-pressure breathing. Sometimes isoproterenol may be given by slow infusion pump for children who do not respond to aminophylline.

Antibiotics are frequently advisable in therapy, since infection may be masked or may not always be evident and is always a threatening complication. Mild sedatives, usually chloral hydrate or a tranquilizing agent, are given with caution to children whose agitation is not caused by hypoxia.

As the attack subsides, fluids and medication are given orally and postural drainage and breathing exercises help remove secretions. Administration of steroids is withdrawn as rapidly as possible.

Medical management: long range

The long-range goal in management of asthma in children is to assist the child to live as normal and happy a life as possible. To accomplish this, efforts are extended to determine the cause of the attacks, prevent or control the attacks, and help the child to deal constructively with the disease. Basic to any therapeutic plan is an evaluation of the child's general health and an assessment of the specific allergenic factors and the nonspecific factors that precipitate symptoms. Specific allergens are identified with protein-allergen extracts, usually by direct skin tests using the scratch or intradermal technique. Other methods, including inhalation tests (bronchial challenge) and controlled exposure, for example, elimination diet, are also available.

Allergen control. Once the specific allergens are identified and confirmed by provocative tests, steps are taken to eliminate or avoid the offending allergens. Often simply removing environmental factors will provide protection from attacks, for example, removal of a dog or cat from the home of a child sensitive to dogs or cats. Allergenic foods are eliminated from the diet. Nonspecific factors that may trigger an attack, such as extremes of temperature, are sometimes controlled by humidifiers or air conditioners, and the child can be helped to develop a tolerance to temperature fluctuations by gradual or systematic exposure to temperature differences.

Medications. Most children do not require medication continuously. Parents and older asthmatic children are taught to implement therapy at the onset of symptoms or when they will be exposed to symptom-provoking situations. Bronchodilators in aerosol sprays provide quick relief and are effective in controlling an attack at the onset, but the child and the parents need careful instruction in their use. The effectiveness of aerosol therapy requires perfect timing of the mist with inhalation, which makes them unsuitable for young children. Oral administration, although somewhat slower, is a safer mode of administration, especially in younger children. Another hazard associated with aerosol therapy is that its use for relief predisposes to overuse. Older children can easily become "spray addicts."

Children with persistent and continuous asthma receive bronchodilators around the clock rather than during acute attacks only. The drug of choice, usually theophylline, is prescribed alone or combined with an expectorant to be taken three times daily and at bedtime. Early morning wheezing can often be controlled by a long-acting preparation for the bedtime dose. Iodide expectorants, such as saturated solution of potassium iodide, are very effective, but prolonged use may produce thyroid enlargement. Corticosteroids are given to the majority of children with chronic asthma. To minimize the undesirable side effects they are administered on intermittent days and the child is gradually weaned over a long period of time after use in an acute attack.

A relatively recent drug used in asthma treatment is *cromolyn sodium*. Neither a bronchodilator nor an anti-inflammatory agent, cromolyn sodium acts superficially to inhibit the release of chemical mediators, especially histamine, in the human lung. The action is essentially prophylactic and is of no value when administered after the allergic reaction. Its chief value is to prevent an attack, and it is especially useful in preventing exercise-induced bronchospasm.

Physical therapy. Physical therapy is one of the standard adjuncts to treatment of chronic asthma. This includes chest physical therapy, breathing exercises, physical training, and inhalation therapy. These therapies help to produce physical and mental relaxation, improve posture, strengthen respiratory musculature, and develop more efficient patterns of breathing. Postural drainage, which includes percussion, vibration, deep breathing, and assisted coughing, helps to clear mucus from the bronchial tree (see p. 1201). For the motivated child, breathing exercises and controlled breathing are of value in preventing overinflation and in improving the strength of respiratory muscles and the efficiency of the cough. Stretch exercises sometimes help to increase the flexibility of the ribs. Sit-ups and leg exercises strengthen abdominal muscles and aid expiration.

Exercise. Vigorous physical activity is frequently followed by an asthmatic attack; therefore, many children choose a sedentary existence. This can seriously hamper peer interaction. It has been found that moderate exercise is advantageous for children with asthma. Selection of activities that do not overtax the respiratory mechanism and use of inhalant bronchodilators prior to activity allow the asthmatic child to participate in a variety of sports and activities. It has been determined that asthmatic children can tolerate exercise that involves stopping and starting activities, such as baseball, skiing, and short sprints, but that they do not tolerate activities that involve endurance exercise, such as running, basketball, or soccer, and strenuous sports, such as wrestling. Swimming, even long-distance swimming, is well tolerated by children with asthma. In part this may be because of the type of breathing it requires. Exhaling underwater prolongs each expiration and increases the end-expiratory pressure within the respiratory tree (essentially, pursed-lip breathing).

The child is advised about the type of exercise that is appropriate and the likelihood of reducing bronchospasm by using inhalant bronchodilators 20 to 30 minutes before the anticipated activity—the length of time depends on the type of medication used. Drugs that have proved effective are isoproterenol (for a limited amount of time), theophylline, atropine (associated vasodilatation with fever and flushing are disadvantages), cromolyn sodium, and salbutamol, which is effective and does not break down into hazardous compounds. All of these drugs except cromolyn sodium can be taken during exercise for relief also.

Asthma camps have become popular in recent years as a means of encouraging physical activity in a more homogeneous, controlled, and less competitive environment. Not all persons subscribe to this practice. There are those who support the positive benefits, which are primarily that the denominator of asthma is removed as a factor. Everyone at the camp has asthma; therefore, no child is different from the others. On the other hand, many believe that such segregation from family and peers serves only to reinforce the sick role.

Hyposensitization. The role of hyposensitization in childhood asthma has not been clarified. In many cases the child demonstrates multiple sensitivities, which makes such therapy impractical. Moreover, the shots hurt. When the allergen can be defined and is one that cannot be avoided or controlled satisfactorily by drugs, specific hyposensitization is seriously considered. Immune therapy is not recommended for allergens that can be eliminated effectively, for example, food sensitivities, drugs, and animal dander. Inhalant allergens such as house dust, pollens, and molds are most often the allergens considered for immune therapy.

Injection therapy is usually limited to clinically significant allergens. The initial dose of the offending allergen(s), based on the size of the skin reaction, is injected subcutaneously. The amount is increased at weekly intervals until a maximum tolerance is reached, after which a maintenance dose is given at 4-week intervals. This may be extended to 5- or 6-week intervals during the off-season for seasonal allergens. Successful treatment is continued for a minimum of 3 years and then stopped. If no symptoms appear, the acquired immunity is said to be retained; if symptoms recur, the treatment is reinstituted.

Prognosis. The outlook for children with asthma varies widely. An impressive number of children lose their symptoms at puberty. The prognosis for control of symptoms or disappearance of symptoms will differ from children who have rare and infrequent attacks to those who are constantly wheezing or some who are subject to status asthmaticus. In general the more severe and numerous the symptoms, the longer they have been present, and the presence of family history of allergy, the poorer is the prognosis for improvement. However, it is impossible to predict which children will outgrow their symptoms of childhood asthma. Many who outgrow them are subject to exercise-induced asthma as adults, and the associated pathologies such as growth impairment, chest deformity, and airway obstruction are maintained throughout life.

Psychologic aspects of childhood asthma

Emotional factors are known to be associated with childhood asthma; however, it is not known whether emotional disturbance is present prior to the onset of asthma and is a probable etiologic factor in its development or if it occurs as a result of the asthma. Although no decisive evidence is available regarding the relative importance of all etiologic factors, the consensus accepts a multicausal etiology for childhood asthma in which hereditary, allergic, infectious, and psychologic factors assume importance independently or, more often, in combination.

Behavioral problems are apt to occur in asthmatic children whose attacks commenced prior to age 2 years and those with continuing asthma and symptoms that are more severe and prolonged. It is unclear whether the emotional disturbances are peculiar to children with asthma or are similar to those that may occur in children with other chronic diseases (Chapter 22). Children with any chronic condition are more likely to develop adjustment problems than are healthy children.

Studies of children with behavioral problems indicate that family interactions play an important role in the child's adjustment to the disease. There is a high correlation between the level of disturbed family relationships and the child's psychosocial adjustments. The severity and course of illness do not appear to be related to the level of family adjustment, however.

Both short- and long-term adaptation of the asthmatic child to his disease depends to a great extent on the family's acceptance of his disorder. The task of living day-to-day with an asthmatic child involves the family continually. There are periodic crises and the ever-present threat of a crisis, requiring parental vigilance, sleepless nights, frequent emergency trips to the hospital, and often overwhelming medical expenses. Throughout these stresses the parents are expected and encouraged to promote as normal a life as possible for the asthmatic child without neglecting the needs of the siblings.

Parental responses to the asthmatic child with emotional disturbances range from rejection to overprotection. A significant number are overprotective, babying the child even during symptom-free periods. Frequently, believing that physical activity precipitates the attacks, the parents attempt to limit the physical activities of their child—in some cases to the point of confining the child to the home. The child appears fearful, is usually physically inactive, and lacks self-confidence. The child has few friends, and the parental protective behavior further alienates him from his peers. On reaching adolescence the overprotected child may rebel against the control to become defiant and overactive, often accompanied by a careless attitude toward the management of his illness that places him at risk for serious respiratory events.

Although encountered less frequently, the child of negligent parents feels insecure and will often associate the nonaccepting behavior of the parents with provoking or worsening an attack of asthma. This may or may not be the case. However, the nonaccepting parental attitudes have usually been present prior to the onset of the child's asthma.

Not uncommonly parents of asthmatic children accuse the child of manipulating his environment by deliberately precipitating an attack to gain his own ends—to gain a special consideration or to avoid a responsibility. This accusation is difficult to verify; however, there are some children who actually claim to have the power of controlling their symptoms and use this as a threat. There is some question that this behavior may represent an effort on the part of these children to master their anxiety regarding attacks by proclaiming to be in control of the onset and course of the asthmatic attacks, particularly when others fail to prevent them.

Where family relationships are determined to produce an adverse effect on the asthmatic child, psychiatric help is recommended and, where disturbances are marked, foster placement or respite care in a residential facility for asthmatic children is advised. A significant finding is that asthmatic symptoms are relieved when the child is removed from the parents, such as when the child is hospitalized or is away from home for other reasons. It is in these rapidly remitting children with asthma, in contrast to the steroid-dependent children, that psychologic factors assume greater significance than allergic or infectious factors in triggering symptoms. For example, an attack can be precipitated by major emotions such as anger, anxiety and worry, sadness and depression, and either pleasurable or nonpleasurable excitement. When a child repeatedly improves during separation from family members, it is strongly suspected that emotional and family interactional factors are contributing to the course of the disease.

Nursing considerations

Nursing care of children with asthma involves both acute and long-term care. Children who are admitted to the hospital with acute asthma are ill, anxious, and uncomfortable. In most instances the child is admitted as an emergency with status asthmaticus and is in acute distress. An intravenous fusion is begun immediately, and medication, usually corticosteroids and aminophylline, is administered to relieve bronchospasm. The child is monitored closely and continuously during aminophylline administration for relief of respiratory distress and signs of side effects or toxicity. The pulse, respiration, and blood pressure are taken and recorded every 5 minutes during rapid infusion and every 15 minutes for at least an hour after the drug has been absorbed.

The child usually prefers the high-Fowler's position, although he may be more comfortable sitting upright or leaning slightly forward. Since oxygen is indicated, he is placed in a mist tent for relief of dyspnea and cyanosis, but an older child may prefer a nasal cannula. Oxygen is not administered indiscriminately but regulated according to the blood gas analysis and objective observation of color, respiratory effort, and sensorium. Associated treatments such as intermittent positive-pressure breathing or postural drainage, and tests, such as blood gases or pulmonary function tests, are often performed by specialized personnel, or they may be the nurse's responsibility.

The child with status asthmaticus is apprehensive and anxious. Moreover, he is usually tired from his respiratory efforts and loss of sleep. The calm, efficient presence of a nurse helps to reassure him that he is safe and will be cared for during this stressful period. It is important to assure the child that he will not be left alone and that his parents are allowed to be near and available when he needs them.

Parents need reassurance too. They want to be informed of their child's condition and the therapies being employed.

Summary of nursing care of the child with status asthmaticus

Goals	Responsibilities
Relieve symptoms immediately	Assist with starting intravenous infusion Initiate oxygen therapy with appropriate equipment Tent Cannula Mask Administer bronchodilators and corticosteroids as prescribed
Relieve bronchospasm	Administer prescribed bronchodilator (usually aminophylline) Carefully regulate flow rate of aminophylline infusion; monitor pulse, respiration, and blood pressure before, during, and after administration
Reduce mucosal inflammation and edema	Administer corticosteroids Provide cool, moist environment Administer antibiotics as prescribed
Detect drug toxicity	Interview parents to determine medications given prior to admission to avoid possible overdose Monitor condition frequently during and after administration of drugs, including oxygen
Liquify secretions	Provide humidified atmosphere Provide adequate hydration Administer expectorants
Promote adequate hydration	Maintain intravenous infusion Measure intake and output Assess urine for concentration and specific gravity Encourage fluids as prescribed Assure adequate humidification of environment Assess for objective signs of adequate hydration
Detect status of respiratory distress	Assess skin color for cyanosis Assess character of respirations Depth Rate Presence of retractions or nasal flaring Effort (inspiratory and expiratory) Lung sounds Collect or assist in collection of blood gases
Correct acidosis	Administer sodium bicarbonate or tromethamine as ordered Administer oxygen to reduce anaerobic metabolism (and subsequent increase in acid metabolites)
Increase ventilatory capacity	Administer bronchodilators, anti-inflammatory agents, expectorants, and oxygen Position for optimum lung expansion High-Fowler's position Provide overbed table with pillows if more comfortable for child Administer or arrange for positive-pressure breathing if ordered Percussion and vibration Postural drainage when condition allows Facilitate removal of secretions with percussion and administration of expectorant drugs

Summary of nursing care of the child with status asthmaticus—cont'd

Goals	Responsibilities
Promote physical comfort	Improve ventilatory capacity by measures on p. 1250 Position for comfort
Promote rest and reduce fatigue	Implement measures to improve ventilation Administer sedation as ordered Organize care to allow for maximum rest Disturb as little as possible when resting or asleep
Reduce anxiety and apprehension	Explain procedures and equipment before use Provide continuous attendance Provide reassurance with calm words and manner Encourage parents to remain near child
Reduce parental anxiety	Provide support and reassurance to parents

They are upset, apprehensive regarding the child's condition, and feeling guilty. Often they feel that they may have in some way contributed to the child's condition or could have prevented the attack. They may even feel, consciously or unconsciously, anger toward the child for continuing to display symptoms despite their efforts to prevent or control the attack. Reassurance regarding their efforts expended on the child's behalf and their parenting capabilities can help alleviate their stress. All efforts to reduce the parental apprehension will, in turn, help reduce the child's distress. Anxiety is easily communicated to the child from parents and members of the staff. (For a summary of nursing care of the child with status asthmaticus, see the boxed material.)

Long-term support. Nurses who are involved with asthmatic children in the home, clinic, or physician's office play an important role in helping the children and their families learn to live with the condition. The disease can be tolerated if it does not interfere with family life, physical activity, or school attendance or if it does not require hospitalization.

Nurses are involved in the initial assessment and workup to determine the cause and extent of the asthma. They assist with diagnostic tests, pulmonary function tests, and general health assessment. Parents need to know the nature of the disease and, when the allergens are determined, how they can avoid and/or relieve asthmatic attacks. The nurse assists the mother in planning and carrying out an elimination diet to detect foods that may precipitate symptoms. When the allergen or allergens are identified, nurses can provide valuable assistance to the parents in modifying the environment to reduce contact with the offending allergen(s).

Removal of causative or potentially troublesome allergens from the home is essential. In the child's bedroom in particular all unnecessary furniture, rugs, curtains, drapes, and stuffed toys need to be removed from the room. Light curtains and throw rugs that can be removed and cleaned weekly are usually permitted. The room will require daily cleaning with a damp mop. Bedding should be free of allergens, for example, foam-rubber pillows or pillows encased in nonallergenic coverings, an allergen-proof covering for mattress and springs, and wool blankets covered with cotton sheeting should be used. Hot-air heating vents should be covered to prevent aeration of dust, especially when the heat is turned on after a summer's accumulation. Another heat source may be necessary for the room. Pets, furry or feathered, should be excluded from the home, and damp areas such as the basement or crawl spaces should be treated with fungicide or dehumidified. Windows should be closed during the pollen season, or an air conditioner should be placed in the window. Electrostatic air filters are often recommended, but high-mist vaporizers are discouraged because they often intensify wheezing and encourage growth of mold. (See p. 489 for a summary of allergy-proofing the home.)

The parents are cautioned to avoid exposing the child to excessive cold, wind, or other extremes of weather and to smoke, sprays, or other irritants. Foods known to provoke symptoms should be eliminated from the diet. The foods most frequently allergenic are eggs, milk, grains, and chocolate. Parents should be advised to read labels on prepared foods and snacks to determine the presence of allergens. For example, a tremendous number of foods contain sodium caseinate or dried milk products.

The parents and the older child need to learn how to use

the medications prescribed to relieve bronchospasm. They are taught to recognize early signs and symptoms of an impending attack so that it can be controlled before symptoms become distressful. Many children are administered theophylline or other medication, and parents should understand the importance of taking the drugs as prescribed. Older children who use a nebulizer or aerosol device to deliver adrenergic drugs need to be taught how to use the device. To be most effective, the spray is inhaled *slowly* for better distribution to narrowed airways. Rapid inspiration causes the drugs to move through unobstructed bronchioles to patent airways where they are less needed. After reaching full lung capacity, the child should count to five slowly before exhaling so that the drugs can be deposited on the obstructed airway.

The child and parents also need to be cautioned about the adverse effects of the drugs and the dangers of overuse. They should know that it is important to use them when needed but not indiscriminately or as a substitute for avoiding the symptom-provoking allergen. Persons can become refractive to the prescribed medication. When a drug is no longer effective, this may be because of altered drug metabolism, a large causative load, or an emotional overlay. If a drug is given long enough, the body frequently develops a resistance to it.

Parents and child are taught to report any changing reaction to a drug or if the drug appears to be losing its effectiveness as evidenced by more frequent need for the drug.

The child should be protected from a respiratory infection that can trigger an attack or aggravate the asthmatic state, especially in young children. Their airways are mechanically smaller and more reactive; therefore, edema from infection causes wheezing and other signs of respiratory obstruction. Also, the equipment used for the child, such as nebulizers, must be kept absolutely clean to decrease the chances of contamination with bacteria and fungi.

Breathing exercises and controlled breathing are taught and encouraged for the motivated youngster (see p. 1203), and the nurse can help him select activities suitable to his capacity. Play techniques can be employed for younger children that extend their expiratory time and increase expiratory pressure, for example, blowing cotton balls or a Ping-Pong ball on a table, blowing a pinwheel, or preventing a tissue from falling by blowing it against the wall. Anything that promotes proper diaphragmatic breathing, side expansion, and generally improved mobility of the chest wall is encouraged. If the child requires segmental drainage and percussion, someone in the family must assume responsibility for carrying out the procedure. It is the responsibility of the physical therapist or the nurse to teach the parent the proper technique (see p. 1201).

Children with emotional overtones associated with their asthma create additional problems. In these children an attack can be triggered by emotional experiences mediated through several central nervous system pathways to precipitate asthmatic symptoms. Even some respiratory behaviors (such as crying, laughing, coughing, and hyperventilation) that accompany strong emotions may trigger a mechanical or reflex narrowing of the airway.

The interactions of members of the family need careful assessment to identify maladaptive behaviors and precipitating factors. A team approach is usually employed, in which family interaction may be a contributing factor in the child's illness. Sometimes all the members of the family need reassurance, education, and referral to persons or agencies that can help meet their needs with continued support and encouragement. Parent groups can be very effective in providing support to parents in dealing with their frustrations.

Sometimes it is necessary to remove the child from the family for short-term respite care and provide the family with crisis therapy. In severe cases long-term respite care is the only satisfactory solution. The children live in one of the residential treatment centers throughout the country in which the needs of the child are met by professionals. The child is removed from the interactional stress of the home environment and educated regarding the nature of his illness and how he can live with it.

The nurse working with asthmatic children can provide them with support in a number of ways. Many asthmatic children voice frustration about the way in which their attacks interfere with their goal achievements and social lives. They need education concerning their disease and to realize that it is not as bad as they might think. Children, their families, and their peers need to know what to do to prevent an attack and what to do during an attack. These children need much reassurance from the health team and reinforcement of their coping mechanisms. Last of all, they need ''grit''—the courage to help them live and cope with their condition one day at a time.

CYSTIC FIBROSIS

Cystic fibrosis of the pancreas, fibrocystic disease of the pancreas, and mucoviscidosis are all terms that are or have been applied to this most common inherited disease of children. Cystic fibrosis is a generalized dysfunction of the exocrine (mucous-producing) glands and is one of the most serious chronic diseases that affect white children. It accounts for a large percentage of lung disease in children; however, the disease affects multiple organ systems in varying degrees of severity, which presents some problems with early recognition.

In the past the mortality rate has been high in young children with the disease, but with early diagnosis and treatment the mortality has decreased significantly. Consequently more persons with the disease reach the reproductive age. Females are able to reproduce, but males are, with few exceptions, sterile.

Etiology and pathophysiology

Cystic fibrosis is believed by most authorities to be inherited as an autosomal-recessive trait, and, as such, the affected child inherits the defective genes from both parents with an overall incidence of 1 in 4 (see inheritance patterns, p. 191). However, there are some who suggest that the disease may be a symptom complex caused by more than one gene. The incidence of the disease is estimated at 1 in 1500 to 2000 births in predominantly white populations. Although the disease is found in all racial and socioeconomic groups, it is almost nonexistent in the Mongoloid races and is far less prevalent in blacks, occurring primarily in areas in which there is apt to be mixed ancestry.

Pathophysiology. The basic biochemical defect in cystic fibrosis is unknown. It is assumed, however, that it is probably caused by alteration in a protein, perhaps an enzyme. The defect gives rise to several apparently unrelated clinical features—increased viscosity of mucous gland secretions, a striking elevation of sweat electrolytes, an increase in several organic and enzymatic constituents of saliva, and suggestive abnormalities in autonomic nervous system function.

There is some evidence for overactivity of the autonomic nervous system, which stimulates the cholinergic glands. This is plausible since this system innervates all exocrine glands. To date, findings are not conclusive. Abnormalities of the nonmucous-producing glands are primarily evidenced in the saliva and sweat. There is an increase in sodium and chloride in both saliva and sweat in children with cystic fibrosis, which forms the basis for one of the most reliable diagnostic procedures, the sweat chloride test.

The sweat electrolyte abnormality is present from birth throughout life and is unrelated to the severity of the disease or the extent to which other organs are involved. The sodium and chloride content of sweat in children with cystic fibrosis is two to five times greater than that of the controls and occurs in 98% to 99% of affected children. The reason for this high level is unclear, although the cause has been postulated to be a substance that inhibits sodium reabsorption.

The primary factor, and the one that is responsible for the multiple clinical manifestations of the disease, is mechanical obstruction caused by the increased viscosity of mucous gland secretions (Fig. 33-6). Instead of forming a thin, free-

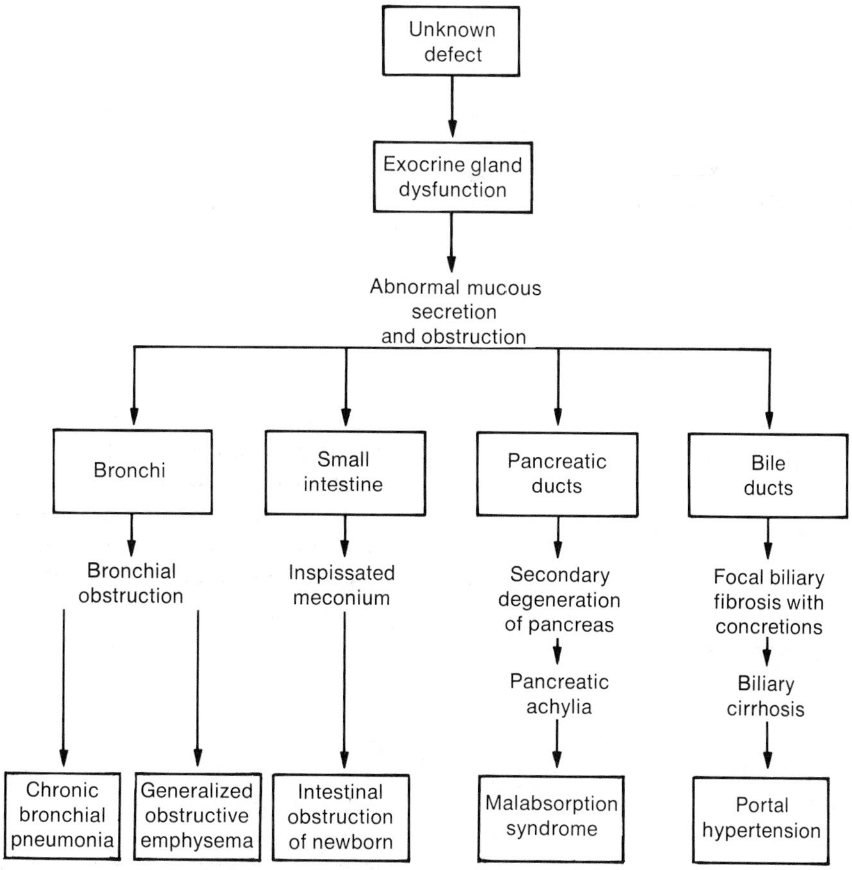

Fig. 33-6. Various effects of exocrine gland dysfunction in cystic fibrosis.

ly flowing secretion, the mucous glands produce a thick, inspissated mucoprotein that accumulates and dilates them. Small passages in organs such as the pancreas and bronchioles become obstructed as secretions precipitate or coagulate to form concretions in glands and ducts.

In the pancreas the thick secretions block the ducts, leading to cystic dilatations of the acini (small lobes of the gland), which then undergo degeneration and progressive diffuse fibrosis. Grossly the pancreas is smaller, thinner, and firmer than normal. Because essential pancreatic enzymes (trypsin, amylase, and lipase) are unable to reach the duodenum, digestion and absorption of nutrients—particularly fats, proteins, and, to a lesser degree, carbohydrates—are markedly impaired. The disturbed absorption is reflected in excessive stool fat (steatorrhea) and protein (azotorrhea). The islands of Langerhans remain unaffected but may decrease in number as pancreatic fibrosis progresses.

In the liver localized biliary obstruction and fibrosis are common and become more extensive with time, eventually giving rise to a distinctive type of multilobular biliary cirrhosis. The gallbladder is small and contains a firm gelatinous material that also fills the cystic duct. Findings similar to those in the pancreas are found in the salivary glands.

Pulmonary complications are present in almost all children with cystic fibrosis and constitute the most serious threat to life. Bronchial and bronchiolar obstruction by the abnormally thick, tenacious mucus causes patchy atelectasis with both lobar and generalized hyperinflation. Because of the increased viscosity of the mucus, there is greater resistance to ciliary action, a slower mucus flow rate, and reduced expectoration, which also contributes to the mucous obstruction. This retained mucus serves as an excellent medium for any bacterial growth. Reduced oxygen–carbon dioxide exchange causes variable degrees of hypoxia, hypercapnia, and acidosis. In severe, progressive lung involvement, compression of pulmonary blood vessels and progressive lung dysfunction frequently lead to pulmonary hypertension and cor pulmonale.

The disease is sometimes expressed in other ways, for example, hypoelectrolytemia caused by massive losses through the sweat, especially in high environmental temperatures or febrile episodes. Infants with cystic fibrosis who fail to thrive frequently demonstrate hypoalbuminemia resulting from diminished absorption of protein, which in severe cases causes generalized edema.

Diagnostic evaluation

Because the disease is variable in severity and extent of manifestations and can simulate a number of clinical entities, the diagnosis is not readily apparent in most cases, especially when there is no familial evidence of disease. Some children display symptoms at birth, whereas symptoms in others are not apparent until several years have passed. Some show only mild forms of the disease with only limited impairment of digestion and respiratory problems, whereas others have severe malabsorption and life-threatening pulmonary complications. Although most affected children display both pulmonary and gastrointestinal symptoms, some may have difficulty with one system only.

Gastrointestinal tract. The earliest manifestation of cystic fibrosis is *meconium ileus* in the newborn. The lumen of the small intestine is blocked with thick putty-like, tenacious, mucilaginous meconium, usually at or near the ileocecal valve, giving rise to signs of intestinal obstruction, including abdominal distention, vomiting, failure to pass stools, and rapid development of dehydration with associated electrolyte imbalance.

As the disease progresses, obstruction of pancreatic ducts and the absence of enzymes (trypsin, amylase, and lipase) in the duodenum prevent conversion of ingested food into compounds that can be absorbed by the intestinal mucosa. Consequently the nondigested food is excreted, chiefly unabsorbed fats and proteins, which increases the bulk of feces two or three times the normal amount. The bulky nature of the stools may go unnoticed at first, but usually by 6 months of age the child passes large, loose stools with normal frequency or unformed stools frequently. As solid foods are added to the diet, the excessively large stools become frothy and extremely foul smelling.

Because so little is absorbed from the intestine, the child compensates with a voracious appetite; however, since he is unable to compensate for the fecal wastage, he loses weight with marked wasting of tissues and failure to grow. The abdomen is distended and the extremities are thin, and the sallow skin droops from wasted buttocks. The impaired ability to absorb fats results in a deficiency of the fat-soluble vitamins A, D, E, and K, and anemia is a common complication.

The most common gastrointestinal complication associated with cystic fibrosis is *prolapse of the rectum,* which occurs most often in infancy and childhood. Affected children of all ages are subject to intestinal obstruction from inspissated or impacted feces.

Respiratory tract. Pulmonary problems are present in almost all children with cystic fibrosis, but the time of appearance is variable. The majority show evidence before 1 year of age; others may not develop symptoms for weeks, months, or years. Initial manifestations are often wheezy respirations and a dry, nonproductive cough. Eventually diffuse bronchial and bronchiolar obstruction lead to irregular aeration with progressive pulmonary disturbance and secondary infection. Dyspnea increases, the cough often becomes paroxysmal, and the mucoid impactions within the small air passages cause a generalized obstructive emphysema and patchy areas of atelectasis.

Progressive pulmonary involvement with hyperaeration

of functioning alveoli produces the overinflated, barrel-shaped chest in which the anteroposterior diameter approaches the lateral diameter. When ventilation is significantly impaired, there is cyanosis and clubbing of fingers and toes. The child suffers repeated episodes of bronchitis and bronchopneumonia, primarily caused by *Staphylococcus aureus* and/or *Pseudomonas aeruginosa*.

Diagnostic tests. The diagnosis of cystic fibrosis is established on the basis of (1) a history of the disease in the family, (2) the absence of pancreatic enzymes, (3) an increase in electrolyte concentration of sweat, and (4) chronic pulmonary involvement. All four criteria are not always present but, for a positive diagnosis, the presence of elevated sweat electrolytes plus either pulmonary disease or pancreatic insufficiency should be present.

Family history. A history of one or more previously affected siblings alerts health personnel to the possibility of the disease in a child born to that family. When diagnosis can be established early, treatment can be initiated to reduce the complications in many instances.

Sweat electrolytes. For a definitive test, the quantitative sweat test is employed. The consistent finding of abnormally high sodium and chloride concentrations in the sweat is a unique characteristic of cystic fibrosis. Mothers frequently observe that their infants taste ''salty'' when they kiss them. For diagnostic purposes the quantitative test is performed on sweat obtained by iontophoresis of pilocarpine in which a small electric current carries the cholinergic drug pilocarpine into a small patch of skin (the forearm in older children; the thigh in infants) to stimulate the sweat glands locally. The sweat is then collected on a filter paper and the chloride content measured in the laboratory. The procedure of applying electrodes and the amount of current and length of its application are carried out according to the manufacturer's instructions. It is important to make certain that the positive electrode is completely covered with gauze and moistened with pilocarpine and that the entire surface of the 4 square inch electrode makes contact with the skin surface. The small amount of current spread over this area is almost indiscernible, but, if contact is poor, the current becomes concentrated in a smaller area and may produce a burn.

Sweat tests are included in the workup of children with recurrent respiratory infections, malabsorption, or failure to thrive. Since sweat glands function inadequately during the first weeks of life, reliable sweat tests are difficult to obtain. Normally the sweat chloride content is less than 40 mEq/liter, with a mean of 18 mEq/liter; a chloride concentration greater than 60 mEq/liter is diagnostic of cystic fibrosis, and levels of 40 to 60 mEq/liter are highly suggestive of the disease. The test is repeated if results are questionable or if results are negative in a case in which clinical symptoms are strongly suggestive.

Several simple screening tests have been developed but are not as reliable for diagnosis. These include measurements of sweat conductivity (shown by increased electrolyte concentrations), silver electrodes, and treated agar plates or filter paper that reacts with the chloride in palmar sweat.

Pancreatic enzymes. Measurements of duodenal enzyme activity may be made to confirm a diagnosis. These enzymes are absent or diminished in children with cystic fibrosis. Usually only trypsin and chymotrypsin are measured. Trypsin is absent in over 80% of patients with the disease.

Fat-absorption tests. Impaired fat absorption in the intestines causes large volumes to be excreted in the stools (steatorrhea). In fat-absorption tests impaired fat absorption is measured in a 5-day stool collection and calculated as a percentage of intake.

Radiographs. Evidence of generalized obstruction emphysema is highly suggestive of cystic fibrosis. With advanced disease, patchy atelectasis and a disseminated infiltrative pattern of bronchopneumonia are observed.

Medical management

Early diagnosis before irreversible pulmonary changes take place and individualized treatment have reduced the morbidity and increased the longevity of children with cystic fibrosis. Pulmonary function tests and blood gas determinations detect lung changes before they are evident on chest x-ray examinations, and new drugs and pulmonary hygiene provide better control of complications. Wherever possible the goals of care are aimed at promoting a normal life for the affected child. This includes maintaining good nutrition, prevention and control of pulmonary infections, and promoting a satisfactory psychologic adjustment to the disease and all of its ramifications.

Diet. The impaired intestinal absorption in cystic fibrosis necessitates a diet significantly higher in calories and protein than is normally required in a child of similar size. Fat content is reduced, although opinions vary regarding the quantities allowed. Fat supplies twice the calories of carbohydrate but may interfere with absorption of other nutrients. However, it is generally regulated according to the degree of pancreatic deficit. High-protein formulas with low-curd tension are recommended during the first weeks of life, followed by low-fat or skim milk and homogenized milk in older children if they are able to tolerate it. Medium-chain triglycerides (MCT) are more readily absorbed than longer chain fats and are sometimes given as a dietary supplement.

Water-miscible preparations of vitamins A, D, and E are provided daily in twice the usually recommended dosage. Vitamin K is indicated if hypoprothrombinemia is present as a result of accompanying liver involvement or in small infants with achylia to prevent hypoprothrombinemia.

Pancreatic enzyme replacement is given in conjunction with meals and snacks and is regulated in order to obtain normal bowel movements, nutrition, and growth. The dosage is determined by the degree of enzyme deficiency, the destruction of the exogenous enzymes by gastric hydrochloric acid, and the food intake. Each enzyme unit will digest only a specific amount of protein, fat, or complex carbohydrate. Simple sugars are absorbed directly. Powdered preparations are administered to infants and young children, and enteric-coated tablets are given to older children and adolescents. An active teenager may require as many as 100 tablets/day. Several preparations are available, but the most commonly used is pancreatin (Viokase).

Since salt depletion through sweating is a hazard, children are allowed to use salt generously. Most children are able to adjust this to their needs, and older children often exhibit a preference for salty foods. Additional salt should be taken during hot weather.

Pulmonary therapy. Management of pulmonary problems is directed toward prevention and treatment of pulmonary infection by (1) removal of mucopurulent secretions and (2) use of antimicrobial agents. Once infection becomes established in relatively defenseless lungs, it is difficult to eradicate, becoming chronic with recurrent episodes of bronchopneumonia sometimes complicated by atelectasis, bronchiectatic abscesses, and stimulating pulmonary fibrosis, which eventually terminates in cor pulmonale.

Pulmonary hygiene is an important aspect of treatment. This is accomplished by (1) physical therapy, (2) expectorant therapy, (3) mucolytic therapy, and (4) mist therapy.

Physical therapy. The purpose of physical therapy is to maintain good pulmonary hygiene by way of postural drainage and breathing exercises. Postural drainage through positioning, clapping with the cupped hand over the lung segment to be drained, and vibration over the segment during exhalation has been described (p. 1201) and is carried out to encourage coughing and assist in removal of mucus and exudate. The procedure should be carried out several times daily prophylactically and, during infections, as often as the child is able to tolerate it without undo fatigue.

Breathing exercises (p. 1203) are recommended for the majority of children with cystic fibrosis, even those with minimal pulmonary involvement. The exercises are usually performed twice daily, preceded by postural drainage. Exercises to improve posture and mobilize the thorax are added, such as swinging the arms and trunk bending and twisting. Children are encouraged to increase physical activity and participate in sports. The ultimate aim of these exercises and activities is to establish a good habitual breathing pattern.

Aerosol therapy. Moisture-laden air is a major modality in pulmonary therapy of cystic fibrosis. It moistens bronchial secretions to assist in their evacuation. Moist air is provided by intermittent inhalation therapy, usually used in conjunction with postural drainage, and by mist tent therapy. In order to be effective, the particles of moisture must be small enough to penetrate to the smaller bronchi; therefore, nebulization must produce particles 0.5 to 5μ in diameter.[12,22]

Intermittent therapy is provided by hand-held nebulizers, either the hand-bulb variety or the jet-aerosal or cartridge-type devices that employ Freon propellants; intermittent positive-pressure breathing devices used in conjunction with deep breaths; and ultrasonic nebulizers that produce smaller droplets of a more consistent size. The recommended schedule for intermittent, or interrupted, therapy to be carried out at least twice daily (morning and evening) and more often if needed consists of three steps:

1. Postural drainage for 5 to 10 minutes
2. Nebulization with appropriate solution
3. Postural drainage for 10 to 20 minutes

Nebulization after postural drainage permits deeper penetration of the droplet particles. There is not total agreement regarding the benefits of bronchodilators or mucolytic agents used in the nebulizing solution. Most favor a solution of 10% propylene glycol and 90% distilled water. Propylene glycol stabilizes the mist in droplet form and prevents vaporization of the droplet. Normal saline is sometimes employed on a short-term basis.[41]

Mist-tent therapy is a controversial issue in treatment of cystic fibrosis. There is evidence that the inhaled droplets are deposited almost entirely in the upper respiratory tract, the esophagus, and stomach. Others believe that the residual volume is considerably less after the mist tent (with propylene glycol in the jet-type nebulizer). If a mist tent is employed in selected cases, it requires a large-capacity nebulizer with a compression or ultrasonic nebulizer and propylene glycol solution. Most mist-tent use is during hospitalization for acute episodes of pulmonary disease. For some children it may be recommended for home use, usually reserved for the sleeping hours. Oxygen therapy is usually recommended for children during acute episodes, and, when lung involvement becomes extensive, it may be needed with nebulization and at night for comfort and to prevent hypoxia. Use of oxygen for nebulization is not recommended for home use. Many of these children have chronic carbon dioxide retention, and the unsupervised use of oxygen for nebulization can be harmful.

Medications. Expectorants, particularly the iodides, which are believed to thin out bronchial secretions are used frequently. Drugs used are saturated solution of potassium iodide, hydriodic acid syrup, and iodopropylidene glycerol (Organidin), an iodinated glycerol. Some children are sensitive to iodides, and excessive use may result in goiter and symptoms of hypothyroidism. Therefore, the drugs are used with caution.[12,41]

Antibiotic therapy. During acute exacerbations of pulmonary disease, intensive antibiotics are employed to control pulmonary infection. Many physicians prefer to use antibiotics only when there is evidence of infection, whereas others prescribe their use as a prophylactic measure. When used therapeutically, it is important that the drugs be given over a long enough period of time and in sufficient dosage to be effective. Oral antibiotics are best selected on the basis of sputum cultures, but in acute situations a broad-spectrum drug is employed pending results of the culture. Antibiotics used for long-term prophylactic therapy are frequently rotated to reduce the chance of developing resistance to any single drug.

The most frequent organism found in sputum is hemolytic *Staphylococcus aureus*. After extended use of antibiotics, the predominant organism is *Pseudomonas*, which is resistant to most oral antibiotics. During acute disease the child is frequently hospitalized and the appropriate antibiotic administered parenterally. Sometimes antibiotics are given by nebulization to provide a high concentration of antibiotic in the respiratory passages, where it can attack the microorganisms directly.

Other complications are treated symptomatically. Rectal prolapse is reduced by gently pressing against the everted rectum with a gloved, lubricated finger while the child is in the knee-chest position. The buttocks are then strapped together with tape. Nasal polyps, to which children with cystic fibrosis are predisposed, are removed surgically to relieve blockage of nasal passages.

Prognosis. It is the pulmonary involvement that determines the ultimate outcome of the disease. Pancreatic enzyme deficiency is less of a problem if adequate nutrition is assured. Hemorrhage from liver cirrhosis and massive salt depletion in hot weather are occasional hazards. With early diagnosis and improved therapeutic measures, the life expectancy has improved. Many more children are reaching adulthood; however, the variation in severity of the disease is an important factor in determining the ultimate outcomes. No exact figures are available regarding the life expectancy of a child with cystic fibrosis. It is estimated to be 15 to 20 years of age. Many still die in infancy and early childhood, but some live to the age of 20 or 30 years.[12,15]

Nursing considerations

Nursing care of infants and children with cystic fibrosis involves both acute and chronic management. These children require regular observation and medical supervision, including ongoing assessment of general health and nutritional and pulmonary status.

The nurse's contact with an affected child usually begins when the child is brought to the hospital or clinic for confirmation of the diagnosis. Perhaps the reason for hospitalization is failure to thrive or recurrent respiratory infections. Later, during recurrent admission to the hospital or during ongoing follow-up in the clinic or at home, the nurse and the child develop a sustained relationship.

Diagnosis. On the initial contact, frequently in the hospital setting, nurses are involved in performing or assisting with diagnostic tests and obtaining primarily sweat for laboratory analysis of chloride content and, less often, of stool specimens for trypsin and fat. The child, usually an infant, needs comfort during the procedures; young children need distraction while they are confined during iontophoresis. Even short periods of inactivity seem long to an active child. Children beyond very early childhood need explanation of the strange, and sometimes painful, procedures and the equipment used for tests and treatments.

At first the respiratory equipment, oxygen mask, mouthpiece, and mist tent are frightening, especially to infants and very young children. The mist tent (if prescribed) can be a source of either fear or comfort and security. The child needs patient support and guidance in using the equipment. Accepting uncharacteristic behavior and explaining this normal stress response to parents are important nursing functions.

Parents are anxious and puzzled. Few of them have any understanding of the disease process and the long-term implications it has for their family. They need patient and careful explanations of the disease, how it might affect their particular family, and what they can do to provide the best possible care for their child.

The shock associated with the diagnosis is overwhelming to parents. They must face the impact of the chronic, life-threatening nature of the disease and the prospect of intensive treatment, for which they must assume a major part of the responsibility and for which they are ill prepared. They often fear that they will be unable to provide the care the child needs. One of the most difficult aspects of the diagnosis is the implications inherent in its etiology, that is, the recognition that each parent contributed the gene responsible for the defect in their child.

Hospital care. When the child is hospitalized for confirmation of the diagnosis or for pulmonary complications, aerosol therapy is instituted or continued. The child may or may not be placed in a mist tent, but nebulization is almost always central to hospital management. Respiratory therapy is usually initiated and supervised by a trained respiratory therapist or physiotherapist. In institutions with large support staffs, they may provide all treatments. If not, it becomes the responsibility of the nurse to perform the prescribed nebulization, postural drainage, percussion, and vibration and to teach supervised breathing exercises.

The child who receives mist therapy requires frequent observation to make certain that the equipment is operating properly and that the reservoir contains the prescribed solution (usually distilled water with a mucolytic agent). The mist should be of sufficient density that the child is barely visible through the moisture. The child requires frequent changes of linen, which becomes wet from the high humidity within the tent or Isolette. Oxygen is cautiously administered to children in respiratory distress but requires frequent assessment. The hazard of oxygen narcosis is a constant threat in children with long-standing disease who receive oxygen (see p. 1199). Intensive aerosol therapy may cause large volumes of sputum to be thinned suddenly in the early hours of treatment; therefore, the child requires close observation to assist him with expectoration and to prevent deeper aspiration. Expectorant drugs are administered orally, which further facilitates the expectoration of mucus.

The diet is implemented for the newly diagnosed child or continued for the child who is hospitalized for pulmonary disease. Enzymes are supplied for each meal or snack, and adequate salt is provided, especially for febrile children. Unless the child is ill, his appetite is usually satisfactory. An ample supply of food should be made available to satisfy the voracious appetite characteristic of many of these children. However, some younger children may object to the extra fluids that are encouraged to promote thinning of mucous secretions.

Special efforts are made to protect the child from further infection, even though a respiratory infection is probably the reason for hospitalization. These children are particularly vulnerable to cross-contamination; therefore, reverse isolation may be implemented for the child's protection.

Frequent skin care is carried out to prevent irritation and skin breakdown over bony prominences. Particular attention is necessary after use of the bedpan or when the diaper is changed. Careful cleansing helps to reduce irritation and odor from offensive stools.

The child will need support for the many treatments and tests that are a necessary part of the hospital therapy. Intravenous fluids, intramuscular injections, and blood tests are almost always a part of the treatment, and the child soon associates hospitalization with these stress-provoking procedures. These children are usually quite thin with little muscle mass, which requires careful selection of injection sites.

Support to both child and family is a vital part of nursing care. The progressive nature of the disease makes each illness requiring hospitalization a potentially life-threatening event. Skilled nursing care and sympathetic attention to the emotional needs of the child and family help them cope with the stresses associated with repeated respiratory infections and hospitalization.

Home care. After the diagnosis is confirmed and a treatment program determined, parents will need help in finding inhalation equipment available for home use that best meets their needs. They will need opportunities to learn about and practice the use of the equipment as well as some of the problems they may encounter.

They need to learn about the preferred diet of nutritious meals with limited fat and ample protein and carbohydrate and the administration of pancreatic enzymes. Children usually adjust well to taking pancreatic enzymes. In powdered form they can be mixed with pureed fruit, such as applesauce, and fed with a spoon. The enteric-coated tablets are more suitable for older children. It is important to stress to parents that the enzymes, in the amount regulated to the child's needs, are to be administered with all meals, including any snacks that may be eaten between meals or at bedtime. They are cautioned about not restricting salt, especially during hot weather.

One of the most important aspects of educating parents for home care is teaching postural drainage and breathing exercises. The success of a therapy program depends on conscientious performance of these treatments regularly as prescribed. The number of times these therapies are performed each day is determined on an individual basis, and, often, parents readily learn to adjust the number and intensity of the treatments to the child's needs. Whether the nurse or therapist instructs the parents, nurses are frequently the persons who can follow up the care in the home and assist the family with innovative approaches to the therapy. For example, using games and normal childhood activities to provide postural drainage reduces the likelihood that treatment will meet with resistance from the child. Simple activities that are fun, such as hanging by the knees from a bar or low-hanging trapeze that can be easily built in the backyard (or indoors), turning somersaults, or playing "wheelbarrow" with the child suspended head down and propelling himself on his hands while the adult holds onto his feet, should be encouraged. Most children respond to a challenge, such as, "How long can you stand on your head?" Small children can "stand on their heads" with their heads on the cushion of a large chair with or without the adult holding onto the feet. Parents soon learn to respond to cues from their children and incorporate spontaneous activities into the treatment regimen.

The nurse can assist the family to contact resources that provide help to families with affected children. The various crippled children's services, many local clinics, private agencies, service clubs, and other community groups often offer equipment and medications either free or at reduced rates. The National Cystic Fibrosis Research Foundation* has chapters throughout the country to provide education and services to families and professionals.

Psychologic support. One of the most important and difficult aspects in providing care for the family of a child with cystic fibrosis is coping with the emotional needs of the child and family. The diagnosis, treatment, and prognosis are fraught with a multiplicity of problems, frustrations, and feelings. The diagnosis with all its implications evokes feelings of guilt and self-recrimination in the parents. These feelings may be particularly marked if the newly diagnosed child is the second affected child in the family and the parents had been counseled regarding the 1 in 4 risk of such an event occurring.

The long-range problems are those encountered in the care of a child with a chronic illness (Chapter 22). Both the

*3379 Peachtree Road, N.E., Atlanta, Ga. 30326.

Summary of nursing care of the child with cystic fibrosis

Goals	Responsibilities
Assist in diagnosis	Perform nursing assessment of child Take family history and health history Encourage medical evaluation for any child who displays suggestive signs of the disease Frequent respiratory infection Large, bulky stools Prolapsed rectum Failure to gain weight Prepare child for diagnostic tests Assist with diagnostic procedures Collect stool specimens Perform sweat test Assist with radiographs
Maintain nutrition	Provide diet high in carbohydrate and protein Discourage use of foods high in fat; provide appropriate fat if recommended by physician Assure adequate intake of salt Administer pancreatic enzyme replacement with meals and snacks Administer water-miscible vitamins and iron supplement
Assist patient to expectorate sputum	Perform postural drainage as prescribed Teach and/or supervise breathing exercises Provide nebulization with appropriate solution equipment as prescribed Place in mist tent as ordered; make certain compressor or ultrasonic mechanism provides very small droplets in ample supply Administer expectorants Administer bronchodilators, if ordered
Prevent infection	Restrict contact with persons who have respiratory tract infections, including family, other children, friends, and members of staff Administer antibiotics as prescribed Manage respiratory infections as in pneumonia
Conserve energy	Provide or encourage activities appropriate to child's developmental level and physical capacity
Improve aeration	Perform postural drainage Supervise breathing exercises Administer medications that promote breathing (bronchodilators, expectorants) Administer oxygen, if indicated and prescribed Provide nebulization Prevent and treat respiratory tract infections Encourage good posture and active exercises suitable to child's needs, capabilities, and preferences
Teach child about disease and treatment	Teach child to assist in his own care Food selection Use of pancreatic enzymes Use of equipment How he can cooperate during treatments and tests

Continued.

Summary of nursing care of the child with cystic fibrosis—cont'd

Goals	Responsibilities
Promote growth and development	Provide or encourage nutritious diet Encourage to maintain usual activities Arrange for continued family contacts during hospitalization Arrange for continued schooling while hospitalized Encourage relationships with peers Promote development of a positive self-image
Provide material support to child and family	Guide to available resources equipped to deal with their special needs Provide counseling services Collaborate with family and health team in assessing family needs and coping mechanisms
Administer optimal home care	Assess home situation Help devise individualized regimen based on assessment Teach family home care Help family acquire needed drugs and equipment Arrange for regular follow-up care to reassess effectiveness of home management Assist family in problem solving
Educate family	Provide accurate information at a rate family can absorb Teach family members physical care of child Use of equipment Exercises and procedures Diet and administration of pancreatic enzymes Administration of drugs Protection from infection Provide or arrange for genetic counseling regarding inherited aspects of the disease
Emotionally support family	Listen to family members—singly or collectively Act on cues that indicate a family member's reaction to child Help family to gain confidence in their ability to cope with child, disability, and its impact on other family members Encourage interaction with other families who have a similarly affected child Help family face possibility of child's death
Participate in community education	Educate community groups regarding disorder Support research efforts Become actively involved in fund raising for cystic fibrosis research and treatment

child and family must make many adjustments, the success of which depends on their ability to cope and also on the quality and quantity of support they receive from sources outside the family. Combined efforts of a variety of health professionals offer the most comprehensive services to families. It is frequently the responsibility of the nurse to organize and coordinate these services, to assess the home situation, and to collect the data needed to evaluate the effectiveness of the services in meeting the needs of the family.

For the family the illness means modification of numerous family activities. Meals require planning in order not to place too many restrictions on the affected child or deprive the other members of the family. Limits on mobility restrict family recreational activities, especially when the child's therapy includes respiratory equipment that is not transportable. Postural drainage must be continued wherever the child may be. Also, members of the family hesitate to take the child too far from familiar and trusted medical care. The illness even determines the family's place of residence and employment, as the child's condition dictates that he should remain near medical care facilities that offer the specialized care he needs.

The persistent need for treatment several times daily also places a strain on the family. Someone must perform the procedures, such as percussion and vibration, even on older children who are able to assume responsibility for their own exercises and respiratory therapy. Children often balk at the treatments, and the parents are placed in the position of insisting on compliance. Sometimes the stress and anxiety related to this continual routine generate feelings of resentment, which are frequently focused on one aspect of the regimen, such as the diet or equipment. When possible, occasional trusted respite care should be made available to the parent or parents to allow them the opportunity to leave the situation for short periods without undo anxiety regarding the child's welfare.

The affected child also may become resentful about his disease, its relentless routine of therapy, and the necessary curtailment it places on his activities and relationships. The child's activities are interrupted or built around treatment, medications, and diet that impose hardships (such as carrying medication to school and other places where they may eat away from home), and growth retardation that is associated with most chronic illness may be trying to the child. Any of these aspects of the disease may be the cause of ridicule from other children.

A constant source of anxiety for both parents and child is the ever-present fear of death. The expected life span, although significantly increased during the past years, offers only limited encouragement regarding prognosis. The future is always uncertain. These families need all the support and skill the nurse can offer to cope with the guarded prognosis (see Chapter 27). (See the boxed material for a summary of nursing care of the child with cystic fibrosis.)

REFERENCES

1. Adair, J. C., and associates: Ten year experience with IPPB in the treatment of acute laryngotracheobronchitis, Anesth. Analg. (Cleve) **50:**649, 1971.
2. Askin, F. B.: Lungs. In Kissane, J. M.: Pathology of infancy and childhood, ed. 2, St. Louis, 1975, The C. V. Mosby Co.
3. Avner, S. E.: Beta-adrenergic bronchodilators, Pediatr. Clin. North Am. **22**(1):129-139, 1975.
4. Bailit, I. W., and Mueller, H. L.: Allergic disorders. In Shirkey, H. C., editor: Pediatric therapy, ed. 5, St. Louis, 1975, The C. V. Mosby Co.
5. Bardana, E. J., Jr.: Modern aspects in diagnosis and treatment of the asthmatic patient, Clin. Notes Respir. Dis. **15**(2): 3-13, Fall 1976.
6. Bennett, R. M.: Drowning and near-drowning, etiology and pathophysiology, Am. J. Nurs. **76:**919-921, 1976.
7. Bierman, C. W., and Pierson, W. E.: Symposium on exercise and asthma, Pediatrics **56**(suppl. 2):843, 1975.
8. Block, R. C., and Block. C. E.: Help, my child is choking, Pediatr. Nurs. **2**(5):48-49, 1976.
9. Cotton, E. K., and Parry, W. H.: Respiratory tract and mediastinum. In Kempe, C. H., Silver, H. K., and O'Brien, D.: Current pediatric therapy, ed. 3, Los Altos, Calif., 1974, Lange Medical Publications.
10. Crawford, L. V.: Allergic diseases. In Hughes, J. G.: Synopsis of pediatrics, ed. 4, St. Louis, 1975, The C. V. Mosby Co.
11. Cropp, G. J. A.: Exercise-induced asthma, Pediatr. Clin. North Am. **22:**63-76, 1975.
12. Crozier, D. N.: Cystic fibrosis: a not-so-fatal disease, Pediatr. Clin. North Am. **21:**935, November 1974.
13. Dees, S. C.: Asthma. In Kendig, E. L., Jr., and Chernick, V., editors: Disorders of the respiratory tract in children, Philadelphia, 1977, W. B. Saunders Co.
14. Dillon, H. C., Jr., and Derrick, C. W., Jr.: Beta hemolytic streptococcal infections. In Shirkey, H. C., editor: Pediatric therapy, ed. 5, St. Louis, 1975, The C. V. Mosby Co.
15. Di Sant'Agnese, P. A.: The pancreas. In Vaughn, V. C., and McKay, R. J., editors: Textbook of pediatrics, ed. 10, Philadelphia, 1975, W. B. Saunders Co.
16. Di Sant'Agnese, P. A., and Darling, R. C.: Cystic fibrosis of the pancreas. In Downey, J. C., and Low, N. L., editors: The child with disabling illness, Philadelphia, 1974, W. B. Saunders Co.
17. Eichenwald, H. F.: Infections of the lower respiratory tract—larynx, trachea, bronchi, lung parenchyma, and pleura. In Shirkey, H. C., editor: Pediatric therapy, ed. 5, St. Louis, 1975, The C. V. Mosby Co.
18. Eichenwald, H. F., and McCracken, G. H., Jr.: The thoracic cavity. In Vaughn, V. C., and McKay, R. J., editors: Nelson's textbook of pediatrics, ed. 10, Philadelphia, 1975, W. B. Saunders Co.
19. Eller, J. J.: Infections: bacterial and spirochetal. In Kempe, C. H., Silver, H. K., and O'Brien, D.: Current pediatric therapy, ed. 3, Los Altos, Calif., 1974, Lange Medical Publications.
20. Fulginiti, V. A., and Sieber, O. F.: Pertussis. In Vaughn, V. C., and McKay, R. J., editors: Textbook of pediatrics, ed. 10, Philadelphia, 1975, W. B. Saunders Co.
21. Graves, S. A.: Drowning and near-drowning. In Vaughn, V. C., and McKay, R. J., editors: Textbook of pediatrics, ed. 10, Philadelphia, 1975, W. B. Saunders Co.
22. Hughes, J. G.: Synopsis of pediatrics, ed. 4, St. Louis, 1975, The C. V. Mosby Co.
23. Johnstone, D. E.: The case for hyposensitization, Pediatr. Clin. North Am. **22:**239-249, 1975.
24. Kissane, J. M.: Pathology of infancy and childhood, ed. 2, St. Louis, 1975, The C. V. Mosby Co.
25. Krugman, S., Ward, R., and Katz, S. L.: Infectious diseases of children, ed. 6, St. Louis, 1977, The C. V. Mosby Co.
26. Lincoln, E. M., and Sewell, E. M.: Tuberculosis. In Krugman, S., and Ward, R.: Infectious diseases of children and adults, ed. 5, St. Louis, 1973, The C. V. Mosby Co.

27. Mascia, A. V.: Rehabilitation of the child with chronic asthma. In Downey, J. A., and Low, N. L., editors: The child with disabling illness, Philadelphia, 1974, W. B. Saunders Co.

28. Mattson, A.: Long-term physical illness in childhood: a challenge to psychosocial adaptation, Pediatrics **50:**801-811, 1972.

29. Mattson, A.: Psychologic aspects of childhood asthma, Pediatr. Clin. North Am. **22:**77-88, 1975.

30. McCracken, G. H., and Eichenwald, H. F.: Acute infections of the larynx and the trachea. In Vaughn, V. C., and McKay, R. J., editors: Textbook of pediatrics, ed. 10, Philadelphia, 1975, W. B. Saunders Co.

31. McLean, J. A., and Ching, A. Y. T.: Follow-up study of relationships between family situation and bronchial asthma in children, J. Am. Med. Child. Psychiatry **12:**142-161, 1973.

32. Middleton, E., Jr.: The biochemical basis for the modulation of allergic reactions by drugs, Pediatr. Clin. North Am. **22:** 111-120, 1975.

33. Modell, J. H.: Pathophysiology and treatment of drowning and near-drowning, Springfield, Ill., 1971, Charles C Thomas, Publisher.

34. Nelson, H. S.: The beta adrenergic theory of bronchial asthma, Pediatr. Clin. North Am. **22:**53-62, 1975.

35. Nelson, J. D.: Pertussis. In Shirkey, H. C., editor: Pediatric therapy, ed. 5, St. Louis, 1975, The C. V. Mosby Co.

36. Norris, C. M.: Foreign bodies in the larynx, trachea, and bronchi. In Vaughn, V. C., and McKay, R. J., editors: Textbook of pediatrics, ed. 10, Philadelphia, 1975, W. B. Saunders Co.

37. Pearlman, D. S., and Sumio, G.: Allergic disorders. In Kempe, C. H., Silver, H. K., and O'Brien, D., editors: Current pediatric therapy, Los Altos, Calif., 1974, Lange Medical Publications.

38. Richards, W.: Differential diagnosis of childhood asthma, Curr. Probl. Pediatr. **4:**1-36, March 1974.

39. Robinson, L. A., Roper, K. E., and Fischer, R. G.: Nursing considerations in the use of non-prescription analgesic-antipyretics: aspirin and acetaminophen, Pediatr. Nurs. **3**(4):18-24, 1977.

40. Sackner, M. A.: Bronchodilator agents, Clin. Notes Respir. Dis. **15**(1):3-14, Summer 1976.

41. Schwachman, H., and associates: Studies in cystic fibrosis, Pediatrics **46:**335, 1970.

42. Sewell, E. M., O'Hare, D., and Kendig, E. L., Jr.: Tuberculin test, Pediatrics **54:**650, 1974.

43. Smith, M. H. D.: Tuberculosis. In Shirkey, H. C., editor: Pediatric therapy, ed. 5, St. Louis, 1975, The C. V. Mosby Co.

44. Weiss, E. B.: Bronchial asthma, Clin. Symp. **27**(1-2):3-72, 1975.

45. Whaley, L. F.: Understanding inherited disorders, St. Louis, 1974, The C. V. Mosby Co.

46. Williams, H. E., and McNichol, K. N.: The spectrum of asthma in children, Pediatr. Clin. North Am. **22:**43-88, 1975.

BIBLIOGRAPHY

Hughes, J. G.: Synopsis of pediatrics, ed. 4, St. Louis, 1975, The C. V. Mosby Co.

Kendig, E. L., Jr., and Chernick, V., editors: Disorders of the respiratory tract in children, Philadelphia, 1977, W. B. Saunders Co.

Krugman, S., Ward, R., and Katz, S. L.: Infectious diseases of children, ed. 6, St. Louis, 1977, The C. V. Mosby Co.

Shirkey, H. C., editor: Pediatric therapy, ed. 5, St. Louis, 1975, The C. V. Mosby Co.

Vaughn, V. C., and McKay, R. J., editors: Textbook of pediatrics, ed. 10, Philadelphia, 1975, W. B. Saunders Co.

Acute respiratory infection

Bishop, B.: How to cool a feverish child, Pediatr. Nurs. **4**(1):19-20, 1978.

Cormier, J. F., and Bryant, B. G.: Treating the common cold, Pediatr. Nurs. **4**(1):7-13, 1978.

Eade, N. R., Taussig, L. M., and Marks, M. I.: Hydrocarbon pneumonitis, Pediatrics **54:**351, 1974.

Glezen, W. P., and Denny, F. W.: Epidemiology of acute lower tract respiratory disease in children, N. Engl. J. Med. **288:**498, 1973.

Griffith, E. W.: Nursing process: a patient with respiratory dysfunction, Nurs. Clin. North Am. **6:**145, March 1971.

Harris, L. C., Pryles, C. V., and Ziai, M.: Pneumonia. In Ziai, M., editor: Pediatrics, ed. 2, Boston, 1975, Little, Brown and Co.

Hsu, K. H. K.: Isoniazid in the prevention and treatment of tuberculosis; a 20 year study of the effectiveness in children, J.A.M.A. **229:**528, 1974.

Kurt, T. L., and associates: Spread of pertussis by hospital staff, J.A.M.A. **221:**264, 1972.

Reeves, K. R.: Acute epiglottitis—pediatric emergency, Am. J. Nurs. **71:**1539-1541, 1971.

Shaw, E. B.: Acute epiglotitis, Am. J. Dis. Child. **130:**782-784, 1976.

Spicher, C.: Nursing care of children hospitalized with infections, Nurs. Clin. North Am. **5:**123-130, 1970.

Pulmonary disturbance caused by noninfectious irritants

Banks, W., and Potsic, W. P.: Elusive unsuspected foreign bodies in the tracheobronchial tree, Clin. Pediatr. **16:**31-35, 1977.

Caudle, J. T.: Emergency nursing of near-drowning victims, Am. J. Nurs. **76:**922-923, 1976.

Clark, E. B., and Niggemann, E. H.: Near-drowning, Heart Lung **4**(6):952, 1975.

Emergency steps in near-drowning, Nurs. Update **7**(7):10-14, 1976.

Fandel, I., and Bancalari, E.: Near-drowning in children: clinical aspects, Pediatrics **58:**573-579, 1976.

Giammona, S. T.: Drowning: pathology and management, Curr. Probl. Pediatr. **1:**3, 1971.

Giammona, S. T., Redding, J., and Snively, W. D.: Keeping the 'saved' from drowning saved, Patient Care **10**(12):81-98, June 15, 1976.

Gooden, B. A.: Drowning and the diving reflex, Can. Med. Assoc. J. **108:**1209, 1973.

Majd, N. S., Mofenson, H. C., and Greensher, J.: Lower airway foreign body aspiration in children, Clin. Pediatr. **16:**13-16, 1977.

Moser, R. H.: Drowning: a seasonal disease, J.A.M.A. **229:**564, July 29, 1974. (Editorial.)

Petty, T. L.: Intensive and rehabilitative respiratory care, ed. 2, Philadelphia, 1974, Lea & Febiger.

Bronchial asthma

Bergner, M., and Hutelmyer, C.: Teaching kids how to live with their allergies, Nursing '76 **6**(8):11-12, 1976.

Biebman, C. W., and Pierson, W. E.: Hand nebulizers and asthma therapy in children and adolescents (commentaries), Pediatrics **54**:668-670, 1974.

Bierman, C. W., Pierson, W. E., and Shapiro, G. G.: Exercise-induced asthma, J.A.M.A. **234**:295, 1975.

Blumberg, M. Z., and associates: Terbutaline and ephedrine in asthmatic children, Pediatrics **60**:14-19, 1977.

Commey, J. O. O., and Levison, H.: Physical signs in childhood asthma, Pediatrics **58**:537-541, 1976.

Committee on Children with Handicaps: The asthmatic child and his participation in sports and physical education, Pediatrics **45**: 150-151, 1970.

Cotton, E. K.: Status asthmaticus, Respir. Care **22**:1077-1083, 1977.

Cotton, E. K., and Parry, W.: Treatment of status asthmaticus and respiratory failure, Pediatr. Clin. North Am. **22**:163-172, 1975.

Dewey, J.: Ways to live with asthma, Nursing '75 **5**:48-51, 1975.

Dyer, B.: Asthmatic kids—independence. One giant step, Pediatr. Nurs. **3**(2):16-23, 1977.

Ellis, E. F.: Allergic disorders. In Vaughn, V. C., and McKay, R. J., editors: Textbook of pediatrics, ed. 10, Philadelphia, 1975, W. B. Saunders Co.

Falliers, C. J., and associates: Psychodynamics of asthmatic children. In Segal, I., editor: The mental health of the child, Public Health pamphlet No. 2168, Washington, D.C., 1971, U.S. Government Printing Office.

Hawkins-Walsh, E., and Pettrone, C. R.: Drugs used in the treatment of pediatric allergy and asthma, Pediatr. Nurs. **3**(2):12-15, 1977.

Hill, M.: Asthmatic child or asthma expert? Pediatr. Nurs. **3**(2): 25-26, 1977.

Lanser, J., and Pancoast, A.: Caring for the asthmatic at home, in school and on the job, Nursing '73 **3**(11):62-64, 1973.

Levison, H., and associates: Asthma: current concepts, Pediatr. Clin. North Am. **21**:951, November 1974.

Lough, M. D., Bolek, J., and Stern, R. C.: Ten year's experience with a camp for children with pulmonary disease, Respir. Care **22**:828-831, 1977.

McFadden, E. R., Jr., Kiser, R., and DeGroot, W. J.: Acute bronchial asthma; relations between clinical and physiologic manifestations, N. Engl. J. Med. **288**:211, 1973.

Moody, L. E.: Nursing care of patients with asthma, Nurs. Clin. North Am. **9**:195-207, 1974.

Nicholson, D. P.: A problem in clinical research: asthma and cromolyn sodium, Heart Lung **5**:71-76, January/February 1976.

Parry, W. H., Martorano, F., and Colton, E. K.: Management of life-threatening asthma with intravenous isoproterenol infusions, Am. J. Dis. Child. **130**:39-42, 1976.

Rebuck, A. S., and Tomarken, J. L.: Pulsus paradoxus in asthmatic children, Can. Med. Assoc. J. **112**:710, 1975.

Souhrada, J. F., and Buckley, J.: Pulmonary function testing in asthmatic children, Pediatr. Clin. North Am. **23**:249-278, May 1976.

Talamo, R. C.: Managing the adolescent asthmatic, Med. Clin. North Am. **59**:1489-1496, 1975.

Tuff, L., and Mueller, H. L.: Allergy in children, Philadelphia, 1970, W. B. Saunders Co.

Weinberger, M. M., and Bronsky, E. A.: Evaluation of oral bronchodilator therapy in asthmatic children, J. Pediatr. **84**:421, 1974.

Weiss, E. B.: Bronchial asthma, Clin. Symp. **27**(1-2):3-72, 1975.

Wilson, A. F., and Galant, S. P.: Recent advances in the pathology of asthma, West. J. Med. **120**:463-490, 1974.

Ziment, I.: The pharmacology of airway dilators, Respir. Ther., pp. 51-56, May/June 1974.

Cystic fibrosis

Bowman, B.: Genetic counseling in cystic fibrosis, Am. Fam. Physician **8**(6):113-118, 1973.

Boyle, I. R., and associates: Emotional adjustment in adolescents and young adults with cystic fibrosis, J. Pediatr. **88**:318, 1976.

Burnette, B. A.: Family adjustment to cystic fibrosis, Am. J. Nurs. **75**:1986-1988, 1975.

Burns, W. T., and associates: Test strip meconium screening for cystic fibrosis, Am. J. Dis. Child. **131**:71-73, 1977.

Di Sant'Agnese, P. A.: Cystic fibrosis (mucoviscidosis), Am. Fam. Physician **7**(3):102-111, March 1973.

Di Sant'Agnese, P. A., and David, P. B.: Research in cystic fibrosis, N. Engl. J. Med. **295**:481, 1976.

Driscoll, C. B., and Lubin, H. A.: Conferences with parents of children with cystic fibrosis, Soc. Casework **53**:140, 1972.

Gayton, W. F., and Friedman, S. B.: Psychosocial aspects of cystic fibrosis, Am. J. Dis. Child. **126**:856-859, 1975.

Grossman, M. L.: The psychosocial approach to the medical management of patients with cystic fibrosis, Clin. Pediatr. **14**:830-833, 1975.

Herron, H. G., and Spock, A.: Mother and daughter with cystic fibrosis, J. Pediatr. **91**:276-277, 1977.

McCollum, A. T., and Gibson, L.: Family adaptation to the child with cystic fibrosis, J. Pediatr. **77**:572-576, 1970.

Motoyama, E. K., Gibson, L. E., and Zigas, C. J.: Evaluation of mist tent therapy in cystic fibrosis, Pediatrics **50**:299, 1972.

Orenstein, D. M., and associates: The effect of early diagnosis and treatment in cystic fibrosis, Am. J. Dis. Child. **131**:973-975, 1977.

Patterson, P. R.: Minocycline in the antibiotic regimen of cystic fibrosis patients: weight gain and clinical improvement, Clin. Pediatr. **16**:60-63, 1977.

Patterson, P. R., and associates, editors: Psychological aspects of cystic fibrosis, New York, 1973, Columbia University Press.

Rosenthal, A., and associates: Echocardiographic assessment of cor pulmonale in cystic fibrosis, Pediatr. Clin. North Am. **23**: 327-344, May 1976.

Selekman, J.: Cystic fibrosis, Pediatr. Nurs. **3**(2):32-35, 1977.

Stadnyk, S., and Bindschadler, N.: A camp for children with cystic fibrosis, Am. J. Nurs. **70**:1691-1693, 1970.

Taussig, L. M., and associates: Fertility in males with cystic fibrosis, N. Engl. J. Med. **287**:586, 1972.

Taussig, L. M., and associates: A new prognostic score and clinical evaluation system for cystic fibrosis, J. Pediatr. **82**:380, 1973.

Tropauer, A., and associates: Psychological aspects of care of children with cystic fibrosis, Am. J. Dis. Child. **119**:431, 1970.

34

The child with a gastrointestinal disorder

PHYSIOLOGY OF DIGESTION AND ABSORPTION

Knowledge of the basic physiology of digestion and absorption is foundational to the understanding of gastrointestinal disorders. For example, the classification of "malabsorption syndrome" relates to a group of diseases or defects of the small intestine, where most of the absorption of nutrients occurs. Obstructive or inflammatory conditions affect digestion and absorption because bowel motility, mucosal functioning, enzymatic activity, and bacterial flora are altered. Specific disorders such as hepatitis or cirrhosis affect these basic processes because liver functions are compromised. The following discussion is meant to serve as an overview of the basic physiology of digestion and absorption. For a review of the major anatomic structures within the abdominal cavity, the reader is referred to Fig. 5-41).

Digestion

Digestion refers to the catabolism of foodstuffs from their original complex form to simple, assimilable nutrients. Foodstuffs are composed of six substances: water, vitamins, mineral salts, carbohydrates, proteins, and fats. The processes of digestion are mainly *mechanical* (mixing and propulsion of food along the alimentary tract) and *chemical* (conversion of carbohydrates, proteins, and fats into assimilable forms, namely, simple sugars, amino acids, and fatty acids and glycerol, respectively).

Mechanical digestion begins in the mouth. The chewing movements of the teeth and tongue mix the food with saliva and reduce the size of the particles into what is called a *bolus*. Besides moistening the food sufficiently to aid in swallowing, saliva initiates digestion. The enzyme ptyalin, also called amylase, catalyzes the more complex carbohydrates or starches into simpler forms, such as maltose. Once the bolus is swallowed, the remainder of mechanical digestion is involuntary.

The pharynx and esophagus are primarily concerned with deglutition, or swallowing. As the tongue pushes the food backward into the pharynx, the food is propelled into the esophagus by two mechanisms, which prevents its entry up into the nasal cavity or respiratory tract. First the soft palate and uvula elevate to block off the nasopharynx. Second the epiglottis closes over the larynx to prevent food from passing into the airway. As food enters the esophagus, it is propelled forward into the stomach by movements called *peristalsis*. These wavelike movements squeeze the food along the entire length of the alimentary tract. The passage of stomach content is controlled by the cardiac sphincter between the esophagus and stomach and the pyloric sphincter between the stomach and duodenum, the beginning of the small intestine.

As the bolus passes into the stomach, gastric movements churn the particles back and forth, mixing them with gastric juice. Gastric juice contains water, pepsin, hydrochloric acid, rennin, lipase, and mucin. Pepsin (also called protease), hydrochloric acid, and rennin partially digest proteins; lipase initiates the digestion of fats. Mucin serves primarily to buffer the strong acid and forms a protective barrier between the acid and stomach. The entire alimentary tract is protected from the digestive action of its various secretions by the production of mucus and the rapid replacement of mucosal cells.

The partially digested food, now called *chyme*, passes from the stomach into the small intestine, where churning movements cause it to mix thoroughly with intestinal juices and to come in contact with the mucosal lining for absorption. Intestinal juice contains the enzymes enterokinase, which activates the pancreatic enzyme trypsin, and amylase. The intestinal epithelial cells contain large quantities of digestive enzymes, which appear to complete digestion while the substances are being absorbed into the cells. These enzymes include (1) peptidases for splitting peptides into amino acids, (2) sucrase, maltase, isomaltase, and lactase for converting disaccharides into the monosaccharides glucose, galactose, and fructose, and (3) lipase for splitting fats into fatty acids and glycerol.

Secretions from the liver and pancreas complete digestion in the small intestine. Bile, formed in the liver, contains no enzymes but is important for digestion because it (1) lowers the surface tension of fat, forming an emulsion that allows the water-soluble lipase to exert its enzymatic effect on the fat globules, and (2) increases the absorption of the end products of fat digestion by the intestinal wall. The absence of bile causes about half of the ingested fat to appear in the feces, a condition called steatorrhea, and impairs the absorption of the fat-soluble vitamins A, D, E, and K.

Pancreatic juice contains three important digestive enzymes: (1) trypsin (also called protease), which converts partially digested proteins, namely proteoses and peptones, and intact proteins into the final end product, amino acids, (2) lipase, which catalyzes the bile-emulsified fats into their final end products, fatty acids and glycerol, and (3) amylase, which hydrolyzes most starches and carbohydrates to the disaccharides maltose, sucrose, and lactose. Each of these three enzymes becomes active only after the inactive forms are secreted into the small intestine. For example, enterokinase is necessary for trypsinogen to be converted into trypsin. If this were not the case, the activated enzymes would digest the pancreas and pancreatic duct.

After the digestion and absorption of the nutritional end product in the small intestine, the remainder of the intestinal contents, namely nondigestible residue and a small amount of undigested fat and protein, pass through the ileocecal valve into the large intestine. Here the contents are prepared for excretion as *feces*. Most of the remaining water and electrolytes is absorbed from the proximal colon. The bacterial flora form vitamin K, vitamin B_{12}, thiamine, riboflavin, and various gases. The odor of feces is primarily the result of the products of bacterial action and depends on the type of colonic flora and ingested food. Defects in digestion or absorption notably alter the odor, as well as the appearance, of feces. The color is caused by the end products of bilirubin, which is converted by bacteria to urobilinogen and then oxidized to urobilin.

As the rectum becomes distended with feces, powerful peristaltic waves are stimulated, which propel the colonic content toward the anus. At the same time the internal anal sphincter relaxes, and, if the external sphincter voluntarily or involuntarily relaxes, defecation occurs.

Absorption

The principal absorbing site in the gastrointestinal system is the small intestine. The inner lining of the small intestine contains may folds called *valvulae conniventes,* which increase the absorptive surface about threefold. In addition the entire surface of these folds is covered with small finger-like projections called *villi,* which greatly increase the absorptive area another tenfold. Millions of *microvilli* make up the luminal surface of the intestinal epithelial cells covering each villi and continue to increase the absorptive surface by another twentyfold. In each villi are *crypts of Lieberkühn,* whose main purpose is to replace the absorptive cells that are constantly being extruded at each villus tip. This process of regeneration is so effective that normally the intestinal epithelium replaces itself every 5 days.

Unlike this type of surface, the stomach and large intestine are devoid of villi. Most of the absorption that takes place there is by *diffusion,* or the movement of substances from an area of higher concentration to one of lower concentration. Absorption in the small intestine may be by simple diffusion or *active transport,* which requires energy to transport a substance across an opposing pressure gradient or against an electric potential. The mechanisms of active transport are not completely understood but are thought to be carried on by the epithelial cells of the intestinal mucosa.

The end products of carbohydrate and protein digestion, the monosaccharides and amino acids, are absorbed into the intestinal capillaries and circulated to the liver by the portal vein, where they are metabolized and either used for energy or stored as the body's reserves. The end products of fat digestion, the fatty acids and glycerol, are absorbed by the epithelial cells of the villi, where they are reconverted to the triglyceride fat molecule, which then moves out of the cells into the lymph capillaries (lacteals) of the villi. The lymphatics carry them to the venous circulation by the thoracic duct to the left subclavian vein, superior vena cava, heart, and general circulation. Some undigested emulsified fats directly enter the circulation by the intestinal capillaries.

All of the vitamins are believed to be absorbed in the small intestine. The fat-soluble vitamins are absorbed along with digested fats in the presence of bile. The water-soluble vitamins, vitamin B complex and C, are quickly absorbed, although absorption of vitamin B_{12} takes place only in the ileum. Water and electrolytes are also absorbed primarily in the small intestine, although some absorption also takes place in the large intestine.

CLASSIFICATION OF MALABSORPTION SYNDROMES

The term "malabsorption syndrome" refers to a long list of disorders associated with some degree of impaired digestion and/or absorption. Most classifications are according to the locations of the supposed anatomic and biochemical defect. For example, pathophysiologic classification divides malabsorptive syndromes into the luminal phase (defects within the lumen of the small intestine, such as cystic fibrosis), the intestinal phase (defects on the surface or within the mucosal cells, such as celiac disease), and the delivery phase (defects in transport of nutrients to the body, such as in congestive heart failure).[2] A more developmental classification groups the disorders according to usual age of onset, whereas a third classification uses the presenting clinical signs of watery, fatty, or normal stools.[1]

Since most of the disorders that affect the main site of absorption, the small intestine, are rare, it is more relevant for the nurse to understand the physiology behind the cause, which guides the main treatment regimens, rather than memorizing a long list of medical conditions.

Digestive defects

Digestive defects mainly include those conditions in which the enzymes necessary for digestion are diminished or absent, such as (1) cystic fibrosis, in which pancreatic enzymes are absent, (2) biliary or liver disease, in which bile production is affected, or (3) lactase deficiency, in which there is congenital or secondary lactose intolerance.

Absorptive defects

Absorptive defects include those conditions in which the intestinal mucosal transport system is impaired. It may be because of a primary defect, such as in celiac disease or gluten enteropathy (discussed below), or secondary to inflammatory disease of the bowel, such as ulcerative colitis. Chronic inflammation results in impaired absorption because bowel motility is accelerated, affecting the rate of propulsion or transit time of food in the bowel. Consequently there is less mixing of food with pancreatic, biliary, and intestinal secretions. As a result bacterial flora is altered, which further disturbs colonic activity. Obstructive disorders, such as Hirschsprung's disease, can also cause secondary malabsorption from enterocolitis, chronic inflammation of the distended small and large bowel.

Absorption is also impaired by a number of biochemical abnormalities, which are generally designated as inborn errors of metabolism. For example, disaccharide deficiency results in the inability to hydrolyze the more complex forms of carbohydrates to simpler, assimilable structures, the monosaccharides. Abnormalities of intestinal lymphatic transport, particularly for fats, are a secondary result of diseases such as lymphoma, leukemia, infectious lymphadenopathy (in parasitic infestations or tuberculosis), and scarring of the submucosa after irradiation. The mechanical blockage of the lymphatics caused by these conditions impairs fat circulation through the lacteals in the villi and results in leakage of plasma proteins into the gastrointestinal tract.

Anatomic defects

Anatomic defects, such as extensive resection of the bowel or ''short bowel syndrome,'' affect digestion by decreasing the transit time of substances with the digestive juices and affects absorption by severely compromising the absorptive surface.

Emotional factors. There are also several disorders that result in malabsorption but for which no specific organic cause can be found. One of the most classic examples is maternal deprivation syndrome or failure to thrive (p. 494), in which malnutrition results despite adequately functioning body systems and is reversed by a program of emotional stimulation rather than medical intervention.

Celiac disease (gluten enteropathy)

The term ''celiac disease'' is often used interchangeably with ''malabsorption syndrome,'' although it includes several different diseases that have four characteristics in common: (1) steatorrhea (fat, foul, frothy, bulky stools), (2) general malnutrition, (3) abdominal distention, and (4) secondary vitamin deficiencies. With advanced knowledge in diagnosis and pathology of malabsorption syndromes, different etiologies have been discovered for several of the ''celiac diseases.''

Presently celiac disease refers to a specific condition, called gluten enteropathy. In adults this same condition is often referred to as nontropical sprue. Tropical sprue is a different disease that has a peculiar propensity for tropical geographic locations. The pathogenesis is unknown, but research suggests that tropical sprue is caused by abnormal bacterial colonization of the upper bowel. Treatment is not dietary, as in nontropical sprue, but antibacterial. Cystic fibrosis of the pancreas is considered a separate disorder, because although the four clinical manifestations are present, the defect is in digestion, not absorption, of fats (see p. 1252). Celiac disease and cystic fibrosis are the two most common malabsorptive disorders in children.

Celiac disease is more common in whites than in blacks or Asians. Although the exact mode of transmission is not known, there is a tendency for the disease to occur in several members of the same family.

Pathology. The exact cause of celiac disease is not known, although the basic defect is believed to be an inborn error of metabolism or an immunologic response. The former theory holds that there is an absence of peptidase in intestinal mucosal cells that results in an inability to hydrolyze the peptides of gliadin, a protein found in gluten. Inability to fully digest gliadin results in accumulation of the amino acid glutamine, which is toxic to the mucosal cells. As a result the newly forming epithelial cells in the crypts of Lieberkühn die before they can migrate to the surface of the villi to replace worn-out cells. This causes the villi to eventually atrophy, thus greatly reducing the absorptive surface of the small intestine and affecting various absorptive processes.

The immunologic theory holds that gliadin acts as an antigen, which evokes an injurious response from the mucosal cells. The resulting peptidase deficiency is a consequence of the antigenic response, rather than the primary defect.

In the early stages of celiac disease fat absorption is primarily affected, resulting in elimination of large quantities of digested fat (soaps and fatty acids) in the stool. The frothy appearance, foul odor, and excessive quantity of stool are the result of altered bacterial flora on the digested, but unabsorbed, fats and proteins. At this time the disease is sometimes called *idiopathic steatorrhea,* which is a general term to describe fat in the stools resulting from unknown causes. However, as the pathologic processes in the villi continue, the absorption of protein, carbohydrates, calcium, iron, folic acid, and vitamins D, K, and B_{12} is greatly impaired and contributes to the typical clinical picture seen in the child (Fig. 34-1).

Severe malnutrition is a result of fecal loss of fat, protein, and carbohydrates and the concurrent anorexia. Generally weight is compromised more than height, although bone growth is also arrested. Muscle wasting is especially severe in the extremities and buttocks, which appear thin, flabby, and wrinkled. The abdomen becomes progressively more distended as a result of a weakened musculature, accumulation of intestinal secretions and gas, altered peristaltic activity, and fluid from altered osmotic pressure resulting from protein loss. Constipation and fecal impaction rather than diarrhea may be present because of decreased peristalsis. Peripheral edema, usually confined to the lower extremities, is also a result of hypoproteinemia.

Anemia is caused by low serum iron and inadequate supplies of vitamin B_{12} and folic acid. *Disturbed blood coagulation* occurs because of inadequate vitamin K and may result in epistaxis, ecchymosis, or intestinal hemorrhage. Low levels of vitamin D impair calcium absorption and result in demineralization of bone *(osteoporosis)* and softening of the bone *(osteomalacia)*. Because bone growth is arrested, actual rickets is not commonly seen.

Clinical manifestations. Symptoms of celiac disease do not begin until the child is ingesting grains (the chief source

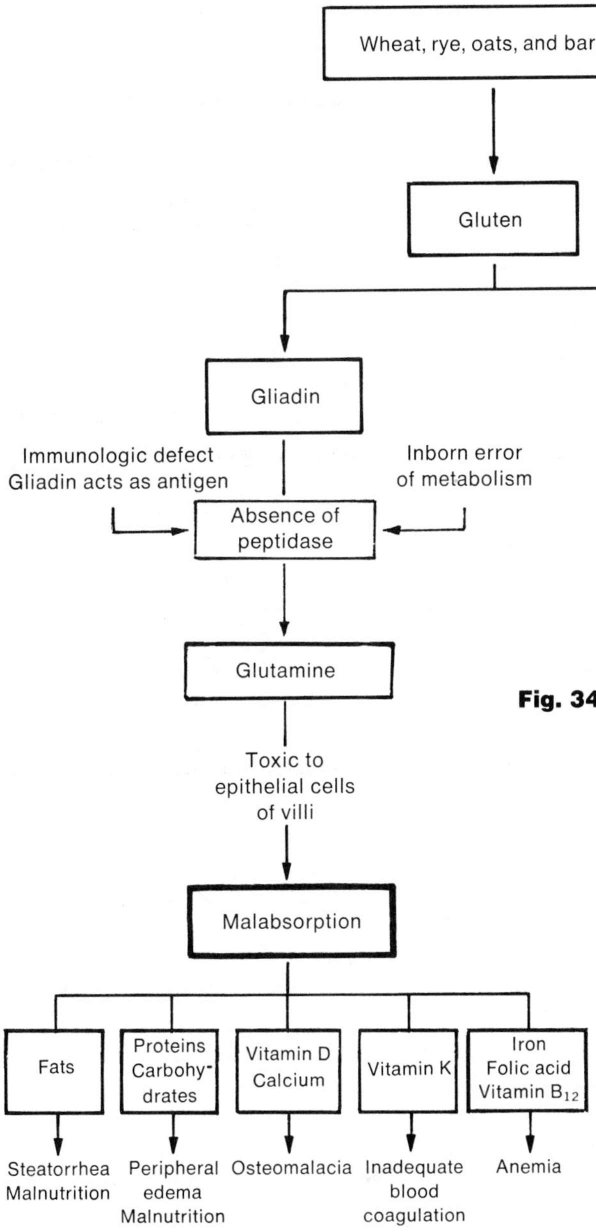

Fig. 34-1. Malabsorptive defect in celiac disease.

of gluten), usually at the addition of cereal during the first year of life. The clinical manifestations are usually insidious and chronic. The first evidence of the disease may be failure to regain weight or appetite after a bout of diarrhea. Behavioral changes, such as irritability, fretfulness, uncooperativeness, or apathy, are common. As the disease progresses, signs of general wasting become evident.

Although steatorrhea is a common symptom, it is absent in 10% to 20% of children. Constipation, vomiting, and abdominal pain may also be initial presenting signs.

Although celiac disease is usually of insidious onset, it may be characterized by acute, severe episodes of profuse watery diarrhea and vomiting, called *celiac crisis*. Such episodes may be precipitated by infections, especially of the gastrointestinal tract, prolonged fasting, dietary sources of gluten, or anticholinergic drugs, such as the preanesthetic agents atropine or scopolamine.

Diagnostic evaluation. Several tests are available for establishing the diagnosis of celiac disease, many of which are based on the expected pathologic findings, such as stool analysis for fecal fat excretion; hematologic studies for hypoproteinemia, anemia, hypoprothrombinemia, serum iron, folic acid, and vitamin B_{12} levels; immunoglobulin levels; x-ray studies for bone age, evidence of osteoporosis and osteomalacia; and bowel studies for dilated, flaccid bowel loops and thickening of the mucosal folds. Pancreatic function studies and a sweat test are usually included in the general laboratory evaluation to rule out the possibility of cystic fibrosis.

However, definitive diagnosis is based on a peroral jejunal biopsy, which demonstrates the atrophic changes in the architecture of the mucosal wall. This procedure is performed by passing a polyethylene tube through the mouth along the alimentary tract to the jejunum of the small bowel. The child is given nothing by mouth for 4 to 8 hours prior to the procedure and is not sedated, because the passage of the tube is slowed as a result of preanesthetic drugs. Older children need preparation for this test in order to enhance their cooperation. Younger children can be prevented from biting the tube by passing it through a rigid plastic tube held between their teeth. In infants the tube can be threaded through a pacifier.

Although bleeding after biopsy is rare, prothrombin time, platelet count, and bleeding time should be evaluated prior to the procedure and vitamin K administered prophylactically. Since hemorrhage and perforation are potential complications, the nurse should observe for signs of shock after the test.

The other essential criterion of diagnosis is dramatic clinical improvement after adherence to a gluten-restricted diet. Within a day or two after instituting the diet, most children with celiac disease demonstrate a favorable personality change. Weight gain, improved appetite, and disappearance of diarrhea and steatorrhea usually do not show improvement for several days or weeks. Since the behavioral changes are commonly seen while the child is hospitalized, but the other signs become evident after discharge, failure to see these expected physical changes is a clue to poor adherence to the diet.

Medical management. Treatment of chronic celiac disease is primarily dietary management. Although the diet is called "gluten free" it is actually low in gluten, because it is impossible to remove every source of this protein. Also, studies demonstrate that most patients are able to tolerate restricted amounts of gluten. Since gluten is found primarily in the grains of wheat and rye, but also in smaller quantities in barley and oats, these four foods are eliminated. Corn and rice become substitute grain foods.

In those children with severe malnutrition, specific deficiencies may be treated with supplemental vitamins, iron, and calories. At times peripheral parenteral alimentation with glucose, amino acids, and fatty acids may be required. Because absorption of fat-soluble vitamins is impaired, these are supplied in a water-miscible form.

Since a celiac crisis is a life-threatening event, prompt medical intervention to correct the dehydration and metabolic acidosis is essential. Usually treatment involves use of a nasogastric tube attached to intermittent suction to decrease abdominal distention; intravenous fluids with supplements of potassium, calcium, and magnesium where indicated; albumin infusions to prevent shock if hypoproteinemia is severe; and intravenous steroids to decrease the inflammation of the bowel. The prompt improvement in response to steroids is believed to support the immunologic theory that gluten acts as an antigen to the mucosal cells.

Nursing considerations. The main nursing consideration is helping the parents and child adhere to diet therapy. This involves considerable time in explaining the disease process to the parents, the specific role of gluten in aggravating the pathology, and those foods that must be restricted. Although the chief source of grain is cereal and baked goods, grains are frequently added to processed foods as thickeners or fillers. To add to the difficulty, gluten is added to many foods but obscurely listed on the label as "hydrolyzed vegetable protein." The nurse must advise parents of the necessity of reading all label ingredients carefully in order to avoid hidden sources of gluten.

Although at first it may appear that eliminating wheat, rye, barley, and oats is a relatively simple matter, one must consider some of the foods aside from cereal in which these ingredients are used, such as bread, cake, cookies, crackers, doughnuts, pies, spaghetti, pizza, prepared soups, some processed ice cream, many types of chocolate candy, milk preparations such as malts, hot dogs, luncheon meats, meat gravy, some prepared hamburgers, and many soups. Many of these products can be eliminated from the infant's or young child's diet fairly easily, but monitoring the diet of a school-age child or adolescent is a much more difficult

Summary of nursing care of the child with celiac disease

Goals	Responsibilities
Prevent celiac crisis	Teach parents specifics of dietary control, especially dangers of prolonged fasting Stress importance of good health in preventing infection and need to avoid known sources of infection Notify other treating physicians of celiac disorder and risk of anticholinergic drugs
Prevent complications from celiac crisis	Monitor intravenous fluids closely Give mouth care during period when nothing is given by mouth Observe child closely for signs of metabolic acidosis (weakness, irritability, decreasing level of consciousness, irregular heartbeat, poor muscular control) Observe child closely for signs of dehydration Monitor nasogastric suctioning and record drainage Observe for signs of shock Administer steroids as ordered; when discontinued by decreasing doses, observe for return of signs suggestive of celiac disease If hyperalimentation is required, observe all precautions to prevent infection (other nursing responsibilities are discussed on p. 1091)
Teach parents dietary control	Explain reason for eliminating gluten from diet Give written list of common food sources of wheat, rye, barley, and oats Emphasize suitable substitutes, especially rice and corn Stress importance of reading labels of prepared food for hidden sources of gluten In addition to gluten-restricted diet, emphasize other dietary principles, such as high calories, high protein, low fat, low residue, and vitamin supplements Make referral to public health nurse for continued dietary counseling after hospital discharge
Help parents and child adjust to life-long adherence to dietary restriction	Allow parents and child opportunity to express discouragement or personal doubt in terms of necessity of diet, especially after symptom-free course Stress positive benefits of diet: remarkable clinical improvement, prevention of crises and complications, such as osteomalacia, delayed growth, anemia, and so on, and decreased risk of gastrointestinal cancer
Promote normal life for child	Help child adjust by focusing on ways he can be normal rather than solely on restrictions that make him feel different Encourage parents to treat child no differently than other siblings; stress need for appropriate limit setting Introduce child to another peer with celiac disease, which may be helpful to all family members Promote positive self-concept; encourage attractive, age-appropriate grooming

situation. Many "favorite" foods, such as hot dogs, pizza, and spaghetti, are chief offenders. Luncheon preparation away from home is particularly difficult, since bread, luncheon meats, and instant soups are not allowed. For families on restricted food budgets, adhering to the diet adds an additional financial burden, since many inexpensive or convenience foods cannot be used.

In addition to restricting gluten, other dietary alterations may also be necessary. For example, in some children who have more severe mucosal damage, the digestion of disaccharides is impaired, especially in relation to lactose. Therefore, these children often need a temporary lactose-free diet, which necessitates eliminating all milk products.

Generally dietary management includes high calories and proteins, low fats, and simple carbohydrates, such as fruits and vegetables. Since the bowel is usually inflamed as a result of the pathologic processes in absorption, coarse, rough foods with high residue, such as nuts, raisins, raw vegetables, and raw fruits with skin, are avoided. Such restrictions further narrow the list of available foods.

Another deterrent to dietary adherence is the recommendation that the child continue it indefinitely. This is especially difficult for parents and children to understand when there have been no symptoms of the disease for an extended period of time and occasional dietary indiscretions probably resulting from increased tolerance to glutens have not caused untoward effects. However, evidence demonstrates that the majority of individuals who relax their diet will eventually have a relapse of their disease and possibly exhibit growth retardation, anemia, or osteomalacia. In addition there is evidence that terminating the diet predisposes affected adults to the risk of developing malignant lymphoma of the small intestine, esophageal cancer, and other gastrointestinal cancers.[2]

When parents and older children are being counseled in regard to the necessity of a lifelong gluten-restricted diet, it is important to stress these long-range complications, as well as reminding parents of the child's physical status prior to dietary treatment and his dramatic improvement after it was begun. For the child, however, these arguments may not be as convincing because the future is less significant than the present, and the past has little meaning. The nurse can be instrumental in allowing the child to express these feelings, while focusing on ways in which the child can still be "normal" like his friends. For example, the usual prepared foods, such as hot dogs and hamburgers, may be restricted, but tacos and other Mexican dishes made with corn tortillas are acceptable. Many children complain that their diet is boring because the parent prepares the same food all the time. One way of dealing with this is encouraging the child to find new recipes using suitable ingredients. With the present emphasis on natural health foods, the nurse can encourage the child to investigate new foods, such as sesame seeds, rice flour, and so on, to enhance their choices, while still being in vogue with peer interests. In some children permanent growth retardation is another emotional crisis.

Since celiac crises can be life-threatening events, the nurse also counsels parents regarding those factors that precipitate a crisis. The need for dietary control has already been discussed. However, the nurse also emphasizes the importance of maintaining good health in order to prevent infections. Whereas avoiding known sources of infection, such as other children who are ill, is certainly sound advice, the nurse also stresses the dangers of excessive overprotection. Since anticholinergic drugs can precipitate a crisis, the nurse advises the parents to inform any other treating physician of the celiac disorder. For example, orthodontic care requiring preanesthetic sedation can be a greater risk to these children, even when the celiac condition is well controlled.

The importance of consistent long-term follow-up care of parents and children with celiac disease cannot be overemphasized. Each phase of child development brings various types of problems related to dietary management and prevention of crises. The nurse is in an optimal position to provide continuous counseling, support, and encouragement to parents and children regarding adjustment to a lifelong disorder. (For a summary of nursing care of the child with celiac disease, see the boxed material on p. 1269.)

OBSTRUCTIVE DISORDERS

Signs and symptoms of intestinal obstruction

Failure of intestinal contents to pass through the bowel is usually the result of *mechanical obstruction,* such as intussusception or pyloric stenosis (see p. 1108), or *inadequate activity* of intestinal muscles, such as Hirschsprung's disease (congenital megacolon). Intestinal obstruction from any cause is characterized by similar signs and symptoms, although the progression may vary greatly. For example, in acute conditions, such as intussusception, the clinical manifestations are apparent within a few hours of the onset of the disorder. In other conditions, such as Hirschsprung's disease, the signs and symptoms may be generally more gradual and may be missed during early stages of the disorder.

One of the nurse's responsibilities is to recognize signs and symptoms of intestinal obstruction. Classically acute mechanical intestinal obstruction is seen by colicky abdominal pain, nausea and vomiting, abdominal distention, and constipation. *Abdominal distention* is the result of accumulation of gas and fluid above the level of the obstruction. The gases are primarily from swallowed air, bacterial action, and diffusion of gases from the bloodstream into the gastrointestinal tract. The fluid is mainly digestive secretions from the stomach and small intestine, fluid and electrolytes from the lumen of the small intestine, and protein from the bloodstream. As these secretions continue to accumulate, the gut becomes excessively irritated and stimulates the vomiting center in the medulla to rid itself of the irritants.

Nausea often precedes vomiting as a conscious recognition that a part of medulla has been stimulated. *Vomiting* is often the earliest sign of a high obstruction and a later sign in lower obstructions. Conversely *constipation* and *obstipation* are early signs of low obstructions and later signs of higher obstructions. For example, a child with a high obstriction can have normal stools for a couple of days as the bowel evacuates itself distal to the defect.

If the obstruction is below the stomach, reflux from the small intestine causes intestinal secretions to flow back into the stomach, where they are vomited along with stomach contents. As this progresses, large quantities of fluid and electrolytes are lost, causing *dehydration*. Electrolyte imbalances can occur as a result of vomiting but are dependent on the location of the obstruction. For example, obstruction at the junction of the stomach and intestines, such as in pyloric stenosis, results in a loss of the highly acidic secretions of the stomach and, therefore, *metabolic alkalosis*. Obstruction high in the small intestines usually does not result in electrolyte imbalance because the highly acidic stomach secretions are neutralized by the alkaline pancreatic, biliary, and intestinal secretions. However, an obstruction near the lower end of the small intestine, such as in intussusception, permits greater amounts of basic than acidic secretions to be loss and thus causes *metabolic acidosis*.

As distention progresses, the abdomen may be rigid and boardlike, with moderate to severe *tenderness*. *Bowel sounds* gradually diminish and cease. In early obstruction high-pitched tinkling sounds are heard best in the dilated loops of the intestine, proximal to the obstruction. In later obstruction the sounds are usually of shorter duration and less intensity, alternating with periods of silence. However, to distinguish these changes, it is necessary to listen for bowel sounds for several minutes. *Respiratory distress* occurs as the diaphragm is pushed up into the pleural cavity. As proteins are lost from the bloodstream into the intestinal lumen, the plasma volume diminishes and *shock* may occur.

Intussusception

Intussusception is one of the most frequent causes of intestinal obstruction during infancy. Half of the cases occur in children younger than age 1 year, more commonly between 3 and 12 months of age, and most of the others occur in children during the second year. Intussusception is three times more common in males than females. Although specific intestinal lesions can be found in a small percentage of the children, generally the cause is not known. The occurrence of intussusception is increased in children with cystic fibrosis and celiac disease.

Pathology. Intussusception is an invagination or telescoping of one portion of the intestine into another. The most common site is the ileocecal valve, in which the ileum invaginates into the cecum and then further into the colon (Fig. 34-2). This type of intussusception is termed *ileocolic*. Other forms include ileoileal (one part of the ileum invaginates into another section of the ileum) and colocolic (one part of the colon telescopes into another area of the colon). The apex of the invagination is usually at the hepatic or splenic flexure or at some point along the transverse colon.

As a result of the invagination, there is an obstruction to

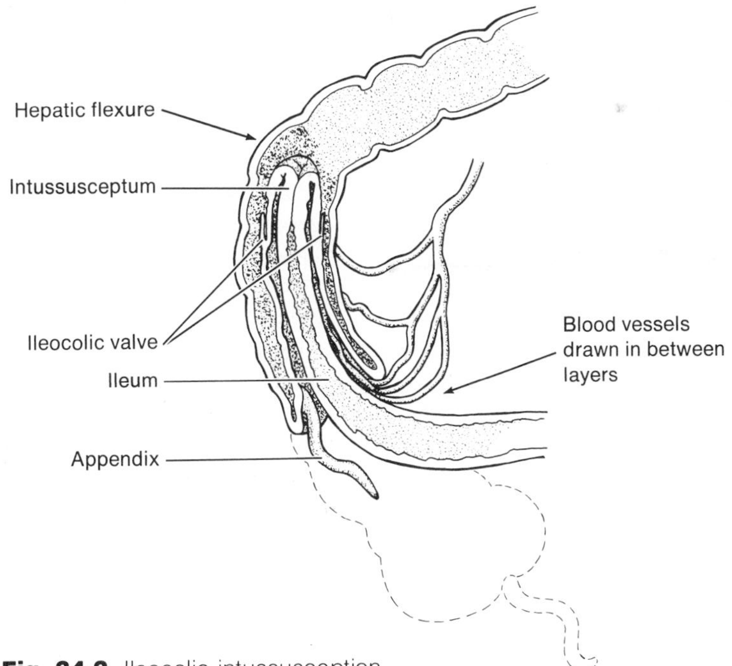

Fig. 34-2. Ileocolic intussusception.

the passage of intestinal contents beyond the defect. In addition the two walls of the intestine press against each other, causing inflammation, edema, and eventually decreased blood flow. As incarceration continues, necrosis results with hemorrhage, perforation, and peritonitis. If untreated this condition is incompatible with life.

Clinical manifestations. The classical presentation of intussusception is a healthy, thriving child, usually between 3 and 12 months of age, who suddenly has an episode of acute abdominal pain. His behavior typically includes screaming and drawing his knees up to his chest. These episodes of severe pain are characterized by intervals in which the child appears normal and comfortable.

During this initial period vomiting usually occurs and the child passes one normal brown stool. However, as the condition worsens, the vomiting increases, the child becomes apathetic, and subsequent stools are red, currant jelly like from the passage of stool mixed with blood and mucus.

The abdomen becomes tender and distended. A sausage-shaped mass may be felt in the upper right quadrant. In contrast the lower right quadrant usually feels empty (Dance's sign) as the bowel distal to the obstruction is less involved and free of contents. If treatment is not sought, the child becomes acutely ill with fever, prostration, and signs of peritonitis (see p. 1279).

Although the classical signs and symptoms of intussusception are intermittent abdominal pain, vomiting, and currant-jelly stools, a more chronic picture may occur, characterized by diarrhea, constipation, occasional vomiting, and periodic colic. Since this condition is potentially life threatening, it is well for the nurse to recognize such signs and closely observe and refer these children for further medical investigation.

Diagnostic evaluation. Frequently the diagnosis can be made on subjective findings alone. However, definitive diagnosis is based on a *barium enema,* which clearly demonstrates the obstruction to the flow of barium. A rectal examination reveals mucus, blood, and occasionally, a low intussusception itself.

Medical and/or surgical management. In most cases the initial treatment of choice is nonsurgical hydrostatic reduction by barium enema. Usually correction of the invagination is carried out at the same time as the diagnostive testing. The principle behind this procedure is that the force exerted by the flowing barium will be sufficient to push the invaginated portion of the bowel into its original position.

Since this procedure is not always successful (about 75% in uncomplicated cases) and is not recommended if there are clinical signs of shock or perforation, the child is also prepared for surgery prior to the barium enema. Surgical intervention involves manually reducing the invagination and, where indicated, resecting any nonviable intestine.

Nursing considerations. Because of the sudden onset of this condition in an otherwise healthy infant, parents are generally totally unprepared for its seriousness and the immediacy of hospitalization and possible surgery. If medical help was not sought early, parents frequently feel guilt and self-reproach for having delayed treatment. In situations in which the presenting clinical manifestations were less definitive and resulted in the physician's decision to delay treatment, parents often feel anger toward the medical personnel. All of these emotions tend to complicate the parents' reactions and adjustments to what may seem to others a benign, correctable disorder.

The nurse can assist in establishing a diagnosis by carefully listening to the parents' history of the child's physical and behavioral symptoms relating to the complaint. Although parents may not know the medical problem, they are astute diagnosticians in detecting that something is wrong. The description of the child's severe colicky abdominal pain combined with vomiting is a significant clue to intussusception. It is not unusual for parents to express that they felt something was seriously wrong with their child before the physician shared their concerns.

As soon as a possible diagnosis of intussusception is made, the nurse begins to prepare the parents for the immediate need for hospitalization, the usual nonsurgical technique of barium enema, and the possibility of surgery. It is important at this time to explain the basic defect of intussusception, which can be easily demonstrated by pushing the end of a finger on a rubber glove back into itself or using the example of a telescoping rod. The principle of reduction by hydrostatic pressure can be simulated by filling the glove with water, which pushes the "finger" into a fully extended position. By using such demonstrations, the parents are aware of why surgery is sometimes necessary. Without this preparation, they may be left with the feeling that the physician "failed" or that their child had "complications."

Since this hospitalization may be the child's first separation from his parents, it is especially important to preserve the parent-child relationship by encouraging rooming-in or extended visiting. It may also be the parents' first experience with hospital care for their child, necessitating their preparation for procedures such as intravenous therapy, frequent vital signs and blood pressure, dressings, and special orders, such as nothing by mouth. Because of the rapidity of the onset, diagnosis, and treatment, parents may be left with the feeling of stunned numbness. They may ask few questions or they may constantly make inquiries, sometimes the same ones several times. If the nurse realizes the circumstances surrounding this condition, the parents' reactions are more likely to be understood and accepted.

Physical care of the child with intussusception differs little from that for any child undergoing abdominal surgery. Even though nonsurgical intervention may be successful, usual preoperative procedures, such as withholding fluids, routine laboratory testing (complete blood count and urinalysis), signed parental consent, and preanesthetic sedation, are done. For the child with signs of electrolyte imbalance, hemorrhage, or peritonitis, additional medical preparation such as replacement fluids, whole blood or plasma, and nasogastric suctioning may be performed. Prior to surgery the nurse monitors all stools. Passage of a normal brown stool usually indicates that the intussusception has reduced itself. This is immediately reported to the physician, who may choose to alter his diagnostic/therapeutic plan of care.

Postprocedural care includes the usual postoperative observations, such as vital signs, blood pressure, intact sutures and dressing, and the return of bowel sounds. In the case of hydrostatic or autoreduction, the nurse observes for passage of barium and the stool patterns, since recurrences of the intussusception are most likely to occur within the first 36 hours after reduction. For this reason the child is kept in the hospital for 2 to 3 days. Overall recurrence of intussusception after nonsurgical or operative reduction is between 4% and 10%.

Hirschsprung's disease (congenital [aganglionic] megacolon)

Hirschsprung's disease is a mechanical obstruction caused by inadequate motility in part of the intestine. It accounts for about one fourth of all cases of neonatal obstruction, although it may not be diagnosed until later in infancy or childhood. It is four times more common in males than females, follows a familial pattern in a small number of cases, and is considerably more common in children with Down's syndrome. Depending on its presentation, it may be an acute, life-threatening condition or a chronic disorder.

Pathology. The term "congenital (aganglionic) megacolon" describes the pathology. The primary defect is absence of autonomic parasympathetic ganglion cells of the submucosal (Meissner's) and myenteric (Auerbach's) plexuses, hence the term "aganglionic," or absence of ganglia. Studies show that the defect is probably the result of defective migration of parasympathetic ganglion cell precursors during embryonic development, therefore, the term "congenital," or present at birth. The functional defect as a result of lack of innervation is absence of propulsive movements (peristalsis), causing accumulation of intestinal contents and distention of the bowel proximal to the defect, hence the term "megacolon," or large colon. In addition there is failure of the internal rectal sphincter to relax, which adds to the clinical manifestations, because it prevents evacuation of solids, liquids, and gas.

The length of aganglionic bowel varies greatly, from only involving the internal sphincter to the entire colon. The latter condition is rare and significantly influences prognosis and mortality. The most common site is the rectosigmoid colon (Fig. 34-3).

Clinical manifestations. Clinical manifestations vary according to the age when symptoms are recognized and the occurrence of complications, such as enterocolitis. In the newborn the chief signs and symptoms are failure to pass meconium within 24 to 48 hours after birth, reluctance to ingest fluids, bile-stained vomitus, and abdominal distention. If the disorder is allowed to progress, other signs of intestinal obstruction, such as respiratory distress and shock, develop.

During infancy the child does not thrive and has constipation, abdominal distention, and episodes of diarrhea and vomiting. The occurrence of explosive, watery diarrhea, fever, and severe prostration is an ominous sign because it often signifies the presence of enterocolitis, which greatly increases the risk of fatality. Enterocolitis

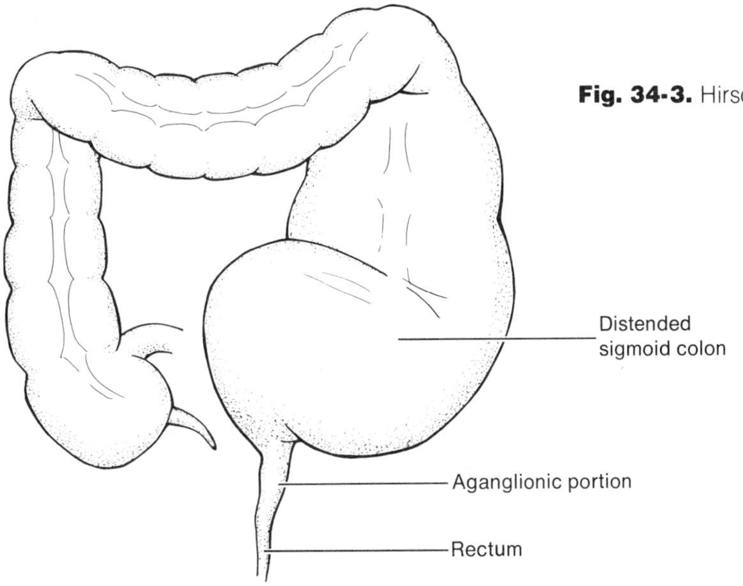

Fig. 34-3. Hirschsprung's disease.

may also be present without diarrhea and is first evidenced with unexplained fever and poor feeding.

During childhood the symptoms are more chronic and include constipation, passage of ribbonlike, foul-smelling stools, abdominal distention, and visible peristalsis. Fecal masses are easily palpable. The child is usually poorly nourished, anemic, and hypoproteinemic from malabsorption of nutrients.

Diagnostic evaluation. In the neonate diagnosis is usually made based on clinical signs of intestinal obstruction and failure to pass meconium. In infants and children the history is an important part of diagnosis and typically details a chronic pattern of constipation. On rectal examination the rectum is empty of feces, the internal sphincter is tight, and there is leakage of liquid, offensive, pale stool and accumulated gas.

Definitive diagnosis is usually based on radiographic studies using a *barium enema,* which demonstrates the transition zone between the dilated proximal colon (megacolon) and the aganglionic distal segment.

However, this typical megacolon and narrow distal segment may not develop until 3 to 4 weeks or even months after birth in some children. In these situations *rectal biopsy* is usually performed and diagnosis is confirmed by histologic evidence of aganglionic cells.

Another procedure that is noninvasive and presents fewer risks to neonates or premature infants than rectal biopsy is *anorectal manometry.* In this test a cylinder with three ballons attached to it is inserted partway into the rectum. Two of the balloons are positioned at the internal sphincter and the third at the external sphincter. The test records the reflex response of the sphincters to distention of the balloons. A normal response is relaxation of the internal sphincter followed by contraction of the external sphincter. In Hirschsprung's disease the external sphincter contracts normally but the internal sphincter fails to relax or contract.

Medical/surgical management. Treatment may be symptomatic in a child with chronic, but not severe, symptoms of megacolon and consists of enemas, stool softeners, and low-residue diet. Only isotonic enemas should be used, since continued use of tap water causes water intoxication, and concentrated salt or phosphate enemas can cause hypertonic dehydration and shock. Low-residue diets decrease the bulk of the stool and cause it to be less irritating to the bowel.

Corrective therapy is surgical intervention to remove the aganglionic bowel and improve functioning of the internal sphincter. In most cases a temporary colostomy of the sigmoid or transverse colon is performed to allow the normal bowel a period of time to rest in order to resume its normal caliber and tonicity.

Two types of temporary colostomies may be performed, the loop or the double-barrel. In the *loop* type an intact segment of bowel is brought through an abdominal incision and sutured onto the abdominal wall. The loop is held above the abdomen by a glass rod placed beneath it. The two ends of the rod are connected by a section of rubber or silicon elastic tubing to prevent it from slipping from the loop. The loop colostomy is opened on the exterior surface (Fig. 34-4).

In the *double-barrel* type the bowel is completely di-

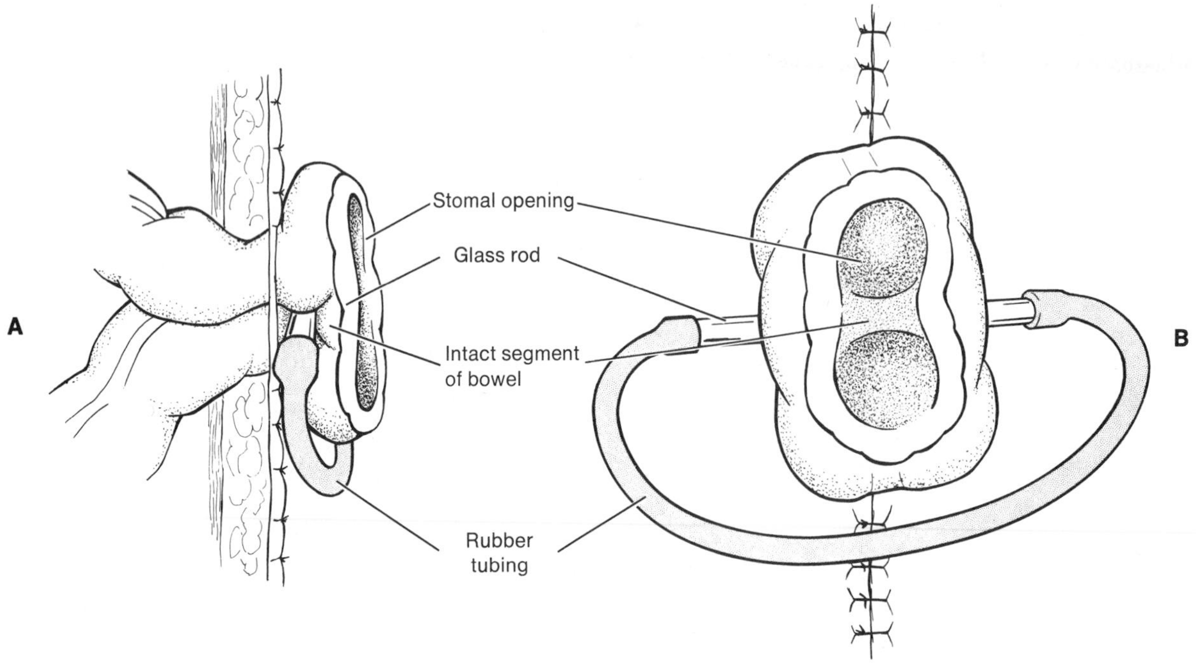

Fig. 34-4. Loop colostomy. **A,** Cross sectional view; **B,** anterior view.

vided and two separate stomas or openings are formed. The proximal stoma (usually positioned higher in the abdomen) drains fecal matter, and the distal stoma (usually positioned below the proximal opening) functions as a fistula for accumulated mucus.

Complete correction with a pull-through anastomosis of the bowel may be done at the time of performing the colostomy or later, especially in those infants or children with preoperative complications. The type of surgical procedure for reanastomosis involves ''pulling'' the end of the intact bowel down to a point usually near the rectum. The most common surgical techniques are Swenson's, the Soave, and the Duhamel operations. In many cases a sphincterotomy of the internal sphincter is done to improve anal control. Closure of the colostomy depends on the physician's evaluation of the child's postoperative progress but is usually performed within a few months to a year. The prognosis after complete surgical repair depends on the child's ability to adjust to a normal diet and to learn bowel control.

Nursing considerations. Many of the nursing concerns depend on the child's age. If the disorder is diagnosed during the neonatal period, the main objectives are helping the parents adjust to a congenital defect in their child, fostering infant-parent bonding, preparing them for the medical/surgical intervention, and assisting them in colostomy care after discharge.

When the disorder is not discovered during this period, the nurse can facilitate establishing a diagnosis by carefully listening to the parents' history, with special emphasis on bowel habits. In Hirschsprung's disease several areas must be investigated: (1) onset of constipation, especially if present since birth, (2) character of stools, particularly ribbonlike and foul smelling, and (3) frequency of bowel movements. Other clues in the history and physical examination include poor feeding habits, fussiness and irritability, a distended abdomen, and signs of undernutrition, such as thin extremities, pallor, muscle weakness, and fatigue.

Preoperative care. Much of the child's preoperative care depends on his age and clinical condition. If the child is malnourished, he may not be able to withstand surgery until his physical status improves. Often this involves symptomatic treatment with enemas, a low-residue, high-calorie and high-protein diet, and, in severe situations, the use of parenteral alimentation.

If the regimen of enemas, stool softeners, and low-residue diet is used, parents need detailed explanation regarding each procedure. The nurse demonstrates proper administration of an isotonic enema and has the parent perform at least one return demonstration. It is important to stress the dangers of using tap water, concentrated salt solutions, soap solutions, or phosphate preparations. Normal saline solution can be purchased without a prescription from a pharmacy. Inexpensive pure sodium chloride tablets are also available. Each 1-g tablet is diluted in 110 ml (almost 4 ounces) of water. An approximate saline solution can be prepared at home by adding 1 level measuring tsp of noniodized salt to 1 pint of tap water. Since the instructions for preparing the solution and administering the enema require several steps, all the directions should be written down as well as verbally explained. Suggested amounts of solution according to the child's age are detailed on p. 947.

Explanation of the low-residue diet includes the reason for its use and a list of foods to avoid (Table 34-1). Since eating difficulties are characteristic of children with Hirschsprung's disease, a dietary history regarding general food habits is essential before planning to alter the diet. In this way favorite low-residue food selections, such as spaghetti, lean broiled hamburger on white bread, broiled chicken, vanilla or chocolate ice cream, crackers, plain cookies, and gelatin desserts, can be stressed as foods to continue serving. Also, specific dietary habits are identified that may influence not only food selection but food preparation as well. For example, the elimination of spices, such as pepper, chili, curry powder, and cayenne pepper, will be especially difficult for children of Mexican or Eastern

Table 34-1. High-residue foods

Food group	Selections
Bread, grains	Whole-grain bread or rolls Whole-grain cereals Most prepared cereals, except cornflakes, Rice Krispies, puffed wheat or rice, and some cooked cereals Pancakes and waffles Muffins with fruit or bran
Dairy products	Highly flavored cheeses Ice cream or yogurt with fruits or nuts Fried eggs
Meats	Fatty or tough meats such as pork Fried or highly spiced meat, rich meat gravy Raw or whole cooked vegetables, except vegetables such as beets, spinach, peas, or squash that must be cooked and strained Fried vegetables such as French fries or potato chips Unrefined (brown) rice
Fruits	Raw fruits, especially those with skins or seeds, other than ripe banana or avocado Raisins, prunes, or other dried fruits Jams, preserves, or marmalade
Miscellaneous	Nuts, spices, highly spiced condiments, vinegar, olives, popcorn

Indian background, where such spices are a staple of food preparation.

Physical preoperative preparation entails the same measures that are common to any surgery (see p. 910). In the newborn, whose bowel is sterile, no additional preparation is necessary. However, in other children emptying the bowel with repeated saline enemas and decreasing bacterial flora with systemic antibiotics and colonic irrigations using antibiotic solution are usually ordered. A nasogastric tube is inserted to prevent abdominal distention, and antibiotic solution may be instilled through the tube to further prepare the gastrointestinal tract. The nurse records all intake and output of irrigant and drainage, particularly noting marked discrepancy in retention or loss of fluid. A rectal tube may also be inserted to allow for escape of accumulated fluid and gas. Because of the rectal tube and to prevent damage to the mucosa, only axillary temperatures are taken.

In children with enterocolitis, emergency preoperative care includes frequent monitoring of vital signs and blood pressure for signs of shock, monitoring fluid replacement with electrolytes, plasma, or other blood derivatives, and observing for symptoms of bowel perforation, such as increasing abdominal distention, vomiting, increased tenderness, irritability, dyspnea, and cyanosis.

Since progressive distention of the abdomen is a serious sign, the nurse measures abdominal circumference by placing a paper tape measure around the largest diameter, usually at the level of the umbilicus. The point of measurement is marked with a pen to assure reliability. In order to lessen any stress to the acutely ill child, the tape measure should be left under the child, rather than removed each time. As a rule of thumb, abdominal measurement can be performed at the same time that vital signs are taken. It is best to record the measurement in serial order so that a change will be readily apparent.

The age of the child dictates the type and extent of psychologic preparation. Since a colostomy is usually performed, the child of at least preschool age is told about the procedure in concrete terms. For example, this can be illustrated by drawing a picture of a child with a stoma on the abdomen and explaining it as ''another opening where bowel movements [or any other term the child uses] will come out. At another time the nurse can draw a bag over the opening to demonstrate how the contents are collected.

Whenever possible, the stoma can also be illustrated by drawing or cutting a small hole on a plastic doll and applying a bag over it. A urine-collecting bag works very well as an example of a colostomy appliance (Fig. 34-5). Since an abdominal dressing is present immediately after

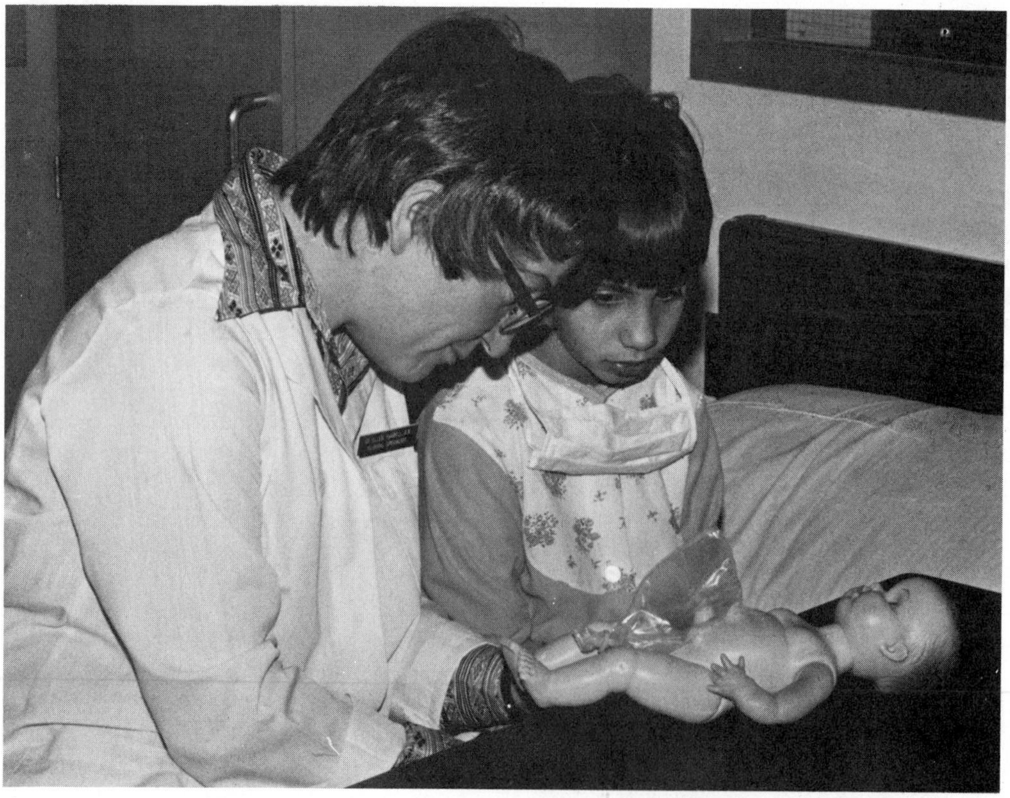

Fig. 34-5. Preparing child for colostomy. Note use of urine-collecting bag as part of colostomy equipment.

surgery, the child should be made aware of this fact. Dressings or "bandages" are especially important to preschoolers, who see them as a form of preserving body integrity. However, it is important to space explanations to prevent anxiety and confusion from too much information.

Parents also need preparation prior to surgery. Since a colostomy represents a change in body function and appearance, the nurse should investigate parents' previous knowledge of this procedure. It is not uncommon for parents to have previous knowledge of a colostomy. For example, one mother related that a friend's father had a permanent colostomy because of cancer. As soon as the mother heard that her child needed this procedure, she was convinced that the mass in her child's abdomen was a cancerous tumor.

It is best not to assume that parents understand a verbal explanation of a colostomy. Drawing a picture or using the doll as described on p. 1276 is excellent for parents as well as children. During this teaching session, the nurse should briefly include basic methods of care. For example, if a sigmoid colostomy is to be performed on an infant, a colostomy appliance is usually not used because the stools are formed and less likely to irritate the skin. Usually only diapers and a nonporous ointment such as zinc oxide around the stoma are used.

It is important to stress to parents and older children that the colostomy for Hirschsprung's disease is temporary, unless so much bowel is involved that a permanent ileostomy must be performed. In most instances the physician is fairly certain of the extent of bowel resection prior to surgery, although the nurse should be aware of those instances when doubt concerning repair exists. The nurse should also keep in mind that, although a temporary colostomy is favorable in terms of future health and adjustment, it also necessitates additional surgery, which may be very stressful to parents and children.

Since feeding and associated behavioral problems are frequently associated with a chronic pattern of megacolon, the nurse should inform parents that although the defect can be corrected, it will take some time for the child's physical status and feeding practices to improve. Although this should not be stated in such a way as to minimize the benefit of surgery, it is necessary to avoid implying that surgical correction is a panacea to all previous physical and behavioral complaints.

Postoperative care. Physical postoperative care usually includes (1) nothing by mouth until bowel sounds return and the colostomy and/or anastomosed bowel are ready for feedings, (2) intravenous fluid to maintain hydration and replace lost electrolytes, (3) nasogastric suctioning to prevent abdominal distention, (4) frequent abdominal dressing changes, and (5) perineal dressing changes, especially if a pull-through procedure was done. To prevent contamination of the abdominal wound with urine, the diaper should be pinned below the dressing. Sometimes a Foley catheter is used in the immediate postoperative period to divert the flow of urine away from the abdomen.

Drainage from the nasogastric tube and the colostomy is measured, since fluid and electrolyte replacement is partially calculated on these losses. In order to accurately measure colostomy drainage before a collecting appliance is applied, the nurse weighs the dry dressing and reweighs it when wet. The difference in weight is calculated as fluid, because 1 g equals 1 ml. For example, if the dressing weighs 40 g when dry and, after soiling, weighs 63 g, the difference is 23g, or 23 ml of fluid output. If formed stool is passed, it is not weighed and calculated as part of fluid loss.

Because the stoma is edematous after surgery, an appliance is usually not fitted for several days. In the instance of a loop colostomy, an appliance is usually fitted after the sutures and glass rod are removed. Once an appliance is in place, drainage is directly measured from the collecting bag.

During the period when the child is not allowed oral fluids, good mouth care is essential. For the infant, sucking needs can be satisfied with a pacifier. To minimize irritation from the nasogastric tube, the tube should be inserted through alternate nostrils and secured to the nose or upper lip with a minimum of tape. The tube should not be taped first to the nose and then to the forehead, because the resulting pressure on the edge of the nostril can cause tissue necrosis. Dried mucous secretions from the nares may need to be removed. Keeping the nostrils lubricated and increasing environmental humidity prevent excessive irritation to the nares.

For the young child who cannot brush his teeth or rinse out his mouth without swallowing fluid, the nurse can institute oral hygience by wiping the teeth, gums, and tongue with a cloth moistened with dilute mouthwash or hydrogen peroxide. It is best to avoid using toothpaste because the foam is difficult to remove without liberally flushing the mouth, in which case the child may ingest or aspirate fluid. Sometimes physicians allow crushed ice after the child is fully alert from anesthesia. If permitted the crushed ice can be offered on a spoon or frozen ice in the form of a Popsicle can be given. If colored ice is used, the colors red and green are avoided, since they can be confused with blood or bile.

When parents initially visit their child postoperatively, they are frequently unprepared for the numerous tubes and intravenous lines attached to various body parts. Even when all the procedures are explained beforehand, the actual visual shock can be great. The nurse should explain the function of each piece of equipment, stressing safety features that permit the child to be safely moved and handled, such as length of tubing, use of armboards at intravenous sites, and tape to secure the nasogastric tube to the nose.

In this way the nurse encourages and assists parents in holding and stimulating their child. The nurse also points out the benefit of frequent handling postoperatively in preventing pulmonary complications and in stimulating gastrointestinal activity.

The nurse emphasizes the expected changes in the appearance of the stoma, which initially is large, protruding, red, and raw looking. If a loop colostomy was performed, the nurse explains the purpose of the glass rod in preventing retraction of the bowel. Since the stomal site appears painful, it is also important to stress that bowel mucosa is nonsensitive but that the surrounding abdominal skin must be protected. During the early postoperative period, including parents and the older child in dressing changes can enhance teaching of colostomy care when an appliance is fitted and promotion of gradual acceptance of the body change.

Discharge care. Postoperatively parents need instruction concerning colostomy care. Even a preschooler can be included in the care by handing articles to the parent, rolling up the colostomy bag after emptying, or applying cream to the surrounding skin. Since these children may have had difficulties with bowel training before surgery because of constipation and erratic stool patterns, the period during the temporary colostomy can relieve the pressures previously associated with bowel control. Although diagnosis of Hirschsprung's disease is less frequent in school-age children or adolescents, if discovered in older children, they should be involved in colostomy care to the point of total responsibility.

In some institutions an enterostomal therapist is available to provide expert assistance in planning procedures for home care, such as preparation of skin, application of the collecting appliance, care of the appliance, control of odor, and signs of stomal complications, such as ribbon-like stools, excessive diarrhea, bleeding, prolapse, or failure to pass flatus or stool. Whenever possible, this person should be utilized in preparing for colostomy care.

If dietary management was not instituted prior to surgery, the nurse needs to explain the role of low-residue foods in keeping the stool less bulky for easier evacuation. The nurse should also emphasize that if a particular food causes gastrointestinal upset, such as diarrhea or excessive flatus, it should also be avoided. The nurse stresses the need for increased fluids to compensate for fecal fluid loss. Sometimes parents mistakenly limit ingested fluids in an attempt to regulate bowel movements. It is important to emphasize that most of the water is absorbed before it reaches the colostomy but that a substantial amount is still lost and must be replaced. Regulation of stool patterns is largely a function of ingested food, especially residue, and the location of the colostomy in the bowel.

Nutritional counseling of children with Hirschsprung's disease often surpasses the limited scope of dietary management regarding the colostomy. Because of their previous anorexia, discomfort after eating from abdominal distention, and the likelihood of combined pressure from parents to eat, these children frequently have feeding problems. Hospitalization provides an excellent assessment period for the nurse to observe parent-child interaction during mealtime. Once specific problems are discovered, the nurse can initiate steps to reverse the pattern. It is important to remember that relearning must take place, because the behavior has probably been reinforced for a long period of time.

Behavior modification techniques tend to be especially effective in changing eating patterns but require a thorough assessment and identification of reinforcement factors. For example, while observing the interaction of a mother and child during mealtime, the nurse identified that all of the mother's attention focused on the child when he did not eat. As soon as he began to eat, she looked away and ignored him. Once the mother was aware of how her attention reinforced poor eating habits, she was able to change her reactions to avoidance when he did not eat and to praise and attention when he did. Other helpful suggestions include establishing regular frequent mealtimes with small servings, avoiding an argument or any type of parental pressure at mealtime, and serving as many of the child's favorite foods as possible.

Referral to a public health nurse establishes continuity of care, especially in relation to colostomy care and dietary management. The community nurse can also assist parents and children in anticipating subsequent surgery. Sometimes families require financial assistance and additional psychologic support. Therefore, a referral to a social worker or other service agency may be necessary.

See the summary of nursing care of the child requiring abdominal surgery on p. 1282.

INFLAMMATORY CONDITIONS

Appendicitis

Appendicitis, inflammation of the vermiform appendix or blind sac at the end of the cecum, is the most common reason for abdominal surgery during childhood. It is rare in children younger than 2 years of age but is associated with increased complications and mortality in children in this age-group. It is most often an acute condition that, if undiagnosed, rapidly progresses to perforation and peritonitis. It is a significant pediatric problem, because early diagnosis is frequently delayed as a result of the child's inability to verbalize and professionals' failure to correctly interpret behavioral clues.

Pathology. The exact cause of appendicitis is poorly understood. It is believed that factors that favor obstruction and infection predispose the bowel to appendicitis. Dietary habits probably play a role, as decreased fiber and residue in the diet slow transit time and result in firmer stools that remain in the bowel longer, thus favoring the development of a fecal obstruction and the growth of bacteria. Fecaliths (hard masses of feces), parasitic infestation, and lymphoid hyperplasia are also contributing factors.

Other physiologic processes peculiar to the infant and young child also influence the pathology of appendicitis. The omentum, which is not fully developed in children in this age-group, is less efficient in walling off the inflammation, sealing perforated viscera, and confining an intraperitoneal disease process. The close proximity of all abdominal and pelvic organs favors the spread of peritonitis to accessory digestive and reproductive organs.

Peritonitis, inflammation of the lining of the peritoneal cavity, generally follows a perforated or ruptured appendix. Since the peritoneum represents a major portion of total body surface, the loss of extracellular fluid to the peritoneal cavity leads to electrolyte imbalance and hypovolemic shock. Progressive peritoneal inflammation results in functional intestinal obstruction of the small bowel, since intense gastrointestinal reflexes severely inhibit bowel motility.

Clinical manifestations. The most common signs and symptoms of appendicitis are abdominal pain, localized abdominal tenderness, and fever. Initially the pain is generalized or periumbilical; however, it usually descends to the lower right quadrant. The most intense site of pain may be at McBurney's point, which is located about 1½ inches above the anterior superior iliac crest along a straight line drawn from this process to the umbilicus. Rebound tenderness (see p. 155), a rigid abdomen, and decreased or absent bowel sounds are important signs of appendicitis.

Vomiting is a common early sign. Although constipation may be present, diarrhea can also occur. Low-grade fever is typically seen early in the disease but can rise sharply once peritonitis has begun. Other signs of peritonitis include sudden relief from pain after perforation, subsequent increase in pain, which is usually diffuse and accompanied by rigid guarding of the abdomen, progressive abdominal distention, tachycardia, rapid shallow breathing as the child refrains from using abdominal muscles, pallor, chills, irritability, and restlessness.

Probably the most significant clinical manifestation is a change in the child's behavior. For the nonverbal child, irritability, a characteristic side-lying position with the knees flexed to the abdomen, and a rigid, motionless posture should alert one to abdominal pain. The older child may exhibit all of these behaviors, while complaining of abdominal pain.

Diagnostic evaluation. Diagnosis is based primarily on history and examination. The chief clues that should alert the practitioner to appendicitis are the progression of abdominal pain, location of abdominal tenderness, decreased peristalsis, pain on rectal examination, and absence of any other symptoms or findings suggesting another disorder, such as pneumonia.

Laboratory evaluation includes a white blood cell count, which is usually elevated but is seldom higher than 15,000 to 20,000/mm^3, and radiographic studies of the abdomen. Although the latter is not always helpful in confirming the diagnosis, it can reveal possible contributing causes of appendicitis, such as fecaliths, or other conditions mimicking this disorder, such as a foreign body.

Surgical management. Treatment of appendicitis is surgical removal of the appendix (appendectomy). For the child with peritonitis, medical management for shock, dehydration, and infection is begun preoperatively. This usually includes intravenous administration of fluid and electrolytes, blood volume replacement with plasma or albumin, systemic antibiotics, oxygen, nasogastric suctioning, and positioning in high-Fowler's position to facilitate drainage into the pelvic area.

Nursing considerations. Because successful treatment of appendicitis is based on prompt recognition of the disorder, a primary nursing objective is assisting in establishing a diagnosis. Even though in many instances nurses may not perform the complete history and examination, they are often in a strategic position to make judgments regarding the child's care. For example, nurses in private physician's offices, ambulatory settings, or emergency units often have the responsibility of counseling parents or triaging patients regarding additional treatment. When the child with a "acute abdomen" (a general term used to describe conditions presenting with acute abdominal pain) is admitted to the pediatric unit, staff nurses usually decide where to place the child, how quickly to arrange for laboratory evaluation, and how much observation and assessment of the child are required and by whom. Even outside the strictly professional relationship, parents may ask nurse friends for advice regarding abdominal pain. Without an appreciation of the signs and symptoms suggestive of appendicitis, these nurses may not make decisions that facilitate rapid diagnosis.

Since abdominal pain is the most common childhood complaint, the nurse needs to make some preliminary evaluation of the severity of pain. One of the most reliable estimates is the degree of change in behavior. A child who stays home from school and voluntarily lies down or refuses to play is much more likely to have considerable pain than the child who is absent from school but plays contentedly at home. In any instance when severe abdominal pain is expected, the nurse must be aware of the danger of administering laxatives, enemas, or applying heat to the area. Such measures stimulate bowel motility and increase the risk of perforation.

For those nurses involved in primary ambulatory care, the responsibility of recognizing a possible instance of appendicitis and prompt medical/surgical referral is particularly great. A detailed history and careful abdominal examination cannot be overstressed. Although the technique for assessment of the abdomen is discussed in Chapter 5, several points justify repetition: (1) inspect the musculature carefully before touching the child, (2) observe the position of most comfort, (3) observe respiratory movements and associated diaphragmatic splinting, (4) encourage the child's trust by palpating nontender areas before attempting to localize pain or elicit rebound tenderness, (5) when palpating possibly painful areas, warn the child beforehand that it may hurt, and (6) use as many distraction techniques as possible when assessing the degree of abdominal rigidity or tenderness.

Preoperative care. Physical preparation of the child with appendicitis is the same as that for any laparotomy (see p. 1282). Any skin preparation, such as shaving the abdomen in an adolescent, must be done very gently because of the area's extreme tenderness. In situations in which medical treatment is required to correct problems associated with peritonitis, the nurse must anticipate expected procedures and set up equipment as quickly as possible to prevent any delay in preparing the child for surgery. This involves having oxygen, nasogastric tubing with a suction machine, syringes, needles, intravenous Solusets, and various electrolyte solutions available for immediate use.

Psychologic preparation of the child and parents is similar to what is employed in other emergency situations (see p. 907). It is important for the nurse to view parents' reactions in light of previous circumstances. For example, parents may react with almost uncontrollable anxiety once they enter the hospital because of fears surrounding "burst appendix" or guilt for having delayed treatment. Once at the hospital they may become outraged that care is not performed quickly enough and continually question personnel regarding the safety of decisions, such as "waiting for blood work" before taking the child to surgery. The emotional contagion of such reactions can greatly influence the child's reaction to expected hospitalization and operative treatment. It is important to take the time to explain to parents and older children why each test is done and the importance of certain preoperative information in assuring the overall safety of surgery.

Postoperative care. Postoperative care for the nonperforated appendix involves the same procedures as for most abdominal operations (see p. 1282). If the appendix was ruptured, Penrose drains are placed in the wound. Positioning in semi-Fowler's position or lying on the right side facilitates drainage from the peritoneal cavity as well as prevents the formation of a subdiaphragmatic abscess. Frequent dressing changes with meticulous skin care are essential to prevent excoriation of the surgical area. Sometimes the abdominal wound is irrigated with antibacterial solution. Parenteral antibiotics are usually infused for 7 to 10 days, and oral preparations may be continued even longer. The course of recovery is considerably longer and may require 2 weeks or more of hospitalization, in contrast to a week or less for an uncomplicated appendectomy.

Parents and older children need an opportunity to express their feelings postoperatively. It is especially important for the nurse to encourage the child to relate all the events he remembers concerning admission and treatment in order to clarify misconceptions. Parents in particular need reassurance that any emotional outbursts during admission are understood and accepted. They should be praised for the right decisions they made regarding the child's care and not be reproached or reprimanded for failing to seek help sooner, except in the rare instance when it represents a continuing pattern of child neglect. However, even in this situation, the anxiety and genuine concern parents feel for their child may be a catalyst for seeking help with intrafamilial problems.

Meckel's diverticulum

Meckel's diverticulum results when the omphalomesenteric or vitelline duct, which connects the midgut to the yolk sac during early embryonic development, fails to completely obliterate. Although several different types of malformations can result, such as cysts, fistulas, or fibrotic cords, Meckel's diverticulum is the most common and consists of an outpouching of the ileum, most commonly in proximity to the ileocecal valve. It may vary in size from a small appendiceal process to a segment of bowel several inches long and wide. At times it may be connected to the umbilicus by a cord.

It is the most common congenital malformation of the gastrointestinal tract and is present in 1% to 2% of the population. It is twice as common in males as in females, and complications are several times more frequent in males. Frequently it exists without causing symptoms. Most symptomatic cases are seen in the first 2 years of life.

Pathology. *Acute diverticulitis* follows the same pathologic process as appendicitis. *Rectal bleeding* is most often the result of ulceration of the mucosa, which in many cases secretes gastric acids. The acid continually irritates the bowel, erodes the surface, and in some instances may lead to perforation.

Mechanical obstruction can occur as a result of volvulus, or twisting of the bowel around the fibrotic Meckel's cord. Intussusception can occur if the diverticulum acts as a lead point for invagination.

Clinical manifestations. Signs and symptoms are based on the specific pathologic process, such as diverticulitis or intestinal obstruction. Rectal bleeding, however, is the chief presenting sign in over half of the cases. Bright red or dark red rectal bleeding is much more common than black tarry stools and represents acute hemorrhage. Usually there is no evidence of abdominal pain. Severe anemia and shock are consequences of the hemorrhage.

Diagnostic evaluation. Diagnosis is usually based on the history. Rectosigmoidoscopy and barium enema are usually performed to eliminate other possible diagnoses, such as anal fissure, polyps, and intussusception. Radiologic studies are frequently not helpful in confirming the diagnosis, because the diverticulum may be too small to be visualized or may fail to fill with barium. Blood studies are usually part of the general laboratory workup to rule out any bleeding disorders and to evaluate the severity of the anemia.

Surgical treatment. Treatment is surgical removal of the diverticulum. In instances in which severe hemorrhage increases the surgical risk, medical intervention to correct hypovolemic shock, such as blood replacement, intravenous fluids, and oxygen, may be necessary. In diverticulitis antibiotics may be used preoperatively to control infection. If intestinal obstruction has occurred, appropriate preoperative measures are used to reverse electrolyte imbalances and prevent abdominal distention.

Nursing considerations

Preoperative and postoperative care. Nursing objectives are similar to those listed in the boxed material on pp. 1282 to 1283. Since the onset is usually rapid, psychologic support parallels that for other conditions, such as appendicitis. It is important to remember that the occurrence of massive rectal bleeding is most often traumatic to both the child and parent and may significantly affect their emotional reaction to hospitalization and surgery.

Specific preoperative considerations when rectal bleeding is present include (1) frequent monitoring of vital signs and blood pressure for shock, (2) keeping the child on bed rest, and (3) recording the approximate amount of blood lost in stools. In the absence of frank rectal hemorrhage, the nurse tests the stools for occult blood.

Ulcerative colitis

Ulcerative colitis is sometimes referred to as "chronic inflammatory bowel disease" but actually is one disease entity under this category. It is characterized by extensive ulceration of the walls of the large intestine. It is basically a disease of young adults, although close to 15% of the cases begin in children younger than 16 years of age. The peak onset in children is between ages 10 and 19 years.

Several genetic and environmental factors influence the incidence of ulcerative colitis: (1) there is a familial tendency in about 5% to 15% of the cases, (2) individuals from higher socioeconomic levels and more whites than nonwhites are affected, (3) the incidence is four times greater in Jewish populations than in the general population; and (4) there is a higher occurrence of allergic disease in relatives of these patients.

Etiology. The exact cause of ulcerative colitis is unknown, although a range of possibilities exists to partially explain the cyclic reaction of inflammation, ulceration, and mucopurulent exudation. One theory holds that *bacterial invasion* produces the inflammatory reaction, although no specific microorganism has been isolated. Another theory supposes that an *immunologic disorder,* specifically an autoimmune reaction, exists.

A controversial etiologic agent is the role of *psychologic factors* in predisposing the individual to the occurrence of the disease process. There have been attempts to stereotype these children as emotionally dependent and immature with mothers who are dominating, overprotecting, and self-centered, but in general such findings are no more peculiar to these families than unaffected ones. Indeed, one must also wonder if the course of the disease has influenced such interactions rather than these behaviors causing the disease. At present the feeling is that ulcerative colitis is an organic disease caused by a combination of physical and emotional factors. Psychologic influences, such as stress, significantly affect the exacerbation and chronicity of the illness.

Clinical manifestations. The major clinical effects of ulcerative colitis are outlined in Fig. 34-6. In addition to these findings, there are generalized nonspecific signs and symptoms of inflammatory disease, such as low-grade fever that peaks in the evening, chills, and elevated white blood cell count. There is also a high incidence of other disorders, such as erythema multiforme, erythema nodosum, aphthous stomatitis, arthralgia or arthritis, chronic active hepatitis, and conjunctivitis.

The clinical course varies markedly in terms of severity, response to therapy, and prognosis. In general the disease follows one of two patterns; acute remitting type or chronic continuous course. The *acute remitting* type is more common and follows a pattern of remissions and exacerbations. During the period of remission, the child is usually well, with few or no symptoms of the disease. However, periods of exacerbation are severe and acute, although they usually respond well to medical treatment. The disease may terminate in a permanent remission or ultimately follow the course of chronic colitis.

In *chronic continuous colitis* there are no definitive periods of severe disease with intermittent good health. Intestinal symptoms tend to be less severe, but chronic malnutrition and anemia are common. Children with this type of colitis often respond poorly to medical therapy and are more likely to suffer from complications, especially carcinoma of the colon.

Children afflicted with either type of colitis have usually been healthy prior to the onset of the disease. Early signs of colitis include (1) frequent passage of loose or watery stools mixed with blood, pus, and mucus or change in bowel habits with constipation rather than diarrhea as the chief symptom, (2) frequent urges to defecate, which are aggravated by ingesting foods but relieved after defecation, (3) tenesmus or the persistent urge to defecate but with little or

Summary of nursing care of the child requiring abdominal surgery

Goals	Responsibilities
Prepare child and parent for expected surgical procedure and postoperative care	Explain reason for surgery; if bowel diversion is to be performed, explain basic principle of ostomy and brief outline of bowel care Explain all preoperative procedures, such as blood work, nasogastric tube, bowel preparation, and any other laboratory test Prepare for postoperative procedures, such as nasogastric tube, intravenous fluids, nothing by mouth, dressing changes, and wound drains if necessary In emergency situation, explain most essential components of surgery, such as where child will be before and after surgery, anesthesia, and dressing on abdomen; accept behavioral reactions of parents and child
Assist in preparing bowel for surgery	Administer colonic enemas as ordered, using only saline antibiotic solution Administer antibiotics as ordered, observing for known side effects (neomycin and kanamycin can cause auditory and renal damage)
Observe for complications Shock	 Monitor vital signs and blood pressure
Intestinal obstruction	Observe for decreased or absent bowel sounds, increasing abdominal distention, vomiting, absence of stools, pain
Perforation and peritonitis	Observe for sudden relief from pain followed by increased diffuse abdominal pain, absence of bowel sounds, tachycardia, pallor, high temperature, abdominal splinting, and rapid, shallow respirations
Prevent and observe for abdominal distention	Give child nothing by mouth Maintain patency of nasogastric tube Check functioning of suction machine Irrigate tube if no drainage is obtained but child vomits around tube Check proper placement of tube (aspirate stomach contents, inject air into tube while listening with stethoscope over stomach, or place free end in water to check for bubbles) Secure tube by taping to nose or upper lip (not forehead) to maintain proper stomach placement Keep child in semi-Fowler's position or as ordered to facilitate drainage of abdominal contents and to promote respiratory expansion Measure abdominal circumference at widest point (mark with pen, usually at umbilicus); record measurements on graph or in sequence to detect changes Check often for bowel sounds
Prevent dehydration	Record all output (urinary, stool, vomiting, or nasogastric) and input (intravenous, oral if allowed, and nasogastric irrigant); notify physician of marked discrepancies Provide environmental humidity (child may be placed in Croupette with humidified room air) Take temperature frequently; notify physician of elevations
Prevent infection	Change dressings (abdominal and/or perineal) whenever soiled; carefully dispose of soiled dressings Pin diapers below abdominal dressing to prevent contamination Maintain respiratory hygiene with coughing, deep breathing, and turning (both preoperatively and postoperatively); suction secretions Use proper hand washing technique, especially if wound drainage is present Place in Fowler's position to prevent subdiaphragmatic abscess formation

Summary of nursing care of the child requiring abdominal surgery—cont'd

Goals	Responsibilities
Prevent skin breakdown	If dressings require frequent changing, use Montgomery straps If ostomy was performed, apply zinc oxide or other ointments as prescribed around stomal area; change dressing often even if not soiled with feces, since intestinal secretions are irritating
Provide comfort measures	Administer mouth care Lubricate nostril to decrease irritation from tube Allow child position of comfort if not contraindicated (usually side lying or prone with legs flexed on chest) Perform procedures (for example, dressing change, deep breathing, and so on) after administering analgesics
Prepare for discharge Wound care	If dressing changes are required at home, teach parent sterile or aseptic procedures; provide written list of necessary equipment and instructions; make referral to public health nurse if necessary
Colostomy care	Begin teaching colostomy care as soon as possible postoperatively Involve enterostomal therapist in teaching plan, if available Include child (even preschooler) in care; older child should eventually assume total responsibility Make referral to public health nurse for continued supervision at home
Dietary management	Discuss purpose of dietary changes, for example, low-residue foods Assess family's food practices before introducing changes; individualize counseling according to cultural/ethnic food practices Provide written list of acceptable/avoidable foods If colostomy was performed, stress need for increased fluids and role of food in regulating bowel movements If gastrectomy was done, discuss ways to prevent "dumping syndrome" Small frequent meals Avoidance of concentrated carbohydrates Limiting fluids (juice, milk, soup, Jell-O) with meals but increasing fluids between meals Eating slowly; avoiding emotional upset; resting after eating

no passage of stool, (4) anorexia, and (5) weight loss.

Diagnostic evaluation. Diagnosis is usually based on a combination of findings from the history, physical examination, and laboratory testing. Specific diagnostic tests to confirm the diagnosis and rule out other possibilities, such as anal fissures, gastrointestinal infections, diverticulitis, and so on, include: (1) radiographic studies of the colon, including a barium enema, which may show loss of haustration (pouches that give the normal colon a scalloped appearance), shortening of its length, and uniform reduction in diameter, all of which give the picture of the so-called leadpipe colon, (2) rectosigmoidoscopy, which demonstrates an inflamed, friable, bleeding, ulcerated mucosa, (3) mucosal biopsy for histologic evidence of the inflammatory process, and (4) stool samples for determining fecal-fat content, presence of pathologic organisms, and malabsorptive defects. Blood studies are done to determine severity of anemia, extent of albumin loss, and immunoglobulin levels.

Medical/surgical management. Medical treatment is based on a combination of therapies: (1) dietary management to allow the colon a rest and improve the child's nutritional status, (2) medication to reduce the abdominal pain and rectal spasm, and (3) steroids to reduce bowel inflammation. The child is usually hospitalized both to ensure proper medical management and to reduce the familial/environmental factors that may be contributing to the disease.

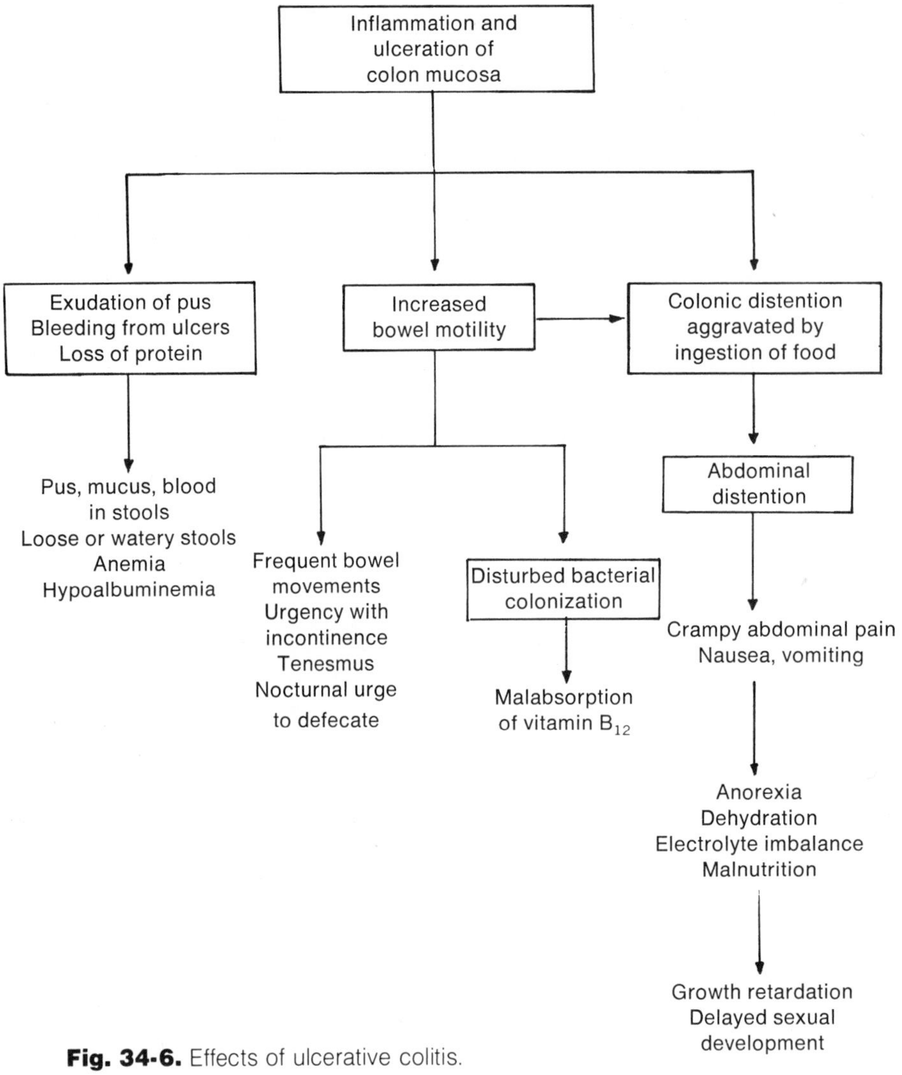

Fig. 34-6. Effects of ulcerative colitis.

Other medical therapies that may be warranted include intravenous fluids to correct dehydration and associated electrolyte imbalances, parenteral alimentation when malnutrition is severe and the colitis is further aggravated by oral diet, and antibiotics to combat secondary colonic infection. Emergency surgical intervention is required for complications such as perforation, massive hemorrhage, or toxic megacolon (fulminating distention of the colon with progressive inflammation).

In some instances a poor response to medical treatment necessitates elective surgery either to allow the bowel a period of rest, in which a temporary colostomy is performed, or to arrest the disease process by removing the entire section of ulcerated bowel, in which case a total colectomy and ileostomy are usually required. The latter procedure is also indicated in those children with chronic colitis of duration of 10 years or more to eliminate the high risk of colonic cancer.

Psychotherapy or family counseling may also prove helpful in reducing stresses that existed prior to the disease and those that have resulted from the colitis. A particularly difficult stress for these children to cope with is the consequent growth retardation and delayed sexual maturation from chronic colitis. Supportive therapy may also be of benefit to those children facing the adjustment of a permanent ileostomy.

Nursing considerations. Many of the nursing considerations relate directly to the medical/surgical interventions in treating colitis. However, the scope of nursing responsibilities extends beyond the immediate period of hospitalization and involves (1) continued guidance of families in terms of dietary management, (2) coping with those factors that increase stress and emotional lability, (3) adjusting to a disease of remission and exacerbations or one of chronic ill health, and (4) when indicated, preparing the child and parents for the possibility of diversionary bowel surgery.

Dietary management. During the acute stage a high-protein, high-calorie, normal-fat, and low- or free-residue diet is recommended. The *high-protein* diet is needed to replace lost protein from the ulcerated bowel, plasma lost through bleeding, and decreased intake resulting from anorexia. The objective is to reverse negative nitrogen balance and promote tissue synthesis. Since lactase activity may be impaired, the limited use of milk products may be necessary. The *high-calorie* diet is needed to restore daily losses in the stool and to combat weight loss. Increasing calories has a protein-sparing effect that promotes positive nitrogen balance. Since *fat* metabolism is generally not impaired, no adjustment in normal requirements is necessary. The *low-residue* diet is to decrease irritation to the bowel. *Vitamin* and *mineral supplements* are usually added to correct the anemia (iron), to promote tissue synthesis (ascorbic acid and vitamin B complex), and to correct deficiencies (vitamin B_{12}).

Encouraging the anorexic child to consume sufficient quantities of this diet while avoiding emotional conflict at mealtime is a nursing challenge. Occasionally the occurrence of aphthous stomatitis further complicates adherence to dietary management. An approach that is more likely to meet with success involves including the child in meal planning, encouraging small, frequent meals or snacks rather than three large meals a day, serving meals around medication schedules when diarrhea, mouth pain, and intestinal spasm are controlled, and preparing high-protein, high-calorie foods, such as eggnog, milk shakes, cream soups, puddings, or custard. Nutritional counseling regarding low-residue foods is similar to that discussed under Hirschsprung's disease (p. 1275). Good mouth care prior to eating and the selection of bland foods help relieve the discomfort of mouth sores.

Reducing stress and facilitating adjustment to chronic illness. Attending to the emotional components of the disease requires a thorough assessment of those stress factors that are disease related or circumstantial. Frequently the nurse can be instrumental in helping these children adjust to the problems of growth retardation, delayed sexual maturation, dietary restrictions, feelings of being "different" or "sickly," inability to compete with peers, and necessary absence from school during exacerbations of the illness.

In the event that a permanent colectomy/ileostomy is required, the nurse can assist the child and family in accepting and adjusting to the change by teaching them how to care for the ileostomy, by emphasizing the positive aspects of surgery, particularly accelerated growth and sexual development, permanent recovery, and eliminated risk of colonic cancer, and by stressing the normalcy of life despite bowel diversion. Introducing the child and parents to other ostomy patients, especially those of the child's age, can be the greatest therapeutic measure in fostering eventual acceptance.

Not infrequently the nurse may identify circumstantial problems, such as marital disharmony, that affect the child's physical condition. In these situations direct intervention may not be possible; however, the nurse can initiate a referral to appropriate sources, such as psychologist, family counselor, clinical nurse specialist, or social worker.

The nurse must also recognize personal feelings toward the child and parents. Indeed, sometimes the dependent child–overprotective mother dyad does exist. The nurse's own feelings toward what is viewed as a "negative relationship" may actually increase stress for the child. For example, if the nurse intervenes to encourage the child's independence and consequently discourages the mother's attempts to care for her child, the nurse may be forcing alterations in the parent-child relationship that are more stressful. Beneficial changes in a relationship are a gradual process. The child needs to be helped to find independence from his parent more rewarding then dependence, and the parent needs assistance in finding a substitute object for his or her attention.

Peptic ulcer

A peptic ulcer is an erosion of the mucosal wall of the stomach, pylorus, or duodenum. Ulcers that arise in the stomach are called *gastric ulcers,* and those that occur in the pylorus or duodenum are termed *duodenal ulcers.* Although peptic ulcers are more common in adults, they are also a significant pediatric problem, occurring most frequently between the ages of 12 and 18 years. Males are affected more than three times as often as females. In children younger than age 6 years gastric ulcers are as common as duodenal ulcers and the majority are secondary to an underlying disease or toxic substance. In children older than 6 years of age, duodenal ulcers are seven times more common than gastric ulcers and the majority are primary, rather than the result of another condition.

Etiology and pathology. The exact cause of peptic ulcer is not known, although one of two mechanisms probably reflects the basic defect: (1) an increase in the rate of production of gastric juice or (2) interference with the normal protective mechanisms of the mucosal lining. As a result of either of these two conditions, the gastric mucosa is highly vulnerable to the digestive effects of gastric juice. Prolonged contact with the highly acidic solution causes an erosion of the mucosal wall, especially in those areas least protected, such as the cardia and lesser curve of the stomach and the area immediately beyond the pylorus. Factors that can result in hypersecretion or decreased protection are outlined in Fig. 34-7. Emotional stress has been implicated as an important contributing factor toward the development, severity, and prognosis of peptic ulcers.

Secondary ulcers are also known to occur after a number of acute disorders, such as encephalitis, meningitis, or sepsis, and several chronic conditions, such as burns, rheuma-

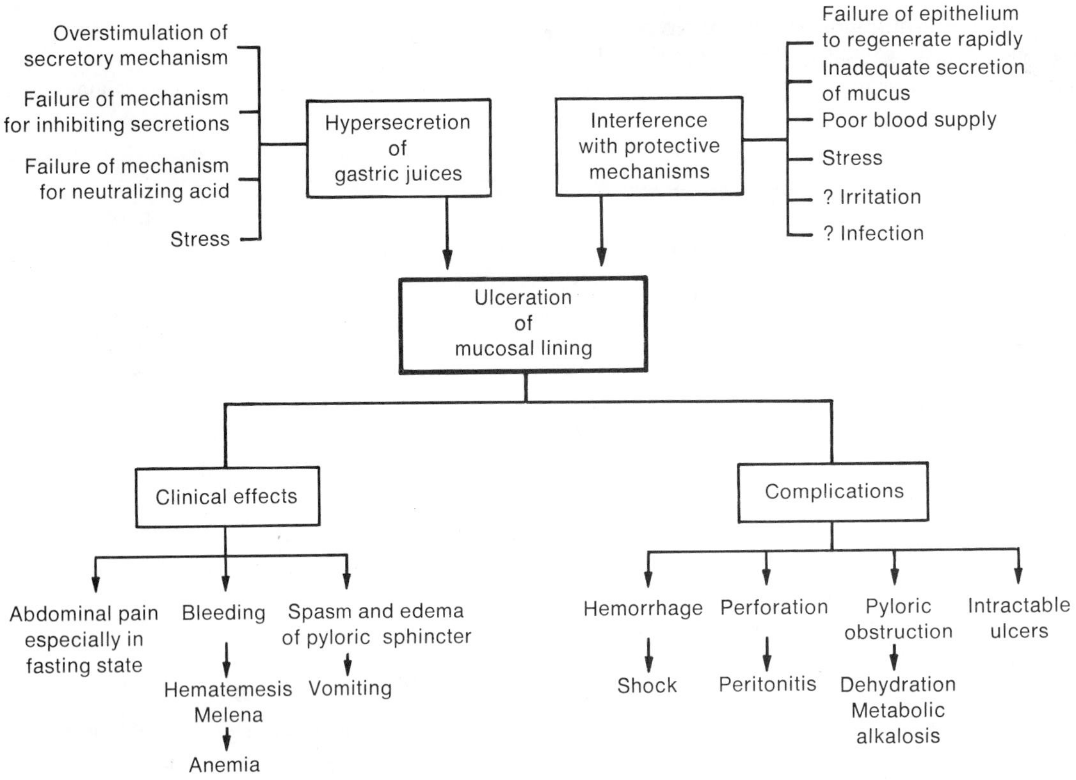

Fig. 34-7. Possible causes and effects of peptic ulcer.

toid arthritis, cirrhosis of the liver, or chronic obstructive lung disease, except cystic fibrosis. They are termed "stress ulcers," although the exact pathology is not known. Certain drugs, particularly aspirin, are ulcerogenic.

Clinical manifestations. Signs and symptoms of peptic ulcers vary according to the age of the child and the location of the ulcer (Table 34-2). The typical pain-food-relief syndrome seen in adults with peptic ulcer is often absent in children. Suggestive symptoms of peptic ulcer include chronic abdominal pain, especially when the stomach is empty, such as during the night or early morning, recurrent vomiting after meals, chronic anemia with occult blood in the stools, and vague gastrointestinal complaints with a positive family history for peptic ulcer.[2]

Diagnostic evaluation. Diagnosis is based on the history (pattern of pain), physical examination (pain in the epigastric area), and diagnostic testing such as radiologic studies, barium swallow, and panendoscopy (visualization of the gastric wall with a fiberoptic instrument). Other tests include blood studies (anemia), stool samples (occult blood), and, occasionally, gastric acid measurements (to isolate hypersecretors).

Medical/surgical management. Management of chronic peptic ulcers is primarily dietary to eliminate acid-producing or irritating foods and to use food in small frequent quantities to neutralize gastric acid. Initially this may involve using the Sippy diet of hourly feedings of milk, cream, and antacids. Anticholinergic drugs, such as propantheline (Pro-Banthine), are helpful in reducing hypersecretion.

A child with an acute ulcer who has developed complications, such as massive hemorrhage, requires emergency care. A nasogastric tube is inserted to remove the blood, prevent abdominal distention, and provide a means of calculating blood loss. Gastric irrigation with cool saline is sometimes used to induce vasoconstriction. Blood replacement, intravenous fluids, and oxygen are usually necessary. Surgical closure of the perforation or bleeding point may be required to stop the hemorrhage.

Management of intractable ulcers (those that do not respond to medical therapy) is either gastric resection or vagotomy with pyloroplasty. A variety of surgical procedures based on the location of the ulcer may be performed for gastric resection. For example, a *subtotal gastrectomy* involves removing 75% to 80% of the lower stomach and anastomosing the remaining upper section to the jejunum. If less of the stomach is removed, too much gastric juice may be secreted, increasing the risk of a marginal ulcer along the site of anastomosis. This is an important fact to stress to the child and parents, who may question the need for removing such a large section of the stomach, when a lesser area is actually involved.

Table 34-2. Clinical manifestation of peptic ulcer

Age-group	Type of ulcer	Signs/symptoms	Comments
Neonates	Usually gastric	Perforation, massive hemorrhage	More likely in infants with hypoxia, sepsis, difficult labor/delivery, or who have a feeding tube inserted Prognosis often poor
Infants to 3-year-old children	Gastric or duodenal, primary or secondary	Poor eating, vomiting, crying spells after feeding, abdominal distention, tarry stools, melena	Primary ulcers more likely to be gastric with slow onset Secondary ulcers more likely to be peptic with acute onset (perforation)
3- to 6-year-old children	Gastric or duodenal	Vomiting related to eating, generalized or periumbilical pain, melena, hematemesis	Perforation more likely in secondary ulcers Nonrecurrence and healing of primary ulcer more favored in infants and young children than among children in older age-groups
6- to 18-year-old children	Usually duodenal and primary	Pain—burning or gnawing sensation in epigastrium related to fasting state, melena, hematemesis, vomiting	More typical of adult type Chances of recurrence greater than 50%

A *vagotomy* (cutting the vagus nerve) temporarily blocks all secretions to the stomach, resulting in dramatic healing of the ulcer usually within a week after surgery. However, stomach secretions usually return after several months. Gastric atony, a consequence of the vagotomy, is a serious complication because the reduced gastric motility greatly retards stomach emptying. Therefore, a *pyloroplasty* is also performed to increase the size of the opening of the pyloris and facilitate stomach emptying into the duodenum.

Nursing considerations. The main nursing objective is to promote healing of the ulcer through dietary management. This involves many of the principles already discussed under ulcerative colitis (p. 1285).

Dietary management. At present there is considerable controversy concerning the benefits of strict, rigid, and slowly advanced dietary control and more liberalized diet therapy. Since children are less likely to comply with a rigid bland diet and power struggles over food restriction are likely to increase emotional tension, a liberal regimen is usually recommended. This includes: (1) avoiding secretagogues (substances that enhance gastric secretion), such as tea, coffee, spices, carbonated beverages, meat extractives (beef broth), fried foods, citrus fruit juices, and alcohol where indicated and (2) eliminating any food that causes the child pain.

The nurse also stresses feeding practices that help neutralize gastric acid, such as (1) eating small frequent meals evenly spaced throughout the day and evening—a typical meal plan may be breakfast at 8:00 AM, a snack of milk and cereal at 10:00 AM, lunch at 12:30 PM, a bowl of soup with crackers at 3:30 PM, dinner at 5:30 PM, and a snack of fruit, ice cream, or pudding and a glass of milk before bedtime; (2) maintaining this regular schedule and especially avoiding prolonged fasting; whenever adhering to a regular meal plan is difficult, such as when traveling, attending school, of working, modifications may be necessary such as carrying packaged foods (instant soups, cheese and crackers, a sandwich, nutritious milk drinks, or fruit) or discussing the importance of in-between meals with the teacher or employer; (3) avoiding overeating, which distends the stomach, thus stimulating the production of increased gastric juice, and (4) drinking small amounts of liquid with meals to avoid diluting stomach contents, thus prolonging emptying time.

Reducing stress and facilitating adjustment to chronic illness. Another nursing responsibility is helping the child and parent reduce stress and adjust to the condition. Many of the suggestions discussed under ulcerative colitis apply here. Sometimes psychotherapy is necessary to prevent recurrence of peptic ulcer as a lifelong problem. When hospitalization is required, manipulating the environment to reduce stress factors, such as separation from parents and home, absence from school, frightening procedures, and possible surgery, can enhance healing of the ulcer.

When surgical intervention is required for intractable ulcers, the nurse can help the child adjust to a gastrectomy. Although the psychologic trauma of losing part of one's stomach is significantly less than that of adjusting to bowel diversion, still there are necessary dietary controls to promote optimum nutrition and prevent a complication called the "dumping syndrome." The dumping syndrome is a physiologic reaction to a high-carbohydrate solution passing directly into the jejunum. The carbohydrates, a hyperosmolar solution, rapidly pull water from the extracellular space into the intestinal lumen. As a result the loss of fluid decreases circulating blood volume, causing symptoms of shock.

To prevent this reaction, carbohydrates, especially simple sugars, are kept to a minimum, small frequent meals are served, proteins and fats are increased to provide sufficient calories and retard bowel emptying, and fluid with meals is kept to a minimum to decrease bowel distention and motility. Ideally the child should eat slowly and regularly, avoid any emotional upset at mealtime, and rest after meals. These instructions can be particularly difficult for adolescents to adhere to, with "fast foods" high in carbohydrates considered a symbol of teenage living. The nurse needs to stress the importance of following dietary instructions for the child to maintain an optimum weight and prevent nutritional deficiencies.

For the child requiring abdominal surgery, see the summary of nursing care on pp. 1282 to 1283.

HEPATIC DISORDERS

The liver is a vital organ that performs several important functions, including (1) secretion of bile, a substance necessary for fat digestion and absorption, (2) assisting in the metabolism of all three food products, secreting several enzymes necessary for their catabolism, (3) serving as a storage depot for glycogen, iron, and vitamins A, D, E, and B_{12}, (4) filtering, detoxifying, and excreting many substances, such as bile pigments (bilirubin), steroids, old red blood cells, and urea, (5) synthesizing several blood proteins, such as prothrombin and fibrinogen for blood clotting, albumins, and many globulins, (6) having a role in maintaining circulation through the synthesis of these proteins, production of heparin to prevent clotting in intact vessels, and storage of large quantities of blood, and (7) from its catabolism, producing considerable heat.

Conditions that affect the liver, either intrahepatically, such as hepatitis or cirrhosis, or extrahepatically, such as biliary atresia or portal vein thrombosis, will affect all or some of these functions. Table 34-3 outlines the usual liver function tests used to diagnose hepatic disorders.

Hepatitis

Etiology. Hepatitis of viral etiology is caused by at least two distinct types of virus, hepatitis virus A or hepatitis virus B. Although the two infectious processes produce the same pathologic changes in the liver and very similar clinical manifestations, they are distinct in their epidemiologic and immunologic characteristics. Table 34-4 compares the various features of both types of viruses.

One of the difficulties in understanding the types of viral hepatitis has been confusion in definition of terms. Prior to the discovery of distinct etiologic agents, the term "infectious hepatitis" was used when a virus could be isolated from feces or blood and no history of possible parenteral contamination could be found. The term "serum hepatitis" was applied when no virus could be isolated but a history of possible contact with contaminated blood, needles, or syringes was positive. Presently these terms are no longer used because the type of virus can be determined in either case (infectious hepatitis caused by virus A and serum hepatitis caused by virus B), and transmission of both can be by the parenteral or oral route.

The term "hepatitis-associated antigen" (HB Ag) or, less frequently, "Australia antigen," is also used synonymously with hepatitis virus B. The term Australia antigen was named because the antigenic factor was first isolated from the serum of an Australian aborigine. The discovery of a specific antigen for hepatitis virus B was a significant breakthrough in identifying the etiologic agent because of the inability to actually cultivate the virus from infected cases. It has also resulted in identifying those asymptomatic individuals who are carriers of the virus and in potentially eliminating the risk of contracting hepatitis virus B from transfused blood of carrier donors.

Although persons in any age-group are susceptible to hepatitis, viral hepatitis type A is most common in children under 15 years of age, especially in low socioeconomic groups, where housing conditions are crowded. Certain groups of people who are in contact with blood products or contaminated equipment are especially at risk for contracting hepatitis type B. With the escalating abuse of parenteral drugs, the incidence of hepatitis type B in the adolescent population has been steadily increasing. It has been reported that as many as 40% to 50% of persons who use illicit drugs have the hepatitis B antigen in their sera.[2] This proportion of possible carriers dramatically increases the reservoir of hepatitis virus B to the general population. In particular, nondrug users who are in close, intimate contact with carriers of hepatitis virus B may contact the virus from oral contamination with semen, saliva, and vaginal secretions, including menstrual blood.

Other groups at risk include persons requiring frequent blood transfusions, such as children who have hemophilia or leukemia or who require hemodialysis, and health personnel who are involved in caring for these patients, who handle blood products, or who are in close contact, such as dentists.

Pathology. The pathologic changes occur primarily in the parenchymal cells of the liver and result in variable degrees of swelling, infiltration of liver cells by mononuclear cells, subsequent degeneration, necrosis, and autolysis. Structural changes within the hepatocyte are thought to account for altered liver functions, such as impaired bile excretion, elevated transaminase and alkaline phosphatase levels, and decreased albumin synthesis.

The pathology is usually self-limiting, with complete

Table 34-3. Liver function tests

Test	Normal function of liver	Abnormal finding and significance
Serum bilirubin level	Conversion of indirect (unconjugated) bilirubin to direct (conjugated) bilirubin for excretion in bile	Increased indirect bilirubin level denotes damage to hepatic cells Increased direct bilirubin level denotes some blockage of bile duct
Urine bilirubin level	Normally, bilirubin excreted in bile, broken down to urobilinogen in stool, and therefore not excreted in urine	Present in urine, produces deep yellow to brown color Reflects direct bilirubin level because only this form is water soluble
Urine urobilinogen level	Normally contains only small amounts from filtration of blood	Increased
Stool sample	Urobilinogen oxidized to pigment urobilin (stercobilin) which gives stool its characteristic color	If bile is not being produced or if its flow is obstructed, stool will be white or clay-colored from lack of bile pigments
Bromsulphalein (BSP) excretion	Filtration and excretion	Removal of this dye is similar to mechanisms used in excreting bilirubin; therefore excess dye in blood stream can indicate problems in hepatic blood flow, liver cells, or bile ducts
Blood ammonia level	Detoxification of ammonia to urea	Increased level reflects poorly functioning hepatic cells and impaired hepatic blood flow
Prothrombin time	Prothrombin manufactured by liver	Prothrombin time is increased, but usually only reflected in severe liver disease
Serum protein levels	Albumin manufactured chiefly by liver; globulins manufactured by liver, spleen, lymphatics, and bone marrow	Albumin usually decreased, whereas globulins increased
Alkaline phosphatase level	Enzyme produced by liver and excreted with bile	Increased level reflects *acute* liver cell disease or bile duct obstruction Not specific because produced by bone as well
Serum glutamic oxaloacetic transaminase (SGOT) level, serum glutamic pyruvic transaminase (SGPT) level, and lactic dehydrogenase (LDH) level	Metabolic enzymes produced by liver	All elevated in *acute* liver destruction as the damaged cells release their enzymes SGOT—found also in heart tissue SGPT—found mostly in liver but a less sensitive indicator than SGOT LDH—found in several organ tissues, therefore not specific for liver disease

Table 34-4. Comparison of types A and B hepatitis

Characteristic	Type A	Type B
Incubation period	15-40 days, average 25 days	6 weeks to 6 months
Period of communicability	Unknown Virus in blood and feces 2 to 3 weeks before onset of jaundice and for at least 1 week after onset of jaundice	Variable Virus in blood (probably in stool but no direct proof) during late incubation period and acute stage of disease; may persist in carrier state for years
Mode of transmission	Principal route—oral-fecal Less frequent route—parenteral Fetal transfer—from transplacental blood during last trimester, but more commonly at time of delivery	Principal route—parenteral Less frequent route—oral, venereal (semen, menstrual secretions, saliva) Fetal transfer—from transplacental blood during last trimester, but more commonly at time of delivery
Onset	Usually rapid, acute Commonly accompanied by fever	More insiduous Less frequently accompanied by fever
Immunity	Present after one attack, but no crossover to type B	Present after one attack, but no crossover to type A
Prophylaxis (passive immunity with immune serum globulin)	Successful, especially during early incubation period	Inconsistent benefits

regeneration of liver cells without scarring occurring within 2 to 3 months. There are, however, forms of hepatitis that do not result in complete return of liver function. These include *fulminant hepatitis,* which is characterized by a severe, acute course with death frequently occurring within 1 to 2 weeks, and *subacute* or *chronic active hepatitis,* characterized by progressive liver destruction and uncertain regeneration with the possibility of scarring.

Clinical manifestations. The clinical manifestations for both types of viral hepatitis are similar except for a more rapid, acute onset in type A and a slower, more insidious onset in type B. Both types may present with flulike symptoms and may never be recognized as actual cases of hepatitis.

However, the classical picture begins with initial symptoms of nausea and vomiting, extreme anorexia, malaise, easy fatigability, and slight to moderate fever. The child may have abdominal pain, especially in the epigastrium or upper right quadrant. He usually acts ill, preferring to rest in bed, and is fretful or irritable. The most significant finding on physical examination is liver tenderness with or without enlargement. This initial anicteric (absence of jaundice) phase usually lasts 5 to 7 days.

Following this period, evidence of jaundice (the icteric phase) is present, beginning with darkening of the urine and the presence of light-colored stools and followed by yellowing of the sclera and skin. Usually as the jaundice worsens the child begins to feel better with improved appetite, behavior, and the absence of nausea, vomiting, and fever. This opposing course of rising bilirubin and improved clinical signs is regarded as a significant diagnostic and prognostic sign of benign viral hepatitis. The appearance of jaundice with worsening constitutional symptoms is regarded as a poorer prognostic sign, with a majority of these children developing fulminant, subacute, or chronic active hepatitis. Some children never develop jaundice; however, although their course is usually milder, they are still infectious.

The icteric phase commonly lasts less than 4 weeks. Complete recovery with return of normal liver function and a feeling of well-being with absence of fatigue or malaise may take 1 to 3 months. Generally children recover promptly. However, it is not unusual for the child to experience a short relapse of slight jaundice and clinical symptoms 10 to 12 weeks after the illness. Unless the symptoms persist and continue to worsen, this relapse is considered benign.

Diagnostic evaluation. Diagnosis is based on history, physical examination, laboratory evidence of the virus, and liver function tests. Besides the history of the chief complaint and present illness, several other factors are significant in confirming exposure to hepatitis virus, such as (1) contact with a person known to have hepatitis, especially a family member, (2) questionable sanitation practices, such as impure drinking water, (3) eating certain foods, such as clams or oysters (especially from polluted water), (4) recent immunizations or blood transfusions, (5) ingestion of hepatotoxic drugs, such as salicylates, sulfonamides, several antineoplastic agents, and many other medications, and (6) parenteral administration of illicit drugs or sexual contact with a person who uses these drugs. The latter event is especially important when hepatitis is suspected in an adolescent and should be coupled with a careful examination for signs of needle marks, especially in the antecubital fossa.

Blood and stool cultures can prove the existence of virus A; however, diagnosis of virus B is usually based on the presence of hepatitis-associated antigen. No liver function test is specific for hepatitis. Serum glutamic-oxaloacetic transaminase (SGOT) and serum glutamic-pyruvic transaminase (SGPT) levels are markedly elevated. Serum bilirubin levels peak 5 to 10 days after clinical jaundice, sodium sulfobromophthalein (Bromsulphalein) test parallels this rise. Urine bilirubin may be elevated before jaundice appears. Serum protein levels may remain normal. Depressed serum albumin and prolonged prothrombin time are indicative of severe liver damage. Lactic dehydrogenase and alkaline phosphatase levels may be slightly elevated.

Medical management

Supportive measures. There is no specific treatment for either type of viral hepatitis. Management is based on palliative treatment of symptoms. For example, antimetics may be helpful to reduce the nausea or vomiting. The value of bed rest in promoting overall recovery is controversial. Since the child feels ill and tired in the anicteric phase, he usually chooses to stay in bed. However, once improvement of physical complaints begins, the child prefers to gradually resume normal activity. The best approach is probably to allow the child to regulate his own pace. Hospitalization is rarely necessary, although proper isolation practices at home are imperative.

Like strict bed rest, a low-fat diet was once recommended for treatment of hepatitis. However, the current trend is to allow the child to choose foods he prefers, especially during the initial stage when anorexia is severe. Generally low-fat foods cause less stomach distention and are better tolerated than foods high in fat content. Carbohydrates should be encouraged to ensure an adequate caloric intake to spare proteins for cell growth. Ingested proteins are restricted only in the event of hepatic coma, which is discussed under cirrhosis. Vitamin K is administered if prothrombin time is prolonged. Other vitamin supplements are not necessary if adequate nutrition can be maintained.

Control measures. An equally important health consideration is control of spread of the infection. Control measures principally include: (1) scrupulous hand washing after toileting and before eating and disposal of feces to eliminate the oral-fecal chain, and (2) disposal of all blood products and associated contaminated articles from the infected person. Isolation or quarantine of the child is not necessary as long as these measures are employed.

At the present time there is no immunization available for viral hepatitis. Prophylactic use of gamma globulin is effective in preventing hepatitis virus A during the early part of the incubation period and, to a lesser extent, before the onset of the disease. It is of inconsistent benefit in preventing type B virus. Although an attack of either virus confers long-lasting immunity to that virus, there is no crossover protection to the other virus.

Nursing considerations. Nursing objectives depend largely on the severity of the hepatitis, the rigidity of medical treatment, and factors influencing the control and transmission of the disease. Since children with benign viral hepatitis are frequently cared for at home, the responsibility of explaining any medical therapies and control measures is frequently left to the clinic or office nurse. In instances in which further assistance is needed for parents to comply with such instructions, a public health nursing referral may be necessary.

Supportive care. During the acute stage when anorexia is severe, the nurse can help parents provide foods that the child may eat, such as small frequent "snacks" rather than actual meals. Since these children are least fatigued and most hungry in the morning the nurse should stress the importance of a nutritional breakfast. As the child tires during the day, the appetite usually wanes as well. If no dietary restriction is medically imposed, the nurse should encourage parents to refrain from forcing foods, since the anorectic phase is generally short.

Many people are aware of the rigid schedule of bed rest frequently ordered for adults with hepatitis. Parents may consequently insist that their child remain in bed, even after the anicteric stage. It is important to discuss a realistic activity schedule early in the course of the illness to prevent this from becoming a parent-child battle. Since hepatitis type A is not infectious within a week or so after onset of jaundice, the child may feel well enough to resume school shortly thereafter.

Because liver function is impaired during the anicteric and early icteric phases, the nurse instructs parents to report immediately any behavioral changes (see Table 34-5) that could indicate prehepatic coma. The parents are also cautioned about administering any medication to the child without the physician's knowledge, since normal doses of many drugs may become dangerous because of the liver's inability to detoxify and excrete them. Common drugs that are affected by hepatic failure include acetaminophen (Tylenol), ferrous sulfate (oral iron), and dextropropoxyphene (Darvon).

In those children with type B virus who have a known or suspected history of illicit drug use, the nurse has the additional responsibility of helping them realize the associated dangers of drug abuse, stressing the parenteral mode of transmission, and encouraging them to seek counseling from a drug program. In these situations the hepatitis may represent a minor aspect of a much larger health problem. For example, members of some drug-using groups view hepatitis as a desirable status symbol. Consequently treatment and concern for prevention and control of transmission are viewed as opposing values, adding to the enormity of preventing the spread of the disease.

Control measures. Hand washing is the single most critical measure in prevention and control of hepatitis. The nurse explains to parents and children the usual ways in which hepatitis virus A (oral-fecal route) and hepatitis virus B (parenteral route) are spread. However, regardless of which type of virus is present, the same general precautions should be followed, since each virus is spread by both modes of transmission. The most important instructions include: (1) always washing hands after toileting and before eating; the child can be reminded of these practices by placing a sign in the bathroom, (2) during menses or if the child wears diapers, discarding all soiled articles by wrapping them first in a plastic bag and employing the same strict hand washing practices, (3) washing the child's eating utensils in a dishwasher or by using *hot* water and detergent; preferably, disposable utensils should be used or the child's eating utensils should be kept separate from those used by the rest of the family, (4) washing or discarding any article soiled with feces or blood, caring for bleeding wounds using strict attention to contaminated objects and hand washing, (5) not allowing any sharing of toothbrushes or razors (accidentally ingested saliva or blood from these objects can transmit the virus), (6) cautioning against any close, intimate contact, such as kissing, and (7) if specific sources of contamination are identified, such as impure water, milk, or foods, eliminating these from the household.

If the child is hospitalized, he is usually isolated in a separate room. All personnel directly caring for him should wear gowns in addition to following other enteric precautions. Special attention must be given to all blood products and invasive equipment. Only disposable needles and syringes should be used. Any contaminated equipment and blood samples are labeled "possibly infectious." The nurse explains to parents and older children the reason for isolation and specific precautions to help them adjust to the experience of hospitalization and to reinforce practice of control measures before and after discharge.

Cirrhosis

Cirrhosis is a result, not a primary cause, of liver dysfunction. The word cirrhosis actually means "yellow" and refers to the typical orange-colored nodules of a fibrotic liver. Hepatic cirrhosis is generally classified according to three types. *Biliary cirrhosis* is characterized by scarring around the bile ducts and lobes of the liver and most often is a result of congenital biliary atresia or, less commonly, a consequence of cystic fibrosis. *Postnecrotic cirrhosis* is characterized by broad bands of connective tissue and is most often the result of neonatal or chronic active hepatitis, Wilson's disease (hepatolenticular degeneration), or, less frequently, sickle cell disease or ulcerative colitis. The third type, *Laennec's cirrhosis,* is characterized by scar tissue around the portal area and is most often a result of protein malnutrition secondary to chronic alcohol ingestion. Although the last type is the most common form found in adults, it is rare in children.

Cirrhosis is becoming an increasingly significant pediatric health problem. With the alarming escalation in the number of adolescents who are at risk for contracting hepatitis type B from illicit parenteral drug use, it is likely that the occurrence of postnecrotic cirrhosis will also increase. Likewise, improved treatment of genetic diseases, such as cystic fibrosis or sickle cell anemia, will also affect the number of children who are at risk for developing this complication. Since the life-threatening complications of severe liver failure, namely, bleeding esophageal varices and hepatic coma, require hospitalization, nurses need to be familiar with their pathologic development and treatment.

Pathology. Cirrhosis is believed to result after some type of injury or insult to the liver. The hepatocellular injury (with or without inflammation) activates fibroblasts that respond by synthesizing collagen, thus forming fibrous connective tissue. The balance among fibrogenesis, the mechanisms for fibrous tissue removal, and hepatocyte regeneration appears to determine the degree of permanent hepatic fibrosis.

Once mature fibrous tissue is formed, a vicious cycle ensues. Vascular pathways form within the fibrotic tissues, depriving hepatocytes of their blood supply. The consequent cellular hypoxia, inflammation, and necrosis stimulate further fibroblastic activity. As a result normal hepatic architecture is sufficiently distorted to affect both hepatocellular function and hepatic blood circulation. These disturbances give rise to the many clinical manifestations of cirrhosis, which are outlined in Fig. 34-8.

Many of the pathophysiologic changes are the result of disturbances in more than one system. For example, the chronic anemia is a consequence of (1) blood loss from gastritis, bleeding varices, and increased tendency toward bleeding resulting from thrombocytopenia and decreased coagulation factors, (2) shortened life span of the erythrocyte as a result of more rapid destruction in the congested spleen, cell membrane alteration, and toxic effects of circulating bile salts, (3) decreased production as a result of poor absorption of iron in the intestine, decreased carrier protein (transferrin) for iron storage, decreased bone marrow activity, and decreased levels of vitamins E and K, and (4) hemodilution, which even in the event of normal circulating red blood cell mass causes proportionally fewer erythrocytes to reach the tissues. As one can readily appreciate, the effects of liver failure are complicated, interrelated, and potentially life threatening.

Clinical manifestations. Clinical manifestations depend on the etiology. In cirrhosis from congenital biliary atresia, jaundice is usually the first sign, although all the pathologic effects eventually become evident, especially since most cases are not amenable to surgical correction. In cirrhosis from other causes, the symptoms are usually vague and the onset insidious. Not infrequently the first evidence of severe liver failure is a complication such as ascites, bleeding esophageal varices, or failure to thrive.

Diagnostic evaluation. Diagnosis rests on (1) the history, especially evidence of prior liver disease, such as hepatitis, (2) physical examination, particularly hepatosplenomegaly, and the cutaneous changes from hemodynamic alterations and increasing hormone levels (see Fig. 34-8), and (3) laboratory evaluation, especially liver function tests. Definitive diagnosis rests on a liver biopsy for evidence of histologic changes.

Medical management. There is no specific therapy for cirrhosis, except in those cases in which a treatable cause, such as an infection, exists. Supportive medical management is concerned with altering the pathologic changes, primarily the nutritional deficiences. A high-calorie diet with low or moderate fats, moderate high-quality protein, and high carbohydrates is recommended. In addition supplements of water-soluble preparations of vitamins A, D, E, and K should be given. In children with vitamin B_{12} deficiency, injectable supplements are necessary. Iron supplements and blood transfusions are sometimes required.

Treatment of complications, such as bleeding esophageal varices and hepatic coma, is discussed on pp. 1294 and 1297.

Nursing considerations. Nursing objectives in caring for the child with cirrhosis depend on several factors, including the precipitating cause of the cirrhosis, the severity of complications, and the prognosis. Overall the latter factor has the greatest impact because the prognosis for life is poor. Since treatment of cirrhosis ideally is treatment of the cause, in many instances a fatal outcome is determined by the inability to surgically correct biliary atresia, reverse hepatitis, or stop the progressive damage as a result of cystic fibrosis. Therefore, nursing care of this child is the same as that for a potentially terminally ill child (Chapter 27). Hospitalization is usually required when complications such as ascites, bleeding esophageal varices, or hepatic coma occur.

Prevention, however, is an important nursing responsibility in terms of those diseases that may ultimately lead to cirrhosis. For example, genetic counseling would reduce the number of children afflicted with many genetic-metabolic disorders, such as galatosemia, sickle cell dis-

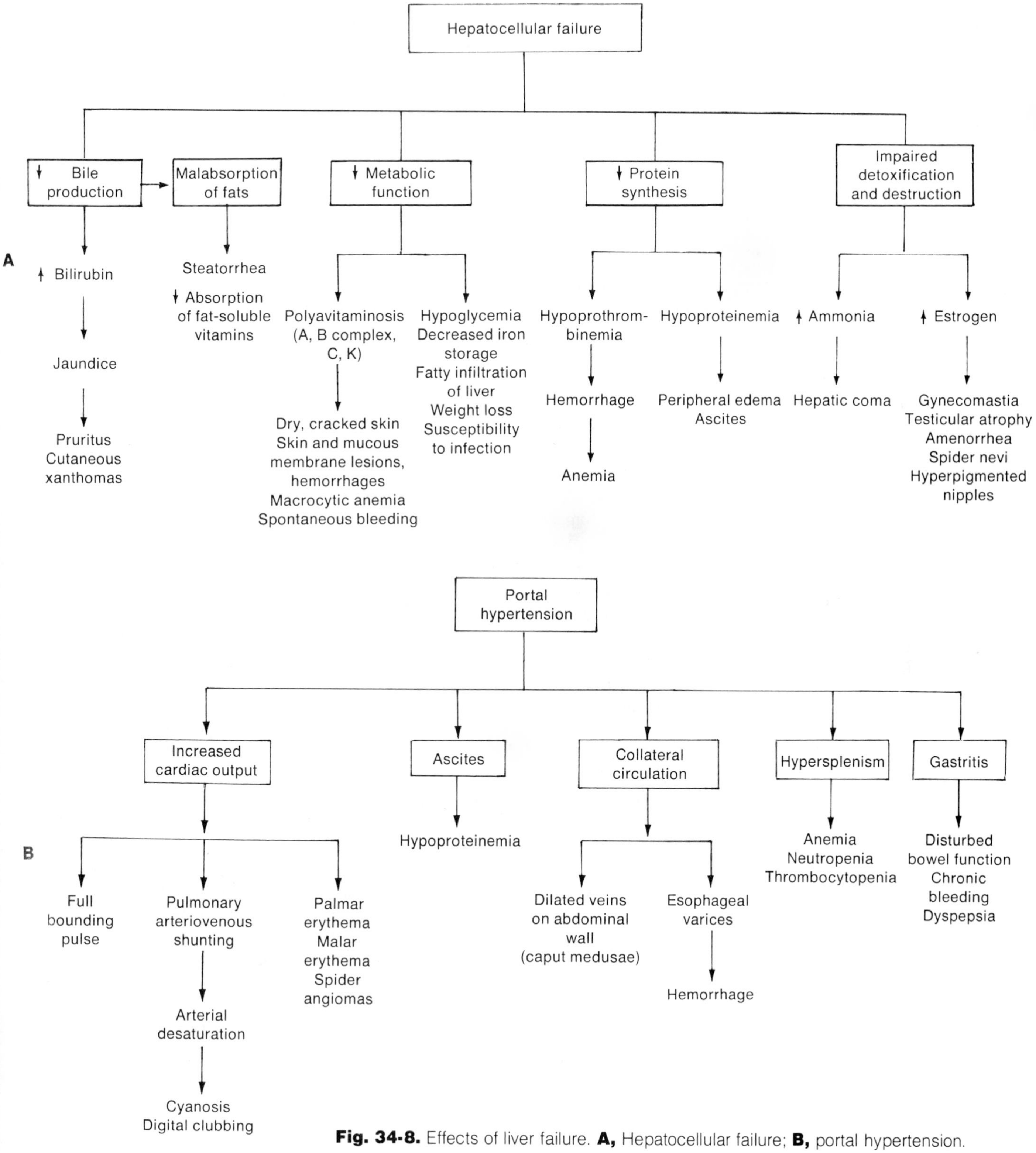

Fig. 34-8. Effects of liver failure. **A,** Hepatocellular failure; **B,** portal hypertension.

ease, or cystic fibrosis. Proper prenatal care can lessen the possibility of neonatal hepatitis from a variety of congenital infections, such as rubella, herpes simplex, syphilis, or cytomegalovirus. Prevention of these diseases may also influence the defect of biliary atresia, which is thought sometimes to be a consequence of in utero infection. Public health education regarding the dangers of hepatitis and in particular the usual modes of transmission of hepatitis virus B may eventually decrease the human reservoir.

Esophageal varices

Pathology. Esophageal varices are the consequence of portal hypertension. Normally almost all of the blood leaving the digestive organs enters the liver from the portal vein. From the central veins of each lobule the blood flows into larger hepatic veins and finally empties into the inferior vena cava. However, in cirrhosis, fibrous tissue surrounds the blood vessels, constricting the diameter and increasing resistance to blood flow. As a result blood backs up into the digestive system.

Normally there are connecting channels that allow blood to flow from the digestive organ to the heart without passing through the liver. The most common site is the cardiac orifice of the stomach, where blood from the esophagus flows directly to the heart and blood from the stomach flows to the liver. However, as resistance to hepatic blood flow increases, blood backs up into the stomach and attempts to leave via the esophageal veins. Consequently these veins dilate, forming varices that may eventually rupture, causing an acute hemorrhage.

Another collateral pathway is at the lower end of the rectum. Venous varices that form here are called *hemorrhoids*. However, hemorrhoidal bleeding is less likely to occur in children than in adults.

Factors that favor variceal bleeding. Exactly what causes the esophageal varices to bleed is still unknown. However, several factors have been postulated that probably account for rupture of the veins. For example, the highly acidic gastric juice may reflux back into the lower esophageal area, eroding the fragile tissue, and initiate a bleeding episode. Foods with a rough texture may cause mechanical irritation and rupture the delicate membrane. A sudden increase in pressure, such as coughing, gagging, vomiting, or straining at stool, may cause the varices to rupture. Drugs, especially aspirin, exert an irritating effect on gastric mucosa and promote bleeding tendencies by interfering with blood clotting.

Clinical manifestations. Bleeding may be acute, beginning with vomiting large amounts of bright red blood, or gradual, with occasional hematemesis or melena. Typically there is abdominal pain with bleeding episodes. In instances of chronic blood loss, anemia may be an early indication of bleeding esophageal varices.

Diagnostic evaluation. To confirm the presence of esophageal varices, a barium swallow is usually done, which demonstrates the dilated veins bulging into the lumen of the esophagus. Direct visualization of the varices can be accomplished through esophagoscopy. Either procedure carries the attendant risk of rupturing a varix and initiating hemorrhage.

In instances of severe bleeding without known liver disease, a battery of tests are usually done to identify the underlying cause. These include liver function tests (see Table 34-3), selective angiography to fluoroscopically view the splenic and portal vein, splenoportography, which involves catheterizing the femoral artery and injecting contrast medium directly into the spleen, and liver biopsy. In the latter two procedures, hemorrhage from the puncture sites is a possible complication.

Medical management. Treatment of esophageal varices is aimed at preventing bleeding by manipulating those factors known to promote rupture. Usual preventive instructions include (1) eating a soft, bland diet and (2) avoiding straining at stool, forceful coughing, strenuous contact sports, and any aspirin or salicylate compound. Occasionally antacids may be given to counteract gastric acidity.

More often, however, medical management is directed at controlling acute hemorrhage. *Vasopressin* (Pitressin), a posterior pituitary hormone, stops the bleeding temporarily. It is usually given by intravenous drip over 20 to 40 minutes. Its main effect seems to be lowering of blood flow to the splanchnic bed (intestinal viscera). Significant side effects of this drug are hypertension, bradycardia, arrhythmias, colicky abdominal pain, defecation, diuresis, and facial pallor.

Local measures to control bleeding include: (1) emptying of the stomach with a nasogastric tube to prevent distention, (2) gastric cooling with cool saline irrigations to promote vasoconstriction and removal of the blood, and (3) gastric compression with a Sengstaken-Blakemore tube. When a nasogastric tube is inserted, the back of the throat should be sprayed with a local anesthetic benzocaine (Cetacaine) to prevent gagging, which can rupture intact varices or reinitiate a bleeding episode. The child is placed in at least a 45-degree sitting position to prevent cardioesophageal reflux. With the tube in place, cool saline irrigations may be done.

Gastric compression is accomplished with a Sengstaken-Blakemore tube. This apparatus includes a nasogastric tube with two inflatable balloons at one end and three connections at the other end. The deflated balloons and tube are passed into the stomach in the same manner as any nasogastric tube. The rounded gastric and elongated esophageal balloons are inflated to exert pressure against the upper part of the stomach and lower portion of the esophagus, respectively. Of the three external connections, one is attached to the gastric balloon, another to the esophageal balloon, and a third to the suction machine. For compres-

Summary of nursing care of the child with bleeding esophageal varices*

Goals	Responsibilities
Control bleeding Provide rest	Place child in quiet room Encourage parents to stay Explain all procedures to allay anxiety and promote cooperation Provide quiet distraction, such as music or television Avoid use of sedatives
Prevent trauma to esophageal varices	Minimize crying episodes (above measures are helpful here) Suction frequently to prevent urge to cough up secretions Instruct child not to cough, clear his throat forcefully, or strain Sengstaken-Blakemore tube Before tube is inserted, inflate balloons to detect any leaks Secure tube to face to maintain traction Restrain child's arms to prevent dislodging tube or partially deflating balloons Deflate balloons at regular intervals (usually 5 to 10 minutes every 6 to 8 hours); observe for bleeding during deflation Periodically check pressure of balloon inflation (attach end of tubing to sphygmomanometer and measure pressure in mm/Hg)
Administer vasopressin	Monitor intravenous infusion closely to infuse drug slowly by Soluset in prescribed length of time Place child on bedpan during drug therapy for possible defecation and diuresis Explain to parents and child expected effects of drug If drug is readministered, failure to observe side effects indicates loss of drug's effectiveness
Monitor for signs of shock	Record vital signs and blood pressure frequently, at least hourly, during acute phase Interpret values in light of side effects of vasopressin (decreased pulse, increased blood pressure, and facial pallor)
Record blood loss	Calculate all drainage from nasogastric or Sengstaken-Blakemore tube; subtract amount of saline irrigation from total output to determine actual fluid loss Check stools for occult blood Record urinary output, especially when vasopressin is administered
Observe for signs of hepatic coma	Since blood in gastrointestinal tract can precipitate coma, observe for mental-neuromuscular changes (Table 34-5) Avoid sedatives
Prevent aspiration	Place child in at least semi-Fowler's position Have large basin at bedside to collect vomitus, especially before nasogastric tube is inserted Sengstaken-Blakemore tube Suction oral secretions frequently Turn head to side to allow secretions to drain from mouth Provide tissues for child to spit out secretions Have scissors attached near bed (but away from small child's reach) to cut tubing in case balloons dislodge against trachea

*NOTE: If emergency or elective surgery is anticipated, see p. 1282 for nursing goals and responsibilities.

Continued.

Summary or nursing care of the child with bleeding esophageal varices—cont'd

Goals	Responsibilities
Administer comfort measures	Administer oral hygiene frequently Moisten lips and tongue with cool cloth to combat severe thirst (child may be receiving nothing by mouth for several days) Remove restraints for younger child whenever supervised Encourage parents to visit or remain with child as much as possible
Prepare for discharge	Teach preventive measures Soft bland diet Avoidance of coughing or straining at stool Avoidance of strenuous contact sports Avoidance of aspirin or aspirin compound; use of acetaminophen (Tylenol) for fever or pain Reporting to physician any evidence of blood in vomitus or stool

sion to be effective, traction must be applied to the tube to keep the balloons in their proper position. Usually this is accomplished by taping the tube to the nose. However, it may also be maintained by attaching the tube to a weight over a pulley. In children a football helmet may be worn and the tube attached to the nose guard. In either instance, maintaining traction severely limits the child's movements.

There are significant dangers to use of the Sengstaken-Blakemore tube. First, constant pressure against the esophagus and stomach can severely impede normal blood flow and lead to ulceration and necrosis. Therefore, the balloons are kept inflated for about 24 hours and, if left in longer, are deflated for 5 to 10 minutes every 6 to 8 hours. Second, airway obstruction can result if the inflated balloons are accidently pulled up against the trachea or if a partially deflated balloon is left attached to traction. Third, because the inflated balloons prevent the child from swallowing oral secretions, saliva can accumulate above the esophageal balloon and be aspirated.

Several supportive measures may also be used to medically treat the child. To facilitate removal of blood in the intestinal tract, repeated saline enemas are given. To prevent the breakdown of the large amounts of plasma protein to ammonia by the colonic bacteria, broad-spectrum antibiotics are given. Although this is helpful in reducing the amount of ammonia in the blood that cannot be detoxified by the liver, it alters bacterial flora, reducing vitamin K synthesis and promoting bacterial and fungal overgrowth.

Whole blood is replaced in the event of shock. However, blood replacement may reinitiate bleeding if it is infused too quickly or in too great a quantity.

To rest the alimentary tract, oral feedings are withheld. If bleeding episodes are frequent, long-term parenteral nutrition may be necessary.

Drug therapy is kept at a minimum, since the liver's ability to detoxify drugs is impaired. Sedation is withheld as much as possible, since it masks signs of hepatic coma.

Surgical treatment. In cases of intractable hemorrhage, emergency surgical intervention may be necessary to ligate the varices. A more drastic approach is to perform an esophagogastrectomy, in which the lower portion of the esophagus and upper section of the stomach are removed. Usually this is a two-stage procedure, in which initially the proximal end of the esophagus is attached to the neck to serve as a fistula and a jejunostomy is done for postoperative feeding. During a subsequent operation, a segment of colon is resected and attached to the proximal end of the esophagus and distal end of the stomach to provide a continuous passageway. However, this procedure has its own complications, such as the dumping syndrome, and bleeding commonly recurs at other sites.

Shunting procedures may be considered as a long-range measure to prevent bleeding episodes by providing another pathway for backed-up blood to reach the systemic circulation. The various bypass procedures include: (1) a *portacaval* shunt in which the portal vein is anastomosed to the inferior vena cava, (2) a *splenorenal* shunt following a splenectomy in which the splenic vein is attached to the left renal vein, and (3) a *mesocaval* shunt, in which the superior mesenteric vein (which branches off to become the portal vein) is anastomosed to the inferior vena cava. In general the portacaval shunt has the greatest success, but it requires a patent portal vein. The splenorenal shunt is only recommended in children more than 10 years old whose splenic vein is large enough to accommodate the large blood flow.

Nursing considerations. Nursing care of the child with bleeding esophageal varices is found in the boxed material on pp. 1295 to 1296. Physical care of the child undergoing emergency surgery requires the usual preoperative and postoperative nursing measures (see Chapter 25). When shunts or an esophagogastrectomy is scheduled, parents and older children need detailed explanations of the purpose and value.

With each procedure's attendant risks, failures, and complications, there may also arise the very difficult ethical consideration of the benefit of such interventions in light of the ultimate prognosis in severe cirrhosis. There are no easy answers to such questions. However, the nurse can be very instrumental in emotionally supporting the child and parents, helping them find solutions by maintaining open channels of communication among all members of the health team, and honestly appraising them of their child's physical condition.

Hepatic coma

Pathology. Normally ammonia (NH_3), a product of protein catabolism, is converted to urea in the liver and excreted by the kidneys in urine. In cirrhosis this process is altered because (1) blood flow to the liver is decreased as a result of portal hypertension and (2) ammonia in blood flowing through the liver cannot be detoxified because of hepatocellular injury. Consequently the ammonia-laden blood reenters the systemic circulation, producing ammonia intoxication or hepatic coma.

The exact role of ammonia toxicity is not known, although the key organ affected is the brain. It is believed that high-ammonia levels interfere with cerebral energy metabolism, resulting in decreased cerebral blood flow and reduced oxygen consumption. This theory partially explains the multiple mental-neuromuscular manifestations of hepatic coma.

Factors that favor hepatic coma. Hepatic coma is more likely to occur when the body's supply of protein and, consequently, ammonia is increased. The chief source of protein is food, although blood proteins, such as from esophageal bleeding, may also be a significant source. Since ammonia is formed mainly from the bacterial action in the small intestine, enteric infections increase this process.

Other conditions that precipitate hepatic coma include fluid and electrolyte imbalance, diuresis, progressive renal failure, sedatives, and anesthetics.

Clinical manifestations. The clinical features of hepatic coma are primarily changes in the mental and neuromuscular state (Table 34-5). Frequently the parent will be the first person to notice the behavioral changes, which are most often described as periods of lethargy alternating with confusion. A characteristic odor, *fetor hepaticus,* similar to the smell of feces, may be evident on the breath and is thought to be a bacterial decomposition product of methionine, which accumulates in the blood.

Table 34-5. Clinical manifestations of hepatic coma

Neuromuscular changes	Mental changes
Incoordination	Confusion
Twitching	Drowsiness
Tremors	Disorientation
Dysarthria (difficulty in articulating)	Restlessness
Asterixis (flapping-like tremor, especially of the hands)	Inappropriate behavior—sucking, crying, disobedience, preoccupation with some activity
Dilated pupils	Apathy
"Faraway" look in eyes	Somnolence
Roving eyes	Stupor (response to noxious stimuli)
Nystagmus	Coma (no response to any stimuli)
Hyperreflexia	
Babinski's sign	
Flexion of legs	

In more advanced stages respirations become deep and forceful. There is progressively more loss of consciousness, beginning with disorientation to time and place and eventually ending in a deep coma and death.

Diagnostic evaluation. Aside from mental and neuromuscular evidence of hepatic coma, the usual laboratory test is blood analysis of ammonia concentration. Other indications of hepatic coma are (1) low blood urea nitrogen levels, since urea is not being formed by the liver, progressing to elevated blood urea nitrogen levels as renal function deteriorates, (2) elevated blood pH (alkalosis), and (3) electrolyte imbalances. An electroencephalogram may be useful in diagnosing precoma states, which are evidenced by slower brain wave activity.

Medical management. The usual approach toward treating hepatic coma is to reduce sources of ammonia by (1) decreasing ingested sources through a low-protein diet and (2) decreasing production of ammonia in the intestine by reducing bacterial flora through administration of large doses of antibiotics, especially neomycin and kanamycin, and high colonic enemas. Since gastrointestinal bleeding is another source of protein, measures to prevent or treat esophageal varices are performed. Any other precipitating causes of coma, such as electrolyte imbalances or infections, are also managed.

More heroic measures to control the coma until liver cells can regenerate include blood exchange transfusions and peritoneal dialysis or hemodialysis. However, since the prognosis of severe liver disease is frequently poor, the ultimate value of such therapies is controversial. In those instances in which there is not evidence of liver cell regeneration, it is believed that medical management of the comatose patient should be the rule, with heroic measures the exception.

Nursing considerations. Many of the nursing considerations depend on the severity of hepatic coma. A priority concern is prevention and detection of impending coma, followed by supportive nursing care of the comatose child and his parents.

Observing behavioral signs. Since most of the children who are candidates for developing hepatic coma are already hospitalized, the nurse observes for neuromuscular and mental changes indicative of ammonia toxicity. When possible, the same nurse should care for the child in order to detect subtle changes. Procedures to identify confusion and disorientation include asking the child about the time of day, where he is, what he did yesterday, to calculate simple arithmetic problems, and so on. To detect dysarthria, the nurse has the child repeat the same phrase or story each day. To identify asterixis, tremor, or incoordination of the hands, a handwriting sample is taken at least daily. With older children who can cooperate with such requests, the nurse can make each task a game. With younger children, the nurse must rely on observation of alertness, motor coordination, and emotional behavior to detect significant alterations. Often this is made more difficult by the other physical problems and medical procedures inflicted on the child, which may evoke emotional reactions. By encouraging parents to stay with their child and to participate in his care, the nurse can validate perceptions of behavioral change with them.

Manipulating factors that influence coma. This involves (1) helping the child adhere to the low-protein diet by including as many allowable "favorites" as possible in the meal plan and explaining to parents and older children why rich sources of protein, such as meat, fish, and dairy products, are eliminated, especially since such foods are usually considered "necessary" items for health, (2) recording all intake and output in order to maintain hydration and weighing the child daily to identify fluid retention, (3) observing for signs of systemic infection, especially a rise in temperature, (4) keeping the child calm and quiet through environmental control to decrease the need for sedation, and (5) administering antibiotics and observing for side effects, namely auditory and renal damage from kanamycin and neomycin.

Supporting parents. Since hepatic coma is often the terminal event following progressive liver failure, the nurse needs to prepare parents for the likelihood of irreversible coma and death. This is sometimes complicated by changing mental statuses in the child. For example, after a period of deep coma, the child may suddenly be alert. Unfortunately these transitory lucid periods do not always mean recovery, and, after renewed hopefulness, the parents are usually forced to see their child relapse into stupor and coma.

Often parents are faced with decisions whether extraordinary measures should be used to keep the child alive despite the grave prognosis. In these situations the nurse's role is one of support, open communication, and honest appraisal of the child's condition. The nurse must also be willing to explore personal feelings regarding this dilemma, since these feelings can affect the parents' decision and adjustment concerning the final outcome of the child's condition.

For a more complete discussion of caring for the comatose child, see Chapter 37.

REFERENCES

1. Ament, M. E.: Malabsorption syndromes in infancy and childhood. Part I, J. Pediatr. **81**(4):685-697, October 1972.
2. Roy, C. C., Silverman, A., and Cozzetto, F. J.: Pediatric clinical gastroenterology, ed. 2, St. Louis, 1975, The C. V. Mosby Co.
3. Willacker, J.: Heard any good borborygmi lately? Nursing '75 **5**(1):36, January 1975.

BIBLIOGRAPHY

Anthony, C. P., and Thibodeau, G. A.: Textbook of anatomy and physiology, ed. 10, St. Louis, 1979, The C. V. Mosby Co.

Barbero, G. J.: Some views on gastrointestinal illness in childhood, Clin. Pediatr. **15**(7):622-624, July 1976.

Brunner, L., and Suddarth, D.: Textbook of medical-surgical nursing, New York, 1975, J. B. Lippincott Co.

Groff, D. B.: Handbook of pediatric surgical emergencies, New York, 1975, Medical Examination Publishing Co., Inc.

Langley, L. L., Telford, I. R., and Christensen, J. B.: Dynamic anatomy and physiology, New York, 1974, McGraw-Hill Book Co.

Ravel, R.: Clinical laboratory medicine, Chicago, 1973, Year Book Medical Publishers, Inc.

Rudolph, A. M., editor: Pediatrics, New York, 1977, Appleton-Century-Crofts.

Widmann, F. K.: Goodales' clinical interpretation of laboratory tests, Philadelphia, 1973, F. A. Davis Co.

Williams, S. R.: Nutrition and diet therapy, ed. 3, St. Louis, 1977, The C. V. Mosby Co.

Classification of malabsorption syndromes

Ament, M. E.: Malabsorption syndromes in infancy and childhood. Part II, J. Pediatr. **81**(5):867-884, November 1972.

Obstructive disorders

Bishop, W. S., and Head, J. J.: Care of the infant with a stoma, Am. J. Maternal Child Nurs. **1**(5):315-319, September/October 1976.

Cooney, D. E., and Grosfeld, J. L.: Care of the child with a colostomy, Pediatrics **59**(3):469-472, March 1977.

Durham, N.: Looking out for complications of abdominal surgery, Nursing '75 **5**(2):24-31, February 1975.

Gibbs, G. E., and White, M.: Stomal care, Am. J. Nurs. **72**(2): 268-271, February 1972.

Gierup, J., Jorulf, H., and Livaditis, A.: Management of intussusception and children: a survey based on 288 consecutive cases, Pediatrics **50**(4):535-546, October 1972.

Gross, L.: Ostomy care: a letter to parents, Am. J. Nurs. **74**(8): 1427-1428, August 1974.

Gutowski, F.: Ostomy procedures: nursing care before and after, Am. J. Nurs. **72**(2):262-276, February 1972.

Lee, C. A., Stroot, V. R., and Schaper, C. A.: What to do when acid-base problems hang in the balance, Nursing '75 **5**(8): 32-37, August 1975.

Literte, J. W.: Nursing Care of patients with intestinal obstruction, Am. J. Nurs. **77**(6):1003-1006, June 1977.

McConnell, E. A.: All about gastrointestinal intubation, Nursing '75 **5**(9):31-27, September 1975.

Suzuki, H., and associates: Nonoperative diagnosis of Hirschsprung's disease in neonates, Pediatrics **51**(2):188-191, February 1973.

Pease, P. W., Corkery, J. J., and Cameron, A. H.: Diagnosis of Hirschsprung's disease by punch biopsy friction, Arch. Dis. Child **51:**541-543, 1976.

Raffensperger, J. G., and Luck, S. R.: Gastrointestinal bleeding in children, Surg. Clin. North Am. **56**(2):413-424, April 1976.

Schnaufer, L.: Hirschsprung's disease, Surg. Clin. North Am. **56**(2):349-359, April 1972.

Stahlgren, L. H., and Morris, N. N.: Intestinal obstruction, Am. J. Nurs. **77**(6):999-1002, June 1977.

Inflammatory conditions

Berger, M., Gribelz, D., and Korelitz, B. I.: Growth retardation in children with ulcerative colitis: the effect of medical and surgical therapy, Pediatrics **55**(4):459, April 1975.

Brunner, L. S.: What to do and what to teach your patient about peptic ulcer, Nursing '76 **6**(11):27-34, November 1976.

Lamb, C., and associates: The G. I. bleeder, Nursing '75 **5**(9): 49-54, September 1975.

Rosenbind, M. L., and Koop, C. E.: Duodenal ulcer in childhood, Pediatrics **45**(2):283-286, 1970.

Hepatic disorders

Altshuler, A.: Esophageal varices in children, Am. J. Nurs. **72**(4): 687-693, April 1972.

Baranowski, K., Greene, H. L., and Lamont, J. T.: Viral hepatitis: how to reduce its threat to the patient and others (including you), Nursing '76 **6**(5):31-39, May 1976.

Committee on Viral Hepatitis: The public health implication of the presence of hepatitis B-antigen in human sera, Morbid. Mortal. **21:**133, 1972.

Dolan, P. O., and Greene, H. L.: Conquering cirrhosis of the liver and a dangerous complication, Nursing '76 **6**(11):44-53, November 1976.

Gillies, D. A., and Alyn, I. B.: How well do you understand cirrhosis? Nursing '75 **5**(1):38-43, January 1975.

Koop, C. E.: Biliary obstruction in the newborn, Surg. Clin. North Am. **56**(2):373-377, April 1976.

Krugman, S., Ward, R., and Katz, S. L.: Infectious diseases of children, ed. 6, St. Louis, 1977, The C. V. Mosby Co.

Surveryer, J. A.: Coma in children: how it affects parents, Am. J. Maternal Child Nurs. **1**(1):17-21, January/February 1976.

UNIT FOURTEEN

The child with problems related to production and circulation of blood

Some of the most common and serious childhood conditions are related to the heart and formed elements of the blood. Many of these disorders are inherited and present at birth, whereas others are acquired. Most of them necessitate medical/surgical intervention to prevent complications and permit normal growth. Nursing care at the time of diagnosis, prior to and during corrective/palliative procedures, and after treatment is essential to promote physical and emotional recovery.

Chapter 35, *The Child with Heart Disease,* discusses the types of congenital and acquired cardiac disorders and the physical consequences of impaired functioning. It focuses on caring for the child with heart disease, preparation of the family for surgery, and postoperative nursing interventions, including discharge planning to help the child and parents adjust to improved physical status. Chapter 36, *The Child with a Problem Related to the Formed Elements of the Blood,* deals with several disorders related to the formed elements of the blood. Since most of these conditions are inherited and chronic, nursing interventions stress helping the family adjust to the disorder and cope with and prevent its complications.

35

The child with heart disease

This chapter focuses on the child with congenital and acquired heart disease. Since the heart is a vital organ, expert medical, surgical, and nursing care are essential for the total physical and psychologic development of the child. Some cardiac defects cause minimal physical limitation, whereas others result in the child's leading a chronically ill existence. For these children surgical repair of the heart defect is only one step toward total recovery. Learning to live a life without overprotection and restriction requires guidance and support from many health professionals, particularly nurses.

CIRCULATORY PHYSIOLOGY AND HEMODYNAMICS

Understanding the effects of congenital and acquired heart defects requires knowledge of the normal heart's functioning. This discussion is primarily concerned with postnatal circulation. The reader is referred to Chapters 7 and 8 for a review of fetal circulation and the cardiopulmonary changes at birth.

Heart

The heart is a muscular four-chambered organ, the primary purpose of which is to pump blood throughout the body. It is located slightly to the left of sternum in the space between the two pleural cavities, called the *mediastinum*. During infancy and early childhood the heart assumes a more horizontal position with the *apex* or lower end of the heart located at the third to fourth intercostal space and lateral to the midclavicular line. With increased chest growth it gradually assumes a more vertical position with the apex at the fifth intercostal and midclavicular line. As a rule, in children over 1 year of age, the width of the heart is less than half the width of the chest.

The heart muscle is covered by a double-walled membrane called the *pericardium*. The outer membrane is the *fibrous pericardium*. The inner membrane, the *serous pericardium,* also consists of two layers, the *parietal* layer, which lines the inside of the fibrous pericardium, and the *visceral* layer *(epicardium),* which lines the heart muscle. Between these two layers is a slight space *(pericardial space),* which is filled with a few drops of serous fluid *(pericardial fluid)*. These layers provide for frictionless movement of the heart muscle.

The muscular wall of the heart is the *myocardium*. Lining the inner surface of the myocardium is the *endocardium,* a thin layer of endothelial tissue.

The interior of the heart is divided into four chambers. The two upper chambers are called *atria* (or auricles), and the two bottom chambers are *ventricles*.* They are separated by a wall called the septum. Because of their different pumping actions, the walls of each chamber differ. The atria are smaller and thinner walled than the ventricles because they receive blood from the systemic (RA) and pulmonary (LA) circulation and only pump blood into the ventricles. The ventricles, on the other hand, pump blood into the lungs (RV) and into the entire systemic circulation (LV). Therefore, they are larger and more thick walled.

Located within the heart chambers are four *valves,* the main function of which is to prevent the back flow of blood (Fig. 35-1). The valves are attached to the heart muscle by several cordlike structures called *chordae tendineae*. The tricuspid valve, named because it has three flaps or cusps of endocardial tissue projecting into the ventricles, is located between the right atrium and ventricle. The *bicuspid* valve (also called the *mitral* valve), which has two flaps is located between the left atrium and ventricle. Together these two valves are often termed *atrioventricular* valves. The *semilunar* valves guard the opening from the right ventricle to the pulmonary artery (pulmonic valve) and from the left ventricle to the aorta (aortic valve). Heart sounds (S_1S_2) are related to the vibrations that result during closing of the valves (see p. 149).

Heart vessels

Five major blood vessels enter and leave the heart, completing the cycle of oxygenating the systemic circulation. The *inferior vena cava* and *superior vena cava* collect

*The following abbreviations are used to describe the chambers: RA, right atrium; LA, left atrium; RV, right ventricle; LV, left ventricle.

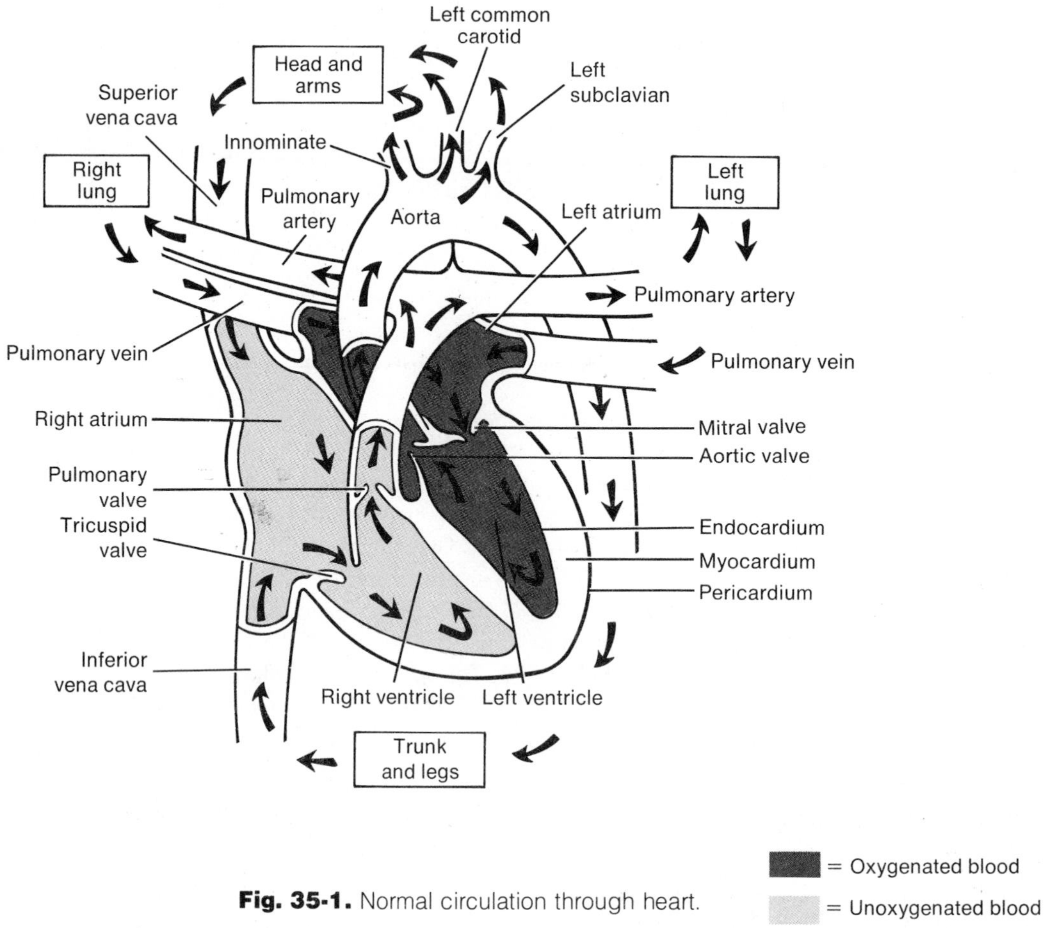

Fig. 35-1. Normal circulation through heart.

blood from the venous circulation and return it to the right atrium. Blood is pumped into the right ventricle, where it flows to the lungs by means of the *pulmonary artery,* which is the only artery to collect unoxygenated blood. However, by definition arteries always carry blood *away* from the heart. After leaving the lungs, oxygenated blood returns to the left atrium by means of the *pulmonary veins,* also the only veins to carry oxygenated blood. From the left ventricle the blood enters the systemic circulation by way of the *aorta* (Fig. 35-1).

Arteries serve primarily the function of distributing blood to the capillaries. Veins function as both collectors and reservoirs. Their function as a reservoir helps maintain normal circulation. For example, under conditions of increased cardiac resistance, blood backs up into the venous circulation, pooling in the liver and thus causing hepatomegaly. The function of the arterioles is mainly to provide resistance to blood flow to maintain blood pressure and circulation.

Although major blood vessels enter and leave the heart, the heart muscle receives its own coronary blood supply. The *right* and *left coronary arteries,* which arise from the aorta just behind the semilunar valve, supply all the myocardium, but most abundantly the left ventricle. *Coronary veins* collect the blood and return it directly to the right atrium or to the coronary sinus, which empties into the right atrium. Anastomoses that form between arteries provide collateral (secondary) circulation to various areas of the heart.

Heartbeat

The conduction system of the heart depends on four structures: (1) the sinoatrial (SA) node located within the right atrial wall near the opening of the superior vena cava, (2) the atrioventricular (AV) node, also located within the right atrium but near the lower end of the septum, (3) the atrioventricular bundle (bundle of His), which extends from the atrioventricular node along each side of the interventricular septum, and (4) Purkinje's fibers, which extend from the atrioventricular bundle into the walls of the ventricles (Fig. 35-2). The electric impulses from this conduction system, which allows the heart to beat in a rhythmic sequence, can be recorded in an electrocardiogram (see p. 1308).

The *sinoatrial node* initiates the heart's conduction system. It also possesses an intrinsic rhythm that maintains a constant heart rate. For these reasons it is called the body's

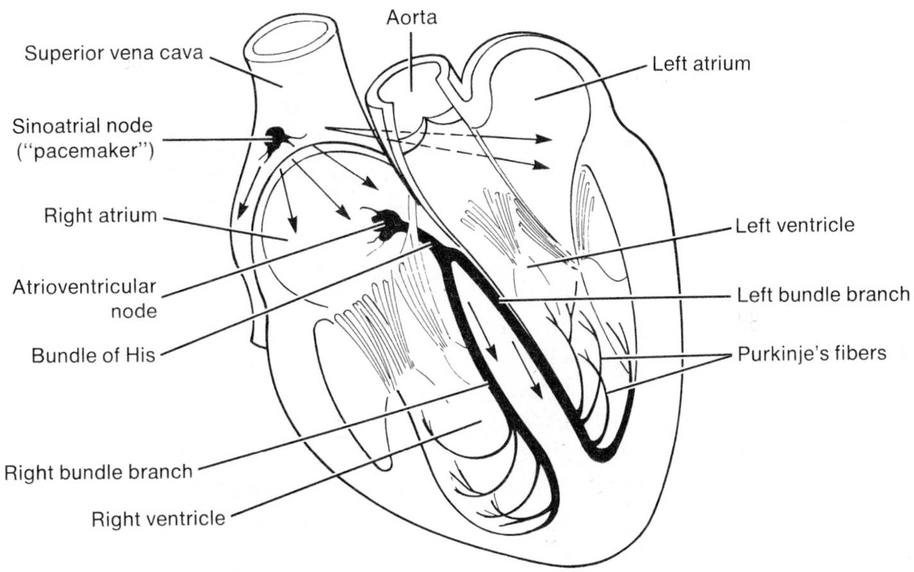

Fig. 35-2. Conduction system of heart.

pacemaker. The sinoatrial impulse spreads throughout the atria to cause contraction (depolarization). As the atria contract, impulses spread to the atrioventricular node to stimulate the ventricles. The atrioventricular node is the only normal pathway by which the impulse from the atria can be transmitted to the ventricles. The impulses then spread to the atrioventricular bundle and Purkinje's fibers to cause simultaneous contraction of the ventricles (depolarization).

A *cardiac cycle* is composed of complete contraction (systole) and relaxation (diastole) of both the atria and ventricles. The phases of contraction-relaxation occur in sequence. First the atria contract, forcing all of their blood into the relaxed ventricles. Then, as the atria relax (repolarization), the ventricles contract to force blood into the pulmonary artery and aorta. During the period of atrial repolarization blood enters the chambers from the systemic and pulmonary veins for emptying into the ventricles, thus completing one cardiac cycle. Although the atria or ventricles contract together, the events on the left side of the heart slightly precede those on the right.

Hemodynamics

The circulation of blood through the heart and the body is a complex process. Only the major events are discussed to facilitate understanding of normal and abnormal circulation.

Blood flows primarily as a result of *pressure* within the circulatory system. Because of resistance in various parts of the system, there exist pressure gradients. Like any fluid, blood flows from an area of high pressure to one of low pressure. If the pressure between two systems becomes equal, blood will no longer flow in a one-way direction. Rather it will pool in the area of least resistance, producing a damming effect. Since veins have a reservoir capacity, blood is most likely to pool in the venous circulation.

Another significant factor in maintaining blood pressure is *peripheral resistance,* or the force imposed by the friction of blood against the vessel walls. Viscosity is the main determinant of resistance and is the result of the formed elements of the blood within the plasma. Of all blood constituents, erythrocytes and, to a lesser extent, plasma proteins are responsible for viscosity. Therefore, hemodilution from anemia will result in lowered viscosity, decreased resistance, lowered pressure, and an increased workload on the pumping action of the heart.

Resistance also develops because of the size of the blood vessels. Resistance is inversely proportion to the diameter of the vessel. Therefore, resistance is greatest in the capillaries and least in the aorta. Any narrowing or constriction of a vessel will result in increased resistance and pressure. Likewise, vascular dilatation will result in lowered resistance and pressure.

Pressure within the veins is fairly constant but varies greatly in the arteries as a result of the contraction and relaxation of the heart. Therefore, blood pressure is measured by means of the arteries. The peak pressure that occurs during systole (ventricular contraction) is called *systolic pressure*. The lowest level reached during relaxation just before ventricular ejection is termed *diastolic pressure*. The difference between these two is the *pulse pressure*. Normally the systolic pressure is equal to the pressure in the left ventricle.

DIAGNOSTIC PROCEDURES

Diagnosis of congenital or acquired heart disease is based on a comprehensive history and physical examination and on a variety of specific and related diagnostic procedures. This discussion is an overview of each of these techniques. Specific findings are included under the discussion of the heart defect.

History

A complete history is essential regardless of the type of heart defect, although the importance of various aspects differs. For example, with congenital cardiac anomalies, a history of previous defects in a sibling, maternal rubella infection during pregnancy, or associated chromosomal abnormalities, such as Turner's or Down's syndrome, are important clues to diagnosis. In rheumatic fever a history of a previous streptococcal infection is of primary importance.

Several symptoms are significant for congenital heart disease (for those during infancy, see the boxed material on p. 1326). The major categories include a history of (1) poor weight gain, poor feeding habits, fatigue during feeding, and difficulty in swallowing or eating solid foods, (2) frequent respiratory infections and difficulties, such as dyspnea, anoxic spells, stridor, and paroxysmal hyperpnea, (3) evidence of persistent or intermittent cyanosis and clubbing of fingers, and (4) evidence of exercise intolerance, such as cyanosis or dyspnea on exertion and characteristic posturing, such as flaccid hyperextension during infancy and squatting during childhood.

Physical examination

Several aspects of the physical examination yield evidence of heart disease. (See Chapter 5 for a discussion of how to assess each of the following characteristics.) The most important is auscultation (1) to assess heart rate and rhythm, normal heart sounds, and adventitious sounds, such as friction rubs or murmurs, (2) to approximate anatomic landmarks for estimating size, such as the point of maximum impulse, and (3) to determine blood pressure.

Palpation and percussion are valuable in assessing the quality and symmetry of all pulses, in locating the cardiac, hepatic, and splenic borders for evidence of enlargement, and in determining adventitious sounds such as thrills.

Inspection of nutritional status, skin color, respiratory rate and rhythm, posturing, chest deformities or asymmetry, distended veins, and abnormal cardiac pulsations may help substantiate evidence of a cardiac defect.

Laboratory tests

Alterations in cardiac function are frequently reflected in compensatory increases in the erythrocyte count, hemoglobin level, and hematocrit. The physiologic basis for polycythemia in cyanotic heart defects is discussed later in this chapter. Thrombocytopenia is frequently associated with cyanotic defects, although the exact relationship between the two is unclear. Because of the lower plasma content to red blood cell count, clot retraction may be altered.

Oxygen saturation tests are done in children with cyanosis to measure the oxygen-carrying capacity of the blood. Normally arterial oxygen saturation is nearly 100%. Oxygen saturation below 92% is indicative of cyanotic heart disease. Oxygen saturation tests are done on arterial blood from femoral artery punctures or heel blood.

If capillary heel blood is used, the nurse first places the foot in warmed towels to increase the circulation of arterial blood. Blood samples are then packed in ice if the test is not done immediately.

Roentgenography

Three noninvasive tests include radiography, fluroscopy, and radiocardiography. In each test the child may be required to drink barium to provide a contrast background for the heart against the barium-filled esophagus. Radiography provides a permanent record of the size and configuration of the heart, its chambers, and the great vessels.

Fluoroscopy provides similar information but also demonstrates changes in function because it provides a dynamic evaluation of the heart in relation to the great vessels and lungs. However, it has the potential hazard of excess irradiation from prolonged exposure. Therefore, the child's eyes and gonads should be shielded and health personnel assisting with the test must wear protective lead devices. A special technique (skiagraphy) can provide a permanent cine film of the fluoroscopy.

Another radiologic technique (radiocardioangiography) is the use of a scintillation camera and intravenous injection of a special radioisotope (usually technetium pertechnetate) to visualize the filling of each chamber and major blood vessels as the blood circulates through the heart. The activity distribution of the radioactive material over the thorax and abdomen is recorded on videotape and serial photos are taken at successive stages in the heart's circulation. This procedure is effective for identifying abnormal pathways of circulation, especially through shunts, and is sometimes done as a preliminary test to cardiac catheterization. It has the advantage of taking only 5 to 10 minutes for the actual procedure and delivering a very low dose of radiation.

Cardiac catheterization

The most diagnostic invasive procedure is cardiac catheterization, in which a radiopaque catheter is inserted through a peripheral blood vessel into the heart. It is usually combined with angiography (angiocardiography), in which radiopaque media are injected through the catheter into the systemic/cardiac circulation. Angiocardiography yields four types of information: (1) oxygen saturation of blood within the chambers and great vessels, (2) pressure changes within these structures, (3) changes in cardiac output or stroke volume (the amount of blood pumped out of the left ventricle into the aorta with each contraction), and (4) anatomic abnormalities, such as septal defects and patent ductus arteriosus.

There are two main types of cardiac catheterizations: (1) right-sided catheterization, in which the catheter is introduced from a vein into the right atrium and (2) left-sided catheterization, in which the catheter is threaded by way of a systemic artery retrograde into the aorta and left ventricle or from a right-sided approach to the left atrium by means of a septal puncture. In children the most common method is a right-sided catheterization, since septal defects permit entry into the left side of the heart.

The catheter is usually introduced by way of the femoral vein through a cutdown procedure in which a small incision is made to expose the vessel or through a percutaneous technique, in which the catheter is threaded through a large-bore needle that is inserted into the vein. The latter approach is associated with fewer complications, such as infection, hemorrhage, or obstruction. The catheter is guided through the heart with the aid of fluoroscopy. As the physician advances the tubing, the child may feel pressure at the insertion site. Once within the heart chambers, the dye is injected and films are taken of the dilution and circulation of the material. At various times blood samples and blood pressure readings are taken for analysis.

Nursing considerations

Preprocedural preparation. The primary nursing consideration is preparation of the child and parents for the test. Although cardiac catheterization has become a routine diagnostic procedure, it is not without risks, especially in neonates, infants, and seriously ill children. Therefore, nursing judgment prior to and after the procedure is essential.

For older children, the nurse explains the basic principles of the test, such as where the "tube" will go and what the physician will see. If the nurse is unaware of the child's concept of the heart, the child should draw a picture so that the nurse can make certain that the explanation coincides with his level of understanding. Taking the time to establish an understanding of basic heart anatomy and physiology in preparation for this test is advantageous if heart surgery is anticipated. The nurse should consider the parents' needs for educational preparation as well.

It is important to explain what the room looks like, because the x-ray machinery can appear frightening. Some institutions routinely take the children on a brief tour of the area the day prior to the test. If this is not permitted, the child can be shown a picture (Fig. 35-3).

The nurse then explains the basic steps in the procedure, namely, that (1) the groin (or sometimes the antecubital

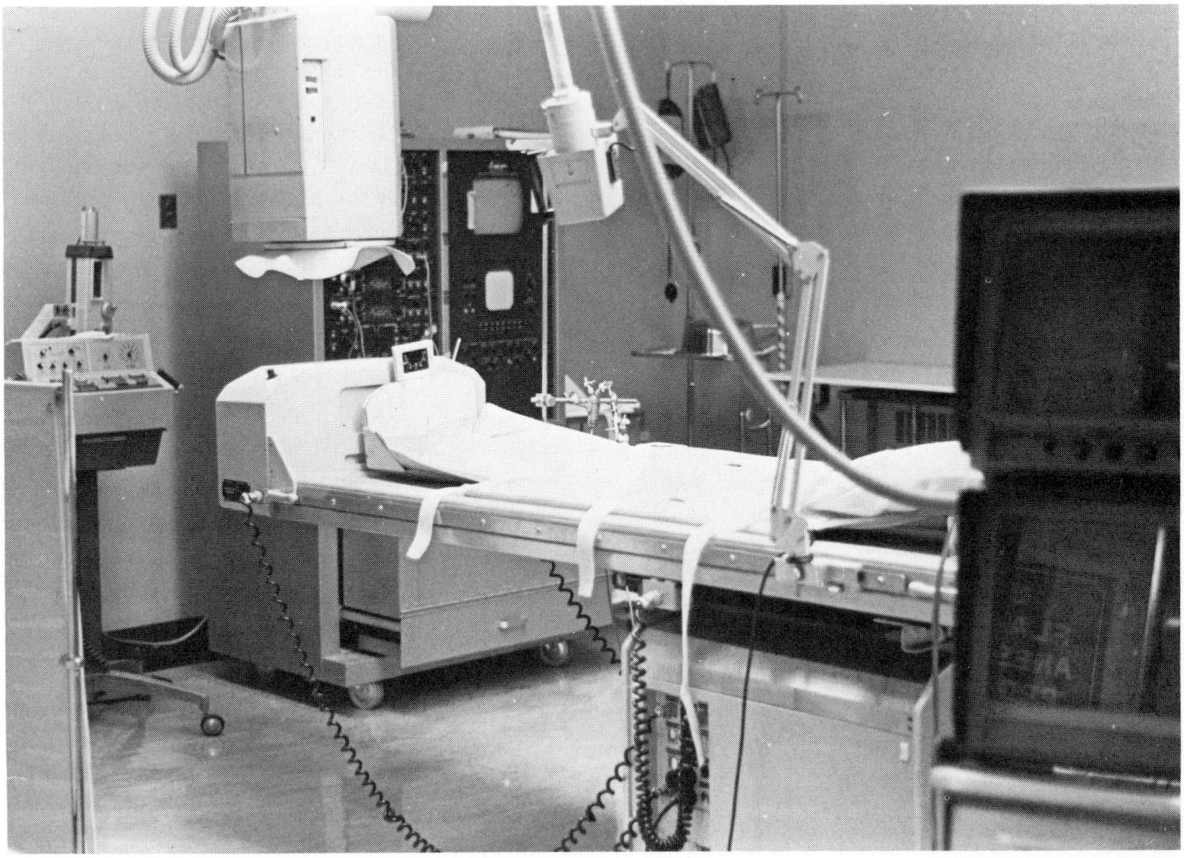

Fig. 35-3. Cardiac catheterization room.

fossa) is cleansed with a special yellow solution, (2) the physician will give him a needle and some medicine lidocaine (Xylocaine) in that area so that the skin will go to sleep, (3) a tube will be placed in a blood vessel, but the child will not feel pain but may feel a little pushing at times, (4) when a special medicine (the dye) is put into the tubing, the child may feel warm for a few seconds, and (5) as soon as the medicine is put in, the lights will go off and a machine will begin to take pictures.

The last point is important to stress because younger children may associate the lights going off with "causing" the warm feeling from the dye. As a result they may become fearful of the dark and the noise from the machines. It is also advisable to avoid using the word "dye" for the radiopaque solution, since children may interpret the word to mean "die." Older children may appreciate a more detailed explanation of how the dye aids in the diagnostic procedure, since this point can be elaborated on during the test to prevent boredom. An adequate explanation is helpful in ensuring the older child's cooperation during the long procedure, which may last from 2 to 5 hours. With a younger child, reading him stories during the test or allowing him to hold a favorite toy is a helpful suggestion for maintaining cooperation.

Other aspects of the test that should be mentioned are the use of electrocardiogram leads on the chest, a rectal or cutaneous electronic thermometer to monitor body heat, and body restraints to maintain immobility. The extent of preparation regarding these procedures depends on the child's age. Overpreparing the child, especially a preschooler, can add to the level of anxiety rather than decrease it.

Since the test is done under sterile conditions, all health personnel wear surgical garb. If the child is unfamiliar with this, he may become frightened by their masked appearance unless prepared beforehand.

Prior to the test the child is given sedation, such as injectable meperidine (Demerol) with promethazine (Phenergan) and chlorpromazine (Thorazine). It is best to leave this fact to the end of the discussion of the procedure, lest the child's anxiety concerning the need for two "needles" increase to the level of selective inattention. One approach toward conveying this point is to prepare the child with the preceding information early in the day and plan to return to evaluate the teaching at a later time. After the nurse is certain that the child understands what will happen during the test, the need for an injection prior to the cardiac catheterization can be introduced. The nurse can explain that this injection is the "I don't care shot" to make the child relaxed and comfortable during the test.[23]

The child is allowed nothing by mouth for 4 to 6 hours before the catheterization. Since young children often wonder why they do not receive breakfast, it is important to explain that this is because of the test and that, after it is over, they can have their breakfast and lunch. Ideally the child should be kept in a room with other children who are receiving nothing by mouth, since watching others eat may make him irritable. Usually the morning dose of oral digoxin is also withheld, although this is clarified beforehand with the physician.

Postprocedural care. There are several potential complications as a result of cardiac catheterization, including arrhythmias, cardiac perforation, hemorrhage, arterial obstruction, reactions to contrast media, infection, phlebitis, and hypoxia. The most important nursing responsibility is observation of the following for signs indicative of these problems: (1) vital signs, which are taken as frequently as every 15 minutes with special emphasis on heart rate counted for 1 full minute for evidence of arrhythmias or bradycardia, (2) blood pressure, especially for hypotension, which may indicate cardiac hemorrhage from perforation or bleeding at the site of initial catheterization, (3) pulses, especially below the catheterization site for equality and symmetry (pulse distal to the site may be weaker for the first few hours postcatheterization but should gradually increase in strength), (4) temperature and color of the affected extremity, since coolness, cyanosis, or blanching may indicate vessel obstruction, and (5) dressing for evidence of bleeding or hematoma formation in the femoral or antecubital area.

Usually the child is kept in bed for up to 24 hours after the procedure. Generally there is only slight discomfort at the cutdown or percutaneous site. The nurse protects the area from possible contamination, such as from soiling if the child wears diapers. If keeping the dressing dry is a problem, the nurse can cover it with a piece of plastic film by sealing the edges of the film to the skin with tape. The nurse must be careful, however, to continue to observe the site for any evidence of bleeding.

It is important at this time to evaluate the child's conception of what occurred during the procedure in order to clarify any misconceptions and allow the child a feeling of triumph and satisfaction in having gone through the experience.

Children's reactions after this procedure suggest that they do not perceive it as innocuous and may actually fear it more than the surgery.[1] One 7-year-old child's drawing of his tiny body on a large examining table with a huge x-ray machine hovering on top of him clearly demonstrated his feeling of powerlessness and insecurity. However, when the nurse remarked, "Look at how small you are next to that big machine," the child proudly answered, "Yes, but I made it!"

Electrocardiography

Electrocardiography (ECG or EKG) measures the electric impulses generated from the heart muscle and provides a graphic illustration of each phase of the cardiac cycle (Fig. 35-4). The *P wave* represents the electric activity associated

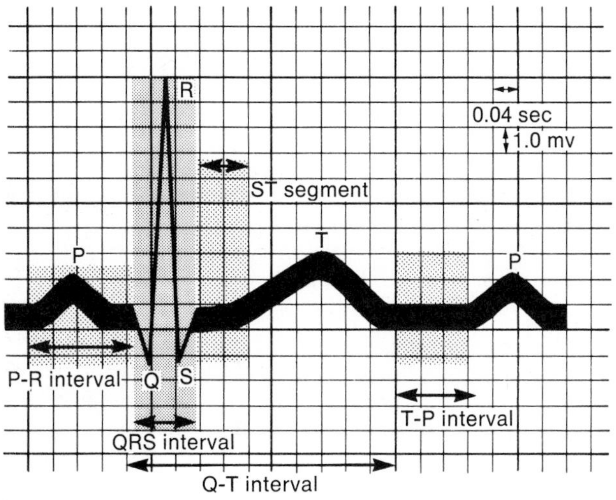

Fig. 35-4. Normal electrocardiogram pattern.

with the sinoatrial node and the spread of the impulse over the atria. It is a wave of depolarization.

The *QRS interval* represents the impulse generated from the atrioventricular node to Purkinje's fibers to cause ventricular contraction. Because there are really two waves of depolarization proceeding in different directions, the electric wave is more complex than the smooth P wave.

The *P-R interval* is measured from the beginning of the P wave to the beginning of the QRS complex. It is termed P-R instead of PQ because frequently the Q wave is absent. This interval represents the time that elapses between the activation of the sinoatrial node and activation of the atrioventricular node or, in other words, the atrioventricular conduction time.

The *T wave* is repolarization of the ventricles. The *Q-T interval* begins with the QRS complex and ends with the T wave. It represents electric systole or the period of electric ventricular contraction and relaxation (depolarization and repolarization). This interval varies with the heart rate. The faster the rate, the shorter the Q-T interval. Therefore, in children this interval is normally shorter than in adults.

The *S-T segment* is normally an isoelectric (flat) line that connects the end of the S wave to the beginning of the T wave. The *T-P interval* represents atrial and ventricular polarization in anticipation of the next cardiac cycle. Table 35-1 summarizes the major electric and mechanical events of the heart cycle and significant changes.

An electrocardiogram is taken by placing leads or electrodes on the skin to transmit electric impulses back to a recording machine. By means of telemetry, the pattern of electric impulses can be demonstrated on an oscilloscope. The position of the electrodes on the body and the manner in which they are attached to the electrocardiogram machine influence the type of recording. In older children and adults, a 12-lead electrocardiogram is usually taken, consisting of three standard leads on the extremities, six chest leads, and three unipolar or augmented leads, attached to one limb. In infants and small children many fewer leads may be used. Usually the electrodes are attached to the body with a rubber strap or a type of adhesive (for continuous monitoring). An electrolyte lubricant for electrolyte-soaked gauze is placed between the skin and lead to increase conductivity.

The PQRST complex is plotted on graph paper. Each small block represents 0.04 second horizontally and 1 mv (millivolt) vertically. By counting the number of squares intersected by the complex, one can calculate the various intervals, such as the P-R or Q-T interval, and the amplitude (height) of each wave. Other information supplied by an electrocardiogram includes heart rate, rhythm, abnormalities of conduction, muscular damage (ischemia), hypertrophy, electrolyte imbalance, effect of various drugs, and pericardial disease.

Vectorcardiography

The vectorcardiogram is a type of electrocardiogram, except that the information is represented differently because three leads yield simultaneous data about the relationship between electric impulses and myocardial function. It reflects both direction and amplitude and is especially helpful in diagnosing congenital defects.

Phonocardiography

A phonocardiogram is a graphic illustration of heart sounds. It may be obtained by placing a sensitive sound receiver directly on the body over the heart and great vessels or by introducing it by means of a catheter into the heart chamber during cardiac catheterization. It yields information about the timing of heart sounds, especially those that are too rapid or low for the human ear to hear.

Echocardiography

Echocardiography is the use of ultrasound to produce an image of the sound waves produced by the heart. It is a noninvasive procedure in which a transducer is placed directly on the chest wall and the sounds are analyzed on paper. It yields information about heart sounds but is more diagnostic in determining the exact location of the defect than the phonocardiogram.

Ultrasonography

Cardiac ultrasonography is the use of echocardiography synchronized with the electrocardiogram to produce a two-dimensional, stop-action image of a section through the heart. It differs from an echocardiogram, which gives a one-dimensional, time-motion recording of the intracardiac structures in the path of the narrow ultrasound beam. From images obtained in a variety of planes, it is possible to evaluate the size and shape of the heart chambers, appear-

Table 35-1. Cardiac cycle

ECG* sequence	Electrical event*	Mechanical action*	Heart sounds*	Significant changes
P wave† (0.03-0.09 second)	Depolarization of atria, impulse approaches atrioventricular node In atrioventricular node, slight delay in impulse conduction	Atrial contraction begins at peak of P wave Ventricles remain relaxed	Fourth heart sound	Enlargement of P wave deflection indicates atrial hypertrophy
P-R segment	Stimulus traverses His bundle and ventricular conductive system and starts into ventricular muscle	Conclusion of atrial contraction Atrioventricular valves remain open		
P-R interval (up to 0.14 second)	All above events	Atrial contraction		Lengthening indicates first-degree heart block resulting from conductive abnormalities
QRS complex (up to 0.08 second)	Orderly depolarization of ventricle: 1. Midseptum, left to right 2. Middle and lower free ventricular walls, endocardium to epicardium 3. Posterobasal or top portion, septum, and left ventricular wall Repolarization of atria	Ventricular contraction begins at peak of R wave: 1. Atrioventricular valves close 2. Isometric contraction of ventricles Beginning of atrial relaxation	First heart sound	Enlargement of R wave deflection indicates ventricular hypertrophy Decrease in amplitude of R wave occurs as a result of compression of the heart by fluid (pericardial effusion)
S-T segment (0.08 second)	Most ventricular cells remain depolarized Few cells begin ventricular repolarization	3. Opening of semilunar valves 4. Rapid systolic ejection 5. Ejection slows Atrial relaxation		Elevation above baseline occurs in pericarditis Depression results from hypoxia or digitalis therapy
T wave	Repolarization of ventricle; generally agreed occurs in opposite direction of depolarization: 1. Epicardium to endocardium 2. Apex to base	Continued slowing of ejection: 6. Closure of semilunar valves	Second heart sound	Enlargement indicates hyperkalemia
Q-T interval (up to 0.32 second)	Ventricular depolarization and repolarization	Ventricular contraction		
T-P interval (variable)	Both atria and ventricles polarized	Isometric relaxation of ventricle Opening of atrioventricular valves Rapid ventricular filling Slow diastolic filling of ventricle	Third heart sound	Lengthening occurs in bradycardia (digitalis therapy) Shortening occurs in tachycardia

*Data from Westfall, U. E.: Electrical and mechanical events in the cardiac cycle, Am. J. Nurs. **76**(2):231-235, February 1976.
†Duration for each segment varies with child's age and heart rate. Approximate values are for children under 3 years of age.

ance of valves, and size, position, and alignment of the great vessels. The technique is limited by the position of the heart against the chest wall, since the ultrasonic beam is impeded by bone or lung. However, like echocardiography, it is a noninvasive, painless, and safe procedure.

CONGENITAL HEART DISEASE (CHD)

The exact incidence of congenital heart disease in children is approximately 8 to 10 per 1000 live births. The sexes are affected differently, depending on the defect (Table 35-2). Heart defects are found in a much higher percentage of stillbirths and spontaneous abortions. The most common heart anomaly is ventricular septal defect. Some studies report that atrial septal defects and patent ductus arteriosus may be as frequent.

Etiology

The etiology of most congenital heart defects is not known. However, several factors are associated with a higher than normal incidence of the disease. These include *prenatal factors* such as (1) maternal rubella or other viruses, such as coxsackie virus, during pregnancy, (2) poor nutrition in the mother, (3) maternal alcoholism, (4) maternal age over 40 years, (5) diabetic women, (6) those taking lithium salts, and (7) possibly those taking progesterone during pregnancy.

Several genetic factors are also implicated in congenital heart disease. There is an increased risk of congenital heart disease in the child who (1) has siblings with a heart defect, (2) has parents with congenital heart disease, (3) has a chromosomal aberration, such as Down's syndrome, or (4) is born with other noncardiac congenital anomalies. Table 35-2 summarizes the incidence and recurrence risks of major cardiac defects and the increased risk in various disorders.

Types of defects

Congenital heart defects are usually divided into two types, based on the alteration in circulation: (1) acyanotic, in which there is no mixing of unoxygenated blood in the systemic circulation, and (2) cyanotic, in which unoxygenated blood enters the systemic circulation, regardless if cyanosis is clinically evident. Clinical manifestations depend on the severity of the defect and the degree of cyanosis more than the specific type of abnormality. In acyanotic defects no associated signs and symptoms may be apparent if the defect is small and the heart is able to compensate for the extra workload.

Altered hemodynamics. To understand the physiology of heart defects, one must recall that blood flows because of pressure and resistance. Normally the pressure on the right side of the heart is lower than that on the left side. Likewise, vessels entering or exiting from these chambers have corresponding pressures. Therefore, if there is an ab-

Table 35-2. Incidence and recurrence risks of congenital heart defects and association with other conditions

Anomaly	Male to female ratio	Risk of recurrence in child having one parent with CHD* (%)	Percentage of incidence of CHD in infants†	Disorders associated with increased incidence
Ventricular septal defect (VSD)	1:1	5.0	28.3	Down's syndrome Holt-Oram syndrome
Patent ductus arteriosus (PDA)	1:3	3.5	12.5	Rubella syndrome Down's syndrome
Atrial septal defect (ASD)	1:3	3.2	9.7	Holt-Oram syndrome Down's syndrome
Coarctation of the aorta	4:1	2.4	8.8	Turner's syndrome Apert's syndrome
Transposition of the great vessels (TGV)	3:1		8.0	Diabetes or prediabetes in the mother
Tetralogy of Fallot	1:1	3.2	7.0	Thalidomide ingestion Down's syndrome
Pulmonic stenosis	1:1	2.9	6.0	Turner's syndrome Rubella syndrome
Aortic stenosis	4:1	2.1	3.5	
Truncus arteriosus	1:1		2.7	Thalidomide ingestion
Other			13.5	

*Data from Nora, J. J., and Nora, A. H.: Recurrence risks in children having one parent with a congenital heart disease, Circulation **53**(4):701-702, April 1976.

†Data from Campbell, M. In Watson, A., editor: Paediatric cardiology, London, 1968, Lloyd-Luke, Ltd., Chapter 5.

normal connection between the heart chambers, such as a septal defect, blood will necessarily flow from an area of higher pressure (left side) to one of lower pressure (right side). This directional flow of blood is termed a left-to-right shunt. If the hole is small and high on the septum, the amount of blood shunted to the atrium or ventricle may be easily compensated for by a moderately increased cardiac effort. In this instance no unoxygenated blood flows directly into the left side of the heart, therefore, the term acyanotic defect (Fig. 35-5).

Severe acyanotic defects are potentially cyanotic, either as a result of pulmonary vascular changes or from associated or secondary defects. As large amounts of blood are shunted to the right side of the heart, the affected chamber enlarges to accommodate the volume and extra workload. At the same time the hypertrophied muscle is delivering the additional blood volume to the lungs, which eventually are unable to compensate for the vascular congestion, thus increasing pulmonary resistance. Blood then backs up into the right ventricle and/or atrium, causing a pressure change that can exceed that in the left side of the heart. As a result blood flow is shifted from the area of high pressure on the right to one of lower pressure on the left, with mixing of unoxygenated blood and, consequently, cyanosis.

Secondary defects that result because of the altered hemodynamics also contribute to the development of cyanosis. For example, enlargement of the right ventricle causes hypertrophy of the infundibulum, that portion of the heart muscle that narrows toward the origin of the pulmonary artery. Infundibular hypertrophy eventually results in pulmonic stenosis, which prevents blood from entering the lungs, causing a buildup of pressure behind the defect and permitting blood to flow across the septal opening of the left side of the heart.

Cyanotic heart defects may be the result of anomalies that cause a change in pressure so that the blood is shunted from the right to the left side of the heart, hence the term right-to-left shunt, because of either increased pulmonic vascular resistance or obstruction to blood flow through the pulmonary valve/artery. Cyanosis may also occur because of a defect that allows direct communication between the pulmonary and systemic circulations, such as an overriding aorta that receives unoxygenated blood from the right ventricle and oxygenated blood from the left ventricle.

Compensatory mechanisms. The body attempts to compensate for the decreased arterial oxygen saturation by increasing the pumping action of the heart, both through *increased force* (cardiomegaly) and *increased rate* (tachycardia). However, the increased workload necessitates a larger coronary blood supply for myocardial metabolism. Eventually a vicious cycle of increased ineffective pumping, increased cardiac oxygen demands, and decreased systemic output results. When the heart is no longer able to compensate, it is said to be in congestive failure. Myocardial hypoxia may result in attacks of angina, especially during exertion. Congestive heart failure is discussed in more detail later in the chapter.

Another compensatory mechanism is *polycythemia*. Decreased tissue oxygenation stimulates erythropoiesis, resulting in the production of large numbers of red blood cells. The theoretic benefit of this compensatory response is to carry supplemental oxygen by means of the increased erythrocytes to all cells. The actual result is a detrimental increase in the viscosity and volume of blood, which further increases resistance to blood flow, forcing the heart to work even harder. Circulation becomes sluggish, especially in the capillaries. As a result, the blood that is able to carry additional oxygen is not able to reach the peripheral circulation. Dehydration presents further hazards to the child because of the increased hemoconcentration.

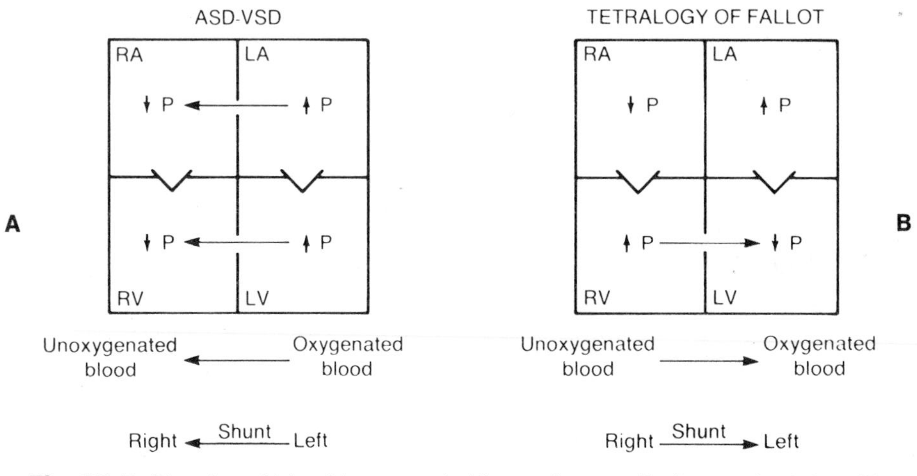

Fig. 35-5. Shunting of blood in congenital heart disease. **A,** Acyanotic defect; **B,** cyanotic defect.

Polycythemia is evident in hematologic tests. The red blood cell count is elevated (above 6 million/mm^3), the hematocrit is high (above 55%) as a result of both the absolute increase in erythrocytes and the increased ratio of red blood cells to plasma, and hemoglobin levels are elevated. However, the change in hemoglobin may be falsely high since the test measures the quantity of hemoglobin per 100 ml of whole blood, which contains excess numbers of red blood cells, not the quantity of hemoglobin within each cell. Because of the body's demand for iron during erythropoiesis, the child may actually be in a state of iron-deficiency anemia despite the usual laboratory findings in polycythemia. The red cell indices, especially the mean corpuscular hemoglobin (MCH), more accurately reflect the true hemoglobin levels. (See p. 1372 for a discussion of these tests.)

Posturing is a compensatory mechanism automatically learned by the child. During infancy the most characteristic positions are either flaccid with the extremities extended or side lying with the knees bent toward the chest (knee-chest position). The former position, in contrast to the normal flexed posturing of infants, is a response to tissue hypoxia. Continual muscle contraction demands additional oxygen supply. Flaccidity is usually a sign of progressive heart failure.

The knee-chest position and, later in childhood, the squatting position serve to decrease venous return by occluding the femoral vein through hip flexion, lessen the workload on the right side of the heart, and increase arterial oxygen saturation, especially to vital organs in the body.

Physical consequences. The general effects of heart malformation may be summarized as (1) increased workload in terms of systolic or diastolic overloading of the chambers, (2) pulmonary hypertension (increased vascular resistance), (3) inadequate systemic cardiac output, and possibly (4) arterial unsaturation from shunting of unoxygenated blood directly into the systemic circulation. The principal physical consequences of these changes, which may vary in severity, are growth retardation, decreased exercise tolerance, recurrent respiratory infections, dyspnea, tachypnea, tachycardia, cyanosis, and tissue hypoxia (Fig. 35-6).

Growth retardation and *decreased exercise tolerance* are direct consequences of inadequate nutrient intake and oxygen supply as a result of decreased cardiac output and/or arterial unsaturation for cellular metabolism. Con-

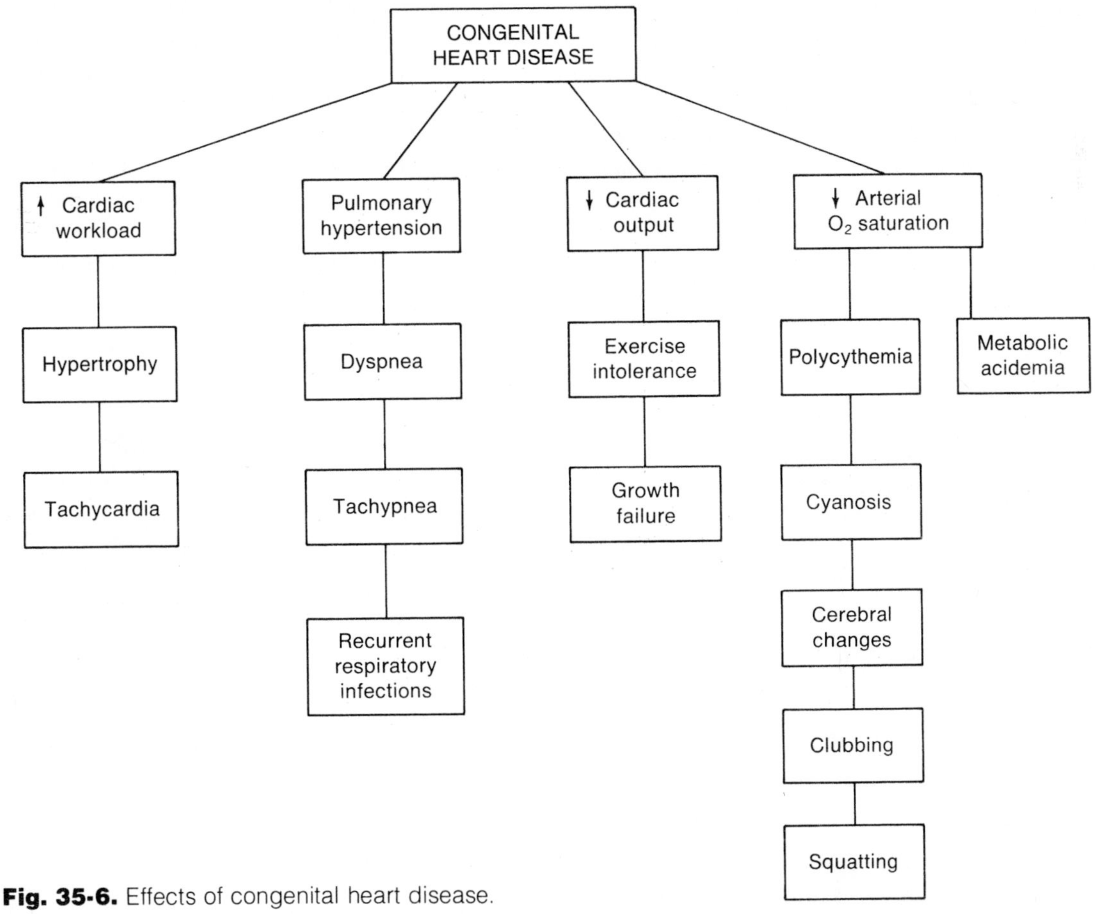

Fig. 35-6. Effects of congenital heart disease.

genital heart disease, especially with heart failure, may also be associated with gastrointestinal malabsorption and protein-losing enteropathy. Failure to gain weight, even during the neonatal period, and poor muscular development, both from decreased metabolism and disuse, are consistent findings. Exercise intolerance is usually first noted by the parent during feedings when the infant is too fatigued to consume the entire formula. The child often chokes, becomes dyspneic, and may turn cyanotic. As the child grows older, he learns to curtail his activity with the severity of the heart defect.

Recurrent respiratory infection is the result of pulmonary vascular congestion as large amounts of blood pool in the lungs, making it readily susceptible to bacterial or viral invasion and growth. The imposed immobility as a result of exercise intolerance also increases the risk of infection, since pulmonary ventilation may be compromised. *Dyspnea* also occurs from increased pulmonary resistance as the lungs are unable to oxygenate adequate supplies of blood, resulting in "air hunger." It may be associated with *tachypnea* as the lungs try to compensate through an increased respiratory effect. *Tachycardia* is the heart's attempt to increase cardiac output by increasing the number of beats per minute.

Cyanosis is the result of deoxygenated hemoglobin in the skin blood vessels, especially in the capillaries. In polycythemia, cyanosis is very common because of the large amount of hemoglobin. Cyanosis, therefore, reflects inadequate arterial blood oxygen saturation. Any event that increases metabolism and thus causes a demand for additional oxygen will result in a more severe degree of cyanosis. (See p. 118 for a discussion of evaluation of skin color.)

Persistent hypoxia may result in tissue changes anywhere in the body. A characteristic finding in cyanotic cardiac lesions is *clubbing* of the fingers, a thickening and flattening of the distal phalanges. Although the exact cause is unknown, some theories include soft tissue fibrosis and hypertrophy from anoxia and formation of increased numbers of capillaries to enhance blood supply. Decreased oxygen to the brain is often manifest in cerebral changes, such as fainting (syncope), mental confusion, seizures, and sometimes mental slowness.

Metabolic acidemia is a direct consequence of tissue hypoxia. If the supply of oxygen is inadequate for metabolic requirements of the cells, changes occur in the metabolic pathways. Normally pyruvic acid ends the glycolytic pathway (conversion of glucose to glycogen and vice versa) and is the gateway to the final common pathway, the Krebs' cycle, in the production of useful energy. However, under reduced arterial oxygen saturation, pyruvic acid is anaerobically converted to lactic acid, which accumulates in the tissue fluids. Lactic acid is incapable of further conversion, and, if steps are not taken to reconvert lactic acid to pyruvic acid by increasing tissue oxygen supplies and/or to reverse the acidemia by administering sodium bicarbonate or other bases, death will occur. In infants with cyanotic heart disease this complication is the most common cause of death.[7]

Murmurs. Another consequence of heart defects is murmurs, abnormal sounds produced by vibrations within the heart chambers or vessels. Auscultation of murmurs has been discussed on p. 150. This discussion is an overview of the types of murmurs heard in heart defects.

The most common cause of murmurs is an abnormal shunting of blood between two heart chambers or between vessels. However, murmurs can also be produced by disturbing the flow of fluid through a vessel as a result of (1) increasing the rate of flow, (2) constricting or dilating

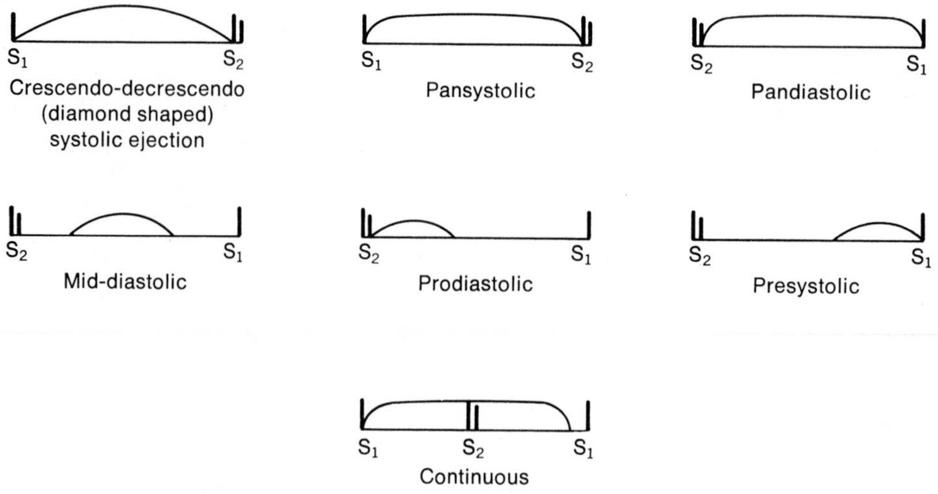

Fig. 35-7. Diagrammatic representation of murmurs.

the lumen, and (3) creating some type of irregularity on the vessel wall, which vibrates as fluid flows past, such as an aneurysm.

Murmurs are classified according to their timing within the cardiac cycle. Murmurs between S_1 and S_2 are *systolic*. Those between S_2 and S_1 are *diastolic*. Murmurs are also divided according to their timing within systole or diastole, namely, early, middle, or late. *Systolic ejection murmurs* begin after the first heart sound, attain a peak during midsystole, and terminate before the second heart sound. They typically have a crescendo-decrescendo quality in terms of intensity. Such a pattern is frequently referred to as diamond shaped. Murmurs that endure during all of systole are *pansystolic* or *holosystolic*. Those last during all of diastole are *pandiastolic* or *holodiastolic*. Early diastolic murmurs are called *prodiastolic,* whereas those occurring late are termed *presystolic*. Murmurs that continue through all of systole and all or part of diastole are *continuous* murmurs (Fig. 35-7).

Murmurs caused by congenital defects involving the septum or great vessels are usually heard best near the sternal borders or over the base of the heart. Those of valvular origin are typically loudest over the respective auscultating valvular area, in the direction of blood flow. Murmurs that originate on the right side of the heart are subject to change during respiration as a result of intrathoracic pressure that prolongs right ventricular filling. Therefore, murmurs originating on the right side of the heart increase during inspiration.

ACYANOTIC DEFECTS

Ventricular septal defect (VSD)

A ventricular septal defect is an abnormal opening between the right and left ventricle (Fig. 35-8). It may vary in size from a small pinhole to absence of the septum, resulting in a common ventricle. It is frequently associated with other defects, such as tetralogy of Fallot, transposition of the great vessels, patent ductus arteriosus, atrial defects, coartation of the aorta, pulmonic stenosis, and heart block. About 50% of the children will experience spontaneous closure of the defect, usually within the first to third years of life, as a result of growth and proliferation of the muscular septum, apposition of a cusp of the tricuspid valve against the defect, or formation of a membranous diaphragm across the opening.

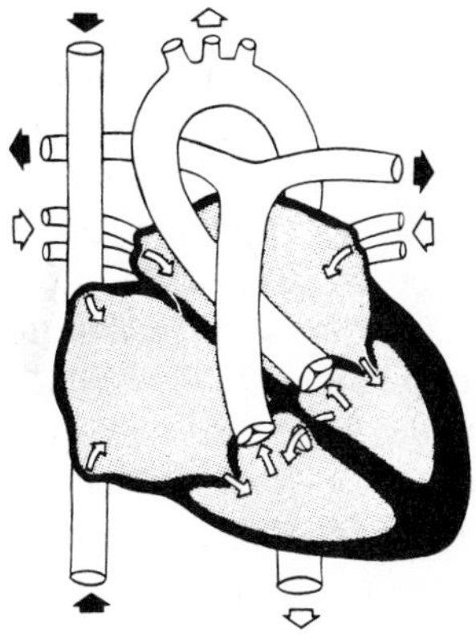

Fig. 35-8. Ventricular septal defects. (From Congenital Heart Abnormalities, Columbus, Ohio, 1968, Ross Laboratories.)

Altered hemodynamics. Because of the higher pressure within the left ventricle, blood flows through the defect to the right ventricle. The increased blood volume is pumped into the lungs, which eventually may become congested with blood, resulting in increased pulmonary vascular resistance. Increased pressure in the right ventricle as a result of left-to-right shunting and pulmonary resistance causes the muscle to hypertrophy. If the pressure is great enough, the right atrium may also enlarge as it attempts to overcome the resistance offered by incomplete right ventricular emptying.

In severe defects the infundibulum hypertrophies, resulting in pulmonic stenosis. Resistance to blood flow within the right ventricle eventually causes shunting of unoxygenated blood across the opening to the left ventricle and directly into the systemic circulation. The physical consequences are similar to those seen in tetralogy of Fallot, except that there is no overriding aorta.

Clinical manifestations. One of the most characteristic signs of a ventricular septal defect is a loud, harsh, pansystolic murmur that is generally heard best at the left lower sternal border and radiating throughout the precordium. The intensity of the murmur is not necessarily an indication of the defect's severity. In neonates the murmur may be absent because of the normally high pulmonary vascular resistance, which tends to equalize the pressure between the two ventricles. A systolic thrill is associated with loud murmurs.

Severe overloading of the right ventricle and occasionally a right atrium causes hypertrophy and an obvious cardiac enlargement. With increased pulmonary vascular resistance, dyspnea and frequent respiratory infections are common. Signs of cyanosis are possible, including a squatting position to decrease venous return.

Diagnostic evaluation. Diagnosis is confirmed with a cardiac catheterization that demonstrates an abnormal communication between the ventricles, possibly an obstruction at the entrance to the pulmonary artery (infundibular stenosis) as well as increased pressure and blood oxygenation in the right ventricle, resulting from shunting of oxygenated blood from the left ventricle. A phonocardiogram or echocardiogram is useful in evaluating the abnormal heart sounds. An electrocardiogram and x-ray examinations reveal right ventricular hypertrophy.

Treatment. Complete ventricular septal defect repair necessitates open-heart surgery and cardiopulmonary bypass to enter the heart chambers. A small defect is sutured with a purse-string approach (sewing around the opening and pulling it closed). Large defects usually require a knitted Dacron patch that is sewn over the opening. The optimum time for an elective complete repair is after 3 to 4 years of age.[10]

In children with large defects who cannot tolerate corrective surgery, a banding procedure is done on the pulmonary artery to decrease the pulmonary blood flow and consequent vascular resistance. The exact value of this palliative approach is controversial, since it combines the mortality rate for banding (in infants less than 3 months, a rate of 5% to 30%) and of complete repair (3% to 5%).[19] However, some physicians believe that it is less hazardous than corrective surgery, which has a mortality rate of 20% in sick infants under age 6 months. Overall survival for ventricular septal defect closure is 95% to 98%.[10]

Complications. Congestive heart failure is a frequent complication of severe ventricular septal defect, especially in infants. Treatment is primarily dependent on controlling the heart failure (see p. 1349). Other complications include infective endocarditis, development of aortic insufficiency or pulmonary stenosis, and progressive pulmonary vascular disease. A potential complication of surgical repair, especially of large defects, is damage to the ventricular conduction system, particularly the branch bundles and Purkinje fibers.

Atrial septal defect (ASD)

An atrial septal defect is an abnormal opening between the two atria (Fig. 35-9). Depending on the phase of arrested embryologic development, the lesion may be one of three types: (1) ostium secundum defects, in which the foramen ovale fails to close, (2) ostium primum defects, in which there is inadequate development of the endocardial cushions, and (3) sinus venosus defects, in which the superior portion of the atrial septum fails to form.

The severity of the defect depends on the size and location. Small defects located high on the septum, such as ostium secundum or sinus venosus defects, may result in no apparent clinical symptoms. However, extensive ostium primum defects are generally associated with mitral and tricuspid valve abnormalities, since both of these structures are derived from the endocardial cushions and may extend to the upper portion of the ventricles, creating a interventricular, as well as interatrial, communication. (This latter instance is often referred to as endocardial cushion defects rather than as atrial septal defects.) Sinus venosus defects may extend to the superior vena cava. In this instance the left atrium may receive unoxygenated blood, resulting in a potentially cyanotic heart condition.

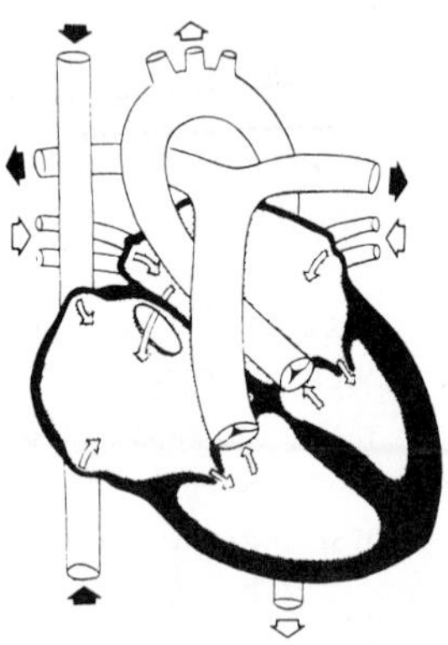

Fig. 35-9. Atrial septal defects. (From Congenital Heart Abnormalities, Columbus, Ohio, 1968, Ross Laboratories.)

Altered hemodynamics. Since pressure in the left atrium exceeds that in the right atrium, blood will flow from left to right, causing an increased flow of oxygenated blood into the right side of the heart. However, this volume is well tolerated by the right ventricle because it is delivered under much lower pressure than in a ventricular septal defect. Although there is right atrial and ventricular enlargement, cardiac failure is unusual in an uncomplicated atrial septal defect, since the pulmonary circulation is less affected by pressure changes.

Clinical manifestations. Atrial septal defects produce a characteristic crescendo-decrescendo type of systolic ejection murmur over the second to third interspace along the left sternal border. The murmur is not produced by blood flow across the defect as in ventricular septal defect because of lower atrial pressures but represents increased ventricular flow through the pulmonic valve to the pulmonary artery. It can be distinguished from innocent murmurs, which are similar, by having the child take a deep breath, hold it, and strain (Valsalva's maneuver). Normally when intrathoracic pressure is increased, systemic venous return and, therefore, right ventricular outflow decrease, in which case the innocent murmur disappears. However, with an atrial septal defect, right ventricular stroke volume is less affected so that the intensity of the murmur is unaltered or only slightly lowered.

Although the heart sounds are normal in intensity, there is a fixed splitting of the second sound. Normally the splitting between the two components of the second sound (aortic and pulmonic valve closure) increases during inspiration because of the delayed closure of the pulmonary valve. However, in atrial septal defect this splitting does not vary with respiration. The probable reason for this effect is that with increased right ventricular stroke volume and a low pulmonary vascular resistance there is consistently delayed pulmonic valve closure.

Children with more severe defects may demonstrate dyspnea and fatigue on exertion. Cyanosis is a possibility with involvement of the superior vena cava (sinus venosus defects) and ventricles (endocardial cushion defects).

Diagnostic evaluation. The most suggestive sign of

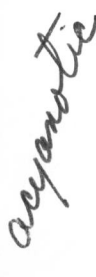

atrial septal defect is fixed splitting of the second sound. Cardiac catheterization definitively demonstrates the abnormal opening in the atrial septum and higher pressures and increased oxygen saturation on the right side of the heart. X-ray findings include right atrial and ventricular hypertrophy and usually pulmonary dilatation from increased blood flow. The electrocardiogram may demonstrate right atrial and right ventricular enlargement.

Treatment. Unless the defect is severe, prophylactic closure is usually postponed until later childhood (prior to entry to school) to prevent possible complications during early adulthood, such as congestive heart failure, pulmonary vascular disease, bacterial endocarditis, and atrial arrhythmias (probably from atrial enlargement and effect on conduction system). Closure involves the same principles as discussed under ventricular septal defect. Postoperative complications are unusual, and survival is greater than 99%.[10] A potential complication following surgical correction, especially of ostium primum defects, is damage to the atrial conduction system.

Patent ductus arteriosus (PDA)

A patent ductus arteriosus is failure of that fetal structure to completely close after birth (Fig. 35-10). In fetal life the ductus arteriosus connects the pulmonary artery to the aorta in order to shunt oxygenated blood directly into the systemic circulation by bypassing the lungs. At birth functional closure of the ductus arteriosus occurs within a few hours as a result of constriction of smooth muscle in its vessel walls from exposure to increased oxygen tension. Complete anatomic closure may take several weeks. However, in premature infants the ductus arteriosus does not respond to the constrictor effect of oxygen; therefore, normally this vessel remains patent until the neonate reaches gestational maturity.

Altered hemodynamics. A patent ductus arteriosus allows blood from the aorta (a vessel of high pressure) to flow into the pulmonary artery (a vessel of lower pressure). The additional blood is reoxygenated in the lungs and returned to the left atrium and left ventricle. The effect of this altered circulation is increased workload on the left side of the heart, increased pulmonary vascular congestion and resistance, and, potentially, increased right ventricular pressure and hypertrophy.

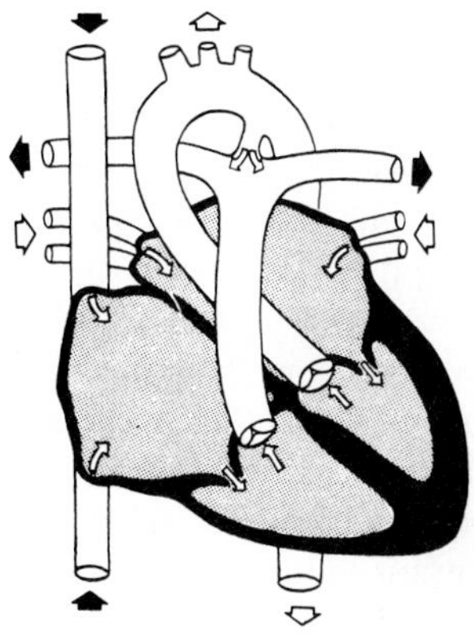

Fig. 35-10. Patent ductus arteriosus. (From Congenital Heart Abnormalities, Columbus, Ohio, 1968, Ross Laboratories.)

Clinical manifestations. The turbulent flow of blood from the aorta through the patent ductus arteriosus to the pulmonary artery results in a characteristic machinery-like murmur, which is heard best at the mid to upper left sternal border. Since there is a continuous flow of blood across the shunt, the murmur is heard during all of systole and most of diastole. It is usually associated with a thrill.

Another common feature is a widened pulse pressure. The systolic pressure rises because the increased left ventricular stroke volume causes a rapid rise in the aortic pressure. The low diastolic pressure is a result of the continuous shunting or runoff of blood through the aortopulmonary communication and reduced peripheral resistance. Cardiomegaly is a consistent finding with enlargement of the left atrium, left ventricle, and possibly right ventricle. The ascending aorta, which receives excess blood under high pressure from the ventricle, is often dilated. Other clinical signs include bounding pulses (from increased systolic pressure), tachycardia, and sometimes a gallop rhythm (caused by rapid filling of the ventricles).

Diagnostic evaluation. The machinery type-murmur is almost diagnostic of patent ductus arteriosus, but it may be absent in neonates or premature infants because of the normally high pulmonary resistance that tends to equalize the pressure between the two vessels. X-ray examinations usually demonstrate left-sided cardiac and right ventricular enlargement, ascending aortic dilatation from increased left ventricular output, and evidence of increased pulmonary vasculature. The electrocardiogram is generally normal, although it may demonstrate left ventricular enlargement. Usually a cardiac catheterization is not necessary to confirm the diagnosis because of the characteristic auscultatory and radiologic findings. An echocardiogram is useful if there is a question of heart changes resulting from the defect or from primary pulmonary disease.

Treatment. Surgical intervention involves surgical division or ligation of the patent vessel. Since the defect is outside the heart chamber, a cardiopulmonary bypass is not necessary. However, it is still a major operative procedure, since the thoracic cavity must be entered. Whenever possible the procedure is delayed until the child is old enough to tolerate surgery and to allow time for spontaneous closure, especially in children born prematurely. The optimum time is after 1 year of age but prior to starting school.[10]

Treatment is recommended even if there are no clinical

indications because of the risk of developing congestive heart failure, pulmonary vascular disease, calcification at the ductal site, and infective endocarditis. In premature infants surgical intervention may be warranted to prevent the complication of necrotizing enterocolitis, which results from chronic intestinal hypoxia. The mortality rate for elective ductal closure is less than 1% but is slightly higher in sick premature infants or newborns.[10]

Coarctation of aorta

Coarctation (*coarct,* to press together) of the aorta is a localized narrowing of the aorta in an otherwise normal vessel (Fig. 35-11). The usual position of the narrowing, called *preductal,* is proximal to the insertion of the ductus arteriosus, commonly between that vessel and the subclavian artery. In the *postductal* type the constriction is distal to the ductus arteriosus. Since in most instances the aortic narrowing is closely related to the ductus arteriosus, the term *juxtaductal coarctation* may be used.

Altered hemodynamics. The effect of a narrowing within the aorta is increased pressure proximal to the defect and decreased pressure distal to it. In the preductal type pressure may increase in the left ventricle, causing left ventricular hypertrophy. If the ductus arteriosus closes gradually, compensary mechanisms, such as myocardial hypertrophy and collateral circulation, may develop to decrease the effect of pressure changes.

Clinical manifestations. Because of the relationship of coarctation of the aorta to the ductus arteriosus, there are two periods of life when clinical manifestation are apparent: (1) early infancy after closure of the patent ductus arteriosus, and (2) early adulthood when growth of the aorta results in a concentric ring of obstruction. The signs and symptoms are directly related to the pressure changes created by the aortic constriction. Those areas of the body that receive blood from vessels proximal to the defect experience high blood pressure and bounding pulses. In the

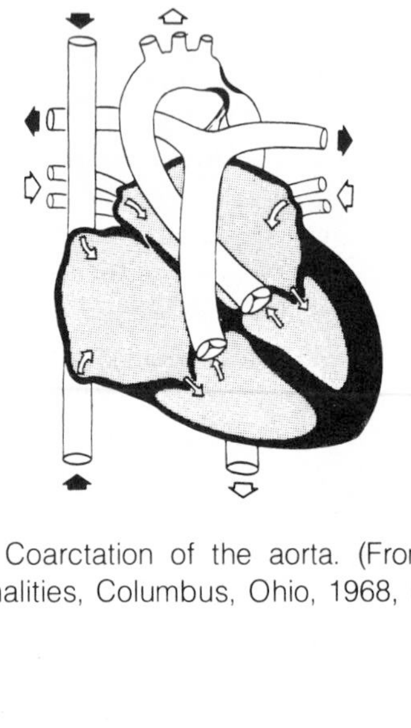

Fig. 35-11. Coarctation of the aorta. (From Congenital Heart Abnormalities, Columbus, Ohio, 1968, Ross Laboratories.)

postductal type these changes occur bilaterally in the upper extremities and head. However, if the constriction is between the insertion of the innominate and left subclavian arteries, the right side will have bounding radial and carotid pulses with high blood pressure readings whereas the left side will have diminished pulses and pressure. Because of the large volume of blood circulating to the head, the child may experience dizziness, headaches, fainting, and epistaxis.

Those areas of the body distal to the defect receive a decreased blood supply. As a result the femoral pulses are weak or absent, the lower extremities may be cooler than the upper ones, and muscle cramps may result during increased exercise from tissue anoxia. If collateral pathways have developed, the only sign may be absent femoral pulses. Therefore, the circulatory changes characteristic of this condition emphasize the importance of routinely assessing the equality of each pulse and comparing blood pressure readings in both arms.

A murmur may or may not be present. A soft high-frequency continuous murmur may be heard high on the sternal border. It represents rapid blood flow through collateral pathways. Notching of the lower margin of ribs may be evident as collateral or enlarged intercostal arteries erode the bone.

Diagnostic evaluation. Diagnosis is based on the characteristic physical findings relating to pressure differences in the upper and lower body. Radiologic studies also demonstrate specific findings, such as notching of the lower end of the ribs, left ventricular hypertrophy, and dilatation of the aorta proximal to the stricture, which is most evident if seen contrasted with a barium-filled esophagus.

Treatment. Surgical treatment is either resection of the coarcted portion with an end-to-end anastomosis of the aorta or replacement of the constricted section using a graft of transplanted aorta. Because the defect is outside the heart chambers, only the thoracic cavity is entered.

The timing of the surgery is significant, since too early intervention may result in excessive strain on the suture line and inadequate diameter of the vessel. The recommended age is between 3 and 5 years.

Complications. Corrective surgery is recommended for children even with minor defects because of the high incidence of complications, including intracranial hemorrhage and stroke, hypertension, a ruptured aorta, hypertensive heart disease, congestive heart failure, the possibility of a ruptured dissecting aortic aneurysm, and infective endocarditis, especially in the dilated poststenotic area of the aorta and the aortic valve. (A dissecting aneurysm is a circumscribed intramural dilatation of the aorta in which blood forces its way between the layers of the walls of the aorta. In coarctation it is the result of degenerative changes within the vessel wall.)[20]

After coarctectomy there are symptoms of gastrointestinal disturbance, especially abdominal pain, distention, and nausea and vomiting. Although the exact reason is not known, it is believed to be caused by increased blood supply to vessels that have previously received blood under lower pressure. Systemic hypertension also occurs. The treatment is to lower blood pressure with antihypertensive medication.

Survival rate after repair in the older child is 96%, but in infants it decreases to 83%.[10]

Pulmonic stenosis

Pulmonic stenosis is a narrowing at the entrance to the pulmonary artery (see Fig. 35-13). Usually the valve is normal, but the raphae (divisions between the cusps) are fused so that movement is restricted. Stenosis may also occur from infundibular hypertrophy.

Altered hemodynamics. In pulmonic stenosis resistance to blood flow causes right ventricular hypertrophy. If the increased pressure is greatly elevated, backup of blood into the right atrium may result in a patent foramen ovale and shunting of unoxygenated blood into the left atrium. If pulmonic stenosis is severe, the right ventricle will be incapable of ejecting the total venous blood into the pulmonary circulation, resulting in systemic cyanosis. An associated defect such as a patent ductus arteriosus partially compensates for the obstruction by shunting blood from the aorta to the pulmonary artery and into the lungs. The resistance to venous return to the heart causes hepatomegaly and prominent pulsating neck veins, as well as eventual right-sided heart failure.

Clinical manifestation. Symptoms depend on the degree of the defect. They can range from only the presence of a murmur to cyanosis and congestive heart failure. A systolic ejection murmur is heard best over the second left intercostal space lateral to the sternum, radiating to the infraclavicular area. It is usually accompanied by a systolic thrill caused by the flow of blood through a narrowed orifice. Because of the delay in right ventricular ejection, the pulmonary component of the second heart sound is widely split. In severe defects the pulmonic component of the second heart sounds becomes less distinct or totally disappears as a result of pulmonic valve insufficiency. Cardiomegaly is a frequent finding from right-sided hypertrophy.

Children with moderate defects generally experience dyspnea and fatigue, especially on exertion, since blood flow to the lungs is insufficient to accommodate demands for increased cardiac output. Children with severe defects will demonstrate signs of cyanosis, congestive heart failure, decreased systemic output, and increased venous resistance.

Diagnostic evaluation. A cardiac catheterization demonstrates the obstruction to the pulmonary artery, any associated defects such as atrial septal defect, and increased pressure in the right side of the heart. Depending on the exact anatomic defects, it may reveal decreased oxygenation in the left side of the heart from a right-to-left shunt (atrial septal defect) and decreased pulmonary blood flow. Radiologic studies show an enlarged heart, usually with normal pulmonary vascular markings (in contrast to other defects in which the lungs receive an overload of blood and become congested) and poststenotic dilatation of the pulmonary artery.

An electrocardiogram may show several changes, including right atrial and ventricular hypertrophy and conduction changes. Echocardiography is useful in analyzing the murmur and changes in the second heart sound.

Treatment. Surgical intervention consists of a pulmonary valvotomy. Entry into the right ventricle is usually required to gain access to the stenotic area, necessitating open-heart surgery. Surgery is recommended for children with severe defects, but the exact criteria for intervention in asymptomatic children are unclear. The indication is a rise in right ventricular systolic pressure that eventually leads to myocardial damage as a result of tissue ischemia from continuous requirements of increased coronary blood flow.

Optimum time for elective surgery is any age past 2 to 3 years. Survival rates for infants and older children are 99% or better.[10]

Aortic stenosis

Aortic stenosis is a narrowing or stricture of the aortic valve. It is usually caused by malformed cusps or fusion of the cusps. Subaortic stenosis is a stricture caused by a fibrous ring below the valve or a membranous diaphragm in the outflow tract of the left ventricle (Fig. 35-12).

Altered hemodynamcis. A stricture at the origin of the aorta causes resistance to blood flow in the left ventricle and decreased cardiac output. The extra workload on the left ventricle causes hypertrophy and increased demands for coronary blood supply. Backup of blood into the left

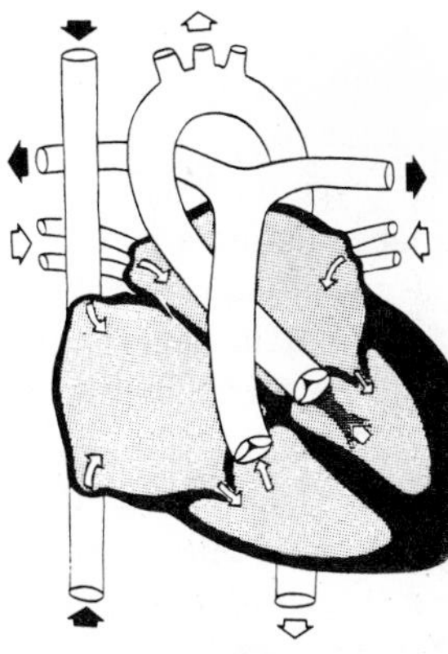

Fig. 35-12. Subaortic stenosis. (From Congenital Heart Abnormalities, Columbus, Ohio, 1968, Ross Laboratories.)

atrium causes increased pressure in that chamber and the pulmonary veins, resulting in pulmonary vascular congestion.

Clinical manifestations. If the stenosis is severe, infants will demonstrate evidence of decreased cardiac output, such as faint peripheral pulses, exercise intolerance, and anginal pain. Children with less severe stenosis may not show signs of the defect until physical growth demands exceed cardiac output. Clinical manifestations such as fainting, epigastric or anginal pain, exercise intolerance, and dizziness after prolonged standing may occur. A serious consequence is sudden death after exertion as a result of a severely ischemic heart.

A murmur is typically heard with aortic stenosis from the regurgitation of blood back into the left ventricle. It varies from a crescendo-decrescendo systolic ejection murmur (in mild defects) to a loud pansystolic murmur (in severe defects). It is heard best at the upper right sternal border to second interspace (aortic space) and radiates to the suprasternal notch, clavicular area, and neck. Sometimes it is transmitted along the left sternal border to the apex. It is usually associated with a thrill.

The second heart sound is characteristically affected. Because the closure of the aortic valve is delayed, the normal splitting of S_2 is narrowed. With severe stenosis the left ventricular ejection may be so prolonged that the closure of the pulmonic valve occurs simultaneously or precedes that of the aortic valve. In the former instance there is no splitting. In the latter event the usual splitting of S_2 narrows with inspiration (the pulmonic component being delayed) and widens with expiration (paradoxical splitting).

Diagnostic evaluation. Diagnosis is rarely made on the history and physical findings alone. A cardiac catheterization is necessary to determine the stenotic area, especially in those children with minimal symptoms who are at risk for acute myocardial ischemia. It is also diagnostic in terms of the surgical approach. If a thin membrance is present, this is easily removed with excellent results.

Radiologic studies may confirm left-sided heart enlargement, increased pulmonary vascularity, and a dilated aorta in the poststenotic area. An electrocardiogram may show left ventricular hypertrophy or may be normal in mild defects unless taken during a period of exercise. Depression of the ST segment indicates myocardial hypoxia. Echocardiography is useful in analyzing the changes in the second heart sound, especially the aortic component.

Treatment. Surgical intervention for valvular aortic stenosis involves opening the valve orifice (commissurotomy). It may be indicated in children with minimal symptoms who demonstrate myocardial ischemia. Unfortunately there is a high incidence in later life of restenosis following a valvotomy, which requires additional surgery on the valve or prosthetic replacement. Survival after a valvotomy is 85% in infants and 97% in older children.[10]

CYANOTIC DEFECTS

Tetralogy of Fallot

Tetralogy of Fallot is the most common cyanotic heart disease in children. The classic form (of which there are several variations) includes four defects: (1) ventricular septal defect, (2) pulmonic stenosis, (3) overriding aorta, and (4) right ventricular hypertrophy (Fig. 35-13). The first three defects are congenital, and the fourth is acquired as a result of the increased pressure within the right ventricle.

Altered hemodynamics. Shunting of blood through the ventricular septal defect is in the direction of right to left because the pulmonic stenosis, which impedes the flow of blood to the lungs, causes an increased pressure in the right ventricle, forcing unoxygenated blood through the septal defect to the left ventricle. The increased workload on the right ventricle causes hypertrophy. The decreased flow of blood to the lungs compounds the amount of unoxygenated blood reaching the systemic circulation.

Alone, the associated defects of pulmonic stenosis and ventricular septal defect produce cyanosis. However, the addition of an aorta that arises from the septal defect or from the right ventricle also adds to the severity of the cyanosis, since it accepts unoxygenated blood directly from the right ventricle. Fortunately the occurrence of this defect varies greatly.

The body attempts to compensate for the anoxia through polycythemia. However, the resultant viscosity of the blood increases pressure, slows circulation, and may lead to complications such as thrombophlebitis, emboli, and cerebrovascular disease.

Clinical manifestations. Newborns usually do not demonstrate cyanosis because of a patent ductus arteriosus that shunts blood to the lungs, bypassing the pulmonic stenosis. Anoxic spells become evident when the infant's oxygen requirements exceed the blood supply, usually

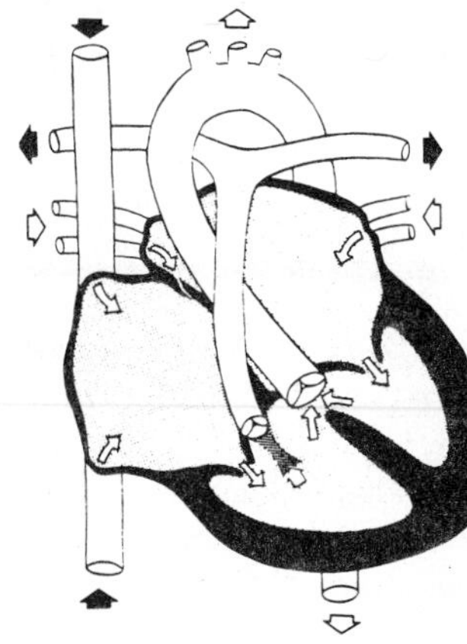

Fig. 35-13. Tetralogy of Fallot. (From Congenital Heart Abnormalities, Columbus, Ohio, 1968, Ross Laboratories.)

during crying or after feeding. The acute severe episodes of cyanosis and hypoxia are often called "blue spells," or the infant is termed a blue baby. The spells may be very brief or prolonged with subsequent limpness, exhaustion, and sleepiness. The infant characteristically assumes a hypotonic extended position.

As the child grows older he learns to limit his activity in accordance with the physical disability. He also learns that squatting helps relieve the chronic hypoxia (Fig. 35-14). He usually prefers this position to standing, sitting, or lying. When reclining he may assume a knee-chest position rather than an extended position. Since such posturing is unusual in children, this should always call attention to a cardiac defect. Children with less severe cyanosis may assume the squat position only after exertion.

Besides physical evidence of cyanosis, the child demonstrates clubbing of the fingers (Fig. 35-15) and markedly delayed physical growth and development. Fainting and/or mental slowness may occur from chronic hypoxia to the brain. Seizures may occur after exertion.

Typically these children do not develop congestive heart failure because the overload of blood in the right ventricle flows freely through the septal defect or the overriding aorta into the systemic circulation. Consequently blood does not back up into the pulmonary circulation by way of left atrial hypertrophy, as in pulmonary stenosis without ventricular septal defect.

A pansystolic murmur is usually heard at the mid to lower left sternal border. It is usually associated with a thrill, which may be felt along the lower left sternal border. Both findings are usually less prominent in severe pulmonic obstruction, since blood flows directly through the septal defect and/or overriding aorta.

Typically the pulmonic component of the second heart sound is faint or absent, as a result of failure of that valve to function. As a result a single second heart sound, caused by closure of the aortic valve, is heard. Cardiomegaly may or may not be obvious, depending on the size of the septal defect in allowing blood to flow into the left ventricle.

Diagnostic evaluation. A diagnosis is usually made on the history and physical findings alone. However, a cardiac catheterization is performed to evaluate the severity of the anatomic defects and cardiac changes. Laboratory tests determine the degree of polycythemia and arterial oxygen unsaturation. These determinations are important in evaluating the child's exercise tolerance.

X-ray examinations may or may not indicate cardiomegaly. However, x-ray studies are helpful in differentiating this defect from others because they demonstrate normal or decreased pulmonary vascularity (in contrast to transposition of the great vessels, for example). They may also reveal a "boot-shaped" heart formed from a concavity

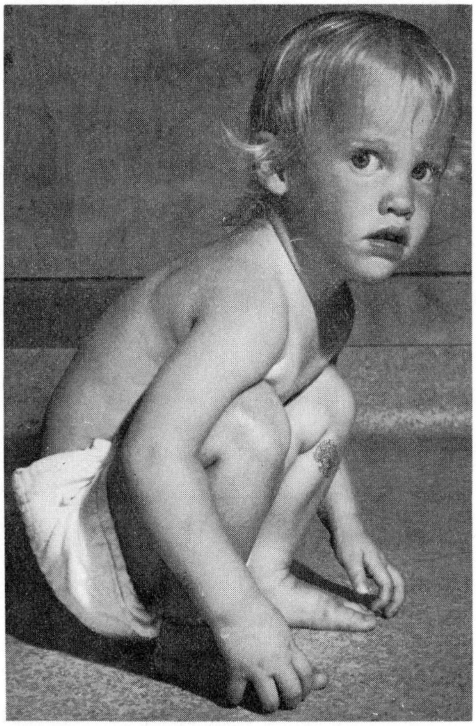

Fig. 35-14. The characteristic squatting position assumed by the child with tetralogy of Fallot. (From Ingalls, A. J., and Salerno, M. C.: Maternal and child health nursing, ed. 3, St. Louis, 1975, The C. V. Mosby Co., p. 587.)

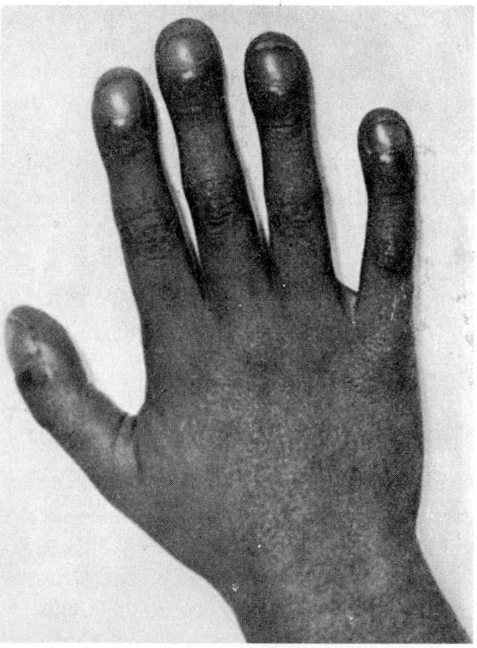

Fig. 35-15. Clubbing of the fingers. (From Ingalls, A. J., and Salerno, M. C.: Maternal and child health nursing, ed. 3, St. Louis, 1975, The C. V. Mosby Co., p. 587.)

in the upper left margin resulting from a hypoplastic main pulmonary artery. An electrocardiogram and echocardiogram are of variable aid in detecting the defect.

Treatment. Supportive treatment usually begins as soon as the defect is diagnosed to decrease tissue hypoxia and prevent complications until the child is old enough to tolerate total corrective surgery. Usually much of the supportive care depends on parental intervention (see summary of nursing care of the child with congenital heart disease, p. 1329).

Several palliative surgical procedures may be performed to increase pulmonary blood flow. The most common systemic-to-pulmonary anastomoses include a side-to-side anastomosis of the ascending aorta to the right pulmonary artery in neonates (Waterston-Cooley shunt) and a subclavian-pulmonary artery anastomosis in older infants and children (Blalock-Taussig operation). The selection of blood vessels to create a type of ductus arteriosus is based on the child's age. For example, an aortopulmonary anastomosis in an older child would allow too much blood to enter the pulmonary circulation, increasing the risk of congestive heart failure. Likewise, a subclavian-pulmonary shunt may be too small in an infant.

A successful systemic-pulmonary anastomosis relieves anoxic spells, cyanosis, and clubbing and increases activity tolerance. It also produces the characteristic machinery-type murmur of a patent ductus arteriosus. In some individuals the shunt may permit adequate functioning for several years.

The preferred surgical intervention is complete repair of the defects, that is, closure of the ventricular septal defect, pulmonic valvotomy, as well as, when it is indicated, correction of the overriding aorta. Many cardiologists believe that this one-stage approach is preferable to palliative and subsequent corrective surgeries that carry a combined mortality rate of 20% to 50% or greater. Recent attempts at complete repair in symptomatic infants have yielded much lower mortality rates.[19] Psychologically it is advantageous because it prevents the development of a "cardiac cripple," a child who continues to live as an invalid despite corrective surgery (see p. 1341). The optimal age for elective repair is after age 3 to 4 years but before school age. Survival after total correction in these children is 90% or better.[10]

Transposition of the great vessels

By definition, transposition of the great vessels refers to a condition in which the pulmonary artery leaves the left ventricle and the aorta exits from the right ventricle (Fig. 35-16). Obviously this type of circulation is incompatible with extrauterine life because there exist two separate circuits of blood flow with no communication between systemic and pulmonary circulations. However, associated defects such as septal defects or a patent ductus arteriosus permit blood to enter the systemic circulation and/or the pulmonary circulation for mixing of unoxygenated and oxygenated blood (Fig. 35-17).

Associated defects and hemodynamics. The most common associated defect is a patent foramen ovale (atrial septal defect). At birth there is also a patent ductus arteriosus, although in most instances this closes functionally and anatomically in the neonate. The other compensatory anomaly is a ventricular septal defect. However, presence of these defects can increase the problems of congestive heart failure as a result of the yet larger amounts of blood flowing through the heart to the lungs.

For example, a large ventricular septal defect will permit blood to flow from the right to the left ventricle, into

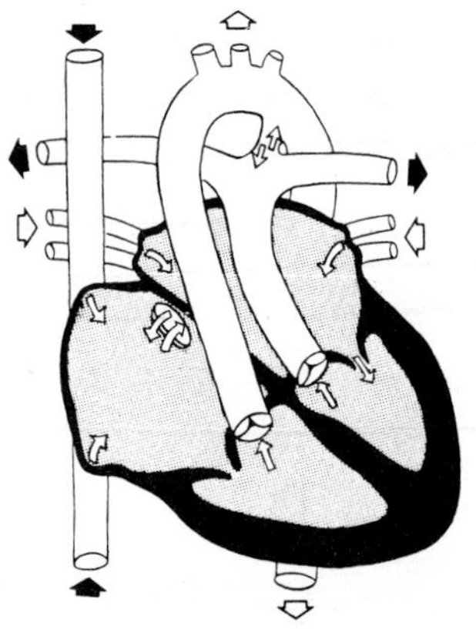

Fig. 35-16. Transposition of the great vessels. (From Congenital Heart Abnormalities, Columbus, Ohio, 1968, Ross Laboratories.)

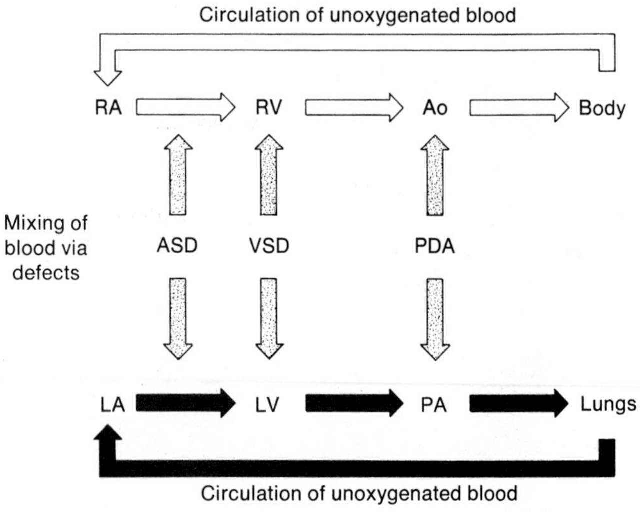

Fig. 35-17. Hemodynamics in transposition of the great vessels.

the pulmonary artery, and finally to the lungs. However, the high pressure within the left ventricle causes pulmonary vascular resistance and greatly increases the risk of congestive heart failure. The same series of events occurs with a large patent ductus arteriosus, since blood directly from the aorta flows under high pressure into the pulmonary artery and lungs.

Clinical manifestations. The severity of the child's condition depends on the type and size of the associated defects. Children with minimal communication are severely cyanotic and depressed at birth. Those with large septal defects or a patent ductus arteriosus may be less severely cyanotic but have symptoms of congestive heart failure. In these infants the only signs at birth may be cyanosis after crying or feeding and progressive hyperpnea in an attempt to compensate for decreased arterial oxygen saturation and in response to developing metabolic acidosis from hypoxia.

The heart sounds vary according to the type of defect present. A murmur usually indicates the presence of a septal defect or a patent ductus arteriosus. Cardiomegaly from right and left ventricular hypertrophy is usually evident a few weeks after birth. Signs of congestive heart failure (see p. 1347) develop rapidly, especially in those infants with a large ventricular septal defect.

Diagnostic evaluation. Definitive diagnosis is based on cardiac catheterization, especially selective angiography of the ventricles to delineate the exact intercommunication between the systemic and pulmonary circulations. Echocardiography is useful in demonstrating the location of the semilunar valves. Radiologic studies may reveal right and left ventricular hypertrophy and increased pulmonary vascularity. An electrocardiogram also demonstrates ventricular enlargement. Laboratory studies are helpful in assessing the degree of cyanosis and acidosis.

Treatment. Both palliative and corrective surgical procedures can be performed. The objective of the palliative approaches is to prevent pulmonary vascular resistance and congestive heart disease until the child is able to tolerate complete cardiac repair. There are several palliative procedures: (1) surgical creation of an atrial septal defect (Blalock-Hanlen operation), (2) enlargement of an existing atrial septal defect by pulling a balloon through the defect (balloon septotomy) during a cardiac catheterization (Rashkind procedure), (3) pulmonary artery banding to decrease blood flow to the lungs, and (4) creation of a ductus arteriosus if pulmonic stenosis is present.

Complete repair of the defect (atrioseptopexy or Mustard's operation) involves removing the entire atrial septum and creating a new atrial septum from existing pericardium or a prothesis that tunnels or baffles blood for more effective oxygenation. The creation of two new *functionally* correct atrial chambers diverts systemic venous blood to the mitral valve, where it enters the left ventricle, pulmonary artery, and lungs. As it returns by means of the pulmonary veins, the oxygenated blood is then diverted to the tricuspid valve, where it enters the right ventricle, aorta, and systemic circulation. Therefore, Mustard's operation does not attempt to transplant the transposed arterial vessels but reverses the function of the atria. Unfortunately there is an increased surgical risk when this procedure is combined with existing pulmonary vascular disease and/or a large ventricular septal defect. However, in the latter instance Mustard's operation offers palliative treatment at low risk if the ventricular septal defect is left unrepaired. Optimal time for repair is between 6 and 18 months of age and is associated with an 85% or higher survival rate (lower if associated defects are present).[2]

Clinical improvement is dramatic after corrective surgery with disappearance of cyanosis, clubbing, and dyspnea and improvement in weight gain, physical growth, activity tolerance, and muscular development. At the present time the long-term effects of atrial diversion are not known. However, complications include atrial arrhythmias from injury to the conduction system, tricuspid regurgitation (blood flowing back through an incompetent valve, probably as a result of high pressure on the right side of the heart), obstruction to systemic or pulmonary blood flow within the diverted atria, and left ventricular outflow obstruction.[3]

Truncus arteriosus

Truncus arteriosus results from failure of normal septation and division of the embryonic bulbar trunk into the pulmonary artery and aorta. As a result this single vessel, which overrides both ventricles, gives rise directly to the pulmonary and systemic circulations (Fig. 35-18).

Altered hemodynamics and physical consequences. Blood ejected from the left and right ventricles enters the common artery and flows either to the lungs or to the aortic arch and body. Since the pressure in both ventricles is

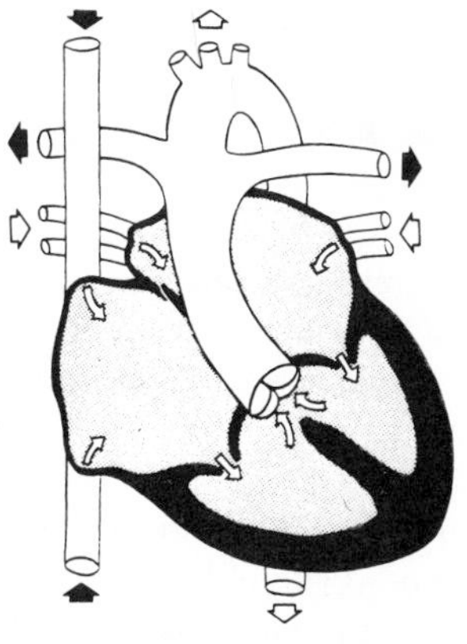

Fig. 35-18. Truncus arteriosus. (From Congenital Heart Abnormalities, Columbus, Ohio, 1968, Ross Laboratories.)

high, the blood flow to the lungs is markedly increased. Prior to the onset of pulmonary vascular congestion, there may be minimal cyanosis. However, as the inefficient circulation progresses, there is marked cyanosis, left ventricular hypertrophy, dyspnea, marked activity intolerance, and retarded growth. Most of these symptoms are evident a few weeks after birth.

Other indications of this defect are a harsh systolic murmur heard at the lower left sternal border and a single second heart sound, caused by the presence of only one semilunar valve. Signs of congestive heart failure usually occur during early infancy.

Treatment. Palliative treatment involves banding both pulmonary arteries as they arise from the truncus arteriosus to decrease the amount of blood flow to the lungs. Corrective treatment involves closing the ventricular septal defect so that the truncus arteriosus originates from the left ventricle and excising the pulmonary arteries from the aorta and attaching them to the right ventricle by means of a prosthetic valved conduit (Rastelli's operation). The success of corrective surgery depends on the child's age and the severity of existing pulmonary vascular disease.

Total anomalous venous return

This rare defect is characterized by no direct communication between the pulmonary veins and the left atrium. Instead the pulmonary veins attach directly to the right atrium or to various veins draining toward the right atrium, such as the superior vena cava, innominate vein, ductus venosus, coronary sinus, and so on. They are classified according to their point of attachment as *cardiac* (direct attachment to the heart, such as to the right atrium or coronary sinus), *infracardiac* (attachment below the diaphragm, such as to the inferior vena cava), or *supracardiac* (attachment above the diaphragm, such as to the superior vena cava). The infracardiac and, to a lesser extent, the supracardiac types are more prone to obstruction by compression from adjacent organs. Usually the pulmonary veins come together to form a channel in close proximity to the left atrium prior to their attachment to the right atrium or vein (Fig. 35-19).

Altered hemodynamics. With the cardiac type, the right atrium receives all the blood that normally would flow into the left atrium. As a result the right side of the heart hypertrophies whereas the left side, especially the left atrium, remains undeveloped. There may be an associated atrial septal defect that shunts blood from the higher pressured right atrium to the left atrium, allowing unoxygenated systemic blood to flow to the left side of the heart. If there is pulmonary vein obstruction, the pressure within the pulmonary circulation rises, restricting blood flow from the pulmonary artery and eventually contributing to heart failure as the pulmonary pressure exceeds the systemic pressure.

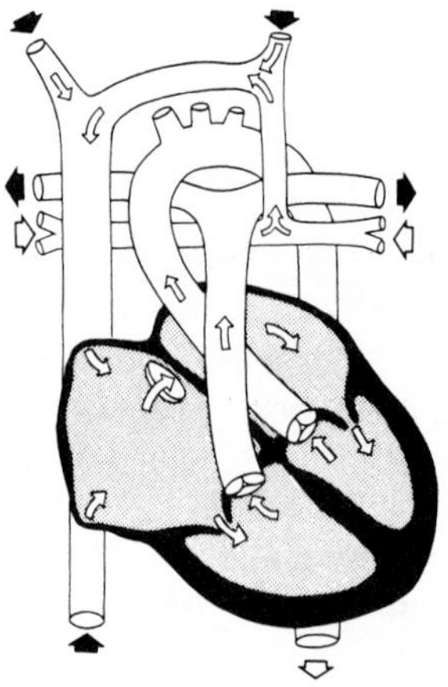

Fig. 35-19. Total anomalous venous return. (From Congenital Heart Abnormalities, Columbus, Ohio, 1968, Ross Laboratories.)

Clinical manifestations. Infants usually develop early signs of cyanosis, pulmonary congestion, and heart failure. If pulmonary obstruction is absent, cyanosis may be minimal since the right side of the heart is shunting blood that is receiving more oxygenated than unoxygenated blood. Once pulmonary obstruction occurs, there is rapid deterioration of the child's physical condition.

Auscultatory findings depend on the hemodynamics. A blowing systolic murmur from tricuspid regurgitation may be heard at the lower left sternal border. A continuous murmur or venous hum may be present from blood rushing through the venous channels. Because the right side of the heart is hyperdynamic, a gallop rhythm is common.

Treatment. There is no palliative procedure for this defect. Surgical correction involves restoring the normal pulmonary venous circulation.

Correction of the coronary sinus type involves forming an opening between the coronary sinus (main coronary vein returning myocardial blood to the general circulation) and the left atrium and closing the sinus with sutures as it enters the right atrium. At the same time any atrial septal defects are repaired. The end result is blood flowing from the pulmonary veins directly into the coronary sinus and to the left atrium. In the infracardiac and supracardiac types, the communicating ascending or descending vein is ligated and the common pulmonary vein is anastomosed to the left atrium. Any associated defects, such as patent foramen ovale, are also repaired.[19]

The success of corrective surgery depends on the location of the defect. Cardiac types are most successful because of ease in restructuring the channels and less chance of pulmonary vein obstruction. The subdiaphragmatic type carries the greatest surgical risk.

Since infants are poor candidates for surgery, the objectives of medical care are to prevent the complication of congestive heart failure and metabolic acidosis. If these children undergo surgery at an optimum age, usually by 2 years, there is a good prognosis.

Tricuspid atresia

Tricuspid atresia is absence of the tricuspid valve, resulting in no opening between the right atrium and right ventricle (Fig. 35-20). It is usually associated with other defects that allow some shunting of blood into the lungs.

Altered hemodynamics. At birth the presence of a patent foramen ovale (or other atrial septal opening) and ductus arterious permits blood to flow across the septum into the left atrium (complete mixing of oxygenated and unoxygenated blood) and through the patent ductus arteriosus to the pulmonary artery for oxygenation into the lungs. A ventricular septal defect allows a modest amount of blood to enter the right ventricle and pulmonary artery for oxygenation. Unless the ventricular septal defect is large, the amount of blood flow is so small that the right ventricle remains hypoplastic. Usually pulmonary blood flow is diminished.

Clinical manifestations. Severe cyanosis, dyspnea, anoxic spells, and signs of right-sided heart failure are evident early during infancy, especially if blood flow to the lungs is restricted by a closing patent ductus arterious. If the child survives later into infancy, all the other signs of a cyanotic lesion are present.

Auscultatory findings depend on the presence of associated defects. A harsh pansystolic murmur usually indicates a ventricular septal defect. The second heart sound may be narrowly split because of decreased blood flow to the pulmonary artery, or the pulmonic component may be absent, when no ventricular septal defect is present. Pulmonary findings of congestive heart failure occur early.

Diagnostic evaluation. Laboratory findings are those of any cyanotic defect (hypoxemia and acidosis). Roentgenographic studies usually reveal a small, undeveloped right ventricle, large atria (which give the heart a rounded or apple-shaped appearance), and decreased pulmonary vascularity. Echocardiography is helpful in confirming absence of tricuspid valve closure. An electrocardiogram shows significant right atrial and left-sided enlargement. Confirmation of the diagnosis is a cardiac catheterization, which reveals total flow of right atrial blood to the left atrium, inability to enter the right ventricle, and presence and adequacy of associated defects.

Treatment. Palliative treatment is the same as for tetralogy of Fallot (pulmonary-to-artery anastomoses) to increase blood flow to the lungs. If the atrial septal defect is small, an atrial septotomy is done during cardiac catheterization.

Total correction is now possible by converting the right atrium into an outlet for the pulmonary artery which involves placing a tubular conduit with a valve between the two and closing the atrial septal defect. This procedure

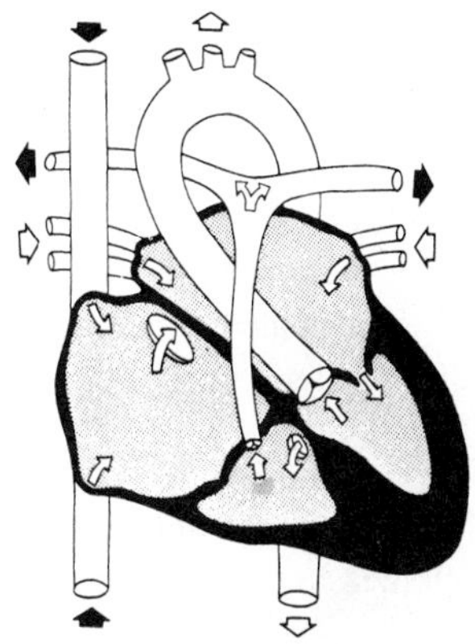

Fig. 35-20. Tricuspid atresia. (From Congenital Heart Abnormalities, Columbus, Ohio, 1968, Ross Laboratories.)

physiologically corrects tricuspid atresia by preventing any mixing of systemic blood in the left atrium and shunting the entire venous blood to the lungs for oxygenation. It has been successful in a limited number of older children.[8]

NURSING CARE OF CHILD WITH CONGENITAL HEART DISEASE

When a child is born with a severe cardiac anomaly, the parents are faced with the immense psychologic and physical tasks of adjusting to the birth of a defective child and raising a child with physical limitations. Although the reactions and nursing interventions in terms of acceptance of a handicapped child differ little from those discussed in Chapter 22, in some situations there is the difficult choice of morally and ethically deciding about treatment for the cardiac problem when the infant has severe chromosomal defects. Although the decision regarding care of severely handicapped persons is far from being reached, nurses involved with these families must be aware of their own feelings and the feelings of parents that shape certain choices.

Although it is not the purpose of this discussion to advance answers to this dilemma, it is hoped that those caring for such families will realize that there are two types of care: the "disease-oriented" approach, in which death is viewed as unacceptable and every known medical technology must be employed toward the preservation of life, regardless of its quality, and the "person-oriented" approach, which attempts to place medical treatment in the perspective of dignity and quality of future life for the patient and family.[6] Each approach has its advantages and risks. Ideally the health team caring for the child should help parents decide by supplying all available knowledge and supporting them unjudgmentally in either choice.

Ideally nursing intervention to prevent congenital heart

formations should begin prenatally whenever possible, such as detecting rubella or other known viral infections early and discussing a therapeutic abortion when feasible, counseling parents of children with heart defects or certain inherited syndromes of the genetic risks in future pregnancies, performing amniocentesis for Down's syndrome on mothers of advanced maternal age (over age 40 years), and counseling diabetic and alcoholic mothers concerning the risks of heart defects in their offspring. Although the relationship of adequate nutrition and prenatal supervision has not been delineated in terms of heart defects, it is known that in general such measures decrease the incidence of birth defects.

This discussion is concerned with the family whose child has a serious heart defect that requires an indefinite period of home care prior to corrective surgery. The goal for this child is normalcy within the limits of his condition. Since the prognosis is often variable, normalcy allows him time to live as a child first and as a patient second. Since many defects are correctable, normalcy prepares the child for leaving behind the sick role and adjusting to the privileges and responsibilities of a well child.

Observation for signs and symptoms of heart defects

Nursing care of the child with a congenital heart defect begins once the diagnosis is suspected. However, in many instances symptoms suggestive of a cardiac anomaly are not present at birth or, if manifest, are so subtle as to be missed. For example, even in the severe condition of tetralogy of Fallot, the only evidence of the disorder in the neonate may be cyanosis during crying or feedings. However, the cyanosis differs from that normally seen in newborns (mainly peripheral) because the lips and tongue, as well as the lower extremities, turn blue. A summary of the signs most indicative of cardiac disease in neonates is listed in the boxed material.

Many heart defects are not evident until the child's growth and/or energy expenditure exceeds the heart's ability to supply oxygenated blood. Since the onset is gradual, the child may curtail his activity so that the signs of exercise intolerance are less obvious. However, a careful history yields important clues to this change. For example, toddlers are normally extremely mobile and their energies are directed toward learning gross motor skills. It is very unusual to hear of a toddler who prefers to sit rather than crawl or walk. Such histories should alert the nurse to assess cardiac function. Likewise, a child who needs frequent rests after limited play periods may also be exhibiting exercise intolerance.

Other clues, which have already been discussed, are a history of retarded weight gain, poor feeding habits, especially the need to pause during feeding, frequent respiratory infections, particularly when the child is well cared for and isolated from known sources of infection, and any unusual posturing, such as squatting. Since parents may not view any of these findings as abnormal, the nurse must specifically ask about them during a physical assessment.

Another indication of heart defects is murmurs. In Chapter 5 the usual distinguishing characteristics between innocent and organic murmurs were discussed. Nurses who perform primary health assessments must be knowledgeable of the differences in order to correctly refer children

Signs and symptoms of cardiac disease in infants

1. Cry: weak and muffled, loud and breathless
2. Color
   a. Cyanotic: usually generalized; increases in supine position; often unrelieved by oxygen, usually deepens with crying; gray, dusky; mild, moderate, severe
   b. Acyanotic: pale, with or without mottling on exertion
3. Activity level
   a. Restless
   b. Lethargic
   c. Unresponsive except to pain
   d. Lack of movement of arms and legs when crying (severe distress)
   e. Arms become flaccid when eating
4. Posturing
   a. Hypotonic: flaccid even when sleeping
   b. Hyperextension of neck
   c. Opisthotonos
   d. Dyspnea when supine
   e. Favors knee-chest position
5. Persistent bradycardia—120 beats/minute—or persistent tachycardia—160 beats/minute
6. Respirations: counted when neonate is sleeping to identify problem early
   a. Tachypnea: 60 breaths/minute
   b. Retractions with nasal flaring or tachypnea
   c. Dyspnea with diaphoresis or grunting
   d. Gasping followed in 2 or 3 minutes by respiratory arrest if not treated promptly
   e. Chronic cough (not often seen)
   f. Grunting with exertion such as crying or feeding by nipple
7. Feeding behavior
   a. Anorexic
   b. Poor suck: from lack of energy or when unable to close mouth around nipple because of dyspnea
   c. Difficulty in coordinating sucking, swallowing, breathing; pulls away from nipple to take breath
   d. Slow, with pauses to rest
   e. Unable to feed by nipple

From Jensen, M. D., Benson, R. C., and Bobak, I. M.: Maternity care: the nurse and the family, St. Louis, 1977, The C. V. Mosby Co.

with heart murmurs of possible organic origin to a cardiologist. There has been controversy over informing parents of innocent murmurs, since some physicians believe that the parent may be unduly worried and transfer that concern to overprotectiveness of the child.[11] However, this problem may actually be that health professionals fail to adequately explain the significance of the finding. If parents are aware that their child has had a murmur, they are able to convey this information to a physician or nurse practitioner unfamiliar with their child who, unaware of a previous history of the murmur, may unnecessarily investigate its origin.

Helping parents and child adjust to diagnosis

Helping families adjust to the diagnosis involves several principles: (1) allowing the family a period of time to grieve for the loss of a perfect child, (2) assessing the level of the parents' and child's understanding of the heart, and (3) fostering family patterns of interaction that enhance the optimum growth and development of each of its members.

Allowing period of grief. Once parents and older children learn of the heart defect, they are initially in a period of shock, followed by high anxiety, especially fear of the child's death. This reaction may occur soon after the child's birth or at a later period in life. Whatever its timing, the family needs a period of grief before assimilating the meaning of the defect. Unfortunately the demands for medical treatment may not allow this, necessitating that the parents be informed of the condition in order to consent to various procedures. However, the nurse can be instrumental by supporting parents in their loss, assessing their level of understanding, supplying information as needed, and helping other members of the health team to understand the parents' reactions.

Severely distressed infants usually remain in the hospital. This can seriously affect parent-infant attachment unless parents are encouraged to hold, touch, and look at their child. With a heart defect, the symptoms of cyanosis, dyspnea, and extreme fatigue may discourage parents from physical contact with the infant. However, every effort must be made by health personnel to foster attachment, especially when parents may be required to continue the care at home. (See Chapter 22 for suggestions in promoting attachment between parents and their hospitalized newborn.)

A congenital heart defect constitutes a chronic family crisis. Even when the child's condition is stabilized or corrected, the family needs to make new adjustments in their life-style. Introducing them to other families with similarly affected children can help them adjust to the daily stresses.* As one mother remarked, ''By the time my child was discharged from the nursery, I felt confident in her care. I thought I had my home organized for her arrival. However, I really didn't know what to expect. I only wish that I could have spoken to another mother who had gone through the experience. Every time I saw my child turn blue or gasp for air, I felt inadequate and scared. That only added to the difficulty of coping with all the physical things I had to do.'' This mother later worked with other parents who had newborns with heart defects.

Assessment of level of understanding. Once parents are ready to hear about the heart condition, it is essential that they be given a clear explanation, based on their level of understanding. One method of simplistically illustrating heart defects is to depict the heart as a four-room structure (house) that normally has exits and entrances (representing the valves and vessels). A septal defect can then be illustrated as an abnormal entrance to one side of the structure that allows mixing of blood that should remain only in that room. Although this explanation may not suffice for all parents, it does allow for clarification of basic information. It is certainly more explanatory than the usual colloquial expression, ''a hole in the heart,'' for septal defects, which is frequently interpreted to mean that blood leaks out of the heart. Parents appreciate receiving written information about the specific defect.*

Another fact to remember is that different health personnel may convey the same information using different medical terms. If this becomes a problem (which often happens when several members of a health team work with a family) the nurse should encourage them to write down the term or ask the informant to clarify it. Sometimes it is helpful to provide the family with a glossary of frequently used words for them to refer to. For example, one mother told the nurse that her child had three heart defects—a hole in the heart, an abnormal opening, and a defect between two ventricles. She understood that the surgeon was to repair all of them at the same time and wondered if her child's heart ''could stand it.'' The nurse clarified that all three terms meant the same thing. However, no expression had any meaning until the nurse showed the mother where the abnormal opening was and how it would be repaired.

Parents are primarily interested in two kinds of information—prognosis and surgery.[14] They are frequently upset about indefinite answers to either. It is helpful if the physician continually mentions that the child's condition can change and that decisions regarding future procedures and treatments may also change. The nurse remains aware of alterations in the plan of therapy in order to convey similar messages to the family.

Children of various ages form different meanings about their heart.[18] Children between 4 and 6 years of age have heard about the heart, know its approximate anatomic location in the chest or back, illustrate it as valentine shaped,

*Some local American Heart Associations have organized parent groups.

*A booklet that can be given to parents is ''If your child has a congenital heart defect,'' New York, 1970, American Heart Association.

and characterize it by the sounds, such as tick-tock, thump, and so on. Children 7 to 10 years of age have a clearer concept of the heart, realizing that it is not shaped like a valentine and that it has vital functions, such as, "It makes you live." However, their knowledge of its integrated functions to pump blood through a system of vessels to all parts of the body is still hazy. By the age of 10 or 11 years, children have a much more involved concept of the heart with knowledge of veins, valves, pumping action, and circulation. They are beginning to appreciate why death occurs when the heart stops.

Information must be tailored to the child's developmental age. Preschoolers need basic information about what they will experience more than what is actually occurring physiologically. School-age children benefit from a concrete explanation of the defect. Using the "house model" can be very effective. Preadolescents and adolescents often appreciate a more detailed description of how the defect affects their heart. Children of all ages need an opportunity to express their feelings concerning the diagnosis.

For example, one 14-year-old girl who had been told that she had an atrial septal defect and was undergoing cardiac catheterization was well informed by her two physician parents. However, no one had asked the adolescent how she felt. Prior to the procedure, the nurse remarked, "I know you are aware of everything that is going to happen, but what do you think about all of this?" The child replied, "I really wonder if I may die." The nurse allowed her to express her unspoken fears. Later, when the nurse mentioned the conversation to her parents, they too remarked that despite all their knowledge of "low risks, complications, and mortality statistics," they too secretly worried for their child's welfare. This opened communication between the parents and child, allowing her to be optimally prepared for open-heart surgery.

Parents also need an explanation regarding the symptoms of the disease. Watching a child turn cyanotic and dyspneic is frightening. However, offering parents suggestions of what to do after such an episode lessens their anxiety by giving them some control. After a cyanotic/dyspneic episode, the child needs to rest and attain a position of comfort, usually side lying with knees flexed and the head and chest elevated. He is kept warm to prevent increased metabolism and vasoconstriction. Most importantly, he should remain calm. This requires treating the cyanotic spell casually to prevent parental emotional contagion to the child. Supplemental oxygen may be helpful but is not always available.

An essential intervention is prevention by tailoring energy expenditure to cardiac output and arterial oxygenation. For older children this involves little difficulty because activity restrictions are self-imposed. However, for the infant it means lessening crying periods as much as possible and feeding him slowly with rest pauses to minimize overexertion. Neither is an easy task. First of all, it is impossible to prevent crying totally. Parents who try are headed for frustration. Rather the approach is to anticipate the infant's needs, realizing his inability to delay gratification. This may involve feeding the child every few hours to prevent excessive hunger, changing wet diapers frequently to avoid irritation, and scheduling play periods to keep the child amused when awake. Although these activities do not differ from those of normal infants, they do vary in degree. For example, the mother of a normal infant may allow him to cry while preparing his formula, but the mother of a child with a cardiac defect would plan to have the formula prepared in advance to prevent prolonged crying.

The infant needs to be fed small amounts of formula every couple of hours to ensure adequate nutrition. This is especially difficult for families because it demands several nighttime feedings for many months. Although there are few ways to avoid this unless the family is financially able to hire outside help, the nurse should discuss with parents the need to share the responsibility and enlist the help of others whenever possible. Often parents do not feel confident leaving the child in anyone else's care because they believe that the child will be upset by a change in routine and that the individual will be unable to cope with the cyanosis and dyspnea. This often sets up a trap for parents, especially mothers, who become locked into the child's care with no relief. Although the parents' fears are justified, they can be minimized by gradually teaching someone (a relative or neighbor) how to care for the child and by seeking baby-sitters who are more familiar with these children, such as nursing students and retired nurses. It also may be helpful to introduce parents to other families with children who have heart disease so that as a group they can share such responsibilities.

Since growth retardation is believed to be a result of inadequate caloric intake, the nurse assists parents in ways of providing highly nutritious foods. Sometimes the physician may order protein/calorie supplements that are mixed with milk or formula. Mixing cereal or other pureed foods in the bottle also enriches the feeding while minimizing the energy needed for ingestion. If thickened feedings are given, the nurse reminds parents to enlarge the nipple hole by cutting a cross in the center to facilitate flow of the formula. If this is not done, the sucking required to feed will be exhausting.

To conserve energy, self-feeding techniques such as the use of a spoon or cup may be delayed. However, the benefit of this practice must be weighed against the consequent lag in development, especially the ability of learning to chew. Parents may wish to encourage finger foods and self-feeding as a method of play rather than at mealtime, when ingesting sufficient nutrients is the priority.

Children with severe cardiac defects are often anorexic. Encouraging them to eat can be a tremendous challenge. Because of the parents' concern over eating, children learn early to manipulate parents through eating, such as making

Summary of nursing care of the child with congenital heart disease

Goals	Responsibilities
Prevent congenital heart disease	Encourage immunization against rubella in all females Detect rubella infection early in pregnant woman; discuss possibility of elective abortion Encourage genetic counseling of parents of child with congenital heart disease regarding subsequent risk to other offspring Discuss risks of congenital heart disease in diabetic or alcoholic women or in women of advanced age Encourage prevention through general measures of optimal nutrition, prenatal supervision, and avoidance of any drugs unless medically indicated
Observe for signs/symptoms of congenital heart disease	For infant, see p. 1326 Take careful history with special attention to poor weight gain, poor feeding habits, exercise intolerance, unusual posturing, or frequent respiratory infections Observe for evidence of cyanosis Carefully evaluate heart murmurs (especially as primary care giver) to distinguish between innocent and organic murmurs Explain insignificance of innocent murmurs to parents; do not investigate them further lest parents doubt examiner's judgment
Help parents and child adjust to diagnosis Allow period of grief	 Accept initial shock and disbelief Repeat information as often as necessary Foster parent-child attachment, especially of newborn Introduce parents to other families who have similarly affected child
Assess level of understanding	Use visual aids to describe heart defect Provide written information Keep technical information simple Convey same information as other health team members Stress that prognosis and plans for surgery may change Base explanation of heart on child's developmental level of understanding: 4- to 6-year-old child: Describes it as valentine shaped Knows approximate anatomic location Characterizes it by sounds 7- to 10-year-old child: Classifies it as vital organ Has beginning concept of function Child over 10 years Has more involved and correct concept of function Relates stopping of heart to death Allow child to express feelings about heart condition
Help parents cope with symptoms of disease	During dyspneic/cyanotic spell, place child in side-lying, knee-chest position, with head and chest elevated Keep child warm; encourage rest and sleep Decrease child's anxiety by remaining calm Feed child slowly Administer small, frequent meals For thickened formula, cut larger hole in nipple Delay self-feeding to minimize exertion Minimize crying by anticipating needs Encourage anorexic child to eat (see p. 1016) Encourage parents to include others in child's care to prevent own exhaustion

Continued.

Summary of nursing care of the child with congenital heart disease—cont'd

Goals	Responsibilities
Foster growth-promoting family relationships	Encourage family members to discuss their feelings about each other Maintain as equal expectations from all the siblings as possible Provide consistent discipline, especially from infancy, to prevent behavioral problems Encourage acceptable pursuits for child Discuss school entry with teacher and school nurse Guide parents to eventual hazards of fostering overdependency Help parents feel adequate in their maternal-paternal roles by emphasizing growth and developmental progress of their child Help parents foster child's development by stimulating child to age-appropriate goals consistent with his activity tolerance Provide social experiences for child
Assist in providing financial support	Investigate state and local agencies that may be able to provide financial assistance, such as state crippled children's services Collaborate with social service agency to ensure optimum utilization of community services

unrealistic demands for foods that are not available. The nurse advises parents of this potential problem, since prevention yields greater success than intervention. For example, the child should be given a choice of available high-quality foods. Suggestions for encouraging anorexic children to eat are discussed on p. 1016.

Fostering growth-promoting family relationships. The effect of a child with a serious heart defect on the family is complex. No member, regardless of the degree of positive adjustment, is unaffected. Mothers frequently feel inadequate in their mothering ability because they are unable to continually satisfy their child. They may view the child's failure to feed well as evidence of their failure, not as a direct consequence of the disease. The usual joys of watching a child grow and thrive are limited. Frequently attainment of gross motor milestones is delayed from physical inability to practice crawling or sitting unsupported. Mothers often feel constantly exhausted from the pressures of caring for these children and the other members of the family.

Likewise fathers and siblings may feel neglected and resentful. Husbands may view their wives' total dedication to the sick child as a rejection of them. If the mother has never shared child-care activities with her spouse, he may feel that they have no activities in common. The consequence is often marital discord. Siblings may feel that they grow in the shadow of their brother or sister because all financial, emotional, and physical resources center on him or her. Even the ill child is not without such feelings. Although he may learn to abuse his condition to attain his own way, he may also feel guilty for draining the family of all their resources, resentment that he is the sick child, and animosity toward his siblings and others who are unrestricted in their physical ability.

These feelings are not abnormal. They are the expected consequences of a chronic illness. However, they can be lessened by encouraging family members to discuss how they feel toward one another, encouraging parents to arrange "time off" from home responsibilities, and fostering normal expectations from all the siblings.

The need to maintain discipline and limit setting cannot be overemphasized. Although it is more difficult because crying must be minimized, using behavior modification techniques, either in the form of concrete awards, such as a favorite food, or social reinforcement, such as approval, can be effective. However, it is most beneficial if employed *before* the child learns to control the family. Therefore, guiding parents toward the need for discipline while the child is in infancy is necessary to prevent problems later on. It also teaches these children how to tolerate frustration and delayed gratification, which so often is lacking because of the immediate satisfaction of all their needs.

Although the child may not be able to participate in physical activity, he should be encouraged toward acceptable pursuits, such as reading, hobbies, needlework, and so on. Allowing the child to watch television as his total means of recreation is not fostering his development. If the child enters school prior to corrective surgery, the parents should discuss with the teacher, school nurse, and principal appropriate activity levels.

Another problem that frequently develops within family relationships is the child's overdependency, especially on his mother. Mothers, in turn, frequently respond to the dependency with overprotectiveness, resulting in a cycle that is mutually satisfying although destructive in terms of developing maturity and responsibility. Like many of the other dilemmas that occur in these families, this one stems first from the need to solve a problem, usually to satisfy the child's needs and to foster the parent's feeling of adequacy. However, guidance to the eventual hazards of continuing dependency and protectiveness as the child grows older assists parents in learning ways to foster optimum development. For example, the nurse should encourage parents to stimulate the infant toward feasible goals, such as holding his own bottle, learning to amuse himself for short periods rather than always being held, picking up finger foods, and so on. Unless parents are helped to see what activities the child can do, they often will only focus on his physical limitations.

The child also needs opportunities for social development. Often these children are isolated from known sources of infection and not allowed to play with other children because of overexertion. This only adds to the dangers of increased dependency on the home environment. Parents need to be encouraged to seek appropriate social activity, especially prior to kindergarten. One approach is to locate families with a similar problem and form a play group. One parent found that her child's first contact with other children was during hospitalization for diagnostic procedures. As she observed the beginning interaction between the children, she introduced herself to the other parents and on discharge continued a friendship with a family who had a child with neurologic impairment. (For a summary of nursing care of the child with congenital heart disease, see the boxed material on pp. 1329 to 1330.)

NURSING CARE OF CHILD UNDERGOING HEART SURGERY

Few surgical procedures demand as much planning for preoperative preparation and postoperative care as heart surgery. Since the general principles for preparing children for surgery are included in Chapter 25, this discussion focuses on those measures specific to the procedure. Although there are technical differences between closed- and open-heart surgery, namely that the latter involves the use of cardiopulmonary bypass (extracorporeal circulation), the type of surgery does not significantly change the preoperative care, although there are some additions to physical care postoperatively in open-heart surgery. Therefore, in general the term heart surgery is used regardless of the actual procedure, except where indicated.

Preoperative care

The child is usually admitted to the hospital 3 or 4 days prior to surgery for diagnostic tests. This time interval is advantageous for preparing the child and parents for surgery. Since a great deal of information is conveyed, it is important to schedule teaching to prevent information overload. Preparation can be divided into three phases: equipment, environment, and procedures. These categories are neither exclusive of each other nor is one always presented before the other. Rather teaching is done following these principles: information is based on the child's level of understanding (developmental age), sensory experiences are emphasized, anxiety-producing information is conveyed last, and teaching is continually evaluated. The following discussion assumes that the child and parents have an understanding of the defect. (Refer to p. 1331 for nursing care of the child with heart disease.)

Introduction of child to his environment. Ideally when the child is admitted he should be assigned to one nurse on each shift. In some institutions the nurse who will care for the child postoperatively in the intensive care unit is also assigned to the child at admission to facilitate forming a relationship with the child and to share preoperative teaching, such as introduction to the recovery room and intensive care unit. To increase familiarity each nurse should call the child by name and refer to herself by name. Wearing an obvious name tag reinforces this point. Postoperatively the child will feel more at ease recognizing familiar names and voices.

The visit to the recovery room and/or intensive care unit should take place when there is least activity in the unit, the parents can accompany the child, and the child is well rested. Usually the day prior to surgery is ample time to allow the child to ask questions and to prevent undue fantasizing about the experience.

When in the intensive care unit, everything that directly affects the child, such as the sounds of electrocardiogram monitors, oxygen tents, placement of the bed, and so on, is pointed out. All positive, nonfrightening aspects of the environment are emphasized, such as the play area, visitors' section, pictures or mobiles in the room, or television. If it is a pediatric intensive care unit, the nurse can introduce the child to other children who may be recovering from surgery. The child and parents are encouraged to ask questions or to explore further any equipment in the room, but this is not insisted on (Fig. 35-21).

Familiarizing child with equipment. Some of the equipment, such as the stethoscope, blood pressure apparatus, and thermometer, will already be familiar to the child. However, the nurse emphasizes that these procedures will

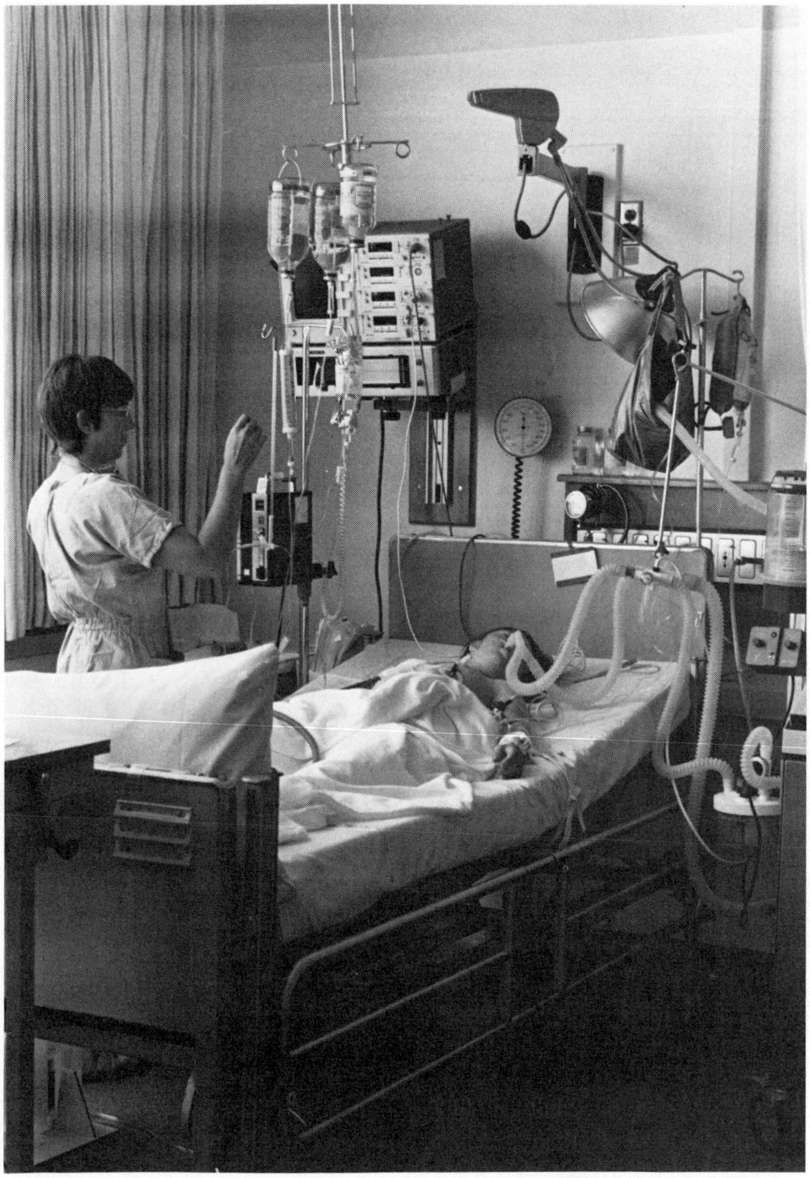

Fig. 35-21. Immediate postoperative setup for open heart surgery. The unfamiliarity of such an environment requires preoperative preparation to decrease the child's and parents' fear and anxiety on arrival at the intensive care unit.

be done more frequently. If continuous monitoring devices are used, such as for temperature, the child is told about the placement of the sensor on his skin. Since blood pressure cuffs are left on, he should also be aware of this.

Pieces of equipment that are new to many children are the oxygen mask, oxygen tent, suction, chest tubes, endotracheal tube, blow bottles, and intravenous tubing. Each of these is shown to the child and demonstrated either on him or on a doll. With a younger child the use of miniaturized equipment that is suitable for use with a doll or puppet is often less anxiety producing than the actual samples. If other children on the unit have an intravenous infusion or are in an oxygen tent, the older child may benefit from seeing them. The more sensations he experiences beforehand, the more likely it is that he will not be frightened by them later. For example, peering through a plastic tent makes the environment look very distorted, especially if one is not prepared for the visual change.

Several intravenous lines are inserted postoperatively: (1) an ordinary line for infusion of fluids, usually inserted in a peripheral vein, (2) a venous pressure line, usually inserted into the right cephalic or basilic vein, and (3) an arterial line for direct measurement of arterial pressure, usually inserted through the femoral or brachial artery. Younger children need only know the location of each tubing, especially that both arms may be restrained to prevent dislodging the tubing. Older children may appreciate knowing the reason for each infusion, especially when venous and arterial measurements are taken. Since the lines are inserted during surgery, they are not painful, only uncomfortable because of the restricted movement.

The nurse also discusses the type and size of dressing the child will have after surgery. Usually one of two types of incision is made: a midline opening from the sternum to the lower abdomen or a transverse incision from the anterior to the posterior midline. In either instance the suture line and dressing are extensive.

The child is told about chest tubes and their purpose in draining fluid from the lungs. He can be shown a picture of the bottles used for drainage, or the setup can be assimilated by attaching one end of the tubes to a doll with a chest dressing and the other end to small bottles (such as empty medicine vials). The nurse stresses that the child must move even though the tubes are in place and that it may hurt. It can be demonstrated on the doll that the tubing is long enough to permit turning. Since this information may be anxiety producing, it is best left to the end of teaching. It is important to be honest about the discomfort because, if the child is unprepared, he may refuse to move for fear of dislodging the tubes.

An endotracheal (ET) tube is inserted during surgery and is usually left in place for ventilatory assistance and deep tracheobronchial suctioning. This tube can be presented as a "breathing tube" that is placed in the nose or mouth. The nurse explains that the child will feel it in his throat (it may feel like a choking sensation) but that nothing is wrong. The nurse demonstrates that the suction catheter will be inserted through the tube. Since talking is difficult with the tube, the nurse suggests that the child learn to express his desires by pointing, such as touching his finger to his lips to indicate thirst. The nurse stresses that the tube will be removed as soon as possible, often during the first postoperative day.

Controversy exists regarding preparing the child for emergency procedures such as a tracheostomy. Each situation must be judged individually. However, considering the anxiety associated with cardiac surgery and the extensive preparation needed for expected postoperative care, forewarning the child of the possibility of a tracheostomy may unduly frighten him. Parents should be aware of the need for such emergency treatment, and, if a tracheostomy is planned, the child is then prepared. The explanation is similar to that for an endotracheal tube except that an opening is made in the neck and a special tube is inserted. The procedure can be demonstrated on a doll.

Practicing postoperative procedures. Several postoperative procedures are imperative to prevent postsurgical complications, especially coughing, turning, deep breathing, postural drainage and percussion, and intermittent positive-pressure breathing. Each of these are practiced several times prior to surgery. Although they can be presented as a game, the nurse tells the child that each procedure will not be as easy after surgery and may cause discomfort. The nurse demonstrates how to relieve the soreness, such as breathing or coughing while splinting the chest with a pillow. The subject of pain is also approached matter-of-factly, stressing that medicine to relieve discomfort can be given to him both before and/or after the procedures.

Deep breathing is demonstrated by having the child watch the nurse's chest rise and fall. The child is told to imitate the nurse's actions, emphasizing that the higher the chest rises, the more air enters the lung. For a young child the nurse can explain that the lungs are like balloons that expand when air is inspired. The use of blow bottles is also demonstrated to encourage breathing. If these are not available, the child can blow bubbles through a straw placed in water. The nurse demonstrates coughing by taking a deep breath and forcibly trying to bring up secretions. It is emphasized that coughing is not the same as clearing the throat. At this time the nurse can also demonstrate the use of suction. If the child resists having the catheter placed in his mouth, the nurse can show him how the suction equipment works by placing the tubing in a glass of water, comparing the effect to a "magic straw."

The child practices turning in bed, usually from side to side while in semi-Fowler's position. The nurse teaches him how to help himself, such as by bending the legs and holding onto the side rails. Although practicing such procedures may seem insignificant at this point, it teaches the child familiar methods of self-help and prepares him for the demands expected of him after surgery.

The nurse also performs postural drainage and percussion, although postoperatively the positioning is fairly restricted. Throughout each demonstration the nurse emphasizes that although the procedure will be uncomfortable, it is essential to the child's recovery. The nurse also clarifies that percussion is not hitting but a special kind of clapping.

Usually intermittent positive-pressure breathing (IPPB) treatments are done by a respiratory therapist who participates in the preoperative teaching. Intermittent positive-pressure breathing is a frightening procedure for many people because the forced air makes one feel as if he cannot breathe. Therefore, it is important that the child learn to breathe with the machine so that postoperatively the procedure is more effortless. The nurse can approach the procedure as special breathing like that used by skin divers or astronauts.

The child also practices using the bedpan or urinal. He should be told that after surgery he will have a special tube (Foley catheter) so that he will not have to urinate but that once the tube is taken out (which does not hurt), he will have to use a bedpan.

The child is also prepared for preoperative procedures, such as nothing by mouth for 12 hours prior to surgery, skin preparation, which includes shaving or the use of a topical depilatory in adolescent males and females, and preoperative sedation medication. Physical preoperative care differs little from that for any type of surgery. Skin preparation may involve a tub bath with special bacteriocidal cleanser the day before surgery. Cleansing enemas are sometimes given to prevent abdominal distention and to lessen the likelihood of straining during defecation in the immediate postoperative period. The nurse clarifies with the physician exactly what preoperative procedures are to be done to avoid the hazard of overpreparing or underpreparing the child.

Preoperative observations

There are several observations, which, when made preoperatively, facilitate care planning postoperatively.

Vital signs. Vital signs and blood pressure are recorded with activity to establish a baseline of the child's energy tolerance. Temperature is carefully evaluated, since an elevation may be the first indication of an infection, which ordinarily is a contraindication to surgery since it increases the risk of infective endocarditis. Any sudden change in vital sign is reported to the physician immediately. For example, an increase in pulse and respirations during periods of rest may be an early sign of congestive heart failure.

Sleep/awake patterns. Sleep and activity are recorded to allow the child optimal rest during the postoperative period and maximum tolerance to stress. With increasing evidence of the importance of identifying an individual's biorhythms, a sleep and activity record illustrates those periods when the child is most tolerant of activity and most in need of sleep. For example, the body's ability to withstand stress is correlated with the usual diurnal pattern of hydrocortisone secretion. Normally hydrocortisone secretion is greatest in the early morning hours and least at night during sleep. By maintaining the usual sleep/awake periods, these levels are maintained so that stressful procedures performed in the morning are best tolerated by the body.[22]

Elimination. Elimination patterns are observed, primarily to avoid constipation postoperatively, which can place excessive strain on the heart muscle and suture line. The child's toilet habits, including expressions for urinating or defecating, are recorded on the care plan. If the child uses a potty-chair, this is also noted to allow the child every opportunity to continue newly learned skills and maintain bodily control. It is often surprising how quickly children recover from extensive heart surgery and how imperative it is for them to remain independent.

Fluid intake. Fluid intake should be recorded prior to surgery to estimate the child's usual fluid consumption and to identify which fluids are preferred. Postoperatively fluids are usually restricted to prevent circulatory overload. By identifying the child's pattern of intake, especially in relationship to sleep/awake periods, intake restrictions can be planned to allow fluids when the child usually prefers them.

Postoperative care

Immediate postoperative care is usually provided by specially trained nurses in intensive care units. Many of the procedures, such as intra-arterial and central venous pressure monitoring and the observations related to vital functions, require advanced educational training. However, nurses caring for the child prior to surgery and during the convalescent period need to be familiar with the major principles of care.

Providing maximum rest. One of the primary objectives after heart surgery is to provide maximum rest to decrease the workload of the heart and promote healing. With a great many procedures and observations to be performed, this objective is met through organized nursing care, which is planned according to the child's usual activity and sleep patterns. The simplest way to assure individualized efficient, high-quality care is to schedule each nursing procedure at the beginning of the shift. For example, each hour is divided into 15-minute intervals and appropriate observations/procedures are scheduled. Periods of rest are identified. Pain medication is tentatively planned when painful procedures are done, such as postural drainage or removing chest tubes. The schedule should be shared with parents to allow them to visit at the most advantageous times, such as after a rest period when no special treatments are anticipated.

Observation of vital signs and arterial/venous pressures. Vital signs and blood pressure are usually taken every 15 minutes for the first 12 to 24 hours. However, they need not disturb the child's rest if the deflated blood pressure cuff is kept in place and an electronic thermometer is used. Heart rate and respirations are counted, compared with the electrocardiogram monitor, and recorded with activity. The heart rate is normally accelerated after surgery. The nurse observes cardiac rhythm and notifies the physician of any changes in regularity.

At least hourly the nurse auscultates the lungs for breath sounds. Diminished or absent sounds most likely indicate an area of atelectasis, which necessitates further medical assessment. Auscultation also guides the nurse's selective use of postural drainage and percussion to those pulmonary lobes most in need of it. It also allows a more objective evaluation of effective pulmonary ventilation vs signs of compromised function.

Temperature changes are usual during the early postoperative period. Hypothermia is expected immediately after surgery from hypothermia procedures, effects of anesthesia, and loss of body heat to the cool environment. During this period the child is kept warm to prevent additional heat loss. Infants may be placed under radiant heat warmers. During the next 24 to 48 hours the body temperature may rise to 37.7°C (100°F) as part of the inflammatory response to tissue trauma.[16] After this period an elevated temperature is most likely a sign of infection and warrants immediate investigation for probable cause.

Intra-arterial monitoring of blood pressure is frequently used in open-heart surgery, because residual vasoconstriction after the use of cardiopulmonary bypass makes indirect blood pressure readings less reliable. A catheter is passed into an artery and the other end is attached to an electronic monitoring system, which provides a continuous recording of the blood pressure on an oscilloscope. The blood pressure readings are compared with those taken indirectly with a sphygmomanometer, since a discrepancy between the two may indicate a change in peripheral vascular resistance or an error in the electronic device. The nurse also observes for potential complications of intra-arterial monitoring, such as arterial thrombosis, infection, air emboli, or blood loss through the catheter. Prevention of each of these hazards is similar to care for any other type of infusion.

The intra-arterial line is irrigated frequently with heparinized saline to prevent clotting. The nurse records the amount of irrigant as intake fluid. Signs of bleeding from the heparin are observed for. The dressing at the site is changed daily. In some institutions a bacteriocidal ointment is applied. If the child's condition remains stable, the arterial catheter is removed in 48 to 72 hours.

Central venous pressure is routinely taken after heart surgery. It is a measurement of the pressure or competency of the right side of the heart. Therefore, it indicates right atrial filling pressure, right ventricular function, the relationship between blood volume (venous return) and cardiac output, and early signs of right-sided congestive heart failure. The central venous pressure catheter is inserted into the right atrium by way of the right basilic, brachial, or cephalic vein, although the jugular vein can also be used. It is attached to an infusion line and a manometer by means of a three-way stopcock. The central venous pressure is taken by positioning the child flat if possible, holding the zero mark of the manometer at the midaxillary line (level of the heart), and turning the stopcock to allow fluid from the manometer to flow into the veins. The drop in the level of fluid in the manometer equals the central venous pressure in the superior vena cava. The normal central venous pressure is approximately 3 to 10 cm of water.

The central venous pressure continually changes according to blood volume, heart rate, and myocardial tone. If the blood volume decreases, such as in shock, the central venous pressure falls. If the efficiency of the left side of the heart decreases, the resistance to right-side systolic ejection will result in an elevated central venous pressure but decreased intra-arterial pressure. Congestive heart failure and/or hypervolemia raise the central venous pressure.

The complications of central venous pressure lines are similar to other infusions, with the addition of atrial arrhythmias from irritation of the atrial wall, hemothorax, pneumothorax, or hydrothorax from accidental puncture as the catheter enters the thorax, and infusion overload, since the intravenous line is kept patent by a continuous drip. The nurse observes for signs and symptoms indicative of each of these risks.

Malpositioning of the central venous pressure catheter past the right atrium can result in life-threatening ventricular arrhythmias and spuriously elevated central venous pressure readings. Signs of malpositioning are vigorous fluctuations of the manometer fluid with the heartbeat, which indicates placement in the right ventricle, or consistently elevated central venous pressure readings without further evidence of hypervolemia or congestive heart failure, which indicates entry into the pulmonary artery. The nurse alerts the physician to these signs.[15] A chest x-ray examination is necessary to confirm misplacement. Treatment is to withdraw the catheter so that it enters only the right atrium. The catheter should be marked with tape close to the site of insertion to readily detect any further advancement.

Maintaining respiratory status. If respirations are impaired, the child may temporarily be placed on a mechanical ventilator. He is kept in a humidified environment, such as a Croupette, to liquify secretions. The nurse ensures that the child is kept warm and dry, since excessive chilling from wet linens causes an increased metabolic need and consequent increased cardiac demand. The child coughs, turns, and deep breathes at least hourly. Every measure is employed to enhance ventilation and decrease pain, such as splinting of the operative site and judicious use of analgesics. Although crying increases heart rate, it is beneficial in promoting deep respirations.

Postural drainage is done frequently, usually every 4 hours. It is helpful to have two nurses work together, one to position the child while the other percusses and vibrates. Since the procedure is uncomfortable, it is important to emphasize to the child the necessity of performing it and to clarify that the percussion, sometimes mistakenly viewed as hitting, is done to loosen secretions in the lungs. Since this procedure may upset parents, it is advisable to do it when they are not visiting. However, if the child is comforted by his parents and they wish to participate, they can be very helpful in positioning him.

Suctioning is done as needed. Infants and young children have a weak cough reflex, necessitating more frequent suctioning. The nurse performs deep suctioning carefully to avoid vagal stimulation (cardiac arrythmias) and laryngospasm. Suctioning is intermittent and maintained for 10 to 20 seconds at a time to prevent depleting the oxygen supply. If the child becomes cyanotic during suctioning, he may need supplemental oxygen with an AMBU bag before and after the procedure. Heart rate is monitored after suctioning to detect changes in rhythm or rate.

Chest tubes are inserted into the pleural space to remove secretions and air in order to allow reexpansion of the lung (Fig. 35-22). One or more catheters may be inserted into each lung and are attached to water-seal drainage bottles. The purpose of the underwater drainage is to prevent air from traveling up the tube into the pleural space. Fig. 35-23 demonstrates three different types of water-seal chest drainage. The following nursing considerations are the same regardless of the drainage system used.

As soon as the child returns from surgery, the nurse checks the placement and patency of the tubes. Since the system must be airtight, every outlet is inspected for leaks: (1) the dressing should be tight around the tubing insertion into the pleural cavity, (2) the chest tube should be securely attached to the bottle, (3) the glass rod inside the bottle should be *under* the water, and (4) the rubber suction cap on the bottle should be tight. At no time does the nurse loosen any attachments to check them, unless the tubing to the chest is clamped.

As a precaution to preserve an airtight seal, all connections are taped closed and the bottles are taped to the floor (they may also be placed in a special metal holder). In case of an accidental break in the system, two Kelly clamps or hemostats for each chest tube, the tips of which are covered with rubber tubing to prevent cutting the catheters, are taped to the bedside. If needed they are clamped to the chest tube as close to the patient as possible. A gauze dressing with one side liberally covered with petrolatum is also taped to the bedside in case the tubes dislodge from the

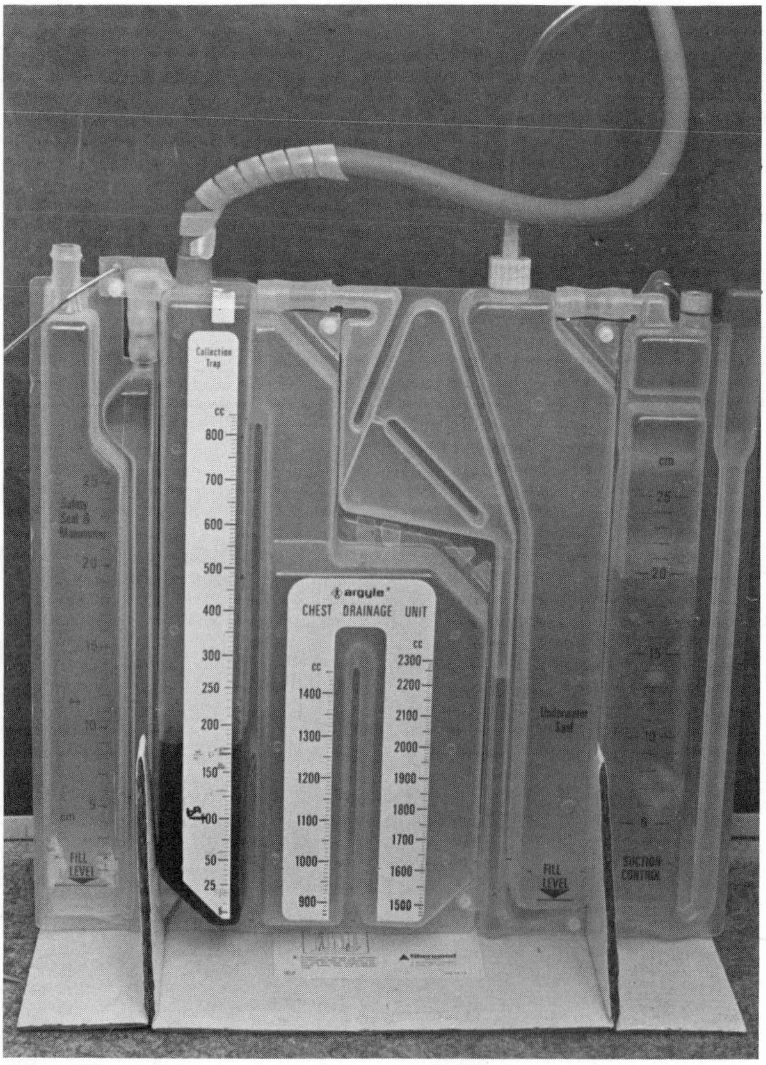

Fig. 35-22. Pleurevac.

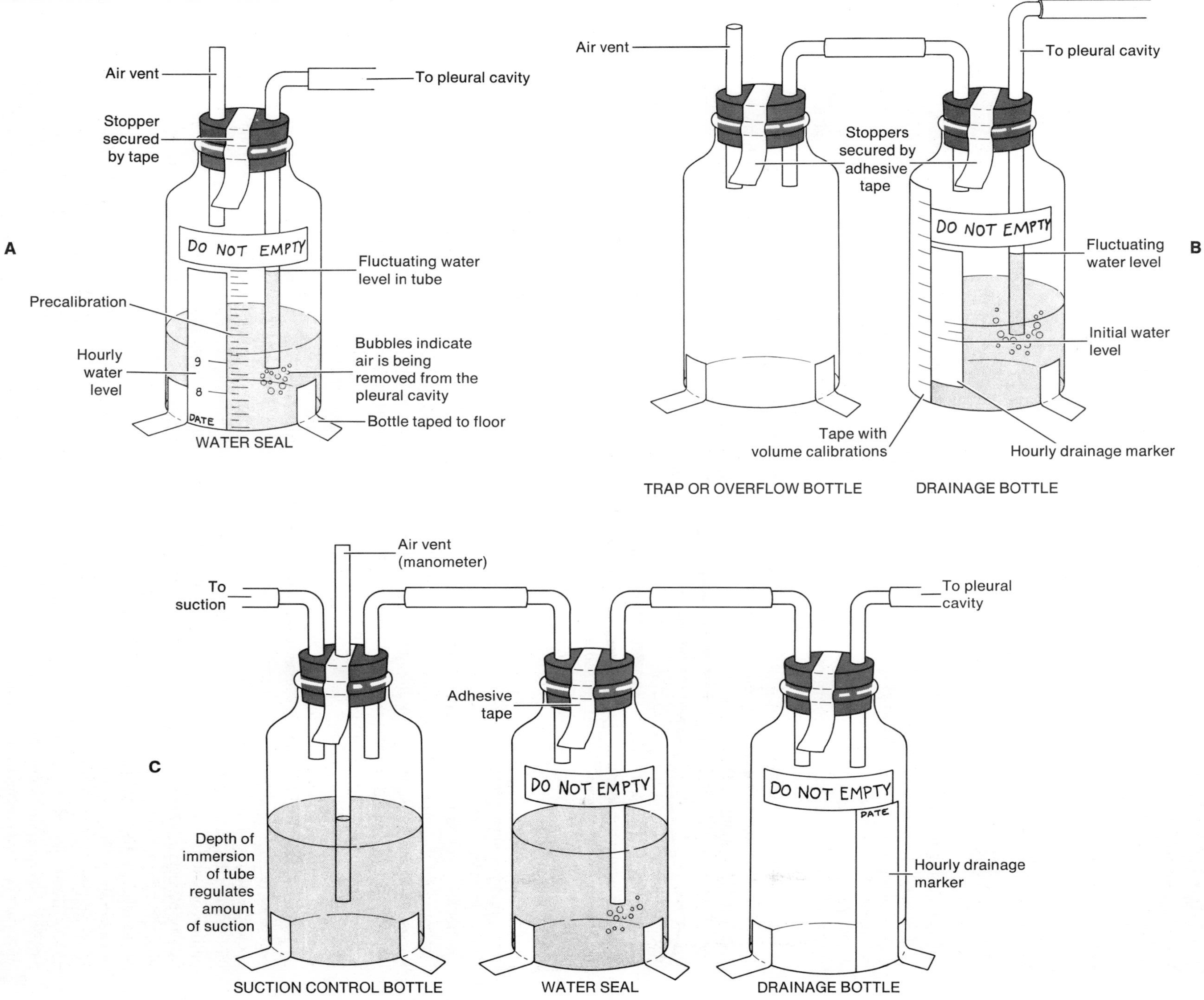
A
Air vent
To pleural cavity
Stopper secured by tape
DO NOT EMPTY
Fluctuating water level in tube
Precalibration
Bubbles indicate air is being removed from the pleural cavity
Hourly water level
9
8
DATE
Bottle taped to floor
WATER SEAL
B
Air vent
To pleural cavity
Stoppers secured by adhesive tape
DO NOT EMPTY
Fluctuating water level
Initial water level
Tape with volume calibrations
Hourly drainage marker
TRAP OR OVERFLOW BOTTLE
DRAINAGE BOTTLE
C
Air vent (manometer)
To suction
To pleural cavity
Adhesive tape
DO NOT EMPTY
DO NOT EMPTY
DATE
Depth of immersion of tube regulates amount of suction
Hourly drainage marker
SUCTION CONTROL BOTTLE
WATER SEAL
DRAINAGE BOTTLE

Fig. 35-23. One-, two-, and three-bottle systems for water-sealed chest drainage.

chest wall. If this occurs the petrolatum side is placed against the skin to maintain an airtight seal. The drainage bottles are labeled "DO NOT EMPTY OR OPEN" to alert everyone to the need for preserving a closed system.

Each of these precautions is instituted prior to the child's return from the operating or recovery room, since accidents during transfer from stretcher to bed may necessitate emergency intervention. In the event that no precautions have been taken and a bottle breaks, the tubing can be clamped by bending it in at least two areas and holding it closed. If the tubes dislodge from the chest, the nurse holds the hand tightly over the site of insertion and summons help without leaving the child. If possible the nurse administers supplemental oxygen, since accidental entry of air may have resulted in a pneumothorax and severely compromised pulmonary function. Signs of pneumothorax are persistent sharp chest pain, sudden dyspnea, tachycardia, rapid, shallow respirations, and cyanosis. Signs of air leaking from the drainage system are evidenced by constant bubbling of air in the water-seal bottle and restlessness, mounting apprehension, progressive dyspnea, and chest pain.

Proper functioning of the tubes is evidenced by fluctuation of water in the long tube. Normally the water rises during inspiration and falls during expiration. Failure to observe this movement may indicate an obstruction in the tubing, such as a kink or a clot. However, it may also signify a fully expanded lung, depending on the length of time the tubes have been inserted. A sudden loss of fluctuation, especially during coughing, which normally causes a sharp fall in the level of water, often indicates loss of patency. The tubing is checked for any kinks, especially from pressure when lying on the affected site. Clots are removed by milking the tubing in the direction of the drainage bottles. This procedure should be done frequently to prevent clot formation. It is important to always be conscious of the pull on the tubing during milking to prevent inadvertently disloding it. One way of avoiding this hazard is to hold the tubing close to the patient with one hand and milk with the other hand.

The child is positioned to facilitate the flow of drainage by gravity. Usually lying on the affected side is most conducive to promoting drainage, but care must be taken to avoid pressure or kinking of the tubing. The length of the tubing must be long enough to facilitate turning without pulling on the insertion site. The tubing is secured to the bed by placing a rubber band around the catheter and pinning the rubber band to the sheet. In this way any tension on the tubing is relieved by the elasticity in the rubber band.

The drainage bottles are always placed below the level of the child's chest to promote drainage and prevent back flow of water and/or secretions to the pleural cavity. This measure is especially important during transportation or ambulation. To prevent cellular injury from accidental back flow, sterile normal saline rather than distilled water should be used to effect the water seal.

Drainage is checked hourly for color and quantity. Immediately postoperatively the drainage may be bright red, but afterward is only blood-tinged. The largest volume of drainage occurs in the first 12 to 24 hours and is more copious in extensive heart surgery.

Some water-seal systems have calibrated markings on the bottles. To chart the time, a piece of adhesive tape is applied next to the calibrations and at each hour the time is recorded next to the level of drainage. If the one-bottle system is used, in which secretions accumulate with the already present sterile saline, the tape is marked to distinguish the level of water from the drainage. For example, if the chest tubes are inserted at 10:00 AM, this time is indicated on the tape at the level of sterile water. The nurse who receives the child from the recovery room checks to ensure that this has been done.

The drainage bottle may be emptied at each shift or not at all, depending on the amount of fluid and the institution's policy. If emptying is necessary, each chest tube is clamped with two hemostats *before* the collecting bottle is opened. If the system is attached to mechanical suction, the machine is turned off. The system is reconnected before the clamps are removed. It is imperative, however, for the nurse to remember this last point. One way of reminding oneself is to write the word "CLAMPS" on the adhesive, which is attached to the bed during disuse. When the clamps are applied, the nurse places the tape on the tubing near its attachment to the collecting bottle. In this way when the chest tube is reconnected, the nurse is automatically reminded of the clamps.

Chest x-ray films are taken when the tubes are inserted to check their location and before removal to evaluate the inflation of the lungs. Chest tubes are usually removed on the second to third postoperative day. Lung expansion is evidenced by decreased fluctuation in the tube and absence of drainage.

Removing chest tubes is a painful and frightening experience. Analgesics should be given 20 minutes prior to the procedure. Children must be told beforehand that they will feel a sharp momentary pain and a shortness of breath. After the suture is cut, the tubes are quickly pulled out during expiration or at the end of full inspiration to prevent intake of air into the pleural cavity. A petrolatum-covered gauze dressing is immediately applied over the wound and securely taped on all four sides to the skin. It is not removed until the opening is healed, usually within 5 to 10 days. It should be checked for signs of drainage, any evidence of infection, or loosening.

Monitoring fluids. Intake and output of all fluids are accurately calculated. Intake is primarily intravenous fluids. However, the nurse must keep a record of fluid used to flush the arterial and central venous pressure lines. Output includes hourly recordings of urine (usually a Foley catheter is inserted and attached to a closed collecting device), drainage from thoracotomy tubes, and blood drawn for analysis. Urine is also analyzed for specific gravity to assess the concentrating ability of the kidneys and to approximately assess the body's degree of hydration. The nurse measures pH to evaluate metabolic acidosis. Kidney failure is a potential risk in open-heart surgery because of tissue ischemia during the cardiopulmonary bypass procedure and from rapid hemolysis of red blood cells, which causes obstruction in the renal tubules and necrosis (the pathologic process is similar to that in blood incompatibility). The signs of kidney failure are decreased urine output (less than 10 ml/hour in an infant and 30 ml/hour in children) and an elevated specific gravity.

Fluids are restricted during the immediate postoperative period to prevent hypervolemia, which places additional demands on the myocardium, predisposing to cardiac failure. Two factors influence increased blood volume. In open-heart surgery the cardiopulmonary pump is primed with a large volume of nonblood fluid (usually electrolyte solution), which greatly dilutes the patient's blood. During circulation through the body, some of this priming fluid diffuses into the interstitial spaces but postoperatively diffuses back into the systemic circulation.[15]

In addition the physiologic changes of open- or closed-heart surgery stimulate the adrenal cortex to secrete aldosterone, which increases renal reabsorption of sodium. This results in water retention but increased excretion of potassium. Concurrently the hypothalamus secretes additional antidiuretic hormone (ADH), which causes the distal and collecting tubules to reabsorb more water.[24] Not only does this process result in hypervolemia, but it also causes electrolyte imbalances, principally, hypokalemia. Decreased potassium affects myocardial function, greatly increasing the risk of arrhythmias. The nurse assesses electrolyte imbalances by observing for signs of hypokalemia and checking all blood electrolyte analysis reports.

Fluid requirements are based on the child's weight and body surface area. The nurse weighs the child daily using the same bed scale at approximately the same time each day to avoid errors in measurement. The child is usually given nothing by mouth for the first 24 hours. If an endotracheal tube is inserted, fluids are not begun until the child is extubated. A fluid restriction is usually imposed even when oral fluids are begun. Therefore, the nurse plans how many milliliters are allowed per 8-hour shift, basing this calculation on the child's preoperative drinking habits. For example, if the child is allowed 1500 ml/24 hours, a typical fluid schedule might be 500 ml during the day shift, 350 to 400 ml during the evening shift, and 150 to 100 ml during the night shift. If additional or less fluid is taken on one shift, an adjustment is made during the next 8-hour period.

Planning for progressive activity. Fatigue and weakness are common after heart surgery, as a result of both the surgical trauma to the heart and sleep deprivation in the immediate postoperative period. However, moderate activity is essential to prevent pulmonary and vascular complications. Initially, turning, coughing, and deep breathing are sufficient to promote respiratory expansion. However, passive range of motion exercises, especially to the lower extremities, are instituted to prevent venous stasis. All infusion sites are inspected for evidence of thrombophlebitis and emboli. The areas are passively exercised to promote circulation.

A progressive schedule of ambulation and activity is planned, based on the child's preoperative activity patterns. For some children the ability to regain independence in self-care may be more of a priority than sitting up to read. Therefore, the nurse conserves the child's energy for what is most important to him. Toys that were enjoyed prior to surgery are provided to encourage movement. It is important to plan the activity at times when the child is well rested, is comfortable (usually has had analgesic medication), and is not scheduled for any strenuous procedure or treatment immediately afterward.

Ambulation is initiated early, usually by the second postoperative day, when chest tubes, arterial lines, and assisted ventilatory equipment may be removed. The nurse begins ambulation for this child as for a child who had undergone any other postsurgical procedure, progressing from sitting on the edge of the bed and dangling the legs to standing up and sitting in a chair. Heart rate and respirations are carefully monitored to assess the degree of cardiac demand imposed by each activity. Tachycardia, dyspnea, cyanosis, and progressive fatigue are signals to limit further energy expenditure. Even if the child is able to ambulate to a chair with a moderate increase in heart rate, the nurse keeps in mind the effort required to return to bed. After ambulation the nurse schedules a rest period.

Providing emotional support. It is not uncommon for older children to become depressed after surgery. This is thought to be caused by preoperative anxiety, postoperative psychologic and physiologic stress, and sensory overstimulation. Typically the disposition of the child improves on leaving the intensive care unit. The nurse should be aware of the possible reasons for such behavioral changes and manipulate the environment to accommodate the child's needs. The following example illustrates this point.

A child in the adult surgical intensive care unit became severely depressed and withdrawn postoperatively. She continually requested that the drapes be kept drawn around her bed. The nurse, realizing the sensory overload from the patient activity around the child, had her transferred to a private room in the unit. Almost immediately the child's mood improved. In 2 days she returned to her own room on the pediatric unit, where she recovered rapidly.

The child may also be angry and uncooperative after surgery as a response to the physical pain and to the loss of control imposed by the surgery and treatments. He needs an opportunity to express his feelings, either verbally or through activity. The nurse can be supportive by reassuring the child that the procedures are difficult to perform, praising him for any effort he makes to cooperate, and refraining from expecting too much "courage" or "bravery." For example, rather than fostering cooperation with statements, such as, "Big boys can stand this pain," the nurse reassures the child that, "Even the bravest of men cry when in pain." With this approach the child is allowed to express his feelings with acceptance from the nurse, regardless of his emotional response.

The nurse also accepts any negative remarks from the child, realizing that pain has been inflicted on him. It is not unusual for children to tell nurses that they hate them during a treatment. Rather than becoming defensive or overly apologetic, nurses should reply that they understand why the child feels that way but that the procedure is necessary for his recovery. They can also help parents and other members of the health team accept the child's negativism by explaining that the outburst is really a response to the treatment, not to the person.

The nurse can support the parents by being available for information and explaining all the procedures to them. The first few postoperative days are particularly difficult because parents see their child in pain and realize the potential risks from surgery. They often feel useless because they can do so little for him. The nurse can minimize such feelings by including parents in care-giving activities if they wish, such as a partial bath, turning, positioning for postural drainage, or the use of blow bottles. The importance of their presence in making the child feel more secure is stressed, even if they cannot physically care for him.

Nurses in the intensive care unit should be aware of statements they make that can be misinterpreted by parents. For example, remarking that the electrocardiogram does not look good can immediately raise parental concern for their child's survival, when actually the nurse may be referring to the machine's functioning. Casual statements or jokes made by nurses and other members of the health team can be viewed as lack of concern for the child. Such miconceptions can be greatly lessened if one nurse assumes responsibility for the child's care and maintains constant communication with the family.

Observation for complications of heart surgery. Several complications can occur after heart surgery, the majority of which are related to open-heart surgery and use of cardiopulmonary bypass. Many of the procedures discussed in the preceding paragraphs are aimed at preventing these problems. Only those that have not already been discussed are included in the following paragraphs.

Hematologic changes. While passing through the heart-lung machine, blood is exposed to substantial trauma by direct contact with oxygen, mechanical action, foreign substances, and massive anticoagulants. The result of this injury is red blood cell hemolysis and potentially renal tubular necrosis, clotting abnormalities from decreased thrombin and prothrombin, as well as heparinization of the blood during extracorporeal circulation, decreased platelets, and altered platelet aggregation.[15]

Hemolysis of red blood cells results in blood loss and anemia, which may require packed red blood cell transfusion. The nurse monitors results of complete blood counts in order to identify the severity of the hemolysis. If transfusions are given, the nurse closely observes for signs of reaction and fluid overload. The necessity of measuring hourly urine output has already been discussed.

Since blood clotting mechanisms are affected, the nurse observes for signs of hemorrhage, especially frank bleeding from the chest tubes and a fall in arterial/venous pressures. Hemorrhage is more likely to occur in cyanotic heart repairs because of the physiologic thrombocytopenia associated with them.

Normally the filter and bubble trap on the machine remove air emboli, tiny clots, fat debris, and organisms from the arterialized (oxygenated) blood prior to its return to the body. However, impure blood entering the systemic circulation can cause fat emboli, thromboemboli, and infection anywhere in the body, but most importantly in the endocardium. Hepatitis from multiple donor transfusions during the bypass procedure is a constant risk.

Cardiac changes. Cardiac failure may result from increased workload on ventricles that have been hypertrophied prior to surgery. For example, in tetralogy of Fallot closure of the ventricular septal defect forces the right ventricle to pump blood only to the pulmonary artery. Inability to meet this new hemodynamic pattern may result in congestive heart failure. Children with congestive heart failure prior to surgery usually continue to show signs of failure and require continued medical treatment with digitalis and diuretics. Heart failure may occur suddenly when there is an obstruction to blood flow secondary to the operative procedure. This complication may require additional surgery to reverse the stricture. The nurse observes for signs of heart failure, including elevation of the central venous pressure.

Low cardiac output syndrome and decreased peripheral perfusion can occur as a result of vasoconstriction after cardiopulmonary bypass and hypothermia or from inability of the left ventricle to maintain systemic circulation. The most important signs of adequate peripheral perfusion are skin color, temperature, and presence of all pulses. Evidence of low cardiac output are similar to those of shock, namely decreased blood pressure, decreased pulse pressure, and oliguria.

Arrhythmias can result from hypokalemia and surgical intervention of the atrial myocardium, especially ostium primum defects. The latter is throught to be the result of injury to the conduction system. The nurse monitors heart rate and rhythm carefully both by observing the electrocardiogram pattern and by counting the apical pulse for 1 full minute.

Cardiac tamponade is compression of the heart by blood and other effusion (clots) in the pericardial sac, which severely restricts the normal heart movement. A characteristic sign is *paradoxical pulse pressure,* in which the systolic pressure drops during inspiration because inhaling causes the accumulated blood to compress the heart, resulting in a drop in cardiac output. Other signs include a rising venous pressure, falling arterial pressure, narrowing pulse pressure, dyspnea, cyanosis, apprehension, and a compensatory posturing of sitting and leaning forward. Any evidence of this potentially fatal complication is immediately reported to the physician. Treatment consists of pericardiocentesis to remove the blood. If active hemorrhage is present, steps are taken to enhance blood clotting.

Pulmonary changes. Areas of atelectasis are not uncommon immediately after surgery as a result of deflation of the lung during cardiopulmonary bypass. Postperfusion lung syndrome is the most serious respiratory problem seen in these patients and is characterized by atelectasis, pulmonary edema, and hemorrhage. Its etiology is unknown, although it may be caused by microemboli in small pulmonary vessels, inhibition of surfactant production, and pulmonary hypoperfusion or hypoxia.[24] The usual respiratory measures employed after surgery to promote ventilation and the use of an endotracheal tube to facilitate ventilatory assistance and deep suctioning of the tracheobronchial tree help to prevent or minimize this complication.

Two other pulmonary complications are pneumothorax, especially caused by faulty chest tubes, and pulmonary edema, from increased pulmonary blood flow or left-sided heart failure. Signs alerting the nurse to pneumothorax have been discussed under chest tubes. Signs of pulmonary edema are the same as those seen in congestive heart failure, namely, rales, wheezing, moist dyspneic respirations, tachycardia, cyanosis, and restlessness.

Neurologic changes. Cerebral edema and brain damage may occur during open-heart surgery. Although the exact cause is unknown, it is thought to be a result of tissue ischemia or emboli. The nurse checks the equality of strength and reflexes in both extremities for evidence of paralysis and assesses the child's orientation to his environment. Any evidence of cerebral damage is immediately reported to the physician.

Postpericardiotomy syndrome. This syndrome of fever, pericardial friction rub, and/or pericardial and pleural effusion can occur anytime the pericardium is opened, either in the postoperative convalescent period or several months after surgery. The cause is unknown, although theories of etiology include a viral infection, autoimmune response to myocardial tissue, or a reaction to blood in the pericardium. It is treated with rest, saliycylates, and sometimes steroids.

Postperfusion syndrome. This syndrome is thought to be an inflammatory/infectious process contracted from donor's blood used in the heart lung machine. It is characterized by fever, hepatosplenomegaly, leukocytosis, malaise, and a maculopapular rash. It commonly occurs between the first and third months after surgery. Treatment is the same as for postpericardiotomy syndrome.

Planning for discharge. Ideally planning for discharge begins on admission when the nurse assesses the parents' and child's readiness and ability to give up the sick role and adjust to the responsibilities and privileges of a healthy child. If parents have been guided in caring for this child with as much normalcy as is shown the other siblings, the transition to full recovery is facilitated. Unfortunately this is not always the case, necessitating that the nurse discuss this phase of recovery with the parents.

One method of approaching this subject is asking parents how they view their child's future. This can vary from one extreme of believing that no surgery can totally correct a heart defect to the belief that now the child can resume all normal activity. Both of these views are harmful. The first preserves the dependent child-parent role and restricts future growth and development. The other places such tremendous demands on the child that he may be forced to resume the sick role in order to cope with unrealistic expectations.

Emotional adjustment involves a gradual resumption of physical ability as well as responsibility. For an older child who has never had the opportunity to develop athletic competence, a sense of competition, or fine muscle coordination, it may be unrealistic to pursue a goal in this direction, despite physical ability to do so. In this instance it is more beneficial to encourage interests that have already been developed. This may be very difficult for fathers who may anticipate that after corrective heart surgery their sons will be able to join them in competitive sports.

Fostering a sense of responsibility is equally difficult. Parents may have a great need to continue a dependent relationship for themselves. Likewise, the child may be unwilling to accept new limits or to give up privileges of the sick role. The nurse investigates the family relationships to identify those roles or needs that may prevent parents or children from establishing a new set of expectations. For example, one mother continued to drive her daughter to school, despite the fact that the child could easily walk the few blocks. When the nurse questioned the mother about this, she became very defensive, stressing that she knew what was best for her child. Rather than pursue this discussion the nurse directed the topic to how the parent's life-style had changed since the child's surgery. The mother readily responded that she had so much more free time. Since her daughter's birth she had stopped working and had severed many former social relationships. The nurse encouraged the mother to pursue some of her former interests. At the next clinic visit, the mother remarked that she had started a part-time job. Out of necessity, she had had to stop driving the child to school. Not only was the parent more contented, but the child had made some new friends and now was "allowed" to play outside after school. The mother stated that she and her husband had gone out to dinner for the first time in years. The nurse encouraged the parent to continue these changes, stressing that they would benefit everyone.

Family relationships extend beyond the parents and child to the siblings as well. Older siblings may tolerate increased responsibility when the child is ill but often become resentful once they know that he can share the chores. Sometimes a sibling becomes very close to the ill child, preferring to care for or play with him rather than seek experiences outside the home. As the child recovers from heart surgery and begins to participate in activities, the other sibling may lag behind. For example, a younger brother of a girl with a severe cyanotic defect was very attached to his sister. He even imitated her behavior to the point of assuming the squat position to be "like her." The parents encouraged the close relationship because the daughter was kept amused and contented by the attention from this child. However, after her surgery at age 5 years, the brother persisted in his behavior toward her as if she were still sick. He viewed her increased physical activity and interests as rejection of him. The parents soon realized they had raised two children with heart disease, one being congenital, the other acquired. The family sought professional advice, which eventually resolved their problems.

The nurse can facilitate adjustment by gradually expecting more from the child in the recovery period and stressing to parents the importance of gradual achievement of new skills and responsibilities. Since the postoperative period is quite short, only 7 to 10 days for an uncomplicated recovery, the nurse should make a referral to a public health nursing agency for follow-up in the home. It is also advisable to discuss plans for enrolling the child in school, including nursery experience. Since social relationships have often been limited prior to corrective surgery, the nurse stresses the importance of providing peer activities. The hospital can serve as an initial experience in meeting and relating to children of various ages. The play therapist may be helpful in structuring group activities appropriate for the child.

Physical care on discharge depends on the child's condition. In an uneventful postoperative convalescence, the only care may be periodic medical examinations. If congestive heart failure is still present, the child may need to continue receiving medication. Since postpericardiotomy and postperfusion syndromes may occur after discharge, the nurse alerts the parents to signs suggesting them, namely, unexplained fever, any chest pain, difficulty in breathing, or a loss of energy. It is best not to place undue emphasis on these syndromes, since anxiety over their occurrence may retard the parents' readiness to foster more realistic expectations from the child. (For a summary of nursing care of the child undergoing heart surgery, see the boxed material on pp. 1343 to 1346.)

Acquired heart disease

CONGESTIVE HEART FAILURE

Congestive heart failure (CHF) is inability of the heart to pump an adequate amount of blood to the systemic circulation to meet the body's metabolic demands. Causes of heart failure can be classified according to the following changes: (1) increased volume, especially with left-to-right shunts that cause the right ventricle to hypertrophy in order to compensate for the additional blood volume, (2) increased pressure, primarily resulting from obstructive lesions, such as valvular stenosis or coartation of the aorta, (3) myocardial factors that affect the contractility of the muscle fibers, such as myocardial ischemia from severe anemia or asphyxia, heart block, acidemia, and low levels of potassium, glucose, calcium, or magnesium, and (4) high cardiac output demands, in which the body's need for oxygenated blood exceeds the heart's cardiac output (even though the volume may be normal), such as in obstructive lung disease, hyperthyroidism, and severe anemia. In children congestive heart failure is most frequently secondary to structural abnormalities that result in increased blood volume and pressure. It is a symptom caused by an underlying cardiac defect, not a disease in itself, since it is usually the result of an excessive workload imposed on a normal myocardium. The majority of children who experience congestive heart failure are infants.

Heart failure is often separated into two classifications: right-sided or left-sided failure. In right-sided failure the right ventricle is unable to pump blood into the pulmonary artery, resulting in less blood being oxygenated by the lungs and increased pressure in the right atrium and systemic venous circulation. Systemic venous hypertension causes edema in the extremities and viscera. In left-sided failure the left ventricle is unable to pump blood into the systemic circulation, resulting in increased pressure in the left atrium and pulmonary veins. The lungs become congested with blood, causing elevated pulmonary pressures and pulmonary edema.

Although each type produces different systemic/pulmonary alterations, clinically it is unusual to observe solely right- or left-sided failure. Since both sides of the heart are dependent on adequate function of the other side, failure of one chamber causes a reciprocal change in the opposite chamber. For example, in left-sided failure increase

Summary of nursing care of the child undergoing heart surgery

Goals	Responsibilities
Preoperative	
Introduce child to environment	Involve intensive care unit nurse who will care for child postoperatively in teaching Introduce intensive care unit nurses to child during visit; use names to increase familiarity Time visit to intensive care unit when most appropriate (child is well rested, parents can accompany him, and unit is quiet), usually day prior to surgery Explain all equipment that will affect child, especially strange noises or sights Emphasize positive aspects of environment (play area, parents' lounge, and so on) Encourage parents and child to ask questions or explore area, but do not insist on either If feasible, introduce child to another young patient recovering from surgery
Familiarize child with equipment	Assess child's familiarity with equipment Acquaint child with equipment used postoperatively Sphygmomanometer and thermometer—taken more frequently, cuff may be left on arm, electronic sensor may be on abdomen Oxygen tent—let child look through plastic; show him another child in tent Oxygen mask—let him try it on Intravenous infusion—emphasize location of each infusion for older child, explain purpose of central venous pressure manometer and/or arterial line; explain that they are inserted during surgery and that only discomfort is from restricted mobility of extremities Dressing—discuss size and location of dressing Chest tubes—leave this to end Explain purpose Demonstrate on doll or show picture Stress that child must move even though it may hurt Endotracheal tube—leave this to end Compare to "breathing tube" placed in nose or mouth Discuss how it feels (something in throat); reassure child that this is normal Can demonstrate use of suction catheter through tube Help child express needs nonverbally Individualize need to discuss emergency procedures with child, but discuss them with parents
Practice preoperative procedures	May be done in conjunction with above If presented as games, clarify that procedures will not be as easy postoperatively Discuss pain matter-of-factly and include measures to reduce pain (splinting operative site and analgesics) Practice each procedure Deep breathing—have child deliberately raise his chest during inspiration to emphasize deep breathing Coughing—demonstrate deep cough, not merely clearing throat Blow bottles—have child practice on one or blow bubbles through straw

Continued.

Summary of nursing care of the child undergoing heart surgery—cont'd

Goals	Responsibilities
Preoperative—cont'd Practice preoperative procedures—cont'd	Suction—demonstrate suction either on child or in glass of water; compare catheter to "magic straw" Turning—have child turn from side to side when in semi-Fowler's position; demonstrate self-help techniques (bending legs and holding side rails) Postural drainage/percussion—demonstrate positions; emphasize that clapping is not hitting IPPB—have respiratory therapist (preferably one who will be working with child postoperatively) demonstrate use of machine; compare breathing to apparatus of skin diver or astronaut Bedpan/urinal—have child practice using them; discuss special tube (Foley catheter) Discuss any other preparatory procedures (nothing by mouth, enema, skin cleansing, sedation medication)
Make preoperative observations	Record vital signs and blood pressure Record with activity Report temperature elevation to physician (infection contraindication to surgery) Report increase in pulse and respiration (may be sign of CHF) Monitor sleep/wake patterns and record to maintain similar schedule after surgery Keep record of elimination Record bowel habits as baseline data for preventing constipation after surgery Record child's specific toilet habits on nursing care plan (use of potty-chair, diapers, expressions for elimination) Measure fluid intake Record daily habits of fluid intake Record fluid preferences
Postoperative Provide maximum rest	Plan procedures to accommodate child's usual sleep/wake pattern Tentatively plan pain medication for when uncomfortable procedures are performed Share schedule with parents for visiting at most opportune time
Observe vital signs and arterial/venous pressures	Record with activity; compare to electronic monitoring devices (pulse and respiration to ECG, intra-arterial line to blood pressure) Report any sudden, unexplained changes in heart rate or rhythm to physician Auscultate lungs for breath sounds; use findings as basis for postural drainage If hypothermic, maintain body heat If hyperthermic, report to physician (after 48 to 72 hours, most likely sign of infection) Observe for complications of arterial lines (thrombophlebitis, emboli, hemorrhage) and central venous pressure (atrial or ventricular arrhythmias or puncture of thorax) Report any changes in arterial/venous pressures to physician

Summary of nursing care of the child undergoing heart surgery—cont'd

Goals	Responsibilities
Postoperative—cont'd	
Maintain respiratory status	Keep child dry and warm if in oxygen tent Have child turn, cough, and deep breathe at least hourly Perform postural drainage/percussion (PD/C) every 4 hours Judge parents' wishes to stay or leave the room Have another nurse (or parent) assist with positioning Schedule analgesics prior to postural drainage/percussion Suction as necessary, being careful not to deplete child's oxygen supply; monitor heart rate after suctioning for changes in rate/rhythm Ensure that chest tubes are functioning Facilitate chest tube drainage Institute precautions against break in water-seal system Be alert to signs of pneumothorax from sudden break in drainage system or slow air leak Persistent short chest pain Sudden dyspnea Tachycardia Rapid, shallow breathing Cyanosis Restlessness and apprehension Check drainage hourly for color and quantity; mark bottle with adhesive tape to accurately record hourly secretions Evaluate readiness for removal of tubes Decreased fluctuation in tube Scanty or absent drainage Prepare child for chest tube removal; emphasize that sharp chest pain is only momentary Have petrolatum covered dressing ready for immediate application over site of insertion; ensure that dressing is airtight
Monitor fluids	Keep accurate record of *all* intake and output, especially irrigating fluid to flush central venous pressure/arterial lines, thoracotomy drainage, and blood drawn for analysis Take daily weight for calculation of fluid requirements Test urine for specific gravity and pH Report decreased urine output (less than 10 to 30 ml/hour) to physician When oral fluids are begun, plan any fluid restriction on child's usual fluid habits Observe for signs of electrolyte imbalance, especially hypokalemia
Plan for progressive activity	Institute coughing, turning, deep breathing, and passive range of motion exercises to extremities Base progressive ambulation on child's preoperative activity tolerance Plan activity when child is well rested and free of pain; do not schedule strenuous procedures after activity but provide for period of rest Monitor vital signs during activity for evidence of overexertion
Provide emotional support	Be aware of environmental factors that may adversely affect child Encourage expression of feelings rather than expectation of bravery or stoicism Praise child for any attempt to cooperate Accept negative remarks without defensiveness or unnecessary apology

Continued.

Summary of nursing care of the child undergoing heart surgery—cont'd

Goals	Responsibilities
Postoperative—cont'd	
Provide emotional support—cont'd	Inform parents of child's progress Include parents in care-giving activities Emphasize importance of parents' presence in emotionally supporting child Refrain from making remarks that can be misinterpreted by parents Encourage parents to discuss their feelings about child's care and progress
Observe for complications	Hematologic Assess blood counts for evidence of anemia or thrombocytopenia Observe for hemorrhage Observe for emboli anywhere in body Cardiac Observe for signs of congestive heart failure Assess peripheral perfusion (skin temperature, color, presence of pulses) Assess cardiac output (if low, signs of shock) Monitor heart rate and rhythm Observe for signs of cardiac tamponade Pulmonary Observe for signs of postperfusion lung syndrome, pneumothorax, and pulmonary edema Institute pulmonary hygiene measures to prevent complications Neurologic Check equality of reflexes and muscular strength Assess orientation to environment Observe for evidence of postcardiotomy and postperfusion syndrome; advise parents to report symptoms such as unexplained fever, rash, chest pain, or malaise to physician
Plan for discharge	Assess parents' and child's readiness to relinquish sick role and gradually assume responsibilities and privileges of healthy child Encourage realistic pursuits for child Identify family-child relationship that may prevent sense of independence in child or other family member Allow family members to discuss their feelings about child's physical improvement During postoperative period, set an example of gradually expecting more participation and independence from child Refer to public health nursing agency for follow-up care in home

in pulmonary vascular congestion will cause back pressure in the right ventricle, resulting in right ventricular hypertrophy, decreased myocardial efficiency, and eventually pooling of blood in the systemic venous circulation.

Compensatory mechanisms

Congestive heart failure is actually failure of compensatory mechanisms to increase cardiac function in accordance with metabolic requirements. Since most of the signs and symptoms result from decompensation, one must first look at the compensatory processes that attempt to preserve cardiac function (Fig. 35-24).

Sympathetic stimulation. When the cardiac output falls, the atrial and venous stretch receptors and the aortic and carotid baroreceptors stimulate the sympathetic nervous system, which exerts two major effects. It increases the

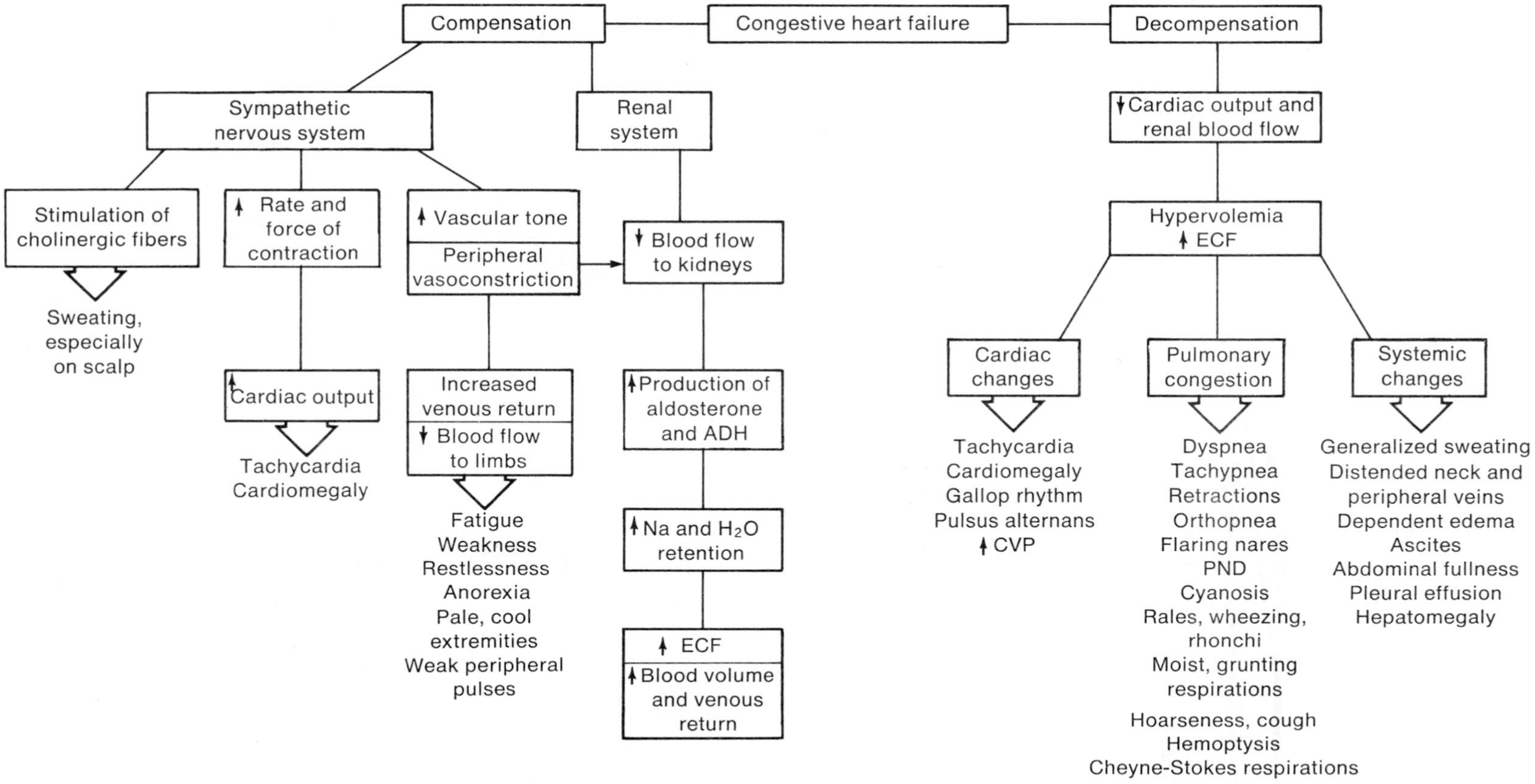

Fig. 35-24. Effects of congestive heart failure.

force and rate of myocardial contraction, resulting in a more efficient pumping action. It also increases venous return by increasing the tone of blood vessels and decreasing peripheral circulation to the limbs. splanchnic bed (viscera), and kidneys.

Stimulation of the sympathetic cholinergic fibers in the skin causes increased sweating, which is especially prominent on the scalp during periods of exertion, such as crying or feeding.

Renal system. Low cardiac output has a profound effect on kidney function because reduced renal blood flow from sympathetic stimulation and decreased arterial pressure result in changes aimed at increasing venous return through increased blood volume. First there is an increase in aldosterone production in response to increased renin secretion from decreased renal blood flow and sympathetic stimulation. Aldosterone increases the rate of sodium reabsorption by the distal tubules, promoting osmosis of water into the blood. The absorbed sodium increases the osmotic concentration of the extracellular fluid, stimulating release of antidiuretic hormone from the hypophysis, which promotes increased water reabsorption by the tubules.

Clinical manifestations of decompensation

If the abnormalities precipitating heart failure are not corrected, the heart muscle becomes damaged. Despite compensatory mechanisms, the heart is unable to maintain an adequate cardiac output. Decreased blood flow to the kidneys continues to stimulate sodium and water reabsorption, leading to hypervolemia, increased workload on the heart, and congestion in the pulmonary and systemic circulations.

Cardiac manifestations. One of the earliest signs of heart failure is *tachycardia* (heart rate above 160 beats/minute in infants), as a direct result of sympathetic stimulation. It is elevated even during rest but becomes markedly rapid during the slightest exertion.

Increased blood volume causes the ventricles to dilate, stretching the myocardial fibers until they are no longer as contractile. Ventricular dilatation results in extra heart sounds, S_3 and/or S_4. The addition of these extra sounds to S_1S_2 produces a *gallop rhythm.* S_3 is believed to be caused by vibrations against the ventricle walls as blood flow is abruptly stopped when the dilated ventricles can no longer accommodate the volume. It is heard immediately after the second heart sound (ventricular diastolic gallop). S_4 is believed to be caused by atrial contraction in response to ventricular resistance during filling of the ventricles. It occurs just before the first heard sound (atrial presystolic gallop). The presence of S_3 and S_4 is called a summation gallop. Each is best heard at the apex.

Variations in the strength of ventricular contraction result in *pulsus alternans,* regular alternation of one strong beat and one weak one. It is best detected by palpating the pulse while taking the blood pressure. The increased pressure from the inflated cuff occludes the weak beats, so that only the stronger beats are counted. As a result the pulse is half the actual rate.

Cardiomegaly results from dilatation of the ventricle to accommodate increasing volumes of blood and from hypertrophy, as a result of persistent lengthening and thickening of the myocardial fibers. Although hypertrophy decreases the contractility of the fibers, it is partially compensated for by an increase in muscle mass.

Pulmonary congestion. As the left ventricle fails, blood volume and pressure increase in the left atrium, pulmonary veins, and lungs. Eventually the pulmonary capillary pressure exceeds the plasma osmotic pressure, pulling fluid into tissues, causing pulmonary edema. The increased pressure also decreases the compliance (expansion) of the lungs.

Dyspnea is one of the earliest signs of failure and is thought to be caused by a decrease in the distensibility of the lungs. As a result additional muscles must be used for respiration, causing *costal retractions.* Dyspnea may initially only be evident on exertion but may progress to the point that only slight activity results in labored breathing. In infants dyspnea at rest is a prominent sign. Other common signs are flaring nares and grunting respirations.

Tachypnea (respiratory rate above 60 breaths/minute in infants) occurs from stimulation of carotid reflexes and the respiratory center in response to decreased arterial oxygenation. Inability to feed with resultant weight loss is primarily a result of tachypnea and dyspnea on exertion.

Cyanosis caused by low arterial oxygen saturation, decreased blood volume, or stasis in the systemic circulation may first be evident in the nail beds, mucous membranes, and conjunctiva. On exertion, such as crying or feeding, the infant may experience mottling of the skin or generalized transient duskiness. Extreme pallor or persistent duskiness is an ominous sign of congestive heart failure.

Orthopnea (dyspnea in the recumbent position) is caused by increased blood flow to the heart and lungs from the extremities. It is relieved by sitting up, because blood pools in the lower extremities, decreasing venous return. In addition this position decreases pressure from the abdominal organs on the diaphragm. In infants orthopnea may be evident in their inability to lie supine and their desire to be held upright.

Paroxysmal nocturnal dyspnea is a severe shortness of breath that occurs shortly after falling to sleep. It is a result of reabsorption of fluid (dependent edema), which increases blood volume, producing more severe pulmonary congestion.

Rales and *moist respirations* are produced by air flowing through abnormal moisture (pulmonary edema). Edema of the bronchial mucosa may also produce *wheezing* and *rhonchi* from obstruction to airflow. Mucosal swelling and irritation result in a persistent, dry, hacking *cough*. As pulmonary edema increases, the cough may be productive from increased secretions. *Hemoptysis* may occur if increased pulmonary venous pressure causes a vessel to break. Pressure on the laryngeal nerve results in *hoarseness*.

A late sign of heart failure is *Cheyne-Stokes respirations* (rapid deep breathing alternating with slow, shallow respirations). It is related to changes in arterial oxygen and carbon dioxide levels and delayed feedback of these changes to the brain because of slowed circulation time.

Systemic congestion. Systemic congestion is a primary consequence of right-sided failure from inability of the right ventricle to eject blood into the pulmonary circulation, resulting in increased back pressure and pooling of blood in the venous circulation. As was explained earlier, it can result as a late consequence of left-sided failure.

Distended neck and peripheral veins, which are more common in older children than infants, result from a consistently elevated central venous pressure. Normally neck and hand veins collapse when the head or hands are raised above the level of the heart, since the blood drains by gravity back to the heart. However, when the venous pressure is high, it prevents the back flow of blood, causing the veins to remain distended.

Edema forms as the sodium and water retention cause systemic vascular pressure to rise. The earliest sign is *weight gain*. However, as additional fluid accumulates, it leads to swelling of soft tissue that is dependent and favors the flow of gravity, such as the sacrum when recumbent, feet or ankles after standing, and loose periorbital tissues. In infants edema is usually generalized and difficult to detect. Gross fluid accumulation may produce *ascites* and *pleural effusions*. Edema within the abdomen produces a feeling of fullness that may cause anorexia and nausea and vomiting.

Hepatomegaly, usually a late sign of failure, occurs from pooling of blood in the portal circulation and transudation of fluid into the hepatic tissues. The liver is usually tender on palpation.

Diagnostic evaluation

Diagnosis may first be made on clinical symptoms such as dyspnea, especially when at rest, flaring nares, moist grunting respirations, subcostal retractions, activity intolerance, particularly during feeding, excessive sweating, and unexplained weight gain from edema. Since the signs of pulmonary congestion from left-sided failure resemble respiratory infections, it is imperative to differentiate between the two. Signs selectively indicative of congestive heart failure are cardiac enlargement, edema, sweating, hepatomegaly, and auscultatory findings such as tachycardia, gallop rhythm, and pulsus alternans.

Definitive diagnosis is based on laboratory tests to confirm cardiac involvement, such as a chest roentgenogram for cardiomegaly and an electrocardiogram for ventricular hypertrophy.

Medical management

Theoretically treatment of congestive heart failure is to remove the cause and allow the heart to compensate for the temporary failure. However, since structural abnormalities commonly precipitate congestive heart failure, this approach is often not possible, especially in infants who may be poor surgical candidates, necessitating medical management to preserve cardiac function. The goals of treatment are (1) improvement of cardiac function, (2) removal of accumulated fluid and sodium, (3) decreased cardiac demands, and (4) improvement of tissue oxygenation.

Improvement of cardiac function. Myocardial efficiency is improved using digitalis glycosides. Digitalis has three major actions: (1) it increases the force of contraction (positive inotropic); (2) it decreases the heart rate (negative chronotropic) and slows the conduction of impulses through the atrioventricular node (negative dromotropic); and (3) it enhances diuresis by increased renal perfusion. The beneficial effects are increased cardiac output, decreased heart size, decreased venous pressure, and relief of edema.

There are two principal preparations: digoxin (Lanoxin) and digitoxin. Their cardiac effects are the same, but their onset and duration of action differ (Table 35-3). In pediatrics digoxin is used almost exclusively because of its more rapid onset and decreased risk of toxicity as a result of a much shorter half-life. It is available as an elixir (0.05 mg/ml) for oral administration. For infants the dose is often calculated in micrograms (1000 μg = 1 mg).

Treatment is based on a digitalizing dose, given intra-

Table 35-3. Comparison of digitalis preparations

Variable	Digoxin	Digitoxin
Onset		
Oral	1 hour	2-4 hours
Intravenous	5-10 minutes	½-2 hours
Peak action		
Oral	6-7 hours	12-24 hours
Intravenous	1-2 hours	8-9 hours
Half-life	28-48 hours	8 days
Absorption and excretion	80%-90%	Complete
	Minimally recycled through liver or bowel	Extensively recycled through liver and bowel
	Poorly bound to serum albumin	Closely bound to serum albumin
	Excreted unchanged in urine	Excreted as cardioinactive metabolites in urine

muscularly as one large dose or in divided doses over a short time span to produce optimum cardiac effects, and a maintenance dose, usually one fourth to one third the digitalizing dose, given orally twice a day to sustain cardiac function. During digitalization the child is monitored by means of an electrocardiogram to observe for the desired effects (prolonged P-R interval and reduced ventricular rate).

Removal of accumulated fluid and sodium. Treatment consists of diuretics, fluid restriction, and sodium restriction. Diuretics are the mainstay of therapy to eliminate excess water and salt to prevent reaccumulation. The most commonly used agents are listed in Table 35-4. Since furosemide and the thiazides cause loss of potassium, potassium supplements and rich dietary sources of the electrolyte are given. A fall in serum potassium enhances the effects of digitalis, increasing the risk of digitalis toxicity. Therefore, serum potassium levels must be carefully monitored.

Fluid restriction may be required in the acute states of congestive heart failure or if fluid retention is accompanied by loss of sodium. In the latter case diuretics would cause additional sodium loss, resulting in hyponatremia, whereas limiting oral fluids would preserve the sodium content. Fluids must be carefully calculated to avoid dehydrating the child, especially if significant polycythemia is present.

Sodium-restricted diets are used less often in children than in adults to control congestive heart failure because of their potential negative effects on appetite. For example, low-sodium milk is unpalatable and poorly tolerated by infants. If salt intake is restricted, the diet usually consists of avoiding additional table salt and highly salted foods.

Decreasing cardiac demands. To lessen the workload on the heart, metabolic needs are kept to a minimum by limiting physical activity (bed rest), preserving body temperature, treating any existing infections, reducing the effort of breathing (semi-Fowler's position), and using medication to sedate an irritable child (usually morphine sulfate, 0.1 mg/kg). Since effectively meeting these objectives depends on nursing intervention, they are discussed in more detail in the next section.

Improvement of tissue oxygenation. All of the preceding measures serve to increase tissue oxygenation either by improving myocardial function or lessening tissue oxygen demands. However, supplemental cool humidified oxygen may also be administered to increase the amount of available oxygen during inspiration. Cool humidification is necessary to counteract the drying effect of oxygen and to cause vasoconstriction and bronchial dilation. The amount of cool humidity is carefully regulated to prevent overhydration and chilling.

Nursing considerations

The objectives of nursing care include (1) assisting in measures to improve cardiac function, (2) decreasing cardiac demands, (3) reducing respiratory distress, (4) maintaining nutritional status, (5) assisting in measures to promote fluid loss, and (6) providing emotional support. Although the objectives are the same, the interventions differ depending on the child's age, especially with infants as compared to older children.

Assisting in measures to improve cardiac function. The nurse's responsibility in administering digitalis includes observing for signs of toxicity, calculating the correct dosage, and instituting parental teaching regarding drug administration at home.

Digitalis is a potentially dangerous drug because the margin of safety of therapeutic, toxic, and lethal doses is very narrow. Many toxic responses are extensions of its therapeutic effects. Therefore, the nurse must maintain a high index of suspicion when administering digitalis for the following signs of toxicity.[25]

Extracardiac signs and symptoms. The earliest manifestation of toxicity is vomiting, usually with anorexia and nausea, caused by stimulation of the emetic control center in the medulla. Although vomiting should alert the nurse to observe for other evidence of cardiac toxicity, one episode of vomiting does not warrant cessation of the drug, because vomiting from other causes is common, especially in infants. However, the nurse reports any emesis to the physician prior to administering the next dose of digitalis.

Other extracardiac signs of toxicity are neurologic symptoms (headache, drowsiness, insomnia, vertigo, confusion, and delirium) and visual disturbances (halos around dark objects, difficulty in reading, glittering spots, or color blindness). Obviously such symptoms are extremely difficult to identify in children and are of little value in assessing toxicity in infants.

Cardiac toxicity. Manifestations of cardiac toxicity are abnormalities in heart rate, rhythm, and conduction. One of the early signs is bradycardia from excessive vagal stimulation. Therefore, the nurse always checks the apical pulse prior to administering digitalis. As a general rule the drug is not given if the pulse is below 90 to 110 beats/minute in infants and young children or below 70 beats/minute in older children (the cutoff point for adults is 60). However, since the pulse rate varies in children in different age-groups, the nurse should have the physician specify with the written drug order at what heart rate the drug should be withheld.

The apical rate is taken because a pulse deficit (radial pulse rate lower than apical) may be present with atrial fibrillation or other arrhythmias. It is counted for 1 full minute to evaluate alterations in rhythm. If the child is monitored by means of an electrocardiogram, the nurse observes the PQRST complex for abnormal lengthening of the P-R interval (more than a 50% increase over predigitalization interval) and signs of ectopic beats, especially premature ventricular contractions (PVCs) (QRS complex is wide and bizarre in shape).

Table 35-4. Diuretics used in congestive heart failure

Drug	Route	Onset	Peak	Duration	Action	Comments	Nursing considerations
Furosemide (Lasix)	Oral IV	20-30 minutes 5 minutes	2-4 hours ½ hour	6-8 hours 2-4 hours	Blocks reabsorption of sodium and water in proximal renal tubule and interferes with reabsorption of sodium in Henle's loop and in the most proximal portion of distal tubule	Drug of choice in severe congestive heart failure Causes excretion of chloride and potassium (hypokalemia may precipitate digitalis toxicity)	Begin to record output as soon as drug is given Observe for dehydration caused by profound diuresis Observe for side effects (nausea and vomiting, diarrhea, ototoxicity, hypokalemia, dermatitis, postural hypotension) Encourage foods high in potassium and/or give potassium supplements Observe for signs of digitalis toxicity
Chlorothiazide (Diuril)	Oral	2 hours	4 hours	6-12 hours	Acts directly on distal tubules and possibly proximal tubules to decrease sodium, water, potassium, chloride, and bicarbonate absorption Decreases urinary diluting capacity	Most commonly used drugs, inexpensive Causes hypokalemia, acidosis from large doses May be given on alternate days or for 4-5 days and stopped for 2 days to allow for reabsorption of potassium	Observe for side effects (nausea, weakness, dizziness, paresthesia, muscle cramps, skin eruptions, hypokalemia, acidosis) Encourage foods high in potassium and/or give potassium supplements
Hydrochlorothiazide (Hydrodiuril)	Same	Same	Same	Same	Same	Effect is ten times more potent than chlorothiazide; therefore, dose is decreased by one tenth	Same
Spironolactone (Aldactone)	Oral	Gradual	72 hours	48-72 hours	Blocks the action of aldosterone, which promotes retention of sodium and excretion of potassium	Has potassium-sparing effect, frequently used with thiazides Poorly absorbed from gastrointestinal tract, expensive Beneficial for children who are resistant to other diuretics	Observe for side effects (skin rash, drowsiness, ataxia, hyperkalemia) Do not administer potassium supplements
Triamterene (Dyrenium)	Oral	2 hours	4-8 hours	12-24 hours	Appears to interfere with exchange of sodium, potassium, and hydrogen in distal tubule	Has a potassium-sparing effect, frequently used with thiazides	Observe for side effects (diarrhea, nausea and vomiting, weakness, headache, dry mouth, rash, hyperkalemia) Do not administer potassium supplements

Treatment of digitalis toxicity consists of immediate discontinuation of the drug and administration of potassium, which has essentially the opposite effects of digitalis since it acts as a myocardial depressant and antiarrhythmic agent. Other antiarrhythmic drugs that may be used are phenytoin (Dilantin), propranolol (Inderal), lidocaine, and procaine amide (Pronestyl). Since digoxin remains in the body 2 to 6 days, the nurse continues to carefully monitor the child for evidence of toxicity as well as for signs of worsening heart failure caused by lack of the drug.

Digitalis toxicity can occur from accidental overdose. To avoid confusion between the two preparations, Lanoxin is usually used to differentiate digoxin from digitoxin. Anyone administering the drug must carefully read the container's label to assure use of the correct preparation. Since margins of safety between therapeutic and toxic doses are narrow, great care must be taken in properly calculating and measuring the dosage. Although the elixir comes with a calibrated dropper for measuring the dose, a tuberculin syringe should be used for greater accuracy. It is essential that the exact number of milliliters be given. When converting milligrams to micrograms to milliliters, the nurse carefully checks the placement of the decimal point, since an error causes a significant change in dosage. For example, 0.1 mg is ten times the dosage of 0.01 mg. To assure safety, the nurse compares her calculations with another staff member prior to giving the drug.

The nurse teaches these same principles to parents, although the correct dose in milliliters is usually specified on the container, thus reducing potential errors in calculation. The nurse observes the parent measure the elixir in the dropper, stressing the level mark as the meniscus of the fluid that is observed at eye level. The necessity of equally dividing doses during the day is also emphasized. Usually maintenance digoxin is given every 12 hours, requiring a schedule such as 6:00 AM and midnight. Although this is an inconvenience, such times should be adhered to as closely as possible to maintain constant blood levels. To minimize forgetting a dose or giving it twice, the nurse makes up a time chart that is completed after each dose is administered.

A problem arises when the child vomits or spits out the medication, since regiving it may result in overdose. In general the physician is notified prior to administering another dose, especially since vomiting may be an early sign of toxicity. To minimize this problem, it is important to administer the drug carefully by slowly squirting it on the side and back of the mouth. It should not be mixed with other foods or fluids, since refusal to consume these substances results in inaccurate intake of the drug.

Parents are also advised of the signs of toxicity. According to the physician's preference they may be taught to take the radial pulse by palpation before giving the drug. Although the apical pulse is more accurate, it is unrealistic to expect parents to purchase a stethoscope. The nurse requests a return demonstration of the procedure from both parents or other principal care giver as part of the teaching plan. Their level of anxiety in counting the pulse is also assessed, since overconcern about the heart rate may result in excessive withholding of the drug.

Decreasing cardiac demands. The infant requires provision of rest and conservation of energy for the task of feeding. Every effort is made to organize care-giving activities to allow for uninterrupted periods of sleep. Whenever possible, parents are encouraged to stay with their infant to provide the holding, rocking, and cuddling that help children sleep more soundly.

To minimize disturbing the infant, changing bedclothes and complete bathing are done only when necessary. Feeding is planned to accommodate the infant's sleep and wake patterns. He is fed as soon as he appears hungry, such as when sucking on his fists rather than when crying for a bottle, since the stress of crying exhausts his limited energy supply. If he is sleeping, he is fed after he awakens.

Usually the older child is placed on complete bed rest to minimize any unnecessary physical activity. This usually means dependency on others for feeding, bathing, and elimination (use of bedpan for older child). Encouraging parents to stay with the child and participate in his care is most beneficial to ensuring bed rest, since the child's physical and emotional needs are anticipated and quickly met. If parents cannot remain, the nurse takes a detailed admission history (see p. 892) in order to individualize care that most satisfactorily meets the child's needs.

Obviously every effort is made to minimize crying or stress. For infants this primarily involves preserving the parent-child relationship and meeting their needs as soon as possible to reduce frustration. Older children need an explanation of what is happening to them to decrease anxiety over their deteriorating physical status. For example, if they are monitored by an electrocardiogram or placed in an oxygen tent, the nurse first explains the procedure. Sometimes the sense of urgency associated with admission of a child in severe congestive heart failure overshadows the need for psychologic preparation. However, the few minutes it takes to reassure a child that electrocardiogram leads do not hurt or to familiarize him with the world through a plastic tent result in lessening physiologic responses to stress.

Temperature is carefully monitored for hyperthermia (a sign of infection) or hypothermia (loss of heat to ambient air). Febrile states are reported to the physician, since infection must be promptly treated. If body temperature is low the nurse keeps the child warm with additional blankets or the use of a radiant heater. Maintaining body temperature is of special importance when the child is receiving cool, humified oxygen and in infants who tend to be diaphoretic and lose heat by way of evaporation.

Causes of infection, such as respiratory infection or skin

breakdown from edema accumulation, are minimized. The child is positioned and turned every 2 hours (from side to side while in semi-Fowler's position), and the skin, especially over the sacrum, is checked for evidence of redness from pressure.

Reducing respiratory distress. To ease the effort of respiration, the child is positioned in semi- to high-Fowler's position in an infant or cardiac seat. Infants and children with cyanotic heart disease often breathe better in the knee-chest position, which decreases venous return and reduces the workload of the right side of the heart. Infants can be maintained in this position by placing them on their side with the knees bent toward the chest and pillows propped behind the back and buttocks. If they must be transported, either position is maintained. Shirts and diapers are pinned loosely to allow maximum chest expansion. Safety restraints, such as those used with the infant seats, are applied low on the abdomen and loosely enough to provide safety and maximum expansion.

Respirations are carefully monitored for 1 full minute during a resting state, since fast labored breathing greatly increases cardiac demands. The nurse immediately reports evidence of Cheyne-Stokes respirations to the physician, since this indicates worsening heart failure. If morphine sulfate is given, the nurse observes for respiratory depression from the drug.

The infant or child is often placed in a Croupette with cool humidified air to help liquify secretions or prevent their formation. Supplemental oxygen may or may not be helpful in relieving the respiratory distress or cyanosis. If a trial period is ordered to determine its effectiveness, the nurse evaluates the child's response by noting the respiratory rate, ease of respiration, degree of cyanosis, and interval of sleep.

Since these children are susceptible to recurrent respiratory infection, they are placed in a room with noninfectious patients. With an older child, it is advantageous to choose a roommate who is also confined to bed and relatively quiet in order to promote a restful environment. Visitors and hospital personnel with active respiratory infection are isolated from the child. Good hand washing is practiced before and after caring for the infant or older child. In some instances prophylactic antibiotics are given to decrease the incidence of respiratory infection. The nurse ensures that the drug is given at equally divided times over a 24-hour schedule to maintain high blood levels of the antibiotic.

Maintaining nutritional status. Many infants with severe cardiac defects are poorly nourished and physically retarded. Because of the dyspnea on exertion, sucking becomes an exhausting activity and the infant is unable to consume his needed nutrients. To minimize the effort of feeding, small frequent mealtimes are scheduled, preferably after the infant is well rested and as soon as he appears hungry. The nipple should be soft with a hole that is large enough to permit entry of milk without the danger of aspiration. If the infant is able to consume solids, these can be mixed with the formula and fed through the bottle. To reduce the respiratory effort, the infant is fed in an upright position and burped only when necessary.

Food selections for older children need to be highly nutritious, easy to ingest, and palatable. They should also provide sufficient fluid to maintain hydration. Blenderized preparations, such as shakes and malted milks, or commercially available food supplements are usually well tolerated by children, especially if prepared with their favorite flavors, such as chocolate or strawberry. The use of a straw, a special cup, or rewards for drinking or eating, such as reading a story or playing a quiet game, can be incentives for the child to eat. Mealtimes should be carefully planned around rest periods and spaced at frequent intervals to minimize the fatigue of eating.

Assisting in measures to promote fluid loss. As soon as diuretics are given, the nurse records fluid intake and output and monitors body weight at the same time each day to evaluate benefit from the drug. Since profound diuresis may cause dehydration and electrolyte imbalance (loss of sodium, potassium, chloride, and bicarbonate), the nurse observes for signs indicative of either complication. Signs and symptoms suggesting reactions to the drugs (Table 35-4) are also observed for. Diuretics should be given early in the day to children who are toilet trained to avoid the need to urinate at night. If potassium-losing diuretics are given, the nurse encourages foods high in potassium, such as bananas, oranges, whole grains, legumes, and leafy vegetables. If potassium supplements are given the elixir is mixed with fruit juice (red punch or grape juice works well) to disguise the bitter taste and to prevent intestinal irritation from a concentrated solution. The nurse observes for signs of hypokalemia (see p. 1077), hyperkalemia from supplemental overdose, and digitalis toxicity (low potassium increases the cardiac effects of digitalis).

Fluid restriction is rarely necessary in infants because of their difficulty in feeding. However, if fluids are restricted, the nurse plans fluid-intake schedules using the same principles as discussed earlier in the chapter under postoperative cardiac care (p. 1339). With toddlers and preschoolers it is psychologically advantageous to give small amounts of liquid in vessels of appropriate size, since young children associate volume with size of the container. Suitable utensils are decorated medicine cups, paper Dixie cups, doll-sized teacups, or measuring cups. It is also important to avoid leaving extra fluids at the bedside, since older children may help themselves to additional servings. The nurse can gain older children's cooperation by placing them in charge of recording fluid intake.

If salt is limited the nurse discusses with the parent food sources of sodium and the necessity of eliminating any additional salt in food preparation. At mealtime the nurse

Summary of nursing care of the child with congestive heart failure

Goals	Responsibilities
Improve cardiac function Administer digitalis	Maintain high index of suspicion regarding toxicity Vomiting (earliest sign) Neurologic symptoms (of questionable value with children) Bradycardia Arrhythmias Pulse deficit Prevent toxicity Count apical pulse prior to giving drug and withhold dose if pulse lower than 90 to 100 (infants) or 70 (older children) Calculate dosage accurately; check with another nurse Use correct preparation (digoxin [Lanoxin]) Monitor serum potassium levels (decrease enhances digitalis toxicity) Teach proper drug administration to parents Evaluate accuracy of measuring dosage Stress importance of equally dividing two daily doses Improvise medication chart to minimize error in forgetting a dose or giving it twice Teach correct administration to prevent vomiting or spitting up of drug Teach parents signs of toxicity Teach technique of taking radial pulse as precaution prior to giving drug
Assist in measures to promote fluid loss Administer diuretics	Record intake, output, and daily weight as soon as diuretics are given Observe for side effects of drug (Table 35-4), especially potassium loss Administer early in day to avoid need for frequent voiding at night Encourage potassium-rich foods to prevent depletion Mix potassium supplements with fruit juice to camouflage bitter taste and prevent intestinal irritation
Restrict fluids	Plan schedule for restricted fluid intake on child's usual drinking habits Administer fluids child prefers in small container Do not leave additional fluid at bedside Gain older child's cooperation in monitoring his fluid intake
Restrict dietary salt	Discuss with parents sources of salt in diet Check meal tray to avoid accidental addition of salt to food
Decrease cardiac and respiratory demands	Maintain bed rest Plan nursing activities to allow for minimum disturbance Place child in room with another quiet child Anticipate child's needs to minimize crying Encourage parents to participate in care Decrease anxiety by preparing child for all procedures Place child in semi- to high-Fowler's position (or infant seat) to lessen respiratory effort Avoid any constricting clothing or restraints around abdomen and chest Report evidence of labored breathing or Cheyne-Stokes respiration to physician Keep child warm Report any evidence of infection to physician

Summary of nursing care of the child with congestive heart failure—cont'd

Goals	Responsibilities

Decrease cardiac and respiratory demands—cont'd	Minimize causes of infection
	  Turn frequently to prevent skin breakdown
	  Place child in room with noninfectious child
	Provide small, frequent meals
	Feed child

Provide emotional support	Keep parents informed of child's condition Reassure family that everything is being done for child Encourage parents to remain with child Demonstrate acceptance of parents' willingness to participate in child's care If this is terminal stage for child, support parents' grief, make child as comfortable as possible, and remain with family

checks the child's tray to make sure that salt was not mistakenly given.

Providing emotional support. Congestive heart failure is a serious, potentially fatal complication of heart disease. Parents and older children are usually acutely aware of the critical nature of the condition. Since stress places additional demands on cardiac function, nurses focus on lessening anxiety through anticipatory preparation, frequent communication with the parent regarding the child's progress, and constant reassurance that everything possible is being done.

The imposed bed rest and placement of the child in an oxygen tent severely limit physical contact between the child and the parents. The nurse can minimize this separation by encouraging parents to participate in care, such as feeding, bathing, positioning, and stimulating the child. As was mentioned earlier, active parent participation also optimally meets the infant's physical and emotional needs with minimal exertion. However, parents must feel comfortable and well accepted by the staff. For example, positioning the child may be cumbersome with the interfering electrocardiogram leads, but, with practice, parents become expert in functioning despite such equipment.

If congestive heart failure is the end stage of a severe heart defect, the nurse cares for this child as for any terminally ill child, using the principles discussed in Chapter 27. (For a summary of nursing care of the child with congestive heart failure, see the boxed material.)

INFECTIVE ENDOCARDITIS

Infective endocarditis (subacute bacterial endocarditis) is an infection of the valves and inner lining of the heart. Although it can occur without underlying heart disease, it most often is a sequela of cardiac anomalies, especially tetralogy of Fallot, ventricular septal defect, patent ductus arteriosus, aortic stenosis, and rheumatic heart disease. The most common causative agents are bacteria (streptococci, especially *Streptococcus viridans,* staphylococci, enterococci, and pneumococci), fungi such as *Candida albicans,* and *Rickettsia*.

Pathophysiology

The microorganisms usually grow on a section of the endocardium that has been subjected to abnormal blood streaming and turbulence, such as occurs when the flow of blood is restricted by an anatomic narrowing or forced through an abnormal opening. Growth may also begin where the abnormal jet of blood strikes the opposing endocardium, causing a thickening of the lining. Changes in the endocardium predispose it to the growth of invading organisms.

Organisms may enter the bloodstream from any site of localized infection. The most common portals of entry are oral from dental work *(S. viridans),* urinary tract, such as from infection after catheterization (gram-negative bacilli), and the bloodstream from long-term infusions. The microorganisms grow on the endocardium forming vegetations (verrucae), deposits of fibrin and platelet thrombi. The lesion may grow to invade adjacent tissues, such as aortic and mitral valves and myocardium and may break off and embolize elsewhere, especially in the spleen, kidney, central nervous system, lung, skin, and mucous membranes.

Clinical manifestations

The onset is usually insidious, with unexplained fever, anorexia, malaise, and weight loss. The most characteristic findings are a result of emboli formation elsewhere in the body, especially splinter hemorrhages (thin black lines) under the nails, Osler's nodes (red, painful intradermal nodes with white centers found on the pads of the phalanges), Janeway's spots (painless hemorrhagic areas on the palms and soles), and petechiae on the oral mucous membranes. A new murmur or a change in a previously existing one may be found as a result of damage to valves or perforation of the myocardium.

Diagnostic evaluation

Several laboratory findings may indicate infectious endocarditis, such as electrocardiographic changes (prolonged P-R interval), x-ray evidence of cardiomegaly, anemia, elevated erythrocyte sedimentation rate, leukocytosis, and microscopic hematuria. However, definitive diagnosis rests on growth and identification of the causative agent in the blood. Usually several blood specimens are drawn for culturing to minimize errors in venipuncture and dilution technique. As soon as an organism is isolated, sensitivity studies are done to determine specific antibiotic therapy.

Medical management

Treatment is administration of high-dose antibiotics (usually penicillin, ampicillin, methicillin, cloxacillin, streptomycin, and gentamicin for specific bacteria or flucytosine for fungi) given intravenously and/or intramuscularly for at least 4 weeks. Blood cultures are taken periodically to evaluate response to antibiotic therapy.

Successful early treatment, especially with bacterial invasion, is almost 100%. However, cases that were diagnosed late or caused by antibiotic-resistant organisms carry a higher mortality rate. Death is most often caused by congestive heart failure, myocardial infarction from coronary emboli, or cardiac perforation. Nonfatal complications result from embolism to other organs, especially to the central nervous system (hemiplegia, aphasia, meningitis, or convulsions), kidney (hematuria and proteinuria), spleen, and bowel.

Prevention of infective endocarditis in susceptible children is achieved by administering prophylactic antibiotic therapy both prior to and for a short period after procedures known to increase the risk of entry of organisms. This includes dental work and any manipulation of the respiratory, genitourinary, or gastrointestinal tract. In female adolescents this also includes childbirth.

Nursing considerations

Ideally the objective of nursing care is counseling parents of high-risk children about the need for prophylactic antibiotic therapy prior to procedures such as dental work. Unless parents are aware of the risk inherent in exposing their child to these events, they may be less inclined to seek medical treatment. The family's regular dentist should be advised of existing cardiac problems in the child as an added precaution to ensuring preventive treatment.

Parents should also have a high index of suspicion regarding potential infectious endocarditis. Without unduly alarming them, the nurses stresses that any unexplained fever, weight loss, and change in behavior (lethargy, malaise, or anorexia) must be brought to the attention of the physician. Such symptoms should not be self-diagnosed as a cold or flu. Early treatment is important in preventing further cardiac damage, embolic complications, and growth of resistant organisms.

Treatment requires long-term hospitalization for the duration of parenteral drug therapy. Nursing goals during this period are (1) preparation of the child for continuous intravenous infusion, possibly multiple intramuscular injections, and several venipunctures for blood cultures, (2) prevention of boredom, especially from restricted mobility caused by intravenous infusion and need for partial bed rest, if required, (3) observation for side effects of antibiotics, and (4) observation for complications, especially from embolism, and the possibility of heart failure. Specific interventions are discussed in the following section on rheumatic fever and the section on congestive heart failure on p. 1350.

RHEUMATIC FEVER

Rheumatic fever is an inflammatory disease affecting the heart, joints, central nervous system, and subcutaneous tissue. It derives its name from involvement of joints and the presence of fever in the acute stage. It is classified as one of the collagen diseases because of its predisposition toward inflammation and damage of connective tissue. The major sequela to rheumatic fever is heart damage, especially scarring of the mitral valve, which is then referred to a rheumatic heart disease.

The exact incidence is not known, although it has been declining during the past 2 decades because of antibacterial control of streptococcal infection and successful treatment of rheumatic fever. It occurs primarily in school-age children with the peak age between 6 and 8 years. Environmental, climatic, and familial factors influence the incidence of the disease in certain individuals. These include: (1) a lower socioeconomic standard of living, (2) crowded housing, (3) cold, humid climate, and (4) parental or personal history of rheumatic fever. Each of these factors also influences the incidence of streptococcal infection. For example, the environmental/familial variables may be related to poor health care practices, which predispose to untreated and transmitted cases of streptococcal infection.

Etiology and pathology

There is strong evidence to support a relationship between infection with group A streptococci and subsequent development of rheumatic fever (usually within 2 to 6

Summary of nursing care of the child with rheumatic fever

Goals	Responsibilities
Prepare family for long-term prophylactic therapy	Emphasize importance of prophylaxis in preventing recurrence of disorder and serious complication of heart damage Investigate family's ethnic beliefs regarding health care that may interfere with preventive therapy Include child in treatment plan, especially if it involves monthly injections Once continuous prophylaxis is terminated, emphasize importance of therapy prior to dental work, childbirth, or certain medical procedures to prevent infectious endocarditis
Encourage bed rest	Discuss frankly with family importance of bed rest to prevent heart damage Provide child with room or bed of his own If in hospital, choose compatible roommate Consult with physician regarding exact limitations imposed by bed rest Include child in planning daily activity schedule Include child's usual activities in daily schedule, such as getting dressed in morning, eating regular meals with family, and so on
Minimize boredom	Include all family members, especially siblings, in child's care Encourage friends to write, call, or visit for brief periods of time Encourage parents to set aside "special time" to be with child Provide appropriate diversional activities, especially those that do not require fine motor skills
Help family adjust to home care	Make referral to public health nurse to help family learn "conveniences" of home care Bed table, bed cradle Commode Wheelchair Footboard Backrest Arrange child's room for ease in helping himself Teach parents how to take vital signs and how to record signs of child's progress Consult with physician regarding resumption of schoolwork Arrange with school to send tutor to child's home Discuss with schoolteacher projects classmates can do to maintain contact with absent member
Encourage adequate nutrition	Encourage parents to be tolerant of anorexia during febrile phase Give parents anticipatory guidance regarding future problems stemming from "forced" feeding Plan highly nutritious diet of soft or liquid foods During convalescence, assess diet's adequacy in terms of protein and calories, especially to prevent excessive weight gain Feed child if choreic movements are severe Permit child as much control in feeding activity as possible Monitor fluid intake to prevent dehydration or overhydration (hypervolemia)
Relieve discomfort	Administer analgesics (aspirin or acetaminophen) for arthralgia Use bed cradle to prevent pressure on joints Position child with pillows Organize care for minimal handling

Continued.

Summary of nursing care of the child with rheumatic fever—cont'd

Goals	Responsibilities
Institute safety measures	Use protective devices if choreic movements are severe (padded bed, mittens on hands, head covering) Assist child in ambulation Use bed rails (improvise with chairs) Restrain child in chair
Provide emotional support	Discuss with child that aside from heart involvement, all other symptoms are temporary Encourage child to discuss feelings concerning chorea Help parents and schoolteachers to understand uncontrollable, sudden nature of choreic movements
Prevent rheumatic fever	Participate in screening programs for group A β-hemolytic streptococcal throat infection Be alert to signs of possible streptococcal throat infection in children Educate parents regarding proper medical treatment of sore throats, especially importance of completing antibiotic therapy after positive throat culture Have high index of suspicion for children with possible undiagnosed rheumatic fever

weeks). In almost all the cases of rheumatic fever a previous infection with group A streptococci can be documented by laboratory evidence of rising antibody titers. Prevention or treatment of group A streptococci infection prevents rheumatic fever.

The mechanism by which group A streptococci initiate connective tissue damage is believed to be an autoimmune process. The streptococci release several different proteins against which antibodies are formed. At some point the body's own proteins or the bacterial antigens initiate an immune response so that specific antibodies are released into the blood and react with many different tissues of the body. For example, the sarcolemma (plasma membrane of a muscle fiber) of cardiac tissue demonstrates susceptibility to reaction with streptococcal antigens.

Clinical manifestations

Although the major manifestations (see the outline on p. 1360) are most diagnostic of the disease, other signs and symptoms may also be present. These include low-grade fever, usually spiking in the late afternoon, unexplained epistaxis, abdominal pain that may be severe enough to simulate appendicitis, arthralgia without arthritic changes, weakness, fatigue, pallor, anorexia, and weight loss (Fig. 35-25).

Carditis. Rheumatic fever produces inflammatory hemorrhagic bullous lesions, called *Aschoff bodies,* which cause swelling, fragmentation, and alterations in the connective tissue of the heart. Subsequent endocarditis produces vegetations, which when healed become fibrous, scarred areas. The structures of the heart most affected are the mitral and aortic valves. If the scar tissue causes fusing of the leaflets (cusps), the valves are stenosed, causing obstruction to blood flow into the left ventricle and/or aorta. If the valve edges are scarred so that they cannot completely close together, regurgitation (valvular insufficiency) or back flow of blood occurs when the valves close.

Signs of carditis are (1) tachycardia, especially during rest or sleep that is out of proportion to the degree of fever, (2) cardiomegaly from increased workload and/or pericardial effusion, (3) a change in preexisting murmurs or new murmurs, (4) muffled heart sounds from pericardial effusion, (5) an accentuated third sound (prediastolic gallop), (6) pericardial friction rub, (7) precordial pain from pericarditis, and (8) changes in the conductivity of the heart, especially prolonged P-R interval (first-degree heart block).

The most common murmur heard is that of mitral insufficiency (apical systolic murmur). It is caused by backward flow of blood through the mitral valve into the left atrium during systole. It is a high-frequency blowing sound that is

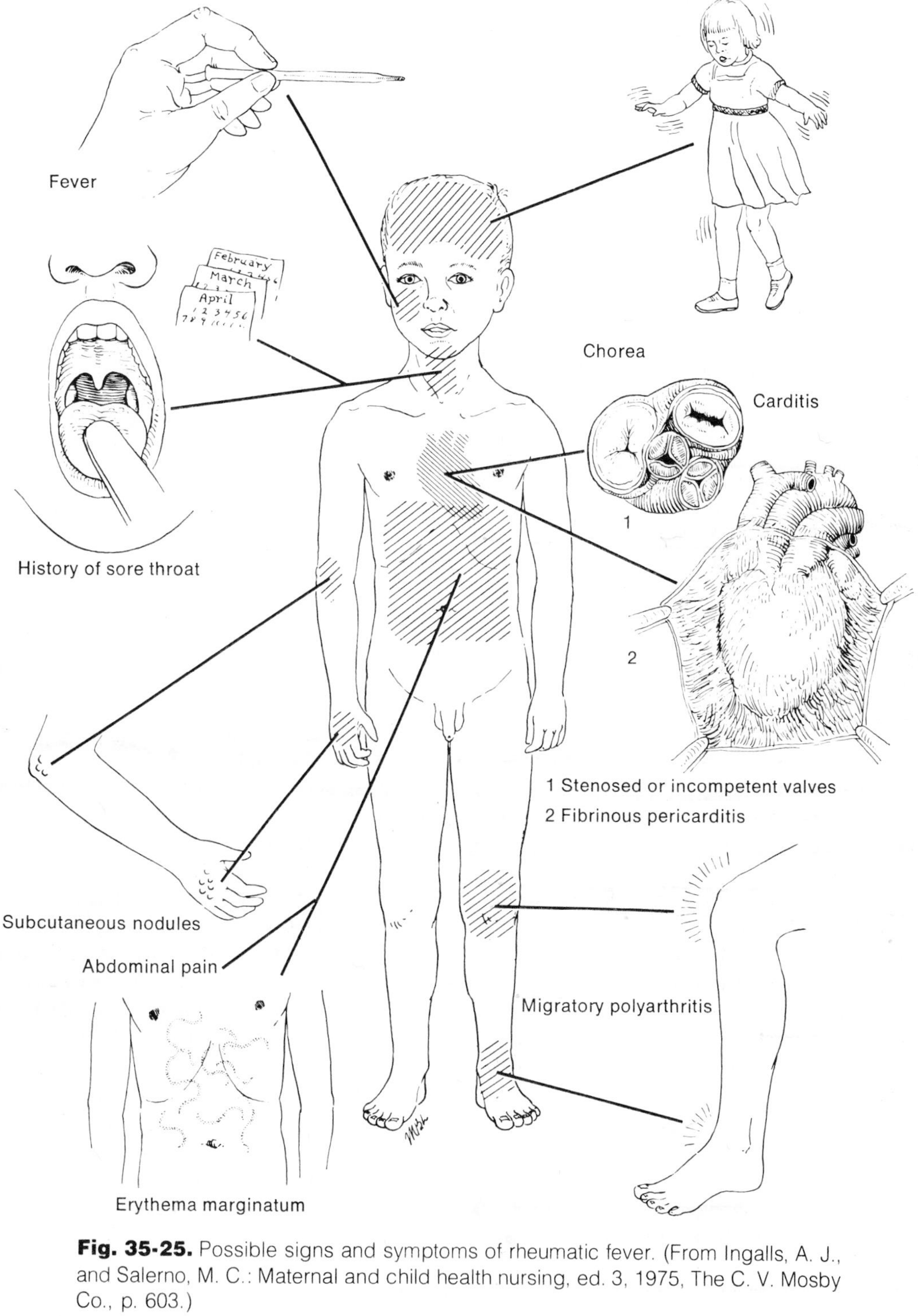

Fig. 35-25. Possible signs and symptoms of rheumatic fever. (From Ingalls, A. J., and Salerno, M. C.: Maternal and child health nursing, ed. 3, 1975, The C. V. Mosby Co., p. 603.)

best heard at the apex, as the sounds are transmitted down the chest wall through the left ventricle. It may be associated with an accentuated third sound. The second most common murmur is of aortic regurgitation. It is the same as mitral insufficiency, except that it occurs during diastole from back flow and turbulence of blood in the left ventricle.

Mitral stenosis is usually a later manifestation of progressive carditis. It is associated with a very weak murmur because severe obstruction to blood flow through the valve into the left ventricle causes minimal vibration of that chamber's walls. However, one may feel a thrill as the flabby ventricular walls reverterate during early systole. Resistance to blood flow causes increased pressure in the left atrium, increased pulmonary venous resistance, and eventually left-sided congestive heart failure. The consequences of aortic stenosis have been discussed earlier in this chapter under congenital heart disease (p. 1319).

Migratory polyarthritis. Pathologic changes in the joints are mainly caused by edema, inflammation, and effusion in joint tissue. They are reversible and migratory in nature, favoring large joints, such as the knees, elbows, hips, shoulders, and wrists. The affected joint is swollen, hot, red, and painful for 1 to 2 days, after which a different joint is affected. The manifestations usually accompany the acute febrile period, usually the first 1 to 2 weeks.

Chorea (St. Vitus' dance or Sydenham's chorea). The exact pathology responsible for changes in the central nervous system is unclear. These changes typically occur after the acute febrile phase and may last for several months, although they are completely reversible. Chorea is characterized by sudden, aimless, irregular movements of the extremities, involuntary facial grimaces, speech disturbances, emotional lability, and muscle weakness that can be profound. They are usually exaggerated by anxiety and attempts at deliberate fine motor activity and relieved by rest, especially sleep.

Subcutaneous nodules. Subcutaneous nodules are small (0.5 to 1.0 cm) nontender swellings that resemble Aschoff bodies in pathology. They are usually found in crops over bony prominences, such as feet, hands, elbows, scalp, scapulae, and vertebrae. They occur during the febrile phase, persist indefinitely after onset of the disease, and gradually resolve with no resultant damage.

Erythema marginatum. The skin manifestation is an erythematous macula with a clear center and wavy well-demarcated border. The transitory, nonpruritic rash is most commonly found on the trunk and proximal extremities.

Diagnostic evaluation

Diagnosis is based on our own modifications of the Jones criteria, as in the following outline.

*Revised Jones criteria for guidance in diagnosis of rheumatic fever**

A. Major manifestations
   1. Carditis
      a. Murmur
      b. Cardiomegaly
      c. Pericarditis
      d. Congestive heart failure
   2. Polyarthritis
   3. Chorea
   4. Subcutaneous nodules
   5. Erythema marginatum

B. Minor manifestations
   1. Clinical
      a. History of previous rheumatic fever or rheumatic heart disease
      b. Arthralgia
      c. Fever
   2. Laboratory
      a. Increased erythrocyte sedimentation rate (ESR)
      b. C-reactive protein
      c. Leukocytosis
      d. Anemia
      e. Prolonged P-R and Q-T intervals on electrocardiogram

C. Supportive evidence
   1. Recent scarlet fever
   2. Positive throat culture for group A β-hemolytic streptococci
   3. Increased antistreptolysin or other streptococcal antibodies

The presence of two major manifestations or one major and two minor manifestations with supportive evidence of recent streptococcal infection indicates a high probability of rheumatic fever. Although there is no one test to definitely confirm the diagnosis, an elevated or rising antistreptolysin-O (ASO) titer is the most objective evidence supporting previous group A streptococcal infection.

Streptolysin O (O because it is oxygen labile) is a streptococcal extracellular product that produces lysis of the red blood cell. Antistreptolysin-O titers measure the concentration of antibodies formed in the blood against this product. Normally the titers begin to rise about 7 days after onset of the infection and reach maximal levels in 4 to 6 weeks. Therefore, a rising titer demonstrated by at least two antistreptolysin-O tests is the most reliable evidence of recent streptococcal infection. Normal values are between 0 and 120 Todd units. Elevations of 333 Todd units indicate recent streptococcal infection in children.

Medical management

The goals of medical management are (1) eradication of hemolytic streptococci, (2) prevention of recurrences of the

*Jones Criteria (revised)—For Guidance in the Diagnosis of Rheumatic Fever, © American Heart Association, 7320 Greenville Avenue, Dallas, Texas 75231. By permission of the American Heart Association, Inc.

disease, (3) prevention of permanent cardiac damage, and (4) providing palliation for the other symptoms. The first two objectives require the use of antibiotic therapy. Penicillin is the drug of choice, with erythromycin as a substitute in penicillin-sensitive children. The usual treatment regimens used include procaine penicillin G, 600,000 U daily, given intramuscularly for 10 days, benzathine penicillin G (Bicillin), 1.2 million U given intramuscularly as a single dose, or erythromycin, 1 g orally for 10 days (dosages are calculated for school-age children).[4]

Prophylactic treatment against recurrence is started after the acute therapy and involves monthly intramuscular injections of benzathine penicillin G (1.2 million U), two daily oral doses of penicillin (200,000 U), or one daily dose of sulfadiazine (1 g).[4] The duration of long-term prophylaxis is still uncertain. The most effective protection is afforded by long-term continuous antibiotic prophylaxis, perhaps for life. However, the risk of recurrence declines with age, with the interval since the most recent attack, and in those patients without cardiac involvement. When regular antibiotic therapy is discontinued, the same treatment used to prevent infectious endocarditis should be instituted here.

Prevention of heart damage depends on adequate antibiotic therapy and bed rest to decrease cardiac demands. Controversy exists regarding the limits of activity restriction. Some physicians advocate complete bed rest for extended periods of time, whereas others believe that moderate activity is preferable after the acute febrile phase to counteract the stress imposed by strict activity limitations on a child who is feeling well. Most agree that increased activity should not begin until signs of a decreased inflammatory reaction, such as falling erythrocyte sedimentation rate and absence of C-reactive protein, are present.

Salicylates are used to control the inflammatory process, especially in the joints. The analgesic and antipyretic actions of salicylates add to their effectiveness in providing palliation of other symptoms. Steroids may be used, but there is controversy over their long-term benefit in preventing heart damage. They are indicated when there is evidence of congestive heart failure. Unfortunately there is no specific treatment for chorea.

Nursing considerations

The objectives of nursing care are in accordance with those of medical management, although the interventions differ. Since the trend is toward home care rather than prolonged hospitalization, this aspect is emphasized and is related primarily to the school-age child.

Preparation of child and parents for long-term antibiotic therapy. If the treatment consists of multiple injections either initially or monthly for a prolonged period, the child needs preparation for the procedure. Deep intramuscular injections of penicillin are painful, and the prospect of receiving one every 4 weeks for years is difficult to accept. Since the school-age child's needs are for control and a sense of accomplishment, these should be emphasized during the treatment. The child can be given the choice of right or left sites, since only the midlateral thigh is recommended. (Gluteal injections of benzathine penicillin G or procaine penicillin G can cause sciatic nerve damage from direct intraneural injection or tissue ischemia from vasospasm as a result of the direct irritant effect of the preparation on nerve fibers.)[5] The child can also assume the responsibility for record keeping of which site was used, the date of injection, and so on. He should be praised for cooperating and given a symbol of achievement, such as a "hero badge."[17] In this way he is made part of the therapy, rather than solely its victim.

The family also needs preparation regarding the necessity of long-term prophylactic therapy. The nurse must take the time to elicit the family's beliefs regarding preventive drugs. Many ethnic groups place little value on medical intervention that yields no visible results. Therefore, once the child has recovered from the disease, they are disinclined to adhere to continuing treatment. Although the nurse does not wish to unduly alarm parents regarding potential complications of rheumatic fever, it is imperative that the seriousness of recurrent attacks and possibility of death from heart disease be stressed. Counseling regarding prophylaxis during certain procedures, such as dental work, is the same as that discussed under infectious endocarditis (p. 1356).

Encouragement of bed rest. One of the greatest challenges of caring for the child with rheumatic fever is maintaining bed rest once the child's physical status improves. For children with mild symptoms, bed rest may be difficult from the day of diagnosis. Therefore, the nurse discusses frankly with the child and parents that with this disease feeling well does not mean that the body is totally recovered. The changes in the heart and the time needed for healing are stressed, realizing that the child at this age is aware of the significance of this vital organ. To encourage active participation in limiting activity, the nurse can demonstrate the change in heart rate during rest and activity, comparing the difference in pulse to the mechanical work required of the heart.

Once the nurse has clarified with the physician the specific confinements imposed by bed rest (for example, bathroom privileges, self-feeding, hygiene, and any ambulation or mental activity, such as schoolwork), a schedule of daily events is planned with the child and parent. It is advisable to base this schedule on as many normal activities in the child's usual day as possible, such as getting dressed in the morning, having an evening bath and periodic shampoo, and taking meals with the family. During the acute stage none of these may be possible, although they can be viewed as markers of progress later on.

At home the child should have a room of his own for the

most restful environment. However, if this is not possible, which frequently occurs in lower socioeconomic housing, the child should have a bed or couch of his own. Although his condition is not contagious, he is susceptible to infection from others who are ill, such as siblings who have colds.

Prevention of boredom. Boredom can be minimized by including other family members in the child's care, encouraging friends to write, telephone, or visit for short periods of time, setting aside a special time for parents to read or participate in a project with the child, and providing activities appropriate to his interests and physical ability. (For the hospitalized child, selecting a compatible roommate who is also confined to bed is tremendously helpful.) Choreic movements may severely limit the child's fine motor skills, since deliberate, purposeful movements exaggerate chorea. Therefore, games that require moving pieces to different blocks, such as checkers or Scrabble, and hobbies, such as needlework, painting, or building models, may be inappropriate and frustrating. Games such as checkers can be made suitable by marking each square with a number and having the opponent move the checkers at the child's request. Card games can be made easier by using a box with slits to hold the cards, rather than using the hands. Often siblings are the best inventors of games, and, by letting them participate, they are less likely to feel left out and neglected.

Helping family adjust to home care. A public health nursing referral should be made to help the family adjust to home care. Simple devices can be made to facilitate activities, such as eating in bed, using a commode, and so on. Although all of these are available commercially, they are fairly expensive, especially for families on a limited budget. Financial assistance is provided by the crippled children's services in some states and should be investigated through local or state departments of health as a potential source of help. However, all of the equipment can be improvised. A bed table is made by cutting out the two long sides and the bottom of a heavy rectangular cardboard box, leaving at least 2 inches around the long sides for added support (this also makes an excellent bed cradle), or by placing a long board across two chairs placed on the side of the bed. A backrest is fashioned by turning a wooden chair so that the back and legs form an incline on the bed. A commode is made by cutting a hole in an old wooden chair (an inexpensive folding chair works well), smoothing out the edges or covering them with tape, and placing a bucket under the hole. A wheelchair can be a play wagon or a chair that has four wheels attached. Other simple conveniences for the child are a bedside bell to call for assistance, an on-off switch attached to the cord of the lamp, and a table or bookshelf placed next to the bed for easy access to books, toilet articles, snacks, and so on.

The visiting nurse (or pediatric nurse if the child is hospitalized) teaches the parents to count the pulse and take an oral or rectal temperature, since these recordings are made during the convalescent period. The nurse also improvises a chart to help parents keep a systematic record of vital signs, daily activity, rest patterns, and oral drug administration. There should also be a space for special comments that may need medical/nursing intervention, such as a change in choreic movements or feeding difficulties.

Once the acute phase is over, the nurse encourages parents to discuss with the physician the feasibility of beginning schoolwork at home with a tutor. Most public school systems automatically provide this assistance for children absent for medical reasons. Continuing learning not only provides the child with purposeful activity but also keeps the child in touch with school activities and classmates. Receiving letters from the students can greatly replace lost social contact. Some classroom projects to send to the absent child can be making a scrapbook of class activities, compiling an album of baby pictures of the students with funny sayings or making up individual "recovery" cards. Such activities also teach the students concern for and interest in a missing member of their group.

Encouragement of adequate nutrition. During the acute phase the child is usually anorexic and too fatigued and ill to eat. The same measures discussed on p. 1353 can be applied here. Small frequent meals, either liquid or soft to minimize chewing, are used initially. The nurse stresses to parents the need to prevent pressuring the child to eat because of the potential problems that can arise over feeding during the convalescent period when the child may use eating and food selection as a controlling mechanism. Once the child's appetite has returned, high-quality nutritious foods are given in accordance with his caloric requirements. Weight gain is a consequence of overfeeding combined with sedentary activity. From boredom, the child may turn to eating for lack of something more constructive to do.

Sometimes the child must be fed to lessen cardiac demands or as a result of choreic movements. To a school-age child this may represent unacceptable dependency. Besides explanations regarding the necessity of needing assistance, the child can be helped to adjust by allowing as much participation as possible, for example, drinking soup through a straw rather than having it fed to him and letting him choose the order in which to consume the food.

Fluids are given according to the child's requirements. During the febrile phase, he may need additional fluid to prevent dehydration, especially if food intake (a source of fluid) is poor. Although fluids are not limited, the nurse bears in mind that excess fluid can lead to hypervolemia and increased cardiac demands.

Relief of discomfort. Arthralgia may be severe. Even the weight of bedclothes or minimal massage can be painful. Aspirin is helpful in managing the pain, but local measures, such as using a bed cradle, minimal handling, and proper body alignment, should also be instituted. The use of massage, passive exercise, or application of heat or cold may aggravate the joint pain. Since no residual deformity occurs and the arthritis is migratory, physical therapy is of less concern than in other rheumatic disorders.

Providing emotional support. The complexity of emotional factors affecting the child and family can be great, including imposed bed rest, forced invalidism, loss of social contact, increased parental responsibility, potential financial burden, and the possibility of permanent heart disease. However, one of the most disturbing and frustrating manifestations of the disease is chorea. The onset is gradual and may occur weeks to months after the illness, sometimes even occurring in children who have not been diagnosed with rheumatic fever. It may be mistaken for nervousness, clumsiness, behavioral changes, inattentiveness, and learning disability. It is usually a source of great frustration to the child because the movements, incoordination, and weakness severely limit physical ability. The child needs an opportunity to verbalize his feelings. Of utmost importance is stressing to parents and schoolteachers the involuntary, sudden nature of the movements. For example, one child was removed from class because the teacher, unaware of the child's condition, mistook the facial grimaces and outbursts of laughter as signs of insolence. Consequently this child refused to attend school, despite a sympathetic apology and reassurance of the teacher that this would not happen again.

The nurse emphasizes that the chorea is transitory and that all manifestations eventually disappear. Some studies have found that children with rheumatic fever and chorea demonstrate postillness emotional problems, such as learning disabilities, low academic achievement, and marital instability.[9] However, other studies refute these findings, stating that postillness maladjustment attributed solely to chorea may be a false assumption.[21] In either case the obvious disruption in daily living imposed by chorea supports the need to help the child adjust during its manifestation to prevent possible future problems.

Institution of safety measures. Occasionally the irregular jerking movements become so violent that the child may actually injure himself. In this case the same precautions as for convulsions are instituted, especially using protective devices such as thick hand mittens or padding on the bed to prevent injury.

Muscle weakness may be profound, necessitating assistance with all care-giving activities. Safety precautions are instituted, such as using bed rails to prevent falling out of bed (these can be improvised by pushing the bed against one wall and placing high-back chairs on the other side with the back of the chair against the bed), restraining the child in a chair during sitting, and assisting him during ambulation. To maintain proper body alignments, pillows can be used to prop him on his side. To prevent footdrop, a footboard is placed at the bottom of the bed. It can easily be improvised by placing a heavy rectangular cardboard box at the end of the bed and securing it to the mattress with tape or a wide piece of cloth. Such a footboard also doubles as a bed cradle.

Prevention. Nurses also have a role in prevention, primarily in screening school-age children for sore throats caused by group A streptococci. This may involve actively participating in throat culture screening programs or in referring children with a possible streptococcal infection to a physician.

The following signs and symptoms should alert the school nurse to the possibility of a streptococcal throat infection: (1) the sore throat began suddenly, (2) the throat hurts when the child swallows, (3) the angle of the jaw is painful and the lymph glands in the neck are swollen and tender, (4) the child has a high fever, usually 38.4° to 40.0°C (101° to 104°F), and (5) the child complains of headache or nausea. In addition any child with a sore throat who has been in contact with another person with streptococcal sore throat or scarlet fever should be suspected of having a streptococcal infection.[12] However, it also entails educating parents to the need for proper medical care of pharyngitis and otitis media. Every sore throat is not caused by streptococci and therefore should not be routinely treated with antibiotics. What etiologic agent is present cannot be known without a throat culture.

After confirmation of a positive hemolytic streptococci culture (available in 24 hours), the child is placed on antibiotic therapy, usually oral penicillin, for 10 to 14 days. The nurse counsels parents regarding the necessity of completing the full course of treatment to totally eradicate the infection. If there is serious concern regarding the parent's compliance with this regimen, one intramuscular injection of benzathine penicillin G is given. Throat culture may be taken after antibiotic therapy to confirm successful treatment.

Nurses working in ambulatory settings, especially as primary care practitioners, must always have a high index of suspicion for undiagnosed rheumatic fever by querying about previous sore throats, especially any with a positive streptococcal culture, identifying high-risk individuals from the history, and asking questions regarding the vague insidious symptoms, namely low-grade fever, malaise, weakness, fatigue, epistaxis (without inciting events such as nose picking or excessively dry mucous membranes), and abdominal pain. Any child with questionable findings is referred for specific laboratory tests to confirm or rule out rheumatic fever. Prophylactic therapy of children with an uncertain present or past history of rheumatic fever is controversial and must be individualized for each child. However, the value of a careful history in identifying major criteria, especially chorea, is an important nursing responsibility, since adequate supportive data are the most useful guidelines for prophylaxis. For a summary of the nursing care of the child with rheumatic fever, see the boxed material on pp. 1357 to 1358.

REFERENCES

1. Aisenberg, R. B., and associates: Psychological impact of cardiac catheterization, Pediatrics **51**(6):1051-1059, June 1973.
2. Champsaur, G. L., and associates: Repair of transposition of the great vessels in 123 pediatric patients, Circulation **47**(5): 1032-1041, May 1973.
3. Clarkson, P. M., and associates: Late postoperative hemodynamic results and cineangiocardiographic findings after Mustard atrial baffle repair for transposition of the great arteries, Circulation **53**(3):525-532, March 1976.
4. Committee on Rheumatic Fever and Bacterial Endocarditis of the Council on Cardiovascular Disease in the Young of the American Heart Association: Rheumatic fever prevention, New York, 1976, American Heart Association.
5. Darby, C. P., Bradham, G., and Waller, C. E.: Ischemia following intragluteal injection of benzathine-procaine penicillin G mixture in a one-year-old boy, Clin. Pediatr. **12**(8):485-487, August 1973.
6. Duff, R. S., and Campbell, A. G.: On deciding the care of severely handicapped or dying persons: with particular reference to infants, Pediatrics **57**(4):487-493, April 1976.
7. Folger, G. M.: Acidemia of cardiogenic origin in young infants with cyanotic congenital heart abnormalities, Clin. Pediatr. **11**(10):573-579, October 1972.
8. Fontan, F., and Baudet, E.: Surgical repair of tricuspid atresia, Thorax **26:**240, 1971.
9. Freeman, J. M., and associates: The emotional correlates of Sydenham's chorea, Pediatrics **35:**42, 1965.
10. Friedberg, D. Z., and Litwin, S. B.: The medical and surgical management of patients with congenital heart disease, Clin. Pediatr. **15**(4):324-333, April 1976.
11. Friedman, S.: Some thoughts about functional or innocent murmurs, Clin. Pediatr. **12**(12):678-679, December 1973.
12. Guide for teachers: children with heart disease, New York, 1971, American Heart Association.
13. Hoffman, J. I.: Ventricular septal defect: indications for therapy in infants, Pediatr. Clin. North Am. **18**(4):1091-1107, 1971.
14. Kupst, M. J., and associates: Improving physician-parent communication, Clin. Pediatr. **15**(1):27-30, January 1976.
15. Long, M. L., Scheuhing, M. A., and Christian, J. L.: Cardiopulmonary bypass, Am. J. Nurs. **74**(5):860-867, May 1974.
16. Marcinek, M. B.: Stress in the surgical patient, Am. J. Nurs. **77**(11):1809-1811, November 1977.
17. McLellan, C. L.: Hero badges mean more than courage, Pediatr. Nurs. **2**(3):7, May/June 1976.
18. Reif, K.: A heart makes you live, Am. J. Nurs. **72**(6):1085, June 1972.
19. Sade, R. M., and Castaneda, A. R.: Recent advances in cardiac surgery in the young infant, Surg. Clin. North Am. **56**(2):451-465, April 1976.
20. Sethi, G. K., Hughes, R. K., and Takaro, T.: Dissecting aortic aneurysms, Ann. Thorac. Surg. **18**(2):201-215, August 1974.
21. Stehbens, J. A., and MacQueen, J. C.: The psychological adjustment of rheumatic fever patients with and without chorea, Clin. Pediatr. **11**(11):638-640, November 1972.
22. Stephenson, C. A.: Stress in critically ill patients, Am. J. Nurs. **77**(11):1806-1809, November 1977.
23. Tesler, M., and Hardgrove, C.: Cardiac catheterization: preparing the child, Am. J. Nurs. **73**(1):80-82, January 1973.
24. Verderber, A.: Cardiopulmonary bypass: postoperative complications, Am. J. Nurs. **74**(5):868-869, May 1974.
25. Winslow, E. H.: Digitalis, Am. J. Nurs. **74**(6):1062-1065, June 1974.

BIBLIOGRAPHY

Andreoli, K. G., and associates: Comprehensive cardiac care, ed. 4, St. Louis, 1979, The C. V. Mosby Co.

Anthony, C. P., and Thibodeau, G. A.: Textbook of anatomy and physiology, ed. 10, St. Louis, 1979, The C. V. Mosby Co.

Guyton, A.: Textbook of medical physiology, Philadelphia, 1976, W. B. Saunders Co.

Rudolph, A. M., editor: Pediatrics, New York, 1977, Appleton-Century-Crofts.

Congenital heart disease

Benzing, G., and Kaplan, S.: Late complications of cardiac surgery, Pediatr. Clin. North Am. **18**(4):1225-1242, 1971.

Breckinridge, I. M., and associates: Mustard's operation for transposition of the great vessels, Lancet **1:**1140, 1972.

Clark, J.: Kelly—an infant with heart defects, Am. J. Nurs. **77**(11):1823-1827, November 1977.

Coats, K.: Non-invasive cardiac diagnostic procedures, Am. J. Nurs. **75**(11):1980-1985, November 1975.

Cogen, R.: Preventing complications during cardiac catheterizations, Am. J. Nurs. **76**(3):401-405, March 1976.

Cortez, A., Mendoza, M., and Muniz, G.: The utilization of nurses in expanded roles to deliver pediatric cardiology health care, Pediatr. Nurs. **1**(3):22-29, May/June 1975.

Day, R. E., and Insley, J.: Maternal diabetes mellitus and congenital malformations, Arch. Dis. Child. **51:**935-938, 1976.

Doyle, E. F., and associates: Sudden death in young patients with congenital aortic stenosis, Pediatrics **53**(4):481-489, April 1974.

Feigenbaum, H.: Newer aspects of echocardiography, Circulation **47**(4):833-842, April 1973.

Friedberg, D. Z., and Caldart, L.: A center for pediatric cardiovascular patients, Am. J. Nurs. **75**(9):1480-1482, September 1975.

Gildea, J. H.: Techniques of cardiopulmonary resuscitation in infants, Am. J. Nurs. **78**(2):265, February 1978.

Gildea, J. H., and associates: Congenital cardiac defects: pre- and postoperative nursing care, Am. J. Nurs. **78**(2):273-278, February 1978.

Gillon, J. E.: Behavior of newborns with cardiac distress, Am. J. Nurs. **73**(2):254-257, February 1973.

Greenwood, R. D., and Nadas, A. S.: The clinical course of cardiac disease in Down's syndrome, Pediatrics **58**(6):893-897, December 1976.

Greenwood, R. D., and associates: Extracardiac abnormalities in infants with congenital heart disease, Pediatrics **55**(4):485-492, April 1975.

Hunt, C. E., and Lucas, R. V.: Symptomatic atrial septal defect in infancy, Circulation **47**(5):1042-1048, May 1973.

King, D. L.: Cardiac ultrasonography: cross-sectional ultrasonic imaging of the heart, Circulation **47**(4):843-847, April 1973.

Kory, R. C.: Cardiac catheterization and related procedures, Cardiovasc. Nurs. **4**(4):17-22, July/August 1968.

Merciondo, K.: C.V.P.: the whys and hows of central venous pressure monitoring, Nursing '74 **4**(1):21-24, January 1974.

McNamara, D.: Management of congenital heart disease, Pediatr. Clin. North Am. **18**(4):1191-1205, 1971.

Neal, W. A., and associates: Operative repair of atrial septal defect without cardiac catheterization, J. Pediatr. **86**(2):189-193, February 1975.

Nicodemus, H. F.: Respiratory failure and airway management in congenital cardiovascular diseases, Clin. Pediatr. **12**(5):259-263, May 1973.

Nielsen, M. A.: Intra-arterial monitoring of blood pressure, Am. J. Nurs. **74**(1):48-53, January 1974.

Nora, J. J.: Multifactorial inheritance hypothesis for the etiology of congenital heart diseases: the genetic environment interaction, Circulation **38:**604-607, September 1968.

Nora, J. J., and Nora, A. H.: Recurrence risks in children having one parent with a congenital disorder, Circulation **53**(4):701-702, April 1976.

Passwell, J., and associates: Abnormal renal functions in cyanotic heart disease, Arch. Dis. Child. **51:**803-805, 1976.

Pickering, D., and associates: Pre- and postoperative growth in persistent ductus arteriosus, Arch. Dis. Child. **51:**562-563, 1976.

Pidgeon, V.: The infant with congenital heart disease, Am. J. Nurs. **2**(67):290-293, February 1967.

Rashkind, W. J.: Transposition of the great vessels, Pediatr. Clin. North Am. **18**(4):1075-1090, 1971.

Reiss, J., and Menashe, V.: Genetic counseling and congenital heart disease, J. Pediatr. **80**(4):655-656, April 1972.

Richardson, R. G.: The scalpel and the heart, New York, 1970, Charles Scribner's Sons.

Roberts, F. B.: A child with heart disease, Am. J. Nurs. **72**(6): 1080-1084, June 1972.

Rosenthal, A., and Castaneda, A.: Growth and development after cardiovascular surgery in infants and children, Prog. Cardiovasc. **18:**27, 1975.

Sacksteder, S., Gildea, J. H., and Dassy, C.: Common congenital cardiac defects, Am. J. Nurs. **78**(2):266-272, February 1978.

Shor, V. Z.: Congenital cardiac defects: assessment and case finding, Am. J. Nurs. **78**(2):256-261, February 1978.

Steele, S.: Nursing care of the child with cardiac conditions requiring long-term care. In Steele, S., editor: Nursing care of the child with long-term illness, New York, 1971, Appleton-Century-Crofts.

Stocker, F. P., and associates: Pediatric radiocardioangiography, Circulation **47**(4):819-826, April 1973.

Strangway, A., and associates: Diet and growth in congenital heart disease, Pediatrics **57**(1):75-86, January 1976.

Tandon, R., and Edwards, J. E.: Cardiac malformations associated with Down's syndrome, Circulation **47**(6):1349-1355, June 1973.

Uzark, K.: A child's cardiac catheterization—avoiding potential risks, Am. J. Maternal Child Nurs. **3**(3):158-161, May/June 1978.

Van Meter, M., and Lavine, P. G.: EKG's. Part 2. Atrial arrhythmias, Nursing '75 **5**(5):37-43, May 1975.

Westfall, U. E.: Electrical and mechanical events in the cardiac cycle, Am. J. Nurs. **76**(2):231-235, February 1976.

Woods, S. L.: Monitoring pulmonary artery pressures, Am. J. Nurs. **76**(11):1765-1771, November 1976.

Acquired heart disease

Albeit, S., and associates: Recognizing digitalis toxicity, Am. J. Nurs. **77**(12):1935-1945, December 1977.

Bauer, J. D., Ackerman, P. G., and Toro, G.: Clinical laboratory methods, St. Louis, 1974, The C. V. Mosby Co.

Blackman, N. S., and Kuskin, L.: Should prophylactic therapy be given to patients with an uncertain history of rheumatic fever? Clin. Pediatr. **11**(1):15-19, January 1972.

Boyle, M. T., and Kaufman, A.: Strep screening to prevent rheumatic fever, Am. J. Nurs. **75**(9):1487-1488, September 1975.

Brownell, K. D., and Bailen-Rose, F.: Acute rheumatic fever in children, J.A.M.A. **224:**1593-1597, June 18, 1973.

Chobin, N., Kangos, J., and Miller, J.: From project to ongoing program, Am. J. Nurs. **75**(9):1489-1491, September 1975.

Committee on Rheumatic Fever and Bacterial Endocarditis of the Council on Cardiovascular Disease in the Young of the American Heart Association: Prevention of bacterial endocarditis, Circulation **46:**3, 1972.

Feeney, R.: Preventing rheumatic fever in school children, Am. J. Nurs. **73**(2):265, February 1973.

Flucytosine, Nursing '72 **2**(10):9-10, October 1972.

Goldring, D., and associates: The critically ill child: care of the child in cardiac failure, Pediatrics **47**(6):1056-1063, June 1971.

Jackson, H.: Prevention of rheumatic fever, Clin. Pediatr. **12**(8): 501-503, August 1973.

Meszaros, W. T.: Lung changes in congestive heart failure, Circulation **47**(9):859-871, April 1973.

Peterson, L. J., and Peacock, R.: The incidence of bacteremia in pediatric patients following tooth extraction, Circulation **53**(4): 676-679, April 1976.

Report on Inter-Society Commission for Heart Disease Resources: Community resources for the diagnosis and acute care of patients with rheumatic fever, Circulation **44:**197-203, July 1971.

Tanner, G.: Heart failure in the MI patient, Am. J. Nurs. **77**(2): 230-234, February 1977.

36

The child with a problem related to the formed elements of the blood

ORIGIN OF FORMED ELEMENTS

Blood is composed of two components: a fluid portion called plasma and a cellular portion known as the formed elements of the blood. The two components are approximately equal in volume. Plasma is about 90% water and 10% solutes. The principal solutes are the proteins albumin, globulin, and fibrinogen. The cellular elements are red blood cells *(erythrocytes),* white blood cells *(leukocytes),* and platelets *(thrombocytes).* The leukocytes are further divided into *granulocytes* and *agranulocytes,* which describes the presence or absence, respectively, of granules within the cytoplasm of the cells.

There are three types of granulocytes: *neutrophils, basophils,* and *eosinophils.* The name of each of these refers to the granule's characteristic staining property during laboratory analysis. Neutrophils stain neutral to the dyes, whereas basophils stain a purple color to the basic methylene blue dye and eosinophils take on a red color to the acidic eosin dye. Because the nuclei of these cells have two or more lobules that are connected by fine chromatin strands, the term *polymorphonuclear* (meaning "many formed nuclei") *leukocytes,* or simply *"polys,"* is collectively used to refer to the granulocytes.

The nongranular leukocytes comprise two cell types, the *monocytes* and *lymphocytes.* Characteristically these cells do not develop granules and the nuclei are not lobulated.

The major blood-forming (hemopoietic) organs of the body are the red bone marrow (myeloid tissue) and lymphatic system. All of the formed elements of the blood, except to some extent the agranulocytes, are believed to be formed in myeloid tissue during postnatal life. During embryonic development the mesenchyme, spleen, liver, thymus, and yolk sac serve as additional sites of blood cell formation. In certain blood disorders these sites, particularly the spleen, can be stimulated to produce blood cells, and constitute *extramedullary hematopoiesis.* In infants and young children all of the bone contains red marrow (so-called because of its color from formation of erythrocytes), but, as bone growth ceases near the end of adolescence, only the ribs, sternum, vertebrae, and pelvis continue to produce blood cells. The remainder of the bone marrow becomes yellow from deposition of fat. However, in conditions of decreased demand for blood cells, the yellow marrow can revert to red marrow as another hemopoietic source.

Although the progressive development of each blood cell is fairly well delineated, there is considerable controversy regarding the origin of the blood cell. One of the most widely held theories (monophylectic) is that each blood cell orginates from a primordial (primitive) cell called a *blast* or *stem* cell. This *hemocytoblast* in turn gives rise to the erythroblast, myeloblast, monoblast, lymphoblast, and megakaryoblast (Fig. 36-1). According to the other theory (polyphylectic), each blood cell is a derivative of a specific precursor, such as the erythrocyte from an erythroblast, and not from the same undifferentiated primordial cell.

Another system that is involved in blood cell production is the *recticuloendothelial* system. Although not a discrete anatomic entity, it refers to widely dispersed cells of mesodermal origin that line the vascular and lymph channels. These cells, called *reticular cells* because they form a network, are capable of phagocytosis (ingestion and digestion of foreign substances), formation of immune bodies, and differentiation into other cells, such as hemocytoblasts, myeloblasts, or lymphoblasts.

Erythrocyte formation

The erythrocyte is formed from the hemocytoblast in the red bone marrow. As illustrated in Fig. 36-1, the *hemocytoblast* forms the proerythroblast. The initial cell of this series has a deep blue (basophilic) staining cytoplasm and therefore is called a *basophilic erythroblast.* The chief change in the erythroblast is accumulation of hemoglobin in the cytoplasm. As the basophilic material decreases and the amount of hemoglobin increases, the cell is called a *polychromatic erythroblast,* which describes its mixture of staining properties. At the same time as the nucleus is decreasing in size, the basophilic material disappears, so that the cell is uniformly stained by eosin dye, hence the

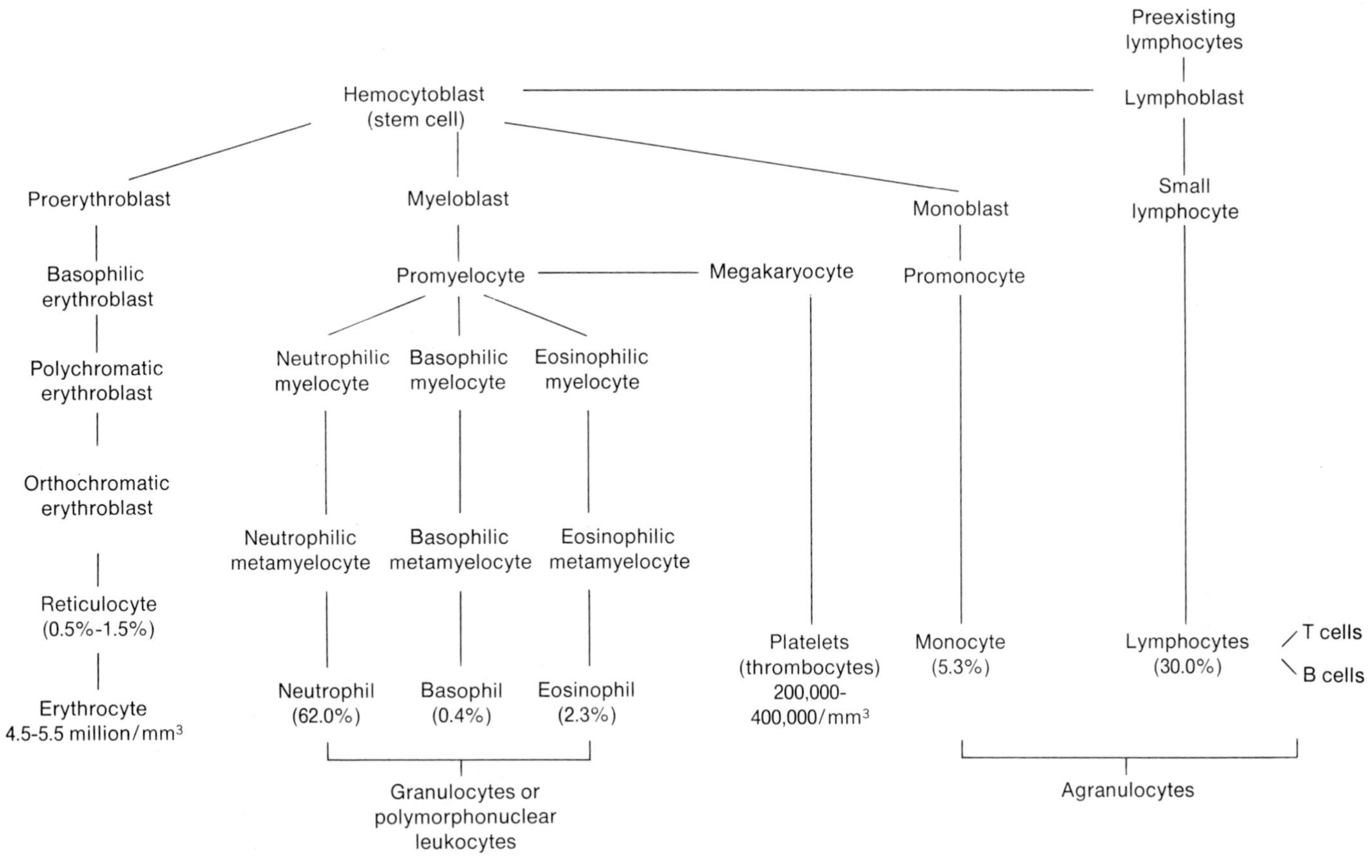

Fig. 36-1. Formation of blood cells. Erythrocyte values are averages for older children. For blood values at each age, see Appendix B, Table B-4.

term *orthochromatic erythroblast* or *normoblast*. Finally the normoblast completely loses its nucleus by a process of extrusion as it squeezes through the pores of the membrane into the capillary. As a result of losing its nucleus, the cell caves on both sides, giving the mature *erythrocyte* its characteristic appearance as a biconcave disc. During each of these stages the different cells continue to undergo mitosis so that increasingly greater numbers of cells are produced.

Normally some of the circulating erythrocytes, called *reticulocytes,* retain a small amount of basophilic reticulum. Ordinarily the total proportion of circulating reticulocytes (known as the reticulocyte count) is between 0.5% and 1.5%. A change in the number of reticulocytes is an indicator of increased red blood cell production or hyperfunctioning of the bone marrow. The *reticulocyte count* is a simple laboratory test frequently used to indirectly analyze hemopoiesis.

Regulation of erythrocyte production

The usual life span of the mature erythrocyte is 120 days. Apparently as red blood cells grow old, their membranes become fragile and eventually rupture. The contents of the cell fragment as they circulate through the blood vessels and are phagocytized by the reticuloendothelial cells in the spleen, liver, and bone marrow. The hemoglobin is broken down into the iron-containing pigment hemosiderin and the bile pigments biliverdin and bilirubin. Most of the iron is reused by the bone marrow for production of new red blood cells or stored in the liver and other tissues for future use. The bile pigments are excreted by the liver in bile.

Normally there is a homeostatic balance between the regulation of red blood cell production and destruction. This balance ensures adequate tissue oxygenation and a blood viscosity that allows the blood to flow freely through the vessels. The basic regulator of erythrocyte production is believed to be tissue oxygenation. In states of tissue hypoxia, *erythropoietin* (also called *erythropoietic stimulating factor* or *hemopoietin*) is released by the kidneys into the bloodstream. As a result the bone marrow is stimulated to produce new red blood cells. The main site of action seems to be an increase in both the maturation rate and mitosis of all stages of erythrocyte production, but primarily at the stem cell level.

During this rapid increase of red blood cell production,

the circulating erythrocytes may not be totally mature. Consequently the number of reticulocytes may increase dramatically (as high as 30% or more of the total red blood cell count). Even normoblasts may appear in the blood. Failure to observe this rise in erythrocyte and reticulocyte count is an indicator of bone marrow failure.

Once tissue oxygenation is met, the production of erythropoietin ceases. Thus tissue oxygen requirements control both the stimulation and termination of erythrocyte production. It is important to note that it is the function of red blood cells within the tissues, not the circulating numbers of erythrocytes, that is the basic regulatory mechanism. This explains why *polycythemia* (increase in the number of erythrocytes) occurs in conditions of prolonged tissue hypoxia, such as cyanotic heart defects (see p. 1312). If the circulating numbers of erythrocytes controlled erythropoietin release, this feedback mechanism would control erythrocyte production at a constant level (4.5 to 5.5 million/mm^3 of blood) regardless of existing tissue hypoxia.

Conditions affecting tissue oxygenation. Increased need for tissue oxygenation can result from several conditions: (1) increased metabolism such as from strenuous physical exercise, infection, or stress, (2) decreased environmental oxygenation, such as living in areas of high altitude or flying in unpressurized aircraft, (3) decreased peripheral circulation, such as in prolonged cardiac failure, (4) inadequate blood oxygenation, such as in cyanotic heart diseases or pulmonary insufficiency, and (5) decreased circulating red blood cells, such as from anemia or hemorrhage.

The tissue oxygenation regulatory mechanism serves to reverse each of these conditions either by restoring the number of erythrocytes to its normal level, such as in hemorrhage or anemia, or by producing additional red blood cells (polycythemia), such as occurs in living in high altitudes or from physiologic disorders.

Functions of erythrocytes

The major function of red blood cells is to transport hemoglobin, which in turn carries oxygen to all cells of the body. However, erythrocytes have other significant functions: (1) they contain quantities of carbonic anhydrase, an enzyme that catalyzes the reaction between carbon dioxide and water, allowing large quantities of carbon dioxide to react with blood for transportation to the lungs, and (2) the hemoglobin, a protein, serves as an effective acid-base buffer, maintaining the blood pH at a constant level. (See also p. 1071.)

Leukocyte formation

Granulocytes. The granulocytes, like erythrocytes, are produced in the bone marrow. For this reason these cells are sometimes referred to as *myelogenous leukocytes*. It is believed that these cells originate from primitive stem cells, which develop into myeloblasts. As Fig. 36-1 illustrates, the genesis of neutrophils, basophils, and eosinophils is similar to the stages observed during erythrocyte production. The differentiation of myeloblasts into various mature white blood cells is primarily the result of specialization within the cytoplasm and degeneration of the nucleus. Unlike the erythrocyte, however, all of the white blood cells are nucleated.

Agranulocytes. The agranulocytes are believed to have their origin in various lymphogenous organs and for this reason are sometimes referred to as *lymphogenous leukocytes*. However, since stem cells and reticular cells are capable of differentiating into monocytes or lymphocytes, the origin of these cells is frequently designated as the lymphomyleloid complex, which includes the bone marrow, lymph nodes, spleen, liver, thymus, subepithelial lymphoid tissue (tonsils, vermiform appendix, and intestinal lymphoid tissues), and connective tissues (mesenchymal cells of the reticuloendothelial system).

The monocytes follow the same sequence of development from the stem cell as the granulocytes (see Fig. 36-1). The monocytes, in turn, have the ability to develop into *macrophages,* large cells that are highly effective phagocytes.

Lymphocyte formation *(lymphocytopoiesis)* is believed to take place anywhere in the lymphomyeloid complex. Lymphocytes may develop from blast cells or preexisting lymphocytes (see Fig. 36-1). Recent research suggests that the thymus gland in the fetus has the important function of producing the original lymphocytes, which then circulate to various lymphomyeloid sites and remain there until the body's need for them triggers further mitosis.

One of the difficulties in delineating the genesis and life history of the lymphocyte is its potentiality to develop into other cells. For example, the lymphocytes produced by the bone marrow (sometimes called B cells) are mainly responsible for immunoglobulin formation, whereas thymic lymphocytes (or T cells) are involved in cell-mediated immunity (or formation of cellular antibodies).

Regulation of leukocyte production

The exact life span of the leukocytes is not as clearly defined as that of the erythrocytes because their existence in the circulation is primarily for transportation to extravascular areas where they reside in reservoirs or where they are needed to resist infection. Therefore, their survival rate has been divided into three phases: (1) the hemopoietic phase, extending from the development of the blast cell to the delivery of the mature leukocyte into the circulation, (2) the intravascular phase, or the period within the circulation, and (3) the extravascular phase, or the period of time spent in the viscera or tissues. The life span of granulocytes up to their entrance into the tissues is estimated as 6½ to 11 days. The average time that granulocytes spend in the circulation is 9 hours.[3]

Agranulocytes probably live for an extended period of time because they remain in inflamed tissue areas longer than the granulocytes. Because monocytes wonder back and forth between the blood and tissues and are capable of becoming macrophages, their life span is still unknown. Lymphocytes probably live as long as 300 days, depending on the body's need for them.

As has already been implied, the regulation of leukocytes is based on the body's need for them. Since the main function of leukocytes is to resist infection, it follows that any tissue damage from bacterial or viral agents promotes leukocyte circulation and production. It is important to note, however, that leukocytosis (increase in leukocytes) results from tissue destruction from almost any factor, such as hemorrhage, neoplastic disease, toxicity, operative procedures, chemical and thermal injury, or tissue ischemia.

After any tissue-damaging process the involved tissues liberate a substance called *leukocytosis-promoting factor*. On diffusing into the blood, it has two actions: (1) it causes large numbers of stored granulocytes, particularly neutrophils, to be released from the bone marrow into the bloodstream, where they are carried to the injured site, and (2) it increases the production of granulocytes within the bone marrow.

At the same time, another substance called *histamine*, which increases local blood and capillary permeability, is released by the injured cells. Large numbers of monocytes and lymphocytes begin to enter the tissues from the blood and begin to change into macrophages for phagocytizing bacteria, necrotic tissue, and other foreign debris.

The leukocytes probably die as a result of their activity at the site of injury and are phagocytized by other newly formed white blood cells. Effective control of the inflammatory process with subsequent tissue recovery most likely results in a feedback mechanism to the bone marrow and lymphogenous organs to cease increased production of white blood cells.

Lymphocyte activity is also controlled by the body's immunologic needs. As has been pointed out earlier, lymphocytes are capable of producing immunoglobulins and cellular antibodies. Therefore, in situations in which invading antigens stimulate the immunologic system, the production of lymphocytes will also be increased.

Functions of leukocytes

Although all of the leukocytes play some role in resisting infection or other tissue-damaging processes, each of the white blood cells plays a specific role. *Neutrophils* and *monocytes* are effective phagocytes and, as a result, are primarily involved in inflammatory reactions. Neutrophilia (increased numbers of neutrophils) is most evident in an acute inflammation, whereas monocytosis (increased number of monocytes) is more evident in chronic conditions. The reason for this is that as the affected area becomes acidic from tissue necrosis, neutrophils, which prefer a neutral environment, become less efficient, and the monocytes, which become macrophages, become more powerful. Since *lymphocytes* have the ability to become monocytes and then macrophages, these cells also increase during chronic inflammation. The other functions of lymphocytes in terms of the immune process have already been discussed.

The function of *eosinophils* is unknown, although eosinophilia (increased numbers of eosinophils) is well documented in a number of conditions: (1) during allergic reactions, (2) in parasitic infestation, (3) in response to foreign proteins, and (4) at the site of blood clots.

It is postulated that eosinophils detoxify proteins, which explains their increase in allergic conditions and possibly in parasitic infections, where the parasites continually produce protein substances. Eosinophils also are thought to release a substance called *profibrinolysin,* which when activated to form fibrinolysin, digest *fibrin,* thereby helping dissolve a clot. (See p. 1391 for a review of the clotting mechanism.)

The function of *basophils* is also poorly understood, although basophilia (increased numbers of basophils) occurs during the healing phase of inflammation and during prolonged chronic inflammation. Since basophils closely resemble mast cells, which liberate heparin (a substance that prevents blood coagulation), it is possible that the basophilia that occurs in these two conditions helps prevent the agglutination process that is peculiar to prolonged inflammation.

Platelet formation

Platelets are actually small fragments of cells. They are smaller than blood cells, do not possess a cellular structure, and consist of a clear ground substance containing granules. The origin of platelets is the megakaryocytes, which are part of the myelogenous group of white blood cells (see Fig. 36-1). It is generally thought that the megakaryocytes fragment in the bone marrow and then pass into the bloodstream. An alternate theory is that the fragmentation occurs after the megakaryocytes are present in the bloodstream, as they attempt to pass through the minute capillaries.

Regulation of platelet production

The life span of platelets is thought to be about 4 days, although it may be as long as a week. Apparently the body regulates platelets to maintain a fairly constant level (between 200,000 and 400,000/mm^3). However, the exact regulatory mechanism and the method of destruction are unknown.

Function of platelets

The term *thrombocyte* means "clot" (thrombo) and "cell" (cyte) and accurately describes the main function of platelets. When there is a break in the continuity of a blood vessel, the platelets, which are normally round or oval discs, come in contact with the wet vessel surface and dramatically change their shape to become swollen spheres with long irregular projections called *pseudopodia* (false feet). As a result the platelets begin to adhere to the wet endothelium and to each other. The initial platelets at the site of injury release substances that attract other thrombocytes to the area. This causes a layering of platelets, which eventually forms a plug. The plug is large enough to partially or totally occlude the opening in the vessel wall but small enough to allow blood flow to continue unimpaired through the vessel.

In small vessel tears, the platelet plug is sufficient to produce hemostasis and additional blood coagulation is not necessary. However, when platelet counts are low, these numerous small ruptures, which occur continually in the body as a result of general functioning, are not repaired. Consequently small hemorrhagic areas called *petechiae* form under the skin.

Platelets also influence hemostasis by releasing a substance called *serotonin* at the site of injury. This substance is a vasoconstrictor that produces vascular spasm to decrease the amount of blood flow to the injured area.

ANEMIAS

Anemia is defined as a decreased number of red blood cells. Actually it is a condition in which the concentration of hemoglobin and/or the number of erythrocytes are below normal. The anemias are the most common hematologic disorders of infancy and childhood. This discussion is primarily concerned with an overview of the classification of anemia. Specific anemic conditions such as iron-deficiency anemia and aplastic anemia are discussed elsewhere (see pp. 473 and 1051, respectively). Later in this chapter the hemoglobinopathies sickle cell anemia and thalassemia are discussed.

Classification

The basic cause of anemia is either (1) an increased loss or destruction of red blood cells or (2) an impaired or decreased rate of production. An etiologic classification is outlined below, based on the various conditions that can lead to either of these results.

Etiologic classification of anemias

I. Excessive blood loss or destruction (hemolysis)
- **A.** Acute or chronic hemorrhage
- **B.** Intracorpuscular defects
  - **1.** Abnormal hemoglobin synthesis (hemoglobinopathies)
    - **a.** Sickle cell anemia
    - **b.** Thalassemia
  - **2.** Red cell membrane abnormalities
    - **a.** Spherocytosis
    - **b.** Stomatocytosis
    - **c.** Elliptocytosis
  - **3.** Enzymatic defects
    - **a.** Glucose-6-phosphate dehydrogenase (G-6-PD) deficiency
    - **b.** Pyruvate kinase deficiency
- **C.** Extracorpuscular factors
  - **1.** Drugs and chemicals
  - **2.** Infections, such as malaria
  - **3.** Antibodies, such as in erythroblastosis fetalis
  - **4.** Burns
  - **5.** Poisoning, such as plumbism
  - **6.** Hypersplenism

II. Decreased or impaired production (erythrogenesis)
- **1.** Nutritional deficiency
  - **a.** Iron
  - **b.** Pyridoxine (vitamin B_6)
  - **c.** Folic acid
  - **d.** Vitamin B_{12}
  - **e.** Ascorbic acid
  - **f.** Protein
- **2.** Depression or inhibition of bone marrow
  - **a.** Infection
  - **b.** Chemicals
  - **c.** Physical agents, such as radiation
  - **d.** Acquired or congenital aplastic anemia
- **3.** Mechanical interference and replacement by abnormal cells
  - **a.** Leukemia
  - **b.** Hodgkin's disease
  - **c.** Generalized malignancies

Blood loss. Acute or chronic hemorrhage results in loss of plasma and all formed elements of the blood. After acute hemorrhage the body replaces plasma within 1 to 3 days, maintaining blood volume. However, this results in a low concentration of red blood cells, which are gradually replaced within 3 to 4 weeks. During this period there is usually a normocytic (normal size), normochromic (normal color) anemia, provided there are sufficient iron stores for hemoglobin synthesis.

In chronic blood loss the actual number of red blood cells may be normal because of continual replacement. However, insufficient iron is available to form hemoglobin as quickly as it is lost. As a result erythrocytes are usually small in size (microcytic) and pale in color (hypochromic).

Excessive destruction. Excessive destruction or hemolysis or erythrocytes can occur from a variety of causes. One of the most common is a result of a defect within the red blood cell (intracorpuscular) that shortens the life span of the cell so that production cannot keep pace with destruction. The two examples discussed in this chapter, sickle cell anemia and thalassemia, have decreased erythrocyte life spans because of a defect in hemoglobin synthesis.

Extracorpuscular factors are those conditions that cause

hemolysis in otherwise normal red blood cells. A classic example is erythroblastosis fetalis, in which Rh-positive red blood cells in the fetus are attached and destroyed by antibodies from the Rh-negative mother (see p. 295). Other causes can be toxic drugs, transfusion reactions, infections such as malaria, and splenic sequestration (hypersplenism). In the latter condition large amounts of blood are sequestered (or pooled) in the spleen, which then proceeds to destroy the red blood cells.

Impaired or decreased production. Production of red blood cells can occur as a result of either bone marrow failure or deficiency of essential nutrients. Bone marrow failure may be caused by (1) replacement of bone marrow by fibrosis or by neoplastic cells, such as in leukemia, (2) depression of marrow activity from irradiation, chemicals, or drugs, or (3) interference with bone marrow activity from other systemic diseases, such as severe infection, chronic renal disease, widespread malignancy (without marrow infiltration), collagen diseases, or hypothyroidism.

The reason for various systemic disorders affecting erythrocyte production varies according to the condition. For example, in severe chronic infection there is evidence that depression of erythropoiesis is caused by a defect in the conversion of protoporphyrin into hemoglobin. In addition there is some degree of hemolysis, although the exact action is not known. In hypothyroidism the anemia is probably a result of decreased metabolic demands of the body. The reverse probably accounts for the anemia of generalized carcinoma.

The most common childhood anemia is a result of deficient iron supply (see p. 473). Besides iron as an essential component of hemoglobin synthesis, red blood cell production is dependent on amino acids, vitamins B_6, B_{12}, and C, folic acid, copper, and possibly cobalt. Chronic malnutrition results in anemia as a result of generalized protein, mineral, and vitamin deficiencies.

Pernicious anemia develops when the gastric mucosa fails to secrete sufficient amounts of intrinsic factor, which is essential for absorption of vitamin B_{12}. This type of anemia is common in the elderly as a result of physiologically decreased gastric secretions. Deprived of vitamin B_{12}, the bone marrow produces fewer but larger (macrocytic) red blood cells. The erythrocytes are usually immature and, because of their extremely fragile cell membranes, are more rapidly destroyed during circulation.

Classification based on morphology. A second classification has been made that is based on the morphologic changes within the red blood cell. The major categories are (1) normocytic, (2) microcytic, and (3) macrocytic. In addition each category may be subdivided according to the amount of hemoglobin in the cell. Since hemoglobin gives the cell its characteristic red color, the usual classifications are (1) normochromic or (2) microchromic. The morphologic classification, as in the outline, is helpful in diagnosing the cause of the anemia. It also enhances one's understanding of the pathologic changes that occur in the erythrocyte and the reason why certain hematologic tests are employed in diagnosing various anemias.

*Morphologic classification of anemias**

- **I.** Normocytic
  - **A.** Hypochromic
    - **1.** Lead poisoning
    - **2.** Anemia caused by some systemic diseases
  - **B.** Normochromic
    - **1.** Acute blood loss
    - **2.** Hemolytic anemia
    - **3.** Bone marrow replacement or hypoplasia
    - **4.** Sickle cell anemia
- **II.** Microcytic
  - **A.** Hypochromic
    - **1.** Iron deficiency
    - **2.** Pyridoxine deficiency
    - **3.** Thalassemia
  - **B.** Normochromic
    - **1.** Uncommon
- **III.** Macrocytic
  - **A.** Hypochromic
    - **1.** Uncommon, except with superimposed iron deficiency
  - **B.** Normochromic
    - **1.** Vitamin B_{12} (pernicious anemia) or folic acid deficiency
      - **a.** Malabsorption defects
      - **b.** Chronic liver disease
    - **2.** Some types of aplastic anemia
    - **3.** Reticulocytosis

Pathology and clinical manifestations

The basic physiologic defect caused by anemia is a decrease in the oxygen-carrying capacity of blood and, consequently, a reduction in the amount of oxygen available to the tissues. Most of the clinical manifestations are directly attributable to tissue hypoxia. Muscle weakness and easy fatigability are common, although children seem to have a remarkable ability to function quite well despite low levels of hemoglobin.

The skin is usually pale to a waxy pallor in severe anemia. Cyanosis is typically not evident, because it is the result of the quantity of deoxygenated hemoglobin in arterial blood. Hemoglobin levels generally must *exceed* 5 g/100 ml before cyanosis is evident. Anemia is caused by decreased hemoglobin and/or red blood cells, not inadequate oxygen saturation of existing hemoglobin. The nurse should also keep in mind that skin pigmentation can alter one's assessment of skin pallor. (For a review of skin assessment, see Chapter 5, p. 118.)

Central nervous system manifestations include headache,

*Adapted from Ravel, R.: Clinical laboratory medicine, Chicago, 1973, Year Book Medical Publishers, Inc.

Table 36-1. Hematologic laboratory tests for anemia

Test	Description	Normal values*	Comments
Red blood cell (RBC) count	Number of RBC/mm³ of blood	4.5-5.5 million/mm³ (Usually expressed in number of millions, for example, 5.3 million, rather than actual count)	Indirectly estimates Hb content of blood
Hemoglobin (Hb) determination	Amount of Hb/100 ml of whole blood	14.5 g/100 ml (May also be expressed as g%) Lower limits of normal 9-11 g	Total blood Hb primarily depends on number of circulating RBCs, but also on amount of Hb in each cell
Hematocrit (Hct)	Percentage or volume of packed RBC to whole blood	40% (May also be expressed as cubic milliliters of RBC per 100 ml of blood or in volumes per 100 ml) Lower limits of normal 27%-33%	Considered a fundamental diagnostic test in anemia because although it depends mostly on the number of RBCs, it is also sensitive to changes in their size, shape, and thickness Indirectly measures Hb content Is approximately three times Hb content
Red blood cell indices			
Mean corpuscular volume (MCV)	Average or mean volume (size) of a single RBC MCV = $\frac{\text{Hct (\%)} \times 10}{\text{RBC count (millions/mm}^3\text{)}}$	Normocytic = 80-94 μ^3 Microcytic < 80 μ^3 Macrocytic > 94 μ^3	MCV and MCH depend on accurate counts of RBCs, whereas MCHC does not; therefore MCHC is often more reliable
Mean corpuscular hemoglobin (MCH)	Average or mean quantity (weight) of Hb of a single RBC MCHC = $\frac{\text{Hb (g)/100 ml} \times 10}{\text{RBC count (millions/mm}^3\text{)}}$	Normochromic = 27-32 $\mu\mu$g Hypochromic <27 $\mu\mu$g Hyperchromic >32 $\mu\mu$g†	All indices depend on *average* cell measurements and do not show individual RBC (anisocytosis) variations
Mean corpuscular hemoglobin concentration (MCHC)	Average concentration of Hb in a single RBC MCHC = $\frac{\text{Hb (g)/100 ml} \times 100}{\text{Hct (\%)}}$	Normochromic = 32%-38% Hypochromic < 32% Hyperchromic > 38%†	
Reticulocyte count	% Reticulocytes to RBCs	0.5%-1.5%	Index of production of mature RBCs by red bone marrow Decreased count indicates depressed bone marrow function Increased count indicates erythrogenesis in response to some stimulus When reticulocyte count is extremely high, other forms of immature RBCs (normoblasts, even erythroblasts) may be present
Stained peripheral blood smear	Visual estimation of amount of Hb in RBCs and overall size, shape, and structure of RBCs	Normochromic and discoid shaped, similar-sized enucleated RBC, occasional reticulocytes	Indirectly estimates hypochromic anemia Shows variation in size and shape of RBCs:—microcytic, macrocytic, poikilocytic (abnormal shapes), anisocytic (variable sizes) Various staining properties of RBC structures may be evidence of immature forms of erythrocyte

*Represent averages during childhood.
†Actually, no cell can be hyperchromic because there is a maximum cell capacity for carrying Hb. However, a macrocyte appears hyperchromic because it contains a proportionately greater amount of Hb, and the thicker density of the cell makes it stain darker.

dizziness, light-headedness, irritability, slowed thought processes, decreased attention span, apathy, and depression. Growth retardation resulting from decreased cellular metabolism and coexisting anorexia is a common finding in chronic severe anemia. It is frequently accompanied by delayed sexual maturation in the older child.

The effects of anemia on the circulatory system can be profound. The viscosity of blood is almost entirely dependent on the concentration of red blood cells. In severe anemia the resulting hemodilution decreases the resistance to blood flow in the peripheral vessels so that far greater quantities of blood return to the heart. Consequently the cardiac workload is markedly increased, as evidenced by tachycardia and tachypnea. Initially this greater cardiac output compensates for the lower oxygen-carrying capacity of the blood, since blood replenished with oxygen returns to the tissues at a faster than normal rate. However, if the body's demand on the pumping action of the heart increases, such as during exercise, infection, or emotional stress, cardiac failure may ensue.

Hematologic evaluation of erythrocytes

Several tests can be used to evaluate the morphologic and quantitative changes resulting from anemia. Table 36-1 summarizes these routine hematologic laboratory procedures and lists normal blood values during childhood. Table B-4 in Appendix B lists more detailed age-specific blood values. Other tests used to diagnose the underlying cause of anemia are included elsewhere in the discussion of the particular disorder.

Medical management

The objective of medical management is to reverse the anemia by treating the underlying cause. For example, in nutritional anemias the specific deficiency is replaced. In blood loss caused by hemorrhage, packed red blood cells or whole blood is given.

In cases of severe anemia supportive medical care may include oxygen therapy, restoration of adequate blood volume, intravenous fluids, and bed rest.

Nursing considerations

Since anemia is not a disorder but a symptom of some underlying problem, nursing care is related to determining the cause, fostering appropriate supportive and therapeutic treatments, and decreasing tissue oxygen requirements. Each of these objectives is discussed and summarized in the boxed material on p. 1374.

Assisting in establishing a diagnosis. Although the physical examination yields valuable evidence regarding the severity of the anemia and some indication of its possible etiology, diagnosis primarily rests on hematologic blood studies and a careful history. In interviewing parents the nurse stresses the following areas that include tentative information regarding common causes of childhood anemia: (1) nutrition, especially dietary intake of iron, (2) past history of chronic, recurrent infection, (3) habits, particularly pica and ingestion of lead-based paint or other toxic agents, (4) bowel habits and presence of frank blood in stools or black, tarry stools, and (5) familial history of hereditary diseases, such as sickle cell anemia or thalassemia.

The nurse should also be aware of the significance of blood tests. For example, if the blood studies show a microcytic, hypochromic anemia suggestive of iron deficiency but the parent reports an iron-rich diet, the nurse needs to pursue the nutritional history for possible discrepancies.

Preparation of child for laboratory tests. Usually a battery of blood tests are ordered, but since they are generally done sequentially rather than all at once, the child is subjected to multiple fingersticks and/or venipunctures. Laboratory technicians frequently are not aware of the trauma that repeated "shots" represent to a child. Therefore, it is the nurse who has the responsibility of preparing the child for the tests by (1) explaining the significance of each test, particularly why the tests are not done at one time, (2) physically being with the child during the procedure whenever possible, and (3) allowing the child to play with the equipment on a doll and/or participate in the actual procedure, for example, by cleansing the finger with an alcohol swab. Older children may appreciate the opportunity to observe the blood cells under a microscope or in photographs. This is an especially important consideration if a serious blood disorder, such as leukemia, is suspected.

Multiple blood samples may present a problem with cumulative blood loss, necessitating blood replacement. This situation occurs most often in infants or young children with severe anemia. To prevent this possibility, blood may be withdrawn through a continuous intravenous line and replaced after the exact amount needed has been tested and discarded. Another measure is to use micromethods of testing that require blood from the heel or finger. However, in the latter case, extravasation of blood into the tissue from multiple punctures causes considerable tenderness at the site. The nurse needs to observe for cumulative effects of blood loss, particularly signs of shock and increased hypoxia, and to explain to parents the reason for blood replacement and the necessity of multiple blood samples.

Bone marrow aspiration is not a routine hematologic test but is essential for definitive diagnosis of the leukemias and aplastic anemias. Preparation of the child for this test is discussed on p. 1013.

Decreasing tissue oxygen needs. Since the basic pathology in anemia is a decreased oxygen-carrying capacity in the red blood cell, a priority nursing responsibility is to minimize tissue oxygen needs. This involves assessing the child's level of tolerance for activities of daily living

Summary of nursing care of the child with anemia

Goals	Responsibilities
Assist in establishing diagnosis	Take careful history regarding common causes of anemia in childhood Be aware of significance of various blood tests
Prepare child for laboratory tests	Explain to older children need for repeated venipunctures or fingersticks for blood analysis, particularly why a sequence of tests is required Allow children to play with laboratory equipment and/or participate with test Older children may enjoy looking at blood smears under a microscope or at pictures of blood cells Observe for signs of shock and hypoxia from repeated blood samples Explain to parents reason for replacing withdrawn blood and necessity of performing tests
Decrease tissue oxygen needs Minimize physical exertion	 Assess child's level of physical tolerance Anticipate and assist child in those activities of daily living that may be beyond his tolerance Provide diversional play activities that promote rest and quiet but prevent boredom and withdrawal Choose an appropriate roommate of similar age and interests and one who requires restricted activity
Minimize emotional stress	Anticipate child's irritability, short attention span, and fretfulness by offering to assist him in activities rather than waiting for him to ask Assess parents' awareness of child's need for dependency to conserve strength Explain to older children and parents reason for behavioral changes caused by anemia Encourage parents to remain with child
Prevent and observe for infection	Place child in room with noninfectious children; restrict visitors with active illnesses Advise visitors (and hospital personnel) to practice good hand washing Report any temperature elevation to physician Observe for leukocytosis Maintain adequate nutrition
Promote safety precautions	Alert ancillary hospital personnel regarding child's physical tolerance and need for assistance during activity Keep side rail raised and use safety restraints when applicable
Observe for complications Cardiac decompensation	 Be alert to signs of heart failure from excessive cardiac demands or from cardiac overload during blood transfusion
Transfusion reaction	Practice all precautions Check blood with another nurse and physician to ensure correct blood group/type with that of child Run blood slowly and remain with child for infusion of initial 50 ml Stop blood immediately if any untoward reaction occurs Attach blood to piggyback setup with normal saline or other intravenous solution to maintain open venous line Observe for signs and symptoms of reaction (see Table 36-2)
Oxygen therapy	Monitor for benefit of oxygen but avoid prolonged use

and play. During periods of rest the nurse takes vital signs and observes behavior to establish a baseline of nonexertion energy expenditure. During periods of activity the nurse repeats these measurements and observations to compare them with resting values. Signs of exertion include tachycardia, palpitations, tachypnea, dyspnea, shortness of breath, hyperpnea, breathlessness, dizziness, lightheadedness, diaphoresis, and change in skin color. The child looks fatigued with sagging limp posture, slow strained movements, and inability to tolerate additional activity.

Once a baseline of physical tolerance has been established, the nurse anticipates those activities that are physically taxing, such as dressing, feeding, or getting out of bed, and allows for conservation of energy by assisting the child as needed. However, since dependency can be threatening to a child, the nurse allows for as much control in the environment as possible. For example, a child with severe anemia may be unable to walk to the bathroom but may be able to use a bedside commode or be transported in a wheelchair to the lavatory rather than have to use a bedpan. Scheduling activities throughout the day with planned rest periods in between maximizes the child's energy potential without causing undue exertion.

Diversional activities are planned that promote rest but avoid boredom and withdrawal. Since short attention span, irritability, and restlessness are common in anemia and increase stress demands on the body, the nurse plans appropriate activities, such as listening to music, using a tape recorder, watching television, reading or listening to stories or comics, continuing a favorite hobby, such as stamp collecting, coloring, or drawing, playing board and card games, or being wheeled in a carriage or chair. Choosing the appropriate roommate, such as a child of similar age with a diagnosis that also requires restricted activity, is a major asset in preventing the boredom of imposed bed rest.

If infants or young children are hospitalized, the importance of avoiding parental separation must be considered. Crying and fretfulness place increased stress demands on the body, which increases oxygen needs. Parents need help in understanding the importance of their presence, even though the child may be less responsive than usual. The nurse also explains the reason for mood changes and the necessity of allowing the child's dependency.

Anemic children are prone to infection because tissue hypoxia causes cellular dysfunction and the disturbed metabolic processes weaken the host's defenses against foreign agents. Infection also worsens the anemia by increasing metabolic needs and, in instances of chronic infection, also interferes with erythropoiesis and shortens the survival time of red blood cells. All the usual precautions are taken to prevent infection, such as appropriate room selection in a noninfectious area, restricting visitors or hospital personnel with active infection, practicing good hand washing, and maintaining adequate nutrition. The nurse also observes for signs of infection, particularly temperature elevation and leukocytosis. However, an elevated white blood cell count sometimes occurs in anemia without the presence of systemic or local infection.

Promoting safety precautions. Children with chronic anemia usually adjust to the low levels of hemoglobin remarkably well. Often it is difficult for others unfamiliar with the child's condition to recognize the actual degree of physical tolerance. The nurse needs to inform all health personnel caring for the child to be alert to signs of overexertion and to anticipate the need for assistance, particularly when getting out of bed or going for a walk. Since young children cannot verbalize their fatigue or weakness, others must rely on observation to prevent accidental injuries. The importance of safety measures such as raised side rails or the use of restraints when the young child is in a high chair or stroller should be emphasized.

Observation for complications. The main complication of anemia is cardiac decompensation, which can result from excessive demands on the heart as a result of increased metabolic needs or of cardiac overload during rapid blood transfusion. The nurse observes for signs and symptoms of heart failure, such as tachycardia, dyspnea, rales, moist respirations, cough, shortness of breath, and sweating. Obviously preventing heart failure through minimizing hypoxia and transfusing blood slowly is of first priority. Packed red blood cells are usually administered to prevent circulatory hypervolemia.

Since blood transfusions are required in severe anemia to increase the hemoglobin level, the nurse practices all the usual precautions for administering blood and observes for signs of transfusion reactions. The major responsibilities are summarized on p. 1389 and discussed in greater detail in Table 36-2.

Oxygen may be administered to provide optimal environmental conditions for hemoglobin saturation. However, oxygen is of limited value because each gram of hemoglobin is able to carry a limited amount of the gas. In addition prolonged supplemental oxygen can decrease erythropoiesis. Therefore, the nurse monitors the child closely for evidence of decreasing benefit from oxygen. One of the first signs of hypoxia is restlessness.

SICKLE CELL ANEMIA

Sickle cell anemia is part of a group of diseases called *hemoglobinopathies,* in which normal adult hemoglobin (hemoglobin A or HbA) is partly or completely replaced by a hemoglobin variant, including fetal hemoglobin (HbF). Sickle cell disease includes all those hereditary disorders, the clinical, hematologic, and pathologic features of which are related to the presence of sickle hemoglobin (HbS). In the United States the most common forms of sickle cell disease are (1) sickle cell trait (also called sicklemia), the heterozygous form of the disease (HbA and HbS or HbSA), (2) sickle cell anemia, the homozygous form of the disease (HbSS), (3) sickle cell–hemoglobin C disease, a variant of sickle cell anemia including both HbS and HbC, and (4) sickle cell–thalassemia disease, a combination of sickle cell trait and β-thalassemia trait.

Sickle cell anemia is found primarily in the black race, although infrequently it affects whites, especially those of Mediterranean descent. The incidence of the disease varies in different geographic locations. Among American blacks, the incidence of sickle cell trait ranges between 7% and 13.4%. In East Africa the incidence is reported to be as high as 45% among native blacks. The high incidence of sickle cell trait in these individuals is believed by some to be the result of selective protection of trait carriers against malaria caused by one specific parasite.

Sickle cell anemia occurs in about 1:400 black Americans. It is estimated that there are at least 75,000 persons in the United States with this disorder. Sickle cell–hemoglobin C disease is the second most frequent form of sickle cell anemia in black Americans.

Mode of transmission

Sickle cell anemia is an autosomal-recessive disorder. The inheritance is described as intermediate because the gene is partially expressed in the heterozygous state and completely expressed in the homozygous state. The expected pattern of transmission from two parents who carry the heterozygous gene HbSA is illustrated on p. 192. In the United States it is estimated that 1 in twelve blacks carries the trait; therefore, the risk of two blacks having a child with the disease is 0.7%.

The occurrence of other forms of sickle cell anemia is the result of union between two individuals who carry the heterozygous form of variants of sickle cell trait. Fig. 36-2 illustrates the inheritance pattern of the various forms of sickle cell anemia.

Basic defect

The basic defect responsible for the sickling effect of erythrocytes is in the globin fraction of hemoglobin, which is composed of 574 amino acids. Hemoglobin S differs from hemoglobin A only in the substitution of one amino acid for another. Valine instead of glutamine resides in the sixth position of the β-polypeptide chain. Under conditions of decreased oxygen tension and lowered pH, the relatively insoluble hemoglobin S changes its molecular structure to form long slender crystals. The rapid growth of these filamentous crystals causes tenting of the cell membrane and the formation of crescent or sickle-shaped red blood cells. The filamentous forms are associated with much greater viscosity than the normal holly-leaf structure of hemoglobin A.

The tendency to sickle is also related to the concentration of hemoglobin within the cell. Since hypertonicity of the blood plasma increases the intracellular concentration of hemoglobin, dehydration promotes sickling.

In most instances the sickling response is reversible under conditions of adequate oxygenation and hydration. During this time the red blood cells are indistinguishable from normal erythrocytes on peripheral examination.

Although the defect is inherited at the time of conception, the sickling phenomenon is usually not apparent until later in infancy. The high levels of fetal hemoglobin prevent sickling of the red blood cells, because fetal hemoglobin is alkali resistant and has a greater affinity for carrying oxygen than hemoglobin A or S. The newborn has from 44% to 89% fetal hemoglobin, but this rapidly decreases during the first year, so that sickling usually becomes apparent after 4 months of age.

Sickle cell trait. Persons with sickle cell trait have the same basic defect, but only about 24% to 45% of the total hemoglobin is hemoglobin S. The remainder is hemoglobin A. Normally these individuals are asymptomatic. However, under conditions of extreme or prolonged deoxygenation, such as strenuous physical exercise, anesthesia, infection,

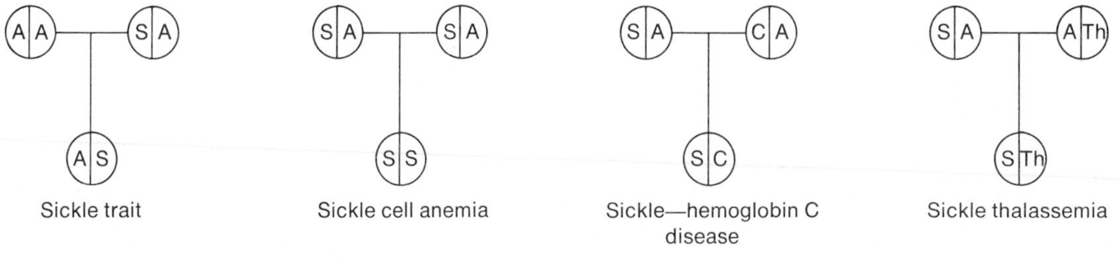

Fig. 36-2. Inheritance pattern of sickle cell hemoglobin and other variants. The letters represent the genes for different types of hemoglobin: *A*, normal hemoglobin; *S*, sickle hemoglobin; *C*, hemoglobin C; and *Th*, thalassemia.

pulmonary disease, anemia, high-altitude environments, underwater swimming, or pregnancy, sickling crises may occur. The higher the percentage of hemoglobin S, the more likely the occurrence of symptomatic responses.

Pathology

The pathologic changes from sickle cell anemia are primarily the result of (1) increased blood viscosity and (2) increased red blood cell destruction (Fig. 36-3). The entanglement and enmeshing of rigid sickle-shaped cells with one another increases the internal friction of the suspension, thus increasing blood viscosity. The thickened blood slows the circulation, causing capillary stasis, obstruction by elongated and pointed erythrocytes, and thrombosis. Eventually tissue ischemia and necrosis result with pathologic changes in the following sites.

Spleen. Initially the spleen becomes enlarged from congestion and engorgement with sickled cells. Eventually the sinuses are compressed and infarctions result. The functioning cells are gradually replaced with fibrotic tissue, until eventually in severe stages of the disease the spleen is decreased in size and totally replaced by a fibrous mass.

As a result of splenic infarction the spleen loses its ability to filter bacteria and to promote the release of large numbers of phagocytic cells. Consequently children with sickle cell anemia are much more susceptible to infection.

Liver. The liver is also altered in form and function. Liver failure and necrosis are the result of severe impairment of hepatic blood flow from anemia and capillary obstruction. The liver is usually enlarged as a result of blood stasis and is occasionally tender. With progressive focal necrosis and subsequent scarring, cirrhosis eventually occurs.

Kidney. Kidney abnormalities are probably the result of the same cycle of congestion of glomerular capillaries and tubular arterioles with sickle cells and hemosiderin, tissue necrosis, and eventual scarring. The principal results of kidney ischemia are hematuria, inability to concentrate urine, enuresis, and, occasionally, nephrotic syndrome.

Bones. The hyperplasia and congestion of the bone marrow results in osteoporosis, widening of the medullary spaces, and thinning of the cortices. As a result of the weakening of bone, especially in the lumbar and thoracic region, skeletal deformities, particularly lordosis and kyphosis, may occur. From chronic hypoxia, the bone becomes susceptible to osteomyelitis, frequently from *Salmonella*. Aseptic necrosis of the femoral head from chronic ischemia is an occasional problem.

Vaso-occlusive crises can result in a variety of skeletal problems. One of the more frequent is the *hand-foot* syndrome, which is caused by infarction of short tubular bones. It is characterized by pain and swelling of the soft tissue over the hands and feet. It usually resolves spontaneously within a couple of weeks. Localized swelling over joints with arthralgia can occur from erythrostasis with sickle cells.

Chronic leg ulcers are common in adolescents and adults and are thought to be the result of thrombosis and decreased peripheral circulation. Many of the skeletal abnormalities that are seen in thalassemia are also present in sickle cell anemia but are usually less prominent (see p. 1385).

Central nervous system. Changes in the central nervous system are primarily intravascular from the same cyclic reaction of stasis, thrombosis, and ischemia. Stroke or cerebrovascular accident is a major complication and can result in permanent paralysis or death. Any number of neurologic symptoms can herald a minor cerebral insult, such as headache, aphasia, weakness, convulsions, or visual disturbances. Loss of vision is usually the result of progressive retinopathy and retinal detachment.

Heart. Cardiac problems are mainly attributable to the stress of chronic anemia, which can eventually result in decompensation and failure. Myocardial infarctions may also occur from stasis and thrombosis.

Blood. With the formation of sickled erythrocytes, mechanical fragility is increased, thereby decreasing the red blood cell's life span. Hemolysis occurs both during intravascular circulation and as a result of stagnation of sickled cells in the congested spleen. Although the body attempts to compensate through stimulated erythropoietic activity, as evidenced by a hyperplasic bone marrow, the rate of destruction exceeds the rate of production. A normocytic, normochromic anemia results.

With increased hemolysis, hemosiderosis (increased storage of iron) is present in the liver, spleen, bone marrow, kidneys, and lymph nodes.

Clinical manifestations

In addition to the effects of sickling on various organ structures, the child with sickle cell anemia may have a variety of complaints, such as weakness; anorexia; joint, back, and abdominal pain; fever; and vomiting. Although sickle cell anemia has been reported during the neonatal period and early part of infancy, it most commonly is recognized after 4 months of age, particularly during the toddler and preschool period. It is frequently first diagnosed during a crisis, after an acute upper respiratory or gastrointestinal infection.

Other generalized effects include growth retardation, both in height and weight, delayed sexual maturation, decreased fertility, and priapism (constant penile erection). If the child reaches adulthood, sexual development and adult height are usually achieved.

Sickle cell crisis. The clinical manifestations of sickle cell anemia vary markedly in severity and frequency. The most acute symptoms of the disease occur during periods of exacerbation called *crises*. There are four types of episodic crises—vaso-occlusive, splenic sequestration, aplastic, and hyperhemolytic crises.

Vaso-occlusive crises are the most common and the only

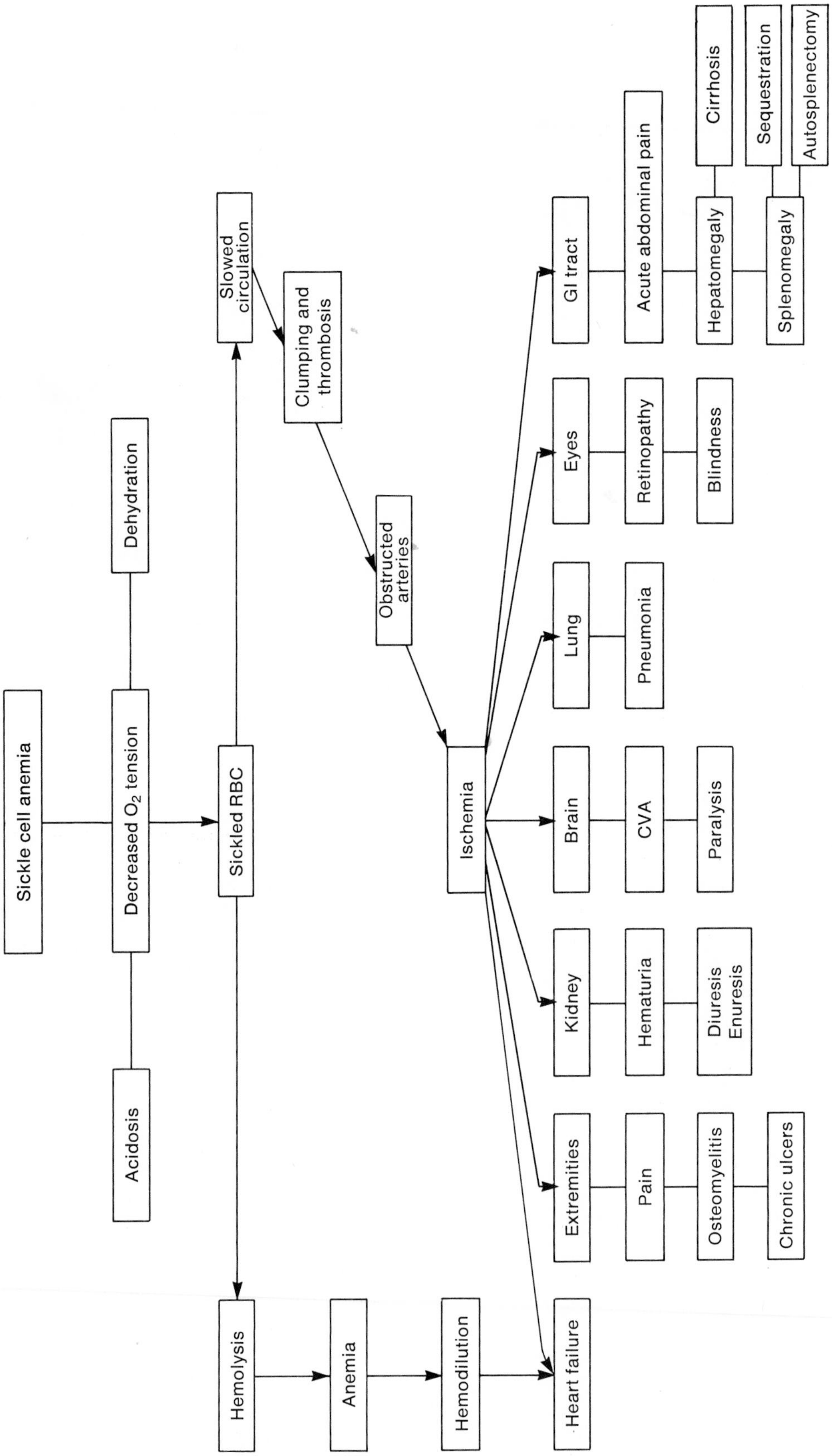

Fig. 36-3. Tissue effects of sickle cell anemia.

painful ones. They are the result of sickled cells obstructing the blood vessels, causing occlusion, ischemia, and potentially necrosis. The major symptoms of this crisis are fever, acute abdominal pain from visceral hypoxia, hand-foot syndrome, and arthralgia, without an exacerbation of anemia.

Splenic sequestration crises are caused by the spleen sequestering (pooling) large quantities of blood, causing a precipitous drop in blood volume and ultimately shock. The crisis may be acute or chronic. The chronic manifestation is termed *functional asplenia*. The acute form occurs most commonly in children between 8 months and 5 years of age and may result in death from profound anemia and cardiovascular collapse.

Aplastic crisis is diminished red blood cell production, usually triggered by a viral or other infection. When superimposed on the existing rapid destruction of red blood cells, a profound anemia results.

Another type of bone marrow crisis is *megaloblastic anemia*, which is attributed to an excess nutritional need for folic acid and/or vitamin B_{12} during periods of pronounced erythropoiesis. Since infection is not always antecedent to aplastic or hypoplastic crises, it is possible that folic acid deficiency is a causative agent.

Hyperhemolytic crisis occurs when there is an even greater rate of red blood cell destruction. It is characterized by anemia, jaundice, and reticulocytosis. It is a rare complication and frequently suggests other coexisting abnormalities, such as glucose-6-phosphate dehydrogenase deficiency, which is also common in blacks.

Diagnostic evaluation

Several tests are available for detecting sickle cell anemia. Although most of the routine hematologic tests described in Table 36-1 are done primarily to evaluate the anemia, this discussion focuses on the four tests specifically used to detect the homozygous or heterozygous form of the disease.

Stained blood smear. Examination of the stained smear of blood may reveal a few sickled red blood cells. However, since the erythrocyte assumes its normal discoid shape under adequate oxygenation, no sickled cells may be present even in the homozygous form of the disease. Whenever sickle cells are found, the diagnosis is usually positive for sickle cell anemia, not sickle cell trait.

Sickling test (sickle cell slide preparation). The simplest method to detect sickling is to place a drop of blood on a slide and cover it with a sealed cover slip to produce deoxygenation. Eventually sickling of the red blood cell occurs. Unfortunately this test may take several hours before results are obtained, and it is not specific for the disease or trait. False negatives for the trait can occur if the blood contains a very small amount of hemoglobin S.

Sickle-turbidity test (Sickledex). In this test anticoagulated blood is mixed with a special solution. Since hemoglobin S is normally much less soluble than hemoglobin A or F (as well as other variants), when mixed with this solution it is insoluble and forms a cloudy or turbid mixture. All other forms of hemoglobin result in a clear suspension. This test is a reliable screening method because it can be done in blood from a fingerstick and yields accurate results in 3 minutes. However, it is not specific for the trait or disease and yields false negatives in anemic children (hemoglobin less than 10 g/100 ml) or in infants less than 4 to 6 months of age who have not completely converted to adult hemoglobin.

Hemoglobin electrophoresis ("fingerprinting"). In this test the blood is specially prepared and separated into various hemoglobins by high-voltage electrophoresis. The resulting pattern of the separated peptides as it appears on paper is referred to as "fingerprinting" of the protein. This test is accurate, rapid, and specific for detecting the homozygous and heterozygous forms of the disease, as well as the percentage of the various hemoglobins.

For screening purposes either the sickling test or the Sickledex is commonly used. If the test is positive, hemoglobin electrophoresis is necessary to distinguish between those children with the trait and those with the disease. Screening for sickle cell trait has become a controversial subject, especially among the black community, since there is no method of preventing the disease other than selective birth procedures. This subject is discussed in more detail under nursing considerations.

Medical management

There is no cure for sickle cell anemia. The aims of therapy are (1) to prevent the sickling phenomenon, which is responsible for the pathologic sequelae, and (2) to treat the medical emergency of sickle cell crisis.

Prevention of sickling. Prevention of sickling involves promoting adequate oxygenation and maintaining hemodilution. The successful implementation of these two goals is often more dependent on nursing intervention as discussed in the following paragraphs than on medical therapies.

A recent treatment aimed at preventing sickling by interfering with the formation of hydrophobic bonds between the hemoglobin S molecules, which result in crystalline formation and the bizarre shapes of the red blood cells, is urea therapy. Urea, a normal constituent of blood from the detoxification of ammonia, is thought to act with cyanate to prevent the sickling phenomenon. However, urea therapy in sufficient therapeutic dosages has its attendant side effects, such as massive diuresis, which promotes dehydration and electrolyte imbalance, subdural hematoma from loss of fluid from the brain, sclerosis and thrombophlebitis at the infusion site, drowsiness, and coma.

Treatment of crisis. More often medical management is

directed at supportive and symptomatic treatment of crises. Although specific treatments are warranted in different types of crises, the main general objectives include (1) bed rest to minimize energy expenditure and oxygen utilization, (2) hydration for hemodilution through oral and intravenous therapy, (3) electrolyte replacement, since hypoxia results in metabolic acidosis, which also promotes sickling, (4) analgesics for the severe abdominal and joint pain, (5) blood replacement to treat anemia and to reduce the viscosity of the sickled blood, and (6) antibiotics to treat any existing infection. The administration of the newly developed pneumococcal and meningococcal vaccine is recommended for these children who are over 2 and 5 years of age, respectively, because of their susceptibility to infection.

Short-term oxygen therapy may be helpful in severe anoxia, especially in children with cardiac failure. Although oxygen may prevent more sickling, it usually is not effective in reversing sickling, because, with the vessels clogged with cells, the oxygen is not able to reach the enmeshed sickled erythrocytes. In addition prolonged administration of oxygen can depress bone marrow activity, further aggravating the anemia.

Oral anticoagulants to relieve the painful vaso-occlusive crises have been somewhat successful but also greatly increase the risk of bleeding tendencies.

Exchange transfusion to reduce the number of circulating sickle cells and therefore slow down the vicious cycle of hypoxia, thrombosis, tissue ischemia, and injury has been successful and is sometimes advocated as a possible preventive technique. However, multiple transfusions carry the risk of hepatitis, hemosiderosis, and transfusion reactions.

In children with recurrent splenic sequestration, splenectomy may be a life-saving measure. However, since the spleen usually atrophies on its own through progressive fibrotic changes, routine splenectomy is not recommended, especially since any surgical procedure has increased risk for these children. Warranted surgical or autosplenectomy has several advantages since the spleen is the major site of sickling, sequestration, and destruction of red blood cells.

Priapism, a painful condition, may be treated with aspiration of the corpora cavernosum. This complication is particularly frequent in vaso-occlusive crises.

Nursing considerations

The primary nursing objectives are (1) preventing sickling and (2) helping the child and parents adjust to a lifelong, potentially fatal, hereditary disease. Many of the measures that prevent sickling are also appropriate when a crisis occurs. In addition special cautions are mandatory when the child undergoes surgery of any kind. Nurses may also be faced with the dilemmas of sickle cell screening and their role in genetic counseling. Each of these subjects is discussed in the following paragraphs. (For a summary of nursing care of the child with sickle cell anemia, see the boxed material.)

Explanation of disease. Since sickle cell anemia is first recognized when the child is a toddler, most of the nurse's counseling is with parents. The nurse explains to parents the basic effect of tissue hypoxia on red blood cells. One simple yet graphic way of illustrating the difference between normal discoid red blood cells and sickle cells is to roll round or oval objects, such as marbles, through a tube to demonstrate normal blood cell circulation and then roll pointed objects such as screws through the tube. The effect of sickling and clumping of the pointed objects is especially noticeable at a bend or slight narrowing of tube. This same idea can be expanded to discuss the importance of increased fluid in keeping the pointed objects suspended away from each other to avoid concentration. Taking time to establish a sound basis of understanding why certain measures are beneficial to the child encourages parents to practice them.

The nurse advises parents to inform all treating physicians of the child's condition. The use of a Medic Alert bracelet is another way of ensuring awareness of the disease. Some people view such identification as "negative labeling." The nurse can stress the positive benefits of displaying this information, especially in emergencies when the use of anesthesia may be required.

Prevention of tissue deoxygenation. Anything that increases cellular metabolism also results in tissue hypoxia. For the child this includes avoiding (1) strenuous physical activity (especially contact sports if the spleen is enlarged, since rupture will cause massive internal hemorrhage), (2) emotional stress, (3) environments of low-oxygen concentration, such as high altitudes or nonpressurized airplane flights, and (4) known sources of infection. If the child has even a mild infection, the parents must seek medical attention at once.

Promotion of hydration. The importance of hemodilution in preventing sickling and later in delaying the stasis-thrombosis-ischemia cycle has already been discussed. The nurse calculates the child's fluid requirements (approximately 100 to 125 ml/kg/day), which is the minimum daily fluid intake. The nurse also assesses the child's usual fluid consumption to evaluate its adequacy and makes adjustments based on this knowledge. It is not sufficient to advise parents to "force fluids" or "encourage drinking." They need specific instructions on how many glasses or bottles of fluid are required. Many foods are also a source of fluid, particularly soups, Jell-O, and puddings, and these can be included as liquid sources.

Children can be encouraged to drink by giving them a "special" cup or glass, using a straw, taking advantage of thirsty times, such as on awakening or after playing, serving frequent, small portions, and leaving the cup in easy reach

Summary of nursing care of the child with sickle cell anemia

Goals	Responsibilities
Explain disease	Inform parents and older children of basic defect and measures that promote sickling Stress importance of informing significant health personnel of child's condition and benefit of Medic Alert tag Explain signs of developing crisis, especially fever, pallor, and pain
Prevent sickling Promote tissue oxygenation	Explain prevention measures Avoidance of strenuous physical exertion Avoidance of emotional stress Prevention of infection Avoidance of low oxygen environment
Promote hydration	Calculate recommended daily fluid intake and base child's fluid requirements on this *minimum* amount Give parents written instructions regarding specific quantity of fluid required Encourage child to drink Teach parents signs of dehydration Stress importance of avoiding overheating as source of fluid loss
Prevent infection	Stress importance of adequate nutrition, protection from known sources of infection, and frequent medical supervision Report any sign of infection to physician immediately
Prevent psychologic problems from enuresis	Stress physical cause of enuresis Encourage parents to view enuresis as one side effect of disease Review possible measures for control such as frequent voiding but emphasize danger of limiting fluid Discuss problem of toilet training
Promote supportive therapies during crisis Pain	Control pain with analgesics, positioning, and application of warmth
Bed rest	Schedule care-giving activities to allow for optimal rest Promote circulation through passive range of motion exercises
Fluid therapy	Record intake and output Monitor intravenous fluids carefully Observe for signs of hydration; diuresis is not a valid indication Observe for electrolyte imbalance
Blood transfusions	Observe for signs of transfusion reactions and cardiac overload
Oxygen	Monitor for evidence of benefit from oxygen Avoid prolonged use
Observe for complications of crises	Monitor for evidence of increasing anemia; utilize appropriate nursing interventions Measure size of spleen; continually monitor for shock Observe mental status for evidence of cerebrovascular accident

Continued.

Summary of nursing care of the child with sickle cell anemia—cont'd

Goals	Responsibilities
Decrease surgical risks	Explain reason for preoperative blood transfusion Keep child well hydrated Decrease fear through appropriate preparation Avoid unnecessary exertion Promote pulmonary hygiene postoperatively Use passive range of motion exercises to promote circulation Observe for signs of infection
Prevent sickle cell anemia	
Screening	Participate in screening programs Be aware of controversial aspects of screening and genetic control
Genetic counseling	Refer all heterozygous (HbSA) parents for genetic counseling Reinforce basics of trait transmission, especially concerning subsequent pregnancies Discuss with parents their feelings regarding selective birth methods
Public education	Participate in education projects, dissemination of literature, and political decisions
Long-term care	Allow parents to express their feelings regarding transmitting disease to offspring Refer to public health nurse for follow-up in home Refer child for medical care through comprehensive sickle cell clinic Discuss prognosis, especially increased chances of survival when sickling is prevented Care for child as one with life-threatening illness

for self-service. Frozen popsicles and flavored ice cubes are sources of fluid commonly accepted by children.

Since the kidney's ability to concentrate urine is impaired, the child is especially prone to dehydration. Dilute urine or low specific gravity is no longer a valid sign of adequate hydration. Parents are taught to observe for other indications of fluid loss, such as dry mucous membranes, weight loss, and sunken fontanel in infants. Also, without the ability to conserve water by concentrating urine, the child is prone to dehydration from environmental factors, particularly overheating. The nurse alerts parents to the need for proper indoor and outdoor clothing and avoiding excess exposure to the sun.

Forced fluids combined with renal diuresis result in the problem of enuresis. Parents who are unaware of this fact frequently employ the usual measures to discourage bedwetting, such as limiting fluids at night, and many revert to punishment and shame to force bladder control. The nurse discusses this problem with parents, stressing the child's inability to master prolonged control. Reminding the child to urinate frequently is helpful during the day, and waking him once during the night may prove beneficial if the child's sleep patterns are not disturbed. Parents who are toilet training their toddlers should be aware of the more frequent pattern of urination and increased difficulty in learning control. It is advisable to treat the enuresis as a complication of the disease, such as joint pain or some other symptom, in order to alleviate parental pressure on the child.

Prevention of infection. Since infection is often a predisposing factor toward a crisis and the body's natural ability to resist infection is compromised, the nurse stresses to parents the importance of adequate nutrition, frequent medical supervision, and isolation from known sources of infection. The latter measure must be tempered with an awareness of the child's need for living a normal life. Overprotection can be equally as devastating emotionally as an infection is physically. Parents need to be aware of the necessity of seeking prompt medical care at the first sign of any infection.

Promotion of supportive therapies during crises. The success of many of the medical therapies relies heavily on nursing implementation. Management of pain is an especially difficult problem and often involves experimenting with various analgesics and schedules before relief is achieved. Frequently heat to the affected area is soothing, as well as passive exercises to promote circulation. Applying cold compresses to the area is avoided because this enhances sickling and vasoconstriction.

Bed rest is usually well-tolerated during a crisis, although actual rest depends a great deal on pain alleviation and organized schedules of nursing care. Although the object of bed rest is to minimize oxygen consumption, some activity, particularly passive range of motion exercises, is beneficial to promote circulation. Usually the best course of action is to let the child dictate his activity tolerance.

If blood transfusions or exchange transfusions are given, the nurse has the responsibility of observing for signs of transfusion reaction (see p. 1387). Since hypervolemia from too rapid transfusion can increase the workload of the heart, the nurse also is alert to signs of cardiac failure.

In splenic sequestration the nurse should gently measure the size of the spleen (for example, 2 cm below the left costal margin), since increasing splenomegaly is an ominous sign. A decreasing spleen denotes response to therapy. Vital signs and blood pressure are also closely monitored by the nurse for impending shock.

If oxygen is administered the nurse notes the child's response in terms of decreased pain and improved physical status. However, since prolonged oxygen can aggravate the anemia, the nurse reports signs of lack of therapeutic benefit, such as restlessness, increased pallor, and continued pain.

Anemia is typically not a presenting complication in vaso-occlusive crises but is a critical problem in other types of crises. The nurse monitors for evidence of increasing anemia and institutes appropriate nursing intervention.

Intake, especially intravenous fluids, and output are recorded. The child's weight should be taken on admission since it serves as a baseline for evaluating hydration. Since diuresis can result in electrolyte loss, the nurse also observes for signs of hypokalemia. The nurse should be familiar with normal serum electrolyte values and report changes to the physician.

Decreasing surgical risks. The main surgical risk is hypoxia from anesthesia. However, emotional stress, the demands of wound healing, and the possibility of infection potentially increase the sickling phenomenon, both in children with the disease and in those with the trait. The primary nursing objectives are aimed at minimizing each of these threats preoperatively and postoperatively. This includes (1) keeping the child well hydrated before and after surgery, (2) preparing the child psychologically to decrease fear, (3) avoiding unnecessary fatigue and exertion, (4) avoiding sedatives and analgesics that depress the respiratory center, (5) promoting pulmonary hygiene with deep coughing, repositioning, administration of oxygen and humidity, and postural drainage if necessary, (6) judicious use of analgesics to control wound pain in order to prevent abdominal splinting and decreased ventilation, (7) passive range of motion exercises to prevent thrombus formation and minimize energy expenditure, and (8) observing vital signs for evidence of infection, especially of the respiratory tract.

Since preoperative transfusions are usually given to prevent anoxia and suppress the formation of new sickle cells and postoperatively to replace lost blood, the nurse observes for signs of transfusion reaction. After major surgery blood gases and electrolytes are monitored. The nurse should be familiar with normal values to detect alterations before they are clinically evident.

Screening and genetic counseling. Although screening children for sickle cell anemia is generally accepted since it allows earlier, more prevention-oriented treatment, there is much controversy concerning the proposed benefits and potential hazards of screening for the trait. One of the basic issues behind this controversy involves genetic counseling. Since the carrier is generally asymptomatic, there is little direct benefit in informing him of his genetic makeup. The advantages of trait identification lie in selective reproduction of offspring not afflicted with hemoglobin SS. Alternate methods of childbearing include artificial insemination, adoption, or abortion of afflicted fetuses. However, presently, many members of the black community and others view such measures as racial genocide.

The nurse needs to be aware of these conflicting views, particularly in understanding why individuals may react negatively to screening measures. To be effective, screening must be combined with genetic counseling and long-term follow-up. The nurse can be instrumental in such programs by conducting parent education sessions, following the family in the home, disseminating correct information about the disease and trait to the community, and rendering support to parents of newly diagnosed children.

A primary consideration in genetic counseling is informing parents who both carry the trait of the chances of having a child with the disease. A frequent misconception is that the "one in four" probability of transmitting the homozygous form of the disease is interpreted to mean that one out of four offspring will be afflicted and that after giving birth to such a child, the next three children will be normal or carriers. It is essential to stress that this interpretation is incorrect and that for each pregnancy there is a 25% chance of transmitting the homozygous genotype (HbSS), a 50% chance of transmitting the sickle cell trait (HbAS), and a 25% chance of having a noncarrier offspring (HbAA) (see Chapter 6).

Long-term care. Besides genetic counseling, parents need the opportunity to discuss their feelings regarding transmitting a potentially fatal, chronic illness to their child. Some parents are able to cope with this fact and decide to have additional children. Some feel great guilt and remorse for giving their child the disease, whereas others regret not knowing that they carried the trait. For many parents the decision regarding subsequent pregnancies is viewed with doubt and ambivalence.

Because of the widely publicized prognosis for children with sickle cell anemia, many parents express their prevalent fear of death. Prognosis varies; usually the greatest risk is in children under 5 years of age, in whom the majority of deaths are caused by overwhelming infection. However, as the child grows older, the crises usually become less severe and less frequent. There is an increasing number of adults who survive with the disease, and, as palliative treatment and antisickling techniques advance, prognosis will also continue to improve. However, since there is no way to predict which child will follow a favorable course, the nurse should care for the family as she would for any family with a child with a life-threatening illness, with particular emphasis on the siblings' reactions, the stress on the marital relationship, and the child-rearing attitudes displayed toward the child (see Chapter 27).

β-THALASSEMIA (COOLEY'S ANEMIA)

The thalassemias include a wide spectrum of inherited syndromes that are characterized by a deficiency in the synthesis of normal adult hemoglobin. Basically there are two chief classifications: thalassemia minor, the heterozygous form, and thalassemia major, the homozygous form. In both the major and minor types there are also varying grades of severity. For example, thalassemia minora, which is also called the trait, has no symptoms, including anemia, whereas the minor type is associated with mild to moderate anemia but usually none of the typical symptoms seen in thalassemia major. Of the major type, at least two forms are described. The intermediate or moderate type is characterized by anemia and the other clinical manifestations of the severe type, but the child functions effectively without transfusions. In the severe type multiple, repeated blood supplements are needed to maintain hemoglobin levels compatible with normal activity. The varying expressions of the disease bear directly on the prospects for survival.

Thalassemia is also classified according to the particular defect in the polypeptide chain of the hemoglobin molecule responsible for its abnormal synthesis. The thalassemias demonstrate differences in four polypeptide chains—alpha, beta, delta, and gamma. However, the most common form and the one discussed here is β-thalassemia or Cooley's anemia, named after the man who first described it. α-Thalassemia, in which the production of α-chains is almost completely suppressed, is a less common form. Its homozygous state is incompatible with fetal survival because insufficient amounts of α-dependent fetal hemoglobin are synthesized. Hydrops fetalis is usually seen in stillbirth.

The term "thalassemia" comes from the Greek word "thalassa" for sea and appropriately refers to those people living near the Mediterranean sea who have the highest prevalence of the disease, namely, Italians, Greeks, and Syrians. There is evidence to suggest that the high prevalence of the disorder among these groups is a result of selective advantage of the trait to malaria, as is postulated in sicklemia.

However, the disorder has a wide geographic distribution, probably as a result of genetic migration through intermarriages or possibly as a result of spontaneous mutation. The exact incidence of the disorder in a country such as the United States is dependent to a large degree on the number of individuals of Mediterranean extraction with the trait who have migrated there. Consequently in areas densely populated with Greeks or Italians, the incidence of this disorder is high.

Mode of transmission

Thalassemia is an autosomal-recessive disorder. The gene has varying expressivity for the severity of anemia. Sometimes the trait is found in only one parent of a child with severe thalassemia. In this situation the likelihood is that the other parent carries a gene for some variant of sickle cell anemia or other hemoglobinopathy. The exact mode of transmission between parents who are heterozygous for thalassemia is illustrated on p. 192. It is important to remember that since there are varying forms of thalassemia minor, the offspring are likely to have a variety of expressions of the major form.

Basic defect

The basic defect in Cooley's anemia seems to be a deficiency in the synthesis of β-chain polypeptides, which results in a decreased *rate* of production of the globin molecule but a structurally normal hemoglobin. The decreased rate of production is compensated for by a hyperplastic bone marrow, which forms defective red blood cells. The body also attempts to balance the low level of circulating hemoglobin A by producing large concentrations of fetal hemoglobin, which normally does not contain β-chains.

Pathology

The clinical effects of thalassemia major are primarily attributable to (1) defective synthesis of hemoglobin A, (2) structurally impaired red blood cells, and (3) shortened life span of the erythrocyte. The major consequences of thalassemia are caused by the pathology, resultant chronic hypoxia, and the existing supportive treatment of multiple blood supplements (Fig. 36-4).

Hemosiderosis and hemochromatosis. *Hemosiderosis* is excess iron storage in various tissues of the body, especially the spleen, liver, lymph glands, heart, and pancreas, but without associated tissue injury. *Hemochromatosis* refers to excess iron storage with resultant cellular damage.

Although the exact mechanism for the conversion of iron storage to tissue destruction is not known, chronic hypoxia is believed to be an important contributing factor.

In thalassemia, excess hemosiderin, the iron-containing pigment from the breakdown of hemoglobin, results from decreased hemoglobin synthesis and increased hemolysis of transfused erythrocytes. Decreased production of hemoglobin results in an excess supply of available iron. In addition the body probably responds to the anemia by increasing the rate of gastrointestinal absorption of dietary iron, since ineffective erythropoiesis is a potent controlling factor regarding exogenous iron utilization. However, the primary source of additional iron is from the hemolysis of supplemental erythrocytes and rapid destruction of defective red blood cells.

Anemia. Anemia results from the body's inability to maintain a level of erythropoiesis commensurate with hemolysis. With the decreased rate of hemoglobin synthesis, the bone marrow compensates by increasing production of structurally defective red blood cells. Although microcytes predominate, there is production of large numbers of immature cells, such as normoblasts and erythroblasts, large cells that are extremely thin and form bizarre shapes, and nonspecific macrocytes called *target cells,* which have abnormal staining properties. As a result of the excessive production of abnormal red blood cells, their life span is severely shortened.

Anemia also is exaggerated by aplastic crises following infection, folic acid deficiencies from demands of bone marrow hyperplasia, splenic sequestration, and progressive hemolysis from repeated blood transfusions.

Skeletal changes. Hyperplasia of the bone marrow results in widening of the medullary spaces, thinning of the cortex, atrophy of the trabeculae, and osteoporosis. The weakened bone is susceptible to pathologic fractures, skeletal deformities, and retarded growth. With regeneration of new bone later in the disease, there is a subsequent thickening, particularly of the skull. The specific bone changes are discussed under clinical manifestations.

Heart. Hemosiderin deposits in the heart cause serious, sometimes fatal, myocardial changes, particularly fibrosis and hypertrophy of the fibers. In addition the chronic anemia greatly increases the cardiac workload, which eventually can lead to decompensation and failure.

Liver. Cirrhosis of the liver is the eventual result of progressive siderosis and consequently fibrosis of the hepatic cells. The high levels of intracellular iron within the liver cells are primarily the result of increased intestinal absorption from hyperactive erythropoiesis and ineffective utilization of the iron in hemoglobin synthesis. Signs of cirrhosis generally develop late in the course of the disorder.

Spleen. The spleen becomes greatly enlarged as a result of extramedullary hemopoiesis, rapid destruction of the defective erythrocytes, and progressive fibrosis from hemosiderin deposits. Splenomegaly may progress until its very size interferes with the function of other abdominal organs and respiratory expansion.

Pancreas. The pancreas becomes fibrotic from progressive hemochromatosis, and eventually the severe degree of scarring may result in diabetes mellitus.

Lymph nodes. The lymph nodes enlarge as a result of their becoming a site for hemopoiesis and also from siderosis.

Growth and sexual maturation. The chronic anemia results in retarded growth and delayed sexual maturation. There is some evidence that both may also be caused by pituitary failure from hemochromatosis in that organ. Children with severe disease usually achieve normal growth rates until puberty, when height becomes markedly retarded. Secondary sexual characteristics are delayed, although maturation is achieved eventually. In females normal menstruation is infrequently achieved. For long-term survivors of Cooley's anemia, bone growth may reach the low normal limits of adult height.

Skin. Hemosiderin deposits in the dermis and jaundice from rapid hemolysis of red blood cells cause the skin to have a tanned, bronzed coloration with fine, dark freckles.

Clinical manifestations

The onset of thalassemia major is usually insidious and not recognized until the latter half of infancy. Signs of anemia, unexplained fever, poor feeding, and a markedly enlarged spleen, particularly in a child of Mediterranean extraction, are descriptive of thalassemia. The bone changes from accelerated medullary hematopoiesis produce characteristic facies in older children: (1) enlarged head, (2) prominent frontal and parietal bosses, (3) prominent malar (cheek bone) eminences, (4) a flat or depressed bridge of the nose, (5) enlargement of the maxilla, with protrusion of the lip and upper central incisors and eventual malocclusion, and (6) a mongoloid appearance to the eyes. Other features that are common to these children are small stature, infantile genitalia, a bronzed freckled complexion, and protrusion of the abdomen from hepatosplenomegaly.

With progressive anemia one can also expect to see signs of chronic hypoxia, namely headache, precordial and bone pain, decreased exercise tolerance, listlessness, and anorexia. Another common symptom in these children is frequent epistaxis, although the exact reason is unknown. Hyperuricemia and gout from rapid cellular catabolism are also seen. In those children who require multiple transfusions for several years, the eventual effects of hemochromatosis in various organs are evident.

Diagnostic evaluation

The classical picture of Cooley's anemia in a child of Mediterranean background provides ample evidence of the disease. Hematologic studies reveal the characteristic

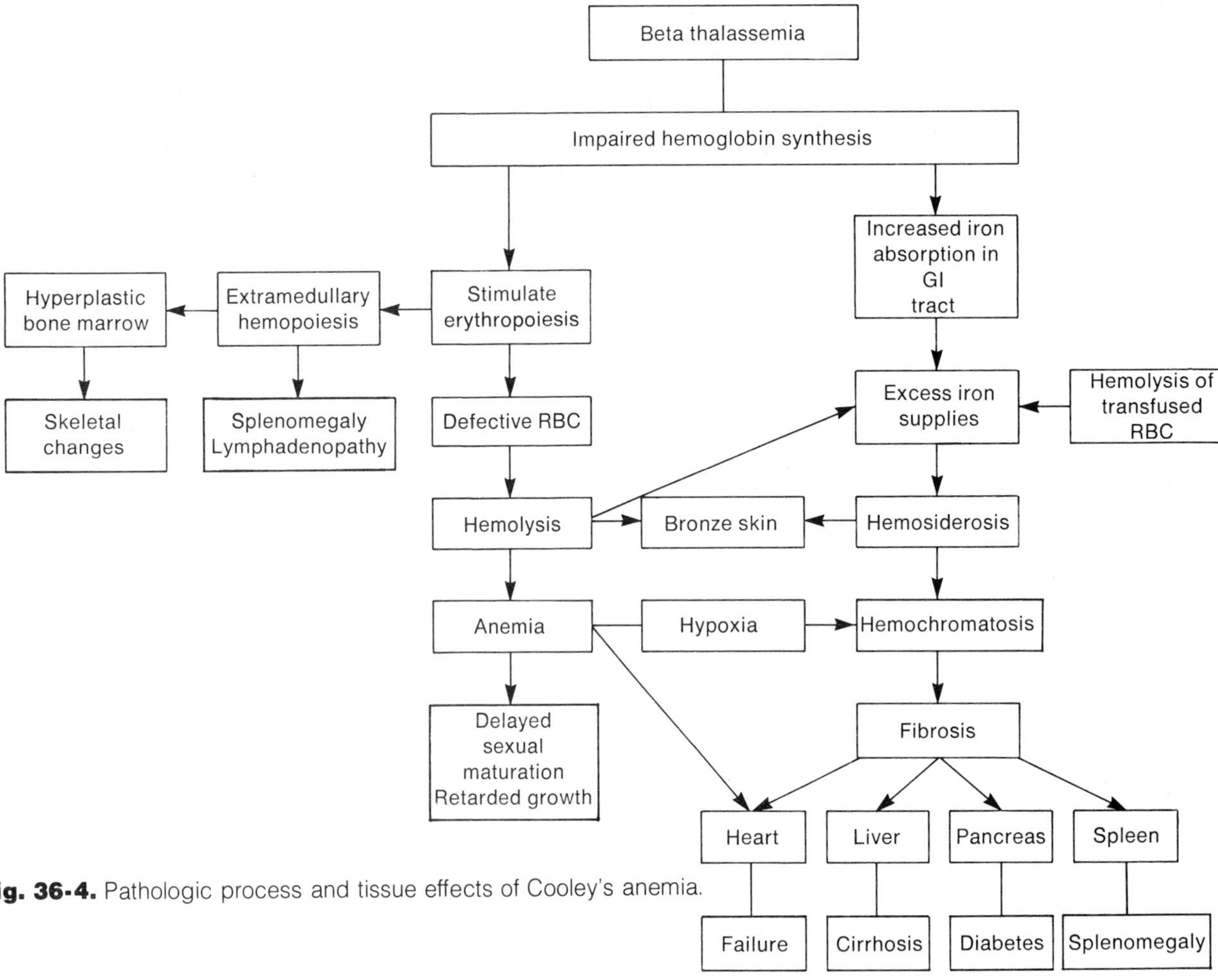

Fig. 36-4. Pathologic process and tissue effects of Cooley's anemia.

changes in the red blood cell, namely microcytosis, hypochromia, anisocytosis, poikilocytosis, target cells, and basophilic stippling of immature erythrocytes of various stages. Low hemoglobin and hematocrit levels are seen in severe anemia, although they are typically lower than the reduction in red blood cell count because of the proliferation of immature erythrocytes.

Hemoglobin electrophoresis is very helpful in diagnosing the type and severity of the various thalassemias because it analyzes the quantity and specific hemoglobin variants found in blood. In β-thalassemia, hemoglobin F and A_2 (a type of normal adult hemoglobin) are elevated because neither is dependent on β-chain polypeptides for synthesis.

Medical/surgical management

There is no specific treatment and no known cure for children with thalassemia major. The objective of supportive therapy is to maintain sufficient hemoglobin levels to prevent tissue hypoxia. Transfusions are the foundation of medical management, although they greatly increase the risk of siderosis. At the present time there is no completely successful method of preventing excessive iron storage, although the use of iron-chelating agents such as deferoxamine (Desferal) has shown promising results.

In some children with severe splenomegaly who require repeated transfusions, a splenectomy may be necessary to decrease the disabling effects of abdominal pressure and to increase the life span of supplemental red blood cells. There is evidence that with repeated blood transfusions, a hemolytic factor develops in the spleen that increases the rate of erythrocyte destruction. After a splenectomy children generally require many fewer transfusions, although the basic defect in hemoglobin synthesis remains unaffected. A major postsplenectomy complication is severe and overwhelming infection. Therefore, these children are usually kept on prophylactic antibiotics with close medical supervision for many years and are considered candidates for the pneumococcal and meningococcal vaccines.

Nursing considerations

The objectives of nursing care involve (1) observing for complications of multiple blood transfusions, (2) assisting the child in coping with the effects of the illness, and (3)

Table 36-2. Nursing care of the child receiving blood transfusions

Complication*	Signs/symptoms	Precautions/nursing responsibilities
Hemolytic reactions (most severe type, but rare) Incompatible blood Intradonor incompatibility in multiple transfusions	Chills Fever Headache Flank pain If progressive, signs of shock and/or renal failure	Positively identify donor and recipient blood types and groups before transfusion is begun; verify with one other nurse or physician Transfuse blood slowly for first 15-20 minutes and/or first 50 ml; remain with patient In event of signs or symptoms, stop transfusion immediately, maintain patent intravenous line, and notify physician Save donor blood to re-cross match with patient's blood Monitor blood pressure for shock Insert urinary catheter and monitor hourly outputs Send sample of patient's blood and urine to laboratory for presence of hemoglobin (indicates intravascular hemolysis) Observe for signs of hemorrhage resulting from intravascular coagulation Support medical therapies to reverse hypovolemia and to prevent renal shutdown and hemorrhages, for example, blood replacement, use of plasma volume expanders, diuresis, alkalinization of body fluids, use of heparin and administration of platelets
Nonhemolytic reactions (pyogenic and febrile reactions most common types) Leukocyte or platelet antibodies Plasma protein antibodies	Fever Urticaria Chills	May give antihistamines or salicylates for prophylaxis Frozen blood, washed red blood cells, or leukocyte-poor blood is less likely to cause reaction Stop transfusion immediately; report to physician for evaluation
Transmission of infection Hepatitis Malaria Syphilis Virus or bacteria	Signs of infection after transfusion, for example, jaundice from hepatitis Bacterial or toxin contamination—high fever, severe headache or substernal pain, hypotension, intense flushing, vomiting/diarrhea	Reject all Australia antigen–positive donors or anyone with history of hepatitis or jaundice Reject donors with history of malaria or syphilis Report any sign of infection, and if occurring during transfusion, stop transfusion immediately, send sample for culture and sensitivity tests, and notify physician
Circulatory overload Too rapid transfusion (even if small quantity) Excessive quantity of blood transfused (even if slowly)	Precordial pain Dyspnea Rales Cyanosis Dry cough Distended neck veins	Transfuse blood slowly Prevent overload by using packed red blood cells or administering divided amounts of blood on successive days Utilize infusion pump to regulate and maintain flow rate If signs of overload, stop transfusion immediately Place child upright with feet in dependent position to increase venous resistance
Allergic reactions—recipient reacts to allergens in donor's blood	Urticaria Flushing Asthmatic wheezing Laryngeal edema	Give antihistamines or steroids for prophylaxis to children with a tendency toward hemolytic, febrile, or allergic reactions Prepare epinephrine for emergency use in severe respiratory distress
Electrolyte disturbances Hyperkalemia	Nausea, diarrhea Muscular weakness Flaccid paralysis Paresthesia of extremities Bradycardia Apprehension Cardiac arrest	Observe blood for signs of clouding or abnormal color, which indicates hemolysis (from extended storage) Use only fresh blood Use blood with plasma removed
"Citrate" intoxication (hypocalcemia)	Tingling in fingers Tetany Muscular cramps Carpopedal spasm Hyperactive reflexes Convulsions Laryngeal spasm Respiratory arrest	Infuse blood slowly (citrate reaction less likely to occur) If signs of tetany occur, clamp tubing immediately, maintain patent intravenous line, and notify physician

*Data from Miller, D. R., and Pearson, H. A.: Smith's blood diseases of infancy and childhood, ed. 4, St. Louis, 1978, The C. V. Mosby Co.

Continued.

Table 36-2. Nursing care of the child receiving blood transfusions—cont'd

Complication	Signs/symptoms	Precautions/nursing responsibilities
Air emboli—may occur when blood is transfused under pressure	Sudden difficulty in breathing Sharp pain in chest Apprehension	When infusing blood under pressure, normalize pressure *before* container is empty If air is observed in tubing, clamp tubing immediately below air bubble, clear tubing of air by aspirating air with syringe or disconnecting tubing and allowing blood to flow until air has escaped
Antibody formation	Signs of allergic reaction and more rapid destruction of red blood cells	Observe for posttransfusion anemia and decreasing benefit from successive transfusions Be prepared for allergic reaction (usually not severe)
Excessive iron deposition Hemosiderosis Hemochromatosis	Bronze-tone skin Progressive organ damage	Restrict transfusion to minimum required for hemoglobin levels compatible with moderate activity
Suppression of erythropoiesis	Anemia	Monitor aftereffects of transfusions closely
Hypothermia	Chills Low temperature Irregular heart rate Possible cardiac arrest	Allow blood to warm at room temperature (less than 1 hour) Use an electric warming coil to rapidly warm blood Take temperature if patient complains of chills; if subnormal stop transfusion

fostering the parents' and child's adjustment to a life-threatening illness. Basic to each of these goals is explaining to parents and older children the defect responsible for the disorder and its effect on red blood cells. Since the prevalence of this condition is high among families of Mediterranean descent, the nurse also inquires regarding the family's previous knowledge about thalassemia. All families with a child with thalassemia should be tested for the trait and referred for genetic counseling.

Observation for complications of blood transfusions. Any blood transfusion carries attendant risks. Some of these, such as hemolytic reactions, are preventable with donor-recipient crossmatching of blood groups and Rh factors. However, others, particularly hemosiderosis, are presently unavoidable in situations of repeated blood supplements. Since the child with thalassemia requires multiple transfusions for several years, the possibility of complications is increased. It is critical for the nurse assisting in this procedure always to be suspicious for signs indicative of a reaction. Table 36-2 summarizes the major hazards of transfusions, the signs and symptoms commonly associated with each, and nursing responsibilities.

Hemolytic reactions. Blood is usually matched between the donor and recipient for blood groups (A, B, AB, or O) and Rh factors (positive or negative). (See p. 296 for a discussion of blood groups and A-B-O and Rh incompatibility.) When blood is mismatched, the A or B antiagglutinin is mixed with red blood cells containing A or B agglutinogens, respectively, and agglutination of the red blood cells occurs. The agglutinins, which are bivalent, attach themselves to two different erythrocytes at the same time, causing the cells to clump together and clog small blood vessels. Over a few hours to days, the entrapped cells degenerate and hemolyze, liberating excessive quantities of hemoglobin into the circulation. The eventual hemolysis of large members of red blood cells decreases the blood volume, causing circulatory failure and *shock*. Treatment is aimed at replacing lost blood and using plasma volume expanders.

Acute kidney shutdown and eventual *renal failure* are the result of renal vasoconstriction from toxic substances released from the hemolyzed blood and tubular blockage from precipitation of hemoglobin. The greatly reduced blood flow causes complete renal failure and death within 7 to 12 days. Treatment involves preventing the precipitation of hemoglobin within the tubules by promoting diuresis with rapid dilute intravenous fluids and diuretics, such as mannitol, and alkalinizing body fluids, which renders hemoglobin more soluble.

Another consequence of hemolysis is the release of large quantities of phospholipids, which are capable of stimulating disseminating intravascular coagulation (DIC). As a result the plasma is depleted of the necessary coagulation factors needed to prevent hemorrhage. Without treatment with heparin to prevent the coagulation and blood components to initiate clotting, death from generalized *hemorrhage* can occur.

Nonhemolytic reactions. The most frequent type of reaction, called a *pyogenic* or *febrile reaction,* is caused by immunization of the recipient to a platelet or leukocyte antigen in the donor blood. Agglutination and hemolysis do not occur, and the reaction is typically allergic in presentation. This type of reaction is common in children with thalassemia.

Transmission of infection. The most common disorder resulting from transfusion is infection with hepatitis, particularly hepatitis type B virus (serum hepatitis). Transmission of malaria is a significant problem in areas in which the disease is endemic. Syphilis is transmitted almost exclusively when fresh blood from an infected donor is used because refrigeration kills the spirochete. Overwhelming infection from grossly contaminated blood is rare, but when it does occur it results in dramatic symptoms and frequently death.

Circulatory overload. Transfusing blood too rapidly may precipitate cardiac failure from circulatory overload. It is most likely to occur in infants, whose body size does not accommodate even small quantities of blood being infused rapidly, or in individuals with severe anemia who already are in danger of cardiac decompensation.

Allergic reactions. Allergic reactions are similar to febrile reactions, but the responsible allergen is not a blood product. For example, if the donor has eaten certain foods to which the recipient is allergic, allergens from the donor's blood can be transmitted to the recipient, who then has an allergic reaction. Such reactions are most likely to occur in allergy-prone children who are receiving multiple transfusions. Anaphylactic shock is a rare but possible complication.

Electrolyte disturbances. In blood that has been stored for prolonged periods of time, hemolysis of the red blood cells occurs, liberating high levels of potassium into the plasma. When such blood is transfused into a recipient, signs of *hyperkalemia* result.

Hypocalcemia occurs when blood containing large quantities of the anticoagulant citrate is administered too rapidly. Citrate acts as an anticoagulant by combining with the calcium ions of plasma; as a result they become nonionizable and, thereby, prevent the coagulation process. If citrated blood is rapidly infused, excess quantities of the recipient's calcium ions in plasma are combined with the anticoagulant and rendered nonionizable.

Air emboli. A large bolus of air entering the circulation during blood transfusion is rare, unless pressurized containers are allowed to empty before the pressure is released. Air emboli are easily prevented by following guidelines for intravenous therapy, observing for any evidence of air in the tubing, and normalizing the pressure bag before the blood is completely infused.

Antibody formation. With repeated transfusions, there is evidence that the recipient develops precipitins (a type of antibody that forms in response to exposure to gradually increasing doses of a foreign protein) to various lipoproteins in the donor's blood. Specific antibodies are also formed against the formed elements of the blood. Signs similar to those of an allergic reaction and more rapid destruction of the blood cells occur.

Excessive iron storage. The role of excess iron storage from the release of hemoglobin in transfused erythrocytes has already been discussed.

Suppression of erythropoiesis. The effect of blood transfusions on erythropoietic mechanisms has previously been alluded to, since reversal of tissue hypoxia through elevated hemoglobin levels sends a negative feedback message to the kidneys and bone marrow. The effect of retarded erythropoiesis is most evident 1 to 3 weeks posttransfusion.

Hypothermia. Hypothermia can result from transfusion of cold blood (usually stored at 1° to 6°C or 34° to 42°F). The main symptom is chills. However, subnormal temperatures place stress on the heart muscle and can lead to cardiac arrhythmias, fibrillation, and eventually arrest. Precautions include allowing the blood to remain at room temperature (less than 1 hour) or using an electric warming coil. If hypothermia is expected, frequent monitoring of vital signs, blood pressure, shivering, and skin color is important.

Besides the nursing precautions and responsibilities outlined in Table 36-2, some general guidelines that apply to all transfusions include: (1) take vital signs and blood pressure before administering blood to establish baseline data for posttransfusion comparison, (2) always check the identification of the recipient with the donor's blood group and type, regardless of the blood product used, (3) never administer drugs by way of the blood, (4) never give ordinary dextrose solutions with the blood because a nonelectrolyte, nonisotonic solution will cause hemolysis, (5) administer blood by means of tubing with a filter to eliminate particles in the blood and prevent the precipitation of formed elements, (6) store blood under refrigeration until needed and then administer within 4 hours because prolonged exposure to room temperature causes blood to decompose, and (7) if a reaction of any type is suspected, stop the transfusion, maintain a patent intravenous line, notify the physician, and do not restart the blood until the child's condition has been medically evaluated.

In adjusting the flow rate it is important to remember that blood administration sets do not use microdrops (60 drops/ml) but regular drops (usually 10 drops/ml). Therefore, when administering the first 50 ml of blood, the nurse should adjust the flow rate to 16 drops/minute to infuse this amount in 30 minutes. If no reaction occurs the flow rate should be increased accordingly to infuse the remainder of blood within 2 hours. For example, if a pint of blood is to be given, a flow rate of 42 drops/minute should permit the remaining 450 ml to be infused in 2 hours. (These calculations are based on 10 drops/ml.)

The best method of maintaining a patent intravenous line is to use a piggyback setup, in which normal saline (or another balanced electrolyte solution) is connected to the tubing by means of a stopcock. If the blood is stopped, the stopcock is turned to open the saline line. In this way blood can be restarted without another venipuncture and emergency drugs can be given intravenously if required during a reaction.

Assisting in coping with effects of disorder. Body image alterations, particularly skeletal changes, skin discoloration, decreased growth, and sexual immaturity, are frequently difficult adjustment problems for older children. These children feel different from their peers, and the added effects of anemia may prevent them from competing in any physically strenuous sport. They need an opportunity to express such thoughts and feelings and to be guided toward activities and scholastic pursuits commensurate with their physical abilities. For girls the adjustment toward physical limitations may be easier than toward acceptance of body image differences.

The nurse can help these children by stressing their abilities and focusing on realistic endeavors, such as quiet hobbies, creative arts and crafts, competitive "thinking" games, and appropriate vocations. Children with less severe forms of thalassemia may benefit from surgery or orthodontic appliances to improve facial structure. Adolescents can learn grooming aides that make them appear more sexually mature, such as up-to-date clothing, new hairstyles, and well-applied makeup.

Since many of these children are frequently overprotected, their ability to interact socially may be less developed, which also segregates them from peers. Discussing this aspect with older children and adolescents may reveal previously hidden ways of fostering group acceptance and meaningful relationships. Introducing such a child to another well-adjusted thalassemic child or using the group process with children who have similar disorders, such as children with sickle cell anemia, often proves very beneficial to all participants. The same approach with parents during the early years of the child's illness can be a way of preventing the cycle of overprotection-dependency–social maladjustment.

The nurse can be instrumental in arranging for blood transfusions and medical supervision at times that interfere least with the child's regular activities. For example, children who state that they dislike school admit to disliking absenteeism even more because it increases the difficulty of feeling like a group member and in keeping up with schoolwork. Also, children are more likely to cooperate with medical treatments that do not interfere significantly with their routine. Probably one of the most adaptive mechanisms for adjusting to a chronic illness is in treating the disorder as an inconvenience and emphasizing the need for a normal life.

Fostering adjustment to life-threatening illness. The prognosis of thalassemia major is variable and relies heavily on the severity of the anemia. Children who do not require repeated transfusions have a better chance for survival than those children dependent on supplemental blood. However, even children in the latter group have increasingly favorable chances with selective transfusions, splenectomy when indicated, prophylactic antibiotics, and greater success with iron-chelating agents. The chief cause of death is heart failure, and, once signs of this complication become evident, death may occur within a year.

Unfortunately it is not possible to predict which severely afflicted child will follow a more favorable course. Since many children with the severe form die before puberty and few survive beyond the third decade, thalassemia is considered a potentially fatal disease. The nurse must care for families of these children in light of this knowledge, be willing to discuss the future prospects with the parents and child as appropriate, and plan realistic, yet growth-promoting goals for the thalassemic child. Long-term follow-up care through a comprehensive health setting or community nurse referral can prevent many problems that are common to families with a chronic illness, such as overprotection, social isolation, lack of discipline, unawareness of the siblings' reactions, and stress on the marital relationship. Attendant financial burdens and unresolved guilt for transmitting a hereditary disorder can disintegrate an already stressed family. Working as a member of the health team to prevent and deal with these problems can help families use the crisis as a growth experience rather than as a destructive event in their lives. (See also Chapter 27.)

Defects in hemostasis

The body controls excessive bleeding through three processes: (1) vascular spasm, (2) platelet aggregation, and (3) coagulation and clot formation. Defects in platelets and clotting factors are the most common causes of bleeding during childhood. The following discussion focuses on the major conditions that require nursing intervention. The reader is urged to apply these principles to other medical conditions that involve similar nursing considerations.

HEMOPHILIA

Hemophilia actually refers to a group of bleeding disorders in which there is a deficiency of one of the factors necessary for coagulation of the blood. Although the symptomatology is similar despite the missing factor, the identification of specific factor deficiencies has allowed definitive treatment with replacement agents. The two most common forms of the disorder are classical hemophilia (hemophilia A or factor VIII deficiency) and Christmas disease (hemophilia B or factor IX deficiency). The following discussion is primarily concerned with the classical form, which accounts for about 75% of all cases.

A major feature of hemophilia is that its expression varies markedly in the degree of bleeding severity. Hemophilia is generally classified into three groups according to the severity of factor deficiency: (1) severe defects with less than 1% of the normal amount of factor, (2) moderate defects with levels of about 5% or more, and (3) mild defects with levels ranging between 25% and 50%. Normal percentages of factor VIII are 60% to 120% and of factor IX, 60% to 130%. Persons with the severe form of hemophilia bleed spontaneously or from minor trauma and literally may die from exsanguination. Those with moderate deficiencies usually bleed after some type of trauma but do not bleed spontaneously. Those with the mild form usually have no manifest bleeding tendencies until they sustain a serious injury or undergo surgery, such as dental extraction or tonsillectomy. The deceptive absence of symptoms in the mild form of hemophilia may present additional risks if these children face such experiences before the disorder is diagnosed.

Modes of transmission

In about 80% of cases of hemophilia, the inheritance is demonstrated as a sex-linked recessive disorder. The most frequent pattern of transmission is between an unaffected male and a trait-carrier female (see p. 193 for an illustration of this type of inheritance). In this situation there is an equal chance that a female offspring will be normal or a carrier and that a male offspring will be normal or affected with the disease.

With improved treatment for persons with hemophilia, it is important to consider the results of mating between an affected male and a normal female or a carrier female. The union of an affected male and normal female results in all carrier female offspring and all normal male offspring. The mating of an affected male with a carrier female results in a one in four chance of producing either an affected son or daughter, a carrier daughter, or a normal son. This is one of the few ways in which a female can become a hemophiliac.

Other reasons for female expression of the disease include (1) a "symptomatic" carrier of classic hemophilia with a moderate defect of factor VIII, (2) a phenotypic female who has inherited the recessive gene for hemophilia but lacks the second normal sex (X) chromosome, as in Turner's syndrome, (3) a female with an autosomally dominant transmitted form of factor VIII deficiency, such as von Willebrand's disease, or (4) a female with severe factor deficiency whose parents are normal.[1] The latter type is probably the result of a spontaneous mutation or chromosomal aberration. It is estimated that about 20% or more of persons with hemophilia have a negative family history and represent a sporadic genetic mutation.

Basic defect

The basic defect of hemophilia A is a deficiency of factor VIII—antihemophilic factor (AHF) or antihemophilic globulin (AHG)—which is necessary for the formation of thromboplastin in phase I of blood coagulation. The degree of severity of the disease is inversely correlated with the amount of antihemophilic globulin found in the blood. The source of the factor in the body is unknown.

Coagulation mechanism. To understand the role that factor deficiencies play in promoting bleeding tendencies, it is necessary to review the normal coagulation process of the blood. Clotting takes place in essentially three phases: (1) a substance called *prothrombin activator* is formed in response to an extrinsic or intrinsic mechanism, (2) the prothrombin activator catalyzes the conversion of *prothrombin* into *thrombin,* and (3) thrombin acts as an enzyme to convert *fibrinogen* into the *fibrin* threads that enmesh the red blood cells and plasma to form a clot (Fig. 36-5).

Phase I. Blood clotting is initiated by either an *extrinsic* mechanism, in which an extract called *thromboplastin* is released from the damaged tissues into the blood, or by an *intrinsic* mechanism, in which the blood itself is damaged and the platelets respond by releasing a substance called *platelet factor 3* into the blood. In both instances several factors, collectively termed a *prothrombin activator,* are present in the plasma, which are necessary to initiate clotting. Table 36-3 lists the various clotting factors and their common synonyms. In addition calcium ions must be available in the plasma for the reactions to take place.

Phase II. After prothrombin activator has been formed, it catalyzes the conversion of prothrombin to thrombin. *Prothrombin* is a plasma protein formed in the liver that is dependent on vitamin K for its synthesis. The rate of formation of thrombin from prothrombin is directly proportional to the amount of prothrombin activator or blood-clotting factors. Therefore, a low level of prothrombin in the blood is potentially an indirect estimate of a factor deficiency, since the prothrombin complex is dependent on factors II, V, VII, and X.

Phase III. Thrombin, a protein enzyme with proteolytic ability, acts on *fibrinogen,* a plasma protein produced by the liver, to form a molecule called *fibrin.* The fibrin molecule polymerizes to form long fibrin threads that run in all directions, shorten, and eventually form a clot by entrapping blood cells and plasma in the web. Phase III factors include factors I and XIII.

After a few minutes following clot formation, the clot retracts, expressing most of the plasma from itself and pulling the broken ends of the blood vessels closer together. Clot retraction is dependent on an adequate number of platelets, which may provide the energy for the fibrin threads to shorten. Since the proteolytic ability of thrombin is capable of initiating more clotting by breaking down prothrombin to form more thrombin in a cyclical reaction, clot formation is controlled by the rate of blood flowing past the injured site to remove excess fibrin. This is also one of the reasons why an injured area is immobilized initially to promote ade-

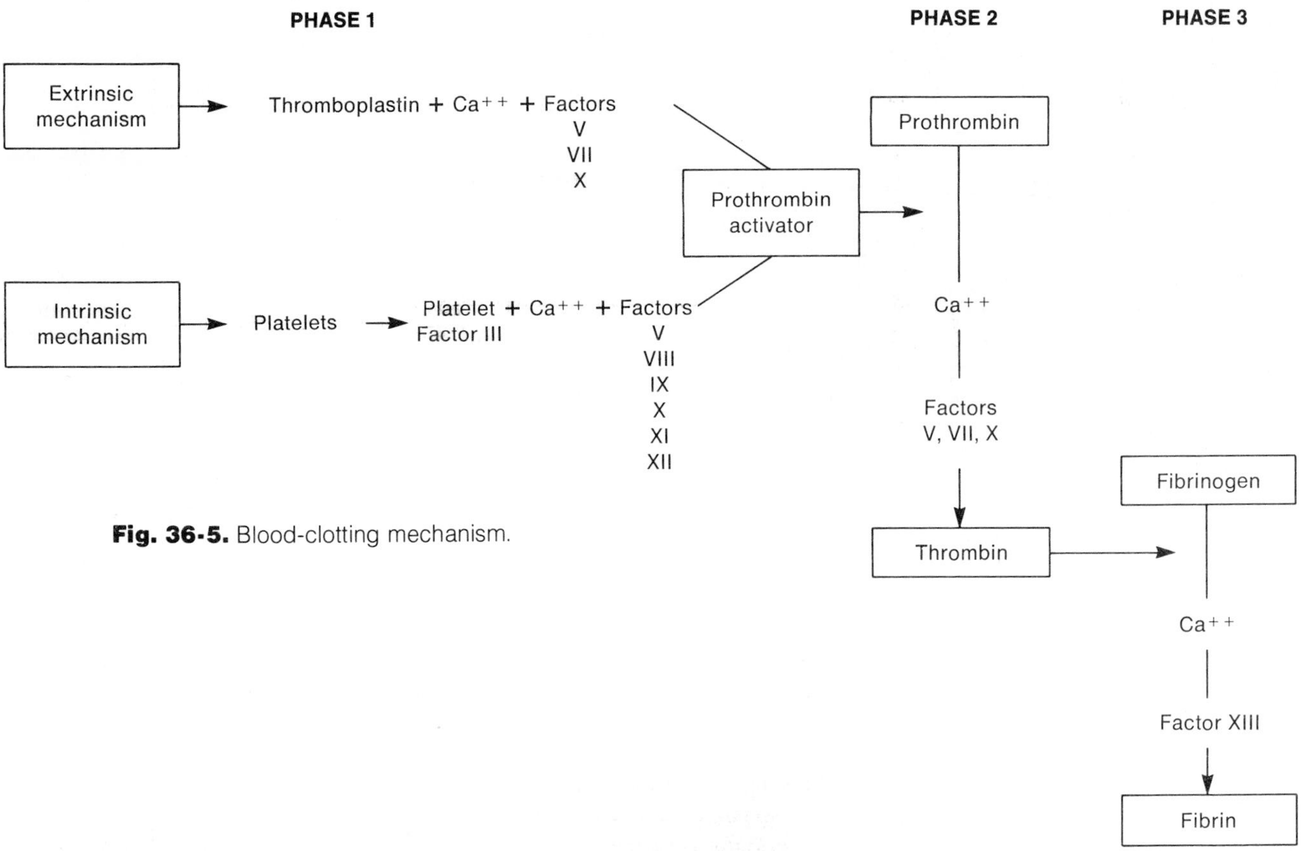

Fig. 36-5. Blood-clotting mechanism.

Table 36-3. Blood-clotting factors

Factor number	Synonyms
I	Fibrinogen
II	Prothrombin
III	Platelet factor 3
IV	Calcium
V	Labile factor, proaccelerin, AC globulin (ACG)
VII	Serum prothrombin conversion accelerator (SPCA), proconvertin, autoprothrombin I
VIII	Antihemophilic factor (AHF), antihemophilic globulin (AHG)
IX	Plasma thromboplastin component (PTC) Christmas factor, autoprothrombin II
X	Stuart-Prower factor, Stuart factor, Prower factor
XI	Plasma thromboplastin antecedent (PTA)
XII	Hageman factor
XIII	Fibrin (protein) stabilizing factor

quate clot formation and why early resumption of too vigorous movement may reinitiate bleeding.

Clinical manifestations

The effect of hemophilia is prolonged bleeding anywhere from or in the body. With severe factor deficiencies hemorrhage can occur as a result of minor trauma, such as after circumcision, during loss of deciduous teeth, or as a result of a slight fall or bruise.

Subcutaneous and intramuscular hemorrhages are common. *Hemarthrosis,* bleeding into the joint cavities, especially the knees, ankles, and elbows, is the most frequent site of internal bleeding and often results in bone changes and, consequently, crippling, disabling deformities. Spontaneous hematuria is not uncommon. Epistaxis may occur but is not as frequent as other kinds of hemorrhage.

Bleeding into the tissue can occur anywhere but is serious if it occurs in the neck, mouth, or thorax, since the airway can become obstructed. Intracranial hemorrhage can result in fatal consequences, although this occurs less frequently than expected because the brain tissue has a high concentration of thromboplastin. Hemorrhage anywhere along the gastrointestinal tract can lead to obstruction, and hematomas in the spinal cord can cause paralysis.

Petechiae are uncommon in persons with hemophilia because repair of small hemorrhages is dependent on platelet function, not on blood-clotting mechanisms.

Diagnostic evaluation

The diagnosis is usually made on a history of bleeding episodes, sex-linked inheritance, and laboratory findings. To understand the significance of various tests of hemosta-

Table 36-4. Laboratory tests for hemostasis

Test	Description	Normal values	Comments
Platelet function			
Bleeding time	Measures time interval for bleeding from small superficial wound to cease	3-6 minutes	Function depends on platelet aggregation and vasoconstriction; two common methods used: Ivy (incision made on forearm) and Duke (incision made on earlobe)
Tourniquet test	Measures platelet function and capillary fragility; apply pressure to forearm with a tourniquet for 5-10 minutes	Absence of petechiae or less than ten	Abnormal in platelet and connective tissue disorders
Clot retraction test	Measures degree to which clot shrinks and expresses serum	Retraction observed in test tube in 2 hours and completed in 24 hours	Depends on platelet function
Blood clotting mechanisms			
Whole blood clotting time	Measures time it takes for clot to form *within* blood	9-12 minutes	Prolonged clotting time indicates problem in thrombin-to-fibrin phase or in any factor in intrinsic clotting mechanism; difficult test to standardize, therefore often unreliable results
Prothrombin time (PT)	Measures activity of prothrombin, as well as factors necessary for its conversion to thrombin and fibrinogen	12-15 seconds (usually measured against control)	Actually does not measure prothrombin levels, but activity; since it bypasses intrinsic-extrinsic mechanism, detects deficiencies of factors V, VII, X, and fibrinogen, as well as prothrombin
Partial thromboplastin time (PTT) test	Similar to PT but measures activity of thromboplastin, which depends on intrinsic clotting factors	39-53 seconds	Specific for factor deficiencies, except factor VII, which results in a normal PTT but prolonged PT
Thromboplastin generation test (TGT)	Measures blood's ability to generate thromboplastin	12 seconds or less	Allows for determination of specific factor deficiencies, especially distinguishing between factors VIII and IX
Prothrombin consumption test	Indirectly measures thromboplastin generation and prothrombin response	Almost complete consumption, with clotting time *above* 20 seconds in serum	Normally as blood clots, prothrombin is converted to thrombin so that serum is depleted of prothrombin; if thromboplastin is decreased (as a result of extrinsic factor deficiencies), not all prothrombin will be converted and removed from serum
Fibrinogen level	Directly measures fibrinogen levels in blood	200-330 mg/100 ml plasma	Not dependent on phase I or II deficiencies

sis, one must recall the usual mechanisms to control bleeding, namely, the function of platelets and of clotting factors. Tests that measure platelet function, such as the bleeding time, tourniquet test, and clot retraction test, are all normal in persons with hemophilia.

Several tests grossly assess clotting functions, the principal ones of which are described in Table 36-4. The tests specific for hemophilia are those that depend on specific factors for a reaction to occur, such as the partial thromboplastin time test, thromboplastin generation test, and prothrombin consumption test. Specific determination of factor deficiencies requires assay procedures normally done by specialized laboratories.

Carrier detection is possible in classical hemophilia and is an important consideration in families in which female offspring may have inherited the trait. The test involves an assay and comparison of factor VIII activity and factor VIII antigen. Factor VIII antigen is a protein found in the plasma that is antigenically similar to factor VIII but has no measurable procoagulant activity. The accuracy of carrier detection by this method is between 77% and 100%.[2]

Medical management

Medical management is aimed at (1) using local or supportive measures to control bleeding and (2) replacing deficient factors to prevent hemorrhage.

Summary of the nursing care of the child with hemophilia

Goals	Responsibilities
Prevent bleeding	Prepare and administer intravenous cryoprecipitate or concentrates as needed
Teach local measures to control bleeding	Apply pressure to area for 10 to 15 minutes Immobilize area Elevate site to about level of heart Apply cold compresses; encourage family to have frozen plastic bags of water prepared in advance
Decrease risk of injury	Make environment as safe as possible Encourage pursuit of intellectual/creative activities Encourage older child to choose activity but accept responsibility for own safety Plan with schoolteacher appropriate activity schedule; confer with school nurse regarding severity of bleeding episodes Discuss with parents appropriate limit-setting patterns Stress need for oral hygiene using soft toothbrush or available substitute Discuss diet, especially effect of overweight on hemarthrosis Advise use of Medic Alert identification in case of emergency During nursing procedures, especially injections, use local measures to control bleeding
Prevent crippling effects of joint degeneration	Use local measures to control bleeding Institute passive range of motion exercises after acute phase Exercise unaffected joints and muscles Administer analgesics prior to physical therapy Avoid use of aspirin or its compounds; substitute acetaminophen for pain relief at home Consult with physical therapist concerning exercise program Refer to public health nurse and/or physical therapist for supervision at home Stress to family serious long-range consequences of hemarthrosis Support any orthopedic measures in joint rehabilitation
Assist in coping with disorder	Provide opportunity for parents and older child to adjust to discovery of diagnosis Assess factors that promote or retard family's adjustment to crisis
Genetic counseling	Refer for genetic counseling, including identification of carrier offspring Assess parents' understanding of sex-linked inheritance Provide opportunity for parents, especially mother, to discuss feelings regarding genetic transmission
Parent discussion groups	Refer to local chapter of National Hemophilia Foundation for parent groups Whenever possible, provide care through comprehensive hemophilia program
Foster independence	Assess family for potential strength in home-care program Institute appropriate teaching Encourage independence and self-help during hospitalizations Introduce child to other hemophiliac children who have adjusted well Encourage parents to promote sense of independence and responsibility in older child Have adolescent investigate job opportunities in appropriate vocation Discuss financial costs, especially insurance coverage at age 21 years Discuss future plans regarding marriage and childbearing; include daughters who carry the trait in discussion

Control measures. Besides the local measures to control bleeding, which are discussed below, certain medical treatments may be beneficial, such as packing the wound with a fibrin foam (Surgicel) or a gelatin sponge (Gelfoam). Topical application of epinephrine (Adrenalin) promotes vasoconstriction. Cauterizing or suturing a wound, which promotes additional bleeding, is avoided, except when absolutely necessary, such as during surgery.

In instances in which blood loss has already been extensive, immediate transfusion with whole blood or packed red blood cells is necessary to prevent shock. In addition the supplemental blood also supplies the body with the deficient factor required to initiate blood clotting.

Preventive measures. Before the discovery of methods for concentrating specific factors from blood, the treatment of choice was to infuse fresh or frozen plasma or whole blood into these children. However, maintaining adequate levels of the factor resulted in hypervolemia from repeated transfusions and carried the attendant risk of transfusion reactions.

Since the discovery of cryoprecipitate in the early 1960s, several commercially prepared products are now available that permit factor replacement in concentrated amounts. *Cryoprecipitate* is made by slowing thawing frozen plasma. Factor VIII remains in the cold-insoluble precipitate. As a standard unit of measure, 1 U of antihemophilic factor is equivalent to the amount of antihemophilic factor found in 1 ml of fresh plasma. In other words, to concentrate 100 U of antihemophilic factor, 100 ml of fresh plasma is required. The dosage of antihemophilic factor units is based on body weight. Examples of commercially prepared factor VIII concentrates are Hemophil, Humafac, and lyophilized concentrate. Factor IX concentrates include Proplex and Konyne. Although these products are very effective in raising factor levels to stop bleeding, the present emphasis is on their prophylactic use in preventing hemorrhage.

Nursing considerations

The objectives for nursing care can be divided into immediate needs and long-term goals. Obviously the most immediate consideration is control of bleeding episodes. However, the ultimate adjustment and prognosis for the hemophiliac person rely heavily on the family's ability to cope with the disorder, to learn effective methods of control and prevention, and to temper child-rearing practices with judicious protection from injury while fostering independence and development. Since the immediate goal is achieved through efforts directed at the long-term needs, the following discussion focuses on this aspect. (For nursing care of the child with hemophilia, see the boxed material.)

Assisting in coping with disorder. Not only is hemophilia a life-long, potentially fatal, hereditary condition, it is also one of unpredictable emergencies. Children with the moderate or mild form may be undiagnosed until an accident or elective medical procedure is performed. At this time coping with the diagnosis may be hindered by the circumstances surrounding its discovery. At other times parents are aware of the severity of the defect from birth and are immediately faced with the birth of a defective child. Whatever the situation, constructive teaching about the disease and measures to control or prevent bleeding must follow a period of parental adjustment to the diagnosis. For the nurse this involves (1) carefully listening to the parents' statements regarding their understanding of the condition, (2) awareness of the parents' feelings, particularly those of the mother concerning transmitting the disorder, and (3) an assessment of those factors that promote or retard coping with a crisis, such as marital stability, previous patterns of coping, and the ability to seek out and use help.

Genetic counseling as soon as possible after diagnosis is essential. Unlike many other disorders in which both parents carry the trait, the feeling or responsibility for this condition rests on the mother. Without an opportunity to discuss these feelings, the marital relationship can suffer. An even more unfortunate event occurs when genetic counseling is not fully understood. For example, in one family the parents had given birth to one normal son and one affected son. Unfortunately the mother had interpreted the statement that only males could have hemophilia to mean that the father had transmitted the disorder. Her blame on her husband created such guilt and discord that the marriage resulted in divorce. After remarrying the mother gave birth to a third son, who also had the disorder. This time, however, she realized that she carried the defective gene. The knowledge of her responsibility in destroying the first marriage and in bearing two hemophiliac children was so great that it resulted in serious emotional problems. The point of this case history is that genetic counseling must include evaluation of parental understanding and counseling of feelings as well as transmission of information.

Teaching local measures to control bleeding. Bleeding that occurs from a wound or close to the skin can be controlled by (1) applying pressure to the area for at least 10 to 15 minutes to allow clot formation, (2) immobilizing and elevating the area above the level of the heart to decrease blood flow, and (3) applying cold to promote vasoconstriction. By teaching parents and older children such measures beforehand, they can be prepared to initiate immediate treatment before blood loss is excessive. Plastic bags of ice should be kept in the freezer for such emergencies. If the bleeding does not stop within 15 minutes, the factor may need to be replaced. In a home-care program this would be done by the child or parent. In other situations the child would require emergency medical treatment.

Preventing bleeding by decreasing risk of injury. Prevention of bleeding through control of behavior is no easy task. During infancy and toddlerhood the normal acquisition of motor skills creates innumerable opportunities for falls, bruises, and minor wounds. Restraining the child from mastering motor development can herald more serious long-term problems than allowing the behavior. However, the environment can be made as safe as possible to minimize the incidental injuries by padding the crib, removing inflexible furniture from the play area and substituting cushions or upholstered chairs, supplying toys that do not have hard, rough, or sharp surfaces, avoiding breakable feeding utensils, using long-sleeved, full-legged clothes, padding the knee and elbow areas, using a helmet to prevent head injury, and maintaining close supervision during playtime.

For older children the family usually needs assistance in preparing for school. A nurse who knows the family can be instrumental in discussing the situation with the school nurse and in jointly planning an appropriate schedule of activity. Since almost all hemophiliacs are boys, the physical limitations in regard to active sports are a difficult adjustment. Encouraging the pursuit of intellectual and/or creative endeavors from early childhood hleps foster a life-style that is fulfilling and less conflicting than one focused on unrealistic goals. Using the group approach with hemophiliac children is often very successful because within the group they can find acceptance, healthy competition, and a sense of camaraderie. In fact, such a setting may be the first time that these children have felt a sense of belonging, because, even with their sibling relationships, they commonly see themselves as outsiders.

Since the mucous membranes bleed easily, the young child is given food that is easily masticated. For the older child food choices need not be limited as long as he understands the necessity of chewing thoroughly and eating slowly. Dental care is very important and may require some readjustment in terms of daily hygiene. For example, the nurse can recommend the use of a Water Pik, softening the toothbrush in warm water before brushing, or using a sponge-tipped disposable toothbrush, which is available in many drugstores. A regular toothbrush should be soft bristled and small in size. Adolescents also need to be advised of the dangers of shaving with a safety razor.

Diet is also an important consideration, because excessive body weight can increase the strain on affected joints, especially the knees, and predispose to hemarthrosis. Since limited activity is frequently the result of a more sedentary life-style and occasional periods of bed rest after tissue bleeding, calories need to be supplied in accordance with energy requirements.

Since any trauma can lead to a bleeding episode, all persons caring for these children must be aware of their disorder. Hemophiliac children should wear Medic Alert identification, and older children should be encouraged to recognize situations in which disclosing their condition is important. During procedures such as dental extraction or intramuscular injections, health personnel need to take special precautions to stop the bleeding. For example, with injections, the nurse injects the solution slowly and applies pressure to the puncture wound continuously for 5 minutes. After releasing pressure the nurse observes the site for at least 1 minute to note rebleeding.

Preventing crippling effects of joint degeneration. From repeated hemarthrosis, incompletely absorbed blood in the joints, and limitation of motion, bone and muscle changes occur that result in flexion contractures and joint fixation. Obviously prevention of bleeding is the ideal goal. However, since spontaneous bleeding is not uncommon in persons with severe hemophilia, definitive measures to limit joint damage are necessary.

During bleeding episodes the joint is elevated and immobilized. Passive range of motion exercises are usually instituted after the acute phase. Physical therapy is beneficial to promote maximum function of the joint and unaffected body parts. If an exercise program is instituted in the home, a physical therapist or public health nurse may need to supervise compliance with the regimen. Occasionally orthopedic intervention such as casting, application of traction, or aspiration of blood may be necessary to preserve joint function. Surgical joint replacement in instances of total disability offers new hope to some persons with hemophilia.

Since many individuals are unaware of the serious effects of joint involvement, the nurse has the responsibility of educating the child and family concerning the long-range consequences of this complication.

Some of the disabling effects on joint mobility and function are caused by voluntary limitation of movement in an effort to avoid pain. Therefore, success of a physical therapy plan involves control of pain. The usual measures of administering analgesics prior to the time of therapy and adjustment of the dose to provide maximum, safe pain relief are foundational. One special caution with hemophiliac children is the need to avoid salicylates and any aspirin-containing compound. Aspirin inhibits platelet aggregation, presumably by altering the cell membrane, and consequently prolongs bleeding time and weakly inhibits prothrombin synthesis. Acetaminophen (Tylenol) is a suitable aspirin substitute, especially for use during control of pain at home.

Fostering independence. The discovery of factor concentrates has greatly changed the outlook for these children. With scheduled infusions of the missing factor, bleeding can be prevented and the child can live a much more normal, unrestricted life. To foster maximum independence, home-care programs that teach the parent and/or child to administer the drug have been instituted. They have been especially successful for persons with severe hemophilia who require frequent transfusions to prevent spontaneous hemorrhage. Home treatment dramatically reduces the cost of hospitalized care and the complications of prolonged hospitalization.

Although the physician generally assumes the responsibility for referring a family for home care, it is the nurse who usually assumes the actual teaching responsibilities. Families selected for such programs should have (1) an adequate knowledge of the disease, (2) sufficient emotional stability to accept the responsibility, (3) a willingness to learn the venipuncture procedure, (4) the ability to follow instructions and to monitor the transfusion, and (5) a willingness to accept the necessity of home care.[4]

The basic preparatory phases for home care include (1) assessment of the family's knowledge of the disorder and their expectations from the program, (2) explanation of aseptic technique in handling the equipment, (3) demonstration and practice of the venipuncture technique, (4) preparation and administration of the concentrate, (5) awareness of signs of transfusion reactions, and (6) recognition of indications regarding the need for subsequent transfusions.

Obviously only a nurse skilled in venipuncture techniques is prepared to implement this phase of teaching program. In addition the nurse must be familiar with the properties of the concentrates. Factor VIII and to a lesser extent factor IX are very labile at room temperature. They must be stored at cool temperatures (slightly above freezing) and administered immediately after their preparation. To hasten the mixing process of reconstituting dried antihemophilic factor with diluent, the solution may be warmed or the vial gently rotated. Excessive heating or shaking of the container will result in loss of active antihemophilic factor. A filtered intravenous setup is usually supplied with the drug to filter any particles in the solution. If the solution is not thoroughly mixed before administration, the filter will also remove the active factor.

Transfusion reactions to cryoprecipitate and, to a lesser degree, the concentrates are possible because anti-A and anti-B isohemagglutinins are present in the solution and the hepatitis virus may have been transferred from the plasma. When cryoprecipitate is given, the plasma should be cross-matched to the recipient's blood type. The nurse teaches the parents and/or child the signs of transfusion reactions and stresses the necessity of notifying a physician of their occurrence.

Not all children with hemophilia are eligible for or have the opportunity of a home-care program. For these hemophiliac children, repeated hospitalizations are the usual outcomes of bleeding episodes. Often these children become familiar boarders on a pediatric unit with the unfortunate consequence that little is done to optimize the potential benefits of the admission. Ideally a core of nurses should work with these children to maintain consistency of care during each hospitalization. Besides the physical goals of controlling bleeding and preventing disability, the nursing objectives should include fostering independence and self-care, providing an opportunity for the children to discuss their feelings regarding the disease, and a continuous re-evaluation of those factors that may influence a bleeding episode.

Long-term goals. The needs of families with hemophiliac children are best met through a comprehensive team approach of physicians (pediatrician, hematologist, orthopedist), nurse, social worker, and physical therapist. Parent-group discussions are beneficial in meeting those needs often best met by similarly affected families. For example, with the improved prognosis for these children, parents and adolescent hemophiliacs are faced with vocational, employment, and financial problems. Once children reach 21 years of age, many insurance companies no longer wish to carry them, which is disastrous in terms of the cost of treatment. A person with severe hemophilia may require factor replacement therapy and other medical treatments in excess of $10,000 a year.

Family-planning choices for the adult hemophiliac are also important future decisions. The nurse who is constantly aware of the long-range consequences of surviving with the disease can help these individuals deal with their feelings regarding a transmittable disorder by precipitating such a discussion. It is also helpful for parents to express their concerns, since aging parents may feel that they can no longer assume total support. One of the advantages of the home-care program is that hemophiliac persons are encouraged to be independent long before the actual need arises.

VON WILLEBRAND'S DISEASE

von Willebrand's disease is a hereditary bleeding disorder characterized by a moderate to severe factor VIII deficiency and vascular abnormalities. Although platelet counts are normal, there is evidence that the platelets fail to adhere to the walls of the ruptured vessel, resulting in a delay in platelet plug formation. Also, the capillaries are coiled and tortuous and fail to constrict after injury.

Comparison with hemophilia

Besides the platelet and vascular defects, von Willebrand's disease differs from hemophilia in the following ways: (1) it affects males and females because its inheritance is autosomal dominant, (2) the most outstanding laboratory finding is a prolonged bleeding time, and (3) severe epistaxis and menorrhagia are common clinical manifestations. However, the treatment and final outcome are similar in both disorders. Control of bleeding is related to replacing factor VIII with plasma or concentrates.

Nursing considerations

The nursing goals are similar to those already discussed under hemophilia; however, a special consideration is its effect on females, especially the severe menorrhagia. Transfusions may be beneficial prior to the menstrual cycle to lessen the flow. Teaching the adolescent methods to prevent embarrassing accidents during menstruation, such as wearing plastic-lined underpants and using double sanitary pads, helps her adjust to the inconvenience. The heavy loss of blood each month may lead to anemia, necessitating whole blood transfusions to replace the red blood cells.

Interestingly these females frequently do not experience excessive bleeding at the time of delivery. This is thought to be because of increased levels of factor VIII during pregnancy. Decisions regarding childbearing are particularly difficult because of the dominant pattern of inheritance, which means that there is a 50% chance that the offspring will be affected.

The nurse also needs to teach parents and older children local measures to control epistaxis. Most of the nosebleeding originates in the anterior part of the nasal septum and can be controlled by applying pressure to the nose with the thumb and forefinger. The child should be kept in a sitting position, not lying down, to prevent aspiration of blood. Pressure is maintained for at least 10 minutes to allow clotting to occur. During this time the child breathes through his mouth. If this method is not successful, inserting dry cotton or tissue into each nostril and applying ice to the bridge of the nose may stop the bleeding. In the event that hemorrhage continues, the child should be evaluated by a physician, who may pack the nose with epinephrine-soaked gauze.

After a nosebleed petroleum jelly can be inserted into each nostril to prevent crusting of old blood and to lessen the likelihood of the child's picking at his nose and restarting the hemorrhage.

The nurse should also forewarn parents that the stools may become tarry in color and that the child may vomit dark material from swallowing blood during the nosebleed. It is important not to confuse these events with occult gastrointestinal bleeding.

THROMBOCYTOPENIA

Thrombocytopenia is defined as a platelet count below $100,000/mm^3$. Decreased platelets can result from (1) bone marrow failure to produce megakaryocytes, (2) failure of megakaryocytes to form platelets, or (3) an unusually rapid rate of platelet destruction. Thrombocytopenic disorders are frequently called ''purpuras'' because of the appearance of characteristic skin hemorrhages (petechiae and ecchymoses). A classification and some of the major causes of the thrombocytopenic purpuras are listed below. The following discussion focuses on the most common form of childhood purpura.

Classification and possible causes of thrombocytopenic purpuras

I. Idiopathic thrombocytopenic purpura (ITP)
- **A.** Viral or bacterial infection
- **B.** Immunoallergic response
- **C.** Hypersplenic sequestration
- **D.** Associated capillary defect

II. Congenital (neonatal) thrombocytopenic purpura
- **A.** Generalized septicemia
- **B.** Congenital rubella, herpes simplex, toxoplasmosis
- **C.** Placental transfer of certain drugs (quinine)
- **D.** Maternal-fetal platelet-type incompatibilities
- **E.** Immunologic disorders in mother
- **F.** Giant hemangioma
- **G.** Skeletal abnormalities

III. Symptomatic thrombocytopenic purpura
- **A.** Infections
- **B.** Chemicals, drugs, physical agents (radiation)
- **C.** Aplastic anemia
- **D.** Bone marrow infiltration (leukemia)
- **E.** Secondary to splenic hyperfunction from other diseases (lupus erythematosus)
- **F.** Massive blood transfusions

Idiopathic thrombocytopenic purpura (ITP)

As the preceding outline illustrates, the etiology of this disorder may result from a variety of pathologic deviations, however, the exact cause is still unknown. The condition is characterized by hemorrhagic tendencies caused by decreased platelet formation, function, or increased destruction.

Clinical manifestations. Idiopathic thrombocytopenic purpura occurs in one of two forms: an acute, self-limiting course or a chronic condition interspersed with remissions. The acute form is most commonly seen after upper respiratory infections or the childhood diseases measles, rubella, mumps, and chickenpox. The most common clinical manifestations of either type include (1) easy bruising with petechiae and/or ecchymoses, particularly over bony prominences, (2) bleeding from mucous membranes, such as epistaxis, bleeding gums, and internal hemorrhage with evidence of hematuria, hematemesis, melena, hemarthrosis, and menorrhagia, and (3) hematomas over the lower extremities that may result in chronic leg ulcers.

Medical/surgical management. The aim of medical management is to reverse the thrombocytopenia by (1) replacing the platelets with transfusions and (2) eliminating or counteracting the pathologic process.

Steroids, especially prednisone, are used to relieve the bleeding symptoms by exerting a hemostatic effect on the blood vessel walls and by stimulating platelet production. Immunosuppressive drugs are employed to interfere with the growth of immunocompetent cells in order to block the autoimmune response. Splenectomy may result in a rapid rise in platelet formation, presumably as a result of eliminating excessive splenic destruction of the cells or by removing a humoral substance that inhibits normal platelet production.

Nursing considerations. The nursing considerations of controlling bleeding, preventing bruising, and preventing crippling effects of hemarthrosis are similar to those discussed under hemophilia. The deleterious effects of using aspirin to control joint pain are critical for these children; therefore, salicylate substitutes should always be used.

Since transfusions of platelet-rich plasma are needed to control bleeding, the nurse observes for transfusion reactions.

The use of more vigorous treatment is variable, since the majority of these children recover spontaneously within 3 to 6 months. However, during this time parents need much support. The physical appearance of the skin, particularly as the hemorrhagic areas become confluent and color changes ensue from degradation of the blood and pigment deposition, is worrisome. Parents may overprotect the child to prevent additional bruising, even though such zealous efforts are not always helpful.

If steroids are used, parents need an explanation of the expected side effects, especially moon face, weight gain, and sometimes hirsutism. Because of the more serious complications, this drug is usually given for a short period of time.

If splenectomy is anticipated, parents and children require the same preparation as for other operative procedures. However, there are additional risks in performing the procedure, such as the stress effects from steroid therapy and the danger of bleeding tendencies. Parents are frequently aware of these hazards and may need additional assistance in coping emotionally. Also, there is no way of predicting which child will benefit from splenectomy, because removing the spleen does not always result in a platelet rise, especially in preadolescents or adolescents. The lack of guarantees is particularly difficult when parents realize that this treatment is a last resource.

After splenectomy there is the danger of overwhelming infection. Most of these children are kept on prophylactic antibiotic therapy for a few years. The nurse needs to reinforce the necessity of strict compliance with antibiotic therapy to prevent this possibly fatal complication, especially in infants and young children.

Immunologic-deficiency disorders

The body's immune system is composed of four components: (1) the phagocytic system, which consists of a variety of mononuclear and polymorphonuclear cells capable of ingesting and digesting foreign agents, (2) antibody-mediated immunity, which consists of several immunoglobulins found in the plasma, interstitial fluid, and body secretions, (3) cell-mediated immunity, which relies on the lymphocytic system to produce cells capable of attacking specific invaders, and (4) the complement system, which consists of substances in the serum that act synergistically to enhance the action of the other three systems.

This discussion is concerned with defects within the antibody- and cell-mediated immune systems. Although a variety of disorders comprise immunologic-deficiency diseases, only two of them are explored. To understand the reason for the particular effects of these conditions, a brief review of the two immune systems follows.

Antibody-mediated immunity

Antibodies, gamma globulins formed in response to specific antigens, are formed from plasma cells. The exact origin of the plasma cell from the original stem cell is not known, although it is believed to be the lymphomyeloid complex. These cells are referred to as B cells and are thought to be lymphocytes. Each B cell is capable of producing a highly specific antibody molecule. All the antibody molecules, now known as G, M, A, D, and E, are collectively termed *immunoglobulins* (Ig) and provide protection against bacteria, viral infection, parasites, allergens, and malignancy. Severe deficiency of antibody-mediated immunity is characterized by absence of all five classes of immunoglobulins and is broadly termed *agammaglobulinemia*.

Cell-mediated immunity

The thymus gland is responsible for the differentiation of stem cells into small lymphocytes that are capable of becoming T cells. The exact mechanism by which the thymus does this is unknown, although it is thought to be the result of various thymic hormones. The small lymphocytes are "seeded" in the lymphoreticular system during fetal life, therefore, cellular immunity is well established before birth. The lymphocytes provide protection against viral, protozoan, and fungal infection, malignancy, graft-vs-host reaction, and autoimmunity. It also appears that T cells may be necessary for normal antibody production of B cells, although the exact interrelationship is unclear.

Cellular immunity differs from antibody immunity in the following ways: (1) once lymphocytes (T cells) have been sensitized to an antigen, they continue to circulate for several years and may even produce new lymphocytes with the same sensitizing properties (this is often referred to as the delayed hypersensitive reaction), and (2) they can develop immunity to minute amounts of antigens that will fail to induce an antibody reaction.

Severe combined immunodeficiency disease (SCID)

Severe combined immunodeficiency disease is a defect characterized by absence of both antibody and cell-mediated immunity. The terms Swiss type lymphopenic agammaglobulinemia, an autosomal-recessive form of disease, and sex-linked lymphopenic agammaglobulinemia have been used to describe this disorder, which, as the names imply, can follow either method of inheritance.

Pathology. The exact cause of severe combined immunodeficiency disease is unknown. The theories include (1) a defective stem cell that is incapable of differentiating into B or T cells, (2) defective organs responsible for the differentiating process, primarily the thymus and lymphoid complex, or (3) an enzymatic defect that suppresses lymphocytic cell function.

The consequence of the immunodeficiency is an overwhelming susceptibility to infection and to the graft-vs-host reaction. The latter occurs when any histoincompatible tissue from an immunocompetent donor is infused into the immunodeficient recipient. For example, in utero the fetus may receive immunocompetent maternal cells. However, because of its immunodeficiency, the fetus is unable to reject the foreign incompatible tissue. Therefore, the antigenic donor cells attack the host's tissues. The graft-vs-host reaction is a serious complication in the only known treatment for severe combined immunodeficiency disease, bone marrow transplant.

Diagnostic evaluation. Diagnosis is usually based on a history of recurrent, severe infections from early infancy, a familial history of the disorder, and specific laboratory findings, which include lymphopenia, lack of lymphocyte response to antigens, and absence of plasma cells in the bone marrow. Documentation of immunoglobulin deficiency is difficult during infancy because of the normally delayed response of the infant to produce his own immunoglobulins and maternal transfer of immunoglobulin G.

Clinical manifestations. Obviously the most common manifestation is susceptibility to infection early in life, most often by 3 months of age when maternal immunity is low. Specifically the children are characterized by chronic infection, failure to completely recover from an infection, frequent reinfection, and infection with unusual agents. In addition the history reveals no logical source of infection. Failure to thrive is a consequence of the persistent illnesses.

If the child should receive a foreign tissue, such as blood supplements, signs of graft-vs-host reaction, such as fever, skin rash, alopecia, hepatosplenomegaly, and diarrhea, are expected. Since the reaction requires 7 to 20 days for tissue damage to become evident, the symptoms may be mistaken for an infection. However, the presence of a graft-vs-host reaction increases the child's susceptibility to overwhelming infection and, therefore, is a grave complication.

Medical management. The only definitive treatment is a histocompatible bone marrow transplant. The perfect donor is an identical twin because the histocompatibility (HL-A) antigens and blood type are exactly the same. The second best choice is a sibling. The procedure consists of aspirating several samples of bone marrow from the donor and infusing the marrow intravenously or injecting it intraperitoneally into the host. However, bone marrow transplants are usually done at medical centers where measures to control postransplantation infection, such as a sterile environment, and other specialized facilities are available. Since the host's immunologic system is incompetent, graft rejection is not a problem. However, a graft-vs-host reaction is always a possibility in a nonidentical twin graft, and, once it occurs, little can be done to reverse the process.

Other approaches to severe combined immunodeficiency disease are providing passive immunity with gamma globulin injections and maintaining the child in a sterile environment. The latter is only effective if instituted prior to the existence of any infectious process in the infant. Other investigational transplant procedures include nonidentical HL-A bone marrow grafts and fetal liver or thymus transplants. However, the results are still uncertain, although they provide potential hope for future children born with the disorder.

Nursing considerations. Since the prognosis for severe combined immunodeficiency disease is very poor if a compatible bone marrow donor is not available, nursing care is directed at supporting the family in caring for a fatally ill child. Genetic counseling is essential because of the modes of transmission in either form of the disorder. Nursing goals are directed at (1) helping parents prevent sources of infection in the child, such as cautious isolation from crowded facilities and individuals with active infection, (2) meticulous skin and mouth care, (3) good general nutrition, and (4) careful supervision during periods of activity to prevent skin trauma. (See also Chapter 27.)

However, even with exacting environmental control, these children are prone to opportunistic infection. Chronic fungal infections of the mouth and nails with *Candida albicans* are frequent problems despite vigorous efforts at prevention or treatment. A hoarse voice may result from repeated esophageal and vocal cord erosions from the fungus. It is important to stress to parents that such conditions are not a result of laxity on their part in preventing them but are the result of the severe immunologic disorder. Parents should be encouraged to immediately notify a physician regarding any evidence of a worsening infection.

Children who receive frequent injections of immune serum globulin (ISG) need support during the procedure because the injections are painful. Infants are best comforted by their parents, but toddlers and preschoolers may benefit from needle play. Immune serum globulin is injected deeply into a large muscle mass, usually the vastus lateralis. To prevent tissue damage and provide maximum absorption, the total amount may be divided into two injections and given in two different sites. If only one injection is required, the nurse keeps a record of the site to ensure a rotating schedule for future injections.

Care of the child undergoing bone marrow transplantation is mainly directed at preventing infection. Because it takes 7 to 20 days before evidence of bone marrow functioning becomes evident, hospitalization is long. It is not the purpose of this discussion to detail the care of the child with a bone marrow transplant, except to emphasize that the psychologic needs of the parents and child are tremendous. For the parents, it represents the last hope for successful therapy and survival. For the child, it means sensory deprivation because of isolation, numerous blood tests, and the possibility of more pain and suffering if a graft-vs-host reaction occurs. To meet these needs, a sensitive, consistent team of nurses who function effectively as members of the total health team is essential.

Wiskott-Aldrich syndrome

The Wiskott-Aldrich syndrome is a sex-linked recessive disorder characterized by several abnormalities: (1) thrombocytopenia, (2) eczema, (3) recurrent infection, (4) an inability to form specific antibodies to polysaccharide antigens, and (5) acquired thymic system deficiency.

Pathology. The exact defect is unknown, although a variety of pathologic findings are evident. The platelets are abnormally small in size and have a shortened life span, possibly because of a metabolic defect in their synthesis. The primary immunologic defect consists of the inability of phagocytes (macrophages) to process foreign antigens, particularly polysaccharides, such as pneumococcus. As a result immunologically competent cells fail to produce normal immunoglobulin patterns. Early in life the immunoglobulin levels may be normal, but later low levels of immunoglobulin M are observed. Typically isohemagglutinins (anti-A and anti-B agglutinins in the blood) are decreased or absent.

The thymus and lymph nodes are normal at birth but become progressively dysfunctional with age, until a profound cellular immunodeficiency results. Consequently these children are highly susceptible to infection and malignancy, especially of the lymphoreticular system.

Clinical manifestation. At birth the major effect of the disorder is bleeding because of the thrombocytopenia. As the child grows older, recurrent infection and eczema become more severe and the bleeding becomes less frequent.

Eczema is typical of the allergic type and easily becomes superinfected. Chronic infection with herpes simplex is a frequent problem and may lead to chronic keratitis of the eye with loss of vision. From infection, chronic pulmonary disease, sinusitis, and otitis media result. In those children who survive the bleeding episodes and overwhelming infections, malignancy presents an additional risk to survival.

Diagnostic evaluation. Diagnosis can usually be made during the neonatal period because of the thrombocytopenia. Specific tests for immunologic function are also useful in confirming the diagnosis.

Medical management. Medical treatment mainly involves (1) counteracting the bleeding tendencies with platelet transfusions, (2) using gamma globulin to provide passive immunity, and (3) administering prophylactic antibiotics to prevent and control infection. Bone marrow transplants have been attempted but, even if successful, do not reverse all the defects of this disorder.

Nursing considerations. Because of the grave prognosis for these children, the main nursing consideration is supporting the family in the care of a fatally ill child. Physical care is directed at controlling the problems imposed by the disorder. The measures used to control bleeding are similar to those discussed under hemophilia (p. 1395) and idiopathic thrombocytopenic purpura (p. 1398). Another major goal is related to preventing or controlling infection, which has been discussed under severe combined immunodeficiency disease (p. 1400). Since eczema is a troublesome problem, nursing measures specific to this condition are especially important (see p. 489).

The genetic implications of this sex-linked recessive disorder differ little from those of hemophilia. However, because of the multiplicity of defects, the emotional adjustment and physical care required for these children are greater than those of many other conditions. The nurse can be especially supportive by providing short-term goals during periods of hospitalization and by focusing on long-range needs through coordinated efforts with a public health nurse.

REFERENCES

1. Czapek, E., and associates: Hemophilia A in a female: use of factor VIII antigen levels as a diagnostic aid, J. Pediatr. **84**(4): 485-489, April 1974.
2. Hathaway, H. J., and associates: Carrier detection in classical hemophilia, Pediatrics **57**(2):251-254, February 1976.
3. Miller, D. R., and Pearson, H. A.: Smith's blood diseases of infancy and childhood, ed. 4, St. Louis, 1978, The C. V. Mosby Co.
4. Sergis, E., and Hilgarten, M.: Hemophilia, Am. J Nurs. **72**(11):2011-2017, November 1972.

BIBLIOGRAPHY

Anthony, C. P., and Thibodeau, G. A.: Textbook of anatomy and physiology, ed. 10, St. Louis, 1979, The C. V. Mosby Co.

Child, J., and associates: Blood transfusions, Am. J. Nurs. **79**(9): 1602, 1605, September 1972.

Guyton, A.: Textbook of medical physiology, Philadelphia, 1971, W. B. Saunders Co.

Langley, L. L., Telford, I. R., and Christensen, J. B.: Dynamic anatomy and physiology, New York, 1974, McGraw-Hill Book Co.

Ravel, R.: Clinical laboratory medicine, Chicago, 1973, Year Book Medical Publishers, Inc.

Rudolph, A. M., editor: Pediatrics, New York, 1977, Appleton-Century-Crofts.

Widmann, F. K., editor: Goodale's clinical interpretation of laboratory tests, ed. 7, Philadelphia, 1973, F. A. Davis Co.

The anemias

Bonner, S. E.: Nursing care of a child with sickle cell disease. In Brandt, P., Chinn, P. L., and Smith, M. E., editors: Current practice in pediatric nursing, vol. 1, St. Louis, 1976, The C. V. Mosby Co.

Byrne, J.: Hematology studies. Part 4. Tips for interpreting the sedimentation rate and reticulocyte count, Nursing '77 **7**(1):9-10, January 1977.

Desforges, J. R., and associates: Sickle cell anemia: improving the odds for your patient, Patient Care **6:**116, February 15, 1972.
Doswell, W.: Sickle cell disease: how it influences preoperative and postoperative care, Nursing '74 **4**(6):19-22, June 1974.
Flynn, D. M., and associates: Hormonal changes in thalassemia major, Arch. Dis. Child. **51:**828-836, 1976.
Fost, N., and Kaback, M.: Why do sickle screening in children? Pediatrics **51**(4):742-745, April 1973.
Foster, S.: Sickle cell anemia: closing the gap between theory and therapy, Am. J. Nurs. **71**(10):1952-1956, October 1971.
Greene, P.: Teaching aid for children with sickle cell disease, Am. J. Nurs. **77**(12):1953, December 1977.
Hegyi, T., and associates: Sickle cell anemia in the new born, Pediatrics **60**(2):213-216, August 1977.
Jackson, D. E.: Sickle cell disease: meeting a need, Nurs. Clin. North Am. **72**(4):727-742, December 1972.
Jackson, R. E., and Short, B. J.: Frequency and prognosis of coexisting sickle cell disease and acute leukemia in children, Clin. Pediatr. **11**(3):183-185, March 1972.
Logothetis, J., and associates: Intelligence and behavior patterns in patients with Cooley's anemia (homozygous beta-thalassemia): a study based on 138 consecutive cases, Pediatrics **48**(5): 740-743, May 1971.
Masera, G., and associates: Role of chronic hepatitis in development of thalassaemic liver disease, Arch. Dis. Child. **51:**680-685, 1976.
McFarlane, J. M.: Everyday care of the child with sickle cell anemia, Pediatr. Nurs. **2**(1):9-11, January/February 1972.
McFarlane, J.: Sickle cell disorders, Am. J. Nurs. **77**(2):1948-1954, December 1977.
McGarry, P., and Duncan, C.: Anesthetic risks in sickle cell trait, Pediatrics **51**(3):507-512, March 1973.
McIntosh, N.: Endocrinopathy in thalassemia major, Arch. Dis. Child. **51:**195-201, 1976.
Pearson, H. A.: Progress in early diagnosis of sickle cell disease, Children **18:**222-226, November/December 1971.
Pearson, H. A., and Diamond, L.: The critically ill child: sickle cell disease crises and their management, Pediatrics **48**(4):629-653, April 1971.
Pochedly, C.: Sickle cell anemia: recognition and management, Am. J. Nurs. **71**(10):1948-1951, October 1971.
Seeler, R. A.: Deaths in children with sickle cell anemia, Clin. Pediatr. **11**(11):634-637, November 1972.
Seeler, R. A., and Shwiaki, M. Z.: Acute splenic sequestration crises (ASSC) in young children with sickle cell anemia, Clin. Pediatr. **11**(12):701-704, December 1972.
Suckett, C.: Caring for children with sickle cell anemia, Children **6:**227-231, Nobember/December 1971.
Vaz, D. D.: The common anemias: nursing approaches, Nurs. Clin. North Am. **7**(4):711-726, December 1972.

Defects in hemostasis

Boutaugh, M., and Patterson, P. C.: Summer camps for hemophiliacs, Am. J. Nurs. **77**(8):1288-1289, August 1977.
Burke, C.: Working with parents of children with hemophilia, Nurs. Clin. North Am. **72**(4):787-798, December 1972.
Chanin, A.: Prevention of recurrent nosebleeds in children, Clin. Pediatr. **11**(12):684, December 1972.
Hathaway, W. E.: Care of the critically ill child: the problem of disseminated intravascular coagulation, Pediatrics **46**(5):767-773, May 1970.
Patterson, P. C.: Hemophilia: the new look, Nurs. Clin. North Am. **72**(4):777-786, December 1972.
Seeler, R. A., Ashenhurst, J. B., and Langehenning, P. L.: Behavioral benefits in hemophilia as noted at a special summer camp, Clin. Pediatr. **16**(6):525-530, June 1977.
Strawczynski, H., and associates: Delivery of care to hemophilic children: home care versus hospitalization, Pediatrics **51**(6): 986-991, June 1973.

Immunologic-deficiency defects

Byers, M. C., and Ventura, J. N.: Care of a baby with bone marrow transplant, Nurs. Clin. North Am. **72**(4):809-816, December 1972.
Dharan, M.: Immunoglobulin abnormalities, Am. J. Nurs. **76**(10): 1626-1628, October 1976.
Donley, D. L.: Nursing the patient who is immunosuppressed, Am. J. Nurs. **76**(10):1619-1625, October 1976.
Nysather, J. O., Katz, A. C., and Lenth, J. L.: The immune system: its development and functions, Am. J. Nurs. **76**(10):1614-1616, October 1976.
Thomas, E. D., and associates: Bone marrow transplantation, N. Engl. J. Med. **292:**832-843, 985-902, April 17, 24, 1975.
Zimmerman, S., and associates: Bone marrow transplantation, Am. J. Nurs. **77**(8):1311-1315, August 1977.

UNIT FIFTEEN

The child with a disturbance of regulatory mechanisms

In an organism such as man, the maintenance of dynamic equilibrium involves a complex interaction of many systems and subsystems. All the activities within the individual cells, tissues, and organs that comprise these systems depend on the function of other systems, and, like all systems, each component part has one or more factors that act on it or affect it. A change in a component part can affect all other component parts. Basic to this interaction are the processes whereby messages are communicated from one area or subsystem to the other and feedback mechanisms by which the system is able to respond to any disturbance that causes a deviation from the normal value by counteracting that disturbance.

Regulation is the function of maintaining automatically an important biologic variable within a narrow range regardless of disturbances that may act on the system and prevent excessive deviations that are incompatible with life. Regulation enables the organism to maintain the function of cells, tissues, organs, and systems within the parameters described as normal for that system despite changes in the internal or external environment. Communication between the various systems and subsystems is carried by chemical or neural mechanisms. Disturbances in the regulatory processes can create disturbances in one or more of the interrelated component parts of the system with consequences that affect other systems and the organism as a whole.

Genetic and numerous chemical regulatory mechanisms, for example, acid-base equilibrium and oxygen-carbon dioxide disturbances, have been discussed in previous segments. The major regulatory mechanisms of the body are the endocrine and neural systems. The portion of the endocrine regulation that involves the pituitary gland is so closely associated with the neurologic system that it is frequently referred to as the neuroendocrine system. It is sometimes difficult to determine if dysfunctions in this interrelated system are caused by impaired function in the target glands that secrete the hormones, the tropic substances that stimulate the target glands to secrete hormones, or the portions of the midbrain that produce releasing factors that stimulate the pituitary gland. Defects within this complex regulatory system and the pancreatic hormones are discussed in Chapter 38, *The Child with an Endocrine Dysfunction,* whereas dysfunction in the central nervous system is discussed in Chapter 37, *The Child with a Disturbance of Cerebral Function*. Defects in the integrity of the peripheral nervous system are elaborated in Unit Sixteen.

37

The child with a disturbance of cerebral function

Neural control of body function is made possible by a complex communication network, and, within this network, control makes integration possible. Any disturbance in this central communication system can produce alterations in the way in which the system receives, integrates, and responds to stimuli entering the system. These disturbances are reflected in a variety of clinical manifestations, depending on the focus of the disturbance and the integrity of the conducting mechanism.

This chapter is concerned primarily with alterations in consciousness caused by seizure activity, infectious processes, and trauma.

REVIEW OF CEREBRAL STRUCTURE AND FUNCTION

The nervous system is composed of three intimately connected and functioning parts: (1) the central nervous system, composed of two cerebral hemispheres, the brain stem, the cerebellum, and the spinal cord; (2) the peripheral nervous system, which consists of the cranial nerves that arise from or travel to the brain stem and the spinal nerves that travel to or from the spinal cord, which may be motor (efferent) or sensory (afferent); and (3) the autonomic nervous system, composed of the sympathetic and parasympathetic systems that provide automatic control of vital functions.

Since this chapter is concerned primarily with disturbances of the brain, the major emphasis will be placed on this system. The structure and function of the spinal cord and autonomic system are elaborated in the discussion of spinal injury in Chapter 40.

Coverings of central nervous system

The bony skull forms the strongest covering and provides the primary protection to the brain. It is an expansible structure in the infant and young child but becomes rigid in the older child and adolescent. Within the skull the brain is covered and protected further by three membranes, the *meninges*—the dura mater, arachnoid membrane, and pia mater (Fig. 37-1). The tough outer membrane, the *dura mater,* is a double layer that serves as the outer meningeal layer and the inner periosteum of the cranial bones. The closeness of this attachment causes slower spread of blood in epidural hemorrhage. Between these layers of dura inside the skull lie large venous sinuses. Sheets of the dura mater also extend downward and inward to form partitions within the cranium. Projecting downward into the longitudinal fissure is the sheet of dura called the *falx cerebri,* separating the cerebral hemispheres, and the *falx cerebelli,* separating the cerebellar hemispheres (see Fig. 9-8). Another segment is a tentlike structure, the *tentorium,* which separates the cerebellum from the occipital lobe of the cerebrum. The large gap through which the brain stem passes is the tentorial hiatus. Brain tissues and nerves pressing through this opening cause many of the symptoms observed in the child with increased intracranial pressure.

The blood supply to the dura mater is supplied by the middle meningeal artery, a branch of the external carotid artery. It enters the skull at a point inferior to the temporal bone, from where it branches over the surface of the dura, usually encased in a groove in the temporal and parietal bones. Damage to this artery or its branches is the frequent cause of an epidural hematoma.

The dura mater is separated from the next membrane, a fine, elastic weblike structure called the *arachnoid* membrane, by a thin subdural space crossed by fine blood vessels, which forms a loose covering for the brain. It is situated close to the dura but is unattached so that any bleeding within the space can spread freely. The vessels that traverse the space have little support and can be shorn easily by trauma to cause extensive bleeding.

The innermost covering layer, the *pia mater,* is a delicate transparent membrane that, unlike the other coverings, adheres closely to the outer surface of the brain conforming to the folds (gyri) and furrows (sulci). The pia is rich in minute blood vessels, and any blood seeping from their rupture becomes rapidly mixed with cerebrospinal fluid. Between the pia mater and the arachnoid membrane is the subarachnoid space, which contains the cerebrospinal fluid that also serves as a protective cushion for the brain tissue.

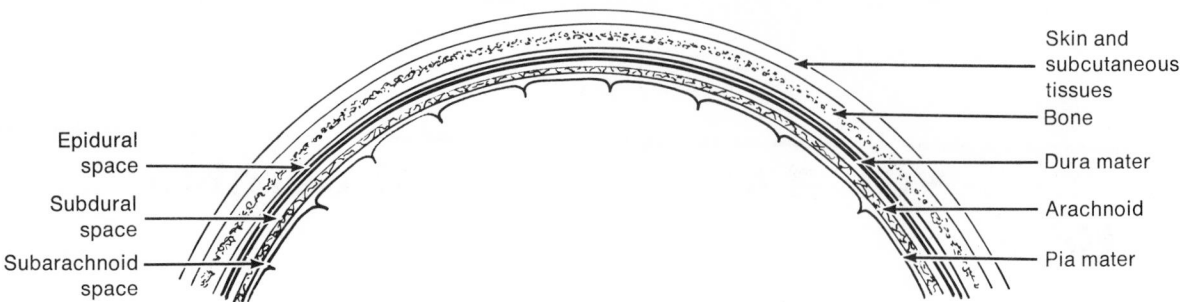

Fig. 37-1. The protective coverings of the brain.

Brain

The brain can be divided into six major divisions, each of which plays a vital role in regulation and control of body function. The two large cerebral hemispheres that occupy the anterior and medial fossae of the skull are separated in the upper part by the *longitudinal fissure*. This separation is complete anteriorly and posteriorly, but centrally the hemispheres are joined by the block of fibers known as the *corpus callosum*. Each hemisphere is artifically divided into lobes. Pressure on or damage to these lobes produces observable signs or symptoms directly related to the area of pathology, which provides clues to the location of the damage.

Situated deeply within each hemisphere and on each side of the midline are the *basal ganglia* (or cerebral nuclei), which serve as vital sorting areas for messages passing to and from the hemispheres. Connected to the hemispheres by thick bunches of nerve fibers is the brain stem, through which all the nerve fibers traverse as they pass from the hemispheres to the cerebellum and spinal cord. The brain stem extends from the base of the hemispheres through the foramen magnum, where it is continuous with the spinal cord. Within the cranium and behind the brain stem is the cerebellum. Any pressure exerted on the intracranial structures can cause compression of the brain stem and prolapse of the cerebellum through the foramen magnum to produce serious consequences.

The major structures of the brain and their functions are briefly outlined in Table 37-1.

The blood supply to the brain tissue is carried by the internal carotid arteries, which branch to supply the various brain segments. The volume of blood to the brain, which constitutes only 15% of the cardiac output, supplies the brain with 20% of the body oxygen. The brain, an ''inactive'' organ, uses ten times the oxygen that is used by the body as a whole. Only the heart uses more oxygen per gram of tissue. The metabolic requirements for oxygen by the brain are not affected by rest or sleep, although they are reduced by narcoses and coma and altered by changes in temperature. Oxygen consumption of the brain is increased by fever and decreased by hypothermia. The brain is dependent on a constant supply of oxygen-rich blood, and, since the oxygen need of the brain is great in relation to the volume of blood supplied, it extracts a greater amount of oxygen from each unit of circulating blood. Oxygen supply to the brain is compromised when the supply is inadequate as a result of impaired respiration, hypotension, increased intracranial pressure, or vascular damage, spasm, or compression.

Neurons are highly susceptible to elevated Pco_2, and the metabolic damage to brain tissue caused by an inadequate supply of well-oxygenated blood can often exceed the effects of trauma. Respiratory acidosis resulting from increased Pco_2 levels can produce symptoms indistinguishable from those of head injury.

Increased intracranial pressure

The brain, tightly enclosed in the solid bony cranium, is well protected but highly vulnerable to pressure that may accumulate within the enclosure. Its total volume, including brain, cerebrospinal fluid, and blood, must remain approximately the same at all times. A change in the proportional volume of one of these components produces an increase in intracranial pressure (ICP). This results in compensatory changes in the other components, which are manifest in neurologic signs and symptoms. An increase in intracranial pressure may be caused by tumors or other space-occupying lesions, accumulation of fluid within the ventricular system, bleeding, or edema of cerebral tissues.[13]

Early signs and symptoms of increased intracranial pressure are often subtle and assume many patterns, such as personality changes, irritability, and fatigue. In older children subjective symptoms are headache, especially when lying flat (such as on awakening in the morning) or when coughing, sneezing, or bending over, and nausea and vomiting. The child may complain of double vision or of blurred vision on movement of the head. Funduscopic examination often reveals papilledema, the most reliable sign of increased intracranial pressure in older children. Seizures are not uncommon. In children prior to closure of the cranial sutures there is an increase in the head circumference and bulging fontanels. As pressure increases, pupils may be dilated and accompanied by an altered level of consciousness that progresses from drowsiness to eventual

Table 37-1. Structure and function of the brain

Structure	Description	Function	Dysfunction
Cerebrum	Two hemispheres Divided (artificially) into lobes	Upper parts divided anteriorly and posteriorly by longitudinal fissure Lower parts joined centrally by block of fibers, corpus callosum	Pressure or damage produces signs and symptoms specific to involved areas
Frontal lobes	Most anteriorly located of all lobes that end posteriorly at fissure of Rolando	Posterior portion contains cells that control motor activity throughout body	Injury or damage to anterior portion may cause personality changes and altered intellectual functioning Impaired movement of body part directly related to motor center for that part
Parietal lobes	Situated posterior to fissure of Rolando	Important for appreciation of sensation, somatic interpretation	
Occipital lobe	At posterior base of skull Most posteriorly placed lobe	Receives stimuli for vision	Injury produces impaired vision
Temporal lobes	Situated anterior to occipital lobe and inferior to parietal lobes	Receives and interprets stimuli for taste, vision, sound, and smell Converts crude visual impressions into recognizable images	Injury or destruction causes inability to interpret meanings of sensory experiences
	Point where temporal, parietal, and occipital lobes converge	Primary interpretive area	Impairment causes inability to interpret sensory stimuli; difficulty in understanding higher levels of meaning of somatic sensory experiences
	Point where temporal, parietal, and frontal lobes converge	Center for speech	Impairment produces aphasia
Cerebellum	Located just below posterior part of cerebrum and separated from it by tentorium Contains two lateral lobes joined by midline portion, vermis	Necessary for refinement and coordination of all muscle movements, including walking, talking, and control of muscle tone and balance	Dysmetria, ataxia, dysarthria, hypotonia
Basal ganglia	Situated deeply within cerebral hemispheres on either side of midline	Unconscious or automatic control of lower motor centers Excitation causes inhibition of muscle tone throughout body	Chorea, athetosis
Diencephalon	Situated between cerebrum and mesencephalon	Contains diffuse fibers that compose reticular activating system	Stupor
Thalamus	Rounded mass that protrudes into lateral ventricles	Major relay station for sensory impulses to cerebral cortex Activates cerebral cortex	Impaired consciousness
Hypothalamus	Lies beneath thalamus Forms floor of third ventricle	Vital control center for involuntary functions, for example, blood pressure, satiety, hunger, rage, feeding, water conservation, temperature Controls secretion of tropic hormones	Impairment causes alterations in vegetative functions Somnolence; coma Endocrine disorders
Brain stem	Extends from cerebral hemisphere to spinal cord	All cranial nerves (except first) arise from brain stem	Stupor, coma
Mesencephalon (midbrain)	Lies below inferior surface of cerebellum and above pons	Main connection between forebrain and hindbrain Contains nuclei for third, fourth, and part of fifth cranial nerves	Impaired consciousness Impaired function of muscles supplied by these nerves
	Ventral portion composed of cerebral peduncles	Control of eye movement	
Pons	Located just above medulla oblongata	Contains pneumotaxic center—control of respiration Cranial nerves V through VIII	Deep, rapid, or periodic breathing
Medulla	Forms attachment of brain to spinal cord Separated from pons by horizontal groove	Contains vital centers, including respiratory and vasomotor Swallowing	Impaired vital functions

coma. Problems related to increased intracranial pressure are discussed in relation to congenital malformation (p. 376), brain tumor (p. 1023), and head injuries (p. 1421).

Physiologic and biochemical changes within the brain vasculature serve to complicate the primary causes of increased intracranial pressure. Initially, especially in cases of trauma, there is often increased blood flow as a result of venous congestion or vasomotor paralysis. If cerebral hypoxia is associated with the cerebral dysfunction, the compensatory vasodilation caused by oxygen deficiency will tend to increase the cerebral flow. However, as intracranial pressure progressively increases, blood flow is reduced with diminished blood supply to the brain tissues.

A marked increase in intracranial pressure will trigger the pressor response, wherein the increased pressure produces an elevation in blood pressure with a reflex slowing of the heart rate.[7] This is an extremely serious sign that requires immediate action. This rise in blood pressure is greater in the systolic than the diastolic pressure, producing an increased pulse pressure. However, the respiratory rate and rhythm are believed to be the most sensitive indicators of increased intracranial pressure. Breathing characterized by periods of hyperpnea that alternate with apena (Cheyne-Stokes respirations) is seen in brain stem damage.

Evaluation of neurologic status

Methods used to evaluate neurologic function are discussed in relation to numerous aspects of child care. The neurologic examination is an integral part of the health assessment (see p. 165), assessment of gestational age (see p. 326), and the newborn assessment (see p. 260). Children younger than 2 years of age are more difficult to evaluate neurologically. In early infancy neurologic responses are primarily reflexive responses that are gradually replaced by meaningful movement in the characteristic cephalocaudal direction of development. This evidence of progressive maturation is a reflection of the more extensive myelinization and changes in neurochemical and electrophysiologic properties. Moreover, children younger than 2 years of age are unable to respond to directions designed to elicit specific responses. Therefore, most information regarding infants and small children is gained through observation of their spontaneous and elicited reflex responses, by their development of increasingly complex locomotor and fine motor skills, and by eliciting progressively more sophisticated communicative and adaptive behaviors.[14]

In evaluating the infant or young child, the pregnancy and delivery history are of greatest importance in determining the possible effect of intrauterine environmental influences known to affect the orderly maturation of the central nervous system. These influences include infections, chemicals, trauma, and metabolic insults. Physical evaluation includes observation of the size and shape of the head, spontaneous activity and postural reflex activity, and sensory responses. The attitude is observed. It is noted whether the infant assumes a normal flexed posture or one of extreme extension, opisthotonos, or hypotonia. Extremities are observed for symmetry of movement. Excessive tremulousness or frequent twitching movements may be significant signs indicating the onset of a seizure disorder. Seizure activity is suspected if holding the extremity snuggly does not stop the activity. An abnormal respiratory cycle such as prolonged apnea, ataxic breathing, paradoxical chest movement, and unilateral expansion of the chest wall may be the result of a neurologic problem. Skin and hair texture may be important in detecting certain neurologic disease. Facial features may suggest a specific syndrome, and a high-pitched, piercing cry is associated with central nervous system disorders. Abnormal eye movements, inability to suck or swallow, lip smacking, asymmetric contraction of facial muscles, and yawning may indicate cranial nerve involvement.

Older children can be evaluated by the usual methods employed in a neurologic examination. In addition, an estimation of the level of development provides essential information about neurologic function. These accomplishments are discussed throughout the book in relation to evaluation for specific disorders such as mental retardation, failure to thrive, minimal brain dysfunction, cerebral palsy, cerebral tumors, and other physical or behavioral problems. The Denver Developmental Screening Test (Appendix F) serves as an excellent screening tool for assessing developmental progress in the young child.

Special diagnostic procedures. Numerous diagnostic procedures are employed for assessment of cerebral function (Table 37-2). Most are carried out with specialized equipment by skilled personnel. The child will need preparation for and support and reassurance during the tests. Children who are old enough to understand require careful explanation of the procedure, why it is being done, what they will experience, and how they can help (see Chapter 25 and p. 1027). It is helpful for nurses to become acquainted with the equipment and the general environment in which the test will take place so that they can better explain the procedure to the child at his level of understanding. Equipment is often strange and ominous to a child and may even appear as a frightening monster. It is especially frightening to young children to experience a large mechanical device coming toward them as if to crush or devour a small helpless child. They need constant reassurance from a trusted companion (Fig. 37-2).

Physical preparation may involve administration of a sedative. If so, the child should be helped through the preparation and administration and assured that someone will remain with him (if this is possible). The child will need continual support and reinforcement during the procedures in which he remains conscious. The child's vital signs and

Table 37-2. Diagnostic procedures

Test	Description	Purpose	Comments
Lumbar puncture (LP)	Long needle is inserted between L3 and L4 vertebrae into subarachnoid space; cerebrospinal fluid pressure is measured, and sample is collected for examination	Diagnostic—measures spinal fluid pressure, obtains cerebrospinal fluid for visualization and laboratory analysis Therapeutic—injection of medication, spinal anesthesia	Contraindicated in patients with increased intracranial pressure, infected skin over puncture site, when test does not contribute to diagnosis or treatment
Subdural tap	Needle is inserted into anterior fontanel or coronal suture	Helps rule out subdural effusions Relieves intracranial pressure	Requires shaving scalp Fluid removed is limited to no more than 15 ml from one side at each tap To and fro movement of needle is avoided to prevent laceration Pressure dressing applied after subdural tap Infant placed in semierect position after subdural tap to minimize leakage from site; avoid crying if possible
Ventricular puncture	Needle is inserted into lateral ventricle via anterior fontanel	Removes cerebrospinal fluid to relieve pressure	Used if lumbar puncture unsuccessful or contraindicated Should be performed by neurosurgeon Risk of intracerebral or ventricular hemorrhage
Electroencephalography	Records changes in electric potential of brain Electrodes are placed at various points on scalp and amplified Impulses are recorded by electromagnetic pen	Measures electric activity of cerebral cortex Detects electric abnormalities—diagnosis of seizures Used to determine brain death	Patient should rest quietly during procedure May require sedation Reduce external stimuli to a minimum during procedure
Computerized tomography	Pinpoint x-ray beam is directed on horizontal or vertical plane to provide series of "cuts" or "slices" that are fed into computer and assembled in image displayed on videoscreen and transferred to permanent record	Visualized horizontal and vertical cross section of brain at any axis Distinguishes density of various intracranial tissues and structures	Noninvasive procedure Requires sedation Can be done on outpatient basis
Brain scan	Intravenous injection of radioactive material that is counted and recorded after fixed time interval	Test material accumulates in areas where blood-brain barrier is defective Identifies focal brain lesions, for example, tumors, abscesses Positive uptake of material with encephalitis and subdural hematoma	Requires sedation in young or uncooperative children and intravenous infusion
Echoencephalography	Pulses of ultrasonic waves are beamed through head; echoes are recorded graphically	Identifies shifts in midline structures from their normal positions as a result of intracranial lesions	Simple, safe, rapid procedure
Radiography	Skull films are taken from several projections—lateral, posterolateral, axial (submentoventrical), half-axial	Shows fractures, dislocations, spreading suture lines, and craniostenosis Shows degenerative changes, bone erosion, and calcifications	Simple, noninvasive procedure
Pneumoencephalography	Introduction of oxygen or air into subarachnoid spaces via lumbar puncture	Visualizes entire ventricular system and subarachnoid spaces Identifies structural abnormalities Localizes intracranial lesions	Requires heavy sedation or anesthesia

Continued.

Table 37-2. Diagnostic procedures—cont'd

Test	Description	Purpose	Comments
Ventriculography	Air introduced into lateral ventricular system by direct ventricular tap in infants, burr hole in older children	Visualizes ventricular system Detects structural anomalies or localizes intracranial lesions Determines patency of ventricular system	May cause some trauma to brain
Cerebral angiography	Percutaneous injection of radiopaque substance into cerebral circulation via carotid system (or by reflux from cannulization of brachial or femoral arteries)	Outlines cerebral arteries and veins—determines size, location, and nature of cerebral vascular disorders and localizes tumors, abscesses, and other space-occupying lesions by detecting distortion of normal vascular patterns	Requires general anesthesia

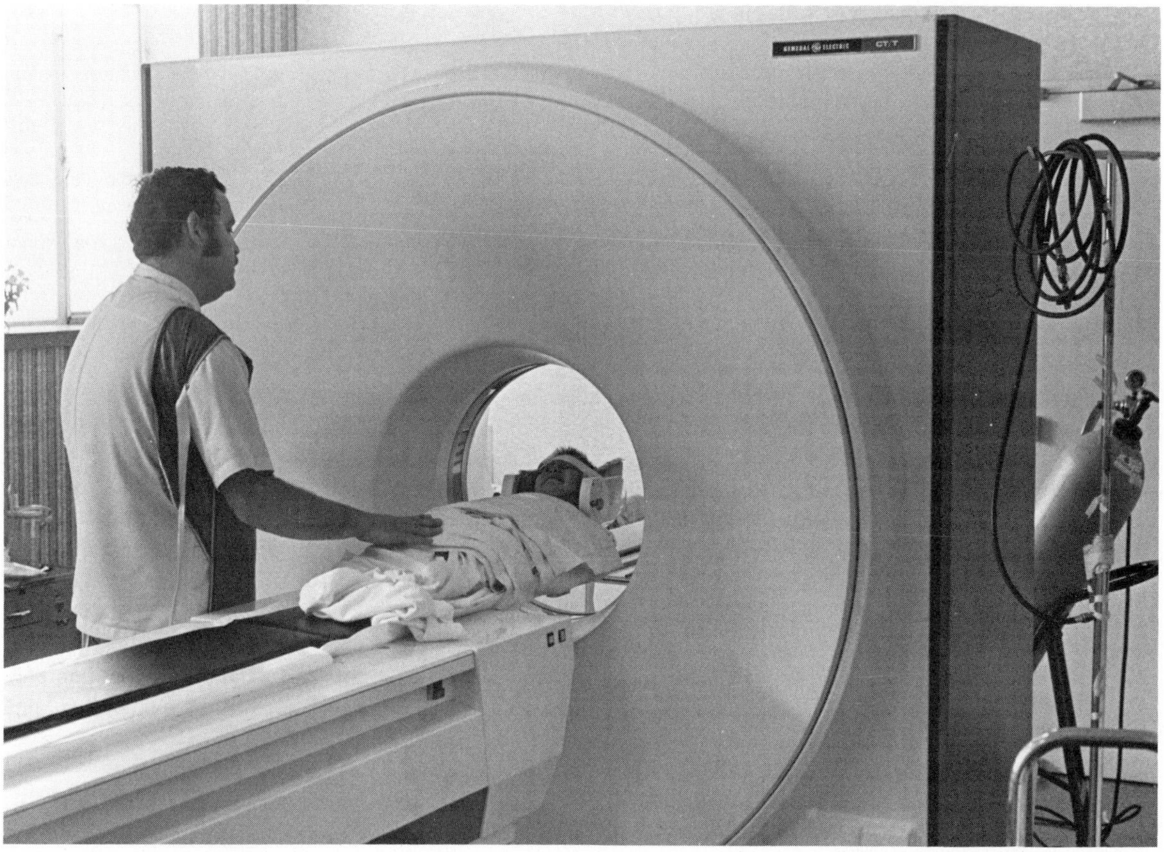

Fig. 37-2. The child reflects the stress and feeling of powerlessness during tomography even when accompanied by a kind and supportive person.

physiologic response to the procedure are monitored throughout. Care after the test depends on the nature of the procedure.

Children who have undergone a procedure with general anesthesia require postanesthesia care, including positioning to prevent aspiration of secretions and frequent assessment of vital signs and level of consciousness. Also, other neurologic functions, such as pupillary responses, motor strength, and movement, are tested at regular intervals. After some procedures, for example, ventriculogram and pneumoencephalogram, the child should be kept flat and at bed rest. Any surgical wound necessitated by the test is checked for bleeding and other complications.

The child's emotional reaction to the procedure is also

considered. He should be allowed to express his feelings about the experience through verbal expression and the use of therapeutic play.

ALTERED STATES OF CONSCIOUSNESS

Consciousness implies certain subjective processes designated as awareness—the ability to respond to sensory stimuli and have subjective experiences that range from simple perceptual discriminations to complex forms of abstraction and thinking. An altered state of consciousness usually refers to varying states of unconsciousness that may be momentary or may extend for hours, days, or indefinitely. *Unconsciousness* is depressed cerebral function—the inability to respond to sensory stimuli and have subjective experiences with modification in cognition and, thus, a change in reaction. *Coma* is defined as a state of unconsciousness from which the patient cannot be aroused even with powerful stimuli.

The seat of consciousness or the "alerting" area of the brain is in the reticular formation of the midbrain and upper pons. The reticular formation receives information from the main afferent pathways and collateral nerves and then projects these impulses diffusely to the thalamus and cortex. The hypothalamus also plays a role in wakefulness. Disturbances of consciousness may occur when any part of the reticular, thalamic, hypothalamic, and cortical circuits is sufficiently impaired. However, the effects may vary according to the areas involved. For example, small lesions of the reticular or hypothalamic regions will produce a profound effect, whereas extensive impairment of the cortex is required to produce quantitatively similar results.

Etiology

An altered state of consciousness may be the outcome of several processes that affect the central nervous system. Some, such as the diffuse changes seen in encephalitis, are directly related to cerebral insult; others are the result of dysfunction to other organs or processes manifest by central nervous system signs. For example, biochemical changes can impair neurologic function without morphologic findings, as in hypoglycemia. In general, coma is produced by focal lesions in the upper brain stem or hypothalamus or by lesions elsewhere that affect these areas secondarily. Somnolence as an early complaint is commonly associated with hypothalamic lesions. The major causes of sudden alteration in consciousness include postictal state, trauma, hemorrhage, infections, metabolic neurotoxins, exogenous neurotoxins, combined causes, anesthesia, and malfunctioning shunt.

Postictal state. Postictal state is the unconsciousness that follows a seizure.

Trauma. Direct trauma to the brain will produce a comatose state. The mechanisms include laceration, contusions, concussions, and epidural, subdural, or intracerebral accumulation of blood. Brain edema is also a contributing factor.

Hemorrhage. Intracerebral bleeding may occur unrelated to trauma. Bleeding may result from vascular malformations, leukemia, hypertension, uremia, or hepatic disease.

Infections. Bacterial, viral, fungal, or other organisms can cause alterations in consciousness as a manifestation of the infectious or postinfectious processes in the brain tissue or meninges.

Metabolic neurotoxins. Cerebral manifestations are often observed in association with other illnesses or conditions. Hypoxia, acidosis (diabetic or other), uremia, hypoglycemia, hyperglycemia, endocrine disturbances, electrolyte imbalances, water intoxication, and hepatic disease may at times produce loss of consciousness. Any space-occupying lesion in the cranium can cause cerebral manifestations by obstructing the ventricular system, exerting direct pressure on vital areas, or exerting the combined effects of increased intracranial pressure.

Exogenous neurotoxins. Substances toxic to brain tissue include drugs such as narcotics, sedatives, alcohol, and salicylates; animal venom or toxins from bites or stings; and various poisonous substances such as lead or other heavy metals, plant poisons (oleander, castor beans), volatile hydrocarbons (glue, benzene), and carbon monoxide.

Combined causes. Sometimes more than one of these factors may be operating, for example, trauma and depressant drugs or poisons.

Anesthesia. General anesthesia is a common cause of temporary loss of consciousness.

Malfunctioning shunt. Hydrocephalic children with shunts sometimes develop a malfunction that causes increased accumulation of cerebrospinal fluid.

Diagnostic evaluation

It is difficult or impossible to determine the subjective state of consciousness; therefore, the phenomena observed or elicited provide the basis of assessment and evaluation. Both observation of clinical signs and objective diagnostic tests are used. Vital signs, observation of posture and movement (both spontaneous and elicited), eye examination, and reflex testing all provide valuable clues regarding the level of consciousness, the site of involvement, and the probable cause.

Level of consciousness. Alteration of consciousness occurs as a continuum and is designated as the *comatose state*. For descriptive purposes this continuum is divided into four grades[7,20]: (1) somnolence, (2) stupor, (3) semicoma (or light coma), and (4) deep coma. The level is determined by observations of the patient's responses to his environment. Other diagnostic tests such as motor activity, reflexes, and vital signs are more variable and do not necessarily directly parallel the depth of the comatose state. Other states of altered consciousness are described as pseudowakeful states and confusion.

Somnolence (grade 1). In this state the patient can be aroused by various stimuli and will then make appropriate verbal and motor responses. The child may be clear mentally or somewhat confused. Somnolence may alternate with delirium. When the stimulus is withdrawn, the patient usually drifts back to sleep. He frequently demonstrates spontaneous movement and spontaneous speech or muttering. He may be restless or display little movement.

Stupor (grade 2). There is often considerable spontaneous movement in stupor. The patient responds to stimuli such as pain, touch, loud sounds, or bright lights. He usually responds by withdrawal behaviors, although a combative response may be elicited. Application of repeated and persistent stimuli often arouses the patient to a sufficient degree that he will respond briefly to questions or follow simple commands. Spontaneous movements are common, including twitching or picking movements. Bowel and bladder control may or may not be present.

Semicoma (light coma; grade 3). At this level painful stimuli will evoke organized (semipurposeful) avoidance or other simple adaptive movements. Sometimes persistent tactile stimulation or shaking may elicit a similar response. Verbal responses are limited to muttering or groaning. Spontaneous movements are uncommon. When the stimulus is removed, the patient resumes his prior state. Reflex responses are present, but there is usually lack of bowel or bladder control.

Deep coma (grade 4). Painful stimuli fail to produce a response, or the patient will, at most, move slightly to a very painful stimulus—usually limited to deep pain, for example, pressure over the styloid process in the neck, the supraorbital nerve, the root of the fingernails, or periosteal surfaces of bone. Squeezing muscle bellies or tendons often produces a similar effect. When attempting to elicit responses with painful stimuli, care must be observed not to harm the patient. Reflexes and pupillary responses are usually absent. No spontaneous movements are observed, muscles are flaccid, and the patient is incontinent. The pulse is usually rapid, respirations are episodic, and blood pressure tends toward shock levels.

Pseudowakeful states. In the fully developed state the patient sits or lies with eyes open but fails to follow objects or lights, does not turn his eyes toward a noise, and does not speak. In less developed states the patient may follow objects or persons with his eyes, turn slowly toward a sound and appear about to speak, but remain silent. This is sometimes described as a "reptilian stare." Response to external stimuli is similar to that of a patient in stupor or light coma. Some of these patients are restless and hyperkinetic; others remain motionless and speechless. These pseudowakeful states may be observed in coma of toxic origin or in focal lesions involving the diencephalon either primarily or secondarily by pressure.

Confusion. The responses of confused patients demonstrate a failure to comprehend their surroundings. They appear to lose their proper bearings. They are unable to estimate direction or location, are apt to be disoriented in time, and may misidentify people. These patients will have difficulty in following even simple directions and tend to misinterpret events. They may be hyperactive or apathetic and immobile. They are usually able to give relevant answers to simple questions such as their age, location of pain, or so on but will give irrelevant and inaccurate answers to more complex questions.

Vital signs.* Pulse, respiration, and blood pressure provide information regarding the adequacy of circulation and the possible underlying cause of altered consciousness. Autonomic activity is most intensively disturbed in deep coma and in brain stem lesions. Body temperature is often elevated, and sometimes the elevation may be extreme. Coma of a toxic origin may produce hypothermia. The pulse is variable and may be rapid, slow and bounding, or feeble. Respirations are more often slow, deep, and irregular. Blood pressure may be normal, elevated, or at shock levels. With increased intracranial pressure, the pressor response causes a slowing of the pulse and an increase in blood pressure. Slow and deep breathing is often seen in the heavy sleep caused by sedatives, after seizures, or in cerebral infections. Slow shallow breathing may result from sedatives or narcotics. Hyperventilation (deep and rapid respirations) is usually the result of metabolic acidosis or of abnormal stimulation of the respiratory center in the medulla as a result of salicylate poisoning, hepatic coma, or Reye's syndrome. Periodic and irregular breathing are signs of brain stem (especially medullary) dysfunction. This is an ominous sign that often precedes complete apnea. The odor of the breath may provide additional clues, for example, the fruity, acetone odor of ketosis, the foul odor of uremia, fetor odor of hepatic failure, or the odor of alcohol.

A fever is most frequently a sign of an acute infectious process or heat stroke but may be caused by ingestion of some intoxicant drugs (especially alcohol and barbiturates) or intracranial bleeding. A fever sometimes follows a cerebral seizure.

Skin. The skin may offer clues to the etiology of unconsciousness. The body surface should be examined for the presence of injury, needle marks, petechiae, bites, and ticks. Evidence of toxic substances may be found on the hands, face, mouth, and clothing—especially in small children.

Eyes. Pupil size and reactivity are assessed. Pinpoint pupils are commonly observed in poisoning, such as opiate or barbiturate poisoning, or in brain stem dysfunction. Widely dilated and reactive pupils are often seen after

*See references 7, 16, 20, and 25.

seizures and may involve only one side. Dilated pupils may also be caused by eye trauma. Widely dilated and fixed pupils suggest paralysis of cranial nerve III secondary to pressure from herniation of the brain through the tentorium. A unilateral fixed pupil usually suggests a lesion on the same side. Bilateral fixed pupils usually imply brain stem damage if present for more than 5 minutes. Dilated and unreactive pupils are also seen in hypothermia, poisoning with atropine-like substances, or prior instillation of mydriatic drugs.

Eye movements are assessed by the doll's head maneuver, in which the child's head is rotated quickly to one side and then to the other. When brain stem centers for eye movement are intact, there is conjugate (paired or working together) movement of the eyes in the direction opposite to the head rotation. Absence of this response suggests dysfunction of the brain stem or oculomotor nerve (cranial nerve III). Downward or lateral deviation is frequently observed in association with pupillary dilatation in dysfunction of cranial nerve III because of tentorial herniation.

The caloric test, or oculovestibular response, is elicited by irrigating the external auditory canal with ice water. This normally causes conjugate movement of the eyes toward the side of stimulation. This is lost when the pontine centers are impaired and, therefore, provide important information in assessment of the comatose patient.

Funduscopic examination reveals additional clues. Papilledema indicates increased intracranial pressure. However, this may not be evident early in the course of unconsciousness since papilledema takes 24 to 48 hours to develop. The presence of preretinal (subhyaloid) hemorrhages in children is almost invariably the result of acute trauma with intracranial bleeding, usually subarachnoid or subdural hemorrhage.[16]

Motor function. Observation of spontaneous activity, posture, and response to painful stimuli provides clues to the location and extent of cerebral dysfunction. Asymmetric movements of the limbs or absence of movement suggests paralysis. In hemiplegia the affected limb lies in external rotation and will fall uncontrollably when lifted and allowed to drop.

In the deeper comatose states there is little or no spontaneous movement and the musculature tends to be flaccid. There is considerable variability in the motor behavior in lesser degrees of coma. For example, the child may be relatively immobile or restless and hyperkinetic; muscle tone may be increased or decreased. Tremors, twitching, and spasms of muscles are common observations. The patient may display purposeless plucking or tossing movements. Combative or negativistic behavior is not uncommon. Hyperactivity is more common in acute febrile and toxic states than in cases of increased intracranial pressure. Convulsions are common in children and may be present in coma as a result of any cause.

As cortical control over motor function is lost in brain dysfunction, primitive postural reflexes emerge. These are evident in posturing and motor movement that are directly related to the area of the brain involved. *Decorticate posturing* is seen when there is severe dysfunction of the cerebral cortex. Typical decorticate posturing includes adduction of arms at the shoulders, the arms being flexed on the chest with the wrists flexed and the hands fisted, and the lower extremities being extended and adducted. *Decerebrate posturing,* a sign of dysfunction at the level of the midbrain, is characterized by rigid extension and pronation of the arms and legs. The posturing may not be evident when the child is quiet but can usually be elicited by applying painful stimuli, such as knuckle pressure to the sternum. Unilateral decerebrate posturing is often caused by tentorial herniation.

Reflexes. Testing of some reflexes may be of limited value. In general the corneal, pupillary, muscle-stretch, superficial, and plantar reflexes tend to be absent in deep coma. The state of reflexes is variable in lighter grades of unconsciousness and depends on the underlying pathologic process and the location of the lesion. The doll's eye reflex maneuver, described previously, reflects paralysis of cranial nerve III. Absence of corneal reflexes and the presence of a tonic neck reflex are associated with severe brain damage. Babinski's reflex, in which the lateral portion of the foot is stroked, may be of value if it is found to be present consistently in children who are older than 1 year of age. A positive Babinski's reflex is significant in assessment of pyramidal tract lesions when it is unilateral and associated with other pyramidal signs. A fluctuating Babinski's reflex is often observed after seizures.

Laboratory examination. Tests that may help to delineate the cause of unconsciousness include blood glucose, urea nitrogen, electrolytes (pH, sodium, potassium, chloride, calcium, and bicarbonate) tests; clotting studies, hematocrit, and a complete blood count; liver function tests; blood cultures if there is fever; and sometimes studies to detect lead or other toxic substances, such as drugs.

Skull x-ray films. Skull radiographs are usually taken to identify possible fractures or other possible etiologic factors.

Lumbar puncture. Examination of spinal fluid is carried out when toxic encephalopathy or infection is suspected. Lumbar puncture is ordinarily delayed if intracranial hemorrhage is suspected and is contraindicated in the presence of increased intracranial pressure. Usual findings are outlined in Table 37-3.

Electroencephalogram. An electroencephalogram provides important information in the assessment of children with impaired consciousness. For example, generalized random slow activity suggests suppressed cortical function; localized slow activity suggests a focal lesion, such as a mass; and generalized projected patterns suggest brain stem

Table 37-3. Significance of cerebrospinal fluid findings in some neurologic disorders

Disorder	Initial pressure	Appearance	Cells	Protein	Glucose
Meningitis					
Bacterial	Increased	Opalescent or purulent	Markedly increased, mostly polymorphonuclear; from 100 to thousands	Increased	Decreased to absent
Viral	Normal or slightly increased	Clear	0 to few hundred	20-125 mg/100 ml	Usually normal
Fungal	Increased	Variable	10-500; early—polymorphonuclear leukocytes, late—monocytes	Elevated and increasing	Decreased
Concussion	Normal	Clear	Normal	Normal	Usually normal
Contusion	Increased or normal	Xanthochromic or bloody	Few to several thousand RBCs	Normal	Usually normal
Hematoma					
Subdural	Increased	Clear in 30%, xanthochromic in 70%	Normal (if fluid clear)	Often normal unless fluid is bloody	Normal
Epidural	Increased	Clear	Same	Same	Same
Hemorrhage					
Cerebral	Usually high	Xanthochromic	Amount and type depend on severity of hemorrhage	Normal or increased	Usually normal
Subarachnoid	Usually high	Xanthochromic or bloody	All cellular elements of blood present	Increased in relation to amount of blood	Usually high initially
Encephalopathies					
Lead, anoxic, uremic, toxic	Increased	Clear to slightly yellow	Normal; occasionally increased, mainly monocytes	Normal or increased	Normal
Parainfectious (measles, varicella, vaccinia)	Usually increased	Usually clear	0-50, mainly monocytes	Increased	Normal

involvement. A flat tracing is now used as evidence of brain death.[20]

Criteria for "brain death."[25] Although there is no standard diagnosis for clinical death, the practice of establishing death by cerebral signs is being employed more frequently in clinical practice. Irreversible coma or a nonfunctioning brain may be suspected when there is absence of spontaneous respirations for 3 minutes after removal of ventilatory support; fixed dilated pupils and absence of other cerebral reflex activity; and nearly total motor and sensory paralysis. Presence or absence of spinal reflexes is not a reliable criterion. Further confirmation can be obtained by electroencephalographic readings. A flat, or isoelectric, tracing at the time of apparent death and a second flat reading 24 hours later are considered reliable indications of brain death. There are two notable exceptions to this rule, however—cases of profound hypothermia and central nervous system depression caused by barbiturates.[25] Therefore, phenobarbital is discontinued prior to electrocardiogram in children receiving the drug therapeutically in order to have a near zero serum phenobarbital level at the time of the test. An early guide to irreversible brain damage is absence of cerebral blood flow as demonstrated by angiography or intravenously injected isotopes.

Medical management

Emergency measures are directed toward assuming a patent airway, treatment of shock, and reduction of intracranial pressure (if present). Delayed treatment often leads to increased damage. A history is very important since it provides valuable cues regarding the etiology of unconsciousness. There may have been an injury or short febrile illness, or the child may be a known diabetic. As soon as emergency measures have been implemented—in many cases concurrently—specific therapies for specific causes are initiated. For example, if diabetic ketoacidosis is suspected, insulin is administered intravenously; a subdural tap is performed to reduce intracranial pressure for a subdural hematoma.

Respiratory status. Respiratory effectiveness is the primary concern in the unconscious child and demands immediate evaluation and intervention. Cerebral hypoxia that extends longer than 4 minutes causes irreversible brain damage. The child is positioned to prevent aspiration of secretions, and the stomach is emptied to reduce the likelihood of vomiting. An endotracheal tube or tracheostomy is frequently needed to assure an adequate airway and to facilitate removal of secretions. Also, upper airway obstruction, that is, laryngospasm, is a frequent complication in comatose children. When the respiratory center is involved, mechanical ventilation is usually indicated (see p. 1203). Blood gas analysis is determined regularly, and oxygen is administered when indicated. Moderately severe hypoxia and respiratory acidosis are often present and are not always evident from clinical manifestations (see p. 1073). Hyperventilation frequently accompanies unconsciousness and may lead to respiratory alkalosis, or it may represent the body's attempt to compensate for metabolic acidosis. Therefore, blood gas and pH determinations are essential guides for electrolyte therapy.

Neurologic assessment. Continual observation of vital signs, pupillary reaction, and level of consciousness is essential to management of central nervous system disorders. Diagnostic tests are performed as indicated for diagnosis and observation of progress.

Sedatives are usually avoided but may be indicated when marked agitation or restlessness may result in further damage. If so, chloral hydrate or diphenhydramine (Benadryl) and, occasionally, paraldehyde are preferred.[25] These drugs are less likely to produce respiratory depression. However, favorable results are achieved with the administration of codeine. Sometimes a large initial dose of phenobarbital is administered, even to the extent that short-term respiratory support is required. Anticonvulsants, primarily phenytoin (Dilantin), are ordered for control of seizure activity.

Increased intracranial pressure. Prompt intervention is lifesaving in the comatose patient who has evidence of marked increase in intracranial pressure (ICP). When increased intracranial pressure is the result of accumulation of cerebrospinal fluid from obstruction of cerebrospinal fluid flow, a ventricular tap will provide relief quickly and effectively. Evacuation of a hematoma reduces pressure from this source.

For increased intracranial pressure resulting from cerebral edema, several medical measures are available. Osmotic diuretics may provide rapid relief in emergency situations. Although their effect is transient, lasting only about 6 hours, they can be lifesaving in emergencies. These substances are rapidly excreted by the kidneys and carry with them large quantities of sodium and water. Mannitol or urea administered intravenously is the drug most frequently employed for rapid reduction. The infusion is given slowly and, because of the profound diuretic effect of the drug, an indwelling catheter is inserted to ensure bladder emptying. Digitalis may be given to improve cerebral circulation. Adrenal corticosteroids are also used to reduce cerebral edema. The effect is less rapid than that of the osmotic diuretics, but high doses can be used over an extended period of time for prolonged control. A tube or other device is sometimes placed into the subarachnoid space or ventricle to monitor intracranial pressure directly. The simplest device is a subdural catheter attached to a standard manometer. Assisted ventilation also helps to reduce intracranial pressure transiently by causing vasoconstriction of cerebral arteries.

Nutrition. Fluids and calories are supplied initially by the intravenous route. Later, if the child remains unresponsive, fluids and nutrition are supplied by nasogastric tube or gastrostomy.

An intravenous infusion is started early, and the type of fluid administered is determined by the general condition of the patient. Fluid therapy requires careful monitoring and adjustment based on neurologic signs and electrolyte determinations. Often the comatose child is unable to cope with the same amounts of fluid that he could handle at other times and overhydration must be avoided to prevent fatal cerebral edema. This altered ability to handle fluid loads is attributed in part to the inappropriate secretion of antidiuretic hormone (ISADH) as a result of hypothalamic dysfunction. This disorder frequently accompanies central nervous system diseases such as head injury, meningitis, encephalitis, brain abscess, brain tumor, and subarachnoid hemorrhage. In the patient with inappropriate secretion of antidiuretic hormone, scant quantities of urine are excreted, electrolyte analysis reveals hyponatremia and hyposmolality, and manifestations of overhydration are evident. It is important to evaluate all parameters, since the reduced urine output might be erroneously interpreted as a sign of dehydration. The treatment of inappropriate secretion of antidiuretic hormone consists of the restriction of fluids until serum electrolytes and osmolality return to normal levels. Since ISADH frequently occurs with meningitis in children, fluid restriction is often prescribed.[16]

Hyperthermia. Fever often accompanies cerebral dysfunction, and, if present, measures are implemented to reduce the temperature to prevent brain damage from hyperthermia. Hypothermia by way of a cooling blanket is frequently prescribed for several days. The body temperature is reduced to 30.5° to 32.2° C (87° to 90° F) to decrease the oxygen demand by the brain.

Specific therapies. The foregoing treatments are nonspecific for comatose children in general. In addition specific therapies for specific disorders are initiated as soon as the diagnosis is determined. For example, if diabetic ketoacidosis is diagnosed or suspected, insulin is administered intravenously, antibiotics are administered for cerebral infections, and tumors or cysts are removed.

Nursing considerations

The unconscious child requires continuous nursing attendance with observation, recording, and evaluation of changes in objective signs. These observations provide valuable information regarding the patient's progress. Often they serve as a guide to diagnosis and treatment. Therefore, careful and detailed observations are essential for the patient's welfare. In addition vital functions must be maintained and complications prevented through conscientious and meticulous nursing care. The outcome of unconsciousness may be early and complete recovery, death within a few hours or days, persistent and permanent unconsciousness, or recovery with varying degrees of residual mental and/or physical disability.

Respiratory status. Maintaining a patent airway is a primary consideration. Children in lighter stages of coma may be able to cough and swallow, but those in deeper states of coma are unable to handle secretions, which tend to pool in the throat and pharynx. A temporary airway can be used for the child who is suffering a temporary loss of consciousness, such as after a seizure or anesthesia. For children who remain unconscious for a period of time, a nasotracheal or orotracheal tube is inserted to maintain the open airway. A tracheostomy is performed in cases in which laryngoscopy for introduction of an endotrachial tube would be difficult or dangerous. Suctioning is used as often as needed to clear the airway. Respiratory status is observed and evaluated regularly. Signs of respiratory embarrassment may be an indication for ventilatory assistance.

Lung physiotherapy is carried out on a regular basis, and the child's position is changed at least every 2 hours to prevent pulmonary complications. In cases of high levels of increased intracranial pressure, nursing procedures tend to trigger reactive pressure waves in many patients. Therefore, procedures such as percussion and suctioning should be carried out to take advantage of therapies that reduce intracranial pressure, such as osmotherapy and sedation.[24] Particular care should be taken in positioning these patients to avoid neck vein compression, which may further increase intracranial pressure by interfering with venous return.

Neurologic assessment. Regular assessment of neurologic signs is a vital part of nursing comatose children. Vital signs are taken and recorded regularly. The frequency depends on the cause of coma, the status, and the progression of the cerebral involvement. The intervals may be as frequent as every 15 minutes or as long as every 2 hours. Significant alterations are reported immediately. Temperature is taken every 2 to 4 hours, depending on the patient's condition.

An elevated temperature is not uncommon in children with central nervous system dysfunction; therefore, a light covering is sufficient. Vigorous efforts are needed, such as tepid sponge baths or application of a hypothermia blanket, to prevent brain damage.

The level of consciousness is assessed periodically, including size, equality, and reaction to light of pupils; signs of meningeal irritation, such as nuchal rigidity; and level of consciousness. This includes response to vocal commands, spontaneous behavior, resistance to care, and response to painful stimuli, such as sternal or supraorbital pressure. Voluntary motions of any kind, changes in muscle tone or strength, and body position are noted. Seizure activity is described according to type and length of seizure and body areas involved (see p. 1438).

Hygienic care. Routine measures for cleansing and maintaining skin integrity are an integral part of nursing care of the unconscious child. Skin folds require special attention to prevent excoriation. Children who are unable to move are prone to develop tissue breakdown and pressure necrosis; therefore, the child is placed on a sheepskin, egg-carton pad, or other resilient appliance (alternating mattresses and water-filled mattresses are also used) to prevent pressure on prominent areas of the body. The goal is prevention by regular change of position and inspection of vulnerable areas, such as the ankle, trochanter, and shoulder. Since supine positioning is seldom employed, the occiput and sacrum are less likely to be involved. Bed linen and any clothing are kept dry and free of wrinkles. Rubbing the back and extremities with lotion or other lubricating preparation stimulates circulation and helps prevent drying of the skin.

Mouth care is performed at least twice daily, since the mouth tends to become dry or coated with mucus. The teeth are carefully brushed with a soft toothbrush or cleaned with gauze saturated with mouthwash. Commerically prepared cleansing devices, such as Toothettes, are convenient for cleansing the mouth and teeth. Mouthwash, glycerine with lemon, or other solutions can be used to cleanse and moisten mucous surfaces. Lips are coated with ointment, glycerine, or other preparations to protect them from drying, cracking, or blistering.

The deeply comatose child is also prone to eye irritation. The corneal reflexes are absent; therefore, the eyes are easily irritated or damaged by linen, dust, or other substances that may come in contact with them. There is excessive dryness as a result of decreased secretions, especially if the child is undergoing osmotherapy to reduce or prevent brain edema, and incomplete closure of the eyes. The eyes should be examined regularly and carefully for early signs of irritation or inflammation. Artificial tears (methycellulose) are placed in the eyes at frequent intervals. Sometimes eye dressings may be needed to protect the eyes from possible damage.

The hair is combed and styled neatly. Long hair is usually braided and secured with rubber bands. The scalp should be kept clean with dry or wet shampoos as needed. The child's head may be shaved for tests or surgical procedures. If so, the hair is saved if possible.

Nutrition and hydration. Initially unconscious children are fed by intravenous infusion or hyperalimentation. Later, nutrition is provided in a balanced formula given by nasogastric or gastrostomy tube. The nasogastric tube is usually taped in place with care to prevent pressure on the nares. The tube is rinsed carefully after each feeding and is replaced frequently (usually every 24 hours) to prevent bacterial growth and to alternate nostrils to prevent nasal irritation and pressure. Overfeeding should be avoided to prevent vomiting with the danger of aspiration. The stomach contents are aspirated and measured prior to feeding to ascertain the amount remaining in the stomach. If the residual volume is excessive (depending on the size of the child), the dietitian and physician should be consulted regarding alteration of the formula composition to provide the needed calories and nutrients in a smaller volume. The aspirated contents should always be refed.

Hydration is maintained in the same manner. When cerebral edema is a threat, the fluids may be restricted to reduce the chance of fluid overload. Skin and mucous membranes are examined for signs of dehydration.

Elimination. A retention catheter is usually inserted in the older child, and a plastic collection bag is placed on the infant or small child. The child with bowel and bladder control is generally incontinent. The collecting devices help keep the skin clean and provide a means for obtaining an accurate intake and output measurement. If the child remains comatose for a long period of time, the indwelling catheter may be removed and periodic bladder emptying accomplished by pressure applied over the suprapubic area (Credé). Stool softeners are usually sufficient to maintain bowel function, but suppositories or enemas may be needed occasionally for adequate elimination.

Positioning and exercise. The unconscious child is positioned to prevent aspiration of saliva, nasogastric secretions, and vomitus and to minimize intracranial pressure. The head of the bed is slightly elevated, and the child is placed on the side or in a semiprone position. A small, firm pillow is placed under the head, and the uppermost limbs are flexed and supported with pillows. The weight of the body should not rest on the dependent arm. In the semiprone position the child lies with the dependent arm at the side behind the body and the opposite side supported on pillows with the uppermost arm and leg flexed and resting on the pillows. This position prevents undo pressure on the dependent extremities. The dependent position of the face encourages drainage of secretions and prevents the flaccid tongue from obstructing the airway.

Normal range of motion exercises are carried out to maintain function and prevent contractures of joints. Exercises should be performed gently and with full range of motion. A small rolled pad can be placed in the palms to help maintain proper position of fingers; footboards or boots can be used to help prevent footdrop, and sometimes splinting may be needed to prevent severe contractures of the wrist, knee, or ankle in decerebrate children.

Medications. The cause of unconsciousness determines specific drug therapies. Children with infectious processes are given antibiotics appropriate to the disease and the infecting organism, and corticosteroids are prescribed for inflammatory conditions and edema. Cerebral edema is an indication for osmotherapy with osmotic diuretics and/or hypertonic glucose solution. Sedatives are often indicated for extreme restlessness, agitation, and hyperresponsiveness to stimuli. Sedatives or anticonvulsants are prescribed for seizure activity. The unconscious child requires stool softeners to maintain bowel function.

Medications such as antibiotics and corticosteroids may be ordered intravenously during the early days of unconsciousness. When nasogastric or gastrostomy feedings are implemented, most medications are given by this route. It is particularly important to be alert to signs of adverse drug reactions, since many of the side effects or toxic effects of drugs involve observation of changes in behavior or responsiveness, which are rendered invalid by the child's unconscious state.

Stimulation. Sensory stimulation is important in the care of the unconscious child, just as it is in the care of the alert child. For the temporarily unconscious or semiconscious child, sensory stimulation helps to arouse him to the conscious state and orient him in terms of time and place. Unconscious children need sensory stimulation as much as conscious children. Auditory and tactile stimulation are especially valuable. Tactile stimulation is not appropriate for the child in whom it may elicit an undesirable response. However, for other children, tactile contact often has a relaxing and calming effect. When the child's condition permits, holding or rocking the child has a soothing effect on the child and provides the body contact needed by young children.

The auditory sense is often present in a state of coma. Hearing is the last sense to be lost and the first sense to be regained; therefore, the child should be spoken to as any other child. Conversation around the child should not include thoughtless or derogatory remarks. A radio playing soft music, a music box, or a record player is frequently employed to provide auditory stimulation. Singing the child's favorite songs or reading a favorite story within his hearing is a tactic used to maintain his contact with a familiar world.

Above all, it is important to remember that this is a child who has all the needs of any ill child.

Parents. Dealing with the parents of an unconscious child is especially difficult. They may demonstrate all the

Summary of nursing care of the unconscious child

Goals	Responsibilities

Maintain patent airway	Position to prevent aspiration
	  Semiprone position
	  Side-lying position
	Aspirate airway as needed
	Insert oral airway if indicated
	Administer care of endotracheal tube or tracheostomy if appropriate; have equipment available for emergency insertion if indicated for respiratory distress

Minimize intracranial pressure	Elevate head of the bed 10 to 15 degrees Avoid pressure on neck veins

Prevent cerebral hypoxia	Maintain patent airway
	Provide oxygen as indicated by objective signs or as ordered
	If on mechanical ventilation
	  Monitor for
	    Correct settings
	    Proper functioning
	  Prepare to provide artificial ventilation in case of ventilatory failure; have AMBU bag at hand
	Administer medications as ordered to prevent cerebral edema and improve cerebral circulation

Detect early signs of cerebral hypoxemia	Monitor vital signs Observe changes in color of face, lips, extremities Observe for changes in responsiveness Observe for seizure activity

Assess neurologic status	Monitor vital signs as ordered
	  Temperature
	  Pulse quality, rate, rhythm
	  Respirations—rate, rhythm, depth
	  Blood pressure
	  Pulse pressure
	Check pupillary reaction
	  Size
	  Reaction to light and accommodation
	  Equality of responses
	Note and describe
	  Voluntary movements of extremities, for example, purposeful, random
	  Changes in muscular tone
	  Changes in position of body and/or head
	  Tremor, twitching
	  Seizure activity, for example, generalized or focal
	  Signs of meningeal irritation, for example, nuchal rigidity, opisthotonos
	In infants measure occipital-frontal circumference
	  Assess status of fontanel—full or sunken, tense or soft

Assess level of consciousness	Observe and record
	  Changes in spontaneous behavior
	  Resistance to care
	  Response to verbal commands
	  Response to noxious stimuli
	  Type of verbalization or crying

Summary of nursing care of the unconscious child—cont'd

Goals	Responsibilities
Prevent cerebral edema	Monitor fluid intake and output Observe for signs of impending overhydration and take appropriate action Administer osmotic diuretics and/or hypertonic glucose as ordered Administer corticosteroids as ordered Weigh daily or as ordered to detect fluid accumulation or reduction
Prevent or control hyperthermia	Assess temperature regularly to detect elevation Remove excess coverings Administer tepid sponge bath for elevated temperature Apply and monitor hypothermia blanket if indicated or ordered
Assist with diagnostic tests	Collect specimens as ordered Carry out examinations as indicated or ordered, such as urine specific gravity, blood samples Prepare for and assist with diagnostic procedures, such as lumbar puncture, x-ray examination Interpret and report results of tests
Prevent respiratory complications	Position for optimum ventilation Turn frequently—at least every 2 hours Avoid contact with persons with upper respiratory infection Maintain patent airway Perform percussion, vibration, and suctioning every 3 to 4 hours Remove accumulated secretions promptly Provide good oral hygiene
Maintain skin integrity	Place child on sheepskin, egg-carton pad, or other resilient surface Change position frequently Protect pressure points, for example, trochanter, sacrum, ankle, shoulder, occiput Inspect skin surfaces regularly for signs of irritation, redness, evidence of pressure Cleanse skin regularly, at least once daily Protect skin folds and surfaces that rub together Keep clothing and linen clean and dry Apply urine collecting device or insert indwelling catheter (if ordered) to prevent irritation from urine Proper care of catheter Carry out good perineal care under collection device Stimulate circulation by gentle rubbing with lotion, cornstarch, or other lubricating substance Protect lips with cream, glycerine, or ointment
Protect from injury	Keep side rails up Pad hard surfaces that may injure extremities during spontaneous or involuntary movements Place protective device between teeth if biting movements occur during seizure Administer sedatives or anticonvulsants as prescribed
Maintain limb flexibility and function	Perform passive range of motion exercises Position to reduce contractures—splint contracting joints if needed
Provide nutrition and hydration	Monitor intravenous feedings when ordered Feed prescribed formula by means of nasogastric or gastrostomy tube

Continued.

Summary of nursing care of the unconscious child—cont'd

Goals	Responsibilities
Assure adequate elimination	Provide sufficient liquid intake, unless contraindicated by cerebral edema or if overhydration is threat Administer stool softener Administer suppositories or enema as indicated
Prevent overstimulation	Avoid stimulation that precipitates undesirable responses Time nursing activities for minimal disturbance
Provide sensory stimulation	Provide tactile stimulation (if it does not wake undesirable muscle response, for example, seizures) Provide auditory stimulation by voice, radio, music box, and so on Provide visual stimuli appropriate for age Provide proprioceptive stimulation by rocking, cuddling, and so on
Support parents	Explain therapies; clarify and reinforce information given to family by physician Interpret child's behaviors and responses Allow expression of feelings and concerns Accept aggressive behavior
Assist in child placement	Provide needed information Answer parents' questions Refer to persons or agencies for further information and clarification Support parents' decision
Arrange for discharge and follow-up care	Teach parents techniques and procedures needed in care of child (if appropriate) Arrange for follow-up visit by appropriate persons, for example, public health nurse

guilt, fear, and anxiety of any parent of a seriously ill child. In addition they are faced with the uncertain outcome of the cerebral dysfunction. The fear of death, mental retardation, or other permanent disability, is present. Nursing intervention with parents depends on the nature of the pathology, the personality of the parents, and the parent-child relationship prior to injury or illness.

The child may regain consciousness within a short period of time. If there is little or no residual effect, the child will be dismissed to home care fairly soon. The parents need the most intensive nursing intervention during the period of crisis and uncertainty. During the recovery phase they are given information, information is clarified, and they are encouraged to become involved in the child's care. Often the child's hospitalization is brief; however, some children require extended hospitalization for intensive therapy and rehabilitation.

The parents of children who succumb within hours or days require the support and guidance that the parents of any dying child would (see Chapter 27) in coping with the reality and resolving their grief.

Probably the most difficult situations are those that involve children who are unconscious permanently or for an indefinite period. Unlike parents who lose a child through death, the finality is lacking for these parents, often leaving them in a state of suspended grief.[31] The presence of the child renders the parents unable to resolve the loss. Like parents of dying children, parents of the comatose child search for any signs of hope. Well-meaning friends and relatives relate instances of miraculous recoveries. The parents seek confirmation and support for such possibilities and assign erroneous meanings to any sign in the child, such as muscle contractions, that might be interpreted as evidence of recovery.

In her observations of families of comatose children, Surveyer[31,32] found that these parents display the feelings and behaviors associated with dying children or the birth of a defective child, including guilt, anger, and hostility.

These feelings may be directed toward the person that the parents believe is responsible for the child's state; toward other children who are well, expressed by envy of the children and their parents; or toward themselves for real or imagined neglect of the unconscious child. Often the aggression is directed toward those who are needed for support, such as the spouse, the child who is unable to respond, or the personnel caring for the child.

Surveyer also observed that, like parents who lose a child through death, the parents of the child lost to their world attempt to reconstitute a representation of the child. They bring items that belong to the child, such as favorite toys, music, and other objects cherished by the child. This is interpreted as an attempt to provide stimulation for the child in the hope of eliciting a response, to let the hospital staff know the child as the unique individual he was so that the parents' distress can be better appreciated, and to reconstitute an image of the child "lost" to them and for whom they mourn. An awareness of these behaviors and coping mechanisms provides nurses with the understanding that helps them support the parents in their grief process.

Superimposed on the process of grieving for the "lost" child, parents may be faced with difficult decisions. First there is the child whose brain is so severely damaged that his vital functions must be maintained by artificial means. When brain death has been determined according to established criteria, the parents must make the final decision to remove the life-support systems. Sometimes parents may even choose to refuse treatment if they believe it to be best for the child and the family (informed dissent).[4] Second there is the child who has survived the illness or injury that produced the brain damage but who is left unconscious permanently. These parents must decide whether to place the child in a rest home or other institution for comatose children or make arrangements to care for the child at home. During these decisions the nurse can listen to their discussions regarding alternatives, provide information where appropriate, and support the family in their decision. Once the decision has been made, the nurse can help the family prepare for the transfer of the child and make referrals to persons or agencies that can provide additional assistance.

The parents who choose to care for their child at home will need education and support in learning to care for the child, regular follow-up observation and assessment of the home management, and planning for some respite care of the child. Parents need to understand that it is important to plan for periodic relief from the continual care of the child.

For a summary of the nursing care of the unconscious child, see the boxed material on pp. 1418 to 1420.

CRANIOCEREBRAL TRAUMA

Accidental injury is the major single cause of death in the pediatric age-group, and, although it cannot be stated with certainty, most of these injuries are probably the result of central nervous system trauma. Whereas serious injury contributes significantly to childhood mortality and morbidity, the majority of accidental head traumas do not leave the injured child with permanent neurologic impairment. Rarely does a child attain adulthood without having sustained a significant bump or blow to the head. Most do not require hospitalization, but it is estimated that 200,000 children are admitted to hospitals each year for evaluation and treatment of head injury. Of these, approximately 5% to 10% exhibit neurologic signs.[6]

Head injury can be defined as any pathologic process involving the scalp, skull, meninges, or brain as the result of mechanical force. The exposed nature of the head renders it particularly vulnerable to external violence, and many of the physical characteristics of children predispose to craniocerebral trauma. For example, infants are frequently left unattended on beds, in high chairs, and in other places from which they can fall. Also, the proportionately larger and heavier head of the infant and toddler is a body part frequently traumatized in a fall. Incomplete motor development contributes to falls at all ages, and the natural curiosity, exuberance, and exploring nature of children frequently place them in situations in which they are more likely to incur an accidental injury.

Falls are the most frequent nonfatal accident in children under 1 year of age, about 75% of which result in some type of head trauma.[21] As in all childhood accidents, head injury involves boys almost twice as often as girls, which is probably a reflection of the more aggressive and venturesome behavior of boys as compared with that of girls. The highest incidence occurs during the ages of 8 to 9 years, with a secondary peak incidence in boys at around 12 to 13 years of age. Because of the relative frequency of craniocerebral injuries in the pediatric age-groups and the potential for damaging sequelae, they present a common and serious clinical entity.

Etiology

Falls are the leading cause of head injury, followed by motor vehicle accidents. Falls are diverse in nature. Some children fall while standing, running, or riding on play equipment such as wagons, skateboards, or tricycles. Others fall from furniture, fences, trees, horses, swings, ladders, or other structures. Motor vehicle accidents involve children as pedestrians who are struck by the vehicle or as passengers who sustain direct trauma or trauma from blows by objects within the vehicle or who fall from the vehicle. Other head injuries are sustained by widely diverse means, such as being hit by a baseball, kicked by a horse, or receiving blows from a variety of objects. Children often run into an object or another person. Bicycle injuries are not uncommon, with the child either falling from the bicycle or being struck by a motor vehicle. There is also a high incidence of head injury associated with other manifestations of battering (see p. 594). Vigorous shaking of an infant can cause central nervous system damage, especially a whiplash type of injury.

Pathophysiology

The skull forms such an excellent protection for the brain that, although nervous tissue is delicate, it usually requires a severe blow to cause significant damage. However, the protective mechanisms vary between individuals and are also influenced by age. For example, a small child's resilient skull may withstand a blow that would be severely damaging to an aged individual. The elastic, pliable skulls of infants and young children absorb much of the direct energy of physical impact to the head and afford some protection to intracranial structures.

Physical forces act on the head through *acceleration, deceleration,* or *deformation.*[22] Injury occurs by way of compression, tearing, or shearing, either singly, in combination, or in succession. Acceleration or deceleration is more descriptive of the circumstances responsible for most head injuries. When the stationary head receives a blow, the sudden acceleration causes deformation of the skull and mass movement of the brain. Continued movement of the intracranial contents allows the brain to strike parts of the skull (such as the sharp edges of the sphenoid or the irregular surface of the anterior fossa) or the edges of the tentorium. Although the brain volume remains unchanged, significant distortion and cavitation take place as it changes shape in response to the force transmitted from the impact to the skull.[6,22] This deformation can cause bruising at the point of impact *(coup)* and/or at a distance as the brain collides with the unyielding surfaces far removed from the point of impact *(contrecoup)* (Fig. 37-3). Part of the changes related to this phenomenon may be a result of a momentary increased pressure that produces a temporary negative pressure with cavitation and vaporization contralaterally. Thus a blow to the occipital region can cause severe injury to the frontal and temporal areas of the brain. Sudden deceleration, such as takes place during a fall, causes the greatest cerebral injury at the point of impact.

Another effect of brain movement is shearing stresses, which are caused by unequal movement or different rates of acceleration at various levels of the brain. A shearing force may tear small arteries that travel from the cerebral surfaces through the meninges to the dural sinuses to cause subdural hemorrhages. Shearing or stretching effects can also be transmitted to nerve fibers. Although shearing forces are maximal at the cerebral surface and extend toward the center of rotation within the brain, the most serious effects are frequently in the area of the brain stem.

Another source of damage occurs when severe compression of the skull causes the brain to be forced through the tentorial opening. This can produce irreparable damage to the brain stem (Fig. 37-4).

As a whole, head injuries can be regarded as localized or generalized. In localized injuries the force is spent on a local area of both skull and underlying tissues; in generalized injuries the force is transmitted to the entire skull, causing widespread movement, distortion, and damage. Local injuries frequently cause hemorrhage and infection, but generalized trauma is associated with a higher mortality. Many head injuries involve both localized and general-

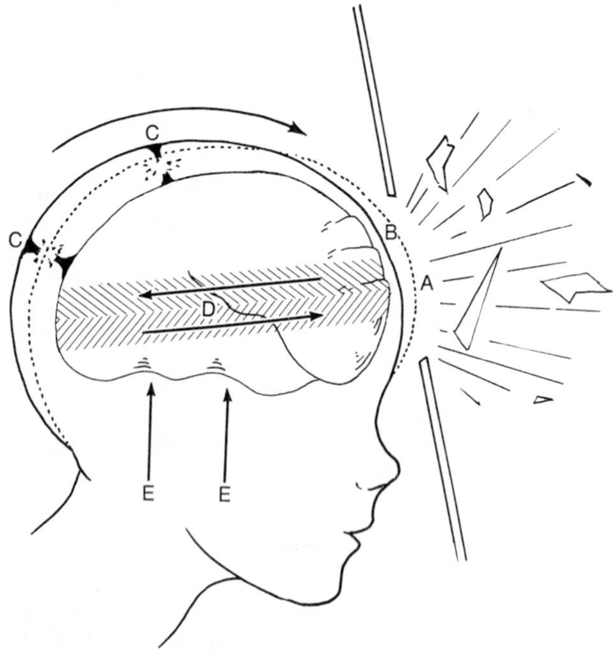

Fig. 37-3. Mechanical distortions of cranium during closed head injury. **A,** Preinjury contour of skull. **B,** Immediate postinjury contour of the skull. **C,** Torn subdural vessels. **D,** Shearing forces. **E,** Trauma from contact with floor of cranium. (Redrawn from Grubb, R. L., and Coxe, W. S.: Central nervous system trauma: cranial. In Eliasson, S. G., Prensky, A. L., and Hardin, W. B., Jr., editors: Neurological pathophysiology, New York, 1974, Oxford University Press.)

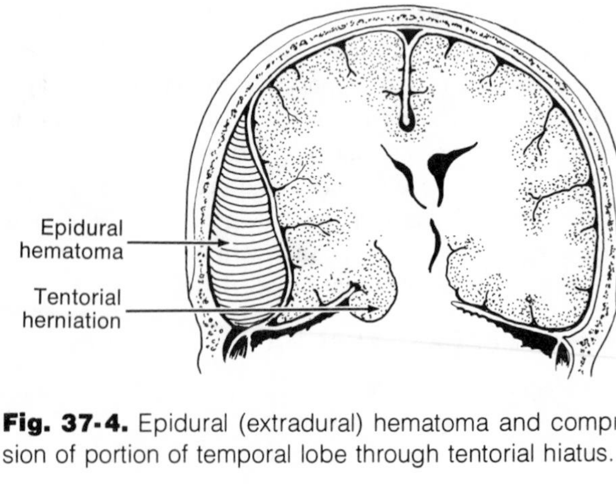

Fig. 37-4. Epidural (extradural) hematoma and compression of portion of temporal lobe through tentorial hiatus.

ized pathology. The physical processes cause numerous pathologic changes that produce several clinical syndromes.

Concussion. The most common head injury is concussion, a transient and reversible neuronal dysfunction with instantaneous loss of awareness and responsiveness from trauma to the head that persists for a relatively short time, usually minutes or hours. It is generally followed by amnesia for the moment of the injury and a variable period prior to the injury. This posttraumatic amnesia is characteristic and reflects the extent and severity of injury to the brain after blunt trauma. Posttraumatic amnesia consists of two parts: (1) retrograde amnesia, the period of time prior to impact for which the patient has no memory, and (2) anterograde amnesia, the period of memory loss after injury. Amnesia in both of these periods tends to lessen with time, although there is some permanent amnesia.[6,21]

The pathogenesis of concussion is still unclear but may be a result of shearing forces that cause stretching, compression, and tearing of nerve fibers, particularly in the area of the central brain stem, the seat of the reticular activating system. It has also been suggested that the anatomic alterations of nerve fibers cause the release of large quantities of acetylcholine into the cerebrospinal fluid and a reduction in oxygen consumption with increased lactate production.[6,22]

Contusion and laceration. The terms contusion and laceration are used to describe visible bruising and tearing of cerebral tissue. Contusions represent petechial hemorrhages along the superficial aspects of the brain at the site of impact (coup injury) and/or a lesion remote from the site of direct trauma (contrecoup injury). In serious accidents there may be multiple sites of injury. The more common points of injury are the poles and undersurfaces of frontal and temporal lobes. Contusions may cause focal disturbances in strength, sensation, or visual awareness. The degree of brain damage in the contused areas varies according to the extent of vascular injury. Signs will vary from mild transient weakness of a limb to prolonged unconsciousness and paralysis. As a rule, contusions are less common in infants and young children than in adults with comparable trauma, and contrecoup injuries are relatively rare in infants.[22]

Cerebral lacerations are generally associated with penetrating or depressed skull fractures. However, they may occur without fracture in small children. When brain tissue is actually torn, with bleeding into and around the tear, there are usually more severe and prolonged unconsciousness and paralysis that leave permanent scarring and some degree of disability.

Fractures. The immature skull, because of its flexibility, is able to sustain a greater degree of deformation than the adult skull before it incurs a fracture. It requires a great deal of force to produce a fracture in the skull of an infant. A fracture may occur with little or no brain damage, or severe and fatal brain injury can take place without fracture. The undersurface of the skull contains grooves in which the meningeal arteries lie. A fracture that runs through one of these grooves may tear the artery and produce severe and damaging hemorrhage.

The majority of skull fractures (about 70%) are linear. The lines of the fracture are predetermined by the site and velocity of the impact as well as the strength of the bone. Linear fractures are often asymptomatic in older children and heal in 3 to 4 months without special treatment, unless they involve a blood vessel, enter the paranasal sinuses, or impinge on the brain stem or cranial nerves. The location of the fracture often provides clues to the possibility of such complications. For example, a fracture that extends through the squamous portion of the temporal bone is more apt to be associated with laceration of the middle meningeal artery, and fractures extending through the base of the skull may cause leakage of cerebrospinal fluid and/or blood into either the auditory or nasal passages. In infants the uneven ossification and the absence of buttresses cause fracture lines to be irregular, following no predictable pattern.[6]

Depressed fractures are those in which the bone is locally broken usually into several irregular fragments that are pushed inward, causing pressure on the brain. The inner portion of the bone is more extensively fragmented than the outer portion, which almost invariably produces tears in the dura. Both linear and comminuted depressed fractures are uncommon before 2 to 3 years of age. In infants and very young children, the soft, malleable bone may become dented in a peculiar rounded or "Ping-Pong ball" depression without laceration of either skin or dura. These are encountered occasionally in difficult deliveries, resulting from either pressure of the head against the pelvis or incorrect application of forceps.

As a rule, the faster the blow, the greater the likelihood of a depressed fracture; a low-velocity impact tends to produce a linear fracture.[22]

Complications of head injuries

The major complications of trauma to the head are hemorrhage, infection, edema, and tentorial herniation. Infection is always a hazard in open injuries, and edema is related to tissue trauma. Vascular rupture may occur even in minor head injuries, causing hemorrhage between the skull and cerebral surfaces. Compression of the underlying brain produces effects that can be rapidly fatal or insidiously progressive.

Epidural hemorrhage. Epidural (extradural) hemorrhage is usually secondary to rupture of the middle meningeal artery, most often as a result of skull fracture that penetrates the groove in the skull occupied by the artery. However, a child's skull can be indented with sufficient force to tear the middle meningeal artery and then rebound intact without causing a fracture. Hemorrhage can also derive from dural veins or the dural sinuses, especially in infants and small children, in whom fracture is less likely to occur. In

20% to 40% of children a skull fracture is not detectable.[22] The blood accumulates between the dura and the skull to form a hematoma, which, because of the difficulty with which dura is stripped from bone, forces the underlying brain contents downward and inward as they expand (Fig. 37-4). Since bleeding is generally arterial, brain compression occurs rapidly. Most often the expanding hematoma is located in the parietotemporal region, forcing the medial portion of the temporal lobe under the edge of the tentorium, where it causes pressure on nerves and blood vessels. Pressure on the arterial supply and venous return to the reticular formation causes loss of consciousness; pressure on cranial nerve III (oculomotor nerve) produces dilatation and (later) fixation of the ipsilateral pupil. Pressure on the fibers of the pyramidal tract is evidenced by contralateral weakness or paralysis and increased deep tendon reflexes. Extreme pressure may extend to the brain stem to cause decerebrate signs and disturbances in the respiratory and other vegetative centers.

The classic clinical picture of epidural hemorrhage is one in which the individual loses consciousness momentarily or is merely stunned by the injury and is then free of symptoms (the lucid period). Within a few minutes or hours (occasionally days), he develops signs and symptoms of intracranial compression. Sometimes signs of increased pressure develop without evidence of a lucid period, however. Clinical signs include headache, vomiting, hemiparesis, and progressive loss of consciousness with focal neurologic signs as described previously. As a rule, the longer the period of consciousness after injury, the slower the accumulation of blood and the better the chances for recovery. Treatment is operative removal of the blood clot.[6]

In children this classic picture is seldom evident. The period of impaired consciousness is frequently lacking, and the symptom-free period is atypical because of nonspecific complaints such as irritability, headache, and vomiting. It frequently lasts longer than 48 hours. Clinically significant epidural hematomas are uncommon in children younger than 4 years of age. These differences may be caused by the decreased tendency of the resilient skull to fracture; the ability of blood to escape through widened sutures, an open fontanel, or a fracture; bleeding from smaller vessels with less rapid and massive bleeding; lower systolic blood pressure in children; and, possibly, the brain being less susceptible to pressure changes in children.[25]

Subdural hemorrhage. A subdural hemorrhage is bleeding between the dura and the cerebrum, usually as a result of rupture of cortical veins that bridge the subdural space (Fig. 37-5). Unlike epidural hemorrhage, which develops inwardly, subdural hemorrhage tends to develop more slowly and spreads thinly and widely until it is limited by the dural barriers—the falx and tentorium. Subdural hematoma is fairly common in infants, frequently as the result of birth trauma.

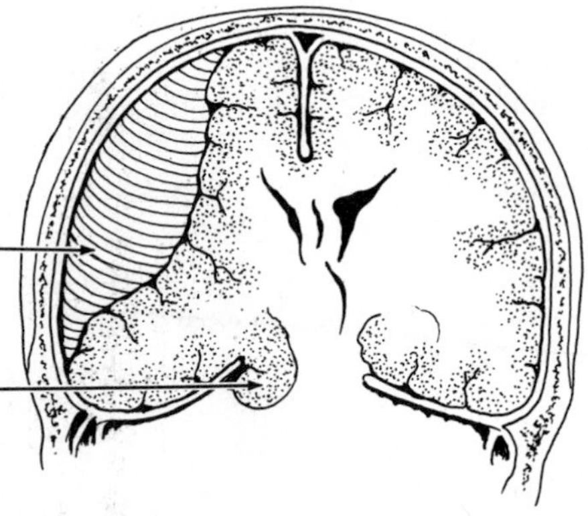

Fig. 37-5. Subdural hematoma.

Subdural hemorrhage can cause either acute or chronic subdural hematoma. Acute subdural hematoma may be associated with contusions or lacerations, but chronic subdural hematoma is more common. The clinical course and manifestations are variable and depend on the damage sustained by the brain substance and the age of the child. Delayed symptoms are common in children with open fontanels and sutures. The most common presenting manifestations in children are seizures, vomiting, and irritability, drowsiness, or other personality changes. Older children may complain of headache. Less common signs are developmental retardation and failure to thrive. Presenting signs include evidence of increased intracranial pressure such as increased head size and bulging fontanels (in the infant), retinal hemorrhages, extraocular palsies (especially cranial nerve VI), hemiparesis, quadriplegia, and sometimes fever. Older children may display an unsteady gait, and papilledema is usually present. In infants the bleeding may be extensive enough to lower the hematocrit significantly.[16,25]

Repeated subdural taps often provide relief in the infant. Surgical evacuation of the hematoma is the treatment in the older child and is frequently required in infants.

Other hemorrhagic lesions. Subarachnoid and intracerebral hemorrhages may occur as the result of head injury. Seizures, nuchal rigidity, and altered consciousness are features of subarachnoid hemorrhage. Manifestations of intracranial bleeding depend on the size and location of the resulting hematoma.

Cerebral edema. Some degree of brain swelling is expected after craniocerebral trauma and often accompanies any of the previous disorders. Cerebral edema caused by direct cellular injury or vascular injury induces vascular stasis, anoxia, and further vasodilatation. Increased tissue pressure within the skull causes venules to collapse, which leads to venous stasis and tissue anoxia. This results in loss of selective permeability of tissue membranes with increased loss of fluid from the vascular compartment to the cerebral tissues, thereby increasing cerebral edema. Thus a self-perpetuating sequence of events is repeated. If this progression continues unchecked, intracranial pressure exceeds arterial pressure and fatal anoxia ensues and/or the pressure causes herniation of a portion of the brain over the edge of the tentorium, compressing the brain stem and occluding the posterior cerebral arteries.[22]

Posttraumatic syndromes. Posttraumatic seizures occur in a number of children who survive a head injury. They are more common in young children and in those who sustain cerebral lacerations. The onset may be in the first 24 hours, usually within the first year, and in most cases within 2 years after the injury.

Structural complications may occur as the result of head injuries. Hydrocephalus is seen when there has been subarachnoid hemorrhage or infection. Focal deficits, including optic atrophy, cranial nerve palsies, motor deficits, diabetes insipidus, or aphasia, may be seen. The type of residual effect depends on the location and nature of the trauma.

Postconcussion syndrome is a common sequela to brain injury, and the manifestations vary with the age of the child. Most often there are behavioral disturbances (such as aggressiveness, withdrawal, and regression), sleep disturbances, phobias, emotional lability, irritability, and alterations in school performance.

Some children younger than 3 years of age develop a fluid-filled cyst, or cephalhydrocele, after a linear fracture. This occurs as a result of a tear in the dura and arachnoid or because a piece of arachnoid is entrapped between bone fragments, causing cerebrospinal fluid to accumulate beneath the scalp.

True mental retardation occurs only after severe injuries.

Diagnostic evaluation

A detailed history, both past and present, is essential in evaluating the child with craniocerebral trauma. It is important to know whether the child suffers from disorders such as drug allergies, hemophilia, diabetes mellitus, or epilepsy, which might assist in diagnosis. Also, events surrounding the injury often supply significant data. For example, if a child stumbles and falls while running and strikes his head on the sidewalk, it is usually safe to assume the neurologic manifestations to be a direct result of the injury. However, if he sinks to the sidewalk and, in doing so, strikes his head, there may be other causes that contributed to the injury. Sometimes a traumatic injury, even a minor one, will aggravate a preexisting disease process, thereby producing neurologic signs out of proportion to the injury.[6]

It is determined whether or not the infant or child exhibited alterations in consciousness. Usually this is easily elicited from older children, but in young children it may be difficult to differentiate from a breath-holding spell or a seizure. The parents of infants are asked if the infant cried immediately after the injury. After a minor injury, initial unconsciousness (if present) is brief and the child will ordinarily exhibit a transient period of confusion, somnolence, and listlessness, most often accompanied by irritability, pallor, and one or more episodes of vomiting.

A severe head injury, such as one sustained in a fall from a significant height or a motor vehicle accident, requires prompt evaluation and treatment. Since head injuries are frequently accompanied by injuries in other areas (for example, spine, viscera, extremities), the examination is performed with care to avoid further injuries.

Initial assessment. The initial assessment of the child with a head injury is carried out quickly in relation to vital signs, level of consciousness, and ocular signs. It is not uncommon for excited and irritable children to have a rapid pulse, hyperventilate, appear pale, and feel clammy shortly after an injury. However, deep, rapid, periodic, or intermittent and gasping respirations, wide fluctuations or noticeable slowing of the pulse, and widening pulse pressure or marked fluctuations in blood pressure are signs of brain stem involvement. Marked hypotension may represent internal injuries.[25]

Ocular signs such as fixed and dilated pupils, fixed and constricted pupils, and pupils that are poorly reactive or unreactive to light indicate increased intracranial pressure or brain stem involvement. Ophthalmic examination may reveal retinal changes. Dilated, nonpulsating blood vessels give evidence of increased intracranial pressure before the appearance of papilledema. Retinal hemorrhages are seen in acute head injuries.

Less urgent but important additional assessments include examination of the scalp for lacerations as well as palpation for depressed skull fractures, widely separated sutures, and the size and tension of fontanels, which indicate intracranial hemorrhage or rapidly developing cerebral edema. Bleeding from the nose or ears (although uncommon in children) needs further evaluation, and a watery discharge from the nose (rhinorrhea) that is positive for glucose, as tested with Dextrostix, suggests leaking of cerebrospinal fluid from a skull fracture. Injury to the skin, extremities, and abdomen is not uncommon after severe blunt head trauma and must be ruled out by sensory examination in children with altered motor function. Testing reflexes provides information about cerebral and pyramidal involvement, although transient abnormalities of the abdominal reflexes and Babinski's sign may be present in children with mild head trauma. Conscious, cooperative children are examined for cerebellar signs such as ataxia. However, it is not uncommon for children to display unsteadiness, clumsiness, and tremor on intentional movement after head injury.

Temperature may be moderately elevated for a day or two following an initial mild hypothermia after injury. A persistent fever may indicate subarachnoid hemorrhage or infection.

An accurate assessment of these various clinical signs provides baseline information. Serial evaluations, preferably by a single observer, help to detect changes in the neurologic status. Alterations in mental status, evidenced by increased difficulty in rousing the child, mounting agitation, development of focal lateral neurologic signs, or marked changes in vital signs, usually indicate extension or progression of the basic pathologic process.

Special tests. After a thorough clinical examination, a variety of diagnostic tests are helpful in providing a more definitive diagnosis of the type and extent of the trauma. Skull x-ray films and other radiographic tests are indicated, especially when the patient has lost consciousness after injury. Echoencephalography, radioisotope scan, and cerebral angiography may contribute to diagnosis and management. Electroencephalography is not particularly helpful for early diagnosis but is useful for defining seizure activity or focal destructive lesions after the acute phase of illness. Lumbar puncture is rarely employed in craniocerebral trauma and is contraindicated in the presence of increased intracranial pressure.

Where available, computerized axial tomography (CAT) is especially valuable in diagnosis of neurologic trauma and usually makes other diagnostic procedures unnecessary. It is easily carried out, is noninvasive, and can be repeated serially for reassessment in the patient who remains unconscious or shows progressive neurologic deterioration.

In the infant or small child a subdural tap through a fontanel or coronal suture may establish the diagnosis of subdural or epidural hemorrhage. In some centers monitoring intracranial pressure is part of the assessment.[7]

Classification. Since the course and prognosis of the child depends on the nature and severity of the craniocerebral trauma, the injuries are sometimes classified as mild, moderate, or severe.[25]

mild craniocerebral trauma alterations or loss of consciousness (if it occurs) is brief, lasting from a few seconds to a few minutes. The posttraumatic period is characterized by mild headache, irritability, drowsiness, and, occasionally, vomiting. The child is easily roused from sleep.

moderate craniocerebral trauma alterations or loss of consciousness lasts several minutes to an hour. Frequently abnormal, but often transient, abnormal neurologic signs are present. The posttraumatic period is characterized by more severe headache, irritability, somnolence, and confusion. Usually mild to moderate fever and vomiting are present for 12 to 36 hours.

severe craniocerebral trauma unconsciousness lasts for an hour or longer; sudden or progressive deterioration of level of consciousness occurs after an initial lucid period. Abnormal neurologic signs persist for hours or are permanent. In the patient who regains consciousness, posttraumatic signs include severe unremitting headache, mental confusion, vomiting, and marked fluctuations in level of consciousness.

Medical management

The majority of children with mild to moderate concussion who have not lost consciousness can be cared for and observed at home after careful examination reveals no serious intracranial injury. The parents are instructed to check the child every 2 hours to determine any changes in responsiveness. The sleeping child should be wakened to see if he can be roused normally. Parents are advised to maintain contact with the attending physician, who usually wishes to examine the child again in 1 or 2 days. The manifestations of epidural hematoma in children do not generally appear until 24 hours or more after injury. The importance of maintaining contact for continued observation and reevaluation when indicated facilitates early diagnosis and treatment of possible complications such as hematoma, hydrocephalus, cysts, and posttraumatic seizures. Children with minor injuries who live a significant distance from medical facilities or whose parents or care giver is not deemed reliable in observing their condition are generally hospitalized for 24 to 48 hours for observation.[6,25]

Children with severe injuries, those who have lost consciousness for more than a few minutes, and those with prolonged and continued seizures or other focal or diffuse neurologic signs must be hospitalized until their condition is stable and their neurologic signs have diminished.

The child is maintained on clear liquids, if he is able to take fluids by mouth, until it is determined that vomiting will not occur. Intravenous fluids are indicated in the child who is comatose or displays dulled sensorium and/or in the child with persistent vomiting. The volume of intravenous fluid is carefully monitored to avoid aggravating any cerebral edema and to minimize the possibility of overhydration in case of inappropriate secretions of antidiuretic hormone. However, damage to the hypothalamus or pituitary may produce diabetes insipidus with its accompanying hypertonicity and dehydration. Fluid balance is closely monitored by daily weight, accurate intake and output measurement, and serum osmolality to detect early signs of water retention, excessive dehydration, and states of hypertonicity or hypotonicity.

Restlessness can be satisfactory managed, if necessary, with diphenhydramine (Benadryl) or chloral hydrate, and headache is usually controlled with aspirin in age-appropriate dosages. Anticonvulsants are employed for seizure control and, frequently, in cases of suspected contusion or laceration. Antibiotics are administered if there are lacerations, cerebrospinal fluid leakage, or excessive cerebral tissue damage. Prophylactic tetanus toxoid is given for open scalp wounds and if the child has not received a booster within 4 years.

Cerebral edema is managed as described for the unconscious child, including administration of corticosteroids and hypertonic solutions. Hyperthermia is controlled with tepid sponges.

Surgical therapy. Scalp lacerations are sutured after careful examination of underlying bone. Depressed fractures require surgical reduction and removal of bone fragments. Torn dura is sutured. Ping-Pong ball skull fractures in very young infants ordinarily correct themselves within a few weeks and do not require specific treatment.

Prognosis. The outcome of craniocerebral trauma depends on the extent of injury and complications. However, the outlook is generally more favorable for children than for adults. Over 90% of children with concussions or simple linear fractures recover without symptoms after the initial period. The incidence of fatalities and neurologic sequelae is lower in children, even in those with severe head injuries.[22]

Nursing considerations

Since all but the most minor head injuries are managed in the hospital, close observation of the child by the nurse is essential. Careful neurologic assessment and evaluation, including vital signs, repeated at frequent intervals provide information needed to establish a correct diagnosis, determine clinical management, and prevent many complications.

The child is placed on bed rest, usually with the head of the bed elevated slightly, and appropriate safety measures, such as side rails kept up for older children and seizure precautions for children of all ages, are implemented. The extremely restless child may require that hard surfaces be padded and the use of restraint to prevent the possibility of further injury. Care is individualized according to the specific needs of the child. The unconscious child is managed as described in the previous section, but most childhood head injuries are those causing momentary stunning or temporary unconsciousness. The child may be restless and irritable, but more often his reaction is to fall asleep when left undisturbed. A quiet environment helps reduce the restlessness and irritability. Bright lights shining directly into the child's face are irritating. This often makes checking the ocular responses more difficult to perform and more aggravating to the child.

Frequent examinations of vital signs, neurologic signs, and level of consciousness are extremely important nursing observations. When possible they should be performed by a single observer in order to better detect subtle changes that may indicate worsening of neurologic status. Pupils are checked for size, equality, and reaction to light. After the initial elevations usually seen after injury, the vital signs generally return to normal unless there is brain stem involvement. A rectal or axillary temperature is the safest method of measuring temperature, since seizures are not uncommon and vomiting is a frequent response in children, especially when the child is disturbed. Hand grasps and motor function, both spontaneous and elicited, are observed, evaluated relative to strength, and compared bilaterally.

Probably the most important nursing observation is assessment of the child's level of consciousness. Alterations in consciousness appear earlier in the progression of an injury than alterations of vital signs or focal neurologic signs (see p. 1411 for evaluation of responsiveness). Some expected responses may be interpreted as deviations from the normal. Frequent examinations of alertness are fatiguing to the child; therefore, he often desires to fall asleep, which may be confused with depressed consciousness. When left alone the child promptly dozes. It is not uncommon to observe ocular divergence through the partially closed eyelids. Also, the child may retch or vomit when aroused.

Observations of position and movement provide additional information. Any abnormal posturing is noted as well as whether or not it occurs continuously or intermittently. Does the movement involve all extremities or is it restricted to one side? Are the child's hand grips strong and equal in strength? Are there any signs of decerebrate or decorticate posturing? What is the child's response to stimulation? Is movement purposeful, random, or absent? Are movement and/or sensation equal on both sides or restricted to one side only?

The child may complain of headache or other discomfort. The child who is too young to describe a headache will be fussy and resist being handled. The child who suffers from vertigo will often assume a position and vigorously resist efforts to move him. Forcible movement causes him to vomit and display spontaneous nystagmus.[27] Seizures, relatively common in children with craniocerebral trauma, may be of any type but are more often generalized regardless of the type of injury. Any seizure activity should be carefully observed and described in detail. This includes type (tonic, clonic, generalized, focal), onset, body parts involved, behavior before and after the seizure, and circumstances that preceded the seizure, such as touching the child (see p. 1437).

Drainage from any orifice is noted. Bleeding from the ear suggests the possibility of a basal skull fracture. The amount and characteristics of the drainage are observed, and, since the auditory canal may be a source of infection, dry, sterile cotton can be placed loosely at the orifice and changed when soiled. Continued drainage of clear fluid from the nose is tested with Dextrostix and the amount and reaction recorded. Head trauma is frequently accompanied by other undetected injuries; therefore, any bruises, lacerations, or evidence of internal injuries or fractures of the extremities is noted and reported. Associated injuries are evaluated and treated appropriately.

The child is usually allowed clear liquids unless fluid is restricted. If the child has an intravenous infusion, it is maintained as prescribed. The diet is advanced to that appropriate for the child's age as soon as his condition permits. Intake and output are measured and recorded, and any incontinence of bowel or bladder is noted in the child who has been toilet trained.

The child should be observed for any unusual behavior,

Summary of nursing care of the child with craniocerebral trauma

Goals	Responsibilities
Protect from bodily injury	Maintain bed rest—head flat or slightly elevated Keep side rails up on beds of older children Apply padding around bed if child extremely agitated Place net over crib if indicated Apply restraints if needed in extremely restless children
Determine neurologic status Vital signs	Take frequently and report changes immediately—serious signs are: Rectal or axillary temperature—hypothermia or hyperthermia Pulse—rapid or slow for age; irregularities Respirations—rapid and shallow; slow and deep; intermittent Blood pressure—decreased (shock) or widening pulse pressure
Ocular signs	Pupil size—dilated; pinpoint; unequal Pupil reaction—sluggish; absent; different Position of globes—divergence; conjugate deviation; skewed Movement of globes—extraocular palsy; nystagmus; fixed gaze
Motor function	Spontaneous—normal but reduced; involuntary Evoked—purposeful; reflex withdrawal Paresis—mild or severe; flaccid, tonic, continuous, or transient Posturing—decerebrate states; any lateralized difference in function
Level of consciousness	Depressed—easily roused Stupor—difficulty in rousing Comatose—unable to rouse; roused only with painful stimuli Crying and speech—present or absent; conversant or confused; monosyllabic; jargon; type of cry—piercing, difficult to hear
Detect additional neurologic data Seizure activity	Observe and record Nature, onset, characteristic Precipitating factors Postictal behavior
Nuchal rigidity	Presence or absence
Drainage from orifice (nose, ear)	Note and record amount and characteristics of drainage Bloody Serosanguinous Clear
Enlarged head (infants)	Measure occipital-frontal circumference Check size and tension of fontanels
Headache	Note presence or absence Note type and location (if this information can be elicited) Determine if continuous or intermittent
Wounds	Describe location, extent, type
Vomiting	Note amount, kind, frequency Determine precipitating factors (such as movement)
Unusual behavior	Note nature and frequency Note circumstances related to behavior
Incontinence (in toilet-trained child)	Bowel; bladder Spontaneous or associated with other phenomena (such as seizure activity)
Cranial nerve dysfunction	Note disturbance of taste, smell, sight, hearing, facial sensation Note inability voluntarily to Roll eyes up, down, or to side Wrinkle forehead
Provide adequate nutrition and hydration	Provide clear liquids as ordered—that is, ad lib or restricted Progress to regular diet as tolerated and condition indicates

Summary of nursing care of the child with craniocerebral trauma—cont'd

Goals	Responsibilities
Prevent overhydration or dehydration	Measure accurately intake and output Provide fluids as prescribed Weigh daily if ordered If child has intravenous infusion, monitor to maintain as prescribed
Assist in definitive diagnosis	Collect specimens as needed Prepare child for diagnostic procedures Assist with procedures as needed Provide supportive care after procedure
Reduce restlessness and anxiety	Provide comfort and reassurance Administer sedatives as ordered
Prevent complications	Observe for early signs of complications, such as Shock—decreasing blood pressure; rapid, weak pulse; reduced sensorium Increased intracranial pressure—increased blood pressure, widening pulse pressure Infection—elevated temperature; nuchal rigidity, redness and swelling at wound site(s) Gastrointestinal bleeding—guaiac all stools and/or nasogastric aspirant Emotional disturbances
Prepare for discharge	Teach parents about observations to be made and what to report Make certain parents know how to contact appropriate persons if needed Instruct in administration of medication if ordered Arrange for follow-up care Appointment with clinic or physician's office Public health nurse referral if needed Refer to appropriate agencies, such as social service, for assistance if indicated

but interpretation of behavior should be made in relation to the child's normal behavior. For example, urinary incontinence during sleep would be of no consequence in a child who routinely wets the bed but would be highly significant for one who is always dry. Also, a child who is subject to nightmares might cry out and demonstrate agitated behavior at night.[27] Parents are valuable resources in evaluating objective behaviors of their children. Information obtained from parents at or shortly after admission is helpful in evaluating the child's behavior, for example, the ease with which the child is roused normally, his usual sleeping position, how much he sleeps during the day, motor activity of which he is capable (rolling over, sitting up, climbing), hearing and visual acuity, appetite, and manner of eating (spoon, bottle, cup). There would be less concern about a child who falls asleep several times during the day if this particular type of behavior is consistent with his usual behavior.

Children may require sedation for severe restlessness, aspirin for headache, and anticonvulsants to control seizure activity. They are rarely given central nervous system depressants.

When the child is discharged the parents are advised of probable posttraumatic symptoms that may be expected. They should understand observations that should be made and how to contact the physician, nurse, or health facility in case the child develops any unusual signs or symptoms. The importance of follow-up evaluation should be emphasized, and it is often advisable to refer the family to a public health agency for home follow-through to be certain that the child receives posthospital evaluation.

For a summary of nursing care of the child with craniocerebral trauma, see the boxed material.

Intracranial infections

The nervous system and its coverings are subject to infection by the same organisms that affect other organs of the body. However, the nervous system is limited in the ways in which it responds to injury. Infectious processes share virtually the same clinical and pathologic features. They differ primarily in the growth and virulence of the specific organism. It is generally difficult to distinguish between the various etiologic agents from clinical manifestations. Laboratory studies are needed to identify the causative agent. The inflammatory process can affect the meninges (meningitis), brain (encephalitis), or the spinal cord (myelitis).

The most common infection of the central nervous system is meningitis. Meningitis can be caused by a variety of organisms, but the three main types are (1) *bacterial,* or pyogenic, caused by pus-forming bacteria, especially the meningococcus, pneumococcus, and the influenza bacillus; (2) *tuberculous,* caused by the tubercle bacillus (see p. 1231); and (3) *viral,* or aseptic, caused by a wide variety of viral agents. Encephalitis is usually caused by a virus, and the discussion is limited to viral encephalitis.

BACTERIAL MENINGITIS

Bacterial meningitis is a potentially fatal disease, and, although the advent of antimicrobial therapy has had a marked effect on the course and prognosis, it remains a significant cause of illness in the pediatric age-groups. Its importance lies primarily in the frequency with which it occurs in infancy and childhood and the unnecessarily high death rates and residual damage caused by undiagnosed and untreated or inadequately treated cases.

Etiology and pathophysiology

Bacterial meningitis can be caused by any of a variety of bacterial agents. *Hemophilus influenzae* (type B), *Streptococcus pneumoniae,* and *Neisseria meningitidis* (meningococcus) organisms are responsible for bacterial meningitis in 95% of children older than 2 months of age. *H. influenzae* is the predominant organism in children 3 months to 3 years of age but is rare in the infant younger than 3 months of age, who is apparently protected by passively acquired bactericidal substances, and in children older than 5 years of age, who are beginning to acquire this protection.[10] Other organisms are the β-hemolytic streptococcus, *Staphylococcus aureus,* and *Escherichia coli.* The leading causes of neonatal meningitis are the group B streptococcus and *E. coli* organisms. *E. coli* infection is seldom seen beyond infancy. Meningococcic (epidemic cerebrospinal) meningitis occurs in epidemic form and is the only form readily transmitted to others.[14] It is transmitted by droplet infection from nasopharyngeal secretions. Although it may develop at any age, the risk of infection increases with the number of contacts; therefore, it occurs predominantly in school-age children and adolescents.

There appear to be some seasonal variations. Meningitis caused by *H. influenzae* is a disease that primarily occurs in autumn or early winter. Pneumococcal and meningococcal infections can occur at any time but are more common in later winter or early spring.

Several factors may predispose the child to the development of bacterial meningitis. Males are affected more often than females, and this ratio is somewhat more pronounced in the neonatal period. The highest incidence of meningitis occurs between ages 6 and 12 months, and the greatest morbidity after meningitis appears to involve children who were afflicted between birth and 4 years of age.[18] In the neonatal period maternal factors, such as premature rupture of fetal membranes, maternal infection during the last week of pregnancy, prolonged labor, and excessive manipulation during labor, have been implicated in the development of septicemia and meningitis. Deficiencies in the immune mechanisms and decreased leukocyte activity may influence the incidence in newborns, children with immunoglobulin deficiencies, and children receiving immunosuppressant drugs. Meningitis appears to occur as an extension of a variety of bacterial infections, probably as a result of the lack of acquired resistance to the various etiologic organisms. The presence of preexisting central nervous system anomalies, neurosurgical procedures or injuries, sickle cell anemia, or primary infections elsewhere in the body are factors related to an increased susceptibility.[10,12]

Pathophysiology. The most common route of infection is by vascular dissemination from a focus of infection elsewhere. For example, organisms from the nasopharynx invade the underlying blood vessels and enter the cerebral blood supply or form local thromboemboli that release septic emboli to the bloodstream. Invasion by direct extension from infections in the paranasal and mastoid sinuses is less common. Organisms also gain entry by direct implantation after penetrating wounds, skull fractures that provide an opening into the skin or sinuses, lumbar puncture or surgical procedures, and anatomic abnormalities such as spina bifida or foreign bodies such as a ventricular shunt. Once implanted, the organisms spread into the cerebrospinal fluid by which the infection spreads throughout the subarachnoid space.

The infective process is that seen in any bacterial infection—inflammation, exudation, white blood cell accumulation, and varying degrees of tissue damage. The brain becomes hyperemic and edematous, and the entire surface of the brain is covered with a layer of purulent exudate. The nature and extent of the exudate vary with the type of organism: meningococcal exudate is most marked over the parietal, occipital, and cerebellar regions; the thick fibrinous exudate of pneumococcal infection is confined chiefly to the surface of the brain, particularly the anterior lobes; and the exudate of streptococcal infections is similar to that of pneumococcal infections, but thinner.

As infection extends to the ventricles, thick pus, fibrin,

or adhesions may occlude the narrow passages, thereby obstructing the flow of cerebrospinal fluid to cause obstructive hydrocephalus. Subdural effusions occur frequently, and thrombosis may occur in meningeal veins or venous sinuses. Destructive changes may take place in the cerebral cortex, and brain abcesses may form by direct extension of the infection or by vascular dissemination. Extension of the infection to the areas of the cranial nerves or compression necrosis from increased pressure may cause deafness, blindness, or weakness or paralysis of facial or other muscles of the head and neck.[11,14,18]

Inappropriate secretion of antidiuretic hormone frequently accompanies meningitis, causing retention of fluid that intensifies the cerebral edema of the acute inflammatory process. This can reach life-threatening proportions.

Meningococcic (epidemic cerebrospinal) meningitis may produce local changes in other areas, the most striking feature of which is petechial or purpuric rash that results from thrombosis, extravasation of red blood cells, and inflammatory changes around the capillaries and other small vessels in the skin. These lesions may also appear in the meninges, joints, and, less often, the eyes, ears, lungs and adrenals.

Diagnostic evaluation

The clinical manifestations of acute bacterial meningitis depend to a large extent on the age of the child. The picture is also influenced to some degree by the type or organism, the effectiveness of therapy for antecedent illness, and whether it occurs as an isolated entity or as a complication of another illness or injury.

Children and adolescents. The illness is likely to be abrupt, with fever, chills, headache, and vomiting that are associated with or quickly followed by alterations in sensorium. Often the initial sign is a seizure, which may recur as the disease progresses. The child is extremely irritable and agitated and may develop delirium, aggressive or maniacal behavior, or drowsiness, stupor, and coma. Sometimes the onset is slower, frequently preceded by several days of respiratory or gastrointestinal symptoms. Occasionally a prior infection treated with antibiotics masks or delays the signs of meningitis.[9]

The child resists flexion of the neck, and, as the disease progresses, the neck stiffness becomes marked until the head is drawn into extreme overextension (opisthotonos). Kernig's and Brudzinski's signs are positive. Reflex responses are variable, although they show hyperactivity.

Other signs and symptoms may appear that are peculiar to individual organisms. Petechial or purpuric rashes usually indicate a meningococcal infection, especially when the eruption is associated with a shock-like state. Joint involvement is seen in meningococcic and *H. influenzae* infection. A chronically draining ear commonly accompanies pneumococcal meningitis. *E. coli* infection may be associated with a congenital dermal sinus that communicates with the subarachnoid space.

Infants and young children. The classic picture of meningitis is rarely seen in children between 3 months and 2 years of age. The illness is characterized by fever, vomiting, marked irritability, and frequent seizures, which are often accompanied by a high-pitched cry. A bulging fontanel is the most significant finding, and nuchal rigidity may or may not be present. Brudzinski's and Kernig's signs are not usually helpful in diagnosis, since they are difficult to elicit and evaluate in children in this age-group.

Neonatal. Meningitis in newborn and premature infants is extremely difficult to diagnose. The vague and nonspecific manifestations, characteristic of all neonatal sepsis, bear little resemblance to the findings in older children. These infants are usually well at birth but within a few days begin to look and behave poorly. They refuse feedings, have poor sucking ability, and may vomit or have diarrhea. They display poor tone, lack of movement, and a poor cry. Other nonspecific signs that may be present include hypothermia or fever (depending on the maturity of the infant), jaundice, irritability, drowsiness, seizures, respiratory irregularities or apnea, cyanosis, and weight loss. The full, tense, and bulging fontanel may or may not be present until late in the course of illness, and the neck is usually supple. Untreated the child will progress to cardiovascular collapse, seizures, and apnea.[11,18]

Diagnostic tests. A diagnosis of acute bacterial meningitis cannot be made on the basis of clinical manifestations. A definitive diagnosis is made only by examination of the cerebrospinal fluid by means of a lumbar puncutre (see Table 37-3). The fluid pressure is measured and samples are obtained for culture, Gram stain, blood cell count, and determination of glucose and protein content. The findings are usually diagnostic. Culture and stain are needed to identify the causative organism. Spinal fluid pressure is usually elevated, but interpretation is often difficult when the child is crying. There is generally an elevated white blood cell count, predominantly polymorphonuclear leukocytes, but it may be extremely variable. The glucose level is reduced, generally in proportion to the duration and severity of the infection. The relationship between the cerebrospinal fluid glucose and serum glucose levels is important in evaluating the glucose content of cerebrospinal fluid; therefore, a serum glucose sample is drawn approximately ½ hour prior to the lumbar puncture. Protein concentration is usually increased.

A blood culture is advisable for all children suspected of meningitis and occasionally proves positive when cerebrospinal fluid culture is negative. Nose and throat cultures may provide helpful information in some cases.

Complications. The incidence of complications from acute bacterial meningitis has been significantly reduced with early diagnosis and vigorous antimicrobial therapy. One of the most dramatic and serious complications usually associated with meningococcal infections is peripheral circulatory collapse, known as the Waterhouse-Friderichsen syndrome, which if untreated is rapidly fatal. Extensive and diffuse intravascular coagulation with marked thrombocytopenia occurs with any form but is most common in meningococcic (epidemic cerebrospinal) meningitis.

Obstruction to the flow of cerebrospinal fluid occurs in the acute phase of illness by clumping of purulent material in the drainage channels and in the chronic phase by adhesive arachnoiditis or fibrotic obstruction through any of the ventricular foramina. Subdural effusions are not uncommon after meningitis. Extension of the inflammation to cranial nerves or compression and destruction of the nerves from intracranial pressure can produce permanent impairment to vision or hearing and other nerve palsies. Auditory nerve damage is usually followed by permanent deafness.

Hemiparesis and quadriparesis may result from damage caused by arteritis and/or thrombosis or other mechanisms. Behavioral changes are noted in some children, and there is evidence to indicate that psychometric and behavioral defects may be a significant concomitant sign of meningitis in childhood, although it is difficult to determine the degree to which meningitis affects the intelligence quotient of children.[28]

Medical management

Acute bacterial meningitis is a medical emergency that requires early recognition and immediate institution of therapy to prevent death and avoid residual disabilities. The initial therapeutic management includes[4a]:

- Isolation
- Initiation of antimicrobial therapy
- Maintenance of optimum hydration
- Maintenance of ventilation
- Reduction of increased intracranial pressure
- Management of bacterial shock
- Control of seizures
- Control of extremes of temperature
- Correction of anemia

The child is isolated from other children. An intravenous infusion is started as soon as the lumbar puncture has been completed in order to facilitate the administration of antimicrobial agents, fluids, anticonvulsive drugs, and blood if needed.

Drugs.[4a] Until the causative organism is identified, the choice of antibiotic is based on the known sensitivity of the organism most likely to be the infective agent in any given situation and the probable interactions with the specific patient. Except under special circumstances, the drugs are administered intravenously throughout the course of treatment. The drugs are given in large doses, and the period of therapy is determined by cerebrospinal fluid findings (normal glucose level and negative culture) and the child's clinical condition.

The drug of choice in older infants and children is the broad-spectrum antibiotic ampicillin, which is effective against the usual causative organisms and is associated with very low toxicity. In areas in which *H. influenzae* has become resistant to ampicillin or in children with well-documented sensitivity to penicillin, chloramphenicol may be the drug of choice for initial treatment. For most organisms ampicillin (often in association with chloramphenicol) or penicillin is continued. For some organisms other drugs may be employed, usually in conjunction with ampicillin, for example, gentamicin and/or kanamycin for *E. coli*.

Nonspecific measures. Maintaining hydration is a prime concern, and intravenous fluids and the type and amount of fluid are determined by the patient's condition. The optimum hydration involves correction of any fluid deficits followed by low maintenance levels to prevent cerebral edema. If indicated, measures are employed to reduce intracranial pressure as described previously (see p. 1415).

Complications are treated appropriately. Subdural effusions in infants are treated by aspirations to relieve symptoms, and heparin therapy may be required for children who develop disseminated intravascular coagulation syndrome. Shock, if it occurs, is managed by restoration of blood volume and maintenance of electrolyte balance.

Lumbar puncture is carried out as needed to determine the effectiveness of therapy. The patient is evaluated neurologically during the convalescent period and at regular intervals during the succeeding year. Prognosis is related to a variety of factors: the age of the child, the type of organisms, the severity of the infection, the duration of the illness prior to the onset of therapy, and the sensitivity of the organism to antimicrobial drugs. The younger the patient, the higher the mortality. Infections caused by *E. coli* and other gram-negative organisms are more difficult to cure than those caused by gram-positive organisms. Infections associated with severe shock syndrome, those that are inadequately treated, and those caused by resistant organisms carry a more serious or ominous outcome. With adequate therapy the chances of recovery are good. Mortality is 5% to 10%, and the incidence of neurologic sequelae has been significantly reduced.[11,18]

Prevention. Two vaccines are now available for types A and C meningococci (a third is currently being developed for type B). At the present time type A is the only one recommended for use in children over 5 years of age who are close contacts of a primary case or who are considered high risk because of asplenia.

Nursing considerations

The child suspected of meningitis is placed on respiratory isolation for at least 24 hours after implementation of antimicrobial therapy. Nurses should take necessary precautions to protect themselves and others from possible

Summary of nursing care of the child with acute bacterial meningitis

Goals	Responsibilities
Prevent spread of infection	Place child in isolation for at least 24 hours after initiation of antibiotic therapy Protect self by observing proper precautions Identify close contacts and high-risk children who might benefit from meningococci vaccinations
Help to establish diagnosis	Assist with diagnostic procedures Order laboratory tests Send obtained specimens, for example, spinal fluid, to laboratory for analysis Obtain specimens, for example, nasopharyngeal smears, as needed
Provide and maintain route for rapid administration of medication	Assist with establishment of intravenous infusion Monitor intravenous infusion Type of fluid Rate of flow Amount of fluid Maintain integrity of infusion Immobilize intravenous site Apply restraint as needed Change tubing and so on as dictated by hospital policy Observe for signs of inflammation at infusion site and along course of vein
Eradicate causative organisms	Administer antibiotics as prescribed
Assess neurologic status	Monitor Vital signs Neurologic signs Level of consciousness Behavior
Detect early signs of complications	Observe for signs of impending Vasomotor collapse or shock Increased intracranial pressure Respiratory distress Altered state of consciousness Intravascular coagulation
Maintain optimal hydration	Regulate intake as prescribed; restrict or encourage fluids as determined by child's status Measure intake and output Weigh daily (if ordered)
Maintain nutrition	Provide diet as ordered; give nothing by mouth or clear liquids initially but appropriate for age as tolerated
Decrease effects of long-term intravenous therapy and immobilization	Remove restraining devices frequently Allow as much freedom of movement as possible and encourage normal activities Provide diversional activities Encourage play

infection. Parents are taught the proper protective procedures and supervised in their application.

The room should be kept as quiet as possible and environmental stimuli kept at a minimum, since most affected children are sensitive to noise, bright lights, and other external stimuli. Most children are more comfortable without a pillow and with the head of the bed slightly elevated. A side-lying position is more often assumed because of nuchal rigidity. The nurse should avoid actions, such as lifting the child's head, that cause pain or increase his discomfort. Measures are employed to assure safety, since the child is often restless and subject to seizures.

The nursing care of the child with meningitis is determined by the child's symptoms and treatment. Observation of vital signs, neurologic signs, level of consciousness, urine output, and other pertinent data is carried out at frequent intervals. The child who is unconscious is managed as described previously (see p. 1411), and all children are observed carefully for signs of complications just described, especially signs of increased intracranial pressure, shock, or respiratory distress.

Fluids and nourishment are determined by the child's status. The child with dulled sensorium is usually given nothing by mouth. Other children are allowed clear liquids initially and progressed to a diet suitable for their age. Careful monitoring and recording of intake and output are needed to determine deviations that might indicate impending shock or increasing fluid accumulation, such as cerebral edema or subdural effusion.

One of the most difficult problems in nursing care of children with meningitis is maintaining the intravenous infusion for the length of time needed to provide adequate antimicrobial therapy. (See the box on p. 1433.) Older infants and small children require restraining devices to maintain the integrity of the infusion site. These children should be released from the restraints as often as possible to reduce the ill effects of long-term immobilization. The children should be allowed ambulation and other normal activities as soon as the condition allows and as often as feasible. In some children, especially older children, a heparin-lock device can be employed to allow for more freedom of movement. The infusion site is monitored for signs of inflammation as well as for patency. Some medications are highly irritating to veins and may tend to produce phlebitis if continued in the same site over a prolonged period of time. These children are particularly in need of attendance and opportunities for play.

NONBACTERIAL (ASEPTIC) MENINGITIS

Aseptic meningitis is a benign syndrome caused by a number of agents, principally viruses, and is frequently associated with other diseases, such as measles, mumps, herpes, and leukemia. Enteroviruses and mumps viruses account for a large number of cases.

The onset may be abrupt or gradual. The initial manifestations are headache, fever, malaise, gastrointestinal symptoms, and signs of meningeal irritation that develop a day or two after the onset of illness. Abdominal pain and nausea and vomiting are common; sore throat, chest pain, and generalized muscular aches or pains are found occasionally. There may be a maculopapular rash. These symptoms usually subside spontaneously and rapidly, and the child is well in 3 to 10 days with no residual effects.

Diagnosis is based on clinical features and cerebrospinal fluid findings, which include increased lymphocytes, predominantly mononuclear cells. It is important to differentiate this benign disorder from the more serious form of meningitis and to diagnose and treat any disease of which it is a manifestation.

Treatment is primarily symptomatic, such as aspirin for headache, moist heat for muscle aches and pains, and positioning for comfort. Antimicrobial agents may be administered and isolation enforced until a definitive diagnosis is made as a precaution against the possibility that the disease might be of bacterial origin.

BRAIN ABSCESS

Localized suppuration in the central nervous system, as elsewhere in the body, constitutes an abscess. The anatomic barriers of the brain define epidural and subdural abscesses. Suppuration within the neuronal substance is an intracranial abscess. Epidural abscesses may form during infections involving the epidural space, usually after trauma or direct spread from purulent otitis media or (rarely) paranasal sinuses. Subdural abscesses usually arise from purulent inflammation of paranasal or mastoid sinuses. Intracerebral abscesses form when pyogenic organisms gain access to neural tissue from the bloodstream from foci of infection or from trauma or surgical procedures. Cerebral abscesses are often due to purulent middle ear infection and mobilization of septic thrombi in children with right-to-left cardiac shunts but can occur secondary to pulmonary suppuration, such as bronchiectasis or pulmonary abscess.[17]

The most common sites of intracerebral abscesses are the temporal and frontal lobes, and the most frequently demonstrated organisms are the streptococci, pneumococci, and staphylococci. Early signs of the disease are rather vague, and the insidious onset often includes vomiting, lethargy, fever, and progression to coma. Specific neurologic signs are related to the area invaded by the infectious process and, as this area enlarges, resemble those produced by an intracranial tumor. Cerebellar abscesses produce signs associated with any posterior fossa mass (see cerebellar tumors, p. 1023).

During abscess formation antibiotic therapy is effective. Fully established abscesses require surgical management, by either open drainage or excision.

ENCEPHALITIS

Encephalitis is an inflammatory process of the central nervous system producing altered function of various portions of the brain and spinal cord. Encephalitis can be caused by a variety of organisms, including bacteria, spirochetes, fungi, protozoa, helminths, and viruses. Most infections are associated with viruses, and this discussion will be limited to these etiologic agents.

Etiology

The disease can occur as the result of (1) direct invasion of the central nervous system by a virus or (2) postinfectious involvement of the central nervous system after a viral disease.[18] Often the specific type of encephalitis in a particular patient may not be identified for some time or not at all. The cause of over half the cases reported in the United States is unknown. The majority of cases of known etiology are associated with the childhood diseases measles, mumps, varicella, and rubella and, less often, the enteroviruses and herpes viruses.

Encephalitis as a result of direct invasion is most often caused by the arboviruses (arthropod-borne viruses) accidentally acquired through an arthropod vector. In the United States there are four arboviruses that are major causes of encephalitis[3]: the eastern equine encephalomyelitis (EEE), Western equine encephalomyelitis (WEE), St. Louis encephalitis (SLE), and California (CE) viruses, each with a characteristic geographic distribution and epidemiologic pattern. The vector reservoir for these arboviruses is the mosquito; therefore, most cases of encephalitis appear during the hot summer months and subside during the autumn.[18] The principal geographic areas of North America in which these varieties are found are eastern equine encephalomyelitis virus in eastern and north central United States and adjacent Canada; western equine encephalomyelitis virus in western United States and Canada and scattered areas further east; St. Louis encephalitis virus in most of the United States with the exception of the northeast sections; and California virus throughout the United States.

Diagnostic evaluation

The clinical features are similar regardless of the agent involved. Manifestations can range from a mild benign form that resembles aseptic meningitis, lasting a few days and being followed by rapid and complete recovery, to a fulminating encephalitis with severe central nervous system involvement. The onset may be sudden or gradual with malaise, fever, headache, dizziness, apathy, stiffness of the neck, nausea and vomiting, ataxia, tremors, hyperactivity, and speech difficulties. In severe cases there is high fever, stupor, seizures, disorientation, spasticity, and coma that may proceed to death. Ocular palsies and paralysis may be seen, also.

The diagnosis is made on the basis of clinical findings, circumstances associated with the disease, and, where possible, identification of the specific virus. Arboviruses are rarely detected in the blood or spinal fluid, but viruses of herpes, mumps, measles, and enteroviruses may be found in cerebrospinal fluid.

Medical management and nursing care

Patients suspected of having encephalitis are hospitalized promptly for skilled nursing care and observation. Treatment is primarily supportive, including conscientious nursing care, control of cerebral manifestations, and adequate nutrition and hydration, with observations and management as for other disorders involving cerebral injury. Follow-up care with periodic reevaluation and rehabilitation are important aspects of survivors with residual effects of the disease.

RABIES

Rabies is an acute infection of the nervous system caused by a virus that is almost invariably fatal. It is transmitted to humans by the saliva of an infected mammal introduced through a bite or skin abrasion. The domestic dog is the principal source of infection, although any animal, including bats, cats, foxes, skunks, coyotes, and raccoons, may be responsible for human infection.

The disease is uncommon in man, but the highest incidence occurs in children under 15 years of age. The incubation period usually ranges from 1 to 3 months but may be as short as 10 days or as long as 8 months. Only 10% to 15% of persons bitten develop the disease, but, once symptoms are present, rabies progresses inexorably to a fatal outcome.[22] The disease is characterized by a period of general malaise, fever, and sore throat followed by a phase of excitement featured by hypersensitivity and increased reaction to external stimuli, convulsions, maniacal behavior, and choking. Attempts at swallowing may cause such severe spasm of respiratory muscles that apnea, cyanosis, and anoxia are produced—the characteristics from which the term ''hydrophobia'' was derived.

Diagnosis is made on the basis of history and clinical features. Once symptoms appear treatment is of little avail, but the long incubation period allows time for induction of active as well as passive immunity before the onset of illness. Active immunity is achieved by one of two types of rabies vaccines: the Pasteur brain-fixed virus vaccine and the duck embryo vaccine, both of which are prepared with inactivated viruses. Passive immunity can be conferred by the administration of hyperimmune antirabies horse serum. There is also a human rabies immune globulin available for persons sensitive to horse serum. Passive immunization should be administered for all severe exposures, regardless of the interval between exposure and treatment by active immunization. Prophylactic immunization is usually not given unless definite exposure has occurred or definite exposure cannot be ruled out with reasonable certainty. Guidelines for treatment have been outlined by the World Health Organization, but most communities employ modifications relative to the conditions present within any given area such as the negligible risk of bites from domestic animals and the reduced contacts between domestic and wild animals.[22]

Prevention should be the major thrust in rabies infection. Ordinances in most areas require vaccination of dogs and, often, other household pets. Children should be taught proper treatment of pets and to avoid unknown animals and seemingly friendly or tame wild animals. Any animal bite should be thoroughly cleansed with mild soap and rinsed with copious amounts of saline solution. Tetanus antitoxin or toxoid is administered and, where indicated, veterinary consultation and field investigation by public health agencies should be carried out.[18] Whenever possible the animal should be captured, confined, and observed by a veterinarian for 5 to 10 days. The importance of determining the health of the animal cannot be overemphasized.

The child who is bitten by a rabid animal or one that has not been apprehended is faced with lengthy and painful prophylactic therapy. Specific prevention in man is vaccination supplemented by passive immunization with hyperimmune serum (especially if the injury is in the area of the head, face, and neck), which must begin as soon as possible after injury. The vaccine is administered subcutaneously each day on 14 consecutive days. The injections are rotated at sites on the abdomen, lower back, and lateral aspect of the thighs. Daily injections of hyperimmune serum are given intramuscularly concurrently with the vaccine for the 21 days or in two separate injections daily for 7 days followed by one daily injection for 7 days. Two booster shots are given—one in 10 days and another in 20 days—after completion of the primary series.

The child will require careful psychologic preparation for this ordeal. Injections of any kind are anxiety-provoking for children and rabies prophylaxis often produces unpleasant side effects including erythema, pruritis, pain, and tenderness in the area of the injections. More unusual symptoms are low-grade fever and possible shock. Since shock is always a possibility, epinephrine should be available at the time of the injections. Parents as well as children are frightened by the urgency and seriousness of the situation. They need anticipatory guidance regarding the therapy and possible side effects and support and reassurance regarding the efficacy of the preventive measures for this dreaded disease.

REYE'S SYNDROME

Acute encephalopathy with fatty degeneration of the liver, first described by Reye in 1963, is a disorder identified with increasing frequency and characterized by fever, profoundly impaired consciousness, and disordered hepatic function. The ages of affected children range from 2 months to adolescence, with peak incidences occuring at 6 and 11 years of age.[34]

Etiology and pathophysiology

The etiology of the disorder is obscure, but several theories have been advanced. There appears to be a relationship between an antecedent viral infection, especially varicella and influenza B. It is suggested that the cause may be either hepatic failure with ammonia intoxication or the interaction between a toxin (such as insecticides and/or herbicides) and a virus, which is foremost at present. Numerous other theories are also being proposed and examined.

The pathologic changes of Reye's syndrome are marked cerebral edema and enlargement of the liver with marked fatty infiltration.

Diagnostic evaluation

The onset of the disease is preceded in most cases by prodromal symptoms, including malaise, cough, rhinorrhea, or sore throat. After about 1 to 3 days, as the child progressively deteriorates, cerebral signs and symptoms appear, accompanied by various physiologic changes. The manifestations of the various clinical stages are[19,34]:

Stage I Vomiting, lethargy, and drowsiness
Stage II Disorientation, delirium, aggressiveness and combativeness, central neurologic hyperventilation (or, sometimes, shallow breathing), hyperactive reflexes, and stupor
Stage III Obtundent, comatose, hyperventilation, and decorticate rigidity
Stage IV Deepening coma, decerebrate rigidity, loss of ocular reflexes, large fixed pupils, and divergent eye movements
Stage V Seizures, loss of deep tendon reflexes, flaccidity, and respiratory arrest

Clinically liver involvement is limited to mild hepatomegaly. Evidence of liver dysfunction is reflected by elevated serum glutamic-oxaloacetic transaminase (SGOT), serum glutamic-pyruvic transaminase (SGPT), and lactic dehydrogenase (LDH) levels. Liver-dependent clotting factors, such as prothrombin time, are diminished. Serum bilirubin and alkaline phosphatase levels are usually unaffected. Blood urea nitrogen and ammonia levels are often elevated, indicating mild renal dysfunction. In the majority of children blood sugar levels fall to below 50 mg/100 ml, with reduced insulin levels and diminished glucagon response. There is a combined respiratory alkalosis and metabolic acidosis.[15,33]

The clinical course of the disease is rapid, and the mortality rate is high (40% to 80% in various studies), particularly in children younger than 2 years of age and in those in whom convulsions are part of the clinical picture.[15] Fortunately recovery is rapid and complete in those who survive, and residual disability is uncommon.

Medical management

Treatment is primarily supportive and directed toward restoring blood sugar levels, controlling cerebral edema, and correcting acid-base imbalances. Intravenous administration of hypertonic (10%) glucose solution with added insulin helps to replace glycogen stores, but it is controlled to avoid overhydration. The pH and electrolytes are monitored and replaced according to regular assessments. Anticonvulsant medication is given for seizure activity. Sometimes corticosteroids are useful, and mannitol may be administered to reduce cerebral edema if the kidneys are not compromised. Endotracheal intubation with respiratory assistance is implemented for respiratory distress, and interventions are initiated to reduce an elevated temperature. Exchange transfusions or peritoneal dialysis has been used in some cases to reduce elevated blood ammonia levels.[30]

Nursing considerations

The child who is acutely ill with Reye's syndrome requires continuous and intensive nursing care. On admission to the hospital numerous procedures and observations must be carried out as quickly as possible. In addition to an appraisal of vital functions and neurologic status, the nurse assists with a lumbar puncture, obtaining blood for laboratory examination, and insertion of various intravenous lines such as peripheral, arterial, and central venous pressure. A retention catheter and a nasogastric tube are inserted, and, when respirations are compromised, an endotracheal tube is inserted and attached to a respirator for controlled respirations. If equipment is available, a line is inserted for continuous monitoring of intracranial pressure.

Care and observations are implemented as for any child with an altered state of consciousness (p. 1416) and increasing intracranial pressure (p. 1427). Accurate and frequent monitoring of intake and output is essential for adjusting fluid volumes to prevent both dehydration and cerebral edema. Since hypovolemic shock is a constant danger in children with Reye's syndrome, vital signs, including central venous pressure, are monitored frequently. Laboratory analysis of serum electrolytes, pH, blood urea nitrogen, glucose, osmolality, and blood gases serves as a guide for therapy, and arranging for their collection is a nursing responsibility. Because of related liver dysfunction, the nurse must observe for signs of impaired coagulation such as prolonged bleeding, petechiae, and so on.

Recovery from Reye's syndrome is rapid, usually without sequelae. However, in her studies Weeks has observed a trend in the behaviors when children waken from the unconscious state. The stress and anxiety they appear to feel in a strange and unfamiliar environment are consistently expressed in silent and withdrawn behavior. They respond to basic questioning but do not display their prehospitalization personality and social behavior until they are transferred from the critical care area.[34]

The children awaken disoriented with no recollection of events that took place during the critical phase of their illness. Strange equipment being used in their care that was started while they were unconscious requires explanation. The appearance of other ill children is puzzling and frightening, increasing their anxiety and stress concerning their own situation. They are powerless to control what is happening to them. Nurses can help these children deal with their stress by orienting them to where they are and the circumstances of their being there, describing what is expected of them, and giving them a sense of control whenever possible. Encouraging parents to visit and providing other items associated with home, such as a favorite toy, a photograph, or other item, help them maintain a link with their lives outside the confines of the critical care environment. Understanding and individualized care help children to weather the stresses and tension of this period of crisis.

CONVULSIVE DISORDERS

Convulsive phenomena are among the most frequently observed neurologic dysfunctions in children and can occur with a wide variety of conditions involving the central nervous system. A *convulsion* is defined as involuntary muscular contractions and relaxation; a *seizure* is a sudden attack. The two words are used synonymously. Convulsive phenomena are characterized by a single or recurrent transient attacks of loss of consciousness, convulsive movements, or disturbed feelings or behavior associated with excessive neuronal discharges. These discharges may be focal or diffuse, and the sites of the discharges determine the clinical manifestations observed during the attack.

Seizure activity can be classified according to (1) etiology, (2) clinical manifestations, or (3) anatomic site or electroencephalographic pattern. In general the term seizure, convulsion, or spell is used to designate a single episode, whereas convulsive disorder is the preferred term for a chronic and recurring disorder. These chronic forms are also known as the *epilepsies*.[22]

Etiology

Convulsive disorders have numerous and varied causes based on idiopathic (unknown) and symptomatic (acquired) factors. Although the cause of idiopathic epilepsy is unknown, it may indicate genetic factors that in some way alter the seizure threshold to influence neuronal discharge. Congenital defects and some genetic disorders (such as tuberous sclerosis) have seizures as a manifestation. Febrile and breath-holding seizures are related to a lowered convulsive threshold that tends to have a higher incidence in certain families. Hereditary electroencephalographic abnormalities have been detected in some families, and there is a higher incidence of seizures among relatives of children with idiopathic convulsive disorders.[14]

A seizure disorder can also be acquired as a result of brain injury during prenatal, perinatal, or postnatal periods.

This injury may be caused by trauma, hypoxia, infections, exogenous or endogenous toxins, and a variety of other causes. A partial list of causative factors is in the boxed material below.

The incidence of causative factors associated with childhood seizures is frequently related to the age of the child. Seizures are more common during the first 2 years of life than during any other period of childhood. In very young infants the most frequent causes are birth injuries, that is, intracranial trauma, hemorrhage, or anoxia, and congenital defects of the brain. Acute infections are a frequent cause of seizures in late infancy and early childhood but become an infrequent cause in middle childhood. In children older than 3 years of age the most common factor is idiopathic epilepsy.

Other contributing factors are fatigue, undo excitement, and stressful situations at home or school. Excessive fluid intake or fluid retention, such as occurs during premenstrual tension, produce alterations in the serum (and brain) concentrations of sodium, potassium, and water, which may precipitate seizures. There appear to be periods of functional instability of the brain, normally when falling asleep or awakening from sleep. At these times seizures are more likely to occur. The hormonal and metabolic changes associated with adolescence can alter the convulsive threshold. Photogenic stimulation by such commonplace things as television, the rays of the sun, or certain kinds of music in susceptible children have been implicated in precipitating seizures in some instances.

Etiology of seizures in children

Nonrecurrent (acute)

- Febrile episodes
- Intracranial infection
- Intracranial hemorrhage
- Space-occupying lesions (cyst, tumor)
- Acute cerebral edema
- Anoxia
- Toxins
  - Drugs
  - Tetanus
  - Lead encephalopathy
  - *Shigella, Salmonella*
- Metabolic alterations
  - Hypocalcemia
  - Hypoglycemia
  - Hyponatremia or hypernatremia
  - Hypomagnesemia
  - Alkalosis
  - Disorders of amino acid metabolism
  - Deficiency states
  - Hyperbilirubinemia

Recurrent (chronic)

- Idiopathic epilepsy
- Epilepsy—secondary to prior
  - Trauma
  - Hemorrhage
  - Anoxia
  - Infections
  - Toxins
  - Degenerative phenomena
  - Congenital defects
  - Parasitic brain disease
  - Hypoglycemia injury
- Epilepsy—sensory stimulus
- Epilepsy-stimulating states
  - Narcolepsy and catalepsy
  - Psychogenic
  - Tetany from hypocalcemia, alkalosis
- Hypoglycemia states
  - Hyperinsulinism
  - Hypopituitarism
  - Adrenocortical insufficiency
  - Hepatic disorders
- Uremia
- Allergy
- Cardiovascular dysfunction or syncopal episodes
- Migraine

Pathophysiology. Regardless of the etiologic factor or the type of seizure, the basic mechanism is the same. There are electric discharges that (1) may arise from central areas in the brain that affect consciousness immediately, (2) may be restricted to one area of the cerebral cortex, producing manifestations characteristic of that particular anatomic focus, or (3) may begin in a localized area of the cortex and spread to other portions of the brain, which, if sufficiently extensive, produce generalized neurologic manifestations.[1]

Seizure activity is believed to be caused by spontaneous electric discharge initiated by a group of hyperexcitable cells referred to as the *epileptogenic focus*. These cells display increased electric excitability but may remain quiescent over a period of time while discharging intermittently as evidenced on electroencephalographic tracings. Normally these discharges are restrained from spreading beyond the focal area by normal inhibitory mechanisms.

In response to any of a variety of physiologic stimuli, such as cellular dehydration, abnormal blood sugar levels, electrolyte imbalance, fatigue, emotional stress, endocrine changes, and so on, these hyperexcitable cells activate normal cells in surrounding areas and in distant, synaptically related cells. When the neuronal excitation from the epileptogenic focus spreads to the brain stem, particularly the midbrain and reticular formation, a generalized seizure develops. These centers within the brain stem, known as the centrencephalic system, are responsible for the spread of the epileptic potentials. The discharges can originate spontaneously in the centrencephalic system or be triggered by a focal area in the cortex. Seizures are designated as focal, focal with rapid generalization, and generalized, on the basis of these characteristic neuronal discharges, as recorded by electroencephalography. In a large proportion of children focal seizures spread to other areas, ultimately becoming generalized with loss of consciousness.[1,22]

Convulsive seizures are described according to several types within the categories of generalized or focal seizures and varied clinical features. The onset of a seizure is abrupt, paroxysmal, and transitory, and signs may vary from behavioral abnormalities to continuous and prolonged motor convulsions.

Features of seizures.[36] There are several features that may be observed during various seizures. A clear description of these phenomena is a valuable aid in localizing the area involved and frequently suggests the underlying pathology.

Aura. The aura is the peculiar sensation experienced

by some persons just prior to the onset of a seizure. The aura serves two useful purposes. It warns the person of the impending attack so that he is able to seek privacy and a safe place to lie down before the seizure begins. The nature of the sensation can also provide the best reliable clue to help localize the origin of the discharge. The most common epileptic aura is a sensation of dizziness or an unusual feeling of ascending abdominal discomfort. Other sensations and the focal areas implicated are visual hallucinations (occipital or temporal lobe), verbal phenomena (the dominant hemisphere), unusual tastes, odors, visceral sensations, or dreamy feelings (temporal lobe).

Eye movement. Discharges in the cortex of one hemisphere tend to cause the eyes to deviate to the opposite side. Bilateral discharges tend to cause the eyes to move upward or straight ahead. However, after the seizure, the eyes will often deviate in the opposite direction. When the child's eyes are closed during the attack, a gentle attempt to open them may provide valuable information.

Muscle contraction. Muscle contraction during the seizure can be one of three types: *clonic, tonic,* or *jacksonian.* Clonic contractions are those in which opposing muscles contract and relax alternately producing rhythmic movements. Tonic contractions are those in which all the muscles are maintained in a contraction for a time causing the person to become rigid. Jacksonian contractions are those in which muscular twitchings begin in one area and spread to another.

Laterality. Seizure activity may involve the entire body, one side, or one or more body parts. The body part or side involved implies an electric discharge in the corresponding area of the opposite cerebral cortex.

Complex motor activity. Seizures may begin with or consist of complex, stereotyped, or repetitive activities. These are often associated with lesions in the temporal lobe.

Loss of consciousness. Loss of consciousness commonly accompanies a seizure and indicates generalized cortical or centrencephalic involvement. The loss of consciousness is frequently shown by various manifestations such as incontinence or injury.

Postictal state. The state of the child in the period after a seizure may be varied. The child may be drowsy, be uncoordinated, and display some sensory or motor impairment. Weakness, hypotonia, or inactivity of a body part may be an indication of an epileptogenic focus in the contralateral corresponding cortical region.

Types of seizures: generalized

Generalized seizures without a focal onset appear to arise in the reticular formation and may occur at any age. Children, as opposed to adults, seldom report an aura or warning. Seizures occur at any time, day or night, and the interval between attacks may be minutes, hours, weeks, or even years. Most affected persons first experience seizures in childhood, and children whose convulsions begin before age 4 years have mental retardation and behavioral and learning problems more frequently than those whose seizures begin after 4 years of age. Later-onset (after age 20 years) convulsive disorders are more apt to be caused by an acquired pathologic condition.[1,14]

Grand mal (major motor). The generalized seizure occurring alone or in combination with other forms and either with or without focal onset is the most common and most dramatic of all seizure manifestations of childhood. The seizure usually occurs without warning. There is a rolling of the eyes upward and immediate loss of consciousness. If the child is standing, he falls to the floor or ground. The child stiffens in a generalized and symmetric tonic contraction of the entire body musculature. The arms usually flex, whereas the legs, head, and neck extend. The child may utter a peculiar piercing cry produced as the jaws clap shut and the thoracic and abdominal muscles contract, forcing air through tightly closed vocal cords. This tonic phase lasts approximately 10 to 20 seconds, during which the child is apneic and may become cyanotic. Autonomic stimulation causes increased salivation.[1,22]

The tonic rigidity is replaced by the violent jerking movements as the trunk and extremities undergo rhythmic contraction and relaxation of the clonic phase. During this time the child may foam at the mouth and be incontinent of urine and feces. As the attack ends the movements become less intense and occur at longer intervals, until they cease entirely. The clonic phase generally lasts about 30 seconds but can vary from only a few seconds to a half hour or longer. A series of seizures at intervals too brief to allow the child to regain consciousness between the time one attack ends and the next begins is known as *status epilepticus.* This requires emergency intervention. A succession of interrupted seizures can lead to exhaustion, respiratory failure, and death.

In the postictal state the child appears to relax but may remain semiconscious and difficult to rouse. He may waken in a few minutes but remains confused for several hours. He is poorly coordinated with mild impairment of fine motor movements. He may have visual and speech difficulties, and he may vomit or complain of severe headache. When left alone, he usually sleeps for several hours. On awakening he is fully conscious but usually feels tired and complains of sore muscles, headache, and no recollection of the entire event.

Petit mal (absences). Petit mal seizures, also called absences or lapses, are characterized by a brief loss of consciousness with minimal or no alteration in muscle tone and may go unrecognized since the child's behavior is altered very little. Attacks almost always first appear during childhood. In most instances the onset occurs between 5 and 9 years of age. Attacks are rarely detected before 5 years of age and usually cease at puberty, although they may be seen in adults. They are more common in girls than in boys.

The onset of petit mal seizures is abrupt, and the child suddenly develops twenty or more attacks daily. Characteristically the brief loss of consciousness appears without warning or aura and usually lasts about 5 to 10 seconds. Slight loss of muscle tone may cause the child to drop objects, but he is able to maintain postural control and seldom falls. There are frequently minor movements such as lip smacking, twitching of eyelids or face, or slight hand movements. The sudden arrest of activity and consciousness is not accompanied by incontinence, and the child is amnesic for the episode but may need to reorient himself to the previous activity. An attack is often mistaken for inattentiveness or daydreaming. Frequent attacks can result in slowed intellectual processes and deterioration in schoolwork and behavior, which is sometimes the first indication of the problem. Attacks can be precipitated by hyperventilation, hypoglycemia, stresses (emotional and physiologic), fatigue, or sleeplessness.

Akinetic. Akinetic seizures are manifest as a sudden, momentary loss of muscle tone and postural control. In infants who are able to sit but not stand, this is observed as a sudden dropping forward of the head and neck—the "salaam spasm." In older children the sudden loss of postural tone and reflexes causes the child to fall to the floor violently. He is unable to break the fall by putting out his hand and may incur a serious injury to the face, head, or shoulder. Loss of consciousness is only momentary. Akinetic attacks recur frequently during the day, particularly in the morning hours and shortly after the child awakens.

Myoclonic. Myoclonic seizures include a variety of convulsive episodes that are characterized by sudden, brief contractures of a muscle or group of muscles, occuring singly or repetitively without loss of consciousness or postictal state. The seizure may or may not be symmetric and may be isolated as benign essential myoclonus or may occur in association with other seizure forms. Myoclonus frequently appears normally in the course of falling asleep or is observed as a nonspecific symptom in many diseases of the nervous system, such as viral encephalitis, uremic encephalopathy, and degenerative diseases of the cerebrum.

Infantile spasms. Infantile myoclonus, massive spasms, or infantile myoclonic spasms most commonly occur between 3 and 12 months of age. They are twice as common in males as in females. The attack consists of a series of sudden, brief, symmetric, muscular contractions by which the head is flexed, the arms are extended, and the legs are drawn up. The eyes may roll upward or inward, and the seizure may be preceded or followed by a cry or giggling. There may or may not be loss of consciousness, and the infant will sometimes flush, turn pale, or become cyanotic. The child may have numerous seizures during the day without postictal drowsiness or sleep.[22]

Less often, alternate clinical forms are observed and include extensor spasms rather than flexion of arms, legs, and trunk and head nodding. Lightening attacks, which involve a single, momentary, shocklike contraction of the entire body, are another variant.

Infantile spasms are almost always associated with cerebral abnormalities, such as structural malformations, chronic edema, and degenerative changes. Microcephaly, choreoathetoid or tonic posture, and abnormal movements are frequently present. There may be a history of maternal infection, prematurity, or birth injury, and development is retarded prior to the onset of seizures. The infantile myoclonic seizures usually disappear spontaneously before age 4 years, but they may be replaced by other seizure forms. The outlook for normal intellectual development is poor, and treatment has no influence on the developmental prognosis.

Types of seizures: partial or focal

Focal or partial seizures are caused by abnormal electric discharges from epileptogenic foci limited to a more or less circumscribed region of the cerebral cortex. There is usually evidence that the irritating focus of the seizure is secondary to an underlying condition that causes damage to brain tissue. Focal lesions include scars from previous craniocerebral trauma, atrophy, malformations, or tumors. Focal seizures may arise from any area of the cerebral cortex, but the frontal, temporal, and parietal lobes are the ones most often affected. The area of cerebral involvement is reflected by clinical manifestations. Partial or focal seizures may spread to other areas and become generalized convulsions. This is known as secondary generalization.

Psychomotor. Partial seizures with complex symptoms are the most difficult to recognize and are among those most difficult to control. Because they involve more organized and higher level cerebral function as well as sensory and motor function, they are termed psychomotor seizures. The attack is characterized by a period of altered behavior for which the individual is amnesic and during which he is unable to respond to his environment.[22] Though the child does not lose consciousness during an attack, he has no recollection of his behavior during the seizure. Drowsiness or sleep usually follows the seizure. Confusion and amnesia may be prolonged.[1]

Psychomotor seizures are observed more often in children from 3 years of age through adolescence and are more common in adults than in children. The seizures are most characteristically associated with focal lesions of the temporal lobe and are sometimes referred to as temporal lobe seizures.

Complex sensory phenomena associated with the beginning of a seizure reflect the complicated connections and integrative functions of that area of the brain. The most frequent sensation is a strange feeling in the pit of the stomach that rises toward the throat. This feeling is often accompanied by odd or unpleasant odors or tastes, complex auditory or visual hallucinations, or ill-defined feelings of elation or strangeness (such as *déjà vu,* a feeling of familiarity in a strange environment). Small children may emit a cry or attempt to run for help as a manifestation of an aura. Strong feelings of fear and anxiety and a distorted sense of time and self may be mental symptoms associated with an episode.[1,36]

A variety of patterns of motor behavior may be observed during a psychomotor attack. The attacks are usually stereotypic and recur in a similar manner with each subsequent seizure. It is sometimes difficult to determine whether the manifestations are related to a seizure disorder or to a nonconvulsive behavioral disturbance.[1] The child may suddenly cease his activity, appear dazed, stare into space, become confused and apathetic, and become limp, stiff, or display some form of posturing. The primary feature may be confusion, and the child may perform purposeless, complicated activities in a repetitive manner (automatisms), such as walking, running, kicking, laughing, or speaking incoherently, most often followed by postictal confusion or sleep. The predominant observations may be oropharyngeal activities, such as smacking, chewing, drooling, swallowing, and nausea or abdominal pain followed by stiffness, a fall, and postictal sleep. In children auras are rarely manifest as rage or temper tantrums and aggressive acts are uncommon during a seizure.

Focal motor seizures. Focal seizures are characterized by localized motor symptoms. The most common focal motor seizure in children is the adversive seizure, in which the eye or eyes and head turn away from the side of the focus. In some children the upper extremity toward which the head turns is abducted and extended and the fingers are clenched, giving the impression that the child appears to look at the closed fist. The child may be aware of the movement or lose consciousness simultaneously with assuming the position.

A common form is the sylvian seizure, in which there are tonic-clonic movements involving the face, salivation, and arrested speech. These are most common during sleep. On rare occasions children display the jacksonian march, an orderly, sequential progression of clonic movements that begin in a foot, hand, or face and, as electric impulses spread from the irritable focus to continuous regions of the cortex, move or "march" body parts activated by these cerebral regions.

Focal motor seizures are particularly common in hemiplegic children. The movements, which are usually clonic, begin in the hemiplegic hand, spread to the entire affected side, and, in many cases, become generalized seizures. Postictal weakness (Todd's paralysis) is common after this type of seizure.[14,36]

Focal sensory seizures. Focal sensory seizures are characterized by various sensations, including numbness, tingling, prickling, paresthesia, or pain that originates in one area (such as the face or extremities) and spreads to other parts of the body. Visual sensations or formed images may be manifestations. Motor phenomena such as posturing or hypertonia may accompany sensory seizures. Sensory focal seizures are uncommon in children under 8 years of age.

Types of seizures: nonepileptic

Febrile convulsions. Febrile convulsions are a transient disorder of children that occur in association with a fever. They are one of the most common neurologic disorders of childhood, affecting 3% to 5% of children. Most febrile convulsions occur after 6 months of age and usually before age 3 years, with increased frequency in children younger than 18 months of age. They are unusual after 5 years of age. Boys are affected about twice as often as girls, and there appears to be an increased susceptibility in families, indicating a possible genetic predisposition.[22,25]

The cause of febrile convulsions is still uncertain. In most children the height and rapidity of the temperature elevation seem to be factors. The fever usually exceeds 38.8°C (101.8°F) and occurs during the temperature rise rather than after a prolonged elevation. Sometimes it constitutes the dramatic beginning of an illness. Febrile convulsions usually accompany an upper respiratory or gastrointestinal infection, and 25% of children with simple febrile convulsion have a recurrence of the seizure with subsequent infections. Since fevers are almost impossible to prevent in children, efforts are directed toward preventing an increase in the temperature.

Treatment consists of controlling the seizure with phenobarbital or diazepam (Valium) in appropriate dosage, reducing the temperature by administration of aspirin and conductive and evaporative cooling of the child, and treatment of the intercurrent infection. Aspirin and cooling sponge baths are administered early as a preventive measure in the event of subsequent infections. Whether or not to implement continuous prophylactic anticonvulsant therapy in children who have experienced their initial febrile convulsion is still controversial. Anticonvulsant therapy is usually reserved for children who have prolonged convulsions or who have experienced a second seizure.

In children who exhibit febrile seizures, there is an increased risk of epilepsy with the increase in the number of seizures. As the number of seizures increases, the severity of the seizures also increases. The chance of developing chronic seizure disorder is increased in children who have a prolonged convulsion, those with focal seizures, those who have a near relative with convulsions, and those with an abnormal electroencephalogram. Recurrences are more likely when the first seizure occurs in the first year of life. Seventy-five percent of recurrences take place within 1 year of the first febrile seizure, and almost 90% within 2 years of onset.

Breath-holding spells (reflex hypoxic crisis). Breath-holding spells are readily recognized and follow a distinct clinical pattern. Not a true convulsive disorder, the typical attack has its onset in infants between the ages of 6 and 18 months of age and may occur up to 4 years of age. The episode is characterized by violent crying and cessation of breathing that is precipitated by fright, frustration, or anger. The breath is usually held on expiration, and the child becomes cyanotic, loses consciousness, and may display a few clonic convulsions of the extremities. The episode ends with a gasp and the color returns promptly. The frequency of attacks varies considerably, but they almost always disappear by 5 to 6 years of age.[22,25]

Breath-holding spells are a benign entity, and drug therapy is generally not indicated. Family therapy may be beneficial, since many children appear to use an attack or the threat of an attack to assert themselves and to express anger. Parents need reassurance that the attacks do not represent a danger to the child, and this knowledge may even help to decrease or eliminate the incidence of attacks.

Migraine. Migraine is the most common paroxysmal disorder that affects the brain. It is characterized by chronic recurrent headache, often preceded by visual disturbances and accompanied by nausea and vomiting. The cause is unknown.

There are two phases in the pathology of migraine, both caused by a functional disturbance of intracerebral circulation. Initially there is a prodromal phase caused by vasoconstriction of intracranial vessels followed by dilatation of the extracranial vessels, which produces a throbbing, pulsating, and pounding headache.[26]

A family history of migraine is elicited in over 50% of the patients, and some observers have noted that children often display a characteristic personality. They tend to be meticulous, compulsive, unusually mature for their age, and high achievers in school and strive to please the family at home. They have difficulty in expressing anger or rage. Boys are affected twice as often as girls.[23]

The diagnosis is seldom made until the child is old enough to relate his symptoms, although one in five children has his first attack before age 5 years. Early in life the symptoms are nonspecific, such as recurrent abdominal pain, car sickness, and restlessness, and the child may display head banging or sudden alterations in personality. The typical attack of migraine begins early in the day, often awakening the child. The prodromal symptoms, induced by vasoconstriction, consist of transient visual disturbances or other neurologic disabilities. In a few minutes or, sometimes, a few hours, the aura is followed by the throbbing unilateral head pain accompanied by nausea and vomiting. Sleep ordinarily terminates an attack.[22]

Treatment is symptomatic. For most patients the vasoconstrictor ergotamine tartrate taken at the onset of symptoms provides relief. Simple analgesics such as aspirin or acetaminophen may be effective and are usually the preferred medication. The outlook for the child with migraine is good, but the child and his parents should be informed that the predisposition to the headaches is lifelong, although benign, and should not interfere with normal activities.

Diagnostic evaluation

The process of diagnosis in a child with a convulsive disorder has two major foci: (1) to ascertain the type of seizure the child has experienced, and (2) to attempt to understand the cause of the attacks. The assessment and diagnosis rely heavily on a thorough history, skilled observation, and employment of several diagnostic tests.[22]

A complete, accurate, and detailed history should be obtained from a reliable and knowledgeable informant. This includes prenatal, perinatal, and neonatal periods, including any instances of infection, apnea, colic, or poor feeding, and information regarding any previous accidents or serious illnesses.

History of the seizure(s) should be equally detailed, including the type of seizure or description of the child's behavior during the attack(s), the age at onset, and the time at which the seizure occurs, that is, early morning, before meals, while awake, or during sleep. Any factors that may have precipitated the seizure are important, including fever, infection, falls that may have caused trauma to the head, anxiety, fatigue, and activity, for example, hyperventilation or exposure to strong stimuli such as bright flashing lights or loud noises. If the child can describe any sensory phenomena, these are recorded. The duration and progression of the seizure (if any) and the postictal feelings and behavior, such as confusion, inability to speak, amnesia, headache, and sleep, are recorded.

A complete physical and neurologic examination, including developmental assessment of language, learning, behavioral, and motor abilities, often provides clues to neurologic disturbances. A family history may offer clues to paroxysmal disorders such as migraine, breath-holding spells, febrile convulsions, or neurologic diseases that may be related to the convulsive disorder.

Laboratory studies that may prove to be of value include a complete blood cell count (for evidence of lead poisoning) and white blood cell count for signs of infection. Blood and cerebrospinal fluid glucose may give evidence of hypoglycemic episodes, and serum electrolytes, blood urea nitrogen, calcium, and other blood studies may indicate metabolic disturbances. Lumbar puncture may confirm a suspected diagnosis of cerebrospinal infection or trauma.[35]

Skull radiographs, computerized tomography, echoencephalograms, brain scans, and other studies help to identify skull abnormalities, separation of sutures, and intracranial calcifications. Invasive procedures such as arteriograms and pneumoencephalograms may be employed.

The electroencephalogram is obtained for all children with convulsive manifestations and is the most useful tool for evaluating seizure disorders. The electroencephalogram is carried out under varying conditions—with the child asleep, awake, awake with provocative stimulation (flashing lights, noise), and hyperventilating. Stimulation elicits abnormal electric activity, which is recorded on the electroencephalogram. Various seizure types produce characteristic electroencephalographic patterns—high-voltage spike discharges are seen in grand mal seizures with abnormal patterns in the intervals between seizures; a 3 per second spike and wave pattern is observed in a petit mal seizure; and absence of electric activity in an area suggests a large lesion, such as an abscess or subdural collection of fluid.[1,35]

Medical management

The objective of treatment of convulsive disorders is to control the seizures or to reduce their frequency, discover and correct the cause when possible, and help the child who has recurrent seizures to live as normal a life as possible. Seizures of a recurrent nature are treated as soon as the diagnosis is established. If the seizure activity is a manifestation of a infectious, traumatic, or metabolic process, the seizure therapy is instituted as a part of the general therapeutic regimen.

Drug therapy. It is known that persons predisposed to epilepsy have seizures when their basal level of neuronal excitability exceeds a critical point or threshold; no attack occurs if the excitability is maintained below this threshold. The administration of anticonvulsive drugs serves to raise this threshold and prevent seizures. Consequently the primary therapy for convulsive disorders is the administration of the appropriate anticonvulsant drug or combination of drugs in a dosage that provides the desired effect without causing undesirable side effects or toxic reactions. Anticonvulsant (antiepileptic) drugs are believed to exert their effect primarily by reducing the responsiveness of normal neurons to the sudden, high-frequency nerve impulses that arise in the epileptogenic focus. Thus the convulsive seizure is effectively suppressed; the abnormal brain waves may or may not be altered. Complete control can be achieved in only 50% to 75% of epileptics, however, even with careful attention to details of therapy.[29]

Therapy is begun with a single drug known to be effective for the child's particular type of seizure, and the dosage is gradually increased until the seizures are controlled or the child develops signs of toxicity. If the drug is effective but does not sufficiently control the seizures, a second drug is added in gradually increasing dose. Once seizures are controlled, the drug or drugs are continued for a prolonged period of time.

Periodic reevaluation of the drug is important to assess the continued effectiveness and to alter the dosage if indicated. The dosage will need to be increased as the child grows. Blood levels often prove valuable in determination of optimum dosage levels. Blood cell counts, urinalysis, and liver function tests are obtained at frequent intervals in children receiving particular anticonvulsant medications. Repeat electroencephalograms are generally obtained every 1½ to 2 years.[25]

When a medication is discontinued the dosage should be reduced gradually over a period of 1 to 2 weeks. Sudden withdrawal of a drug can cause an increase in the number and severity of seizures, often precipitating status epilepticus. If the time for reducing the medication coincides with puberty or, in younger children, during periods when the child is subject to frequent infections, the drug is continued for a longer period of time.

The drugs used for control of seizures are outlined in Table 37-4. Side effects of continued use of anticonvulsant medications are sometimes distressing to the child and his family. Phenytoin (Dilantin) causes gingival hyperplasia that can be cosmetically undesirable. Frequent gum massage and careful attention to good oral hygiene are recommended. Application of steroid cream is effective in some instances, but, in severe cases of overgrowth, surgical removal of excess gingiva may be required. Ataxia and rashes often disappear when drug dosages are reduced, and drowsiness from some drugs can be counteracted by judicious use of dextroamphetamine (Dexedrine) (see p. 804).

Status epilepticus is managed by supportive measures, including maintaining an adequate airway, administration of oxygen, and hydration, and by the intravenous administration of either diazepam or phenobarbital. Most physicians prefer diazepam for its dramatic effect on persistent seizures. The child must be closely monitored during administration to detect early alterations in vital signs that may indicate impending cardiac arrest or respiratory depression. When diazepam is ineffective, phenobarbital (intravenously), often in extremely high levels that may require respiratory support, is given as the initial medication. Occasionally paraldehyde (intramuscularly or rectally) is administered. Cases that do not respond to drug therapy may require the use of intravenous lidocaine, general anesthesia, or a potent skeletal muscle relaxant such as curare. This should be administered by an anesthesiologist.

Dietary therapy. The beneficial effects of fasting have been known to be effective in reducing seizures for decades. A ketogenic diet that simulates the ketosis and acidosis of starvation has been advocated as therapy for epilepsy. The diet restricts protein and carbohydrate intake and supplies 80% of the caloric requirements in fats. It appears that the ketones have a tranquilizing effect and that they raise the

Table 37-4. Drugs used for control of convulsive disorders

Seizure	Drug	Side effects	Comments
All seizures	Phenobarbital	Drowsiness Irritability, hyperactivity Skin rash Hyperpyrexia Mild ataxia Vitamin D and folic acid deficiencies	Safest overall drug Most useful in combination with other drugs Bitter taste
	Mephobarbital (Mebaral)	Same as above	Tasteless Requires twice quantity of phenobarbital
	Primidone (Mysoline)	Drowsiness Ataxia, diplopia	Effective with phenobarbital in mixed-type seizure patterns
Adjunctive medication to use with phenobarbital, mephobarbital, and primidone	Acetazolamide (Diamox)	Anorexia Numbness and tingling of extremities Increased urinary output Drowsiness	Supplement to other medications Especially useful in petit mal and other minor motor seizures Often given to control seizures associated with menstrual cycle
	Diazepam (Valium)	Somnolence Ataxia Rash Dysarthria	Useful in minor motor seizures and infantile spasms Often ceases to be effective after a time
	Dextroamphetamine (Dexedrine)	Insomnia Agitation Nervousness Anorexia Palpitations	Used to combat sedative effects of other drugs
	Amphetamine (Benzedrine)	Same as above	Same as above Less potent but better tolerated than dextroamphetamine
Grand mal	Phenytoin (Dilantin)	Gum hyperplasia Hirsutism Ataxia Rash Nystagmus, diplopia Anorexia Nausea and vomiting Nervousness Peripheral neuropathy Vitamin D and folate deficiency Severe toxicity: Pseudodementia Liver damage Macrocytic anemia Lupus erythematosus	Generally effective and safe, especially combined with phenobarbital or primidone Not apt to cause behavioral disturbances in children Gum hyperplasia reduced with good dental hygiene May aggravate petit mal and myoclonic seizures
	Mephenytoin (Mesantoin)	Rash Drowsiness Ataxia Severe toxicity: Aplastic anemia Granulocytosis	Effective anticonvulsant Risk of bone marrow depression limits usefulness Take monthly blood count
Petit mal	Ethosuximide (Zarontin)	Nausea Gastric discomfort Anorexia Vomiting Headache Rare effect: bone marrow depression	Drug of choice for petit mal Occasionally aggravates generalized seizures Administer with food
	Methsuximide (Celontin)	Folate deficiency	Monthly blood count

Table 37-4. Drugs used for control of convulsive disorders—cont'd

Seizure	Drug	Side effects	Comments
Akinetic and myoclonic	Trimethadione (Tridione)	Rash Photophobia Nausea Irritability Drowsiness Severe toxicity: Leukopenia Agranulocytosis Nephrosis Lupus erythematosus	Useful in petit mal absences if ethosuximide fails May aggravate generalized seizures Monthly blood counts and urinalysis
	Paramethadione (Paradione)	Same as above	Same as above
	Phensuximide (Milontin)	Drowsiness Headache Dizziness Nausea Slight nephroxicity	Less effective May be used when others fail Monthly urinalysis

seizure threshold. Reduction of fluid intake to create a negative fluid balance also tends to increase the ketogenic effect. The ketogenic diet has proved most effective in controlling myoclonic seizures and is of value in grand mal seizures, particularly in younger children. It does not influence petit mal seizures or psychomotor attacks.[2,14,22]

The diet is most effective in children between ages 2 and 5 years. In older children, who respond less well, it is usually employed for those children with poor response to anticonvulsant therapy. The diet requires strict control of intake, including careful weighing and measuring of foods, and it becomes monotonous over a period of time. These practical difficulties limit its usefulness in most instances, especially for older children.[8]

Surgical therapy. Obviously when seizure activity is determined to be caused by a hematoma, tumor, or other progressive cerebral lesion, surgical removal is the treatment. When medication is unsuccessful and accumulated evidence indicates a single, distinct epileptogenic focus in a surgically removable and functionally silent area of the brain, excision of the involved tissue is sometimes considered. Persons most likely to benefit are patients with grand mal or psychomotor seizures. Surgical excision of the epileptogenic focus does not eliminate the need for continuation of drug therapy. Drug administration is restarted as soon as the patient regains consciousness and is continued until he is free of seizures for at least 4 years.[22]

Nursing considerations

Nursing care of the child with a convulsive disorder involves both acute care during a seizure and long-term management, including support to the child and his family and education of the child, family, and community regarding the disorder.

Acute care. Nurses, when they first witness a child in a generalized cerebral seizure, are often frightened, puzzled, and immobilized. These reactions are normal but can reduce the effectiveness of care for the child and of significant observations of the event. The child must be protected from injury during the seizure, and nursing observations that are made during the attack provide valuable information for diagnosis and management of the disorder.

It is impossible to halt a seizure once it has begun, and no attempt should be made to do so. The nurse must remain calm, stay with the child, and prevent him from sustaining any harm during the attack. If possible the child should be isolated from the view of others by closing a door or pulling screens around him. A seizure can be very upsetting to visitors and to other children and their families. If other persons are present they should be assured that the affected child is in no danger, and, after the attack, they can be provided with a simple explanation to meet their needs.

The convulsing child should not be moved or forcefully restrained, and force should not be exerted in an attempt to place a solid object between his teeth. If it is possible at the beginning of an attack, a rubber wedge, padded tongue depressor, or the corner of a collar, blanket, wallet, or similar item can be used if it can be placed without difficulty. Nurses should never place their own fingers in the child's mouth during a seizure since the forceful muscular contractions can produce a serious bite. If the child is standing and the nurse is able to reach him in time or if he is seated in a chair (including a wheelchair), he should be eased to the floor immediately. The nurse can protect the child from injury by supporting his head and gently restraining his hands to decrease the likelihood of injury from violent movements against the floor. After the attack the child should be placed on his side in his bed or a similar place to allow him to sleep until he awakens. If he is at school or away from his home, the parents should be contacted so that he can be taken home to rest.

A child who is known to have convulsive attacks or one who is under observation for seizures will require special precautions. The extent of these measures will depend on the type and frequency of the seizure. The child who is subject to daily seizures should not be permitted to engage in activities in which he might be injured, such as climbing, swimming, or handling sharp implements, and most of these children are advised to wear lightweight protective helmets. They should have side rails on beds with the hard surfaces padded if there is danger that they could hurt themselves. A padded tongue depressor or rubber wedge should be in a convenient spot so that it can be quickly placed between the child's teeth, if possible.

A child who has infrequent seizures or who is relatively free of seizures will have few restrictions on his activities. When he is hospitalized appropriate precautions should be implemented, such as side rails kept up when he is sleeping or resting, especially if his seizures are of the grand mal variety, since many of these children are subject to nocturnal attacks. The bed should be protected with a waterproof mattress or sheeting.

An important nursing function during a convulsion is to observe the seizure and describe its pertinent features. This includes the child's behavior before, during, and after the attack. Grand mal seizures and other seizures with dramatic manifestations are easily detected, but petit mal episodes may be more difficult to detect. They are easily misinterpreted as inattention. Any unusual behavior, even seemingly inconsequential behavior such as a momentary interruption of activity, staring, or mental blankness, should be described. The more detailed these descriptions, the more valuable they are for purposes of assessment.

The nurse should note the time that the seizure began and time the length of the seizure. This is especially important if the child becomes cyanotic.

For a summary of nursing care during a generalized convulsive seizure, see the boxed material.

Long-term care. Care of the child with a recurrent convulsive disorder involves the physical care and instruction regarding the importance of the drug therapy and, probably more importantly, the problems related to the emotional aspects of the disorder. There are few diseases that generate as much anxiety among relatives as epilepsy. Fears and misconceptions about the disease and its treatment abound in the lay person's mind. For many it represents the archetype of severe hereditary affliction. Therefore, the foci of nursing care are directed toward helping the child and his family to deal with the psychologic and sociologic problems related to the disorder and to educate the child, his family, his peers, and the public in general toward a more realistic and liberal view of the disease.

Physical aspects. Children subject to seizures are placed on some type of drug therapy. The nurse can help the parents plan the administration of the medication at convenient times in order to disrupt the family routine as little as possible. Once a sufficient blood level of the drug has been achieved, the daily dosage can be given at less frequent intervals to reduce the interruptions in the parents' and the child's daily activities. This also increases the likelihood of compliance. The most convenient times for administration seem to be with meals or at bedtime. Although the anticonvulsant drugs are available in liquid extracts or emulsions, the tablet form is preferred by neurologists. The unequal distribution of the drug in the solute and the increased likelihood of inaccurate measurements make liquid medication less desirable. For small children the tablet of the proper dosage can be crushed and administered in syrup, jelly, or other palatable substances.

It is important to impress on the family the necessity of continuing the medication regularly without interruption for as long as required. This is usually 2 to 3 years after the last seizure, after which the drug is discontinued slowly over a period of time to avoid the possibility of precipitating a seizure. Planning ahead to replace a nearly empty bottle will prevent the risk of running out of the medication. It is sometimes easy to skip doses or omit them for any of a variety of reasons, especially when the child is free of seizures most of the time. This is particularly so when the child is older and assumes the responsibility for his medication. Omitting medication is the most frequent cause of status epilepticus.

The parents and the child will need to know the side effects of the drug prescribed. They should understand the common side effects so that they can report any unusual observations that might indicate unfavorable reactions. These should be known in detail. Parents should understand that the child needs periodic physical assessment and laboratory studies if he is taking phenytoin, primidone, ethosuximide, or methsuximide. Possible adverse effects on the hematopoietic system, liver, and kidneys may be reflected in symptoms such as fever, sore throat, enlarged lymph nodes, jaundice, and bleeding manifestations such as easy bruising, petechiae, ecchymoses, and epistaxis.

Parents need to be warned of possible behavioral changes as the convulsions are controlled in children taking primidone, phenobarbital, or phenytoin. Changes in personality, indifference to school activities and family, hyperactivity, or even psychotic behavior is sometimes observed.

The degree to which activities are restricted is individualized for each child and depends on the type, frequency, and severity of the seizures, the child's response to therapy, and the length of time the seizures have been controlled. Normal healthy activities are encouraged for children, and participation in competitive sports is determined on an individual basis. With encouragement most

Summary of nursing care during a generalized convulsive seizure

Goals	Responsibilities

Protect child during seizure	If child is standing or sitting in wheel-chair at beginning of attack, ease child down so that he will not fall; when possible place cushion or blanket under child
	Remain with child
	Loosen restrictive clothing
	Prevent child from hitting hard or sharp objects that might cause injury
	  Remove object(s)
	  Pad object(s)
	  Gently support child
	Do not force hard object between the teeth when jaw is tightly closed

Observe seizure	Describe and record
	  Only what is actually observed
	  Order of events
	  Duration of seizure

Onset	Describe and record
	  Significant preseizure events
	    Bright lights
	    Noise
	    Excitement
	    Emotional outbursts
	  Behavior
	    Change in facial expression such as of fear
	    Cry or other sound
	    Stereotyped or automatous movements
	    Random activity
	  Position of head, body, extremities
	    Head turned to side or straight
	    Unilateral or bilateral posturing of one or more extremities
	    Body deviation to side
	  Time of onset

Movement	Describe and record
	  Change of position, if any
	  Site of commencement
	    Hand, thumb, mouth
	    Generalized
	  Tonic phase, if present
	    Length
	    Parts of body involved
	  Clonic phase
	    Twitching or jerking movements
	    Parts of body involved
	    Sequence of parts involved
	    Generalized
	    Change in character of movements
	  Lack of movement of any extremity

Face	Describe and record
	  Color change
	    Pallor
	    Cyanosis
	    Flushing
	  Perspiration
	  Mouth
	    Position
	    Deviating to one side
	    Teeth clenched
	    Tongue bitten
	    Frothing at mouth
	    Flecks of blood or bleeding

Continued

Summary of nursing care during a generalized convulsive seizure—cont'd

Goals	Responsibilities
Eyes	Describe and record Position Straight ahead Deviation upward Deviation outward Conjugate or divergent Pupils (if able to assess) Change in size Equality Reaction to light and accommodation
Respiratory effort	Describe and record Presence and length of apnea Presence of stertor
Other	Describe and record Involuntary urination Involuntary defecation
Observe postictally	Describe and record Method of termination State of consciousness Unresponsiveness Drowsiness Confusion Orientation to time, place, persons, and so on Sleeping but able to be roused Motor ability Any change in motor power Ability to move all extremities Any paresis or weakness Ability to whistle (if appropriate to age) Speech Changes Peculiarities Type and extent of any difficulties Sensations Complaint of discomfort or pain Any sensory impairment of hearing, vision Recollection of preseizure sensations, warning of attack Awareness that attack was beginning
Promote rest	Make child comfortable Allow child to rest after seizure Reduce sensory stimuli Record length of postictal sleep Notify physician if seizure is followed by other seizures in rapid succession or if duration of seizure is excessive
Reduce anxiety	Provide calm, relaxed atmosphere

older children can accept the restrictions placed on activities. Contact sports such as football, karate, or wrestling are to be avoided, but basketball, baseball, and tennis are allowed. Climbing trees or apparatus from which the child might fall and be seriously injured is not usually permitted. The well-controlled epileptic child can ride a bicycle or swim if accompanied by a companion.

Because the child is encouraged to attend school, camp, and other normal activities, the school nurse and his teacher should be made aware of his condition and his therapy. They can help to ensure regularity of medication and any special care the child might need. The child's teacher should be instructed regarding care of the child during a seizure so that he or she can act in a calm manner for the welfare of the child and to influence the attitude of his classmates.

Parents of epileptic child. Parental attitudes and management of a child with a convulsive disorder are as varied as those of other parents of children with a chronic disorder, and they are subject to the same long-term problems (see Chapter 22). Whether the seizures result from illness, injury, or unknown etiology, the parents may feel guilt, anxiety, and, often, humiliation. In the past epilepsy has had a derogatory connotation. The parents want to know if it will affect the child's mental capacities. To many persons epilepsy is erroneously associated with mental deficiency. Seizures do frequently accompany other manifestations of severe brain damage from disease or injury, but the majority of children with seizures, like any population of healthy children, display a wide range of intelligence.

Parents also wonder how the illness will affect the child's future and need reassurance that the illness will not shorten the life of the child and that he can attend school, marry, and have the right to elect to have children. The child will need vocational guidance, and the parents will need to become familiar with the laws in their state regarding any limitations that might be imposed on the child because of the disorder. It should be emphasized that the seizures can be controlled or greatly reduced in the large majority of affected children and that new studies hold the promise of progress in treatment in the future. Parents need reassurance that in this enlightened day and age there is less stigma attached to the disease than there has been in the past.

It is important to encourage a healthy attitude toward the child and his disease and to help the parents feel competent in their ability to meet their responsibilities to the child. The child should be reared as any normal child with natural concern tempered by the understanding of his need not to be overprotected. Many parents refrain from correcting or punishing the child, especially if they have had the experience of such an emotional stress precipitating an attack. The child should not be made to feel that he is different. Parents should be encouraged to be honest and open about the disorder to the child and others. Some parents are tempted to try to conceal the nature of the child's illness because of the belief that the disorder is shameful or a disgrace to the family.

Restrictions on the child's activities will be necessary for his safety, but this area can be approached in a positive way in terms of what he *can* do rather than what he cannot do. Sometimes parents curtail the child's activities more than necessary. The child needs to experience the maturing influences of play and work. The Epilepsy Foundation of America* is a national organization that works toward and for the welfare of epileptic persons and their families, helps with employment and legal problems, and provides education to patients, families, and communities.

Child. The adjustment of the child who is provided the security of a loving family, rewards and punishments no different from those of other children, and support in acquiring self-esteem is more apt to be positive about his disease. Development of normal emotional maturity is inhibited by parental overprotection, indulgence, and restrictions. Maladaptation and a negative self-image are stimulated by peer and family rejection, embarrassment and humiliation, teasing by playmates, and social segregation.

The child derives his self-concept and self-esteem from his observations of others' reactions to him and his own perception of his capabilities. When others consider him to be different, inferior, or an object of ridicule, he comes to view himself as different, inferior, and incapable. He may become frustrated because his activities are limited or because he is excluded from activities in which he feels capable of participating but is segregated from them by others, including his family. Such children are encouraged in dependency.

Behavioral problems are common in children with epilepsy and can become a more serious problem than the seizures. Much of the behavioral difficulties, especially aggressive or delinquent behaviors, has been attributed to the child's reaction to parental rejection. Feelings of guilt, frustration, depression, and self-negation can contribute to antisocial behaviors.

The suddenness and unpredictability of the attacks and the reactions of others further influence his feelings. The child needs to learn about his disease and the role that the medication plays in contributing to his prolonged well-being. As soon as he is old enough, the child should assume responsibility for taking his own medication. He should be advised to carry a card or a Medic Alert bracelet with pertinent information about his condition. Planning activities with the child and emphasizing those in which he can engage rather than those in which he cannot participate help the child to succeed and to gain satisfaction in his achievements. He should be offered opportunities and encouraged to exercise judgment in his daily life.

The adolescent period may prove to be a trying time for

*1828 L Street NW, Suite 406, Washington, D.C. 20036.

the epileptic child. The normal changes and emotional responses may be confused with symptoms of the disease. Normal rebellious attitudes and behavior may cause the more insecure adolescent, angry at being different, to stop taking medication. Sudden withdrawal of the drug together with the accelerated metabolic needs and the increased stress of his period of life will often cause a resumption of or an increase in seizures. Normally the adolescent with a convulsive disorder will need his dosage increased to meet the new growth needs. Limits imposed on his activities at a time when he desires freedom and independence may bring his handicap into sharp focus. For example, some states do not allow epileptic persons to obtain a driver's license, even when the disease is controlled; in others there are restrictions on employment, insurance, and, in a few isolated instances, a marriage license.

Epilepsy should not be a severe handicap to most youngsters, and the nurse, by assuming the role of patient advocate, helping to educate the public regarding the disease, working toward making opportunities available to persons with the disorder, and lobbying for legislation that recognizes the needs of the individual with a seizure disorder, can help to erase the stigma that still remains regarding the disease.

REFERENCES

1. Bruya, M. A., and Bolin, R. H.: Epilepsy: a controllable disease. Part I. Classification and diagnosis of seizures, Am. J. Nurs. **76:**389-392, 1976.
2. Bruya, M. A., and Bolin, R. H.: Epilepsy: a controllable disease. Part II. Drug therapy and nursing care, Am. J. Nurs. **76:**393-397, 1976.
3. Butler, I. J., and Johnson, R. T.: Central nervous system infection, Pediatr. Clin. North Am. **21:**649-668, 1974.
4. Campbell, A. G. M.: Infants, children, and informed consent, Br. Med. J. **3:**334-348, August 1974.

4a. Committee on Infectious Diseases of the American Academy of Pediatrics: Statement, 1974.

5. Conway, B. L.: Pediatric neurologic nursing, St. Louis, 1977, The C. V. Mosby Co.
6. DeVivo, D. C., and Dodge, P. R.: Diagnosis and management of head injury. In Smith, C. A., editor: The critically ill child, Philadelphia, 1977, W. B. Saunders Co.
7. Ducker, T. B., Blaylock, R. L. D., and Perot, P. L., Jr.: Emergency care of patients with cerebral injuries, Postgrad. Med. **55:**102-110, 1974.
8. Farmer, T. W.: Convulsive disorders, syncope, and headache. In Farmer, T. W., editor: Pediatric neurology, ed. 2, New York, 1975, Harper & Row, Publishers.
9. Farmer, T. W.: Intracranial infections. In Farmer, T. W., editor: Pediatric neurology, ed. 2, New York, 1975, Harper & Row, Publishers.
10. Feigin, R. D., and Dodge, P. R.: Bacterial meningitis: newer concepts of pathophysiology and neurologic sequelae, Pediatr. Clin. North Am. **23:**541-556, 1976.
11. Fulginiti, V. A., and Seiber, O. F., Jr.: Acute bacterial meningitis. In Vaughn, V. C., and McKay, R. J., editors: Textbook of pediatrics, ed. 10, Philadelphia, 1975, W. B. Saunders Co.
12. Hambleton, G., and Davies, P. A.: Bacterial meningitis: some aspects of diagnosis and treatment, Arch. Dis. Child. **50:**674, 1975.
13. Hinkhouse, A.: Craniocerebral trauma, Am. J. Nurs. **73:** 1719-1722, 1973.
14. Hughes, J. G.: Synopsis of pediatrics, ed. 4, St. Louis, 1975, The C. V. Mosby Co.
15. Huttenlocher, P. R.: Reye's syndrome: relation of outcome to therapy, J. Pediatr. **80:**845, 1972.
16. Huttenlocher, P. R.: The nervous system. In Vaughn, V. C., and McKay, R. J., editors: Textbook of pediatrics, ed. 10, Philadelphia, 1975, W. B. Saunders Co.
17. Kissane, J. M.: Pathology of infancy and childhood, ed. 2, St. Louis, 1975, The C. V. Mosby Co.
18. Krugman, S., Ward, R., and Katz, S. L.: Infectious diseases of children, ed. 6, St. Louis, 1977, The C. V. Mosby Co.
19. Lovejoy, F. H., and associates: Clinical staging in Reye syndrome, Am. J. Dis. Child. **128:**36-41, 1974.
20. Mayo Clinic and Mayo Foundation: Clinical examinations in neurology, ed. 4, Philadelphia, 1976, W. B. Saunders Co.
21. McLaurin, R. L.: Head injury. In Farmer, T. W., editor: Pediatric neurology, ed. 2, New York, 1975, Harper & Row, Publishers.
22. Menkes, J. H.: Textbook of child neurology, Philadelphia, 1974, Lea & Febiger.
23. Menkes, M. M.: A study of family dynamics in children with migraine, Pediatrics **53:**560-564, 1974.
24. Mickell, J. J., and associates: Intracranial pressure: monitoring and normalization therapy in children, J. Pediatr. **59:**606-613, 1977.
25. Nellhaus, G.: Neuromuscular disorders. In Kempe, C. H., Silver, H. K., and O'Brien, D., editors: Current pediatric therapy, ed. 5, Los Altos, Calif., 1978, Lange Medical Publications.
26. Prensky, A. L.: Migraine and migrainous variants in pediatric patients, Pediatr. Clin. North Am. **23:**461-471, 1976.
27. Reeves, K. R.: Children's reactions to head injuries, Am. J. Nurs. **70:**108-111, 1970.
28. Sell, S. W., and associates: Psychological sequelae to bacterial meningitis: two controlled studies, Pediatrics **49:**212-217, 1972.
29. Sibley, W. A.: Diagnosis and treatment of epilepsy: overview and general principles, Pediatrics **53:**531-535, 1974.
30. Silverman, A., Ray, C., and Dubois, R. S.: Liver and pancreas. In Kempe, C. H., Silver, H. K., and O'Brien, D., editors: Current pediatric diagnosis and treatment, Los Altos, Calif., 1978, Lange Medical Publishers.
31. Surveyer, J. A.: Coma in children: how it affects parents, Am. J. Maternal Child Nurs. **1**(1):17-21, January/February 1976.
32. Surveyer, J. A.: The emotional toll on nurses who care for comatose children, Am. J. Maternal Child Nurs. **1:**243-247, 1976.
33. Thaler, M. M.: Metabolic mechanisms in Reye syndrome: end of a mystery? Am. J. Dis. Child. **130:**241, 1976.
34. Weeks, H. L.: What every ICU nurse should know about Reye's syndrome, Am. J. Maternal Child Nurs. **1:**231-238, 1976.

35. Williams, A.: Classification and diagnosis of epilepsy, Nurs. Clin. North Am. **9:**747-760, 1974.

36. Willis, J. K., and Oppenheimer, E. Y.: Children's seizures and their management, Issues Comprehensive Pediatr. Nurs. **2**(2):56-67, 1977.

BIBLIOGRAPHY

Bachman, D. S., Hodges, F. J., and Freeman, J. M.: Computerized axial tomography in neurologic disorders of children, Pediatrics **59:**352-363, 1977.

Bellam, G.: The nursing challenge of the child with neurological problems, Nurs. Forum **11**(4):396-418, 1972.

Blount, M., and Kinney, A. B.: What to remember about EEG, Nursing '74 **4**(8):36-40, 1974.

Blount, M., Kinney, A. B., and Donohoe, K. M.: Obtaining and analyzing cerebrospinal fluid, Nurs. Clin. North Am. **9:**593-610, 1974.

Bolin, K. L.: Assessing the status of neurological patients, Am. J. Nurs. **77:**1478-1479, 1977.

Conway, B. L.: Carini and Owens' neurological and neurosurgical nursing, ed. 7, St. Louis, 1978, The C. V. Mosby Co.

Dodge, P. R.: Neurologic history and examination. In Farmer, T. W., editor: Pediatric neurology, ed. 2, New York, 1975, Harper & Row, Publishers.

Donohoe, K. M., Blount, M., and Kinney, A. B.: Cerebral circulation and cerebral angiography, Nurs. Clin. North Am. **9:**623-632, 1974.

Farmer, T. W., editor: Pediatric neurology, ed. 2, New York, 1975, Harper & Row, Publishers.

Ford, F. R.: Diseases of the nervous system in infancy, childhood, and adolescence, ed. 6, Springfield, Ill., 1973, Charles C Thomas, Publisher.

Mendoza, S. A.: Syndrome of inappropriate antidiuretic hormone secretion (SIADH), Pediatr. Clin. North Am. **23:**681-690, 1976.

Mitchell, P. H., and Mauss, N.: Intracranial pressure: fact and fancy, Nursing '76 **6**(6):53-57, 1976.

Ouellette, E.: The child who convulses with fever, Pediatr. Clin. North Am. **21:**2, 1974.

Rosman, N. P.: Increased intracranial pressure in childhood, Pediatr. Clin. North Am. **21:**483-499, 1974.

Rudy, E.: Early omens of cerebral disaster, Nursing '77 **7**(2):59-62, 1977.

Shearer, D., Collins, B., and Creel, D.: Preparing a patient for EEG, Am. J. Nurs. **75:**63-64, 1975.

Teasdale, C., and Jennett, B.: Assessment of coma and impaired consciousness, Lancet **2:**81-84, 1974.

Tilbury, M. S.: The intracranial pressure screw: a new assessment tool, Nurs. Clin. North Am. **9:**642-645, 1974.

Craniocerebral trauma

Alexander, E.: Medical management of closed head injuries, Clin. Neurosurg. **19:**240, 1972.

Ambrose, J., Gooding, M. R., and Uttley, D.: E.M.I. scan in the management of head injuries, Lancet **1:**847, 1976.

Craft, A. W., Shaw, D. A., and Cartlidge, N. E. F.: Head injuries in children, Br. Med. J. **4:**200, 1972.

Dowman, C. E.: Early management of head injuries in children, South. Med. J. **63:**992-997, 1970.

Feuer, H.: Early management of pediatric head injury: physiologic aspects, Pediatr. Clin. North Am. **22:**524-532, 1975.

Hafey, L. W., and Keane, B. A.: Patients with acute insult to the central nervous system, Nurs. Clin. North Am. **8:**743-749, 1973.

Harwood-Nash, D. C.: Cranio-cerebral trauma in children, Curr. Probl. Radiol. **3:**3, 1973.

Hekmalpanah, J.: The management of head trauma, Surg. Clin. North Am. **53:**47, 1973.

Hendrick, E. B., Hoffman, H. J., and Humphreys, R. P.: Trauma of the central nervous system in children, Pediatr. Clin. North Am. **22:**415-424, 1975.

Javid, M.: Current concepts: head injuries, N. Engl. J. Med. **291:** 890, 1974.

Jennett, W. B.: Head injuries in children, Dev. Med. Child. Neurol. **14:**137, 1972.

Johnson, M. R.: Emergency management of head and spinal injuries, Nurs. Clin. North Am. **8:**389-400, 1973.

Kinney, A. B., Blount, M., and Donohoe, K. M.: Cerebrospinal fluid circulation and encephalography, Nurs. Clin. North Am. **9:**611-622, 1974.

Klonoff, H.: Head injuries in children: predisposing factors, accident proneness, and sequelae, Am. J. Public Health **61:**2405-2417, 1971.

Knox, C., and Kimura, D.: Cerebral processing of nonverbal sounds in boys and girls, Neuropyschologia **8:**227-237, 1970.

Mandrillo, M. P.: Brain scanning, Nurs. Clin. North Am. **9:**633-640, 1974.

Meachum, W., and McPherson, W.: The diagnosis and treatment of subdural fluid collection in infants, Pediatr. Clin. North Am. **17:**363-372, 1970.

Mealey, J., Jr.: Infantile subdural hematomas, Pediatr. Clin. North Am. **22:**433-442, 1975.

Nezamis, F. K.: The child with a head nurse, Issues Comprehensive Pediatr. Nurs. **2**(2):29-37, 1977.

Norsworthy, E.: Nursing rehabilitation after severe head trauma, Am. J. Nurs. **74:**1246-1250, 1974.

Nursing Grand Rounds: Epidural hematoma, Nursing '75 **5**(3):35-38, 1975.

Parsons, L. C.: Respiratory changes in head injury, Am. J. Nurs. **71:**1287-1291, 1971.

Rosman, N. P.: Increased intracranial pressure in childhood, Pediatr. Clin. North Am. **21:**483-499, 1974.

Stover, S. L., and Zeiger, H. E.: Head injury in children and teenagers: functional recovery correlated with the duration of coma, Arch. Phys. Med. Rehabil. **57:**201, 1976.

Swift, N.: Head injuries, essentials of excellent care, Nursing '74 **4**(9):26-33, 1974.

Tate, G.: Assessment and direction of nursing care for patients with acute central nervous system insult, Nurs. Clin. North Am. **6:**165-171, 1971.

Tindall, G. T., Meyer, G. A., and Iwata, K.: Current methods of monitoring patients with head injury, Clin. Neurosurg. **19:**98, 1972.

Wiley, L.: Hazardous head injury, Nursing '72 **2**(2):11-16, 1972.

Yarzaguray, L.: Craniocerebral trauma in children, Surg. Clin. North Am. **53:**59, 1973.

Young, J. F.: Recognition, significance and recording of the signs of increased intracranial pressure, Nurs. Clin. North Am. **4:** 223, 1969.

Intracranial infections

Bell, W. E., and McCormick, W. F.: Neurologic infections in children, Philadelphia, 1975, W. B. Saunders Co.

Gehrz, R. G., and associates: Meningitis due to combined infections, Am. J. Dis. Child. **130:**877-879, 1976.

Haltalin, K. C., and Wilson, H. D.: Bacterial meningitis beyond the neonatal period. In Shirkey, H. C., editor: Pediatric therapy, ed. 5, St. Louis, 1975, The C. V. Mosby Co.

Jacob, J., and Kaplan, R. A.: Bacterial meningitis, Am. J. Dis. Child. **131:**46-56, 1977.

Kindit, G. W., and associates: Intracranial pressure in Reye's syndrome; monitoring and control, J.A.M.A. **231:**822-825, 1975.

Langner, B. E., and Schott, J. R.: Nursing implications of central nervous system infections in children, Issues Comprehensive Pediatr. Nurs. **2**(2):38-53, 1977.

Murray, J. D., and associates: Acute bacterial meningitis in childhood: an outline of management, Clin. Pediatr. **11:**455-464, 1972.

Murray, J. D., and associates: The continuing problem of purulent meningitis in infants and children, Pediatr. Clin. North Am. **21:** 967, November 1974.

Oppenheimer, E. Y., and Rosman, N. P.: Bacterial meningitis in childhood: neurological complications and their management, Pediatr. Ann. **5:**10, 1970.

Smith, D. H.: The challenge of bacterial meningitis, Hosp. Pract. **11:**71, 1976.

Smith, D. H., and associates: Bacterial meningitis, Pediatrics **52:** 586-600, 1973.

Reye's syndrome

DeVivo, D. C., Keating, J. P., and Haymond, M. W.: Reye syndrome: results of intensive supportive care, J. Pediatr. **87:**875, 1975.

Flammang, M., and Hohm, J.: The child with Reye's syndrome, Nursing '76 **6:**80C-80E, 1976.

Haller, J. S.: Letter: Reye syndrome protocol, Am. J. Dis. Child. **129:**137, 1975.

Page-Goertz, S. S., and Lansky, L. L.: Reye's syndrome: an overview of nursing and medical management, Issues Comprehensive Pediatr. Nurs. **1**(6):41-56, May 1977.

Reeves, K. R.: Beware of Reye's syndrome, Am. J. Nurs. **74:** 1621-1622, 1974.

Samaha, F. J., and associates: Reye's syndrome: clinical diagnosis and treatment with peritoneal dialysis, Pediatrics **53:**336-339, 1974.

Shaywitz, B. A., and associates: Prolonged continuous monitoring of intracranial pressure in severe Reye's syndrome, Pediatrics **59:**595-605, 1977.

Sinatra, F., Yoshida, T., and Sunshine, P.: Reye syndrome, Am. J. Dis. Child. **130:**781-782, 1976.

Thaler, M. M.: Pathogenesis of Reye's syndrome: a working hypothesis, Pediatrics **56:**1081, 1975.

vanCaillie, M., and associates: Reye's syndrome: relapses and neurological sequelae, Pediatrics **59:**244-249, 1977.

Convulsive disorders

Berman, P. H.: Management of seizure disorders with anticonvulsive drugs: current concepts, Pediatr. Clin. North Am. **23:** 443-460, 1976.

Bogdanoff, B. M., and associates: Computerized transaxial tomography in the evaluation of patients with focal epilepsy, Neurology **25:**1013, 1975.

Carozza, V. J.: Understanding the patient with epilepsy, Nurs. Clin. North Am. **5:**13-22, 1970.

Castle, G. F., and Fishman, L. S.: Seizures, Pediatr. Clin. North Am. **20:**819-836, 1973.

Cooper, C. R.: Anticonvulsant drugs and the epileptic's dilemma, Nursing '76 **6**(1):45-50, 1976.

Dodson, W. E., and associates: Management of seizure disorders: selected aspects, J. Pediatr. **89:**527-554 (Part I), 695-703 (Part II), 1976.

Douglas, E. F., and White, P. T.: Abdominal epilepsy—a reappraisal, J. Pediatr. **78:**59-67, 1971.

Gastaut, H.: Computerized transverse axial tomography in epilepsy, Epilepsia **17:**325-328, 1976.

Gold, A. P., and Carter, S.: Pediatric neurology. In Shirkey, H. C., editor: Pediatric therapy, ed. 5, St. Louis, 1975, The C. V. Mosby Co.

Harkness, L.: Bringing epilepsy out of the closet, Am. J. Nurs. **74:**875-876, 1974.

Harrison, H. E.: Convulsive disorders. In Vaughn, V. C., and McKay, R. J., editors: Textbook of pediatrics, ed. 10, Philadelphia, 1975, W. B. Saunders Co.

Kutt, H.: The use of blood levels of antiepileptic drugs in clinical practice, Pediatrics **53:**557, 1974.

Lerman, P., and Kivity, S.: Benign focal epilepsy of childhood, Arch. Neurol. **32:**261-264, 1975.

Levine, I.: Getting to know the epilepsies, Patient Care **10:**102-136, April 1977.

Livingston, S.: Comprehensive management of epilepsy in infancy, childhood, and adolescence, Springfield, Ill., 1972, Charles C Thomas, Publisher.

Livingston, S., Pauli, L. L., and Pruce, I. M.: Epilepsy! Diagnosis and treatment, Pediatr. Nurs. **2**(3):23-27, 1976.

Menkes, J. H.: Diagnosis and treatment of minor motor seizures, Pediatr. Clin. North Am. **23:**435-442, 1976.

Nelson, K., and Ellenberg, J.: Predictors of epilepsy in children who have experienced febrile seizures, N. Engl. J. Med. **295:** 1029, 1976.

Ozmon, B.: Convulsive seizures: a guide to immediate nursing care, Nursing '74 **4**(1):104-105, 1974.

Priehard, J. S.: Convulsive disorders in children: some notes on the diagnosis and treatment, Pediatr. Clin. North Am. **21:**981, November 1974.

Richardson, D. W., and Friedman, S. B.: Psychosocial problems of the adolescent patient with epilepsy, Clin. Pediatr. **13:**121-126, February 1974.

Shope, J. T.: The clinical specialist in epilepsy. Patients, problems and nursing intervention, Nurs. Clin. North Am. **9:**761-772, 1974.

Singer, H. S., and Freeman, J. M.: Seizures in adolescents, Med. Clin. North Am. **59:**1461-1472, 1975.

Wiley, L.: The stigma of epilepsy, Nursing '74 **4**(1):36-45, 1974.

Zwang, H. J.: Epilepsy, Crit. Care Update **4**(7):5-15, 1977.

38

The child with an endocrine dysfunction

The major chemical regulators of the body are the internal secretions and their secreting cells, which are collectively known as the endocrine system. The function of the endocrine system is to secrete intracellularly synthesized hormones into the circulation where they are transported to nearby or distant sites to stimulate, catalyze, or serve as pacemaker substances for metabolic processes. Together with the closely related but more rapidly reacting nervous system, they serve to integrate the various physiologic functions of the organism in adjusting to external and internal environmental demands. Endocrine substances even in extremely small concentrations are effective in modifying metabolism, behavior, and development.

The endocrine system consists of three components: (1) the cell, which sends a chemical message by means of a hormone; (2) the target cells, or end organs, which receive the chemical message; and (3) the environment through which the chemical is transported (blood, lymph, extracellular fluids) from the site of synthesis to the sites of cellular action. Some hormones, such as acetylcholine, have specific local effects; others are secreted by specific endocrine glands and then transported by the fluids to create their effects on target tissues at locations distant from the secreting glands. Some of the general hormones, such as thyroid hormone and growth hormone, affect most cells of the body, whereas the effect of others, such as the tropic hormones, is chiefly restricted to some specific tissues. This chapter is primarily concerned with problems associated with oversecretion or undersecretion of the major hormones or defective responses in those organs and tissues that are sensitive to these hormones. The initial discussion is devoted to disorders of the large interrelated neuroendocrine system. The most common endocrine disturbance in childhood, diabetes mellitus, caused by defective pancreatic hormone (insulin) secretion, will be discussed at length.

NEUROENDOCRINE INTERRELATIONSHIPS

Homeostasis is maintained by two regulatory systems: the endocrine and the autonomic nervous system (also called collectively the neuroendocrine system). The endocrine system traditionally consists of seven glands located throughout the body. Three additional structures are also considered endocrine glands, although for the following reasons they are not usually included. The functions of the *pineal body* (epiphysis cerebri), which is located in the cranial cavity behind the midbrain and third ventricle, are largely speculative. The *thymus,* located behind the sternum and below the thyroid gland, plays an important role in immunity, but only during fetal life and early childhood. The *placenta,* which secretes ovarian hormones and chorionic gonadotropin, is only a temporary endocrine gland. The endocrine glands secrete chemicals known as *hormones* directly into the bloodstream. Because the glands have no ducts, they are sometimes called ductless glands, in contrast to exocrine or duct glands.

The autonomic nervous system consists of the sympathetic and parasympathetic systems. It controls nonvoluntary functions, specifically of smooth muscle, myocardium, and glands. The parasympathetic system is primarily involved in regulating digestive processes, whereas the sympathetic system functions to maintain homeostasis during stress. The higher autonomic centers, located in the hypothalamus and limbic system, help control both sympathetic and parasympathetic functioning. The autonomic chemical transmitters are acetylcholine, released by cholinergic fibers, and norepinephrine, released by adrenergic fibers. Neural release of norepinephrine into the plasma produces the same effects as secretion of this substance by the adrenal medulla. This similarity in chemical activity demonstrates the interrelatedness between the two systems.

The neuroendocrine system acts by synthesizing and releasing various chemical substances that regulate body functions. Information is carried by means of neural impulses in the autonomic system and by the blood in the endocrine system. In general, neural responses are more rapid and localized; endocrine responses are more lasting and widespread. The two systems function synergistically because neural impulses transmitted to the central nervous system stimulate the hypothalamus to manufacture and release several releasing or inhibiting factors. These substances are transferred to the anterior pituitary gland, where they lead to the release of certain tropic hormones.

Control of endocrine system

The endocrine system controls or regulates metabolic processes governing energy production, growth, fluid and electrolyte balance, response to stress, and sexual reproduction. Hormones (chemical transmitters) are released by the endocrine gland into the bloodstream, in which they are carried to tissues that are responsive to them (target cells). The target may be another endocrine gland or an organ or tissue. Regulation of hormonal control is based on a feedback system. Usually the feedback control is one of negative function, which means that an increase in one hormone results in a decrease in another substance.

The main endocrine gland controlling the release of other hormones is the pituitary gland (hypophysis). For this reason it is often called the ''master gland.'' The anterior lobe of the pituitary secretes tropic (which literally means ''turning'') hormones that regulate the secretion of hormones from various target organs (Fig. 38-1). Decreased levels of target cell hormones result in increased secretion of tropic hormones. As blood concentrations of the target hormones reach normal levels, a negative message is sent to the anterior pituitary to inhibit its production of the tropic hormone. For example, thyroid-stimulating hormone (TSH) responds to low levels of circulating thyroid hormone (TH). As blood levels of thyroid hormone reach normal concentrations, a negative feedback message is sent to the anterior pituitary, resulting in a diminished release of thyroid-stimulating hormone.

The pituitary gland is under the influence of the hypothalamus. Especially in times of stress, the hypothalamus receives messages from the central nervous system that result in the synthesis and secretion of certain hypothalamus chemicals called neurosecretions or releasing factors. These chemicals are transported by way of the pituitary portal system to the anterior pituitary, where they stimulate the secretion of tropic hormones. An example of this is the secretion of corticotropin releasing factor (CRF) by the hypothalamus, which stimulates the pituitary to secrete adrenocorticotropic hormone (ACTH). In this instance the anterior pituitary is the target of the hypothalamus and secondarily effects a response from another target gland, the adrenals. The adrenals in turn secrete glucocorticoids, which have multiple target sites throughout the body.

Not all hormones are dependent on other hormones for their release. For example, insulin production is dependent on blood glucose concentrations. Other hormones not under the control of the pituitary gland are glucagon, parathyroid hormone (PTH), antidiuretic hormone (ADH), and aldosterone.

As one can readily appreciate, the activity of the endocrine glands is highly interdependent and interrelated to each other. Consequently a malfunction in one gland produces effects elsewhere in the body. Endocrine dysfunction may result because of an intrinsic defect in the target gland (primary) or because of a diminished or elevated level of tropic hormones (secondary). Endocrine problems occur from hypofunction or hyperfunction of the glands. Primary hypofunction is usually associated with a more profound deficiency of the target gland hormone because little or no hormone is secreted. In secondary dysfunction the target glands secrete some of their hormones but in smaller

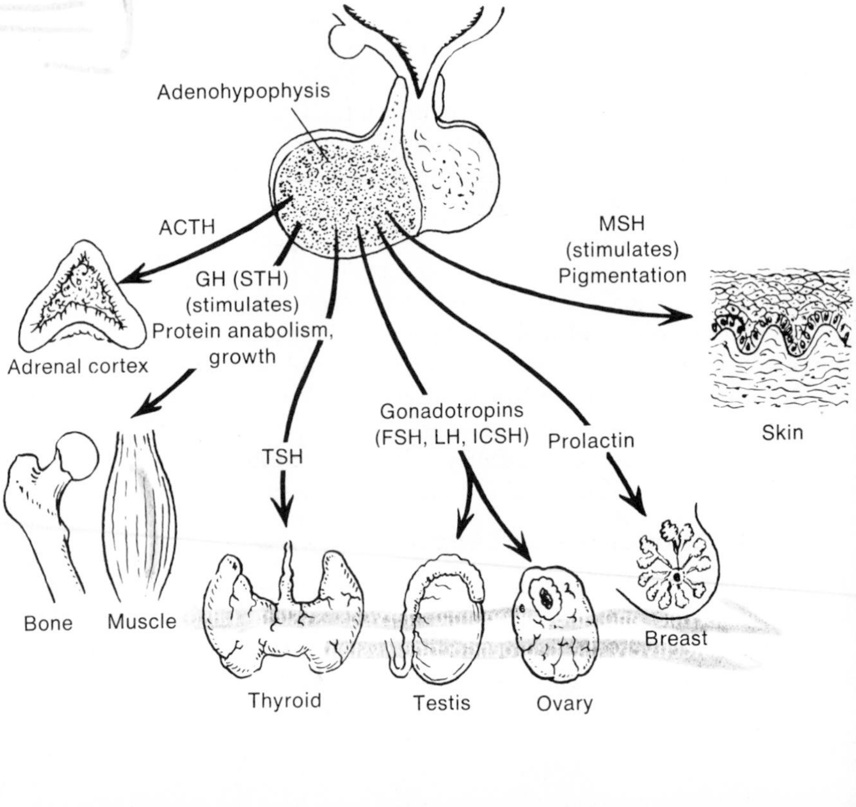

Fig. 38-1. Anterior pituitary hormones and their target organs. Tropic hormones: ACTH (adrenocorticotropic hormone); TSH (thyroid-stimulating hormone); FSH (follicle-stimulating hormone); LH (luteinizing hormone); ICSH (male analogue of LH); MSH (melanocyte-stimulating hormone); GH (STH) (growth hormone [somatotropic hormone]). (From Anthony, C. P., and Thibodeau, G. A.: Textbook of anatomy and physiology, ed. 10, St. Louis, 1979, The C. V. Mosby Co.)

amounts and less rapidly. Hyperfunction may result in an increase of the tropic hormones (primary) and a consequent increase in the target gland hormones (secondary). The pituitary gland (hypophysis) actually consists of two separate glands: the anterior pituitary (adenohypophysis) and the posterior pituitary (neurohypophysis). Since each of these lobes secretes different hormones, they are discussed separately. In general, the more common pituitary disorders during childhood affect one lobe rather than the entire hypophysis. A summary of the endocrine glands, their functions, and the primary effects of oversecretion or undersecretion are summarized in Table 38-1.

Table 38-1. Summary of the endocrine system

Gland	Location	Hormones	Function	Target sites	Disorders
Pituitary (hypophysis)	Embedded within base of brain in sella turcica (saddlelike depression in sphenoid bone)				
Adenohypophysis (anterior lobe)		Growth hormone (GH, somatotropin)	Promotes growth of bone and soft tissues Promotes protein anabolism Promotes fat mobilization and catabolism Has hyperglycemic effect (anti-insulin action)	Bones Soft tissues	Hypofunction Dwarfism Pituitary cachexia (Simmonds' disease) Hyperfunction Gigantism (childhood) Acromegaly (adult)
		Thyrotropin (thyroid-stimulating hormone [TSH])	Stimulates thyroid gland to secrete its hormones thyroxine and triiodothyronine	Thyroid	Hypothyroidism Hyperthyroidism
		Adrenocorticotropin (ACTH)	Stimulates adrenal cortex to secrete glucocorticoids	Adrenal cortex	Hypofunction (Addison's disease)—acute adrenocortical insufficiency Hyperfunction—Cushing's syndrome
		Gonadotropins:			Hypofunction—delayed sexual maturity Hyperfunction—precocious puberty
		Follicle-stimulating hormone (FSH)	Stimulates growth and development of graafian follicles and of follicle cells to secrete estrogen	Ovary	
			Stimulates development of seminiferous tubules and promotes spermatogenesis	Testes	
		Luteinizing hormone (LH)	Promotes complete maturation of follicle Promotes ovulation and formation of corpus luteum Stimulates corpus luteum to secrete estrogen and progesterone	Graafian follicle	
		Interstitial cell–stimulating hormone (ICSH)	Stimulates interstitial cells to develop and secrete testosterone	Interstitial cells (testes)	
		Prolactin (luteotropic hormone)	Maintains corpus luteum and progesterone secretion during pregnancy	Corpus luteum Breast	Inappropriate lactation

Continued.

Table 38-1. Summary of the endocrine system—cont'd

Gland	Location	Hormones	Function	Target sites	Disorders
Adenohypophysis (anterior lobe)—cont'd			Stimulates milk secretion		
		Melanocyte-stimulating hormone (MSH)	Promotes increased pigmentation of skin	Skin	Hyperfunction—increased skin pigmentation
Neurohypophysis (posterior lobe)		Antidiuretic hormone (ADH) (vasopressin)	Acts on distal and collecting tubules, making them more permeable to water, thus increasing reabsorption	Distal/collecting tubules of kidney	Hypofunction—diabetes insipidus
		Oxytocin	Stimulates powerful contractions of uterus	Uterus	
			Causes ejection of milk from alveoli into breast ducts (let-down reflex)	Breasts	
Thyroid	In neck just below larynx; two lateral lobes are connected by a portion called the isthmus	Thyroid hormone, thyroxine, triiodothyronine	Regulates metabolic rate; controls rate of growth of body cells Promotes mobilization of fats and gluconeogenesis	Multiple sites	Hypofunction Cretinism Myxedema Hashimoto's thyroiditis Hyperfunction—exophthalmic goiter (Graves' disease)
		Thyrocalcitonin	Regulates calcium and phosphorus metabolism	Skeleton	
Parathyroid glands	Attached to posterior surfaces of lateral lobes of thyroid gland	Parathyroid hormone (PTH)	Promote calcium reabsorption from blood, bone, and intestines Promote excretion of phosphorus in kidney tubules	Bone, kidney, gastrointestinal tract	Hypofunction—hypocalcemia (tetany) Hyperfunction Hypercalcemia (bone demineralization) Hypophosphatemia
Adrenal glands	Situated on superior poles of each kidney				
Cortex		Mineralocorticoids	Primarily involved in salt metabolism	Kidneys	Hypofunction Adrenogenital syndrome (some types) Adrenocortical insufficiency
Zona glomerulosa		Aldosterone	Stimulates renal tubules to reabsorb sodium, thus promoting water retention but potassium loss		Hyperfunction—aldosteronism
Zona reticularis		Sex hormones (androgens, estrogens, progesterone)	Influences development of bone, reproduction organs, and secondary sexual characteristics	Gonads	Hypofunction—male feminization Hyperfunction—adrenogenital syndrome
Zona fasciculata and reticularis		Glucocorticoids Cortisol (hydrocortisone and compound F) Corticosterone (compound B)	Promote normal fat, prc tein, and carbohydrate metabolism In excess, tend to accelerate gluconeogenesis and protein and fat catabolism Mobilize body defenses during period of stress Suppress inflammatory reaction	Multiple sites	Hypofunction Addison's disease Acute adrenocortical insufficiency Hyperfunction—Cushing's syndrome
Medulla		Epinephrine (Adrenalin), norepinephrine (noradrenalin)	Produces vasconstriction of heart and smooth muscles (raises blood pressure) Increases blood sugar via glycolysis	Multiple sites	Hypofunction—none Hyperfunction—caused by Pheochromocytoma Neuroblastoma Ganglioneuroma

Table 38-1. Summary of the endocrine system—cont'd

Gland	Location	Hormones	Function	Target sites	Disorders
Medulla—cont'd			Stimulates ACTH production, which in turn prolongs sympathetic effects Inhibits gastrointestinal activity Activates sweat glands		
Pancreas Islands of Langerhans	Lies behind stomach with its head near duodenum and its tail adjacent to spleen				
Beta cells		Insulin	Promote glucose transport into the cells (lowered blood glucose concentrations) and increase glucose utilization and glycogenesis Promote fatty acid transport into the cells and lipogenesis Promote amino acid transport into the cells and protein synthesis	Multiple sites	Hypofunction—diabetes mellitus Hyperfunction—hyperinsulinism
Alpha cells		Glucagon	Act as antagonist to insulin, thereby increasing blood glucose concentration by accelerating glycogenolysis	Multiple sites	Hypofunction—hypoglycemia
Ovaries	Located on either side of uterus and behind fallopian tubes	Estrogens	Accelerate epithelial cells, especially in uterus following menses Promote protein anabolism Promote epiphyseal closure of bones Promote breast development during puberty and pregnancy Play role in sexual function Stimulate water and sodium reabsorption in renal tubules	Multiple sites	Hypofunction—lack of or repression of sexual development Hyperfunction—precocious puberty, early epiphyseal closure
		Progesterone	Prepares uterus for nidation of fertilized ovum and aids in maintenance of pregnancy Aids in development of alveolar system of breasts during pregnancy Inhibit myometrial contractions Have effect on protein catabolism Promote salt and water retention, especially in endometrium	Primarily uterus and breasts	
Testes	Lie within each scrotum	Testosterone	Accelerate protein anabolism for growth Promote epiphyseal closure Promote development of secondary sex characteristics Play role in sexual function	Multiple sites	Hypofunction—delayed sexual development or eunuchoidism Hyperfunction—precocious puberty, early epiphyseal closure

Disorders of pituitary function

Anterior pituitary hormones

The anterior pituitary secretes seven hormones: growth hormone (GH), adrenocorticotropic hormone (ACTH), thyrotropin or thyroid-stimulating hormone (TSH), two gonadotropins—follicle-stimulating hormone (FSH) and luteinizing hormone (LH) in females or interstitial cell–stimulating hormone (ICSH) in males, prolactin, and melanocyte-stimulating hormone (MSH). With the exception of melanocyte-stimulating hormone, each of these hormones controls somatic and sexual development.

Growth hormone (GH) or somatotropin. Growth hormone promotes growth of bone and soft tissues without affecting sexual development. Its direct effect on protein anabolism promotes cellular growth. It accelerates fat catabolism and utilization for energy. Although its exact effect on carbohydrate metabolism is not known, it tends to increase the blood glucose concentration—a hyperglycemic response. Therefore, long-term oversecretion of growth hormone may result in diabetes mellitus, an opposite effect of the hormone insulin.

The secretion of growth hormone is under the influence of somatotropin releasing factor (SRF) from the hypothalamus. Hyposecretion of growth hormone during the years of skeletal growth results in a condition called *dwarfism*. If it occurs after epiphyseal closure (during late adolescence) it causes a rare condition known as *Simmonds' disease* (pituitary cachexia). Hypersecretion during the years of active bone growth produces *gigantism,* whereas excess growth hormone during adult life results in a condition known as *acromegaly*.

Adrenocorticotropic hormone. The main function of adrenocorticotropic hormone is to control the adrenal gland's secretion of the glucocorticoids and, to a lesser extent, of androgen. The control of adrenocorticotropic hormone secretion is under the influence of the hypothalmic chemical corticotropin releasing factor. Hyposecretion or hypersecretion of adrenocorticotropic hormone results in clinical manifestations directly attributable to a lack or excess of hormones from the target gland, the adrenal cortex.

Thyrotropin or thyroid-stimulating hormone. As its name infers, thyroid-stimulating hormone promotes and maintains growth of the thyroid gland and stimulates its secretion of thyroid hormone (thyroxine and triiodothyronine). The secretion of thyroid-stimulating hormone is controlled by thyrotropin-releasing factor (TRF) from the hypothalamus. Hyposecretion or hypersecretion of thyroid-stimulating hormone produces symptoms directly attributable to a lack or excess of thyroid hormone.

Gonadotropic hormones. The gonadotropic hormones follicle-stimulating hormone, luteinizing hormone, interstitial cell–stimulating hormone, and prolactin are responsible for the growth and maturation of the gonads at puberty and for the ongoing stimulation of germ cell production during adulthood. The function of these hormones has been discussed in relation to puberty and will not be elaborated here (see p. 689).

ANTERIOR PITUITARY HYPOFUNCTION

Deficiencies of the anterior pituitary hormones may be the result of organic defects or of idiopathic etiology. The most common organic cause is craniopharyngiomas (p. 1024). These tumors usually invade the anterior as well as the posterior pituitary lobes and the hypothalamus and may cause panhypopituitarism, a generalized state of hypopituitarism. The effects of panhypopituitarism are outlined in Table 38-2.

Table 38-2. Effects of panhypopituitarism

Hormone	Clinical effects
Growth hormone (GH)	Short stature but proportional height and weight Delayed epiphyseal closure Retarded bone age proportional to height Premature aging Increased insulin sensitivity
Thyroid-stimulating hormone (TSH)	Short stature with infantile proportions Dry, coarse skin, yellow discoloration, pallor Cold intolerance Constipation Somnolence Bradycardia Dyspnea on exertion Delayed dentition, loss of teeth
Gonadotropins	Absence of sexual maturation or loss of secondary sex characteristics Atrophy of genitalia, prostate gland, breasts Amenorrhea without menopausal symptoms Decreased spermatogenesis
Adrenocortico-tropic hormone (ACTH)	Severe anorexia, weight loss Hypoglycemia Hypotension Hyponatremia, hyperkalemia Adrenal apoplexy, especially in response to stress Circulatory collapse
Antidiuretic hormone (ADH)	Polyuria Polydipsia Dehydration
Melanocyte-stimulating hormone (MSH)	Decreased pigmentation
Prolactin, oxytocin	Effects of deficiency not evident because of delayed sexual development

Most often various deficiencies of pituitary hormones are idiopathic, occurring as a single hormonal problem or in combination with other hormonal deficiencies. The clinical manifestations are dependent on the hormones involved and the age of onset. If the tropic hormones are involved, the resulting disorder is related to the target gland. For example, if thyroid-stimulating hormone is deficient, the sequela is hypothyroidism.

Hypopituitary dwarfism

Idiopathic hypopituitarism is most frequently associated with growth hormone deficiency. A small number of the cases appear to be the result of an autosomal-recessive trait. In the majority of instances the cause is unknown and the defect is limited to a lack of somatotropin. However, sometimes gonatropins, adrenocorticotropic hormone, and thyroid-stimulating hormone are also deficient.

Clinical manifestations. The usual presenting complaint with dwarfism is short stature. These children generally grow normally during the first year and then follow a slowed growth curve that is below the third percentile. Height may be retarded more than weight because with good nutrition these children can become overweight or even obese. In fact, their well-nourished appearance is an important diagnostic clue to differentiation from other disorders such as anorexia nervosa.

Their body proportions and facial structure are normal but remain immature. Consequently they appear younger than their chronologic age. However, later in life premature aging is common. The appearance of fine wrinkles about the eyes and mouth gives them a peculiar impression of immaturity combined with presenility.

Usually primary teeth appear at the expected age, but the eruption of the permanent teeth is delayed. Because of the underdeveloped jaw, the teeth are overcrowded and malpositioned. Sexual development is usually delayed but is otherwise normal. Even without growth hormone replacement, dwarf adults are able to reproduce normal offspring. However, if the gonadotropins are deficient, sexual maturation is absent.

Most of these children have normal intelligence. In fact, during early childhood they often appear precocious in their learning because their ability seems to exceed their small size. However, emotional problems are not uncommon, especially as they near puberty when their smallness becomes increasingly apparent compared to their peers.

It is difficult to predict their eventual height. Because the period of growth is prolonged past adolescence into the third or fourth decade, many of them reach a permanent height of 4 to 5 feet.

Diagnostic evaluation. Only a small number of children with delayed growth or short stature have hypopituitary dwarfism. In the majority of instances the cause is constitutional delay (see p. 710). Diagnostic evaluation is aimed at isolating organic causes, which in addition to growth hormone deficiency may include hypothyroidism, hypersecretion of cortisol, gonadal aplasia, chronic illness, or nutritional inadequacy.

A complete diagnostic workup includes a family history, a history of the child's growth patterns and previous health status, physical examination, radiologic surveys, and endocrine studies.

Family history. A family history is of utmost importance in relating short stature to genetic background. Children with constitutional delays frequently are the products of parents who experienced similar slow growth patterns and delayed sexual maturation. Likewise a small percentage of those with hypopituitary dwarfism have a family history that can be traced to demonstrate an autosomal-recessive inheritance pattern for the disorder. Height and weight of siblings are taken and compared to the child's growth patterns at comparable age periods.

Child's history. A thorough prenatal history is significant in ruling out maternal disorders, which may have influenced the child's growth retardation, such as malnutrition. Birth height and weight are compared to gestational age. Children with hypopituitary dwarfism are usually of normal size and gestational age at birth.

The child's past health history is investigated for evidence of chronic illness that may have influenced growth patterns. Usually, however, the diagnosis of a chronic illness, such as congenital heart disease, malabsorptive disorders, severe anemia, or neurologic impairments, has been identified long before the growth problem becomes a concern. Of importance is assessment of signs and symptoms suggesting a tumor, such as visual disturbances, headache, and signs of increasing intracranial pressure. Such symptoms have often preceded the slowed growth rate but may not have been regarded as significant at the time. With lesions involving the hypothalamus, the history may also reveal characteristic manifestations of dysfunction such as somnolence, thermodysregulation, epilepsy, and hyperphagia, resulting in obesity. Since a craniopharyngioma can affect the secretion of any of the pituitary hormones, assessment for hypothyroidism, hypoadrenalism, and hypoaldosteronism is also included.

Whenever possible the child's growth patterns since birth are evaluated. A progressive retardation in height and weight since early childhood is suggestive of idiopathic hypopituitary dwarfism, whereas a recent change from normal growth is indicative of a tumor. Therefore, age of onset of short stature is a significant diagnostic clue. In addition these children are usually well nourished, ruling out other causes of growth failure, such as malnutrition, chronic illness, or emotional deprivation.

Physical examination. Obviously, accurate measurement of height and weight and comparison to standard growth charts are essential. Other measurements may include crown-to-pubis and pubis-to-heel length to compare body proportions. A funduscopic examination and testing for visual acuity should be performed to detect evidence of ocular damage from a tumor. Sexual development is assessed and compared to age-appropriate development (see p. 691). Observation of general appearance yields valuable clues, especially signs of premature aging and infantile facial features.

Radiologic surveys. Radiographic examination of the wrist for centers of ossification is an important procedure in evaluating growth. In pituitary dwarfism epiphyseal maturation is retarded but is in proportion to the retardation in height. This is in contrast to hypothyroidism, in which bone maturation is greatly retarded, or gonadal dysplasia, such as Turner's syndrome, in which bone age is near normal. Radiographic studies also include a skull series to detect enlargement of the sella turcica, which may permit recognition of a craniopharyngioma.

Endocrine studies. Definitive diagnosis is based on radioimmunoassay of plasma growth hormone levels. Since children's levels of growth hormone are normally so low that they cannot be reliably differentiated from abnormal concentrations, the testing is done by first stimulating growth hormone secretion and then measuring blood levels. One method employs giving insulin to produce hypoglycemia. Since growth hormone has a hyperglycemic effect, low blood glucose levels should stimulate the secretion of growth hormone. An intravenous injection of arginine has the same stimulatory effect. In hypopituitary dwarfs neither of these substances results in increased levels of growth hormone.

Endocrine studies to detect tropic hormone deficiencies are also performed if there is evidence of hypothyroidism or hypoadrenalism. Tests for these hormones are discussed under the discussion of thyroid and adrenal disorders.

Medical management. Treatment involves replacement of growth hormone. Unfortunately the supplies of growth hormone are limited because they must be obtained from human cadavers. In addition not all children benefit from hormone replacement. A small number demonstrate circulating antibodies to growth hormone that inhibit its activity. Children who respond to the therapy eventually achieve a normal adult height. They continue to experience a growth spurt past adolescence because epiphyseal closure is delayed.

Children with other tropic hormone deficiencies require replacement therapy to correct the specific disorders. This may involve administration of thyroid extract, cortisone, testosterone, or estrogens and progesterone. The sex hormones are usually begun during adolescence to promote normal sexual maturation.

If an organic cause is discovered, appropriate therapy is indicated. In most instances this involves partial or total removal of a craniopharyngioma. Such treatment is discussed in more detail in Chapter 28 under brain tumors.

Nursing considerations. The principal nursing consideration is identification of children with growth problems. Despite the fact that the majority of growth problems are not a result of organic causes, any delay in normal growth and sexual development poses special emotional adjustments for these children.

Assisting in establishing diagnosis. The nurse must be aware of signs of growth retardation and participate in history taking to establish a diagnosis. For example, if serial height and weight records are not available, the nurse can question the parent about the child's growth in comparison to that of siblings, peers, or relatives. Investigating dress sizes is often helpful in determining growth at different ages. Parents of these children frequently comment that the child wore out his clothes before he grew out of them or that, if the clothing fit the body, it often was too long in the sleeves or legs.

The nurse also questions parents about symptoms suggestive of a tumor. Because the behavioral or physical changes are insidious, they are frequently overlooked. It is important to correlate the onset of any positive findings with the initial evidence of growth retardation. For example, visual problems and headache are not uncommon in school-age children and can coincidentally occur after a growth problem is recognized. In fact, the headache may represent the emotional trauma caused by the short stature rather than a symptom of a tumor. The nurse pursues this line of questioning cautiously to avoid unduly alarming parents about the possibility of a brain tumor.

Providing emotional support. Once a diagnosis confirming an organic cause of the problem is made, the parents and child need an opportunity to express their thoughts and feelings. Not infrequently a growth problem that was present since birth is missed until adolescence, at which time the child's difference in body development becomes dramatically evident when compared to his peers. Family members may feel anger and resentment toward members of the health staff for not detecting the problem sooner. Parents may experience guilt for not seeking medical attention earlier, especially if the child had been miserable from experiencing ridicule and criticism from his associates. Each family member needs a sympathetic listener who is aware of his needs and realizes the importance of remaining objective and not defensive or overly apologetic. Appropriate emotional support from the nurse can include an affirmation of each person's justified feelings, such as anger or guilt, and emphasis on the treatment plan and prospects for improvement in the future.

Nursing interventions for children with constitutional delays are discussed on p. 716.

Children require additional support because even when hormone replacement is successful, their eventual adult height is attained at a slower rate than that of their peers. They need assistance in setting realistic expectations regarding improvement. For example, increases in height of

3 to 5 inches are common during the first year of therapy, but increases are less dramatic during the subsequent years. Both sexes but especially males need guidance toward appropriate vocational goals. For example, children with aspirations for athletic sports such as basketball would be better advised to explore other activities not dependent on excessive height.

Since these children appear younger than their chronologic age, others frequently relate to them in infantile or childish ways. Parents and teachers benefit from guidance directed toward realistic expectations of the child, based on his age and abilities. For example, in the home the child should have the same age-appropriate responsibilities as his siblings. As he approaches adolescence he should be encouraged to participate in group activities with his peers. He should wear styles that accentuate his actual age—not his size. If his abilities and strengths are emphasized rather than his physical size, he is more likely to develop a positive self-image.

ANTERIOR PITUITARY HYPERFUNCTION

An overproduction of the anterior pituitary hormones may result in gigantism from excess growth hormone during childhood, hyperthyroidism, hypercortisolism (Cushing's syndrome), and precocious puberty from excessive gonadotropins. The cause is thought to be caused by hyperplasia of the pituitary cells, which may eventually progress to a tumor (adenoma), or a primary hypothalamic defect that results in excess of the hormone's respective releasing factor. Although the initial clinical manifestations are a result of pituitary hypersecretion, eventually pituitary insufficiency occurs and the signs of panhypopituitarism become evident (Table 38-2).

Pituitary gigantism and acromegaly

Excess growth hormone prior to closure of the epiphyseal shafts results in proportional overgrowth of long bones, until the individual reaches a height of 8 feet or more. Vertical growth is accompanied by rapid and increased development of muscles and viscera. Weight is increased but is usually in proportion to height. Proportional enlargement of head circumference also occurs and may result in delayed closure of the fontanels. Children with a pituitary secreting tumor may also demonstrate signs of increasing intracranial pressure, especially headache.

If hypersecretion of growth hormone occurs after epiphyseal closure, growth is in the transverse direction, producing a condition known as *acromegaly*. Typical facial features include overgrowth of head, lips, nose, tongue, jaw, and paranasal and mastoid sinuses, separation and malocclusion of the teeth in the enlarged jaw, disproportion of the face to the cerebral division of the skull, increased facial hair, and thickened, deeply creased skin.

Diagnostic evaluation. Diagnosis is based on a history of excessive growth during childhood and evidence of increased levels of growth hormone. Radiologic studies may reveal a tumor in an enlarged sella turcica, normal bone age, enlargement of bones, such as the paranasal sinuses, and evidence of joint changes. Endocrine studies to confirm excess of other hormones, namely thyroid, cortisol, and sex hormones, is also included in the differential diagnosis.

Medical management. If a lesion is present, surgical treatment, including cryosurgery or hypophysectomy, may be warranted to remove the tumor whenever feasible. Other therapies aimed at destroying pituitary tissue include external irradiation and radioactive implants. Depending on the extent of surgical extirpation and the degree of pituitary insufficiency, hormone replacement with thyroid extract, cortisone, and sex hormones may be necessary.

Nursing considerations. The primary nursing consideration is early identification of children with excessive growth rates. Although medical management does not make the child shorter, it does retard height. The earlier the treatment, the more control one has in predetermining a normal adult height. Nurses in ambulatory settings who are frequently involved in growth screening should refer children who demonstrate excessive linear growth for a medical evaluation. They should also observe for signs of a tumor, especially headache, and evidence of concurrent hormonal excesses, particularly the gonadotropins, which cause sexual precocity.

These children require the same emotional support as those with short stature. However, girls may suffer from the effects of excessive height much more than boys. In fact, males may find the tallness an asset when pursuing sports such as basketball. Children and their parents need an opportunity to express their thoughts. A compassionate nurse can be very supportive to these children, especially prior to adolescence when they are larger than their peers. The nurse can emphasize to a tall girl that as boys grow older they become taller and that she will not always be looking down at them. Since early adolescence is a time of idol worship, the nurse can point out marriages of celebrities in which the woman is taller than the man to help the girl gain a perspective that not all heterosexual relationships must follow stereotypic models.

Precocious puberty

Normally at the time of puberty the hypothalamic releasing factors stimulate secretion of the gonadotropic hormones from the anterior pituitary. In the male interstitial cell—stimulating hormone stimulates Leydig's cells of the testes to secrete testosterone. (The effects of testosterone on sexual development are discussed on p. 690.) In the female follicle-stimulating hormone and luteinizing hormone stimulate the ovarian follicles to secrete estrogens (see p. 690 for the effect of estrogen on sexual development). This sequence of events is known as the hypothalamic-pituitary-gonadal axis. If for some reason there is premature activation of this cycle, precocious puberty occurs (see p. 715).

In most cases the etiology is unknown and treatment chiefly involves psychologic support to the child and family (see p. 716). Despite early sexual development, maturation of the gonads and the appearance of secondary sexual characteristics proceeds normally. The most difficult time for the child is usually the school years prior to adolescence. Once in adolescence, the child's physical differences from his peers are no longer present.

Although the child's heterosexual behavior is appropriate for his chronologic age, the nurse should emphasize to parents that the child is fertile. Usually no form of contraception is necessary, unless the child is sexually active. In this situation proper counseling is important because forms of birth control such as estrogen pills will prematurely initiate epiphyseal closure, resulting in stunted linear growth.

POSTERIOR PITUITARY HYPOFUNCTION

Diabetes insipidus

The principal disorder of the posterior pituitary is hyposecretion of antidiuretic hormone, producing a condition known as diabetes insipidus. Primary diabetes insipidus may result from genetic transmission or from idiopathic causes. The secondary type is the result of damage to the posterior pituitary, usually as a result of head trauma or neoplasms (cranipharyngioma). Another form of diabetes insipidus (nephrogenic) is caused by unresponsiveness of the renal tubules to the hormone, not to hyposecretion of antidiuretic hormone, by the pituitary. Nephrogenic diabetes insipidus is a rare hereditary disorder that primarily affects males. (See also p. 1168.)

Clinical manifestations. The cardinal signs of diabetes insipidus are polyuria and polydipsia. In the older child excessive urination accompanied by a compensatory insatiable thirst may be so intense that the child does little else other than go to the toilet and drink fluids. Not infrequently the first sign is enuresis. In the infant the initial symptom is irritability that is relieved with feedings of water but not milk. The infant is also prone to dehydration, electrolyte imbalance, hyperthermia, azotemia, and potentially circulatory collapse.

Dehydration is usually not a serious problem in older children who are able to drink larger quantities of water. However, any period of unconsciousness, such as after trauma or anesthesia, may be life threatening because the voluntary demand for fluid is absent. During such instances careful monitoring of urine volumes and blood concentration and intravenous fluid replacement are essential to prevent dehydration.

Diagnostic evaluation. The simplest test used to diagnose this condition is restriction of oral fluids and observations of consequent changes in urine volume and concentration. Normally reducing fluids results in concentrated urine and diminished volume. In diabetes insipidus fluid restriction has little or no effect on urine formation but causes weight loss from dehydration. Accurate results from this procedure require strict monitoring of fluid intake, urine output, measurement of urine concentration (specific gravity or osmolality), and frequent weight checks. A weight loss of between 3% and 5% is indicative of moderate dehydration and necessitates termination of the fluid restriction.

If this test is positive the child is given a test dose of injected aqueous vasopressin (Pitressin), which should alleviate the polyuria and polydipsia. Unresponsiveness to exogenous vasopressin usually indicates nephrogenic diabetes insipidus.

Other tests employed in the diagnostic evaluation include a skull x-ray film to detect a tumor, kidney function tests and blood electrolyte levels to assess renal failure, and specific endocrine studies to isolate associated problems. In rare instances a psychologic consultation may be warranted to confirm the possibility of compulsive water drinking because of psychogenic causes.

Medical management. The usual treatment is hormone replacement, either with an intramuscular or subcutaneous injection of vasopressin in peanut oil or nasal sprays of aqueous vasopressin (lypressin). The injectable form has the advantage of lasting for 48 to 72 hours, which affords the child a full night's sleep. However, it has the disadvantages of requiring frequent injections as well as proper preparation of the drug. To be effective the active material must be thoroughly resuspended in the oil by holding it under warm running water for 7 minutes and shaking it vigorously prior to drawing it into the syringe. If this is not done the oil is injected minus the antidiuretic hormone.

The nasal spray has the benefit of a simple, painless route of administration. However, applications must be repeated every 2 to 6 hours to prevent recurrence of symptoms. To provide longer relief during the night, a cotton pledget moistened with the spray can be inserted into the nostril. However, mucous membrane irritation caused by a cold or allergy renders this route unreliable. Although the vaginal and buccal mucosa are substitute routes for the spray, they can be inconvenient.

Children with the nephrogenic type do not benefit from antidiuretic hormone replacement. The polyuria can be controlled by reducing the solute load on the kidney, both with dietary restriction of salt and protein and the use of diuretics, such as chlorothiazide, which diminish reabsorption of sodium and chloride ions. These children still require frequent oral intake of fluids to prevent dehydration.

Nursing considerations. The initial objective is identification of the disorder. Since an early sign may be sudden enuresis in a child who is toilet trained, the nurse investigates the occurrence of excessive thirst with the bedwetting. Another clue is persistent irritability and crying in an infant that is relieved only by bottle-feedings of water.

Once the diagnosis is suspected, the nurse participates

in diagnostic procedures. Accurate measurements of weight, intake and output, and urine concentration are essential for reliable results. In children who are not toilet trained, collection of urine specimens may necessitate bagging the child with a urine-collecting device (see p. 930) or placing the undiapered child on a special frame called a metabolic bed. The apparatus allows for collection of urine through a special opening in the center of the mattress.

After confirmation of the diagnosis, parents need a thorough explanation regarding the condition with specific clarification that diabetes insipidus is a different condition than diabetes mellitus. They must realize that treatment is lifelong. If the child is to receive the injectable vasopressin (Pitressin), ideally both parents should be taught the correct procedure for preparation and administration of the drug. Once the child is old enough he should be encouraged to assume full responsibility for his care. (See the discussion of diabetes mellitus on p. 1490 for helping the child learn to give his own injections.)

For emergency purposes these children should wear Medic Alert tags. Older children should carry the nasal spray with them for temporary relief of symptoms. School personnel need to be aware of the problem in order that they can grant the child unrestricted use of the lavatory. Failure to permit this may result in embarrassing accidents that often result in the child's unwillingness to attend school.

Disorders of thyroid function

The thyroid gland secretes two types of hormones: thyroid hormone and thyrocalcitonin. Thyroid hormone actually consists of two hormones: thyroxine (T_4) and triiodothyronine (T_3). The synthesis of these hormones is dependent on available sources of dietary iodine and tyrosine. The thyroid is the only endocrine gland capable of storing excess amounts of the hormone and releasing it as needed for oxidative purposes. During circulation in the bloodstream thyroxine and triiodothyronine are bound to carrier proteins (thyroxine-binding globulin [TBG]). They must be unbound before they are able to exert their metabolic effect.

The main physiologic action of thyroid hormone is to regulate the basal metabolic rate and thereby control the processes of growth and tissue differentiation as listed below.

*Physiologic effects of thyroid hormone**

- Regulates metabolic rate of all cells; protein, fat, and carbohydrate catabolism; and nitrogen excretion.
- Regulates body heat production and heat-dissipating mechanisms.
- Regulates protein synthesis and catabolism, amino acid incorporation into protein, and transcription of messenger RNA.
- Increases gluconeogenesis and peripheral utilization of glucose.
- Maintains appetite and secretion of gastrointestinal substances.
- Maintains calcium mobilization.
- Stimulates cholesterol synthesis and hepatic mechanisms that remove cholesterol from the circulation. Stimulates lipid turnover and free fatty acid release.
- Regulates hepatic conversion of carotene to vitamin A.
- Maintains growth hormone secretion, skeletal maturation, and tissue differentiation.
- Is necessary for muscle tone and vigor and normal skin constituents.
- Maintains cardiac rate, force, and output.
- Affects respiratory rate, depth of oxygen utilization, and carbon dioxide formation.
- Affects central nervous system development and cerebration during first 2 to 3 years.
- Affects milk production during lactation and menstrual cycle fertility.
- Maintains sensitivity to insulin and insulin degradation.
- Affects red cell production.
- Affects cortisol secretion, probably due to direct effect on adrenal glands and by increasing ACTH secretion.

*From Krueger, J. A and Ray, J. C.: Endocrine problems in nursing: a physiologic approach, St. Louis, 1976, The C. V. Mosby Co.

Unlike somatotropin, thyroid hormone is involved in many more diverse activities influencing the growth and development of body tissues. Therefore, a deficiency of thyroid hormone exerts a more profound effect on growth than that seen in pituitary dwarfism.

The secretion of thyroid hormone is controlled by thyroid-stimulating hormone of the anterior pituitary, which in turn is regulated by the hypothalamic thyrotropin-releasing factor (TRF). This negative feedback mechanism follows the same principles as were described earlier. Consequently hypothyroidism or hyperthyroidism may result from a defect in the target gland or from a disturbance in the secretion of thyroid-stimulating hormone or thyrotropin-releasing factor.

Thyrocalcitonin helps maintain blood calcium levels by decreasing the calcium concentration. Its effect is opposite that of parathormone, in that it inhibits skeletal demineralization and promotes calcium deposition in the bone.

THYROID HYPOFUNCTION

Hypothyroidism is one of the most common endocrine problems of childhood. It may be either congenital, such as in cretinism, or acquired, such as from autoimmunization (Hashimoto's thyroiditis). Hypothyroidism from dietary insufficiency of iodine is now rare in the United States because the use of iodized salt has permitted a readily available source of the nutrient.

Congenital hypothyroidism (cretinism)

Cretinism is usually caused by failure of embryonic development of the thyroid gland, but it may also be a result of inborn enzymatic defects in the synthesis of thyroxine. The severity of the disorder is dependent on the amount of thyroid tissue present. Usually the neonate does not exhibit obvious signs of hypothyroidism, probably because of the exogenous source of thyroid hormone supplied by means of the maternal circulation. In addition breast-fed infants may not demonstrate the more severe complications of the disorder, such as mental retardation, because human milk contains sufficient thyroid hormone to attenuate and prevent some of the more tragic consequences.[3] However, in another type of cretinism, transfer of goitrogens (substances that can induce a goiter), such as the antithyroid drugs phenylbutazone, para-aminosalicylic acid, and cobalt, may inhibit thyroid secretion, thereby resulting in the condition of congenital cretinism. Although the latter is a self-limiting condition, because once the maternal supply is terminated the thyroid will produce its own hormones, it is a potentially fatal situation. A large goiter in a neonate may cause total blockage of the airway.

Diagnostic evaluation. The symptoms of cretinism usually become apparent by 3 to 6 months of age in bottle-fed infants. However, prior to this time the earliest symptoms indicating hypothyroidism include prolonged physiologic jaundice, feeding difficulties, inactivity (excessive sleeping and minimal crying), anemia, and problems resulting from hypotonic abdominal musculature, such as constipation, diastasis recti, protruding abdomen, and umbilical hernia. The behavioral characteristics often lead parents to describe the infant as exceptionally "quiet and good."

Impaired development of the nervous system leads to mental retardation. The severity of the intellectual deficit is related to the degree of hypothyroidism and the duration of the condition prior to treatment. With adequate thyroid hormone replacement by 3 months of age, the chance for a normal intelligence quotient is increased.[18,24] Other nervous system manifestations include slow, awkward movements, somnolence, lethargy, and abnormal deep tendon reflexes (often referred to as "hung-up" because the relaxation phase after the contraction is slow).

Because skeletal growth is severely stunted, the child is short. Unlike pituitary dwarfism, infantile proportions persist in that the length of the trunk remains long in relation to the legs. The decreased metabolic rate results in weight gain and often leads to obesity. Characteristic infantile facial features from myxedema include a short forehead, wide, puffy eyes, wrinkled eyelids, broad, short upturned nose, and a large protruding tongue. The hair is often dry, brittle, or lusterless and follows a low hairline. Dentition is delayed and usually defective. Such facial features give the child a characteristic dull expression.

The skin is yellowish from carotenemia as a result of the depressed hepatic conversion of carotene to vitamin A. Loss of heat from reduced metabolism is reflected in a cool skin. Cold intolerance is another common consequence. Anemia results in pallor, fatigue, and lethargy, and vitamin A deficiency causes thickened, coarse, dry, scaly skin.

The cardiovascular changes are slow pulse, decreased circulation, mottling, and decreased pulse pressure. The decreased cardiac rate and output are directly related to the decreased oxygen requirements from a low metabolic rate. Respiratory changes include exertional dyspnea and decreased respiratory effort.

In breast-fed infants the clinical manifestations may be delayed until the child is weaned, at which time the facial features, skin and hair changes, growth retardation, muscular hypotonia, and cardiovascular alterations become evident. Because breast milk contains suboptimal amounts of thyroid hormone, bone age is greatly retarded, usually comparable to that of a newborn. Significantly, however, intellectual functioning remains near normal.[3]

Diagnostic tests. Several tests are available to assess thyroid activity. The more common ones are measurement of protein-bound iodine (PBI), free thyroxine, thyroid-stimulating hormone, and thyrotropin-releasing factor and radioimmunoassay of thyroxine and triiodothyronine. These tests measure the amount of thyroid hormone secreted and the intactness of the homeostatic mechanisms. Tests of thyroid gland function usually involve an oral infusion of a radioactive isotope of iodine (^{131}I) and measurement of the iodine uptake by the thyroid, usually within 24 hours. In congenital cretinism protein-bound iodine, thyroxine, triiodothyronine, and free thyroxine levels are low and thyroid uptake of ^{131}I is decreased. Neonatal screening is now possible with a highly sensitive and specific radioimmunoassay for thyroxine or thyroid-stimulating factor.[6,17] Diagnosis rests on the detection of a high serum level of thyroid-stimulating factor and a low level of thyroxine during the early days of life.

Medical management. Treatment involves indefinite replacement therapy with desiccated thyroid to abolish all signs of hypothyroidism and reestablish normal physical and mental development. If started before 3 months of age the chance for completely normal growth is possible.[18]

To avoid the risk of overdosage of thyroid hormones, regular evaluations of thyroxine and triiodothyronine levels should be assessed. Bone age surveys are also done to ensure optimal growth.

Nursing considerations. The most important nursing objective is early identification of the disorder. Nurses caring for neonates and those in ambulatory settings for well-infant care need to be aware of the earliest signs of cretinism. Parental remarks about an unusually "good" baby coupled with any of the early physical manifestations should lead the nurse to suspect hypothyroidism and refer the child for specific tests. Unfortunately many parents harbor guilt about their impressions of the infant prior to the diagnosis because the child's inactivity may not have alerted them to a problem, resulting in delayed treatment.

Once the diagnosis is confirmed, parents need an explanation about the disorder and the necessity of lifelong treatment. They should be aware of signs indicating overdose, namely, rapid pulse, dyspnea, irritability, insomnia, fever, sweating, and weight loss. Ideally they should know how to count the pulse and be instructed to withhold a dose and consult the physician if the pulse rate is above a certain value.

If the diagnosis was delayed past early infancy, the chance of permanent mental retardation is great. Parents need the same guidance in caring for their child as others who have a retarded offspring (Chapter 23). They need an opportunity to discuss their feelings regarding late recognition of the disorder. Although treatment will not reverse the intellectual deficit, it will prevent further damage. Helping the parents deal with future prospects for the child, encouraging them to stimulate him to his potential, and directing their focus to his strengths rather than disabilities can promote an earlier and more positive adjustment to the diagnosis of mental retardation.

Goiters

A goiter is an enlargement or hypertrophy of the thyroid gland. It may occur in hypothyroid, hyperthyroid, or euthyroid (normal) states. When thyroid hormone production is impaired, such as in congenital cretinism resulting from enzymatic defects or from autoimmune disease (Hashimoto's thyroiditis), thyroid-stimulating hormone stimulation results in hypertrophy and hyperplasia of the gland. The size of the gland can cause severe respiratory distress. Thyroid hormone replacement is necessary to treat the hypothyroidism and reverse the thyroid-stimulating hormone effect on the gland.

Hashimoto's thyroiditis

Thyroiditis is the most common cause of goiters and acquired hypothyroidism in children. High serum titers of antibodies suggest that this disease is an autoimmune process. Treatment is replacement of thyroid hormone.

Nursing considerations. Identification of large goiters is facilitated by their obvious appearance. Smaller nodules may only be evident on palpation. Nurses in ambulatory settings need to be aware of the possibility of goiters and report such findings to a physician. Benign enlargement of the thyroid gland may occur during adolescence and should not be confused with pathologic states. Nodules rarely are caused by a cancerous tumor but always require evaluation. Since they are frequently associated with a history of exposure to irradiation of the neck or upper thorax, the nurse inquires about this possibility as part of the assessment.

If an infant is born with a goiter, immediate precautions are instituted for emergency ventilation, such as supplemental oxygen and a tracheostomy set. Positioning the child with the neck hyperextended often facilitates breathing. Immediate surgery to remove part of the gland may be lifesaving.

When thyroid replacement is necessary, parents have the same needs regarding its administration as were discussed for the parents of children who have cretinism. Since the effects of hormone replacement are cumulative, the parents need guidance regarding care of the child with symptoms of hypothyroidism. Since the child's movements are slow, he benefits from an unhurried environment that allows him to proceed at his own pace. Often this requires the cooperation of school personnel to modify academic requirements until the child's condition is stabilized. Provision of rest during the night and periodically during the day is important. Dietary requirements are regulated to meet the child's growth needs but to avoid obesity. A high-protein but moderate carbohydrate and fat diet is recommended.

Thyroid hyperplasia of adolescence

It is not uncommon for teenagers, especially girls, to develop an enlarged thyroid gland, or goiter, during the prepubertal changes. The incidence of all types of goiter rises at this time, although the reasons for this increased incidence are unclear. However, the occurrence of diffuse thyroid hyperplasia (nontoxic goiter) appears to be related to the intense endocrine demands of adolescence and is not associated with iodine insufficiency or excess or with hypofunction or hyperfunction of the thyroid gland.

The presence of the enlarged thyroid gland is usually detected by the physician or pediatric nurse practitioner during a routine examination, although it may be noted by parents when the youngster swallows. The entire gland is enlarged symmetrically with one side usually more dominant than the other, but it is extremely rare for nontoxic diffuse goiter to enlarge to the extent that its size causes mechanical symptoms. Most often the goiter is transient, asymptomatic, and regresses spontaneously within a year or two. Laboratory studies of thyroid function are usually sufficient to establish the diagnosis or to determine whether further tests should be carried out for more complex thyroid pathology.

Therapy of nontoxic diffuse goiter is usually simple, uncomplicated, and effective. Oral administration of thyroid hormone will decrease the size of the gland significantly. Therapy is based on the fact that the simple goiter results from compensatory pituitary thyrotropic stimulation. When the thyroid gland is unable to secrete sufficient amounts of thyroid hormone, the feedback mechanism to the hypothalamic-pituitary system is triggered to release pituitary thyroid-stimulating hormone. In response to this stimulation the thyroid gland is unable to respond adequately enough to inhibit further release of thyroid-stimulating hormone. The gland enlarges in an attempt to supply sufficient hormone. Supplemental oral thyroid extract provides the feedback needed to suppress thyroid-stimulating hormone stimulation, and the hyperplastic thyroid gland regresses in size. Surgery is contraindicated in this disorder. Nursing care consists of identifying the youngster with thyroid enlargement, reassuring him that the condition is probably only temporary, and reinforcing the physician's instructions for thyroid therapy.

THYROID HYPERFUNCTION

Hyperthyroidism (Graves' disease)

Hyperthyroidism is much less common in children than hypothyroidism. It occurs more frequently in females and demonstrates a significant increase in incidence prior to and during puberty. It may be caused by overstimulation of the thyroid by a pituitary tumor that results in excess thyroid-stimulating hormone or by long-acting thyroid stimulator (LATS), a substance found primarily in the serum of persons with this disease.

Diagnostic evaluation. Graves' disease is characterized by a triad of goiter, thyrotoxicosis, and exophthalmos (protrusion of the eyeballs). The signs and symptoms caused by excess thyroid hormone are opposite those seen in deficient states. The principal clinical manifestations are those of excessive motion, such as irritability, hyperactivity, short attention span, tremors, insomnia, and emotional lability. Gradual weight loss despite a voracious appetite is common. Linear growth and bone age are usually accelerated. Muscle weakness often occurs. Hyperactivity of the gastrointestinal tract may cause vomiting and frequent stooling. Cardiac manifestations include a rapid pounding pulse even during sleep, widened pulse pressure, systolic murmurs, and cardiomegaly. During slight exertion, such as climbing stairs, dyspnea occurs.

Exophthalmos is accompanied by a wide-eyed staring expression, increased blinking, lid lag, lack of convergence, and absence of wrinkling of the forehead when looking upward. As protrusion of the eyeball increases, the child may not be able to completely cover the cornea with the lid. Visual disturbances may include blurred vision and loss of visual acuity.

The skin is warm, flushed, and moist. Heat intolerance may be severe and is accompanied by diaphoresis. The hair is unusually fine and unable to hold a wave.

Thyroid crises may occur from sudden release of the hormone. Although unusual in children, they can be life threatening and cause circulatory collapse. These "storms" are characterized by severe irritability and restlessness, vomiting, diarrhea, hyperthermia, hypertension, and prostration. They are precipitated by acute infection, surgical emergencies, and discontinuation of antithyroid therapy, especially after the use of iodine.

Diagnostic tests. Protein-bound iodine, thyroxine, and free thyroxine levels are increased. ^{131}I uptake by the thyroid gland is accelerated. Not infrequently the white count shows granulocytopenia. A goiter is usually present.

Medical management. The major forms of therapy are aimed at retarding the rate of hormone secretion. Antithyroid drugs, which interfere with the biosynthesis of thyroid hormone, include propylthiouracil (PTU), methimazole (Tapazole), and carbimazole. An effective response to these drugs occurs after a latent period, since they inhibit production of additional thyroid hormone but do not retard secretion of stored supplies. Generally some improvement is noted within the first 2 weeks, with evidence of decreased nervousness, less fatigue, increased strength, a lowered pulse, and weight gain. In many children an initial treatment course of 1 to 2 years will be followed by a complete remission of the disorder. Those who relapse may benefit from a second course of therapy but may also be candidates for surgical intervention.

The most serious side effect of these antithyroid drugs is agranulocytosis (pronounced leukopenia), which generally occurs within the initial weeks or months of therapy. It is usually accompanied by a sore throat and fever. Treatment involves immediate discontinuation of the drug, isolation of the child, and administration of antibiotics and glucocorticoids.

An antithyroid formerly used for treatment of thyrotoxicosis but now reserved primarily for preparation of the child prior to surgery or during a thyroid crisis is iodine. The major action of iodine is rapid, making it suitable for use in emergency situations. It is not used for maintenance therapy because of its several disadvantages, including exacerbation of thyrotoxicosis once the drug is stopped, interference with treatment by radioactive iodine since the saturated thyroid will have no affinity for the isotope, and an incomplete or temporary effectiveness of the drug in some patients. Iodine is available in oral preparations (Lugol's solution or saturated potassium iodide solution [SSKI]). When it cannot be given by mouth, it may be administered by means of the nasogastric route or intravenously (sodium iodide).

Other drugs used in conjunction with antithyroid preparations are sympathetic antagonists. Since catecholamines have a stimulatory effect on the basal metabolic rate, especially during states of thyrotoxicosis, drugs that deplete tissues of their catecholamine content (reserpine or guanethidine) or block the response to catecholamines at the receptor site (propranolol) decrease the sympathetic manifestations of hyperthyroidism. Consequently sweating, tremors, and tachycardia are relieved. Reserpine is a beneficial agent because of its antihypertensive and sedative actions. It is frequently administered during thyroid crises.

Definitive treatment involves surgical ablation of the thyroid (thyroidectomy). Although this approach has the advantage of being a long-lasting form of therapy, it also has a number of serious disadvantages, namely, the postoperative risks of hypothyroidism, hypoparathyroidism, and laryngeal nerve damage. Therefore, surgery is reserved for those children who do not respond to or comply with the use of antithyroid drugs or who are prone to recurrences.

Another form of treatment that permanently destroys thyroid tissue is radioiodine therapy. However, it is not recommended for children because of the increased risk of subsequent carcinoma of the thyroid and the possibility of genetic damage.

Nursing considerations. The initial nursing objective is identification of children with Graves' disease. Since the clinical manifestations often appear gradually, the goiter and ophthalmic changes may not be noticed and the excessive activity may be attributed to behavioral problems. Nurses in ambulatory settings, particularly those caring for children in school, need to be alert to signs suggestive of this disorder, especially weight loss coupled with an excellent appetite, academic difficulties resulting from short attention span and inability to sit still, unexplained fatigue and sleeplessness, and difficulty with fine motor skills, such as writing.

Much of the child's care is related to the physical symptoms. He needs a quiet, unstimulated environment that is conducive to rest. Sometimes hospitalization is necessary during the immediate treatment phase to remove the child from a troubled home. A regular routine is beneficial in providing frequent rest periods, minimizing the stress of coping with unexpected demands, and meeting the child's needs promptly.

Since the nervous manifestations often interfere with schoolwork, a consultation with the child's teachers is important in advising them of the medical reason for the problem and suggesting ways of helping the child adjust. For example, he may benefit from a shortened school day or at least study periods in a quiet area. Limiting demands on the child, such as reciting in class or participating in extracurricular activities, may help him conserve his strength for academic studies. Despite the excessive activity of these children, they tire easily, experience muscle weakness, and are unable to relax to recoup their strength.

Emotional lability is often manifest by sudden episodes of crying or elation. Such behavior, coupled with irritability, disrupts interpersonal relationships, creating difficulties within and outside the home. Parents need help in understanding the uncontrollable nature of these outbursts and ways of minimizing them through decreased environmental stimulation, stress, and frustration. The child should be encouraged to express his feelings about his behavior and the effect that it has on others. The nurse can encourage him to concentrate on friendships with one special peer rather than a group until such time as his condition is stabilized.

Heat intolerance may produce considerable family conflict. Since the child prefers a cooler environment than others, he is likely to open windows, complain about the heat, wear minimal clothing, and kick off blankets while sleeping. Although he should dress in accordance with climatic conditions, the use of light cotton clothing in the home, good ventilation, frequent baths, and adequate hydration is helpful in providing comfort. Hygiene should be stressed because of the excessive sweating.

Dietary requirements are regulated to meet the child's increased metabolic rate. Although his need for calories is increased, these should be provided in wholesome foods rather than ''junk'' foods. He may require vitamin supplements to meet his daily requirement. Rather than three large meals, the child's appetite may be better satisfied by five or six moderate meals throughout the day. Family members should refrain from making remarks about the child's appetite, lest he voluntarily restrict his eating to avoid such attention.

Once therapy is instituted, the nurse explains the drug regimen, emphasizing the importance of observing for side effects of antithyroid drugs. Untoward effects of propylthiouracil and related compounds include skin rash, drug fever, enlargement of the salivary and cervical lymph glands, diminished sense of taste, hepatitis, and edema of the lower extremities. Since sore throat and fever accompany the grave complication of leukopenia, these children should be seen by a physician if these occur. Parents should also be aware of the signs of hypothyroidism, which can occur from overdose of the drugs. The most common indications are lethargy and somnolence.

If surgery is anticipated, iodine is usually administered for a few weeks prior to the procedure. Since oral iodine preparations are unpalatable, they should be mixed with a strong tasting fruit juice, such as grape or punch flavors, and given through a straw. Compliance with iodine therapy is essential because of the danger of thyroid crisis after sudden discontinuation. Since this form of therapy produces dramatic improvement in the child's condition, the nurse should forewarn parents of the expected change to prevent their questioning the necessity of surgery. Iodine is given to improve the child's physical status and reduce the size of the goiter, thereby reducing the risks of operating.

Psychologic preparation of the child for thyroidectomy is similar to that for any other surgical procedure (Chapter 25). However, of special consideration is the site of the incision. The fear of cutting one's throat is very real and in older children is associated with death. The nurse explains that the throat is not cut, only the skin, to allow for removal of the gland. Showing the child a picture of the anatomic location of the thyroid around the trachea is often helpful (see Fig. 5-14). The child should be prepared for the dressing around the neck and the possibility of an endotracheal or ''breathing'' tube after surgery.

Postoperative care involves observation for bleeding into the operative site, which can rapidly lead to asphyxiation. The nurse inspects the dressing for bleeding and checks behind the neck for accumulation of draining blood.

Any signs of hemorrhage and respiratory distress are reported. The child should be positioned with the neck slightly flexed to avoid strain on the sutures.

Another complication is damage to the recurrent laryngeal nerve. If damage is bilateral, airway obstruction will usually occur within a few hours, producing severe stridor. Any evidence of stridor is reported immediately, and a tracheostomy set is placed at the bedside. Unilateral injury to the nerve causes dysphonia. Although the hoarseness often improves in a few weeks, the child may have a permanent speech defect.

Since hypothyroidism and/or hypoparathyroidism may result, the nurse observes for signs of these conditions. The earliest indication of hypoparathyroidism may be anxiety and mental depression, followed by paresthesia and evidence of heightened neuromuscular excitability, such as Chvostek's and Trousseau's signs and carpopedal spasm (tetany). The nurse notes such signs and correlates them with serum calcium levels. The behavioral manifestations, including those of hypothyroidism, must be differentiated from emotional depression as a reaction to the stress of surgery. Each of these conditions may require appropriate chemical replacement, which is discussed with the family prior to discharge.

Disorders of parathyroid gland

The parathyroid glands secrete parathormone (PTH), whose main function is to maintain homeostasis of blood calcium concentration. The principal effects of parathormone on its target sites include the following: (1) in the *bone* it increases the release of calcium and phosphate by increasing osteoclastic activity, resulting in bone demineralization, (2) in the *kidney* it increases the absorption of calcium and the excretion of phosphate, and (3) in the *gastrointestinal tract* it promotes calcium absorption. The net result of these actions is to increase the plasma calcium concentration while lowering the plasma phosphate concentration. As was noted earlier, the effect of parathormone on calcium is opposite that of thyrocalcitonin.

The secretion of parathormone is controlled by a simple negative feedback system involving the serum calcium ion concentration. A low calcium level stimulates parathormone secretion, resulting in absorption of calcium by the target tissues.

Parathyroid hypofunction

Hypoparathyroidism may result from a number of conditions, including removal of the glands during parathyroid or thyroid surgery; during the neonatal period from high phosphorus to calcium ratio in cow's milk, immature functioning of the kidneys (see p. 303), maternal hyperparathyroidism, or idiopathic causes. Regardless of the cause, the clinical manifestations, treatment, and nursing considerations are similar.

Diagnostic evaluation. The most common presenting sign is generalized convulsions. Other manifestations of neuromuscular excitability are described on p. 304. In addition the child may exhibit abnormalities of the teeth, such as delayed dentition, premature loss of teeth, enamel hypoplasia, and caries, cracking and ridging of the nails, alopecia, dry, scaly skin, and eye disorders, including blepharospasm, photophobia, keratoconjunctivitis, and cataracts. Digestive symptoms caused by irritability of the gastrointestinal tract include nausea and vomiting and diarrhea or constipation.

Since hypoparathyroidism results in decreased bone resorption and inactive osteoclastic activity, skeletal growth is retarded. Developmental abnormalities include short stature, round face, short neck, and stocky body build.

Physical assessment may yield clues to the diagnosis, such as positive Trousseau's and Chvostek's signs (p. 304). Laboratory tests include serum assays of calcium, phosphate, and parathormone. Kidney function tests are included in the differential diagnosis to rule out renal insufficiency. Although bone radiographs are usually normal, they may demonstrate increased bone density and suppressed growth.

Medical management. The objective of treatment is to maintain normal serum calcium levels (8.5 to 10 mg/100 ml). Ideally this would involve replacement of parathormone. However, the hormone extract can only be given parenterally since the oral form is inactivated by digestive enzymes, treatment is painful and expensive, and the development of antibodies to the exogenous supply is frequent. Because of these disadvantages, calcium is replaced with the administration of oral calcium salts and high doses of vitamin D, which facilitates absorption of the mineral. In acute instances of hypocalcemia, intravenous calcium gluconate is administered.

Nursing considerations. The initial objective is recognition of hypocalcemia. Unexplained convulsions, irritability, especially to external stimuli, gastrointestinal symptoms, and positive signs of tetany should lead the nurse to suspect this disorder. Much of the initial nursing care is related to the physical manifestations and includes (1) institution of seizure and safety precautions, (2) reduction of environmental stimuli, such as minimal holding of the infant, dim lights, and decreased noise, and (3) observation for signs of laryngospasm, such as stridor, hoarseness, and a feeling of tightness in the throat. A tracheostomy set and injectable calcium gluconate should be placed near the bedside for emergency use. If calcium gluconate is administered the nurse takes precautions against extravasation of the drug.

After initiation of treatment, the nurse discusses with the

parents the need for continuous daily administration of calcium salts and vitamin D. If a low-phosphorus diet is recommended, the nurse advises parents to eliminate foods such as milk, cheese, and eggs. Restriction of dairy products may necessitate formula substitutions in infants. The benefit of commercial formulas and breast milk in neonatal hypocalcemia is discussed in Chapter 9. Since high doses of vitamin D (25,000 to 200,000 U) may be needed daily to maintain normal calcium levels, parents need to be advised of the side effects of hypervitaminosis (see p. 485) and to report such findings to the physician.

Parathyroid hyperfunction

Hyperparathyroidism may be caused by primary defects, such as idiopathic hyperplasia of the parathyroid gland, a tumor (adenoma), or secondary defects that decrease the serum calcium ion concentration, resulting in a compensating parathyroid hyperplasia. The most common cause of secondary hyperparathyroidism is chronic renal failure (see renal rickets, p. 1178).

Diagnostic evaluation. Increased parathyroid hormone causes retention of calcium. The clinical manifestations are produced by hypercalcemia and include (1) bone resorption that results in signs of rickets (p. 484), skeletal pain, and pathologic fractures, (2) hypercalciuria, which is associated with deposition of calcium in the kidney, producing renal calculi, (3) decreased neuromuscular irritability, such as muscular weakness, constipation, bradycardia, and cardiac irregularities, and (4) central nervous system disturbances, especially lethargy, stupor, and sometimes psychosis. The most common symptoms are caused by renal involvement, particularly polyuria, polydipsia, dysuria, nocturia, and renal colic. Advanced renal destruction may cause kidney failure.

Diagnostic tests. Blood studies to confirm the presence of elevated calcium and lowered phosphorus levels are routinely done. Measurement of parathormone, as well as several tests to isolate the cause of the hypercalcemia, such as renal function studies, are included. Other procedures employed to substantiate the physiologic consequences of the disorder include electrocardiography and radiographic bone surveys.

Medical treatment. Treatment depends on the etiology of hyperparathyroidism. The treatment of primary hyperparathyroidism is surgical removal of the hyperplasic tissue. Whenever possible the underlying cause contributing to secondary hyperparathyroidism is treated, which consequently restores the serum calcium balance. However, in some instances the underlying disorder is irreversible, such as in chronic renal failure. In this instance treatment is aimed at raising serum calcium levels in order to inhibit the stimulatory effect of low levels on the parathyroids. This includes oral administration of calcium salts, high doses of vitamin D to enhance calcium absorption, a low-phosphorus diet, and administration of aluminum hydroxide to reduce phosphate absorption.

Nursing considerations. The initial nursing objective is recognition of the disorder. Since secondary hyperparathyroidism is a consequence of chronic renal failure, the nurse is always alert to signs suggestive of this complication, especially bone pain and fractures. Since the urinary symptoms are the earliest indication of this disorder, the nurse should assess other body systems for evidence of high calcium levels when polyuria and polydipsia coexist. Change in behavior, especially toward inactivity, unexplained gastrointestinal symptoms, and cardiac irregularities should lead the nurse to suspect this problem.

Much of the initial nursing care is related to the physical symptoms and prevention of complications. To minimize renal calculi formation, hydration is essential. Fruit juices that maintain a low urinary pH, such as cranberry or apple juice, are encouraged, since acidity of body fluids promotes calcium absorption. All urine should be strained for evidence of renal casts.

Safety precautions, such as side rails in place at all times and assistance with ambulation, are instituted because of the tendency toward fractures and muscular weakness. Children with renal rickets (osteodystrophy) may wear braces to correct skeletal deformities. These should be worn as prescribed. If the child is confined to bed, the nurse consults with the physical therapist regarding proper use of orthopedic appliances.

Vital signs are taken frequently, and the pulse is counted for 1 full minute to detect irregularities. A decrease in pulse rate is reported, since it may signal severe bradycardia and cardiac arrest. The diet needs supervision to ensure compliance with low-phosphate foods, particularly dairy products. The nurse instructs parents regarding foods that need to be avoided and the necessity of administering calcium and vitamin D.

If surgery is anticipated the care is similar to that discussed for the child with hyperthyroidism (p. 1467). Since hypocalcemia is a potential complication, the nurse observes for signs of tetany, institutes seizure precautions, and has calcium gluconate available for emergency use.

Disorders of adrenal cortex

The adrenal glands consist of two distinct portions: the cortex, or outer section, and the medulla, or inner core. Each produces different hormones. The cortex secretes three main groups of hormones that are collectively called steroids and are classified according to their biologic activity: (1) glucocorticoids (cortisol, corticosterone), (2) mineralocorticoids (aldosterone), and (3) sex steroids (androgens, estrogens, and progestins). The glucocorticoids and mineralocorticoids are essential for survival, influencing metabolic regulation and stress adaptation. The sex steroids influence sexual development but are not essential because the gonads secrete additional supplies of the hormones.

The medulla produces the catecholamines epinephrine and norepinephrine. Since these chemicals are also produced by the sympathetic nervous system, absence of the adrenal supply is not incompatible with life.

Adrenal cortex hormones

Glucocorticoids. The most important glucocorticoids in man are cortisol and corticosterone. Their principal effects include (1) stimulation of gluconeogenesis by the liver (a hyperglycemic effect), (2) increased protein catabolism with a resultant reduction in protein stores, except in the liver, (3) increased mobilization and utilization of fatty acids for energy, (4) increased storage of adipose tissue in certain sites, (5) decreased inflammatory and allergic actions, (6) regulation of fluid and electrolytes through promotion of sodium retention and potassium excretion by the kidneys and through water diuresis by direct antagonistic action against antidiuretic hormone, (7) increased gastric acid and pepsin production, and (8) suppression of lymphocytes, eosinophils, and basophils but elevation of neutrophils, erythrocytes, and thrombocytes.

The secretion of the glucocorticoids is directly controlled by adrenocorticotropic hormone from the anterior pituitary. For example, a decrease in circulating levels of cortisol results in an increased secretion of adrenocorticotropic hormone, which stimulates the adrenal cortex to secrete additional glucocorticoids. In times of stress the anterior pituitary is stimulated by corticotropin releasing factor from the hypothalamus, which causes the release of increased amounts of adrenocorticotropic hormone. Stressful stimuli capable of provoking this response include trauma, anesthesia, surgical intervention, sepsis, acute anoxia, hypothermia, hypoglycemia, and emotional states, especially panic, anxiety, or anger. Stress has been implicated in the pathogenesis of ulcer, possibly through increased production of cortisone and its effect on gastric acid secretion (p. 1285).

Secretion of the glucocorticoids is also regulated by body rhythms. Blood levels of cortisol demonstrate a typical diurnal or circadian pattern. In individuals who follow a regular routine of nighttime sleeping, cortisol levels are highest in the early morning hours after arising and lowest in the evening hours prior to bedtime.

Mineralocorticoids. The most important mineralocorticoid is aldosterone. Like cortisol, it promotes sodium retention, as well as the anions chloride and bicarbonate, and potassium excretion in the renal tubules. However, its effect is many times more potent than that of the glucocorticoids in maintaining extracellular fluid volume, acid-base balance, and normal potassium levels.

Aldosterone secretion is primarily under control of the renin-angiotensin system. The juxtaglomerular cells of the kidney respond to decreased arterial pressure and/or blood volume and to decreased sodium concentrations by secreting the enzyme renin into the blood. Renin in turn converts angiotensinogen to angiotensin I and then to angiotensin II. Increased levels of angiotensin stimulate the adrenal cortex to secrete aldosterone, which preserves sodium, thereby retaining water. The renin-angiotensin mechanism also results in increased blood pressure.

Sex steroids. Except for the first few days of life, the sex hormones are normally secreted in only minimal amounts until adolescence, at which time they play a role in pubertal changes. Their actions are the same as those of the gonadal hormones on internal and external sexual structures and skeletal growth.

ADRENOCORTICAL HYPOFUNCTION

Acute adrenocortical insufficiency

The acute form of adrenocortical insufficiency (adrenal apoplexy) may result from a number of causes during childhood. Although a rare disorder, some of the more common etiologic factors include hemorrhage into the gland from trauma, including a prolonged, difficult labor; fulminating infections, such meningococcemia, which result in hemorrhage and necrosis (Waterhouse-Friderichsen syndrome); abrupt withdrawal of exogenous sources of cortisone or failure to increase exogenous supplies during stress; and in congenital adrenogenital hyperplasia of the salt-losing type.

Diagnostic evaluation. Early symptoms include increased irritability, headache, diffuse abdominal pain, weakness, nausea and vomiting and diarrhea. Generalized hemorrhagic manifestations are present in the Waterhouse-Friderichsen syndrome (p. 1432). Fever increases as the condition deteriorates and is accompanied by signs of central nervous system involvement, such as nuchal rigidity, convulsions, stupor, and coma. The child is in a shock-like state with a weak, rapid pulse, decreased blood pressure, shallow respirations, cold clammy skin, and cyanosis. Circulatory collapse is the terminal event.

In the newborn adrenal apoplexy is accompanied by extreme hyperpyrexia, tachypnea, cyanosis, and convulsions. Usually there is no evidence of infection or purpura. However, hemorrhage into the adrenal gland may be evident as a palpable retroperitoneal mass.

There is no rapid, definitive test for confirmation of acute adrenocortical insufficiency. Routine procedures such as measurement of plasma cortisol levels are too time consuming to be practical. Therefore, diagnosis is usually made on clinical presentation, especially when a fulminating sepsis is accompanied by hemorrhagic manifestations and signs of circulatory collapse despite adequate antibiotic therapy. Since there is no real danger in administering a cortisol preparation for a short period of time, treatment should be begun immediately. Improvement with this therapy confirms the diagnosis.

Medical management. Treatment involves replacement of cortisol, replacement of body fluids to combat dehydration and hypovolemia, administration of glucose solutions to correct hypoglycemia, and specific antibiotic therapy in the presence of infection. Initially intravenous hydrocortisone (Solu-Cortef) is administered. Normal saline containing 5% glucose is given parenterally to replace lost fluid, electrolytes, and glucose. If hemorrhage has been severe, whole blood may be replaced. In the event that these measures do not reverse the circulatory collapse, vasopressors such as phenylephrine (Neo-Synephrine), levarterenol (Levophed), or metaraminol (Aramine) are used for immediate vasoconstriction and elevation of blood pressure.

Once the child's condition is stabilized, oral doses of cortisone, fluids, and salt are given, similar to the regimen used for chronic adrenal insufficiency. To maintain sodium retention, aldosterone is replaced by synthetic salt-retaining steroids, such as fludrocortisone (Florinef) or desoxycorticosterone acetate (Doca).

Nursing considerations. Because of the abrupt onset and potentially fatal outcome of this condition, prompt recognition is essential. Vital signs and blood pressure are taken every 15 minutes to monitor the hyperpyrexia and shocklike state. Seizure precautions are instituted, since convulsions from the elevated temperature are not uncommon. As soon as therapy is instituted the nurse monitors the child's response to fluid and cortisol replacement. Too rapid administration of fluids can precipitate cardiac failure, whereas overdosage with cortisol produces hypotension and a sudden fall in temperature. The nurse regulates intravenous infusions carefully to guard against too rapid administration of drugs. Intake and urinary output are recorded.

Once the acute phase is over and the hypovolemia is corrected, the child is started on oral fluids, such as small quantities of ginger ale, fruit juice, or salted broth. Too rapid ingestion of oral fluids may induce vomiting, which increases dehydration. Therefore, the nurse plans a gradual schedule for reintroducing liquids. For children who refuse to drink, the prospect of having the intravenous infusion removed once oral fluids are increased is often a motivating factor.

An ascending flaccid paralysis may occur on the second to third day of treatment because of an abnormally low serum potassium level secondary to overtreatment with cortisol and sodium chloride. The nurse observes for signs of hypokalemia, such as cardiac irregularities and poor muscle control, and evaluates serum electrolyte levels. The condition is rapidly corrected with intravenous and oral potassium replacement. When the oral preparation is given, it should be mixed with a small amount of strongly flavored fruit juice to disguise its bitter taste.

The sudden, severe nature of this disorder necessitates a great deal of emotional support for the child and family. The child may be placed in an intensive care unit where the surroundings are strange and frightening. Despite the need for emergency intervention, the nurse must be sensitive to the family's psychologic needs and prepare them for each procedure, even if this is as brief as a statement, such as, "The intravenous infusion is necessary to replace fluid that the child is losing." Since recovery within 24 hours is often dramatic, the nurse keeps the parents apprised of the child's condition, emphasizing signs of improvement such as a lowered temperature and elevated blood pressure. If paralysis occurs the nurse assures them that this condition is temporary and quickly reversed.

If treatment needs to be continued past the acute stage, parents require the same preparation as those of children with chronic adrenal insufficiency. Preparation for discharge should begin as soon as possible after the child's condition has stabilized.

Chronic adrenocortical insufficiency (Addison's disease)

This disorder is rare in children. When it does occur, it is usually caused by a destructive lesion of the adrenal glands, neoplasms, or an idiopathic etiology. At one time generalized tuberculosis was the leading cause of adrenal gland destruction.

Evidence of this disorder is usually gradual in onset, since 90% of adrenal tissue must be nonfunctional before signs of insufficiency are manifest. However, during periods of stress when demands for additional cortisol are increased, symptoms of acute insufficiency may appear in a previously well child.

Diagnostic evaluation. The cardinal signs and symptoms are (1) muscular weakness and mental fatigue, which are aggravated by slight additional exertion or minor illness; (2) pigmentary changes of previous scars, palmar creases, mucous membranes, and hair; hyperpigmentation over pressure points (elbows, knees, or waist); or, less frequently, loss of pigmentation (vitiligo); (3) weight loss resulting from dehydration and anorexia from impaired gastrointestinal functioning (decreased hydrochloric acid); (4) hypotension and small heart size, which predispose to dizziness and syncopal (fainting) attacks; (5) irritability, apathy, and negativism; and (6) signs of hypoglycemia, such as headache, hunger, weakness, trembling, and sweating. Other signs seen in some children are recurrent unexplained convulsions, an intense craving for salt, and acute abdominal pain.

Definitive diagnosis is based on measurements of functional cortisol reserve. The procedure involves a 24-hour urine collection for measuring levels of 17-hydroxycorticoids, the excretable end product of cortisol, and/or levels of 17-ketosteroids, the metabolic breakdown product of adrenal androgen. After this initial 24-hour period, an infusion of adrenocorticotropic hormone is given over a period of 8 hours and urinary levels of 17-hydroxycorticoids or steroids are again measured. In normal individuals the test dose of adrenocorticotropic hormone causes a severalfold increase above urinary control levels. However, in children with chronic adrenal insufficiency there is less of a rise in 17-hydroxycorticoids than in normal subjects.

During this test an eosinophil count is taken prior to and at the end of the adrenocorticotropic hormone infusion. Circulating eosinophils are depressed by increased levels of cortisol. Therefore, absence of or a marked fall in eosinophils after adrenocorticotropic hormone administration is diagnostic of adrenal insufficiency.

Medical management. Treatment involves replacement of glucocorticoids (cortisol) and mineralocorticoids (aldosterone). Some children are able to be maintained solely on oral supplements of cortisol (cortisone or hydrocortisone preparations) with a liberal intake of salt. Cortisone acetate is given in three daily doses and should be taken with meals to minimize gastric irritation. During stressful situations, such as infection, emotional upset, or surgery, the dosage must be tripled to accommodate the body's increased need for glucocorticoids. Failure to meet this requirement will precipitate an acute crisis. Overdosage produces appearance of cushingoid signs.

Children with more severe states of chronic adrenal insufficiency require mineralocorticoid replacement to maintain fluid and electrolyte balance. Since aldosterone is not available, a synthetic salt-retaining steroid is administered. The preferred treatment is daily oral doses of fludrocortisone. The dosage is controlled by taking daily prebreakfast weights. Weight loss despite adequate food intake indicates the need for additional replacement, whereas continuous weight gain signifies overdose. Other forms of therapy include monthly injections of desoxycorticosterone acetate or implantation of desoxycorticosterone acetate pellets subcutaneously every 9 to 12 months.

Nursing considerations. Once the disorder is diagnosed, parents need guidance concerning drug therapy. They must be aware of the continuous need for cortisol replacement. Sudden termination of the drug because of inadequate supplies or inability to ingest the oral form because of vomiting places the child in danger of an acute adrenal crisis. Therefore, parents should always have a spare supply of the medication in the home. Ideally they should have a prefilled syringe of hydrocortisone in the home and be instructed in proper technique for intramuscular administration of the drug in case of a crisis. As was mentioned earlier, unnecessary administration of cortisone will not harm the child but, if needed, may be lifesaving. Any evidence of adrenal apoplexy is reported to the physician immediately.

Parents also need to be aware of side effects of the drugs. Undesirable side effects of cortisone include gastric irritation, which is minimized by ingestion with food or the use of an antacid, increased excitability and sleeplessness, weight gain that may require dietary management to prevent obesity, and, rarely, behavioral changes, including depression or euphoria. Parents should be aware of signs of overdose (see Table 38-3) and report these to the physician.

The side effects of mineralocorticoids are primarily caused by overdosage and include generalized edema, which is first noticed around the eyes; hypertension, which may cause headaches; cardiac arrhythmias; and signs of hypokalemia. Ideally the child should be evaluated periodically for evidence of excessive medication. Emphasizing the importance of routine follow-up care is a significant nursing responsibility.

Since the body cannot supply endogenous sources of cortical hormones during times of stress, the home environment should be stable and relatively unstressful. Parents need to be aware that during periods of emotional or physical crisis the child requires additional hormone replacement. The child should wear a Medic Alert tag to permit medical personnel to adjust his requirements during emergency care.

ADRENOCORTICAL HYPERFUNCTION

The disorders of adrenocortical hyperfunction may be related to an excessive production of any of the hormones, such as cortisol (Cushing's syndrome), androgens (adrenogenital syndrome), or aldosterone (primary hyperaldosteronism). Since the adrenocortical cells are capable of producing any of the steroids, pathologic conditions may result in an excess of more than one type of hormone.

Cushing's syndrome

Cushing's syndrome is caused by excessive production of cortisol. It may arise from excessive production of adrenocorticotropic hormone, which causes adrenal hyperplasia, such as in anterior pituitary tumors, an adrenocortical tumor, overdosage of exogenous cortisol preparations, or chronic stress without any pathologic change in the adrenal gland. Cushing's syndrome is rare in children and when seen is often caused by excessive or prolonged steroid therapy that produces a cushingoid appearance. This condition is reversible once the steroids are gradually discontinued. Abrupt withdrawal will precipitate acute adrenal insufficiency. Gradual withdrawal of exogenous supplies is necessary to allow the anterior pituitary an opportunity to secrete increasing amounts of adrenocorticotropic hormone to stimulate the adrenals to produce cortisol.

Diagnostic evaluation. Because the actions of cortisol are widespread, clinical manifestations are equally profound and diverse (Table 38-3). Those symptoms that produce changes in physical appearance occur early in the disorder and are of considerable concern to older children. The physiologic disturbances, such as diabetes mellitus,

Table 38-3. Clinical manifestations of Cushing's syndrome

Signs/symptoms	Physiologic cause
Centripetal fat distribution Truncal obesity Supraclavicular fat pads Fat pads on neck and back ("buffalo hump") Rounded or "moon" face	Increased appetite and deposition of fat
Muscular wasting Thin extremities Pendulous abdomen Muscle weakness Thin skin and subcutaneous tissue Poor wound healing	Increased protein catabolism resulting in negative nitrogen balance
Increased susceptibility to infection Decreased inflammatory response	Decreased production and circulating levels of antibodies by lysis of fixed plasma cells and lymphocytes
Excessive bruising Petechial hemorrhages	Capillary weakness resulting from loss of protein
Facial plethora ("red cheeks") Reddish purple abdominal striae	Thin skin allows capillary blood to be visible, increased color from polycythemia
Hypertension—arteriosclerosis	Increased salt and water retention (hypervolemia)
Hypokalemia Alkalosis	Increased excretion of potassium and hydrogen ions
Osteoporosis Compression fractures of vertebrae Kyphosis Backache Retarded linear growth Hypercalciuria—renal calculi	Increased glomerular filtration rate and excretion of calcium and decreased absorption of calcium from intestinal tract
Psychoses Irritability Insomnia Euphoria Depression Frank psychoses	Cause unknown
Peptic ulcer	Increased production of hydrochloric acid and pepsin and decreased gastric mucous production
Hyperglycemia Glycosuria Latent or overt diabetes	Increased gluconeogenesis by liver and decreased rate of glucose utilization by cells
Virilization Hirsutism Acne Deepening of voice Clitoral enlargement Tendency toward male physique in female Amenorrhea Impotence	Excess production of androgens

susceptibility to infection, hypertension, and hypokalemia may have life-threatening consequences unless recognized early and treated successfully.

Several tests are helpful in confirming excess cortisol levels, such as fasting blood glucose levels for hyperglycemia, serum electrolyte levels for hypokalemia and alkalosis, 24-hour urinary levels of elevated 17-hydroxycorticoids and 17-ketosteroids, and radiographic studies of the bone for evidence of osteoporosis and of the skull for enlargement of the sella turcica. Another procedure used to establish a more definitive diagnosis is the dexamethasone (cortisone) suppression test. Administration of an exogenous supply of cortisone normally suppresses adrenocorticotropic hormone production. However, in individuals with Cushing's syndrome, cortisol levels remain elevated. This test is helpful in differentiating between children who are obese and those who appear to have cushingoid features.

Medical/surgical management. Treatment depends on the cause. In most cases surgical intervention involves bilateral adrenalectomy and postoperative replacement of the cortical hormones (the therapy for this is the same as that outlined for Addison's disease). If a pituitary tumor is found, surgical extirpation or irradiation may be chosen. In either of these instances, treatment of panhypopituitarism with replacement of growth hormone, thyroid extract, antidiuretic hormone, gonadotropins, and steroids may be necessary for an indefinite period.

Nursing considerations. Nursing care also depends on the cause. When cushingoid features are caused by steroid therapy, the effects may be lessened with administration of the drug early in the morning and on an alternate-day basis. Giving the drug early in the day maintains the normal diurnal pattern of cortisol secretion. If given during the evening it is more likely to produce symptoms because endogenous cortisol levels are already low and the additional supply exerts more pronounced effects. An alternate-day schedule allows the anterior pituitary an opportunity to maintain more normal hypothalamic-pituitary-adrenal control mechanisms.

If an organic cause is found, nursing care is related to the treatment regimen. Although a bilateral adrenalectomy permanently solves one condition, it reciprocally produces another syndrome. Prior to surgery parents need to be adequately informed of the operative benefits and disadvantages. Postoperative teaching regarding drug replacement is the same as discussed previously in Addison's disease.

Postoperative complications of adrenalectomy are related to the sudden withdrawal of cortisol. The nurse observes for signs of a shocklike state, especially hypotension and hyperpyrexia. Anorexia and nausea and vomiting are very common and may be improved with the use of nasogastric compression. Muscle joint pain may be severe, requiring use of analgesics. The psychologic depression can be profound and may not improve for months. Parents should be aware of the physiologic reasons behind these symptoms in order to be supportive of the child. Facial changes that occur rapidly often help to improve family members' disposition but may not affect the child's behavior until his physiologic state is stabilized.

Congenital adrenogenital hyperplasia

In broad terms adrenogenital syndrome may be defined as a condition resulting from increased production of adrenal androgens. Although hyperfunction of the adrenal gland can occur from a number of causes, such as a virilizing adrenal tumor, in children the most common is congenital adrenogenital hyperplasia (CAH), an inborn deficiency of various enzymes necessary for the biosynthesis of cortisol. Congenital adrenogenital hyperplasia is inherited as an autosomal-recessive disorder.

Pathophysiology. Interference in the biosynthesis of cortisol during fetal life results in an increased production of adrenocorticotropic hormone, which stimulates hyperplasia of the adrenal gland. Depending on the enzymatic defect, increased quantities of cortisol precursors and androgens are secreted. There are six major types of biochemical defects. The most common is partial or complete 21-hydroxylase deficiency. With partial deficiency, enough aldosterone is produced to preserve sodium and adequate cortisol is produced to prevent signs of adrenocortical insufficiency. In the complete or "salt-losing" form, insufficient amounts of aldosterone and cortisol are produced, so that circulatory collapse occurs without immediate replacement of the mineralocorticoids and glucocorticoids. In 11-hydroxylase deficiency there is an increase in the mineralocorticoid 11-desoxycorticosterone, which leads to hypertension. In each of these types there is excess production of androgens. Other forms of congenital adrenogenital hyperplasia do not result in excess production of androgens but cause various degrees of hypoaldosteronism or hyperaldosteronism.

Diagnostic evaluation. Excessive androgens cause masculinization of the urogenital system during the twelfth and twentieth weeks of fetal development. The most pronounced abnormalities occur in the female, who is born with varying degrees of ambiguous genitalia (pseudohermaphrodite). Masculinization of external genitalia causes the clitoris to enlarge so that it appears as a small phallus. Fusion of the labia produces a sac-like structure resembling the scrotum without testes. However, no abnormal changes occur in the internal sexual organs, although the vaginal orifice is usually closed by the fused labia (see also p. 417).

In the male enlargement of the genitals (macrogenitosomia precox) and frequent erections are the principal signs. When androgen production is not excessive, virilizing effects in the female may be minimal or absent and the male may have evidence of pseudohermaphroditism, such as microphallus, hypospadias, and incompletely fused scrotum.

Untreated congenital adrenogenital hyperplasia results in early sexual maturation, with enlargement of the external sexual organs; axillary, pubic, and facial hair; deepening of the voice; acne; and marked increase in musculature with changes toward an adult male physique. However, in contrast to precocious puberty, breasts do not develop in the female, and she remains amenorrheic and infertile. In the boy the testes remain small and spermatogenesis does not occur. In both sexes linear growth is accelerated and epiphyseal closure is premature, resulting in short stature by the end of puberty.

Diagnostic tests. Clinical diagnosis is initially based on congenital abnormalities that lead to difficulty in assigning sex to the newborn and on signs and symptoms of adrenal insufficiency or hypertension. Definitive diagnosis is confirmed by evidence of increased 17-ketosteroid levels in most types of congenital adrenogenital hyperplasia. Usually the level of 17-hydroxycorticoids is low or near normal. In complete 21-hydroxylase deficiency, blood electrolytes demonstrate loss of sodium and chloride and elevation of potassium. In older children bone age is advanced and linear growth is increased. A buccal smear for positive sex determination should always be done in any case of ambiguous genitalia.

Another test that can be used to visualize the presence of pelvic structures is ultrasonography, a noninvasive, painless imaging technique that does not require anesthesia or sedation. It is especially useful in congenital adrenogenital hyperplasia because it readily identifies the absence or presence of female reproductive organs in a newborn or child with ambiguous genitalia. Because it yields immediate results, it has the advantage of determining the child's gender long before the more complex laboratory results for chromosomal analysis or steroid levels are available.[20]

Medical management. The initial medical objective is to confirm the diagnosis and assign a sex to the child, usually in accordance with the genotype (see also p. 422). In both sexes cortisone is administered to suppress the abnormally high secretions of adrenocorticotropic hormone. As a result the signs and symptoms of masculinization in the female gradually disappear and excessive early linear growth is slowed. Puberty occurs normally at the appropriate age. In those children with the salt-losing type of congenital adrenogenital hyperplasia, the replacement of aldosterone as is outlined under chronic adrenal insufficiency is instituted. Because these children, particularly infants, are prone to adrenal crises during periods of stress, they may require the same emergency treatment as discussed for acute adrenal apoplexy.

Depending on the degree of masculinization in the female, reconstructive surgery may be required to reduce the size of the clitoris, separate the labia, and create a vaginal orifice. This should be done after the infant is physically able to withstand the procedure and before she is old enough to be aware of the abnormal genitalia. Plastic surgery is generally done in stages and yields excellent cosmetic results. Reports concerning sexual satisfaction after partial clitoridectomy indicate that the capacity for orgasm and sexual gratification is not necessarily impaired.

Unfortunately not all children with congenital adrenogenital hyperplasia are diagnosed at birth and raised in accordance with their genetic sex. Particularly in the case of affected females, masculinization of the external genitalia may have led to sex assignment as a male. Diagnosis is usually delayed until early childhood, when signs of virilism appear. In these situations it is advisable to continue rearing the child as a male in accordance with his assigned sex and phenotype. Hormonal replacement may be required to permit linear growth and to initiate male pubertal changes. Surgery is usually indicated to remove the female organs and reconstruct the phallus for satisfactory sexual relations. Obviously these individuals are not fertile.

Nursing considerations. Of major importance is recognition of ambiguous genitalia in newborns (Table 5-8). If there is any question regarding assignment of sex, the parents need to be told immediately to prevent the embarrassing situation of informing family members of the child's sex and then having to change the pronouncement. As with any congenital defect, the parents require an adequate explanation of the condition and a period of time to grieve for the loss of perfection. In this instance they may also need to grieve for the loss of the desired sex child. For example, the birth of a phenotypically male infant may fulfill their wish for a son. Knowledge of the child's actual sex may leave them disappointed. Such situations may also lead them to discuss the possibility of raising the child as a male despite the actual sex. This is a difficult question that requires thoughtful discussion among the parents and members of the health team. In general rearing the child as a female is preferred because of the satisfactory results with hormones in reversing the virilism, the prospect of a normal puberty, ability to conceive, and success of surgical intervention. This is in contrast to the choice of rearing the child as a male, in which case the child is sterile and may never be able to function satisfactorily in heterosexual relationships. If the parents persist in their decision to assign a male sex to the child, a psychologic consultation should be requested to explore their motivations and ensure their understanding of the child's future consequences.

Parents need an explanation regarding this disorder that facilitates their explaining it to others. Prior to confirmation of the diagnosis and sex, the nurse should refer to the infant as "child" or "baby" rather than by the pronouns "he" or "she" and definitely not "it." When referring to the external genitalia, it is preferable to refer to them as sex organs and to emphasize the similarity between the penis/clitoris and scrotum/labia during fetal development. In this way one can explain that the sex organs were overdeveloped because of secretion of too much male hormone. Using a correct vocabulary allows parents to explain the abnormalities to others in a straightforward manner, just as if the defect involved the heart or an extremity.

The nurse also stresses that sex assignment and rearing is dependent on psychosocial influences, not on genetic sex or hormonal influences during fetal life. Parents often fear that the infant will retain "male behavioral characteristics" because of prenatal masculinization and will not be able to develop "feminism." Using the word "hermaphrodite" often confuses parents because they interpret this term to mean that the child is "half male–half female." Since the prognosis for normal isosexual development is excellent after early treatment, the nurse fosters identification with the child as solely one sex. It is also beneficial to mention that ambiguous genitalia have no relationship with homosexual or bisexual activity later in life.

As soon as the sex is determined, parents are informed of the fact and encouraged to choose an appropriate name. From this point on, the child should be identified as a male or female, with no reference to ambiguous sex. If the appearance of the enlarged genitalia in a female child concerns parents, they should be encouraged to discuss their feelings. Suggesting ways of avoiding questioning remarks from visitors, such as diapering the child in a separate room, is also helpful. If surgery is anticipated the nurse can show parents photographs of before and after reconstruction to reinforce the expected cosmetic benefits.

Nursing considerations regarding cortisol and aldosterone replacement are the same as those that are discussed under chronic adrenocortical insufficiency. However, since parents may be overwhelmed with the diagnosis and obvious abnormalities at the time of birth, they may not hear all the discharge instructions regarding the medication schedule. A follow-up visit by a public health nurse is ideal to ensure that parents understand and comply with the treatment regimen. Likewise nurses in well-child facilities should assume the responsibility for guidance and supervision regarding this aspect of care during each visit. Since infants are especially prone to dehydration and "salt-losing crises," parents need to be aware of signs of dehydration and the necessity of immediate medical intervention to stabilize the child's condition.

In the unfortunate situation in which sex is erroneously assigned and later diagnosed, parents need a great deal of help in understanding the reason for the incorrect sex identity and the options for sex reassignment and/or medical/surgical intervention. Since children become aware of their sexual identity by 18 months to 2 years of age, it is believed that any reassignment after this period can cause tremendous psychologic conflicts in the child. Therefore, sex rearing should be continued as previously established with medical/surgical intervention as required. The dilemma often arises, however, regarding what the child should know about his condition. Because the knowledge that one has been reared opposite his genetic gender can initiate profound psychologic problems, it is recommended that the child not be told this fact but rather be given an explanation regarding his physical disabilities, such as infertility, and need for hormone replacement and plastic surgery. Parents, in turn, must believe that the child has been raised his "true sex," which is absolutely honest, since sex is not solely a biologic entity but an expression of multiple environmental influences.

Since congenital adrenogenital hyperplasia is an autosomal-recessive disorder, parents are referred for genetic counseling prior to conceiving another child. The nurse's role is to ensure that parents understand the probability of transmitting the trait or disorder with each pregnancy (see p. 191). Affected offspring also require genetic counseling since both sexes are generally able to reproduce. (See Chapter 6 for recurrence risks and genetic counseling.)

Hyperaldosteronism

Excessive secretion of aldosterone may be caused by an adrenal tumor or, in some types of adrenogenital syndromes, may be a result of enzymatic deficiency. The signs and symptoms are caused by increased sodium levels, water retention, and potassium loss. Hypervolemia causes hypertension and resultant headaches. Paradoxically, funduscopic changes resulting from increased blood pressure and edema from water retention are minimal. Hypokalemia results in muscular weakness, paresthesia, episodes of paralysis, and tetany and may be responsible for polyuria and consequent polydipsia.

The clinical diagnosis is suspected on the findings of hypertension, hypokalemia, and polyuria that fails to respond to antidiuretic hormone administration. Renin and angiotensin titers are abnormally low. Urinary levels of 17-hydroxycorticosteroids and 17-ketosteroids are normal in primary hyperaldosteronism because of an aldosterone-secreting tumor but are usually abnormal in adrenogenital syndrome.

Medical/surgical treatment. Temporary treatment of the disorder involves replacement of potassium and administration of spironolactone (Aldactone), a diuretic that blocks the effects of aldosterone, thereby promoting excretion of sodium and water while preserving potassium. Definitive treatment involves removing the tumor or performing a bilateral adrenalectomy. In the latter instance the postoperative treatment is similar to that of chronic adrenocortical insufficiency.

Nursing considerations. An important nursing consideration is recognition of this syndrome, particularly in children who demonstrate high blood pressure. Other clues include bed-wetting, excessive thirst, and unexplained weakness. After the diagnosis nursing care is related to the treatment regimen. If diuretics are used they should be administered in the morning to avoid accidents during the night. Children need unrestricted use of lavatory privileges at school. Potassium supplements should be mixed with fruit juice to increase their acceptability, and potassium-rich foods are encouraged. The parents need to be aware of the signs of hypokalemia and hyperkalemia.

After an adrenalectomy the nursing care is similar to the principles discussed under chronic adrenocortical insufficiency.

Disorders of adrenal medulla

The adrenal medulla secretes the catecholamines epinephrine and norepinephrine. Both hormones have essentially the same effects on different organs as those caused by direct sympathetic stimulation, except that the hormonal effects last several times longer. Their major actions include: (1) increased cardiac activity, (2) vasoconstriction of blood vessels (elevation of blood pressure), (3) increased rate and depth of respirations, (4) bronchial dilatation, (5) inhibition of gastrointestinal activity, (6) increased muscular contraction, (7) pupillary dilatation, (8) increased metabolic rate, (9) heightened sensory awareness, and (10) diaphoresis.

Although the catecholamines exert similar responses from target sites, there are some important differences. Epinephrine has a greater effect on cardiac activity than norepinephrine, but it causes only weak constriction of the blood vessels of muscles in comparison to the effect of norepinephrine. As a result norepinephrine elevates blood pressure, whereas epinephrine increases cardiac output. Another important difference is their effect on metabolism. Epinephrine increases the metabolic rate to a much greater extent than norepinephrine. These differences in action have been attributed to the catecholamines' effects on α- or β-adrenergic receptors. Supposedly norepinephrine can only affect those effector cells that contain α-receptors, which are mostly excitatory in nature (constriction and contraction). Epinephrine, however, can affect both α- and β-receptors, and β-receptors are mostly inhibitory (dilatation and relaxation).

Control of the secretion of the catecholamines is primarily in response to physiologic or emotional stress through the hypothalamus. Stimulation of the sympathetic nervous system results in the release of epinephrine and norepinephrine from the sympathetic nerves and adrenal medulla. Both systems support each other and can be substituted for the other. For this reason there is no condition attributable to hypofunction of the adrenal medulla. Even in bilateral adrenalectomy, catecholamine replacement is not necessary because the sympathetic release of these chemicals is sufficient to meet all the physiologic functions required to cope with stressful events.

HYPERFUNCTION OF ADRENAL MEDULLA

Pheochromocytoma

Catecholamine-secreting tumors are the primary cause of adrenal medullary hyperfunction. In children the most common neoplasms of this type are pheochromocytoma, neuroblastoma, and ganglioneuroma. Pheochromocytomas most commonly arise from the chromaffin cells of the adrenal medulla but may occur wherever these cells are found, such as along the paraganglia of the aorta or thoracolumbar sympathetic chain. Approximately 10% of these tumors are located in extra-adrenal sites. In children they are frequently bilateral or multiple and are generally benign. Often there is a familial transmission of the condition as an autosomal-dominant trait that tends to favor males.

Ganglioneuromas are thought to be neuroblastomas (see p. 1038) that have undergone maturation into a benign tumor composed of ganglion cells. These tumors are associated with less abnormal catecholamine secretion than the other two types, but persons with ganglioneuromas may have a clinical picture of chronic diarrhea, failure to thrive, skin rash, hypokalemia, persistent cough, and abdominal distention. The exact reason for these symptoms is unknown, although they are attributable to the tumor since they disappear after surgical extirpation of the mass.

Diagnostic evaluation. The clinical manifestations of pheochromocytoma are caused by an increased production of the catecholamines, producing hypertension, tachycardia, headache, decreased gastrointestinal activity with resultant constipation, increased metabolism with anorexia, weight loss, hyperglycemia, polyuria, polydipsia, hyperventilation, nervousness, and diaphoresis. In severe cases signs of congestive heart failure are evident (p. 1348).

The clinical manifestations mimic those of other disorders, such as hyperthyroidism, diabetes mellitus, or functional hyperventilation. Therefore, several tests specific to these conditions may be performed as part of the differential diagnosis. In only a small number of instances is a palpable tumor suggestive of the diagnosis. Definitive tests include measurement of urinary levels of the catecholamine metabolites, especially vanillylmandelic acid (VMA) (see p. 1038), histamine stimulation, which will provoke a hypertensive attack from sudden release of large amounts of catecholamines, and α-blocking agents (phentolamine [Regitine]), which will produce a hypotensive episode from inhibiting the action of circulating catecholamines.

Medical/surgical management. Definitive treatment consists of surgical removal of the tumor. However, in those situations in which surgery is contraindicated, such as in a debilitated child, medical management aimed at inhibiting the effects of catecholamine is employed. The major group of drugs used are the α-adrenergic blocking agents, such as phentolamine, a short-acting preparation, and phenoxybenzamine (Dibenzyline), a longer-acting medication. Success of therapy is judged by lowering of the blood pressure to normal, absence of hypertensive attacks (flushing or blanching, fainting, headache, palpitations, tachycardia, nausea and vomiting, and profuse sweating), decrease in perspiration, and disappearance of hyperglycemia. A disadvantage of these drugs is their inability to block the effects of catecholamines on β-receptors.

Nursing considerations. An initial nursing objective is identification of children with this disorder. Outstanding clues are the hypertension and hypertensive attacks. Because of the behavioral changes (nervousness, excitability, overactivity, and even psychosis), the increased cardiac and respiratory activity may appear to be related to an acute anxiety attack. Therefore, a careful history of onset of symptoms and association with stressful events is helpful in distinguishing between an organic and psychologic cause for the symptoms.

Prior to surgical extirpation the nurse monitors vital signs frequently and observes for evidence of hypertensive attacks and congestive heart failure. Once pharmacologic agents are given, the nurse checks for therapeutic effects as evidenced by normal vital signs and absence of glycosuria. Urine should be tested at least daily for sugar and acetone. The nurse also notes signs of hyperglycemia and reports these immediately.

The environment should be conducive to rest and free of emotional stress. This requires adequate preparation during hospital admission and prior to surgery. Parents should be encouraged to room-in with their child and to participate in his care. Play activities need to be tailored to the child's energy level but should not be overly strenuous or challenging, since these can increase metabolic rate and promote frustration and anxiety.

After surgery the child is observed for signs of shock from removal of excess catecholamines. If a bilateral adrenalectomy was performed, the nursing interventions are those discussed under chronic adrenocortical insufficiency.

Disorders of pancreatic hormone secretion

The islets of Langerhans of the pancreas have three major functioning cells: the alpha cells, which produce glucagon, the beta cells, which produce insulin, and the delta cells, which produce somatostatin. Glucagon causes an increase in the blood glucose by stimulating the liver and other cells to release stored glucose (glucogenolysis). Glucagon acts as an emergency supplier of glucose whenever the blood glucose falls too low and is believed to function more independently when insulin is lacking.[25] Somatostatin, although secreted by the islet cells, is found in greater supply in the hypothalamus, where it prevents the release of growth hormone. In the islets of Langerhans it is believed to regulate the release of insulin and glucagon. The discussion of disorders of pancreatic hormone secretion is limited to diabetes mellitus.

DIABETES MELLITUS

Diabetes mellitus has been diagnosed since antiquity. Even in early times it was recognized that people affected with the disease ''melted'' away, that flies were attracted to their urine, and that the urine tasted ''sweet.'' Prior to the discovery of insulin, developing diabetes in childhood was considered a death sentence. Even today, many reports indicate that the life expectancy of the child with diabetes is limited. The life span of a diabetic person is estimated to be only two thirds that of a nondiabetic person, which adds a psychologic burden to the affected child and his family. However, new data support the concept that life expectancy in the diabetic child is lengthened if the body is maintained in as normal a physiologic state as possible. Promotion of good health, a balance of adequate rest and exercise, and good nutrition along with close management of the disease will allow the person with diabetes to live as long if not longer than the nondiabetic person, who may not develop health and nutrition habits as good as those of the properly managed diabetic person.

There were 10 million people in the United States with diabetes in 1971 according to the National Diabetes Commission, and the incidence of the disease is increasing at the rate of 6% per year.[26] It has been found that 1 of every four families has a history of diabetes. The older the individual, the greater the chance of developing some type of diabetes. The exact prevalence of diabetes in children is not known. One study reports that 1 out of 529 school-age children have diabetes mellitus.[19] Children younger than school age have a lower incidence of the disease than school-age children; therefore, the overall prevalence in children is probably less but greater than the old studies that indicated an incidence of 1 in 2500.

Etiology and pathophysiology

Heredity is unquestioned as a prominent factor in the etiology of diabetes mellitus, although the mechanism of inheritance is unknown. Diabetes may be actually a syndrome rather than a specific disease. A variety of genetic mechanisms have been proposed, but most favor a multifactorial inheritance or a recessive gene somehow linked to the tissue-typing antigens, the human leukocyte–A (HL-A) system. However, the inheritance of maturity-onset diabetes (MODM) and juvenile-onset diabetes (JODM) appears to be different. Nearly 100% of offspring of parents who both have maturity-onset diabetes develop that type of diabetes, but only 45% to 60% of the offspring of both parents who have insulin-dependent (juvenile-onset) diabetes will develop the disease. There is also an increased risk of diabetes with obesity. The incidence of the disease doubles with every 20% of excess weight, and this figure applies to the young as well as to the older diabetic person. Diabetes is now the third leading cause of death by disease and the first leading cause of new cases of blindness.

Viruses have been implicated in the etiology of diabetes. The viral theory states that the beta cells of some individuals (most specialists believe that the beta cells are genetically susceptible because of the defects in the HL-A system) are attacked by certain viruses, causing cell damage or death. The body reacts to this damaged or changed tissue in an autoimmune phenomenon, forming antibodies that ''attack'' the beta cells, resulting in cell death. When there are not enough available beta cells to supply sufficient insulin to meet the needs of the body, insulin-dependent diabetes results. Tumors of the pancreas, pancreatitis, stress drugs such as steroids, stress diseases that involve other endocrine organs such as acromegaly, heredity, and viral diseases are now believed to play a part in causing diabetes.

Diabetes mellitus is characterized by a deficiency (relative or absolute) of the hormone insulin, which is normally produced by specialized cells in the islets of Langerhans of the pancreas. Insulin deficiency brings about metabolic adjustments or physiologic changes in almost all areas of the body. In maturity-onset diabetes (more correctly termed noninsulin dependent, nonketosis-prone, or type II diabetes), disturbed carbohydrate metabolism may be a result of a sluggish or insensitive secretory response in the pancreas or a defect in body tissues that requires unusual amounts of insulin, or the insulin secreted may be rapidly destroyed, inhibited, or inactivated in affected persons. A lack of insulin because of reduction in islet cell mass or destruction of the islets is the hallmark of the person with insulin-dependent (ketosis-prone or type I diabetes) or juvenile-onset diabetes.

Pathophysiology. Insulin is needed to support the metabolism of carbohydrates, fats, and proteins, primarily by facilitating the entry of these substances into the cell. Insulin is needed for the entry of glucose into the muscle and fat cells, for the prevention of mobilization of fats from fat cells, and for storage of glucose as glycogen in the cells of liver and muscle. Insulin is not needed for the entry of glucose into nerve cells or vascular tissue.

Although knowledge of insulin has advanced greatly over the last 20 years, there is much left to determine regarding its function, mode of action, and secretion. The chemical composition and molecular structure of insulin are such that it carries out its function by fitting into receptor sites on the cell membrane.[7] Here it initiates a sequence of poorly defined chemical reactions that alter the cell membrane to facilitate the entry of glucose into the cell and stimulate enzymatic systems outside the cell that metabolize the glucose for energy production.

With a deficiency of insulin, glucose is unable to enter the cell and its concentration in the bloodstream increases. The increased concentration of glucose (hyperglycemia) produces an osmotic gradient that causes the movement of body fluid from the intracellular space to the extracellular space and into the glomerular filtrate in order to "dilute" the hyperosmolar filtrate. Normally the renal tubular capacity to transport glucose is adequate to reabsorb all the glucose in the glomerular filtrate. When the glucose concentration in the glomerular filtrate exceeds the threshold (180 mg/100 ml), glucose "spills" into the urine along with water. This osmotic diversion causes polyuria, one of the cardinal signs of diabetes. The urinary fluid losses are the cause of the excessive thirst, polydipsia, observed in diabetes. As might be expected, this water washout results in a depletion of other essential chemicals from the body.

Ketoacidosis. When the cells are unable to take up glucose, the body chooses alternate sources of fuel, principally fat. If insulin is deficient, glucose is unavailable for cellular metabolism. Consequently fats break down into fatty acids and glycerol in the fat cells and in the liver and are converted to ketone bodies (β-hydroxybutyric acid, acetoacetic acid, and acetone). The ketone bodies are used as the alternative to glucose as a source of fuel but are utilized in the cells at a limited rate. Any excess is expelled from the body in the urine (ketonuria) or the lungs (acetone breath). Protein is also wasted during insulin deficiency. Since glucose is unable to enter the cells, protein is broken down and converted to glucose by the liver (glucogenesis). This new glucose contributes further to the hyperglycemia. These mechanisms are similar to those seen in starvation when substrate (glucose) is absent. In effect, during insulin deficiency, the body is in a state of starvation. Without the use of carbohydrates for energy, fat and protein stores are depleted as the body attempts to meet its energy needs. The hunger mechanism is triggered, but the increased food intake enhances the problem by further elevating the blood glucose.

Ketones are organic acids that readily produce excessive quantities of free hydrogen ions, causing a fall in plasma pH. The respiratory buffering system is activated in an effort to excrete the excess hydrogen ions and raise the pH. The carbonic acid is broken down in the respiratory system, in which the carbon dioxide is excreted by Kussmaul's respirations, the hyperventilation characteristic of metabolic acidosis. The ketones are buffered by sodium and potassium in the plasma. The kidney attempts to compensate for the increased pH by increasing tubular secretion of hydrogen ions and ammonium ions in exchange for fixed base. Thus the base buffer is depleted.

Potassium is also a problem and was once the cause of unexplained deaths shortly after insulin therapy was instituted. With cellular death, potassium is released from the cell into the bloodstream and is excreted by the kidney. The total body potassium is then decreased, even though the serum potassium level may be increased as a result of the decreased fluid levels in which it may be residing. Alteration in serum and tissue potassium can result in cardiac arrest.

If these problems are not reversed, progressive deterioration occurs with dehydration, electrolyte imbalance, acidosis, coma, and death. The deterioration can be reversed by insulin therapy in combination with correction of the fluid deficiency and electrolyte imbalance. Diagnosis of diabetic ketoacidosis should be carried out promptly in a seriously ill patient and therapy instituted that includes insulin, fluids, and electrolytes, such as sodium, potassium, and bicarbonate, as appropriate.

Long-term pathology. In addition to the acute problem of diabetic ketoacidosis as outlined in the preceding paragraphs, the long-term problems of the disease are intimately connected to the basic pathologic defects (that is, insulin deficiency and hyperglycemia).

The problems that shorten life in the individual with diabetes are related to damage to the vascular and nervous system (retinopathy, nephropathy, and neuropathy). There has for some time existed a major controversy as to the etiology of these long-term problems. One school of thought holds that the long-term problems of diabetes are a *concomitant* of the disease, genetically predetermined and unalterable by control of the blood glucose. The other theory holds that the long-term problems are *complications* somehow related to the reduction of insulin and/or hyperglycemia and are thus preventable by careful and meticulous control of the blood glucose level.

Assisting the body to become physiologically normal takes time and determination. Some have said that the effort to closely control the disease would psychologically damage the child, that vascular problems would develop no matter what one did, and that, therefore, control is not only not helpful but on the other hand might be harmful.[1,29] It has been determined that loving discipline is a supportive measure for any child; however, it has been shown that children with poorer diabetic control come from predominantly disruptive family units with little or no discipline as part of the family life-style and that control is not psychologically harmful.

Some researchers have recognized the importance of providing adequate amounts of insulin in prevention of vascular disease and have not seen any vascular changes prior to the time of onset of carbohydrate intolerance. With poor diabetic control, vascular changes appear as early as 2½ to 3 years after diagnosis; however, with good to excellent control, changes have been postponed for 20 or more years. Changes prior to puberty are uncommon, but after puberty the poorer the control, the more rapid the vascular changes. The result is damage to the kidney as well as blindness and neuropathy. The damage in the young diabetic person is to the small blood vessels (microangiopathy), and it has been demonstrated that the elevated blood glucose level—not the genetics—causes the vascular disease. It has been a goal of many investigators to determine a more accurate parameter to determine the level of control of diabetes. Urine tests and blood glucose levels do not give optimal information about overall control.[14,16]

Diagnostic evaluation

The diagnosis of diabetes mellitus may be quite obvious or quite elusive. The sequence of chemical events described previously results in hyperglycemia and acidosis, which in turn produce the three "polys" of diabetes—polyphagia, or frequent eating associated with weight loss; polydipsia, or frequent water drinking; and polyuria, or frequent urination—the cardinal symptoms of the disease. Other symptoms are dry skin, blurred vision, and sores that are slow to heal. More commonly in children, tiredness and bed-wetting are the chief complaints that prompt parents to take their child to the physician.

The symptomatology of diabetes is more readily recognizable in children than in adults, so it is surprising that the diagnosis may sometimes be missed or delayed. Diabetes is a great imitator: influenza, gastroenteritis, and appendicitis are the conditions most often diagnosed, only to find that the disease was really diabetes.

Observation and testing are important to the diagnosis of diabetes in children. Those families with a strong family history of diabetes should suspect diabetes, especially if there is one child in the family with diabetes. If children demonstrate glycosuria, are overweight, or exhibit symptoms of hypoglycemia, they are candidates for glucose tolerance testing. It is difficult to do glucose tolerance testing in children younger than 3 years of age, since norms for children in this age-group have not been established. The glucose load for oral glucose tolerance testing in children should be determined by body weight. The glucose load in children is 1.75 g/kg of ideal body weight for height.[11] To make the information more meaningful, insulin values should also be obtained during glucose tolerance testing.

The urine test will show positive glucose only when the disease is actually manifest. A negative urine test does not necessarily rule out early diabetes, nor does a positive test necessarily indicate diabetes. Renal glycosuria, unrelated to diabetes, can result in glucose in the urine. The fasting blood glucose test may miss the diagnosis of early diabetes (called chemical diabetes) and has been known to miss as many as 85% of children who had an abnormal glucose tolerance test with asymptomatic disease. The 4-hour glucose tolerance test has been found to be the most useful test for the diagnosis of early or chemical diabetes, whereas the 6-hour glucose tolerance test is most helpful for the diagnosis of hypoglycemia. Based on norms established for normal, nondiabetic children of various ages, the criteria for the diagnosis of early diabetes is two or more abnormal tests with two or more values in each test that are outside the normal range.[23] However, standardization of food intake before the test may be important and those preparing for the test should emphasize the importance of following the directions for diet supplied by the physician or laboratory.

Stages of diabetes in children

Prediabetes. Prediabetes is a state of genetic susceptibility, with no signs or symptoms, during which all tests of glucose tolerance are normal. If both parents have diabetes, if there is a strong family history of diabetes, if the mother has had infants with birth weights of more than 9 pounds, if the mother has had frequent stillbirths or miscarriages, or if signs of microvascular disease have been noted without abnormal findings in glucose tolerance, the classification of prediabetes may be made.

Chemical diabetes. Chemical diabetes is found in an individual who has a normal fasting blood glucose level but an abnormal glucose tolerance test. Chemical diabetes may be stable, may be slowly progressive, or may progress rapidly to overt diabetes. In time the mildly abnormal tests may return to normal. Early chemical diabetes may produce a rapid elevation of the blood glucose level with a delayed output in insulin release followed by a dramatic drop in blood glucose and insulin levels. This type of response is often symptomatically followed by shakiness, weakness, fainting, or headache. Except for symptomatic hypoglycemia occurring as a side effect of having to take injectable insulin, this type of hypoglycemia is the most common cause of hypoglycemia.

A home stress test has been found useful in the decision to repeat the glucose tolerance test or to determine if more acute or overt diabetes has occurred:

1. Have the child go to the bathroom and empty the bladder.
2. Give the child a loading dose of sugar consisting of:
   a. Younger than 6 years of age: 1 tbsp of sugar in 4 ounces of orange juice or 2 ounces of grape juice, followed in 20 minutes by 3 ounces of a cola drink.

b. Six years of age and older: 2 tbsp of sugar in 8 ounces of orange juice or 4 ounces of grape juice, followed in 20 minutes by 6 ounces of a cola drink.
3. On the first voiding, hopefully 2 hours or more later, check for glucose.

Note: If the child is taking cephalosporin drugs, a false-positive result may be seen on Clinitest, in which case a tape test would be more useful. The tape test is more useful when the testing is done during a febrile illness. Glucose in the urine indicates the need for more definitive diagnostic measures.

The diagnosis of chemical diabetes should be established only by serial testing, and the child should not be labeled until the tests are conclusive because of the problems often encountered by an individual labeled ''diabetic.'' Treatment for mild alterations of glucose tolerance are being researched, but at present the only course is restriction of concentrated sweets, maintaining ideal body weight for height, and small frequent feedings (three meals and three or more between-meal snacks). The frequency of feedings decreases the challenge of boluses of food, resulting in less demands of insulin release from the pancreas, and giving the child a small amount of food more frequently keeps the glycogen stores ready and the release of insulin less dramatic.

Overt diabetes. Overt diabetes is symptomatic diabetes with an elevated fasting blood glucose level. In adult-type diabetes (noninsulin dependent diabetes, which has also been found in older children), the insulin values are found to be elevated and 80% to 90% of this population have been found to be overweight. The insulin-dependent diabetic person has markedly decreased insulin levels. When the diabetes becomes complete, there is no demonstrable insulin at all. Symptomatology in the adult is often tiredness and frequent infections (such as monilial infections in females). The child may start wetting the bed, become grouchy and ''not himself,'' or act overly tired. Abdominal discomfort is common. Weight loss, though quite observable on the charts, may be a less frequent presenting complaint because of the fact that the family might not have noticed the change. Another outstanding sign of overt diabetes is thirst. One couple reported that their child, during a trip from California to Kansas, drank the contents of a gallon jug of water between each gas station stop. At a certain point in the illness the child may actually refuse fluid and food, adding to the increasing state of dehydration and malnutrition. The child may be *hyperglycemic,* with elevated blood glucose levels and glucose in the urine; may be in *diabetic ketosis,* with ketones as well as glucose in the urine but not noticeably dehydrated; or may be in *diabetic ketoacidosis,* with dehydration, electrolyte imbalance, and acidosis.

Problem of diagnosis. Signs, symptoms, and chemical tests may lead to the conclusion that the child has diabetes, when, in reality, another condition may be present. This is true in salicylate intoxication, which can be ruled out easily by boiling the urine. The acetone, if present, will boil out of the urine, leaving a negative Acetest if related to diabetes and a positive Acetest if related to salicylate intoxication. Temporary hyperglycemia may accompany such stressful conditions as burns, hyperalimentation, pancreatitis, and encephalitis. The glucose tests usually return to normal once the stress is reversed; however, insulin may be needed for a short period of time in the stress illnesses, especially when the child is undergoing hyperalimentation. Other abnormal conditions that may cause glucose to be found in the urine are certain renal diseases, some other endocrine disorders, and lead encephalopathy.

Medical management

The management program for any child with diabetes mellitus should involve flexibility and 24-hour insulin coverage and should be able to fit into the child's life-style. The insulin treatment should be determined by the recognition that the effective duration of action of insulin in children may be somewhat different from that in adults.[22] The effective action of insulin is described as the effect of a certain amount of insulin in lowering the blood glucose level over a period of time. Ideally the blood glucose level is maintained at less than 140 mg/dl and no lower than 60 mg/dl during the time of specific action of the insulin, based on past information regarding the duration of action of the intermediate-acting insulins. The accepted duration of action of intermediate-acting insulins is 24 hours or more. In animals or noninsulin-dependent people this may be so, but in insulin-dependent children it does not appear to be the case. The duration of effective action for intermediate-acting insulin has been found to be 12 to 14 hours.[12] Lente insulin is the longest acting of the intermediate-acting insulins, but even it lasts only 14 to 16 hours (Table 38-4).[21]

In working with these insulins, it is wise to remember that Lente insulin is 30% semilente and 70% ultralente. Lente insulins that mix with no other insulins other than regular derive their action from the size and number of crystals—small and numerous crystals = semilente insulin; large and less numerous crystals = ultralente insulin. Protamine zinc insulin (PZI) is seldom used today because of its very long duration of action and its very low tissue insulin levels, which may not saturate receptor sites on the cell membrane sufficiently well to effectively help the body utilize the glucose that may be present. The potential overlap of insulin action is unsuited for children, who are active one minute and very inactive the next. The balance that needs to be achieved between insulin, diet, and activity is most difficult when using this type of insulin. The intermediate-acting insulins (other than lente insulin) derive their delayed action from a protein tag. The most commonly used insulins are the intermediate-acting insulins, principally NPH, which are usually given in a single

Table 38-4. Onset, peak, and duration of action for various insulin preparations

Type of insulin	Onset (hours after administration)	Peak (hours)	Effective duration of action (hours)
Short acting			
Crystalline zinc (regular insulin)	½-1	2-4	6-8
Semilente (prompt insulin zinc suspension)	½-1	2-4	8-10
Intermediate acting			
Globin zinc (globulin zinc insulin)	1-2	6-8	12-14
Isophane (neutral protamine Hagedorn [NPH])	1-2	6-8+	12-14
Lente (insulin zinc suspension; 30% Semilente and 70% Ultralente)	1-2+	8-12	14-16
Longer acting			
Ultralente (extended insulin zinc suspension)	4-6	8-12	24-36
Protamine zinc (protamine zinc insulin suspension [PZI])	4-6	18+	36-72

early morning dose combined with a small amount of short-acting insulin (usually regular).

Acute-care setting. The parents, as well as other family members, of the child with newly diagnosed diabetes mellitus experience various emotional responses to the crises just as the physiologic responses affect the child with diabetes. Care in the acute setting is short but may create fears and frustrations. Episodes of diabetic ketoacidosis or hypoglycemia bring about a fear of loss and dread of reoccurrence that are not soon forgotten and may alter a person's approach to control of his disease.

Diabetic ketoacidosis. Diabetic ketoacidosis (DKA), the most complete state of insulin deficiency, is a life-threatening situation that was once synonymous with death. Management with adequate insulin, along with fluids and appropriate electrolytes, can reverse the ketoacidosis within a few hours. The insulin is administered in one of two ways:

1. The initial dose of 2 U/kg of regular insulin is administered as a bolus followed by subcutaneous injections. Since the half-life of insulin is only 3 to 4 minutes, half the initial dose of insulin is given intravenously and half is administered subcutaneously or intramuscularly. This initial dose is followed in 3 to 4 hours with a dose of 1 U/kg and again in 3 to 4 hours by a dose of 0.5 U/kg, all subcutaneously. The patient then receives 0.5 U/kg of regular insulin every 6 hours until ketoacidosis is relieved.
2. In perfused insulin, a more recent technique, 0.1 U/kg/hour of regular insulin is infused intravenously and the dose is controlled at a rate to lower the blood glucose about 100 mg/dl/hour until a blood glucose level of about 200 mg/dl is reached.[8] Subcutaneous insulin is then instituted. The perfused insulin may be placed in a 20-ml syringe, diluted to equal units of insulin/cm^3 of fluid, and infused with a syringe-type pump.

Vital signs, hourly tests of urine for sugar and acetone, and cardiac monitoring are other parameters to observe. The cardiac monitor is employed to determine changes in the potassium levels of the child (a U wave after the T wave will indicate hypokalemia; an elevated and spreading T wave indicates increasingly abnormal hyperkalemia). Hourly Dextrostix blood sugar determinations are a useful adjunct to therapy. This or other bedside tests can give quick, although not completely accurate, information. The Dextrostix is best read in the Eyetone reflectance meter.* The manufacturer's directions, as found on the Dextrostix package, must be explicitly followed to ensure accuracy of the test.

Plasma expanders may be administered during the initial phase of treatment of diabetic ketoacidosis in order to establish renal blood flow. The fluids may then be changed to balanced solutions with dextrose as soon as plasma expansion is accomplished. Potassium is added as soon as renal output is established. Bicarbonate is added if the pH and/or serum bicarbonate levels are quite low.

Once the child has recovered from the most acute state, insulin is administered on a proportional basis as follows: 35% of the total daily amount of insulin is given before breakfast, 22% before lunch, 28% before supper, and 15% before a bedtime snack. Only regular insulin is used during this early phase. As oral feedings are tolerated, clear liquids are advanced to soft foods and then to a regular diet, in a three-meal, midnight snack pattern of six eighteenths for breakfast, six eighteenths for lunch, five eighteenths for supper, and one eighteenth at bedtime. Urine samples are collected as fractionals or block specimens, from before breakfast to before lunch, from before lunch to before supper, from before supper to about 11 PM, and from 11 PM to before breakfast. A Clinitest, Acetest, and total urine volume are recorded for each fraction. Insulin dosages are adjusted according to the previous day's total urine tests. U100 insulin is used but can be diluted for readability and accuracy to U50, U25, or U10, as necessary. It is especially useful to dilute regular insulin (by use of diluting fluid that may be obtained through a physician from Eli Lilly & Co. in Indianapolis, Ind.), for very young children who are sensitive to very small insulin changes.

The total quantity of insulin should be increased or decreased based on the previous 24-hour urine results, not

*The Ames Co.

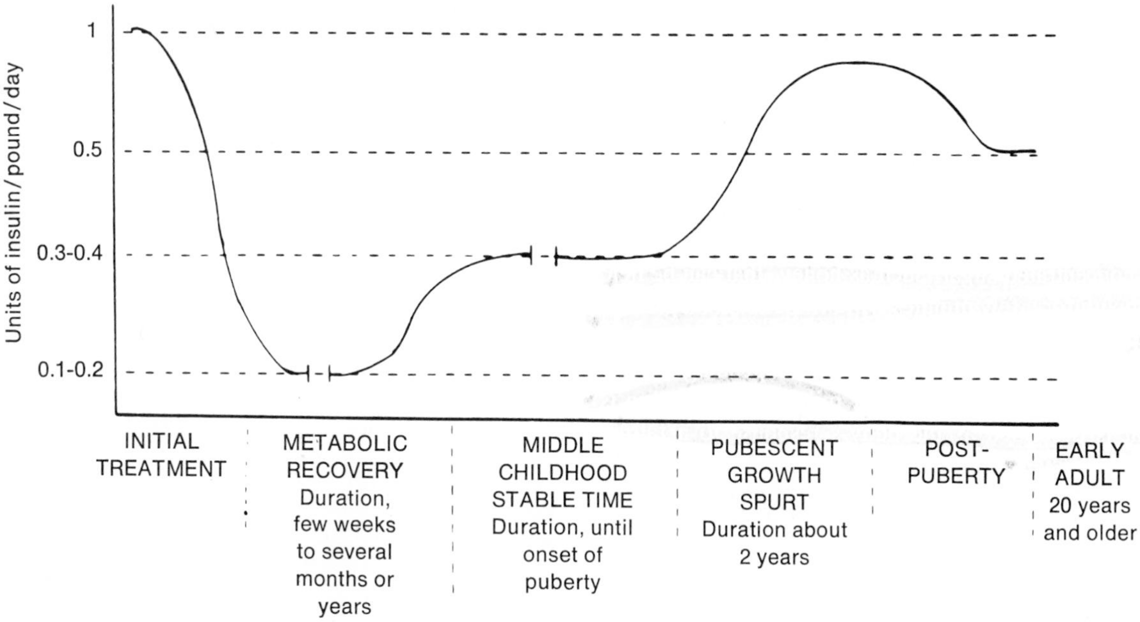

Fig. 38-2. Management of newly diagnosed juvenile diabetes. Insulin requirements related to age, activity, and growth needs.

just on the previous specimen, as is done in many cases. This is a time of repletion when weight loss is reversed and body stores are replenished; therefore, the children are given as much food as they feel comfortable eating in order to accomplish the repletion as quickly as possible. Insulin requirements will be high in order to metabolize the ingested food. Initially the insulin doses may be near 2 U/kg/day with a gradual decline (Fig. 38-2).

Once the child is stabilized on regular insulin, the total amount of insulin is gradually decreased. A split-dose insulin schedule and a three-meal, three-snack feeding pattern is begun. Two thirds of the total daily dose of insulin is given about ½ hour before breakfast, and one third is given ½ hour before supper. The morning insulin is usually two thirds NPH and one third regular insulin. The evening insulin is either 1 part NPH and 1 part regular or 2 parts NPH and 1 part regular. If the child is less active after supper, the 1:1 dosage is given. (For example, if a total of 54 U is given, two thirds, or 36 U of mixture is given before breakfast and 18 U of mixture is given before supper.) Once tissue stores are replenished and weight regained, there is a gradual lowering of insulin requirements since some endogenous insulin secretion returns.[30] Hypoglycemia should be avoided at this time, since a severe insulin reaction may destroy the confidence of the parents. In most instances the child's dosage decreases about 5% to 10% per day until dosages of about 0.1 to 0.2 U/kg/day are required. The better the insulin secreting ability is preserved, the more stable the diabetes is to manage and the better off the child will be. This period of time when the child is able to secrete some endogenous insulin, which is called by many the "honeymoon," or the period of time with the most stability of the diabetes, can last months or even years.

Hypoglycemia. The other end of the scale is low blood glucose levels. Just as getting insulin into the individual with diabetic ketoacidosis is an emergency, so is getting glucose into the individual with hypoglycemia. The brain depends on glucose, the lack of which can cause coma and even permanent brain damage. Neurologic signs and symptoms appear when the blood glucose drops below about 30 mg/dl (more than 20 mg/dl). Interestingly enough, some (few) individuals with 20 mg/dl blood glucose levels may experience nothing more than irritability and slowed mental function, whereas others experience more severe symptoms with a blood glucose level of 40 to 50 mg/dl. The first rule of diabetes therapy is prevention of hypoglycemia. The balance of food, exercise, and insulin with the manipulation of food intake with changing activity is the best preventative.

The causes of hypoglycemia are exactly the opposite of diabetic ketoacidosis. They include the ingestion of too little food, the increase in exercise without adequate food support, or the increase in insulin, whether accidental or on purpose, without adequate support by additional food. Gastroenteritis, in which there is a gastric stasis, may impede the absorption of food, resulting in hypoglycemia, and is probably the most threatening cause of hypoglycemia. It is possible to eat reasonably well and still have an insulin reaction, unaware that the food is not being absorbed. Another sometimes baffling occurrence may happen when the blood glucose level is low to the point of causing gastric stasis. The child then may eat a meal or snack and, after the meal or snack, have an insulin reaction. Continued feeding does not seem to alter the blood glucose level, as a result of both the gastric stasis and the simple glucose or sugar being diluted in the stomach contents. In the majority of cases, simple concentrated sugar, such as honey, that can be held in the mouth for a few minutes will bring the blood glucose level up.

Treatment of hypoglycemia varies, depending on the severity of the insulin reaction. A mild insulin reaction is one that is described as the body's response to a falling blood sugar level. Epinephrine is released, causing the feelings of hunger, increased pulse rate, hyperactivity, increased respiratory rate, and weakness. Epinephrine triggers a glycogenolysis, which will raise the blood glucose level. If the blood glucose level falls further, cerebral function may be affected. Symptoms include yawning, lethargy, and increasing difficulty in the thought process, along with irritability and belligerence. Food taken when the initial symptoms appear in their mildest form reverses the lowered blood glucose level. Milk is a very good food to use in children. It supplies them with lactose or milk sugar as well as a more prolonged action from the protein and fat (aids in decreased absorption). Forty to 80 kcal are about all the food that is needed to reverse the blood glucose level at this state.

Moderate insulin reactions result from more severe lowering of the blood glucose level with a decline in cerebral activity and a more profound sympathetic response. Sweating, if not generalized, becomes noticeable on the extremities, the back of the neck, and the axilla area. Extreme nervousness and tremors may be noted. Stomachache and headache are common complaints. Vomiting may shortly follow. The pulse rate will usually increase and become stronger. Blood pressure may become lower, leading to faintness or dizziness. Blurring of vision may be noted at this state. Treatment must be with a simple sugar, preferably in the form of concentrated sugar. The simpler the sugar, the more rapidly it is absorbed. Ten to 20 kcal for preteenagers and 20 to 40 kcal for teenagers is all that is usually needed. It is better to overtreat than to undertreat, but overtreatment should be kept to a minimum whenever possible. The treatment may be repeated in 10 to 15 minutes if the initial response is not satisfactory. With good response to the simple sugar, the pulse rate should show a noticeable change in 2 to 3 minutes. Rest and the addition of food should be part of the plan.

The severe insulin reaction is often the most feared aspect of having diabetes, since severe brain symptoms may develop. Each of the areas of the brain is responsible for various physiologic responses, and the activity of one brain center may be greater than the activity of another. The various areas of the brain respond in sequence: the forebrain with increased drowsiness and perspiration; the hypothalamus and thalamus with tachycardia and loss of consciousness; the midbrain with seizure activity that may be started from stimulation initially from the hypothalmus; and finally the hindbrain with respones of deeper coma and decreasing reflexes. The treatment of choice is 50% glucose administered intravenously.[27]

Glucagon is sometimes prescribed for home treatment of hypoglycemia. It is available as a tablet to be mixed with diluting fluid from its accompanying bottle and is administered intramuscularly or subcutaneously. It requires about 15 to 20 minutes to elevate the blood glucose level by releasing the stored glucose from the liver. Once the child is responsive, the lost glycogen stores are replaced by small amounts of sugar-containing fluid administered frequently until the child feels comfortable about trying solid foods.

Prevention of hypoglycemia is the best procedure to follow. More food is needed for more activity, and less food is needed for less activity. The extra food for activity is given preferably before the activity and repeated for increased activity every 45 to 60 minutes if activity continues. The only ''excuse'' for a severe insulin reaction is the development of unknown gastroenteritis. All other causes of hypoglycemia are preventable.

Somagyi's reflex should be recognized as a separate response, although not actually an acute emergency. This phenomenon is a physiologic reflex that occurs when the blood glucose level decreases to the point that the release of counterregulatory hormones—epinephrine, growth hormone, and corticosteroids—is triggered. The blood glucose level then rises, often overshooting, causing an elevated blood glucose level. Instead of the expected decrease in blood glucose level with exercise, the blood glucose level is raised as demonstrated by a positive urine test for glucose after the exercise. Since the increased blood glucose level is caused by not enough food or too much insulin, the treatment is to increase the food and/or decrease the insulin. Hyperglycemia and glycosuria will subside as hypoglycemia and the counterregulatory hormonal response subside.

Intermediate-care setting. Intermediate-care problems are those that happen out of the ordinary and are not associated with the acute-care settings.

Illness management. Illness alters diabetes management, usually according to the seriousness of the illness. If the diabetes is well controlled, illness will run its course in the child with diabetes as it will in the nondiabetic child. The goal during illness is to maintain some glucosuria but to keep the urine free of acetone. In most illnesses, even if the child is not eating well, he will spill glucose and some acetone. This is an indication for increased insulin. As the child is less hungry during illness, a 20% decrease in caloric intake, simpler foods along with fluids and simple sugars, may reduce the need for insulin in the child.[13] It is important that the calories ingested be simple ones, especially in severe illness or in children in whom gastrointestinal tract problems are present. Keeping up with the insulin needs is the major factor in preventing ketoacidosis during the illness. The illness itself should be handled as if the child did not have diabetes and the appropriate increases or adjustment in insulin given to cover the rising or changing blood or urine sugar level.

Surgery. Another stress that requires alteration in treatment for the diabetic child is surgery. The physiologic and emotional stresses related to surgery require careful adjustment of insulin during this time. Since the child receives intravenous glucose during surgery and the stress of the surgery itself will also raise the blood glucose level, the risk of an insulin reaction is very slight. Regular insulin only is given during surgery and continued until the child is able to tolerate oral feedings and his routine pattern of insulin dosages may be resumed.

Psychosocial adjustment. Perhaps the most important intermediate-care problem is the child's adjustment to having a chronic illness. Children in the years prior to preadolescence probably accept their condition most easily. Adolescents appear to have the most difficulty in adjusting to a chronic illness. Adolescence is a time when there is much stress toward being perfect and being like their peers and, no matter what others say, having diabetes is being different. If children can accept the difference as a part of life, in other words, that each person has something different about him, then with adequate parental support they should be able to adjust well. Parent relationships may vary from no support (it is your disease) to a smothering kind of support that produces a totally dependent, immature person. The most frustrating kind of support is the one in which the parents say they will do all they can to help and then do not recognize that they are actually not doing anything, for example, the parent who states that "anything our child needs he will get," and then does not attend diabetes education classes to learn what those needs are. This is often caused by the parents having suppressed feelings of rejection and/or their choice of priorities.

There is a grief process that the older child and most parents must go through. Some aspects of the grief process, such as denial, may, in some people, last for months or even years, before they progress to a form of acceptance. The initial anger, on diagnosis, may be fought with feelings of guilt, especially if lack of knowledge causes the parents to blame one or the other. Doubt becomes most manifest when the parents try to find other alternatives or question the diagnosis or the need for lifetime insulin. An individual or parent may never truly accept the disease or adjust to the regimen that is imposed on the child's life-style by the diabetes.

Overall management of diabetes should be flexible enough that it can be altered to fit almost any life-style. This flexibility motivates greater acceptance of the disease. Twenty-four–hour control of the disease is important, but it is also important to use a flexible regimen to achieve that control. If a flexible program that fits into the life-style of the patient is followed, there is better compliance with fewer psychologic problems.

Certain fears may develop in the parents and children as a result of past experiences with the disease. A severe insulin reaction with seizures is certainly one experience that contributes to fear of a repeat. Once parents experience a seizure or the adolescent has one in a public place, the desire to maintain better control is reinforced. Families need education about regulated control and the prevention of problems such as hypoglycemia. They must understand how to prevent problems and how to handle problems calmly and coolly if they occur. They must understand the complexities of the body, the disease, and its complications.

Chronic-care setting. Chronic care is daily care, usually supervised on an outpatient basis. Flexible programs are individualized for day-to-day care. The more frequent use of short-acting insulin adds more flexibility to the individual's program, and the intermediate-acting insulins administered with an adequate overlap give satisfactory 24-hour insulinization. The split-dose insulin schedule, using mixtures of regular and intermediate-acting insulins twice daily, is the closest approximation of a four-dose schedule of regular insulin without giving four shots per day (Fig. 38-3). Some children respond more favorably to two doses of regular insulin, one before breakfast and one before lunch, with a mixture of intermediate- and short-acting insulin before supper. Parents and children should never be psychologically locked in to any given number of injections but should be prepared to accept frequent administration of medication if that best meets the needs of the child.

A three-meal, three-snack feeding pattern is the most common pattern used for young children. The intake is divided as follows: four eighteenths of the total daily food at breakfast, two eighteenths for a midmorning snack, five eighteenths for lunch, one eighteenth for the mid-afternoon snack, five eighteenths for supper, and one eighteenth as a bedtime snack. This distribution of calories can be altered to fit the activity pattern of any individual child. For example, the child who is more active in the afternoon will need the larger snack at that time. This larger snack might also be split to allow some food at school and some food after school. Alterations in food intake should be made so that food, insulin, and exercise are balanced. Extra food is needed for extra activity.

The food intake may be planned in a variety of ways. The family may follow the more conventional exchange system approved by the American Diabetes Association (ADA) or the approach called the point system, which is based on 75

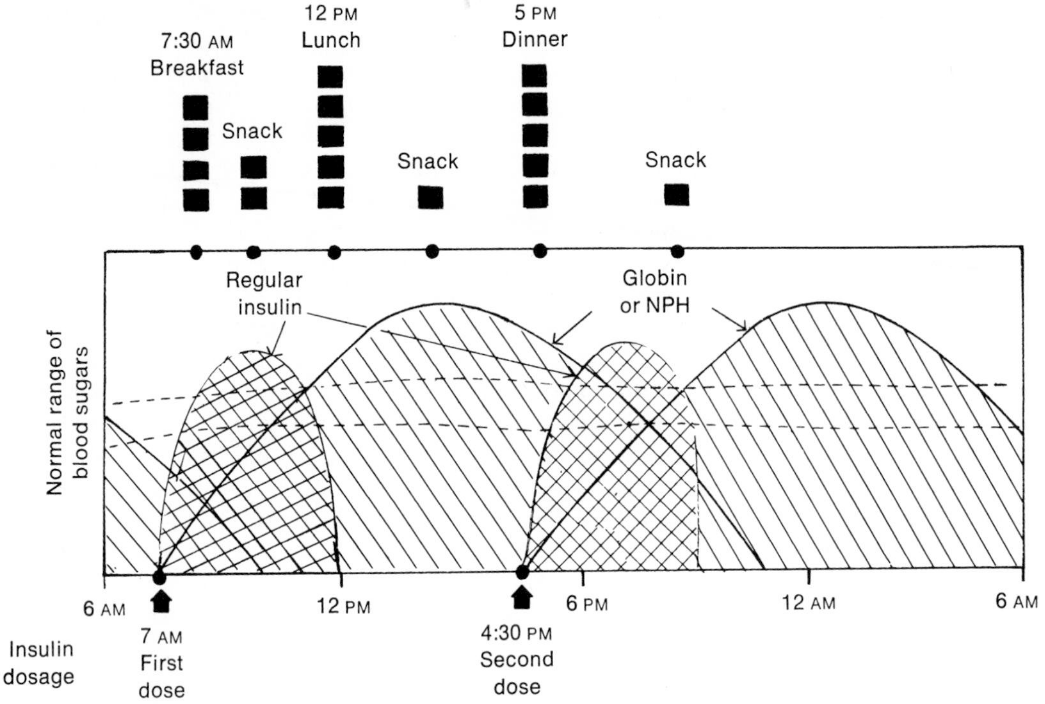

Fig. 38-3. Twenty-four–hour insulin action two dose schedule. Split insulin dose schedule using regular and NPH insulins.

kcal equaling 1 point. Concentrated sweets are eliminated, and foods are chosen from food groups similar to the basic four. Since the carbohydrate content of the diet per se does not have in the majority of instances a specific effect on blood glucose level elevation, carbohydrates are not restricted except for simple sugars.

The exchange system (revised June 1976) uses the following six food groups: milk, meat, vegetables, fat, fruit, and bread. This allows a more precise calculation of calories and nutritional needs in the diet. Correctly used, it allows for flexibility in the diet and the incorporation of preferred foods in most instances.[31]

In the diabetic child food restriction should never be used for diabetic control. If the child is overweight, food restriction may be used for weight control, but not for diabetic control. In general the child's appetite should be the guide for the amount of calories needed with the total calorie intake increased as appetite and activity increase. A rough rule for expected calorie intake is 30 kcal/pound for prepubescent children, and 30 kcal/kg for pubescent and postpubescent children. More calories per pound or kilogram should be added for weight gain or increased activity; fewer calories per pound or kilogram should be used for weight loss or decreased activity. However, very small children and infants may need 40 to 50 kcal/pound of body weight.

Exercise should be encouraged and never restricted unless other health conditions necessitate it. Insulin in children should not be reduced for increased activity unless the needed increase in food cannot be tolerated. It is better to eat extra food when one is more active. This is also true with the child with diabetes. The only factor that is different in the diabetic child is the need to preplan the food intake before and during the activity whenever possible. For the less active child, such activities as bicycle riding, stationary or otherwise, jumping rope, and a planned exercise program may be more acceptable. In addition to a feeling of well-being, the exercise aids in the utilization of food and often necessitates less insulin.

Urine records should be reviewed by the family weekly. At these times they look for frequent, even if insignificant, insulin reactions and plan to increase food or decrease the insulin. For patterned urinary glucose spills, alterations of food or insulin are planned for the period prior to the spill rather than after the spill period. Urine tests are based on first-voided urine specimens, as it is difficult to obtain a second-voided specimen from a child. The first-voided urine test provides information about how the food is being handled by the insulin in relation to the exercise over a period of time rather than at a point in time.[10] Looking at urine records objectively and at frequent intervals will help both the parents and the appropriately understanding child to learn from their experiences as well as to maintain a very high degree of control of the disease.

Nursing considerations: acute care

Diabetic children in the hospital are generally admitted at the time of their initial diagnosis, during illness or surgery, or for episodes of ketoacidosis, which may be precipitated by any of a variety of factors. Most diabetic children are able to keep the disease under control with periodic assessment and adjustment of insulin, diet, and activity as needed under the supervision of the physician. Under most circumstances these children can be managed very well at home and require hospitalization only for a serious illness or upset. However, there are a small number of diabetic children who exhibit a degree of metabolic lability and who have repeated episodes of diabetic ketoacidosis that require hospitalization, which interferes with education and social development. These children appear to display a characteristic personality structure. They tend to be unusually passive and unassertive and to come from families that are inclined to smooth over conflicts without resolution. Children in this type of setting experience emotional arousal with little, if any, opportunity or ability to bring about its termination. This emotional stress causes an increased production of endogenous catecholamines, which stimulates fat breakdown leading to ketonemia and ketonuria.[15]

It is often difficult to distinguish between ketoacidosis and a hypoglycemic reaction (Table 38-5). Since the symptoms are similar and usually begin with changes in behavior, the simplest way to differentiate between the two is to obtain a urine sample and test for glucose content. The urine will be negative for glucose in hypoglycemia, or hyperinsulinism, whereas in hyperglycemia the glucose content will be excessive. The young child may not be able to void on command. However, urine output is diminished in hypoglycemia and there is increased urine formation in hyperglycemia. This should provide an additional clue to the alert observer. In doubtful situations and when a urine specimen cannot be obtained for analysis, it is safer to give the child some simple sugar. This will help alleviate the symptoms in the case of hypoglycemia but will do little harm if the child is hyperglycemic. Severe hyperinsulinism and hyperglycemia constitute emergencies and require hospitalization.

The child with diabetic ketoacidosis requires intensive nursing care. On admission to the hospital an intravenous infusion is started immediately to hydrate the child and to administer insulin either as a single bolus or as a continuous infusion (see medical management, p. 1482). The blood glucose level is monitored at regular intervals by Hemostix or Dextrostix or laboratory analysis, and the insulin dosage is adjusted accordingly. Insulin is also administered subcutaneously or intramuscularly as ordered.

Sodium, potassium, and bicarbonate levels are monitored and replaced as indicated. Since potassium and sodium reenter the cells rapidly after administration of insulin, depletion of these electrolytes can be a serious consequence. Bicarbonate is rapidly depleted to buffer acid metabolites, chiefly ketoacids.

The child is carefully observed for circulatory complications. He is generally attached to a cardiac monitor for continuous assessment of cardiac status, especially when potassium levels are markedly altered. Vital signs are observed and recorded frequently. Hypotension caused by the contracted blood volume of the dehydrated state may cause decreased peripheral blood flow, which can be particularly hazardous in the heart, lungs, and kidneys. An elevated temperature may indicate the presence of infection and should be reported so that treatment can be implemented immediately.

Table 38-5. Comparison of manifestations of hypoglycemia and hyperglycemia

	Hypoglycemia	Hyperglycemia
Onset	Rapid	Gradual
Cause	Too much insulin Increased exercise with no increase in food intake Diminished food intake	Too little insulin Improper diet Reduced exercise with no reduction in food intake Emotional stress Physical stress such as infection, injury Drugs such as thiazides or corticosteroids
Manifestations	Lability of mood Irritability Shaky feeling Headache Impaired vision Hunger Convulsions	Weakness Increased thirst Frequent urination Signs of dehydration such as dry mucous membranes or soft eyeballs Nausea and vomiting Abdominal pain Acetone breath Rapid, deep respirations
Ominous features	Shock—coma—death	Acidosis—coma—death
Urinary findings		
Glucose	Negative	Positive
Acetone	Usually negative	Positive
Diacetic acid	Negative	Positive
Blood findings		
Glucose	Decreased (60 mg/100 ml or less)	Increased (250 mg/100 ml or more)
Acetone	Negative	Usually positive
Bicarbonate (CO_2)	Usually normal	Decreased (less than 20 mEq/liter); leukocytosis present

Careful and accurate records are maintained, including vital signs (pulse, respiration, temperature, and blood pressure), intravenous fluids, electrolytes, insulin, blood glucose level, and intake and output. A urine collection device or retention catheter is used to obtain the urine measurements, which include volume, specific gravity, and glucose and acetone values. The volume relative to the glucose content is important, since 5% glucose in a 300 ml sample is a significantly greater amount than a similar reading from a 75 ml sample. A diabetic flow sheet maintained at the bedside provides an ongoing record of the vital signs, urine and blood tests, amount of insulin given, and intake and output of the patient. The level of consciousness is assessed and recorded at frequent intervals. The comatose child generally regains consciousness fairly soon after initiation of therapy but is managed as any unconscious child during that time.

When the critical period is over, the task of regulating insulin dosage to diet and activity is begun. The same meticulous records of intake and output, urine glucose and acetone levels, and insulin administration are maintained. The capable child is actively involved in his own care and is given responsibility for keeping the intake and output record, testing the urine, and, when appropriate, administering his own insulin—all under the supervision and guidance of the nurse (Figs. 38-4 and 38-5).

Nursing considerations: long-term care

Once the diabetic child is diagnosed and insulin therapy initiated, the major nursing responsibility is the education and reinforcement of information for the family and the child who is old enough to participate in the self-management of the disease. In the case of the diabetic child, the parents must supervise and manage the child's therapeutic program, but the child should assume responsibility for self-management as soon as he is capable. Children can begin to test their own urine at a relatively young age, and most should be able to administer their own insulin at about 9 years of age. In situations in which the parents are inconsistent and/or unreliable, the child is taught self-care at an earlier age.

Children and their families vary in educational background and the capacity to learn and understand the various aspects of the therapeutic program. Some families respond

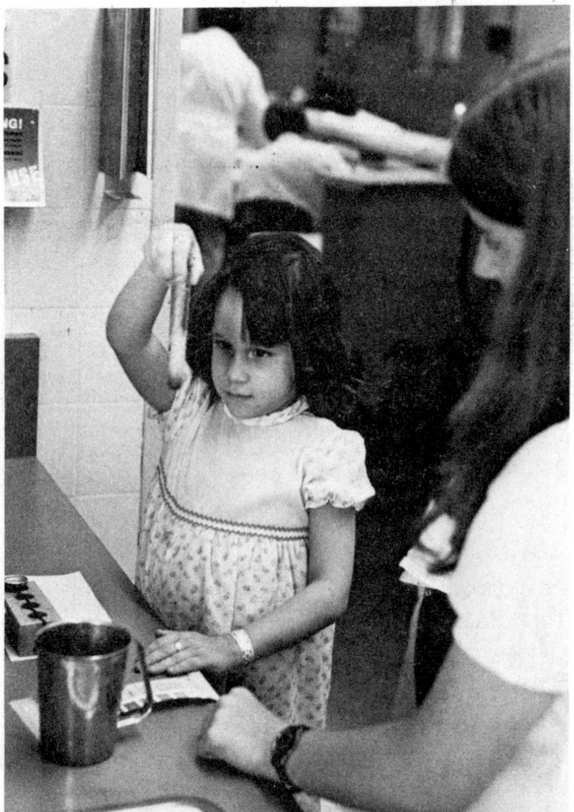

Fig. 38-4. School-age children are able to take responsibility for urine testing.

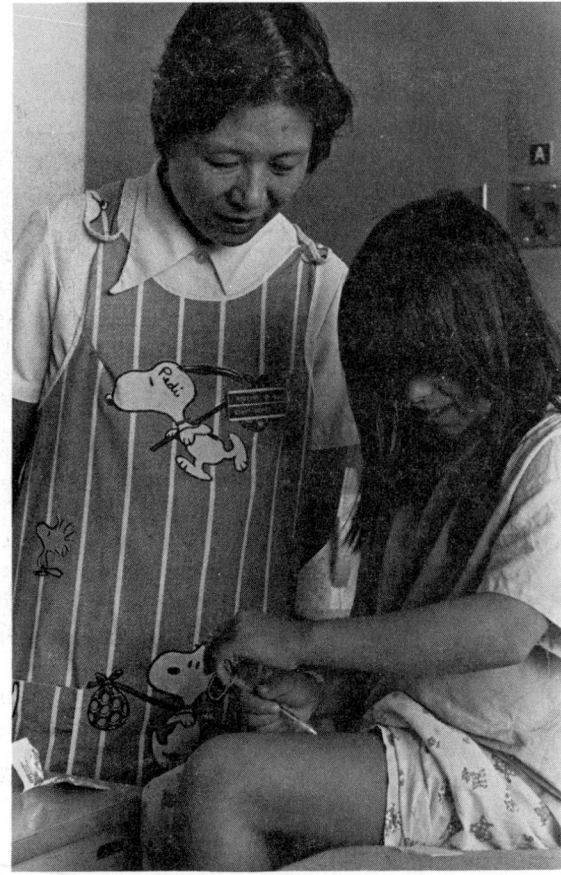

Fig. 38-5. School-age children are able to administer their own insulin.

best to very simple explanations and directions, whereas others expect thorough, in-depth information about the physiologic processes and responses associated with the disease and its therapy. All the principles of teaching and learning are applied in the educational process, and, before beginning, the nurse must determine the optimal time, place, method, and content to be taught. Properly educated, any family should be able to follow a program of regulated control satisfactorily.

When to teach a diabetic family is best judged by the psychologic state of the family and/or the child and the time of initial diagnosis. If a child is newly diagnosed, the psychologic adjustment to the disease can block the learning process completely, for example, members of the family who in a follow-up visit state that it is the first time that they have heard a certain bit of information when, in reality, the specific material had been covered several times in the course of teaching. Certainly the first 3 or 4 days after diagnosis are not an optimum time for learning. In fact, the later the more complex material is presented, the better. For example, one successful program teaches only essential, or survival, information first and intense information a month later. The choice of time for teaching in another program is a week after diagnosis followed by a review of survival techniques 2 weeks after discharge. Probably the most inopportune and ineffective time for teaching is the day or so after diagnosis when the education must be compressed into a few hours or days so that the child can be discharged early. Whether teaching is done on an outpatient basis or in a preparatory, in-depth manner on an inpatient basis, the ability of the individuals involved to learn must be accurately assessed. This includes assessment of the educational background and emotional stability of the individual(s) involved and the use of appropriate measurement tools, such as a pretest or an objective assessment of the learner's educational level.

The setting for the educational process can facilitate the learning process. An environment that is too hot or too cold or one in which there is too much noise will distract the learner. Bedside education may be necessary in some cases, but the coming and going of a number of people are also distracting. There are times in the educational process when individual instruction is needed, but contact with other children and/or parents will assist in adjustment to the reality of the disease and the implications of having a chronic condition. Supplementary material such as audiovisual aids enhances the learning process and promotes retention of information.

A child learns best when sessions are kept short, no more than 15 to 20 minutes. The parents do best in periods of 45 to 60 minutes and, often, longer if they are inquisitive.[9] Education should involve all the senses, and, although visual aids are valuable tools, participation is the most effective method for learning. For example, to teach urine testing, the technique is explained, the procedure is demonstrated, the learner is allowed to perform the procedure followed by a review of the material by visual aids, and the learning is validated by some testing method that includes a feedback. A variety of teaching methods and teaching aids can be employed. Some visual aids may be beautifully illustrated but miss a major point; therefore, materials should be previewed for accuracy and appropriateness. Varying the presentation with a variety of audiovisual materials including motion pictures, slide-tape programs, and books stimulates the senses and helps the individual to learn. The American Diabetes Association, Inc.,* is a valuable resource for educational material.

The content of the educational course must include the various aspects of the disease as they relate specifically to the individual child. There are many aspects of the disease that may not be covered in an initial educational course but postponed until subsequent office or clinic visits or through referral sources such as the American Diabetes Association. The minimal information is that which will help the family survive from one day to the next; expanded information helps the individual in the bio/psycho/social adjustment basic to in-depth knowledge about the disease. The more an individual understands the disease in relation to body needs, the better he is able to maintain a high degree of control. The following information will allow the family to manage the daily aspects of care.

Nature of diabetes. The better the parents understand the pathophysiology of diabetes and the function and action of insulin and glucagon in relation to calorie intake, the better their understanding of the disease and its effect on the child. Parents have a number of questions (voiced or unvoiced) that give them an increased feeling of mental adjustment when answered. They want to know about the procedures performed on their child, such as what is being put in the intravenous bottle and the expected effect.

Meal planning. Normal nutrition is a major aspect of information included in order that the family can learn how the meal plan relates to the requirements of normal development and the disease process. Diet instruction is usually conducted by the dietitian with reinforcement and guidance from the nurse. Learning about foods within specific food groups helps in choices. Weights and measures of foods, used as eye-training devices in defining food volumes, should be practiced for about 3 months with gradual conversion to estimating foods. Even though the child and/or parents become astute in estimating food volumes, rechecking should take place weekly or monthly and certainly when there is any change of brands. Members of the family are also guided in reading labels for the nutritional value of foods and food contents.

Family members should also become familiar with the

*1 W. 48th Street, New York, N.Y. 10020.

concept of calories. Calorie changes may be necessary in case a food is not available in sufficient quantity or if they wish to eat foods that may be more difficult to calculate because they lack specific exchanges (such as pizza or other fast-food items). Discussion should include situations the child might encounter in the classroom and in the school cafeteria (the kindergarten or first-grade student might like to have a special box from which he can choose items that are sugar free for occasions when treats containing excess sugar are brought to the classroom). Role playing and discussion help the teenager to choose foods when out on dates, with friends in their home, or on a food break after school.

Medication. Families need to understand the treatment method. They need to learn about the effective duration, onset, and peak action of the insulin prescribed. They also need to know the characteristics of the various types of insulins, the proper mixing and dilution of insulins, and how to substitute another type when their usual brand is not available.

Injection procedure. Learning to give the insulin injections is a source of anxiety for the parents and the child. It is helpful for the learner to know that this important aspect of care will become as routine as brushing the teeth. First the basic injection technique is taught using an orange or similar item for practice. To gain the confidence of the child, the nurse demonstrates the technique by giving a skillful injection to the parent and then the parent returns the demonstration by giving the nurse an injection. Thus with practice the parents soon are able to give the insulin injection to the child and he will trust them. Both parents should participate, and as little time as possible should elapse between instruction and the actual injection, especially with parents and the teenage learner.

Insulin can be injected into any area in which there is skin over muscle with fatty tissue in between. The length and angle of the needle is altered according to the thickness of the skin.[4] Usually the smaller the child, the thinner the skin. The pinch technique is the most effective method for obtaining skin tightness to allow easy entrance of the needle to subcutaneous tissues in children. The parents and child are helped to work out a rotation pattern. The site selected will sometimes depend on whether the child or parent administers the insulin. The arms, thighs, hips, and abdomen are usual injection sites for insulin. The child can reach the thighs, abdomen, and part of the hip and arm easily but may require help to inject other sites. For example, a parent can pinch a loose fold of skin of the arm while the child injects the insulin. Injections are rotated to various areas of the body to enhance absorption, since insulin absorption is slowed by the fat pads that develop in overused areas of injection. A rotation plan involves giving about four or five injections in one area (each injection about 1 inch from the previous injection) and then moving to another area. In this way injection sites for an entire month can be worked out in advance on a simple chart. Insulin absorption is enhanced by exercise so that injection into the legs might be avoided prior to excess exercise involving the legs.[32] It is a good idea for the parent to give a couple of shots a week in the areas that are difficult to reach in order to keep in practice.

The same basic methodology is employed when teaching the child to give his own insulin injections. He should practice first on an orange or a doll, building his courage gradually. His first attempt will undoubtedly be awkward as he tends to slowly push the needle through the skin rather than using a quick approach. It is best not to pressure the child into assuming this responsibility until he is ready. When he participates in a group-learning situation or has an opportunity to observe his peers giving their own injections, he is more strongly motivated. The parents should be warned that at some time he will give himself an uncomfortable injection at home and will need their support and encouragement. Otherwise he may not wish to give himself another injection for some time.

The teaching includes the proper way to equalize pressure in the bottle by injecting an amount of air equal to the amount of solution withdrawn and removal of air bubbles from the syringe. When insulin dosages are small an air bubble in the syringe can displace a signifiicant amount of medication. The parents and the child are taught always to remove insulin from the same bottle first so that only one bottle is apt to be adulterated by the contents of the other. The recommended procedure is to withdraw regular insulin first, then the modified insulin. Some physicians advocate premixing the insulins in the bottle both for convenience and to reduce the chance for contamination of one insulin with the other. This option should not be taught unless the child's physician approves it and the person who mixes the insulins is reliable. Some types of insulin (such as regular and NPH) cannot remain mixed for an extended period of time. The NPH insulin may be added to the regular insulin in any ratio desired, but the mixing should take place immediately before its use to prevent physiologic changes that can lead to unpredictable activities of the combination over a period of time.* Insulin syringes should be compared for accuracy, comfort, strength, and the family and/or child should be able to choose both "their" insulin and "their" syringe from a variety of samples.[33] Use of the same syringe (even during hospitalization) is recommended to prevent errors in dosage due to varying amounts of dead space among syringes.

Urine testing. Urine testing is easily taught and should include all methods of urine testing, not just the test to be used for the particular child. Use of the copper reduction test (Clinitest) includes instruction of the 5-, 2-, and 1-drop

---

*Lilly Research Laboratories, Indianapolis, Ind.

methods. The range for the 5-drop method (5 drops of urine, 10 drops of water, and 1 tablet) is 0% to 2%; the range for the 2-drop test (2 drops of urine, 10 drops of water, and 1 tablet) is 0% to 5%; and the range for the 1-drop test (1 drop of urine, 11 drops of water, and 1 tablet) is 0% to 10%, obtained by doubling the results on the 2-drop test. Instruction also includes the pass-through phenomenon, which occurs when there is more glucose in the specimen than the test can record. It responds by "going backward" on the color scale or "passes through" the bright orange color at the top of the scale. This may occur during the "boiling" or during the 15-second waiting period. The likelihood for this pass-through to occur is much less with the 2-drop test, since it is able to show more glucose in the urine than the 5-drop test. More programs are using the 2- and 1-drop method when there is pass through on the 5-drop method. The copper reduction test may give false-positive results when certain antibiotics are being taken and with the introduction of sugars other than glucose. Shaking the test tube during the "boiling" will increase the addition of oxygen and cause an alteration in the test results; therefore, shaking of the test tube should not occur until after the 15-second wait.[2] Families should be cautioned about handling the tablet, which contains lye, and to keep the bottle out of reach of small children.

The glucose oxidase tests (Diastix, Clinistix, and Tes-Tape) are more sensitive tests and are responsive to glucose only. These tests are very useful for travel and for school but are a little too sensitive for daily control. Directions for interpreting the tests should be read carefully. The percentage readings are the same as those for the Clinitest, but there are differences in the plus values.

The tests for acetone are the Ketostix and the Acetest. The test is read after a 30-second wait. The acetone tests are not done daily, as the glucose tests are, but should be performed during times of illness or high sugar spills.

Moisture will cause changes to take place in the tablets. Families should be instructed to discard tablets that are discolored, that have been open for a specified period of time, or after an expiration date.

Hyperglycemia. Severe hyperglycemia is most often caused by illness, growth, or emotional upset. Parents who are accustomed to seeing negative urines respond immediately when they see their child start to spill some sugar in the urine. If the child is receiving less than 0.2 U/pound/day of insulin, the pancreas is probably producing some endogenous insulin and it is desirable to preserve this function for as long as possible. The parents should understand how to adjust food, activity, and insulin at the time of illness and when the child is treated for an illness with a medication known to raise the blood glucose level. The hyperglycemia resulting from growth is managed by increasing insulin soon after the increased spill is noted.

Hypoglycemia. Hypoglycemia is caused by imbalances of food intake, insulin, and activity. Ideally hypoglycemia should be prevented and parents need to be prepared to prevent, recognize, and treat the problem. They should be familiar with the signs of hypoglycemia and instructed in treatment, including care of the child with seizures (see p. 1445). Hypoglycemia can be managed effectively as follows:

Mild reaction—treat with food
Moderate reaction—treat with simple sugar followed by food
Severe reaction—treat with glucagon (or simple sugar administered rectally) followed by simple sugar in 15 to 20 minutes

It is a good idea for parents to plan for extra excitement or exercise. Also, gastroenteritis will often decrease insulin slightly if vomiting and/or diarrhea occur or if the appetite is depressed from nausea. If the urine is negative for glucose but acetone is present, the family should be aware of the increased need for simple sugar.

All diabetic children should be provided with identification that explains their condition so that it will be noticed in times of emergency. This will bring aid to the child more quickly. Identification is noticed more readily if it is in the form of a bracelet rather than a necklace or dog tag.

Hygiene. All aspects of personal hygiene are emphasized for the child with diabetes. The child has not had time to develop the blood vessel disease that causes a decrease in peripheral circulation; therefore, foot care is not as important in the child as it is in the adult with diabetes. However, the correct method of nail and extremity care instituted for each particular child (with the guidance of a podiatrist) can begin health practices that last a lifetime. Eyes should be checked once a year unless the child wears glasses and then as directed by the ophthalmologist. Regular dental care is emphasized, and cuts and scratches should be treated with plan soap and water unless otherwise indicated.

Exercise. Exercise should be planned, as may be necessary for the sedentary teenager, or observed, as is found in most active children. If the child is more active at one time of the day than at another, food and/or insulin can be altered to meet the activity pattern of the individual child. Food should be increased in the summer when children tend to be more active. Decreased activity on return to school may require a decrease in food intake. The child who is active in team sports will need an increase in food intake on the days of activity, and races or other competition may call for a slightly higher food intake than practice times. Food will usually need to be repeated for prolonged activity periods, often as frequently as every 45 minutes to 1 hour. Families should be informed that if increased food is not tolerated, decreased insulin is the next course of action. If the timing of the exercise is changed so that the supper meal is delayed, the insulin in the second or third dose of the day may be moved back to precede the mealtime. Sugar may sometimes be needed during exercise periods for quick response. Parents should be aware that if sugar is seen in the urine after extreme activity it may represent Somagyi's reflex (see p. 1484).

Record keeping. Keeping information about food, insulin, and glucosuria is useful to the physician as well as to the family. The record should contain information on insulin doses and variations in urine tests that include as many urine tests as possible. Both glucose and acetone should be recorded when the glucose spill is high, especially during illness or during wellness when there are continued glucose spills of 2% or more. Insulin reactions should be noted, including the time, severity, treatment, and response to treatment. Dietary variations are noted so that an increased glucose spill can be analyzed in relation to insulin dose, food intake, and activity level. The record should contain types and variations in activity that are markedly above or below the expected activity levels, dietary variations, and illnesses. If slips in the management occur (such as eating a candy bar), the child should be encouraged to note it and not be condemned for the transgression.

Complications. It is debatable whether or not knowledge of potential hazards of poor control should be shared with the family and child. If so, the implications of the disease are presented in a tactful, clear, and nonfearful manner. Knowledge of the complications of diabetes and their relationship to control provides a basis for knowledgeable decision making. Eye and kidney disease are the greatest threats, with neurologic complications close behind. Clear explanations of these problems clarify false information often given by well-meaning friends. By this time the nurse has developed a rapport with the patient and family and knows at what level and how openly the problem can be discussed. The information should include discussion of research so that the family is left with the positive impression that others are concerned about finding answers and preventing complications. It also gives them hope that somehow, someway, a prevention and/or cure are possible.

Self-management. Self-management is the key to close control. Being able to make changes at the time they are needed rather than waiting until the next contact with health professionals is important for self-management and gives the individual and family the feeling that they have control over the disease. Psychologically this helps the family members feel that they are useful and participating members of the team. Learning to look at records objectively gives the child support. The child will not be accused of cheating every time a spill occurs. As children grow and assume more and more responsibility for self-management, they develop confidence in their ability to manage their disease and in themselves as persons. They grow to respond to the disease and to make more accurate interpretations and changes in self-management when they become adults. Self-management techniques to be mastered are the alteration of insulin and diet with exercise, illness, emotional upset, surgery, and so on. However, limitations are set regarding how many alterations should be made without consulting with the health professionals. The degree of control prior to the illness is a determining factor in seeking medical help during illness. In an individual with poor control it takes but a few hours before the trouble is severe, whereas if control is good prior to illness several days may elapse before help is needed. Patients and families are cautioned to seek assistance if the urine has elevated glucose levels and has not become free of acetone after 24 hours of self-management.

Problem solving. In any educational program psychologic needs are just as important as the physical needs of the child. Adjustment to a chronic illness is difficult and follows the grief process (see Chapter 22). A noticeable adjustment cycle occurs during the week-long education course. First there is interest and perhaps some anger and doubt, followed by denial and accompanied by the overwhelming feeling of "Why me?" There are doubts regarding the ability to absorb so much essential information. Then there are the acceptance and synthesis of material as the learners realize that they are able to state and demonstrate their understanding of the material.

School and associated activities need to be discussed. The parents are encouraged to visit their child's school and talk to the appropriate people, such as the principal, homeroom teacher, and the school nurse. In younger children it is often helpful to educate their classmates, who may think that the disease is catching and, therefore, shun the child with diabetes. Snack areas should be identified, and lunchroom personnel are sometimes included in planning for the diabetic child. Another helpful aid is a card, available from the diabetes association, that can be filled out and placed where it is readily visible to a substitute teacher.

Camping and other special groups are very useful. In the camp for children with diabetes, these children learn that they are not alone. As a result they become more independent and resourceful in the nondiabetic camp setting, especially if they have had experience in a diabetic camp. Useful information about such camps and organizations can be obtained from the American Diabetes Association. Many families find solace and comfort from their religious faith, and, where appropriate, a representative of the faith should be contacted to help provide for this very special need.

Nursing considerations: psychosocial adjustment

Children have changing needs associated with the developmental processes, and many of the problems of illness and adjustment are related to the age of the child. Physiologic development is not a smooth, consistent process but one that takes place in spurts and plateaus. Growth data that consistently fit the established norms are one indicator of disease control. Poor control is reflected by an erratic or retarded growth curve. Psychologic development is a continuous process, and satisfactory adjustment is reflected in good control of the disease, healthy activities and relationships, and the child's ability to talk about his disease comfortably. Many of the psychologic adjustments are related to the age of the child at the time of diagnosis as well as the attitude and support provided by the family.

Infant. At this age problems of adjustment are not those of the infant but of the parents. Medical management problems are most difficult at this age. The most rapid increase in growth, activity, and diet changes takes place during this period. Urine is tested by touching a test strip or stick to a wet diaper or by placing cotton balls inside the diaper to catch urine, from which a few drops are squeezed for testing. Frequent doses of short-acting insulin are preferred at this age, and the administration poses few problems once the parents adjust to the initial reluctance. Dilutions of insulin to U10 or other convenient amount offer more security to the parents regarding accuracy of the dose. Food intake in infants is fairly regular and evenly spaced. Adequacy of hydration during illness is important because increased concentration of the urine can alter test results and the infant can become acidotic more quickly.

Baby K has been diabetic since 3 days of age. She had her pancreas removed because of beta cell hyperplasia that caused severe hypoglycemia, which had been responsible for the death of an older sibling shortly after birth. Pancreatic enzymes were administered to aid digestion. Since the infant was quite sensitive to insulin, she was given small doses of regular insulin diluted to a strength of U1, but within 3 months the insulin was adjusted to U10 and then the amount gradually increased with growth. The parents learned to recognize hypoglycemia by signs of irritability and a cold, clammy feeling of the infant's skin. The increased activity resulting from crying sometimes led to hypoglycemia, but this was gradually alleviated when the proper balance of food, activity, and insulin was achieved. With three insulin injections per day the urine was kept free of sugar 60% to 80% of the time without significant hypoglycemia. A consistent rate of growth attests to her satisfactory control, and the parents appear to be adjusting well to the challenges the infant presents.

Toddler. The toddler is at greater risk for problems related to the adjustment of his disease. A major problem is the acceptance of insulin injections without fear. Others include the variable activity pattern and appetite characteristic of children in this age-group (see Chapter 14). If hospitalization is required, separation anxiety is also present.

An erratic activity pattern in children in this age-group is quite common as naps become shorter and activity becomes more variable. One minute the child will be extremely active, and the next he will sit quietly reading a book. Erratic food intake will also occur during this time. Except for times of lowered or elevated blood sugar levels, these children will easily eat in response to activity. Unless they are overinsulinized, they will not usually overeat, but restriction of food without an adequate decrease in insulin can lead to hypoglycemia. The child who dawdles or plays in his food, takes too long to eat, or refuses to eat may be subconsciously using food as a means of gaining attention. The more attention the parents give by force feeding, punishing, and cajoling, the less the child will cooperate. Children of this age are best fed in small amounts and by allowing them to ask for more rather than serving so much food that they refuse to eat.

Parents are helped to observe the activity and to adjust food intake accordingly. The normal decrease in growth rate during the second year and changes in food intake are accompanied by changes in insulin dosage. Accurate recording of observations and adjustments provide a reference for future alterations.

One tactic used to break the cycle of poor eating to gain attention is to lower the insulin dosage so that there is no danger of hypoglycemia and then to place the food on the plate for a specified period of time and praise the child for bites taken. All other behaviors should be ignored. At the end of the specified period of time, about 30 minutes, the food is removed without fuss. It usually requires a number of days to break the cycle, but the child should not be forced to eat every last bite. Mealtimes should be positive times.

Insulin injections can also be used by the child as an attention-getting device, for example, when the child runs and the parents respond to the "game" by chasing the child around the house at injection time. This is often followed by the need to hold the child down for the injection, which creates a negative atmosphere at this time. Acceptance of the procedure as part of the daily routine is the goal. The injection must become as habitual as brushing the teeth or combing the hair. Following the injection time with some special and positive attention such as reading, talking, or other pleasant activity is one way to convert the child who refuses injections to one who accepts them.

Another source of toddler rebellion is refusal to void or, less often, psychogenic drinking of large amounts of fluid. In the first instance the psychologic response of the child may be, "You want something from my body by which you can control me and I am not going to give it to you." In the other case it may be, "You see me going to the bathroom frequently or drinking a lot and you think I'm sick all over again so I get attention." Parents are instructed to relax and take off the pressure (which should not have been there in the first place). Bathroom visits should be appropriately scheduled before and after meals and at bedtime. If the results are not obtained within a few minutes, the parents should nonchalantly allow the child to go on with play or other activities without special attention but with approval when a specimen is obtained. The toddler should be able to sit on the potty for a specified period of time, but the time should not be prolonged. For the frequent voider who is not being tested for sugar and/or acetone, ignoring the frequent trips to the water faucet or bathroom is usually the best approach.

K. R. was a precocious 2-year-old child who was the first child of intelligent but overanxious parents. The parents expected a perfect child, and diabetes tarnished this perfect image. In the hospital the child cooperated after the first few days in getting her injections, but 2 weeks after discharge she became a "shot refuser." The data gathered revealed that during the first few days after discharge from the hospital the parents played a "peekaboo" game that was expanded to "catch-me-if-you-can." K. R. continued to run and refused to cooperate. Based on the family assessment, it was recommended that the parents use a firm approach, without chasing, and have the child's favorite book or toy available at injection time. The parents, who talked to the toy or read the book aloud until the child quietly sat at their side, were amazed at the positive response. The child came to understand that this was expected behavior.

Preschool child. The preschool child has problems similar to those of the toddler but of less erratic nature. Preschoolers can recognize that candy is not good for them unless eaten at special times as a medicine, and their ability to recognize some colors helps them to relate them to colors on the urine test color charts. They may also have a beginning understanding of the concept that the food they eat needs a key (insulin) in order to get into the boxes (or cells) inside the body, where it supplies the body's energy needs. They may be somewhat resistant to injections but should be developing an interest in self-care and general acceptance of their particular life-style.

The preschool child will have a more active but slightly less erratic activity pattern than the toddler. Naps take less time or are abandoned completely. The attention span will be slightly longer, and the child will spend longer periods in quiet activities. Food intake will be less erratic, but food likes and dislikes may become rigid and pronounced, which can cause some problems with the diabetes management. The individual pattern of activity is identified and the insulin and diet structured around that pattern. The nurse can help the parents to recognize increased or lowered insulin needs related to the amount of overall level of food intake. Eating time is made a neutral time with praise given after meals or at specific instances for positive responses during the meal. Forced feeding, which contributes to poor food habits and reinforces negative attention behaviors, is discouraged.

Poor eating habits established earlier in the child's life become more ingrained during this period but may be continued in order to gain attention. However, they may be caused by listlessness or other disabilities related to poor control of the disease. They may also represent negative feelings toward food and toward the parents and used as a mechanism of getting attention. The goal is to encourage the child to eat an appropriate amount of food by providing foods acceptable to the child initially and then gradually to expand his horizons to new tastes at weekly or monthly intervals.

Children at this age are able to accept that it is time for an insulin injection but may attempt to get attention by refusing the injection. This problem is perhaps more difficult to control at this age than at any other and becomes worse if the parents believe that they must participate in some kind of game playing or chasing in order to get the child to cooperate. If there is a definite fear of the injection procedure, the child should be given a chance to play out the feeling with syringes and dolls or, if he is unable to handle syringes without discomfort, to express his feelings in drawings. By working through these feelings fear of the injection procedure can be lessened, but first it must be determined whether the child is afraid of the injection or is merely using the refusal as an attention-getting device. The best approach is for the parents to announce at the appointed time that it is time for the insulin injection.

Collecting urine specimens can be frustrating to both parents and child, although the child is more responsive at this age than he was as a toddler. He should be toilet trained by this time but may recognize that withholding specimens can create anxiety. Needed specimens should not be obtained by pressure, but the child should develop a habit pattern of supplying a specimen before mealtimes and at bedtime. Any difficulty with toilet training may be related to other medical problems, such as diabetes out of control, urinary tract infection, or other systemic infections.

A well-managed child produces needed specimens at the appropriate times and takes injections without any particular discomfort or fear the majority of the time. The family should be able to alter food needs with activity and be able to recognize patterns in the excretion of urinary sugar. The child should demonstrate a healthy and a consistent growth pattern with good control of the disease.

T. M. is 4 years old and has had diabetes for 3 years. She has been fairly ill during much of this period. In play she constantly refers to the dolls as being sick with frequent emesis, having to stay in bed, and requiring glucagon to treat insulin reactions. She is able to count to 10; therefore, she is able to count drops needed to do her own urine testing. She relates this to the ten fingers on her hands for the water, her two hands for the 2 drops of urine, and her one head for the 1 tablet. She has learned to recognize negative or positive urine and that when she has negative urines she feels better and could continue to feel better if her tests remain negative most of the time. The nurse helps her to play through the idea with the use of puppets that "they" feel better because they have enough insulin to keep them from becoming ill as frequently as before.

The parents were instructed in self-management of the child, who is now much better managed, is in much more stable control, and appears to be much happier. The whole concept of illness that was part of the family's expected philosophy has diminished and has been replaced by a concept of wholeness and health.

School-age child. School-age children should be able to

understand the basic concepts regarding their disease and its treatment—that they are unable to get sugar into the cells without insulin, that there must be a balance of food and activity, and the relationship between food, activity, and insulin. The child should be able to test urine, recognize food groups, give injections, start record keeping, and recognize various feelings so that he can differentiate among fear, excitement, and hypoglycemia. He should understand how to recognize, prevent, and treat hypoglycemia.

Elementary school children should become aware of themselves and what they are feeling. There should be a normal psychologic acceptance of injections, even though there will be times when there are negative feelings concerning them. School-age children usually have questions about the disease and are more involved mentally as well as physically in self-care. They respond much more acutely to pain and discomfort and, if uncomfortable injections have occurred, may become quite negative about self-administration of insulin.

School-aged children, also, may use their diabetes for secondary gain. They sometimes fake insulin reactions or may actually cause an insulin reaction to occur in order to get negative attention. Not eating or eating too much of certain foods is also guaranteed to get some kind of feedback. Some children may eat some or all of the meal or eat forbidden foods and then vomit. Such children may have fears, may be seeking attention, may be ill, or may have an imbalance of food or insulin. Another problem is complaining that "my tummy hurts." As children enter the middle years of childhood, there is a greater awareness of self-image. Pain and discomfort becomes more intense. Body feelings and body parts are now recognized as part of the integrated whole. Abdominal pain is a common form of internalization of feeling and tension seen in nondiabetic, as well as diabetic, children in this age-group.

Parents need to learn how to help the child to seek other outlets for acting out. Parents can be guided into providing opportunities for positive behaviors so that child will not have to resort to the diabetes for gaining attention. Some children have difficulty in channeling their attention seeking. Nurses can help parents analyze their child's behavior and choose certain alternate ways in which to provide the needed attention. For example, if the child is playing or reading quietly in another part of the house, the parents can make an effort to find the child and say, "I missed you," or show an interest in what the child is doing. As children begin to feel loved, they will feel more secure in their needs or other types of attention. Although "using diabetes" occurs in children in all age-groups, it appears more frequently in the school-age child and may be a reflection of insecurity and an increased need for attention. The ability of the family to support the changing emotional needs during growth and development may be assessed by the frequency of abnormal episodes over a period of time.

When periodic or cyclic vomiting becomes a problem, as it often does, many parameters such as fear, tension, and imbalance in food and insulin need to be explored so that one may determine the cause of vomiting and deal with it accordingly. If the problem is simple psychogenic vomiting, insulin needs to be decreased to a minimum amount to cover a minimum amount of food, and retraining is in order. In other words, this child should be retrained to accept small amounts of food comfortably before more appropriate amounts of food intake for the child's height and weight can be accepted. It is possible that retraining may have to be started from the beginning, repatterning types and amounts of food eaten. Pressure at mealtime must be eliminated. A calm, peaceful atmosphere should prevail. Sometimes soothing, cheerful music can be a positive distraction from the vomiting actions.

For the "my tummy hurts" response, the child's feelings should be discussed and the timing of the pain should be determined. Ways in which to relieve the tension and ease the "pain" under the pain should be investigated. Then, if unsuccessful, referrals for counseling or medication can be planned if needed. The nurse should assist the parents in recognizing the problem and whether there is a specific need for treatment. If the actual problem is hypoglycemia, it should be treated promptly and without any added attention. The parents should help the child learn to differentiate between psychogenic and physiologic symptoms of hypoglycemia. The nurse's intervention through education and support plus counseling will help in progress toward behavioral change. The goal is to decrease these periods of discomfort and to give understanding as to the cause so that it may become a learning experience to the child.

Evaluation of the problems of the school-age child may be made from the history or by keeping records concerning each manipulation. The simplest method of evaluation of response in the child is the use of a point or token system. A point or token is given to the child each time he is able to pinpoint the moment when he feels like using his diabetes. If the parent catches the child using diabetes, then a point or token is removed. This is done in cooperation with the child and will show the child when he feels like using diabetes to get his way. It gives him another mechanism for attention getting other than having to use the diabetes in ways that might be harmful to his own health.

G. T. was 7 years old and ready to enter the second grade. He became quite fearful of his injections shortly after the procedure was begun. It required four nurses to catch and hold this pint-sized child down for his injections. Use of play revealed a very fearful child who would have nothing to do with syringes in the play case (Fig. 38-6). He was given some crayons and paper and asked to draw pictures of himself. His drawings showed a stick man with angrily made spots or dots over the center section of the paper, many of them touching the man. On questioning the child insinuated that he was a pincushion. After this self-image awakening

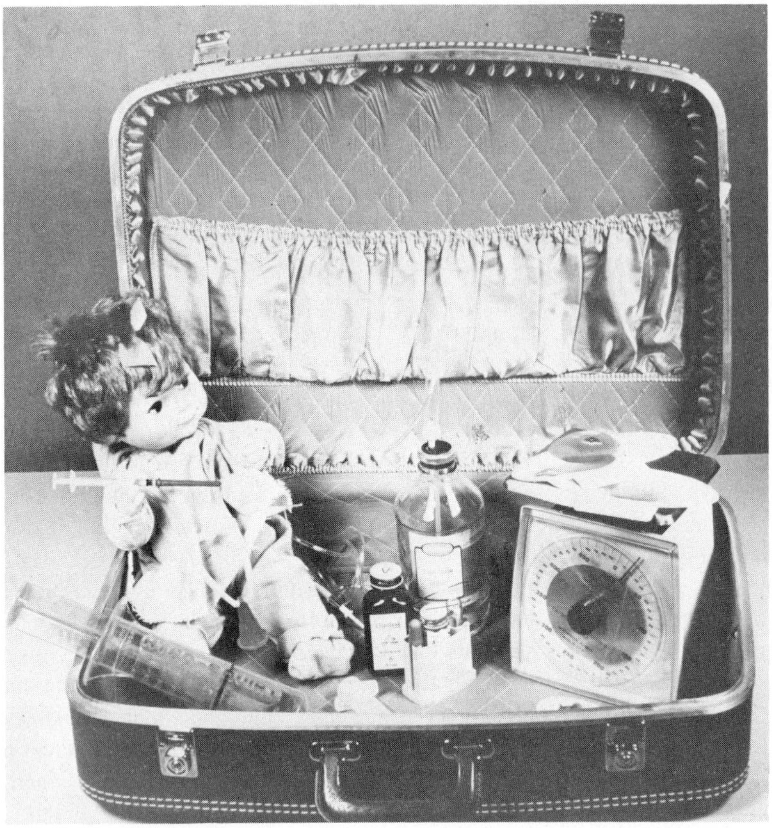

Fig. 38-6. Diabetic play equipment conveniently collected and stored in a small suitcase.

and without any outside interference, he began to play with the syringes in the play kit and started to accept his injections without fuss.

After he went home from the hospital, he began using his diabetes by acting out imaginary hypoglycemic episodes, but he always improved just seconds after he ate something containing simple sugar. His pulse did not change, and he was caught opening his eyes when he apparently thought his parents were not looking. When the parents recognized that the child was using his diabetes, they sought counseling. They soon realized that the only time they had given this child attention in the past was when he was doing something that he should not be doing. As they learned to handle his fears and his desires for attention, the need became less and less and his pattern of using diabetes decreased without any direct intervention. He is now a very well-adjusted boy, and the parents have become very supportive in a protective but comfortable manner.

Early teenage child. The child in junior high school can usually understand his disease and the methods of determining food amounts. He is able to test urine correctly, to give injections and rotate the sites, to keep records and understand why it is requested for him to do so, and to contribute to decisions on alterations of diabetes management. Children in this age-group should begin to recognize that there are complications associated with the disease and that close control of the disease will retard or prevent these problems.

Conflict and self-doubt are characteristic of the junior high school student. Rebellion is a normal reaction, and resolution is desirable. Variations in diet will begin to occur as the child "tries out" the diabetes. The adolescent should have knowledge of normal, expected nutritional intake so that he can assess the adjustment of food and insulin with changes in activity. Urine testing becomes a mechanical, boring, and time-consuming reminder of diabetes, a restriction resented by many youngsters. Children soon recognize that negative urine tests bring on smiles and feelings of acceptance, whereas positive urine tests may bring about disapproval and recrimination; therefore, they may feel that giving false urine tests brings approval, even though they recognize that such a practice is harmful to themselves. Failure to do the tests is the most common problem of early adolescence, doing the tests but not recording them is next most common, and frank falsification of tests is the least common problem related to urine testing. Also, urine tests may be adulterated by water, fruit juice, or other substances.

Teenagers do not want to feel different or be different from their peers. If they do not tell anyone about the disease, they may believe that it will go away and not make them different. They wish to be acceptable to others and not appear as freaks, but they must recognize that the disease is going to continue to be present until a cure is found. If the disease is accepted by all family members, the affected child will see less reason to hide or deny the disease. Youngsters who are taught to reach out rather than to withdraw in both thought and action have less difficulty in accepting the disease and less reason for denial of the diabetes. The goal is to help the youngsters to learn that they are accepted for who they are and that they are loved. Group rap sessions provide them with the opportunity to express their feelings to others. Counseling and diabetic camps are most appropriate for children in this age-group so that they can see that they are not the only ones with problems, which will help them to adjust to their life-style.

Bitterness and resentment may be a part of the thoughts of insulin-dependent teenagers. Such bitterness may also result as a response to complications caused by poor control of blood glucose. Food (other than concentrated sweets) should never be restricted as a means of diabetic control in the child or adolescent diabetic. Calories may on occasion need to be restricted to prevent or control obesity, but this is restriction for weight control, not diabetic control.

Learning about the disease and how it affects others is a hard but realistic approach. As prepubescent teenagers the likelihood of complications is something that they may be looking at and that may be especially magnified if their control has not been adequate. Helping the individuals to make choices while learning about all aspects of the disease may help in further determination of choices as they go into the later years of adolescence. This also gives them an opportunity to feel that they have control over their future.

Cheating on the diet is really a sign of mismanagement. If a child is getting an adequate amount of food, there is no need to cheat. Certainly a candy bar or some other forbidden food may be eaten, but this may become a problem if it is not handled appropriately by the child's parents and/or his peers. Foods should be adequate for activity and needs for normal growth and development, and, if the diet is adequate, cheating will not be necessary and will rarely occur. Adequate information should be made available to help the teenager understand about the rapid absorption rate of simple concentrated sugar vs the slow absorption of insulin from the tissue. The decision to restrict concentrated sweets must come from the youth directly. The family may support the child by keeping these temptations out of the home.

Frequent hospitalizations may be necessary because of poor management or may be used as attention-getting devices when the youngster is not receiving the attention at home that he gets in the hospital. It may also be used as a "cop-out" from responsibility in school or at home. Hospitalization may make the youngster feel more accepted when there is a negative self-image at home. Frequent hospitalizations may be decreased by improving control through medical management, education, individual motivation, and improved compliance. The frequent hospitalizations may be a result of environmentally negative factors. Improvement of the home environment by counseling and appropriate therapy may alter the youth's attention-seeking behaviors manifest by self-caused hospitalization. Once the cause is determined, counseling that includes parental influence may be carried out in individual or group therapy type situations. Understanding actions of the insulin on the body may assist the youngster in making judgments, especially if the child has acquired a more positive self-image.

There is no answer to the question, "Why me?" One can only supply support and help the youngster to recognize that the disease has occurred and that existence must go on from that point. Thoughts must be positively directed so that the child will believe that life has much to offer and that he has much to offer life.

M. T. is a junior high school student who has had diabetes for 6 years. Her parents divorced over a year ago and the mother was beginning to date and the child was resentful of this. It was found that every time the mother dated, M. T. would alter her medical management and end up in the hospital. During these hospitalizations she was happy, cheerful, cooperative, and the ideal patient. When the discovery that this was her mechanism for coping with both her disease and her family was made, counseling was provided by the nurse specialist. M. T. was able to recognize that she needed the support of her mother but that her mother needed friends just as she did. The mother was counseled regarding the needs of her child. On discharge this patient became a little more understanding of her own and her mother's needs, and the hospitalizations ceased. Although she still has other problems, especially the "Why me?," she has made a better adjustment in the home situation and is meeting her own needs for adequate growth and development and acceptance of the disease appropriate for her age level.

Later teenage child. Children in the later teenage years should be able to perform all the mechanical tasks related to diabetes self-care and have an understanding of the physiology of the disease that facilitates knowledgeable self-management. These youngsters are in the late stages of the rebellion of adolescence. A concern over self-image will be most apparent as they try to find where they fit into society, and one of the biggest problems is recognizing and accepting the various tasks of self-care as part of self-management. This is the age when greatest falsifying of records occurs. As diabetic persons progress from the last year of high school into the first year of college, they should have developed some major conclusions about themselves and begun to adjust in relation to knowledge and life goals. Feelings of self-fears and doubts should be dealt with progressively with the support of adequate counseling and/or psychiatric intervention when needed. Feelings concerning self and the preservation of self are major problems. This is the age in which there is the highest suicide rate for those having this disease.

For senior high school students, urine testing is a hassle. Taking time to do the test, even though it takes just a few minutes each day, will seem too much, too "heavy," too cumbersome, and too bothersome. They should be able to test urine carefully and accurately and to understand the results of these tests as part of the total self-management program. They should be able to recognize that they may intelligently alter the medical management in various ways and that the urine test may be an indicator of overall control and serve as feedback from the positive approach to the disease.

Denial can be expressed by not taking insulin, not performing urine tests, and not eating correctly. Denial of the disease should decrease during this period of time as the diabetic youngsters begin to feel their worth. During denial nurses can offer counseling directed toward helping the youngsters or their parents recognize the mechanisms used to deny the disease, recognize the feelings within themselves as they associate with their peers and their families, and overcome these negative feelings. The "Why me?" question may become very intense and severe at this age, since adolescents are intolerant of body imperfections and diabetes is a defect that emphasizes their vulnerability and imperfection. The ability to look beyond themselves and recognize that they may be of service to others is a goal.

Inaccurate doses of insulin may occur as an error or, if done frequently, an attention-seeking device, or, in a number of cases, a subconscious but socially accepted method of suicide. Inaccurate intake of food leads to overweight, which may also represent a subconscious death wish. The nurse can attempt to determine the true feelings of the child and/or parents and assist them to recognize these feelings and the alternatives for coping, such as professional counseling or alternate courses of action. The nurse, aware of the psychologic needs of the youngster, can guide the youngster to appropriate counseling resources that may be supportive, as offered by the nurse; testing, assessment, and counseling as offered by the psychologist; or specific therapy as offered by the psychiatrist. Behavioral alterations will be needed if suicidal tendencies are amplified by the diabetes.

Rehospitalizations are most often related to poor control of the disease, although it is also possible that they are indirectly related to noncoping and become a method of getting away from the pressures caused by family and peers. The hospital may represent an environment that is peaceful and free of stress. The goal for this problem is to determine the cause of the hospitalization. It may be poor control or self-management or the need for better supportive management at home. Evaluation should be based on both the physiologic as well as the psychologic adjustment of the child and the family.

T. T. was a 15-year-old boy whose life goal was to become a pilot. He soon found, however, that an insulin-dependent diabetic person cannot pilot a motorized aircraft. When he found that he could not become a pilot, he started denying his disease, refused to take any urine tests, would not follow his meal plan, and on occasion would not take his insulin. After a number of episodes of diabetic ketoacidosis that required hospitalization, he began to recognize that the only individual he was hurting was himself. Through counseling, alternative life-styles were discussed. The counselor found that a diabetic person can pilot a motorless aircraft such as a glider or sailplane.

T. T. has now learned to become a glider pilot, which fulfilled his desire to be involved in aviation, and he is now able to fly in both national and international meets. In order to fly well, he has to feel well, so he has assumed more control over his disease and is now in very good control of his diabetes. He has become much better adjusted, is goal oriented toward improved control of his disease, and is also becoming more of an expert in his field of interest.

Parents. Parents develop guilt feelings when they have a child with any chronic disease, especially if it has a heredity component. They deal with these feelings in a number of ways. They may respond by being overprotective or neglectful. Parents may choose various ways in which to cope with the internal feelings of guilt and hurt. Guilt-ridden parents blame the disease on themselves consciously or subconsciously. They must come to realize through education and counseling that there was nothing they could have done to prevent the child from having the disease and that it was not their fault, since environmental as well as hereditary factors may be involved in the development of the disease.

When parents become overprotective this usually results from feelings of guilt as well as feelings of fear of the unknown. Overprotection is a mechanism that alters the guilt responses to justify their own needs, for example, "If the child is in my sight, nothing worse will happen than what has already happened by the child getting diabetes. Therefore, I am going to watch this child every single minute because I will let nothing further happen to him." The overprotective mother becomes the smothering mother, one that hampers the growth, development, and maturation of the affected child.

The neglectful parents, on the other hand, have a different problem. This response is a mechanism developed to block feelings that give them pain. Thus there is a relief from their guilt feelings. "This is your disease and I have no responsibilities related to what is your disease; therefore, if anything bad happens to you as a result of you having this disease, it is not my fault." The neglectful mother or father gives the child responsibilities before he is mature enough to accept the more adult role.

Threatened parents look at the disease as a way in which to keep the child tied to them. If the child learns to be independent, such as is expected by the child in the camping experience, the parent may feel threatened and thus place obstacles in the child's path to independent development. If there are individual problems within the parental response, it is a challenge to the nurse to assist by counseling or, if severe enough, to appropriately refer the parents to other resources developed to help them alter their feelings. When the children are mature enough, the health professional may see them alone. The mother and/or father should not be made to feel that they are being left out. If the child is seen alone, times, either during the child's clinic visit or afterward, should be set up to meet the parents' needs. Parents should be included in special sessions so that they may keep up with the child's management, continue to participate in the child's care, and have an opportunity to express their own feelings concerning their own or their child's adjustment to the disease. The amount of information that they can give at this particular time may show their level of support of the child and may also be of assistance in decisions concerning the medical management of the child. This will help in guiding the child through the most disruptive time of life, the teenage years.

The health professionals must be aware of parents who say that they are supporting the child and appear to be supporting the child to the optimum level but who, with deeper interview techniques, may be found to be supporting the child in word but not in deed. These parents may not see the need for following through from verbalization to fulfill the real needs of the child and unknowingly put obstacles in the path of the child without realizing what they are doing. They may be assisting the child in growing up too fast and, therefore, insecurely. Counseling is urgently needed. The parents should be enlightened about the effect they are having on the child. The classroom experience, group therapy, or parenting programs help guide the parents' responses toward their children. All parents should be made to recognize that as children grow and develop they are persons first and individuals with diabetes second. The parents may then be guided to more supportive roles and to become more communicative individuals who help with the developmental process of their children in a more acceptable manner.

REFERENCES

1. Ack, M.: Psychological problems in long standing, insulin dependent diabetic patients, Kidney Int. **1:**141-143, 1974.
2. Ames Co., Inc.: Chart: factors affecting urine chemistry, Elkhart, Ind., 1977.
3. Bode, H. H., Vanjonack, W. J., and Crawford, J. D.: Mitigation of cretinism by breast-feeding, Pediatrics **62**(1):13-16, July 1978.
4. Burke, E. L.: Insulin. In Guthrie, D. W., and Guthrie, R. A., editors: Nursing management of diabetes mellitus, St. Louis, 1977, The C. V. Mosby Co.
5. Cahill, G. F., Etzwiller, D., and Freinkel, N.: Control and diabetes, N. Engl. J. Med. **294:**1004, 1976.
6. Dussautt, J. H., Coulombe, P., and Laberge, C.: Preliminary report on a mass screening program for neonatal hypothyroidism, J. Pediatr. **86:**670, 1975.
7. Fritz, I. B.: A review of the mode of action of insulin, Mod. Med. Can. **27:**17, 1972.
8. Genuth, S. M.: Constant intravenous insulin infusion in diabetic ketoacidosis, J.A.M.A. **223:**1348, 1973.
9. Guthrie, D. W.: Exercise, diets, and insulin for children with diabetes, Nursing '77 **7**(2):48-54, 1977.
10. Guthrie, D. W., Guthrie, R. A., and Hinnen, D.: Single vs. double void technique for urine testing. Diabetes **26**(suppl. 1): 357, 1977.
11. Guthrie, R. A., and Murthy, D. Y. N.: Oral glucose tolerance tests and their reliability, Metabol. Clin. Exp. **22:**237-245, 1973.
12. Jackson, R. L., and Guthrie, R. A.: The child with diabetes, Curr. Concepts, 1975.
13. Jackson, R. L., Guthrie, R. A., and Guthrie, D. W.: The child with diabetes: parents manual, Columbia, Mo., 1970, University of Missouri Press.
14. Jackson, R. L., and associates: Muscle capillary basement membrane changes in normal and diabetic children, Diabetes **24**(suppl. 2):400, 1975.
15. Kaye, R.: Juvenile diabetes. In Shirkey, H. C., editor: Pediatric therapy, ed. 5, St. Louis, 1975, The C. V. Mosby Co.
16. Kilo, C., Vogler, N., and Williamson, J. R.: Muscle capillary membrane changes related to aging and diabetes mellitus, Diabetes **21:**881, 1972.
17. Klein, A., Meltzer, S., and Kenny, F.: Successful laboratory screening for congenital hypothyroidism, Lancet **2:**77, 1974.
18. Klein, A. H., and associates: Improved prognosis in congenital hypothyroidism treated before age 3 months, J. Pediatr. **81:**912, 1972.
19. Kyllo, C. J., and Nuttall, F. Q.: Prevalence of diabetes mellitus in school age children in Minnesota, Diabetes **27:**57, 1978.
20. Lippe, B. M., and Sample, W. F.: Pelvic ultrasonography in pediatric and endocrine disorders, J. Pediatr. **92**(6):897-902, June 1978.
21. Metz, R., and Bowers, M.: Plasma insulin glucose and free fatty acid relationships in insulin treated diabetes, Diabetes **21**(suppl. 1):325, 1972.
22. Molnar, D. G., Taylor, W. F., and Longworthy, A. L.: Plasma immuno reactive insulin pattern in insulin treated diabetes: studies during blood glucose monitoring, Mayo Clin. Proc. **47:**709, 1972.
23. Pickens, J. M., Burkeholder, J. N., and Womack, W. N.: Oral glucose tolerance test in normal children, Diabetes **16:** 11, 1967.
24. Raiti, S., and Newns, G. H.: Cretinism: early diagnosis and its relation to mental prognosis, Arch. Dis. Child. **46:**692, 1971.
25. Rasken, D., Fumita, Y., and Unger, R.: Alpha cell dysfunction in human diabetes, Diabetes **24:**410, 1975.
26. Report of the National Commission on Diabetes **3:**93-354, 1975, U.S. Government Printing Office.
27. Schumann, D.: Insulin reactions: fighting fear and fact. In

Managing diabetes properly, Horsham, Pa., 1977, Nursing Skillbooks, Intermed Communications.

28. Simond, J. F.: Psychiatric status of diabetic youth matched with a control group, Diabetes **26:**921, 1977.
29. Siperstein, M. D., Unger, R. H., and Madison, L. L.: Studies of muscle capillary basement membranes in normal subjects, diabetic and pre-diabetic patients, J. Clin. Invest. **47:**1973, 1968.
30. Steiner, D. F., and associates: Isolation and properties of proinsulin, intermediate forms and other minor components from crystalline bovine insulin, Diabetes **17:**725, 1968.
31. Stucky, V.: The meal plan. In Guthrie, D. W., and Guthrie, R. A., editors: Nursing management of diabetes mellitus, St. Louis, 1977, The C. V. Mosby Co.
32. Vieikho, A. K., and Felig, P. L.: Effects of exercise on insulin release from injection sites in diabetic man, Diabetes **26**(suppl. 1):357, 1977.
33. Wolfe, L. W.: Insulin: easing the daily routine. In Managing diabetes properly, Horsham, Pa., 1977, Nursing Skillbooks, Intermed Communications.

BIBLIOGRAPHY

Driscoll, A. E.: A teaching aid for endocrine disorders, Am. J. Nurs. **73**(11):1944-1945, November 1973.

Gardner, L., editor: Endocrine and genetic disorders of childhood, Philadelphia, 1975, W. B. Saunders Co.

Krueger, J. A., and Ray, J. C.: Endocrine problems in nursing, St. Louis, 1976, The C. V. Mosby Co.

Wilkins, L.: The diagnosis and treatment of endocrine disorders in childhood and adolescence, Springfield, Ill., 1965, Charles C Thomas, Publisher.

Williams, R. H., editor: Textbook of endocrinology, Philadelphia, 1974, W. B. Saunders Co.

Disorders of pituitary function

Bell, M.: Preoperative teaching and postoperative care of the hypophysectomy patient, J. Neurosurg. Nurs. **4:**165-171, December 1972.

Coping with problems in human growth, Roche Image Med. Res. **14:**1-4, November 1972.

Hobdell, E. F.: Growing up without growing: the child with growth hormone deficiency, Am. J. Maternal Child Nurs. **2:** 299-303, 1977.

Howe, A.: The mammalian pars intermedia: a review of its structure and function, J. Endocrinol. **59:**385-409, 1973.

Lovinger, R. D., Kaplan, S. L., and Grumbach, M. M.: Congenital hypopituitarism associated with neonatal hypoglycemia microphallus: four cases secondary to hypothalamic hormone deficiencies, J. Pediatr. **87:**1171, 1975.

Thyroid and parathyroid disorders

Blalock, J. B.: Surgical treatment of parathyroid disease, A.O.R.N. **20:**696-697, 1974.

Delange, F., and associates: Transient hypothyroidism in the newborn infant, J. Pediatr. **92**(6):974-976, June 1978.

Emmanuel, S.: Surgery of the thyroid and parathyroid glands. Part III, RN **37:**1-2, November 1974.

Fisher, D. A., and associates: Recommendations for screening programs for congenital hypothyroidism. Report of a committee of the American Thyroid Association, J. Pediatr. **89:**692, 1976.

Hollingsworth, D. R., Mabry, C. C., and Ekerd, J.: Hereditary aspects of Graves' disease in infancy and childhood, J. Pediatr. **81:**446, 1972.

Mackin, J. F., Canary, J. J., and Pittman, L. S.: Thyroid storm and its management, N. Engl. J. Med. **291:**1396-1398, 1974.

McGaan, M.: Function and care of the patient with hyperparathyroidism, RN **37:**48-51, November 1974.

Rallison, M., and associates: Occurrence and natural history of thyroiditis in children, J. Pediatr. **86:**675, 1975.

Adrenal disorders

Bennett, A. H., and Morse, F. P.: Tumors of the adrenal gland, Hosp. Med. **9:**108-111, October 1973.

Blount, M., and Kinney, A. B.: Chronic steroid therapy, Am. J. Nurs. **74**(9):1626-1631, September 1974.

Danon, M., and associates: Cushing syndrome, sexual precocity, and polyostotic fibrous dysplasia (Albright syndrome) in infancy, J. Pediatr. **87:**917, 1975.

Dluhy, R. G., Lauler, D. P., and Thorn, G. W.: Pharmacology and chemistry of adrenal glucocorticoids, Med. Clin. North Am. **57:**1155, 1973.

Gray, D.: Adrenogenital syndrome, Nurs. Times **68:**1408-1410, 1972.

Hill, S.: The child with ambiguous genitalia, Am. J. Nurs. **77**(5): 810-814, May 1977.

Jones, H. W., and Verkauf, B. S.: Congenital adrenal hyperplasia: age at menarche and related events at puberty, Am. J. Obstet. Gynecol. **109:**292, 1971.

McFarlane, J.: Congenital adrenal hyperplasia, Am. J. Nurs. **76**(8):1290-1292, August 1976.

McGann, M.: Cushing's syndrome: its complexities and care, RN **38:**40-43, August 1975.

Money, J.: Sex errors of the body, Baltimore, 1968, The Johns Hopkins Press.

Munro, D. S., and Duthie, H. L.: The management of Cushing's syndrome, Nurs. Mirror **137:**12-15, September 21, 1973.

Strobele, B.: How to counsel patients on cortisone, RN **38:**57-60, July 1975.

Diabetes mellitus

Bauer, R., and associates: Treatment for uncontrolled juvenile diabetes, Pediatr. Psychol. **2:**2-3, Summer 1974.

Burke, E.: Insulin injection; the site and the technique, Am. J. Nurs. **72:**2194-2196, 1976.

Collier, B. N., Jr., and Etzwiler, D. D.: Comparative study of diabetes knowledge among juvenile diabetics and their families, Diabetes **20:**51-57, 1971.

Drash, A.: Diabetes mellitus in childhood: a review, J. Pediatr. **78:**919-914, 1971.

Ehrlich, R. M.: Diabetes mellitus in childhood, Pediatr. Clin. North Am. **21:**871, 1974.

Felig, P.: Insulin: rates and routes of delivery, N. Engl. J. Med. **291:**1031, 1974.

Friedland, G. M.: Learning behaviors of a preadolescent with diabetes, Am. J. Nurs. **76:**59-61, 1976.

Garner, A. M., and Thompson, C. W.: Facts in management of juvenile diabetes, Pediatr. Psychol. **2:**6-7, Summer 1974.

Guthrie, D. W., and Guthrie, R. A.: Juvenile diabetes mellitus, Nurs. Clin. North Am. **8:**587-604, 1973.

Guthrie, D. W., and Guthrie, R. A.: Diabetes in adolescence, Am. J. Nurs. **75:**1740-1744, 1975.

Guthrie, D. W., and Guthrie, R. A., editors: Nursing management of diabetes mellitus, St. Louis, 1977, The C. V. Mosby Co.

Jackson, R. L.: The child with diabetes, Nutr. Today **6**(2):2-9, 1971.

Kaufman, R. V., and Hersher, B.: Body image changes in teenage diabetics, Pediatrics **48:**123-127, 1971.

Kaye, R.: Diabetic ketoacidosis: the bicarbonate controversy, J. Pediatr. **87:**156-159, 1975.

Kennell, C.: Outpatient management of the juvenile diabetic, Pediatr. Nurs. **2**(6):19-24, 1976.

Kogut, M. D.: Pathogenesis, diagnosis and treatment of diabetic ketoacidosis, Curr. Prob. Pediatr. **6**(4):1-35, February 1976.

Laron, Z.: Treatment of diabetes in children; revisited, Pediatr. Ann. **3:**63-77, 1974.

Managing diabetes properly, Horsham, Pa., 1977, Nursing Skillbooks, Intermed Communications.

Martin, M. M., and associates: Obesity, hyperinsulinism, and diabetes mellitus in childhood, J. Pediatr. **82:**192-201, 1973.

McFarlane, J.: Children with diabetes: special needs during growth years, Am. J. Nurs. **73:**1360-1365, 1973.

O'Connor, M. L.: Glucose tolerance test, Nursing '75 **5**(7):10-14, 1975.

Pagliara, A. S., and associates: Hypoglycemia in infancy and childhood. Part II, J. Pediatr. **82:**558, 1973.

Roundtable: Juvenile diabetes, Patient Care **9**(9):16-67, May 1, 1975.

Seasonal variation in the onset of diabetes in children: commentary, Pediatrics **59:**113-115, 1977.

Sperling, M. A., Kyrieckos, A., and Voina, S.: Suppressibility of glucagon secretion by glucose in juvenile diabetes, Pediatrics **90:**543-547, 1977.

Thompson, R. G.: The management of diabetes mellitus in the adolescent, Med. Clin. North Am. **59:**1349-1358, 1975.

Wolfe, L.: Insulin: paving the way to a new life, Nursing '77 **7**(11):38-41, 1977.

Wood, F. C., and Bierman, E. L.: New concepts in diabetic dietetics, Nutr. Today **7**(3):4-12, 1972.

UNIT SIXTEEN

The child with a problem that interferes with locomotion

Childhood is the age of onset for a variety of physically disabling conditions that are caused by hereditary, infectious, or traumatic etiologies. Many disorders that interfere with locomotion are present at birth, a few of which have been discussed previously, including congenital defects (Chapter 11) such as myelomeningocele, congenital dislocation of the hip, and congenital foot deformities. Others appear later in childhood. Of these, some can occur at any age, such as fractures, and others make their appearance at ages characteristic for the specific condition, such as muscular dystrophy during early childhood and slipped epiphysis at puberty.

Some locomotor disabilities are acquired in an instant, such as amputation or spinal cord injury, whereas others develop over an extended period, such as tuberculosis or progressive muscular atrophy. Some need only short-term therapy, such as fractures; others require long-term therapy and a longer term of adjustment and involve the whole problem of daily living activities, such as spinal cord injuries and cerebral palsy.

The physical limitations may involve only temporary inconvenience, or they may be permanent with the need to substitute an alternative form of locomotion. Some are helped by specific treatments; for others therapy is merely supportive. A large number of these disabilities require a health team approach with contributions from a variety of specialists. Concomitant problems associated with permanent disabilities, particularly those acquired in later childhood, are emotional adjustment and alterations in self-image.

Chapter 39, *The Child With a Disorder of Neuromuscular, Musculoskeletal, or Articular Function,* is concerned primarily with congenital and acquired disorders involving neurologic, muscular, skeletal, and articular systems, whereas Chapter 40, *The Child Immobilized With a Traumatic Injury,* deals with the consequences of traumatic injury. The coverage is by no means comprehensive, but representative examples are used to illustrate specific problems.

39

The child with a disorder of neuromuscular, musculoskeletal, or articular function

Defects in locomotion can be associated with diseases or deficits in the supporting structures (the skeleton), the movement-producing structures (muscles or their innervation), or the articulating structures (joints) of the body. Defects in bones are readily identified in most instances, but disorders involving muscular function offer more difficult problems of diagnosis. All interfere in some way with adequate locomotion. The first part of this Chapter is devoted to the child with neuromuscular dysfunction, whereas the second part deals with defects primarily caused by musculoskeletal and articular disorders.

Muscle dysfunction: general considerations

Weakness of skeletal muscle may represent a defect in the muscle itself or reflect a pathologic disorder at some point along the neural pathway from the cortex of the brain to the neuromuscular junction. The identification of the source of muscle dysfunction includes not only the testing of muscle function but also the systematic elimination of possible disorders of neural structures on which muscle function depends for its stimulus. In a few disorders muscle disease may be accompanied by a neural disorder.

Some clinical features are shared by muscle disease (myopathy), which differs in many ways from muscle dysfunction resulting from disorders of neuronal structures—brain, cranial nerve nuclei, long nerve tracts, anterior horn cells of the spinal cord, and peripheral nerves. Motor function is accomplished by means of the simple reflex arcs or by way of impulses transmitted from the cerebral cortex and other centers in the brain through the various nerve pathways of the central nervous system. The upper motor neurons consist of cells that lie in the cerebral cortex and fibers that transverse the brain stem and spinal cord to terminate at their synapses with the anterior horn cells. The anterior horn cells, axons, and peripheral nerve branches constitute the lower motor neurons. The motor unit consists of the lower motor neuron, the neuromuscular junction, and the muscle fibers it supplies (Fig. 39-1). The upper motor neuronal pathways from the cerebrum to the lower motor neuron are described as (1) pyramidal—those whose fibers extend from the cortex, come together in the medulla, cross from one side to the other, then extend down the cord to synapse with anterior horn motor neurons; and (2) extrapyramidal—a complex network of motor neurons that comprise relays between motor areas of the cortex, basal ganglia, thalamus, cerebellum, and brain stem.[6]

The site of pathology determines the type of muscular dysfunction. In general, upper motor neuron lesions produce weakness associated with spasticity, increased deep tendon reflexes, and abnormal superficial reflexes; lesions of lower motor neurons cause weakness associated with hypotonia or flaccidity, diminished or absent deep tendon reflexes, and preservation of normal superficial reflexes. Pathology of the extrapyramidal pathway and the cerebellum rarely produces muscle weakness. Lower motor neuron involvement is usually symmetric (except that of poliomyelitis and single peripheral nerve disease), whereas disorders of the pyramidal tract are more often asymmetric. Muscle wasting is characteristic of lower motor neuron lesions and more marked than in diseases of muscles. Deep tendon reflexes are briskly active in upper motor neuron disease, are diminished or absent in lower motor neuron disease, and depend on the progress of muscle degeneration in the myopathies.[6]

The primary upper motor neuron dysfunction is cerebral palsy, which will be discussed first, followed by the neuropathies caused by lower motor neuron dysfunction and diseases of muscles.

CEREBRAL PALSY

Cerebral palsy is a nonspecific term applied to impaired muscular control resulting from a nonprogressive abnormality in the pyramidal motor system (motor cortex, basal ganglia, and cerebellum). The etiology, clinical features, and course are variable, characterized by abnormal muscle tone and coordination as the primary disturbances. It is the most frequent permanent physical disability of childhood, and, although the incidence is not known, various studies suggest that it varies from 1.5 to 5 per 1000 live births.[21]

Etiology and pathophysiology

A variety of prenatal, perinatal, and postnatal factors contribute to the etiology of cerebral palsy, singly or in combinations. Cerebral anoxia, which has long been associated with cerebral damage, is an important cause during the prenatal and perinatal periods. Any complication of pregnancy in which there is a risk of anoxia to the fetus can cause prenatal brain damage. Recent studies indicate that a large percentage of children with cerebral palsy weighed less than 2500 g at birth. The following is a list of some known causes of cerebral palsy[6,11,21]:

Prenatal factors
- Genetic factors
- Developmental anomalies of brain
- Maternal metabolic disease
- Maternal anemia
- Radiation
- Intrauterine infection (rubella, toxoplasmosis, cytomegalic inclusion disease)
- Blood incompatibilities
- Maternal bleeding
- Toxemia
- Trauma
- Drugs

Perinatal factors
- Immaturity at birth
- Mechanical trauma or other factors during birth process
- Anesthesia and/or analgesia during labor and delivery
- Cardiorespiratory problems in newborn
- Metabolic disturbances
- Electrolyte disturbances (hypoglycemia, hypernatremia)
- Hyperbilirubinemia

Postnatal factors
- Head trauma
- Toxicoses
- Cerebrovascular accident
- Infections (meningitis, encephalitis)

Pathophysiology. It is difficult to establish a precise location of neurologic lesions based on etiology or clinical signs because there is no characteristic pathologic picture. In some cases there are gross malformations of the brain. In others there may be evidence of vascular occlusion, atrophy, loss of neurons, and laminar degeneration that produce narrower gyri, wider sulci, and low brain weight. Anoxia plays the most significant role in the pathology of brain damage, which frequently is also secondary to other causative mechanisms.[19,21]

There are a few exceptions. In some cases the manifestations or etiology can be related to anatomic areas. For example, cerebral palsy associated with prematurity is usually spastic diplegia caused by hypoxic infarction or hemorrhage in the area adjacent to the lateral ventricles. In the athetoid type of cerebral palsy caused by kernicterus and hemolytic disease of the newborn, there are pigment deposits in the basal ganglia and some cranial nerve nuclei. Hemiparetic cerebral palsy is frequently associated with mechanical trauma to the cortex or cerebrovascular accident of the middle cerebral artery. Cerebral hypoplasia and, sometimes, neonatal hypoglycemia are related to ataxic cerebral palsy. Generalized cortical and cerebral atrophy have been shown to cause severe quadriparesis with mental retardation and microcephaly.

Diagnostic evaluation

The neurologic examination and history are the primary modalities for diagnosis. A thorough knowledge of normal variations of motor development is required for detecting abnormal progress, and a careful history is elicited to detect possible etiologic factors. The child's spontaneous movements and behavior are observed, including posture, attitude, and muscle size, function, and tone.

Supplemental diagnostic tests may be employed, such as electroencephalography, pneumoencephalography, tomography, screening for metabolic defects, and serum electrolyte values. The possibility of slowly progressive degenerative disease and early onset, slowly growing brain tumors must be ruled out.

Early recognition. Infants at risk based on known etiologic factors associated with cerebral palsy warrant careful assessment during early infancy in order to identify signs of muscular dysfunction as soon as possible. Careful assessment of the infant who had a low birth weight or was prematurely born, the infant with a low Apgar score at 5 minutes, and the infant who demonstrated other perinatal or neonatal abnormalities such as seizures, intracranial hemorrhage, or metabolic disturbances should be carried out. Early recognition is made more difficult by lack of reliable neonatal neurologic signs. Cortical control of movement does not occur until later in infancy; therefore, motor impairment associated with voluntary control is usually not apparent until after 2 to 4 months of age at the earliest. More often the likelihood of a diagnosis cannot be confirmed until the second half of the first year. Motor dysfunction in some mildly affected infants may be overlooked until they exhibit delay or abnormality of some advanced motor skills such as standing or walking.

The alert observer may be suspicious when a child demonstrates some of the following groups of manifestations.[21]

Delayed gross motor development. This is a universal manifestation of cerebral palsy. The child shows delay in all motor accomplishments, and the discrepancy between motor ability and expected achievement tends to increase with successive developmental milestones as growth advances. It is especially significant if other developmental behavior, such as language and personal-social achievement, is normal.

Abnormal motor performance. Neuromotor dysfunction is particularly evident in motor performance. An early sign is preferential unilateral hand use that may be apparent at about 6 months of age. Hand dominance does not normally develop until 18 months to 2 years of age. Abnormal crawl with progression by hand movements only and with lower extremities and hips hiked along, much like a "bunny hop," is seen in diplegia. Children with hemiplegia use an asymmetric crawl using the unaffected arm and leg to propel themselves on either the buttocks or abdomen. Spasticity may cause the child to stand or walk on the toes. Uncoordinated or involuntary movements are characteristic of dyskinetic cerebral palsy, and facial grimacing and writhing movements of the tongue, fingers, and toes are signs of athetosis. Other significant signs of motor dysfunction are poor sucking and feeding difficulties with persistent tongue thrust. Head staggering, tremor on reaching, and truncal ataxia may be observed, also.

Alterations of muscle tone. Increased or decreased resistance to passive movements is a sign of abnormal muscle tone. The child may exhibit opisthotonic postures (exaggerated arching of the back), he may feel stiff on handling or dressing, and there is difficulty in diapering him because of spasticity of hip adductor muscles and lower extremities. When the child is pulled to a sitting position, he may extend the entire body, rigid and unbending at the hip and knee joints. This is an early sign of spasticity.

Abnormal postures. Children with spastic cerebral palsy assume abnormal postures at rest or when their position is changed. From an early age a child lying in a prone position will maintain the hips higher than the trunk with the legs and arms flexed or drawn under the body. In the supine position spasticity is evident by scissoring and extension of legs and with the feet plantar flexed. This posture is exaggerated when the child is suspended vertically or when others try to make him bear weight. It may be mild or severe depending on the degree of impairment. A persistent infantile resting and sleeping posture, that is, arms abducted at shoulders, elbows flexed, and hands fisted, is a sign of spasticity when it remains constant after 4 to 5 months of age. The hemiparetic child may rest with the affected arm adducted and held against the torso with the elbow pronated, slightly flexed, and the hand closed.

Reflex abnormalities. Persistence of primitive infantile reflexes is one of the earliest clues to cerebral palsy, for example, obligatory tonic neck reflex at any age or nonobligatory persistence beyond 6 months of age and the persistence or even hyperactivity of the Moro, plantar, and palmar grasp reflexes. Hyperreflexia, ankle clonus, and stretch reflexes can be elicited on many muscle groups on fast passive movements, for example, resistance to passive abduction when hips are suddenly separated (adductor catch).

Clinical classification. Cerebral palsy has been classified in several ways, but the most useful classification is based on the nature and distribution of neuromuscular dysfunction.

Spastic cerebral palsy. The most common clinical type, spastic cerebral palsy, represents an upper motor neuron type of muscular weakness. The reflex arc is intact and the characteristic physical signs are increased stretch reflexes, increased muscle tone, and, often, weakness. Early neurologic manifestations are usually generalized hypotonia or decreased tone that lasts for a few weeks or may extend for months or even as long as a year.

Spastic cerebral palsy consists of the following clinical features[21]:

Hypertonicity
Uneven tone distribution
Persistent primitive reflexes
Lack or delay of normal postural control
Spastic paresis

Because of these characteristics, the child has poor control of posture, balance, and coordinated motion, and impairment of fine and gross motor skills. Active attempts at motion increase abnormal postures and are accompanied by an overflow of movement to other parts of the body.

Hypertonic muscle groups are in a state of continuous reflex contraction, which, in time, become tight and shortened as a result of permanent chemical changes in their elastic properties. At the same time antagonistic muscle groups are overstretched and eventually develop disuse weakness. In time the spastic muscle imbalance produces joint and bone deformities, causing limitation of mobility and progressive functional deterioration. The most common contractures in spastic cerebral palsy are heel-cord tightening with equinus foot position (extreme plantar flexion), coxa valga and anteversion of the femoral neck with eventual hip dislocation, scoliosis, hip anteversion with toeing-in gait, and hip and knee flexion.

Spastic cerebral palsy can be classified according to the distribution of muscles involved, and the characteristics of each are described as follows:

Hemiparesis—one side of body affected
- Motor deficit usually greater in upper extremity
- Most common form of spastic cerebral palsy
- Most children able to walk
- Pattern of spasticity
  - Leg—increased tone of calf, hamstring, and hip adductor muscles
  - Gait—walk with foot inverted and plantar flexed, knee flexed, and leg adducted
  - Arm—increased tone in shoulder adductor and internal rotator muscles, elbow flexor and pronator muscles, and wrist and finger flexor muscles
- Parietal lobe syndrome—impairment of cortical sensory function (absence or inability to recognize size, shape, or tex-

ture of objects held in affected hand); impaired two-point discrimination and position sense

Underdevelopment of affected limbs

Quadriparesis or tetraparesis—all four extremities involved

Upper and lower limbs equally affected

Same physical manifestations as hemiparesis bilaterally except lower extremities are more involved than in hemiparesis, which causes considerable tightness of hip adductor muscles; there is difficulty in separating legs or even crossing them over one another ("scissor" gait)

Highest incidence of severe disability

One fourth only mildly affected with minimal functional limitations on ambulation, self-care, and other activities; one half moderately impaired and impeded in self-care and independence in a sheltered situation; and one fourth severely damaged and require almost total care

Delay in attaining development milestones proportionate to degree of motor deficit

Speech is dysarthric, swallowing may be impaired, and tongue protrusion is incomplete

Emotions are more labile with inappropriate laughing or crying

Diplegia—all four extremities involved

Spasticity in legs greater than in arms

Late attainment of gross motor milestones, sitting, standing, and walking; development of hand skills generally appropriate for age

Monoplegia—involving only one extremity*

Triplegia—involving three extremities*

Paraplegia—pure cerebral paraplegia of lower extremities*

Dyskinetic cerebral palsy. Dyskinesis implies abnormal involuntary movements. These movements originate in the basal ganglia, especially the globus pallidus, and the nuclei of cranial nerve VIII and of other cranial nerves. Movements disappear in sleep and are aggravated by stress. The major manifestation is athetosis, characterized by slow, worm-like, writhing movements that usually involve all extremities, the trunk, neck, facial muscles, and tongue. Dyskinetic movements of tongue and other pharyngeal, laryngeal, and oral muscles cause drooling and dysarthria (imperfect speech articulation), which makes it difficult to understand what the child is saying. There is often high-frequency hearing loss or deafness and conjugate upward gaze palsy, in which the eyes are converged toward the midline and displaced upward.[19,21]

Involuntary movements may take on choreiform (involuntary irregular, jerking movements) and dystonic (disordered muscle tone) manifestations that increase in intensity under emotional stress and around adolescence. Deformities rarely develop as a result of continuous uncontrollable movements that maintain joint mobility.

Ataxic cerebral palsy. The least common type of cerebral palsy, ataxia, is caused by a defect in the cerebellum or its pathways and is characterized by nonprogressive failure of muscle coordination and irregular muscle action. Affected children have a wide-based gait and perform rapid repetitive movements poorly. There is disintegration of movements of the upper extremities when the child reaches for objects. Cerebellar coordination tends to improve as the child grows, but there is very slow development in the first 3 to 5 years of life.

Mixed-type cerebral palsy. A combination of spasticity and athetosis is described as mixed-type cerebral palsy. Many affected children are severely disabled. This combination is sometimes observed after traumatic postnatal head injury.

Rigid, tremor, and atonic types. These types are uncommon. Both rigid and atonic types have a poor prognosis with deformities and lack of active movement. Tremors as a leading manifestation in cerebral palsy are rare. The tremor is seen at rest and on movement, but motor accomplishments are favorable and musculoskeletal complications do not occur.

Associated disabilities. Some of the disabilities associated with cerebral palsy are subnormal learning and reasoning capacity (mental retardation), impaired behavioral and interpersonal relationships (minimal brain dysfunction), seizures, and impairment of special senses.[19]

Mental retardation. The most serious handicap is mental retardation. One third of the children with cerebral palsy have normal intelligence (fewer have high normal or superior intelligence compared with the normal population); one third are mildly retarded; and one third are moderately retarded or below (low-grade deficiency is more common in persons with cerebral palsy than in the general population). As a group children with athetosis and ataxia are intellectually superior to those with other types of cerebral palsy. Incidence of severe or profound retardation is highest in rigid, atonic, and quadriparetic cerebral palsy.

Seizures. Seizures are more apt to accompany postnatally acquired hemiplegia. They are an unusual finding in athetosis and diplegia. The most common type is grand mal seizures, and the peak incidence of commencement is between 2 and 6 years of age. Approximately 50% of children with cerebral palsy have some type of seizure.[21]

Minimal brain dysfunction (MBD). The manifestations of minimal brain dysfunction may occur in children with cerebral palsy. The primary presenting symptoms are poor attention span, marked distractibility, hyperactive behavior, and defects of integration (see minimal brain dysfunction, p. 641).

Sensory impairment. Abnormalities of vision occur more often in cerebral palsy, and hearing loss is frequently an associated handicap. Strabismus is much higher in spastic children and hearing loss is often seen in athetosis.

Medical management

The goals of therapy for children with cerebral palsy are early recognition and promotion of an optimal developmental course in order that the child may realize his potential

*Rare occurrences.

within the limits of his brain dysfunction. The disorder is permanent, and therapy is chiefly symptomatic and preventive. To be effective it requires the services of an organized team of health professionals that considers (1) the nature of the physical handicap, (2) defects associated with the disorder, and (3) the interpersonal and social influences encountered by the affected child.[17]

The beneficial influences of a habilitation program on both child and family are based on recognition of the disability as early as possible and implementation of treatment. Parents are essential to a treatment program, and their cooperation and confidence are considered in all aspects of management. With early diagnosis parents can begin to provide sensorimotor experiences that are essential for cognitive development, since central nervous system structures depend on stimulation and use to maintain their functional integrity.

The broad aims of therapy are (1) to establish locomotion, communication, and self-help; (2) to gain optimal appearance and integration of motor functions; (3) to correct associated defects as effectively as possible; and (4) to provide educational opportunities adapted to the individual child's needs and capabilities.[17] Each child is evaluated and managed on an individual basis. The plan of therapy may involve a variety of settings, facilities, and specially trained persons, including the parents. The scope of the child's needs may require, in addition to the pediatrician and nurse, such professionals as a psychologist and/or psychiatrist, orthopedist, physical therapist, teacher, social worker, speech pathologist and/or therapist, neurologist, orthotist, audiologist, and occupational therapist.

Braces are often used to help prevent or reduce deformity, and orthopedic surgery may be required to decrease or abolish spastic muscle imbalance. This includes tendon lengthening procedures (especially heel-cord lengthening), release of spastic wrist flexor muscles, and correction of hip and adductor muscle spasticity or contracture to improve the child's locomotion. Surgical intervention is usually reserved for the child who does not respond to the more conservative measures but is also indicated for the child whose spasticity causes progressive deformities. Surgery is primarily used to improve function rather than for cosmetic purposes and is followed by physical therapy. Neurosurgical procedures are used only in selected cases.

Drugs to decrease spasticity have little usefulness in improving function in cerebral palsy. Antianxiety agents have been used to some extent to relieve excessive motion and tension, particularly in the athetoid child. Skeletal muscle relaxants, such as dantrolene, which has a direct influence on spastic hypertonicity, have been tried with encouraging results in decreasing stiffness and, thus, facilitating ease of motion. Local nerve block to motor points of a muscle with a neurolytic agent such as phenol solution reduces spasticity temporarily. Recently cerebellar stimulation through an implanted electric pacemaker has been suggested as a means for reducing spasticity.

Children with seizures should receive anticonvulsant medications, and hyperactive, dyskinetic children perform better when given dextroamphetamine or other drugs used for the child with minimal brain dysfunction (see p. 641). Care of visual and auditory deficits requires the attention of appropriate specialists, and speech therapy involves the services of a speech therapist (see Chapter 24).

Physical therapy

Physical therapy is one of the most frequently employed conservative treatment modalities. It requires the specialized skills of a qualified therapist with an extensive repertoire of exercise methods who can design a program to stimulate each child to achieve his functional goals. In general, physical therapy is directed toward good skeletal alignment for the spastic child; training in purposeful acts, even in the face of involuntary motion, for the athetoid child; and maximum development of proprioceptive sense in ataxia. An active therapy program involves the family, the physical therapist, and, often, other members of the health team, especially the nurse. Basically there are two conceptual approaches to reaching the goals of optimal function. Each is founded on sound principles, advocates early implementation, and is directed toward improving motor function. The first approach attempts to alleviate the motor dysfunction in relation to specific muscle groups. The goals are accomplished through traditional types of therapeutic exercises that consist of stretching, passive, active, and resisted movements applied to specific muscle groups or joints to maintain or increase range of motion, strength, or endurance.[21]

The second approach deals with motor dysfunction from a broader perspective that involves all components of abnormal and deranged movements. The techniques used are known collectively as sensorimotor, reflex therapeutic, or neuromuscular facilitation methods. Instead of focusing specifically on muscle groups and joints, these methods attempt to alter abnormal tone and posture and to elicit desired movements through positional manipulation or other means of modifying or augmenting sensory output. Very briefly the major methods advanced are:

Bobath a neurodevelopmental method directed toward the inhibition of abnormal reflex activity and the facilitation of normal automatic movement.

Kabat; Knott and Voss a system of resistive exercises that facilitate voluntary control of movements through increased proprioceptive input to the brain.

Rood muscles are activated through application of an array of sensory stimuli such as heat, cold, and brushing.

Brunnstrom use of synergistic reflex movements to bring about active motion.

Doman-Delacato an outgrowth of a theory proposed by Fay, this method training is carried out in basic patterns of movement according to an evolutionary sequence that progresses from fish-like swimming motions onward to the cross-pattern creeping of the anthropoid.

No matter what approach is employed, none is able to achieve spectacular changes in the ultimate outcome of motor disability. Therefore, the most practical approach is to select a mode of intervention that is most appropriate for the specific problem and that best suits the need of the individual child at any given time. Early efforts are focused on alleviating abnormal postures and positions by positioning and range of motion exercises. For example, rather than pulling a spastic infant to a sitting position by the arms, hypertonic extensor muscles of the back are not as likely to be stimulated when he is slowly pushed forward by hands placed posteriorly on the child's trunk. Extensor spasticity and scissoring of legs can be avoided if the infant straddles a thigh or hip when carried in the sitting position.

Passive range of motion exercises and stretching are valuable at any age, even at early ages when the child is unable to cooperate. They are of particular value for postural abnormalities around various joints. For example, stretching of the gastrocnemius muscle and its tendon helps to prevent tightness and spasticity that leads to toe walking and equinus position of the ankle. When the child is old enough to cooperate, some active extension can be performed with passive motion applied to complete joint extension. Prevention of contracture deformity is a prime function of physical therapy.

Functional and adaptive training (occupational therapy). Training in manual skills and activities of daily living proceeds along developmental lines and according to the child's functional level. Sitting, balance, crawling, and walking are encouraged at appropriate ages, accompanied by stimulation of protective extension and equilibrium reactions. When standing is attempted, therapy may be needed to strengthen and improve balance, which is sometimes facilitated by the use of braces, especially to control plantar flexion and, less often, to prevent knee flexion caused by hamstring muscle spasticity and inadequate control of hip and knee extensor muscles. Walking, using reciprocal leg motion, should be attempted at the appropriate age even if the child requires considerable assistance from braces and other persons, and the child should be encouraged to progress to parallel bars or other ambulatory aids as soon as possible.

Hand activities are begun early to improve motor function and provide the child with sensory experiences and information about his environment. Use of extremities requires some stability of the trunk; therefore, a gross motor position in which the child has some active control is selected. Objects and toys are selected to provide needed sensory input, using a variety of shapes, forms, and textures. The child will electively use the less affected or unaffected hand as the dominant one, and there are differing opinions about whether or not the child should be therapeutically encouraged to use the deficient extremity. Undue insistence often provokes an adverse emotional reaction. Play that encourages the use of hands for unimanual and bimanual activities is initiated early. Large balls, a doll carriage to push, or other toys that require some manner of manipulation are accepted without resistance and promote assistive use of both hands. Play is a valuable tool in a therapeutic program and is selected to combine therapy with the child's ability and interest. This often requires a great deal of ingenuity and inventiveness on the part of those involved in the child's care.

The child may need considerable help (and patience) in learning to feed, dress, and care for his personal hygiene needs, the most important and earliest tasks on which to concentrate. Children should be fed in the normal eating position. When they have difficulty with sucking and swallowing, it is a temptation to hold them in a semireclining posture to make use of gravity flow. This method does not promote active swallowing, however, and the neck hyperextension may even interfere with swallowing. A more flexed sitting position with arms brought forward to decrease the tendency toward back and neck extension is more natural during bottle- or spoon-feeding and encourages active swallowing.

As the child progresses from simple feeding and self-care activities, training is extended to include other tasks that are within his developmental and functional capabilities, such as cooking or typing. It should be remembered that a child should not be expected to learn a task until he is at the developmental stage at which it would be accomplished in a normal state. In all activities of daily living it is important to capitalize on the child's assets and compensate for his liabilities. For example, a child with visual-motor dysfunction would be helped by substituting an electric typewriter for the laborious task of handwriting. Learning one-handed tying of shoelaces would be needed by a hemiparetic child. The level of expected independence is related to both gross and fine motor manipulation, and even when complete independence in a specific activity is not realistic the child should learn any part of the task that he can master. However, motor function is not the sole purpose of learning as much independence as possible. Any accomplishment promotes self-reliance and self-esteem for healthier personality development.[21]

Speech training under the supervision of a speech therapist is begun early before the child learns poor habits of communication. Parents and others can help by following the directions of the speech therapist and by talking to the child slowly and using pictures or handling objects about which the adult is speaking. Feeding techniques, such as forcing the child to use his lips and tongue in eating, help to facilitate speech, for example, placing food at the side of the tongue, first one side then the other; making the child use his lips to take food from a spoon rather than placing it directly on his tongue; and avoiding using the teeth to remove the food from the utensil. If severe dysarthria prevents articulate speech and the child has reasonable intelligence, nonverbal communication is taught.

Education and recreation. As in all aspects of care, educational requirements are determined by the child's needs and potential. This includes the severity of the child's disease and the presence and degree of associated conditions that affect learning and participation, such as learning impairment, abnormal actions or behavior, impaired vision and/or hearing, and seizures. Children with mild physical handicap, normal intelligence, and no associated learning disability should attend regular school, although this is sometimes difficult because of the physical structure of the school. When attendance at regular school is not appropriate for the child, special classes or school facilities designed to meet the special needs of handicapped children are available in most larger communities. For those who are unable to benefit from formal education, a training program may be appropriate. At adolescence prevocational and vocational counseling and guidance are arranged. At any phase or in any setting, education is geared toward the child's assets.

Recreational opportunities are also a necessary part of growing up. Recreational outlets and after-school activities should be considered for the child who is unable to participate in the regular athletic and other peer activities. Some can compete in athletic and artistic endeavors, and there are many games and pastimes that are suited to their capabilities. When they are unable to participate with normal children, there are many special programs for handicapped children. If these are not available, they should be instigated. Recreational activities serve to stimulate the child's interest and curiosity, help them adjust to their handicap, improve their functional abilities, and build self-esteem.[6]

Nursing considerations

Nurses in a community setting, especially public health nurses, nurses in physicians' offices and clinics, and nurses in schools, are more likely to become involved with a family in which there is a child with cerebral palsy. Both the child and family need the help, support, and encouragement that nurses are prepared to offer, and nurses can be involved in all aspects of the child's management. Nurses who know the family and their special needs and problems are in the best position to provide guidance and support to that family.

Early recognition of cerebral palsy is often a result of alert observation by the nurse. Detection begins at birth, and the nurse should be especially observant for signs in an infant who has a history that includes any of the prenatal and perinatal conditions that predispose to brain damage. An infant in the nursery who displays any sign that may indicate that all is not well, for example, poor feeding, rigidity, tenseness, or hypotonia, merits closer scrutiny and evaluation. Unusual manifestations in a newborn can be signs of a variety of conditions, but a history of these unexplained signs is cause for repeated assessment. The disorder is not readily identifiable in the early months of life; often evidence is not apparent until the child begins to walk.

Delayed attainment of developmental milestones is one of the most valuable clues to recognizing cerebral palsy; therefore, slow development in a child is cause for concern. Nurses working with children need to be well acquainted with normal child growth and development and the tools of assessment. The earlier any deviation from the normal is detected, the better the outlook for therapeutic intervention. This is true for cerebral palsy or any childhood disorder. It is also important that the child receive appropriate therapy from persons or agencies qualified to provide such services. Parents are sometimes tempted to follow advice from unreliable sources. Nurses who are acquainted with services and facilities can refer the family to qualified practitioners.

Nurses who work directly with the child in the home or in the therapeutic setting are members of the health team who plan and carry out a program of therapy. Since children are being treated at an earlier age, mothers are participating earlier in treatment programs for their handicapped child. They are now commonly taught the proper handling and home care of young children with cerebral palsy. Mothers need carefully programmed steps so that their change of role from mother to therapist can be melded into an already established relationship. The nurse or therapist needs to have documented data about the mother-child relationship before teaching the mother how to facilitate the child's posture or inhibit certain reflex patterns.

Mothers are instructed by therapists concerning how to posture children, how to introduce and carry out appropriate exercises, and how to place children in appropriate positions for play, dressing, eating, bathing, toileting, and other daily activities. Nurses are acquainted with the special needs of the child and the physical therapy objectives and modalities; thus they are able to reinforce the plan and assist the family in devising and modifying equipment and activities to follow through and reinforce the therapy program in the home, for example, modifying eating utensils by building up spoon handles for easier grasp and modifying clothes to facilitate self-help (see also Chapter 23).

Mothers are sometimes very preoccupied with their ability to perform activities such as positioning the child; as a result the child's personal comfort and satisfaction may be overlooked. They often perceive their child's inability to perform or behave to be a direct result of their own inadequacy in working with the child. The mothers are so intent on achieving a desired goal, such as flexing the child's knees, that they repeatedly remind the child of his errors but fail to acknowledge or support his less-than-successful efforts to comply, even though he is willing. Nurses can help mothers integrate therapy into play activities in more natural and less frustrating ways.

Some children have difficulty in keeping their heads upright. Because of this they cannot explore much of their environment and process the information. Parents need to be complimented on their efforts to provide a stimulating environment for these children. These infants are "at risk" for delayed development in holding up their heads, righting their shoulders and trunks for stable posture, sitting, pulling, standing, and crawling. Most mothers of children with impaired movements benefit from support and practical suggestions for feeding, moving, holding, and encouraging the infant to explore his hands and feet and to begin to play. Although practical advice is important, the nurse or physical therapist should not bombard the mother with suggestions. This may make her feel more inadequate in her parenting abilities. The nurse should have the mother define her concern, acknowledge the concern as genuine, and ask the mother how long she has tried a certain approach. In this way the nurse is able to find out what works, what does not work, and *what the mother* would like to try next. The mother should be given positive feedback for her observations of her infant, the progress *she* notes, and how *she* differentiates the child's needs. Sometimes mothers need support simply because the demands made on them are very fatiguing. It is probably better for mothers of young children with cerebral palsy to reduce the *quantity* of involvement with their child, rather than reduce the *quality* of the interactions. As the normal preschool child acquires autonomous skills, language, and mobility, he spends less time with his parents and is less dependent.

Probably the nursing interventions most valuable to the family are support and help in coping with the emotional aspects of the disorder, many of which have been discussed in relation to the handicapped child (Chapter 22). Initially the parents need supportive counseling directed toward understanding the implications of the diagnosis and all the feelings that it engenders. Later they need clarification regarding what they can expect from the child and from health professionals. Having a child with cerebral palsy implies numerous problems of daily management and changes in the life of the family. There are constant demands with few rewards, and the day-by-day changelessness of these demands is trying to parents. Many find that their child with cerebral palsy gives them little pleasure. The nurse needs to support the mother in her frustration, her problem solving, her concerns, her approaches to helping the child, and her lack of gratification, as well as the positive approaches she uses. All of these aspects must be explored and discussed. Parents as well as other members of the family require a great deal of support and counseling. Siblings of a handicapped child are affected and may respond to the presence of the child with overt or less evident behavioral problems. The family needs a relationship with nurses who can provide the continued contact with the family and who can provide support and encouragement through the long process of habilitation.

Parents can also find help and solace from parent groups with whom they can share problems and concerns and from whom they can derive comfort and practical information. The national organization, United Cerebral Palsy Association,* has branches in most communities that are listed in the telephone directory, and the address of the nearest branch can be obtained from a local agency directory or a local health department or by writing to the national headquarters. The association provides a variety of services for children and families.

Hospitalized child. Cerebral palsy is not a disorder that requires hospitalization; therefore, when children with cerebral palsy are hospitalized they are usually admitted for another reason or for corrective surgery. Consequently many nurses are not accustomed to handling these children. Nurses who have never been associated with a child with cerebral palsy may react in a variety of ways, including fear, repulsion, or overwhelming pity. The basic concept to keep in mind when caring for these children is that they are, first of all, children who happen to be afflicted with a disorder that limits their capacities in performing some activities of daily living and, for some, communicating with others. They should be approached and treated the same as any child in the hospital. The nurse's actions should convey acceptance, affection, and friendliness and promote a feeling of trust and dependability in the child. This is especially true with older children who have normal intelligence but who may have communication problems. All too frequently nurses tend to "talk down" to these children and do things for them that they are perfectly capable, though not as adeptly, of doing for themselves. This is especially humiliating to a teenager who values his independence and self-esteem.

To faciliate the care and management of the child, the therapy program should be continued, insofar as his condition allows, during the time he is hospitalized. This should be incorporated into his nursing care plan and every effort expended to make certain that the ground that has been so laboriously gained is not lost. Encouraging the parent to room in and actively participate in the child's care facilitates a continuation of the home therapy program and helps the child adjust to an unfamiliar environment.

The child with cerebral palsy frequently displays behavioral problems. In some of these children the emotional disturbance is probably a reflection of the brain lesion. However, in most cases the behavioral problem is the result of conscious or unconscious rejection by others, particularly the parents. This is not surprising since this condition is

*66 E. 34th Street, New York, N.Y. 10016.

often frightening and unpleasant to others and because some of these children are socially unacceptable, which may cause a parent to reject the child. When parents are helped to accept the child, the behavioral problems are significantly reduced.

Neuromuscular deficit

Abnormal muscle performance may result from defects within the muscle itself, defective transmission of nerve impulses to muscles, or dysfunction of peripheral motor or sensory nerves. These disorders are known collectively as neuromuscular diseases and involve one or more of the structures that compose the spinal reflex arc. These include the anterior horn of the spinal cord, the motor and sensory nerve fibers, the myoneural junction, and the muscle fiber (see Fig. 39-1). Since a defect in any of these structures interrupts the reflex arc, there is weakness and atrophy of the skeletal muscles involved with associated depression

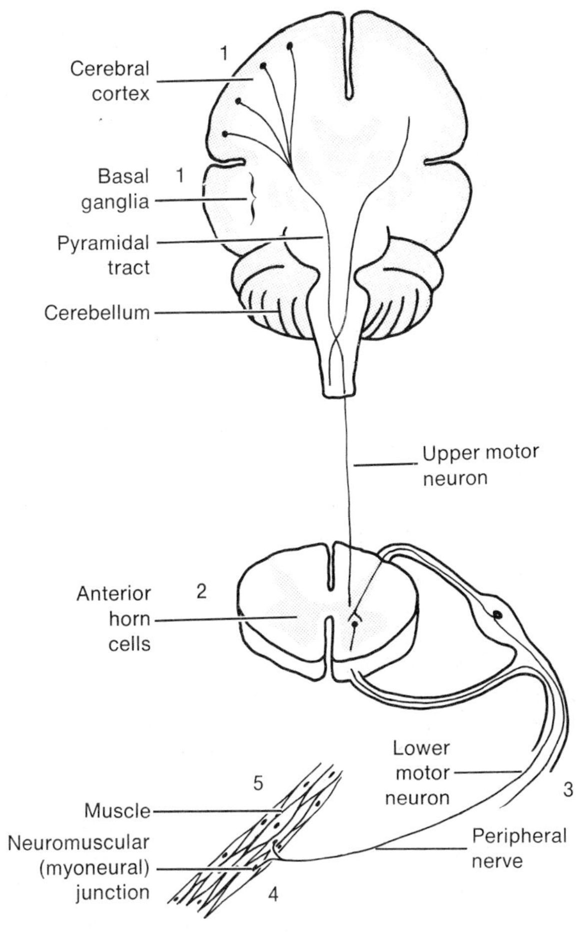

Fig. 39-1. Site of origin for neuromuscular disorders. (1) Cerebral palsy. (2) Poliomyelitis, spinal muscular atrophy. (3) Mononeuropathies, polyneuropathies. (4) Myasthenia gravis, neurotoxic disorders. (5) Muscular dystrophies.

of the related deep tendon reflexes. Consequently the predominant feature in all of these disorders is flaccid paralysis and manifestations, including muscle weakness and wasting, which eventually progress to atrophy with varying degrees of contracture deformity.

The neuromuscular disorders are often classified according to the source of the pathologic lesion[11]:

1. *Diseases of anterior horn cells.* In anterior horn cell disease there is destruction or atrophy of the anterior horn of the spinal column with the inability to transfer impulses from sensory neurons to motor neurons.
2. *Neuropathies.* Disorders affecting peripheral nerves may be *mononeuropathies,* involving a single nerve and the muscles it innervates, or *polyneuropathies,* which involve multiple nerves and the muscles they supply.
3. *Diseases of neuromuscular junction.* Disorders involving a neurohormonal deficiency interfere with transmission of nerve impulses to muscles at the neuromuscular junction.
4. *Diseases of muscles.* Disorders that affect the muscles directly may be a result of inflammatory, degenerative, or metabolic causes.

These disorders can also be categorized according to onset: those in which there is acute onset of flaccid paralysis and those with more gradual onset and progressive degeneration.

In most instances the sudden appearance of flaccid paralysis in a previously healthy child can be attributed to an infectious process. Neurotoxins (for example, botulism, tick paralysis, or heavy metal poisoning), pressure on the spinal cord from tumors or abcesses, or spinal cord injury are less likely causes. Hereditary factors and metabolic disease are more often responsible for muscular weakness and atrophy of gradual onset.

Diagnostic tools

To aid in differentiating between diseases with similar manifestations, several general diagnostic tools are employed. In addition a number of more definitive tests are used to establish a specific diagnosis. The neurologic examination is a basic test that helps to assess the extent of motor and sensory responses. Muscle biopsy is frequently used to confirm a diagnosis.

The electromyogram (EMG) measures the electric potentials generated in individual muscles. A small metal disc is placed on the skin overlaying the muscle to be tested, or a sterile needle electrode is inserted directly into the muscle. The electric activity generated in the skeletal muscles is measured at rest, with slight voluntary contraction, and with maximal contraction. The electric activity is amplified and displayed on a cathode-ray oscilloscope. Needle electrodes are sensitive enough to pick up the activity of a single muscle fiber, and this is usually the method of choice.

Serum enzyme measurements are helpful in diagnosis

and monitoring the course of muscular disease. These include:

creatine phosphokinase (CPK) found in skeletal muscle and a few other organs and elevated in skeletal muscle disease. This is the most specific test.
aldolase present in skeletal and heart muscle and significantly elevated in muscle damage.
serum glutamic-oxaloacetic transaminase (SGOT) elevated in muscle disease but has wider distribution in organs.
lactic dehydrogenase (LDH) elevated in muscle disease but has wider distribution.

Diseases of anterior horn cells

Diseases and disorders that affect the anterior horn cells of the spinal cord impair motor function to the muscles supplied by these nerves. Enteroviruses with a worldwide distribution are prominent etiologic agents that selectively affect anterior horn cells. These include the polioviruses, of which there are three types: coxsackie viruses, groups A and B, and the ECHO viruses. Since the development and widespread use of active immunization against the poliovirus, the incidence of the disease has been drastically reduced throughout the world (see p. 456). Degeneration of the anterior horn cells is caused by inherited disorders, primarily the spinal muscular atrophies.

POLIOMYELITIS

Although the incidence of poliomyelitis has been virtually eliminated as a threat in most areas, there are still reported cases in persons who are not adequately immunized. In many parts of the world poliomyelitis still occurs frequently and results in chronic handicaps and permanent disabilities.[19]

Etiology and pathophysiology

Poliovirus types I, II, and III have been identified as the causative organisms in poliomyelitis, but factors related to the host influence susceptibility to the disease. Oral poliovirus vaccine confers active immunity. Although the disease can affect persons of all ages, the majority of affected persons with paralytic manifestations are younger than 10 years of age, usually younger than 5 years of age.[10]

Factors that appear to influence the susceptibility and may affect the severity of some forms are[25]:

1. The rate of paralytic involvement is twice as high in prepubertal boys as girls.
2. The incidence and severity of paralytic disease is higher in pregnant than nonpregnant women.
3. The clinical severity of the disease increases with the age of the affected person.
4. Stresses such as muscular exhaustion, chilling, and surgical procedures increase the susceptibility.

The disease is transmitted from person to person through oropharyngeal secretions or fecal contamination. The virus gains access to the host by way of the oropharynx, multiplies in the alimentary tract, and spreads by means of lymph and other reticuloendothelial structures. Direct access to nerve structures or the bloodstream can occur if the virus is encountered when there is a fresh or healing wound such as after a tonsillectomy.

The neuronal damage is a result of viral multiplication, and the type and extent of clinical manifestations depend on the number and location of affected neurons. The regions most frequently invaded in spinal paralytic poliomyelitis are the anterior horn cells of the spinal cord with a typical irregular and asymmetric distribution. Since the cervical and lumbar regions contain more anterior horn cells, the extremities are involved more frequently than the trunk. The lower extremities seem to be more commonly and more severely involved than the upper extremities and the proximal muscle groups more than distal groups. Intercostal involvement frequently accompanies upper extremity paralysis.

Less frequent but more serious is bulbar poliomyelitis involving the brain stem. Sites most often affected are motor cranial nerve nuclei, particularly of cranial nerves IX and X, with the potential consequences of dysphagia, dysphonia, and palate and vocal cord paralysis. Involvement of the brain stem and higher centers is unusual; the combined bulbar and spinal paralytic forms are more common than bulbar poliomyelitis.

Diagnostic evaluation

The following are four possible responses in susceptible persons, in order of frequency of occurrence[10,25]:

1. *Asymptomatic infection,* in which the affected person exhibits no clinical features.
2. *Abortive poliomyelitis,* in which there is minor illness, including fever, malaise, headache, nausea and vomiting, sore throat, and vague abdominal discomfort.
3. *Nonparalytic poliomyelitis,* in which the manifestations are those of the abortive response plus meningeal signs such as pain and stiffness of the posterior muscles of the neck, back, and legs.
4. *Paralytic poliomyelitis,* in which the symptoms of the abortive response are seen followed by a symptom-free period of several days, after which there are recurrence of symptoms and development of paralysis.

In spinal paralytic poliomyelitis the peak of paralysis is usually reached within a week. Anterior horn cells that are destroyed are lost permanently; those that are swollen and inflamed may recover function. The earlier the function returns, the better the prognosis. Pain and muscle spasm occur early. The discomfort plus the asymmetry of muscle weakness cause hesitancy to move, which enhances the tendency toward deformity.

Laboratory studies that help establish the diagnosis include identification of poliovirus from oropharyngeal washings (early in the disease) and feces and a rising complement fixation titer to poliovirus.

Medical management

Treatment of the abortive and nonparalytic forms is symptomatic, consisting of bed rest until the child is afebrile, good nutrition, and mild sedation if indicated. Strenuous activity or overexertion should be avoided for at least 2 weeks if the illness is believed to be the abortive form or if there are diagnosed cases of poliomyelitis in the community.

The child with the paralytic response is hospitalized where he can be closely observed for possible advancing disease. Heat has proved beneficial. Hot packs or baths and range of motion exercises are started early. The child with respiratory involvement requires assisted ventilation, and the general supportive measures are the same as those for any paralyzed child. After the acute phase of the disease, the child with residual paralysis is launched on a comprehensive rehabilitation program.

Nursing considerations

Nursing care of the child with paralytic poliomyelitis is the same as for any child immobilized with a paralytic disorder (see p. 1589). The functional outcome of muscle paralysis depends on the degree of paralysis, the extent of musculoskeletal deformity, and the psychologic adjustment of the child. Those with bulbar poliomyelitis involving vital centers of respiration and circulation usually remain dependent on a respirator or require some other artificial device. Rehabilitation may require several years and is best accomplished in a facility with a comprehensive rehabilitation program. With adequate support from the rehabilitation team and sufficient motivation, many affected persons are able to live productive lives.

One of the most important aspects of the nursing care for children with spinal paralytic poliomyelitis is the long-term support and encouragement of both child and family. Initially the threat of death is the predominant psychologic stress with all its implications. Later there are the multiple problems associated with a child who suffers from a chronic illness (Chapter 22). Throughout all phases of acute and rehabilitative care, the nurse serves as a key member of the health team. (See also Table 16-1, p. 562.)

Although the reported incidence of this dread disease is now infrequent, infection still occurs in areas in which there are a number of children who have not been vaccinated. With few reported cases some parents become complacent regarding active immunization of their children. There is increasing concern among public health officials that the decreasing number of immunized children may result in a poliomyelitis epidemic. An important nursing role is health teaching with emphasis on immunization against this serious but preventable disease.

SPINAL MUSCULAR ATROPHY

The disorders designated as the spinal muscular atrophies are characterized by progressive weakness and wasting of skeletal muscles caused by progressive degeneration of anterior horn cells. These diseases are inherited as autosomal-recessive traits (p. 191) that occur primarily in infancy.

Progressive spinal muscular atrophy of infants (Werdnig-Hoffmann paralysis)

The most severe form of neurogenic atrophy and the most common paralytic form of the ''floppy infant syndrome'' is Werdnig-Hoffmann paralysis. The site of pathology is the anterior horn cells of the spinal cord and the motor nuclei of the brain stem, but the primary effect is atrophy of skeletal muscles.

The disorder is manifest early, usually at birth, frequently in utero, and almost always prior to age 2 years. Inactivity of the infant is the most prominent feature. The child lies with legs in the frog position; breathing is diaphragmatic with sternal retractions caused by intercostal muscle paralysis; and there are weakness and limited movements of the shoulder and arm muscles. The cry and cough are weak, and secretions tend to pool in the pharynx. The facies are alert, and sensation and intellect are normal.

The diagnosis is established from electromyography demonstrating a denervation pattern and is confirmed by muscle biopsy.

Early death from respiratory failure or infection is usual. The most common complication is pneumonia. Few children with this type of paralysis live beyond 4 or 5 years of age. For nursing considerations, see below.

Juvenile spinal muscular atrophy (Kugelberg-Welander disease)

This disorder is also characterized by anterior horn cell and motor nerve degeneration. The onset of proximal muscle weakness (especially of the pelvic girdle) appears later, in early childhood or adolescence, and the progression is slower. Muscles of the lower arms and legs are involved relatively late, and muscles of the trunk and those supplied by the cranial nerves are usually unaffected. Many affected persons have a normal life expectancy.

Nursing considerations

The infant and small child with extensive paralysis requires frequent change of position to prevent complications, especially pneumonia. The pharynx requires frequent suctioning to remove secretions, and feeding must be carried out slowly and carefully to prevent aspiration. Since these children are intellectually normal, verbal, tactile, and auditory stimulation are important aspects of care. Supporting them so that they can see the activities around them and transporting them in a buggy to provide them with a change of environment provide stimulation and a broader scope of contacts.

Parents of a chronically ill or potentially fatally ill child require a great deal of support and encouragement (see Chapters 22 and 27). The parents of a child with a genetically transmitted disorder also need to be encouraged to seek genetic counseling (see p. 200).

Neuropathies

Disorders that feature single or multiple peripheral nerve paralysis are caused by a number of hereditary diseases, traumatic injury, infections, poisons, and, secondarily, some metabolic diseases. Polyneuropathy can be restricted to specific areas, as in diabetes, and some hereditary diseases involve skeletal muscles extensively. Usually distal limbs (feet and hands) are affected first, with gait disturbance and footdrop as early manifestations. The involvement gradually progresses medially as the disorder becomes more severe.

In some polyneuropathies there is segmented or patchy loss of the myelin sheath of nerve fibers; in others the primary process appears to be progressive degeneration of nerve fibers. Examples of acute and chronic polyneuropathies are infectious polyneuritis and peroneal atrophy, respectively.

INFECTIOUS POLYNEURITIS (GUILLAIN-BARRÉ SYNDROME)

Infectious polyneuritis, also known as infectious neuronitis and Landry's or Guillain-Barré syndrome, is probably the most common form of polyneuritis and may occur at any age. It is an acute polyneuropathy in which motor dysfunction predominates over sensory disturbance and in which there is bilateral facial paresis or paralysis and, occasionally, weakness of the bulbar and respiratory musculature. Although children are less often affected than adults, the incidence in the pediatric age-group appears to be increasing, with higher susceptibility in children between ages 4 and 10 years. Both sexes are affected with equal frequency.

Etiology and pathophysiology

The precise etiologic agent is unknown. Since the disease has been associated with a number of viral infections or the administration of vaccines, it has been suggested that it may be a toxic sequela of an original infection, an activated latent virus, or a manifestation of an acute infection. Some believe that it may represent an autoimmune response. Pathologic changes show inflammation and segmented demyelination of peripheral nerves.[22]

Diagnostic evaluation

The paralytic manifestations are usually preceded by a mild influenza-like illness or sore throat. In 3 to 12 days neurologic symptoms appear, initally involving muscle tenderness, sometimes accompanied by paresthesia and cramps. Symmetric muscle weakness progressing to paralysis starts in the periphery and rapidly ascends from the lower extremities, frequently involving the muscles of the trunk, upper extremities, and those supplied by cranial nerves. Paralysis is flaccid with loss of reflexes and may include variable degrees of sensory impairment. Paralysis of facial, extraocular, labial, lingual, pharyngeal, and laryngeal muscles may be affected. Evidence of intercostal and phrenic nerve involvement includes breathlessness in vocalizations and shallow, irregular respirations. Most patients complain of muscle tenderness or sensitivity to slight pressure. Urinary incontinence or retention and constipation are frequently present.

Cerebrospinal fluid analysis reveals an increased protein concentration, but other laboratory studies are noncontributory. The symmetric nature of the paralysis helps differentiate this disorder from spinal paralytic poliomyelitis, which usually affects sporadic muscles.

Course. The general health of the child and the extent of paralysis influence the outcome of the illness. Almost all deaths are caused by respiratory failure; therefore, early diagnosis and access to respiratory support are especially important. Muscle function begins to return 2 days to 2 weeks after the onset of symptoms, and recovery is complete in most cases. The rate of recovery is usually related to the degree of involvement, which may extend from a few weeks to months. The greater the degree of paralysis, the longer the recovery phase.

Medical management

Treatment of Guillain-Barré syndrome is symptomatic. Corticosteroid therapy has been of benefit in the early stages. Respiratory and pharyngeal involvement require assisted ventilation, frequently with tracheostomy.

Nursing considerations

Nursing care is essentially supportive and is the same as that required for quadriplegia from any etiology. Since the care of the quadriplegic child is discussed extensively in Chapter 40 (p. 1589), it will not be considered at length here. The emphasis of care is on close observation to assess the extent of paralysis and prevention of complications.

During the acute phase of the disease the child's condition should be carefully observed for possible difficulty in swallowing and respiratory involvement. There should be a respirator on standby, with a cardiac monitor attached, and suction apparatus, tracheostomy tray, and vasoconstrictor drugs available at the bedside. Vital signs and level of consciousness are monitored frequently.

Throughout the recovery phase special emphasis is

placed on prevention of complications, including good postural alignment, frequent change of position, and passive range of motion exercises. Children with oral and pharyngeal involvement are usually fed by means of a nasogastric tube to assure adequate feeding. Bowel and bladder care are needed to avoid constipation and urine retention. Sensory impairment makes the child susceptible to burns and trophic ulcers.

Physical therapy is limited to passive range of motion exercises during the evolving phase of the disease. Later, as the disease stabilizes and recovery begins, an active physical therapy program is implemented to prevent contracture deformities and facilitate muscle recovery. This may include active exercise, gait training, and bracing.

PROGRESSIVE NEUROPATHIC (PERONEAL) MUSCULAR ATROPHY (CHARCOT-MARIE-TOOTH DISEASE)

Progressive neuropathic (peroneal) muscular atrophy is a slowly progressive disorder characterized by gradual wasting of distal limb musculature. The disease is usually inherited by autosomal-dominant transmission, although exceptions have been reported. The age of onset is late childhood or adolescence, and muscle wasting involving first the intrinsic foot muscles and those of the anterolateral aspect of the lower leg is seen. In time the wasting extends proximally to include the entire lower leg and sometimes the lower thigh. This distal wasting gives the "stork leg" appearance to the lower extremities, and the footdrop leads to the high-stepping, foot-slapping gait. No specific treatment is available. The disease is slowly progressive but has no effect on the life span. With orthopedic assistance it usually causes little disability.

MONONEUROPATHIES

Defects involving a single nerve may be congenital or acquired as a secondary effect of inflammation, trauma, or injection of irritant materials.

Seventh nerve palsy

Bell's palsy, paralysis of cranial nerve VII, is often associated with a recent history of otitis media or herpes zoster and may be related to swelling, constriction, and congestion of the nerve in the facial canal. However, the etiology is obscure. It seldom occurs in children younger than 3 years of age and occurs with increased frequency in children with hypertension and those with diabetes mellitus. The weakness of the muscles on the affected side cause the face to be pulled toward the normal side by the unopposed muscles. The nasolabial fold is flattened, and the child is unable to close the eye on the affected side. Therapy is supportive with special protection of the cornea of the eye on the affected side and administration of corticosteroids to reduce inflammation.

Paralysis of cranial nerve VII is also caused by birth trauma from either pressure of the cheek against the sacral prominence in spontaneous delivery or pressure from forceps. Paralysis, which is usually transient, requires only symptomatic treatment (see also p. 311).

Brachial paralysis

For information on brachial paralysis, see p. 312.

Peripheral nerve trauma

Significant for nurses working with children is the damage that can result from improper technique and management. Incorrect intramuscular injection in the buttocks is an important cause of sciatic nerve damage in childhood that can produce paralysis of knee flexion and movements below the knee. Permanent damage in early childhood can result in considerable disability. In well-nourished adults an injection site in the upper, outer quadrant of the buttocks is relatively safe, but in infants and young children the distance from the sciatic nerve is insufficient to prevent possible sciatic injury. Some drugs tend to be more neurotoxic than others when deposited in this area, especially streptomycin and tetracycline.[19] (See also p. 1361.)

Pressure from casts and arm boards can injure peripheral nerves, for example, footdrop from peroneal nerve injury, wristdrop from radial nerve damage, and clawhand from damage to the ulnar nerve. Consequently meticulous attention to the assessment of sensory and motor function is an important aspect in the care of children with devices that can produce pressure on vulnerable nerves.

DISEASES OF NEUROMUSCULAR JUNCTION

Several diseases are responsible for muscle weakness or paralysis as a result of a defect in transmission of nerve impulses at the myoneural junction. Normally nerve impulses are transmitted to skeletal muscles across the neuromuscular junction by acetylcholine. This is accomplished in three steps[11]: (1) acetylcholine is released from vesicles in the terminal nerve endings, (2) it then diffuses across the junction and contacts receptor sites in the muscle membrane, stimulating the muscle to contract, and (3) it is removed by the action of cholinesterase. Interference at any of these three steps will block transmission of nerve impulses and prevent muscular contraction.

Neurotoxins

Several toxic substances act at the myoneural junction to inhibit nerve impulses to the skeletal muscles. Examples of toxins that prevent release of acetylcholine are those that produce the paralysis of botulism and tick paralysis. Action at receptor sites is blocked by the drug curare. Paralysis caused by inhibition of cholinesterase release is caused by poisoning with organic phosphate insecticides.[11]

Botulism. Botulism is a serious food poisoning that results from ingestion of the preformed toxin produced by the anaerobic bacillus *Clostridium botulinum.* The most common source of the toxin is improperly sterilized home-canned foods. Nervous system symptoms appear abruptly about 12 to 36 hours after ingestion of contaminated food and may or may not have been preceded by acute digestive disturbance. There is weakness, dizziness, headache, difficulty in talking and speaking, diplopia, and vomiting. Progressive respiratory paralysis is life threatening.

Treatment consists of intravenous administration of botulism antitoxin and general supportive measures. Respiratory support is often needed, and, since the toxin has a relatively short half-life and does not bind to tissues firmly, therapy is continued until paralysis abates.[4]

Tick paralysis. Saliva from ticks contains a neurotoxin that inhibits the release of acetylcholine, producing a rapidly ascending paralysis that is often accompanied by pain and hypersensitivity. Diagnosis is established on discovery of the imbedded tick. Total removal of the tick is followed by rapid improvement and recovery; otherwise death may result from respiratory paralysis.

Tetanus

Tetanus, or lockjaw, is an acute, preventable, and often fatal disease caused by the exotoxin produced by the anaerobic spore-forming, gram-positive bacillus *Clostridium tetani*. It is characterized by painful muscular rigidity primarily involving the masseter and neck muscles.

Etiology and pathophysiology. There are four requirements for the development of tetanus: (1) presence of tetanus spores or vegetative forms of the bacillus, (2) injury to the tissues, (3) wound conditions that encourage multiplication of the organism, and (4) a susceptible host.

Tetanus spores are found in soil, dust, and the intestinal tracts of man and animals, especially herbivorous animals. The organisms are more prevalent in rural areas but are readily carried to urban areas by the wind. The organisms are not invasive but enter the body by way of wounds, particularly a puncture wound, burn, or crushed area. They may enter through a very minor, unnoticed break in the skin such as a thorn or needle prick, bee sting, or scratch. In the newborn, infection may occur through the umbilical cord, usually in situations in which infants are delivered in contaminated surroundings. The disease has the greatest incidence in months when persons are more involved in outdoor activities. Drug addicts are especially susceptible from poor injection technique and the use of street heroin, which is often mixed with quinine, a protoplasmic poison that favors the growth of the organism.

When conditions are favorable, the organisms proliferate and elaborate two exotoxins, (1) tetanospasmin, a potent toxin that affects the central nervous system to produce the clinical manifestations of the disease, and (2) tetanolysin, which appears to have no significance. The ideal conditions for growth of the organisms are devitalized tissues without access to air, such as wounds that have not been washed or kept clean and those that have crusted over, trapping pus beneath. The exotoxin appears to reach the central nervous system by way of either the neuron axons or the vascular system. The toxin becomes fixed on nerve cells of the anterior horn of the spinal cord and the brain stem. The toxin acts at the myoneural junction to produce the muscular stiffness and lower the threshold for reflex excitability.

Diagnostic evaluation. The incubation period for tetanus varies from 1 to 54 days but is generally less than 14 days. The more extensive the injury, the shorter the incubation period and the more severe the symptoms.

The manner of onset varies, but the initial symptoms are usually a progressive stiffness and tenderness of the muscles in the neck and jaw. The characteristic difficulty in opening the mouth (trismus), caused by sustained contraction of the jaw-closing muscles, is evident early and gives the disease its common name, lockjaw. Spasm of facial muscles produces the so-called sardonic smile (risus sardonicus). Progressive involvement of the trunk muscles causes opisthotonos and a boardlike rigidity of abdominal and limb muscles. There is difficulty in swallowing, and the patient is highly sensitive to external stimuli. The slightest noise, a gentle touch, or bright light will trigger convulsive muscular contractions that last seconds to minutes. The paroxysmal contractions recur with increased frequency until they become almost continuous. The mentation is unaffected; therefore, the patient remains alert and reflects his pain and distress with rapid pulse, sweating, and an anxious expression. Laryngospasm and tetany of respiratory muscles and accumulated secretions predispose to respiratory arrest, atelectasis, and pneumonia. Fever is usually absent or only mild; presence of fever generally indicates a poor prognosis.

The mortality rate is about 30%, but the disease is almost invariably fatal in the newborn infant. As the child recovers from the disease, the paroxysms become less and less frequent and gradually subside. Survival beyond 4 days usually indicates recovery, but complete recovery may require weeks.

Medical management: prevention. Preventive measures are based on the immune status of the affected child and the nature of the injury. Specific prophylactic therapy after trauma is administration of either tetanus toxoid or tetanus antitoxin. Children who have completed the immunization series (see p. 456) are given a tetanus toxoid booster prophylactically if none has been given in the prior 3 years or, if there is a heavily contaminated wound, if none has been given in the previous year. Protective levels of antibody are maintained for at least 5 years; therefore, antitoxin is not indicated for the fully immunized child. (See also Table 12-12, p. 461.)

The unprotected or inadequately immunized child who sustains a "tetanus-prone" wound (contaminated soil, crush injury, burn, compound fracture, retained foreign body, or a wound unattended for 24 hours, for example) should receive human tetanus immune globulin (TIG). Human tetanus immune globulin is preferred to bovine or horse tetanus antitoxin (TAT) because of its absence of sensitivity reactions and longer half-life. Once the toxin has bound to central nervous system tissue, antitoxin has no effect, but if the binding has taken place only peripherally, administration of human tetanus immune globulin or bovine or horse tetanus antitoxin will prevent binding in the central areas. Concurrent administration of both human tetanus immune globulin and toxoid at separate sites is recommended both to provide protection and to initiate the active immune process. Completion of active immunization is carried out according to the usual pattern.

Proper surgical cleansing and débridement of contaminated wounds reduce the chance of infection.

Medical management: treatment. The affected child is best treated in an intensive care facility where he can be closely and constantly observed and where equipment for monitoring and respiratory support are readily available. A quiet environment is preferred to reduce external stimuli. Neonates are placed in an open unit or Isolette in which a constant environmental temperature can be maintained and oxygen supplied.

General supportive care, including maintenance of adequate fluid and electrolyte balance and caloric intake, is indicated. Indwelling oral or nasogastric feedings are used whenever possible, but severe laryngospasm may be an indication for intravenous alimentation or gastrostomy feeding. Recurrent laryngospasm or excessive accumulation of secretions may require endotracheal intubation.

Antitoxin therapy to neutralize toxins not yet bound to nervous tissue is the most specific therapy for tetanus. Human tetanus immune globulin is preferred, but, if unavailable, bovine or horse tetanus antitoxin is given. Antibiotics are administered to control the proliferation of the vegetative forms of the organism at the site of infection. When the child recovers, active immunization should take place since the disease does not confer a permanent immunity.

Local care of the wound by surgical débridement and cleansing helps reduce the numbers of proliferating organisms at the site of injury. An antibacterial agent such as pHisoHex or povidone-iodine (Betadine) followed by a dilute solution of hydrogen peroxide has proved effective. The cleansing should be repeated several times during the first 48 hours, and deep infected lacerations are usually exposed and débrided.

Sedatives or muscle relaxants are administered to help reduce muscle spasm and prevent convulsions. The most widely used is diazepam (Valium), but phenobarbital, chloral hydrate, the phenothiazines, and paraldehyde may be employed. Patients with severe tetanus and those who do not respond to other sedatives may require the administration of a neuromuscular blocking agent, usually tubocurarine. Because of their paralytic effect on respiratory muscles, use of these drugs requires mechanical ventilation and constant attendance by trained personnel until muscle spasms are controlled.

Tracheostomy is often indicated and should be performed before severe respiratory distress develops. Administration of corticosteroid preparations has met with success in some instances.

Nursing considerations. In caring for the child with tetanus, every effort should be made to control or eliminate stimulation from sound, light, and touch. Although a darkened room is ideal, sufficient light is essential in order that the child can be carefully observed. Also, light appears to be less irritating than vibratory or auditory stimuli. The infant or child is handled as little as possible, and extra effort is expended to avoid any sudden and/or loud noise.

Medications are administered as prescribed, and vital signs are observed and recorded at frequent intervals. The location and extent of muscle spasms and assessment of their severity are important nursing observations. Respiratory status is carefully evaluated for any signs of embarrassment, and appropriate emergency equipment is kept available at all times. Muscle relaxants and sedatives that may be prescribed can also cause respiratory depression; therefore, the child must be assessed for excessive central nervous system depression. Blood gases are obtained frequently to evaluate the respiratory status. Attention to hydration and nutrition may involve monitoring an intravenous infusion, monitoring nasogastric or gastrostomy feedings, and suctioning oropharyngeal secretions when indicated.

Although most affected children are neonates and receive the nursing care and assessment of any high-risk infant (Chapter 10), the older child may acquire a tetanus infection. Since the child's mental status is clear, he is aware of what is happening to him and is often in a state of terror. He should not be left alone, and all efforts should be made to reduce his anxiety, which can contribute to muscular spasms. A calm and reassuring manner and sympathetic understanding can help immeasurably in getting the child through this crisis situation.

Myasthenia gravis

Myasthenia gravis is relatively uncommon in childhood but may appear in two forms: neonatal and juvenile. The precise mechanism has not been determined, although the abnormality is associated with altered function of cholinesterase on the acetylcholine released at the neuromuscular junction. An autoimmune response has also been implicated.

Neonatal myasthenia gravis. A *transient* form of myasthenia gravis occurs in infants born to mothers with myasthenia gravis who may not be aware that they have the disease. These infants display generalized weakness and hypotonia at birth with a depressed Moro reflex, ptosis, ineffective sucking and swallowing reflexes, and weak cry. There is no evidence of neurologic damage. In this form the symptoms usually disappear within 2 to 4 weeks.

Persistent neonatal myasthenia gravis appears indistinguishable from the transient form, but the mother usually does not have the disease. The disease persists throughout life, and more than one sibling may be affected, which suggests a genetic etiology. Sex distribution is equal. The disorder is relatively resistant to drug therapy, and the eyelid and extraocular muscles seem to be the muscles most severely affected.

Juvenile myasthenia gravis. Juvenile myasthenia gravis appears to be identical to that seen in adults and usually has its onset after age 10 years but may appear as early as age 2 years. Girls are affected six times as often as boys. The most common symptoms are general paralysis of the optic muscles with ptosis and diplopia. Difficulty in swallowing, chewing, and speaking are also prominent, accompanied by weakness and paralysis of all skeletal muscles. The signs and symptoms are more pronounced in the late afternoon and evening. They are relieved by rest and made worse by exercise.

The diagnosis is made on the basis of the characteristic distribution of muscle weakness and the progressive weakness on repeated or sustained muscular contraction. The diagnosis is established by observation of the response to the anticholinesterase drugs. Intravenous administration of a small test dose of edrophonium (Tensilon) or neostigmine (Prostigmin) produces a beneficial effect in 1 minute but lasts for less than 5 minutes. Electromyography is helpful in diagnosis and reveals high amplitude muscle responses followed by contractions of rapidly diminishing amplitude.

Treatment consists of the oral administration of anticholinesterase drugs, the least toxic of which is pyridostigmine (Mestinon). The initial dose is 30 mg every 4 hours in the older child and 5 mg every 4 hours in the infant. The dosage is gradually increased until a satisfactory result is obtained. The child must be observed for signs of parasympathetic stimulation from overmedication. These include lacrimation, salivation, abdominal cramps, sweating, diarrhea, vomiting, bradycardia, and weakness of respiratory muscles.

These children need continuous medical and nursing supervision. The parents are taught the importance of accurate administration of medications, with special emphasis on recognizing side affects with the dangers of choking, aspiration, and respiratory distress.

Parents are counseled regarding promoting a life-style that minimizes stress and maximizes relaxation. Strenuous activity is discouraged. They are also warned of the possibility of a sudden exacerbation of symptoms during times of physical or emotional stress (myasthenia crisis) that requires immediate medical attention. They should receive instruction in providing respiratory assistance until help arrives or the child can be transported to medical aid.[6]

The prognosis in persistent congenital myasthenia gravis is usually good. Although there is gradual worsening of symptoms with age, the life span is not affected significantly. A high percentage of persons with childhood-onset (juvenile) myasthenia gravis become resistant or unresponsive to medication, with the danger of exacerbation and respiratory failure. Spontaneous remissions are infrequent.

Diseases of muscles

Skeletal muscles are subject to a large number of disorders that cause degeneration of muscle fibers with subsequent loss of function. In most there is fibrous connective tissue replacement of muscle fibers, proximal muscles are affected more severely than distal ones, and the lower extremities are affected to a greater extent than the upper extremities. Children with muscle disease characteristically develop a waddling gait and have difficulty in running, climbing, and rising from a sitting position. Innervation is not affected.

In addition to the electromyogram, measurement of serum enzyme activity, especially creatine phosphokinase, is often helpful in differential diagnosis of muscle disease. The intracellular enzyme creatine phosphokinase is present in muscle tissues and very few other organs and is released in large amounts in some diseases of muscles such as muscular dystrophy. Creatine phosphokinase is not elevated in neurogenic disease. Although the treatment in a large number of muscle disorders is palliative and symptomatic rather than curative, an accurate diagnosis is essential for purposes of rehabilitation, counseling, and treatment in those amenable to specific therapy.

Diseases of skeletal muscles can be inflammatory, such as polymyositis, caused by endocrine dysfunction, such as hypothyroidism and hyperthyroidism, and caused by congenital defects, such as absence of muscle, periodic paralysis, and the various muscular dystrophias and myotonias.

INFLAMMATORY DISEASES OF MUSCLES

Inflammation occurs in a number of infectious illnesses such as trichinosis, toxoplasmosis, and those caused by coxsackie virus and is seen in collagen diseases including lupus erythematosus, periarteritis nodosa, dermatomyositis, rheumatoid arthritis, and polymyositis.

Polymyositis and dermatomyositis

Polymyositis and one of its forms, dermatomyositis, are remarkably similar in manifestations and are often difficult

Table 39-1. Summary of the primary myopathies with onset in childhood

Primary myopathy	Inheritance pattern	Age of onset	Initial manifestations	Progression	Therapy
Muscular dystrophies					
Pseudohypertrophic (Duchenne's)	X-linked recessive; sporadic	Early childhood; age 1-3 years	Lordosis Waddling gait Difficulty in rising from floor and climbing stairs Fat deposits replace wasted gastrocnemius muscles	Rapid Ultimately involves all voluntary muscles Death usually occurs between ages 15 and 25 years	Supportive Physical therapy to prevent disuse atrophy of unaffected muscles
Limb-girdle	Autosomal recessive (usually)	Late childhood or during adolescence; over age 8 years	Weakness of proximal muscles of both pelvic and shoulder girdles	Variable but usually slow Most become incapacitated within 20 years of onset; in some, disability may remain slight	Supportive Physical therapy to prevent disuse atrophy of unaffected muscles
Facioscapulohumeral (Landouzy-Déjerine)	Autosomal dominant	Early adolescence; over age 8 years	Lack of facial mobility Difficulty in raising arms over head Forward slope of shoulders	Very slow May be intervals with no progression Considerable disability in time but life span unaffected	Supportive
Congenital dystrophy	Unknown but familial tendency	At birth	Small, weak muscles May be multiple contracture deformities	Rapid Death in early infancy	None
Ocular myopathy (ophthalmoplegia)	Autosomal dominant	Late childhood; over age 10 years	Weakness of extraocular muscles, causing ptosis Gradually spreads to pharyngeal muscles with difficulty in swallowing and speaking	Slow	Corticosteroids may be useful Plastic surgery to correct ptosis
Myotonic dystrophies					
Myotonia congenita (Thomsen's disease)	Autosomal dominant	Early childhood	Difficulty in relaxing muscles after contraction Aggravated by cold and emotional excitement	None Mild, lifelong disability	Drug therapy—phenytoin
Myotonic dystrophy (Steinert's disease)	Autosomal dominant	Adolescence or older May manifest at birth	Weakening of hand and forearm muscles Inability to relax handgrip Eye, tongue, and masseter muscles often affected In infants, difficulty in nursing and proximal muscle weakness Aggravated by cold	Variable Reaches severe stage of disability 15 to 20 years after onset Normal life span rarely attained	Symptoms may be relieved by drugs—procainamide orally three times daily or phenytoin

to differentiate from muscular dystrophy. There is proximal limb and trunk muscle weakness and loss of reflexes. Neck muscles are frequently affected, and the child may have difficulty in lifting the head or supporting it in an upright position. Muscles tend to be stiff and sore. Distal muscle strength and reflex response remain unaffected. Dermatomyositis, frequently classified as a collagen disease, is characterized by red, indurated skin lesions over the malar areas and nose and a violet discoloration of the eyelids. The skin over extensor muscle surfaces may be erythematous, scaly, and atopic.

Polymyositis and dermatomyositis respond to corticosteroid therapy, and with early and vigorous treatment most affected children recover. Physical therapy is essential to prevent contracture deformity and to rebuild muscle strength. Bracing or splinting may be needed.

Myositis ossificans

Soft tissue injury is relatively common in children, and trauma of major degree may cause hematoma formation with subsequent organization and ossification in the areas adjacent to the bone, which appear 2 to 3 weeks after injury. The quadriceps muscle of the thigh and the triceps muscle of the upper arm are the muscles most frequently affected. Treatment consists of immobilization of the part in a plaster cast until the ossification ceases to progress, after which gentle exercises, which help to regain function, are carried out. Muscles do not regain normal strength and size.

Myositis ossificans progressiva is a rare progressive disease of connective tissue that appears to be inherited by autosomal-dominant inheritance. Gradual and widespread ossification of tendons and fascia causes progressive disability until death from respiratory failure occurs in early adulthood.

MYOTONIAS

The myotonias are a group of muscle disorders characterized by increased irritability and contractility of skeletal muscles with decreased power of relaxation and either wasting or hypertrophy of the affected muscles. All are aggravated by cold. Myotonia is also a symptom of other disorders, such as familial hyperkalemia periodic paralysis and McArdle's disease, a glycogen storage disease caused by deficiency of muscle phosphorylase (see Table 39-1).

Muscular dystrophies

The muscular dystrophies constitute the largest and most important single group of muscle diseases of childhood. They all have a genetic origin in which there is gradual degeneration of muscle fibers and are characterized by progressive weakness and wasting of symmetric groups of skeletal muscles with increasing disability and deformity. In all forms of muscular dystrophy there is insidious loss of strength, but each differs in regard to muscle groups affected, age of onset, rate of progression, and inheritance patterns.[27]

The basic defect in muscular dystrophy is unknown, although it appears to be caused by a metabolic disturbance unrelated to the nervous system. Serum creatine phosphokinase is consistently increased in affected individuals, which assists in diagnosis and affords a means for early detection of the disorder in asymptomatic children in families at risk.

Treatment of the muscular dystrophies consists mainly of providing supportive measures, including physical therapy, orthopedic procedures to minimize deformity, and assisting the affected child in meeting the demands of daily living.

The various forms of muscular dystrophy are summarized in Table 39-1, and the initial sites of muscle involvement in the major types are illustrated in Fig. 39-2. The most common form, pseudohypertrophic or Duchenne's muscular dystrophy, is discussed below.

PSEUDOHYPERTROPHIC (DUCHENNE'S) MUSCULAR DYSTROPHY

The most severe and the most common muscular dystrophy seen in childhood is pseudohypertrophic muscular dystrophy. The incidence is approximately 0.14 per 1000 children, and an X-linked inheritance pattern is identified in 50% of cases; the remainder appear as sporadic cases and probably represent fresh mutations.[11] As in all X-linked disorders, males are affected almost exclusively and the incidence is approximately 4 per 100,000 persons.[6]

The clinical course is characteristic.[28]

1. Early onset, usually between 3 and 5 years of age
2. Progressive muscular weakness, wasting, and contractures
3. Calf muscle hypertrophy in most cases
4. Loss of independent ambulation by 9 to 11 years of age
5. Slowly progressive generalized weakness during teenage years
6. Relentless progression until death from respiratory or cardiac failure

Diagnostic evaluation

Evidence of muscle weakness usually appears during the third year, although there may have been a history of delay in motor development, particularly walking. Difficulty in running, riding a bicycle, and climbing stairs are usually the first symptoms noted. Later abnormal gait on a level surface becomes apparent. In the early years rapid developmental gains may mask the progression of the disease. Questioning of parents may reveal difficulty in rising from a sitting or supine position. Occasionally enlarged calves may be noticed by parents.

Typically the affected male has a waddling gait and

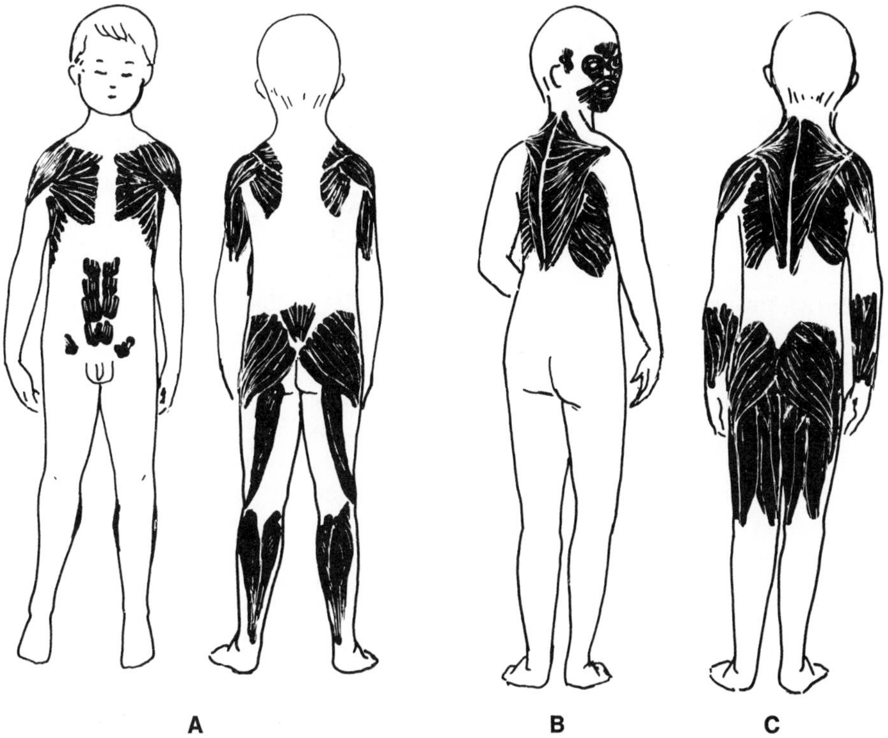

Fig. 39-2. Initial muscle groups involved in the muscular dystrophies. **A,** Pseudohypertrophic; **B,** facioscapulohumeral; **C,** limb-girdle. (From Whaley, L. F.: Understanding inherited disorders, St. Louis, 1974, The C. V. Mosby Co., p. 67.)

lordosis, falls frequently, and develops a characteristic manner of rising from a squatting or sitting position on the floor (Gowers' sign)—he turns onto his side or abdomen, flexes his knees to assume a kneeling position, then with knees extended gradually pushes his torso to an upright position by "walking" his hands up his legs. The muscles, especially of the thighs and upper arms, become enlarged from fatty infiltration and feel unusually firm or woody on palpation. The name pseudohypertrophy is derived from this muscular enlargement. Profound muscular atrophy occurs in later stages, and, as the disease progresses, contractures and deformities involving large and small joints are common complications. Ambulation usually becomes impossible by 12 years of age. Facial, oropharyngeal, and respiratory muscles are spared until the terminal stages of the disease. Ultimately the disease process involves the diaphragm and auxiliary muscles of respiration, and cardiomegaly is common. The cause of death is usually respiratory tract infection or cardiac failure.

Mild mental retardation is commonly associated with muscular dystrophy. The mean intelligence quotient is about 20 points below the normal, and frank mental deficit is present in 25% of these children.[11]

The disease is confirmed by serum enzyme measurement, muscle biopsy, and electromyography. The serum creatine phosphokinase, aldolase, and serum glutamic-oxaloacetic transaminase levels are extremely high in the first 2 years of life prior to clinical weakness. They diminish with muscle deterioration but do not reach normal levels until severe muscle wasting and incapacitation have occurred. Muscle biopsy reveals degeneration of muscle fibers with fibrosis and fatty tissue replacement. Electromyography shows decrease in amplitude and duration of motor unit potentials. Diagnosis poses few problems in children 2 to 7 years of age, but in older children the similarity of symptoms to those of limb-girdle muscular dystrophy and some other myopathies confuses the diagnosis.[6]

Medical management

There is no effective treatment for childhood muscular dystrophy. Maintaining function in unaffected muscles for as long as possible is the primary goal. It has been found that children who remain as active as possible are able to avoid wheelchair confinement for a longer period of time. Early recourse to a wheelchair accelerates deconditioning and promotes the development of lower extremity contractures. Maintenance of function often includes range of motion exercises, surgery to release contracture deformities, bracing, and performance of activities of daily living (ADL). Genetic counseling is recommended for parents, female siblings, and maternal aunts and their female offspring (see p. 200).

Complications

The major complications of muscular dystrophy include contractures, disuse atrophy, infections, obesity, and cardiopulmonary problems.

Contracture deformities of hips, knees, and ankles occur from early selective muscle involvement and often exaggerate the weakness. Passive range of motion exercises, stretching, and active exercises under the supervision of a physical therapist are effective in treating reducible contractures. Nonreducible contractures require wedge casting or surgical reduction. Scoliosis caused by muscle imbalance is common and tends to progress even when the child becomes dependent on a wheelchair. Bracing with a rigid corset may be needed for support, although it may interfere with mobility. Frequent rest periods in the recumbent position are often beneficial. For correction of deformities it is essential to select a procedure that immobilizes the child for as short a period as possible to minimize the chances of developing disease atrophy.

Atrophy of disease from prolonged inactivity occurs readily when the child is immobilized or confined to bed with illness, injury, or surgery. To minimize this complication, physical therapy should be implemented if bed rest extends beyond a few days. A daily goal for the well child should be at least 3 hours ambulation when disability is moderate to maintain muscle strength.

Infections become increasingly frequent as the dystrophic process produces a progressive decrease in vital capacity resulting from weakness of primary, secondary, and associated muscles of respiration. Consequently even minor upper respiratory infections may become serious problems in these children. Prompt and vigorous antibiotic therapy supplemented by postural drainage and intermittent respiratory therapy are effective therapy. Because these children are unable to cough, secretions collect easily.

Obesity is a frequent complication that contributes to premature loss of ambulation. Children with restricted opportunity for physical activity and who suffer from boredom easily consume calories in excess of their needs. This is compounded by overfeeding by well-meaning family and friends. Proper dietary intake and a diversified recreational program help reduce the likelihood of obesity and enable the child to maintain ambulation and functional independence for a longer period of time.

Cardiac manifestations are usually late events but may occur in the ambulatory child. Most significant of these, cardiac failure, is difficult to correct in advanced cases, but treatment with digoxin and diuretics is often beneficial in the early stages of the disease.

Nursing considerations

The care and management of a child with muscular dystrophy involves the combined efforts of a comprehensive health team, and nurses can help clarify the roles of these health professionals to family and others. The major emphasis of nursing care is to assist the child and his family cope with the progressive, incapacitating, and fatal nature of the disease, to help design a program that will afford a greater degree of independence and reduce the predictable and preventable disabilities associated with the disorder, and to assist them to deal constructively with the limitations the disease imposes on their daily lives.

Working closely with other team members, nurses help the family in developing the child's self-help skills to give the child the satisfaction of being as independent as possible for as long as possible. It is all too tempting for parents to overprotect their affected children. Children derive pleasure and build self-esteem from performing actions that produce visible pleasure in their parents. Even the physical weakness that prevents the child from physical competition with other children has little effect on the child as long as it does not affect the parents' attitude toward him as an individual. Therefore, parents must be helped to develop a balance between limiting the child's activity because of muscular weakness and allowing him to accomplish things by himself. This requires continual evaluation of the child's capabilities, which are often difficult to assess. It is not always possible to know when the child seeks parental assistance because he wants a little extra attention or because his muscles are overtired. Fortunately most children with muscular dystrophy instinctually recognize this need to be as independent as possible and strive to do so.

Practical difficulties faced by families are physical limitations of housing and mobility. Families often live in houses or apartments that are unsuited to wheelchairs, many with no street-level entrance, and upstairs bedrooms and bathrooms, many with no tub. Many of these families have no independent means of transportation. Assisting with these problems involves team problem solving. Parents also need help in buying and modifying clothing for their disabled child. It is difficult to find clothing and footwear to wear comfortably in a wheelchair, to fit over contracted limbs, and to fit an obese child. Parent's social activities are also restricted, and the family's activities must be continually modified to the needs of the affected child (see Chapter 22). The child cannot be left with an ordinary teenage baby-sitter but requires a specially trained person, such as a student nurse. Consequently parents, too, tend to lead more isolated lives.

Each child's therapy program is tailored to his individual needs and capabilities, and families should be active participants. Parents need assistance with the physical therapy program and education regarding a home regimen of exercises and activity. Many parents erroneously believe that if the child expends himself sufficiently it will overcome the weakness and prevent progression of the disease process. They should also be advised to notify the nurse or other designated person when the child becomes even temporarily bedridden so that the exercise program can be continued, although modified, during this time.

A prominent feature of children with muscular dystrophy is their relative absence of emotional problems. As their physical condition deteriorates to the point that they can no longer keep up with friends and classmates, they learn behaviors that bring them the rewards of other children's company. These friends are often children who have been rejected by more able-bodied classmates. The greater the dependency of children with muscular dystrophy, the more they tend to become socially isolated. However, most appear to be outgoing and cheerful.

No matter how successful the program and how well the family adapts to the disorder, superimposed on the physical and emotional problems associated with a child with a long-term disability is the constant presence of the ultimate outcome of the disease. All the manifestations seen in the child with a fatal illness are encountered in these families (see Chapter 27). The guilt feelings of the mother may be particularly pronounced in this disorder because of the mother-to-son transmission of the defective gene.

Nurses are especially valuable health professionals as they come to know the family and the family's problems. Nurses can be alert to problems and needs of the families and make necessary referrals when supplementary services are indicated. The Muscular Dystrophy Association of America, Inc.* has branches in most communities to provide assistance to families in which there is a member with muscular dystrophy.

Musculoskeletal disorders

The disorders affecting the skeletal structures and associated musculature are primarily congenital, traumatic, secondary to metabolic dysfunction, or iodiopathic in origin. Some appear at any age, such as fractures (p. 1558), whereas others have a predilection for a different stage of the childhood span of growth and development. There are those detected at birth or shortly after, such as congenital foot and hip deformities (see Chapter 11); Legg-Calvé-Perthes disease affects children in middle childhood; and slipped femoral capital epiphysis and scoliosis are more characteristic of late childhood and adolescence.

LEGG-CALVÉ-PERTHES DISEASE

Legg-Calvé-Perthes disease, sometimes called coxa plana or osteochondritis deformans juvenilis, is a self-limited disorder in which there is aseptic necrosis of the femoral head. The disease affects children 3 to 12 years of age, but most cases occur in males between 4 and 8 years of age as an isolated event. In approximately 10% to 15% of cases the involvement is bilateral, and most of the affected children have a skeletal age significantly below their chronologic age.[14] The male : female ratio is 4 or 5 to 1, and white children are affected ten times more frequently than black children.[5]

Etiology and pathophysiology

The cause of the disease is unknown, but there is a disturbance of circulation to the femoral capital epiphysis that produces an ischemic aseptic necrosis of the femoral head. This circulatory impairment seems to extend to the epiphysis and acetabulum as well.

The pathologic events seem to take place in three stages, each usually consisting of 9 months to 1 year. First there is aseptic necrosis of the femoral capital epiphysis with degenerative changes producing flattening of the upper surface of the femoral head, the *initial* or *avascular stage*. Second revascularization takes place with fragmentation (vascular resorption of the epiphysis) that gives a mottled appearance on roentgenograms, the *fragmentation* or *revascularization phase*. Third is the *reparative* or *regeneration stage* with new bone formation and gradual reformation of the head of the femur. The entire process may encompass as little as 18 months or continue for several years. The reformed femoral head may be severely altered or appear entirely normal.

Diagnostic evaluation

The child usually complains of persistent pain that may be accompanied by joint dysfunction with limp and limitation of motion and may or may not have been preceded by trauma. The diagnosis is established by x-ray examination.

Medical management

Since deformity occurs early in the disease process, the aim of treatment is to keep the head of the femur in the acetabulum and maintain a full range of motion. This can be accomplished by nonweight-bearing devices such as an abduction brace, leg casts, or a leather harness sling that prevents weight bearing on the affected limb; use of abduction-ambulation braces or casts after a period of bed rest and traction; and surgical reconstructive and containment procedures. Conservative therapy must be continued for 2 to 4 years, whereas surgical correction, although a relatively recent advance and subject to additional risks (such as anesthesia, infection, and blood transfusion), returns the child to normal activities in 3 to 4 months.

The disease is self-limited, but the ultimate outcome of therapy depends on early and efficient treatment and the age of onset of the disorder—the younger the child, the more complete the recovery appears to be. In most cases the prognosis is excellent.

*810 Seventh Avenue, New York, N.Y. 10019

Nursing considerations

Nursing care of the child with Legg-Calvé-Perthes disease depends on the therapy implemented. Care of the child in immobilization devices is discussed in Chapter 40, and the reader is referred to this for more definitive nursing interventions. Nurses are often the first health professionals to identify affected children and to refer them for medical evaluation. They are also persons on whom the child and his family can rely to help them to understand and adjust to the therapeutic measures.

One of the most difficult aspects associated with the disorder is coping with a normally active boy who feels well but must remain relatively inactive. Suitable activities must be devised to meet the needs of the child in the process of developing a sense of initiative or industry. Activities that meet his creative urges are well received. This is also an opportune time to encourage the child to begin a hobby such as collections, model building, or crafts.

SLIPPED FEMORAL CAPITAL EPIPHYSIS

Slipped femoral capital epiphysis, or coxa vara, refers to the spontaneous displacement of the proximal femoral epiphysis in a posterior and inferior direction. It develops most frequently shortly before or during accelerated growth and the onset of puberty (children between the ages of 10 and 16 years—median age, 13 years for boys, 11 years for girls) and is most frequent in obese children. Bilateral involvement has been reported variously as 16% to 40%.

Etiology and pathophysiology

The etiology is unknown, but it occurs most often in "overlarge" youngsters or very tall, thin, rapidly growing children. There has been some evidence to implicate hormonal factors, for example, resistance of the growth plate to sheer stress is decreased by growth hormone and increased by sex hormone, suggesting that the disorder may be related to excess sex hormone in the tall child and decreased sex hormone in the obese child.[15] It has also been associated with endocrine abnormalities, renal osteodystrophy, and growth hormone therapy.[5]

The pathologic processes as seen in x-ray films involves first a rarefaction of bone on the lower femoral side of the epiphysis with widening of the growth plate. After trauma or slight injury the femoral portion of the epiphysis slides upward. As slipping increases, the epiphyseal displacement becomes posterior and inferior.

Diagnostic evaluation

Slipped femoral epiphysis is suspected when an adolescent or preadolescent youngster, especially one who is obese or tall and lanky, begins to limp and complains of pain in the hip continuously or intermittently. The pain is frequently referred to the groin, anteromedial aspect of the thigh, or knee. Physical examination reveals early restriction of internal rotation on adduction and external rotation deformity with loss of abduction and internal rotation as the severity increases. The diagnosis is confirmed by x-ray examination.

The following different varieties of clinical behavior have been observed: (1) an episode of trauma in which the epiphysis is acutely displaced in a previously functional joint; (2) gradual displacement without definite injury with progressively increased hip disability; (3) intermittent bouts of displacement alternating with periods of well-being with gradual appearance of symptoms associated with ambulation (such as external rotation); and (4) a combined gradual and traumatic displacement, in which there is gradual slippage with further displacement caused by injury.[15,26]

Medical management

The treatment varies with the degree of displacement but involves surgical stabilization and correction of deformity. In mild cases simple pin fixation is sufficient. More extensive displacement requires skeletal traction followed by pin fixation or osteotomy. The prognosis depends on the degree of deformity and on whether or not complications, such as avascular necrosis and cartilaginous necrosis, affect the progress. As in other disorders, early diagnosis and implementation of therapy increase the likelihood of a satisfactory cure.

Nursing considerations

Nursing care is the same as that for a child in a cast or a child in traction, discussed in Chapter 40.

KYPHOSIS AND LORDOSIS

Kyphosis is an abnormally increased convex angulation in the curvature of the thoracic spine (Fig. 39-3). The most common form of kyphosis is "postural." Children, especially during the time when skeletal growth outpaces growth of muscle, are prone to exaggeration of tendency toward kyphosis. They assume bizarre sitting and standing positions. This is particularly common in self-conscious adolescent girls who assume a round-shouldered slouching posture in the attempt to hide their developing breasts.

Postural kyphosis is almost always accompanied by a compensatory postural lordosis, an abnormally exaggerated concave lumbar curvature. Treatment consists of postural exercises to strengthen shoulder and abdominal muscles and bracing for more marked deformity. Unfortunately treatment is difficult because of the nature of the adolescent personality. The normal rebellious tendencies of the adolescent together with continual parental nagging to "stand up straight" often interfere with compliance to a therapeutic regimen. The best approach is to emphasize the cosmetic value of corrective therapy and to place the responsibility on the adolescent himself for carrying out an exercise program at home with regular visits to and assessments by a

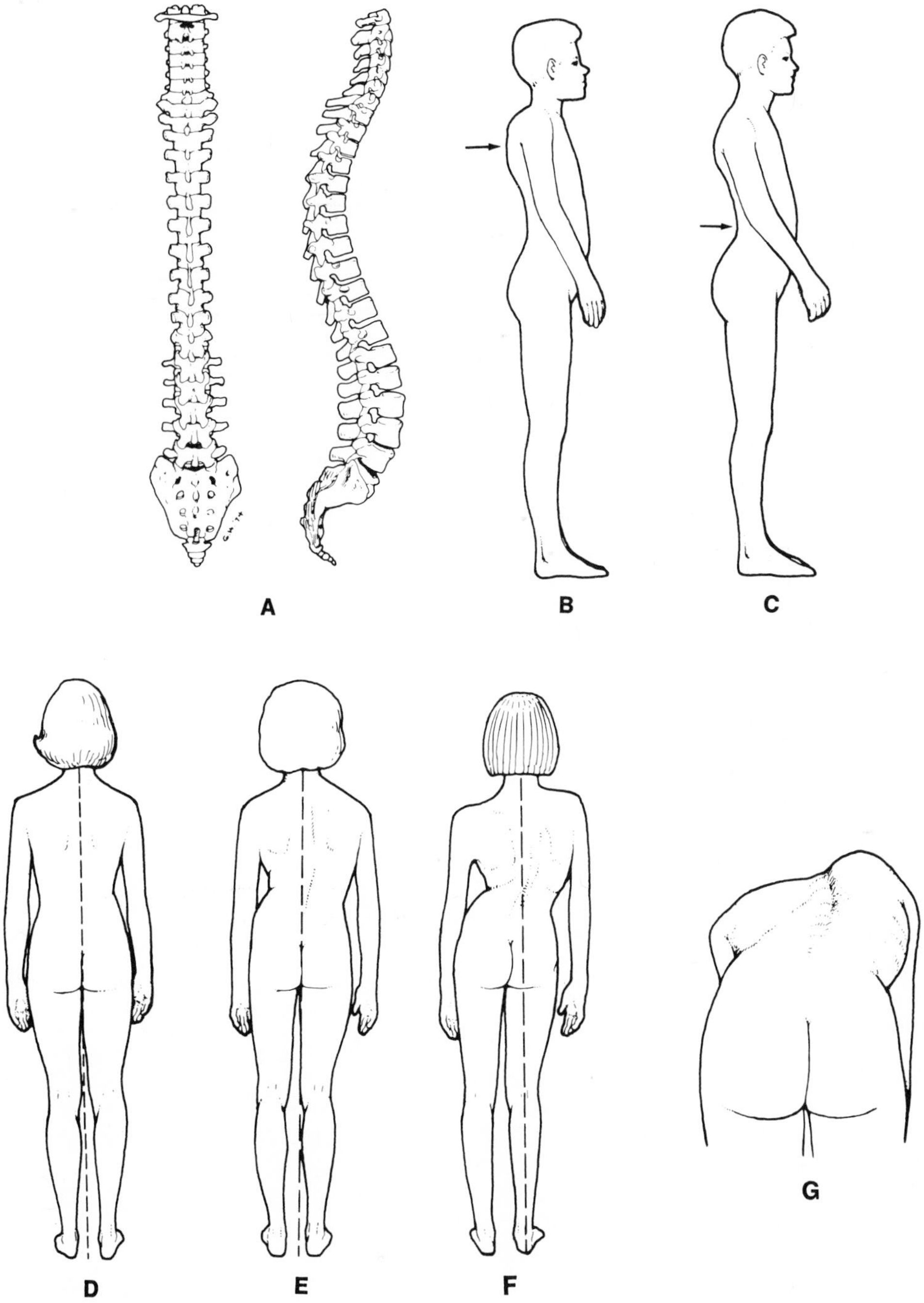

Fig. 39-3. Defects of the spinal column. **A,** Normal spine. **B,** Kyphosis. **C,** Lordosis. **D,** Normal spine in balance. **E,** Mild scoliosis in balance. **F,** Severe scoliosis, not in balance. **G,** Rib hump and flank asymmetry seen in flexion due to rotary component. (From Hilt, N. E., and Schmitt, E. W.: Pediatric orthopedic nursing, St. Louis, 1975, The C. V. Mosby Co., p. 34.)

therapist. Most adolescents respond well to selected sports as a supplement to regular exercise. Boys prefer weight lifting (preferably performed from a prone or supine position on a bench) and track sports. Girls respond well to dancing classes (ballet or modern dancing). Swimming is excellent and has the added advantages of exercising all muscles, eliminating gravity, and teaching breath control.[16]

SCOLIOSIS

Scoliosis is a lateral curvature of the spine usually associated with a rotary deformity that eventually causes cosmetic and physiologic alterations in the spine, chest, and pelvis. It can appear at any age but is most frequent in adolescent girls.[16]

Etiology and pathophysiology

Scoliosis can be caused by a number of etiologic agents and may occur spontaneously or in association with other diseases or deformities. When the curve is flexible and corrects by bending, it is called a "nonstructural" curve. When the curve fails to straighten on side-bending, it is termed a "structural" curve and is characterized by changes in the spine and its supporting structures.

Nonstructural scoliosis may be postural with a slight curve that disappears when the child lies down or to compensate for a leg-length discrepancy. A transient scoliosis may be produced by pressure on a nerve root or inflammation. Structural scoliosis, on the other hand, is characterized by loss of flexibility and noncorrectable deformity. The cause in 70% of cases is "idiopathic" without apparent cause; however, evidence indicates that it is probably genetic and transmitted as an autosomal-dominant trait with incomplete penetrance (pp. 191 and 194) and onset during three peak periods of childhood: infantile, juvenile, and adolescent. Other causes include congenital, neurogenic, myopathic, acquired with other diseases, and trauma[16] (see the boxed material).

Diagnostic evaluation

Diagnosis is made by observation and x-ray examination. There are rarely discomfort and few outward signs until

Structural scoliosis

Idiopathic (genetic) scoliosis

- Infantile
  - Age of onset—birth to 3 years of age
  - More common in males
  - Usually left thoracic curve
  - Poor prognosis
- Juvenile
  - Age of onset—4 to 10 years of age
  - More equal distribution between sexes
  - Usually right thoracic curve
  - Severity increases with growth
- Adolescent
  - Age of onset—10 years of age to skeletal maturity
  - Predominant in females, about 7 to 1
  - Right thoracic and thoracolumbar curves more common

Congenital scoliosis

- Associated with myelomeningocele or other dysrhaphism
- Hemivertebrae

Neuromuscular (paralytic) scoliosis

- Caused by muscular imbalance
- Neurogenic
  - Lower motor neuron disease such as poliomyelitis, spinal muscular atrophy
  - Upper motor neuron disease such as cerebral palsy
- Myogenic
  - Progressive disease such as muscular dystrophy
  - Static disease such as amyotonia congenita
- Mixed—weakness and overpull by stronger trunk muscles such as Friedeich's ataxia

Neurofibromatosis

- Short sharp thoracic curve often associated with kyphosis

Traumatic

- Thoracogenic—result of thoracotomy and thoracoplasty with rib resection
- Spinal trauma
  - Irradiation such as tumor therapy
  - Fractures

Spinal irritation

- Spinal cord tumor
- Nerve root irritation

Miscellaneous

- Secondary to irritation
  - Tumor
  - Inflammation
- Nutritional—rickets
- Metabolic—renal osteodystrophy

Mesenchymal disease

- Congenital disorders
  - Dwarfism
  - Disease of connective tissue such as arachnoidactyly, arthrogryposis multiplex congenita
  - Disease of bone such as osteogenesis imperfecta
- Acquired disorders—rheumatoid arthritis

the deformity is well established. Early detection and treatment are essential to successful management. The undressed child viewed from the posterior side will often reveal primary curvature and a compensatory curvature that places the head in alignment with the gluteal fold (Fig. 39-3, *E*). In uncompensated scoliosis the head and hips are not in alignment (Fig. 39-3, *F*). In advanced cases with rotary deformity, rib hump and flank asymmetry are observed when the child bends from the waist unsupported with the arms (Fig. 39-3, *G*). X-ray films taken in the standing position establish the state of deformity.

Medical management

A thorough examination, history, and assessment of the child are carried out in order to evaluate the status of the deformity, factors contributing to the defect, and factors that may influence the outcome of therapy. Treatment is best undertaken in a center in which a team is available that specializes in management of scoliosis.

Bracing and exercise. Exercises can often help postural scoliosis but are rarely of value with structural defects. Nonoperative treatment by application of a properly constructed and well-fitted external bracing device and close supervision are successful in halting the progression of most curvatures.[16] The most commonly used device is the Milwaukee brace, an individually adapted steel and leather brace that extends from a chin cup and neck pads to the pelvis, where lumbar pads rest on the hips (Fig. 39-4). The brace is used for minimal curvatures and is worn 23 hours a day but offers little interference with normal activity. Supplemental exercises are employed daily both in and out of the brace. The brace is adjusted at regular trimonthly intervals and, when x-ray examinations reveal bone maturity, the child is gradually weaned from the brace over a 1- to 2-year period. The brace is then worn only at night until the spine is absolutely mature.[1]

Surgery. For many curvatures surgical intervention is needed. Spinal fusion techniques followed by casting for a period of 6 months to a year produce satisfactory results. For the most severe scoliotic curvatures, traction devices are employed for a time prior to spinal fusion. The traction is applied to the spine by way of a metal ring, or halo, attached to the skull and pins inserted into either the distal femur or the iliac wings of the pelvis. With halo-pelvic traction the child is placed on a special Stryker frame and traction is applied by weight. Halo-pelvic traction is applied by means of turnbuckles and the child can remain ambulatory. After traction a spinal fusion is performed and an

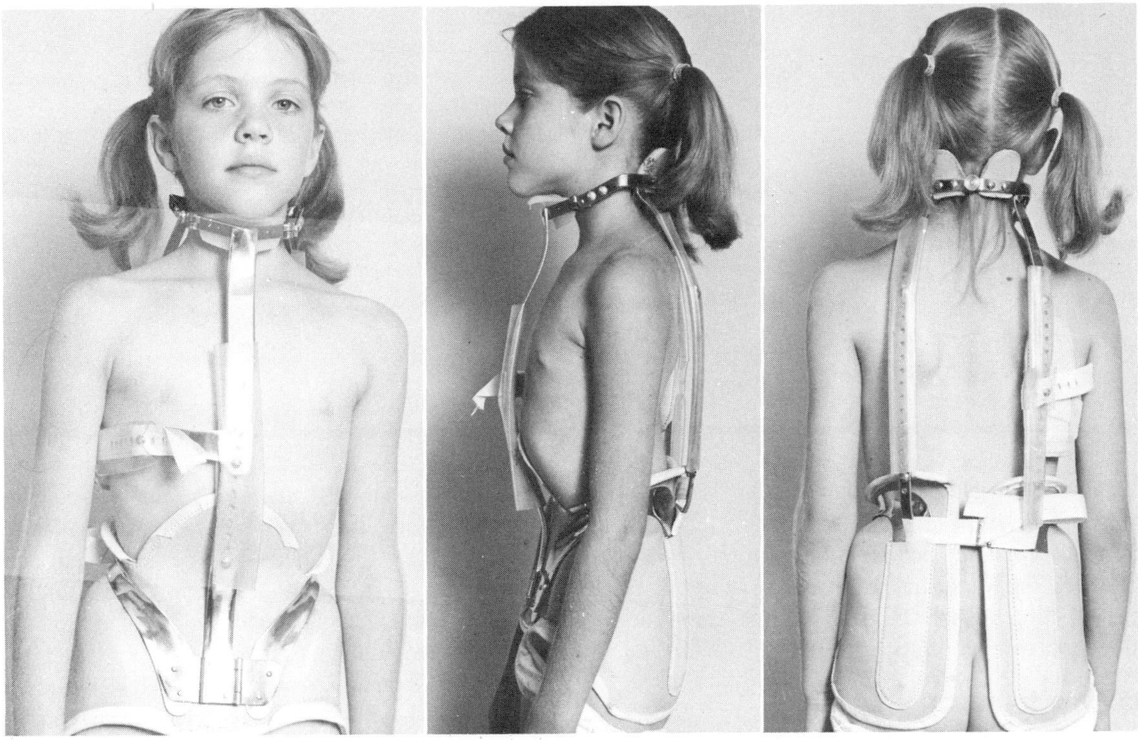

A B C

Fig. 39-4. Milwaukee brace. **A,** Front view. **B,** Side view. **C,** Rear view. (From Blount, Walter P., and Mueller, Karl H.: Orthopädische Praxis **8:**139-149, June 1972.)

Summary of nursing care of the adolescent with mild structural scoliosis

Goals	Responsibilities
Recognize deformity	Check spine alignment as part of child assessment Be alert to comments by child or parent that indicate possible problems such as Clothes do not fit right Skirt hems are uneven One hip seems higher than other Recommend screening for other family members
Assist in medical evaluation	Encourage child and parents to seek medical evaluation Refer to family physician and/or specialized services Determine if referrals were utilized
Prepare for application of brace	Reinforce and clarify explanations provided by orthopedist—explanations of Appliance Plan of care Activities allowed/restricted Child's and parents' responsibilities in therapy
Provide for supportive services	Refer to social services and/or crippled children's services for financial assistance, transportation, and so on, if needed
Assist in physical adjustment to appliance	Assess brace and its fit Attempt to determine source of any discomfort Refer to orthotist for needed adjustment and service Examine skin surfaces in contact with brace for signs of irritation; implement corrective action to treat or prevent skin breakdown Assist with plan for personal hygiene Help in selection of appropriate wearing apparel to wear over brace and footwear to maintain proper balance Reinforce teaching regarding removal and reapplication of appliance Investigate any complaints of discomfort
Help child adjust to restricted movement	Demonstrate alternative modes of accomplishing tasks such as Getting in and out of bed Dressing Help devise alternatives for restricted activities and coping with awkwardness

immobilizing plaster jacket is applied from occiput to pelvis, which is worn for 8 months to 1 year.[1]

Surgical implantation of metal (Harrington) rods by way of clips to hold the vertebrae is sometimes an effective means for correcting the deformity. Metal rods are used in combination with external support methods.[17]

Nursing considerations

Treatment for scoliosis extends over a significant portion of the affected child's period of growth. In adolescents this period is the one in which their identity, physical and psychologic, is formed. For some youngsters much of this time is spent in the hospital sitting immobilized in complex, unattractive appliances. For those treated on an outpatient basis it means a modified life-style and being "different" from their peers, even though they are usually able to engage in many activities enjoyed by other youngsters.

When the child first faces the prospect of a prolonged period in a brace, cast, or other device, the therapy program and the nature of the device must be explained thoroughly to the child and parents so that they will have an understanding of the anticipated results, how the appliance corrects the defect, the freedoms and constraints imposed by the device, and what they can do to help

Summary of nursing care of the adolescent with mild structural scoliosis—cont'd

Goals	Responsibilities
Prevent injury	Assess environment for hazards Teach safety precautions such as using hand rail on stairways, avoiding slippery surfaces, and so on Help develop safe methods of mobilization
Encourage compliance to regimen	Establish communication with child and family Assess understanding of plan of care Instruct child and family in various aspects of therapy and care as needed Provide feedback and praise for positive behavior Provide assistance and encouragement when needed Arrange appointments Assist family with transportation to appointments Identify goals with achievable outcomes Include family in setting goals Allow to express discouragement at what appears to be slow progress and interference with activities
Support normal growth and development	Encourage independence where appropriate Allow for dependence when needed Involve in scheduling appointments and other aspects of care Encourage school attendance and socialization with peers Encourage involvement in activities compatible with limitations
Help child develop positive self-image	Accentuate positive aspects of appearance Motivate to good habits of personal hygiene Encourage to wear attractive clothes and hairstyle Emphasize positive long-term outcome Help devise positive ways to deal with reactions of others

achieve the desired goal. The management involves the skills and services of a team of specialists, including the orthopedist, physical therapist, orthotist (a specialist in fitting orthopedic braces), nurse, social worker, and sometimes pulmonary specialists.

It is difficult for a child to be restricted at any phase of development, but the teenager needs continual positive reinforcement, encouragement, and as much independence as can be safely assumed during this time. Socialization with peers should be encouraged and every effort expended to help the adolescent feel attractive and worthwhile.

Since many persons view any handicap as deviant, the child will need help in learning how to deal with reactions of others to the appliance. Preparation for such responses places the child at an advantage. The best approach is usually to initiate the interaction by mentioning the device and its purpose. This alleviates the ambiguity surrounding the appliance and its purpose and reduces the anxiety on the part of the child and the other person. Most important, the child should be helped to view the condition and appliance in a positive way and avoid seeing them as a stigma.[13]

For a summary of nursing care of the adolescent with mild structural scoliosis, see the boxed material.

Orthopedic infections

OSTEOMYELITIS

Osteomyelitis is an infectious process of bone that can occur at any age but that occurs most frequently between 5 and 14 years of age. It is twice as common in boys as in girls.

Etiology and pathophysiology

Any organism can cause osteomyelitis, and there is some relationship between the age of the child and the type of organism responsible. In older children staphylococci are the most common organisms, approximately 80% of which are *Staphylococcus aureus;* in younger children other organisms predominate, especially *Hemophilus influenzae*. In children with sickle cell anemia *Salmonella* organisms are frequently responsible for osteomyelitis. Osteomyelitis can be acquired from *exogenous* or *hematogenous* sources.

Exogenous osteomyelitis. Exogenous osteomyelitis is acquired by direct invasion of the bone by direct extension from the outside as a result of a penetrating wound, open fracture, contamination during surgery, or secondary extension from an overlying abscess or burn.

Hematogenous osteomyelitis. Hematogenous spread of organisms from a preexisting focus is the most common source of infection. Common sources of foci include furuncles, skin abrasions, impetigo, upper respiratory tract infection, acute otitis media, tonsillitis, abscessed teeth, pyelonephritis, or infected burns. Other factors that predispose to development of osteomyelitis are poor physical condition, nutrition, and surroundings that are not hygienic.

Pathophysiology. Infective emboli from the focus of infection travel to the small end arteries in the bone metaphysis, where they set up an infectious process. The infection does not spread to the epiphysis since it has a blood supply separate from the metaphysis. The infectious process leads to local bone destruction and abscess formation. The abscess with its collected necrotic debris exerts pressure within the rigid, unyielding bone and ruptures into the subperiosteal space, where the pressure lifts and strips the periosteum. The infection spreads beneath the periosteum, thrombosing vessels and adding further to the bony necrosis. In infants and very young children the elevated periosteum attempts to wall off the infection by forming new bone, *involucrum*. Underneath, the cortex, deprived of blood supply, dies and the necrotic bone that cannot be absorbed continues to produce more intraosseous tension and necrosis. Granulation forms around the dead bone. This dead bone is called *sequestrum*. Sinuses may form between the sequestra and the skin surface or into a joint to create a suppurative arthritis. Small areas of sequestrum may be absorbed, but larger areas surrounded by dense bone become honeycombed with sinuses that retain infective material and cause exacerbations for years (the chronic stage of osteomyelitis).

Diagnostic evaluation

The signs and symptoms of *acute* hematogenous osteomyelitis begin abruptly and build up to a maximum intensity during the first few days of the disease, usually less than 1 week. There is frequently a history of trauma to the affected bone.

The child with acute osteomyelitis appears very ill. He is irritable and restless with elevated temperature, rapid pulse, and dehydration. There is usually localized tenderness, increased warmth, and diffuse swelling over the involved bone. The extremity is painful, especially on movement. The child holds it in semiflexion, and the surrounding muscles are tense and resist passive movement. Most cases involve the femur or tibia and to a lesser extent the humerus and hip. In infants the diagnosis is more difficult because of lack of systemic symptoms and may involve multiple bones or joints because of the difficulty in confining an infectious process in children in this age-group.

In *subacute* hematogenous osteomyelitis, symptoms have been present for a longer period of time and the child sometimes has been treated with antibiotics, often for another infection, which modify the clinical symptoms. In some instances the infection may produce a walled-off abscess rather than a spreading infection.

In acute osteomyelitis there is marked leukocytosis and an elevated erythrocyte sedimentation rate. Blood culture is usually positive during the early stage, but radiographic findings are often negative or show only soft tissue swelling for 10 to 14 days. After this time the radiographic findings reveal new bone formation. Tomography may reveal bone changes at an early stage.

Similar symptoms are observed in rheumatic fever, rheumatoid arthritis, leukemia and other malignant lesions, cellulitis, erysipelas, and scurvy. Sometimes the osteomyelitis may be unrecognized if it occurs as a complication of a severe toxic and debilitating illness.

Medical management

As soon as blood cultures have been drawn, prompt and vigorous intravenous antibiotic therapy is initiated. The choice of antibiotic is influenced by age, and the dosage determined is sufficient to ensure high blood and tissue levels. Since most cases of osteomyelitis are caused by staphylococci, large doses of penicillin G are administered and supplemented by methicillin or oxacillin. In children younger than 3 years of age, the infectious agents are more apt to be penicillin-resistant staphylococci or gram-negative organisms; therefore, the agents of choice are usually methicillin, nafcillin, or clindamycin in conjunction with ampicillin. Neonates in whom coliform organisms are likely to be involved are given kanamycin or gentamicin, either intramuscularly or *slowly* by the intravenous route in addition to intravenously administered ampicillin.

When the infective agent is identified, the appropriate antibiotic is usually continued for at least 3 to 4 weeks, but the length of therapy is determined by the duration of symptoms, the initial response to treatment, and the sensitivity of the organism in the specific case. Because of prolonged high-dose therapy, it is important to monitor hematologic, renal, hepatic, and other organ systems that might be adversely affected by the drugs.

Antibiotic therapy is accompanied by local treatment. The child is placed on complete bed rest, and immobilization of the affected extremity with a splint or bivalved cast is continued throughout therapy to limit the spread of infection and, when it is a complication of a fracture, to maintain alignment of bone fragments.

Opinions differ regarding surgical intervention, but many advocate sequestrectomy and surgical drainage to decompress the metaphyseal space before pus erupts and spreads to the subperiosteal space to form abscesses that strip the periosteum from bone or form draining sinuses. When these complications occur a chronic infection usually persists. When surgical drainage is carried out, polyethylene tubes are placed in the wound—one tube instills an antibiotic solution directly into the infected area by gravity, and the other, connected to a suction apparatus, provides drainage.

Nursing considerations

During the acute phase of illness any movement of the affected limb will cause discomfort to the child; therefore, he should be positioned comfortably with the affected limb supported. Moving and turning are carried out carefully and gently to minimize discomfort. The child may require pain medication or sedation. Vital signs are taken and recorded frequently, and measures are implemented to reduce a significant temperature elevation.

Antibiotic therapy requires careful observation and monitoring of the intravenous equipment and site (p. 1084). Since more than one antibiotic is usually administered, the compatibility of the drugs must be determined and care must be taken to avoid mixing noncompatible drugs. A double, or piggyback, setup is safest so that there is less opportunity for the two drugs to come in contact with each other. The stability of the drugs is also considered when determining the rate of administration.

The child with an opened wound is placed on complete or wound isolation precautions, depending on the policies of the institution. The wound is managed according to the directions of the physician. Antibiotic solution administered directly into the wound is most efficiently accomplished with a regular intravenous infusion setup that is prepared and regulated as an intravenous infusion. The drainage tubes are connected to low Gomco or wall suction for continuous removal. Intake and output are measured and recorded, and the character of the wound drainage is noted. The amount and character of drainage on wound dressing are also noted.

Casts are sometimes employed for immobilization, and, if so, routine cast care is carried out. The extremity is examined for sensation, circulation, and pain, and the area over the inflammation is usually left open for observation. The affected area, casted or uncasted, is assessed for color, swelling, heat, and tenderness.

The child usually has a poor appetite and may be subject to vomiting. Nourishment in the form of high-calorie liquids such as fruit juices, gelatin, and juice bars should be encouraged until the child begins to feel better. The appetite returns as the acute symptoms subside. During convalescence adequate nutrition must be maintained to aid healing and reconstitution of new bone.

When the acute stage subsides, the child begins to feel better, his appetite improves, and he becomes interested in his surroundings and relationships. He wishes to move about in bed and is allowed to do so. However, weight bearing on the affected limb is not permitted until healing is well under way in order to avoid pathologic fractures.[8] Diversional and constructive activities become important nursing interventions. The child is usually confined to bed for some time after the acute phase but may be allowed about the unit on a gurney or in a wheelchair when isolation and bed rest are no longer necessary. At this stage the continuous intravenous infusion may be replaced by a heparin lock to allow greater freedom (see p. 1013).

As the infection subsides physical therapy is instituted to ensure restoration of optimal function. The child is usually discharged with oral antibiotics, and his progress is followed closely for some time.

SEPTIC (SUPPURATIVE, PYOGENIC, PURULENT) ARTHRITIS

The source of infection of the joints, like infection of bone, is usually by hematogenous dissemination and spread from another focus. Occasionally it may result from direct extension of a soft tissue infection. The infection occurs predominantly in males, especially in the adolescent age-group. In infancy the age distribution is more nearly equal. Any joint may be involved, but the hip, knee, shoulder, and other large joints are more commonly affected. It usually affects only one joint.

The signs and symptoms of suppurative arthritis, unlike osteomyelitis, are usually characteristic. The presence of a warm and tender joint, painful on even gentle pressure, is sufficient to differentiate it from osteomyelitis, in which gentle passive motion is tolerated. When superficial joints are involved they are exquisitely painful and swollen; deep-seated joints show little superficial evidence. In most instances there is history of a traumatic injury to the affected joint. Fever, leukocytosis, and increased erythrocyte sedimentation rate are present but may not be demonstrated in affected infants.

The most common pathogens are *Staphylococcus aureus*, group A streptococci, and *Hemophilus influenzae*. Diagnosis is made from blood culture, joint fluid aspirate, and radiographs.

Treatment consists of open surgical drainage of hip and shoulder joint disease and repeated needle aspirations of the joint space in other joints. The goals are (1) to cleanse the joint to avoid destruction of articular cartilage, (2) to decompress the joint to avoid interference with the blood supply to the epiphysis, (3) to eradicate the infection with adequate antibiotic therapy, and (4) to prevent secondary bone infection and hematogenous spread. Therapy is similar to that for osteomyelitis: intravenous antibiotic therapy, relief of pain, immobilization of the joint, and prohibition of weight bearing until healing is complete. Nursing care is the same as that for osteomyelitis.

TUBERCULOSIS

Tubercular infection of the bones is acquired by hematogenous dissemination from a primary tubercular focus. The most common sites in infants and small children are the carpals and phalanges and corresponding bones of the feet. A single bone or several bones may be involved with spindle-shaped swelling and tenderness as soft tissues are affected. The process, relatively painless, persists with intermittent symptoms for several months and may leave a permanent deformity. The affected areas are immobilized with a splint or cast.

Tuberculosis of spine (Pott's disease)

In older children the infection attacks the body of one or more vertebrae, destroying the bone, and spreads to all the articular tissues (Pott's disease), producing a kyphotic deformity. The lower thoracic spine is most frequently affected. Symptoms are insidious. The child will be irritable and complain of persistent or intermittent pain over the areas innervated by spinal nerves that arise adjacent to the affected vertebrae. There is muscle splinting and pain on increased pressure on the head, and the child assumes a position that best eases the weight on the diseased vertebrae, such as avoiding bending, walking stiffly and carefully on the toes, and prefers to rest on the abdomen or across a chair or a lap.

Treatment is immobilization with extension on a Bradford frame until there is no evidence of active infection followed by spinal fusion. Antimicrobial therapy and drainage of tubercular abcess are standard therapies. The reparative process is slow, but, in most instances, recovery takes place with little or no deformity.

Tuberculosis of hip

The hip is the most common joint affected by tuberculosis, but the process usually begins in the epiphysis of the femoral head and then erupts into the joint capsule. The initial manifestation is a limp that occurs intermittently, most often on arising in the morning or after exercise. There is progressive destruction of the femoral head with symptoms of pain, and the thigh gradually becomes fixed and adducted with internal rotation. There may be swelling around the hip and abscess formation.

Treatment involves bed rest, traction to reduce muscle spasm, and appropriate drug therapy. Hip fusion may be necessary in severe cases.

SKELETAL DISORDERS

Fractures of bones are relatively common in childhood and are discussed in Chapter 40. Rickets is less common but is still a preventable disease in most instances (p. 484). Uncommon disorders of bone and connective tissue such as arachnodactyly (Marfan's syndrome) and achrondroplasia do not cause immobilization and have been briefly mentioned (p. 195). There are other rare disorders, but only one—osteogenesis imperfecta—will be elaborated further.

Osteogenesis imperfecta

Osteogenesis imperfecta is a rare hereditary disorder characterized by increased fragility of bones that are easily fractured by the slightest trauma. The disorder is inherited as an autosomal-dominant trait. Although there is some thought that a more severe form may be autosomal recessive, this is not entirely accepted. The disorder may be apparent at birth—*osteogenesis imperfecta congenita*—and is characterized by multiple intrauterine or perinatal fractures with considerable deformity and, often, early death. The disease of later onset—*osteogenesis imperfecta tarda*—runs a milder course. The tendency to fracture appears later (at variable ages) and disappears after puberty. During childhood the shafts of long bones are slender with reduced cortical thickness resulting from defective periosteal bone formation. Features associated with the disease are blue sclera, thin skin, hyperextensibility of ligaments, hypoplastic and deformed teeth, and a tendency toward development of otosclerosis with hearing loss. Tendency to recurrent epistaxis, excess diaphoresis, tendency to bruise easily, and mild hyperpyrexia are also common manifestations. The disease shows variable expressivity, that is, the number and extent of pathologic features present in any individual range from severe to minimal involvement.[2,27]

The treatment is primarily supportive. These children require careful handling to avoid fractures. Even changing a diaper may cause a fracture in severely affected infants. Oral administration of magnesium oxide appears to decrease the fracture rate, diaphoresis, hyperpyrexia, and constipation in many affected children. Infants and children with this disorder require careful handling to prevent fractures. Both parents and the affected child need education regarding the child's limitations and guidelines in planning suitable activities that promote optimum development as well as protect him from harm. Realistic occupational planning and genetic counseling are part of the long-term goals of care.

JUVENILE RHEUMATOID ARTHRITIS

Clinically and pathologically juvenile rheumatoid arthritis (JRA) is an inflammatory disease for which the inciting agent is not known. There are two peak ages of onset: between 2 and 5 years of age and between 9 and 12 years of age. Females are affected somewhat more frequently than males, and the incidence has been estimated variously as 1 in 1000, 1 in 5000, and 3 in 100,000. In many instances the disease remains undiagnosed for years.[3]

Definitions[3]

arthritis clinical evidence of joint inflammation in the form of (1) swelling caused by effusion and/or synovial thickening or (2) definite loss of function because of pain and/or swelling.

monoarticular involving one joint.

pauciarticular or **oligoarticular** involving few joints, usually less than five.

polyarticular simultaneous involvement of four or more joints.

''wet'' arthritis painful, tender swelling and synovial thickening associated with laxity of ligaments and loss of joint cartilage; less tendency to contracture; more characteristic of adult disease but is seen in children with severe, progressive polyarthritis.

''dry'' arthritis painless contractures in the absence of significant swelling or loss of joint cartilage; restriction of movement secondary to contraction of capsule and pericapsular tissues; more characteristic of juvenile disease.

Juvenile rheumatoid arthritis is, in many ways, similar to adult disease, but there are many features that are quite distinct. A distinguishing characteristic is its tendency to occur in the prepubertal child. Characteristics of juvenile rheumatoid arthritis include negative results in the latex fixation test in 90% of cases; classic symptoms of spiking fever, skin rash, or pericarditis in 5% to 10% of cases; tendency to be very mild in 70% of cases with few joints involved; tendency toward the ''dry'' form of contracting arthritis that involves large rather than small joints; development of iridocyclitis as a complication in 8% to 20% of milder forms; and ''burning itself out'' over 2 to 3 years in milder forms and over 8 to 10 years in most other forms.[3]

Etiology and pathophysiology

The etiology of juvenile rheumatoid arthritis is unknown. Both infectious and autoimmune theories have been presented, but there is no convincing evidence to establish either one as an etiologic agent. There is a slight tendency to occur in families.

Pathophysiology. The rheumatic process is characterized by a chronic inflammation of the synovium with joint effusion and eventual erosion, destruction, and fibrosis of the articular cartilage. Adhesions between joint surfaces and ankylosis of joints occur if the process persists long enough.

Diagnostic evaluation

Whether a single or multiple joints are involved, there is development of stiffness, swelling, and loss of motion in the affected joints. They are swollen and warm to the touch but seldom red. The swelling results from edema, joint effusion, and synovial thickening. The affected joints may be tender and painful to the touch or relatively painless. The limited motion, early in the disease, is the result of muscle spasm and joint inflammation; later it is caused by ankylosis or soft tissue contracture. Morning stiffness or ''gelling'' of the joint(s) is characteristic and present on arising in the morning or after inactivity. Infections, injuries, or operations often precipitate a flare-up of the arthritis; therefore, prompt recognition and treatment of infections are necessary.[24]

Growth may be retarded during periods of active disease, usually with growth spurts during remissions. In severe long-standing cases growth is significantly retarded. Corticosteroid therapy is also a contributing factor. There may be growth disturbances, either overgrowth or undergrowth, adjacent to the inflamed joints, for example, altered leg length after knee involvement and micrognathia (receding chin) from temporomandibular arthritis.

Each child with juvenile rheumatoid arthritis has a unique combination of signs and symptoms; however, the major manifestations can be generalized in semidistinct categories that help to predict the possible duration of the disease, the degree of disability during the course of the disease, and the eventual functional outcome. These are based on such general criteria as the nature of the onset, the number of joints involved, the type of arthritis, and the nature and extent to which other systems are involved.

Onset. The onset may be acute or gradual. An acute and painful onset when only a few joints are involved is usually associated with a short course of only a few months, whereas acute, painful onset of widespread polyarthritis is more apt to be a long-lasting illness of 8 to 10 years. Gradual onset with few involved joints tends to resolve in 2 to 3 years with mild disability, whereas polyarthritis with gradual onset usually does not clear for 8 to 10 years, and the degree of disability is variable.

Age at onset. In very small children there is frequently acute febrile onset and widespread systemic changes but little joint involvement. In small children the onset tends to be severe and more likely to involve many joints. In older children joint involvement is more often restricted to one or two large joints without significant systemic manifestations, and the course tends to be more quiet and abates in the early teen years. Disease that begins during adolescence is usually the adult variety.[23]

Number of joints. The disability during the course of the disease and the residual disability is much less in monoarticular and pauciarticular disease and is usually associated with more mild systemic reaction. In polyarticular disease there is more apt to be a severe systemic reaction and a prolonged course.

Systemic involvement. There are two categories of systemic involvement—classic and general. In the classic form the symptoms are specific to the disease, that is, daily spiking fever, typical rheumatoid rash, and pericarditis. When these symptoms are associated with severe polyarthritis the clinical course is usually prolonged and progressive. When these symptoms are associated with few involved joints there is a good chance that the process will subside with a favorable outcome.

General systemic involvement is not specific to the disease but resembles symptomatology seen in most childhood illness—low-grade fever, anorexia, failure to gain weight, anemia, lymphadenopathy, and generalized fatigue. These manifestations, with long-standing polyarthritis, are associated with long duration and extensive disability. When generalized systemic involvement occurs with monoarticular and pauciarticular arthritis, the symptoms may be those of a multisystem disease such as lupus erythematosus, ulcerative colitis, periarteritis, and so on.

Polyarticular arthritis. Polyarticular juvenile rheumatoid arthritis is characterized by multiple joint involvement accompanied by classic or general systemic involvement. Any joints may be affected. Involvement is usually symmetric and frequently begins in large joints such as knees, ankles, wrists, and elbows. Joints of fingers and toes become swollen and inflamed and assume a spindle, or fusiform, shape. Hip, cervical, and temporomandibular joint involvement is common. The onset of joint symptoms may be acute or gradual with painful "wet" or "dry" arthritic manifestations. A small number of children gradually develop a painless, "dry" arthritis, usually morning stiffness, over a period of months or years without definable systemic manifestations.

Monoarticular and pauciarticular arthritis. Isolated arthritis is most commonly seen in the knee, ankle, wrist, hip, and proximal interphalangeal joint; it occurs least often in the shoulder. Polyarticular disease often begins in a single joint, becoming polyarticular in 3 to 6 months. If spread occurs after 6 months, it is usually mild and limited to one or two joints. Pauciarticular arthritis of five joints or less is more common in children 2 or 3 years of age and tends to have the most favorable prognosis.

Diagnostic tests. Radiologic findings are variable, but the earliest manifestations are widening joint spaces followed by gradual evidence of fusion and articular destruction.

There are no specific diagnostic tests for juvenile rheumatoid arthritis. The erythrocyte sedimentation rate may or may not be elevated, depending on the degree of inflammation present. Leukocytosis is generally present in the early stages of classic systemic disease. Latex fixation test, the most common test used to detect the presence of "rheumatoid factor" in adults, and antinuclear antibodies are seldom positive in children with juvenile rheumatoid arthritis and, if positive, are not diagnostic.

Medical management

There is no specific cure for juvenile rheumatoid arthritis. The major goals of therapy are to preserve joint function, prevent physical deformities, and relieve symptoms without therapeutic harm. Whenever possible the child is treated at home under the supervision of the health team and intermittent treatment by qualified professionals is administered. Hospitalization may be needed during severe exacerbations or when intercurrent illness warrants. Iridocyclitis (inflammation of the iris and ciliary body), which is unique to juvenile rheumatoid arthritis, is not an uncommon complication that requires the attention of an ophthalmologist.

Drugs.[3,9] Several drugs, including salicylates, corticosteroids, and gold salts, are effective in suppressing the inflammatory process and relieving pain. Acetylsalicylic acid (aspirin) is administered to maintain a blood level of 20 to 30 mg/100 ml, approximately 100 mg/kg of body weight. Since there is a narrow margin between effective and toxic doses, the levels are monitored regularly until the dosage is sufficient to maintain the optimal level and a satisfactory clinical response. The total daily dose is divided into four doses to be administered with each meal and at the parent's bedtime, around 10:00 or 11:00 PM. To avoid the acute gastritis and bleeding associated with large amounts of aspirin, especially when administered with daily corticosteroids, it may be given in an enteric-coated form or accompanied by an antacid.

Corticosteroids are the most potent anti-inflammatory agents available. However, they do not cure the disease or prevent joint damage, and their chronic side effects are undesirable. They are administered in the lowest effective dose, given on alternate days rather than daily, and used for the shortest period of time possible. Indications for daily corticosteroid (prednisone) therapy are life-threatening disease (such as pericarditis), incapacitating systemic disease unresponsive to other anti-inflammatory therapy, and iridocyclitis.

Gold salts such as gold sodium thiomalate are often useful in severe forms of the disease.

Physical management. Programs of physical management are individualized for each child and designed to reach the ultimate goal—the preservation of function. Physical therapy is directed toward (1) specific joints, focusing on strengthening muscles, mobilizing restricted joint motion, and preventing or correcting deformities and (2) generalized mobility and performance of activities of daily living.[3]

General treatment or maintenance programs seldom requires the close supervision of a trained physiotherapist. Strength is frequently lost around the involved joints, and inactivity leads to generalized weakness. However, normal activities of daily living and the child's natural tendencies to be active are usually sufficient to maintain muscle strength and joint mobility. Exercising in a pool is excellent, since it allows freedom of movement with support and minimal gravitational pull. When joints are inflamed, heavy resistance aggravates the pain, and, at these times, simple isometric or tensing exercises that do not involve joint movement are generally tolerated and should be encouraged. Range of motion exercises are an important aspect of therapy and are continued after evidence of disease has disappeared in order to detect any signs of recurrence.[12]

Use of splints is controversial, but most therapists recommend splinting and positioning during rest to help minimize pain and prevent or reduce flexion deformity. Joints most frequently splinted are knees, wrists, and hands. Positioning during rest is also important. The children rest on a firm mattress with no pillow or a very low one and have no support under the knee. Loss of extension in the knee, hip, and wrist causes special problems and requires vigilance to detect the earliest signs of involvement and vigorous attention to prevent deformity with specialized passive stretching, positioning, and resting splints.

Surgery. The benefits of synovectomy, an established preventative and therapuetic procedure in adults, are questionable in the child with rheumatoid arthritis. Some older children have benefited from it, but it is seldom recommended for younger children. To be of value the child must be able to cooperate in vigorous preoperative and postoperative physical therapy; therefore, surgery is reserved for the older and very cooperative child.

Nursing considerations

The child with rheumatoid arthritis presents a challenge to himself and his family and to the professionals who help them cope with this prototype of chronic illness. The effects of the disease are felt in every aspect of the child's life—in physical activities, social experiences, and personality development. Much of the child's adjustment to the stresses and demands of the disease and level of functioning he achieves is directly related to the reaction and support he receives from his family and the health professionals concerned with his care and management.

Promoting general health. The general health of the child must be considered and is frequently overlooked as parents and health personnel concentrate on the disease. A well-balanced diet and assessment of nutritional status are integral parts of health supervision. The discomfort and increased need for rest may create problems of weight control. Excess weight causes additional strain on inflamed joints, especially those of the lower extremities. Excessive fatigue and overexertion should be avoided with regular periods of rest, especially during acute flare-ups of arthritis. The child is susceptible to frequent upper respiratory infection, which should receive prompt treatment.

Posture and body mechanics are important for the child with juvenile rheumatoid arthritis, both when he is at rest and when he is active. He must have a firm mattress to maintain good alignment of spine, hips, and knees and no pillow or a very thin one. The child who is confined to bed either at home or in the hospital may require sandbags, other support, or splints to maintain positioning. Lying in the prone position is encouraged to straighten hips and knees, such as during rest periods or television viewing. The family is instructed in the principles and purposes of splints so that they can use them judiciously.

School-age children are allowed to attend school, even on days when there may be some pain or discomfort. The aid of the school nurse is enlisted so that the child is permitted to take the prescribed aspirin at school and to arrange for rest in the nurse's office during the day.

Heat and exercise. Heat has been shown to be beneficial to children with arthritis. Moist heat is best for relieving pain and stiffness, and the most efficient and practical method is in the bathtub. The temperature and duration of the bath are specified by the therapist but usually do not exceed 10 minutes at 37.8°C (100°F). Sometimes a daily whirlpool bath, paraffin bath, or hot packs may be used as needed for temporary relief of acute swelling and pain. Hot packs are easily applied at home using a Turkish towel wrung out after being immersed in hot water, applied to the area, and covered with plastic for 20 minutes. Painful hands or feet can be immersed in a pan of water for 10 minutes two or three times daily in addition to tub baths.

Pool therapy is the easiest method for exercising a large number of joints. Swimming activities strengthen muscles and maintain mobility in larger joints. Most children have access to a therapy pool, although transportation may be a problem for some families. Very small children who are frightened of the water can carry out their exercises in the bathtub. Small children love to splash, kick, and throw things in the water.

Activities of daily living provide satisfactory exercise for older children to maintain maximum mobility with minimum pain. They should be encouraged in their efforts and patiently allowed to dress and groom themselves, to assume daily tasks, and to care for their belongings. It is often difficult for stiff fingers to manipulate buttons, comb or brush hair, and turn faucets, but parents and other care givers should refrain from assisting them. Also, the child should learn and understand why others do not help him. Many helpful devices, such as Velcro fasteners, tongs for manipulating difficult items, and grab bars installed in bathrooms for safety, can be employed to facilitate tasks. A raised toilet seat often makes the difference between dependent and independent toileting, since weak quadriceps muscles and sore knees inhibit the ability to raise the body from a low sitting position.

The child's natural affinity for play offers many opportunities for incorporating therapeutic exercises. Throwing or kicking a ball, hanging from monkey bars, and riding a tricycle (with the seat raised to achieve maximum leg extension) are excellent moving and stretching exercises for preschool children. These are especially important for the very young child whose daily living activities are physically limited.[3]

An effective approach to beginning the day's activities is to awaken the child early to give him his medication and then to allow him to sleep for an hour. On arising the child takes a hot bath (or shower) and carries out a simple ritual of limbering-up exercises, after which he commences the activities of the day, such as going to school. Exercise, heat, and rest are spaced throughout the remainder of the day according to individual needs and schedules. Parents are instructed in exercises that are designed to fit the needs of the child.[12]

The parents are instructed regarding administration of medications as well as the value of a regular schedule of administration to maintain a satisfactory drug level in the body. They need to know that aspirin should not be given on an empty stomach and to be alert for signs of aspirin toxicity, which include hyperventilation as a sign of acidosis, bleeding from decreased clotting capacity, tinnitus (ringing in the ears) as a sign of cranial nerve VIII involvement, and undue drowsiness that may indicate central nervous system depression.

The Arthritis Foundation* provides services for both parents and professionals, and nurses should refer families to this agency as an added resource.

Child. Rheumatoid arthritis affects every aspect of the child's daily life. The physical pain and limitations interfere with performance of normal tasks and provision of self-care. Even simple tasks, such as dressing, hair combing, use of the bathroom, cutting food, climbing stairs, manipulating doors and faucets, and using public transportation, are difficult or impossible. There may be school difficulties related to transportation to and from school, stairs, and loss of time as a result of exacerbations and hospitalization. Physical limitations interfere with participation in many activities, both curricular and extracurricular, which limits peer contacts and interaction and increases social isolation. These problems are especially critical for adolescents, for whom peer acceptance and relationships are so vital to their personality development. These children increasingly turn to solitary activities and to the family at a time when they are expected to move into increasing independence and relationships with peers.[20]

Changes in personality usually accompany juvenile rheumatoid arthritis as in any child with a chronic illness. They may be temporary, such as demanding, irritable behavior, or may be manifest in a more permanent way, such as passive hostility, uncommunicativeness, and manipulativeness. Efforts should be made to break through the child's defenses and to identify his anxieties, concerns, and conflicts in order to intervene early to prevent the development of permanent personality problems[3] (see Chapter 22 for problems of the child with chronic illness).

*1212 Avenue of the Americas, New York, N.Y. 10036.

Parents. The beginning of the disease is often sudden and frightening, and its variable course with cycles of remissions and exacerbations is discouraging. Many parents become susceptible to unorthodox cures advanced by well-meaning friends and advertisers. These should be carefully evaluated. Obviously harmless measures such as wearing a copper bracelet need not be discouraged, but parents must be dissuaded from questionable or conspicuously harmful practices such as active exercising of swollen, feverish joints. Parents' understanding of the disease and their attitude toward the child are the key to the success or failure of a treatment program, and major foci of nursing intervention are parental education and support.

Nurses are alert to cues that signal undue anxiety and guilt that may lead to an unhealthy degree of overprotection, such as preoccupation with causative factors, constant analysis of effects of various therapies, experimenting with diets, and continually searching for a magical cure.[18] The dangers of parental overprotection and overindulgence can be especially detrimental to the progress of the child with rheumatoid arthritis. Sometimes parents are hesitant to give prescribed medications, keep him home from school unnecessarily, restrict his interaction with agemates, may be reluctant to discipline the child, and assume self-care activities that are best performed by the child.

A visit to the home to observe the family in their own setting helps provide clues to their resources and promotes a more comfortable, relaxed atmosphere for discussing problems. The family's strengths and weaknesses are assessed, as well as their reaction to the diagnosis and the prospect of coping with a chronically ill child and all its implications. Help prior to the development of problems can be anticipated by a careful home assessment and supplying support, assistance, and reassurance. It also provides an outlet for anxiety and an opportunity for members of the family to express feelings of guilt and hostility constructively.

Most of the reactions, problems, and concerns of parents of a child with juvenile rheumatoid arthritis are those of any parents of a chronically ill and/or handicapped child. The impact of the diagnosis is felt most acutely by the parents, who demonstrate anxiety, guilt, and all the manifestations of the grief process. The problems and relationships with parents of a chronically ill or handicapped child are discussed extensively in Chapter 22, and the reader is directed to this chapter for additional guidance in planning care.

REFERENCES

1. Anderson, B., and D'Ambra, P.: The adolescent patient with scoliosis, Nurs. Clin. North Am. **11**:699-708, 1976.
2. Berstrom, W. H., and Gardner, L. I.: The bones and joints. In Vaughn, V. C., and McKay, R. J., editors: Nelson's textbook of pediatrics, ed. 10, Philadelphia, 1975, W. B. Saunders Co.

3. Boone, J. E., Baldwin, J., and Levine, C.: Juvenile rheumatoid arthritis, Pediatr. Clin. North Am. **21:**885, November 1974.
4. Chisolm, J. J., Jr.: Poisoning from food, chemicals, drugs and metals. In Vaughn, V. C., and McKay, R. J., editors: Nelson's textbook of pediatrics, ed. 10, Philadelphia, 1975, W. B. Saunders Co.
5. Chung, S. M. K.: Identifying the cause of limp in childhood, Clin. Pediatr. **13:**769-771, 1974.
6. Chutorian, A. M., and Meyers, S. J.: Diseases of muscle. In Downey, J. A., and Low, N. L., editors: The child with disabling illness, Philadelphia, 1974, W. B. Saunders Co.
7. Conway, B. L.: Pediatric neurologic nursing, St. Louis, 1977, The C. V. Mosby Co.
8. Haltalin, K. C.: Acute bacterial osteomyelitis. In Shirkey, H. C., editor: Pediatric therapy, ed. 5, St. Louis, 1975, The C. V. Mosby Co.
9. Hanissian, A. S.: Arthritis in childhood. In Hughes, J. G.: Synopsis of pediatrics, ed. 4, St. Louis, 1975, The C. V. Mosby Co.
10. Hughes, J. G.: Synopsis of pediatrics, ed. 4, St. Louis, 1975, The C. V. Mosby Co.
11. Huttenlocher, P. R.: Neuropathies and muscular disorders. In Vaughn, V. C., and McKay, R. J., editors: Nelson's textbook of pediatrics, ed. 10, Philadelphia, 1975, W. B. Saunders Co.
12. Jacobs, J. C., and Downey, J. A.: Juvenile rheumatoid arthritis. In Downey, J. A., and Low, N. L., editors: The child with disabling illness, Philadelphia, 1974, W. B. Saunders Co.
13. Jones, S. L.: Orthopedic injuries: illness as deviance, Am. J. Nurs. **75:**2030-2033, 1975.
14. Kamhi, E.: Legg-Calvé-Perthes disease, Postgrad. Med. **60**(4):125-130, 1976.
15. Katz, J. F., and Challenor, Y. B.: Childhood orthopedic syndromes. In Downey, J. A., and Low, N. L., editors: The child with disabling illness, Philadelphia, 1974, W. B. Saunders Co.
16. Keim, H. A.: Back deformities, Pediatr. Clin. North Am. **24:**871-880, 1977.
17. Larson, C. B., and Gould, M.: Orthopedic nursing, ed. 9, St. Louis, 1978, The C. V. Mosby Co.
18. Levy, D. M.: Maternal overprotection, New York, 1966, W. W. Norton & Co., Inc.
19. Low, N. L., and Downey, J. A.: Lower motor neuron diseases. In Downey, J. A., and Low, N. L., editors: The child with disabling illness, Philadelphia, 1974, W. B. Saunders Co.
20. McAnarney, E. R., and associates: Psychological problems of children with chronic juvenile arthritis, Pediatrics **53:**523-528, 1974.
21. Molnar, G. E., and Taft, L. T.: Pediatric rehabilitation. Cerebral palsy and spinal cord injuries, Part I, Curr. Probl. Pediatr. **7**(3):6-46, 1977.
22. Nelson, J. S.: Peripheral nerves and skeletal muscle. In Kissane, J. M.: Pathology of infancy and childhood, ed. 2, St. Louis, 1975, The C. V. Mosby Co.
23. O'Brien, D.: Connective tissue or "immune complex" diseases. In Kempe, C. H., Silver, H. K., and O'Brien, D., editors: Current pediatric diagnosis and treatment, ed. 3, Los Altos, Calif., 1974, Lange Medical Publications.
24. Schaller, J. G., and Wedgewood, R. J.: Rheumatic diseases. In Vaughn, V. C., and McKay, L. J., editors: Nelson's textbook of pediatrics, ed. 10, Philadelphia, 1975, W. B. Saunders Co.
25. Steigman, A. J.: Poliomyelitis. In Vaughn, V. C., and McKay, R. J., editors: Nelson's textbook of pediatrics, ed. 10, Philadelphia, 1975, W. B. Saunders Co.
26. Stewart, M. J.: Pediatric orthopedics. In Hughes, J. G.: Synopsis of pediatrics, ed. 4, St. Louis, 1975, The C. V. Mosby Co.
27. Whaley, L. F.: Understanding inherited disorders, St. Louis, 1974, The C. V. Mosby Co.
28. Ziter, F. A., and Allsop, K. G.: The diagnosis and management of childhood muscular dystrophy, Clin. Pediatr. **15:**540-548, 1976.

BIBLIOGRAPHY

Aegerter, E., and Kirkpatrick, J. A.: Orthopedic diseases, ed. 4, Philadelphia, 1975, W. B. Saunders Co.

Bellum, G.: The nursing challenge of the child with neurological problems, Nurs. Forum **11:**396, 1972.

Bleck, E. E., and Nagel, D. A., editors: Physically handicapped children, New York, 1975, Grune & Stratton, Inc.

Conway, B. L.: Carini and Owens' neurological and neurosurgical nursing, ed. 7, St. Louis, 1978, The C. V. Mosby Co.

Farmer, T. W., editor: Pediatric neurology, ed. 2, New York, 1975, Harper & Row, Publishers.

Frykman, G. K.: Peripheral nerve injuries in children, Orthop. Clin. North Am. **7:**701-716, 1976.

Hilt, N. E., and Schmitt, E. W., Jr.: Pediatric orthopedic nursing, St. Louis, 1975, The C. V. Mosby Co.

Kelsey, J. L., Keggi, K. J., and Southwick, W. O.: The incidence and distribution of slipped capitol femoral epiphysis in Connecticut and southwestern United States, J. Bone Joint Surg. **52-A:**1203-1216, 1970.

Kempe, C. H., Silver, H. K., and O'Brien, D., editors: Current pediatric diagnosis and treatment, ed. 3, Los Altos, Calif., 1974, Lange Medical Publications.

Larson, C. B., and Gould, M.: Orthopedic nursing, ed. 9, St. Louis, 1978, The C. V. Mosby Co.

Lichtenstein, L.: Diseases of bone and joints, ed. 2, St. Louis, 1975, The C. V. Mosby Co.

Low, N. L., and Downey, J. A.: Lower motor neuron diseases. In Downey, J. A., and Low, N. L., editors: The child with disabling illness, Philadelphia, 1974, W. B. Saunders Co.

Miles, J. S., and Solomons, C. C.: Bones and joints. In Kempe, C. H., Silver, H. K., and O'Brien, D., editors: Current pediatric diagnosis and treatment, Los Altos, Calif., 1974, Lange Medical Publications.

Moffat, H. L.: Pediatric infectious diseases, Philadelphia, 1975, J. B. Lippincott Co.

Schaller, J. G.: Arthritis and infections of bones and joints in children, Pediatr. Clin. North Am. **24:**775-790, 1977.

Sullivan, D. B.: Prognosis in childhood dermatomyositis, J. Pediatr. **80:**555, 1972.

Tachdjian, M.: Pediatric orthopedics, Philadelphia, 1972, W. B. Saunders Co.

Tilkian, S. M., and Conover, M. H.: Clinical implications of laboratory tests, St. Louis, 1975, The C. V. Mosby Co.

Wolfish, M. G., and McLean, J. A.: Chronic illness in adolescents, Pediatr. Clin. North Am. **21**:1043-1050, 1974.

Cerebral palsy

Bleck, E. E.: Locomotor prognosis in cerebral palsy, Dev. Med. Child Neurol. **17**:18, 1975.

Blockley, J., and Miller, G.: Feeding techniques with cerebral-palsied children, Physiotherapy **57**:300-308, 1971.

Bobath, B.: Motor development, its effect on general development and application to the treatment of cerebral palsy, Physiotherapy **57**:526-532, 1971.

Eggland, E. T.: Locus of control and children with cerebral palsy, Nurs. Res. **22**:329, 1973.

Hanson, R., Byers, B., and Berenberg, W.: Changing motor patterns in cerebral plasy, Dev. Med. Child Neurol. **12**:309, 1970.

Knapp, M. E.: Cerebral palsy I, Postgrad. Med. **47**:229-232, 1970.

Knapp, M. E.: Cerebral palsy II, Postgrad. Med. **47**:247-252, 1970.

Lepler, M.: Having a handicapped child, Am. J. Maternal Child Nurs. **3**(1):32-33, 1978.

Low, N. L., and Downey, J. A.: Cerebral palsy. In Downey, J. A., and Low, N. L., editors: The child with disabling illness, Philadelphia, 1974, W. B. Saunders Co.

Menkes, J. H.: Textbook of child neurology, Philadelphia, 1974, Lea & Febiger.

Mitchell, R. G.: The prevention of cerebral palsy, Dev. Med. Child Neurol. **13**:137, 1971.

Pothier, P. C.: Therapeutic handling of the severely handicapped child, Am. J. Nurs. **71**:321-324, 1971.

Robinson, R. O.: The frequency of other handicaps in children with cerebral palsy, Dev. Med. Child Neurol. **15**:305, 1973.

Shere, E. S.: Patterns of child rearing in cerebral palsy; effects upon the child's cognitive development, Pediatr. Digest **23**:28, 1971.

Wright, T., and Nicholson, J.: Physiotherapy for the spastic child: an evaluation, Dev. Med. Child Neurol. **15**:146, 1973.

Neuromuscular deficit

Bell, W. E., and McCormick, W. F.: Neurologic infections in children, Philadelphia, 1975, W. B. Saunders Co.

Glenn, J. D., and Karels, R. G., Sr.: Pediatric paralysis in Bogota, Am. J. Nurs. **73**:299-301, 1973.

Kealy, S. L.: Respiratory care in Guillain-Barré syndrome, Am. J. Nurs. **77**:58-60, 1977.

Kealy, S. L.: The patient with Guillain-Barré syndrome, Crit. Care Update **5**(1):5-12, 1978.

Masucci, E. F., and Kurtzke, J. F.: Diagnostic criteria for the Guillain-Barré syndrome, J. Neurol. Sci. **13**:483, 1971.

Murphy, E. G., and Waisburg, H.: Chronic peripheral neuromuscular disorders in childhood, Pediatr. Clin. North Am. **21**:917-926, 1974.

Nursing Grand Rounds: Coma: hope makes a difference in nursing care, Nursing '74 **4**(5):24-29, 1974.

Sibley, W. A.: Polyneuritis, Med. Clin. North Am. **56**:1299, 1972.

Siegel, I. M.: Charcot-Marie-Tooth disease: a diagnostic problem, J.A.M.A. **228**:873, 1974.

Stockhouse, J.: Myasthenia gravis, Am. J. Nurs. **23**:1544-1547, 1973.

Muscular dystrophies

Chutorian, A. M., and Myers, S. J.: Disease of muscle. In Downey, J. A., and Low, N. L., editors: The child with disabling illness, Philadelphia, 1974, W. B. Saunders Co.

Eyring, E. J., Johnson, E. W., and Burnett, C.: Surgery in muscular dystrophy, J.A.M.A. **222**:1056, 1972.

Guinter, R. H., Hernried, L. S., and Kaplan, A. M.: Infantile neurogenic muscular atrophy with prolonged survival, J. Pediatr. **90**:95-97, 1977.

Mearig, J. S.: Some dynamics of personality development in boys suffering from muscular dystrophy, Rehabil. Lit. **34**:226-228, 1973.

Murphy, E. G., and Waisburg, H.: Chronic peripheral neuromuscular disorders in childhood: principles of diagnosis and management, Pediatr. Clin. North Am. **21**:917, November 1974.

Taft, L. T.: The care and management of the child with muscular dystrophy, Dev. Med. Child Neurol. **15**:510, 1973.

Musculoskeletal disorders

Cantrell, D.: Osteogenesis imperfecta, Orthop. Nurs. Assoc, J. **3**:163, 1976.

Chung, S.: Disease of the developing hip joint, Pediatr. Clin. North Am. **24**:857-870, 1977.

Cordell, L. D.: Slipped capitol femoral epiphysis, Postgrad. Med. **60**(4):135-141, 1976.

Karadimas, J. E.: Conservative treatment of coxa plana: a comparison of the early results of different methods, J. Bone Joint Surg. **53B**:315-325, 1971.

Kelsey, J.: Epidemiology of slipped capitol femoral epiphysis: a review of the literature, Pediatrics **51**:1042-1049, 1973.

Rang, M. C., Rogers, L. F., and Zimmerman, R. C.: Growth plate injuries: treat or refer? Patient Care **10**(9):60-94, May 1, 1976.

Solomons, C. C., and Millar, E. A.: Osteogenesis imperfecta: new perspectives, Clin. Orthop. **96**:2, 1973.

Specht, E.: Epiphyseal injuries in childhood, Am. Fam. Physician **10**:102, 1974.

Scoliosis

Baker, E. A., and Zangger, B.: School screening for idiopathic scoliosis, Am. J. Nurs. **70**:766, 1970.

Barrett, M. J.: Surviving adolescence in a back brace: Laura's experience, Am. J. Maternal Child Nurs. **2**:160-163, May/June 1977.

Blount, W. P.: Use of the Milwaukee brace, Orthop. Clin. North Am. **3**:3, 1972.

Bowring, V. N.: Electro-spinal instrumentation: a new look at pediatric scoliosis, Orthop. Nurs. Assoc. J. **3**:172, 1976.

Cowell, H. R., Hall, J. H., and Mac Ewen, G. D.: Genetic aspects of idiopathic scoliosis, Clin. Orthop. **86**:121, 1972.

Dadich, K.: An eleven year old girl's use of control while immobilized in halo-femoral traction, Maternal-Child Nurs. J. **1**(1):67-74, 1972.

Harrington, P. R.: Technical details in relation to the successful use of instrumentation in scoliosis, Orthop. Clin. North Am. **3:**49-68, 1972.

Hill, P. M., and Romm, L. S.: Screening for scoliosis in adolescents, Am. J. Maternal Child Nurs. **2:**156-159, May/June 1977.

Holhne, D.: The child with scoliosis: nursing intervention. In Steele, S., editor: Nursing care of the child with long-term illness, New York, 1971, Appleton-Century-Crofts.

Hungerford, D. S.: Spinal deformity in adolescence: early detection and nonoperative management, Med. Clin. North Am. **59:** 1517-1526, 1975.

Katz, J. F.: Scoliosis. In Downey, J. A., and Low, N. L., editors: The child with disabling illness, Philadelphia, 1974, W. B. Saunders Co.

Keim, H.: Scoliosis, Clin. Symp. **24**(1):1-32, 1972.

Mol, J. H.: Methods of correction and surgical techniques in scoliosis, Orthop. Clin. North Am. **3:**17-48, 1972.

Neff, J. A.: Feminine identity concerns of girls undergoing correction for scoliosis, Maternal-Child Nurs. J. **1**(1):9-18, 1972.

Perry, J.: The halo in spinal abnormalities: practical factors and avoidance of complications, Orthop. Clin. North Am. **3:**69-80, 1972.

Raynolds, N.: Teaching parents home care after surgery for scoliosis, Am. J. Nurs. **74:**1090-1092, 1974.

Rodriguez, W., and associates: Clindamycin in the treatment of osteomyelitis in children, Am. J. Dis. Child **131:**1088-1093, 1977.

Seigil, C.: Current concepts in the management of scoliosis, Nurs. Clin. North Am. **11:**691-698, 1976.

Sells, C. J., and May, E. A.: Scoliosis screening in public schools, Am. J. Nurs. **74:**60-62, 1974.

Shifrin, L. Z.: Scoliosis: current concepts, Clin. Pediatr. **11:** 594, 1972.

Strong, C., and Gavaghan, M.: Scoliosis and its implications, Issues Comprehensive Pediatr. Nurs. **2**(4):33-45, 1977.

Weiler, D. R.: Scoliosis screening, J. Sch. Health **44:**563, 1974.

Wilson, R.: The MUD bed and its implications for nursing care, Nurs. Clin. North Am. **11:**725-730, 1976.

Osteomyelitis

Boland, A. L., Jr.: Acute hematogenous osteomyelitis, Orthop. Clin. North Am. **3:**225-240, 1972.

Chung, S. M. K., and Pollis, R. E.: Diagnostic pitfalls in septic arthritis of the hip in infants and children, Clin. Pediatr. **14:** 758-767, 1975.

Curtiss, P. H., Jr.: The pathophysiology of joint infections, Clin. Orthop. **96:**129, 1973.

Ferguson, A. B., Jr.: Acute and chronic osteomyelitis: osteomyelitis in children, Clin. Orthop. **96:**51, 1973.

Gledhill, R. B.: Subacute osteomyelitis in children, Clin. Orthop. **96:**27, 1973.

Morrey, B. F., and Peterson, H. A.: Hematogenous pyogenic osteomyelitis in children, Orthop. Clin. North Am. **6:**935-951, 1975.

Morrey, B. F., Bianco, A. J., and Rhodes, K. H.: Septic arthritis in children, Orthop. Clin. North Am. **6:**923-934, 1975.

Nelson, J. D.: The bacterial etiology and antibiotic management of septic arthritis in infants and children, Pediatrics **50:**437, 1972.

Nelson, J. D., and Haltalin, K. C.: Septic arthritis. In Shirkey, H. C., editor: Pediatric therapy, ed. 5, St. Louis, 1975, The C. V. Mosby Co.

Rhodes, K. H.: Antibiotic management of acute osteomyelitis and septic arthritis in children, Orthop. Clin. North Am. **6:**915-921, 1975.

Weissberg, E. D., Smith, A. L., and Smith, D. H.: Clinical features of neonatal osteomyelitis, Pediatrics **53:**505, 1974.

Juvenile rheumatoid arthritis

Ansell, B.: Rheumatoid arthritis—medical management, Nurs. Mir. **133**(11):20-23, 1971.

Baden, A. M.: Children with arthritis: some everyday help, Nursing '73 **3**(12):22-24, 1973.

Brewer, E. J., Jr.: Juvenile rheumatoid arthritis, Philadelphia, 1970, W. B. Saunders Co.

Calabro, J. J.: Management of juvenile rheumatoid arthritis, J. Pediatr. **77:**355-365, 1970.

Calabro, J. J.: The three faces of juvenile rheumatoid arthritis, Hosp. Pract. **9**(2):61-68, 1974.

Grossman, B. J., and Mukhopadhyay, D.: Juvenile rheumatoid arthritis, Curr. Probl. Pediatr. **5**(12):3-65, October 1975.

Hymovich, D. P.: Bobby—a very difficult little boy, Nursing '73 **3**(2):44-45, 1973.

Kornreich, H., Koster, K., and Hanson, V.: The rheumatic disease in adolescence, Pediatr. Clin. North Am. **20:**911-932, 1973.

Lindsley, C. B.: The child with arthritis, Issues Comprehensive Pediatr. Nurs. **2**(4):23-32, 1977.

Millender, L. H., and Sledge, C. B., editors: Symposium on rheumatoid arthritis, Foreword, Orthop. Clin. North Am. **6**(3):601-602, July 1975.

Pendleton, T., and associates: Rehabilitating children with inflammatory joint diseases, Am. J. Nurs. **74:**2223-2226, 1974.

Schaller, J., and Wedgewood, R.: Juvenile rheumatoid arthritis: a review, Pediatrics **50:**940-953, 1972.

Schubert, W. K.: Collagen diseases. In Shirkey, H. C., editor: Pediatric therapy, ed. 5, St. Louis, 1975, The C. V. Mosby Co.

Sills, E. M.: Juvenile rheumatoid arthritis and systemic lupus erythematosus in the adolescent, Med. Clin. North Am. **59:** 1497-1506, 1975.

40

The child immobilized with a traumatic injury

Traumatic injuries are common in childhood. Most are relatively minor and cause little disruption in the daily life of the child and produce only minor discomfort. However, accidents are the leading cause of death in the pediatric age-group. Every year thousands of children die and many thousands more are permanently disabled as a result of trauma. Some injuries, such as those involving the musculoskeletal system, heal in a short period of time, whereas others, such as fractured femurs and spinal cord injuries, require long-term care and a rehabilitative team approach throughout the acute and restorative stages of the child's care.

Immobilization is a major therapy for injuries to soft tissues, long bones, ligaments, vertebrae, and joints. Restriction of motion for a period of time at the site at which muscle or bone integrity has been disrupted allows tissue and bone to heal. However, prolonged immobilization, whether for therapy or because of disability, can produce severe complications, many of which are preventable. The nurse's awareness and implementation of appropriate actions during this restrictive state can significantly reduce the adverse effects of immobilization. Therefore, nursing care plans must focus not only on tissue and bone healing but also on regaining functional use of the injured part to the greatest extent possible.

This chapter is concerned with the common types of musculoskeletal traumas of childhood, their complications, and nursing responsibilities. The related problems of multiple trauma, which include cardiovascular and pulmonary collapse, rupture of internal organs, and head injury, although frequently associated with trauma, will not be included in this chapter. The last section of this chapter will deal with the complex problems of spinal cord pathology, focusing primarily on the teenager with a spinal injury.

IMMOBILIZED CHILD

One of the most difficult aspects of illness is the immobility it often imposes on a child. The child's natural tendency to be mobile influences all the elements of growth and development—physical, social, psychologic, and emotional. It is also an important means for expression and for dealing with anxiety and frustration. For these reasons children are immobilized only when necessary and for the shortest time possible.

Etiology of immobilization

The usual reason for immobilizing or restricting the activity of a child is illness or injury. Bed rest or mechanical restraining devices are frequently prescribed to aid in the healing and restorative processes. When children are ill they are content to remain quiet, and most of them instinctively reduce their activity. It is children who are forced to remain inactive because of physical limitations or therapy who display the multiple effects of restricted movement. The most frequent reasons for immobility are congenital defects (such as spina bifida), degenerative disorders (such as muscular dystrophy), and infections or accidents that impair the integumentary (severe burns), musculoskeletal (fractures or osteomyelitis), or neurologic systems (spinal cord injury, poliomyelitis, polyneuritis, head injury, and so on). Sometimes therapies, such as traction and spinal fusion, are responsible for prolonged immobilization.

Physiologic effects of immobilization

Although the bulk of information about the effects of immobility has been obtained from studies on adults, it is assumed that similar results occur in children. Many clinical studies, including space program research, have documented predictable consequences that occur following immobilization and the absence of gravitational force. Functional and metabolic responses to restricted movement can be noted in most of the body systems, all of which have a direct influence on the child's growth and development, since homeostatic mechanisms thrive on normal use and need feedback to maintain dynamic equilibrium. Inactivity leads to a decrease in the functional capabilities of the whole body as dramatically as the lack of physical exercise leads to muscle weakness.

Most of the pathologic changes that take place during immobilization arise from decreased muscle strength and mass, decreased metabolism, and bone demineralization, which are closely interrelated with one change leading to or affecting another. Some results of immobilization are primary and produce a direct effect; other pathophysiologic consequences occur frequently but seem to be more indirect and are, therefore, secondary effects. Many pathophysiologic changes affect more than one body system, with the primary or secondary effect being demonstrated in both systems.

Children who are confined to bed during a disease process or who are immobilized with an injury are usually restricted in movement for a relatively short time or are sufficiently active to avoid the physical consequences of immobility. Most physical and biologic effects of immobilization are the result of complete immobility, usually as a result of paralysis caused by trauma to the brain or spinal cord or nervous system infection such as poliomyelitis, encephalitis, or polyneuritis. Partial paralysis or weakness may be caused by birth defects (usually myelomeningocele), trauma, infection, or degenerative disease such as muscular dystrophy or muscular atrophy.

The major effects of immobilization (Fig. 40-1) are related directly or indirectly to decreased muscle activity, which produces numerous primary changes in both muscular and bone structures with secondary alterations in the cardiovascular, respiratory, metabolic, and renal systems. The major consequences are:

Significant loss of muscle strength, endurance, and muscle mass (atrophy)
Bone demineralization leading to osteoporosis
Loss of joint mobility and contractures

The larger the portion of the body immobilized and the longer the immobilization, the greater the hazards of immobility.

Muscular system. Inactive muscle loses strength at the rate of 3% per day and, in cases without primary neuromuscular deficit, sometimes requires several weeks or months to regain function. A stretching can occur as muscle loses its tone or as excessive strain is put on weakened muscle, for example, stretching by tight covers or poor body position that produces wristdrop or footdrop seen in debilitated children. The disuse leads to tissue breakdown and loss of the muscle mass (atrophy). The chief intracellular muscle enzyme, creatine, is released into the serum as the muscle atrophies; therefore, serum levels provide an indication of the amount of muscle mass undergoing degeneration. Inactive muscle also affects the cardiovascular system by decreasing venous return and cardiac output.[15,19,31]

Skeletal system. The daily stresses on bone created by motion and weight bearing maintain the balance between bone formation (osteoblastic activity) and bone resorption (osteoclastic activity). When these stresses are diminished, bone formation ceases, whereas the bone destruction continues, thus disrupting the state of equilibrium. Calcium becomes severely depleted, and there is increased secretion of phosphorus and nitrogen. This demineralization of the bone (osteoporosis) makes the skeletal structures prone to pathologic fractures.

In children who are unable to move, such as the child who is unconscious or paralyzed or the child with rheumatoid arthritis, joint mobility becomes restricted, because, in the absence of normal structural stretching, collagen fibers

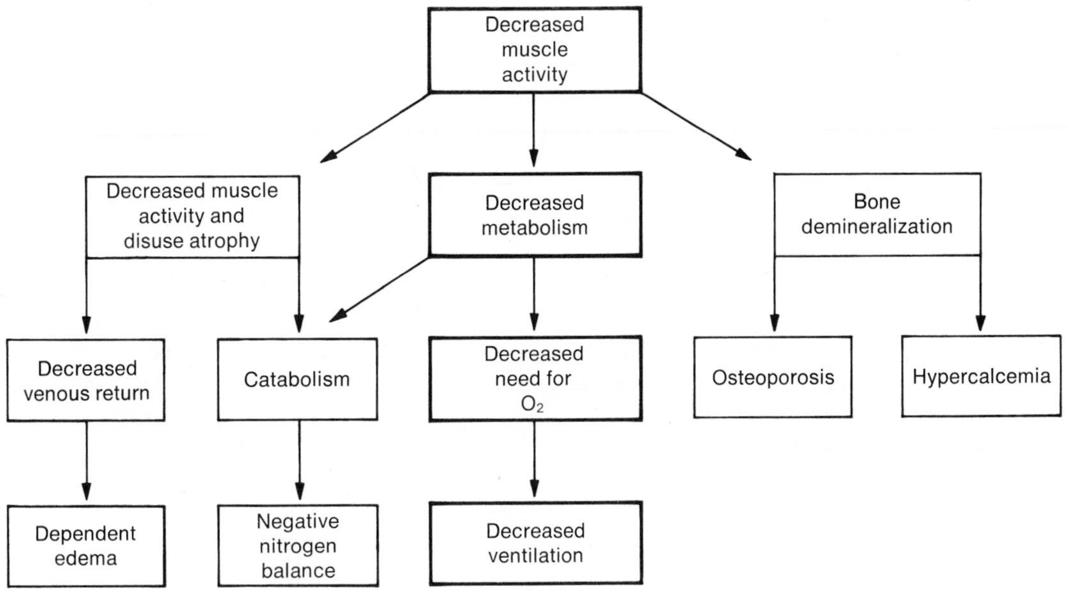

Fig. 40-1. Effects of immobilization.

generating within the joint become fibrotic and further limit movement. This tissue fibrosis creates a shortening of the muscles and a contracture of the joint. Any decrease in circulation to the joint by edema, inflammation, or restrictive positioning will contribute to further fibrotic changes. The problem rapidly becomes cyclic as the contracture leads to muscle fatigue and pain, which causes the child to splint the site, thus leading to more fibrosis. This process is further exaggerated because body flexor muscles are stronger than the extensor muscles, and, unless range of motion is instituted within 3 to 7 days, contractures will develop. Frequent disabling contractures are hip flexion, knee flexion, shoulder stiffness, and plantar flexion of the feet.

Cardiovascular system. There are three major cardiovascular consequences of immobility: orthostatic hypotension, increased workload of the heart, and thrombus formation. During movement muscle contraction causes pressure on peripheral veins, which, in turn, causes the venous valves to close, thus assisting return of the blood to the heart when the individual is in an upright position.[19,31] In the absence of this assistance blood tends to pool in the dependent areas, reducing the blood supply to trunk and brain. Also, direct reflex stimulation to the splanchnic and peripheral vessels causes them to constrict when a person is upright. Impairment of this neurovascular orthostatic reflex activity from lack of motion causes further interference with venous return. The individual displays signs of excessive autonomic activity, that is, pallor, sweating, and restlessness that is frequently followed by fainting. The child with a spinal cord injury has unique problems with orthostatic hypotension, which will be discussed later in this chapter.[19,31]

Changes in vascular resistance caused by the horizontal position and immobility alter the distribution of blood within the body. The reduction in gravity pressure to the extremities causes much of the total blood volume to be redistributed from the lower extremities to other parts of the body. Consequently there is an increase in the venous return and the volume of blood to be handled by the heart. Therefore, the cardiac output and stroke volume are increased as well as a progressive increase in heart rate. When immobilization extends over a period of time, there is a compensatory decrease in blood volume and a decrease in heart rate.

Without muscle contraction the venous stasis and increased intravascular pressure in the extremities lead to dependent edema. If undue pressure is exerted on the major veins by positioning or mechanical devices, the likelihood of interstitial edema is increased. Most frequently this situation is seen when the child is placed on his side with one leg resting on the other or when the youngster is permitted to sit for a long time with pressure on the large veins behind the knee and in the groin. Edematous tissue is prone to infection and trauma, especially tissue located over an area that receives much of the body's weight.

Circulatory stasis combined with hypercoagulability of the blood resulting from factors such as increased serum calcium or damage to the inner walls of blood vessels by trauma or infection can lead to thrombus and embolus formation. Bed rest alone will not produce the blood-clotting problems, but debilitated persons often have one or more of these other contributing factors. Sudden chest pain and dyspnea, the symptoms of pulmonary edema, or pain and swelling in the lower extremities, which indicates deep vein thrombosis, are constant concerns of the nurse.

The deconditioned state of cardiac function, caused by skeletal muscle inactivity, can produce a variety of secondary problems in other systems. However, the major clinical manifestation is increased pulse and heart rate in response to an active exercise program. After prolonged immobility the child should build up his activity tolerance slowly to allow the heart to regain its optimal capabilities.

Respiratory system. Initially the effects of immobilization are compensatory or adaptive. The basal metabolic rate is decreased, since, with reduced expenditure of energy, the cells require less oxygen and produce less carbon dioxide. Lessened demand for oxygen–carbon dioxide exchange causes the respirations to become slower and more shallow. Chest expansion may be limited by the supine posture; by abdominal distention caused by accumulation of feces, gas, or fluid; and by mechanical restriction such as a body cast, brace, or tight binders. Reduced muscle power and coordination secondary to altered innervation can also hinder respiratory movement. More effort is required to expand the lungs in the supine position.

Prolonged immobility also reduces the normal movement of secretions from the tracheobronchial tree, particularly in the presence of impaired muscle function and positional changes that facilitate their removal. A weak and ineffectual cough reflex contributes to stasis of secretions and the possibility of airway obstruction. Shallow respirations and obstruction of the airway with thick mucus contribute to the development of secondary complications such as atelectasis, hypostatic pneumonia, and respiratory acidosis.

Gastrointestinal system. Prolonged immobility produces a state of negative nitrogen balance resulting from the increased catabolic activity related to muscle atrophy. This and the reduced energy requirements contribute to a diminished appetite and a resulting decrease in ingestion of nutrients. The mechanisms of eating and feeding become more difficult with immobility, and the risk of aspiration is increased. Intake is further influenced by associated psychologic factors.

The process of elimination depends on the integration of smooth and skeletal muscle activity and on visceral reflex patterns. Immobility may interfere with these mechanisms as well as the gravitational effect on stool passing through the intestines. Slowing of stool in the colon causes the feces to become hard, and the bowel wall is not stimulated to further its peristaltic movement down the tract to the rectum. Weakened muscles used in defecation (diaphragmatic and abdominal muscles) decrease intra-abdominal pressure needed for elimination. Sometimes embarrassment in using the bedpan may be the cause of not responding to the urge to defecate.

Urinary system. The structure of the urinary system is designed to function in an upright posture. When the gravitational force is altered by the reclining position, the peristaltic contractions of the ureters are insufficient to overcome gravitational resistance. Consequently there may be stasis of urine in the kidney pelves, and any particulate matter that settles in the calyces may serve as nuclei for calculi formation or as foci for infection.[15]

In the horizontal position the individual has difficulty in relaxing the perineal musculature and external sphincter sufficiently to initiate the integrated reflex micturition mechanism that involves the external sphincter, the internal sphincter, and the detrusor muscle of the bladder wall. If adequate intra-abdominal pressure is exerted, voiding can occur, but, if the individual does not respond to the sensation to void, bladder distention leads to stasis and its complications add to overflow incontinence, a source of embarrassment. In time reflex and back pressure may impair renal function, and urinary tract infection is always a hazard with urine retention.

Normally the kidney is able to handle the increased metabolites from protein breakdown and bone demineralization. However, the increased level of calcium excreted may predispose to the formation of calculi. Calculi formation is further favored by urinary stasis, infection, and an alkaline urine caused by the decreased production of the acid by-products of metabolism.

Metabolism.[17,19] Immobility or severe restriction of activity is often accompanied by decreased or inappropriate nutritional intake that often leads to decreased basal metabolic rate, a negative nitrogen balance associated with catabolism, and a high-calcium serum level.

All body systems are influenced by a decrease in metabolism. The altered energy level leads to further fatigue and lack of motivation for moving. Although less of a problem in children, immobilized persons often feel sluggish and have a poor appetite, particularly for protein foods. The protein breakdown in the body related to a loss of muscle and other tissues is more apt to be severe after injury or surgery. Protein breakdown produces nitrogenous wastes, and, on the fifth or sixth day of catabolic protein metabolism, an increase in urinary nitrogen appears that contributes to delayed healing and anemia.

Another metabolic problem is hypercalcemia associated with bone catabolism.[37] Completely immobilized youngsters are especially prone to hypercalcemia. Symptoms include nausea and vomiting, polydipsia, polyuria, and lethargy that usually appears 4 to 8 weeks after immobilization. In quadriplegia it may occur within 10 days and last for as long as 6 months. The accelerated rates of bone metabolism in youngsters make the bone demineralization a greater hazard. Larger amounts of calcium are released into the blood than the kidney can excrete, and calcium continues to accumulate in the serum. High levels of serum calcium decrease neuronal permeability that can lead to a depression of the central and peripheral nervous systems. Symptoms including smooth and skeletal muscle fatigue, diminished reflexes, and atony of the gastrointestinal tract are the result of the depressed nervous system.[37]

Medical treatment for hypercalcemia consists of restricting dietary calcium, increasing weight bearing where this is possible, and, most importantly, vigorous hydration (for example, 3000 to 4000 ml/day for a teenager). Electrolyte imbalances are corrected, and diuretics are administered to promote removal of calcium. Sometimes pharmacologic agents, such as corticosteroids, oral phosphates, and thyrocalcitonin, may be used to lower serum calcium levels. Any urinary tract infection is treated.

A child with bone demineralization may not develop hypercalcemia, but the excess amount of calcium that his kidneys are required to excrete may produce a negative calcium balance with more calcium than citric acid lost in the urine. This imbalance causes the urine to become alkaline with the potential danger of renal calculi, especially if there is an accompanying retention of urine.

Integumentary system.[20,28] Circulation to the skin is reduced during inactivity and may be further impeded by dependent edema. Circulation is especially compromised in places where the bone surface is near the skin, such as areas over the sacrum, occiput, trochanter, and ankle, and continued impairment causes rapid necrosis with ulcer formation. Mechanical irritation from appliances, such as straps, rods, ropes, and so on, and the friction of bedclothes during turning or other movement can produce skin breakdown. Healing capacity is also impaired by the poor circulation, negative nitrogen balance, and anemia. Immobilization often makes it difficult to carry out adequate cleansing and hygienic measures, which may also contribute to tissue breakdown in areas that are difficult to reach. Children with neurologic deficit should be guarded against extremes of heat and cold in direct contact with the skin.

Cellular breakdown caused by prolonged pressure can be identified by several characteristics. Normally, when pressure is applied to the skin, the skin appears pale but becomes very red, or hyperemic, after pressure is removed. This reactive hyperemia should disappear within 5 to 15 minutes. Prolonged redness (over 30 minutes) indicates that a pressure area is developing, and treatment should be instituted. Other manifestations of tissue ischemia include an increase in temperature in the area, blistering, swelling, or dark purple or black areas. The pressure area may be limited to the skin and subcutaneous layers or may be deeper and more extensive. The skin changes observed may represent the top of a cone-shaped area with widespread tissue destruction, beneath which tissue rapidly ulcerates and creates a large hole that sometimes extends to the bone. The skin may be broken or even accompanied by a purulent drainage. Fig. 40-2 illustrates the sequence of events in tissue breakdown.

Neurosensory system. Studies indicate that immobilization does not produce neurosensory consequences directly; however, two occurrences—loss of innervation and sensory and perceptual deprivation—are common.

Peripheral nerves, in contrast to skeletal muscles, do not degenerate with disuse, but loss of innervation takes place if nerves are damaged by pressure or if their blood supply is disrupted. Improper body positioning or poorly applied casts or restraints can place unwarranted pressure on nerves and blood vessels that can lead to ischemia and nerve degeneration. Frequent sites of this compression phenomenon are pressure on the peroneal nerve, resulting in footdrop or on the radial nerve, leading to wristdrop. These complications significantly interfere with attempts to regain functional use of extremities, but they can be prevented by conscientious nursing assessment and intervention. Preventing pressure on vulnerable areas and preventing unnatural positions of flexion and extension that apply inappropriate pressure on nerves and blood vessels reduce the likelihood of compression injury. Periodic plantar flexion and dorsiflexion of the feet and hands will stimulate circulation and keep nerves from becoming pinched. Numbness and tingling are symptoms of neurologic impairment and should be evaluated immediately.

Psychologic effects of immobilization

For children one of the most difficult aspects of illness is immobilization. Throughout childhood physical activity is an integral part of daily life and is essential for physical growth and development. It also serves children as an instrument for communication and expression and as a means for learning about and understanding their world. It helps them deal with a variety of feelings and impulses and provides a mechanism by which they can exert control over inner tensions. Children respond to anxiety with increased activity. Removal of this power deprives them of necessary input and a natural outlet for their feelings and fantasies. Through movement children also gain sensory input that provides an essential element for developing and maintaining a body image.[4,8,27]

In daily life children's activity is restricted in many ways: limits are set on behavior and expression, activity is restricted by physical and verbal barriers, and neuromuscular function is affected directly by disease or injury. The child perceives restraint by persons or inanimate objects as either comforting or stressful. Adult controls on behavior often provide the child with a sense of security in frightening situations or when he fears loss of control. On the other hand, forced inactivity deprives him of one of his most valuable means for dealing with stress. A child who is confined to bed may become a victim of his fears and fantasies without the physical means for stress reduction. Sometimes a child will impose restrictions on himself, particularly in

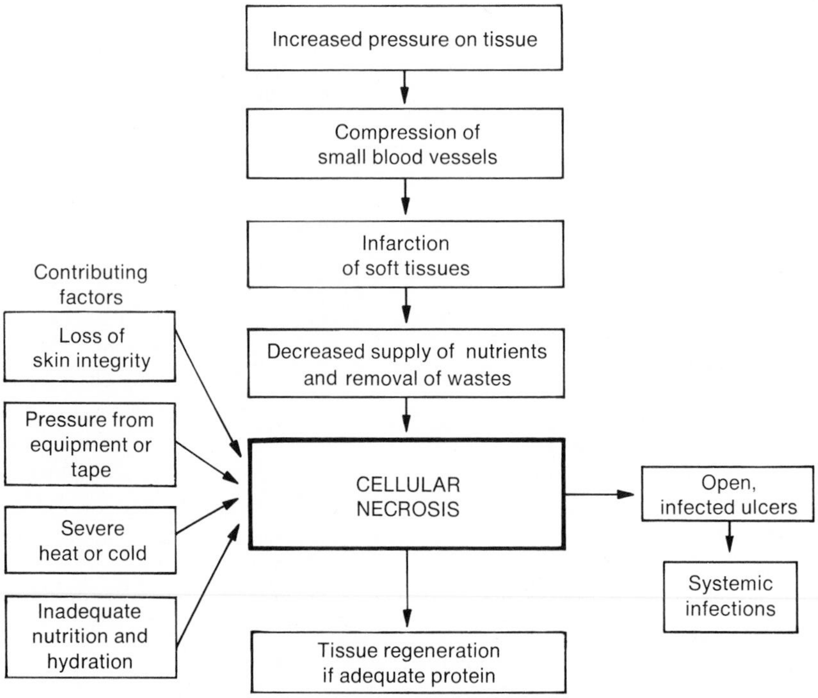

Fig. 40-2. Sequence of events in tissue breakdown.

interaction with others, by confining himself to his bed with blankets pulled about him or by retreating into sleep in the presence of stimulation.[23]

The active child has many opportunities for input from a wide variety of settings. When he is immobilized by disease or as a part of a treatment regimen, he experiences diminished environmental stimuli with a loss of tactile input and an altered perception of himself and his environment. Sudden or gradual immobilization narrows the amount and variety of environmental stimuli he receives by means of all of his senses: touch, sight, hearing, taste, smell, and proprioception—a feeling of where he is in his environment. This sensory deprivation frequently leads to a feeling of isolation, boredom, and being forgotten, especially by his peers.

Sensorimotor activity is a predominant mode of activity in infants; even newborn infants respond with rage when they are physically restrained. Physical interference with the activity of infants and young children gives them a feeling of helplessness. It has also been found that speech and language skills require sensorimotor activity and experience. There appears to be a significant relationship between physical restraint and the incidence of language problems. Children who are restrained by casts, splints, or straps during the first 3 years of life have more difficulty with language than children whose activities remain unrestricted. Language delay is even more marked in children with neurologic impairment.[29]

Observations of children's behavior during restraint indicate some differences between infants and older children. Initially infants temporarily freed from physical restraint remain immobile and then submit without protest to restoration of restraint. However, with subsequent release, their activity level progressively increases as does their protesting behavior after reapplication of restraints. In contrast toddlers and preschool children show a decrease in protest with each subsequent removal and restoration of restraint. It is uncertain whether this diminished protest in these children reflects inhibitions developed as a result of frustration or a development of trust that the nurse will return to release the restraint.[8]

The struggle for independence is thwarted by imposed immobility. For the toddler, exploration and imitative behaviors are essential to developing a sense of autonomy; the preschooler's expression of initiative is evidenced by his penchant for vigorous physical activity; the school-age child's development is strongly influenced by physical achievement and competition; and the adolescent relies on mobility to achieve independence. The quest for mastery at every stage of development is related to mobility. To the child the inability to move is threatening to self-preservation and reactivates the struggle between activity and passivity and between dependence and independence. "To move is to be *alive;* to be still is to be dead."[4,9]

Behavioral changes are noted when a child experiences prolonged sensory deprivation. These behaviors are demonstrated by a higher than normal level of anxiety: restlessness, difficulty in problem solving, inability to concentrate on activities, and egocentrism. The monotony of the situation can lead to sluggish intellectual and psychomotor responses, decreased communication skill, increased fantasizing, and even hallucinations and disorientation. The child is likely to become depressed over his loss of ability to function or the marked changes in his body image. His significant others are apt to notice regressive behavior and a greater reliance on them for tasks he is able to perform as he seeks their attention by reverting to earlier developmental behaviors, such as wanting to be fed, bed-wetting, and baby talk. In many ways the immobilized child is realistically dependent on others; therefore, intelligent and sensitive care is required to prevent major growth and developmental regressions during the period of immobility.

Limbs in casts or traction transmit less than normal sensory data. The presence of sensory impairment may be a concomitant problem of the involved part. Numbness or loss of feeling markedly alters proprioception. A child who has limited ability to feel others touching him not only experiences less tactile stimuli in a physical sense but is also deprived of warm, loving feelings that arise from being touched. The loss of feeling derived from touch can further add to his sense of being isolated and unwanted.

The type and extent of immobilization influence the emotional response. When children are able to see the reason for their restraint (such as a cast or intravenous infusion) they are less likely to be resistant. The child whose activity is restricted because of a nonvisible disorder (such as rheumatic fever) finds it difficult to understand the reason for adult restrictions on activity, imagines the worst, and may react with noncompliance and overactivity when unobserved. Children may react to immobility by active protest, anger, and aggressive behavior, or they may become quiet, passive, and submissive. Often the child believes that the immobilization is a justified punishment for misbehavior. Children should be allowed to discharge their anger, but it should be within the limits of safety to their self-esteem and not damaging to the integrity of others. For example, providing an object to attack rather than a person or a valued possession is safe and therapeutic.

Unfortunately most adults resent and find it difficult to deal with the acting-out behavior of children. Too often this behavior is considered "bad" even when it is obviously a release of tension. In some cases, such as the paralyzed child, nurses may feel inadequate to cope with the child's profound distress and feelings of hopelessness, and the professional help of a psychologist or psychiatrist is needed.

The most difficult situations are those involving major injuries and diseases that produce a disfigurement or a severe loss of function that directly affects a child's self-image, such as burns, amputation, or the sudden catastrophic effects of an accident that leaves a healthy, athletic child paralyzed for life. Feelings of anger and hostility are difficult for the child to express when he is at the mercy of his environment. He dares not speak out against or defy the authorities on whom he depends so completely. Consequently his aggression may be masked by cheerfulness or rigidity. When he is unable to express his anger, the aggression is often displayed inappropriately in regressive behavior and outbursts of crying or temper tantrums over insignificant irritations, such as warm milk, a wrinkled collar, or a delay in routine.[9]

Effect on families. Brief periods of immobilization have few effects on the family; however, catastrophic illness or disability severely taxes the resources of the family. In general emotionally mature families with financial resources and satisfactory problem-solving skills handle the crises well. Their needs are often very specific, primarily in the areas of instruction concerning medical and nursing care, community resources to contact, and emotional support as they go through the grief process. However, many families are unstable, are already plagued by unmet needs, operate from crisis to crisis, and are often unable to use outside help appropriately. For these families the new situation can disrupt the entire family; therefore, the rehabilitation team must help the family members identify unmet needs and problems and actively help in the family's problem-solving process. Commonly occurring problems are[24]:

1. Financial strains that may decrease or totally eliminate the family's resources.
2. The focus of attention is placed, at least temporarily, on the affected member; therefore, other members of the family may feel neglected or their needs may not be met.
3. The family may have difficulty in accepting the child's altered body image.
4. Individual family members may be unable to express their feelings and become immobilized in the face of the crisis.

The family's needs can often be met by the physician and nurse but may also require the services of other professionals, such as a social worker, psychiatrist, or marriage counselor. In preparation for discharge, home visits are advisable and home management is frequently planned weeks in advance of the actual discharge, including special considerations for economic, physical, and psychologic needs. A severely disabled child is very dependent, and care givers need rest periods to revitalize themselves. Individual and group counseling are very beneficial for pre-problem-solving situations and providing an emotional support system. Parent groups are also helpful and often provide nonthreatening social contact. The families of permanently handicapped children need long-term resources, since some of the most difficult problems arise as they try to sustain high-quality care for many years (see Chapter 22).

Nursing considerations

The effects of immobilization can be minimized and, in many cases, prevented by conscientious nursing care. The major goals in care of the immobilized child are to prevent the pathophysiologies associated with immobility and to utilize measures for regaining function and remobilization within the limitations of the therapeutic regimen or the physical disabilities of the child.

Frequent position changes help to prevent dependent edema and fluid movement and to stimulate circulation, respiratory function, gastrointestinal motility, and neurologic sensations. When the child's condition allows, periodically assuming the upright position on a tilt table or similar device stimulates gastrointestinal and renal function and increases the stress on bones.

Each metabolic disturbance is treated specifically. Metabolism is increased by activity within the limitations of the disability and capabilities of the child. High-protein, high-calorie foods are encouraged for correction of negative nitrogen balance. This may be difficult to correct by diet, especially if anorexia is present. Stimulating the appetite with small servings of attractively arranged preferred foods may be sufficient. Sometimes supplementary nasogastric feedings or hyperalimentation may be needed.

Diet modification for the child with increased serum calcium presents problems, since the diary foods that children often desire are high in this mineral. Acid ash foods, such as cereals, meats, poultry, fish, and cranberry juice are encouraged. Lying in a prone position may precipitate problems with swallowing or self-feeding. Therefore, offering small bites, controlling swallowing with semi-solid food, and using a straw for fluids are nursing behaviors that will prevent choking. A suction machine should be in the vicinity for emergencies. The primary nursing measure for hypercalcemia is conscientious hydration and active remobilization as soon as possible.

Adequate hydration promotes bowel and kidney function and helps prevent complications in these systems. A knowledge of the child's previous bowel habits and determining a way to get him up to a commode helps promote elimination and will be valuable data if needed for a bowel program. Embarrassment can be avoided by a mutually satisfactory communication system. Whenever possible, the child should be helped into a sitting position so that he can use a fracture urinal or bedpan. Providing privacy for toileting and encouraging the child to participate in solving toileting problems will increase the chances of a successful program.

Children should be encouraged to be as active as their condition and restrictive devices allow. This poses few problems in children, whose innate ingenuity and natural inclination toward mobility provide them with the impetus for physical activity. They need the opportunity, the materials or objects to stimulate activity, and the encouragement and participation of others. Those who are unable to move will need passive exercise and movement.

Whenever possible, transporting the child by stretcher, stroller, or wagon from the confines of his room will increase environmental stimuli and provide social contact with others. While hospitalized, frequent visitors, clocks and calendars, and a program of diversional therapy will help the child to function in a more normal way. As soon as possible he should wear ''street clothes'' and resume school and preinjury hobbies. Play is the most useful tool of nursing (p. 947), and activities, which are selected on the basis of interest, ability, and limitations, should include some form of physical activity that encourages the use of uninvolved muscles and joints. Any activity that is tolerated, even turning in bed or changing the position of a bed in the room, helps to alter the monotony of immobilization and dissipate tension and frustration.

Using dolls to illustrate and explain the restraining method is a valuable tool for small children. Placing a cast, tubing, or other restraining equipment on the doll offers the child a nonthreatening opportunity to express, through the doll, his feelings concerning the restrictions and the nurse and provides a means for anticipatory teaching and explanation of needed restraining devices.

One of the most useful interventions to help children cope with immobility is participation in their own care. Self-care to the maximum extent is usually well received by most children. They can help plan their daily routine, select their diet (where possible), and choose the clothes they are to wear, including innovative adornment, such as a baseball cap, brightly colored stockings, or other items of apparel that express each child's autonomy and individuality. They should be encouraged to do as much for themselves as they are able in order to keep muscles active and their interest alive. Where possible, they should be placed where they can benefit from the company of other children who are immobilized to assure them that they are not singled out for this treatment.

It is important for the child to understand behavioral limitations or rules, and his questions should be answered. For example, he needs to know the reasons for medical, nursing, occupational, and physical therapy and to know that schedules are necessary. In some areas he has a choice; in others he does not. He may or may not be permitted to sleep late, but he can choose his own clothing. A major part of a child's activity of daily living is play; therefore, therapies that incorporate this concept as much as possible are more apt to gain his cooperation.

Visits from significant persons, such as family and friends, offer occasions for emotional support and also provide opportunities for learning the child's care. A severely disabled child's needs can be very complex, and family members require time to assimilate the teachings and demonstrations that are needed to understand his situation and care.

Some privacy is needed, particularly by the teenager, and most long-term health care facilities recognize that rooms shared by two to four youngsters are better environments for habilitation or rehabilitation. When roommates are selected according to age and companionship, a chance is available to safely test out thoughts and feelings with others. If a traumatic incident caused the child's disability, guilt feelings may be displayed overtly or masked behind regressive or aggressive behavior. The feeling that, ''I must have been bad'' to receive this fate is common, and honest feedback stating, ''It just happened—it was an accident'' needs repeating many times. Additional aspects of grieving are involved if there was a loss of another in the accident. All of these feelings need to be brought out and dealt with. In addition, professional persons working with the severely disabled child must not baby or overprotect him but help him to cope with the altered body image and reestablish his self-esteem.

For a child with markedly restricted movement, for example, the quadriplegic child or the child with a large bilateral hip spica cast, nursing care is a challenge. These situations require long-term care either in the hospital or at home, but, wherever the care occurs, consistent planning and coordinating of activities with professionals and significant others are vital. Nursing assessment includes psychosocial data as well as physical manifestations, since long-term immobilization has a profound effect on the child and his family. Nursing approaches are evaluated frequently and continued, discontinued, or modified to meet the changing problems and goals.

Mobilization devices

Children usually respond well to mobilization and require little encouragement, but they need instruction in correct use of appliances, their operation, and precautions for their safe usage.

Braces. Paralyzed or markedly weakened extremities can sometimes be stabilized by metal braces that facilitate walking. Some are designed to stabilize the extremities and offer support during ambulation. Special joint hinges permit the hip, knee, and ankle to flex during sitting, whereas the leg is held rigid during ambulation. Meticulous skin care and the wearing of protective clothing under the brace are necessary. Well-fitted braces promote ambulation, whereas ill-fitting braces are dangerous to the balance of the child and frequently cause muscle stress and tissue breakdown. Braces on the growing child will need frequent adjusting and replacement by the orthotist if long-term use is necessary.

The Milwaukee brace (see Fig. 39-4, p. 1529) and the Jewett-Taylor brace are frequently used to support the spine and trunk during ambulation in conditions such as scoliosis and spinal cord injury. The brace must fit each body curvature to avoid undue pressure on tissues and imbalance between muscle groups. Bony prominences where the brace has contact, such as along the spine, chin, and iliac crests, are observed closely for pressure or irritation and are padded as necessary. A corset with metal stays may provide the needed torso support, especially in a paraplegic child. Generally the corset is more comfortable than the metal and leather brace and presents fewer problems with dressing.

Parallel bars. Parallel bars provide secure hand rails on both sides of the child as he is learning to walk again with or without braces. As he becomes more proficient, a walker with or without wheels is substituted for the bars and the child is no longer confined to a limited territory. He then progresses to crutches.

Crutches and canes. Crutches are used when a child is not allowed to bear weight or can only place part of his body weight on an extremity. This begins immediately in most lower leg injuries. A variety of crutches are employed, and the selection is determined by the individual needs of the child. *Axillary* crutches are used most frequently as temporary assistance. *Forearm* crutches are the usual selection for children who anticipate permanent use, such as the paraplegic child who is able to use braces. For children with limited hand and arm strength or function, *trough* crutches allow the weight to be assumed by the elbow. For habilitating small children who have not yet learned to walk or who are unsteady, special crutches stabilized with three or four legs provide needed stability for the child to maintain an upright position and learn to walk (Fig. 40-3).

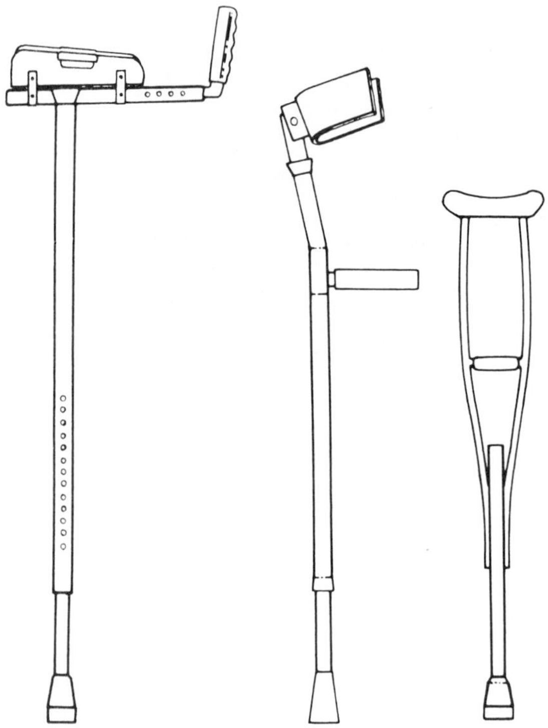

Fig. 40-3. Types of crutches. (From Hilt, N. E., and Schmitt, E. W.: Pediatric orthopedic nursing, St. Louis, 1975, The C. V. Mosby Co., p. 198.)

The child must be properly fitted for the crutch or cane to prevent poor posture and crutch pressure on the axilla during ambulation. Teaching crutch and cane use is usually assumed by the physical therapist in most institutions but is also the responsibility of nurses, especially those in physicians' offices, outpatient departments, and schools. Nurses are the persons who supervise the use of crutches in pediatric units and in the home. The type of crutch gait taught to the child depends on his degree of stability, whether or not the knees can be flexed, and the specific goal established for the child.

Bed exercises for strengthening arms and shoulders are important if immobilization has been prolonged. The youngster gains confidence in ambulating by wearing a safety belt held onto by the therapist. The types of gaits used and instructions to the child are similar to those given adults. They are conveyed with language the child understands and with demonstration. Most children grasp the techniques readily.

Special beds. Older quadriplegic children often require a special bed to immobilize the head and spine during the early phases of spinal cord injury care. Some rehabilitation units use a regular bed for the patient in cervical traction, whereas others use a Stryker frame or one of the Roto-rest beds. Whatever special bed is used, the success of its use is greatly influenced by the preparation of the child. Explanations of how the bed works and, when possible, showing the child someone being turned in the bed, are needed. Nursing personnel need in-service practice in the operation of these beds to ensure the safe handling of the equipment.

A Stryker frame employes two frames, one anterior and one posterior, to turn the child horizontally. The Stryker wedge frame was designed to allow prone-supine turning by one person. Cervical traction can easily be attached to the stationary frame and presents no discomfort when turning as long as the weights are prevented from swinging. Prior to turning, the child's arms and legs are aligned within the frame and straps are wrapped around the entire ''sandwich'' of frames. All of the skin areas should be checked with each turning.

The Roto-rest bed operates electrically; with the person's entire body securely immobilized by firm bolsters, he is slowly and constantly rotated from side to side. Traction can be attached to this bed, and various parts can be re-

A 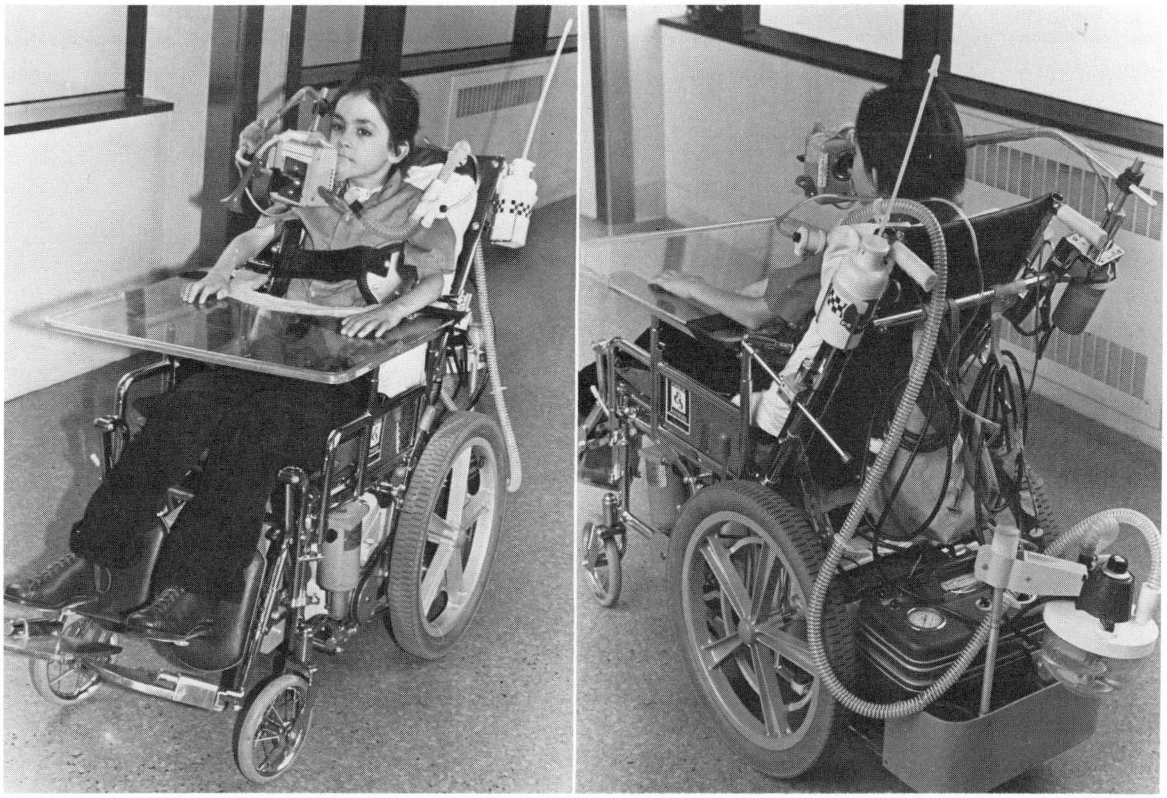 B

Fig. 40-4. Motorized wheelchair for quadriplegic child. **A,** Front view, **B,** Back view. Note the portable respirator.

moved to permit care and physical therapy. The continuous changes of position decrease the problems of pressure areas and promote venous circulation. The bed has a major advantage over a Stryker frame for teenagers with tracheostomies or other conditions that do not allow placing them in the prone position. The bed is made in an adult size and is suited only for large children.

Wheelchairs. Wheelchairs are used temporarily or permanently as a means of transportation. For temporary use, a wheelchair should fit the child and contain any adaptations needed, such as an elevating leg rest or reclining back. The child is taught how to transfer in and out of the chair and how to propel it safely. Prescribing a wheelchair for permanent use is the joint responsibility of physician and therapist after an assessment of home and surroundings. A wheelchair should be neither too small nor too large, preferably one that can be adapted to the child's growth needs. Detachable or rotating armrests, which permit easy transfer in and out, are needed for children with spinal cord injuries. Other desirable features are detachable and swing-away footrests and detachable desk arms. Elevating leg rests are required for children who are prone to contractures, and a reclining back rest is needed for those who may have poor trunk balance. A proper cushion with adequate padding should be provided for the child who has decreased sensation. Hand rim and brake lever projections are helpful for the child with upper extremity weakness. The paraplegic child will require upper arm strengthening exercises and instruction on transfer techniques prior to wheelchair mobilization. Often a tilt table must be used to overcome the problems of orthostatic hypotension before wheelchair sitting can be tolerated. Various motorized chairs are available for marked upper extremity weakness, and mouth- or cheek-operated models are available for children who do not have use of upper extremities so that the children can operate them independently (Fig. 40-4). Very small children who have permanent paralysis of lower extremities are provided with specially designed units that allow independent mobility (Fig. 40-5). A detachable handle on these units permits their conversion to strollers.

For a summary of physical effects of immobilization with nursing interventions, see Table 40-1.

Table 40-1. Summary of physical effects of immobilization with nursing interventions

Primary effects	Secondary effects	Nursing considerations
Muscular system		
Decreased muscle strength, tone, and endurance	Decreased venous return and decreased cardiac output Decreased metabolism and need for oxygen Decreased exercise tolerance Bone demineralization	Use elastic stockings or wrap legs with Ace bandages to promote venous return Place in upright posture when possible
Disuse atrophy and loss of muscle mass Loss of joint mobility	Catabolism Loss of strength Contractures, ankylosis of joints	Give range-of-motion, active, passive, and stretching exercises Maintain correct body alignment Use splint joints as indicated to prevent further deformity
Weak back muscles Weak abdominal muscles	Secondary spinal deformities Impaired respiration	Maintain body alignment See nursing considerations for respiratory system
Skeletal system		
Bone demineralization—osteoporosis, hypercalcemia	Negative calcium balance Pathologic fractures Calcium deposits Extraosseous bone formation, especially at hips, knee, elbows, and shoulder Renal calculi	In paralysis, use upright posture on tilt table Handle extremities carefully when turning and positioning Administer calcium-mobilizing drugs (diphosphonates) if ordered Ensure adequate intake of fluid Acidify urine Promptly treat urinary tract infections
Negative calcium balance	Life-threatening electrolyte imbalance	Monitor blood levels of calcium and electrolytes Give electrolyte replacement as indicated
Metabolism		
Decreased metabolic rate	Slowing of all systems Decreased food intake	Mobilize as soon as possible Give active and passive resistive and deep breathing exercises Ensure adequate food intake Provide a high-protein diet
Negative nitrogen balance	Decline in nutritional state Impaired healing	Encourage small, frequent feedings with protein and preferred foods Prevent pressure areas
Hypercalcemia	Electrolyte imbalance	See nursing considerations for skeletal system
Decreased production of stress hormones	Decreased physical and emotional coping capacity	Identify etiologies of stress Implement appropriate interventions to lower physical and psychosocial stresses
Cardiovascular system		
Decreased efficiency of orthostatic neurovascular reflexes	Inability to adapt readily to upright position Pooling of blood in extremities in upright posture	Monitor peripheral pulses and skin temperature changes Wrap legs in elastic bandage or stockings to decrease pooling when upright
Diminished vasopressor mechanism	Orthostatic hypotension with syncope—hypotension, decreased cerebral blood flow, tachycardia	Give abdominal support In severe cases, use antigravitational suit Administer peripheral sympathetic stimulating agents such as ephedrine, if ordered Position horizontally
Altered distribution of blood volume	Decreased cardiac work load Decreased exercise tolerance	Monitor hydration and urine output
Venous stasis	Pulmonary emboli and/or thrombi	Have frequent position changes Elevate extremities without knee flexion Ensure adequate fluid intake Give active or passive exercises or movement, if ordered Prescribe routine wearing of antiembolic stockings or wrap lower extremities from metatarsus to gluteal folds

Table 40-1. Summary of physical effects of immobilization with nursing interventions—cont'd

Primary effects	Secondary effects	Nursing considerations
Venous stasis—cont'd		Measure circumference of extremities periodically Give anticoagulant drugs if ordered until mobilization possible Promptly intervene to maintain adequate oxygen if signs and symptoms of pulmonary emboli
Dependent edema	Tissue breakdown and susceptibility to infection	Administer good skin care Turn every 2 hours Monitor skin color, temperature, and integrity
Respiratory system		
Decreased need for oxygen	Altered oxygen–carbon dioxide exchange and metabolism	Exercise as tolerated Use position for chest expansion
Decreased chest expansion and diminished vital capacity	Diminished oxygen intake Dyspnea and inadequate arterial oxygen saturation; acidosis	Use prone positioning without pressure on abdomen to allow gravity to aid in diaphragm excursion When sitting, be certain of good alignment to prevent pressure on respiratory mechanism
Poor abdominal tone and distention	Interference with diaphragmatic excursion	Avoid restriction of chest and abdominal musculature Supply torso support to promote chest expansion
Mechanical or biochemical secretion retention	Hypostatic pneumonia Bacterial and viral pneumonia Atelectasis	Frequently change position Carry out percussion, vibration, and drainage (or suctioning), as necessary
Loss of respiratory muscle strength	Poor cough	Encourage coughing and deep breathing Support chest wall when coughing Use special devices such as a rocking bed, Ambu bag, incentive spirometers, intermittent positive-pressure breathing Observe for signs of acute respiratory distress with blood gas levels measured as necessary
	Upper respiratory infection	Avoid contact with infected persons Provide adequate hydration
Gastrointestinal system		
Distention caused by poor abdominal muscle tone	Interference with respiratory movements	Use abdominal binder if indicated Monitor bowel sounds Encourage small, frequent feedings
	Difficulty in feeding in prone position	Sit in upright position if possible
No specific primary effect	Gravitational effect on feces through ascending colon or weakened smooth muscle tone may cause constipation	Carry out bowel training program with hydration, stool softeners, and mild laxatives if necessary
	Anorexia	Stimulate appetite with favored foods
Urinary system		
Alteration of gravitational force	Difficulty in voiding in prone position	Position as upright as possible to void
Impaired ureteral peristalsis	Urinary retention in calyces and bladder Infection Renal calculi	Hydrate to adequate urinary output for age Collect specimens as needed Stimulate bladder emptying with warm water, running water, striking suprapubic area Catheterize only for severe retention
Integumentary system		
No specific primary effect	Decreased circulation and pressure leading to tissue injury	Turn and position at least every 2 hours
	Difficulty with personal hygiene	Frequently inspect total skin surface Eliminate mechanical factors causing pressure, friction, or irritation Assess ability to perform hygienic care and assist with bathing, grooming, and toileting as needed

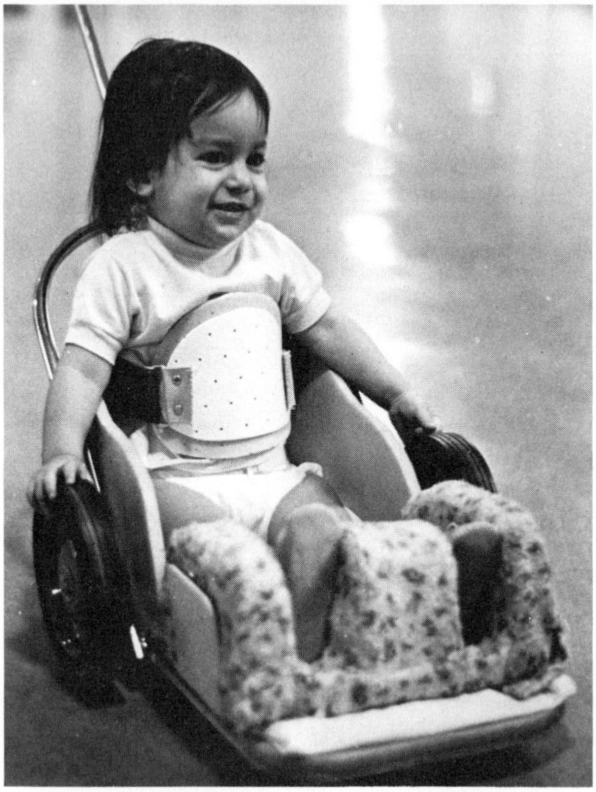

Fig. 40-5. Mobilization device for very young child.

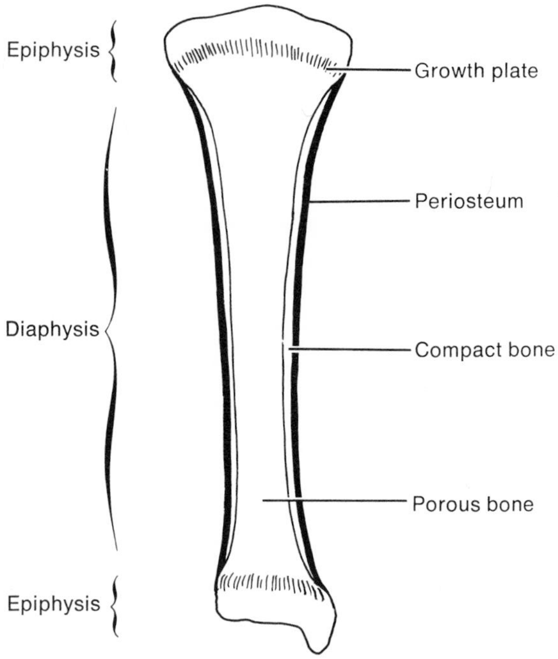

Fig. 40-6. Long bone.

CHILD AND TRAUMA

Musculoskeletal structures

A variety of structures constitute the musculoskeletal system. Each component part of the musculoskeletal system is essential for the mobility needed to perform activities of daily living, such as walking, feeding, dressing, and playing. The skeleton or bony framework provides the support; the muscles, tendons, ligaments, and joints allow for active movement. Muscles are attached to bones by tendons, and strong, fibrous bands called ligaments attach the bone ends to an articulated joint. Muscles are innervated by sensory and motor fibers from the central nervous system. Any or all of these structures can be involved in a traumatic injury and may alter the course of healing in certain situations.

The musculoskeletal system, as all the body systems of the newborn, is immature, and the specific functions of the system develop slowly so that the muscles, bones, tendons, and ligaments can function in an integrated fashion to perform complex tasks. The process of ossification, the gradual conversion of precursor substances (namely cartilage) to bony structures, begins in the embryo and continues until the child is 18 to 21 years of age. In long bones this process progresses outwardly from the diaphysis, the hard shaftlike portion that constitutes the major portion of the bone. Within this hard, compact shaft is the hollow medullary canal composed of the bone marrow. The epiphysis, located at the ends of long bones, consists of layers of cartilage, subchondral bone, and spongelike cancellous bone. Situated between the diaphysis and epiphysis is the epiphyseal plate, which plays a major role in the longitudinal growth of the developing child. The periosteum, the thin, tough membrane covering all bones, contains blood vessels that nourish the living bone (Fig. 40-6). Damage to this thin membrane can be a major problem in bone growth and healing.

Types of trauma

In many ways childhood trauma differs little from trauma in adults. However, many aspects of injury are affected by the developmental stage of the child in both the type of injury that is incurred and the physiologic response to injury.

Accidents. Among the leading causes of morbidity in children are medical problems resulting from traumatic incidents at home, at school, in an automobile, or associated with recreational activities. Children's everyday activities include vigorous play, such as climbing, falling, running into immovable objects, and receiving blows to any part of their bodies. All of these activities make them prone to injury. Adolescents are vulnerable to multiple and severe trauma because they are mobile on bikes and motorcycles and active in sports. Speed and congested surroundings often intensify the impact. Young children and teenagers usually do not calculate risks as they learn to manipulate their environment and achieve developmental goals. Therefore, accidents are a part of most childhood experience. Fortunately, when children fall or are hit, their body resilience protects them from incurring serious damage to soft tissue, the musculoskeletal system, or other body organs. Their bones are more flexible and, therefore, do not resist the external forces that are likely to cause fractures.

Child abuse injury.[14] Unfortunately careless handling of an infant or child, in some instances intentional physical abuse, is not uncommon in our society. A multitude of different types of bone and soft tissue injuries are inflicted on children by adults (see p. 597), and the smaller children who are unable to protect themselves are most vulnerable. It is estimated that perhaps 25% of fractures in children under 3 years of age are the result of child abuse.[14] Emergency room and pediatric office personnel should be alert to situations in which the child's injuries are not congruent with the parent's description of the incident; in which the child's behavior, such as lack of crying or fearful mannerisms are not the expected ones; or in which x-ray films show multiple healed fractures. For example, toddlers do not readily fall and break bones or catch a leg in the crib and break it. Reporting these incidents will aid in securing help for the child and parents. A traumatic incident that produces physical injury to an infant or child may be the outcome of an accident that was no one's fault or may be associated with child abuse. A well-documented history is essential to determine the cause of the injury.[25]

Birth injuries. During the birth process fractures, dislocations, and/or nerve damage may be sustained. These injuries are most often seen when the baby is large, when the presentation is breech, or when forceful extraction is used because of fetal distress. The two most common types of musculoskeletal injuries are fractured clavicle and brachial plexus injury. The presence of a qualified person at delivery will aid in reducing the complications of a difficult delivery. Complete postdelivery assessment of the newborn is essential for early detection of neurologic and/or musculoskeletal problems. Brachial plexus injury is discussed on p. 312.

Fractured clavicle. A fractured clavicle in a newborn may be asymptomatic. The problem should be suspected when an infant demonstrates limited use of the affected arm, shows a malposition of the arm, has local swelling or tenderness, or cries in pain when his arm is moved. Crepitus (the crackling sound produced by rubbing together of fractured bone fragments) is often heard on further examination, and x-ray films usually reveal a complete fracture with overriding of the fragments. Damage to the brachial plexus may accompany this injury.

Conservative treatment is gentle handling of the infant and immobilization with a triangular sling or figure-of-8 bandage. Parents need careful instruction about supporting the baby's shoulders when caring for him so that they are not afraid of hurting the infant and feel comfortable holding and moving him.

Prevention of injuries

Hazardous environmental factors play a major role in the number of serious accidents incurred by children. The stairway without hand rails or a gate at the top, the cluttered walkways, the waxed floors, or throw rugs can contribute to a severe fall. Playground equipment should be checked periodically for hazards, and play areas should be supervised. Adults in charge of sports are encouraged to promote the use of safety-tested equipment and follow game rules to prevent trauma and overplaying of a young athlete whose immature musculoskeletal system and lack of coordination cannot tolerate excessive abuse.

Musculoskeletal trauma is most likely to occur in contact sports, with sprains being very common. Certain contact sports, such as football, tend to produce joint damage, especially knee injuries. Severe hyperflexion of the neck from diving, trampoline activities, or football produces spinal cord injury and quadriplegia. Protective head and shoulder gear are helpful, but youngsters usually do not consistently wear appropriate protection unless they are well supervised.

An effective infant or child car seat is a must for children riding in a car to avoid their being thrown during a sudden stop or the impact of an accident. If this practice is begun when the child is an infant, the young child will be more likely to develop the habit of securing safety belts before the engine is started. In their everyday life observant nurses are a valuable community resource in giving suggestions to parents and schools that might prevent at least some very serious injuries.

See accident prevention segments in health supervision of children in various age-groups.

ASSESSMENT OF TRAUMA

Priority interventions

The site of the accident usually influences the order of priority interventions when instituting emergency care. The safety of both the victim and his "Good Samaritan" rescuers must be considered in order to prevent further injury. For example, removing a child from a burning building or the bottom of a swimming pool is the obvious action to the logically thinking person, but an anxious rescuer may not consider this to be of prime importance. The major reason for thinking through steps to be taken in an emergency prior to the actual incident is to have a mental reservoir of preplanned actions available at a stimulus-response level. The following guide will help establish emergency priorities[12,30]:

1. Make certain that the child and rescuer are not in immediate danger of additional trauma. Do not move the child unless absolutely necessary. Keep him flat unless injury or symptoms specifically indicate otherwise, such as obvious or suspected head injury (elevate head slightly) or vomiting (turn to side).

2. Assess cardiovascular and respiratory function and begin cardiopulmonary, or mouth-to-mouth, resuscitation if indicated.

3. Treat any severe bleeding by removing gross debris from the wound, such as glass, but not if a large object is impaled in the victim, in which case the wound should be covered with a sterile or clean dressing. Apply direct pressure over the wound or at appropriate pressure points. Apply a cold pack and elevate the extremity if possible. Tourniquets are used only when bleeding cannot be stopped by any other means and are not removed until a physician is present.

4. Assess for further injury. In children shock is rarely caused by fractures and, if present, usually indicates internal injury. Decrease anxiety by maintaining a calm manner, remaining close to the reclining infant or child, and touching him. If head injury is present, elevate the head slightly without flexing the neck.

5. Determine if the infant or child is conscious and alert by observing his behavior and talking to him. Observe the pupils for equality and size.

6. Observe the child from head to toes, since a major problem in assessing injuries in an infant or young child is his inability to verbalize except by crying, a nonspecific communication.

7. Check for evidence of decreased motor or sensory function in extremities. In an infant and young child the lack of spontaneous movement in any extremity is a significant observation. An older child can be asked if he has any feeling or if he can wiggle his fingers or toes. Do not encourage the child to move all extremities until after cervical films are taken.

8. Evaluate the severity of pain and try to decrease it by supporting extremities.

9. Assess the pulses in the extremity distal to the injuries. Check for color and changes in skin temperature. This provides data concerning circulatory disturbances.

10. Splint any extremity in which there is evidence of fracture or dislocation. The joints above and below the fracture site must be immobilized so that the fracture ends do not move when the extremity is moved in transport. Do not attempt to realign a fracture or dislocation, and move an injured joint or extremity as little as possible. Paramedics are taught to gently reduce or realign fractures only if distal pulses and sensation are absent. The fractured arm or dislocated shoulder can best be immobilized or supported by a folded towel, jacket, or small pillow secured in place during transport. When a leg is involved and there is no traction splint available, the other leg can be used as a splint with a pillow or jacket placed between the legs and the legs secured together. In that way they can be lifted log fashion with the rest of the child.

11. A spinal cord injury is suspected if there is loss of sensation, no motor function, or lack of a Babinski's reflex response. The child must be moved only if necessary and then in log fashion with the head and neck held firmly in a neutral position. Do not attempt to transport a person with a spinal cord injury until adequate help can be obtained to keep the body in straight alignment throughout and after the repositioning. Pain at the level of the injury, local muscle spasms, and sensorimotor loss are the oustanding features of this type of injury.

12. Look for identification and seek information from anyone who knows the child to identify possible existing health problems.

13. Ask witnesses for details about the incident to aid in the assessment of the child's physical and emotional responses.

14. In cases of serious injury, emergency attendants are necessary to treat shock and to appropriately transport the child to the nearest hospital.

Hospital emergency departments have protocols for starting an intravenous infusion, establishing an airway, giving oxygen as necessary, monitoring vital signs, taking appropriate x-ray films, and ordering laboratory tests. If the child's fracture has created an open wound, tetanus toxoid booster or antitoxin will be administered.

INJURY TO JOINTS AND SOFT TISSUE

A variety of injuries can result when an external force is exerted with severe stress on tissue, muscle, and skeletal structures. The body structures attempt to accommodate the force, but, when unable to do so, injuries occur. Various types of injuries are associated with each structure (Fig. 40-7). Learning the site of injuries and correct terminology aids in understanding and recording the signs and symptoms and medical descriptions.

Contusion

A contusion is damage to the soft tissue, subcutaneous structures, and muscle. The tearing of these tissues and small blood vessels and the inflammatory response lead to hemorrhage, edema, and associated pain when the child attempts to move the extremity. The escape of blood into the tissues will be observed as *ecchymosis,* a black and blue discoloration.

Early treatment of a contusion with cold packs decreases the pain threshold and triggers a local vasoconstriction resulting in decreased hemorrhage and edema. Local cold therapy has the additional advantage of lessening muscle spasm, probably by decreasing muscle irritability and the responsiveness of muscle spindles to stretch. Adjunctive therapy to cold is compression bandaging and elevation of the extremity.

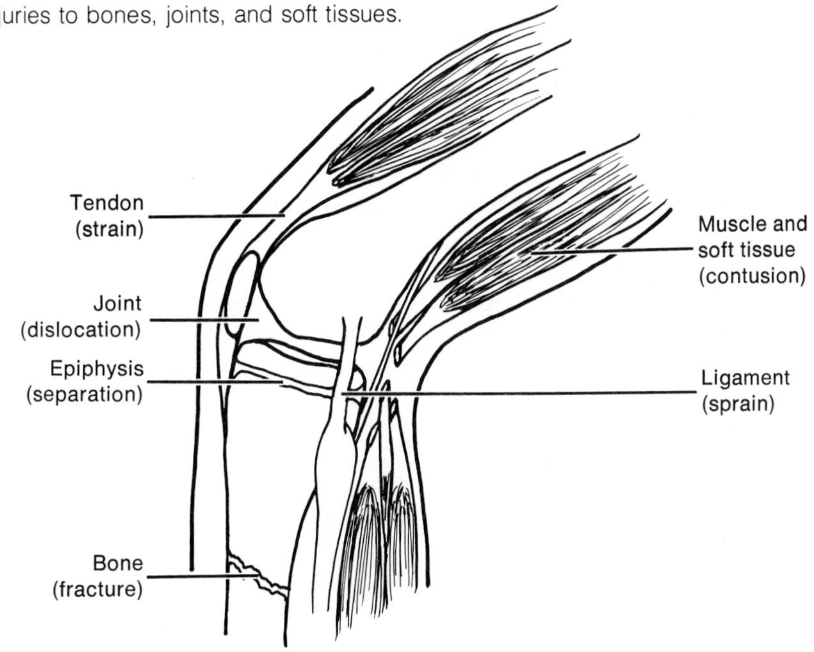

Fig. 40-7. Sites of injuries to bones, joints, and soft tissues.

Sprains and strains

When trauma is so severe that a ligament is partially or completely torn or stretched by the force created as a joint is twisted or wrenched, a *sprain* develops, often accompanied by damage to associated blood vessels, muscles, tendons, and nerves. A microscopic tear to the musculotendinous unit is called a *strain*. The area is painful to touch and swollen. Application of cold, immobilization with elastic bandage, and elevation of the extremity will help alleviate these symptoms. Major sprains or tears to the ligamentous tissue rarely occur in growing children. Ligaments are stronger than bone, and the epiphysis and growth plate are the weakest areas of the bone; therefore, the more usual sites of injury are at the growth plate. Torn ligaments, especially those in the knee, are usually treated by immobilization with a cast for 3 to 4 weeks or strapping of the joint with adhesive or Elastoplast bandage. Passive leg exercises, gradually increased to active ones, are begun as soon as sufficient healing has taken place. Generally strains require only support, heat, and muscle relaxants with occasional use of intermittent traction.

Dislocations

Long bones are held in approximation to one another at the joint by ligaments. A dislocation occurs when the force of stress on the ligament is so great as to displace the normal position of the opposing bone ends or the bone end to its socket. The predominant symptom is pain that increases with attempted passive or active movement of the extremity. In dislocations there may be an obvious deformity and the child usually loses the ability to move the joint. Temporary restriction of the joint, such as with a sling or bandage that secures the arm to the chest in a shoulder dislocation, provides sufficient comfort and immobilization until the child can receive medical help. The physician will manipulate the joint, often under anesthesia, to replace the bones in anatomic alignment. Immobilization for 3 weeks or more is necessary for healing of the torn ligaments.

Dislocations are less common in children than in older persons. Before final closure of the epiphyses, injuries to the joints are more likely to cause epiphyseal separation than dislocation. For example, shoulder dislocation is seen only in older adolescents, and dislocation unaccompanied by fracture is rare. However, dislocation of the hip is probably the most common dislocation and occurs more frequently than femoral neck fracture (seen often in persons in the older age-groups). In children younger than 5 years of age the hip is usually dislocated by a fall, but trauma is minimal because of the largely cartilaginous acetabulum and general joint laxity. With increasing age the degree of violence also increases, and the cause of dislocation between 6 and 10 years of age is more often an athletic injury. Thereafter, automobile accidents are the most frequent cause. Treatment is immediate reduction of the dislocation and immobilization for approximately 3 weeks, followed by gentle, graduated exercises without stretching, usually performed by the child himself.[25]

Dislocation of the patella is a recurrent episode in some children; in others it is the result of injury. It is quite common in adolescent girls. The patella is always dislocated laterally. Most dislocations are reduced either spontaneously or by a companion before the child is seen by a physician.

Therapy is immobilization for 3 to 4 weeks. Surgery may be needed for recurrent dislocations.

The most common dislocation injury, often handled by a pediatrician, is subluxation of the head of the radius in the elbow that occurs when a child between ages 1 and 4 years stumbles or is pulled along while holding onto the hand of an adult. The child is jerked upward by the adult while his arm is in a position of extension. The child has pain in the elbow and wrist, refuses to move the arm, and holds it slightly flexed and pronated. The physician manipulates the arm by applying firm finger pressure to the head of the radius and then supinates and flexes the forearm to return the bone structures to normal alignment. A click is heard, and functional use of the arm returns.[25]

Children with naturally lax joints, such as children with Down's syndrome, are more prone to recurrent dislocation of the hip.

FRACTURES

Bones fracture when the resistance of the bone against the stress being exerted yields to the stress force. Fractures are a common injury at any age but are more likely to occur in children and aged persons. The natural tendency toward active mobility and their limited gross motor coordination make children more susceptible to physical injury. Because of the characteristics of the child's skeleton there are some differences in the pattern of fractures, problems of diagnosis, and methods of treatment.

Etiology and pathophysiology

The etiology of fracture injuries in children are those just described for general traumatic injuries in childhood. Fractures in infancy are more often the result of birth trauma, accidents, or child abuse. Aside from automobile accidents, true accidents rarely occur in infancy; therefore, injury in children in that age-group warrants further investigation. In any small child x-ray evidence of fractures at various stages of healing are, with few exceptions, the result of physical abuse. Most often early bone trauma in infants consists of periosteal bleeding in the long bones of arms and legs, usually caused by rough handling, twisting, and pulling, which is not evident on x-ray examination until 3 to 6 weeks after the injury. Unfortunately child abuse is not uncommon in the United States.

Fractures of the forearm are common bone injuries in childhood and are usually caused when the child extends the palm of the hand to break a fall. The clavicle is probably the bone most frequently broken in children, approximately half in children under 10 years of age. Hip fractures are rare in children and require a great deal of violence to produce. A femoral neck fracture may be sustained in children 6 or 7 years of age whose hip height is on a level with the automobile bumper. In older children the femur and in adolescents the knee are the most likely targets.

Children fall from heights (trees, roofs, and so on) as their insatiable curiosity and immature judgment lure them to places of danger. Fractures in school-age children are often the result of bicycle-automobile or skateboard accidents. At all ages motor vehicle accidents are a frequent cause of bone injury. Most children who are hit by an automobile are between 4 and 7 years of age and sustain a triad of injuries, which must be kept in mind when making an assessment of injuries: (1) the child's femur, which is at the level of the bumper, is fractured, (2) the hood of the automobile produces trunk injuries, and (3) a contralateral head injury is usually sustained when the child is thrown to the ground by the impact. Therefore, a child with any of these injuries who was struck by an automobile should be examined for evidence of the other two.

Children are different. The anatomic, biomechanical, and physiologic nature of children's skeletons causes differences in the pattern of fractures, the problems of diagnosis, and the methods of treatment. The bones of the adult are strong and require a violent traumatic force to fracture and are accompanied by massive injury to surrounding soft tissues. In children the bones are more easily injured and may result from minor falls or twists and, thus, are likely to be accompanied by damage. As a result features of children's fractures that are not observed in the adult include the following.[26]

Growth plate. The portion of the bone at which growth takes place is a thick, elastic plate that serves to absorb shock and protect joint surfaces from injury and is the means by which the limb is able to grow and to straighten itself. Growth is stimulated by a fracture in the diaphysis, whereas damage to the growth plate can cause shortening and, often, a progressive angular deformity.

Thick periosteum. Compared with the adult, the periosteum of children's bone is thicker, is stronger, and has more active osteogenic potential.

More plastic bone. The bones of growing children are more porous than those of the adult, which allows them to bend, buckle, and break in a "greenstick" manner. The increased porosity increases the flexibility of the bone and dissipates and absorbs a significant amount of the force of impact.

Rapid healing. Healing is more rapid in children, and the rapidity is inversely related to the age of the child. The younger the child, the more rapid the healing process. Nonunion of bone fragments is almost unknown in children.

Stiffness is unusual. Unlike adults, an uninjured joint in children can be immobilized for a long period of time without producing stiffness that lasts longer than a few minutes. Injured joints do become stiff, however, and the current trend is toward early mobilization and active range of motion exercises as preventive measures.

Complaint. Children only complain when something is wrong. Unreasonable crying, restlessness, and calling for the mother are usually indications that something is amiss and require investigation.

Types of fractures. A fractured bone consists of fragments—the fragment closer to the midline, or the proximal fragment, and the fragment farthest from the midline, or the distal fragment. When fracture fragments are separated, the fracture is *complete;* when fragments remain attached it is said to be *incomplete*. The fracture line can be:

transverse crosswise, at right angles to the long axis of the bone.
oblique slanting but straight, between a horizontal and a perpendicular direction.
spiral slanting and circular, twisting around the bone shaft.

All affect the entire cross-section of the bone. The twisting of an extremity while the bone is breaking results in the spiral break. If the fracture does not produce a break in the skin, it is a *simple,* or *closed,* fracture. *Open,* or *compound,* fractures are those with an open wound through which the bone is or has protruded. If the bone fragments cause damage to other organs or tissues (such as the lung or bladder), the injury is said to be *complicated*. When small fragments of bone are broken from the fractured shaft and lie in the surrounding tissue, the fracture is called *comminuted*. This type of fracture is rare in children. The types of fractures seen most often in children are shown in Fig. 40-8.[25]

bends a child's flexible bone can be bent 45 degrees or more before breaking. However, if bent, the bone will straighten slowly, but not completely, to produce some deformity but without the angulation seen when the bone breaks. Bends occur more commonly in the ulna and fibula, often associated with fractures of the radius and tibia.
buckle fracture compression of the porous bone produces a *buckle,* or *torus,* fracture. This appears as a raised or bulging projection at the fracture site. Torus fractures occur in the most porous portion of the bone near the metaphysis (the portion of the bone shaft adjacent to the epiphysis) and are more common in young children.
greenstick fracture a greenstick fracture occurs when a bone is angulated beyond the limits of bending. The compressed side bends and the tension side fails, causing an incomplete fracture similar to the break observed when a green stick is broken.
complete fracture complete fractures are those that divide the bone fragments. They often remain attached by a periosteal hinge, which can aid or hinder reduction.

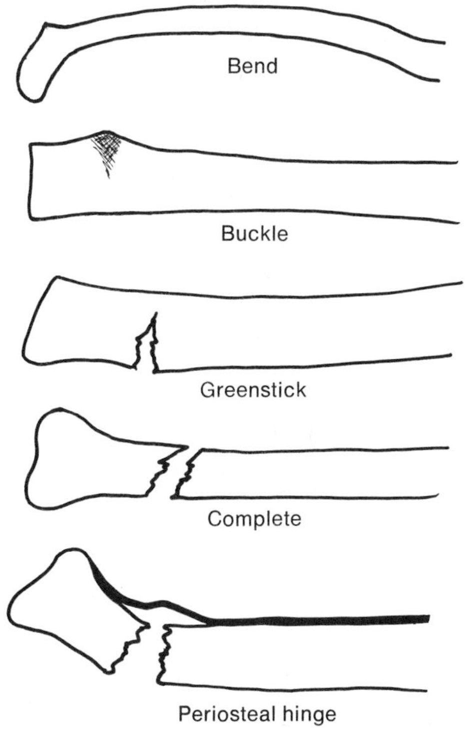

Fig. 40-8. Types of fractures in children.

Epiphyseal injuries. The weakest point of long bones is the cartilage growth plate or epiphyseal plate. Consequently this is a frequent site of damage during trauma. Under most conditions, fractures in this area proceed along the zone of degenerating cartilage cells, before the cartilage begins to ossify, without damage to the growth plate to cause little damage. Healing is usually prompt. When fracture lines deviate from a transverse direction through the degenerating cells, more serious damage to the epiphysis and the plate may occur. Fig. 40-9 illustrates the types of epiphyseal injuries in order of increasing risk of permanent epiphyseal damage and possible growth disturbance.

Detection of epiphyseal injuries is sometimes difficult, and they may be mistaken for dislocations or ligamentous injuries. Fractures involving the epiphysis or epiphyseal plate present special problems in determining whether or not bone growth will be affected. Early and correct assessment are essential to minimize the incidence of longitudinal growth problems and angular deformities. The medical management of these injuries is different than that for other fractures in that open reduction and internal fixation are often employed to prevent complications. If the affected limb is shorter, epiphyseal surgery is done either to stimu-

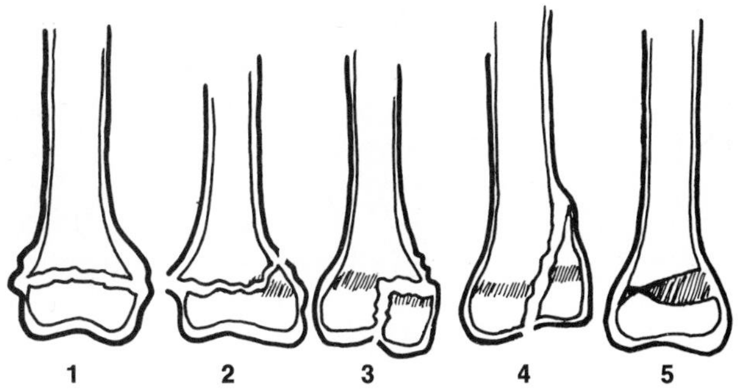

Fig. 40-9. Types of epiphyseal injuries in children in order of increasing risk.

late the involved epiphysis or to retard growth in the unaffected leg.

Associated problems. Immediately after a fracture occurs the muscles contract and physiologically splint the injured area. This phenomenon accounts for the muscle tightness observed over a fracture site and the deformity that is produced as the muscles pull the bone ends out of alignment. This muscle response must be overcome by traction or complete muscle relaxation, that is, anesthesia, in order to realign the distal bone fragment to the proximal bone fragment.

Contusions of the soft tissues frequently accompany fractures, especially of femurs, and severe hemorrhage into the tissues is not uncommon. Both the bleeding and pain are major contributors to shock associated with this injury; therefore, suspected musculoskeletal injury should be treated as a fracture until x-ray confirmation can be made. The surrounding tissue will be swollen, and a hematoma is usually present. The soft tissue injury must be treated as any contusion. Since the injury may cause damage to essential structures, the circulatory and neurologic status of tissues distal to the fracture are carefully assessed. This is especially true in femoral and supracondylar fractures of the elbow.

A

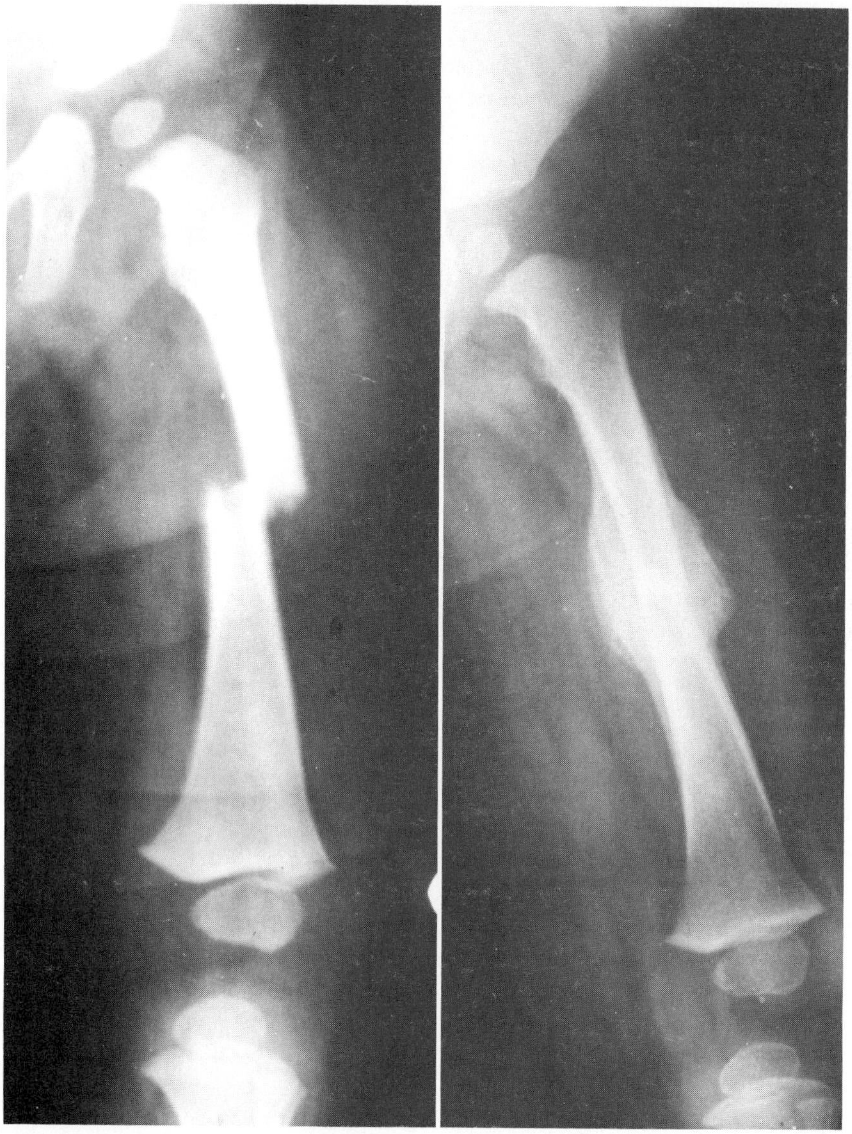

B

Fig. 40-10. Fractured femur. Most fractured femurs in childhood are of spiral type shown here. Note comparison of original x-ray films, **A,** with the 6-month postfracture film, **B,** showing callus formation. (Courtesy Henrietta Egleston Hospital for Children, Atlanta, Ga.) (From Hilt, N. E., and Schmitt, E. W.: Pediatric orthopedic nursing, St. Louis, 1975, The C. V. Mosby Co., p. 43.)

Bone healing and remodeling. Bone healing is characteristically rapid in children because of the thickened periosteum and generous blood supply. When there is a break in the continuity of bone, the periosteal and intraosseous osteoblasts are in some way stimulated to maximum activity. New osteoblasts are formed in immense numbers almost immediately after the injury and, in time, are evidenced by a bulging growth of osteoblastic tissue and new bone matrix between the fractured bone fragments. This is followed by deposition of calcium salts to form a *callus* (Fig. 40-10).[15,32]

Bone healing follows a patterned sequence of events as outlined in Table 40-2. A hematoma and available fibroblasts, osteoblasts, and calcium are essential to the formation of a callus. Fractures heal more quickly in children than in adults. In the young child, for example, there is frequently a solid union of the femoral shaft in 3 to 4 weeks, whereas in the adult callus sufficient to avoid deformities from constant muscle contraction associated with movement may not take place in less than 10 to 16 weeks. The approximate healing times for a femoral shaft are[32]:

Neonatal period—2 to 3 weeks
Early childhood—4 weeks
Later childhood—6 weeks
Adolescence—8 to 10 weeks

Table 40-2. Bone healing process*

Time†	Physiologic events
3-5 minutes	Bone and tissue bleeding after injury *Hematoma forms and clots;* fibrin assists in clotting periosteal membrane, which aids in repair
After 24 hours	Blood supply increases, bringing available calcium, phosphate, and fibroblasts, which convert to osteoblasts (bone-forming cells)
Next few days	Hematoma becomes *granulation tissue;* forms framework for deposition of bone-forming substances Osteoblasts produce intercellular substance or matrix, in which calcium and phosphate is deposited (beginning of callus)
2-3 days	*Halisteresis* (softening of bone ends) 1/8-1/4 inch absorption of bone cells
6-10 days	*Provisional callus develops;* holds bone fragments together but will not support body weight
14-21 days	*True callus develops;* seen on x-ray; usually more than needed but with remodeling, excess callus absorbs; gradual weight bearing
3-10 weeks	*Callus to bone,* which grows beneath periosteum of fragments; fuses defect by ossification; no intermedullary canal
Over 9-month period	Bone marrow cavity restored; fracture line can always be seen on x-ray film

*Total healing time depends on age, type of bone, and complications.
†Process in infants and young children is more rapid.

Remodeling is a unique process that occurs in the healing of fractures of long bone prior to epiphyseal closure. When a bone remodels, the irregularities produced by the fracture become indistinct as hallows are filled in and angles are rounded off in the healing process, which gives the bone a straighter appearance. It does not alter the alignment of the bone. The buildup of new bone or callus will restore a portion of the normal bone structure in most cases despite observable malalignment. The younger the child and the closer the proximity of the fracture to the growth plate, the more likely it is that spontaneous correction will take place. In some cases a 90-degree angle will straighten in a year, but rotational deformities do not correct themselves. Various factors such as the type and location of the fracture, the age of the child, and the amount of fragment angulation or rotation will influence the degree of correction in alignment that can be obtained by remodeling.[11,32]

Wolff's law is applied to treating children with orthopedic problems. Paraphrased, it states that bone will grow in the direction in which stress is placed on it. Examples of the use of this law are the hip spica cast with an abduction bar for treating congenital hip disorders or application of casts or traction at a selected angle to influence the direction of bone healing.

Bone healing in persons in any age-group is greatly influenced by the general health of the traumatized person. The child with a fracture requires adequate nutrition, including supplementary vitamins. No special dietary changes need to be made except to correct nutritional deficiencies. Monitoring of fluid and electrolyte balance, renal function, and possible anemia are equally important to promote wellness of the child.

Diagnostic evaluation

A history is often lacking in childhood injuries. Infants are unable to communicate, and older children are unreliable informants and seldom volunteer information (even under direct questioning) when the injury occurred during forbidden activities. Unless they are witnesses to the injury, parents may misinterpret what the child is trying to say. In cases of child abuse parents may give false information deliberately in order to protect themselves.

Children demonstrate the usual signs of injury—generalized swelling, pain or tenderness, and diminished functional use of the affected part. There may be bruising, severe muscular rigidity, and sometimes crepitus (a grating sensation at the fracture site), which are also frequent signs in adults. More often the fracture is remarkably stable because of the frequently intact periosteum. The child may even be able to use an affected arm or walk on a fractured leg. However, a fracture should be strongly suspected in a small child who refuses to walk.[16]

Although neurologic and vascular damage are much less frequent in children than in adult patients, the integrity of these structures must be accurately assessed. This is often difficult in infants and young children who are unable to cooperate. Vascular injury is most likely to occur with supracondylar fractures of the humerus and femur. Femoral and popliteal vessels and the sciatic nerve are prone to trauma in femoral fractures; humeral fractures may cause damage to the medial, ulnar, or radial nerves and to the brachial artery. The three ''Ps'' of ischemia from a vascular injury—pain, pulselessness, and paralysis—should be kept in mind when making an assessment.[16]

Radiography. Radiographic examination is the most useful diagnostic tool for assessing skeletal trauma. The calcium deposits in bone make the entire structure radiopaque. However, in normal growth and development bony structures ossify from precursor substances, usually cartilage, to form true bone from the shaft or diaphysis toward the epiphysis. This ossification process begins in the embryo and continues until bone formation is completed by 18 to 21 years of age. Ossification centers alter the appearance of the bone, and much of the skeleton of infants and young children is composed of radiolucent growth cartilage that does not appear on radiographs. Also, the epiphyseal cartilage and undisplaced separations of the epiphysis, which often occur, are not easily detected on radiographs. Many physicians obtain a film of the uninjured limb for a direct comparison to help identify minor alterations in alignment and configuration of the epiphysis and associated injuries that might be missed. Radiographic films are taken after fracture reduction and, in some cases, may be taken during the healing process to determine satisfactory progress.

Blood studies.[35] Severe soft tissue, muscle, and bone injury often result in a destruction of red blood cells with a rise in bilirubin and a fall in the hemoglobin or hematocrit reading. The child's homeostatic mechanisms are activated to correct the problem, and generally only supportive therapy with high-protein diet and iron replacement is needed. When muscle integrity is disrupted, enzymes normally contained within muscles are released into the bloodstream. Serum levels of alkaline phosphatase, serum glutamic-oxaloacetic transaminase (SGOT), and lactic dehydrogenase (LDH) may increase in proportion to the amount of muscle damage.

A normal physiologic response to tissue injury is the inflammatory process with a slight elevation of white blood cells, especially neutrophils. When infection occurs the rise in leukocytes is anticipated and the accompanying symptoms of fever and lethargy develop.

Electromyography. The response of a muscle to electric stimuli can be a valuable tool in determining if the muscular weakness or paralysis is neurologic or muscular in origin. Stimulation of the muscle is accomplished by inserting a sterile needle electrode into the muscle and visualizing the amplified response on an oscilloscope. If no response is recorded the presence of intrinsic muscle disease is suspected. About 1 to 2 weeks after complete denervation of a muscle, the oscilloscope will show reflex response that is recorded differently than when the nerve is intact. The muscle without nerve supply shows a spastic type of reaction unless there is muscle atrophy or fibrosis as well.

Medical management

The majority of children's fractures heal well, and nonunion is rare. Most are readily reduced by simple traction and immobilization until healing takes place. However, the position of the bone fragments in relation to one another influences the rapidity of healing and the residual deformity. A gap between fragments delays (or prevents) healing (Fig. 40-11, *A*). Healing is prompt and complete with end-to-end apposition (Fig. 40-11, *B*), but the fracture stimulates accelerated growth of the neighboring epiphysis, which causes bony overgrowth and increased length of the extremity. When the fragments overlap in a bayonet-type reduction, there is sufficient bone contact to allow for rapid healing and the lost length compensates for overgrowth as a result of epiphyseal stimulation (Fig. 40-11, *C*). The length that can be compensated for depends on the age of the child. Approximately 1 cm of overlap can be allowed in a young child, but in a child who is near the end of the growth period, correction will be less; therefore, overlap must be less. Angulation deformity caused by an incomplete fracture (Fig. 40-11, *D*) may remodel in the young child, but the degree of residual deformity depends on the relationship of the angulation of the bone fragments to the angle of the joint. This requires careful evaluation and reduction to prevent permanent deformity.[26]

The goals of fracture management are[15]:

1. To regain alignment and length of the bony fragments (reduction)

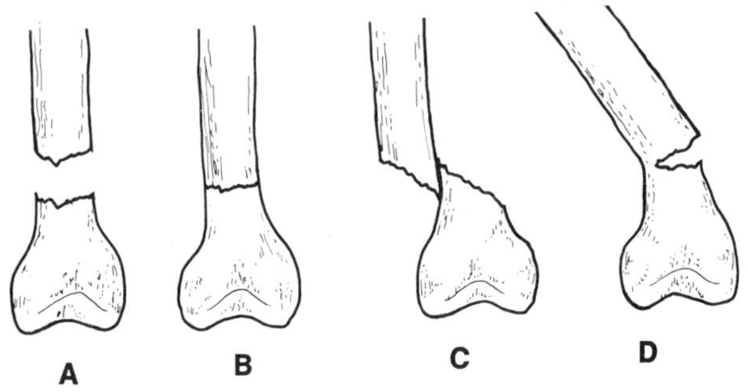

Fig. 40-11. Relationships of fracture fragments. **A,** Gap between fragments. **B,** End-to-end apposition. **C,** Bayonet apposition or overlap. **D,** Angulation of an incomplete fracture.

2. To retain alignment and length (immobilization)
3. To restore function to the injured parts

In children the bone fragments are usually realigned and immobilized by traction or by closed manipulation and casting until adequate callus is formed. Weight bearing and active movement for the purpose of regaining function can begin after the fracture site is stable. The child's natural tendency to be active is usually sufficient to restore normal mobility, and physical therapy is rarely needed. Open reduction is seldom required and is limited to fractures that cannot be maintained by conservative methods and when there is interposed tissue or injury to arteries or nerves. However, surgical reductions are more apt to delay normal healing and often predispose to nonunion. In most cases children's fractures can be managed by closed reduction and plaster immobilization, which is most often provided on an outpatient basis with reevaluation in 7 to 10 days.

Children are most frequently hospitalized for fractures of the femur and the supracondylar area of the distal humerus. If simple reductions cannot be achieved or a neurovascular problem is detected after injury, observation on a hospital unit is indicated. Severe contusions with profound swelling cannot be treated with a cast, which would act as a tourniquet on the extremity, and badly malaligned fractures will require traction for a period of time before a cast is applied. Table 40-3 outlines the various fractures and their usual management.

Table 40-3. Common fractures in children and their usual management

Bone	Method of immobilization	Comments
Clavicle		
Anterior displacement of distal fragment	Figure-of-eight bandage or cast—arms free	
Posterior displacement of distal fragment	Shoulder and arm on affected side immobilized with bandage and/or sling suspended from opposite shoulder	
Humerus		
Neck	Minimal—arm and shoulder immobilized with Stockinette collar and sling; frequently reinforced with plaster to last Severe—collar and cuff sling or shoulder spica cast or bandage; sometimes Dunlop traction followed by use of shoulder spica cast	Reduction assisted by gravitational force May require anesthesia for reduction May require application of light traction
Shaft	U-slab of plaster to immobilize arm against chest with elbow at 90- or 45-degree angle Thoracobrachial box cast incorporating arm, shoulder, and chest	Reduction assisted by gravity; may incorporate a lead weight in elbow portion of cast to increase traction
Elbow	Collar and cuff sling for undisplaced fracture Dunlop traction followed by collar and cuff sling	Reduction under general anesthesia Elbow mobilization as soon as feasible Risk of complications—stiffness, ischemic contractures, nerve damage—greater
Lower arm		
Radius only	Cast from below forearm to metacarpal head	
Radius and ulna	Cast from midhumerus to metacarpals	
Phalanges	Aluminum finger splint Splint to adjacent finger	
Femoral shaft	Spica cast Traction type determined by location and manner of displacement; followed by use of spica cast	May require anesthesia if extensive manipulation Seldom requires open reduction
Tibia and fibula	Plaster cast from groin to toes	Weight bearing possible after second week

Medical problems and interventions. The method of fracture reduction is determined by:

- Age of child
- Degree of displacement
- Amount of overriding
- Degree of edema
- Condition of skin and soft tissue
- Sensation and circulation distal to fracture

Some problems that are associated with fracture injury and involve both the physician and nurse are:

- Control of pain, hemorrhage, and edema
- Relief of muscle spasms
- Realignment of fracture fragments
- Promotion of bone healing
- Immobilization of fracture until adequate healing has begun
- Prevention of secondary complications
- Limitation of disuse syndrome
- Restoration of function

The specific interventions and nursing responsibilities in the general management directed toward restoring bone integrity and functional use are summarized in the following paragraphs.

Surgical intervention. When surgical intervention is necessary to realign a fracture, the child needs physical and psychologic preparation. The preoperative teaching is the same as for any other surgical procedure, except that orthopedic surgery utilizes a variety of rods, screws, and plates and the child needs to know about these unfamiliar things and how they will appear when he returns from the operation. The fixating devices are made of substances that do not act as foreign proteins to the body and, therefore, are not rejected. Usually the rods are driven down the shaft of the long bones, whereas screws and plates are attached to the side of the bone shaft. Postoperatively the bone healing proceeds as a new fracture with the callus formation process. Generally the child with an internal fixation device can be mobilized to a chair and to a walker or crutches within a few hours or days. The most common postoperative complications are infections and slippage of the fixation device. The nurse's responsibility includes close monitoring of neurovascular changes in the involved extremity and the prevention of postanesthesia problems.

Child in cast

Nurses are frequently in a position where they must make the initial assessment of a child with a suspected fracture. The child and his parents are frightened and upset, the child is in pain, and, since most fractures are obvious, the parents and (frequently) the child are already convinced of the diagnosis. Therefore, if the child is alert and there is no evidence of hemorrhage, the initial nursing interventions are directed toward calming and reassuring the child and his parents so that a more extensive assessment can be more easily accomplished.

Maintaining a calm manner and speaking in a quiet voice, the parents can be asked to describe what happened and how they feel about it. Since the child usually arrives with the limb supported in some manner, this minute or two does not delay or endanger the treatment. It is best not to touch the child initially but to ask him to point to the painful area and to wiggle his fingers or toes. By this time he usually feels relatively safe and will allow someone to gently touch him just enough to feel the pulse and test for sensation. However, the child needs to be told what will happen and what he can do to help. A child's anxiety is greatly influenced by previous experiences with injury and health personnel. The affected limb need not be palpated and should not be moved unless properly splinted. If the child is at home or if the physician is not present to examine the child, some type of splint should be applied carefully for transport to the hospital and to the radiography department and cast room.

Cast application. The completeness of the fracture, the type of bone involved, and the amount of weight bearing influence how much of the extremity must be included in the cast to immobilize the fracture site completely. In most cases the joints above and below the fracture are immobilized to eliminate the possibility of movement that might cause displacement at the fracture site. The types of casts used for the more common fractures are illustrated in Fig. 40-12.

When a cast is being applied by a physician, it is often the nurse's role to set up the cast materials and hold the extremity in alignment, Fig. 40-13. Special cast tables that hold the child's body are used for applying large hip spica casts. If possible, the child should be allowed to play with a small doll that has a cast so that he understands what will be done.

A tube of stockinette is stretched over the area to be casted, and bone prominences are padded with soft cotton sheeting. Dry rolls of gauze impregnated with plaster of Paris are immersed in a pail of cold water with the open end of the roll downward to allow soaking of the bandage. The wet plaster rolls are put on in a bandage fashion and molded to the extremity. A heat-producing chemical reaction occurs between the plaster and water as the plaster becomes a crystalline gypsum. During application of the cast the underlying stockinette is pulled over the raw edges of the cast and secured with a layer of wet plaster ½ to 1 inch below the rim to form a smooth padded edge to protect the skin.

If the physician does not form such a protective edge with stockinette, the raw edges of the cast can be protected by a "petaled" edge. Small pieces approximately 2 to 3 inches long are cut from 1- or 1½-inch wide adhesive tape. The edges are rounded with scissors, and each of these "petals" is placed over the edge of the cast, each petal slightly overlapping the previous petal to form a smooth, neat edge. It is easier to apply the petal to the underside of the cast first

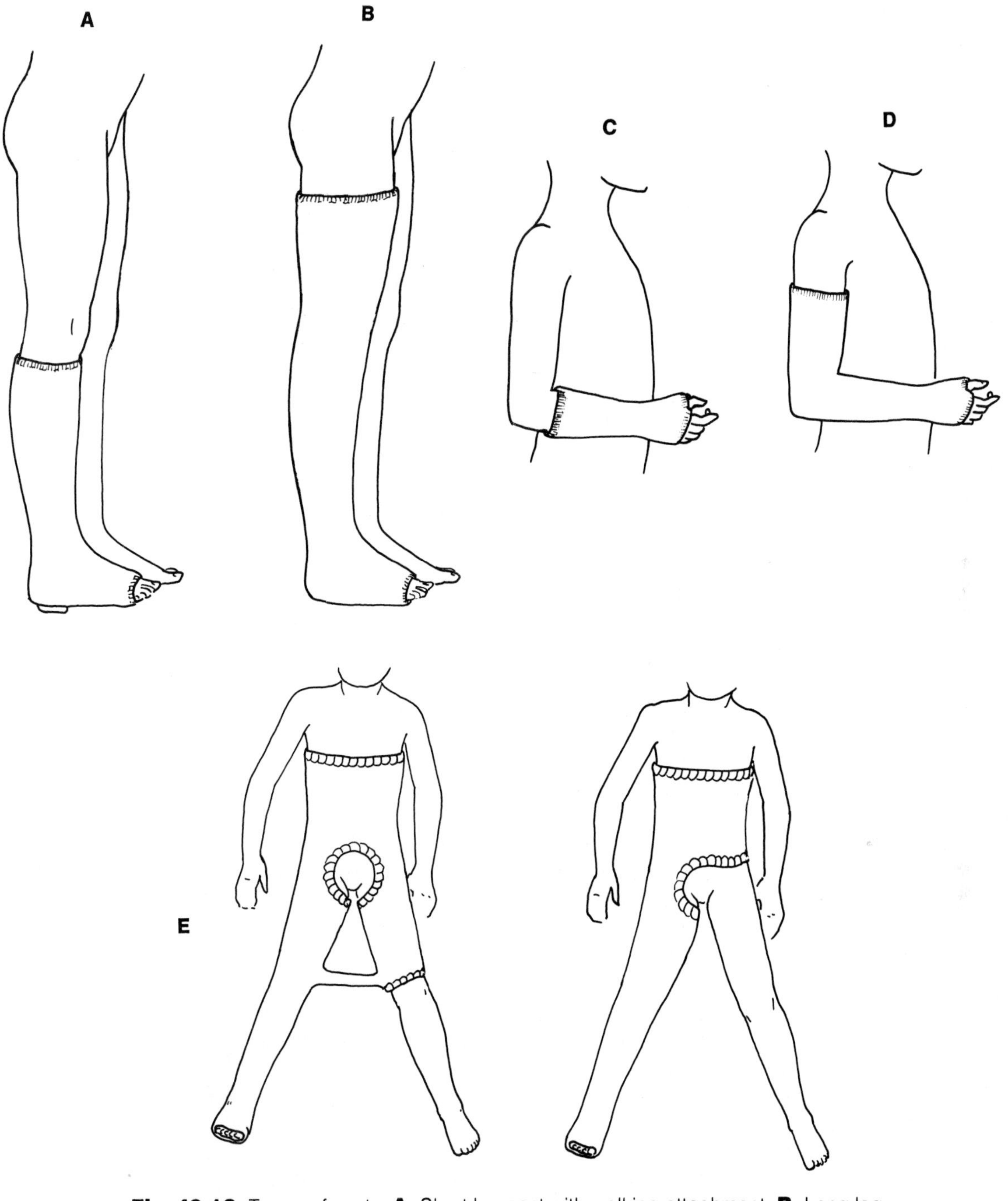

Fig. 40-12. Types of casts. **A,** Short leg cast with walking attachment. **B,** Long leg cast. **C,** Short arm cast. **D,** Long arm cast. **E,** Hip spica casts.

and then bring the unadhered edge to the front, pressing firmly so that the edges remain securely attached.

Fiberglass, plastic, and resin materials are being used as casting materials with increasing frequency. They are lightweight, can tolerate more contact with water, and can be lightly sponged when they become soiled.

Nursing care of child with cast. The complete evaporation of the water from a hip spica cast can take 24 to 48 hours when older types of plaster materials are used. Drying occurs within 8 to 10 hours with new quick-drying substances. Turning the child at least every 2 hours will help to dry the cast evenly. The cast must remain uncovered to allow the cast to dry from the inside out. A regular fan to circulate air may be helpful during high-humidity weather.

A

B

C

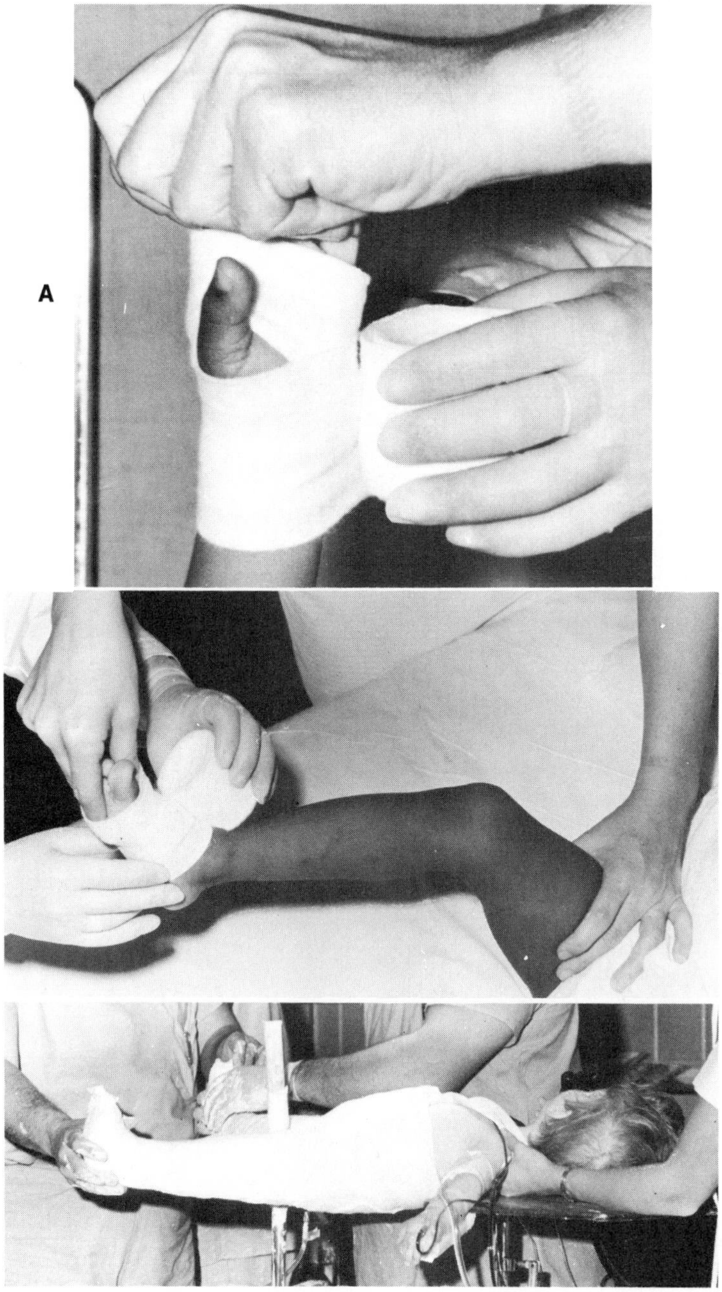

Fig. 40-13. Proper methods of holding a child for a cast application. **A,** Arm cast: arm should be held by the fingers (and the upper arm, if necessary) and off the side of the table or bed to permit exposure of entire arm. **B,** Leg cast: grasp the foot and toes with one hand as shown, and the upper thigh with the other hand; maintaining the knee in flexion will discourage kicking. **C,** Hip spica cast: one individual maintains the desired leg position; another individual pushes the child at the shoulder level toward the perineal post; the child's shoulders and pelvis should remain level. (From Hilt, N. E., and Schmitt, E. W.: Pediatric orthopedic nursing, St. Louis, 1975, The C. V. Mosby Co., p. 76.)

Summary of nursing care of the child with a cast

Goals	Responsibilities
Maintain optimal temperature	Check temperature; imbalance can be produced by Chemical reaction in cast drying process, which generates heat Water evaporation, which causes heat loss
Prevent circulatory impairment	Elevate cast extremity Place leg cast on pillows, making certain that leg is well supported and that there is no pressure on heel Elevate arm on pillows or support in stockinette sling suspended from intravenous infusion pole—either in bed or during ambulation; triangular arm sling is adequate for lesser elevation and support Monitor cardiovascular status Monitor peripheral pulses Blanch skin on extremity distal to fracture to ascertain adequate circulation to the part Feel cast for tightness; cast should allow insertion of fingers between skin and cast after it has dried Assess for increase in Pain Swelling Coldness Cyanosis Assess finger movement and sensation Request child to move fingers Report signs of impending circulatory impairment immediately Instruct child to report any feelings of numbness or tingling
Detect signs of infection	Smell cast for foul odor Be alert to increased temperature, lethargy, and discomfort
Detect respiratory impairment	Assess child's chest expansion Observe respiratory rate Observe color and behavior
Prevent skin from becoming irritated	Make certain that all edges are smooth and free from irritating projections; trim and/or pad as necessary; petal cast edges if needed Keep crumbs and other items from getting between cast and skin Inspect skin for irritation or pressure areas In small children, inspect beneath cast for items that child may place there In older children, caution not to place items under cast Keep exposed skin clean and free of irritants
Maintain cast integrity	Do not allow weight bearing until cast is completely dry—even if weight-bearing device is attached Change position of child in body cast or hip spica cast periodically; small child can be managed easily; adolescent may require one or two persons; eventually children become very adept at moving themselves Do *not* use abduction stabilizer bar between legs of hip spica as handle for turning Position with buttocks lower than shoulders during toileting to prevent urine from flowing under cast at the back; body can be supported on pillows Protect rim of cast around perineal area of body cast with plastic film, oil silk, or Saran wrap to prevent soiling during toileting For infants and small children who are not toilet trained or who are prone to "accidents," use plastic-backed disposable diaper with edges tucked underneath rim of cast; a sanitary napkin can also be used if waterproof material is placed between pad and cast Place small child on Bradford frame Caution against activities that might cause physical damage to cast

Continued.

Summary of nursing care of the child with a cast—cont'd

Goals	Responsibilities
Maintain muscle use of unaffected areas	Encourage to ambulate as soon as possible Support casted arm in sling Teach use of mobilizing devices such as crutches for casted leg (walking device is applied when weight bearing allowed) With newer devices, encourage to ambulate as soon as general condition allows Provide and encourage use of muscles in play activities and diversions If affected limbs are paralyzed, carry out range of motion exercises
Provide comfort	Position for comfort; use pillows to support dependent areas Alleviate itching underneath cast by alcohol swabs, cool air blown from Asepto syringe or fan Avoid using powder or lotion under cast, since these substances have tendency to "ball" and produce irritation Sometimes piece of tape is placed lengthwise beneath stockinette prior to cast application so that it can be moved up and down to "scratch" skin Soiled areas of cast can be removed with damp cloth and small amount of white, low-abrasive cleanser
Educate parents	Teach cast care and support of casted part Make certain that parents understand signs of circulatory impairment and infection Help parents plan suitable activities Help parents in problem solving of modification of clothing to fit over casted area Help parents devise supportive devices and modification of furniture for positioning (such as pillows, pads, and so on) Help parents in problem solving of means of transporting child
Support child during cast removal	Explain procedure Demonstrate safety of equipment Provide reassurance

Heated fans or dryers should not be used, since they cause the cast to dry on the outside and remain wet beneath or cause burns from heat conduction by way of the cast to the underlying tissue.

A wet cast should be supported by a pillow covered with plastic and handled by the palms of the hands to prevent indenting the cast and creating pressure areas. A dry plaster of Paris cast produces a hollow sound when it is tapped with the finger. If "hot spots" are felt on the cast surface, which usually indicate an infection beneath the area, this should be reported so that a window can be made in the cast to observe the site.

Frequently the child will be discharged to home care after a cast is applied in the emergency room or clinic. Parents need instructions on care of the cast and symptoms that indicate that the cast is too tight. They should also be told to bring the child for attention if the cast becomes too loose, since a loose cast no longer serves to maintain its purpose. During the first few hours after a cast is applied, the chief concern is that the extremity may continue to swell to the extent that the cast becomes a tourniquet, shutting off circulation and producing neurovascular complications. A measure for reducing the likelihood of this potential problem is to elevate the body part, thereby increasing venous return. If edema is excessive, casts are bivalved, that is, cut to make an anterior and a posterior half that are held together with an elastic bandage.

When casting an extremity that has sustained an open fracture, a window is often left over the wound area to allow for observation and for dressing of the wound. A surgical reduction is usually casted as for a closed fracture. For the first few hours after surgery there may be substantial bleeding that will soak through the cast. Periodically the circumscribed blood-stained area should be outlined with a ball-point pen or pencil and the time indicated to provide a guide for assessing the amount of bleeding.

Cutting the cast to remove the cast or relieve tightness is frequently a frightening experience for a child. He fears the sound of the cast cutter and is terrified that his flesh as well as the cast will be cut. Since it works by vibration, a cast cutter cuts only the hard surface of the cast. This can be demonstrated on the nurse or person removing the cast. However, the vibration generates heat that may be felt by the child, and this should be explained to him. Preparation for the procedure will help reduce his anxiety, especially if a trusting relationship has been established between the child and his nurse. Many young children come to regard the cast as a part of themselves, which intensifies their fear of removal. Using the analogy of having fingernails or hair cut sometimes helps reduce their anxiety. They need continual reassurance that all is going well and that their behavior is accepted.

For a summary of nursing care of the child with a cast, see the boxed material on pp. 1567 to 1568.

After the cast is removed the skin surface will be caked with desquamated skin and sebaceous secretions. Simple soaking in a bathtub is usually sufficient for its removal over a period of several days. Application of olive oil or lotion may provide comfort. Parents and child should be instructed not to pull or forcibly remove this material with vigorous scrubbing, which may cause excoriation and bleeding.

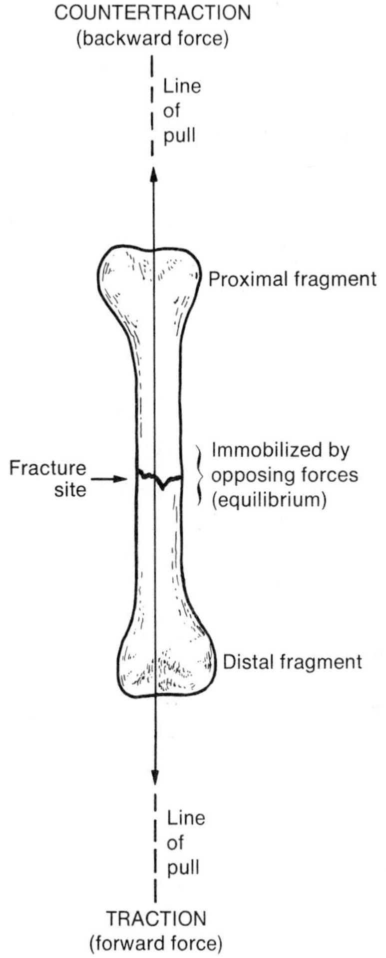

Fig. 40-14. Application of traction for maintaining equilibrium.

Child in traction

Bone fragments that cannot be aligned initially by simple traction and stabilization with a cast require the extended pulling force offered by continuous traction. Traction may be used for other purposes also: to provide rest for an extremity, to help correct or prevent contracture deformity, or, rarely, to reduce muscle spasms. In these cases the traction may be applied at night and intermittently during the day. Muscle relaxants may be administered for muscle spasms.

Purposes of traction. When forces having both direction and magnitude act on an object at the same point simultaneously from opposite directions, the object either changes its state of rest or motion or remains in equilibrium. The use of traction in the management of fractures is the direct application of these forces to produce equilibrium at the fracture site. A forward force (traction) is produced by attaching weight to the distal bone fragment, which is balanced by the backward force of the muscle pull (countertraction) and the frictional force between the patient and the bed. Thus the three essential components of traction management are traction, countertraction, and friction.[10] (Fig. 40-14).

To reduce or realign a fracture site, traction is provided by weights applied to the distal bone fragment; body weight provides countertraction. By adjusting the line of pull upward or downward or by adducting or abducting the extremity, the physician uses these forces to align the distal and proximal bone fragments. To attain equilibrium, the amount of forward force is adjusted by adding weight to or subtracting weight from the traction, and/or countertraction can be increased by elevating the foot of the bed to create a greater gravitational pull to the backward force. A bed board placed under the mattress of heavy children prevents sagging, which can change the direction of the forces applied to the fracture.

The three primary purposes for use of traction are:

1. To fatigue the involved muscle and reduce muscle spasm so that bones can be realigned
2. To position the distal and proximal bone ends in desired realignment to promote satisfactory bone healing

3. To immobilize the fracture site until realignment has been achieved and sufficient healing has taken place to permit casting or splinting

Fatiguing of a muscle is accomplished by applying constant stress to the muscle so that the buildup of lactic acid will produce muscle relaxation. The all-or-none law, characteristic of muscle contractability, influences the complete relaxation. When muscle is stretched, muscle spasm ceases and permits the realignment of the bone ends. The continuous maintenance of traction is important during this phase because releasing the traction allows the muscle's normal contracting ability to again cause a malpositioning of the bone ends.

The realignment of the fragments is a gradual process that is achieved more rapidly in infants, who have limited muscle tone, than in muscular teenagers. The desired line of pull and callus formation are checked periodically by x-ray examination. The traction pull to some degree immobilizes the fracture site; however, adjunctive immobilizing devices such as splints or casts are sometimes used with skeletal traction. In injuries in which there is severe soft tissue swelling or vascular and nerve damage, it is customary to use traction until these complications have been resolved and it is safe to apply a cast. A cast can act as a tourniquet if swelling occurs beneath it. Immobilization with traction will be maintained until the bone ends are in satisfactory realignment, after which a less-confining type of immobilization, usually a cast, will be applied.

Types of traction (general).[34] The pull needed for traction can be applied to the distal bone fragment in several ways:

manual traction traction applied to the body part by the hand placed distally to the fracture site. Nurses frequently provide manual traction during cast application.

skin traction pull applied directed to the skin surface and indirectly to the skeletal structures. The pulling mechanism is attached to the skin with adhesive material or an elastic bandage.

skeletal traction pull applied directly to the skeletal structure by a pin, wire, or tongs inserted into or through the diameter of the bone distal to the fracture.

Manual traction is used by the physician in uncomplicated arm or leg fractures in which there is little overriding of the bones and minimal muscle pull to overcome. Manual traction is used to realign bone fragments for immediate cast application. Skin traction is applied when there is minimal displacement and little muscle spasticity but is contraindicated when there is associated skin damage. Skin traction has specific limits of weight that it can pull without causing tissue breakdown. Skeletal traction is employed when significant traction pull must be applied in order to achieve realignment and immobilization. By inserting a pin or wire into the bone, the stress is placed on the bone and not on the surrounding tissue.

The type of traction applied is determined primarily by the age of the child, the condition of the soft tissues, and the type and degree of displacement of the fracture. The fractures most commonly treated by application of traction are those involving the humerus, femur, and vertebrae.

Upper extremity traction. Treatment of fractures of the humerus by traction is accomplished either by overhead suspension, in which the arm, bent at the elbow, is suspended vertically by skin or skeletal attachment and traction is applied to the distal end of the humerus, or by Dunlop traction.

Dunlop traction. With Dunlop traction (Fig. 40-15) the arm is suspended horizontally, using either skin or skeletal attachment. When skin traction is used, straps are placed on the lower and upper arm with the arm flexed to accomplish pull in two directions: one along the longitudinal direction of the upper arm and one to maintain alignment of the lower arm. In instances such as supracondylar frac-

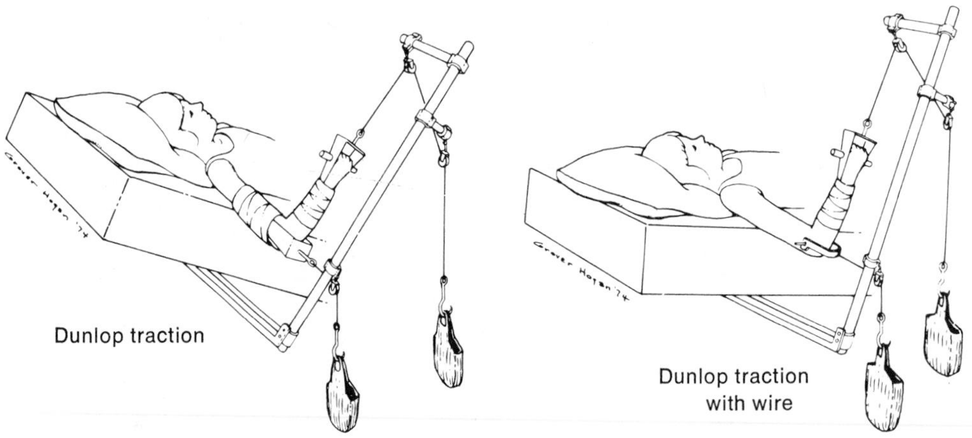

Fig. 40-15. Upper extremity traction used in treatment and care of children. (From Hilt, N. E., and Schmitt, E. W.: Pediatric orthopedic nursing, St. Louis, 1975, The C. V. Mosby Co., p. 121.)

tures, the amount of traction pull needed to align the site more critically necessitates that the Dunlop traction have a skeletal wire placed in the upper arm to allow the additional weight.[13]

Fractures of the humerus, which are usually the result of a fall with the arm in extension, frequently involve the supracondylar portion. There are three major complications associated with this injury: Volkmann's contractures (described on p. 1578), traumatic injury to the median, ulnar, or radial nerves, and angulation deformities. The fracture must be carefully reduced, sometimes under anesthesia, and because of the danger of complications, children with closed reduction of supracondylar fractures are frequently hospitalized for observation. In severely malaligned fractures closed reduction under anesthesia is followed by application of skeletal traction for 2 to 3 weeks, after which a long arm cast is applied for an additional 2 to 3 weeks.

Lower extremity traction. The frequent site for a femoral fracture is in the middle one third of the shaft as pictured by the x-ray film in Fig. 40-10. With this fracture there is significant overriding but minimal displacement. In a fracture in the lower one third of the shaft, the pull of the gastrocnemius muscle causes the distal fragment to become downwardly displaced. The severity of the fracturing force and the ability of the muscles to hold the fracture out of alignment will determine the fracture type and amount of overriding of the fragments. The periosteum may remain intact, but a spiral fracture with much displacement often occurs.

Fractures of the femur can often be reduced with immediate application of a hip spica cast in young children. When traction is required several types may be employed, based on the initial assessment.

Bryant's traction. When a traction pulls only in one direction it is called running traction. Bryant's traction is this type of traction (Fig. 40-16). Adhesive traction strips are applied to the child's legs and secured with elastic bandages wrapped from the foot to the groin. Both of the child's hips are flexed at a 90-degree angle with the knees in extension and the legs suspended by pulleys and weights. The child's weight supplies the countertraction; therefore, the buttocks are slightly elevated off the bed. By applying the same amount of traction to both legs and restraining the torso, the pelvis and hips are prevented from rotating and equal stress is placed on the growing extremities. The ankle bones are protected with stockinette or cotton wadding. This type of traction is used for children younger than 2 years of age whose weight is not sufficient to provide ade-

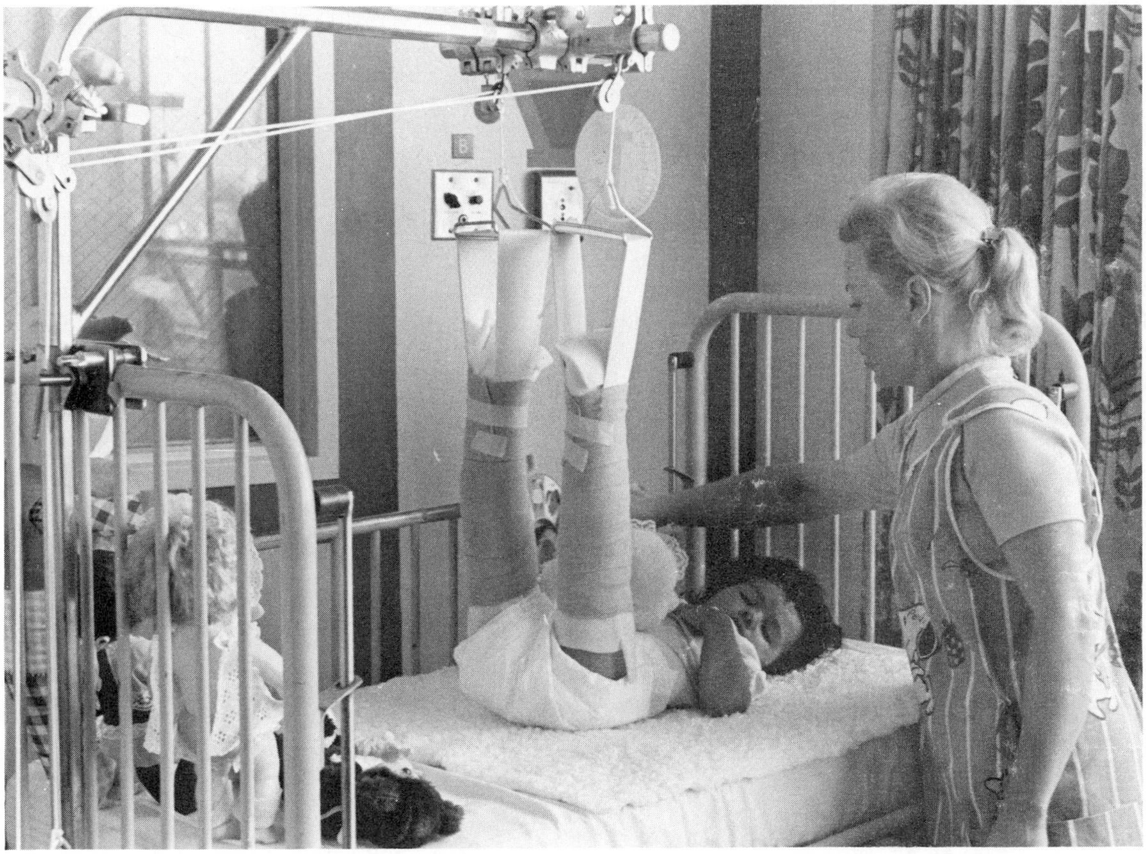

Fig. 40-16. Bryant's traction.

quate countertraction without the additional gravitational force. Both legs are suspended, even though only one may be involved. Bryant's traction is unsuited to older children and is usually limited to children who weigh less than 12 to 14 kg (26 to 30 pounds) because of the risk of postural hypertension and to those without spasticity or contractures of the hamstring muscles. The child's position needs to be monitored, and the alignment of the fracture is checked by periodic x-ray films with needed traction adjustments made by the physician. Remodeling and callus formation occur rapidly, within 2 to 3 weeks, after which the child is placed in a hip spica cast for an additional 3 to 9 weeks.

A specific complication of overhead traction is impairment of circulation with Volkmann's syndrome (see p. 1578). This is especially a problem in Bryant's traction because there is gravitational vascular draining of the elevated extremities, the possible tourniquet effect of the bandages, and the effect of the traction, which can trigger vasospasms.

A child younger than 2 years of age normally has his hips in flexion a good deal of the time; therefore, the mild contracture that might develop from this position is easily corrected. The youngster is permitted sufficient room between his foot and the traction foot plate to move his foot and prevent ankle problems. The legs must be maintained perpendicular to the trunk, and the buttocks should not be allowed to rest on the mattress. Sometimes the child, especially the very active child, is placed in a jacket restraint or on a Bradford frame to prevent his turning and twisting out of alignment.

Buck's extension. Buck's extension (Fig. 40-17) is also a running skin traction with the legs in an extended position, but it differs from Bryant's traction in that the hips are not flexed. The postural hypertension that could develop as a result of Bryant's traction is avoided, and this traction allows for greater mobility. Careful turning from side to side is permitted with the involved leg kept in alignment. Buck's extension is used primarily for short-term immobilization or, frequently, for correcting contracture or bone deformities such as Legg-Calvé-Perthes disease (p. 1525).

Russell traction. Russell traction (Fig. 40-18) uses skin traction on the lower leg and a padded sling under the knee. Two lines of pull, one along the longitudinal line of the lower leg and one perpendicular to the leg, are produced. This combination of pulls allows realignment of the lower extremity and immobilizes the hip and knee in a flexed position. The hip flexion must be kept at the prescribed angle to prevent fracture malalignment, since there is no direct support under the fracture and the skin traction may slip. Because the traction is set up to have two ropes pulling in the same direction at the foot plate, the traction pull will be twice the amount of weight at the end of the bed. For example, 5 pounds of weight produces 10 pounds of pull. Special nursing measures include carefully checking the position of the traction so that the amount of desired hip flexion is maintained and damage to the common peroneal nerve under the knee does not produce footdrop.

Ninety-degree–90-degree traction. The most common skeletal traction is 90-degree–90-degree traction (Fig. 40-19), in which the lower leg is put in a boot cast and a skeletal Steinmann's pin or Kirschner wire is placed in the distal fragment of the femur. This traction:

- Achieves the desired line of pull for reducing the fracture by means of the skeletal traction
- Allows a 90-degree flexion of both the hip and knee
- Supports the lower extremity in a desired position with good venous return
- Provides adequate immobilization of the fracture site

From a nursing standpoint this traction easily facilitates position changes, toileting, and prevention of traction complications.

Balance suspension traction. Balance suspension traction (Fig. 40-20) may be used with or without skin or skeletal traction. Unless used with another traction, the balanced suspension merely suspends the leg in a desired flexed position to relax the hip and hamstring muscles and does not exert any traction directly on a body part. A Thomas' splint extends from the groin to midair above the foot and a Pearson attachment supports the lower leg. Towels or

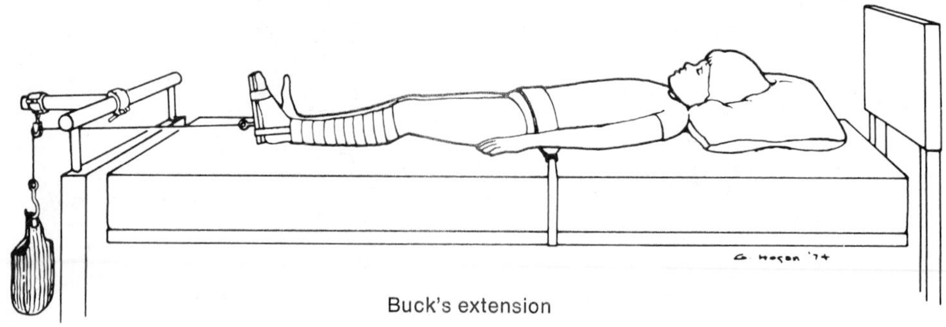

Fig. 40-17. Buck's extension. (From Hilt, N. E., and Schmitt, E. W.: Pediatric orthopedic nursing, St. Louis, 1975, The C. V. Mosby Co.,. p. 122.)

pieces of felt, covered with stockinette, are clipped or pinned to the splints for leg support. Note that the ropes are attached to create a balanced traction. If the child is lifted off the bed, the traction will lift with him and no alignment will be lost. The Pearson attachment will stay wherever positioned. Many times the physician will put a rope between the end of the Pearson attachment and the end of Thomas' splint to prevent any knee flexion alteration while the child is moved. This traction requires very careful checking of splints and ropes to make certain that no slippage or fraying has occurred. The traction is of great value in an older and heavier child when lifting the patient for care is essential.

Cervical traction. The cervical area is a vulnerable site for flexion or extension injuries to muscle, vertebrae, and/or the spinal cord. Cervical muscle trauma without other

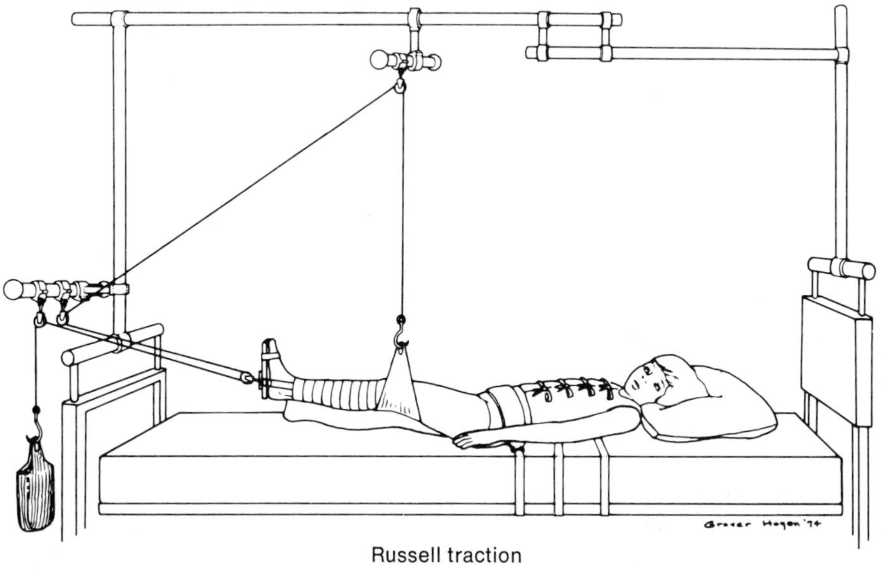

Fig. 40-18. Russell traction. (From Hilt, N. E., and Schmitt, E. W.: Pediatric orthopedic nursing, St. Louis, 1975, The C. V. Mosby Co., p. 123.)

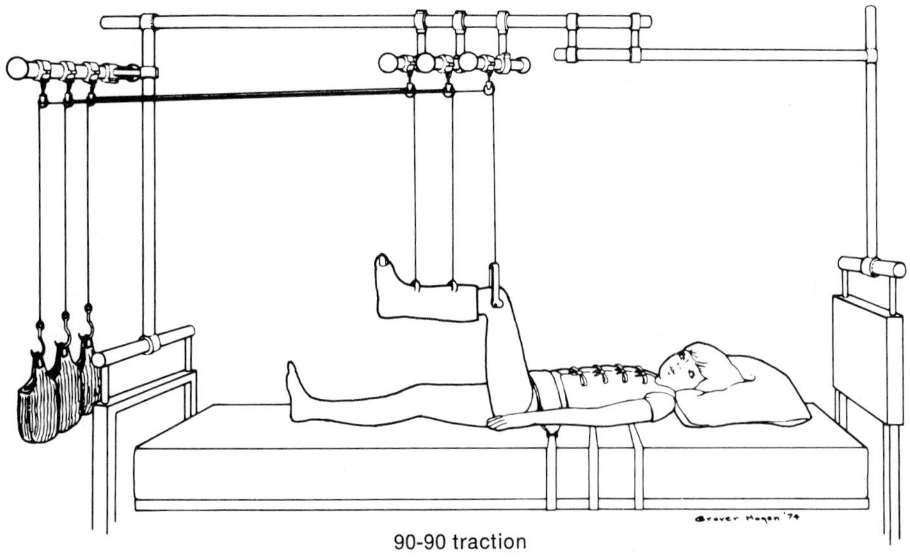

Fig. 40-19. Ninety-degree–90° traction. (From Hilt, N. E., and Schmitt, E. W.: Pediatric orthopedic nursing, St. Louis, 1975, The C. V. Mosby Co., p. 124.)

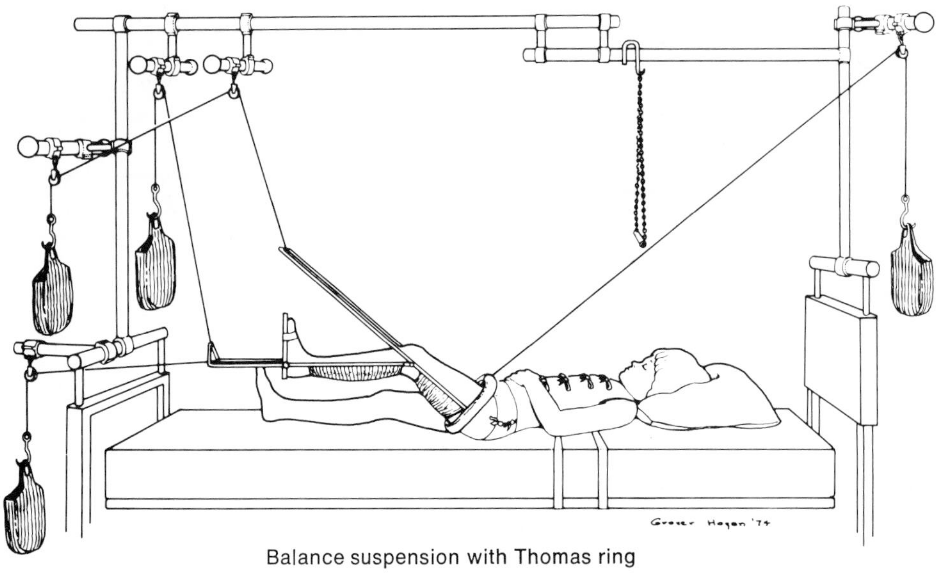

Balance suspension with Thomas ring splint and Pearson attachment

Fig. 40-20. Balance suspension. (From Hilt, N. E., and Schmitt, E. W.: Pediatric orthopedic nursing, St. Louis, 1975, The C. V. Mosby Co., p. 124.)

complications is treated with a cervical soft or hard collar to relieve the weight of the head from the fracture site. Intermittent cervical skin traction might be employed with a chin halter and weight to decrease muscle spasms (Fig. 40-21). The injuries limited to cervical muscles can be very uncomfortable but, with prompt medical care, usually resolve with conservative treatment.

When a child displaces or fractures a cervical vertebra, it is necessary to reduce and immobilize the site with cervical skeletal traction. The spinal cord runs through the intravertebral canal, and dislocation or fracture of the vertebrae can also cause spinal cord trauma.

Physical examination, especially a neurologic assessment, and roentgenographic studies are essential diagnostic aids to determine:

- Presence of vertebral fracture
- Degree of vertebral dislocation
- Displacement of intravertebral disc
- Compression of spinal cord and other neurologic structures
- Sensory, motor, and autonomic nerve deficits

Cervical traction is usually accomplished by making burr holes in the skull and inserting Crutchfield or Cone-Barton tongs. The head is placed in a hyperextended position, and, as the neck muscles fatigue with constant traction pull, the vertebral bodies gradually are pulled apart and the cord is no longer pinched between the vertebrae. Immobilization until fracture healing can occur is a second goal of cervical traction. If the injury has been limited to a vertebral fracture without neurologic deficit, a halo cast can be applied to permit earlier ambulation.

Nursing care of child in traction. Traction is a valuable therapy if the purposes for the traction are achieved without complications. Generally the child in traction is hospitalized under the direct care of nurses who develop individualized nursing care plans based on an understanding of correct traction management. Evaluating the therapeutic effects and possible negative consequences is essential to good patient care. Many of the nursing problems associated with a child in traction are related to immobility. However, there are a number of physical needs that require attention and vigilance. First of all it is important that nurses understand the basic principles of traction and their role in its maintenance. Skeletal traction is never released by the nurse, but, under certain circumstances, such as the child with Legg-Calvé-Perthes disease or scoliosis, nonadhesive skin traction may be removed by the nurse. In these cases intermittent traction is periodically released and reapplied as ordered. When skin traction must be constantly maintained, such as in fractures, nurses may occasionally remove and reapply the Ace bandage if this is approved by the attending physician, provided that *someone manually maintains the traction during the rewrapping process*. It is not uncommon for a child to have several types of traction at one time, and each traction must be assessed separately to avoid problems.

When the child is first placed in traction he may have an increase in discomfort as a result of the traction pull fatiguing the muscle. Analgesics and muscle relaxants will help during this phase of care, but helping the child cope with the confinement and new experience requires more than medications. At the child's level of development an explanation should be given of what is happening and why he must

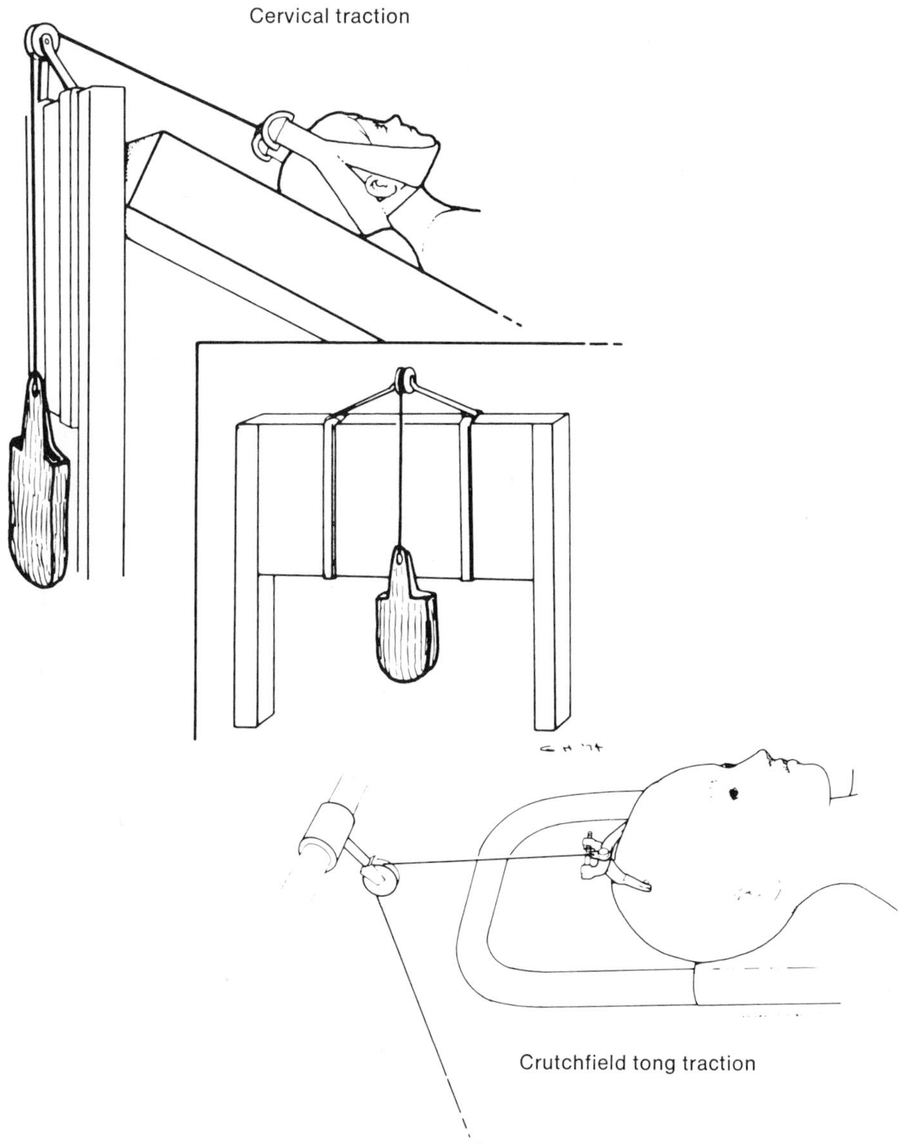

Fig. 40-21. Cervical traction. (From Hilt, N. E., and Schmitt, E. W.: Pediatric orthopedic nursing, St. Louis, 1975, The C. V. Mosby Co., p. 125.)

remain in the device, and he should be reassured of the presence of someone who will aid him in adjusting to the traction and coping with the problems of immobilization.[11]

The specific nursing responsibilities for the patient in cervical traction include:

1. Watching for any changes in neurologic signs and symptoms that indicate that traction is benefiting or causing more problems.
2. Carrying out meticulous skin care around the tong sites often. The nursing protocol is to clean the sites several times a day with saline solution or hydrogen peroxide and then apply a topical antiseptic such as povidone-iodine (Betadine). Sloughing of the pin site and osteomyelitis of the skull bone are potential dangers.
3. Use of the guidelines in the summary of nursing care for a child in traction as outlined in the following section. (See the boxed material.)
4. Log rolling the child's body without flexion of neck or spine at least every 2 hours. Stryker frames are often used with cervical traction to facilitate maintaining alignment.
5. Placing supporting pillows beside the neck prior to turning and having necessary pillows available to support the back, arms, and legs.
6. Use of nursing approaches for persons with spinal cord injuries as elaborated later in this chapter.

Summary of nursing care of the child in traction

Goals	Responsibilities
Decrease anxiety and gain cooperation	Explain traction apparatus to child Explain to child what his nursing care will be Determine with child how he can participate in his care Make certain that child knows how to call for help Assure child that he will not be left totally helpless
Maintain traction	Understand purpose of traction Understand function of traction in each specific situation Check desired line of pull and relationship of distal fragment to proximal fragment Check whether fragment is being directed upward, adducted, or abducted Check function of each component part Position of bandages, frames, splints Ropes In center track of pulley Taut No fraying Knots tied securely Pulleys In original position on attachment bar; have not slid from original site Wheels freely movable Weights Correct amount of weight Hanging freely In safe location Check bed position—head or foot elevated as directed for desired amount of pull and countertraction Do not remove skeletal traction or adhesive traction straps on skin traction
Skin traction	When permitted and/or absolutely necessary, replace nonadhesive straps and/or Ace bandage on skin traction, but make certain that traction on limb is maintained by someone during procedure Assess bandages to ascertain if they are correctly applied (diagonal or spiral), not too loose or too tight, which could cause slippage and malalignment of traction
Skeletal traction	Check pin sites frequently for signs of bleeding, inflammation, or infection Cleanse and dress pin sites as ordered Apply topical antiseptic or antibiotic daily as ordered Cover ends of pins with protective cord or padding to prevent child's being scratched by pin Note pull of traction on pin; pull should be even Check pin screws to be certain that screws are tight in metal clamp that attaches traction apparatus to pin
Maintain alignment	Observe for correct body alignment with emphasis on alignment of shoulders, hip, and leg(s) Check after child has moved Apply restraints when indicated Maintain correct angles at joints, for example: Bryant's traction—90-degree angle at hip Russell traction—20-degree angle at hip

Summary of nursing care of the child in traction—cont'd

Goals	Responsibilities
Prevent complications	Assess child's behavior to determine if traction causes pain or discomfort
Pressure	Change position at least every 2 hours to relieve pressure and stimulate circulation with gentle massage over pressure areas Provide sheepskin or alternating pressure mattress underneath hips and back Make total body skin checks for redness or breakdown, especially over areas that receive greatest pressure; wash and dry skin at least twice daily Assess circular dressings for excessive tightness Assess restraining devices Make certain that they are not too loose or too tight Remove periodically and check for pressure areas Encourage deep breathing frequently with maximal inspiratory chest expansion Note any neurovascular changes, such as Color in skin and nail beds Alterations in sensation Alterations in motor ability Take immediate action to correct problem or report to physician if neurovascular change found Record findings of neurovascular changes Carry out passive, active, or active-with-resistance exercises as prescribed Note if any tightness, weakness, or contractures are developing in uninvolved joints and muscles Take measures to correct or prevent further development, such as applying foot plate to prevent footdrop Move involved joint or muscle frequently to avoid contractures Encourage child in activities that provide exercise for uninvolved muscles and joints
Provide adequate nutrition and hydration	Encourage fluid intake so child stays well hydrated Provide nourishing, nonconstipating diet with preferred foods when possible and foods that child can manage unassisted Make certain that child ingests sufficient amount of calcium-rich foods
Promote elimination	Check frequency and consistency of bowel movements Adjust fluid and food intake according to stools, for example, increase fluids, fruits, grains for constipation Administer stool softeners as indicated Administer rectal suppository or mild laxative if indicated Use fracture pan for bowel movements Assure adequate renal output by increasing fluids when indicated
Relieve pain and discomfort	Administer pain medication as needed during first 2 or 3 days after fracture Use pads, pillows, and rolls to position for comfort

Fracture complications

Complications associated with fractures and immobilization are varied and have some problems in common. In addition to problems related to immobilization, the major complications of fractures include the following.

Inadequate circulation. If the trauma or immobilizing device restricts veins or arteries in the affected extremity, bone healing will be seriously impaired. Careful assessment of the pulses, skin color, and temperature is an important nursing responsibility. After injury swelling of tissues occurs more rapidly in children than in the adult. In the upper extremity brachial, radial, ulnar, and digital pulses are felt. In the leg femoral, popliteal, posterior tibial, and dorsalis pedis pulses are checked. When circulatory impairment is evident (absence of pulse, discoloration, swelling, and pain), the nurse takes quick action to relieve the problem, that is, the situation is reported immediately. If the physician is unable to come and release the pressure, the nurse must be able to cut the cast in half to form a bivalve cast or make a large window in it to decrease the pressure.

Closely associated with an inadequate blood supply is a low hematocrit value, which can result from the initial blood loss or surgically induced anemia. Although the blood flow may be adequate, a lowered amount of hemoglobin will not provide sufficient oxygen for tissue repair.

Volkmann's syndrome.[32] Elbow and knee injuries are prone to arterial blood vessel obstruction, which can lead to Volkmann's syndrome. This type of ischemia is a pathologic process that begins with arterial occlusion and then progresses to muscle anoxia and reflex vasospasms. Finally the lack of blood supply leads to muscle necrosis, paralysis, and contractures. Any fracture that requires excessive traction, especially Bryant's traction, can be complicated by Volkmann's syndrome.

The neuromuscular symptoms are severe pain, pallor or cyanosis, absence of pulses in the extremity, paresthesia, and paralysis. Unrelieved, the occlusive hypoxic process can do a great deal of muscle damage within 12 to 24 hours with muscle fibrosis and contractures in 5 to 10 days.

The immediate treatment is aimed at removing any mechanically obstructive materials such as tight bandages and extending the joint to free the blood vessels. If the symptoms do not improve within a few hours, arteriography is done in anticipation that surgery may be needed to decrease arterial spasms and to improve the blood supply by separation of the fascial sheaths of the involved muscles. Secondary complications of Volkmann's syndrome are muscle contractures that severely limit function and nerve damage leading to paralysis.

Local nerve damage. Nerve damage can take place at the time of injury, develop in the process of realignment, or be a complication of an immobilizing apparatus. Peroneal nerve damage can result in footdrop, and radial nerve impairment produces wristdrop. Both of these disabilities can significantly interfere with activities of daily living. Sensory testing with touch and pinprick and evaluating motor strength by asking the child to move the unaffected joint distal to the injury are common means of determining neurologic involvement. The physician determines whether correcting the alignment will alleviate pressure on the nerve or if surgical intervention is necessary. At times sensory or motor changes indicate ischemia and the treatment is to correct the vascular problem.

Epiphyseal damage. Growth of bone occurs from the epiphyseal plate, and damage to this structure could result in an unequal extremity length. Surgical intervention to the epiphysis on the affected leg or to the epiphyseal line on the opposite leg is the usual treatment.[16,26]

Nonunion. Bone healing and callus formation can span and repair only a limited space between fragments. When inadequate reduction, poor immobilization, or a damaged or softened cast cannot maintain the bone fragments in correct alignment for repair, bone healing is impaired. Based on the physiologic needs for bone healing, the factors most likely to interfere with bone healing and cause delayed union or nonunion are:

- Loss of hematoma
- Interposition of tissue
- Infections
- Poor nutrition
- Interruption of blood supply
- Diseases that influence calcium metabolism (such as thyroid disorder)
- Cancer of bone
- Administration of steroids

The hematoma, which becomes the matrix for bone deposition in the break, must be free of infection or bits of adipose or connective tissue. The constant supply of nutrients and bone-forming cells brought to the area by way of the bloodstream provide the vital ingredients for repair.

Sometimes artificial means are employed to facilitate bone healing. Bone grafting becomes necessary when bone nonunion occurs. The donor sites are usually the tibia or the iliac crest. Bleeding of bone ends may need to be created, and at times holes are drilled near the bone ends in an attempt to increase circulation. Postsurgical immobilization of the recipient area is crucial to a successful graft.

Malunion. Unsatisfactory reduction is the usual reason for malunion. A cast or splint that allows fracture movement will also likely result in malunion. Periodic x-ray examinations will help detect this possible complication and avoid its becoming a major problem over a long period of time.

Osteomyelitis.[32] Osteomyelitis, infection of the bone, is often secondary to a bloodstream infection but is a potential problem in open fractures or when bone surgery has been performed (see p. 1531). Any bacterial organism can cause this infectious process; however, *Staphylococcus aureus* is the most frequent pathogen.

Kidney stones. Although uncommon in children, renal calculi are a potential risk whenever the child is nonweight bearing for a period of time, especially if the circumstances also produce urinary stasis. An associated problem, hypercalcemia, is reviewed under problems of the immobilized child. Preventative measures for renal calculi are to maintain good hydration, to mobilize the child as much as possible, and to check closely the amount and characteristics of urinary output. Any urinary tract infection should be treated promptly with appropriate antimicrobials and urine acidification because the nucleus of the calculi is often composed of bacterial debris or calcium and the buildup of stone is precipitated by alkaline urine.

Pulmonary emboli.[25,32] Blood, air, or fat emboli can be a hazard to the child with a fracture. As the postinjury bleeding and clotting occur, a small piece of the clot can travel to vital organs such as the lung, heart, or brain and produce a life-threatening vascular obstruction and ischemia. Generally the pulmonary system is the most frequent site for emboli deposition, but it may not occur until 6 to 8 weeks postinjury.

Fat emboli are the greatest threat to an individual with multiple fractures, particularly in fractures of the long bones such as the femur. Fat droplets from the marrow are transferred to the general circulation by means of venous-arterial route where they can be transported to the lung or brain. This type of emboli phenomenon occurs within the first 24 hours, generally in the second 12 hours after the injury occurs.

Emboli in the vital organs produce the classic signs and symptoms of shock. Petechial hemorrhages of the chest and shoulders are the outstanding signs that differentiate this condition from other etiologies of shock. In the immobilized child who suddenly develops chest pain and dyspnea when turned, pulmonary embolism should be suspected. The severe dyspnea must be treated immediately by elevating the head when possible and administering oxygen by means of mask, cannula, or hood. Deep breathing, coughing, and mechanical respiratory assistance are important to maintain adequate alveolar gas exchange. An intravenous infusion is established to treat the shock and administer medications such as heparin and corticosteroids.

Amputation. A child may be born with the congenital absence of a body part (p. 394), have a traumatic loss of an extremity, or need a surgical amputation for a pathologic condition such as osteogenic sarcoma (p. 1049). With today's surgical technology and the quick thinking of a bystander who saves a traumatically amputated body part, some children have had fingers and arms sewn back on with variable degrees of functional use regained. A severed part should be wrapped in a clean cloth or placed in saline if possible and taken to the hospital with the victim.

Operative amputations or the surgical repair of a permanently severed limb focuses on constructing an adequately nourished stump. A smooth, healthy, padded stump, free of nerve endings, is important in prothesis fitting and subsequent ambulation. In some situations in which there is no vascular or neurologic deficit, a cast is applied to the stump immediately postoperatively and a pylon, metal extension, and artificial foot are attached so that the patient can walk on the temporary prothesis within a few hours.

Stump shaping is done postoperatively with special elastic bandaging using a figure-of-8 bandage, which applies pressure in a cone-shaped fashion. This technique decreases stump edema, controls hemorrhage, and aids in developing desired contours so that the child will bear weight on the posterior aspect of the skin flap rather than on the end of the stump. Stump elevation may be used during the first 24 hours, but after this time the extremity should not be left in this position since contractures in the proximal joint will develop and seriously hamper ambulation. Monitoring proper body alignment will further decrease the risk of flexion contractures.

For older children and adolescents, arm exercises and bed pushups, as well as parallel bars, which are used in prothesis-training programs, help to build up the arm muscles necessary for walking with crutches. Full range of motion of joints above the amputation must be performed several times daily, using active and isotonic exercises. Young children are spontaneously active and require little encouragement.

Depending on the child's age, he or his parent will need to learn stump hygiene with careful soap and water washing every day and checking for skin irritation, breakdown, or infection. A tube of stockinette, cornstarch, or talcum powder is used to slide the prosthesis on more easily. A careful skin check must be done every time the prosthesis is removed, and prosthesis tolerance time must be adjusted to prevent skin breakdown.

Phantom limb sensation is an expected experience for the child who has had an amputation because the nerve-brain connections are still present. Gradually these sensations fade. Preoperative discussion of this phenomenon will aid the child in understanding his "usual feelings" and not hide his experiences from others. Limb pain, especially pain that increases with ambulation, should be evaluated for the possibility of a neuroma at the free nerve endings in the stump. Psychogenic phantom limb pain is a complex problem involving the child's response to the altered body image and the coping mechanisms he is using to handle the new experience. The problem of amputation, particularly the psychologic aspects, is discussed on p. 1049.

SPINAL CORD INJURIES

Spinal cord injuries with major neurologic involvement are not a common cause of physical handicap in childhood.

However, there are a sufficient number of children with these injuries admitted to major medical centers and, because of the increased survival as the result of improved management, nurses are more likely to become involved with such children. In addition the catastrophic nature of spinal cord injury with its serious sequelae and the importance of preventative and functional rehabilitation justify a discussion of the topic. Also, the principles of management and nursing care apply to all spinal cord lesions regardless of etiology, particularly myelomeningocele, the most common cause of paraplegia in the pediatric age-group (p. 369).

No comprehensive studies are available to indicate the incidence of spinal cord injury in children. Isolated reports indicate the highest incidence to be in young adults, whereas major rehabilitation centers report from two to four new cases per year in children.

However, it is not rare to have a number of teenagers in the population of rehabilitation centers, and their care is complex since it involves nursing activities associated with vertebral fracture healing, immobilization for a prolonged period of time, psychosocial disruption of the child and his family, and a neurologic deficit.

The first part of this chapter focused on musculoskeletal trauma and care of the immobilized child, which is applicable to the child with damage to the spinal cord. The child with a spinal cord injury presents additional problems, namely the complications of the neuropathology of the central and autonomic nervous systems.

Definitions: quadriplegia and paraplegia. *Paraplegia* is defined as a paralysis in two extremities, usually the lower limbs. A high level of paraplegia may create major problems in being able to sit upright without support, whereas paraplegic children with lower level injuries can walk with minimal assistance. The extent of paralysis is determined by both neurologic and clinical assessment. Although the majority of children with spinal cord injuries are paraplegic, many are quadriplegic. In medical terminology *quadriplegia,* or *tetraplegia,* means functional disuse in all four extremities. Some quadriplegic children are able to move only their face and neck muscles, whereas others are able to lift and bend their arms but are unable to perform fine hand movements. This word usually evokes a mental picture of a completely limp person, but this is not generally the case. Whereas a layman, on hearing the terms quadriplegia and paraplegia, generally focus on the loss of sensation and motor ability of the child, the professional who has cared for a child with a spinal cord injury is aware of the full extent of the problem. Almost every physiologic system is disrupted in a child with high-level quadriplegia. Not only are the central and peripheral nerves impaired, but there is also autonomic nervous system dysfunction. Vital structures such as blood vessels, lungs, bladder, and bowel are affected. Therefore, an understanding of neuromuscular physiology is essential to care effectively for the child with damage or injury to the spinal cord.

Review of essential neuromuscular physiology

The spinal cord extends from the medulla oblongata to the lower border of the first lumbar vertebra and contains millions of nerve fibers (Fig. 40-22). However, because of its protected location, a considerable amount of direct trauma is required to cause injury. Anteriorly the cord is protected by the spinous processes, which are stabilized by related ligaments and muscles. It is further protected by the spinal fluid, which surrounds it and absorbs some of the shock.

The spinal cord is subdivided into thirty-one segments—cervical (eight), thoracic (twelve), lumbar (five), sacral (five), and coccygeal (one). The eight cervical cord segments lie within the first seven vertebrae, and the remaining cord segments extend from the first thoracic vertebra to the lower level of the first lumbar vertebra; therefore, the cord segments do not match anatomically by number the thirty associated vertebrae. However, nerves that arise from the cord segments exit from the spinal column at the numerically corresponding vertebrae. Nerve tracts that extend downward from the end of the cord within the spinal column and exit through the lumbar and sacral vertebrae to innervate the lower extremities are called the cauda equina. In describing injuries to the spinal cord, the highest point at which there is normal function is referred to in relation to these segments, for example, an intact cord at the sixth cervical segment is designated as a C6 injury. In order for a cord segment to be normal it must have its reflex arc, sensory pathway, and motor response intact. For example, a child with a T8 injury would have reflexes, sensorium, and motor power at the thoracic 8 cord level but a neurologic deficit at the thoracic 9 level.

Certain areas of the curved vertebral column are less stable and more prone to damage from severe flexion and twisting. These sites are the cervical area, especially C5, C6, and C7, and the junction of the thoracic and lumbar regions, T12, L1, and L2. The rib cage and torso provide support to the thoracic portion; therefore, injuries to these segments occur less often. However, when spinal cord damage occurs in the thoracic area it usually produces irreparable damage. For example, injuries at levels T1 through T12 will cause decreased vital capacity as a result of nerve disruption to intercostal muscles. The cervical vertebrae are the most frequently fractured, and this high level of injury can produce many associated neurologic problems. For example, injuries to the C5 level or above involve the phrenic nerve leading to the diaphragm; high cervical levels (C1 through C3) may have brain stem involvement with tachycardia or bradycardia, respiratory insufficiency or failure, and stimulation of the vomiting center. Cervical and high thoracic segment injuries (T4 level and above) produce

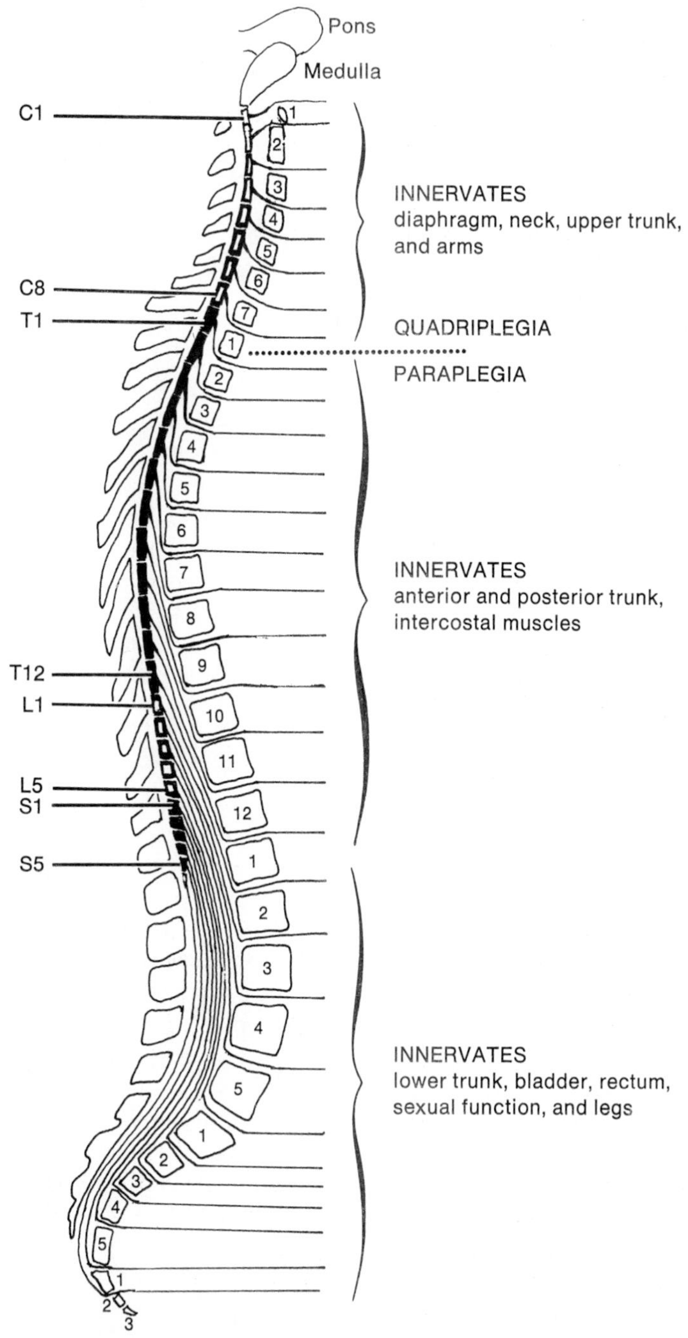

Fig. 40-22. Relationship of spinal cord segments and spinal nerves to vertebral bodies. Cervical nerves exit through intervertebral foramina above their respective vertebral bodies (seven cervical vertebrae and eight cervical nerves). The spinal cord ends at the L1 to L2 vertebral level. (Modified from Mayo Clinic: Clinical examinations in neurology, Philadelphia, 1971, W. B. Saunders Co.)

sweating, blood pressure problems, respiratory disturbances, and autonomic hyperreflexia. Horner's syndrome (changes in the eyeball and ptosis of the upper lid) results from sympathetic nervous system involvement. Damage to sacral cord segments produces mobility problems of varying degrees; S2, S3, S4, and S5 involvement leads to bladder, bowel, and sexual problems (especially in the male).

The spinal cord is nourished by branches of the vertebral and radicular arteries, specifically the anterior spinal artery and two posterior spinal arteries. Traumatic tearing or embolic occlusion of these vessels can markedly jeopardize the cord tissue. When this rich blood supply is impaired, the result is frequently severe neurologic deficit, extending even to complete loss of cord function at that level.

Cell bodies of interneurons and motor neurons within the spinal cord are identified as H-shaped gray matter surrounded by columns of white myelinated nerve fibers, each column serving as a route for a specific type of impulse, such as touch, vibration, pain, and temperature (Fig. 40-23). Nerve pathways in the spinal cord transmit sensory and motor impulses between peripheral receptors and the brain, conduct impulses through the reflex arc, and transmit sympathetic and parasympathetic nerve impulses from the brain to peripheral structures. (See also Fig. 39-1, p. 1513.)

Thirty-one pairs of spinal nerves, one pair for each spinal cord segment, conduct impulses from receptor end-plates to the spinal cord. Sensory transmission begins in the peripheral receptors where sensory receptors pick up a wide variety of stimuli and transfer the impulses, by means of peripheral nerves, to the spinal nerves where they make ganglionic connections and enter the cord posteriorly. At this point the impulses travel in two directions: (1) across the intraneuron connection and then to the motor neurons (reflex arc), and (2) up the spinal cord to the brain. The motor fibers of the reflex arc are *lower motor neurons,* an important point to remember when making a neurologic assessment. The relative dominance of the higher central nervous system over the reflex arcs suppresses some of the reflex responses and explains some of the spastic responses observed in spinal cord injury when the central centers no longer exert an influence. The sensory impulses are carried to various predetermined areas of the brain where a response is elicited.

With motor cortex stimulation in the brain, impulses are transmitted to the medulla, where nerve tracts cross, and then proceed down the descending motor pathways of the spinal column. When the impulses reach the desired level within the spinal cord, they connect with the anterior horn cells and are transmitted to the muscle fibers by means of the lower motor neurons, which are part of the spinal nerves. The spinal nerves synapse with the peripheral nerves and then complete the impulse conduction to a group of muscles to complete a meaningful movement, such as lifting an arm. A network of nerves that serves the major muscle groups constitutes a plexus. Total involvement of any one of these plexuses seriously impairs function to the areas it innervates. The three major plexuses are:

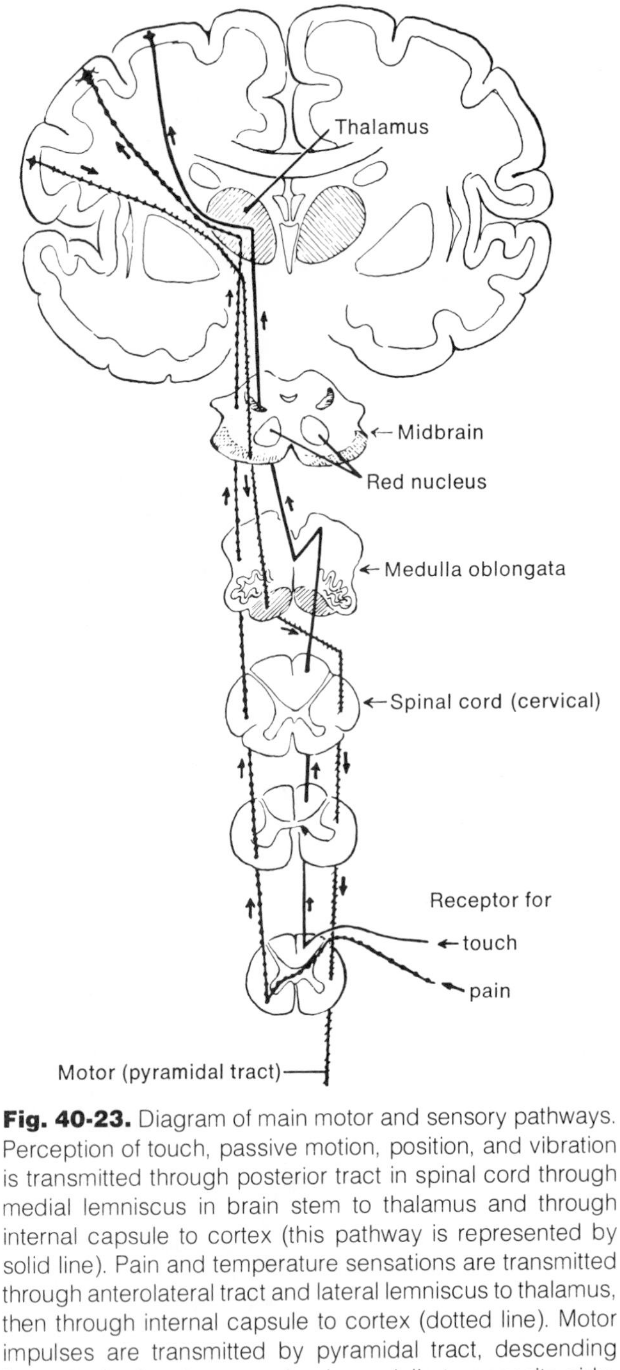

Fig. 40-23. Diagram of main motor and sensory pathways. Perception of touch, passive motion, position, and vibration is transmitted through posterior tract in spinal cord through medial lemniscus in brain stem to thalamus and through internal capsule to cortex (this pathway is represented by solid line). Pain and temperature sensations are transmitted through anterolateral tract and lateral lemniscus to thalamus, then through internal capsule to cortex (dotted line). Motor impulses are transmitted by pyramidal tract, descending from cerebral cortex, crossing in medulla to opposite side, and continuing to anterior horns of spinal cord. (From Conway, B. L.: Carini and Owens' neurological and neurosurgical nursing, ed. 7, St. Louis, 1978, The C. V. Mosby Co., p. 65.)

Cervical plexus (C1 through C4), which innervates the neck and diaphragm

Brachial plexus (C4 through T1), which supplies the shoulders, chest, and arms
Lumbosacral plexus (L1 through S4), which transmits impulses to the lower trunk and legs

Upper vs lower motor neuron. Upper motor neurons are those that extend from cerebral centers to the cells in the spinal column; lower motor neurons consist of the anterior horn cells and the spinal and peripheral nerves. In spinal cord injury the trauma is referred to as an upper or lower motor neuron injury; therefore, an understanding of the basic anatomy and physiology of these nerve pathways is essential for intelligent nursing care of the child with a spinal cord injury. For example, if a cord is injured at the C7 level, all upper motor neurons at and below that point and the specific reflex arcs at the C7 level would be involved. A child with lower motor neuron damage suffers a neurologic deficit in the anterior horn cell or in the spinal and peripheral nerves that contain the lower motor neurons. For example, a child with only a cauda equina injury would have involvement limited to the lower motor neurons. Most persons with spinal cord injuries have upper motor neuron injuries; children born with spinal cord defects primarily have lower motor neuron deficits. Table 40-4 illustrates the differences between upper and lower motor neuron syndromes.

Effect on sensory and motor tracts. Voluntary muscle control is lost when complete transection of the cord occurs. In partial transection function is altered in varying degrees, depending on the areas innervated by the nerves involved. Because of the crossing at various levels it is possible for an injured person to have motor paralysis in one leg but retain pain and temperature sensation to that leg while losing these sensations in the opposite leg, which retains its motor function.

Although a transected cord injury leads to sensory loss, it is not uncommon for the injured person to have pain experiences. Smooth or skeletal muscle spasms may cause pain. Other etiologies of pain are destruction of the myelin sheath with impulses crossing over to adjacent nerves and scar formation or irritation of nerve endings. The pain suffered by a quadriplegic or paraplegic person is often intensified because of the loss of sensation in other parts. Narcotics should be used with discretion, and, when possible, tranquilizers (which are good muscle relaxants) such as diazepam (Valium), should be used. Severe and prolonged pain should be medically evaluated for treatable pathology.

Effect on autonomic system. The cell bodies of the sympathetic nervous system are located in the lateral gray columns of the twelve thoracic and first three or four lumbar cord segments, and the preganglionic fibers, or axons, travel a short distance by way of the spinal nerves to the ganglionic chains lying on each side of the spinal cord. From the ganglionic chains the long post-ganglionic fibers terminate in a wide variety of organs. There are many interconnections within the ganglionic chains that produce the numerous effects of an activiated sympathetic nervous system called the ''mass response.''

Table 40-4. Differences in clinical manifestations between upper and lower motor neuron syndromes

Upper motor neuron syndrome	Lower motor neuron syndrome
Spastic paralysis in muscle groups below lesion (reflex arcs below lesion are intact)	Flaccid paralysis caused by muscle atonia (reflex arcs are permanently damaged)
Hyperreflexia with tendon reflexes exaggerated, Babinski reflex present	Reflex with associated muscle response absent
No wasting of muscle mass due to increased muscle tone	Marked atrophy of atonic muscle
Flexion contractures and spasms of mucle groups below lesion level common	Fasciculations (local twitching of muscle groups) common No flexor spasms
No skin or tissue changes	Loss of hair Skin and tissue changes Cornified nails

Parasympathetic cell bodies arise in the nuclei of the brain stem and in the lateral gray columns of the sacral cord. The long preganglionic fibers are contained in cranial nerves III, VII, IX, X, and XI and some pelvic nerves. The ganglia of the parasympathetic nerves lie near the effector organ, and a parasympathetic stimulus is relatively confined to a local organ response.

The sympathetic and parasympathetic systems receive both excitatory and inhibitory stimuli from the autonomic centers in the cerebral cortex, limbic system, and hypothalamus. These stimuli are transmitted by means of the white matter in the anterior portion of the cord with a feedback mechanism within the ascending fibers of the cord that normally control descending input. Axons of the many central nervous system neurons synapse with the autonomic preganglionic fibers and, thus, are able to alter their patterned responses. The most significant effects of autonomic disruption are:

1. Decreased muscle tone and impairment of vasoconstrictive effects of sympathetic innervation that cause venous pooling, diminished venous return to the heart, decreased cardiac output, and hypotension, especially orthostatic hypotension
2. Disruption between the thermoregulatory center in the hypothalamus and the skin receptors. Blood vessels remain dilated during the initial stage, the child is unable to sweat in response to increased environmental temperature, and elevated body temperature occurs rapidly
3. Loss of voluntary control of bowel and bladder function because of damage to L1, L2, and L3 levels and parasympa-

thetic fibers from S2, S3, and S4 levels, which innervate these organs

4. Altered sexual function, such as lack of erection, ejaculation, and orgasm resulting from interference with numerous nerve fibers and plexuses of sympathetic and parasympathetic nerves

Etiology and pathophysiology

The most common cause of serious spinal cord damage in children is congenital defects of the spinal cord. Postnatal causes are primarily accidental injury, especially motor vehicle accidents (including automobile-bicycle accidents), sports injuries (especially from diving, trampoline activities, and football), and birth trauma.

Mechanisms of injury. In automobile accidents most spinal cord injuries in children are the result of indirect trauma caused by sudden hyperflexion or hyperextension of the neck, often combined with a rotational force. Trauma to the spinal cord without evidence of vertebral fracture or dislocation is particularly apt to occur in motor vehicle accidents when proper restraints are not used. An unrestrained child becomes a projectile during sudden deceleration and subject to injury from contact with a variety of objects inside and outside the automobile. Falling from heights occurs less often in children than in adults, but vertebral compression of the spine from blows to the head or buttocks occurs in water sports (diving and surfing) or falls from horses or other athletic injuries. Birth injuries may occur in breech delivery from traction force on the cord during delivery of the head and shoulders. A number of teenagers receive cord injuries when they are accidentally shot or stabbed in the back.[20]

Common sites of injury in children are levels T12, L1, C5 and C6, and C1 and C2. Fracture dislocation is the most frequent immediate cause of spinal cord injury, particularly in the lower cervical region, because of the marked mobility of the neck. Spinal cord injury without fracture, although unusual in adults, is not uncommon in the child whose spine is more mobile than that of the adult, so that the force is more easily dissipated over a larger number of segments. In children the vertebral column, composed of cartilaginous rings, is capable of considerable elongation, whereas the cord itself, its meninges, and its vascular supply are unable to withstand the same degree of traction.[21,25]

Pathophysiology. The severity of the force, the mechanisms of the injury, and the degree of the individual's muscular relaxation at the time of the injury greatly influence the extensiveness of the trauma. Compression, contusion, laceration, or anatomic transection are the basic types of cord injuries and usually involve the following four interrelated pathologic changes:

1. Cellular damage to cord tissue
2. Hemorrhage and vascular damage
3. Structural changes of white and gray matter related to vascular disruption, inflammation, and edema
4. Local biochemical response to trauma

These changes are interrelated in that one can lead to the other. For example, an acute injury produces a decreased blood supply to the cord tissue with resultant ischemia that can lead to cellular necrosis. Acid metabolites accumulate with the hypoxic state and can contribute to further cellular damage. A concurrent inflammatory process produces cord edema above and below the traumatized segment, which further decreases the blood supply. Experimental spinal cord trauma indicates that the neurotransmitters norepinephrine and dopamine can be markedly altered in the first few hours postinjury, which causes further development of hemorrhagic necrosis in the central gray matter.

Clinical manifestations

As a result of these pathologic responses to the initial injury, spinal cord injury manifests two stages; therefore, the extent and severity of damage cannot be determined initially. Immediate loss of function is caused by both anatomic and impaired physiologic function, and improved function may not be evident for weeks or even months.

First stage. Manifestations of the initial response to acute injury is flaccid paralysis below the level of the damage.[24] This stage is known as diaschisis or *spinal shock syndrome* and is caused by the sudden disruption of central and autonomic pathways. The local effects of cord edema and ischemia produce a physiologic transection with or without an anatomic severance. The signs and symptoms will depend on the location and severity of the cord damage, but most children with a spinal cord injury experience some spinal shock. These symptoms are:

Absence of reflexes at or below the cord lesion, resulting in flaccidity or limpness of the involved muscles
Loss of sensation and motor function
Autonomic dysfunction manifest by hypotension, low or high body temperatures, loss of bladder and bowel control, and autonomic dysreflexia (p. 1591)

These symptoms occur soon after the injury and last 1 to 6 weeks with much autonomic reflex cord function returning in about 3 weeks. The length of this stage is, to some degree, indicative of the extent of later recovery. In general, the shorter the duration of spinal shock, the more neurologic return can be anticipated. In children with cauda equina injuries at or below level L1, flaccid paralysis persists unless there is subsequent recovery. It may also remain in cases in which there is extensive damage below the level of injury because of severe vascular compromise.

The problems related to this first stage are the serious consequences of prolonged immobility: atrophy of both paralyzed and noninvolved muscles caused by inactivity;

negative nitrogen balance resulting from loss of appetite, partially as a result of depression; calcium loss from bone caused by lack of weight bearing with subsequent urinary calculi; urinary retention; risk of decubiti from prolonged pressure; reduced cardiac output and plasma volume; atonic bladder with urinary retention; and respiratory compromise, especially in children with high-level involvement. Autonomic paralysis also affects thermoregulatory functions. Afferent impulses from the skin temperature receptors are not integrated; therefore, the patient is subject to alterations in the environmental temperature. Body temperature rises or falls as the ambient temperature changes; therefore, hyperthermia can result from excessive ambient temperature, such as too many bedclothes.

Second stage. Except in the situations previously mentioned, flaccid paralysis is replaced by spinal reflex activity and increasing spasticity or, in partial lesions, greater or lesser degree of neurologic recovery. At this stage diagnosis may be confused in infants. Spinal reflexes that occur in paralyzed limbs may be misinterpreted as the normal movements in the infant. Even minor stimuli, such as rubbing the mattress, are sufficient to elicit spinal reflexes. Concurrent crying may also lead to the erroneous impression that sensation is intact. Absence of spontaneous leg movement of the extremities when the infant is held vertically suspended under the axilla is highly suggestive. Reflex withdrawal or extension of the limb after tactile or pinprick stimulus confirms a diagnosis.[2,20]

Spasticity leads to different problems than those associated with flaccid paralysis. Spasticity predisposes to contractures, especially of the hip adductor and hip and knee flexor muscles and the heel cords. Frequent contraction of muscles in spastic paralysis plus increased activity and assisted weight bearing reduce the progress of bone demineralization and nitrogen loss. The previously flaccid, atonic bladder now becomes hypertonic, and, instead of continuous dribbling, the urine is expelled involuntarily at intervals by reflex action.

The paralytic nature of autonomic function is replaced by *autonomic hyperreflexia,* especially when the lesions are above the midthoracic level. With disturbed central inhibitory control, sensory stimuli may produce a sudden generalized increase in sympathetic activity manifested by flushing of the face, sweating of the forehead, pupillary constriction, marked hypertension, headache, and bradycardia. The precipitating stimulus may be merely a full bladder or rectum or other internal or external sensory input. It can be a catastrophic event; therefore, nurses must be alert to this possibility and take immediate action to eliminate the stimulus.

Third stage. In the final stage of spinal cord injury the neurologic signs are stabilized regarding loss and recovery of function. The major emphasis is on rehabilitation. Table 40-4 outlines the differences in the physical effects of upper and lower motor neuron dysfunction.

A problem unique to injury in childhood is progressive spinal deformity (see p. 1528) that is usually not seen in adults or in adolescents near the end of the growth period. Scoliosis develops in a high percentage of children with high thoracic and cervical lesions and is almost certain to occur in the quadriplegic child whose injury occurred in infancy or early childhood. Consequently affected infants and children are placed in a carefully constructed trunk support. Kyphosis usually appears locally at the site of initial injury, especially injuries resulting from hyperflexion-type injuries. Proper immobilization during vertebral healing helps to prevent progressive deformity. Increasing lordosis occurs with the development of hip contracture caused by spasticity or by prolonged sitting in the nonambulatory child.[2]

Diagnostic evaluation

A history is a vital part of diagnostic evaluation of all accidental injuries and is the basis of any assessment. The nature of the injury provides valuable clues regarding the possible type of damage incurred and provides direction for proceeding with further assessment without the risk of additional damage.

A complete neurologic examination is performed on any child suspected of having a spinal cord injury to determine if damage was incurred and, if so, the level and extent of any impairment in the central and autonomic nervous systems.[33]

In order for a neurologic unit of the central nervous system to be considered normal, it must be determined that:

1. The reflex arcs are functioning.
2. The sensory tracts are intact when each dermatome is examined separately.
3. The voluntary motor response demonstrates ability to move a body part against gravity on command.

The last completely normal cord segment identifies the diagnostic level of injury. For example, a C5 level of injury has neurologic deficits beginning with the C6 segment, and sensory motor tracts are intact at level C5.

Testing of a reflex arc is done by stimulating the peripheral receptors at a specific site, such as eliciting the patellar reflex. Reflexes are often graded on a 0 to 4+ scale: 0 indicates no response, 2+ indicates a normal reflex response, and 4+ means hyperactive reflexes, usually associated with upper motor neuron disease. Symmetric testing is performed to ascertain whether the neurologic deficit involves the cord bilaterally or unilaterally. A sufficient number of reflexes are tested to test motor function thoroughly.

Peripheral sensory receptors are widely distributed throughout the body. Some structures such as the skin are more abundantly supplied than the deep visceral structures. Sensory tracts are tested with the blunt end of a safety pin to assess pressure sensitivity and with the sharp point to elicit

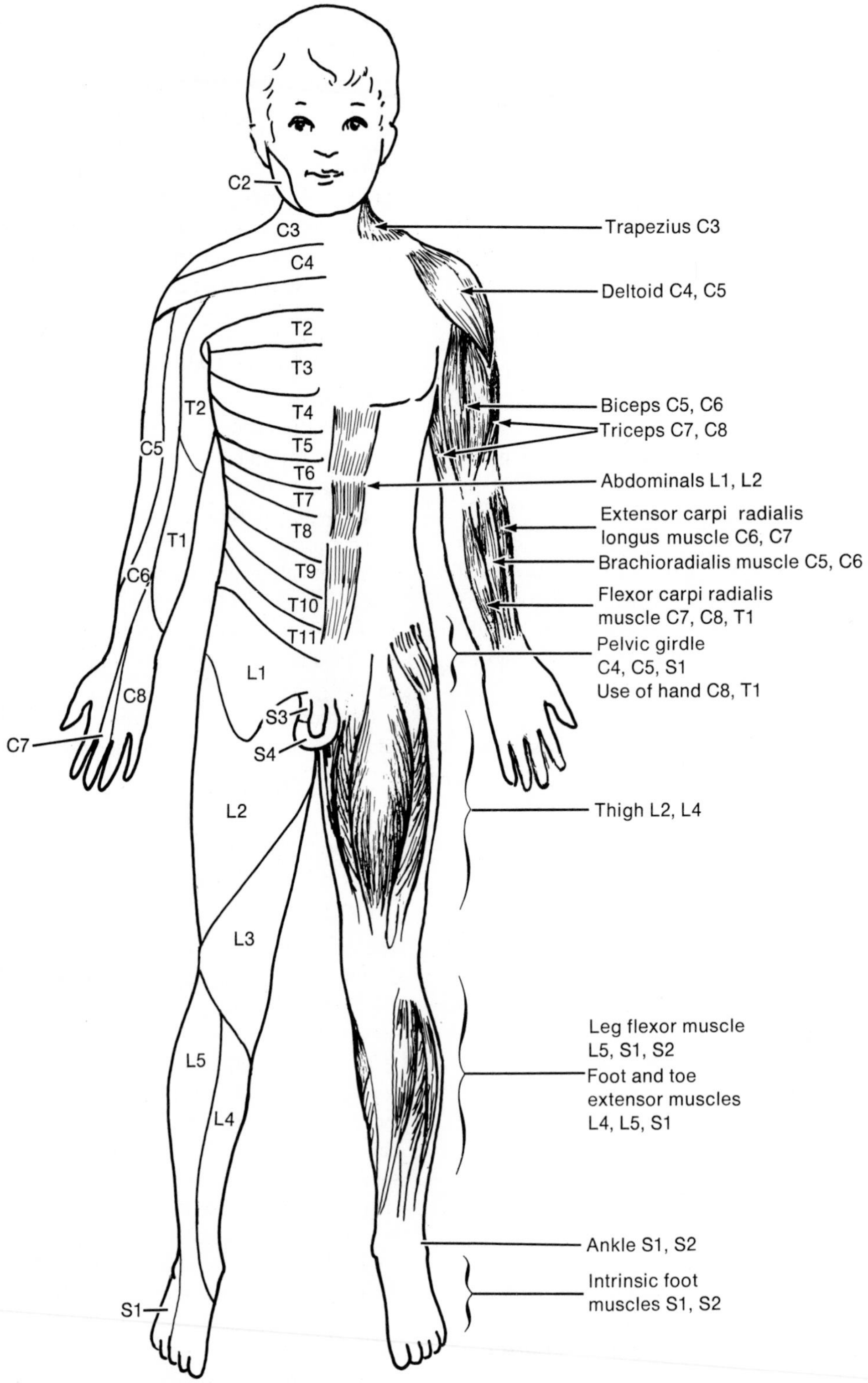

Fig. 40-24. Dermatomes and muscle innervation of major muscles needed for performing activities of daily living.

pain. Hot and cold water, a tuning fork, and cotton may also be used to determine specific sensory loss, for example, temperature, vibration, and light touch. The body surface has delineated zones or dermatomes that accurately correspond to the spinal cord segment receiving the sensory input from the peripheral nerves in that zone. Systematically pinpricking the body surface in each zone can determine if the sensory pathways are intact. Fig. 40-24 shows the zones and the spinal cord segments they represent. The examiner tests for each specific sensory fiber in the dermatome areas in which there is a suspected neurologic deficit. Proprioception, or knowing where one's extremities are, is a very vital sense for ambulating safely.

Motor system testing includes observing the child's gait if he is able to walk, noting if he can maintain balance with his eyes open and closed, and asking him to lift, flex, and extend his arms and legs. Testing muscle strength with and without resistance and against gravity will give cues to the specific nature and degree of motor dysfunction. Fig. 40-24 identifies the major muscles needed for performing activities of daily living with the cord segment that supplies each muscle group. The number of muscles in any muscle group that remain completely intact in the upper extremities makes a marked difference in the individual's ability to provide self-care, especially at the C5 and C6 levels. The presence of abdominal muscles is valuable in bladder and bowel training and in maintaining an upright sitting position. Hip movement is necessary if ambulation with braces and crutches is to be accomplished.

The degree to which supportive aids are needed for ambulation is determined by the strength, stability, and movement of the pelvis, trunk, hip flexors muscles, and quadriceps muscles. A general guideline for determining the capacity for self-help is that a paraplegic person who has function down to and including the quadriceps muscle or muscle function below the L3 level will have little difficulty in learning to walk with or without braces and crutches. It is especially vital that children with lumbar levels of injury be taught to walk functionally so that they are weight bearing at least part of the time to minimize the risk of problems with osteoporosis and hypercalcemia. The functional significance of spinal cord lesion level is summarized in Table 40-5.

If a physician detects central nervous system pathology, a body system assessment is begun to determine the degree to which the pathology has disrupted the autonomic innervations. Because the cord and central nervous system directly influence the function of the autonomic nerves, the specific sympathetically related organ systems examined are skeletal muscle and vascular tone and body temperature regulation. For example, bladder and gastrointestinal function have sympathetic and parasympathetic innervation and local reflexes.

Radiographic examination is important for localizing the lesion, but the nature of the spine in childhood frequently creates difficulty in interpretation. Radiographs must be taken carefully and with sufficient help to prevent further damage to the spine. Several persons may be needed to log roll the patient and to support the head during turning or transfer.

Prognosis

The ultimate outlook for spinal cord function after injury depends on the completeness of the cord transection, the site of injury, and complicating damage to the neuronal tissue. Healing of the injury and return of neurologic function are related to two factors:

1. Although individual nerve fibers do regenerate, they do not necessarily reconnect or make synaptic connections with the distal portion of the severed fibers, and the chance of numerous fibers reconnecting is highly unlikely.
2. The damage resulting from cord ischemia produces necrosis in the gray and white matter of the cord tissue, which does not regenerate if the axon cylinder is not intact.

In general, recovery in thoracic lesions is usually hopeless for motor function and victims are relegated to life in a wheelchair. Cervical injuries are variable in extent of damage. Incomplete lesions produce hemiplegia, and complete transection implies some involvement of all extremities from partial use of upper extremities to complete paralysis, including the need for artificial maintenance of respiration. Lumbar injury may involve partial or complete loss of function in lower extremities and bladder.

Medical management

The management of spinal cord injury is complex and controversial. Initial care begins at the scene of the accident; therefore, education and training of rescue personnel in stabilization and transfer techniques to prevent or reduce the severity of injury are of utmost importance. In any situation in which spinal cord injury is suspected or a possibility, the child should be calmed, reassured, and advised not to move, and no one should be allowed to move him unless they are able to do so carefully. He should be lifted gently and without undue haste (preferably by a coordinated team) to avoid twisting or bending the spine. If conscious he is placed supine on a rigid surface to prevent sagging. Because of the complexity and relative infrequency of these injuries, it is usually recommended that these persons be transferred to a spinal injury center for care by a coordinated team of specially trained personnel.

Management during the first stage is primarily supportive with efforts directed toward preventing further neuronal damage, preventing complications, and maintaining vital functions. Children with cervical lesions often have compromised respiratory function and may require ventilatory assistance by means of endotracheal tube or tracheostomy.

Table 40-5. Functional significance of spinal cord lesions

Highest intact cord segment	Muscle innervation	Functional capacity	Functional goals
C1-3	None below chin, including phrenic nerve to diaphragm	No voluntary control below chin Respiratory paralysis complete May cause brady- or tachycardia, vomiting	Artificial respiration; can be taught glossopharyngeal breathing to be used for short periods Electric wheelchair Adaptive equipment for special tasks in bed or wheelchair using mouth stick
C4 (high quadriplegia)	Intact sternocleidomastoid, trapezius, upper cervical paraspinous muscles	No voluntary function of upper extremities, trunk, or lower extremities All neck movements Respirator dependent	Electric wheelchair Externally powered devices and adaptive equipment for special tasks in bed or wheelchair with mouth stick, such as turning pages, using electric typewriter Totally dependent for activities of daily living
C5	Partial deltoid, biceps, major muscles of rotator cuffs of shoulders Diaphragm	Abduction, flexion, and extension of arm Flexion and extension of forearm Unable to roll over or attain sitting position Abdominal respiration Poor respiratory reserve	Electric wheelchair Requires attendant to assist in moving and transfer to wheelchair Adaptive devices for self-feeding, grooming, using electric typewriter Vocational potential with adaptive devices
C6	Pectoralis major, serratus anterior, latissimus dorsi muscles Complete deltoid and brachioradialis muscles Partial triceps muscle	Significant increase in function over that with lesion at C5 level Adduction and medial rotation of arm Wrist extension Good elbow flexion	Cuff strapped to hand permits use of implements for self-care and other activities Able to assist in dressing and transfer Hand rim extension permits independence in wheelchair
C7	Triceps and finger flexor and extensor muscle Shoulder depressor muscles Still nerve disruption to intercostal muscles	With elbow stabilized in extension and intact shoulder depressor muscles able to lift body weight Grasp and release still weak; dexterity lacking	Almost complete independence within limitations of wheelchair Requires some assistance in transfer and lower extremity dressing Hand splints helpful Can roll over in bed, sit up in bed, and eat independently Homebound employment possible Outside work usually not feasible
T1-10 (high paraplegia)	Full innervation of upper extremity muscles	Full use of upper extremities, including intrinsic muscles of hand Trunk balance poor May have difficulty in lifting sufficiently to put on lower extremity clothing Considerable energy expenditure to put on long leg braces with extensive attachments	Completely wheelchair dependent Trunk balance benefits from training Able to drive automobile with hand controls May be braced for standing May hold job away from home Cannot manage public transportation
T10-L2	Full abdominal and upper back muscle control	Good trunk balance Good respiratory reserve Can accomplish moderate hip-hiking using external oblique and latissimus dorsi muscles	Ambulation with bilateral long braces using four-point or swing-through crutch gait Usually able to negotiate curbs Some able to use public transportation Few vocational limitations as long as does not require much walking or standing
L3 or below	Quadriceps muscle Partial gluteus and hamstring muscles	May be lumbar lordosis Floppy ankles	Ambulates well, often with short leg braces with or without cane Difficulty in getting out of wheelchair May never require wheelchair

Cervical lesions may require halter or skeletal traction and sandbags to maintain position, and corticosteroids are administered in an attempt to prevent destructive edema. Drainage of urine from the atonic bladder is ensured by periodic application of external suprapubic pressure (Credé's maneuver), intermittent catheterization, or an indwelling catheter. Operative intervention may be necessary to remove bone fragments and debris, but routine surgical exploration is not usually recommended.

The focus of the second phase is primarily rehabilitative and is aimed at returning the patient to the home and community. The focus is on maximizing the potential for self-help, education, and, for the older child, vocational counseling.

Nursing considerations

The nursing care of the paraplegic or quadriplegic child is complex and challenging. As a member of the acute care and the rehabilitation teams, the nurse is involved in all aspects of care. Ideally initial care takes place in a special intensive care unit with personnel trained to handle spinal cord injuries and nursing management is concerned primarily with prevention of complications and maintenance of functions.

Once the acute period is over, the lesion is usually static and nonprogressive, regardless of whether the paralysis is secondary to trauma, congenital defects, infection, treated tumor, or surgery. In treatment of children with spinal cord injuries, the nurse is a member of a team of specialists including physicians from a number of speciality areas, physical and occupational therapists, psychologists, social workers, teachers, and vocational counselors. Each team member has a unique contribution to make, and mutual agreement for specific areas of responsibility is determined during regularly scheduled team conferences. Periodic evaluation of the team's progress is discussed in subsequent conferences.

Although care of the child with a spinal cord injury is, in most aspects, the same as that of any immobilized child, there are some important differences.

Respiratory care. The child with a high injury (quadriplegia) will require continuous respiratory assistance. In most instances a tracheostomy is the method of choice for greater ease in clearing secretions and for less trauma to tissues for long-term respirator dependence. Respiratory therapy personnel are responsible for establishing and maintaining the equipment, but the nurse must understand how it works and recognize deviations from the prescribed rate and volume and mechanical malfunction. In case of malfunction the nurse must be prepared for maintaining respirations manually with a ventilation bag. In some youngsters breathing pacemaker devices (phrenic nerve stimulators) are implanted to stimulate the phrenic nerve and produce diaphragmatic contractions and lung expansion without a ventilator. If the child has a pacemaker, part of the nursing function is understanding its function and operation.

Children with lesions below the C4 level are seldom dependent on respirators, but their vital capacity is significantly reduced. They should be positioned for optimal chest expansion and a variety of breathing exercises, and assistive devices are employed to stimulate deep breathing. Intermittent positive-pressure breathing by machine may be needed, and vital capacity and blood gases are monitored periodically. Percussion and vibration, with suction as necessary, are performed several times daily, and nebulized oxygen may be needed occasionally. Regular routine monitoring of breath sounds to assess for adequate ventilation in all lobes is part of routine care.

The cough reflex is markedly diminished and, together with weak intercostal muscles, the youngster may have difficulty with secretions. Increasing the elastic qualities of the lung by exercise will help to achieve a productive cough.

Temperature regulation. Vital signs and other general assessments are carried out periodically, with particular attention to alterations that might indicate adverse autonomic responses. Temperature regulation usually creates few problems, although environmental conditions can influence the body temperature. During the spinal shock stage the dilated capillaries conducting body heat to the subcutaneous tissues cause heat loss to the environment. In hot weather, without the capacity to sweat, heat is retained. Consequently clothing and blankets are added or removed according to the body temperature. An elevated temperature that cannot be corrected by environmental measures should be evaluated for urinary tract or upper respiratory infection. However, excessive perspiration observed in sentient areas usually indicates an elevated ambient temperature.

Skin care. In cases in which spinal cord injury is associated with vertebral fracture, cervical traction with Crutchfield tongs is maintained for several weeks until there is sufficient evidence of bone healing. Initially the child is turned every 2 hours around the clock by specially trained personnel. An alternating pressure mattress, egg carton mattress, or sheepskin is kept underneath the child, and the skin is thoroughly inspected at least once a day for signs of pressure, especially over bony prominences. Prevention of decubiti is much easier than treatment. A number of factors contribute to the risk of skin breakdown in these children: decreased sensation, poor nutrition from negative nitrogen balance, low hemoglobin level, spasticity, and improper positioning. The areas most apt to be affected are the sacrum, scapulae, heels, and occiput when in a supine position; the trochanters and the lateral aspect of the ankles, heels, and knees when in a side-lying position; and the ischial tuberosities when in a sitting position. The common type of pressure lesion begins in deeper tissues and is only visible on the surface at a later stage; therefore, areas that feel firm, irregular, warm, or appear to be only slightly reddened require careful evaluation. Keeping the skin clean and dry is particularly important in these children, especially those who are incontinent. Treatment of pressure areas or decubiti is instituted early, according to the protocol of the institution.

Physical therapy. Physical therapy is a vital part of nursing care. Maintaining good body alignment, preventing pressure from bedclothes, providing proper support, and applying splints as ordered and padded booties to hold the feet in correct position are important in daily care. Range of motion, passive, and active exercises are carried out under the guidance of a physical therapist (see Table 40-6). In children with upper motor neuron involvement, the spasticity that develops may require administration of an antispasmodic, usually diazepam. Decreasing stimuli to the muscles also helps reduce spasticity. For example, tight clothing and bedclothes should be avoided, and extremities should be handled by the joints rather than by the belly of the muscle. Anticipating the possibility of spasms when the child is moved and providing the necessary safety precautions prevent possible injury during transport.

Table 40-6. Types of exercises and their uses

Type of exercise	Uses
Joint range of motion exercise—three to five times for each joint, two to three times per day; done either passively or actively	Maintain range of motion of each involved joint during periods of inactivity and gradually increase motion of affected joints Prevention of contractures Increase range of motion in contracted joint by stretching muscle and tendons
Passive exercise with therapist moving child's extremity because of weakness or paralysis	Used when doing joint range of motion exercise Stimulates circulation but does not strengthen muscles
Active exercise with child voluntarily moving extremity per request	Builds up and maintains muscle strength Stimulates circulation
Active exercise against resistance, that is, therapist exerts some opposing force	Builds up muscle strength and endurance
Coordination	Develops a number of muscle groups to improve smooth patterns for normal function
Isometric exercise where child is taught to put his extremity in a specified position and then tighten and relax specific muscle groups	Strengthens muscle groups Often used for quadriceps or forearm muscle strengthening

During the period of immobilization, unless there are contraindications, exercises are aimed at maintaining and increasing strength of the child's intact musculature. Upper extremity strengthening is especially important to the paraplegic child who must rely on these muscle groups for turning, transferring, dressing, crutch walking, and other activities. Children are usually eager to use their muscles and respond to interesting and innovative activities.

Neurogenic bladder. When the bladder is denervated, as in the acute stage of spinal shock syndrome or after lower motor neuron damage, the bladder wall is flaccid. The danger in this type of neurogenic bladder is overextension. This lack of tone causes a deficiency in the ability of the bladder to respond to changes in passive pressure. That is, if the bladder is filled, emptied, and filled again, the pressure observed the second time will be less than the pressure noted after the first filling. Therefore, it is important to prevent overdistention by periodic emptying, even though there may be dribbling between emptying. In contrast the upper motor neuron lesion causes an increase in tone and bladder contractions that often includes the urinary sphincter. Thus, even though the bladder empties periodically by reflex action, complete emptying is prevented, causing urinary retention and ureteral reflex.

The intervals of urination depend on many factors, including patterns of fluid intake and perspiration. Most children require some type of external collecting device. This is relatively simple in boys, but no satisfactory device is available for girls, who usually must rely on diapers and incontinent pants. As early as possible attempts are made to keep the child relatively dry by regulating fluid intake and output and periodically emptying the bladder by manual expression by applying downward pressure on the bladder (Credé's maneuver), intermittent catheterization, or both. The older paraplegic child can be taught to express urine manually and to perform self-catheterization.[1] Bladder-training programs usually begin with intermittent bladder emptying at regular intervals, which are gradually increased. Periodic urine cultures and, in manual emptying, periodic catheterization for residual volume are performed until the child achieves regular, complete emptying.

The urine is kept acidic to decrease the likelihood of stone formation and to inhibit bacterial growth. Ascorbic acid, 1 to 4 g daily, is most effective. The traditional cranberry juice may also be advised. Oral antimicrobials are frequently administered prophylactically. Maintenance of bladder dynamics and control of urinary tract infections are of utmost importance. Pyelonephritis and renal failure are the most significant causes of death in long-standing paraplegia.

Bowel training. Successful bowel training is easier to institute than bladder management. The aim is to control defecation until an appropriate time and place are found. A diet with sufficient roughage for adequate stool bulk and insertion of a glycerin or bisacodyl (Dulcolax) suppository at a convenient time, either morning or evening, are often all that are necessary to induce a bowel movement within a short time. The probability of an accident betweentimes is diminished once the bowel is completely evacuated. Stool softeners, such as dioctyl sodium sulfonsuccinate (Colace), are usually prescribed, and manual anal stimulation may help initiate evacuation, especially in spastic paraplegia. Sometimes an oral laxative such as bisacodyl may be necessary. Once an appropriate regimen is established, little modification is required.

Autonomic hyperreflexia. Children with high lesions are very susceptible to the development of autonomic hyperreflexia, which requires prompt action to prevent encephalopathy and shock. As soon as a quick assessment has ruled

Table 40-7. Specific neurogenic problems related to spinal cord lesions with associated interventions

Problem	Structural innervations	Specific problem	Intervention
Neurogenic bowel	Parasympathetic (mostly vagal)—increases smooth muscle mobility, tone, and secretions	Atony of gastric and upper intestinal segment—paralytic ileus	Nothing given by mouth; decompression with nasogastric tube
	Sympathetic—decreases gastrointestinal motility	Development of stress ulcer from excessive vagal stimulation	Antacids; diet control
	Voluntary central nervous system control—control of external sphincter and timing of defecation	Fecal incontinence or constipation	Bowel training program with diet regulation, suppositories, mild laxative, stool softeners, manual evacuation
Neurogenic bladder	Parasympathetic—contraction of bladder wall to facilitate emptying of bladder, relaxing of sphincter muscle	Lower motor neuron damage or spinal shock—urinary retention with overflow incontinence	Evaluation of kidney function Use of Foley catheter if necessary
	Sympathetic—maintains internal sphincter tone and relaxes wall of bladder	Uppor motor neuron damage after shock—bladder spasms, external sphincter paralysis, internal sphincter spasm	Intermittent catheterization program
Autonomic hyperreflexia	Visceral distention or irritation, particularly bowel or bladder, triggers sensory impulses, which travel to cord lesion and are blocked to activate excessive sympathetic reflex reaction; not controlled by higher centers Usually occurs in persons with a lesion at T4 level or above	Hypertension (vasoconstriction below lesion) Occipital pounding headache Flushed face (vasodilatation above lesion) Tachycardia Sweating below lesion level Can lead to cerebrovascular accident or epilepsy	Bowel or bladder emptied gently Topical anesthetic (tetracaine [Pontocaine]) instilled in bladder or rectum to reduce irritability (prophylactic) Parasympatholytic drugs (methantheline [Banthine]) given, as well as drugs to lower blood pressure and prevent seizures
Orthostatic hypotension	Sympathetic—stimulates vascular tone to maintain blood pressure	Pooling of blood in dependent areas Syncope when head elevated or body in upright position	Ambulating activities performed *slowly* Sitting tolerance time recorded and gradually increased Antistasis support with elastic stocking or Ace bandage wraps Head lowered if orthostatic episode occurs
Thermoregulation	Hypothalamic and autonomic regulation to control peripheral sweating and evaporative heat loss	Faulty adaptation to changes in environmental temperatures	Frequent monitoring of body temperature Environmental temperature adjusted by raising or lowering, especially cooling ambient temperature Clothing suitable for environment High fevers lowered slowly with cool sponges
Sexual dysfunction	Nerves at S2 to 4 levels innervate sensory and motor components of genitalia	Inability to feel sexual stimuli Inability to have and maintain an erection and/or ejaculation, particularly in lower motor neuron damage	Touch approach Alternative methods for sexual gratification Referral to qualified sex therapist for long-term sexual adjustment

out other causes, such as orthostatic hypertension, someone should take the blood pressure while the bladder is checked for distention (the usual precipitating cause). The bladder is drained slowly, and, if symptoms are not relieved, any tight clothing is loosened and the bowel is checked for the pressure of impacted feces. If removal of the causative agent is unsuccessful in controlling the syndrome, intravenous administration of an antihypertensive drug is indicated followed by oral maintenance doses. Antispasmodics may also be administered.

The specific neurogenic problems related to spinal cord lesions are listed in Table 40-7 with the associated nursing interventions.

Remobilization. As soon as his condition warrants, the child is moved from a reclining to an erect position. Cardiovascular deconditioning and impaired autonomic responses below the level of injury will cause pooling of blood in the extremities because of peripheral vasodilatation, a drop in blood pressure, and a feeling of light-headedness, dizziness, or fainting on sudden assumption of an upright posture. Therefore, this must be accomplished gradually by first placing him on a tilt table and securing him by passive restraint, after which the table is slowly elevated from a horizontal to a 30-degree semireclining position. This is performed twice daily for 20 to 30 minutes, gradually increasing the angle until the vertical angle is reached. During the procedure the vital signs are monitored and the behavior is observed for subjective symptoms of syncope. Elastic hose or wrapping the lower extremities with elastic bandage from instep to groin and applying an abdominal binder reduce the pooling of blood. The process of achieving upright posture may require several weeks. After tolerance is achieved, the child will be ready to begin to use a wheelchair. Each time the child gets up this should be accomplished slowly by gradually elevating the bed over a period of 20 to 30 minutes before placing him in the wheelchair, then gradually lowering the legs after he has been in the chair a short time.

All adaptive devices help children increase their mobility, function, and endurance. The paraplegic child with some lower extremity function progresses to parallel bars and then to a walker; the quadriplegic child learns to use a wheelchair. The wheelchair is among the most valuable aids available to the child with a spinal cord injury, and its selection should be made carefully in relation to where it will be used, architectural barriers, and the functional capacity of the child. For lower extremity paralysis the wheelchair described on p. 1551 is applicable. For children with severe upper extremity paralysis, a variety of motorized wheelchairs are used, but the more complex they are, the greater their cost, weight, and tendency to break down (see Fig. 40-4). Wheelchair tolerance is gained over a period of time accompanied by measures to prevent orthostatic hypotension and pressure sores.

A variety of braces and other appliances can be adapted for use by many children with spinal cord injuries. The primary purpose of lower extremity bracing in the child with a spinal cord injury is for ambulation, although correction of deformities may be attempted. However, the efficacy is limited because of the tendency to develop pressure lesions over insensate areas. The higher the lesion, the more support required, with the accompanying difficulties of getting into the brace and the greater energy expended in using the appliance. The energy required in ambulating with crutches and braces is two to four times greater than that required for normal walking.[20] Children with their natural and overwhelming propensity for mobility usually attain, or may even surpass, the maximum expectation in ambulation. However, as they approach adulthood, the increasing weight and energy cost usually cause them to resort to predominant use of the wheelchair for mobility and the pursuit of more intellectual and vocational interests. Wheelchair mobility has the advantage that it requires no more energy than normal walking and allows the paraplegic person to maintain the speed of other pedestrians on level ground.[21]

Rehabilitation

Physical rehabilitation has been briefly described in the foregoing segments, and the major aims are to prepare the child and family to resume life at home and in the community. Members of the rehabilitation team work collaboratively to identify the child's problems and to plan realistic interventions. This is one of the more complex health teams, and the integration of activities is coordinated by one team member, most often the physician who is a specialist in physical medicine and rehabilitation (Fig. 40-25). Through mutual trust, good communication, professional respect, and sincere interest in the child and his family, members of the team attempt to achieve their collaborative goals. Training in the rehabilitation center involves achieving the maximum expected accomplishments commensurate with the physical capacities. Instruction for home routine is stressed and includes all the precautions and management implemented in the hospital, that is, skin care, nutrition, bladder and bowel training, and an exercise program.

The overall goals of rehabilitation of the child with an acquired spinal injury and habilitation of the child with a congenital defect are:

- Maximizing function and minimizing the handicapping effects of the pathology
- Assisting the child and family in setting realistic goals for him, learning to be good problem solvers, and using the assets he has
- Helping the child to cope with the stigma of being different and to build a valued self-concept

Physical rehabilitation of the quadriplegic child takes

approximately 6 months; a paraplegic child can achieve these goals in 1 to 3 months, but he requires constant vigilance to avoid complications. Emotional adjustments take longer, especially in the older child and adolescent. In most children the outlook is favorable unless life-threatening consequences of urinary pathology are severe or emotional adjustment is poor.[20]

A restorative program is begun as soon as possible after injury. Frequent changes in body position while in bed are essential, using positioning aids such as splints and pillows to support body parts after turning. One of the primary goals is to use interventions for regaining function and remobilization within the limitations of the therapeutic regimen and the child's physical disabilities. An overhead trapeze bar and side rails aid a larger child with upper extremity use to move about in bed. Exercises to develop his ability to bend the elbow and raise the lower arm may need additional therapies to enable him to perform self-feeding or self-dressing. The child is encouraged to become involved in activities appropriate to his developmental level and physical capabilities.

Exercise therapy is the focal point of all restorative interventions. It is important to maintain the movement, tone, and strength in uninvolved joints and muscles and to exercise affected musculoskeletal structures as soon as possible. There are many types of exercises with various purposes, and the guiding principle is that the child should perform the type of exercise that will accomplish the major goal of active movement against resistance (See Table 40-6). Exercise programs must be scheduled at least two times each day with approximately ten repetitive movements during each exercise. A complete exercise program takes time, since each major joint and muscle group requires several movements to accomplish full range of motion and strengthening. The normal ranges of motion for major joints are:

1. Wrist—flexion and extension; medial (ulnar) and lateral (radial) deviation
2. Elbow—pronation and supination; flexion and extension
3. Shoulder—adduction and abduction; rotation with arm at side; forward and backward flexion and extension; horizontal flexion and extension
4. Hip—abduction and adduction; rotation and extension of hip joint; flexion of hip joint
5. Knee—flexion and extension
6. Ankle—flexion and extension

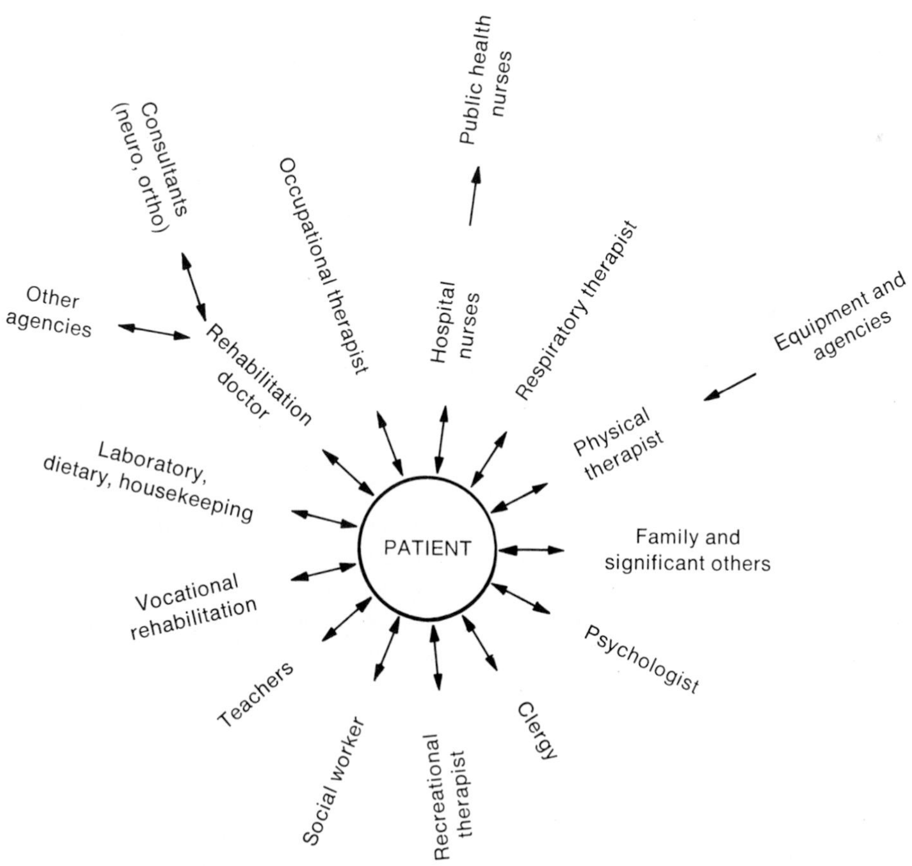

Fig. 40-25. Rehabilitation team.

The child will be more enthusiastic if toys and play strategies can be incorporated into the therapy. Exercises can be a part of other nursing care such as hygienic procedures and dressing. To perform an activity of daily living such as bathing, feeding, or dressing, the child may require an adaptive device to compensate for functional loss. Velcro straps replace zippers and buttons, a spoon handle is enlarged when the grip is poor, or a hand splint is provided with a strap to hold the utensil. Environmental adaptations include ramps, lowered furniture, or special hydraulic lifts for transferring larger children. Most adaptive aids do not encourage muscle strengthening but assist the child in the functional use of whatever movement remains.

Psychosocial rehabilitation. Early acquired or congenital disability is usually more readily accepted by the child than paralysis that appears later in childhood. Rehabilitation includes not only the child's emotional responses but also those of the persons who maintain the closest contacts with the child. It involves intensive education so that members of the family understand the nature of the disability, the therapeutic regimen, and complications so that they are able to provide the physical and emotional support needed by the child. As with any disability, the child should be treated as normally as possible and encouraged in developmental tasks at the age at which he would normally be expected to acquire abilities and perform activities. However, goals must be realistic, and the child should not be forced beyond his capabilities. The child's and the family's routines and the parents' child-rearing practices will be significantly altered.

As he becomes aware of the impact of the disability and its implications, the youngster may become self-effacing and begin to think of himself as very different, ugly, undesirable to others, less than human, or a useless cripple. When his appearance and physical capacity have changed markedly, the responses of peers, family, professionals, and even strangers who come in contact with him influence his perception of himself and can significantly alter his self-concept. Any loss related to his preinjury state is a severe threat to the development of a positive identity. All disabled youngsters grieve their losses, and the way in which they are able to weather the crisis and adjust to their new physical state depends on the way in which they deal with adversity and the help they receive from others. Satisfactory adjustment is not necessarily related to the extent of the disability. Sometimes children with marked impairment make a better adjustment than those with only minimal disability. All must go through the process of grieving their loss. The typical sequence in the grief process is:

1. Preshock or unawareness of what has happened or is happening to him. His perception of reality is fuzzy, his responses may be "automatic" or inappropriate, and he seems somewhat detached.
2. Shock and disbelief, as he becomes more aware of his losses and feels the threat to his being. Panic and anxiety are common feelings coupled with thoughts, such as "It didn't really happen."
3. Some form of denial, which is often resorted to when normal coping mechanisms are inadequate to handle the situation. Attitudes associated with denial include, "I'm not really unable to move," or "I'll be okay in a short time." The denial may be manifest by withdrawal behaviors such as sleeping a great deal or by focusing on less threatening concerns such as toys or food.
4. Confrontations of the reality of the situation continue to have an impact on the child, and he begins to acknowledge what is occurring. This usually provokes anger and depression.

Severe depression can be emotionally and intellectually immobilizing, but it indicates that the child is no longer hiding behind denial. It is desirable in a child's rehabilitation for him to begin to express his negative feelings toward the situation, since these feelings, redirected by efforts of the rehabilitation team, are the ones that will motivate him toward learning a new way of life.

The multiple problems related to altered self-image, especially in the older child and adolescent, have been discussed in relation to the handicapped child (Chapter 22). The severely disabled child may need to alter some concepts about self and social roles. If he describes an adult as someone with complete control over his body and the ability to do what he wants when he wants to, he will need to develop a more realistic definition of interdependent adult living. The needs of the permanently disabled youngster must be reevaluated periodically by the total rehabilitation team, including the youngster and his family. As a young adult the disabled teenager may not be financially independent, which alters his choice of occupation or profession. Vocational rehabilitation involves not only helping the permanently disabled teenager to find meaningful work activities but also to assist him in enrolling in formal educational programs.

The problems of self-concept are particularly marked when the child with a spinal cord injury reaches puberty and are likely to be even more intense if the disability occurs during adolescence. Sexual development and awareness and changing perceptions of body image are prominent aspects of adolescence, and loss in these areas is a severe blow to the youngster. Development of secondary sex characteristics does not seem to be altered by spinal cord injury, and it is now believed that, with comprehensive rehabilitation, well-motivated young people can look forward to successful participation in marital and family activities.

In girls, if the injury occurs after the onset of menstruation, there is usually a temporary cessation and irregularity of menstrual flow, but in the majority of girls menstruation usually resumes. Ovulation and conception are possible, but they will not experience vulval or clitoral orgasms although they can learn to use other errogenous zones for a sexual experience. This is important to emphasize in sex education, because many girls have the misconception that because they lack sensation, they are unable to conceive. Also, the pregnant paraplegic or quadriplegic girl may be unaware that she is in labor, and those with a high-level injury are subject to autonomic hyperreflexia during labor.

As soon as the adolescent male becomes aware of his functional loss, he will be concerned about his sexual capacities regardless of the type of sexual experiences he had prior to spinal cord injury. The physician and/or psychologist will provide him with information about what he can expect regarding erection, ejaculation, and other sexual experiences. The health professional should take the initiative in discussing sexuality with the child and his family. Parents of younger children will want to know about their child's potential. As his interest and understanding increase, the child needs to know the specifics of physiology, prognosis, and sexual techniques related to his particular problems.

The male with an upper motor neuron lesion may be capable of reflex erections and, with penile stimulation, may maintain the erection for a time. However, ejaculation is possible only with intact innervation at S2, S3, and S4 levels, which is seldom present. Erection is usually absent in lower motor neuron dysfunction. Only a small percentage of males with complete lesions have children because of loss of ejaculation and the decreased incidence of successful intercourse.

Erection can be achieved psychogenically or reflexogenically. Psychogenic stimulation can be visual, olfactory, somatesthetic, and/or auditory with subsequent integration of the sensory input and autonomic nerve response. An individual must have a functional cervicothoracolumbar cord to have a psychogenic erection. Reflexogenic erections occur when the lower motor neuron reflexes in the sacral region are intact and local skin or penal stimulation produces an erection. In general the male with an incomplete upper motor neuron injury will be very successful in having psychogenic and reflexogenic erections and coitus. Those with complete upper motor neuron injuries are usually able to have reflexogenic erections; males with complete lower motor neuron injuries or damage are least likely to have erections and coitus.

A knowledgeable rehabilitation team will be valuable to the child as he experiences loss as a sexual being. This is especially true of the paraplegic or quadriplegic teenager. Most sexual counseling for the adolescent with a spinal cord injury focuses on developing the idea that sex means different things to individuals, and the youngster is encouraged to discuss his ideas. Most rehabilitation teams have an active program in sexual counseling to help the child learn intimacy and how to function sexually within his limitations. Through individual and group counseling he gains new attitudes concerning his sexuality. Knowledge that sexual gratification comes from giving and sharing assist him to look at alternative ways to achieve sexual gratification for himself and his partner. For example, he learns the value of masturbation as a means to determine if he can have and sustain an erection. As he adjusts to trials and successes, he develops his own ways of achieving sexual experiences exclusive or inclusive of intercourse.

While in the hospital the teenage youngster may display aggressive sexual behavior toward the nurses. Flirtatious behavior is a way of checking out with others his or her acceptance as a sexual being. This behavior can be handled easily by setting behavioral limits. Approaches that help nurses cope with the youngster with the prospect of altered sexual roles include:

1. Exploring their own attitudes toward sex and being aware of their abilities and limitations in relating with the youngster on this topic.
2. Use of resource people to answer questions that they are unable to answer or feel uncomfortable in handling.
3. Respecting another's attitudes and sexual behaviors, unless they are self-destructive, and trying to be nonjudgmental while maintaining their own attitudes and beliefs.
4. Reinforcing that sexual roles are learned and that there is more to sex than functioning in a "prescribed" physical manner.

The outlook for children is favorable for integration into society. Increased awareness of the needs of handicapped persons has removed many structural and occupational barriers. The success of a rehabilitation program is not judged by how well the child manages within the rehabilitation setting but by how well he functions on the outside. In addition to agencies that offer assistance to handicapped children in general, some agencies provide specific assistance to paralyzed persons, including children. Some of these are The National Paraplegia Foundation,* The Paralyzed Veterans of America,† The National Wheelchair Athletic Association,‡ and The National Association of Physically Handicapped.§

REFERENCES

1. Altshuler, A., Meyer, J., and Butz, M. K.: Even children can learn to do clean self-catheterization, Am. J. Nurs. **77:**97-101, 1977.
2. Babcock, J. L.: Spinal injuries in children, Pediatr. Clin. North Am. **22:**487-500, 1975.
3. Beall, M. S., Jr.: Evaluation of the musculoskeletal system in the pediatric patient, Issues Comprehensive Pediatr. Nurs. **2**(4):1-13, 1977.
4. Blake, F. G.: Immobilized youth, a rationale for supportive nursing intervention, Am. J. Nurs. **69:**2364-2369, 1969.

*Chicago, Ill. 60601.
†Washington, D.C. 20010.
‡Woodside, N.Y. 11377.
§Lincoln Park, Mich. 48146.

5. Burke, D. C.: Traumatic spinal paralysis in children, Paraplegia **11:**268-276, 1974.
6. Conway, B.: Pediatric neurologic nursing, St. Louis, 1977, The C. V. Mosby Co.
7. Deyoe, F. S.: Marriage and family patterns with long term spinal cord injury, Paraplegia **110:**219-224, 1972.
8. Dowd, E. L., Novak, J. C., and Ray, E. J.: Releasing the hospitalized child from restraints, Am. J. Maternal Child Nurs. **2**(6):370-373, 1977.
9. Erickson, F.: When 6- to 12-year olds are ill, Nurs. Outlook **17:**48-50, 1965.
10. Flitter, H. H.: An introduction to physics in nursing, ed. 7, St. Louis, 1976, The C. V. Mosby Co.
11. Hilt, N. E., and Schmitt, E. W.: Pediatric orthopedic nursing, St. Louis, 1975, The C. V. Mosby Co.
12. Hinkhouse, A.: Physical assessment: multiple trauma, Crit. Care Update **3**(12):15-19, 1976.
13. Hogan, K., and Sawyer, J.: Fracture dislocation of the elbow, Am. J. Nurs. **76:**1266-1268, 1976.
14. Hopkins, J.: The nurse and the abused child, Nurs. Clin. North Am. **5:**589-598, 1970.
15. Larson, C. B., and Gould, M.: Orthopedic nursing, ed. 9, St. Louis, 1978, The C. V. Mosby Co.
16. Lindseth, R. E., and DeRosa, G. P.: Fractures in children, Pediatr. Clin. North Am. **22:**465-486, 1975.
17. Maynard, F., and Imai, K.: Immobilization hypercalcemia in spinal cord injury, Arch. Phys. Med. Rehabil. **58:**16-24, 1977.
18. Melzak, J.: Paraplegia among children, Lancet **2:**45-48, 1969.
19. Mitchell, P. H.: Concepts basic to nursing, ed. 2, New York, 1977, McGraw-Hill Book Co.
20. Molnar, G. E., and Taft, L. T.: Pediatric rehabilitation. Cerebral palsy and spinal cord injuries. Part I, Curr. Prob. Pediatr. **7**(3):46-55, 1977.
21. Myers, S. J.: The spinal injury patient. In Downey, J. A., and Low, N. L., editors: The child with disabling illness, Philadelphia, 1974, W. B. Saunders Co.
22. O'Boyle, C. M.: Sports injuries in adolescents: emergency care, Am. J. Nurs. **75:**1732-1739, 1975.
23. O'Grady, R. S.: Restraint and the hospitalized child. In Bergerson, B. S., and associates: editor: Current concepts in clinical nursing, vol. 2, St. Louis, 1969, The C. V. Mosby Co.
24. Pierce, D., and Nichel, V.: The total care of spinal cord injuries, Boston, 1977, Little, Brown & Co.
25. Rang, M.: Children's fractures, Philadelphia, 1974, J. B. Lippincott Co.
26. Rang, M. C., and Willis, R. B.: Fractures and sprains, Pediatr. Clin. North Am. **24:**749-773, 1977.
27. Riddle, I.: Nursing intervention to promote body image integrity in children, Nurs. Clin. North Am. **7:**651-661, 1972.
28. Sather, M., Weber, C., and George, J.: Pressure sores and the spinal cord injury patient, Drug Instill. Clin. Pharmacol. vol. 2, 1977.
29. Sibinga, M. S., and Freedman, C. J.: Restraint and speech, Pediatrics **48:**116-122, 1971.
30. Siner, E.: Emergency care update. Skeletal trauma, Crit. Care Update **4**(2):20-23, 1977.
31. Stryker, R.: Rehabilitation aspects of acute and chronic nursing care, ed. 2, Philadelphia, 1977, W. B. Saunders Co.
32. Tachdjian, M.: Pediatric orthopedics, Philadelphia, 1972, W. B. Saunders Co.
33. Thomas, S.: Guide to reflexes in neurologic diagnosis, Hosp. Med., 1977.
34. Thompson, M. A.: Traction fundamentals, San Jose, Calif., 1973, The Lansford Publishing Co.
35. Tilkian, S., and Conover, M.: Clinical implications of laboratory tests, St. Louis, 1975, The C. V. Mosby Co.
36. Trigiano, L. L.: Independence is possible in quadriplegia, Am. J. Nurs. **70:**2610-2613, 1970.
37. Tripp, A.: Hyper and hypocalcemia, Am. J. Nurs. **76:**1142-1145, 1976.
38. Tudor, L. L.: Bladder and bowel retraining, Am. J. Nurs. **70:** 2391-2393, 1970.

BIBLIOGRAPHY

Altshuler, A., and Seidl, A. H.: Teen meetings: a way to help adolescents cope with hospitalization, Am. J. Maternal Child Nurs. **2**(6):348-350, 1977.

Anderson, N.: Rehabilitative nursing practice, Nurs. Clin. North Am. **6:**303-309, 1971.

Anthony, C. P., and Thibodeau, G. A.: Textbook of anatomy and physiology, ed. 10, St. Louis, 1979, The C. V. Mosby Co.

Bates, B.: A guide to physical examination, Philadelphia, 1974, J. B. Lippincott Co.

Beaumont, E.: Wheelchairs, Nursing '73 **3**(11):48-57, 1973.

Bellack, J. P.: Helping a child cope with the stress of injury, Am. J. Nurs. **74:**1491-1494, 1974.

Bickerstaff, E.: Neurology for nurses, London, 1965, The English Universities Press, Ltd.

Boeriche, P.: First aid for open wounds, severe bleeding, shock and closed wounds, Nursing '75 **5**(3):40-47, 1975.

Brower, P., and Hicks, D.: Maintaining muscle function in patients on bed rest, Am. J. Nurs. **72:**1250-1253, 1972.

Bruis, M., and Innes, B.: Assessment: essential to prevent pressure sores, Am. J. Nurs. **76:**1762-1764, 1976.

Ciuca, R.: Range of motion exercises, active and passive: a handbook, Nursing '73 **3**(12):25-37, 1973.

Drury, J. H., Jr.: Handbook for range-of-motion exercises, Nursing '72 **2**(4):19-22, 1972.

Foss, G.: Breaking the architectural barrier with crutches, wheelchairs, and walkers, Nursing '73 **3**(10):17-31, 1973.

Guyton, A. C.: Textbook of medical physiology, ed. 5, Philadelphia, 1976, W. B. Saunders Co.

Hirschberg, G., Lewis, L., and Vaughan, P.: Promoting mobility, Nursing '77 **7**(5):42-47, 1977.

Howell, S.: Psychiatric aspects of habilitation, Pediatr. Clin. North Am. **20:**203, 1973.

Hyman, L. R., and associates: Immobilization hypercalcemia, Am. J. Dis. Child. **124:**723-727, 1972.

Jordan, H. S., and Kavchak, M. A.: Transfer techniques, Nursing '73 **3**(3):19-22, 1973.

Kern, F. C., and Poole, L.: Transfer techniques, Nursing '72 **2**(7): 25-28, 1972.

Kinley, A. E.: Night report, orthopedics, Am. J. Nurs. **69:**2417-2419, 1969.

McFarlane, J. M.: Pediatric care in the emergency room, Pediatr. Nurs. **2**(2):22-25, 1976.

McMaster, W. C.: When to use ice for injuries, Consult. **17**(4):83-85, 1977.

May, C. M.: Wheelchair patient for a day, Am. J. Nurs. **73:**650-651, 1973.

Menkes, J. H.: Textbook of child neurology, Philadelphia, 1974, Lea & Febiger.

Mitchell, P. H.: Concepts basic to nursing, ed. 2, New York, 1977, McGraw-Hill Book Co.

Penalver, M.: Helping the child handle his aggression, Am. J. Nurs. **73:**1554, 1973.

Ranalls, J.: Crutches and walkers, Nursing '72 **2**(12):21-24, 1972.

Smith, E. C., and associates: Reestablishing a child's body image, Am. J. Nurs. **77:**445-447, 1977.

Tachdjian, M.: Pediatric orthopedics, Philadelphia, 1972, W. B. Saunders Co.

Webb, K.: Early assessment of orthopedic injuries, Am. J. Nurs. **74:**1048-1052, 1974.

Young, C.: Exercise: how to use it to decrease complications in immobilized patients, Nursing '75 **5:**81, 1975.

Ziai, M., and associates: The musculoskeletal system. In Aiai, M., editor: Pediatrics, ed. 2, Boston, 1975, Little, Brown & Co.

Fractures

Aitken, G. T.: The child amputee: an overview, Orthop. Clin. North Am. **3:**447-472, 1972.

Alt, P.: Nursing care of a child in traction, Orthop. Nurs. Assoc. J. **3:**40, 1976.

Deyerle, W. M., and Crossland, S. A.: Broken legs are to be walked on, Am. J. Nurs. **77:**1927-1930, 1977.

The dos and don'ts of traction care, Nursing '74 **4**(11):35-41, 1974.

Felman, A. H.: Bicycle spoke fractures, J. Pediatr. **82:**302, 1973.

Griffin, P. P.: Supracondylar fractures of the humerus: treatment and complications, Pediatr. Clin. North Am. **22:**277-286, 1975.

Hohl, J. C., editor: Symposium on fractures and other injuries in children, Orthop. Clin. North Am. **7**(3), 1976.

Hubbard, D. D.: Injuries of the spine in children and adolescents, Clin. Orthop. **100:**56-65, 1974.

Kurth, J. S.: Correct application of the Thomas splint and Pearson attachment, Nursing '73 **3**(7):20-24, 1973.

Lane, P. A.: A mother's confession; home care of a toddler in a spica cast: what it's really like, Am. J. Nurs. **71:**2141-2143, 1971.

Lindseth, R. E., and DeRosa, G. P.: Fractures in children: general consideration and treatment of open fractures, Pediatr. Clin. North Am. **22:**465-476, 1975.

Meyers, S. J.: The spinal injury patient. In Downey, J. A., and Low, N. L., editors: The child with disabling illness, Philadelphia, 1974, W. B. Saunders Co.

Nursing Grand Rounds: Battered body, Nursing '78 **8**(1):36-41, 1978.

O'Boyle, C. M.: Sports injuries in adolescents: emergency care, Am. J. Nurs. **75:**1732-1739, 1975.

Perry, J.: The halo in spinal abnormalities. Practical factors and avoidance of complications, Orthop. Clin. North Am. **3:**69-80, 1972.

Rang, M.: Children's fractures, Philadelphia, 1974, J. B. Lippincott Co.

Ritchie, J.: Body image changes following amputation in an adolescent girl, Maternal Child Nurs. J. **1:**39, 1972.

Ryan, J.: Compression in bone healing, Am. J. Nurs. **74:**1998-1999, 1974.

Siner, E.: Skeletal trauma, Crit. Care Update **4**(1):32-33, 1977.

Stein, A., Mandell, D., and Ferguson, J.: Multiple fractures, Nursing '74 **4**(11):26-32, 1974.

Whitehead, D. J.: Emergency care in orthopedic injuries, Nurs. Clin. North Am. **8:**435-440, 1973.

Spinal cord injuries

Burke, D. C.: Spinal cord trauma in children, Paraplegia **9:**1, 1971.

Coffey, H., and Koch, C. R.: Psycho-social care of the paralyzed child, Pediatr. Nurs. **1:**21, 1975.

Delchanty, L., and Stravino, V.: Achieving bladder control, Am. J. Nurs. **70:**312-316, 1970.

Feuer, H.: Management of acute spine and spinal cord injuries, Arch. Surg. **3:**638-644, 1976.

Feustel, D.: Autonomic hyperflexia, Am. J. Nurs. **76:**228-230, 1976.

Ford, J. R., and Duckworth, B.: Moving a dependent patient safely, comfortably. Part I. Positioning, Nursing '76 **6**(1):27-36, 1976.

Ford, J. R., and Duckworth, B.: Moving a dependent patient safely, comfortably. Part 2. Transferring, Nursing '76 **6**(2): 58-65, 1976.

Hanlon, K.: Maintaining sexuality after spinal cord injury, Nursing '75 **5**(5):58-62, 1975.

Henderson, G. M.: Teaching-learning for rehabilitation of the spinal cord–disabled individual, Nurs. Clin. North Am. **6:**655-668, 1971.

Hubbard, D. D.: Injuries of the spine in children and adolescents, Clin. Orthop. **100:**56-65, 1974.

Johnson, M. R.: Emergency management of head and spinal injuries, Nurs. Clin. North Am. **8:**389-400, 1973.

Larrabee, J.: The person with a spinal cord injury, physical care during early recovery, Am. J. Nurs. **77:**1320-1329, 1977.

Lindh, K., and Richerson, G.: Spinal-cord injury. You can make a difference, Nursing '74 **4**(2):41-45, 1974.

Mach, E., and Dawson, W.: Injury to the spine and spinal cord, Hosp. Med. **12**(7):23-41, 1976.

Martinez, J. W.: Merry Christmas, David, Am. J. Nurs. **77:**1931, 1977.

Nursing Grand Rounds: Caring for the totally dependent patient, Nursing '76 **6**(7):38-43, 1976.

Pepper, G. A.: The person with a spinal cord injury: psychological care, Am. J. Nurs. **77:**1330-1336, 1977.

Protocols for G.U. team. Spinal Cord Injury Unit, Santa Clara Valley Medical Center, San Jose, Calif.

Scanlan, M., and associates: Quadriplegic adolescent, Nursing '72 **2**(6):28, 1972.

Shearer, J. D.: The adolescent wheelchair athlete, Pediatr. Nurs. **3**(5):20-22, 1977.

Smolock, M. A.: The nurse's role in rehabilitations of the handicapped child, Nurs. Clin. North Am. **5:**411, 1970.

Appendixes

A

Normal pulse, respiration, and blood pressure readings for children

Table A-1. Average pulse rates at rest*

Age	Lower limits of normal	Average	Upper limits of normal
Newborn	70	120	170
1-11 months	80	120	160
2 years	80	110	130
4 years	80	100	120
6 years	75	100	115
8 years	70	90	110
10 years	70	90	110
12 years			
Girls	70	90	110
Boys	65	85	105
14 years			
Girls	65	85	105
Boys	60	80	100
16 years			
Girls	60	80	100
Boys	55	75	95
18 years			
Girls	55	75	95
Boys	50	70	90

*Rates given in beats/minute.

Table A-2. Average respiratory rates at rest

Age	Rate (breaths/minute)
Newborn	35
1-11 months	30
2 years	25
4 years	23
6 years	21
8 years	20
10 years	19
12 years	19
14 years	18
16 years	17
18 years	16-18

Table A-3. Normal blood pressure values at various ages

Age (years)	Systolic		Diastolic	
	Mean	Range	Mean	Range
½-1	90	65-115	61	42-80
1-2	96	69-123	65	38-92
2-3	95	71-119	61	37-85
3-4	99	76-122	65	46-84
4-5	99	78-112	65	50-80
5	94	80-108	55	46-64
6	100	85-115	56	48-64
7	102	87-117	56	48-64
8	105	89-121	57	48-66
9	107	91-123	57	48-66
10	109	93-125	58	48-68
11	111	94-128	59	49-69
12	113	95-131	59	49-69
13	115	96-134	60	50-70
14	118	99-137	61	51-71
15	121	102-140	61	51-71

Table A-4. Mean blood pressure at wrist and ankle in infants (flush technique)*

Age	Blood pressure at wrist		Blood pressure at ankle	
	Mean	Range	Mean	Range
1-7 days	41	22-66	37	20-58
1-3 months	67	48-90	61	38-96
4-6 months	73	42-100	68	40-104
7-9 months	76	52-96	74	50-96
10-12 months	57	62-94	56	102

From Moss, A. J.: Indirect methods of blood pressure measurement, Pediatr. Clin. North Am. **25:**3-14, 1978.
*Data from Moss, A. J., and Adams, F. H.: Problems of blood pressure in childhood, Springfield, Ill., 1962, Charles C Thomas, Publisher.

B

Tables of normal laboratory values*

Table B-1. Blood chemistry

Determination	Specimen*	Age/sex†	Normal value‡		
Acetone					
Qualitative			Negative		
Quantitative			0.3-2.0 mg/dl		
Albumin—see Electrophoresis, protein					
Aldolase (fructose-1, 6-diphosphate, 37°C)		Infant	1.5-18.8 IU/liter		
		Child	2.3-13.5 IU/liter		
		Thereafter	2.3-11.3 IU/liter		
Alpha-1-antitrypsin			0.8-1.6 mg inhibition/dl		
Amino acids (maximum normal levels)			*Neonatal (μm/dl)*	*Child (μm/dl)*	*Thereafter (μm/dl)*
Alanine			52	41	67
α-Amino-n-butyric acid			7	3	4
Arginine			12	12	20
Aspartic acid			2	2	5
Citrulline			4	3	6
Cystine			8	8	19
Glutamic acid			26	20	25
Glutamine			210	75	61
Glycine			52	52	56
Histidine			13	12	12
Isoleucine			12	8	10
Leucine			22	12	18
Lysine			35	30	27
Methionine			8	5	4
Ornithine			22	15	13
Phenylalanine			20	12	12
Proline			48	40	44
Serine			30	24	19
Taurine			22	22	20
Threonine			34	32	25
Tryptophan			7	7	7
Tyrosine			21	15	9
Valine			35	35	32
Ammonia	Whole blood	Premature/jaundiced infant	100-200 μg/dl		
		Newborn	90-150 μg/dl		
		Child	40-80 μg/dl		
		Thereafter	20-120 μg/dl		

From Vaughn, V. C., and McKay, R. J., editors: Textbook of pediatrics, Philadelphia, 1975, W. B. Saunders Co.

*Serum or plasma unless otherwise indicated.

†Age ranges are defined as follows: premature, birth-1 month; newborn, birth-1 week; neonatal, 1 week-1 month; infant, 1 month-2 years; child, 2 years-puberty; adolescent, puberty-adult; adult, > 18 years.

‡dl = 100 ml.

Table B-1. Blood chemistry—cont'd

Determination	Specimen	Age/sex	Normal value
Amylase (starch, 37°C)		Newborn Infant/child Thereafter	0-2500 IU/liter 160-3700 IU/liter 1200-3200 IU/liter
Ascorbic acid			0.5-1.5 mg/dl
Bilirubin, total		 Cord 0-1 day 1-2 day 3-5 day Thereafter	Premature/full term <2 <2 mg/dl <8 <6 mg/dl <12 <8 mg/dl <16 <12 mg/dl <2 <1 mg/dl
Bilirubin, direct			0-1 mg/dl
Bromsulphalein (BSP), 5 mg/kg			$<5\%$ at 45 minute
Calcium, total		Newborn Infant Child Thereafter	3.7-7.0 mEq/liter 5.2-6.0 mEq/liter 5.0-5.7 mEq/liter 4.5-5.7 mEq/liter
Calcium, ionized			2.1-2.6 mEq/liter
Carbon dioxide (CO_2) content	Venous (arterial 2 mEq/l less)	Cord Newborn Infant Child Thereafter	14-22 mEq/liter 19-27 mEq/liter 20-28 mEq/liter 18-27 mEq/liter 23-29 mEq/liter
Carbon dioxide, partial pressure (P_{CO_2})	Whole blood, arterial Whole blood, venous		35-45 mm Hg 40-50 mm Hg
Carboxyhemoglobin	Whole blood		$<5\%$
Carotene		Infant Child Thereafter	0-40 μg/dl 40-130 μg/dl 50-300 μg/dl
Ceruloplasmin (p-phenylenediamine dihydrochloride, 37°C)		Newborn-6 months 6 months-1 year 1-12 years Thereafter	1-30 mg/dl 15-50 mg/dl 30-65 mg/dl 22-50 mg/dl
Chloride		Cord Newborn Infant Child Thereafter	96-104 mEq/liter 93-112 mEq/liter 95-110 mEq/liter 101-108 mEq/liter 98-108 mEq/liter
Cholesterol, total		Cord Newborn Infant Child Thereafter	45-100 mg/dl 45-170 mg/dl 70-175 mg/dl 120-240 mg/dl 150-250 mg/dl
Cholesterol, esters		Newborn Child Thereafter	42%-71% of total 55%-65% of total 70%-78% of total
Copper		Newborn Infant/child Child/adolescent Thereafter	20-70 μg/dl 30-150 μg/dl 90-240 μg/dl 70-120 μg/dl
Cortisol AM specimen PM specimen			 15-25 μg/dl 5-10 μg/dl
Creatine		Male Female	0.2-0.6 mg/dl 0.6-1.0 mg/dl
Creatine phosphokinase (CPK) (creatine phosphate, 30°C)		Newborn Thereafter Male Female	10-300 IU/liter 0-70 IU/liter 0-50 IU/liter
Creatinine			0.3-1.1 mg/dl

Continued.

Table B-1. Blood chemistry—cont'd

Determination	Specimen	Age/sex	Normal value
Creatinine clearance (endogenous)	Serum and urine	Newborn	40-65 ml/minute/1.73 m^2
		Child	
		Male	98-150 ml/minute/1.73 m^2
		Female	95-123 ml/minute/1.73 m^2
		Thereafter	
		Male	91-119 ml/minute/1.73 m^2
		Female	77-113 ml/minute/1.73 m^2
Electrophoresis, protein (cellulose acetate)—see protein			

	Total protein	*Albumin*	*α_1-globulin*	*α_2-globulin*	*β-globulin*	*γ-globulin*	*Units*
Premature	4.3-7.6	3.1-4.2	0.1-0.5	0.3-0.7	0.3-1.2	0.3-1.4	g/dl
Newborn	4.6-7.4	3.6-5.4	0.1-0.3	0.3-0.5	0.2-0.6	0.2-1.2	g/dl
Infant	6.1-6.7	4.4-5.3	0.2-0.4	0.5-0.8	0.5-0.8	0.3-0.7	g/dl
Thereafter	6.2-8.1	4.0-5.8	0.1-0.3	0.4-1.0	0.5-0.9	0.3-1.0	g/dl

Determination	Specimen	Age/sex	Normal value
Fatty acids, free			0.4-0.9 mEq/liter
Fibrinogen		Newborn	150-300 mg/dl
		Thereafter	200-400 mg/dl
Folate			5-20 mg/dl
Galactose		Newborn/infant	0-20 mg/dl
Globulins—see Electrophoresis, protein			
Glucose, fasting (FBS)		Premature	20-60 mg/dl
		Newborn	30-80 mg/dl
		Child	60-100 mg/dl
		Thereafter	70-110 mg/dl
Haptoglobin (as hemoglobin-binding capacity)		Neonatal	0-20 mg/dl
		Thereafter	20-200 mg/dl
Hemoglobin	Serum		<5 mg/dl
Immunoglobulin levels	Serum		

	IgG (mg/dl)	*IgM (mg/dl)*	*IgA (mg/dl)*	*Total Ig (mg/dl)*
Newborn	645-1244	5-30	0-11	660-1439
1-3 months	272-762	16-67	6-56	324-699
4-6 months	206-1125	10-83	8-93	228-1232
7-12 months	279-1533	22-147	16-98	327-1687
13-25 months	258-1393	14-114	19-119	398-1586
25-36 months	419-1274	28-113	19-235	499-1418
3-5 years	569-1597	22-100	55-152	730-1771
6-8 years	559-1492	27-118	54-221	640-1725
9-11 years	779-1456	35-132	12-208	966-1639
12-16 years	726-1085	35-72	70-229	833-1284
Adult	569-1919	47-147	61-330	730-2365

Determination	Specimen	Age/sex	Normal value
Iodine, total serum organic (PBI)		Newborn	4-14 μg/dl
		6 weeks-16 years	5-9 μg/dl
		Thereafter	4-8 μg/dl
Iodine, butanol extractable (BEI)		Newborn	3-13 μg/dl
		6 weeks-16 years	4-8 μg/dl
		Thereafter	3.2-6.4 μg/dl
Iodine, T_3 (Triosorb)			
Normal			25%-35%
Hyperthyroidism			>35%
Hypothyroidism			<25%

Table B-1. Blood chemistry—cont'd

Determination	Specimen	Age/sex	Normal value
Iodine, T_4-by-column (thyroxine)		Newborn	3-12 μg/dl
		Thereafter	3.4-6.2 μg/dl
Iodine, T_4/comp. protein binding (thyroxine)		Newborn	3-12 μg/dl
		Thereafter	3-7 μg/dl
Iron		Newborn	100-200 μg/dl
		4 months-2 years	40-100 μg/dl
		Thereafter	85-150 μg/dl
Iron-binding capacity (IBC)		Newborn	60-175 μg/dl
		4 months-2 years	100-400 μg/dl
		Thereafter	350-450 μg/dl
Lactic acid	Whole blood, venous		5-20 mg/dl
Lactic dehydrogenase (LDH) (pyruvate, 30°C)		Newborn	300-1500 IU/liter
		Thereafter	
		Male	50-150 IU/liter
		Female	40-140 IU/liter
Lead, normal	Whole blood, venous		0-40 μg/dl
Abnormal, nontoxic			40-80 μg/dl
Toxic			>80 μg/dl
Lipase (olive oil, 37°C)		Infant	9-105 IU/liter
		Thereafter	20-136 IU/liter
Lipids, total		Newborn-2 years	170-450 mg/dl
		2-14 years	490-1000 mg/dl
		Thereafter	400-800 mg/dl

Lipoproteins

	Total	*Alpha*	*Beta*	*Chylo*	*Units*
Newborn	170-440	70-180	50-160	50-110	mg/dl
Infant	240-800	70-280	120-450	50-250	mg/dl
Thereafter	500-1100	150-330	225-540	100-270	mg/dl

Determination	Specimen	Age/sex	Normal value
Magnesium		Newborn	1.4-2.9 mEq/liter
		Infant	1.2-2.7 mEq/liter
		Thereafter	1.2-2.6 mEq/liter
Malic dehydrogenase (MDH) (oxalacetic acid, 37°C)		Cord	41-68 IU/liter
		Thereafter	32-48 IU/liter
Methemoglobin	Whole blood		0.0-0.3 gm/dl
premature infants (at higher level)			(0.4)
Osmolality			270-285 mOsm/liter
Oxygen, partial pressure (Po_2)	Whole blood, arterial		75-100 mm Hg
	Whole blood, venous		20-50 mm Hg
Oxygen, % saturation	Whole blood, arterial	Newborn	40%-95%
		Thereafter	95%-98%
	Whole blood, venous	Newborn	30%-80%
		Thereafter	35%-85%
pH (37°C)*	Whole blood, arterial	Premature (cord)	7.15-7.35
		Premature (48 hours)	7.35-7.50
		Newborn	7.27-7.47
		Thereafter	7.35-7.45
Phenylalanine			0.5-2.0 mg/dl

*Arterial blood is approximately 0.03 pH units greater than circulating venous blood.

Continued.

Table B-1. Blood chemistry—cont'd

Determination	Specimen	Age/sex	Normal value
Phosphatase, acid		Newborn-2 weeks	10.4-16.4 IU/liter
(phenylphosphate, 37°C)		2 weeks-13 years	8.6-12.6 IU/liter
		Thereafter	
		Male	0.5-11.0 IU/liter
		Female	0.2-9.5 IU/liter
Phosphatase, alkaline		Newborn	50-275 IU/liter
(p-nitrophenylphosphate,		Infant	100-330 IU/liter
AMP buffer, 37°C,		Child	90-230 IU/liter
Auto-Analyzer)		Adolescent	100-250 IU/liter
		Thereafter	30-90 IU/liter
Phosphorus		Newborn	3.5-8.6 mg/dl
		Infant	4.5-6.7 mg/dl
		Child	4.5-5.5 mg/dl
		Thereafter	2.5-4.8 mg/dl
Phospholipids		Newborn	75-170 mg/dl
(lipids P × 25)		Infant	100-275 mg/dl
		Child	180-295 mg/dl
		Thereafter	150-380 mg/dl
Potassium		Premature (cord)	5.0-10.2 mEq/liter
		Premature (48 hours)	3.0-6.0 mEq/liter
		Newborn (cord)	5.6-12.0 mEq/liter
		Newborn	5.0-7.7 mEq/liter
		Infant	4.1-5.3 mEq/liter
		Child	3.5-4.7 mEq/liter
		Thereafter	3.4-5.6 mEq/liter
Protein, total		Premature	4.3-7.6 gm/dl
		Newborn	4.6-7.6 gm/dl
		Child	6.2-8.1 gm/dl
		Thereafter	5.5-7.8 gm/dl
Sodium		Premature (cord)	116-140 mEq/liter
		Premature (48 hours)	128-148 mEq/liter
		Newborn (cord)	126-166 mEq/liter
		Newborn	139-162 mEq/liter
		Infant	139-146 mEq/liter
		Child	138-145 mEq/liter
		Thereafter	135-151 mEq/liter
Thiamine	Whole blood		5.5-9.5 μg/dl
Transaminases			
Glutamic oxaloacetic (GOT)		Newborn/infant	5-70 IU/liter
(aspartate, 30°C)		Thereafter	5-20 IU/liter
Glutamic pyruvic (GPT)		Newborn/infant	5-50 IU/liter
(alanine, 30°C)		Thereafter	5-30 IU/liter
Transferrin			0.2-0.3 gm/dl
Triglycerides		Newborn/infant	5-40 mg/dl
		Thereafter	10-190 mg/dl
Urea nitrogen (BUN)		Newborn/infant	5-15 mg/dl
		Thereafter	10-20 mg/dl
Uric acid		Child	2.0-5.5 mg/dl
		Thereafter	
		Male	2.1-7.7 mg/dl
		Female	1.8-6.6 mg/dl
Vitamin A			16-60 μg/dl
Vitamin B_{12}			100-700 pg/ml
Vitamin E (tocopherols)			0.5-1.5 mg/dl

Table B-2. Special chemistry

Determination	Specimen*	Age/sex	Normal value
Aldosterone			2-26 μg/24 hour
Ammonia		Infant	10-50 mEq/24 hour
		Child	15-50 mEq/24 hour
		Thereafter	20-70 mEq/24 hour
Amylase		Neonatal	0-1000 IU/hour
		Thereafter	700-5200 IU/hour
Calcium			2.5-20 mEq/24 hour
Catecholamines			
	Norepinephrine	*Epinephrine*	*Units*
Newborn	2-4	0-1	μg/24 hour
Neonatal	2-12	1-2	μg/24 hour
Infant	3-60	1-15	μg/24 hour
Child	20-70	1-15	μg/24 hour
Adolescent	30-80	5-15	μg/24 hour
Adult	40-100	5-15	μg/24 hour
Chloride		Infant	2-10 mEq/24 hour
		Child	15-40 mEq/24 hour
		Thereafter	150-250 mEq/24 hour
Chloride	Sweat		
Normal			0-30 mEq/liter
Marginal (that is, asthma, Addison's disease, malnutrition, etc.)			30-70 mEq/liter
Cystic fibrosis			70-200 mEq/liter
Creatinine		Infant	8-20 mg/kg/24 hour
		Child	8-22 mg/kg/24 hour
		Adolescent	8-30 mg/kg/24 hour
		Thereafter	14-26 mg/kg/24 hour
Fat, fecal	Feces		<5 gm/24 hour
5-Hydroxyindoleacetic acid (5-HIAA)			0-10 mg/dl
17-Ketogenic steroids (17-KGS)		Birth-2 years	2-4 mg/24 hour
		2-6 years	3-6 mg/24 hour
		6-10 years	6-8 mg/24 hour
		10-14 years	8-14 mg/24 hour
		Adult: Male	10-20 mg/24 hour
		Female	6-17 mg/24 hour
17-Ketosteroids (17-KS)		0-14 days	0.5-2.5 mg/24 hour
		14 days-2 years	0-0.5 mg/24 hour
		2-6 years	0-2.0 mg/24 hour
		6-8 years	0-2.5 mg/24 hour
		8-10 years	0.7-4.0 mg/24 hour
		10-12 years: Male	0.7-6.0 mg/24 hour
		Female	0.7-5.0 mg/24 hour
		12-14 years: Male	1.3-10.0 mg/24 hour
		Female	1.3-8.5 mg/24 hour
		14-16 years: Male	2.5-13.0 mg/24 hour
		Female	2.5-11.0 mg/24 hour
		Adult: Male	9.0-22.0 mg/24 hour
		Female	6.0-15.0 mg/24 hour

From Vaughn, V. C., and McKay, R. J., editors: Textbook of pediatrics, Philadelphia, 1975, W. B. Saunders Co.
*Urine unless otherwise indicated.

Continued.

Table B-2. Special chemistry—cont'd

Determination	Specimen	Age/sex		Normal value	
		Normal	*Abnormal, nontoxic*	*Toxic*	*Units*
Lead and metabolites					
Lead	Whole blood	0-40	40-80	>80	µg/dl
Lead	Urine	0-80	80-150	>150	µg/dl
Coproporphyrin	Urine	0-150	150-500	>500	µg/dl
δ-Aminolevulinic acid (ALA)	Urine	0.1-0.6	0.6-2.0	>2.0	µg/dl
Lipase (olive oil, 37°C)	Duodenal drainage (intestinal juice)			8-35 IU/ml	
Phosphorus				0.7-1.1 gm/24 hour	
Pituitary gonadotropins (FSH)		Child		0 mouse u	
		Female			
		Premenopausal		25-40 mouse u	
		Pregnant		2,000-50,000 mouse u	
		Postmenopausal		20-50 mouse u	
		Male		0-20 mouse u	
Porphyrins					
Porphobilinogen				0 µg/24 hour	
Uroporphyrin				0-30 µg/24 hour	
Coproporphyrin		Male		130-248 µg/24 hour	
		Female		92-176 µg/24 hour	
Potassium				25-100 mEq/24 hour	
Pregnanetriol		Newborn		0 mg/24 hour	
		Infant		0-0.2 mg/24 hour	
		Child		0.3-1.1 mg/24 hour	
		Thereafter		0.5-4.0 mg/24 hour	
Protein, total (albumin)				2-8 mg/dl	
				10-100 mg/24 hour	
Sodium		Child		40-180 mEq/24 hour	
		Thereafter		80-220 mEq/24 hour	
Titratable acidity†	Gastric juice				
Basal acid output (BAO)				0-6 mEq/hour	
Maximal histamine stimulation acid output (MAO)		Male		10-35 mEq/hour	
		Female		5-30 mEq/hour	
Trypsin (N-benzoyl-arginine ethyl ester, 25°C)	Duodenal drainage (intestinal juice)			160-180 µg/ml	
Urobilinogen				<3 mg/24 hour	
Vanillylmandelic acid (VMA)		Newborn		0-1 mg/24 hour	
		Neonatal		0-1 mg/24 hour	
		Infant		0-2 mg/24 hour	
		Child		1-5 mg/24 hour	
		Adolescent		1-5 mg/24 hour	
		Thereafter		2-7 mg/24 hour	
Xylose absorption				<20% retention of dose in 5 hours	

†At birth the neonate usually has gastric acidity similar to that of adults. Within a few days after birth, however, and for several weeks thereafter, the ability to secrete acid may become impaired. The response to histamine stimulation in older children (when corrected for body weight or surface area) closely resembles that in adults.

Table B-3. Cerebrospinal fluid

Determination	Age	Normal value	
Calcium		2-3 mEq/liter	
Cell count		*WBC's/mm³*	*RBC's/mm³*
	Premature	0-18	0-500
	Newborn	0-15	0-500
	Infant	0-8	0-10
	Thereafter	0-5	0-10
Chloride	Neonatal	108-122 mEq/liter	
	Thereafter	112-130 mEq/liter	
Glucose*	Newborn	20-40 mg/dl	
	Infant/child	70-90 mg/dl	
	Thereafter	50-80 mg/dl	
Lactic dehydrogenase (LDH) (pyruvate, 30°C)	Newborn	5-80 IU/liter	
	Thereafter	5-30 IU/liter	
Magnesium		2.8-3.3 mg/dl	
Pandy's test (for excess globulins)		Negative	
pH (37°C)		7.33-7.42	
Phosphorus, inorganic		1.5-3.0 mg/dl	
Potassium		2.8-4.1 mEq/liter	
Protein, total	Newborn-1 month	20-120 mg/dl	
	Thereafter	15-45 mg/dl	
Albumin		52%	
$Alpha_1$		5%	
$Alpha_2$		14%	
Beta		10%	
Gamma		19%	
Sodium		130-165 mEq/liter	
Specific gravity		1.007-1.009	
Transaminase Glutamic oxaloacetic (GOT) (aspartate, 30°C)		2-10 IU/liter	
Volume (increases with age to adult figure)	Newborn	Up to 5 ml	
	Adult	100-150 ml	

From Vaughn, V. C., and McKay, R. J., editors: Textbook of pediatrics, Philadelphia, 1975, W. B. Saunders Co.
*Glucose levels in CSF vary with those of serum glucose. CSF value is approximately one half to two thirds the serum glucose level.

Table B-4. Hematology

Determination*	Age/sex	Normal value
Hematocrit (PCV)	Newborn	44%-64%
	Neonatal	35%-49%
	Infant	30%-40%
	Child	31%-43%
	Thereafter: Male	40%-54%
	Female	37%-47%
Hemoglobin†	Newborn	14-24 gm/dl
	Neonatal	11-20 gm/dl
	Infant	10-15 gm/dl
	Child	11-16 gm/dl
	Thereafter: Male	14-18 gm/dl
	Female	12-16 gm/dl
Hemoglobin, fetal (Hb F)	Newborn	40%-70% of total
	Neonatal	20%-40% of total
	Infant	2%-10% of total
	Thereafter	1%-2% of total
Nucleated RBCs	Cord	250-500/mm^3
	Day 1	200-300/mm^3
	Day 2	20-30/mm^3
	Thereafter	0
Osmotic fragility		0.44%-0.40% NaCl
50% hemolysis		0.5%-1.5% NaCl
Platelet count	Premature	100-300,000/mm^3
	Newborn	140-300,000/mm^3
	Neonatal	150-390,000/mm^3
	Infant	200-473,000/mm^3
	Thereafter	150-450,000/mm^3
Red blood cell (RBC) count	Newborn	4.8-7.1 mil/mm^3
	Neonatal	4.1-6.4 mil/mm^3
	Infant/child	3.8-5.5 mil/mm^3
	Thereafter: Male	4.6-6.2 mil/mm^3
	Female	4.2-5.4 mil/mm^3

From Vaughn, V. C., and McKay, R. J., editors: Textbook of pediatrics, Philadelphia, 1975, W. B. Saunders Co.
*Specimen is whole blood unless otherwise indicated.
†During the neonatal period, hemoglobin measurements from capillary blood are 2-3 gm/dl greater than those in blood obtained by venipuncture.
‡Eosinophilia (up to 20% of WBC count) may occur normally in infancy.

Table B-4. Hematology—cont'd

Determination	Age/sex	Normal value
Blood indices		
MCH	Newborn	32-34 $\mu\mu$g
	Thereafter	27-31 $\mu\mu$g
MCV	Newborn	96-108 μ^3
	Thereafter	82-91 μ^3
MCHC	Newborn	32%-33%
	Thereafter	32%-36%
Reticulocyte count	Newborn	2.5%-6.5% total RBC
	Neonatal	0.1%-1.5% total RBC
	Infant	0.5%-3.1% total RBC
	Thereafter	0%-2.0% total RBC
Sedimentation rate (ESR) (uncorrected)	Newborn	0-2 mm/hour
	Neonatal/puberty	3-13 mm/hour
	Adult: Male	10-15 mm/hour
	Female	15-25 mm/hour
White blood cell (WBC) count‡	Newborn, total	9000-30,000/mm³
	%Neutrophils	≃ 61%
	%Lymphocytes	≃ 31%
	1 week, total	5000-21,000/mm³
	%Neutrophils	≃ 45%
	%Lymphocytes	≃ 41%
	4 weeks, total	5000-19,500/mm³
	%Neutrophils	≃ 35%
	%Lymphocytes	≃ 56%
	6-12 months, total	6000-17,500/mm³
	%Neutrophils	≃ 32%
	%Lymphocytes	≃ 61%
	2 years, total	6200-17,000/mm³
	%Neutrophils	≃ 33%
	%Lymphocytes	≃ 59%
	Thereafter, total	5000-10,000/mm³
	%Neutrophils	≃ 60%
	%Lymphocytes	≃ 30%

Table B-5. Coagulation*

Determination	Specimen†	Age/sex	Normal value
Activated clotting time (ACT)	Plasma		<2.16 minute
Bleeding time (Ivy)	Whole blood	Premature	1-8 minute
		Newborn	1-5 minute
		Thereafter	1-6 minute
Clot retraction	Whole blood		Complete at 4 hours
Clotting time	Whole blood		
Two tubes			5-8 minute
Three tubes			5-15 minute
Fibrinogen	Plasma	Newborn	150-300 mg/dl
		Thereafter	200-400 mg/dl
Fibrinolysin (plasminogen)	Plasma		Lysis of clot
Partial thromboplastin time (PTT)‡	Plasma	Premature	<120 second
		Newborn	<90 second
		Thereafter	<60 second
Prothrombin time, one stage (PT)‡	Plasma	Premature	12-21 second
		Newborn/neonatal	12-20 second
		Thereafter	12-14 second
Thromboplastin generation test (TGT)‡	Plasma	Premature	8-24 second at 6-minute tube
		Newborn	8-20 second at 6-minute tube
		Thereafter	8-16 second at 6-minute tube

From Vaughn, V. C., and McKay, R. J., editors: Textbook of pediatrics, Philadelphia, 1975, W. B. Saunders Co.
*Coagulation factors (I to XIV) are low in the newly born, rising to adult levels during the first months of life.
†Anticoagulants and collection instructions vary for individual laboratories.
‡Moderate deficiency of coagulation factors dependent on vitamin K (II, prothrombin; VII, proconvertin; IX, plasma thromboplastin component; X, Stuart-Prower factor) occurs during the first days of life. Values return to near normal levels within 1 week. This deficiency may account for prolonged PTT, PT, and TGT during this period.

Table B-6. Serology

Determination	Specimen*	Value
Alpha-1-fetoprotein		None detected
Antistreptolysin O titer (ASO)		
Normal		12-100 Todd units
Recent streptococcal infection†		200-2500 Todd units
Antihyaluronidase titer (AHT)		<1:256
Colloidal gold curve	CSF	
Normal		Flat curve (1,1,1,1,0,0,0,0,0,0,0)
Central nervous system syphilis, multiple sclerosis		First zone curve (5,5,5,5,4,3,2,1,1,0,0)
Abnormal spinal fluid		Mid zone curve (0,1,2,3,3,3,2,1,0,0,0)
Acute purulent meningitis		End zone curve (0,0,0,1,1,2,3,3,3,3,0)
Cold agglutinins		0-1:32
C-reactive protein (CRP)		None detected
Febrile agglutinins		
Typhoid O		0-1:40‡
Typhoid H		0-1:20‡
Brucella		0-1:20
Rickettsia (Proteus OX 19)		0-1:40
Tularemia		0-1:40
Hepatitis-associated (Australia) antigen		None detected
Heterophil antibody		
Mono "spot" test		Negative
Thyroid autoantibodies		
Thyroglobulin antibody (tanned red cell method)		0-1:32

From Vaughn, V. C., and McKay, R. J., editors: Textbook of pediatrics, Philadelphia, 1975, W. B. Saunders Co.
*Serum unless otherwise indicated.
†Convalescent specimen should be examined to demonstrate rise in titer.
‡May be higher in individuals who have received typhoid vaccine.

Table B-7. Urinalysis

Determination	Age/sex	Normal value		
Addis count				
Leukocytes		<1,000,000/12 hours		
Erythrocytes		<250,000/12 hours		
Casts		<5,000/12 hours		
Protein		<20 mg/12 hours		
Colony count, colonies/ml urine (fresh specimen)		*Clean catch, midstream**	*Catheterization*	*Suprapubic bladder puncture*
	Infant/child	<1,000	<100	0
	Thereafter	<10,000	<100	0
Gastric analysis/Diagnex Blue titration		>0.6 mg Azure A excreted		
Microscopic				
Leukocytes		0-4 per high-power field		
Erythrocytes		Rare per high-power field		
Casts		Rare per high-power field		
Osmolality	Premature/newborn	100-600 mOsm/liter		
	Thereafter	50-1400 mOsm/liter		
pH	Newborn/neonatal	5-7		
	Thereafter	4.5-8		
Specific gravity	Newborn/infant	1.001-1.020		
	Thereafter	1.001-1.030		
Volume	Newborn	30-300 ml/24 hour		
	Neonatal	250-450 ml/24 hour		
	Infant	400-600 ml/24 hour		
	Child	500-1000 ml/24 hour		
	Adolescent	500-1500 ml/24 hour		
	Adult	500-2000 ml/24 hour		

From Vaughn, V. C., and McKay, R. J., editors: Textbook of pediatrics, Philadelphia, 1975, W. B. Saunders Co.

*Pure cultures with colony counts >100,000 are considered diagnostic in adults, whereas colony counts of >10,000 are usually considered diagnostic in children. Intermediate counts must be interpreted relative to the clinical situation. For females, the physician must be aware of the cleanliness and care used in collecting the specimen. Urine obtained by means of a plastic collection device or by voiding into a container without prior preparation of the patient is usually contaminated and has limited usefulness in evaluating the possibility of urinary tract infection.

Table B-8. Radioisotopic procedures

Determination	Specimen	Normal value
^{51}Chromium		
Cell survival (T/2)	Whole blood	25-35 days ½-time
Red cell mass	Whole blood	28-32 ml/kg
^{51}Chromium-albumin		
Normal	Urine	10%-15% of dose in 72 hours
Exudative enteropathy	Urine	6%-12% of dose in 72 hours
Normal	Stool	0-1% of dose in 72 hours
Exudative enteropathy	Stool	2%-20% of dose in 72 hours
Iodine (^{131}I) uptake	Neck scan	6%-17% of dose in 6 hours
	Neck scan	10%-30% of dose in 24 hours
Rose bengal-^{131}I		
Normal	Urine	5%-30% of dose in 72 hours
Hepatocellular obstruction	Urine	10%-20% of dose in 72 hours
Biliary obstruction	Urine	15%-25% of dose in 72 hours
Normal	Stool	40%-70% of dose in 72 hours
Hepatocellular obstruction	Stool	10%-50% of dose in 72 hours
Biliary obstruction	Stool	0-5% of dose in 72 hours

From Vaughn, V. C., and McKay, R. J., editors: Textbook of pediatrics, Philadelphia, 1975, W. B. Saunders Co.

C

Conversion tables

Table C-1. Conversion of pounds to kilograms for pediatric weights

Pounds → ↓	0	1	2	3	4	5	6	7	8	9
0	0.00	0.45	0.90	1.36	1.81	2.26	2.72	3.17	3.62	4.08
10	4.53	4.98	5.44	5.89	6.35	6.80	7.25	7.71	8.16	8.61
20	9.07	9.52	9.97	10.43	10.88	11.34	11.79	12.24	12.70	13.15
30	13.60	14.06	14.51	14.96	15.42	15.87	16.32	16.78	17.23	17.69
40	18.14	18.59	19.05	19.50	19.95	20.41	20.86	21.31	21.77	22.22
50	22.68	23.13	23.58	24.04	24.49	24.94	25.40	25.85	26.30	26.76
60	27.21	27.66	28.12	28.57	29.03	29.48	29.93	30.39	30.84	31.29
70	31.75	32.20	32.65	33.11	33.56	34.02	34.47	34.92	35.38	35.83
80	36.28	36.74	37.19	37.64	38.10	38.55	39.00	39.46	39.91	40.37
90	40.82	41.27	41.73	42.18	42.63	43.09	43.54	43.99	44.45	44.90
100	45.36	45.81	46.26	46.72	47.17	47.62	48.08	48.53	48.98	49.44
110	49.89	50.34	50.80	51.25	51.71	52.16	52.61	53.07	53.52	53.97
120	54.43	54.88	55.33	55.79	56.24	56.70	57.15	57.60	58.06	58.51
130	58.96	59.42	59.87	60.32	60.78	61.23	61.68	62.14	62.59	63.05
140	63.50	63.95	64.41	64.86	65.31	65.77	66.22	66.67	67.13	67.58
150	68.04	68.49	68.94	69.40	69.85	70.30	70.76	71.21	71.66	72.12
160	72.57	73.02	73.48	73.93	74.39	74.84	75.29	75.75	76.20	76.65
170	77.11	77.56	78.01	78.47	78.92	79.38	79.83	80.28	80.74	81.19
180	81.64	82.10	82.55	83.00	83.46	83.91	84.36	84.82	85.27	85.73
190	86.18	86.68	87.09	87.54	87.99	88.45	88.90	89.35	89.81	90.26
200	90.72	91.17	91.62	92.08	92.53	92.98	93.44	93.89	94.34	94.80

Table C-2. Conversion of pounds and ounces to kilograms for pediatric weights

Pounds	Kilograms	Ounces	Kilograms	Pounds	Kilograms	Ounces	Kilograms
1	0.454	1	0.028	9	4.082	9	0.255
2	0.907	2	0.057	10	4.536	10	0.283
3	1.361	3	0.085	11	4.990	11	0.312
4	1.814	4	0.113	12	5.443	12	0.340
5	2.268	5	0.142	13	5.897	13	0.369
6	2.722	6	0.170			14	0.397
7	3.175	7	0.198			15	0.425
8	3.629	8	0.227				

Table C-3. Conversion of pounds and ounces to grams for pediatric weights

Pounds	Ounces 0	1	2	3	4	5	6	7	8	9	10	11	12	13	14	15	Pounds
0	—	28	57	85	113	142	170	198	227	255	283	312	430	369	397	425	0
1	454	482	510	539	567	595	624	652	680	709	737	765	794	822	850	879	1
2	907	936	964	992	1021	1049	1077	1106	1134	1162	1191	1219	1247	1276	1304	1332	2
3	1361	1389	1417	1446	1474	1503	1531	1559	1588	1616	1644	1673	1701	1729	1758	1786	3
4	1814	1843	1871	1899	1928	1956	1984	2013	2041	2070	2098	2126	2155	2183	2211	2240	4
5	2268	2296	2325	2353	2381	2410	2438	2466	2495	2523	2551	2580	2608	2637	2665	2693	5
6	2722	2750	2778	2807	2835	2863	2892	2920	2948	2977	3005	3033	3062	3090	3118	3147	6
7	3175	3203	3232	3260	3289	3317	3345	3374	3402	3430	3459	3487	3515	3544	3572	3600	7
8	3629	3657	3685	3714	3742	3770	3799	3827	3856	3884	3912	3941	3969	3997	4026	4054	8
9	4082	4111	4139	4167	4196	4224	4252	4281	4309	4337	4366	4394	4423	4451	4479	4508	9
10	4536	4564	4593	4621	4649	4678	4706	4734	4763	4791	4819	4848	4876	4904	4933	4961	10
11	4990	5018	5046	5075	5103	5131	5160	5188	5216	5245	5273	5301	5330	5358	5386	5415	11
12	5443	5471	5500	5528	5557	5585	5613	5642	5670	5698	5727	5755	5783	5812	5840	5868	12
13	5897	5925	5953	5982	6010	6038	6067	6095	6123	6152	6180	6209	6237	6265	6294	6322	13
14	6350	6379	6407	6435	6464	6492	6520	6549	6577	6605	6634	6662	6690	6719	6747	6776	14
15	6804	6832	6860	6889	6917	6945	6973	7002	7030	7059	7087	7115	7144	7172	7201	7228	15
16	7257	7286	7313	7342	7371	7399	7427	7456	7484	7512	7541	7569	7597	7626	7654	7682	16
17	7711	7739	7768	7796	7824	7853	7881	7909	7938	7966	7994	8023	8051	8079	8108	8136	17
18	8165	8192	8221	8249	8278	8306	8335	8363	8391	8420	8448	8476	8504	8533	8561	8590	18
19	8618	8646	8675	8703	8731	8760	8788	8816	8845	8873	8902	8930	8958	8987	9015	9043	19
20	9072	9100	9128	9157	9185	9213	9242	9270	9298	9327	9355	9383	9412	9440	9469	9497	20
21	9525	9554	9582	9610	9639	9667	9695	9724	9752	9780	9809	9837	9865	9894	9922	9950	21
22	9979	10007	10036	10064	10092	10120	10149	10177	10206	10234	10262	10291	10319	10347	10376	10404	22
	0	1	2	3	4	5	6	7	8	9	10	11	12	13	14	15	

Table C-4. Conversion factors for temperature

Celsius	Fahrenheit	Celsius	Fahrenheit
34.0	93.2	38.6	101.5
34.2	93.6	38.8	101.8
34.4	93.9	39.0	102.2
34.6	94.3	39.2	102.6
34.8	94.6	39.4	102.9
35.0	95.0	39.6	103.3
35.2	95.4	39.8	103.6
35.4	95.7	40.0	104.0
35.6	96.1	40.2	104.4
35.8	96.4	40.4	104.7
36.0	96.8	40.6	105.2
36.2	97.2	40.8	105.4
36.4	97.5	41.0	105.9
36.6	97.9	41.2	106.1
36.8	98.2	41.4	106.5
37.0	98.6	41.6	106.8
37.2	99.0	41.8	107.2
37.4	99.3	42.0	107.6
37.6	99.7	42.2	108.0
37.8	100.0	42.4	108.3
38.0	100.4	42.6	108.7
38.2	100.8	42.8	109.0
38.4	101.1	43.0	109.4

(°C) × (9/5) + 32 = °F
(°F − 32) × (5/9) = °C
°C = temperature in Celsius (centigrade) degrees
°F = temperature in Fahrenheit degrees

D

Recommended daily dietary allowances

Table D-1. Food and Nutrition Board, National Academy of Sciences–National Council Recommended healthy people in the United States)

	Age (years)	Weight		Height		Energy (kcal)†	Protein (g)	Fat-soluble vitamins			
								Vitamin A activity		Vitamin D (IU)	Vitamin E activity‖ IU
		kg	lb	cm	in			RE‡	IU		
Infants	0.0-0.5	6	14	60	24	kg × 117	kg × 2.2	420§	1,400	400	4
	0.5-1.0	9	20	71	28	kg × 108	kg × 2.0	400	2,000	400	5
Children	1-3	13	28	86	34	1300	23	400	2,000	400	7
	4-6	20	44	110	44	1800	30	500	2,500	400	9
	7-10	30	66	135	54	2400	36	700	3,300	400	10
Males	11-14	44	97	158	63	2800	44	1,000	5,000	400	12
	15-18	61	134	172	69	3000	54	1,000	5,000	400	15
	19-22	67	147	172	69	3000	54	1,000	5,000	400	15
	23-50	70	154	172	69	2700	56	1,000	5,000		15
	51+	70	154	172	69	2400	56	1,000	5,000		15
Females	11-14	44	97	155	62	2400	44	800	4,000	400	12
	15-18	54	119	162	65	2100	48	800	4,000	400	12
	19-22	58	128	162	65	2100	46	800	4,000	400	12
	23-50	58	128	162	65	2000	46	800	4,000		12
	51+	58	128	162	65	1800	46	800	4,000		12
Pregnant						+300	+30	1,000	5,000	400	15
Lactating						+500	+20	1,200	6,000	400	15

*The allowances are intended to provide for individual variations among most normal persons as they live in the United States under usual environmental defined.
†Kilojoules (kJ) = 4.2 × kcal.
‡Retinol equivalents.
§Assumed to be all as retinol in milk during the first 6 months of life. All subsequent intakes are assumed to be half as retinol and half as β-carotene
‖Total vitamin E activity, estimated to be 80% as α-tocopherol and 20% other tocopherols.
¶The folacin allowances refer to dietary sources as determined by *Lactobacillus casei* assay. Pure forms of folacin may be effective in doses less
#Although allowances are expressed as niacin, it is recognized that on the average 1 mg of niacin is derived from each 60 mg of dietary tryptophan.
**This increased requirement cannot be met by ordinary diets; therefore the use of supplemental iron is recommended.

aily Dietary Allowances (revised 1974)* (designed for the maintenance of good nutrition of practically all

Water-soluble vitamins							Minerals					
Ascorbic acid (mg)	**Folacin¶ (μg)**	**Niacin# (mg)**	**Riboflavin (B_2) (mg)**	**Thiamine (B_1) (mg)**	**Vitamin B_6 (mg)**	**Vitamin B_{12} (μg)**	**Calcium (mg)**	**Phosphorus (mg)**	**Iodine (μg)**	**Iron (mg)**	**Magne-sium (mg)**	**Zinc (mg)**
35	50	5	0.4	0.3	0.3	0.3	360	240	35	10	60	3
35	50	8	0.6	0.5	0.4	0.3	540	400	45	15	70	5
40	100	9	0.8	0.7	0.6	1.0	800	800	60	15	150	10
40	200	12	1.1	0.9	0.9	1.5	800	800	80	10	200	10
40	300	16	1.2	1.2	1.2	2.0	800	800	110	10	250	10
45	400	18	1.5	1.4	1.6	3.0	1200	1200	130	18	350	15
45	400	20	1.8	1.5	2.0	3.0	1200	1200	150	18	400	15
45	400	20	1.8	1.5	2.0	3.0	800	800	140	10	350	15
45	400	18	1.6	1.4	2.0	3.0	800	800	130	10	350	15
45	400	16	1.5	1.2	2.0	3.0	800	800	110	10	350	15
45	400	16	1.3	1.2	1.6	3.0	1200	1200	115	18	300	15
45	400	14	1.4	1.1	2.0	3.0	1200	1200	115	18	300	15
45	400	14	1.4	1.1	2.0	3.0	800	800	100	18	300	15
45	400	13	1.2	1.0	2.0	3.0	800	800	100	18	300	15
45	400	12	1.1	1.0	2.0	3.0	800	800	80	10	300	15
60	800	+2	+0.3	+0.3	2.5	4.0	1200	1200	125	18+**	450	20
80	600	+4	+0.5	+0.3	2.5	4.0	1200	1200	150	18	450	25

resses diets should be based on a variety of common foods in order to provide other nutrients for which human requirements have been less well

hen calculated from international units. As retinol equivalents, three fourths are as retinol and one fourth as β-carotene.

an one fourth of the recommended dietary allowance.

E

Growth measurements

Table E-1. Weight and height measurements for girls

Age*	Weight distribution by percentile†						Height distribution by percentile†					
	3†		50†		97†		3†		50†		97†	
	lb	kg	lb	kg	lb	kg	inches	cm	inches	cm	inches	cm
Birth	5.8	2.63	7.4	3.36	9.4	4.26	18.5	47.1	19.8	50.2	21.1	53.6
3 months	9.8	4.45	12.4	5.62	14.9	6.76	22.0	55.8	23.4	59.5	24.8	63.1
6 months	12.7	5.76	16.0	7.26	20.0	9.07	24.0	61.1	25.7	65.2	27.1	68.8
9 months	15.1	6.85	19.2	8.71	24.2	10.98	25.7	65.4	27.6	70.1	29.2	74.1
1	16.8	7.62	21.5	9.75	27.1	12.29	27.1	68.9	29.2	74.2	31.0	78.8
1¼	18.1	8.21	23.0	10.43	29.0	13.15	28.3	71.9	30.5	77.6	32.6	82.8
1½	19.4	8.80	24.5	11.11	30.9	14.02	29.5	74.9	31.8	80.9	34.1	86.7
2	21.6	9.80	27.1	12.29	34.4	15.60	31.5	80.1	34.1	86.6	36.7	93.3
2½	23.6	10.70	29.6	13.43	38.2	17.33	33.3	84.5	36.0	91.4	38.9	98.7
3	25.6	11.61	31.8	14.42	41.8	18.96	34.8	88.4	37.7	95.7	40.7	103.5
3½	27.5	12.47	33.9	15.38	45.3	20.55	36.2	92.0	39.2	99.5	42.5	108.0
4	29.2	13.25	36.2	16.42	48.2	21.86	37.5	95.2	40.6	103.2	44.2	112.3
4½	30.7	13.93	38.5	17.46	50.9	23.09	38.6	98.1	42.0	106.8	45.7	116.2
5†	32.1	14.56	40.5	18.37	52.8	23.95	39.4	100.0	42.9	109.1	46.8	118.8
5†	33.7	15.29	41.4	18.78	51.8	23.50	40.4	102.6	43.2	109.7	46.5	118.0
6	37.2	16.87	46.5	21.09	58.7	26.63	42.5	108.0	45.6	115.9	49.4	125.4
7	41.3	18.73	52.2	23.68	67.3	30.53	44.9	114.0	48.1	122.3	51.9	131.7
8	45.3	20.55	58.1	26.35	78.9	35.79	46.9	119.1	50.4	128.0	54.1	137.4
9	49.1	22.27	63.8	28.94	89.9	40.78	48.7	123.6	52.3	132.9	56.5	143.4
10	53.2	24.13	70.3	31.89	101.9	46.22	50.3	127.7	54.6	138.6	58.8	149.3
11	57.9	26.26	78.8	35.74	112.9	51.21	52.1	132.3	57.0	144.7	62.0	157.4
12	63.6	28.85	87.6	39.74	127.7	57.92	54.3	137.8	59.8	151.9	64.8	164.6
13	72.2	32.75	99.1	44.95	142.3	64.55	56.6	143.7	61.8	157.1	66.3	168.4
14	83.1	37.69	108.4	49.17	150.8	68.40	58.3	148.2	62.8	159.6	67.2	170.7
15	89.0	40.37	113.5	51.48	155.2	70.40	59.1	150.2	63.4	161.1	67.6	171.6
16	91.8	41.64	117.0	53.07	157.7	71.53	59.37	150.8	63.9	162.4	67.7	172.0
17	93.9	42.59	119.1	54.02	159.5	72.35	59.45	151.0	64.0	162.5	67.8	172.2
18	94.5	42.87	119.9	54.39	160.7	72.89	59.45	151.0	64.0	162.5	67.8	172.2

Adapted from studies by Howard V. Meredith, Iowa Child Welfare Research Station, The State University of Iowa. In Vaughan, V. C., and McKay, R. J., editors: Nelson's textbook of pediatrics, Philadelphia, 1975, W. B. Saunders Co.

*Years unless otherwise indicated.

†The figures for the several percentiles for age 5 years differ slightly because they were obtained from a different population of children.

Table E-2. Weight and height measurement for boys

Age*	Weight distribution by percentile						Height distribution by percentile†					
	3†		50†		97†		3†		50†		97†	
	lb	kg	lb	kg	lb	kg	inches	cm	inches	cm	inches	cm
Birth	5.8	2.63	7.5	3.4	10.1	4.58	18.2	46.3	19.9	50.6	21.5	54.6
3 months	10.6	4.81	12.6	5.72	16.4	7.44	22.4	56.8	23.8	60.4	25.1	63.7
6 months	14.0	6.35	16.7	7.58	20.8	9.43	24.8	63.0	26.1	66.4	27.7	70.4
9 months	16.6	7.53	20.0	9.07	24.4	11.07	26.6	67.7	28.0	71.2	29.9	75.9
1	18.5	8.39	22.2	10.07	27.3	12.83	28.1	71.3	29.6	75.2	31.6	80.3
1¼	19.8	8.98	23.7	10.75	29.4	13.33	29.3	74.4	30.9	78.5	33.1	84.2
1½	21.1	9.57	25.2	11.43	31.5	14.29	30.5	77.5	32.2	81.8	34.7	88.2
2	23.3	10.57	27.7	12.56	34.9	15.83	32.6	82.7	34.4	87.5	37.2	94.6
2½	25.2	11.43	30.0	13.61	37.0	16.78	34.2	86.9	36.3	92.1	39.2	99.5
3	27.0	12.25	32.2	14.61	39.2	17.78	35.7	90.6	37.9	96.2	40.5	102.8
3½	28.5	12.93	34.3	15.56	41.5	18.82	37.1	94.3	39.3	99.8	41.9	106.5
4	30.1	13.65	36.4	16.51	44.3	20.09	38.4	97.5	40.7	103.4	43.5	110.4
4½	31.6	14.33	38.4	17.42	47.4	21.50	39.6	100.6	42.0	106.7	45.0	114.3
5†	33.6	15.24	40.5	18.37	50.4	22.86	40.2	102.0	42.8	108.7	46.1	117.1
5†	34.5	15.65	42.8	19.41	53.2	24.13	40.2	102.1	43.8	111.3	47.0	119.5
6	38.5	17.46	48.3	21.91	61.1	27.71	42.7	108.5	46.3	117.5	49.7	126.2
7	43.0	19.5	54.1	24.54	69.9	31.71	44.9	114.0	48.9	124.1	52.5	133.4
8	48.0	21.77	60.1	27.26	79.4	36.02	47.1	119.6	51.2	130.0	55.2	140.2
9	52.5	23.81	66.0	29.94	89.8	40.73	48.9	124.2	53.3	135.5	57.2	145.3
10	56.8	25.76	71.9	32.61	100.0	45.36	50.7	128.7	55.2	140.3	59.2	150.3
11	61.8	28.03	77.6	35.20	111.7	50.67	52.5	133.4	56.8	144.2	60.8	154.4
12	67.2	30.48	84.4	38.28	124.2	56.34	54.4	138.1	58.9	149.6	63.7	161.9
13	72.0	32.66	93.0	42.18	138.0	62.60	56.0	142.2	61.0	155.0	66.7	169.5
14	79.8	36.20	107.6	48.81	150.6	68.31	57.6	146.4	64.0	162.7	69.7	177.1
15	91.3	41.41	120.1	54.48	161.6	73.30	59.7	151.7	66.1	167.8	71.6	181.8
16	103.4	46.90	129.7	58.83	170.5	77.34	61.6	156.5	67.8	171.6	73.1	185.6
17	110.5	50.12	136.2	61.78	175.6	79.65	62.6	159.0	68.4	173.7	73.5	186.6
18	113.0	51.26	139.0	63.05	179.0	81.19	62.8	159.6	68.7	174.5	73.9	187.6

Adapted from studies by Howard V. Meredith, Iowa Child Welfare Research Station, The State University of Iowa. In Vaughan, V. C., and McKay, R. J., editors: Nelson's textbook of pediatrics, Philadelphia, 1975, W. B. Saunders Co.

*Years unless otherwise indicated.

†The figures for the several percentiles for age 5 years differ slightly because they were obtained from a different population of children.

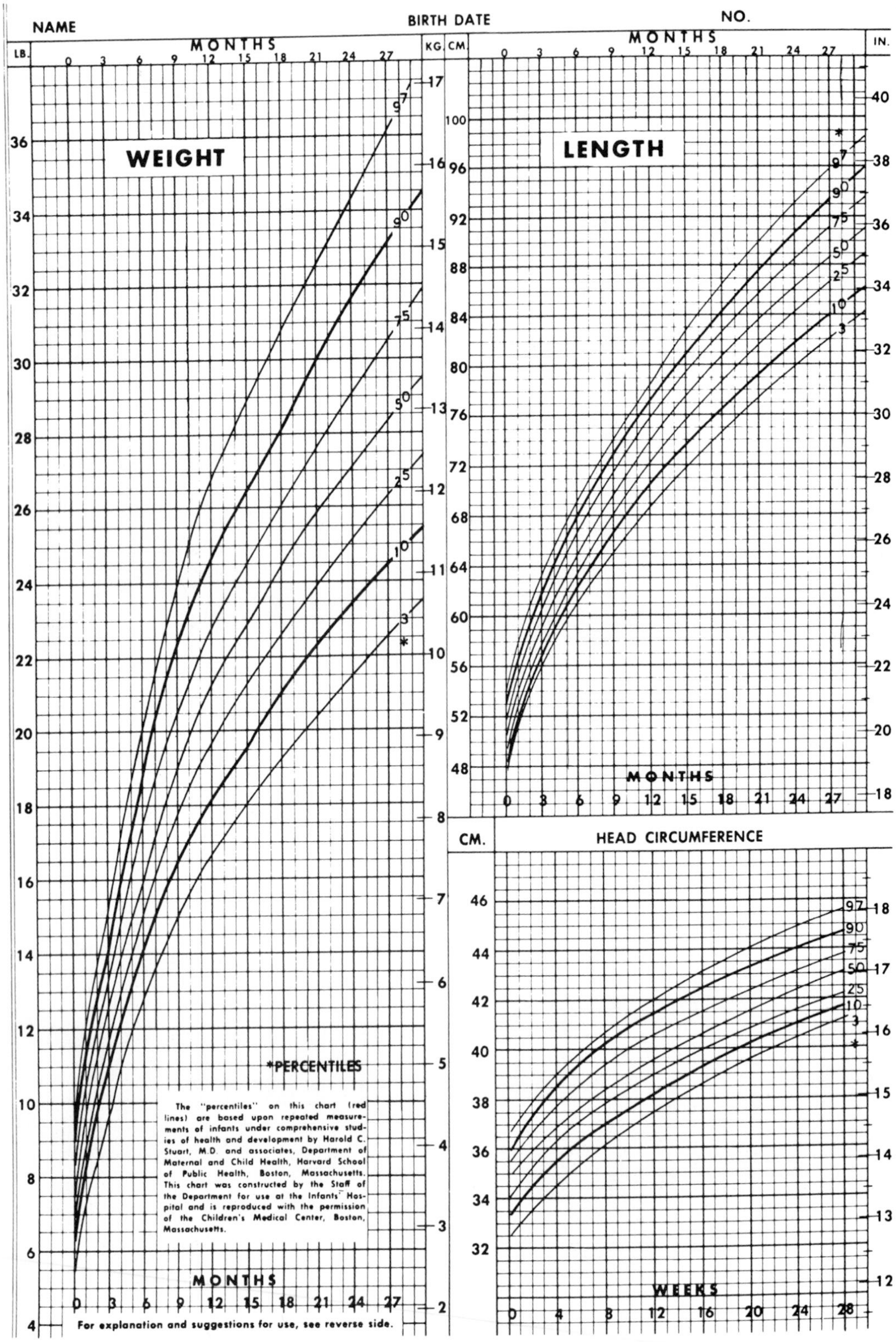

Fig. E-1. Percentile chart for measurements of infant girls. (From The Children's Hospital Medical Center, Boston, Mass. Reprinted by permission.)

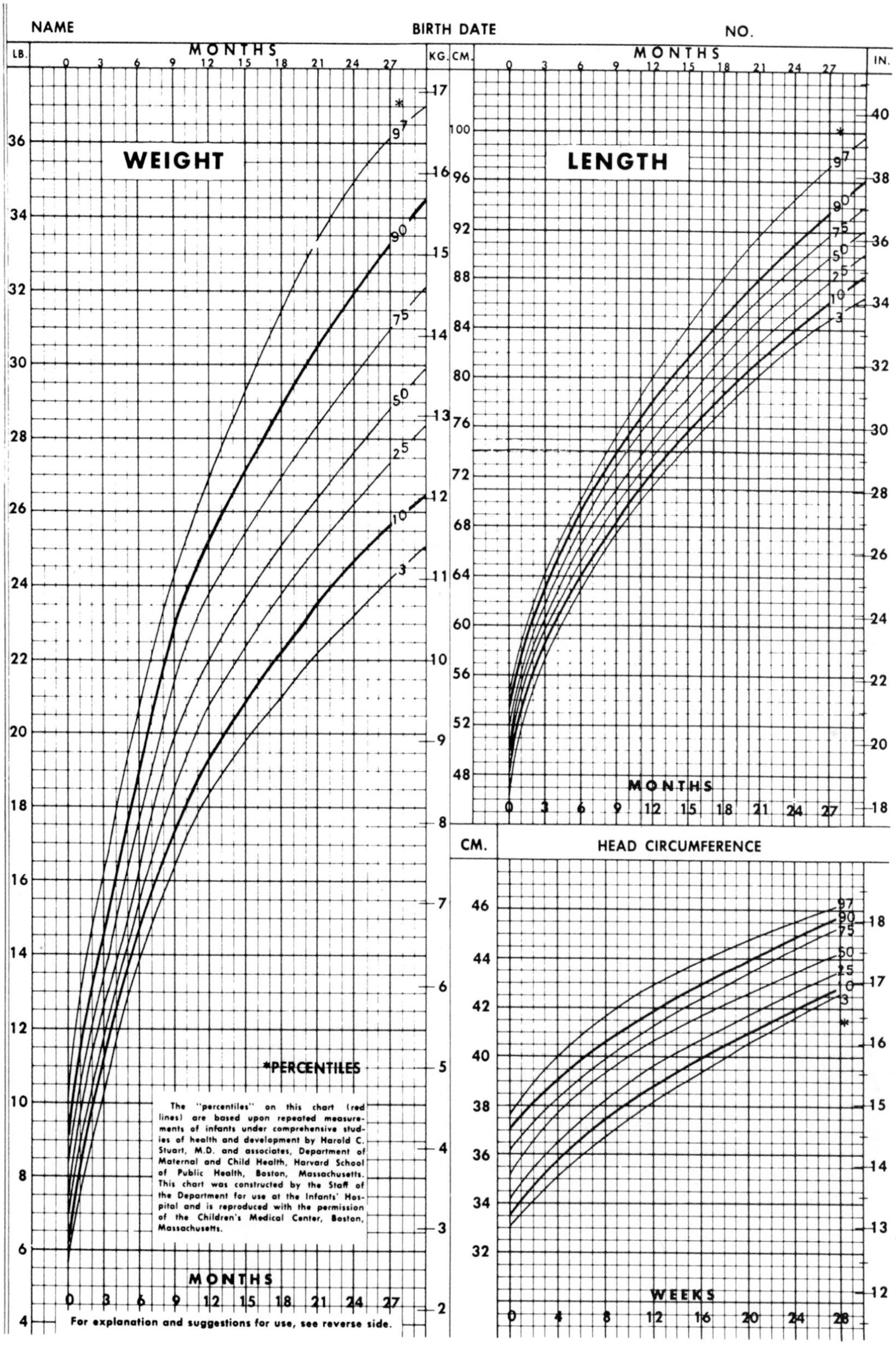

Fig. E-2. Percentile chart for measurements of infant boys. (From The Children's Hospital Medical Center, Boston, Mass. Reprinted by permission.)

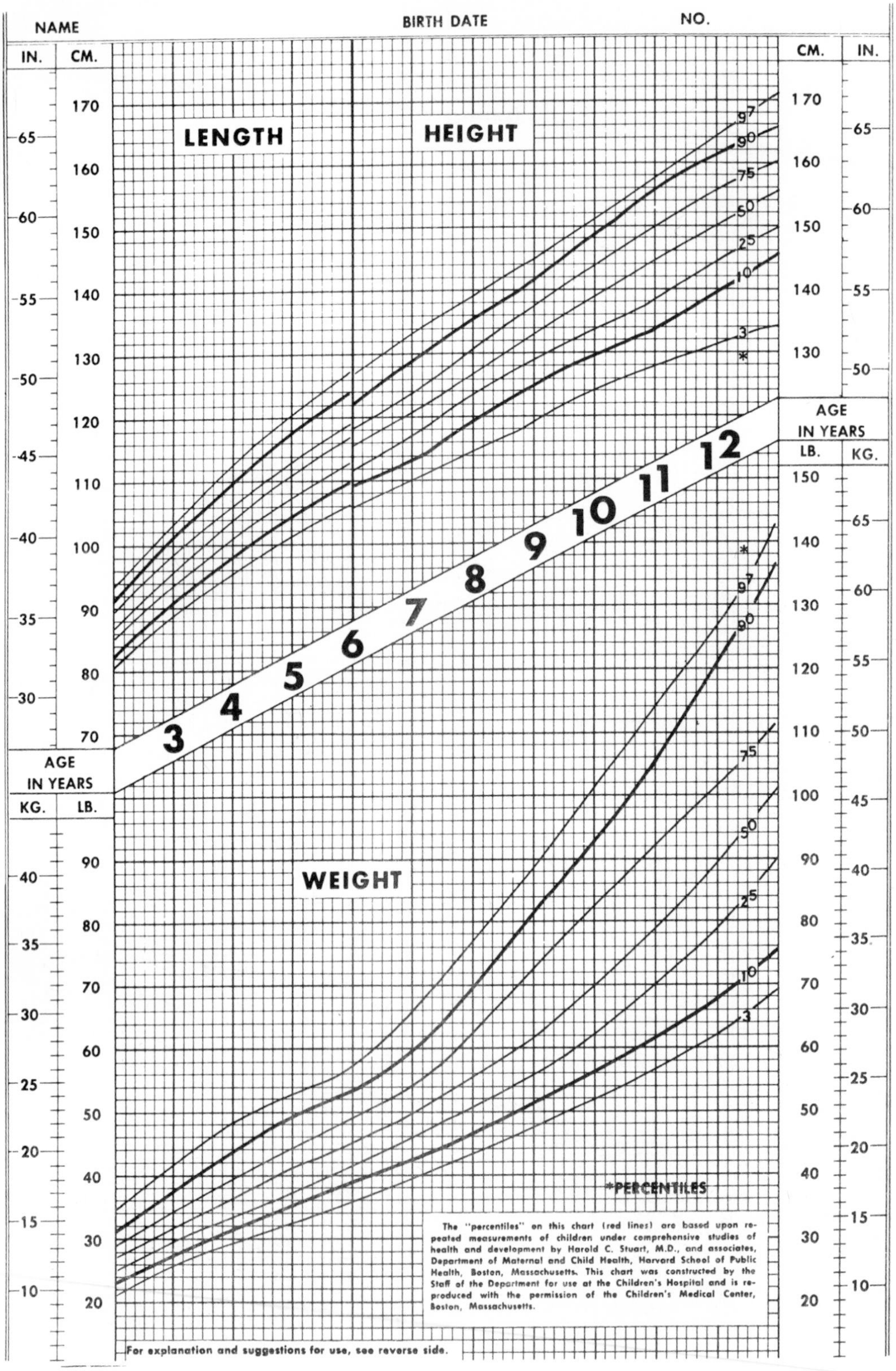

Fig. E-3. Percentile chart for measurements of girls. (From The Children's Hospital Medical Center, Boston, Mass. Reprinted by permission.)

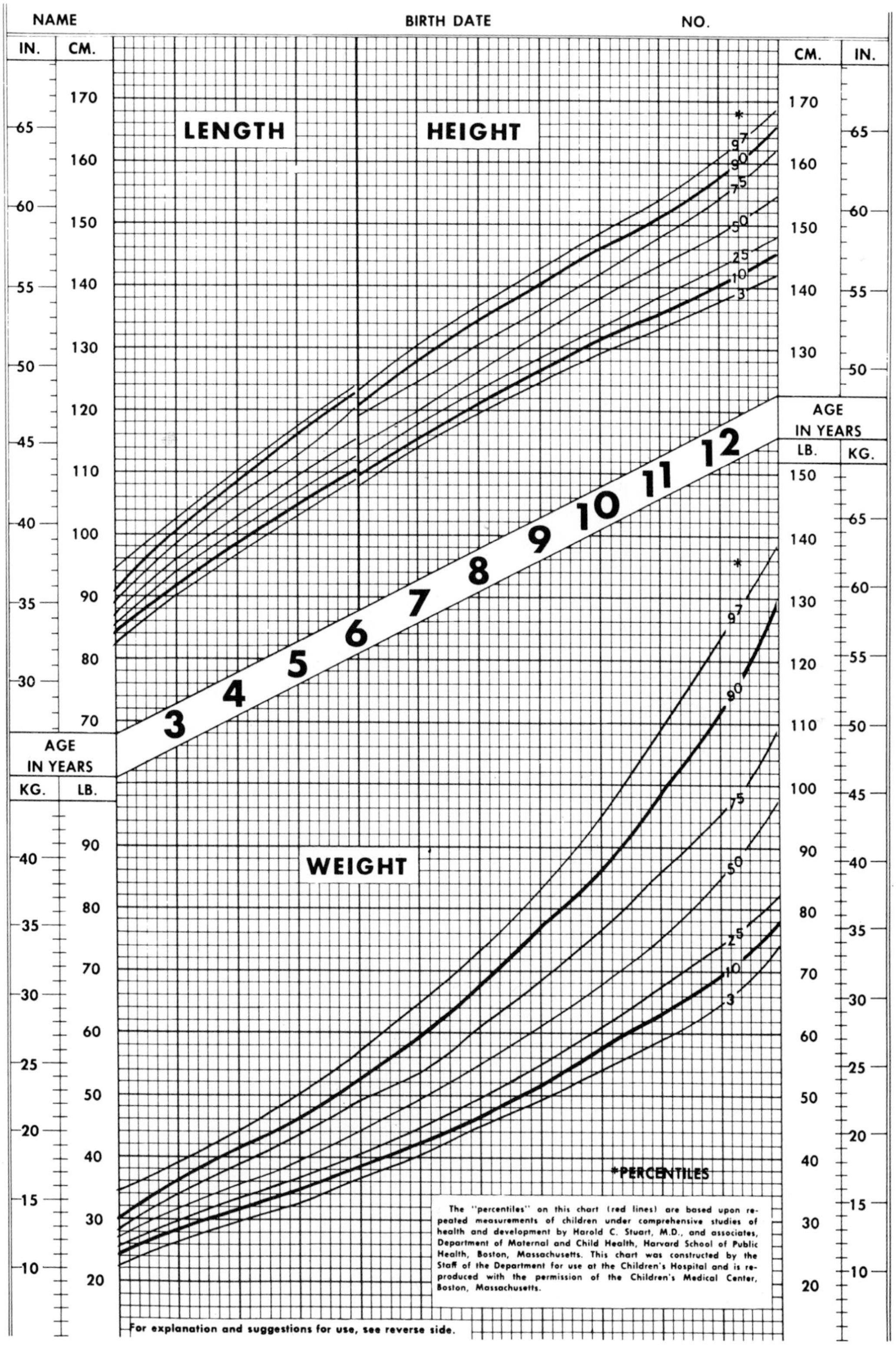

Fig. E-4. Percentile chart for measurements of boys. (From The Children's Hospital Medical Center, Boston, Mass. Reprinted by permission.)

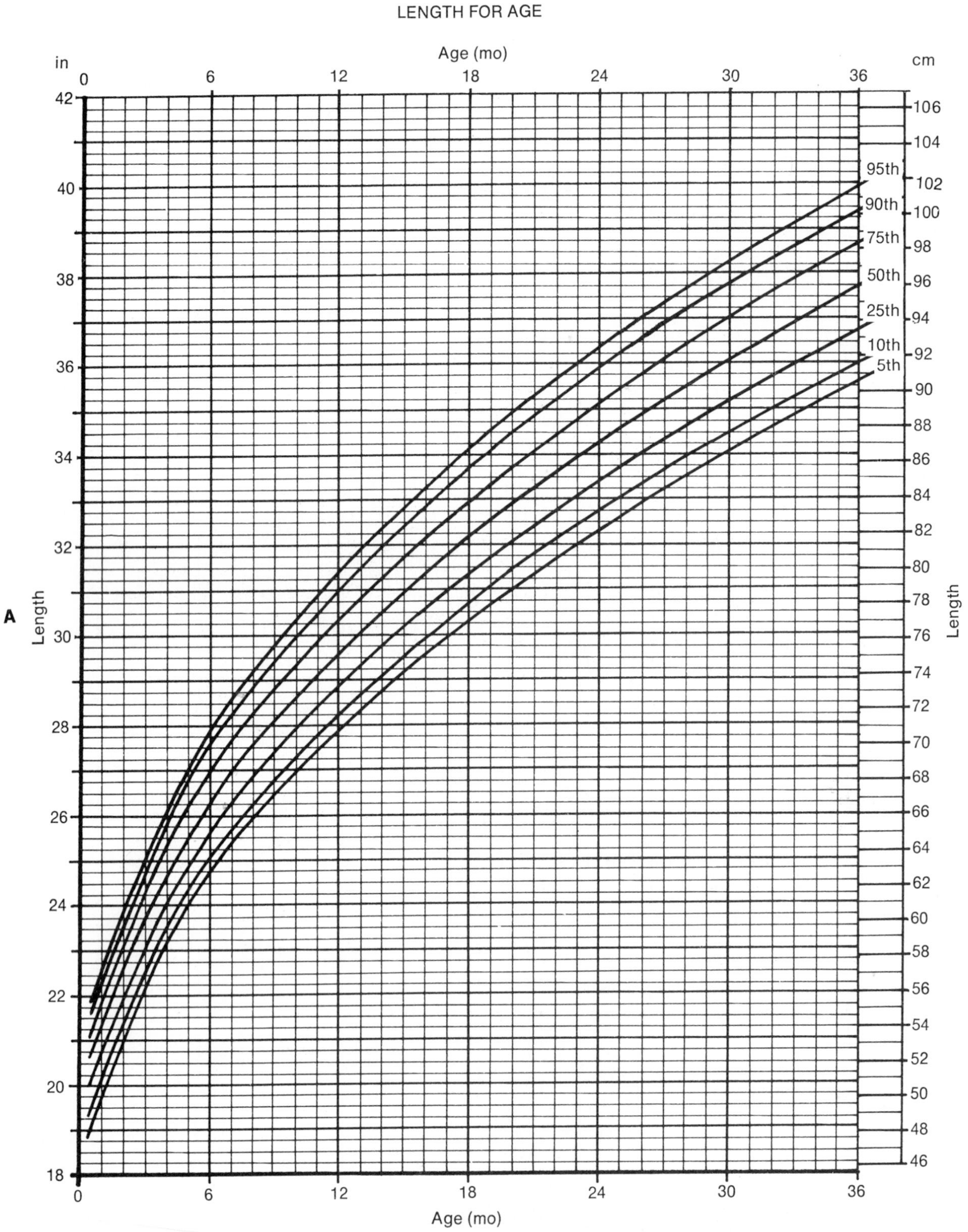

Fig. E-5. Growth charts with reference percentiles for girls birth to 36 months of age. **A,** Length for age; **B,** weight for age; **C,** head circumference for age and weight for length. (From Department of Health, Education and Welfare, Public Health Service Health Resources Administration, National Center for Health Statistics, and Center for Disease Control.)

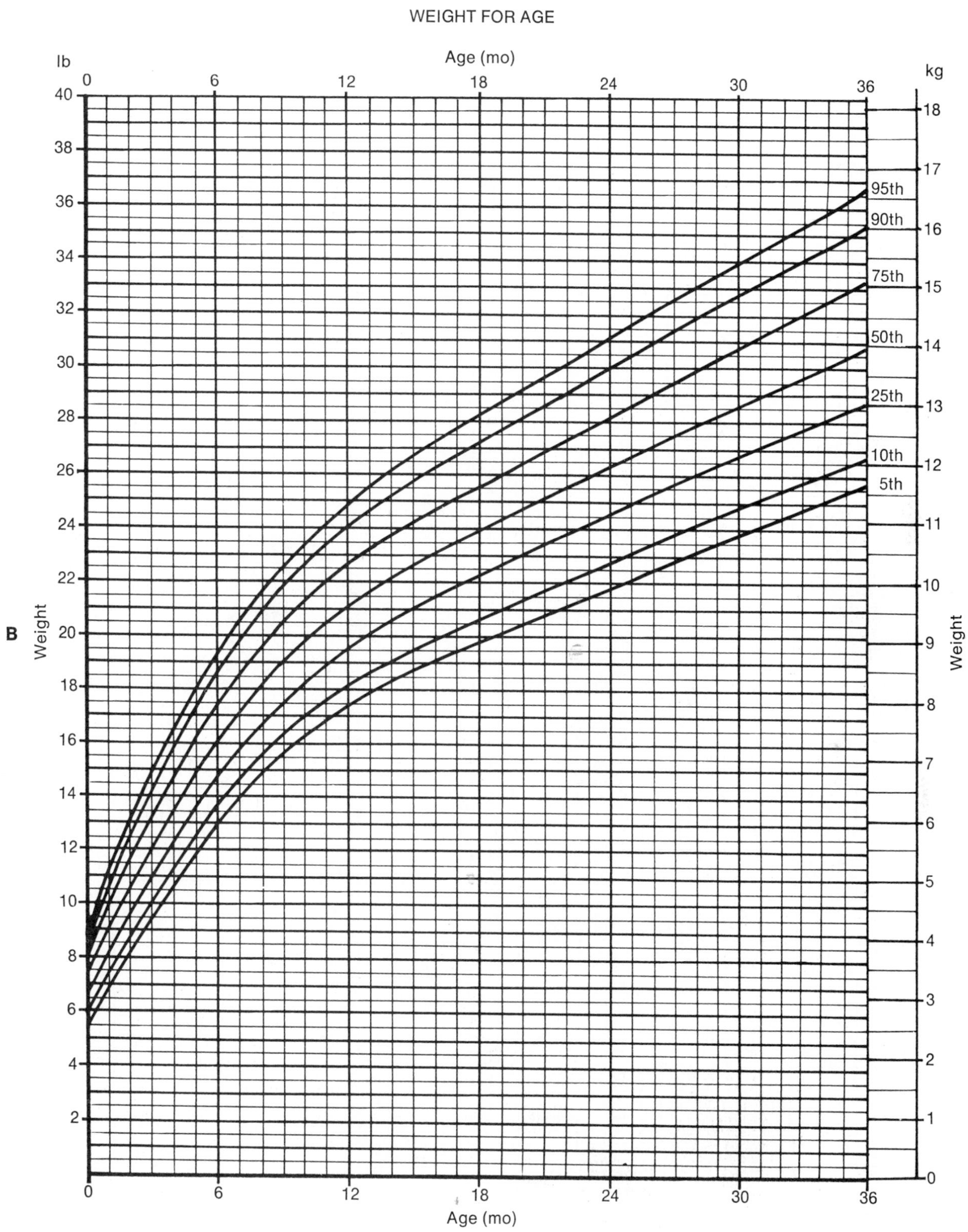

Continued.

Fig. E-5, cont'd. For legend see opposite page.

C

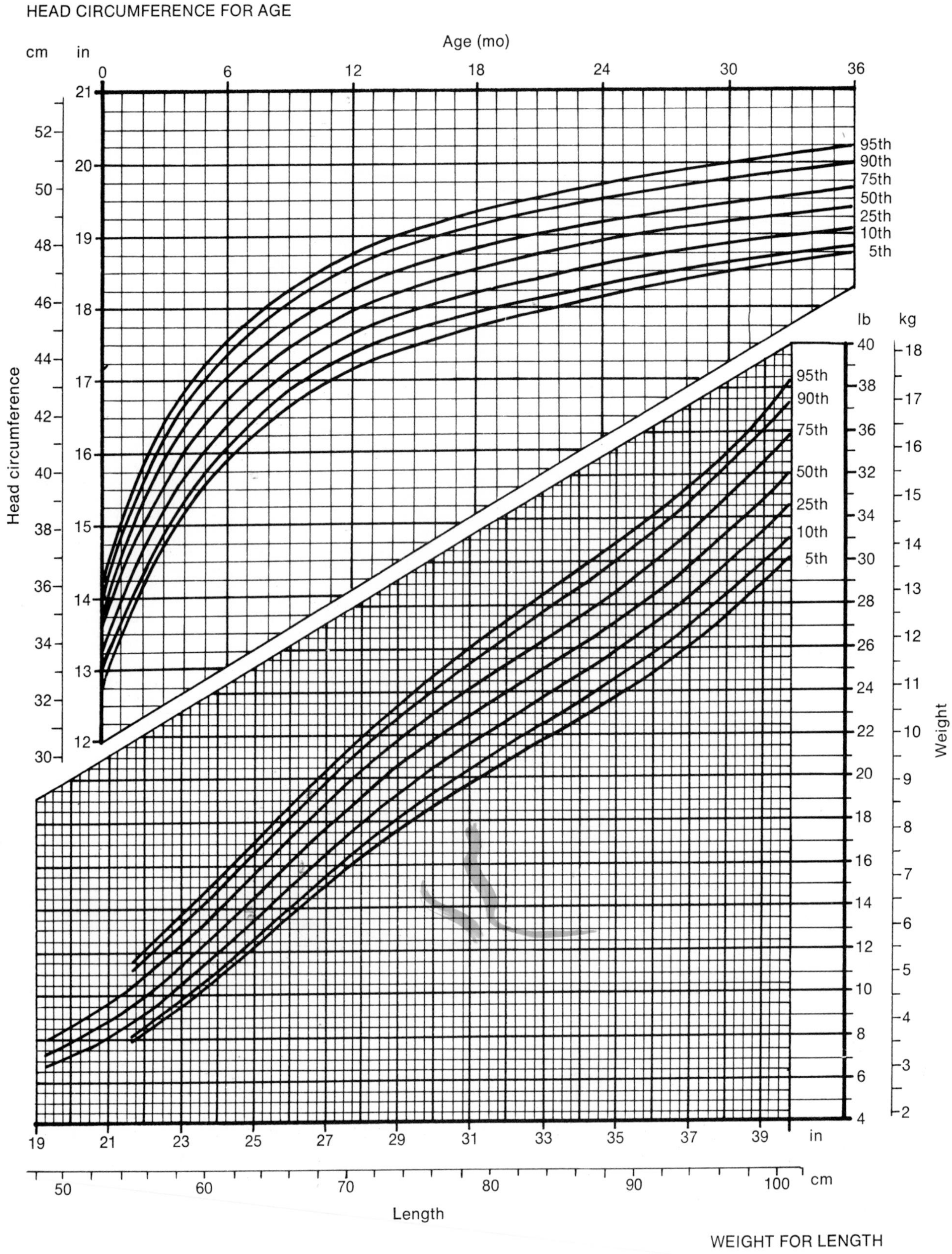

Fig. E-5, cont'd. For legend see p. 1624.

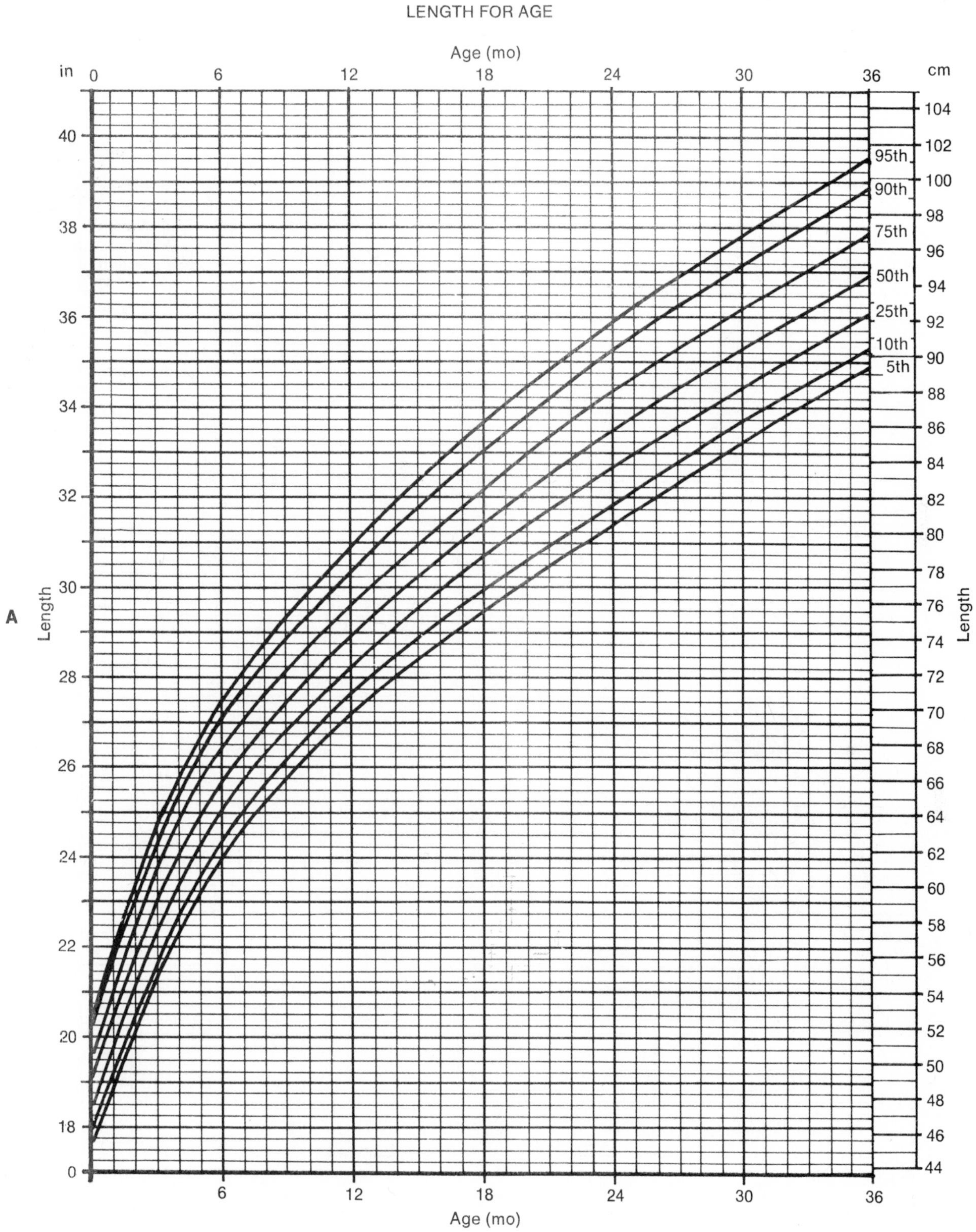

Continued.

Fig. E-6. Growth charts with reference percentiles for boys birth to 36 months of age. **A,** Length for age; **B,** weight for age; **C,** head circumference for age and weight for length. (From Department of Health, Education and Welfare, Public Health Service Health Resources Administration, National Center for Health Statistics, and Center for Disease Control.)

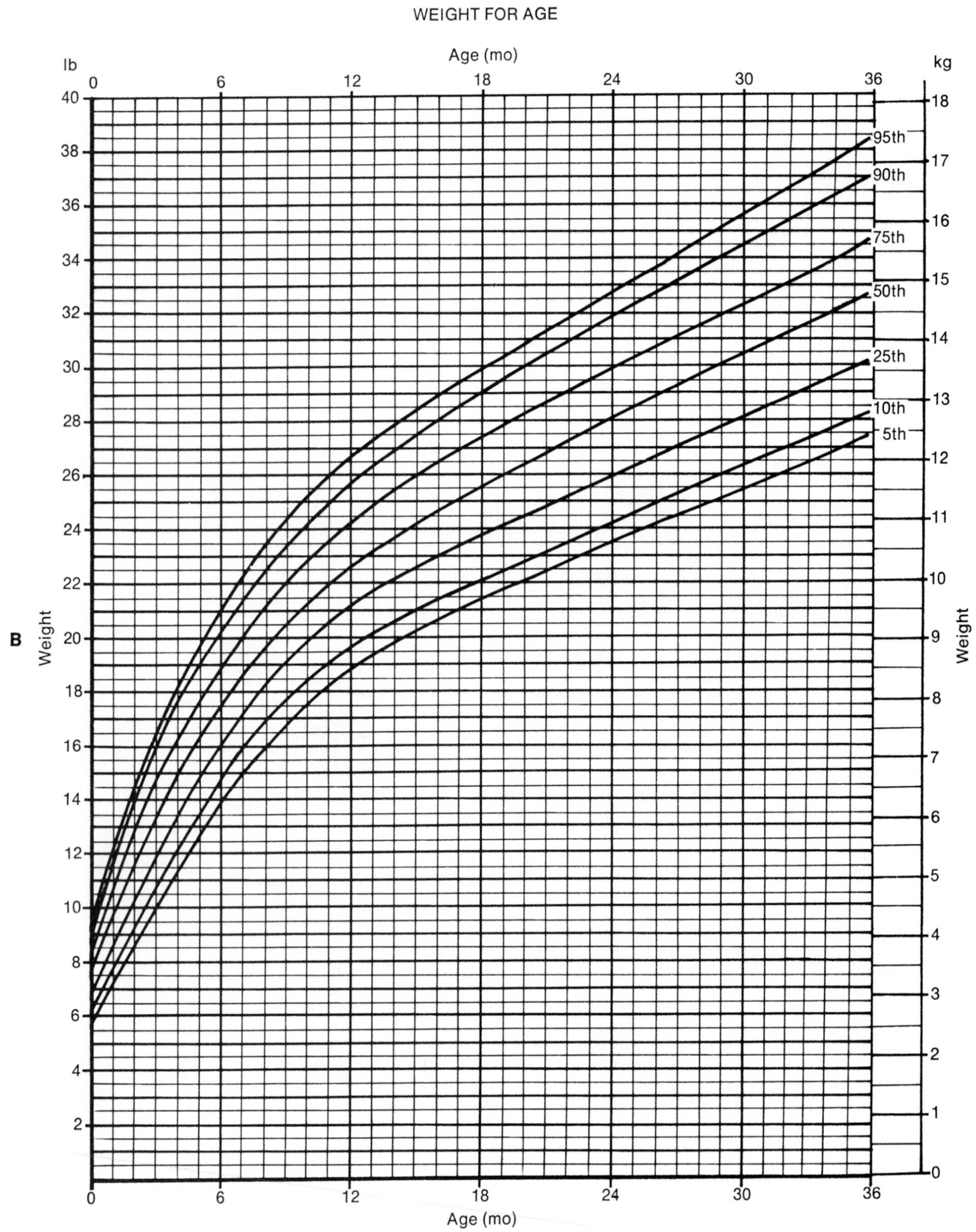

Fig. E-6, cont'd. For legend see p. 1627.

C

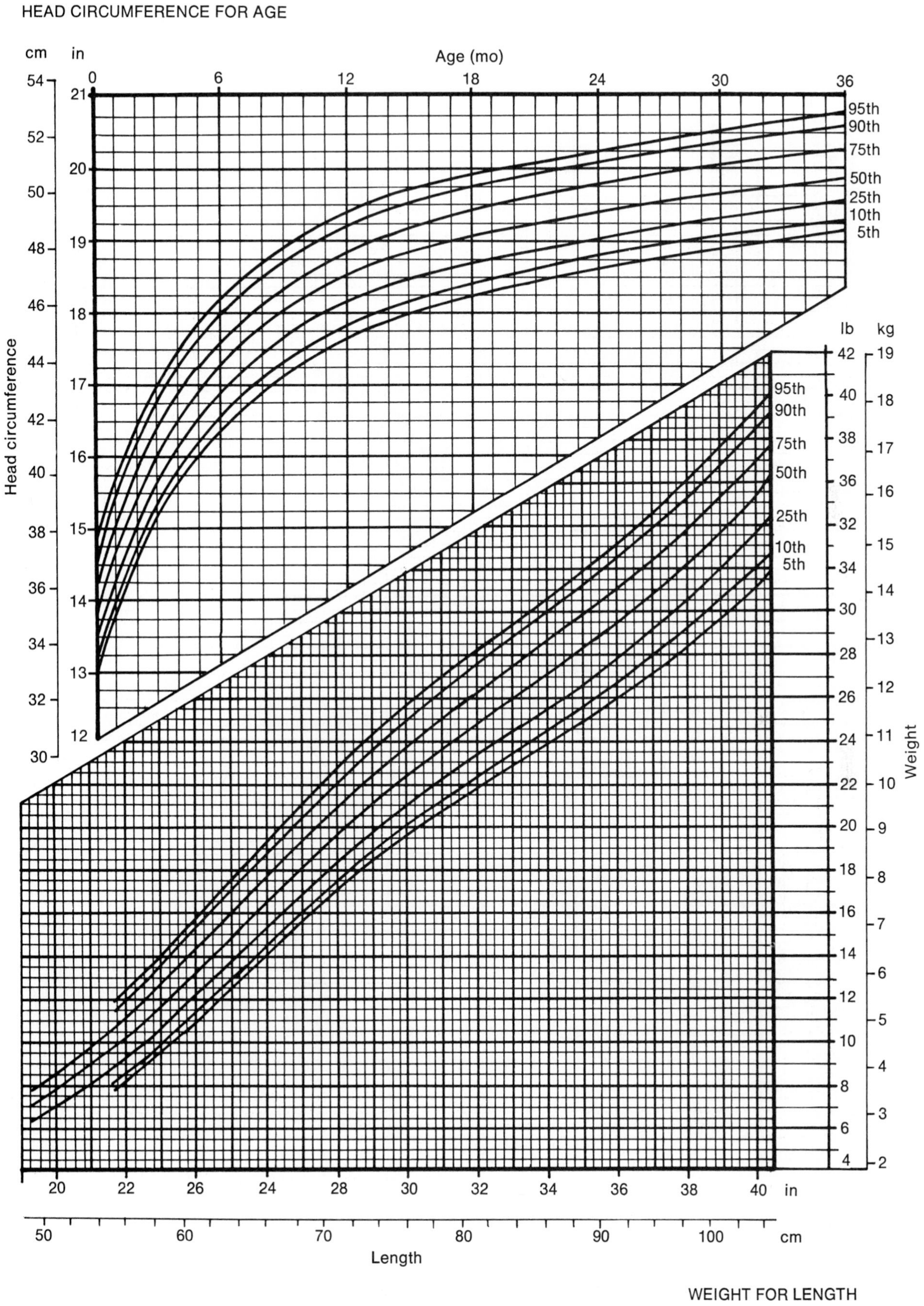

Fig. E-6, cont'd. For legend see p. 1627.

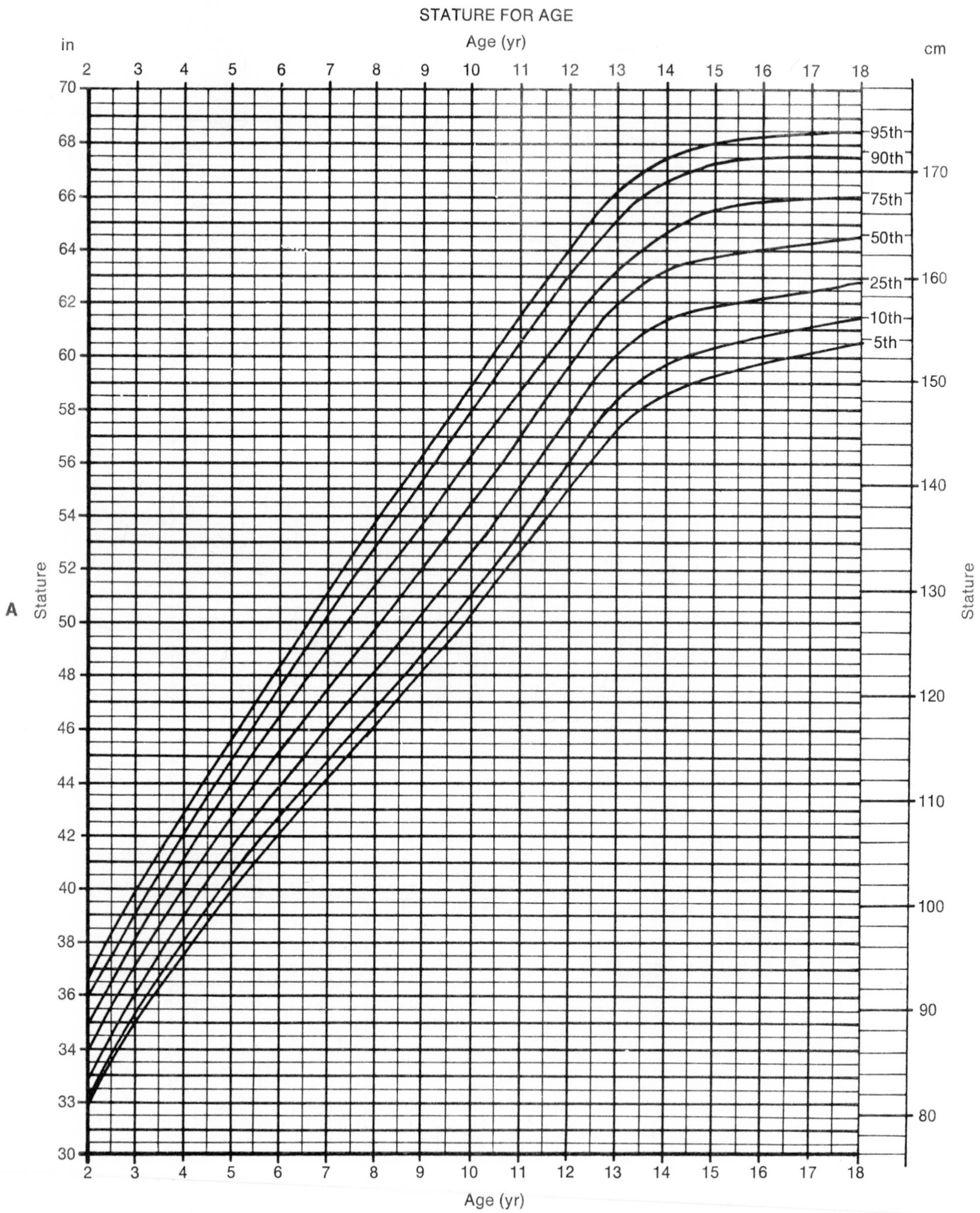

Fig. E-7. Growth charts with reference percentiles for girls 2 to 18 years of age. **A,** Stature for age; **B,** weight for age. (From Department of Health, Education and Welfare, Public Health Service Health Resources Administration, National Center for Health Statistics, and Center for Disease Control.)

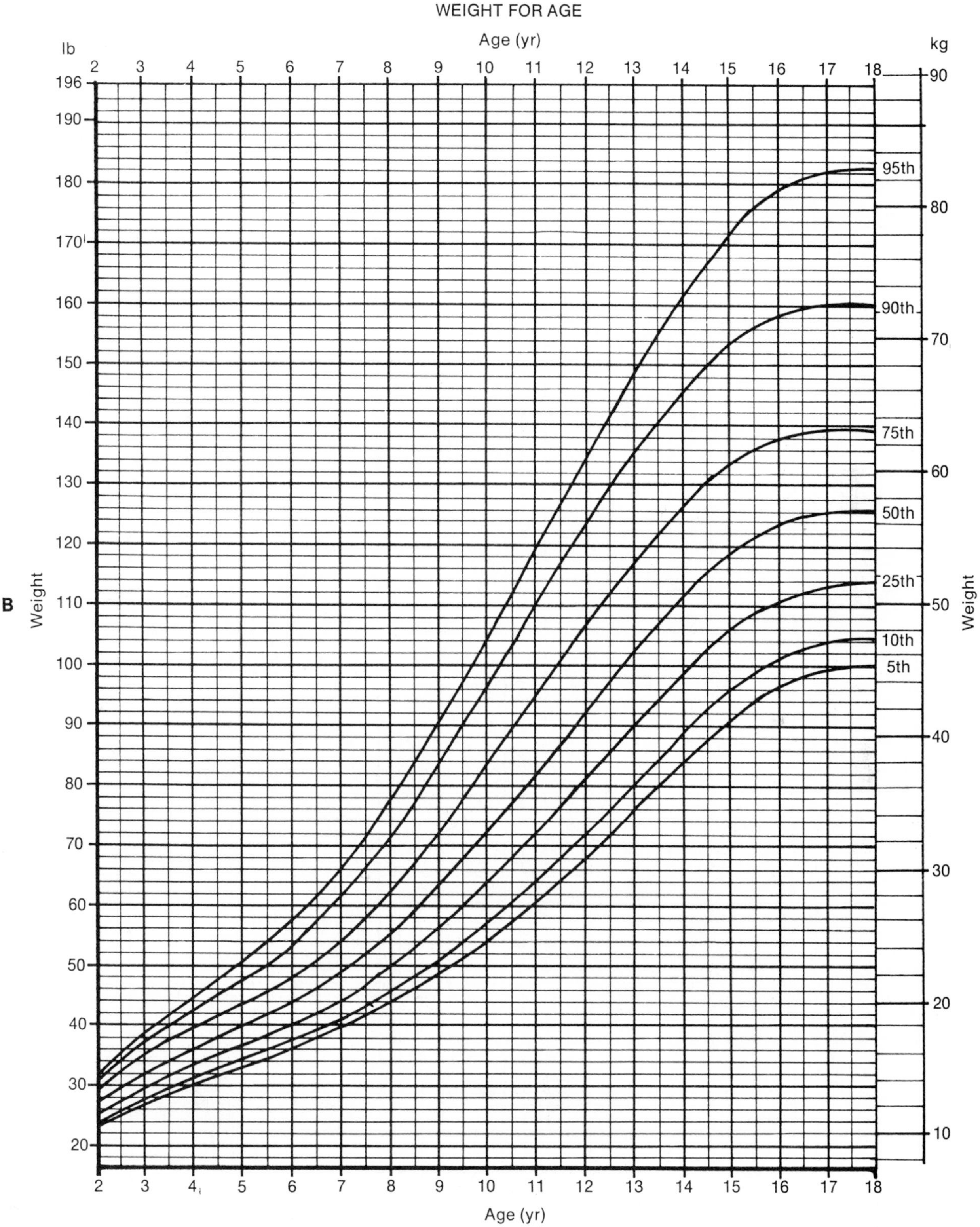

Fig. E-7, cont'd. For legend see opposite page.

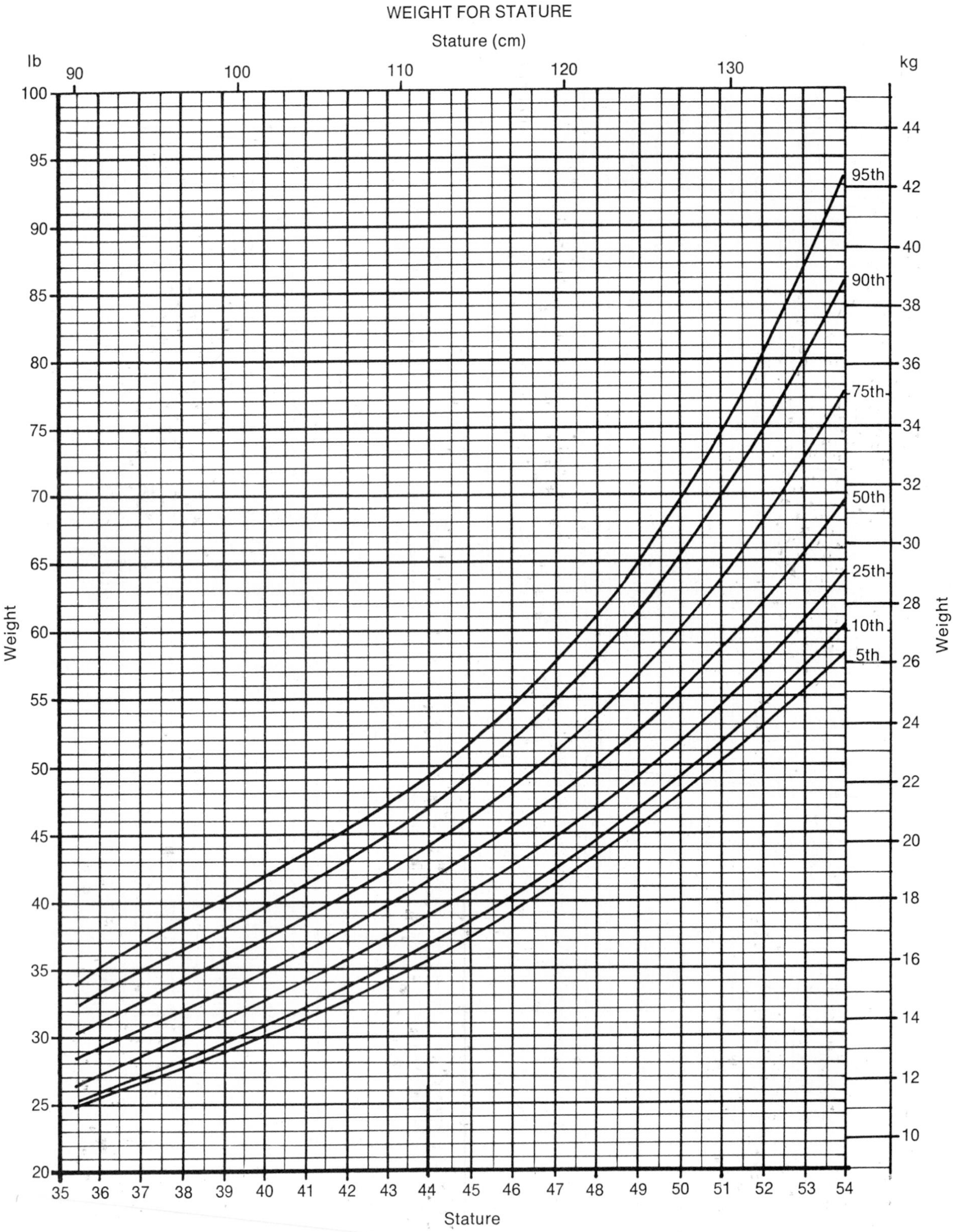

Fig. E-8. Growth chart with reference percentiles for prepubertal girls from 2 to 10 years. Weight for stature. (From Department of Health, Education and Welfare, Public Health Service Health Resources Administration, National Center for Health Statistics, and Center for Disease Control.)

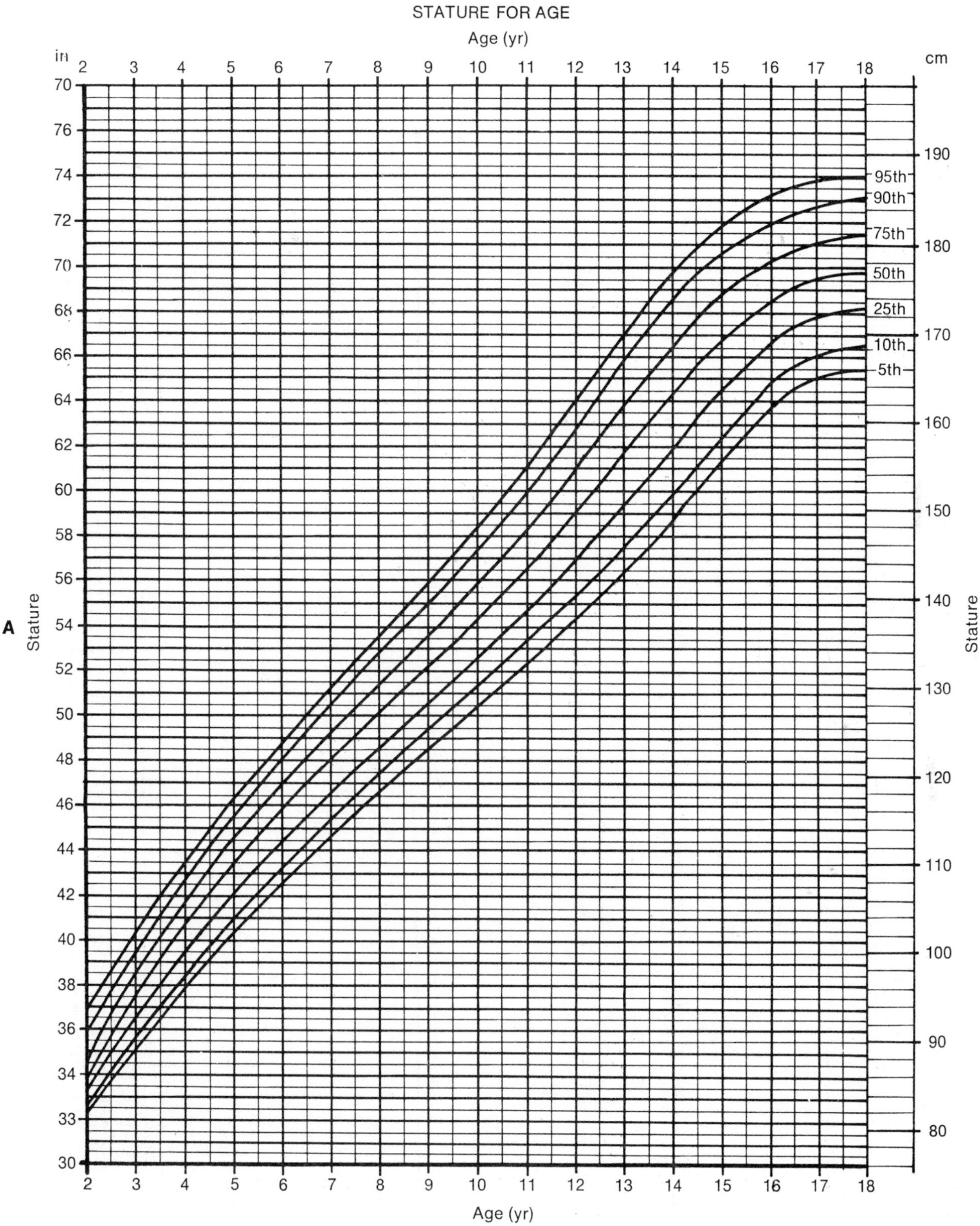

Continued.

Fig. E-9. Growth charts with reference percentiles for boys 2 to 18 years of age. **A,** Stature for age; **B,** weight for age. (From Department of Health, Education and Welfare, Public Health Service Health Resources Administration, National Center for Health Statistics, and Center for Disease Control.)

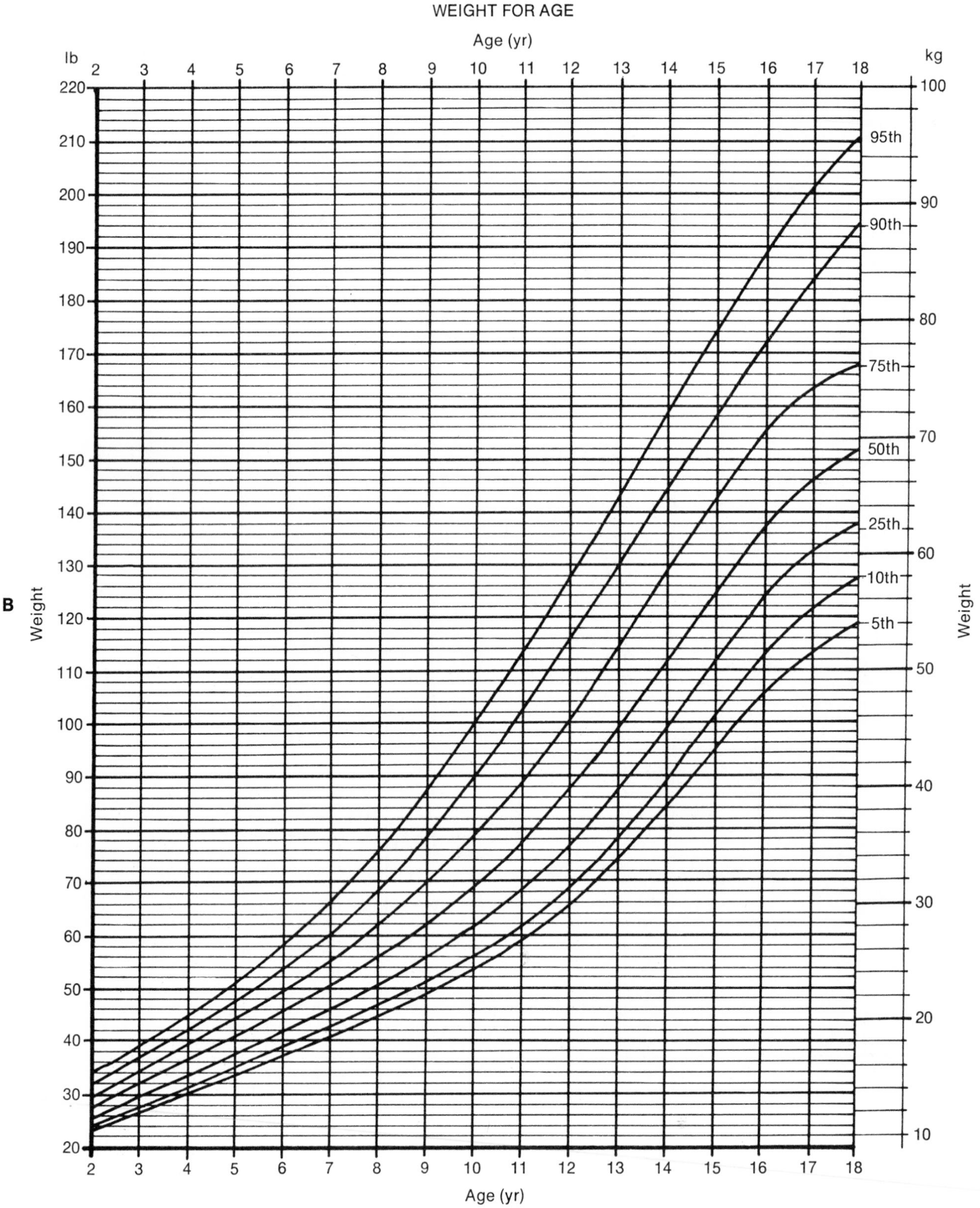

Fig. E-9, cont'd. For legend see p. 1633.

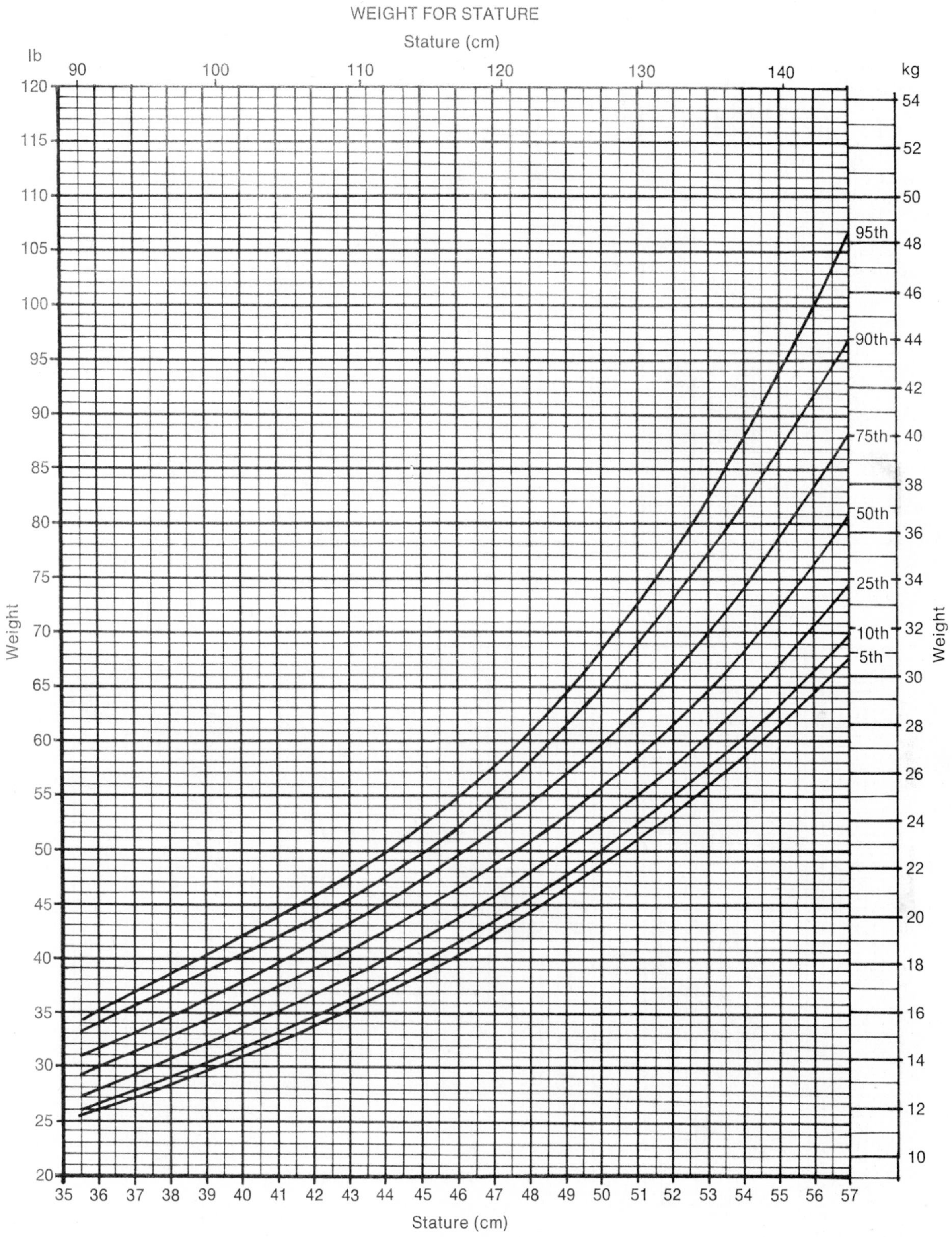

Fig. E-10. Growth chart with reference percentiles for prepubertal boys from 2 to 11½ years of age. Weight for stature. (From Department of Health, Education and Welfare, Public Health Service Health Resources Administration, National Center for Health Statistics, and Center for Disease Control.)

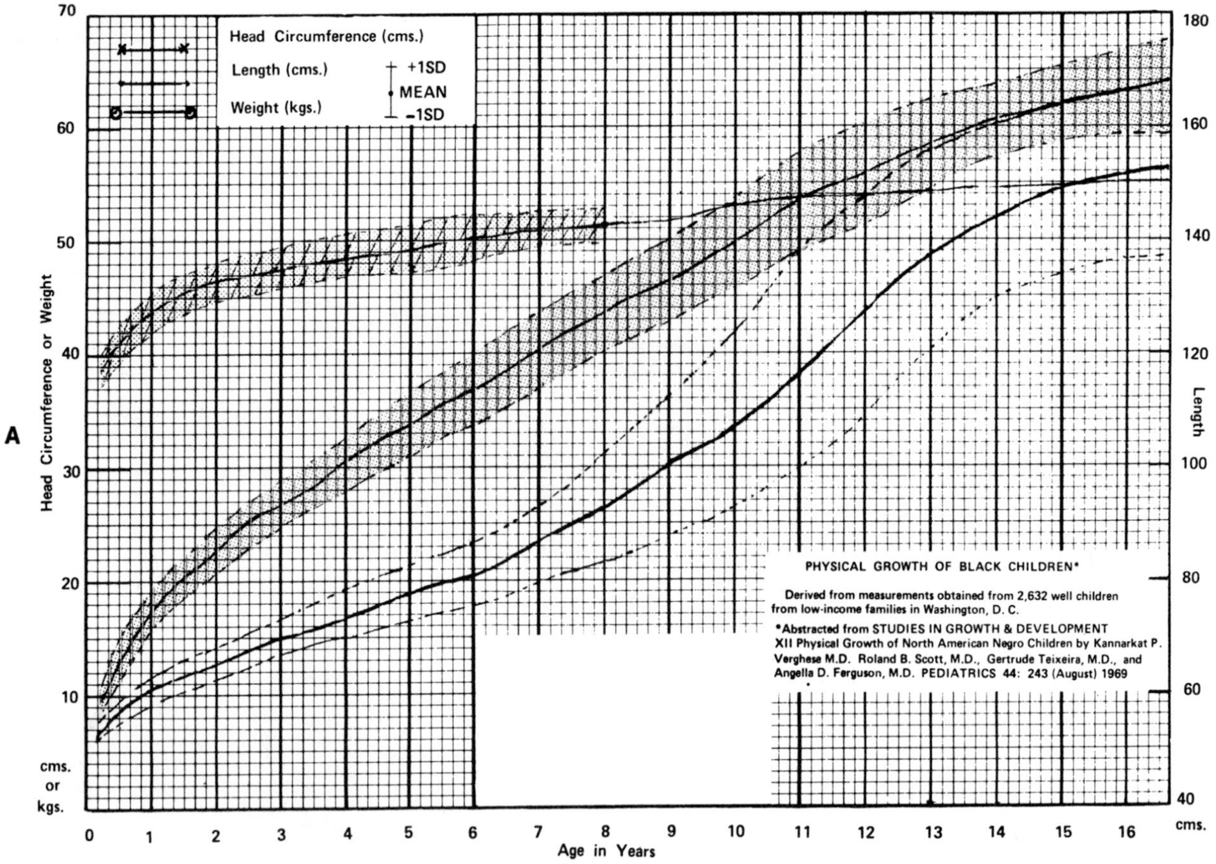

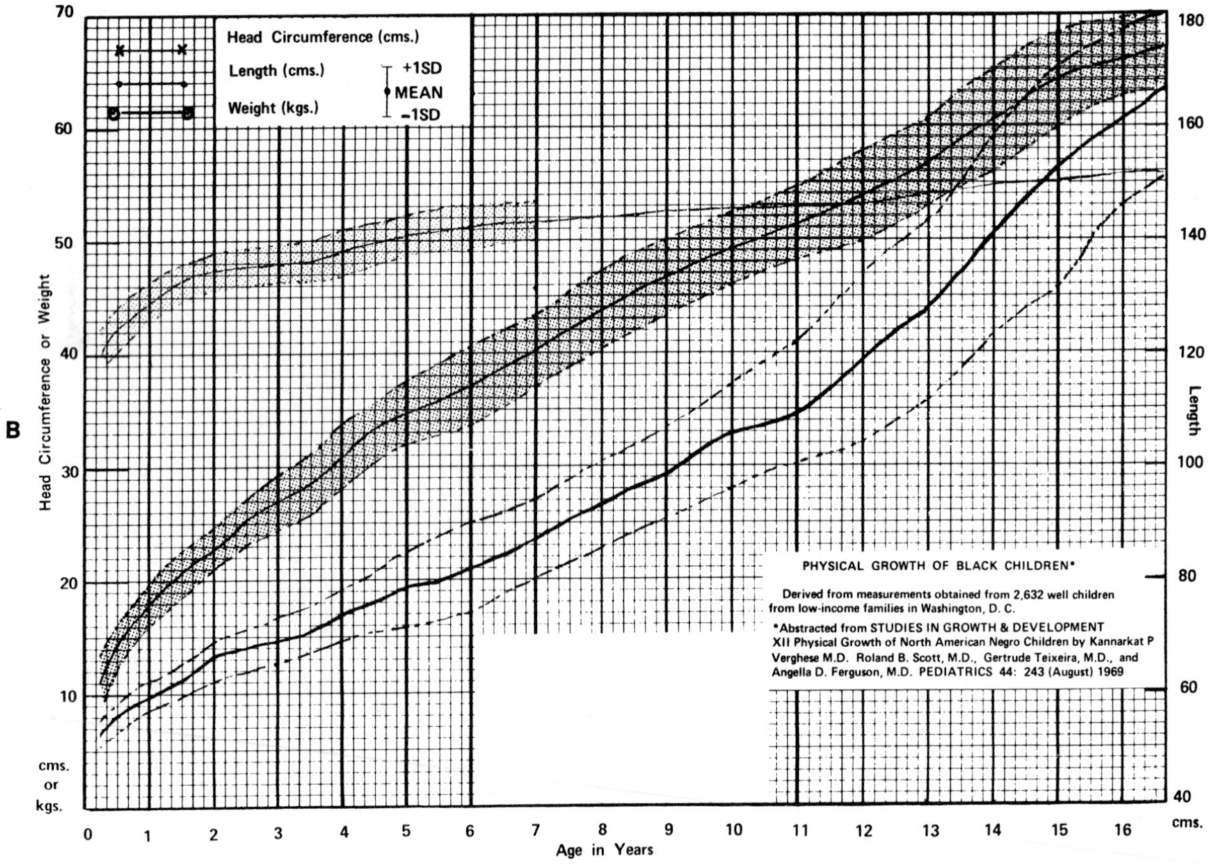

Fig. E-11. Physical growth of black children. **A,** Girls; **B,** boys. (Abstracted from Verghese, K. P., and associates: Studies in growth and development. XII. Physical growth of North American Negro children, Pediatrics **44:**243, August 1969. Copyright American Academy of Pediatrics, 1969.)

A

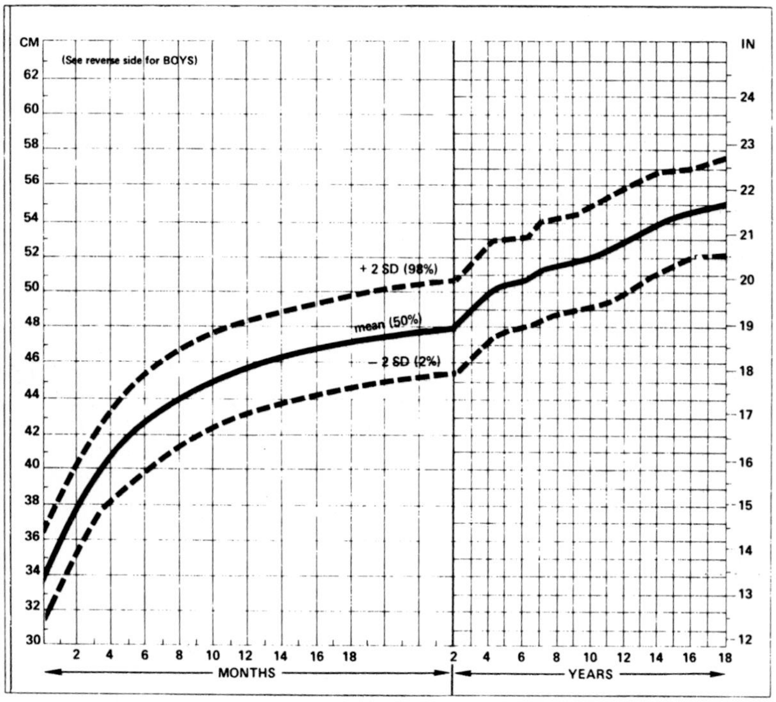

B

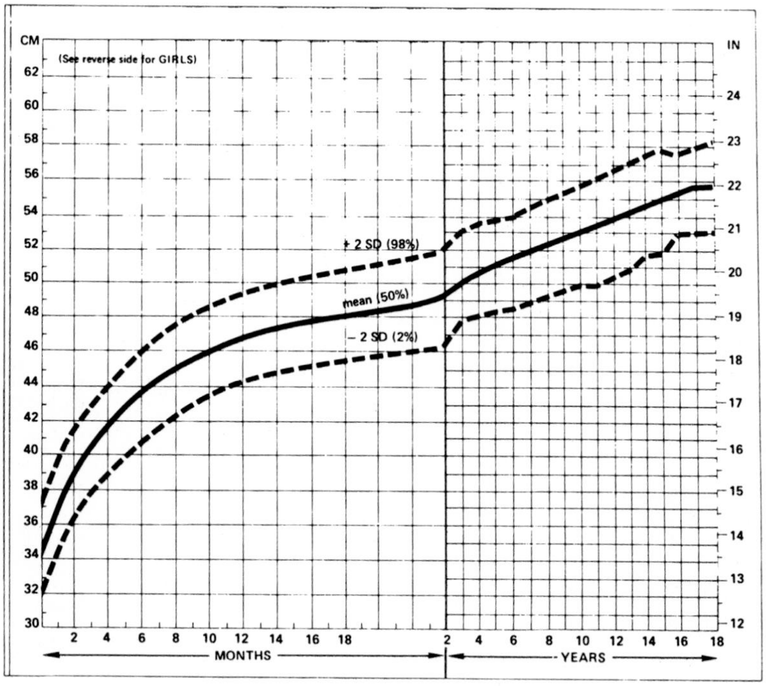

Fig. E-12. A, Head circumference chart for girls; **B,** Head circumference chart for boys. (From Nellhaus, G.: Composite international and interracial graphs, Pediatrics **41:**106, 1968. Reprinted by permission. Copyright American Academy of Pediatrics, 1968.)

F

Developmental assessment

A

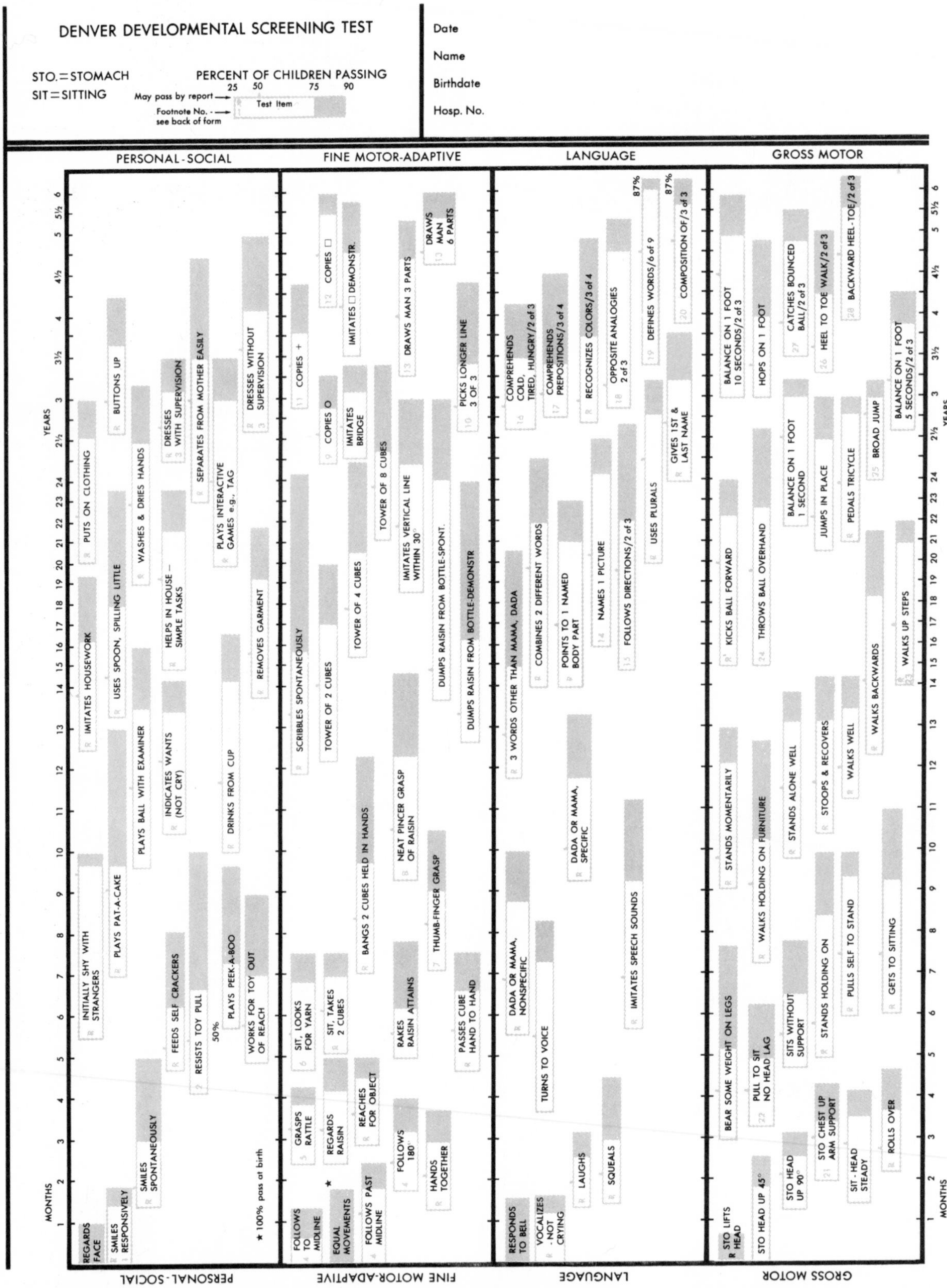

Fig. F-1. For legend see opposite page.

DATE
NAME
DIRECTIONS BIRTHDATE
HOSP. NO.

1. Try to get child to smile by smiling, talking or waving to him. Do not touch him.
2. When child is playing with toy, pull it away from him. Pass if he resists.
3. Child does not have to be able to tie shoes or button in the back.
4. Move yarn slowly in an arc from one side to the other, about 6" above child's face. Pass if eyes follow 90° to midline. (Past midline; 180°)
5. Pass if child grasps rattle when it is touched to the backs or tips of fingers.
6. Pass if child continues to look where yarn disappeared or tries to see where it went. Yarn should be dropped quickly from sight from tester's hand without arm movement.
7. Pass if child picks up raisin with any part of thumb and a finger.
8. Pass if child picks up raisin with the ends of thumb and index finger using an over hand approach.

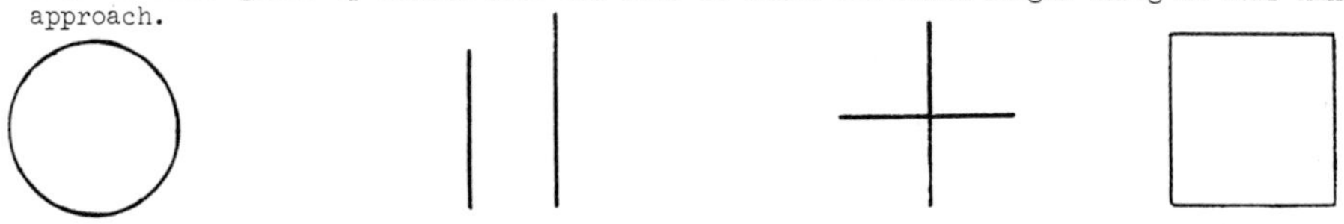

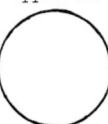

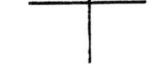

9. Pass any enclosed form. Fail continuous round motions.
10. Which line is longer? (Not bigger.) Turn paper upside down and repeat. (3/3 or 5/6)
11. Pass any crossing lines.
12. Have child copy first. If failed, demonstrate

When giving items 9, 11 and 12, do not name the forms. Do not demonstrate 9 and 11.

13. When scoring, each pair (2 arms, 2 legs, etc.) counts as one part.
14. Point to picture and have child name it. (No credit is given for sounds only.)

B

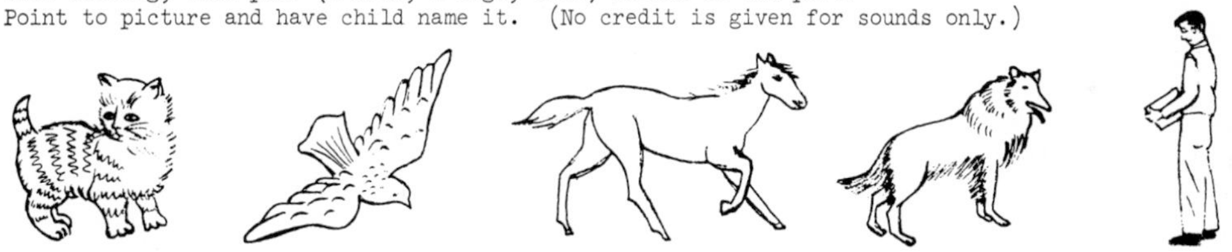

15. Tell child to: Give block to Mommie; put block on table; put block on floor. Pass 2 of 3. (Do not help child by pointing, moving head or eyes.)
16. Ask child: What do you do when you are cold? ..hungry? ..tired? Pass 2 of 3.
17. Tell child to: Put block <u>on</u> table; <u>under</u> table; <u>in front</u> of chair, <u>behind</u> chair. Pass 3 of 4. (Do not help child by pointing, moving head or eyes.)
18. Ask child: If fire is hot, ice is ?; Mother is a woman, Dad is a ?; a horse is big, a mouse is ?. Pass 2 of 3.
19. Ask child: What is a ball? ..lake? ..desk? ..house? ..banana? ..curtain? ..ceiling? ..hedge? ..pavement? Pass if defined in terms of use, shape, what it is made of or general category (such as banana is fruit, not just yellow). Pass 6 of 9.
20. Ask child: What is a spoon made of? ..a shoe made of? ..a door made of? (No other objects may be substituted.) Pass 3 of 3.
21. When placed on stomach, child lifts chest off table with support of forearms and/or hands.
22. When child is on back, grasp his hands and pull him to sitting. Pass if head does not hang back.
23. Child may use wall or rail only, not person. May not crawl.
24. Child must throw ball overhand 3 feet to within arm's reach of tester.
25. Child must perform standing broad jump over width of test sheet. (8-1/2 inches)
26. Tell child to walk forward, 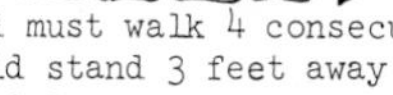 heel within 1 inch of toe. Tester may demonstrate. Child must walk 4 consecutive steps, 2 out of 3 trials.
27. Bounce ball to child who should stand 3 feet away from tester. Child must catch ball with hands, not arms, 2 out of 3 trials.
28. Tell child to walk backward, 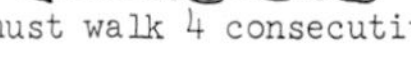 toe within 1 inch of heel. Tester may demonstrate. Child must walk 4 consecutive steps, 2 out of 3 trials.

<u>DATE AND BEHAVIORAL OBSERVATIONS</u> (how child feels at time of test, relation to tester, attention span, verbal behavior, self-confidence, etc,):

Fig. F-1. A, Denver Developmental Screening Test; **B,** directions for numbered items on testing form. (From W. K. Frankenburg and J. B. Dodds, University of Colorado Medical Center, 1969.)

A

DENVER ARTICULATION SCREENING EXAM
for children 2 1/2 to 6 years of age

Instructions: Have child repeat each word after you. Circle the underlined sounds that he pronounces correctly. Total correct sounds is the Raw Score. Use charts on reverse side to score results.

NAME

HOSP. NO.

ADDRESS ____________

Date: __________ Child's Age:________ Examiner: ______________________ Raw Score:__________
Percentile:________ Intelligibility:______________ Result:____________________

1. table	6. zipper	11. sock	16. wagon	21. leaf
2. shirt	7. grapes	12. vacuum	17. gum	22. carrot
3. door	8. flag	13. yarn	18. house	
4. trunk	9. thumb	14. mother	19. pencil	
5. jumping	10. toothbrush	15. twinkle	20. fish	

Intelligibility: (circle one) 1. Easy to understand 2. Understandable 1/2 the time. 3. Not understandable 4. Can't evaluate

Comments:

Date: __________ Child's Age:__________ Examiner:____________________ Raw Score ________
Percentile:__________ Intelligibility:______________ Result:____________________

1. table	6. zipper	11. sock	16. wagon	21. leaf
2. shirt	7. grapes	12. vacuum	17. gum	22. carrot
3. door	8. flag	13. yarn	18. house	
4. trunk	9. thumb	14. mother	19. pencil	
5. jumping	10. toothbrush	15. twinkle	20. fish	

Intelligibility: (circle one) 1. Easy to understand 2. Understandable 1/2 the time. 3. Not understandable 4. Can't evaluate

Comments:

Date: ____________ Child's Age: ________ Examiner:____________________ Raw Score____________
Percentile: ___________ Intelligibility:______________ Result:____________________

1. table	6. zipper	11. sock	16. wagon	21. leaf
2. shirt	7. grapes	12. vacuum	17. gum	22. carrot
3. door	8. flag	13. yarn	18. house	
4. trunk	9. thumb	14. mother	19. pencil	
5. jumping	10. toothbrush	15. twinkle	20. fish	

Intelligibility: (circle one) 1. Easy to understand 2. Understandable 1/2 the time. 3. Not understandable 4. Can't evaluate

Fig. F-2. A, Denver Articulation Screening Examination for Children 2½ to 6 years of age; **B,** percentile rank. (From A. F. Drumwright, University of Colorado Medical Center, 1971.)

To score DASE words: Note Raw Score for child's performance. Match raw score line (extreme left of chart) with column representing child's age (to the closest previous age group). Where raw score line and age column meet number in that square denotes percentile rank of child's performance when compared to other children that age. Percentiles above heavy line are ABNORMAL percentiles, below heavy line are NORMAL.

PERCENTILE RANK

B

Raw Score	2.5 yr.	3.0	3.5	4.0	4.5	5.0	5.5	6 years
2	1							
3	2							
4	5							
5	9							
6	16							
7	23							
8	31	2						
9	37	4	1					
10	42	6	2					
11	48	7	4					
12	54	9	6	1	1			
13	58	12	9	2	3	1	1	
14	62	17	11	5	4	2	2	
15	68	23	15	9	5	3	2	
16	75	31	19	12	5	4	3	
17	79	38	25	15	6	6	4	
18	83	46	31	19	8	7	4	
19	86	51	38	24	10	9	5	1
20	89	58	45	30	12	11	7	3
21	92	65	52	36	15	15	9	4
22	94	72	58	43	18	19	12	5
23	96	77	63	50	22	24	15	7
24	97	82	70	58	29	29	20	15
25	99	87	78	66	36	34	26	17
26	99	91	84	75	46	43	34	24
27		94	89	82	57	54	44	34
28		96	94	88	70	68	59	47
29		98	98	94	84	84	77	68
30		100	100	100	100	100	100	100

To Score intelligibility:

	NORMAL	ABNORMAL
2 1/2 years	Understandable 1/2 the time, or, "easy"	Not Understandable
3 years and older	Easy to understand	Understandable 1/2 time Not understandable

Test Result: 1. NORMAL on Dase and Intelligibility = NORMAL

2. ABNORMAL on Dase and/or Intelligibility = ABNORMAL

* If abnormal on initial screening rescreen within 2 weeks. If abnormal again child should be referred for complete speech evaluation.

Fig. F-2, cont'd. For legend see opposite page.

DIRECTIONS FOR SNELLEN SCREENING*

Preparation

1. Hang the Snellen chart on a light-colored wall so that the 20- to 30-foot lines are at eye level when children 6 to 12 years old are tested in the standing position.

2. Secure the chart to the wall with double-stick tape on the back side at all four corners. If the chart must be reversed for use of the letter or E chart, secure it at the top and bottom with tacks. Make sure that the chart does not swing when in place.

3. The illumination intensity on the chart should be 10 to 30 footcandles, without any glare from windows or light fixtures. The illumination should be checked with a light meter.

4. Mark an exact 20-foot distance from the chart. Mark the floor with a piece of tape or ''footprints'' positioned so that the heels touch the 20-foot line.

Procedure

1. Place the child at the 20-foot mark, with the heel edging the line if child is standing or with the back of the chair placed at the marker if the child is seated.

2. If the E chart is used, accustom the child to identifying which direction the ''legs of the E'' are pointing. Use a demonstration E card for this purpose.

3. Teach the child to use the occluder to cover one eye. Instruct him to keep both eyes open during the test. Provide a clean cover card for each child and then discard after use.

4. If the child wears glasses, test only with glasses on.

5. Test both eyes together, then right eye, then left eye.

6. Begin with the 40- or 30-foot line and proceed with test to include the 20-foot line.

7. With the child suspected of low vision, begin with the 200-foot line and proceed until the child can no longer correctly read three out of four or four out of six symbols on a line.

8. Use covers on the Snellen chart to expose only one symbol or one line at a time. When screening kindergarten or younger children, expose one line but use a pointer to point to one symbol at a time.

Recording and referral

1. Record the last line the child read correctly (three out of four or four out of six symbols).

2. Record visual acuity as a fraction. The numerator represents the distance from the chart, and the denominator represents the last line read correctly. For example, 20/30 means that the child read the 30-foot line at a 20-foot distance.

3. Observe the child's eyes during testing and record any evidence of squinting, head tilting, thrusting the head forward, excessive blinking, tearing, or redness.

4. Only make referrals after a second screening has been made on children who are potential candidates for referral.

5. The following children should be referred for a complete eye examination:

- **a.** All children who consistently present any of the signs of possible visual disturbance, regardless of visual acuity.
- **b.** Any child with a one-line difference between each eye.
- **c.** Three-year-old children with visual acuity of 20/50 or less (inability to read the 20/40 line).
- **d.** Four-year-old children through grade 3 with visual acuity of 20/40 or less (inability to read the 20/30 line).
- **e.** All children in grade 4 and up with visual acuity of 20/30 or less (inability to read the 20/20 line).

---

*From National Society for the Prevention of Blindness: Vision screening of children, New York, 1971, The Society.

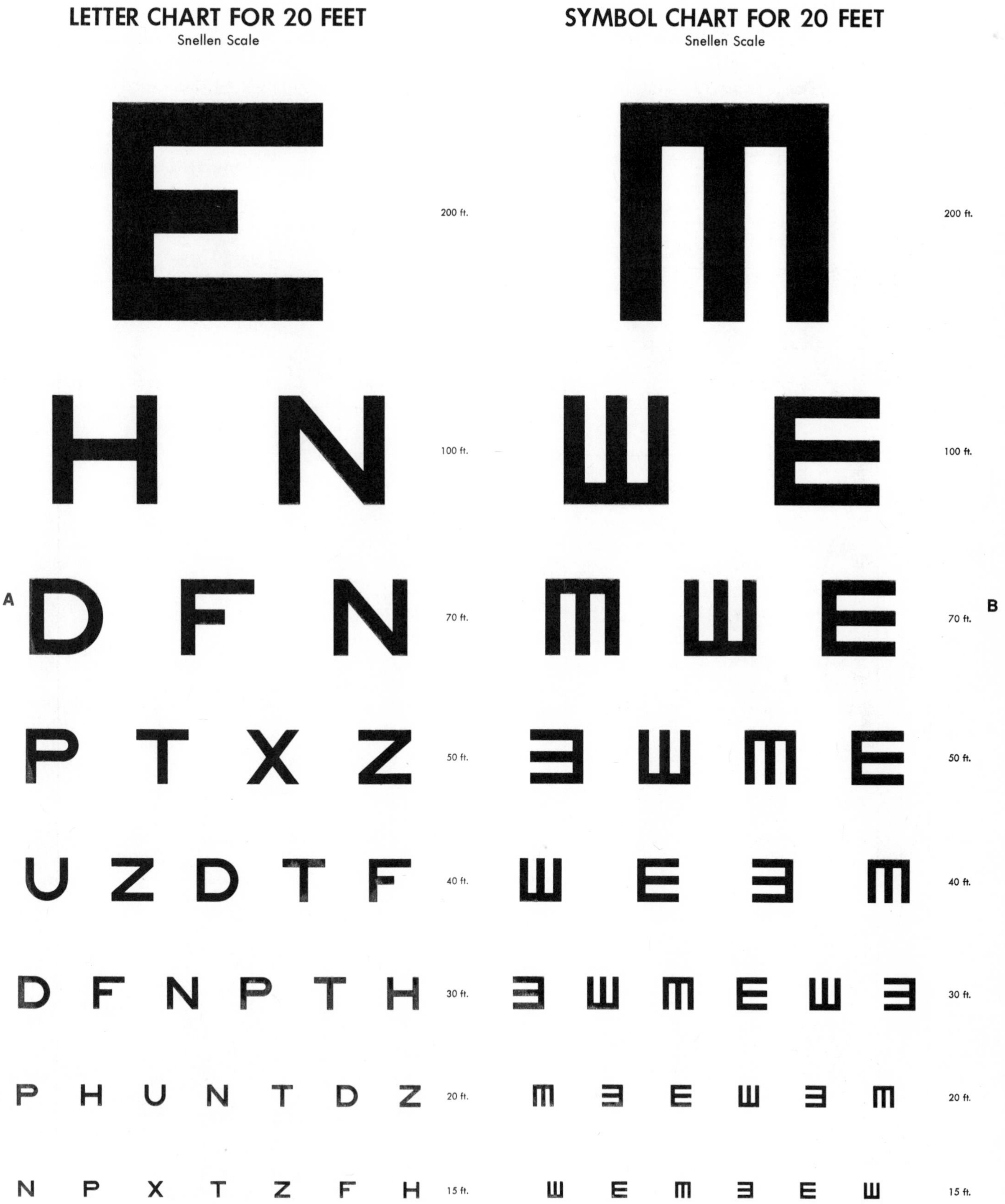

Fig. F-3. Snellen Chart. **A,** Letter chart for 20 feet–Snellen scale; **B,** symbol chart for 20 feet–Snellen scale. (From National Society to Prevent Blindness, Inc., New York. Member of National Health Council.)

Lit. 217

DENVER EYE SCREENING TEST

Name
Hospital No.
Ward
Address

Vision Tests	1ST SCREENING:DATE						RESCREENING:DATE					
	Right Eye			Left Eye			Right Eye			Left Eye		
	Normal	Abnormal	Untestable	Normal	Abnormal	Untestable	Normal	Abnormal	Untestable	Normal	Abnormal	Untestable
1. "E" (3 years and above-3 to 5 trials)	3P	3F	U	3P	3F	U	3P	3F	U	3P	3F	U
2. Picture Card (2 1/2 - 2 11/12 yrs.-3 to 5 trials)	3P	3F	U	3P	3F	U	3P	3F	U	3P	3F	U
3. Fixation (6 months - 2 5/12 years)	P	F	U	P	F	U	P	F	U	P	F	U
4. Squinting		yes			yes			yes			yes	

Tests for Non-Straight Eyes	1ST SCREENING: Normal	Abnormal	Untestable	RESCREENING: Normal	Abnormal	Untestable
1. Do your child's eyes turn in or out, or are they ever not straight?	NO	YES	U	NO	YES	U
2. Cover Test	P	F	U	P	F	U
3. Pupillary Light Reflex	P	F	U	P	F	U

Total Test Rating (Both Eyes)	1ST SCREENING	RESCREENING
Normal (passed vision test plus no squint, plus passed 2/3 tests for non-straight eyes)	Normal	Normal
Abnormal (abnormal on any vision test, squinting or 2 of 3 procedures for non-straight eyes)	Abnormal	Abnormal
Untestable (untestable on any vision test or untestable on 2/3 tests for non-straight eyes)	Untestable	Untestable
Future Rescreening Appointment for Total Test Rating (Abnormal or Untestable)	Date:	Date:

Fig. F-4. Denver Eye Screening Test. (From W. K. Frankenburg and J. B. Dobbs, University of Colorado Medical Center, 1969.)

G

The Washington Guide to Promoting Development in the Young Child*

MOTOR SKILLS

Expected tasks	Suggested activities
1 to 3 months	
1. Holds head up briefly when prone 2. Head erect and bobbing when supported in sitting position 3. Head erect and steady in sitting position 4. Follows object through all planes 5. Palmar grasp 6. Moro reflex	1. Place infant in prone position 2. Support in sitting position with his head erect 3. Pull infant to sitting position 4. Provide with opportunity to observe people or activity 5. Hang bright-colored objects and mobiles within reach across crib 6. Provide with opportunity to observe objects or people while in sitting position 7. Use infant seat 8. Alternate bright shiny objects with dark and light visual patterns
4 to 8 months	
1. Sits with minimal support, with stable head and back 2. Sits alone steadily 3. Plays with hands, which are open most of time 4. Grasps rattle or bottle with both hands 5. Picks up small objects, for example, cube 6. Transfers toys from one hand to other 7. Neck-righting reflex	1. Pull up to sitting position 2. Provide opportunity to sit supported or alone when head and trunk control are stabilized 3. Put bright-colored objects within reach 4. Give toys or household objects: rattles, teething ring, cloth animals or dolls, 1-inch cubes, plastic objects such as cups, rings, and balls 5. Offer small objects such as cereal to improve grasp 6. Offer a variety of patterns or textures to play with 7. Use squeak toys
9 to 12 months	
1. Rises to sitting position 2. Creeps or crawls, maybe backward at first 3. Pulls to standing position 4. Stands alone 5. Cruises 6. Uses index finger to poke 7. Finger-thumb grasp 8. Parachute reflex 9. Landau reflex	1. Provide playpen, allow child to pull himself to standing 2. Give opportunity and space to practice creeping and crawling 3. Have child practice moving on knees to improve balance prior to walking 4. Have child use walker or straddle toys 5. Play airplane with child; have child practice catching himself while rolling on large ball 6. Provide with objects such as spoons, plastic bottles, cups, ball, cubes, finger foods, saucepans, and lids
13 to 18 months	
1. Walks a few steps without support 2. Balanced when walking 3. Walks upstairs with help, creeps downstairs 4. Turns pages of book	1. Provide opportunity to practice walking, climbing stairs with help 2. Give toys that can be pushed around 3. Supervise activity with paper and large crayons 4. Provide toys such as cubes, cups, saucepans, lids, rag dolls, and other soft, cuddly toys 5. Begin introducing child to swing

*From Barnard, K. E., and Erickson, M. L.: Teaching children with developmental problems: a family care approach, ed. 2, St. Louis, 1976, The C. V. Mosby Co.

Continued.

MOTOR SKILLS—cont'd

Expected tasks	Suggested activities
19 to 30 months	
1. Runs 2. Walks up and down stairs, one at a time (not alternating feet) 3. Imitates vertical strokes 4. Imitates building tower of four or more blocks 5. Throws ball overhand 6. Jumps in place 7. Rides tricycle	1. Provide opportunity to practice and develop activities 2. Provide pattern for child while he watches and then encourage him to try 3. Provide tricycle or similar pedal toys; secure foot on pedal if necessary
31 to 48 months	
1. Walks downstairs (alternating feet) 2. Hops on one foot 3. Swings and climbs 4. Balances on one foot for 10 seconds 5. Copies circle 6. Copies cross 7. Draws person with three parts	1. Continue with blocks, combining materials, toy cars, and trains 2. Provide clay and other manipulating materials 3. Give opportunities to swing and climb 4. Provide with activities such as finger painting, chalk, and blackboard
49 to 52 months	
1. Balances well 2. Skips and jumps 3. Can heel-toe walk 4. Copies square 5. Catches bounced ball	1. Provide with music and games to synchronize hand and foot, tapping with music, skipping, hopping, and dancing rhythmically to improve coordination

FEEDING SKILLS

Expected tasks	Suggested activities
1 to 3 months	
1. Sucking reflex present 2. Rooting reflex present 3. Ability to swallow pureed foods 4. Coordinates sucking, swallowing, and breathing	1. Consider a change in nipple or posturing if there is difficulty in swallowing 2. Introduce solids, one kind at a time (use small spoon, place food well back on infant's tongue) 3. Hold in comfortable relaxed position while feeding 4. Pace feeding tempo to infant's needs
4 to 8 months	
1. Tongue used in moving food in mouth 2. Hand-to-mouth motions 3. Recognizes bottle on sight 4. Gums or mouths solid foods 5. Feeds self cracker	1. Give finger foods to develop chewing, stimulate gums, and encourage hand-to-mouth motion (cubes of cheese, bananas, dry toast, bread crust, cookies) 2. Encourage upright supported position for feeding 3. Promote bottle holding 4. Introduce junior foods
9 to 12 months	
1. Holds own bottle 2. Drinks from cup or glass with assistance 3. Finger feeds 4. Beginning to hold spoon	1. Bring child in highchair to table and include in part of or entire meal with family 2. Have child in dry comfortable position with trunk and feet supported 3. Encourage self-help in feeding; use of table foods 4. Offer spoon when interest is indicated 5. Introduce cup or glass with small amount of fluid

FEEDING SKILLS—cont'd

Expected tasks	Suggested activities
13 to 18 months	
1. Holds cup and handle with digital grasp 2. Lifts cup and drinks well 3. Beginning to use spoon, may turn bowl down before reaching mouth 4. Difficulty in inserting spoon into mouth 5. May refuse food	1. Continue offering finger foods (wieners, sandwiches) 2. Use nontip dishes and cups; dishes should have sides to make filling of spoon easy 3. Give opportunity for self-feeding 4. Provide fluids between meals rather than having child fill up on fluids at mealtime
19 to 30 months	
1. Drinks without spilling 2. Holds small glass in one hand 3. Inserts spoon in mouth correctly 4. Distinguishes between food and inedible material 5. Plays with food	1. Encourage self-feeding with spoon 2. Do not rush child 3. Serve foods plainly but in attractive servings 4. Small servings of food will encourage eating more than large servings
31 to 48 months	
1. Pours well from pitcher 2. Serves self at table with little spilling 3. Rarely needs assistance 4. Interest in setting table	1. Encourage self-help 2. Give opportunity for pouring (give rice and pitcher to promote pouring skills) 3. Encourage child to help set table 4. Have well-defined rules about table manners
49 to 52 months	
1. Feeds self well 2. Social and talkative during meal	1. Socialize with child at mealtime 2. Have child help with preparation, table setting, and serving 3. Include child in conversations at mealtimes by planning special times for him to tell about events, situations, or what he did during the day

SLEEP

Expected tasks	Suggested activities
1 to 3 months	
1. Night: 4- to 10-hour intervals 2. Naps: frequent 3. Longer periods of wakefulness without crying	1. Provide separate sleeping arrangements away from parents' room 2. Reduce noise and light stimulation when placing in bed 3. Have room at comfortable temperature with no drafts or extremes in heat 4. Reverse position of crib occasionally 5. Place child in different positions from time to time for sleep 6. Alternate from back to side to stomach 7. Keep crib sides up
4 to 8 months	
1. Night: 10 to 12 hours 2. Naps: 2 to 3 (1 to 4 hours in duration) 3. Night awakenings	1. Keep crib sides up 2. Refrain from taking child into parents' room if he awakens 3. Check to determine if there is cause for awakenings: hunger, teething, pain, cold, wet, noise, or illness 4. If a baby-sitter is used, attempt to find some person with whom infant is familiar. Explain bedtime and naptime arrangements
9 to 12 months	
1. Night: 12 to 14 hours 2. Naps: one to two (1 to 4 hours in duration) 3. May begin refusing morning nap	1. Short crying periods may be source of tension release for child 2. Observe for signs of fatigue, irritability, or restlessness if naps are shorter 3. Provide familiar person to baby-sit who knows sleep routines

Continued.

SLEEP—cont'd

Expected tasks	Suggested activities
13 to 18 months	
1. Night: 10 to 12 hours 2. Naps: one in afternoon (1 to 3 hours in duration) 3. May awaken during night crying (associated with wetting bed) 4. As he becomes more able to move about, he may uncover himself, become cold, and awaken	1. Night terrors may be terminated by awakening infant and offering reassurance 2. Check to see that child is covered 3. Avoid hazardous devices to keep child covered, including blanket clips, pins, and garments that enclose child to neck
19 to 30 months	
1. Night: 10 to 12 hours 2. Naps: one (1 to 3 hours in duration) 3. Doesn't go to sleep at once—keeps demanding things 4. May awaken crying if wet or soiled 5. May awaken because of environmental change of temperature, change of bed, change of sleeping room, addition of sibling to room, absence of parent from home, hospitalization, trip with family, or relatives visiting	1. Quiet period of socialization prior to bedtime—reading child book or telling story 2. Holding child—talking quietly with him 3. Ritualistic behavior may be present; allow child to carry out routine; helps him overcome fear of unexpected or fear of dark; for example, child may wish to arrange toys in certain way 4. Explain bedtime ritual to baby-sitter 5. Give more reassurance, spend more time before bedtime preparation 6. Provide familiar bedtime toys or items 7. Allow crying-out period if he is safe, comfortable, and tucked in 8. Place in bed before he reaches excessive state of fatigue, excitement, or tiredness 9. Eliminate sources of stimulation or fear 10. Maintain consistent hour of bedtime
31 to 48 months	
1. Daily range: 10 to 15 hours 2. Naps: beginning to disappear 3. Prolongs process of going to bed 4. Less dependent on taking toys to bed 5. May awaken crying from dreams 6. May awaken if wet	1. Television programs may affect ability to go to sleep; avoid violent television programs 2. Anxiety about going to bed and desire to stay up with parents—requires limits 3. Regularity and consistency important to promote good sleeping habits 4. Reassurance—night light or leaving door ajar 5. Do not use bedtime or naptime as punishment 6. Encourage naps if signs of fatigue or irritability are evidenced
49 to 52 months	
1. Daily range: 9 to 13 hours 2. Naps: rare 3. Quieter during sleep	1. Encourage napping if excessive or strenuous activity occurs and child is overly tired 2. Explain to child if baby-sitter will be there after child is asleep

PLAY

Expected tasks	Suggested activities
1 to 3 months	
1. Quieted when picked up 2. Regards face of others	1. Encourage holding and touching of child by mother 2. Provide with cradle gyms and mobiles, brightly colored, visually interesting objects within arm's distance
4 to 8 months	
1. Plays with own body 2. Differentiates strangers from family 3. Seeks out objects 4. Grasps, holds, and manipulates objects 5. Repeats activities he enjoys 6. Bangs toys or objects together	1. Begin patty-cake and peekaboo 2. Provide for periods of solitary play (playpen) 3. Encourage holding and touching of child by mother 4. Provide variety of multicolored and multitextured objects that child can hold 5. Encourage exploration of body parts 6. Provide floating toys for bath
9 to 12 months	
1. Puts objects in and out of containers 2. Examines objects held in hand 3. Plays interactive games (peekaboo) 4. Extends toy to other person without releasing 5. Works to get toy out of reach	1. Continue mother-infant games 2. Give opportunity to place objects in containers and pour out 3. Provide large and small objects with which to play 4. Encourage interactive play
13 to 18 months	
1. Plays by himself—may play near others 2. Has preferred toys 3. Enjoys walking activities, pulling toys 4. Throws and picks up objects, throws again 5. Imitates, for example, reading newspaper, sweeping	1. Introduce to other children even though child may not play with them 2. Provide music, books, and magazines 3. Encourage imitative activities—helping with dusting, sweeping, stirring
19 to 30 months	
1. Parallel play—not interactive but plays alongside another child 2. Uses both large and small toys 3. Rough-and-tumble play 4. Play periods longer than before—interested in manipulative and constructive toys 5. Enjoys rhymes and singing (television programs)	1. Provide with new materials for manipulating and feeling—finger paints, clay, sand, stones, water, and soap Wooden toys—cars and animals Building blocks of various sizes, crayons, and paper Rhythmical tunes and equipment—swing, rocking chair, rocking horse Children's books—short, simple stories with repetition and familiar objects; enjoys simple pictures, brightly colored 2. Guide child's hand to actively participate with specific activities, for example, using crayons, hammering
31 to 48 months	
1. In playing with others, beginning to interact, sharing toys, taking turns 2. Dramatizes, expresses imagination in play 3. Combining playthings; more use of constructive materials 4. Prefers two or three children to play with; may have special friend	1. Encourage play with small groups of children 2. Encourage imaginative and dramatic play activities 3. Music: singing and experimenting with musical instruments 4. Group participation in rhymes, dancing by hopping or jumping 5. Drawing and painting (seldom recognizable)
49 to 52 months	
1. Dramatic play and interest in going on excursions 2. Fond of cutting and pasting, creative materials 3. Completes most activities	1. Painting and drawing (objects will be out of proportion; details that are most important to child are drawn largest) 2. Encourage printing of numbers and letters 3. Clay: making recognizable objects 4. Cutting and pasting 5. Provide with materials, for example, boxes, chairs, barrels, for building sturdy structures

Continued.

LANGUAGE

Expected tasks	Suggested activities
1 to 3 months	
RECEPTIVE ABILITIES 1. Movement of eyes, respiration rate, or body activity changes when bell is rung close to child's head 2. Smiles when socially stimulated 3. Has facial, vocal, and generalized bodily responses to faces 4. Reacts differentially to adult voices EXPRESSIVE ABILITIES 1. Makes prelanguage vocalizations that consist of cooing, throaty sounds, for example, gu 2. Makes "pleasure" sounds that consist of soft vowels 3. Makes "sucking" sounds 4. Crying can be differentiated for discomfort, pain, and hunger as reported by mother 5. An "A" sound as in cat is commonly heard in distress crying	1. Observe facial expressions, gestures, bodily postures, and movements when vocalizations are being produced 2. Smile and talk softly in pleasant tone while holding, touching, and handling infant 3. Hold, touch, and interact frequently with infant for pleasure 4. Refrain from letting infant engage in prolonged and incessant crying
4 to 8 months	
RECEPTIVE ABILITIES 1. Eyes locate source of sound 2. Responds to "hi, there" by looking up at face that is across and in front of him 3. Head turns to sound of cellophane held and crunched 2 feet away and at a 135-degree angle on either side of head 4. Will turn head to locate sound of "look here" when spoken at a 90-degree angle from head 2 feet away* 5. Turns head to sound of rattle 6. Responds differently to vacuum cleaner, phone, doorbell, or sound of dog barking: may cry, whimper, look toward sound, or mother may report change in body tension 7. Responds by raising arms when mother reaches toward child and says "come up" EXPRESSIVE ABILITIES 1. Uses different inflectional patterns: ah ah uh 2. Laughs aloud when stimulated 3. Has differential patterns of crying when hungry, in pain, or angry 4. Produces vowel sounds and chained syllables (baba, gugu, didi) 5. Makes "talking sounds" in response to others talking to him 6. Babbles to produce consonant sounds: ba, da, m-m 7. Vocalizes to toys 8. Says "da-da" or "ma-ma" but not specific to presence of parents	1. Engage in smiling eye-to-eye contact while talking to infant 2. Vocalize in response to inflectional patterns and when infant is producing babbling sounds; echo the sounds he makes 3. Observe for subtle communication clues such as eye aversion, struggling to move away, flushing of skin, tension of body, or movement of arms 4. Vocalize with infant during handling, while feeding, bathing, dressing, diapering, bedtime preparation, and holding 5. Stimulate laughing by light tickling 6. Observe child's reactions to bells, whistles, horns, phones, laughing, singing, talking, music box, noisemaking toys, and common household noises 7. While talking to infant, hold in position so that he can see your face 8. Have infant placed at position of eye level while talking to him throughout the day 9. If crying or laughing sounds are not discerned at this stage, report to family physician, pediatrician, public health nurse, or well-child clinic
9 to 12 months	
RECEPTIVE ABILITIES 1. Ceases activity when name is pronounced or "no-no" is said 2. Gives toys on request when accompanied by facial and bodily gestures 3. Attends to simple commands EXPRESSIVE ABILITIES 1. Imitates definite speech sounds such as tongue clicking, lip smacking, or coughing 2. Should have two words that are *specific* for parents: "ma-ma," "dada," or equivalents	1. Gain child's attention when giving simple commands 2. Accompany oral directions with gestures 3. Vocalize with child during feeding, bathing, and playtimes 4. Provide sounds that child can reproduce such as lip smacking and tongue clicking 5. Repeat direction frequently and have child participate in action: open and close the drawer; move arms and legs up and down 6. Have child respond to verbal directions: stand up, sit down, close door, open door, turn around, come here

*Do not test for localization of sound by producing sound directly behind infant's head.

Expected tasks	Suggested activities
13 to 18 months	
RECEPTIVE ABILITIES 1. Attends to person speaking to child 2. Finds "the baby" in picture when requested, for example, on baby food jar, in magazine, or in storybooks 3. Indicates wants by gestures 4. Looks toward family members or pets when named EXPRESSIVE ABILITIES 1. Uses three words other than mama and dada to denote *specific* objects, persons, or actions 2. Indicates wants by naming object such as cookie	1. Incorporate repetition into daily routine of home a. Feeding: name baby's food and eating utensils; ask if he is enjoying his dessert; concentrate on reviewing day's events in simple manner b. Household duties: mother names each item as she dusts; pronounces word while cooking and preparing foods c. Playing: identify toys when using them; explain their function 2. Let child see mouthing of words 3. Encourage verbalization and expression of wants
19 to 30 months	
RECEPTIVE ABILITIES 1. Points to one named body part 2. Follows two or three verbal directions that are not accompanied by facial or body gestures, for example, put ball on table, give it to mommy, or put toy in box EXPRESSIVE ABILITIES 1. Combines two different words, for example, "play ball," "want cookie" 2. Names object in picture, for example, cat, bird, dog, horse, man 3. Refers to self by pronoun rather than by name	1. Continue to present concrete objects with words; talk about activities child is involved with 2. Include child in conversations during mealtimes 3. Encourage speech by having child express wants 4. Incorporate games into bathing routine by having child name and point to body parts 5. As child gains confidence in remembering and using words appropriately, encourage less use of gestures 6. Count and name articles of clothing as they are placed on child 7. Count and name silverware as it is placed on table 8. Sort, match, and name glassware, laundry, cans, vegetables, and fruit with child 9. Have child keep scrapbook and add new picture every day to increase recognition of vocabulary words 10. Spend 15 to 20 minutes per day going through booklets and naming pictures; have child point to pictures as objects are named 11. Help child develop functional core vocabulary to express safety needs and information about neighborhood 12. Whenever possible, use word (for example, paper), show object, have child handle and use it, encourage him to watch your face while you say the words, and suggest that he repeat it; refrain from undue pressure
31 to 36 months	
RECEPTIVE ABILITIES 1. Takes turns when asked while playing, eating 2. Attends longer to stories and television programs 3. Demonstrates understanding of two prepositions by carry-out two commands one at a time, for example, "put the block under the chair" 4. Can follow commands asking for two objects or two actions 5. Demonstrates understanding of concepts of big and little, for example, selects larger of two balls when asked for big one 6. Points to additional body parts EXPRESSIVE ABILITIES 1. Uses regular plurals, for example, adds "s" to apple, box, orange (does not use irregular plurals, for example, mouse to mice) 2. Gives first and last name 3. Names what he has drawn after scribbling 4. On request, tells you his sex, for example, are you a little boy or a little girl? 5. Can repeat a few rhymes or songs 6. On request, tells what action is going on in picture, for example, the kitten is eating	1. Read stories with familiar content but with more detail: nonsense rhymes, humorous stories 2. Expect child to follow simple commands 3. Give child opportunity to hear and repeat his full name 4. Listen to child's explanation about pictures he draws 5. Encourage child to repeat nursery rhymes by himself and with others 6. Address child by his first name

Continued.

LANGUAGE—cont'd

Expected tasks	Suggested activities
37 to 48 months	
1. Expresses appropriate responses when asked what child does when tired, cold, or hungry 2. Tells stories 3. Common expression: I don't know 4. Repeats sentence composed of twelve to thirteen syllables, for example, "I am going when daddy and I are finished playing" 5. Has mastered phonetic sounds of p, k, g, v, tf, d, z, lr, hw, j, kw, l, e, w, qe, and o	1. Provide visual stimuli while reading stories 2. Have child repeat story 3. Arrange trips to zoo, farms, seashore, stores, and movies and discuss with child 4. Give simple explanations in answering questions
49 to 52 months	
RECEPTIVE ABILITIES 1. Points to penny, nickel, or dime on request 2. Carries out in order command containing three parts, for example, "pick up the block, put it on the table, and bring the book to me" EXPRESSIVE ABILITIES 1. Names penny, nickel, or dime on request 2. Replies appropriately to questions such as, "What do you do when you are asleep?" 3. Counts three objects, pointing to each in turn 4. Defines simple words, for example, hat, ball 5. Asks questions 6. Can identify or name four colors	1. Play games in which child names colors 2. Encourage use of please and thank you 3. Encourage social-verbal interactions with other children 4. Encourage correct usage of words 5. Provide puppets or toys with movable parts that child can converse about 6. Provide group activity for child; children may stimulate each other by taking turns naming pictures 7. Allow child to make choices about games, stories, and activities 8. Have child dramatize simple stories 9. Provide child with piggy bank and encourage naming coins as they are handled or dropped into bank

DISCIPLINE

Expected tasks	Suggested activities
1 to 3 months	
1. Draws attention by crying	1. a. Needs should be identified and met as promptly as possible b. Every bit of fussing should not be interpreted as emergency requiring immediate attention c. Infant should not be ignored and permitted to cry for exhaustive periods
2. Infant desires whatever is pleasant and wishes to avoid unpleasant situations	2. Begin to present limit of having to wait so that infant can learn that tension and discomfort are bearable for short periods
3. Beginning to "wiggle" around	3. Place infant on surfaces that have sides to protect him from falling off
4 to 8 months	
1. Begins to respond to "no-no"	1. a. Reserve "no-no" for times when it is really needed b. Be consistent with word "no-no" for same activity and event that requires it; be friendly and firm with verbal control of limit setting
2. Infant who is left alone for long periods of time may become bored or fretful; learns that crying and whining result in attention	2. Make special efforts to attend to infant when he is quiet and amusing himself
3. Beginning to show signs of timidity and fretfulness and may whimper and cry when mother separates from him or when strangers pick him up	3. a. Gradually introduce strangers into infant's environment b. Refrain from promoting frightening situations with strangers during this stage c. Play hiding games like peekaboo in which mother disappears and reappears d. Allow infant to cling to mother and get used to persons a little at a time e. If baby-sitter is used, find person familiar to infant or introduce for brief periods before mother leaves infant in her care f. Encourage gentle handling by mother, father, and siblings. Discourage rough handling, particularly by strangers

DISCIPLINE—cont'd

Expected tasks	Suggested activities
4. Beginning to grasp objects and bring to mouth, but unable to differentiate safe from hazardous items	4. a. Provide toys that do not have small detachable parts b. Check frequently for small objects in his line of reach 5. When traveling in car, place in crib or seat with safety belts securely fastened
9 to 12 months	
1. Beginning to respond to simple commands, for example, "pick up the ball, put the toy in the box"	1. a. Avoid setting unreasonable number of limits b. Give simple commands one at a time c. Once limit is set, adhere to it firmly each time and connect it immediately with misbehavior d. Respond with consistency in enforcing rule e. Allow time to conform to request f. Gain child's attention
2. Ready to go places on his own and is trying out newly developing motor capacities (not to be confused with naughtiness, "spoiled," or stubbornness)	2. a. Begin setting and enforcing limits on where child is allowed to travel and explore b. Remove tempting objects c. Remove sources of danger such as light sockets, protruding pot handles, hanging table covers, sharp objects, and hanging cords d. Keep child away from fans, heaters, and certain drawers and do not place vaporizer close to infant's crib e. Keep high chair at least 2 feet away from working and cooking surfaces in kitchen f. Use gate to keep child out of kitchen when it is being used g. Be certain that pans, basins, and tubs of hot water are never left unattended h. Remove all possible poisons or substances that are not food that can be eaten or drunk off floor, low-level cabinets, and under sink i. Keep child from objects or surfaces that he may chew, for example, porch rails, windowsills, *repainted* toys or cribs that may contain lead j. Instruct baby-sitter on all safety items
3. Has emerging desires to look at, handle, and touch objects	3. a. Experiment with diversionary measures b. Provide child with own play objects
4. Explores objects by sucking, chewing, and biting	4. a. Remove household poisons, cosmetics, pins, and buttons that he could put in his mouth b. Be certain that objects that go into mouth are hygienic c. Check toys for detachable small parts
5. Beginning to test reactions to certain parental responses during feeding and may become choosy about food	5. a. Once problem behaviors are defined, plan to work on changing only one behavior at a time until child behaves or conforms to expectations b. Be certain that child understands old rules before adding new ones c. Respond with consistency in enforcing old rules: enforce each time, do not ignore next time d. Provide regular pattern of mealtimes e. Refrain from feeding throughout day f. Allow child to decide what he will eat and how much g. Introduce new foods gradually over period of time h. Continue to offer foods that may have been rejected first time i. Do not force food j. Refrain from physically punishing child for changes in eating habits
6. Beginning to test reactions to parental responses at bedtime preparation	6. a. Provide regular time for naps and bedtime b. Avoid excessive stimulation at bedtime or naptime c. Ignore fussing and crying once safety and physical needs are satisfied and usual ritual is carried out d. Keep child in own room e. Refrain from picking up and rocking and holding if needs seem satisfied

Continued.

DISCIPLINE—cont'd

Expected tasks	Suggested activities
13 to 18 months	
1. Understands simple commands and requests	1. a. Begin with one rule; add new ones as appropriate b. In selecting new rules, choose on the basis of being able to clearly define it to self and child, having it reasonable and enforceable at all times; demand no more than fulfillment of defined expectations c. Plan decisive limits and plan to give consistent attention to them
2. In learning mastery over impulses and self-control, child begins testing out limit setting	2. a. Immediately correct errors in behavior as they occur b. Use consistent enforcement of short-term rules (which are given as verbal commands) and long-term rules (which pertain to chores and family routines) c. Ignore temper tantrums d. Show child when you approve of his behavior and praise for obedience throughout day
3. With increasing fine motor control, child can manipulate objects that may be hazardous	3. a. Set limits regarding play with doorknobs and car door handles b. Keep away from open windows; latch screens c. Supervise around pools and ponds or drain or fence them d. Lock cabinets e. Keep open jars and bottles out of reach f. Use gate to protect child from falling down stairs
19 to 30 months	
1. Attention span increasing	1. a. Gain attention before giving simple commands, one at a time; praise for success b. Add new rules as child conforms to old ones c. Refrain from expecting *immediate* obedience
2. Begins simple reasoning—asks question why; may be repetitive	2. Make special efforts to answer questions; give simple explanations; gauge need for simplicity by number of times act is repeated or question asked
3. Interested in further exploration of environment; may lack physical control	3. a. Supervise on stair rails and waxed floors b. Set rules about crossing streets and carrying knives, sharp objects, or glass objects c. Have outdoor play area securely fenced or supervised d. When riding in car, secure child safely by seat belt or insist on his sitting in back seat; do not permit standing on car seats e. Keep matches out of reach f. Shield adult tools such as knives, lawnmowers, sharp tools
4. Negativistic behavior is expected; responds more frequently with word "no"; may show more resistance at bedtime preparation and during mealtime	4. a. Practice consistency in responding to behavior b. Allow more time to conform to expectation
5. Behavior may change if new sibling is introduced into family unit	5. a. Explain verbally or through play that new child is expected b. Exercise more patience with child c. Set special times aside for parental attention to child d. Allow child to help with special care tasks of new sibling

DISCIPLINE—cont'd

Expected tasks	Suggested activities
31 to 48 months	
1. Displays more interest in conforming	1. a. Exercise consistency in parental demands; enforce each time and avoid ignoring behavior next time b. Show concrete approval and give immediate recognition for acceptable behavior c. Refrain from use of threats that produce fearfulness
2. Shows greater understanding when simple reasoning is communicated	2. a. Give simple explanations; allow child chance to demonstrate understanding by talking about event, situation, or rule b. Eliminate unnecessary and impractical rules c. Refrain from constant verbal reprimands d. Denial of privileges should not be excessive or prolonged
3. Will respond to simple commands such as putting toys away	3. a. Assign simple household tasks that child can carry out each day; show approval for performance and success b. Decide if child is capable of doing what is asked by observing him c. Determine how much time is necessary to complete a chore or activity before expecting maximum performance
4. Displays a greater independence in general activities	4. a. Be extra cautious about supervising riding tricycles in streets and watching for cars in driveways b. Do not permit dashing into street while playing c. Do not allow child to follow ball into street d. Areas under swings and slides should not be paved e. Provide an imitative model that child can copy, for example, do not jaywalk f. Provide scissors that are blunt tipped
49 to 52 months	
1. Can be given two or three assignments at one time; will carry out in order 2. Complies readily with reasonable, well-defined, and consistent requirements 3. Understands reasoning	1. Give more opportunities to be independent 2. Use simple explanations and reasoning 3. Ask child to define role if he disobeys 4. Have child correct mistakes as they occur 5. Do not use punishment without warnings 6. Praise for successful performance 7. Use gold stars on chart for rewards 8. If leaving for social obligation, vacation, or visiting away from home, let child know 9. Avoid making promises that cannot be kept 10. Avoid bribing, ridicule, shaming, teasing, inflicting pain, using unfavorable comparison with other children, and exhibition of behavior by parents they are trying to stop in child 11. Remember that child may be imitating models of behavior set up by parents, brothers, sisters, a neighborhood child, or maybe a television hero 12. Recognize that there are stress periods in family or child's life that may result in changes in child's behavior including accidents, illness, moving into new neighborhood, separation from friends, death, divorce, and hospitalization of child or parents (be more patient with child's behavior, give more time to conform, show more approval for mastery of tasks, and exercise consistency in handling problems as they occur)

Continued.

TOILET TRAINING

Expected tasks	Suggested activities
9 to 12 months	
1. Beginning to show regular patterns in bladder and bowel elimination 2. Has one to two stools daily 3. Interval of dryness does not exceed 1 to 2 hours	1. Watch for clues that indicate child is wet or soiled 2. Be sure to change diapers when wet or soiled so that child begins to experience contrast between wetness and dryness
13 to 18 months	
1. Will have bowel movement if put on toilet at approximate time 2. Indicates wet pants	1. Sit child on toilet or potty chair at regular intervals for short periods of time throughout day 2. Praise child for success 3. If potty chair is used, it should be located in bathroom 4. Training should be started when social disruptions are at minimum 5. Respond promptly to signals and clues of child by taking him to bathroom or changing pants 6. Use training pants, once toilet training is commenced 7. Plan to begin training when disruptions in regular routine are minimized, that is, do not begin on vacation
19 to 30 months	
1. Anticipates need to eliminate 2. Same word for both functions 3. Daytime control (occasional accident) 4. Requires assistance (reminding, dressing, wiping)	1. Continue regular intervals of toileting 2. Reward success 3. Dress in simple clothing that child can manage 4. Remind occasionally, particularly after mealtime, juicetime, naptime, and playtime 5. Take to bathroom before bedtime 6. Bathroom should be convenient to use, easy to open door
31 to 48 months	
1. Takes responsibility for toilet if clothes are simple 2. Continues to verbalize need to go; apt to hold out too long 3. May have occasional accident 4. Needs help with wiping	1. May still need reminding 2. Dress in simple clothing that child can manage 3. Ignore accidents; refrain from shame or ridicule
49 to 52 months	
1. General independence (anticipates needs, undresses, goes, wipes, washes hands)	1. Praise child for his accomplishment

DRESSING

Expected tasks	Suggested activities
13 to 18 months	
1. Cooperates in dressing by extending arm or leg 2. Removes socks, hat, mittens, shoes 3. Can unzip zippers 4. Tries to put shoes on	1. Encourage child to remove socks, etc. after task is initiated for him 2. Do not rush child 3. Have him practice with large buttons and with zippers
19 to 30 months	
1. Can undress 2. Can remove shoes if laces are untied 3. Helps dress 4. Tries to unbutton 5. Pulls on simple clothes	1. Provide opportunities to button with extra-large–sized buttons 2. Encourage and allow opportunity for self-help in getting drink, removing clothes with help, hand washing, unbuttoning, etc. 3. Simple clothing 4. Provide mirror at height child can observe himself for brushing teeth, etc.
31 to 48 months	
1. Greater interest and ability in dressing 2. Intent on lacing shoes (usually does incorrectly) 3. Does not know back from front 4. Washes and dries hands, brushes teeth 5. Can button	1. Provide with own dresser drawer 2. Simple garments encourage self-help; do not rush child 3. Provide large buttons, zippers, slipover clothing 4. Self hand washing but help with brushing teeth 5. Provide regular routine for dressing, either in bathroom or bedroom
49 to 52 months	
1. Dresses and undresses with care except for tying shoes and buckling belts 2. May learn to tie shoes 3. Combs hair with assistance	1. Assign regular task of placing clothes in hamper or basket 2. Continue to use simple clothing 3. Encourage self-help in dressing and undressing 4. Allow child to select clothes he will wear

H

United Nations Declaration of the Rights of the Child

PREAMBLE

Whereas the peoples of the United Nations have, in the Charter, reaffirmed their faith in fundamental human rights, and in the dignity and worth of the human person, and have determined to promote social progress and better standards of life in larger freedom,

Whereas the United Nations has, in the Universal Declaration of Human Rights, proclaimed that everyone is entitled to all the rights and freedoms set forth therein, without distinction of any kind, such as race, color, sex, language, religion, political or other opinion, national or social origin, property, birth or other status,

Whereas the child, by reason of his physical and mental immaturity, needs special safeguards and care, including appropriate legal protection, before as well as after birth,

Whereas the need for such special safeguards has been stated in the Geneva Declaration of the Rights of the Child of 1924, and recognized in the Universal Declaration of Human Rights and in the statutes of specialized agencies and international organizations concerned with the welfare of children,

Whereas mankind owes to the child the best it has to give

NOW THEREFORE THE GENERAL ASSEMBLY PROCLAIMS

This Declaration of the Rights of the Child to the end that he may have a happy childhood and enjoy for his own good and for the good of society the rights and freedoms herein set forth, and calls upon parents, upon men and women as individuals and upon voluntary organizations, local authorities and national governments to recognize these rights and strive for their observance by legislative and other measures progressively taken in accordance with the following principles:

PRINCIPLE 1

The child shall enjoy all the rights set forth in this Declaration. All children, without any exception whatsoever, shall be entitled to these rights, without distinction or discrimination on account of race, color, sex, language, religion, political or other opinion, national or social origin, property, birth or other status, whether of himself or of his family.

PRINCIPLE 2

The child shall enjoy special protection, and shall be given opportunities and facilities, by law and by other means, to enable him to develop physically, mentally, morally, spiritually and socially in a healthy and normal manner and in conditions of freedom and dignity. In the enactment of laws for this purpose the best interests of the child shall be the paramount consideration.

PRINCIPLE 3

The child shall be entitled from his birth to a name and a nationality.

PRINCIPLE 4

The child shall enjoy the benefits of social security. He shall be entitled to grow and develop in health; to this end special care and protection shall be provided both to him and to his mother, including adequate pre-natal and post-natal care. The child shall have the right to adequate nutrition, housing, recreation and medical services.

PRINCIPLE 5

The child who is physically, mentally or socially handicapped shall be given the special treatment, education and care required by his particular condition.

PRINCIPLE 6

The child, for the full and harmonious development of his personality, needs love and understanding. He shall, wherever possible, grow up in the care and under the responsibility of his parents, and in any case in an atmosphere of affection and of moral and maternal security; a child of tender years shall not, save in exceptional circumstances, be separated from his mother. Society and the public authorities shall have the duty to extend particular care to children without a family and to those without adequate means of support. Payment of state and other assistance toward the maintenance of children of large families is desirable.

PRINCIPLE 7

The child is entitled to receive education, which shall be free and compulsory, at least in the elementary stages. He shall be given an education which will promote his general culture, and enable him on a basis of equal opportunity to develop his abilities, his individual judgment, and his sense of moral and social responsibility, and to become a useful member of society.

The best interests of the child shall be the guiding principle of those responsible for his education and guidance; that responsibility lies in the first place with his parents.

The child shall have full opportunity for play and recreation, which shall be directed to the same purposes as education; society and the public authorities shall endeavor to promote the enjoyment of this right.

PRINCIPLE 8

The child shall in all circumstances be among the first to receive protection and relief.

PRINCIPLE 9

The child shall be protected against all forms of neglect, cruelty and exploitation. He shall not be the subject of traffic, in any form.

The child shall not be admitted to employment before an appropriate minimum age; he shall in no case be caused or permitted to engage in any occupation or employment which would prejudice his health or education, or interfere with his physical, mental or moral development.

PRINCIPLE 10

The child shall be protected from practices which may foster racial, religious and any other form of discrimination. He shall be brought up in a spirit of understanding, tolerance, friendship among peoples, peace and universal brotherhood and in full consciousness that his energy and talents should be devoted to the service of his fellow men.

Index

S